6 EDITION

PRIMARY CARE

INTERPROFESSIONAL COLLABORATIVE PRACTICE

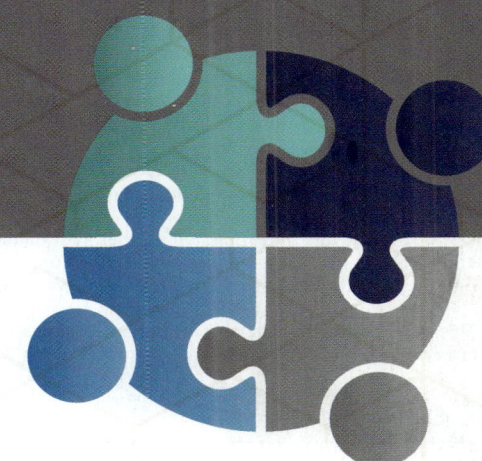

Terry Mahan Buttaro, PhD, AGPCNP-BC, FAANP, FNAP

Clinical Assistant Professor
Coastal Medical Associates
Salisbury, Massachusetts;
University of Massachusetts Boston
Boston, Massachusetts

Patricia Polgar-Bailey, PsyD, MPH, FNP-BC, CDE, BC-ADM

Family Nurse Practitioner and Integrative Care Provider
Charlottesville Free Clinic
Charlottesville, Virginia;
Clinical Psychologist
Blue Mountains Health
Charlottesville, Virginia

Joanne Sandberg-Cook, MS, APRN, ANP/GNP-BC

Adult/Gerontologic Nurse Practitioner (retired)
Dartmouth-Hitchcock Medical Center
Dartmouth-Hitchcock at Kendal
Hanover, New Hampshire;
Director
Community Nurse of Thetford, Inc
Thetford Center, Vermont

JoAnn Trybulski, PhD, ARNP, FNAP

Formerly, Director, DNP Program
Chamberlain College of Nursing
Miami, Florida

Associate Editor
John Distler, DPA, MBA, MS, FNP-C, FAANP

Family Nurse Practitioner
Maryland Asthma and Allergy Center
Baltimore, Maryland;
Professor
Nurse Practitioner Programs
Chamberlain University
Downers Grove, Illinois

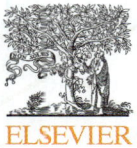

ELSEVIER

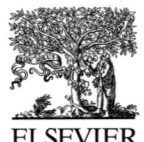

ELSEVIER

3251 Riverport Lane
St. Louis, Missouri 63043

Notices

Knowledge and best practice in this field are constantly changing. As new research and experience broaden our understanding, changes in research methods, professional practices, or medical treatment may become necessary.

Practitioners and researchers must always rely on their own experience and knowledge in evaluating and using any information, methods, compounds, or experiments described herein. In using such information or methods they should be mindful of their own safety and the safety of others, including parties for whom they have a professional responsibility.

With respect to any drug or pharmaceutical products identified, readers are advised to check the most current information provided (i) on procedures featured or (ii) by the manufacturer of each product to be administered, to verify the recommended dose or formula, the method and duration of administration, and contraindications. It is the responsibility of practitioners, relying on their own experience and knowledge of their patients, to make diagnoses, to determine dosages and the best treatment for each individual patient, and to take all appropriate safety precautions.

To the fullest extent of the law, neither the Publisher nor the authors, contributors, or editors, assume any liability for any injury and/or damage to persons or property as a matter of products liability, negligence or otherwise, or from any use or operation of any methods, products, instructions, or ideas contained in the material herein.

Previous editions copyrighted 2017, 2013, 2008, 2003, and 1999.

Library of Congress Control Number: 2019953331

Executive Content Strategist: Lee Henderson
Senior Content Development Specialist: Heather Bays
Publishing Services Manager: Julie Eddy
Senior Project Manager: Cindy Thoms
Design Direction: Renee Duenow

Printed in Canada

Last digit is the print number: 9 8 7 6 5 4 3 2 1

Working together
to grow libraries in
developing countries

www.elsevier.com • www.bookaid.org

A Special Tribute

To JoAnn Trybulski, a teacher, a mentor, a colleague, a friend. We miss her laughter, her generosity, and her willingness to give everyone the benefit of the doubt. Mainly we miss her!

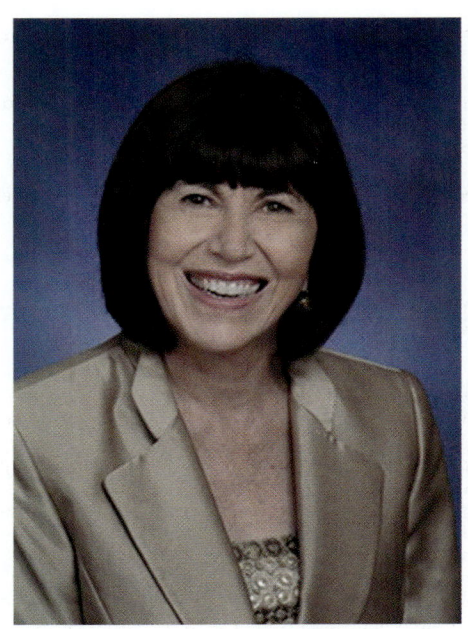

Contributors

Karen S. Abate, PhD, FNP-BC, FNAP
Nurse Practitioner
Hope Clinic
Dover, Delaware

Lisa V. Adams, MD
Associate Dean for Global Health
Medicine
Geisel School of Medicine at
 Dartmouth;
Director
Center for Health Equity
Geisel School of Medicine at
 Dartmouth;
Director
Global Initiatives
Office of the Provost
Dartmouth College
Hanover, New Hampshire

Imatullah Akyar, PhD, MsN, RN
Visiting Scholar
School of Nursing
University of Alabama at Birmingham
Birmingham, Alabama;
Assistant Professor
Faculty of Nursing
Hacettepe University
Ankara, Turkey

Traci Alberti, PhD, FNP-BC
Assistant Professor
School of Health Sciences
Merrimack College
North Andover, Massachusetts;
Family Nurse Practitioner
Urgent Care
Winchester Hospital Urgent Care,
 Wilmington
Wilmington, Massachusetts

Zubair Ansari, BS, MD
Resident Physician
Department of Ophthalmology
The University of Miami Bascom
 Palmer Eye Institute
Miami, Florida

Alex Bahadori, DNP, MS, FNP-C
Associate Dean
Graduate Program, FNP
Chamberlain University
Downers Grove, Illinois;
Dermatology Specialist
Spring Hill, Florida

Marie A. Bakitas, DNSc, NP-C, FAAN
Professor, Marie O'Koren Endowed
 Chair
School of Nursing
University of Alabama at Birmingham;
Associate Director
Center for Palliative and Supportive
 Care
University of Alabama at Birmingham,
Birmingham, Alabama

James T. Banta, MD
Associate Professor of Clinical
 Ophthalmology
Bascom Palmer Eye Institute
University of Miami Miller School of
 Medicine
Miami, Florida

Jodie A. Barkin, MD
Assistant Professor of Clinical Medicine
Division of Gastroenterology
Leonard M. Miller School of Medicine
University of Miami
Miami, Florida

Bethany Meyers Bartlett, M.S. Ed., M.D.
Lieutenant
Family Medicine
Naval Hospital Camp Pendleton,
Camp Pendleton, California

Jillian C. Belmont, DNP, FNP, AGACNP, SCRN
Nurse Practitioner
Neurology
Dartmouth Hitchcock Medical Center;
Assistant Professor in Neurology
Neurology
Dartmouth Geisel School of Medicine
Lebanon, New Hampshire

Lindsay E. Bergmann, MS, APRN, FNP-BC
Advanced Practice Registered Nurse
Department of General Surgery
Division of Surgical Oncology
Dartmouth-Hitchcock Medical Center
Lebanon, New Hampshire

Courtney L. Betts, MSN, ANP-BC
Adult Nurse Practitioner
New England Community Medical
 Services
North Andover, Massachusetts

Glen Blair, BS, MSN
Program Coordinator
Deptartment of Dermatology
Harvard Vanguard Medical Associates;
Lecturer
Graduate School of Nursing and Health
 Professions
University of Massachusetts
Boston, Massachusetts

Daniel A. Blaz, DNP
Chief of Clinical Operations
Surgeon Directorate
U.S. Army Central
Shaw AFB, South Carolina;
Adjunct Assistant Professor
Daniel K. Inouye Graduate School of
 Nursing
Uniformed Services University
Bethesda, Maryland

Maureen Bell Boardman, BSN, MSN
Clinical Assistant Professor of
 Community and Family Medicine
Community and Family Medicine
Geisel School of Medicine at
 Dartmouth
Hanover, New Hampshire;
ARNP/Director of Clinical Quality
Little Rivers Healthcare
Bradford, Vermont

Marie Elena Botte, MSN
Family Nurse Practitioner, CDE
Endocrinology
Boston Children's Hospital
Boston, Massachusetts

Elizabeth Bouley, ARNP-BC, MS, FNP-BC
Advanced Registered Nurse Practitioner
Internal Medicine Department
Dartmouth-Hitchcock
Nashua, New Hampshire;
Advanced Registered Nurse Practitioner
Family Practice
Keady Family Practice
Claremont, New Hampshire

Nicole Bove, BSOP, MSEM
Orthotics and Prosthetics
Tampa, Florida

Susan Bove, MSN, ARNP, FNP-BC
Nurse Practitioner
Family Care Center
Winchester Physician Associates
Stoneham, Massachusetts;
Adjunct Professor
Family Nurse Practitioner Program
Endicott College
Beverly, Massachusetts

Jennifer C. Braimon, MD
Endocrinologist
Department of Endocrinology
Lahey Hospital and Medical Center
Peabody, Massachusetts;
Assistant Clinical Professor
Tufts University School of Medicine
Boston, Massachusetts

Susan Culbertson Brighton, MS, APRN, AOCNP
Nurse Practitioner
Hematology and Oncology
Dartmouth Hitchcock Medical Center
Lebanon, New Hampshire

Cindy Broholm, MS, MPH, FNP-BC
Assistant Professor of Nursing
Harriet Rothkopf Heilbrunn School of
    Nursing
Long Island University/Brooklyn
Brooklyn, New York;
Family Nurse Practitioner
Callen-Lorde Community Health
    Center
New York, New York

Lin A. Brown, MD
Clinical Professor of Medicine
Geisel School of Medicine at
    Dartmouth
Hanover, New Hampshire;
Staff Rheumatologist
Medicine
New London Hospital
New London, New Hampshire

Jacqueline Rosenjack Burchum, DNSc, FNP-BC, CNE
Associate Professor
College of Nursing Department of
    Advanced Practice and Doctoral
    Studies
University of Tennessee Health Science
    Center
Memphis, Tennessee

Michael S. Calderwood, MD, MPH
Regional Hospital Epidemiologist
Section of Infectious Disease and
    International Health
Dartmouth-Hitchcock Medical Center
Lebanon, New Hampshire;
Assistant Professor of Medicine
Geisel School of Medicine (Dartmouth)
Hanover, New Hampshire

Virginia Curtin Capasso, PhD, ANP-BC, ACNS-BC, CWS, FACCWS
Advanced Practice Nurse
Institute for Patient Care
Massachusetts General Hospital;
Nurse Scientist
Munn Center for Nursing Research
Massachusetts General Hospital;
Instructor in Surgery
Harvard Medical School
Boston, Massachusetts

Stephanie Cassone, MSN, FNP-BC, ACHPN
Nurse Practitioner
Palliative Care
Brigham and Women's Hospital
Boston, Massachusetts

Benjamin P. Chan, MD, MPH
Clinical Assistant Professor of Medicine
Infectious Disease and International
    Health
Dartmouth-Hitchcock Medical Center
Lebanon, New Hampshire;
State Epidemiologist
New Hampshire Department of Health
    & Human Services
Division of Public Health Services
Concord, New Hampshire

Vicki Chandler, DNP, FNP-BC, MSN, BSN
Assistant Professor
Health Promotion and Disease
    Prevention
University of Tennessee Health Sciences
    Center
Memphis, Tennessee

Emma Virginia Clark, MHS, MSN
Certified Nurse Midwife
Family Health and Birth Center
Community of Hope;
Director
Maternal, Newborn, and Child Health
Chemonics International;
Adjunct Faculty
School of Nursing
NM/WHNP Program
Georgetown University
Washington, DC

Jean Sheerin Coffey, PhD, APRN
Associate Professor/Director
Nursing
Plymouth State University
Plymouth, New Hampshire

Michelle Collins, PhD, CNM, FACNM, FAAN
Professor, Director
Nurse-Midwifery Program
Vanderbilt University School of Nursing
Nashville, Tennessee

Karen F. Cotler, DNP, FNP
Clinical Assistant Professor
Family Nurse Practitioner
University of Illinois College of
    Nursing;
Clinical FNP Practitioner
Miles Square Health/COIP
University of Illinois Health
Chicago, Illinois

Ashley H. Cotter, PT, DPT, MS, OCS, COMT
Orthopedic and Manual Clinical
    Specialist Physical Therapist
Rehabilitation Services
Brigham and Women's Hospital
Health Care Center
Foxborough, Massachusetts

Jennifer L. Culgin, ANP ACHPN
Care Dimensions
Needham, Massachusetts

Lauren Curtis, APRN FNP-BC
Structural Heart
Hartford Hospital
Hartford, Connecticut

Lindsey Cushing, APRN, WHNP-BC
Advanced Practice Registered Nurse
Women's Health
Dartmouth Hitchcock Keene
Keene, New Hampshire

David de Gijsel, MD, MSc
Instructor
Medicine
Geisel School of Medicine at
    Dartmouth
Hanover, New Hampshire;
Physician
Infectious Diseases
Dartmouth-Hitchcock Medical Center
Lebanon, New Hampshire

Teresa Denk Smajda, BS, MN, FNP
Family Nurse Practitioner
Primary Care
Saint Luke's Medical Group
Kansas City, Missouri

Martha DesBiens, MD
Physician
Infectious Disease and International
    Health
Dartmouth Hitchcock Medical Center
Lebanon, New Hampshire

Kevin Dholaria, MD
Fellow
Gastroenterology
University of Miami
Miami, Florida

Karen Dick, PhD, GNP-BC, FAANP
Associate Dean for Advanced Practice
    Programs
Graduate School of Nursing
UMASS Medical School
Worcester, Massachusetts;
Nurse Practitioner
Hebrew Senior Life
Boston, Massachusetts

**John Distler, DPA, MBA, MS, FNP-C,
FAANP**
Professor
Family Nurse Practitioner Track
Chamberlain College of Nursing
Downers Grove, Illinois

Leigh Dobbs, BS, RN, MSN, FNP-BC
Family Nurse Practitioner
Primary Care
Thundermist Health Center
Woonsocket, Rhode Island

**Catherine Marie Duffy, MSN,
APRN-BC, ACHPN**
Nurse Practitioner
Palliative Care
Care Dimensions
Danvers, Massachusetts

Evelyn Duffy, BS, MS, DNP
Associate Professor
Frances Payne Bolton School of Nursing
Case Western Reserve University;
Adult Gerontology Nurse Practitioner
Geriatric Medicine
University Hospitals of Cleveland
Cleveland, Ohio

Jacob Starr Duker, MD
Resident Physician
Ophthalmology
Bascom Palmer Eye Institute
Miami, Florida

**Joel Dulaigh, MSN, ACNP-BC,
FAANP**
Chief of Staff
Office of the Surgeon General
U.S. Department of Health and Human
    Services
Washington, DC

Andrea Efre, DNP, ARNP, FNP
Owner, Nurse Practitioner and Educator
Nurse Practitioner Consultant
Healthcare Education Consultants
Tampa, Florida

Vickie K. Ernste, DNP, MSN, RN
Nurse Manager
Emergency Department
Mayo Clinic
Rochester, Minnesota

Linda Evans, PhD
Assistant Professor
Nursing
Nova Southeastern University
Ft. Lauderdale, Florida

**Kathy J. Fabiszewski, PhD, RN,
A/GNP, BC**
Nurse Practitioner
Extended Care Facilities Program
Atrius Health
Harvard Vanguard Medical Associated
Peabody, Massachusetts;
Adjunct Clinical Faculty
College of Nursing
Endicott College
Beverly, Massachusetts

Mary Lynn Fahey, DNP, MS, ARNP
Assistant Clinical Professor;
Family Nurse Practitioner Program
    Director
School of Nursing
Northeastern University
Boston, Massachusetts

Kenneth C. Fan, MD, MBA
Ophthalmologist
Ophthalmology
Bascom Palmer Eye Institute
Miami, Florida

**Heidi Collins Fantasia, PhD, RN,
WHNP-BC**
Associate Professor
Zuckerberg College of Health Sciences
Solomont School of Nursing
University of Massachusetts, Lowell
Lowell, Massachusetts

A. Susan Feeney, BS, MS, DNP
Assistant Professor;
Family Nurse Practitioner Program
    Coordinator
Graduate School of Nursing
University of Massachusetts Worcester
Worcester, Massachusetts;
Family Nurse Practitioner Senior
    Associate
Wright and Associates Family Health
    Care
Amherst, New Hampshire;
Senior Faculty
Fitzgerald Health Education Associates,
    Inc.
N. Andover, Massachusetts

Henrique J. Fernandez, MD, FACP
Director, Gastroenterology Fellowship
Gastroenterology
Parkview Medical Center
Pueblo, Colorado

Carey J. Field, MD
Assistant Professor of Rheumatology
Rheumatology
White River Junction Veterans Affairs
    Medical Center
White River Junction, Vermont;
Assistant Professor of Rheumatology
Rheumatology
Dartmouth-Hitchcock Medical Center
Lebanon, New Hampshire

Julia A. Ford, MD
Clinical Fellow
Rheumatology
Brigham and Women's Hospital
Boston, Massachusetts

**Jessica Helen Fortunak, RN, BS,
MSN, CPNP, FNP-C**
Nurse Practitioner
Primary Care
HealthNet
Brownsburg, Indiana

Catherine Franklin, MSN, DNP
Clinical Administrative Director
Department of Family Medicine
East Boston Neighborhood Health
   Center
East Boston, Massachusetts

Brad E. Franklin, DNP, RN, FNP-C
Officer in Charge
Byrd Medical Home
Blanchfield Army Community Hospital
Fort Campbell, Kentucky

**Michelle Freshman, MPH, MSN,
APRN, FNP-BC**
Nurse Practitioner
Department of Medicine
Newton-Wellesley Hospital
Newton, Massachusetts

Megan Carol Gallagher, MD
Physician
Infectious Diseases and International
   Health
Dartmouth-Hitchcock Medical Center
Lebanon, New Hampshire

Anthony S. Gemignani, MD
Cardiologist
Cardiology
White River Junction Veterans Affairs
   Medical Center,
White River Junction, Vermont;
Assistant Professor of Medicine
Geisel School of Medicine at
   Dartmouth
Hanover, New Hampshire

Sarah Hauke Given, MSN, ANP-BC
Nurse Practitioner
Psychosocial Oncology and Palliative
   Care
Dana Farber Cancer Institute
Boston, Massachusetts

Donna M. Glynn, PhD, RN, ANP
Associate Dean Pre-Licensure Nursing
School of Nursing
Regis College
Weston, Massachusetts;
Nurse Scientist
Nursing
VA Boston Healthcare System
West Roxbury, Massachusetts

Meghan Glynn, MSN, FNP-BC
Clinical Nurse Educator
Pediatric Nursing
Franciscan Children's
Brighton, Massachusetts

**Randy Michael Gordon, DNP,
FNP-BC**
Associate Professor
Graduate Program
Family Nurse Practitioner Track
Chamberlain College of Nursing
Downers Grove, Illinois

Sharon L. Grantham, MSN, DNP
Doctor Grantham
Family Practice
Dr. Grantham & Assoc, LLC
Fort Myers, Florida

Glen P. Greenough, M.D.
Associate Professor
Psychiatry, Medicine and Neurology
Geisel School of Medicine at
   Dartmouth
Lebanon, New Hampshire

John S. Groundland, MD, MS
Clinical Instructor
Department of Orthopedic Surgery
Huntsman Cancer Institute;
Primary Children's Hospital;
University of Utah;
Salt Lake City, Utah

Patricia Hadidian, MSN
GNP-BC
HouseCalls
Optum
Columbia, Maryland

Wendy L. Halm, DNP, APNP, FNP-BC
Clinical Associate Professor
School of Nursing
University of Wisconsin Madison
Madison, Wisconsin

**Wanda J. Handel, MSN, RN,
ACCNS-AG, CNRN**
Clinical Nurse Specialist
Neuroscience
Center for Nursing Excellence
Dartmouth-Hitchcock Medical Center
Lebanon, New Hampshire

**Margaret Thorman Hartig, PhD,
APRN-BC, FAANP**
Professor
Advanced Practice and Doctoral Studies
College of Nursing
University of Tennessee Health Science
   Center
Memphis, Tennessee

**Brittany Blair Hay, DNP, APRN,
ANP-BC, FNP-BC**
Assistant Professor
College of Nursing
University of South Florida
Tampa, Florida

Simon M. Helfgott, MD, CM
Associate Professor of Medicine
Medicine
Harvard Medical School;
Director of Education & Fellowship
   Training
Division of Rheumatology
Brigham and Women's Hospital
Boston, Massachusetts

Eric R. Henderson, MD
Assistant Professor
Orthopaedics
Dartmouth College
Hanover, New Hampshire;
Section Chief
Orthopaedic Surgery
White River Junction Veterans Affairs
   Medical Center
White River Junction, Vermont

John W. Hinkle, MD
Physician
Ophthalmology
Bascom Palmer Eye Institute
Miami, Florida

James Peter Ioli, DPM
Chief
Division of Podiatry
Department of Orthopedics
Brigham and Women's Hospital;
Assistant Professor of Orthopedic
   Surgery
Harvard Medical School
Boston, Massachusetts

Zacharia Isaac, MD
Division Chief
Pain and Spine Care
Department of Physical Medicine and
   Rehabilitation
Harvard Medical School;
Associate Chairman
Physical Medicine and Rehabilitation
Brigham and Women's Hospital
Boston, Massachusetts

Robyn M. Jennings, MD, MPH
Family Medicine Resident
North Colorado Family Medicine
   Residency Program
Greeley, Colorado

Tamara K. Jo, NP, WHNP, MSN, RN
Nurse Practitioner
Hematology Oncology
Mount Auburn Hospital
Cambridge, Massachusetts

Dorothy K. Johnson, FNP, PhD
Nurse Practitioner
Rheumatology
LAC/USC Heathcare Network
Los Angeles, California

Brooke G. Judd, MD
Section Chief
Sleep Medicine
Dartmouth-Hitchcock Medical Center
Lebanon, New Hampshire;
Assistant Professor
Medicine
Geisel School of Medicine at
    Dartmouth
Hanover, New Hampshire

Kevin D. Kerin, MD
Physician
Rheumatology
University of Vermont Health Network
    Central Vermont Medical Center
Berlin, Vermont

Amelia Siani Kerner, PA-C, MMSc
Lead Associate Provider
Medical ICU
Dartmouth Hitchcock Medical Center
Lebanon, New Hampshire

Elizabeth Kimtis, BA, BSN, MSN, APRN
Nurse Practitioner
Hematology/Oncology
Dartmouth Hitchcock Medical Center
Lebanon, New Hampshire

Nancy B. Kuemmerle, DO, PhD
Staff Physician
Medicine, Section of Hematology/
    Oncology
White River Junction Veterans Affairs
    Medical Center
White River Junction, Vermont;
Assistant Professor
Medicine
Geisel School of Medicine at
    Dartmouth
Hanover, New Hampshire

Patrick LaRose, DNP, MSN/Ed, RN
Associate Professor
Doctor of Nursing Practice (DNP)
    Program
College of Nursing
Chamberlain University
Downers Grove, Illinois

Diana M. Laura, MD
Resident
Ophthalmology
Bascom Palmer Eye Institute
Miami, Florida

Nancy McQueen Le, BA, MSN
Nurse Practitioner
Neurology
Boston University Department of
    Neurology
Braintree, Massachusetts

Leslie Lezell Levitan, BSN, MSN, FNP, ACHPN
Palliative Care Nurse Practitioner
Hospice and Palliative Care
Care Dimensions
Danvers, Massachusetts

Catherine Gaines Ling, PhD, FNP-BC
Associate Dean
Graduate Clinical Programs
University of South Florida College of
    Nursing
Tampa, Florida

Sharon Little, DNP, FNP-BC
Assistant Professor
Health and Disease Promotion (DNP/
    FNP Program)
College of Nursing
University of Tennessee Health Science
    Center
Memphis, Tennessee

Rene Love, PhD, DNP, PMHNP
DNP Director / Clinical Associate
    Professor
Nursing
University of Arizona
Tucson, Arizona

Jason R. Lucey, MSN, FNP-BC
Assistant Professor
School of Nursing
MGH Institute of Health Professions
Boston, Massachusetts

Erin A. Lyden, MSN, BSN, BS, FNP-C
Northport, Florida

Alan Ona Malabanan, MD
Staff Physician
Endocrinology, Diabetes and
    Metabolism
Beth Israel Deaconess Medical Center
Boston, Massachusetts

Maura A. Malone, MSN, RN
Clinical Nurse Specialist, Hemophilia
    and Thrombosis
Hematology
Dartmouth Hitchcock Medical Center
Lebanon, New Hampshire

Ann H. Maradiegue, PhD, FNP-BC, FAANP
Adjunct
School of Nursing
The George Washington University
Washington, DC

Priscilla Marsicovetere, JD, PA-C
Director
Master of Physician Assistant Studies
    Program
Franklin Pierce University
Lebanon, New Hampshire;
Assistant Professor
Department of Medical Education
Geisel School of Medicine at
    Dartmouth
Hanover, New Hampshire

Roselyn Cristelle I. Mateo, MD MSc
Endocrinology
Beth Israel Deaconess Medical Center
Boston, Massachusetts

Varghese Mathai, MPAS, MDiv
Physician Assistant
Lymphoma/Myeloma
MD Anderson Cancer Center
Houston, Texas

Elizabeth B. McCabe, MS, APRN
Nurse Practitioner
Surgical Oncology
Dartmouth Hitchcock
Lebanon, New Hampshire

Ellen M. McCafferty-O'Connell, GNP, DCNP
NP, Clinical Nurse Manager
Dermatology
Atrius Health;
Nurse Practitioner, Educator
Nursing
University of Massachusetts,
Boston, Massachusetts

Tracy McClinton, DNP, AGACNP-BC
Assistant Professor
College of Nursing
University of Tennessee Health Science
Center
Memphis, Tennessee

Talli McCormick, BS, MSN
Clinical Assistant Professor
School of Nursing
MGH Institute of Health Professions
Boston, Massachusetts

Laurel McKernan, RN, MSN
Hemophilia Clinical Specialist
Section of Hematology
Dartmouth Hitchcock Medical Center
Lebanon, New Hampshire

Sheila Ann Medina, MAJ Sheila Ann Medina, DNP, FNP-C, MBA
Family Nurse Practitioner
Chief of Hospital Education
Carl R. Darnall Army Medical Center
Fort Hood, Texas

Ashley Moore-Gibbs, DNP, RN, AGPCNP-BC, CHFN
Nurse Practitioner
Adult Cardiology
Sanger Heart & Vascular Institute;
ACP Cardiovascular Fellowship Director
Center for Advanced Practice
Atrium Health
Charlotte, North Caroline

Deanne Munroe, JD, MSN
Pre-surgical Nurse Practitioner
Hospitalist
PIH Health Hospital
Whittier, California

David Patrick Murphy, MD, FCCP
Head, Pulmonary / Critical Care
Medicine
Internal Medicine
Naval Hospital Camp Pendleton
Camp Pendleton, California

Amelia Nelson Nadler, DNP, FNP-C
Clinical Nurse Practitioner
Emergency Department
Winchester Hospital
Winchester, Massachusetts

Leslie Neal-Boylan, PhD, RN, CRRN, APRN, FAAN
Associate Dean for Academic Affairs
and Program Innovation and
Professor
Nursing
MGH Institute of Health Professions
Boston,
Massachusetts

Patrice K. Nicholas, DNSc, DHL (Hon.), MPH, MS, RN, ANP, FAAN
Professor
School of Nursing
MGH Institute of Health Professions;
Director and Senior Nurse Scientist
Division of Global Health Equity and
Center for Nursing Excellence
Brigham and Women's Hospital
Boston, Massachusetts

Meaghan E. O'Leary, MSN, AGACNP-BC
Nurse Practitioner, Gerontology
Surgical Care Group
Catholic Medical Center
Manchester, New Hampshire

Lisa M. O'Neal, MSN, MS, BSN, BA, ACNP-BC, ANP-BC
Nurse Practitioner
Surgical Intensive Care/ICU
Baptist Health
Miami, Florida

Daniel W. O'Neill, MD, ThM
Assistant Clinical Professor
Family Medicine
University of Connecticut School of
Medicine,
Farmington;
Managing Editor
Christian Journal for Global Health
Putnam, Connecticut

Deborah L. Ornstein, MD
Medical Director
Comprehensive Hemophilia &
Thrombosis Center
Dartmouth-Hitchcock Medical Center
Lebanon, New Hampshire

Tracia L. O'Shana, MSN, APRN
Advanced Practice Registered Nurse
Gastroenterology and Hepatology
Dartmouth Hitchcock Medical Center
Lebanon, New Hampshire

Diane Todd Pace, PhD, APRN, FNP-BC, NCMP, IF FAANP, FAAN
Professor/Director, Special Academic
Programs
College of Nursing
University of Tennessee Health Science
Center;
Associate Professor
College of Medicine
Department of Obstetrics and
Gynecology
University of Tennessee Health Science
Center
Memphis, Tennessee

Duellyn Pandis, DNP, MS, BSN
Professor
College of Nursing
University of South Florida
Tampa, Florida;
President
Family Nurse Practitioner
Passport Health of Tampa Bay,
Tampa, Florida

Nimesh A. Patel, MD
Doctor
Ophthalmology
Bascom Palmer Eye Institute
Miami, Florida

Donna Jenell Pease, BSN, MSN, ANP, GNP, CDE, BC-ADM
Diabetes Nurse Practitioner
Gold Medical Home
Blanchfield Army Community Hospital
Fort Campbell, Kentucky

Pamela Sue Porter, DNP, APRN, FNP-BC, CNS, PHN, PA-C
Associate Professor
Graduate Nursing
Chamberlain University
Downers Grove, Illinois;
FNP II
School of Medicine Medical
Surveillance
University of California, Davis
Davis, California

Marcia Potter, DNP, FNP-BC
Nurse Practitioner
Malcolm Grow Medical Clinics &
Surgery Center
Joint Base Andrews, Maryland

Jill M. Price, PhD, MSN, RN
Senior Director
Post Licensure College of Nursing
    Programs
Post-Licensure Online
Chamberlain University
Downers Grove, Illinois

Magen M. Price, FNP-BC
Family Nurse Practitioner
Family Medicine
Upham's Corner Health Center
Boston, Massachusetts

Richard Matthew Prior, DNP, FNP-BC, FAANP
Associate Professor
College of Nursing
University of Cincinnati
Cincinnati, Ohio

Emily Proulx, MSN, APRN
Women's Health Nurse Practitioner
OB/GYN
Dartmouth Hitchcock
Nashua, New Hampshire

Anthony Provenzano, MD
Nephrology Fellow
Duke Medical Center
Durham, North Carolina

Francisco P. Quismorio, Jr., MD
Professor of Medicine and Pathology
Medicine
Keck School of Medicine
University of Southern California,
Los Angeles, California

Laura A. Rabin, PhD
Professor
Department of Psychology
Brooklyn College and The Graduate
    Center of CUNY
Brooklyn, New York

Paula K. Rauschkolb, DO
Assistant Professor
Medicine
Geisel School of Medicine at
    Dartmouth
Hanover, New Hampshire

Laura Reed, DNP, APRN, FNP-BC
Assistant Professor
Advanced Practice and Doctoral Studies
The University of Tennessee Health
    Science Center
Memphis, Tennessee

Geri Cage Reeves, PhD, APRN, FNP-BC
Assistant Professor
School of Nursing
Vanderbilt University
Nashville, Tennessee

Elizabeth Remo, BSHSE, MS, DNP, APRN, FNP-BC
Assistant Professor
College of Nursing
University of South Florida
Tampa, Florida

Katherine McCabe Reyad, MSN, FNP-BC
Nurse Practitioner
Primary Care/Cardiology
Plymouth Heart Center
Plymouth, Massachusetts

Janet Rico, BSN, MSN, MBA, PhD
Assistant Dean Northeastern University
    Graduate Nursing Programs
Nursing
Northeastern;
Nurse Practitioner
Emergency Services
Massachusetts General Hospital
Boston, Massachusetts

Suzanne M. Rieke, MD
Endocrinologist; Assistant Clinical
    Professor
Department of Endocrinology
Lahey Hospital and Medical Center
Tufts University School of Medicine
Peabody, Massachusetts

Marylou Virginia Robinson, PhD, FNP-C
Associate Professor
School of Nursing
Pacific Lutheran University
Tacoma, Washington

Maria Isabel Romano, MSN
Associate Vice President
Medical Informatics
Premise Health
Brentwood, Tennessee

Andrew J. Rong, MD
Doctor
Ophthalmology
Bascom Palmer Eye Institute
Miami, Florida

Dionna C. Rookey, MPAS, MS, BS
Physician Assistant
Family Medicine
Dartmouth Hitchcock Medical Center
Lebanon, New Hampshire

Barbara G. Rosato, DNP, CNP, ANP-BC, CDE
Adult Nurse Practitioner
General Internal Medicine & Primary
    Care
Beth Israel Deaconess Medical Center
Boston, Massachusetts

Sule Steve Salami, MD, FACC
Medical Director
Chest Pain Program
Cardiac Catheterization Lab
Cardiology
Adventhealth Waterman;
Tavares, Florida

Susan Sanner, PhD, APRN, FNP-BC
Associate Professor of Nursing
MSN FNP Program
Chamberlain College of Nursing,
Downer's Grove, Illinois

Anna D. Schaal, MS, ARNP
Nurse Practitioner
Hematology
Norris Cotton Cancer Center
Dartmouth Hitchcock Medical Center;
Lebanon, New Hampshire

Naomi Schlesinger, MD
Professor of Medicine;
Chief, Division of Rheumatology
Rutgers Robert Wood Johnson Medical
    School
Rutgers University
New Brunswick, New Jersey

Lindsay M. Schommer, BS, BSN, MSN
Instructor in Neurology
Neurology
Dartmouth Medical School
Hanover, New Hampshire;
Nurse Practitioner
Neurology
Dartmouth Hitchcock Medical Center
Lebanon, New Hampshire

Karen L. Secore, MS, APRN, CNRN
Nurse Practitioner/Coordinator
Dartmouth Hitchcock Epilepsy Center
Dartmouth Hitchcock Medical Center
Lebanon, New Hampshire

Diane C. Seibert, PhD, WHNP-BC, FAANP, FAAN
Associate Dean for Academic Affairs
Graduate School of Nursing
Uniformed Services University
Bethesda, Maryland

Christopher Joseph Shaw, MSN, ANP, PMHNPc, CARN AP
Nurse Director
Substance Use Disorder Initiative
The Massachusetts General Hospital
Boston, Massachusetts;
Psychiatric Mental Health NP
Outpatient Psychiatry
Waltham Behavioral Health
Waltham, Massachusetts

Emily Karwacki Sheff, MS, RN
Assistant Professor
Nursing
Rivier University
Nashua, New Hampshire

Ani Sinanyan, MSN-Ed, FNP-BC
Nurse Practitioner
Glendale, California

Sharon Smart, BSN, MS, FNP
Nurse Practitioner
New England Community Medical
    Services
North Andover, Massachusetts

Sara Smoller, MSN, ANP-BC
Instructor
School of Nursing
MGH Institute of Health Professions
Boston, Massachusetts;
Adult Nurse Practitioner
Family Doctors, LLC
Swampscott, Massachusetts

Hannah Steere, MD
Resident Physician
Physical Medicine and Rehabilitation
Spaulding Rehabilitation Hospital
Charlestown, Massachusetts

Julie G. Stewart, DNP, MPH, MSN, FNP-BC, FAANP
Associate Professor
College of Nursing
Sacred Heart University
Fairfield, Connecticut

Melissa C. Storms, MSN
Hematology/Oncology Nurse
    Practitioner
Norris Cotton Cancer Center
Dartmouth-Hitchcock Medical Center
Lebanon, New Hampshire

Swarup S. Swaminathan, MD
Resident Physician
Ophthalmology
Bascom Palmer Eye Institute
Miami, Florida

Kathryn D. Swartwout, PhD, APRN, FNP BC
Associate Professor
Community, Systems and Mental
    Health Nursing
Rush University
Chicago, Illinois

Elizabeth A. Talbot, MD
Associate Professor
Medicine
Geisel School of Medicine at
    Dartmouth
Hanover, New Hampshire;
Deputy State Epidemiologist
New Hampshire Department of Health
    and Human Services
Concord, New Hampshire

Richard Anthony Taylor, DNP, CRNP, ANP-BC
Assistant Professor
Acute, Chronic and Continuing Care
University of Alabama at Birmingham
    School of Nursing
Birmingham, Alabama

Thomas H. Taylor, MD, MS
Chief Infectious Diseases and
    Rheumatology
Medicine
White River Junction Veterans Affairs
    Medical Center
White River Junction, Vermont;
Associate Professor of Medicine
Geisel School of Medicine at
    Dartmouth
Hanover, New Hampshire

Lynsey P. Teulings, MS, APRN
Nurse Practitioner
Hematology Oncology
Dartmouth Hitchcock Medical Center
Lebanon, New Hampshire

Derrick J. Todd, MD, PhD
Staff Physician
Rheumatology, Immunology, and
    Allergy
Brigham and Women's Hospital
Boston, Massachusetts

Ann Q. Tran, MD
Resident in Ophthalmology
Ophthalmology
Bascom Palmer Eye Institute
Miami, Florida

Grace Ellen Urquhart, DNP, MSN, BSN, ADN, FNP-C
Nurse Practitioner
Family Practice
Frontier Nursing University
Hyden, Kentucky

Denise A. Vanacore-Chase, PhD, CRNP, ANP-BC, PMHNP-BC
Director DNP & NP programs
Graduate Nursing
Gwynedd Mercy University
Gwynedd Valley, Pennsylvania

Nandini Venkateswaran, MD
Resident Physician
Department of Ophthalmology
Bascom Palmer Eye Institute
Miami, Florida

Erin R. Voelschow, BA, MS
Medical Student
Rocky Vista University,
Parker, Colorado

John David Wagner, MD
Family Medicine
Naval Hospital Camp Pendleton,
Camp Pendleton, California

Jill S. Walsh, DNP, MS, BSN
Dean
Doctor of Nursing Practice (DNP)
    Program
Chamberlain College of Nursing
Downers Grove, Illinois

Lauren Jean Welton, MS, PA-C
Physician Assistant
General Surgery
Dartmouth-Hitchcock;
Clinical Faculty
Physician Assistant Program
Massachusetts College of Pharmacy and
    Health Sciences;
Physical Assistant
Trauma, Vascular and General Surgery
Elliot Hospital
Manchester, New Hampshire

Karen J. Whitt, PhD, RN, FNP-C, AGN-BC, FAANP
Associate Professor
School of Nursing
George Washington University
Washington, DC

Alicia Wierenga, MSN, NP
Nurse Manager
Hematology/Oncology BMT Inpatient
    Nurse Manager
Umass Memorial Medical Center
Worcester, Massachusetts

**Dawn Williamson, RN, DNP,
PMHCNS-BC, CARN-AP**
Addiction Psychiatry Consultation
Emergency Department
Massachusetts General Hospital
Boston, Massachusetts

**Yvette T. Wilson, MSN, DNP,
FNP-BC**
Associate Dean of Faculty;
Adjunct Professor
Chamberlain University
Downers Grove, Illinois

**Christine Wilson, PhD, ANP-BC,
FNP-BC**
Director of Medical Scientific Liaisons
Medical Affairs
E Pharma
Tampa, Florida

**Chris Winkelman, PhD, ACNP-BC,
CCRN, CNE, FAANP, FCCM**
Associate Professor
Frances Payne Bolton School of Nursing
Case Western Reserve University
Cleveland, Ohio

**Mary E. Wood, RN, MS, CDE,
BC-ADM**
Diabetes Clinical Nurse Specialist
Nursing Practice
Dartmouth-Hitchcock Medical Center,
Lebanon, New Hampshire;
Instructor
Community and Family Medicine
The Geisel School of Medicine at
    Dartmouth
Hanover, New Hampshire

**Charles Yingling, DNP, FNP-BC,
FAANP**
Clinical Assistant Professor—FNP
    Program Director
Department of Health Systems Science
University of Illinois at Chicago College
    of Nursing,
Chicago, Illinois

**Mary Young-Breuleux, MSN, APRN,
BC, CNE**
Adult Nurse Practitioner
Adult Health
Good Neighbor Health Clinic
White RIver Junction, Vermont

Susan Yuditskaya, MD
Assistant Professor of Medicine
Endocrinology
Dartmouth-Hitchcock Medical Center
Lebanon, New Hampshire

Leo R. Zacharski, MD
Emeritus Professor of Medicine
Medicine
Geisel School of Medicine at
    Dartmouth College
Lebanon, New Hampshire

Elke Zschaebitz, DNP, FNP-BC
Nurse Practitioner
General Medicine
University of Virginia,
Charlottesville, Virginia;
Faculty
Department of Nursing and Health
    Science
Georgetown University
Washington, DC

Reviewers

Deborah A. Bristol, PA-C
VA Medical Center
Home Based Primary Care
White River Junction, Vermont

Caitlin Greenberg, DO
Hospitalist
Department of Internal Medicine
University of Vermont Medical Center
Burlington, Vermont

A. Susan Feeney, DNP, FNP-BC
Assistant Professor
Family Nurse Practitioner Program
    Coordinator
Graduate School of Nursing
University of Massachusetts School of
    Medicine
Worcester, Massachusetts

Amelia Nelson Nadler, DNP, FNP-C
Clinical Nurse Practitioner
Emergency Department
Winchester Hospital
Winchester, Massachusetts

Anthony Provenzano, MD
Nephrology Fellow
Duke Medical Center
Durham, North Carolina

Sule Steve Salami, MD, FACC
Medical Director
Cardiac Catheterization Lab
Cardiology
Florida Hospital Waterman
Tavares, Florida

Preface

Since the first edition of *Primary Care: A Collaborative Practice*, our vision has been to emphasize the value of professionals working together to improve patient care and well-being. In the past twenty years, hundreds of healthcare professionals from a wide geographic range have shared that vision and worked jointly with us and others in this intellectual endeavor. We are now acknowledging this work by changing the title of the book to *Primary Care: Interprofessional Collaborative Practice* to clearly state our commitment to collaborative practice.

We, as editors, work together respecting one another's unique talents and strengths, solving problems together, just as healthcare professionals do each day. In the clinical setting collaboration is the essence of interprofessional care, and team-based care is a fundamental component of complex care management. Most important, though, is the collaborative partnership between patient and provider. These relationships are the foundation of high-performing primary care practices.

NEW CHAPTERS

In the sixth edition of this text we have added new chapters and expanded on others. In Chapter 1, we address the challenges and opportunities of interprofessional collaboration in a turbulent health care environment. Patient-centered care, quality care objectives, and the changing landscape of primary care are explored. Chapter 2, *Translating Research into Clinical Practice*, addresses the relationship of primary care to research initiatives and how research translates and impacts clinical practice. The increasing incidence of chronic illness and the growing responsibilities of caring for patients across the continuum of care are discussed in Chapter 4, *Coordinated Chronic Care*. Our hope in providing this chapter is that understanding the challenges that patients and families face when entering or leaving a healthcare facility will aid in preventing adverse events, stress, and re-hospitalizations. In chapter 5, *Introduction to Health Literacy, Health Care Disparities, and Culturally Responsive Primary Care*, the disparities in care experienced by specific at risk populations and other factors impacting patient health are explored.

Other new chapters are included in the sixth edition. Each of these chapters recognizes aspects of clinical practice that are fundamental yet at times perhaps not fully considered. Because many of our patients prefer a more holistic approach to health and well-being, we have added a Wellness Chapter that explores the scope of wellness and recommended interventions. This edition also recognizes the serious issues associated with human trafficking (Chapter 12) and some of the health issues that are associated with this hidden, criminal and exploitive trend. Information about alternative therapies in which many patients and caregivers are interested are mentioned in the individual clinical chapters enabling nurse practitioners and other primary care providers to more fully understand the risks and benefits of the supplements and alternative approaches that patients are using. *Risk Management*, **Chapter 8,** identifies

the attitudes and relationship skills in healthcare settings that can positively or negatively impact the patient's perceptions of the patient-provider relationship. The chapter author addresses the legal risks inherent in practice and recommends strategies to improve care, patient satisfaction, and risk management. **LGBTQ Patient Care** reflects the editors' concern about disparities in healthcare, with the hope that the information in this chapter will aid all of us in improving care for all patients.

FORMAT

The format of the sixth edition of *Primary Care: Interprofessional Collaborative Practice is* purposefully similar to the systematic approach used in primary care practice and is designed and organized to promote improved clinical reasoning skills. Each section is an important building block in the assessment and diagnosis of each patient's presentation. Understanding the **Epidemiology** and **Pathophysiology** of illness is integral to understanding a patient's symptoms and the consideration of possible causes. The **Clinical Presentation** and **Physical Examination** sections in each chapter address the cognitive, physical, or psychosocial features and physical exam findings that can be associated with the patient's complaint. Attention to the patient's concerns and detection of pertinent positive and negative findings are the clues that create the list of possible **Differential Diagnoses.** The Differential Diagnosis requires clinical reasoning, a decision-making process that considers the "do not miss" differentials, and helps determine the most likely diagnosis and necessary **Diagnostics.** To aid in this process, the Differential Diagnosis sections discuss the possible differentials, and the Diagnostics boxes list the appropriate essential tests that should be considered. These include initial tests (tests that may be performed in the office setting, such as peak flow measurement or pulse oximetry), laboratory tests, imaging studies (radiographic, ultrasound, nuclear, or magnetic resonance imaging), or other miscellaneous studies that may be necessary in the evaluation of the disorder (such as EEGs or biopsies). Because the clinical presentation differs with each patient, not all diagnostic tests listed may be necessary in each circumstance. An asterisk is placed beside those tests that may be indicated by clinical presentation and physical examination findings. For more detailed information, the reader should refer to the "Diagnostics" and "Differential Diagnosis" sections included with each disorder.

The **Management** section of each chapter addresses goals of treatment and therapeutic interventions based on current evidence and guidelines. Pharmacologic agents are included, as are recommendations for non-pharmacologic therapies. The management sections make every attempt to incorporate the research contributions that create an evidence base for practice. Authoritative management guidelines, as well as current ongoing research findings, are incorporated whenever available. As with any evolving science, recommendations can be in a state of flux. Management recommendations may change, and new recommendations for practice supersede the management recommendations presented in this textbook. In addition, the reader is directed to check drug indications, dosages, and potential drug-drug interactions in medication product information before prescribing or administering any medication.

Complications associated with the disease and treatments are described, and clear recommendations for **Patient and Family Education** are included throughout the textbook. This information is crucial in promoting health literacy and assisting healthcare providers in interpreting information about the illness and management to patients and caregivers.

This edition continues to provide clear guidelines for referrals, and the **Emergency and Physician Referral Icons** highlight conditions that may require immediate consultation. The reader should be aware that more comprehensive referral or consultation criteria are contained in the text of the chapters that contain these special icons. The reader should also realize that the emergency icons might not represent all of the conditions requiring emergency referral. The editors are also aware that experienced providers may not require consultation for all the specified circumstances. In addition, state practice regulations may mandate referral under certain circumstances; these regulations supersede any consultation recommendations detailed in this text.

The sixth edition again provides a collection of Instructor Resources on an Evolve website (http://evolve.elsevier.com/Buttaro), available via your Elsevier Education Solutions Consultant for programs adopting classroom quantities of the book. The Instructor Resources consist of a Test Bank, Power-Point Collection, and Image Collection. The Test Bank includes approximately 685 test items delivered in Evolve Assessment Manager for easy exam construction and administration. The PowerPoint Collection consists of approximately 685 slides for classroom or online instruction. The Image Collection includes all original images from the textbook. We trust that these frequently requested resources will help to facilitate high-quality instruction of Nurse Practitioner students.

THE FUTURE

It is evident that an aging population, globalization, science, and technology continue to impact healthcare and clinical practice. An aging population with multiple co-morbidities has already impacted healthcare expenditures and unless we are able to identify and control these diseases earlier and effectively, morbidity, mortality, and healthcare costs will continue to rise. Global travel and an increase in transnational businesses have increased the risk of disease spread and the importance of vigilant awareness of global threats to the public health. Every day, scientific breakthroughs affect disease management, healthcare quality, and health information management. It is clear that to meet the healthcare needs of the future, innovative technology will be needed to relieve the cognitive burden created by these new discoveries. It is the editors' hope that *Primary Care: Interprofessional Collaborative Practice*, will provide a solid foundation on which tomorrow's primary care providers can help patients to lead increasingly healthy lives.

ACKNOWLEDGMENTS

This textbook represents a strong collaborative effort. We remain indebted to our contributors, past and present. They generously provided their time and expertise to make this textbook the trusted resource that it is. We welcome and are appreciative of the contributions made by our patients, students, and colleagues. We continue to try to incorporate their suggestions to make this book a useful one for students and practicing clinicians alike.

We greatly appreciate the support of everyone at Elsevier. Still, we are particularly thankful for the guidance of Heather Bays throughout the editing and production process, and for Lee Henderson, who encouraged us through the fourth, fifth, and now the sixth edition.

Finally, our families, friends, and colleagues deserve our eternal thanks. Their patience and understanding throughout this endeavor is greatly appreciated!

Contents

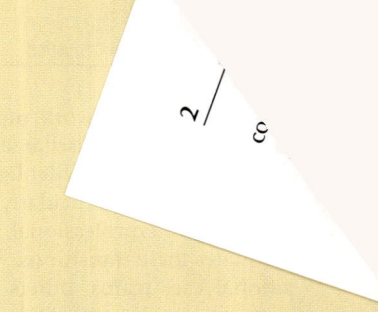

CHAPTER 1

INTERPROFESSIONAL COLLABORATIVE PRACTICE: WHERE WE ARE TODAY

Terry Mahan Buttaro • Joanne Sandberg-Cook

We continue to live and work in a world of volatility, uncertainty, complexity, and ambiguity (VUCA). Based on theories developed by Warren Bennis and Burt Nanus to characterize the world at large, VUCA is certainly applicable to the current state of interprofessional collaborative practice and primary care.[1] Primary care practice with well-defined rules and roles, time for each patient, fewer documentation requirements, and lower costs has been replaced by new rules, complicated insurance, and new types of health care professionals. There is unchallenged recognition of the importance of an evidence base for practice decisions, disease prevention, health promotion, maintenance of well-being, involvement of patients in their health decisions, and coordination of care given by a team of health care providers. Interprofessional collaboration throughout the continuum of care is essential for successful, cost-effective care. However, the American health care system is increasingly challenged by (1) an aging population with multiple chronic conditions that often require several (expensive) medications, (2) inadequate financial and social resources, and (3) health care providers pressed for time and resources. The medical workforce is also aging and retiring, leaving gaps in the provision of service and increased demands on those remaining practitioners. Provisions of the Affordable Care Act are constantly challenged, with a resultant decrease in coverage for many people who initially benefited. This is especially true in states that refused to expand Medicaid, those states that instituted new requirements for work in order to qualify for Medicaid benefits, or in those that have removed the preexisting condition clause.[2] The type of insurance and policy level carried by a patient and family can determine the health care providers and hospitals where a patient or family member can receive covered care, diagnostics, medications, and other prescribed treatments. The current landscape of primary care is in a constant state of chaos with patients at the center.

CURRENT FORCES SHAPING THE PRIMARY CARE LANDSCAPE

Evidence-Based Practice

The evidence-based practice (EBP) movement is especially relevant for primary care providers (PCPs). Research findings inform health care practice across the transitions of care. In primary care, clinical practice guidelines, best practice, and the accessibility of information technology (IT) at our fingertips promote a culture of EBP providing resources to improve patient outcomes. Guidelines are also increasingly updated more frequently contributing to standardized evidence-based care. Insurers use this information to create reimbursement structures, driving providers and patients to treatments that have been found to be efficacious and cost effective, based on available evidence as opposed to those that provide no benefit. See Chapter 2, Translating Research into Clinical Practice, for background on how clinical evidence is created, evaluated, and disseminated.

Value-Based Purchasing

Value-based purchasing (VBP)[3] is a Centers for Medicare and Medicaid Services (CMS) initiative that affects all providers who practice in or admit Medicare patients to a hospital setting. VBP is part of the Affordable Care Act of 2009; its goal is improving care quality by linking payment by the CMS for inpatient services to successful outcome measures. VBP measures hospital performance on an approved set of measures grouped into four domain areas of care: safety, clinical care, efficiency and cost reduction, and patient- and caregiver-centered experience of care/care coordination (to be renamed person and community engagement as of fiscal year 2019). Private insurers are using similar metrics when negotiating contracts with institutions and PCPs. We have entered a "pay for performance" world where contracts are negotiated based on quality metrics. As a result, the field of practice analytics has arisen. There are currently sophisticated computer programs modeling financial opportunities for hospital service lines and individual health care practices based on payer mix per-case cost and contribution margin. Providers currently have a crucial opportunity along with inpatient care management to affect not only the quality of care delivered to their patients but also the financial state of organizations in which their patients receive care, as well as their own financial opportunities.

Management of Care Transitions

VBP is further shaping primary care delivery by reducing Medicare payments for all patients by a small percentage in a hospital where the unplanned readmission rate within 30 days of discharge exceeds the hospital's expected rate for patients with the selected conditions of acute MI, heart failure, coronary artery bypass graft surgery, pneumonia, chronic obstructive pulmonary disease (COPD), hip arthroplasty, and knee arthroplasty.[4] This program, known as Hospital Readmissions Reduction Program (HRRP), provides hospitals with a financial incentive to improve their communication and care rdination and work more successfully with patients and aregivers on post-discharge planning.[4]

This new reality highlights the importance of managing care transitions, particularly the transition from inpatient care to home. Interprofessional collaboration and communication facilitates these transitions. Many institutions have created transitional care teams, others make post discharge phone calls, and some make post-discharge home visits often by nurses or nurse practitioners. See Chapter 4, Coordinated Chronic Care, for a more in-depth exploration.

PATIENT-CENTERED MEDICAL HOME

The Institute of Medicine (IOM) has developed a commonly accepted definition of primary care which is as follows: "Primary care is the provision of integrated, accessible health care services by clinicians who are accountable for addressing a large majority of personal health care needs, developing a sustained partnership with patients, and practicing in the context of family and community."[5] The term *integrated* in the IOM definition encompasses "the provision of comprehensive, coordinated, and continuous services that provide a seamless process of care."[5] Using the six aims of patient-centered care as a framework gives providers easily measurable care goals resulting in improved care.[6] Primary care should be:

- **Safe**: Avoiding harm to patients from the care that is intended to help them.
- **Effective**: Providing services based on scientific knowledge to all who could benefit and refraining from providing services to those not likely to benefit (avoiding underuse and misuse, respectively).
- **Patient centered**: Providing care that is respectful of and responsive to individual patient preferences, needs, and values and ensuring that patient values guide all clinical decisions.
- **Timely**: Reducing waits and sometimes harmful delays for both those who receive and those who give care.
- **Efficient**: Avoiding waste, including waste of equipment, supplies, ideas, and energy.
- **Equitable**: Providing care that does not vary in quality because of personal characteristics such as race, gender identity, gender, sexual orientation, ethnicity, geographic location, or socioeconomic status.

The patient-centered medical home model of patient care meets each of the aforementioned aims using a team approach with continuous participation of the patient and where appropriate, the family. This model provides increased access to medical providers and coordinated care between providers. The goal of the patient-centered medical home (PCMH) is to coordinate health care for a patient, prevent possible medical situations from arising, and provide increased quality and safety of medical care by approved practitioners. The model requires considerable practice resources and is often not appropriately reimbursed.

Accountable Care Organizations

Accountable Care Organizations (ACOs) are groups of doctors, hospitals, and other health care providers, who come together voluntarily to give coordinated high-quality care to the Medicare patients they serve. Coordinated care helps ensure that patients, especially the chronically ill, get the right care at the right time, with the goal of avoiding unnecessary duplication of services and preventing medical errors. When an ACO succeeds

in both delivering high-quality care and spending health care dollars more wisely, it will share in the savings it achieves for the Medicare program."[7] The vision of primary care as a collaborative practice is realized with the advent of ACOs, which potentially form the centerpiece of health care reform efforts. There are multiple models for ACOs, including one that defines an ACO as a group of patient-centered medical homes (see earlier) resulting in a medical "neighborhood."[8] There are three levels, or tiers, of an ACO, each with its distinct requirements for organizational structure, performance measures, IT requirements, and payment models.

Level 1 ACOs have the least amount of financial risk and fewest requirements. The organization's structure may be just a legal entity, and the ACO may have the IT capability to track a limited number of performance measures. Level 1 ACOs receive shared savings bonuses based on achievement of benchmarks for quality measures and expenditures.[9]

Level 2 ACOs have the potential to capture a greater portion of below-target spending amounts but have accountability for above-budget spending. The level 2 ACO has an evolved infrastructure, with advanced IT systems and care coordination for chronic diseases such as asthma, diabetes, and heart failure. Performance measures are linked to outcomes for chronic diseases and reduction in health risks. These organizations must make financial projections and have minimum cash reserve standards.[9]

Level 3 ACOs offer a full range of services and have the infrastructure to provide comprehensive health care services. They have electronic medical records (EMRs) linking all components and report on health-related outcomes, care experiences, and quality of life in multiple patient populations in the system. Level 3 ACOs have strict requirements for financial reporting and maintain larger cash reserves.[9]

High-quality primary care is essential to the success of ACOs. In addition, there must be sufficient technical capability and support, innovation in payment and reimbursement systems (bundled payments), and establishment of performance measures using practice analytics that reflect improved health state in patients, all of which can be a financial burden for smaller practices. In an ACO, there are care navigators to assist patients with care access and sophisticated technology to communicate with and monitor patients. Nurses have various roles—system administrators, service line managers, practice managers, case managers, PCPs, educators, and home health providers. Recent studies have demonstrated shorter hospital stays, decreased readmission rates, and decreased Medicare spending when patients are a part of an ACO.[10] The downside may be that many community practices do not have the financial resources or enough patients to statistically reflect improvement in care and cost savings. When smaller practices join together to form a super ACO the patient numbers increase and cost savings become measurable.[11]

The super ACO alliance is created to expand the reach of the smaller systems in the alliance to create initiatives that enhance the care experience for patients and providers, control costs, and maximize reimbursement potential.[12]

NEW LOOK OF PRIMARY CARE

In a 2014 survey conducted by the Advisory Board Company, 4000 consumers were asked questions about primary care preferences. Patients' preferences for low-acuity complaints in primary care included 24/7 access to care, a walk-in setting with the ability to be seen within 30 minutes, and close proximity to home.[13] The retail health movement, with urgent care walk-in clinics associated with pharmacy chains and department stores, is currently an accepted component of the health care delivery system and is part of the new look of primary care. Retail clinics have expanded services beyond minor acute emergencies and currently include several components of primary care (e.g., annual physicals, some chronic disease management, and medispa services) in response to documented patient preferences for close proximity to home and readily accessible primary care.[13] Primary care practices are responding to this emerging trend by opening urgent care centers, some in and near retail locations that are linked to the primary care practices, providing needed care continuity while meeting patient preferences. Other previously traditional primary care practices have converted to direct primary care or concierge practices, where patients pay an additional yearly fee directly to the practice for 24/7 rapid access to the PCP and house calls.

The new look of primary care has spawned new collaborative health care partner roles. As older physicians retire, primary care will be increasingly delivered by nurse practitioners and physician assistants. Many health care systems have community health resource specialists, sometimes called community workers, who assist patients with obtaining a variety services, care navigators who help patients with coordinating care appointments and services, and practice-based clinical pharmacists who assist both providers and patients with medication regimens. Community and parish nurses provide care coordination and education especially helpful during care transitions and provide primary care coordination to frail elders and others in need of support. Emergency medical services (EMS) providers in some communities now participate in the delivery of primary care and preventive services such as falls risk home evaluations and basic health monitoring. Community nurses, community workers, and community first responders not only monitor patients identified as high risk by hospitals and medical practices but also provide valuable community and individual social and demographic information to referring institutions.

CHALLENGES AND OPPORTUNITIES
Opioid Crisis

The opioid crisis in America continues to escalate, with 72,000 overdose deaths (200/day) in 2017. This number of deaths is more than the number who died in the Vietnam and Iraq wars combined. The escalating crisis can be partially blamed on poor access to addiction treatment, with only approximately 20% of those who would benefit actually getting the care. The number of overdose deaths is currently so high that for the first time since the 1960s the average age of death has decreased.[14]

PCPs including NPs and PAs are in the perfect position to relieve the crisis, but there are barriers and myths to overcome. Currently federal law requires time-consuming training and limited PCP access to medications that are proven to reduce overdose deaths (e.g., buprenorphine, methadone, and naltrexone). Other barriers which may prevent more PCPs from in-office addiction care include the erroneous belief that drugs such as methadone and buprenorphine substitute one addiction for another, that detox and rehab work are more successful options, that reducing the number of opioid prescriptions written will reduce overdoses (patients turn to the illicit market increasing the risk), and that in-office addiction treatment is

time consuming and burdensome (protocols are the likely solution to this concern).[15]

Enlisting PCPs and relaxing access to training and life-saving addiction medications will be a straightforward and achievable first step in addressing the crisis and reducing overdose deaths.

Advanced Practice Registered Nurse Compact License Movement

In May 2015, the National Council of State Boards of Nursing (NCSBN) took an unprecedented step forward in potentially shaping the landscape of primary care. The NCSBN created rules and a model for the advanced practice registered nurse (APRN) Compact legislation, modeled after the successful nurse compact model, currently in effect in 25 states.[16] The purpose of the APRN Compact is to allow APRNs within the compact states who meet the compact requirements to obtain a multistate license, thereby expanding advanced nursing practice and mobility for APRNs, fostering the use of technologies to monitor and communicate with patients, and increasing the safety of and access to health care. The proposed legislation under the compact mode includes provisions for independent APRN practice and prescriptive authority for controlled substances but can be implemented only when 10 states have enacted this legislation.[16] There is ongoing discussion about a similar compact model for medical licenses. PCPs interested in fostering collaborative efforts to increase access to high-quality health care should advocate for legislation to make the APRN Compact license a reality.

Building Interprofessional Collaborative Practice Initiatives

Interprofessional collaboration is a crucial element in the current changing health care landscape. Collaboration is a requirement for funding in research and program support. Collaborative research is exponentially productive because it combines resources, expertise, and thinking in the creation of knowledge for practice and should include a focus on patient outcomes. Collaborative leadership of health care initiatives allows more individuals to participate, and the outcome derives from a collective of minds. Collaboration in clinical practice offers improved quality of care for patients and significant others as professionals share expertise.

The Interprofessional Education Collaborative (IPEC), composed of representatives from the major care delivery disciplines in health care, models collaboration that is advancing the practice.[17] An IPEC expert panel produced guidelines for collaborative practice core competencies that begin with interprofessional education to enable collaboration and improve outcomes. The IPEC report advocates for components of professional education of the various disciples to occur together, in interprofessional teams, to build the core collaboration competencies of values and ethics needed for interprofessional practice, roles and responsibilities in collaborative practice, interprofessional team communication, and knowledge of teams and teamwork.[17] The interprofessional educational efforts should instill the core competencies by following guiding principles of being patient centered; having a community or population focus; emphasizing relationships and processes; containing developmentally appropriate activities and assessments; and being outcome driven.[18]

A recent study with results published in 2015 explored the experiences of collaboration among physicians, nurses, and unlicensed assistive personnel.[19] Findings from this qualitative exploration indicate that we have much work to do in the area of collaboration. Most participants in this study indicated that they experienced a hierarchical feel to communication and decision-making. When there was collaboration between physicians and nurses, they failed to solicit input from unlicensed assistive personnel.[19] We also know that longer shifts, increasingly mandated by hospitals, negatively affect collaboration.[20] Patient care involves activities apportioned among physicians, nurses, and unlicensed assistive personnel; seamless coordination is required to prevent errors and a siloed experience for the patients and their families. Creating a model without a hierarchical structure requires that members of the team (1) understand the roles and expected contributions of each member, (2) encourage one another to meet team expectations, and (3) make the outcomes desired for patients and families the center of focus.[19]

CONCLUSION

The landscape of the health care system is ever changing. PCPs are delivering care in new venues with new technologies, with new types of collaborators, and in new kinds of health care systems. Health care reform continues to evolve and shape the vision for primary care. Health promotion and wellness is currently and will be an integral component of health care for all our patients and families. The current focus on wellness and primary care continues to provide opportunities for physician assistants and nurse practitioners to improve patient access to care and impact the direction and structure of health care delivery systems.

The vision of primary care as a collaborative practice remains timely and important. Although there are challenges, interprofessional collaborative practice represents the commitment that a team of expert clinicians from a variety of disciplines will offer patients and families optimal primary care even as primary care models continue to evolve.

REFERENCES

1. Johnson, R. (2012). *Leaders make the future: Ten skills for an uncertain world* (2nd ed.). San Francisco: Berrett-Koehler Publishers.
2. Medicaid Work Requirements. (2018). Renewed threats to ACA consumer protections. Policy and politics. *American Journal of Nursing*, 118(8), 22–23.
3. Value Based Purchasing. https://www.cms.gov/Outreach-and-Education/Medicare-Learning-Network-MLN/MLNProducts/downloads/Hospital_VBPurchasing_Fact_Sheet_ICN907664.pdf. (Accessed August 26, 2018).
4. https://www.cms.gov/Medicare/Quality-Initiatives-Patient-Assessment-Instruments/Value-Based-Programs/HRRP/Hospital-Readmission-Reduction-Program.html. (Accessed August 26, 2018).
5. Donaldson, M. S., Yordy, K. D., Lohr, K. N., et al. (Eds.). (1996). *Institute of Medicine (US) Committee on the Future of Primary Care*. Washington, DC: National Academies Press.
6. https://www.ahrq.gov/professionals/quality-patient-safety/talkingquality/create/sixdomains.html. (Accessed August 22, 2018).
7. Accountable Care Organizations. https://innovation.cms.gov/initiatives/aco/. (Accessed August 26, 2018).
8. Accountable Care Organizations vs patient centered medical homes. https://www.curemd.com/aco-vs-pcmh/. (Accessed September 7, 2018).
9. McClellan, M., McKethan, A. N., Lewis, J. L., et al. (2010). A national strategy to put accountable care into practice. *Health Affairs (Project Hope)*, 29(5), 982–990.
10. Divyansh, A., & Werner, R. (2018). Effect of hospital and post-acute care provider participating in accountable care organizations on patient outcomes and Medicare spending. *Health Services Research*, https://doi.org/10.1111/1475-6773.1323. (Accessed August 26, 2018).
11. Betbeze, P. (2018). Regional "Super" ACOs may relieve small ACO risk problem. https://www.healthleadersmedia.com/strategy/regional-super-acos-may-relieve-small-aco-risk-problem.
12. Anderson, D. G., & Morris, D. E. (2015). Characteristics of successful "super ACOs". *Healthcare Financial Management: Journal of the Healthcare Financial Management Association*, 69(6), 98–100.
13. Advisory Board Company. (2014). What do consumers want from primary care? Retrieved from www.AdvisoryBoardCompany.
14. https://www.vox.com/science-and-health/2018/8/16/17698204/opioid-epidemic-overdose-deaths-2017.
15. Wakeman, S., & Barnett, M. (2018). Primary care and the opioid overdose crises—Buprenorphine myths and realities. *The New England Journal of Medicine*, 379, 1–4. https://www.nejm.org/doi/full/10.1056/NEJMp1802741.
16. National Council of State Boards of Nursing. APRN compact model. Retrieved from www.ncsbn.org/APRN_Compact_Final_050415.pdf. (Accessed May 4, 2015).
17. Interprofessional Education Collaborative (IC) Expert Panel. (2011). *Core competencies for interprofessional collaborative practice: Report of an expert panel*. Washington, DC: Interprofessional Education Collaborative.
18. World Health Organization. (2010). Framework for action on Interprofessional education and collaborative practice 2010. http://whqlibdoc.who.int/hq/2010/WHO_HRH_HPN_10.3_eng.pdf. (Accessed September 7, 2018).
19. Lancaster, G., Kolakowsky-Hayner, S., Kovacich, J., & Greer-Williams, N. (2015). Interdisciplinary communication and collaboration among physicians, nurses and unlicensed assistive personnel. *Journal of Nursing Scholarship*, 47(3), 275–283.
20. Ma, C., & Stimpfel, A. W. (2018). The association between nurse shift patterns and nurse-nurse and nurse-physician collaboration in acute care hospital units. *The Journal of Nursing Administration*, 48(6), 335–341.

CHAPTER **2**

TRANSLATING RESEARCH INTO CLINICAL PRACTICE

Jill Walsh • Patrick LaRose

INTRODUCTION

Primary care providers are at the forefront of identifying practice problems and are pivotal in translating research recommendations into practice, bringing innovation from "bench to bedside." In the true spirit of interprofessional practice, the identification and solving of practice problems are a group effort, requiring the expertise of all members of the health care team.

Nursing Research as an Exemplar for the Evolution of Knowledge Development in Health Care Professions

Over the years, nursing research has had multiple evolutions in terms of what role nurses play in the discovery of empirical research-driven information and, most notably, how nurses should use this information to rightfully impact practice, the provisions of care, and patient outcomes. To truly understand the role of nurses in relationship to research, one needs to go back in history and review the role of Florence Nightingale. Often considered the first nurse researcher, Nightingale was one of the first nurses to actually use evidence, from her practice, to make clinically relevant decisions based on the care of patients.[1] In her book *Notes on Nursing*, published in 1859, Nightingale discusses the importance of cleanliness, warmth, clean air, and personal hygiene as a means of improving outcomes for patients. Much of what Nightingale did during this time was groundbreaking. Sadly, her efforts to use evidence as a means to influence practice would not be recognized until many years after her death. However, much of what Nightingale did during her professional career as a nurse served as a foundation for the research nurses currently do.

Medical research is focused on the discovery of information and evidence used to help patient outcomes or serves to provide the foundation for practice changes that improve clinical care guidelines, enhance practice in public health, or provide evidence to serve the larger population in our country. Medical care providers currently look to evidence-based guidelines to help frame their practice as they work to improve the health and safety of clients (patients) within their communities.[1] Evidence-based guidelines are most often derived from systemic reviews of random clinical trials where the evidence of this research is compiled statistically to bring meaning to the large amount of data available on the clinical subject being studied. The Agency for Healthcare Quality and Research (AHRQ)[2] identifies clinical guidelines as the synthesis of empirical studies where the clinical guidelines, recommendations, and empirical information from random clinical trials can be brought together as cohesive evidence on best practice for care. The AHRQ publications clearing house closed in the fall of 2018, but publications and resources will continue to be available online at: https://www.ahrq.gov/research/publication/index.html. These guidelines serve to help nurse practitioners, physician assistants, physicians, and other primary care providers provide patients with clinical care that is evidence based and consistent with best practice across the country.

Evidence-Based Practice. Evidence-based practice (EBP) is an approach to practice that uses a problem-solving approach in which individual patient care decisions are made using best available evidence. The evidence-based practice movement began in the 1970s and 1980s, partly in response to observations made by Archibald Cochrane, considered to be the father of evidence-based medicine (EBM), that treatment decisions used in medicine were being made without evidence to demonstrate the effectiveness of interventions.[3] In 1992, the EBM movement was launched with the breakthrough article in the *Journal of the American Medical Association* (*JAMA*) from the EBM Working Group. They stated that EBM "de-emphasises intuition, unsystematic clinical experience, and pathophysiologic rationale as sufficient grounds for clinical decision making and stresses the examination of evidence from clinical research."[4] As EBP evolved, the definition has been broadened to include a life-long problem-solving approach to how health care is delivered that integrates the best evidence from high-quality studies with a clinician's expertise and also a patient's preferences and values.[5]

Congruent with the use of evidence to drive clinical outcomes, evidence is also used to promote changes to clinical practice. Years ago, much of nursing practice was governed by traditions, textbook, and the guidance from clinical specialists/experts where a more experienced nurse would hand down the practice standards to newer nurses entering the profession. There was little room for newer nurses to question practice standards during this time. However, as nursing research began to take shape and more nurses were conducting empirical studies and adding to the scientific body of nursing knowledge, this information would trickle down to clinical practice. Although EBP was not the standard at this time, nurses who were forward thinking and progressive would read articles, often generated from medical research that described best practice, and would secretly implement these standards into their own clinical practice.[1]

Advancements in medical care and the use of technology continued to propel the use of evidence as a means to define best practice into the late 20th century. These changes, coupled with increasing educational standards of many health care professions, led to a paradigm shift in the way nurses thought about nursing practice and how this practice should look into the future.

Translational Research for Practice Change

New knowledge from research is being generated at an accelerated rate. In fact, some research articles would even say there has been an explosion of new medical knowledge. The true challenge is how to move this knowledge from the bench to bedside through translational research.[6] Translational research simply means moving empirically based understanding into clinical practice.[7] Although the concept of moving empirically based information into clinical practice may sound simple, it does require a skill set that allows the PCP to understand how to translate evidence through a system of grading and critique to determine the validity of the evidence, the scope in which the evidence is applicable to a specific practice change, and the practicality of the intervention for the practice environment.[7]

Defining Practice Change and Appraising the Evidence. The first step for the utilization of translational research is defining what needs to be changed. For PCPs, this step is often generated by a single provider asking a question of why a policy or procedure is done a certain way. In the past, policies and procedures were developed by clinical experts where tradition framed the practice policy. Currently, evidence from empirical research findings is used to frame or shape professional practice standards. Within the context of this understanding, translational research allows providers to develop a better understanding of the evidence and how the evidence can help change practice. Qidwai says, "Application of the latest research into clinical practice is a mandatory requirement for improving healthcare delivery."[8(p453)]

Once the practice issue has been defined, the PCP will begin a search of the evidence to determine evidence-based interventions used to inform best practice standards. Searching the evidence can often be tedious and can result in many research studies that have little to do with needed information. Conducting a strong and accurate search of the literature requires a skill set where the PCP can filter through hundreds of research articles that have little to do with the needed information. This is where working with the medical science librarian or the librarian from the local university can be very helpful. Librarians have an excellent skill set for conducting scholarly searches and can provide nurses with assistance and key pointers for sifting through the large amount of information and filtering to collect studies that support the data set needed for the practice change.

Once the evidence for the practice change has been located and the research has been read and understood, it is time to determine the applicability of the research for the change and grade the evidence for strength and lack of bias. These actions are most often the biggest challenge for those who have little experience in determining the types of evidence that is appropriate for a practice change.[9] However, there is a standard for grading the evidence that provides health care providers with a framework for helping determine evidence that is valid for the practice change and evidence that would not serve to support the practice change.

Grading evidence requires the PCP to develop an understanding of the different types of research studies that are available and determining the strength of the evidence. The first level in grading the evidence is focused on evidence that is derived from random clinical trials. This evidence is often considered the most scientific and most reliable (Table 2.1).[11] A high level of confidence is provided with the strength of this evidence because it is normally evaluated based on systematic reviews. According to Cochran Collaboration, "a systematic review summarizes the results of available carefully designed healthcare studies (controlled trials) and provides a high level of evidence on the effectiveness of healthcare interventions."[10(para 1)] This type of information allows the PCP to determine the related strength of the evidence in support of the interventions. Systematic reviews are most often used with the development of clinical guidelines to promote a standard of care.[10]

The next level of strength is cohort and case studies. These types of studies are often considered observational or analytical studies and identify the causality and effect on the participants.[11] Cohort or case studies provide excellent empirical information and evidence that is considered as reliable as those found in random clinical trials. Level III evidence is expert opinion. Although this level of evidence is often questioned, experience of a clinician can be used to frame a practice change where this experience has provided the clinician with a reasonable opportunity to understand how the practice change may or may not positively impact the population. Furthermore, with the absence of clear evidence to support the practice change, the role of expert opinion from clinicians that are change agents can often provide sufficient experiential or qualitative data to support the practice change.[12] Weighing the evidence basically informs the PCP of the strength of the research design and provides a structured and methodical approach to deciding which pieces of evidence should be considered for the literature review of support and which pieces of evidence do not have the inherent design or strength/trust to be included. The use of a systematic and logical evaluation system is helpful in the process and provides the PCP with a method and structure that can help make sense of all the data. Of course, no system of evaluation is perfect, and it is highly important for the PCP to understand the shortfalls and limitations of any system of ranking. According to Evans, "From this perspective, it acknowledges that, when evaluating an intervention, a variety of research methods can contribute valid evidence."[13(p82)]

One approach that provides a structure methodology is identified in Table 2.2 Within this structure, researchers can order evidence based on level of the empirical question (discovery), by purpose of the research, methodology (or research design), types of analysis, and application. "Evidence on effectiveness, appropriateness and feasibility provides a sounder base for evaluating healthcare interventions, in that it acknowledges the many factors that can have an impact on success."[13(p79)] For the PCP researcher, the most important aspect of this evaluation

---

TABLE 2.1 Canadian Task on the Periodic Health Examination's Levels of Evidence

Level	Type of Evidence
I	At least 1 RCT with proper randomization
II.1	Well-designed cohort or case-control study
II.2	Time series comparisons or dramatic results from uncontrolled studies
III	Expert opinions

From Canadian Task Force on the Periodic Health Examination. (1979). The periodic health examination. *Canadian Medical Association Journal*, 121, 1193–1254.

TABLE 2.2 Summary of Study Parameters

Level of Question	Purpose	Methods	Analysis	Application
I. What is it?	To describe or to define a phenomenon of interest To identify pertinent variables or characteristics	Qualitative methods Structured interviews Questionnaires Surveys	Content analysis Ethnography Nonparametric statistics Measures of central tendency	May suggest assessment parameters (Do you experience …?)
II. What is happening here?	To identify relationships between variables—associations and differences	Epidemiologic studies Cross-sectional studies Correlational studies Studies of group-wise differences	Correlations among variables Differences between variables or groups Mann-Whitney U test; analysis of variance; t test	Suggests avenues of further assessment (If you observe x, what is the likelihood that y will occur?)
III. What is the nature of the relationship among variables (cause-and-effect relationship)?	To determine cause-and-effect relationships among variables To explicate mechanisms mediating the phenomenon of interest	Experimental designs Quasi-experimental designs	Analysis of variance Regression analysis	Suggests underlying pathologic conditions that may be treated
IV. What is the therapeutic effect of a proposed intervention? What is the proper dose of a treatment to achieve a predictable outcome?	To determine predictability of hypothesized outcome at specific dose in selected population	Randomized clinical trial	Intent-to-treat analysis Analysis of variance Regression analysis	Demonstrates usefulness of particular treatment for patient population; with sufficient replication, clinician may be reasonably sure that treatment will be effective

may relate to applicability of the evidence. In this case, weighing the ability to operationalize the recommended interventions may be the primary purpose of this evaluation. If the evidence or recommendations are challenging or difficult to operationalize (perhaps related to cost, structure, or availability of resources), this would preclude the provider from including this evidence in the supportive literature. Conversely, evidence that had strong applicability and could be easily implemented might rise to the top of the ranking based on the weight of this review and the ease of applicability.

Primary care providers who use an evidence ranking system such as the one in Table 2.2 can better understand how the evidence can be used to support practice change, inform policy development or revision, and best influence patient outcomes.

Grading the Evidence. Once the evidence has been appraised for applicability and the strength of the evidence has been reviewed, the PCP can apply this knowledge to the grade of the evidence. Table 2.3 provides a summary of grading which is a standardized nomenclature for the applicability of the evidence for the practice change.[14]

Grading the evidence provides the PCP with the opportunity to declare confidence in the strength and reliability of the evidence collected. For the high category, the PCP has full confidence in the research and believes the evidence gained is sufficient to promote the practice change. From here the PCP does not believe there is a need for additional support. Each level of the grading tool demonstrates the PCP's overall confidence with the evidence and the applicability of the evidence for use in the practice change with the lowest level being insufficient; where there is no evidence to support a change.

Within the context of appraising and grading evidence, the PCP demonstrates his or her knowledge and understanding of the need for change and the empirical support that can be located to support change. Once empirical support is located within the evidence, a framework for theoretical change can be established. This includes providing a theoretical context to the change by assigning a model that represents either a nursing grand theory or a mid-range theory and the theory for change.

THEORIES OF CHANGE AND ADOPTION OF INNOVATIONS

Planned change is a common thread that runs throughout health care and is necessary for many reasons, but it can be challenging to implement. Primary care providers and change agents therefore must have knowledge of change theories in order to implement planned change in nursing. It is important also to understand how an innovation (i.e., new idea, practice, or object) gains momentum over time, diffuses (or spreads), and is adopted by a culture.

As early as the 1940s, Kurt Lewin originated the term *planned change* to distinguish the process from accidental or imposed change[15] Lewin's theory is a time-tested easy-to-use change theory that is applicable for individual, group, and organizational change. Lewin considered behavior to be a dynamic balance of forces working in opposing directions that can affect change, which he called *force-field analysis*. He assumed that there are both driving and restraining forces that influence change. Successful organizational change is achieved by either strengthening the driving forces (facilitators) in the desired direction or weakening the restraining forces (barriers) that impede change. Therefore, to shift the balance in the direction of the planned change, the forces need to be first analyzed and understood. Lewin's change theory consists of a three-step model of change: unfreezing, movement, and refreezing. The first step is the unfreezing of the old pattern of doing things. Unfreezing is then replaced with the moving phase of change, followed by refreezing as people adjust to the new ways of doing things (Box 2.1).

In health care, there are many evidence-based innovations; however, knowledge disseminates slowly. The diffusion of innovation (DOI) theory developed by E. M. Rogers in 1962 is a classic theory that seeks to explain how, why, and at what rate new ideas and technology spread through a specific population or social system. Rogers[16] proposed four fundamental elements of the diffusion process that affect the spread of a new idea: the innovation (an idea, practice, or object perceived as new by an individual), communication channels (the process for

TABLE 2.3	Strength of Evidence Grades and Definitions
Grade	**Definition**
High	We are very confident that the estimate of effect lies close to the true effect for this outcome. The body of evidence has few or no deficiencies. We believe that the findings are stable (i.e., another study would not change the conclusions).
Moderate	We are moderately confident that the estimate of effect lies close to the true effect for this outcome. The body of evidence has some deficiencies. We believe that the findings are likely to be stable, but some doubt remains.
Low	We have limited confidence that the estimate of effect lies close to the true effect for this outcome. The body of evidence has major or numerous deficiencies (or both). We believe that additional evidence is needed before concluding either that the findings are stable or that the estimate of effect is close to the true effect.
Insufficient	We have no evidence, we are unable to estimate an effect, or we have no confidence in the estimate of effect for this outcome. No evidence is available or the body of evidence has unacceptable deficiencies, precluding reaching a conclusion.

From Berkman, N. D., Lohr, K. N., Ansari, M. T., Balk, E., Kane, R., McDonagh, M. S., et al. (2015). Grading the strength of a body of evidence when assessing health care interventions: An EPC update. *Journal of Clinical Epidemiology*, 68(11), 1312–1324.

BOX 2.1

Lewin's Change Theory

Unfreezing	**Moving or Changing**	**Refreezing**
• Recognize need for change • Prepare the desired change • Identify and increase driving forces for change • Identify and decrease resisting forces against change	• Develop new attitudes or behaviors • Implement the desired change	• Reinforce and stabilize change to make permanent • Solidify the desired change • Hardwire the desired change through new norms and operating procedures

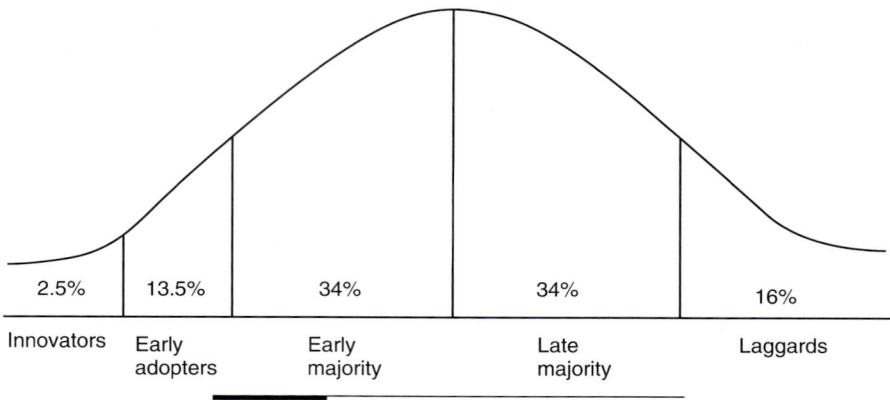

| 2.5% | 13.5% | 34% | 34% | 16% |
| Innovators | Early adopters | Early majority | Late majority | Laggards |

F I G . **2.1**   Roger's diffusion of innovation theory.

messages to travel from one individual to another), time (time it takes for individuals to get used to an idea and the rate of adoption), and the social system (groups that join together to solve problems for a common goal).

Rogers modified and expanded Lewin's change theory and described five stages through which individuals (or larger decision-making groups) pass during the adoption of a new idea—the "innovation-decision" process. The five stages include knowledge, persuasion, decision, implementation, and confirmation. Knowledge is the process whereby the individual is exposed to a new idea and has some information about how the innovation works. Persuasion is the process in which the individual is interested in the idea and develops an attitude about the innovation. In the decision phase, the individual decides to either adopt or reject the innovation. In the implementation phase, the individual puts the innovation into use and may seek out additional evidence. Lastly, the confirmation phase is when the individual evaluates the results of the innovation and decides to continue the innovation.

Rogers proposed that there are also personal characteristics that influence how rapidly people adopt an innovation. He identified five categories of adopters: innovators, early adopters, early majority, late majority, and laggards (Fig. 2.1). Innovators are people who are willing to take risks and are the first to adopt. Early adopters are likely to be opinion leaders who embrace change opportunities and are comfortable adopting new ideas. The majority of the population or the critical mass is in the early majority and late majority categories. The early majority adopt new ideas slower than the previous groups, will adopt if practical, and are rarely leaders. The late majority adopt an innovation after it has been proven and often not by choice but rather out of necessity. Lastly, the laggards are change averse, very conservative, and very skeptical of change.

Rogers identified attributes of innovations that help decrease uncertainty about the innovation and influence decisions to adopt or reject. Rogers asserted that individual's perceptions about the five characteristics of innovations: relative advantage, compatibility, complexity, trialability, and observability predict the rate of adoption of innovations.

USE OF THEORETICAL APPROACHES IN IMPLEMENTATION SCIENCE

Use of a framework, theory, or model to systematize and guide the planning, implementation, and evaluation of practice change projects supports successful implementation of EBP. There are many models for implementation of EBP available for use in clinical settings. However, selection is dependent on the setting and type of practice change proposed.

Nilsen[17] identified five categories of theoretical approaches used in implementation science. Process models are used to describe and/or guide the research-to-practice process. Determinant frameworks, classic theories, and implementation theories aim to understand and or explain what influences implementation outcomes. Evaluation frameworks provide a structure to evaluate implementation efforts.

Four commonly used process models that focus on the implementation process from both the practitioner and organizational perspectives will be presented, including: (1) the Iowa Model of Evidence-Based Practice to Promote Quality Care,[18] (2) the ACE Star Model of Knowledge Transformation,[19] (3) the Johns Hopkins Nursing Evidence-Based Practice Model (JHNEBP),[20] and the (4) the Stetler Model of Evidence-Based Practice.[21]

The Iowa Model of Evidence-Based Practice to Promote Quality Care[18] is a widely used, very practical model for the systematic implementation of EBP. The Iowa model is applicable in diverse settings, including academic settings and health care institutions, and is intended for nurses and other clinicians at the point of care.

The Iowa model consists of a flowchart to guide decision-making that includes problem-solving steps and feedback loops to guide the change process. The first step in the Iowa model is determining if the topic is a problem-based or knowledge-based trigger and if it is a priority for the organization. A team of stakeholders with consideration of interprofessional involvement is then formed to develop, implement, and evaluate the practice change. The team first searches, critiques, and synthesizes the literature to determine if the research evidence is sufficient. At this decision point, if the research evidence is not sufficient, the team can recommend conducting more research or using lower levels of evidence. If sufficient evidence is found, a pilot of the practice change is initiated. The team then evaluates the pilot for feasibility and effectiveness and decides whether to adopt the change in practice. Ongoing monitoring and dissemination of results are further elements of the model.

The Iowa Model Collaborative convened in 2012 to review and revise the Iowa model based on changes in health care and feedback from users. The Iowa Model-Revised: Evidence-Based

Practice to Promote Excellence in Health Care was validated and made available in 2015. Important additions to the revised model include the explicit inclusion of patient and family values and preferences, more detail based on user feedback about the "design and pilot the change" step, and the "integrate and sustain the practice change" step (Fig. 2.2).[18]

The ACE Star Model of Knowledge Transformation[19] was developed in 2004 and revised in 2012 and is another process model created from the nursing-led field of research use/utilization to guide change. The Star model is useful as a simple yet comprehensive framework to translate evidence into practice. The model has been used in both educational and clinical practice and can be used by both individual practitioners and organizations to guide practice change in a variety of settings. The major focus of the Star model is knowledge transformation.

The five stages of the Star model depict the stages of knowledge transformation as research evidence is incorporated into practice. The five stages include: (1) discovery research, (2) evidence summary, (3) translation to guidelines, (4) practice integration, and (5) process, outcome evaluation. In the first stage, discovery, the literature is searched using databases such as CINAHL for primary research studies. The next stage is evidence summary in which the large amount of available evidence is synthesized and integrated in summary forms (e.g., evidence synthesis and systematic reviews) so that the review of available evidence is more manageable. The third stage is translation into action where the evidence is translated into a practice document or tool that guides practice, such as an evidence-based clinical practice guideline. Practice integration is the fourth stage and is where the evidence is implemented and there is a change in practice. The final stage, evaluation, is the stage in which the impact of the practice change on outcomes is evaluated (Fig. 2.3).

The ACE Star Model of Knowledge Transformation provides an organized and practical framework for implementing best evidence into clinical practice. As new knowledge is transformed through the five stages, the final outcome is evidence-based quality improvement of health care.[19]

The JHNEBP[20] was developed jointly by a collaborative group of leaders in nursing education and practice at Johns Hopkins Hospital and the Johns Hopkins University School of Nursing and implemented in 2004 to address the identified need for a process to implement EBP in the hospital setting. The model was updated in 2013 and again in 2017. The JHNEBP model is a process model specifically designed as a practical guide for clinicians to use for implementation of best evidence for care decisions. The three-step model called PET is composed of three components: (1) the practice question, (2) evidence, and (3) translation.

The aim of the JHNEBP model is to assist clinicians to rapidly and appropriately incorporate the latest research findings and best practices into patient care. The 2017 revised model reflects a change to the conceptual model itself and offers updated tools for question development, rating the evidence and appraising research and nonresearch evidence. New tools include a stakeholder analysis tool, action-planning tool, and dissemination tool.

The revised conceptual model currently has "inquiry" as the starting point. Individuals or teams raise the question as to whether the current practice reflects evidence-based best practice. Inquiry as the starting point ignites a dynamic,

interactive process for practice change, creating an ongoing cycle of inquiry, practice, and learning (Fig. 2.4).

The Stetler Model of Evidence-Based Practice[21] was first developed in 1976, refined in 1994, and updated in 2001. The Stetler model is a process model that is practitioner oriented and emphasizes the critical thinking process. The model links research use, as a first step, with evidence-informed practice and promotes use of both internal and external sources of evidence. Stetler's model consists of five phases: (1) preparation, (2) validation, (3) comparative evaluation/decision-making, (4) translation/application, and (5) evaluation. Each phase is designed to facilitate critical thinking about the practical application of research findings and related evidence; result in the use of evidence in the context of daily practice; and mitigate some of the human errors made in decision-making.[22] The last two versions of this model consist of two parts: five phases of research/evidence use and clarifying information and options for each phase (Figs. 2.5 and 2.6).

The Promoting Action on Research Implementation in Health Services (PARIHS) framework,[23] originally developed in 1998, is a determinant framework that is useful for clinicians and researchers to understand the nature of complex interventions and how new knowledge moves into practice. The PARIHS framework is a multidimensional conceptual framework that proposes that key factors and the interplay and interdependence of these factors influence successful implementation of EBPs. This framework presents successful implementation as a function of the quality and type of evidence; the characteristics of the setting or context; and the way in which the evidence was introduced or facilitated into practice.

The PARIHS framework was refined in 2015 and is currently called the integrated-PARIHS (i-PARIHS) framework.[24] In the revised framework, the core constructs are facilitation, innovation, recipients, and context (Fig. 2.7). In this approach, facilitation is the active element that promotes successful implementation of new knowledge in the clinical setting active element through assessing, aligning, and integrating the other three constructs. The framework identifies three core facilitation roles—the beginner or novice facilitator, experienced facilitator, and expert facilitator—and provides structured interventions they need to undertake as they move out to different layers of context.

The Advancing Research & Clinical Practice through Close Collaboration (ARCC) model: A Model for System Wide Implementation and Sustainability of EBP[25] is an organized conceptual framework that provides health care institutions with a guide for system-wide implementation of EBP to achieve quality outcomes. The model was developed using nurse input about the barriers and facilitators of using EBP and is based in control theory and cognitive behavioral theory. A considerable amount of research exists to support the ARCC model.[24]

The central constructs of the model include: (1) assessment of organizational culture and readiness for EBP, (2) identification of strengths and barriers to EBP, (3) development and use of EBP mentors, (4) EBP implementation, and (5) outcome evaluation (Fig. 2.8). Research findings showed that a key strategy to sustain EBP is the presence of an EBP mentor and that having a mentor leads to stronger beliefs and greater implementation of evidence-based care by nurses.[26]

The ARCC model emphasizes organizational environment and factors that support EBP. This model includes several scales to measure organizational culture and measurement

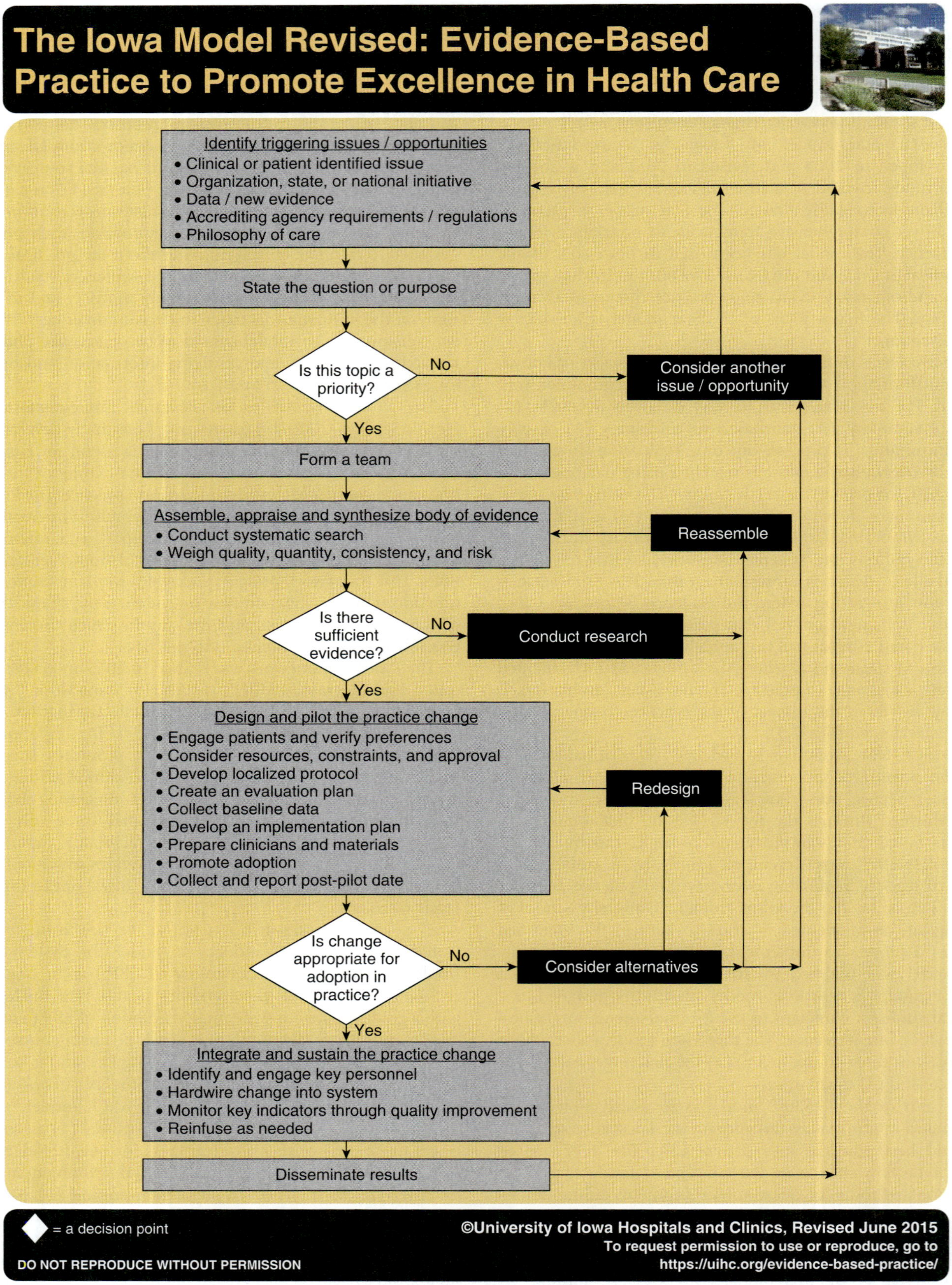

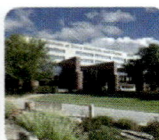

The Iowa Model Revised: Evidence-Based Practice to Promote Excellence in Health Care

Identify triggering issues / opportunities
- Clinical or patient identified issue
- Organization, state, or national initiative
- Data / new evidence
- Accrediting agency requirements / regulations
- Philosophy of care

State the question or purpose

Is this topic a priority? — No → Consider another issue / opportunity

Yes ↓

Form a team

Assemble, appraise and synthesize body of evidence
- Conduct systematic search
- Weigh quality, quantity, consistency, and risk

← Reassemble

Is there sufficient evidence? — No → Conduct research

Yes ↓

Design and pilot the practice change
- Engage patients and verify preferences
- Consider resources, constraints, and approval
- Develop localized protocol
- Create an evaluation plan
- Collect baseline data
- Develop an implementation plan
- Prepare clinicians and materials
- Promote adoption
- Collect and report post-pilot date

← Redesign

Is change appropriate for adoption in practice? — No → Consider alternatives

Yes ↓

Integrate and sustain the practice change
- Identify and engage key personnel
- Hardwire change into system
- Monitor key indicators through quality improvement
- Reinfuse as needed

Disseminate results

◆ = a decision point

DO NOT REPRODUCE WITHOUT PERMISSION

©University of Iowa Hospitals and Clinics, Revised June 2015
To request permission to use or reproduce, go to
https://uihc.org/evidence-based-practice/

FIG. 2.2 The Iowa Model Revised: Evidence-based Practice to Promote Excellence in Health Care (2017). (From Iowa Model Collaborative. [2017]. Iowa model of evidence-based practice: Revisions and validation. *Worldviews on Evidence-Based Nursing*, 14[3], 175–182. Used/reprinted with permission from the University of Iowa Hospitals and Clinics, copyright 2015. For permission to use or reproduce, please contact the University of Iowa Hospitals and Clinics at 319-384-9098.)

cf effectiveness of EBP in practice. These include the EBP beliefs (EBPB) scale, Organizational Culture and Readiness for System-Wide Implementation of EBP (OCRSIEP), EBP Knowledge Assessment Questionnaire (EBP-KAQ), and the EBP implementation (EBPI) scale.

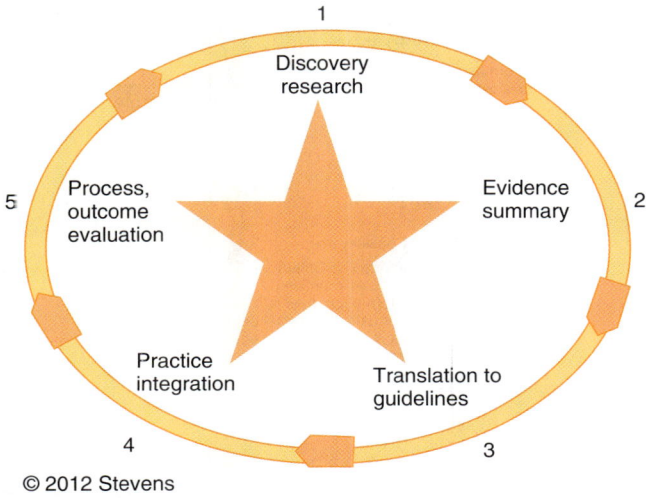

FIG. **2.3** The ACE star model of knowledge transformation. (From Stevens, K. R. [2012]. *Star Model of EBP: Knowledge Transformation*. Academic Center for Evidence-Based Practice. The University of Texas Health Science Center at San Antonio.)

Developing an Evidence-Based Practice Change—the Final Piece

It is widely acknowledged that EBP improves the quality and reliability of health care, improves patient outcomes, and reduces variations in care and costs.[27] Primary care providers are leading, implementing, and evaluating practice change projects and quality improvement (QI) initiatives with a goal of improving patient outcomes and organizational effectiveness.

The Plan-Do-Study-Act (PDSA) cycle is an improvement-science model commonly used for testing a change. The steps include: "P" Plan—plan a change or test of how something works; "D" Do—carry out the plan or test; "S" Study—observe and learn from the consequences and analyze the data; and "A" Act—decide what actions should be taken to improve. The model is summarized in three simple questions: (1) What are we trying to accomplish? (2) How will we know that a change is an improvement? (3) What changes can we make that will result in improvement?[28]

It can sometimes be challenging to identify whether an activity involving human participants and data collection falls in the realm of QI or human subjects research due to subtle differences and frequent overlap. The Department of Health and Human Services (DHHS) definition of research (from 45 CFR 46.102) is: "A systematic investigation, including research development, testing and evaluation, designed to develop or contribute to generalizable knowledge. Activities that meet this definition constitute research for purposes of this policy, whether or not they are conducted or supported under a program that is considered research for other purposes. For example, some demonstration and service programs

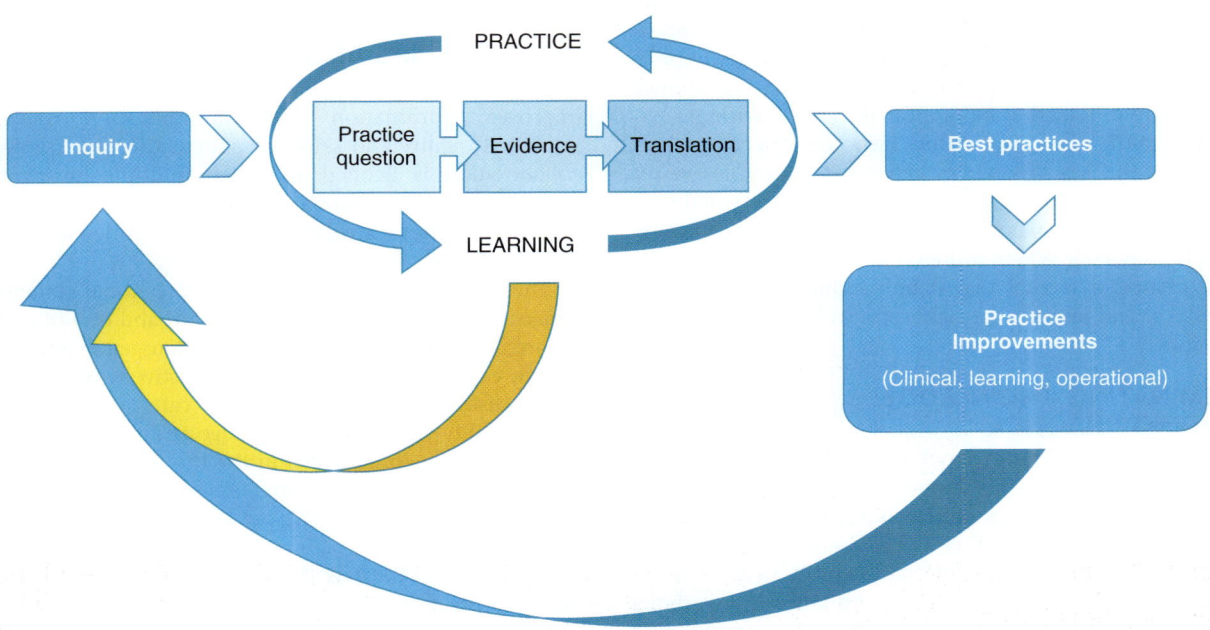

© The Johns Hopkins Hospital / Johns Hopkins University School of Nursing

FIG. **2.4** The Johns Hopkins Nursing Evidence-Based Practice Model (JHNEBP) (2017). (© The Johns Hopkins Hospital/The Johns Hopkins University School of Nursing.)

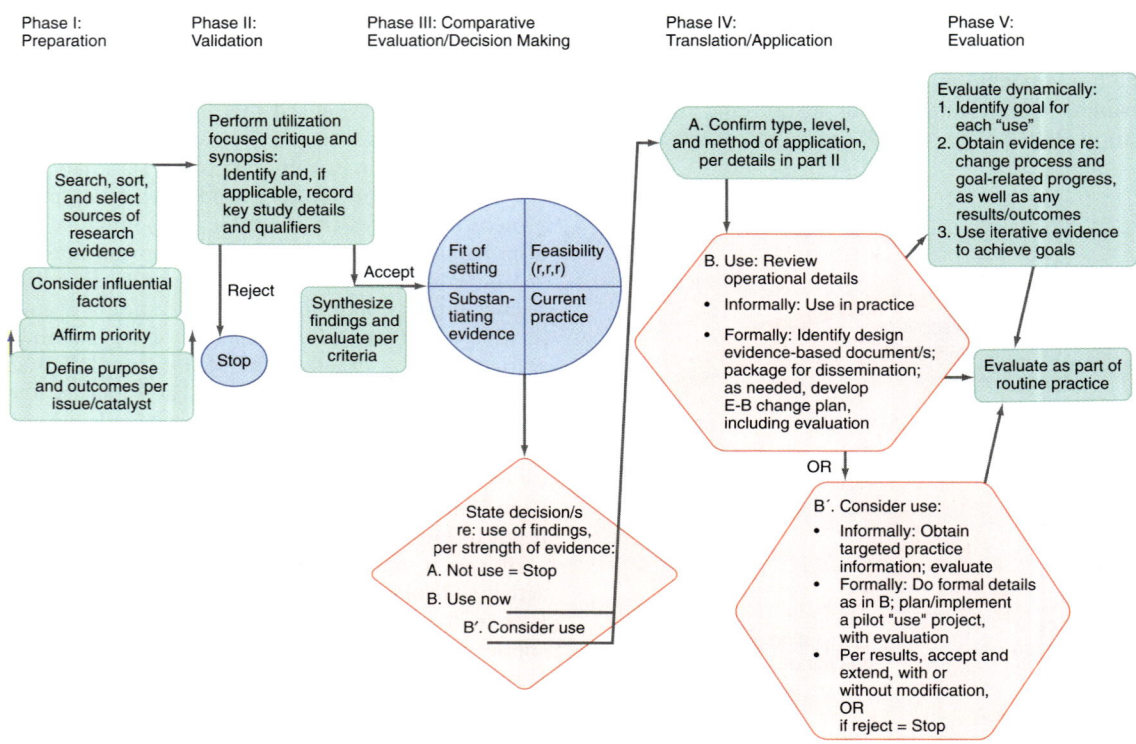

FIG. 2.5 Stetler model, Part I. Shown are the steps of research utilization to facilitate evidence-based practice. (From Stetler, C. B. [2001]. Updating the Stetler model of research utilization to facilitate evidence-based practice. *Nursing Outlook, 49*[6], 276.)

may include research activities."[29] Important in this definition are the words "designed to contribute to generalizable knowledge." To be considered "generalizable knowledge," the activity would include the following concepts: knowledge contributes to a theoretical framework of an established body of knowledge; results are expected to be generalized to a larger population beyond the site of data collection or population studied; and results are intended to be replicated in other settings.

Many health care institutions have developed policies that describe the key differences between QI activities versus research and provide guidance for determining whether a project constitutes human subjects research (and subsequently requires IRB review). Whether the QI activity is human subject research or not, it is vital that it be conducted in a manner that is ethical and respects the rights and welfare of the human participants.

DISSEMINATING KNOWLEDGE: CHANGING PRACTICE

APNs and their interprofessional colleagues are publishing findings of studies or practice change projects that use evidence to improve either practice or patient outcomes that contribute to the body of medical and nursing knowledge.[30]

Chronic diseases and conditions such as heart disease, stroke, cancer, type 2 diabetes, obesity, and arthritis are among the most common, costly, and preventable of all health problems.[31] The management of chronic diseases and health problems is rapidly becoming the major component of primary care. The use of evidence-based guidelines to manage these conditions has become standard practice. Primary care providers can

influence the closing of the research–evidence–practice gap by implementing clinical practice guidelines within their own practice setting and disseminating information about guideline implementation strategies for other organizations.

PARTNERSHIPS AND COLLABORATION

Research has shown that interprofessional collaboration improves coordination and communication resulting in improved quality and safety of patient care. Interprofessional collaboration is defined as "when multiple health workers from different professional backgrounds work together with patients, families, caregivers, and communities to deliver the highest quality of care."[32]

There are many benefits to interprofessional collaboration. Patient outcomes, quality of care, safety, and cost of care delivery are improved when disciplines work together and approach patient care from a team-based perspective with a shared goal that focuses on the patient. Primary care providers must take responsibility to gain the knowledge and develop the skills to lead interprofessional teams in the implementation of EBP to improve patient, organizational, and system outcomes.

SUMMARY

Translational research is the movement of research from the bench to practice with the understanding of how the research supports the practice change to improve outcomes. Advancements in technology and health care research are changing the way nurses practice. Although large amounts of research evidence are continually being produced, it sometimes takes more than a decade to implement research into clinical practice.

Phase 1: Preparation	Phase II: Validation	Phase III: Comparative Evaluation/Decision Making	Phase IV: Translation/Application	Phase V: Evaluation
Purpose, Context, & Sources of Research Evidence	Credibility of Findings & Potential for/Detailed Qualifiers of Application	Synthesis & Decisions/ Recommendations per Criteria of Applicability	Operational Definition of Use/Actions for Change	Alternative Types of Evaluation

• Potential Issues/ Catalysts = *a problem, including unexplained variations or less-than-best practice; or routine update of knowledge: or validation/routine revision of procedure, policy, etc.; or innovative program goal*
• Affirm perceived problems, with internal evidence
• Focus on high priority issues
• Decide if need to form a team or involve formal "structures"/ key stakeholders
• Consider other influential internal and external factors, such as beliefs, resources, or timeliness
• Define desired, measurable outcomes
• Seek out systematic reviews
• Determine need for an explicit type of research evidence, if relevant
• Select research sources with conceptual fit
	• Critique & synopsize essential component, operational details, and other qualifying factors, per source
	  o *See instructions for use of utilization-focused review tables to facilitate this task; fill in the tables for group decision making or potential future analysis*
	• Critique systematic reviews
	• Re-assess fit of individual sources
	• Rate the level & quality of each evidence source per a "table of evidence"
	• Differentiate statistical and clinical significance
	• Eliminate non-credible sources
	• End the process of there is no evidence or there is clearly insufficient credible research evidence that meets your need
		• Synthesize the cumulative findings:
		  o *Logically organize & display the similarities and differences across multiple findings, per common aspects or sub-elements of the topic under review*
		  o *Evaluate degree of substantiation of each aspect/sub-element; reinforce any qualifying conditions*
		• Evaluate degree & nature of the other criteria: feasibility (r,r,r = risk, resources, readiness); pragmatic fit; & current practice
		• Make a decision whether/what to use:
		  o *Can be personal practitioner-level decision or a recommendation to others*
		  o *Judge the strength of this decision; and indicate if primarily "research-based" or per use of supplemental information, "evidence-based", qualify the related level of strength of decision/ recommendations per related table*
		  o *For formal recommendations, determine degree of stakeholder consensus*
		• If decision = *"Not use"* research findings:
		  o *May conduct own research or delay use all additional research done by others*
		  o *If still decide to act now, e.g. on evidence of consensus or another basis for practice,* STOP use of model *but consider need for planned change and evaluation*
		• If decision = *"Use/Consider Use"*, can mean a recommendation for or against a specific practice
			• Types = *cognitive, symbolic &/or instrumental*
			• Methods = *informal or formal; direct or indirect*
			• Levels = *individuals, group or department/organization*
			• Direct instrumental use: *change individual behavior (vis-à-vis assessment; plan/intervention options; implementation details; &/or evaluation) or change policy, procedure, protocol, algorithm, program components, etc.*
			• Cognitive Use: *validate current practice: change personal way of thinking: increase awareness: better understand or appreciate conditions or experiences*
			• Symbolic use: *develop position paper or proposal for change; or persuade others regarding a way of thinking*
			• CAUTION: Assess whether translation/ product or use goes beyond actual findings/evidence:
			  o *Research evidence may or may not provide various details for a complete policy; procedure, etc.; indicate this fact to users and note differential levels of evidence therein*
			• Formal dissemination & change strategies should be planned per relevant research:
			  o *Simple, passive education is rarely effective as an isolated strategy. Consider multiple strategies, e.g., interactive education, opinion leaders, educational research, etc.*
			• Consider need for appropriate, reasoned variation
			• WITH B' where made a decision to use in the setting:
			  o *With formal use, may need a dynamic evaluation to effectively implement & continuously improve/ refine use of best available evidence*
			• *WITH B'* where made a decision to *consider use & thus obtain additional, pragmatic information before a final decision*
			  o *With formal consideration, need a pilot project*
			  o *With a pilot project, must assess if need IRB review, per relevant institutional criteria*
				• Evaluation can be formal or informal; individual or institutional
				• Consider cost-benefit of various evaluation efforts
				• Use RU-as-process to enhance credibility of evaluation data
				• For both dynamic pilot evaluations; include two types of evaluative information:
				  o *formative, regarding actual implementation & goal progress*
				  o *summative, regarding Phase I outcomes and goal results*

NOTE: Model applies to all forms of practice, i.e. educational, clinical, managerial, or other
See Stetler, C., Morsi, D., Rucki, S., Broughton, S., Corrigan, B., Fitzgerald, J., Giuliano, K., Havener, P., & Sheridan E.A. (1998). Utilization-focused integrated reviews in a nursing service, *Applied Nursing Research*, 11 (4), 195-206 for noted tables, reviews, and synthesis process.

FIG. **2.6** Stetler Model, Part II: Additional, per phase details. (From Stetler, C. B. [2001]. Updating the Stetler model of research utilization to facilitate evidence-based practice. *Nursing Outlook*, 49[6], 276.)

Primary care providers need to have an understanding of empirical evidence and how to use this evidence to improve patient and systems outcomes. Knowledge of appraisal and grading of the evidence is needed to determine the strength and confidence in the evidence for use with a practice change.

Use of a framework, theory, or model to systematize and guide the planning, implementation, and evaluation of practice change projects supports successful implementation of EBP. There are many models for implementation of EBP available for use in clinical settings; however, selection is dependent on the setting and type of practice change proposed.

Primary care providers can influence the closing of the research–evidence–practice gap by gaining the knowledge and developing the skills to lead interprofessional teams in the implementation of EBP to improve patient, organizational, and system outcomes.

Facilitator focus and activity

What the facilitator looks at
What the facilitator does

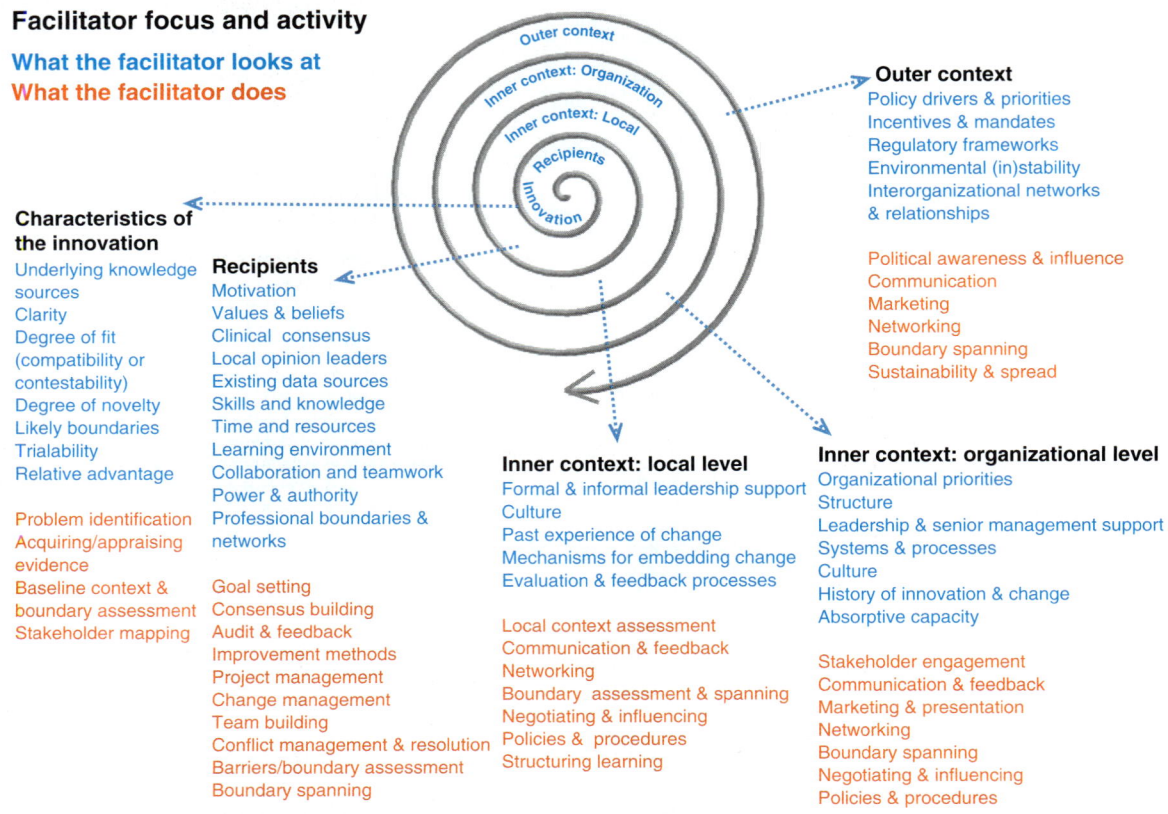

Outer context
Policy drivers & priorities
Incentives & mandates
Regulatory frameworks
Environmental (in)stability
Interorganizational networks
& relationships

Political awareness & influence
Communication
Marketing
Networking
Boundary spanning
Sustainability & spread

Characteristics of the innovation
Underlying knowledge
sources
Clarity
Degree of fit
(compatibility or
contestability)
Degree of novelty
Likely boundaries
Trialability
Relative advantage

Problem identification
Acquiring/appraising
evidence
Baseline context &
boundary assessment
Stakeholder mapping

Recipients
Motivation
Values & beliefs
Clinical consensus
Local opinion leaders
Existing data sources
Skills and knowledge
Time and resources
Learning environment
Collaboration and teamwork
Power & authority
Professional boundaries &
networks

Goal setting
Consensus building
Audit & feedback
Improvement methods
Project management
Change management
Team building
Conflict management & resolution
Barriers/boundary assessment
Boundary spanning

Inner context: local level
Formal & informal leadership support
Culture
Past experience of change
Mechanisms for embedding change
Evaluation & feedback processes

Local context assessment
Communication & feedback
Networking
Boundary assessment & spanning
Negotiating & influencing
Policies & procedures
Structuring learning

Inner context: organizational level
Organizational priorities
Structure
Leadership & senior management support
Systems & processes
Culture
History of innovation & change
Absorptive capacity

Stakeholder engagement
Communication & feedback
Marketing & presentation
Networking
Boundary spanning
Negotiating & influencing
Policies & procedures

FIG. 2.7 The integrated Promoting Action on Research Implementation in Health Services framework. (From *Implementing evidence-based practice in healthcare: A facilitation guide*, G. Harvey & A. Kitson. Copyright [© 2015] and Routledge. Reproduced by permission of Taylor & Francis Books, United Kingdom.)

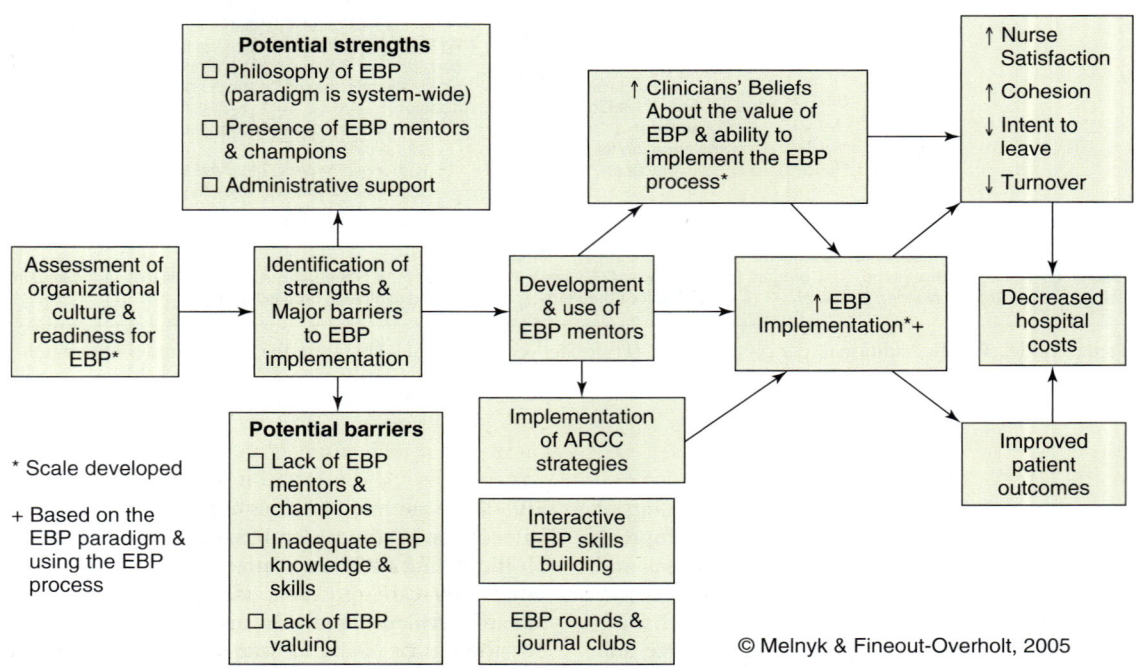

Potential strengths
☐ Philosophy of EBP
   (paradigm is system-wide)
☐ Presence of EBP mentors
   & champions
☐ Administrative support

↑ Nurse
Satisfaction
↑ Cohesion
↓ Intent to
leave
↓ Turnover

↑ Clinicians' Beliefs
About the value of
EBP & ability to
implement the EBP
process*

Assessment of
organizational
culture &
readiness for
EBP*

Identification of
strengths &
Major barriers
to EBP
implementation

Development
& use of
EBP mentors

↑ EBP
Implementation*+

Decreased
hospital
costs

* Scale developed

+ Based on the
EBP paradigm &
using the EBP
process

Potential barriers
☐ Lack of EBP
   mentors &
   champions
☐ Inadequate EBP
   knowledge &
   skills
☐ Lack of EBP
   valuing

Implementation
of ARCC
strategies

Improved
patient
outcomes

Interactive
EBP skills
building

EBP rounds &
journal clubs

© Melnyk & Fineout-Overholt, 2005

FIG. 2.8 Advancing Research and Clinical Practice Through Close Collaboration *(ARCC)* model. (© 2005, Melnyk and Fineout-Overholt.)

REFERENCES

1. Mackey, A., & Bassendowski, S. (2017). Original Article: The history of evidence-based practice in nursing education and practice. *Journal of Professional Nursing, 33,* 51–55. doi:10.1016/j.profnurs.2016.05.009.

2. Agency for Healthcare Quality & Research, (AHRQ). (2018). Guidelines synthesis. Updated July 13, 2017. https://www.guideline.gov/syntheses/index. (Accessed 28 December 2017).

3. Cohen, A. M., Stavri, P. Z., & Hersh, W. R. (2004). A categorization and analysis of the criticisms of evidence-based medicine. *International Journal of Medical Informatics, 73,* 35–43.

4. Evidence Based Medicine Working Group. (1992). Evidence-based medicine. A new approach to teaching the practice of medicine. *JAMA: The Journal of the American Medical Association, 268,* 2420–2425.

5. Melnyk, B. M., & Fineout-Overholt, E. (2015). *Evidence-based practice in nursing & healthcare. A guide to best practice* (3rd ed.). Philadelphia, PA: Wolters Kluwer.

6. Cowman, S. (2018). Bedside to bench: Re-thinking nursing research. *Journal of Advanced Nursing, 74,* 235–236. doi:10.1111/jan.13254.

7. Lopes Júnior, L. C. (2015). Translational research and nursing: The lab bench to bedside. *Revista De Enfermagem UFPE online, 9*(12), 1328. doi:10.5205/01012007.

8. Qidwai, W. (2016). Translational research and complexity of clinical practice: Issues, challenges, and way forward. *Journal of the College of Physicians and Surgeons–Pakistan, 26*(6), 453–454. doi:2339.

9. Murad, M. H., Almasri, J., Alsawas, M., & Farah, W. (2017). Grading the quality of evidence in complex interventions: A guide for evidence-based practitioners. *Evidence-Based Medicine, 22*(1), 20. http://dx.doi.org.chamberlainuniversity.idm.oclc.org/10.1136/ebmed-2016-110577.

10. What is a systematic review? Cochran Collaboration. Published 2018. http://consumers.cochrane.org/what-systematic-review. (Accessed 4 January 2018).

11. Song, J. W., & Chung, K. C. (2010). Observational studies: Cohort and case-control studies. *Plastic and Reconstructive Surgery, 126*(6), 2234–2242. http://doi.org/10.1097/PRS.0b013e3181f44abc.

12. Titler, M. G. (2008). The evidence for evidence-based practice implementation. In R. G. Hughes (Ed.), *Patient safety and quality: An evidence-based handbook for nurses.* Rockville, MD: Agency for Healthcare Research and Quality (US). Retrieved from https://www.ncbi.nlm.nih.gov/books/NBK2659/.

13. Evans, D. (2002). Hierarchy of evidence: A framework for ranking evidence-evaluating healthcare interventions. *Journal of Clinical Nursing, 12*(1), 77–84.

14. Berkman, N. D., Lohr, K. N., Ansari, M. T., Balk, E., Kane, R., McDonagh, M. S., et al. (2015). Grading the strength of a body of evidence when assessing health care interventions: An EPC update. *Journal of Clinical Epidemiology, 68*(11), 1312–1324. doi:10.1016/j.jclinepi.2014.11.023.

15. Burnes, B., & Bargal, D. (2017). Kurt Lewin: 70 years on. *Journal of Change Management, 17*(2), 91–100.

16. Rogers, E. (2003). *Diffusion of innovations* (5th ed.). New York, NY: Simon and Schuster.

17. Nilsen, P. (2015). Making sense of implementation theories, models, and frameworks. *Implementation Science, 10,* 53. doi:10.1186/s13012-015-0242-0.

18. Iowa Model Collaborative. (2017). Iowa model of evidence-based practice: Revisions and validation. *Worldviews on Evidence-Based Nursing, 14*(3), 175–182. doi:10.1111/wvn.12223.

19. Stevens, K. R. (2012). Star Model of EBP: Knowledge Transformation. Academic Center for Evidence-based Practice. The University of Texas Health Science Center at San Antonio.

20. Dang, D., & Dearholt, S. (2017). *Johns Hopkins nursing evidence-based practice: Model and guidelines* (3rd ed.). Indianapolis, IN: Sigma Theta Tau International.

21. Stetler, C. (2001). Updating the Stetler model of research utilization to facilitate evidence-based practice. *Nursing Outlook, 49*(6), 272–279. doi:10.1067/mno.2001.120517.

22. Stetler, C. B. (2010). Stetler model. In J. Rycroft-Malone & T. Bucknall (Eds.), *Models and frameworks for implementing evidence-based practice: Linking evidence to action* (pp. 51–88). West Sussex, UK: Wiley-Blackwell.

23. Rycroft-Malone, J. (2004). The PARIHS framework—A framework for guiding the implementation of evidence-based practice. *Journal of Nursing Care Quality, 19*(4), 297–304.

24. Harvey, G., & Kitson, A. (2016). PARIHS revisited: From heuristic to integrated framework for the successful implementation of knowledge into practice. *Implementation Science, 11,* 33. doi:10.1186/s13012-016-0398-2.

25. Melnyk, B. M., & Fineout-Overholt, E. (2014). *Evidenced based practice in nursing and healthcare* (3rd ed.). Philadelphia, PA: Wolters Kluwer.

26. Melnyk, B., Fineout-Overholt, E., Giggleman, M., & Choy, K. A. (2017). A test of the ARCC® model improves implementation of evidence-based practice, healthcare culture, and patient outcomes. *Worldviews on Evidence-based Nursing, 14*(1), 5–9. doi:10.1111/wvn.12188. [Epub 2016 Dec 21].

27. Melnyk, B. M., Fineout-Overholt, E., Gallagher-Ford, L., & Kaplan, L. (2012). The state of evidence-based practice in US nurses: Critical implications for nurse leaders and educators. *The Journal of Nursing Administration, 42*(9), 410–417.

28. Science of Improvement. Institute for Healthcare Improvement. Published 2018. http://www.ihi.org/about/Pages/ScienceofImprovement.aspx. (Accessed 5 January 2018).

29. Regulations and Policy. HHS.gov. Office for Human Research Protections. Published on February 16, 2016. http://www.hhs.gov/ohrp/humansubjects/guidance/45cfr46.htm#46.102. (Accessed 20 December 2017).

30. Broome, M., Riner, M., & Allam, E. (2013). Scholarly publication practices of doctor of nursing practice-prepared nurses. *The Journal of Nursing Education, 52*(8), 429–434. doi:10.3928/01484834-20130718-02. [Epub 2013 Jul 18].

31. Chronic Disease Overview. Centers for Disease Control and Prevention (CDC). Published June 28, 2017. https://www.cdc.gov/chronicdisease/overview/index.htm. (Accessed 28 December 2017).

32. Framework for Action on Interprofessional Education & Collaborative Practice. World Health Organization. Published 2010. http://apps.who.int/iris/bitstream/10665/70185/1/WHO_HRH_HPN_10.3_eng.pdf. (Accessed 5 January 2018).

CHAPTER **3**

EMPOWERING PATIENTS AS COLLABORATIVE PARTNERS: A NEW MODEL FOR PRIMARY CARE

Marcia Potter

CURRENT CHALLENGES

The past decade has produced a sea change of health care regulations, access to care, patient satisfaction, and reimbursement issues. Coupled with decreasing numbers of physicians entering primary care, increased numbers of physicians leaving primary care, the aging population, and growing disease burden, many Americans remain underserved by the US health care system.[1,2] Although the implementation of the Affordable Care Act in 2010 increased the number of Americans with access to insurance, gaining access to care services has been more elusive.[3] Significantly, the cost of care continues to impose a major burden on individuals and the US economy, reaching more than $3 trillion in 2015, equating to nearly $10K per person in the United States.[1,4]

SOLUTIONS FOR CURRENT CHALLENGES: ANY SUCCESSFUL SOLUTION MUST EMPOWER PATIENTS

To reverse the current health care crisis, policy experts across multiple domains within the health care system have advocated for primary care transformation.[1,5,6] Based on the broad goals of the Quadruple Aim and set within the Institute of Medicine's definition of high-quality health care, paradigms for transformation have gained traction in primary care.[7–9] The Quadruple Aim is an expansion of the Institute for Health Care Improvement's Triple Aim, adding the fourth aim, to improve patient care team (or clinician's) experience to the previous three aims: (1) improve patient satisfaction with health care, (2) reduce per capita costs, and (3) improve population health.[7] All of these are important contributors of high-quality health care: safe, patient centered, efficient, effective, timely, and equitable.[9] However, none of these initiatives can reach optimal success without the inclusion and empowerment of the most important member of the health care team, the patient. Designing care processes around the patient has been referred to as patient-centered care, but even this perspective falls short of the full partnership and empowerment required of patients.[1,10]

As health care transforms, the awareness of the need to personalize health care to individuals became the rallying cry for many, including Congress. Patient-centered care sought to put patients at the center of their health care, include them in all decision-making, cocreate shared goals, and improve health outcomes. Unfortunately, this has remained an elusive goal, partly because even in patient-centeredness, human beings are constrained by the medicalization of their perception of their own health; this does not foster the patient empowerment that is needed to make care truly patient centered.[10]

What is emerging is the idea that patients are *persons* throughout their experience of their health state. Indeed, because people cannot be separated from their health state, their wishes, goals, and desires should account for more than simply the navigation of a particular condition—it should reflect respect for the holistic needs and life force of each human being. For these reasons, empowering patients to be full participants in their health care is integral to improving their health and the health of the health system. The goal of health care is to create high-quality health capability for patients. In turn, this capability creates capacity to live a high-quality life, to liberate energy allowing people to pursue their goals and desires, and to enable personal freedom. In professional practice, the shift to person-centered caring also encompasses the professional development of each team member. As health care is transforming, so must health care team members transform their perspective about their work, their patients, and themselves.[1,10]

Two concepts are integral to the perspective of person-centered care and empowering patients: activation and engagement. Activation is the belief that a particular choice is important; engagement is the belief that choice can be carried out, even in adverse circumstances.[11,12] Although activation and engagement for the patient empowerment and collaboration is key, so is the activation and engagement of the health care staff. After all, one cannot expect full partnership without full participation of each partner. But how is this partnership created? What structures, processes, and outcomes should be included to optimize this concept? What framework provides the foundation to guide decision-making?

One of the most studied and well-supported paradigms for transforming the health care team from patient centered to person centered is the Chronic Care Model (CCM).[13] Of course, paradigms alone will not transform a complex adaptive system such as health care. To optimize the potential of a paradigm, evidence must provide the foundation and theory should guide decision-making.[14] Health care providers are uniquely educated and situated to both transform practice and influence health policy using multiple levels of evidence applied across all levels of the health system.[6] Therefore it is imperative to apply theory as the foundation for practice transformation.

So why is it important to begin with a theory? Theory not only guides practice; it frames how we view the world, our professions, and our decision-making and supports practice

situates within health care at all levels. When choosing a theory to guide practice, the unique needs of all stakeholders within the health system must be addressed. Bureaucratic Caring Theory (BCT), a grounded, phenomenological theory, seeks synthesis between the thesis of caring and the antithesis of bureaucracy, essentially seeking to humanize an inherently bureaucratic system, such as health care systems (Fig. 3.1).[15] This humanization is key to the transformation of health care delivery models from a productivity-driven business model to one of human caring and relationship-building that empowers patients as partners in their care.

Bureaucratic Caring Theory

Originally developed by Dr. Marilyn Ray in 1989, the BCT seeks to synthesize the inherently humanistic and bureaucratic needs within health care organizations. Because health care is situated within systems, the health of the system must be balanced with the needs of the individuals who cocreate the system. Health care, as a complex adaptive system, changes and evolves at decision points, leading to increasing order or disorder.[16] As a complex adaptive system, health care organizations reside at these bifurcation points in nearly every domain of existence. BCT is composed of eight domains of caring (Table 3.1). It is important to know that it is not a choice of whether or not to care but how caring is accomplished.[17]

Expanded Chronic Care Model

Originally developed by Edward Wagner, Director at the MacColl Institute for Healthcare Innovation, Group Health Cooperative of Puget Sound, Washington, the CCM was designed to meet the health care needs of patients and populations with complex chronic conditions.[18] The CCM focuses on longitudinal needs of the patient's health condition, rather than fragmented, episodic visits. Evidence strongly supported four interventions that led to the greatest improvement in health outcomes: use all staff at the top of their skillset levels; educate and support patients; planned, proactive, team-based care; and better use of registry-based information.[18] The CCM, in use for two decades, has robust evidence to support its effectiveness in improving care and health outcomes at all levels of the health care system.[18,19] In 2003, the CCM was expanded to include the components of preventive care and renamed the Expanded Chronic Care Model (ECCM).[20] This focus on prevention as well as chronic condition management is more aligned to the nursing perspective of holistic nursing care: reducing pain and suffering and preventing disability. Six components comprise the ECCM: organizational support, clinical information systems, delivery system design, decision support, self-management support, and community resources. We can build a new model for primary care that empowers patients by leveraging the caring domains that relate to the components of the ECCM.

BUILDING PATIENT EMPOWERMENT BY USING COMPONENTS OF THE EXPANDED CHRONIC CARE MODEL AND CARING DOMAINS OF THE BUREAUCRATIC CARING THEORY

Organizational Support

With any process improvement, optimization occurs when leaders at all levels of the organization cocreate a culture that supports evidence-based practice (EBP). For these improvements to come to fruition, leaders must value not just

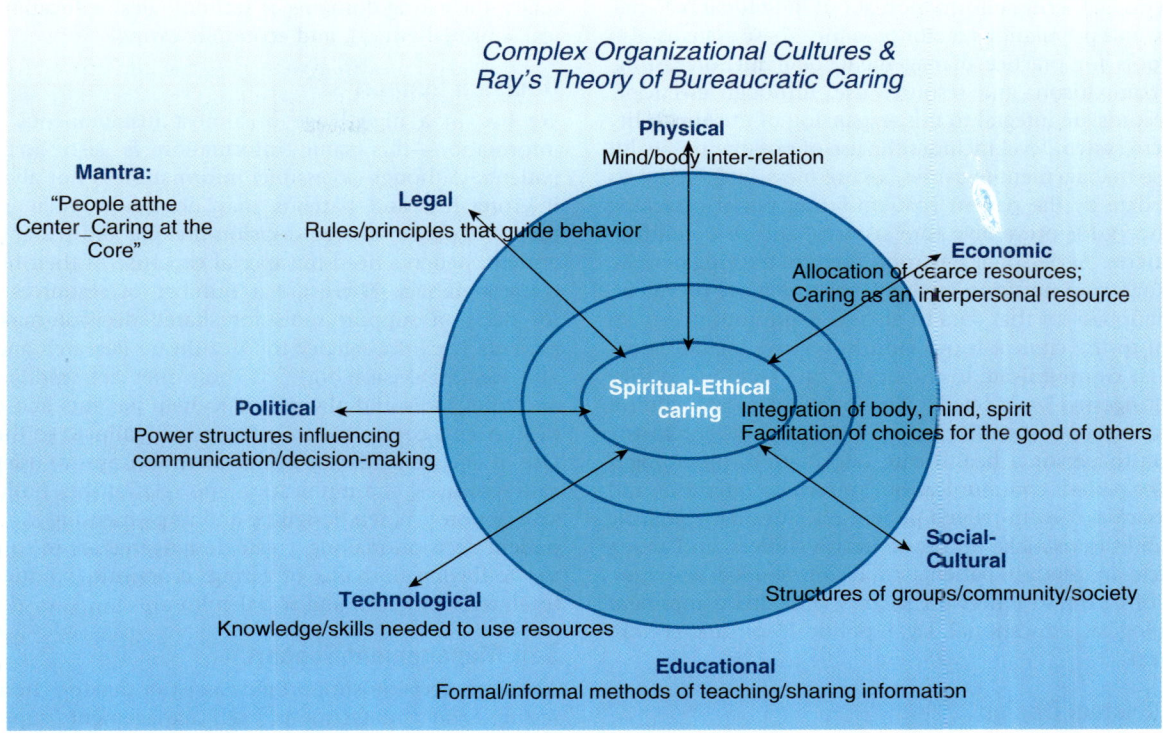

FIG. 3.1 Bureaucratic Caring Theory. (From Ray, M., & Turkel, M. [2015]. Marilyn Ann Ray's theory of bureaucratic caring. In M. Smith & M. Parker [Eds.], *Nursing theories and nursing practice* [4th ed.]. Philadelphia: F. A. Davis Company, with permission.)

TABLE 3.1	Bureaucratic Caring Theory Caring Domains[15]
Spiritual-ethical caring	Facilitating choices of good for others. It is the domain of body-mind-spirit, viewing human as spiritual beings and founded in the ethical principles of autonomy, beneficence, and nonmaleficence.
Physical caring	Physical and mental well-being of humans. Encompasses all of the physical ways in which caring is expressed to another, as well as biologic and mental patterns.
Legal caring	Caring through justice and fairness. All of the laws and regulations we follow in our profession.
Technological caring	The nonhuman ways in which caring is expressed. Includes information technology, information technology systems, medications, and care delivery processes and procedures. Encompasses the knowledge and skills to use those resources.
Political caring	Power and the use of legitimate authority to convey caring. Political caring is the process for and outcomes of policy decisions, workplace relations, and lines of authority.
Economic caring	Monetary and fiscal health of organizations. The economic ability to provide care for patients as well as funds for health care resources and decisions on coverage inclusions/exclusions/limits
Educational caring	How we teach patients, what we teach. Includes the essential knowledge and skills needed to provide health care services.
Social-cultural caring	Relationships forged as individuals, teams, and organizations cocreate bonds, affiliations, and partnerships with one another and in the wider community. All of the social relationships as well as the expression and meaning of health to the individual.

From Ray, M., & Turkel, M. (2015). Marilyn Ann Ray's theory of bureaucratic caring. In M. Smith & M. Parker (Eds.), *Nursing theories and nursing practice* (4th ed.). Philadelphia: F. A. Davis Company, with permission.

outcomes but the process of innovation and change, and they must provide resources needed for this change. For the implementation and success of the ECCM, this will also include the resource of time.[19] In the design and implementation of any process improvement, we encourage empowerment by ensuring the initiatives reflect the caring domains of political, social-cultural, spiritual-ethical, economic, technological, legal, physical, and educational caring.

Clinical Information Systems

Clinical information systems bridge the gap between data creation and storage to high-quality health services. Without these systems, gathering information about individual patients, aggregates, and populations is not possible. These systems also serve as tools for practice management, demand forecasting, outcome comparison, and resource use. Although electronic medical records are integral to this, expansion of this capability to the macro system level includes the use of population health and disease management registries, secure messaging, access to electronic data by the patient (patient-facing portal), tracking and reminders for preventive care services, and risk stratification of patients. As personal electronic medical tracking devices, such as fitness and nutrition tracking, become more prevalent, the expectation is for that data to also be communicated from the patient to the clinical team. Futuristic views include medications that communicate to the health care team when they have been ingested or injected.[21] Key functions of any clinical information system should empower patients by enhancing their access to personal health care information, providing a platform for patient communication concerning questions and requests, tracking health-related patient activities/data, guiding patients' abilities to make optimum health choices, and acting as a vehicle to remind patients of recommended activities. Domains of caring to reflect for success with this component are technological, educational, legal, political, spiritual-ethical, and physical.

Delivery System Design

The roles and tasks of each team member, including the patient, how they interact, how visits are structured, and how follow-up is managed, comprise delivery system design. New initiatives focus on engaging patients in delivery system design, emphasizing the need for their voice in cocreating a system that will meet their needs. In this component, each team member performs to the top of their skills and training, works collaboratively, and is respected for their knowledge. Hallmarks are frequent communication, ongoing training, and strong leadership. In each encounter, the team is both patient focused and practice focused, ensuring the right care is delivered to the right person at the right time.

In the traditional model of care, the physician may not engage with the physician assistant, nurse practitioner, nurse, or other support team members except in complex cases. In the ECCM, each member of the team is needed to provide care services in some capacity for each patient. In complex cases, there is often a need to engage nurses, medical assistants, health coaches, and administrative staff to provide planned outreach to patients in between office visits. Using staff resources in this way facilitates improved access to care, health outcomes, and patient and staff satisfaction, while decreasing the overall cost of care.[19]

The structure of the health care visit is integral to delivery system design. Planned visits for the management of chronic health conditions and for preventive visits should be separate from acute care visits. Although this may seem counterintuitive, evidence supports that adults retain only approximately 30% of what they have heard.[22] Trying to address too many issues in a single visit leads to increased fragmentation, frustration, and poorer outcomes in all caring domains.[13] Although in-person appointments remain the majority of encounters, virtual visits, group visits, and secure messaging (asynchronous visits) are becoming more prevalent.[21] The goal must be to build empowerment patients by ensuring that care delivery system designs reflect the caring domains of technological, educational, political, spiritual-ethical, and economic caring.

Decision Support

We live in a digital age of almost instantaneous access to information—this same information is also accessible to patients. Although accessible, information is not always easily interpretable, and patients may not know what applies to them. As part of shared decision-making and patient empowerment, patients need the special expertise of their health care team members. There are a number of resources available for decision support tools for shared decision-making with patients (e.g., the Agency for Healthcare Research and Quality and HealthDecision.org).[23,24] These sites are readily available and offer tools and algorithms to help patients and clinicians determine a course of care relevant and tailored to the patient. Use of decision aids has been shown to improve use of health care resources, communication and relationship building, and satisfaction.[24] When designing and implementing initiatives for patient decision-making, create designs that are in concert with the following domains of caring: economic, spiritual-ethical, legal, technological, and social-cultural.

Self-Management Support

Although decision support aids assist in making choices about testing and interventions, self-management support aids assist the patient to navigate the experiences of their health condition, foster activation and engagement, and enable personal freedom. Self-management is founded on the idea of self-efficacy and the ability to complete tasks and reach goals.[11,12] A patient's self-efficacy is subject to change over time and can be highly influenced by the health care team's support and engagement with the patient. Building patient empowerment in this component uses the spiritual-ethical, technological, political, social-cultural, educational, and economic caring domains.

Community Resources

Patients and health care teams do not exist in vacuums but are part of a larger community system. This system of resources enables or impedes patient self-efficacy, health outcomes, and health care team effectiveness. Health care systems often develop outreach programs within the communities they serve, to project the effectiveness of the clinical encounter into the patient's social environment. This is important for a variety of reasons: access to health services, ongoing support to improve health, and improvement of population health. Although a discussion of this is beyond the limits of this chapter, community resources are integrally linked with community and population health efforts, needs, and outcomes. Incorporate information from the caring domains of spiritual-ethical, economic, political, social-cultural, and physical when establishing the network of community resources.

INCORPORATING BUREAUCRATIC CARING THEORY AND THE ENHANCED CHRONIC CARE MODEL TO EMPOWER PATIENTS AS COLLABORATORS IN A NEW MODEL FOR PRIMARY CARE

Theory-guided, EBP underpins the health of the health system and ensures that patients and their health care team

TABLE 3.2 **Solutions to Practice Design Problems**

Problem	Solutions	Key Stakeholders
Engaging Patients and Team members	Build trust by respect, reliability, and relational caring in every encounter. Prior experience with the organization affects trust.	Patients, team members, organization leaders
Patients nonadherent to care	Use social-culture domain of caring to respect patient's values. Explore reasons for nonadherence.	Patients, team members
Leading health care delivery	Treat as a complex adaptive system. Understand the interplay in any organization of the BCT domains of caring. Identify sources of resistance; engage stakeholders in seeking a better way. Frame daily work using the ECCM. Communicate linkages of ECCM to Caring Domains. Engage team members in authentic dialogue about their perspective of how the ECCM affects and reflects their practice. Be open to their observations and discoveries. Coach them in best practices of caring behaviors. Remember that change can begin with only small number that grows.	Team members, organization leaders
Frustration with Requirements for Mentoring/ Professional Development (peer review, performance reports and administrative)	Expand the view of what nursing is as a profession and what are professional obligations. As practitioners of a profession, we have an obligation to educate and insure adherence to ethical standards. Peer Review is a method to ensure quality care, fulfilling professional as well as legal requirements for monitoring safety and quality of nursing services. Performance reports are a critical component of professional development, mentoring and leadership development. Monitoring a person's quality performance should lead to authentic feedback about their goals, potential, and actual capabilities. People are integral to a human system, so we want to be sure we provide them the caring they need. In these tasks we see the expression of caring in the educational, legal, technological, social-cultural, and spiritual-ethical domains.	

Grounded in BCT from the Take Your Theorist to Lunch series developed by the author and based on work by Melrose.
BCT, Bureaucratic Caring Theory.
Data from Melrose, S. (2006). Lunch with the theorists: A clinical learning assignment. *Nurse Educator, 31*(4), 147–148.

partners cocreate the circumstances for optimal health outcomes. Although health care organizations are complex adaptive systems, so are people. Patients and health care team members are all human; the potential for complexity multiplies exponentially. Each decision point in creation of health initiatives has the potential to lead to increasing order or disorder, improved health, or increased disability. Using the BCT to frame practice system designs and quality improvement initiatives humanizes health care system designs, leverages knowledge about the effects domains of caring have on the health care system, clinical teams, and patients, and provides a roadmap for successful care delivery modes that empowers patients as collaborators. Table 3.2 addresses the application of the BCT to some current challenges in primary care practices, with possible solutions in critical areas of patient care, practice leadership, and mentoring and by imagining a conversation over lunch with the Dr. Marilyn Ray, the BCT theorist, to energize ideas for solutions to primary care practice issues.[25] Framing primary care model decisions within the BCT enables caring to flourish in all domains without compromising any particular domain, empowering patients and creating individualized practice-based solutions for providers. Incorporating the ECCM into a primary care practice creates a model that empowers patients and health care team members to collaborate, engage, and grow in capability and capacity.

A new model for primary care that empowers patients as collaborators starts with the delivery system design. Overarching characteristics of the delivery system in the new model has each team member's understanding that they cocreate the patient experience in every interaction each of them has with a patient. Team members have a commitment to enabling

planned, caring, proactive patient visits and practice to the full extent of their education and training. Leaders in the new model ensure there are adequate human, financial, technological (includes analytics), physical, and educational resources. Leaders act to hold team members accountable for performance of their assigned duties, the quality of their patient communication, response times within patient visits, and response times to patient requests. The structure of the health care visit is integral to delivery system design. Begin by restructuring practice templates and schedules to allot 30 minutes for well and established appointments and 15 minutes for acute and routine appointments. Institute team huddles at the beginning of each day to discuss what is needed for each patient from team members. There are critical activities for the NP, RN, and medical technician and administrative staff for each patient visit: previsit, at the time of visit, and post visit. (Table 3.3).

As both team leaders and team members, practitioners are uniquely positioned to shape the design and delivery of health care as we progress in health care reform. Using the BCT and the ECCM in a new model for primary care, practitioners cocreate innovative, person-centered systems to improve the health of individuals, populations, and the health system. Understanding how each of our patients experience their health states differently reflects the holistic view of patient as person. Framing practice as person centered empowers patients as collaborators and offers the opportunity to embrace the beautiful mural of human experiences and interactions, cocreating relationship-based care and moving beyond the medical to the humanistic. This is a new model for primary care that will truly reform our current health care system.

TABLE 3.3 **Planned Visit Protocol in the New Model for Primary Care**

Stage	Team Member	Critical Activities
Previsit	Registered nurse	Consult chronic disease/preventive services registries for patient's record
		Assess: How is the patient tolerating medications; exercise type/frequency; dietary measures; barriers to self-management: social, physical, psychological, spiritual; successes with self-management: social, physical, psychological, spiritual
		Plan: Labs, supply refills, bridge medication refills, appointment with primary care; consults to specialty clinics per standing orders; prevention needs: immunizations: flu, shingles, pneumonia; general: mammogram, pap smear, colorectal cancer screening, sexually transmitted infection screening
		Implement: Order needed labs, supplies, bridge medications per standing orders; enter consult requests per standing orders; reinforce lifestyle measures; remind patient to bring all medications to planned visit
		Evaluate: Patient's understanding of plan; patient's acceptance of plan; patient's follow-up with scheduled/recommended interventions
		Document in patient's electronic health record
	Medical technician	Reviews clinician schedule 4 weeks in advance
		Assess: Are labs completed and in the record? Has patient picked up medication (if needed)? Is patient enrolled in patient portal?
		Are primary prevention services completed or scheduled?
		Plan: Ensure labs transferred to electronic health record encounter; ensure any primary preventive services updated in EHR encounter
		Implement: For any services not completed, contact patient to remind them to complete services
		Document in patient's electronic health record.
At the Visit	Primary care provider	Assess: Review all lab data, nursing information, screening data with patient
		Conduct needed physical exam
		Plan: Medication or lifestyle adjustments; community resources that may be required
		Implement: Tailor plan of care to patient's needs based on:
		Nursing evaluation; primary care provider evaluation and judgment; patient-identified goals and desires; decision aids and shared decision-making
		Enter/sign appropriate orders
		Enter any further consults needed
		Provide information on community resources
		Create checkout sheet for patient (discharge instructions)
		Evaluate: Patient's understanding and agreement with cocreated plan of care
		Ensure patient knows: When to follow-up; how to follow-up (appointment, virtual visit, secure messaging); how to engage in community resources; clarify any questions patient has before visit ends
		Document in patient's electronic health record
	Administrative staff	Assess: Review checkout sheet with patients
		Plan/Implement: Schedule patient for follow-up as directed by clinician (face to face, virtual, telephone); review patient demographics; ensure patient signed up for patient portal
		Evaluate: Does the patient have any questions prior to leaving?
Post visit	All team members	Team huddle to debrief any issues with specific patients or processes as needed
		Ensure team members aware of any community resources needed and how to engage patient with these
		Ensure all orders signed

REFERENCES

1. National Academy of Medicine. Vital Directions for health and health care. 2017. Washington, DC: National Academy of Medicine. Retrieved Dec 2017. Retrieved from https://nam.edu/initiatives/vital-directions-for-health-and-health-care. (Accessed 12 Dec 2017).
2. Dickson, V. (2014). Underinsured ACA enrollees strain community health centers. *Modern Healthcare.* Retrieved from http://www.modernhealthcare.com/article/20140925/NEWS/309259947. (Retrieved Nov 2017).
3. The Center for Consumer Information & Insurance Oversight (CCIIO). Young adults and the affordable care act: Protecting young adults and eliminating burdens on family and businesses. 2017.Centers for Medicare & Medicaid Services (CMS). Retrieved from https://www.cms.gov/CCIIO/Resources/Files/adult_child_fact_sheet.html.
4. National Center for Health Statistics. (2017). Health Expenditures. Retrieved from https://www.cdc.gov/nchs/fastats/health-expenditures.htm. (Accessed 15 Dec 2017).
5. Berwick, D. M. (2008). The triple aim: Care, health, and cost. *Health Affairs, 27*, 759–769.
6. Institute of Medicine of the National Academies. The future of nursing: Leading change, advancing health. 2010. Retrieved from http://www.nationalacademies.org/hmd/Reports/2010/The-Future-of-Nursing-Leading-Change-Advancing-Health.aspx. (Accessed 3 Nov 2017).
7. Bodenheimer, T., & Sinsky, C. (2014). From triple aim to quadruple aim: Care of the patient requires care of the provider. *Annals of Family Medicine, 12*(6), 573–576.
8. The Institute of Medicine (IOM). (2001). *Crossing the quality chasm: A new health system for the 21st century.* Washington, DC: National Academy Press.
9. Agency for Healthcare Research and Quality (AHRQ). (2015). The six domains of health care quality. Retrieved from https://www.ahrq.gov/professionals/quality-patient-safety/talkingquality/create/sixdomains.html. (Accessed 3 Dec 2017).
10. Miles, A., & Ashbridge, J. (2014). The European Society for person centered healthcare (ESPCH)—raising the bar of health care quality in the century of the patient. *Journal of Evaluation in Clinical Practice, 20*, 729–733.
11. Hibbard, J. H., Mahoney, E. R., Stock, R., & Tusler, M. (2007). Self management and healthcare utilization. *Health Services Research, 42*(4), 1443–1467.

12. Bandura, A. (1977). Self efficacy theory: Toward a unifying theory of behavior change. *Psychological Review*, 84(2), 191–215.

13. Coleman, K. A., Austin, B. T., Brach, C., & Wagner, E. H. (2003). Evidence on the chronic care model in the new millenium. *Health Affairs*, 28(1), 75–85.

14. American Academy of Nursing. Nursing Theory Guided Practice. 2001. http://www.aannet.org/expert-panels/ep-nursing-theory-guided-practice. (Accessed 14 Nov 2017).

15. Ray, M., & Turkel, M. (2015). Marilyn Ann Ray's theory of bureaucratic caring. In M. Smith & M. Parker (Eds.), *Nursing theories and nursing practice* (4th ed.). Philadelphia, PA: F. A. Davis Company.

16. Davidson, A. W., Ray, M. A., & Turkel, M. C. (2011). *Nursing, caring and complexity science: For human-environment well-being*. New York, New York: Springer Publishing.

17. Ray, M., & Turkel, M. (2014). Caring as emancipatory practice: The theory of relational caring complexity. *Advances in Nursing Science*, 37(2), 132–146.

18. Stellefson, M., Dipnarine, K., & Stopka, C. (2013). The chronic care model and diabetes management in US primary care settings: A systematic review. *Preventing Chronic Disease*, 10, doi:http://dx.doi.org/10.5888/pcd10.120180.

19. Potter, M. A., & Wilson, C. (2017). Applying bureaucratic caring theory and the chronic care model to improve staff and patient self-efficacy. *Nursing Administration Quarterly*, 41(4), 310–320.

20. Barr, V. J., Robinson, S., Martin-Link, B., Underhill, L., Dotts, A., Ravensdale, D., et al. (2003). The expanded chronic care model: An integration of concepts and strategies from population health promotion and the chronic care model. *Hospital Quarterly*, 7(1), 73–82.

21. Topol, E. (2015). *The patient will see you now*. Philadelphia, PA: Basic Books.

22. Kessels, R. (2003). Patients' memory for medical information. *Journal of the Royal Society of Medicine*, 219–222.

23. Agency for Healthcare Research and Quality. (2015). Clinical decision support. Retrieved from https://www.ahrq.gov/professionals/prevention-chronic-care/decision/clinical/index.html. (Accessed 1 Dec 2017).

24. Health Decision support and shared decision making. 2015. Retrieved from https://www.healthdecision.com. (Accessed 28 Nov 2017).

25. Melrose, S. (2006). Lunch with the theorists: A clinical learning assignment. *Nurse Educator*, 31(4), 147–148.

CHAPTER **4**

COORDINATED CHRONIC CARE

Laura Reed

A chronic disease or illness is defined as diagnosed illness, functional limitation, or cognitive impairment that lasts at least a year, places limits on a person's daily activities, and requires regular attention and medical care.[1] The Centers for Disease Control and Prevention (CDC) states that chronic diseases and conditions such as asthma, heart disease, stroke, cancer, type 2 diabetes, obesity, HIV/AIDS, and arthritis are among the most common and costly of all health problems. As of 2012, approximately half of all adults in the United States—117 million people—had one or more chronic conditions. One in four adults had two or more chronic health conditions[2] Seven of the top 10 causes of death in 2015 were from chronic diseases. Heart disease and cancer together accounted for almost 46% of all deaths.[2]

Chronic diseases impact lives in many ways. Many people with chronic illnesses experience a reduced quality of life and limitations in the activities of daily living. People with chronic illnesses have increased numbers of hospitalizations and emergency room visits and higher medical expenses compared with those who do not have a chronic illness. In the United States, 86% of the nation's $2.7 trillion annual health care expenditures are for people with chronic physical and mental health conditions.[2] Decreasing the incidence of chronic illnesses can reduce these costs.

Cardiovascular disease, diabetes, arthritis, and obesity are chronic conditions that may be prevented or delayed by life style changes such as increased exercise, improved nutrition, tobacco cessation, and reduced alcohol intake.[2] Risky health behaviors and health disparity issues, such as income, education, community resources, and access to health care, contribute to higher rates of chronic illness, poorer health outcomes, and increased medical costs among minority communities.

The prevalence of chronic diseases is steadily increasing, and it is estimated that by 2030 the number of adults living with one chronic illness will be in excess of 171 million. In clinical practice, chronic illness management must include effective communication between team members and coordination of care across different health care settings to improve the overall care of the chronically ill.[3]

COMPREHENSIVE CARE COORDINATION

As the incidence of chronic illnesses continues to rise internationally, strategies have been developed to address the optimal care of these patients. Care coordination is the deliberate organization of patient care activities between two or more participants (including the patient) involved in a patient's care to facilitate the delivery of health care services. This involves the gathering of personnel and other resources needed and communication between all parties involved including the patient.[4] The Chronic Care Model (CCM) was originally developed by Edward Wagner to organize the care of the chronically ill. This model incorporated six key components necessary to ensure improved clinical and functional outcomes. These six areas are: community resources, health system support, self-management support, delivery system support, decision support, and clinical information systems. The model was developed when the focus of care was the hospitalized patient. More recently, the focus of illness care is moving from hospital-based to community-based care, and the need for integration of health promotion into the prevention and treatment of chronic diseases model is obvious. The Expanded Chronic Care Model (ECCM), developed in 2003,[5] includes a community portion to address the influence of social determinants of health on the prevention and management of individuals with chronic diseases. It is believed that the combination of population health promotion and improved disease management as described in the ECCM will be a game-changer in addressing the burden of chronic disease on the health care system.[5]

Primary care offices and clinics are the gateway to coordinated care for many individuals with complex mental health disorders and substance use issues, as well as a variety of chronic health illnesses. Often patients do not seek early treatment because of the challenges associated with their medical needs, the complexity of the health care system, and financial and transportation challenges. To address these needs, integrated health care programs have been developed often as part of a population health initiative.

Over the past few decades, there have been many attempts to establish a health care system that could effectively care for patients with chronic illnesses. Because the majority of these patients are insured by Medicare and Medicaid, the Centers for Medicare and Medicaid Services (CMS) has worked diligently to find a health care system that will address all the needs of these patients while reducing hospitalizations, emergency room visits, and cost.

Several models of care are worth mentioning. These models can be organized in several different ways: by diagnosis, population served, age of population served, type of provider offering services, and payment sources. All models, regardless of structure, will benefit from assigning an "integrater" to each patient.

Berwick and associates identified the need for an "integrater" as a critical component of any CCM—one individual who would formulate a care plan with the patient and all those involved in his care, guide the patient through the technological nightmare of acute care, advocate for the patient and family, and interpret complex instructions and systems.[6]

MODELS OF CARE

Several models of care have been established, including Patient-Centered Medical Homes (PCMHs), self-management programs, house call or home-based primary care programs, and distance chronic disease programs (telehealth), to address the care of those with chronic illnesses who live in rural areas or are homebound. PCMH are based on the CCM and provide comprehensive primary care using a team approach to deliver patient-centered coordinated care.[6,7]

Self-management programs were designed to encourage the patient as an active participant in his or her own care. These programs initially started in rehabilitation settings but are currently being used in the primary care setting to include the patient as a partner in the management of his or her chronic illnesses. Distance chronic disease programs were designed to allow patients who live in rural areas access to care via internet or telephone to address their chronic disease processes.

House call programs are gaining in popularity and are available in many communities. The Veterans Health Administration (VHA) has a long-established home-based primary care programs using MDs, NPs, and PAs to deliver primary care to older or homebound veterans using house calls and phone calls.

First introduced at the Massachusetts General Hospital in 2006 as a Medicare demonstration project, the Integrated Care Management Program (iCMP) matches high-risk patients with a nurse care manager who works closely with patients and their families to develop a customized health care plan that addresses the specific health care needs of the patient. The care is individualized and relationship based and includes biopsychosocial care planning, multidisciplinary case rounds, outcomes accountability, and a standardized electronic health information platform. This program focuses on early identification and aggressive management of the most complex, highest-risk patients to control costs and improve the quality of care and quality of life of the individual. These programs are guided by an interdisciplinary team of professionals including primary care providers, mental health providers, nurses, licensed clinical social workers, and an array of other key personnel. Each patient is assigned a case manager who works with other team members to ensure all areas of care coordination are addressed. Outcomes have been impressive: lower costs, lower readmission rates, and lower mortality. Although the initial investment is high, subsequent cost reductions have resulted in savings (see https://www.partners.org/Innovation-And-Leadership/Population-Health-Management/Current-Activities/Integrated-Care-Management-Program.aspx).

Several small communities in rural New Hampshire and Vermont have established community nurses or are recognizing the work of parish nurses working from local churches. These registered nurses, often recently retired or no longer working full time, are practicing as care coordinators for frail older adults in their towns. The nurse functions in the "integrator" role as an educator, advocate, and coordinator of care. There is no charge for services, and services are delivered in patient's homes. The nurse is paid by a creative system of small town and private grants and donations, thereby keeping insurers and government payers completely out of the loop. The goals are similar to all community-delivered health services: keep people out of the emergency room and hospital, reduce medication errors and cost, improve patient confidence and satisfaction with care, and promote aging with dignity. See https://www.uvcnp.org.

The explosion in availability of personal electronic monitoring devices is potentially useful to many patients with chronic disease and others hoping to maintain good health. Millions of Americans currently use devices to monitor their health and fitness. These include scales, activity monitors (Fitbit, Apple Watch, Microsoft Band, with more being developed every day), heart rate, anticoagulant monitoring, and blood sugar monitors that do not require finger sticks, and more. Data are recorded and can help people have more control over their health and lifestyle. It can also help health care providers keep track of their patients' health status, because information from these devices can be uploaded into apps and electronic health records. These devices are becoming more affordable and some are covered by Medicare. Coupled with telehealth, e-mail or other electronic communication with health care providers allow patient problems to be recognized early and lives and dollars saved.

TELEHEALTH MEDICINE

Telehealth/telemedicine use is rapidly increasing in the United States. This use of technology allows increased access to care for patients who live in rural areas with limited health care access or those who are homebound. Telehealth or telemedicine is the use of electronic communication, ideally an interactive audio-video communication system, to provide medical services and monitoring to patients without them having to travel to the health care facility. Telehealth services are further divided into two categories: synchronous and asynchronous.

Synchronous or real-time telehealth requires the presence of both parties at the same time and a communication link between them that allows a real-time interaction to take place. Videoconferencing equipment is one of the most common forms of technologies used in synchronous telehealth. There are also peripheral devices that can be attached to computers or the videoconferencing equipment, which can aid in an interactive examination.

Asynchronous telehealth involves acquiring medical data (e.g., medical images, biosignals, voice recordings) and then transmitting these data to a doctor or medical specialist at a convenient time for assessment offline. It does not require the presence of both parties at the same time.

These services are being used effectively to monitor patients with diabetes, heart failure, and chronic obstructive lung disease, as well as dermatologic conditions. Telemedicine is also providing consulting services to intensive care unit ICU patients and staff in small hospitals and remote locations that may not have access to highly trained intensivists. The ability to provide care to a chronically or acutely ill patient from a distance can have a positive influence on the patient's overall health status and quality of life. Telehealth/telemedicine programs are currently available in all 50 states and the VA and are increasing in popularity across the United States as the technology becomes more available and less expensive.

The VHA has one of the largest telehealth programs in the United States. This program coordinates care for more than 490,000 veterans with chronic illnesses across the country. The goal of the program is to increase access to care and improve patient outcomes of those living with chronic diseases. Each participant has a home health device that collects the data and transmits it to the VHA electronic record system. This system allows health care providers to manage chronic diseases such as diabetes, congestive heart failure, depression, and chronic lung disease. The VHA also has a telehealth in the primary care clinic that allows rural outreach clinic to connect with specialists at larger VHA medical centers. Researchers at the VHA investigated the long-term effect of home telehealth on hospitalization rates. The study showed that there was statistically significant reduction in hospitalizations in the patients who participated in the telehealth program.[8]

There are issues with training patients to use equipment, meeting patient expectations of 24-hour care, understanding which health markers are most helpful in monitoring to prevent exacerbation of disease, and maintaining equipment. Studies are mixed regarding cost effectiveness, but the potential impact is considerable.

CMS restricts reimbursement of telehealth services to patients who reside in either a health provider shortage area (HPSA) or a US census–defined micro statistical area (MSA). These services are being reevaluated by CMS currently, and new guidelines have been published in 2018. See https://www.cms.gov/Outreach-and-Education/Medicare-Learning-Network-MLN/MLNProducts/downloads/TelehealthSrvcsfctsht.pdf.

In 2015, CMS recognized chronic care management as a critical component of primary care. CPT codes were assigned, and Medicare currently reimburses clinicians, including MDs, NPs, and PAs, for 20 to 60 minutes of time devoted to the coordination of care of medically complex individual patients with two or more chronic conditions that place the patient at risk of death, decompensation, or functional decline.

The use of integrated care programs has increased nationwide with the Affordable Care Act of 2010, especially in the Medicare/Medicaid-eligible patient population, although these services are still scarce and resources supporting them are also sparce.[9]

CHRONIC CARE CONDITIONS

Adolescents and children with medical complexity (CMC) are defined as a group with chronic medical conditions or neurodevelopmental impairments in need of complex coordinated care. Although these individuals make up 0.4% to 0.7% of all US children (approximately 320,000 to 560,000 children), their health care costs account for 15%–30% of pediatric health care costs.[10,11] These children require comprehensive complex care that most primary care clinicians or community pediatricians have limited experience in providing. Specialist pediatricians are scarce and usually practice in large children's hospitals that are often located at great distance from families. Other barriers to caring for CMC include decreased time to spend with the patient and his or her family in settings that require high patient volumes, limited resources including staff, and poor reimbursements.

Care of CMC requires care coordination between primary care and specialty providers and health care agencies, as well as addressing the developmental, educational, dental, social, and family financial concerns. Frequent communication with the family allows for early identification of any illness, social, or financial issue that, if not addressed, could result in complications and/or hospitalization. All aspects of care, including caregiver needs, should be addressed to ensure optimal health of the CMC and the family.[1,3,10]

Care coordination for CMC is integral to the long-term outcomes. Close cooperation with the school and development of an individualized education plan (IEP) should be a part of the overall plan of care. The care plan should also include addressing physical, social, and psychological aspects of the child's life, including the family's psychological support system and financial status. When care coordination is instituted in the primary care setting, the family of CMC report increased patient satisfaction, improved quality of life, and decreased health care costs.[10]

NPs and physician assistants have the skills and competencies to effectively manage the health care needs for CMC. Pediatric NPs in particular can provide comprehensive care in schools and various health care settings. Research has shown that care provided by NPs and PAs as part of a multidisciplinary team results in better health outcomes and patient/family satisfaction.[12]

TRANSITIONAL CARE

Transitional care is defined as a set of activities that ensures coordination and continuity of care of patients as they move from one level of care to another or one setting to another.[13] Transitional points include: home or nursing home to emergency room to inpatient settings, hospital discharge to a rehab facility, nursing home, or care transferred from primary care providers to specialists, hospitalists or home care agencies and back. These transition periods are associated with increased rates of adverse events (AEs) and rehospitalizations that can be avoided if risks are properly identified and anticipatory measures taken. Some common AEs include unnoticed laboratory abnormalities or outstanding lab tests at the time of discharge, adverse drug effects, infections, falls with injuries, and surgical complications. Older patients and patients with complex medical conditions are at the highest risk for transitional complications or an AE (Box 4.1). Transitional care, including care coordination with primary care providers, communication with home care agencies, and careful written and verbal discharge directions, in a language understood by the patient and family, should be in place for all patients with complex medical or surgical conditions. Provider ambiguity has been identified as an impediment to patient safety during transitions, particularly in the immediate post–hospital discharge period. Conflicting instructions from specialists and the primary care provider can be confusing and lead to a variety of AEs.

There are penalties associated with inadequate care transitions that result in complications and rehospitalizations. The component of the Affordable Care Act that resulted in the Readmissions Reduction Program requires that CMS reduce payments to Acute Care Hospital Inpatient Prospective Payment System (IPPS) hospitals for readmissions to the

BOX **4.1**

Potential Risks for Adverse Events

- Use of high-risk medication (antibiotics, glucocorticoids, anticoagulants, narcotics, antiepileptic medications, antipsychotics, antidepressants, and hypoglycemic agents)
- Polypharmacy
- More than six chronic conditions
- Cognitive impairment
- Physical frailty
- Prior hospitalization within the last 6–12 months
- Older age
- Black race
- Low health literacy
- Reduced social network indicators (e.g., being alone most of the day with limited or no family or friend contact by phone or in person)
- Lower socioeconomic status
- Hospital discharge against medical advice

same or another IPPS-associated hospital within 30 days of discharge.

Multiple research studies have shown that transitional care provided by advanced practice nurses (APNs) or registered nurses improves patient outcomes and reduces health care expenditures. Hirschman and colleagues conducted a randomized study with high-risk older adults that revealed transitional care provided by APNs decreased cost and readmission rates. In this study, transitional care was initiated with hospital discharge planning and continued at home after discharge. Patients were first visited in the hospital within 48 hours of admission. After discharge, two home visits were conducted. The first one was conducted within the first 48 hours after discharge and the second was with in the first 7 to 10 days. The APNs were available 7 days a week by telephone and called the patients at least weekly.[14] Coleman et al. conducted a study that used transitional coaches who were APNs, specifically master's degree–prepared geriatric NPs who performed home visits within the first 24 to 72 hours after discharge. The APNs performed medication management and reconciliation, evaluation or worsening symptoms, and communicated with health care providers regarding the patient's condition.[14,15] APNs and PAs are both qualified providers for these services because of their knowledge of medications and medication management, their ability to assist the patient in transitioning from the hospital to home, and an awareness of self-management tools needed by the patient and families to adapt to their new daily routines at home.

Any time a patient moves from one setting to another, the risk for an AE is raised, especially when caring for older adults and/or the medically complex patient. The most common reason for the AE is poor communication, both verbal and written. Many of these events can be avoided with detailed patient and family education before discharge from a health care setting or between health care settings and careful monitoring after discharge. Clear communication between providers, including the primary care provider and other specialists participating in the care of the chronically ill patient, should also include all members of the care team such as nursing, physical therapy, home health services, and social work.

Communication is most effective when there are verbal interactions between care team members, as well as written forms such as discharge summaries and medicine reconciliation sheets. When electronic records are not transferable from one setting to the next, printed copies can be sent with the patient or faxed to the receiving facility. Ideally, discharge summaries and written instructions arrive at the same time as the patient.

Polypharmacy is responsible for many of the issues that arise after discharge, especially if new medications have been prescribed without adequate education. In older adults, high-risk medications such as insulin, warfarin, oral antiplatelet agents, and oral hypoglycemic medications, as well as benzodiazepines and opioids, are the most likely culprits for an AE and/or readmission.[16]

Primary care providers play a crucial role in transitional care. The recently discharged complex patient should be seen within 48 to 72 hours of discharge to review the discharge plan and evaluate the patient's medication list to ensure all changes are in writing and that the patient and family understand the medication instructions. Ideally, a house call is made for this purpose. Studies have shown that care coordination by a nurse, communication with the primary care providers upon discharge, and a nurse home visit within 3 days significantly reduced readmission rates.[17] A written list of the current medications and instructions using large print at a third-grade reading level should be given to the patient at the end of the appointment. Patients should be reminded that medications taken before hospitalization may no longer be on the current list or be listed at a different dosage. A discussion of polypharmacy can be found in Chapter 13.

Other impediments to successful transitions between levels of care are cognitive impairment, depression, physical frailty, and delirium that developed as a result of the hospitalization. Care coordinators should establish the patient's cognitive and physical baseline before the current illness by interviewing family or caregivers in order that the most appropriate discharge plan is established.

Healthy People 2020 defines social determinants of health as "conditions in the environments in which people are born, live, learn, work, play, worship, and age that affect a wide range of health, functioning, and quality-of-life outcomes and risks."[18] These conditions can be social, economic, and/or physical. People in lower socioeconomic brackets and/or who have lower educational levels are at higher risk for chronic illnesses because of lack of insurance, limited access to health care, or language barriers. Health care providers need to incorporate awareness of health disparities when planning the transition of care. These health disparities all influence the chronically ill patient's access to primary care, ability to follow a prescribed care plan, and make these patients more likely to experience AEs. Acknowledging a patient's health beliefs and incorporating those beliefs into the care plan are elements of cultural competent care and an important part of successful transitional care planning.

Several models of care proposed over the past decade were designed to avoid hospital readmission. Most include a pre-discharge interview with a nurse or social worker, a home visit within 72 hours, and periodic home visits and phone calls to monitor medications and functional status. Basic primary care services delivered at home as well as restorative services such as physical, occupational, and speech therapy can be features of a successful transition model. House call programs, parish nurses, and community nurses are becoming more popular as communities look for better ways to care for homebound residents. Assisting patients to navigate the complex medical system reduces confusion and likely improves compliance with the medical plan, hopefully resulting in fewer health crises and hospital admissions.

Concerns about patient safety mandate improved health literacy assessment, uncomplicated medication instructions, and safer transitions for patients from hospital to home. Improved medication reconciliation and more expedient follow-up after hospitalizations may promote successful transitions.

CARE OF THE PATIENT WITH END OF LIFE ISSUES

As the population ages, the number of people dealing chronic health problems is rapidly rising. Chronic and eventually terminal health issues such as heart disease, cancer, chronic respiratory disease, and dementia can have prolonged courses with a gradual decline and long periods of disability. These patients can benefit from palliative care in collaboration with regular medical care.

Palliative care is defined as patient- and family-centered care that optimizes quality of life by anticipating, preventing, and treating suffering. Palliative care throughout the continuum of illness involves addressing physical, intellectual, emotional, social, and spiritual needs and facilitating patient autonomy, access to information, and choice. Patients with chronic medical conditions such as heart disease, cancer, stroke, diabetes, renal disease, and Alzheimer disease can be treated with palliative care. Research has shown that patients who received early palliative care had less depression, better quality of life, and increased survival time (see Chapter 14 for an in-depth discussion of Palliative Care and End of Life discussions).

The care of the chronically ill patient is complex, time consuming, and expensive. It requires the coordination of multiple providers, health care systems, and reimbursement systems. This care is constantly challenged by the high cost of care and medications, lack of public transportation to office visits, unstable living situations, food insecurity, poor communication between health care providers, and myriad other social issues without clear solutions. As the population of the United States continues to age, there will continue to be an increase in the number of patients with complex medical conditions who need these services making the need for universally applied models imperative.

REFERENCES

1. Martyn, H., & Davis, K. (2014). Care coordination for people with complex care needs in the U.S.: A policy analysis. *International Journal of Care Coordination*, 17(3–4), 93–98. doi:10.1177/2053434514559721.
2. Mitchell, F. M. (2015). Racial and ethnic health disparities in an era of health care reform. *Health & Social Work*, 40(3), e66–e74. doi:10.1093/hsw/hlv038.
3. Center for Disease Control and Prevention. (2018). Chronic Disease Overview. Retrieved July 12, 2018 from https://www.cdc.gov/chronicdisease/overview/index.htm.
4. Scholz, J., & Minaudo, J. (2015). Registered nurse care coordination: Creating a preferred future for older adults with multimorbidity. *Online Journal of Issues in Nursing*, 20(3), 4. doi:10.3912/OJIN.Vol20No03Man04.
5. Barr, V., Robinson, S., Marin-Link, B., Underhill, L., Dotts, A., Ravensdale, D., et al. (2003). The expanded Chronic Care Model: An integration of concepts and strategies from population health promotion and the Chronic Care Model. *Hospital Quarterly*, 7(1), 73–82.
6. Berwick, D., Nolan, T., & Whittington, J. (2008). The triple aim: Care, health and cost. *Health Affairs*, 27(3).
7. Gee, P., Greenwood, D., Paterniti, D., et al. (2015). The health enhanced chronic care model: A theory derivation approach. *Journal of Medical Internet Research*, 17(4), e86.
8. Darkins, A. Telehealth services in the United States Department of Veterans Affairs (VA). https://myvitalz.com/wp-content/uploads/2016/07/telehealth-services-in-the-united-staates.pdf. (Accessed 11 July 2018).
9. Kennedy, M. (2013). Community based health plans take the (complex) path to integrated care. *Generations (San Francisco, Calif.)*, 37(2), 30–32.
10. Samuels, C., et al. (2017). The case for the use of nurse practitioners in the care of children with medical complexity. *Children (Basel)*, 4(4), 24. doi:10.3390/children4040024. EBSCOhost.
11. Berry, J., Hall, M., Neff, J., Goodman, D., et al. (2014). Children with medical complexity and Medicaid: Spending and cost savings. *Health Affairs*, 33(12).
12. Cady, R. G., Kelly, A. M., Finkelstein, S. M., Looman, W. S., & Garwick, A. W. (2014). Attributes of advanced practice registered nurse care coordination for children with medical complexity. *Journal of Pediatric Health Care*, 28(4), 305–312. doi:10.1016/j.pedhc.2013.06.005.
13. Verhaegh, K. J., MacNeal, V., Roomen, J. L., Eslame, S., et al. (2014). Transitional care intervention prevents hospital readmissions for adults with chronic illness. *Health Affairs (Project Hope)*, 33(9), 1531–1539.
14. Hirschman, K., Shaid, E., McCauley, K., Pauly, M., & Naylor, M. (2015). Continuity of care: The transitional care model. *OJIN: The Online Journal of Issues in Nursing*, 20(3), 1.
15. Coleman, E. A., Mahoney, E., & Parry, C. (2005). Assessing the quality of preparation for posthospital care from the patient's perspective: The care transitions measure. *Medical Care*, 43(3), 246.
16. Pavon, J. M., Zhao, Y., McConnell, E., & Hastings, S. N. (2014). Identifying risk of readmission in hospitalized elderly adults through in-patient medication exposure. *Journal of the American Geriatrics Society*, 62(6), 1116–1121.
17. Forster, A. J., Murff, H. J., Peterson, J. F., Gandhi, T. K., & Bates, D. W. (2005). Adverse drug events occurring following hospital discharge. *Journal of General Internal Medicine*, 20(4), 317–323. doi:10.1111/j.1525-1497.2005.30390.x.
18. Healthy People. (2020). [Internet]. Washington, DC: U.S. Department of Health and Human Services, Office of Disease Prevention and Health Promotion [cited [02/26/2018]]. Retrieved from https://www.healthypeople.gov/2020/topics-objectives/topic/social-determinants-of-health. (Accessed 10 July 2018).

CHAPTER **5**

AN INTRODUCTION TO HEALTH CARE DISPARITIES AND CULTURALLY RESPONSIVE PRIMARY CARE

Catherine Gaines Ling

The Quadruple Aim is a framework for improving health at a systems level. The four areas of focus are: improving population health, decreasing cost of care, improving patient experience, and attending to the health and well-being of the care team.[1] Social factors or determinants of health have a significant impact on all of these areas and are an increasingly critical part of primary care delivery. Social determinants of health include race, socioeconomic status, gender, education, occupation, and sexual orientation.[2] These factors are integral to delivery of holistic, quality, and safe care. Failure to integrate or acknowledge factors that affect health care behaviors and health care decisions creates a significant cost, both for the individual and for society as a whole. At its core, caring for another human being involves communication. For that communication to be health promoting, health literacy and an understanding and awareness of disparities and culturally relevant care delivery are essential for health care providers. This chapter provides an introduction to the topics

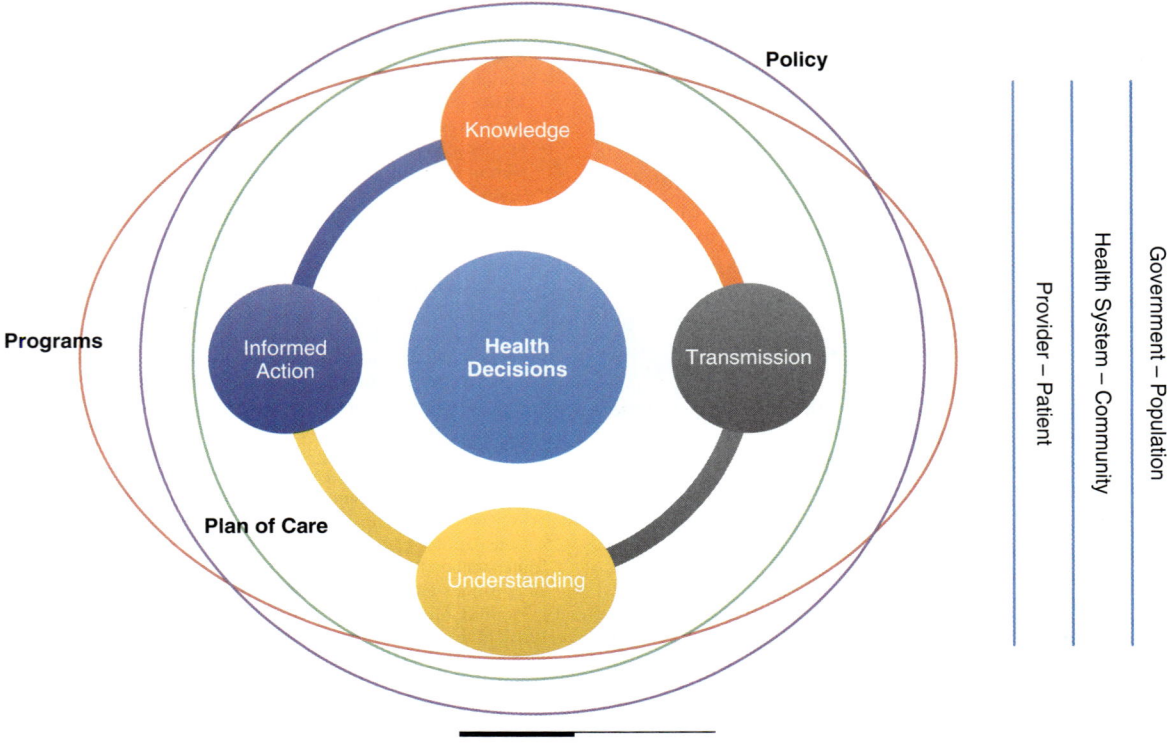

FIG. 5.1 Health literacy.

of health care literacy, health care disparities, and culturally responsive care.

HEALTH LITERACY

Health literacy is a person's capacity to find, discuss, and comprehend health information and health systems and also to be able to use that knowledge to make informed decisions about all aspects of his or her health.[3–5] That ability to make informed decisions is critical for health promotion and self-monitoring. These are key skills for managing chronic diseases like diabetes and hypertension. There are several factors (knowledge, transmission, understanding, and informed action) that interact to inform health decisions that are the core of all aspects of care from the individual to the societal level (Fig. 5.1).[3–9]

Healthy People 2020 is the blueprint for the United States to achieve aspects of the Quadruple Aim. This blueprint has three objectives focused on improving health literacy.[10] These objectives state that delivery systems, organizations, and providers need to:

1. Increase the proportion of persons who report that their health care provider always gave them easy-to-understand instructions about what to do to take care of their illness or health condition.
2. Increase the proportion of persons who report that their health care provider always asked them to describe how they will follow the instructions.
3. Increase the proportion of persons who report that their health care providers' office always offered help in filling out a form.[10]

The most recent estimate of financial costs of inadequate health literacy is $106 to $238 billion annually.[11] The Health Literacy of America's Adults report from the National Assessment of Adult Literacy survey (NAAL) stated that only 12% of

BOX 5.1

Risks Associated With Low Health Literacy

Delays in accessing care
Higher emergency department use
Higher hospitalization and re-hospitalization rates
Limited knowledge about personal health conditions
Limited self-management
Limited use of preventive health measures, including screenings and immunizations
Misunderstanding of follow-up recommendations
Misunderstanding of treatment options and medications
Misunderstood forms
Poor/limited or no follow-up care

Americans had a proficient level of health literacy, with 53% having an intermediate level.[12] This leaves approximately 88 million Americans with a basic or below-basic level of health literacy. Factors associated with high health literacy included being female, having an education beyond high school, and speaking primarily English, whereas low health literacy was associated with belonging to a minority, living in poverty, and being older than age 65.[12,13]

HEALTH LITERACY AND HEALTH CARE OUTCOMES

Individuals with low health literacy are at risk for myriad poor health outcomes that impose increased fiscal and societal costs (Box 5.1).[14–17] These poor outcomes start in childhood. Children with parents who have low health literacy are more prone to be seen in the emergency department, have increased severity of conditions (e.g., asthma), and are less likely to be fully immunized.[16,18-20] Adolescents have not been as thoroughly studied as some other populations, but it stands to reason that this dynamic stage in life presents an opportunity to improve health literacy. It is posited that poor health literacy contributes to increased mortality, as noted in suicide and untreated depression.[21,22] During adulthood, low health literacy is related to inadequately treated conditions (e.g., hypertension, influenza, HIV, heart failure, and mental health issues), which, in turn, lead to increased morbidity.[14,15,23-25] Systematic reviews found that low health literacy is associated with increased emergency department use and hospitalizations, inappropriate use of medications, misunderstanding of follow-up instructions, and decreased use of preventative services such as mammograms.[14,15] Older adults are particularly vulnerable to poor health outcomes related to low health literacy and have a higher risk of all-cause mortality even when lower cognition is not a consideration.[14]

HEALTH LITERACY—FROM MODEL TO ACTIONABLE COMPONENTS

Health literacy does not refer solely to the general ability to read and write. However, those with low general literacy rates will often have low health literacy rates. Knowledge refers to the baseline understanding of how the body and disease processes work. While this ability to understand physiology and pathology are facets of health literacy, even patients who are highly literate and educated can have low health literacy. Transmission and understanding refer to the delivery and receipt of key pieces of information. These data can be given verbally (requires adequate hearing and language comprehension), in written format (requires adequate eyesight and reading comprehension, including numeracy), or via technology (requires ability to use and understand technology). Successful understanding leads to informed action, often defined by providers as self-management.[7,24] For more information, see Chapter 6. Identifying strategies for improving communication with patients can have a positive impact on health outcomes.

Strategies to Improve Oral Communication

Oral communication (sending and receiving) is the cornerstone of health care delivery. Conversations with patients with low literacy can be affected by four different qualities: (1) use of medical terminology, (2) complex speech content, (3) abstract context, and (4) dense, rapid discussion.[6,26,27] Providers need to use plain speech and avoid cramming multiple abstract and complex concepts into a fast-paced discussion. Additionally, they need to check with the patient and see what message was received. One method for accomplishing this is known as teach-back.[28,29] Teach-back will be discussed in more detail in a subsequent section.

Strategies to Improve Written Communication

Every handout, prescription, or written referral is provided with the assumption of a certain level of patient reading comprehension. The average American has an eighth-grade reading level; however, the suggested reading level for health information is fifth grade.[30] There are several tools for determining the reading level expectation of written material. Two that are integrated into Microsoft Word are the Flesch Reading Ease test and the Flesch Kincaid Reading Ease level. The Centers for Medicare

and Medicaid Services has an 11-part toolkit for gauging the reading comprehension level of a provider's written materials, along with tools and tips to clarify those materials and make them more user-friendly for patients (www.cms.gov/Outreach-and-Education/Outreach/WrittenMaterialsToolkit).

Strategies to Improve Communication Using Technology

Electronic health or eHealth materials that have successfully reached individuals with low health literacy through a number of different platforms include audio files, videos, and voiceover slides, along with read-only materials and non–internet-dependent DVDs.[31] It is critical to gauge the patient's technologic literacy as a component of their health care literacy in using the various technology programs and platforms as electronic health records, self-monitoring applications, and communication via smart phones and computers become more integrated into health care delivery.[7,32,33] Health care providers should inquire about patients' familiarity with using the various technology programs and platforms utilized by their practices.

INTRODUCTION TO HEALTH LITERACY ASSESSMENT

The first step in addressing the needs of low–health-literacy patients is to do an assessment. Although there are a variety of tools for gauging health literacy, there are four that are readily translatable into primary care settings: (1) the Patient Education Materials Assessment Tool (PEMAT),[34,35] (2) Rapid Estimate of Adult Literacy in Medicine–Short Form (REALM-SF)[36]; (3) Ask Me 3[37]; and the (4) Newest Vital Sign[38-40] or ice cream label assessment (see Chapter 6).

An Overview of Health Literacy Interventions

It is not only patients and materials that need to be assessed for health literacy. Providers need to develop the awareness, knowledge, and interventions to effectively meet the needs of patients with less-than-optimal health literacy. Patients should be routinely assessed for health literacy levels using one of the methods listed previously. Previous research has found that using images and symbols and decreasing the overall amount of text broaden the health literacy scope of materials.[41] Teach-back is another patient-centered intervention. This method involves asking a patient to verbally relate their understanding of a plan, instructions, or a routine.[29]

In addition, use of native language materials, disease- or condition-specific information, and print-only alternate formats (like podcasts, videos, or infographics) can help address information needs of patients with low health literacy.[4,33,42,43] Box 5.2 provides measures to reduce the impact of health literacy. For further information, see Chapter 6.

Organization-Centered Interventions

Organizations should systematically review materials and navigation procedures to gauge the health literacy expectation of users and then involve employees and community members in planning, implementing, and evaluating steps to address health literacy needs.[44] The Centers for Disease Control and Prevention provides health literacy toolkits emphasizing the use of plain language in all written, audio, video, and virtual materials; these toolkits can be found by accessing www.cdc.gov/healthliteracy. The Ask Me 3 website (www.npsf.org/?page=askme3) offers

BOX **5.2**

Measures to Reduce Health Literacy Impact

1. Routinely assess patients for health literacy level.
2. Routinely assess providers for communication skills.
3. Use the teach-back method in patient interactions.
4. Provide written patient education materials at reading level appropriate for every patient.
5. Use pictographs and symbols to convey information in patient education materials.
6. Minimize the use of text in written materials.
7. Provide alternative formats of information (e.g., audio, video).

helpful resources for providers and ideas for making primary care settings more user-friendly for patients with lower health literacy (see Chapter 6).

HEALTH CARE DISPARITIES

Along with health literacy, disparities in care are a key social determinant impacting health outcomes. Disparities occur when one group has barriers to the standard of care and poorer health outcomes than another group.[43] The inability to access high-quality and timely care results in increased morbidity and mortality. The direct cost of health care disparities is estimated to be over $229 million.[8] Specific populations are particularly vulnerable to disparities in accessing adequate care and resources. Patients with decreased mobility, those in lower socioeconomic strata, and minorities face existing or worsening health care disparities.[43] These care inequities also impact lesbian, gay, bisexual, and transgendered individuals and are found to be more prevalent in certain zip codes and geographic regions.[43,45–47] The Office of the Surgeon General, the Department of Health and Human Services Office of Minority Health, National Partnership for Action to End Health Disparities, and the Centers for Disease Control and Prevention are a few of the federal agencies involved in addressing health care disparities.

Although disparities in health care would seem to be a system- or organizational-level concern, it is incumbent on health care providers to know who the vulnerable populations are in their communities, identify the disparities those patients face, and implement programs to address those disparities. Examples include a traditional foods project for diabetes prevention in partnership with indigenous tribes and a community-based asthma exacerbation and prevention project.[43,48] The initial efforts providers make to address disparities start through self-examination for personal biases. This is essential because unintended or implicit biases in a health care professional affect clinical decision-making.[49,50]

AN OVERVIEW OF CULTURALLY RESPONSIVE CARE

Like disparities and health literacy, an individual's cultural context determines how, when, and to what degree he or she will seek care and what interventions are considered acceptable. Cultural context determines what is considered to be health, what are normative treatments, and what is illness behavior. Providers must provide culturally responsive care in patient-centered environments, maximizing communication and minimizing bias.

OBLIGATIONS IN CULTURALLY RESPONSIVE PRIMARY CARE

Address Cultural Variations Among Diverse Patient Groups

With increases in globalization and increasing access to health care services, the diversity of patient populations in the United States has increased. Health care professionals might not be familiar with all the cultural views represented in a practice; however, this knowledge is essential to provide high-quality care. In a patient-centered environment, health care professionals inquire about beliefs regarding health, illness, and treatment; are responsive to individual preferences; and work with patients and their families to devise treatment plans that are acceptable and actionable and therefore have an increased likelihood of adherence.[51]

Create a Patient-Centered Environment

Clinicians must always ask and not assume a patient's cultural, racial, ethnic, or gender context. A discussion of health concerns should include the patient's perspective because that perspective factors greatly into the approach to and success of the treatment plan. That plan should be negotiated within the framework of the patient's worldview. Culturally responsive patient-centered environments seek a culturally relevant understanding of health from the patient and other sources.[52] The resources available from the AHRQ give a road map to assessing and developing culturally competent care (https://www.ahrq.gov/cahps/quality-improvement/improvement-guide/6-strategies-for-improving/communication/strategy6kcultural competence.html).

Minimize Clinician Bias

The personal views and professional and personal experiences of health care providers can also create bias and impede culturally responsive care. Recognition of bias begins in training through self-reflection, observed clinical encounters, and simulation (see Chapter 6).[50]

Overcome Patient Barriers: Language Environment

Increasingly, health care providers deliver care to culturally diverse populations of individuals who are not native English language speakers. Only approved, professional interpreters experienced in health care interpretation should be allowed to interpret for patients. Family members or friends should *not* be used as interpreters. Use of family members or friends may create misinterpretation or misunderstanding between the clinician and the patient. Family members may not understand medical terms or may interpret only what they feel is important, or patients might feel uncomfortable divulging personal information to the person interpreting.

Every effort should be made to use a certified, professional interpreter, with bilingual staff members used as interpreters only in emergency situations. When interacting with a patient through an interpreter, clinicians should still speak directly to the patient and refrain from discussing the patient in the third person with the interpreter. The patient should feel that the clinician is directly interacting with him or her and not with the interpreter. Pausing every two or three sentences, especially in discussing or describing complex diseases or treatments, will ensure that the interpreter is able to correctly interpret all of the information discussed with the patient. Disease information, brochures, and consent for treatment and procedures should be printed in the patient's language. Federal law regarding Medicaid and Medicare federally funded programs mandates access to linguistic services. Certified translation services are available by phone 24 hours a day from multiple vendors.

CONCLUSION

In today's changing and challenging health care environment, primary care providers are called to improve health care literacy, reduce health care disparities, and deliver care to culturally diverse populations. This challenge is accomplished by assessing and improving health care literacy, delivering culturally responsive primary care, and addressing disparities. Key components of culturally responsive primary care include addressing cultural variations among diverse patient groups, creating patient-centered friendly environments, recognizing clinician bias, and overcoming patient language and social barriers.

REFERENCES

1. Bodenheimer, T., & Sinsky, C. (2014). From triple to quadruple aim: Care of the patient requires care of the provider. *Annals of Family Medicine, 12,* 573–576.
2. Braveman, P., Egerter, S., & Williams, D. R. (2011). The social determinants of health: Coming of age. *Annual Review of Public Health, 32,* 381–398.
3. Hernandez, L. M., & Institute of Medicine (U.S.). (2013). *Health literacy: Improving health, health systems, and health policy around the world: workshop summary.* National Academies Press.
4. US Department of Health and Human Services Office of Disease Prevention and Health Promotion. (2010). *National action plan to improve health literacy.* Department of Health and Human Services.
5. Sørensen, K., et al. (2012). Health literacy and public health: A systematic review and integration of definitions and models. *BMC Public Health, 12,* 80.
6. Harrington, K. F., & Valerio, M. A. (2014). A conceptual model of verbal exchange health literacy. *Patient Education and Counseling, 94,* 403–410.
7. Suri, V. R., Majid, S., Chang, Y.-K., & Foo, S. (2016). Assessing the influence of health literacy on health information behaviors: A multi-domain skills-based approach. *Patient Education and Counseling, 99,* 1038–1045.
8. US Department of Health and Human Services Office of Disease Prevention and Health Promotion. (2013). CDC Health disparities and inequities report 2013. *MMWR. Morbidity and Mortality Weekly Report, Supplement 62.*
9. Anderson, R. M., & Funnell, M. M. (2010). Patient empowerment: Myths and misconceptions. *Patient Education and Counseling, 79,* 277–282.
10. HealthPeople.gov. (2017). Healthy people 2020. Social Determinants of Health.
11. Vernon, J. A., Trujillo, A., Rosenbaum, S., & DeBuona, B. (2007). *Low health literacy: Implications for national health policy.* George Washington University.
12. Kutner, M., Greenberg, E., Jin, Y., & Paulsen, C. (2006). *The health literacy of America's Adults: Results from the 2003 National Assessment of Adult Literacy.* Department of Education.
13. Johnson, J. L., Moser, L., & Garwood, C. L. (2013). Health literacy: A primer for pharmacists. *American Journal of Health-System Pharmacy: AJHP: Official Journal of the American Society of Health-System Pharmacists, 70,* 949–955.
14. Berkman, N. D., Sheridan, S. L., Donahue, K. E., Halpern, D. J., & Crotty, K. (2011). Low health literacy and health outcomes: An updated systematic review. *Annals of Internal Medicine, 155,* 97–107.
15. Herndon, J. B., Chaney, M., & Carden, D. (2011). Health literacy and emergency department outcomes: A systematic review. *Annals of Emergency Medicine, 57,* 334–345.
16. DeWalt, D. A., & Hink, A. (2009). Health literacy and child health outcomes: A systematic review of the literature. *Pediatrics, 124,* S265–S274.
17. Ventura, H. O., & Piña, I. L. (2018). Health literacy: An important clinical tool in heart failure. *Mayo Clinic Proceedings. Mayo Clinic, 93,* 1–3.
18. Fry-Bowers, E. K., Maliski, S., Lewis, M. A., Macabasco-O'Connell, A., & DiMatteo, R. (2014). The association of health literacy, social support, self-efficacy and interpersonal interactions with health care providers in low-income Latina mothers. *Journal of Pediatric Nursing, 29,* 309–320.
19. Morrison, A. K., Myrvik, M. P., Brousseau, D. C., Hoffmann, R. G., & Stanley, R. M. (2013). The relationship between parent health literacy and pediatric emergency department utilization: A systematic review. *Academic Pediatrics, 13,* 421–429.
20. Perry, E. L., et al. (2017). Health literacy in adolescents with sickle cell disease. *Journal of Pediatric Nursing, 36,* 191–196.
21. Perry, E. L. (2014). Health literacy in adolescents: An integrative review: Health Literacy in Adolescents: An integrative review. *Journal for Specialists in Pediatric Nursing, 19,* 210–218.
22. Hart, S. R., et al. (2014). Achieving depression literacy: The adolescent depression knowledge questionnaire (ADKQ). *School Mental Health, 6,* 213–223.
23. Aboumatar, H. J., Carson, K. A., Beach, M. C., Roter, D. L., & Cooper, L. A. (2013). The impact of health literacy on desire for participation in healthcare, medical visit communication, and patient reported outcomes among patients with hypertension. *Journal of General Internal Medicine, 28,* 1469–1476.
24. Heijmans, M., Waverijn, G., Rademakers, J., van der Vaart, R., & Rijken, M. (2015). Functional, communicative and critical health literacy of chronic disease patients and their importance for self-management. *Patient Education and Counseling, 98,* 41–48.
25. Pellowski, J. A., Kalichman, S. C., & Grebler, T. (2016). Optimal treatment adherence counseling outcomes for people living with HIV and limited health literacy. *Behavioral Medicine (Washington, D.C.), 42,* 39–47.
26. Nouri, S. S., & Rudd, R. E. (2015). Health literacy in the 'oral exchange': An important element of patient–provider communication. *Patient Education and Counseling, 98,* 565–571.
27. Roter, D. L. (2011). Oral literacy demand of health care communication: Challenges and solutions. *Nursing Outlook, 59,* 79–84.
28. Green, J. A., Gonzaga, A. M., Cohen, E. D., & Spagnoletti, C. L. (2014). Addressing health literacy through clear health communication: A training program for internal medicine residents. *Patient Education and Counseling, 95,* 76–82.
29. Porter, K., et al. (2016). Using Teach-Back to understand participant behavioral Self-Monitoring skills across health literacy level and behavioral condition. *Journal of Nutrition Education and Behavior, 48,* 20–26.e1.
30. DuBay, W. (2013). Plain language at work newsletter: Know your readers.
31. Jacobs, R. J., Lou, J. Q., Ownby, R. L., & Caballero, J. (2014). A systematic review of eHealth interventions to improve health literacy. *Health Informatics Journal,* doi:10.1177/1460458214534092.
32. Neter, E., & Brainin, E. (2012). eHealth literacy: Extending the digital divide to the realm of health information. *Journal of Medical Internet Research, 13,* e19.
33. Agency for Healthcare Research and Quality. (2014). Health literacy measurement tools (revised): fact sheet.
34. Shoemaker, S. J., Wolf, M. S., & Brach, C. (2017). The Patient Education Materials Assessment Tool (PEMAT) and User's Guide: An Instrument To Assess the Understandability and Actionability of Print and Audiovisual Patient Education Materials.
35. Shoemaker, S. J., Wolf, M. S., & Brach, C. (2014). Development of the Patient Education Materials Assessment Tool (PEMAT): A new measure of understandability and actionability for print and audiovisual patient information. *Patient Education and Counseling, 96,* 395–403.
36. Arozullah, A. M., et al. (2007). Development and validation of a short-form, rapid estimate of adult literacy in medicine. *Medical Care, 45,* 1026–1033.
37. National Patient Safety Foundation. (2014). Ask Me 3.
38. Pfizer Inc. (2017). The newest vital sign: A health literacy assessment tool for patient care and research.
39. Weiss, B. D. (2005). Quick assessment of literacy in primary care: The newest vital sign. *Annals of Family Medicine, 3,* 514–522.
40. Shealy, K. M., & Threatt, T. B. (2016). Utilization of the Newest Vital Sign (NVS) in Practice in the United States. *Health Communication, 31,* 679–687.
41. Sheridan, S. L., et al. (2011). Interventions for individuals with low health literacy: A systematic review. *Journal of Health Communication, 16,* 30–54.
42. Boston University. Health literacy tool shed.
43. US Department of Health and Human Services Office of Disease Prevention and Health Promotion. (2014). Strategies for reducing health disparities—Selected CDC-Sponsored interventions, United States, 2014. *MMWR. Morbidity and Mortality Weekly Report, Supplement 63.*
44. Willis, C. D., et al. (2014). Improving organizational capacity to address health literacy in public health: A rapid realist review. *Public Health, 128,* 515–524.
45. Gonzales, G., & Blewett, L. A. (2013). Disparities in health insurance among children with same-sex parents. *Pediatrics, 132,* 703–711.
46. Gonzales, G., & Blewett, L. A. (2014). National and state-specific health insurance disparities for adults in same-sex relationships. *American Journal of Public Health, 104,* e95–e104.
47. Adler, N. E., et al. (2016). *Addressing social determinants of health and health disparities. Discussion paper, vital directions for health and health care series.* National Academy of Medicine.

48. Ayanian, J. Z., Landon, B. E., Newhouse, J. P., & Zaslavsky, A. M. (2014). Racial and ethnic disparities among enrollees in Medicare Advantage plans. *The New England Journal of Medicine, 371,* 2288–2297.

49. Chapman, E. N., Kaatz, A., & Carnes, M. (2013). Physicians and implicit bias: How doctors may unwittingly perpetuate health care disparities. *Journal of General Internal Medicine, 28,* 1504–1510.

50. Jernigan, V. B. B., Hearod, J. B., Tran, K., Norris, K. C., & Buchwald, D. (2016). An examination of cultural competence training in US medical education guided by the tool for assessing cultural competence training. *Journal of Health Disparities Research and Practice, 9,* 150–163.

51. Campinha-Bacote, J. (2011). Delivering patient-centered care in the midst of a cultural conflict: The role of cultural competence. *Online Journal of Issues in Nursing, 16.*

52. Douglas, M. K., et al. (2011). Standards of practice for culturally competent nursing care: 2011 update. *Journal of Transcultural Nursing, 22,* 317–333.

CHAPTER **6**

PATIENT/FAMILY EDUCATION AND HEALTH LITERACY

Jill M. Price

Part of primary care delivery involves educating patients and families on health promotion and disease prevention. Determining the readiness of a person's ability to learn is critical in the delivery of information and comprehension of knowledge.[1] If patients and families do not have a grasp of health literacy, then information taught by primary care providers is meaningless.[2] All health care providers need to assess the learning needs and health literacy levels of patients while delivering culturally responsive care as required by The Joint Commission (TJC).[3] The basic components of learning begin with the theoretical foundations of knowing or constructivism. Understanding constructivism and how primary care providers can use it as a foundation to educate patients and families is essential in increasing health literacy and delivery of holistic, culturally responsive care.

CONSTRUCTIVISM

Learning occurs at various stages of human development. Piaget (1972) claimed knowledge is constructed over time.[4] Constructivism focuses on getting people involved in their own learning through active learning, versus just teaching.[5] Primary care providers can provide patient and family education by keeping the learning focused on something relevant to the patient and/or family where new ideas or constructs can be built. Additionally, having patients and families take an active role in their own learning is critical to the paradigm shift toward being a proactive versus a reactive health care consumer.[2] Patients and families should also be health literate in order to play an active role and make their own decisions in health promotion and disease prevention. Moreover, primary care providers need to be aware of how societal factors can influence health literacy.[6]

SOCIETAL FACTORS

Social determinants of health are individual and societal factors, including race, socioeconomic status, education, language, literacy, and culture.[7] Failure to integrate all factors that affect health care behaviors and health care decisions creates a significant cost, both for the individual and for society as a whole. Two specific social determinants of concern for providers are health literacy and culturally responsive care.

HEALTH LITERACY

Health literacy is the capacity of a person to find, discuss, and comprehend health information and the ability to use that knowledge to make informed decisions about all aspects of his or her health.[8-10] *Healthy People 2020* has a goal focused on improving health communication that addresses the need to "increase the proportion of the people who report that their health care providers always explain things so they can understand them."[7] Health care providers generally communicated with patients and families at a college level in terms of terminology, while most adults in the United States read at an eighth-grade level and some adults read at a lower level than that.[11] The Health Literacy of America's Adults report from the National Assessment of Adult Literacy survey (NAAL), last calculated in 2003, stated that only 12% of Americans had a proficient level of health literacy, with 45% having an intermediate level, 29% basic, and 14% below basic.[11] Factors associated with high health literacy included being female, having an education beyond high school, and speaking primarily English, whereas low health literacy was associated with belonging to an ethnic minority, living in poverty, and being older than age 65.[12,13]

HEALTH LITERACY COMPONENTS

Health literacy refers to the general ability to read and write basic health-related words and equate numbers to solve problems related to health care medical needs.[11] Furthermore, those with low general literacy rates will often have low health literacy rates. During the course of caring for a patient, key pieces of information are given verbally, in written format, and now via technology. These require adequate hearing and language comprehension, adequate eyesight and reading comprehension, including numeracy, and an ability to use and understand technology. Examining these components identifies strategies for improving communication with patients and can have a positive impact on health promotion and disease prevention.

Oral Communication

Oral communication (sending and receiving) is the cornerstone of health care delivery. In any interaction with patients and their family members, providers should understand first the role(s) of the family member(s) present in the interaction. Providers need to not only determine the readiness of patients and their family members to learn from a constructivist perspective but also use plain speech and avoid cramming multiple abstract and complex concepts into a fast-paced discussion. To increase health literacy in patients and their family members, educational material can be presented in various forms, including teach-back (asking the patient and/or his or her caregiver family member to repeat the information taught), readable pamphlets at a low readability index, and videotapes with transcripts.[14]

Reading Comprehension

Every handout, prescription, or written referral is provided to patients with the assumption of a certain level of patient reading comprehension. The average American has an eighth-grade reading level; the suggested reading level for health information is fifth grade.[15] However, some patients have an even lower reading level and require simpler written instructions. The Office of Disease Prevention and Health Promotion established a website, http://health.gov/healthliteracyonline, in 2015 to assist health care providers in the development of health websites and educational material (digital and written) that assists in enhanced health literacy.

Numeracy

Numeric literacy is the capacity to comprehend quantitative data in all forms and use it to make health care decisions.[16] Data forms range from statistical to epidemiologic to simple number use and include numeric data that is presented graphically.[17] From the patient perspective, numeric literacy can include telling time and knowing what time they need to take their medication or even self-administer insulin. When delivering health care education to a patient and/or his or her caregiver family member, gauging his or her interpretation of numeric data is a key component in individually tailoring digital, oral, and written communication to their health literacy needs.

Technology

Educational materials are now often delivered electronically and involve literacy expectations that transcend reading comprehension. The patient and/or his or her caregiver family member must know how to use technology devices by taking an active role in learning and navigating through virtual materials.

Electronic health or eHealth materials that have successfully affected individuals with low health literacy through a number of different platforms include audio files, videos, and voice-over slides, along with read-only materials and non–Internet-dependent DVDs.[18] It will become more and more critical to gauge the patient's and/or his or her caregiver family member's technologic literacy as electronic health records and communication via smart phones and computers become more integrated into health care delivery.[19]

HEALTH LITERACY ASSESSMENT

A health literacy assessment is the first step in addressing the needs of low–health-literacy patients. Although there are a variety of tools for gauging health literacy, there are three that are readily translatable into primary care settings. These include the Rapid Estimate of Adult Literacy in Medicine–Short Form (REALM-SF); Ask Me 3; and the Newest Vital Sign or ice cream label assessment.

REALM-SF

The REALM-SF is a seven-item instrument that has been validated and used with a variety of populations.[11] It is easy and fast to administer; a drawback is that it looks only at medical word recognition—not comprehension or numeracy. The full instrument and instructions on how to administer it is available on the Agency for Healthcare Research and Quality (AHRQ) website (https://www.ahrq.gov/professionals/quality-patient-safety/quality-resources/tools/literacy-toolkit/index.html).

Ask Me 3

Another tool, Ask Me 3, encourages patients and/or their caregiver family members to ask health care providers three primary questions to enhance patient-provider communication:

1. What is my main problem?
2. What do I need to do?
3. Why is it important for me to do this?

This simple yet effective framework helps patients and caregivers initiate communication with the health care provider about health concerns. These are great prompts to start dialogue but do not help gauge the health literacy of the patient and/or his or her caregiver family member—that is, his or her understanding of the answers that providers will give to those questions.

Newest Vital Sign

The Newest Vital Sign instrument, distributed by Pfizer, is also known as the ice cream label test.[20] A patient and/or his or her caregiver family member are asked to look at the nutrition label from a container of ice cream and answer six questions. These questions include numeracy skills (calculating the number of calories in the container) and general knowledge (should a patient who is allergic to peanuts eat this ice cream?). The toolkit containing the instrument and administration and scoring instructions is available on the Pfizer website https://www.pfizer.com/health/literacy/public-policy-researchers/nvs-toolkit.

HEALTH LITERACY INTERVENTIONS
Patient-Centered Interventions

To meet the needs of patients and/or their caregiver family members with less-than-optimal health literacy, providers must develop the awareness, knowledge, and interventions required to address low or inadequate health literacy. Patients and/or their caregiver family members should be assessed for health literacy levels. Research has found the use of alternate formats to print (podcasts, videos, tables) can help address information needs of patients and/or their caregiver family members with low health literacy.[9] Box 6.1 provides measures to reduce health literacy impact.

Provider and Organizational Interventions

It is not the job of the provider alone to do the work of reducing low health literacy's barrier to optimal care. Health care organizations should review materials and navigation procedures to assess the health literacy expectation of users. Then employees and community members should be involved in planning, implementing, and evaluating steps to address health literacy needs.[21] The Centers for Disease Control and Prevention provides health literacy toolkits emphasizing the use of plain language in all written, audio, video, and virtual materials; these

---

BOX **6.1**

Measures to Reduce Health Literacy Impact

1. Assess patients and/or their caregiver family members for health literacy level.
2. Provide written patient education materials at reading level appropriate for every patient and/or their caregiver family member.
3. Use pictographs and symbols to convey information in patient education materials.
4. Minimize the use of text in written materials.
5. Provide alternative formats of information (e.g., audio, video).

Health Literacy Resources

Agency for Healthcare Research and Quality's Health Literacy Universal Precautions Toolkit provides a plethora of resources for improving health literacy communication. Available at: www.ahrq .gov/professionals/quality-patient-safety/quality-resources/tools/ literacy-toolkit/index.html.

Centers for Disease Control and Prevention's Health Literacy website provides tools and information for providers and organizations. Available at: www.cdc.gov/healthliteracy.

Institute of Medicine: Roundtable on Health Literacy (2014) provides updates on the latest discussions and reports from the Institute of Medicine examining health literacy. Available at: www.iom.edu/ Activities/PublicHealth/HealthLiteracy.aspx.

National Action Plan to Improve Health Literacy is an initiative from the Department of Health and Human Services to assist health care systems, organizations, and providers in reducing the barrier to care posed by health literacy issues. Available at: www.health.gov/ communication/hlactionplan/pdf/Health_Literacy_Action_Plan.pdf.

toolkits can be found at www.cdc.gov/healthliteracy. Box 6.2 has a list of some additional resources for individual providers and organizations.

CULTURALLY RESPONSIVE CARE

Like assessing health care learning and health literacy needs, cultural awareness is paramount in primary care providers delivering culturally responsive care. An individual's cultural context determines how, when, and to what degree he or she will seek care and what interventions are considered acceptable. Cultural context determines what is considered to be health, what are normative treatments, and what is illness behavior. Providers must provide culturally responsive care in patient-centered environments, maximizing communication and minimizing bias.

Create a Patient-Centered Environment

Primary care providers must always ask and not assume a patient's cultural, racial, ethnic, or gender context. A discussion of health concerns should include the patient's perspective because that perspective factors greatly into the approach to and success of the treatment plan. That plan should be negotiated within the framework of the patient's worldview. Culturally responsive patient-centered environments seek a culturally relevant understanding of health from the patient and other sources.[22]

Minimize Clinician Bias

The personal views and professional and personal experiences of health care providers can also create bias and impede culturally responsive care. Provider bias (e.g., regarding race, ethnicity, size, socioeconomic class, gender, age, physical disabilities, and sexual orientation) can be an unconscious influence on a provider's plan of care. Primary care providers need to recognize and address personal bias. Patient care decisions should be evidence-based, individualized, and not based on supposition or assumption. Available treatment options should also

be openly discussed with patients and/or their caregiver family members. Primary care providers may share a preferred treatment, but they need to decipher if this is a personal preference or if the treatment decision is based on evidence-based practice principles.

Overcome Patient Barriers: Language Environment

Increasingly, primary care providers deliver care to culturally diverse populations of individuals who are not native language speakers. Only approved, professional interpreters experienced in health care interpretation are appropriate interpreters for patients. Family members or friends should *not* be used as interpreters. Use of family members or friends may create misinterpretation or misunderstanding between the provider and the patient. Family members may not understand medical terms or may interpret only what they feel is important, or patients might feel uncomfortable divulging personal information to the person interpreting.

Every effort should be made to use a certified, professional interpreter, with bilingual staff members used as interpreters only in emergencies. Disease information, brochures, and consent for treatment and procedures should be printed in the patient's language.[11] Federal law regarding Medicaid and Medicare federally funded programs mandates access to linguistic services. Certified translation services are available by phone 24 hours a day from multiple vendors.

CONCLUSION

In today's challenging health care environment, primary care providers are called to educate patients and families on health promotion and disease prevention, improve health care literacy, and deliver holistic care to culturally diverse populations. This challenge is mastered by educating patients and families using a constructivist active learning approach; using tools to improve digital, oral, and written health care literacy; and delivering culturally responsive primary care. Moreover, the ultimate goal of increased health promotion and decreased disease prevention can be accomplished.

REFERENCES

1. Merriam, S. B., & Bierema, L. L. (2013). *Adult learning: Linking theory and practice.* Somerset, MA: John Wiley & Sons.
2. Truccolo, I. (2016). Providing patient information and education in practice: The role of the health librarian. *Health Information and Libraries Journal* [serial online], 33(2), 161–166. Available from: MEDLINE Complete, Ipswich, MA. (Accessed December 16, 2017).
3. The Joint Commission. (2017). Facts about patient-centered communications. Oakbrook, IL: Joint Commission Resources, Inc. Available from: https:// www.jointcommission.org/facts_about_patient-centered_communications/. (Accessed December 16, 2017).
4. Piaget, J. (1972). *The principles of genetic epistemology.* New York, NY: Routledge & Kegan Paul.
5. Billings, D. M., & Halstead, J. A. (2015). *Teaching in nursing: A guide for faculty* (5th ed.). St. Louis, MO: Elsevier Saunders.
6. Pétré, B., Gagnayre, R., De Andrade, V., Ziegler, O., & Guillaume, M. (2017). From therapeutic patient education principles to educative attitude: The perceptions of health care professionals—a pragmatic approach for defining competencies and resources. *Patient Preference and Adherence, 11,* 603–617. [serial online]. 2017;603. Available from: Directory of Open Access Journals, Ipswich, MA. (Accessed December 17, 2017).
7. HealthyPeople.gov. Healthy People 2020. Soc. Determinants Health 2015. Retrieved from www.healthypeople.gov/2020/topics-objectives/topic/social -determinants-health. (Accessed December 16, 2017).
8. Hernandez, L. M., Institute of Medicine (U.S.). (2013). *Health literacy: Improving health, health systems, and health policy around the world: Workshop summary.* Washington, DC: National Academies Press.

9. U.S. Department of Health and Human Services Office of Disease Prevention and Health Promotion. (2010). *National action plan to improve health literacy.* Washington, DC: Department of Health and Human Services.

10. Sørensen, K., Van den Broucke, S., Fullam, J., Doyle, G., Pelikan, J., Slonska, Z., et al. (2012). Health literacy and public health: A systematic review and integration of definitions and models. *BMC Public Health, 12*(1), 80.

11. Engelke, Z. (2016). Patient Education: Caring for Patients with Low Health Literacy. CINAHL Nursing Guide [serial online]. July 1. Available from: Nursing Reference Center Plus, Ipswich, MA. (Accessed December 17, 2017).

12. Kutner, M., Greenberg, E., Jin, Y., & Paulsen, C. (2006). *The health literacy of America's adults: Results from the 2003 National Assessment of Adult Literacy.* Washington, DC: Department of Education.

13. Johnson, J. L., Moser, L., & Garwood, C. L. (2013). Health literacy: A primer for pharmacists. *American Journal of Health-System Pharmacy, 70*(11), 949–955.

14. Veenker, H., & Paans, W. (2016). A dynamic approach to communication in health literacy education. *BMC Medical Education* [serial online], *16*(1), 280. Available from: MEDLINE Complete, Ipswich, MA. (Accessed December 18, 2017).

15 DuBay, W. (2013). Plain language at work newsletter: Know your readers. Retrieved from www.impact-information.com/impactinfo/literacy.htm. (Accessed December 16, 2017).

16. Ferme, E. (2014). What can other areas teach us about numeracy? *The Australian Mathematics Teacher* [serial online], *70*(4), 28–34. Available from: ERIC, Ipswich, MA. (Accessed December 18, 2017).

17. Rodríguez, V., Andrade, A. D., García-Retamero, R., Anam, R., Rodríguez, R., Lisigurski, M., et al. (2013). Health literacy, numeracy, and graphical literacy among veterans in primary care and their effect on shared decision making and trust in physicians. *Journal of Health Communication, 18*(Suppl. 1), 273–289.

18. Jacobs, R. J., Lou, J. Q., Ownby, R. L., & Caballero, J. (2016). A systematic review of eHealth interventions to improve health literacy. *Health Informatics Journal, 22*(2), 81–98.

19. Neter, E., & Brainin, E. (2012). eHealth literacy: Extending the digital divide to the realm of health information. *Journal of Medical Internet Research, 13*(1), e19.

20. Pfizer. (2015). The Newest Vital Sign: a health literacy assessment tool for patient care and research. Retrieved from www.pfizer.com/health/literacy/public_policy_researchers/nvs_toolkit. (Accessed December 16, 2017).

21. Willis, C. D., Saul, J. E., Bitz, J., Pompu, K., Best, A., & Jackson, B. (2014). Improving organizational capacity to address health literacy in public health: A rapid realist review. *Public Health, 128*(6), 515–524.

22. Schub, T., & Uribe, L. (2017). Health Literacy. *CINAHL Nursing Guide* [serial online]. June 9. Available from: Nursing Reference Center Plus, Ipswich, MA. (Accessed December 18, 2017).

CHAPTER **7**

GENETIC CONSIDERATIONS IN PRIMARY CARE

Ann H. Maradiegue • Diane C. Seibert • Karen J. Whitt

INTRODUCTION

Over the past 50 years, genetic science has expanded from a small, quiet scientific discipline into a key component in clinical medicine. The number of genomic tools, resources, and guidelines has exploded in the past decade and primary care providers are now expected to conduct genomic risk assessments, counsel patients; make referrals to appropriate specialists; select the correct diagnostic or genetic test; consider the ethical, legal, and social implications of genomic health care; and do it all in a primary care appointment. Many providers practicing today learned little about genetics and rarely encountered patients in which genetic concepts needed to be considered, but now genetic concepts should be woven into

each patient encounter. Providers working in primary care settings are perfectly positioned to provide genomic health care because they assess risk, implement prevention strategies, and manage disease.[1]

Several technological advances have made genetic health care possible: (1) the cost of genetic testing has plummeted as a result of expanding computing speed, increased data storage capability, and evolving gene sequencing technologies; (2) more is known about gene–gene and gene–environment relationships in single-gene (i.e., cystic fibrosis) and complex conditions (e.g., hypertension, diabetes); and (3) more is now known about how to treat genetic disorders. As sequencing costs continue to drop and knowledge expands, more and more people will be treated on the basis of their unique genetic risk, and truly personalized health care will become a reality.[2]

A Genomic Primer

The health/illness continuum includes genes, the environment (lifestyle, behaviors, exposures), and the interaction between genes and the environment. The term *genetics* refers to the influence of specific genes on particular conditions (i.e., single-gene disorders). The term *genomics*, coined in 1987,[3] describes the interaction of many genes and reflects the influence of the psychosocial, cultural, and physical environments in which humans live, and is more accurate when assessing an individual's risk for disease because humans interact in highly complex ways with one another and with their environments. A *genomic assessment* captures not only the evaluation of a particular genetic disorder, but also takes into account an individual's overall health.

Single-gene disorders (i.e., sickle cell anemia, Huntington disease) are often fairly well understood because their inheritance patterns are straightforward and symptoms can be traced back to a single genetic variation. Although single-gene disorders individually are rather rare, collectively they affect millions of Americans.[4] Complex conditions such as heart disease, behavioral health disorders (depression, anxiety, addictions), cancer, and diabetes develop as a result of interaction between multiple genes and the environment.[5] Understanding the genetics of single-gene and complex diseases is essential if patients and families are to be appropriately assessed for disease risk, diagnosed, managed, referred, and educated. Providers need to have a basic knowledge of genetic disorders, understand the risks and benefits of genetic testing, be able to counsel and refer patients and families, and design personalized management plans based on genetic information.

The terms *personalized* and *precision* medicine are both used in health care settings. *Personalized medicine* involves the use of genetic or genomic information to guide decision-making with regard to prevention, diagnosis, and treatment of disease.[6] Personalized medicine is already widely used in clinical settings, particularly in oncology (e.g., molecular tumor testing for breast and colon cancers) and in tailoring drug doses for individuals (pharmacogenomics). *Precision medicine* expands the concept of personalized medicine by including genomic, epigenomic, exposure, behavioral, and other data.[7,8] Epigenomics, a part of precision medicine, refers to the study of the process of modifications to cellular DNA that influence gene expression without alteration of the primary DNA sequence (e.g., methylation, histone modification).[9,10]

Genomic testing strategies (e.g., exome sequencing) that are faster, cheaper, and more accurate also have the potential to change health care delivery. The exome is the protein coding portion of the genome. Whole exome sequencing (WES) is currently being studied for use in clinical settings to uncover disease predisposition in newborns, though some clinical, ethical, and technical concerns have been raised about the implications inherent in possible findings.[11] WES may have other clinical uses in genetic or genomic diagnosis, disease treatment, screening, disease management, drug discovery, and prenatal diagnosis.[12,13] This is in contrast to most genetic testing in the past, which focused on a single-gene disorder and tested one gene at a time. Multigene panel tests are also currently available and can provide genetic sequencing for genes involved in more than one disease or syndrome. These panel tests are now being offered to individuals suspected to have hereditary breast, colon, or other cancer syndromes, or cardiomyopathy, and can simultaneously test many genes often associated with these specific disorders. This is a more cost-effective testing approach than stepwise testing, which evaluates one potential gene at a time.[14] Careful counseling should be done prior to multigene panel testing and WES, because this type of testing may identify unanticipated genetic conditions or variants of uncertain clinical significance, making clinical interpretation and management challenging.[14,15]

Many health care providers admit to feeling poorly prepared to provide genomic health care[16,17] because genomic content was not emphasized in their basic clinical preparation programs. As a result, providers may struggle to integrate medical findings with physical findings, the family medical history, cultural preferences, and the patient's and family's psychological readiness for genomic information.[16,17] Clinicians should be familiar with the benefits and limitations of genetic testing, understand testing options, facilitate referrals, communicate test results to patient and at-risk family members, formulate a plan for disclosure of additional or secondary findings, re-assess genomic data as new information becomes available, and counsel patients and families to help them make informed decisions.[18]

In 2012, the American Nurses Association (ANA) issued the "Essential genetic and genomic competencies for graduate nurses," which outlines the essential genomic competencies expected from nurses prepared at the graduate level. The document, established by a consensus panel, contains 38 competencies nested within 2 domains: Professional Practice (risk assessment and interpretation; genetic education, counseling, testing, and results interpretation; clinical management; ethical, legal, and social implications) and Professional Role (leadership; research).[19] A detailed discussion of genetic and genomic principles and disorders is beyond the scope of this chapter, but two key principles—risk assessment and family history collection—are discussed in this chapter in detail because they are the foundation for genomic health care. Two other important genomic issues are discussed, the 2008 passage of the Genetic Information Nondiscrimination Act (GINA) because it may affect the way genomic health care is perceived and/or delivered and direct-to-consumer (DTC) genetic testing because it has significant ethical, legal, and social implications.

If genomics is to take its rightful place in health care, clinicians must expand their view of health and disease. As the largest group of health professionals in the United States, nurse practitioners are on the front lines of health care and have the power to improve health care outcomes.

RISK ASSESSMENT

If optimal outcomes are to be achieved, clinicians must be prepared to assess and identify patients at increased risk for gene–gene and gene–environment interactions.[20,21] Analysis of a patient's risk for developing a disease, or *risk assessment*, is essential in health care. Broadly defined, risk assessment is a systematic process used to determine whether a potential hazard exists and/or to evaluate the extent of possible risk to human health, safety, or the environment. Risk assessment incorporates the nature, duration, intensity, and frequency of the hazard or exposure.[20-25] Risk assessment in health care is used in a variety of ways that includes potential environmental hazards or external factors. In assessing risk in a health care setting, genetic/genomic and biologic factors (e.g., age, race, ethnic background, ancestry, country of origin), individual behaviors (e.g., smoking, alcohol abuse), and environmental factors (e.g., radiation exposure, dietary preferences) must all be combined to accurately evaluate an individual's risk for developing a particular disease, disability, or behavior.[23-25] Health care risk assessment includes gathering data about the patient, his or her immediate and multigenerational family members, and their environmental exposures.[20,21] These data are then evaluated in the context of emerging research and epidemiologic studies to predict the likelihood that an adverse event or illness will occur.[22,24] Risk assessment therefore is a process used to assist clinicians in making a medical decision.[23,25] Assessment of risk may also involve the use of empirical and/or probability risk assessment models—tools that can provide valuable information in the form of a risk estimate because they compare an individual's risk with the population risk. Two commonly used empirical risk models are the Gail model,[26] used to calculate breast cancer risk, and the Framingham model,[27] used to predict heart disease. Other probability models—for example, BRCAPRO, the Breast and Ovarian Analysis of Disease Incidence and Carrier Estimation Algorithm (BOADICEA), and PENN II—are used in genetic specialty clinics by trained professionals to assess an individual's risk for having an inherited predisposition to a genetic condition such as breast and/or ovarian cancer.[28-30]

The overarching goal of risk assessment is to recognize disease early or identify asymptomatic individuals at increased risk so that appropriate preventative measures (e.g., chemoprevention, prophylactic medications), enhanced surveillance (e.g., more frequent mammograms for individuals at high risk for breast cancer), or risk-reduction surgery (e.g., bilateral mastectomy or oophorectomy for individuals at high risk for breast or ovarian cancer) can be initiated to improve health care outcomes. If an individual is suspected to be at high risk for a particular genetic condition, collaboration with another health professional is often indicated. For example, a genetic specialist (e.g., geneticist, genetic counselor, APN trained in genetics) should be consulted if the personal or family history is suspicious for an inherited cancer predisposition syndrome, such as that of hereditary breast and ovarian cancer (HBOC) syndrome. These specialists will often perform additional risk assessment and will gather and interpret personal and family histories, offer education about disease inheritance, discuss risks and benefits of genetic testing, discuss management and prevention strategies, and provide resources, information, and counseling.[20,21,25] Genetic counseling services are used to help both the individuals and their families understand and adapt

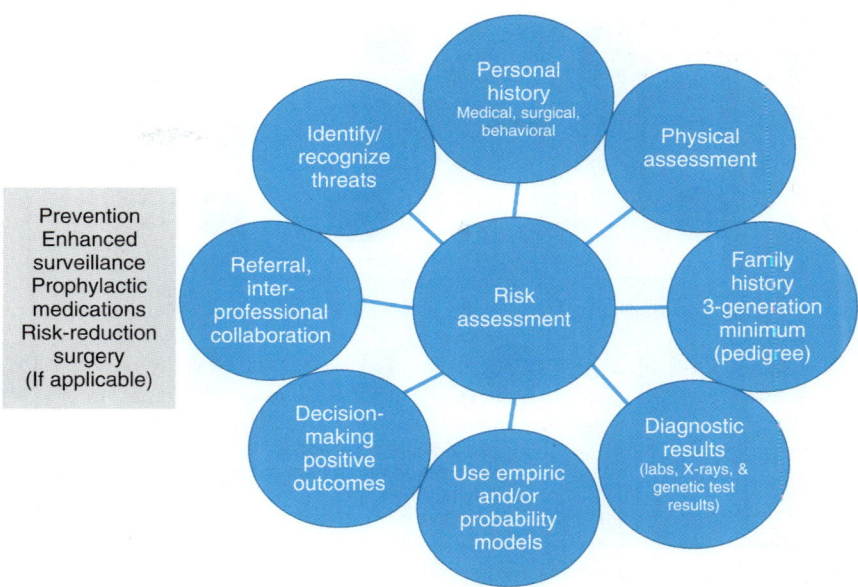

F I G . 7.1   Risk assessment model. Risk assessment model denoting important elements in the process of analyzing clients' disease risk, including factors associated with decision-making and need for interprofessional collaboration.

to the stressful medical, psychological, and familial issues[20,25] that often arise during the process of testing for or diagnosing a genetic disorder.

Although risk assessment is a process involving numerous dimensions and elements for identifying patients who may be at risk for a particular disease (Fig. 7.1), the most valuable components of risk assessment are thorough personal and family histories. The personal history and family histories can assist a clinician in recognizing: (1) single-gene or chromosomal disorders; (2) susceptibilities that may pose future risk for health problems because of increased familial risk of common chronic disorders (e.g., diabetes, hypertension); (3) increased susceptibility to cancers; and (4) "red flags" that warrant referral, consultation, or genetic testing, all important for personalized care.[31–35] See Box 7.1 for an example of how family and personal medical histories influence risk assessment.

FAMILY HISTORY

A first step to assessing risk for the individual and family members is to take a good family history. Family history is so important that it has often been called the "first genetic test," because when done correctly it can highlight common diseases and disease clusters within a family. This information can then be used to guide the kind of genetic or diagnostic testing that might be needed for clinical decision-making.[20]

Personal and Family History

A personal history should include the current age of the patient, their race and/or ethnicity, a history of their current concern or problem, and any pertinent past medical, surgical, or ancillary history. A detailed reproductive and obstetric or infertility history should also be collected from female patients. Confirmatory documentation of medical, laboratory, or ancillary tests should be obtained if possible,[20] and a focused physical examination should be conducted based on the physical, laboratory, and family history findings.[21]

BOX **7.1**

Case Scenario

J.D. is a 34-year-old Caucasian male of Northern European descent on both the maternal and paternal lineage. He comes to the primary care clinic with a 3-month history of a facial lesion that he is afraid may be skin cancer. His medical history is unremarkable, but his family history is significant for a 43-year-old brother who was diagnosed a year ago with colon cancer and a father who was diagnosed with colon cancer twice—at ages 45 and 49—and who died of the disease at age 51. His paternal grandparents' histories are unknown, and his maternal lineage is uneventful (Fig. 7.2). The nurse practitioner (NP) suspects that the facial lesion is a sebaceous adenoma, which, when combined with the "red flags" in the family history (i.e., early-age onset of colon cancer; two first-degree relatives with colon cancer), raises the suspicion for Muir-Torre syndrome (MTS), a subtype of a familial hereditary colon cancer syndrome known as Lynch syndrome.[32] The facial lesion was biopsied with a confirmatory diagnosis of sebaceous adenoma, and further testing revealed microsatellite high lesion (MSI-H) and absence of MutS Homolog 2 (MSH2) protein staining consistent with a history of MTS.[32] A colonoscopy was performed on J.D., and two benign adenomatous polyps were found in the right colon. The patient and his brother went for genetic counseling on advice of the NP, and both tested positive for Lynch syndrome caused by a deleterious mutation in the *MSH2* gene. Additional interprofessional collaboration with the surgeon, genetic counselor, gastrointestinal specialists, oncologists, and mental health counselors, based on the patient's history, is now in progress. Sebaceous adenomas, particularly with this pattern of genetic changes, are often found in individuals with Lynch syndrome.[33,34]

In this example, the NP integrated the patient's personal and family histories, his physical examination findings, his ancillary test results, and the NP's knowledge of hereditary syndromes to identify the genetic red flags in the scenario. The NP suspected that J.D. might be at increased risk for a high-risk cancer syndrome, initiated appropriate early colon cancer screening, and initiated referral for additional genetic counseling and consultation.

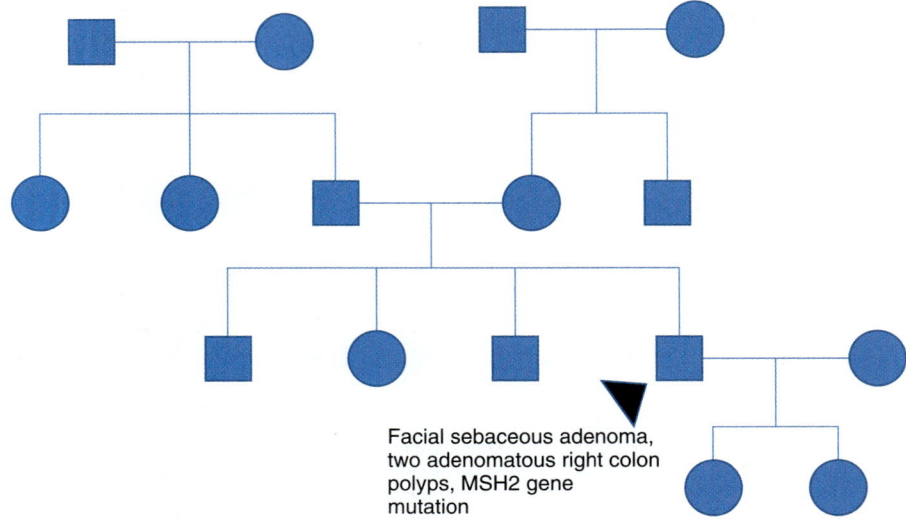

Facial sebaceous adenoma, two adenomatous right colon polyps, MSH2 gene mutation

F I G . **7.2** Four-generation pedigree of fictitious patient J.D. *(arrowhead)*, with biopsied confirmed facial sebaceous adenoma, two adenomatous right colon polyps, and deleterious *MSH2* gene mutation.

Family history, collected in the form of a three-generation pedigree on maternal and paternal sides, often reveals information that is better evaluated than a text-based history because it's presented graphically, so relationships, family size, and disease risk patterns can be more easily seen. Family members who may be at increased risk are also more easily identified,[22–24] and environmental (e.g., asbestos) and behavioral (e.g., alcohol, tobacco) risk factors may also be recognized. Once a complete family history has been obtained, it can be used to calculate risk, guide screening, intervention, and surveillance.[25]

Disease risk is divided into three categories: average or population risk, moderate risk, and increased or high risk.[18] Prevention guidelines were designed to assess risk in the average or population risk group. U.S. Preventive Services Task Force (USPSTF) guidelines, for example, recommend colon cancer screening (i.e., colonoscopy) begin at age 50 in individuals with no personal or family history of colorectal cancer (in other words people who are at average risk for developing colon cancer)[31]; guidelines from the American Cancer Society now recommend screening for people of average risk to start at age 45.[32] Earlier routine colorectal cancer screening beginning at age 45 years for African Americans is recommended by the American College of Gastroenterology.[33] Individuals with a personal or family history of colon cancer are not at average risk, and screening recommendations are significantly different. Individuals at moderate risk for developing colon cancer may need earlier or more frequent screening based on a personal history of adenomatous polyp(s) or sessile serrated polyp(s); personal history of inflammatory bowel disease; family history of colorectal cancer; and/or a first-degree relative with advanced adenomas.[34] Deciding when to start and how often to screen for colorectal cancer is based on which family member has cancer (i.e., first-degree, second-degree), his/her age at diagnosis, and the type of tumor (advanced adenoma[s]).[35] People at high risk for colon cancer, such as those with Lynch syndrome or polyposis syndromes (i.e., classic familial adenomatous polyposis [FAP]; attenuated FAP; *MUTYH*-associated polyposis; Peutz-Jeghers syndrome; juvenile polyposis syndrome; serrated polyposis syndrome), require enhanced colorectal surveillance and should be screened and monitored for other disorders as well, depending on the syndrome.[33] Enhanced surveillance may also be warranted for those with no inherited syndromes but the presence of significant personal or familial risk. Referral to a genetic specialist should be considered for individuals with a strong personal and/or family history or a genetic predisposition to the disease.

Gathering a Family History

For appropriate assessment of risk, the family history has to be taken in a systematic fashion. Clinicians are usually taught to take a family history and how to record it in the form of a pedigree, however in actual practice they often ask just a single question: "Do you have a family history of heart disease, cancer, or diabetes?" Although all of these are important health care concerns, gathering information in this way is not systematic; there is no information about who has had the disease, how many people have been affected, at what age the disease manifested, or whether a family member has died from the disease. In addition, by merely asking about a specific disorder, the clinician may miss pertinent conditions that may be caused by an inherited syndrome. Completing a family history by using a pedigree provides a means to ensure that all members in both lineages are included in the assessment and that the pattern of disease(s), if present, can be identified.[36]

Drawing a pedigree is not a difficult process, and several tools are available to assist in gathering and recording an accurate pedigree. For example, asking patients to complete the Surgeon General's family history tool online and bring the pedigree with them to an appointment greatly facilitates both the collection process (saves time) and accuracy (they can call family members for additional information) of this critical information.[37] It also involves patients in the process, which may illuminate familial patterns that were not visible to them before, and may encourage adherence to lifestyle recommendations (e.g., smoking cessation) once the patient sees the impact of shared genetic and lifestyle factors in disease(s) affecting the family.

Standard Pedigree Symbols

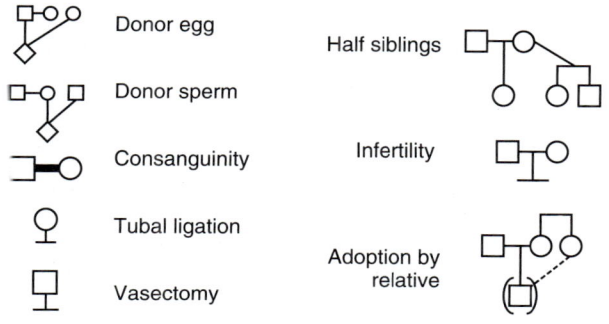

□	Male	Proband	
○	Female		
◇	? Gender or pregnancy	Mating	
▲	Pregnancy loss	Sibship	
(□)	Adopted		
■	Affected	Dizygotic twins	
⊘	Deceased	Monozygotic twins	

Less Common Pedigree Symbols

	Donor egg	Half siblings	
	Donor sperm		
	Consanguinity	Infertility	
	Tubal ligation		
	Vasectomy	Adoption by relative	

F I G . 7.3 Example of commonly used standardized pedigree symbols. (With permission from Bennett, R. [2010]. *The practical guide to the genetic family history* [2nd ed.]. Malden, MA: Wiley-Blackwell.)

The systematic nature of a pedigree collection is critical and facilitates the gathering and recording of complete health information about each family member. Standard pedigree figures have been developed and should be used so that other health professionals can quickly interpret the pedigree (Fig. 7.3).[20] When drawing a pedigree, the affected individual (the proband)[36] is identified by an arrow. If the person reporting the family history is not the proband (e.g., a parent of an affected child), then the proband is identified on the pedigree and a note is made on the form regarding the individual who provided the history. The term "consultand" is also used when conducting a pedigree when the individual is not affected with a disorder of concern but is undergoing history-taking or seeking medical attention or has other family members with a specific disorder(s)[36] Information on all of the proband's or consultand's first-degree (i.e., parents, siblings, children, stillborn fetuses, and miscarriages) and second-degree (i.e., grandparents, aunt and uncles, and cousins) relatives, both living and deceased, should be collected and recorded (Fig. 7.4). At a minimum, each family member's information should include significant health history, the age of disease onset, and the cause and age of death (Box 7.2). Environmental exposures (e.g., smoking) should also be included. For example, if a first-degree relative died of lung cancer at a young age, the interviewer would want to establish whether or not this relative was a smoker.[37]

It is important to indicate how family members are related to one another, whether the relatives are in the maternal or paternal lineage, and what other type of relationships exist

in the family, such as adoption (in or out), half-siblings, and twins, either dizygotic (fraternal) or monozygotic (identical). These relationships may have a significant impact (monozygotic twins) or no impact at all (nonbiologic adopted sibling). It is also important to recognize that some family histories are limited in structure because of few family members by history, early-age onset of death among family members, limited number or few members of a specific gender, or lack of information from birth parents (e.g., adoption). This limited structure may result in interpretation of the pedigree as challenging because of difficulty in identifying patterns when there are few or no informative family members to evaluate. For example, an autosomal dominant (AD) pattern of inheritance for breast cancer may be masked when assessing a patient for a HBOC cancer syndrome such as that resulting from a deleterious mutation in the *BRCA* genes because of a small family size or transmission through males via sex-limited expression.[38,39]

Pertinent family health information, when possible, should be verified through medical records, pathology reports, and/or laboratory results. Verification is an important part of the risk assessment process because family members do not always have accurate health information (e.g., reported history of prostate cancer, but medical record reveals benign prostatic hypertrophy). In addition, family history is a living document that needs to be updated regularly. Family health history is a dynamic process, and regular updating is required to annotate births, deaths, and change in health status of individuals as well as family members.

Interpreting a Family History

Once the three-generation pedigree has been collected, interpretation can begin. Interpretation is done by identifying patterns and red flags in the pedigree as shown in Figs. 7.5 and 7.6. Red flags include early age of disease onset (e.g., colon cancer at age 38); disease across multiple generations; disorders occurring predominantly in one gender (only males affected); disease in the absence of known risk factors (e.g., hyperlipidemia in an individual of normal weight with adequate diet and exercise); or uncommon disease presentation (e.g., breast cancer in a male).[40] The acronym *GENES* may be useful in identifying red flags. For this acronym, G = groups of anomalies; E = early or extreme presentation of common diseases; N = neurodevelopmental or neurodegenerative conditions; E = exception or unusual pathology; and S = surprising laboratory findings—any of which may be indicative of an underlying genetic condition.[41] In addition, some genetic disorders are more common among certain ethnic groups (e.g., sickle cell anemia and African Americans), and families with a history of consanguinity among members are at increased risk for autosomal recessive (AR) conditions.[40] Often pedigrees are complex and may be difficult to interpret. Consultation and/or referral to experts in genetics should be sought if interpretation of the pedigree is uncertain and there is a potential for a disease or syndrome. Important online resources, such as locating a genetic counselor for high-risk patients, are listed in Table 7.1.

Common Inheritance Patterns

Autosomal Dominant Disorders. Pedigree interpretation requires that clinicians be able to recognize inheritance patterns. In an AD disorder, only one parent has to have a gene mutation to pass on the disease to the next generation. These

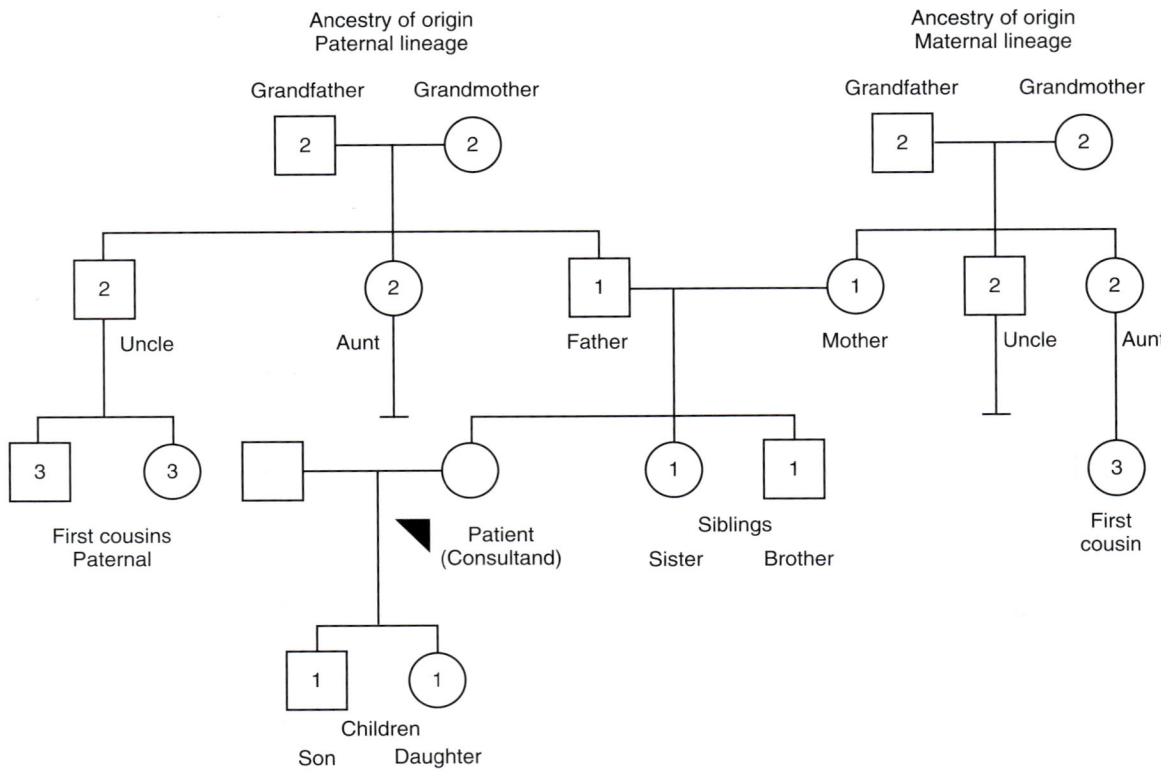

FIG. 7.4 A four-generation pedigree depicting first-, second-, and third-degree relatives of the consultand (unaffected individual or patient seeking care as noted per *arrowhead*).

"Red Flags" and Collection Guidelines

INDIVIDUAL MEDICAL HISTORY

Dysmorphic features (especially with a learning disorder)
Learning disabilities or behavioral problems
Movement disorders—hypotonia, ataxia
Unexplained infertility
Congenital or juvenile deafness, blindness, or cataracts
Environmental or lifestyle risk factors (smoking, alcohol use, and dietary preferences)
Patient's occupation and the occupation of relatives with chronic conditions
Protective environmental or lifestyle modifications, such as regular exercise

FAMILY MEDICAL HISTORY

Multiple affected family members with same or related conditions
Earlier age at onset than expected (e.g., myocardial infarction at age 40)
Condition in the less-often-affected sex (breast cancer in a male)
Disease in the absence of known risk factors (hyperlipidemia in a young, athletic, normal-weight individual)
Ethnic predisposition to certain diseases (Tay-Sachs in an Ashkenazi Jewish infant)

Close biologic relationship between parents (consanguinity)
Three or more pregnancy losses

PEDIGREE SHOULD INCLUDE

Legend
- Pedigree key (e.g., darkened circle indicates breast cancer)
- Date recorded or updated
- Name of the person reviewing the history with the patient

Race or ethnicity; country or countries of family origin for maternal and paternal lineage
Gender
Age and age at diagnosis
Age and cause of death
Primary site for any cancer
Pregnancy losses
Chronic or long-term conditions (noting the condition[s] of interest)
Surgical history and/or relevant interventions or procedures
Increased risk, or unusual diagnosis; validate by reviewing medical records, pathology reports, death certificates
Surgical history

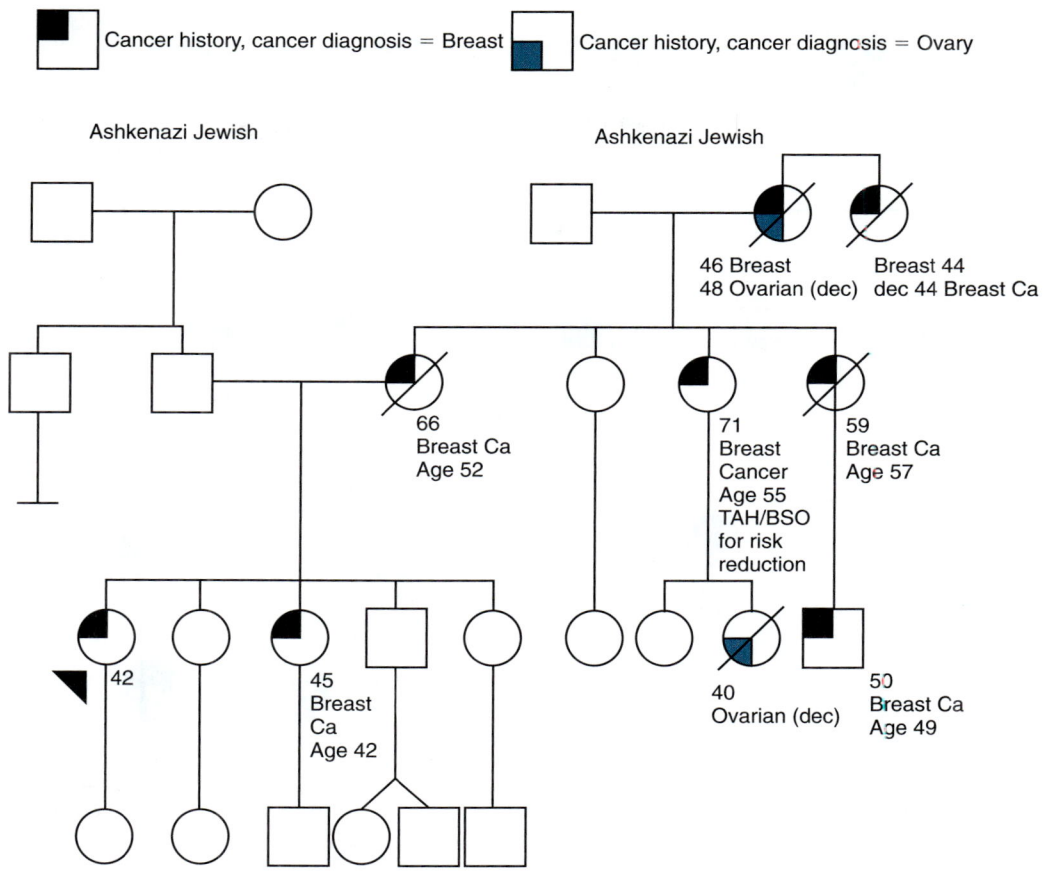

Cancer history, cancer diagnosis = Breast

Cancer history, cancer diagnosis = Ovary

Ashkenazi Jewish

Ashkenazi Jewish

46 Breast
48 Ovarian (dec)

Breast 44
dec 44 Breast Ca

66
Breast Ca
Age 52

71
Breast
Cancer
Age 55
TAH/BSO
for risk
reduction

59
Breast Ca
Age 57

42

45
Breast
Ca
Age 42

40
Ovarian (dec)

50
Breast Ca
Age 49

FIG. 7.5 Fictitious four-generation pedigree of family members with inherited breast and ovarian cancer (positive for deleterious *BRCA1* mutation, an autosomal inherited syndrome). Pedigree displays "red flags," including early age of onset of breast and ovarian cancer among family members; male breast cancer; multiple generations affected with breast cancer; and breast and ovarian cancer in a family in the same lineage (maternal), raising suspicion for an inherited breast cancer syndrome.

mutations are carried on autosomes (chromosomes 1 to 22) not on the sex chromosomes (X and Y), so both genders are equally affected. Examples of AD disorders include many of the hereditary cancer syndromes (e.g., Lynch syndrome, HBOC), Marfan syndrome, familial hypercholesterolemia, polycystic kidney disease, and Huntington disease. Features of AD inheritance include individuals affected in each generation (with the exception of some families with limited structure) and males and females equally affected. The usual pattern of inheritance seen on the pedigree is one of vertical transmission (see Fig. 7.6). At conception there is a 50% chance of the infant inheriting the condition when the gene mutation has an AD pattern.

Autosomal Recessive Disorders. A genetic disease that appears to emerge suddenly in one generation raises suspicion for an AR disorder. The pedigree in AR disorders usually has a horizontal pattern of inheritance (Fig. 7.7) rather than the vertical pattern of transmission found frequently in AD disorders. Like AD disorders, AR disorders are also carried on autosomes (chromosomes 1 to 22), so they affect both sexes equally. In the case of a recessive disorder, however, both parents are typically unaffected carriers. Children of two carrier parents fall into one of three categories: (1) they receive two normal genes, one from each parent, and are not carriers, nor are they affected; (2) they receive one copy of the mutation from one parent and a normal gene from the other and are carriers like

their parents; or (3) they receive two copies of the mutation, one from each parent, and are affected. In many AR disorders, carrier frequencies (individuals in the population who carry a copy of the mutation) can be high, but the number of affected individuals (people with two copies of a mutation) can be relatively low. In certain cultural and ethnic groups, however, AR disorders may be more common because marriages to close relatives (consanguineous relationships) are sanctioned, increasing the likelihood that both parents carry the same AR mutation. Examples of AR disorders include sickle cell disease, cystic fibrosis, and thalassemia disorders.

X-Linked Disorders. Another form of genetic inheritance causes X-linked disorders. X-linked disorders should be ruled out if the disease appears to manifest exclusively in male family members (Fig. 7.8). Men are affected by mutations on the X chromosome because they have only one copy of the X chromosome, and there is no "backup" X chromosome to produce even a small amount of normal gene product. Depending on the type of X-linked mutation, female carriers may be asymptomatic or may have very mild symptoms because their other X chromosome is producing normal gene products. Males with an X-linked gene disorder do not pass the mutation on to any of their sons because their sons get only the Y chromosome from the male parent. Fathers will, however, pass the mutation along to each of their daughters. Daughters of men

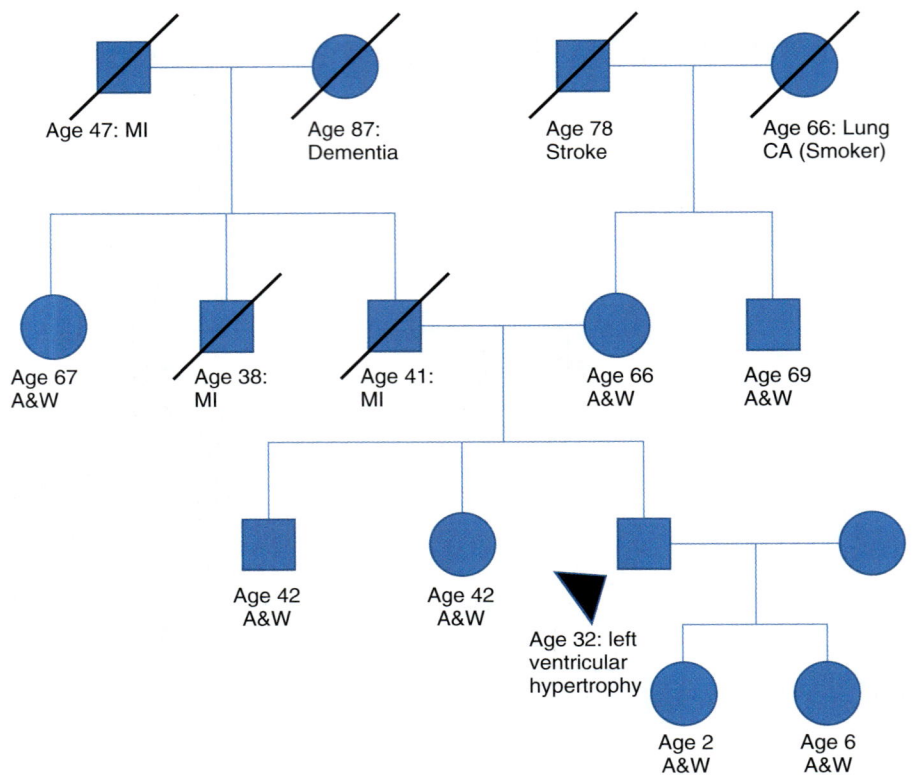

F I G . 7.6 Fictitious four-generation pedigree of proband (noted with *arrowhead*) diagnosed with early-age onset of left ventricular hypertrophy and family history of early-age sudden cardiac death in father, paternal uncle, and paternal grandfather, raising suspicion for hypertrophic cardiomyopathy.

TABLE 7.1	**Examples of Online Genetic Resources**
Patient information and support groups—provides assistance and support to patients, families, and clinicians caring for individuals with rare disorders	FORCE—Facing Our Risk of Cancer Empowered (information regarding hereditary breast and ovarian cancer): www.facingourrisk.org/index.php National Organization for Rare Disorders: www.rarediseases.org/patients-and-families/patient-assistance GeneTests (select "Resources" link): www.genetests.org Genetic and Rare Diseases Information Center: http://rarediseases.info.nih.gov/resources/5/support-for-patients-and-families March of Dimes "Family Teams": www.marchforbabies.org/FamilyTeams?intnav=MFB_PUB_HDR_FAMTEAMS
Professional and public education about birth defects and other health complications for mothers and babies	March of Dimes: http://www.marchofdimes.org/complications/birth-defects-and-health-conditions.aspx
Family history tools	Centers for Disease Control and Prevention (family history fact sheet, tools, resources): www.cdc.gov/genomics/famhistory/index.htm American Medical Association (collecting family history): https://www.ama-assn.org/delivering-care/precision-medicine/collecting-family-history
General genetics resources	National Human Genome Research Institute: www.genome.gov/Education Dolan DNA Learning Center: www.dnalc.org Genetic Science Learning Center: http://learn.genetics.utah.edu Genetics Education Center: www.kumc.edu/gec
Resources to help clinicians integrate genetics into patient care	National Coalition for Health Professional Education in Genetics: www.nchpeg.org GeneTests (select "Educational Materials" and "Genetic Tools"): www.genetests.org March of Dimes Genetics and Your Practice: www.marchofdimes.com/professionals/pregnancy-and-health-profile.aspx National Cancer Institute: Prevention, Genetics, Causes: www.cancer.gov/cancerinfo/prevention/genetics

TABLE **7.1**	**Examples of Online Genetic Resources—cont'd**
Clinical genetics specialist professional organizations	American College of Medical Genetics: www.acmg.net National Society of Genetic Counselors: www.nsgc.org International Society of Nurses in Genetics: www.isong.org American Board of Medical Genetics: www.abmg.org American Board of Genetic Counseling: www.abgc.net (Can be searched by name, city, or state but does not currently differentiate genetics researchers from clinicians, unless one cross-checks individual entries with certification status.)

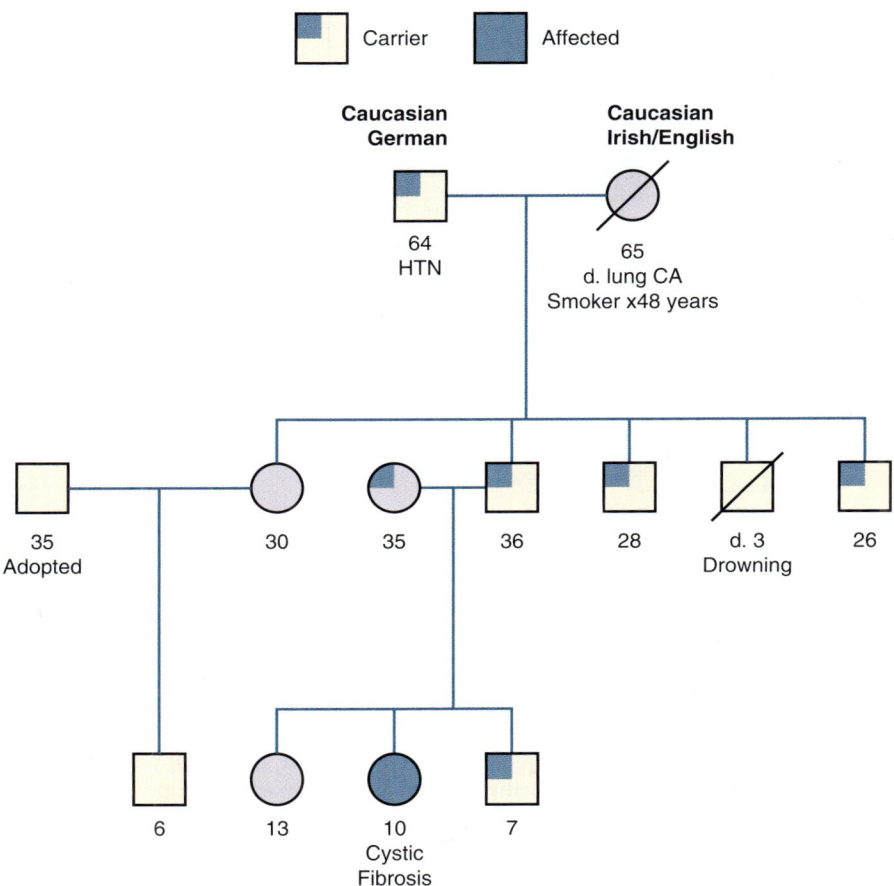

FIG. 7.7   Example of a fictitious three-generation pedigree of a 10-year-old girl with cystic fibrosis and family members who are carriers of the disease. A horizontal pattern of inheritance is revealed, consistent with autosomal recessive genetic disorders.

with X-linked diseases are therefore considered "obligate carriers" (one normal X and one affected X chromosome), and every one of their children has a 50% chance of inheriting the affected X chromosome. If the carrier female passes the affected X chromosome along to her daughter, the daughter, like her mother, will be a carrier. If the carrier female passes the affected X chromosome along to her son, however, he will be affected with the disease. It should be noted that X-linked disorders can also be inherited in a dominant or recessive pattern. X-linked dominant disorders are relatively rare and since only one copy of the mutation is required to express the phenotype, females can be affected in these disorders. For example, if a father is affected with an X-linked dominant disorder all daughters but none of the sons will be affected with the disorder unless the mother is also affected. Also, a mother with an X-linked

dominant disorder may have both affected and non-affected sons. Examples of X-linked disorders include hemophilia, fragile X syndrome, red-green color blindness, and Duchenne muscular dystrophy.

GENETIC INFORMATION NONDISCRIMINATION ACT

Gathering a complete health history, recognizing genetic red flags, and referring patients to appropriate genomics resources is essential, but it is only the beginning for many patients and their families. As part of a genomics workup, genetic testing may be recommended and concerns may arise about who will have access to the results and how those results will be used. Individuals have a legitimate concern about employment or health insurance discrimination. It is one thing to have a genetic

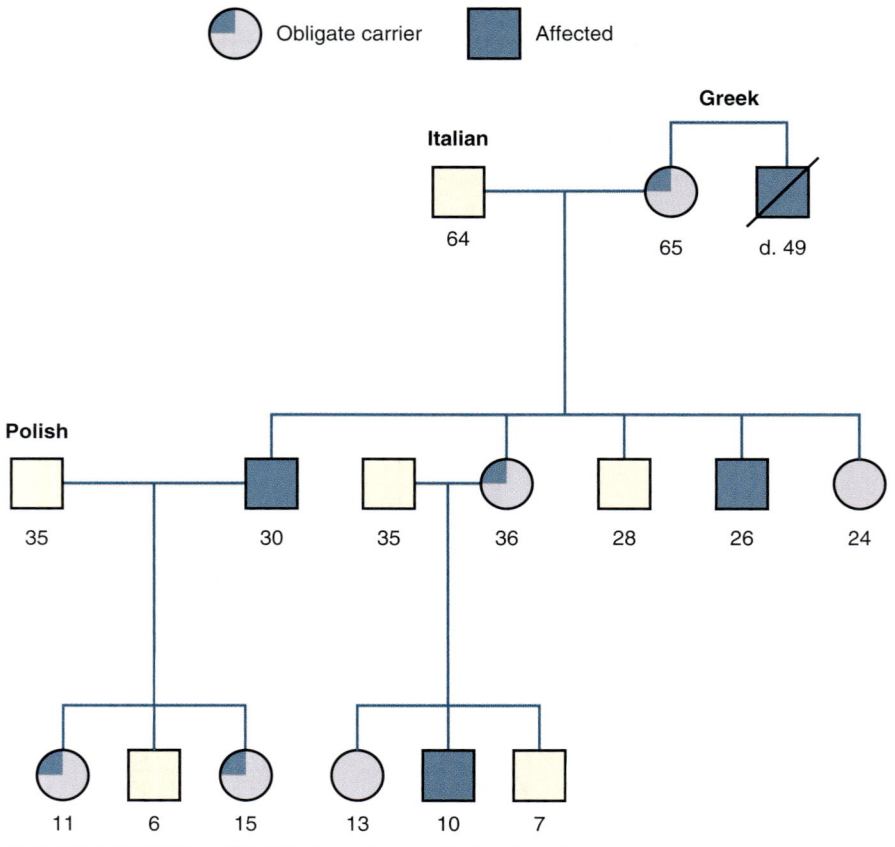

○ Obligate carrier   ■ Affected

FIG. **7.8**   Example of a three-generation pedigree depicting an X-linked genetic disorder with female carriers and affected males.

disorder but another to be asymptomatic and know that one might be at increased risk because of a strong family history of a genetic disease. When someone has a genetic disease, health insurance companies usually know about it because these individuals use specific health care resources (e.g., children with cystic fibrosis are typically hospitalized once a year and their medications are expensive). These individuals often pay higher insurance premiums; however, under the Affordable Care Act (ACA), people with preexisting health conditions could not be denied health insurance.[42] For otherwise healthy individuals considering genetic testing based solely on a strong family history, misuse of genetic information is a significant concern.

Legal protections from genetic discrimination took a long time to secure. Genetic nondiscrimination language was first proposed in the US House of Representatives in 1995 and in the US Senate the following year. Neither bill passed, but advocates were persistent, and the bills were brought forward every year for over a decade. Finally, in April 2007 GINA passed in the House and in April 2008 the legislation passed in the Senate. GINA was signed into law by President George W. Bush on May 21, 2008, and all aspects of GINA went into effect on November 21, 2009.[42,43]

All health care providers should be knowledgeable about GINA and its prohibitions related to discrimination in health coverage and employment based on genetic information. Table 7.2 provides a summary of important information about GINA pertaining to health insurance and employment. For additional information on GINA, a resource pertaining to case studies involving GINA in clinical settings can also be found on the Jackson Laboratory website at https://www.jax.org/ education-and-learning/clinical-and-continuing-education/ ccep-non-cancer-resources/gina-overview/case-studies-of-gina -in-clinical-settings.[43–45]

There have been many scientific advances since GINA and ACA were enacted. Proposed changes to ACA could potentially make your genes a preexisting condition. While GINA protects individuals from discrimination based on a genetic finding, once there is an abnormal mammogram or EKG, for example,[46] this is no longer considered a genetic finding. In March 2017 the House Committee on Education and the Workforce approved HR 1313,[47] which would allow employers to force employees to disclose their genetic information and loosen the current ACA requirements, regardless of other legal restrictions such as GINA.[48] HR 1313 would allow employers to offer insurance rebates to employees who take part in wellness programs that may include submitting to health risk assessments incorporating genetic screening, charging more for employees who decline to take part in the genetic screening process.[46–48] Disability advocates (ADA) and the genetic community are strongly opposed to the proposed legislation HR 1313. The ADA and GINA rules protect employees from being coerced into sharing sensitive health information about themselves or family members.

DIRECT-TO-CONSUMER GENETIC TESTING

Several companies market genetic testing services directly to consumers, providing individuals with an opportunity to order and receive genetic test results without involving a health care

TABLE 7.2 **Overview of the Genetic Information Nondiscrimination Act**

Health Insurance Protections

General protections	Genetic information regarding an individual and his or her family members.
	DOES NOT cover an individual who is symptomatic, is being treated for, or has been diagnosed with a genetic condition.
	An insurer may *request* genetic information if coverage may be appropriate only if there is a known genetic risk.
Health insurers may NOT:	Require an individual to provide genetic information about himself or herself or a family member for eligibility, coverage, underwriting, or premium-setting decisions.
	Use genetic information to make enrollment or coverage decisions.
	Request or require a genetic test.
	Use genetic information as a preexisting condition in the Medicare supplemental and individual health insurance markets.
Research exceptions	For research activities conducted jointly by health insurers and external research entities, a health insurer may request, but not require, in writing that an individual undergo a genetic test.
	The individual may voluntarily choose to undergo such genetic testing, but noncompliance will not have a negative effect on his or her premium or enrollment status. This information may be used only for research and not for underwriting purposes.

Employment Protections

General protections	Covers genetic information of an individual and his or her family members.
	DOES NOT cover an individual who is symptomatic, is being treated for, or has been diagnosed with a genetic condition.
Employers and/or unions may NOT:	Use genetic information in making decisions regarding hiring, promotion, terms or conditions, privileges of employment, compensation, or termination.
	Limit, segregate, or classify an employee or member or deprive that employee or member of employment opportunities on the basis of genetic information.
	Request, require, or purchase genetic information about the individual or a family member of the individual, except when:
	• Inadvertently provided as part of the medical history.
	• Information is publicly available.
	• Obtained as part of an occupational assessment.
	• Employer offers health or genetic services, including services offered as part of a wellness program.
	• Employer operates as a law enforcement entity and requires the individual's DNA for quality control purposes in the forensic laboratory or human remains identification settings.
	Fail or refuse to refer an individual for employment on the basis of genetic information.
	Use genetic information in making decisions regarding admission to or employment in any program for apprenticeship or training and retraining, including on-the-job training.
	Exclude or expel from membership, or otherwise discriminate against, an individual because of genetic information.

GINA Limitations

Insurance	Does not protect individuals from discrimination based on genetic information:
	• When qualifying for life insurance
	• Disability insurance
	• Long-term care insurance
	• Participants of the US Military's Tricare program
	• US veterans obtaining health care through the Veteran's Administration
	• Health care obtained through the Indian Health Service
Affordable Care Act (2010)	Conflict with a provision in Title II of GINA that limits employers from using an employee's genetic information in employer-sponsored wellness programs.

GINA, Genetic Information Nondiscrimination Act.

provider or insurance company. As the cost for DTC testing continues to decline, this may be a viable option for many consumers. Supporters of DTC testing believe this is part of the consumer's right to exercise autonomy in health care decisions. The benefits of DTC genetic testing include the private nature of the testing (e.g., insurance companies will not find out the results), an increased awareness of genetic diseases, and the ability of interested consumers to take a test to explore their ancestral origins.

Despite these benefits, professional groups have raised concerns about the type of genetic information that is provided by DTC testing companies and the lack of counseling for consumers.[49] Consumers may receive information they are not prepared to deal with such as a risk for disease for which there is no treatment or prevention (e.g., Alzheimer).[50,51]

DTC testing encompasses a wide variety of genetic testing including both single-gene disorders and susceptibility to common complex disorders based on genome-wide association study (GWAS) data, which provide relatively small contributions to disease prediction[52] including results of studies that still need to be confirmed by the scientific community. Because much of the evidence provided for the markers tested is inconclusive at this time, interpretation of the DTC results is difficult[53] and does not necessarily signify that those markers are the strongest indicators for a disease or that patients who have the same mutations will manifest the same health condition clinically. For complex diseases, the family history in the form of a three-generation pedigree provides a first-line measure to evaluate potential risk based on first-degree relatives (parents and siblings), which is not part of most DTC testing processes. Although some DTC testing centers reportedly offer to consumers the assistance of a genetic counselor for an additional fee to assist with understanding of the results, most do not provide any form of genetic counseling.[53]

Concerns about the genetic risk information being provided to consumers by one DTC center, as well as the validity and usefulness of their platform and risk algorithms, came to the attention of the US Food and Drug Administration (FDA), which is responsible for DTC testing oversight. This prompted a letter to be issued in 2013, requiring the DTC site to stop dispensing genetic health risk reports to consumers until the company complied with an order to provide FDA-requested materials.[54]

DTC health care is highly dynamic, so clinicians should pay close attention to developments in this area. Two recent developments in the area of DTC testing include the FDA granting approval to 23andMe to resume disease-based susceptibility testing, and a November 2017 request from Senator Chuck Schumer (D-New York) to the Federal Trade Commission to review DTC testing for privacy policies and standards.

CONCLUSION

This chapter sets the stage for thinking about health and disease through a genomics lens. Genomics is becoming increasingly important in health care as "personalized health care" is becoming a reality. The very first step in genomic health assessment is to collect a structured, complete personal and family history, looking for genetic red flags, and referring to an appropriate genetics consultant if indicated. Risk assessment and interpretation are part of the ANA's genetic core competencies for nurses with graduate degrees. Advanced genomic technologies such as molecular profiles and genetic testing offer clinicians the opportunity to identify disease risk and provide more personalized screening and surveillance,[55] but none of this technology is helpful if the people who need this surveillance are not identified. Risk assessment starts with assessment but genetic education, counseling, testing, results interpretation, and appropriate referral and management are also critical pieces of care. As genetic knowledge continues to expand through the use of powerful genomic tools, including gene editing (repair) technologies such as CRISPR (Clustered Regularly Interspaced Short Palindromic Repeats), the term *genomics* will gradually replace the word *genetics* in the clinician's lexicon.[56] The underlying genetic contributions to common disorders such as diabetes, hypertension, arthritis, Alzheimer disease, and mental health disorders are becoming more understood, and the hope of more effective treatment for all of them is on the horizon. With better understanding of basic biologic processes, more accurate diagnostic tools, better drugs, and new treatments will all emerge, moving humanity toward the promise of "precision medicine."

RESOURCES

Resource Name	Description	Url
Genetic Alliance	A national, nonprofit health advocacy organization committed to transforming health through genetics and promoting an environment of openness centered on the health of individuals, families, and communities. The Alliance chaired the Coalition for Genetic Fairness, a multistakeholder coalition of more than 500 organizations committed to passing federal genetic nondiscrimination legislation.	www.geneticalliance.org
Jackson Laboratories	Founded in 1929, The Jackson Laboratory (JAX) is an independent, nonprofit biomedical research institution with more than 1900 employees who are passionate about our mission: to discover precise genomic solutions for disease and empower the global biomedical community in the shared quest to improve human health. The Laboratory is a world leader in mammalian genetics and human genomics and generating the development of scientific breakthroughs and improved therapies with ever-greater precision and speed. We also educate current and future scientists and provide critical resources, data, tools, and services to researchers worldwide.	https://www.jax.org/education-and-learning/clinical-and-continuing-education/clinical-topics
Genetics and Public Policy Center	Created to help policymakers, the press, and the public understand and respond to the challenges and opportunities of genetic medicine and its potential to transform global public health	http://www.pewtrusts.org/en/archived-projects/genetics-and-public-policy-center
National Institutes of Health, National Human Genome Research Institute (NHGRI)	Supports the development of resources and technology that will accelerate genome research and its application to human health. A critical part of the NHGRI mission is the study of the ethical, legal, and social implications of genome research. NHGRI also supports the training of investigators and the dissemination of genome information to the public and to health professionals. Website includes information on research and research funding; health information for patients, the public, and professionals; a calendar of events and media information; information on education, issues in genetics, and careers and training; and specialized information for students, educators, patients, health professionals, grant applicants, and news media.	www.genome.gov

Resource Name	Description	Url
Genome Magazine	A free, very readable magazine appropriate for clinicians and patients	http://genomemag.com
	Genome is a quarterly magazine for the public at large: patients, family, caregivers, and health care professionals on the education frontlines. The magazine's mission is to empower readers to make informed health decisions that will help them live better and longer.	
	The magazine explores complicated subjects concerning genomics and medicine—and the associated ethical, legal, and social issues—but tells those stories in a relevant, easy-to-understand manner.	
Genetics Home Reference	Genetics Home Reference is the National Library of Medicine website for consumer information about genetic conditions and the genes or chromosomes associated with those conditions. The content includes information on direct-to-consumer genetic testing	https://ghr.nlm.nih.gov/

REFERENCES

1. Scott, J., & Trotter, T. (2013). Primary care and genetics and genomics. *Pediatrics*, 132(Suppl. 3), S231–S237.
2. Collins, F. S. (2010). *The language of life: DNA and the revolution in personalized medicine*. New York, New York: HarperCollins.
3. McKusick, V. A., & Ruddle, F. H. (1987). A new discipline, a new name, a new journal. *Genomics*, 1, 1–2.
4. Genetic, A., & District of Columbia Department of Health. (2010). Understanding genetics: A district of columbia guide for patients and health professionals.
5. Nicol, N., Skirton, H., Feero, W. G., & Green, E. (2013). Relevance of genomics to nursing practice. *Journal of Nursing Scholarship*, 45, 1–2.
6. National Human Genome Research Institute. (2014). Talking glossary of genetic terms: Personalized medicine. Retrieved from www.genome.gov/glossary/idex.cfm?textonly=&search=personalized+medicine.
7. 2011). Editorial. Moving toward precision medicine. *Lancet*, 378(9804), 1678.
8. National Institutes of Health (NIH). About the *All of Us* Research Program, a key element of the Precision Medicine Initiative (PMI). Retrieved from https://allofus.nih.gov/about/about-all-us-research-program. (Accessed 12 November 2017).
9. 2016). Cell editorial team. A cornucopia of advances in human epigenomics. *Cell*, 5, 1139.
10. Moran, S., Martinex-ardus, A., Boussiss, S., & Esteller, M. (2017). Precision medicine based on epigenomics: The paradigm of carcinoma of unknown primary. *Nature Reviews. Clinical Oncology*, 14, 682–694.
11. Berg, J. S., Agrawal, P. B., Bailey, D. B., Beggs, A. H., Brenner, S. E., Brower, A. M., et al. (2017). Newborn sequencing in genomic medicine and public health. *Pediatrics*, e20162252.
12. Johnston, J. J., Rubinstein, W. S., Facio, F. M., et al. (2012). Secondary variants in individuals undergoing exome sequencing: Screening of 572 individuals identifies high penetrance mutations in cancer susceptibility genes. *American Journal of Human Genetics*, 91, 97–108.
13. Rabbani, B., Tekin, M., & Mahdieh, N. (2014). The promise of whole-exome sequencing in medical genetics. *Journal of Human Genetics*, 59, 5–15.
14. LaDuca, H., Stuenkel, A. J., Dolinsky, J. S., Keiles, S., Tandy, S., Pesaran, T., et al. (2014). Utilization of multigene panels in hereditary cancer predisposition testing: Analysis of more than 2,000 patients. *Genetics in Medicine*, 16, 830–837. Retrieved from www.nature.com/gim/journal/vaop/ncurrent/full/gim201550a.html.
15. McKusick-Nathans Institute of Genetic Medicine JHUB, MD, National Center for Biotechnology Information NLoMB, MD. Online Mendelian Inheritance in Man, OMIM.
16. Maradiegue, A., Edwards, Q. T., & Seibert, D. (2013). 5-Years later—have faculty integrated medical genetics into nurse practitioner curriculum? *International Journal of Nursing Education Scholarship*, 10, 245–254.
17. Maradiegue, A., Edwards, Q. T., & Seibert, D. (2013). Erratum. 5-years later—have faculty integrated medical genetics into nurse practitioner curriculum? *International Journal of Nursing Education Scholarship*, 10, 245–254.
18. Facio, M., Lee, K., & O'Daniel, J. M. (2014). A genetic counselor's guide to using next-generation sequencing in clinical practice. *Journal of Genetic Counseling*, 23, 455–462.
19. Greco, K. E., Tinley, S., & Seibert, D., American Nurses Association. (2012). Essential genetic and genomic competencies for graduate nurses. www.nursingworld.org/MainMenuCategories/EthicsStandards/Genetics-1/ANA-and-ISONG-Announce-New-Publication.html.
20. Bennet, R. L. (2010). *The practical guide to the genetic family history* (2nd ed.). Hoboken: John Wiley & Sons.
21. Doerr, M., & Teng, K. (2012). Family history: Still relevant in the genomics era. *Cleveland Clinic Journal of Medicine*, 79(5), 331–336. Retrieved from http://www.mdedge.com/ccjm/article/95739/genetics/family-history-still-relevant-genomics-era.
22. South, C. D., Hampel, H., Comeras, I., Westman, J. A., Frankel, W. L., & de la Chapelle, A. (2008). The frequency of Muir-Torre syndrome among Lynch syndrome families. *Journal of the National Cancer Institute*, 100(4), 277–281.
23. Abbas, O., & Mahalingam, M. (2009). Cutaneous sebaceous neoplasm as markers of Muir-Torre syndrome: A diagnostic algorithm. *Journal of Cutaneous Pathology*, 36(6), 613–619.
24. Bhaijee, F., & Brown, A. S. (2014). Muir-Torre syndrome. *Archives of Pathology & Laboratory Medicine*, 138, 1685–1689. doi:10.5858/arpa.2013-0301-RS.
25. Edwards, Q. T., & Maradiegue, A. H. (2017). *Genetics and genomics in nursing: Guidelines for conducting a risk assessment*. New York: Springer.
26. National Institute of Health, National Cancer Institute. (Updated May 2011). Breast cancer risk assessment tool. Retrieved from www.cancer.gov/bcrisktool.
27. National Institute of Health, National Heart, Lung and Blood Institute. Risk assessment tool for estimating your 10-year risk of having a heart attack. Retrieved from www.nhlbi.nih.gov/health-pro/guidelines/current/cholesterol-guidelines/quick-desk-reference-html/10-year-risk-framingham-table.
28. Panchal, S. M., Ennis, M., Canon, S., & Bordeleau, L. J. (2008). Selecting a *BRCA* risk assessment model for use in a familial cancer clinic. *BMC Medical Genetics*, 9, 116.
29. Ståhlbom, A. K., Johansson, H., Liljegren, A., von Wachenfeldt, A., & Arver, B. (2012). Evaluation of the BOADICEA risk assessment model in women with a family history of breast cancer. *Familial Cancer*, 11(1), 33–40.
30. University of Cambridge, Centre for Cancer Genetic Epidemiology, Department of Public Health and Primary Care/Department of Oncology. (2017). BOADICEA Web application. Retrieved from ccge.medschl.cam.ac.uk/boadicea/boadicea-web-application.
31. U.S. Preventive Services Task Force. (2014). Screening for colorectal cancer. Retrieved from https://www.uspreventiveservicestaskforce.org/Page/Document/final-research-plan54/colorectal-cancer-screening2. (Accessed 15 November 2017).
32. American Cancer Society. Guideline for Colorectal Cancer Screening. For people of average risk. Retrieved from https://www.cancer.org/cancer/colon-rectal-cancer/detection-diagnosis-staging/acs-recommendations.html. (Accessed 27 March 2019).
33. Rex, D. K., et al. (2017). Colorectal cancer screening: Recommendations for physicians and patients from the US Multi-Society Task Force on Colorectal Cancer. *The American Journal of Gastroenterology*, 112(7), 1016–1030. https://gi.org/guideline/colorectal-cancer-screening-recommendations-for-physicians-and-patients-from-the-u-s-multi-society-task-force-on-colorectal-cancer/. (Accessed 15 November 2017).
34. National Comprehensive Cancer Network. (2017). Colorectal cancer screening. NCCN Clinical Practice Guidelines in Oncology (NCCN Guidelines), Version 2. Online. https://www.nccn.org/professionals/physician_gls/pdf/colorectal_screening.pdf. (Accessed 15 November 2017).
35. National Comprehensive Cancer Network. (2017). Genetic/familial high-risk assessment: colorectal, NCCN Clinical Practice Guidelines in Oncology (NCCN Guidelines) Version 3. Retrieved from https://www.nccn.org/

professionals/physician_gls/pdf/genetics_colon.pdf. (Accessed 15 November 2017).

36. Genetic Alliance; The New England Public Health Genetics Education Collaborative. (2010). Pedigree and family history taking. In *Understanding genetics: A New England guide for patients and health professionals*. Washington (DC): Genetic Alliance. Retrieved from www.ncbi.nlm.nih.gov/books/ NBK132175/.

37. United States Department of Health and Human Services. (2016). My Family Health Portrait Tool. Retrieved from https://www.hhs.gov/programs/ prevention-and-wellness/family-health-history/family-health-portrait-tool/ index.html.

38. Pagon, R. A., Adam, M. P., Ardinger, H. H., et al. (Eds.). GenReviews (pp. 1193–2014). Seattle (WA): University of Washington, Seattle. Retrieved from www.ncbi.nlm.nih.gov/books/NBK5191/. (Accessed 15 November 2017).

39. Weitzel, J. N., Lagos, V. I., Cullinane, C. A., Gambol, P. J., Culver, J. O., Blazer, K. R., et al. (2007). Limited family structure and BRCA gene mutation status in single cases of breast cancer. *JAMA: The Journal of the American Medical Association*, 297(23), 2587–2595.

40. The Jackson Laboratory. Genetic Red Flags Checklist. Retrieved from https:// www.jax.org/education-and-learning/clinical-and-continuing-education/ cancer-resources/genetic-red-flags-checklist. (Accessed 15 November 2017).

41. Whelan, A. J., Ball, S., Best, L., Best, R. G., Echiverri, S. C., Ganschow, P., et al. (2004). Genetic red flags: Clues to thinking genetically in primary care practice. *Primary Care*, 31(3), 497–508.

42. Zamosky, L. (2014). *Health care reform and pre-existing conditions: FAQ*. WebMD. Retrieved from www.webmd.com/health-insurance/health-reform -insurance-for-pre-existing-conditions.

43. Genetic Information Nondiscrimination Act (GINA) of 2008. March 2012. Retrieved from https://www.genome.gov/10002328/.

44. Genetic Alliance. Understanding GINA the Genetic Information Nondiscrimination Act. Retrieved from http://www.ginahelp.org/GINA_you.pdf. (Accessed 16 October 2017).

45. The Jackson Laboratory. (2017). GINA-case studies. Retrieved from https:// www.jax.org/education-and-learning/clinical-and-continuing-education/ ccep-non-cancer-resources/gina-overview/case-studies-of-gina-in-clinical -settings.

46. Zhang, S. (March 13, 2017). The loopholes in the law prohibiting genetic discrimination. The Atlantic. Retrieved from https://www.theatlantic.com/ health/archive/2017/03/genetic-discrimination-law-gina/519216/. (Accessed 16 October 2017).

47. Ramos, G. A., & Curevac, Z. (2017). House Committee passes H.R. 1313 allowing employers to collect genetic information under workplace wellness programs. The National Law Review. Retrieved from https://www.natlawreview .com/article/house-committee-passes-hr-1313-allowing-employers-to-collect -genetic-information. (Accessed 16 October 2017).

48. Lewis, R. (March, 9, 2017). Saving GINA: Is genetic privacy in peril? DNA Science Blog. Retrieved from http://blogs.plos.org/dnascience/2017/03/09/ saving-gina-is-genetic-privacy-imperiled/. (Accessed 16 October 2017).

49. American College of Obstetricians and Gynecologists. (2008). ACOG committee opinion No. 409: Direct-to-consumer marketing of genetic testing. *Obstetrics and Gynecology*, 111, 1493–1494.

50. Hahn, E. S. (2016, February 24). Is direct-to-consumer genetic testing right for you? Blog, National Society of Genetic Counselors. Retrieved from https://www.nsgc.org/p/bl/et/blogid=53&blogaid=577.

51. O'Daniel, J. (2010). The prospect of genome-guided preventive medicine: A need and opportunity for genetic counselors. *Journal of Genetic Counseling, 19*, 315–327.

52. Kalf, R. R. J., Mihaescu, R., Kundu, S., de Knijff, P., Green, R. C., & Janssens, A. C. J. W. (2014). Variations in predicted risks in personal genome testing for common complex diseases. *Genetics in Medicine, 16*, 10. doi:10.1038/ gim.2013.80.

53. Harris, A., Kelly, S. E., & Wyatt, S. (2013). Counseling consumers: Emerging roles for genetic counselors in direct-to consumer-testing. *Journal of Genetic Counseling, 22*, 277–288.

54. U.S. Food and Drug Administration (FDA). (2014). Inspections, compliance, enforcement, and criminal investigations: warning letter, 23andme, Inc. Retrieved from www.fda.gov/ICECI/EnforcementActions/WarningLetters/ 2013/ucm376296.htm.

55. Filipski, K. K., Murphy, J. D., & Helzlsouer, K. J. (2017). Updating the landscape of direct-to-consumer pharmacogenomic testing. *Pharmgenomics Pers Med, 10*, 229–232. doi:10.2147/PGPM.S140461.

56. National Library of Medicine. Genetics Home Reference, What are genome editing and CRISPR-Cas9. https://ghr.nlm.nih.gov/primer/genomicresearch/ genomeediting. (Accessed 15 November 2017).

CHAPTER **8**

RISK MANAGEMENT

Deanne Munroe

 Physician referral for any patient seen twice for the same complaint(s) without resolution.

Primary care providers and other health care providers need to understand the malpractice risks inherent in caring for patients in office practices, nursing homes, hospitals, and the community. Unfortunately, despite the best of intentions, health care providers sometimes do not understand how easily a simple error or omission can negatively affect a career, as well as professional and personal relationships and personal well-being. Not every patient concern, unexpected or adverse patient outcome is related to a provider error. However, if a patient care error or unexpected patient outcome occurs, risk management team members should be notified as soon as possible. The purpose of this chapter is to introduce primary care providers to risks associated with clinical practice, provide knowledge that will empower primary care providers, and improve patient care.

NURSE PRACTITIONER MALPRACTICE CLAIMS

Data related to claims asserted against nurse practitioners (NPs) are difficult to determine. Malpractice carriers possess the best information and statistics on malpractice claims and the factors involved in those cases. A malpractice claim is the "tip of the iceberg." Each malpractice claim contains multiple process failures that culminate in the malpractice claim. In outpatient care, the primary allegations are associated with diagnosis, medications, and medical and surgical treatment.[1] Handoff communication and electronic health records (EHRs) play a role in cases with adverse patient outcomes and are discussed later.

The Nurse Practitioner Claim Report

The fourth edition of the Nurse Practitioner Claim Report (NPCR) was published in 2017 and provides an opportunity to learn areas of risk in clinical practice. Areas of the report include closed claims (resolution of the case has occurred) and average aesthetic or cosmetic payout amount. The closed claim area of the report is divided into diagnostic, treatment, and medication prescription sections.

Overall Claims. Four specialties accounted for 80.9% of outpatient NP closed claims: adult and family primary care practice, behavioral health practice, gerontology primary care practice, and aesthetic and cosmetic practice. Of those, 35.9% occurred in the physician office practice setting, 16.4% occurred in the nurse practitioner office practice setting, and 13% occurred in the skilled nursing facility setting. Many involved failure to order a diagnostic test, failure to review the result, and failure to act on the result when appropriate.[1]

Adult primary care closed cases accounted for 41.2% of outpatient NP closed cases with an average payout of $267,476. Family practice accounted for 12.5% of outpatient NP closed cases with an average payout of $251,848.[1]

Gerontology closed claims increased from 10.5% reported in 2012 to 11.9% in 2017.[1]

Behavioral health closed claims accounted for 15.3% of the 30.9% of closed claims and involved improperly prescribed medications and failure to address behavioral health with the average payout of $204,182.[1]

Average Aesthetic or Cosmetic Payout. The average aesthetic or cosmetic payout increased from $51,944 in 2012 to $205,278 in 2017 largely due to one case involving a nurse practitioner who did not follow up on the results of a shave biopsy for more than 1 year, resulting in aggressive squamous cell carcinoma that resulted in the patient's death.[1]

Diagnosis-Related Claims. Diagnosis-related closed claims are subdivided into the following categories: (1) failure to identify observation findings or change in condition, (2) failure to order appropriate tests to establish a diagnosis, (3) delay in establishing a diagnosis, (4) failure to diagnose, and (5) failure to order or address diagnostic test results.[1] The failure to diagnose subcategory accounted for the largest percentage of the claims and involved a failure or delay in the diagnosis of an infection, abscess, sepsis, or cancer. Lung cancer was the most often missed diagnosis, followed by similar rates for missing the diagnoses of pelvic, colon, skin, and breast cancers.[1] In this category, failure to identify changes in condition or new findings had almost double the average payout amount ($500,000) compared to the other categories in the diagnosis-related closed claims.[1]

Treatment-Related Claims. Treatment-related closed claims involve (1) failure to establish or order proper treatment appropriately or in a timely manner, (2) the improper or negligent performance of a treatment or test, and (3) the improper or untimely management of an elderly resident, a medical patient, or a medical complication.[1]

Medication-Prescribing Claims. Medication-prescribing closed claims involving allegations increased to 29.4% in 2017 from 16.5% in 2012. These closed claims involved (1) failure to properly instruct patient on medication instructions, (2) failure to recognize a known complication or adverse interaction of prescribed medications, and (3) improper prescription or management of medication.[1]

IMPORTANT AREAS OF RISK IN PATIENT CARE
Medications

As demonstrated in the NPCR data presented earlier, adverse events related to medication prescription and monitoring are areas that require careful focus in primary care. A 12-year study published in Clinical Toxicology analyzed data from the National Poison Control System and found that every 2 minutes someone calls a United States poison control center regarding a medication error. Approximately 14 of those calls involve a serious medication error requiring medical treatment.[2]

Outpatient medication errors doubled between 2000 and 2012. Errors cited were taking the wrong dose, inadvertently taking a medication twice, and taking someone else's medication, among others. The most common medications involved in serious errors were cardiovascular drugs (accounted for 20.6%), pain medication (e.g., opioids and acetaminophen accounted for 12% of serious errors), and 11% involved hormone therapy, predominantly insulin.[2] To reduce risk when prescribing medications, see best practices in Box 8.1.

Multiple Diagnostic Failures

When a patient sees multiple providers, there is an increased risk that the health care provider(s) will fail to identify the

---

BOX **8.1**

Best Practices to Reduce Risk When Prescribing Medications

- Obtain complete medication history, including prescription medicines, over-the-counter preparations, herbal supplements, or nutritional preparations.
- Before prescribing any new medication, screen medication history for potential interactions with the medication you are considering.
- Give careful instructions how to take the medication, including any food substances or medications (including over-the-counter medications) that should be restricted when taking the prescribed medication.
- Instruct patients about signs and symptoms that indicate a medication reaction and review actions the patient should take if these occur.
- Review with the patient the necessary ongoing monitoring that is required with the medication.
- Establish with the patient parameters for follow-up and what to do if there is no improvement.
- Ascertain the health care literacy of the patient and tailor instructions to individual patients.

BOX **8.2**

Best Practices to Reduce Risk With Collaborative Practice

- Review existing records carefully and completely when seeing a patient who has seen multiple providers for care of the condition.
- Update the family history, personal history, treatment history, and medication history each time you see the patient. At each patient visit, confirm the information on the chart and ask if there are any additions to the record.
- Physician referral is indicated for patients seen for the second time for the same complaint.
- Refer patients to specialist care appropriately.
- Ensure patient follow through with referrals and with ordered diagnostic tests. Document efforts made to ensure patient follow through.
- Review patients who are non-responsive to prescribed management with another provider to identify any additional evaluation or treatment that may be indicated.
- Establish communication with all providers caring for patients.

patient's problem and an even greater possibility that the patient's problem will be overlooked or mismanaged. This type of episodic patient care increases the risk of a malpractice claim for all providers. Some of the factors involved in these types of diagnostic failures include (1) failure to update the family history or to indicate a recent treatment or preexisting disease, (2) failure to make a referral or ensure patient follow-through with a referral or a diagnostic test, (3) failure to require a different evaluation, and (4) failure to communicate with all providers.[3] Multiple diagnostic process failures frequently culminate in multiple claims. Best practices in the area of collaborative care to reduce risk are found in Box 8.2.

DISCLOSURE OF ERRORS AND ADVERSE MEDICAL EVENTS

In 2002, the University of Michigan Health System adopted a policy of sharing investigative findings of adverse events with patients and families. A process of apologizing and offering compensation was initiated when deemed appropriate based on the organization's inquiry. The University of Michigan Health System has reported that this policy succeeded in decreasing litigation costs by half, and new claims fell by more than 40%.[4]

To ensure that the patient and family will receive a consistent message, one person on the health care team is designated as spokesperson to be certain that one message is communicated. Mistrust of the health care team can occur when patients and families hear different information from multiple providers or spokespersons.

Determining the root cause of an adverse event requires effort and time. The Harvard School of Medicine's affiliated teaching hospitals developed the following approach for communicating adverse events to patients and families immediately after the occurrence of the adverse event.[5,6]

- Acknowledge that the event occurred.
- Express regret and empathize with the patient's situation.
- Apologize if appropriate.
- Take appropriate steps to minimize further harm.
- Explain to the patient and family what will happen next.
- Communicate that an investigation will commence to determine how the adverse event occurred.

Discussion of the results of the internal investigation includes the following:

- Disclose the results of the internal investigation.
- Apologize if there has been an error or systems failure.
- Make changes to prevent the failure from recurring.
- Provide continuing emotional support to the patients and health professionals involved.[5,6]

In a situation involving an adverse event, the practitioner may assume an adverse outcome was the result of an error on his or her part and may feel guilt or overwhelming shock. The provider should avoid blaming another practitioner, blaming a piece of equipment, or blaming the system. An appropriate response to patient or family is "I am sorry for your loss. We are doing everything in our power to investigate the facts surrounding this event." The practitioner should continue to demonstrate appropriate empathy when a family's grief or fear manifests as anger or threats of legal action.[6]

Many states have enacted "I'm sorry" laws that bar the admissibility of statements, writings, or gestures expressing apology or condolences. Communication protected by law differs from state to state. "I'm sorry" laws allow the practitioner to apologize without fear of legal repercussions.[7] The provider should know his or her state law; some practitioner statements are admissible in malpractice claims.

THE "SECOND VICTIM"

Practitioners are often the overlooked second victim of a serious medical error that results in permanent serious injury or patient death. The practitioner experiences stress-related psychological and physical reactions. Emotions can range from sadness to anger to despair. Practitioners may fear losing their job; a medical malpractice claim; loss of licensure; and being viewed as incompetent by colleagues, their family, and

the patient's family.[8-13] A wide range of emotions including self-doubt, loss of professional confidence, intrusive thoughts, and embarrassment may surface in the weeks after an event.[8-13]

Signs of post-traumatic stress disorder may develop in the months after an adverse event and manifest as sleep disturbances, flashbacks, insecurity, and thoughts of suicide.[14] Immediate intervention after an event includes debriefing and counseling and is proactive in preventing post-traumatic stress disorder. Some organizations also have informal peer support networks that can be helpful. Potential consequences to the practitioner include leaving the profession,[10] isolation, and deterioration of professional and personal relationships, which may lead to divorce, substance misuse, and suicide.[13,14]

THE NATIONAL PRACTITIONER DATA BANK FOR NURSE PRACTITIONER

The National Practitioner Data Bank collects information disclosed by state boards against NP licensure and certification. Medical malpractice payouts, judgments, and negative actions by peer review and private accreditation organizations are also collected and reported. Also reported are adverse actions taken by state Medicaid fraud units, state agencies administering or supervising the administration of state health care programs, and state law enforcement agencies; civil judgments; and criminal convictions. The preceding reportable information is disclosed upon initial credentialing and at each credentialing cycle thereafter. Information reported by the National Practitioner Data Bank can potentially affect employment as well as licensure.[15]

DEALING WITH BOARD OF NURSING COMPLAINTS

If an NP receives a letter from the board of nursing advising the NP of a complaint, the NP should immediately contact his or her malpractice insurance carrier and then contact an attorney experienced in administrative law (if not provided by the malpractice carrier). Board of nursing complaints usually involve a violation of the nurse practice act related to incompetent, unsafe, or negligent nursing practice that places the patient at risk. Violations include but are not limited to practicing under the influence of drugs or alcohol, practicing beyond the NP's scope of practice, falsifying records, engaging in criminal conduct, or crossing professional boundaries, including emotional, physical, or sexual abuse of a patient. NPs have been falsely accused of misconduct by patients, families of patients, and employers.[16]

Filing a board of nursing complaint against an NP is not complicated. Many board of nursing websites contain a link for submitting a complaint online. The name of the complainant is kept confidential in most cases to protect his or her identity unless the complainant is a key witness to the conduct of the NP. When the board of nursing complaint is unfounded, the complainant is protected from civil liability in most states if the complaint was made in good faith.[16]

The board of nursing will notify the NP in writing of a complaint and the commencement of an investigation. If an investigator or attorney for the board contacts the NP, it is best, from a risk perspective, to obtain that person's contact information, because any statement made by the NP can be used against him or her. The primary role of the board of nursing is to protect the public through regulation of nursing practice, and the board's formal inquiry is analogous to a criminal investigation. A board of nursing complaint may result in the loss of licensure, loss of a career, and fines.[16]

The NP should carry his or her own malpractice insurance. An employer may provide malpractice insurance; however, a conflict of interest may arise, and the NP could then be unprotected.[16] In this situation, the following questions should be asked and answered in writing by any attorney the employer retains to represent the NP in a matter:

- "Who are you working for, me or my employer?"
- "If there is a conflict between my defense and my employer's defense, will you continue to represent me or will you represent my employer?"

The American Association of Nurse Attorneys (TAANA), the American Health Lawyers Association (AHLA), or the state bar association referral service can assist with an appropriate attorney referral. Representing oneself before the board of nursing may result in an unfavorable outcome for the practitioner.[16]

CURRENT NURSE PRACTITIONER LICENSE PROTECTION TRENDS

The 2017 Nurse Practitioner Claim Report analyzed 404 closed cases against nurse practitioner and reported license protection claims affecting CNA/NSO-insured NPs. Two hundred forty claims resulted in license defense cost. The majority of defense fund claims involved medication prescribing and/or management (27.1%), scope of practice (22.1%), treatment and care management (13.3%), and professional conduct (8.8%.)[1]

Legal costs, which included attorney fees, associated travel costs, and reimbursable wage loss under the policy, were averaged at $5987. Legal defense paid claims were made for medical and non-medical regulatory board complaints against nurse practitioners.[1]

TELEMEDICINE

The American Telemedicine Association defines telemedicine as "the use of medical information exchanged from one site to another via electronic communications to improve a patient's clinical health status." Telemedicine has been available for decades formally and informally, and includes a growing variety of applications and services using two-way video, e-mail, smart phones, wireless tools, and other forms of telecommunications technology.[17]

Telemedicine is used to improve access to care and the health of patients in rural and underserved communities. Practitioners must be licensed in the state in which the patient is located; the state of California criminally prosecuted a Colorado practitioner who prescribed medications over the Internet to a patient in California.[18] The primary care practitioner who dispenses advice over the phone or receives a picture of a wound or rash via cellular phone or by electronic mail is participating in telemedicine.

Devices other than traditional landline telephones must meet the compliance requirements of the Health Insurance Portability and Accountability Act (HIPAA) and the Health Information Technology for Economic and Clinical Health (HITECH) Act, including the security of point-to-point contact and the use of encryption-protected devices.[19,20] Protocols and guidelines for telemedicine patient encounters are required.

Professional liability may not cover the exposures inherent to telemedicine: (1) privacy breaches; (2) disruption of telemedicine communication; and (3) errors and omissions of telemedicine practice. Product liability insurance must be considered for equipment failures. Good communication between the practitioner and patient are imperative because breakdowns in communication can lead to patient claims of abandonment.

MEDICAL MALPRACTICE RISK MANAGEMENT STRATEGIES
Patients First

"Patients first" is a value espoused by many organizations emphasizing patient-centered care. However, unless this value is embraced and modeled by health care providers and administrators, patients may not experience the compassionate care and service that strengthens the provider-patient relationship.

Ambulatory medicine should be "customer-centric," emphasizing patient experience and satisfaction. Risk management begins with the patient's first interaction with office staff. The patient should feel valued with his or her initial experience, whether it is a phone call to a receptionist or a call-center operator to schedule an appointment. Policies and procedures for triaging urgent matters requiring a same-day appointment are essential to ensure patient safety and satisfaction. Then, when a patient arrives in the office, front office staff should acknowledge the patient, smile, make eye contact, and maintain a welcoming, professional demeanor.

The patient's experience with office personnel affects the patient's perception of the clinician. Their interpersonal skills and ability to work together as a team decrease liability risk. Treating patients with empathy and kindness is always important. The acronym SHARE[21] encompasses the attitude and skill set that each office staff member should possess:
Sense patients' needs before they ask (initiative)
Help one another (teamwork)
Acknowledge people's feelings (empathy)
Respect the dignity and privacy of everyone (courtesy)
Explain what is happening (communication)

Patient Communication

First Impressions. Communication with patients in all health care settings is an important factor in patient satisfaction and safe care. In ambulatory care, patients should be informed when the practitioner is running behind—ideally at the time of check-in—and then given the option to reschedule the appointment with another provider or for another date and time. This practice communicates respect for the patient's time. Once a patient is roomed, practitioner delays should be communicated to the patient at least every 15 minutes. Staff can use a variety of means to track patient communication about practitioner delays (e.g., a sticky note with the patient's rooming time placed on the door or on a wall-mounted whiteboard or medical chart holder outside the patient's room).

The first few seconds a provider spends with a patient are crucial and are the cornerstone of the patient-practitioner relationship. The first impression made by a health care professional should communicate professionalism and genuine regard for the patient. It is important to recognize that greetings in some cultures may vary. The provider should smile, make eye contact, extend his or her hand, and as a rule shake the patient's hand firmly and confidently. It is important to be aware, however, that handshake culture around the world can vary. For example, in some cultures a gentler handshake is indicated, or it might not be appropriate at all. If the patient has been waiting, apologize and thank the patient for his or her patience.

Although it is important that patients have a favorable experience, patient satisfaction can have unfavorable consequences. We want patients to be happy with the care provided, but patient satisfaction should not override evidence-based practice. For example, taking time to explain to patients why they do not need an antibiotic for acute bronchitis and making an effort to manage patient expectations are important.[22] A prescription for an antibiotic in this example might produce high patient satisfaction scores on a survey; however, prescribing antibiotics inappropriately is not proper and does not aid the patient or society.

Communication Issues. The patient-provider relationship and patient-provider communication are often cited as factors in litigation claims. Having good interpersonal skills and establishing effective communication with the patient and family are paramount in providing safe and effective patient care. More than 20 years ago, Beckmam (1994) found that the patient or family decision to sue was based on problematic physician-patient communication issues that fell into four categories: (1) deserting the patient; (2) devaluing patient and/or family views; (3) poor delivery of information; and (4) failure to recognize or understand the patient and/or family views.[23] Despite this knowledge, there continues to be a positive correlation between patient complaints and malpractice claims.[24]

A review of malpractice claims asserted against CRICO-insured health care providers and the Harvard Medical Institutions from 2006 to 2010 revealed that ineffective communication among practitioners, nurses, residents, or specialists about patients occurred in 42% of cases.[24] Half of these litigation claims involved outpatient cases. Patient communication included issues surrounding informed consent.[24]

Similarly, Levinson and colleagues identified communication behaviors of primary care physicians without malpractice claims. Positive behaviors included managing patients' expectations, using humor and laughter, actively seeking the patients' opinion, encouraging a dialogue with the patient, and confirming patients' understanding of their care. In addition, the length of time spent with the patient during routine visits was a positive predictor of malpractice claims. Physicians without malpractice claims spent more time with their patients.[25]

Listening to patients and families is integral to assessing the patient's clinical condition as well as meeting the patient's needs and expectations. Meeting, anticipating, and managing patient expectations are basic risk management skills and are essential elements in patient satisfaction and patient safety.

In addition, effective patient communication should be stated in a positive manner. For example, the provider should state, "It's my pleasure" or "You're welcome," rather than "It's not a problem." This change may seem small but is significant in setting a positive tone for communication with the patient.

Patient Concerns. Referring to a patient complaint as a *concern* has a more positive connotation. Patient concerns are a great opportunity to view an experience through the patient's eyes, then review and improve processes. In general, patient concerns are handled from an administrative perspective, but there are a variety of ways to review a clinical concern (e.g., a quality-of-care perspective or peer review). A referral to risk management specialists is appropriate when a patient requests a refund or waiver of a balance owed or insurance copayment.

BOX 8.3

Checklist for Handling Patient Concerns

- By phone: Instruct staff to prioritize patients calling and asking for the manager. If the manager is unavailable to take the call, ask staff to document the best time to return the call and the phone number.
- **INTRODUCTION:** In person—Introduce yourself.
  - Discuss the patient's concerns in a private area.
  - Sit down—this communicates to the patient that you are not in a hurry and the conversation can take as long as the patient needs.
- **ACKNOWLEDGE/DESCRIBE:** "I understand we did not meet your needs with _____ (e.g., returning phone calls, scheduling an appointment, getting back to you with your test results). Can you tell me about it?" Take notes as necessary. Listen to the patient until the patient has finished speaking.
- **APOLOGIZE:** "I would like to apologize on behalf of the practice and the staff that we did not meet your needs. This is not the experience we want for our patients."
- **EXPECTATIONS:** Review the patient's concerns and ask questions to ensure you understand what happened. "We take your concerns seriously. If possible, what do you think could be done?"
- **REVIEW CONCERNS:** Tell the patient you will review his or her concerns, and ask what form of response the patient would like. Document this information in an event report.
  - Letter   □ Phone call   □ None
- **INTERVIEW:** Talk to all staff and physicians involved in the incident. Take notes, and update the RDE with either staff or physician statements or results of your interviews.
- **FOLLOW-UP:** Contact the patient in the manner in which the patient previously stated. Most patients will be satisfied to receive a call back and hear that their complaint has been discussed.
  - Offer your direct phone number to patients and invite them to call you if they have any further concerns.
  - If the concern is taken over the phone, tell the patient to ask for you when they come in next for an appointment so you can meet them face to face.
- **EVENT REPORT DOCUMENTATION:** All patient concerns should be entered into an event report.
- **REFER** any patient concern that cannot be addressed immediately to Patient Services if that is an option.[26]

Acknowledging the patient's concern in a positive manner is important—for example, by saying, "I understand that we did not meet your needs or "I am sorry that we did not meet your expectations." Do not assume blame or liability but emphasize that all patient concerns are taken seriously.[26]

Every patient concern should be entered into an event report or an electronic event reporting system designed to track patient concerns and trends over time. Box 8.3 is a checklist for use in addressing a patient concern.

Informed Consent

Informed consent is based on the ethical principle of autonomy and is required for any invasive patient procedure done in an office or health care facility (e.g., joint aspiration, joint injection, biopsy, or lesion excision; may be appropriate for complex medical treatment plans as well). Every competent adult has the fundamental right to self-determination over his or her body.[27] Minors or incompetent adults have the right to be represented by a competent adult who will protect their interests and preserve their basic rights. Informed consent applies to the treating practitioner and the patient unless otherwise stated and documented. A well-written, signed informed consent form serves as evidence that the patient received the appropriate information and is crucial to defending a malpractice claim. Informed consent is just as important in managing the patient's expectations. Malpractice claims may arise when the patient's expectations do not align with treatment outcomes.[28]

A certified medical interpreter should be used for non–English-speaking patients for the informed consent discussion.[29] There is no guarantee that a family member is interpreting correctly. Avoid assumptions of medical literacy based on language fluency. There may be cultural barriers or family dynamics that prevent a family member from interpreting certain medical diagnoses or treatment options. Documentation of the interpreter's name is included either on the informed consent form or in the medical record.

Documentation of informed consent includes the following elements as well as the patient's understanding of the procedure. Procedure-specific informed consent forms can be used that include (1) the nature of the procedure; (2) risks, complications, and expected benefits or effects of the procedure; (3) reasonable alternatives and relevant risks, benefits, and side effects related to such alternatives, including the possible results of receiving no care or treatment; and (4) disclosure of potential conflicts of interest such as financial or research interests.

Excision, shave, and punch biopsies of lesions should be documented with photographs of the marked sites. Photographs should be taken from a distance to give context to the location of a lesion. If a biopsy is positive and requires a referral to a dermatologist or plastic surgeon, the picture taken in the primary care office provides an extra layer of safety in confirming the site for further treatment.

Informed consent is effective until the patient revokes it or until the patient's circumstances materially change. A material change can be a new diagnosis, decompensation in physical status, or a recent update in family history. The material change may alter the risks of the procedure and/or the alternatives to the procedure to which the patient initially consented. Material patient changes require a new informed consent discussion with the patient along with documention.[1,28] Informed consent may be done once for a series of injections—for example, as in a planned series of joint injections. Informed consent is a process that requires thorough documentation.

Universal Protocols and Timeouts

Universal protocols or "timeouts" serve to maximize patient safety and minimize clinical risk. Elements include use of two patient identifiers, involvement of the patient in confirming the correct site, and confirmation of the procedure.[30]

The procedure note contains the following elements:

- Name of procedure
- Location of the procedure
- Skin preparation
- Anesthesia
- Description of the procedure
- Medications used
- How the patient tolerated the procedure

Informed Refusal

Informed refusal is a concept built on informed consent. A patient may not initially fully comprehend the consequences of his or her decision. The health care provider has a duty to discuss the medical consequences of treatment refusal with the patient. Documentation of the informed refusal discussion should include the specific clinical consequences disclosed to the patient. A treatment refusal form confirms that the patient acknowledges the medical consequences of refusing treatment and is aware of the risks of not proceeding with the proposed treatment.[31]

Patient Adherence and Compliance

Missed appointments, failure to follow up with a referral or a diagnostic test, and failure to comply with dietary, medication, or exercise recommendations are all obstacles to improved patient health and safety. When appropriate, missed appointments should be followed up with a letter to the patient that summarizes the clinical consequences of follow-up failure. Concerns regarding patient lifestyle or medication recommendations require exploration to determine factors that may be a barrier to compliance. Patient discussions require specific documentation in the medical record and should include the clinical consequences of continued nonadherence. These discussions should be followed up with a letter describing the clinical consequences of continued noncompliance.

From a medical–legal perspective, the ordering practitioner is responsible for patient completion of referrals, laboratory testing, and diagnostic studies. The practitioner needs to develop a suitable system of monitoring referrals, tests, and other diagnostic studies to be certain they are completed. Each type of health record system, whether paper, electronic, or a hybrid (paper and electronic), poses its own challenges in terms of monitoring when patients complete provider recommendations. The EHR can be optimized to monitor for ordered referrals and tests.[32]

These recommendations are important because in the event of a poor patient outcome, the practitioner's failure to address a patient's noncompliance may be construed by a plaintiff's attorney as condoning the behavior. Patient letters should be sent with a Return Receipt requested and via First-Class Mail. Sending a letter by First-Class Mail creates a legal presumption that the patient received it in the event that the patient does not collect the Return Receipt letter from the post office.

Patient letters should be written at a Flesch-Kincaid level as close to grades 6 to 8 as possible. Grade level can be checked with Microsoft Word. The ease with which a letter can be read should be considered and checked in Word simultaneously with grade level.[32]

Patient Dismissal

Allegations of abandonment can result when a patient is dismissed. To avoid the allegation, certain rules are followed. Patient dismissals may be regulated by the board of medicine, the state department of public health, or individual health plans. It is important to develop an office policy that incorporates applicable regulations and contractual health plan agreements.

Dismissal of patients is done for defined patient behaviors that result in undermining the patient-practitioner relationship.

Behavior ranges from chronic tardiness for appointments that inconveniences other patients and upsets the workflow of staff and practitioners to missed appointments or disruptive behavior. All patient noncompliance and disruptive behavior is documented in an objective manner in the medical record. Documentation supports the practitioner's dismissal decision and is the best evidence to protect against charges of abandonment or medical malpractice.[33]

From a risk perspective, a patient dismissed from one practitioner in a practice is dismissed from the entire practice or group, whichever the circumstances dictate. Otherwise, there is the likelihood that the practitioner will encounter the dismissed patient in the future while covering for another provider within the group practice.

The patient dismissal letter is sent with a Return Receipt requested and by First-Class Mail and should include the following information:

- The last day the practitioner will be available to render emergency medical care, ensuring that the patient will receive emergency care for 30 days
- Indication that medication refills will be provided during this period
- Alternative sources of medical care (e.g., refer to a local medical society's referral service if available)
- Information necessary to obtain the medical records

Patient Handoffs

Patient handoff is the transfer of care of a patient from one practitioner to another. Handoff is a vulnerable time for patients as well as practitioners. Inadequate assessment or communication can result in a poor patient outcome.[34] Checklists help ensure that all pertinent patient information is communicated correctly. Checklists should be standardized and include major diagnoses, recent hospitalizations, procedures, medications, allergies, and pending laboratory and diagnostic studies with the facilities' contact information.[35]

Interruptions should be limited during handoff. Tools such as *SBAR* (situation, background, assessment, recommendations) should be used to keep the communication focused. A "read-back" to confirm that the correct information was received and understood is necessary.[35,36]

ELECTRONIC MEDICAL RECORDS

Offices and other health care facilities may have paper medical records, EHRs, or a combination of both. The HITECH Act mandated adoption of computerized EHRs for patient continuity of care and patient safety. There are differences in EHR software depending on the vendor. Unfortunately, there are possible inherent risks in software that can limit the tasks that can be completed electronically (e.g., entering patient information electronically on a laboratory or pathology order form versus a paper form). The more steps needed to complete a task, the more likely an error can occur. In addition, medical information in the ambulatory or inpatient medical record may not be available because of a lack of an interface or because the information entered is incorrect.

The ECRI Institute Patient Safety Organization (formerly the Emergency Care Research Institute) ranked electronic data hazards as the No. 1 patient safety concern in 2018. The Pennsylvania-based nonprofit indicates electronic health care networks may be vulnerable to ransomware as well as cyber-security threats that can impact patient safety.[37] Infiltration of networks can be accomplished through personal e-mail as well as unregulated use of the Internet.[1]

The Doctors Company conducted a study of EHR-related claims between January 2007 and June 2014 that contributed to professional liability. The EHR Closed Claims Study analyzed 97 EHR-related claims.

System factors included (1) fragmented EHR; (2) system technology/design including lack of HELP Desk support and an outdated medication formulary; (3) failure or lack of alerts, alarms, and clinical decision support; (4) failure to ensure security; (5) lack of provider access during system/technical failure. User factors involved (1) hybrid records, paper and electronic; (2) prepopulating fields or copy and pasting information; and (3) incorrect data entry and user error.[38]

Another risk is the overreliance on system alerts, resulting in alert fatigue from the false-positive warnings and missing real warnings requiring action. "Overlays" may exist between two separate systems that may or may not interface. The expectation of toggling back and forth between systems increases the likelihood of missing information germane to the care of the patient.[38]

The autofill capability of the EMR system should be used cautiously. Bringing all available patient information into a note and not addressing each item is done at the practitioner's peril. This practice results in "note bloat" and the presumption that everything in the problem list was acknowledged and addressed by the practitioner.

EMRs have produced challenges and opportunities to effectively communicate with the patient during an office visit, over the telephone, or through a patient portal. Facing the patient with both provider and patient at eye level is essential to frame and sustain the provider-patient relationship. Providing the patient undivided attention when communicating over the telephone or electronically is a practice that improves patient safety.

The use of speech recognition software to dictate into the electronic record does not eliminate the practitioner's responsibility for reviewing the dictated note. Spelling errors can change the context of the HPI, problem list, assessment, or plan and result in nonsensical words or phrases as well as incorrect information in the EHR.

Release of Information

Release of information (ROI) to third parties requires authorization by the patient or his or her legal representative. Specially protected information, such as information related to drug and alcohol abuse, mental health, and human immunodeficiency virus (HIV) and acquired immunodeficiency syndrome (AIDS) as well as care received under workers' compensation requires specific authorization by the patient or legal representative before release.

Reasonable efforts must be taken to limit the use or disclosure of, and requests for, protected health information to the minimum amount necessary to fulfill the authorized request.[39] The minimum necessary standard does not apply to the following:

- Disclosures to or requests by a health care practitioner for treatment purposes
- Disclosures to the individual who is the subject of the information
- Uses or disclosures made with the individual's authorization
- Uses or disclosures required for compliance with HIPAA Administrative Simplification Rules

- Disclosures to the Department of Health and Human Services (HHS) when disclosure of information is required under the Privacy Rule for enforcement purposes
- Uses or disclosures required by other law[39]

Patient Portals

Patient portals offer secure non-urgent, non-emergency communication between the practitioner and the patient. Depending on the size of the practice or group, a staff member or department may be assigned to follow up on prescription refills and to triage appropriate communication, thus freeing up the practitioner. Consequences regarding patient abuse of the portal should be included in the office or organizational policy.

Patient Request to Amend or Make an Addendum to the Medical Record. Many portals allow patients access to their problem list and the health information contained in their medical records. Patient access has led to an increase in the number of requests for amendments to the medical record or addendum. Aside from the organization's policy and procedures, there may be laws regarding medical record amendment and addendum. Changes should be made based on the presence of an error in the record and not because the patient disagrees with what is written.

Meaningful Use and Automatic Technology

Some organizations are using automatic technology to communicate with patients through voice calls, e-mails, and text messages. An entry is automatically made into the patient's medical record after delivery of the communication. Documentation serves as an attestation for the Preventative Care Reminders measure for both Stage 1 and Stage 2 Meaningful Use. The measure states that reminders for follow-up and preventative care are to be sent to patients by the mechanism the patient chooses, including but not limited to telephone, mail, and secure messaging.[39]

The preceding paragraph sets the stage for the potential risk with the expanded use of this automatic technology for appointment reminders, referral reminders, laboratory reminders, and any other order. The health care provider is ultimately responsible for anything he or she orders and therefore should be notified of missed appointments and patient failure to follow through on laboratory orders, diagnostic studies, and referrals. It is imperative that the health care provider be notified of missed appointments, laboratory tests, referrals, and other diagnostic evaluations.

Electronic Mail Communication With Patients

Private electronic mail does not afford the security mandated by HIPAA to transmit personal health information. Electronic mail communication must be secure. An alternative method of communication with the patient must be established—for instance, a telephone number or address.[40]

The practitioner should refrain from giving medical advice through electronic mail. This recommendation is based on the following scenario: Consider the patient who customarily communicates with the practitioner via private electronic mail. One day the patient e-mails complaining of chest discomfort, but the practitioner is on vacation with no one monitoring his or her private electronic mail. The patient dies 2 days later from a myocardial infarction.[40]

Practitioners are responsible for preserving e-mail communication with or regarding their patients. Electronic mail is electronically stored information (ESI) and as such is subject to discovery. An obligation to retain electronic mail may be triggered by an adverse event, by a notice of a malpractice claim against the practitioner, or in some states by a notice of intent to sue. The practitioner has an obligation to preserve evidence as spelled out in the Federal Rules of Civil Procedure. One must ask, who has control over the practitioner's electronic mail (e.g., Google, Yahoo, or other Internet provider)?[40]

SOCIAL MEDIA

Many office practices have an Internet presence for marketing purposes. It is important that the website not contain false advertisements. Disclaimers are necessary when any medical information appears on the website. The disclaimer must specify that the information posted does not constitute medical advice, nor is the accuracy of the information guaranteed. Users are advised to seek medical attention in the event of a medical emergency.

As data becomes more transparent and more accessible to the public, plaintiff's attorneys will use these data along with The Joint Commission's standards to support allegations and theories of malpractice claims.

Removal of Social Media Posts

The majority of social media sites have a privacy complaint process. The individual whose recognizable appearance is posted is the one who can make the request to have the image removed from the site. An organization cannot ask to have an image removed on behalf of an individual because the organization does not have the same standing.

Threats on Social Media

All threats should be taken seriously. Local law enforcement should be notified, as well as the individual targeted in the threat. A duty to protect or to warn the intended victim has been established by case law and by statute that varies from state to state.[41]

Responding to Negative Comments

Negative comments should be addressed with the individual who posted, if appropriate. The practitioner should not respond publicly to a negative post, nor should protected health information be divulged publicly to answer a post. Avoid responding publicly by attacking the negative poster. Do not ask patients to sign an agreement not to post on social media.

SURREPTITIOUS RECORDING BY PATIENTS

The patient is required to obtain authorization to record an office visit before recording any interaction. Thorough clinical summaries provided to the patient negate the need to tape an office visit. If a staff member believes he or she is being recorded, it is within his or her rights to ask the patient directly, "Are you recording this conversation?" If the patient responds yes, then the staff member may ask the patient to stop and tell the patient, "I do not authorize you to record my conversation with you." If the patient refuses to stop, then the staff member should leave the situation and find the manager. It would be helpful to have staff practice this dialogue ahead of time so that if the situation arises the words will flow easily.[42]

Documentation of the patient recording without permission and the practitioner's discussion with the patient should be placed in the medical record. A follow-up letter sent to the patient reiterating the discussion serves as notice to the patient that the behavior will not be tolerated and evidence for dismissal if needed. Secretly recording is not legal; individual staff members have to consent to having their images or voice recorded. Secret recording makes staff feel uncomfortable and undermines the patient-practitioner relationship. The patient may be made aware of office policies regarding photography and recording via posted signage and through the notice of Patient's Rights and Responsibilities.

NURSE PRACTITIONER SCOPE OF PRACTICE

NPs are nationally certified health care providers licensed by the state in which they practice. As a health care provider caring for patients in a nursing home or in primary, acute, or specialty care, NPs are accountable for patients' well-being and health care outcomes. The scope of practice for NPs varies from state to state. In 23 states and Washington D.C., NPs have full authority to practice independently; 15 states grant reduced practice authorities to NPs requiring regulated collaboration agreement with a physician; and 12 states restrict NP practice by requiring physician supervision, delegation, or team management by a physician. Knowing the scope of practice as prescribed by the board of nursing in the state in which he or she practices is each NP's responsibility.

Ancillary staff mix is a consideration when assessing any practitioner's medical legal risk. NPs work with individuals with a variety of clinical and nonclinical training in the ambulatory setting and need to be aware if staff are practicing within their scope of practice.[43,44] Scope of practice for licensed personnel is defined by the appropriate state board. Medical assistants are not licensed; however, the board of medicine defines the scope of practice for medical assistants in many states.

NPs in independent practice who employ staff may be responsible for the negligent acts or omissions of employees based on the legal theory of *respondeat superior*. The employee must be acting within the course and scope of his employment. The finding of liability is based on the concept of *vicarious liability*, which states that the employer is responsible for the employee's acts of negligence or omissions and not based on anything the employer may have done improperly. Liability attaches to the employer regardless of employee hiring, training, or proof of competencies.[45]

From a risk management perspective, professional liability insurance should cover the NP as well as nursing and all staff in the office. An example of a malpractice claim arising from nonclinical staff is a scheduler failing to recognize the urgency of the patient's stated reason for the appointment, resulting in a delay in care and patient injury. Additional examples include misfiled laboratory and diagnostic study results and failure to communicate patient complaints to the practitioner.

Employees must be held accountable for their actions and behavior. Employee issues must be addressed in a timely manner and documented in the employee file. Problematic employees should not be retained.

LEGAL DOCUMENTS

Legal documents are time sensitive. Subpoenas or letters of intent to sue should be served directly to the named practitioner. Legal documents may also be served by First-Class Mail. There is no prerequisite for them to arrive in an envelope with an attorney's return address. Patients may become plaintiffs, or the party who sues, in a medical malpractice action. When the patient (plaintiff) sues without retaining an attorney, he or she is referred to as a *pro se litigant*. A pro se litigant may download a legal document from the Internet and serve the notice of intent to sue or the subpoena by First-Class Mail, giving the recipient no indication as to the contents of the envelope.

Open all mail immediately. Notify the malpractice carrier and/or risk management at once on receipt of any legal document involving professional practice.

THIRD-PARTY CASES

Third-party cases are those cases in which the health care provider is not a named party in the lawsuit but cared for one of the parties in the legal case who was a patient. The patient may be either the plaintiff—the party bringing the legal action—or the defendant—the party defending against the legal action. Examples of third-party cases include employment discrimination, workers' compensation, motor vehicle liability, and slip and fall cases. Although the NP is not a party to these cases, it is advisable to have an attorney prepare the NP for the deposition.

A plaintiff's attorney may name the treating health care provider as a non-retained expert witness in a third-party case. The health care provider forms his or her opinion based on the injured party's medical history, independent physical examination, diagnostic studies, and so on. A treating health care provider is not hired specifically to testify regarding the injured party's injuries but is sought by the injured party or patient to treat his or her injuries at the time.

In contrast, a retained expert witness is hired by the attorney of the injured party to examine the injured party or other documents and deposition testimony to form opinions outside the realm of the treating health care provider, such as rendering an opinion in response to the other party's retained expert witness.

AGAINST MEDICAL ADVICE

Occasionally a patient has a clinical condition that warrants a transfer to an emergency department by emergency medical services. A patient with the capacity to make medical decisions who has all the information needed to make an informed decision to go against sound medical advice may do so. However, each situation is different. The patient's decision does not relieve the practitioner from the duty of contacting emergency services when the patient is driving himself or herself. The patient cannot refuse to have the NP call emergency services; rather, the patient must refuse emergency services once they arrive on scene. The NP has a duty to a third party in the event that the patient crashes a car and injures someone else or destroys property.

A patient with capacity may leave against medical advice (AMA) when accompanied by someone to drive. The practitioner has an obligation to discuss the risks of leaving AMA. Documentation of the patient's decision should include specific risks, either on an AMA form or in the medical record.[45]

Transportation of Patients to the Emergency Department

Health care providers working on the campus of a hospital should insure transport of patients requiring emergency services by emergency medical personnel. Many hospital campuses have patient transport services through buses, trams,

TABLE 8.1 Overview of Claims by Outpatient Setting

Outpatient Setting	% Claims
Physician Offices & Hospital Clinics	78
Ambulatory & Day Surgery	10
Emergency Department	9
Patient's Home	3

TABLE 8.2 Overview of Claims by Narcotic

Narcotic Pain Medication	% Claims
Dilaudid	34
Morphine	24
Fentanyl	16
Methadone	16
Oxycodone	9

cr gators similar to a golf cart. No patient should be sent for further emergency evaluation by any of the modes of transportation mentioned previously. Drivers are not trained emergency medical technicians and could not provide proper care should a patient require those services during transport.

AREAS OF HEIGHTENED RISK

Narcotic Medications

Medication closed claims were discussed previously. Of the 1770 claims analyzed by The Doctor's Company that closed between 2007 and 2015 involving patient harm due to medication factors, 272 claims or 15% were related to narcotic pain medication. The outpatient setting accounted for 64% of the narcotic pain medication claims. The following tables illustrate the setting and specific pain medication involved in the claims (Tables 8.1 and 8.2).

The claims analysis revealed practitioners prescribed narcotics for pain of undocumented origin (24%), pain related to the spine (22%), joint- or extremity-related pain (9%), mental health issues (6%), and drug abuse/dependence (4%).

Patient allegations involved improper pain management or treatment (70%), wrong medication dose (9%), and wrong medication (3%). Of the 66% of narcotic pain medication patient injury claims, 60% represented death.

Thirty-nine percent of patient contributing factors included noncompliance with the treatment plan, failure to follow instructions, failure to keep or make follow-up appointments and communication issues accounted for 32% of closed claims.[46] Additional risk management of issues involving medication are as follows.

Medication Reconciliation When There Are Multiple Providers

Patients receive health care from various practitioners. One of the biggest risks to patient safety is multiple prescribers. Primary care providers are expected to coordinate care and are responsible for reconciling medications.[47–49] The Joint Commission identifies medication reconciliation as one of their 2018 Ambulatory Health Care National Patient Safety Goals.[47]

Medication Samples and Dispensing

A system of accounting for medication samples and controlling staff access is required. Each sample dispensed should be tracked in a log or documented in the medical record; otherwise there is no way of accounting for patients who may have been given medication that has been recalled by the manufacturer. The health care provider is responsible for educating the patient and explaining the risks and benefits of medications he or she is dispensing.[50] Documentation of the specific education provided is required by many states that place the duty of educating patients about medications with the pharmacist.

Office Medication Administration Safety

The Joint Commission has identified improving medication safety as an Ambulatory National Patient Safety Goal for 2018. Medications should be labeled when withdrawn from the original packaging. Single-dose vials should be used whenever possible. In spite of "the five rights of medication administration," medication administration errors continue to occur. Each wrong medication, wrong dose, wrong route, or patient error should be reviewed from a process standpoint rather than a punitive provider perspective.[47] This perspective advocated by the Institute of Medicine in its 1999 report "To Err Is Human" does not eliminate personal responsibility for errors.[51] Each situation is unique and requires a thoughtful approach to preventing the same error from coming close to or reaching the patient.

Prescription Pad Security

The health care provider is responsible for the security of his or her prescription pads. The pads should be secured at all times when not in use. Patients and staff should not have free access to a prescription pad. Practitioner identity theft as evidenced by fraudulently obtained controlled substances is reportable to the Drug Enforcement Administration (DEA).[52]

Detecting Suicide Risk

Depression should be screened for using the Patient Health Questionnaire (PHQ-9).[53] In addition, behaviors that indicate a serious or immediate risk of suicide that may be precipitated by a recent loss, a painful event, or a major change in the patient's life should be addressed.

Serious risk behaviors for suicide include:
- Talking about feeling trapped or in unbearable pain
- Talking about being a burden to others
- Demonstrating extreme mood swings
- Too little sleep or prolonged sleeping
- Increasing the use of alcohol or drugs
- Isolation or withdrawal
- Agitation, behaving anxious or recklessly
- Showing rage or talking about seeking revenge
- Displaying extreme mood swings
  Immediate risk behaviors for suicide include:
- Voicing feelings of hopelessness
- Statements of having no reason to live
- Searching for a method of killing oneself, obtaining a weapon, or online searches
- Statements regarding wanting to die or kill oneself

Additional considerations include but are not limited to a history of suicide attempt, mental health issues, and family history of suicide.[54,55]

Risks With Chronic Pain Management

The Centers for Disease Control and Prevention (CDC) reports a steady annual increase in drug overdose deaths involving opioids. Opioid overdose deaths have been referred to as a crisis in the United States with politicians and the media calling for action. According to the Diversion Control Division of the Drug Enforcement Administration, opioids were involved in 63,632 deaths in 2016, 174 deaths per day, 1 death every 8.28 minutes with 42,249 or 66.4% of those due to opioids. Opioid overdose deaths have increased five times since 1999.[56] See Chapter 15, Acute, Chronic, End of Life and Oncologic Pain Management, for additional information.

Practitioner's Duty to Prescribe Responsibly. The DEA relegates pain management to the practitioner's judgment, cautioning about prescribing for a "legitimate medical purpose" and in the "usual course of professional practice." The DEA revokes prescribers' registrations for "failure to conform to minimal standards of care of similar practitioners."[57] The DEA's guidance is vague and open to interpretation. The Department of Justice has been active in recent years in shutting down "pill mills"—health care providers or clinics that prescribe opioids without supporting documentation of medical need.

Evaluation of the Patient in Chronic Pain. The CDC has published guidelines for prescribing opioids for chronic pain with the intent to improve a patient's understanding of the risks and benefits of opioid treatment for chronic pain; improve the safety of treatment; and reduce the risks of long-term use including opioid use disorder, overdose, or accidental death. The guidelines present a challenge in defending a malpractice claim or criminal charge, particularly when state boards of medicine have issued chronic pain management guidelines.[58] These guidelines can potentially transform the standard of care when a plaintiff's attorney enters settlement negotiations or argues before a jury.

Establish a Chronic Pain Diagnosis and Medical Necessity. A diagnosis with documentation of medical necessity for chronic pain management must exist for malpractice claims or criminal prosecution to be avoided. The diagnosis is established with a thorough patient assessment, the administration of appropriate risk tools, a careful review of past medical records, and the ordering of new diagnostic studies as appropriate. Nonopioid treatment options must be considered in addition to opioid therapy in developing a treatment plan. Regular reviews of goals, determination of whether goals are met, and therapy adjustment to meet the patient's needs are required. Elements of documentation follow in the next section.[58]

The CDC recommends alcohol screening and brief intervention before prescribing opioids to reduce the risk of accidental death. Risk assessment tools predict opioid abuse and the extent of the substance use problem. Screener and Opioid Assessment for Patients with Pain–Revised (SOAPP-R) predicts possible opioid abuse in chronic pain patients. The Opioid Risk Tool (ORT) predicts aberrant behavior in patients receiving chronic pain management. The CAGE questionnaire evaluates the extent of substance misuse. A patient experienced in diversion will complete the tools without raising a "red flag" with the practitioner.

Similarly, it is just as important to gain insight into how the patient measures his or her own pain and its impact on daily living. There are numerous patient-rated measurement scales—for example, the Wong-Baker Faces Pain Rating Scale, the 0-to-10 numeric pain rating scale, and the Sheehan Disability Scale.[58]

A pain management agreement between the practitioner and the patient establishes documented expectations of opiate use. Pain management agreements should be employed at the third visit within 2 months, for all long-acting opiates, and for pain management that is anticipated to be required for more than 3 months.[58]

The pain management agreement includes but is not limited to addressing safe medication use, frequency of refills, establishment of the one pharmacy that will be used for medication refills, random toxicology screens, and the patient's obligation to inform all health care providers of the medication agreement. From a risk management perspective, the agreement should be formatted to allow the patient to initial each element of the agreement. Patient violation of the pain management agreement provides documentation and establishes the foundation for patient dismissal.[58]

The practitioner has a duty to counsel patients on the risk of overdose. Family members and friends should be involved in education to recognize the signs of overdose. This counseling equates to the patient's informed consent for treatment and should be documented thoroughly.[1,58]

Medical Record Documentation. Medical record documentation of chronic pain assessment and treatment should include the following elements:

- Patient's medical history
- Physical examination findings
- Results of laboratory and diagnostic tests
- Pain management agreement
- Risk assessment results, including screening tools used
- Treatments provided, including medications prescribed or administered (date, type, dose, and quantity)
- Instructions to patients, including discussions of risks and benefits with patient and significant others
- Results of ongoing monitoring of patient progress (or lack of) in terms of pain management and functional improvement
- Consultations
- Any other information used to support initiation, continuation, revision, or termination of treatment and the steps taken in response to aberrant medication use behavior
- Authorization for ROI to other treatment providers
- Results from the Prescription Drug Monitoring Program (PDMP), a statewide database that collects information pertaining to controlled substances
- Treatment plan and objectives, with regular reviews
- Patient consent form
- Patient management agreement
- Documentation of counseling on overdose risk[1,58]

Patient compliance tools are essential to patient safety, as well as practitioner protection should a malpractice claim arise. Compliance tools include (1) random pill counts; (2) random urine toxicology screens; and (3) use of the PDMP. Compliance applies to *all* patients, not just patients thought to have a drug problem. All patients must be treated in the same way to avoid claims of discrimination.[59]

FALLS

The consequences of a patient fall can be devastating. Up to 30% of falls result in moderate to severe injuries such as lacerations, hip fracture, and head trauma. In older individuals, the

BOX 8.4

Falls

Factors That Increase Risk of a Fall	Fall Prevention Methods
Use of an assistive device—for example, walker, cane	Remove obstacles in the waiting and patient care areas
Sensory deficits—poor vision, hearing loss	Offer a wheelchair if appropriate
Impaired judgment	Education of staff on identification of individuals at risk for fall
Altered mental status—confusion, anxiety	Alert in the scheduling or EMR
Medications—narcotics, benzodiazepines, diuretics, stool softeners	Assist patients with transfers into and out of chairs and onto and off of examination tables
History of previous fall[46,60]	

results of a fall may lead to permanent disability or death. A fall may result in a loss of independence or in self-limitation of activity, leading to decreased physical fitness and thus increasing the risk of another fall.[46,60] See Chapter 13, Aging and Common Geriatric Syndromes, for additional information.

A fall in the outpatient setting may result in a general liability claim for injuries to either a patient or visitor. A fall prevention program identifies individuals at risk for a fall. Placing a sign or a symbol such as a falling star similar to those seen in the hospital on the door of a patient alerts everyone in the office of the patient risk. Risk reduction includes employing interventions for high-risk fall patients and educating staff, patients, and families on falls and injury prevention (Box 8.4).[60]

Managing Risk in the Nursing Home

Risk management in the nursing home is complicated by the pervasive cognitive deficits and complex medical problems of the patients. Patients can be very frail and are often taking multiple medications, which increases the risk of adverse events. Areas of concern include preventing falls (see earlier); decreasing use of restraints, both chemical and mechanical; ensuring adequate nutrition and hydration; preventing pressure sores; preventing medication errors and overuse, especially of antipsychotic medication; monitoring residents who are prone to wandering or elopement; and addressing medical concerns on a timely basis. These are the most vulnerable of patients, who are often living in these facilities for extended periods of time. Staff turnover is high, and there is often no medical provider on site. This combination of circumstances requires open and honest communication with residents and families regarding the current condition and concerns as well as solid policies in place to ensure a culture of safety.[61]

CURBSIDE CONSULTATIONS

A curbside consultation is an informal discussion between practitioners regarding a patient. The curbside "consultant" must be clear in his or her communication that opinions rendered are general and not based on a review of the patient's medical record or an examination of the patient. The practitioner seeking advice should not rely on the consultant's opinion for a treatment decision. The name of any curbside consultant is not to be entered into the medical record. If the practitioner insists on the consultant rendering a treatment decision, then a request for a formal consultation is necessary.[62]

It is important to understand the risks inherent in curbside consultations: a plaintiff's attorney may be able to establish a duty to the patient through a curbside consultation when an audit of the EMR reveals the electronic footprint of the practitioner. A plaintiff must prove four elements in a malpractice claim. First, was there a duty to the patient? Was a practitioner-patient relationship established? Second, was the duty breached? Third, was the patient harmed? And last, was the practitioner the proximate cause of the patient's harm?

STAFF AS PATIENTS

Before a provider makes the decision of whether or not to accept as a patient an employee who works in the same office, the provider should consider the following from a risk perspective:

- Patient privacy and HIPAA and confidentiality concerns may be issues.
- Roles may blur between the NP (or any health care provider) and the employee/patient.
- Basic rules should be established to prevent certain circumstances (e.g., an employee approaching a prescriber with a request for a prescription without the expectation of a proper assessment).
- Any medical care or advice rendered to an employee/patient must be documented in the medical record.
- The practitioner may be placed in an uncomfortable situation that affects the practitioner's ability to maintain a professional work relationship with the employee/patient.

PATIENT REQUESTS FOR WAIVER, WRITE-OFF, OR REIMBURSEMENT OF FEES FOR SERVICES

There are occasions when the NP will be asked to write off, waive, or reimburse the fee for their services. There are many reasons for this type of patient request. The practitioner's rationale for considering the patient's request is often based on a patient outcome or the fear of being sued. However, a patient's decision to sue will not be negated by the waiving of a $10.00 insurance copayment; the patient will sue regardless.

From a risk perspective, the routine waiver of copayments may (1) constitute violation of Medicare and Medicaid anti-kickback statutes, false claims, or abuse; (2) expose the organization as well as the practitioner to potential charges of fraud, jeopardizing nonprofit status; and (3) affect contractual obligations with the insurer to collect copayments, as well as the contractual obligation between the insurer and the insured to pay the copayment. In addition, there is no guarantee that the patient will not file a formal complaint or file legal action. Waiver of copayments may be construed by a plaintiff's (patient's) attorney as an indication that an error or mistake was made by the practitioner (i.e., an admission of guilt). Some insurance companies require explanation of why the copayment was waived. An expectation can be created that the patient is entitled to reimbursement of other monies paid for related hospital or outpatient services.

CHAPERONES

Chaperones should be available to make the patient feel comfortable during examinations. The practitioner shows respect for a patient's dignity by providing a comfortable atmosphere as well as appropriate gowns and drapes. Female breast, genital, or anorectal examinations and male genital and anorectal examinations call for the use of a chaperone. Each aspect of an examination should be explained to the patient before any of these physical examinations. Discussions of a sensitive nature should be done privately outside the presence of the chaperone.[63]

Signage displayed prominently in the examination room communicates the policy of providing chaperones. Health care professionals rather than friends or family members should serve as chaperones; this practice helps to protect the practitioner against accusations of physical, emotional, or sexual abuse.[64]

Chaperones should be available to patients of both genders and not withheld because the practitioner is the same gender as the patient. Documentation of the examination includes the presence of and the full name of the chaperone. The offer of a chaperone, any refusal of a chaperone, and subsequent informed refusal discussion should be documented in the patient's record.[65]

POLICIES

Office policies provide guidance for the operation of an office, whereas procedures outline steps in carrying out tasks in the most efficient manner. Procedures create consistency and uniformity in the way that tasks are carried out—for example, answering the telephone or filing. The Joint Commission's Ambulatory Health Care National Patient Safety Goals should be incorporated into office policies and procedures regardless of whether the office is accredited through The Joint Commission.[47] Policies and procedures should be reviewed annually. Revised policies are to be archived and retained. Policies and procedures are retained for the purpose of discovery should a malpractice or general liability suit occur. Policy and procedure retention periods vary.

The following is a list of basic policies for the medical office:
- Medical emergency action plan
- Office safety precautions
- HIPAA policies and procedures
- Release of Information, ROI
- Scheduling policy
- No-shows and cancelled appointments
- Billing and collection policies
- Tracking and filing incoming laboratory and diagnostic study results
- Abnormal laboratory and diagnostic study results—patient notification
- General consent to treat
- Informed consent—for all invasive procedures
- Patient portal
- Disclosure
- Chaperones
- Patient complaints or grievances
- Securing prescription pads
- Medication refills
- Telephone guidelines for issues that require immediate notification of the practitioner
- Chronic pain management guidelines
- Counseling and dismissal of patients
- Medical record retention policy
- Business record retention policy
- Patient request to amend the medical record
- Workplace violence

REFERENCES

1. CNA and NSO Nurse Practitioner Claim Report: 4th Edition. Retrieved from https://www.nso.com/Learning/Artifacts/Claim-Reports/Nurse-Practitioner-Claim-Report-4th-Edition-A-Guide-to-Identifying-and-Addressing-Professional-Liability-Exposures. (Accessed 29 March 2019).
2. Hodges, N., Spiller, H., Casavant, M., et al. (2018). Non-healthcare facility medication errors resulting in serious medical outcomes. *Clinical Toxicology (Philadelphia)*, 56, 43–50.
3. Bradley, J. Failure to connect the dots. CRICO. Retrieved from www.rmf.harvard.edu/Clinician-Resources/Case-Study/2009/Failure-to-Connect-the-Dots-During-Multiple-Visits. (Accessed 29 March 2019).
4. Boothman, R., Blackwell, A., Campbell, D., Jr., Commiskey, E., & Anderson, S. (2009). A better approach to medical malpractice claims? The University of Michigan experience. *Journal of Health and Life Sciences Law*, www.med.umich.edu/news/newsroom/Boothman%20et%20al.pdf. (Accessed 29 March 2019).
5. LaValley, D. (January 1, 2009). Guidelines for disclosure. CRICO. Retrieved from https://www.rmf.harvard.edu/Clinician-Resources/Article/2012/~/link.aspx?_id=1F382144EA8941459E4F0B9D5A4AF037&_z=z. (Accessed 14 February 2018).
6. Keyes, C. Responding to an adverse event. Volume 18 Number 1 April 1997 Forum. Risk Management Foundation of the Harvard Medical Institutions. Retrieved from https://www.rmf.harvard.edu/~/media/Files/_Global/KC/Forums/1997/ForumApr1997.pdf#page=2. (Accessed 14 February 2018).
7. Leape, L. The power of apology, presented May 11, 2006, at the NPSF Patient Safety Congress. Retrieved from www.amednews.com/article/20060612/profession/306129957/7/. (Accessed 14 February 2018).
8. February 14, 2018). Second victims of medical errors and the disclosure movement. The SorryWorks Coalition. Retrieved from www.sorryworks.net/2nd-victims-of-medical-errors-and-the-disclosure-movement-cms-286.
9. Wolf, Z. R. (2007). Health care providers' experiences with making fatal medication errors. In M. Cohen (Ed.), *Medication errors* (2nd ed., pp. 43–51). Washington, DC: American Pharmacists Association.
10. Scott, S. D., Hirschinger, L. E., & Cox, K. R. (2008). Sharing the load. Rescuing the healer after trauma. *RN, 12*, 38–43.
11. Scott, S. D., Hirschinger, L. E., Cox, K. R., McCoig, M., et al. (2010). Caring for our own: Deploying a systemwide second victim rapid response team. *Joint Commission Journal on Quality and Patient Safety, 36*(5), 233–240. Retrieved from http://psnet.ahrq.gov/resource.aspx?resourceID=18023. (Accessed 14 February 2018).
12. Denham, C. (2007). TRUST: The 5 rights of the second victim. *Journal of Patient Safety, 3*(2), 107–119.
13. Rassin, M., Kanti, T., & Silner, D. (2005). Chronology of medication errors by nurses: Accumulation of stresses and PTSD symptoms. *Issues in Mental Health Nursing, 26*, 873–886.
14. Augello, T. (January 1, 2010). Helping clinicians cope after adverse events. CRICO. Retrieved from www.rmf.harvard.edu/Clinician-Resources/Article/2010/Helping-Clinicians-Cope-after-Adverse-Events.
15. National Practitioner Data Bank (NPDB). NPDB research statistics. Adverse actions taken against an advanced practice nurse. Retrieved from www.npdb.hrsa.gov/resources/npdbstats/npdbStatistics.jsp#contentTop. (Accessed 29 March 2019).
16. Nester, M. (May 21, 2004). Defending yourself against a BON complaint. Advance Healthcare Network for Nurses. Retrieved from http://nursing.advanceweb.com/article/defending-yourself-against-a-bon-complaint.aspx. (Accessed 21 October 2014).
17. American Telemedicine Association. (2012). What is telemedicine? American Telemedicine Association. Retrieved from www.americantelemed.org/about-telemedicine/what-is-telemedicine.
18. Hageseth, V. The Superior Court of San Mateo County, 59 Cal. Rptr.3d 385 (Cal. Ct. App. 2007). Law Link. Retrieved from www.lawlink.com/research/CaseLevel3/84446.
19. Department of Health and Human Services (HHS), Office of the Secretary. 45 CFR Parts 160, 162, and 164. [CMS-0049-F] RIN 0938-AI57; Health Insurance Reform: Security Standards. 8334 Fed Reg Vol. 68, No. 34 / Thursday, February 20, 2003 / Rules and Regulation. Retrieved from www.hhs.gov/ocr/privacy/hipaa/administrative/securityrule/securityrulepdf.pdf.
20. Department of Health and Human Services (HHS), Office of the Secretary. 45 CFR Parts 160, 162, and 164. [CMS-0049-F] RIN 0938-AI57;

Health Insurance Reform: Security Standards. 8334 Federal Register / Vol. 68, No. 34 / Thursday, February 20, 2003 / Rules and Regulation. Retrieved from www.hhs.gov/ocr/privacy/hipaa/administrative/securityrule/securityrulepdf.pdf.

21. Lee, F. (2014). Introduction. In *If Disney ran your hospital* (pp. 1–7). Bozeman, MT: Second River Healthcare.

22. Kravitz, R. (1998). Patient satisfaction with health care: Critical outcome or trivial pursuit? *Journal of General Internal Medicine, 13*(4), 280–282. Retrieved from www.ncbi.nlm.nih.gov/pmc/articles/PMC1496942. (Accessed 5 March 2019).

23. Beckman, H., Markakis, K., Suchman, A., & Frankel, R. (1994). The doctor-patient relationship and malpractice. Lessons from plaintiff depositions. *Archives of Internal Medicine, 154*(12), 1365–1370. Retrieved from www.ncbi.nlm.nih.gov/pubmed/800268. (Accessed 14 February 2015).

24. Hoffman, J., & Raman, S. (2012). Communication factors in malpractice cases. Retrieved from www.rmf.harvard.edu/Clinician-Resources/Article/2012/Insight-Communication-Factors-in-Mal-Cases. (Accessed 29 March 2019).

25. Levinson, W., Roter, D., Mullooly, J., Dull, V., & Frankel, R. (1997). Physician-patient communication. The relationship with malpractice claims among primary care physicians and surgeons. *JAMA: The Journal of the American Medical Association, 277*(7), 553–559.

26. Texas Medical Association. How to handle patient complaints. Retrieved from www.texmed.org/Template.aspx?id=4110. (Accessed 14 March 2019).

27. American Nurses Association (ANA). Short definitions of ethical principles and theories: familiar words, what they mean? Retrieved from www.nursingworld.org/MainMenuCategories/EthicsStandards/Resources/Ethics-Definitions.pdf. (Accessed 1 January 2015).

28. Morton, R. Informed consent: Substance and signature. The Doctors Company. Retrieved from www.thedoctors.com/KnowledgeCenter/PatientSafety/articles/CON_ID_000333. (Accessed 12 March 2015).

29. U.S. Food and Drug Administration (FDA), U.S. Department of Health and Human Services (HHS). (2014). Non–English speaking subjects. in A guide to informed consent—information sheet. Guidance for institutional review boards and clinical investigators. Retrieved from www.fda.gov/RegulatoryInformation/Guidances/ucm126431.htm#illiterate. (Accessed 29 March 2019).

30. American College of Obstetricians and Gynecologists (ACOG). (2004). Committee on professional liability. *Obstetrics and Gynecology, 104*(6), 1465–1466.

31. Crane, M. Best ways to deal with noncompliant patients. The Doctors Company. Retrieved from www.medscape.com/viewarticle/703674_3. (Accessed 2 May 2015).

32. U.S. Department of Health and Human Services (HHS), Centers for Medicare and Medicaid Services (CMS). Toolkit for making written material clear and effective. Section 4: Special topics for writing and design. Part 7: Using readability formulas: a cautionary note. Retrieved from www.cms.gov/Outreach-and-Education/Outreach/WrittenMaterialsToolkit/Downloads/ToolkitPart07.pdf. (Accessed 29 March 2019).

33. Dixon, L. Terminating patient relationships. The Doctors Company. J8729 4/12. Retrieved from www.thedoctors.com/KnowledgeCenter/PatientSafety/articles/CON_ID_000326. (Accessed 27 March 2015).

34. Schuldt, L. (Ed.), (2010). *The Joint Commission. Improving communication during transitions of care* (p. 3). Joint Commission Resources, Inc.

35. Agency for Healthcare Research and Quality (AHRQ). Handoffs and signouts. Retrieved from www.psnet.ahrq.gov/primer.aspx?primerID=9. (Accessed 29 March 2019).

36. Boyle, D. (2013). Course notes for communicating in the office. COPIC Insurance. Retrieved from www.callcopic.com/resources/Eduction%20Course%20Materials/323132_Comm.%20Tech.%20in%20the%20Office%20course%20notes.pdf. (Accessed 14 April 2015).

37. ECRI Institute. 2015 Top 10 health technology hazards. Retrieved from www.ecri.org/Pages/Thank-You-2015-Hazards.aspx. (Accessed 22 July 2014).

38. The Doctors Company. Electronic Health Record Closed Claims Study. Retrieved from https://www.thedoctors.com/the-doctors-advocate/fourth-quarter-2017/electronic-health-record-closed-claims-study/. (Accessed 20 December 2017).

39. U.S. Department of Health and Human Services (HHS). Minimum necessary requirement. 45 CFR 164.502(b), 164.514(d). Retrieved from www.hhs.gov/ocr/privacy/hipaa/understanding/coveredentities/minimumnecessary.html. (Accessed 2 September 2017).

40. U.S. Department of Health and Human Services (HHS). Health information privacy. Does the HIPAA Privacy Rule permit health care providers to use e-mail to discuss health issues and treatment with their patients? Retrieved from www.hhs.gov/ocr/privacy/hipaa/faq/health_information_technology/570.html. (Accessed March 2019).

41. 45 CFR Part 164, Subpart C. Security standards for the protection of electronic protected health information. Retrieved from www.ecfr.gov/cgi-bin/text-idx?SID=66ebc4ad481f8b758a4cc747c17d258b&mc=true&node=se45.1.164_1318& rgn=div8. (Accessed 7 October 2015).

42. Chesanow, N. (February 17, 2015). Should patients be permitted to record doctor visits? Retrieved from www.medscape.com/viewarticle/838207.

43. American Nurses Association (ANA). Scope of practice. Nursing World. Retrieved from www.nursingworld.org/sop. (Accessed 29 March 2019).

44. American Nurses Association (ANA). State law and regulation. Nursing World. Retrieved from www.nursingworld.org/statelawandregulation. (Accessed 15 January 2015).

45. Levy, F., Mareiniss, D., & Iacovelli, C. (2012). The importance of a proper against-medical-advice (AMA) discharge. How signing out AMA may create significant liability protection for providers. *The Journal of Emergency Medicine, 43*(3), 516–520.

46. U.S. Department of Health and Human Services (HHS), the Agency for Healthcare Research and Quality (AHRQ). National Center for Patient Safety Falls Toolkit 2004. National Center for Patient Safety Falls Toolkit. (Accessed 9 May 2018).

47. The Joint Commission (TJC). Ambulatory health care: 2018 national patient safety goals. Introduction to reconciling medication information. Retrieved from https://www.jointcommission.org/assets/1/6/2018_AHC_NPSG_goals_final.pdf. (Accessed 14 February 2018).

48. Agency for Health Care Quality and Research (AHQR), U.S. Health and Human Services. Medication reconciliation. Retrieved from http://healthit.ahrq.gov/ahrq-funded-projects/emerging-lessons/medication-reconciliation. (Accessed 29 March 2019).

49. Klein, C. (2006). Dispensing pharmaceutical samples: A few reminders. The Nurse Practitioner. Retrieved from www.nursingcenter.com/lnc/pdfjournal?AID=639809an=00006205-200604000-00004&Journal_ID= & Issue_ID. (Accessed 26 February 2015).

50. The Joint Commission (TJC). (November 14, 2014). Ambulatory health care: 2015 national patient safety goals. Improve the safety of using medications. Retrieved from www.jointcommission.org/assets/1/6/2015_NPSG_AHC1.PDF. (Accessed 29 March 2019).

51. Institute of Medicine. (November 1999). To err is human. Retrieved from http://iom.edu/~/media/Files/Report%20Files/1999/To-Err-is-Human/To%20Err%20is%20Human%201999%20%20report%20brief.pdf. (Accessed 26 February 2015).

52. Drug Enforcement Administration (DEA), Department of Justice. Dispensing of controlled substances for the treatment of pain. FR Doc 04-25469. Federal Register: November 16, 2004 (Volume 69, Number 2200.) Notices Page 67170-67172. From the Federal Register Online via GPO Access [wais.access.gpo.gov]. Retrieved from www.deadiversion.usdoj.gov/fed_regs/rules/2004/fr1116.htm. (Accessed 14 April 2015).

53. Patient Health Questionnaire (PHQ-9)—US Preventive Services Task Force Retrieved from https://www.uspreventiveservicestaskforce.org/Home/GetFileByID/218.

54. Suicide Prevention Resource Center. Warning Signs for Suicide. Retrieved from https://www.sprc.org/sites/default/files/resource-program/RS_warningsigns.pdf. (Accessed 25 March 2018).

55. American Foundation for Suicide Prevention. Risk Factors and Warning Signs. Retrieved from https://afsp.org/about-suicide/risk-factors-and-warning-signs/. (Accessed 25 March 2018).

56. Centers for Disease Control and Prevention. Understanding the Epidemic. Retrieved from https://www.cdc.gov/drugoverdose/epidemic/index.html. (Accessed 25 March 2018).

57. U.S. Department of Justice. Drug Enforcement Administration. Diversion Control Diversion. Practitioner's Manual. Section V. Valid Prescription Requirements. Retrieved from https://www.deadiversion.usdoj.gov/pubs/manuals/pract/section5.htm.

58. CDC Guideline for Prescribing Opioids for Chronic Pain—United States, 2016. Retrieved from https://www.cdc.gov/drugoverdose/prescribing/resources.html. (Accessed 5 March 2018).

59. The Doctors Advocate First Quarter 2017/ Prescription Opioid Abuse Epidemic. Analysis of Medication Related Claims from The Doctor's Company. Retrieved from https://www.thedoctors.com/the-doctors-advocate/first-quarter-2017/analysis-of-medication-related-claims-from-the-doctors-company/. (Accessed 25 March 2018).

60. Centers for Disease Control and Prevention (CDC). Falls among older adults. Retrieved from www.cdc.gov/HomeandRecreationalSafety/Falls/adultfalls.html. (Accessed 2 May 2015).

61. Weinberg, A., & Levine, J. (2015). Clinical areas of liability. Risk management concerns in long term care. *Annals of Longterm Care, 13*(1), 26–32.

62. Shepard, S. Curbside consultations. The Doctor's Company. Retrieved from www.thedoctors.com/KnowledgeCenter/PatientSafety/articles/CON_ID _001610. (Accessed 22 July 2014).

63. American Medical Association (AMA). Opinion 8.21—Use of Chaperones during physical exams. Retrieved from www.ama.assn.org/ama/pub/ physician-resources/medical-ethics/code-medical-ethics/code-medical-ethics/ opinion821.page. (Accessed 2 September 2017).

64. American Academy of Pediatrics (AAP). (2011). American Academy of Pediatrics (AAP) policy statement—use of chaperones during the physical examination of the pediatric patient. *AAP News, 32*(5), 1. Retrieved from http://www.ama-assn.org/ama/pub/physician-resources/medical-ethics/ code-medical-ethics/opinion821.page. (Accessed 2 September 2014).

65. American Society of Healthcare Risk Management. Risk management pearls on principles for developing safe and effective policies and procedures 2011 Edition.

Primary Care: Adolescence Through Adulthood

CHAPTER 9

ADOLESCENT ISSUES

Jean Sheerin Coffey

Adolescence spans the age range from the start of puberty to the transition to young adulthood. There is variation in the progression through the adolescent years as each child experiences the physical and emotional changes at their own unique pace. It is a period of rapid growth with significant physical, cognitive, emotional, and psychosocial development. The age range generally stated for adolescence is between 11 and 21 years of age.[1] In recent years the endpoint of adolescence has come into question and is not as well defined, with stated ranges anywhere from 20 to 24. The variation is due to recent societal changes related to this phase of life. These include young adults remaining in their childhood home well into their 20s.[2]

Despite some of the challenges associated with this life stage, most adolescents develop typically without major difficulties. The role of the clinician is to support the young person and their caregivers through this transition with a focus on both physical and emotional health. Adolescent- and youth-friendly care, as described by adolescents, includes: a clinician attitude of respect as well as friendliness, high-quality clinical communication skills, medical competency, accessibility, confidentiality, teen-oriented materials, opportunity for self-directed care, and support for transition to adult health care.[3] The clinician must also support parents and caregivers as their role and interactions with the adolescent evolve and change. The parent/caregiver role is to continue to offer guidance while providing independence to the youth.

It is incumbent on the clinician to assure confidentiality for the adolescent visit while respecting parents and caregivers. The clinician must be well versed in the state and federal parental notification laws. Consequently, the clinician must be vigilant to potential threats to confidentiality, such as billing statements and insurance notification. Adolescents are more likely to seek care if they feel they will be afforded a confidential visit. However, in a recent integrative literature review it was estimated that as many as 40% of US adolescents do not receive confidential care. The same review indicated that the providers' assurance of confidential care seemed to prompt the adolescent to share sensitive information with that clinician.[4]

Adolescence is a time when youth may engage in risky behaviors that can lead to significant consequences. The brain at this age does not resemble that of an adult and will not until the early 20s. As scientists continue to study the adolescent brain, it is clear that the part of the brain responsible for top-down control matures last. In addition, the adolescent's emotional responses are heightened, and their ability to keep emotional impulsive responses in check is decreased, contributing to risk-taking behavior.[5] The challenges facing youth include substance use, interpersonal violence, mental illness, questioning of sexual orientation, sexually transmitted diseases, eating disorders, poor school performance, injury, housing instability, and food insecurity. The clinician must work to identify the risks as well as protective factors that can support the adolescent during this challenging time.[1]

The transformation in adolescence is gradual and is often delineated by three stages: early (ages 10 to 14), middle (15 to 17), and late (18 to 21), with each stage having physical, emotional, cognitive, and psychosocial-emotional developmental milestones that vary with each youth.

Individuals in early adolescence challenge authority, experience wide mood swings, reject the activities and ideation of childhood, can be argumentative or disobedient, and desire more privacy. This period is marked by tremendous physical growth that is rapid ("growth spurt"). Secondary sex characteristics and puberty accompany preoccupation with normal body changes such as menses or nocturnal emissions ("wet dreams"). Greater sexual interest occurs during this stage. An imaginary audience may influence behavior and increase insecurities.[6] Peer groups, manifested by close friendships with those of the same sex along with contact with members of the opposite sex in groups, may become more important than parental influence. These adolescents may express future plans and an emerging value system; although these ideations are initially idealistic, they may change frequently. During this stage, health promotion should focus on the immediate impact of behaviors. Priorities for health promotion in this age group include evaluating physical growth and development, social and academic connectedness, and emotional well-being. Risk reduction with regard to substance use, tobacco use, and sexual activity (pregnancy and sexually transmitted infections [STIs]), along with violence and injury prevention, is important.[1]

Individuals in middle adolescence (those aged 15 to 17 years) are strongly influenced, positively or negatively, by peer groups. Physical growth slows for females but continues for males, and puberty is typically completed during this stage. In addition, the "tired teenager" surfaces, sexual drive heightens, and fad behavior predominates. This is the age of experimentation with sex, drugs, different types of friends, and risk-taking behaviors. However, as abstract thought continues to develop, consideration of the future and goal setting increase, as does intellectual ability. Health promotion goals outside of physical growth and development continue to include risk reduction related to tobacco and substance use and an increased focus on safer sexual activity. As youths spend more time away from their families and develop more independence, an increased emphasis on injury prevention, avoidance of texting while driving, substance use, and evading interpersonal violence is of utmost importance.[1]

As they become emancipated from the nuclear family, individuals in late adolescence (those over age 18) begin to assimilate adult roles. At this age, adolescents are becoming more comfortable with their body image, and abstract thinking matures. Peer influences remain important. Adolescents pursue realistic goals, understand the consequences of their behavior, and may be able to delay gratification by the end of this period. However, parts of the brain develop at different times, in particular the prefrontal cortex, and impulse control may not fully develop until young adulthood.[4] Physical growth and development are complete in females; however, males continue to gain height, muscle mass, and body hair. Priorities for this stage include evaluation of physical growth and development, use of substances, reproductive health, and transitions to adult care.[1]

PHYSICAL DEVELOPMENT

Although growth occurs over a continuum, adolescence is marked by a 15% to 18% growth spurt, during which time about 95% of the adult size is reached.[1] Before that growth spurt occurs, other specific pubertal physical changes take place. These changes are regulated by the endocrine feedback systems, including the somatotropic, the adrenal, and the hypothalamic-pituitary-gonadal axes, as well as by interplay with the thyroid axis. For girls, physical changes typically begin with breast development or breast buds around the age of 10 years.[7] For boys, testicular enlargement at an average age of 11.5 years marks the initiation of puberty.[8]

The average age at menarche, which follows a growth spurt, is 12.5 years, with more than 95% of girls experiencing menarche between 10.5 and 14.5 years of age. African-American girls may experience an earlier menarche. Dysmenorrhea is rare during the first few periods as they are usually anovulatory. Girls acquire fat during puberty because a body fat composition of at least 17% is needed for menarche, and 22% to maintain regular ovulatory cycles. Girls may have asymmetric breast development in the early stages. Physiologic leukorrhea, which begins several months before menarche, may continue for several years. Puberty for female adolescents is completed with the sculpting of the body, resulting in the familiar adult shape.[7]

For boys, the first sign of puberty is around age 11 and begins with testicular enlargement. Nocturnal emissions begin after testicular and penile growth is under way and dreams become more sexual in nature under the influence of hormones. Male adolescents may have tender or non-tender gynecomastia or unilateral breast buds, which may be present for about 1 year. Testicular asymmetry is also common. These adolescents may need reassurance that the size of the penis is not an indication of sexual functioning, and they should be made aware that impregnation is a possibility because the testicles are probably capable of producing a few sperm at ejaculation. The remaining male physical developmental changes include voice deepening, axillary hair, and facial hair.[8]

Pubertal changes in adolescents should be tracked with each physical examination by use of the Sexual Maturation Scale (SMS) or Tanner stages. The family history will often dictate the timing of puberty, but it is worrisome for boys when testicular enlargement occurs before the age of 9.5 to 10 years (precocious) or when no changes have occurred by the age of 13.5 years (delayed). It is equally worrisome for girls when breast buds appear before the age of 8 to 8.5 years (precocious) or when no breast buds have appeared by the age of 13 years (delayed). An easy and inexpensive intervention to evaluate these variations is the bone age radiograph. If the bone age (wrist) is less than the chronologic age but is still appropriate for height, no further diagnostic testing is necessary.[7] For adolescents who have not reached puberty and for whom an evaluation of the hypothalamic-pituitary-gonadal axis is being considered, referral to a pediatric endocrinologist is warranted because interpretation of hormone test results and treatment require a specialist.

COGNITIVE DEVELOPMENT

A distinguishing feature of adolescent thought is abstract reasoning. By late adolescence, many youth can understand and create general principles or formal rules to explain many aspects of human experience. Piaget called this last stage of cognitive development, which is ideally attained by approximately 15 years of age, formal operational thought. However, many adolescents arrive at this cognitive stage later than the age of 15 years. One of the qualities of adolescence that is most exasperating to parents is that adolescents are able to reason well in academic subjects but at the same time exhibit illogical thinking about their own lives. It is normal for youths to argue and go on tangents, jump to conclusions, and be self-centered and dramatic. It is important for caregivers and clinicians to understand this as a normal part of growth and development, which may help them to understand adolescent behavior. Simply listening and not correcting, unless there is risk involved, is the best approach to use with adolescents.[9]

The capacity of a person to learn will never be greater than during adolescence. However, with increasing sophistication and mental agility, an egocentric attitude emerges and peaks at about 13 years of age. The belief that they can handle anything and that adults do not understand them can lead adolescents to engage in risk-taking behaviors such as drug use and unprotected sex. It is important to note that despite this higher level of thinking, adolescents continue to need guidance from adults to develop and make rational decisions. Adults can also assist adolescents to make better decisions by helping them to weigh their options and consider consequences, as opposed to telling them which decision is the correct one.[4]

EMOTIONAL DEVELOPMENT

Throughout adolescence, the parts of the brain involved in keeping emotional, impulsive responses under control are still reaching maturity.[4] A major task for youths is to learn to manage their emotions and cope with common emotions such as disappointment, stress, and anger. The quest for identity, a major task of adolescence, is accomplished in part by the development of new goals and the abandonment of childhood aspirations. The successful management of emotions combined with increased moral development is referred to as an individual's "emotional intelligence" (EI). A high degree of EI helps the adolescent master skills in building relationships and getting along well with others.[10]

SOCIAL DEVELOPMENT

Successful identity formation depends on the support of family and friends. Peer groups are important not only to social development, but also to development of the transition between childhood dependency and adult independence. This is a period of heightened self-consciousness, and adolescents are often preoccupied with other people's thoughts and opinions of them.[11] This has been termed *egocentrism* and was described as the "imaginary audience" and the "personal fable" by psychologist David Elkind and is a normal part of adolescent development.[6]

Given the developmental tasks of increasing independence, some parental conflict is inevitable. A consistent and fair parenting style can help alleviate the ongoing conflict. Parents can be influential, especially if family members respect one another and engage in rational discussion. If parents recognize and become more comfortable with the growing autonomy of their adolescent, the difficulties will usually diminish with time. Adults can engage adolescents with questions that are nonthreatening and open ended. It is essential to be nonjudgmental and refrain from asking "why," which can put adolescents on the defensive. Neighborhoods, faith institutions, school, and work are also important influences on development. "Rites of passage" such as bar or bat mitzvahs, achievement awards, proms, parties, driver's licenses, voter registration, and graduations foster, focus, celebrate, and further the attainment of adult identity.[1]

THE ADOLESCENT HEALTH VISIT

A comprehensive health history should be taken at the visit. The provider must take into account the family structure and support system as well as the socioeconomic and cultural background of the youth. Anticipatory guidance for health promotion, safety, and risk issues is also addressed. The focus of these guidelines varies with each stage of adolescence. Therefore, modifications based on variations of patient populations are recommended.

The comprehensive adolescent health visit should begin with the parent present for the initial interview to assess the family and patient medical, mental health, and surgical history. Family practices such as household smoking, rules, meals, and safety are discussed in addition to routine health screening questions. The parent's presence at the beginning of the adolescent interview affords the opportunity to observe the relationship between the adolescent and the parent. The adolescent should remain dressed at this stage of the visit. Careful explanation of the changing provider-patient relationship for adolescents and the safeguarding of their privacy are stressed. At this time, parents should be asked about their current concerns or stressors. Once these have been addressed, parents should be asked to leave the room to provide the adolescent privacy for the remainder of the visit.

Adolescents may delay medical care if privacy is not ensured, so the interview continues in private with the adolescent. The format of the visit should also be explained, and confidentiality should be maintained. Before proceeding, inform adolescent patients of what the limits of confidentiality are, such as not sharing answers to personal questions unless someone is hurting them or they are hurting themselves. After information about the patient's diet, elimination, and sleep habits has been elicited and screening has been done for hearing and vision, the remainder of the health history can be organized around the mnemonic *HEADSS FIRST*. In this assessment, adolescents are asked about home, education, activities, drugs, sexual activity, suicide or depression, friends, image, recreation, safety issues, and threats.[12]

BOX **9.1**

CRAFFT Questions

- Ever ridden in a car driven by someone who was high or had been using drugs (including yourself)?
- Ever use alcohol or drugs to relax, feel better about yourself, or fit in?
- Ever use alcohol or drugs while you are alone?
- Ever forget things you did while using alcohol or drugs?
- Do family or friends ever tell you to cut down on your drinking or drug use?
- Ever in trouble while using alcohol or drugs?

From Martin, J., & Sokol, B. (2011). Generalized others and imaginary audiences: A neo-Meadian approach to adolescent egocentrism. *New Ideas in Psychology, 29*(3), 364–375.

ADOLESCENT SUBSTANCE USE

Research has shown that approximately 46% of middle school and 77% of senior year high school adolescents have used alcohol.[1] Affirmative answers to questions concerning the use of drugs or alcohol can be further explored with a useful mnemonic: *CRAFTT* (cars, relax, alone, forget, friends, trouble) (Box 9.1).[1,13,14] Smoking, drinking, and illicit drug use are the leading causes of injury and death in this population. Misuse of prescription drugs is highest among adolescents in the 18- to 25-year-old age range. In addition 80% to 90% of adult smokers began during adolescence. Protective factors to help prevent adolescent substance use include connectedness to parents and participation in extracurricular activities. Clinicians are best to refer positive screens for substance use to a counselor or targeted program for youth.[1]

ADOLESCENT MENTAL HEALTH

Mental health problems affect a large number of adolescents. Teens frequently present in primary care with symptoms of anxiety and depression. Screening patients for these diagnoses using established instruments is the most reliable approach to care, as some teens do not present with classic symptoms of either illness.

Screening for depression can be done with the Patient Health Questionnaire (PHQ)-2. If the results are positive the teen can be given the PHQ-9 which is more specific and can be used to assess depression severity. A referral for immediate psychiatric assessment is indicated if the adolescent has made a suicide plan or has actually attempted suicide (Box 9.2).[15]

Attention deficit disorder is a chronic health condition that must be treated in the adolescent years. Adequate treatment can reduce school dropout rates and increase success in setting and attaining goals in school. Adolescents who are treated for their illness are less likely to abuse drugs and alcohol than their peers.[8]

Adolescence is a time where mental illness symptoms may become more apparent, leading to diagnoses such as anxiety and bipolar illness. Youth may also exhibit symptoms of eating disorders and disordered eating during this time.[8] Screening for anxiety in the primary care setting can be done with the generalized anxiety disorder (GAD)-7.[16] If the youth is positive for anxiety, referral to psychotherapy is the preferred treatment. The clinician will make a referral to a psychiatrist for more complex mental illness diagnoses, such as suspected bipolar illness.

Suicide Risk Factors

- Recent loss of a family member
- Social isolation
- Family history of affective disorders
- Interpersonal problems with peers
- Sexual identity concerns
- Abuse or neglect
- Exposure to suicide
- Prior attempts
- Suicidal ideation with a plan
- Physical illness or injury
- Intense life stresses
- Poor coping skills

ADOLESCENTS AND INTERPERSONAL VIOLENCE

Interpersonal violence refers to being a victim of, perpetrator of, or witness to harmful behaviors that are physical or emotional and can start early and continue into adulthood. This includes behaviors that range from bullying, slapping, or hitting to robbery and assault, as well as emotional harm. Given that the need to belong is so prevalent during adolescence, joining a gang may inappropriately fulfill that need.[17] Some children and adolescents are motivated to join a gang for a sense of connection or to define a new sense of who they are. Others are motivated by peer pressure, a need to protect themselves and their family because a family member also is in a gang, or to make money.[16,17] Teen bullying is another cause of interpersonal violence and a major societal issue. In the wake of school-related violence, it warrants screening and intervention efforts. Bullying is the use of power to cause distress to another.[18] A referral to appropriate professionals for conflict resolution, anger management, or assertiveness training should be considered. A suspicion of abuse mandates reporting according to the laws in each state.

ADOLESCENTS AND SEXUAL ACTIVITY

Sexually active adolescents need counseling regarding safer sexual activity, including reducing the risks of STI and human immunodeficiency virus (HIV) infection. The use and limitations of condoms should be explained. Contraception options are also addressed during this discussion. All 50 states and the District of Columbia have confidentiality laws regarding sexual health in teens. Adolescents should be made aware that they are able to seek care without parental consent and should be informed about confidentiality laws as they pertain to sexual health.[7]

BODY PIERCINGS AND TATTOOS

The need for self-expression during adolescence is manifested in many ways including body piercings and tattoos. These practices afford the youth the opportunity for uniqueness, however the permanence of the decision and the risks are typically not considered by the adolescent. The phrase *think before you ink* may help the adolescent in the decision-making process.[18] Avoidance of infection and blood borne illness can be the greatest challenge when getting a tattoo. Assessment of the tattoo business's reputation and cleanliness may mitigate the risk. Body piercings are also permanent and can pose a risk for infection and blood borne illness. Healing of piercings depends on the site. The range of time to heal is about 4 weeks for the tongue and up to nine months for a piercing in the navel. The clinician can provide guidance on how to reduce the risks associated with body art during the health visit.[19]

PHYSICAL EXAMINATION

Annual adolescent preventive visits continue to the age of 21 to 25 years and include appropriate anticipatory guidance and a complete physical examination.[1] The abbreviated preparticipation visit for sports is no longer recommended as the youth is better served with the benefits of a complete physical exam that includes screening questions for sports participation risk.[8] Height, weight, vital signs (including blood pressure), and body mass index are obtained and graphed appropriately for age and gender. The findings from these examinations should be explained to the patient. Privacy should be respected to the extent possible, and parents should remain out of the room during the exam.

The routine gynecological exam with cervical cell sampling and Papanicolaou (PAP) testing begins at age 21. The initial reproductive visit is important because it sets the tone for future visits. Routine testing for STI including chlamydia and HIV are done at the adolescent visit.[7]

Precollege visits are an opportune time to update the adolescent's records, including the evaluation of immunization status, and to offer anticipatory guidance regarding sexuality (e.g., contraception, risks and prevention of STIs and HIV infection, responsible sexual behavior, prevention of sexual assault), cardiovascular health (e.g., nutrition, exercise, smoking), injury prevention (e.g., automobile and campus safety), obesity prevention, and mental health (e.g., stress, substance use, eating disorders). This visit is also a good time to begin the discussion regarding the transition to adult care.

HEALTH MAINTENANCE AND HEALTH PROMOTION

Unlike for younger children, health promotion as a focus of anticipatory guidance should shift from the parent to the adolescent. Although working with parents is also essential, it is important to build autonomy in the adolescent patient and to address risk factors in balance with strengths and assets.

Immunizations are an important part of health promotion and should be reviewed and updated at these annual visits per the published Centers for Disease Control guidelines. This includes recommendations on tuberculosis (TB) screening which is not usually performed unless the patient has risk factors for TB or the test is required for college admission or employment. High-risk groups include close contacts of a person with infectious disease, foreign-born persons from areas where TB is common, and persons from medically underserved and low-income populations.

Adolescence is a challenging time for providers, parents, and adolescents themselves. However, this is an important transitional period of rapid growth and development; health habits, attitudes, and beliefs can carry into adulthood, and the provider's role should not be underestimated. Providers are in an opportune place to provide comprehensive health promotion, education, and care to youths, and to have a positive impact and influence on the emerging adult during this important life stage (Box 9.3).

BOX **9.3**

Resources for Caring for Adolescents

American Academy of Child and Adolescent Psychiatry
3615 Wisconsin Ave., NW
Washington, DC 20016-3007
800-333-7636
www.aacap.org
American Academy of Pediatrics
141 Northwest Point Blvd.
Elk Grove Village, IL 60007
847-434-4000
www.aap.org
American Psychological Association Parenting
http://www.apa.org/topics/parenting/
Bright Futures
Family Tip Sheets
www.brightfutures.org/TipSheets/index.html
Center for Young Women's Health, Boston Children's Hospital
333 Longwood Ave., 5th Floor
Boston, MA 02115
617-355-2994
www.youngwomenshealth.org
www.youngmenshealth.org
PFLAG: Parents, Families, and Friends of Lesbians and Gays
1726 M St., NW, Suite 400
Washington, DC 20036
202-467-8180
www.pflag.org
Society for Adolescent Health and Medicine (SAHM)
www.adolescenthealth.org
Suicide Prevention Hotline
800-621-4000

Transition from adolescence to adulthood results in a firmer sense of identity and emotional stability and involves the attainment of economic and emotional independence from parents. As adolescents transition into adulthood, they have established sexual identity and the development of meaningful relationships. This life stage often culminates with a concern for the future and interest in moral reasoning and the hallmark milestones of the adolescent period: an increased capacity for abstract thinking.[20]

REFERENCES

1. Bright Futures Guidelines for Health Supervision of Adolescents. Fourth Edition 2017.
2. Sawyer, S., Szzoparedi, P., Wickremarathne, D., & Patton, G. (2018). The age of adolescence. *The Lancet, 2*(3), 223–228.
3. Ambresin, A. E., Bennett, K., Patton, G., Sanci, L., & Sawyer, S. (2013). Assessment of youth-friendly health care: A systematic review of indicators drawn from young people's perspectives. *Journal of Adolescent Health, 52,* 670–681.
4. Baldridge, S., & Symes, L. (2018). Just between us: An integrative review of confidential care for adolescents. *Journal of Pediatric Health Care, 32*(2), e45–e58.
5. The teen brain: Still under construction-national institute of mental health. Retrieved from https://infocenter.nimh.nih.gov/pubstatic/NIH%2011-4929/NIH%2011-4929.pdf. (Accessed May 2018).
6. Elkind, D. (1967). Egocentrism in adolescence. *Child Development, 38*(4), 1025–1034.
7. Emans, J., & Laufer, M. (2012). *Pediatric and adolescent gynecology.* Philadelphia: Wolters Kluwer.
8. Burns, C. E., Dunn, A. M., Brady, M. A., Starr, N. B., & Blosser, C. G. (2012). *Pediatric primary care* (5th ed.). St. Louis: Elsevier.
9. Young woman's health, be there for teens: A guide for parents. Retrieved from https://youngwomenshealth.org. (Accessed 13 June 2018).
10. Mavroveli, S., Petrides, K. V., Rueffe, C., & Bakker, F. (2007). Trait emotional intelligence, psychological wellbeing and peer rated social competence in adolescence. *British Journal of Developmental Psychology, 25,* 263–275.
11. Martin, J., & Sokol, B. (2011). Generalized others and imaginary audiences: A neo-Meadian approach to adolescent egocentrism. *New Ideas in Psycholology, 29*(3), 364–375.
12. Cohen, E., Mackenzie, R. G., & Yates, G. L. (1991). HEADSS, a psychosocial risk assessment instrument: Implications for designing effective intervention programs for runaway youth. *Journal of Adolescent Health, 12*(7), 539–544.
13. Center for Adolescent Substance Abuse Research (CaASAR). The CRAFFT screening tool. Retrieved from www.ceasar-boston.org/CRAFFT/index.php. (Accessed 13 June 2018).
14. Pilowsky, D., & Wu, L. (2013). Screening instruments for substance use and brief interventions targeting adolescents in primary care: A literature review. *Addictive Behaviors, 38,* 2146–2153
15. Sahni, A., & Agius, M. (2017). The use of the PHQ9 self rating scale to assess depression within primary. *Psychiatria Danubina, 29*(Suppl. 3), 615–618.
16. Spitzer, R. (1960). A brief measure for assessing generalized anxiety disorder: The GAD-7. *Archives of Internal Medicine, 166*(10), 1092–1097.
17. American Academy of Child Adolescent Psychiatry Gangs and Children. Retrieved from https://www.aacap.org/AACAP/Families_and_Youth/Facts_for_Families/FFF-Guide/Children-and-Gangs-098.aspx. (Accessed 13 June 2018).
18. Seylor, C., et al. (2012). Bullying and ostracism scales BOSS; development and application. *Journal of Children's Health, 41*(4), 322–343.
19. Young Men's Health. Retrieved from http://youngmenshealthsite.org. (Accessed 13 June 2018).
20. American Psychological Association and Maternal and Child Health Bureau, Health Resources and Services Administration, U.S. Department of Health and Human Services. (2002). The developing adolescent. Retrieved from www.apa.org. (Accessed 13 June 2018).

CHAPTER **10**

LGBTQ PATIENT CARE: CARE OF SEXUAL AND GENDER MINORITY PEOPLE

Charles Yingling • Karen F. Cotler • Cindy Broholm

INTRODUCTION

Sexual and gender minority (SGM) people live, work, and receive health care throughout the country. Census data demonstrate that gay, lesbian, bisexual, and transgender people are part of the communities of every state in the nation.[1,2] This chapter provides an introduction to providing primary care for SGM communities, including understanding the terminology used to describe SGM communities, using appropriate language to describe and interact with SGM patients, applying the minority stress theory to understand health disparities in SGM communities, and developing treatment plans to promote health and prevent disease in SGM populations.

DEFINITIONS

Often, SGM communities are referred to by acronyms such as LGBT, LGBTQ, or LGBTQIA. These initials represent an expanding understanding of the different groups (lesbian, gay, bisexual, transgender, queer/questioning, intersex, and asexual) that make up SGM populations. Tables 10.1 through 10.4 introduce the terminology associated with SGM populations.

TABLE 10.1   Sexual Minority Terminology

Social/Community Term	Definition	Comparable Behavioral Term
Lesbian (adjective or noun)	Women who form romantic and/or sexual relationships with other women	Women who have sex with women (WSW) An exclusively behavioral term, primarily for clinical and public health data
Gay (adjective)	Men or women who form romantic and/or sexual relationships with people of the same sex	Men who have sex with men (MSM) Women who have sex with women (WSW) An exclusively behavioral term, primarily for clinical and public health data
Bisexual (adjective)	People with the capacity for romantic and/or sexual relationships with both men and women	Same as social/community term
Asexual	A person who does not feel sexual attraction towards others	N/A

TABLE 10.2   Gender Minority Terminology

Term	Definition
Transgender (adjective)	A person whose gender identity differs from their assigned biological sex
Cisgender (adjective) Note—this term is used for parity in communication when discussing gender identity and is not considered a gender minority	A person whose gender identity is the same as their assigned biological sex
Intersex (adjective)	A person who has discordance in their sexual organs (e.g., having both a penis and ovaries)
Genderqueer Gender nonconforming Gender fluid Gender non-binary	Terms that some people may use to describe fluidity in gender as well as an expression of gender that is neither male nor female

TABLE 10.3   Terms That May Be Used in Both Sexual Minority and Gender Minority Communities

Term	Definition	Comments
Queer (adjective)	A term that describes a sexual orientation or gender identity different from the majority	While many people may describe themselves as queer, the term may be pejorative to other SGM people
Questioning (adjective)	A term that describes an individual who is developing their sexual or gender identity	

SGM, Sexual and gender minority.

TABLE 10.4   Inappropriate or Outdated Terminology

Community	Term	Rationale
Sexual minority people	Homosexual	Outdated term that can be offensive
	Alternative lifestyle	Inaccurate term that implies deviation from an unstated norm
	Dyke, queen, fag	Slang terms that may be used by sexual minority people to describe themselves, but should never be used by clinicians
	Sexual preference	Inaccurate term that implies choice in sexual orientation
Gender minority people	Transvestite	Outdated, inaccurate term that implies pathology
	Cross-dresser	Inaccurate term to refer to transgender people
	Transsexual	Outdated term to describe transgender people
	Hermaphrodite	Outdated term to describe intersex people

In any community, individuals' definitions of themselves may vary from the definitions and descriptions placed on them. For example, some men who have sex with men (MSM) do not identify as gay men. So as you approach the content in this chapter, be mindful that patients may use their own terminology to describe themselves. We provide these definitions here so that health care professionals may approach an understanding of this material from a common starting point.

Many people think of the SGM population as an aggregate. However, this often leads to confusion for clinicians who may be new to caring for patients in these communities. Sexual minority people are people whose capacity for romantic attraction and formation of intimate relationships (i.e., sexual orientation) is something other than exclusive attraction to people of the opposite sex. Gender minority people are people whose sense of being male, female, or another gender entirely (i.e., gender identity) is something other than their assigned biological sex. Sexual orientation and gender identity (SO/GI) are mutually exclusive constructs.

While there are common challenges facing many SGM people (e.g., stigma, discrimination), there is no cohesive experience of being an SGM person. The *intersectionality* of race, class, gender, culture and geography can serve to exacerbate or mitigate the stresses associated with being a member of an SGM group. For example, a white gay man from an affluent community will likely have a very different experience with how his sexual orientation affects his health and well-being than an African American lesbian woman from the same affluent community. While both individuals may experience prejudice or stigma as sexual minorities, an African American lesbian woman will face additional experiences of prejudice based on her race and gender.

CULTURAL HUMILITY

In proceeding with this unit on SGM health care, it is helpful to view these communities through the lens of *cultural humility*. In nursing education and professional development, it is common to hear the phrase *cultural competence* when approaching content about caring for populations other than the majority. However, this approach is flawed in that it falsely connotes an endpoint at which the learner becomes competent in the care of this population. A cultural humility approach[3] urges the learner to accept that their own culture and background permanently affect the way they view others. Rather than trying to master a checklist of common cultural traits that may or may not apply to the community of interest, the cultural humility framework urges learners to look inward and be aware of their own beliefs, values and biases that may affect the care they provide. Further, the cultural humility framework invites respectful questions and embraces the reality that no person is a representative of any given culture.

MINORITY STRESS THEORY

In the remainder of this chapter, the concentration will be focused on understanding the health needs of select sexual minority communities: gay men/MSM, lesbian women/women who have sex with women (WSW), bisexual people and asexual people, and gender minority communities (transgender people and intersex people). Each of these communities has unique health needs that are driven, in part, by the health disparities they face.

The Minority Stress Theory[4] provides a framework to understand the health disparities in SGM communities. While developed with a focus on sexual minority people, the Minority Stress Theory helps to understand the experiences of gender minority people in many ways as well. The Minority Stress Theory posits that health disparities in sexual minority people are due to societal prejudice and hostility towards gay, lesbian, and bisexual people. *Experiences of prejudice* (e.g., anti-gay words or actions), *internalized homophobia* (i.e., the belief that there is something inherently wrong with one's sexual orientation), and *expectations of rejection* (e.g., a lesbian adolescent's fear that her family will shun her) can lead to *hiding and concealing* (e.g., denying one's sexual orientation) and a great deal of psychological stress. In an effort to relieve that stress, sexual minority people may seek out *ameliorative coping processes* to feel better. Some of these processes may be helpful, such as finding a network of friends to provide emotional support. Other efforts to relieve this stress can be harmful, such as overuse of alcohol and other drugs or engaging in high-risk sexual practices. Ultimately it is the cumulative effects of stress and negative ameliorative coping processes that explain many of the health disparities faced by SGM communities.

GENERAL PRINCIPLES OF CARING FOR SEXUAL AND GENDER MINORITY PEOPLE

Entry-level competencies for primary care providers include the independent provision of patient-centered, culturally sensitive care that incorporates a patient's values, beliefs and preferences.[5] These competencies include the ability to identify personal biases that may affect the quality of care.[5] This section of the chapter will aid providers in preparing themselves and their practice setting to care for SGM patients by learning to identify their own biases that may affect care, familiarizing themselves with practice-level strategies to create a safe and welcoming climate for SGM patients, and improving communication strategies.

Biases

All people have biases that inform their interactions with others.[6] *Implicit biases* are unconscious, automatic, and pervasive responses to people or situations.[6] Implicit biases form during childhood in response to prevailing family and societal values.[6] Due to a societal preference for heterosexuality and cisgender identity, most people, including people who are themselves members of an SGM group, exhibit biases against SGM people.[7] It is common for implicit biases to be in conflict with one's stated values or beliefs.[6] Even a provider who expresses an openness to caring for SGM groups can have implicit biases that may affect the quality of care.

Knowledge of one's own biases allows one to be aware when those biases are affecting the care they give. Evolving science suggests that awareness of a bias can facilitate it being "unlearned."[6] A helpful tool to identify biases is the Implicit Association Test (IAT). There are several tests and they are freely available from Harvard University's Project Implicit program (https://implicit.harvard.edu/).

PRACTICE-LEVEL STRATEGIES TO IMPROVE CARE OF SEXUAL AND GENDER MINORITY PEOPLE

In addition to staff familiarity with SGM communities, there are strategies that can improve the experience of care for SGM patients. The Joint Commission and the Gay and Lesbian Medical Association both provide resources that can lead to the creation of welcoming practices for SGM people.[8,9] These strategies include visual cues to SGM patients, work processes that are sensitive to SGM people's needs, physical facilities, and communication strategies that promote inclusivity.

Visual Cues

Visual cues that SGM patients are welcome in the practice can include the display of welcoming iconography (e.g., rainbow flag or pink triangle). A clearly posted nondiscrimination statement that includes references to SO/GI can serve as another cue that the practice welcomes all patients. Inclusion of images of same sex couples and families as well as transgender people in online and print materials (e.g., brochures, patient education) are other cues to SGM people that the practice is a welcoming one.

Work Processes

Work processes that impact SGM people are typically intake forms and interviewing tools. The U.S. Department of Health and Human Services requires that all electronic health records certified under stage 3 of the Meaningful Use program have the ability to capture data about a patient's SO/GI.[10] Asking these questions is not only welcomed by most patients, but also serves as a cue to SGM patients that the practice is sensitive to their needs.[11] Fig. 10.1 illustrates the two-step strategy to asking SO/GI questions on intake forms. Additionally, intake forms should solicit a patient's preferred gender pronouns (e.g., she/her/hers) so that those pronouns can be used when interacting with or discussing that patient.

Physical Facilities

Physical facilities that promote inclusivity include access to all-gender restrooms in both waiting areas and clinical areas. Labeled all-gender restrooms provide a visual cue to gender minority patients that the practice is sensitive to their needs.

Do you consider yourself to be:
- ☐   Straight
- ☐   Lesbian or gay
- ☐   Bisexual
- ☐   Other
- ☐   Don't know/Not sure
- ☐   Decline to Answer

Additional Information:_____

What is your current gender identity?
(Check all that apply)
- ☐   Male
- ☐   Female
- ☐   Female-to-Male (FTM)/Transgender Male/Trans Man
- ☐   Male-to-Female (MTF)/Transgender Female/Trans Woman
- ☐   Genderqueer, neither exclusively male nor female
- ☐   Additional Gender Category/(or Other), please specify
- ☐   Decline to Answer

Additional Information:_____

What sex were you assigned at birth on your original birth certificate?
(Check one)
- ☐   Male
- ☐   Female
- ☐   Decline to Answer

Additional Information:_____

F I G. 10.1 Sexual Orientation and Gender Identity Questions With 2-Step Gender Identity Question.

Additionally, these facilities assure that gender nonconforming people are not compelled to use a restroom that does not feel appropriate to their gender identity.

Communication Strategies

Effective clinical communication with SGM patients requires two strategies: use of normalizing statements to introduce sensitive questions and avoidance of heteronormative language and assumptions. *Normalizing statements* frame the question that is to follow and give the patient permission to answer honestly. An example of this when collecting a sexual history would be: "Sexuality is an important part of human health, so I talk to all my patients about sexual practices and sexual orientation. Would it be alright if we talked about that topic now?" Assuming an affirmative response, a follow-up question may be, "Are you sexually active?" and to that question, "Are your sex partners men, women or both?" The Centers for Disease Control and Prevention (CDC) provides a comprehensive guide to sexual history taking.[12]

Avoidance of *heteronormative language* means that the health care provider does not make assumptions about a patient's sexual orientation or behaviors. Examples of heteronormative language include [to an adolescent male], "Have you asked a girl to the dance yet?" or [to an adult man at his child's well-child check], "You and your wife must be delighted to have such a beautiful child." At a minimum, heteronormative language can be dissatisfying to a patient. At its worst, heteronormative language can fuel mistrust in the health care system and avoidance of needed care.

CARE OF SEXUAL MINORITY PEOPLE

It is difficult to precisely quantify the number of people in the United States who identify as gay, lesbian, or bisexual. In recent national surveys, between 3.5% and 4%[13,14] of adults identified as gay or lesbian, and 5.5% of women and 2% of men self-reported a bisexual identity.[15] However in one study, between 8.1% and 10.6% of adult male respondents ($n = 866$) and between 9.8% and 16.7% of adult female respondents ($n = 1269$) reported having had sexual contact with someone of the same sex at least once in their life.[16]

It is important for the primary care provider to distinguish identity (gay, lesbian, bisexual) from behavior (MSM or WSW). As evidenced in the statistics above, many people who have had same sex partners do not identify as gay, lesbian, or bisexual. There are a variety of reasons that people who have same-sex partners may not identify as being a sexual minority. Some reasons include community or familial intolerance of an LGB identity, internalized homophobia, or sexual activity during incarceration. Therefore, it is essential to consider both the patient's stated sexual orientation as well as sexual behaviors when developing a plan of care.

Care of Gay Men/MSM

Health Disparities. Gay men suffer a disproportionate burden of mental health and behavioral health problems as compared to straight men. These problems include an excess burden of depression, eating disorders, substance use, and intimate partner violence.[17] When examined through the lens of the Minority Stress Theory, the primary care provider should consider that many of these problems are rooted in the constructs of minority stress and negative ameliorative coping mechanisms. Further, gay male communities are marketing targets for tobacco and alcohol makers.[18,19]

MSM suffer a disproportionate burden of sexually transmitted infections (STIs), including HIV. Amplifying this excess burden is the intersectionality of race and sexual orientation. If current infection rates continue, one in two black MSM and one in four Latino MSM will be infected with HIV in their lifetime.[20] Among MSM overall, the risk of HIV infection is one in six.[20]

Among all patients, there are specific sexual behaviors that increase the risk of STIs. Receptive anal sex confers a greater risk for contracting an STI than penetrative anal sex. So when quantifying risk for MSM, it is important to fully understand the patient's sexual practices. The CDC provides a tool for taking a structured sexual history that includes specific sexual practices.[12]

Lifespan Considerations in Primary Care.

Adolescence. A sense of one's sexual orientation typically becomes clear in early adolescence.[17] Though it may take a number of years until a gay or bisexual male adolescent affirms his identity, the primary care provider can support his emotional and physical health until that time. Primary care recommendations for gay or bisexual male adolescents are no different than any other patient. However, the primary care provider should be particularly aware of mental health risks including depression and suicidality due to minority stress. In particular, gay adolescents may experience bullying in school[21] which can lead to excessive absenteeism and mental health consequences.

The US Preventive Services Task Force (USPSTF) recommends screening for depression in all adolescents.[22] However, the primary care provider should be mindful that gay male adolescents have higher rates of depression than their straight counterparts.[21] This excess rate of depression is highly correlated to experiences of rejection in the home and in school.[21]

While depression can cause significant morbidity in gay adolescents, it is also associated with higher rates of suicidality.[23] An important role of the primary care provider in caring for gay male adolescents is not just to affirm and support the adolescent's sexual identity, but to educate the family as well on the negative mental health effects of rejection.

Young Adults/Adults. Young adult and adult gay men and MSM should receive all the same age-appropriate preventive services as their heterosexual counterparts. However, there are certain preventive services to which the primary care provider should be attentive when caring for gay men and MSM.

Substance Use. Gay men have higher rates of substance use than age-matched heterosexual peers.[17] This includes tobacco, alcohol, and recreational drug use. The drivers of this problem include ameliorative coping processes, previously discussed, as well as targeted marketing to gay men by the tobacco and alcohol industries.[18,19] The USPSTF recommends screening all adults for tobacco use[24] and alcohol use,[25] but does not find sufficient evidence to screen all adults for recreational drug use.[26] Nevertheless, we recommend that all clinicians caring for SGM patients screen for recreational drug use given higher rates of substance use in these communities.

Vaccinations. In an effort to prevent the spread of the human papillomavirus (HPV), the 9-valent *HPV vaccine* is recommended for all children beginning as early as age 9.[27] However, for individuals that did not receive the vaccine in childhood, MSM are among the priority groups to receive the vaccine at any time until age 26.

In the United States, 10% of new hepatitis A cases and 20% of new hepatitis B cases occur in MSM.[28] Though *hepatitis A and hepatitis B vaccines* are part of the routine childhood vaccine schedule, the CDC recommends both vaccines be offered to adult MSM who have not been vaccinated.

Anal Dysplasia Screening. Screening for anal dysplasia (anal Pap smear) is a consideration among MSM as well as women who have anal sex. Currently, there is insufficient data to support a program of universal screening for anal dysplasia in MSM.[29,30] However, among MSM with HIV, there is growing consensus among HIV providers to screen for anal dysplasia using Pap testing.[31] If a practice implements a screening program for anal dysplasia, it is essential to have a referral mechanism to a facility with high resolution anoscopy for follow up. There is no consensus guideline for the frequency of anal dysplasia screening.

HIV and STI Prevention. Beginning in adolescence, all young people should receive counseling and resources to prevent HIV and other STIs. Since STIs and HIV occur at higher rates in MSM populations,[32] it is important for health care providers to tailor screening and prevention strategies to these communities. Screening for STIs among MSM includes routine testing for HIV, syphilis, gonorrhea, and chlamydia. It is essential that specimen collection for gonorrhea and chlamydia be from all sites of possible exposure—oropharyngeal, anorectal, urethral.

Any MSM who is at high risk for HIV infection should be offered HIV pre-exposure prophylaxis (PrEP).[33] HIV PrEP is a comprehensive program of HIV prevention which includes once daily tenofovir/emtricitabine. HIV PrEP can prevent up to 92% of new cases of HIV and at the 22nd International AIDS conference in 2018, it was revealed that on-demand PrEP (day before and after high risk behavior) and daily PrEP were equivalent. The PARTNER-2 Study, also presented at the 22nd International AIDS conference, indicated that an undetectable HIV viral load is equivalent to no HIV infection.

Family Planning. Many gay men will choose to start families. While family planning for gay men will typically occur outside of the primary care setting, the primary care provider can be a resource for family planning tools including adoption resources and assisted fertility resources (e.g., surrogacy). There is a very limited body of research on family planning for SGM populations,[34] but excellent resources outside of the health care literature[35] exist for providing care to these communities.

Geriatric Considerations. The primary care of gay and MSM elders does not differ from the care of any other older adult. However, the primary care providers should be mindful that sexual minority elders face a multitude of challenges that are unique. Social isolation for older adults who never had families, stigma surrounding sexual orientation, and financial barriers are all factors that can adversely affect healthy aging in sexual minority people.[36] Further, the phenomenon of "re-closeting" (concealing one's sexual orientation after coming out) is reported in long-term care settings and can dramatically affect quality of life in gay elders.[37] Comprehensive resources are available for providing care to these communities.[36]

Care of Lesbian Women/WSW

Health Disparities. Similar to gay men, lesbian women may exhibit disproportionately higher rates of mental and behavioral health problems as compared to straight women. These issues include tobacco use, alcohol and drug use, depression and eating disorders.[38] These behaviors are likely developed as a means to ameliorate stress associated with being a sexual minority (as described by the Minority Stress Theory). However, when considering health disparities in WSW, it is important to recognize the great diversity in this population and the intersectionality of other factors such as race and class and their impact on the health of individuals.

Some research suggests lesbian women may have increased rates of ovarian and breast cancer.[39] Other research suggests that any excess cancer risk in sexual minority populations is limited to cancers related to HPV or HIV.[40] All research in this area is limited by inconsistency in data collection of sexual orientation. If there is an excess risk of breast or ovarian cancer in lesbian women, it is likely related to later age of first pregnancy or nulliparity.[41] But all cancer risk is exacerbated by discrimination or negative experiences with the health care system that reduce lesbian women's access to preventive services such as mammography and cervical cancer screening.[42]

Lifespan Considerations in Primary Care.

Adolescence. Health promotion recommendations for lesbian and bisexual adolescents are no different than for straight or questioning adolescents. However, because of discrimination and social attitudes, lesbian and bisexual teens, like their gay male and transgender counterparts, are at increased risk of being bullied, physically and sexually assaulted, and ostracized, leading to disproportionate rates of depression, anxiety, and suicide.[43] Family rejection or fear of rejection can further compound the toll on the adolescent's mental health. The primary care provider can play an important role in the patient's physical and emotional health by providing an accepting environment, identifying youth at risk, and making prompt referrals to supportive agencies.

It is important to remember that the development of sexual orientation is a process and identity and behavior can differ.

While a teen may identify as lesbian, she may also be sexually active with males. There is some evidence that bisexual teen girls may be at higher risk for STIs as they may be less likely to use condoms or other barrier methods, have multiple sex partners, and experience more coercion in sexual contact as compared to heterosexual teen girls.[44] STI screening and education should be based on behavior rather than identity. As mentioned earlier, it is important to avoid heteronormative language and not assume, for instance, that a teenage girl needs contraception. Asking if the patient is having sex with men, women, or both rather than asking whether she needs birth control normalizes the possibility that she can be sexually active and that you are willing to hear with whom she chooses to be sexual.

Young Adult/Adult. Any woman who has had any sexual contact with another person is at risk for HPV-related disease. It is recommended that screening for cervical cancer begin after 21 years of age.[45] For women who have never had penetrative intercourse (whether with a man or with sex toys), this may be an uncomfortable procedure. The health care provider should be aware that for any woman, a pelvic examination can resurface memories of past trauma or abuse. The recommendations for cervical cancer screening are evolving and it is important to be aware of current guidelines that may provide varied options for screening such as HPV testing without cervical cytology.[46]

Health promotion and screening activities are related to behavior regardless of sexual orientation. As mentioned before, women who identify as lesbians may also be having sex with men and be at risk of pregnancy and STIs. For women who exclusively have sex with women, there is a lack of evidence regarding the ease of transmission of some STIs, however, there is clear evidence that herpes simplex virus (HSV), HPV, syphilis, and hepatitis can be transmitted between women.[44] Shared sex toys and active herpes lesions can increase the risk of STI transmission and acquisition. There is evidence that bacterial vaginosis, while not generally considered an STI, can be transmitted between female partners.[44]

Family planning involves pregnancy prevention as well as planning for becoming pregnant. Many WSW choose to become pregnant through sperm donation (either known or anonymous) or with a male partner. It is important to ask about goals and plans for children in order to provide appropriate recommendations and referrals (e.g., folic acid supplementation and referral for assistive reproductive technologies).

Geriatric Considerations. The primary care of older adult lesbian women and WSW does not differ from caring for all older adults except in being mindful of potential differences in family structures and social supports. Lesbian women who have never had children are at risk for social isolation.[36] Additionally, stigma and discrimination can adversely impact the health of elderly sexual minorities. As with gay male elders, older lesbian women can face the risk of "re-closeting" in health care settings.[37]

Care of Bisexual People

Bisexual people are people who have the capacity for sexual attraction to people of both sexes. Some people who are attracted to others regardless of their sex or gender identity may prefer the terms pansexual or omnisexual. Others may use the terms such as fluid sexuality to describe the capacity for attraction to different genders. Regardless of the words one uses to identify themselves, it is important to know that sexual orientation occurs on a continuum.[47]

Health Disparities. Bisexual people face similar, if not worse, health disparities than gay men and lesbian women.[44,48] Many of these disparities arise from specific sexual behaviors. But others are due to antibisexual bias (biphobia) from both heterosexual and gay and lesbian people.[49] As with other SGM populations, bisexual people face an excess burden of Minority Stress-related mental health problems: substance use, depression, eating disorders, and emotional stress.[48]

Physical health disparities among bisexual people mirror the disparities seen in lesbian women and gay men. Many are due to specific sexual behaviors (e.g., higher risk of STIs among bisexual men). Others are due to systemic factors that make the health care system unwelcoming to sexual minority people (e.g., underutilization of mammography and cervical cancer screening among bisexual women).

Principles of Caring for Bisexual People. More than one-third of bisexual people report never disclosing their sexual identity to a health care provider.[48] Creating a welcoming clinical environment can help a patient feel safe in disclosing their sexual orientation and behaviors to the primary care provider. Once a patient discloses their bisexuality, the primary care provider should consider the patient-specific risks and behaviors in developing a plan of care.

Care of Asexual People

Asexuality refers to a lack of sexual attraction.[50,51] It is an orientation in the same way that some people are attracted to the opposite sex and some are attracted to the same sex. A person who is asexual does not feel attraction to either gender and this lack of attraction is persistent.[52] However, lack of sexual attraction does not mean that there is a lack of romantic attraction. Sex researchers have distinguished between sexual attraction/lust and romantic/affectionate attraction for others.[51]

MacInnis and Hodson[53] document negative attitudes towards asexual people in which they were viewed as "less human" and less valued as well as a willingness to discriminate against this sexual minority. Although there is little research on this topic, it is likely that asexual people experience sexual minority stress and prejudice as do LGBT people. Scholars in the field of asexuality challenge the notion of asexuality as a disorder and argue that any increased incidence of mental health problems among asexual people may be a result of minority stress rather than being asexual.[54]

Primary care providers should be mindful that sexual attraction is not a universal phenomenon and its absence is not inherently unhealthy. The absence of sexual attraction is only unhealthy if it causes distress for a patient.

CARING FOR GENDER MINORITY PEOPLE
Care of Transgender People

In approaching the care of transgender people, it is important to begin with a common lexicon. Gender is a person's sense of being male or female.[17] Sex, on the other hand, is assigned at birth based on an individual's anatomy.[17] A person who is *cisgender* has concordance between their gender and sex (e.g., a person identifies as a woman and has female anatomy). A person who is *transgender* has discordance between their gender and sex. A transgender man is an individual who identifies as a man but who was assigned a female sex at birth. A transgender woman is an individual who identifies as a woman but was assigned a male sex at birth. Gender nonconforming and gender non-binary people are people who may not identify as exclusively male or female or may identify as something other than the binary gender narrative.

There are approximately 1.4 million people in the United States who self-identify as transgender.[2] This number doubled in the period from 2011 to 2016, in part due to increased societal acceptance of a transgender identity. A lack of consistent data collection methods as well as the diversity and hidden nature of transgender communities makes it difficult to accurately report the true transgender population.

Transgender identity has existed around the world for millennia.[55] Many ancient cultures were open to the idea of a "third gender" and fluidity of gender. It is only in relatively recent history that a strict view of binary genders came to be.[56] In 1917, Dr. Alan Hart was the first documented transgender man in the United States to undergo a hysterectomy and live as a man.[56] In 1931, Lill Elbe was one of the first transgender women to undergo what was then called sex reassignment surgery in Copenhagen.[56] Surgical procedures to facilitate a person's gender transition are now called *gender-affirming surgeries.*

It is only recently that health care professionals ceased to view transgender identity as a disorder, but rather as a normal variant of human gender. In 2013, the American Psychiatric Association's Diagnostic and Statistical Manual of Mental Disorders (DSM-5) eliminated the term "Gender Identity Disorder" in reference to transgender people. The pathology surrounding gender identity is not that a transgender identity itself is pathological, rather the distress resulting from the conflict between gender and assigned sex (i.e., gender dysphoria) is the problem. Gender-affirming therapies are the treatments that can alleviate the distress associated with gender dysphoria.

Transgender people have long been included in the LGBTQIA grouping. This has led to a misunderstanding in some that all transgender people identify as lesbian or gay and engage in same sex behavior, which is untrue. Transgender people represent the full range of sexual identities and behaviors.

Health Disparities. Transgender people experience unique health disparities separate from the sexual minority community.[57] These disparities include a higher burden of depression and suicidality, victimization, negative experiences with health care, and housing instability.[17] In one recent study of transgender health ($n = 5885$), 46% of transgender men and 42% of transgender women had attempted suicide. More than half of respondents reported bullying and discrimination at school or work. Sixty percent of respondents reported being refused treatment by a health care provider, and 69% of respondents reported having been homeless at least once.[58] Intersectionality can serve to amplify these disparities. For example, transgender people of color are more likely to have attempted suicide than white transgender people.[58]

Institutionalized discrimination against transgender people leads to negative health outcomes in these communities.[58,59] In many localities it is legal to deny a transgender person access to public accommodations (e.g., restaurants, retail establishments). In other localities it is legal to fire a person from their job or deny them housing for being transgender.[59] These realities impact the health and wellness of transgender people and illustrate the interplay between the social determinants of health and an individual's health.

Lifespan Considerations in Primary Care. Comprehensive primary care of transgender people is within the scope of any primary care nurse practitioner. This section of the chapter provides an overview of this care. Detailed resources for providing comprehensive services, including hormone therapy, are available.[17,60,61]

General Principles. As discussed above, there are a number of practice-level strategies to improve the experience of care for SGM people. Using the 2-step approach to collect sex and gender demographics is an important practice-level strategy to improve quality of care (Fig. 10.1). Additionally, solicitation of every patient's preferred gender pronouns can communicate acceptance as well as facilitate communication.

Misgendering occurs when a transgender person's gender identity is either intentionally or unintentionally misstated. For instance, referring to a transgender woman as "him" is an example of misgendering. To prevent misgendering, use a patient's preferred gender pronouns when speaking to or about them. Another strategy to avoid misgendering is to avoid terms like "ma'am" and "sir." In the event that a primary care provider inadvertently misgenders a patient, the most appropriate course of action is an apology.

Childhood. The most common situation in which a primary care provider would address gender identity issues with a child would be when a parent expresses concern about their child's gender identity. It is common for a parent to express concerns about a male child who prefers pink clothing or a female child who likes trucks and rough play. Many children have normal interests and behaviors that are different than societal gender norms. The primary care provider role in these conversations is to clarify whether a child's perceived gender atypical behavior is merely a part of the child's self-expression or, rather, is a pervasive and distressing issue for the child.

Gender dysphoria can be seen in children as early as age 4 and is not an element of the child's play. Rather, it is an insistence across all contexts that the child is a different gender.[62] The role of the primary care provider when gender dysphoria is present is to affirm the family's concerns while educating them that forcing the child to express gender in a way that is not comfortable for the child is, in fact, harmful to the child's health. Additionally, if the primary care provider is not experienced in the care of transgender children, linkage with behavioral health and specialty providers is appropriate.

Adolescence. Not uncommonly, gender dysphoria worsens with the onset of puberty. The development of secondary sex characteristics can cause considerable anxiety, depression, social isolation, or self-harm.[62] While there is considerable controversy about whether children have the right to determine their gender identity, it is clear that allowing people to express gender as they experience it is curative of the symptoms of gender dysphoria.[61] The role of the primary care provider in helping families negotiate this complicated issue is to serve as an advocate for the adolescent, while being sensitive to the parents' concerns.

In order to avoid the development of undesired secondary sex characteristics and delay the onset of puberty, a model protocol was developed in the Netherlands that includes gonadotropin-releasing hormone (GnRH) analogues. Behavioral problems and general psychological functioning improve when youth age 12 and older delay puberty with suppression therapy.[63] Delaying puberty allows time for the child and their family to participate in comprehensive services to develop a plan of care, which may include gender-affirming treatments and procedures.

Young Adults/Adults. Health promotion activities for transgender and gender nonconforming people are the same as for cisgender people and are based on behavior and anatomy. For instance, transgender men should have cervical cancer screening according to the current guidelines if they still have a cervix, and mammogram if they have not had gender affirming surgery to remove their breasts. While the data is limited, expert recommendation is for transgender women receiving estrogen therapy to begin breast cancer screening 5 years after the start of estrogen therapy and performed within the current age and risk factor recommendations for the general population of women.[60] Transgender women who have not had prostate removal or orchiectomy should be screened according to the recommended guidelines for cisgender men.

The use of hormonal therapies in transgender people may contribute to cardiovascular (CV) risk, but there is limited evidence in this area. Some studies have shown that transgender men who use testosterone do not have any excess CV risk as compared to cisgender women.[64] Among transgender women who use estrogen, there is the possibility of excess CV risk due to estrogen therapy. But this risk may be mitigated by using transdermal rather than oral estrogen treatment.[64] When stratifying CV risk for a transgender patient, the primary care provider may wish to consider using the risk estimator associated with the sex hormones to which the individual has had the longest exposure. For example, a 50-year-old transgender woman who began estrogen supplementation in her 40s would use the male risk assessment. A 50-year-old transgender woman who began estrogen in her 20s would use the female risk assessment due to longer exposure to estrogen.

Transgender women are at high risk for all STIs, including syphilis and HIV.[65] This is due to a variety of factors, including higher rates of need-based transactional sex (due to employment discrimination and housing instability) and unprotected receptive anal sex.[66] The health care provider caring for sexually active transgender women should be mindful of offering HIV prevention services such as PrEP as well as screening for STIs from all sites of sexual contact (i.e., oral, anal, vaginal, urethral).

Hormone Therapy and Gender-Affirming Surgeries. Gender identity is expressed in a range of ways and is individual to each person. Many transgender and gender nonconforming people choose to take hormones and/or have surgery so that their physical appearance aligns with their gender identity. Two important principles to understand when caring for transgender people are that surgery is not an endpoint and inquiries regarding gender-affirming surgeries or the status of one's genitalia can be traumatic. Discussions around an individual's genitourinary anatomy should be limited to times when it is relevant to care being rendered (e.g., treatment for an STI) or after such time as a rapport and trust between the primary care provider and patient is established.

When a primary care provider is involved in helping a patient obtain gender-affirming therapies, extensive resources are available.[17,60,61] When surgical intervention is being considered, encourage patients to seek out services from a surgeon with expertise in these procedures. Common gender-affirming surgeries are presented in Table 10.5.

CARE OF INTERSEX PEOPLE

In countries around the world, intersex infants, children, and adolescents are subjected to medically unnecessary surgeries, hormonal treatments, and other procedures in an attempt to forcibly change their appearance to be in line with societal

TABLE 10.5	Gender-Affirming Surgical Procedures	
Feminizing procedures	Augmentation mammoplasty	Creation of breasts
	Vaginoplasty	Creation of a vagina
	Orchiectomy	Removal of testes
	Penectomy	Removal of penis
	Facial feminization procedures	Series of procedures to feminize the face and neck
Masculinizing procedures	Hysterectomy	Removal of the uterus
	Oophorectomy	Removal of the ovaries
	Vaginectomy	Removal or closure of the vagina
	Metoidioplasty	Creation of genital tissue (neophallus) from existing clitoral tissue
	Phalloplasty	Creation of a penis
	Scrotoplasty	Creation of a scrotum

expectations about female and male bodies. When, as is frequently the case, these procedures are performed without the full, free, and informed consent of the person concerned, they amount to violations of fundamental human rights…[67]

Intersex is a term used for a broad range of conditions in which the appearance of the external genitalia is either atypical or does not match the gonadal or chromosomal sex of the individual. Historically this was called hermaphroditism, now considered a pejorative term. There is controversy surrounding the terminology associated with intersex. The health care community typically refers to intersex conditions as *disorders of sex development* (DSD).[68] Intersex advocates suggest that the terms *intersex* or *differences of sex development* be used instead of "disorders" to still allow for the continued use of DSD.[69]

Differences do not necessarily constitute pathology. However, the health care community has historically been quick to "fix" atypical appearing genitals in infants or remove gonads that are incongruent with the assigned sex. Unfortunately, the surgeries can interfere with sexual function and fertility, require lifelong hormonal replacement, and often have to be revised as the child ages. There are many anecdotal reports by intersex individuals of the abuse, shame and trauma experienced as a result of unnecessary surgery and intervention.[70] What was historically considered a medical necessity to correct atypical genitalia, is increasingly being recognized as a social intervention that has long-term negative consequences. For instance, there are no long-term outcome data on the functional capacity of the clitoris even with newer nerve sparing procedures.[68] In a 2014 study of parents whose infants underwent hypospadias repair, a condition more prevalent in intersex children, over half reported decisional regret a year later.[71]

Best practices for the care of intersex infants, children, and their families include a multidisciplinary team approach with care continuing throughout the lifespan.[72] If a primary care provider has a patient that is identified as intersex, it is imperative that there is involvement of a team specializing in the care of intersex persons and that provides support for the parents while advocating for the infant or child. Lee and colleagues[73] cite a number of ethical, legal, and cultural considerations that are key to guiding the clinical management of intersex patients: preserving potential fertility; protecting the individual's right to participate in decisions and therefore avoid irreversible decisions that are not medically necessary; supporting the individual's healthy sexual and gender identity development; and sharing decision-making that respects the individual's parents' wishes and beliefs. However, there may be conflict in these goals as in the case of parents that wish for early genital surgery to "normalize" genitalia. So while parental wishes are important, the Intersex Society of North America asserts that, "parents' distress should not be treated by surgery on the child."[74]

For a health care provider approaching the care of a newborn who has intersex genitalia, the only urgent clinical concern is to rule out congenital adrenal hyperplasia (CAH). This is the most common cause of atypical genitalia and comprises different adrenal disorders, some of which can result in salt-wasting adrenal crises. CAH should be ruled out in any virilized newborn without palpable testes as an adrenal crisis can lead to shock and death if not recognized and treated within the first days of life.[69]

Humans, gender, gender identity, and sexuality are all complex and there is more diversity than society often chooses to recognize. The problems associated with intersexuality are not necessarily problems of gender or gender identity. Rather, they are problems of trauma and stigma.[74]

CONCLUSION

Most primary care providers will, knowingly or unknowingly, provide care for SGM people throughout their career. While these communities have historically faced discrimination and adverse health outcomes, the next generation of primary care providers is poised to meet the needs of these communities and redress these health inequities.

REFERENCES

1. Gallup Inc. Vermont Leads States in LGBT Identification. (2016). Retrieved from http://news.gallup.com/poll/203513/vermont-leads-states-lgbt-identification.aspx. (Accessed 24 November 2017).
2. Flores, A. R., Herman, J. L., Gates, G. J., & Brown, T. N. T. How many adults identify as transgender in the United States? The Williams Institue. 2016;(June):1–13. Retrieved from https://williamsinstitute.law.ucla.edu/wp-content/uploads/How-Many-Adults-Identify-as-Transgender-in-the-United-States.pdf. (Accessed 24 November 2017).
3. Tervalon, M., & Murray-García, J. (1998). Cultural humility versus cultural competence: A critical distinction in defining physician training outcomes in multicultural education. *Journal of Health Care for the Poor and Underserved, 9*(2), 117–125. Retrieved from http://www.ncbi.nlm.nih.gov/pubmed/10073197. (Accessed 17 January 2018).
4. Meyer, I. H. (2003). Prejudice, social stress, and mental health in lesbian, gay, and bisexual populations: Conceptual issues and research evidence. *Psychological Bulletin, 129*(5), 674–697. doi:10.1037/0033-2909.129.5.674.
5. Thomas, A. C., Crabtree, M. K., Delaney, K. R., et al. (2017). Nurse practitioner core competencies. Washington, D.C. Retrieved from http://c.ymcdn.com/sites/www.nonpf.org/resource/resmgr/competencies/2017_NPCoreComps_with_Curric.pdf. (Accessed 3 October 2017).
6. Staats, C., Capatosto, K., Tenney, L., & Mamo, S. (2017). State of the science: Implicit bias review 2017 edition. Retrieved from http://kirwaninstitute.osu.edu/wp-content/uploads/2017/11/2017-SOTS-final-draft-02.pdf. (Accessed 17 January 2018).
7. Westgate, E. C., Riskind, R. G., & Nosek, B. A. (2015). Implicit preferences for straight people over lesbian women and gay men weakened from 2006 to 2013. *Collabra, 1*(1). doi:10.1525/collabra.18.
8. The Joint Commission. (2011). Advancing effective communication, cultural competence, and patient- and family-centered care for the lesbian, gay, bisexual, and transgender (LGBT) community: A field guide. Oak Brook, IL. Retrieved from https://www.jointcommission.org/assets/1/18/LGBTFieldGuide_WEB_LINKED_VER.pdf. (Accessed 17 January 2018).
9. Gay and Lesbian Medical Association. (2006). Guidelines for the care of lesbian, gay, bisexual and transgender patients. Retrieved from http://glma.org/_data/n_0001/resources/live/GLMA guidelines 2006 FINAL.pdf. (Accessed 17 January 2018).
10. Sweeney Anthony, E., & Lipinski, M. L. (2015). 2015 edition final rule improvements to the ONC health IT certification program and the 2015 edition health IT certification criteria division of federal policy and regulatory affairs. Retrieved from https://www.healthit.gov/sites/default/files/onc2015editionfinalrulepresentation_10-9-15.pdf. (Accessed 31 January 2018).
11. Asking patients questions about sexual orientation and gender identity in clinical settings. Retrieved from http://thefenwayinstitute.org/wp-content/uploads/COM228_SOGI_CHARN_WhitePaper.pdf. (Accessed 17 January 2018).
12. Centers for Disease Control and Prevention. A guide to taking a sexual history. Retrieved from https://www.cdc.gov/std/treatment/SexualHistory.pdf. (Accessed 21 November 2017).
13. Gates, G. J. (2011). How many people are lesbian, gay, bisexual, and transgender? Retrieved from https://williamsinstitute.law.ucla.edu/wp-content/uploads/Gates-How-Many-People-LGBT-Apr-2011.pdf. (Accessed 17 January 2018).
14. Gallup Corporation. Americans greatly overestimate percent gay, lesbian in U.S. Retrieved from http://news.gallup.com/poll/183383/americans-greatly-overestimate-percent-gay-lesbian.aspx. (Accessed 17 January 2018).
15. Copen, C. E., Chandra, A., & Febo-Vazquez, I. (2016). Sexual behavior, sexual attraction, and sexual orientation among adults aged 18–44 in the United States: data from the 2011–2013 National Survey of Family Growth. *Natl Health Stat Report., 87*(January), 1–14. Retrieved from https://www.cdc.gov/nchs/data/nhsr/nhsr088.pdf. (Accessed 31 January 2018).
16. Villarroel, M. A., Turner, C. F., Eggleston, E., et al. (2006). Same-gender sex in the United States: Impact of T-ACASI on prevalence estimates. *Public Opinion Quarterly, 70*(2), 166–196. doi:10.1093/poq/nfj023.
17. Makadon, H. J., Mayer, K. H., Potter, J. P., & Goldhammer, H., American College of Physicians (2003). The fenway guide to lesbian, gay, bisexual, and transgender health.
18. Smith, E. A., & Malone, R. E. (2003). The outing of Philip Morris: Advertising tobacco to gay men. *American Journal of Public Health, 93*(6), 988–993. http://www.ncbi.nlm.nih.gov/pubmed/12773366. (Accessed 31 January 2018).
19. National Public Radio. Advertisers come out of the closet, openly courting gay consumers: NPR. Retrieved from https://www.npr.org/2014/06/29/326524942/advertisers-come-out-of-the-closet-openly-courting-gay-consumers. (Accessed 31 January 2018).
20. Centers for Disease Control and Prevention. Lifetime risk of HIV diagnosis. Retrieved from https://www.cdc.gov/nchhstp/newsroom/2016/croi-press-release-risk.html. Published 2016. (Accessed 3 October 2017).
21. Lee, C., Oliffe, J. L., Kelly, M. T., & Ferlatte, O. (2017). Depression and suicidality in gay men: Implications for health care providers. *Am J Mens Health, 11*(4), 910–919. doi:10.1177/1557988316685492.
22. United States Preventative Services Task Force. (2016). Final recommendation statement—depression in children and adolescents: Screening. Retrieved from https://www.uspreventiveservicestaskforce.org/Page/Document/RecommendationStatementFinal/depression-in-children-and-adolescents-screening1. (Accessed 31 January 2018).
23. Russell, S. T., & Joyner, K. (2001). Adolescent sexual orientation and suicide risk: Evidence from a national study. *American Journal of Public Health, 91*(8), 1276–1281. Retrieved from http://www.ncbi.nlm.nih.gov/pubmed/11499118. (Accessed 17 January 2018).
24. United States Preventative Services Task Force. Final update summary: Tobacco smoking cessation in adults, including pregnant women: behavioral and pharmacotherapy interventions—US Preventive Services Task Force. Retrieved from https://www.uspreventiveservicestaskforce.org/Page/Document/UpdateSummaryFinal/tobacco-use-in-adults-and-pregnant-women-counseling-and-interventions1. (Accessed 31 January 2018).
25. United States Preventative Services Task Force. Final recommendation statement: Alcohol misuse: screening and behavioral counseling interventions in primary care—US preventive services task force. https://www.uspreventiveservicestaskforce.org/Page/Document/RecommendationStatementFinal/alcohol-misuse-screening-and-behavioral-counseling-interventions-in-primary-care. (Accessed 31 January 2018).
26. United States Preventative Services Task Force. Final recommendation statement: Drug use, illicit: screening—US preventive services task force. Retrieved from https://www.uspreventiveservicestaskforce.org/Page/Document/RecommendationStatementFinal/drug-use-illicit-screening. (Accessed 31 January 2018).
27. CDC, Ncird. (2016). HPV vaccine information for clinicians. https://www.cdc.gov/hpv/hcp/need-to-know.pdf. (Accessed 22 January 2018).
28. Centers for Disease Control. Viral hepatitis and men who have sex with men. https://www.cdc.gov/hepatitis/populations/msm.htm. (Accessed 22 January 2018).
29. Centers for Disease Control. Screening—Q & A—2015 STD treatment guidelines. Retrieved from https://www.cdc.gov/std/tg2015/qa/screening-qa.htm. (Accessed 22 January 2018).

30. Leeds, I. L., & Fang, S. H. (2016). Anal cancer and intraepithelial neoplasia screening: A review. *World J Gastrointest Surg, 8*(1), 41–51. doi:10.4240/wjgs.v8.i1.41.

31. Aberg, J. A., Gallant, J. E., Ghanem, K. G., Emmanuel, P., Zingman, B. S., & Horberg, M. A. (2014). Primary care guidelines for the management of persons infected with HIV: 2013 update by the HIV medicine association of the infectious diseases society of America. *Clinical Infectious Diseases: an Official Publication of the Infectious Diseases Society of America, 58*(1), e1–e34. doi:10.1093/cid/cit665.

32. Centers for Disease Control. STDs in men who have sex with men—2016 STD surveillance report. Retrieved from https://www.cdc.gov/std/stats16/msm.htm. (Accessed 22 January 2018).

33. Centers for Disease Control and Prevention. (2014). Preexposure prophylaxis for the prevention of HIV infection in the United States—2014 clinical practice guideline. Retrieved from https://www.cdc.gov/hiv/pdf/prepguidelines2014.pdf. (Accessed 3 October 2017).

34. Klein, D. A., Berry-Bibee, E. N., Baker, K. K., Malcolm, N. M., Rollison, J. M., & Frederiksen, B. N. (2018). Providing quality family planning services to LGBTQIA individuals: A systematic review. *Contraception,* doi:10.1016/j.contraception.2017.12.016.

35. National LGBT Health Education Center. Pathways to parenthood for LGBT people. Retrieved from https://www.lgbthealtheducation.org/wp-content/uploads/Pathways-to-Parenthood-for-LGBT-People.pdf. (Accessed 22 January 2018).

36. LGBT Movement Advancement Project (MAP) & Services and Advocacy for Gay, Lesbian B and TE (SAGE). (2010). Improving the lives of LGBT older adults. Retrieved from https://www.sageusa.org/files/Improving the Lives of LGBT Older Adults—Snapshot report.pdf. (Accessed 22 January 2018).

37. Steelman, R. E. (2018). Person-centered care for LGBT older adults. *Journal of Gerontological Nursing, 44*(2), 3–5. doi:10.3928/00989134-20180110-01.

38. Przedworski, J. M., McAlpine, D. D., Karaca-Mandic, P., & VanKim, N. A. (2014). Health and health risks among sexual minority women: An examination of 3 subgroups. *American Journal of Public Health, 104*(6), 1045–1047. doi:10.2105/AJPH.2013.301733.

39. Mattingly, A. E., Kiluk, J. V., & Lee, M. C. (2016). Clinical considerations of risk, incidence, and outcomes of breast cancer in sexual minorities. *Cancer Control: Journal of the Moffitt Cancer Center, 23*(4), 373–382. doi:10.1177/107327481602300408.

40. Saunders, C. L., Meads, C., Abel, G. A., & Lyratzopoulos, G. (2017). Associations between sexual orientation and overall and site-specific diagnosis of cancer: Evidence from two national patient surveys in England. *Journal of Clinical Oncology: Official Journal of the American Society of Clinical Oncology, 35*(32), 3654–3661. doi:10.1200/JCO.2017.72.5465.

41. Schonfeld, S. J., Pfeiffer, R. M., Lacey, J. V., et al. (2011). Hormone-related risk factors and postmenopausal breast cancer among nulliparous versus parous women: An aggregated study. *American Journal of Epidemiology, 173*(5), 509–517. doi:10.1093/aje/kwq404.

42. Knight, D. A., & Jarrett, D. (2017). Preventive health care for women who have sex with women. *American Family Physician, 95*(5), 314–321. Retrieved from http://www.ncbi.nlm.nih.gov/pubmed/28290645. (Accessed 28 January 2018).

43. Russell, S. T., & Fish, J. N. (2016). Mental health in lesbian, gay, bisexual, and transgender (LGBT) youth. *Annual Review of Clinical Psychology, 12*, 465–487. doi:10.1146/annurev-clinpsy-021815-093153.

44. Marrazzo, J. M., & Gorgos, L. M. (2012). Emerging sexual health issues among women who have sex with women. *Current Infectious Disease Reports, 14*(2), 204–211. doi:10.1007/s11908-012-0244-x.

45. United States Preventative Services Task Force. (2012). Cervical cancer screening: Final recommendation statement. Retrieved from https://www.uspreventiveservicestaskforce.org/Page/Document/RecommendationStatementFinal/cervical-cancer-screening.

46. Wright, T. C., Stoler, M. H., Behrens, C. M., Sharma, A., Zhang, G., & Wright, T. L. (2015). Primary cervical cancer screening with human papillomavirus: End of study results from the ATHENA study using HPV as the first-line screening test. *Gynecologic Oncology, 136*(2), 189–197. doi:10.1016/j.ygyno.2014.11.076.

47. Kinsey, A., Pomeroy, W., & Martin, C. The Kinsey Scale. Retrieved from https://www.kinseyinstitute.org/research/publications/kinsey-scale.php. (Accessed 31 January 2018).

48. Human Rights Campaign. Health disparities among bisexual people. Retrieved from https://assets2.hrc.org/files/assets/resources/HRC-BiHealthBrief.pdf?_ga=2.235177345.1060495272.1517432349-1229058356.1517432349. (Accessed 31 January 2018).

49. Dodge, B., Herbenick, D., Friedman, M. R., et al. (2016). Attitudes toward bisexual men and women among a nationally representative probability sample of adults in the United States. Hoffmann H, ed. *PLoS ONE, 11*(10), e0164430. doi:10.1371/journal.pone.0164430.

50. AVEN. Overview: The asexual Visibility and Education Network. Retrieved from asexuality.org.

51. Bogaert, A. F. (2015). Asexuality: What it is and why it matters. *Journal of Sex Research, 52*(4), 362–379. doi:10.1080/00224499.2015.1015713.

52. Bogaert, A. F. (2012). *Understanding asexuality.* Rowman & Littlefield Publishers.

53. Macinnis, C. C., & Hodson, G. (2012). Intergroup bias toward "Group X": Evidence of prejudice, dehumanization, avoidance, and discrimination against asexuals. *Gr Process Intergr Relations, 15*(6), 725–743. doi:10.1177/1368430212442419.

54. Bogaert, A. F. (2015). Asexuality: What it is and why it matters. *Journal of Sex Research, 52*(4), 362–379. doi:10.1080/00224499.2015.1015713.

55. Bolich, G. G. (2007). *Transgender history & geography: Crossdressing in context* (Vol. 3). Psyche's Press.

56. Frey, J. D., Poudrier, G., Thomson, J. E., & Hazen, A. (2017). A historical review of gender-affirming medicine: Focus on genital reconstruction surgery. *The Journal of Sexual Medicine, 14*(8), 991–1002. doi:10.1016/J.JSXM.2017.06.007.

57. Institute of Medicine. (2011). *The health of lesbian, gay, bisexual, and transgender people.* Washington, D.C.: National Academies Press. doi:10.17226/13128.

58. Haas, A. P., Rodgers, P. L., & Herman, J. L. (2014). Suicide attempts among transgender and gender non-conforming adults findings of the national transgender discrimination survey. Retrieved from https://williamsinstitute.law.ucla.edu/wp-content/uploads/AFSP-Williams-Suicide-Report-Final.pdf. (Accessed 2 February 2018).

59. Reisner, S. L., Hughto, J. M. W., Dunham, E. E., et al. (2015). Legal protections in public accommodations settings: A critical public health issue for transgender and gender-nonconforming people. *The Milbank Quarterly, 93*(3), 484–515. doi:10.1111/1468-0009.12127.

60. Deutsch, M. Guidelines for the primary and gender affirming care of transgender and gender nonconforming people. UCSF Center of Excellence for Transgender Health. Retrieved from http://transhealth.ucsf.edu/pdf/Transgender-PGACG-6-17-16.pdf. Published 2016. (Accessed 31 January 2018).

61. World Professional Association for Transgender Health. Standards of care for the health of transsexual, transgender, and gender nonconforming people. Retrieved from https://s3.amazonaws.com/amo_hub_content/Association140/files/Standards of Care V7—2011 WPATH (2)(1).pdf. (Accessed 2 February 2018).

62. Ilana Sherer, M., Joel Baum, M., Diane Ehrensaft, P., Stephen, M., & Rosenthal, M. Affirming gender: Caring for gender-atypical children and adolescents. *Contemp Pediatr.* January 2015. Retrieved from http://contemporarypediatrics.modernmedicine.com/contemporary-pediatrics/news/affirming-gender-caring-gender-atypical-children-and-adolescents?page=full. (Accessed 2 February 2018).

63. Cohen-Kettenis, P. T., Steensma, T. D., & de Vries, A. L. C. (2011). Treatment of adolescents with gender dysphoria in the netherlands. *Child and Adolescent Psychiatric Clinics of North America, 20*(4), 689–700. doi:10.1016/j.chc.2011.08.001.

64. Gooren, L. J., Wierckx, K., & Giltay, E. J. (2014). Cardiovascular disease in transsexual persons treated with cross-sex hormones: Reversal of the traditional sex difference in cardiovascular disease pattern. *European Journal of Endocrinology, 170*(6), 809–819. doi:10.1530/EJE-14-0011.

65. Baral, S. D., Poteat, T., Strömdahl, S., Wirtz, A. L., Guadamuz, T. E., & Beyrer, C. (2013). Worldwide burden of HIV in transgender women: A systematic review and meta-analysis. *The Lancet Infectious Diseases, 13*(3), 214–222. doi:10.1016/S1473-3099(12)70315-8.

66. Deutsch, M. B., Glidden, D. V., Sevelius, J., et al. (2015). HIV pre-exposure prophylaxis in transgender women: A subgroup analysis of the iPrEx trial. *Lancet HIV, 2*(12), e512–e519. doi:10.1016/S2352-3018(15)00206-4.

67. United Nations Office of the High Commissioner on Human Rights. Intersex Awareness Day. Retrieved from http://www.ohchr.org/EN/NewsEvents/Pages/DisplayNews.aspx?NewsID=20739&LangID=E. Published 2016. (Accessed 31 January 2018).

68. Houk, C. P., Baskin, L. S., & Levitsky, L. L. Management of the infant with atypical genitalia (disorder of sex development)—UpToDate. UpToDate.

69. Indyk, J. A. (2017). Disorders/differences of sex development (DSDs) for primary care: The approach to the infant with ambiguous genitalia. *Transl Pediatr., 6*(4), 323–334. doi:10.21037/tp.2017.10.03.

70. Baratz, A., & Karkazis, K. (2015). Cris de Couer and the Moral Imperative to Listen to and Learn from Intersex People. *Narrat Inq Bioeth, 5*(2), 127–132.

71. Lorenzo, A. J., Ao, J., Pippi Salle, L., et al. (2014). Hypospadias decisional regret after distal hypospadias repair: Single institution prospective analysis of factors associated with subsequent parental remorse or distress. *The Journal of Urology, 191*, 1558–1563. doi:10.1016/j.juro.2013.10.036.

72. Moran, M. E., & Karkazis, K. (2012). Methodology report developing a multidisciplinary team for disorders of sex development: Planning, implementation, and operation tools for care providers. *Advances in Urology*, 1–12. doi:10.1155/2012/604135.

73. Lee, P. A., & Houk, C. P. (2016). Changing and unchanging perspectives regarding intersex in the last half century: Topics presented in the Lawson Wilkins lecture* at the 2015 Pediatric Endocrine Society meeting. *Pediatric Endocrinology Reviews*, 13(3), 574–584. Retrieved from http://www.ncbi.nlm.nih.gov/pubmed/27116845. (Accessed 31 January 2018).

74. Intersex Society of North America. What does ISNA recommend for children with intersex? Retrieved from http://www.isna.org/faq/patient-centered. Published 2016. (Accessed 31 January 2018).

CHAPTER **11**

PREGNANCY, PRENATAL CARE, AND LACTATION

Emma Virginia Clark

PREGNANCY AND PRENATAL CARE: A HISTORICAL OVERVIEW

Pregnancy, beginning at conception, moving through embryologic and fetal development to parturition, is a period of dynamic change for a mother, baby, and family.[1] This makes pregnancy a unique opportunity to identify and minimize health risks, promote health, and provide necessary psychosocial support and medical follow-up for the whole family, in and beyond the pregnancy.[2]

Prenatal care has routinely been offered only since the early 1900s. Initially, prenatal care did not result in improvements in high rates of infant or maternal mortality because many women did not attend prenatal care or received care that was poorly performed with excessive or inappropriate intervention. In the decades that followed, knowledge of pregnancy grew and medical advancements allowing the close observation of maternal and fetal health throughout pregnancy, labor, and delivery brought about a decline in infant and maternal mortality rates.[3]

In 1985 the Institute of Medicine (IOM) acknowledged the relationship between adequate prenatal care utilization and low birth weight and infant mortality.[4] Four years later, the USPHS released a landmark report defining the number of visits and the content of each visit, and it was recommended that women be offered preconception counseling before pregnancy.[2] In the 1990s, additional social programs were created, increasing services to address health care disparities for women of lower socioeconomic status.[4]

Despite this progress, the United States lags behinds other high-income countries in maternal mortality and morbidity, with maternal mortality ratios increasing from 16.9 deaths per 100,000 live births in 1990 to 26.4 deaths per 100,000 live births in 2015.[5] Although the neonatal mortality rate has dropped in recent years, it has declined more slowly and remains approximately 83% higher than the comparable country average. In 2014, 38% of infant deaths were attributable to congenital malformations, deformations, and chromosomal abnormalities and to short gestation and low birth weight disorders. Maternal complications of pregnancy were also a major cause of infant mortality.[6] Racial and ethnic disparities in both maternal and neonatal morbidity and mortality are an issue of major concern; black women in the United States are two to three times more likely than white women to die from pregnancy-related complications, and the neonatal mortality rate for non-Hispanic blacks was almost twice that for non-Hispanic whites.[6] The causes of these disparities are not fully understood, but are generally attributed to a combination of patient, provider, and system-level factors.[7] Prenatal care has a critical, if not yet fully understood, role to play in improving neonatal and maternal morbidity and mortality rates and addressing health disparities. Largely given this, currently, one of *Healthy People 2020's* objectives to improve the health and well-being of women, infants, children, and family is to increase the proportion of pregnant women who receive early and adequate prenatal care in order to reduce risk of maternal and infant mortality and pregnancy-related complications.[8]

GOALS OF PRENATAL CARE

Although inadequate prenatal care has been clearly associated with increased complications, because of mixed evidence and unclear relationships between prenatal care and such critical issues as preterm birth and low birth weight, there continues to be discussion about what, exactly, the goals, critical elements of prenatal care, and education are.[9] For most women, pregnancy and birth are fundamentally health and normal functions, not physiologic processes. However, pregnancy does present the possibility of problematic conditions, and providers must be vigilant about identifying the small but critical subgroup of women who will have pregnancy-related complications that affect fetal or maternal health.[10] Prenatal care acts as an opportunity to do so, while also providing critical education to the woman and her family on pregnancy, overall health, and care of the newborn.

However, there remains a need to determine which components of care are most beneficial for a targeted outcome and to clearly evaluate current practices through evidence-based research to establish a future course for prenatal care.[11]

FACTORS IMPACTING USE OF PRENATAL CARE

Use of prenatal care can be broken down into two concepts: motivation to use services and facilitation of service providers in helping women access prenatal care.[12] Facilitation of access can improve motivation and ultimately improve use of prenatal care, resulting in the improved maternal and fetal outcomes associated with prenatal care use. This is especially critical given that women with the lowest motivation to seek care are highly correlated with those at risk for poor outcomes, such as those with unplanned pregnancies. Facilitation of access by clinics and providers includes making facilities physically accessible (e.g., located on bus routes, no parking fees), financially accessible (e.g., acceptance of a variety of payment options, low out-of-pocket costs for care), culturally accessible (e.g., immigration status blind, multiple languages spoken), temporally accessible (e.g., evening appointments, reasonable wait times, initial appointments soon after first contact), and practically accessible (e.g., safe play areas for children).

PRENATAL CARE RECOMMENDATIONS

In the United States, a number of different organizations have published recommendations for the delivery of prenatal care, although it has received little attention or updating in recent years. Perhaps the most traditional format for care begins with an initial visit at 8 to 10 weeks (or earlier if patient is at risk) every 4 weeks until 28 weeks, every 2 to 3 weeks until 36 weeks, and weekly visits until delivery, totaling 13 visits.[1,11] The USPHS diverged from this recommendation in its outdated but unfortunately not updated 1989 report, suggesting that nine visits are adequate, omitting weeks 20 and 28 in an uncomplicated pregnancy. The USPHS expert panel also recommended bimonthly instead of weekly appointments beginning at 36 weeks until delivery.[2]

In an effort to improve access to and quality of prenatal care, an innovative model called CenteringPregnancy was initiated in 1993. In CenteringPregnancy, a woman attends 10 2-hour group sessions with the same cohort, assuming responsibility for self-monitoring of blood pressure, weight, and fundal height, and participating in group discussion and education.[13] This method has been shown to increase the satisfaction with and use of prenatal care, improve perinatal knowledge, decrease preterm birth rates, and promote higher breastfeeding initiation rates.[13] Providers are also more satisfied. It is important to note that when compared with standard prenatal care, CenteringPregnancy is notable for its ability to recruit and retain a demographic of women who have historically had the poorest pregnancy and birth outcomes and to improve not only outcomes but overall mental health and well-being of participants.[14]

CONTENT OF PRENATAL VISITS

Standard components of an initial prenatal visit are a complete history, a comprehensive physical examination including ensuring that clinical information correlates to dating of the pregnancy, baseline laboratory and diagnostic tests, and educational and anticipatory guidance about the expected pregnancy course. Subsequent visits are to track progress of the pregnancy and to assess gestational milestones, to follow up on tests, and to provide ongoing education and support both about the pregnancy and in preparation for the postpartum period and parenthood. Table 11.1 details the content and timing of prenatal care.

Diagnosis of Pregnancy

The diagnosis of pregnancy is the gateway to initiation of prenatal care. For the diagnosis of pregnancy to be made, either a urine or serum pregnancy test or ultrasound study may be used. Serum pregnancy tests can detect β human chorionic gonadotropin (β-hCG) levels as low as 1.0 mIU/mL as early as 8 to 9 days after ovulation and before the onset of menses. Urine pregnancy tests are also highly accurate but are not as sensitive as serum tests, and very few can detect β-hCG levels lower than 12.5 mIU/mL, making them subject to a higher false-negative rate.[1] In experienced hands, a pelvic ultrasound study (ideally with a vaginal probe) can detect a pregnancy as early as 4 to 5 weeks of gestation, with β-hCG levels as low as 1000 to 2000 mIU/mL.[1]

Assumptions should not be made about a woman's desire for or plans for pregnancy. A woman with an unplanned pregnancy should be offered unbiased, nonjudgmental, direct information regarding her reproductive options, tailored to her stage of gestation at diagnosis of pregnancy.[10] These include medical or surgical elective termination of pregnancy or continuation of pregnancy with plans to either keep the baby or place it up for adoption. Appropriate referrals should be given as necessary.

Estimated Date of Delivery (EDD)

An accurate menstrual history assists in determining the estimated due (delivery) date (EDD), which facilitates clinical decision-making, particularly determining viability or post dates.[15] In addition, trimester of first visit is a standard, if incomplete, clinical quality indicator of access to prenatal care and requires accurate calculation of pregnancy dates.[8] An EDD is calculated based on the first day of the last normal menstrual period (LNMP). A traditional way to calculate the EDD is called the Nägele rule, which is done by subtracting 3 months and adding 7 days to the LNMP. If the LNMP is unsure or unknown, an ultrasound study may be used to determine the EDD. As a last resort, clinical data such as fundal height can be used to provide a rough estimate of pregnancy dating. As a word of caution, ultrasound dating becomes increasingly less accurate as the pregnancy advances and the fetus becomes susceptible to genetic and environmental influences.[1,15] Ultrasound dating is most accurate up to 13 5/7 weeks' gestation.[11]

Gravidity and Parity

Gravidity and *parity* are terms used to describe a woman's obstetric history. *Gravidity* describes the total number of pregnancies (including the current one) that a woman has experienced in her lifetime. *Parity* is the total number of pregnancies that have progressed beyond 20 gestational weeks in a woman's lifetime. Parity is about the uterus being empty; it is not about the number of babies born (i.e., in the situation of multifetal deliveries [twins, triplets], parity is still a single event).

Gravidity and parity are often strung together as a form of obstetric shorthand to communicate a woman's obstetric history. Gravidity, G, is usually listed first, followed by a series of four numbers (TPAL) to communicate what happened during each pregnancy: T, the number of term (>37 completed gestational weeks) deliveries; P, the number of preterm (20 to 36 5/7 completed gestational weeks) deliveries; A, abortion (elective or spontaneous delivery before 20 completed gestational weeks); and L, living children.[1,15]

As an example, a woman arrives for prenatal care and reports that she has had four previous pregnancies: one delivery at 38 weeks (child is living), one miscarriage at 9 weeks, one elective termination at 10 weeks, and a delivery of twins at 36 weeks (both living). Her G/TPAL is G5 and P1123 (one full-term delivery, one preterm delivery, two abortions, and three living children).

Health History in Prenatal Care

In addition to the menstrual and obstetric history, thorough medical, surgical, family, and social histories are vital to prenatal care. A medication history identifies therapies that should be changed to reduce risk of teratogenicity.[10] All women should be screened for use of tobacco, alcohol, and illicit substances. As studies indicate that the rate of domestic violence may increase during pregnancy, a woman's current safety and abuse history should be evaluated at her initial visit, at least once per trimester, at the postpartum checkup, and as indicated by behavioral and physical signs throughout pregnancy, using direct, specific questions about abuse.[16] Weight gain goals for pregnancy should be set at the initial visit based on prepregnancy body mass index (BMI); dietary and exercise patterns should be reviewed regularly, especially if excessive or insufficient weight gain is noted.[17] An awareness of preexisting

TABLE 11.1 Content and Timing of Routine Prenatal Care

Prenatal Care	First Trimester (6–12 Weeks)	Second Trimester (13–27 Weeks)	Third Trimester (28–39 Weeks)	Post Dates (40–42 Weeks)
HISTORY				
Menstrual, establish gestational age	X			
Obstetric (complications)	X			
Medical and surgical	X			
Medications and immunizations (influenza, tetanus, and diphtheria)	X	X	X	X
Family and genetics	X			
Social (habits, abuse, stress, work)	X			
PHYSICAL EXAMINATION				
Periodontal	X			
Blood pressure	X	X	X	X
Weight, body mass index	X	X	X	X
Pelvic	X			
Fundal height	X[a]	X	X	X
Fetal heart tone, position	X[a]	X	X	X
LABORATORY AND DIAGNOSTIC TESTS				
Pregnancy test	X			
Ultrasound examination	X[a]	X[a]	X[a]	X[a]
Blood type, Rh	X			
Antibody screen	X		X[a]	
Hemoglobin and hematocrit	X		X[a]	
Glucose tolerance test			X	
Urine	X			
Urine culture	X			
Pap smear	X[a]			
Chlamydia and gonorrhea, if indicated	X		X[a]	
RPR, VDRL (syphilis screen)	X		X[a]	
Hepatitis B surface antigen	X			
HIV infection	X[b]			
Herpes simplex	X			
Rubella	X			
Varicella	X			
Tuberculosis	X[a]			
Group B *Streptococcus*			X	
Fetal aneuploidy screen		X[c]		
Neural tube defect screen		X[c]		
Cystic fibrosis screen	X[b]			
COUNSELING, EDUCATION, AND SCREENING				
Physical and emotional changes, self-care	X	X	X	X
Preterm labor, blood pressure precautions	X	X	X	X
Fetal movement		X[a]	X	X
Nutrition and exercise	X	X	X	X
Tobacco, alcohol, drug use	X	X	X	X
Safety (seat belt, avoid teratogens)	X	X	X	X
Domestic violence	X	X	X	X
Depression, social	X	X	X	X
Breastfeeding	X	X	X	X
Sexuality	X	X	X	X
Family planning			X	X
Labor preparation			X	X

[a]If indicated.
[b]Offer or counsel.
[c]Offer or counsel early in trimester.
HIV, Human immunodeficiency virus; *RPR*, rapid plasma reagin; *VDRL*, Venereal Disease Research Laboratory.

Data from Corton, M., Leveno, K., Bloom, S., et al. (2014). *Williams obstetrics* (24th ed.). New York: McGraw-Hill; Callahan, T., & Caughey, A. (2017). *Blueprints Obstetrics and Gynecology* (7th ed.). Philadelphia, PA: Wolters Kluwer; U.S. Public Health Service. (1989). *Caring for our future: The content of prenatal care*. Washington, DC: U.S. Government Printing Office; American College of Obstetricians and Gynecologists (ACOG), American Academy of Pediatrics, American College of Obstetricians and Gynecologists. (2017). *Guidelines for perinatal care* (8th ed.). Elk Grove Village, IL: AAP; Washington, DC: ACOG; U.S. Department of Veterans Affairs and Department of Defense. (2009). *VA/DoD clinical practice guideline: management of pregnancy*. Washington, DC. Retrieved from www.healthquality.va.gov/up/mpg_v2_1_sumc.pdf; and U.S. Department of Health and Human Services, Centers for Disease Control and Prevention. *2015 Sexually transmitted diseases treatment guidelines*. Retrieved from http://www.cdc.gov/std/tg2015/default.htm. Accessed December 27, 2017.

TABLE 11.2	Considerations for Genetic Counseling or Testing
Chromosomal abnormalities	Trisomy 21 Trisomy 18 Trisomy 13
Sex chromosomal abnormalities	Turner syndrome Klinefelter syndrome
Autosomal dominant disease	Achondroplasia Polycystic kidney disease Huntington chorea Marfan syndrome Neurofibromatosis types 1 and 2
Autosomal recessive disease	Cystic fibrosis Sickle cell disease Tay-Sachs disease Thalassemia syndrome
X-linked disease	Duchenne and Becker muscular dystrophy Hemophilia A and B Fragile X syndrome
Congenital anomalies	Neural tube defect (spina bifida, anencephaly) Cardiac defects Potter syndrome
Other conditions	Advanced maternal or paternal age Abnormal genetic screening, ultrasound abnormalities Consanguinity Stillbirth or neonatal death Mental retardation Ambiguous genitalia, dysmorphic disease

Data from Corton, M., Leveno, K., Bloom, S., et al. (2014). *Williams obstetrics* (24th ed.). New York: McGraw-Hill; Callahan, T., & Caughey, A. (2017). *Blueprints Obstetrics and Gynecology* (7th ed.). Philadelphia, PA: Wolters Kluwer; and Bienstock, J. L., Fox, H. E., Wallach, E. E., et al. (2015). *The Johns Hopkins manual of gynecology and obstetrics* (5th ed.). Philadelphia, PA: Lippincott Williams & Wilkins.

physical and mental health conditions, such as depression, helps to tailor management during the prenatal and postpartum period (see Chapter 226 for depression screening). If there is a personal or family history of genetic disease, the pregnant woman can be offered individual counseling and testing (Table 11.2).[1,10,15] With recognized safety of vaginal birth after cesarean section, a woman with a previous cesarean section should be counseled on vaginal and repeat cesarean delivery options, depending on the indications for previous cesarean sections, type of uterine incision, coexisting medical conditions, and plans for future pregnancies.[18]

Oral health should also be assessed, including presence of swollen or bleeding gums or other mouth problems and date of last dental visit.[19] Prenatal oral disease and adverse pregnancy and birth outcomes have been linked, although evidence on how effective dental treatment during pregnancy may improve outcomes is mixed. However, pregnancy does represent an important time for oral health promotion, both education and dental care services. All women should be counseled on good oral hygiene and dental care–seeking behaviors. Any woman who has oral health problems or has not had a dental examination in more than 6 months should be referred for dental care and should receive reassurance that diagnosis and treatment of dental conditions, including radiographs with shielding of abdomen and use of local anesthesia (lidocaine with or without epinephrine) are safe.[19]

A vaccination history can help to determine if any immunizations will be required during pregnancy. Common vaccinations contraindicated or not recommended in pregnancy include measles, mumps, and rubella (MMR); varicella; herpes zoster; live, attenuated influenza; and human papillomavirus (HPV).[20] The inactivated influenza vaccine is safe and strongly recommended to receive at any point in pregnancy.[20] The tetanus, diphtheria, and acellular pertussis (Tdap) vaccine is similarly safe, and pregnant women should receive a Tdap vaccine in every pregnancy, optimally between 27 and 36 weeks' gestation, to provide the infant with critical short-term protection via passive antibody transfer.[20] Family members and others who will have close contact with the newborn should also be counseled to receive the flu vaccine annually and be up to date on their Tdap vaccine.[20] Women who are at risk for hepatitis B (have had more than one sex partner during the previous 6 months, been evaluated or treated for a sexually transmitted infection [STI], have a history of recent or current injection drug use, or have a sex partner with hepatitis B) should receive the hepatitis B vaccine.[20] Pregnant women who are not immune to rubella and varicella should be vaccinated immediately after delivery.[20]

Nutrition and Weight Gain in Pregnancy

Nutritional requirements during pregnancy range from 1800 to 2400 kcal/day, and daily protein intake increases to 60 to 75 g/day,[15,21] depending on the physical stature and exercise habits of an individual woman. Most women overestimate the number of additional calories. Dietary recommendation must be personalized to the woman's age, her prepregnant BMI, and her rate of weight gain.[21] Women are encouraged to eat a variety of foods to ensure adequate intake of folic acid, vitamin B_{12}, iron, calcium, and vitamin D.[21]

Poor maternal weight gain is associated with fetal undernutrition, which affects fetal survival and poor health outcomes later in life.[21] Women with inadequate weight gain should be evaluated for food security and, as necessary, referred to food assistance programs (such as the Special Supplemental Nutrition Program for Women, Infants, and Children [WIC]), many of which target pregnant women. Thyroid-stimulating hormone (TSH) levels, toxicology, serum albumin, and hepatitis screening should be considered as clinically indicated, as well as ultrasound to evaluate for intrauterine growth restrictrion.[10]

On the flip side, excessive weight gain in pregnancy and being overweight or obese before the start of pregnancy are also associated with a number of health problems and poor outcomes, including miscarriage, preeclampsia, gestational diabetes mellitus (GDM), perinatal depression, large-for-gestational-age fetus, further excess weight gain, risk of preterm birth, stillbirth, birth injury, neural tube defects, postpartum hemorrhage, delayed lactogenesis, and need for labor induction and operative birth.[10,22] In addition, pregnancy can worsen preexisting diabetes and hypertension (HTN), and obesity can complicate surgical interventions such as cesarean section.[22] Because of the significant risks associated with obesity in pregnancy, the IOM revised its recommendations for weight gain in pregnancy (Table 11.3). Overweight and obese women should undergo a 1-hour oral glucose tolerance test (OGTT) at their first visit and a repeat OGTT at 24 to 28 weeks, a urine dipstick at every visit

TABLE 11.3 Recommendations for Total and Rate of Weight Gain During Pregnancy, by Prepregnancy Body Mass Index

Prepregnancy BMI	BMI[a] (kg/m^2)	Total Weight Gain Range (lb)	Rates of Gain[b] in Second and Third Trimesters (Mean Range in lb/week)
Underweight	<18.5	28–40	1 (1–1.3)
Normal weight	18.5–24.9	25–35	1 (0.8–1)
Overweight	25.0–29.9	15–25	0.6 (0.5–0.7)
Obese (includes all classes)	≥30.0	11–20	0.5 (0.4–0.6)

[a]Based on the World Health Organization cutoff points. To calculate body mass index (BMI), go to www.nhlbisupport.com/bmi/.
[b]Calculations assume a 0.5- to 2-kg (1.1- to 4.4-lb) weight gain in the first trimester.
From Rasmussen, K. M., & Yaktine, A. L., (Eds.). (2009). Committee to Reexamine IOM Pregnancy Weight Guidelines; Institute of Medicine; National Research Council: *Weight gain during pregnancy: Reexamining the guideline.* Washington, DC: National Academies Press.

for glucose and protein related to the increased risk of GDM and preeclampsia, and monitoring of fetal growth and should receive careful nutritional counseling and support.[10]

Women who have undergone malabsorptive or restrictive gastric bypass surgeries, such as Roux-en-Y and laparoscopic gastric banding, could experience micronutrient deficiencies, and close monitoring and supplementation with micronutrients may be indicated.[23]

Activity in Pregnancy

Regular physical activity in pregnancy has minimal risks and many benefits, including weight management, reduced risk of gestational diabetes in obese women, overall improvements in psychological well-being, potentially decreased cesarean and operative vaginal delivery, prevention of preeclampsia, and reduced postpartum recovery times.[24] Women with uncomplicated pregnancies should be encouraged to initiate or continue approximately 150 minutes of moderate intensity aerobic activity per week, spread throughout the week and adjusted as medically necessary. Vigorous-intensity physical activity (e.g., running) can continue for women who were already engaged in these activities before pregnancy, although they should be counselled on remaining healthy and adjusting level of activity over time.[24] Those beginning physical activity for the first time during pregnancy should be encouraged to start slowly and gradually increase over time, with activities such as swimming.[24]

The American College of Obstetricians and Gynecologists (ACOG) advises a clinical evaluation before initiation of an exercise regimen and provides guidelines for absolute and relative contraindications to aerobic exercise in pregnancy. Certain activities (scuba diving; activities that increase the risk for trauma, such as mountain climbing) should be avoided during pregnancy. Women should be instructed to stop exercising if they experience preterm labor signs (contractions, bleeding, leakage of amniotic fluid), chest or head pain, calf pain, or decreased fetal movement. Women should also be reminded that they need to consider their shifting center of gravity, the additional effort that the extra weight of pregnancy requires,

and the effect of pregnancy hormones on relaxing all ligaments, especially in later pregnancy.[24]

Sexual activity in pregnancy is considered safe. Anticipatory guidance should be offered to women about physical changes and sexual positions that may influence sexual comfort during pregnancy. Women at risk for preterm labor, placenta previa, or recurrent pregnancy loss may be advised to avoid sexual activity.[1] Therapeutic bed rest is no longer recommended for most women because it has been proven ineffective at prevention of preterm birth and is associated with multiple risks including venous thromboembolism, bone demineralization, and deconditioning.[24]

Physical Examination and Laboratory and Diagnostic Tests

The purpose of the physical examination and laboratory and diagnostic tests is to establish baselines, to detect abnormalities, and to monitor underlying chronic conditions. The pelvic examination should evaluate the size and position of the cervix and uterus, and the remainder of the physical examination (heart, lungs, thyroid, abdomen) is focused on identification of any previously unrecognized disorders.[15] Assessment of the breast and nipple, best done during the first trimester, can identify potential anatomy-related issues for breastfeeding such as lack of changes in the breast, primary hypoplasia of the breasts, or breast augmentation or reduction.[25] These women should be referred to a lactation consultant, or close follow-up in the early postpartum period should be planned. Laboratory tests are routinely conducted in pregnancy to identify conditions that could affect maternal or fetal outcomes (see Table 11.1).[11]

Although ultrasound imaging has a place in obstetric care, commercial ultrasound examinations used for the specific purpose of imaging to "see the baby," to preserve keepsakes, or to determine the sex of the unborn child are increasing in popularity. The American Institute of Ultrasound in Medicine and ACOG advise that fetal ultrasound examinations be conducted only by trained professionals, based on medical necessity, and done in a way that the clinical question is answered.[1,11]

Counseling and Education in Prenatal Care

Counseling and education are fundamental components of prenatal care. Counseling and education should be individualized and timely and should empower the woman and her family to make healthy decisions.[11] Historically, the primary focus of education and counseling in pregnancy has been the prenatal course and preparation for labor and delivery. However, this focus misses critical opportunities to prepare a woman for the postpartum period and motherhood, including breastfeeding education and postpartum birth control options. The prevalence of postpartum contraceptive use is highest when both prenatal and postpartum counseling is done.[26]

There is increasing evidence that prenatal education and support for breastfeeding by clinicians increases breastfeeding rates.[27] Written and verbal information should be provided starting at the initial prenatal visit and continuing throughout pregnancy. This information should include the value of exclusive breastfeeding for both short-term and long-term health (Box 11.1), discussion of social supports breastfeeding, as well as barriers and concerns, and a discussion about what to expect in the immediate postpartum period. Mothers should be taught to nurse frequently in the first days after birth to minimize breast engorgement and optimize milk supply, effective latch

BOX **11.1**

Ten Steps to Successful Breastfeeding

CRITICAL MANAGEMENT PROCEDURES

1a. Comply fully with the International Code of Marketing of Breast-milk Substitutes and relevant World Health Assembly resolutions.

1b. Have a written infant feeding policy that is routinely communicated to staff and parents.

1c. Establish ongoing monitoring and data-management systems.

2. Ensure that staff have sufficient knowledge, competence and skills to support breastfeeding.

Key Clinical Practices

3. Discuss the importance and management of breastfeeding with pregnant women and their families.

4. Facilitate immediate and uninterrupted skin-to-skin contact and support mothers to initiate breastfeeding as soon as possible after birth.

5. Support mothers to initiate and maintain breastfeeding and manage common difficulties.

6. Do not provide breastfed newborns any food or fluids other than breast milk, unless medically indicated.

7. Enable mothers and their infants to remain together and to practise rooming-in 24 hours a day.

8. Support mothers to recognize and respond to their infants' cues for feeding.

9. Counsel mothers on the use and risks of feeding bottles, teats and pacifiers.

10. Coordinate discharge so that parents and their infants have timely access to ongoing support and care.

From World Health Organization, UNICEF. (2018). The ten steps to successful breast-feeding. Available at https://www.who.int/nutrition/bfhi/ten-steps/en/.

BOX **11.2**

Provider Checklist for Patient Education in Prenatal Care

Pregnant women are educated on the following topics:
- Benefits of breastfeeding for mother and child
- The importance of exclusive breastfeeding for the first 6 months
- Early initiation of breastfeeding
- Early skin-to-skin contact
- Rooming-in on a 24-h basis
- Baby-led feeding
- Promotion of milk supply through frequent feeding
- Effective positioning and latch techniques
- Continuation of breastfeeding after introduction of appropriate complementary foods

BOX **11.3**

Significant Maternal and Infant Health Benefits Associated With Breastfeeding

BENEFITS OF BREASTFEEDING FOR INFANT
- Optimal immune system development and establishment of gut health
- Decreased risk of hospitalization in first year of life
- Decreased frequency and severity of communicable diseases: diarrhea, otitis media, and respiratory tract infections
- Decreased risk of chronic noncommunicable disease, including respiratory and gastrointestinal allergies, obesity, diabetes, hypertension, cancer, and Crohn disease
- Improved motor and intellectual development

BENEFITS OF BREASTFEEDING FOR MOTHER
- Decreased risk of ovarian cancer
- Decreased risk of osteoporosis
- Decreased blood loss in the postpartum period
- Decreased risk of some types of breast cancers
- Promotion of postpartum weight loss

Data from Lutter, C., Ross, J., & Martin, L. (2002). *Quantifying the benefits of breast-feeding: A summary of the evidence.* Washington, DC: Pan American Health Organization (PAHO).

and positioning techniques, and to avoid bottles and supplements unless their use is medically indicated.[28] Health providers can use the Ten Steps to Successful Breastfeeding, Checklist for Patient Education in Prenatal Care, and Significant Maternal and Infant Health Benefits Associated with Breastfeeding to guide mothers in thorough planning for successful breastfeeding (Boxes 11.2 and 11.3; see Box 11.1).

COMMON PROBLEMS IN PREGNANCY
Anemia

Iron deficiency anemia (IDA) is very common in pregnancy—approximately 20% of pregnant women are affected in industrialized countries. IDA increases risks of preterm labor, low birth weight, and infant mortality.[21] It is usually detected through routine complete blood count (CBC) testing at the initial visit and repeat testing early in the third trimester, although a woman may also be symptomatic with fatigue, dizziness, pica (eating of nonfood items such as starch or clay or ice chewing), dyspnea, or tachycardia or palpitations, depending on severity and maternal tolerance.[10] Iron replacement therapy with 60 to 120 mg of elemental iron daily is indicated if hemoglobin is less than 11 g/dL, along with an increase in iron-rich food intake.

Infections

Some infections may occur more frequently or pose increased risk during pregnancy. See Table 11.4 for an overview of the important infections in pregnancy.[1,15,29]

Urinary Tract Infections. Pregnant women are at increased risk for urinary tract infections (UTIs), which are the most common bacterial infection in pregnancy[1,15] and are implicated in premature deliveries and low birth weight. UTIs are also much more likely to progress to pyelonephritis in pregnant women. UTIs in pregnant women include asymptomatic bacteriuria, acute cystitis, and acute pyelonephritis. Asymptomatic bacteriuria occurs in 2% to 13% of pregnant women, but if it is identified and treated early, the risk of pyelonephritis can be reduced from 30% to 40% to 3% to 4%, possibly also decreasing the risk of preeclampsia, premature birth, and low neonatal birth weight.[30] Pregnant women should have a urine culture (ideally including sensitivity of any identified bacteria to various antibiotics) at 12 to 16 weeks' gestation, or at the first prenatal visit if later, to screen for asymptomatic bacteriuria and should be treated with antibiotics if colony counts are 100,000 or higher.[30,31] Women should also receive treatment for symptomatic UTIs on the basis of symptoms and

TABLE 11.4	Infections in Pregnancy			
Infection	**Organism**	**Symptoms**	**Diagnostics**	**Treatment Options**
Urinary tract infection	*Escherichia coli* *Klebsiella pneumoniae* *Enterococcus* *Proteus* *Staphylococcus* Group B *Streptococcus*	May be absent Dysuria Frequency Urgency	Suprapubic tenderness Urinalysis Culture Repeat 1–2 weeks after treatment	Amoxicillin Ampicillin Nitrofurantoin Trimethoprim-sulfamethoxazole[a] Cephalexin
Vulvovaginal candidiasis	*Candida albicans* *Candida* species Yeast	Pruritus Dyspareunia Abnormal vaginal discharge	Wet mount Hyphae or buds Normal pH	Topical azoles only
Bacterial vaginosis	*Gardnerella vaginalis* *Mobiluncus* species *Bacteroides* *Mycoplasma hominis* *Prevotella* species *Ureaplasma* *Mycoplasma*	May be absent Odor Irritation	Wet mount Clue cells Whiff pH >4.5	Metronidazole (oral)[b] Clindamycin (oral) Avoid douching
Trichomoniasis	*Trichomonas vaginalis*	Odor Yellow-green discharge Irritation	Wet mount *T. vaginalis* Whiff *Trichomonas* rapid test Culture	Metronidazole (oral)[b] Counseling for sexually transmitted disease

[a]Avoid in first and third trimesters.
[b]Use with consultation only.
Data from Corton, M., Leveno, K., Bloom, S., et al. (2014). *Williams obstetrics* (24th ed.). New York: McGraw-Hill; U.S. Department of Health and Human Services, Centers for Disease Control and Prevention. 2015 Sexually transmitted diseases treatment guidelines. Retrieved from http://www.cdc.gov/std/tg2015/default.htm; Callahan, T., & Caughey, A. (2017). *Blueprints obstetrics and gynecology* (7th ed.). Philadelphia, PA: Wolters Kluwer; Lyons, P. (2015). *Obstetrics in family medicine: a practical guide* (2nd ed.). Switzerland: Springer International.

bacterial colony counts as low as ≥10^2 to 10^3 colony-forming units (CFU)/mL. Nitrofurantoin and sulfonamides are the first line agents for treatment and prevention of UTI in the second and third trimesters and are appropriate for use in the first trimester if no alternative antibiotics are available.[32] If antibiotics are given for a UTI or other infections, a prescription for yeast treatment to be taken as needed at completion of antibiotic treatment may also be given, particularly for women who are prone to yeast infections.[10] Women should undergo a test of cure after treatment and have a repeat urine culture every 6 to 12 weeks for the remainder of the pregnancy, and a urine dipstick should be performed at every visit to evaluate for blood, nitrites, and leukocytes.[10] After two positive cultures, suppressive therapy should be given.[30]

Group B *Streptococcus*

Approximately 25% of pregnant women are colonized with group B *Streptococcus* (GBS) in their rectum and/or vagina and are considered GBS positive.[33] Universal screening of pregnant women at 35 to 37 weeks' gestation by sterile rectovaginal swab is used to identify GBS in pregnant women.[34] Although not generally considered clinically significant for women, they are at risk for passing the GBS bacteria to their babies during birth, causing neonatal GBS disease—commonly sepsis, pneumonia, or, less frequently, meningitis. Antibiotic treatment for GBS-positive women during labor is highly effective, reducing the chances of a GBS-positive woman delivering a baby with GBS disease from 1 in 200 to 1 in 4000.

If GBS is identified in urine in any number at any time in pregnancy, a woman should be considered GBS positive.[10,33] As with bacteriuria caused by other organisms, pregnant women who have GBS colony counts less than 100,000 CFU/mL and are asymptomatic should not receive antibiotics at time of culture.[35] However, treatment with antibiotics in labor or after rupture of membranes to prevent early-onset neonatal GBS disease is indicated, and additional vaginal and rectal screening at 35 to 37 weeks' gestation is not necessary. Women who have previously given birth to an infant with GBS disease should automatically be given antibiotics in labor and do not need the vaginal and rectal screening at 35 to 37 weeks.[34]

Zika Exposure. Since 2015, transmission of the Zika virus has spread quickly around the world, making it increasingly likely that a health care provider will care for patients who have lived in or travelled to an area of Zika transmission. Zika is primarily transmitted through mosquito bites and sexually. Although pregnant women are not more susceptible to Zika or more severely affected, there is strong evidence that maternal-fetal transmission of the virus occurs and can cause devastating birth defects, particularly microcephaly.[36] Because of this, pregnant women should be advised against travel to Zika transmission areas. If travel is unavoidable, pregnant women should vigorously protect themselves again mosquito bites and sexual transmission. Women should be asked about Zika exposure at all prenatal visits. All pregnant women with possible Zika exposure and Zika symptoms (fever, headache, muscle or joint pain, conjunctivitis, rash), as well as pregnant women with ongoing Zika exposure but no Zika symptoms, should be tested. Health care providers should contact their local or state health department to facilitate testing.[37] Women with confirmed or suspected Zika exposure should have serial ultrasounds every 3 to 4 weeks that include detailed fetal anatomy, particularly fetal neuroanatomy.[37] For addition information, see Chapter 215, Mosquito-Borne Illnesses.

Vaginitis. Vaginitis can be caused by yeast, bacteria, or protozoa, and symptoms may vary by the cause; common symptoms are itching, burning, and/or increased or malodorous discharge. Vaginitis can be a common but often overlooked cause of mild bleeding in pregnancy, particularly after intercourse, because vaginal infections can cause the cervix to become friable.[10] Due to hormonal changes from pregnancy, yeast infections are very common in pregnancy. In pregnancy, the most appropriate first-line treatment for vaginal yeast infections in pregnancy is a 7-day topical vaginal azole cream, due to lack of information about short-term use of low-dose (150 mg) oral azole antifungal agents (fluconazole) in pregnancy and concerns about increased risk of spontaneous abortion (SAB) and, possibly, stillbirth.[38]

Bacterial vaginosis (BV) is also common in pregnancy. BV is correlated with adverse pregnancy outcomes because if it is left untreated, bacteria can ascend into the uterus, inducing preterm labor, preterm premature rupture of membranes (PPROM), intrauterine infection, and postpartum endometritis. Despite this association, current recommendations do not support routine screening for BV, because this approach has not consistently yielded a reduction in preterm births for those at high or low risk for preterm delivery.[29] There is some evidence that if treatment of BV is given early in pregnancy (<22 completed weeks' gestation), the rate of preterm birth decreases, presumably because treatment prevents irreversible inflammatory damage, but there is currently lack of consensus regarding this.[29] Treatment is recommended for all symptomatic women to reduce the signs and symptoms. Standard treatment is with either 250 or 500 mg of oral metronidazole (Flagyl) twice a day for 7 days, which has been shown to be safe in pregnancy. However, 5 mg of 0.75% vaginal metronidazole gel intravaginally once a day for 5 days or 5 g of 2% clindamycin cream intravaginally at bedtime for 7 days are also both effective and acceptable in pregnancy.[29]

Vaginitis caused by the protozoan *Trichomonas vaginalis* manifests similarly to BV in pregnancy, although the symptoms may be much more severe and discharge may be more diffuse and yellowish-green. Its impact on pregnancy outcomes is also similar to BV. Like BV, routine screening is not currently recommended due to no effect of treatment on adverse outcomes of pregnancy. However, trichomoniasis is an STI, and symptomatic women and their partners should both be treated at any point in pregnancy. The pregnant woman receives a single 2-g oral dose, and her partner can be treated with either a single 2-g oral dose or 500 mg of oral metronidazole twice daily for 7 days.[29]

With all of the aforementioned vaginal infections, patients should be counseled to refrain from douching, frequently wash hands with soap and water, wear cotton underwear and loose clothing, keep underwear dry, promptly change wet underwear, avoid scented panty liners and pads, avoid wearing panty liners or pads every day, avoid the use of scented products on the vaginal area, and eat yogurt or use probiotics to promote the growth of "good bacteria" that keep yeast in check.[39] In addition, women should avoid scratching, which can make symptoms worse and introduce infection. Cold yogurt or petroleum jelly or a freezer gel pack can soothe itchy, irritated areas, as can a tepid bath.

For additional information, please see Chapter 153, Vulvar and Vaginal Disorders.

Nausea and Vomiting

Approximately 75% of women experience some nausea and/or vomiting in pregnancy, and 1% will develop hyperemesis gravidarum, which may require evaluation for underlying causes (e.g., a hydatidiform mole, metabolic or gastrointestinal disorders) and hospitalization for rehydration therapy and parenteral nutrition.[40] Although usually not life threatening and usually self-limiting by 12 to 16 weeks of pregnancy, nausea and vomiting can negatively affect a woman's quality of life. Initial treatment consists of emotional support and reassurance of normalcy. Recommend dietary changes include small, frequent meals (with food eaten first thing in the morning before rising), bland foods high in carbohydrates and low in fat, high-protein foods that promote level blood sugar, and avoidance of "trigger" or strong-smelling foods and sour foods; carbonated beverages can bring relief in some women. If nausea or vomiting persists, ginger, acupressure, and vitamin B_6 (25 mg PO q8h) may be introduced.[11,41]

If nonpharmacologic treatment is not effective, a combination of doxylamine and pyridoxine (vitamin B_6) is the first line pharmacologic treatment. A medication combining 10 mg of doxylamine and 10 mg of pyridoxine (Bendectin) was pulled from the market in 1983 owing to safety concerns, despite multiple studies showing no increased risk of birth defects, but remained on the market in Canada. This combination was reintroduced in 2013 in the United States as Diclegis, a US Food and Drug Administration (FDA)-approved category A drug for the management of nausea and vomiting (two tablets PO hs for mild symptoms; up to four tablets PO hs for more severe symptoms).[40] Alternatively, the combination can be replicated with an over-the-counter histamine H_1 blocker (Unisom) and vitamin B_6 (25 mg PO q8h B_6 plus 12.5 mg Unisom PO hs). If this is not adequate, antiemetics are the second-line treatment, including prochlorperazine (Compazine), chlorpromazine (Thorazine), trimethobenzamide (Tigan), or ondansetron (Zofran).[40] Other H_1 blockers that have been used include diphenhydramine (Benadryl), hydroxyzine, and meclizine. If a patient reports that she has been unable to eat or drink for more than 24 hours or has signs of dehydration or significant weight loss, evaluation of the urine for ketones and specific gravity and blood tests for electrolytes, blood urea nitrogen (BUN), and creatinine can provide valuable information about the need for further intervention.[10]

Gastroesophageal Reflux

High progesterone levels, which relax the gastroesophageal sphincter, and pressure on the diaphragm from an enlarging uterus combine to cause reflux of hydrochloric acid into the esophagus. This gastroesophageal reflux produces an unpleasant, midsternal burning sensation. Raising the head of the bed; eating small, bland meals; and avoiding lying flat after eating can reduce symptoms.[42] If lifestyle changes are inadequate, antacids are first line treatment, but bicarbonate-containing antacids should be avoided to reduce the risk of metabolic acidosis and fluid overload. Antacids containing aluminum, calcium, and magnesium are recommended, but women should be counseled to limit intake to 1.0 g because doses higher than 1.4 g of calcium carbonate have been associated with an increase in milk-alkali syndrome. The H_2 blockers cimetidine and ranitidine and the proton pump inhibitor omeprazole have been shown to be safe and effective in pregnancy.[1,15] For women hoping to avoid medication, papaya enzymes may be suggested as an herbal alternative.[10]

Constipation and Hemorrhoids

Approximately one-third of women will experience constipation during pregnancy, with the worst symptoms occurring during the third trimester. This is believed to result from a combination of hormonal and metabolic changes, the relaxation effect of progesterone on bowel motility, the increasing compression of the bowel as the fetus enlarges, dehydration, decreased physical activity, and dietary changes (small, more frequent meals with inadequate fiber intake).[15]

Management of constipation begins with dietary and behavioral changes, starting with increased water and fiber intake, intake of foods with laxative properties (e.g., prunes, decaffeinated coffee), and moderate physical activity. Bulking agents (psyllium, methylcellulose) have been shown to be safe in pregnancy, even for long-term use, and are first line treatments, usually 1 tablespoon in 8 ounces of fluid 1 to 3 times a day. Polyethylene glycol is not approved by the FDA for use in pregnancy, but toxicity is unlikely because of its reduced absorption. However, they are more likely to cause side effects such as flatulence and bloating. Stimulant laxatives such as anthraquinones, senna, and cascara are safe to use intermittently but not routinely in pregnancy. Prolonged use could lead to electrolyte imbalances. The stool softener docusate sodium is also considered safe in pregnancy. Mineral oil, castor oil, and saline should be avoided during pregnancy.[43]

Straining to pass bowel movements when constipated combined with increased pressure on the rectum and perineum can lead to hemorrhoids in pregnant women. If this occurs, the woman should be counseled in the aforementioned measures to prevent constipation. Cold witch hazel compresses, sitz baths with baking soda, and Tucks pads can be used for symptomatic relief as needed.[10] Topical anesthetics may be used unless otherwise contraindicated, although evidence regarding the efficacy of these is lacking.[10] Hemorrhoids typically resolve spontaneously postpartum.

PREGNANCY COMPLICATIONS
Bleeding in Pregnancy

Twenty percent to 25% of women will experience bleeding during the first trimester, and only half of these pregnancies will result in a live infant.[1] The causes of first trimester bleeding are numerous, including cervical, uterine or chromosomal abnormalities, ectopic pregnancy, hormonal or nutritional imbalance, trauma, poorly controlled diabetes, maternal infection, and substance use. Diagnosis is based on ultrasound examination to evaluate viability and rule out ectopic or trophoblastic pregnancy, and laboratory studies. Laboratory tests should include serial β-hCG measurements 48 hours apart, CBC with platelets, blood type and Rh, antibody screen, coagulation studies if a missed abortion is suspected, and type and crossmatch if surgery is being considered.[10] To reduce risk of isoimmunization, women who are Rh negative should receive RhoGAM.[1,10]

 First Trimester Bleeding

Rule out:
- Threatened or spontaneous abortion
- Cervical or uterine abnormalities
- Ectopic implantation
- Maternal infection
- Chromosomal abnormalities
- Implantation bleeding
- Molar pregnancy
- Hormonal or nutritional imbalance
- Substance use
- Poorly controlled diabetes
- Trauma

Data from Tharpe, N. L., Farley, C. L., & Jordan, R. G. (2013). *Clinical practice guidelines for midwifery and women's health* (5th ed.). Burlington, MA: Jones & Bartlett; 2013; and Corton, M., Leveno, K., Bloom, S. et al. (2014). *Williams obstetrics* (24th ed.). New York: McGraw-Hill.

If a nonviable pregnancy is located within the uterus and there are no signs of infection, a woman may be offered expectant, medical, or surgical management. With expectant management, the expulsion of the uterine contents can be allowed to proceed spontaneously. A woman should be counseled to maintain pelvic rest; be prepared for significant bleeding lasting up to 7 to 10 days; return for care if uterine contents have not passed within 7 days; and call if bleeding increases or is accompanied by pain, adnexal pain, or fever occurs, or heavy bleeding with pain lasts for longer than 1 hour.[10] Medical management with 800 mcg of vaginal or 600 mcg of oral misoprostol is very safe for incomplete SAB at less than 13 weeks' gestation and results in less pain, but more bleeding, than surgical intervention.[10,44] If expulsion of uterine contents has not occurred by day 3, the dose should be repeated, and if it has still not occurred by day 8, surgical management is indicated. Surgical intervention (dilation and curettage) may be necessary if the products of conception are not completely evacuated (incomplete) or are not evacuated at all (missed) or the woman develops sepsis, or if desired by the woman at any point.[1] Antibiotics are not indicated unless there are signs of sepsis. A repeat β-hCG measurement should be done 4 to 6 weeks after an SAB to ensure that β-hCG has returned to nonpregnant levels.[10]

An ectopic pregnancy, or pregnancy with implantation outside of the uterus, should be suspected with slowly rising or continued positive β-hCG levels after no intrauterine pregnancy is seen on an ultrasound.[10] The ultrasound should be repeated in 2 to 7 days to confirm. Transvaginal ultrasound may be more accurate in diagnosing ectopic pregnancy than transabdominal ultrasound, particularly if β-hCG levels are less than 1500 to 2000 mIU/mL.[1] An ectopic pregnancy may or may not be accompanied by severe lower abdominal pain, spotting, and diaphragmatic irritation, particularly with rupture. Management of ectopic pregnancy is very different from management of SAB; watchful waiting is not an option. Medical management with methotrexate can be offered, but surgical intervention for an ectopic pregnancy is often used, depending on the location of the ectopic products of conception and the hemodynamic status of the woman.[1]

Bleeding in the second and third trimesters may be related to benign causes such as bloody show in term labor, postcoital or postexamination spotting, or vaginal or cervical infection or to more serious conditions such as placenta previa, preterm labor, or placental abruption.[10] For benign causes, reassurance, review of danger signs, and treatment of any underlying causes (e.g., BV) should be provided. Placenta previa is caused by implantation of the placenta near or across the cervical os, and although it typically occurs early in gestation, serial ultrasound examinations are important because the condition often resolves as the uterus enlarges. Although complete previa occurs in a very small (0.5%) number of pregnancies, it contributes to 20% of all antepartum hemorrhages. Bleeding is painless and usually occurs after the 28th week.[1] If previa is suspected, vaginal examination should be delayed until location of the placenta has been confirmed.[10] If bleeding stops and the fetus is not compromised, delivery may be delayed until the pregnancy reaches term with strict pelvic rest. For complete previa, a cesarean section is scheduled at term; for marginal previa with minimal or no bleeding and if the fetus remains healthy, a vaginal birth can be attempted, with monitoring of the fetus. If the fetus status becomes compromised and bleeding continues, immediate delivery by cesarean section is indicated.

Placental abruption occurs when part of or the entire placenta separates inappropriately from the uterine wall. Abruption occurs in approximately 0.5% to 1.5% of pregnancies, and accounts for up to 25% of third trimester bleeding.[45] Risk factors that have been associated with abruption include increased age and parity, maternal HTN, PPROM, multiple gestation, smoking, and cocaine use.[1,10,15] Diagnosis is clinical, with the classic presentation including blackish metrorrhagia with severe abdominal and/or back pain and uterine hypertonia, although in reality this "classic" triad was found to be present in only 9.7% of abruption cases.[45] Symptoms can vary by the degree of placental separation, and the bleeding can be concealed and discovered only on examination of the placenta after delivery. Bleeding was the only clinical presenting sign in 60% of cases in one study.[45] If the placental separation is abrupt and complete or nearly complete, hemorrhage and hypovolemic shock can occur.[45] Abruption significantly increases the risk for fetal hypoxia and is the underlying cause in 15% of perinatal mortality.[45]

Emotional support is critical, regardless of the trimester in which unexpected bleeding occurs. Exploring all options with the pregnant woman and her family can assist them in making informed, empowered decisions for the best physiologic and psychological outcomes.[10,44]

Preterm Labor

Preterm labor, defined as spontaneous rupture of membranes and/or uterine contractions that cause cervical change and dilation before 37 weeks of gestation, is a serious pregnancy complication that often (45% of the time) leads to premature delivery.[1] Approximately 70% of neonatal deaths are related to prematurity, and those infants who survive face potential lifetime consequences including 50% of the long-term neurologic disabilities in the United States.[46] Factors associated with preterm labor include socioeconomic status, genetic conditions, periodontal disease, uterine or cervical abnormalities, multiple gestation, substance use, maternal infections, and diseases such as preeclampsia.[1,10]

Of women with preterm labor, only approximately 10% will give birth within 7 days.[47] Fetal fibronectin (fFN) testing and cervical length assessment can help to predict which women with premature uterine contractions are the most likely to progress to premature delivery, with positive fFN and cervical length less than 25 mm being strong predictors of preterm birth,[10] although they should be used in conjunction with other information to direct management.[44] fFN testing must be done before digital examination of the cervix and can be affected by recent sexual activity or bleeding.[10] Taking fFN, gestational age, fetal status, and cervical length variables into account, timely identification and treatment of high-risk women including cerclage or tocolytics (β-mimetics, calcium channel blockers, magnesium sulfate, or prostaglandin inhibitors) can prolong pregnancy and reduce morbidity and mortality associated with preterm birth.[1,10,47] Tocolytics are effective for only 48 hours and are thus usually reserved for cases in which the fetus is viable and would benefit from an additional 48 hours, such as for the administration of corticosteroids.[47] They are not indicated after 34 weeks' gestation or if contractions are not leading to cervical change, and are not recommended for maintenance therapy to prevent preterm birth.

If delivery appears possible in the next 7 days, injectable steroids (i.e., betamethasone, dexamethasone) should be used at 24 to 34 weeks' gestation to mature fetal lungs and to prevent neurologic and gastrointestinal complications associated with extreme prematurity.[1,44] Antibiotics are recommended only to prevent GBS infection and to conservatively manage PPROM when the fetus is very immature.[44] Women with a history of preterm birth may be candidates for treatment with 17-hydroxyprogesterone to prevent preterm birth in subsequent pregnancies.[46]

OTHER MEDICAL CONDITIONS IN PREGNANCY

 Physician consultation, collaborative management, or referral is indicated for many preexisting and emergent disorders associated with pregnancy. Common conditions that may indicate the need for this include severe HTN, preeclampsia, or eclampsia; gestational, type 1, or type 2 diabetes; new-onset hyperthyroidism; vaginal bleeding; pyelonephritis; congenital or suspected heart disease; renal disease; ectopic pregnancy; or asthma exacerbation. The initial visit should include screening for prepregnancy conditions that could affect pregnancy, and a plan of care with appropriate levels of care should be developed and put into action as soon as possible to ensure adequate management.

Asthma

Given that the prevalence of asthma continues to increase in the United States, it is critical to understand asthma in pregnancy.[48] Approximately 4% to 8% of women have a history of asthma when they become pregnant, and some additional women will first receive an asthma diagnosis during pregnancy.[49] Of these women, approximately one-third will have their asthma improve, one-third will have no change, and one-third will have their asthma worsen, and there is no good way of predicting which will occur with any given woman.[48] However, it is clear that women with mild or well-controlled moderate asthma are not at increased risk for adverse pregnancy outcomes, but women with poorly controlled or severe disease are likely to have more exacerbations[1] and are at increased risk for premature delivery, preeclampsia, intrauterine growth restriction (IUGR), and cesarean section. Thus, to reduce maternal and fetal morbidity and mortality, preconception care should focus on ensuring that women with asthma enter pregnancy with well-controlled disease, and prenatal care should focus on closely monitoring asthma and taking

TABLE 11.5 Stepwise Therapy for Chronic Asthma During Pregnancy

Asthma Severity	Medication
Mild intermittent	No daily medications Short-acting β_2 agonist (if needed)
Mild persistent	Low-dose inhaled corticosteroid Alternative: cromolyn, leukotriene receptor antagonist, or theophylline[a]
Moderate persistent	Low-dose inhaled corticosteroid and salmeterol; or Medium-dose inhaled corticosteroid; or Medium-dose inhaled corticosteroid and salmeterol[b] Alternative: low- or medium-dose inhaled corticosteroid + leukotriene receptor antagonist or theophylline[a]
Severe persistent	High-dose inhaled corticosteroid and salmeterol[b] and (if needed) oral corticosteroid Alternative: high-dose inhaled corticosteroid + theophylline[a] and oral corticosteroid (if needed)

[a]Check therapeutic level, 5 to 12 mcg/mL.
[b]Add-on use of salmeterol is preferred to add-on use of leukotriene receptor antagonist or theophylline.
From American College of Obstetricians and Gynecologists. (2008). Practice bulletin no. 90: Asthma in pregnancy. *Obstetrics and Gynecology, 111*, 457–464. Reaffirmed 2016.

necessary steps to maintain control to reduce maternal and fetal morbidity and mortality.[49]

Diagnosis and monitoring of asthma are done through tracking of symptom frequency, timing, and severity (such as by using a daily asthma symptom diary) and spirometry to measure peak expiratory flow rate twice daily, with a goal range of 380 to 550 L/min.[1] Management goals are reinforced through education, reduction of environmental triggers, routine monitoring of pulmonary function, and use of pharmacologic management as indicated.[1] A stepwise approach to management of asthma medication is listed in Table 11.5.[49] The most commonly used classes of asthma medications in pregnancy are inhaled corticosteroids, long-acting β_2 agonists, a combination of these two, and short-acting β_2 agonists.[48] According to the National Asthma Education and Prevention Program, albuterol is the short-acting β_2 agonist drug of choice, and the preferred inhaled corticosteroid is budesonide. However, a woman should continue taking the same inhaled corticosteroid used before pregnancy if possible. Pregnant women should be counseled that use of asthma medications during pregnancy is safer for both the woman and the fetus than are the consequences of uncontrolled asthma and exacerbations.[10] ACOG recommends fetal surveillance for women with poorly controlled, moderate, or severe asthma or women recovering from a severe exacerbation, with serial ultrasound examinations and antenatal fetal testing beginning at 32 weeks' gestation.[49] Stepdown of corticosteroid inhalers should be done only postpartum.[48]

Hypertension

There are four categories of HTN in pregnancy: chronic HTN, gestational HTN, and, most dangerous, preeclampsia and eclampsia, and preeclampsia superimposed on chronic HTN.[1,10]

Collectively, these conditions affect 5% to 10% of pregnancies, making HTN the most common medical condition in pregnancy.[1] Diagnostic criteria are outlined in Table 11.6.[15,50]

Risk factors for the development of preeclampsia are preexisting HTN, chronic renal disease, multiple gestations, molar pregnancy, African or Asian race, maternal age younger than 20 years or older than 35 years, nulliparity, previous preeclampsia, new paternal partner, obesity, pregestational diabetes, and antiphospholipid antibody syndrome.[1,15,51] Uteroplacental insufficiency can result in fetal consequences, including fetal distress, IUGR, and iatrogenic prematurity. Maternal consequences of HTN include increased risk for preterm labor, placental abruption, disseminated intravascular coagulopathy, and HELLP syndrome (hemolytic anemia, elevated liver enzymes, low platelet count), making HTN one of the leading causes of maternal mortality worldwide.[10] Given the tremendous potential for devastating effects, careful antenatal surveillance, evaluation of symptoms, and prompt treatment are indicated.

For women with chronic HTN, baseline laboratory testing includes urine dipstick for proteinuria, hematocrit and hemoglobin, platelet count, serum creatinine, and electrolytes; liver function tests may be useful in later differentiation of onset of preeclampsia.[10] Chronic HTN is associated with increased risk of cesarean section, postpartum hemorrhage, GDM, preeclampsia, and increased severity of HTN during pregnancy. Home monitoring of BP is recommended for women with chronic HTN.[51] Treatment of mild to moderate chronic HTN in pregnancy does not appear to decrease fetal risk or prevent development of preeclampsia, so management remains controversial, but antihypertensive treatment is recommended if maternal blood pressure is higher than 160/105 mm Hg.[51] Nifedipine is the recommended antihypertensive, although labetalol and methyldopa are reasonable second line alternatives.[52] Consultation is recommended if use of one of these is not effective. BP levels should be maintained in the range of 120 to 160/80 to 105 to prevent compromised uteroplacental flow with pharmacologically induced low BP levels.[52] Ultrasonography to screen for fetal growth restriction is recommended, and antenatal fetal testing should be performed if there is evidence of growth restriction.[51]

Management of gestational HTN and mild preeclampsia (including superimposed preeclampsia) is expectant management, with delivery at 37 weeks' gestation recommended if mother and fetus are stable. Antenatal testing for the fetus should be performed twice weekly for preeclampsia and once weekly for gestational HTN.[51] The fetus is monitored by daily kick counts, ultrasonography to assess growth every 3 weeks, and amniotic fluid assessment weekly. The mother is monitored by BP assessment twice weekly and CBC and liver enzyme and serum creatinine levels once a week. Women with gestational HTN should also be evaluated for proteinuria at each visit. Women should be counseled to report immediately symptoms of severe preeclampsia: severe headaches that do not resolve with rest, acetaminophen, fluids, and food; right upper quadrant pain; visual changes; or shortness of breath.

If severe features are present or develop, expectant management beyond 34 weeks is not recommended and referral is indicated. Parenteral magnesium sulfate for seizure prevention is recommended, as are antenatal corticosteroids for fetal lung development if less than 34 weeks' gestation, and delivery is deferred for 48 hours if the fetus is viable and the mother and

TABLE 11.6	Diagnostic Criteria for Hypertension in Pregnancy		
Classification	**Blood Pressure**[a]	**Laboratory Values**[b]	**Symptoms**
Chronic	BP >140/90 mm Hg <20 weeks Persistent >12 weeks PP	No urine protein	Asymptomatic
Gestational	BP >149/90 mm Hg >20 weeks Normal by 12 weeks PP	No urine protein	Asymptomatic
Preeclampsia[c,d]	Mild: ≥140/90 mm Hg Severe: ≥160/110 mm Hg Normal by 12 weeks PP	Mild: urine protein >2 g/24 h or ≥1+ dipstick Severe: urine protein ≥5 g/24 h or ≥3+ dipstick Platelets <100,000 mm³ AST and ALT elevated LDH elevated Serum creatinine >1.2 mg/dL	Altered mental status Headaches Visual disturbances Pulmonary edema Epigastric pain <500 mL urine output per day Thrombocytopenia Hemolytic anemia
Superimposed preeclampsia	BP ≥140/90 mm Hg <20 weeks Persistent >12 weeks PP	New onset: urine protein ≥2 g (300 mg)/24 h >20 weeks Sudden increase in BP Sudden increase in urine protein Low platelet count <20 weeks	Same as preeclampsia
Eclampsia			Seizures (other causes ruled out)

[a]To reduce artifact, take BP on two separate occasions no more than 7 days apart.
[b]Use 24-hour urine protein for diagnosis.
[c]May progress to HELLP (hemolytic anemia, elevated liver enzymes, low platelet count), a subcategory of preeclampsia.
[d]Unless previously elevated.
ALT, Alanine transaminase; *AST*, aspartate transaminase; *BP*, blood pressure; *LDH*, lactate dehydrogenase; *PP*, postpartum.
Data from Callahan, T., & Caughey, A. (2017). *Blueprints obstetrics and gynecology* (7th ed.). Philadelphia, PA: Wolters Kluwer; and National Institutes of Health, National High Blood Pressure Education Program. (2000). *Working group report on high blood pressure in pregnancy.* U.S. Department of Health and Human Services, National Heart, Lung, and Blood Institute. Retrieved from www.nhlbi.nih.gov/guidelines/archives/hbp_preg/hbp_preg_archive.pdf.

fetus are stable. Eclampsia (status epilepticus) requires emergent delivery, regardless of the age of the fetus.[1,51,53]

Pharmacologic management of gestational HTN and preeclampsia is the same as for chronic HTN. Low-dose aspirin (75 mg/day) for women at high risk of developing preeclampsia is recommended, as is calcium supplementation (1.5 to 2.0 g of elemental calcium per day) to increase placental blood flow in pregnancies complicated by preeclampsia.[53] However, calcium supplementation appears to decrease risk only in women with poor dietary calcium intake.[53] Bed rest; restricted salt intake; supplementation with vitamins C, D, and/or E; diuretics; magnesium; omega-3 fatty acids; and antioxidants have not proven to be effective in reducing maternal blood pressure or improving fetal outcomes.[1,53]

Diabetes

Diabetes mellitus (DM) is classified as type 1 diabetes (insulin deficiency), type 2 diabetes (decreased insulin secretion and insulin resistance), diabetes from other causes including cystic fibrosis and medication therapy, or GDM (diabetes diagnosed during pregnancy).[54] Approximately 6% to 9% of pregnancies are complicated by DM, 90% of them by GDM, and with increasing prevalence of obesity and sedentary lifestyles globally, GDM prevalence is growing.[55]

In addition to women who have been diagnosed with DM before pregnancy, some women will be diagnosed with overt (nongestational) DM at their first prenatal visit based on a fasting blood glucose followed by a 75-g glucose load and a 2-hour plasma glucose measurement, or by the 50-g two-step screening process noted later.[55] Women with a high risk of

overt DM, including previous GDM, having given birth to a large-for-gestational-age infant, and strong family predisposition, should be screened at their first prenatal visit and diagnosed with overt diabetes if results are positive. Given a lack of evidence regarding this type of screening, providers must use their clinical judgment to determine who requires first trimester or early pregnancy screening.[54] The American Diabetes Association (ADA) supports diagnosis of women with pregestational (overt) diabetes rather than GDM when they meet diagnostic criteria at the initial prenatal visit.[54]

The risks to a fetus of a mother who has been diagnosed with DM (type 1 or type 2) vary greatly depending on how well controlled her sugars are in the first trimester, which underscores the need for preconception counseling and care for women with diabetes and early identification of previously undiagnosed diabetes whenever possible.[54] Even mild levels of hyperglycemia have the potential to cause fetal malformations including anencephaly, microcephaly, and congenital heart disease, with the risk of a major birth defect directly proportional to the degree of blood sugar control in the first trimester. In caring for the patient with preexisting diabetes, a clinician should carefully evaluate the patient for use of drugs commonly prescribed for patients with diabetes including statins, angiotensin-converting enzyme inhibitors, and angiotensin receptor antagonists, all of which are contraindicated and should be discontinued during pregnancy.[54]

GDM is typically diagnosed at 24 to 28 weeks' gestation. Risk factors for GDM include race (i.e., Hispanic/Latino, Asian/Pacific Islander, Native American), obesity, sedentary lifestyle, family history, previous history of GDM, delivery of a macrosomic infant, polycystic ovarian syndrome or other signs of insulin resistance, and history of cardiovascular disease. If a woman has HTN, high-density lipoprotein level less than 35 mg/dL, triglyceride level greater than 250 mg/dL, hemoglobin A1c (HbA1c) greater than 5.7%, signs of impaired glucose tolerance, or impaired fasting glucose on a previous test, she is also at risk for GDM during pregnancy.[55]

Like pregestational DM, GDM is associated with poor maternal and fetal outcomes. Although congenital malformations are less common in pregnancies complicated by GDM, adverse fetal effects do include macrosomia, neonatal hypoglycemia, hyperbilirubinemia, shoulder dystocia birth trauma, and stillbirth; maternal complications include preeclampsia, cesarean section, and, of greatest concern, an increased risk of developing diabetes later in life.[1,55] Interestingly, maternal hyperglycemia during pregnancy is a risk factor for childhood obesity and later development of type 2 diabetes.[55]

Current recommendations are for all women, regardless of risk status, to be screened for GDM at or beyond 24 weeks' gestation.[55,56] This includes women who had a negative early screening result. Most health care providers in the United States use the 50-g, 1-hour test, with those who exceed the screening threshold undergoing a diagnostic 100-g, 3-hour test. GDM is diagnosed if a woman has two or more abnormal values on the 3-hour test.[55] However, an increasing number of health care providers are using the single 75-g, 2-hour glucose tolerance test proposed by the Fifth International Workshop-Conference on GDM. Cutoffs vary, and a single cutoff is typically set by an institution or practice for consistency.[55]

To reduce the development of fetal and maternal complications, women are counseled to maintain tight glycemic control without becoming hypoglycemic during pregnancy. For women diagnosed with GDM, the initial strategy should be achievement of normoglycemia through dietary management and moderate exercise.[55] If possible, dietary counseling with a registered dietitian and development of a personalized nutrition plan should occur shortly after diagnosis. The focus of nutritional counseling is total caloric allotment (30 to 35 kcal/kg/day), carbohydrate intake as 33% to 40% of calories, and remaining calories distributed between protein (20%) and fat (40%). Complex carbohydrates rather than simple carbohydrates should be eaten when possible, and caloric intake should be spread over three meals and two snacks to reduce glucose fluctuations. Continued surveillance of blood glucose levels is necessary to ensure that glycemic control is consistently achieved with diet management alone. Daily fasting and 2-hour postprandial testing can be used for this, with the goal to have 75% of glucose readings (no more than one abnormal value per day) within normal range of fasting glucose of 95 or less and 2-hour postprandial glucose of 120 or less.[54]

If dietary management of GDM to control hyperglycemia is inadequate, pharmacologic management is indicated. Pharmacologic management is adjusted to the type of diabetes and level of disease. Although insulin has historically been the preferred treatment option for all women in pregnancy, oral medications (glyburide, metformin) are equally effective, may be used as first-line therapy, and are not associated with increased short-term adverse maternal and neonatal outcomes as compared with insulin.[55] Insulin is required for all type 1 diabetes patients, although their levels may require adjustment in pregnancy. Women with preexisting type 2 diabetes may continue to use any oral medications they were using before pregnancy.

Women with preexisting diabetes and GDM with poor glycemic control should receive antenatal fetal testing related to the increased risk of fetal demise. This usually starts at 32 weeks' gestation but may be started earlier as indicated. Because there is little agreement on the role of fetal surveillance for women with well-controlled GDM, the type, timing, and requirements of fetal surveillance are largely be dictated by local practice. Due to risks for polyhydramnios, it typically includes serial measures of hypoglycemia. Induction of labor at 39 weeks may decrease risk of perinatal mortality without increasing risk of cesarean section for women with good glycemic control; induction at 37 to 38 weeks may be considered for those with poorly controlled GDM.[55]

All women diagnosed with GDM should have follow-up at 4 to 12 weeks postpartum with a 75-g, 2-hour OGTT to identify those who have impaired glucose fasting glucose or glucose tolerance or diabetes.[55]

Thyroid Dysfunction

Thyroid disease is increasingly being seen in women of childbearing age.[57] However, identification of thyroid disorders in pregnancy can be challenging; symptoms can mimic those of pregnancy itself, and significant metabolic changes occur very early in pregnancy.[58]

Hypothyroidism during pregnancy affects approximately 03% to 0.5% for overt hypothyroidism (high TSH and low FT_4 levels) and 2% to 3% for subclinical hypothyroidism (high TSH and normal FT_4 levels). When left undiagnosed or untreated, it is associated with increased fetal risk of anemia, neurocognitive deficits, gestational HTN, low birth weight, miscarriage, placental abruption, preeclampsia, and preterm birth.[57] Despite the risks associated with hypothyroidism, there is insufficient evidence to recommend for or against universal screening for thyroid dysfunction in early pregnancy. However, at the initial prenatal visit all women should be verbally screened for factors that could make them high risk for thyroid disease, including personal or family history of thyroid disease, history of type 1 diabetes or other autoimmune disorder; history of pregnancy loss, infertility, or preterm delivery; morbid obesity; two or more previous pregnancies; age older than 30 years; and symptoms of thyroid dysfunction. Women who are identified as high risk should receive testing for serum TSH with reflux thyroid peroxidase antibody (TPOAb) if TSH is 2.5 to 10 mU/L. If initial serum TSH testing is greater than 10 mU/L, then the woman should be treated with levothyroxine.[58] Women with a positive TPOAb result should be treated with levothyroxine if their TSH is the upper limit of the reference range (ULRR)-10 mU/L. If TPOAb is positive and TSH is 2.5 mU/L-ULRR, or if TPOAb is negative but TSH is ULRR-10 mU/L, then consider starting patient on levothyroxine. No treatment is necessary if the TPOAb is negative and TSH is 2.5 mU/L-ULRR.

The typical dosage of levothyroxine is 100 to 150 mcg/day orally, adjusted as necessary. The goal of treatment is a target TSH in the lower half of the trimester-specific reference range, or if this is not available, a target TSH concentration less than 2.5 mU/L. Due to significant variation in serum TSH between populations, it is recommended that population-based trimester-specific reference ranges for serum TSH should be defined by a health provider's practice population.[58] Patients on levothyroxine should have their TSH measured every 4 to 6 weeks until 20 weeks' gestation, or until the patient is on a stable medication dose and again at 24 to 28 weeks and 32 to

34 weeks' gestation. Treatment reduces the risk of miscarriage and preterm birth and fetal intellectual development but has not been shown to have impact on the development of maternal hypertensive disorders and placental abruption.[57]

Hyperthyroid disease, or low TSH levels and elevated FT_4 levels, in pregnancy is less common than hypothyroidism, affecting approximately 0.2% of pregnancies, 95% of them due to the autoimmune disorder Graves disease. Overt hyperthyroid disease predisposes the woman to heart failure, placental abruption, preeclampsia, and preterm delivery, and the fetus to goiters, IUGR, small for gestational age, stillbirth, and thyroid dysfunction related to maternal treatment.[57] Subclinical hyperthyroid disease (low TSH but normal FT_4 levels) is somewhat more common, estimated to affect 1.7% of pregnancies, but contributes minimally to adverse maternal or neonatal effects and so no treatment is recommended.[1] Diagnosis is made based on TSH and FT_4 levels and the presence of antithyroid antibodies; the radioactive iodine uptake scan typically used in diagnosis of hyperthyroidism is contraindicated in pregnancy. Unfortunately, treatment for hyperthyroid disease has potential teratogenic effects. Health care providers should consider discontinuing all antithyroid medication for women who are euthyroid in early pregnancy, taking into consideration disease history, recent thyroid function tests, duration of therapy, and other clinical factors. If medication is discontinued, maternal thyroid function testing (TSH and FT_4) should be done every 1 to 2 weeks to ensure the woman remains euthyroid. If she does, test intervals can increase to 2 to 4 weeks in the second and third trimester. However, if a woman is at high risk of developing thyrotoxicosis if antithyroid drugs are discontinued, propylthiouracil (PTU) is preferred in the first trimester, because methimazole is associated with birth defects, but should be switched to methimazole at 16 weeks when the risk of liver failure associated with PTU outweighs the risk of congenital anomalies.[57] The goal of PTU therapy is to maintain a serum fT_4 level in the upper one-third level of normal. Serum TSH and fT_4 levels are evaluated every 2 weeks until the woman is on a stable dose to achieve this. Monthly ultrasounds from 20 weeks should be done for women on antithyroid medication or with poorly controlled hyperthyroidism to assess fetal thyroid dysfunction, as well as weekly antenatal testing beginning at 32 to 34 weeks.[57] The use of radioactive iodine is contraindicated in pregnancy because it can cross the placenta and destroy the fetal thyroid as well.[1,58]

LACTATION

The evidence in support of breastfeeding as a primary health practice for both mother and baby is strong. Research into the human microbiome and epigenetics shows that breastfeeding increases physical and emotional well-being across the life span.[59] Optimal breastfeeding duration has been defined by the World Health Organization (WHO) and the American Academy of Pediatrics (AAP) as exclusive breastfeeding for 6 months and continued breastfeeding for a year or longer.[60] Primary care providers are in a unique position to protect, support, and promote breastfeeding. There are many resources to assist the health care provider in this work. The health care professional promotes and supports lactation, engages in open dialogue with the patient or family, provides information based on clinical assessment and knowledge, and coordinates care appropriately. Health care professionals consider cultural and situational contexts for each family while eliminating barriers to breastfeeding whenever possible. The Academy of Breastfeeding Medicine provides evidence-based protocols for use by primary care providers: www.bfmed.org.

Prenatal recommendations for breastfeeding teaching and physical assessment are discussed earlier. Postpartum mothers are taught to position the baby for correct latching and to assess whether the baby is getting enough milk. A feeding log will help mothers record feeding frequency and understand stooling and voiding patterns. Feeding requirements for breastfed infants depend on many factors such as gestational age, size for gestational age, birth history, and early adaptation to extrauterine life. Preterm infants have fewer reserves and are vulnerable to complications, such as hypoglycemia and low weight gain.[61] Infants who are large for gestational age or small for gestational age require careful observation of feeding as well. Signs of good feeds include the mother's breasts softening after feeding; the infant is satisfied and may fall asleep after suckling. The second breast should be offered, but in the early days, the baby may fall asleep after one breast and feed at more frequent intervals. As the baby becomes accustomed to larger milk volumes, feeding on both sides is more common, as are longer feeding intervals.[62]

Mothers are encouraged to feed the baby on demand and to wake a sleepy baby to ensure that the newborn has 8 to 12 good feedings in 24 hours. It is important to provide reassurance to women that the first 2 weeks, when an infant feeds frequently, can be very demanding and, in general, the infant will begin to space out feedings thereafter.[63] Mothers should be supported during this transition and reassured that mother-infant dyads sustained through the first 2 weeks of breastfeeding typically go on to meet the mother's breastfeeding goals.[62]

At the time of discharge, instructions should be provided in writing and reviewed with the mother to assess her understanding. These materials should include information about expected feeding and voiding patterns and the normal progression of the stool. Expected goals for feeding and elimination are reviewed and parents taught to report concerns rather than being taught "danger" signs. Use of language that associates breastfeeding with danger should be avoided. Parents should be taught to recognize and to report when an infant is not meeting the standard for a "good" intake, because early intervention is critical.[62]

Infants should be evaluated 1 to 3 days after discharge to assess weight and check for jaundice. Mothers should be instructed to call the provider before the scheduled visit if the infant develops jaundice or has difficulty feeding. Infants may lose up to 8% to 10% of their birth weight during the first week of life. A supplemental feeding plan should be initiated for infants who lose more than 10% of their birth weight (Box 11.4).[64]

Mothers should be provided with a list of community-based lactation resources; problems that threaten continued lactation should be referred to lactation consultants.[65,66]

Common Breastfeeding Issues

Jaundice. Most newborns become mildly jaundiced during the third to fifth days of life. Breastfed babies commonly appear jaundiced into the third or fourth week of life and less commonly for 8 to 12 weeks. Bilirubin levels decrease as the endocrine and digestive systems mature. Hyperbilirubinemia, or persistent or excessive jaundice, may be a result of

Components of a Plan to Improve Breast Milk Intake

- Evaluate the breastfeeding and correct any problems with attachment technique or positioning.
- Suggest the appropriate feeding frequency and duration based on individual assessment.
- Use a hospital-grade breast pump with a double-pump setup (pumping both sides at once) to increase breast emptying and stimulation. Use the pumped milk to supplement breastfeeding.
- Assess adequacy of feeding by closely following weight gain. If the maternal supply is adequate, weight gain should be approximately 1 oz/day. If the supply is less than required, supplemental feedings of formula or banked human milk may be required temporarily. Taper supplemental volumes as soon as the supply is increased and weight gain is improved.
- Slowly taper the pumping sessions after the infant has gained the appropriate weight and is breastfeeding without supplement.
- If the breastfeeding problem is not resolved by improving technique and supply, contact the referral network for expert help. Continue to maintain contact with the mother and specialists.

inadequate fluid intake or complicating conditions.[67] Frequent feedings usually result in frequent stools, and bowel movements are the primary excretion route for bilirubin. When feedings and associated stools are infrequent, the bilirubin in the meconium stool is reabsorbed into the bloodstream, which raises the serum bilirubin level and results in clinical jaundice. Newborn care providers must familiarize themselves with AAP neonatal jaundice guidelines and develop follow-up plans to assess the baby during the most vulnerable period, 3 to 5 days of age. The AAP has developed hyperbilirubinemia phototherapy treatment guidelines based on the rate of rise of the bilirubin levels plotted against the baby's age in hours. See http://bilitool.org. Frequent breastfeeding, once the mother's milk is in, will usually improve the jaundice. Formula supplementation may be required in cases of low milk supply. If the baby is lethargic, the mother may extract the milk with a breast pump and feed it to the baby with a supplemental nursing system, cup, or bottle until the baby regains the vigor to extract milk directly from the breast.[68] Babies with high levels of unconjugated bilirubin who meet criteria established by AAP guidelines are treated with phototherapy to prevent kernicterus, also called chronic bilirubin encephalopathy.

Poor Latch. If the baby is having difficulty latching on, positioning strategies can improve comfort for the mother and milk transfer for the baby. Mothers should be taught how to bring the baby to the breast to prevent the infant from sucking on the nipple tip. Shallow latch causes pain and poor let-down.[69] It is important that the mother be positioned comfortably. A seated, cross-legged position with pillows for back and thigh support is comfortable for most women, even those who have had a cesarean section. An upright seated position may require a stool under the feet to create some hip flexion. The infant should be positioned at the breast in an open position, so that the upper body is slightly extended. The infant's head should not be cradled in the crook of her arm or cupped in the mother's hand if doing so causes the baby's head to be flexed forward

with the chin tucked in. Instead, the infant is held in the cradle position with the head allowed to fall over mother's arm, so the baby is looking up to the breast. The baby is held very close to the mother's body, tucked under the opposite breast.

For women with sore nipples, the cross-cradle position provides more control of attachment. In the cross-cradle position, the mother holds the baby in the arm opposite the breast by grasping the baby's shoulders and upper back and tucking the baby closely under both breasts; this allows the head to fall through the web space in her hand. The baby's head will tip back, creating plenty of room between the chin and chest so that the mouth can gape. The baby will be able to open the mouth widely if the mother entices him or her by moving the baby, not the breast. The mother's hand should grasp the breast well behind the areola, compressing and projecting the breast forward so that when the infant latches on with flanged lips, he or she connects deeply with the tissue behind the areola to extract colostrum or milk. The infant should be attached asymmetrically, with more of the underside of the breast laid on the baby's gaping lower jaw and the nipple tucked into the baby's mouth last, disappearing just under the upper gum line. The baby is drawn into the mother's body deeply. Latching asymmetrically allows the baby to strip the breast effectively, minimizing nipple trauma and maximizing colostrum or milk transfer.[70] Helpful materials for health care providers, mothers, and families are available at Coffective.com.

Breast Engorgement. Breast engorgement may occur on the third or fourth postpartum day in first-time mothers and sooner in women who have had previous births. It can usually be minimized by feeding the infant 8 to 12 times each day in the days leading up to the milk coming in. Mothers should be taught to evaluate the difference between sustained and intermittent suckling, grazing at breast, and milk or colostrum removal. Babies who are gulping with feeds and having copious wet diapers with yellow stools do not need to be awakened to feed to meet their own needs but may be awakened after 2 to 3 hours to assist the mother to manage engorgement. Some women with engorgement may need to express some milk manually or with a pump to soften the areola enough to allow the infant to latch on. To prevent nipple damage and extract milk, infants need to latch deeply onto engorged breasts. A mother with engorgement may need to compress the breast manually to form it for the infant's mouth.

Deep asymmetric latch-on and sustained suckling will resolve most engorgement. If engorgement persists, ice packs may be applied to the breasts between feedings to reduce edema, and hot packs may be applied right before feedings to soften the areola. Pumping for a minute or two before latch-on may also help. If the mother cannot get her infant to latch on, direct observation of feeding is required. When an engorged breast is not well emptied, the resulting backpressure on the milk glands can result in decreased milk production.[71]

Delayed Let-Down. Let-down, or milk ejection, results from smooth muscle contraction of the myoepithelial cells surrounding the secretory alveoli of the breast. Oxytocin produced in response to the infant's suckling as well as to the sight, sound, and smell of the infant causes this contraction and the resultant milk flow. Stress, pain, and alcohol inhibit let-down. The let-down response is enhanced through thoughts about the infant, breast massage, and relaxation. Although all mothers should be informed about inhibiting and enhancing factors for let-down, this information may be especially important for mothers who need to pump milk from their breasts, including mothers of premature infants or mothers returning to work.[72]

Low Milk Production. Low milk supply is the most common reason for discontinuing breastfeeding. Lactogenesis is a complex and not completely understood biochemical and psychosocial process. Mothers who have suboptimal milk production must be assessed for physiologic, psychological, and social support variables that may be influencing milk supply.[73]

Low milk production usually results from inadequate suckling and breast emptying, low prolactin levels, inadequate mammary glandular tissue, delayed or inadequate lactogenesis, or undetermined causes. Uniformly low prolactin levels suggest an endocrine basis for low milk supply. Inadequate mammary glandular tissue can result in low milk production despite normal prolactin levels. Breast glandular tissue should be assessed prenatally and may also be assessed during the breastfeeding newborn's first office visit, if the health care provider has any concern about milk supply.

Double pumping in addition to nursing produces the best results for increasing supply. If lactogenesis is delayed or inadequate, the infant should receive supplemental feedings while breast stimulation is increased with a breast pump.[73] Close follow-up of mother and baby is required. The Academy of Breastfeeding Medicine recommends caution when considering medication or herbs to enhance milk production, because neither pharmaceutical nor herbal lactogogues have produced consistent results.[73] For additional information, see Box 11.4, Components of a Plan to Improve Breast Milk Intake.

Low Infant Weight Gain. Infants who have lost 8% or more of their birth weight must be closely monitored to prevent problems. Infants who are feeding well should have four or more milk curd stools per day by the fourth day and at least six wet diapers per day. To assess an infant with low weight gain, providers must observe a breastfeeding session. Strategies to increase success include breast pumping to increase the milk supply and increased feeding frequency. Mothers may also use techniques to arouse sleepy infants, such as stroking the infant's back, talking softly to the infant, stroking the feet, rocking the baby from sitting position to lying (supported baby sit-ups), changing the diaper, and placing the infant on the mother in skin-to-skin contact.

A supplemental nursing system can deliver supplemental formula or pooled pasteurized human milk while the infant is breastfeeding. Supplemental nursing systems offer an important alternative to bottles; breastfed babies who are offered bottles sometimes have difficulty returning to the breast, especially when the mother's milk supply is low. The supplemental nursing system offers increased flow at the breast to keep the baby interested and engaged while increasing stimulation and extraction at the breast.

Significant infant weight loss or difficult management problems require careful evaluation and follow-up. Health care providers should consider consultation with lactation consultants or physicians experienced with breastfeeding management and care of infants with failure to thrive.[66]

Cracked Nipples. Cracked nipples are usually caused by attachment or latch-on problems. The nipple becomes abraded when the infant latches only to the tip of the nipple, instead of to the underside of the breast followed by the nipple. Mothers should be taught the asymmetric latch-on technique. Treatment of cracked nipples includes correcting the attachment and supporting milk extraction.

Nipple damage and pain are sometimes so severe that mothers temporarily stop breastfeeding and maintain lactation by pumping or hand expression. Twenty-four hours of nipple rest and pumping may allow enough healing of the irritated nipples for breastfeeding to be resumed. Close-interval assessment of mother-infant dyad breastfeeding sessions will limit the need for nipple rest.

Sore nipples can heal while the baby is breastfeeding if the attachment is corrected. The mother should be taught to listen for audible swallowing to determine when the infant is actively feeding. She can remove the infant from the breast after the nursing rhythm changes from active deep suckling that removes milk to leisurely comfort sucking. The mother should be taught to use her finger to detach the baby by sliding her finger over the baby's lips, over the gum line, all the way back to the hinge of the baby's jaw. This will protect the nipple from further damage.

Medical-grade lanolin may improve breastfeeding comfort if the nipples are dry and cracked. For severely damaged nipples, hydrogel dressings are useful to maintain a moist wound healing environment. In addition, mothers must avoid overdrying their nipples and should apply warm, moist compresses after feedings to soothe and promote healing. Nipple soreness typically improves after a rest from breastfeeding for 24 hours and institution of the correct attachment position. Mothers will need to pump every 3 hours while not breastfeeding. In general, it takes 10 days for sore nipples to heal completely. If improvement is not progressive, the health care provider should reevaluate the breastfeeding technique and treatment plan. A referral to a lactation specialist may be indicated. Bacterial infection or yeast overgrowth should be considered and treated appropriately with topical or oral antibiotics or antifungal medication.[72,74]

Mastitis

Mastitis, or cellulitis of the interlobular connective tissue of the breast, is often a marker of breastfeeding problems. Mastitis usually manifests with fever, generalized malaise, influenza-like symptoms, local erythema, and breast warmth and tenderness. Bacteria often gain entry to breast tissue through a combination of unrelieved breast engorgement with cracked or abraded nipples.

Treatment of mastitis includes the application of warm packs to the breast and frequent breastfeeding or pumping. In addition to these nonpharmacologic interventions, the infection is treated with antibiotics such as amoxicillin-clavulanate, dicloxacillin, or a broad-spectrum cephalosporin to cover a probable staphylococcal or streptococcal infection. The infant's sucking technique and the mother's breastfeeding pattern and support system should also be evaluated. Mastitis can progress to abscess if early intervention is not instituted. Therefore any occurrence of influenza-like symptoms in a breastfeeding mother requires an evaluation for mastitis.[74]

Other Lactation Considerations

Referrals. Expectant and new mothers may be referred to breastfeeding support groups such as La Leche League International, Nursing Mothers Council, and WIC services. Patients who need additional assistance or specialized help during prenatal or postpartum periods should be referred to breastfeeding or lactation specialists. Lactation consultants can be found through the International Lactation Consultant Association. The AAP, Academy of Breastfeeding Medicine, La Leche League

International Medical Associates, and International Board of Lactation Consultant Examiners are resources for health care providers.

Weaning

Weaning is a natural process. It is physically and emotionally less painful when it is done gradually and the infant leads the process. As the infant grows, other activities and other foods often replace the need to breastfeed. Babies who wean before 1 year of age should continue to use formula until their first birthday. Weaning may happen as late as 2 or 3 years of age. Some mothers and infants choose to breastfeed into the toddler years, and there is no reason to oppose a continuation of this bond. The ethnographic literature suggests that before the widespread use of artificial infant formulas, children were traditionally nursed for 3 to 4 years.[75]

When mothers desire to wean, feedings should be replaced by supplemental milk or formula (depending on the infant's age), one feeding at a time, for a period of a few weeks until all feedings have been replaced. Cow's milk should be withheld until infants are older than 1 year. When weaning toddlers, mothers may replace some feedings with activities instead of food.

INTEGRATED HEALTH CARE FOR WOMEN

Although an emphasis remains on prenatal care for improving health outcomes, over the past decade *Healthy People 2020* and other guiding documents have increasingly recognized the role that preconception and interconception care can play. This has been driven in part by the increasing number of women facing chronic health conditions during their childbearing years as well as by a slowing of progress in improvement of pregnancy outcomes, particularly the key indicators of low birth weight, premature birth, and infant mortality, and an improvement in understanding of the way that chronic diseases contribute to these.[8] Although a woman and her partner's health itself should be the primary goal of prepregnancy health care, improving her prepregnancy health has a great deal of potential to improve her reproductive health. In general, preconception care that focuses on reducing unintended pregnancies, and identifying and modifying biomedical, behavioral, and social risks before she becomes pregnant are likely to have the greatest impact on pregnancy outcomes.[76,77] However, awareness of need for this type of care remains low, and there are little data on the efficacy of preconception care in improving outcomes; many opportunities remain to understand and improve preconception care and access.

REFERENCES

1. Corton, M., Leveno, K., Bloom, S., et al. (2014). *Williams obstetrics* (24th ed.). New York: McGraw-Hill.
2. U.S. Public Health Service. (1989). *Caring for our future: The content of prenatal care.* Washington, DC: U.S. Government Printing Office.
3. U.S. Department of Health and Human Services, Health Resources and Services Administration, Maternal and Child Health Bureau. Maternal child health timeline. Retrieved from: https://mchb.hrsa.gov/about/timeline/. (Accessed December 27, 2017).
4. Institute of Medicine. (1985). *Preventing low birthweight.* Washington, DC: National Academy Press.
5. Global Burden of Disease Maternal Mortality Collaborators. (2016). Global, regional, and national levels of maternal mortality 1990–2015: A systematic analysis for the Global Burden of Disease Study 2015. *Lancet, 388,* 1775–1812.
6. Kaiser Family Foundation. (2017). How does infant mortality in the U.S. compare to other countries? Retrieved from https://www.healthsystemtracker .org/chart-collection/infant-mortality-u-s-compare-countries/#item-start. (Accessed December 27, 2017).
7. Jain, J. A., Temming, L. A., D'Alton, M. E., et al. (2017). SMFM special report: Reducing racial and ethnic disparities in maternal morbidity and mortality: A call to action. *American Journal of Obstetrics and Gynecology,* [accepted for publication].
8. U.S. Department of Health and Human Services. *Developing Healthy People 2020: Maternal, infant, and child health.* Retrieved from www.healthypeople .gov/2020/topicsobjectives2020/overview.aspx?topicid=26. (Accessed December 21, 2017).
9. Zolotor, A. J., & Carlough, M. C. (2014). Update on prenatal care. *American Family Physician, 89*(3), 199–208.
10. Tharpe, N. L., Farley, C. L., & Jordan, R. G. (2013). *Clinical practice guidelines for midwifery and women's health* (5th ed.). Burlington, MA: Jones & Bartlett.
11. American Academy of Pediatrics, American College of Obstetricians and Gynecologists. (2017). *Guidelines for perinatal care* (8th ed.). Elk Grove Village (IL): AAP. Washington, DC: ACOG.
12. Phillippi, J. C., & Roman, M. W. (2013). The motivation-facilitation theory of prenatal care. *Journal of Midwifery and Women's Health, 58,* 509–515.
13. Tilden, E. L., Hersh, S. R., Emeis, C. L., et al. (2014). Group prenatal care: Review of outcomes and recommendations for model implementation. *Obstetrical and Gynecological Survey, 69*(1), 46–55.
14. Benediktsson, I., McDonald, S. W., Vekved, M., et al. (2013). Comparing CenteringPregnancy to standard prenatal care plus prenatal education. *BMC Pregnancy and Childbirth, 13*(Suppl. 1), S5.
15. Callahan, T., & Caughey, A. (2017). *Blueprints obstetrics and gynecology* (7th ed.). Philadelphia, PA: Wolters Kluwer.
16. Chisholm, C. A., Bullock, L., & Ferguson, J. E. (2017). Intimate partner violence and pregnancy: Screening and intervention. *American Journal of Obstetrics and Gynecology, 217*(2), 141–144.
17. American College of Obstetricians and Gynecologists. (2013). Committee opinion no. 548: Weight gain during pregnancy. *Obstetrics and Gynecology, 121*(1), 210–212.
18. American College of Obstetricians and Gynecologists. (2017). Practice bulletin no. 184: Vaginal birth after cesarean delivery. *Obstetrics and Gynecology, 130*(5), 1167–1169.
19. Vamos, C. A., Thompson, E. L., Avendano, M., et al. (2015). Oral health promotion interventions during pregnancy: A systemic review. *Community Dentistry and Oral Epidemiology, 43,* 385–396.
20. U.S. Department of Health and Human Services, Centers for Disease Control and Prevention. (2016). Guidelines for vaccinating pregnant women. www.cdc.gov/vaccines/pubs/preg-guide.htm. (Accessed December 22, 2017).
21. Academy of Nutrition and Dietetics. (2016). Position of the Academy of Nutrition and Dietetics: Obesity, reproduction, and pregnancy outcomes. *Journal of the Academy of Nutrition and Dietetics, 116*(4), 677–691.
22. Academy of Nutrition and Dietetics. (2014). Practice paper of the Academy of Nutrition and Dietetics: Nutrition and lifestyle for a healthy pregnancy outcome. *Journal of the Academy of Nutrition and Dietetics, 114*(7), 1099–1103.
23. Willis, K., Lieberman, M. D., & Sheiner, E. (2015). Pregnancy and neonatal outcome after bariatric surgery. *Best Practice and Research. Clinical Obstetrics and Gynaecology, 29,* 133–144.
24. American College of Obstetricians and Gynecologists. (2015). Committee opinion no. 650: Exercise during pregnancy and the postpartum period. *Obstetrics and Gynecology, 126,* e135–e142, reaffirmed 2017.
25. Schiff, M., Algert, C. S., Ampt, A., Sywak, M. S., & Roberts, C. L. (2014). The impact of cosmetic breast implants on breastfeeding: A systematic review and meta-analysis. *International Breastfeeding Journal, 9*(1), 1–8.
26. Zapata, L. B., Murtaza, S., Whiteman, M., et al. (2015). Contraceptive counseling and postpartum contraceptive use. *American Journal of Obstetrics and Gynecology, 212*(2), 171.e1–171.e8.
27. Kornides, M., & Kitsantas, P. (2013). Evaluation of breastfeeding promotion, support, and knowledge of benefits on breastfeeding outcomes. *Journal of Child Health Care: For Professionals Working With Children in the Hospital and Community, 17*(3), 264–273.
28. Centers for Disease Control and Prevention (CDC). (2013). *Strategies to prevent obesity and other chronic diseases: The CDC guide to strategies to support breastfeeding mothers and babies.* Atlanta: U.S. Department of Health and Human Services.
29. U.S. Department of Health and Human Services, Centers for Disease Control and Prevention. 2015 Sexually transmitted diseases treatment guidelines. Retrieved from http://www.cdc.gov/std/tg2015/default.htm. (Accessed December 27, 2017).
30. Matuszkiewicz-Rowinska, J., Malyszko, J., & Wieliczko, M. (2015). Urinary tract infections in pregnancy: Old and new unresolved diagnostic and therapeutic problems. *Archives of Medical Science: AMS, 11*(1), 67–77.

31. United States Preventive Services Task Force. (2014). Final recommendation statement: Asymptomatic bacteriuria in adults: screening. *Annals of Internal Medicine, 149,* 43–47.

32. American College of Obstetricians and Gynecologists. (2017). Committee opinion no. 717: Sulfonamides, nitrofurantoin, and risk of birth defects: Interim Update. *Obstetrics and Gynecology, 130,* e150–e152.

33. Centers for Disease Control and Prevention. (2010). Prevention of perinatal Group B streptococcal disease, revised guidelines from CDC, 2010. *MMWR. Recommendations and Reports: Morbidity and Mortality Weekly Report. Recommendations and Reports, 59,* RR-10.

34. American College of Obstetricians and Gynecologists. (2011). Committee opinion no. 485: Prevention of early-onset Group B Streptococcal disease in newborns. *Obstetrics and Gynecology, 117*(4), 1019–1027, reaffirmed 2016.

35. Allen, V. M., Yuddin, M. H., Bouchard, C., et al. (2012). Management of group B streptococcal bacteriuria in pregnancy. *Journal of Obstetrics and Gynaecology Canada, 34*(5), 482–486.

36. Meaney-Delman, D., Rasmussen, S. A., Staples, J. E., et al. (2016). Zika virus and pregnancy: What obstetric health care providers need to know. *Obstetrics and Gynecology, 127,* 642–648.

37. Centers for Disease Control. (2017). Zika and pregnancy for healthcare providers: Caring for Pregnant Women. Retrieved from https://www.cdc.gov/pregnancy/zika/testing-follow-up/pregnant-woman.html. (Accessed December 29, 2017).

38. Mølgaard-Nielsen, D., Svanström, H., Melbye, M., et al. (2016). Association between use of oral fluconazole during pregnancy and risk of spontaneous abortion and stillbirth. *JAMA: The Journal of the American Medical Association, 315*(1), 58–67.

39. American College of Nurse Midwives. (2012). Vulvar care. *Journal of Midwifery and Women's Health, 57*(3), 311–312. Retrieved from http://www.midwife.org/ACNM/files/ccLibraryFiles/Filename/000000002192/Vulvar%20Care.pdf. (Accessed December 27, 2017).

40. Herrell, H. E. (2014). Nausea and Vomiting of Pregnancy. *American Family Physician, 89*(12), 965–970.

41. American College of Nurse-Midwives. Share with women: Nausea and vomiting during pregnancy. Retrieved from http://www.midwife.org/ACNM/files/ccLibraryFiles/Filename/000000000650/Nausea%20and%20Vomiting%20During%20Pregnancy.pdf. (Accessed December 22, 2017).

42. Phupong, V., & Hanprasertpong, T. (2015). Interventions for heartburn in pregnancy. *The Cochrane Database of Systematic Reviews,* (9), CD011379.

43. Trottier, M., Erebara, A., & Bozzo, P. (2012). Treating constipation during pregnancy. *Canadian Family Physician, 58*(8), 836–838.

44. Breeze, C. (2016). Early pregnancy bleeding. *Australian Family Physician, 45*(5), 283–286.

45. Boisrame, T., Sananes, N., Fritz, G., et al. (2014). Placental abruption: Risk factors, management and maternal-fetal prognosis. Cohort study over 10 years. *European Journal of Obstetrics, Gynecology, and Reproductive Biology, 179,* 100–104.

46. American College of Nurse Midwives. (2012). Position statement: Prevention of preterm labor and preterm birth. Retrieved from http://www.midwife.org/ACNM/files/ACNMLibraryData/UPLOADFILENAME/000000000274/Prevention%20of%20Preterm%20Labor%20and%20Preterm%20Birth%20June%202012.pdf. (Accessed December 22, 2017).

47. American College of Obstetricians and Gynecologists. (2016). Practice bulletin 171: Management of preterm labor. *Obstetrics and Gynecology, 128*(4), e155–e164.

48. Mihaltan, F. D., Antoniu, S. A., & Ulmeanu, R. (2014). Asthma and pregnancy: Therapeutic challenges. *Archives of Gynecology and Obstetrics, 290*(1).

49. American College of Obstetricians and Gynecologists. (2008). Practice bulletin no. 90: Asthma in pregnancy. *Obstetrics and Gynecology, 111,* 457–464. Reaffirmed 2016.

50. National Institutes of Health, National High Blood Pressure Education Program Working Group on High Blood Pressure in Pregnancy. (2000). Report of the National High Blood Pressure Education Program Working Group on High Blood Pressure in Pregnancy. *American Journal of Obstetrics and Gynecology, 183*(1), S1–S22.

51. American College of Obstetricians and Gynecologists Task Force on Hypertension in Pregnancy. (2013). Hypertension in pregnancy. Washington, DC: American College of Obstetricians and Gynecologists. Retrieved from https://www.acog.org/~/media/Task%20Force%20and%20Work%20Group%20Reports/public/HypertensioninPregnancy.pdf. (Accessed on December 22, 2017).

52. Firoz, T., Magee, L. A., MacDonell, K., et al. (2014). Oral antihypertensive therapy for severe hypertension in pregnancy and postpartum: A systematic review. *BJOG: An International Journal of Obstetrics and Gynaecology, 121*(10), 1210–1218.

53. World Health Organization. (2011). Recommendations for prevention and treatment of preeclampsia and eclampsia. Geneva: World Health Organization. Retrieved from http://whqlibdoc.who.int/publications/2011/9789241548335_eng.pdf?ua=1. (Accessed December 26, 2017).

54. American Diabetes Association. (2018). Management of diabetes in pregnancy: Standards of medical care in diabetes—2018. *Diabetes Care, 41*(S1), S137–S143.

55. American College of Obstetricians and Gynecologists. (2017). Practice Bulletin no. 180: Gestational diabetes mellitus. *Obstetrics and Gynecology, 130,* e17–e31.

56. United States Preventive Services Task Force. Final Recommendation Statement: Gestational Diabetes Mellitus, Screening. 2016. Retrieved from https://www.uspreventiveservicestaskforce.org/Page/Document/RecommendationStatementFinal/gestational-diabetes-mellitus-screening. (Accessed December 26, 2017).

57. Carney, L. A., Quinlan, J. D., & West, J. M. (2014). Thyroid disease in pregnancy. *American Family Physician, 89*(4), 273–278.

58. Alexander, E. K., Pearce, E. N., & Brent, G. A. (2017). 2017 Guidelines of the American Thyroid Association for the diagnosis and management of thyroid disease during pregnancy and the postpartum. *Thyroid, 27*(3), 315–389.

59. Yatsunenko, T., Rey, F. E., Manary, M. J., Trehan, I., Dominguez-Bello, M. G., Contreras, M., et al. (2012). Human gut microbiome viewed across age and geography. *Nature, 486*(7402), 222–227.

60. American Academy of Pediatrics (AAP). (2012). Section on Breastfeeding: Breastfeeding and the use of human milk. *Pediatrics, 129*(3), e827–e841.

61. Protocol, A. B. M. (2016). ABM clinical protocol #10: Breastfeeding the late preterm infant (34 [0/7] to 36 [6/7] weeks gestation) and early term infants 37-38 [6/7] week gestation)(second revision 2016). *Breastfeeding Medicine: The Official Journal of the Academy of Breastfeeding Medicine, 11*(10), 494–500.

62. Holmes, A. V., McLeod, A. Y., & Bunik, M. (2013). ABM clinical protocol# 5: Peripartum breastfeeding management for the healthy mother and infant at term, revision 2013. *Breastfeeding Medicine: The Official Journal of the Academy of Breastfeeding Medicine, 8*(6), 469–473.

63. Grawey, A. E., Marinelli, K. A., & Holmes, A. V., the Academy of Breastfeeding Medicine. (2013). ABM clinical protocol #14: Breastfeeding-friendly physician's office: optimizing care for infants and children, revised 2013. *Breastfeeding Medicine: The Official Journal of the Academy of Breastfeeding Medicine, 8*(2), 237–242.

64. Evans, A., Marinelli, K. A., & Taylor, J. S. (2014). ABM clinical protocol #2: Guidelines for hospital discharge of the breastfeeding term newborn and mother: "The going home protocol," revised 2014. *Breastfeeding Medicine: The Official Journal of the Academy of Breastfeeding Medicine, 9*(1), 3–8.

65. Holmes, A. V., McLeod, A. Y., & Bunik, M. (2013). ABM clinical protocol #5: Peripartum breastfeeding management for the healthy mother and infant at term, revision 2013. *Breastfeeding Medicine: The Official Journal of the Academy of Breastfeeding Medicine, 8*(6), 469–473.

66. Holmes, A. V. (2013). Establishing successful breastfeeding in the newborn period. *Pediatric Clinics of North America, 60,* 147–168.

67. American Academy of Pediatrics (AAP). (2004). Subcommittee on Hyperbilirubinemia: Management of hyperbilirubinemia in the newborn infant 35 or more weeks of gestation. *Pediatrics, 114,* 297–316.

68. Academy of Breastfeeding Medicine Protocol Committee. (2017). ABM clinical protocol #22: Guidelines for management of jaundice in the breastfeeding infant equal to or greater than 35 weeks' gestation. *Breastfeeding Medicine: The Official Journal of the Academy of Breastfeeding Medicine, 12*(5), 250–257.

69. Blair, A., Cadwell, K., Turner-Maffie, C., et al. (2003). The relationship between positioning, the breastfeeding dynamic, the latching process, and pain in breastfeeding mothers with sore nipples. *Breastfeeding Review: Professional Publication of the Nursing Mothers' Association of Australia, 11*(2), 5–10.

70. Neifert, M. (2004). Breastmilk transfer: Positioning, latch-on, and screening for problems in milk transfer. *Clinical Obstetrics and Gynecology, 47*(3), 656–675.

71. Buhimschi, C. S. (2004). Endocrinology of lactation. *Obstetrics and Gynecology Clinics of North America, 31*(4), 963–979.

72. Centuori, S., Burmaz, T., Ronfani, L., et al. (1999). Nipple care, sore nipples, and breastfeeding: A randomized trial. *Journal of Human Lactation, 15*(2), 125–130.

73. Academy of Breastfeeding Medicine Protocol Committee. (2011). ABM clinical protocol #9: Use of galactogogues in initiating or augmenting the rate of maternal milk secretion (first revision January 2011). *Breastfeeding Medicine: The Official Journal of the Academy of Breastfeeding Medicine, 6*(1), 41–49.

74. Amir, L. H., & Academy of Breastfeeding Medicine Protocol Committee. (2014). ABM clinical protocol #4: Mastitis, revised March 2014. *Breastfeeding*

Medicine: The Official Journal of the Academy of Breastfeeding Medicine, 9(5), 239–243.

75. Sellen, D. W. (2010). Feeding in human evolution. In *Human diet and nutrition in biocultural perspective: Past meets present* (Vol. 5). New York: Berghahn.

76. American College of Nurse-Midwives. (2013). Position statement: The role of the certified nurse-midwife/certified midwife in preconception health and health care. Retrieved from http://www.midwife.org/ACNM/files/ACNM LibraryData/UPLOADFILENAME/000000000081/Preconception%20Health %20and%20Health%20Care%20Feb%202013.pdf. (Accessed December 21, 2017).

77. St. Fleur, M., Damus, K., & Jack, B. (2016). The future of preconception care in the United States: Multigenerational impact on reproductive outcomes. *Upsala Journal of Medical Sciences, 121*(4), 211–215.

CHAPTER **12**

HUMAN TRAFFICKING

Vickie K. Ernste

DEFINITION AND EPIDEMIOLOGY

Human trafficking is a form of modern-day slavery that exists throughout the United States and globally. Within the United States, human trafficking has been reported in all 50 states and the District of Columbia. Human trafficking is the trade of a human for profit and is defined as the recruitment, transportation, transfer, harboring, or receipt of a human via force, deception, coercion, abuse of power, or position of vulnerability with the purpose to exploit the human. Exploitation includes prostitution or other forms of sexual exploitation, forced labor or services, slavery or practices similar to slavery.[1] Human trafficking includes the forced trading of sexual acts, labor, or commercial sexual exploitation in exchange for profit. Within the United States, human trafficking is a crime as traffickers use violence, threats, lies, debt bondage, and other forms of coercion to compel adults and children to engage in commercial sex acts or forced labor against their will. Victims need not be transported from one place to another to be considered trafficked victims. The federal definition identifies sex trafficking as a commercial sex act induced by force, fraud, or coercion, or in which a person induced to perform such an act has not attained the age of 18 years.[2] Under United States law, force, fraud, or coercion need not exist for children (under 18 years old) to be considered a trafficking victim. While that is the federal definition, individual states do not always require the element of force, fraud, or coercion to demonstrate sex trafficking for either adults or youth.

Human trafficking is a growing public health concern within the United States and is the second largest criminal industry within the world, surpassing illegal arms trading.[3] Many human trafficking victims remain unidentified as trafficked victims. While it is difficult to ascertain the actual number of trafficked victims worldwide, the International Labour Organization estimates there are 20.9 million victims at any one given time. Among the 20.9 million victims, there are 11.4 million females and 9.5 million males. Of these, approximately 945,000 are children.[4] Human trafficking victims can be of any age, race, sex, socioeconomic status, sexual orientation, or citizenship. Within the United States, labor trafficking victims typically are undocumented (67%) or legal (28%) immigrants who are aged 25 years or older. In contrast, 83% of sex trafficking victims are US citizens and are under 25 years old.[5] The

average age of entry for sex trafficking within the United States is 12 to 14 years of age.

In a study of sex trafficking survivors, 87.8% of sex trafficking survivors state they encountered a health care provider.[6] Health care may be the only opportunity for intervention for human trafficking victims. The suffering of victims of human trafficking increases the longer they are in captivity. Health care providers need to have a keen awareness to human trafficking, including what comprises human trafficking. Box 12.1 provides resources to promote awareness. The effects of human trafficking are a public health concern.

CLINICAL PRESENTATION AND PHYSICAL EXAMINATION

Human trafficking victims are unlikely to identify themselves as human trafficking victims due to fear of their trafficker, distrust of authority, inability to understand language, or sense of shame for their situation. Trafficked victims may present alone or in the presence of the trafficker, who may represent him- or herself as a family member or trusted friend. The trafficker can appear very caring and empathetic to the victim. Traffickers, male or female, often present in a professional manner and are well-spoken to avoid suspicion.[3]

Human trafficking victims will access health care services for a range of chief complaints. There are no specific chief complaints presenting with trafficked victims. As it can be challenging to identify trafficked victims, health care providers should be astute to "red flags" and vulnerable populations.

Red Flags	Vulnerable Populations
Avoids eye contact	Business employees in ethnic communities (e.g., massage)
Appears younger than stated age	History of childhood abuse/neglect
Appears submissive	Justice system involvement
Disoriented to time or place	Learning disabilities
Incongruent expensive items	Mental health issues
Inconsistent story	No address
Presence of controlling person	Impoverished
Profound fearfulness	Runaway or throwaway youth
Signs of abuse	
Substance use	
Unusual tattoo(s)	

Provider suspicion should elevate when the accompanying individual doesn't allow for the victim to be alone or they answer all questions for the victim. Victims may display a profound fearfulness during examination. Similar to domestic abuse victims, trafficking victims may provide vague or inconsistent stories for the injury or illness.

Victims of sex trafficking, in particular, may appear younger than their stated age and have unusual tattoos. Traffickers are known to brand their victims, via tattoo, with a barcode, a monetary symbol, or the trafficker's name. Oftentimes the victim will not be able to provide their address or identification documents, and they can be unaware of their location or the date. Like any abuse victim, human trafficking victims may have varying signs of abuse, such as cut marks, cigarette burns, or bruises.

Vulnerable populations for human trafficking include runaway or throwaway youth. Adults and children of the justice system and welfare system are high risk for trafficking. A history of childhood abuse and neglect as well as poverty and learning disabilities can be predictors for human trafficking victims.

DIAGNOSTICS (SCREENING TOOLS)

Once a provider has potentially identified a trafficked victim, a complete screening needs to occur. First and foremost, the provider will want to make sure the patient is alone before asking any questions. Build time to speak with the victim as he or she needs to know the provider can be trusted, is safe, and empathizes with the victim. Victims view providers as smart individuals and have a sense when judgment occurs. Trust, safety, and empathy are important components to display to the potential victim as these core components have been lost through the process of victimization. When asking questions of the patient, it remains important to ask questions in a compassionate manner, in a conversational style. If the victim needs an interpreter, use a professional neutral interpreter. The National Human Trafficking Resource Center has created *Framework for a Human Trafficking Protocol in Healthcare Settings* to assist health care providers (Box 12.2).

If the victim answers yes to any of the screening questions or if other indicators of human trafficking are present, the provider can call the National Human Trafficking Resource Center (NHTRC) hotline at 1-888-373-7888. The hotline resources can assist the provider with the next steps, including local resources available to assist the victim. The provider should ensure compliance with HIPAA (Health Insurance Portability and Accountability Act of 1996) and mandatory reporting regulations during any interactions with outside agencies, including the hotline. If the victim answers no, the provider should refer the patient to the local social services as appropriate. If the provider highly suspects trafficking, however the patient does not screen positive, it can be helpful to provide the patient with a phone number to call if they or any of their friends ever need help. It can be beneficial to have the patient program

the phone number into their cell phone under a name (e.g., 373-7888 under the name "Amy").

PHYSICAL EXAMINATION

The patient may exhibit signs similar to those described. Ask the patient what their primary concern is for the visit, being careful to make them feel comfortable. After establishing trust and comfort, try to get a basic history and review of systems (ROS). Physical examination of suspected human trafficking patients includes a detailed examination comprised of both a thorough physical examination and a thorough mental health examination. Additional examinations should include a detailed social history.

Perform the physical assessment in a systematic way, starting with vital signs to include weight, body mass index (BMI), and general appearance. Oftentimes, victims go without proper professional health care services, including dental visits. As a result, they may have untreated chronic medical conditions, scarring from home procedures, acute and remote signs of abuse, and poor dentition. A thorough skin assessment is essential. Protected areas of the body, such as the torso, genitals, neck, and medial thighs, may display signs of inflicted trauma, such as cigarette burns, cuts, and scars. The presence of unexplained tattoos, especially of names, initials, gang signs, or money bags located in unusual locations, such as the back of the neck, underarm, lower back, or inner thigh, can indicate an individual is trafficked.

Proceed with HEENT examination (head, eyes, ears, nose, and throat) and each body system with an emphasis placed on skin and gynecological conditions. If the patient indicates they have a medical history, it will be important to review that body system (e.g., asthma) as it is likely untreated. Review history of sexually transmitted infections (STIs) and check for STIs while explaining that we encourage everyone to be checked routinely. If the patient endorses unwanted sexual assaults, consider proceeding with a sexual assault examination. In cases with sex trafficking, retained foreign objects may be found in the vaginal vault.

After your physical assessment, a thorough psychosocial assessment is imperative (Box 12.3). First, ask the patient if they have identification and have access to their identification (e.g., passport, visa). Ascertain their current living arrangements and who else lives with them (i.e., do they live with their "boyfriend/girlfriend" and many other people). Inquire if they are able to come and go as they please. Seek to understand their financial situation, and phrase it in a way stating you are always worried about health care costs so you need to ask. Substance use is common among trafficked individuals. At times,

---

BOX **12.2**

Screening Questions

1. Have you been forced to engage in sexual acts for money or favors?
2. Is someone holding your passport or identification documents?
3. Has anyone threatened to hurt you or your family if you leave?
4. Has anyone physically or sexually abused you?
5. Do you have a debt to someone you cannot pay off?
6. Does anyone take all or part of the money you earn?

BOX **12.3**

Physical Assessment	Psychosocial Assessment
Weight, BMI, general appearance	Identification
Overall nutritional status and hydration	Living history
Dentition	Level of freedom
General hygiene	Financial situation
Thorough skin assessment	Substance use
Signs of abuse (burns, scars, cuts)	Sexual partners
Acute/remote injuries	
History of STIs	

BMI, Body mass index; *STI,* sexually transmitted infections.

BOX **12.4**

Physical and Mental Health Consequences

Physical Health	Mental Health
Communicable diseases, including sexually transmitted infections	Dissociative disorders
Homicide	Memory loss
Malnutrition and dehydration	Overdose
Poor dentition	Psychosomatic syndromes
Skin disorders	Posttraumatic stress disorder
Sterilization	Self-injurious behaviors
Traumatic injuries	Sleep disorders
Vaginal, perineal, and rectal injuries	Stockholm syndrome
Unsafe abortion complications	Substance use
Untreated chronic health conditions	Suicide

BOX **12.5**

Human Trafficking Components

Sexual Exploitation	Labor Trafficking
Cyber exploitation	Construction workers
Massage parlors	Domestic workers in private homes
Prostitution	Farm laborers
Pornography	Manufacturing workers
Stripping	Restaurant workers
	Servitude

the substance use is forced upon them and at other times, they endorse substance use as a way to cope with their situation.

INTERPROFESSIONAL COLLABORATIVE MANAGEMENT

In 2013, the United States federal government passed the Stop Exploitation Through Trafficking Act, which is a law that encourages states to pass Safe Harbor laws. Safe Harbor laws allow trafficked individuals to receive services to assist them in transitioning to independent living. Some state Safe Harbor laws also allow trafficked individuals to be protected as victims rather than criminalized. Depending upon the state, the state anti-trafficking infrastructure is housed through the public health or social work entity.

If you are unaware of how to connect with your local agencies and resources, the National Human Trafficking Hotline can assist you in connecting with the appropriate individuals. The multilingual 24/7 hotline can be accessed by health care providers, trafficking victims, law enforcement, or anyone with an interest in trafficking information. Engaging system professionals, such as victim advocates, early in the identification process allows the trafficked individual to receive optimal ongoing follow-up and care.

COMPLICATIONS (MENTAL/PHYSICAL HEALTH CONSEQUENCES)

Both physical and psychological health consequences exist with trafficked individuals (Box 12.4). Trafficked individuals typically do not seek routine health care as they may be held in captivity and/or manipulated through psychological, physical, or sexual control antics. Furthermore, they may not be familiar with the area or know the local culture, which further prohibits them from seeking necessary health care.[7] There is a direct correlation between the length of captivity and the severity of consequences. Physical health consequences for sex trafficking victims include untreated chronic health problems, broken bones, bruises, burns, and scars. The most common physical symptoms of sex trafficked victims include headache, back pain, stomach pain, memory problems, traumatic brain injury (TBI), and STIs. Mental health complaints include anxiety, depression, post-traumatic stress disorder (PTSD), self injury (SI), panic attacks, and substance use.

PATIENT AND FAMILY EDUCATION

Providing appropriate resources, including safety, shelter, medical care, legal assistance, and other critical service resources, to the patient and family members is crucial. Sharing information and allowing safety for the patient can lead to success. If a patient screens negative for trafficking, however the provider has high suspicions, it is good practice to provide information to the patient in a confidential manner.

HEALTH PROMOTION

Health care providers who intervene or provide preventative education to at-risk individuals potentially prevent future trafficking victimization. Focusing efforts on at-risk populations and those individuals who are exposed to at-risk populations can increase awareness and serve as a preventative health measure (Box 12.5). Youth are a particularly vulnerable population due to their immature brain development and limited life experiences, which lead to impulsive and risky behaviors. Promoting abstinence of drugs and alcohol is important as use of these mind-altering substances decrease inhibition and impair judgment, which can lead to risky behaviors or dangerous situations.[4]

REFERENCES

1. United Nations Office on Drugs and Crime website. (n.d.). Retrieved from https://www.unodc.org.
2. Orme, J., & Ross-Sheriff, F. (2015). Sex trafficking: Policies, programs, and services. *Social Work, 60*(4), 287–294. http://dx.doi.org/Retrieved, http://dx.doi.org/Retrieved, https://www.unodc.org. from Peters, K., Clutter, P., & Rush, C. (2013). The growing business of human trafficking and the power of emergency nurses to stop it. *Journal of Emergency Nursing, 39*(3), 280–288, from United Nations Office on Drugs and Crime website. (n.d.).
3. Becker, H. J., & Bechtel, K. (2015). Recognizing victims of human trafficking in the pediatric emergency department. *Pediatric Emergency Care, 31*(2), 144–147. Retrieved from Emergency Nurses Association. (2014). *Human trafficking patient awareness in the emergency setting* [Position Statement]. Des Plaines, IL: Author.
4. Varma, S., Gillespie, S., McCracken, C., & Greenbaum, V. J. (2015). Characteristics of child commercial sexual exploitation and sex trafficking victims presenting for medical care in the United States. *Child Abuse & Neglect, 44*, 98–105.
5. Macias-Konstantopoulos, W. (2016). Human trafficking: The role of medicine in interrupting the cycle of abuse and violence. *Annals of Internal Medicine, 165*(8), 582–588.
6. Greenbaum, V. J., Dodd, M., & McCracken, C. (2018). A short screening tool to identify victims of child sex trafficking in the health care setting. *Pediatric Emergency Care, 34*(1), 33–37.
7. Ahn, R., Alpert, E. J., Purcell, G., Macias Konstatntopoulos, W., McGahan, A., Cafferty, E., et al. (2013). Human trafficking: Review of eduational resources for health professionals. *American Journal of Preventive Medicine, 44*(3), 283–289.

CHAPTER 13

AGING AND COMMON GERIATRIC SYNDROMES

Patricia Hadidian

We live in a society that is rapidly aging. Between 2007 and 2016 the population of people aged 65 and older increased by 30%. Population projections predict that by 2020, one in six Americans will be over 65 and by 2050 that number will increase to one in five.[1] An understanding of the issues that affect the health of older adults is vital to any health care practice.

Because of this anticipated increase in numbers of older adults, as well as their ethnic diversity, this age group will have an unprecedented need for services and goods. Heart disease and cancer remain the two top causes of death and disability among older adults. Alzheimer's disease (AD) continues as the fifth leading cause of death in the United States in adults older than 65 and the incidence has increased by almost 40% in the same time period. People aged 85 and older are five times more likely to die from AD than those aged 75 to 84.[2] Unintentional accidents and chronic respiratory infections now rank as the third and fourth leading causes of death in older adults. Older individuals are now living with multiple chronic conditions, adding to the complexity of their care.[1]

CHALLENGES IN PRIMARY CARE

The goal of geriatric primary care is to maintain independence, function, and comfort of the individual. The challenges in achieving this goal include ageism, the paucity of geriatric education in the nation's health professional schools, the low numbers of health care providers choosing geriatrics, the complexity of illness in older adults, the increasing numbers of older adults, and cost.

Robert Butler coined the term *ageism* in 1965 to describe the culturally rooted discomfort with growing older. He observed not only revulsion on the part of young people but also fear of losses associated with aging.[3] Despite the fact that attention was brought to this bias more than 40 years ago, ageism in practice still exists. As noted in a recent symposium of the American Association of Geriatric Psychiatry, ageism is prevalent in society and can result in substandard care and poor health outcomes for elders. Undertreatment can result as complaints may be dismissed as being due to "old age," and overtreatment results due to a lack of understanding of the effects of aging on pharmacokinetics or because of a poor understanding of the patient's goals or anticipated longevity.[4]

Research demonstrates that the presentation of disease is often atypical in an aging patient. Treatment must be based on an understanding of the body's ability to adapt to aging and the effect of aging on pharmacokinetics. Although the human body demonstrates remarkable resiliency with aging, physiologic and psychological stress disrupts this adaptation.

An individual experiencing the usual aging pattern is increasingly vulnerable to multiple health problems and experiences losses that affect stamina, motivation for self-care, and the ability to function effectively. Functional problems affecting the older adult's mental and physical status and care are aggravated by many factors, including a lack of exercise, nutritional deficiencies, constipation, infection, sleep disturbances, failing cognition, social isolation, and depression. Nonprescription drugs and prescriptions from multiple medical specialists can result in a dangerous mix of medications, which must be identified to avoid adverse reactions and interactions. Reduced memory, slowed mental processing of new information, and impaired sensory input further complicate diagnosis and treatment plans. Additional challenges arise from the use of alcohol and tobacco.

MENTAL STATUS AND FUNCTIONAL ASSESSMENTS

There are multiple assessment tools available to screen for dementia syndromes and differentiate mild cognitive impairment from dementia (see Chapter 174) as well as document the progression of cognitive impairment. These include the Folstein Mini-Mental State Examination, the Mini-Cog screen for dementia, the Short Portable Mental Status Questionnaire, the AD8 Dementia Screening Interview, and the Montreal Cognitive Assessment (MoCa). These tools are screening tools at best and can be misleading in individuals with higher educational levels, lower socioeconomic levels, or vision, hearing, or speech impairments.[5] A detailed history of cognitive change and lifelong habits most often provided by family or friends are vital elements in the differential diagnosis of dementia syndromes. Maintaining a record of the patient's baseline mental status, ruling out depression as a factor in impaired mental status, and tracking the results of subsequent mental status testing are helpful for accurate diagnosis and management. The value of screening for dementia is controversial and while it is a requirement of the Medicare Annual Wellness visit, the US Preventive Services Task Force (USPSTF) concluded there is insufficient evidence to recommend for or against screening so generally testing should be done only after concern for cognitive impairment is raised.[5]

Tools for the assessment of functional status, including the Barthel Index, the Physical Self-Maintenance Scale, and the Katz Index, are also well developed, validated, and easily administered. Function is addressed on two levels: (1) basic activities of daily living, including feeding, bathing, dressing, ambulation, and toileting; and (2) the more complex, instrumental activities of daily living, including cooking, shopping, using the telephone, reading, writing, and managing money. Poor performance on functional or mental status testing might explain a failure to respond to medications, noncompliance with exercise or diet recommendations, falls and injuries, or the occurrence of depression or anxiety.[5] The provider should never rely solely on assessment tools to determine an older adult's functional or cognitive capacity because many older adults, even those with impairment, can do very well on testing or are only partially truthful, therefore skewing the results in their favor.

HEALTH SCREENING

Routine screening of older adults for disease remains controversial simply because few outcome data exist for this population. Guidelines for cutoff ages for various screenings vary among entities (Table 13.1). For example, the USPSTF recommends mammograms only to the age of 74, whereas the American Cancer Society recommends no upper age limit. More recently, the American Board of Internal Medicine Choosing Wisely initiative lists evidence-based recommendations for tests and screenings to help providers and patients make

TABLE 13.1 **Recommended Screening and Immunizations for Older Adults**			
Service	**USPSTF Rating**	**CDC**	**Medicare Benefit**
IMMUNIZATIONS			
Prevnar 13	NR	Y	Y
Pneumovax 23: one time after age 65	NR	Y	Y
Influenza (age appropriate): annually	NR	Y	Y
Herpes zoster, RZV5 (Shingrex): 2 doses, 2–6 months apart after age 50	NR	Y	Y
Tetanus (Tdap): once	NR	Y	Y
Td: every 10 years	NR	Y	Y
CARDIOVASCULAR SCREENING			
Abdominal aorta ultrasound: once in males who have ever smoked after age 65	A	Y	Y
Hypertension: at each office visit, no age restriction	A	Y	Y
Height and weight at each office visit	A	Y	Y
Blood glucose in overweight/obese until age 70	B	Y	Y
Fasting lipid panel every 5 years unless levels are high or other CV risk factors present.	B	Y	Y
CANCER SCREENING			
Colorectal screening: The USPSTF recommends screening for colorectal cancer starting at age 50 years and continuing until age 75 years. The risks and benefits of different screening methods vary. The decision to screen for colorectal cancer in adults aged 76 to 85 years should be an individual one, taking into account the patient's overall health and prior screening history.	A	Y	Y
Cervical cancer screening: none after age 65	A	Y	Y
Breast mammogram: every 2 years until age 74	B	Y	Y
Prostate-Specific Antigen (PSA): Screening in men age 55–70 based on symptoms, preference and discussion with provider; not recommended for age >70	C	NR	Y
BONE MASS			
Once at age 65 (women); once age 70 (men)	B	Y	
OTHER SCREENINGS			
Dementia	I		Y
Hearing	I		N
Vision	I		N
Glaucoma	I		N
Falls	B	Y	Y

Y means yes.
Ratings:
A: Recommended service—usually covered by Medicare.
B: Recommended service—usually covered by Medicare.
C: USPSTF recommends against routine use of this service.
D: USPSTF discourages the use of this service.
I: Insufficient evidence for recommendations.
NR: No recommendations.
CDC, Centers for Disease Control and Prevention; *USPSTF,* US Preventive Services Task Force.
Data from Centers for Disease Control and Prevention. (2018). *Recommended immunization schedule for adults aged 19 years or older, by vaccine and age group-United States, 2018.* From https://www.cdc.gov/vaccines/schedules/hcp/imz/adult-compliant.html; U.S. Preventative Services Task Force. (2018). *Recommendations for adults.* From https://www.uspreventiveservicestaskforce.org.

decisions on appropriate care based on the individual's general health, predicted longevity, and personal and family history.[6] These tests should focus on the function, comfort, and safety of the individual. It is reasonable to assess and discuss with the older adult his or her anticipated life expectancy, considering all comorbidities, and his or her personal preferences before embarking on routine screening. Many older patients refuse invasive and even routine screening or treatment regimens,

choosing comfort and quality of life over longevity. Explanation to older adults who are accustomed to years of routine screening for issues that are no longer of concern must be carefully undertaken and can be difficult. Annual examinations should be comprehensive, are necessarily time-consuming, and should include responsible family members; however, time should be set aside to discuss care preferences and current recommendations and when to stop screening, especially for cancer.

COUNSELING ELDER DRIVERS

Providing useful assessment and counseling to the older adult driver often falls to primary health care providers. Older adults, especially those who live in rural areas or continue to work past retirement, rely on driving to remain mobile and independent. Traffic fatalities involving older adults declined between 2005 and 2016, yet 18% of all traffic fatalities involve individuals 65 and older and motor vehicle accidents prove to be more harmful to older adults than other populations due to the fragility that accompanies aging. Some older adults will comfortably report difficulty with selected driving situations, including driving in bright sunlight or at dusk or transitions from light to darkness (e.g., driving into a parking garage, driving in bad weather, and driving at night) and self-regulate their driving.[7] However, some older adults may lack insight into the extent of their driving impairment and continue to drive when no longer safe thereby putting themselves and others at great risk.[8] Assessment of cardiovascular status, mental and cognitive status, vision, hearing, balance, gait, range of motion, and strength of hips and knees can provide information regarding the older adult's ability to drive. Reports from family members or friends are very informative. Those drivers judged at risk should be referred to the registry of motor vehicles for a road test or to a private rehabilitation facility where trained screeners, usually occupational therapists, can test the older adult's driving skills in a safe environment. Frank discussions with patients, families, and supportive peers that elaborate the risks of driving can be difficult, especially if the recommendation is to discontinue driving, but are essential to protect the safety of the older driver and the public at large. Mandatory reporting of unsafe drivers is the law in many states.

IMPORTANCE OF ADVANCE DIRECTIVES

The primary care of older adults includes a discussion of advance directives and the identification of a health care proxy or durable power of attorney for health care. A living will or similar document, which describes in detail the patient's wishes with regard to resuscitation, hospitalization, treatment goals and limits, and a health care proxy, should be part of each patient's health care record. The goal in completion of advance directives is to provide the individual autonomy in decisions regarding his or her manner and location of death as well as relieving family burden and conflict while the older individual is mentally competent to do so.

Silveira and colleagues in two retrospective cohort studies measured trends over time of advance directive completion and compared hospitalizations before death and death in hospital. They found an increase in completion of advance directives from 47% in 2000 to 72% in 2010. There was also a coincident finding of a decrease in the proportion of patients dying in the hospital from 45% to 35%, although it is difficult to prove completion of an advance directive as a causative factor.[9]

In January 2016 the Centers for Medicare and Medicaid Services updated the Medicare Physician Fee Schedule to establish payment for advance care planning services under the Medicare Fee-For-Service Program. This allows for reimbursement of up to 30 minutes of time for this important discussion with patients.[10] Time to discuss choices and offer explanations of terminology can be set aside in an office visit; ideally, the named health care proxy is included. Individual states are now offering forms online and are keeping this information in statewide registries. A lawyer is usually not necessary for the completion of these documents; witnesses and notarization are all that are typically required. Typically emergency medical technicians are unable to implement advance directives. Once emergency services are called, stabilization and transport to the nearest hospital are required. Once the patient has been evaluated, advance directives can be activated.

The Physician Orders for Life-Sustaining Treatment (POLST) or Medical Orders for Life-Sustaining Treatment (MOLST) Paradigm programs are designed to improve the quality of care people receive at the end of life. These programs are based on effective communication of patient wishes, documentation of medical orders, and a promise by health care professionals to honor these wishes. Recent studies confirm that patients with POLST Paradigm instructions were less likely to die in the hospital and more likely to receive the care specified than those without such orders.[11] These are typically printed on a brightly colored form, often pink, as well as on wallet-sized cards for portability. The existence and regulation of POLST Paradigm programs vary from state to state. The website www.polst.org can be used to check for a local POLST Paradigm program.

THE CHALLENGE OF GERIATRICS

The challenge for any health care provider who treats older adults is to recognize the individual aging process, promote optimum health and functioning, provide care and comfort during illness, minimize the length and severity of the premorbid illness and disability period, and finally, ensure a comfortable and dignified death.

To this end, several models of care have been proposed over the past decade designed to shorten or avoid hospital admission, avoid hospital readmission after discharge, reduce overtreatment, provide older adults and their families with information specific to their individual situation and preferences, and provide care in the preferred setting, allowing aging in place. The most studied and successful are transitional care models designed to help older adults with multiple comorbidities transition from hospital to home or nursing home or from nursing home to home (see Chapter 4). The 2010 Affordable Care Act established a variety of transitional care programs designed to improve quality and reduce costs. Often these services are managed by an advanced practice nurse and frequently include discharge planning, case management services, counseling or coaching, and assistance with navigating the health care system.[12] Basic primary care services delivered to individuals at home as well as restorative services such as physical and occupational therapy can also be features.[13] House-call programs are gaining in popularity and availability because care delivered at home is timely, less expensive, and more acceptable to frail elders.[14] Town or parish nurses are becoming more common as communities look for better ways to care for their aging population. The value of caring for vulnerable older adults in their homes is substantiated in multiple studies and is confirmed as preferable in most surveys of older adults.[15]

Continuity of primary care services as the end of life approaches is the key to avoiding overdiagnosis, unnecessary hospitalizations, and overtreatment of acute problems when the outcome is generally acknowledged as death regardless of the intensity of treatment.

COMMON GERIATRIC SYNDROMES

Primary care, including health promotion and disease prevention, as well as the prevention of disease exacerbation, complications, and disability, must continue in all settings in which older adults live and is ideally provided by a coordinated team of health care professionals. Geriatric syndromes are complex, multicausal entities that test the diagnostic prowess of the health care provider. Chaos may reign, but therein lays the challenge in meeting the primary care needs of older patients. This section discusses six common syndromes seen in older adults: polypharmacy, cognitive impairment, dehydration, falls, failure to thrive (FTT), and elder abuse.

POLYPHARMACY
Definition and Etiology

Polypharmacy is the use or misuse of multiple drugs (usually defined as more than five per person or any not medically indicated), both prescription and nonprescription, and their interaction with one another. It is a common cause of iatrogenic illness in older adults, including a higher risk of falls and drug-related changes in mental status.[16] Polypharmacy arises from many sources, including multiple comorbidities, multiple prescribers for the same patient, fear of accusation of ageism or cultural bias, changing medical guidelines for treatment of specific conditions, medication advertising, and good intentions to treat the side effects of one medication with another.[17]

Pathophysiology

Drug distribution and clearance are affected by normal aging changes, including a reduction in lean body mass and blood flow to the kidney and liver and an increase in body fat. These issues are compounded in frail older adults because, in addition to normal aging changes, disease alters the function of specific organ systems and affects pharmacokinetics. Abnormalities in the cardiac conduction system, decreased gastric acid production, decreased total body water, and increased total body fat all affect drug absorption and metabolism. Age-related renal changes lead to increased drug levels and potentially toxic effects of renally excreted drugs.[17]

Consequences of Polypharmacy

The most prevalent consequence of polypharmacy is an adverse drug reaction leading to a change in mental status, sedation, falls, and other serious outcomes (Box 13.1). The risk of adverse drug reactions increases precipitously as the number of medications an individual takes increases.[18] A drug-related side effect should be considered for any presenting symptom until proven otherwise. Drug-drug interactions and poor adherence because of the complexity of a medication regimen or cost are other consequences of polypharmacy.

Management

To avoid the negative consequences of polypharmacy, it is important to review all medications at each patient contact and to maintain good communication with consultants. There are a number of tools available to assist with evaluating for polypharmacy. The Beers list is the most familiar for practicing providers in the United States.[19] It provides a list of potentially inappropriate medications in all patients age 65 and older as well as a list of potentially inappropriate medications for those

---

Medication Analysis: General Considerations

1. Common adverse drug effects in older adults:
   - Constipation or diarrhea
   - Indigestion
   - Delirium
   - Dizziness
   - Depression
   - Dermatologic effects
2. Specific problems of older adults that increase the risk of medication AEs:
   - Dehydration
   - Drug cost
   - Malnutrition
   - Poor compliance
   - Renal failure

---

older adults with specific conditions. Although not 100% foolproof, this tool enables providers to plan interventions that may minimize drug-related problems and reduce costs.

Other tools, more often used in Europe and Canada, are the Improved Prescribing in the Elderly Tool (IPET), Screening Tool to Alert Doctors to the Right Treatment (START), and Screening Tool of Older Persons and Potentially Inappropriate Prescriptions (STOPP).[20] Patients should be encouraged to carry an up-to-date list of their medications and have one readily available to give emergency medical providers in the event of an emergency. Patients should be encouraged to order drugs from a pharmacy with computerized drug data whenever possible. As an educator for both the patient and the health care provider, the pharmacist plays an important role in preventing poor outcomes from polypharmacy. In fact, most pharmacies are equipped with programs that can review a list of medications and immediately detect potential drug-drug interactions and alert prescribers. Providers also can subscribe to affordable, point-of-care, technologic clinical tools that aid in identifying potential drug-drug interactions and safety concerns.

The drug risk/benefit ratio should be determined when considering the use of any new drug. The general principles of drug therapy in geriatrics are first considered, such as the pharmacodynamics of the drug class and common adverse effects experienced by older adults (see Box 13.1). For example, older adults are more susceptible than younger adults to the anticholinergic effects of drugs. Second, the specific side effect profiles of a drug class and a patient's history of previous adverse effects, morbidity, and general nutritional state are considered. The known or suspected risk is weighed against the presumed benefit of administering the drug. "Start low and go slow" is common advice when prescribing for older adults. The prescription of any drug regardless of clinical indication must be balanced against the patient's functional and cognitive capacity as well as predicted longevity. The ongoing medical necessity of all drugs should be reviewed at each visit, with strong consideration given to discontinuing those that are marginally effective, may be causing an adverse effect, and are poorly tolerated by the patient or being administered to a patient with a limited life span.

COGNITIVE IMPAIRMENT
Definition and Etiology

The most common and feared cause of a decline in cognition is dementia, and the most prevalent form of dementia is AD (see Chapter 174). The cost of treating AD approaches $100 billion annually in the United States. The incidence of AD doubles every 5 years after age 65, approaching 30% by age 85 and 50% by age 90.[21]

Clinical Presentation

AD is a chronic, irreversible illness with a gradual onset and a steady decline in cognition. Short-term memory loss is the primary symptom in AD, along with one or more of the following: disorientation; disturbance in executive functioning (planning, organizing, and abstract thinking); problems with activities of daily living; and one of three common neurologic disorders—aphasia, apraxia, or agnosia. Day-night sleep cycles are often reversed; consciousness and psychomotor changes are not evident until late in the disease. Irritability, withdrawal, and apathy may be exhibited in the early stages of the disease. Psychotic symptoms such as paranoia, hallucinations, delusions, and agitation can be seen later in the disease (see Chapter 174).

Delirium, a common cause of cognitive change in the sick or hospitalized older adult, is a transient waxing and waning level of consciousness. It is characterized by acute onset and fluctuations in orientation and attention. The incidence in hospitalized older adults is high and associated with longer lengths of stay and increased rates of admission to nursing homes. Delirium is more likely seen in the hospitalized cognitively impaired older adult. Some providers believe that in-hospital delirium may actually be the unmasking of a previously undiagnosed dementia (see Chapter 174).

DEHYDRATION
Definition and Etiology

Dehydration is more prevalent in older adults and has a greater likelihood of a negative outcome than in younger adults. It is defined as a state of fluid intake deprivation and/or excess fluid loss. Accompanying electrolyte imbalances may ensue. The most significant electrolyte abnormality is sodium imbalance (see Chapter 190). Because of this, dehydration is further categorized by the associated relationship between free water and sodium.[22]

In older adults, dehydration is often multifactorial (Box 13.2 and Table 13.2). Environmental issues, polypharmacy, and diseases prevalent in older adults predispose this group to dehydration, as do age-related changes in plasma osmolality and thirst response.

Pathophysiology

Three principal changes in the homeostatic mechanism that controls the volume and osmolality of extracellular fluids occur in older adults. These normal changes result in a reduced adaptability and reserve to deal with system stressors. First, the thirst response, which is stimulated by dehydration, is diminished and results in an increased solute/water ratio. Second, decreased renal plasma flow may be responsible for a decline in the body's ability to concentrate urine. The inability to concentrate urine prevents the body from retaining enough fluid to avert dehydration. Finally, vasopressin release stimulated

---

BOX **13.2**

Common Causes of Dehydration

INADEQUATE INTAKE (FLUID DEPRIVATION)
Environmental Factors
- Restricted mobility/ambulation
- Decreased hearing or vision
- Poorly fitting dentures
- Esophageal lesions
- Dysphagia

Increased Metabolic Demands
- Infections (resulting in malaise, reduced appetite, and poor intake)
- Neurologic disease

Pharmacologic Factors
- Narcotics
- Sedatives
- Neuroleptics
- Anticholinergics

Normal Aging Changes
- Ineffective water conservation
- Decreased thirst drive

Poor Appetite
- Fatigue
- Constipation
- Depression

Fluid Limitations
- Before a procedure or operation
- Prevention of urinary incontinence
- Management of heart failure
- Management of hyponatremia

OUTPUT (FLUID EXCESS)
Environmental Factors
- Hot weather
- Alcohol intake

Increased Metabolic Demands
- Infections (resulting in tachypnea and sweating)
- Diarrhea
- Vomiting
- Sweating

Endocrine Disorders
- Diabetes insipidus
- Hyperglycemia or glycosuria

Pharmacologic Factors
- Diuretics
- Laxatives

Normal Aging Changes
- Ineffective salt conservation

TABLE 13.2 **Dehydration Management**				
	Low Risk[a]		High Risk[a]	
Setting	Treatment	Comfort	Treatment	Comfort
Office practice	OR[b]	OR	NA	OR
Home	OR, clysis	OR	NA	OR
Nursing home	OR, clysis	OR	Clysis, IV	OR
Hospital	OR	OR	IV	OR

[a]Risk is defined by clinical parameters and may include severity of electrolyte imbalance. High risk may be defined as a serum sodium ≥150 mEq/L, an inability to take sufficient fluids by mouth, or comorbid conditions that increase the risk of complications from rehydration (e.g., congestive heart failure). This definition of risk is not research based.
[b]OR is used when fluids by mouth are possible.
NA, Not applicable; *OR,* oral rehydration; *IV,* intravenous

by low fluid volume is diminished. Therefore the inherent homeostatic mechanism that prevents the sequelae of hypovolemia is blunted.[23]

Clinical Presentation

The presenting symptoms of dehydration are often vague and nonspecific. These include confusion, lethargy, rapid weight loss, and functional decline. Dehydration is often a feature of FTT. The history should include an assessment of fluid intake, functional status, weight, and cognition. The presence of constipation may indicate a lack of water intake (see Box 13.2).

Physical Examination

The physical examination includes a cardiovascular assessment and may reveal an orthostatic drop in blood pressure and a rise in pulse, indicating volume depletion. Temperature may be elevated as a result of dehydration or an inflammatory or infectious process. Mucous membranes are often not noticeably dry until severe dehydration is present. Because of changes in skin collagen, poor skin turgor, often used as a sign of dehydration in younger individuals, is unreliable in older adults. The tongue may be swollen and furrowed.

DiagnosticsLaboratory data include a review of serum electrolytes, blood urea nitrogen (BUN)/creatinine ratio, osmolality, hematocrit and hemoglobin, and glucose. A BUN/creatinine ratio of 25:1 or more suggests dehydration. Dehydration is present when the sodium level is greater than 148 mEq/L.[22] However, with isotonic or hypotonic dehydration, serum sodium is normal or low, respectively. Hematocrit is elevated compared with the level of hematocrit when the patient is well hydrated. Respiratory and genitourinary infections are common, and a urinalysis and chest x-ray studies may be appropriate.

Differential Diagnosis

 Acute changes in mental status, a serum sodium >148.

Fever, poor fluid intake, iatrogenic drug use, and gastrointestinal fluid losses are the most common causes of dehydration in older adults. Other causes of dehydration should be pursued if electrolyte imbalances persist after treatment, with a focus on the endocrine system. However, older adults respond slowly to the treatment of severe electrolyte abnormalities.

BOX **13.3**

Dehydration Prevention

- Drink six to eight 8-ounce glasses of water or juice daily.
- Take a full glass of water or juice with medications.
- Drink more than usual in hot weather or when you have a fever.
- Keep a fluid intake record for 2 days.
- Poor dental hygiene, missing teeth, or poorly fitting dentures will interfere with food and fluid intake.
- People with memory problems need fluid monitoring.

Management

Management is determined by the severity of the electrolyte imbalance, the treatment setting, and the patient's treatment goals. Fluid deficit is determined by establishing the pre-illness weight minus the current weight:[23]

$$\text{Pre-illness weight (kg)} - \text{Current weight (kg)} = \text{Fluid deficit (L)}$$

A "prescription" for oral fluid replacement can then be recommended to include half of the calculated fluid deficit plus ongoing losses in the first 24 hours, totaling at least 1500 mL/day.[13] Although oral hydration may be the preferred route, patients who are vomiting, drowsy, or cognitively impaired may not be able to comply. In that case, especially if the patient resides in a nursing facility, hypodermoclysis (clysis) may be a good alternative.[24] This is a subcutaneous administration of fluid into the upper arm or abdomen using a standard subcutaneous needle or "button." Maximum volume of (isotonic) fluid administered subcutaneously is 1500 mL per site per 24 hours. There are many advantages to the subcutaneous route for hydration. The cost is substantially lower, there are fewer side effects, it can be administered in a variety of settings including the office or nursing facility, and it may result in avoidance of hospital admission. Clysis should not be used in an emergency situation.

Intravenous administration of fluid remains the fastest method for rehydration, but comes with a cost. The fluid type used depends on the serum sodium level, which depends on the availability of a laboratory. The administration and monitoring of the fluid and intravenous site requires specialized training often not available outside the hospital setting. It is often difficult and painful to insert a cannula into dehydrated, older patients, and the process may not be consistent with the patient's advance directives.

Complications include fluid overload, heart failure, or cerebral edema; there can be pain or infection or infiltration of fluid at the insertion site. After dehydration has been treated, it may take weeks or months for the older adult to regain functional or cognitive losses.

Education

Education focuses on the prevention of dehydration (Box 13.3). When it occurs, the amounts and types of fluids to ingest are included in the educational plan. Fluids high in sodium (e.g., tomato juice, bouillon, or sports drinks) are appropriate for those with low sodium levels, whereas water is appropriate for those with high sodium levels. Caffeinated and alcoholic beverages, especially beer, have a mild diuretic effect and should be avoided.

FALLS

Definition and Etiology

Falling is an unintentional loss of balance that results in a position change and contact with the ground. The most feared sequela of a fall is a fracture. Quality of life may also be severely affected by a "fear of falling," with self-imposed isolation and immobility causing a vicious cycle of risk. Fall assessment focuses on known risk factors, including sensory abnormalities and abnormalities of the central and peripheral nervous system, musculoskeletal system, and cognition.[25,26]

In a community sample, one-third to one-half of older adults fell each year. The probability of falling increases with age. In long-term care, the annual fall incidence per resident is greater than 50%. Approximately 20% to 30% of falls result in major injuries, including lacerations, contusions, and head injuries; 3% to 5% result in fractures. Falls are a major contributor to death in the older population and contribute to 40% of nursing home admissions.[27]

Pathophysiology

Falls are multifactorial in origin. The majority occur during walking, stepping, or position changes and not during more hazardous activities. Contributing factors are lower extremity weakness, poor balance, orthostatic hypotension, central nervous system disease, cognition and sensory abnormalities, and unsafe environments. The role of lower extremity weakness as a marker of preclinical disability has been well demonstrated.

Sensory input from vision, hearing, vestibular function, and proprioception is important in preventing falls. Visual impairment increases as a result of normal age-related changes and the increased prevalence of ocular diseases. Normal age-related changes cause glare intolerance and slower adaptation to changes in light levels than in younger adults.

Balance depends on sensory cues and vestibular function, both peripheral and central. Disequilibrium and unsteadiness are common in older adults and are related to aging changes and disease of the inner ear, as well as to changes in the transmission of signals from the periphery. Acute and chronic changes in mental status and depression contribute to falls, but the mechanism of action is unclear. Drugs causing sedation, postural hypotension, and electrolyte imbalance have been implicated in the risk for falls. The use of four or more medications increases the risk for falls, regardless of the type of medication.[26]

Normal aging changes in the cardiovascular system blunt the homeostatic mechanisms that maintain adequate organ perfusion and blood pressure control, causing hypotension and threatening the ability to maintain balance. Musculoskeletal and joint diseases affect balance and gait, as do environmental factors, such as loose rugs, cords, and clutter in the home. A fall erodes the self-confidence of older adults and intensifies their fear of dependence and loss of control over their lives. This may result in more cautious behavior and reduced activity and ambulation because of a fear of falling again. Ironically, the fear of falling is an independent risk factor for further falls.

Clinical Presentation

The clinical presentation of falling is varied. The health history should focus on previous falls and events surrounding a fall, including episodes of syncope, unsteadiness, and dizziness. The mnemonic *DDROPP* (diseases, drugs, recovery, onset, prodrome, and precipitants) helps ensure a complete post fall assessment. The assessment should also focus on any history of coronary artery disease or arrhythmias, vision and hearing problems, neurologic dysfunction, lower extremity joint pain or foot problems, fractures, cognitive changes, and medications.

Self-reported functional scales quickly supplement the history with information on mobility, self-care abilities, mood, hospitalizations, and nutrition. It is important to ask questions in reference to current activities. The reply to "How did you get to this appointment?" is immensely informative, as is simply watching how a patient enters the examination room and with whom.

Physical Examination

A complete physical examination with a focus on postural vital signs is necessary and should include a cardiovascular and neurologic examination, including Romberg test with a sternal nudge and a check for nystagmus. Mobility (including gait and balance), upper extremity function and strength, cognition, vision, and hearing are also examined. Quick and easy mobility and gait tests are now available and correlate positively with the risk for falls and a decline in self-care ability. With the timed up and go (TUG) test, the patient is timed as he or she gets up from a chair with his or her arms folded across the chest, walks 10 feet, returns to the chair, and sits down using regular footwear and any regular walking aid.[28] The ease of gait, balance, position change, and turning are evaluated. Completion of the task in 20 seconds or less correlates with functional independence; those taking 30 seconds or more are considered at high risk of falling.

Lower extremity balance is tested by evaluating the patient standing with the feet side by side, semi-tandem and tandem, and balancing for 10 seconds. The functional reach test for balance is completed by asking the individual to reach forward in a parallel plane without taking a step.[29] Patients with a reach of less than 17.8 cm (7 inches) are considered very frail and at higher risk of falling. Patients should be closely monitored by a member of the clinical team while performing any activity that may be associated with falling.

Diagnostics

Most falls are mechanical, but frequent fallers may benefit from additional testing including complete blood count (CBC) (to rule out anemia and infections), electrolytes, BUN, creatinine (to look for dehydration and electrolyte imbalance), serum glucose, and a stool occult blood test. An electrocardiogram (ECG) can help rule out rhythm disturbances. If syncope and ECG abnormalities are present, a myocardial infarction must be excluded, and a careful examination and diagnostic workup for ischemic disease are indicated. If the neurologic examination is positive, magnetic resonance imaging (MRI) will rule out brain or spinal cord lesions or other abnormalities. The patient with true vertigo is most likely to have inner ear disease. Benign positional vertigo (BPV) is common in older adults. The vertigo of BPV is episodic and is provoked by position changes (see Chapter 175).

Management

The goal of treatment and education is to alter modifiable risk factors (Box 13.4). The American Geriatrics Society and the

British Geriatrics Society have collaborated on the development of evidence-based fall prevention guidelines.[25-27] If lower extremity weakness is present, a referral to a physical therapist for strength training is recommended. Resistance training benefits even those of advanced age and frailty.[27] If balance is altered, balance training consists of having the patient stand on one foot for 10 seconds and gradually increase the time and frequency. Low-intensity tai chi has been demonstrated to improve balance.[30] Balance may also be improved by proper footwear and the use of assistive devices including canes, walking sticks, or walkers. Medication reduction and the avoidance of alcohol are important if hypotension is present. A home safety evaluation or checklist is indicated if trips and falls are prevalent (Fig. 13.1).

Complications

Serious complications of falls (e.g., subdural hematoma, hip fracture, or cervical fracture) occur 3% to 5% of the time. Because of the high incidence of osteoporosis in older adults, fractures requiring surgical intervention occur with falls. The most feared fractures are of the hip, but wrist, humerus, and compression fractures of the spine are common and disabling. Soft tissue injury is a more common outcome. Consultation should be considered if complications are suspected, particularly if fracture, syncope, true vertigo, or abnormal cardiovascular or neurologic findings are present.

Fall prevention is an excellent example of success through the collaborative effort of a multidisciplinary team.[31] Physical and occupational therapists provide appropriate exercise, balance, and gait-training programs and teach patients about environmental hazards. Physicians, nurse practitioners, and physician assistants assess medication usage and monitor the treatment of orthostatic hypotension, peripheral vascular disease, and incontinence (a few of the immediate causes of falls). Nutritionists prevent dehydration and anemia through teaching sessions. Community exercise and

---

BOX **13.4**

Fall Prevention

- Evaluate the home to eliminate loose cords, clutter, trip hazards, and slippery surfaces.
- Install and use bathroom and stair rails.
- Change position slowly.
- Treat foot problems and wear well-fitting, low-heeled footwear.
- Light the environment well.
- Exercise to maintain lower leg strength.
- Join a tai chi class for balance training.
- Bring all medications, including nonprescription medications, to your health care provider at each visit.
- Have regular hearing and vision testing.

Check Your Risk for Falling

Please circle "Yes" or "No" for each statement below.			Why it matters
Yes (2)	No (0)	I have fallen in the last 6 months.	People who have fallen once are likely to fall again.
Yes (2)	No (0)	I use or have been advised to use a cane or walker to get around safely.	People who have been advised to use a cane or walker may already be more likely to fall.
Yes (1)	No (0)	Sometimes I feel unsteady when I am walking.	Unsteadiness or needing support while walking are signs of poor balance.
Yes (1)	No (0)	I steady myself by holding onto furniture when walking at home.	This is also a sign of poor balance.
Yes (1)	No (0)	I am worried about falling.	People who are worried about falling are more likely to fall.
Yes (1)	No (0)	I need to push with my hands to stand up from a chair.	This is a sign of weak leg muscles, a major reason for falling.
Yes (1)	No (0)	I have some trouble stepping up onto a curb.	This is also a sign of weak leg muscles.
Yes (1)	No (0)	I often have to rush to the toilet.	Rushing to the bathroom, especially at night, increases your chance of falling.
Yes (1)	No (0)	I have lost some feeling in my feet.	Numbness in your feet can cause stumbles and lead to falls.
Yes (1)	No (0)	I take medicine that sometimes makes me feel light-headed or more tired than usual.	Side effects from medicines can sometimes increase your chance of falling.
Yes (1)	No (0)	I take medicine to help me sleep or improve my mood.	These medicines can sometimes increase your chance of falling.
Yes (1)	No (0)	I often feel sad or depressed.	Symptoms of depression, such as not feeling well or feeling slowed down, are linked to falls.
Total_____		Add up the number of points for each "yes" answer. If you scored 4 points or more, you may be at risk for falling. Discuss this brochure with your doctor.	

FIG. **13.1** Algorithm for fall risk assessment and interventions. (From CDC.org. *Stay independent brochure.* Available at http://www.cdc.gov/homeandrecreationalsafety/pdf/steadi-2015.04/Stay_Independent_brochure-a.pdf. Accessed October 26, 2015.)

educational programs are fun and effective at improving strength and balance.[32] When falls are prevented, pain, disability, and hospitalization with iatrogenic complications are also prevented.

FAILURE TO THRIVE (FRAILTY)
Definition and Etiology

FTT is a syndrome described as a progressive loss of energy, strength, and stamina leading to decreased function and general physical and cognitive deterioration. A physiologic vulnerability results from reduced reserve and capacity to withstand stress. Patients exhibit signs of anorexia, weight loss, skeletal muscle loss (sarcopenia), and functional decline. There may be accompanying depression and impaired immune function. The results of these signs can be weakness, osteopenia, balance and gait disorders, undernutrition, deconditioning, and slow gait speed.[33]

Pathophysiology

FTT, also known as *frailty*, is strongly associated with age and is seen in the late stages of decline. Weight loss and sarcopenia are strongly associated with age and undernutrition. The results are decreased strength and endurance, weakness, and fatigue. Loss of muscle mass may result in decreased bone density and slowing of metabolic rate, thereby disrupting thermoregulation and leading to heat and cold intolerance. Age-related changes in lean body mass are partially caused by changes in growth hormone, estrogen, and androgen secretion. Administering these hormones increases lean body mass but does not necessarily improve functional capacity and strength, and the associated risks of lower high-density lipoprotein (HDL), metabolic syndrome, and possibly prostate cancer seem to outweigh the potential benefit.[34] The immune system changes with age, including an overall decline in T cells and decreased effectiveness of T memory cells. This decline may explain the shorter duration of effectiveness of immunizations in older individuals and their increased vulnerability to infections.[35] End-stage chronic diseases (e.g., heart failure, pulmonary disease, renal disease) and malignancy cause weight loss, general weakness, and debility.

Clinical Presentation

Patients with FTT may be seen by their health care provider with any of the following symptoms: weakness, inability to care for self, dizziness, weight and memory loss, and depression. Weight loss in FTT is often gradual. The health history focuses on chronic diseases with signs of organ failure, the presence of gastrointestinal malabsorption, cancer risk factors, infection, thyroid abnormalities, depression, and changes in memory. Nutritional intake and the progression of weight loss are calculated. Adverse reactions to medications, including confusion or anorexia, may be partially responsible for FTT. A history of smoking and alcohol use may be helpful in discovering cause. Reversible causes of FTT are sought (Box 13.5).[36]

Physical Examination and Diagnostics

 An unplanned loss of 10% or more of body weight in less than a year.

The diagnostic evaluation of FTT seeks to differentiate reversible from irreversible causes. A complete physical examination should focus on symptoms, organ failure, infections, and

---

BOX **13.5**

Failure-to-Thrive Causes

DISEASE
- Organ failure
- Metastases
- Infection
- Stroke
- Thyroid disease
- Fractures

MEDICATION (CAN CAUSE)
- Cognitive changes
- Anorexia
- Dehydration

ENVIRONMENTAL CAUSES
- Isolation
- Neglect
- Poverty

PSYCHIATRIC CAUSES
- Depression
- Dementia
- Psychosis
- Delirium

GASTROINTESTINAL CAUSES
- Malabsorption
- Dysphagia
- Dental problems
- Diarrhea
- Vitamin deficiency

---

malignancy. A skin, mucous membrane, and eye examination may reveal muscle wasting; ulcerative lesions; and signs of vitamin deficiency, anemia, and dehydration. A complete oral examination, including an evaluation of the dentition and denture fit, is necessary. Tests of swallowing ability and the gag reflex are included in the neurologic examination. Many older women have not had a vaginal or breast examination for years, if ever; thus it is important to consider these as indicated by symptoms to rule out malignancy. Mammography continues to be recommended by the American Cancer Society as long as a woman is in reasonable health and a good candidate for treatment.[37] Pap smears are generally discontinued after age 65, especially if previously screened and negative. Bimanual pelvic examination may be indicated.

Screening tests should include a CBC, electrolytes, kidney and thyroid studies, fasting blood glucose, liver function tests, calcium levels, urinalysis, stool for occult blood ×3, and possibly a chest X-ray examination. Additional diagnostics may be indicated, depending on initial testing, examination, and patient preference.[33]

Any discovered explanation for FTT, such as malignancy or end-stage organ disease, should prompt careful discussion with the older adult and family. The patient, family, or both need to be involved in any decision to perform further or invasive diagnostic testing. The patient or proxy may not always desire treatment of potentially life-threatening conditions, making expensive and invasive diagnostic testing moot. End-of-life support and comfort may be a reasonable approach after discussion and preliminary evaluation.

A lifelong history of anorexia because of body image concerns has been reported in the literature. Older adults may have lifelong patterns of dieting and anorexia nervosa–like symptoms, which can be overlooked as a cause of weight loss in this population.

Management

Adequate protein and caloric intake is mandatory. Meals on Wheels, community meals and other community support organizations may be necessary if isolation or functional decline is present. High-calorie and high-protein supplements may be beneficial.[38-40] A daily multivitamin supplement and 800 IU of vitamin D is recommended. https://ocs.od.nih.gov/factsheets/VitaminD-HealthProfessional/ Appetite stimulants are not recommended. Depression can be treated with antidepressants and counseling for the older adult and/or caregivers.

Creative solutions to prevent malnutrition in nursing home residents have been proposed and include small group dining for dementia patients, the use of volunteer or family assistants at dinner time, and ethnically appropriate foods.

Regular exercise is possible and helpful in building strength in even the very old, deconditioned nursing home patient. In one study, weight training coupled with nutritional supplements over a 10-week period in nursing home patients ages 85 and older improved muscle strength by more than 125% compared with 3% in the control group.[41-43]

Families need to be included in education and support measures when older adults begin to fail. Often families are the first ones to urge patients to seek health care when the patients themselves are reluctant to do so. Concerned families can be encouraged to set up appointments with health care providers and accompany the older adult to these appointments as a witness and provider of information that may not otherwise be revealed. Patient autonomy can be preserved as long as dementia and depression are not found to be contributing to the frailty. If explanations for FTT are not found, it may be the natural course of life's end.

ELDER ABUSE
Definition

Recent studies indicate that 1 in 6 adults over the age of 60 worldwide have experienced abuse for more than 1 year.[44] Elder abuse is defined by the Centers for Disease Control and Prevention (CDC) as "any abuse and neglect of persons age 60 and older by a caregiver or another person in a relationship involving expectation of trust." *Self-neglect* refers to the behavior of an older person that results in being unable to provide for his or her needs. There are seven kinds of elder abuse: physical, sexual, psychological, financial exploitation, neglect, abandonment, and self-neglect.[45] Older adults with disabilities and dementia are at particular risk. One literature review concluded that 26% to 90% of adult men and women with disabilities experience abuse in their lifetime.[46,47] The vast majority of abusers are family members.[45] Older adults whose family members are overwhelmed by caregiving responsibilities or who have problems with mental illness or substance use are at higher risk for abuse.[48,49]

Clinical Presentation

Older adults who come into the health care provider's office or hospital with bruises, pressure or rope marks, broken bones, or burns may be suffering physical abuse. Bruising of the breasts or genital area may indicate sexual abuse.[46] Sudden withdrawal from usual activities or a change in behavior or alertness may indicate psychological abuse. A change in financial situation or checks signed by unauthorized persons raises suspicions of financial exploitation. Bedsores, unattended medical needs, poor hygiene or nutritional status, hoarding, or inappropriate clothing for the weather can be signs of neglect or self-neglect.[48] The suffering is often in silence, but an alert health care provider will notice subtle changes and start to question causes.

Management

In the home setting, any suspicion of abuse is reported to the state adult protective services. Concern for abuse in the long-term setting is reported to the long-term care ombudsman, or, if the risk is immediate, the police. Older adults and their caregivers can reduce the risk of abuse by seeking professional help for medical, psychological, and substance use problems. Residents of long-term care facilities, knowing their rights as patients and individuals, can report abuse either personally experienced or witnessed to the state long-term care ombudsman. Choosing a trusted person to hold durable power of attorney or to be a guardian reduces the risk of financial exploitation. Unfortunately, many older adults in abusive situations are cognitively impaired or mentally ill and often cannot advocate for themselves. In this case, concerned families or friends, health care providers, or religious or community organizations should call state adult protective services. The Elder Justice Act (EJA) was passed into law as part of the Affordable Care Act in 2010.[50] Features of this law include penalties to long-term care facilities that punish whistle-blowers, increased funding for adult protective services, grants for long-term care staff training, and civil and monetary consequences for failing to report abuse in long-term care facilities.

More information on elder abuse can be found on the National Center on Elder Abuse website (https://ncea.acl.gov/); on the American Bar Association Commission on Law and Aging website (www.americanbar.org/groups/law_aging.html); and through adult protective services and long-term care ombudsman program laws by state.

SUMMARY

Comprehensive assessment of geriatric syndromes by an interdisciplinary team may be the preferred approach to problems that clearly involve medical, mental, and social disability (Box 13.6). Annual examinations should be comprehensive, are necessarily time-consuming, and should include responsible family members. Time should be set aside to discuss care preferences and when to stop screening, especially for cancer. Patients and families should be asked to bring all medications and supplements to the examination and to be prepared with a list of concerns.

Specialized geriatric assessment focuses on prioritizing problems and approaches, improving functional capacity, and minimizing invasive and expensive medical care, with goals focused on high quality of life with the very shortest premorbid period possible and a comfortable, dignified death.

BOX **13.6**

Components of a Comprehensive Outpatient Geriatric Evaluation

1. Medical history and physical examination
2. Medication and supplement review
3. General assessment of dentition, hearing, and vision
4. Pain assessment
5. Bowel and bladder function
6. Nutritional status
7. Frequency of falls
8. Cognitive status
9. Emotional status
10. Functional status (activities of daily living [ADLs]; instrumental activities of daily living [IADLs])
11. Balance and gait
12. Social history, alcohol use, home environment (living situation, safety, financial)
13. Advance directive, health care proxy
14. Care preferences

Modified from Reuben, D., Herr, K., Pacala, J., et al. (2017). *Geriatrics at your finger-tips* (19th ed.). New York: American Geriatrics Society.

REFERENCES

1. Reference Bureau. Retrieved from www.prb.org (Accessed December 2017).
2. Kochanek, K. D., Murphy, S. L., Xu, J., & Arias, E. Mortality in the United States, 2016. National Center for Health Statistics December 2017 Retrieved from cdc.gov (Accessed December 2017).
3. Butler, R. (1969). Ageism: Another form of bigotry. *The Gerontologist, 9*(4), 243–246.
4. Ageism in Medicine Must Stop Experts Say. Medscape, 3/19/2018.
5. Reuben, D., Herr, K., Pacala, J., et al. (2017). *Geriatrics at your fingertips* (19th ed., p. 72). New York: The American Geriatric Society.
6. American Geriatrics Society. 10 things physicians and patients should question. Retrieved from www.choosingwisely.org; Released Feb, 2013, revised April, 2015. (Accessed April 8, 2019).
7. Clinicians guide to Assessing and Counseling Older Drivers 3rd edition Chapter 1—The Older Adult: An Overview 2015 American Geriatrics Society. Retrieved from geriatricscareonline.org (Accessed March 2018).
8. National Center for Statistics and Analysis: Traffic safety facts DOT HS 812 372: older population. Retrieved from http://www.nhsta. (Accessed March 2018).
9. Silveira, M., Wirtola, W., & Piette, J. (2014). Advance directive completion by elderly Americans: a decade of change. *Journal of the American Geriatrics Society, 62*(4), 706–710.
10. Centers for Medicare and Medicaid Services. Advance Care Planning. ICN 909289 August 2018. https://www.cms.gov/Outreach-and-Education/Medicare-Learning-Network-MLN/MLNProducts/Downloads/AdvanceCarePlanning.pdf (Accessed March 1, 2018).
11. Schmidt, T., Zive, D., Fromm, E., Cook, J., & Tolle, S. (2014). Physician Orders for Life Sustaining Treatment (POLST): Lessons learned from analysis of the Oregon POLST registry. *Resuscitation, 85*(4), 480–485.
12. Naylor, M. D., Aiken, L. H., Kurtzman, E. T., & Olds, D. M. (2011). The importance of transitional care in achieving health reform. *Health Affairs, 30*(4), 746–754.
13. Reuben, M. D., & Tinetti, M. (2012). Goal-oriented patient care—an alternative health outcomes paradigm. *The New England Journal of Medicine, 366,* 777–779.
14. Finn, M. Want better health care? Have doctors make house calls. *Los Angeles Times.* 2014.
15. Rauch, J. The Home Remedy for Old Age. *The Atlantic,* December, 2013.
16. Compton, R. D. (2013). Polypharmacy Concerns in the Geriatric Population. *Osteopathic Family Physician, 5*(4), 147–152.
17. Maher, R., & Hanlon, J. (2014). Hajjae E. Clinical consequences of Polypharmacy in Elderly. *Expert Opinion on Drug Safety, 13*(1), 57–65.
18. Davies, E. A. (2015). Adverse drug reactions in special populations—the elderly. *British Journal of Clinical Pharmacology, 80*(4), 796–807.
19. AGS 2015 Beers Criteria Update Expert Panel (2015). Updated Beers Criteria for potentially inappropriate medication use in older adults. *Journal of the American Geriatrics Society, 63*(11), 2227–2246.

20. O'Mahony, D., O'Sullivan, D., Byrne, S., et al. (2015). Stopp/Start Criteria for potentially inappropriate prescribing in older people: Version 2. *Age and Ageing, 47*(2), 213–218.
21. The Alzheimer's Foundation. Alzheimer's Disease Facts and Figures. Retrieved from www.alzheimers.org. (Accessed September 9, 2014).
22. Hooper, L., Bunn, D., Jimoh, F., & Fairweather-Tart, S. (2014). Water-loss dehydration and aging. *Mechanisms of Ageing and Development, 136-137,* 50–58.
23. An Evidence Based Review of Dehydration in the Pediatric Patient. Retrieved from www.ebmedicine.net/topics. (Accessed Sept 10, 2014).
24. Dalton, C. The resurgence of an old Hydration Technique—Hypodermoclysis. Pedagogy. Infusion. Retrieved from http://pedagogyeducation.com. (Accessed June 26, 2014).
25. Gale, C., Cooper, C., & Sayer, A. A. (2016). Prevalence and risk factors for falls in older men and women. The English Longitudinal Study and Ageing. *Age and Ageing, 45*(6), 789–794.
26. Ambrose, A. F., Geet, P., & Hausdoff, J. M. (2013). Risk factors for falls among older adults: A review of the literature. *Maturitas, 75*(1), 51–61.
27. American Geriatric Society. (2010). *Guideline for falls prevention.* AGS. Retrieved from www.americangeriatrics.org/health_Care_prevention_of_falls_summary_of_recommendations. (Accessed September 10, 2014).
28. Podsiadlo, D., & Richardson, S. (1991). The timed "up and go": A test of basic functional mobility for frail elderly persons. *Journal of the American Geriatrics Society, 39*(2), 142–148.
29. Weiner, D. K., Duncan, P. W., Chandler, J., et al. (1992). Functional reach: A marker of physical frailty. *Journal of the American Geriatrics Society, 40,* 203–207.
30. Herrington, C., Michaleff, Z. A., Fairhall, N., et al. (2017). Exercise to prevent falls in older adults: An updated systematic review and meta-analysis. *British Journal of Sports Medicine, 51,* 1750–1758.
31. Hopewell, S., Adedire, O., Copsey, B. J., et al. (2018). Multifactorial and multiple component interventions for preventing falls in older people living in the community. *The Cochrane Database of Systematic Reviews,* (7), CD012221, doi:10.1002/14651858.cd12211pub2.
32. US Preventive Services Task Force. (2018). Interventions to prevent falls in community-dwelling older adults: US Preventive Services Task Force recommendation statement. *JAMA: The Journal of the American Medical Association, 319*(16), 1696–1704. doi:10.1001/jama.2018.3097.
33. Clegg, A., Iliffe, S., Rikkert, M. O., & Rockwood, K. (2013). Frailty in elderly people. *Lancet, 38*(9868), 752–762.
34. Spitzer, M., Huang, G., Basara, S., et al. (2013). Risks and benefits of testosterone therapy in men. *Nature Reviews. Endocrinology, 9,* 414–424.
35. Haq, K., & McElhaney, J. (2014). Immunosenescence: influenza vaccine and the elderly. *Current Opinion in Immunology, 29,* 38–42.
36. Gaddey, H. L., & Holder, K. (2014). Unintentional weight loss in older adults. *American Family Physician, 89*(9), 718–722.
37. American Cancer Society. Guidelines for the early detection of cancer. Retrieved from www.cancer.org/healthy/findcancerearly/ca.
38. Cruz-Jentoft, A. J., Kiesswetter, E., Drey, M., & Sieber, C. C. (2017). Nutrition, frailty and sarcopenia. *Aging Clinical and Experimental Research, 29*(1), 43–48.
39. Park, Y., Chou, J. E., & Hwang, H. S. (2018). Protein supplementation improves muscle mass and physical performance in undernourished, prefrail and frail elderly subjects: A randomized, double-blind, placebo controlled trial. *The American Journal of Clinical Nutrition, 108*(5), 1026–1033.
40. Mangels, A. (2018). Malnutrition in older adults. *The American Journal of Nursing, 118*(3), 34–41.
41. Fiatarone, M. A., O'Neil, E. F., Ryan, N. D., et al. (1994). Exercise training and nutritional supplements for physical frailty in very old people. *The New England Journal of Medicine, 330,* 1769–1775.
42. Matsuda, P. N., Shumway-Cook, A., & Ciol, M. A. (2014). The effects of a home based exercise program on physical function in frail older adults. *Journal of Geriatric Physical Therapy, 33*(2), 78–84.
43. Landi, F., Marzette, E., Martone, A. M., Bernaber, R., & Onder, G. (2014). Exercise as a remedy for sarcopenia. *Current Opinion in Clinical Nutrition and Metabolic Care, 17*(1), 25–31.
44. Elder Abuse Facts. Retrieved from https://www.ncoa.org/public-policy-action/elder-justice/elder-abuse-facts/ (Accessed April 9, 2019).
45. Yon, Y., Miktin, C., Gassoumis, Z., & Wilbur, K. (2017). Elder abuse prevalence in community settings: Systematic review and meta-analysis. *The Lancet Global Health, 5*(2), e147–e156.
46. Dong, X. (2015). Elder abuse: Systematic review and implications for practice. *Journal of the American Geriatrics Society, 63*(6), 1214–1238.
47. Beach, S. R., Carpenter, C. R., Rosen, T., Sharps, P., & Gelles, R. (2016). Screening and detection of elder abuse: Research opportunities and lessons learned from emergency geriatric care, intimate partner violence, and child abuse.

Journal of Elder Abuse & Neglect, 28, 4–5, 185–216. doi:10.1080/08946566.2016.1229241.

48. Lach, M., & Pillemer, K. (2015). Elder abuse. *The New England Journal of Medicine, 375*, 1947–1956.

49. Stall, N., Kim, S., Hardacre, K., et al. (2018). Association of informal caregiver distress with health outcomes of community-dwelling dementia care recipients: A systematic review. *Journal of the American Geriatrics Society, 67*(3).

50. Colello, K. (2017). *The Elder Justice Act: Background and issues for congress.* Congressional Research Service. Retrieved from https://fas.org/sgp/crs/misc/R43707.pdf. (Accessed April 10, 2019).

CHAPTER **14**

PALLIATIVE CARE

Margaret Firer Bishop • Richard Anthony Taylor • Imatullah Akyar • Marie A. Bakitas

DEFINITION AND EPIDEMIOLOGY

The National Consensus Project (NCP) endorses the Centers for Medicare and Medicaid definition: Palliative care means patient- and family-centered care that optimizes quality of life by anticipating, preventing, and treating suffering. Palliative care throughout the continuum of illness involves addressing physical, intellectual, emotional, social, and spiritual needs and to facilitate patient autonomy, access to information, and choice.

Palliative care is specialized medical care for people with serious illness. This type of care is focused on providing patients with relief from the symptoms, pain, and stress of a serious illness—whatever the diagnosis. The goal is to improve quality of life for both the patient and the family. Palliative care is provided by a team of doctors, nurses, and other specialists who work with a patient's other doctors to provide *an extra layer of support.* Palliative care is appropriate at any age and at any stage in a serious illness, and can be provided together with curative treatment."

A preponderance of positive evidence about quality of life, symptom mood, caregiver burden, health care use, and in some cases patient survival outcomes have led to multiple professional guidelines recommending that palliative care should begin early in the trajectory of serious or life-limiting illness.[1,2] However, health care providers and consumers have long associated palliative care only with end of life hospice care. The National Consensus Project (NCP) for Quality Palliative Care first released *clinical practice guidelines* (with subsequent editions in 2009, 2013, and 2018) to provide a national standard for development of palliative care programs in all settings and offer a benchmark for established programs.[3] The NCP guidelines emphasize that palliative care is a critical dimension of health care for any patient with a serious illness regardless of care setting or disease. Box 14.1 lists the Centers for Medicare and Medicaid Services' definition of palliative care endorsed by the NCP.

The exponential growth of hospital-based palliative care programs has resulted in increased availability for most US citizens. More than 90% of US hospitals with 300 or more beds reported a palliative care program.[4] However, there are still disparities in access in smaller, rural areas that often serve minority populations. Additionally, patients who could benefit

---

BOX **14.1**

Definitions and Underlying Tenets of Palliative Care

TENETS OF PALLIATIVE CARE

- Care is provided and services coordinated by an interdisciplinary team.
- Patients, families, and palliative and nonpalliative health care providers collaborate and communicate about care needs.
- Services are available concurrently with, or independent of, curative or life-prolonging care.
- Patient and family hopes for peace and dignity are supported throughout the course of illness, during the dying process, and after death.
- There is an emphasis on coordinated assessment and continuity of care across health care settings. There should be an interdisciplinary team with specialty education, training, and certification.
- Management of physical and psychological symptoms is multidimensional and includes pharmacologic, interventional, behavioral, and complementary interventions.
- Bereavement is a necessary aspect of every palliative care program.
- Interdisciplinary engagement and collaboration with patients and families to identify, support, and capitalize on patient and family strengths are essential to social support.
- Spiritual care includes exploration, assessment, and attention to spiritual issues of the patient and family, including spiritual and religious rituals and practices for comfort and relief.
- Culture is recognized as a course of resilience and strength for the patient and family, with particular attention given to cultural and linguistic competence including plain language, literacy, and linguistically appropriate service delivery.
- Care of the patient at the end of life focuses on the meticulous assessment and management of pain and other symptoms; family guidance as to what to expect during the dying process; and the postdeath period, which is emphasized.
- It is recognized that palliative care includes advance care planning ethics and legal aspects of care.

Data from National Consensus Project for Quality Palliative Care. (2013). *Clinical practice guidelines for quality palliative care* (3rd ed.). Pittsburgh, PA: National Consensus Project and the Center to Advance Palliative Care (www.capc.org).

---

from palliative care services but are not hospitalized may have difficulty receiving services as an outpatient, in a nursing home, or in their home. Innovations such as providing palliative care via telehealth and increasing community-based programs are beginning to reduce such disparities in care.[5]

Despite national efforts, patient and provider misconceptions about the broader focus of palliative care compared to hospice inadvertently created barriers to early access to palliative care. Hospice is a specific type of palliative care provided to individuals with a life expectancy measured in months, not years. Hospice teams provide patients and families with expert medical care, medications and equipment as well as emotional, and spiritual support, focusing on improving patient and family quality of life. An opinion poll found that 70% of the general public were "not at all knowledgeable" about palliative care.[6] In an effort to improve acceptance of palliative care, a series of consumer focus groups were convened that resulted in a more patient- and family-centered definition

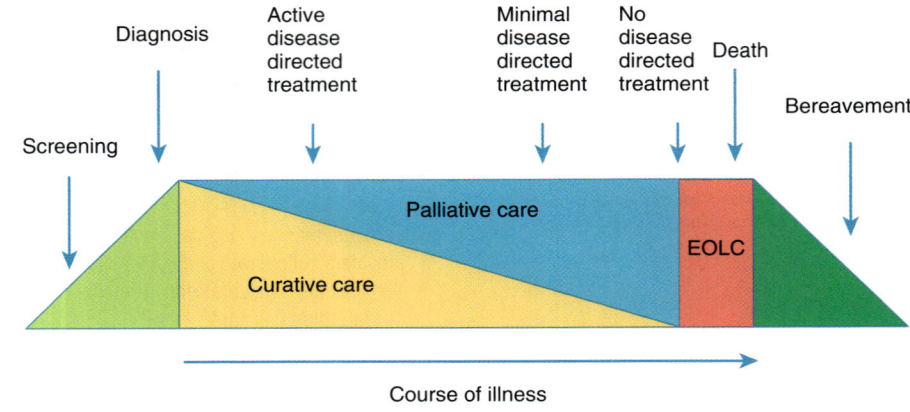

F I G . 14.1   The Palliative Care Continuum. (Modified from http://depts.washington.edu/pallcare/training/ppt.shtml.)

Data from Aslakson, R., Dy, S. M., Wilson, R. F., Waldfogel, J., Zhang, A., Isenberg, S. R., et al. (2017). Patient- and Caregiver-Reported Assessment Tools for Palliative Care: Summary of the 2017 Agency for Healthcare Research and Quality Technical Brief. *Journal of Pain and Symptom Management, 54*(6), 961–972; Quill, T. E., & Abernethy, A. P. (2013). Generalist plus specialist palliative care—creating a more sustainable model. *New England Journal of Medicine, 368*(13), 1173–1175; and Weissman, D. E., & Meier, D. E. (2011). Identifying patients in need of a palliative care assessment in the hospital setting: A consensus report from the Center to Advance Palliative Care. *Journal of Palliative Medicine, 14*(1), 17–23.

BOX **14.2**

Palliative Care Web Resources

American Academy of Hospice and Palliative Medicine
  (www.aahpm.org)
Americans for Better Care of the Dying *(www.abcd-caring.org)*
Center to Advance Palliative Care (CAPC) *(www.capc.org)*
Growth House *(www.growthhouse.org)*
Hospice and Palliative Nurses Association (HPNA) *(www.hpna.org)*
Hospice Foundation of America *(www.hospicefoundation.org)*
National Board for Certification of Hospice and Palliative Nurses
  (www.nbchpn.org)
National Consensus Project for Quality Palliative Care
  (www.nationalconsensusproject.org)
National Hospice and Palliative Care Organization *(www.nhpco.org)*
National Palliative Care Research Center (NPCRC) *(www.npcrc.org)*
VITALtalk *(http://vitaltalk.org/)*

BOX **14.3**

Primary Versus Specialty Palliative Care

Primary Palliative Care
Palliative care delivered by health care professionals who are not palliative specialists, including:
- Basic management of pain, depression, anxiety, and other symptoms
- Basic discussions regarding code status, identifying goals of care, patient's understanding of illness, prognosis, and treatment options

Specialty Palliative Care
Palliative care delivered by palliative care specialists to include:
- Management of refractory pain/symptoms
- Management of complex depression, anxiety, grief, and existential distress
- Assisting in conflict resolution within families, between staff and families, or among treatment teams regarding goals or treatment options
- Assisting in addressing cases of near futility

provided in Box 14.1. Of note, the consumer definition does not include stigmatizing words such as "death," "dying," "emotional," or "psychosocial" and clarifies that this type of care is provided as "an extra layer of support" along with other medical care. This latter clause emphasizes that accepting palliative care does not mean that a patient must "give up" familiar care providers or standard life-prolonging or curative care, but rather palliative care is provided concurrently with these treatments. Armed with this new definition, frontline primary care providers are in a prime position to translate this philosophy into evidence-based care for their seriously ill patients and the family and friend care partners of these patients. Box 14.1 lists additional Tenets of Palliative Care and Fig. 14.1 illustrates the overall principles of this care model. The key concept is to replace a dichotomous "either/or" model of cure versus palliation with one that focuses on integrating palliative strategies early and concurrently with disease-modifying treatments. As Fig. 14.1 illustrates, palliative care is appropriate at the time of diagnosis with a serious illness; as the disease progresses and disease-modifying treatments diminish, the palliative focus enlarges. Resources for learning about palliative care approaches and locating specialists are listed in Box 14.2. This chapter compares the role of the palliative care specialist

with the role of the primary care clinician, with a special focus on the primary palliative care skills that are important for all clinicians who care for adults with life-threatening illnesses from the time of diagnosis through the end of life and family bereavement.

PRIMARY VERSUS SPECIALTY PALLIATIVE CARE

Palliative care delivery is increasingly characterized as either primary (also called basic or generalist) palliative care or specialty palliative care.[7] Core elements of primary palliative care, such as aligning treatment and patient goals or basic symptom management are seen as routine aspects of care delivered by any practitioner. Routine palliative care problems (e.g., uncomplicated symptom management) are more likely to be managed by primary care clinicians in the same way that they handle routine cardiac problems (e.g., prescribing cardiac medications) rather than referring to cardiologists. Box 14.3

BOX **14.4**

When to Consider Requesting a Palliative Care Consult

When a patient has a potentially life-limiting or life-threatening condition and one or more of the following:

- Distressing physical, psychological, or spiritual symptoms that are difficult to manage
- Poor understanding from the patient/family/surrogate of the current illness, prognostic trajectory, and treatment options
- Unresolved conflict between patient and family/surrogate regarding wishes
- Treatment options that do not seem to be aligned to patient goals
- Complex care requirements (functional dependence, home ventilator/antibiotics/feedings)
- Decisions regarding the following interventions are being considered:
  - Feeding tube placement
  - Tracheostomy
  - Dialysis
  - Left Ventricular Assist Device or Implantable Cardioverter-Defibrillator placement
  - Bone marrow or stem cell transplant
- Lack of advance care planning despite persistent efforts
- Past hospice program enrollee
- Increasing frequency of emergency room visits and/or hospital admissions

Data from from Hui, D., & Bruera, E. (2015). Integrating palliative care into the trajectory of cancer care. Nature reviews. Clinical oncology, 13(3), 159–171; Weissman, D. E., & Meier, D. E. (2011). Identifying patients in need of a palliative care assessment in the hospital setting: A consensus report from the Center to Advance Palliative Care. *Journal of Palliative Medicine, 14*(1), 17–23.

BOX **14.5**

Components of a Palliative Care Consultation

- Past medical history
- Past social/spiritual/emotional history
- Review of symptoms
- Recommendations for refractory or challenging symptom management
- Consideration of advance care planning including Advance Directives and Resuscitation Wishes
- Discussion of understanding of illness, treatment options, and patient's values—particularly as to how they impact treatment decision-making
- Identification of goals of care
- Identification of points of conflict

identifies the key components of primary versus specialty palliative care.

Access to specialty palliative services can be limited, particularly on an outpatient basis. Even though inpatient palliative care services are more readily available, the need far exceeds the availability of services. Prospectively identifying local inpatient and outpatient palliative care services, either through a medical center or sometimes through a local hospice, is valuable. Recognizing that outpatient palliative services are scarce, advocating for an inpatient palliative care consult in the event a patient in need is hospitalized can be highly beneficial. Even in the absence of an outpatient palliative program, inpatient palliative specialists may be able to provide follow-up resources or phone consultation once the patient is discharged. Box 14.4 describes some criteria to consider in selecting appropriate patients for a palliative care consult. Another strategy that has shown promise is the use of the "surprise question." This simple screener, "Would you be surprised if this patient died within the next year?" has been found to be sensitive and specific in identifying patients who could benefit from a primary or specialty palliative care approach.[8]

MODELS OF PALLIATIVE CARE AND PRIMARY COLLABORATION

In the event that palliative specialty care is needed it is important to be aware of what the primary care provider can expect. Box 14.5 describes the standardized components of a comprehensive palliative care consultation. However, specialty palliative care practices may differ regarding which aspects of the patient's care they will assume relative to the primary care provider. The three most common models are consultative, co-management, and primary management models. When the consultative model is used, the palliative team, after conducting an initial assessment as described in Box 14.5, will act solely in the consultant role and will provide recommendations rather than assume any of the ordering (medications, labs or radiology requests, for example). In this case, the primary provider maintains prescriptive/ordering responsibility. The co-management role can be more active. For example, after discussion and in agreement with the primary provider, the palliative care specialist may assume management of one or more aspects of the patient's palliative care plan (e.g., pain management). Rarely, palliative care specialists may assume the overall care of the patient. This may happen if the patient has been followed by a specialist service such as oncology or cardiology and there has not been a primary provider regularly involved in the patient's care.

PRIMARY PALLIATIVE CARE COMMUNICATION STRATEGIES

Good communication skills are the foundation of both primary and specialty palliative care. Many useful communication tools have been developed and applied in the practice of palliative care. Three of the most common strategies that are used are SPIKES, NURSE, and Ask-Tell-Ask. SPIKES is a mnemonic to describe a six-step communication protocol (Box 14.6).[9] NURSE is a mnemonic to assist with addressing the emotions in difficult discussions (Box 14.7). Ask-Tell-Ask is a strategy to encourage an interactive, two-way conversation ensuring that information is not only relayed, but also received and understood (Box 14.8).[10–13]

EXPLORING GOALS OF CARE AND MAKING RECOMMENDATIONS

After establishing setting (the "S" in the SPIKES protocol), all goals of care conversations must start with establishing the common ground around what is known and understood about the patient's illness. Asking what the patient/family understand (the "P" in SPIKES, as well as the ASK-TELL-ASK protocol), asking permission to share information (the "I" in SPIKES), and sharing information (the "K" in SPIKES) lays the groundwork

BOX **14.6**

SPIKES

- Setting
  - Confirm the medical facts and review what will be discussed
  - Identify who needs to be present—who does the patient want there
  - Ensure privacy and adequate seating
  - Hold calls, silence pagers, allow adequate time for encounter
- Perception
  - Determine what the patient knows about their illness
  - "What do you understand about your illness?"
  - "How would you describe your medical condition?"
  - "What have the other doctors told you about what's happening?"
- Invitation
  - Determining how much the patient wants to know
  - Asking permission to share information
  - "Are you the type of person who likes to know the details of their condition or just the general points?"
  - "Some people don't want to know the specifics of their illness and would rather their families be told instead."
  - "Is it okay if I tell you what I understand about what is happening right now?"
- Knowledge
  - Share the information in a sensitive but straightforward way
  - Start by letting the patient know you have bad news (warning shot)
    - "I have some difficult news to share."
  - Keep language simple, avoid technical jargon or euphemisms
  - Pause between chunks of information to allow for comprehension
- Empathize
  - Allow time for expression of feelings without rushing
  - Validate and normalize their feelings
  - Resist the temptation to make things better, fix things, or keep talking
    - "Tell me more about how you are feeling."
    - "I imagine this is difficult news."
    - "You appear to be angry, what are you thinking right now?"
- Summary
  - Summarize what has been discussed
  - Establish a plan for next steps and follow up
  - Consider additional support needed
  - Reassure family they are not being abandoned
  - Allow time for questions

Data from Hauser, J. (2017). Communication in heart failure and palliative care. *Heart Failure Reviews, 22*(5), 535–542; Hollyday, S. L., & Buonocore, D. (2015). Breaking bad news and discussing goals of care in the intensive care unit. *AACN Advanced Critical Care, 26*(2), 131–141; McEwan, A., & Silverberg, J. Z. (2016). Palliative care in the emergency department. *Emergency Medicine Clinics of North America, 34*(3), 667–685; and van Vliet, L. M., Lindenberger, E., & van Weert, J. C. (2015). Communication with older, seriously ill patients. *Clinics in Geriatric Medicine, 31*(2), 219–230.

BOX **14.7**

NURSE

- Name the emotion: "Some people feel frustrated in a situation like this."
- Understand the emotion: "It must be hard to depend on others when you've been so independent."
- Respect the patient: "I'm impressed you've been able to stay so determined."
- Support the patient: "We are here to help you feel as well as possible."
- Explore the emotion: "Tell me more about what you meant by being sad."

Data from Hauser, J. (2017). Communication in heart failure and palliative care. *Heart Failure Reviews, 22*(5), 535–542; McEwan, A., & Silverberg, J. Z. (2016). Palliative care in the emergency department. *Emergency Medicine Clinics of North America, 34*(3), 667–685; and van Vliet, L. M., Lindenberger, E., & van Weert, J. C. (2015). Communication with older, seriously ill patients. *Clinics in Geriatric Medicine, 31*(2), 219–230.

BOX **14.8**

Ask-Tell-Ask

- Ask
  - Ask the patient/surrogate to tell you their understanding of the current situation
- Tell
  - Relay the information in an understandable, jargon-free manner
- Ask
  - Ask patient/surrogate if they understand
  - Consider asking them to tell you what they understand
    - "Just so I can make sure I was clear, can you tell me what you understand from what I just said?"

Data from Hauser, J. (2017). Communication in heart failure and palliative care. *Heart Failure Reviews, 22*(5), 535–542; Hollyday, S. L., & Buonocore, D. (2015). Breaking bad news and discussing goals of care in the intensive care unit. *AACN Advanced Critical Care, 26*(2), 131–141; and McEwan, A., & Silverberg, J. Z. (2016). Palliative care in the emergency department. *Emergency Medicine Clinics of North America, 34*(3), 667–685.

for further discussion. Responding with empathy and addressing emotions establishes trust and conveys support (the "E" in SPIKES, as well as the NURSE mnemonic). It is also helpful to spend some time exploring the context of the patient's life, who they are as an individual and what is of value to them. What they identify as most important to them will drive their personal hopes and goals. Eliciting patients' hopes and fears can structure what their goals might be and inform medical decision-making.

For example, you have a patient that tells you they are fiercely independent. The idea of losing functional ability is completely unacceptable to them. Understanding this value will inform the discussion you have with them around resuscitation wishes, life support, or even their desire for rehospitalization. Patients' hopes, and therefore their goals, change over time. They may initially hope for life prolongation or cure. As the illness progresses, hopes may shift to symptom management or quality time spent with a loved one.

After better understanding who a patient is and what his/her values and goals are, reviewing the benefit versus burden of potential medical interventions takes on fuller meaning. You now have an idea of how this patient defines his/her quality of life. If the patient's initial goal is cure or life prolongation, then interventional choices will become centered on that goal. Weighing the benefit of medical interventions that support that goal (life prolongation) against the burden of those choices (e.g., high risk of being bedbound) is often not considered. You may be the first clinician to introduce this framework.

Taking into account an individual's definition of quality of life and how that fits into medical decision-making may be a completely new consideration for that patient. Having these conversations upstream and proactively is ideal, allowing time for contemplation and discernment. As clinicians, as much as possible we must look ahead to future medical decision-making points and help patients and families consider them in noncrisis moments versus waiting until there is an emergency.

Discussion regarding prognosis is another aspect when considering goals of care. Clinicians often wait for patients to introduce this topic and patients often wait for clinicians. Proactively introducing discussion around prognosis can be useful. Using a statement such as, "Some patients want to know about their prognosis, or life expectancy, and some do not. If we had some information regarding this, would you want to know?" This allows the patient control over the information and, again, we ask permission to share information. Definitive answers such as "You have 6 months" or being too vague, such as "I don't know," are less helpful than talking about prognosis in ranges. Ranges can encompass what we know medically about life expectancy as well as the uncertainty inherent in prognostication. "Hours to days," "Days to weeks," "Weeks to months," and "Months to years" are better ways to convey prognosis. It is useful to include a caution regarding the unpredictability of illness and the possibility of the unexpected. Exploring with patients why they are asking about prognosis or why they want this information can help determine the level of detail to provide. Patients who want to plan for their future may want more detailed information. Patients who are frightened might want more generalized information.[12]

Finally, summarizing (the last "S" in SPIKES) and making recommendations is an important step following a "goals of care" discussion. First, confirm a shared understanding of the patient's goals which allows for reflection of what you understand, summary of what was discussed, and validation that you were listening and alignment between you and the patient (the ASK-TELL-ASK technique). Again, asking permission to give recommendations (similar to the "I" in SPIKES) is crucial. Making a statement such as, "I have some ideas about what steps to take next. Is it okay if I share them with you?"[13]

PRIMARY PALLIATIVE CARE
Eliciting Patients' Values and Preferences

Advance Care Planning. An important and first step in primary or specialty palliative care support is to understand the patient's preferences and help him/her to identify goals of care, recognizing that goals may change as the disease status changes.[14] This voluntary discussion and planning for future health care between an individual and a health care provider is called advance care planning (ACP). The ACP process supports adults at any age or stage of health in understanding and sharing their personal values, life goals, and preferences about future health. It should be a component of the initial history for all patients and be revisited at least annually and any time the patient has a change in condition. The main goal of ACP is to help medical care be consistent with the patient's values. It is the result of a conversation and shared understanding between the patient and his/her health care provider and results in the documentation of an ACP plan, usually in the form of a document called an Advance Directive (AD), and through the appointment of a surrogate decision-maker, also called a durable power of attorney for health care (DPOA-HC).

Advance Care Planning in summary:
- Involves the patient, health care professionals, and family/caregivers
- Is the articulation of wishes, preferences, values, and goals in regard to current and anticipated medical status including potential treatment options
- Respects personal autonomy and medical reality
- Needs a patient with decision-making capacity to participate
- Should take place early in the course of the illness but can happen at anytime
- Should be used to inform decision-making, even in acute medical emergencies
- Is open to change, revision, and cancelation
- Should be regularly reviewed and updated whenever a patient's health status or life goals change
- Is not confined to medical issues—may include spiritual or interpersonal issues

The Role of the Primary Care Provider in Completing Advance Directives. Following the Patient Self-Determination Act (PSDA) of 1991, all states adopted AD legislation. An AD serves as a mechanism for an individual's wishes for medical care to be known and followed when he/she lacks decisional capacity to make a medical decision. A number of AD instruments have evolved over past years and are available to patients. They include an instructional directive and identification of a *durable power of attorney for health care* (DPOA-HC). Instructional directives are sometimes referred to as a "living will" or the medical directive and provide direction about the type and amount of medical care desired when the person becomes incapacitated. The DPOA-HC is the person identified to serve as a surrogate for decision-making (Table 14.1). Other instruments listed among ADs are combined directives, do not resuscitate (DNR) orders, and physician orders for life sustaining treatment/medical order life sustaining treatment (POLST/MOLST).

Advance Directives: When, How and Who to Use. As legal documents, ADs must be executed by an individual with decision-making capacity. Determining whether an adult has decisional capacity includes assessing if they have the ability to understand information, weigh risks and benefits, consider consequences, and make and communicate decisions. If there is no AD, an authorized person is identified who can make decisions on behalf of the person/patient. This person is usually determined by state law, most often starting with relatives. (Current individual state laws should be consulted to determine the priority of surrogates in the absence of an appointed agent for health care; e.g., https://www.americanbar.org/content/dam/aba/administrative/law_aging/2014_default_surrogate_consent_statutes.authcheckdam.pdf.)

A living will, or medical directive, is a document explaining whether or not a person wants to be on life support if he/she falls terminally ill and will die shortly without life support, or falls into an irreversible coma or persistent vegetative state and lacks decisional capacity. It describes wanted, limited, or unwanted interventions with detailed (e.g., continuation or termination of artificial nutrition or hydration), general (e.g., no extraordinary measures), or personal values and goals (e.g., avoid suffering). It may also include other preferences and instructions for care and designate persons with whom providers may discuss the person's condition.[14]

The health care proxy or DPOA-HC is the person who makes health care decisions for the patient when the patient

TABLE 14.1   **Advance Directives**

Instructional Directives	Living Wills and Medical Directives	Do-not-resuscitate or CPR Directives	Five Wishes
	Describe wishes for life-sustaining treatment including wanted, limited, or unwanted interventions. Allows patients to specify their desires for, or refusals of, specific treatments under certain circumstances should the patient become incapacitated. Instructional directives usually include a designated proxy.	If the patient suffers cardiopulmonary arrest, the health care team will not make any attempt to stop the process or bring the patient back to life. Refusal of CPR.	(1) The person I want to make care decisions for me when I can't (2) The kind of medical treatment I want or don't want (3) How comfortable I want to be (4) How I want people to treat me (5) What I want my loved ones to know
Proxy Directives	**The Durable Power of Attorney for Health Care (DPOA-HC)** Patients designate another person to make health care decisions if they are incapacitated. This person can be referred to as health care proxy, health care agent, surrogate, or durable power of attorney for health care. Proxy designation is usually combined with an instructional directive.		
Instructional Directives SPECIAL FORMS Forms vary by state and include: **POLST** Provider Orders for Life Sustaining Treatment **POST** Physician Orders on Scope of Treatment **MOLST** Medical Orders for Life Sustaining Treatment **MOST** Medical Orders for Scope of Treatment **COLST** Clinical Orders for Life Sustaining Treatment **TPOPP** Transportable Physician Orders for Patient Preferences	**Single Page Medical Order** Documents conversation between a provider and the patient. Summarizes patient's wishes in the form of medical orders. A form of "treatment wishes"	Actionable throughout the entire community. Immediately recognizable and can be used first hand with any involved health care providers. Valid across all health care facilities.	www.polst.org

CPR, Cardiopulmonary resuscitation.
Data from National POLST Paradigm: POLST and Advance Care Planning, Matzo M, Sherman D, eds. Palliative Care Nursing: Quality Care to the End of Life, 3e, Springer, 2010, New York. https://polst.org/polst-advance-care-planning/.

lacks decision-making capacity or if the patient defers to the proxy. The DPOA-HC is fully empowered to consult with physicians, view medical records, and make all decisions related to health care according to the wishes of the patient. Health care proxies cannot override a valid living will or cardiopulmonary resuscitation (CPR) directive, nor are they authorized to make any decisions other than those directly related to health care.

The DNR order, or CPR directive, instructs emergency medical service personnel, health care providers, and health care facilities on administration of CPR. Typically, this instruction is a refusal of CPR. In the absence of a DNR order, consent for CPR is presumed. DNR orders remain in effect following the patient's discharge from the hospital as long as the durable DNR order is signed by the clinician and patient.

Most standardized AD forms are written in a defensive tone, indicating the type of care a patient does not want. An exception is the *Five Wishes* tool which addresses the type of care a patient wants as disease progresses. Five Wishes offers choices and opportunities for direction around health and personal care, such as desire for visitors, preferred place of death, comfort measures, funeral plans, documentation of values, memories, spiritual and personal legacy, etc. This type of care involves minimizing procedures that do not contribute to comfort. It does not provide authoritative instructions on administration of CPR.

Physician Orders for Life Sustaining Treatment. Unlike traditional ADs, *POLST* is a medical order completed by a medical provider after discussion with the patient or surrogate. The POLST acts as an order for other health care providers in support of patients' preferences. This form is more uniform and comprehensive and provides a portable method of documentation of patients' treatment desires. It is intended to stay with person/patient (especially chronically or seriously ill person who is in frequent contact with health care providers) among various health care facilities and settings. These directives are summarized in Table 14.1.

Advance Care Planning Discussions and Advance Directive Communications. Most patients and end-of-life care experts recommend conducting ACP discussions during routine office visits with primary care clinicians when patients are medically stable and after establishing rapport. Communication starts with introducing the concept of ACP, providing AD or related materials, and asking the patient to consider proxy preferences. Using the strategies described earlier in the chapter are good models to initiate and address these issues. The patient will need some reflective time to read the materials and consider who they would elect as their preferred proxy. The next step is helping the patient to identify personal values, goals, and specific treatment wishes. This is done through exploring what makes their life worthwhile, how they experience enjoyment in life, and what thoughts they have about life-sustaining treatments. The discussions and statements should be summarized as much as possible using the patient's own words, should be signed by the patient, and copies distributed to the medical record, the patient, and the proxy decision maker decision-maker. The patient's wishes, preferences, and goals should be reviewed, and any needed updates should be recorded.

Reimbursement for Conducting Advance Care Planning Discussions in Primary Care. Since January 1, 2016, Medicare is reimbursing providers for ACP discussions. Reimbursement lowers barriers and offers compensation for the process.

Details for billing include:
- Code 99497 (for initial 30-minute voluntary consultation), 99498 (an add-on code for additional 30-minute time blocks needed)
- ACP discussions need to be face-to-face with patients and/or their surrogates to be billed
- Completion of legal ADs is not needed
- Providers billing the codes must be the patient's "managing physician" or must be providing direct supervision to the qualified health professional conducting the ACP conversation

Ethical/Legal Considerations

Medical Futility, Withdrawal Versus Withholding Treatment. Advances in medical therapies and life-support technologies intend to benefit patients and restore them to well-functioning lives. However, in some situations, these treatments do not provide net benefit to the patient and questions arise around the benefit versus burden of proposed medical interventions. Specifically, are life-prolonging measures improving the quality of life or prolonging suffering and postponing the dying process?

The concept of medical futility evolved in response to patients and families who insisted on life-prolonging treatments which were seen as inappropriate by providers.[15] In cases where there is concern for futility, interventions primarily focus on negotiation with the patient/family and on-going communication. This approach highlights the importance of understanding the patients', families' and health care professionals' concerns; acknowledging families' wish that all that can be done is being done; and having careful conversation around points of conflict.

When is a treatment futile? Whether a treatment's effects are deemed desirable or beneficial will depend on the patient's and/or the clinician's perspective. There is clinical agreement that a particular therapy can be futile for one patient yet not for another. It is recommended to avoid using the phrasing "futility" and instead using precise descriptions of the patient's clinical situation.[15]

The criteria for withdrawing interventions is the same as the criteria for withholding them: the interventions are considered burdensome or are against the expressed wishes of the patient. Withholding treatment involves never beginning an intervention; and benefit/burden analysis determines whether a proposed treatment should be withheld. Withdrawing an intervention entails stopping an artificial measure so that the disease process comes to a natural end; no lethal act is committed to bring about death. The clear consensus about when life-sustaining treatment may be withheld or withdrawn is when its use is against the patient's wishes, when it will or has begun to harm the patient, or when it does not or will not benefit the patient in the future.[15]

Historically withholding or withdrawing life-prolonging treatments started with CPR, but currently it can involve the use of ventilators, dialysis, cardiac assist devices (implantable cardioverter-defibrillator, pacemaker, and ventricular assist devices), chemotherapy, and sophisticated intensive care unit technologies.

Conversations about "futility" awaken patient fears of being abandoned by health professionals. It is important to emphasize that care will not be withdrawn, and that symptom management and patient care will continue. Only the treatments lacking benefit for the patient are halted. Communication regarding nonbeneficial therapies may include the following:[15]
- Giving time and providing a proper atmosphere of privacy for the family to digest the reality of illness and being aware of imminent grieving of family
- Documenting the basis for a judgment that further "curative efforts" are deemed "nonbeneficial", including clinical and quality of life judgments about burdens and benefits for the patient
- Demonstrating that the health care team has partnered with the family in trying to make the right decision for the patient
- Providing understanding and reassurance for the family that all comfort needs and pain management will be carefully provided
- Making every effort to accommodate the religious perspective of the patient and family

Palliative Sedation

At the end of life patients may experience refractory, intractable, or intolerable symptoms, including pain, that are impossible to control in the absence of sedation. Palliative sedation is an option for these patients. Palliative sedation is a recent concept with inconsistent definitions but has the same goals as palliative care: ensuring comfort, relief of suffering, and respecting patient wishes.[16] Beginning in the late 1980s, palliative sedation has been defined as the use of sedative medications to relieve (or prevent) intolerable and refractory distress by inducing unconsciousness. Drugs used for sedation are typically sedatives and anesthetics. Palliative sedation should be supervised or provided by palliative care specialists, it often requires the signing of informed consent, and sometimes requires an evaluation from the ethics committee as well. The choice to use palliative sedation is a careful one and decided only after all other symptom management options have been exhausted. It is important to recognize that the intention of palliative sedation is to relieve symptoms, not to hasten death.

Physician Assisted Death

Physician assisted death (PAD) also known as "aid in dying" has been a controversial topic amongst patients with serious illness, as well as within state legislatures. PAD requires the patient be able to consent, a physician be able to prescribe the life-ending medication, and the patient to independently be able to ingest it.[17] PAD is distinct from euthanasia, a practice that is not legal in the United States, in which the physician actually administers the lethal dose of medication.

In the United States, Oregon was the first state to legalize PAD. The criteria to be eligible for PAD are: the patient must be older than 17, reside legally in Oregon, be terminally ill with a remaining life expectancy less than 6 months, and be able to communicate and make decisions. PAD is still considered illegal in 44 states.

Clinical evaluation of patients potentially receiving assisted death includes:[17]

1. Does the patient have full decision-making capacity, and is he or she aware of all alternative approaches?
2. Is the patient's suffering being fully addressed with all reasonably available palliative treatments?
3. Is the patient's illness fully defined, including its degree of reversibility?
4. Is the degree to which the patient is terminally ill fully understood?

Health care professionals should assess patients for thoughts of suicide and dissatisfaction about his/her circumstances, which can lead to a desire for assisted death. Clinicians need to intensify symptom relief or make referrals when necessary. Above all, clinicians should check for legality of assisted death in their state, if so they understand and meet all requirements of practice. Congress has not authorized the use of federal funds (Medicare, Veterans Administration) to pay for drugs used for PAD, however some state Medicaid programs reimburse the cost of these drugs.

PRIMARY PALLIATIVE CARE
Managing Spiritual Distress

The spiritual and religious dimensions of a person are relevant in their care and important for clinical providers to acknowledge and incorporate into routine clinical practice, especially in care of persons' with a serious illness or during the end of life.[18,19] Spirituality and religion are often used interchangeably; these concepts are separate and distinct, but not mutually exclusive. Spirituality has no commonly accepted definition; it is an evolving, dynamic multidimensional concept intermingled into all dimensions of the whole person (body-mind-spirit). Spirituality broadly encompasses a person's search for the sacred or significant meaning in life, purpose, and a connection or relationship with a higher being, the sacred, self, nature, or others.[20,21] Religion is an organized system of beliefs, practices, and behaviors grounded in the doctrine of a religious denomination.[21,22]

A person's spirituality and or religion can inform medical decision-making while having a positive influence on coping with illness, well-being, optimism, self-care, resiliency, life satisfaction, and health.[23] Negative religious/spiritual coping is associated with low quality of life, poorer mental well-being, higher levels of depression, anger, anxiety, and distress.[23,24] It is important for providers to be aware when providing care, especially symptom management for a serious illness or at the end of life, that religious beliefs or customs can influence the types and level of aggressiveness of interventions or medications permitted, resulting in under or overtreatment.[25,26] Providers can experience personal discomfort and fear of addressing spiritual matters. They may feel unprepared by their education or training to meet the needs of a patient, leading to moral distress, uncertainty, and apprehension about treatment options.[27]

Patients and caregivers that are well supported by a religious community, have a high positive religious coping, or belong to certain racial/ethnic minority groups and are more likely to receive aggressive end-of-life interventions, die in the intensive care unit, and have lower hospice enrollments.[28,29] Many of these patients opt for aggressive interventions in hopes of medically prolonging life until God heals them through a miracle. This core religious belief is common to multiple religions and provides a sense of comfort and hope to people. Understanding these religious/spiritual beliefs, exploring religious interpretations of meaning and hope, and avoiding the natural urge to convince a change of mind, can help mitigate the experience of loss and suffering.[29–31] When discussing end-of-life care it is important to acknowledge the patient's or caregiver's hope for a miracle, but also express your worries or concerns about the clinical situation. Acknowledging their beliefs first can demonstrate empathy and spiritual support without taking away hope.[32] Patients and families that endorse religion or spirituality as important to them strongly desire to discuss these beliefs with their primary health care providers when framing their health care, especially surrounding end-of-life or serious illness discussions, but this rarely occurs.[27,33,34] When health care providers give attention to spiritual concerns during these discussions, patients and families report more satisfaction with care and goal concordant care, improved quality of care, appropriate levels of hope, increased referrals to hospice, and decreased anxiety and stress with decision-making.[21,33,35] Involvement of a chaplain or the palliative care team during challenging and complex spiritual conversations can be helpful, but with a shortage of both of these in some settings or communities, it is important that all health care professionals have some basic skills to explore religious and spiritual concerns in the clinical setting.[33]

Existential Distress

Individuals that do not identify as spiritual or religious do have an "existential" domain that is part of their personhood, their wholeness. The term existential, like spiritually, does not have a consistent definition. It is a dynamic, abstract, and multidimensional concept.[36,37] The term is frequently associated with spirituality, but is not the same; spirituality is a subcomponent of the existential. Existential relates to one's sense of connectedness with self and others, wholeness, self-identity, purpose in life, and autonomy.[36–38] A threat to life or an injury to the integrity of the existential self, results in distress or existential suffering manifested as grief, a loss of meaning or purpose, a sense of helplessness and hopelessness, isolation, sadness, desire to hasten death, anxiety, inadequacy, and depression.[36,39,40]

Under the strain of a serious or life-limiting illness, patients can develop significant spiritual or existential distress, especially at the end of life.[38,41,42] This distress is expressed in questions such as "Why me?" "What did I do to deserve this?" or "Why would God let this happen to me? I've been faithful all my life!" Actively listening for these distress "cues," not trying to "fix" the situation, and acknowledging to one's self and the person asking them that such questions have no answers is imperative. They reflect a search for meaning in the experience, an effort to align their beliefs with the experience and to make sense of the incomprehensible.[37,43] Patients may begin to question their sense of connectedness to a higher power or to relationships that they consider important. The challenge is to act as an intuitive, compassionate listener who remains present with the patient. The healing begins in the telling of the story.[31,42]

If a sense of hopelessness emerges in the patient, it is incumbent on the health care provider to determine meaningful, empowering interventions. Attempting to ease spiritual distress and suffering, as one would a physical symptom, is a moral and ethical imperative of health care providers and is a required domain of palliative care.[42] Investigating spiritual or religious beliefs in the clinical setting falls into three broad categories: spiritual screening, spiritual history-taking, and spiritual assessment. Balboni et al.[44] describe many spiritual well-being screening and assessment tools that can be used in the clinical setting. Being mindfully present and in the moment with the patient or family and not avoiding or running from the uncomfortableness of their spiritual/existential distress communicates empathy and validates their feelings. Health care providers should avoid the pitfalls of trying to "fix" the distress or focusing exclusively on the physical symptoms by escalating anxiolytics or other medications.[43] Identifying prior coping strategies, and family, social and community support available to the patient and family is important. These connections with others provide a basis for new hope.[44] Patients who have relied more on cognitive coping strategies often find information or anticipatory guidance useful in alleviating anxiety and providing a new source of hope. Patients and families may wish to know what to expect as they approach the end of life and to have their decisions and beliefs regarding end-of-life experiences validated. As body, mind, and spirit are interwoven together, formal interventions such as meaning-centered psychotherapy, meaning-making intervention, chaplaincy care, palliative care, life review interventions, acupuncture, therapeutic touch, biofeedback, music, massage, etc., address the connection between these areas of personhood.[44,45] The provision of spiritual and existential support of patients and family by health care providers centers around the provider's mindful presence during conversations and open, honest, and supportive communication.[43] Strategies for intervention that intentionally include spiritual and existential care encourage the patient's search for meaning in life, decrease distress, improve quality of life and coping, and decrease suffering.[36,40,45]

REFERENCES

1. Ferrell, B. R., Temel, J. S., Temin, S., et al. (2016). Integration of palliative care into standard oncology care: American Society of Clinical Oncology clinical practice guideline update. *Journal of Clinical Oncology, 0*(0), JCO.2016.2070.1474.
2. Kavalieratos, D., Corbelli, J., Zhang, D., et al. (2016). Association between palliative care and patient and caregiver outcomes: A systematic review and meta-analysis. *JAMA: The Journal of the American Medical Association, 316*(20), 2104–2114.
3. National Consensus Project. (2018). Clinical Practice Guidelines for Quality Palliative Care; Fourth Edition. Brooklyn, NY: National Consensus Project for Quality Palliative Care.
4. Meier, D. E., Back, A. L., Berman, A., Block, S. D., Corrigan, J. M., & Morrison, R. S. (2017). A national strategy for palliative care. *Health Affairs (Project Hope), 36*(7), 1265–1273.
5. Bakitas, M. A., Clifford, K., Dionne-Odom, J. N., & Kvale, E. (2015). Rural palliative care. In B. R. Ferrell & N. Coyle (Eds.), *Oxford textbook of palliative nursing* (4th ed., pp. 812–822). Oxford: Oxford University Press.
6. Center to Advance Palliative Care. (2011). 2011 Public Opinion Research on Palliative Care: A Report Based on Research by Public Opinion Strategies. New York: Center to Advance Palliative Care and American Cancer Society Action Network.
7. Quill, T. E., & Abernethy, A. P. (2013). Generalist plus specialist palliative care—creating a more sustainable model. *The New England Journal of Medicine, 368*(13), 1173–1175.
8. Romo, R. D., & Lynn, J. (2017). The utility and value of the "surprise question" for patients with serious illness. *Canadian Medical Association Journal, 189*(33), E1072–E1073.
9. Baile, W. F., Buckman, R., Lenzi, R., Glober, G., Beale, E. A., & Kudelka, A. P. (2000). SPIKES—A six-step protocol for delivering bad news: Application to the patient with cancer. *The Oncologist, 5*(4), 302–311.
10. McEwan, A., & Silverberg, J. Z. (2016). Palliative Care in the Emergency Department. *Emergency Medicine Clinics of North America, 34*(3), 667–685.
11. Hollyday, S. L., & Buonocore, D. (2015). Breaking bad news and discussing goals of care in the Intensive Care Unit. *AACN Advanced Critical Care, 26*(2), 131–141.
12. Hauser, J. (2017). Communication in heart failure and palliative care. *Heart Failure Reviews, 22*(5), 535–542.
13. van Vliet, L. M., Lindenberger, E., & van Weert, J. C. (2015). Communication with older, seriously ill patients. *Clinics in Geriatric Medicine, 31*(2), 219–230.
14. Institute of Medicine. (2014). *Dying in America: Improving quality and honoring individual preferences near the end of life.* Washington, DC: The National Academies Press.
15. Aghabarary, M., & Dehghan Nayeri, N. (2016). Medical futility and its challenges: A review study. *Journal of Medical Ethics and History of Medicine, 9*, 11.
16. Blinderman, C. D., & Billings, J. A. (2015). Comfort care for patients dying in the hospital. *The New England Journal of Medicine, 373*(26), 2549–2561.
17. Snyder Sulmasy, L., & Mueller, P. S., for the E, Professionalism, Human Rights Committee of the American College of P. (2017). Ethics and the legalization of physician-assisted suicide: An American College of Physicians position paper. *Annals of Internal Medicine, 167*(8), 576–578.
18. Osório, I. H. S., Gonçalves, L. M., Pozzobon, P. M., et al. (2017). Effect of an educational intervention in "spirituality and health" on knowledge, attitudes, and skills of students in health-related areas: A controlled randomized trial. *Medical Teacher, 39*(10), 1057–1064.
19. Lucchetti, G., & Lucchetti, A. L. G. (2014). Spirituality, religion, and health: Over the last 15 years of field research (1999–2013). *International Journal of Psychiatry in Medicine, 48*(3), 199–215.
20. Mishra, S., Togneri, E., Tripathi, B. & Trikamji, B. (2017). Spirituality and religiosity and its role in health and diseases. *Journal of Religion and Health, 56*(4), 1282–1301.
21. Steinhauser, K. E., Fitchett, G., Handzo, G. F., et al. (2017). State of the science of spirituality and palliative care research part I: Definitions, measurement, and outcomes. *Journal of Pain and Symptom Management, 54*(3), 428–440.
22. Delgado-Guay, M. O. (2014). Spirituality and religiosity in supportive and palliative care. *Current Opinion in Supportive and Palliative Care, 8*(3), 308–313.
23. Ng, G. C., Mohamed, S., Sulaiman, A. H., & Zainal, N. Z. (2017). Anxiety and depression in cancer patients: The association with religiosity and religious coping. *Journal of Religion and Health, 56*(2), 575–590.
24. Smith-Macdonald, L., Norris, J. M., Raffin-Bouchal, S., & Sinclair, S. (2017). Spirituality and mental well-being in combat veterans: A systematic review. *Military Medicine, 182*(11), e1920–e1940.
25. Chakraborty, R., El-Jawahri, A. R., Litzow, M. R., Syrjala, K. L., Parnes, A. D., & Hashmi, S. K. (2017). A systematic review of religious beliefs about major end-of-life issues in the five major world religions. *Palliative & Supportive Care, 15*(5), 609–622.
26. Mitchell, D. (2015). Spiritual and cultural issues at the end of life. *Medicine (United Kingdom), 43*(12), 740–741.
27. Best, M., Butow, P., & Olver, I. (2016). Doctors discussing religion and spirituality: A systematic literature review. *Palliative Medicine, 30*(4), 327–337.
28. LoPresti, M. A., Dement, F., & Gold, H. T. (2016). End-of-life care for people with cancer from ethnic minority groups. *The American Journal of Hospice & Palliative Care, 33*(3), 291–305.

29. Balboni, T. A., Balboni, M., Enzinger, A. C., et al. (2013). Provision of spiritual support to patients with advanced cancer by religious communities and associations with medical care at the end of life. *JAMA Internal Medicine,* *173*(12), 1109–1117.

30. Blackler, L. (2017). Hope for a Miracle. *Journal of hospice and palliative nursing: JHPN: the official journal of the Hospice and Palliative Nurses Association, 19*(2), 115–121.

31. Ellington, L., Billitteri, J., Reblin, M., & Clayton, M. F. (2017). Spiritual care communication in cancer patients. *Seminars in Oncology Nursing, 33*(5), 517–525.

32. Llewellyn, H., Jones, L., Kelly, P., et al. (2015). Experiences of healthcare professionals in the community dealing with the spiritual needs of children and young people with life-threatening and life-limiting conditions and their families: Report of a workshop. *BMJ Supportive Palliative Care, 5*(3), 232–239.

33. Ernecoff, N. C., Curlin, F. A., Buddadhumaruk, P., & White, D. B. (2015). Health care professionals' responses to religious or spiritual statements by surrogate decision makers during goals-of-care discussions. *JAMA Internal Medicine, 175*(10), 1662–1669.

34. Best, M., Butow, P., & Olver, I. (2015). Do patients want doctors to talk about spirituality? A systematic literature review. *Patient Education and Counseling, 98*(11), 1320–1328.

35. Partain, D. K., Ingram, C., & Strand, J. J. (2017). Providing appropriate end-of-life care to religious and ethnic minorities. *Mayo Clinic Proceedings. Mayo Clinic, 92*(1), 147–152.

36. Bates, A. T. (2016). Addressing existential suffering. *British Columbia Medical Journal, 58*(5), 268–273.

37. Grech, A., & Marks, A. (2017). Existential suffering part 1: Definition and diagnosis #319. *Journal of Palliative Medicine, 20*(1), 93–94.

38. Alesi, E. R., Ford, T. R., Chen, C. J., et al. (2015). Development of the CASH assessment tool to address existential concerns in patients with serious illness. *Journal of Palliative Medicine, 18*(1), 71–75.

39. Moonen, C., Lemiengre, J., & Gastmans, C. (2016). Dealing with existential suffering of patients with severe persistent mental illness: Experiences of psychiatric nurses in Flanders (Belgium). *Archives of Psychiatric Nursing, 30*(2), 219–225.

40. Bueno-Gómez, N. (2017). Conceptualizing suffering and pain. *Philosophy, Ethics, and Humanities in Medicine, 12*(1).

41. Velosa, T., Caldeira, S., & Capelas, M. L. (2017). Depression and spiritual distress in adult palliative patients: A cross-sectional study. *Religions, 8*(8).

42. Gillilan, R., Qawi, S., Weymiller, A., Puchalski, C., & Weymiller, A. J. (2017). Spiritual distress and spiritual care in advanced heart failure. *Heart Failure Reviews, 22*(5), 581–591.

43. Grech, A., & Marks, A. (2017). Existential suffering part 2: Clinical response and management #320. *Journal of Palliative Medicine, 20*(1), 95–96.

44. Balboni, T. A., Fitchett, G., Handzo, G. F., et al. (2017). State of the science of spirituality and palliative care research part II: Screening, assessment, and interventions. *Journal of Pain and Symptom Management, 54*(3), 441–453.

45. Guerrero-Torrelles, M., Monforte-Royo, C., Rodríguez-Prat, A., Porta-Sales, J., & Balaguer, A. (2017). Understanding meaning in life interventions in patients with advanced disease: A systematic review and realist synthesis. *Palliative Medicine, 31*(9), 798–813.

CHAPTER **15**

ACUTE, CHRONIC, ONCOLOGIC, AND END-OF-LIFE PAIN MANAGEMENT IN PRIMARY CARE

Jennifer L. Culgin • Catherine Marie Duffy • Leslie Lezell Levitan

Primary Care Providers play an important role in managing their patients' pain. Providers are also responsible for using best practice when prescribing potentially addictive medications, monitoring pain medication usage, and identifying inappropriate substance use. In this chapter, the key components of pain, including the pathology, types of pain,

and treatment options will be discussed; the goal always for pain and symptom management is improving the patient's quality of life. Special attention will be given to the differences between acute, chronic, oncologic, and end-of-life pain so that health care providers can manage each of these conditions appropriately.

PAIN

DEFINITION AND EPIDEMIOLOGY OF PAIN

Pain is an unpleasant sensation unique to each individual. The International Association for the Study of Pain (IASP) defines pain as "an unpleasant sensory and emotional experience associated with actual or potential tissue damage, or described in terms of such damage."[1-3] Margo McCaffrey developed the classic definition of pain as "whatever the experiencing person says it is, existing whenever the experiencing person says it does."[4] Pain is a normal physiologic response that is protective in nature, warning of actual or potential tissue damage in response to a chemical, thermal, or mechanical stimulus.[5]

Most people experience some form of pain on a daily basis, from a stubbed toe to a paper cut to pulled hair. The type of pain that would be considered minor is usually seen as "just part of life," and there is an innate assumption that the minor pains will improve or resolve fairly quickly. When moderate to severe pain is noted on a daily basis, with or without an obvious cause, most people will want some form of intervention leading to pain reduction or resolution, prompting a visit for urgent or emergent care.[4] Pain can lead to serious compromises in health, loss of independence, loss of mobility, and can decrease one's quality of life.[6]

Despite this common problem, there are still many barriers that providers face in their efforts to effectively manage pain. Some of these include inadequate attention given to pain mechanisms and treatment modalities in most medical, nursing, and pharmacy program curricula; reluctance to prescribe opioids based on the prescriber's fear of addiction, abuse, diversion, and misuse; poor pain assessment, including discrepancies between perception of pain culturally and within one's gender; and patient adherence issues with a treatment regimen.[7] Impediments also include monitoring and regulatory controls, as well as the challenge of insurance payment for expensive medications, requiring timely prior authorization paperwork or phone calls by the provider.

PATHOPHYSIOLOGY OF PAIN

Pain is categorized as either organic or idiopathic. Organic pain is further delineated as nociceptive (somatic or visceral) or neuropathic. Nociceptive pain is the most common type of pain, and is a normal function of the central nervous system (CNS). Nociceptors are receptors that respond to noxious stimuli and transmit a message through the peripheral nerves to the spinal cord and then up to the cerebral cortex where the message can be interpreted. Some motor responses (e.g., withdrawal of an extremity from intense heat) are initiated from the spinal cord, whereas others are initiated by higher brain centers.[8] Nociceptive pain is further differentiated as **somatic** (i.e., pain from soft tissue and musculoskeletal structures) or **visceral** (i.e., pain arising from the internal organs). Somatic pain is often described as dull, sharp, aching, crushing, or heavy, although other adjectives might be used. In contrast, visceral pain is usually poorly localized and often is not attributable to the involved organ (i.e., referred pain). It may be described as dull, crampy, or deep. Visceral nociceptive pain can be referred to other areas in a dermatomal distribution because often the autonomic fibers innervate the organs or hollow viscera found in the dermatome.[9-11]

Neuropathic pain occurs as a result of injury or disease, causing damage to the peripheral nerves, spinal cord, nervous system, or brain tissue. Nerves can be injured or damaged by direct trauma (laceration, compression, stretching, crushing, burning, freezing, or exposure to toxic agents such as chemotherapeutic drugs or viruses), repetitive movements (typing), or diseases (e.g., polio, diabetes, multiple sclerosis). The result of the injury is a cascade of events that creates both anatomic and neurochemical changes in the neurons. Once the damage has occurred, the regeneration process of the nerve may result in incomplete healing, which can lead to chronic pain or reduced function.[8] Common examples of neuropathic pain syndromes that result in chronic pain include postherpetic neuralgia, phantom pain, postthoracotomy pain, intercostal neuralgia, and peripheral neuropathy. Because it follows the distribution of peripheral nerves in a dermatomal pattern, neuropathic pain is most often described as burning, numbness, tingling, shocking, electric, and jolting and may have a delayed onset from the time of the injury. For example, postherpetic neuralgia can occur and persist months to years after the skin lesions of a herpes zoster virus (HZV) have healed. In that time, the perception of normally mild and nonpainful stimuli (e.g., touch or wearing clothing) can change to an exquisitely sensitive or painful sensation (allodynia or hyperestesia). In moderate to severe cases, neuropathic pain may be accompanied by regional sympathetic dysfunction, whereby an injured nerve may develop an electrical or a chemical interaction with sympathetic nerve fibers, providing continuous painful stimuli to peripheral nerves.[8,10,12,13] Central neuropathic pain, however, is caused by damage of the nerves in the CNS.[11]

Idiopathic pain may not demonstrate any clinical evidence of an associated organic cause, but might include additional psychological elements at the time of presentation. Nonetheless, as previously stated, the experience of pain is purely subjective. Subsequently, the reality of a patient's idiopathic pain is comparable to that of organic pain, and therefore it must be treated.

CLINICAL PRESENTATION OF PAIN

Since pain is subjective, a patient's report is the most reliable means of establishing the degree or intensity of the pain. The most convenient method, and one that most patients can use, is the Numeric Rating Scale (NRS) for pain. The patient rates his or her pain from 0 to 10, where 0 indicates no pain and 10 indicates the worst pain imaginable. Other scales can be used, such as the Visual Analog Scale (VAS), the McGill Pain Questionnaire (MPQ), and the Wong-Baker FACES Scale. The Wong-Baker FACES Scale is used frequently and uses a series of faces depicting comfort level, which can be useful for children (3 years of age and older) and for patients with communication difficulties (e.g., a language barrier or a problem with speech), as they can simply point to the face that matches how they feel.[4] As there are multiple scales available for use, it is important for providers to use one scale consistently with the patient so that a sense of change in status or an impact of your interventions over time can be determined.

While performing the pain assessment, it is important to review other symptoms that may have an impact on a patient's pain level and treatment plan. Tools used to assess multiple symptoms include the Edmonton Symptom Assessment System (ESAS) and the MD Anderson Symptom Inventory (MDASI).[14,15]

To interpret the ratings from the various scales, providers must remember that these are subjective measures and therefore there are no "normal" values. In general, ratings of 1 to 3 are considered to be mild pain; 4 to 6, moderate; and 7 or greater, severe.[4] A very useful assessment tool is to ask the patient what pain level can be tolerated, as this will help the provider establish the treatment goal. One could expect to see a decrease in reported pain scores when patients are given an effective means for pain reduction.[3] As there is considerable individual variation in the way patients use these scales, comparison among patients should be avoided except for aggregate analysis for research and quality assurance purposes.

Objective findings also exist when determining a patient's level of pain. A nonverbal pain assessment is essential for those who are unable to effectively communicate, may be sedated, or comatose. Some objective findings include facial grimacing (especially with movement), diaphoresis, shaking, restlessness, crying, moaning, fidgeting, hypertension, tachycardia, and tachypnea. Body language can also be helpful with a nonverbal pain assessment. Additional signs of pain can include clenched fists, hitting, biting, kicking, guarding a sore area, and laying with the knees pulled to the chest.[16]

PHYSICAL EXAMINATION FOR PAIN

Pain is frequently undermanaged because of poor clinical assessment by clinicians, and under reporting by patients. It is critical that pain assessment be integrated into a detailed history and physical exam, with reassessment at each visit. An initial comprehensive clinical pain history should include past relevant health issues, psychiatric history, psychosocial factors, addiction risk, social and occupational functional assessment, goals of treatment, and pain beliefs. Previous treatments and outcomes, both traditional and alternative therapies, should be explored. A thorough review of current medications, including over-the-counter and complementary medications, should be included.[17]

Pain assessment can be aided by the mnemonic PQRST.[18] P stands for provocative-palliative factors, such as specific movement, temperature, or activities that improve or worsen the pain. Q stands for quality and is a description of the pain, such as sharp, dull, aching, burning, stabbing, or shooting. R stands for the region or site of pain. S stands for severity, measured by rating the pain over time. To quantify their pain, patients are often asked to use a scale of 1 to 10, a scale of calm to distressed faces, or a scale of description of no pain to worst imaginable pain. No one scale applies to all patients; rather, the important issue is to choose one scale that is appropriate for a patient and use it consistently. T is for temporal or the timing of the pain during day or night, in which the pain is more constant or the duration is longer. Box 15.1 offers sample questions for assessment.

PHARMACOLOGIC MANAGEMENT OF PAIN

Pain management can be challenging and should always be multifactorial with use of both nonopioid and opioid medications

Questions for Assessment of Distress

What is your day like?
How does your pain interfere with your life?
What are your expectations of pain relief?
What are your past experiences of pain?
How did you cope with pain in the past?
How is this pain different?
What is the meaning of pain?
How are you coping with this pain?
How has your life changed?
Does culture or religion have any influence over expression of pain or pain management?

INITIAL DIAGNOSTICS

Oncology Pain

ESSENTIAL DIAGNOSTICS FOR ONCOLOGY PAIN
Imaging
- Radiography[a]
- Computed tomography[a]
- Magnetic resonance imaging[a]
- Bone scan[a]
- Electromyography[a]

Blood Tests (Complete Blood Count With Differential)

———
[a]If clinically indicated.

as appropriate. There are numerous drugs commonly used to manage the symptoms of pain. These include nonsteroidal antiinflammatories, steroids, muscle relaxants, and opioid and nonopioid pain medications. The World Health Organization (WHO) developed a three-step analgesic ladder to help guide clinicians in choosing and prescribing pain medications (https://www.who.int/cancer/palliative/painladder/en/). This ladder was originally developed to treat cancer pain, however it is now commonly used by providers to help guide pain relief stemming from many other causes. Step 1 begins with the use of nonopioids and adjuvant medications. These include nonsteroidal antiinflammatory drugs (NSAIDs), tricyclic antidepressants (TCAs), selective serotonin reuptake inhibitors (SSRIs), and adjuvants such as anticonvulsants. Step 2 of the three-step analgesic ladder includes mixed opiate products including codeine, acetaminophen and codeine phosphate, and tramadol. These medications can be used alone or in combination with step 1 to treat mild to moderate pain. Step 3 medications are recommended when step 1 and step 2 drugs are not effective in relieving pain or when the pain is moderate to severe in intensity. Step 3 medications include pure opioid compounds such as morphine, fentanyl, oxycodone, methadone, and hydromorphone. Ongoing concerns about opioid abuse and addiction have led to underdosing and underprescribing of opioids.[18,19] However, the risk of not properly managing pain appropriately is that this can result in chronic pain, its associated complexities, and increased morbidity and mortality.

Opioid Medications

In light of the national crisis of opioid addiction and overdoses, it is imperative that best practices are followed not only when prescribing and dosing opioids, but also in management, abuse and addiction. This section focuses on proper opioid use and management. Opioids are classified as pure agonists, mixed agonist-antagonists, or partial agonists. The pure agonists can be relied on to produce effective analgesia and can be titrated to pain relief without having a ceiling effect.

The mixed agonist-antagonist opioids produce analgesia but can also reverse analgesia. These drugs are also associated with a high incidence of psychotomimetic side effects. When agonist-antagonists are given to a patient who has been taking a pure agonist opioid, the agonist-antagonist acts as an antagonist by displacing the agonist from the opiate receptors, which precipitates withdrawal and reverses analgesia.[20]

Unfortunately, pure agonist opioids remain misunderstood by many health care providers. To use these opioids effectively, it is important to distinguish between key terms that are often misapplied in practice: addiction, dependence, and tolerance. The phenomenon known as pseudoaddiction must also be recognized so patients can be properly educated about their treatment. Pseudoaddiction is a real and complex phenomenon in which patients may exhibit drug seeking behaviors and appear aggressive when requesting to increase pain medications when, in fact, they are inadequately treated for their actual pain. These patients may be labeled as "difficult," "drug seeking," and "clock watchers." Although these actions may serve as warning signs to alert the practitioner to abuse, the adequacy of treatment must also be assessed before a judgment can be made.

The key principle for effective pain control with opioids is to titrate the dose to achieve the desired pain reduction without side effects.[21,22] Considerable variability in dosage exists between patients. Tolerance will be seen with chronic dosing of any opioid, however this does not happen at the same rate for each patient.[20] While some opioids (e.g., morphine and hydromorphone) are classified as strong, and others (e.g., codeine and hydrocodone) are classified as weak, these opioids are all actually capable of producing equally effective analgesia when given in equianalgesic doses. Some weak opioids are combined with an NSAID or acetaminophen to enhance pain reduction. Dosing with these combined medications is limited by the potential for renal and hepatic problems related to the nonopioid drug.

There are numerous preparations widely available allowing for different routes of administration for opioid medications. These include oral, sublingual, buccal, intravenous, subcutaneous, transdermal, rectal, and intraspinal (epidural and intrathecal).[23] The oral route of administration is the route of choice in most situations because of ease, comfort, and cost-effectiveness. The choice of route and drug depends on a variety of patient factors, including the nature and stability of the pain, the functional status of the gastrointestinal (GI) tract, the abilities of the patient and caregiver to manage the regimen (e.g., cognitive function, psychomotor skills), the side effects, the dosage forms and availability, and the cost. More invasive routes of administration, such as parenteral and intraspinal, increase the risk for complications (e.g., infection and displacement of the needle), are usually more costly, and should be reserved for carefully selected patients. The subcutaneous, transdermal, and rectal routes can also deliver excellent pain control in patients who cannot tolerate oral medications but who want to be managed at home.

Short-acting opioids are clinically indicated to treat postoperative pain and for moderate isolated painful incidents. Short-acting opioids can also be helpful as a preventative approach to pain control with breakthrough pain associated with activity, treatments, or other obvious factors. When an event or activity (e.g., ambulation) is known to provoke pain, the as-needed (PRN) dose should be taken about 30 to 45 minutes prior to that activity whenever possible. For moderate to severe pain that is poorly managed, however, long-acting opioids should be administered around-the-clock based on their expected duration of action. PRN opioid dosing with these patients can lead to greater peaks and valleys in analgesic blood levels between doses, especially if patients wait until the pain is severe before taking the medication. The short-acting opioid dose should be between 10% and 15% of the total daily dose of the long-acting opioid.[21] If two or three breakthrough doses are required routinely, the case can be made for the long-acting medication to be titrated upward.

Short-term or long-term use of parenteral or subcutaneous administration of opioids may also be necessary for some patients. Use of patient-controlled analgesia pumps can be ideal for patients looking at end-of-life comfort care, as these pumps give continuously programmed drug delivery. Pumps can also be very helpful for patients in an acute pain crisis, with the goal being to ultimately wean off the pump and restart oral medications once the pain is more manageable. The on-demand patient-administered dose, used as needed with or without a continuous (basal) infusion, allows for individualized dosing and sustained analgesia. If the patient shows evidence early on of delirium, somatization, or chemical coping, the on-demand patient-administered dose should be avoided because of the possibility of opioid-induced neurotoxicity.[24]

Morphine is often used in varied equivalent dose tables for comparison to other opioids because it is the most widely used opioid and there is extensive existing research about its pharmacokinetics. The route of administration must be considered when calculating equianalgesic doses. For example, opioids administered through the GI tract are subject to a first-pass effect, whereby a portion of the drug is metabolized to nonanalgesic substances as it is routed through the hepatic circulation before being circulated systemically. If a patient is receiving adequate analgesia from 10 mg of morphine sulfate given parenterally, it takes 30 mg to achieve the same effect if it is given orally because approximately 20 mg is metabolized before reaching the systemic circulation. The parenteral-to-oral ratio also varies from drug to drug. In addition, the longer a patient is taking an opioid, the less accurate these relationships can be due to cross-tolerance with similar substances. It must be noted that the relationship between different opioids is not absolute; it is always important to use the same equianalgesic table as other health care providers in your organization to assure consistent dosing. With opioid rotation it is always important to err on the side of caution, as the risk of overdose does not outweigh risk of transient discomfort.

Side Effects of Opioid Medications

Vigilant oversight is critical to the successful treatment of patients with pain. Side effects are among the most common reasons cited for opioid failure and premature abandonment of therapy. A patient who experiences nausea, sedation, or clouded thinking may be improperly labeled as being allergic to opioids. A true allergy to opioid medications is actually rare. Some side effects, particularly nausea and sedation, are usually transient and improve once tolerance develops. Respiratory depression can also happen from opioids, however there is usually a rapid onset with this and often after a few days of drug exposure, this reduces. Most patients develop a tolerance to the emetic and sedating effects over several days. One cause of sedation seen with taking opioids is actually due to sleep deprivation, which one can rationalize is to be expected in patients who have experienced long periods of unrelieved pain. Sedation usually abates within 72 hours on a stable dose of opioids, and once sleep is restored. Pain also contributes to weight loss and cachexia, as patients who are uncomfortable often have a decreased appetite.

Nausea and vomiting from opioids can be managed with antiemetics on a scheduled basis initially and then as needed once the opioid dose is stabilized. Nausea is often directly related to decreased bowel function, which may resolve once constipation is alleviated. Unfortunately, patients do not develop a tolerance to the constipating effects of opioids, so most patients will need an aggressive bowel management program.[25] Opiate drugs bind to receptors on the smooth muscle of the bowel, slowing intestinal motility and increasing fluid absorption. A patient who has not had a bowel movement in more than 3 to 5 days should be monitored for proper hydration and given a diet with foods rich in fiber. However, when patients are prescribed opioids for chronic use, they will likely need to routinely use stool softeners and laxatives just to maintain a normal bowel regimen. If this does not work, more aggressive therapies, such as polyethylene glycol (MiraLax), lactulose, bisacodyl (Dulcolax) suppositories, prepared enemas, or magnesium citrate can be used. Caution should be used with polyethylene glycol since constipation may worsen if not enough water is consumed with it. In a refractory situation, laxatives and enemas may need to be repeated every 12 hours. Once proper bowel function has been restored, a prophylactic regimen should be initiated with a combination of a senna laxative and stool softener.[25] The bowel regimen is similar to the pain regimen with standard around-the-clock medications (laxative with stool softener) and a more aggressive preparation (suppository or enema) for breakthrough if no bowel movement occurs within 3 days. If, at any time, there is concern that an ileus or malignant bowel obstruction is present, the patient needs to be medically evaluated, including appropriate diagnostic tests (e.g., X-ray, computed tomography [CT]).

All opioids have the potential to cause delirium. Patients who have rapid escalation of opioids develop renal or hepatic failure, or have other pathophysiologic causes of delirium are at higher risk. Identification of the cause of the delirium and then reversal of it, if possible, is the appropriate treatment. If opioids are suspected to be the cause, an opioid rotation is required. Refer to the delirium section of this textbook for further discussion of delirium.

Less common opioid side effects include urinary retention and myoclonus (the intermittent muscle jerking that occurs especially during sleep). Urinary retention is often transient and can be temporarily relieved with straight catheterization or rotation to another opioid. Myoclonus is usually seen at higher opioid doses and with long-term opioid use. It is important to monitor for myoclonus because it can lead to seizures if untreated. If myoclonus persists, the opioid should be decreased or changed. Other complications to be aware of in pain management are an increased risk for GI bleeding with the prolonged use of NSAIDs, and hepatotoxicity with high doses of acetaminophen. Always be aware of how many milligrams of these medications patients are taking daily, whether alone or combined with prescribed opioids.

NONPHARMACOLOGIC PAIN MANAGEMENT

Nonpharmacologic interventions for pain should be used in addition to, not instead of, pharmacologic management, both physical and psychological methods. Some physical interventions include chiropractic techniques, thermal modalities (e.g., heat or cold application), physical therapy, massage, elevation, and rest. Psychological interventions include education, meditation, biofeedback, psychotherapy, and coping skills training. Traditional and complementary therapies (e.g., nutritional and herbal supplements, spiritual healing, acupuncture, Reiki) can also be effective as well.[19,26] It is important to ask patients about use of supplements as there may be potential interactions with prescription medications.

PRESCRIBING GUIDELINES FOR PAIN

Management of patients with pain is complex and may require a combination of both nonpharmacologic and pharmacologic modalities, and often an interdisciplinary approach. If pain is inadequately managed with nonpharmacologic options, the addition of pharmacologic interventions may be beneficial. If appropriate, nonpharmacologic options should be tried initially, but require patient participation and motivation. Examples of nonpharmacologic options are discussed previously in this chapter.

When pharmacologic options are needed, primary care providers should refer to the WHOs ladder for guidance on prescriptive practices. A general first rule is to begin with nonopioid medications such as acetaminophen, NSAIDS and aspirin. These medications can be used alone or in addition to adjuvant pain medications such as anticonvulsants and antidepressants as discussed previously in this chapter. When nonopioid options are inadequate, the introduction of opioid medications may be necessary. Opioids vary in potency and a general rule of thumb when treating pain unrelieved with nonpharmacologic or nonopioid options is to begin with what is considered a weaker opioid. If these prove ineffective or the patient's pain is considered severe in nature, stronger opioids may be needed.[27] As with nonopioid options, opioid medications can be used with or without adjuvant medications in an effort to best control the patient's pain.

Prescribing Opioids

When considering opioids to treat a patient's pain, it is important to weigh the risks and benefits of initiating opioid therapy. While short-term opioid therapy for acute pain is well supported, there is limited benefit for opioid use when treating chronic noncancer pain. Of course, each patient's situation is different, and each patient should receive individualized therapy. When initiating use of opioids, a risk assessment should always be performed to evaluate for risk of overdose, opioid misuse, or opioid use disorder. Patient education should be provided, and close follow-up planned.[28] When prescribing opioids for acute pain, the lowest effective dose should be used, and a general timeline of 3 days or less is usually sufficient. Opioid use for more than 1 week is rarely needed.

TABLE 15.1	Side Effects and Adverse Effects of Opioid Therapy
Misuse	Androgen deficiency
Substance use disorder	Cardiovascular events
Overdose	Hyperalgesia
Sedation	Tolerance
Withdrawal	Depression, anxiety
Constipation	Pruritis
Nausea, vomiting	Liver toxicity
Urinary retention	Preterm delivery
Congenital defects	Neonatal abstinence syndrome

Always start with immediate-release opioids before initiating extended-release medications.[29]

Fear of overdose is always a concern for primary care providers, patients and families. Some patients with comorbidities (sleep apnea, lung disease, heart disease), those with prescriptions for sedative-hypnotics, and those with problematic alcohol use or psychiatric comorbidities are at higher risk. Opioid misuse is nontherapeutic use, such as taking more than prescribed or by an alternate route. Opioid use disorder is a diagnosis defined by out of control use, compulsive use, and continued use despite adverse consequences. To screen for misuse and use disorder one should look at requests for early refills, prescriber "shopping," urine toxicology screens, and checking the state prescription monitoring program. Use a formal screening tool such as Opioid Risk Tool, Screener Opioid Assessment for Patients with Pain, and others.[28,30] If a patient appears to have developed misuse or use disorder, do not hesitate to refer to a substance use specialist. See Chapter 227, Substance Use Disorders, for more information. Patient education should be provided prior to initiating therapy and in a way that the patient can understand. Side effects and adverse effects should be reviewed. See Table 15.1 for more details on side effects and adverse effects.[28,30]

For patients who are on continuing opioid therapy, a follow-up appointment should occur at least every 3 months to evaluate efficacy and ongoing risk assessment. In addition, a controlled substance agreement should be signed between the patient and provider with clearly delineated guidelines and expectations. There are many opioid contracts available online including with American Academy of Family Physicians/Family Practice Management or Kaiser Permanente.[28,30] The Centers for Disease Control and Prevention (CDC) developed comprehensive guidelines for prescribing opioids for chronic pain, which can also be applied to acute pain.[31] See Box 15.2 for a summary.

When a decision is made to discontinue opioid therapy, opioids should be slowly decreased to avoid withdrawal. Dose should be decreased by 5% to 10% every 1 to 4 weeks, but again, this should be individualized to each patient's need. When pain is not improving, is worsening with opioid therapy, or the patient is requiring escalating doses of narcotics, a referral to an appropriate specialist should be considered. Patients on long-term therapy should also be periodically evaluated by a pain specialist for alternative therapies or new management options.[30]

BOX **15.2**

Centers for Disease Control and Prevention Guidelines for Opioid Prescribing

- Consider nonpharmacologic and nonopioid pharmacologic therapy first.
- Establish treatment goals with patient and discuss risks of opioids and benefits.
- Start with immediate-release opioids at lowest effective dose.
- Prescribe for 3 days or less. More than 7 days rarely needed.
- Reevaluate within 1 month of starting therapy or dose change.
- Continue to evaluate at least every 3 months and evaluate risk.
- Use state prescription monitoring program.
- Consider urine testing prior to initiation and at least annually.
- Avoid prescribing opioids and benzodiazepenes concurrently.

Data from Dowell, D., Haegerich, T. M., & Chou, R. (2016). CDC Guideline for Prescribing Opioids for Chronic Pain—United States, 2016. *MMWR Recommendations and Reports, 65* (No. RR-1), 1–49. doi: 10.15585/mmwr.rr6501e1.

ACUTE PAIN

DEFINITION AND EPIDEMIOLOGY OF ACUTE PAIN

Acute pain is generally short-lived, less than 3 months in duration, and is relieved when the underlying injury has resolved. It is associated with hypertension, sweating, tachycardia, and vasoconstriction. Acute pain often follows a trauma, disease process, or invasive intervention, and is often severe enough for the patient to seek health care.[5,32] The lifetime prevalence of acute pain is 100%, with 66% of the population worldwide suffering from a headache at least once in their lives.[33] One study found that prevalence of pain in hospitalized patients ranged from 37% to 84%.[34]

PATHOPHYSIOLOGY OF ACUTE PAIN

Acute pain is caused by signals from nociceptors at the end of sensory neurons warning of potential or actual injury. This increased activity can sometimes change the operation of neuronal circuits which leads to chronic pain.[35]

CLINICAL PRESENTATION AND PHYSICAL EXAMINATION OF ACUTE PAIN

As previously mentioned, acute pain often follows a trauma, disease process or invasive intervention, and can be nociceptive or neuropathic in nature. The clinical presentation will be related to the underlying cause, and some of the most common reasons for emergency room visits are abdominal pain, chest pain, headache, back pain and injury.[36]

A thorough physical examination is necessary in the assessment of a patient presenting with acute pain to identify any obvious causes. However, given that pain itself is subjective, patient report is the gold standard, and severity of pain may not match with physical findings.

DIAGNOSTICS FOR ACUTE PAIN

The specific injury and location of acute pain will often direct the diagnostic studies. No specific diagnostics are indicated for acute pain without a source, though ultrasound, X-rays, CT scans, magnetic resonance imagings (MRIs), blood work, or other diagnostic tests may be ordered to identify the cause of the pain.

INTERPROFESSIONAL COLLABORATIVE MANAGEMENT OF ACUTE PAIN

Acute pain may be unexpected (e.g., trauma), or expected, as in a planned surgery or childbirth. Thus the management of acute pain may be by the primary care provider, or the specialist managing the underlying disorder. The goal of management is always to intervene early, reduce pain levels, and encourage recovery. While pharmacologic management is general first line management of acute pain, nonpharmacologic methods also play an important role.[19]

PHARMACOLOGIC AND NONPHARMACOLOGIC MANAGEMENT OF ACUTE PAIN

Pharmacologic and nonpharmacologic management of acute pain have been discussed previously. Refer to the previous pain management sections of this chapter.

PATIENT AND FAMILY EDUCATION OF ACUTE PAIN

- Explanation of injury and expected time of healing
- Medication teaching including importance of following prescription guidelines
- Side effects and adverse effects of medications

HEALTH PROMOTION FOR ACUTE PAIN

The goal of health promotion is to improve the health of individuals and their communities through a multidisciplinary approach of education and change. Depending on the cause of the acute pain, different approaches to behavioral change or education may be appropriate. Health promotion around physical activity, risk-taking behaviors, or substances use may help a patient avoid future injuries.

CHRONIC PAIN

DEFINITION AND EPIDEMIOLOGY OF CHRONIC PAIN

Chronic pain may be instigated by injury but is ongoing for reasons often unrelated to the initial cause.[5,32] It may also occur in the absence of injury, has no known physical benefit, and carries significant morbidity and mortality. Chronic pain affects more than 100 million people in the United States and has associated health care costs of up to $635 billion.[37] Due to the complexities of chronic pain, complete pain relief is often unlikely and strategies for pain control include local repair of injury as well as a global management strategy of rehabilitation. Therapy focuses on promoting optimum functioning, coping, and quality of life with use of a full-dimensional approach of interdisciplinary care and community support in decision-making and goals.[38]

Multiple conditions may result in the development of chronic pain. The most common is low back pain, followed by headaches, neck pain and facial pain. But abdominal or pelvic pain, noncardiac chest pain, pain syndromes, neuropathies, and conditions that are vascular, cutaneous, musculoskeletal, cancerous, or psychological in nature can also be chronic.[37,38] Pain can also be related to other diseases including cardiac, pulmonary, or neurologic conditions. When individuals with chronic pain start to develop symptoms beyond the pain, such as depression, anxiety, or insomnia, this becomes a chronic pain syndrome. Additionally, well-known psychological sequelae to chronic pain include depression, anxiety, and anger. In 2010 the concept of mental defeat was described as an aspect of catastrophizing strongly associated with functional and psychosocial disability, emotional distress, self-reported pain interference, and sleep disturbance in patients with chronic pain. Additional studies found significant disability among those seeking treatment for their pain, and it is believed that early identification of mental defeat can help with early intervention for depression and anxiety.[39,40]

PATHOPHYSIOLOGY OF CHRONIC PAIN

Chronic pain is caused by a "chronic pathologic process in somatic structures or viscera, or by prolonged and sometimes permanent dysfunction of the peripheral and central nervous system or both."[32] The physiologic, affective, and behavioral responses to chronic pain are quite different from the responses to acute pain.

CLINICAL PRESENTATION AND PHYSICAL EXAMINATION OF CHRONIC PAIN

There are hundreds of identified chronic pain states, thus the patient presentation will vary widely.[41] Often the clinical picture may be nonspecific and noted only in terms of a retrospective review, in which certain patterns may emerge. Both physical and psychological elements must be considered in a patient with chronic pain. As established, chronic pain is pain that continues for a prolonged period and beyond a reasonable healing time for a specific injury. Just a few years ago, the majority of patients with chronic pain were managed by their primary care provider; now only about half are followed by their primary care provider for their pain issues. The majority of the remainder of patients are typically seeing a specialist that manages the underlying diagnosis, or a pain specialist.[42] In addition to physical manifestations, it is also important to ask about mental health issues as it is well documented that chronic pain and depression often coexist. Additionally, patients may have work difficulties or be on disability, problems in relationships, or financial issues all stemming from their chronic pain.[4]

The physical examination of a patient with chronic pain should be thorough and multifactorial. It should include a general examination of appearance, gait, neurologic and mental status, cranial nerve testing, motor and musculoskeletal strength, reflexes, and a full joint and myofascial examination.[26]

DIAGNOSTICS FOR CHRONIC PAIN

No specific diagnostics are indicated for chronic pain. However, electrocardiography, imaging, blood work, nerve conduction studies, or other diagnostic tests may be ordered to rule out causes of the pain.

DIFFERENTIAL DIAGNOSIS FOR CHRONIC PAIN

Because of the lack of specificity of the many symptoms associated with chronic pain, other diagnoses must be considered. Neurologic, nonneurologic, and psychiatric causes should be acknowledged and evaluated.

INTERPROFESSIONAL COLLABORATIVE MANAGEMENT OF CHRONIC PAIN

As previously mentioned, patients are seeing a variety of specialists for chronic pain management, ranging from a primary provider, to a diagnosis specific specialist, to pain specialists in clinics. These providers may be managing the chronic pain in addition to the psychosocial comorbidities, and thus a multidisciplinary approach is often the key to improved management. This may include social workers, psychiatric providers, or substance use counselors.

PHARMACOLOGIC MANAGEMENT OF CHRONIC PAIN

It is likely that a patient with chronic pain has been treated with multiple medications in the past with varying degrees of success. It is important to obtain a complete prescriptive history prior to adding, changing, or increasing any medications. The WHO three-step analgesic ladder is an appropriate tool to guide clinicians in choosing and prescribing pain medications. Refer to section Pharmacologic Management of Pain for further details.

If medication management is unsuccessful or results in unwanted side effects, evaluation by an interventional pain specialist may provide alternative pain relief recommendations (e.g., nerve block—an anesthetic injected to prevent painful conduction of pain at the nerve ending, site point injection—a steroid injection to reduce inflammation, and trigger point injections to help with muscle spasticity). Results from these procedures vary; however, many patients obtain some degree of pain relief for weeks or months, and these injections may decrease the need for medication or unwanted side effects associated with pain medications.

NONPHARMACOLOGIC MANAGEMENT OF CHRONIC PAIN

Nonpharmacologic measures are important adjuvants in chronic pain. Refer to section on "Nonpharmacologic Management of Pain" for further details.

LIFESPAN CONSIDERATIONS FOR CHRONIC PAIN

Pain issues are common in older adults, affecting 50% to 65% of the population, especially those with expected comorbidities of obesity, arthritis, osteoporosis, hip fractures, and mental health issues. In addition, chronic pain may be more common in older women and in older adults with lower levels of education and socioeconomic status. Untreated pain in older adults can lead to increased falls and cognitive issues, but often these patients underreport pain to avoid admitting deficits, functional decline, or cognitive changes. Some older adults report interference with nutrition, sleep, and social and recreational activities, as well as depression and anxiety, and exhibit greater need for health care use.[43–45]

Management of chronic pain in older adults is complicated by multiple health issues and the underprescribing of analgesics because of both prescriber and patient concerns. Also, the majority of older adults are treated for single sites of pain, when in reality widespread pain is very common. Because some pain medications can have adverse effects in elders, current guidelines encourage pharmacologic and nonpharmacologic interventions.[46,47]

Young adults and children with pain have a 30% chance of developing chronic musculoskeletal chronic pain issues, with up to 20% of children in the United States being affected by chronic pain. There are psychosocial, psychiatric, and biological long-term effects, and a multidisciplinary approach is encouraged.[48,49] It has been well documented that young adults and children of parents with chronic pain are more likely to have pain issues themselves, and overall poorer outcomes in life.[50]

PATIENT AND FAMILY EDUCATION OF CHRONIC PAIN

- Explanation of pathophysiologic changes associated with chronic pain
- Medication teaching including importance of following prescription guidelines
- Side effects and adverse effects of medications
- Goals of management, which may include reduction of pain to tolerable level, improvement in function, improved quality of life.

HEALTH PROMOTION FOR CHRONIC PAIN

Health promotion activities for patients with chronic pain include strategies that promote activities of daily living and coping, with the goal of maintaining or improving both physical and psychological function. Educating a patient about using a comprehensive approach that focuses on both the physical and psychological dimensions of quality of life is now the standard of care, and patients may need encouragement to stay involved with their interdisciplinary team.

ONCOLOGY PAIN

DEFINITION AND EPIDEMIOLOGY OF ONCOLOGY PAIN

Experiencing pain and suffering is one of the most common fears of patients and caregivers of patients undergoing cancer treatment. While pain is largely subjective in nature, there are both subjective and objective findings one can use to determine the severity of the oncologic pain experience. The impact of cancer pain is unique to the individual and may be affected by a multitude of other symptoms that cancer patients also experience, both physically and emotionally.[51]

PATHOPHYSIOLOGY OF ONCOLOGY PAIN

The key to treating cancer pain effectively is to identify the underlying cause whenever possible. Cancer pain can be aggravated by factors such as infection, trauma, and tumor growth, therefore careful assessment and physical examination are essential.[52] Factors such as inflammation and myofascial pain may also contribute to the overall pain perception. Cancer pain often exhibits a classic referral pattern, depending on the cancer pathology. For example, pain associated with cancer of the pancreas can be experienced as pain in the middle or upper back, or as shoulder pain. Associated swelling also causes pressure on the nerves or other sensitive structures, which will contribute to the severity of the pain. Tumors can cause mechanical injury, compression, ischemia, and injury to sensory and sympathetic fibers, leading to neuropathic pain.[53]

CLINICAL PRESENTATION OF ONCOLOGY PAIN

Pain associated with cancer has many presentations. It can evolve slowly from an awareness of discomfort with increasing intensity, or it may be acute and severe at the onset. The patient's chronic cancer pain may seem well managed for a length of time, and then a sudden worsening in the pain or a completely different type of pain is reported by the patient or caregiver.[52] Because it is possible for pain to be experienced prior to tumor detection, it is paramount when treating someone with a history of cancer to rule out tumor growth from metastases in the list of differential diagnoses, even if the patient has been disease-free for some time. Patients who experience a sudden worsening of pain, or a new pain, might also fear relapse or disease progression and may insist on referral back to the oncologist.[54]

A careful and thorough history includes identification of the pattern, characteristics, severity, and impact of the pain. The provider should always ask the patient the specific location(s) of the pain. Primary care providers should remember that cancer patients often have pain in multiple body areas from several sources, therefore the pain relief regimen needs to accommodate these characteristics.[2]

Because pain is a subjective complaint, cancer pain can be influenced by or distorted by delirium, somatization, and chemical coping. It is imperative to assess not only the pain complaint but also the patient's cognitive status and coping mechanisms. Cognition can be assessed by standardized tools designed to detect delirium and evaluate overall mental status. Somatization and chemical coping can be difficult to detect, but a careful medical history with a patient or caregiver may help detect these.

 Red Flag includes a pain complaint which may be influenced by one of the following: rapid opioid escalation, continued complaints of severe pain despite aggressive titration, and history of substance use.

PHYSICAL EXAMINATION OF ONCOLOGY PAIN

Patients can experience significant cancer pain without giving the appearance of suffering. Coping abilities vary widely among individuals. With persistent pain, physiologic and psychosocial adaptations usually occur, which can be confusing on exam.[54] The physical examination should focus initially on the painful areas to identify any lesions, inflammation, vascular changes, edema, or pain on palpation. Sensory changes in the affected part or new areas should also be carefully assessed. Changes between exams can often be attributed to new disease pathology or injury from other sources, such as radiation therapy and chemotherapy. Joint range of motion and muscle strength should also be observed for changes in motor function. Watch the patient during ambulation, whenever possible, to determine the impact of pain on movement and functional ability. Complaints of back and leg pain warrant a high suspicion of impending cord compression from primary tumor growth or metastases. Assessment questions for possible cord compression include a history of sensory changes (leg weakness, numbness/tingling), autonomic dysfunction (loss of bladder or bowel function), and back or leg pain (usually sudden onset).

DIAGNOSTICS FOR ONCOLOGY PAIN

There are no specific imaging or laboratory techniques that exist with which to directly study pain. The diagnostic evaluation should, therefore, be guided by the location and nature of the patient's report of pain, and an understanding of the pathophysiology of the underlying cancer(s). Relevant imaging is essential, however, and should be reviewed and repeated periodically. CT scans may be indicated to identify masses that involve the vital organs or lymphadenopathy. Bone scans and plain X-ray films should be obtained if bone metastases are suspected. A bone scan is a sensitive test used to image disease before it is visible on X-ray, but it is not specific and may be positive for other inflammatory processes, which can be confusing.

Since MRI can identify nerve root or spinal cord compression, patients with a history of tumors that tend to metastasize to the bone, especially lung, prostate, multiple myeloma, breast, renal, and non-Hodgkin lymphoma, should promptly undergo MRI to exclude cord impingement in the setting of back and leg pain.[50] Spinal cord compression is a true medical emergency since the earliest possible intervention (steroids, surgery, and/or radiotherapy) is critical to preserve neurologic function. Consider electromyography (EMG) to assist with determining if there is nerve compression or nerve root injury that is not identified on a scan. Blood tests can also be obtained, including a complete blood count (CBC), which can help evaluate for relapse of disease, particularly with cancers of the blood. There is increasing concern with the rising costs of health care and unnecessary, costly tests ordered for oncology patients where results of these tests may not provide any additional information needed for the patient's overall management. The primary care provider should always be mindful when ordering any test as to whether this will assist in decision-making regarding the patient's care.[55]

DIFFERENTIAL DIAGNOSES OF ONCOLOGY PAIN

Pain is a significant problem for the majority of cancer patients at some point during the course of their disease and treatment. Researchers have found that 24% to 60% of patients undergoing active cancer treatment report pain, and 62% to 86% of patients with advanced cancer report pain.[56] While oncology pain can occur at any time and may be related to a tumor, the incidence and severity of pain will often increase as the disease progresses. Common treatment-related cancer pain syndromes include those associated with surgery, chemotherapy, radiotherapy, and biologic therapy. For example, surgical patients may develop postmastectomy, postthoracotomy, or phantom pain. Some chemotherapeutic agents, such as the vinca alkaloids and cisplatin, can cause peripheral neuropathies, while extravasational agents can cause significant tissue and nerve damage. Radiation effects can be early (e.g., mucositis) or late (e.g., brachial plexopathy or osteoradionecrosis). Biologic agents such as interferon can cause peripheral neuropathy and joint pain, both of which can be transient or chronic in nature. Tumor-related pain can result from the compression of pain-sensitive structures by a mass (e.g., epidural cord compression, organ),[57] or can be related to direct infiltration, especially of the nervous and musculoskeletal systems. Pain resulting from bone metastasis is one of the most severe and disabling types of oncology pain.[58]

Oncology patients may experience pain that is unrelated to the oncological problem, which the primary care provider must also address in their treatment plan. Patients may have a documented, preexisting chronic pain problem, such as chronic low back or neck pain, migraine headaches, or diabetic peripheral neuropathy. An infection can cause sudden and severe pain that is easily improved with appropriate antimicrobial medications. HZV can be contracted in immunocompromised oncology patients. It presents with a localized rash following a dermatomal dissemination and is accompanied by sharp, burning, and/or aching pain that can resolve or persist. Obstruction, constipation, ileus, peptic ulcer disease, gallbladder disease, pancreatitis, diverticulitis, and appendicitis are all examples of other diseases and conditions that can each cause acute or chronic abdominal pain requiring intervention.

MANAGEMENT OF ONCOLOGY PAIN

Effective pain management, particularly for the patient with advanced cancer, requires a comprehensive approach that often involves the use of multiple modalities. A thorough assessment, physical examination, and careful review of medical records are important to determine the type of pain and pathology of the pain so that an appropriate treatment plan can be established. Opioid pain medications and adjuvant treatments (e.g., muscle relaxants, NSAIDs, antidepressants, anticonvulsants, thermal modalities, relaxation techniques) are all utilized to improve the oncology patient's quality of life.[6,52,59]

Opioids, the preferred term for narcotic analgesics, are effective and well-tolerated when used to relieve many forms of cancer pain (Box 15.3).[3,60] The most commonly used opioid medications for the treatment of cancer pain include morphine, oxycodone, oxymorphone, hydrocodone, hydromorphone, methadone, and fentanyl. The mixed agonist-antagonist opioids produce analgesia but can also reverse analgesia. These drugs are associated with a high incidence of psychotomimetic side effects and not recommended for routine use in critically ill patients. When agonist-antagonists are given to a patient who has been taking a pure agonist opioid, the agonist-antagonist acts as an antagonist by displacing the agonist from the opiate receptors, which precipitates withdrawal and reverses analgesia.[20] Withdrawal and exacerbation of pain can not only reduce one's quality of life but also poses a considerable risk to critically ill and debilitated patients. For this reason, the injudicious use of naloxone, a pure opioid antagonist, should be avoided with oncology patients.

Patients may also be reluctant to take opioid medications in the early stages of their cancer diagnosis because they may have the belief that morphine is "for dying patients only." Fears of becoming "immune," or that the drug will not work when it is "really needed," can also account for reluctance to take opioid medications. There are patients with stable cancer pain who may stay on the same dose of pain medication for years without a decreased efficacy, but this is not the norm. One can certainly become more tolerant to opioid medication with prolonged use, therefore patients should be educated on dose escalation which can be used to counter this. Progression of the patient's disease is the most common reason for dose escalation, especially when a rapid increase is needed.[2,61] Other causes of dose escalation can include delirium, somatization,

---

BOX **15.3**

Opioid Agonists Used for Cancer Pain

- Codeine (Tylenol #3[a] or #4[a])
- Fentanyl (Actiq, Fentora, Duragesic[b])
- Hydrocodone (Vicodin,[a] Lortab,[a] Zohydro[b])
- Hydromorphone (Dilaudid)
- Oxymorphone (Opana, Opana ER[b])
- Methadone (Dolophine)
- Morphine (MSIR, Roxanol, MS Contin,[b] Oramorph,[b] Avinza,[b] Kadian[b])
- Oxycodone (Percocet,[a] Percodan,[c] Roxicodone, OxyContin[b])

NOTE: The following medications are not recommended for the relief of cancer pain: mixed agonist-antagonist, partial agonists, and placebos.[21]
[a]Combination containing acetaminophen.
[b]Sustained- or controlled-release delivery system.
[c]Combination containing aspirin.

and chemical coping. Opioid medications do not have a ceiling dose, therefore, these medications can be continually titrated on the basis of the patient's need. The possible development of tolerance is often concerning to prescribers as well as patients, especially when solely looking at the total amount of medications the patient is taking.[7]

The WHO recommends a step approach to managing cancer pain, which begins when the patient first experiences pain. Initially a nonopioid medication such as an NSAID can be used for minor pain (1 to 3 on the pain scale of 1 to 10). If pain persists, initiation of a mild opioid is then indicated, followed by a stronger opioid. Titration of opioid medications is done until the patient experiences tolerable pain, with the understanding patients may never be truly "free" of pain. Adjuvant medications can enhance pain control (e.g., muscle relaxants, antidepressants, antianxiety and anticonvulsant medications). Throughout the step process, adjuvant medications are used to help with fear and anxiety.[18,62]

INDICATIONS FOR REFERRAL OR HOSPITALIZATION FOR ONCOLOGY PAIN

A pain management or palliative care specialist can certainly be consulted by the primary care provider if efforts to titrate the opioid dose to the desired effect are not successful or to manage the opioid-related side effects. Consultation is also appropriate whenever an invasive route of opioid administration is indicated and needs more oversight. Referral to a pain center should be considered for procedures such as epidural steroid injections, trigger point injections, and local nerve blocks. Hospitalization may be necessary if the patient's pain is so severe that despite all efforts the pain will not abate and high doses of intravenous opioid medication with close monitoring becomes necessary until the pain is more tolerable.

PATIENT AND FAMILY EDUCATION OF ONCOLOGY PAIN

Education regarding side effects will help the oncology patient anticipate problems that may arise, and allow for active participation. Involving oncology patients in the care plan can also promote optimal pain control.[7] Patients should be aware that most side effects from opioid medications will improve with tolerance and that treatment can be given without sacrificing pain reduction. General education about the differences between "around-the-clock" dosing and "as-needed" dosing also needs to be provided. Patients and care givers should be instructed to contact the health care provider if medication regimens are no longer helping to keep the pain manageable, if constipation is poorly managed, or if there are signs and symptoms of opioid-induced neurotoxicity. Opioid-induced neurotoxicity is a phenomenon whereby patients may experience symptoms of sedation, delirium, hallucinations, and myoclonus, and require immediate dose reduction of the opioid.[24] Patients and care givers should also be encouraged to discuss with the health care provider their concerns about pain management, including the fear of pain, the fear of addiction, and possible misconceptions about pain management for oncology-related pain.

The primary care provider has the essential role of identifying problems and coordinating care within the oncology team, as cancer patients will need medical, psychological, psychosocial, and spiritual support throughout their treatment.

END-OF-LIFE PAIN

DEFINITION AND EPIDEMIOLOGY OF END-OF-LIFE PAIN

Pain is a highly prevalent symptom in those with a terminal disease, especially in the 4 months before death. This makes it one of the most feared symptoms at the end of life.[63] Dame Cicely Saunders, key contributor to the modern hospice movement, coined the term *total pain* and suggested that pain be understood as having physical, psychological, social, emotional, and spiritual components.[64] Despite recent advances in the understanding of pain control, pain is still often untreated or undertreated. Consequently, a significant number of patients needlessly suffer physical pain and mental distress at end of life.[65]

Unrelieved pain at the end of life is unnecessary and with few exceptions is treatable. Practical issues can be the most challenging, including the loss of the oral route for medication administration, a wish to die at home, nonopioid-responsive total pain or suffering, and fear that pain treatment may hasten death. With the skill and expertise of hospice or home care support, all of the previously mentioned issues can be overcome and expert pain relief can occur at home or in long-term care settings.

DIAGNOSTICS FOR END-OF-LIFE PAIN

Obtaining a comprehensive pain assessment is essential and should be the first step in diagnosing and treating one's pain. When possible, it is ideal to obtain the history directly from the patient, however, patients nearing end of life are often in varying degrees of consciousness and with varying abilities to communicate which may make giving a history difficult. In these cases, the primary care provider should consider behavioral cues such as grimacing and posturing in the patient, caregiver/family/proxy report, and previous pain issues.[66]

In conjunction with the pain assessment, diagnostic tests (radiographic imaging, radiation therapy, etc.) can prove to be helpful in diagnosing and treating one's pain. However, as patients near end of life, it is appropriate for the primary care provider to review goals of care with patients and families (prior to obtaining any diagnostic imaging) to ensure that imaging is in conjunction with the goals of care and assess the benefits that imaging would provide.

DIFFERENTIAL DIAGNOSIS FOR END-OF-LIFE PAIN

If the patient did not previously have pain, but now appears to be in pain, or seems to have changes in pain behaviors, excluding the other potential causes of distress is imperative. These potential causes may include constipation, bladder distention, hypoxemia, infections, delirium, decubitus ulcers (check bony prominences), mucositis (especially if the patient is neutropenic), and opioid toxicity (associated with increasing analgesic use).[66]

BARRIERS TO OPTIMAL END-OF-LIFE PAIN MANAGEMENT

Barriers to optimal pain management at the end of life come in many forms and are often categorized into three groups: Patient and Family, Health Care Providers, and Health Care System.[67]

- Patient and Family
  - Denial by patient and/or family, causally linking pain as a sign of deterioration
  - Fear that increasing pain is a herald of disease progression
  - Patients' and families' beliefs that pain is a natural part of illness and cannot be relieved
  - Fear of addiction and abuse
- Health Care Providers
  - Nonrecognition of pain, including denial of its presence
  - Nonrecognition of the global nature of pain, including psychological, social, and cultural aspects
  - Fear of doing harm, causing adverse effects, and/or tolerance to opioid use
  - Fear of diversion
  - Exclusion of effective concurrent nonpharmacological measures
- Health Care System
  - Restrictive formularies or cost prohibitions which prevent appropriate treatment

PHARMACOLOGIC MANAGEMENT OF END-OF-LIFE PAIN

There are three general principles that should be followed when providing pain control at the end of life. First, pain can be controlled in most patients by following the WHO's step-care approach. See "Pharmacologic Management of Pain" section in this chapter. Second, acute, escalating or intractable pain is a medical emergency that requires prompt attention. A delay in responding to this pain will make it more difficult to control. Third, addiction should not be considered an issue in patients with a terminal illness. When pain is treated appropriately, addiction problems are rare.[65]

For most patients with terminal illness, opioid therapies often provide the greatest analgesic relief. There are a variety of medications which can be utilized and multiple routes of administration depending on the needs of your patient. Collaboration with a pain/palliative care specialist can often prove beneficial. Constant assessment and reassessment of pain status as well as the patient's ability to ingest the medications is necessary and there is frequently a need to adjust medication dosages, formulations, and routes of administration as one nears the end of life.

NONPHARMACOLOGIC MANAGEMENT OF END-OF-LIFE PAIN

Nonpharmacologic management of pain has been presented previously in this chapter. See Nonpharmacologic management of pain section of this chapter.

COMPLICATIONS IN END-OF-LIFE PAIN
Loss of Oral Route

There are many alternatives to oral opioid administration, and routes of administration should be modified as needed. Medications can be provided rectally (including enteric-coated tablets or suppositories), transdermally, sublingually (by high-concentrate solutions administered to the oral cavity), or subcutaneously (continuously, intermittently, or by a patient-controlled pump). Given these options, there rarely is a need for intravenous or intrathecal catheters, which can be painful to insert and provide interrupted analgesia when infiltrated. There is no ceiling dose of opioids. Balancing analgesia against reduced level of consciousness can be based on patient preference.[68]

Fear of Hastening Death

There is great fear that the administration of opioids at the end of life will hasten death. This misunderstanding has unfortunately resulted in inadequate pain management at the end of life. Many professionals believe that opioid doses require extensive escalation during the last days to hours of life and fear that providing these doses will result in hastening death. In reality, several studies indicate that for the majority of patients in their last 24 hours of life, the opioid dose remained low. For patients who did require significant increases, their survival was no different than patients who remained on stable dosing.[66]

As the front line in patient care, primary care providers, nurses and caregivers often voice a fear regarding administration of opioids to patients at end of life. The common fear is that they will hasten death. However, no one involved in the patient's care wants to see the patient/loved one suffer. This can be a major dilemma and cause much anxiety. The American Nurses Association (2010) position statement, "Registered nurses' roles and responsibilities in providing expert care and counseling at the end of life" supports the nurse in this role, as does the Hospice and Palliative Nurse Association (2013), *The ethics of opioid use at end of life.* Often, this is considered the rule of double effect: if the intent is good (i.e., relief of pain and suffering), then the act is morally justifiable even if it causes a foreseeable but unintended result (e.g., hastening of death). Thus, nurses and caregivers should provide pain relief without fear of sedation or respiratory depression limiting the use of opioids.[66] A retrospective study of patients cared for at home found that the use of opioids, even high-dose opioids or escalating doses, did not shorten survival.[69] Patients develop enormous tolerance to the respiratory depressant effects of opioids, and high doses of opioids can be both appropriate and safe in terminally ill patients with pain.[4] Patients who have a life-limiting illness should continue to receive opioids for pain relief or dyspnea until the time of death. Respiratory depression from opioids can occur but is most often noted in the opioid-naive person. Careful upward titration in response to pain rarely causes respiratory depression because pain is a natural stimulant to the respiratory center. Patients, families, and nursing staff should be educated about the appropriate use of pain medications for symptom control. For further information, see Chapter 14, Palliative Care.

OTHER COMPLICATIONS

Complications included here are adverse effects of opioids. Constipation is a common and expected side effect of opioid use. Stimulants should be started concurrently with standing opioid regimens with a note to hold for diarrhea. If patients experience nausea and vomiting while taking opioids, antiemetics are prescribed on a schedule for the first 3 to 5 days after opioid use is initiated. Undesirable sedation may occur with use of opioids. Discussing with the patient and/or family what an acceptable level of sedation is may be helpful. If the patient or family is distressed with the level of sedation, low-dose methylphenidate (Ritalin) can be utilized.

LIFE SPAN CONSIDERATIONS FOR END-OF-LIFE PAIN

Pain in older patients is often undertreated with patterns of low doses of analgesics or the use of only nonopioids. Guidelines from the APS, the National Comprehensive Cancer Network (NCCN), and the American Geriatric Society recommend application of the same pharmacologic approaches as for younger adults, with the direction to "start low and go slow" as the general rule of opioid titration and to compensate for potentially diminished drug metabolism. Geriatric oncologists emphasize the importance of individual assessment rather than treatment based solely on age.[70]

PATIENT AND FAMILY EDUCATION FOR END-OF-LIFE PAIN

Pain at the end of life is a commonly held fear by both patients and families. Reassurance needs to be provided that pain will be managed and that medication dosages, formulations, and routes of administration can be altered depending on the patient's needs.

PAIN MANAGEMENT IN PRIMARY CARE

There exists an ethical imperative to achieve proper pain management while enhancing patients' quality of life. The American Nurse's Association's Board of Directors adopted a position statement in 2018 entitled *The Ethical Responsibility to Manage Pain and the Suffering It Causes*.[71] In this position statement, the authors recognize the challenge the current opioid crisis presents to nurses to manage pain while fulfilling their duty to protect patients from harm; recommendations include developing individualized pain management plans in concert with other health care professionals, dealing with personal bias(es) and practice setting issues that prevent nurses from adequately managing patients' pain, guarding against moral disengagement when managing patients in pain, and resolving economic limitations that prevent patients from accessing the full spectrum of modalities that relieve pain beyond pharmacologic preparations.[71] Nurses are encouraged to work collaboratively with other professional organizations to develop ethical policies and legislation to improve pain management for patients, as well as developing knowledge through nursing research to establish best practices in opioid use, addiction treatment, and pain management.[71]

The opioid epidemic has raised concerns about opioid pain management in primary care. Patient education must include the appropriate use of opioids in pain management (e.g, short term for fractures or post operative pain or for end-of-life care). Appropriate storage of opioids, misuse and the risk of diversion to other family members are concerns that need to be discussed with any patient prescribed an opioid. Additionally, all primary care practices should have narcotic contract with every patient prescribed an opioid. The contract should be discussed with the patient and both patient and provider should sign the contract. Patients and families should be made aware that the CDC Prescription Monitoring Program will be checked by the prescriber before a narcotic prescription is renewed. To avoid weekend issues regarding opioids, it is recommended that the maximum monthly prescription for a narcotic only be for 28 days.

Patients should also be educated on the importance of appropriate storage of opioids (to avoid diversion) and how to destroy or dispose of left over opioids.

SUMMARY

Primary care providers are often the front line when it comes to treating pain in their patients. Whether it is acute pain, chronic pain, oncologic pain, pain at the end of life, or any combination thereof, it is important to first understand the pathophysiology behind the different types of pain, and the

treatment options available. Poorly controlled pain can lead to unnecessary suffering and long-lasting sequelae. However, with comprehensive histories and assessments, ongoing review of symptoms, use of appropriate medications, appropriate interdisciplinary referrals, and by assessing patients' physical as well as emotional reasons for pain, primary care providers can ensure proper management of pain and enhanced quality of life for patients.

REFERENCES

1. International Association for the Study of Pain: IASP taxonomy. (2011). Retrieved from www.iasp-paino.rg/AM/Template.cfm?Section=General_Resource.Links &Template=/CM/HTMLDisplay.cfm&ContentID=3058. (Accessed 27 October 2017).
2. Pergolizzi, J., Gharibo, C., & Ho, K. Y. (2015). Treatment considerations for cancer pain: A global perspective. *Pain Practice*, 15(8), 778–792.
3. Arslan, M., Albaş, S., Küçükerdem, H., et al. (2016). "The evaluation of the effectiveness of palliative pain management in cancer patients with visual analogue scale. *FamPrac and Pall Care*, 1(1), 5–8.
4. Pasero, C., & McCaffery, M. (2011). *Pain assessment and pharmacologic management*. St. Louis: Elsevier.
5. Nagda, J., & Bajwa, Z. (2017). Definitions and classification of pain. In Z. H. Bajwa, R. Wootton, & C. A. Warfield (Eds.), *Principles and Practice of Pain Medicine* (ed. 3). New York, NY: McGraw-Hill. Retrieved from http://accessanesthesiology.mhmedical.com/content.aspx?bookid=1845&sectionid=133682578. (Accessed 15 October 2017).
6. Chang, H. Y., Daubresse, M., Kruszewski, S. P., et al. (2014). Prevalence and treatment of pain in EDs in the United States, 2000 to 2010. *The American Journal of Emergency Medicine*, 32, 421–431.
7. Kwon, J. H. (2014). Overcoming barriers to pain management. *Journal of Clinical Oncology: Official Journal of the American Society of Clinical Oncology*, 32, 1727–1733.
8. Mitchel, W. M., & Von Gunten, C. F. (2011). Approach to the management of cancer pain. In H. T. Benzon, R. N. Srinivasa, S. S. Liu, et al. (Eds.), *Essentials of pain medicine* (ed. 3, pp. 511–519). Philadelphia: WB Saunders.
9. Panchal, S. J., & Grami, V. (2014). Pain, nociceptive vs. neuropathic. In *Encyclopedia of the Neurological Sciences* (ed. 2, pp. 749–752). Elsevier Inc.
10. Todd, A. J., & Koerber, H. R. (2013). Neuroanatomical substrates of spinal nociception. In *Wall &Melzack's textbook of pain* (ed. 6, pp. 77–93). Saunders.
11. Arnstein, P. (2010). *Clinical coach for effective pain management*. Philadelphia: FA Davis.
12. International Association for the Study of Pain (IASP). (2012). IASP taxonomy. https://www.iasp-pain.org/Taxonomy?navItemNumber=576. (Accessed 22 October 2017).
13. Devor, M. (2013). Neuropathic pain: Pathophysiological response of nerves to injury. In *Wall &Melzack's textbook of pain* (ed. 6, pp. 861–888). Saunders.
14. Ferrell, B., & Nessa, G. (2010). Pain assessment. In *Oxford textbook of palliative nursing*. New York: Oxford University Press.
15. The MD Anderson Symptom Library. (2017). Retrieved from https://www.mdanderson.org/research/departments-labs-institutes/departments-divisions/symptom-research/symptom-assessment-tools/md-anderson-symptom-inventory.html. (Accessed 5 December 2017).
16. Pasternak, G. W. (2014). Opiate pharmacology and relief of pain. *Journal of Clinical Oncology: Official Journal of the American Society of Clinical Oncology*, 32(16), 1655–1661.
17. Price, C., Lee, J., Taylor, A., & Baranowski, A. (2014). Initial assessment and management of pain: A pathway for care developed by the British Pain Society. *British Journal of Anaesthesia*, 112(5), 816–823.
18. Kumar, N. (2007). WHO normative guidelines on pain management: Report of a Delphi Study to determine the need for guidelines and to identify the number and topics of guidelines that should be developed by WHO. Retrieved from www.who.int/medicines/areas/quality_safety/delphi_study_pain_guidelines.pdf. (Accessed 17 November 2017).
19. The American Pain Society. Management of acute pain and chronic noncancer pain. Retrieved from http://americanpainsociety.org/uploads/education/section_4.pdf. (Accessed 18 November 2017).
20. Pasternak, G. W. (2014). Opiate pharmacology and relief of pain. *JCO*, 32(16), 1655–1661.
21. McPherson, M. L. (2010). Equianalgesic opioid dosing. In *Demystifying opioid conversion calculations: A guide for effective dosing*. Bethesda: American Society of Health-System Pharmacists: Special Publishing.
22. Smith, H. S. (2012). Rapid onset opioids in palliative medicine. *Annals of Palliative Medicine*, 1(1), 45–52.

23. 2014). Narcotic analgesics, and Nonnarcotic analgesics. In J. Ko, et al. (Eds.), *MPR nurse practitioners' edition* (Vol. 21(2), pp. 200–220). New York: Haymarket Media, Inc.

24. De Stoutz, N. D., Bruera, E., & Suarez-Almazor, M. S. (1995). Opioid rotation for toxicity reduction in terminal cancer patients. *Journal of Pain and Symptom Management, 10*(5), 378–384.

25. Casey, G. (2014). Constipation: Motility and the gut. *Kai Tiaki Nursing New Zealand, 19*(11), 20–24.

26. Benzon, H. T., Rathmell, J. P., Wu, C. L., et al. (2014). History and physical exam of the pain patient. In *Practical management of pain* (pp. 151–161). St Louis: Mosby.

27. Jackman, R., Purvis, J., et al. (2008). Chronic non-malignant pain in primary care. *American Family Physician, 78*(10), 1155–1162.

28. Lembke, A., Humphries, K., & Newmark, J. (2016). Weighing the risk and benefits of chronic opioid therapy. *American Family Physician, 93*(12), 982–990.

29. Opioid prescribing. Where you live matters. Retrieved from www.cdc.gov/vitalsigns/opioids. (Accessed 24 January 2018).

30. Munzing, T. (2017). Physician guide to appropriate opioid prescribing for noncancer pain. *The Permanente Journal, 21*, 16–169.

31. Dowel, D., Haegerich, T., & Chou, R. (2016). CDC guideline for prescribing opioids for chronic pain. *MMWR. Recommendations and Reports: Morbidity and Mortality Weekly Report. Recommendations and Reports / Centers for Disease Control, 65*(1), 1–49.

32. Turk, D., & Okifuji, A. (2010). Pain terms and taxonomies of pain. In S. M. Fishman, J. C. Ballantyne, & J. P. Rathmell (Eds.), *Bonica's management of pain* (ed. 4, pp. 13–23). Philadelphia: Lippincott Williams & Wilkins.

33. Diener, H., Schneider, R., & Aicher, B. (2008). Per-capita consumption of analgesics: A nine country survey over 20 years. *The Journal of Headache and Pain, 9*(5), 225–231.

34. Gregory, J., & Mcgowan, L. (2016). An examination of the prevalence of acute pain for hospitalized adult patients: A systematic review. *Journal of Clinical Nursing, 25*(5–6), 583–598.

35. Cohen, S. (2017). Pathophysiology of pain. In Z. H. Bajwa, R. Wootton, & C. A. Warfield (Eds.), *Principles and Practice of Pain Medicine* (ed. 3). New York, NY: McGraw-Hill. Retrieved from http://accessanesthesiology.mhmedical.com/content.aspx?bookid=1845&sectionid=133682578. (Accessed 15 October 2017).

36. The Centers for Disease Control. (2014). National hospital ambulatory medical care Survey. Retrieved from https://www.cdc.gov/nchs/data/nhamcs/web_tables/2014_ed_web_tables.pdf. (Accessed 29 October 2017).

37. The American Academy of Pain Medicine. (2011). AAPM facts and figures on pain. Retrieved from www.painmed.org/patientcenter/facts-on-pain. (Accessed 15 October 2017).

38. Irving, G., & Squire, P. (2010). Medical evaluation of the chronic pain patient. In S. M. Fishman, J. C. Ballantyne, & J. P. Rathmell (Eds.), *Bonica's management of pain* (ed. 4, pp. 209–223). Philadelphia: Lippincott Williams & Wilkins.

39. Tang, N., Goodchild, C., Heste, J., et al. (2010). Mental defeat is linked to interference, distress, and disability in chronic pain. *Pain, 149*(3), 547–554.

40. Tang, N., Shum, S., Leung, P., et al. (2013). Mental defeat predicts distress and disability in Hong Kong Chinese with chronic pain. *The Clinical Journal of Pain, 29*(9), 830–836.

41. IASP. Classification of chronic pain (ed 2). Retrieved from https://www.iasp-pain.org/PublicationsNews/Content.aspx?ItemNumber=1673&navItemNumber=677. (Accessed 29 October 2017).

42. Dubois, M., & Follett, K. (2014). Pain medicine: The case for an independent medical specialty and training programs. *Academic Medicine: Journal of the Association of American Medical Colleges, 89*(6), 863–868.

43. The American Academy of Pain Medicine. (2011). AAPM facts and figures on pain. Retrieved from www.painmed.org/patientcenter/facts-on-pain. (Accessed 15 October 2017).

44. Arnstein, P., & Herr, K. (2010). Pain in the older person. In S. M. Fishman, J. C. Ballantyne, & J. P. Rathmell (Eds.), *Bonica's management of pain* (ed. 4, pp. 782–790). Philadelphia: Lippincott Williams & Wilkins.

45. Patel, K., Guralnik, J., Dansie, E., & Turk, D. (2013). Prevalence and impact of pain among older adults in the United States: Findings from the 2011 National Health and Aging Trends Study. *Pain, 154*, 2649–2657.

46. Stewart, C., Leveille, S., Shmerling, R., et al. (2012). Management of persistent pain in older adults: The MOBILIZE Boston study. *Journal of the American Geriatrics Society, 60*(11), 2081–2086.

47. Eggermont, L., Leveille, S., Shi, L., et al. (2014). Pain characteristics associated with the onset of disability in older adults: The MOBILIZE Boston study. *Journal of the American Geriatrics Society, 62*(6), 1007–1016.

48. Holley, A., Wilson, A., & Palermo, T. (2017). Predictors of the transition from acute to persistant musculoskeletal pain in children and adolescents: A prospective study. *Pain, 158*(5), 794–801.

49. Mahrer, N., Gold, J., Luu, M., & Herman, P. (2017). A cost-analysis of an interdisciplinary pediatric chronic pain clinic. *The Journal of Pain.*

50. Higgins, K., Birnie, K., Chambers, C., et al. (2015). Offspring of parents with chronic pain: A systematic review and meta-analysis of pain, health, psychological, and family outcomes. *Pain, 156*(11), 2256–2266.

51. Corli, O., Martoni, A. A., Porcu, L., et al. (2016). Non-clinical factors influencing pain intensity in cancer patients: Socio-cultural–economic status, awareness of disease and the relation with the oncologist. *European Journal of Internal Medicine, 33*, e18–e19.

52. Paice, J., Portenoy, R., Lacchetti, C., et al. (2016). Management of chronic pain in survivors of adult cancers: American society of clinical oncology clinical practice guideline. *Journal of Clinical Oncology: Official Journal of the American Society of Clinical Oncology, 34*, 3325–3345.

53. Mantyh, P. W., Clohisy, D. R., Koltzenburg, M., et al. (2002). Molecular mechanisms of cancer pain. *Nature Reviews. Cancer, 2*, 201–209.

54. Brant, J., Eaton, L. H., & Irwin, M. M. (2017). Cancer-related pain: Assessment and management with putting evidence into practice interventions. *Clinical Journal of Oncology Nursing, 21*(3), 4–6.

55. Sima, C. S., Panageas, K. S., & Schrag, D. (2010). Cancer screening among patients with advanced cancer. *JAMA: The Journal of the American Medical Association, 304*(14), 1581–1594.

56. Van den Beuken-van Everdingen, M. H. J., de Rijke, J. M., Kessels, A. J., et al. (2007). Prevalence of pain in patients with cancer: A systematic review of the past 40 years. *Annals of Oncology: Official Journal of the European Society for Medical Oncology / ESMO, 18*(9), 1437–1449.

57. White, N. (2016). Metastatic spinal cord compression. *Hospital Medicine Clinics, 5*(3), 452–465.

58. Von Moos, R., Costa, L., Ripamonti, C. I., et al. (2017). Improving quality of life in patients with advanced cancer: Targeting metastatic bone pain. *European Journal of Cancer, 71*, 80–94.

59. 2014). Narcotic analgesics, and Nonnarcotic analgesics. In J. Ko, et al. (Eds.), *MPR nurse practitioners' edition* (Vol. 21(2), pp. 200–220). New York: Haymarket Media, Inc.

60. Wickham, R. J. (2017). Cancer pain management: Opioid analgesics, part 2. *Journal of the Advanced Practitioner in Oncology, 8*(6), 588–602.

61. Hammer, K., Segal, E., Alwan, L., et al. (2016). Collaborative practice model for management of pain in patients with cancer. *American Journal of Health-System Pharmacy, 73*(18), 1434–1441.

62. World Health Organization. WHO's cancer pain ladder for adults. World Health Organization, Geneva, Switzerland. Retrieved from http://www.who.int/cancer/palliative/painladder/en/. (Accessed 27 October 2017).

63. Smith, A., Cenzer, I. S., Knight, S. J., et al. (2010). The epidemiology of pain during the last 2 years of life. *Annals of Internal Medicine, 153*(9), 563–569.

64. Saunders, C. (1993). Introduction: History and challenge. In C. Saunders (Ed.), *The management of terminal malignant disease* (pp. 1–14). London, Great Britain: Hodder and Stoughton.

65. Miller, K., Miller, M., et al. (2001). Challenges in pain management at the end of life. *American Family Physician, 64*(7), 1227–1235.

66. ELNEC-Core Curriculum. (2016). Module 8: Final Hours: [Powerpoint slides].

67. Reynolds, J., Drew, D., et al. (2013). American Society for Pain Management Nursing Position Statement: Pain management at the end of life. *Pain Management Nursing, 14*(3), 172–175.

68. National Comprehensive Cancer Network (NCCN). (2014). NCCN palliative care guidelines for pain version 1. Retrieved from www.nccn.org/professionals/physician_gls/pdf/palliative.pdf. (Accessed 29 August 2014).

69. Bengoechea, I., Vrotsou, K., et al. (2010). Opioid use at the end of life and survival in a hospital at home unit. *Journal of Palliative Medicine, 13*(9), 1079–1083.

70. Paice, J., & Ferrell, B. (2011). The management of cancer pain. *CA: A Cancer Journal for Clinicians, 61*(3), 157–182.

71. ANA Center for Ethics and Human Rights. The ethical responsibility to manage pain and the suffering it causes. Retrieved from https://www.nursingworld.org/~495e9b/globalassets/docs/ana/ethics/theethicalresponsibilitytomanagepainandthesufferingitcauses2018.pdf. (Accessed 20 April 2018).

CHAPTER 16

WELLNESS: AN INTEGRATED PERSPECTIVE

Joanne Sandberg-Cook

Wellness is simply defined by Merriam-Webster as "the state of being in good health, especially as an actively pursued goal."[1] There are several dimensions of wellness, including emotional, occupational, social, intellectual, spiritual, financial, and environmental. Each dimension requires specific attention and direction. Becoming aware of and making choices toward a healthy and fulfilling life is the goal. Wellness is more than being free from illness; instead, it is a dynamic process of change and growth.[2]

Substantial gains have been made in reducing death rates and improving the health and well-being of the US population. Implementation of public health initiatives to improve health and wellness and national goal setting to reduce the burden of morbidity continue to be top priorities. Inappropriate nutrition, inadequate physical activity, and a lack of stress management are dominant lifestyle factors that contribute to leading causes of death in the United States. Heart disease, cancer, accidents, diseases of the lower respiratory tract, and stroke persisted as the top five leading causes of death in 2017.[3] Physical inactivity, diet, obesity, stress, social isolation, substance use including tobacco, alcohol, and opioids all remain high on the lists of independent risk factors for morbidity and mortality.

The US Department of Health and Human Services (HHS) examines evidence-based studies and national health trends on an ongoing basis. The Office of Disease Prevention and Health Promotion communicates these data, as well as the national health improvement objectives, via the federal prevention initiative *Healthy People*. Overarching goals of the *Healthy People 2020* initiative are to increase quality and length of life; to be free of preventable disease, disability, injury, and premature death; to achieve health equality by eliminating disparities; to create social and physical environments that promote proper health; and to promote increased quality of life, healthy development, and healthy behaviors across all life stages, all goals that are consistent with the definition of wellness (https://www.healthypeople.gov/2020/topics-objectives).

DOMAINS OF WELLNESS

Intellectual Wellness

Intellectual wellness is being open to new ideas, thinking critically, and seeking out new challenges. It is being creative, curious, and engaged in ongoing learning inside and outside the classroom by:

- Identifying projects, organizations, and classes that are exciting and rewarding
- Engaging one's intellect in new areas (attending a cultural event, theater, reading a book on something you know nothing about, learning about a friend's favorite sport, learning a new language).

Emotional Wellness

Emotional wellness is being aware of and able to navigate a wide range of emotions in a constructive, supportive way and having the tools and resources to navigate life's ups and downs by:

- Talking to someone (counselor, advisor, clergy, friend, or family) about how you are doing and feeling.
- Considering pet ownership.
- Making time for regular reflection, perhaps through journaling.
- Taking technology breaks—time away from texting, email, and social media—to meaningfully reconnect with yourself or others.

Social Wellness

Social wellness includes enjoying strong personal connections with others, managing interpersonal conflict effectively, and connecting with community and the people around you by:

- Striving toward healthy relationships while getting to know new people through classes, *club activities*, church and civil volunteerism, and other social activities.
- Using FaceTime, Skype, and telephone calls to stay connected with important people in your life.
- Exploring opportunities for building community and making connections.

Spiritual Wellness

Spiritual wellness is making meaning of life events, having and understanding purpose, and being compassionate towards oneself and others by:

- Finding a spiritual connection or community.
- Cultivating a *mindfulness practice*.
- Experiencing awe, perhaps with *nature* or music
- Choosing projects and service opportunities that align with personal values.

Environmental Wellness

Environmental wellness is characterized by awareness of the interactions among ourselves, our environment, and our community. This dimension recognizes the influence that environment (home, school, town, etc.) has on an individual, as well as the individual impact on the environment. Suggestions could include:

- Walking or biking instead of driving when going short distances.
- Carpooling where possible.
- Bringing your own reusable bags, utensils, mugs, and cups.
- Reduce, reuse, recycle
- Consider donating unneeded furniture or clothing.
- Checking online sites for buying used instead of buying new.
- Participating in groups and causes that support protecting and preserving the environment.

Financial Wellness

Financial wellness is developing skills for managing resources, as well as an understanding of the process of sustaining oneself financially for the short and long term by:

- Saving a portion of each pay check.
- Ensuring financial literacy with the goal of managing your finances now and in the future. Consider using community classes and *online educational resources* to improve your financial literacy.
- Making a budget and tracking spending regularly. Consider an online tool such as *Mint* (https://www.mint.com/) or You need a budget (https://www.youneedabudget.com/).

Occupational Wellness

- Gaining personal satisfaction and enrichment from one's work.

Physical Wellness

Physical wellness is caring for the body to allow for optimal health and functioning, including making intentional choices with respect to alcohol and other drug use, nutrition, illness prevention, physical activity and movement, sexual health, sleep, stress management, and safety.

- Choose a variety of delicious, nutrient-rich whole foods regularly.
- Explore the resources for healthy eating.
- Consult with a *dietitian,* if you have questions or concerns.
- Move your body! Dance, swim, run, walk, play sports, kayak—any activity that you find fun that gets you moving!
- Check into exercise classes in your community.
- Consider joining a *club* or *intramural* sports team.
- Explore opportunities to experience being outside.
- Rest and hydrate when you are feeling under the weather and get medical care when needed.
- Ask about an age-appropriate immunization schedule. Get a flu shot annually.
- Maintain a regular sleep schedule, aiming for 7 to 8 hours a night. Avoid screen time before bed.

WELLNESS EXAMINATION, ROUTINE HEALTH SCREENINGS, AND IMMUNIZATIONS

An annual visit to the primary care provider is an opportunity to become aware of your patients' successes and challenges. Each annual visit should include a measurement of height, weight, and blood pressure; heart, lung, and abdominal examinations; an ear exam; and a vision screening. Chronic conditions can be updated, as well as family and social history. A discussion of the patient's personal stress management strategies, including the use of alcohol, drugs, and tobacco, as well

as healthy alternative approaches, such as meditation, massage, exercise, yoga, or tai chi. Asking about relationships, social supports, hobbies, interests, occupation, and any current or history of intimate partner violence or sexual assault is often revealing. A history of combat stress might explain unhealthy reactions to stressful situations, failed personal relationships, or excessive drug or alcohol use.

The status of routine health screenings must be reviewed and updated. Because these recommendations may change from time to time, patients are often confused about what they need, what they have already had, and how recommendations have changed over the years. Health screenings and immunization schedules are specific to age and gender and are available online. See the US Preventative Task Force website at https://www.uspreventiveservicestaskforce.org/BrowseRec/Index/browse-recommendations for screening recommendations as of 2018.

Immunizations are continuously developed or improved so patients may need the latest version of a specific immunization or be made aware of the availability of others. In general, all persons older than 6 months of age should be immunized against influenza annually (see Chapter 210). A schedule of immunizations for both adults and children is available at: https://www.cdc.gov/vaccines/schedules/hcp/imz/adult.html and https://www.cdc.gov/vaccines/schedules/hcp/imz/child-adolescent.html.

Medicare currently covers an initial "Welcome to Medicare physical examination" and an "Annual Wellness exam." These visits include all information mentioned previously, plus areas of screening specific to older adults, including a cognitive screen and time allotted for a discussion of advance directives. A booklet published by CMS describing the individual points to be covered in an annual visit as well as billing and coding guidelines is available at https://www.cms.gov/Outreach-and-Education/Medicare-Learning-Network-MLN/MLNProducts/Downloads/AWV_Chart_ICN905706.pdf. Any comprehensive assessment of lifestyle includes screening for and assisting patients with nutritional status, weight management, stress management, wellness promotion across the life span, safety issues, and substance use. Most negative effects of poor lifestyle choices are cumulative. Providers must recognize that patients are not always forthcoming in their discussion of personal lifestyle matters. Primary care providers often need to use their history taking and physical examination skills to identify lifestyle factors needing further elaboration. A detailed family history may uncover health problems responsive to lifestyle management. Observant providers can uncover clues throughout the interview and physical examination encounter, which may help to identify lifestyle concerns needing additional attention. For example, cigarette smoke odor often lingers on a patient's clothing. In addition, tobacco-stained fingertips or other signs of substance use such as skin integrity manifestations or altered affect may be observed while conversing with the patient. Providers who prioritize lifestyle factors in the overall assessment of their patients are more likely to have a positive impact of the wellness of their patients.

INTERVENTIONS FOR THE PHYSICAL DOMAIN
Nutrition

The wellness exam will provide important clues to lifestyle, including those related to cultural and religious practices that influence food preparation and consumption. Eating habits such as frequency of eating and types of food consumed should be identified. For an individual with weight management problems, the provider should evaluate dietary intake of sugar and fats, high-fiber foods including fruits and vegetables, overall caloric intake, and consumption of alcohol and caffeinated products. Patterns such as "stress" or "bored" eating should be elicited, and alternative activities suggested.

Food insecurity is defined as households that were uncertain of having, or unable to acquire, enough food to meet the needs of all their members because they had insufficient money or other resources for food. Food-insecure households include those with *low food security* and *very low food security*. At-risk households include those living at the poverty level, single women living alone, and households with children, especially those with children younger than age 6 years of age. In 2017, 11.8% of households in the United States were food insecure at some time during the year (https://www.ers.usda.gov/topics/food-nutrition-assistance/food-security-in-the-us/key-statistics-graphics.aspx).

Nutritional recommendations for the United States are updated every 5 years, with the next update due in 2020. Current recommendations suggest looking at patterns of eating rather than specific amounts of individual food groups. The 2015 to 2020 guidelines are summarized as follows; details and the entire repost are available at: https://health.gov/dietaryguidelines/2015/.

- Follow a healthy eating pattern across the life span. All food and beverage choices matter.
- Focus on variety, nutrient density, and amount.
- Limit calories from added sugars and saturated fats and reduce sodium intake.
- Shift to healthier food and beverage choices.
- Support healthy eating patterns for all.

Physical Activity

Physical activity must also be considered a part of any wellness assessment. Many more Americans are working at sedentary occupations and engage in less-active leisure activities. Insufficient exercise produces harmful consequences, not only for cardiovascular health and flexibility but also for psychological well-being. Sedentary lifestyles predispose individuals to fatigue, low self-esteem, and a host of health problems, including sleep disorders, obesity, prediabetes, and metabolic syndrome. The lifestyle assessment should include information about the type, frequency, and duration of physical activity during work and leisure time.

The Physical Activity Guidelines for Americans, released by the HHS, provides a comprehensive set of recommendations for Americans on the amounts and types of physical activity needed each day (https://health.gov/paguidelines/second-edition/report/). Adults need at least 150 minutes of moderate-intensity physical activity and should perform muscle-strengthening exercises on 2 or more days each week. Youth ages 6 to 17 years need at least 60 minutes of physical activity per day, including aerobic, muscle-strengthening, and bone-strengthening activities. Individuals can engage in regular physical activity in a variety of ways throughout the day and by choosing activities they enjoy. A list of federal resources, including handouts, online assessments, trackers, and interactive websites, is available at the aforementioned website. These can be used to help motivate patients to make healthy physical activity choices.

A concern for all patients as they age is a progressive loss of skeletal muscle mass and strength known as sarcopenia. Sarcopenia is most significant in older adults, and it contributes to an increased rate of falling with fracture, as well as functional loss that can impair ambulation and self-care. Sarcopenia is often associated with frailty, poor nutrition, and/or the cachexia of chronic disease. The problems associated with sarcopenia can be mitigated by regular strength training regardless of age. A short in-office screen for sarcopenia can be found at: https://www.researchgate.net/publication/243966215_SARC-F_A_Simple_Questionnaire_to_Rapidly_Diagnose_Sarcopenia.[4]

Stress. An individual's response to stress has the potential to produce detrimental effects on cardiovascular health and other organ systems. Understanding the nature of a particular stressor is an important process that can assist both patients and providers to plan more effective interventions. The provider should explore attributes of stress with the patient. What is the source of the stress? Is there a single stressor, or are there multiple stressors? What is the acuity level of the stress? Is the stress long-standing or newly acquired? Does the patient have prior experience in coping with the particular stressor? How effective are the patient's usual means of managing stress and what in particular has been effective?

Behavioral signs of stress manifest physically by rigidity and tightness of the body, such as folded or crossed arms or legs. Fists may be clenched to indicate anxiety, or the forehead may be furrowed to signify worry. Direct behavioral distress symptoms reflect internal states and include teeth grinding, irritability, compulsiveness, rapid speech, stuttering, verbal aggression, a withdrawn demeanor, and crying spells. Addictive and escape behaviors may be less obvious reactions to stress. An elevated level of stress can increase the frequency of unhealthy behaviors. Addictions may be observed in increased smoking, excessive alcohol consumption, and the use of drugs to mitigate tension or to induce sleep.

When questioned about stress in their lives, patients are often forthcoming with evidence and usually can identify their most significant stressors. Stress related to overload (even children are reporting feeling overloaded) is common and is characterized by an urgency about time. Other common sources of stress are interpersonal relationships, relationships within social or work domains, financial worries, and major life changes.

In general, stress is associated with negative or unpleasant situations. However, happy events and occasions can create a type of stress known as eustress. These events may include a marriage, the birth of a baby, buying a home, or winning the lottery. The stress accompanies the modifications in behavior required to adapt and to adjust to the change. The stress associated with the changes accompanying these pleasant events is often not consciously acknowledged but can nevertheless manifest as physical signs.

Many stress-relieving activities are available and can be very useful. These include maintaining a positive attitude, learning what stresses you personally, limiting alcohol and caffeine, getting enough sleep, meditation, deep breathing, regular exercise that incorporates gentle, mindful exercise programs such as yoga and tai chi, and maintaining close personal relationships. Establishing a realistic expectation of what can be accomplished in a day then practicing good time management can help to relieve anxiety and a feeling of being overburdened.

The relaxation response is an antidote to the physiologic alterations triggered by exposure to a stressor. Blood glucose levels decrease with relaxation, as do heart rate, respiration rate, and blood pressure. Muscles relax as well. Psychological advantages may include decreased anxiety and an enhanced ability to cope with fearful situations. Napping, walking, stroking a pet, participating in a hobby, listening to soothing music, and other activities can elicit the relaxation response. Breathing techniques are also effective for decreasing stress. Deep breathing involves two steps: (1) inhaling through the nose with the intention of inflating the lungs, and (2) exhaling through the mouth at a slower rate than inhaling. This is the "cleansing breath" many individuals learn in Lamaze classes. Another technique involves diaphragmatic breathing (i.e., using the diaphragm to regulate respiration). This is sometimes called "belly breathing," which can be observed in the way an infant breathes. The belly is thrust outward as a long, deep breath is taken. Because the relaxation occurs on exhalation, the exhalation should be long and slow.

INTERVENTIONS FOR THE EMOTIONAL DOMAIN

There is considerable overlap between those interventions that benefit the physical domain and the emotional domain. One area of great importance in all domains is the presence of healthy relationships in our lives. Relationships based on coercive or controlling behaviors exercised by one person over another can lead to stress and violence. Behaviors can range from economic control, social isolation, emotional abuse, and stalking and cyber stalking to sexual assault and threats of or actual physical violence and death. Domestic violence (aka intimate partner violence) or elder abuse occurs in all ages, racial, socioeconomic, and sexual orientation groups. This is a significant public health care problem with widespread and devastating effects for patients, their children, their families, and their communities. Individuals who experience these types of violent insults are at significant risk for physical injury, poor mental health, and chronic physical health problems.[5]

Psychosocial Indicators of Domestic Violence/Abuse

In addition to physical injuries and complaints, patients may experience a variety of psychosocial problems. A study supports the need for better understanding of the effects of nonphysical forms of abuse. Victims may be treated for symptoms of depression, anxiety or even recurring physical injuries without assessment for interpersonal violence (IPV); if these symptoms are taken out of context of the abuse, treatment may be ineffective. Psychologically, the victim can experience a complex traumatic stress response, which includes the symptoms of posttraumatic stress disorder—intrusive thoughts, nightmares, dissociative flashbacks, psychic numbness, hypervigilance, and exaggerated startle response. Victims commonly experience depression, anxiety, and their related symptoms, including anhedonia, difficulty concentrating, changes in sleep and eating patterns, depressed mood, somatization, decreased self-esteem, and suicidal ideations. There may be an alteration in affect (predominantly depressed or restricted), an alteration in perceptions of the perpetrator (seeing the abuser as omnipotent), and an alteration in the sense of self (disappearance of self and increased feelings of self-blame). This complex traumatic response can be immobilizing and can prevent the victim from escaping the abusive relationship or seeking help.

All patients seen in primary care should be screened for age-appropriate neglect or abuse, and help should be offered to address this growing threat. There are local resources available in every state, and a national hotline at 1-800-799-7233 (https://www.thehotline.org/).

SUBSTANCE USE

Focusing on health and wellness is particularly important for people with, or at risk for, behavioral health conditions. Behavioral health is a critical aspect of maintaining physical health and wellness. People with mental and/or substance use disorders typically die years earlier than the general population. The use of prescription drugs and/or illicit street drugs is a crisis of epidemic proportion in the United States.[6] In 2017 there were 72,000 overdose deaths. A 2006 nationally representative survey reported that individuals with mental disorders died an average of 8.2 years younger than the rest of the population.[6] Individuals with substance use conditions are often at higher risk for HIV and AIDS and hepatitis C due to intravenous drug use. Substance use is discussed extensively in Chapter 227.

Smoking continues to be a major health risk for Americans. Smoking cessation programs are available to all, often at the state level, with Medicaid reimbursement for pharmacologic aides such as nicotine gum and patches. Assistance with prescription drugs such as Chantix is also often available. It is never too late to stop smoking, and patients should be supported through this difficult transition, with all available resources. Prevention programs aimed at teens also need the support of medical and educational professional, as well as parents and peers. See https://www.cdc.gov/tobacco/quit_smoking/how_to_quit/resources/index.htm or websites in your state.

While great strides have been made in the United States regarding reducing the numbers of cigarette smokers, the use of e-cigarettes, sometimes known as "vaping," has reached epidemic proportions among teens and young adults. Marketed in a variety of flavors, this nicotine delivery system is especially appealing to young people. In 2018, more than 3.6 million U.S. middle and high school students used e-cigarettes in the past 30 days, including 4.9% of middle school students and 20.8% of high school students (https://www.cdc.gov/tobacco/basic_information/e-cigarettes/about-e-cigarettes.html#references). The surgeon general has issued a report discussing the dangers of e-cigarettes and recommending strategies for reducing their use especially among young people who may not understand the toxic risk and addiction potential of these benign appearing devices (https://e-cigarettes.surgeongeneral.gov).[7]

SAFETY

Home safety consists of opportunities to prevent accidents and provide a safe environment in which to live. According to the National Safety Council, there were 161,374 unintentional injury–related deaths in 2016, most in the home, making this the third leading cause of death in the United States (https://www.safetyandhealthmagazine.com/articles/16581-unintentional-injuries-third-leading-cause-of-death-nsc). Securing a safe home requires focusing in several key areas:
- Preventing poisoning from chemicals, gases, and, most importantly, prescription drug use and abuse.
- Screening homes for fall risks, especially where older adults are living.
- Preventing drowning, especially of children left unsupervised in the bathtubs or pools.

- Preventing fires associated with faulty electrical systems, fireplaces, space heaters, and so forth.
- Understanding when and how to intervene if someone is choking on food.
- Establishing your personal and family disaster plan and your community disaster planning.
- Locking unloaded guns securely and storing ammunition separately.
  Home safety checklists are available from many organizations, including:
  https://www.nsc.org/home-safety.
  https://www.usfa.fema.gov/downloads/pdf/home_safety_checklist.pdf.
  https://assets.aarp.org/external_sites/caregiving/checklists/checklist_homeSafety.html.

Part of securing a safe environment is planning for natural or other community disasters. Individuals must know what disasters and hazards could affect your area, how to get emergency alerts, and where you would go if you and your family need to evacuate. Disasters recently experienced by many Americans include floods, hurricanes, tornados, wildfires, landslides, volcanos, pandemics, and active shooters. Talking with family members about plans for communicating and a central meeting place is essential. Some families may want to keep a "go" bag or disaster preparedness kit stocked and ready in the event of an unexpected event. Being familiar with community disaster plans, including safe evacuation sites, makes the entire community safer. See https://www.ready.gov/be-informed for detailed plans and recommendations.

INTEGRATIVE HEALTH CARE AND ALTERNATIVE THERAPIES

Many patients will choose to add alternative therapies to Western medical approaches to wellness or even use these approaches exclusively. This is known as integrative medicine and defined as the "practice of medicine that reaffirms the importance of the relationship between practitioner and patient, focuses on the whole person, is informed by evidence, and makes use of all appropriate therapeutic approaches, healthcare professionals, and disciplines to achieve optimal health and healing" (https://www.abpsus.org/integrative-medicine-defined).

This approach recognizes the biologic, psychological, sociological, and spiritual dimensions inherent in each patient and each patient encounter. This approach combines Western and Eastern health practices, energy therapies and nutritional recommendations, dietary supplements, and environmental health recommendations into health care decisions by:

- Educating and empowering people to be active participants in their own care.
- Integrating the best of Western medicine science with a broader understanding of the nature of illness, healing, and wellness.
- Supporting the individualization of care within healing partnerships between patient and provider.
- Creating a culture of wellness.

General good health and well-being depends on the integration of wellness strategies and reliable access to primary care providers. Primary care providers can act as coaches, cheerleaders, and educators about physical and mental health issues and our patient's access to and acceptance of healthy lifestyle options.

STAYING WELL WHILE TRAVELING

As international travel and studying abroad, as well as medical volunteerism with aide groups traveling to disaster sites, become more common, health care providers will need to become more knowledgeable about travel medicine and the relevant health care issues for international travel. At the very least, providers should have fully explored the travel health care options around them and should be prepared to make referrals for travelers who require additional services. Travelers with any underlying or chronic illness should be well prepared to manage the common minor complications or manifestations of their illness for themselves and should know which signs and symptoms should prompt them to seek professional medical care. All travelers should attend to their routine health care maintenance needs before travel and should be educated about how to improve their personal safety and reduce their risk from injury in a motor vehicle accident. Travelers should receive the vaccines that are required (e.g., yellow fever or meningococcal vaccine) or recommended (e.g., hepatitis A and B, typhoid fever, rabies, Japanese encephalitis) for their itinerary, preferably 4 to 6 weeks before departure. They also must be offered appropriate information about mosquito and other vector transmitted diseases, malaria prophylaxis, and malaria education if there is any risk of malaria at their destination (see Chapter 215). Travelers should also clearly understand basic food and water precautions and how to manage traveler's diarrhea (see Chapter 211) if it occurs. They should know how to protect themselves against sexually transmitted infections and pathogens spread person-to-person through the respiratory tract. Finally, travelers should be advised to understand their own health care plan benefits when traveling, research the best sources of medical care in the countries they will be visiting, and make informed decisions about whether they will obtain travel or medical evacuation insurance before departure. The CDC maintains an excellent website that provides information on immunizations for a particular destination, travel alerts, travel resources for travelers and clinicians, and other important useful information. See https://wwwnc.cdc.gov/travel/.

REFERENCES

1. Wellness defined. Retrieved from https://www.merriam-webster.com.
2. https://www.samhsa.gov/wellness-initiative/eight-dimensions-wellness.
3. Heron, M. (2018). Deaths: Leading causes for 2016. *NVSS*, 67(6).
4. Malmstrom, T., & Morley, J. (2013). SARC-F: A simple questionnaire to rapidly diagnose sarcopenia. *Journal of the American Medical Directors Association*, *14*, doi:10.1016/j.jamda.2013.05.018.
5. Smith, S. G., Zhang, X., Basile, K. C., et al. (2018). The National Intimate Partner and Sexual Violence Survery (NISVS): 2015 Data Brief—Updated Release. Atlanta, GA: National Center for Injury Prevention and Control, Centers for Disease Control and Prevention.
6. Schiller, E. Y., & Mechanic, O. J. Opioid overdose. [Updated 2019 Mar 2]. In: StatPearls [Internet]. Treasure Island (FL): StatPearls Publishing; 2019 Jan-. Retrieved from https://www.ncbi.nlm.nih.gov/books/NBK470415/.
7. https://e-cigarettes.surgeongeneral.gov/documents/surgeon-generals-advisory-on-e-cigarette-use-among-youth-2018.pdf.

CHAPTER 17

OBESITY AND WEIGHT MANAGEMENT

Sharon L. Grantham

DEFINITION AND EPIDEMIOLOGY

Obesity is a worldwide problem of epidemic proportions. Globally, nearly 2.5 billion adults are affected by overweight (OW) or obesity (OB) (body mass index [BMI] of 25 kg/m^2 and 30 kg/m^2 or greater, respectively). It is associated with an estimated 3.4 million deaths, 3.9% years of life lost, and 3.8% of disability-adjusted life-years (DALYs).[1] From 1975 to 2014 the global age-standardized BMI increased from 21.7 kg/m^2 to 24.2 kg/m^2 in men, and from 22.1 to 24.4 kg/m^2 in women. These averages increased to 1.5 kg per decade across all populations. The mean men's and women's adults' BMIs in American Samoa, Polynesia, and Micronesia, as well as the mean women's BMI in some Middle Eastern and north African countries and the Caribbean, is over 30 kg/m^2. In developed countries, the increase in adult OB has slowed due to public health concern and efforts. However, the global increase in BMI has not slowed. The probability of global OB reduction, as targeted, is virtually zero, according to predicted trends.[2]

In the United States, the estimated crude prevalence of adults with OB was 39.8% according to data from the 2015 to 2016 National Health and Nutrition Examination Survey (NHANES).[3]

OB affects different ages and populations variably. OB rates are lowest (12.7%) among non-Hispanic Asians. Hispanics (47%) and non-Hispanic blacks (46.8%) are higher than non-Hispanic white adults (38%). By age, adults age 40 to 59 years have higher OB prevalence in men (40.8%) and women (44.7%). Among US non-Hispanic black women, 54.8% have OB compared with 50.6% of Hispanic and 38% of non-Hispanic white women.[4] Food insecurity is modestly associated with higher OB rates in US women but not in men, and the relationship is stronger in non-white women.[5] Level of education is inversely related to OB and OW.[5] In immigrant adults born outside the United States, OB rates increase with time lived in the United States and vary among countries of origin. US adults born in Mexico, South America, Europe, Russia, Africa, and the Middle East have a three-times-higher odds ratio (OR) of being OW after 15 years compared with their counterparts who have resided less than 5 years in the United States. Among immigrants from the Indian subcontinent and Southeast Asia, excess weight increases begin earlier. In young women migrants from Africa and the Indian subcontinent, the OR of being OW is higher than in those from Europe.[6] Of US military veterans, 78% are affected by OB or OW.[7]

Body Mass Index and Waist Circumference

BMI is a proxy measure of body fatness, more accurate than weight alone, and is easy and inexpensive to use in clinical settings. It is a simple numeric calculation of weight in kilograms divided by height in meters squared (BMI = kg/m^2). English measurement conversion involves a multiplier of 703: BMI = (pounds/inches^2) × 703.

BMI is a screening tool, with low specificity, and is to be used as a screening tool rather than a definitive diagnostic standard. There are limitations in using BMI as a standard for determining excess body fat in association with increased disease risk, OW, and OB. The BMI measurement does not account for body fat percentage, body fat distribution, body frame size, capacity for metabolic activity, and amount of lean tissue, such as muscle and bone. A BMI calculation does not account for muscularity resulting from physical training, puberty or menopause status, race or ethnicity, gender, limb length, limb amputations, spinal deformities, or sarcopenia related to aging.[8] For example, physically fit individuals with increased muscle mass may have a high BMI measurement indicating erroneously that they are OW and at risk for the complications of OB. Patients with BMI under 25, and of Asian descent, especially when accompanied by excess abdominal fat and enlarged waist circumference, may have OB-associated metabolic disturbances. Despite its limitation, screening for OB through use of BMI is recommended for all adults.[7,8]

Waist circumference as a reliable surrogate adipose measure is clinically practical because of its low cost, portability, and ease of use. Even with variable user techniques and guideline differences about tape measure locations for waist circumference, the strong association of central adiposity with higher morbidity and mortality is maintained. This waist circumference relationship is strongest for adverse cardiovascular and cancer outcomes and is more robust in women than in men. Waist-to-hip ratios indicate increasing cardiometabolic disease risk as the ratio increases in men and women (larger waist compared with smaller hips), and the risk increases with circumference. In North American adults with BMI between 25 and 35 kg/m^2, waist measurement circumference of 102 cm (40 inches) or greater in men and 89 cm (35 inches) or greater in women indicates increased cardiometabolic risk. These cutoff values are lower in individuals of European, South Asian, Chinese, or Japanese origin as compared with North American cutoffs with regard to cardiometabolic disease risks.[9] Annual measurement is indicated. However, in individuals with a BMI above 35, elevated waist circumference is not likely to provide additional information regarding disease risk.[9]

Reliable measures of adiposity include hydrodensitometry (underwater weighing), air displacement plethysmography, dual-energy X-ray absorptiometry (DXA), computed tomography (CT) scan, and magnetic resonance imaging (MRI), which are used in research settings but are not practical in routine clinical use.

Bioimpedance Analysis

Bioimpedance analysis (BIA) predicts body fat and lean mass by use of alternating current that passes through the body. BIA is noninvasive, portable, safe, and inexpensive. It allows practitioners to estimate body fat in a clinic setting and is often used in weight loss research; patients may be familiar with it because BIA instruments are present in some fitness centers and available for consumer home use. Results are comparable to those of DXA and hydrostatic weighing and are reliable. BIA has disadvantages that include variable results according to hydration status and recent physical activity. Its use in elders, children, and those with high levels of physical fitness are not as reliable. Men with body fat higher than 25% and women with body fat higher than 30% are considered to have OB.[10] Guidelines for treatment of OW and OB do not recommend the use of BIA in routine clinical application because it adds no more information than BMI and waist circumference and requires additional resources.[9]

PATHOPHYSIOLOGY

Determinants of energy balance and OB are many, complex, interrelated, and not fully elucidated; determinants alone do not fully explain OB's prevalence, severity, or unequal distribution. Understanding this can facilitate a more compassionate approach to people with OB and OW. The causes of common OB are multifactorial with two commonalities: increased energy intake and reduced energy expenditure. These obesogenic factors—kilocalorie abundance in a sedentary environment—interact with genetic predispositions in complex obesogenic systems favoring increasing adiposity storage. Excess body weight and OB result when the energy intake and conserving energy expenditure forces are greater than the opposing forces.

In those with OB, the homeostatic balance between energy intake and energy expenditure is dysfunctional, resulting in excess energy stored in adipose tissue to the extent that this excess adipose negatively affects health with signs, symptoms, harm, and morbidity. An obesogenic environment has myriad contributors, including genetic factors, excess calorie intake, reduced physical activity, increased sedentary behavior, gut microbiome, environmental contributions, prenatal conditions, hyper-palatable food, and food industry promotion to increase consumption. OB is considered a chronic disease disorder. As such, it requires chronic disease management, perpetual care, support, and follow-up.[8,9,11]

Adipose tissue is composed of adipocytes (fat cells that store energy as triglycerides plus glycerol), preadipocytes, vascular structures, fibroblasts, endothelial cells, and macrophages.[12] The size and number of adipocytes vary across body regions; more deleterious health consequences are linked with hypertrophied fat cells in the intra-abdominal area visceral fat depots compared with subcutaneous or femoral-hip fat deposits. Adipose tissue functions include energy storage, body structure cushioning, and complex endocrine, exocrine, paracrine, inflammation, and immune roles. Adipose tissue has embryonic origins and may contain only one lipid droplet in the immature state.

Individual appetite, satiety, and meal size are driven by neuroendocrine factors, adipocyte size and number, gut factors, food availability, society norms, and nutrient interactions that occur in the context of cultural, economic, and genetic environments. An abundance of food is needed for OB to develop, but variations occur across genotypes, age at exposure, source and quality of food, conscious efforts to control kilocalorie intake, hormone status, endocrine disruptors, medications, and as yet undefined environmental interactions. In theory, an extra 100 kcal/day taken in or not expended can result in a gain of 4.5 kg (10 pounds) per year. But research has proven complex interactions of OB that cannot be explained by simple kcal equations. Acknowledging these can foster more compassionate care for those with OB.

Individual energy intake and output balance factors are of great interest to OB researchers. The central nervous system (CNS) controls energy intake through appetite, hunger, and satiety; the drive for energy expenditure occurs mainly in the hypothalamus, with feedback from adipose tissue, muscle, liver, pancreas, and gut signals. Insulin and leptin signal adequacy of food and adipose tissue; gut hormones send satiety signals during meals. A competing system between anorexic neuron and orexigenic neuron activity controls in the arcuate nucleus of the hypothalamus regulates food intake, energy expenditure, and glucose homeostasis. The orexin pathway is mediated by agouti-related protein/neuropeptide Y (AgRP/NPY) neurons; they promote hunger and increased food intake and conserve energy by inhibiting activities that use energy. Anorexic neurons, pro-opiomelanocortin (POMC) and cocaine-amphetamine–regulated transcript (CART), drive anorexia and energy-expending, catabolic processes. Both neuron populations signal alternatively through the melanocortin receptors (MC4R and MC3R).

The competing systems are asymmetric, with redundancy in the mechanisms regulating hunger and conservation of energy as well as stronger drivers in the orexigenic hunger and energy-conserving pathways. Overriding of the satiety system's homeostasis can occur with hyper-palatable, hedonic foods, which have high neurally mediated rewarding properties. Highly rewarding sights and sounds and palatable layering of flavors contribute to hedonic rewards of food. The hedonic pathway is especially activated with the combination of sweet plus fatty foods. Hedonic hunger occurs when there is no physiologic basis for perceived energy needs. The amount of work needed to obtain food, the food's hedonic qualities, and the quantity of food available override homeostatic energy balance mechanisms.[13,14]

Dopamine- and opioid-mediated pleasure and reward pathways in the brain can become fixed and hardwired to crave sweet plus high-fat foods. Hyperinsulinemia, common in people with OB and metabolic syndrome, prevents dopamine clearance from the pleasure centers, so pleasure from food is enhanced and intake continues beyond energy needs.[15] People with OB also have lower dopamine D_2 receptor activity in negative correlation with BMI when it is measured by positron emission tomography. Motivation to eat and pleasure or reward may be dysfunctional, inhibitory satiety processes may be disrupted, and increased eating with OW and OB results.

Lesions—chemically caused, inherited, or arising from structural damage to the hypothalamus—can induce hyperphagia by suppressing POMC and CART neurons and MC3R and MC4R, so satiety signaling is impaired, energy output is reduced, and hunger increases. Causes of hypothalamic OB include head trauma, cranial surgery, ventriculoperitoneal shunt placement, hypothalamic radiation therapy, antipsychotic medications, and tumors; they are associated with rapid weight gain, uncontrolled eating, reduced energy expenditure, and hyperinsulinemia.[16]

Adipocytes in white adipose tissue store extra energy through insulin, affecting lipid and glucose uptake by glucose transporter type 4 (GLUT4) and other transporters. Insulin is the hormonal central controller of energy balance. Higher insulin levels, whether endogenous or exogenous, promote greater uptake of energy (glucose) in fat and muscle cells and inhibit lipolysis, or fat breakdown. Pancreatic β cells secrete insulin in response to food intake, glucose and fatty acid uptake is facilitated, and glycogenesis (glucose storage in muscle or hepatic tissue) is inhibited. In a fasted state, glucagon is released from pancreatic α cells to maintain euglycemia by stimulating hepatic gluconeogenesis and glycogenolysis.[17] Insulin, whether it is endogenous or exogenous, not only inhibits lipolysis (the use of stored lipids) but also stimulates de novo free fatty acid synthesis.[17] Decreased pancreatic insulin secretion occurs in the absence of dietary carbohydrates, and lower insulin levels will increase the use of stored fat.[18] Insulin, along with leptin, crosses the blood-brain barrier and signals satiety in the lateral hypothalamus.[17] Central, CNS administration of insulin antibodies results in increased food intake and weight gain, and inactivated insulin receptors plus excess food results in OB. In addition to lower insulin levels, adrenal epinephrine and norepinephrine released during exercise promote use of stored fat.[18]

Leptin, a hormone secreted by adipocytes, acts as a long-term "lipostat"; it communicates the amount of stored body fat to the hypothalamus. Leptin secretion by adipocytes increases in parallel with increases in fat mass. Leptin and insulin receptors in the hypothalamus are saturable, contributing to central leptin and insulin resistance in OB. In leptin resistance, higher levels fail to initiate an anorectic plus increased energy expenditure effect that should follow an overabundance of stored energy. Leptin is also secreted by gastric mucosa, along with cholecystokinin, and relays gut information to the CNS that results in satiety and controls meal size.[17] Leptin levels reflect subcutaneous fat more than visceral adipose tissue and are higher in women. Adipokines are cytokines of adipose tissue origin and include leptin, adiponectin, and tumor necrosis factor-α (TNF-α) among others.[12] Adiponectin secreted by adipocytes is inversely proportionate to fat mass; higher fat masses are associated with lower serum levels. Adiponectin has beneficial effects on glycemic control, insulin sensitivity, and nonatherogenic lipid profiles and has anti-inflammatory properties. Visceral adipose tissue secretes less adiponectin than subcutaneous depots do. TNF-α is an inflammatory cytokine secreted from resident macrophages of adipose tissues in proportion to BMI.[12]

Gut hormones involved with energy homeostasis include ghrelin, a potent gastric orexigen that signals hunger through arcuate nucleus–released AgRP/NPY to drive increased food intake. Cholecystokinin, in response to protein and fat ingestion, is secreted from the small bowel; it stimulates pancreatic digestive enzymes and gallbladder contraction and sends satiety signals through the vagus nerve to the hindbrain. Glucagon-like peptide 1 (GLP-1) from the bowel also acts as a CNS satiety signal, slows gastric emptying, and regulates glucose by alternating insulin and glucagon activity.[17]

Energy Output

Energy is needed for physical activity, digestion of food, heat liberation from brown adipose tissue, and maintenance of the minimal essential functions of body organs. These essential energy needs constitute 50% to 70% of a sedentary person's energy output and collectively make up the basal metabolic rate (BMR). BMR varies according to gender, thyroid activity, smoking status, growth hormone levels, skeletal muscle mass, and fever. The remaining energy output is expended in purposeful physical activity (25%), nonexercise activity (7%), and the thermic effect of food (8%).[18] Processing, digesting, absorbing, and storing of food after meals raise the metabolic rate. This increased metabolic, thermogenic effect of food can be about 4% after a high-carbohydrate meal and as much as 30% after ingestion of a high-protein meal.[18]

Insufficient Physical Activity

Lack of physical activity is risk factor for OB and its related comorbidities, type 2 diabetes mellitus (T2DM), cardiovascular disease, hypertension, stroke, breast and colon cancer, and other health concerns.[19] Moderate to vigorous levels of recommended activity are based on promotion and maintenance of health. Recommended endurance (aerobic) exercise minimums are 30 min/day for moderate-intensity or 20 min/day for vigorous-intensity physical activity, in bouts of 10 minutes or more. Brisk walking at 3 mph, bicycling at 10 to 12 mph, and dancing are moderate, expending 3.0 to 6.0 metabolic equivalents (METs). Jogging, shoveling, and bicycling at 12 to 16 mph are vigorous activities that expend more than 6.0 METs. The health benefits of physical activity are dose dependent. For preventing weight gain, maintaining weight loss, or relying on physical activity as a primary means to weight loss, more than the minimum (150 minutes of moderate or 60 to 75 minutes of vigorous physical activity accumulated per week) may be necessary. Most studies and recommendations support as much as 300 minutes of moderate-intensity activity per week, or about 1 h/day, to avoid weight gain or to prevent regain after weight loss.[20] Less than half of US adults get the recommended minimum level of physical activity, and more than one in five have no leisure-time activity.[19] Physical activity energy expenditure is frequently distorted, and even among adults educated in guidelines, distortions persist about actual activity performed. It is common to overestimate the relative kilocalories expended in various physical activities and also to overestimate the amount of one's physical activity.[21]

Energy Intake

Energy intake has increased by 150 to 300 kcal/day during the last 30 years, with about half of these calories from sugar-sweetened beverages. Liquid kilocalories do not have the stronger satiety signaling properties of solid foods, and sugar-sweetened beverages may contribute to hedonic rewards that mediate greater kilocalorie ingestion.[21] Factors contributing to this include media consumption, food exposure, more food-efficient consumption, nutritional quality of food and drink, variety, and grazing habits. Observation of the proximate and conventional approaches to OB management and those links that promote greater intake of energy highlights the pressing number of factors to be overcome in managing persons with OB.

Genetics

OB genes are those that influence BMI, waist-to-hip ratio, eating behaviors, energy expenditure, and abdominal fat, with overlap for genes that influence lipids, blood pressure, insulin, and nutrient partitioning. Putative loci are on all chromosomes except Y. The understanding of gene-environment contributions to obese phenotypes is continuing to expand, as is discovery of how genes can be silenced or activated by environmental triggers. Genome-wide association studies support theories that interactions of multiple genes contribute to OB.[22]

Adiposity is a heritable, quantitative trait. BMI, as a measure of adiposity, can vary quantitatively. For example, a 5-foot, 8-inch person's BMI can range from 16 to 60 kg/m^2 (105 to 400 pounds). Gene pool shifts cannot account for the sharp increase in global OB; a gene-environment effect offers more likely explanations, with abundant food supply a necessary component. Family and twin studies have confirmed strong heritable factors in BMI, accounting for as much as 45% to 75% variance. Maternal OB has a stronger effect than paternal

OB, perhaps from the prenatal and postnatal environment, with sex difference correlations in offspring OB. Genetic contributions for macronutrient preferences, restrained and binge eating, meal size, and activity levels have been studied.[23]

Monogenic causes of OB are rare and are associated with MC4R-mediated appetite control center disruption involving satiety and energy expenditure signaling dysfunctions. Normally, adiposity increases coincide with increased circulating leptin from adipose tissue, which signals satiety. In *MC4R* mutations, rising leptin levels fail to signal satiety by MC4R mechanisms. More than 130 *MC4R* mutations are known; most confer extra OB risk.

Inborn leptin deficiency is rare, but treatment with recombinant leptin results in substantial fat loss as hyperphagic, all-day eating patterns cease. Mutations for leptin, leptin receptor, and prohormone convertase 1 and *POMC* genes result in early, severe OB, along with specific phenotype characteristics. The two most common syndrome obesities are Prader-Willi and Bardet-Biedl.[24]

Polygenic OB, the most common type, is caused by expression of additive and nonadditive effects of multiple alleles that control the quantitative BMI phenotype. Perhaps 100 polygenic variants, each with small effect sizes of less than 100 g, are present uniquely in individuals with OB.[23,24] The fat mass and OB gene, *FTO*, is recognized as the strongest OB signaling gene; yet the *FTO* BMI effects are small, accounting for less than 0.5% variance, about 6 pounds.[22]

Maternal and Early-Life Influences

Metabolic programming begins at least in utero and during the preconception period. It may begin sooner in maternal grandmothers' gestation. The hypothalamic appetite center, adipocytes, and insulin-glucose homeostasis are sensitive to the gestational environment. High maternal glucose concentration—130 mg/dL or higher—even in healthy BMI mothers without gestational diabetes, is associated with a doubled risk for OW or OB in toddlers compared with gestational glucose concentration below 100 mg/dL.[25] Excessive maternal weight during pregnancy is associated with higher childhood and adult OB in the offspring.[5] After birth, early feeding practices continue to influence BMI. Breastfeeding may confer a decreased risk for childhood, adolescent, and adult OB, and has been associated with reduced maternal cardiometabolic risks decades later[26] during the mother's menopause years. Breastfeeding infants are self-regulators of their intake and do not ingest more even when maternal milk supplies are intentionally increased. Leptin from maternal mammary secretion may signal infant satiety and affect hypothalamic appetite. In addition to leptin, the hormones adiponectin, insulin-like growth factor 1, resistin, and obestatin are found in human milk and may be part of early nutritional programming in developing hypothalamic appetite and energy output control centers. These human milk peptides could have effects beyond the time of lactation. Formula-fed infants have higher serum ghrelin (hunger hormone) levels.[5] Timing of solid food introduction may have variable effects on weight gain based on formula feeding versus breastfeeding. Formula-fed infants had greater odds of OB at the age of 3 years when solid foods were introduced before 4 months of age compared with breastfed infants.[27] Cortisol levels in human milk may contribute to intestinal villi maturation and early metabolic programming that confers protection against later OB.

Famine, resulting from natural causes or war, has given evidence of long-lasting effects on offspring OB that manifest in toddlerhood and midlife, preferentially in female children, from poorly nourished mothers during gestation. These children are shorter and, as adults, remain short with a greater risk of OB 50 years later.[28] Maternal smoking during pregnancy is associated with 50% increased odds of OB in children and young adults, ages 3 to 33 years.[29]

Smoking Status and Smoking Cessation

The BMIs of cigarette smokers tend to be lower than those of nonsmokers, but their visceral fat stores are greater even without increased waist circumferences. Weight gain related to smoking cessation occurs in the majority of quitters, occurs mostly in the early months after cessation, and is typically 10 pounds or less. Weight gain predictors after cessation include younger age, higher baseline BMI, smoking more than 25 cigarettes per day, African-American race, pregnancy, and genetic predisposition. Weight gain concerns can be barriers to smoking cessation, especially in women. Nicotine also acts as an appetite suppressant, more so when it is combined with caffeine.[30] Further effects of nicotine include increased metabolic rate, about 200 kcal/25 cigarettes, decreased NPY and orexin (both increase food intake), suppression of fat storage effects from adipose tissue protein lipase, and changes in leptin levels. Weight gain from smoking cessation tends to involve visceral, centrally located adipose tissue and is accompanied by worsening of other metabolic syndrome components, except high-density lipoprotein cholesterol (HDL-C). The risk for diabetes increases in early years after smoking cessation, and this seems to be associated with weight gain. However, diabetes risk drops significantly in subsequent years. Nicotine replacement therapy with bupropion or varenicline may delay weight gain associated with smoking cessation, but the gain typically occurs when these therapies are discontinued. Some individuals use cigarette smoking, and possibly electronic cigarettes (e-cigarettes), as a means of weight control. In past years the tobacco industry promoted smoking as "slimming" and as an alternative to snacking.[31] The health benefits of smoking cessation exceed the short-term metabolic weight gain and in general take priority over weight concerns. Use of other nicotine delivery methods, such as the increasingly popular e-cigarettes, should be discussed as possible unhealthy weight control strategies used by individuals.

Pharmaceuticals Associated With Weight Gain

Genetic variations contribute to different metabolic responses to the weight gain effects of pharmaceuticals. CNS-mediated weight gain is associated with antidepressants, antipsychotics, anticonvulsants, mood stabilizers, and migraine prophylaxis agents. Many anti-diabetic medications are associated with significant weight gain, which compromises health and increases risk factors for cardiovascular disease.[32–34]

Diabetes Medications. *Insulin and insulin analogues increase weight more than other anti-diabetic drugs, through multiple means.* Prandial and bi-phasic regimens are associated with greater weight gains than basal insulins. Glycosuria calories are recovered, lipolysis is inhibited, triglyceride and glucose storage in adipocytes is upregulated, appetite increases, and anabolic protein and adipose synthesis increases. Expected weight gain trends along with expected improvement in hemoglobin A1C (HbA_{1c}): additional 2 to 10 kg for 1.5% to 2.5%

improvements. Insulin secretagogues—sulfonylureas especially, but also meglitinides—have a similar effect; as insulin levels increase, the anabolic effects result from more insulin. Thiazolidinediones increase appetite, fat mass through the adipogenic effects of peroxisome proliferator-activated receptor γ (PPAR-γ), and fluid retention and may cause 0.5 to 1.4 kg weight gain. Metformin may be weight negative (−0.5 to −4.5 kg) initially because of gastrointestinal (GI) side effects, but also because of reduced hepatic glucose output and stimulation of GLP-1 endogenous release without an increase in insulin output. GLP-1 receptor agonists and amylin analogues are associated with weight loss. Dipeptidyl peptidase 4 inhibitors and α-glucosidase inhibitors are weight neutral.[32,35] Sodium-glucose-linked transporter-2 (SGLT-2) medications are associated with weight loss.[34]

Antidepressants, Neuroleptic and Seizure Medications. Tricyclic antidepressants (TCAs) are hypothesized to increase carbohydrate craving because of anti-histaminergic effects, altering hypothalamic neuromodulated food-energy balance toward increasing fat stores and decreasing energy expenditures. Amitriptyline is associated with the highest gain. Resting metabolic rate decreases during TCA treatment. Irreversible monoamine oxidase inhibitors (MAOIs) are also associated with weight gain. Selective serotonin reuptake inhibitors (SSRIs) are commonly prescribed. SSRIs disrupt appetite stimulation through changes in 5-hydroxytryptamine type 2 C and histamine H_1 receptors and may induce carbohydrate cravings. These agents may result in an initial weight loss, followed by weight gain. Paroxetine is the most weight-positive SSRI, especially in women. Mirtazapine has been associated with 11% weight gain, mostly in the early time period. Lithium weight gain tends to peak within the first 2 years and is greater in those with greater baseline BMI. Lithium's weight gain effects possibly result from increased carbohydrate craving, increased storage of carbohydrates and lipids, and lower BMR from reduced thyroid function. The antidepressant venlafaxine is weight neutral, and bupropion is associated with 1.0- to 4.4-kg weight loss.[32,33,35]

Atypical antipsychotics have potent orexigenic effects of reversing leptin's hypothalamic anorectic effect, upregulating adenosine monophosphate-activated protein kinase, blocking a histamine receptor, stimulating appetite, and causing central insulin resistance, all of which contribute to weight gain of 2 to 17 kg, impaired glucose handling, diabetes, and dyslipidemia. Clozapine and olanzapine cause the greatest weight gains, which tend to be dose dependent. Risperidone and quetiapine weight gains are more modest and possibly dose dependent. Aripiprazole, olanzapine, and zotepine are associated with less weight gain.[32,33]

Valproic acid elevates leptin and insulin levels and decreases gluconeogenesis, β-oxidation of fatty acids, albumin binding with long-chain fatty acids, and energy expenditure, all of which contribute to weight gain that continues even after years of treatment. Carbamazepine, pregabalin, and gabapentin are associated with weight gain. Lamotrigine, levetiracetam, and oxcarbazepine are weight neutral, whereas topiramate and zonisamide promote weight loss.[32,33]

Antihistamines. The weight gain effects of antihistamines are mediated by blockade of H_1 receptors. H_1 activity promotes satiety; hence, blockade increases appetite with possible increased carbohydrate cravings. Antihistamine users have higher BMIs, waist circumferences, and insulin levels.

Cyproheptadine is especially appetite stimulating. Loratadine and desloratadine are associated with little or no weight gain. Weight gain is proportionate to CNS effect, and less sedating agents less weight positive.[32,33,35]

Human immunodeficiency disease treatment with antiretroviral therapy has been associated with a weight gain of 8.6 kg, in one study. The metabolic effects of antiretrovirals lead to redistribution of fat from subcutaneous to visceral depots as well as insulin resistance, resulting in unavoidable weight gain, lipodystrophy, and increased waist circumference.[33,35]

Hormonal Preparations. Combined hormone contraceptives and menopause hormone replacement are not associated with weight gain in population studies, but individual responses could vary. Women using oral contraceptives (OC) do not respond to a higher protein diet's increase in postprandial energy that is present in women not taking OC and men.[34] Progesterone-only contraceptive medroxyprogesterone injections may increase fat gains without increasing appetite, but the effect may be limited to adolescents with preexisting OW condition.[32] The levonorgestrel-releasing intrauterine system also lists weight gain as a side effect in its provider information. Megestrol stimulates appetite. Tamoxifen and aromatase inhibitors have mixed reports about weight gain. Corticosteroids increase weight, especially centrally located fat, by impairing glucose tolerance. All administration routes, including inhaled corticosteroids, have been implicated in weight gains.[32]

Cardiac Medications. β blockade inhibits β-adrenergic satiety effects and lipolysis, reduces thermogenic responses to food, reduces BMR, and reduces energy expenditure. β blockers also increase insulin resistance and serum triglycerides, and because visceral fat depots have more β-adrenergic receptors, visceral fat could increase.[32] Blockade of sympathetic activity was researched in hypertensive, β blocker–treated participants compared with weight-matched controls. Results demonstrated that treated individuals had higher BMI, 50% lower thermogenic responses to food, 32% lower fat oxidation rate, and 30% lower energy expenditure from physical activity. β blockers with a vasodilating effect, carvedilol and nebivolol, are associated with less weight gain and perturbed glucose.[35] Calcium channel blockers can increase edema but not fat gains. Central-acting $α_2$-adrenergic receptor agonists can decrease metabolic rate and increase appetite.[32]

Environmental Factors

An endocrine-disrupting substance is defined by the US Environmental Protection Agency as "an exogenous agent that interferes with synthesis, secretion, transport, metabolism, binding action, or elimination of natural hormones that are present in the body and are responsible for homeostasis, reproduction, and developmental process."[36] Endocrine disrupters acting as obesogens may be pharmaceuticals, environmental toxins, and food components that promote fat accumulation through several pathways. The disruptions can occur in metabolic sensing, sex steroid regulation, central (hypothalamic) energy balance, adipogenesis, and metabolic set-points.[37] The exposure effects vary according to timing of exposure (perinatal and developmental periods), levels of exposure, and synergistic interactions with multiple endocrine disrupters; the effects may have latent expression and in some cases be transmitted across multiple generations. Adipose tissue stores and concentrates many fat-soluble compounds, and a positive correlation exists between BMI and endocrine disrupter burden.

Environmental estrogens can affect lipogenesis, lipolysis, adipocyte production of leptin, and estrogen receptors. Genistein, found in soy, in low concentrations seems to inhibit lipogenesis through its binding with estrogen receptors, but in high concentrations, genistein promotes lipogenesis through PPAR-γ receptors. Bisphenol A (BPA) has an impact on pancreatic β cell function, is associated with hyperinsulinemia, inhibits adiponectin (thus reducing insulin sensitivity), and increases susceptibility to OB comorbidities, metabolic syndrome, and T2DM. BPA may increase estrogen receptor expression in the hypothalamus, and it is highly concentrated in amniotic fluid. Endocrine disrupters appear in the food supply, including human milk, which concentrates substances, and soy-based formulas that are packaged in BPA-lined cans.[36] The effects may be synergistic because endocrine-disrupting substances act as obesogens, interacting with other genetic and behavioral factors and a food supply rich in highly palatable, rewarding foods to disrupt regulation of energy balance.[37]

Sleep Factors

Sleep deprivation contributes to OB and OW (as well as diabetes mellitus Type 2) and can interfere with both weight loss and weight maintenances. It is associated with lower levels of physical activity, less desire to be active, and lowers the energy used for activity. Inadequate sleep is associated with disturbed orexin-A, increased ghrelin, decreased leptin, disturbed glucose-insulin homeostasis, increased appetite with preference for high-carbohydrate foods, and more opportunities for food intake, which may contribute to its association with OB in many populations.[38,39] Sleep habits may be an overlooked factor in weight gain and weight loss efforts. A small study of short duration reported better fat loss and sparing of lean tissue and better fat oxidation in those sleeping 8.5 hours compared with those with short sleep conditions (5.5 hours) during a kilocalorie-restricted diet.[40]

Gut Microbiota

Intestinal flora, or gut microbiota, in persons with OB tends toward a greater proportion of gram-negative Firmicutes and fewer gram-negative Bacteroidetes compared with lean individuals. These differences may provide a gut environment that favors greater calorie extraction from carbohydrates ingested, enhances lipogenic effects favoring fat storage, and provides a source of endotoxins that support a chain of events involving low-grade inflammation, insulin resistance, adverse atherosclerotic environments, and nonalcoholic fatty liver disease (NAFLD).[41] Gut microbiota changes may predate or be the result of OB, and alterations are associated with antibiotics, non-nutritive artificial sweeteners, and cesarean section birth methods that bypass the vaginal flora exposure for neonates.[42]

Psychosocial Stress and Cortisol

Stress is a risk factor for modest adiposity gains, but the effect size was small in meta-analysis of 14 longitudinal cohort studies. Men experiencing major life events and acute stressors showed a greater effect, possibly related to the higher cardiovascular, neuroendocrine, and elevated cortisol responses to stressors compared with women. Studies with follow-up of 5 years or longer showed stronger effects than those with follow-up of less than 5 years.[43] Chronic exposure, as measured by hair cortisol concentrations, was found to be positively correlated with weight, BMI, and raised waist circumference and

OB persistence in 2527 older adults in the English Longitudinal Study of Ageing.[44]

Food Quality, Nutrients, and Availability

The nutritional content or lack of nutritional content of food affects weight status. Nutrient-poor but energy-dense foods are less expensive than nutrient-rich foods and more abundant in most settings.[5] Deficiencies in micronutrients are common in OB. In preoperative nutritional evaluations, bariatric surgery (BS) patients commonly have deficiencies of vitamins D, A, E, and C and some B vitamins, as well as calcium, iron and ferritin, zinc, and selenium.[45] Deficiencies occur across countries of varying income status, and although the relationship between cause and effect is not solid, the deficiencies seem to precede OB in populations with greater deficiencies. US families with food insecurity eat foods that are less nutrient rich, get less dietary calcium, eat fewer vegetables and consume more kilocalories from nutrient-poor foods, have greater access to market outlets for such foods ("food swamps"), and may have less access to market outlets for nutrient-rich foods ("food deserts").[5]

A report to Congress examined availability and affordability of nutritious food—such as access to fruits, vegetables, whole grains, and milk, and grocery stores—in relation to their impact on health, including OB. Food deserts are areas of low access to nutritional high-quality food,[46] and food swamps are areas replete with energy-dense food of low nutritional value. Food swamps seem to have a greater association with increased energy intake and OB than food deserts do.[5,46]

Food pricing and government policy have both short- and long-term effects on food choices, and future policy decisions propose greater integration of health outcomes.[5] If the nation's individuals decided to follow nutrition guidelines, there would be a shortfall in fruits, vegetables, whole grains, and milk. A national mismatch occurs between what is produced and what is recommended for health.[47]

Food density—the proportion of nutrients to water and air—is correlated with greater BMI in population studies, and lower–food density diets have been shown to be effective in weight loss.[48]

Differences in food quality can have variable effects on metabolic health, weight gain, and fat gain. For example, recent trends indicate that monounsaturated fats, such as those found in peanuts and olives, may increase metabolism and assist weight loss. Dairy products intake seems to be protective against OB in children and adults. In a systematic review of long-term (average 3-year) dairy consumption and childhood OB, children with the highest dairy consumption were 35% less likely to have OB compared to the lowest dairy consumers. Each 1 serving/day reduced body fat and risk of OW/OB.[49] In adults, yogurt consumption has been associated with lower body fat and healthy waist circumferences and BMIs. Possible mechanisms include GLP and peptide YY (PYY), known anorexins; lower plasma ghrelin (hunger hormone); fermentation benefits to the gut microbiota favoring lean habitus; calcium's effect on switching from fat accretion to lipogenesis; fecal fat loss attributed to calcium; and well-documented satiety benefits of casein and whey protein.[50] In Midwestern US firefighters, greater adherence to the Mediterranean diet improved weight loss, weight loss maintenance, and metabolic parameters (blood pressure, blood sugar, triglycerides, total cholesterol). It is a myth that all kilocalories are the same.[51]

CLINICAL PRESENTATION AND HISTORY

OW and OB affect more US adults than are not affected, and measurement of BMI is indicated in all adults. OB comorbidities are major (increased waist circumference, established coronary artery disease [history of myocardial infarction, angioplasty, coronary artery bypass graft surgery, or acute coronary event], peripheral vascular disease, abdominal aortic aneurysm, symptomatic carotid artery disease, Type 2DM, and obstructive sleep apnea [OSA]) or minor (cigarette smoking, hypertension or use of antihypertensives, dyslipidemia, elevated glucose concentration or impaired glucose handling, and family history of premature coronary artery disease). Osteoarthritis, gallbladder disease, gout, PCOS, stress incontinence, and fatty liver diseases are common, less life-threatening conditions. Direct specific OSA queries about loud snoring, witnessed periods of apnea, morning headache, and daytime sleepiness. Depression and eating disorder screening is indicated. Beliefs about healthy weight, food, and physical activity and health consequences of OB are diverse and need to be queried with open-ended questions. Current nutrition and physical activity levels need to be quantified as part of the assessment, including portions, nutrients overconsumed or underconsumed, meal replacements, supplements, timing of meals and snacks, and eating disorder behaviors. Review all medications, including supplements. Attend to sleep patterns, shift work, current smoking status or other nicotine use, country of birth, and support system information gathered in the social history. Medical and surgical history, patterns of weight gain, associations with childbirth, life-changing events, smoking and tobacco cessation history, and medications must be thoroughly investigated. Any previous attempts to lose weight, diets, medications, supplements, and surgeries should be investigated from the patient's perspective, clarifying details and perceptions as needed. Permit the patient to identify anything that is perceived to contribute to excess weight (food intake, physical activity level, weight-based discrimination or stigma, and weight-associated comorbidities) without judgment. A questionnaire can facilitate the history gathering and can be completed before the appointment. Determine readiness for change in areas of weight loss, prevention of weight gain, physical activity dietary improvements, and participation in lifestyle weight loss interventions.

Treatment of comorbidities may not improve weight status but must be addressed. If the history reveals more pressing concerns, such as bulimia with purging or untreated substance use, these take priority. Smoking cessation is also considered a priority over weight loss.

PHYSICAL EXAMINATION

Every encounter should be nonjudgmental, nonbiased, and free of stereotypes. Language and other communications by staff should have no negative connotations. Weighing can be sensitive for many and should be private, with efforts made to avoid embarrassment. Medical equipment must be size appropriate, including armless, wide chairs; sturdy examination tables; step stools to approach examination tables; gowns; blood pressure cuffs; and speculums. The waiting room environment, including reading material, should reflect the needs of every size patient. All office people, processes, protocols, and standards should incorporate a team approach that is therapeutic. The provider must accept the task of compassionately treating patients who have OW/OB with no condemnation,

BOX **17.1**

Body Mass Index Calculations and Classification

METRIC
Weight in kilograms/(height in meters)^2

AMERICAN STANDARD
Weight in pounds/(height in inches)$^2 \times 703$

CLASSIFICATION
Underweight: BMI less than 18.5 kg/m^2
Normal weight: BMI 18.5–24.9 kg/m^2
Overweight: BMI 25–29.9 kg/m^2
Obesity class 1: BMI 30–34.9 kg/m^2
Obesity class 2: BMI 35–39.9 kg/m^2
Obesity class 3: BMI ≥40 kg/m^2 (formerly *morbid obesity*)
Obesity class 4: BMI 50–59.9 kg/m^2
Obesity class 5: BMI 60 kg/m^2 and above

BMI, Body mass index.

judgment, or weight-based stereotypes. Comfort should be facilitated as much as possible by ensuring adequate lighting, warmth, and draping.

Weight status is categorized by obtaining an accurate height (measured, not stated), weight, and abdominal circumference (Box 17.1). Discern BMI. Abdominal girth is measured above the iliac crest, with an inelastic tape placed parallel to the ground. Hip circumference is measured at the widest area across the gluteus, but this measurement is not necessary according to some guidelines. Only discuss or announce the number on the scale in strict privacy.

Intertriginous areas susceptible to maceration should be inspected—under breasts, under an abdominal pannus (apron), in the groin, between buttocks, and between toes. Acanthosis nigricans, a velvety maculopapular condition, occurs mostly in the neck, axilla, and groin. It indicates insulinemia and insulin resistance and is more prevalent in black and Hispanic populations. Skin tags are common. Acne, male pattern hirsutism, and linea nigra may indicate PCOS. Carotenemia noted on the palms or soles may indicate low thyroid hormone level, as can absent eyebrows in the lateral third margin.[52] An obese abdomen is evaluated no differently from a non-obese abdomen.

A neck circumference of more than 17 inches in men or 16 inches in women increases the risk of OSA and may also be associated with scleral injection and leg edema. Leg edema may also be related to a large pannus or right-sided heart congestion. An upper back fat pad indicates hypercortisolism. Rectal examination is best approached from the left Sims position, with the patient's assistance in holding up the upper buttock, or the lithotomy position. Search for indications of other common OB-related conditions: osteoarthritis, mobility limitations, gout, and diabetic neuropathies. Ensure staff uses proper body position and cuff size for obtaining blood pressure.

DIAGNOSTICS

Essential laboratory tests for individuals with OB are consistent with common comorbidities of OB. Include fasting serum glucose, hemoglobin A1C, lipid profile (total cholesterol, low-density lipoprotein [LDL], high-density lipoprotein [HDL], triglycerides); uric acid, blood urea nitrogen, and creatinine concentrations; complete blood count (CBC); thyroid-stimulating hormone (TSH) level; liver function tests, including alanine aminotransferase (ALT), aspartate aminotransferase (AST), alkaline phosphatase, and total and direct bilirubin; and urinalysis and urine for microalbumin. Indications for electrocardiography (ECG) are coronary disease risk factors, T2DM, family history of cardiovascular disease, diuretic medications, and consideration of anorectic medications.[52]

Suspect OSA if neck and/or waist circumference is enlarged and history reveals daytime sleepiness, load snoring, gasping or choking during sleep, and morning headaches. Consider polysomnography with oxygen saturation, apneic and hypopneic events. Cushing syndrome findings include moon facies, thin skin, violaceous stria, and easy bruising. Consider 24-hour free cortisol, salivary cortisol, and overnight dexamethasone suppression test.

Screen for depression. Eating disorders common in persons with OB/OW include binge-eating disorder (BED) and night eating syndrome (NES). BED in the DSM-5 is characterized by frequent episodes of eating larger than normal amounts of food more than 1/week for at least 3 months; there is no purging or excessive exercise; it involves an overwhelming loss of control; and there is shame or guilt about food intake. It is possibly the most common eating disorder in the United States. Among people with OB/OW seeking treatment, the prevalence was 32%.[53]

NES is characterized by eating at least 25% of daily food after the evening meal, recurrent wakening from sleep with eating to go back to sleep, and morning anorexia. NES in US military veterans seeking OB treatment was over 10%.[54]

Additional diagnostics depend on history and physical (H&P) exam findings and index of suspicion. Diagnostics to consider are: 2-hour oral glucose tolerance test with insulin levels; gallbladder ultrasonography for gallstones; ultrasound or hepatic CT or MRI if hepatomegaly is found or NASH or NAFLD is suspected as indicated by liver study laboratory results.[52] Routine mammography and colorectal screenings are often neglected in those with OB, even though OB increases breast and colon cancer risk; schedule for these screenings are according to age and risk profile.

DIFFERENTIAL DIAGNOSIS

 Priority differentials include (1) hormonal OB syndromes, (2) genetic OB syndromes, (3) neurological OB causes.

Polycystic Ovarian Syndrome

H&P may reveal oligomenorrhea, amenorrhea, or menses may be regular. Other clinical findings include infertility, hyperandrogenism, hirsutism, acne from androgen excess, or acanthosis nigricans related to insulin resistance or T2DM. When PCOS is suspected, order: serum testosterone (morning, free and weekly), DHEAS (dehydroprogesterone sulfate), and prolactin, and consider testing while off OC, TSH. Imaging tests recommended include transvaginal ultrasound of pelvis.

Hypothyroidism

H&P reveals mild weight gain, fatigue, lethargy, weakness, slow speech, slow cerebration, cold intolerance. Skin findings include dryness, carotenemia, and non-pitting edema in hands and eyelids (myxedema). Hair characteristics are brittle and coarse,

with loss of lateral eyebrows. Patients can exhibit a dull facies, thick tongue, and coarse speech. Other physical exam findings can be distant heart sounds, bradycardia, delayed deep tendon relaxation (DTR), cerebellar ataxia, peripheral neuropathies with paresthesia, musculoskeletal weakness, stiffness, carpal tunnel syndrome. There may be a history of hyperthyroidism treatment, menorrhagia, secondary amenorrhea or decreased libido. Order the following laboratory tests: TSH, and possibly free T_4, free T_3, serum thyroxine-binding globulin (TBG).

Cushing Syndrome

H&P findings reveal central adiposity, muscle wasting, moon face, thin skin, easy bruising, poor wound healing, severe fatigue, red-purple abdominal striae. There can be a history of long-term glucocorticoid therapy. Laboratory tests that are indicated: overnight dexamethasone suppression test, and 24-hour urine for free cortisol, repeated twice.

DRUG-INDUCED OBESITY (SEE SECTION, PHARMACEUTICALS ASSOCIATED WITH WEIGHT GAIN)
Genetic Obesity Syndromes

Prader-Willi Syndrome. Findings include OB, reduced fetal activity, hypotonia at birth, short stature, hypogonadism, small hands and feet, mental retardation, and early onset hyperphagia between 12 and 24 months of age. It is the most common OB syndrome.

Bardet-Biedl Syndrome. Findings include trunk OB during infancy, dysmorphic extremities (syndactyly, polydactyly, brachydactyly), retinal-caused impaired vision, hypogonadism, mental retardation, and abnormal kidney structure and function.

Alström Syndrome. Findings include early onset truncal OB, cone-rod dystrophy, progressive hearing loss, cardiomyopathy, and insulin resistance.

Secondary Neurological Obesity Causes

Hypothalamic injury-associated OB are rare. These include history of tumor, cranial radiation, craniopharyngioma, trauma, inflammatory disease, increased intracranial pressure, and pituitary resection.

INTERPROFESSIONAL COLLABORATIVE MANAGEMENT
Motivational Interviewing and the Transtheoretical Model for Change

The five As of motivational interviewing (MI), adapted from smoking cessation counseling, are useful for providers who may feel unprepared to give OB counseling.

Ask: Ask permission to discuss weight in a nonjudgmental manner and explore readiness for change.

Assess: Assess the person's BMI and OB stage, waist circumference, and contributing factors of excess weight.

Advise: Advise on the individual health risks associated with having OB and the benefits of modest weight loss; set the stage for long-term treatment strategy that emphasizes health.

Agree: Agree on realistic goals and specific treatment options.

Assist: Assist in locating resources, addressing barriers, making consultations, and arranging follow-up.

Principles and strategies of MI incorporate resisting directing of the patient; understanding the individual's motivation; listening with empathy; asking open-ended questions that lead to improved understanding and change talk; and using affirmations, reflections, and summaries that foster a therapeutic relationship while supporting motivation to change.[7,55]

Identification of the individual's stage of change, according to the transtheoretical model, can help integrate MI with patients at any level of motivation. The stages of change are precontemplation; contemplation; preparation; action; and maintenance, relapse, or recycling. The stages are nonlinear, tend to cycle, and do not necessarily predict behavior changes.[56]

As of February 2018, the US Preventive Health Service Task Force (USPHSTF) recommended that clinicians offer or refer adults with a BMI of 30 or higher to intensive, multicomponent behavioral interventions.

These guidelines are available at: https://www.uspreventiveservicestaskforce.org/

Strategies for Weight Loss

Cardiovascular diseases' risk factors, T2DM, hypertension, OSA, stress incontinence, osteoarthritis, and menopause symptom reduction improve with intensive lifestyle weight loss interventions. Diagnosis, gender, ethnicity, culture, and language should be considered in forming weight loss groups to foster social interaction as part of the therapeutic milieu.

Three components—an energy deficit from reduced kilocalories, physical activity, and behavioral changes—are interrelated for all weight loss and management efforts. The trio combined is known as *lifestyle intervention*. Individualization of the right strategy depends on assessment of severity of OB and presence of comorbidities, contributing components, willingness to change, and desire to learn new skills to create patient-centered goals. A decrease in energy intake is needed to create a deficit sufficient for weight loss efforts to succeed; behavioral and lifestyle changes and physical activity together are rarely sufficient to achieve weight loss when energy intake is not also reduced. Typically, a 500- to 1000-kcal deficit must be created through a combination of decreased intake and increased physical activity for excess weight to be lost. Intentional weight loss success definitions vary and are not concrete or consistent historically. Recent guidelines advocate using percent body weight lost from the initial starting weight.

Clinical health benefits begin at 5% weight loss, especially in patients with greater cardiometabolic risk factors. Improvements are noted specifically in blood pressure, blood lipid profiles, waist circumference, glycemic control, lower medication burden, and less hospitalizations and medical costs. The benefits begin at 5% and increase as weight losses become more dramatic.[57] Nonsurgical weight loss is based on percentage difference from beginning weight, with target set at 10%. This can be higher, depending on the patient's desire. A 10% weight loss, with 7% kept off during maintenance, is associated with decreased risk of OB-associated comorbidities.[58] Successful weight loss maintenance, according to the 1998 National Heart, Lung, and Blood Institute (NHLBI) guideline, is weight regain of less than 6.6 pounds in 2 years and a sustained reduction in waist circumference of 4 cm (1⅗ inches). When an initial weight loss goal is not agreeable to an individual, alternative goals can be improved dietary composition, physical activity, and avoidance of weight gain.[59]

Weight loss resulting from BS views and measures success differently and is based on excess body weight (the amount of weight above a BMI of 25). Surgically achieved "success" is the loss of more than 50% of excess body weight. Successful maintenance after BS is a minimum of 80% loss kept off 3 to 5 years after weight loss stabilizes. Surgical weight loss failure is weight loss that is less than 50% of excess body weight.

Reducing Energy Intake. Reducing energy intake is primary among the three components for weight loss. Kilocalories or calories are supplied mainly by three macronutrients: protein, carbohydrates, and fats.

Proteins. Protein provides 4 kcal/g. Essential amino acids are the protein building blocks that must be ingested, as the body cannot synthesize them. Major protein sources are animal (meat, poultry, fish, milk) and non-animal (legumes, nuts, and seeds). US Department of Agriculture (USDA) 2010 guidelines recommend that men and women consume 56 g and 46 g of protein per day, respectively, and typically represent the need as a percentage of kilocalories.[47] However, protein needs are unchanged when kilocalories are reduced, and protein intake should not be lowered during weight loss. Rather, protein needs during weight loss should be met first, with fats and carbohydrates added to meet calorie needs.[60] Protein's primacy during weight loss is based on its tendency to protect lean body mass, help stabilize blood glucose concentration, improve lipid profile, provide greater satiety properties (compared with carbohydrates or fats), and to increase postmeal thermogenic effects.[60] Breakfast protein intake is especially important after an overnight fast, with optimal benefits from 30 g. Other protein intake suggested is 20 to 30 g per meal spread over the day to prevent sarcopenia.[61] Post-BS protein intake is recommended as a minimum of 60 to 120 g/day for the short and long term to prevent loss of lean body tissue and to avoid protein malnutrition, with supplements used if dietary sources are not tolerated.[60] Protein supplements and meal replacement package labeling should indicate protein sources, not just total grams. High-quality protein sources supply all essential amino acids and may come from eggs, whey, or soy. Collagen sources are inferior sources and should not be solely relied on to supply protein needs. Protein ingestion is associated with improved weight loss maintenance, and a combination of protein sources (low-fat animal and nonanimal) may have the best effects when protein sources are low in saturated fat.[62]

Carbohydrates. Carbohydrates supply 4 kcal/g, are a major energy source, and may come from simple or complex glucose polymers. Plants are the major carbohydrate source, except for lactose from dairy.[63] A *simple carbohydrate* refers to a monosaccharide or a disaccharide. Simple carbohydrates occur in fruit, milk, beets, and honey naturally and in processed added sugar products, table sugar, and corn syrup. Americans average more than 22 teaspoons of added sugars, or 355 kcal, per day. Added sugars supply no nourishment with their energy and are associated with dyslipidemias (low HDL, high triglycerides), insulin-glucose disruption, higher blood pressure, T2DM, and poorer overall nutrition.[15] Complex carbohydrates are larger polymers, an important fiber source, and are mainly supplied by cereal grains. Other sources are legumes, fruits, and vegetables. Whole grains are associated with lower BMI and other long-term health benefits compared with refined grains.[64] Whole grains supply 1.1 g fiber per 10 g carbohydrates. Reducing simple carbohydrate sugar energy intake is appropriate for people of all ages and is a general recommendation in the 2010 USDA guidelines. The American Heart Association (AHA) recommendations are more specific: maximum added sugar intake for men is 150 kcal/day and for women is 100 kcal/day. These should be lower to meet weight loss goals.[15]

Fats. Fats are the most energy dense among the macronutrients, supplying 9 kcal/g. They supply essential fatty acids and the fat-soluble vitamins A, D, E, and K; they slow gastric emptying and can reduce satiety, leading to more intake. About one-third of Americans' energy intake is from fats. Sources include animal products, grain oils, vegetable oils, seeds, and nuts. α-linolenic and linoleic acids must be obtained from the diet to avoid deficiency. Reduced-fat diets are considered conventional for weight loss.[63] The Mediterranean diet pattern is moderate in fat content, supplied mostly from olive oil. Preferred sources of monounsaturated and polyunsaturated fats are olive oil, nuts, seeds, and fatty fish.[63]

Alcohol. Although it is a considered a macronutrient, alcohol has 7 kcal/g and is a large energy source for some adults. It is not an important source of nutrients and may be combined with sugar-sweetened mixers and contribute to greater kilocalorie intake. Moderate alcohol use is defined as two and one drinks per day for men and women, respectively. It is a component of the Mediterranean dietary pattern. About half of Americans do not drink alcohol. For those who do not drink, it is not recommended that alcohol consumption be initiated for health benefits.

Eating for Weight Loss "Diets." Dietary patterns for weight loss have one commonality: reduced kilocalories to create an energy deficit. The macronutrient proportions used in achieving the kilocalorie deficit are variable, and these variable proportions are debated. Discretionary calories in excess from sugar, solid fats, and alcohol should be limited for general and cardiovascular health benefits across most populations, regardless of weight status, and are generally agreed to be the starting point for creating an energy deficit to treat (or to prevent) OB.

Balanced Energy Deficit Diets. These diets reduce overall kilocalories by approximately 500 to 1000 across all macronutrients and follow USDA nutrition guidelines for macronutrient percentages. They are low in fat (<30%), high in carbohydrates (>55%), moderate in protein (10% to 15%), high in fiber (25 to 30 g/day), and very low in alcohol. Weight loss is slow, about 1 and 2 pounds/week in women and men, respectively.[65]

Low-Calorie Diets, Portion-Controlled, Meal Replacement. These diets are similar to balanced energy deficits but supply only 1000 to 1500 kcal/day, which creates a greater energy deficit. They are considered traditional weight loss diets.[63]

Portion-controlled servings and meal replacements facilitate weight loss by providing individuals with predetermined foods having a known kilocalorie and nutrient content.

Low-fat diets have been a traditional approach for decades and guide the preponderance of weight loss intervention studies. Reducing fat intake alone is not sufficient for clinically significant weight loss without reducing overall kilocalories.[65] When there is a medical history of high triglycerides, glucose intolerance, PCOS, and/or and body habitus (central adiposity) a low-fat diet should not be advocated as the best choice since lowering fat proportion typically results in higher carbohydrate intake.

Low-Carbohydrate Diets. These diets have variable carbohydrate restrictions, some as low as 20 g/day, typically supplied from green vegetables. The remaining macronutrient percentages are high for protein, and the fat content varies according to protein sources. A popular low-carbohydrate diet is the Atkins diet. Low-carbohydrate intervention studies have used the Atkins protocol and found the weight loss method safe in adults and adolescents, with supervision.[66] Older versions of Atkins diets were high in saturated fat, but newer protocols have modified the protein sources to be leaner. There are also vegetarian Atkins variations. Low-carbohydrate diets produce rapid weight loss in the early months. Non–weight loss uses of low-carbohydrate diets are higher in kilocalories and useful in treatment of PCOS, resistant epilepsy in children, and some glycolytic cancers.

Very-Low-Calorie Diets. These diets typically contain approximately 800 kcal/day and 70 to 100 g of protein; they use meal replacement products solely or in combination with lean protein food sources. Vitamin and mineral supplementation is essential, and health care supervision is warranted. Weight loss is rapid with very-low-calorie diets (VLCDs). They may be used preoperatively for BS patients.[65]

The diabetes in remission study, DiRECT, delivered VLCD via primary care providers to people with OW or OB and T2DM. The 12-month intervention involved 850-calorie VLCD and intensive lifestyle intervention (ILI) for 12 months. The control group continued with standard care. The control group had less than 1 kg weight loss or no weight changes and no T2DM remissions, whereas the VLCD and intense lifestyle participants had weight loss and T2DM remissions in a dose-dependent manner:

- Less than 5 kg weight loss, 7% remission;
- 5 to 10 kg weight loss, 34% remission;
- 10 to 15 kg weight loss, 57% remission;
- 15 kg + weight loss, 86%;

Remission of T2DM was defined as achieving an HgA1c < 6.5% without use of anti-diabetic medication for a minimum of 12 months.[67]

The Mediterranean Diet. This diet is plant based and composed of fruits, vegetables, whole grains, nuts, and legumes; it has olive oil for its main source of fat. Animal protein sources are low-fat fish and poultry consumed in low to moderate amounts. Red meat consumption is low, and wine intake is moderate. When this diet is used along with exercise, it is effective as a weight loss method, even though its fat content is much higher than that of conventional weight loss diets. The carbohydrate proportion is lower at 45%, fat is 35% to 40%, and protein is 15% to 20% of kilocalories. The Mediterranean diet pattern is associated with treatment and reduction of the risk for development of metabolic syndrome.[68]

Weight Loss Maintenance Diet and Other Factors. Dansinger and coworkers[66] compared the Atkins, Ornish, Weight Watchers, and Zone diets for weight loss and heart disease risk factor reduction in a 1-year, random assignment study. Because of high attrition rates and waning adherence to assigned dietary patterns, the 12-month comparisons were similar across all groups. Those who adhered to their diet assignment had better weight loss and improvements in cardiovascular risk factors.

After weight loss, adherence to a long-term reduced energy intake is necessary indefinitely. Weight loss and reduced energy expenditure are not proportionate: Weight-reduced individuals have lower resting metabolic rates compared to similar individuals whose weight has been stable. Research has supported the importance of implementing the skills and behaviors learned in lifestyle interventions. Ongoing research is examining meal timing (restricting the hours for eating), intermittent fasting, and macronutrient components and how these can best be manipulated to maintain weight loss long term. Successful individuals consistently adhere to reduced dietary intake, whether lower kcal, fat, or carbohydrate; self-monitor their weight, usually daily; eat home-prepared foods; exercise greater than one hour per day; and watch little television.

Look Actions in Health and Diabetes

The Look AHEAD (Actions in Health and Diabetes) was the largest RCT to observe ILI evaluating weight loss. The 9.6-year study observed 5145 participants with T2DM and OB. Participants were randomly assigned to ILI (with goals of at least 10% weight loss and at least 175 minutes of moderate physical activity per week), or to diabetic support and education as the control. Diabetes Prevention Program (DPP) materials were adapted for the group delivery format of Look AHEAD. Primary outcomes included cardiovascular deaths, nonfatal myocardial infarctions, and hospitalizations for cardiac events during a prolonged follow-up after intensive weight loss and other ILI.[69] The study was stopped after 9.6 years. (Although weight loss was greater in the ILI intervention group, cardiovascular events were not reduced.)[70] The Look AHEAD participants' ILI was delivered in group meetings and reinforced with homework and handouts. MI and cognitive restructuring guided the ILI and weight loss coaches. ILI and weight loss topics fell into five categories: knowledge (nutrition, safe exercise, controlling kilocalories); motivation (increasing self-efficacy built on successes); self-regulatory skills (keys to weight loss and long-term success, self-monitoring, cognitive restructuring, relapse plans); group and individual experience (social support); and environmental factors (overcoming barriers with practical advice). These are critical components within an individual's control to succeed at weight loss and long-term management within the current obesogenic system.[69] The length of the intervention, over multiple years, helped establish new behaviors that develop into new neurally reinforced habits. The ILI delivery format included multiple weekly, then monthly, visits and these ILI components collectively are becoming a standard of care for weight loss.

The diet chosen for the Look AHEAD study is low fat, 1200 to 1800 kcal/day or less if necessary; it supplies a minimum of 15% calories from protein and provides meal replacements three times per day during the first 6 months. Meal replacement continues for one meal and one snack per day for 4 years. If weight loss is not realized after 6 months of participation, orlistat may be used by those who choose. Both exercise and increasing lifestyle physical activity are priorities in the weight loss intervention. A weekly goal of at least 175 minutes of moderate-intensity physical activity is set as a means of improving cardiovascular risk factors, improving lipids, reducing blood glucose and serum insulin levels, and facilitating maintenance of weight loss. It is not the primary means of creating a kilocalorie deficit for weight loss.[69] The Look AHEAD protocol, leader and participant manuals, and publications are also available (www.lookaheadtrial.org/). They are evidence-based intervention tools to help individuals successfully navigate an obesogenic environment. The Look AHEAD publication topics relate aggressive weight loss as part of the ILI.[71] The intervention methods and materials can be appropriated in the health care and larger community settings.

Side Effects of Weight Loss

Side effects of weight loss are generally mild and self-limited.[66] However, iatrogenic effects from diabetic medications are more serious, and reduction or discontinuation of insulin

and insulin secretagogues (sulfonylureas, repaglinide, and nateglinide) should be done preemptively before weight loss. Home glucose monitoring is expected. Antihypertensives and diuretics likewise require astute blood pressure monitoring and appropriate medication alterations.[58] It is the responsibility of the provider to anticipate and prevent dangerous episodes of hypoglycemia, hypovolemia, and hypotension from prescribed medications when patients are losing weight, especially in the early days and weeks of rapid weight loss.[7,72]

Patients with a history of gout may experience an increase in uric acid during early weight loss, and prophylactic prescription of allopurinol may be appropriate. Cholestasis can be prevented by ensuring that dietary fat is at least 20 g/day. Prophylactic use of ursodeoxycholic acid may be considered in those predisposed to gallstones. Side effects from VLCDs tend be greater than in patients reducing carbohydrates while keeping calorie restriction to 1200 to 1500 kcal/day.

Resources for Weight Loss, Physical Activity, and Overweight and Obesity

Competence in manipulating medications associated with weight gain is essential for providers. A Pharmacological Management of OB: An Endocrine Society Clinical Practice Guideline overviews commonly prescribed agents associated with weight gain and alternative prescribing suggestions. Share the pharmaceutical decisions and quantify any expected weight changes.[34]

Veterans Affairs MOVE! A comprehensive resource, MOVE!, from the Department of Veterans Affairs (VA) and Department of Defense's clinical practice guideline for screening and management of OW and OB, version 2.0 2014,[7] is accessible by providers outside the VA system. It contains a provider guideline, including OB screening, MI information, dietary approaches, physical activity approaches, behavioral change components, pharmacotherapy, BS, evidence for interventions, treatment cards, evidence ratings for approaches, and research summaries in about 200 pages that clinicians may find valuable. It has more than 100 patient handouts for group or individual counseling covering standard components: food and activity diaries, goal setting, and cognitive changes; nutrition components (30 handouts); and physical activity components (38 handouts).[7] The materials are comprehensive for weight loss, physical activity, behavior modification, and cognitive restructuring. Group application is intended, but it can be adopted for individuals. The materials consider health needs unique to older veteran populations, address issues not relevant in Look AHEAD research protocols (pain and physical activity, psychiatric diagnoses, smoking cessation), and does not require high reading skills.[73]

American Society of Bariatric Physicians. Additional resources are available from the American Society of Bariatric Physicians (https://obesitymedicine.org). Available materials include an OB algorithm, fact sheets, patient information, and PowerPoint presentation that is updated.[31]

American Medical Association and the American College of Sports Medicine

Exercise and physical activity counseling from a health care provider has a dose-dependent effect. The website ExerciseIsMedicine.org has public access resources created by the American Medical Association (AMA) and the American College of Sports Medicine for providers; these resources include exercise prescriptions, a readiness for change overview, office brochures on myriad exercise-related topics, fliers, and patient handouts for physical activity in specific health conditions. (http://www.exerciseismedicine.org/support_page.php/health-care-providers/.)

National Heart, Lung, and Blood Institute (NHLBI) National Institutes of Health. The NHLBI National Institutes of Health (NIH) website has materials for its Aim for a Healthy Weight available to download, or hardcopies can be purchased. Information is accessible for both patients and providers.[74]

Group lifestyle intervention for WL is an effective and economical format. The MOVE! and Look AHEAD materials can also guide weight loss in groups with OB-related comorbidities.

Pharmaceutical Options

Pharmaceutical treatment for weight loss can target centrally mediated appetite, satiety, neural pathways of reward, and peripheral gastric absorption of nutrients. All agents are associated with weight loss plateaus; none is indicated as monotherapy without lifestyle changes, and all are associated with weight regain on discontinuation if lifestyle changes are not adopted. No pharmaceutical treatment increases weight loss via long-term thermogenesis or metabolic rate changes. Intensity of lifestyle intervention is proportional to desired results, with 16 face-to-face visits over 12 months demonstrating best results across clinical trials. Several pharmaceuticals have been approved and labeled for long-term weight loss maintenance, in keeping with a chronic disease model wherein OB is a chronic condition.[75]

Sympathomimetic Medications in Weight Loss. The older sympathomimetic monotherapy drugs phentermine, 15 to 30 mg/day; diethylpropion (Tenuate), 25 mg three times per day or sustained release (SR) 75 mg/day; benzphetamine (Didrex), 25 to 50 mg one to three times a day; and phendimetrazine (Bontril), 17.5 to 70 mg three times per day, inhibit norepinephrine and dopamine uptake at nerve endings, resulting in hypothalamically mediated anorexia. Bontril dose is 25 mg two to three times a day. The SR form of phendimetrazine (Bontril) is 105 mg, once a day, taken 30 to 60 minutes before breakfast. These medications are Schedule III and IV drugs because of US Drug Enforcement Administration (DEA) concerns regarding abuse. The medications were labeled for short-term use for weight loss. These medications were approved before OB was recognized as a chronic condition. Abrupt withdrawal is associated with increased appetite. Some providers prescribe them intermittently, or alternatively, because of concerns about short-term use.[58] There exists a possibility for dependence and withdrawal. The most widely prescribed sympathomimetic agent, phentermine, is indicated for exogenous OB in adults or children older than 16 years, with BMI of 30 kg/m^2 or higher, or 27 kg/m^2 or higher with comorbidities.[57,75,76] Common side effects of sympathomimetic weight loss drugs are CNS stimulation, insomnia, and nervousness, which may abate with use. Tremor and dry mouth are common. Other adverse effects are pulmonary hypertension, valvular heart disease, psychosis, tachyarrhythmias, euphoria, dysphoria, GI complaints, and blood marrow suppression (diethylpropion). As a precaution, baseline cardiac evaluation, including echocardiogram, may be warranted in some patients. These agents are not recommended in patients with valvular heart disease or heart murmur. Diabetic medications and antihypertensives require astute monitoring. Phentermine

is contraindicated in patients with glaucoma, or within 14 days of MAOI agents. None are to be used in pregnancy.[57,72] Always consider medication's effect on weight, quantify expected weight gain, and select medications that do not have weight gain as a side effect, whenever possible in shared decision-making.[35,77,78]

Orlistat. Orlistat (Xenical, 120 mg, by prescription and Alli, 60 mg, over the counter [OTC]) is an irreversible pancreatic lipase inhibitor than prevents dietary fat from hydrolysis and absorption. Fecal fat loss, as undigested triglycerides, occurs in a dose-dependent manner, with up to 30% of dietary fat not absorbed. It was approved in 1999 as an adjunct to a low-fat diet (30% kilocalories from fat) for WL and has shown minimal benefit in weight maintenance. The indication is BMI 30 kg/m^3 or higher, or 27 kg/m^3 or higher with comorbidities. Dose is 60 mg (OTC) or 120 mg (by prescription) taken with a fat-containing meal (about 15 g) or up to 1 hour after meal ingestion. Orlistat raises GLP-1 and C-peptide but lowers an acute cholecystokinin response to meals. It has been implicated in rare cases of liver-related adverse events in reports to the US Food and Drug Administration (FDA). Patients may develop increased urinary oxalate; use cautiously in patients with a history of calcium oxalate kidney stone. It must be accompanied by vitamin supplementation containing fat-soluble vitamins A, D, E, and K and β carotene, given at bedtime or a minimum of 2 hours before or after the medication, to reduce fat-soluble vitamin deficiency risks. Weight loss results with orlistat peak at about 8% to 9% after 35 weeks when it is combined with dietary restrictions, followed by partial weight regain. Final weight reductions are approximately 7%, compared with approximately 5% for placebo, after 2 years. Mean weight loss in three 1-year studies was 3.45 kg more than placebo at 120 mg three times per day. GI side effects are common and include defecation urgency, flatus with discharge, diarrhea, abdominal discomfort, and oily fecal leakage. These GI side effects are reduced when dietary fat intake is restricted to less than 50 to 60 g/day or 30% of the dietary kilocalories distributed over 3 meals. Drug interactions include the need to separate doses of orlistat and levothyroxine by 4 hours and orlistat and cyclosporine by 3 hours. Warfarin and anticonvulsant drug monitoring is recommended.[8,72,76,79]

Cetilistat. Cetilistat is a lipase inhibitor, similar to orlistat, approved in Japan (but not in the United States) for weight loss. It has been found in contaminated weight loss products (Herbal Xenicol).[80]

Lorcaserin (Belviq). Lorcaserin (Belviq) was approved by the FDA in 2012 as an adjunct to a reduced-calorie diet and exercise for chronic weight management in adults with initial BMI of 30 kg/m^2 or higher, or BMI 27 kg/m^2 or higher with at least one weight-related condition. Dose is 10 mg PO twice daily, without regard to food. It is contraindicated in pregnancy (FDA Category X). Clinical trials included only 2.5% (135 participants) adults older than age 65, and it was not determined if dose or response was different from that in younger subjects. Dosage used in those older than 65 years should be based on renal function. No dose adjustment for mild renal impairment; use lorcaserin with caution in patients with moderate renal impairment. Lorcaserin is not recommended for patients with severe renal impairment or in end stage renal disease. No dose adjustment is required in patients with mild hepatic impairment (Child-Pugh score 5 or 6) to moderate hepatic impairment (Child-Pugh 7 to 9). Use lorcaserin with caution in patients with severe hepatic impairment.

Discontinue lorcaserin after 12 weeks if 5% weight loss is not achieved.[35,77,81]

Common adverse effects in nondiabetic patients include nausea, diarrhea, constipation, dry mouth, vomiting, fatigue, headache, and dizziness; and in diabetic patients, hypoglycemia, headache, back pain, cough, and fatigue. Suspected adverse drug reactions should be reported (Eisai, 1-888-274-2378; FDA, 1-800-FDA-1088 or www.fda.gov/medwatch).[81]

Monitoring includes weight; blood pressure (especially in patients taking antihypertensive medication); monthly pregnancy tests (in office or at home) in women of childbearing potential if deemed appropriate; glucose and hypoglycemia in diabetics; signs and symptoms of valvulopathy; signs and symptoms of depression or suicidal thoughts or behavior; prolactin excess; pulmonary hypertension; CBC changes; and cognitive impairment or mood changes. Heart rate may be decreased, and hence this medication should be used with caution in patients with a history of bradycardia or heart block greater than first degree.[81]

Warnings and precautions include possible serotonin syndrome (agitation, hallucinations, coma, autonomic instability, hyperreflexia, incoordination, and/or GI symptoms) or neuroleptic malignant syndrome–like reactions. Valvulopathy has been reported with other 5-HT$_{2B}$ receptor agonists, because these receptors are located on cardiac interstitial cells, and is theoretically possible with lorcaserin, a 5-HT$_{2C}$ agonist. In clinical trials, 2.4% of patients taking lorcaserin and 2.0% receiving placebo developed echocardiographically determined changes, with none noted to be symptomatic. The drug should be discontinued if any valvular heart disease signs or symptoms develop, including dyspnea, dependent edema, congestive heart failure (CHF), or a new cardiac murmur, and the appropriate evaluations should be performed. Lorcaserin is used with caution in combination with other serotonergic or antidopaminergic drugs or MAOIs.[81]

Priapism is a potential result of 5-HT$_{2C}$ receptor agonism, and lorcaserin should be used with caution in men with predisposition to priapism (e.g., those with sickle cell anemia, multiple myeloma, or penile anatomic deformations). Lorcaserin is used with caution when combined with phosphodiesterase type 5 inhibitors. Moderate prolactin level elevations occurred in clinical trials in a subset of patients; serum prolactin should be measured when prolactin excess is suspected or if patients develop galactorrhea or gynecomastia.[81]

Lorcaserin is a serotonergic agonist that activates the 5-HT$_{2C}$ receptors. It is believed to decrease food intake and promote satiety by activation of these receptors, creating an anorexigenic effect via opiomelanocortin neurons located in the hypothalamus.[82] It is a DEA Schedule IV controlled substance with low incidence of euphoria and hallucination in patients with OB. Clinical trial weight loss in nondiabetic patients taking lorcaserin was 3.3% greater than with placebo, with 47.1% of patients losing 5% or more of their initial body weight compared with 22.6% in the placebo group. Mean WL at 52 weeks for lorcaserin-treated patients was 7.9 kg compared with 3.7-kg weight loss in the placebo group.[81]

Phentermine/Topiramate Sustained Release (Qsymia). Phentermine combined with topiramate SR (P/T), branded as Qsymia, received approval in 2012 for long-term use in OB or OW with weight-related complications. Phentermine's known anorectic properties reduce appetite and food consumption. Topiramate's mechanism of action is not known, but the drug

has been shown to reduce appetite and enhance satiety. These effects may be the result of the central augmentation of neurotransmitter γ-aminobutyric acid (GABA); topiramate is associated with weight loss when used as monotherapy.[72,82]

Qsymia capsules come in formulations of 3.75 mg/23 mg, 7.5 mg/46 mg, 11.25 mg/69 mg, and 15 mg/92 mg to titrate upward during initiation; titration should be used during discontinuation as well, to prevent possible seizures from sudden withdrawal of topiramate. Administration is begun with 3.75 mg/23 mg in the morning for 14 days; the dosage is increased to 7.5 mg/46 mg each morning for 12 weeks. If a 3% weight loss is not achieved with the 7.5 mg/46 mg formulation, the dose is increased to 11.25 mg/69 mg. If the patient is not responding and if the drug is to be withdrawn, alternate-day administration for a minimum of 1 week is used to avoid precipitation of seizures. Maximum dose is 15 mg/92 mg. Use in older adult patients should begin with low doses and increased cautiously.[83]

Qsymia is DEA Schedule C-IV due to the phentermine component. Teratogenicity—topiramate's association with cleft lip and cleft palate in infants born to mothers taking the drug during pregnancy—is a safety risk for which a Risk Evaluation and Mitigation Strategy (REMS) has been required by the FDA. Provider training is available on the website http://qsymiarems.com, along with downloadable files, including a dose-management chart; full prescribing information; a patient brochure on the risk of birth defects; and links to certified pharmacies participating in Qsymia's REMS program. If a patient becomes pregnant while using Qsymia, this should be reported by the patient and the provider to the Qsymia pregnancy surveillance program.

Qsymia warnings and precautions include the risk of fetal toxicity in females of reproductive potential. Cranial facial and cleft palate abnormalities are associated with topiramate. A negative pregnancy test result should be obtained before initiation of therapy and monthly (in office or at home) during therapy, and effective contraception use should be assessed. Heart rate may increase. The possibility of suicidal behavior and ideation necessitate close monitoring for depression or suicidal thoughts. If acute myopia and secondary angle-closure glaucoma occur, the drug should be discontinued; if mood and sleep disorders occur, the dose should be reduced or the drug discontinued. Cognitive impairment including disturbed attention or memory can occur, so patients should be cautioned. Metabolic acidosis and elevated creatinine may occur, requiring monitoring before and during treatment. The most common adverse reactions are paresthesia, dizziness, dysgeusia (altered taste), insomnia, constipation, and dry mouth. Patients taking OC may experience irregular bleeding or spotting, but the risk of pregnancy is not increased. Combination with alcohol should be avoided because of CNS depressant effect. Hypokalemia may occur when used with non–potassium-sparing diuretics. Reduced urinary citrate excretion and elevated urinary pH may promote kidney stone formation, and the risk may increase with a diet-induced ketogenic environment. Qsymia is contraindicated in pregnant patients, in those with glaucoma or hyperthyroidism, during or with MAOI use, and in those with known hypersensitivities to sympathomimetic amine drugs.[81]

Sustained Release Bupropion/Naltrexone (Contrave). The combination agent containing SR bupropion and naltrexone (Contrave)[84] was approved in 2014 for chronic weight management. It is indicated for treatment of patients with OB or OW with weight-related comorbidities. A boxed warning includes increased risk of suicidal thinking and behavior; the provider should monitor for worsening and emergence of depression or other psychic disorders. Serious neuropsychiatric events have been associated with use of bupropion for smoking cessation, and study data in pediatric patients are lacking. Contraindications include uncontrolled hypertension; seizure disorders; anorexia nervosa or bulimia; abrupt alcohol cessation; use of benzodiazepines, barbiturates, and/or antiepileptic drugs; use with other bupropion-containing products; chronic opioid use; use of MAOIs currently or within previous 14 days; known allergies to ingredients; and pregnancy. Tablets are a combination of extended-release naltrexone 8 mg and bupropion 90 mg to be administered incrementally over 4 weeks: 1 tablet in the morning during week 1, adding a second tablet in the evening in week 2, increase to 2 tablets in the morning during week 3, and from week 4 onward, 2 tablets twice daily, morning and evening.[84]

Drugs metabolized by CYP2D6 (SSRIs, TCAs, antipsychotics, β blockers, propafenone) may have increased concentration owing to bupropion's action and require dose reduction. Drugs metabolized by CYP2B6 (ticlopidine or clopidogrel) (CYP2B6 inhibitors) may increase bupropion's concentration; hence bupropion/naltrexone should be given at the lower dose, 1 tablet twice per day (bid). CYP2B6 inducers (ritonavir, carbamazepine, phenobarbital, phenytoin) may reduce bupropion effect and should not be used with bupropion/naltrexone.[84]

Common Medications That Have Weight Loss as a Side Effect. Pharmacologic agents that are approved for indications other than weight loss but are associated with weight loss include bupropion, extended-release exenatide, pramlintide, metformin, topiramate, and zonisamide. Agents under investigation include bupropion SR combined with zonisamide SR; pramlintide with metreleptin; and tesofensine.[7,57,72]

Exenatide and Liraglutide. The GLP-1 receptor agonists exenatide and liraglutide, currently used in treatment of T2DM, are associated with weight loss independent of their side effect of nausea. These have boxed warnings for an increased pancreatitis and thyroid tumor risk. Liraglutide, under the name Saxenda (Novo Nordisk), is a GLP-1 receptor agonist given by subcutaneous injection for the chronic treatment of OB in nondiabetics.[7,72] Weight loss should be monitored and liraglutide discontinued if a minimum of 4% weight loss has not occurred. Liraglutide is contraindicated in pregnancy (Category X) and in patients with multiple endocrine neoplasia syndrome.

Medications Without Current FDA Approval for Weight Loss. Sibutramine (Meridia) was voluntarily removed from US and Canadian markets in 2010 for adverse cardiovascular risk associations.[76] Rimonabant (Acomplia) blocks endocannabinoid receptors but has been associated with neuropsychiatric side effects, including suicide, and has never been approved for use in the United States.[85] Fenfluramine-phentermine ("fen-phen") combination therapy and dexfenfluramine were voluntarily withdrawn in 1997 after cardiac valvulopathy side effects were attributed to fenfluramine.[76] Human chorionic gonadotropin (hCG) injections have been prescribed with a 500-kcal diet (i.e., Dr. Simeon's protocol) but are not FDA approved for weight loss and have not been shown to benefit weight loss, fat redistribution, appetite suppression, or improvement in mood when compared with placebo injections.[86] The

US FDA, the AMA, and Obesity Medicine Association (OMA) have denounced hCG as ineffective for treating OB.

Other pharmaceutical options *not* recommended for inducing weight loss include testosterone replacement in hypogonadal or eugonadal men with OB; cyanocobalamin (vitamin B_{12}); and levothyroxine or liothyronine thyroid use in euthyroid patients.[72]

Consensus Pharmacologic Recommendations: the Endocrine Society, the European Society of Endocrinology, and the Obesity Society

In 2015, a consensus process among members of the Endocrine Society, the European Society of Endocrinology, and the OB Society produced a clinical practice guideline on the pharmacologic management of OB. A summary of the recommendations for management of OW/OB includes the following:

1. Work with all patients to reduce food intake, increase physical activity, and engage in behavior modification techniques.
2. For patients with BMI of 25 kg/m² or higher, use diet, exercise, and behavior modification techniques alone.
3. Reserve pharmacotherapy for weight loss in patients with BMI of 27 kg/m² or higher with comorbidity, or BMI of 30 kg/m² or higher.
4. Consider BS as an adjunct in patients with BMI of 35 kg/m² or higher with comorbidity, or BMI of 40 kg/m² or higher.
5. Patients may be candidates for weight loss medications if they have a history of lack of success with weight loss and maintenance of the weight loss and if they meet medication label requirements.
6. Consider use of weight loss medications to promote long-term weight maintenance in patients with a BMI of 30 kg/m² or higher, or a BMI of 27 kg/m² or higher with one comorbidity such as hypertension, dyslipidemia, T2DM, or OSA.
7. Assess patients monthly for the first 3 months, then reassess need for medication every 3 months.
8. In patients with an adequate response (weight loss of 5% body weight or more in 3 months), continue weight loss medication. If response is not adequate or if safety or tolerability concerns arise, discontinue medication and consider alternative medications or referral for alternative therapies.
9. Start medication at a low dose and escalate while monitoring for side effects; do not exceed recommended doses.
10. Do not use sympathomimetic agents such as phentermine and diethylpropion in patients with a history of heart disease or uncontrolled hypertension; consider lorcaserin or orlistat.
11. In patients who have OW and T2DM, choose oral antidiabetic medications that are weight neutral or promote weight loss (GLP-1 analogues or sodium-glucose linked transporter-2 inhibitors) in addition to metformin.
12. If individual with OB and T2DM requires insulin therapy, add at least one of the following: metformin, pramlintide, or GLP-1 agonists to offset insulin-induced weight gain. Use basal (long-acting) insulin instead of insulin alone or in combination with sulfonylurea.
13. For individuals with OB and hypertension, angiotensin-converting enzyme inhibitors, angiotensin receptor blockers, and calcium channel blockers are preferred over β-adrenergic blockers for first-line therapy.[77,78]

Dietary Supplements

Dietary supplements during weight loss are commonly used to replace missing dietary vitamins and minerals. However, some supplements are also proposed to contribute to weight loss as an intended effect above that attributed to reduced kilocalories and increased energy expenditure. They may be viewed as more "natural" than pharmaceuticals. Nutraceuticals, botanicals, amino acids, and trace elements have been marketed for weight loss effects. A systematic review of weight loss supplements found that clinical studies are small, are of poor quality, have variable measurements that are not consistent, and do not control for covariables. No weight loss above 5% was achieved. Nine supplements, their associated weight loss findings, and some proposed mechanisms of actions were reviewed and reported on by Onakpoya and colleagues.[87] Ephedrine is associated with significant short-term weight loss effects but can have serious side effects. It works by enhancing thermogenesis. Glucomannan studies showed significant weight loss in persons with OB; the proposed effect is by increasing satiety through slowing of gastric emptying. *Camellia sinensis* (green tea) demonstrated efficacy for weight loss and maintenance by fat oxidation stimulus and increased energy expenditure. Chromium picolinate was associated with a relatively small weight loss effect by increasing BMR and insulin sensitivity. Chitosan had inconclusive short-term weight loss effects. The authors concluded that conjugated linoleic acid, calcium supplements, *Citrus aurantium* (bitter orange), and guar gum were not efficacious for weight loss.[76,87]

Weight loss supplements are frequently a target of FDA actions. Supplements for weight loss have been tainted with many ingredients, including sibutramine (an appetite-suppressant drug removed in 2010 from the US market), the diuretic bumetanide, rimonabant, phenytoin, and the suspected carcinogen phenolphthalein.[88]

Bariatric Surgery and Endoluminal Therapies

Approximately 216,000 metabolic and BSs were performed in 2016, and primary care, endocrine, and gastroenterology providers will follow patients for decades after surgery as the need for postoperative care is lifelong.[89] BS does not cure OB or guarantee weight loss results. Weight regain is a common problem, and nutritional and metabolic complications routinely occur.[60] BS is an effective tool, with results that can be durable.

Indications and Contraindications. Indications for BS are BMI of 40 kg/m² or higher, or 35 kg/m² or higher with OB-associated comorbidity; failure of previous weight loss attempts; commitment to postoperative care, supplements, and testing; and exclusion of reversible endocrine or other causes of OB. In 2011 the FDA approved use of the Lap-Band for those with BMIs of 30 to 40 kg/m² or higher with one OB-related comorbidity. Suggested contraindications are current substance use; uncontrolled, severe psychiatric illness; lack of understanding of surgical risks and benefits, expected outcomes, alternative weight loss options, and lifestyle changes required after BS; and extremely high operative risk.[90]

Bariatric Surgery. BS accomplishes weight loss for those unable to obtain or maintain weight loss via non-surgical means. This tool, BS, is accompanied by ILI, and can lead to durable weight loss along with improvement and even resolution of comorbid conditions. In the recent past, BS were divided into categories based on size restriction of the gastric pouch or malabsorption, or a combination. This division oversimplifies the evidence for weight loss from neural, gut hormone, and endocrine signals that change eating behaviors and food preferences, reduce appetite, enhance satiety, reduce caloric intake, change intestinal microbiota, and maybe change energy expenditure post BS. Hence, BS may be referred to as a metabolic intervention.[80]

Laparoscopic Adjustable Gastric Banding. In laparoscopic adjustable gastric banding (LAGB) or (AGB), an adjustable gastric band is placed around the upper stomach, creating a 15- to 30-mL pouch. A subcutaneous port is placed to adjust the amount of constriction by injecting or removing saline.[91] WL at 3 years has been reported to be 15% total body weight.[91] AGB placement has decreased substantially worldwide and in the United States from over 35% of BS in 2011 to less than 4% in 2016.[92] Compared with Roux-en-Y gastric bypass (RYGB), weight loss from AGB is less and control of T2DM less dramatic, but LAGB results in fewer long-term nutritional and metabolic complications and is associated with less lean tissue loss during weight loss. AGB is more likely to need reversal because of band-related complications, and it may require conversion to a more malabsorptive procedure. Complications include band slippage, band erosion, balloon failure, port dilation, and port infections. Regurgitation, vomiting, and gastric dysmotility may occur.[60] Greater weight loss success with LAGB is associated with a starting BMI of 45 or higher, postprandial satiety after placement, and frequent band adjustments in the first year.[90]

Roux-en-Y Gastric Bypass. RYGB was previously the most frequently performed surgery in the United States and worldwide, but is no longer.[92] In the United States, 18.7% of BS procedures were RYGB in 2016, down from over 37% in 2012. In RYGB, the upper section of the stomach is transected, creating a small 10- to 30-mL pouch. This gastric pouch is attached to the proximal jejunum, leaving some of the jejunum, the duodenum, and the remaining stomach "bypassed" and not available for nutrient absorption. The length of the limb determines the extent of malabsorption. RYGB results in greater loss of excess body weight, faster weight loss, and quicker T2DM improvements and resolution compared with AGB.[90] RYGB is considered a metabolic surgery. In addition to its mechanical restrictive and malabsorptive properties, it is associated with changes in gut hormones GLP-1, ghrelin, and PYY and improvements in T2DM independent of weight loss.[93]

Sleeve Gastrectomy. Laparoscopic vertical sleeve gastrectomy (VSG) reduces the stomach size by 80% and has a complication rate of less than 1%. In this procedure, the greater curvature of the stomach is stapled and removed. A tubular shaped lesser curvature stomach remains. There is no intestinal anastomosis. This is a restrictive, irreversible procedure involving a distinct anatomic change to the alimentary canal with associated physiologic implications.[94] The resection of the greater curvature of the stomach results in a lack of ghrelin hormone, causing increased satiety. Over 58% of BS in the United States were VSG in 2016, making it the most widely used surgical technique.[92] Long-term data are not available. Increased risk for Barrett esophagus is significant for long-term monitoring.

Biliopancreatic Diversion. Biliopancreatic diversion (BPD) is not commonly performed (0.6% of BS during 2016 in the United States) due to its high risk of nutritional and other complications, both short and long term. It is a more complex procedure compared to other BS. A sleeve gastrectomy is done which is then anastomosed to the proximal duodenum. This large bypass of intestine is responsible for a high degree of nutrient malabsorption.[91,92]

Vagal Nerve Blocking. Vagal nerve blocking is proposed to help reduce hunger and stimulate satiety. This procedure has had less than anticipated weight loss outcomes, and is performed sparsely in the United States.[90,91]

Bariatric Surgery Outcomes. Surgically induced weight loss is rapid. Comorbidities improve or may be resolved. Mortality from all causes is reduced, with reductions greatest in cardiovascular deaths.[95] Weight loss is more durable in BS compared with no treatment or presently available nonsurgical treatments. Secondary procedures are for BS reversal, revision, or conversion to another surgical weight loss technique.

Long-term LAGB outcomes of 12 years or longer in 151 Belgian patients were 0% operative mortality and 3.7% long-term mortality (not surgically related); 22% had minor complications, and 39% experienced major complications, including 28% with band erosions. Seventeen percent had the LAGB converted to RYGB, and 51% retained their band. A BS meta-analysis found that excess body weight loss was 50% after LAGB and 76% after RYGB.[60]

The Swiss multi-center bypass of sleeve study randomly assigned 217 surgical candidates to SG or RYGB with a 5-year follow up. Excess BMI losses were similar in both groups: SG 61 1% vs. RTGB 69.3%. Gastric reflux remission was observed more often in RYGB (60.4%) than in SG (31.8%), and gastric reflux worsened more often in SG (31.8%) compared to RYBG (22%).[96]

Operative mortality varies from 0.1% to 2% after RYGB.[97] Complications are related to complexity of the surgical procedure, surgeon experience, bariatric center experience, number of comorbidities, higher BMIs, and size of visceral fat stores.[97] Early perioperative complications include thromboembolism, pulmonary insufficiency, hemorrhage, peritonitis, postoperative leaks, and wound infection. Nutritional deficiencies, anastomotic stenosis, internal hernia, diarrhea, bacterial overgrowth, and dumping syndrome may follow RYGB later. Dumping syndrome symptoms include abdominal pain, cramping, lightheadedness, flushing tachycardia, and syncope. It is commonly related to ingestion of simple carbohydrates and occurs in as many as three of four patients after RYGB. It typically improves with time and can be mitigated with small, slow meals (30 minutes' duration), avoiding liquids with meals, avoiding simple carbohydrates, and increasing protein intake.[60]

Endoscopic Bariatric Therapies for Weight Loss. Endoscopic bariatric therapies (EBTs) are less invasive than BS, may be used to obtain weight loss and improve control of metabolic comorbidities, may be used in place of surgical revision to treat weight regain post BS, and may be viewed as filling a large gap between lifestyle intervention, pharmaceutical, and BS (Table 17.1). EBTs are performed endoscopically (under general anesthesia or under light sedation) and may be space occupying,

TABLE 17.1 Selected Endoscopic Bariatric Therapies

Device	Procedure	Mechanism	Regulatory Status	
Orbera	Intragastric saline-filled balloon	Space-occupying device	FDA approved	Retrieved at 6 months
Integrated dual balloon	Intragastric balloon	Space-occupying device	FDA approved	Retrieved at 6 months
OverStitch	Endoscopic sleeve gastroplasty	Gastric remodeling-anastomosis	FDA approved (for tissue apposition)	
Incisionless operating platform	Primary OB endoluminal surgery	Gastric remodeling	FDA approved (for tissue apposition)	
Articulating circular endo. stapler	Gastroplasty	Gastric remodeling	In human trials	
AspireAssist	Aspiration therapy percutaneously	Aspiration of stomach contents after meals	FDA approved	Can be reversed by removal
Self-assembling magnet	Endoscopic and colonic placed; enteral anastomosis	Dual-path enteral bypass	In human trials	Type 2 diabetes treatment; magnets pass naturally
OverStitch	Transoral outlet reduction for revision of GB	Anastomotic reduction	FDA approved (for tissue apposition)	
Incisionless operating platform POSE	Revision OB surgery endoluminal for revision of GB	Anastomotic and pouch reduction	FDA approved (for tissue apposition)	
Elipse swallowable balloon	Swallowed capsule attached to catheter	Space-occupying device	Not evaluated by FDA	Auto deflation at 4 months; passes naturally
TransPyloric Shuttle	Placed thru overtube	Intermittently blocks pylorus	In human trials	Retrieved at 12 months
EndoBarrier	60-cm Teflon sleeve lines duodenum to jejunum	Sleeve creates bypass similar to RYGB		

FDA, US Food and Drug Administration; *GB*, gastric bypass surgery; *OB*, obesity; *RYGB*, Roux-en-Y gastric bypass.
Data from Kumar, N. (2016). Weight loss endoscopy: Development, applications, and current status. *World Journal of Gastroenterology, 22*(31):7069–7079. doi: 10.3748/wjg.v22.i31.7069; Thompson, C. C., Dayyeh, B. K., Kushner, R. Sullivan, S., Schorr, A. B., Amaro, A., et al. (2017). Percutaneous gastrostomy device for the treatment of class II and class III obesity: Results of a randomized controlled trial. *American Journal of Gastroenterology, 112*:447–457. doi: 10.1038/ajg.2016.500.

remodel gastric mucosa, create bowel anastomosis, provide outlet for post-meal food removal, achieve both weight loss and metabolic benefits, and serve as a bridge therapy to reduce surgical risk before bariatric or other major surgery. Space occupying devices (balloons) and are removed after six months, with lifestyle interventions continued for another 6 months. Methylene blue is added to the balloon in one device (Orbera) for leak detection; should the device rupture, urine will turn green. Long-term weight loss in a study of 500 patients with OB was 23 kg at 12 months and 7.3 kg at 5 years for those available to follow-up. Comorbidities such as T2DM, hypertension, and dyslipidemia improved in addition to improved quality of life.

Aspiration Therapy. Aspiration therapy (AspireAssist) involves a 30-French percutaneous endoscopic gastrostomy (PEG) placed through the abdominal wall. Twenty to thirty minutes after meals, water is infused and the stomach contents subsequently drained. About 30% of ingested kcal are removed. Dietary and lifestyle interventions are to be ongoing. In a randomized control trial, total weight loss at 12 months was 18% in the aspiration group compared to 6% in the dietary and lifestyle intervention alone. A VLCD used in a small study 4 weeks prior to tube placement resulted in greater weight loss compared to the group without a VLCD. Contraindications include BED, night eating disorder, or other eating disorders. Improved eating behaviors include eating slower, chewing food thoroughly (large pieces will not pass through the tube), increased water consumption during meals, better dietary choices, and meal planning. T2DM markers are improved: lower fasting blood glucose and hemoglobin A1C, with some patients able to discontinue diabetic medication. Adverse effects include perioperative abdominal pain, post-procedure granulation tissue, peristomal irritation, abdominal fluid collection, and skin infection.

Post-Procedure Nutritional Supplementation. In addition to a chewable multivitamin, vitamin B_{12} (by various routes), folate, iron as ferrous sulfate with vitamin C, calcium as calcium citrate, and vitamin D supplementation are needed lifelong. Thiamine supplementation may be indicated for some patients, particularly if neuropathy occurs, or for patients with significant emesis or weight loss after BS.[98] For post-BS patients with thinning hair, zinc is a supplement consideration.[98] Prenatal vitamins, products from bariatric nutrition suppliers, and specially compounded medications may be combined to meet individual needs. Therapy changes are based on laboratory analysis, physical signs of deficiency, dietary shortfalls, and nutritionist recommendations.[60]

Monitoring After Bariatric Surgery. Lifelong testing after BS includes vitamin D, calcium, phosphorus, parathyroid hormone (PTH); alkaline phosphatase levels and bone density DXA (after 2 years) every 6 months until weight is stable; and perhaps urinary C-peptide for bone health monitoring. A full annual mandatory test list includes these in addition to CBC, liver function tests, glucose, creatinine, electrolytes, iron, vitamin B_{12}, folate, calcium, intact PTH, 25-hydroxyvitamin D, and optionally albumin or prealbumin, vitamin A, zinc, and vitamin B_1.[60] Testing is more frequent in the first 24 postoperative months.

OB is a risk factor for gallstones and gout, and any rapid weight loss may incite acute gout attacks and cholelithiasis. During early postsurgical weight loss months, prophylactic therapy may be indicated.[90]

Medications After Bariatric Surgery. Medications to avoid after BS are nonsteroidal anti-inflammatory drugs, salicylates, corticosteroids, oral bisphosphonates, ethanol, and extended-release formulations, which can irritate the GI tract, injure the pouch, or result in altered absorption. To minimize dumping syndrome, medications with sucrose, corn syrup, maltose, and sorbitol should be avoided. Calcium channel blockers, β blockers, nitrates, anticholinergics, and some antihistamines may increase gastroesophageal reflux and thus should be avoided if possible. Pills and tablets may not be tolerated; liquid or nonenteric delivery options may be pursued. Diuretics should be held any time liquids are not tolerated and if vomiting or diarrhea persists.[90] Tobacco should also be avoided.[97]

Pregnancy After Bariatric Procedures. Women should delay pregnancy 12 to 24 months after BS but may have variable responses to OC and should rely on non-hormonal or non–oral hormone delivery methods. Gestational diabetes and preeclampsia are reduced in post-BS pregnancies in comparison to pre-surgery pregnancies. Rates of cesarean delivery and premature rupture of membranes may be higher in comparison to nonsurgical women with OB. Higher BS is not an indication for cesarean delivery. The bariatric surgeon should be consulted if adjustment to the LAGB is indicated. Nutritional evaluation must be thorough, with parenteral supplementation if deficiencies are not responsive to oral replacements. Common GI complaints of pregnancy, such as nausea and vomiting, may warrant investigation for anastomotic leaks, bowel obstructions, internal or ventral hernias, and band migration or erosion. Dumping syndrome may preclude tolerance of oral glucose tolerance testing. Consider home glucose monitoring.[99]

Weight Regain Post-Procedure. Weight regain is common after any weight loss, but special considerations after surgical weight loss include evaluation for GI anastomosis, fistula, or loss of band integrity in LAGB.[60] Expected weight regain 10 years after BS is commonly 20% to 25% of weight lost, but the true prevalence is not known because patients are not typically followed up long term or are lost to follow-up.[60]

Psychological Results After Bariatric Surgery. Improved health-related quality of life is typically expected after BS. Body image, sexual functioning, and marital relationships have been reported to improve. Not all enjoy these benefits, and some may find the life-changing experience negative and the nutritional and GI side effects problematic; overall, they may perceive themselves as being greatly restricted because of these changes. In a qualitative study, participants' concerns, chronic pain, low energy levels, and lower social functioning were dismissed by practitioners, and patients reported feeling shame and stigma because of their less-than-ideal responses to surgery.[100] In Pennsylvania, the suicide risk among post-BS individuals was alarmingly high compared with the state average. The first 3 years after surgery were found to be the most critical period; 70% of the suicides occurred in this time frame.[101] Lifelong caring for the whole person requires understanding of these possibilities and appropriate intervention after astute assessment for depression and suicide ideation.

Preoperative Management. Preoperative management includes optimization of nutritional status, a psychological evaluation with clearance, initiation of a physical activity program, and control of comorbidities. Weight loss before surgery improves operative risks and comorbidity management and aids in the technical aspects of the procedure. A VLCD may be used to reduce liver volume. Patients requiring coronary artery bypass grafting or stent placement before surgery may also require an aggressive VLCD before the needed cardiac intervention.[90] Some third-party insurance payers require preoperative weight loss.

Indications for Referral or Hospitalization

Patients with OB may be referred to sleep specialists for OSA or OB hypoventilation syndrome evaluations. Bedtime eating disorder responds best to cognitive behavioral therapy or structured self-help, and may warrant referral. Other eating disorders such as bulimia should be referred to an experienced provider.

When BS is considered, evaluation by a nutritionist is suggested. A referral should be made to a bariatric center of excellence that performs large numbers of bariatric procedures. Specific performance data should be reviewed. Preoperative and postoperative involvement with a full bariatric surgical team is correlated with success, and the primary care provider should encourage full engagement. An ongoing relationship with the primary care provider and experienced bariatric surgeons begins before referrals are made and continues long term.[60] The American Society for Metabolic and BS website (www.asmbs.org) and the OB Society website (www.obesity.org) can facilitate locating BS and non-surgical OB specialist providers.

A post-BS complication that requires inpatient treatment is severe protein deficiency, which requires hospitalization for parenteral nutrition in about 1% of malabsorption cases.[60] Surgical revision may be indicated if weight loss is inadequate, significant weight regain occurs, or malnutrition therapy is not amenable to medical intervention. Revision is considered after medical options have failed.[90] Frequent vomiting should be evaluated with a contrast study before an endoscopic examination. A radionuclide gastric emptying study should be ordered if gastroparesis is suspected. Other indications for endoscopic examination include stoma stricture, reflux, inflammation, and stoma erosion. Outpatient management is indicated for dilation of strictures.[60]

LIFE SPAN CONSIDERATIONS

OB has perinatal and multigenerational origins. Maternal health and nutrition, gestational weight gain, cigarette smoking, environmental toxin exposures, exercise, and early infant feedings affect short- and long-term energy balance in offspring, with durable manifestations spanning developmental phases from birth weight to midlife weight. Appropriate BMI during preconception, limiting of pregnancy weight gain to less than 40 pounds, promotion of breastfeeding, delay of food introduction in formula-fed infants, and avoiding unnecessary antibiotics are only a few early preventive measures. In adults, prevention applies to a minority, as two-thirds of US adults are above a healthy BMI. Avoiding future weight gain, improving dietary intake, and increasing physical activity are minimal goals for populations and individuals.

Older adults can increase physical activity and reduce excess weight safely. Nearly 300 older adults—with an average age of 67 years, OB, cardiovascular or cardiometabolic disease, and limitations in mobility and who were not physically active—were assigned to successful aging education, physical activity, or weight loss plus physical activity intervention groups for 18 months in a community center. The weight loss and physical activity treatment group had clinically significant improvements in physical walking performance, decreased weight by 8.5%, and maintained a weight loss of 7.7% at 18 months. The successful aging and physical activity groups had similar but minimal improvement in walking performance scores, with weight decreases about 1% from baseline after 18 months. The greatest treatment effects were in those with poorest baseline mobility. The side effects were mostly minor, temporary musculoskeletal effects with two serious side effects (not specified) and not statistically significant between groups.[102]

Individuals with sarcopenia, muscle loss occurring after the age of 30 years, can accumulate a 30% reduced muscle mass by the age of 60 years. Sarcopenia may be mitigated by physical activity and adequate protein ingestion. Protein synthesis, which contributes to gains in muscle mass, immune components, and wound healing, may be maximized by sufficient high-quality dietary protein intake of 25 to 30 g at each meal combined with resistance training.[103] Weight loss in older adults is associated with body composition changes comparable to changes in younger weight loss individuals. Typically, losses consist of about 25% lean and 75% fat tissue. Metabolic abnormalities and cardiac risk factors improve with intentional weight loss in older adults, and physical function is best improved in combination with physical activity.

COMPLICATIONS OF OBESTIY
Increased Medical Costs

OB-related deaths account for 5% to 15% of deaths in the United States. Increased health care spending for persons with OW and OB (class I, II, and III) is estimated to be 10%, 23%, 45%, and 80%, respectively, compared to those with normal weight.[104] US spending in 2017 for health care and societal cost was calculated at $3.88 million dollars. Additional private and public spending for lifetime medical costs in a 20-year-old person with OB, with no metabolic disease apparent, is calculated at $14,059 in addition to $14,141 for societal costs, totaling over $28,000, compared to a person with normal weight. For a metabolically healthy 50-year-old person with OB these costs are $15,925 plus $20,120, totaling $36,278 compared to a metabolically healthy person with a normal BMI. Higher BMIs are associated with incremental costs across the lifespan, peaking at age 50 years. Weight loss is associated with likewise incremental cost savings.[105] Understanding, treating, and preventing OB has a substantial economic impact for the country.

Social Stigma and Discrimination

Significant social stigma and discrimination affect people with OB. The stigma of OB is pervasive and may profoundly affect many individuals. OB stigma is the devaluation of individuals with OB as members of a group. It can manifest externally as weight-based discrimination or internally as prejudice. Stigma can also be self-directed as devaluation, guilt, and shame. Discrimination based on weight status affects opportunities for housing, career, education, and parental support; it is associated with bullying and harassment, and it contributes to health care disparities in provider expectations, recommendations, and preventive screenings ordered by practitioners.

Increased Morbidity and Mortality

Compared with a reference BMI of 22 to 24.9, mortality increases as BMI increases in nonsmoking adults without prevalent disease. This relationship is strongest when the higher

BMI is noted before age 79 years. Significant health consequences associated with excess adiposity include increased mortality, chiefly from cardiovascular disease and cancers, but also from all other causes.[48] Cancers of the uterus, gallbladder, kidney, cervix, thyroid, liver, colon, and ovaries, leukemia, and postmenopausal breast cancer are associated with BMIs above 22 kg/m^2.[106] Other OB-related conditions are gallbladder disease, non-alcohol fatty liver disease (NAFLD) and nonalcoholic steatohepatitis (NASH), dyslipidemias, hypertension, atrial fibrillation, infertility, erectile dysfunction, asthma, chronic back pain, eye diseases (cataracts, glaucoma, age-related maculopathy, and retinopathy), osteoarthritis, decreased functioning in elderly, OSA, and pulmonary embolism.

Relative risk for death from respiratory, cardiovascular, and cancer causes increased as waist circumferences increased above 90 cm in men and 75 cm in women. NAFLD represents the liver's response to OB and is a hepatic component of metabolic syndrome. Steatosis, increased liver fat, begins the process of inflammation, hepatic cell death, and fibrotic scarring, leading to end-stage liver disease or hepatic cancer. Excess liver fat is an independent cardiovascular disease risk factor.[107]

OB and insulin resistance occur in half of women with polycystic ovary syndrome (PCOS); women with OB have a 12% PCOS prevalence.[36] Fertility is impaired with OB, mainly from oligo-ovulation and anovulation, and there is a reduced response to gonadotropin ovulation therapy. When pregnancy occurs in women with OB, risks for miscarriage, spontaneous preterm birth, gestational diabetes, preeclampsia, cesarean delivery, and infectious complications are greater. Vaginal birth after cesarean delivery is less likely to be successful in women with OB. Surgical times are increased, recovery from anesthesia is longer, greater blood loss occurs, and incidence of thromboembolism is higher in obese maternal surgeries. Labor is more likely to be prolonged. Fetal risks for congenital anomalies, growth abnormalities, defects of the neural tube and cardiac system, and cleft palate are increased. Stillbirth rates can be two to four times greater in mothers with OB compared with normal-weight mothers.[99] Infants small and large for gestational age are associated with maternal OB, and these children face an increased risk of childhood OB.

Osteoarthritis risk is increased, not only in the weight-bearing joints of people with OB, but also in non–weight-bearing joints. Disability and reduced quality-adjusted life-years in people with OB affected by knee osteoarthritis are much higher than in individuals with healthy BMIs. Black and Hispanic women with OB experience even greater reduced quality-adjusted life-years because of knee osteoarthritis than white women with OB.[108] A dose-dependent response between BMI above 22.5 kg/m^2 and knee osteoarthritis was noted in a meta-analysis of studies from seven countries. BMIs at 25, 30, and 35 kg/m^2 were associated with increased relative risks of 1.59, 3.55, and 7.45, respectively.[109]

OSA prevalence in those with OB is 41% to 58% and markedly higher when BMI is above 40 kg/m^2.[38] Chest wall compliance is reduced, work of breathing is increased, a higher minute ventilation accommodates a higher metabolic rate, and reduced lung volumes lend mechanical contributions to OB hypoventilation. Insulin resistance with an altered hypothalamic response to orexins may contribute to neuroendocrine components of OSA in people with OB. In women who have OB and PCOS, OSA prevalence may be as high as 44% to 70%.[38]

OB-related impaired immunity function creates increased susceptibility for infectious disease from tuberculosis, influenza, coxsackievirus, *Helicobacter pylori*, and encephalomyocarditis virus and reduces antibody responses to vaccinations.[12] Risks for surgical wound infection, community-acquired pneumonia and other respiratory tract infections, in-hospital septicemia, and severe H1N1 influenza outcomes, including death, are increased.[12]

PATIENT AND FAMILY EDUCATION

Encourage active engagement in supportive resources for all ages:
- Aim for a Healthy Weight (NIH) https://www.nhlbi.nih.gov/health/educational/lose_wt/index.htm
- Losing Weight and Getting Healthier (AHA) http://www.heart.org/HEARTORG/HealthyLiving/WeightManagement/Obesity/Losing-Weight-and-Getting-Healthier_UCM_447778_Article.jsp#.Wmp4zzdOk2w
- Obesity Action Coalition http://www.obesityaction.org/

HEALTH PROMOTION

Patients and families should be educated about the benefits of maintaining a healthy weight, engaging in regular exercise, and getting adequate sleep. Encourage, support, and offer comprehensive weight loss and weight loss maintenance efforts. OB by its chronic nature is difficult to treat and presents a lifelong struggle for many adults. Early diagnosis and intensive treatment are essential. Ideal intervention programs are intensive, incorporate family members, and include education about healthy eating, sleep, and the importance of daily physical activity. Encourage a skilled lifestyle that implements these.

Practitioners can develop MI techniques. Include questions regarding weight control behaviors, dietary habits, and physical activity in routine health assessments. Effective OB prevention involves the providers' knowledge and skill regarding proximate contributions of OW and obesity. Embrace a long-term, lifelong approach for intensive, comprehensive weight management with other health care professionals. Maintain a non-judgmental environment. Keep abreast of resources and new research that relates to promoting healthy weight, weight loss, and weight management.

REFERENCES

1. Ng, M., Fleming, T., Robinson, M., et al. (2014). Global, regional, and national prevalence of overweight and obesity in children and adults during 1980–2013: A systematic analysis for the Global Burden of Disease Study 2013. *Lancet, 384*(9945), 766–781.
2. NCD Risk Factor collaboration. (2016). Trends in adult body-mass index in 200 countries from 1975 to 2014: A pooled analysis of 1698 population-based measurement studies with 19.2 million participants. *Lancet, 387*(10026), 1377–1396. DOI: http://dx.doi.org/10.1016/S0140-6736(16)30054-X.
3. Ogden, C., Carroll, M., Kit, B. K., & Flegal, K. (2014). Prevalence of childhood and adult obesity in the United States, 2011–2012. *JAMA: The Journal of the American Medical Association, 311*(8), 806–814.
4. Hale, et al. (2017). Prevalence of obesity among adults and youth: United States, 2016-2016. US Dept of Health & Human Services. NCHS Data Brief, No. 288.
5. Troy, L. M., Miller, E. A., & Olson, S. (2011). Hunger and obesity: Understanding a food insecurity paradigm: workshop summary. Washington, DC: National Academies Press. Retrieved from www.nap.edu/catalog/13102.html. (Accessed November 2017).
6. Oza-Frank, R., & Narayan, K. M. (2010). Effect of length of residence on overweight by region of birth and age at arrival among U.S. immigrants. *Public Health Nutrition, 13*, 868–875.

7. U.S. Department of Veteran Affairs and Department of Defense. (2014). VA/DoD clinical practice guideline for screening and management of overweight and obesity. Version 2.0. Retrieved from http://www.healthquality.va.gov/guidelines/CD/obesity/VADoDCPGManagementOfOverweightAndObesityFinal.pdf. (Accessed 28 November 2017).

8. Mechanick, J. I., Garber, A. J., Handelsman, Y., & Garvey, W. T. (2012). American Association of Clinical Endocrinologists' position statement on obesity and obesity medicine. *Endocrine Practice, 18*(5).

9. Jensen, R., Donato, D., Donato, K., et al. (2014). AHA/ACC/TOS prevention guideline: 2013 AHA/ACC/TOS guideline for the management of overweight and obesity in adults: A report of the American College of Cardiology/American Heart Association Task Force on Practice Guidelines and The Obesity Society. *Circulation, 129*(25 Suppl. 2), S102–S138.

10. Cooper, J. T. (2010). Evaluation of the obese patient. In G. M. Steelman & E. C. Westman (Eds.), *Obesity: Evaluation and treatment essentials*. New York: Informa.

11. American Medical Association (AMA). (2013). Council on Science and Public Health Report 3-A13. Is obesity a disease? Resolution 115-A-12. AMA House of Delegate Annual Meeting. (Chicago, IL). Retrieved from www.ama-assn.org/assets/meeting/2013a/a13-addendum-refcomm-d.pdf. (Accessed 12 September 2014).

12. Karlsson, E. A., & Beck, M. A. (2010). The burden of obesity on infectious disease. *Experimental Biology and Medicine, 235*(12), 1412–1424.

13. Finucane, M. M., Stevens, G. A., Cowan, M. J., et al. (2011). National, regional, and global trends in body-mass index since 1980: Systematic analysis of health examination surveys and epidemiological studies with 960 country-years and 9.1 million participants. *Lancet, 377*(9765), 557–567.

14. Butland, B., Jebb, S., Kopelman, P., et al. (2007). *Foresight: Tackling obesities: Future choices—project report* (2nd ed.). United Kingdom: Government Office for Science.

15. Johnson, R. K., Appel, L. J., Brands, M., et al. (2009). American Heart Association Nutrition Committee of the Council on Nutrition, Physical Activity, and Metabolism and the Council on Epidemiology and Prevention: Dietary sugars intake and cardiovascular health: A scientific statement from the American Heart Association. *Circulation, 120*(11), 1011–1020.

16. Lee, M., & Korner, J. (2009). Review of physiology, clinical manifestations, and management of hypothalamic obesity in humans. *Pituitary, 12*(2), 87–95.

17. Beckerman, M. (2009). *Cellular signaling in health and disease*. New York: Springer.

18. Guyton, A. C., & Hall, J. E. (2006). *Textbook of medical physiology* (11th ed.). Philadelphia: Elsevier Saunders.

19. Haskell, W. L., Lee, I. M., Pate, R. R., et al. (2007). Physical activity and public health: Updated recommendation for adults from the American College of Sports Medicine and the American Heart Association. *Medicine and Science in Sports and Exercise, 39*(8), 1423–1434.

20. Lee, I. M., Djoussé, L., Sesso, H. D., et al. (2010). Physical activity and weight gain prevention. *JAMA: The Journal of the American Medical Association, 303*(12), 1173–1179.

21. International Association for the Study of Obesity. (2010). Obesity: understanding and challenging the global epidemic: 2009–2010 report from the International Association for the Study of Obesity. London: IASO.

22. McCarthy, M. I. (2010). Genomics, type 2 diabetes, and obesity. *The New England Journal of Medicine, 24*, 2339–2350.

23. Farooqi, I. S., & O'Rahilly, S. (2007). Genetic factors in human obesity. *Obesity Reviews: An Official Journal of the International Association for the Study of Obesity, 8*, 37–40.

24. Hinney, A., Vogel, C. I. G., & Hebebrand, J. (2010). From monogenic to polygenic obesity: Recent advances. *European Child and Adolescent Psychiatry, 19*(3), 297–310.

25. Deierlein, A. L., Siega-Riz, A. M., Chantala, K., et al. (2011). The association between maternal glucose concentration and child BMI at age 3 years. *Diabetes Care, 34*(2), 480–484.

26. Schwarz, E. B., Ray, R. M., Stuebe, A. M., et al. (2009). Duration of lactation and risk factors for maternal cardiovascular disease. *Obstetrics and Gynecology, 113*(5), 974–982.

27. Huh, S. Y., Rifas-Shiman, S. L., Taveras, E. M., et al. (2011). Timing of solid food introduction and risk of obesity in preschool-aged children. *Pediatrics, 127*(3), e544–e551.

28. Wang, Y., Wang, X., Kong, Y., et al. (2009). The great Chinese famine leads to shorter and overweight females in Chongqing Chinese population after 50 years. *Obesity, 18*(3), 588–592.

29. Ino, T. (2010). Maternal smoking during pregnancy and offspring obesity: Meta-analysis. *Pediatrics International, 52*(1), 94–99.

30. Oza-Frank, R., & Narayan, K. M. (2010). Overweight and diabetes prevalence among US immigrants. *American Journal of Public Health, 100*(4), 661–668.

31. Claire, C., Gonseth, S., Cornuz, J., & Berlin, I. (2014). Tobacco use, smoking cessation, and obesity. In G. Bray & C. Bouchard (Eds.), *Handbook of obesity: Clinical applications* (4th ed., Vol. 2, pp. 339–348). Boca Raton: CRC Press Taylor and Francis Group.

32. Davtyan, C., & Ma, M. (September 10, 2008). Drug-induced weight gain: clinical vignette. Proceedings of UCLA HealthCare. UCLA Department of Medicine.

33. Hsieh, A., Sweeting, A., Suryawanshi, A., & Caterson, I. D. (2014). Drugs that cause weight gain and clinical alternatives to their use. In G. Bray & C. Bouchard (Eds.), *Handbook of obesity: Clinical applications* (4th ed., Vol. 2, pp. 219–232). Boca Raton: CRC Press Taylor and Francis Group.

34. Duhita, M., Schutz, Y., Montani, J., et al. (2017). Oral contraceptive pill alters acute dietary protein-induced thermogenesis in young women. *Obesity, 25*(9), 1482–1485. doi:10.1002/oby.21919.

35. Apovian, C. A., Aronne, L. J., Bessesen, D. H., et al. (2015). Pharmacological management of obesity: An Endocrine Society clinical practice guideline. *The Journal of Clinical Endocrinology and Metabolism, 100*(2), 342–362. doi:10.1210/jc.2014-3415.

36. Diamanti-Kandarakis, E., Bourguignon, J. P., Giudice, L. C., et al. (2009). Endocrine-disrupting chemicals: An Endocrine Society scientific statement. *Endocrine Reviews, 30*(4), 293–342.

37. Grün, F., & Blumberg, B. (2009). Endocrine disrupters as obesogens. *Molecular and Cellular Endocrinology, 304*(1–2), 19–29.

38. Spiegel, K., Tasali, E., Leproult, R., et al. (2009). Effects of poor and short sleep on glucose metabolism and obesity risk. *Nature Reviews. Endocrinology, 5*, 253–261.

39. Canuto, R., Pattussi, M. P., Macagnan, J. B. A., Henn, R. L., & Olinto, M. T. A. (2014). Sleep deprivation and obesity in shift workers in southern Brazil. *Public Health Nutrition, 17*(11), 2619–2623. doi:10.1017/S1368980013002838. [Epub 2013 Oct 29].

40. Nedeltcheva, A. V., Kilkus, J. M., Imperial, J., et al. (2010). Insufficient sleep undermines dietary efforts to reduce adiposity. *Annals of Internal Medicine, 153*(7), 435–441.

41. Manco, M., Putignani, L., & Bottazzo, G. F. (2010). Gut microbiota, lipopolysaccharides, and innate immunity in the pathogenesis of obesity and cardiovascular risk. *Endocrine Reviews, 31*(6), 817–844.

42. Devaraj, S., Hemarajata, P., & Versalovic, J. (2013). The gut microbiome and body metabolism: Implications for obesity and diabetes. *Clinical Chemistry, 59*(4), 617–628.

43. Wardle, J., Chida, Y., Gibson, E. L., et al. (2011). Stress and adiposity: A meta-analysis of longitudinal studies. *Obesity, 19*(4), 771–778.

44. Jackson, S. E., Kirschbaum, C., & Steptoe, A. (2017). Hair cortisol and adiposity in a population-based sample of 2,527 men and women aged 54 to 87 years. *Obesity, 25*(3), 539–544. doi:10.1002/oby.21733.

45. Aills, L., Blankenship, J., Buffington, C., et al. (2008). ASMBS allied health nutritional guidelines for the surgical weight loss patient. *Surgery for Obesity and Related Diseases, 4*(5), S73–S108.

46. ver Ploeg, M., Breneman, V., Farrigan, T., et al. (2009). Access to affordable and nutritious food: Measuring and understanding food deserts and their consequences: A report to Congress. U.S. Department of Agriculture. Retrieved from http://www.ers.usda.gov/media/242675/ap036_1_.pdf. (Accessed 30 January 2018).

47. Krebs-Smith, S. M., Reedy, J., & Bosire, C. (2010). Healthfulness of the U.S. food supply: Little improvement despite decades of dietary guidance. *American Journal of Preventive Medicine, 38*(5), 472–477.

48. Patel, A., Hildebrand, J., & Gapstur, S. (2014). Body mass index and all-cause mortality in a large prospective cohort of white and black U.S. adults. *PLoS ONE, 9*(10), e109153.

49. Lu, L., Xun, P., Wan, Y., et al. (2016). Long-term-association between dairy consumption and risk of childhood obesity: A systematic review and meta-analysis of prospective cohort studies. *European Journal of Clinical Nutrition, 70*, 414–423.

50. Tremblay, A., Doyon, C., & Sanchez, M. (2015). Impact of yogurt on appetite control, energy balance, and body composition. *Nutrition Review, 73*(sup1), 23–27. https://doi.org/10.1093/nutrit/nuv015.

51. Korre, M., Sotos-Prieto, M., & Kales, S. N. (2017). Survival Mediterranean style: Lifestyle changes to improve the health of the US Fire Service. *Frontiers in Public Health, 5*(article 331), doi:10.3389/fpubh.2017.00331.

52. Cooper, J. T. (2010). Evaluation of the obese patient. In G. M. Steelman & E. C. Westman (Eds.), *Obesity: Evaluation and treatment essentials*. New York: Informa.

53. Kornstein, S. (2017). Epidemiology and recognition of Binge-Eating Disorder in psychiatry and primary care. *The Journal of Clinical Psychiatry, 79*(suppl1), 3–8.

54. Dorflinger, L. M., Ruser, C. B., & Masheb, R. B. (2017). Night eating among veterans with obesity. *Appetite, 117,* 330–334. doi:10.1016/j.appet.2017.07.011.

55. Vallis, M., Piccinini-Vallis, H., Sharma, A., & Freedhoff, Y. (2013). Modified 5 As: Minimal intervention for obesity counseling in primary care: Clinical review. *Canadian Family Physician, 59,* 27–31.

56. Van Nes, M., & Sawatzky, V. (2010). Improving cardiovascular health with motivational interviewing: A nurse practitioner perspective. *Journal of the American Academy of Nurse Practitioners, 22*(12), 654–660.

57. Bray, G. (2013). Why do we need drugs to treat the patient with obesity? *Obesity, 21*(5), 893–899.

58. Wadden, T. A., West, D. S., Delahanty, L., et al. (2006). Look AHEAD Research Group: The Look AHEAD study: A description of the lifestyle intervention and the evidence supporting it. *Obesity, 14*(5), 737–752.

59. National Heart, Lung, and Blood Institute. (1998). Practical guide: Identification, evaluation, and treatment of overweight and obesity in adults, NIH Publication Number 00–4084, Washington DC.

60. Heber, D., Greenway, F. L., Kaplan, L. M., et al. (2010). Endocrine and nutritional management of the post-bariatric surgery patient: An Endocrine Society Clinical practice guideline. *The Journal of Clinical Endocrinology and Metabolism, 95*(11), 4823–4843.

61. Symons, T. B., Sheffield-Moore, M., Wolfe, R. R., et al. (2009). A moderate serving of high-quality protein maximally stimulates skeletal muscle protein synthesis in young and elderly subjects. *Journal of the American Dietetic Association, 109,* 1582–1586.

62. Lin, P. H., Wang, Y. G., Grambow, S. C., et al. (2012). Dietary saturated fat intake is negatively associated with weight maintenance among the PREMIER participants. *Obesity, 20*(3), 571–575.

63. International Association for the Study of Obesity (IASO). (2010). Obesity: understanding and challenging the global epidemic: 2009–2010 report from the International Association for the Study of Obesity. London: IASO.

64. Sun, Q., Spiegelman, D., van Dam, R., et al. (2010). White rice, brown rice, and risk of type 2 diabetes in U.S. men and women. *Archives of Internal Medicine, 170*(11), 961–969.

65. Wadden, T. A., Byrne, K. J., Krauthamer-Ewing, S., et al. (2006). Obesity management. In M. E. Shils, M. Shike, & A. C. Ross (Eds.), *Modern nutrition in health and disease* (10th ed.). Philadelphia: Lippincott Williams & Wilkins.

66. Dansinger, M. L., Gleason, J. A., Griffith, J. L., et al. (2005). Comparison of the Atkins, Ornish, Weight Watchers, and Zone diets for weight loss and heart disease risk reduction: A randomized trial. *JAMA: The Journal of the American Medical Association, 293*(1), 43–53.

67. Lean, M. E., Leslie, W. S., Barnes, A. C., et al. (2017). Primary care-led weight management for remission of type 2 diabetes (DiRECT): An open-label, cluster-randomised trial. *Lancet,* doi:10.1016/S0140-6736(17)33102-1.

68. Kastorini, C. M., Milionis, H. J., Esposito, K., et al. (2011). The effect of Mediterranean diet on metabolic syndrome and its components: A meta-analysis of 50 studies and 534,906 individuals. *Journal of the American College of Cardiology, 57*(11), 1299–1313.

69. Protocol: action for health in diabetes: Look AHEAD clinical trial. (2009). Retrieved from https://www.lookaheadtrial.org/public/LookAHEADProtocol.pdf. (January 8, 2018).

70. The Look AHEAD Research Group. (2013). Cardiovascular effects of intensive lifestyle intervention in type 2 diabetes. *The New England Journal of Medicine, 369,* 145–154.

71. Look AHEAD: action for health in diabetes, (Internet). Retrieved from www.lookaheadtrial.org/public/home.cfm. (Accessed 30 January 2018).

72. Bray, G., & Ryan, D. (2014). Drugs that modify fat absorption and alter metabolism. In G. Bray & C. Bouchard (Eds.), *Handbook of obesity: Clinical applications* (4th ed., Vol. 2, pp. 243–250). Boca Raton: CRC Press Taylor and Francis Group.

73. MOVE! Weight management program. Retrieved from www.move.va.gov. (Accessed 30 January 2018).

74. Aim for a healthy weight: information for health professionals. (Internet). Retrieved from http://www.nhlbi.nih.gov/health/educational/lose_wt/profmats.htm. (Accessed 30 January 2018).

75. Bray, G. A., & Greenway, F. L. (2007). Pharmacological treatment of the overweight patient. *Pharmacological Reviews, 59*(2), 151–184.

76. Balkon, N., Balkon, C., & Zitkus, B. S. (2011). Overweight and obesity: Pharmacotherapeutic considerations. *Journal of the American Academy of Nurse Practitioners, 23*(2), 61–66.

77. Apovian, C. M., Aronne, L. J., Bessessen, D. H., et al. (2015). Pharmacological management of obesity: An Endocrine Society clinical practice guideline. *The Journal of Clinical Endocrinology and Metabolism, 100*(2), 342–362. doi:10.1210/jc.2014-3415. (Accessed 5 January 2018).

78. Apovian, C. M., Aronne, L. J., Bessessen, D. H., et al. (2015). Corregendum for pharmacological management of obesity: An Endocrine Society clinical practice guideline. *The Journal of Clinical Endocrinology and Metabolism, 100*(5), 2135–2138. (Accessed 5 January 2018).

79. Xenical (orlistat). (2013). Highlights of prescribing information. Genentech USA, Inc, a Member of the Roche Group. San Francisco.

80. US Food & Drug Admin. (2017). Tainted weight loss products. Retrieved from https://www.fda.gov/Drugs/ResourcesForYou/Consumers/BuyingUsingMedicineSafely/MedicationHealthFraud/ucm234592.htm. (Accessed 11 January 2018).

81. Belviq, lorcaserin HCl. (2012). Highlights of prescribing information. Arena Pharmaceuticals: Zofingen, Switzerland.

82. Bray, G., & Ryan, D. (2014). Drugs that modify fat absorption and alter metabolism. In G. Bray & C. Bouchard (Eds.), *Handbook of obesity: Clinical applications* (4th ed., Vol. 2, pp. 243–250). Boca Raton: CRC Press Taylor and Francis Group.

83. Qsymia: phentermine and topiramate extended-release. Full prescribing information. Vivus, Mountain View, CA 9/2013. https://qsymia.com/pdf/prescribing-information.pdf.

84. Contrave. Bupropion and naltrexone. Prescribing information, Takeda Pharmaceuticals America, Inc. Retrieved from http://general.takedapharm.com/content/file.aspx?filetypecode=CONTRAVEPI&cacheRandomizer=b19a05a0-3a85-4f8b-8e03-eaa87db9ea36. (Accessed 30 January 2018).

85. Topol, E. J., Bousser, M. G., Fox, K. A., et al. (2010). Rimonabant for prevention of cardiovascular events (CRESCENDO) a randomized, multicentre, placebo-controlled trial. *Lancet, 376*(9740), 517–523.

86. Lijesen, G. K., Theeuwen, I., Assendelft, W. J., et al. (1995). The effect of human chorionic gonadotropin (HCG) in the treatment of obesity by means of the Simeons therapy: A criteria-based meta-analysis. *British Journal of Clinical Pharmacology, 40*(3), 237–243.

87. Onakpoya, I. J., Wider, B., Pittler, M. H., et al. (2011). Food supplements for body weight reduction: A systematic review of systematic reviews. *Obesity, 19*(2), 239–244.

88. US Food & Drug Admin. Beware of products promising miracle weight loss. Retrieved from www.fda.gov/ForConsumers/ConsumerUpdates/ucm246742.htm. (Accessed 11 Jan 2018).

89. American Society for Metabolic and Bariatric Surgery. Estimate of bariatric surgery numbers, 2011-2016. Retrieved from https://asmbs.org/resources/estimate-of-bariatric-surgery-numbers. (Accessed May 13 2017).

90. Mechanick, J. I., Kushner, R. F., Sugerman, H. J., et al. (2008). American Association of Clinical Endocrinologists, the Obesity Society, and American Society for Metabolic and Bariatric Surgery medical guidelines for clinical practice for the perioperative nutritional, metabolic, and nonsurgical support of the bariatric surgery patient. *Endocrine Practice, 14*(Suppl. 1), 1–83.

91. Wolfe, B. M., Kvach, E., & Eckel, R. H. (2016). Treatment of obesity: Weight loss and bariatric surgery. *Circulation Research, 118*(11), 1844–1855. doi:10.1161/CIRCRESAHA.116.307591.

92. Estimate of bariatric surgery numbers, 2001-2016. (July 2016). American Society of Bariatric and Metabolic Surgery. https://asmbs.org/resources/estimate-of-bariatric-surgery-numbers. (Accessed 3 January 2018).

93. Chebli, J. E. (2009). The current state of obesity, metabolism, and bariatric surgery. *Bariatric Nursing and Surgical Patient Care, 4*(4), 295–297.

94. Gagnon, L., & Karwacki Sheff, E. J. (2012). Outcomes and complications after bariatric surgery. *The American Journal of Nursing, 112*(9).

95. Pontiroli, A. E., & Morabito, A. (2011). Long-term prevention of mortality in morbid obesity through bariatric surgery. A systematic review and meta-analysis of trials performed with gastric banding and gastric bypass. *Annals of Surgery, 253*(3), 484–487.

96. Peterli, R., Wolnerhanssen, B. R., Peters, T., et al. (2018). Effect of laparoscopic sleeve gastrectomy vs laparoscopic Roux-en-Y gastric bypass on weight loss in patients with morbid obesity: The SM-BOSS randomized clinical trial. *JAMA: The Journal of the American Medical Association, 319*(3), 255–265. doi:10.1001/jama.2017.20897.

97. Poirier, P., Cornier, M. A., Mazzone, T., et al. (2011). The American Heart Association Obesity Committee of the Council on Nutrition, Physical Activity, and Metabolism: Bariatric surgery and cardiovascular risk factors: A scientific statement from the American Heart Association. *Circulation, 123*(15), 1683–1701.

98. Mechanick, J. I., Youdim, A., Jones, D. B., et al. (2013). Clinical practice guidelines for the perioperative nutritional, metabolic, and nonsurgical

support of the bariatric surgery patient—2013 update: Cosponsored by American Association of Clinical Endocrinologists, the Obesity Society, and American Society for Metabolic and Bariatric Surgery. *Endocrine Practice, 19*(2), 337–372.

93. Kominiarek, M. A. (2009). Bariatric surgery and pregnancy: ACOG practice bulletin: Clinical management guidelines for obstetrician-gynecologists, Number 105, June 2009. *Obstetrics and Gynecology, 105*, 1405–1413.

100. Groven, K. S., Raheim, M., & Engelsrud, G. (2010). Living with chronic problems after weight loss surgery: "My quality of life is worse compared to my earlier life." *International Journal of Qualitative Studies on Health and Well-Being, 5*, 5553.

101. Tindle, H. A., Omalu, B., Courcoulas, A., et al. (2010). Risk of suicide after long-term follow-up from bariatric surgery. *The American Journal of Medicine, 123*(11), 1036–1042.

102. Rejeski, W. J., Brubaker, P. H., Goff, D. C., et al. (2011). Translating weight loss and physical activity programs into the community to preserve mobility in older, obese adults in poor cardiovascular health. *Archives of Internal Medicine, 171*(10), 880–886.

103. Paddon-Jones, D., & Rasmussen, B. B. (2009). Dietary protein recommendations and the prevention of sarcopenia. *Current Opinion in Clinical Nutrition and Metabolic Care, 12*(1), 86–90.

104. Healthcare cost of the consequences of overweight, primarily from failing to treat obesity.

105. Fallah-Fini, S., Adam, A., Cheskin, L., et al. (2017). The additional costs and health effects of a patient having overweight or obesity: A computational Model. *Obesity, 25*, 1809–1818. doi:10.1002/oby.21965.

106. Bhaskaran, K., Douglas, I., Forbes, H., dos Santos-Silva, I., Leon, D., & Smeeth, L. (2014). Body-mass index and risk of 22 specific cancers: A population-based cohort study of 5.24 million UK adults. *Lancet, 384*(9945), 755–765.

107. Brunt, E. M. (2010). Pathology of nonalcoholic fatty liver disease. *Nature Reviews. Gastroenterology & Hepatology, 7*(4), 195–203.

108. Losina, E., Walensky, R. P., Reichmann, W. M., et al. (2011). Impact of obesity and knee osteoarthritis on morbidity and mortality in older Americans. *Annals of Internal Medicine, 154*(4), 217–226.

109. Zhou, Z., Liu, Y., Chen, H., & Liu, F. (2014). Body-mass index and knee osteoarthritis risk: A dose-response meta-analysis. *Obesity, 22*(10), 2180–2185.

CHAPTER **18**

PRINCIPLES OF OCCUPATIONAL AND ENVIRONMENTAL HEALTH IN PRIMARY CARE

Grace Ellen Urquhart

OCCUPATIONAL HEALTH, ENVIRONMENTAL HEALTH, AND HEALTH PROMOTION IN THE WORKPLACE

According to the World Health Organization (WHO) a health-promoting workplace results in a healthy workforce.[1] The workplace has been identified as one of the priority settings for health promotion in the 21st century as it influences the physical, mental, social, and economic well-being of workers and the health of their families, communities, and society.[2] Occupational health is a multidisciplinary activity designed to promote the wellness of workers.[3] The primary goals of the Occupational Safety and Health Administration (OSHA) are to promote health and safety through the prevention of injury/disease using early detection and health promotion.[4] Occupational health is unique in that the hazards and disease potentials are often identified long before the injury or exposure occurs. Many of these are addressed in workplace safety policies and OSHA regulations.[4]

Achieving optimal health and safety in the workplace requires employers and employees working together to achieve goals that are mutually beneficial. Reducing the risk of injury and disability requires employers to develop and prioritize safety measures and workers to observe and follow safety practices.[5] The employer should openly disclose any potential risks and/or hazards associated with the job and the employee should provide an honest and forthright health history including any past illnesses and/or injuries.[6,7] (See Box 18.1 for Occupational Health History.)

PREPLACEMENT HEALTH EVALUATION

Achieving optimal health promotion in the workplace should include a complete physiological and psychological evaluation. Preemployment testing has been shown to reduce the risk of future debilitating injuries.[8] Functional capacity testing may be one of the best predictors of employment longevity and injury prevention. While many employers require a physical examination at the onset of employment, few provide specific fitness parameters for the state of health as a condition of employment.[5–7]

Job-specific physical and psychological requirements are one way to ensure appropriate preemployment health assessments are completed on employees. These forms and examinations can be tailored to include a history and physical based on the potential for injury and/or exposure.[9] A focused, job-specific physical exam will provide better assurance the candidate has the physical functional capacity to perform (without injury) the work for which they were hired.[10] Functional testing is performed post-employment offer but prior to starting work.[10]

Any complete health evaluation of a patient should include an occupational and environmental health history and assessment for risks associated with a patient's occupation. A thorough occupational and environmental health history should include at least the following[2,3]:

- Current and past positions held
- Previous employers; years employed; type of industry or employer; and products manufactured, developed, or used in production process
- A brief description of the position requirements
- Known health hazards in the workplace
- Any current or past exposure to chemicals or other hazardous substances, noise, radiation, heat, vibration, or repetitive motion
- Use of personal protective equipment (PPE)
- Significant time off work for a health problem or injury
- Changed residence because of health problems
- Household member with dust or chemical contact at work
- Use of pesticides in gardens or around the home
- Recreational activities and exposure to noise, radiation, repetitive motion, heat, vibration, and chemicals in these activities

The Department of Transportation (DOT) has developed a standardized method of medically evaluating commercial vehicle drivers. Some conditions and/or use of certain medications will disqualify a person from this workforce.[11] This is just one example of fit-for-duty testing. In order to perform these evaluations, medical providers must take a certification examination and be listed on the registry. Some medical conditions have become regulated by the DOT (Table 18.1) and may limit or disqualify a person from obtaining or renewing a commercial driver's license (CDL).[12]

BOX **18.1**

Occupational Health History

PAST MEDICAL HISTORY
- Hospitalizations
- Surgeries
- Past injuries
- Worker's comp claims
- Exposure to hazardous materials
- Any unexplained illnesses

MEDICATIONS
- Current medications
- Allergies
- Past medications
  - Chronic illness medications
  - Pain medications
  - Over-the-counter or herbal medications

SOCIAL HISTORY
- Past occupational history
- Use of tobacco products
- Use of illicit drugs
- Recreational activities
- Exercise

FAMILY HISTORY
- Genetic history of sudden cardiac death
- Single or married (life partner)
- Children

REVIEW OF SYSTEMS
General
- Sleep disorder
- Diet and exercise
- Fatigue
- Fever or night sweats
- Unintentional weight loss/gain

Head, Eyes, Ears, Nose, and Throat
- Color blind
- Wear corrective lenses
- Use of safety glasses or shields
- Any eye injuries in the past
- Any problems with vision
- Difficulty with hearing; use of hearing aids
- Use of earplugs or other ear protection
- Sinus or allergy problems

Skin
- Rashes, lesions, burns
- Past injuries to skin that did or did not require treatment

- Use of protective gloves, sunscreen, gowns, other skin protective equipment

Respiratory
- Cough
- Shortness of breath
- Wheezing
- Exercise intolerance
- Use of respirator or face mask in the past
- Hazardous material/environmental exposures in the past (occupational and recreational)

Cardiac
- Chest pain
- Palpitations
- Hypertension (treated or untreated)

Musculoskeletal
- Fractured bones
- Soft tissue injuries (sprain, strain, tendon or ligament tear or rupture)
- Back pain
- Joint pain
- Muscle cramps
- Muscle pain
- Weakness
- MS injuries in the past (back, neck, upper/lower extremities)
- Use of compression, neutralizing or stabilizing braces for back or extremities

Neurological
- Numbness or tingling in extremities
- Headache
- Dizziness
- Problems maintaining balance
- Problems with independent mobility
- Syncope

Psychological
- Depression
- Anxiety
- Anger
- Self-harm
- Auditory or visual hallucinations
- Behavioral problems

Allergies
- Food
- Environmental
- Drugs

Fit-for-Duty Testing

Health care providers perform fit-for-duty health assessments to:
- Certify eligibility for a newly hired employee
- Ensure the employee is maintaining proper health at regular intervals

- Determine if an employee is well enough to return to work after an illness or an injury
- Evaluate for ill effects of work hazards on the employee's health. This requires the examiner have a thorough understanding of the potential risks and hazards of the job.
- Fit-for-duty pre-employment exams need to closely simulate the worker's expected performance or job duty.[13]

TABLE 18.1	Department of Transportation Physical Requirements	
Condition	**Requirements**	**Plan**
Diabetes	No needle insulin	Oral medications are permitted
Blood sugar	Hemoglobin A1C < 10%	Oral medications are permitted
Blood pressure	140–159/90–99 = 1-year certificate 160–179/100–109 = 3-month temp certificate >180/110 = Disqualifying	
Heart problems	Any history of syncope, cardiac insufficiency, failure, disease	Any cardiac issue requires an annual stress test and release from cardiologist
Sleep apnea	Must demonstrate it is under control	Provide a readout from machine/annual sleep study and release from provider
Vision	20/40 in each eye 70-degree peripheral vision	May use corrective lenses to achieve
Hearing	Must be able to hear forced whisper from 5 feet in at least one ear	May use hearing aid to achieve
Medications	All medications must be prescribed and certified by a licensed medical provider	See list at www.fmcsa.dot.gov

INJURY AND DISEASE PREVENTION IN THE WORKPLACE

The US Department of Health and Human Services (HHS) reports the most common workplace illnesses and injuries result from musculoskeletal, respiratory, skin, ear, and eye exposures to hazardous conditions or materials. Some workers may also be at risk for communicable diseases or psychological and circulatory problems.[14]

Occupational health promotion is primarily focused on the prevention of occupational injury and disease. This is accomplished primarily by reducing exposures to hazardous materials, identifying disease before it becomes clinically apparent (disease surveillance), and minimizing the adverse effects of a known exposure.[15] Reducing worker exposure is best accomplished by first eliminating the potential hazard through engineering controls, renovating the workstation, redesigning the job, and improved administrative controls, and second by the rotation of workers. The use of PPE and regular periodic screenings are integral to protecting the worker from injury and the early detection of health problems. Health exams and screenings should include diagnostic, physical, and functional capacity testing depending on the potential hazard or exposure.[15] The goal of occupational medicine is early detection and intervention through health promotion and injury prevention.

Musculoskeletal Injuries and Injury Prevention

Musculoskeletal disorders (MSDs) are a major cause of absence from work with an estimated 70 million injuries annually.[16,17] This accounts for 130 million health care encounters in outpatient clinics, emergency rooms, and hospitals at an estimated cost of $50 billion in lost wages, lost productivity, and compensation costs.[16]

MSDs include injuries involving bones, muscles, tendons, cartilage, ligaments, and nerves. Most MSDs are the result of a sudden injury or the overuse of a specific region of the body.[18] Usually, these injuries correlate to occupational hazards such as working in an awkward position, exposure to vibratory stimuli, sitting/kneeling/standing in a static position for long periods of time, repetitive motions, or lifting/carrying heavy loads.[18]

Musculoskeletal injuries are classified as acute or chronic. An acute injury is generally caused by a sudden and/or heavy overload to a particular region of the body, resulting in acute pain.[19] A chronic or lingering injury is the result of long-term overstressing, overloading, or repetitive use.[19] Persistent overuse may result in cumulative trauma disorders (CTDs), repetitive strain injuries (RSIs), and repetitive motion injuries (RMIs).[20] The prevention of chronic, lingering, overuse injuries may be achieved through the use of ergonomics and limiting repetitive exposure to an activity.[20]

Factors affecting the occurrence and illness course of MSDs include personal body characteristics and workplace hazards. Age, gender, body mass index, and physical condition impact a worker's response to physiological, emotional, and psychological stressors in the work environment.[20] Recent studies point out psychosocial factors may play a larger than expected role in musculoskeletal injuries. Some studies suggest a strong relationship between low back disorders and job satisfaction, interpersonal relationships, job performance, pace of work, and stress as well as a worker's perceived ability to work.[17] Age and gender seem to impact the extent to which a person can tolerate continued exposure before injury occurs.[17] Factors such as repetition, vibration, load force, and amount of exposure over time also play a role in low back injuries. Recent studies also suggest a link between upper extremity injuries and nonwork stress, tension, and anxiety.[17] Repetition and nonneutral wrist positions contribute to the changes in nerve structure and function of the upper extremities.[20] Controlling the risk of injury involves primary and secondary interventions. Primary includes reducing the biomechanical stress load[20] while secondary focuses on the modification of workstations and individual factors such as exercise and job rotation.[20]

Ergonomics. Ergonomics is a process by which a job is matched to a worker, not a worker to a job.[20] The aim is to optimize the health and safety of the worker by integrating principles of anatomy, physiology, and psychology with the mental and functional capacities of the worker.[20] Ergonomic principles may reduce the risk of injury in the workplace by utilizing proper body mechanics for certain activities (work technique) along with the use of assistive devices (such as workstations). The end goal of ergonomics is to reduce the stress load and decrease the risk of injury.[20]

Ergonomic parameters exist for different types of activities including sitting, standing, lifting, bending, reaching, and computer use.[20] According to OSHA, work-related MSDs are mostly preventable. Ergonomics is the process of fitting a job to a person which helps lessen muscle fatigue, increases productivity, and reduces the number and severity of work-related MSDs.[20] OSHA has developed a toolkit for the prevention of MSDs. The publication can be accessed at: https://www.osha.gov/Publications/osha3465.pdf.

Musculoskeletal Exam. The initial musculoskeletal exam should include a thorough evaluation of the musculoskeletal and neurological systems. Testing should include:
- Musculoskeletal system
  - Passive and active range of motion (ROM) of the upper and lower extremities
  - Strength and functional testing of upper and lower extremities
  - Movement, agility, coordination of upper and lower extremities and spine
- Nervous system
  - Cranial nerve tests
  - Deep tendon reflexes of upper and lower extremities
  - Sensory perception testing of upper and lower extremities

If an illness or injury occurs, the same exam should be performed with clear documentation of any changes or deficits. (See Table 18.2 for musculoskeletal injuries and treatment.)

Skin Injury Prevention

Skin is the largest organ in the body and accounts for approximately 10% of the body mass. It assists with water preservation, shock absorption, temperature control, tactile sensation, lubrication, waterproofing, and vitamin D synthesis.[21] Though skin provides protection to other organs of the body, it is itself susceptible to occupational exposures from chemical, mechanical, biological, and physical/environmental hazards.[21,22] The most effective methods of skin injury prevention includes the utilization of avoidance and barrier protection (protective/proper clothing, masks, and gloves).[21] Health care workers and those working with humans, animals, or human/animal substances have increased risk of exposure to bacterial, viral, parasitic, and fungal infections.[22]

When avoidance is impossible, prevention of skin injuries is then best accomplished through barrier protection. However, if an injury occurs, proper treatment should be initiated as soon as possible to limit the loss of healthy tissue and scarring. An initial physical examination of the skin should note:
- Any scars, lesions, masses, moles, warts, bruises
- Color
- Texture
- Temperature
- Turgor

Documentation should include any changes, exposures, or risk factors.

Occupational skin diseases (OSDs) are the second most common type of occupational disease.[21] Physical exposures to the skin may result in contact dermatitis, skin cancer, skin injury, or infection. Mechanical trauma may result in lacerations, abrasions, burns, contusions, and calluses.

Treatment for these may include cleaning the area of debris, suturing if necessary, application of topical antimicrobials, and covering the area affected. Analgesics may be needed depending on the degree of injury.

The National Institute for Occupational Safety and Health (NIOSH) has developed a system called Skin Notations (SK) to assist in the delineation of direct, systemic, and immune-mediated effects of skin exposure to heat or chemicals.[22] The skin notation profiles provide information directly related to the type of hazards associated with the exposure. The online NIOSH Pocket Guide to Chemical Exposures can be accessed at: https://www.cdc.gov/niosh/npg/.

Treatment of Burns, Sunburns, Frostbite. Protection from cumulative sun exposure through the use of proper clothing, head covering, and sunscreen will reduce the long-term risk of skin cancer.[22,23] Prevention of exposure to freezing temperatures will decrease the risk of frostbite and skin injury from overexposure.[23] Workers in agriculture, fishing, construction, and mechanics are at higher risk for sun and cold exposure injuries.[23,24]

Sunburn injury	• Cool baths • Application of moisturizers containing soy or aloe vera • Aspirin or ibuprofen to reduce pain, redness, and swelling
Frostbite injury	• Check for hypothermia • Gently rewarm the skin with warm water until it becomes red and warm • Avoid refreezing or re-exposure • Avoid walking on frostbitten feet or toes • Take pain medicine

Eye Injury Prevention

Ocular injuries can result from exposure to a foreign body, mechanical trauma, chemical or heat burn, or human/animal contact. These injuries may cause severe pain, redness, drainage, decreased visual acuity, photosensitivity, conjunctivitis, infection, and changes in pH. The normal pH of the eye is between 7.0 and 7.3.[25]

Proper use of safety glasses and shields will prevent most eye injuries. Some workers may require corrected vision safety glasses which will necessitate an examination and proper fitting by an optometrist or ophthalmologist.

Occupational eye strain may result from any concentrated close-up work including excessive reading and computer usage. This can result in dry eyes, blurred vision, light sensitivity, neck tension, and headaches. Proper lighting and visual acuity are interrelated and play a role in posture. Workers should have an annual eye exam and employ visual ergonomics in the workplace.[16,20] Proper use of corrective lenses, computer glasses, and regular breaks will help decrease eye strain.

The initial eye examination should include[25]:
- Visual acuity
- Pupillary response
- Visual field testing including confrontation
- Extraocular movement (EOM)
- Complete physical examination including palpation and inspection of the orbit, eyelid, conjunctiva, cornea, sclera, and retina
- Color blindness test (Ishihara test)

Documentation should include any abnormal findings, changes, deficits, hazardous exposures, and use of corrective lenses.

TABLE 18.2   **Musculoskeletal Disorders Causes and Treatment**

Illness or Injury	Cause	Physical Exam and Diagnostics	Treatment
Carpal Tunnel syndrome	RMI, RSI	Test for thenar atrophy Evaluate ↓ sensation Phalen maneuver Tinel test 2-point discrimination >5 mm Electrophysiologic testing	• Rest/reduce repetitive movement • Nonsteroidal anti-inflammatory drugs (NSAIDs) naproxen or ibuprofen • Ice or cold packs applied 3–4 times/day • Splinting at work and during sleep • Physical or occupational therapy • Surgery if all other treatments fail
Tendonitis	RSI, RMI, CTD	Contralateral comparison Point of maximal tenderness Strength testing Neuromuscular exam X-ray, bone scan, or MRI	• Rest/reduce or eliminate repetitive movement • NSAIDs naproxen or ibuprofen • Ice or cold packs applied 3–4 times/day • Splinting to reduce strain in daytime and at sleep
Muscle strain	RSI, RMI, CTD	Inspect for swelling, tenderness, ecchymosis Point of maximal tenderness Examine joint stability Palpate for a defect in muscle X-ray, MRI	• Rest • Ice applied to affected area • Compression • Elevation of extremity • Analgesics/NSAIDs/muscle relaxers may be prescribed
Rotator cuff injuries	RSI, RMI, CTD	Passive ROM normal Active ROM limited Unable to raise arm or unable to hold arm up Tenderness to palpation over greater tuberosity X-ray, MRI	• Rest—avoid straining activities • Ice applied to affected area • Physical therapy • NSAIDs naproxen or ibuprofen
Epicondylitis	RSI, RMI	Localized tenderness Lift a chair or stool palm up + pain is lateral epicondylitis Press a chair with palm down + pain is medial epicondylitis X-ray to rule out arthritis MRI to confirm diagnosis	• Identify cause and stop activity • Ice applied to affected area • Elbow strap to reduce or eliminate elbow strain • NSAIDs naproxen or ibuprofen
Trigger finger	RSI, RMI	Tenderness in the palm Locked finger Tendon nodule Full flexion of digit may not be possible No diagnostics needed	• Rest/reduce repetitive movement • NSAIDs naproxen or ibuprofen • Steroid injections in digital flexor sheath • Splinting to limit use • Ice to reduce swelling • Warm water soak to relax tendon • May require surgical repair with 1–2-week recovery
Low back strain	RSI, RMI, CTD	Mechanical pain aggravated by activity Pain relieved with lying down Pain may radiate to one or both buttocks Lumbar or sacroiliac tenderness Range of motion tenderness with turning and bending Waddell signs should be negative • Straight leg raise • Axial stimulation • Non-organic tenderness • Sensory exam • X-ray	• Rest • Ice applied to affected area 3–4 times/day • Compression (back brace) • Heat after 2–3 days 3–4 times/day • Physical therapy—gentle stretching exercises • NSAIDs naproxen or ibuprofen • Muscle relaxers for associated spasms • Corticosteroids

Chemical exposures to the eye may result from being sprayed or splashed by a substance or by rubbing the eye.[25,26] Typically acidic solutions will cause more pain and redness than alkaline but are more easily removed with flushing. Alkaline substances are not as painful and thus may cause more damage due to the delay in seeking medical attention.[25,26] Patients with chemical exposures will often complain of foreign body sensation, blurred vision, photophobia, and moderate to severe pain.[25,26]

Traumatic eye injury should be treated as a medical emergency and the patient should be referred to the closest hospital with emergency ophthalmology services.[25] A protective shield

TABLE 18.3   **Eye Injuries**

Illness or Injury	Initial Treatment	Follow-Up or Referral
Foreign body (FB) exposure	• Gentle flush with sterile normal saline • Gentle removal with a cotton tipped swab from cornea, sclera, conjunctiva, or under the eyelid • Antibiotic ointment	Follow-up: Ophthalmology
Chemical exposure	• Copious irrigation of up to 20 L with normal saline or lactated ringers • pH testing until normal 7.0–7.3	Referral: Emergency room Follow-up: Ophthalmology
Orbital fracture	• Ice to reduce swelling • Head and neck in neutral position • Sitting up at 45 degrees if possible • CT scan	Referral: Maxillofacial surgeon Referral: Ophthalmology; may use scoring system
Laceration	• Wound washed with sterile normal saline • Ice applied to reduce swelling • Suture if >25% of eyelid area is involved • Antibiotic ointment applied • Tetanus and oral antibiotics dependent on mechanism of injury • CT dependent on mechanism of injury	Referral: Ophthalmology for complicated lacerations
Traumatic or mechanical injury	• Ice applied • CT scan	Referral: Ophthalmology
Global fracture or penetration	• Eye shield • CT head and orbits • Analgesia and antiemetics • Systemic antibiotics initiated within 6 h of the injury.	Referral: Emergency room Follow-up: Ophthalmology
Eye strain	• Visual acuity with corrective lenses • Computer glasses	Referral: Optometrist if corrective lenses are needed
Corneal abrasion	• Confirm diagnosis with fluorescein and wood's lamp • Remove foreign bodies • Topical antibiotic ointment ciprofloxacin or ofloxacin • No contact lenses until healed, usually 2–4 weeks • Topical nonsteroidal antiinflammatories such as ketorolac 0.5%	Referral: Ophthalmology if: • Symptoms worsen or do not resolve in 48–72 h • Large abrasions • Unable to remove FB • >20/40 vision loss • Chemical burn injury • Rust ring

should be placed over the affected eye and caution should be exercised to avoid any strenuous activity in the event a global fracture has occurred.[25] Antibiotics should be administered systemically within 6 hours of the injury.[25] Recommendations for initial therapy include oral or parenteral administration of fluoroquinolones, aminoglycosides, and cephalosporins. Conjunctival lacerations greater than 1 cm should be referred to an ophthalmologist for suture placement and further evaluation for a possible global fracture.[25]

All eye injuries should be treated as potential emergencies, but not all injuries require emergency room evaluation.[27] Prompt and appropriate care should be provided including diagnostics, follow-up, and referrals. The American Academy of Family Physicians has developed a guide for eye injuries in primary care (Table 18.3). Additional information may be available at https://www.aafp.org. See Part 6, Evaluation and Management of Eyes Disorders, for other pertinent information.

Occupational Lung Disease and Respiratory Injury Prevention

Occupational lung disease results from continued exposure to contaminants such as inhaled dusts, powders, fibers, solvents, gases, or fumes.[28] These can adversely affect the upper and lower respiratory tract and may result in diseases or injuries such as asthma, chronic obstructive pulmonary disease, lung cancer, lung infections, and pleural disease. Most of these illnesses and injuries are caused by repeated, long-term exposure and are preventable (Table 18.4).[29] Because many exposures do not result in acute symptoms, workers may be unaware that they have been exposed to potentially hazardous materials. The challenge for health care providers, especially those unfamiliar with occupational medicine, is to maintain a high index of suspicion that a symptom or cluster of symptoms may have a connection with a patient's job or work history.

Although the true scope of occupational lung disease is difficult to quantify, it is recognized that a small percentage of chronic occupational respiratory diseases is correctly associated with work-related exposures. Asthma is the most common type of occupational pulmonary disease in the industrialized world. As many as 15% of all asthma cases in adults may be work related.[30] Occupational asthma may be related to specific antigens in the workplace (e.g., psyllium or latex) or to chemical irritants.[30] Interstitial pulmonary fibrosis, which results from workplace exposure to asbestos and silica, persists throughout the world despite knowledge of the potential hazard. Though the death rate for silicosis has declined by approximately 70%,

TABLE 18.4 **Respiratory Injury**	
Airway Disease	**Cause and Effect**
Asthma	• Inflammatory disease of the bronchi • Exposure to inhaled agents may cause or exacerbate disease • Triggers may include allergens, irritants, temperature or humidity changes, isocyanates
COPD	• Risk for smokers and nonsmokers • Chronic exposure to metal fumes, organic dust and fibers, exhaust fumes, chemical gases or vapors, metal fumes, mineral dusts
Interstitial fibrotic lung disease	• Exposure to asbestos, coal dust, mineral dust, or metals • Inflammatory disease that leads to scarring • Includes asbestosis, chronic beryllium disease (CBD), silicosis, coal workers pneumoconiosis
Hypersensitivity pneumonitis	• Immune inflammatory reaction • Includes exposure to bird proteins, mold, bacteria • Acute reaction that can become chronic with repeated exposures • May lead to interstitial lung disease
Lung cancer	• Risk for smokers and nonsmokers • Exposure to asbestos, silica, diesel exhaust fumes
Lung infections	• Exposure to infectious agents by human carrier, contaminated humidifiers, air handlers and includes environmental bacteria, mold, fungus, virus • Influenza, legionella, tuberculosis, community acquired pneumonia (CAP)
Bronchiolitis obliterans/airway destruction	• Damage to bronchioles results in scarring and chronic airflow obstruction • Exposure to some flavoring chemicals

asbestosis has increased by nearly 400%.[31] As many as 65,000 workers in the United States may have work related asbestosis. In the United States alone, 85,000 cotton mill workers are partially or fully disabled as a result of exposure to cotton dust[32] and the prevalence of latex hypersensitivity, including latex-induced asthma, is as high as 14% among health care workers.[33]

These statistics seem staggering, yet the number of affected individuals captured in any occupational surveillance system may be a gross underestimate because many cases are undiagnosed, under reported, or are not attributed to workplace exposure.[31]

Military Personnel and Veterans: Overlooked Populations. The short- and long-term health effects of war-related exposures on military service personnel are a growing concern. Exposures to toxins during the past two decades have been different from those of previous wars. The Centers for Disease Control and Prevention and other organizations, such as the Agency for Toxic Substances and Disease Registry, have been studying the post-service morbidity and mortality of veterans who have served in the Vietnam, Gulf, and Iraq wars, as well as in the conflict in Afghanistan. There is some evidence that Gulf War veterans with previous respiratory illnesses, such as asthma, experienced more respiratory symptoms than did veterans without a history of illness. However, this may not be unique to Gulf War veterans and may be similar to the experience of veterans of other wars, despite the exposure to spilled oil and smoke plumes unique to Gulf War veterans. At this point, it is unclear whether there is a connection between war-related exposures and specific health outcomes that remain long after the exposure.[33,34]

Pathophysiology

Inhaled noxious substances affect the respiratory tract in several ways. Direct irritation results in increased mucus production, cough, and airway hyperreactivity that may cause bronchospasm, chest tightness or pain, dyspnea, pneumonitis, or pulmonary edema. The full effect of certain irritants may not be realized until 12 to 24 hours after the exposure. Small particles (≤5 mm) may remain in the lung to induce a fibrotic or granulomatous response. A latency period of 15 to 20 years between exposure and onset of clinical disease often obscures the causal relationship, which makes the diagnosis of occupational lung disease more difficult. Hypersensitivity and abnormal functioning of the immune system may contribute to the development of certain occupational respiratory diseases, including bronchitis, asthma, hypersensitivity pneumonitis, asbestosis, and chronic beryllium disease. The presence of certain host factors, such as cigarette smoking and exposure in the home environment (e.g., proximity to sources of pollutants), play a role in the development of work-related lung disease.

Occupational respiratory diseases include obstructive airway diseases (asthma, byssinosis), interstitial lung disease (coal workers' pneumoconiosis, asbestosis, silicosis, acute and chronic beryllium disease, hypersensitivity pneumonitis), industrial bronchitis, cancer, and noncardiogenic pulmonary edema. Asthma, one of the most common types of occupational respiratory disease, has been associated with at least 250 specific workplace exposures. In comparison to many other occupational illnesses, asthma produces more persistent, even permanent, effects.[35] Byssinosis is another obstructive airway disease associated with exposure to cotton, hemp, and flax processing. It is characterized by shortness of breath and chest tightness. Prolonged exposure may cause irreversible byssinosis, which is associated with fixed airway obstruction. Cigarette smoking significantly increases the risk of irreversible byssinosis. Bronchitis is a common manifestation of airway irritation and inflammation associated with many occupational exposures. Chronic bronchitis is defined as the presence of cough and sputum on most days for 3 months or longer per year and for 2 or more consecutive years.

Some health care professionals are at increased risk for occupational respiratory problems as a result of their exposure to specific pathogens and toxins. Occupational asthma (as well as latex-related dermatitis and life-threatening anaphylaxis) resulting from latex allergy is becoming an increasing problem. Establishing a diagnosis of latex-related asthma is essential to avoid permanent respiratory compromise. With the resurgence of tuberculosis (TB) in this decade, increasing numbers of health care workers have become infected with TB. The risk for infection is compounded by the convergence of immunocompromised individuals in various settings staffed by health care workers, including long-term care facilities, hospitals, homeless shelters, correctional facilities, and drug treatment centers. A number of TB outbreaks have occurred in these settings, resulting in approximately 300 cases of TB. These outbreaks were characterized by transmission of both isoniazid-resistant TB and in some cases multidrug-resistant TB.[36]

History and Clinical Presentation

A thorough history should be obtained from patients, including any known environmental or occupational exposure (past and present), smoking habits, and careful review of respiratory symptoms. Sometimes workers are unaware of hazardous exposures in which case the medical examiner should review the entire occupational history of the worker.[28,29] Detailed information about the jobs performed (including an outline of a typical workday), work habits, materials used (dyes, solvents, dusts, powders, acids, alkalis, gases, metals), and use of protective equipment must be elicited. All workers should be questioned about any potential safety or health concerns they might have.

The review of symptoms should include questions about onset of any symptoms (rhinitis, conjunctivitis, cough, sputum production, wheezing, dyspnea, chest tightness or pain) and a history of allergies, asthma, or respiratory infections. In addition, it is important to elicit the relationship of symptoms to time spent at work. For example, an improvement of symptoms during periods away from work or intensification during periods at work might suggest an occupational exposure.

Exposure to noxious substances may cause various types of reactions in both the upper and lower respiratory tract. Acute symptoms of upper respiratory tract irritation include nasal and paranasal sinus irritation, sinus congestion, frontal headaches, rhinorrhea, and occasionally epistaxis. A dry cough and hoarseness may indicate pharyngeal and laryngeal inflammation, respectively. Mid–respiratory tract irritation and inflammation often result in bronchospasm, of which asthma is an example. Acute irritation of the deep respiratory tract causes pulmonary edema and pneumonitis.

Chronic respiratory exposure may result in various permanent pulmonary reactions. Chronic bronchitis is one of the most common pulmonary responses to long-term occupational exposure and results from excessive mucus production in the bronchi. Toxic workplace substances that can cause chronic bronchitis include mineral dusts and fumes (e.g., from coal, fibrous glass, asbestos, metal, and oils), organic dusts (e.g., from cotton, grains, and wood), gases (e.g., ozone and nitrous oxide), plastic compounds (isocyanates), acids, and smoke. Fibrosis or pneumoconiosis (localized and nodular) is usually caused by small particles of inorganic dust and

produces symptoms that initially include a nonproductive cough and shortness of breath; in the later stages, there is a productive cough, distant breath sounds, and right-sided heart failure. Pleural plaques and diffuse pleural thickening are manifestations of asbestos exposures. Emphysema-related changes, which include destruction of alveolar walls and air trapping, result from chronic exposure to coal dust or cadmium. The formation of pulmonary granulomas is a less common response to inhaled work-related exposures but can occur from chronic exposure to metal dust.[32] In addition, catastrophic exposures, such as occurred during the World Trade Center collapse, have been implicated in the development of granulomatous pulmonary disease.[37]

Physical Examination

Many workplace exposures do not cause acute respiratory symptoms, and therefore the physical examination findings may be entirely normal. The physical examination is most helpful when the results are abnormal because normal physical examination findings do not negate the possibility of work-related respiratory disease. In fact, once an occupational exposure results in obvious acute symptoms, the disease may have already progressed to the point that symptomatic relief, rather than a cure, is all that is possible. However, it is important always to consider occupational asthma when an adult suddenly develops asthma.

A thorough physical examination with special attention to the respiratory system is necessary. Auscultation can provide helpful diagnostic clues. For example, fine basilar crackles and a pleural friction rub are more common in certain interstitial lung diseases such as asbestosis. Wheezes may suggest asthma. Digital clubbing in conjunction with a positive history of asbestos exposure might suggest asbestosis, especially in the presence of other manifestations of the disease.

A cardiac examination is also important. Ventricular failure may reflect underlying lung disease. Left ventricular failure may manifest as dyspnea, and right ventricular failure may denote severe or advanced lung disease.[35] In addition to assessing the respiratory and cardiac systems, the health care provider should perform a complete physical examination to identify manifestations of chronic or acute occupational exposure in order to provide clues to the cause of the specific respiratory problem being evaluated.

The physical assessment of the respiratory system includes:
- Examination of upper respiratory system
  - Nasal passages (turbinate, septum, mucous membranes)
  - Sinuses (frontal, maxillary, ethmoid)
- Examination of lower respiratory system
  - Lung sounds (adventitious or clear breath sounds in all fields)
  - Ratio of inspiratory and expiratory phase (should be 1:1)
  - Spirometry or pulmonary function tests (PFT)

Additional PFTs include the measurement of residual volume, pulmonary diffusion lung capacity, and arterial blood gases (PaO_2, PCO_2, and pH) and exercise testing. Pulmonary compliance measures the distensibility of the lungs, which is reduced when lungs stiffen.

Skin testing can be helpful in identifying specific antigens. A diagnosis of occupational asthma is a strong consideration if the result of skin testing is positive and the patient has been having bronchospasms. The addition of sputum cytology eosinophil counts to serial peak expiratory flow (PEF) measurement can enhance the diagnosis of occupational asthma.[30] In one study, sputum eosinophil counts were found to increase by 1% to 2% when subjects with occupational asthma were at work.[38]

Diagnostics

Important diagnostic studies include chest radiography and PFTs. A chest X-ray examination can help identify early evidence and progression of parenchymal and pleural disease, including opacities, calcifications, and pleural thickening. In addition to a standard reading, chest radiographs should be interpreted according to the International Labour Organization (ILO) nomenclature and classification system. The ILO system provides a standardized set of comparison radiographs that can be used to classify X-ray films at one point in time or to observe an individual or group for changes over time.[35] Although chest radiographs do reveal evidence of abnormalities, they do not provide information about the degree of disability or impairment, nor do they provide an accurate assessment of lung function.

> ### INITIAL DIAGNOSTICS
> #### Occupational Disease
>
> **IMAGING**
> - Chest X-ray studies
> - CT scan
>
> **OTHER DIAGNOSTICS**
> - Pulmonary function tests
> - Arterial blood gases
> - Skin testing
> - Sputum cytology for eosinophils

PFTs are used to assess lung function. They are of value in determining the type and extent of lung disease, observing the progression of disease for changes in severity or response to therapy, and fulfilling legal and compensatory purposes. The basic tests of ventilatory function can be performed with a spirometer, which can provide an accurate assessment of the relationship between chronic respiratory symptoms and diminished ventilatory capacity.[17,39] Although spirometry provides many measures, the most useful for evaluation of work-related respiratory disease are forced vital capacity (FVC), forced expiratory volume in 1 second (FEV_1), and the ratio of these two measurements (FEV_1/FVC). FVC refers to the maximum volume of air that is exhaled after a maximum inspiration. FEV_1 is an estimate of the flow rate and is obtained by measuring the volume exhaled during the first second. Results are compared with expected values, which are derived from a healthy population of nonsmoking adults, and are expressed as a percentage of the expected value.[35]

Obstructive diseases such as asthma involve an obstruction in airflow without a reduction in lung volume. Therefore measurements of FVC remain within 80% to 120% of the population standard and are considered normal. However, measurements of both FEV_1 and FEV_1/FVC are decreased in asthma and other obstructive diseases. In contrast, restrictive disease, including silicosis, asbestosis, and coal workers' pneumoconiosis, is characterized by reductions in both FEV_1 and FVC, resulting in a normal or greater ratio of FEV_1/FVC. Mixed pulmonary conditions may also be present; this occurs when cigarette smoking or multiple environmental exposures coexist with a given occupational exposure and may confuse the results of the PFTs. Nonetheless, PFTs are a useful instrument for considering the general characteristics of work-related lung disease. The response to bronchodilator inhalation is another method for differentiating between obstructive and restrictive airway disease.[35]

DIAGNOSIS

To accurately diagnose and manage occupational disease, health care providers must familiarize themselves with their patients' social and occupational environments. However, much more is involved than simply knowing an individual's work history. Accurately diagnosing occupational asthma is imperative. If overlooked, continued exposure can increase symptoms and contribute to persistent asthma, even when exposure to precipitants has been eliminated.[30] Conversely, making an error in the diagnosis of occupational disease may have serious economic and psychological implications for workers and employers.[30]

MANAGEMENT

The management of occupational respiratory diseases is a multifaceted process and should include general guidelines and specific instructions for modifying hazardous work conditions. Important steps include elimination of the exposure source, referral to a specialist, early diagnosis, effective treatment, and worker's compensation (if indicated).[39]

It is useful to distinguish among exposures that cause acute symptoms, those that may produce irreversible symptoms after prolonged exposure, and those that produce disease that manifests only after a long latency period. Workers whose exposure produces airway changes that are acute or reversible once the exposure has been removed benefit the most from environmental controls (e.g., an exhaust system), alteration of work practices (e.g., wetting asbestos before removing it), and substitution of a nonhazardous substance for a hazardous one. Other preventive measures that benefit workers to a lesser extent include education about specific work hazards, use of PPE, administrative measures (e.g., job rotation), and screening for early detection of disease.

INTERPROFESSIONAL COLLABORATIVE MANAGEMENT

The management of occupational respiratory disease depends on the specific respiratory illness treated. It is essential that the patient be removed from the exposure as promptly as possible after symptoms have developed. For many occupational respiratory diseases, the most important prognostic determinant is the length of exposure before diagnosis. The principles of managing occupational symptomatic asthma are the same as for nonoccupational asthma.[40] Treatment modalities specific to the disease and close monitoring of symptoms and lung function must be maintained for every individual with an occupational respiratory disease.

LIFE SPAN CONSIDERATIONS

Certain occupational respiratory toxins affect both the female and male reproductive processes, compromising the health of both the workers and their children. Information about pregnant women's work activities and those of their partner (including work done at home) and all related exposures should be obtained as part of the perinatal history. Although household work is performed by more women in American society than in any other, it is often forgotten as a source of potential respiratory toxins. Products used routinely in the home—including scouring powders, chlorine bleaches, furniture polish, drain cleaners, furniture or paint strippers containing organic solvents, glues, paints, epoxies, and pesticides—are all potential hazards, especially when they are used in a small or poorly ventilated area.[41]

Another important life span consideration related to occupational respiratory disease involves latency in older adults. Many occupational respiratory diseases are characterized by long asymptomatic periods from the time of exposure to the clinical evidence of disease. The manifestation of certain cancers may not appear for 10 to 20 years or more after an occupational exposure occurred. The screening of workers at risk for certain diseases must take into consideration such latency issues. In addition, the differential diagnoses for a constellation of signs and symptoms must reflect the possibility the occupational exposure may have occurred many years before.

COMPLICATIONS

Documentation of the respiratory exam should include the normal and abnormal findings of the upper and lower respiratory system, the inspiratory/expiratory ratio, and any diagnostic findings. The results of spirometry testing and PFTs provide a good baseline of lung function. This diagnostic tool is well utilized for interval lung function testing and is beneficial in the evaluation of a worker's ability to safely use a respirator.[42]

COMPLICATIONS

Complications of occupational respiratory disease are dependent on the specific disease process. TB and fungal infections are a complication peculiar to silica pneumoconiosis. In recent years, the increased risk of mortality associated with certain chronic respiratory exposures has become much better recognized. For example, asbestos-related pleural thickening can cause respiratory failure. Multiple occupational exposures, including those to arsenic, chromium, vinyl chloride monomer, asbestos, and radiation, have been causally identified with respiratory tract cancers.

INDICATIONS FOR REFERRAL OR HOSPITALIZATION

Most health care providers are unfamiliar with occupational medicine. Patients should be referred to an occupational medicine specialist if a diagnosis is not clear or if symptoms are unresponsive to treatment. Chronic work-related respiratory tract illnesses are often best managed by an occupational medicine or pulmonary specialist. This includes the management of many respiratory diseases resulting from chronic exposures (e.g., asbestosis or byssinosis) and may also include the management of acute problems, such as silicosis-related TB.

PATIENT AND FAMILY EDUCATION

Education must include an explanation of diagnostic tests and the specific treatment modalities being considered and used. The specifics depend on the specific respiratory disease involved. Occupational medicine is at its best preventive health care. Patients need to be educated about the relationship of their symptoms to workplace exposure, the consequences of continued exposure, and their rights and responsibilities as employees. Employers are required by law to maintain MSDSs, which describe toxic substances, their proper handling, and the symptoms that may arise from contact with them. However, many workers are unaware of the existence of MSDSs and need to be encouraged to read those that are relevant to their jobs.

BOX 18.2

Occupational Safety and Health Administration Respirator Use Requirements

A medical examination is required before a worker can be declared safe to use a respirator.

The medical evaluation consists of:

- Evaluation by a professional licensed health care provider (PLHCP) using the OSHA Medical Evaluation Questionnaire[a] and/or an initial medical examination which includes spirometry.
- The information obtained by the questionnaire and/or examination must answer the questions laid out under the OSHA Guidelines Appendix C of 1910.134.

Regardless of how a contractor chooses to have employees evaluated, the worker is required to provide supplemental information to the PLHCP before the final determination can be made. This supplemental information includes:

- Type and weight of respirator to be used · Duration and frequency of use · Expected physical work effort
- Whether additional personal protective equipment is to be worn
- Temperature and humidity extremes
- A copy of the written program and the medical evaluation portion of the standard
- A follow-up medical examination is required if certain questions are answered "yes" on the questionnaire,[a] or the initial examination warrants it. Further evaluations are needed when any of the following occurs:
- An employee reports medical symptoms that are related to ability to use a respirator. A PLHCP, supervisor, or program administrator informs the contractor that the employee needs reevaluation.
- Information from the respiratory protection program, including observations made during fit-testing and program evaluation, indicates a need for reevaluation.
- There is an increase in the physiological burden placed on the employee from temperature changes, changes in PPE, etc.

[a]A copy of the OSHA Medical Evaluation Questionnaire is available at: https://www.osha.gov/dte/grant_materials/fy09/sh-18796-09/respiratoryprotection.pdf.

Education needs to include information about the importance of PPE and workplace hygiene. A list of resources, such as those offered through OSHA and the NIOSH, should be made available to the patient.

Respiratory exposure to dust, fibers, asbestos, silicon, smoke, gas, fumes, chemicals, or other airborne contaminants may necessitate the use of respirators. OSHA requires persons using respirators have a medical evaluation by a professional licensed health care provider (PLHCP).[29,42] The use of respirators places an increased demand on the human body, particularly the cardiovascular system. Persons with any history of heart or pulmonary disease or smokers (past or present) should be medically evaluated and cleared before using these devices (Box 18.2).[42,43]

Noise Injuries and Ear Injury Prevention

OSHA reports an estimated 22 million workers are exposed to potentially damaging noise each year.[44] The National Institute of Occupational Safety and Health recommends limiting worker exposure to sudden or sustained levels that exceed 85 dB for longer than 8 hours.[45] To put this in perspective, normal conversation occurs at 60 dB and is not loud enough to cause damage.[45] Noise-induced hearing loss (NIHL) may result in as little as one day when exposed to high levels of noise that are either sudden or sustained.[45] Hearing loss is considered a preventable work hazard and employers are encouraged to develop a hearing conservation plan in the workplace.[45,46]

Utilization of PPE will protect workers against potential hearing loss in environments that exceed the acceptable level of noise.[45,46] High levels of noise will damage the hair cells in the middle ear and result in irreparable hearing loss.[44] Symptoms of NIHL include ringing or humming in the ears or temporary hearing loss when leaving the workplace.[44] While employers should test the work environment for noise pollution, workers should also be evaluated for exposure and the risk of NIHL. A medical evaluation should be done at regular intervals and include[43,45]:

- A complete history of exposure and the use of PPE including ear muffs and ear plugs
- Inspection and palpation of outer structures of the ear
- Otoscopy exam of the ear canal and tympanic membrane
- Hearing test
  - Whisper test
  - Weber and Rinne
  - Audiometry

Documentation should include any reported symptoms of tinnitus, difficulty hearing normal conversations, or muffled sounds along with the physical exam findings of the ear structures and hearing tests.[43,46]

Personal Protective Equipment

Some jobs require the use of PPE. These may include:
- Barrier protection (clothing, shoe covers, gloves)
- Safety glasses/shields
- Medical/surgical masks
- Respirators
- Ear protection (earplugs or ear muffs)

Use of these protection devices should be included in the documentation of the patient history. Some protective devices will require additional medical evaluation or screening.

WORKER'S COMPENSATION

The US Bureau of Labor Statistics defines a work-related injury as any damage to the body that results from an event occurring in the work environment. Work-related illnesses and injuries that require medical attention beyond first aid, modified duty or time away from work, loss of consciousness, or death are considered recordable.[46]

Worker's compensation (WC) is a state-mediated insurance program.[47] If an employee sustains a workplace injury or exposure on the job which requires medical attention, a WC form should be completed and filed with the state agency. The employee is responsible for reporting the event to the employer accurately and in a timely manner.

WC forms are filed by both the employee and provider. Provider reports of treatment, specialty referrals, assessment of disability level, and findings of permanency should conform to the state guidelines when applicable. Fit-for-duty may include a full release to return to work or an order of modified duty. This recommendation is at the discretion of the medical provider.[47] Additional state-specific WC information is available at the following website: https://www.irmi.com/free-resources/insurance-industry-links/workers-comp-agencies

REGULATORY AGENCY AND OTHER REQUIREMENTS IN OCCUPATIONAL AND ENVIRONMENTAL HEALTH

Primary health care providers who choose to provide evaluation for employment and other occupational health–related issues need to be familiar with other regulations and recommendations for screening and treatment. Copies of these regulations can be obtained through the respective agency responsible for the regulation, or they can be found on the Internet. There are several sources to consult when primary care providers include occupational or environmental health issues as part of their practice. The major agencies with regulations affecting workplace surveillance and worker's compensation are OSHA and NIOSH. In addition, the Americans with Disabilities Act has provisions that apply to workers disabled in the workplace. Finally, many professional organizations have specific recommendations for maintaining the health of their members in the workplace.

Occupational Safety and Health Administration

Created by Congress in 1970, OSHA requires each employer to provide "a place of employment, which is free from recognized hazards that are causing or are likely to cause death or serious physical harm to employees."[48] OSHA functions under the Department of Labor. It has the authority to fine or to imprison employers who are found to be in violation of its regulations. Although most of OSHA's regulations deal with safety-related concerns, this organization has also issued a number of standards that specify medical evaluations and the testing of employees who may be exposed to certain workplace hazards.[48] Testing is required when exposures meet or exceed a certain level. Other standards require that employees receive medical clearance before using required protective equipment. Providers granting medical clearance for the use of protective equipment must be familiar with these standards.

National Institute for Occupational Safety and Health. NIOSH was established under the Occupational Safety and Health Act of 1970 and is part of the HHS. Its function is to conduct research and to advise OSHA on issues about hazards in the workplace. NIOSH provides educational information to health care providers, employers, and employees.

Americans With Disabilities Act

Congress enacted the Americans with Disabilities Act in 1990 to protect disabled workers from discrimination in the workplace. This Act must be considered in offering many occupational health–related evaluations. The Act requires that an employer make reasonable accommodations so that the disabled employee is able to perform those job functions considered essential to the position.[49] In addition, it is necessary to determine whether disabled employees can perform the job without posing a "direct threat" to the health and safety of themselves or others.[49]

Professional Organizations. Professional organizations such as the American College of Occupational and Environmental Medicine,[50] the American Association of Occupational Health Nurses,[51] and the American Conference of Governmental Industrial Hygienists[52] offer texts, guidelines, and other information that can assist the health care provider with occupational health–related cases.

Provider resource services are available at the following websites:

Occupational Safety and Health: OSHA.gov

https://search.osha.gov/search?affiliate=usdoloshapublicweb site&query=injuries

Center for Disease Control: National Institute for Occupational Safety and Health

https://search.cdc.gov/search/?query=occupational+health& utf8=%E2%9C%93&affiliate=cdc-main

National Institute of Health: Occupational Health

https://search.nih.gov/search?utf8=%E2%9C%93&affiliate=nih &query=Occupational+health&commit=Search

World Health Organization: Occupational Health

http://search.who.int/search?q=Occupational+health&ie=utf8 &site=who&client=_en_r&proxystylesheet=_en_r&output =xml_no_dtd&oe=utf8&getfields=doctype

Department of Labor: Workers Compensation

https://www.dol.gov/general/topic/workcomp

Department of Transportation: Certified Drivers Licensing

https://www.fmcsa.dot.gov/medical/driver-medical-require ments/dot-medical-exam-and-commercial-motor-vehicle -certification

REFERENCES

1. Workplace Health Promotion. Retrieved from http://www.who.int/ occupational_health/topics/workplace/en/. (Accessed 12 January 2018).
2. (2012). American College of Occupational and Environmental Medicine position statement—Optimizing health care delivery by integrating workplaces, homes, and communities. How occupational and environmental medicine can serve as a vital connecting link between accountable care organizations and the patient-centered medical home. *Journal of Occupational and Environmental Medicine, 54*(4), 504–512.
3. Work related musculoskeletal disorders. Retrieved from http://www.who .int/occupational_health/publications/oehmsd3.pdf?ua=1. (Accessed 5 April 2018).
4. The Public Health Impact of Chemicals: Knowns and Unknowns. Retrieved from http://apps.who.int/iris/bitstream/handle/10665/206553/WHO_FWC_ PHE_EPE_16.01_eng.pdf?sequence=1. (Accessed 25 March 2018).
5. Recommended Practices for Safety and Health Programs. Retrieved from https://www.osha.gov/shpguidelines/management-leadership.html#ai1. (Accessed 1 March 2018).
6. Thompson, J. N., Brodkin, C. A., Kyes, K., Neighbor, W., & Evanoff, B. (2000). Use of a questionnaire to improve occupational and environmental history taking in primary care physicians. *Journal of Occupational and Environmental Medicine, 42*(12), 1188–1194.
7. Rosenstock, L., Logerfo, J., Heyer, N. J., & Carter, W. B. (1984). Development and validation of a self-administered occupational health history questionnaire. *Journal of Occupational Medicine: Official Publication of the Industrial Medical Association, 26*(1), 50–54.
8. Serra, C., Rodriguez, M. C., Delclos, G. L., et al. (2007). Criteria and methods used for the assessment of fitness for work: A systematic review. *Occupational and Environmental Medicine, 64,* 304–312.
9. Schaafsma, F. G., Mahmud, N., Reneman, M. F., Fassier, J. B., & Jungbauer, F. H. W. (2016). Pre-employment examinations for preventing injury, disease and sick leave in workers. *The Cochrane Database of Systematic Reviews,* (1), CD008881, doi:10.1002/14651858.CD008881.pub2.
10. Cordes, D. H., & Rea, D. F. (1994). Work site risk assessment. *Primary Care, 21*(2), 267–274.
11. Department of Transportation Medical Evaluation Instructions and Forms. Retrieved from https://www.fmcsa.dot.gov/medical/driver-medical -requirements/medical-applications-and-forms. (Accessed 22 March 2018).
12. Department of Transportation CDL Medical Requirements. Retrieved from https://www.fmcsa.dot.gov/faq/Medical-Requirements. (Accessed 22 March 2018).
13. Sluiter, J. K., & Frings-Dresen, M. H. W. (2007). What do we know about ageing at work? Evidence-based fitness for duty and health in fire fighters. *Ergonomics, 50*(11), 1897–1913. doi:10.1080/00140130701676005.
14. National Institute for Occupational Safety and Health. Retrieved from https://www.cdc.gov/niosh/about/default.html. (Accessed 28 March 2018).
15. National Institute for Occupational Safety and Health. Workplace safety and health topics. Retrieved from https://www.cdc.gov/niosh/topics/default.html. (Accessed 30 March 2018).
16. Work-related musculoskeletal disorders evaluation measures. Retrieved from https://www.cdc.gov/workplacehealthpromotion/health-strategies/musculo skeletal-disorders/evaluation-measures/index.html. (Accessed 23 April 2018).
17. Musculoskeletal disorders and the workplace: Low back and upper extremities. Retrieved from https://www.ncbi.nlm.nih.gov/books/NBK222446/. (Accessed 25 April 2018).
18. Musculoskeletal disorders in Health and Safety Executive. Retrieved from http://www.hse.gov.uk/msd/index.htm. (Accessed 24 April 2018).
19. Low Back Pain Fact Sheet. Retrieved from https://www.ninds.nih.gov/ Disorders/Patient-Caregiver-Education/Fact-Sheets/Low-Back-Pain-Fact -Sheet. (Accessed 1 May 2018).
20. Ergonomics. Retrieved from https://www.osha.gov/SLTC/ergonomics/. (Accessed 25 April 2018).
21. Skin exposures and effects. Retrieved from https://www.cdc.gov/niosh/topics/ skin/. (Accessed 30 April 2018).
22. Skin notation profiles. Retrieved from https://www.cdc.gov/niosh/topics/ skin/skin-notation_profiles.html. (Accessed 30 April 2018).
23. Skin cancer. Retrieved from https://www.cdc.gov/cancer/skin/basic_info/ prevention.htm. (Accessed 30 April 2018).
24. Shaunnessey, T. (Feb 2015). Combating Cold Stress Professional Safety, Des Plaines. Vol. 60, Iss. 2: 23.
25. Pokhrelp, P. K., & Loftus, S. A. (2007). Ocular emergencies. *American Family Physician, 76*(6), 829–836.
26. Singh, P., Tyagi, M., Kumar, Y., Gupta, K. K., & Sharma, P. D. (2013). Ocular chemical injuries and their management. *Oman Journal of Ophthalmology, 6*(2), 83–86. http://doi.org/10.4103/0974-620X.116624.
27. al-Qurainy, I. A., Dutton, G. N., Ilankovan, V., Titterington, D. M., Moos, K. F., & el Attar, A. (1991). Midfacial fractures and the eye: The development of a system for detecting patients at risk of eye injury—a prospective evaluation. *The British Journal of Oral and Maxillofacial Surgery, 29*(6), 368–369.
28. American Thoracic Society. Work related lung diseases. Retrieved from https://www.thoracic.org/patients/patient-resources/resources/occupational -lung-disease.pdf. (Accessed 28 April 2018).
29. Occupational respiratory disease surveillance. Retrieved from https:// www.cdc.gov/niosh/topics/surveillance/ORDS/. (Accessed 30 April 2018).
30. Malo, J. L., & Taylor, A. N. (2007). Defining occupational asthma and confirming the diagnosis: What do experts suggest? *Occupational and Environmental Medicine, 64*(6), 359–360.
31. Iossifova, Y., Bailey, R., Wood, J., & Kreiss, K. (2010). Concurrent silicosis and pulmonary mycosis at death. *Emerging Infectious Diseases, 16*(2), 318–320. https://dx.doi.org/10.3201/eid1602.090824.
32. Wang, X. R., Eisen, E., Zhang, H. X., et al. (2003). Respiratory symptoms and cotton dust exposure: Results of a 15-year follow-up observation. *Occupational and Environmental Medicine, 60,* 935–941.
33. Centers for Disease Control and Prevention. Veterans' health activities. Retrieved from www.cdc.gov/nceh/veterans/vet_hlth_actvy.pdf. (Accessed 26 January 2015).
34. Agency for Toxic Substances and Disease Registry. Congressional testimony: Potential adverse effects of service in the Persian Gulf War. Retrieved from www.atsdr.cdc.gov/testimony/testimony-1992-09-16.html. (Accessed 26 January 2015).
35. Centers for Disease Control. (2017). Occupational respiratory disease surveillance. Retrieved from https://www.cdc.gov/niosh/topics/surveillance/ ORDS/. (Accessed 30 July 2018).
36. Centers for Disease Control. All workplace safety and health topics. Tuberculosis. Last updated March 22, 2016. Retrieved from https://www.cdc.gov/ niosh/topics/. (Accessed 30 July 2018).
37. Safirstein, B., Klukowicz, A., Miller, R., et al. (2003). Granulomatous pneumonitis following exposure to the World Trade Center collapse. *Chest, 123*(1), 301–304.
38. Bandyopadhyay, A., Roy, P. P., Saha, K., Chakraborty, S., Jash, D., & Saha, D. (2013). Usefulness of induced sputum eosinophil count to assess severity and treatment outcome in asthma patients. *Lung India: Official Organ of Indian Chest Society, 30*(2), 117–123. http://doi.org/10.4103/0970-2113.110419.
39. Centers for Disease Control. All workplace safety and health topics. Work related asthma. Last updated January 26, 2018. Retrieved from https:// www.cdc.gov/niosh/topics/. (Accessed 30 July 2018).
40. Wu, M., McIntosh, J., & Liu, J. (2016). Current prevalence rate of latex allergy: Why it remains a problem? *Journal of Occupational Health, 58*(2), 138–144. doi:10.1539/joh.15-0275-RA.
41. Carlo Di Renzo, G., Conry, J., Blake, J., DeFrancesco, M., DeNicola, N., & Martin, J. (2015). International Federation of Gynecology and Obstetrics

opinion on reproductive health impacts of exposure to toxic environmental chemicals. *International Journal of Gynaecology and Obstetrics*, 131(3), https://doi.org/10.1016/j.ijgo.2015.09.002.

42. Belafsky, S., Vlach, J., & McCurdy, S. A. (2013). Cardiopulmonary fitness and respirator clearance: An update. *Journal of Occupational and Environmental Hygiene*, 10, 5–277.

43. Desautels, N., Singh, J., Burrell, J., & Rosenman, K. D. (2016). What should be the content and frequency of performing a medical evaluation to determine fitness to wear a respirator? *Journal of Occupational and Environmental Medicine*, 58, 9–892.

44. Occupational noise exposure. Retrieved from https://www.osha.gov/SLTC/noisehearingconservation/. (Accessed 1 May 2018).

45. Masterson, E. A., Bushnell, P. T., Themann, C. L., & Morata, T. C. (2016). Hearing impairment among noise-exposed workers—United States, 2003–2012. *MMWR. Morbidity and Mortality Weekly Report*, 65, 389–394. http://dx.doi.org/10.15585/mmwr.mm6515a2.

46. Fausti, S. A., Wilmington, D. J., Helt, P. V., Helt, W. J., & Konrad-Martin, D. (2005). Hearing health and care: The need for improved hearing loss prevention and hearing conservation practices. *Journal of Rehabilitation Research and Development*, 42(4 Suppl. 2), 45–62.

47. Workers Comp Agencies. Retrieved from https://www.irmi.com/free-resources/insurance-industry-links/workers-comp-agencies. (Accessed 5 May 2018).

48. U.S. Department of Labor, Occupational Safety and Health Administration. General industry OSHA safety and health standards. Retrieved from https://www.osha.gov/pls/oshaweb/owastand.display_standard_group?p_toc_level=1&p_part_number=1910.

49. Employment Rights Under the Americans with Disabilities Act (and other related laws). Fourth Edition. April 2010, publication #5068.01. Retrieved from www.disabilityrightsca.org/pubs/506801.htm. (Accessed 24 January 2015).

50. (2014). American College of Occupational and Environmental Medicine guidance statement. American College of Occupational and Environmental Medicine's Occupational and Environmental Medicine competencies—2014. *ACOEM OEM Competencies Task Force. Journal of Occupational and Environmental Medicine*, 56(5), e21–e40. Retrieved from www.acoem.org. (Accessed 11 December 2014).

51. American Association of Occupational Health Nurses (AAOHN). Retrieved from www.aaohn.org/component/content/?view=featured. (Accessed 25 January 2019).

52. American College of Governmental Industrial Hygiene (ACGIH). Retrieved from http://www.acgih.org/about/orgchart.htm. (Accessed 13 December 2014).

CHAPTER **19**

COLLEGE HEALTH

Elizabeth Remo • Brittany Blair Hay

INTRODUCTION

Students in colleges and universities face many challenges, including a newly defined independence and making autonomous decisions that can impact their personal growth and development, both socially and professionally. College health focuses on the diverse needs of these students, which can greatly impact health and well-being. Student health services across colleges and universities provide an avenue for addressing the challenges and opportunities many students face while advancing their education. These may range from emotional concerns driven by class assignments or personal/family issues to physical illnesses secondary to the body's reaction to internal and environmental stressors. Recognizing the impact of student health on personal, social, and academic domains led to the formation of the national organization known as the American College of Health Association (ACHA) in 1920. This organization continues to address the health needs

of students and promotes advancement of student health initiatives within colleges and universities to better serve this unique population.

Student health services offer primary care services comparable to primary care clinics within a local community. Although the amount and variety of available services may vary depending on the campus size and location (i.e., urban or rural setting), interprofessional partnerships between health care providers, including mental health and public health team members, can provide increased access to quality health care for this population.

ROLES OF COLLEGE HEALTH CARE PROVIDERS

Students enrolled in college today represent a diverse cadre of race, ethnicity, identities, and ages as both traditional and nontraditional populations matriculate. Health care providers are in a key position to partner with students and positively impact health, growth, and development at whatever life stage they may be in during this time. From adolescence through adulthood, these students will not only need medical attention but will also need a partner to help guide them in their treatment or care decisions, a teacher to educate them on health promotion and disease prevention, a counselor to listen and provide them with appropriate resources, a guide to help them navigate the confusing world of health insurance coverages, and a provider who will continue to advocate for their actual and potential health care needs.

The health services provided in colleges and universities may vary, with the programs structured to fit the need and culture of the campus. Wellness programs may be housed in athletic facilities or student unions, in addition to the student health clinic site. Health education programs may be provided in different departments and may be designed in collaboration with mental health counselors, athletics department staff, health educators, alcohol and drug counselors, peer educators, and residential life staff. In addition, program design should also focus on current campus trends, top college health issues, gender differences, risk-taking behaviors, safety concerns, and emergency preparedness. To support these efforts, the ACHA-National College Health Assessment research survey is periodically conducted to assess health needs and critical issues relevant to those in colleges and universities. Data from this survey includes smoking habits, contraceptive use, mental health issues, relationship difficulties, sexual behaviors, exercise habits, preventive health practices, and perceptions of drugs and alcohol use and their impact on academic performance.[1]

Confidentiality

Privacy and confidentiality of personal and health information are critical in the partnership of a provider and student. Confidentiality of health information and exchange of private information disclosed by the younger students and their parents/guardian impacts access to health care and the outcome of care. For this reason, the Health Insurance Probability and Accountability Act (HIPPA) of 1996 was developed in response to the need to federally protect personal health information and respect of patients' right to that information.[2]

Students older than 18 years of age are legally able to make health care decisions without parental involvement. However, the age of students varies across colleges and universities. Nevertheless, parental involvement does not dictate the age of the students and the need to highlight the importance of confidentiality and privacy. The formation of the Privacy Rule allowed disclosure of patient information if needed for patient care and other defined important purpose.[2]

Obtaining a student's written permission to discuss a specific illness episode with a parent, professor, or administrator affirms respect for the student's privacy. Circumstances such as serious or life-threatening illnesses can be made known to parents at the discretion of the professional staff. The American College Counseling Association for University and College Counseling Center Directors collaborated with the Campus Litigation and Privacy Act of 2015 to assure better protection of student medical records.[2] Students under their parents' health insurance may face additional challenges with privacy. If a student is covered by a parent's medical insurance plan, confidential information may be inadvertently revealed to the policyholder (parent) because of routine billing procedures and documents. Barriers to obtaining services related to gynecological care, contraception, or treatment for STDs may occur if students do not have their own policies. Establishing open communication between individual students, providers, affiliated staff, and other responsible parties is critical in maintaining confidentiality and respecting their rights as a patient.

Health Insurance

Access to care issues present challenges and opportunities in college health reflecting that of the national health care landscape. Financing student health services, whether per capita or as part of general funds, can impact access to preventative and primary care services. Although the goal is to provide primary care services for free to students, it is not always financially feasible. Clear communication to students regarding out-of-pocket costs and/or additional fees needs to occur. Affordable options should be available for students to meet their needs while in school, especially when coverage under parental insurance plans is not available.

HEALTH TOPICS
Mental Health

Student health services can be involved in medical maintenance, treatment, referral, or co-management of students with mental health needs. Organizations such as ACHA have partnered with the Higher Education Mental Health Alliance to provide leadership in the advancement of college health to address mental health needs that can greatly impact student success.[3] Students with mental health needs may be identified through the information they provide on a health intake form or brief screening questions, such as PHQ-2 and GAD-7, especially if they provide a listing of their psychiatric medications. Transfer or coordination of mental health care from home to the college setting can be challenging, as students may already have established a therapeutic relationship with their mental health provider and may be reluctant to establish a new relationship with an unfamiliar therapist. Student health and counseling services must collaborate when necessary to provide optimum care for these students while maintaining confidentiality.

Student health services can serve as a conduit to campus counseling services when asked by the athletic or dance department to evaluate a student with a potential eating disorder, substance use disorder, or other mental health issue. The academic or student life department may also refer a student with a potential mood, thought, or adjustment disorder. Health care providers must be sensitive to the possible perception of a stigma in seeking mental health services as this can be a barrier to care for some students. A gesture of acceptance and availability may give students comfort to seek access to mental health–related care.

Stress and Anxiety

Several factors surrounding college life can be stressful, especially during the first year of transition. Students bring certain expectations and mixed emotions. These factors can tremendously affect educational opportunities and learning. These emotional barriers can hinder programmatic success, and personal and professional growth and development.

Depression

Transition to college life may present acutely stressful situations and be accompanied by periods of hopelessness for some students. It is essential that college and university health providers and counselors maintain a high level of vigilance for suicide or depression risk in assessing all students. Safety is critical in students battling depression, as some may socially withdraw or exhibit atypical symptoms, preventing early detection and intervention.

Sleep

Assessment of sleep behaviors should be included when possible during clinical visits. Sleep disturbance or lack of adequate sleep can contribute to unpleasant personal and health outcomes. Responsibilities related to academic, athletic, social, and work life all contribute to students' inadequate sleep. By resetting their biologic clocks, sleep-deprived students can develop concentration difficulties, impaired immune systems, anxiety, irritability, and possibly increased drug or alcohol use.[4] It can also be a contributing factor to or a result of mental health conditions, such as depression or anxiety. Visible and reported signs and symptoms, such as fatigue, illness, or depression, should trigger further investigation of sleep habits and sleep disorders.

Infectious Diseases

Health and well-being in general can directly impact academic performance. Missed classes because of an illness can potentially delay a student's progress. Primary prevention of infectious disease is key, however secondary prevention is of equal importance, with early treatment and management of clinical diagnoses.

Upper Respiratory Disease

Influenza and/or influenza-like illnesses (ILI) can greatly impact college health as it affects not just the individual student but holds potential to spread campus-wide. The CDC describes ILI as a medical condition that presents with fever (temperature of 100°F or greater) and cough, with or without sore throat, of unknown cause other than influenza.[5] The H1N1 flu pandemic in 2009 brought to light its potential impact in the college setting. This led to a surveillance project initiated by ACHA to determine disease burden and attack rates related to ILI.[5] Data collected provided information regarding the epidemiology of the H1N1 outbreak, vaccine availability, and supported tracking of vaccination trends. This event made clear the importance of being prepared, addressing current and future management, and preventing pandemic concerns related to ILI.

Measles

Presence of a contagious viral illness on campus is worrisome because of its potential ease of spread with students in close contact, especially those within classrooms and dormitories.[6] Measles is particularly contagious as it can inoculate others through its presence on surfaces and in the air.[6] It can lead to serious illnesses and complications including pneumonia, encephalitis, and death.[6] Clinically, students may present with a rash. However, symptoms of cough and sneezing may appear before the rash and obfuscate early recognition. Transmission can easily be prevented through vaccination. Therefore, review of immunization status of enrolled students is essential in preventing an outbreak. Unvaccinated students should be highly encouraged to update their immunization status prior to matriculation. Regardless, colleges and universities should have an emergency plan established to mitigate the risk of spread in the event of an outbreak.

Meningitis

Adolescents 11 to 18 years of age and college students living in dormitories are at high risk for contracting meningococcal disease and should consider vaccination prior to arrival on campus.[7] Immunization with both the traditional conjugate (Menactra and Menveo) and newer serogroup B (Bexsero and Trumenba) vaccines may be advisable for this population as outbreaks of serogroup B meningococcal disease have been documented on campuses from New England to the West Coast.[8]

SCREENINGS AND IMMUNIZATIONS

Pre-matriculation immunizations are mandated by colleges, universities, and state law. Student health services are responsible for ensuring student compliance with these mandates, including documentation of students who remain unimmunized due to religious beliefs. Evidence of immunity or current immunization to measles, mumps, and rubella is usually required for college enrollment. Immunization or evidence of immunity to hepatitis B, chickenpox, meningococcal disease, and tetanus is recommended. The Centers for Disease Control and Prevention Advisory Committee on Immunization Practices and ACHA recommend that both students and parents be educated about the risks of meningococcal disease in the college, and that vaccination is encouraged.[9] Current meningococcal prevention mandates for specific colleges and universities by state can be found at the Immunization Action Coalition website at www.immunize.org/laws/menin.asp.

Students arriving from tuberculosis-endemic countries within the past 5 years must typically receive tuberculin skin testing before enrollment.[10] For those traveling from countries where BCG immunizations are routinely given, interferon-gamma release assays may be substituted (e.g., QuantiFERON-TB Gold In-Tube or T-SPOT.TB tests).[11] Students planning to study abroad during college will also need advice on travel immunizations and information relevant to appropriate infectious disease prevention well in advance of travel dates. Students returning from travel to tuberculosis-endemic countries will require rescreening. If college health clinics are unable to provide this type of service, referral to a local health department or suitable community agency is advisable.

SEXUAL HEALTH

Developmentally, transition to college for young adults occurs during a time when good decision-making is challenged by peer influence and contributes to risky sexual behavior. The behavioral decisions made in adolescence can impact health and well-being for a lifetime.[12] Thus, educational outreach to support primary prevention of sexually transmitted infections (STI), unintended pregnancy, and intimate partner violence paired with age-appropriate screenings and confidential treatment when indicated are paramount for those providing care to this population.

Sexually Transmitted Infections

According to the CDC, nearly half of all new STIs occur in people 15 to 24 years of age.[13] These infections may present in an asymptomatic or symptomatic manner depending on the pathogen and, if untreated, convey a significant threat to general health and future fertility. Therefore, yearly STI screening with or without the presence of symptoms is recommended by the CDC and intensive behavioral counseling for all sexually active adolescents and at-risk adults is recommended (Grade B: high certainty to be of moderate benefit) by the United States Preventive Services Task Force (USPSTF).[13]

Partnerships with local, state, and national agencies can assist with efforts to provide STI screening through campaigns such as *Get Yourself Tested* (GYT) and are supported by the American College Health Association, Kaiser Family Foundation, National Coalition of Sexually Transmitted Disorders (STD) Directors, Music Television (MTV), and Planned Parenthood, along with the CDC.[13] Free STI testing on college campuses can serve to optimize screening and early treatment efforts while bypassing barriers to testing such as concerns that adolescents and younger adults may have regarding parental notification through insurance carriers.[14]

Human Papilloma Virus

Human papillomavirus (HPV) has been linked to oral, esophageal, cervical, and anorectal cancers, which represent approximately 5% of the global burden of cancer.[15] Immunization, as recommended by the Advisory Committee on Immunization Practices (ACIP) for all preadolescent children, can prevent approximately 90% of associated cancers, however, college-age immunization rates remain low, especially in males.[1,15,16] Reasons for this gap are multifactorial as college students may be unaware of the importance of this vaccine, recommendations for catch-up vaccination schedules or the availability of low-cost or free vaccinations.[17] Although age restrictions may apply in some cases, HPV vaccination cost is currently covered through private insurance plans, Medicaid, the Children's Health Insurance Program (CHIP), or the Vaccines for Children (VFC) Program.[18] Additionally, pharmaceutical manufacturers may provide vaccines to eligible patients through patient assistance programs.

Human Immunodeficiency Virus/Acquired Immune Deficiency Syndrome

The CDC reported in 2016 that 80% of the 8451 new youth human immunodeficiency virus (HIV) diagnoses occurred in young adults ages 20 to 24. Of these cases, the majority were attributable to male-to-male sexual contact. Yet, in the National College Health Assessment report, only 25.8% of college students report ever being tested for HIV infection.[1] Adding further complexity to the problem, sexually active students report use of condoms with vaginal intercourse at a rate of 46.2% and only 25.9% for higher-risk anal intercourse.[1] These findings parallel a trend noted by the CDC: those at highest risk for HIV are not being tested, primarily influenced by low perceived risk and lack of provider recommendation.[19]

HIV screening ought to be part of annual STI screening practices for all sexually active youth and adults, with more frequent testing for those at high risk (USPSTF recommendation A: high certainty that net benefit is substantial).[20] Today many people are living with acquired immune deficiency syndrome (AIDS) despite the absence of a cure, as appropriately timed therapies have lowered the risks for clinical progression, complications, and transmission.[20] Persons with HIV/AIDS at college will need access to regular medical care, supportive therapies, and protective immunizations including: TdAP (tetanus and diphtheria), influenza (flu), hepatitis B, HPV, meningococcal, and pneumococcal formulations.[21]

Contraception

Undesired pregnancy is a common concern among college students and a priority for college health providers. If not planned, pregnancy can cause significant stress and negatively impact individual academic performance. Both heterosexual and sexual minority women are at risk of unintended pregnancy.[1,22] The top three methods of contraception used by young adults include male condoms (60.1%), birth control pills (55.5%), and withdrawal (32.9%), with 49.4% of students using a male condom plus another method.[19] Providers ought to be knowledgeable regarding the efficacy, nuances, and cultural and/or religious implications of contraceptive methods to support informed choice.

National, state, and local programs exist to support education of young adults in contraceptive measures. Local health departments and nonprofit women's centers may provide free services to those in need. The *Power to Decide* program is an example of a national and higher education partnership providing young people with the information and skills to take charge of their sexual health while in college.[23]

WEIGHT MANAGEMENT
Nutrition and Eating Disorders

All students, particularly women, who visit student health services should be observed for evidence of an eating disorder. Diagnosis and management of anorexia nervosa or bulimia are addressed elsewhere in this text (see Chapter 207). However, diagnosis and treatment in the college setting has unique aspects.

Female students are acutely aware of the myth of the "freshman 15," which purports that women will gain 15 pounds during their first year on campus.[24] Students with an eating disorder in remission who find college life stressful are prone to regression. Women pressured to compete socially or athletically may respond with disordered eating while at college, which may progress to a full eating disorder. Adding to the problem, the use of social networking sites, a staple for many college students, is associated with increased body image concerns and disordered eating.[25]

Students living in dorms or sororities and students participating in activities such as athletic teams, dance, or theater groups may notice fellow students exhibiting behavior indicative of an eating disorder. Students, as well as coaches, professors, or student leaders, may approach student health services to seek advice regarding concern for a friend or classmate.[25] Whether working alone or in concert with student counseling services, the student health services staff must proceed carefully to protect the individual while listening to those concerned about their friend or classmate.[25] Depending on the clinical situation, remaining in treatment and meeting established goals to remain in college can serve as strong motivating factors for the student with an eating disorder. Unfortunately, health service personnel are often powerless to intervene if the student never seeks treatment on his/her/their own. Mandated visits have limited value beyond possible initial diagnosis and can sabotage future treatment.

TOBACCO, ALCOHOL, AND DRUG USE

Alcohol use in the college population continues to be a problem despite institutional efforts to curb it.[26] Secondary effects of binge drinking include academic failure, sexual assault, violence, property damage, motor vehicle accidents, and death. Among the strategies most often used to curb alcohol consumption are alternative late-night alcohol-free events, increased sanctions, student involvement in campus policies and adjudication, and peer education. Student health services treat both the acute and secondary effects of alcohol intoxication. This encounter affords the opportunity to educate the student on issues connected with alcohol use. In addition, referrals to counseling services, on-campus alcohol education programs, or community alcohol treatment programs may be appropriate.

Tobacco use on college campuses also continues to be an issue. Almost 19% of college students smoke, with new opportunities arising in the availability of hookah, vaporizers, e-cigarette, or other nicotine delivery systems, and subsequent risks relating to parties, socializing, and weekend use.[27,28] College health care providers have a role both in advocating for policies that restrict smoking and in promoting smoking prevention and cessation. Tobacco use should be the "fifth vital sign" in students' sick visit encounters to initiate the opportunity to discuss smoking cessation. Even when there is little student demand for formal cessation programs, these programs must remain part of the wellness and health promotion initiatives for this population.

Other Drugs of Abuse and Prescription Abuse

College health providers will inevitably encounter students who abuse prescription or illicit drugs. Educating individual students on the health, mental health, and academic consequences of drug abuse may be beyond the scope of the provider and merit a referral to a specialist. Students who are prescribed neurostimulants must be advised of the consequences of giving or selling prescription medication to others (a felony) and, if these medications are prescribed by the college health center, must engage in a written or verbal contract regarding their appropriate use and safekeeping. Legalization of previously controlled substances, such as marijuana in some jurisdictions, warrants knowledge of school polices and health concerns for use of those substances related to school performance and overall health risks.

CHRONIC HEALTH CONDITIONS

Today, college health clinic services are not only sought for management of acute episodic illness but increasingly for support of ongoing chronic conditions. Owing to advances in medical and surgical care, an increasing number of college students with chronic health conditions (e.g., cancer, diabetes, auto-immune disorders, congenital heart disease, etc.) are now matriculating.[29] Approximately 6% of respondents in the National Center for Health Statistics (NCHS) 2017 study report having a chronic illness, demonstrating a 2.2% increase over the past decade. Furthermore, chronic health problem(s) or serious illness within the past 12 months was noted by 4.2% of respondents to negatively impact academic performance either thorough (1) receipt of a lower exam, project, or course grade; (2) contributing to an incomplete or dropped course; or (3) causing a significant disruption in thesis, dissertation, research, or practicum work.[29]

Adolescents with chronic health conditions may require additional support as they navigate the usual developmental tasks of becoming more autonomous while managing additional vital requirements of monitoring and attending to health needs.[30,31] Successful management of college students with chronic health needs requires providers to engage in care coordination across transitions to and from college involving navigation of multiple health care systems and linkages to needed resources including referrals for specialty services where applicable. Ongoing communication across these transitions of care is needed between patients, their families (or caretakers), and providers to minimize threats to safe care.

DIVERSITY AND CULTURAL COMPETENCY

Cultural competency is crucial to the success of student health services in caring for a diverse student population. Cultural competency is more than cultural awareness (knowledge) and cultural sensitivity (knowledge plus some experience with the culture). It encompasses the ability to think about power differentials in relationships and respond with varied skills to establish rapport with diverse individuals.[32] Student health care providers must be sensitive to voice, body language, and gestures as they communicate with patients. There may be culture-specific meanings in populations of patients for aspects of health care such as pain and reproductive issues. College health providers can expect to experience multiple cultures on their campus and must be leaders in modeling and fostering cultural competency.

HEALTH CARE ISSUES: POPULATION SPECIFIC
Female Students

Distance from home may provide an opportunity for more intimate sexual relationships and lack of daily parental oversight. These new experiences come with concomitant responsibilities. The first well-woman visit at student health services should include a thorough lifestyle assessment and allow sufficient time for a first pelvic examination (if appropriate), a thorough sexual history, STD education, and contraceptive counseling. Some institutions may schedule this as a two-part visit.

Reproductive, Substance, and Safety Issues. Appointments requested specifically for STD screening or emergency contraception create opportunities for the provider to explore the college woman's sense of control in a sexual situation, the impact of drug or alcohol use on her decisions, and any sense of guilt or regret connected to her sexual experience. Although sexual assault is covered elsewhere within this textbook, it must be noted that research suggests college women are at greater risk for sexual assault than are women of a comparable age in the general population. In a survey conducted by the ACHA, 5% of college women reported an attempted or completed rape in 2009.[33] Other studies put the annual (9-month) incidence at 3%.[34] Discrepancies in numbers may be based on underreporting resulting from barriers including: fears about confidentiality or sanction, guilt over alcohol use, cultural differences in definitions of dating, violence, sexual assault, or rape, or institutional misunderstanding/ignorance regarding reporting guidelines. Several legislative acts from 1990 to 1998, including the Clery Act, have mandated that colleges and universities make available statistics on campus crime, including sexual assault, and that schools have policies in place to address sexual assault.[35] Student health services are an active participant in reporting such crimes and in developing programming to prevent sexual assault and contributors. As a supportive member of the college community, student health services must have a thorough understanding of the institution's policies and procedures for reporting rape, sexual misconduct, and sexual harassment. Understanding the level of risk-taking behavior enables the provider to guide a student in appropriate health screenings and contraceptive care, refer to student counseling services and alcohol or drug programs if warranted, and schedule follow-up appointments for continuation of care.

Male Students

Males 16 to 20 years of age have far fewer health care visits than younger males (11 to 15 years old) or their female contemporaries.[36] Male college students visit the health center only episodically for sick visits or injuries. This results in fewer opportunities for health education or risk-reduction counseling than for college-age women. Efforts to connect with this population through outreach programs in dormitories, fraternities, or athletic teams can help bridge the gap.

Reproductive, Substance, and Safety Issues. Young men may also come to a student health center for STD screening. This occasion provides an opportunity to screen for high-risk behaviors, including drug and alcohol use, violence, nonrelational sexual activity, and condom use. The STD screening visit is an excellent opportunity for one-on-one teaching of college men. Because testicular cancer is more prevalent in this age group, education about testicular cancer and self-examination should be offered to the individual and promoted in wellness efforts. The proper use of condoms can also be taught at an STD screening visit.

Injuries related to violence because of male clubs, organizations, or initiation rites are a cause for concern and must be discussed with college students, particularly if coupled with substance use. However, the student may be conflicted about giving information, particularly if the student took an oath of confidentiality. Understanding the institution's policies regarding these activities may help guide the provider's response. All forms of campus violence or abuse—sexual, psychological, physical, or verbal—impede the educational mission of a college campus. Providers in college health play a critical role in preventing, reporting, and caring for victims of violence. Those working in college health also must be aware of signs that a student may be at high risk for perpetrating a violent act on campus. Reporting these concerns in a timely manner to appropriate authorities is needed while prioritizing safety and balancing the need for disclosure versus privacy. Campuses should have in place clear policies and guidelines for handling situations that hold potential to place students and staff at risk as well as contingency plans for disaster. Periodic trainings and drills to improve readiness for such untoward events ought to be implemented.

Lesbian, Gay, Bisexual, and Transgender Students

Lesbian, gay, bisexual, and transgender (LGBT) students face multiple challenges on college campuses, ranging from health to safety issues. Student health services may need to initiate outreach to LGBT student communities as gender and sexual minority students are often hesitant to initiate contact and seek services. Services provided by the student health center must be visible and appropriate for these diverse communities. Specific health concerns of LGBT students include but are not limited to HIV or AIDS care, STD prevention, identifying and reducing suicide risk, help in "coming out," school anti-bullying policies, smoking prevention and cessation, and culturally competent care.[37] Speaking with student LGBT organizations and requesting feedback on the state of health services and programming may be of benefit in efforts to provide an LGBT-friendly environment with valued services.

RESOURCES

A student health advisory committee is a useful tool for student feedback on student perception of services, cultural competency, sponsored insurance plans, and other issues related to delivery of service. A reasonable representation should include athletes, LGBT students, underrepresented minority students, users of student health insurance, and student government members. Students not only can provide critical feedback on health services, but can also advocate to the administration for needed funding of improvements of programs and services. In addition, the ACHA, with membership representing more than 2500 health care providers and 920 institutions of higher education, provides useful standards and guidelines for college health programs and services. Its website can be accessed at www.acha.org.

REFERENCES

1. American College Health Association. (2018). *American College Health Association—national college health assessment II: Reference group executive summary fall 2017*. Hanover, MD: American College Health Association.
2. American College Health Association. (2018). HIPPA/medical records. Retrieved from http://www.acha.org/ACHA/Resources/Topics/HIPAA.aspx.
3. American College Health Association. (2018). Mental health. Retrieved from http://www.acha.org/ACHA/Resources/Topics/MentalHealth.aspx.
4. Kadison, R., & DiGeronimo, T. (2004). *College of the overwhelmed*. San Francisco: Jossey-Bass.
5. American College Health Association. (2018). ACHA pandemic influenza surveillance. Retrieved from http://www.acha.org/ACHA/Resources/ILI_Project.aspx.
6. American College Health Association. (2018). Measles update 2015: implications for the college setting. Retrieved from http://www.acha.org/ACHA/Programs_and_Services/CE_Activities/Measles_Update_2015.aspx.
7. American College Health Association. (2018). Update on meningococcal disease. Retrieved from http://www.acha.org/ACHA/Programs_and_Services/CE_Activities/Update_on_Meningococcal_Disease.aspx.
8. Centers for Disease Control and Prevention. (2018). Meningococcal disease. Retrieved from https://www.cdc.gov/meningococcal/index.html.
9. Centers for Disease Control and Prevention. (2000). Meningococcal disease in college students. Recommendations of the advisory committee on immunization practices (ACIP). *MMWR. Recommendations and Reports: Morbidity and Mortality Weekly Report. Recommendations and Reports, 49*(RR-7), 13-20.
10. American College Health Association. (2014). ACHA guidelines: tuberculosis screening and targeted testing of college and university students. Retrieved from www.acha.org/documents/resources/guidelines/ACHA_Tuberculosis_Screening_April2014.pdf.
11. Centers for Disease Control and Prevention. (2016). Tuberculosis. Retrieved from https://www.cdc.gov/tb/publications/factsheets/testing/tb_testing.htm.
12. Calamidas, E. G., & Crowell, T. L. (2017). A content analysis of college students' health behaviors. *American Journal of Health Education, 49*(3), 133-146.
13. Centers for Disease Control and Prevention. (2016). College health and safety. Retrieved from https://www.cdc.gov/family/college/.
14. Leichliter, J. S., Copen, C., & Dittus, P. J. (2017). Confidentiality issues and use of sexually transmitted disease services among sexually experienced persons aged 15-25 years, 2013-2015. *MMWR Morb Mortal Wkly Report, 66*(9), 237-241. doi:10.15585/mmwr.mm6609a1.
15. Razzaghi, H., Saraiya, M., Thomson, T. D., Henley, S. J., Viens, L., & Wilson, R. (2018). Five-year relative survival for human papillomavirus-associated cancer sites. *Cancer, 124*(1), 203-211.
16. Lee, H. Y., Lust, K., Vang, S., & Desai, J. (2018). Male undergraduates' HPV vaccination behavior: Implications for achieving HPV-associated cancer equity. *Journal of Community Health, 43*(3), 459-466.
17. Radecki Breitkopf, D., Finney Ruten, L. J., Findley, V., Jacovson, D. J., Wilson, P. M., Albertie, M., et al. (2016). Awareness and knowledge of human papillomavirus, HPV-related cancers, and HPV vaccines in an uninsured adult clinic population. *Cancer Medicine, 5*(11), 3346-3352.
18. Kaiser Family Foundation. (2017). The HPV vaccine: access and use in the U.S. Retrieved from https://www.kff.org/womens-health-policy/fact-sheet/the-hpv-vaccine-access-and-use-in/.
19. Febo-Vazquez, I., Copen, C. E., & Daugherty, J. (2018). Main reasons for never testing for HIV among women and men aged 15-44 in the united states, 2011-2015. *National Health Statistics Report, 107*, 1-12.
20. U.S. Preventative Services Task Force. (2014). Published recommendations for primary care. Retrieved from https://www.uspreventiveservicestaskforce.org/Page/Document/RecommendationStatementFinal/sexually-transmitted-infections-behavioral-counseling1.
21. Health and Human Services. (2018). AIDS info: Offering information on HIV/AIDS, treatment, prevention, and research. Retrieved from https://aidsinfo.nih.gov.
22. Blunt-Vinti, H. D., Thompson, E., & Griner, S. B. (2018). Contraceptive use effectiveness and pregnancy prevention information preferences among heterosexual and sexual minority college women. *Women's Health Issues, 28*(4), 342-349.
23. Power to Decide. (2018). What we do. Retrieved from https://powertodecide.org/contact-us.
24. Klein, D. (2008). The freshman 15: Is it real? *Journal of American College Health: J of ACH, 56*(5), 531-534.
25. Holland, G., & Tiggemann, M. (2016). A systematic review of the impact of the use of social networking sites on body image and disordered eating outcomes. *Body Image, 17*, 100-110.
26. Wechsler, H., Lee, J. E., Kuo, M., et al. (2002). Trends in college binge drinking during a period of increased prevention efforts. *Journal of American College Health, 50*(5), 203-217.
27. Johnston, L. D., O'Malley, P. M., Bachman, J. G., & Schulenberg, J. E. (2007). Monitoring the future: national survey results on drug use, 1975-2006: Volume II, College students and adults ages 19-45. (NIH Publication No. 07-6206). Bethesda, MD.
28. Cronk, N. J., Harris, K. J., Harrar, S., et al. (2011). Analysis of smoking patterns and context among college student smokers. *Substance Use Misuse, 46*(8), 1015-1022.
29. Centers for Disease Control and Prevention. (2018). National Center for Health Statistics National Health Interview Survey 2017 Data Release. Retrieved from https://www.cdc.gov/nchs/nhis/nhis_2017_data_release.htm.
30. Hardy, R. Y., Gurvitz, M., Jackson, J. L., May, S., Miller, P., Daskalove, R., et al. (2018). College students with congenital heart disease: A critical time frame for transition. *Journal of American College Health, 66*(4), 324-328.
31. Ravert, R. D., Russell, L. T., & O'Guin, M. B. (2017). Managing chronic conditions in college: Findings from prompted health incidents diaries. *Journal of American College Health, 65*(3), 217-222.
32. American College Health Association. (2011). ACHA Guidelines: Cultural competency statement. Retrieved from www.acha.org/documents/resources/guidelines/ACHA_Cultural_Competency_Statement_Feb2011.pdf.
33. American College Health Association. (2009). *American College Health Association: National college health assessment II: Reference group executive summary, Spring 2009*. Linthicum, Md: ACHA.
34. Fisher, B. S., Cullen, F. T., & Turner, M. G. (2000). *The sexual victimization of college women, (NCJRS Publication No. 182369)*. Washington, DC: U.S. Department of Justice, National Criminal Justice Reference Service.

35. Clery Center. (2018). Summary of the Jeanne Clery Act. Retrieved from https://clerycenter.org/policy-resources/the-clery-act/.
36. Marcell, A. V., Klein, J. D., Fischer, I., et al. (2002). Male adolescent use of health care services: Where are the boys? *Journal of Adolescent Health, 30,* 35–43.
37. U.S. Department of Health and Human Services. (2016). Lesbian, gay, bisexual, and transgender health. Retrieved from https://www.hhs.gov/programs/topic-sites/lgbt/index.html.

CHAPTER **20**

PRESURGICAL CLEARANCE

Lindsay E. Bergmann

SIGNIFICANCE OF THE PRESURGICAL EVALUATION

Presurgical evaluation is the process of examining a patient prior to a surgical procedure to identify any previously undiagnosed disease and/or risk factors that have the potential to increase the individual patient's surgical risk, and thus provides an opportunity for any necessary intervention that might help minimize the risk to the patient.[1] Primary care providers may work in an environment where they are asked to participate in or complete presurgical evaluations. Therefore understanding the importance of the presurgical evaluation, as well as how to accurately perform this type of encounter (e.g., obtaining a history, completing a physical exam, deciding what—if any—testing is warranted, knowing when to refer, and providing preoperative patient education), is crucial for all primary care providers.

Advanced practice nurses completing presurgical evaluations must be aware of the pathophysiologic changes of a patient's underlying and concurrent medical problems, and the effect that surgery and anesthesia may have on these problems. Ideally, patients planning for an upcoming surgery will have their underlying medical conditions well managed. However, there are patients who present for presurgical evaluations that do not have regular primary care, have difficulty managing comorbid diseases, or are not adhering to recommended treatments. It is important that health care providers take the opportunity at the presurgical visit to educate the patient and their family about the importance of having regular primary care, particularly after surgery when their care needs are greater and potentially more complex.

Although there is potential risk with any surgical procedure, it is helpful to know that there are some "low-risk" procedures. These include cataract removal, carpal tunnel release, breast biopsy, and inguinal hernia repair.

OBTAINING A PRESURGICAL HISTORY

Important information and history to obtain from the patient to determine appropriateness for surgery includes the following[2]:

- The type of surgical procedure and expected date.
- The social supports for the patient after surgery and the possible need for rehabilitation or home services.
- A thorough medication list including any over-the-counter medications and herbal products.
- A detailed list of allergic reactions and adverse effects to any medications.

- Personal and family history of adverse reactions to anesthesia (e.g., malignant hyperthermia), blood clots, or bleeding problems.
- Past medical history, including patient comorbidities and status (e.g., previous history of myocardial infarction, uncontrolled diabetes, asthma, chronic lung disease, hypertension, hypothyroidism, or malignancy).
- Past surgical history.
- Quantification of daily intake of alcohol, tobacco (including pack years for smokers), marijuana, vaping, or other substance use.

In the United States, adults older than the age of 65 account for roughly one-third of inpatient surgeries.[2] While age alone does not increase the risk for a person undergoing surgery, the number and type of chronic diseases an individual has and how optimized the disease state is will have an effect on the morbidity and mortality in the postoperative period. Overall, the more chronic the disease and the older the individual, the more likely the life expectancy will be negatively affected.[3] Because older adults may be at increased risk for changes in cognition, delirium, functional decline, polypharmacy, and comorbid disease, the optimum preoperative evaluation should be designed to capture issues specific to the medically complex older adult. Therefore, a comprehensive presurgical evaluation of the geriatric patient should include screening and assessment for the following[2]:

1. Functional status and frailty
2. Cognition
3. Sensory impairment
4. Mental health
5. Medication management (including indication, dose, adverse events, and adherence)
6. Pain management
7. Cardiovascular risk stratification
8. Pulmonary risk assessment
9. Obstructive sleep apnea

KEY ASPECTS OF THE PRESURGICAL EVALUATION

There are no evidence-based guidelines indicating when the appropriate time to conduct a presurgical evaluation is, but typically it is done within the 30 days prior to surgery. It is important that the visit occur with time enough in advance of the surgical procedure to allow necessary specialist consultations and referrals, if these are indicated. For example, if a patient scheduled for an open, elective abdominal aortic aneurysm repair develops new-onset angina, it is important that there be enough time to schedule cardiac stress testing and to review the results with the surgeon and anesthesia team.

Medication Reconciliation

Medication reconciliation is a crucial part of any encounter with a patient, but is particularly important during a presurgical evaluation. A complete list of the patient's medications, including prescription, over the counter, vitamins, and herbal supplements should be obtained. The surgeon and anesthesia team will use that information to determine if and when any medications (e.g. aspirin, anticoagulants, morning insulin) should be held prior to surgery. Depending on the type of surgery, the patient's risk factors, and the indication for a particular prescribed medicine, the parameters as to when to hold that medication before surgery may vary. As the nature and purity of herbal medications is somewhat unclear, and have the potential to interact adversely with perioperative medications, it is recommended that patients stop any herbal supplements at least one week prior to surgery.[4]

Review of Systems

A full review of systems, with careful attention paid to cardiac and pulmonary systems, as well as the system that incorporates the area undergoing surgery is warranted.

Cardiovascular evaluation should include asking about symptoms (e.g., chest pain or "angina," dyspnea, syncope, and palpitations) as well as a history of heart disease, including ischemic, valvular, or cardiomyopathic disease. Cardiac functional status should be determined to aid in assessing the risk of cardiopulmonary complications postoperatively. A simple screening of cardiac functional status may be done by simply asking if the patient can walk four blocks or climb two flights of stairs.[5] A history of hypertension, diabetes, chronic kidney disease, and cerebrovascular or peripheral artery disease is also necessary to discern and document.[5]

Pulmonary evaluation should include asking about exercise intolerance, cough, or unexplained dyspnea as these symptoms may suggest undiagnosed heart failure or chronic lung disease.[6] Patient-related risk factors for pulmonary complications post-operatively include: age, chronic obstructive pulmonary disease, asthma, smoking, general health issues, obesity, pulmonary hypertension, heart failure, upper-respiratory infection, and metabolic and nutritional factors. Obstructive sleep apnea is an increasing concern in healthcare and many patients are undiagnosed. Thus this information is essential to elicit in the ROS to enable presurgical management and avoid potential adverse outcomes during the surgical procedure or post operatively. Procedure-related risk factors for pulmonary complications post-operatively include the surgical site, the duration of surgery, the type of anesthesia, and the type of neuromuscular blockade.[6]

Physical Exam

Physical examination of a patient for presurgical evaluation should be focused on the presenting surgical problem and expected type of anesthesia. It should include objective data such as baseline vital signs (including oxygen saturation), height, weight, and overall general appearance and functional status of the patient. Evaluation of mental status, airway, dentition, and range of motion of the head and neck is also necessary. Any abnormalities of the appearance of neck veins or the presence of bruits, as well as any abnormalities on auscultation of the heart, lungs, and abdomen should be noted. Further evaluation for any abdominal masses, genitourinary or rectal problems, of peripheral pulses, cranial nerves, and for any neurologic changes may also be warranted depending on the reason for presentation, the medical history, and the anesthetic plan. For example, the physical examination of a healthy 32-year-old man with a herniated lumbar disc should include all of the evaluations listed because this patient may manifest neurologic or peripheral vascular changes as a presenting symptom associated with his back problem or may develop them postoperatively as a complication of surgery.

PRESURGICAL TESTING

Diagnostic testing for presurgical clearance is variable and depends on several factors: (1) the presenting diagnosis,

(2) the patient's age, (3) the patient's comorbidities, (4) the type of anesthesia agent planned, and (5) the surgeon's preference. Over time, presurgical testing has evolved from everyone getting a standard chest X-ray, EKG, labs, and urinalysis to a more conservative approach where perioperative risk assessment drives the need for select testing on individuals. The rationale behind this paradigm shift is that healthy individuals have a low overall risk with surgery. Routine preoperative testing leads to "false-positive results, unnecessary costs, and a potential delay in surgery," therefore the general consensus is that testing should only be performed when there is a clear clinical indication.[1] Guidelines for determining if presurgical testing is indicated for a patient is often based on risk stratification and the American Society of Anesthesiologists (ASA) anesthesia classification (Table 20.1).

There are several surgical risk assessment calculators that aid in assessing each patient's risk for complications. These include the National Surgical Quality Improvement Program (NSQUIP) Surgical Risk calculator, a detailed overview of potential surgical complications available at https://riskcalculator.facs.org/RiskCalculator/PatientInfo.jsp, and the Heart Score for Major Cardiac events, available at https://www.mdcalc.com/heart-score-major-cardiac-events. Though not appropriate for ambulatory, vascular, or low risk surgical procedures, the Revised Cardiac Risk Index (RCRI) available at https://qxmd.com/calculate/calculator_195/revised-cardiac-risk-index-lee-criteria is another risk assessment tool that can be helpful in some situations.

If laboratory tests are indicated, it is often acceptable to use previously resulted normal lab results if they were done within the past four months and if there has not been any changes in the patient's clinical picture.[1] If an electrocardiogram is indicated, the imaging should be reviewed for any Q-waves or significant ST-segment depression or elevation, as these findings may be concerning for possible myocardial infarction or ischemia, QTc prolongation, bundle-branch block, arrhythmia, or left ventricular hypertrophy.[5]

WHEN TO REFER

Estimating the perioperative risk of adverse cardiac events helps determine whether (1) the patient should proceed to surgery, (2) the surgery should be delayed to obtain further testing, (3) the procedure should be changed to one with less risk (if possible), or (4) medical management that does not include surgery is indicated. Surgery should be cancelled if a more pressing issue (e.g., if heart valve replacement is indicated) needs to take place first.[5]

Optimal management of patients with hemodynamically important valvular disease (particularly aortic stenosis), high-grade arrhythmias, decompensated heart failure, recent MI, or unstable angina may warrant a cardiology referral due to the elevated risk of perioperative MI, ventricular fibrillation, primary cardiac arrest, heart failure, complete heart block, and cardiac death in these patients.[5] Cardiology referral may also be indicated in patients with an intermediate or high cardiovascular risk for a major cardiac event or those patients with a functional capacity less than 4 metabolic equivalents (inability to climb a flight of stairs).

PREOPERATIVE PATIENT EDUCATION

As primary care providers providing presurgical evaluations, it is important to have a basic understanding of the potential

TABLE 20.1	**Presurgical Testing**

Test	Indications for Performing Test
Chest radiograph	• History of cardiovascular or pulmonary diseases • Patients older than 50 years of age who are undergoing abdominal aortic aneurysm surgery or upper abdominal/thoracic surgery
Electrocardiography	• For patients with known coronary artery disease, significant arrhythmia, peripheral arterial disease, cerebrovascular disease, or other significant structural heart disease electrocardiography is indicated within 30 days of a non-low risk surgical procedure; *excludes* patients undergoing low-risk surgery (risk of major adverse cardiac event <1%). • Asymptomatic patients undergoing surgery with elevated risk (risk of major adverse cardiac event ≥1%)
Pulmonary function testing	• Those undergoing lung resection • Patients with known or suspected pulmonary disease (e.g., reduced exercise intolerance, unexplained dyspnea, cigarette smoking >20 years, chronic obstructive pulmonary disease [COPD], interstitial lung disease)
Complete blood count	• All patients 65 years of age or older who are undergoing major surgery. • Younger patients undergoing surgery that is expected to result in significant blood loss • Any patient whose history suggests anemia
Coagulation studies	• Patients whose history, physical examination, or family history suggests the presence of a bleeding disorder
Electrolytes	• Patients with a history that increases the likelihood of an abnormality (e.g., known chronic kidney disease, use of diuretics, angiotensin-converting enzymes [ACE] inhibitors, or angiotensin receptor blockers [ARB])
Renal function (creatinine)	• Patients over the age of 50 undergoing intermediate or high-risk surgery • Younger patients suspected of having renal disease, when hypotension is likely during surgery, or when nephrotoxic medications will be used
Urinalysis or urine culture and sensitivity	• Not recommended in the absence of clinical symptoms of a urinary tract infection
Pregnancy test	• All reproductive-age women prior to surgery

Data from Smetana, G. W. (2017a). Evaluation of preoperative pulmonary risk. *UpToDate*. Retrieved from https://www.uptodate.com/contents/evaluation-of-preoperative-pulmonary-risk?search=preoperativepulmonary%20risk&source=search_result&selectedTitle=4~150&usage_type=default&display_rank=4. Accessed December 30, 2017; and Smetana, G. W. (2017b). Preoperative medical evaluation of the adult healthy patient. *UpToDate*. Retrieved from https://www.uptodate.com/contents/preoperative-medical-evaluation-of-the-adult-healthy-patient?search=preoperative%20evaluation&source=search_result&selectedTitle=2~150&usage_type=default&display_rank=2. Accessed December 30, 2017.

risks and complications of anesthesia in order to educate the patients. Complications related to anesthesia are multiple and range from major, life-threatening events (rare) to the more common benign and easily resolved occurrences. Complications vary by anesthetic type, but comorbid conditions can increase risk. For general anesthesia, complications include nausea, vomiting, sore throat, fatigue, stroke, myocardial infarction, allergic reaction, and death. For spinal or other regional anesthesia, complications can include headache, nerve damage, infection, and limb loss.[7] All potential complications are considered in the presurgical evaluation to stratify risk and to minimize perioperative morbidity and mortality.[7] The potential risks and complications will be discussed again in further detail with the patient by the anesthesiologist or anesthetist providing care on the day of surgery before consent is obtained.

Patient and family education at the presurgical evaluation should be focused on the surgical and anesthesia care plan, as well as on areas of health promotion that may affect the patient's surgical and hospital course. The culture, language, and individual learning style of the patient should be assessed and teaching should be done accordingly, then evaluated with the "teach back" method. Preoperative and postoperative teaching, as well as expectations about the patient's care on discharge either to home or to another facility. Reviewing the anesthesia care plan and possible complications, as well as effects of anesthesia, and pain management concerns for during and after surgery may also be discussed at this time. The presurgical evaluation provides the health care provider an opportunity to encourage lifestyle changes and appropriately refer the patient to programs that address substance use (i.e., alcohol or drug), smoking cessation, stress management, nutritional counseling, exercise, home safety, and/or domestic violence. Smoking alone can increase a patient's risk of pneumonia, intubation, cardiac arrest, stroke, myocardial infarction, infections, and sepsis in the perioperative period.[8] Taking the time to address these individual lifestyle changes prior to surgery has the potential to positively impact the patient's surgical course.

Patients going to the hospital for surgery are unique, and the ways in which they each cope cannot be predicted or assumed. Anxiety levels and coping styles are not foreseeable in this setting and are often related to current life stresses, perceived level of support, and psychosocial development issues. Therefore, a careful assessment of these factors is necessary to accurately evaluate and plan for each individual's care.

PERIOPERATIVE SURGICAL HOMES: THE FUTURE

The aims of health care in the United States continue to be (1) improve quality and (2) contain costs. As a result, a new practice model (i.e., the Perioperative Surgical Home [PSH]) is evolving. PSHs are defined as "patient-centered and physician-led multidisciplinary and team-based system[s] of coordinated care that guides the patient throughout the entire surgical experience ... (preoperative, intraoperative, postoperative, and post-discharge)."[9] By using standard protocols for each phase of the surgical experience, the surgical home model hopes to reduce the fragmentation of care across the perioperative community.

The role of the anesthesia providers has changed with the surgical home model to include oversight of the entire perioperative process. Benefits of this change are multifactorial. These include tailored optimization for medical conditions, early identification of surgical risk complications, initiation of evidence-based practice (EBP) protocols to address the risk of delirium and venous thromboembolism (VTE), initiation and oversight of quality metrics (e.g., Surgical Care Improvement project [SCIP] measures, methicillin-resistant *Staphylococcus aureus* [MRSA] precautions, and first case starts), and individually tailored patient recovery plans to reduce length of stay, emergency department visits, and readmissions by using early remote monitoring with teletechnology.[10]

By reducing variability in perioperative care, the PSH model aims to improve patient outcomes by decreasing complications and errors while providing overall better care at a lower cost.[9] Since this is still a relatively newer conceptual framework in perioperative care delivery, and therefore not standard practice throughout, presurgical evaluation will continue to be the responsibility of the surgeon, anesthesia care team, specialists, and/or primary care provider. However, the surgical home approach offers exciting opportunities for health care providers to collaborate across the care continuum in the future.

REFERENCES

1. Smetana, G. W. (2017b). Preoperative medical evaluation of the adult healthy patient. *UpToDate*. Retrieved from https://www.uptodate.com/contents/preoperative-medical-evaluation-of-the-adult-healthy-patient?search=preoperative%20evaluation&source=search_result&selectedTitle=2~150&usage_type=default&display_rank=2. (Accessed 30 December 2017).
2. Marwell, J. G., Heflin, M. T., & McDonald, S. R. (2018). Preoperative screening. *Clinics in Geriatric Medicine*, 34, 95–105. https://doi.org/10.1016/j.cger.2017.08.004.
3. DuGoff, E., Canudas-Romo, V., Buttorff, C., Leff, B., & Anderson, G. (2014). Multiple chronic conditions and life expectancy. *Medical Care*, 52(8), 688.
4. Muluk, V., Cohn, S. L., & Whinney, C. (2017). Perioperative medication management. *UpToDate*. Retrieved from https://www.uptodate.com/contents/perioperative-medication-management?search=perioperative%20medication%20management&source=search_result&selectedTitle=1~53&usage_type=default&display_rank=1. (Accessed 30 January 2018).
5. Cohn, S. L., & Fleisher, L. A. (2017a). Evaluation of cardiac risk prior to noncardiac surgery. *UpToDate*. Retrieved from https://www.uptodate.com/contents/evaluation-of-cardiac-risk-prior-to-noncardiac-surgery?search=preoperative%20cardiac%20risk&source=search_result&selectedTitle=1~150&usage_type=default&display_rank=1. (Accessed 30 December 2017).
6. Smetana, G. W. (2017a). Evaluation of preoperative pulmonary risk. *UpToDate*. Retrieved from https://www.uptodate.com/contents/evaluation-of-preoperative-pulmonary-risk?search=preoperativepulmonary%20risk&source=search_result&selectedTitle=4~150&usage_type=default&display_rank=4. (Accessed 30 December 2017).
7. Gupta, A. (2009). Preoperative screening and risk assessment in the ambulatory surgery patient. *Current Opinion in Anaesthesiology*, 22(6), 705–711. doi:10.1097/ACO.0b013e3283301fb3.
8. Turan, A., Koyunco, O., Egan, C., You, J., Ruetzler, K., Sessler, D. I., et al. (2017). Effect of various durations of smoking cessation on postoperative outcomes; A retrospective cohort analysis. *European Journal of Anaesthesiology*, 34, 1–10. doi:10.1097/EJA.0000000000000701.
9. Kain, Z. N., Vakharia, S., Garson, L., Engwall, S., Schwarzkopf, R., Gupta, R., et al. (2014). The perioperative surgical home as a future perioperative practice model. *Anesthesia and Analgesia*, 118(5), 1126–1130. doi:10.1213/ANE.0000000000000190.
10. Warner, M. A., & Kain, Z. (2014). Perioperative home summit presentation. *ASA-AHA-PHS webinar*. Newport Beach, California.

CHAPTER 21

PREPARTICIPATION SPORTS PHYSICAL

Susan Sanner

The American Heart Association (AHA) recommends cardiovascular preparticipation screening with a history and physical examination for all athletes participating in high school and college sports.[1] However, the AHA also states that these recommendations are applicable to other populations.[1] For secondary school and college athletes, an annual sports physical is a prerequisite for student participation in school-related sports, but sports medicine physicians recommend that middle school and junior high school students also have a physical examination for school-related sports activities. Despite the recommendations to screen athletes, the actual requirements of this examination remain controversial and are not clearly defined. The primary purpose of the sports physical is to determine the patient's health status and physical fitness for participation in sports, yet the concerns about cardiovascular death among young athletes heighten concerns about the consistency of these examinations. Nurse practitioners should be aware of their state's requirements, and be attentive to emerging research and recommendations related to preparticipation physical examinations.[2,3]

The primary goal for these examinations is to identify athletes at risk for an adverse event (e.g., cardiovascular event), but it is also necessary to identify other medical problems and to provide appropriate treatment before the athlete participates in any athletics. Determining the athlete's overall health, providing counseling, and strengthening the provider-patient relationship are other objectives. The preparticipation sports physical is an excellent opportunity to provide education related to healthy behaviors and injury prevention, in addition to identifying risk factors that affect well-being.[2,4,5] Still, the importance of the sports preparticipation examination cannot be overstated. The examiner must be skilled and have significant experience in performing both cardiovascular and musculoskeletal examinations to identify any condition that would prohibit participation in the chosen sport. Despite these screening precautions, it is not possible to completely eliminate injuries, particularly in contact or collision sports.

It is preferable to perform the examination in the office so that adequate time can be spent ascertaining the personal and family health history and performing the examination. If possible, the examination should be performed at least 6 weeks before the beginning of the sports activity.[6,7] For student athlete sports physicals, it is essential that a parent accompany the student to the examination to fully establish the family history and cardiovascular risk factors.[3,7] It is often helpful to have the student and parent complete and sign a preparticipation health history form before the examination. It is then necessary that the provider review the form with the student and parent and specifically question the parent and student about each item on the health history form.

HISTORY

Allergies, current and past medications, and the personal and family history should be carefully assessed. Answers to the following questions should be determined before the examination commences.[7]

1. Medical history, including the following:
   - Anaphylaxis or allergic or untoward reactions to exercise, medications, pollens, foods, and stinging insects (including the specific nature of the reaction)
   - Current medications, including vitamins or herbal supplements, prescribed or over-the-counter medications, and nutritional supplements
   - Habits such as smoking, vaping, caffeine, and alcohol or drug use
   - Immunization history: tetanus status, hepatitis, chickenpox, and MMR (measles, mumps, rubella)
   - Previous surgeries (particularly orthopedic, genital, kidney, or eye surgeries)
   - Previous hospitalizations
   - Loss of an organ such as eye, kidney, or testicle
2. Present or past illness, including the following:
   - Recent viral illness, such as mononucleosis or myocarditis
   - Recent weight loss or gain
   - Previous sports restriction
   - History of heat-related illness
   - Skin piercings or reactions (hives, rashes, infections)
   - Head injury, concussion, neck injury, loss of consciousness, fainting, concussion, dizziness, headaches, seizures
   - Previous eye injury, visual problems, such as blurred vision or a history of detached retina; whether the patient wears glasses or contacts
   - History of heart surgery, hypertrophic cardiomyopathy, myocarditis, mitral valve prolapse, prior embolic event, commotio cordis, or coronary artery abnormalities; history of chest pain, dizziness, fatigue or weakness, syncope, near syncope, or palpitations (heart racing or skipped heart beats) with or after exercise; history of hypertension; history of heart murmur[1,3,4]
   - Breathing problems, such as wheezing, coughing, excessive exertional and unexplained dyspnea associated with exercise; history of asthma[3]
   - History of musculoskeletal injury, such as fracture or dislocation; injury or pain in neck, shoulder, back, elbow, hand, finger, knee, ankle, foot, or toe that caused missed work, school, or practice
   - History of use of special equipment for sports-related activities
   - History of numbness or tingling in the upper or lower extremities
   - History of "burners" or "stingers" (injury to arm nerve supply) caused by contact or collision sport activity[5]
   - History of eating disorder, excessive fatigability, diabetes, bleeding problems, anemia, hepatitis, mononucleosis
   - History of stress, anxiety, or depression
   - Menstrual history: menarche, last menstrual period, frequency of menses (number of menstrual periods in the past year), history of amenorrhea or other menstrual dysfunction
   - History of anemia or sickle cell disease
3. Family history, including the following:
   - History of premature or sudden death before the age of 50 years, ion channelopathies, short QT syndrome,[a]

long QT syndrome, Wolff-Parkinson-White syndrome, arrhythmias, hypertrophic or dilated cardiomyopathy, Marfan syndrome, or Brugada syndrome[b]
   - Family history of coronary artery disease
   - Disabling heart disease in a close relative

PHYSICAL EXAMINATION

The physical examination should be focused and thorough to determine the presence of an acute infection or any impairment that would prohibit participation in the selected sport. General appearance, posture, overall health, height, weight, and percentage of body fat should be determined. It is vital to note congenital deformities, such as arachnodactyly or other signs of Marfan syndrome. Additional components of the physical examination include the following:

1. Visual acuity with Snellen chart (corrected visual acuity should be 20/40 or better)[3]
2. Vital signs including bilateral brachial blood pressure and heart rate sitting at rest, 3 minutes after exercise, and again 6 minutes after exercise
3. Skin evaluation for signs of fungal, candida, scabies, or other infection
4. Head, eye (including documentation of pupil reactivity or anisocoria), ear, nose, and throat (HEENT) evaluation to determine infectious processes and to evaluate any lymphadenopathy
5. Cardiovascular examination

The cardiovascular exam is a key component of the preparticipation sports physical. When screening for genetic or congenital cardiovascular abnormalities, the AHA and American College of Cardiology (ACC) recommend the AHA 14-point screening guidelines along with a thorough history and physical (Boxes 21.1 and 21.2).[1]

The cardiac examination will include the following:
- Pectus deformity of the anterior chest; evaluate for Marfan syndrome.
- Assess the heart sounds with the patient in the supine, standing, and squatting positions with a Valsalva maneuver. Special emphasis is necessary to determine the presence of any murmurs or arrhythmias. Arrhythmias, extra heart sounds (S_3, S_4), a new murmur, a diastolic murmur, a systolic murmur grade 3/6 or higher, a left sternal border systolic murmur that increases in intensity with standing or Valsalva maneuver, or a mitral valve click accompanied by a murmur requires further evaluation before clearance for sports participation can be given.[1,3]
- Radial and femoral pulses should be symmetric to exclude coarctation of the aorta.
- Blood pressure must be compared with age-adjusted tables. Elevated blood pressure requires treatment, and it must be within the accepted range before medical clearance is given. The use of beta blockers, which can be considered to be performance enhancers, or diuretics may preclude athletic participation in some states.

The AHA/ACC does not recommend universal screening of the general population of young persons with 12-electrocardiography (ECG), regardless of their athletic status due to possible false-positive or negative results and cost.[1]

---

[a]Sudden death in individuals with structurally normal hearts associated with short QT interval.[3]

[b]Sudden death in individuals with normal hearts associated with ST-segment elevation in right precordial leads.[3]

BOX **21.1**

Personal, Family History, and Physical Examination Components

PERSONAL AND FAMILY HISTORY

- A family history of at least one relative who prior to age 50 was disabled by heart disease or died unexpectedly from heart disease
- A family history of hypertrophic or dilated cardiomyopathy (enlarged heart cavity or wall), Marfan syndrome (fragility of cardiac arteries or walls), prolonged QT syndrome (potentially fatal dysrhythmia), or alarming cardiac rhythm or dysrhythmia
- A previous, personal history of sports participation restriction in the past
- A previous personal history of prior cardiac testing (ordered by a health care provider)
- Chest pressure or pain associated with exertion
- Exercise-induced fatigue that is unexplained and disproportionate
- Syncope or near-syncope

PHYSICAL EXAMINATION COMPONENTS

- Brachial artery blood pressure (checked while patient is sitting)
- Hypertension
- Heart murmur
- Femoral pulses to exclude narrowing of the aorta
- Physical appearance of Marfan syndrome

BOX **21.2**

AHA 14-Point Screening Guidelines for Genetic or Congenital Cardiovascular Abnormalities

- Chest pain/discomfort upon exertion
- Unexplained fainting or near-fainting
- Excessive and unexplained fatigue associated with exercise
- Heart murmur
- High blood pressure
- One or more relatives who died of heart disease (sudden/unexpected or otherwise) before age 50
- Close relative under age 50 with disability from heart disease
- Specific knowledge of certain cardiac conditions in family members: hypertrophic or dilated cardiomyopathy in which the heart cavity or wall becomes enlarged, long QT syndrome which affects the heart's electrical rhythm, Marfan syndrome in which the walls of the heart's major arteries are weakened, spontaneous coronary artery dissection, or clinically important arrhythmias or heart rhythms
- Heart murmur
- Femoral pulses to exclude narrowing of the aorta
- Physical appearance of Marfan syndrome
- Brachial artery blood pressure (taken in a sitting position)
- If individual has been restricted from participation in sports in the past
- If individual has had prior testing for the heart, ordered by a health care provider

From Maron, B.J., Friedman, R.A., Kligfield, P., Levine, B.D., Viskin, S., Chaitman, B.R., ... American College of Cardiology. (2014). Assessment of the 12-lead ECG as a screening test for detection of cardiovascular disease in healthy general populations of young people (12–25 Years of Age): a scientific statement from the American Heart Association and the American College of Cardiology. *Circulation, 130*, 1303–1334.

6. Pulmonary examination; an assessment of lung sounds anteriorly and posteriorly.

Athletes who have asthma that is well-controlled and are asymptomatic at rest and with exertion can be cleared after a thorough physical exam. Participation should be restricted in athletes who are actively wheezing or are recovering from an asthma exacerbation until symptoms have subsided. A rescue inhaler may be required as a condition for participation.[8]

7. Abdominal examination; further evaluation if organomegaly is detected[c]
8. Genitourinary examination
   - Tanner staging.
   - The testes must be descended.
   - The presence of inguinal hernias must be determined.

Genital examination is not recommended in females but may be indicated in males with a history or symptoms of genitourinary problems.[8]

9. Musculoskeletal examination
   - Is there neck pain on examination or with range of motion (ROM)?[c]
   - With the patient standing, the back should be evaluated for scoliosis, flexibility, and pain with ROM.[c]
   - All extremities, muscles, and joints, including the shoulders and arms, elbow and forearm, wrist and hand, hip and thigh, knee, leg and ankle, foot, and acromioclavicular joint, must be evaluated for muscle atrophy, flexibility, symmetry, tenderness, and full ROM. Resisted shoulder shrug plus shoulder abduction, internal and external rotation, and resisted flexion and extension must be determined.[c] Heel-toe walking, knee extension, and patellar tracking should be assessed. Asymmetry or pain with ROM requires further evaluation.
   - The physical signs of Marfan syndrome should be excluded.
   - Can the patient "duck walk" at least four steps?
   - Can the patient hop on each foot several times?
   - A brief standardized orthopedic screening is adequate for most asymptomatic athletes. A more focused physical exam is reserved for individuals with a history of musculoskeletal injury.[8] Athletes with a known orthopedic injury should receive a thorough joint-specific examination. Clearance is provided based on functional status. In general, if the athlete has full ROM, full strength, and no disabling pain in the affected area and passes functional tests in a supervised sports setting, clearance to participate may be provided.[8]
10. Neuromuscular examination
    - Cranial and sensory nerves
    - Deep tendon reflexes
    - Cerebellar function

MEDICAL CLEARANCE

Physician consultation or referral is indicated and medical clearance deferred if there is a family history of the following:
- Sudden or unexpected death before the age of 50 years[1,3]
- Disabling cardiac disease in a family member younger than 50 years[1,3]

---

[c]Any pain or deficit requires further evaluation before medical clearance is given for sports participation.

DIAGNOSTICS

Diagnostics are not usually necessary for student preparticipation sports physicals, although some states require urinalysis to determine the presence of protein or glucose in the urine. Further diagnostics are dependent on the history and physical examination findings. In some countries, a 12-lead electrocardiogram (ECG) is a routine part of the diagnostic evaluation. ECG screening is not currently recommended by the AHA.[1-3] An ECG is warranted to determine QT prolongation when the patient is taking a medication known to prolong the QT and for patients who note palpitations. If an arrhythmia is not identified on ECG, a Holter monitor, event recorder, or continuous telemetry ambulatory cardiac event monitor is indicated with a history of palpitations.[3] A complete blood count with differential, electrolyte determinations, and thyroid-stimulating hormone level are also necessary for patients who note palpitations.[3] Other diagnostics such as exercise stress testing, echocardiography, lipid panel, or fasting glucose concentration are necessary if the history and physical examination suggest that there is risk of coronary artery disease or cardiac abnormalities or if there is a family history of hypertrophic cardiomyopathy. Hemoglobin and hematocrit should be determined as necessary in female athletes. Athletes with hemophilia and other bleeding disorders may be restricted from contact or collision sports. Individuals with sickle cell disease are limited to low-intensity activities except in those with sickle cell trait who are cleared to participate in all activities.[8] Although athletes have the option to decline, The National Collegiate Athletic Association (NCAA) mandated in 2010 that the sickle cell trait of all incoming athletes must be determined.[8]

- Cardiomyopathy, long QT syndrome or ion channelopathies, Marfan syndrome, significant arrhythmias (e.g., Wolff-Parkinson-White syndrome)[1,3]

Physician consultation or referral is indicated and medical clearance deferred if there is a personal history or physical finding of the following:
- Abdominal organomegaly
- Absence of an eye, kidney, or testicle (these conditions usually prohibit participation in any contact sport)
- Acute systemic infection
- Asthma, uncontrolled
- Asymmetric femoral pulses[1,3]
- Antoaxial instability[1]
- Audible heart murmur in standing position or with Valsalva maneuver[1,3]
- Bleeding disorder[1]
- Cardiac history of hypertension,[1] heart murmur,[1] structural heart disease
- Detached retina or visual acuity less than 20/40 in both eyes
- Diabetes, uncontrolled
- Down syndrome
- Eating disorder[3]
- Exercise-related chest discomfort, dyspnea,[1,3] or fatigue[1,3]
- Fever
- Hypertension[1,4]
- Inability to perform duck walk maneuvers
- Lymphadenopathy (significant)
- Marfan syndrome stigmata[1,3]
- Neck pain or cervical stenosis
- Neurologic deficit

- Obesity
- Palpitations or dysrhythmias
- Previous history of hypertension,[1,3] heart murmur,[1,3] structural heart disease
- Post-traumatic convulsive disorder
- Shoulder asymmetry, joint tenderness, or pain with ROM
- Unexplained syncope or near-syncope[1,3]

Physician consultation or referral is indicated if the athlete or athlete's family refuses diagnostic testing and specialist referral or does not understand the risk of sports participation.[7]

PATIENT AND FAMILY EDUCATION

- Students, parents, and coaches can exert considerable pressure on the health care provider to provide medical clearance for the athlete. However, the health care provider's fundamental responsibility is to protect the student from harm.
- Any concerns elicited during the history or physical examination must be carefully explained to both the parent and the student.
- It is important that both the parent and student understand that medical clearance cannot be given until the results of diagnostic testing and specialist evaluation are known.
- The parent and student should also understand that a preparticipation sports physical examination has limitations and cannot completely eliminate the risks inherent in any athletic activity.
- Parents of all children should be educated on the signs and symptoms associated with a head injury or concussion and referred to the CDC's HEADS UP to Youth Sports (https://www.cdc.gov/headsup/youthsports/parents.html).

REFERENCES

1. Maron, B. J., Zipes, D. P., & Kovacs, R. J. (2015). Eligibility and disqualification recommendations for competitive athletes with cardiovascular abnormalities: Preamble, principles, and general considerations: A scientific statement from the American Heart Association and American College of Cardiology. *Circulation, 132,* e256–e261. doi:10.1161/CIR.0000000000000236.
2. Roberts, W. O., Lollgen, H., Matheson, G., et al. (2014). Advancing the preparation physical evaluation (PPE): An ACSM and FIMS joint consensus statement. *Current Sports Medicine Reports, 13*(6), 395–401.
3. Conley, K. M., Bolin, D. J., Carek, P. J., et al. (2014). National Athletic Trainers' Association position statement: Preparticipation physical examinations and disqualifying conditions. *Journal of Athletic Training, 49*(1), 102–120.
4. American Heart Association. (2012). Preparticipation cardiovascular screening of young competitive athletes: policy guidance. Retrieved from www.heart.org/idc/groups/ahaecc-public/@wcm/@adv/documents/downloadable/ucm_443945.pdf.
5. Whitfield, G. P., Pettee, G., Kelley, K., et al. (2014). Application of the American Heart Association/American College of Sports Medicine adult preparticipation screening checklist to a nationally representative sample of U.S. adults aged (40 years from the National Health and Nutrition ExamMination Survey 2001 to 2004). *Circulation, 129,* 1113–1120.
6. Madsen, N. L., Drezner, J. A., & Salerno, J. C. (2014). The preparticipation physical evaluation: An analysis of clinical practice. *Clinical Journal of Sport Medicine, 24*(2), 142–149.
7. American Academy of Family Physicians, American Academy of Pediatrics, American College of Sports Medicine, American Medical Society for Sports Medicine. (2010). *Preparticipation physical evaluation* (4th ed.). American Academy of Pediatrics.
8. Mirabelli, M. H., Devine, M., Singh, J., & Mendoza, M. (2015). The preparticipation sports evaluation. *American Family Physician, 92*(5), 371–376.

PART 4 — Office Emergencies

CHAPTER 22

ACUTE BRONCHOSPASM

Tracy McClinton

 Immediate emergency department referral or physician consultation is indicated for patients in acute respiratory distress or with an SaO2 of less than 92% on room air, failure to improve with nebulizer treatment given 3 times or epinephrine injection administered 3 times, or a peak flow less than 80% of predicted.

DEFINITION AND EPIDEMIOLOGY

Asthma that is not appropriately managed may lead to exacerbations requiring emergent care.[1] Bronchospasm, a symptom of asthma, is also referred to as *bronchial spasm* and is defined as a sudden constriction of the muscles of the bronchial walls that leads to a temporary narrowing of the bronchi. When muscle tightening and inflammation of the bronchioles occur, the result is coughing, wheezing, shortness of breath, and thicker mucus production.[2]

The actual incidence of bronchospasm is difficult to determine because it be can intermittent and the conditions that cause bronchospasm are myriad. It is estimated that 24.6 million Americans have been diagnosed with asthma. The 2015 prevalence rate for females was reported to be higher than in males, and it is reported that the prevalence in the African American population is higher than in the Caucasian population.[3] Acute bronchospasm when associated with asthma is responsible for an estimated 14.2 million outpatient visits, 1.8 million emergency department visits, 439,000 hospital admissions, and approximately 4000 deaths annually.[2,3] Young adults are considered a high-risk population as they are less likely to seek or adhere to preventive care and may face challenges with filling their asthma prescriptions.[1]

Bronchospasm usually occurs as a response to a specific trigger, the most common identified as asthma. Clinical conditions that are associated with bronchospasm include any precipitating factors that cause airway inflammation, airway obstruction, or narrowing of the airway.[2] These factors include but are not limited to: anaphylactic reactions to medications, allergens (indoor, outdoor, or food), asthma, chronic obstructive pulmonary disease, cardiac conditions, respiratory tract infections, bacterial or viral infections, exercise, mechanical airway obstruction (usually aspirated) by anatomic changes or tumor, tracheal stenosis, pulmonary embolism, and vocal cord dysfunction.[2,4,5] Allergenic triggers include "house dust mites (HDMs), molds, pets, cockroaches, and rodents."[6]

Nonallergenic exposures include "viral infections, active and passive smoking, meteorological changes, and occupational exposures."[6]

Proper assessment for severe bronchospasm is vital. A patient who speaks in words instead of phrases, sits in a hunched position, and uses accessory muscles is in severe respiratory compromise.[5] Further indications of distress include a respiratory rate greater than or equal to 30, a pulse rate greater than or equal to 120, and a peak expiratory flow (PEF) less than or equal to 50, predicted or best.[5] A patient who is drowsy, confused, or poorly controlled in addition to the compromised vital signs previously mentioned has reached a life-threatening state.[5] Patients in severe or life-threating respiratory distress should be transferred to the emergency department immediately. While waiting for transport, the patient should be given inhaled short-acting β_2-agonists (SABAs), ipratropium bromide, systemic corticosteroids and, if available, supplemental oxygen.[5] For patients unable to coordinate a metered-dose inhaler (MDI) or who show no improvement, epinephrine and terbutaline, if available, are indicated.[7]

During a severe exacerbation, arterial blood gases (ABGs) are necessary to monitor for hypoxemia, hypercapnia, and respiratory acidosis. Recommendations are that PaO_2 be kept above 60 mm Hg. An arterial saturation greater than 90% is needed to prevent tissue hypoxia and to preserve tissue cellular oxygenation.[2]

PATHOPHYSIOLOGY

Bronchospasm results when hyperreactivity of the airways, caused by inflammatory substances, produces airway bronchoconstriction, edema, and obstruction. On exposure to causative agents, substances that are released from basophils or mast cells lead to an allergic reaction that causes constriction and inflammation.[2,4] Airway hyperresponsiveness (AHR) occurs along with inflammation. AHR is the contraction of small muscles surrounding the airways, and this can limit the individual's ability to move air throughout the lungs.[4] The bronchospasm may be intermittent and resolve without treatment, or the obstruction may progress to respiratory arrest, with potential for death.

CLINICAL PRESENTATION

Patient presentations can vary from mild anxiety to acute respiratory distress. Symptoms may occur spontaneously or be precipitated by a trigger.[5,7] The most common symptom of bronchospasm is wheezing. However, the patient with acute bronchospasm may have breathlessness, chest tightness, and coughing. Symptoms may vary in degree of severity.

A repetitive, spasmodic cough may be the only sign of bronchospasm. The patient's inability to speak a full sentence without pausing to breathe indicates severe bronchospasm.

Patients' psychological states vary according to their previous experience with this condition and the severity of symptoms. Patients with a history of asthma may have experienced bronchospasm frequently and may even have come to accept this as a usual daily pattern, whereas patients who experience their first episode or a severe episode may understandably be anxious.

PHYSICAL EXAMINATION

The skin color of a patient with acute bronchospasm may be normal, flushed, or pale. The presence of pruritus or a rash suggests an allergic cause. In addition, the patient may have tachypnea, tachycardia, and a normal or slightly elevated blood pressure. Hypotension occurs in an allergic reaction with anaphylaxis. Pulsus paradoxus (a change in blood pressure during inspiration) of greater than 20 mm Hg is a uniform indicator of severe respiratory compromise.[7]

Proper assessment for severe bronchospasm is vital. Wheezing may be audible or detected during auscultation on inspiration or expiration. With audible wheezing, the trachea should be auscultated to discern whether these sounds are indicative of laryngospasm or partial airway obstruction with a foreign body. A patient who speaks in words instead of phrases and sits in a hunched position using accessory muscles is experiencing severe respiratory compromise.[5] Further indications of distress include a respiratory rate greater than or equal to 30, a pulse rate greater than or equal to 120, and a PEF less than or equal to 50, predicted or best.[5] A patient who is drowsy, confused, or poorly controlled in addition to the compromised vital signs previously mentioned is in a severe life-threatening state and requires immediate emergency department transfer.[5]

While waiting for transport, the patient should be given inhaled SABAs, ipratropium bromide, systemic corticosteroids and, if available, supplemental oxygen.[5] For patients unable to coordinate a MDI or who show no improvement, epinephrine and terbutaline, if available, are indicated.[7]

DIAGNOSTICS

Peak flow measurements will be less than expected for the patient's age and height or reduced from the patient's baseline. Pulse oximetry values below 90% in adults indicate more severe bronchospasm. ABG analysis is best performed in an emergency department and during a severe exacerbation is necessary to monitor for hypoxemia, hypercapnia, and respiratory acidosis. Recommendations are that PaO_2 be kept above 60 mm Hg. An arterial saturation greater than 90% is needed to prevent tissue hypoxia and to preserve tissue cellular oxygenation.[2]

Chest radiographs may assist in determining the cause of the bronchospasm. With asthma or allergy, the chest radiograph can be normal or show hyperinflation. Serology may reveal eosinophilia and elevated immunoglobulin E levels, suggesting an allergic cause.

INITIAL DIAGNOSTICS

Acute Bronchospasm

INITIAL
- Pulse oximetry
- Peak flow

LABORATORY
- ABGs[a]

IMAGING
- Chest radiograph[a]

---

[a]If indicated.
ABG, Arterial blood gases.

DIFFERENTIAL DIAGNOSIS

The history and clinical presentation indicate the origin of the respiratory failure. Potentially fatal conditions require immediate exclusion. The presence of a urticarial rash with decreasing blood pressure is a sign of anaphylaxis, necessitating immediate treatment with supplemental oxygen through nasal cannula or mask and diphenhydramine (Benadryl), 25 or 50 mg intravenously (no faster than 25 mg per minute) or intramuscularly; or epinephrine, 0.3 to 0.5 mg of a 1 : 1000 (1 mg/mL) solution intramuscularly in the vastus lateralis muscle (middle-outer aspect of the thigh), anterolateral aspect for the adult patient.

Cardiac failure may manifest as bronchospasm in the setting of known cardiac disease. A history of paroxysmal nocturnal dyspnea associated with distended neck veins or pedal edema on examination confirms the diagnosis. Vascular redistribution or pleural effusion may be seen on chest radiographs, but treatment for cardiac failure should not be delayed to obtain chest radiographic studies.

Bronchospasm with acute dyspnea may herald impending respiratory failure in patients with chronic lung disease. Other causes of respiratory failure include depressed respiratory drive, pneumonia, atelectasis, asthma, airway obstruction, pulmonary edema, pulmonary hemorrhage, pulmonary contusion, and acute respiratory distress syndrome. Bronchospasm is also a potential complication of intubation during general anesthesia.

Pulmonary embolization should be suspected when bronchospasm occurs in a patient at risk for a pulmonary embolus (i.e., smokers and patients with signs of vascular thrombosis, a history of atrial fibrillation, a history of oral contraceptive use, obesity, or other risk factors).

Recurrent bronchospasm or a poor response to bronchodilation medication indicates the need for reassessment and thorough evaluation for mechanical airway obstruction caused by anatomic changes or tumor as well as for vocal cord dysfunction, a missed case of heart failure, or pulmonary embolus.

INITIAL STABILIZATION AND MANAGEMENT

The ultimate goal of both expert care and patient self-management is to reduce the impact of acute bronchospasm and asthma on related morbidity, functional ability, and quality of life. Treatment goals include facilitating expectoration, eliminating airway irritation, and suppressing the stimulation of cough receptors.[5] Acute bronchospasm occurring in the setting of lower respiratory tract infection, asthma, or chronic obstructive pulmonary disease is initially managed by supplemental oxygen through nasal cannula or mask and inhalation of a beta agonist through an MDI or nebulizer. Short-acting β_2 agonists include medications such as albuterol, levalbuterol (Xopenex), metaproterenol (Alupent), and pirbuterol (Maxair). Other medications include anticholinergics, such as ipratropium bromide (Atrovent), and systemic corticosteroids, such as methylprednisolone, prednisolone, and prednisone.

There are several delivery device mechanisms: MDIs, dry powdered inhalers, and spacer or valved-holding chambers and nebulizers.[5] Treatment to reverse bronchospasm by an MDI (90 mcg/puff) consists of 4 to 10 puffs of albuterol every 20 minutes for the first hour. "After the first hour, the dose of SABA required varies from 4–10 puffs every 3–4 hours up to 6–10 puffs every 1–2 hours, or more often," as long as tachycardia does not increase or palpitations are not precipitated by the treatments.[5] As an alternative, nebulizer treatments with 2.5 to 5 mg of albuterol can be administered every 20 minutes for up to three treatments, and then 2.5 to 10 mg every 1 to 4 hours if necessary.[7] Alternatively, a continuous nebulizer treatment with albuterol at a rate of 10 to 15 mg/h can be used.[7] For best results, the albuterol should be diluted with saline to a volume of at least 3 mL and delivered at an oxygen flow rate of 6 to 8 L/min.[7] Ipratropium bromide 0.5 mg may be added to the nebulizer solution with saline for administration every 30 minutes for three doses, then given every 2 to 4 hours as needed to augment and to prolong bronchodilation.

Investigations continue to center on alternative routes and improvements for albuterol and other bronchodilator administration. A small study concluded that endotracheal liquid bolus administration of albuterol may be an option in reversing bronchoconstriction in patients who are intubated.[8] Another study investigated percentage deposition in patients following inhalation with soft mist inhalers compared to pressurized metered–dose inhalers.[9] Due to the harm to the ozone layer caused by chlorofluorocarbon (CFC) propellants, the FDA phased out CFC-containing inhalers as of December 2013.[9]

Worsening respiratory status, increased respiratory difficulty, decreasing pulse oximetry values, and failure to respond to beta agonist therapy indicate impending respiratory failure. The health care provider should be prepared to support respiration by intubation and mechanical ventilation with an ambu bag while transferring the patient to the nearest emergency department for other therapeutic modalities. The treatments may include but are not limited to: "SABAs, ipratropium bromide, oxygen therapy to maintain saturations of 93–95% (children 94% to 98%), oral or intravenous corticosteroids, intravenous magnesium (single 2 GM infusion over 20 minutes), and high-dose inhaled corticosteroids."[5]

Once acute bronchospasm is resolved, oral prednisone "burst" in a single dose of 40 to 60 mg daily or a divided dose twice a day for 5 to 10 days should be prescribed.[7] Not only do systemic corticosteroids speed up the resolution of acute bronchospasm, they are also effective in preventing relapse. Oral and intravenous corticosteroids are found to be just as effective and less expensive.[5] Studies also using nebulizer-administered lidocaine have shown it to be safe and effective in treating refractory cough.[10]

DISPOSITION AND REFERRAL

The health care provider should be acquainted with the capabilities of the local emergency medical services (EMS) system and have a plan for the emergency transport of patients. Patients who fail to respond to treatment or who do not improve with initial therapy should be transported to an emergency treatment facility.

PREVENTION AND PATIENT EDUCATION

Clinicians should take every opportunity to reinforce the patient's understanding of bronchospasm. Patient education should include reinforcing the difference between quick-release medications and long-term control medications, reviewing how to take medications correctly, reviewing device usage, and advising on how to avoid environmental exposures that trigger bronchospasm. Review of self-monitoring and an action plan benefits the patient's self-management skills to prevent or to control exacerbations and to reduce urgent care

visits, hospitalizations, and health care costs.[1,5] In addition to regular assessment by a consistent clinician, a written action plan should be provided. Written action plans can be based on either symptoms or peak flow measurements when asthma is the cause of the bronchospasm. These written action plans should include three important concepts: (1) management of daily medications; (2) actions to control environmental factors that trigger bronchospasm; and (3) how to recognize symptoms and necessary actions to take when rescue medications fail. Several action plans are available from professional sources, such as the National Institutes of Health and the American Lung Association.

The health care provider needs to be prepared to manage acute bronchospasm in the office setting and must have a plan for emergency medical support. Equipment and supplies needed in initial management of the patient include pulse oximetry, peak flow meters (disposable or capable of being decontaminated), β-agonist inhalers (albuterol), anticholinergic medication (ipratropium), epinephrine, and oxygen. If an emergency department is not readily available, additional recommended supplies include a handheld nebulizer, parenteral steroids, intravenous access capability, and intubation equipment.

When evaluating the patient in primary care, the clinician should also address preventive health care measures. Patient and family education includes the importance of yearly influenza vaccination, good handwashing practice, avoidance of those who are sick, maintenance of optimal weight, and smoking cessation if indicated. In addition, for those patients taking corticosteroids, bone density measurement should be performed, and calcium with vitamin D supplementation should be prescribed.[11]

REFERENCES

1. Hamburger, R., Berhane, Z., Gatto, M., Yunghans, S., & Turchi, R. (2015). Evaluation of a statewide medical home program on children and young adults with asthma. *Journal of Asthma, 52*(9), 940–948. Retrieved from www.tandfonline.com/doi/full/10.3109/02770903.2014.999282. (Accessed 20 February 2018).
2. Chatburn, R., Kallet, R., et al. (2017). *Egan's fundamentals of respiratory care.* St. Louis, Missouri: Mosby.
3. Centers for Disease Control and Prevention. Retrieved from https://ftp.cdc.gov/pub/Health_Statistics/NCHS/NHIS/SHS/2015_SHS_Table_A-2.pdf. (Accessed 19 February 2018).
4. Kasper, D. L., & Fauci, A. S. (2015). *Asthma. Harrison's principles of internal medicine.* New York, NY: McGraw-Hill. 19e Eds. Ch. 309.
5. Global strategy for asthma management and prevention 2018. Retrieved from https://ginasthma.org/wp-content/uploads/2018/04/wms-GINA-2018-report-V1.3-002.pdf. (Accessed 17 April 2019).
6. Gautier, C., & Charpin, D. (2017). Environmental triggers and avoidance in the management of asthma. *Journal of Asthma and Allergy, 10,* 47–56. http://doi.org.ezproxy.uthsc.edu/10.2147/JAA.S121276.
7. Cydulka, R. K. (2016). Acute asthma. In J. E. Tintinalli, J. Stapczynski, O. Ma, D. M. Yealy, G. D. Meckler, & D. M. Cline (Eds.), *Tintinalli's emergency medicine: A comprehensive study guide, 8e.* New York, NY: McGraw-Hill. http://accessmedicine.mhmedical.com.ezproxy.uthsc.edu/content.aspx?bookid=1658&sectionid=109429684. (Accessed 27 February 2018).
8. Johnston, D. A., Gilmore, T. W., & Gosselin, K. P. (2015). A comparison of metered-dose inhaled albuterol versus endotracheal liquid bolus albuterol for the treatment of bronchoconstriction. *Respiratory Care, 60*(5), 627–635. doi:10.4187/respcare.03494.
9. MacGregor, T., ZuWallack, R., et al. (2016). Efficiency of Ipratropium Bromide and Albuterol Deposition in the lung delivered via a soft mist inhaler or Chlorofluorocarbon metered-dose inhaler. *Clinical and Translational Science, 9*(2), 105–113. http://doi.org.ezproxy.uthsc.edu/10.1111/cts.12387.
10. Özyiğit, L. P., Erer, A., et al. (2016). Nebulized lidocaine as an alternative therapy for reactive airway dysfunction syndrome. *Turkish Thoracic Journal, 17*(2), 82–83. http://doi.org.ezproxy.uthsc.edu/10.5578/ttj.17.2.017.

11. Solidoro, P., Bellocchia, M., Aredano, I., et al. (2017). Asthmatic patients with vitamin D deficiency have decreased exacerbations after vitamin replacement. *Nutrients, 9*(11), 1234. doi:10.3390/nu9111234.

CHAPTER **23**

ANAPHYLAXIS
Karen S. Abate

 Immediate referral is indicated for patients with angioedema, respiratory distress, and vascular collapse. If anaphylaxis in an adult is suspected, aqueous epinephrine: 1:1000 dilution (1 mg/mL), 0.2 to 0.5 mg intramuscularly in the anterolateral aspect of the mid-thigh is indicated.

DEFINITION AND EPIDEMIOLOGY

Anaphylaxis is an acute life-threatening systemic event associated with a potentially life-threatening hypersensitivity reaction. Manifestations of an anaphylactic reaction occur across multiple organ systems, including the cardiovascular, respiratory, integumentary, gastrointestinal, and central nervous systems. Reactions may occur within seconds to days after exposure to the offending allergen.[1-3] It is imperative that an anaphylactic reaction be immediately recognized and treated appropriately to prevent an untoward outcome. As many as 57% of anaphylactic events are unrecognized or under recognized by urgent care and emergency room staff.[4] It is estimated that there is a lifetime prevalence of anaphylaxis range of 1.6% to 5.1%.[4] Common offending allergens include food, medication, insect venom, latex, occupational or inhaled allergens, radiocontrast media, cold air, exercise, heat, blood products, and potentially any substance (Box 23.1).[1,3,5]

PATHOPHYSIOLOGY

An anaphylactic reaction occurs when there is a rapid release of immunoglobulin E in an immune hypersensitivity reaction, resulting in the activation of mast cells and basophils.[2,6,7] On activation, histamine, platelet-activating factor, prostaglandins, leukotriene, and heparin are released.[6-8] The clinical presentation is reflective of the systemic effects of these inflammatory mediators. The release of histamine stimulates vasodilation, increases vascular permeability, increases heart rate and force of contraction, and increases glandular secretions.[7] The release of prostaglandins results in bronchoconstriction, coronary vasoconstriction, and peripheral vasodilation.[7] Leukotriene release further stimulates bronchoconstriction and increases vascular permeability.[7] The result can be a potentially life-threatening upper or lower airway obstruction causing bronchospasm, hypoxemia, or respiratory distress. All of these, as well as vascular collapse and angioedema (Fig. 23.1), are indicative of a severe reaction.

CLINICAL PRESENTATION AND PHYSICAL EXAMINATION

Anaphylactic reactions differ in how long they take to manifest. Uniphasic and biphasic reactions can occur anywhere from minutes to up to 10 to 12 hours after exposure.[1-3] Protracted reactions can be severe, lasting from 24 to rarely 72 hours.[1-3] The intensity of previous hypersensitivity reactions is

BOX **23.1**

Potential Anaphylaxis-Inducing Allergens

Foods
- Peanuts
- Tree nuts (walnuts, almonds, hazelnuts, Brazil nuts)
- Shellfish (lobster, shrimp)
- Fin fish (tuna, salmon, cod)
- Cow milk
- Eggs
- Soy
- Wheat
- Preservatives

Drugs
- β-Lactam antibiotics
- Penicillin
- Cephalosporin
- Vancomycin
- Ciprofloxacin
- Angiotensin-converting enzyme inhibitors
- Insulin
- Nonsteroidal anti-inflammatory drugs
- Vaccines (rare)
- Aspirin
- Vitamin K
- Ibuprofen
- Anesthetics
- Oversulfated chondroitin sulfate–contaminated heparin
- Contrast media (iodine, fluorescein)
- Blood products

Insect venom
- Bees
- Wasps
- Hornets
- Yellow jackets
- Fire ants

Latex
Allergen immunotherapy injections
Occupational allergens (various chemicals, hair dye)
Red meat
Inhaled allergens (animal dander, grass, pollen)

Nonimmunologic triggers
- Cold air
- Cold water
- Exercise
- Heat
- Radiation
- Ethanol
- Exercise

No known cause

not an indication of intensity of subsequent occurrences.[1] In addition, clinical presentation may vary in severity from pruritic dermal rashes to more severe systemic manifestations. A comprehensive history and physical examination are invaluable. This information should be obtained from the patient as well as the family and those who have witnessed an anaphylactic event whenever possible.[3] The clinician must determine the following:

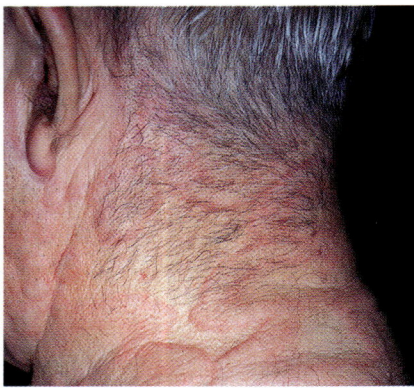

FIG. **23.1** Angioedema affects the face, lips, palms, soles, or a portion of the extremity. It may become confluent and cover wide areas. The color is uniform. Hives vary in color. (From Habif, T. P., Campbell J. L., Dinulos, J., Chapman, M. S., & Zug, K. [2011]. *Skin disease: Diagnosis and treatment* [3rd ed.]. St Louis: Saunders.)

- History of past reactions including current and former triggers
- Significant past medical history and comorbidities
- Any domestic or international travel history
- Detailed past and current exposure history
- Presence of risk factors
- Onset and severity of presenting symptoms
- The exact nature of the occurrence
- Medications or herbal supplements used as well as over-the-counter preparations
- Alternative or home remedies utilized
- Vaccination history
- Recent activities that were occurring relative to this event
- Location and timing of the event including duration
- Known exposures, i.e., heat, cold, stings, bites, plants, food stuffs
- Food and drug consumption over last several hours
- What medical care might have been provided
- The recovery from occurrence

The rapid and accurate identification of anaphylaxis is imperative. The presentation of an individual having an anaphylactic reaction depends on the organ system affected. Physical findings related to the cardiovascular system and associated increases in vascular permeability may include tachycardia, hypotension, arrhythmias, diaphoresis, syncope, or cardiopulmonary arrest.[9] Pulmonary examination may reveal bronchospasm, hoarseness, wheezing, dyspnea, or nasal congestion. The oropharynx should be examined for edema, itchy throat, or stridor.[1,3,7,9] Common findings include the presence of urticaria, erythema, pruritus, and cutaneous wheals.[1,3,7,9] These cutaneous manifestations can be localized or systemic; therefore, the entire body surface area should be examined. Angioedema, coryza, nausea, cramping, vomiting, vertigo, flushing, substernal pain, and weakness may also occur.[1,3,7,9] Central nervous system manifestations can include headache, confusion, seizure, and a sense of unease.[9,10] Any of these manifestations can occur at various times after allergen exposure based on whether the reaction is uniphasic, biphasic, or protracted.[1,2,3]

DIAGNOSTICS

Diagnostics should be used to monitor as well as to eliminate any other conditions that may mimic this presentation. Cardiac monitoring and pulse oximetry can be used to monitor cardiopulmonary status. Analysis of arterial blood gases (ABGs) can be used to exclude a pulmonary embolism, foreign body obstruction, or acute asthma attack. Chest X-ray examination is indicated for patients with underlying pathologic processes or respiratory compromise. Electrocardiography is beneficial for individuals with chest pain or cardiac symptoms.

INITIAL DIAGNOSTICS

LABORATORY
- Pulse oximetry
- Arterial blood gases
- Electrocardiogram (ECG)[a]
- Serum glucose to assess for hypoglycemia
- Additional diagnostics
- 24-h urine specimen for histamine metabolites[9,a]
- Plasma histamine level[9]: to confirm anaphylaxis[a]
- Serum tryptase level—elevation is indicative of mast cell activation[9,a]

IMAGING
- Chest radiograph

[a]Any laboratory testing or diagnostics needed to establish a diagnosis similar in-patient presentation to anaphylaxis.

DIFFERENTIAL DIAGNOSIS

The diagnosis of anaphylaxis is based on clinical presentation, history, and physical examination.

Priority differentials include myocardial infarction, foreign body aspiration, pulmonary embolism, seizure disorder, hypoglycemia, and shock.

In children, clinicians should consider foreign body aspiration, acute poisoning, congenital malformations, or sudden infant death syndrome. Acute asthma, syncope, panic or anxiety attack, pulmonary embolism, hyperventilation, and vasovagal reaction should be considered. Inflammatory mediators can cause coronary artery spasms that can resemble a myocardial infarction. Septic and cardiogenic shock as well as hypoglycemia can present with similar manifestations as an anaphylactic occurrence.

INTERPROFESSIONAL COLLABORATIVE MANAGEMENT
Pharmacologic Management

Intramuscular epinephrine is always first-line pharmacologic treatment in an anaphylactic event because of the maximum pharmacodynamic effect that occurs within minutes of administration in the lateral aspect of the thigh.[1,3,9,10]

Epinephrine dose for pregnant or non-pregnant adults:
- Aqueous epinephrine: 1:1000 dilution (1 mg/mL), 0.2 to 0.5 mg intramuscularly in the anterolateral aspect of the mid-thigh as the preferred site. Repeat every 5 to 15 minutes as needed to a maximum dose of 1 mg.[9]

Epinephrine dose for children and infants:
- Aqueous epinephrine: 1:1000 dilution (1 mg/mL), 0.01 mg/kg per dose in children, maximum of 0.3 mg,

intramuscularly or subcutaneously; repeat every 5 to 20 minutes as needed with a maximum dose of 0.3 mg.[3,9]

Intramuscular injection in the mid-anterolateral thigh (vastus lateralis) is preferred. The vastus lateralis provides for faster absorption and less variability than a subcutaneous injection. Endotracheal epinephrine administration can be used if intravenous access is unattainable.

H_1 and H_2 antagonists are commonly used as a second line of treatment for less severe or cutaneous anaphylactic reactions but should not ever be used as a first-line modality due to the delay in onset of action.[2,9] For adults, diphenhydramine 25 to 50 mg may be given parenterally; the dose for children would be 1 to 2 mg/kg.[2,9]

The use of ranitidine as a second-line agent may be considered as well. Ranitidine 50 mg for adults and 1 mg/kg for children intramuscularly or through slow intravenous as the onset of action is similar.[3,9] The use of ranitidine and diphenhydramine in combination has demonstrated improved efficacy over stand-alone therapy. Once again, this would be a second-line therapy and should not be used alone in the treatment of anaphylaxis.[2,9]

If respiratory symptoms persist after administration of epinephrine, the administration of inhaled β_2 agonists may be useful.[2,9] These will not have any effect on obstruction or shock; however, they can be useful with bronchospasm. Patients who take a β blocker may experience alterations in epinephrine effect and as such glucagon 1 to 5 mg intravenously over 5 minutes could be appropriate.[9] Identification and removal of the offending allergen is imperative.

Nonpharmacological Management. In an emergent anaphylactic reaction, it is imperative to assess and to maintain airway patency. Continuous maintenance of airway, breathing, circulation, and level of consciousness is vital. Monitoring of vital signs and mental status is essential. Individuals experiencing an anaphylactic event must be immediately transported to a local emergency facility. Intravenous access must be promptly established and isotonic saline administered to support volume expansion. If it is not contraindicated, supplemental oxygen should be administered, and preparation should be made for potential endotracheal intubation as warranted.

Consultations. Any individual having an anaphylactic reaction should be immediately transported to an emergency facility for treatment monitoring and should be observed for a minimum of 6 to 8 hours relative to the reaction type to monitor for additional incidents or complications.[1,9] Individuals with severe anaphylactic reactions or cardiovascular or respiratory compromise should be observed for a more extensive period in the emergency department or admitted to the hospital as warranted.

Follow-up with a primary care provider is recommended. In addition, referral to an allergist or immunologist is warranted for potential identification of triggers and the development of appropriate treatment plans.[1,2,3,9]

LIFE SPAN CONSIDERATIONS

Vigilant lifetime avoidance of the precipitating allergen is the primary goal. Management of comorbid disorders is advisable.

COMPLICATIONS

Most individuals recover from an anaphylactic event without incident; however, monitoring for sequelae is warranted.

HEALTH PROMOTION

All individuals who have experienced or are at risk for anaphylaxis should wear a medical identification bracelet. Printed information should be provided about trigger identification and avoidance.[3,9] Instruction should be provided surrounding reading food labels to determine potential allergen exposures in processed food. Children should have an emergency action plan in place in schools, camps, and other regularly attended places. In addition, individuals attending college should be in close contact with campus health services, staff, and faculty to develop an emergency treatment plan.[10]

All at-risk individuals should be equipped with at least two epinephrine auto-injectors.[1,3,9,10] Epinephrine auto-injectors are commercially available devices that provide a single premeasured epinephrine dose; they should be prescribed for individuals with a known history of allergen sensitivity or past anaphylactic reaction. Instruction in proper use is key. It is imperative that patients, friends, family, coworkers, and others understand that epinephrine auto-injectors should be used without delay before emergency personnel arrive on the scene.[1,3,9,10]

There are four automatic epinephrine injectors available for use in the United States.[9] It is vital that prescribed self-administration epinephrine injectors for children be the appropriate dosage based upon the child's weight. Epinephrine auto-injectors for children come in two fixed doses: 0.15 mg and 0.3 mg. The 0.15-mg dose is appropriate for use in infants and young children weighing less than 25 kg.[11] For children weighing 25 to 30 kg, the 0.3-mg auto-injector should be prescribed.[11] Injection can be repeated with one additional dose. There is no commercially available auto-injector preparation for infants and small children weighing less than 10 kg.[11]

For adults, the 0.3-mg auto-injector should be prescribed for one-time use intramuscularly. Injection can be repeated with one dose.

Most states allow students and children to self-carry an epinephrine auto-injector with proper consent and a prescription.[11] It is recommended that providers and patients check their own state regulations regarding children self-carrying epinephrine auto injectors in schools, camps, and other venues.

The American Academy of Allergy, Asthma, and Immunology recommends the development of an individual emergency action plan for those at risk for anaphylaxis.[1,9]

REFERENCES

1. Lieberman, P. (2014). Recognition and first-line treatment of anaphylaxis. *The American Journal of Medicine, 127*(1), S6–S11.
2. Steinberg, P. (2017). Anaphylaxis: 36 practical pointers for reducing the risk of reaction. *Consultant, 57*(10), 588–595.
3. Lieberman, P., Nicklas, R. A., Oppenheimer, J., et al. (2010). The diagnosis and management of anaphylaxis practice parameter: 2010 update. *The Journal of Allergy and Clinical Immunology, 126*(3), 477–480.
4. Fromer, L. (2016). Prevention of anaphylaxis: The role of the epinephrine auto injector. *The American Journal of Medicine, 129*, 1244–1250.
5. Wood, R. A., Camargo, C. A., Lieberman, P., et al. (2014). Anaphylaxis is in America: The prevalence and characteristics of anaphylaxis in the United States. *The Journal of Allergy and Clinical Immunology, 133*(2), 461–467.
6. Moriber, N. A. (2014). Disorders of the immune response. In S. Grossman & C. M. Porth (Eds.), *Porth's pathophysiology* (9th ed., pp. 341–350). Philadelphia: Lippincott Williams & Wilkins.
7. Grossman, S. (2014). Inflammation, tissue repair, and wound healing. In S. Grossman & C. M. Porth (Eds.), *Porth's pathophysiology* (9th ed., pp. 306–319). Philadelphia: Lippincott Williams & Wilkins.

8. Bethel, J. (2013). Anaphylaxis: Diagnosis and treatment. *Nursing Standard*, 27(41), 49–56.

9. Lieberman, P., Nicklas, R. A., Randolph, C., et al. (2015). Anaphylaxis—a practice parameter update 2015. *Annals of Allergy, Asthma and Immunology*, 341–384.

10. Gupta, R. S. (2014). Anaphylaxis in the young adult population. *The American Journal of Medicine*, 127(1A), S17–S24.

11. Sicherer, S. H., & Simons, F. E. R., AAP section on Allergy and Immunology. (2017). Epinephrine for first aid management of anaphylaxis. *Pediatrics*, 139(3), e20164006.

CHAPTER **24**

BITES AND STINGS

Terry Mahan Buttaro • Joanne Sandberg-Cook

INSECT BITES AND STINGS

 Immediate emergency department referral or physician consultation is indicated for anaphylaxis and suspected black widow or brown recluse spider bites.

DEFINITION AND EPIDEMIOLOGY

More species of insects are in existence than any other form of multicellular life. Insects that bite and infest include mosquitoes, flies, bedbugs, kissing bugs, fleas, lice, blister beetles, centipedes, millipedes, scabies, chiggers, and ticks. Stinging insects include vespids, bees, and ants. The medical importance of insects is that they bite, sting, and envenomate; they are vectors for infectious pathogens, and they cause hypersensitivity reactions. Insect bites and stings can cause toxic reactions that range from local and mild to life-threatening.

PATHOPHYSIOLOGY AND CLINICAL PRESENTATION

Although many insect bites and stings are simply a nuisance, some patients can have severe skin or systemic reactions. Vespids (yellow jackets, hornets, and wasps), bees (honeybees and bumblebees), and ants inject venom with a stinger. The sting results in immunoglobulin E–mediated systemic reactions that cause the release of mediators (histamines, the slow-reacting substance of anaphylaxis, and eosinophil chemotactic factors of anaphylaxis)[1] from mast cells, culminating in local inflammation involving many cell types and numerous mechanisms.[1,2]

These stings induce local, toxic, systemic, and delayed reactions. A local reaction consists of erythema, edema, and pruritus at the sting site. A toxic reaction is initially seen as gastrointestinal distress, lightheadedness, syncope, headache, fever, drowsiness, muscle spasms, edema, and occasionally seizures. A systemic reaction is anaphylaxis, which can occur within 15 minutes, and manifests initially as itchy eyes, facial flushing, generalized urticaria, and dry cough.[1] Anaphylaxis can quickly intensify to respiratory distress, and may deteriorate to respiratory or cardiovascular failure.[1] A delayed reaction can occur 10 to 14 days after the sting and cause fever, malaise, headache, urticaria, lymphadenopathy, polyarthritis, or more systemic autoimmune illnesses (i.e., leukocytoclastic vasculitis or Henoch-Schönlein purpura).[1,2] Table 24.1 describes the

TABLE 24.1	Summary of Insect Bites and Stings	
Insect	**Clinical Presentation**	**Pathophysiology**
Wasps, bees, ants, hornets, yellow jackets	Local reaction Toxic reaction Systemic reaction Delayed reaction	Inject venom with stinger
Fire ants	Papule progressing to sterile pustule in 6–24 h	Inject venom with stinger
Mosquitoes, flies	Pruritic, painful papule Secondary infection common	Inject salivary material
Bedbugs, kissing bugs	Clustered, erythematous, pruritic nodules	Painlessly suck blood
Fleas	Pruritic grouped welts, papules, vesicles Secondary infection common	Deposit saliva in bite
Lice	Pruritus Nits in scalp, body, or pubic hair	Deposit saliva in bite
Blister beetles	Large blisters	Release hemolymph
Centipedes	Pain and itching with local necrosis	Inject venom with fangs
Millipedes	Brown-stained area with blistering	Excrete toxic chemicals
Scabies	Burrow lesion with pruritus Secondary infection common	Burrow in epidermis
Chiggers	Pruritic papules or vesicles Secondary infection common	Release digestive substances in bite
Ticks	Pruritic papule with tick present Secondary infection common	Attach to victim with painless bite

pathophysiology and clinical presentation of other insect bites and stings.

PHYSICAL EXAMINATION

The initial assessment of bites and stings should determine any compromise in airway, breathing, and circulation (i.e., evidence of anaphylaxis). A thorough examination is necessary to determine location of the bite or sting. The surrounding area should be assessed to determine the extent of envenomation and any associated infection.

DIAGNOSTICS

Adults with systemic allergic reactions should be considered for venom immunotherapy, which is successful in virtually all patients. The diagnosis of insect sting allergy can be made on the basis of a history of anaphylaxis with a sting and/or positive skin test results.[1] Otherwise, no specific laboratory evaluation is required unless it is indicated by the clinical course.

DIFFERENTIAL DIAGNOSIS

The diagnosis of all insect bites and stings is made by obtaining a careful history. It is helpful if the patient brings in the insect. Insect bites are commonly confused with contact dermatitis and viral exanthems. Flea bites may resemble varicella. Reactions to blister beetles may resemble bullous impetigo, burns, contact dermatitis, and viral exanthems. Because of such similarities, a history of exposure may be the only diagnostic clue.[3]

INTERPROFESSIONAL COLLABORATIVE MANAGEMENT

- Evidence of a systemic reaction must be immediately treated as anaphylaxis with IM (preferably the lateral thigh as most effective) or subcutaneous epinephrine. For adults the dosing recommendation is 0.3 to 0.5 mg (0.3 to 0.5 mL of 1:1000 concentration [1 mg/mL]). In children the recommended dose is 0.01 mg/kg (up to 0.3 mg).[1] The patient should be immediately be brought to the nearest emergency room for further evaluation.[1]
- All insect bites and stings require local wound care, removal of the stinger, cleaning the area with soap and water, ice packs, antihistamines (H_1 and H_2 blockers) for itching, topical steroids for inflammation, topical or systemic antibiotics for secondary infection, and nonsteroidal anti-inflammatory drugs to relieve discomfort.[1,3]
- Management also includes eradication of the insect. For flea infestation, it is necessary to vacuum thoroughly, treat pets, wash the rugs and beds, and use an insecticide. Lice can be eradicated by shampooing 30 mL of lindane to dry hair for 4 minutes, then adding a small amount of water, continuing the shampoo, then rinsing the hair and using a small-toothed comb to remove the lice. Permethrin (Nix, Elimite) is another effective scabies treatment. Long-standing or crusted scabies infestation may require oral Ivermectin, although this is off-label use.
- Bedbugs have become an increasingly prevalent problem in institutional settings, including dormitories, assisted-living and nursing home facilities, and hotels. These pests are difficult to eradicate and travel easily, "hitching" rides in suitcases and sleeping bags. Although their bites do not carry disease and often go unnoticed, they can cause significant psychological and economic distress.[4]
- Ticks are effectively removed with blunt, angled, medium-tipped forceps or a specific tick-removal instrument. The tick should be removed as soon as possible by grasping it close to the mouth, flipping the tick so the backside is closest to the skin, and pulling the tick straight up.[5] After removal of the tick, the health care provider should inspect the bite area for retained mouth parts, remove if possible, then carefully clean the area with an antiseptic.[5] Antibiotic prophylaxis may be indicated where Lyme disease is endemic or if the length of time the tick has been imbedded is not known. A tick needs to be embedded and feeding for more than 36 hours to infect with Lyme disease (see Chapter 213).

DISPOSITION AND REFERRAL

Systemic reactions to bites and stings may be life-threatening. Thus, any systemic or anaphylactic reaction requires a referral to the emergency department for definitive management including epinephrine, antihistamines, and possible hospitalization.

PREVENTION AND PATIENT EDUCATION

Preventive management against bites and stings includes avoidance and protective clothing. Repellents can be used, including diethyltoluamide (DEET), dimethyl phthalate, dimethyl carbate, ethyl hexanediol, butopyronoxyl (Indalone), and benzyl benzoate.[6] Any person with a history of anaphylaxis from wasp or bee stings should understand the importance of wearing medical warning tags, carrying and learning to use an epinephrine injector kit safely, and be referred to an allergist or immunologist for venom immunotherapy.[1,7,8]

Bedbugs are a serious problem worldwide, probably because of increasing global travel and resistance to insecticides. Bedbugs are not known to carry any pathogen but are serious pests. Sleeplessness is a common problem for people in known infested settings. Because bedbugs are visible, travelers should be advised to look for them in the crevices of mattresses, behind headboards, and in the folds of bed linens and curtains. Luggage should be thoroughly vacuumed and cleaned if it is suspected of being infested. Clothing and bed linens are washed in hot water and dried on the hottest setting the fabric can withstand to eradicate the bedbugs. Serious infestations should be managed by professional exterminators.[4,9]

SPIDER BITES

DEFINITION AND EPIDEMIOLOGY

About 40,000 species of spiders, very few of which are medically important to humans, are found worldwide.[1] In the United States, problems are caused by the bites of two spiders: brown recluse spiders (*Loxosceles reclusa*), and black widow spiders (*Latrodectus*).[1] Most bites thought to be spider bites are actually caused by other insects. However, urticating hairs of the tarantula can be associated with stinging, inflammation, and even anaphylaxis.[10]

The brown recluse spider is a six-eyed nocturnal spider that avoids people. Its bite is always unintentional. It is yellow, brown, or black with thin legs that are five times the body length; the entire spider is approximately the size of a quarter. It has a violin-shaped marking on its back. A native of the United States, it is commonly found in the central Midwest south to the Gulf of Mexico. These spiders do travel in boxes and packages, exposing people in other parts of the country to potential bites. In its natural environment, the brown recluse spider is found in warm, dry areas such as abandoned buildings, woodpiles, and cellars.[1]

The female black widow spider is the most venomous of all spiders and has a body size of approximately 1.5 cm.[1] This spider is found in temperate climates all over the world. In the United States, although they are seen everywhere, they are most common in the South and West. Despite the name *black widow*, these spiders may be black, brown, tan, or variegated.[11] The classic orange-red, hourglass-shaped marking is actually found on only one species (*Latrodectus mactans*) and may be merely an indistinct yellow or orange spot. The male spider is only one-third the size of the female; its bite cannot penetrate human skin. Black widow spiders are aggressive toward other insects; humans are not their usual prey, and bites tend to be defensive only. They tend to live in basements, gardens, woodpiles, and garages.[1]

PATHOPHYSIOLOGY AND CLINICAL PRESENTATION

The venom of the brown recluse spider is chemotactic, which results in endothelial injury and subsequent thrombosis.[11] It is a neurotoxin that causes the release of acetylcholine and norepinephrine at the neurosynaptic junction.[2] The bite of the brown recluse spider is almost painless and most commonly manifests as a mild, erythematous lesion that may become firm and then heal over the course of several days to weeks. The bite can also be more severe, causing erythema, blistering, and a bluish discoloration within 24 hours and possibly becoming necrotic within 3 to 4 days.[1] The lesions can vary in size from 1 to 30 cm and take 6 weeks to 4 months to heal. The victim may have a systemic response and experience fevers, chills, nausea, vomiting, myalgia, arthralgia, petechiae, hemolysis, or seizures within 24 to 48 hours of the bite.[1] Severe systemic manifestations can lead to hemoglobinuria, renal failure, disseminated intravascular coagulation, and death.[11,12]

The bite of the black widow spider is mildly to moderately painful; erythema, swelling, and muscle cramps begin at the site within 30 minutes to 12 hours. The muscle cramping progresses to large muscle groups and the abdomen and can mimic peritonitis.[1] The muscle pain can subside in a few hours but can flare during the following 2 to 3 days, with muscle weakness and intermittent spasms persisting for weeks to months. Hypertension can be a serious complication. Anxiety or confusion can also occur. Severe envenomation may lead to shock, coma, or respiratory failure secondary to muscle paralysis. The bite can be fatal to small children, elders, and those with cardiovascular disease.[11,12]

HISTORY AND PHYSICAL EXAMINATION

The history and physical examination of the patient should be thorough. The history is important to elicit associated symptoms such as fever, nausea, or pain in addition to information on when and where the suspected bite occurred. In areas where spider bites are not endemic, a recent history of travel should be determined if a spider bite is suspected. It is most helpful if the actual spider is captured and brought for identification.

The primary survey should determine any compromise of the airway, breathing, or circulation (i.e., evidence of anaphylaxis). Assessment of vital signs and a thorough examination, including a careful evaluation of the bite and surrounding area, are then necessary to determine the extent of envenomation and any associated infection.

DIAGNOSTICS

If a brown recluse spider bite is suspected, complete blood count (CBC), blood urea nitrogen (BUN), electrolytes, blood glucose, creatinine, coagulation profile, and urinalysis (for hemoglobinuria) should be ordered. No specific laboratory tests are indicated for a suspected black widow spider bite.[1] However, CBC, urinalysis, BUN, creatinine, glucose, electrolytes, and an acute abdominal series may be indicated because the presentation may mimic an acute abdomen.

DIFFERENTIAL DIAGNOSIS

Brown recluse and black widow spider bites should be included in the differential diagnosis of any spider bite. However, the diagnosis of either of these spider bites can be difficult, and errors in diagnosis are common, especially in the absence of the actual spider. Very few necrotic skin lesions are the result of a spider bite. The unusual presentation of acute abdominal pain requires that all causes of acute abdomen be considered in the differential diagnosis.

INITIAL STABILIZATION AND MANAGEMENT

The bite of the brown recluse spider requires no medications, and no antivenom is currently available. Tetanus prophylaxis

and supportive measures should be provided. Antibiotics are indicated only if infection is suspected. Pain relief may be required in some cases. Daily wound care is important for necrotic lesions, and surgical debridement may be required for necrotic lesions larger than 2 cm.[1]

The initial therapy for black widow spider bites is basic supportive care—airway, breathing, and circulation. Local wound care and tetanus prophylaxis should always be provided. Narcotic analgesics, benzodiazepines, and intravenous 10% calcium gluconate are all effective means of pain relief and muscle relaxation. Tetanus prophylaxis is recommended. Antivenom is available and reasonably safe, although not always readily available and has been associated with allergic reactions.[11,12] Antivenom is indicated only for a confirmed severe bite because of the risk of anaphylaxis and serum sickness, and it can be given only to patients who have not previously had exposure to horse serum.[11]

Wolf spiders, of which the tarantula is the most common, cause bites the equivalent of a wasp sting without necrosis. These bites usually require only supportive care.[3]

INTERPROFESSIONAL COLLABORATIVE MANAGEMENT
Disposition and Referral

 Immediate hospital referral and close observation for adults and children with evidence of significant systemic reactions. Patients with black widow spider bites that require antivenom should always be referred to the emergency department or for hospital admission.

PREVENTION AND FAMILY EDUCATION

People living in endemic areas should be taught to recognize the brown recluse spider and to avoid its habitats. Clothing, bed linens, attics, closets, and woodpiles should be examined closely in endemic areas because the spider is aggressive only if it is forced into contact with humans.

- Black widow spiders are more commonly found in their webs at night. Therefore, the webs should be cleaned cautiously at night and the spider mechanically destroyed. Everyone in endemic areas should be taught to recognize the black widow spider. Protective sleeves and gloves are recommended in handling wood and brush in infested areas.[11,13]

REPTILE BITES AND SCORPION STINGS
DEFINITION AND EPIDEMIOLOGY

In the United States, the venomous snakes include the pit vipers and coral snakes. Pit vipers include rattlesnakes, copperheads, cottonmouths (water moccasins), and bushmasters. Worldwide, 100,000 to 125,000 deaths occur each year from snake bites, but in the United States, about 10,000 snakebites are reported annually.[14] Only one-third to one-half of these bites are caused by venomous snakes. The most severe envenomations tend to occur with rattlesnakes (also known as crotaline or pit viper snakes), but copperheads (also pit vipers though not quite as venomous), coral snakes, and snakes imported from other countries and kept as pets are other causes of snakebites. Of the venomous snakebites, 20% result in no envenomation and 40% result in only mild envenomation.[15]

Other reptiles to consider are Gila monsters, which are slow-moving lizards in the deserts of the southwestern United States. Gila monsters do more than bite, they continue chewing and often have to be forcefully removed from the victim.[16] Medically significant scorpion stings also occur in the southwestern United States.

PATHOPHYSIOLOGY

The venom of the pit viper is a complex mixture of cytotoxic, hemotoxic, and neurotoxic enzymes that cause local tissue injury, systemic vascular damage, hemolysis, fibrinolysis, and neuromuscular dysfunction.[17] Coral snake venom is neurotoxic.[17,18] Gila monster venom is as toxic as rattlesnake venom, but Gila monsters do not have the apparatus to effectively inject the venom; they have short, grooved teeth, and require a prolonged bite for envenomation.[17,18] Gila bites are not often deadly, but can cause significant edema, toxicity, and hypertension.[18] Scorpion venom is primarily neurotoxic and is composed of proteins and polypeptides that activate sodium channels to produce a hyperadrenergic state.[16]

CLINICAL PRESENTATION AND PHYSICAL EXAMINATION

The history is particularly important in identifying the type of bite. An attempt should be made to determine whether the bite is venomous. Venomous rattlesnakes have fangs, whereas nonvenomous rattlesnakes do not.[17] Poisonous coral snakes also have fangs and are easily identified by their red and yellow bands.[17] Information about associated symptoms, such as pain, dizziness, nausea, vomiting, or paresthesias, is important to elicit.

For the bites in which there is no envenomation, the only clinical finding is the puncture wound. The clinical picture of patients who are envenomated depends on several factors: the amount of venom introduced; the anatomic location of the bite; and the patient's size, age, and overall health. The bites are classified by the degree of envenomation: none, minimum, moderate, or severe. The presentation of no envenomation is minimum pain and no significant swelling. Minimum envenomation manifests as local swelling of less than 15 cm (6 inches) from the bite wound and no systemic manifestations. Moderate envenomation has local swelling of 15 to 30 cm (6 to 12 inches) with systemic signs and symptoms. Severe envenomation has local swelling of more than 30 cm with severe systemic signs and symptoms, including coagulation abnormalities.[15]

Coral snake bites resemble scratch marks and are somewhat painful. Patients are initially seen with neurologic symptoms such as tremors, salivation, dysarthria, diplopia, dysphagia, dyspnea, and seizures. These symptoms, which are usually delayed 1 to 6 hours or even up to 12 hours, may progress to respiratory muscle paralysis and death.[15] In most cases, the bite of the Gila monster causes only local pain and swelling that worsens during several hours and then subsides in the next several hours. Only occasionally will a systemic reaction occur, with weakness, lightheadedness, paresthesias, diaphoresis, or hypertension.[2] Scorpion stings may cause mild symptoms with only local pain or paresthesias, or they may progress to somatic or cranial nerve dysfunction. Cardiovascular dysfunction including conduction abnormalities can be seen. Autonomic nervous system symptoms including hypersalivation, hypotension, and diaphoresis can occur. Motor nerve

effects include roving eye movements, fasciculations, dysphagia, and the autonomic effects of tachycardia and excessive secretions.[16]

The physical examination of the patient should be thorough. First, any compromise of the airway, breathing, or circulation (i.e., anaphylaxis) should be determined. This is followed by assessment of vital signs; evaluation of the patient for bleeding; and thorough examination of the bite and surrounding area to determine the extent of envenomation, tissue damage, and associated lymphadenopathy. A careful neurologic examination and documentation are necessary initially and should be routinely repeated to assess for neurologic involvement.

DIAGNOSTICS: REPTILE BITES AND SCORPION STINGS

Several corroborating laboratory studies are needed, including CBC, coagulation studies (PT/PTT, clotting time, fibrinogen level), serum glucose, serum electrolytes, BUN, creatinine, creatine kinase, and urinalysis. A type and crossmatch for blood, an arterial blood gas analysis, and an electrocardiogram are needed if the envenomation is severe.[16]

DIFFERENTIAL DIAGNOSIS

The diagnosis is made on the basis of a history of a snakebite or scorpion bite, with a clinical presentation consistent with envenomation. It is helpful if the victim can identify the snake or scorpion with use of a picture or photograph. Patients should be discouraged from bringing the actual snake in for identification as snakes can reflexively bite immediately after death.

INTERPROFESSIONAL COLLABORATIVE MANAGEMENT

 First aid measures must be instituted first, but all patients bitten by venomous snakes or scorpions must be taken to a health care facility. For snakebites, consultation with a physician or poison control center familiar with envenomation is always recommended

- Further first aid measures include retreating beyond striking range, remaining calm, immobilizing the extremity involved, minimizing physical activity, wiping the bite site, identifying the snake if it can be done safely, and closely observing the patient's respiratory status.[19]
- In the prehospital or office setting, management includes providing advanced cardiac life support as appropriate, immobilizing the limb, establishing intravenous access, and administering oxygen. The wound should be cleaned and tetanus prophylaxis administered.[17]
- Incision of the wound, suction of the wound, and tourniquets are not recommended.[17]
- The limb should not be elevated above the level of the heart.
- The major determinant of the required therapy is the degree of envenomation; the mainstay of therapy for moderate to severe venomous snakebites is antivenom.[15]
- For Gila monsters, local wound care is probably sufficient and must include the removal of any teeth in the wound; no antivenom is available.[1]
- For scorpion bites, management is supportive with analgesics and wound care; there is antivenom for severe bites, but it is available only in Arizona and is rarely used.[16]

DISPOSITION AND REFERRAL

- All bites by venomous snakes and scorpions need to be observed for a minimum of 12 hours, because the clinical symptoms can be delayed. The patient must be in an emergency department or hospital setting in which antivenom is available.

PREVENTION AND PATIENT EDUCATION

Most snake bites occur in April through October when outdoor activities are popular. Snakes are most often found in tall grass or brush, rocky outcrops, fallen logs, swamps, and deep holes. Patients should be given the following advice:

- In an area where snakes are likely to live, walk with a stick tapping ahead of you to scare the snakes away.
- Be watchful where you step, swim, and sit when outdoors.
- Wear loose, long pants and high, thick leather or rubber boots.
- Shine a flashlight on your path when walking outside at night.
- Never handle a snake, even if you think it is dead. Recently killed snakes may still bite by reflex.
- Regularly trim hedges, keep lawns mowed, and remove brush from your yard and any nearby vacant lots. This will reduce the number of places where snakes like to live.
- Don't allow children to play in vacant lots with tall grass and weeds.
- Always use tongs when moving firewood, brush, or lumber. This will safely expose any snakes that may be hidden underneath.
- Always sleep on a cot when camping.
- Be aware of snakes if you are swimming or wading in rivers, lakes, or other bodies of water (this includes areas covered with water because of flooding).
- Learn to identify poisonous snakes and avoid them.[20]

REFERENCES

1. Schneier, A., & Clark, R. (2016). Bites and stings. In J. E. Tintinalli (Ed.), *Emergency medicine: A comprehensive study guide* (8th ed.). New York: McGraw-Hill.
2. Golden, D. B. (2013). Advances in diagnosis and management of insect sting injury. *Annals of Allergy, Asthma and Immunology, 111*(2), 84–89.
3. Vetter, R., & Isbister, G. (2008). Medical aspects of spiders bites. *Annual Review of Entomology, 53*, 400–429.
4. Fong, D., Bos, C., Stuart, T., et al. (2013). Prevention, identification and treatments options for the management of bed bug infestations. National Collaborating Centre for Environmental Health. Retrieved from www.ncceh.ca/sites/. (Accessed 30 September 2014).
5. Due, C., Fox, W., Medlock, J. M., et al. (2013). Tick bite prevention and tick removal. *British Medical Journal, 347*.
6. Krau, S. D. (2013). Bites and stings: Epidemiology and treatment. *Critical Care Nursing Clinics of North America, 25*(2), 143–150.
7. Casale, T. B., & Burks, A. W. (2014). Clinical practice, hymenoptera sting hypersensitivity. *The New England Journal of Medicine, 370*, 1432–1439.
8. Hahlbohm, D. (2013). Stinging Insect Allergy: Avoidance and access to epinephrine are essential. *Advance for NPs & PAs, 4*(4), 20–22.
9. McNeill, C., et al. (2011). Bed bugs: Current treatment guidelines. *The Journal for Nurse Practitioners, 13*(6), 381–388.
10. Ruha, A. M. (2014). Spider bites and scorpion stings. In E. T. Bope, R. E. Rakel, & R. Kellerman (Eds.), *Conn's current therapy 2014*. Philadelphia: Elsevier.
11. Isbister, G., & Fan, H. W. (2011). Spider bites. *Lancet, 378*(9808), 2039–2047.
12. Schwartz, R. A., & Steen, C. J. (2012). Arthropod bites and stings. In L. A. Goldsmith, S. I. Katz, B. A. Gilchrest, A. S. Paller, D. J. Leffell, & K. Wolff (Eds.), *Fitzpatrick's dermatology in general medicine* (8th ed.). New York, NY: McGraw-Hill. Chapter 210.
13. Lavonase, E. J., Ruha, A. M., Banner, W., et al. (2011). Unified treatment algorithm for the management of crotaline snakebite in the United States, results of an evidence informed consensus workshop. *BMC Emergency Medicine, 11*, 2.
14. Spyres, M., Ruha, A., Seifert, S., Onisko, N., Padilla-Jones, A., & Smith, E. (2016). Occupational snake bites: A prospective case series of patients reported to the ToxIC North American Snakebite Registry. *Journal Of Medical Toxicology* [Serial Online], *12*(4), 365–369.
15. Daley, B. J., & Torres, J. (2014). Venomous snakebites. *JEMS: A Journal of Emergency Medical Services, 39*(6), 58–62.
16. Isbister, G. K., & Bawaskar, H. S. (2014). Scorpion envenomations. *The New England Journal of Medicine, 371*(5), 457–463.
17. Evans, D. D., & Nelson, L. W. (2013). Treating venomous snakebites in the United States: A guide for nurse practitioners. *Nursing Practice, 38*(7), 13–22.
18. Dart, R. C., & White, J. (2015). Reptile bites. In J. E. Tintinalli, J. Stapczynski, O. Ma, D. M. Yealy, G. D. Meckler, & D. M. Cline (Eds.), *Tintinalli's emergency medicine: A comprehensive study guide* (8th ed.). New York, NY: McGraw-Hill.
19. Wall, C. (2012). British military snake bite guidelines: Pressure immobilization. *Journal of the Royal Army Medical Corps, 158*(3), 194–198.
20. Prevention of Snake Bites. Retrieved from https://familydoctor.org/avoiding-snakebites/; www.familydoctor.org. (Accessed 22 June 2018).

CHAPTER **25**

BRADYCARDIA AND TACHYCARDIA

Terry Mahan Buttaro • Amelia Nelson Nadler

BRADYCARDIA

 Immediate emergency department referral or physician consultation is indicated for patients with symptomatic bradycardia or Mobitz Type II or third-degree heart block.

DEFINITION AND EPIDEMIOLOGY

Absolute bradycardia is defined as a heart rate of less than 60 beats/min. Athletes, older adults, and other individuals may have normally slow heart rates, and bradycardia may not be pathologic during sleep or after a Valsalva maneuver or other vagal stimulation.[1] Relative bradycardia occurs when the heart does not respond as expected to trauma, hypovolemia, or an infectious process.[1] Other reversible causes of bradycardia include drug toxicity, electrolyte abnormality, periatrioventricular node inflammation (Lyme disease), and transient injury to the conduction system as during open heart surgery.[2]

Numerous medications, cardiac disease, hypothyroidism, electrolyte abnormalities, sleep apnea, infections, increased intracranial pressure, hypothermia, hypoxemia, acidemia, and other disease states can also produce bradycardia. Asymptomatic bradycardia does not require urgent intervention. However, careful monitoring and therapy are indicated if the bradycardia causes symptoms (e.g., angina, change in mental status, dizziness associated with hypotension, hypertension, heart failure, or syncope) or if the bradycardia is related to type II second-degree (Mobitz type II) or third-degree atrioventricular (AV) block.

PATHOPHYSIOLOGY

Bradycardia may result from sinus node dysfunction or AV block.[3] Sinus node dysfunction can be a result of increased vagal tone, as seen in athletes or conditioned young people, or in older adults as the result of underlying disease processes, medications, or toxicity.[4] AV block is also associated with various disease processes, including myocardial infarction, coronary artery spasm, digitalis toxicity, cardiac mesotheliomas, and infectious processes. Medications, particularly beta blockers and calcium channel blockers, may induce sinus node or AV dysfunction.

CLINICAL PRESENTATION AND PHYSICAL EXAMINATION

Some symptoms may be nonspecific, but dizziness, fatigue, and syncope are complaints commonly identified with bradycardia.[3] Nausea, vomiting, and confusion have also been correlated with bradycardia. Any bradyarrhythmia associated with chest pain, shortness of breath, exercise intolerance, decreased level of consciousness, hypotension, seizure, congestive heart failure, or myocardial infarction is considered a prearrest condition. A careful symptom analysis and review of the patient's medical history, including allergies and prescribed and over-the-counter medications, is necessary to discern the cause of the bradycardia so that appropriate treatment can be initiated.

The physical examination is often guided by the patient's symptoms, but a focused history and physical examination are necessary. The patient's level of responsiveness and vital signs (including temperature, blood pressure, pulse, respiratory rate, and oxygen saturation) are significant and should be continually reassessed. Hypotension, altered mental status, and pulmonary congestion are serious signs indicating the need to identify the cardiac rhythm and to institute rapid, appropriate treatment.

 Immediate physician consultation is indicated for patients with pretibial edema, the hallmark exam finding for myxedema coma.

 Immediate physician consultation is indicated for patients with hypothermia as SA and AV node dysfunction can cause sinus bradycardia and heart block.

DIAGNOSTICS
Essential Diagnostics

The first and most essential diagnostic test is an electrocardiogram (ECG). Once performed, proper interpretation of the ECG is imperative in the diagnosis of any arrhythmia. In reviewing the ECG, careful attention to the rhythm and rate can help identify the likely arrhythmia and guide necessary treatment. Analysis of the ECG should be focused on looking for ischemic changes, heart block, and signs of ST segment elevation myocardial infarction.

Additional Diagnostics

All diagnostic testing should be determined based on close review of the history and physical exam. Glucose levels should be checked on any symptomatic bradycardic patient. Further diagnostics are guided by the history and physical examination but can include drug levels, electrolyte values, blood urea nitrogen (BUN) level, creatinine concentration, liver function, complete blood count (CBC), troponin T or troponin I level,

thyroid studies, and chest X-ray studies. Troponin T and I can be used as measure of cardiac strain and indicate myocardial infarction.

If there is concern for myocardial infarction, an echocardiogram should be performed to evaluate for ejection fraction and heart wall motion. Bradycardia can also occur in relation to ingestion of prescribed or illicit drugs, so patients with an altered sensorium and bradycardia should have toxicology screens for substance use drugs.

Patients with hepatic or renal dysfunction may be unable to clear their normal medications (e.g., digoxin); therefore, for patients on digoxin, digoxin levels should be done to determine the presence of digoxin toxicity.

If the history or physical exam raises concern for a pulmonary or cardiac abnormality, a chest X-ray may show cardiomegaly that could suggest more advanced structural changes requiring further investigation. Finally, any patient presenting with a Mobitz Type II heart block or complete heart block in areas with endemic Lyme disease should have Lyme panels sent.[2]

INITIAL DIAGNOSTICS

Bradycardia

INITIAL
- Electrocardiogram

LABORATORY
- Drug levels[a]
- Serum glucose electrolytes, blood urea nitrogen, Creatinine[a]
- Creatine kinase muscle-brain[a]
- Troponin T or I[a]
- Complete blood count and differential[a]
- Thyroid-stimulating hormone[a]

OTHER
- Chest radiograph[a]
- Echocardiogram[a]
- Lyme Titers[a]

———
[a]If indicated.

DIFFERENTIAL DIAGNOSIS

The most common differential diagnoses for bradycardia include medication induced (β blocker, calcium channel blockers, digoxin, illicit drugs), vasovagal response, and sick sinus syndrome. However, there are a number of diagnoses related to bradycardia that should not be missed including myocardial infarction, sepsis, digitalis toxicity, Mobitz type II heart block, complete heart block, hypothermia, and head trauma.

Determination of the arrhythmia and associated disease is essential for treatment. Herbals and medications can also be a common cause of bradycardia, but infections, vasovagal syncope, myocardial infarction, digitalis toxicity, sick sinus syndrome, bradycardia-tachycardia syndrome, hypothyroidism, and other disease states are also possible reasons.[3]

INTERPROFESSIONAL COLLABORATIVE MANAGEMENT
Nonpharmacological Management

Initial management depends largely on the history and physical exam. No intervention is necessary if the patient is stable and asymptomatic, but continued monitoring is indicated to ensure the patient's well-being and safety. The American Heart Association recommends cardiac monitoring, intravenous (IV) access, and continuous assessment of the patient (including airway, breathing, vital signs, oxygen saturation, and supplementary oxygen) when indicated.[4]

Pharmacologic Management

Patients with suspected myocardial infarction should be treated for acute coronary syndrome according to the 2015 American Heart Association guidelines (with oxygen, if indicated); aspirin (162 to 325 mg chewed, if not aspirin allergic); nitroglycerin; morphine; and, if appropriate, reperfusion therapy.[4]

For adult patients with symptomatic bradycardia, especially if the bradycardia is associated with Mobitz type II second-degree heart block or third-degree heart block, the American Heart Association recommends atropine, 0.5 mg intravenously every 3 to 5 minutes (up to a total dose 3 mg), until a transcutaneous or transvenous pacer (class I intervention) is available.[4] However, atropine can induce cardiac ischemia, precipitate ventricular tachycardia (VT) or fibrillation, and be deleterious for patients with a history of cardiac transplantation.[4] In the presence of Mobitz type II second-degree heart block or third-degree heart block associated with wide-complex ventricular escape beats, atropine should be avoided and treatment with a transcutaneous or transvenous pacer applied as soon as possible.[4] Some defibrillator monitors may also have a transcutaneous pacer component.

If the bradycardia is drug induced (e.g., β blocker or calcium channel blocker overdose), a pacer is not available, atropine is contraindicated, or the patient is unresponsive to atropine or pacing, IV epinephrine 2 to 10 mcg/min can be used to treat critical bradycardia.[4] A dopamine infusion of 2 to 20 mcg/kg/min can also improve cardiac output and increase blood pressure and may be used alone or in conjunction with an epinephrine infusion.[4]

Indications for Referral and Hospitalization

Patients with syncope who have had suspected ventricular arrhythmias should be hospitalized for evaluation and monitoring.[5] Symptomatic patients with worsening clinical symptoms or prearrest conditions related to the bradycardia may require urgent intervention before a definitive underlying condition is identified. Therefore, any patient who is unstable with bradycardia should be promptly sent to the emergency department. Patients with signs of ischemia on ECG should be transferred to the emergency department for further evaluation. If ECG is concerning for ST elevation myocardial infarction, the patient should be transferred by ambulance immediately to the closest hospital with a catheterization lab for expedited reperfusion therapy.

Prevention, when possible, may avert complications or serious injury. Patients who complain of syncope, fatigue, or other symptoms that may be related to bradycardia require diagnostic assessment. A permanent pacemaker may be indicated for bradycardia associated with sinus node dysfunction and certain heart blocks (e.g., fascicular block or acquired AV block).[2,3,5]

Further evaluation in collaboration with a cardiologist is warranted for patients experiencing ongoing symptoms related to bradycardia.

Lifespan Considerations

Most patients live long lives with bradycardia when the underlying etiology is diagnosed and treated effectively. Patients may require pacemaker placement for lifelong support and prevention of symptoms related to bradycardia. Patients with recurrent syncopal events have decreased quality of life.[5] Therefore, it is imperative that patients with symptomatic bradycardia be carefully evaluated with expert consultation to improve quality of life.

COMPLICATIONS

Complications vary for bradycardia based on the potential causes. Those that are treated appropriately for infectious or structural causes can experience a low number of complications. For those patients who have complications that go undiagnosed, complications may include ischemia, hypoperfusion, and possibly death.

PATIENT AND FAMILY EDUCATION

- Patients should understand the importance of calling their health care provider if they experience syncope, lightheadedness, or a slow heart rate that hinders activities.
- Both patients and caregivers should know how to activate the emergency medical system (911) if these symptoms occur with chest discomfort or shortness of breath.
- Careful education on the required medication regimens, understanding of mechanism of actions, common side effects, and reasons to seek medical attention are important components of patient understanding and adherence to recommendations.

TACHYCARDIA

 Emergency room referral or physician consultation is indicated for new-onset atrial fibrillation, atrial flutter, sick sinus syndrome, ventricular tachycardia, or supraventricular tachycardia.

DEFINITION AND EPIDEMIOLOGY

Tachycardia is described as a heart rate exceeding 100 beats/min. Normal sinus tachycardia does not usually require medical intervention, but other tachyarrhythmias can result in hemodynamic compromise and warrant urgent treatment. A rapid assessment of airway, breathing, and circulation, and a complete history, physical examination, and 12-lead ECG are indicated.

Asymptomatic individuals with tachycardia can have stable cardiac rhythms that do not require emergent treatment. Fever, nicotine, exercise, stimulants, medications, and anxiety can precipitate normal sinus tachycardia. Pregnancy, coronary heart disease, congestive heart failure, valvular heart disease, pulmonary embolus, pericardial disease, valvular disorders, ischemia, metabolic and electrolyte abnormalities, medications, toxins, infection, and volume depletion should be considered possible precipitants identified with atrial and ventricular arrhythmias as well as tachycardia.

PATHOPHYSIOLOGY

The pathology of tachycardia is varied. Sinus tachycardia is a normal physiologic response and should not be considered pathologic. Atrial fibrillation and flutter, the narrow-complex tachycardias (ectopic atrial tachycardia, multifocal atrial tachycardia, junctional tachycardia, and paroxysmal supraventricular tachycardia [SVT]), the stable wide-complex tachycardias of unknown type, and monomorphic-polymorphic VT are tachyarrhythmias that can cause hemodynamic instability (see Chapter 100). In narrow-complex tachycardia, such as paroxysmal tachycardia, the heart rate increases suddenly and rapidly and then decreases suddenly. The attack may last seconds or days, during which time the ventricular rate is rapid and regular, usually between 150 and 225 beats/min. This pathologic condition is most likely related to an aberrant reentry involving the AV node, although an obscure bypass tract near the AV node may cause the aberrant conduction (as in Wolff-Parkinson-White syndrome).[5]

Atrial fibrillation and atrial flutter are rhythm disturbances characterized by rapid atrial stimulation and varied ventricular response. These atrial stimulation arrhythmias can vary from paroxysmal to permanent. In fibrillation, it can be related to stress. However, atrial arrhythmias are commonly related to varied disease states. These include coronary heart disease, rheumatic fever, mitral stenosis, thyrotoxicosis, infection, metabolic abnormalities, pulmonary embolism, and chronic lung disease. Atrial arrhythmias can develop with age and typically progress over time.[6]

Whether monomorphic or polymorphic, VT is a rhythm disturbance that arises in the ventricles. The arrhythmia is life-threatening if the patient is pulseless, but the patient can be hemodynamically stable when VT is associated with a pulse.

CLINICAL PRESENTATION AND PHYSICAL EXAMINATION

Some tachyarrhythmias are well tolerated, but chest discomfort, anxiety, restlessness, shortness of breath, weakness, fatigue, dizziness, and palpitations are commonly presented symptoms.[5] Any tachycardia associated with chest pressure, acute myocardial infarction or cardiac ischemia, alteration in consciousness, hypotension or shock, shortness of breath, dyspnea on exertion, heart failure, or dizziness requires emergency care and potentially urgent synchronized cardioversion.[5] A careful history of the presenting event; past medical history; and review of allergies, medications, and excessive use of caffeine, alcohol, or stimulants can help determine whether an underlying pathologic condition is causing the tachycardia and will facilitate appropriate treatment.

An ECG or "quick look" with a conventional or external defibrillator is necessary to determine the cardiac rhythm and presence of arrhythmias or ischemia. Because tachycardia can precipitate hemodynamic instability, cardiac monitoring and assessment of vital signs (including temperature, blood pressure, heart rate, respirations, and oxygen saturation) should be continuous. The physical examination should be focused and exact with particular attention to the patient's respiratory and oxygenation status, because tachycardia is frequently related to hypoxemia.[5] The assessment will help determine the precipitating pathologic condition, establish whether the patient is stable or unstable, and determine whether the tachycardia has precipitated serious signs and symptoms.

DIAGNOSTICS
Essential Diagnostics

As with bradycardia, the most essential initial diagnostic test is an ECG. A 12-lead ECG is necessary for correct identification

of the tachyarrhythmia and requires careful review for signs of ischemia and ST segment changes indicative of myocardial infarction.

 Immediate transfer to the emergency department is indicated for signs of myocardial ischemia, cardiac strain, or infarction.

Additional Diagnostics

A chest X-ray and laboratory studies, including drug levels, electrolyte values, CBC, and thyroid studies (thyroid-stimulating hormone [TSH], T_3, free T_4) may also be indicated, but are usually deferred to emergency department evaluation. A chest X-ray should be performed if heart failure, cardiomegaly, pneumothorax, or pneumonia is suspected.[6] A CBC should be evaluated if the patient's history and physical exam raise concerns for infection or acute blood loss. Abnormalities in electrolytes can also be a reversible cause of tachycardia. If a patient appears to be having torsades de points, a serum magnesium is indicated. Patients with likely ventricular arrhythmias should have an echocardiogram to evaluate for structural heart disease and cardiac function.[5]

INITIAL DIAGNOSTICS

Tachycardia

INITIAL
- Electrocardiogram
- Laboratory
- Drug levels[a]
- Serum glucose, electrolytes, magnesium, BUN, and creatinine[a]
- Complete blood count and differential[a]
- Thyroid-stimulating hormone, T_3, Free T_4[a]

IMAGING
- Chest radiograph[a]
- Echocardiogram[a]

---
[a]If indicated.

DIFFERENTIAL DIAGNOSIS

 Immediate evaluation of patients with tachycardia with associated chest pain, shortness of breath, or hypoxia for pulmonary embolism (especially those on exogenous estrogen, during pregnancy, or those with a history of hypercoagulability).

The most common differential diagnoses in tachycardia are atrial fibrillation, atrial flutter, and narrow-complex tachycardias or sinus tachycardia. However, VT and stable wide-complex tachycardias may also be seen. All tachyarrhythmias can have potentially serious consequences.

The 2010 to 2015 American Heart Association guidelines for emergency cardiovascular care recommend classifying patients as stable or unstable, identifying whether serious signs and symptoms are present, and determining whether the arrhythmia has caused these signs and symptoms.[4] Patients with unstable tachycardia may complain of chest discomfort, be hypotensive, or display cognitive changes or signs of shock.[4]

Identification of the tachycardia and its related pathologic condition is essential for appropriate treatment. For prevention of inappropriate therapy, the patient's condition and the etiology of the tachycardia should be carefully considered before treatment is initiated. Medications, substance use (e.g., cocaine), pregnancy, hyperthyroidism, acute myocardial infarction, congestive heart failure, pulmonary embolus, hypotension, hypoxia, hypovolemia, infection, electrolyte abnormalities, energy drinks, alcohol withdrawal, and other disorders (e.g., Wolff-Parkinson-White syndrome) may precipitate a rapid heart rate and its resultant symptoms. Treatment of the specific disorder may result in resolution of the tachycardia.

INTERPROFESSIONAL COLLABORATIVE MANAGEMENT

Nonpharmacologic Management

A 12-lead ECG, oxygen when indicated, and continuous monitoring of the patient's oxygen saturation and blood pressure are critical. The ECG will permit identification of the rhythm and enable appropriate treatment. The advanced cardiovascular life support guidelines do not recommend treatment of tachycardia if the patient is stable and does not have chest pressure, acute myocardial infarction, change in mental status, hypotension, shortness of breath, congestive heart failure, or other signs and symptoms indicating instability.[4] Hemodynamically unstable patients should have electrical cardioversion emergently. In patients who are more stable but with persistent atrial fibrillation, cardioversion may be performed to restore sinus rhythm if the patient is known to have been in atrial fibrillation for less than 48 hours. If the patient has been in atrial fibrillation for more than 48 hours, anticoagulation is indicated for 3 weeks before the patient is cardioverted and continued for 4 weeks after cardioversion.[6] In stable patients with SVT, vagal maneuvers should be attempted while other methods of conversion are being prepared.[4] These maneuvers can include Valsalva or carotid sinus massage.

Pharmacologic Management

IV access with a large-bore catheter and isotonic normal saline solution (with the IV fluid running at "keep open rate" to maintain catheter patency) is recommended.[4]

Any patient who is unstable and symptomatic from their tachycardia should have IV access established and maintained in case medication administration is necessary. Suction, intubation, and defibrillation equipment should be readily available. Patients with pulseless VTs should be treated based on advanced cardiac life support (ACLS) protocols. This includes cardiopulmonary resuscitation (CPR), administration of epinephrine, and immediate defibrillation in wide-complex tachycardias.[4] Synchronized electrical cardioversion should be used in unstable patients in narrow-complex tachycardias.[5] In patients in SVT, adenosine should be used.[7]

Sinus Tachycardia. For those patients with stable tachycardias due to secondary causes such as infection, heart failure, or respiratory distress, the underlying cause should be determined and treated rather than treating the heart rate.

Narrow-Complex QRS Tachycardia. Reentry supraventricular rhythm; narrow-complex QRS (<0.12 seconds) with or without P waves.

If vagal maneuvers are unsuccessful, consider adenosine 6 mg rapid IV push. If rhythm continues, give adenosine 12 mg IV rapid push. Reentry SVT is the probable rhythm if the rhythm converts to normal sinus rhythm (patient will require monitoring for recurrence). If rhythm does not convert with adenosine by rapid IV push, reevaluate rhythm (consider atrial flutter, ectopic atrial tachycardia, or junctional tachycardia). Amiodarone (150 mg IV over 10 minutes; can repeat every 10 minutes to maximum dose of 2.2 g) is also recommended for narrow-complex QRS tachycardias (reentry SVT rhythms) unresponsive to vagal maneuvers or adenosine.[7]

Irregular Narrow QRS Tachycardia. Atrial fibrillation, atrial flutter, or multifocal atrial tachycardia.

The focus of treatment for atrial fibrillation and flutter is on rate control and the prevention of thromboembolism. Rate control in these patients is essential to improve quality of life, prevent cardiomyopathy, and has been shown to decrease morbidity and mortality.[8] Though the goal heart rate for patients with AF is not clear, the range (80 to 110) is more lenient than in the past and considers the individual patient and their activity.

For a patient with rapid atrial fibrillation and hemodynamically unstable, immediate direct current cardioversion is indicated.[8] For hemodynamically stable patients requiring rate control, the recommended first-line medication for control of ventricular rate is now an intravenous β blocker (metoprolol 2.5 TO 5 mg IV every 2 to 5 minutes) provided they do not have heart failure or bronchospasm.[8] Intravenous nondihydropyridine calcium channel blockers (diltiazem 0.25 mg/kg IV over 2 minutes [may repeat 0.35 mg/kg in 15 minutes if necessary]) are a second choice, but with the caveat that the patient is not hemodynamically unstable or in heart failure.[8] Other options for rate control include amiodarone or digoxin. However, these agents should be used in collaboration with a cardiologist. These medications are used intravenously during the acute phase and orally for daily control.

With regard to anticoagulation for patients with AF, the decision is based on shared decision making based on the relative risk of the patient for thromboembolic event. Use of the CHA2DS2-VASc is recommended for the assessment of stroke risk in patients with nonvalvular atrial fibrillation.[8] Options for anticoagulation in patients with new onset AF (less than 48 hours) includes heparin, warfarin, a direct thrombin inhibitor or a factor Xa inhibitor.[8] Dabigatran can also be used in nonvalvular atrial fibrillation.[8]

Regular Stable Wide-Complex Tachycardia. QRS >0.12 seconds.

This is most likely VT or SVT. If SVT, treat with adenosine (as in narrow-complex QRS tachycardia). If monomorphic, stable VT, treat with synchronized cardioversion or procainamide 20 to 50 mg/min. Procainamide therapy is discontinued if the arrhythmia resolves, the QRS is prolonged more than 50% compared with the original QRS, the patient develops hypotension, or the maximum dose is given (17 mg/kg). Amiodarone 150 mg IV over 10 minutes (may repeat if needed up to 2.2 g/24 h) is an alternative antiarrhythmic, as is sotalol 1.5 mg/kg IV over 5 minutes. Sotalol is not appropriate for patients with QT prolongation.[4]

Polymorphic (Irregular) Ventricular Tachycardia. Immediate defibrillation. Consider cause of polymorphic VT (e.g., ischemia, Brugada syndrome, torsades de pointes, or long QT syndrome) and treat appropriately.

Amiodarone or other antiarrhythmic medications, wearable defibrillators, implantable cardioverter-defibrillators, pacemakers, or ablation therapy may be indicated for the prevention of recurrent symptomatic tachycardia.[4-7]

Indications for Referral and Hospitalization

Ideally, symptomatic patients with tachycardia should be stabilized with initial management and transferred to the nearest emergency department. Immediate transfer by ambulance to an emergency department is indicated for patients requiring continued assessment and management. Patient with symptomatic tachycardias that do not resolve should be immediately transferred to the emergency department for further evaluation and stabilization.

In healthy patients, urgent cardioversion is rarely necessary when the heart rate is less than 150 beats/min, but for patients with coronary artery disease or other comorbid illnesses, an elevated heart rate may cause significant compromise. Prompt attention must be paid to anyone who is symptomatic from the arrhythmia. Patients experiencing altered mental status, chest pain, or hypotension should receive rapid assessment and treatment in the emergency department. Immediate synchronized cardioversion is indicated if the patient is unstable because of the tachycardia.[4] Consult with a physician experienced in ACLS for synchronized cardioversion of unstable reentry SVT, unstable atrial flutter or fibrillation, unstable monomorphic VT, and polymorphic (irregular) tachycardia (Box 25.1). If the patient is stable, certain medications can also be used to treat specific tachyarrhythmias.

BOX **25.1**

Cardioversion and Defibrillation of Unstable Patients With Tachycardia

STABLE ATRIAL FIBRILLATION
- Synchronized cardioversion with monophasic waveform: 200 J.[a]
- Synchronized cardioversion with biphasic waveform: 120–200 J.

ATRIAL FLUTTER
- Synchronized cardioversion with monophasic waveform: 50–100 J.[a] Increase as necessary in step increments.
- Synchronized cardioversion with biphasic waveform: 50–100 J.[a] Increase as necessary in step increments.

MONOMORPHIC VENTRICULAR TACHYCARDIA
- Synchronized cardioversion with monophasic waveform: 100 J.[a] Increase as necessary in step increments.
- Synchronized cardioversion with biphasic waveform: 100 J. Increase as necessary in step increments.

POLYMORPHIC VENTRICULAR TACHYCARDIA
- Treat as ventricular fibrillation with unsynchronized shocks.
- If monophasic defibrillator: one shock at 360 J, then resume chest compressions and CPR for five cycles before checking rhythm and delivering a repeated shock.
- If biphasic defibrillator: one shock at 120–200 J, then resume chest compressions and CPR for five cycles before checking rhythm and delivering a repeated shock.

[a]If a second shock is necessary, the number of joules can be increased as needed. *CPR*, Cardiopulmonary resuscitation.
Data from Neumar, R. W., Shuster, M., Callaway, C. W., Gent, L. M., Atkins, D. L., Bhanji, F., et al. (2015). Part 7: Adult Advanced Cardiovascular Life Support: 2015 American Heart Association Guidelines Update for Cardiopulmonary Resuscitation and Emergency Cardiovascular Care. *Circulation, 132*, S444–S464. American Heart Association. (2016). Advanced Cardiovascular Life Support.

Lifespan Considerations

Tachyarrhythmias can cause significant complications, especially in patients with preexisting cardiomyopathy, heart failure, or coronary artery disease. Younger, healthy patients may be able to tolerate elevated heart rates, but sustained tachyarrhythmias can place the patient at increased risk of heart failure.[8] Tachycardia should be carefully evaluated for secondary causes. The treatment of the underlying cause and reduction in heart rate can improve patient symptoms, well-being, and prevent long-term cardiovascular compromise.

Complications

There exists a wide range of complications from tachyarrhythmias including temporary symptoms, cardiac ischemia, heart failure, cardiomyopathy, and death. Tachycardias should be carefully evaluated for underlying causes and managed promptly to prevent further sequelae.[8] The management of tachycardias should be focused on decreasing the heart rate to prevent long-term complications.

PATIENT AND FAMILY EDUCATION
- Tachyarrhythmias often recur. Careful explanation of the specific disorder and how to recognize untoward symptoms is an important part of patient education.
- Electrolyte disturbances and medications can precipitate some tachyarrhythmias. It is important that health care providers discuss the medication regimens and medication safety with patients.
- Patients and family members should receive education on when to seek medical care emergently and when to call their primary care provider for less-emergent follow-up.

HEALTH PROMOTION

Promoting overall health should continue to be a focus after the initial acute phase of any bradycardic or tachycardic event. Because these patients may be at increased cardiovascular risk, they will require ongoing continued monitoring for hypertension and hyperlipidemia. Promoting patient autonomy is essential, as always, with shared decision-making and encouraging healthy behaviors (e.g., smoking cessation, exercise, etc.). Patients may experience exercise intolerance related to medication regimens. It is important to discuss this with the patient and attempt to titrate medications for improved patient well-being. A tachycardic or bradycardic event may be life-threatening. Some patients may need more emotional support than others and should be screened for depression and anxiety regularly.

REFERENCES

1. Heuer, A. J. (2014). Interpretation of electrocardiogram tracings. In *Wilkins clinical assessment in respiratory care* (7th ed.). St Louis: Mosby.
2. Tracy, C. M., Epstein, A. E., Darbar, D., et al. (2013). 2012 ACCF/AHA/HRS focused update incorporated into the ACCF/AHA/HRS 2008 guidelines for device-based therapy of cardiac rhythm abnormalities: A report of the American College of Cardiology Foundation/American Heart Association Task Force on Practice Guidelines and the Heart Rhythm Society. *Journal of the American College of Cardiology, 61*(3), e6–e75.
3. Semelka, M., Gera, J., & Usman, S. (2013). Sick sinus syndrome: A review. *American Family Physician, 87*(10), 691–696. Retrieved from www.aafp.org/afp/2013/0515/p691.html. (Accessed February 8, 2015).
4. Link, M. S., et al. (2015). Part 7: Adult advanced cardiovascular life support: 2015 American Heart Association Guidelines update for cardiopulmonary

resuscitation and emergency cardiovascular care. *Circulation, 132*(18 Suppl. 2), S444–S464.

5. Shen, W. K., et al. (2017). 2017 ACC/AHA/HRS guideline for the evaluation and management of patients with syncope: A report of the American College of Cardiology/American Heart Association Task Force on Clinical Practice Guidelines and the Heart Rhythm Society. *Heart Rhythm, 14*(8), e155–e217.

6. January, C. T., Wann, L. S., Alpert, J. S., et al. (2014). AHA/ACC/HRS guideline for the management of atrial fibrillation: A report of the American College of Cardiology/American Heart Association Task Force on Practice Guidelines and the Heart Rhythm Society. *Journal of the American College of Cardiology.*

7. 2015 ACC/AHA/HRS guideline for the management of adult patients with supraventricular tachycardia: A report of the American College of Cardiology/American Heart Association Task Force on Clinical Practice Guidelines and the Heart Rhythm Society. (2016). *Journal of the American College of Cardiology, 67,* e27–e115.

8. January, C. T., Wann, L. S., Calkins, H., et al. (2019). 2019 AHA/ACC/HRS focused update of the 2014 AHA/ACC/HRS guideline for the management of patients with atrial fibrillation. *Circulation,* CIR0000000000000665. Web.

CHAPTER **26**

CHEMICAL EXPOSURE

Terry Mahan Buttaro

 Immediate emergency department referral, physician consultation, and contact with poison control is indicated for a chemical exposure.

DEFINITION AND EPIDEMIOLOGY

Chemical exposures can occur by inhalation, ingestion, injection, or absorption through the skin and mucous membranes. Although a chemical exposure can be related to a biologic, radioactive, or chemical toxin, harmful chemicals are ubiquitous and occur at home, at work, and at play.[1] Smoke, fumes, pesticides, solvents, lead, mercury, phthalates, bisphenol A, and frequently used household and beauty products all have potential long-term health ramifications.[1] Unfortunately, in some instances, the patient may be unaware of the exposure, especially if the experience occurred over a long period of time (e.g., a workplace exposure involving inhalation, heavy metals, or other types of contaminants).

Common household chemicals that are a concern include shoe polishes, cosmetics, over-the-counter and prescription medications, alcohols (isopropyl alcohol, methanol, and ethanol), detergents, cleaning products (especially chlorine, ammonia, and lye-containing cleaners), rodent and insect poisons, common yard chemicals, and paints and paint products. Household chemicals are often associated with poisonings in children, but chemical exposures in the home affect people of all ages. Unfortunately, chemical exposures are not always accidental. Hydrocarbons, solvents, and similar volatile substances that are readily available in household and workplace products are often being inhaled for their pleasurable, though potentially fatal effects.[2] Exposure to wood or cigarette smoke, fumes, or other compounds can cause nausea, dizziness, cough, difficulty concentrating, and other symptoms that cause patients to seek care.

Chemicals also abound in the workplace, and many of these cause irritation or toxicity if the human body is exposed to them. The Occupational Safety and Health Administration (OSHA) requires that all employers and employees be advised of chemical hazards by means of a hazards communication program, which includes having a Material Safety Data Sheet (MSDS) for each chemical used in the workplace. The employer must ensure that MSDSs are readily accessible to employees during each work shift when they are in the work area.[3] MSDSs are fact sheets provided by chemical manufacturers that list chemical, physical, and health hazard data for a particular substance.[3] Health hazard data include routes of entry, acute and chronic effects, signs and symptoms of exposure, and emergency and first aid procedures. For safety reasons and because federal law requires accurate labeling on chemical containers, it is wise to avoid the unnecessary transfer of potentially dangerous chemicals into any other containers. If transfer to another container is necessary, OSHA labeling requirements must be followed.[4]

Accidental poisonings are increasing, but many poisoning deaths are related to the increasing numbers of opioid-related overdoses and deaths.[5] Medication-related poisonings in adults are frequently associated with prescription medications (pain medications, sedatives, antipsychotics, hypnotics, antidepressants, cardiac medications, stimulants), cosmetics, and personal care products. In young children, the causes continue to be related to personal care products, cosmetics, pain medications, and cleaning compounds. Carbon monoxide poisoning is another common cause of poisoning in the United States.[1] Other sources of continued concern include e-cigarettes and the potential for nicotine toxicity, the use of synthetic cannabinoids, the risk of poisoning in children by ingestion of laundry detergent packs, and energy drink toxicity.

PATHOPHYSIOLOGY

The pathophysiologic and systemic effects of a chemical exposure depend on the characteristics and effects of the substance, the degree and route of exposure, and the patient's comorbidities.

CLINICAL PRESENTATION AND PHYSICAL EXAMINATION

When the chemical exposure is a poisoning, the history needs to address the five W's: who, the patient's age, weight, sex, and relationship to others present; what, the name and dose of the substance, congestents, and amount ingested; when, the time and date of ingestion; where, both the route if poisoning and the geographic location in which the poisoning occurred; and why, whether the ingestion was intentional or unintentional, plus any associated details. A comprehensive medical history should include previous poisonings, comorbid medical conditions, and concurrent medications that might affect the patient's response to and the metabolism or elimination of ingestants. Additional information should include a history of psychiatric illness, alcohol or substance use, and presence of hepatic or renal disease. The review of systems can aid in identifying the extent of the toxicity and the possible exposure.

The patient who has experienced a toxic exposure may be affected in many different ways. The presentation of chemical exposures is varied and can be particularly challenging, ranging from a headache to respiratory distress to coma or death.[2] In children, there is often physical evidence (e.g., a smell of cleaning products, pill or plant fragments, nonfood stains, open bottles or containers). In acute chemical exposures, adults commonly know the type of exposure unless they are incapacitated by it, in which case witnesses may be able to identify the exposure. If the exposure is occupational, the chemical may be readily identifiable. Review of the MSDS for pertinent information after an occupational exposure may also be helpful.

The clinical presentations of chemical exposures are related to the specific toxins involved. Medications such as dimenhydrinate, diphenhydramine, astemizole, loratadine, meclizine, promethazine, and tricyclic antidepressants, as well as household and wild plants such as mandrake, jimsonweed ("loco weed"), and nightshade are anticholinergics. Anticholinergics cause a syndrome that is often remembered by the mnemonic "hot as Hades, blind as a bat, red as a beet, dry as a bone, mad as a hatter," which describes, respectively, the following effects: hyperthermia, mydriasis, flushed skin, dry mucous membranes, urinary retention, decreased bowel motility, and hallucinations or frank psychosis.

Alkalis are found in numerous household cleaning products (e.g., detergents, drain cleaners, dishwashing fluids), batteries, and other substances, and cause irritation to the oral mucosa, esophagus, and stomach. This irritation ranges from mild to extremely severe. Both acids and alkalis cause extensive tissue damage to mucous membranes and the gastric system. The alkalis, however, are associated with a much more serious prognosis because they tend to penetrate tissues more deeply and rapidly than do the acids, particularly if the eye is involved.[6]

Hydrocarbons and metals are potential toxins that can cause poisoning acutely or chronically. Hydrocarbons are the basis of many industrial chemicals, yet they are also often found in products in many garages and sheds. These substances cause a host of reactions, including coughing, choking, tachypnea, fever, vomiting, a chemical odor to the breath, and, in severe exposure, unconsciousness and coma.[2] Metals such as iron, arsenic, aluminum, lead, mercury, and cadmium are also potentially poisonous. Aluminum poisoning can affect welders; lead and cadmium are sometimes found in jewelry. Arsenic, mercury, and lead are found almost everywhere in the environment.

Even drinking water should be suspect because of the increasing numbers of drinking water outbreaks over the past few years. These include not only parasite- or disease-related illnesses (e.g., Giardia or Legionella), but also chemicals, lead, and other toxins.[7]

Patients with chronic chemical exposure present to primary care with a variety of complaints, and the cause of the patient's concerns may not be obvious. Because chemical exposure can be so pervasive, it is always important to consider hydrocarbon exposure, heavy metals, and other sources of poisoning as a potential cause of the patient's symptoms.

The physical exam for a possible chemical exposure must initially be rapid, focused, but also comprehensive. Airway, breathing, and circulation must be supported and cardiac function monitored. Temperature, heart and respiratory rates, blood pressure, oxygen saturation, blood glucose concentration, and cardiopulmonary function should be assessed and then frequently reassessed, and a possible deterioration in the patient's status should be anticipated. The examination must focus on systems (e.g., cognitive status, responsiveness, restlessness, agitation, or seizure activity), skin appearance (e.g., needle marks, contusions, petechiae, bullae, skin color, flushed appearance, or diaphoresis), pupil appearance and reactivity, nares, mucous membranes (odor, excessive salivation), cardiac rhythm and rate, pulmonary congestion, bowel sounds or abdominal rigidity, and motor tone (e.g., fasciculations, tremors, or other neuromuscular abnormalities) to help

determine clues to the chemical exposure and on adjuvant diagnostic laboratory studies.[8]

DIAGNOSTICS AND DIFFERENTIAL DIAGNOSIS

Useful diagnostic studies in the evaluation of a chemical exposure include complete blood count (CBC), serum glucose, an electrolyte panel to calculate the anion gap, liver function tests (LFTs), blood urea nitrogen (BUN), and creatinine. If an inhalation injury is suspected, analysis of arterial blood gases (ABGs) is indicated to assess ventilation or perfusion problems related to the possible exposure. Other diagnostics should be ordered as the history warrants. These may include drug and alcohol levels; methemoglobin level for possible carbon monoxide toxicity; carboxyhemoglobin, if methylene chloride contamination; blood serum measurements of specific chemicals, such as lead, arsenic, or mercury; and, if indicated, serum levels of acetaminophen, aspirin, or other drugs.[2] An electrocardiogram (ECG) is necessary, as is urinalysis for drug screening.

The differential diagnosis depends on the type, length, and route of exposure, and on the patient's presenting signs and symptoms. Causes not related to the exposure (e.g., head trauma in a patient with altered mental status) and comorbid conditions should be considered in the differential diagnosis. The poison control center and appropriate references should be consulted for specific recommendations.

INITIAL DIAGNOSTICS

Chemical Exposure

INITIAL
- Pulse oximetry, if inhalation exposure

LABORATORY
- Complete blood count and differential
- Serum glucose, electrolytes, blood urea nitrogen, creatinine
- Anion gap
- Liver function tests
- Prothrombin time/partial thromboplastin time (PT/PTT)
- Arterial blood gases, if inhalation exposure
- Methemoglobin for carbon monoxide
- Ethylene glycol test[a]
- Serum ammonia, lead, arsenic, mercury, or other specific chemical tests[a]
- Carboxyhemoglobin[a]
- Blood and urine toxicology (alcohol and drug levels)[a]

IMAGING
- Chest radiograph for inhalation exposure[a]
- Abdominal X-rays[a]

OTHER
- Electrocardiogram

---

[a]If indicated.

INTERPROFESSIONAL COLLABORATIVE MANAGEMENT
Initial Stabilization

The initial objective in the treatment of any chemical exposure or poisoning is to ensure circulation and protect or establish an airway and breathing for adequate oxygenation. Oxygenation and intubation are recommended for obtunded or comatose patients if gastric lavage is considered. Once circulation, airway, and breathing have been established, the nearest poison control center should be contacted, the patient carefully examined (including a cautious search of clothing and belongings), and transfer arranged to the nearest emergency department. Poison control center personnel are able to help identify the chemical and guide appropriate treatment. The main poison control telephone number (800-222-1222) will direct callers to their specific regional centers, and all health care providers should be aware of the location of the main telephone number or the number of their regional poison control center.

Intravenous access should be obtained as soon as possible. Naloxone and thiamine are usually given immediately. Intravenous dextrose is administered if the patient is hypoglycemic. Physical examination findings may indicate the type of toxicologic emergency and expedite appropriate treatment. Vital signs and an ECG are particularly important because chemical exposures and poisonings may cause significant hypertension, hemodynamic instability, cardiac arrhythmias, conduction defects, respiratory depression, or coronary ischemia. It is essential to determine the patient's state of consciousness and presence of agitation; ocular, throat, or facial burns; and cardiopulmonary status. Toxin decontamination depends on the type of exposure and should be expeditious.

Ingestions

For ingestions, therapy depends on the material ingested. It is essential to check toxicologic clinical guidelines and poison control for specific recommendations based on the substance. Gastrointestinal decontamination through gastric lavage or with activated charcoal is rarely recommended, because all ingestion decontamination procedures are associated with potentially serious complications and in some instances are absolutely contraindicated (i.e., a hydrocarbon or corrosive substance).[9] Orogastric lavage (accomplished by insertion of an orogastric tube through the mouth to the stomach) may be acceptable for some ingestions (e.g., a potentially life-threatening amount of poison) and should be initiated within 60 minutes of ingestion and only by a provider skilled in the procedure.[1,9] The procedure often initiates vomiting in the victim; thus, adequate airway protection must always be ensured. Aspiration, esophageal or gastric perforation, and hypoxemia are some of the potential complications.

Though previously used in the management of poisoned patients, ipecac is no longer recommended, and in large or repeated doses, can cause toxicity.[9,10] Ipecac should be avoided in patients with a decreased level of consciousness and in patients who have[10] ingested a corrosive substance or hydrocarbon with high aspiration potential.[10]

The efficacy of activated charcoal is also controversial, though in specific situations can be used for gastrointestinal decontamination.[11] It can be taken orally or administered through an orogastric or nasogastric tube. The charcoal absorbs ingested substances, thereby reducing absorption by the gastrointestinal tract but is also associated with vomiting and aspiration, and is not helpful for caustic acids and alkalis, alcohols, petroleum distillates, lithium, iron, potassium, or heavy metals.[11] Caution and endotracheal intubation are necessary for unconscious patients.[11]

In specific circumstances, enhancing bowel motility to reduce the body's absorption of specific toxins may be indicated. Whole bowel irrigation with polyethylene glycol (e.g., GoLYTELY) may be helpful in selected poisonings (e.g.,

medications that are enteric coated or prepared for sustained release, alcohols, acids, alkalis, heavy metals, and body packer ingestions).[1,11]

Agitated patients with anticholinergic exposure will require sedation (e.g., lorazepam or haloperidol) to prevent rhabdomyolysis and hyperthermia.[11] Medications with anticholinergic effects should be avoided. Physostigmine, 0.5 to 1 mg IV, is appropriate for central and peripheral anticholinergic syndrome but not for tricyclic overdose.[11] Caution and discussion with a physician skilled in emergency medicine is necessary as is cardiac monitoring because asystole, bradycardia, heart block, and seizure activity are possible sequelae.[11]

Other treatments can include antidotes for specific poisons (e.g., acetylcysteine within 10 hours—as early as possible—for acetaminophen overdose)[11] or hemodialysis, which is beneficial for some drug overdoses (e.g., severe salicylate poisoning).[11]

Age is an important consideration in toxicologic emergencies because the treatment for an infant or child can differ from that for an adult. In addition, specific toxins have specific antidotes. The poison control center is the single best source to quickly determine these antidotes.

Skin Exposure

Most skin exposures to chemicals must be treated immediately with copious irrigation with water (i.e., "dilution is the solution to pollution"). Removal of saturated clothing and vigorous showering to wash the chemical off the skin with large quantities of water are essential to prevent further damage to the patient. Exposed areas should be irrigated for at least 15 to 30 minutes. This minimizes the time the offending agent is in direct contact with the skin, thus limiting the damage caused by the chemical agent. Provider caution during any decontamination procedure is strongly advised.

DISPOSITION AND REFERRAL

Once a patient's condition has been initially stabilized, he or she should be referred for definitive care. If the exposure has been minimal, follow-up with the primary care provider may be all that is necessary. Severe intoxication may warrant admission to the intensive care unit. Hospital admission should be considered if the extent of exposure is unknown or significant; this is especially true for older adults and the very young.

PATIENT AND FAMILY EDUCATION

Toxic and chemical exposure can be easily prevented by using appropriate personal protective equipment and correctly labeling, storing, and locking up potentially harmful agents. Patients should frequently be reminded to handle and to dispose of hazardous chemicals appropriately, and they should be able to recognize the signs and symptoms of chemical exposure: dizziness, headache, blurred vision, unsteady gait, clumsiness, poor coordination, difficulty breathing, nausea, abdominal cramping, skin discoloration or irritation, and eye or mucous membrane irritation. MSDSs are available online.

Careful storage of alcohol and medications (prescribed and over-the counter), should be discussed with all adults but especially parents and grandparents. All patients should also know how to dispose of medications safely. The National Take Back Drugs Initiative occurs twice a year, but some pharmacies and primary care practices also will take back drugs and dispose of them safely.

The telephone number for the local poison control center should be posted in everyprimary care office and near every home and business telephone for ready access if required. The U.S. national Poison Control helpline is 1-800-222-1222.

RESOURCES

U.S. Environmental Protection Agency: *Integrated risk information system*. Available at www.epa.gov/IRIS/.

REFERENCES

1. Dillon, B. E., & Morrissey, R. P. (2017). Poisoning. In C. Stone & R. L. Humphries (Eds.), *CURRENT diagnosis & treatment: Emergency medicine, 8e.* New York, NY: McGraw-Hill.

2. Heise, C., & LoVecchio, F. (2016). Hydrocarbons and volatile substances. In J. E. Tintinalli, J. Stapczynski, O. Ma, D. M. Yealy, G. D. Meckler, & D. M. Cline (Eds.), *Tintinalli's emergency medicine: A comprehensive study guide, 8e.* New York, NY: McGraw-Hill.

3. Occupational Safety and Health Administration. OSHA Hazard communication. Retrieved from https://www.osha.gov/dsg/hazcom/. (Accessed 3 December 2017).

4. Occupational Safety and Health Administration. Regulations standards. Retrieved from https://www.osha.gov/law-regs.html. (Accessed 3 December 2017).

5. Centers for Disease Control and Prevention.(2017). Prescription opioid overdose data. Retrieved from https://www.cdc.gov/drugoverdose/data/overdose.html. (Accessed 3 December 2017).

6. Greenberg, R. D., & Dippold, A. L. (2017). Eye emergencies. In C. Stone & R. L. Humphries (Eds.), *CURRENT diagnosis & treatment: Emergency medicine, 8e.* New York, NY: McGraw-Hill.

7. Morbidity and Mortality Weekly Report 1216 MMWR / November 10, 2017 / Vol. 66 / No. 44 US Department of Health and Human Services/Centers for Disease Control and Prevention Surveillance for Waterborne Disease Outbreaks Associated with Drinking Water—United States, 2013–2014 Katharine M. Benedict, DVM, PhD1,2; Hannah Reses, MPH2; Marissa Vigar, MPH2; David M. Roth, MSPH2; Virginia A. Roberts, MSPH2; Mia Mattioli, PhD2; Laura A. Cooley, MD3; Elizabeth D. Hilborn, DVM4; Timothy J. Wade, PhD4; Kathleen E. Fullerton, MPH2; Jonathan S. Yoder, MPH, MSW2; Vincent R. Hill, PhD2. Retrieved from https://www.cdc.gov/mmwr/volumes/66/wr/pdfs/mm6644-H.pdf.

8. Mycyk, M. B. (2014). Poisoning and drug overdose. In D. Kasper, A. Fauci, S. Hauser, D. Longo, J. Jameson, & J. Loscalzo (Eds.), *Harrison's principles of internal medicine, 19e.* New York, NY: McGraw-Hill.

9. Greene, S. (2016). General management of poisoned patients. In J. E. Tintinalli, J. Stapczynski, O. Ma, D. M. Yealy, G. D. Meckler, & D. M. Cline (Eds.), *Tintinalli's emergency medicine: A comprehensive study guide*, (8th ed.). New York, NY: McGraw-Hill.

10. Brunton, L. L., Hilal-Dandan, R., & Knollmann, B. C. (Eds.), (2018). *Goodman & Gilman's: The pharmacological basis of therapeutics*, (13th ed.). New York, NY: McGraw-Hill.

11. Olson, K. R. (2018). Poisoning. In M. A. Papadakis, S. J. McPhee, & M. W. Rabow (Eds.), *Current medical diagnosis & treatment 2018.* New York, NY: McGraw-Hill.

CHAPTER **27**

ELECTRICAL INJURIES
Terry Mahan Buttaro

 Immediate emergency department referral or physician consultation is indicated for patients with electrical injuries.

DEFINITION AND EPIDEMIOLOGY

Injuries from an electrical accident can be minor or can result in severe damage, electrocution, and even death. In the United States, there are approximately 1000 electricity-related deaths each year.[1] In 2015, 134 electrical fatalities were work-related;

most were related to electrocution and occurred in the construction industry.[1,2] Fortunately, work-related electrical deaths seem to be decreasing; unfortunately, electrical injuries and electrical fires continue. The actual number of accidental and environmental electrical injuries is uncertain, but the result of an electrical injury can be electricity-related trauma, burns, shock, seizures, cardiac arrhythmias, and respiratory arrest.[3]

Electrical injuries and death can be caused by lightning as well as low-voltage and high-voltage alternating or direct electrical current.[4] Household electrocutions and electrical injuries involve 110- or 220-V currents and are usually the result of failure to ground tools or appliances, the use of hair dryers or other electrical devices (e.g., plugged-in cell phones or curling irons) near water, and even electronic cigarettes.[5] A common cause of electrical injury in young children (<6 years) is oral or hand contact with electrical cords or wall sockets and the placement of conductive bodies in wall sockets,[1] while teens and young adults are injured climbing trees or poles.

Lightning is a common natural phenomenon that can cause injury in a variety of ways (e.g., directly striking an individual or indirectly causing injury by striking the ground or nearby area).[1] Fatality statistics associated with lightning strikes are varied and range from 50 to up to 500 each year.[1,3] Not all lightning strikes cause death, but the voltage is significantly greater and the sequelae different.

PATHOPHYSIOLOGY

Electrical injuries result from the direct effects of current and from the conversion of electrical energy into thermal energy as current passes through body tissues. Factors that determine the severity and distribution of injury include the type of current, voltage, amperage, tissue resistance, surface contacted, pathway of current, duration of contact, and other associated trauma.[1,3] Alternating current (AC), the more common cause of electrical injuries, is more dangerous than direct current (DC) because it can produce tetanic skeletal muscle contractions and prevent the victim from letting go of the energized source, thus increasing current delivery to the victim. AC voltage at 25 to 300 Hz and 25 to 220 V, the common household current level, can easily cause ventricular fibrillation if the pathway of the current includes the heart. Low-voltage contact, although potentially lethal, does not result in the magnitude of tissue necrosis seen with high-voltage injury. The voltage in a lightning strike is in the range of 10 million to 2 billion volts, but the duration of a lightning strike is short.

Heat generation is responsible for most burns seen with electrical injuries and is associated with high-voltage and electric-arc injuries, rather than low-voltage contact.[3] Heat damage is proportional to tissue resistance. Tissues with high fluid and electrolyte content conduct electrical current better than others do. Listed in decreasing order of magnitude of tissue necrosis are nerves, blood vessels, muscle, skin, tendon, fat, and bone. Nerve tissue has the least resistance to direct flow and therefore is most easily damaged. Electrical current passing through the head or crossing the thorax is more likely to cause respiratory arrest or ventricular fibrillation than is current passing through the leg. Skin, the initial barrier to current flow, is an effective insulator to deeper tissues. As current flows from the contact point, tissue with the least electrical resistance sustains the greatest current density and destructive injury. The most severe cutaneous and deep injuries are adjacent to contact sites, and the damage decreases with increasing distance from damage points.

CLINICAL PRESENTATION AND PHYSICAL EXAMINATION

Scene safety is paramount with any trauma, and there can be considerable risks if a natural disaster strikes a community and electricity is involved. Some patients will require scene resuscitation, and it is essential that all health care providers are aware of the risks involved when electrical wires are down.

The history of the patient's electrical injury (i.e., lightning or low- or high-voltage injury) is important to discern, as is the sequelae the patient experienced which could range from a transient unpleasant sensation to instantaneous death. Since the patient may be unable to relate what exactly occurred, bystander witness and first responder report is invaluable. Injuries from electricity occur by three mechanisms: (1) the direct effect of current on tissue; (2) the conversion of electrical energy to heat, causing burns; and (3) a mechanical injury caused by muscle contraction, falling, or a direct lightning strike. Cardiopulmonary arrest and fatal arrhythmias are primary causes of immediate fatalities from electrical injury and common in patients with high-voltage electrical and lightning injury. In lightning injuries, cardiac activity can spontaneously return, but chest wall paralysis is a possibility and an associated respiratory arrest and death is possible.[1] Common lightning-related sequelae include auditory and visual changes; hypertension; tachycardia; cardiac muscle necrosis; respiratory paralysis; burns; fractures; ruptured tympanic membrane; hyphema; vitreous hemorrhage; and injuries to the brain, spinal cord, peripheral nervous system, and vascular systems.[3]

Myoglobinuria is more often associated with high-voltage electrical injuries and indicates massive acute muscle necrosis and impending renal failure.[3] Disseminated intravascular coagulation can result from massive trauma. Neurologic deficits are sometimes evident immediately after the current exposure. However, complications such as reflex sympathetic dystrophy and motor neuron disease may not be readily apparent for days to months after the electrical trauma. Long bone fracture often occurs with falls, and fractures (particularly of the vertebral column) can result from tetanic muscle contraction at the time of electrocution.

The *physical examination* of any electrical injury requires a rapid, but thorough, evaluation as patient airways can be impacted and intubation may be indicated. The neck should initially be treated as being unstable and the neurologic exam assessment include cranial, spinal, or other neurological trauma and injury. The patient should always be completely undressed to determine entry and exit wounds, associated injuries (including scalp, hands, feet, etc.), and possible sequelae (e.g., compartment syndrome). Cardiopulmonary presentations vary, and patients can lack the characteristic chest discomfort indicative of myocardial ischemia, but arrhythmic conduction disturbances and infarct patterns can be present on the electrocardiogram (ECG). Abdominal injuries are also possible sequelae of an electrical injury, so careful examination and possibly imaging are necessary.[3] Transient, mild paresthesias and complete and irreversible impairment of sensory or motor function, or both, can be present in patients with electrical injuries. Absent pulses, decreased peripheral perfusion, and impaired neurologic function are also seen in patients with acute vascular complications from electrical trauma.

Circulatory integrity is best judged with Doppler ultrasound of distal peripheral pulses.

Injuries consistent with findings of blunt trauma to the head, spinal cord, and musculoskeletal, intrathoracic, and intra-abdominal areas are possible in patients who were thrown from the energized current source, had forceful tetanic muscle contractions associated with AC injuries, or fell after losing consciousness and muscle control.[3] Skin wounds are typically leathery or charred areas of full-thickness skin loss, but the size, degree, or even absence of burns does not exclude serious internal injury.[1] The entry and exit sites can be depressed, giving the appearance that current exploded the tissue. Underlying injury to a major muscle compartment is accompanied by edema formation.

Periodic reassessment will be necessary even if the initial assessments are within normal limits, because injury associated with high-voltage electricity can be delayed.[3]

DIAGNOSTICS

Initial studies include complete blood count (CBC), electrolytes, glucose, blood urea nitrogen (BUN), creatinine, coagulation profile, serum creatine phosphokinase, troponin I/T, myoglobin level, urinalysis, and arterial blood gas (ABG) analysis.[1,3] A 12-lead ECG and continuous cardiac monitoring are necessary for all patients with electrical injury. Fetal monitoring is necessary if the victim is pregnant. Patients with suspected spinal injuries should undergo cervical spine radiography. Other imaging studies are indicated to exclude fracture if localized edema and pain are present. Consideration of other diagnostic studies should be coordinated with the consulting specialists.

INITIAL DIAGNOSTICS

Electrical Injuries

INITIAL
- ECG

LABORATORY
- Complete blood count and differential
- Serum glucose, electrolytes, blood urea nitrogen, creatinine
- Coagulation studies
- Arterial blood gases

- Serum creatine phosphokinase
- Creatine kinase muscle-brain fraction
- Myoglobin
- Urinalysis

IMAGING
- As indicated by physical examination findings

DIFFERENTIAL DIAGNOSIS

Priority differentials of an electrical injury include cardiopulmonary arrest, arrhythmias, peripheral neuropathies, seizures, cerebral vascular accident, syncope, and nonelectrical trauma or burns. The diagnosis of electrical injury may be unclear, particularly in unwitnessed cases in which the victim is confused, amnestic, or unconscious or if external signs of injury are absent. Circumstances surrounding the electrical injuries should also be sought to determine the possible mechanism of the injury. Precipitating factors such as intoxication, suicidal intention, or foul play should be considered.

A person struck by lightning may appear to be comatose or dead and have no physical injury. Other lightning victims may be close by with a similar appearance. After ensuring that the environment is safe (e.g., no downed power lines), immediate resuscitation is advised because the person likely is in respiratory or cardiac arrest.

The Taser is a conducted electrical weapon used by law enforcement to subdue violent or dangerous individuals. Injuries associated with the use of Tasers are generally mild skin burns, but serious injuries, including fractures, injuries to the face or eyes, and head injuries related to falls are possible.[3] Death from cardiac arrest has also been reported.[3] The use of conducted electrical weapons is not recommended for pregnant women, individuals with low body weight, or those with obvious medical issues such as seizures.

Interprofessional Collaborative Management

Emergency room evaluation, hospitalization, and prompt specialist consultation are indicated and dependent on each patient's injuries. All patients who have lost consciousness or sustained cardiac or respiratory arrest as well as those with ischemic chest pain, myoglobinuria, or significant burn wounds should be hospitalized. Referral to a burn center is often necessary for electrical burns because considerable injury to deeper neurovascular and musculoskeletal structures may not be obvious until several days after the injury.

INITIAL STABILIZATION AND MANAGEMENT

Patients who have experienced an electrical injury are treated as trauma patients. Immediate priorities include restoration of circulation, airway, and breathing (i.e., basic life support and advanced cardiac life support).[6] The cervical spine should be immobilized and the airway secured while respiration is supported, with adequate oxygenation and stabilization of circulation if required. Cardiopulmonary resuscitation must be initiated, and the emergency medical services system should be activated.[6] Defibrillation is indicated for ventricular tachycardia or ventricular fibrillation, and early intubation is recommended for patients with facial or neck burns.[6] Continued thermal damage can be limited by removal of affected clothing. Intravascular volume is initially managed per the Parkland formula.[3] Increased intravenous fluid resuscitation and monitoring of serum electrolytes, serum pH, and urine output (goal 1 to 2 mL/kg/h) is indicated if myoglobinuria develops.[3]

Wound care involves treatment of both cutaneous and the resultant deep soft tissue injuries related to entry wounds and burns. Consultation with a surgeon is recommended to evaluate the need for formal wound exploration, debridement, and, if compartment syndrome is suspected, fasciotomy.[3] Tetanus prophylaxis should be updated. Management of other complications resulting from electrical trauma generally follows standard emergency therapy.

PATIENT AND FAMILY EDUCATION

All discharged patients should have reliable home support. Patients should be advised to return immediately to their health care provider if any symptoms occur. A specific follow-up visit should be arranged with a health care provider familiar with electrical injuries, and patients should receive careful explanation of the injury and recuperative process.

HEALTH PROMOTION

Open sockets and outlets must be covered with childproof devices, and children must be watched carefully. Older children should be aware of the dangers of climbing near high-tension wires. Plug-in electrical appliances should be kept away from water sources. Safety education reminders regarding downed electrical poles and wires during storms and before natural disasters is important. Community education programs, particularly at school and at work, are necessary to help prevent accidents. Safety standards in industry and in the community must be constantly updated and enforced.

REFERENCES

1. Foris, L. A., & Huecker, M. R. Electrical Injuries. [Updated 2017 Oct 9]. In: StatPearls [Internet]. Treasure Island (FL): StatPearls Publishing.
2. Electrical Safety Foundation International. Workplace fatalities and injuries 2003–2015. Retrieved from http://www.esfi.org/resource/workplace-fatalities-and-injuries-2003-2015-571. (Accessed 11 December 2017).
3. Bailey, C. (2016). Electrical and lightning injuries. In J. E. Tintinalli, J. Stapczynski, O. Ma, D. M. Yealy, G. D. Meckler, & D. M. Cline (Eds.), *Tintinalli's emergency medicine: A comprehensive study guide* (8th ed.). New York, NY: McGraw-Hill.
4. Nemer, J. A., & Juarez, M. A. (2018). Disorders related to environmental emergencies. In M. A. Papadakis, S. J. McPhee, & M. W. Rabow (Eds.), *Current medical diagnosis & treatment.* New York, NY: McGraw-Hill.
5. Campbell, R. (2016). Electronic cigarettes, explosions and fires. The 2015 Experience. National Fire Protection Association. Retrieved from http://www.nfpa.org/News-and-Research/Fire-statistics-and-reports/Fire-statistics/Fire-causes/Electrical-and-consumer-electronics/Electronic-Cigarette-Explosions-and-Fires-The-2015-Experience. (Accessed 11 December 2017).
6. Vanden Hoek, T. L., Morrison, L. J., Shuster, M., et al. (2010). Cardiac arrest in special situations: 2010 American Heart Association guidelines for cardiopulmonary resuscitation and emergency cardiovascular care. *Circulation, 122*(18 Suppl. 3), S829–S861.

CHAPTER **28**

ENVIRONMENTAL AND FOOD ALLERGIES

John Distler

 Immediate referral to an emergency department and/or allergy practice is required in cases of severe urticaria, anaphylaxis, and uncontrolled asthma that does not respond to home or in-office bronchodilation.

ENVIRONMENTAL ALLERGIES

DEFINITION AND EPIDEMIOLOGY

Environmental allergens are responsible for a wide range of atopic signs and symptoms including rhinitis, eczema, urticaria, and bronchospasm to anaphylaxis. With repeated exposure, immediate type 1 hypersensitivity reactions may occur through the development of immunoglobulin E (IgE). Allergens can be found both indoors and outdoors and fluctuate among households, with the change of seasons, weather patterns including heat and humidity, and by the area in which one lives in the United States. Common indoor allergens include dust mites, indoor molds, and animal dander. The more common outdoor allergens are pollen (i.e., grass, trees, and weeds) and outdoor molds, including mold smuts in wheat, corn, oat, and barley fields.[1] The incidence of environmental allergies with subsequent symptom development has been on the rise.[2] Allergic rhinitis may affect up to 20% of the US population and up to 40% of children.[1] Atopic dermatitis was found to have a direct cost to the US health care system ranging from $1 to $4 billion, with an average cost per patient of approximately $609.[3] The potential psychosocial effects of atopic dermatitis are also staggering.

Allergic rhinitis is often considered the first step in the development of allergic asthma.[4] The Centers for Disease Control and Prevention (CDC) reported a steady increase in the development of asthma in both adults and children from 2001 to 2010.[5] However, symptom development may be secondary to other non–IgE-mediated environmental factors, such as urbanization, toxins, air pollution, viral illness, exercise, cold air, and tobacco smoke exposure.[1] Occupational exposure has also become an increasingly important patient consideration.[6] It is important to make the clinical distinction between a true IgE-mediated cause and those symptoms that result in irritation and subsequent inflammation of the mucous membranes in the nose, lungs, and skin.[7]

PATHOPHYSIOLOGY

With repeated exposure to an environmental allergen through the respiratory tract, genetically predisposed people begin to develop IgE as an inappropriate means to protect the body from the protein allergen (antigen). Antigen-specific T cells are activated through the lymphatic system in response to the antigen. The activated antigen-specific T cells then activate B cells, and IgE is created in lymphoid tissue or at local tissue sites.[3,8] The newly created antigen-specific IgE is released by plasma cells and binds to high-affinity IgE receptors located on the basophils and mast cells. This leads to the sensitization of the cells in the tissues of the nose, lung, or skin.[4,8]

Although other immunoglobulins, such as IgG, IgA, and IgM, are produced that appropriately protect the body, circulating levels of IgE and the attachment of the allergen to target cells is responsible for the atopic reaction.[8] With repeated exposure and further sensitization, IgE binds with the antigen protein and degranulation of the mast cells and basophils begins, starting the allergic cascade. Mediators, including histamine, proteoglycans, enzymes, cytokines, and many others, are released as a result of the degranulation. The chain in the release of mediators is responsible for the immediate and late-phase responses of the cells. Histamine may be fully released within 30 minutes of degranulation, whereas cytokines may be released over many hours.[1,8,9] Depending upon the allergen, the reaction may be immediate (e.g., animal dander), and others more delayed (up to 4 hours; e.g., grass, trees, weeds). Reactions that occur days after exposure are rarely IgE mediated.[8]

Atopic diseases are typically genetically determined, yet individual responses to antigen exposure are also based on environmental factors and susceptibility of the host as well. For instance, the timing of the exposure to an allergen may affect the exposure response. High-level exposure to allergens early on may predispose a person to develop a more severe atopic response. The period of sensitivity is highly variable among people. Some may exhibit symptoms after one exposure, while others require multiple exposures until the onset of symptoms.[8] In addition, exposure to cigarette smoke and pathogens may also alter the body's immune response, modifying the level of IgE activation.

COMMON ENVIRONMENTAL ALLERGENS

Recurrent exposure to an environmental allergen and subsequent sensitization result in the typical presenting signs and symptoms of patients with a genetically determined atopic disorder. Environmental allergens may be either indoor or outdoor and are influenced by a variety of factors.

Common indoor allergens include molds, dust mites, cockroaches, and animal dander. Prominent indoor molds include *Penicillium*, *Alternaria*, *Cladosporium*, and *Aspergillus*. Indoor molds are fungi and are found in warm, moist, and humid environments of bathrooms, basements, and laundry rooms.[10] Molds thrive in these conditions and spread through the production of spores. The mold spores become airborne in certain conditions, resulting in exposure to the host. Molds are hearty in that they can survive environmental conditions adverse to their growth, such as dry air and exposure to sunshine. No growth occurs under these conditions, but molds also do not die. Dust mites are microscopic relatives of the spider and are common in all households. Two common dust mites responsible for triggering of an atopic reaction are *Dermatophagoides pteronyssinus* and *Dermatophagoides farinae*. Like molds, dust mites also thrive in warm, moist environments; they survive through the ingestion of flakes of skin from humans and live in bedding, mattresses, carpets, curtains, and upholstered furniture.[10] The total eradication of dust mites from the home is impossible. Pet dander is created by the oil glands, saliva, and urine of animals, not the fur. In combination, these excreted substances become allergenic to some individuals. An important consideration for patients with animal dander allergy is that dander is a sticky allergen and may remain in the home weeks or months after an animal has been removed. Cat dander and dog dander are among the most common allergens in schools, brought in by students with an animal in their home.[10] Animals such as rabbits, gerbils, hamsters, guinea pigs, horses, and cows are also potentially allergenic, depending on exposure. Cockroaches are another indoor allergen and can cause severe asthma reactions in children living in crowded urban environments and older dwellings. The allergenic protein that cockroaches create is from their saliva and feces.[10]

Outdoor allergens consist mainly of pollen from trees, grass, and weeds in addition to molds and mold smuts. Tree pollen, grass pollen, and weed pollen are the only seasonal environmental allergens. The pollination season varies from one area of the United States to another. In the spring, trees are typically the first to shed their pollen. Southern states may have detectable levels of tree pollen as early as late January, whereas northern states may not have measurable levels until May or June. Not all tree pollen is allergenic. Trees that release allergenic pollen include oak, elm, maple, hickory, poplar, willow, box elder, and walnut.[10] In some southern states, pine trees may cause an IgE mediated reaction in patients, while in the northern states they are less likely to cause symptoms.

As with trees, only a small number of the many species of grass are allergenic. For the most part, grass pollen season tends to follow tree season, and again the variability is dependent on the area of the United States. Some common grasses that release allergic pollen are Kentucky bluegrass, Johnson grass, Bermuda grass, orchard grass, sweet vernal grass, and timothy. Grass pollen levels are affected by temperature, moisture, humidity, and time of day. Weeds are typically fall pollen producers and may begin to pollinate as early as August and into November, depending on the type of weed and location in the United States. Common allergenic weeds include ragweed, pigweed, plantain, sheep's sorrel, sagebrush, and lamb's quarters. Like grass pollen counts, weed pollen counts are higher at dawn and dusk and also on hot, dry, windy days.[10] Flower pollens are rarely allergenic because their pollen is heavier and is dispersed by insects that carry the pollen from plant to plant.[9] Outdoor molds tend to be more allergenic than indoor molds. Common outdoor molds include *Alternaria*, *Hormodendrum*, and *Cladosporium*. *Alternaria* is a common mold that can be brought indoors by humans and pets. Like indoor molds, outdoor molds produce spores for growth and are found commonly on fallen leaves and rotting vegetation. Mold smuts grow in the soil and roots of wheat, corn, oat, and barley fields. Mold counts tend to be higher from July into late summer, depending on the geographic location. In the colder months, mold becomes dormant but does not die with snow or frost. When it is covered with snow or ice, mold is less likely to release its spores into the wind.[10] Therefore a warmer, more humid late fall and early winter may produce more mold spores.

CLINICAL PRESENTATION AND PHYSICAL EXAMINATION

Patients with environmental allergies may have a variety of signs and symptoms. Typical presenting signs and symptoms include rhinitis, eczema, urticaria, bronchospasm, and anaphylaxis.[1] Exposure to environmental allergens may also exacerbate other non–IgE-mediated symptoms as discussed previously. The combination of IgE mediated and non–IgE-mediated triggers increases a patient's likelihood of symptom exacerbation.

A cause-and-effect relationship must be determined; a patient may have rhinitis because of grass pollen, bronchospasm from cat exposure, or urticaria from dust mite sensitivity.[11] An important diagnostic consideration is to determine whether a patient's symptoms are seasonal or perennial or both. A patient may live with dust mite sensitivity and have subclinical symptoms, yet their symptoms become bothersome only during the spring when the seasonal flare results in further IgE activation. Similarly, patients may become symptomatic only in the winter when doors and windows are closed and their exposure to dust mites and animal dander increases. Understanding of the patient's individualized IgE activation triggers and the environmental timing is essential in helping patients control their symptoms.

A detailed history is required to determine a cause-and-effect relationship of environmental allergen exposure and the development of symptoms. Standard history questions include current medications, medication allergies, past medical history, family history, and surgeries and hospitalizations. In addition, further atopy, including the potential for stinging insect venom allergy and food allergies, must be understood; the presence of these conditions may trigger further IgE activation, potentially increasing a patient's physical response.

To understand the entire allergic presentation, additional questions must be asked about the environment. The type of home in which one lives and the age of the dwelling may indicate the potential for mold or cockroaches. Heating and cooling sources must be identified because the use of forced hot air may add to the disbursement of dust mite and animal dander. Radiant heat may increase the humidity of the home, resulting in an increase in mold spore production and dust mites. The presence of a crawl space or unfinished damp basement may also increase the potential for indoor mold. Dust mites may be present in bed linens, older pillows, mattresses, and stuffed animals. The frequency of laundering of bed linens must also be recorded. Determination of the number and type of animals in the home and the area of the house in which they are allowed is essential. Recent renovations to the home could modify mold or dust mite exposure. Ideally, the humidity in the home should be 35% to 40% to decrease indoor mold spore growth and to control dust mite propagation.[3]

A thorough physical examination must be performed after the environmental allergy history. The examination should always include a careful head, eyes, ears, nose, and throat (HEENT) examination to look for allergic symptoms of the nose and eyes, including sclera erythema and injection, allergic shiners from venous engorgement, swollen pink nasal turbinates, and tonsillar enlargement. Small, nontender movable posterior cervical nodes in the neck are a common finding in children. Direct visualization of the skin with ambient lighting should be performed to look for cutaneous symptoms of urticaria and eczema. Encouraging the patient and parents to take pictures of the cutaneous response would also be helpful in cases of intermittent symptoms. A complete cardiopulmonary exam is required. Pulmonary function tests (PFTs) should be performed, if they are available, to look for reversibility (obstructive versus restrictive disease) of symptoms and PFT results after bronchodilation. An abdominal examination should also be conducted for each patient, looking for other diagnostic clues.

DIAGNOSTICS
Essential Diagnostics

- Skin testing
  - A skin prick test (SPT) can be performed by either the scratch or intradermal method. Both histamine and normal saline controls are placed on patients at the time of testing. The reaction to histamine must be positive and the reaction to saline negative to ensure reliability of the test results.[12]
  - Certain medications, such as antihistamines, H_2 blockers, and tricyclic antidepressants, must be discontinued for up to 5 days before skin testing because these may interfere with test result reliability.
  - Skin tests are placed on the back, upper arm, or ventral surface of the forearms, depending on the amount of testing to be performed and the age of the patient.[13] The use of the back in children is recommended because pruritus from a positive test result may make the patient scratch the area. Scratching of the area may mix allergens placed on the skin, interfering with evaluation of the results. Results are read within 15 to 20 minutes.
  - Scratch testing involves scratching the surface of the skin with a single stylus for each allergen.[12] This form of allergy testing is safer, more rapid, and less uncomfortable to patients than intradermal testing but is not as sensitive as intradermal testing. Depending on the practice, providers may begin with scratch testing and proceed to

intradermal testing if the results are negative.[13] Scratch testing is also associated with a lower potential for anaphylaxis than intradermal testing.

- Intradermal testing is more sensitive and reproducible than scratch testing. This test involves the use of a 25-gauge needle with a small drop of allergen (0.02 to 0.05 mL) placed beneath the skin.[9] Depending on the practice and the type of allergen, the concentration placed beneath the skin may be 1:10 or as high as 1:1000.[12] If the patient reacts to the allergen, that particular allergen (e.g., grass pollen) is not tested further, and the test result is considered positive. If the test result is negative, higher concentrations are used. A stepwise approach to intradermal testing should be taken to ensure safe patient outcomes. All providers and staff must be trained to handle any potential systemic reactions, including urticaria, bronchospasm, and full anaphylaxis.
- **Serum IgE levels** may be of benefit in some patients such as those with dermographism, multiple tattoos, and uncooperative pediatric patients. However, the results are not reliable for definitive diagnosis as the results may be falsely positive or negative as a result of cross-reactivity of multiple allergens.

DIFFERENTIAL DIAGNOSIS

The differential diagnoses for atopic rhinitis, eczema, urticaria, bronchospasm, and anaphylaxis are extensive and may require additional referrals to a dermatologist, otolaryngologist, or pulmonologist for further workup.[11] Some of the more common differential diagnoses in order of priority include vasomotor rhinitis, idiopathic urticaria, and non-allergic asthma. The diagnosis can be determined by the history, the causal relationship, response to treatment, and the results of allergy testing. Urticaria or eczema may be more difficult to diagnose, and biopsy may be indicated to confirm the diagnosis.[11] Discontinuation of the potential offending agent (e.g., removal of animals and other control measures) is also diagnostic. Depending on the results of the workup, allergy immunotherapy may be indicated.

INTERPROFESSIONAL COLLABORATIVE MANAGEMENT
Non-Pharmacologic Management

Control of reactions to seasonal pollen from trees and grass in the spring and weeds in the summer and fall can be effective with use of simple measures. It is essential that patients keep their windows closed and air conditioning (seasonally) on during periods of high pollen counts, especially from 5 AM to 10 AM.[10] Pollen easily enters the screens of windows and is deposited on furniture and bedding.[14] Therefore, bed linens should be changed weekly and washed in hot water.

High-efficiency particulate air (HEPA) filters can be used in bedrooms and living areas. Patients should also be encouraged to shower and change their clothes when coming in from the outside. Clothes should be dried in an automatic dryer, not outdoors.

Outdoor mold exposure can be decreased by avoiding areas of decaying plants, rotting leaves, and other debris. Wearing a mask when working outside might also be of benefit. Indoor mold can best be controlled by increasing light and ventilation in damp areas of the home and by keeping the humidity levels between 35% and 40%. This also helps control dust mite growth. Diluted bleach can be used in bathrooms to remove mold and mildew from surfaces.

Dehumidifiers in the basement and other potentially moist areas of the home help remove dampness.[14] Indoor plants may also contain mold in the soil, but the spores become airborne only if the soil is disturbed.

The control of dust mite sensitivity is focused on the bedroom because of the time spent in that room. Hardwood floors are best, with no scatter rugs or clutter. Carpets should be vacuumed routinely with use of a HEPA cleaner. Pillows should be hypoallergenic and both the pillow and mattress covered with hypoallergenic covers. Stuffed animals and books should be covered in the room in storage bins. Homes with forced hot air and central air conditioning should have the filters changed every 2 to 3 weeks.

Patients with animal dander sensitivity can be more difficult to treat if the family's decision is to keep the pet. Pets must be kept out of the patient's room at all times, and a HEPA filter should be run in the bedroom. Because animal dander is sticky, bedclothes should be clean before entering the bedroom. Washing the hands and face after pet exposure is also advised.[10]

It is imperative to control a patient's exposure to environmental allergens that cause an atopic reaction, but non-allergic triggers can also add to the clinical picture. Exposure to cigarette smoke in the home or vehicle can cause exacerbations of rhinitis or asthma and should be prohibited. Air pollution including perfumes, paints, carpet off-gassing, diesel or other industrial fumes, or wood smoke can cause reactions. Weather conditions, such as hot, humid days or extremes of cold temperatures, can also exacerbate symptoms.[9] Patients should be advised of these non-allergic triggers and their potential for increasing symptoms. Finally, viral syndromes can also exacerbate symptoms of rhinorrhea and asthma.

Pharmacologic Management

In addition to prescriptive and over-the counter (OTC) medications used to treat allergic rhinitis, urticaria, and asthma, subcutaneous desensitization may further enhance management of patient's symptoms. Subcutaneous injections to desensitize patients to environmental allergies (allergy immunotherapy) began in 1911.[15] Before that, an oral route was used. Desensitization may prevent the development of allergic asthma in patients with allergic rhinitis.[15] Allergy immunotherapy is proposed to work through the lymphocyte response by decreasing the T-cell response to the allergen. Mast cell and eosinophil responses are decreased by upregulation of antigen-specific T-regulatory cells. IgG4 antibodies that are protective to the body may be produced and inhibit basophil histamine release. The result is a decrease in the binding mechanism of the antigen to IgE and therefore the inhibition of the allergic cascade.

Allergy immunotherapy is started with weekly injections of allergens according to the results of skin testing. Depending on the practice, dilutions of either 1:1000 or 1:10,000 are given in minute quantities (e.g., 0.05 mL). The amount is increased weekly until the patient reaches the maintenance dose, typically within 4 to 6 months.[15] If a patient has a reaction to the dose, the next dose is typically decreased, and it is only increased once the patient tolerates it without reaction. Once this dose is reached, maintenance continues for 4 to 6 years on an every 2- to 3-week schedule. Patients must remain in the office for 20 minutes after their allergy injection to be sure that they do not have a significant reaction. Patients must also be advised that there is a potential for delayed reactions and must be given instructions for intervention should this occur.[14] Rush schedules are also used in some settings; however, the probability of systemic reactions is much greater than with standard therapy.

Allergy immunotherapy is contraindicated in patients with poorly controlled, severe persistent asthma and in those with comorbid conditions, such as unstable angina or uncontrolled hypertension. Patients taking beta blockers are also not candidates for allergy immunotherapy because these medications can block the effect of epinephrine if it is given as a result of a systemic side effect.[14]

Sublingual therapy, another form of allergy immunotherapy, has been used in Europe with some documented positive results.[15] Data available in the United States on the efficacy of sublingual therapy show mixed results and are limited in terms of patient outcomes. There is less standardization of sublingual extract than of intradermal extract.[16] Therefore, results of studies cannot be used for extracts manufactured in the United States. The Food and Drug Administration has approved two forms of sublingual tablets as immunotherapy to treat both grass and ragweed pollen allergic rhinitis symptoms with or without conjunctivitis. Treatment is initiated at least 12 weeks before the expected onset of the pollen season and continues throughout the season. The dose is 1 tablet daily under the tongue. The initial dose of the sublingual tablet must be given under the supervision of trained medical personnel, and patients must remain in the practice for 30 minutes after the initial dose.[16]

Management of environmental allergies depends on the patient's presenting signs and symptoms in addition to the results of the allergy workup. In the primary care practice, management begins with environmental control and appropriate medications. Antihistamines including the non-sedating forms, steroid nasal sprays, topical steroids for skin reactions, and oral steroids for severe reactions are commonly used medications. Asthma may need to be diagnosed and treated (see Chapter 85). Patients whose symptoms are not controlled with these initial actions may need to be referred to an allergy practice for consideration of allergy immunotherapy, especially if perennial or seasonal flares are severe.

Indications for Referral and Hospitalization

Specialty Consultation. When environmental control and medications are not controlling a patient's symptoms, a referral to an allergy practice may be indicated.[15] This is especially true if the patient has more than one atopic disorder, such as allergic rhinitis and allergic asthma, or if there is also the potential for food or stinging insect sensitivity.

Skin testing can be performed in patients with atopic disorders. However, desensitization can be performed only in patients with environmental allergies and stinging insect sensitivity, not food allergies. Referral to an allergy, asthma, and immunology specialist will assist in determining true IgE sensitization and therefore a management plan that is tailored to the patient's specific sensitivities. Hospitalization may be required for some atopic patients such as urticaria that requires parenteral steroids and has been unresponsive to oral medication management. In addition, hospitalization is required for patients with bronchospasm that does not respond to home or office bronchodilation or in cases with suspected comorbidity

including sinopulmonary infections such as asthmatic bronchitis or pneumonia. This is especially more common in the pediatric and geriatric population.[12]

COMPLICATIONS

Complications of allergy immunotherapy are cause for concern and must be treated appropriately. Allergy extract must be checked for its expiration date as well as to make certain that the right patient is receiving the correct dose. Documentation of reactions to allergy immunization must be performed routinely, and patients must be given clear instructions on what to expect from their allergy immunotherapy as well as potential side effects and systemic reactions. Providers and staff must be thoroughly trained to effectively deal with systemic reactions in their practices.

PATIENT AND FAMILY EDUCATION

- Much of what has been discussed in the section on management must be given to the patient in written format, and the patient should verbalize understanding of these avoidance modalities. This should be performed at each subsequent patient encounter to ensure continued proper treatment.
- Medications used in the treatment of rhinitis, eczema, urticaria, bronchospasm, and anaphylaxis must be reviewed at each visit.
- Emergency action plans in the case of systemic reactions must be reviewed and documented at each patient visit. Those in allergy specialty practices must be certain that communication with the primary care provider is ongoing and up to date to prevent duplicate services.

FOOD ALLERGIES

DEFINITION AND EPIDEMIOLOGY

The incidence of food allergies in children has risen dramatically over the past decade. In 2010, the CDC reported that 5 of every 100 children in the Unites States had some form of food allergy.[5] An 18% increase was reported from 1997 to 2007 for children younger than 18 years. From 2006 to 2008, hospital discharge rates for children with a food allergy–related diagnosis were nearly 9500 per year. In addition, children with food allergies were also more likely to have other IgE-mediated disorders such as asthma, allergic rhinitis, and eczema.[17]

Although an allergy may develop to a wide variety of foods, 90% of all allergic reactions occur from the ingestion of just eight foods. These foods are cow's milk, hen eggs, peanuts, tree nuts, fish, shellfish, soy, and wheat.[18] Whereas these eight foods are responsible for the majority of reactions, cow's milk, hen eggs, and peanuts account for nearly 80% of these reactions in children.[3] In adults, shellfish, peanuts, tree nuts, and fish are the more common allergens.[19]

While these eight foods are responsible for the majority of atopic reactions in children and adults, other foods may also cause symptoms with a much lower incidence rate.[18]

The allergic reactions patients may exhibit range from rhinorrhea to full anaphylaxis.[20] Other possible reactions include asthma exacerbations, eczema, urticaria, gastrointestinal pain, and possibly nausea and vomiting. Patients may also exhibit a combination of symptoms caused by specific foods (e.g., eczema to milk and anaphylaxis to peanuts). Adults are less likely to develop food allergies later in life as compared to children. Many children tend to outgrow their allergic reactions to some foods within the first decade of life. Nearly two-thirds of children with egg allergy will outgrow the allergy by 5 years of age. With milk allergy, 85% to 90% will no longer have an allergic response after 3 years of age.[17] In children, only 20% tend to outgrow their allergy to peanuts by 6 years of age. Peanuts, tree nuts, and shellfish have a higher incidence of lifetime allergy.[21]

PATHOPHYSIOLOGY

The development of food sensitivity is dependent on many factors. After ingestion of the food, the body undergoes an abnormal response through the mucosal immune system. The mucosal immune system "sees" a large quantity of food and in genetically predisposed people develops an inappropriate immune response to the protein antigens present in foods.[22] The breakdown or lack of development of oral tolerance starts the sensitivity process, resulting in food-specific IgE production. IgE-mediated interactions occur with mast cells and basophils on target organs.

Once stimulated by further food protein ingestion, IgE antibodies bind the food protein antigen to high-affinity FcεRI receptors on mast cells and basophils and low-affinity FcεRII receptors on macrophages, monocytes, lymphocytes, eosinophils, and platelets.[23] As in other IgE-mediated disorders, inflammatory mediators are released including histamine, prostaglandins, leukotrienes, and cytokines. The inflammatory cascade continues with vasodilatation, smooth muscle contraction, mucus secretion, and potential for petechial hemorrhage. Specific symptoms result depending on the target organ affected.[22]

This period of increasing sensitivity is highly variable among patients. Reactions do not occur until the immune response has developed to a degree that the IgE levels are elevated sufficiently to cause some form of allergic reaction. In some patients, a reaction may occur after the second ingestion; others may need 100 or more exposures to develop an allergic response.[23]

DIAGNOSTICS

Prior to age 5 or 6, in most pediatric patients with persistent rhinorrhea, eczema, or urticaria, the condition is secondary to food allergies as their exposure to IgE-mediated environmental triggers has not resulted in IgE production. At this age, asthma is commonly caused by non-allergic triggers such as viral syndrome. The diagnosis is based on the patient's history of food ingestion and the subsequent field reaction, SPT, and the results of ImmunoCAP laboratory testing.[20,21]

Essential Diagnostics

SPT is performed at the scratch level (i.e., the strongest dilution scratched on the skin). A positive SPT results in erythema, pruritus, and elevation at the test site with both a flare and wheal.[24] Histamine and saline controls are placed simultaneously on another area of the body (e.g., the back or upper arms). Readings of SPTs are done 15 minutes after placement. The histamine should cause a positive reaction and the saline should cause no reaction for the results to be considered reliable.

It is important that patients be reminded to stop all antihistamines, H_2 blockers, and tricyclic antidepressants before testing, because these will interfere with the allergic response.

Negative SPT reactions are most likely accurate, and SPT is more sensitive than serum IgE ImmunoCAP testing. Positive results may be falsely positive, indicating patient tolerance. IgE levels may also be elevated because of a cross-reactivity of environmental pollen and food proteins.

An important clinical pearl is that patients are allergic to a food only if they develop symptoms after ingestion. If the skin test and/or ImmunoCAP indicates a positive result and the patient eats the food routinely without reaction, then this indicates clinical tolerance.[23]

When testing for potential food allergies, it is essential that a careful dietary history be obtained. If the patient rarely or never ingests a particular food, it is highly unlikely that he or she is allergic to the food protein. The body must "see" the food in sufficient quantity to build up the IgE–food protein response.

Additional Diagnostics

Component-resolved diagnostics (CRD) testing can also be considered in the diagnosis of food allergies. This serum blood test provides a molecular view of the individual protein components of an allergenic source. This allows valuable knowledge of IgE sensitization patterns to specific allergen components and cross-reactive allergen components.[25]

DIFFERENTIAL DIAGNOSES

Nearly 20% to 25% of parents believe that their child has a food allergy based on observed signs and symptoms. However, the actual prevalence is much lower, with approximately 4% of adults and 6% to 8% of children affected. Therefore, it is important to distinguish a true IgE-mediated allergic reaction from adverse food reactions.[20,21]

The differential diagnoses of IgE-mediated food allergies include:
- Cell-mediated food hypersensitivities such as food-induced enterocolitis and colitis, malabsorption syndrome, and celiac disease.
- Dietary protein–induced enterocolitis or colitis is seen in infants from 1 week to 3 months of age after milk and soy ingestion. Symptoms typically resolve by 1 to 2 years of age as the child develops tolerance.
- Malabsorption syndrome is also self-limited but may result in failure to thrive (FTT). In addition to milk and soy, wheat is also commonly implicated in this disorder. Resolution is typical by 6 to 18 months of age.[22]
- Celiac disease results in FTT and is often lifelong. The offending foods with celiac disease include wheat, rye, and barley.
- Other non–IgE-mediated food intolerances include lactase deficiency, psychological aversions to particular foods, and toxic reactions to foods (e.g., sulfites, aspartame).[22,26]

INTERPROFESSIONAL COLLABORATIVE MANAGEMENT
Non-Pharmacologic Management

Once the diagnosis of food allergy has been made, the mainstay of therapy involves strict removal of all foods causing allergic reactions. The majority of patients have an IgE-mediated allergy to one food. In others, multiple foods may be allergenic, especially in patients younger than 5 years. The literature also makes note of food families—for example, legumes include peanuts, string beans, and peas. Although a patient may develop an allergy to one food in the food family, it is unlikely that one would be allergic to all foods in the same family.

Two exceptions to food family allergies include tree nuts and crustaceans (i.e., shrimp, crab, and lobster). Patients may react clinically to only one food in the family; however, because of the high allergenicity of these foods and potential for anaphylaxis, patients should be advised to avoid all foods in the family. It is also imperative to point out that the protein in tree nuts is entirely different from the protein in peanuts. An allergic response to one does not indicate an allergy to both foods.[19]

Strict avoidance of foods must be considered a therapeutic intervention. When recommending the avoidance of a food, it is imperative that an alternative be recommended.[21] In children, coordinated efforts must be in place with the patient's primary care provider to be certain that there is appropriate height and weight gain. The nutritional requirements for patients with food allergies are not different from those without food allergies. When withholding foods as a result of an allergy, one must consider total calories, carbohydrates, fat, and protein requirements, as well as minerals and vitamins. Consultation with a registered dietitian may be required.[21]

The length of time a food must be avoided to produce tolerance is dependent on the severity of the reaction, the patient's age, and the results of SPT and serum IgE testing. In children with milk, egg, or wheat allergy who have rhinorrhea or eczema, withholding the food for 3 to 6 months may result in clinical tolerance. Reintroduction of foods one at a time is required as parents monitor symptoms. The return of symptoms necessitates further food avoidance. With egg allergy, it is best to have the patient eat egg in cooked and baked products as a means of developing tolerance.[21]

Patients who have more severe symptoms such as urticaria, facial swelling, or anaphylaxis may require a longer length of time for avoidance and may require lifelong avoidance as discussed earlier. The results of IgE testing become important in this clinical situation. A patient with a peanut IgE of less than 2.0 may safely undergo a food challenge to test for food tolerance or sensitivity. Any IgE result above this level is not considered safe for food challenge, especially in light of past anaphylaxis. Oral food challenge (OFC) remains the gold standard in the evaluation of food allergies.[26]

In the case of true anaphylaxis, parents must undergo substantial education regarding accidental ingestion and the need for a written emergency action plan. Parents need to be encouraged to have a healthy respect for the food allergy, not a fear of the reaction. Parents who are adequately prepared can educate the child about reading food labels and checking food content when eating out or at a friend's house. Accidental ingestions can occur even in the most vigilant families. This is an important period of time for patient education because those with a lifelong allergy will need to be prepared to handle accidental ingestion once they leave the home.

Pharmacologic Management

Oral diphenhydramine in either tablet, dissolvable, or liquid form is the preferred antihistamine used in cases of accidental ingestion and the development of symptoms. Diphenhydramine is used with symptoms of pruritus, urticaria, or eczema.

The development of respiratory compromise, facial flushing, abdominal pain, and nausea and vomiting indicate the possibility of impending anaphylaxis. Most cases of anaphylaxis occur within 1 hour of ingestion, but latent reactions up to 4 hours after ingestion are possible.[26] Epinephrine (1:1000 solution) is given immediately via the subcutaneous route. Doses may be repeated at 5- to 15-minute intervals two or three times.[17] The emergency management system is also activated.

One important clinical pearl is that the only way to predict anaphylaxis is to have had prior anaphylaxis. Patients with a past history of pruritus, urticaria, or facial swelling may progress to anaphylaxis with future ingestions. Finally, death is most frequent in the late teenage years, after the individual has left the home, when epinephrine is not given rapidly with the onset of early signs of anaphylaxis.

The New England Journal of Medicine published new peanut allergy guidelines in early 2015.[24] These new guidelines were a result of the LEAP-On study (Learning Early about Peanut Allergy) and have dramatically changed past practices in children with food allergies and published in the 2010 "Guidelines for the diagnosis and management of food allergy in the United States." This randomized trial was the first to look at early allergen introduction in children.[24] The 2010 guidelines recommended withholding potentially allergenic foods in children with either a genetic predisposition to the development of food allergies or past reactions to other foods.

The new guidelines now recommend the introduction of peanuts in patients as early as 4 to 6 months of age. These patients include those with severe eczema, documented egg ingestion reaction, or both. They also recommend the introduction of other foods prior to peanut to ensure the infant is developing normally.[24] An allergy workup including serum IgE measurement and skin prick-testing must be performed prior to introduction of foods that contain peanut. The goal of early introduction is to assist the infant in the development of food tolerance in the gastrointestinal tract early on. Of course, those patients with a known reaction to peanut must adhere to strict avoidance.[24]

REFERENCES

1. Shaker, M. (2014). New insights into the allergic march. *Current Opinion in Pediatrics, 26*(4), 516–520.
2. Burbank, A. J., et al. (2017). Reviews and feature article: Environmental determinants of allergy and asthma in early life. *The Journal of Allergy and Clinical Immunology, 140*, 1–12. doi:10.1016/j.jaci.2017.05.010. EBSCOhost.
3. Ostrov, B., & Robbins, L. (2014). A146: Strategies for assessment and management of severe environmental allergies at 'Camp JRA'. *Arthritis & Rheumatology, 66*, S189. (Accessed 17 October 2017). [Serial online], Retrieved from CINAHL Complete, Ipswich, MA.
4. Garg, N., & Silverberg, J. (2014). Association between childhood allergic disease, psychological comorbidity, and injury requiring medical attention. *Annals of Allergy, Asthma and Immunology, 112*(6), 525–532.
5. Centers for Disease Control and Prevention. Asthma: A presentation of asthma management and prevention. Retrieved from https://www.cdc.gov/nchs/fastats/asthma.htm. (Accessed 17 October 2017).
6. Campbell, D. E., et al. (2015). Mechanisms of Allergic Disease—Environmental and Genetic Determinants for the Development of Allergy. *Clinical and Experimental Allergy, 45*(5), 844–858. doi:10.1111/cea.12531. EBSCOhost.
7. Blaiss, M., Dykewicz, M., Allen-Ramey, F., et al. (2014). Diagnosis and treatment of nasal and ocular allergies: The Allergies, Immunotherapy, and RhinoconjunctivitiS (AIRS) surveys. *Annals of Allergy, Asthma & Immunology, 112*(4), 322–328, e1.
8. Lood, L. (2016). Manual of allergy and clinical immunology for otolaryngologists. *Journal of Laryngology & Otology, 130*(3), 322. (Accessed 18 October 2017). [Serial online], Retrieved from CINAHL Complete, Ipswich, MA.
9. Cardona, V., & Ansotegui, I. (2016). Component-resolved diagnosis in anaphylaxis. *Current Opinion in Allergy and Clinical Immunology, 16*(3), 244–249. (Accessed 18 October 2017). [Serial online], Retrieved from CINAHL Complete, Ipswich, MA.

10. Wright, L. S., & Phipatanakul, W. (2014). Environmental remediation in the treatment of allergy and asthma: Latest updates. *Current Allergy and Asthma Reports, 14*(3), 419. doi:10.1007/s11882-014-0419-7. EBSCOhost.

11. Mudd, K. (1995). Indoor environmental allergy: A guide to environmental controls. *Pediatric Nursing, 21*(6), 534–574. (Accessed 17 October 2017). [Serial online], Retrieved from CINAHL Complete, Ipswich, MA.

12. Geisler, S. (2003). The AAAAI adherence guidelines: Taking control of asthma therapy … American Academy of Allergy, Asthma and Immunology. *JAAPA: Official Journal of the American Academy of Physician Assistants, 16*(11), 35–50. (Accessed 17 October 2017). [Serial online], Retrieved from CINAHL Complete, Ipswich, MA.

13. Nierengarten, M. (2017). Asthma and food allergies associated with early-onset AD: New research looked at subtypes of atopic dermatitis for clues to other allergic diseases. *Contemporary Pediatrics, 34*(9), 30–31. (Accessed 17 October 2017). [Serial online], Retrieved from CINAHL Complete, Ipswich, MA.

14. Thompson, C. (2014). Sublingual immunotherapy approved for grass pollen allergies. *American Journal of Health-System Pharmacy,* 770.

15. Distler, J. (2011). Environmental allergens: Diagnosis and management of IgE-mediated disorders. *Am J Nurs Pract, 15*(9–10), 14.

16. Gupta, R., Warren, C., Blumenstock, J., Kotowska, J., Mittal, K., & Smith, B. (2017). OR078 The prevalence of childhood food allergy in the United States: An update. *Annals of Allergy, Asthma & Immunology, 119,* S11. (Accessed 17 October 2017). [Serial online], Retrieved from CINAHL Complete, Ipswich, MA.

17. Rance, K., & O'Laughlen, M. (2014). Managing food allergies in primary care. *Clinical Advisor, 17*(2), 53–60.

18. Schroer, B., Bjelac, J., & Leonard, M. (2017). What is new in managing patients with food allergy? Almost everything. *Current Opinion in Pediatrics, 29*(5), 578–583. (Accessed 17 October 2017). [Serial online], Retrieved from CINAHL Complete, Ipswich, MA.

19. Jones, S., & Burks, A. (2017). Food allergy. *The New England Journal of Medicine, 377*(12), 1168–1176. (Accessed 17 October 2017). [Serial online], Retrieved from CINAHL Complete, Ipswich, MA.

20. Sicherer, S., Allen, K., Lack, G., Taylor, S., Donovan, S., & Oria, M. (2017). Critical issues in food allergy: A National Academies consensus report. *Pediatrics, 140*(2), 1–8. (Accessed 17 October 2017). [Serial online], Retrieved from CINAHL Complete, Ipswich, MA.

21. Sicherer, S. H., Allen, K., Lack, G., Taylor, S. L., Donovan, S. M., & Oria, M. (2017). Critical issues in food allergy: A National Academies consensus report. *Pediatrics,* e20170194. doi:10.1542/peds.2017-0194.

22. Berdanier, C. (2017). Food sensitivity versus food allergy. *Nutrition Today, 52*(4), 174–178. (Accessed 17 October 2017). [Serial online], Retrieved from CINAHL Complete, Ipswich, MA.

23. Greenhawt, M. (2016). Early allergen introduction for preventing development of food allergy. *Journal of the American Medical Association, 316*(11), 1157–1159. (Accessed 17 October 2017). [Serial online], Retrieved from CINAHL Complete, Ipswich, MA.

24. Peanut Allergy Prevention. (2017). Guidelines from the NIAID. *American Family Physician, 96*(2), 13. (Accessed 17 October 2017). [Serial online], Retrieved from CINAHL Complete, Ipswich, MA.

25. Ramesh, M., & Lieberman, J. (2017). Adult-onset food allergies. *Annals of Allergy, Asthma & Immunology, 119*(2), 111–119. (Accessed 17 October 2017). [Serial online], Retrieved from CINAHL Complete, Ipswich, MA.

26. Leibel, S., Alsaggaf, A., & Murphy, J. (2017). OR073 Cost-effectiveness of confirmatory oral food challenges in the diagnosis of children with food allergy. *Annals of Allergy, Asthma & Immunology, 119,* S9–S10. (Accessed 17 October 2017). [Serial online], Retrieved from CINAHL Complete, Ipswich, MA.

CHAPTER **29**

HEAD TRAUMA

Mary Lynn Fahey

 Immediate emergency department referral or physician consultation is indicated for head trauma with alteration in level of consciousness, paralysis, paresthesia, rhinorrhea, raccoon sign (ecchymosis beneath both eyes), Battle sign, otorrhea, or hemotympanum.

DEFINITION AND EPIDEMIOLOGY

A traumatic brain injury (TBI) is caused by a bump, blow, or jolt to the head that disrupts the normal function of the brain. Forceful impact can cause movement of the brain in the skull. This sudden movement of the brain can lead to the creation of chemical and inflammatory changes in the brain and potential damage to the brain cells.

The Centers for Disease Control and Prevention (CDC) estimates reveal that serious TBIs contributed to about 30% of all injury deaths, with an estimated 153 deaths each day in 2017 in the United States from injuries that included TBI.[1] Falls have been a number one cause of TBI in children younger than age 14 and in adults older than age 65.[1] Intentional self-harm was the second leading cause of TBI-related deaths (33%) in 2013,[1] while motor vehicle crashes were the third most common cause of TBI death.[1] Fortunately, most head injuries are concussions, are relatively mild, and not associated with significant trauma.[2] Many individuals who incur a sports or recreational brain injury are not hospitalized, nor do they even seek emergency department treatment.[2] In general, patients who lose consciousness for more than 10 minutes or have a focal neurologic deficit are considered to have a major brain injury, whereas those who are unconscious for less than 10 minutes and have no neurologic deficit are classified as having a minor TBI.[3]

An ever-increasing number of older patients present with TBI.[4] These older patients can also incur serious injury even when the head injury is minor. Older adults require more hospitalizations and have a higher mortality rate than other age groups for TBI. Falls from a height, or falls in the home, are the most common cause of older adult TBIs. Medical comorbidities, age-related brain atrophy, anticoagulant therapy, and decreased free radical clearance all contribute to making TBIs more severe in older adults.

TBI is also a common injury for active duty military personnel and can range from mild to severe depending on the type of injury.[5] There is increased concern about the number of mild traumatic brain injuries (MTBI) and undiagnosed TBIs that occur not only in combat but also in sports and recreational activities.[2] Repetitive brain trauma or chronic traumatic encephalopathy is usually related to repeated injuries and is often associated with sports. Although chronic head trauma does not result in immediate death, there are chronic brain changes that cause depression and other personality changes, as well as Alzheimer or Parkinson disease. In MTBI, imaging studies may be normal, but patients may complain of a variety of symptoms that affect sleep patterns, daily work, and life activities for weeks to months after the injury.[2,6]

The injury can be mild, or severe enough to dramatically affect a patient's intellectual and physical capacity as well as his or her psychological, social, and economic well-being. Long-term effects of TBI not only affect the injured individual, but also his or her family and community.[1]

Patients with MTBI may not lose consciousness, and patients with epidural bleeding may have only brief loss of consciousness, then be alert and behave appropriately before clinical deterioration rapidly ensues.[2] It is essential that health care providers be aware of the "talk and deteriorate" syndrome. Patients with this syndrome utter recognizable words after the head injury and then deteriorate to a severe, brain-injured condition within 48 hours. The most common neurologic findings

TABLE 29.1 Glasgow Coma Scale

Sign	Score
EYE OPENING	
Spontaneous	4
To verbal command	3
To pain	2
No response	1
BEST MOTOR RESPONSE	
Obeys verbal commands	6
Localizes pain	5
Movement or withdrawal to pain	4
Flexion response to pain (decorticate)	3
Extension response to pain (decerebrate)	2
No response	1
BEST VERBAL RESPONSE	
Alert and oriented	5
Converses but confused or disoriented	4
Nonsensical or inappropriate words	3
Nonspecific sounds	2
No response	1

Modified from Teasdale, G., & Jennett, B. (1974). Assessment of coma and impaired consciousness. A practical scale. *Lancet*, *304*(7872), 81–84.

are altered mental status and focal hemispheric deficits. For these patients, early and appropriate use of computed tomography (CT) scanning is necessary to detect significant intracranial lesions before clinical neurologic deterioration occurs.

In acute injury, the severity of damage can be described by an injury-rating system such as the Glasgow Coma Scale (GCS) score (Table 29.1).[4] The GCS assesses eye opening responses, motor responses, and verbal responses. Numbers are assigned for the level of function attained in each category and then totaled. A normal patient has a score of 15, whereas a patient who is brain dead has a score of 3. Minor head trauma is defined as an initial GCS score of 13 to 15 and a period of unconsciousness of less than 20 minutes. Moderate head injury refers to an initial GCS score of 9 to 12 with or without loss of consciousness. Severe head trauma is defined as an initial GCS score of less than 8 or a comatose state for 6 hours or more.[4]

The older adult with TBI may have an initial GCS that does not accurately reflect the severity of injury. Although this may be more apparent in cases of more severe injury, elders with TBI may score higher on the GCS than a younger person with the same level of injury.[7] It is important to be alert to this possibility.

PATHOPHYSIOLOGY

The cranial vault is a fixed space that contains the brain, cerebrospinal fluid (CSF), and blood. Because the skull limits intracranial volume, neurologic damage after head injury can be directly related to cerebral edema that causes increased intracranial pressure (ICP), which in turn decreases cerebral blood flow and causes cerebral ischemia. Head trauma can

consist of soft tissue injury, skull fracture, and/or hemorrhage. Brain injury from trauma can occur in two stages: primary and secondary. Primary injury is sustained in the initial insult and may result from blunt or blast trauma, penetrating injury, coup-contrecoup lacerations or contusions of the brain, or direct disruption of brain tissue by the shearing of axons. Secondary injury may occur from increased ICP, cerebral hypoxia, systemic hypotension, decreased cerebral blood flow, and oxygen free radicals resulting in cellular death. The secondary sequelae may cause further neuronal damage, which can compromise an already injured brain. In mild TBI, the primary cause of injury is the dysfunction of brain metabolism rather than structural injury.[7]

CLINICAL PRESENTATION

It is important to have a structured approach to assessing the individual with TBI. A thoughtful history and thorough assessment is necessary and includes both a primary and a secondary assessment.[8] The history should include timing and mechanism of the injury (determining the mechanism of injury can alert the clinician to possible non-accidental trauma). It is critical to determine if the injury resulted from blunt or penetrating trauma, or high-energy—high-impact trauma. The stability and progression of the patient's symptoms, as well as any prior conditions, significant medical history including current medications (especially antiplatelet or anticoagulant therapy), and allergies are essential to discern. The cause and exact location of the injury should be determined: Was it accidental or intentional? Changes in mentation and any loss or change in level of consciousness should be learned; elicited from the patient, when possible, but also from witnesses. A history of amnesia (retrograde or anterograde) concerning the traumatic event, even if fleeting, often indicates altered consciousness and needs to be quantified.[8] It is also necessary to learn the patient state of consciousness before the head injury to identify other pathologic conditions, such as stroke, myocardial infarction, or respiratory distress. Additional causes of altered mental status, such as hypoglycemia, drug overdose, hyperthermia, or arrhythmias, must also be investigated. Alcohol intoxication and substance use may mask the signs and symptoms of a head injury; therefore it is important to determine if these were involved. The history should also elicit any previous history of concussion or other brain trauma, complaints of seizure activity, confusion, drowsiness, dizziness, headache, visual changes, blurred vision, tinnitus, slurred speech, neck pain, nausea, vomiting, upper or lower extremity weakness, difficulty concentrating, and emotional lability such as increased irritability or other change in behavior.[2]

In older patients, the first sign of brain injury may be confusion or a change in behavior rather than a reported fall or other injury. The patient may not remember a fall or injury or may believe that the injury was insignificant. Family members or caregivers may also not be aware that an event occurred.

PHYSICAL EXAMINATION

Patients with head trauma can fluctuate from being awake and alert to being comatose and in respiratory distress. The initial evaluation should follow the standard protocol developed for all trauma patients. The patient's circulation, airway, and breathing and the cervical spine must be evaluated and stabilized. Focus on the patient's level of consciousness, oxygen saturation, vital signs, and determination of GCS score is necessary. The skull must be examined for fractures, penetrating injuries, lacerations, or CSF drainage; clinical signs of skull fracture include raccoon sign (bruising around the orbit), Battle sign (mastoid ecchymosis), and blood in the external auditory canal. The extremities are assessed for injuries and symmetric movement. A quick, thorough neurologic examination is necessary to determine brain injury, focal deficits, and stability of the patient, as well as mental status, memory, concentration, cranial nerves, motor strength and tone, deep tendon reflexes, and, when possible, finger-to-nose test, deep tendon reflexes gait, and Romberg test. Repeated neurologic examinations are required to determine whether the patient's condition is stable, improving, or deteriorating. However, normal neurologic examination findings do not eliminate the possibility of brain injury. The severity of injury and prognosis are indicated by the amount of retrograde or post-traumatic amnesia.

DIAGNOSTICS

- Pulse oximetry and continuous vital signs.
- Cervical spine X-ray examination, because patients with head injury can have an associated cervical spine fracture.
- Non-enhanced head CT scan, multislice CT, or X-ray study is indicated for:
  - Patients with a depressed or deteriorating level of consciousness, skull fracture, neurologic deficit, open head wound, penetrating head injury, amnesia, or high risk of intracranial injury.
  - Older patients and patients who are receiving anticoagulants or antiplatelet therapy.
  - Patients with MTBI (loss of consciousness for less than 5 minutes or amnesia accompanied by GCS score <15, headache, post-traumatic seizure, focal neurologic deficit, impaired short-term memory, depressed skull fracture, trauma above clavicle, age older than 60 years, or presence of alcohol or drug intoxication).[9,10]
  - Patients with concussion and age 65 or older, alcohol intoxication, coagulopathy, continued headache or vomiting, focal neurological deficit, GCS < 15, retrograde amnesia 30 minutes or more, seizure, or skull fracture or soft tissue injury of head or neck.[9,10]
  - Repeated head CT scans may be necessary if neurologic deficits develop.[9,11,12]
- Magnetic resonance imaging has a limited role in head injury but may be indicated after CT scan in some instances for more specific anatomic detail and identification of diffuse axonal injury.
- Laboratory studies.
  - Complete blood count (CBC)
  - Serum glucose, electrolytes, magnesium, blood urea nitrogen (BUN), creatinine
  - Urinalysis, arterial blood gases (ABGs)
  - Coagulation panel
  - Blood alcohol level and drug screen, if indicated
  - Type and crossmatch for blood transfusion in cases of severe trauma

DIFFERENTIAL DIAGNOSIS

 Priority differentials include (1) penetration injuries, (2) skull fracture, (3) concussion, (4) cerebral contusion, (5) epidural or subdural hematoma, (6) subarachnoid or intracerebral bleeding, and (7) cerebral edema.

Cerebral concussion is defined as the loss of consciousness without significant anatomic damage to the brain. The severity of the injury is quantified by the duration of amnesia—the length of amnesia concerning the time before impact (antegrade amnesia) plus the length of amnesia after impact (retrograde amnesia). It is helpful to determine the time interval between the first thing and the last thing remembered. Cerebral contusions usually occur on the undersurface of the poles of the frontal lobes or on the poles of the temporal lobes. The patient is typically awake and alert after the initial injury, but increasing ICP, decreased level of consciousness, and focal neurologic deficits may develop as the contusion mass increases in size.

INITIAL STABILIZATION AND MANAGEMENT
Traumatic Brain Injury

- First priority for patient with traumatic head injury: Manage circulation, airway, breathing, and cervical spine.
- Second priority: Correct hypoxia with 100% high-flow oxygen (in adults, PaO_2 < 60 mm Hg) and hypotension (in adults, systolic blood pressure <90 mm Hg). This is essential to decrease the risk of secondary brain injury (and associated morbidity and mortality) related to hypoxia and hypotension.[13]
- Third priority: Assess primary injury and rapidly recognize surgically correctable lesion.
- Further evaluation for evidence of lacerations and other trauma (e.g., depressed skull fracture) is necessary.
- Ongoing assessment for increasing ICP (i.e., decreasing GCS, abnormal posturing) to avoid further cranial injury.

Minor Head Trauma

- Although CT scans are usually not indicated for most patients with minor head trauma or a GCS score of 15, diagnostic testing is dependent on the patient's history and physical examination findings. In general, it is important to assess and treat for alcohol ingestion, hypoglycemia, hypothermia, and/or narcotic overdose.
  - CT scan should be a consideration in patients with alcohol intoxication and those with amnesia, severe headache, loss of consciousness or short-term memory deficit, seizure, or vomiting. Anticoagulant use, patient history of coagulopathy, definitive external evidence of injury above the clavicles, or neurologic deficit is an additional concern. Available tools that offer reassurance when determining appropriate CT scanning include:
    - The PECARN Pediatric Head Injury/Trauma Algorithm available at https://www.mdcalc.com/pecarn-pediatric-head-injury-trauma-algorithm
    - The New Orleans/Charity Head Trauma/Injury Rule indicated for use in patients who did lose consciousness after a head injury but are deemed neurologically normal available at https://www.mdcalc.com/new-orleans-charity-head-trauma-injury-rule
    - CDC Updated Mild Traumatic Brain Injury Guideline for Adults available at https://www.cdc.gov/traumaticbraininjury/pdf/TBI_Clinicians_Factsheet-a.pdf
- Patients *without* agitation, amnesia, behavior change, confusion, continued nausea and vomiting, depressed skull fracture, drowsiness, focal neurologic deficits, loss of consciousness, slurred speech, weakness, worsening headache, or seizures do not require a CT scan.[14]

- Patients may be discharged home if observation is available and instructions are given on proper patient evaluation.
- Patients with mild TBI and a negative head CT are also able to be discharged home with appropriate discharge instructions.
- In the future, laboratory biomarkers (e.g., plasma total tau) may be able to predict which patients with a concussion will require specific clinical therapy.[15]

DISPOSITION AND REFERRAL

- Patients may be discharged home with proper instructions if the CT scan is normal and if a family member or friend can provide close observation for 24 hours.
- If no one is available to monitor the patient or if there is evidence of a pathologic condition, the patient should be admitted to the hospital for observation.
- A patient who has had more than 5 minutes of unconsciousness, post-traumatic seizures, a GCS score of 12 to 14, focal neurologic deficits, a lesion on the CT scan, or a moderate head injury (a GCS score of 9 to 12) should be hospitalized, stabilized, and closely observed for any neurologic deterioration; a neurosurgical evaluation is also indicated.
- Patients with severe head trauma (a GCS score of 8 or less, penetrating skull injuries, or compound skull fractures) should be evaluated at the nearest hospital and have a neurosurgical evaluation.

PATIENT AND FAMILY EDUCATION

Specific instructions must be provided to those who will be observing the patient who is discharged home. The patient should remain in the care of a competent caregiver and rest in a quiet environment for the first 24 hours after discharge, because the first 24 hours after the injury are the most important.

Aspirin (and medications that contain aspirin), alcohol, and narcotics should not be taken for 1 week after the injury.

The patient should return for treatment if any of the following develop: drowsiness or difficulty awakening (the patient should be awakened every 2 hours during sleep), continuous nausea, vomiting more than twice, seizures or convulsions, visual disturbances or pupillary changes, slurred speech, new-onset weakness or an inability to move body parts, severe headache, confusion, personality changes, unusual restlessness, difficulty breathing, dizziness, or difficulty walking.[5,16]

Patients should also be informed about the post-traumatic or postconcussion syndrome, which is not life-threatening but may disable a patient for weeks to months to even years. Symptoms can last 2 to 6 weeks in most cases, but can be present for longer and include headache, tinnitus, memory loss, dizziness, giddiness, poor concentration, emotional lability, irritability, nervousness, disturbed sleep, fatigue, and decreased libido. Treatment consists of rest, reassurance, and analgesics. It is also extremely important that patients return to work as soon as possible, even if a reduced workload is necessary.

Athletes diagnosed with a concussion should not be permitted to return to physical activity until the concussion has resolved (Level B evidence).[16] Neurocognitive testing or other evidence of concussion resolution is necessary before these patients return to practice or play sports (Level B evidence).[16]

Physical therapy, occupational therapy, psychotherapy, and speech therapy may benefit some patients, whereas others may require cognitive behavioral therapy if anxiety is a concern.[17] If the injury was related to substance use, the patient is encouraged to seek treatment.[17]

Patients and families should understand that a potential complication is the development of post-traumatic epilepsy, which is defined as two or more seizures after head trauma.[11] Additionally, patients, families and coaches should be aware of Second-impact Syndrome, brain edema that can occur (and may be lethal), if a second concussion is incurred before the first concussion has completely resolved.[18]

Patients must be educated about safety issues, such as the proper use of bicycle helmets, seat belts, and car seats for infants and children. Safety issues in the home should also be reviewed (e.g., staircases, gates, throw rugs, cluttered environment, and lighting) in an attempt to reduce falls in children and older adults.[19]

REFERENCES

1. Centers for Disease Control and Prevention. Injury prevention and control: Traumatic brain injury. Retrieved from http://www.cdc.gov/traumaticbraininjury/get_the_facts.html. (Accessed 26 April 2019).
2. Centers for Disease Control and Prevention. Heads up: The basics. Retrieved from https://www.cdc.gov/headsup/basics/concussion_whatis.html. (Accessed 26 April 2019).
3. Roosen, G., Vandenbussche, N., & Depreitere, B. (2013). Traumatic brain injury in the elderly: Beyond the tip of the iceberg. Aging Health., 9(1), 81–87.
4. Teasdale, G. The Glasgow structured approach to assessment of the Glasgow Coma Scale. Retrieved from http://www.glasgowcomascale.org/. (Accessed 26 April 2019).
5. Heltemes, K. J., Dougherty, A. L. MacGregor, A. J., & Galarneau, M. R. (2010). Inpatient hospitalizations of U.S. military personnel medically evacuated from Iraq and Afghanistan with combat-related traumatic brain injury. Military Medicine, 176(2), 132–135.
6. Schreiber, S., et al. (2008). Long-lasting sleep patterns of adult patients with minor traumatic brain injury (mTBI) and non-mTBI subjects. Sleep Medicine, 9(5), 481–487.
7. Kehoe, A., Rennie, S., & Smith, J. (2015). Glasgow Coma Scale is unreliable for the prediction of severe head injury in elderly trauma patients. Emergency Medicine Journal: EMJ, 32(8), 613–615.
8. Prasad, G. L. (2017). Outcome of Head Injury in the Elderly. World Neurosurgery, 103, 944.
9. Diagnostic Imaging Pathways. Canadian CT Head Rules. Retrieved from http://www.imagingpathways.health.wa.gov.au/index.php/imaging-pathways/musculoskeletal-trauma/trauma/adult-with-head-injury#pathway. (Accessed 26 April 2019).
10. Centers for Disease Control and Prevention. Updated mild traumatic brain injury guideline for adults. Retrieved from https://www.cdc.gov/traumaticbraininjury/mtbi_guideline.html. (Accessed 26 April 2019).
11. Stippler, M., Smith, C., McLean, A. R., et al. (2012). Utility of routine follow-up head CT scanning after mild traumatic brain injury: A systematic review of the literature. Emergency Medicine Journal, 29, e528–e532.
12. Aminoff, M. J., & Douglas, V. C. (2018). Nervous system disorders. In M. A. Papadakis, S. J. McPhee, & M. W. Rabow (Eds.), Current medical diagnosis & treatment. New York, NY: McGraw-Hill.
13. Brain Trauma Foundation. (2016). Guidelines for the management of severe traumatic brain injury; 4th edition. Neurosurgery. Retrieved from https://braintrauma.org/uploads/07/04/Guidelines_for_the_Management_of_Severe_Traumatic.97250__2_.pdf. (Accessed 26 April 2019).
14. Centers for Disease Control. Concussion signs and symptoms checklist. Retrieved from https://www.cdc.gov/headsup/basics/concussion_symptoms.html. (Accessed 26 April 2019).
15. Gatson, J., & Diaz-Arrastia, R. (2014). Tau as a biomarker for concussion. JAMA Neurol.
16. Giza, C. C., Kutcher, J. S., Ashwal, S., Barth, J., et al. (2013). Summary of evidence-based guideline: Evaluation and management of concussion in sports. Report of the Guideline Development Subcommittee of the American Academy of Neurology. Neurology, 80(24), 2250–2257.
17. Torrence, C. B., DeCristofaro, C., & Elliott, L. (2010). Empowering the primary care provider to optimally manage mild traumatic brain injury. J Am Acad Nurs Pract., 23(2011), 638–647.

18. American Association of Neurological Surgeons. Concussion. Retrieved from https://www.aans.org/en/Patients/Neurosurgical-Conditions-and-Treatments/Concussion. (Accessed 26 April 2019).
19. Roy, H., & Richards, P. (2017). The management of traumatic brain trauma. *Paediatrics and Child Health* September 2017.

CHAPTER **30**

HYPOTENSION

Ashley Moore-Gibbs

 Immediate emergency department referral is indicated for patients with significant symptoms and evidence of end-organ damage such as altered mental status, chest discomfort, or shortness of breath.

DEFINITION AND EPIDEMIOLOGY

Hypotension, or low blood pressure, is defined as a systolic blood pressure of 90 mm Hg or less.[1] Blood pressure readings should always be interpreted in the context of the patient's prior measurements. In patients with preexisting hypertension, a significant reduction from baseline with accompanying symptoms may represent relative hypotension, despite a reading above 90 mm Hg.

The causes of hypotension are numerous, ranging from relatively benign to life-threatening. Therefore it is important for health care providers to determine the etiology of hypotension through a methodical approach using broad categories; that is, cardiovascular, endocrine, gastrointestinal, immunologic, infectious disease, neurologic, pulmonary, renal, vascular, and traumatic. *Cardiovascular* causes of hypotension include cardiac pump failure (e.g., myocardial infarction, heart failure, negative inotropic medications), dysrhythmia, pericardial tamponade, vasovagal reactions, and inadequate intravascular volume.[1] *Pulmonary* causes of hypotension include acute pulmonary embolus and decompensated pulmonary hypertension.[1] *Gastrointestinal* causes of hypotension include gastrointestinal bleeding and increased volume loss from vomiting and/or diarrhea.[1] *Endocrinologic* causes of hypotension include adrenal insufficiency, diabetic ketoacidosis, and hypothyroidism.[1] Anaphylaxis is the most important *immunologic* cause of hypotension.[1] *Neurologic* causes of hypotension include autonomic dysfunction and peripheral neuropathy.[1] *Renal* causes of hypotension include volume loss from renal tubular dysfunction or overzealous use of diuretics.[1] *Vascular* causes of hypotension include ruptured abdominal aortic aneurysm, ruptured ectopic pregnancy, and the use of vasodilator medications. *Traumatic* causes of hypotension are traditionally divided into hemorrhagic causes and nonhemorrhagic causes. Hemorrhage can be external, or into several body cavities: chest, abdomen, pelvis, and long bones. Nonhemorrhagic causes of traumatic hypotension include pericardial tamponade, tension pneumothorax, myocardial contusion, and spinal shock.[1]

Orthostatic hypotension is commonly seen in the ambulatory and emergency department settings and is defined by a sustained reduction in systolic blood pressure of more than 20 mm Hg or in diastolic blood pressure of more than 10 mm Hg within 3 minutes of standing.[2] It is the second most common cause of syncope and frequently affects older adults.[2]

PATHOPHYSIOLOGY

When hypotension occurs, there is an alteration in one or more of the three components necessary for the maintenance of normal blood pressure. The first component is the state of contraction of the muscles in the blood vessel wall. Vasodilator medications, sepsis, anaphylaxis, autonomic nervous system dysfunction, and certain endocrine disorders may cause abnormal blood vessel relaxation and a decrease in blood pressure.[2] The second component is intravascular volume. When intravascular volume is reduced as a result of bleeding, vomiting, diarrhea, or inadequate fluid intake, hypotension may result.[2] The third component is the adequacy of cardiopulmonary function.[2] A decrease in cardiac function resulting from pump failure or dysrhythmia will cause a reduction in cardiac output and blood pressure. Understanding of these three fundamental mechanisms of hypotension will help generate a differential diagnosis. Abnormalities of more than one of these three components may occur simultaneously in the same patient.

Common in older adults, orthostatic hypotension occurs most frequently in those with diseases involving the peripheral autonomic nervous system (diabetes mellitus and amyloidosis), neurodegenerative disorders (Parkinson disease and autonomic failure), and those taking vasoactive medications.[3,4] Orthostatic hypotension is associated with increased morbidity and mortality due to the consequences of multiple falls that contribute to fractures, head injuries and their associated complications.[5]

Orthostatic hypotension may result from either neurogenic or nonneurogenic causes. In turn, neurogenic orthostatic hypotension can be caused by abnormalities of either the central nervous system or peripheral nervous system. Peripheral autonomic dysfunction is the most frequent cause of orthostatic hypotension in older adults.[6] With aging, there is a decrease in baroreflex sensitivity. This blunts the normal physiologic response to standing (i.e., vasoconstriction and a modest increase in heart rate), with a resultant drop in blood pressure. In addition to decreased baroreflex sensitivity, older individuals have diminished heart rate responses and impaired alpha$_1$-adrenergic vasoconstriction.[3] Age-related reductions in parasympathetic tone also occur and result in less cardioacceleration during vagal withdrawal on standing.[3] Orthostatic hypotension is more common in patients with degenerative neurologic diseases and some peripheral neuropathic syndromes.[3] Medications, including diuretics, antihypertensives, alpha blockers, nitrates, calcium channel blockers, antidepressants, and opiates, may provoke or worsen orthostatic hypotension.[7]

Neurogenic orthostatic hypotension involves the central nervous system and is well associated with increased mortality rates in patients with diabetes, hypertension, or Parkinson disease, and those receiving dialysis.[8] Patients with neurogenic orthostatic hypotension may be symptomatic or asymptomatic during episodes of orthostatic hypotension. Symptoms emerge during postural changes, after prolonged standing, with dehydration, after alcohol ingestion, after carbohydrate-heavy meals, with heat exposure or fever, during stressful events, or with Valsalva maneuvers from straining.[8]

Nonneurogenic causes of orthostatic hypotension include cardiac functional impairment, dehydration, and vasodilation. A transient drop in blood pressure occurring with an abrupt change in position and resolving rapidly suggests a nonneurogenic cause.[8]

Postprandial hypotension is another potential cause of hypotension in the elderly. It should be suspected when there is a decrease in blood pressure within 2 hours after eating.[6] The mechanism of postprandial hypotension is poorly understood. Current evidence suggests that the cause of postprandial hypotension is multifactorial, including autonomic and neural dysfunction, changes in gastrointestinal hormones, meal composition, gastric distention, and the rate of delivery of nutrients to the small intestine.[6] Multiple factors contribute to a postprandial fall in blood pressure, and this manifests with inadequate cardiovascular compensation for meal-induced splanchnic blood pooling.[6] Postprandial changes in diastolic blood pressure are not as marked as systolic blood pressure changes. Typically there is a fall in systolic blood pressure of more than 20 mm Hg, or a decrease to 90 mm Hg or lower when the preprandial blood pressure is 100 mm Hg or higher within 2 hours of a meal.[6]

Younger patients experiencing symptoms concerning for hypotension may maintain their systolic blood pressure and exhibit an increased pulse with a position change in conjunction with symptoms of cerebral hypoperfusion (fatigue, lightheadedness, exercise intolerance, or cognitive impairment); this represents postural orthostatic tachycardia syndrome (POTS).[9] There is an absence of orthostatic hypotension; however, the standing heart rate is often 120 beats/min or higher.[9] POTS is more common in women aged 15 to 25 years. Up to half of those diagnosed with POTS have antecedent viral illness, and 25% have a family history of similar complaints.[9] Pathophysiologic mechanisms of POTS are multifactorial and include hypovolemia, venous pooling, hyperadrenergic states, and restricted adrenergic neuropathies in the lower limbs.[9]

CLINICAL PRESENTATION AND PHYSICAL EXAMINATION

Although the symptoms of hypotension vary greatly, those related to the brain and heart predominate. Lightheadedness and dizziness are common symptoms of hypotension. In addition, some individuals may experience blurred or tunnel vision and a dull pain in the back of the neck and shoulders.[7] Symptoms are more pronounced with positional changes such as standing, and do not occur while the patient is supine.[7] Neurologic symptoms of hypotension include lightheadedness, dizziness, confusion, focal neurologic deficits, and loss of consciousness.[7] Cardiopulmonary symptoms of hypotension include shortness of breath, dyspnea on exertion, chest pain, palpitations, and syncope.[7]

In addition to identification of the physical symptoms that result from hypotension, careful attention should be paid to symptoms that may reveal the underlying cause. Inquiry should be made about fluid intake, nausea and vomiting, diarrhea, rectal bleeding or melena, polyuria, and any antecedent cardiopulmonary symptoms.

Obtaining vital signs with orthostatic blood pressure readings, heart rate, temperature, respiratory rate, and oxygen saturation level should be performed in addition to evaluation of capillary refill and skin temperature. The heart should be auscultated for rate, rhythm, murmurs, and extra sounds, and the chest for air movement and visualized bilateral chest wall rise. Abdominal auscultation evaluates bowel sounds in all quadrants and palpation is performed to assess for tenderness and pain. Peripheral pulses should be palpated for timing and contour. When abnormal, these physical exam findings provide insight into the possible underlying cause of the patient's hypotensive episode.[10]

DIAGNOSTICS
Essential Diagnostics

When hypotension is identified, diagnostic testing is guided by the patient's history and physical examination findings. Hypotension may be evident on simple blood pressure measurement or after an assessment of orthostatic vital signs. A decrease in systolic blood pressure of 20 mm Hg and/or a decrease in diastolic blood pressure of 10 mm Hg taken at 3 minutes of standing is diagnostic of orthostatic hypotension.[7] In those with hypertension, a reduction of systolic blood pressure readings of 30 mm Hg may be more appropriate when determining a diagnosis of orthostatic hypotension, depending on the patient's baseline.[7]

A low blood pressure, absolute or in comparison with the patient's normal pressure when the patient is supine, confirms the diagnosis, particularly if the decrease is associated with dizziness, lightheadedness, or tachycardia when the patient is in the standing position.[7]

Measurement of heart rate concomitantly with blood pressure is important because failure of the pulse to increase with a decrease in blood pressure is indicative of neurogenic hypotension or central or peripheral nervous system diseases resulting in autonomic failure.[7] Tachycardic heart rates that are exaggerated suggest underlying volume depletion such as dehydration.[7] In elders, age-related reduction in baroreflex sensitivity decreases the ability for an appropriate heart rate response and is less useful as a diagnostic tool for measurement of heart rate.[7]

Relatively simple bedside tests with a high diagnostic yield include electrocardiography (ECG), serum hemoglobin, serum electrolytes, serum blood urea nitrogen and creatinine levels, and stool testing for occult blood. Performing a urine or serum pregnancy test in women of childbearing age may provide guidance in the management of a young woman with a ruptured ectopic pregnancy. A careful review of the patient's medical regimen is fundamental because numerous drugs may cause or worsen hypotension.

Additional Diagnostics

The detection of hypotension may require multiple measurements performed on different days and at different times. Orthostatic measurements are more sensitive early in the morning when the patient awakens because of nighttime pressure natriuresis.[2] Ambulatory automated blood pressure monitors may be useful in detecting orthostatic changes, but the patient must be able to recall specific times symptoms were noted with a change in posture.

Additional testing should be based on the differential diagnosis. If cardiac dysfunction is suspected, additional studies (e.g., echocardiography, cardiac monitoring) may be indicated. When a pulmonary embolus is suspected, a D-dimer test and, if positive, a computed tomography (CT) scan of the chest should be performed. If intraabdominal bleeding is the presumed cause, a CT scan of the abdomen may be required.

DIFFERENTIAL DIAGNOSIS

The differential diagnosis is based upon the patient's history and physical exam. Patients with hypotension may present

INITIAL DIAGNOSTICS

Hypotension

LABORATORY
- Hemoglobin
- Serum electrolytes, BUN and creatinine, glucose
- Stool testing for occult blood
- Urine or serum pregnancy test (all women of childbearing age)
- D-dimer test (when pulmonary embolus is suspected)
- Urinalysis and blood cultures (when sepsis is suspected)

IMAGING
- Electrocardiogram
- Echocardiography, cardiac monitoring (when cardiac dysfunction is suspected)
- CT imaging of the chest (when pulmonary embolus is suspected)
- CT imaging of the abdomen (when intraabdominal bleeding is suspected)
- Chest X-ray study (when sepsis is suspected)

with varying degrees in their symptoms. Several factors including age, underlying medical conditions, and the cause of their hypotension contribute to the potential severity of symptoms. Determining if there is an alteration in one or more of the three components necessary for the maintenance of normal blood pressure (outlined in the pathophysiology section) is an important approach in distinguishing the etiology of hypotension. Considering broad categories contributing to hypotension can assist the clinician in generating an appropriate differential diagnosis for the underlying etiology(ies) of hypotension and direct definitive management strategies.

By asking the following questions, the clinician may ascertain information needed to provide definitive and effective treatment for the hypotensive patient:

- Is the patient volume depleted?
- Is the patient bleeding?
- Does the patient have cardiac dysfunction?
- Does the patient have an acute infection?
- Is the patient having an allergic reaction?
- Does the patient have adrenal failure?

 Priority differentials include (1) sepsis, (2) cardiovascular causes, (3) gastrointestinal bleeding, and (4) dehydration. For women of childbearing age, pregnancy should always be considered.

INTERPROFESSIONAL COLLABORATIVE MANAGEMENT

The causes of hypotension are numerous; therefore the treatment strategies will also be broad. The astute clinician performing a good physical examination and using limited diagnostic testing is often able to target the most likely cause of hypotension at the bedside.

Pharmacologic Management

The Volume Depleted Patient. Historical features that suggest volume depletion include a history of poor fluid intake, vomiting, diarrhea, or polyuria. In addition to hypotension, the physical exam may reveal tachycardia, dry mucous membranes, and decreased skin turgor. In this situation, the administration of fluids by mouth or intravenously may be all that is needed to correct hypotension.[1] Treatment of the underlying cause will also be important.

The Bleeding Patient. In the ambulatory patient the most common causes of blood loss leading to hypotension are gastrointestinal and vaginal bleeding. Gastrointestinal bleeding may be gradual or acute, and in the former scenario the patient may not be aware that this is occurring. For this reason, Hemoccult stool testing should be a routine step in the assessment of the hypotensive patient. When a gastrointestinal bleed is suspected or proven, a complete blood count should be obtained. Current guidelines recommend packed red blood cell transfusion in patients with a hemoglobin of <7 g/dL.[11]

The Patient With Cardiac Dysfunction. This should be considered in the older patient and in all those complaining of chest pain, shortness of breath, orthopnea, and worsening peripheral edema.[12,13] The physical exam may reveal pulmonary congestion, tachycardia, dysrhythmia, and/or new murmurs. In this situation, a bedside ECG should be obtained and referral to an acute care facility is advisable.[13]

The Patient With an Acute Infection. Hypotension in the septic patient is an ominous finding that is predictive of significant morbidity and mortality. The mostly likely causes of a patient experiencing hypotension from an infection in the ambulatory setting include pneumonia, urinary tract infection, soft tissue infection, and intraabdominal sources.[1] Prompt administration of fluids and referral for appropriate testing to identify the underlying pathogen are important.[1]

The Patient Having an Allergic Reaction. Always ask the hypotensive patient about new medications and/or exposures. If anaphylaxis is suspected, the cornerstone of therapy includes intravenous fluids and the administration of epinephrine by a trained health care provider.[14]

The Patient With Adrenal Failure. While rare, adrenal failure is important to consider in the right patient because it is almost always refractory to traditional shock therapy.[15] In the ambulatory setting the most common cause of adrenal failure is noncompliance with, or rapid tapering of, chronic oral corticosteroids. If this is suspected, the patient will benefit from the prompt administration of hydrocortisone, typically given as a 100 mg IV dose.[15]

CONSULTATIONS

Emergency medicine evaluation is indicated for patients with suspected sepsis/acute infection, cardiopulmonary dysfunction, active gastrointestinal bleeding, allergic reaction, or adrenal failure.

Cardiology evaluation is indicated for patients with orthostatic hypotension, structural heart disease, acute coronary syndrome, or heart failure.

Geriatric specialist referral is recommended to evaluate older patients with fall tendency, cognitive impairment, and/or dementia.

Endocrinologist consultation is recommended to evaluate patients with endocrine disorders (e.g., hypothyroidism or adrenal disease).

LIFE SPAN CONSIDERATIONS

Postural and postprandial hypotension are both common in older adults for a number of reasons. Postural hypotension is potentiated by impaired compensatory mechanisms to rapid changes in position (i.e., vascular tone and increases in heart rate), limited cardiovascular reserve, poor fluid intake, and concomitant use of vasoactive medication.[16] Postprandial hypotension is more likely a result of autonomic and neural dysfunction, changes in gastrointestinal hormones, gastric distention, and the use of antihypertensive medications before eating a high-carbohydrate meal. Both postural and postprandial hypotension care have serious consequences in older adults, including syncope, cardiovascular complications, and injuries secondary to falls.[16]

PATIENT AND FAMILY EDUCATION

Patient education is essential in the prevention and control of orthostatic hypotension. Patients should be educated to recognize the factors that precipitate low blood pressure, such as prolonged standing, alcohol consumption (causing vasodilation), heat exposure (hot weather or hot bath or shower), sudden postural changes, prolonged recumbency, early morning orthostatic hypotension related to nocturnal diuresis and arising from bed, and high-carbohydrate meals (causing postprandial orthostatic hypotension).[2] Patients taking medications that cause orthostasis should be taught to change positions slowly.

Instructing patients to keep a log of supine and upright blood pressure readings during symptomatic episodes can aid in identifying whether worsening symptoms are related to a mechanism other than orthostatic hypotension.[2]

REFERENCES

1. Winters, M. E., DeBlieux, P., Marcolini, E. G., Bond, M. C., & Woolridge, D. P. (2017). *Emergency department resuscitation of the critically ill.* Gwynn Oak, MD: United Book Press, Inc.
2. Ricci, F., De Caterina, R., & Fedorowski, A. (2015). Orthostatic hypotension epidemiology, prognosis, and treatment. *Journal of the American College of Cardiology, 66*(7), 848–960.
3. Arnold, A. C., & Raj, S. R. (2017). Orthostatic hypotension: A practical approach to investigation and management. *The Canadian Journal of Cardiology, 33,* 1725–1728.
4. Arnold, A. C., & Shibao, C. (2013). Current concepts in orthostatic hypotension management. *Current Hypertension Reports, 15*(4), 304–312.
5. Low, P. A., & Tomalia, V. A. (2015). Orthostatic hypotension: Mechanisms, causes, management. *Journal of Clinical Neurology, 11*(3), 220–226.
6. Trahair, L. G., Horowitz, M., & Jones, K. L. (2014). Postprandial hypotension: A systematic review. *Journal of the American Medical Directors Association, 15*(1), 394–409.
7. Shibao, C., Lipsitz, L. A., & Biaggianoi, I. (2013). ASH position paper: Evaluation and treatment of orthostatic hypotension. *Journal of Clinical Hypertension, 15*(3), 147–153.
8. Arbique, D., Cheek, D., Welliver, M., & Vongpatanasin, W. (2014). Management of neurogenic orthostatic hypotension. *Journal of the American Medical Directors Association, 15*(1), 234–239.
9. Benarroch, E. (2012). Postural tachycardia syndrome a heterogeneous and multifactorial disorder. *Mayo Clinic Proceedings. Mayo Clinic, 87*(12), 1214–1225.
10. Richards, J. B., & Wilcox, S. R. (2014). Diagnosis and management of shock in the emergency department. *Emergency Medicine Practice, 16*(3), 1–22.
11. Villanueva, D., Colomo, A., Bosch, A., et al. (2013). Transfusion strategies for acute upper gastrointestinal bleeding. *The New England Journal of Medicine, 368*(1), 11–21.
12. Fisher, E. S., & Burns, B. (2017). Acute decompensated heart failure: New strategies for improving outcomes. *Emergency Medicine Practice, 19*(5), 1–24.
13. Hollander, J. E., Than, M., & Mueller, C. (2016). State-of-the-art evaluation of emergency department patients presenting with potential acute coronary syndromes. *Circulation, 134,* 547–564.
14. Singer, E., & Zodda, D. (2015). Allergy and anaphylaxis: Principles of acute emergency management. *Emergency Medicine Practice, 17*(8), 1–24.
15. Cutright, A., Ducey, S., & Barthold, C. L. (2017). Recognizing and managing adrenal disorders in the emergency department. *Emergency Medicine Practice, 19*(9), 1–24.
16. Eliopoulos, C. (2018). *Gerontological nursing* (9th ed.). Philadelphia: Wolters Kluwer/Lippincott Williams & Wilkins.

CHAPTER **31**

POISONING

Elizabeth Bouley • Terry Mahan Buttaro

 Immediate emergency department referral is indicated for victims of poisoning.

DEFINITION AND EPIDEMIOLOGY

Poison is defined as a chemical capable of causing illness by entering the body through ingestion, inhalation, intravenous administration, radiation, transdermal absorption, or venom transmitted by stings or bites. Poisonings can be accidental (e.g., contact with concentrated chemicals or industrial agents, taking the wrong medication) or intentional (e.g., illicit drug use). Poisonings can also be industrial (e.g., spraying field workers with pesticides) or an act of war or terrorism (e.g., chemical weapons). Whatever the means or cause, poisoning can be life-threatening and in many cases is best treated in an ED that has decontamination and isolation resources (if required), diagnostic laboratory services immediately available, and intensive care monitoring.

In the United States there is a national system of 55 regional poison control centers that provide rapid threat assessment for poisonings, as well as a major database for understanding poisoning trends. In 2017 about 2.7 million calls were fielded by the centers. In 2016, of the cases involved, 46.4% were children younger than 6 years of age, and 99.4% of these exposures were unintentional.[1] A total of 77.8% of exposures were determined to be accidental.[1] Cosmetics and personal care products are listed as the most common substances affecting the pediatric population, but fumes, gases, and vapors are the single most common cause of pediatric fatalities.[1] Pain medications led the most common substances implicated in the adult poisonings.[1]

Some patients with poison exposures can be safely observed at home and not require an ER visit. In 2016, 66.6% of poison exposures were observed without medical intervention.[1]

That same year, 85.1% of children age 6 or under with a poison exposure were observed at home and did not require physician or emergency room treatment, while 47.1% of adults with a poison exposure did not require physician or emergency room management.[1]

PATHOPHYSIOLOGY

The pathophysiologic process is dependent on the poisonous substance and on the route, duration, and amount of exposure. A patient's underlying physical condition and initial first aid measures will also impact the effect of the toxin.

CLINICAL PRESENTATION AND PHYSICAL EXAMINATION

The presentation of poisoning can have differing signs and symptoms depending on the patient and type of poisoning. Some patients will look fine, but caution is paramount because poisoning can be deadly.[2] Ideally the patient or patient's family can provide accurate information about the situation, but often poisoning is assumed based on circumstantial findings such as a sleeping person who will not wake up and, perhaps, empty acetaminophen bottles are found nearby.

Providers should suspect poisoning in patients with unexplained and sudden respiratory wheezing or dyspnea, acute agitation, progressive somnolence, hallucinations or delusions, seizures, areas of erythema or rash that appear suddenly, acute onset of epigastric pain, vomiting, diarrhea, hypertension, hyperthermia, and sudden and unexplained mental status changes or loss of consciousness. Cardiac concerns include hyper/hypotension, bradycardia/tachycardia, and electrocardiogram changes.[2]

The clinical evaluation begins with a detailed history. Special attempts are made to obtain information from family and first responders. Learning recent activities and the time period in which the poisoning may have occurred is crucial. This is especially important in acetaminophen or aspirin poisonings because treatment is based on exposure time. Attempts must be made to recover medication bottles and over-the-counter medicines. Recovery of any chemicals used at the site of overdose or exposure is important. Material Safety Data Sheets should be available at any site where chemicals are in use. These provide vital information on the chemicals' composition and phone numbers for additional information.

Previous exposures, medical conditions including chronic illnesses, and current medications should be obtained. Psychiatric issues will be important in assessment of stress reaction to the poisoning, as well as previous suicide attempts, mental health interventions, and hospitalizations.

The *physical examination* should be thorough as any body system can be affected. The approach should be systematic and ongoing as in any emergency situation:

- Airway, breathing, circulation, vital signs (temperature, heart rate, respiratory rate, blood pressure, pulse oximetry), serum glucose. Careful attention should be paid to assessing the pharynx and oral mucosa for erythema, edema, soot, or any other abnormality.
- Mood, emotions, mental status, issues of depression, anxiety, suicidality, sleep disturbance, substance use, and hallucinatory or delusional processes must be explored.
- The neurologic examination should note pupillary reaction, nystagmus, deep tendon reflexes, gait, station, Romberg test result, and pronator drift. The Glasgow Coma Scale score is recorded on arrival to determine mental status and monitor the patient for change,[3] available at http://www.glasgowcomascale.org/what-is-gcs/.
- Skin temperature and color are noted. The patient should be completely undressed in order to be assessed for rashes, burns or irritations, bruising, and needle marks suggestive of injection drug use. The provider must observe for areas of discoloration or frank necrosis as well as blistering.
- Cardiovascular (CV) considerations include an ECG to determine presence of tachycardia, bradycardia, arrhythmias, widening QRS, and prolonged QT. The peripheral circulation should be evaluated.
- The respiratory system must be evaluated for good air movement and oxygen saturation; carbon monoxide and carbon dioxide should be tested at bedside when available; and secretions, color, retractions, rales, and wheezing should be noted.
- Gastrointestinal examination includes observation of vomitus and feces, watching especially for bleeding. Guaiac testing of stool and vomitus should be done. Bowel sounds must be noted and their character reported.

INITIAL DIAGNOSTICS

Laboratory values are an important aspect of the diagnostic evaluation and aid in management. Diagnostic tests are dictated by the toxicologic exposure. Some substances, including alcohol, aspirin, acetaminophen, illicit drugs, iron, lead, mercury, carboxyhemoglobin, and ethylene glycol, can be measured directly. Assessment of arterial blood gases, the anion gap, the osmolar gap, and the oxygen saturation gap may provide additional information.

Other laboratory studies are helpful in assessing end-organ involvement. These should include a complete blood count (CBC), serum electrolytes, serum glucose, liver function tests with gamma-glutamyl transferase (GGT), and blood urea nitrogen (BUN) and creatinine concentrations. Urine screens are indicated if a drug overdose, cocaine, opiates, or marijuana is suspected, or the ingested substance is unknown. Urine myoglobin is necessary if rhabdomyolysis, a potential result of alcohol and varied drugs, is a consideration. A pregnancy test should be obtained, if indicated. An ECG is necessary with specific poisons, and assessment will need to be repeated in some instances. Further evaluation is indicated if abnormalities such as acidosis and hypoxia are discerned.

INITIAL DIAGNOSTICS

Poisoning

LABORATORY
- CBC
- Serum glucose, electrolytes, BUN, Creatinine
- Liver function tests including GGT
- Serum levels for specific medications (e.g., digoxin, lithium, valproic acid)[a]
- Carboxyhemoglobin (carbon monoxide)[a]
- Methemoglobin[a]
- Serum ammonia
- Serum lactate

- Blood gases (arterial if respiratory distress)[a]
- Acetaminophen or salicylate level (if ingestion)
- Ethanol and toxicology levels (urine or blood)
- Serum hCG (female patients)[a]
- Prothrombin time/partial thromboplastin time/international normalized ratio (PT/PTT/INR)

INITIAL
- ECG
- Capnography

[a]If indicated.

DIFFERENTIAL DIAGNOSIS

- Other causes of a change in status should always be considered, especially if there is not clear evidence of poisoning. Allergies, anaphylaxis, carbon monoxide, electrolyte abnormalities (e.g., hypo/hypernatremia, hypo/hyperkalemia), methemoglobin, renal or liver failure, seizures, and iron overload are considerations other than alcohol or drug overdose. Other differentials are myriad, and in addition to those already discussed, include, but are not limited to, arsenic, acute onset dementia, cyanide, heavy metals, lead, infection, medications (prescribed, over-the-counter, herbals or illicit) seizure, sepsis, stroke, or terrorism.
- A more recent poisoning concern is electronic cigarettes (ECs), a nicotine delivery method with unclear safety and not regulated by the U.S. Food and Drug Administration. The primary concerns are the potential release of higher

quantities of chemical aerosols than in traditional cigarettes and exposure to children—especially those younger than age 6. The resultant nausea and vomiting are common symptoms that bring children to the ER. Adult exposures include ingestion, skin and eyes related to ingredients that include propylene glycol (antifreeze), nicotine (addictive), polycyclic aromatic hydrocarbons, tobacco-specific nitrosamines, volatile organic compounds, and inorganic compounds. ECs impact the respiratory and cardiovascular systems potentially causing lipoid pneumonia from aspiration, diminished lung function, high blood pressure, rapid heart rate, and myocardial effects, as well as hypertension, tachycardia, change in mitral flow velocities, and myocardial effects.[4]

- Synthetic cannabinoids (K2/Spice) have chemical properties similar to marijuana and can be inhaled or smoked, are human-made, mind-altering chemicals that can be sprayed, dried so they can be smoked, or sold as liquids to be vaporized and inhaled in ECs. Effects of these easily obtained psychoactive products include suicidality, tachycardia, vomiting, and violent behavior. Withdrawal in patients who regularly use these products is associated with anxiety, depression, headaches, and irritability.[5]

INTERPROFESSIONAL COLLABORATION AND MANAGEMENT

- Mobilize the emergency medical services (EMS) system (911).
- Contact Poison Control (United States only) for treatment guidance: 1-800-222-1222.
- The initial and frequent reassessment of the poisoned patient requires attention to airway, breathing, and circulation, disability (cognitive), and toxidrome exposure (ABC).[6]
- Oxygen and continuous airway maintenance are critical. The patient should be carefully monitored in a critical care area for potential need for intubation, and the provider should be ready to secure the airway with an endotracheal tube.
- Intravenous access is also necessary.
- Transport must be arranged to the closest appropriate facility by use of transport ambulance capable of critical care intervention.
- Determine the identity of the poison or substance, how it entered the person's system, why it was used or encountered, and when the contact was made. Transmit the substance with the patient to the emergency department if the patient has stable vital signs and is alert and oriented, and if this information is believed to be reliable. The provider can initiate a call to the poison control center for further instruction.
- In general, skin and eye decontamination are done immediately on hospital arrival (should be started prehospital, if possible, and completed on hospital arrival). Immediate contact is made with poison control for expert guidance in management. Poison control should be alerted at the first notice of the arrival of a potential poisoning patient. Any volatile or toxic chemical exposure requires decontamination of the patient and the patient's EMS caregivers. The patient should not be allowed into a hospital or clinic without decontamination. The facility should have in place a system for avoiding contact with the patient and

isolating the patient until decontamination can be set up. This is vitally important in mass casualties. Workers trained in decontamination technique are appropriately garbed in self-contained breathing apparatus and protective clothing. The water used to decontaminate must be segregated and not allowed to enter public drainage systems. All of these issues are addressed in training of the decontamination team. The goal is to prevent rescuers from becoming victims and extension of the contamination to others. The next steps will occur simultaneously in the emergency department. In an unconscious or obtunded patient, a standard cocktail will be given to treat hypoglycemia, Wernicke encephalopathy, and opioid overdose: glucose, 25 to 50 g intravenously (1 amp $D_{50}W$ is 25 grams); thiamine, 100 mg intravenously; and naloxone, 2 mg intravenously, intramuscularly, or subcutaneously.[6]

- If the airway is compromised, it should be emergently secured with endotracheal intubation and ventilation. After the ABCs are managed, attention returns to decontamination or reversal of the poison's effect. Activated charcoal is rarely indicated but sometimes helpful in specific ingestions. It should be given under the direction of a toxicologist in discussion with poison control. For ingested components, activated charcoal, the usefulness of which is dependent on the length of time since ingestion (within one hour of poison ingestion is recommended), may be indicated for patients whose airway is intact or protected. Charcoal dosing is based on body weight, the type of ingestion (some substances are not well absorbed by charcoal), and patient status (must be awake and is not considered a candidate for endoscopy, nor be suspected of a gastrointestinal perforation).[6] Whole bowel irrigation with polyethylene glycol electrolyte solution is sometimes indicated, but cautiously.[6]
- Considering the large number of substances that could potentially act as toxins, a relatively small number of antidotes are available.

Some commonly used antidotes for adults include the following:

- N-acetylcysteine for acetaminophen. N-acetylcysteine is available orally and intravenously and preferably used soon after ingestion (within 8 hours). Dosing is somewhat individualized depending on the time of ingestion and time of presentation. The initial oral dosing is 140 mg/kg by a standard protocol based on a nomogram to determine the necessity of treatment for acetaminophen overdoses. Further doses at 70 mg/kg p.o. every 4 hours, continued for up to 72 hours.[7]
- Flumazenil for benzodiazepines. Though there are concerns about, flumazenil it can administered intravenously in 0.2 mg dose every minute to a maximum of 1 mg Flumazenil can reverse the effects of benzodiazepines, but could be detrimental if it is given to patients with benzodiazepine dependence, mixed substance overdose, alcohol overdose, or seizure history.[8]
- Naloxone for opioids. Naloxone is an opiate antagonist and is available intranasal, SQ, and IV and given in doses of 0.4 mg intravenously, repeated every 2 to 3 minutes in the non–opiate-dependent patient.[8] For opiate dependent patients, a smaller dose is recommended to prevent withdrawal syndrome. As a result the lowest effective dose is now recommended for opiate dependent patients.[9]

TERRORISM

Varied biologic and chemical weapons continue to remain a potential threat throughout the world. State and national planning efforts are attempting to prepare an emergency response. Additionally, the Centers for Disease Control and Prevention (CDC) has medical information addressing specific biological weapons available at https://emergency.cdc.gov/bioterrorism/. Information systems are being developed to alert health care providers when a crisis occurs, and training programs in managing poisonings are under way. At this time, the existing systems for hazardous materials decontamination and basic and advanced life support measures remain the standard of care. Although all health care providers must maintain vigilance for suspicious presentations and clusters of patients with the same toxidrome, it will remain a complex system of identification of the chemical or biologic used and dissemination of antidotes, vaccines, and response plans. The first priority is to contain the exposures and to prevent expansion of the event; the second priority is basic life support; and the third priority is close communication with authorities charged with managing such emergencies.

PATIENT AND FAMILY EDUCATION

Since many poisonings occur in children younger than 6 years, prenatal and well-child counseling is an excellent opportunity to provide education and prevention advice. Families with young children need to survey their home for chemicals and medications. All need to be stored in areas inaccessible to children (with the caveat that few areas remain inaccessible to determined and curious children). These visits also provide the opportunity to discuss home and over-the-counter medications and treatments. Acetaminophen, a common fever and pain reliever, is a valuable medication, but dangerous at improper doses. A careful review of age-appropriate dosage and when to use acetaminophen can help parents prevent accidents. Increasing attention must also be addressed to various forms of nicotine and caffeine ingestion, as well as awareness that marijuana is now legally available in many jurisdictions. Alerting parents to the potentially deadly effects of drugs and other substances (e.g., alcohol, vaping) should be part of early childhood counseling. In addition, many homes have other "recreational" drugs, from which children must also be protected.

Time spent with adults in reviewing potentially dangerous substances (e.g., energy drinks), new prescriptions, and proper scheduling is important to prevent poisoning or drug overdose. Equipping patients with a basic understanding of each drug's intended effect, the expected outcome, and symptoms or reaction of toxicity is valuable.

Education becomes increasingly important with older patients, too. Confusion and misunderstandings about prescribed and over-the-counter medications can result in accidental overdose. Establishing a system and engaging family, pharmacist, and caregivers in organizing medications can be invaluable. All patients require a careful medication reconciliation at each office visit and leave with a medication list that reflects the name of the medication as distributed from the pharmacy so that there are no misunderstandings. Older adults should also be reminded to keep medications in a safe environment—away from children and adolescents. All patients should be advised to dispose of unused medications safely.

REFERENCES

1. Poisoning Statistics. National data 2016. Retrieved from https://www.poison.org/poison-statistics-national-data-from-2016. (Accessed 6 June 2018).
2. Comprehensive evaluation and treatment. In K. R. Olson, I. B. Anderson, N. L. Benowitz, P. D. Blanc, R. F. Clark, T. E. Kearney, et al. (Eds.), Poisoning & drug overdose (7th ed.). New York, NY: McGraw-Hill.
3. Lominadze, G., Kazzi, M. G., & Shiloh, A. L. (2016). Pre-ICU syndromes. In J. M. Oropello, S. M. Pastores, & V. Kvetan (Eds.), Critical care. New York, NY: McGraw-Hill. Retrieved from http://accessmedicine.mhmedical.com.ezproxy.simmons.edu/content.aspx?bookid=1944&sectionid=143515747. (Accessed 14 June 2018).
4. Know the risks: E-cigarettes and young people. Retrieved from https://e-cigarettes.surgeongeneral.gov/. (Accessed 14 June 2018).
5. National Institute of Drug Abuse Synthetic Cannabinoids. Retrieved from https://www.drugabuse.gov/publications/drugfacts/synthetic-cannabinoids-k2spice. (Accessed 14 June 2018).
6. Erickson, M. A., & Penning, T. M. (2018). Drug toxicity and poisoning. In L. L. Brunton, R. Hilal-Dandan, & B. C. Knollmann (Eds.), Goodman & Gilman's: The pharmacological basis of therapeutics (13th ed.). New York, NY: McGraw-Hill.
7. Olson, K. R. (2018). Poisoning. In M. A. Papadakis, S. J. McPhee, & M. W. Rabow (Eds.), Current medical diagnosis & treatment (57th ed.). New York, NY: McGraw-Hill.
8. Mihic, S., Mayfield, J., & Harris, R. (2018). Hypnotics and sedatives. In L. L. Brunton, R. Hilal-Dandan, & B. C. Knollmann (Eds.), Goodman & Gilman's: The pharmacological basis of therapeutics (13th ed.). New York, NY: McGraw-Hill.
9. Rzasa, L. R., & Galinkin, J. L. (2017). Naloxone dosage for opioid reversal: Current evidence and clinical implications. Therapeutic advances in drug safety, 9(1), 63–88. doi:10.1177/2042098617744161.

CHAPTER **32**

SEXUAL ASSAULT
Julie G. Stewart

DEFINITION AND EPIDEMIOLOGY

Sexual violence consists of a variety of crimes including rape, sexual assault, and sexual harassment.[1] Sexual harassment includes many types of unwelcome sexual advances, remarks, and gestures. The legal definition of rape according to the Federal Bureau of Investigation (FBI) is "penetration, no matter how slight, of the vagina or anus with any body part or object, or oral penetration by a sex organ of another person, without the consent of the victim." The National Incident-Based Reporting System (NIBRS) defines rape as, "The carnal knowledge of a person, without the consent of the victim, including instances where the victim is incapable of giving consent because of his/her age or because of his/her temporary or permanent mental or physical incapacity."[2] Sexual assault has a much broader definition. It is defined as any sexual act that is forced or coerced without the consent of the victim and includes any victim who is unable to consent.[3] Rape and sexual assault are not sexually motivated acts; rather, they are motivated by rage, aggression, and the determination to dominate another human being.

In the United States, a person is a victim of sexual assault every 98 seconds.[4] According to the National Crime Victimization Survey, 321,500 rapes and sexual assaults of persons aged 12 years or older are reported on average every year.[5] Further surveys indicate that 1 of 5 women and 1 of 59 men in the United States experience an attempted or completed rape at some point in their lifetime.[6] Half of all the perpetrators of sexual violence are over the age of 30, and 57% are white.[7] The rates of sexual assault are higher for females and males aged 18–24 years, with sexual assault the most commonly reported crime on campuses. Transgender, genderqueer, and nonconforming college students have higher rates of sexual assault.[7] These statistics reflect only reported incidents. Sixty percent of sexual assaults are not reported to the police.[4] The incidence of rape is about 10 times higher for women than for men, although men are less likely to report the occurrence. (For the purpose of this chapter, the term *she* is used, although this information can also apply to men who have been victims of sexual assault.)

There are no known absolute risk factors for becoming a victim of sexual assault. In fact, anyone can be a victim regardless of age, race, gender, or socioeconomic status. However, sexual assault victims are predominantly female, and the perpetrators are almost always heterosexual males. Female victims are more likely to be assaulted by someone they know, and reports indicate that 63% of sexual assault victimizations involve offenders with whom the victim had a relationship as a family member, intimate, or acquaintance.[4] Among developmentally disabled adults, up to 83% of women and 32% of men are victims of sexual violence; of these victims of sexual violence, 49% will experience 10 or more abusive incidents.[9]

Sexual assault can also occur in the context of any intimate partner relationship. This includes marital, nonmarital, gay, lesbian, or past relationships. However, these sexual assaults are often recurring and one of the symptoms of a larger domestic violence problem that needs to be addressed. Consequences for ongoing sexual violence by an intimate partner are severe and require ongoing monitoring and attention by the health care provider.

CLINICAL PRESENTATION AND PHYSICAL EXAMINATION

The physical presentation of a patient in the clinic or office setting who has been sexually assaulted is immensely varied. Some patients may report a chief complaint of sexual assault to their health care provider, whereas others may not mention that a sexual assault has occurred. Likewise, the presentation of psychological effects of trauma also varies among victims, ranging from visibly shaken and crying to appearing calm. Some patients may choose to disclose that a sexual assault occurred if they are asked by a trusted health care provider. However, other patients may deny that violence occurred despite evidence of trauma. Whatever the reasons for the patient's denial, the health care provider must respect it and offer compassionate support. Reassuring the patient that sexual assault is always an act of control and violence and is never something anyone "deserves" or "asked for" is crucial for emotional support.

The health care provider does not need to make a final determination whether sexual assault has occurred; that must be left to the court to decide if the patient opts to report the assault. However, reporting to the police should be encouraged. It is helpful for the provider to let the patient know that sexual assault is, unfortunately, a common experience and that it is a problem the provider may be able to assist with. This may leave the door open should the patient decide in the future to disclose what happened. Unfortunately, in a national study, most rape and sexual assault victims were not treated for their injuries.[5] According to this study, only approximately 30% of victims received treatment, with 20% of this total receiving care

at a physician's office or clinic.[5] Health care providers are mandated to report sexual assault of children (state laws vary on age limit), the elderly, and the disabled.

If the patient does disclose a sexual assault, the provider should defer a physical examination and refer the patient to the emergency department if the sexual assault occurred within the past 5 days, preferably within 72 hours. A referral to the emergency department will ensure that the appropriate measures are taken to collect evidence and to comply with standardized protocol. This is essential to support the patient's current or future desire for legal pursuits, because some patients may decide later to report the incident to the police. This specialized forensic examination should be free of charge because federal and state funds are available. Having this examination and collection of evidence completed does not require the patient to press criminal charges or to report the incident to law enforcement. Testing for drugs that might have been used to render the patient unaware of what was happening can also be done at no cost to the patient. Furthermore, the emergency department will also be able to provide the patient with comprehensive and compassionate services, including crisis intervention, rape counseling, and referrals to appropriate community agencies. In many emergency departments, there are specially trained nurses (sexual assault nurse examiners [SANEs] and sexual assault forensic examiners [SAFEs]) who help provide the patient with appropriate sensitive care.

The health care provider can prepare the patient for what to expect in the emergency department. It is not necessary that the provider request specific information about the assault; this information will be gathered in the emergency department. Retelling of the story can be traumatizing for the patient. Rather, providers can attentively listen and document what the patient desires to express, using exact quotes whenever possible. The health care provider should carefully note emotional responses (e.g., crying, restlessness, anxious behavior, shaking, withdrawal) because this would be useful in court as an adjunct to the emergency department records. It is important to advise the patient not to shower, urinate, brush teeth, or wash clothing that might contain evidence.

If the patient does not desire to pursue an examination in the emergency department or if more than 5 days have passed since the assault, medical care can be managed in the office setting. The provider needs to obtain a detailed history including the patient sexual history and any history of prior abuse, and then perform a full physical and gynecologic examination. About 40% of rape victims sustained a collateral injury; 5% sustained a major injury, such as severe lacerations, fractures, internal injuries, or unconsciousness.[10] Injuries are most common among victims aged 30 years or older.[10] Possible gynecologic injuries include vaginal or anal tearing, rectal bleeding, bruising, and soreness. Other physical symptoms associated with trauma include gastrointestinal irritability, dysmenorrhea, pelvic pain, and urinary tract infection.

When the patient prefers to have a physical examination in the primary care office, the provider should assure her that the examination can stop at any time and that there is time to take a break if needed. The examination to be performed is a complete head-to-toe examination observing for any injuries because the patient may not be aware of abrasions or bruising in areas not visible to her. If any injuries are discovered, it is important to measure them with a ruler for documentation.

Using the face of a clock to reference areas in the genitalia with the clitoris at the 12-o'clock position and the anus at the 6-o'clock position, the provider documents any abnormal findings. In particular, the health care provider should closely examine the posterior fourchette because it is frequently an area in which injuries such as lacerations and abrasions occur.[10,11] Culture specimens are obtained for gonorrhea and chlamydia testing; serum testing for syphilis, hepatitis B and C, and human immunodeficiency virus (HIV) infection; and pregnancy is discussed as appropriate.

DIAGNOSTICS

Potential consequences of sexual assault include the risk of pregnancy and sexually transmitted diseases (STDs), including HIV infection. If it has been more than 72 hours since the sexual assault, it is not feasible to offer pregnancy or STD prophylactics or antiretroviral therapy for postexposure prophylaxis.[12] A pregnancy test should be completed, with appropriate counseling pending the results. Testing for STDs should be determined individually. If the patient seeks treatment within 72 hours after the assault, the presence of an infection may indicate that the STD was present before the assault, even though laws in the United States limit the use of prior infections and sexual history as evidence in court. The patient may express fears about having contracted HIV infection; testing should be done 6 weeks and 3 and 6 months after the assault because of the length of time for seroconversion to occur. If the appropriate time has passed, patients should have pretest and posttest education and counseling. Education should include risks of acquiring the infection, potential transmission of the virus, and instruction about safe sex practices at least until testing is complete, or longer if the results are positive.

Documentation

Accurate and precise documentation of the patient's physical and emotional signs and symptoms of sexual assault are always necessary, but especially so when there is a possibility that the documentation will corroborate the patient's testimony in court. It is essential that health care providers use medical rather than legal terminology. For example, calling the assault the "alleged rape" should be avoided; rather, it should be described as the "reported sexual assault." Likewise, the word "patient" should be used rather than "victim." The connotation of words must be considered. *Penetration* is a better word than *intercourse* because the latter may sound as though the act were consensual. If the patient does not wish to have a certain part of the examination completed, it should not be documented as "refused" because this makes the patient sound uncooperative; rather, the provider should write that the patient "declined" the examination. Use of the patient's own words in quotation marks whenever possible best captures the description of the incident and is extremely helpful in court. The provider should avoid writing "no weapons used" but should describe exactly what happened because there may have been verbal or implied threats. It is also important to be wary of using medical terminology that could be misinterpreted. For example, if the patient appears calm and collected, it is better to document that than to say, "No apparent distress." Documentation of unnecessary history that is not related to the chief complaint (e.g., psychiatric history, substance use history) could be used in court to discredit the patient's testimony.[11]

Primary Care Management

When a patient reports that she has been a victim of sexual assault and it has been determined that she will be treated in the primary care setting, it is important to assess more than the patient's physical well-being. Patients may seek care soon after the assault or after an extended period. The patient's account of the assault will aid the provider in understanding the patient's experience and what type of services may be of benefit.

Patients who seek care shortly after the assault may display a range of emotions or may show a lack of emotions. Some may appear frightened, shocked, or angry. Regardless of their demeanor, these patients need understanding and support. The patient's emotional presentation is not indicative of the level of trauma that has been experienced. A review of the patient's home environment and support system is appropriate. Because of the stigma associated with sexual assault, it is sometimes difficult for victims to inform significant people in their life about their victimization. Some fear that their intimate partner or parent may seek physical revenge against the perpetrator, if the perpetrator is known to them. As a result, they may be reluctant or unwilling to disclose information in an effort to protect their partner or parent from potential legal problems. Unfortunately, some patients are afraid to inform someone about the assault because they think that no one will believe them or that they are to blame for the assault. This is especially true if the patient consumed alcohol or drugs before the assault, or if she thought she was dressed in provocative attire. As a result, the patient may not receive adequate support.

The provider can assist patients in identifying people in their lives to whom they can disclose the assault and who can provide support. Patients may also benefit from a discussion of the various ways in which to talk with their family or partner about the assault. Patients may experience a high degree of fear over the potential for further harm and may be afraid to be alone or to return home. Assistance must be offered in determining how to appropriately address their fears.

Patients who wait a while after the assault to initially seek care may be prompted to do so because of physical complaints, such as STDs or pregnancy, or because of psychological difficulties. Some patients may experience symptoms of distress consistent with posttraumatic stress disorder. One study revealed that almost one-third of rape victims develop posttraumatic stress disorder at some point after the rape; this rate is six times higher than the rate for women who have not been raped.[13]

Reactions of people who have been sexually assaulted vary according to a variety of factors, including age, gender, ethnicity, and circumstances surrounding the assault. Regardless of when the patient seeks care after a sexual assault, it is important for the provider to gain an accurate understanding of the patient's concerns, level of functioning, and support system before developing an appropriate treatment plan. The health care provider's comfort level with the subject matter may affect the patient's willingness to disclose information that would provide insight into the patient's needs. The provider is in a pivotal role to aid the patient in identifying the need for additional services, including mental health services.

INTERPROFESSIONAL COLLABORATIVE MANAGEMENT

- *Emergency department:* It is strongly advised that the patient be treated in a specially equipped emergency department by trained SANEs, SAFEs, or other appropriate health care providers if the examination occurs within several days of the assault.

- *Mental health services:* The patient should always be referred to mental health services that explicitly address issues surrounding sexual assault. Most areas have sexual assault crisis services available 24 hours/day, 7 days/week.
- *Legal services or police:* If the patient is treated in the primary care setting, an assessment must be made to determine her or his legal needs, level of functioning, and willingness to pursue additional services.
- *Other services:* Clearly, appropriate referral needs to be made for any symptoms, illnesses, or injuries for which treatment is beyond the scope of the office setting.
- *Mandated reporting:* Any sexual assault perpetrated on a victim who is younger than 18 years or on any adult who is physically dependent or cognitively impaired must be reported to the local child or adult protective agency as well as to law enforcement. Health care providers are mandated to report any suspicion of sexual assault in these populations, regardless of whether the patient reports that sexual assault has occurred. Although it is not the provider's responsibility to prove that the violence occurred, it is his or her responsibility to act on the clinical evidence presented. Because laws vary among states, providers should become familiar with the laws within their area.

LIFE-SPAN CONSIDERATIONS
Children and Adolescents

Sexual abuse of children and adolescents is a serious and complicated issue that requires specialized training in interviews and physical examinations whenever abuse is suspected. Guidelines for caring for children and adolescents and collaboration with agencies that are child and adolescent specific should be the goal for this population in an effort to avoid lifelong complications related to the abuse.

Older Adults

Older patients are particularly vulnerable because of age-related illness and an overall decrease in physical strength. In fact, people over the age of 60 account for 18% of sexual assault victims.[14,15] In a study of older adult female sexual abuse victims, 81% of abuse was perpetrated by the victim's primary caregiver.[14] Seventy-eight percent was perpetrated by family members, of whom 39% were sons.[14]

Older adults may sustain more injuries and specifically more genital injuries. Older women are also unlikely to report being sexually assaulted; they may feel extreme embarrassment, humiliation, and shame because they were raised during a time when issues related to sex were not discussed. Some patients may be concerned that reporting the assault will result in a loss of their independence. Risk factors for being sexually assaulted include impaired hearing, diminished physical strength, limited mobility, reliance on others for help, and memory issues.

SPECIFIC POPULATIONS
Male Patients

Although male victims represent a minority of sexual assault victims, it is critical that they be treated the same as female patients. Male victims may experience rectal or penile trauma, bleeding or discharge, infection, or trauma to the mouth and pharynx. The patient may receive frontal injuries from being in a prone position during the assault. Men are usually assaulted by other men. For many reasons, men are less likely than women to seek services after being sexually assaulted, although they commonly experience similar physical and emotional reactions. Men may feel that they are "less of a man," may experience shame about not being able to defend themselves, and may be confused about their sexuality. If the assailant was a woman, the patient may feel particularly weak or inferior. Anxiety, depression, alienation, and insomnia are some of the psychological effects for men who have been sexually assaulted. As with all victims of sexual assault, it is important for the patient to receive mental health services.

Disabled Adults

Among the most vulnerable populations are individuals who are developmentally and/or physically disabled. Interpersonal violence against women and men with disabilities ranges from 26% to 90%.[16] Among developmentally disabled adults, up to 83% of women and 32% of men are victims of sexual violence.[16] Of those victims of sexual violence, 49% will experience 10 or more abusive incidents.[16] From 97% to 99% of their attackers are known to the victims.[16] Health care providers who provide medical services to the developmentally disabled need to assess for any signs and/or symptoms of abuse (physical and/or sexual). Examples of signs and symptoms include unexplained bruises, genital lacerations, STDs, regression, acting out, sleep disturbances, and depression.

Homeless or Marginally Housed

The intersection between lack of adequate housing and sexual violence occurs on a variety of levels. It is vital for the health care provider to be sensitive and to assess for any history of sexual assault in patients who are either homeless or living in inadequate housing. Being homeless or marginally housed increased the risk for being sexually assaulted, particularly for lesbian, gay, bisexual, and/or transgender (LGBT) youth. According to data from the National Sexual Violence Resource Center, over 60% of young women left their homes because they had been sexually abused.[17] For those youths, and adults who sought to relocate after being abused by their landlords or whose perpetrator lived nearby, over 70% to 80% were unable to move because of lease or legal issues or a lack of housing options.[17]

Transgender

Transgender individuals are often victims of sexual violence, with one out of two reporting a history of sexual assault at least once in their lives.[18] Transgender persons of color, youths, and the disabled are at highest rates of victimization in addition to those who are homeless. Transgender females of color are at the highest risk of all forms of interpersonal violence. Perpetrators can be any type of individual, including those working as health care professionals and police.

The Office for Victims of Crime suggests *Five Keys to Service* when caring for transgender victims of sexual assault.[18] These are: (1) Don't categorize; use your client's terms; (2) know why you are asking, and explain why; (3) consider the whole person; (4) partner with your client; and (5) manage your curiosity. Comprehensive discussion related to this population and how best to help are found on the Office for Victims of Crimes: Responding to transgender victims of sexual assault website.

Immigrants

Many immigrants have difficulty accessing care because of limited resources, language barriers, and lack of awareness about how to access services; however, additional concerns arise with respect to receiving services for sexual assault. Some patients may be afraid to report the sexual assault to authorities because they are concerned that it may have a negative impact on their immigration status, especially if the patient is an undocumented alien. They also may not understand that it is illegal for them to be assaulted and that they have a right to report the crime. Another significant factor for immigrants in accessing services to address sexual assault is their cultural beliefs. Some may think it is inappropriate for them to discuss intimate matters with a professional, although they may not have the means or methods to address their issues within a cultural context. It is important for health care providers to be aware of cultural factors when providing care, to modify their treatment to the extent that they are able, and to ensure that the patient is aware of his or her rights and the availability of services.

PATIENT EDUCATION AND HEALTH PROMOTION

Sexual assault occurs in a variety of settings and may victimize people of all ages, races, religions, and socioeconomic backgrounds. Providers can give patients various tips to promote their general safety; however, there is no known prevention for sexual assault. All health care providers should assess every patient for any history of sexual abuse or assault; they should educate their patients about the dynamics of sexual assault, including the fact that it is an act of violence; and they should encourage patients to seek mental health services if a positive history is uncovered.

REFERENCES

1. National Institute of Justice. Rape and sexual violence. Retrieved from www.nij.gov/topics/crime/rape-sexual-violence/pages/welcome.aspx.
2. Federal Bureau of Investigation (FBI). New definition of rape. Frequently asked questions, May, 2013. Retrieved from www.fbi.gov/about-us/cjis/ucr/recent-program-updates/new-rape-definition-frequently-asked-questions.
3. U.S. Department of Justice (DOJ). (2019). Sexual assault. Retrieved from https://www.justice.gov/ovw/sexual-assault.
4. Rape, Abuse and Incest National Network (RAINN). RAINN Statistics, 2016. Retrieved from https://www.rainn.org/statistics. (Accessed 28 April 2019).
5. National victimization survey: criminal victimization. (2015). NCJ 227777, Washington, DC, U.S. Department of Justice, Office of Justice Programs.
6. Centers for Disease Control (CDC). (2014). Sexual violence surveillance. Retrieved from https://www.cdc.gov/violenceprevention/pdf/sv_surveillance_definitionsl-2009-a.pdf.
7. Rape, Abuse and Incest National Network (RAINN). (2016). RAINN Statistics. Retrieved from https://www.rainn.org/statistics. (Accessed 29 April 2019).
8. Deleted in proofs.
9. Connecticut Sexual Assault Crisis Service (CONNSACS). (2012). Sexual assault in Connecticut. Fact sheets and statistics. Retrieved from www.connsacs.org/learn/stats.htm.
10. An analysis of data on rape and sexual assault. Washington, DC: U.S. Department of Justice, Office of Justice Programs; 1997.
11. Ledray, L., Burgess, A., & Giardina, A. Medical response to adult sexual abuse: A resource for clinicians and related professionals. St Louis: STM Learning; October 26, 2010.
12. Centers for Disease Control and Prevention. (2006). Sexually transmitted diseases treatment guidelines, 2006. MMWR. Recommendations and Reports: Morbidity and Mortality Weekly Report. Recommendations and Reports, 55(RR–11), 1–94.
13. Hodgson, J., & Kelley, D. (2002). Sexual violence: Policies, practices. and challenges in the United States and Canada. Westport, Conn: Praeger.
14. Connecticut Sexual Assault Crisis Service (CONNSACS). (2014). National statistics on sexual violence. fact sheet. Retrieved from www.connsacs.org/learn/stats.htm.
15. Burgess, A. W., Hanrahan, N. P., & Baker, T. (2005). Forensic markers in elder female sexual abuse cases. Clinics in Geriatric Medicine, 21(2), 399–412, NCJ 245450.
16. National Center on Elder Abuse and Neglect. Abuse of adults with a disability. Research Brief. Retrieved from http://ncea.aoa.gov/Resources/Publication/docs/Disabilities_ResearchBrief_508web.pdf. (Accessed 26 June 2015).
17. National Sexual Violence Resource Center (NSVRC). Link between housing and sexual violence. Retrieved from www.nsvrc.org/sites/default/files/nsvrc_infographic_link-between-housing-sexual-violence.pdf.
18. Office for Victims of Crime. Responding to transgender victims of sexual assault. Retrieved from https://www.ovc.gov/pubs/forge/tips_five_keys.html.

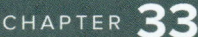

CHAPTER **33**

SYNCOPE
Magen M. Price

 Immediate emergency department referral or physician consultation is indicated for syncope in a patient with a family history of sudden death or for syncope associated with exercise, chest pain, congestive heart failure, palpitations, acute hemorrhage, trauma, transient ischemic attacks, seizures, or abnormal electrocardiogram (ECG) recording or chest X-ray study.[1] Patients with syncope and a medical history of anatomic heart disease or previous surgical repair of a cardiac lesion also require emergency department referral or physician consultation. Patients who may have new-onset seizure disorder should be considered for hospital admission to a unit with appropriate monitoring capabilities.

DEFINITION AND EPIDEMIOLOGY

Syncope is defined as a temporary loss of consciousness and postural tone that is followed by spontaneous complete recovery and does not require resuscitation. Presyncope or near-syncope is a sensation of lightheadedness or faintness in which the patient senses that true syncope may be imminent but complete loss of consciousness never occurs.

The true incidence of syncope in the general population is not well known owing to differences in definition, under-reporting, and variations within age groups or special populations. There is a similar incidence for men and women until 70 years of age, after which there is a sharp increase in incidence that favors women.[2] Women are therefore twice as likely as men to experience syncope during their lifetime.[3] Syncope is more common in older patients than in other age groups and is often associated with falls and greater risk for adverse outcomes.[4] The increase in syncopal events is likely to be related to the number of comorbidities and prescribed medications in this cohort.[2] In addition, the physiologic changes of aging increase an older adult's risk for syncope.[2]

PATHOPHYSIOLOGY

Syncope is a symptom of an underlying process or processes (Box 33.1). These processes result in syncope by one of two pathophysiologic mechanisms: deprivation of nutrients to the brain or deprivation of oxygen to the brain. Deprivation of nutrients most often results from decreased blood

BOX **33.1**

Causes of Syncope

CARDIAC

Mechanical or Obstructive Processes
- Cardiac valvular diseases
- Atrial myxoma
- Hypertrophic or obstructive cardiomyopathy
- Pulmonary hypertension
- Pulmonary embolism
- Pericardial disease
- Cardiac tamponade
- Myocardial infarction or ischemia

Arrhythmias
- Sick sinus syndrome
- Atrioventricular conduction disturbances
- Supraventricular or ventricular tachycardia
- Prolonged or shortened QT syndrome
- Pacemaker malfunction

NEUROLOGIC

Reflex or Neuromediated
- Autonomic failure
- Vasovagal (common faint)
- Situational (micturition, cough, swallow, defecation)
- Carotid sinus hypersensitivity (primarily found in older adults)

Cerebrovascular
- Vertebrovascular transient ischemic attack

MISCELLANEOUS
- Hypoglycemia
- Hypovolemia (especially in older patients who are taking antihypertensive medications)
- Postprandial hypotension
- Psychiatric disease (panic disorder, hysteria, depression)

flow secondary to hypovolemia, cardiac outflow obstruction, cardiac arrhythmias, or neurovascular causes. Deprivation of oxygen is most often associated with hypoxia or anemia. It is important to distinguish true syncope from seizure disorders or other conditions that might result in altered levels of consciousness, such as iatrogenic syncope from medication therapy, drug or alcohol intoxication, concussions, amnesia, or metabolic causes (e.g., hypoglycemia). Seizure-like activity may be present with syncope; this is secondary to generalized cerebral hypoxia.

There are three main classifications of syncope: (1) neurally mediated or reflex, (2) orthostatic hypotensive, and (3) cardiac.[5] The most common cause of syncope is vasovagal; however, cardiac causes have an increased incidence of sudden death and must be evaluated early.[5] The cardiac causes consist of two major categories: (1) mechanical or ventricular outflow obstructive processes and, more commonly, (2) arrhythmias. Possible mechanical or obstructive processes responsible for syncope include cerebrovascular disease, cardiac valvular disease, atrial myxoma, hypertrophic or obstructive cardiomyopathy, pulmonary hypertension, pulmonary embolism, pericardial disease or tamponade, acute myocardial infarction or

ischemia, and possible prosthetic valve malfunction. Possible rhythm disturbances include sick sinus syndrome, atrioventricular conduction disturbances, supraventricular and ventricular tachycardias, long QT syndrome, and pacemaker system malfunction. Tachycardias can also trigger vasovagal syncope.[5]

Neurally mediated syncope is the most common type of syncope and is primarily seen in young adults.[3] Situational syncope, carotid sinus syncope, and others are also classified as neurally mediated. Although different in their provocation, these disorders share a reflex response that causes vasodilation, bradycardia, and paradoxical systemic hypotension, eventually leading to decreased blood flow to the brain.[5] In carotid sinus syncope, the trigger sites are thought to be peripheral receptors that respond to mechanical stimuli (such as neck stretching or tight collars); this type of syncope occurs most often in older adults.[5]

Finally, orthostatic stress can cause insufficient peripheral vasoconstriction, leading to syncope. Orthostatic hypotension is rare in patients younger than 40 years, yet is one of the most common causes of syncope in patients older than 70 years.[6] Classic orthostatic hypotension is defined as a drop in systolic blood pressure (BP) of greater than 20 mm Hg or of diastolic BP of greater than 10 mm Hg within 3 minutes of transition from supine to standing.[6] This can be triggered by blood loss, dehydration, or autonomic dysfunction. In the older adult population, syncope is often reported in the morning after taking medications.[2] It is important to note that orthostatic stress can be present with both cardiac and neurally mediated syncope.[5]

Several miscellaneous causes of syncope are not easily classified into any of the previously mentioned categories. Hypoglycemia is a possible metabolic cause of syncope and is usually found in individuals with diabetes who have taken too much of a particular hypoglycemic agent. Hyperventilation is another possible cause. Several psychiatric causes, including depression, hysteria, and panic attacks, may subsequently result in hyperventilation, which can lead to hypocapnia and cerebral vasoconstriction compounded by possible peripheral vasodilation.

CLINICAL PRESENTATION AND PHYSICAL EXAMINATION

The patient's past medical history, family history, and history of present illness are essential in determining the cause of the event and whether the patient requires hospitalization. The history needs to detail the syncopal episode, including presyncopal and postsyncopal signs and symptoms.[7] In many cases, a witness is needed for the specific details of the event to be determined. It should be established what the patient was doing before the syncopal episode and whether there were any preceding symptoms. Syncope is an important differential for any geriatric patient presenting for fall, given up to 40% of older patients will present with amnesia for loss of consciousness and up to 60% without witness to the fall.[8]

A history of syncope during exercise should raise concern for a cardiac cause such as an arrhythmia or hypertrophic cardiomyopathy, especially in patients younger than 40 years.[5] In addition, abrupt syncope without warning, the presence of chest pain or palpitations, or a positive family history of sudden death, coronary artery disease, arrhythmias, Wolff-Parkinson-White syndrome, prolonged QT, or Brugada syndrome also necessitates exclusion of a cardiac cause.[7]

A report of defecating, swallowing, coughing, shaving, neck straining or pressure, pain, or stressful event before syncope is suggestive of a form of neurally mediated syncope. However, older patients may have difficulty recalling any presyncopal symptoms, in part because of retrograde amnesia, which is common with vasovagal syncope.[5] If the provider is unable to evoke an accurate presyncopal history, postsyncopal symptoms can aid in differentiation of cardiac and vasovagal episodes. Patients with cardiac syncope may experience a rapid recovery, whereas vasovagal syncope often results in fatigue and nausea for up to several hours after consciousness is regained.[5]

If the patient is able to relate the presyncopal or syncopal episode to a change from a horizontal to a vertical position, the episode may be a result of hypovolemia or orthostatic hypotension. Numbness and tingling in the face and hands suggest hyperventilation.

The patient may also have noted nausea, diaphoresis, or warmth just before losing consciousness; however, the presence of an aura, such as a peculiar smell, might be a clue to an underlying seizure disorder. Differentiation among a seizure, postsyncope symptoms, and seizure-like activity can be difficult. Therefore determining how the patient acted while unconscious is important. Signs most suggestive of a seizure include tongue laceration, head turning, and abnormal posturing. Signs less likely to indicate seizure include presyncope spells, diaphoresis, and loss of consciousness after an extended period of standing or sitting.[2] Most syncopal events are brief; patients often recover once they are in the horizontal position, which allows the resumption of blood flow to the brain. Postictal symptoms during the recovery phase are more consistent with seizures.

Younger patients who report frequent syncopal episodes with vague symptoms and no injury history should be evaluated by a specialist for psychiatric disorders.[2] Psychogenic pseudosyncope is a conversion disorder involving somatic responses to psychological stress. This disorder should not be confused with malingering or Munchausen syndrome as the "syncopal" response is involuntary.[2] Certain medications may be the underlying or contributing cause. Antihypertensive medications may aggravate orthostatic symptoms, especially in older adults. Antiarrhythmic drugs may have proarrhythmic side effects. It is important to know if the patient is being treated for a seizure disorder, any psychiatric disorders, or diabetes, and if the patient has been taking medications as prescribed.

The importance of thoroughly reviewing the patient's past medical history and current medications, especially recently prescribed medications, herbals, and over-the-counter medications, cannot be overstated. The social history should include alcohol use, possible illicit drug use, and the patient's occupation. In patients suspected of having an underlying cardiac problem, the presence of any cardiac risk factors for coronary artery disease should be determined. Risk factors include male gender, a family history of premature coronary artery disease or sudden death, hypercholesterolemia, hypertension, smoking, and diabetes.

The initial physical evaluation begins once it is established that the patient is stable and needs to focus on the cardiovascular system. The presence of bruits indicates cardiovascular disease.[5] Cardiac auscultation may reveal murmurs (e.g., a midsystolic ejection murmur radiating to the right side of the neck suggests aortic stenosis), gross rhythm disturbances, or extra heart sounds such as an S_3 or S_4. The pulmonary evaluation might suggest heart failure, possibly secondary to an acute myocardial infarction or pulmonary disease. Other signs of heart failure include jugular venous distention, hepatojugular reflux, and edema.

Orthostatic vital signs (i.e., BP and pulse) should be measured to determine the presence of hypovolemia.[5] These measurements are obtained by having the patient lie in the supine position for at least 5 minutes and then measuring the BP and pulse. The BP and pulse are checked while the patient is sitting up and then on standing. A drop in systolic pressure by at least 20 mm Hg, a drop in diastolic pressure by at least 10 mm Hg, or an increase in the pulse rate by at least 20 beats per minute within the first 3 minutes of assuming a more upright position is considered a positive test result.[6]

In patients older than 40 years with an unknown cause of syncope, carotid sinus massage can assist with diagnosis.[5] Carotid sinus massage should not be performed in patients with carotid bruits, or within 3 months after myocardial infarction or stroke. Massage is ideally performed with continuous ECG monitoring and beat-to-beat BP monitoring. It should be initiated in the supine position, with gentle rhythmic massage to the right and then to the left of the carotid body for 5 to 10 seconds each.[5] The current diagnostic criteria for carotid sinus hypersensitivity require an asystolic pause of 3 seconds or more, or a fall in systolic BP of 50 mm Hg or more; however, suggested revisions to these criteria recommend diagnosis if asystole exceeds 6 seconds or if systolic BP falls below 60 mm Hg.[5]

Evidence suggests that routine neurological testing is of limited value as a part of a comprehensive syncope evaluation, as the diagnostic yield is low.[2] However, a complete neurologic examination including a funduscopic examination may be helpful if a clear cause is not determined. A rectal examination will help determine if gastrointestinal bleeding is present.

DIAGNOSTICS

Essential Diagnostics. Initial evaluation for all patients reporting syncope should include a standard 12-lead ECG and orthostatic BP monitoring.[5] An ECG is necessary to detect ischemia, arrhythmias, pacemaker failure, prolonged QT, or other congenital cardiac syndromes. Broad-panel laboratory testing is not recommended, however initial testing of serum glucose test, complete blood count (CBC), and pregnancy test for women of childbearing age is recommended.[2]

Additional Diagnostics. An electroencephalogram (EEG) should be obtained if there is concern for seizure disorder.[6] Cardiac enzyme levels should be measured if the patient has cardiac risk factors, if the patient has a history of chest pain, or if physical findings are consistent with heart failure. A chest radiograph and brain natriuretic peptide level will help determine the presence of heart failure or cardiomegaly (i.e., a heart shadow that takes up more than half of the chest cavity on the posteroanterior view). If a cardiac obstructive cause is suspected, echocardiography may be indicated.[2] Further diagnostics may also be indicated because the cause of the event can be difficult to determine. These include an exercise stress test, continuous ECG monitoring (i.e., Holter, event, or implantable loop recorder), electrophysiologic studies, tilt-table testing, EEG, head computed tomography (CT) or magnetic resonance imaging (MRI), and carotid Doppler evaluation.[2,5]

INITIAL DIAGNOSTICS

Syncope

INITIAL
- Electrocardiogram
- Orthostatic blood pressure
- Pulse oximetry

LABORATORY
- Complete blood count and differential
- Serum glucose
- Urine hCG[a]

---
[a]If indicated.

DIFFERENTIAL DIAGNOSIS

The list of differential diagnoses for syncope is extensive.

 Primary differentials include (1) cardiovascular disease with obstruction, (2) transient ischemic attack, (3) pulmonary embolism, (4) cardiac arrhythmia, and (5) hypovolemia.

Additional differentials include vasovagal syncope, orthostatic hypotension, seizure disorder, autonomic failure, alcohol or substance use, concussion, hypoglycemia, anemia, and hypoxia. In addition, syncope may be related to medication therapy or a psychogenic disorder.

INTERPROFESSIONAL COLLABORATIVE MANAGEMENT

The treatment of neurally mediated and orthostatic hypotension syncope is largely supportive.[1] During a witnessed event, the patient should be placed in a supine position. Tight clothing should be loosened and the patient's head turned to the side. If the history and diagnostic testing indicate that an initial episode of syncope was not secondary to a cardiac pathologic condition, therapy can be directed at the underlying disorder. Low-risk patients can be evaluated safely in an outpatient setting.[9] If the patient's condition is unstable, the appropriate advanced cardiac life support and advanced trauma life support protocols need to be followed.

DISPOSITION AND REFERRAL

In older patients, a thorough history should be taken to determine whether some other problem in their home environment is preventing them from staying hydrated or taking their medications properly. These patients may need a visiting nurse, a social worker, or a health benefits adviser. For neurally mediated syncope, and especially with recurring episodes, the patient should be referred to a neurologist for possible tilt-table testing and, if indicated, tilt-training treatment.[5] Other therapies that may be helpful for patients with recurrent syncope include compression stockings, isometric physical counterpressure maneuvers, or treatment with salt tablets, fludrocortisone, desmopressin, or pressor agents.

All patients need to understand the importance of adequate hydration and need to avoid circumstances that might precipitate syncope. They should be told to return to the clinic if the syncope recurs. Depending on the suspected underlying cause, a referral to either a neurologist or a cardiologist is appropriate at this time.

PREVENTION AND PATIENT EDUCATION

Patients and families should receive a careful explanation regarding the cause of the syncopal event. Prevention of injury is an important goal for older adults because many falls are related to a syncopal event.[4] In the case of vasovagal, carotid sinus, and situational syncope, patients need to be made aware of the particular behaviors, activities, or circumstances that might result in syncopal episodes, and they should be given adequate avoidance strategies. Prevention of orthostatic changes necessitates that patients learn to rise slowly from the bed or chair, exercising the leg muscles before standing. Although syncope is often not recurrent, patients with syncope should be advised not to operate motorized equipment until the cause of the event has been determined and treated.

REFERENCES

1. Runser, L., Gauer, R., & Houser, A. (2017). Syncope: Evaluation and differential diagnosis. *American Family Physician, 95*(5), 303–312.
2. Shen, W., Sheldon, R., Benditt, D., Cohen, M., Forman, D., & Goldberger, Z. (2017). 2017 ACC/AHA/HRS guideline for the evaluation and management of patients with syncope. *Journal of the American College of Cardiology, 70*(5), e25–e59.
3. Kenny, R. A., Bhangu, J., & King-Kallimanis, B. L. (2013). Epidemiology of syncope/collapse in younger and older Western patient populations. *Progress in Cardiovascular Diseases, 55*(4), 357–363.
4. Grossman, S. A., Chiu, D., Lipsitz, L., Mottley, J. L., & Shapiro, N. I. (2014). Can elderly patients without risk factors be discharged home when presenting to the emergency department with syncope? *Archives of Gerontology and Geriatrics, 58*(1), 110–114.
5. Saklani, P., Krahn, A., & Klein, G. (2013). Contemporary reviews in cardiovascular medicine: Syncope. *Circulation, 127*, 1330–1339.
6. Rafanelli, M., Morrione, A., Landi, A., Ruffolo, E., Chisciotti, V., & Brunetti, M. (2014). Neuroautonomic evaluation of patients with unexplained syncope: Incidence of complex neutrally mediated diagnoses in the elderly. *Clinical Interventions in Aging, 9*, 333–339.
7. Koenig, T., Duncker, D., Hohmann, S., et al. (2014). Clinical evaluation and risk stratification in patients with syncope. *Herz, 39*(4), 429–436.
8. Bhangu, J., McMahon, G., Hall, P., Bennett, K., Rice, C., & Crean, P. (2016). Long-term cardiac monitoring in older adults with unexplained falls and syncope. *Heart (British Cardiac Society), 102*, 681–686.
9. Grossman, S., Chiu, D., Lipsitz, L., Mottley, L., & Shapiro, N. (2014). Can elderly patients without risk factors be discharged home when presenting to the emergency department with syncope? *Archives of Gerontology and Geriatrics, 58*(1), 110–114.

CHAPTER **34**

THERMAL INJURIES

Karen S. Abate

HEAT-RELATED ILLNESS

 Immediate emergency department referral is indicated for any individual with heat stroke, heat exhaustion, or frost bite.

DEFINITION AND EPIDEMIOLOGY

Heat-related illnesses are a continuum of conditions related to sensitivity and acclimation to heat. In all heat-related illnesses, there is an acute inability to adjust to elevations in the core temperature.[1] The manifestations of this inability vary with the type of heat-related condition. Heat stroke is an emergent medical condition in which the core body temperature potentially is greater than 104°F and in which central nervous system (CNS) abnormalities occur.[1-5] Heat exhaustion is a less severe condition that is the result of excessive sweating, sodium, electrolyte, and water loss.[1-3] Heat exhaustion can rapidly progress to the more severe and potentially fatal heat stroke. Heat syncope is dizziness or fainting that occurs with standing for long periods, or on sudden rising during heat exposure.[2,3] Heat cramps are involuntary muscle pains or spasms occurring in individuals performing physical activity and result from low sodium levels and volume loss.[2,3,6]

Risk factors for heat-related illnesses are varied. Whether young or old, the risk of developing a heat-related illness is real,[2,5] as is the risk for athletes, individuals who work outdoors, and for those persons taking specific medications (e.g., diuretics, anticholinergics, psychotropics).[5,6] It is imperative that heat-related illnesses be properly recognized and treated to prevent additional complications.

PATHOPHYSIOLOGY

The body maintains homeostasis by efficiently balancing heat gains and losses. Thermoregulatory centers of the CNS, including the hypothalamus and spinal cord, address heat gains by increasing blood flow to the skin, dilating peripheral blood vessels, increasing eccrine gland production, and increasing heart rate and cardiac output.[2] Ineffective heat regulation can be caused by numerous factors, resulting in the core temperature being elevated beyond the capabilities of the thermoregulatory compensatory systems.[2] Escalating ambient environmental temperatures and humidity can overwhelm the body's natural ability to dissipate heat. Increases in internal heat production related to disease processes or hypothermic dysfunction, as well as impaired heat dissipation caused by medications or age, can result in deficient heat regulation.[2,5]

In heat stroke, an extremely elevated core body temperature can result in cerebellar and liver dysfunction. Heat exhaustion, heat syncope, and heat cramps are caused by dehydration and electrolyte depletion associated with heat exposure.[1,4]

CLINICAL PRESENTATION AND PHYSICAL EXAMINATION

Heat-related illnesses can develop rapidly or over a period of several days. Physical symptoms may differ in the amount of time they take to manifest. Rapid diagnosis and treatment are imperative. A comprehensive history and physical examination are invaluable. The clinician must determine the following:

- Significant past medical history
- Travel history
- Onset of presenting symptoms
- Medications or herbal supplements that can contribute
- Alternative or home remedy exposure history and severity

Heat stroke is considered a medical emergency in which core body temperature rises above 104°F.[2,5,6] Patients with heat stroke will have CNS abnormalities, which can include hallucinations, confusion, slurred speech, and headache.[1-3] Dehydration, tachycardia, and hypotension can occur. Red, hot, dry skin is a key characteristic of heat stroke. Heat stroke can rapidly deteriorate to hepatocellular damage or multiorgan system failure.[1,6]

Symptoms are milder in patients with heat exhaustion. These patients may have generalized fatigue, weakness, profuse sweating, nausea, vomiting, diarrhea, irritability, and potentially hypotension, but no CNS involvement.[1-4,6] Skin will be pale and flushed, which is significantly different from the red, hot, dry skin of patients experiencing heat stroke.[1] Patients

with heat exhaustion will have a pulse that is fast and breathing that is rapid and shallow, as well as headache, nausea, dizziness, decreased urine output, and diaphoresis.[1,2]

The presentation of patients with heat syncope will involve vertigo, lightheadedness, and syncope.[1-4] Heat cramps will involve pain or spasms in muscles of the abdomen, arms, or legs.[2,3,6] These symptoms are caused by dehydration and electrolyte depletion.

Rapid identification of heat stroke and heat exhaustion is imperative to prevent complications and untoward outcomes. A complete comprehensive history and physical examination, including past extent and severity of exposure is required.[1] Evaluation of airway, breathing, and circulation (ABC) is warranted. Physical examination findings related to the neurologic system include inappropriate behavior, impaired judgment, vertigo, delirium, seizures, and other symptoms of CNS dysfunction.[1] A baseline Glasgow Coma Scale score should be obtained and reassessed throughout treatment.

Cardiovascular findings may include tachycardia; hypotension may occur because of vasodilation and dehydration. Patients with a heat-related illness could manifest symptoms associated with decreased preload, decreased peripheral vascular resistance, increased stroke volume, and increased cardiac output.[1] It is possible to have normotensive findings in some patients as well, because of compensatory mechanisms. Musculoskeletal examination may demonstrate muscle tenderness, cramping, or weakness.

DIAGNOSTICS

Essential Diagnostics. Diagnostics should be based on the patient's exposure and severity history, the clinical presentation, and past medical history. Testing should be used in conjunction with physical examination findings. Diagnostics should also be used to monitor treatment, as well as to determine the presence of associated complications. Cardiac monitoring and pulse oximetry may be indicated to obtain baseline and monitor hemodynamic status. Arterial blood gas (ABG) analysis and chest X-ray examination can be beneficial for patients with shallow breathing. Computed tomography or magnetic resonance imaging may be indicated for patients with altered mental status. A urine sample should be obtained to assess kidney function. Laboratory tests that may be indicated include a complete blood count (CBC) with differential, coagulation studies, an electrolyte panel, blood urea nitrogen (BUN), and creatinine.

Additional Diagnostics. The following values are necessary to assess for disease progression or complications: BUN, creatinine, sodium, potassium, calcium, lactate dehydrogenase, aspartate aminotransferase, alanine aminotransferase, creatine kinase, and bilirubin. Liver function test (LFT) results can be elevated, in some cases, 12 hours after initial injury.[1] Creatine kinase should be measured if there are concerns surrounding potential rhabdomyolysis.[1]

DIFFERENTIAL DIAGNOSIS

The diagnosis of heat-related illness is based on clinical presentation, history, and physical examination. The differential should include infections, head trauma or CNS injury, epilepsy, thyroid storm, acute cocaine intoxication, malignant hyperthermia, pheochromocytoma, anticholinergic poisoning, serotonin syndrome, drug-associated toxicity, and environmental exposure.[1]

INTERPROFESSIONAL COLLABORATIVE MANAGEMENT

- In an emergent heat-related illness, it is imperative to assess and maintain airway patency. Continuous maintenance of the ABCs is vital. Monitoring of vital signs and mental status is essential. Individuals experiencing heat stroke or heat exhaustion must be immediately transported to a local emergency facility, and physician consultation should be obtained. Intravenous access must be promptly established and intravenous solutions administered for rehydration. If not contraindicated, supplemental oxygen should be administered, and preparation should be made for potential endotracheal intubation as warranted.

- The goals of treatment are the lowering of core body temperature, rehydration, and electrolyte replenishment. Patients with any heat-related illness should be moved to a cool, well-ventilated area with most clothing removed to allow for increased surface area exposure. This will facilitate heat evaporation.[1,4] Increased air flow can be provided with fans and a cool mist. Shivering can occur when some rapid cooling techniques are implemented. Shivering is the result of peripheral vasoconstriction and heat production; therefore caution must be used with cooling. Antipyretics are ineffective in heat stroke. Core temperature should be regularly monitored. Complications and sequelae should be treated accordingly. Electrolytes such as sodium and potassium should be replenished as warranted.

- Individuals with heat syncope or heat cramps who are not responding to treatment should be reassessed at an emergency facility. Referral to specialists will be required on the basis of the patient's response to treatment and long-term sequelae.

LIFE-SPAN CONSIDERATIONS

Select populations are more prone to heat-related injury. Older adults and those with hypertension or poor cardiac function are prone to heat exhaustion.[2] This includes people who regularly take β-blocker medications because of an inability to increase cardiac output relative to the demands in a heat-related illness.[1] Individuals on diuretics are at risk for

dehydration, and those on anticholinergics have a diminished capacity to perspire, increasing their risk for thermal illness.[1] Outdoor workers, those without air-conditioning, and patients with obesity and other comorbidities, such as diabetes and hypertension, are also at risk.[2]

COMPLICATIONS

Complications related to heat stroke include rhabdomyolysis and renal, hepatic, or cardiac failure.[3,4] There is potential for the occurrence of multiorgan dysfunction syndrome, which includes disseminated intravascular coagulation, encephalopathy, acute respiratory distress syndrome, myocardial injury, intestinal ischemia or injury, pancreatic injury, and thrombocytopenia.[1,4]

PATIENT AND FAMILY EDUCATION

All heat-related illnesses are preventable. Education to increase awareness and early identification of heat-related conditions is invaluable. Individuals who are at risk for heat-related illnesses should be instructed in how to properly maintain adequate hydration. Strenuous outdoor activities, including work and exercise, should be monitored and limited. Heat-related prevention plans should be developed and implemented during heat waves. The consumption of alcohol should be deterred, whereas the use of fans or air-conditioning should be encouraged.

COLD INJURY

DEFINITION AND EPIDEMIOLOGY

Cold injuries can range from minor to life-threatening. In thermal injuries related to cold exposure, transitional physiologic changes occur as the patient's core body temperature progressively decreases. Decreases in core body temperature can be caused by environmental cold exposure or abnormal thermoregulation.

Frostbite may potentially occur on any exposed area; however, the structures at high risk of frostbite injuries occur on the fingers, toes, nose, cheeks, chin, and ears.[7–9] Frostbite can be classified on the basis of severity as simply superficial or deep.[10] Superficial frostbite is limited to the skin, with epidermal sloughing and superficial skin vesiculation.[10] Deep frostbite involves the reticular dermis, dermal vascular plexus, complete dermis, muscle, tendon, bone, and deep tissue.[10]

PATHOPHYSIOLOGY

The pathophysiologic process associated with frostbite involves the freezing of exposed tissues. There are four pathologic phases to frostbite. Prefreeze, freeze-thaw, vascular stasis, and late ischemic phases often overlap.[7,10] In the prefreeze stage, there is superficial tissue cooling and associated vasoconstriction.[7,10] In the freeze-thaw phase, ice crystals form in the intracellular and extracellular tissue.[7,10] Vasoconstriction alternates with vasodilation in the vascular stasis phase, resulting in microvascular sludging and stasis with potential leakage.[7,10] Finally, the ischemic phase involves inflammation and hypoxia, ultimately leading to potential necrosis.[7,10] Peripheral vasoconstriction and decreased blood flow occur. These progressive changes ultimately can result in ischemic changes and tissue necrosis.[8]

As the core body temperature decreases, progressive changes associated with hypothermia occur. These changes vary in severity by the extent of core body temperature reduction. Cardiovascular response is initially tachycardia followed by atrial fibrillation, bradycardia, ventricular dysrhythmia, and ultimately asystole. Cardiac output and blood pressure gradually diminish. Respiratory response to the hypothermic state involves increased oxygen consumption, depressed respiratory drive, and, ultimately, acidosis. Ataxia, slurred speech, loss of deep tendon reflexes, loss of consciousness, and coma are neurologic occurrences for hypothermic patients.

CLINICAL PRESENTATION AND PHYSICAL EXAMINATION

Presentation of the individual with frostbite will vary according to the severity of exposure. Hypothermia presentation also corresponds to the extreme lowering of core body temperatures. Severity can range from ataxia and slurred speech to absent reflexes and asystole. Hypothermia can be life-threatening and manifestations can be seen in multiple body systems depending upon the extent of exposure.

A comprehensive history and physical examination are imperative for any patient with a potential cold-related injury. The clinician must determine the exposure history, including length and severity, the significant past medical history, presence of risk factors, current medications taken, and any treatments or therapies that have already taken place.

The physical examination requires rapid identification of cold-related injuries. The presentation of an individual having a cold-related injury depends on the severity of core body temperature drop. Core temperature should be accurately measured on initial presentation and at regular intervals during treatment. In severe hypothermia, delirium, bradycardia, hypotension, hypopnea, hypotonia, oliguria, thrombocytopenia, and pancreatitis are potential findings.[11]

Physical findings related to the integumentary system vary according to exposure and severity. In mild or moderate frostbite, the affected area will potentially demonstrate edema and manifestations of vasoconstriction.[11] Deep frostbite manifests as skin that is bluish-gray in appearance with hemorrhagic blisters and potential necrosis to underlying structures.[9] During the course of several days, there is a progression from edema, non-blanching surface, cyanosis, and hemorrhagic blisters to tissue necrosis. It is important for the clinician to examine all limbs and the entire surface for affected areas.

Cardiovascular effects may include arrhythmias, dysrhythmias, hypotension, fibrillation, and asystole. The neurologic examination may reveal sensory changes, ataxia, progressive loss of deep tendon reflexes, changes in level of consciousness, and decreased response to noxious stimuli. Respiratory drive will be steadily diminished as the core temperature is lowered in hypothermia.[11]

DIAGNOSTICS

Diagnostics are not warranted in frostbite. In patients with hypothermia, diagnostics are indicated to assess the severity of hypothermia and subsequent response to ongoing treatment. Cardiac monitoring and pulse oximetry may be indicated. ABG analysis can be used to assess for acidosis. Chest X-ray examination is indicated for patients with underlying pathologic changes or respiratory compromise. Electrocardiography (ECG) is beneficial for individuals with cardiac symptoms. Blood work should include a CBC, electrolytes, BUN, creatinine, and clotting factors.

INITIAL DIAGNOSTICS

Cold-Related Injuries

INITIAL
- Electrocardiography, cardiac monitoring
- Pulse oximetry

LABORATORY
- Complete blood count with differential
- Serum glucose, electrolytes, blood urea nitrogen, creatinine
- Coagulation studies (prothrombin time/partial thromboplastin time [PT/PTT])
- Cardiac isoenzymes[a]
- Arterial blood gases[a]

IMAGING
- Chest X-ray[a]

---

[a]If indicated.

DIFFERENTIAL DIAGNOSIS

The diagnosis of cold-related conditions is based on clinical presentation, history, and physical examination. The differential diagnosis of individuals with frostbite should include frostnip and chilblains, commonly known as trench foot.[8] The differential diagnosis of individuals with hypothermia should include hypoglycemia, drug intoxication, myxedema, coma, cerebral vascular attack, allergic reactions, and compartment syndrome.[9]

INTERPROFESSIONAL COLLABORATIVE MANAGEMENT

Any individual with a cold-related injury should immediately be removed from the cold exposure. A patient with frostbite or hypothermia should be immediately transported to an emergency facility for evaluation and treatment. Hospitalization may be warranted for deep frostbite or hypothermia patients. Referral to a surgeon can be advantageous for possible amputation.

Frostbite management focuses on stabilization of the patient and rewarming of the affected area once in an environment where potential reexposure is not possible.[12] Wet or constrictive clothing should be removed once the individual is out of the cold environment. Rewarming can be achieved with warm blankets or immersion in a warm water bath for repeated short periods when in a medical facility.[10,12] Spontaneous rewarming once the patient has been removed from the cold exposure might be sufficient; however, he or she should be assessed relative to the extent of the injury.[10] The affected area can be elevated or splinted as needed, but it should not be massaged or rubbed.[8,10,12] Rewarming near a fire runs the risk of potential burn.[12] Pain control may be needed.[10] Antibiotics are needed only for contaminated areas. Postthaw management follows traditional principles of wound management. Debridement, physical therapy, or amputation may be needed.

In patients with hypothermia, it is imperative to assess and to maintain airway patency. Continuous maintenance of the ABCs is vital, and monitoring of vital signs and mental status is essential. In the severely hypothermic individual, peripheral pulses may not be palpable; therefore the cardiac electrical rhythm should be obtained before chest compressions are initiated. Individuals experiencing hypothermia must be immediately transported to a local emergency facility, and physician consultation should be obtained. Intravenous access must be promptly established. If it is not contraindicated, supplemental oxygen should be administered, and preparation should be made for potential endotracheal intubation as warranted.

COMPLICATIONS

Individuals who have experienced a cold-related thermal injury may maintain lifetime sensitivity to cold. The sequelae associated with superficial frostbite include long-term neuropathic pain, sensory deficits, edema, or hair and nail deformities. Tissue necrosis can occur with deep frostbite.[10]

PATIENT AND FAMILY EDUCATION

Awareness of weather conditions to avoid illness or injury should be encouraged in all populations. Individuals who have experienced a cold-related injury should be instructed in the proper identification of cold-related conditions. Patients should be advised to stop smoking because of the vasoconstrictive effects. In addition, patients should refrain from alcohol intake, especially with exposure to cold conditions. The use of protective clothing in cold environments should be stressed. Clothing should be well ventilated and loose to limit perspiration during activity.

REFERENCES

1 Atha, W. F. (2013). Heat related illness. *Emergency Medicine Clinics of North America, 31*(4), 1097–1108.
2. Raukar, N., Lemieux, R., Finn, G., Stearns, R., & Casa, D. (2015). Heat illness—A practical primer. *Rhode Island Medical Journal, 98*(7), 28–31.
3. Centers for Disease Control and Prevention (CDC). (2016). Heat stress—Heat related illness, *NIOSH fast facts*. Retrieved from https://www.cdc.gov/niosh/topics/heatstress/heatrelillness.html. (Accessed 29 April 2019).
4. Pryor, R. R., Casa, D. J., Holschen, J. C., O'Connor, F. G., & Vandermark, L. W. (2013). Exertional heat stroke: Strategies for prevention and treatment from the sports field to the emergency department. *Clin Pediatr Emerg Med, 14*(4), 267–278.
5. Yan, W., Bobb, J., Di, Q., et al. (2016). Heat stroke admissions during heat waves in 1,916 US counties for the period from 1999–2010 and their effect modifiers. *Environmental Health: A Global Access Science Source, 15*, 1.
6. Noonam, B., Bancroft, R., Kines, J. S., & Bedi, A. (2012). Heat- and cold-induced injuries in athletes: Evaluation and management. *The Journal of the American Academy of Orthopaedic Surgeons, 20*(12), 744–754.
7. Zonnoor, B., (2018). Frostbite. Retrieved from https://emedicine.medscape.com/article/926249-overview. (Accessed 29 April 2019).
8. Centers for Disease Control and Prevention (CDC). (2018). Cold stress. Retrieved from www.cdc.gov/niosh/topics/coldstress. (Accessed 29 April 2019).
9. Rivlin, M., King, M., Kruse, R., & Ilyas, A. M. (2014). Frostbite in an adolescent football player: A case report. *Journal of Athletic Training, 49*(1), 97–101.
10. McIntosh, S. E., Opacic, M., Freer, L., Grissom, C. K., Auerbach, P. S., Rodway, G. W., et al. (2014). Wilderness Medical Society practice guidelines for the prevention and treatment of frostbite: 2014 Update. *Wilderness and Environmental Medicine, 25*, S43–S54.
11. Cheshire, W. P. (2016). Thermoregulatory disorders and illness related to heat and cold stress. *Autonomic Neuroscience: Basic and Clinical, 196*, 91–104.
12. Fudge, J. (2016). Exercise in the cold: Preventing and managing hypothermia and frostbite injury. *Sports Health, 8*(2), 133–139.

CHAPTER **35**

EXAMINATION OF THE SKIN AND APPROACH TO DIAGNOSIS OF SKIN DISORDERS

Maria Isabel Romano

DEFINITION AND EPIDEMIOLOGY

Skin problems occur often in the general population and are the presenting complaint in many primary care patients.[1] A large number of skin diseases manifest in similar ways. Factors such as age, ethnic and genetic makeup, risk factors, body habitus, skin surface, and self-care practices may complicate a diagnosis by altering the appearance and distribution of lesions that are characteristic of the skin disorder. Underlying systemic pathologic conditions may also contribute to the difficulty of making a definitive diagnosis of skin lesions.

OVERVIEW OF SKIN FUNCTION, ANATOMY, AND STRUCTURES

The primary functions of the skin are protection of the underlying body structures from the entrance of microorganisms, control of body heat and elimination of body waste through perspiration, and prevention of injury to core body structures. The skin protects the body from infectious agents; protects against loss of body heat through conduction, convection, and radiation; and provides a first-line defense against mechanical, chemical, and thermal injury. Glands in the dermal layer of the skin secrete a substance that lubricates the body surface and assists with a variety of body functions. The peripheral sense receptors contained in the skin alert the body to pain, temperature changes, pressure, and touch.

The skin is composed of three layers: the epidermis, the dermis, and the hypodermis or subcutis. The outer epidermal, or cuticle, layer is avascular and is divided into an outer horny layer (the stratum corneum) and an underlying horny layer (the stratum mucosum). The stratum corneum consists of keratinocytes—cells that originate in the basal cell layer of the epidermis and migrate upward to the stratum corneum and slough off as dead cells, called *squames*. As long as the stratum corneum (the outer horny layer) is intact, normal skin bacteria are prevented from invading deeper skin and gaining access to the bloodstream. The lower layer of the epidermis contains the Langerhans cells, which function as antigen-presenting cells that migrate to the lymph nodes and play an important role in the allergic skin response. Melanocytes found in the basal

layer of the epidermis constitute the body's principal protection against ultraviolet (UV) radiation.[2]

The second layer of the skin, the dermis (also termed the *cutis, corneum,* or *true skin*), holds the epidermis in place. The dermis is composed of an outer papillary layer and an inner reticular layer that contains connective tissue and the blood supply, as well as lymphatic vessels, peripheral nerves, elastic tissue, and a reservoir of water and electrolytes. The dermal appendages are contained within the reticular layer and include the eccrine sweat glands that serve to control body temperature by evaporation, the sebum-producing sebaceous glands that lubricate the stratum corneum through openings in the skin (called *pores*), the hair follicles, and the nail bed. Other appendages include apocrine glands attached to hair shafts located in the axillary, perianal, and genital areas. These glands respond to the increased hormone levels associated with puberty, adolescence, and young adulthood, and decrease their activity with normal aging. A variation of the apocrine gland is the cerumen-producing glands lining the external auditory canal. The oily substance, cerumen, serves to protect the skin lining the ear canal from bacterial invasion.

A third layer of the skin, the hypodermis or subcutis, functions to store fat, to insulate the body from extremes in temperature, and to provide a cushion against injury. It also contributes to the skin's mobility over underlying body parts.

CHANGES IN THE SKIN ASSOCIATED WITH AGING

With age, both structural and functional changes occur in the skin. These changes include decrease in the number of Langerhans cells; variation in size, shape, and staining of the keratinocytes; decrease in the thickness of the dermis; and loss of elastic tissue. There is a decrease in the number of sweat glands, hair follicles, and specialized nerve endings, as well as decreased vascularity and increased fragility of existing capillaries. Functional changes in the skin include a decreased inflammatory response; increased time for wound healing; thinning of the skin, resulting in increased fragility and risk of injury; decreased sweat capacity; and increased dryness secondary to reduced sebum production.[3]

SKIN ASSESSMENT

Formulation of a differential diagnosis for skin lesions is based on an in-depth knowledge of various common skin disorders and their characteristic physical properties, including location and morphologic appearance. In addition, knowledge of the associated history typical of common rashes is essential. Variations in color, texture, and continuity of a patient's skin may be a normal genetic or ethnic variant, an indicator of a local skin pathologic condition, or an indicator of an underlying systemic disease process. A proper assessment forms the basis

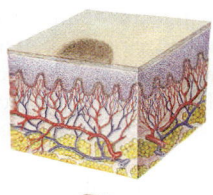

MACULE: Skin color change without elevation, i.e., flat (freckles or petechia). Described as a "patch" if greater than 1 cm (vitiligo).

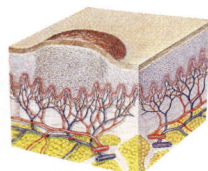

PAPULE: Elevated, solid lesion of less than 1 cm, varying in color (warts or elevated nevus).

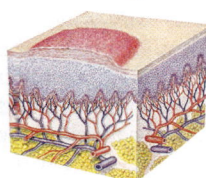

PLAQUE: Raised, flat lesion formed from merging papules or nodules.

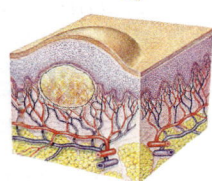

NODULE: Larger than a papule. Raised solid lesion extending deeper into the dermis. A large nodule is referred to as a tumor.

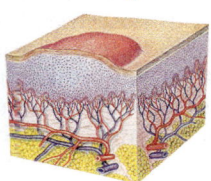

WHEAL (hive): Fleeting skin elevation that is irregularly shaped because of edema (mosquito bite or urticaria).

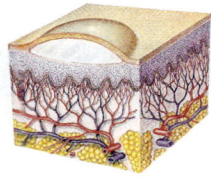

VESICLE (blister): Elevated, sharply defined lesion containing serous fluid. Usually less than 1 cm (blister, chickenpox, or herpes simplex).

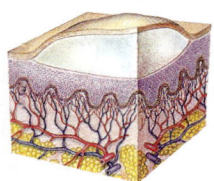

BULLA (plural, bullae): Large, elevated, fluid-filled lesion greater than 1 cm (partial-thickness burn).

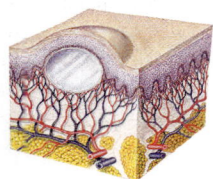

CYST: Elevated, thick-walled lesion containing fluid or semisolid matter.

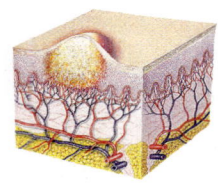

PUSTULE: Elevated lesion less than 1 cm containing purulent material. Lesions larger than 1 cm are described as boils, abscesses, or furuncles (acne or impetigo).

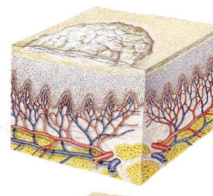

SCALE: Dried fragments of sloughed epidermal cells, irregular in shape and size and white, tan, yellow, or silver in color (dandruff, dry skin, or psoriasis).

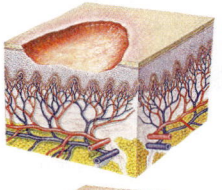

EROSION: A moist, demarcated, depressed area due to loss of partial- or full-thickness epidermis. Basal layer of epidermis remains intact (ruptured chickenpox vesicle).

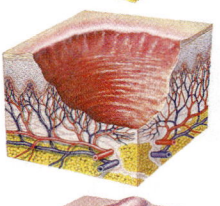

DEEP ULCER: Irregularly shaped, exudative, depressed lesion in which entire epidermis and all or part of dermis are lost. Results from trauma and tissue destruction (pressure ulcer).

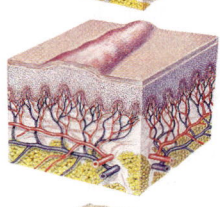

SCAR: Mark left on skin after healing. Replacement of destroyed tissue by scar tissue.

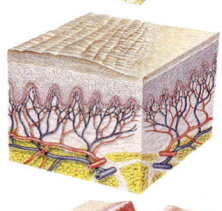

LICHENIFICATION: Epidermal thickening resulting in elevated plaque with accentuated skin markings. Usually results from repeated injury through rubbing or scratching (chronic atopic dermatitis).

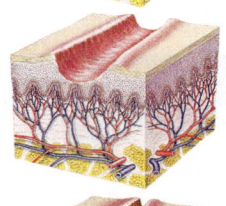

EXCORIATION: Superficial, linear abrasion of epidermis. Visible sign of itching caused by rubbing or scratching (atopic dermatitis).

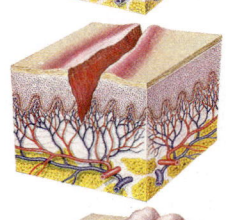

FISSURE: Deep linear split through epidermis into dermis (tinea pedis).

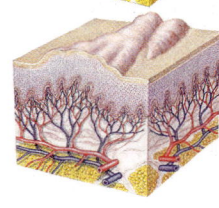

KELOID: Irregularly shaped, elevated, progressively enlarging scar; extends beyond the boundaries of the wound; and caused by excessive collagen formation during post-surgical healing.

FIG. 35.1   *Left,* Primary lesions: visually recognizable structural changes in the skin that have specific characteristics. *Right,* Secondary lesions: primary lesions that have changed because of the natural progression of the lesion or because of physical change (scratching, irritation, or secondary infection). (From Black, J. M., & Hawks, J. H. [2009]. *Medical-surgical nursing: Clinical management for positive outcomes* [8th ed.]. St Louis: Saunders.)

for an appropriate care plan, patient education for self-care of acute and chronic skin lesions, and prevention of recurrence. Assessment begins with a careful history and physical examination of basic features, including skin turgor, pigmentation, and degree of photodamage to sun-exposed surfaces.[2] Additional investigative techniques, such as Wood light examination, laboratory data, and microscopic skin scraping examination, may be necessary to ensure a definitive diagnosis.

Clinical Presentation and Physical Examination

Subjective components of a dermatologic history include taking a history from the patient or caregiver regarding the onset and progression of the rash, associated symptoms, any prior skin disorder, medications, over-the-counter medications, herbal preparations, nutritional supplements, travel history, lesions in close contacts, social and occupational factors, and dietary practices. The health care provider should inquire about self-care practices, such as homeopathic remedies, lotions, skin care products, soaps, any change in laundry products, new clothing or fabrics, use of rubber gloves, cosmetics, sunbathing, tanning salons, and the humidity of the patient's typical ambient environment. In addition, a family history or self-history of skin disorders, allergy, atopy, asthma, or eczema in childhood is reviewed.

The use of a contact dermatoscope or a noncontact microscope that uses cross-polarized light is an important adjunct to the objective examination of skin lesions. Dermoscopy affords the examiner the advantage of visualizing the epidermis and superficial dermis and can reveal changes in pigmentation throughout the lesion, such as in a melanoma.[4] It can also be used to determine whether the lesion's borders are regular or irregular. When a contact dermatoscope is used, the application

of immersion oil or ultrasound gel to the skin further enhances the translucency of the stratum corneum and permits better visualization of skin fissures, hair follicles, and pores in the lesion.[4] The presence of scaling and inflammation can also be determined. A listing of primary and secondary lesions is provided in Fig. 35.1.

A freestanding light that can be adjusted to provide direct or oblique lighting is a necessary adjunct. Darkening of the ambient lighting allows greater illumination and contrast of the involved lesion. Overillumination, however, may wash out important details of a lesion. Direct lighting with an intense penlight or the ophthalmoscope head with a halogen light permits visualization of closed vesicles or pustules and differentiation of fluid or cystic masses.

Another form of lighting is the Wood light, or black light, which emits long wavelengths (>365 nm) of UV rays through a filter made of nickel oxide and silica, rendering UV rays harmless to the skin. The advantage is that under this lighting method, skin diseases such as tinea versicolor fluoresce white to yellow, and erythrasma, a scaly skin condition caused by *Corynebacterium minutissimum*, fluoresces a bright coral red.[5] Even small amounts of decreased melanin, such as vitiligo, are accentuated under Wood light and appear stark white. *Pseudomonas* infections appear pale blue, and the presence of dermatophytes such as *Microsporum canis* will appear yellow.[6]

Palpation of skin lesions provides information on the extent of the lesion below the skin surface, its consistency, its exact size, and associated pain. Certain lesions, such as dermatofibromas, will indent with lateral palpation, a distinguishing characteristic known as the *Fitzpatrick sign*. Dermatographism is a phenomenon that occurs when the skin of a person with urticaria is lightly rubbed with a pointed object, such as the

---

BOX **35.1**

Skin Examination Techniques and Procedures

Diascopy can be performed with use of a flat microscope slide or other clear instrument, such as a magnifying glass. Blanching of blue to red lesions followed by a gradual refilling indicates blood in the capillaries; absence of blanching indicates blood leaching outside of the capillaries, as in petechiae.

Gram stain of exudates from lesions is helpful in distinguishing the cause as either a gram-positive or gram-negative organism.

The Tzanck test with Wright or Giemsa stain can uncover multinucleated giant cells that are typical of herpes simplex or varicella-zoster virus. The top of the vesicle must be removed to obtain fresh fluid from the base of the lesion.

A 10% to 30% potassium hydroxide (KOH) stain determines the presence of hyphae and spores consistent with candidiasis or uncovers the spaghetti-and-meatball appearance of tinea versicolor, caused by the skin fungus *Malassezia furfur* or *Malassezia ovalis*. Attempts should be made to obtain scrapings from the top of a lesion or from the advancing edge of a lesion. The skin lesion is aligned vertical to the microscopic slide, and a gentle scraping of the lesion with the side of a slide or a scalpel loosens skin debris, collected on the slide below. KOH is applied directly to the scale debris, and a coverslip is placed over the skin scraping, or the KOH is applied alongside the edge of the coverslip, and the KOH then gravitates to cover the specimen by capillary action. Heating of the preparation over a low flame will allow the hyphae to separate from

the epithelial cells. The specimen is then set under the microscope for examination, first using 10× power and then proceeding to 40× for finer detail. The examiner must be certain to close the condenser diaphragm and turn the condenser down to enhance the detail of hyphae that are embedded in the scaly debris.

Culture for herpesvirus, *Streptococcus*, *Staphylococcus*, or *Pseudomonas* organisms requires removal of the outer crust or cuticle of the lesion to obtain fluid for culture. The fluid at the base of the lesion is most likely to be positive for the contributing organisms and free of contamination from the skin surface. A special collecting device for a viral culture specimen must be used in accordance with laboratory specifications. Bacterial culture specimens for streptococci and staphylococci can be collected with a regular throat-culture–collecting swab. *Candida* organisms can be grown on Sabouraud agar in a 2- to 6-day period, whereas dermatophytes take up to 2 to 4 weeks to grow on the same agar. The organisms of tinea versicolor grow only on special media.

In *scabies preparation*, a superficial skin shaving from a skinfold area is obtained from the top of a burrow and examined under oil immersion. Oil or KOH solution should be placed on the lesion first. With a scalpel, the top is shaved off the lesion, and the debris is placed on a microscopic slide. Additional oil and a coverslip are added, and the specimen is examined under 10× magnification. The presence of adult mites, eggs, or feces in the burrows is sufficient in the diagnosis of scabies.

Data from Habif, T. P. (2016). *Clinical dermatology: A color guide to diagnosis and therapy* (6th ed.). Edinburgh: Elsevier; and Klauss, W., Johnson, R. A., Saavedra, A. P., & Roh, E. K. (2017). *Fitzpatrick's color atlas and synopsis of clinical dermatology* (8th ed.). New York: McGraw-Hill.

back of a fingernail; histamine is released under the skin surface, and the skin becomes raised and red where the object touched it.

DIAGNOSTICS

Diagnosis involves a close evaluation of the lesion's distribution or location, configuration, borders, size, shape, color, and surface characteristics or appearance. A cluster of lesions may appear in various stages of evolution, as with varicella and dermatitis herpetiformis, whereas others, such as warts, will remain the same for the duration of their existence.[7] Documentation includes a description of the lesion's size, color, shape, surface characteristics, distribution, and configuration. A discussion of skin examination techniques is provided in Box 35.1.

INTERPROFESSIONAL COLLABORATIVE MANAGEMENT

Primary care providers may be the initial and continuing contact with health care for dermatologic problems. Quality of care is enhanced when providers develop strong interpersonal relationships with patients. The patient's satisfaction has been shown to be related to the provider's ability to teach patients about their condition and to show concern and caring for their problem. This, in turn, may lead to enhanced compliance and better treatment outcomes.[8] Primary care providers should develop good referral relationships with dermatology providers to facilitate optimum patient handoff and continuity of care.

REFERENCES

1. St. Sauver, J. L., Warner, D. O., Yawn, B. P., et al. (2013). Why patients visit their doctors: Assessing the most prevalent conditions in a defined American population. *Mayo Clinic Proceedings. Mayo Clinic, 88*(1), 56–67.
2. Goldman, L., & Schafer, A. (2015). *Cecil medicine* (25th ed.). New York: Elsevier.
3. Farage, M. A., Miller, K. W., Elsner, P., et al. (2013). Characteristics of the aging skin. *Advances in Wound Care: The Journal for Prevention and Healing, 2*(1), 5–10.
4. Unlu, E., Akay, B. N., & Erdem, C. (2014). Comparison of dermatoscopic diagnostic algorithms based on calculation: The ABCD rule of dermatoscopy, the seven-point checklist, the three-point checklist and the CASH algorithm in dermatoscopic evaluation of melanocytic lesions. *The Journal of Dermatology, 41*(7), 598–603.
5. Habif, T. P. (2016). *Clinical dermatology: A color guide to diagnosis and therapy* (6th ed.). Edinburgh: Elsevier.
6. LeBlond, R. F., Brown, D. D., Suneja, M., & Szot, J. F. (2015). *DeGowin's diagnostic examination* (10th ed.). New York: McGraw-Hill.
7. James, W. D., Berger, T. G., & Elston, D. M. (2016). *Andrews' diseases of the skin: Clinical dermatology* (12th ed.). Philadelphia: Elsevier.
8. Alagheband, S. J., Miller, J. J., & Clarke, J. T. (2015). Individualizing patient education for greater patient satisfaction. *Cutis; Cutaneous Medicine for the Practitioner, 95*(5), 291–292.

CHAPTER 36

SURGICAL OFFICE PROCEDURES

Randy Michael Gordon

INDRODUCTION

The skin is the largest organ of the human body and the only organ that is nearly completely visible by the naked eye.

Cutaneous diseases such as rashes, infections, benign and malignant tumors, and lesions represent a sizeable portion of the skin complaints of patients seen in primary care, yet many providers are not comfortable with diagnosis or treatment of cutaneous disease.[1]

Concurrently, multiple forces are at work that will influence the provision of dermatologic care in the future. Demand for dermatology services is predicted to increase, but the supply of dermatology providers is predicted to remain low, despite the influx of nonphysician providers.[2,3] The need to restrain the growth of health care spending is likely to place greater pressures on primary care providers to treat common dermatologic issues in the office rather than to refer patients for more expensive specialty services. Providers of primary care services will be challenged to be selective in which patients to refer and which patients to treat. Dermatologists delivering telemedicine can work with primary care providers to determine whether dermatology services are needed or to assist with diagnosis. The education of primary care providers to perform skin biopsies for diagnosis in primary care could conceivably help prioritize requests for high-demand specialty services, especially in the early age of teledermatology.

Performance of primary care office-based procedures for the treatment of benign lesions such as warts, skin tags, and irritated seborrheic keratoses is one way to try to meet this challenge while also reducing the cost to the patient. Cryosurgery, electrocautery, curettage, punch biopsy, shave biopsy, and scissor excision are common dermatology office procedures. Primary care providers can safely perform these procedures with proper education and training.

A note on the treatment of benign lesions: patients may request treatment of benign lesions that are painful or irritating, such as plantar warts, but at times they may seek treatment because they find the lesion unattractive. Although the treatment of benign lesions that are causing physical discomfort is usually a covered expense, patients are often distressed to discover that many insurance carriers do not cover dermatology treatment performed for cosmetic concerns.

CRYOSURGERY

Cryosurgery or cryotherapy is the application of cold, such as nitrogen in its liquid state, to produce therapeutic tissue necrosis.[3] Liquid nitrogen, which has a boiling point of −196°C (−321°F), is the coldest and most commonly used cryogen. It is administered with a cryosurgical canister with a spray tip attachment or sometimes manually with a cotton-tipped applicator. A 30-second spray of liquid nitrogen will result in tissue temperatures of −25°C to −50°C (−13°F to −58°F). Most benign lesions will be destroyed at a tissue temperature of −20°C to 30°C. Further destruction occurs during the thaw phase. Maximum destruction occurs with repeated freeze-thaw cycles.

Cryosurgery is indicated in the treatment of myriad skin conditions, and its use is ubiquitous in dermatology.[3] In primary care, it is used typically in the destruction of benign lesions that are easily recognizable, such as acrochorda (skin tags), warts, and seborrheic keratosis. It is also used for the treatment of actinic keratosis—scaly, erythematous patches on habitually sun-exposed surfaces that are considered precancerous. Cold intolerance, cold urticaria, and cryoglobulinemia are relative contraindications to cryosurgery, as is treatment of digits in patients with a history of Raynaud disease. Patients who are darkly pigmented are at risk for depigmentation resulting from destruction of melanocytes or postinflammatory hyperpigmentation (PIH) after tissue injury. Alternative treatments should be considered. Avoid the use of cryotherapy at the vermilion border of the lips, oral commissures, eyebrows, canthi, and nasal ala because of the risk of scarring. Freeze time and the duration of cooling varies from lesion to lesion.

When performing cryosurgical therapy, position the nozzle of the spray tip 1 to 1.5 cm from the lesion to be treated. Spray the lesion until a 2 mm rim of frost develops around the lesion and then continue spraying for 5 to 30 seconds, depending on the thickness, diameter, and location of the lesions. For larger lesions, this can be done in spiral or paintbrush pattern. Actinic keratosis generally requires 5- to 20-second application time delivered in 1 or 2 freeze-thaw cycles, depending on the location and size of the lesion; seborrheic keratosis requires 5 to 10 seconds for thin, flat lesions; warts require 10 seconds, although plantar warts may require a second freeze cycle; and skin tags require only 5 seconds or less per lesion. Cover the eyes, nostrils, and exterior auditory canal with gauze or cotton if cryosurgery is done near those sites. Care should also be taken not to deeply freeze the skin near the digital nerves on the medial and lateral aspects of the fingers and toes.

Inform the patient that cryotherapy is painful during and sometimes for several minutes after the procedure. As mentioned, hypopigmentation may be more prominent in individuals with darker skin types. Scarring can occur if the freezing extends into the dermis. Patients can expect some redness and swelling during the healing process. Bullae, sometimes hemorrhagic, may develop. Patients should be advised to protect the bullae from trauma until healing is complete, but they can be drained if uncomfortable. Posttreatment care includes keeping the area clean with soap and water and using petrolatum if the patient desires. Unless patients use them routinely and without issue, topical antibiotic ointments such as bacitracin should be avoided, owing to the high incidence of contact dermatitis.

ELECTROSURGERY

Electrosurgery is a technique that uses the transmission of electricity to cut tissue, destroy tissue, and cauterize vessels. Variations in current wavelength result in different biologic effects on tissue. For cutaneous procedures, electrosurgery can be categorized into six different treatment modalities: (1) electrofulguration, (2) electrodesiccation, (3) electrocoagulation, (4) electrosection, (5) electrocautery, and (6) electrolysis.[4]

Electrofulguration uses a damped sine wave, high-voltage, low-amperage alternating current to generate a spark from a monoterminal electrode to the tissue via the air. There is no contact between the electrode and the tissue. This modality is the least tissue damaging of all of the high-frequency electrosurgery techniques, resulting in rapid tissue healing. Most of the tissue damage is superficial, primarily involving the epidermis.

Electrodessication is the direct application of the tip to the skin or lesion surface to deliver the current and is the preferred method for treatment of most lesions. Electrodesiccation uses a damped sine wave, high-voltage, low-amperage alternating current to generate a current from direct contact of a monoterminal electrode to the tissue. Superficial tissue damage occurs as heat is transferred to tissue, causing cell death.

Electrocoagulation uses a moderately damped sine wave, low-voltage, high-amperage alternating current to generate a current from direct contact of a biterminal electrode to the tissue. Tissue damage is deeper than with electrofulguration and electrodesiccation, providing tissue coagulation through the generation of heat in the tissue.

Electrosection uses an undamped or slightly damped sine wave, low-voltage, high-amperage alternating current to cut tissue with minimal peripheral heat damage. The "Bovie" knife incorporates a blended undamped and damped sine wave that provides both cutting and coagulation at the same time.

Electrolysis uses low-voltage, low-amperage direct current from a negative electrode to the positive electrode. The negative electrode is applied to the target tissue where electrons are released. The electrons interact with the tissue to produce sodium hydroxide and hydrogen gas, resulting in tissue liquefaction. Acids are produced at the positive electrode resulting in tissue coagulation. The main use of electrolysis is for hair removal.[4] With the exception of electrocautery, the previously mentioned electrosurgical procedures are not discussed in this chapter.

Electrocautery uses a heating filament tip connected to a low-voltage, high-amperage direct current—usually a battery. In primary care, electrocautery can be used for the treatment of acrochorda, actinic keratosis, small angiomata, compound nevi, warts, and seborrheic keratoses. Heat is transferred from the filament to the target tissue, causing protein denaturation and tissue coagulation. There is no electric current transfer to the target tissue, and the patient is not part of the circuit loop. Electrocautery is preferable to other modalities of electrosurgery for patients with pacemakers or implantable cardiac defibrillators (ICDs). Electrocautery is useful for nonconductive tissue areas of the body, such as the cartilage, bone, and nails.[4]

Electrosurgical current will ignite flammable substances like alcohol. When prepping the patient before electrosurgery, nonflammable disinfectants such as iodine or chlorhexidine should be used. If an alcohol-based disinfectant is used, the surgical area must be allowed to dry for at least 90 seconds prior to electrosurgery. In addition, electrosurgery should not be used near the presence of nasal cannulas, masks, or endotracheal anesthesia administering oxygen. Finally, care should be taken not to ignite paper surgical drapes in the surgical field.

Once the skin is prepped, 1% or 2% lidocaine, with or without epinephrine, can be used in those cases when significant pain is anticipated. Treatment of small lesions without anesthesia is often preferable to the discomfort of the anesthesia itself. Vascular lesions may become less identifiable because of the vascular effects of the anesthetic agent, so they are best treated without local anesthesia. The electrocautery tip is passed lightly and repeatedly over the treatment surface until the degree of desired tissue destruction has been achieved.

Electrocautery is an attractive alternative to cryotherapy when pigmentation issues are of concern and is more useful in the treatment of vascular lesions. Complications are rare. In combination with curettage (i.e., electrodessication and curettage), it is one of several standard treatment options available for nodular basal cell and invasive squamous cell carcinomas.

CURETTAGE

Curettage is a technique that uses a scraping instrument, a curet, to remove soft and superficial skin lesions. These include seborrheic keratoses, some warts, and molluscum, as well as some types of skin cancers. The curet has a sharp oval ring that

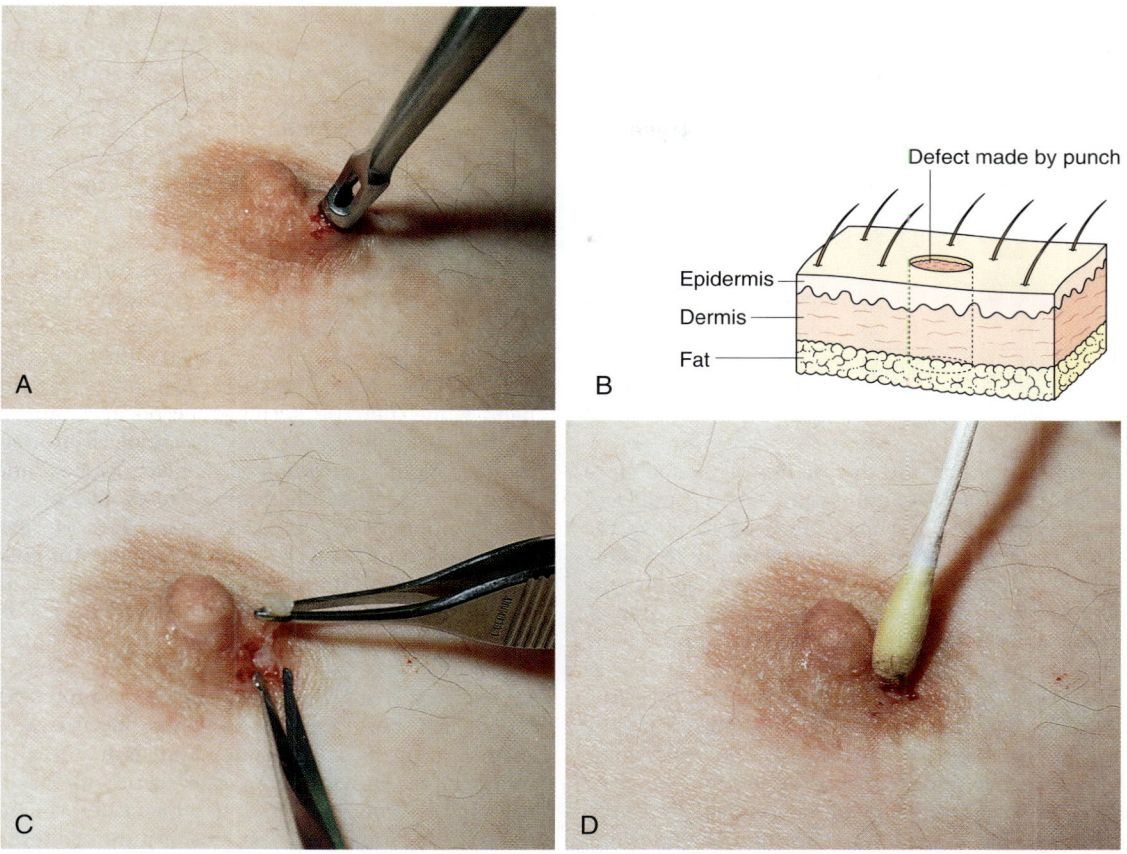

F I G .   36.1   Punch biopsy. (A) The dermal punch is rotated back and forth while gently advancing it through the dermis into the subcutaneous tissue. (B) The punch should be introduced through the dermis and into the fat. (C) The cylindrical piece of tissue is gently supported with forceps and cut deep to include subcutaneous tissue. (D) Bleeding is controlled with Monsel solution. (From Habif, T. [2016]. *Clinical dermatology: A color guide to diagnosis and therapy* [6th ed.]. Philadelphia: Elsevier.)

separates the lesion from the dermis. The area is cleaned. Local anesthesia is usually required. The skin is stabilized with the nondominant hand. The curet is pressed against the skin until firm resistance is met, and the soft area is removed with multiple strokes of the curet. The specimen is placed in a fixative and submitted to the pathology laboratory to confirm its histologic nature. Local hemostasis is achieved with electrocautery or the application of a hemostatic solution such as aluminum chloride. Curets come in various sizes, and single-use, sharp disposables are available.

BIOPSY

A biopsy is appropriate when the nature of the lesion or dermatitis is in question. Primary care offices are seeing increasing numbers of patients with suspicious melanocytic lesions, and some practices have begun to perform skin biopsies if the provider has education in this procedure.[1] In addition, the provider performing the biopsy must be able to establish a differential diagnosis, be prepared to interpret the pathology report, be able to recognize whether the pathologic process is consistent with the clinical presentation, and be able to arrange for appropriate treatment.[1] With a federal push toward computerized medical records and the advent of teledermatology, it is conceivable that images will be shared more routinely with specialists who will be available for consultation from remote sites.

A punch biopsy (Fig. 36.1) is performed when knowledge of the depth of the lesion is required, such as with pigmented lesions, for which the depth of the lesion is one of the most important prognostic indicators of malignant melanoma.[2] Punches are also useful when the lesion is small and can be entirely removed. They are available as single-use, disposable tools that are fitted with a sharp, round blade and available in increments of 1 mm; they range in size from 2 to 10 mm in diameter.[5] The most commonly used sizes for diagnostic biopsies are 3 to 4 mm. When removal cannot be accomplished with a punch, an elliptical excision of the entire lesion with a 1- to 3-mm border is recommended.[6] Referral is recommended for large lesions. For those occasions when options are limited, multiple smaller samples can be obtained from the most unusual portions of the lesion, knowing that a negative finding on pathologic examination is not necessarily a negative diagnosis.

To perform a punch biopsy procedure, the provider measures the pigmented lesion to choose the appropriate diameter of the biopsy punch; the punch should remove the lesion with at least a 1-mm margin, because any portion of a lesion that remains, as well as the adjacent skin, may contain pathologic changes.[1,6] First, the provider dons clean gloves and prepares the area with an alcohol wipe before infiltrating with the appropriate local anesthesia; in general, 1% to 2% lidocaine with or without epinephrine is used. Lidocaine should not

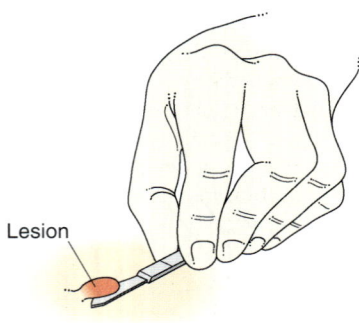

Lesion

F I G . **36.2**   Shave biopsy. (From Habif, T. [2016]. *Clinical dermatology: A color guide to diagnosis and therapy* [6th ed.]. Philadelphia: Elsevier.)

be used with epinephrine at the tips of the digits and nose and the glans penis. A small-volume syringe (1 to 3 mL) and a small-gauge needle (e.g., 31 gauge) are used to inject the anesthetic into the dermis by producing a wheal. A visible wheal indicates that the anesthetic has been deposited into the dermis. The area intended to be sampled should be draped, and the provider should don sterile gloves and position the punch over the lesion. The punch is pushed into the skin as the provider rotates it between thumb and forefingers. The punch is inserted until resistance eases, indicating that the punch has reached the subcutaneous fat. The provider must ensure that the punch is inserted into the subcutaneous fat layer; this ensures that the entire lesion is sampled. The cylinder of skin is gently removed with forceps without crushing the sample. The specimen is cut with sterile scissors deep enough to include subcutaneous fat, and the sample is placed in a container with a standard fixative. The defect is closed with suture material suitable for the area of the body and the strength of the surrounding tissue: 5.0 or 6.0 for the face and genitalia; 5.0 for the dorsa of the hands, ventral forearms, and breasts; 4.0 or 5.0 for the torso and extremities; and 3.0 or 4.0 for the scalp, palms, and soles. The wound is dressed with petrolatum and a dry sterile bandage. The patient should be instructed to keep the area clean with soap and water, to monitor the wound for signs of infection, and to change the bandage daily until the sutures are removed. As general guidelines, suture removal occurs typically after 3 to 5 days for the face and neck; 7 days for the scalp, chest, abdomen, and upper extremities; 10 days for the back; and 10 to 14 days for the lower extremities and the feet.[6]

A shave biopsy (Fig. 36.2) is used when a full-thickness specimen is not required for diagnosis. This includes nonmelanocytic lesions such as actinic keratoses, basal and squamous cell carcinomas, warts, and seborrheic keratosis. To perform a shave biopsy, the provider cleans the skin area with an alcohol wipe and anesthetizes as described previously. A No. 15 scalpel is selected; razor blades are also used. The blade is obliquely pressed through the skin to remove all or part of the lesion. If the lesion is small, the lesion can sometimes be removed entirely. Removal of larger lesions through a shave, though, is

likely to leave a visible scar. The goal of a shave biopsy is to produce a saucer-shaped skin defect that has smooth edges.[1] The specimen is removed with forceps and placed into a container with fixative. Bleeding can be controlled with direct pressure, light electrocautery, or hemostatic solutions such as aluminum chloride. The biopsy site is dressed with a small amount of petrolatum and a bandage. The patient should be instructed to clean the wound daily with soap and water, to monitor for signs of infection, and to apply a small amount of petrolatum and a clean bandage daily for 2 or 3 days.

Scissor excision should be performed on pedunculated lesions such as skin tags. With these lesions, anesthesia is rarely needed. The area should be cleaned with an alcohol wipe. The lesion should be grasped with forceps by the nondominant hand while the base is snipped with sterile iris scissors held in the dominant hand. Bleeding can be controlled by direct pressure, light electrocautery, or hemostatic solutions such as aluminum chloride. The biopsy site should be dressed with a small amount of petrolatum and a bandage. The patient should be instructed to clean the wound daily with soap and water, to monitor for signs of infection, and to apply a small amount of petrolatum and a clean bandage daily for 2 or 3 days.

SUMMARY

Cryosurgery, curettage, electrocautery, punch biopsy, shave biopsy, and scissor excision are common office procedures used in the diagnosis and treatment of dermatologic conditions. Primary care providers can safely perform these procedures with proper education and training. Referral to or consultation with a dermatology specialist is indicated for large lesions, lesions that do not respond to treatment, malignant lesions, lesions whose diagnosis cannot be established, and lesions that the provider is not knowledgeable enough to manage.

REFERENCES

1. Endrizzi, B., & Souter, C. (2013). Dermatologic procedures. In C. Soutor & M. K. Hordinsky (Eds.), *Clinical dermatology*. New York, NY: McGraw-Hill.
2. Usatine, R. P., Smith, M. A., Chumley, H. S., & Mayeaux, E. J., Jr. (Eds.). (2013). Squamous cell carcinoma. In *The color atlas of family medicine, 2e*. New York, NY: McGraw-Hill. Retrieved from http://accessmedicine.mhmedical.com .chamberlainuniversity.idm.oclc.org/content.aspx?bookid=685&sectionid =45361237. (Accessed 29 November 2017).
3. Usatine, R. P., Smith, M. A., Chumley, H. S., & Mayeaux, E. J., Jr. (Eds.). (2013). Flat warts. In *The color atlas of family medicine, 2e*. New York, NY: McGraw-Hill. Retrieved from http://accessmedicine.mhmedical.com .chamberlainuniversity.idm.oclc.org/content.aspx?bookid=685&sectionid =45361190. (Accessed 30 November 2017).
4. Vujevich, J. J., & Goldberg, L. H. (2012). Cryosurgery and electrosurgery. In L. A. Goldsmith, S. I. Katz, B. A. Gilchrest, A. S. Paller, D. J. Leffell, & K. Wolff (Eds.), *Fitzpatrick's dermatology in general medicine, 8e*. New York, NY: McGraw-Hill. Chapter 246. Retrieved from http://accessmedicine.mhmedical .com.chamberlainuniversity.idm.oclc.org/Content.aspx?bookid=392&sectionid =41138986. (Accessed 30 November 2017).
5. Urba, W. J., & Curti, B. D. (2014). Cancer of the skin. In D. Kasper, A. Fauci, S. Hauser, D. Longo, J. Jameson, & J. Loscalzo (Eds.), *Harrison's principles of internal medicine, 19e*. New York, NY: McGraw-Hill. Retrieved from http:// accessmedicine.mhmedical.com.chamberlainuniversity.idm.oclc.org/content .aspx?bookid=1130&sectionid=79729820. (Accessed 30 November 2017).
6. Habif, T. (2016). *Clinical dermatology: A color guide to diagnosis and therapy* (6th ed.). Philadelphia: Elsevier.

PRINCIPLES OF DERMATOLOGIC THERAPY

Ellen M. McCafferty-O'Connell

A variety of topical and systemic medications are used to treat dermatologic conditions. This chapter will review the most common topical agents used in dermatologic conditions, topical corticosteroid preparations. In addition, an overview of therapy principles and other medications used to treat patients with dermatologic conditions will be provided.

SKIN STRUCTURE

The skin is the largest organ of the body. The primary function of the skin is to provide a barrier to passage of substances into and from the body and to maintain internal homeostasis.[1] Three main layers form this barrier.[1] The stratum corneum is the most superficial section of the epidermis, or outer layer. The stratum corneum consists of enucleated keratinocytes, which are filled with keratin and an interfilamentous matrix. The middle layer is the vascularized dermis, which contains connective tissue and skin appendages. The innermost layer is the subcutaneous layer, composed of adipose tissue.

The thickness and permeability of the stratum corneum vary on different areas of the body. When the stratum corneum is irritated and inflamed, the protective skin barrier is interrupted. These characteristics have clinical implications for dermatologic therapy because they affect drug absorption. The skin structure in older adults is dryer, thinner, and less elastic, which needs to be considered when prescribing for older adults.

ESTABLISHING THE DIAGNOSIS AND SELECTING TREATMENT: AN OVERVIEW

The critical first step in treating any dermatologic condition is accurate diagnosis. Other important components are the type of lesion to be treated, the medication, the vehicle of the active medication, and the method used to apply the medication. A thorough history is the most important step in the assessment of dermatologic problems.

The history of present illness should include questions regarding routine skin care regime. These should include: How often do you bathe? Do you use soap or cleanser—and if so, which one? Do you lather from head to toe? Moisturize?

Often a minor itch is exacerbated by what a patient does or doesn't do. Review any skin products being used and treatments tried, including OTC medicated and nonmedicated creams, as well as frequency and duration. Also be aware of any natural or botanicals products that a patient may have tried.

In dermatologic therapy, the type of lesion guides therapy. Moist, weeping lesions are treated with Burow solution to hasten drying while providing soothing relief. Wet dressings are beneficial when treating exudative skin diseases because they help suppress inflammation through vasoconstriction of superficial vessels, as well as promote drying of lesions and wound debridement.[1] In dry dermatitis, therapeutic agents incorporated into creams or ointments increase moisture in the skin and provide relief from pruritus.

For each patient, general skin care advice is an essential component of dermatology therapy. Recommend a warm, not hot, comfortable shower daily or every other day only cleansing routinely soiled areas, avoiding excessive soaping of the back, arms, and legs. If a patient prefers to bathe twice a day, one shower should be a rinse only, without using soap. Avoiding harsh soaps and abrasive washing implements should be discussed, as these can increase skin irritation.[1] Recommending more frequent moisturizing for older patients, patients taking medications that cause dry skin, and patients with health conditions that produce dry skin is also important. Ointments and oils are soothing to the skin although patients may not like the greasy texture. Petroleum jelly is often used and recommended by dermatologists on biopsy sites, skin fissures, and irritated skin.[1] Ointments provide the most hydration, offer the greatest barrier of protection, and are especially effective for thick, dry, scaly skin. Next in the order of dermatological preference are creams, then lotions.

DERMATOLOGY THERAPY

Medications for dermatologic therapy can be administered topically, intralesionally, and systemically.[2] Lesions, if appropriate, may be treated by biopsy, surgery, electrocautery, or cryotherapy. Within a dermatology setting, other treatment modalities include ultraviolet (UV) radiation, ionizing radiation, and laser therapy.

Topical Corticosteroids

Topical corticosteroids (TCS) are the mainstay of dermatology care. The major effects of corticosteroids are the reduction of the inflammatory response, vasoconstriction, and a decrease in collagen synthesis.[3] They are available in several classes based on potency (Table 37.1), and they come in a variety of strengths and vehicles. The health care provider should be familiar with several medication types in each corticosteroid class for ease in prescribing and should prescribe the correct recommended potency for patients, as underprescribing will prolong therapy and cause frustration for the patient. It is important that class 1 to IV corticosteroids never be used on the face or genitals. The suggested potencies for specific diagnoses are listed in Table 37.2. The health care provider should be familiar with several medication types in each class of corticosteroid for ease in prescribing, and prescribe the correct recommended potency for patients, as underprescribing will prolong therapy and cause frustration for the patient.

TCS are exceptionally useful in treating various dermatologic diseases, but they are not without potential adverse effects. Common side effects with TCS or their vehicle include contact dermatitis, acne-like eruptions, and hypopigmentation.[1] Higher corticosteroid potency, improper body location, and prolonged use can contribute to the development of non-reversible adverse effects. Collagen synthesis is affected, which results in striae and tissue atrophy. Telangiectasia, which are visible capillaries, and purpura may result from a thinning of the epidermis. Systemic side effects can be avoided when TCS are prescribed and used appropriately. Important patient education includes reviewing gentle skin care instructions, explaining to patients that corticosteroid prescriptions should not be filled indefinitely, and that nonsteroidal alternatives may be a better option for some individuals.[1] TCS work best in conjunction with OTC moisturizers.

TABLE 37.1 Topical Corticosteroids Ranked by Potency

Class	Concentration and Generic Name (Selected Brand Names and Vehicle)
Class 1— Superpotent	• Clobetasol propionate (Temovate) 0.05% ointment/cream • Betamethasone dipropionate (Diprolene) 0.05% ointment/lotion/gel • Fluocinonide (Vanos) 0.1% cream
Class 2—Potent	• Mometasone furoate (Elocon) 0.1% ointment • Halcinonide (Halog) 0.1% cream • Fluocinonide (Lidex) 0.05% ointment/cream • Desoximetasone (Topicort) 0.25% ointment/cream • Betamethasone dipropionate (Diprolene) 0.05% cream
Class 3—Upper midstrength	• Fluticasone propionate (Cutivate) 0.005% ointment • Halcinonide (Halog) 0.1% ointment • Betamethasone valerate (Valisone) 0.1% ointment
Class 4— Midstrength	• Mometasone furoate (Elocon) 0.1% cream • Triamcinolone acetonide (Kenalog) 0.1% ointment/cream • Fluocinolone acetonide (Synalar) 0.025% ointment
Class 5—Lower midstrength	• Fluocinolone acetonide (Synalar) 0.025% cream • Hydrocortisone valerate (Westcort) 0.2% ointment
Class 6—Mild	• Desonide (DesOwen) 05% ointment/cream/lotion • Alclometasone dipropionate (Aclovate) 0.05% ointment/cream
Class 7—Least potent	• Hydrocortisone (Hytone) 2.5%, 1%, 0.5% ointment/cream/lotion

Modified from Kliegman, R. M., Stanton, B. F, St Geme, J. W., & Schor, N. F. (2016). *Nelson textbook of pediatrics* (20th ed.). St. Louis: Elsevier.

TABLE 37.2 Suggested Strength of Topical Steroids to Initiate Treatment

Groups I and II	Groups III to V	Groups VI and VII
Psoriasis	Atopic dermatitis	Dermatitis (eyelids)
Lichen planus	Nummular eczema	Dermatitis (diaper area)
Discoid lupus[a]	Asteatotic eczema	Mild dermatitis (face)
Severe hand eczema	Stasis dermatitis	Mild anal inflammation
Poison ivy (severe)	Seborrheic dermatitis	Mild intertrigo
Lichen simplex chronicus	Lichen sclerosus et atrophicus (vulva)	
Hyperkeratotic eczema	Intertrigo (brief course)	
Chapped feet	Tinea (brief course to control inflammation)	
Lichen sclerosus et atrophicus (skin)	Scabies (after scabicide)	
Alopecia areata	Intertrigo (severe cases)	
Nummular eczema (severe)	Anal inflammation (severe cases)	
Atopic dermatitis (resistant adult cases)	Severe dermatitis (face)	

[a]Use on the face may be justified.
Stop treatment, change to less potent agent, or use intermittent treatment once inflammation is controlled.
From Habif, T. P. (2015). *Clinical dermatology* (6th ed.). St Louis: Elsevier.

If the patient is not improving, it is important to consider the following: Noncompliance or contact dermatitis from the TCS or preservative is a possible cause. Although controversial, tachyphylaxis may occur in response to the repeated use of a topical agent, thus requiring a decrease in the amount of topical agent used, as well as an increase in dosing interval times. If there is worsening of a rash being treated with a TCS, consider an undiagnosed fungal or yeast infection.[1]

Variables to Consider When Prescribing Steroids

Body location and safety are the most important variables to consider when prescribing TCS. The thickness of the stratum corneum, known as a diffusion barrier, will influence the variation in drug absorption and effectiveness. Steroids are categorized in seven classes—the strongest in class I and the weakest in class VII.[3] An example of class VII is OTC hydrocortisone 1% (see Table 37.1). There is increased skin permeability in the very young and old, or when the skin is broken down by disease, trauma, and chemical agents such as soaps and detergents.[1]

Vehicle refers to the base of the active ingredient; the types range from very thin to very thick. Research has found that the effectiveness of the active ingredient varied with a different vehicle.[2] Note on Table 37.1 that the active ingredients of fluocinonide, halcinonide, fluocinolone acetonide, and mometasone furoate are located in more than one class, based on preparation vehicle and strength. Creams are semisolid emulsions of oil in water that vanish when rubbed into the skin.[2] Preservatives are added to prevent the growth of bacteria and fungi and may cause a contact dermatitis in some individuals.[2] Hairy areas are difficult to penetrate, so in these areas, a solution, foam, spray, or gel may work better. These preparations are formulated by dissolving the active ingredient in alcoholic vehicles that evaporate to leave the active agent on the skin.[2] Other vehicles include combinations of powders, oils, and liquids in varying proportions. Powders aid in absorbing moisture, decrease friction, and help cover wide areas. Oils provide an emollient function and, because of their occlusive properties, often enhance drug absorption. Liquids provide a cooling, soothing sensation by evaporation while helping exudative lesions to dry.

All types of dermatologic medications are applied in a single thin layer. Thicker applications do not increase skin penetration or effectiveness of the medication.[1]

Always take into consideration the body surface area that the prescription needs to cover. One gram typically covers an area of 10 × 10 cm; ointments cover a slightly larger area.[1] For example, to treat scabies properly, the patient needs enough permethrin to cover the entire body from the neck down on day 1 and day 7. The amount needed for a single application for the entire body is approximately 30 g, so it would be necessary to prescribe a 60 g tube of permethrin. Another practical way to measure topical application is the fingertip unit (FTU). An FTU is defined as the amount of ointment expressed from a tube with a 5-mm nozzle to cover from the tip of the index finger to the distal skin crease. This is approximately 0.5 g.[1]

Systemic Corticosteroids

Systemic glucocorticosteroid therapy should be reserved for short-term treatment of self-limited rashes, as the risks of systemic corticosteroids frequently outweigh the benefits.[4] Some dermatitis (e.g., psoriasis) will flare after a course of oral prednisone.

ANTIFUNGAL MEDICATIONS

Topical antifungal solutions and creams are available to treat dermatophyte infections. The products should be continued 1 week after clearing of the lesions to discourage recurrence; however, recurrence of tinea infections is common.[4-6]

Systemic antifungal medications are used for widespread tinea or infections that involve the nails or scalp. Certain systemic antifungals need to be taken with a high-fat food for complete absorption. The use of oral medications requires careful dosage calculation and monitoring for potential side effects. Oral ketoconazole (Nizoral) should be avoided because of risks of hepatotoxicity and serious drug interactions.[5] Terbinafine is not recommended for patients with a history of renal or liver dysfunction. Monitoring of liver function is required every 6 weeks or if the patient experiences nausea, anorexia, or fatigue during therapy. Neutropenia has been reported as a side effect of terbinafine therapy; therefore, a complete blood count should be performed every 6 weeks or if there are symptoms suggestive of neutropenia.[4] A careful and complete drug history should be taken before therapy is initiated with itraconazole; itraconazole is metabolized by the cytochrome P-450 3A4 (CYP3A4) system and affects the cytochrome P-450 enzyme system, creating many drug interactions.[1] Neither the oral nor the topical form of oral terbinafine or oral itraconazole is recommended for pregnant or nursing women. A variety of agents—powders, intravaginal agents, oral suspensions, creams, and tablets—are commonly used for the treatment of candidal infections

ANTIVIRAL MEDICATIONS

Both topical (e.g., penciclovir cream and Xerese, a combination of acyclovir and hydrocortisone) and systemic antivirals (e.g. acyclovir, famciclovir, or valacyclovir) are used with herpetic outbreaks. Antiviral theory is administered acutely and for suppression of disease. Suppressive therapy is needed for individuals with recurrent outbreaks more than six times per year.[7]

BIOLOGIC AGENTS

Biologic agents target immune-mediated inflammation. Classes of these medication include TNF antagonists, such as infliximab, etanercept, adalimumab, and others, that have been approved for the treatment of moderate to severe psoriasis. Several other biologic agents are approved for use in patients with psoriatic arthritis. The medications are typically prescribed by dermatology or rheumatology and administered as a self-administered subcutaneous or intramuscular injections or as intravenous infusions. These medications are costly, as much as $25,000

per year. Insurance companies often require that other treatment modalities have been attempted and have failed before patients are approved for the biologics.[8] Several agents come with a US Food and Drug Administration–mandated "black box" warning for safety concerns relative to increased susceptibility to infection from fungi, viruses, bacteria, and mycobacteria, and a possible connection to lymphoma; hematologic diseases such as aplastic anemia, melanoma, nonmelanoma skin cancers; and other solid organ cancers. Conflicting data exist about whether or not there is increased risk of infection or malignancy in patients with psoriasis who use biologics. Each medication has its own particular safety profile; thus it is good practice that patients be screened for tuberculosis and hepatitis B before initiation of therapy to avoid latent disease activation. Histories of multiple sclerosis or other demyelinating disease and congestive heart failure are relative contraindications. Monitoring parameters include psoriasis lesion and surface area reduction, QOL assessments, periodic liver function tests and complete blood counts, and assessment for evidence of infectious disease.[9,10]

Patients who receive biologics are essentially considered to be immunocompromised. Prior to starting biologics titers should be checked and the patient's immunization status updated because live vaccines are contraindicated during treatment. They can, however, be administered 2 weeks to a month before treatment. It is important that inactivated influenza vaccines are received yearly. Pneumococcal vaccines should be considered, even in those under 65 years of age.[11]

RETINOID MEDICATIONS

Retinoid medications, often prescribed for acne, wrinkles, or psoriasis are available in both topical and systemic formulations. Retinoid medications are vitamin A analogs and are thought to inhibit sebum production, to decrease follicular obstruction, and to have an antiinflammatory effect. Use of oral systemic retinoids for therapy is best managed by a dermatologist or dermatology nurse practitioner. With some oral systemic retinoid medications, patients need monthly monitoring of triglyceride levels and hepatic function. Oral systemic retinoids have teratogenic potential, and careful contraceptive measures must be taken. Sexually active women of childbearing age must use two forms of birth control and be monitored for pregnancy monthly; depending on the systemic retinoid preparation, contraception and avoidance of pregnancy is recommended for varying length of times post treatment. For some of the newer preparations, the time frame may be as long as 3 years.[4]

PATIENT AND FAMILY EDUCATION

The first guideline of dermatologic therapy is to keep the treatment as simple as possible. Health care providers should prescribe enough medication to complete therapy and should provide realistic expectations.

The provider should write out the specific application procedures and ensure that the patient fully understands the instructions. Important information to review with the patient includes how much topical medication to apply, exactly where to apply it, and how often to moisturize. Patients should be instructed not to apply the dermatologic medication to areas other than where instructed. In addition, patients should be aware of possible adverse reactions and should know when to call the office and return for follow-up evaluation.

Patients taking systemic preparations must understand that additional monitoring is required and that follow-up will be necessary. Patients (and families when indicated) need to be informed about all potential side effects, as well as actions to take if any side effects are noted. In addition, this information should be documented in the patient's medical record.

Medications with teratogenic potential require further education, as some products require special precautions when handling (e.g., gloves). Women of childbearing age require careful, consistent education detailing the risks of becoming pregnancy while on any teratogenic medication, as well as monthly surveillance for pregnancy. Teratogenic medications are not commonly prescribed in primary care, and some medications (e.g., isotretinoin) can only be prescribed by specific prescribers.

REFERENCES

1. Bobonich, M. A., & Nolen, M. E. (2015). *Dermatology for advanced practice clinicians*. Philadelphia: Wolters Kluwer.
2. Marks, J. G., & Miller, J. J. (2013). *Lookingbill and Marks' principles of dermatology* (5th ed.). London: Elsevier.
3. Habif, T. P. (2015). *Clinical dermatology* (6th ed.). St Louis: Elsevier.
4. Bolognia, J. L., Schaffer, J. V., & Cerroni, L. (2017). *Dermatology* (4th ed.). St. Louis: Elsevier.
5. Cellulitis, common warts, genital warts; impetigo; herpes simplex virus infection; measles, rubella, varicella; vaginitis; [monograph]. In: Epocrates [online]. San Francisco, CA: Epocrates, Inc.; 2018. Last updated: November 13, 2017. Retrieved from http://www.epocrates.com. (Accessed 17 January 2018).
6. Goldsmith, L. A., Katz, S. I., Gilchrest, B. A., Paller, A. S., Leffell, D. J., & Wolff, K. (Eds.). (2012). *Fitzpatrick's dermatology in general medicine* (8th ed.). New York, NY: McGraw-Hill.
7. Centers for Disease Control and Prevention. (2015). Sexually transmitted diseases treatment guidelines, 2015. *MMWR. Recommendations and Reports: Morbidity and Mortality Weekly Report. Recommendations and Reports, 64*(3), 27–32. Retrieved from https://www.cdc.gov/mmwr/pdf/rr/rr6403.pdf. (Accessed 23 February 2018).
8. Polat, M., & İlhan, M. N. (2015). The prevalence of interdigital erythrasma: A prospective study from an outpatient clinic in Turkey. *Journal of the American Podiatric Medical Association, 105*(2), 121–124.
9. Ferri, F. (2018). *2018 Ferri's clinical advisor: 5 books in 1*. Philadelphia: Elsevier.
10. McCann, S. A., & Huether, W. E. (2014). Structure, function, and disorders of the integument. In K. L. McCance & S. E. Huether (Eds.), *Pathophysiology: The biologic basis for disease in adults and children* (ed. 7). St. Louis: Elsevier. Ch 46.
11. Stern, S. C., Cifu, A. S., & Altkorn, D. (Eds.). (2014). *Symptom to diagnosis: An evidence-based guide* (3rd ed.). New York, NY: McGraw-Hill. Retrieved from http://accessmedicine.mhmedical.com.ezproxy.hsc.usf.edu/content.aspx?bookid=1088&sectionid=61696294. (Accessed 21 January 2018).

CHAPTER **38**

SCREENING FOR SKIN CANCER
Randy Michael Gordon

DEFINITION AND EPIDEMIOLOGY

Although early detection and treatment of skin cancer can improve patient outcomes, the evidence base for practice does not contain any randomized clinical trials for total body skin examination (TBSE) during routine office visits, and studies in the literature utilize poor and inconsistent research methodology.[1] Only limited evidence was identified for routine skin cancer screening, particularly regarding potential benefit of skin cancer screening on melanoma mortality. As a result, the US Preventive Services Task Force (USPSTF) concluded that while there was insufficient evidence to recommend routine screening for early detection, that the benefits of skin cancer screening may be greatest among subgroups most likely to develop fatal melanoma, and future research on skin cancer screening should focus on evaluating the effectiveness of targeted screening in those considered to be at higher risk for skin cancer.[1] In light of the incomplete evidence base for practice in this critical area, many professional organizations support skin cancer screening of high-risk individuals. Both the National Cancer Institute and the American Cancer Society recommend monthly self-skin examinations (SSEs).[1] A purpose of routine skin cancer screening during an office visit is to educate both the patient and the provider how to identify the characteristic changes associated with skin cancer.

Approximately 5.4 million cases of basal cell carcinoma (BCC) and squamous cell carcinoma (SCC) are diagnosed each year, occurring in about 3.3 million Americans, as some people have more than one.[1] Although BCC is the most common form of skin cancer, malignant melanoma (MM) is by far the most fatal. Based on reports from 2010 to 2014, the age-adjusted incidence rate of melanoma is 22.3/100,000 men and women per year according to the national Surveillance, Epidemiology, and End Results (SEER) database.[2] Of the estimated 77,110 new cases of melanoma of the skin that occur annually, 9730 deaths are expected.[3] One person dies of melanoma every hour (every 54 minutes).[3] In 2014, there were an estimated 1,169,351 people living with melanoma of the skin in the United States.[3] Overall, MM incidence rates are higher in white women than in men before age 50—a higher probability of developing melanoma than any other cancer except breast and thyroid cancers. However, MM incidence rates in men versus women are twice as high by age 65, and nearly triple by age 80.[3] The differences in risk by age and sex primarily reflect differences in occupational and recreational sun exposure, which have changed over time. The rising incidence of skin cancer during the past 3 decades may also be attributed to increased sun exposure associated with societal and lifestyle shifts in the US population and to depletion of the protective ozone layer.[4]

Ninety percent of all skin cancers are caused by the sun.[5] Acute sunburns place the patient at increased risk, and the effects of sun damage are cumulative. Second-degree burns before the age of 18 years can double the incidence of non-melanoma skin cancer (NMSC) and greatly increase the risk for MM. Fair-skinned men and women older than 65 years, patients with atypical moles, and those with more than 50 nevi constitute known groups at substantially increased risk for development of melanoma.[3] In addition, skin cancers appear to have a hereditary component. Xeroderma pigmentosum is the prototype syndrome of genetically determined increased skin cancer risk.[4]

Multiple risk factors exist for all types of skin cancer, including endogenous factors (phototype, skin and eye color, number of melanocytic nevi, presence of dysplastic nevi, and individual or family history of skin cancer) and exogenous factors (type and degree of cumulative sun exposure, history of sunburn, and sun protection behavior).[3–5] Primary care providers should devote more time to screening patients with multiple risk factors. Providers must learn to identify high-risk patients for targeted assessment by incorporating patient risk assessment tools into their practice.[4]

PATHOPHYSIOLOGY

The pathogenesis of skin cancer is multifactoral. Heavy sun exposure is a significant risk factor for MM.[4] Ultraviolet radiation (UVR) in sunlight is the main causative agent in the development of MM and NMSC. UVR produces DNA damage, gene mutations, immunosuppression, oxidative stress, and inflammatory responses, all of which play a pivotal role in photoaging of the skin and skin cancer genesis. Researchers have suggested an association between skin cancer genesis and UVR-induced immunosuppression. UVR is a complete carcinogen in that it not only initiates tumorigenesis by inducing mutations in tumor suppressor genes, but also promotes tumor development. When UVR penetrates the skin, much of its energy is absorbed by the DNA of epidermal keratinocytes. Another major mechanism of carcinogenesis is UVR-induced free radical damage, and genetically determined ability to metabolize free radicals may also predispose patients to skin cancer.[4] Repeated and unprotected exposure to ultraviolet light causes photoaging of the skin over time.

Normal skin aging begins by age 30 to 35 and is characterized by thinning, atrophy, decreased elasticity, and fragility that leads to wrinkling. Skin that is photoaged from sun damage may be coarse with yellow discoloration (solar elastosis), irregularly pigmented, rough, or atrophic with deep wrinkling. Reactive hyperplasia of melanocytes results in persistent hyperpigmentation or hypopigmentation of the hands, forearms, legs, chest, and back.[4] Chronic exposure disrupts the maturation of the outer layer of the epidermis, resulting in scaling, roughness, seborrheic keratoses, actinic keratoses, and NMSCs.[6] Tanning beds and sun lamps provide additional sources of ultraviolet light exposure and should be avoided.[3] The International Agency for Research on Cancer has classified indoor tanning devices as "carcinogenic to humans" based on an extensive review of scientific evidence.[3]

CLINICAL PRESENTATION AND PHYSICAL EXAMINATION

Primary care providers must solicit a detailed patient history, including a social, family, and UVR-exposure history, to identify patients with the highest risk of developing skin cancer. Questions about the patient's use of sunscreens, repeated sun exposure without protection, tendency to burn, outdoor employment, or family history of melanoma are beneficial to estimate the risk for NMSC and MM.[4] Patients scheduled for routine physical examinations should be queried about any changes in the appearance or size of skin lesions (Table 38.1). Warning signs for skin cancer include (1) an open sore that does not heal for 3 weeks; (2) a spot or sore that burns, itches, stings, crusts, or bleeds; and (3) any mole or spot that changes in size or texture, develops irregular borders, or appears pearly, translucent, or multicolored. Important clinical signs of cutaneous carcinoma include changes in size, shape, color, or texture of a mole or other skin lesion or the appearance of a new growth on the skin. Changes that occur over a few days are usually not cancer, but changes that progress over a month or more should be evaluated by a health care provider.[4]

The physical examination consists of a complete and thorough TBSE, the most commonly advocated screening test for skin cancer. With the patient disrobed, the examiner must systematically inspect the entire skin surface, including the scalp, nails, and palms of the hands and the soles of the feet.[1] Detection of a suspicious skin lesion, such as BCC, warrants biopsy or referral. NMSC lesions such as BCC may vary from a normal flesh-colored lesion to a slightly pigmented lesion (Fig. 38.1). These are characterized by a raised, shiny appearance, often

TABLE 38.1 Signs Suggesting Malignant Transformation in Pigmented Lesions

Sign	Implication
CHANGE IN COLOR	
Sudden darkening; brown, black	Increased number of tumor cells, the density of which varies within the lesion, creating irregular pigmentation
Spread of color into previously normal skin	Tumor cells migrating through epidermis at various speeds and in different directions (horizontal growth phase)
Red	Vasodilation and inflammation
White	Areas of regression or inflammation
Blue	Pigment deep in dermis; sign of increasing depth of tumor
CHANGE IN CHARACTERISTICS OF BORDER	
Irregular outline	Malignant cells migrating horizontally at different rates
Satellite pigmentation	Cells migrating beyond confines of primary tumor
Development of depigmented halo	Destruction of melanocytes by possible immunologic reaction and inflammation
CHANGES IN SURFACE CHARACTERISTICS THAT SHOULD PROMPT EVALUATION FOR SKIN CANCER	
Scaliness	
Erosion	
Oozing	
Crusting	
Bleeding	
Ulceration	
Elevation	
Loss of normal skin lines	
DEVELOPMENT OF SYMPTOMS THAT SHOULD PROMPT EVALUATION FOR SKIN CANCER	
Pruritus	
Tenderness	
Pain	

From Habif, T. P. (2016). *Clinical dermatology* (6th ed.). Philadelphia: Elsevier.

with pearly borders. An SCC lesion is a roughened, scaling area that does not heal and readily bleeds when scraped (Fig. 38.2). Keratinization of these can lead to a heaped-up appearance that flakes. MM is characterized by a lesion that is best described by the *ABCDEs* of MM (Fig. 38.3).[1,3,4] These include *a*symmetry (of the entire lesion), *b*order (irregularities), *c*olor (variability within the lesion from a brown to black discoloration), *d*iameter (>6 mm [1/4 inch]), and *e*levation (recently raised). As mentioned, other symptoms suggestive of skin cancer include nonhealing skin areas, ulceration, bleeding, and

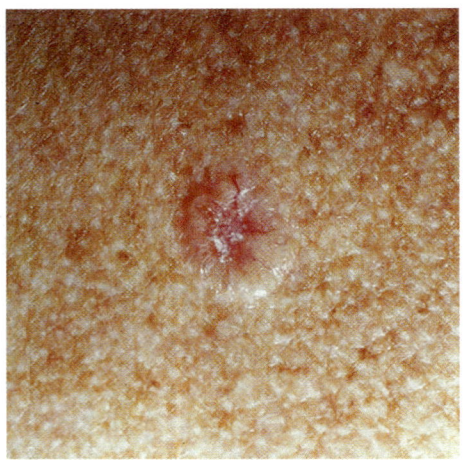

F I G . **38.1** Nodular basal cell carcinoma. (From Ignatavicius, D. D., & Workman, M. L. [2016]. *Medical-surgical nursing: Patient centered collaborative care* [8th ed.]. St. Louis: Mosby.)

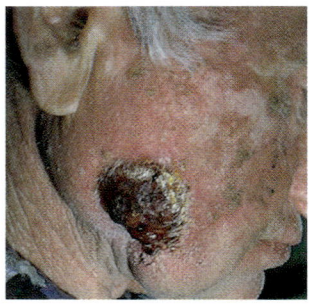

F I G . **38.2** Squamous cell cancer. (From Ignatavicius, D. D., & Workman, M. L. [2016]. *Medical-surgical nursing: Patient centered collaborative care* [8th ed.]. St. Louis: Mosby.)

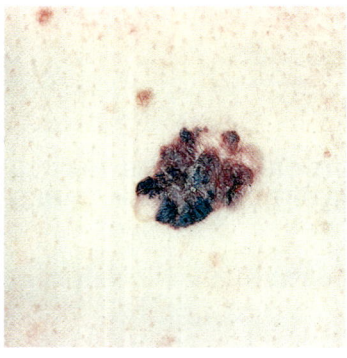

F I G . **38.3** Superficial spreading melanoma. (From Ignatavicius, D. D., & Workman, M. L. [2016]. *Medical-surgical nursing: Patient centered collaborative care* [8th ed.]. St. Louis: Mosby.)

weeping sores. In African Americans, Asian Americans, and dark-skinned individuals, abnormal lesions of the nails, hands, or feet should also be evaluated because these are common sites for melanomas in these populations (Fig. 38.4).[5,7]

ESSENTIAL DIAGNOSTICS

Skin biopsy is the definitive diagnostic test and is best performed by an experienced heath care provider. A shave or

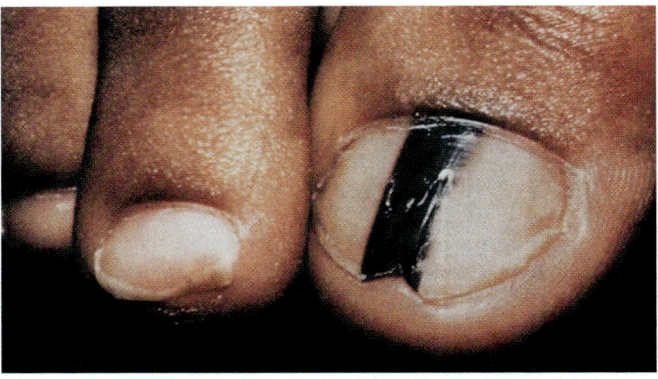

F I G . **38.4** Acral-lentiginous melanoma. It occurs most often on hands, feet, or nail beds of dark-skinned individuals. Very common in African Americans and Asian Americans. (From Habif, T. P., Campbell, J. L., Chapman, M. S., et al. [2011]. *Skin disease: Diagnosis and treatment* [3rd ed.]. St Louis: Saunders.)

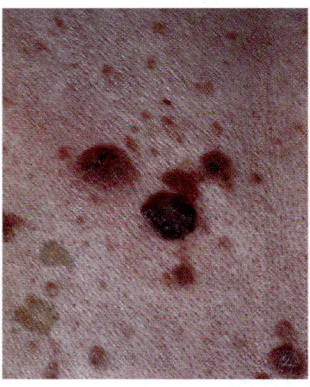

F I G . **38.5** Seborrheic keratosis (mimicking melanoma). (From Kumar, V., Cotran, R. S., & Robbins, S. L. [2003]. *Robbins basic pathology* [7th ed.]. Philadelphia: Saunders.)

punch biopsy technique is appropriate for diagnostic evaluation of suspected NMSC (see Chapter 36). Excisional biopsy (total removal) of suspicious MM lesions should be followed by a wider excision if MM is diagnosed.

INITIAL DIAGNOSTICS

Skin Cancer

- Skin biopsy (shave, punch, or excisional)

DIFFERENTIAL DIAGNOSIS

Screening for skin cancer includes the evaluation of skin for all atypical-appearing lesions.

 Priority differentials include (1) malignant melanoma, (2) squamous cell carcinoma, and (3) basal cell carcinoma.

Skin lesions may range from a seborrheic keratosis (Fig. 38.5) to a premalignant solar (actinic) keratosis to BCC, SCC, or MM. An actinic keratosis is a persistent or recurrent reddened and roughened area that scales or crusts. These lesions are effectively treated with liquid nitrogen by a freeze-thaw technique to obtain a 1- to 3-mm (0.04- to 0.12-inch) rim of freeze, which allows appropriately slow thawing during 20 to 40 seconds.[5,7] See Chapter 36.

INTERPROFESSIONAL COLLABORATIVE MANAGEMENT
Treatment

BCC is treated with electrodessication and curettage.[5,7] Definitive treatment of SCC is total excision.[7] An experienced dermatologist or surgeon is best equipped to treat an MM lesion based on the stage of the disease with a wide excision. If an NMSC or MM is recognized early by the patient or provider, surgical cure is close to 100%.

An annual skin examination of sun-exposed areas is recommended for patients with the diagnosis of BCC or SCC. A primary care provider or dermatology specialist can accomplish this. A TBSE by an experienced clinician is recommended for patients diagnosed with MM lesions.

Complications and Life-Span Considerations

Despite the tendency of NMSC lesions to grow slowly, failure to diagnose them can result in disfigurement. There is indirect evidence that the shift to screening and recognition of melanoma at earlier tumor stages may be associated with better clinical outcomes.[1] The survival rate at 5 years is inversely proportional to the depth of the MM at the time of diagnosis—the deeper the lesion at diagnosis, the lower the survival rate at 5 years.[2] There are minimum risks from TBSE; however, the examination may be embarrassing to some patients and could lead to unnecessary treatment as a result of misdiagnosis or detection of lesions that might not have caused clinical consequences but were sampled by biopsy.[1,4]

INDICATIONS FOR REFERRAL OR HOSPITALIZATION

The identification of atypical-appearing skin lesions warrants referral or a biopsy. If the biopsy reveals an NMSC or MM, a trained primary care provider, dermatology specialist, or surgeon should provide the definitive treatment.

PATIENT EDUCATION AND HEALTH PROMOTION

The incidence of melanoma has increased 15 times in the last 40 years.[2] In 2014, the US Surgeon General released *Call to Action to Prevent Skin Cancer*, citing the elevated and growing burden of this disease.[3] The purpose of this initiative is to increase awareness and encourage all Americans to engage in behaviors that reduce the risk of skin cancer. Knowing that damage to the skin caused by the sun is cumulative may help patients take precautions against sun exposure and thereby reduce their risk; 80% of lifetime sun exposure occurs before the age of 18 years.[1] Precautions include avoiding the sun, wearing protective clothing, and using sunscreens to prevent solar damage to the skin, both for young children and for adults. Prevention of sunburns, which carry a high risk of malignant transformation over time, is paramount. Education of patients at higher risk is crucial. (See the Clinical Presentation section for factors that place patients at higher risk.)

Sun exposure for longer than 15 minutes requires protection with a sunscreen that has a sun protection factor (SPF) of at least 15. Sunscreens should be applied before sun exposure and reapplied every 2 hours or after swimming.

It is important for patients to know that they should seek medical attention for nonhealing sores (sores usually heal within 4 to 6 weeks) or for any lesion that changes in size, shape, texture, or color. Early identification of atypical-appearing skin lesions results in timely referral and effective treatment.

Strategies to improve skin cancer screening by health care providers in the primary care setting include (1) increasing clinicians' skin cancer awareness and understanding, (2) training providers to target high-risk patient populations for screening, and (3) empowering nonphysician providers to gain confidence and competence in their screening skills. By increasing skin cancer and screening comprehension, clinicians can improve screening practices and promote early detection.[3,8]

REFERENCES

1. Wernli, K. J., Henrikson, N. B., Morrison, C. C., Nguyen, M., Pocobelli, G., & Blasi, P. R. (2016). Screening for skin cancer in adults updated evidence report and systematic review for the US Preventive Services Task Force. *JAMA: The Journal of the American Medical Association, 316*(4), 436–447. doi:10.1001/jama.2016.5415.
2. SEER. Cancer stat facts: Melanoma of the skin. National Cancer Institute. Bethesda, MD. Retrieved from http://seer.cancer.gov/statfacts/html/melan.html. (Accessed 29 November 2017).
3. American Cancer Society (ACS). (2017). Cancer facts and figures. Retrieved from https://www.cancer.org/content/dam/cancer-org/research/cancer-facts-and-statistics/annual-cancer-facts-and-figures/2017/cancer-facts-and-figures-2017.pdf. (Accessed 29 November 2017).
4. Gordon, R. M. (2014). Increasing skin cancer awareness and screening in primary care. *The Nurse Practitioner, 39*(5), 48–54.
5. Wolff, K., Johnson, R. A., Saavedra, A. P., & Roh, E. K. (2017). *Fitzpatrick's color atlas and synopsis of clinical dermatology* (8th ed.). New York, NY: McGraw-Hill.
6. McDaniel, D., Farris, P., & Valacchi, G. (2018). Atmospheric skin aging—Contributors and inhibitors. *Journal of Cosmetic Dermatology, 17*, 124–137. https://doi.org/10.1111/jocd.12518.
7. Habif, T. P. (2016). *Clinical dermatology* (56th ed.). China: Elsevier.
8. Loescher, L. J., John, M. H., & Curiel-Lewandrowski, C. (2011). A systematic review of advanced practice nurses' skin cancer assessment barriers, skin lesion recognition skills, and skin cancer training activities. *Journal of the American Academy of Nurse Practitioners, 23*(12), 667–673.

CHAPTER **39**

ADNEXAL DISEASE
Duellyn Pandis

DEFINITION AND EPIDEMIOLOGY

The epidermis is composed of appendages also known as an adnexal structure.

The word *adnexa* is a Latin verb defined as "bind to, attach, connect, or join." The term *adnexal* refers to the parts of a structure that are connected. Specifically, the adnexal structures of dermatology include the pilosebaceous unit, which includes the hair follicle, sebaceous glands, eccrine gland, apocrine sweat gland, and the arrector pili muscle. Example of these include skin, hair, and nails. These are a direct extension of the epidermis. Any injury or disease associated with this type of structure is considered adnexal disease.[1] Adnexal diseases that are discussed in the chapter are acne vulgaris, acne rosacea, perioral dermatitis, folliculitis, hidradenitis, and hyperhidrosis.

ACNE VULGARIS
Definition and Epidemiology

Acne vulgaris is the most common dermatologic disorder in the United States. Although first observed in the pediatric age group, the condition can persist well into the adult years. Whereas it is not usually a serious medical problem, acne should never be dismissed as a minor condition that will eventually be outgrown. The psychological effects of prolonged acne and scars include poor confidence, impaired social contact, embarrassment, shame, anxiety, and difficulty with employment.[2] Advances in acne treatment enable management of this disease for many patients.

Acne vulgaris is a disorder of the pilosebaceous follicles resulting in increased sebum production, altered keratinization, inflammation, and bacterial colonization. Acne is characterized by the formation of comedones, erythematous papules and pustules, and nodules.[2]

Up to 80% of individuals with a first-degree relative with acne may have acne.[3] Acne affects nearly all people 15 to 17 years of age.[3,4] Up to 85% of people aged 12 to 24 have acne. Severity has been correlated with pubertal maturity. Of adults in their 20s and 30s, respectively, up to 64% and 43% of individuals have acne. Women beyond the age of 25 tend to have acne related to circulating androgens.[3] Although acne is not clearly associated with ethnicity, black individuals are more prone to postinflammatory hyperpigmentation.[4]

Pathophysiology

There are four key processes in the development of acne: inflammation (inflammatory mediators are released into the skin); abnormal desquamation of keratinocytes, which plugs the pilosebaceous follicles; increased or altered sebum production; and colonization with *Propionibacterium acnes*.[3,5] Before and during puberty, hormonal stimulation increases production of the sebaceous glands in the pilosebaceous follicles. Abnormally adherent keratinocytes cause plugging of the pilosebaceous follicles, which contributes to the formation of the primary lesion (the comedone). The open comedone (blackhead) is an obstruction at the follicular mouth, which is filled with a plug of stratum corneum cells. The black color is a result of compacted follicular cells, not dirt.[6] Closed comedones (whiteheads) are a result of cystic swelling of the follicular duct below the epidermis. These closed comedones are the precursors of inflammatory papules and pustules (Fig. 39.1). Inflammation, increased sebum production, altered

keratinization, and bacterial colonization with *P. acnes* lead to the production of chemotactic factors and proinflammatory cytokines.[6] The inflammatory material around the comedone creates inflammatory papules and pustules.

Self-inflicted trauma such as scratching and squeezing of the lesions may result in scars, appearing as pits or hypopigmented spots. Furthermore, the rupture of cystic acne lesions may also result in scar formation without any manipulation of the lesions. Another potential aftereffect of acne is the formation of keloids, especially over the sternum and upper back. In patients with darker skin, inflammatory lesions often resolve with postinflammatory hyperpigmentation. Patients can be reassured that this "staining" is not scarring and usually clears spontaneously after several months.[2,4,5] For comparison of Adnexal diseases, see Table 39.1.

Clinical Presentation and Physical Examination

The duration of acne, past treatments, use of topical products for acne, menstrual history and contraceptive method, family history of acne, allergies, past medical history and review of systems, and current medications should be included in the patient's history. It is important to document how long previous treatments were used and any side effects. One frustrating fact of acne therapy is that most treatments require 6 to 12 weeks to take effect; shorter treatment therapies may not have been given an adequate trial.[2,5]

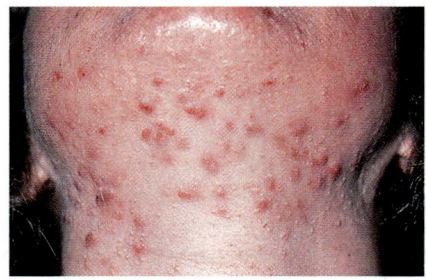

FIG. 39.1 Pustular acne. (From Gawkrodger, D. J., & Ardern-Jones, M. R. [2017]. *Dermatology: An illustrated text* [6th ed.]. Edinburgh: Elsevier, Ltd.)

TABLE 39.1	Adnexal Disease Comparison	
Disease	**Physical Exam Findings**	**Occurrence**
Acne	In general, occurs on face, neck, and upper trunk. Appears as comedones, inflammatory papules, and/or pustules or nodules.	Begins after puberty could extend into adulthood
Rosacea	Occurs centrally on the face. Appears as erythema, telangiectasia, inflammatory papules, and/or pustules on central face. There are no comedones.	Usually begins after age 30. Chronic course.
Perioral dermatitis	Occurs around the lower face region. Periorificial dermatitis may be seen occurring around the eyes, the nostrils, as well as the mouth. Presenting with erythematous base with or without scale. Could present with papules and/or pustules.	Commonly seen in females aged 20–45. Recurrence often.
Folliculitis	Occurs in hair-bearing areas as inflammatory papules or pustules.	Begins after puberty, may recur intermittently. Can become chronic.
Hidradenitis suppurativa	Occurs in the axillae and the inguinal areas. Presenting as inflammatory papules with abscesses. Sinus tracts and scarring may be present.	Early 20s onset. Chronic condition.

Drugs That Induce or Aggravate Acne

Anabolic steroids
Adrenocorticotropic hormone
Bromides
Dehydroepiandrosterone (DHEA)
Glucocorticoids
Hydantoins
Iodides
Isoniazid
Lithium
Oral contraceptives with high progestin androgenic activity
Phenobarbital
Phenytoin
Rifampin
Trimethadione

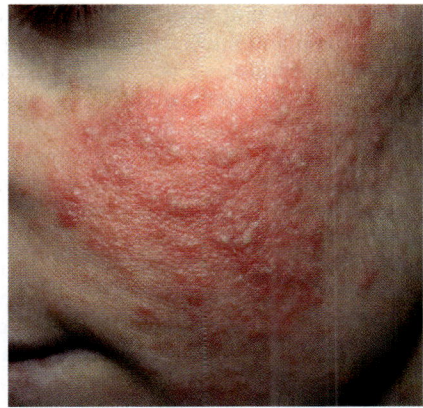

F I G . 39.2   Rosacea. (From Tüzün, Y., Wolf, R., Kutlubay, Z., Karakuş, Ö., & Engin, B. [2014]. Rosacea and rhinophyma. *Clinics in Dermatology, 32*[1], 35–46.)

While obtaining the history, the provider must consider that seasonal and hormonal factors may affect acne flares. More severe lesions occur during the winter months when there is less sunlight because acne is an inflammatory condition that improves with exposure to ultraviolet light.[7]

A careful history should include an inquiry about exposure to cosmetic and hairstyling products. Cosmetic acne can result from oil-based cosmetics, lotions, and hair products. It is usually worse in the areas in contact with the cosmetic. Pomade acne is seen on the forehead and neck as the result of oily lotions and creams used to style the hair.[3,5]

Mechanical acne can result from friction from headbands, hats, helmets, chin straps, collars, and tight bras. This presentation typically demonstrates acneiform lesions in the area where these devices contact the body, whereas other locations are spared. Acne excoriée is a subtype of acne in which the primary lesions have been scratched. Patients with acne excoriée must be encouraged to stop manipulating or scratching these lesions as an important part of successful therapy for this acne condition.[6]

Certain medications can induce or aggravate acne (Box 39.1).[7] Typically, drug-induced acne has a rapid onset and may involve the usual acne areas as well as unusual areas, such as the postauricular area, upper arms, lower back, abdomen, and legs.[6]

Lifestyle factors may play a role in acne exacerbations. Although diet has not been shown to cause acne, diets with high glycemic loads and dairy have been associated with an increase in acne exacerbations.[7] In addition, stress has been shown to be a major trigger for exacerbations. Although smoking and poor hygiene have not been shown to cause or worsen acne, clinicians are encouraged to promote a healthy lifestyle for their patients.[4]

A physical examination should include the type, location, and extent of acne lesions.[5] The highest concentration of sebaceous glands occurs on the face, chest, back, and shoulders. Patients may be seen with a variety of lesions, including comedones, papules, pustules, and nodules. Surprisingly, the skin of a patient with acne will not necessarily be oily.[3] Mild acne covers less than a fourth of the face without the presence of nodules or scarring. Moderate acne involves half of the face with some nodules and few scars. Severe acne involves at least three quarters of the face with multiple nodules and scars.[5]

Diagnostics

Essential Diagnostics. Acne is diagnosed by physical examination. Laboratory blood testing is necessary only if adrenal or gonadal dysfunction is a possible cause.[5] Other conditions may be misdiagnosed as acne. These include milia, rosacea (Fig. 39.2), the adenoma sebaceum lesions of tuberous sclerosis, nevus comedonicus, miliaria of the newborn, flat warts, and molluscum contagiosum.

INITIAL DIAGNOSTICS

Acne Vulgaris

LABORATORY
- Total testosterone
- Dehydroepiandrosterone sulfate (DHEAS)
- Androstenedione
- Luteinizing hormone
- Follicle-stimulating hormone
- Lipid profile
- Glucose tolerance testing.[2]

Differential Diagnosis

The differential diagnosis must include diseases that should be considered and excluded when appropriate. These can be narrowed down with the patient history, patient's age, recent activity, and/or exposure.

 Priority differentials include (1) closed comedonal acne, milia, and sebaceous hyperplasia; (2) open comedonal acne, dilated pore of Winer, and Favre–Raccuchot syndrome; (3) inflammatory acne, rosacea, and perioral dermatitis; (4) fungal, flat warts, molluscum contagiosum, folliculitis; (5) tuberous sclerosis; (6) facial angiofibromas; (7) adnexal tumors; (9) keratosis pilaris; (10) acne keloidalis nuchae; (11) pseudofolliculitis barbae; (12) sebaceous hyperplasia.[7]

Interprofessional Collaborative Management

Pharmacologic Management. Therapy should be individualized according to the severity of acne. Goals of treatment include normalizing keratinization of the follicular epithelium, decreasing sebum production, reducing *P. acnes* proliferation, reducing inflammation, and minimizing scarring.[6]

Topical Therapy. Topical therapy is considered first-line therapy. Topical medications reduce inflammation, inhibit the growth of *P. acnes*, and regulate keratinocyte desquamation to prevent comedone formation, reduce existing lesions, and decrease the formation of new lesions. Topical preparations include tretinoin (Retin-A), adapalene (Differin), tazarotene (Tazorac), azelaic acid (Azelex), benzoyl peroxide, and salicylic acid. These agents are applied to clean skin once daily, usually before bedtime. Side effects include erythema, dryness, and sun sensitivity. Patients should be warned that acne may worsen before skin clears. Patients should continue to use a noncomedogenic moisturizer and sunblock.[8]

Several topical agents are available to decrease *P. acnes* proliferation and inhibit the production of inflammatory mediators. These agents include erythromycin, clindamycin, metronidazole, sulfonamide, azelaic acid, and benzoyl peroxide. Topical antibiotics are not recommended in monotherapy. There are combination products with benzoyl peroxide and erythromycin or clindamycin, usually applied once or twice a day after cleansing. Although these agents may be used alone, they also work synergistically with keratolytics.

Oral Antibiotics. Oral antibiotics are effective in treating inflammatory acne by decreasing *P. acnes* and by reducing the concentration of free fatty acids, thereby inhibiting comedogenesis. Oral antibiotics are reserved for severe cases, lesions unresponsive to topical therapy, patients at risk for scarring, and lesions on the trunk or back.[3] Treatment is necessary for a minimum of 6 to 8 weeks for improvement to be obvious and may continue for several months with a reevaluation period at 12 to 18 weeks. Antibiotic therapy should include the use of benzoyl peroxide to reduce resistance.[5] The most commonly used oral antibiotics include erythromycin, tetracycline, doxycycline, and minocycline.[3] Minocycline may be more effective than doxycycline.[2] Less commonly used antibiotics include clindamycin, trimethoprim-sulfamethoxazole, azithromycin, cephalexin, ampicillin, and amoxicillin.[3] Once acne improvement is achieved, antibiotics should be discontinued, and retinoids should be continued for maintenance.[5]

Hormone Therapy. Androgen induces sebum production, which in combination with keratin leads to comedone formation. Antiandrogen medications that cause sebaceous gland suppression include combined oral contraceptives (COCs), spironolactone, and drospirenone.[3] A Cochrane review found that COCs were effective in reducing inflammatory and noninflammatory acne. Yaz (drospirenone and ethinyl estradiol), Ortho Tri-Cyclen (ethinyl estradiol and norgestimate), and Estrostep (norethindrone acetate and ethinyl estradiol) are the only COCs with a labeled use for acne treatment at the time of publication.[9] Progesterone-only contraceptives may worsen acne.[3] Spironolactone and drospirenone are additional antiandrogens that reduce sebum production. Drospirenone is available as a combination oral contraceptive pill. According to the US Food and Drug Administration (FDA), patients taking drospirenone may have an increased risk of blood clots.[9] Combination oral contraceptives and spironolactone are contraindicated in pregnant and lactating women and in the presence of thromboembolic disorders, renal impairment, and hyperkalemia.

Retinoid Therapy. Isotretinoin is restricted to the treatment of recalcitrant nodulocystic acne that has been unresponsive to

standard therapies. Its use is best managed by a dermatologist, dermatology nurse practitioner, or dermatology physician's assistant. It is thought to inhibit sebum production, to decrease follicular obstruction, and to have an anti-inflammatory effect. Patients need monthly monitoring of triglyceride levels and hepatic function. Isotretinoin is teratogenic, and careful contraceptive measures should be taken. Sexually active women of childbearing age must use two forms of birth control and be monitored for pregnancy monthly. Treatment usually lasts 4 to 6 months. Approximately 60% of patients who complete a course of isotretinoin therapy will experience a long-term remission. Of the other 40%, some require further courses of isotretinoin, but some have acne that is controllable with simpler forms of acne therapy.[2,3,5]

Nonpharmacologic Management

Mild Cleansers. Mild cleansers and cleansing bars are helpful to remove sebum from the surface of the skin. They do not alter sebum production. Harsh soaps, astringents, "buff puffs," and grainy washes should be avoided because they may dry the skin or aggravate inflammatory lesions. Moisturizers, makeup, and hair products should be water-based and labeled noncomedogenic or nonacnegenic.[5]

Indications for Referral. All patients with recalcitrant or severe nodulocystic acne should be referred to a dermatologist for treatment. Considering that suicide is one of the five leading causes of death in the adolescent population, patients with issues related to depression and self-esteem should be referred to a mental health professional.

Life-Span Considerations

Scarring, hyperpigmentation, and keloids are complications associated with acne. Complications can also result from therapy. Serious side effects are associated with some systemic therapies, particularly isotretinoin, which not only is teratogenic but may also cause hypertriglyceridemia and hepatic dysfunction. Patients need monthly monitoring of triglyceride levels and hepatic function. Isotretinoin is teratogenic, and careful contraceptive measures are necessary. Sexually active women of childbearing age must use two forms of birth control and be monitored for pregnancy monthly.

Complications

Patients with darker skin pose a challenge because of their increased tendency to develop postinflammatory hyperpigmentation. Keloid formation is also more prevalent in blacks compared with other ethnicities. Concomitant therapy is important in patients with darker skin to reduce the risk of permanent skin alterations from acne.[10]

According to the US FDA, patients taking drospirenone may have an increased risk of blood clots.[9] Combination oral contraceptives and spironolactone are contraindicated in pregnant and lactating women and in the presence of thromboembolic disorders, renal impairment, and hyperkalemia.

Emerging Management Trends

Several trends are currently being used to help with the treatment of acne vulgaris. Intense pulse light therapy for inflammatory acne vulgaris has been seen as effective with minimal reversible side effects.[11] Additional therapies include the use of tea tree oil, which was comparable to benzoyl peroxide but was better tolerated. Additional agents that have shown promise include topical and oral ayurvedic compounds, oral barberry extract, and gluconolactone solution.

Patient and Family Education

- Acne treatment may take several weeks to months before improvement is appreciated.
- Patience and understanding of the prescribed treatment regimen are crucial.
- Phone contact and periodic office visits will help evaluate improvement and compliance. This type of support is often important for this frustrating and often long-term or recurrent disorder.

Health Promotion

Patients are encouraged to gently wash the involved skin once or twice a day. Increasing patient awareness that non–water-based cosmetic and hair products may cause acne is important. Patients may have jobs that require them to wear protective headgear and should be encouraged to maintain a careful face cleansing routine to minimize the occurrence of mechanical acne.

ROSACEA

 Immediate referral is indicated for ocular rosacea. Ocular rosacea can cause patients to have light sensitivity, blurred vision, and foreign body sensation.[11,12]

    If corneal ulcers are suspected, the patient should be referred to an ophthalmologist immediately.[7]

Definition and Epidemiology

Rosacea often coexists with acne vulgaris and may closely mimic it. Sometimes called *acne rosacea* (see Fig. 39.2), this condition is rare in adolescents and occurs most often between the ages of 30 and 50 years. It is more common in women. However, men are more severely affected.[5,6] The primary distinction between acne vulgaris and rosacea, however, is that comedones do not occur in rosacea. Rosacea may newly arise or may follow acne, sometimes by years. There are four types of rosacea; these include erythematotelangiectatic, papulopustular, phymatous, and ocular.[6,13] To date there is no cure for rosacea. Rosacea treatment may take several weeks to months before improvement is appreciated. Patience and understanding of the prescribed treatment regimen are crucial. Phone contact and periodic office visits will help evaluate improvement and compliance. This type of support is often important for this frustrating and often long-term or recurrent disorder. Patients with rosacea can contact the National Rosacea Society at www.rosacea.org for more information. For comparison of adnexal diseases, see Table 39.1.

Pathophysiology

The cause of rosacea is unknown. It is possibly linked to immune-mediated inflammation.[6] Additional factors involved include nerve innervation, vascularization of the skin, and the presence of dense sebaceous glands.[14] It is thought that the basic mechanism to create rosacea is increased sebum production, hyperproliferation of the keratinocyte along with inflammation, and altered bacterial colonization with propionibacterium acne.[8] Situations that are nonresponsive to treatment may be the result of Demodex folliculorum.[13] Facial flushing and the development of rosacea has a causal relationship. The flushing reaction is usually seen in the early stages and may progress to a more persistent state and eventually may be permanent. These may be in response to triggers such as response to heat, hot drinks, spicy foods, alcohol, and emotional situations.[5]

Clinical Presentation and Physical Examination

Hallmark characteristics of rosacea include flushing, facial erythema, inflammatory papules and pustules, telangiectasia, edema, and watery or irritated eyes.[11] Rosacea has four subtypes; these include subtype 1 erythematotelangiectatic, subtype 2 papulopustular rosacea, subtype 3 phymatous rosacea, and subtype 4 ocular (Table 39.2). The patient may present with one or more of these.[15]

Diagnostics

Essential Diagnostics
- None

> ## INITIAL DIAGNOSTICS
>
> ### Rosacea
>
> **ADDITIONAL DIAGNOSTICS**
> - Consider skin biopsy to reveal nonspecific granulomatous or lymphohistiocytic infiltrate; associated edema, telangiectases, sebaceous hyperplasia; and increased number of Demodex mites in the hair follicle.
> - ANA if there is a question of lupus erythematosus

Differential Diagnosis

 Priority differentials include (1) adult acne vulgaris, (2) photodermatitis, (3) seborrheic dermatitis, and (4) contact dermatitis.

Less common differential conditions should include systemic lupus erythematosus, atopic dermatitis, sun damage, folliculitis, bromoderma, and mastocytosis. On occasion, rosacea is confused with perioral dermatitis, which is much more common in the younger population.[14]

Interprofessional Collaborative Management

Pharmacologic Management. Papules and pustules are best treated with topical or oral antibiotics. These medications help disrupt the link between flushing and papules. See Table 39.2 for specific treatment of the four subtypes of rosacea.

Topical Treatments

Metronidazole. Metronidazole 1% or 0.75% gel, cream, or lotion is applied twice daily for an average of 3 to 4 months and up to 2 years; treatment should be stopped if there is no clinical improvement. Metronidazole has been shown to be effective in treating the erythema associated with rosacea.[16]

Topical Azelaic Acid. Topical azelaic acid 15% gel or cream (depending on patient preference) is applied twice a day for 2 months. If there is no clinical improvement within 4 weeks, the medication should be discontinued. Topical azelaic acid has been shown to be effective in treating the erythema associated with rosacea.[16]

Plexion Cleanser. Plexion cleanser (sodium sulfacetamide 10% and sulfur 5%) has also been shown to help reduce erythema, as well as papules.[16]

TABLE 39.2	Rosacea Table Physical Exam Findings and Treatment Regimen	
Type	**Physical Exam Findings**	**Treatment Regimen**
Subtype 1: Erythema-totelangiectatic	Persistent history of flushing and erythema over the central facial region. Mostly on nose and cheeks lasting greater than 10 min. Telangiectasia and small papules may be present. Often occurs after triggers have been engaged.	**Primary:** *Topical:* metronidazole, azelaic acid and sulfacetamide/sulfur, brimonidine *Oral:* doxycycline, tetracycline **Secondary:** *Topical:* erythromycin, clindamycin, metronidazole *Oral:* ampicillin *May add:* benzoyl peroxide *May add:* laser treatment ± tacrolimus for telangiectasias and erythema **Tertiary:** *Topical:* terbinafine *Oral:* minocycline, azithromycin, clarithromycin, trimethoprim/sulfamethoxazole In conjunction with Benzoyl Peroxide *Additional:* laser treatment ± tacrolimus for telangiectasias and erythema Improvement can be seen after 4 weeks but can take up to 12 weeks
Subtype 2: Papulopustular	Same as Subtype 1 with an increase of telangiectasias, transient papules, pustules in the distributed in the central facial area including the forehead. Resembles acne; however, no comedones are present.	**Primary:** *Topical:* metronidazole, azelaic acid and sulfacetamide/sulfur, Ivermectin *Oral:* doxycycline, tetracyclines **Secondary:** *Topical:* erythromycin, metronidazole, clindamycin *Oral:* ampicillin **Tertiary:** *Topical:* terbinafine *Oral:* minocycline, azithromycin, clarithromycin, trimethoprim/sulfamethoxazole *Additional:* laser treatment ± tacrolimus for telangiectasias and erythema Improvement can be seen after 4 weeks but can take up to 12 weeks
Mild form Subtype 3: Phymatous	Occurs mostly in men. Presents very slowly with thick, pink plaques with enlarged, irregular, nodular surface considered classic rhinophyma but may also see in eyelids, ears, and other areas of the face.	Same treatment at Subtype 2. May also use topical Benzoyl peroxide and brimonidine.
Severe Subtype 3: Phymatous	More prominent features mild Subtype 3	**Primary:** invasive procedures: electrosurgery, laser, or cryotherapy In conjunction with oral isotretinoin or topical tacrolimus
Subtype 4: Ocular	May precede or occur with cutaneous presentation. Ocular should be considered with watery or bloodshot appearance, dryness, foreign body sensation, blurred vision, burning or stinging, itching, dryness, light sensitivity. May also have telangiectases of the conjunctiva, lid margin, and periocular erythema. These conditions may also be present: blepharitis, conjunctivitis, Meibomian gland inflammation.	**Primary:** artificial tears, lid hygiene, *Topical:* metronidazole topical, cyclosporine *Oral:* tetracyclines, azithromycin **Secondary:** *Oral:* metronidazole, ampicillin **Tertiary:** *Oral:* minocycline, azithromycin, clarithromycin, trimethoprim/sulfamethoxazole

Data from Bhate, K., & Williams, H. C. (2012). Epidemiology of acne vulgaris. The British Journal of Dermatology, 168, 474–485; Jablonski, N. G. (2017). The Anthropology of Skin Colors: An Examination of the Evolution of Skin Pigmentation and the Concepts of Race and Skin of Color. In N. Vashi & H. Maibach (Eds.), Dermatoanthropology of Ethnic Skin and Hair. Cham: Springer; Oussedik, E., Bourcier, M., & Tan, J. (2017). Psychosocial Burden and Other Impacts of Rosacea on Patients' Quality of Life. Dermatologic Clinics, doi:10.1016/j.det.2017.11.005.

Oral Medication

Tetracycline Antibiotics. Tetracycline is prescribed for rosacea, 250 to 500 mg twice daily. Doxycycline, 100 to 200 mg/day, or minocycline, 50 to 100 mg/day, can be used. Tetracycline antibiotics are typically prescribed for 3 months but may continue long term.

Isotretinoin. Isotretinoin is occasionally used, under the care of a dermatologist, in recalcitrant or severe cases. Isotretinoin is effective in low doses.[2]

Other Medications. The flushing associated with rosacea may be reduced with a trial of oral contraceptives, beta-blockers, clonidine, spironolactone, naloxone, ondansetron, aspirin, or selective serotonin reuptake inhibitors (SSRIs). None of these products has evidence-based data to support its use in this manner.

Nonpharmacologic Management

Skin Care. Proper skin care will help improve symptoms. Mild emollient-based cleansers along with light, nongreasy facial moisturizers promote health and repair of the skin through gentle cleansing and hydration without further aggravating the inflamed and sensitive skin. Cleansers and moisturizers should have a neutral pH; surfactants that do not strip the natural lipids, proteins, and moisture from the skin barrier; and formulas without potential irritants or allergens. Oil-based products are to be avoided. Patients do not need to avoid makeup.[14]

Complementary Approaches. Treatment is aimed at managing the signs and symptoms and improving the patient's quality of life.[3,17] Persistent erythema and inflammation are difficult to treat. Erythema with minimal inflammatory lesions and telangiectasias, often the result of constant flushing, may respond to a series of intense pulsed light (IPL) or laser treatments.[3,18]

Recent studies have shown promise with using botanicals as treatment for rosacea. Quassia Amara, bitterwood, a tree from Jamaica. This therapy showed improvement in inflammation when using a 4% topical gel for 6 weeks. Chrysanthellum indicum, a flower from West Africa, was used and proven to have decreased erythema in the subjects that used the 1% cream. However, this cream is hard to find.[3]

Indications for Referral. Patients with severe rosacea not responsive to topical or oral antibiotics should be referred to a dermatologist. A dermatologist should manage complications such as rhinophyma, lymphedema, or ocular involvement. Rosacea cases causing psychological distress should also be considered for referral.[17]

Life-Span Considerations

When taking oral isotretinoin, extra steps are needed to ensure the protection of those taking the medication. Women should have pregnancy tests before and monthly while taking isotretinoin. This drug is considered teratogenic. It may only be prescribed through the iPledge system. Providers, pharmacies, and patients are required to register with iPledge before the drug is dispensed.[19]

Complications

The most serious medical complication of rosacea is the ocular form, which causes watery eyes, telangiectasia of the conjunctiva and lid margin, and periocular erythema. Blepharitis, conjunctivitis, and keratitis are common presentations. Ocular rosacea can cause patients to have light sensitivity, blurred vision, and foreign body sensation.[20] In addition to the dermatologist, an ophthalmologist consultation should be sought for ocular symptoms that are not responsive to treatment in primary care. If corneal ulcers are suspected, the patient should be referred to an ophthalmologist immediately.

Patient and Family Education

- Acne treatment may take several weeks to months before improvement is appreciated.
- Patience and understanding of the prescribed treatment regimen are crucial.
- Phone contact and periodic office visits will help evaluate improvement and compliance. This type of support is often important for this frustrating and often long-term or recurrent disorder.

- Patients with rosacea can contact the National Rosacea Society at www.rosacea.org for more information.[15]

Health Promotion

The use of topical steroids and any products used on the face that may cause irritation should be discontinued. Avoidance of trigger factors (e.g., alcohol, hot fluids, spicy foods) is essential.

Sun exposure should be avoided, especially midday; the use of sunscreens and head coverings that offer shaded protection is encouraged.[20]

PERIORAL DERMATITIS
Definition and Epidemiology

Perioral dermatitis, also known as *periorificial dermatitis*, usually occurs in young women aged 20 to 45, resembling acne. It has been seen in patients as young as 6 months. It affects all races equally. The exact etiology is unknown but specific triggers are suspect.[21] For comparison of adnexal diseases, see Table 39.1.

Pathophysiology

Triggers include but are not limited to cosmetics, skin care moisturizers, fluorinated toothpaste, steroids both topical and inhaled, oral contraceptives, menstruation, pregnancy, and emotional stress. It is possible that Candida and Demodex mites have also been isolated from lesions, but it not clear that these cause the disease.[21]

Clinical Presentation and Physical Examination

Perioral dermatitis has a classic presentation. Resembling acne, it presents with papules and pustules with diffuse erythema, which may or may not have scale. Pustules are rare. Often there is a cleared vermilion border, sparing the lips. Generally perioral dermatitis is confined to the chin and occasionally the nasolabial folds.[20] The lesions are often symmetric; however, in periorificial dermatitis, the presentation may be seen in the perioral, perinasal, and periocular areas unilaterally.[2] Patients may complain of itching or a burning sensation.[21]

Diagnostics

Essential Diagnostics. None.

Additional Diagnostics. Skin scrapings have proven to be nonbeneficial in diagnosis and treatment.

Differential Diagnosis

 Priority differentials for nongranulomatous perioral dermatitis should include granulomatous rosacea. For granulomatous perioral dermatitis, include (1) rosacea, (2) seborrheic dermatitis, (3) allergic contact dermatitis, (4) irritant contact dermatitis, and (5) lip-licking cheilitis.

Additional considerations for nongranulomatous differentials should include (1) acne vulgaris, (2) psoriasis, (3) impetigo, (4) tinea facei, (5) Gram-negative folliculitis, (6) demodex infestation. For granulomatous perioral dermatitis, the following should be considered: (1) fungal or mycobacterial infection, (2) blau syndrome, (3) lupus miliaris, and (4) zirconium dermatitis.[7]

Interprofessional Collaborative Management

Pharmacologic Management

Topical Therapy

Metronidazole. Topical metronidazole is used for milder cases and may help resolve the condition with this use alone.

However, a systemic antibiotic can be added for more difficult cases. Most cases respond well to 0.75% metronidazole applied twice each day or 1% metronidazole daily. A nongreasy formulation is best for topical applications.[2]

Pimecrolimus Cream. Pimecrolimus, 1% cream, has been found to be very effect for steroid induced dermatitis.[2,21]

Antiacne Topical Therapy. Antiacne medications alone are effective. These include benzoyl peroxide 5%/clindamycin 1% gel, benzoyl peroxide 5%/erythromycin 3% gel, and benzoyl peroxide alone. Azelaic acid 20% or 15% gel applied twice a day is also effective.[2,21]

Oral Therapy

Doxycycline. Tetracyclines, both minocycline and doxycycline, have been effective when taken on a daily basis.

Minocycline 50 to 100 mg orally twice a day or doxycycline 100 mg orally once or twice a day is the usual dosage for treatment of perioral dermatitis. The course of therapy may take 6 to 8 weeks to completely resolve and may include combination therapy.[2,21]

Erythromycin. Erythromycin, 250-500 mgs twice a day or clindamycin 400 mg orally three times a day is an alternative for unresponsive therapy or for those where doxycycline is contraindicated.[2,21]

Nonpharmacologic Management. Avoid topical steroid creams and occlusive type creams on the face. Use of these preparations is associated with perioral dermatitis.

Indications for referralPersistent perioral dermatitis requires referral to dermatology for more extensive treatment. Topical steroids or corticosteroids should be discontinued; it may be beneficial to taper the dose to prevent a flare-up.

Life-Span Considerations

Doxycycline and other antibiotics that cross the placenta or may be present in breast milk should not be prescribed to adolescents, pregnant, or breastfeeding women.

Complications

The most common complication from perioral dermatitis is the use of topical corticosteroids resulting in reoccurrence. The patient may find compliance with of length of treatment difficult.

Patient and Family Education

- The best prevention is avoidance of topical steroids, occlusive face creams, makeup, and oily sunscreen.
- Perioral dermatitis may recur after treatment has stopped.
- Recurrence should use the same treatment regimen.[21]

Health Promotion

The patient should be encouraged to taper off any steroid creams. When the rash is present, wash with water only. After cleaning, choose a nonsoap or liquid face cleanser. When choosing sunscreen, encourage a nongreasy liquid or gel.

FOLLICULITIS
Definition and Epidemiology

Folliculitis, an inflammation of the hair follicles, is a common occurrence caused by varied factors. These include bacterial and fungal organisms, as well as chemical irritation or injury to the follicle. Most cases are the result of an infection. The classic presentation is erythematous papules or pustules around the hair follicle. Folliculitis, both superficial and deep, commonly occurs in regions with hair that is thick, long, and dark, preferring an area under occlusion, but can involve head, neck axillae, groin, and buttocks.[2,12,20]

Pathophysiology

Folliculitis, an infection or inflammation of the hair follicule, can have non infectious and infectious etiologies.. Depending on the cause, inflammatory cells can permeate the walls of the hair follicles. The inflammation of the upper part of the hair follicle is affected superficially, while deeper involvement affects the entire follicle. Fungal infections are caused by an infection with dermatophytes, Candida, and Pityrosporum orbicular. These may become chronic if left untreated. Demodex folliculorum mites in high numbers may cause a rash on the face and other body areas.

Mechanical folliculitis or traction folliculitis is caused by hair being pulled tightly back and frequent hair removal techniques such as waxing, plucking, and shaving. Mechanical folliculitis may also result from chronic friction associated with tight clothing.

Infections in human immunodeficiency virus individuals or transplant recipients result in eosinophilic folliculitis. The most common form is bacterial folliculitis caused by *Staphylococcus aureus* (*S. aureus*), *Pseudomonas aeruginosa*, and other gram-negative organisms. Viral types of folliculitis include Herpes simplex, Varicella zoster, and Molluscum contagiosum.[12]

Clinical Presentation and Physical Examination

Patients with folliculitis typically present with multiple erythematous, follicular papules, and pustules in regions where there is hair. Most cases of superficial folliculitis are associated with pruritus and only mild discomfort. When it becomes more extensive and the inflammation infiltrates, furuncles or carbuncles can form. Physical examination reveals erythematous papules, pustules, or cysts around the opening of the hair follicles. Large carbuncles may form when hair follicles coalesce. Resolution can take months to years to completely fade in darkly pigmented individuals.

Folliculitis caused by *S. aureus* is commonly seen around the upper lip and within beards. This superficial form presents as eroded or crusted erythematous papules and pustules. When it presents as deeper indurated, erythematous nodules, and plaques in and around the follicle, the condition is called *sycosis barbae*.

Gram-negative types of folliculitis include Klebsiella, Enterobacter, and Proteus. These appear as tiny pustules on the cheeks, chin, and perinasal areas.

P. aeruginosa folliculitis occurs as the result of swimming in contaminated water. Commonly called *hot tub folliculitis*, occurring about 3 days after immersion, this type presents as multiple, large, erythematous papules and pustules on the trunk or area where swimwear fits snuggly.

Fungal folliculitis presents in several different forms. One form is candida, as well as dermatophytic folliculitis, which includes, tinea capitis, tinea barbae, and Majocchi granuloma. Presentation of Tinea capitis is seen as alopecia, brittle hair breaking at the scalps surface. The scalp will have scaling, erythema, and boggy plaque. Tinea barbae frequently occurs in warmer, more humid climates and is usually transferred from animals to humans. This type affects the upper lip, chin, and neck area. Majocchi granuloma involves the entire hair follicle caused by *Trichophyton rubrum*. The subcutaneous nodular form is more commonly found in in immunocompromised hosts who have been on long-term suppressive therapy, bone marrow, or organ transplants.

Viral folliculitis may be caused by Herpes simplex 1 or Herpes simplex 2. Men typically will present in the beard region and may spread as a result of shaving. Molluscum sycosis is a result of Molluscum contagiosum and appears as multiple skin-colored papules. Varicella-zoster may also affect the hair follicles presenting with itchy tender erythematous plaques with small, red papules or blisters filled with pus following a dermatomal distribution pattern.

Demodex folliculitis is caused by a mite and typically occurs on the face as scaling, erythematous papules, or pustules. It resembles rosacea or acne.[12]

Diagnostics

Additional Diagnostics. However, cultures or a scraping may be obtained to help distinguish the cause and aid in prescribing the appropriate medication.[2,16,22]

Differential Diagnosis

The differential diagnosis must include diseases that should be considered and excluded when appropriate. These can be narrowed down with the patient history, patient's age, and recent activity.

 Priority differentials include (1) acne vulgaris, (2) pseudofolliculitis barbae, (3) miliaris, (4) superficial or dermatophyte fungal infections, (5) keratosis pilaris, and (6) cutaneous candidiasis.[22]

Consideration for additional differentials includes Fox-Fordyce disease, fire ant bites, impetigo, papular urticaria, and sea bather's eruption.

Interprofessional Collaborative Management

Pharmacologic Management

Topical Benzoyl Peroxide. Topical benzoyl peroxide should be applied twice daily until cleared. This is the first line of treatment for uncomplicated superficial folliculitis. Benzoyl should be used for the treatment of gram negative organisms, *S. aureus*, *P. aeruginosa*; however, many times the organism is unknown.[2,12,22]

Dicloxacillin. Dicloxacillin is used for recurrent folliculitis possibly caused by resistant *S. aureas* and is prescribed as 250 mg orally four times daily for 10 days. Dosage needs to be adjusted for patients with renal impairment. Also, dicloxacillin may decrease the effectiveness of oral contraceptives.[2,12,22]

Cephalexin. Cephalexin is a penicillinase-resistant antibiotic commonly used to treat *S. aureus* infections. The dosage is prescribed as 250 to 500 mg orally four times daily for 10 days. This is the most commonly prescribed medication for soft tissue infections.[2,12,22]

Ampicillin. For mild to moderate courses of gram-negative folliculitis, ampicillin 250 mg orally four times a day for 10 to 14 days should be considered. Individuals may experience some gastrointestinal discomfort.[2,12,22]

Ciprofloxacin. P. aeruginosa, also known as hot tub folliculitis, is usually self-limited and treated with ciprofloxacin 500 mg orally twice a day for 10 days. Common ciprofloxacin side effects have included tinnitus, blurred vision, and gastrointestinal discomfort. Prescribe with caution in individuals with previous tendon rupture.[2,12,22]

Antifungals. Antifungals are used to treat Dermatophytic folliculitis. The primary treatment is itraconazole 100 mg by mouth twice a day for 4 days or terbinafine 250 mg by mouth daily for 14 days. Treatment may extend for up to 3 weeks. For the treatment of Candida species, treatment is fluconazole 100 to 200 mg orally for 14 to 21 days or itraconazole, as described for Dermatophytic folliculitis. It is important to monitor liver function while taking these medications. There is a potential for QT prolongation and exfoliative dermatitis to occur. Individual concomitant medications may be altered if they are affected by the metabolism of the P450 enzyme.[2,12,22]

Demodex. Demodex folliculitis is treated with antiparasitic therapy. A topical application of permethrin cream 5% to the affected area nightly for 7 days or a single oral dose of ivermectin 200 micrograms/kg.

Pain Management. Acetaminophen or NSAIDs can be used to manage discomfort with folliculitiss.[2,12,22]

Nonpharmacologic Management. Superficial folliculitis if left untreated usually resolves on its own. Patient education is key in prevention of folliculitis. Important factors include avoidance of chemical or mechanical skin irradiation. Swimming pools, hot tub, or spas should be checked for adequate chlorination. The use of new razors as well as good hygiene is helpful to prevent and control folliculitis recurrence.[2,12,22]

Complementary Approaches.

Hair Removal. Individuals who have recurrent folliculitis may consider laser hair removal or use of depilatories.

Indications for Referral. Dermatological consultation should be considered in individuals who have severe recurrent or persistent cases of folliculitis.

Life-Span Considerations. When prescribing the appropriate therapy, it is important to obtain a complete history. Caution is necessary when prescribing certain medications to pregnant or nursing women, individuals who may have compromised livers or prolonged QT intervals, as well as potential interactions with concomitant medications.[12]

Complications

Extensive scarring could result in cases of deep folliculitis, which are difficult to treat or if left untreated. Individuals who are immunocompromised are at a greater risk of developing systemic infections. Fungal folliculitis may recur if not treated aggressively. Adverse reactions or side effects from prescribed medications may occur.

Patient and Family Education

- Treatment of folliculitis should begin with explaining how to prevent the recurrence.
- Focus should be on good personal hygiene, avoidance of clothes that are too tight.
- Proper chlorination of pools and hot tubs are essential.
- Discuss hair removal practices. Use clean razors that are effective to prevent folliculitis. Clean electric razors with alcohol. Avoid shaving over problem areas to prevent recurrence.

Health Promotion

Properly washed clothing, sheets, and linens are important to aid in preventing reinfection. It is also important to remind patients to wear proper fitting clothes and maintain a healthy lifestyle.

HIDRADENITIS SUPPURATIVE (ACNE INVERSA)
Definition and Epidemiology

Hidradenitis suppurativa (HS), historically known as *Verneuil disease*, also referred to as *acne inversa*.[23] HS has long been considered a disease of the apocrine glands. Histopathologic research indicates that the primary lesion is infundibular hyperkeratosis of the sebaceous gland follicles with a secondary infection of the apocrine glands.[24] The presence of inflamed perifollicular and subepidermal infiltrate, especially CD8 lymphocytes, indicates a cell-mediated cause of this disorder.[24] This chronic disease is characterized by recurrent abscesses, draining sinus tracts, and comedones and may be found in association with severe nodulocystic acne and pilonidal sinuses.[24] The prevalence of the disease is greater in females, with genitofemoral lesions being most common; axillary lesions are found equally in males and females, and anogenital lesions are found more commonly in males.[24] Case studies indicate that the onset of hidradenitis is associated with the production of adrenal androgens, dehydroepiandrosterone, and androstenedione at the time of adrenarche until menopause.[20,24] No studies have identified distribution between race or ethnic groups. HS has been connected to multiple comorbidities. A genetic predisposition has been noted 40% of patients, specifically in females, with mother-daughter transmission being most common; a familial autosomal dominant tendency also exists.[24] Studies reveal an increased risk among cigarette smokers as well as an association between HS and inflammatory bowel disease. This is particularly seen with perianal involvement.[7,22,25] A convenient way of grading the severity of HS is by using the Hurley system. See Box 39.2.

Pathophysiology

The exact cause of hidradenitis is not known and is controversial. Theories of causation include keratin plugging of the apocrine ducts, a primary failure of the apocrine glands to drain effectively, and hormonal involvement, given the occurrence is between puberty to menopause with flareups around menses. An association with immunosuppression is cited in the literature.[7,24] With keratin plugging, the apocrine duct and hair follicle are occluded by keratin, which causes increased ductal pressure and inflammation. Bacteria cause the ducts to rupture and, with extension of infection, lead to cyst, sinus tract, and fistula formation. *Acne inversa* is proposed as a more appropriate name for this disease because in the early stages, the pathogenic change occurs in the pilosebaceous ducts, similar to the pathogenesis of acne.[3,4] Deep cultures of active lesions in HS are often polymicrobial. The most commonly isolated bacteria are *S. aureus*, *Staphylococcus epidermidis*, and *Staphylococcus hominis*.[7,22] Other organisms implicated include *Escherichia coli*, *Proteus mirabilis*, *P. aeruginosa*, and streptococci.[7] HS is often seen with obesity but is unlikely to be the cause, as it is considered an exacerbating factor. Other triggers include tight-fitting clothes, deodorants and depilation, and certain drugs—specifically lithium, contraceptives, and isotretinoin—which may initiate flares.[7,24,25]

Clinical Presentation and Physical Examination

The hallmarks of HS are single or multiple areas of swelling, pain, and erythema accompanied by acute abscess formation. The active phase of the disease is preceded by the appearance of double or triple black comedones on the affected skin surface (Fig. 39.3). The condition often progresses to a chronic

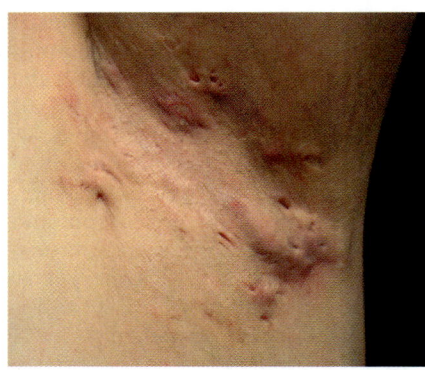

FIG. 39.3 Hidradenitis suppurative (acne inversa). Erythematous papules, cysts, nodules, and sinus tracts are seen in the axilla. (From Robinson, J. K., Hanke, C. W., Siegel, D. M., Fratila, A., Bhatia, A. C., & Rohrer, T. E. [2015]. *Surgery of the skin* [3rd ed.]. Philadelphia: Elsevier.)

BOX **39.2**

Hurley Stages

Stage I: Abscess formation (single or multiple) without sinus tracts and cicatrization
Stage II: One or more widely separated recurrent abscesses with tract formation and scars
Stage III: Multiple interconnected tracts and abscesses throughout an entire area

---

state of pain, sepsis, sinus tract and fistula formation, purulent discharge, and keloids. Disfiguring scar formation marks long-standing hidradenitis. Patients usually give a history of multiple episodes of repeated abscesses that have been drained and treated with antibiotic medications for a period of years. Unlike acne, the disease is unrelenting and often progressive, leaving hypertrophic scars that form a basket-weave configuration accented by marked erythema beneath the breast and in the axillary, suprapubic, groin, and anogenital regions. Sinus tracts form under the skin in which connecting, inflamed, and plugged glands drain into one another and trap bacteria. Patients are concerned about the cause of the problem and may fear they have a malignant disease.[1,6] Predisposing factors include obesity, dissecting cellulitis of the scalp, smoking, hirsutism, history of acne, use of lithium, and hyperandrogenism.[22,24] Remissions of a spontaneous nature are noted in patients older than 35 years.[23]

The lesions are palpated to determine their readiness for incision and drainage. The axillae, groin, perianal region, buttocks, chest, inframammary area, and back are examined to determine the involvement and extent of the disease. Disease classification models include the qualitative Hurley staging system, which is the most common. An additional method is the HS specific severity index (HSSI). Both are used to classify the severity of the disease (Box 39.2). Quantitative model types include the modified Sartorius score (MSS), Hidradenitis Suppurative Physician Global Assessment (HS-PGA), and the Suppurativa Clinical Response (HiSCR).[25]

Diagnostics

Essential Diagnostics. The initial diagnosis is based on clinical observation and chronicity. Lesions that are actively discharging are cultured, and sensitivity tests are performed. A skin biopsy is indicated for patients with stubborn cases or suspicious lesions. Laboratory tests may be necessary to exclude other, more serious underlying diseases.

INITIAL DIAGNOSTICS

Hidradenitis Suppurativa

LABORATORY
- Culture and sensitivity of lesions with discharge
- Skin biopsy
- C-reactive protein
- CBC[a]
- Lipid panel[a]
- LFTs[a]

IMAGING
- Sonography

[a]Should regularly be monitored if on Isotretinoin.

Differential Diagnosis

 Priority differentials include (1) bacterial folliculitis, (2) bacterial furunculosis, (3) cat-scratch disease, (4) lymphadenitis, and (5) erysipelas.

The differential diagnosis should take into consideration the patient's past medical history and recurrence of the disease. It is critical to differentiate between early-stage HS, which includes furuncle, carbuncle, lymphadenitis, and inclusion cyst, and the later stages, which include granuloma inguinale, lymphogranuloma venereum, regional enteritis, scrofuloderma, squamous cell carcinoma, cutaneous tuberculosis, sinus tracts, and fistulas associated with ulcerative coliti.[22,24]

Interprofessional Collaborative Management

Pharmacologic Management.

Oral Antibiotics. Treatment of HS should be done in collaboration with a dermatologist. Treatment of an acute abscess may require a 6- to 8-week course of therapy. Primary options include a choice of twice daily oral administration of tetracycline 500 mg, doxycycline 100 mg, minocycline 100 mg orally, or amoxicillin 500 mg, twice daily.

When treating Hurley Stage 1 disease, antibiotic consideration should be based on the results of the culture sensitivities. Primary options include a choice of twice daily oral tetracycline 500 mg, doxycycline 100 mg, or minocycline for 8 weeks.

Hurley stage II can also be treated with twice daily oral doxycycline 100 mg. Additional choices include clindamycin 300 mg and rifampin 300 mg; both taken orally twice daily. Should an additional therapy option be needed, twice daily sulfamethoxazole/trimethoprim, 800/160 mg topical antibiotic, or antibacterial therapy needs to be included with the use of oral therapy.

Prescribing antibiotics for Hurley stage III needs to occur over a longer period. As with Stage II, the primary antibiotics are the same; however, the treatment length for clindamycin should be over 10 weeks while doxycycline and sulfamethoxazole/trimethoprim are taken over 8 weeks After the initial treatment, a 10-week course of rifampin, 300 mg twice daily, and clindamycin, 300 mg twice daily, has shown remission of up to 4 years.[2,12]

Topical Antibiotic or Antibacterial Therapy. Mild disease, Hurley stage I, II, and III are all treated with topical therapy over the course of 8 weeks. Topical clindamycin 1% twice daily to the affected area has been shown to be as effective as oral tetracycline. Additional options include twice daily application of metronidazole 1%, or chlorhexidine 4%. These can be used in conjunction with the tetracycline class of oral antibiotics.[2,12]

Pain Management.

Nonsteroidal Anti-Inflammatory Medications. Pain associated with HS is dependent on the degree of inflammation. Treatment of all stages include NSAID therapy and should be used before any other type of pain medication. Initial treatment involves ibuprofen 600 to 800 mg po every 6 to 8 hours as needed, but no more than 3200 mg/day. A caveat is that NSAIDs impact renal function especially in older adults and have been shown to increase the patient's risk of cardiovascular disease, including myocardial infarction and stroke.[2,12] An additional option would be acetaminophen 325 to 1000 mg orally every 4 to 6 hours with a maximum dose of 3000 mg daily if there are no contraindications (e.g., warfarin therapy).

Use of Other Antiinflammatory Medications. Antiinflammatory medications such as Dapsone, a miscellaneous antiinfective, and Prednisone have effectively reduced inflammation in both Stage II and III. If the standard first and second line of therapy fail, dapsone therapy, 50 to 150 mg/day orally, should be initiated. Prednisone, maximum 80 mg orally, should be considered for 2 or 3 days and tapered during a 14-day period.[2,12]

Other Adjunctive Medications.

Spironolactone. Women with Stage II and III who have a premenstrual flare can be treated with spironolactone as an effective antiandrogen adjunct. The dosing is 50 to 100 mg orally once a day over 8 weeks. This treatment is limited to women who are on adequate birth control.[2,12,23]

Oral Retinoid. Individuals with concomitant acne vulgaris in either Stage II or III can use topical isotretinoin cream 0.05%, which may be efficacious in relieving keratin plugging of the apocrine glands.[2,14] Isotretinoin, 0.5 to 1 mg/kg/day for 20 weeks, may be tried under co-management with a physician in the early stages of the disease or as an adjunct to surgical intervention, although it has a very limited therapeutic effect when it is used as monotherapy.[2,12] Because of the teratogenic effects of this medication, all women must be screened for pregnancy before taking isotretinoin and protected against pregnancy while taking the medication. (See section on "Acne Vulgaris" for precautions regarding isotretinoin therapy.) Retinoid therapy is best initiated and monitored by a dermatologist or dermatology nurse practitioner or physician's assistant.

Tumor Necrosis Factor-α Inhibitors. Tumor necrosis factor-α (TNF-α) inhibitors are not considered standard of care for patients with HS. However, in individuals with a comorbidity of inflammatory bowel disease, they have been particularly successful. These medications are potent antiinflammatory and can be used in conjunction with systemic antibiotics. Because TNF-α inhibitors are immunosuppressive, caution is advised with prescribing this for individuals with a history of malignancy and tuberculosis. Currently adalimumab 80 mg subcutaneously on day 1, followed by 40 mg every other week starting 1 week after initial dose is the only medication of this type approved by the FDA for HS. The treatment course should last at least 12 weeks.[2,12,22]

Finasteride. Finasteride, an anti-androgenic agent, is an inhibitor of II5 α-reductase. It appears to alter end-organ sensitivity of the folliculopilosebaceous component. A 5 mg daily dose has been used as an effective monotherapy or adjunctive therapy in men and women for advanced HS. Caution is advised with use in women of childbearing age due to the teratogenic effects.[26,27]

Nonpharmacologic Management. The patient's quality of life must be considered. A questionnaire called the Dermatology Life Quality Index (DLQI) tool is an excellent instrument to determine how the disease has impacted the individual. Mental health plays a crucial role in how a patient responds to treatment. Proper mental health therapy as well as encouraging a healthy lifestyle, weight reduction, and metabolic syndrome control will aid in the reduction of disease recurrence.[23] Additional measures include smoking cessation, avoidance of tight-fitting clothing, or friction. The application of warm compresses to affected areas aids in drainage of purulent lesions.[22]

Surgical Incision. Fluctuant abscesses in which the skin has become thin and the underlying mass is soft can be surgically incised and drained in the health care provider's office. A local anesthetic with 1% to 2% lidocaine with or without epinephrine is provided through a 30-gauge needle and a 1- to 3-mL syringe. The sting of lidocaine can be buffered by preparing a mixture of 1 mL of sodium bicarbonate with 9 mL of lidocaine. A pointed, lance-shaped No. 11 surgical blade is recommended for incision. The blade is inserted parallel to the skin lines, cutting across the thin area of skin and creating an opening through which purulent material can drain. Pressure is applied to the surrounding tissue to facilitate drainage. A curet drawn back and forth through the abscess will loosen adhesions and aid in the removal of necrotic material. A semiocclusive sterile dressing with a thin film of topical bacitracin should then be applied. Care must be taken to cleanse the area daily with soap and water; the dressing is reapplied for 3 to 5 days.

Smaller nodules can be injected with triamcinolone acetonide, 3 to 5 mg/mL diluted with lidocaine, followed by a course of oral antibiotics. Larger cysts can be injected with triamcinolone, 3 to 5 mg/mL, directly into the wall of the lesion, and later incised. Low-grade inflammation is responsive to oral antibiotics, but long-term treatment is necessary before clinical remission is evident.[27]

Indications for Referrals. A referral to a dermatologist is recommended for patients with hidradenitis that is recalcitrant to traditional oral therapy or for patients with recurrent lesions after incision and drainage. Newer treatment approaches used by these specialists include carbon dioxide (CO_2) laser therapy and infliximab (Remicade), a chimeric monoclonal antibody with high affinity for TNF-α. Laser treatment of moderate-stage HS is an effective noninvasive alternative for patients who wish to avoid systemic therapies.[23] Patients treated with oral isotretinoin, 1 mg/kg/day for 20 weeks, may also be co-managed with a nurse practitioner or physician assistant to determine treatment response and monitoring side effects (see section on "Acne Vulgaris" for precautions regarding isotretinoin therapy).

Surgical excision is recommended for patients with chronic, recurrent HS that involves sinus tracts and fibrotic scarring. Complete excision of the involved glands and skin grafting may be necessary. CO_2 laser therapy can be performed by a qualified dermatologist skilled in this technique. If surgery will involve extensive surgical resection and reconstruction of the female genitals, the services of a gynecologic oncologist may be required.[23]

A variety of treatment measures to include topical, oral, and surgical may be needed to treat HS effectively. A combination approach to treatment is advocated, including steroids, antibiotics, traditional surgery, CO_2 laser surgery, monoclonal antibody therapy, and isotretinoin.

Life-Span Considerations

Onset of HS is usually between the second and fifth decades, with onset as early as puberty in some individuals. Many cases of hidradenitis disappear after patients reach 35 years of age.[24,27,28]

Complications

The health care provider should be aware of the impact of body image changes on patients with this disease, especially young adolescents. As with any chronic illness, an assessment for clinical depression and threats to self-esteem should be included as part of the ongoing care. Patients may become progressively less social in moderate to severe disease because of embarrassment, foul odor, and chronic pain.[24] The most common complication is chronicity. Additional complications include formation of a fistula from the groin area to the urethra and bladder, dermal contraction, spread of microorganisms resulting in local or systemic infection, arthritis as a result of inflammation, squamous cell carcinoma located within the sinus tracts, lymphedema occurring from inflammation, and scarring.[24] Cases of reactive arthritis have been identified in the literature.[25] Vigilant follow-up monitoring is necessary to uncover those patients who fail to respond to treatment. Cases of anogenital squamous cell carcinoma have been diagnosed in patients with long-term hidradenitis. Patients taking large doses of erythromycin may experience damage to their auditory nerve and deafness.[24]

Emerging Management Trends

Current trends that aid in diagnosis include ultrasound to identify subclinical lesions. Using ultrasound helps identify widening hair follicles, dermal thickening, fluid collections, and fistula tracts. A clinical sonographic scoring system is currently being developed but is not yet validated.[24,27] Emerging therapy currently being used to treat HS includes the Nd:YAG laser, IPL, as well as photodynamic therapy. These new therapies show promise; however, additional studies are needed to establish therapeutic guidelines.[23]

Patient and Family Education

- Explain that a clear cause of the disease is not known. Hypothetical causes of the disease process should be discussed.
- Topical isotretinoin may cause skin irritation, and caution should be exercised to avoid excessive use.
- Stress sun sensitivity with the use of isotretinoin and encourage patients to wear appropriate protective clothing while in the sun.
- Educate patients on the side effects of the prescribed antibiotics, including photosensitivity and interaction with oral contraceptives.
- Advise patients to avoid concurrent ingestion of terfenadine, astemizole, and ketoconazole.
- Patients should also be aware that surgical removal of all affected tissues may be the only effective treatment.
- Support and additional information can be found on the HS Foundation website (www.hs-foundation.org).

Health Promotion

Providers need to be thorough in assessing for psychological and psychosocial issues associated with the disease process, as well as comorbidities of the disease. Referrals to a dermatologist or surgeon for treatment of extreme cases are indicated. HS support groups and therapists will be beneficial in helping the patient deal with this chronic debilitating disease. Encouragement and educational support to help deal with triggers of the disease will be beneficial.[28]

HYPERHIDROSIS

Definition and Epidemiology

Hyperhidrosis is estimated to affect 3% of the population. It is a condition marked by excessive sweating, abnormal wetness, sweaty palms, excessive axillary sweating, gustatory-stimulated sweating, wet shoes, and offensive body odor. Most cases are idiopathic or primary in nature, caused by sympathetic overstimulation of the eccrine sweat glands. More easily treated is secondary hyperhidrosis, as there is an underlying cause that is responsive to medication.[29]

Pathophysiology

Perspiration is one of the body's mechanisms for thermal regulation and fluid and electrolyte balance. The center for body temperature regulation is located in the hypothalamus. Cooling perspiration is under hypothalamic control, whereas emotional perspiration is under cerebral control.[30] Sweat glands are located in the hypodermis of the skin. The eccrine duct opens directly onto the surface of the skin. Millions of sweat glands are located in the hypodermis throughout the body, with the largest concentration in the palms, soles, and axillae. Secretions from the eccrine glands function to cool the body. Neural control is anatomically sympathetic. However, sweating is subject to cholinergic control mediated by acetylcholine, not epinephrine.[31] Overactivity of the thoracic sympathetic ganglion may be the underlying cause of non–medically related excessive sweating.

A common cause of generalized increased sweating is a decline in ovarian function. Changes in neurohumoral function lead to increased stimulation of the hypothalamic thermal regulatory center, leading to the hot flashes associated with menopause. Other factors include fever, underlying infection or malignant disease, peripheral neuropathy or surgical damage to the autonomic nervous system, thyrotoxicosis, Parkinson disease, alcohol abuse, and a variety of medications (including insulin, meperidine, propranolol, physostigmine, pilocarpine, tricyclic antidepressants, and serotonin reuptake inhibitors and pilocarpine).[31,32]

Clinical Presentation and Physical Examination

The presentation of primary hyperhidrosis is excessive sweating unrelated to ambient heat or humidity. Areas most commonly affected include the palms, soles, and axillae, but the condition may involve any body surface or may take on a unilateral distribution. Concern about the social consequences of this disorder (and its resulting body odor) and embarrassment may create a barrier to intimate relationships or affect the patient's choice of occupation. When the soles are involved, widespread fungal infections of the skin and nails are accompanied by foot odor. More generalized body sweating is associated with an underlying condition, whereas localized sweating confined to the palms, soles, and axillae is more often a response to anxiety or heat or is idiopathic. Episodic sweating may be associated with hypoglycemia. A history of medications, including oral hypoglycemic agents and SSRIs, and alcohol intake is an important consideration.[33]

To properly diagnose hyperhidrosis, the patient must present with focal and visible sweating over a 6-month history not as a result of a secondary cause. In addition, two of the following conditions must be met: bilateral and symmetric hyperhidrosis, disruption of activities of daily living, prior to age 25, at one or more episodes occurring weekly, familial history of the disease, or not having episodes during sleep. Hyperhidrosis Disease Severity Scale, a validated tool, has been used effectively to determined how hyperhidrosis affects the quality of life.[33]

Based on the history and presenting complaint, the health care provider should try to locate evidence of any underlying disease process. A complete history is taken and a thorough physical assessment is performed, searching for signs and symptoms of hyperthyroidism. Blood pressure should be measured to exclude high blood pressure associated with pheochromocytoma.[31] Heat intolerance associated with sweating in the upper half of the body and absence of sweating in the lower half of the body is evidence of diabetic peripheral autonomic neuropathy.[32]

Visual inspection during the physical examination is important in diagnosing the patient with generalized sweating; the examiner should look for miliaria rubra, an abnormal blocking of the sweat ducts. In this condition, sweat is trapped in the stratum corneum, creating tiny, pinpoint, clear papules that with pressure rupture the sweat ducts, creating an erythematous maculopapular rash. Other associated presentations include dyshidrotic eczema. This is a simple eczema promoted by the retention of sweat in the stratum corneum.[34]

Diagnostics

Essential Diagnostics. Thyroid and fasting blood glucose studies are indicated to exclude thyroid disease and diabetes. If night sweats are present, a purified protein derivative test or interferon-γ release assay (QuantiFERON-TB Gold In-Tube [QFT-GIT] test; T-SPOT) is necessary to exclude tuberculosis. For perimenopausal women with hyperhidrosis, tests for follicle-stimulating hormone and luteinizing hormone are recommended to document menopause and to provide reassurance to the patient. SSRIs may provoke night sweats. A different SSRI should be considered before the drug class is changed.

A common cause of excessive perspiration is a sympathetic-mediated response to stress. A careful history and examination will indicate the necessity to exclude hyperthyroidism with an ultrasensitive test for thyroid-stimulating hormone (TSH) and thyroxine (T4). A patient symptom diary of provoking factors, response to foods, body temperature, and amount and location of perspiration is a helpful adjunct in determining the cause of sweating. If infection or malignant disease is suspected, a thorough evaluation is mandated. A tuberculin skin test should be performed for those with complaints of night sweats. A fasting blood glucose study is performed to exclude diabetes mellitus. In women with variations in the length and amount of menses, a search for accompanying symptoms of vasomotor hot flashes and objective evidence of ovarian failure is necessary. Symptoms of sweating and flushing accompanied by marked hypertension require an evaluation for pheochromocytoma. Evidence of central nervous system disease or autonomic peripheral neuropathy warrants referral to a neurologist.[32]

Additional Diagnostics. Gravimetry may also be measured by weighing sweat that is accumulated on filter paper. In addition, an ECG or echocardiogram may be beneficial to ensure there are no cardiac issues that may be causing the hyperhidrosis. Urine for drug screen may be obtained if substance use is suspected.[12]

INITIAL DIAGNOSTICS

Hyperhidrosis

LABORATORY
- Thyroid-stimulating hormone, thyroxine
- Purified protein derivative[a]
- Fasting blood glucose
- Follicle-stimulating hormone, luteinizing hormone
- Iodine-starch test
- Urinary catecholamines
- Uric acid
- Other tests as indicated to exclude systemic conditions

IMAGING
- Chest radiography

---

[a]If indicated.

Differential Diagnosis

Priority differentials include (1) hyperthyroidism, (2) infection, (3) diabetes mellitus, and (4) menopause.

Additional considerations include tuberculosis, pheochromocytoma, alcoholism, central nervous system diseases, autonomic peripheral neuropathy, malignant diseases, and other hormonal imbalances.

Interprofessional Collaborative Management

Pharmacologic Management

Topical Aluminum Chloride. The first line of treatment should include topical applications of a 20% alcoholic solution of aluminum chloride hexahydrate (Drysol, Keralyt). These work by blocking the openings of the sweat duct. Mucopolysaccharides combine with metal ion precipitates damaging the cells along the lumen of the duct, thereby creating a plug that blocks sweat. A less potent solution of 6.25% aluminum chloride hexahydrate (Xerac) can be prescribed for patients who have more sensitive skin. The perspiring area is coated lightly with the solution and allowed to dry. An occlusive wrap is then applied, or vinyl gloves can be worn on the hands and left on for 8 hours, followed by a complete soap-and-water wash of the affected areas. Applications are repeated every 2 or 3 days as tolerated. With satisfactory dryness, maintenance requires a once-weekly application.[31,34]

Oral Medications. Oral medications such as anticholinergic agents, antihypertensive agents, anxiolytics, and antidepressants are rarely used in the management of primary hyperhidrosis and should be used only as a second- or third-line therapy. More recently, a practice guideline was released, stating there was minimal compelling evidence that would support the use of systemic anticholinergic agents in a safe and efficacious manner.[12,34]

Injectable Therapy. Botulinum toxin is an effective treatment an effective option, although temporary, for those who do not respond to topical or oral agents. The anticholinergic effects make it a viable option. This type of treatment has proven to reduce axillary sweat between 4 to 8 months. Other studies have had positive results for palmar and plantar hyperhidrosis. Multiple injections are required at the injection site. The use of topical anesthetics has proven beneficial in reducing pain associated with the procedure.[33,34]

Nonpharmacologic Management. Using the DLQI scale to determine quality of life severity, referral to mental heal providers, as well as the International Hyperhidrosis Society support groups (https://www.sweathelp.org), can prove to be an effective coping mechanism, along with proper medical treatments.[33]

Mechanical and Surgical. Iontophoresis is a procedure that allows electrical current to pass across intact skin. The mechanism of action remains unclear. Treatments consist of eight sessions over a 28-day time frame and provide a sweat reduction of 81%. Improvement lasted 16 weeks. However, to maintain effectiveness, repeat sessions are required. Microwave thermolysis (MiraDry) is another type of treatment that has proven effective in reduction sweat for those with hyperhidrosis. A reduction of 89% was shown after treatment after 12 months 69% continued to have reduced sweating. It has shown minimal side effects. The device permanently ablates the axillary sweat and odor glands. A second treatment may be needed for a small percentage. The Nd:YAG laser has also proven effective for the treatment of hyperhidrosis. Other treatments include liposuction of the axillary sweat glands, sympathectomy, and surgical excision of axillary tissue. Persistent primary palmar hyperhidrosis has shown a positive response to thoracic endoscopic surgery. Bilateral interruption of the upper dorsal sympathetic chain of D2 and D3 can provide a cure for primary hyperhidrosis.[32–34]

Indications for Referral. Consultation with a dermatologist may be useful for patients with hyperhidrosis that is refractory to topical treatments. The dermatologist may try a number of other remedies, including iontophoresis, microwave thermolysis. Administration of botulinum toxin has been found to be effective for hyperhidrosis affecting the axillae and palms and for gustatory sweating.[32] Referral to the surgeon may be indicated should liposuction or sympathectomy be chosen. Consideration of these and other treatments warrants consultation with an appropriate specialist. Sweating associated with anxiety or panic attacks warrants co-management with a mental health specialist or neuropsychiatrist.

Life-Span Considerations

Hyperhidrosis is a condition that affects the individual over their life span. While not associated with mortality, it can create serious quality of life issues.

Complications

Patients with hyperhidrosis may experience difficulty functioning in social or occupational situations as a result of this disorder, significantly affecting their quality of life. Other complications are rare, although patients with sensitive skin may develop reactions to the topical solutions prescribed for treatment. In most instances, decreasing the concentration of the solution will decrease skin irritation. Patients who undergo sympathectomy may experience compensatory sweating.

Other complications are directly related to the treatment of the disease, including medication side effects, infection or microfractures of damaged joints, and failure of prosthetic components.

Evidence of an underlying medical condition leading to secondary hyperhidrosis, such as pheochromocytoma, warrants referral. Patients with primary hyperhidrosis refractory to topical treatments are referred for evaluation to a surgeon experienced in thoracoscopic sympathicolysis, liposuction, or axillary dissection. Patients with excessive perspiration associated with anxiety or panic disorders can benefit from mental health counseling.[32-34]

Emerging Management Trends

Medical advances continue to treat this condition. More studies are needed to evaluate the benefits of laser, iontophoresis, and microwave thermolysis.

Patient and Family Education

- Education is critical to assist patients in coping with and understanding this socially stigmatizing condition.
- Provide each patient with a complete explanation of the etiology of primary hyperhidrosis and an explanation of sympathetic overactivity.
- Reassure patients you have searched for any underlying pathologic reasons for the disorder; provide and discuss results of laboratory tests.
- Support patients by providing education for their family members and significant others as an important aspect of comprehensive care.

Health Promotion

Good personal hygiene is encouraged for those with axillary sweating. Both open-toe and canvas shoes with cotton socks promote evaporation of foot perspiration while decreasing foot odor and preventing fungal infections of the feet. Occupational environments should be well ventilated and include air conditioning.

REFERENCES

1. Learning module: Basic science of the skin. *Learning module: Basic science of the skin. American Academy of Dermatology*, American Academy of Dermatology. Retrieved from www.aad.org/education/basic-derm-curriculum/suggested-order-of-modules/basic-science-of-the-skin. (Accessed 19 January 2018).
2. Habif, M. D., & Thomas, P. (2016). *Clinical dermatology: A color guide to diagnosis and therapy* (6th ed.). Edinburgh: Elsevier. Chapters 7, 9, 13.
3. Grobel, H., & Murphy, S. A. (2018). Acne vulgaris and acne rosacea. In D. Rakel (Ed.), *Integrative medicine* (4th ed., pp. 759–770.e5). Philadelphia: Elsevier. Chapter 77. https://doi.org/10.1016/B978-0-323-35868-2.00077-3.
4. Bhate, K., & Williams, H. C. (2012). Epidemiology of acne vulgaris. *The British Journal of Dermatology*, 168, 474–485.
5. McCall, C. O., & Lawley, T. J. (2015). Eczema, psoriasis, cutaneous infections, acne, and other common skin disorders. In D. Kasper, A. Fauci, S. Hauser, D. Longo, J. Jameson, & J. Loscalzo (Eds.), *Harrison's principles of internal medicine* (19th ed.). New York: McGraw-Hill.
6. Nicol, H. N., & Huether, W. E. (2014). Alterations of the integument in children. In K. L. McCance & S. E. Huether (Eds.), *Pathophysiology: The biologic basis for disease in adults and children* (7th ed., pp. 1653–1654). St. Louis: Elsevier Mosby.
7. Zaenglein, A. L., Pathy, A. L., Schlosser, B. J., Alikhan, A., Baldwin, H. E., Berson, D. S., et al. (2016). Guidelines of care for the management of acne vulgaris. *Journal of the American Academy of Dermatology*. Retrieved from https://www.aad.org/practicecenter/quality/clinical-guidelines/acne. (Accessed 3 January 2018).
8. Titus, S., & Hodge, J. (2012). Diagnosis and treatment of acne. *American Family Physician*, 86(8), 734–740.
9. Trivedi, M. K., Shinkai, K., & Murase, J. E. (2017). A review of hormone-based therapies to treat adult acne vulgaris in women. *International Journal of Women's Dermatology*, 3(1), 44–52. PMC. Web. 4 Jan. 2018.
10. Jablonski, N. G. (2017). The anthropology of skin colors: An examination of the evolution of skin pigmentation and the concepts of race and skin of color. In N. Vashi & H. Maibach (Eds.), *Dermatoanthropology of Ethnic Skin and Hair*. Cham: Springer.
11. Picardo, M., Eichenfield, L., & Tan, J. (2017). Acne and rosacea. *Dermatology and Therapy*, 7(S1), 43–52. doi:10.1007/s13555-016-0168-8.
12. Rosacea; folliculitis [monograph]. (2018). In *Epocrates [online]*. San Francisco, CA: Epocrates, Inc. Retrieved from http://www.epocrates.com. (Accessed 6 January 2018). Last updated: November 13, 2017.
13. Abokwidir, M., & Fleischer, A. B., Jr. (2015). Additional evidence that rosacea pathogenesis may involve demodex: New information from the topical efficacy of ivermectin and praziquantel. *Dermatology Online Journal*, 21, 13030/qt13v249f5.
14. Oge', L. K., Jr., Muncie, H. L., & Phillips-Savoy, A. R. (2015). Rosacea: Diagnosis and treatment. *American Family Physician*, 92(3), 187–196. Web. 5 Jan. 2018.
15. The many faces of rosacea. Rosacea.org., 2012. Web. (Accessed 8 January 2018).
16. Layton, A. (2017). Pharmacologic treatments for rosacea. *Clinics in Dermatology*, 35(2), 207–212. doi:10.1016/j.clindermatol.2016.10.016. [Epub 2016 Oct 27].
17. Oussedik, E., Bourcier, M., & Tan, J. (2017). Psychosocial burden and other impacts of rosacea on patients' quality of life. *Dermatologic Clinics*, doi:10.1016/j.det.2017.11.005. Retrieved from http://www.sciencedirect.com/science/article/pii/S0733863517301638. (Accessed 5 January 2018). IN PRESS 2017 November 29.
18. Grove, J. (2017). The use of intense pulsed light therapy in the treatment of acne vulgariss. *Journal of Aesthetic Nursing*, 6(8), 400–405.
19. iPledge. Retrieved from https://www.ipledgeprogram.com/. (Accessed 6 January 2018).
20. Holmes, H. (2013). Acne, rosacea, and related disorders. In C. Soutor & M. K. Hordinsky (Eds.), *Clinical dermatology*. New York, NY: McGraw-Hill. Retrieved from http://accessmedicine.mhmedical.com.ezproxy.hsc.usf.edu/content.aspx?bookid=2184&sectionid=165459903. (Accessed January 04, 2018).
21. Tolaymat, L., & Hall, M. R. (2019). Dermatitis, perioral. [Updated 2018 Oct 27]. In *StatPearls [Internet]*. Treasure Island (FL): StatPearls Publishing. Retrieved from https://www.ncbi.nlm.nih.gov/books/NBK525968/.
22. Ferri, F. F. (2018). *2017 Ferri's clinical advisor: 5 books in 1*. Philadelphia: Elsevier.
23. Zouboulis, C. C., Desai, N., Emtestam, L., Hunger, R. E., Ioannides, D., JuHasz, I., et al. (2015). European S1 guidelines for the treatment of hidradenitis suppurativa/acne inversa. *Journal of the European Academy of Dermatology and Venereology*, 29(4), 619–644. doi:10.1111/jdv.12966.
24. Martorell, A., García-Martínez, F. J., Jiménez-Gallo, D., Pascual, J. C., Pereyra-Rodriguez, J., Salgado, L., et al. (2015). Actualización en hidradenitis supurativa (I): Epidemiología, aspectos clínicos y definición de severidad de la enfermedad. *Actas Dermo-Sifiliograficas*, 106(9), 703–715.
25. Napolitano, M., Megna, M., Timoshchuk, E. A., et al. (2017). Hidradenitis suppurativa: From pathogenesis to diagnosis and treatment. *Clinical, Cosmetic and Investigational Dermatology*, 10, 105–115. doi:10.2147/CCID.S111019. PMCID: PMC5402905.
26. Khandalavala, B. N., & Do, M. V. (2016). Finasteride in hidradenitis suppurativa: A 'male' therapy for a predominantly 'female' disease. *The Journal of Clinical and Aesthetic Dermatology*, 9(6), 44–50.
27. Saunte, D. M. L., & Jemec, G. B. E. (2017). Hidradenitis suppurativa advances in diagnosis and treatment. *JAMA: The Journal of the American Medical Association*, 318(20), 2019–2032. doi:10.1001/jama.2017.16691.
28. Gill, L., Williams, M., & Hamzavi, I. (2014). Update on hidradenitis suppurativa: Connecting the tracts. *F1000prime Reports*, 6, 112. doi:10.12703/P6-112. (Accessed 14 January 2018).
29. Singh, S., Davis, H., & Wilson, P. (2015). Axillary hyperhidrosis: A review of the extent of the problem and treatment modalities. *The Surgeon: Journal of the Royal Colleges of Surgeons of Edinburgh and Ireland*, 13(5), 279–285.
30. Goldman, L., & Schafer, A. I. (2015). *Goldman-Cecil medicine* (25th ed.). Philadelphia: Elsevier.
31. Kliegman, R. M., Stanton, M. D., & St. Geme, J. (2015). *Nelson textbook of pediatrics* (20th ed.). Philadelphia: Elsevier.
32. Semkova, K., Gergovska, M., Kazandjieva, J., & Tsankov, N. (2015). Hyperhidrosis, bromhidrosis, and chromhidrosis: Fold (intertriginous)

dermatoses. *Clinics in Dermatology*, *33*(4), 483–491. doi:10.1016/j.clindermatol.2015.04.013.

33. Grabell, D. A., & Hebert, A. A. (2017). Current and emerging medical therapies for primary hyperhidrosis. *Dermatology and Therapy*, *7*(1), 25–36. doi:10.1007/s13555-016-0148-z.

34. Owen, K. (2016). Excessive sweating: Are patients suffering unnecessarily? *The Journal for Nurse Practitioners*, *12*(1), 35–40. doi:10.1016/j.nurpra.2015.09.015.

CHAPTER **40**

ALOPECIA

Maria Isabel Romano

DEFINITION AND EPIDEMIOLOGY

Alopecia is a term used to describe abnormal hair loss. There are varied causes of hair loss. Medications, chemotherapy, radiation therapy, diabetes, trichotillomania, and hair loss from hair dyes or hairdos are possible causes, but alopecia is also related to congenital hair abnormalities and the more commonly observed alopecia from androgenetic or pattern hair loss. Whatever the cause, hair loss is a disturbing and highly emotional issue for many patients.

PATHOPHYSIOLOGY

Alopecia, except for congenital alopecia, can be divided into two types of alopecia: scarring (cicatricial alopecia) and non-scarring (noncicatricial alopecia).[1] In noncicatricial alopecia, the hair follicles are still present and there is no sign of inflamed tissue, scarring, or atrophy.[1] Alopecia areata, androgenetic alopecia, lupus erythematosus, syphilis, telogen effluvium, and tinea capitis are all potential causes of noncicatricial alopecia.[2] Cicatricial alopecia—scarring alopecia—is usually the result of an intense inflammatory process of the scalp, with resultant skin atrophy and scarring.[1] Chronic cutaneous discoid lupus, folliculitis decalvans, lichen planus, linear scleroderma, sarcoidosis, and cutaneous metastasis are potential causes of scarring alopecia.[2]

Each hair follicle goes through a highly programmed cycle over and over again throughout its life. The cycle of hair growth involves three phases—anagen, catagen, and telogen—which represent the growth, involution, and rest phases.[1] The anagen (growth) phase varies according to the location of the follicle on the body. This phase is longest on the scalp (producing long hairs) and much shorter on the eyebrows (producing short hairs). During the catagen phase, the hair involutes. This is the shortest of the three stages. During the telogen phase, the mature hair is shed, resulting in the loss of 50 to 150 scalp hairs each day.

Anagen Phase Disturbances

Three common types of hair loss are a result of anagen phase disturbance: androgenetic alopecia, anagen effluvium, and alopecia areata. Androgenetic alopecia, the most common type of hair loss, is the hereditary thinning of hair in susceptible men and women, and is related to an androgen receptor variation.[3] This condition results from the sensitivity of hair on certain portions of the scalp to androgens. Testosterone, an androgen, is converted to dihydrotestosterone (DHT) peripherally. DHT binds to receptors on scalp hair follicles, causing

a series of events that leads to the shortening of the anagen or growth part of the cycle. As a result, hair follicles that previously produced thick, pigmented terminal hairs begin to make thin vellus hairs. This process, called miniaturization, produces the fine hair seen in androgenetic alopecia, or pattern hair loss.

Anagen effluvium is the term used to describe the alopecia from the diffuse, rapid, and dramatic loss of anagen hairs. The most common cause is chemotherapy. Chemotherapeutic agents prevent the rapid division of the hair matrix cells. Hair production stops, and the hairs that are already present become frail, break off, and are shed. Normal hair production resumes when the antineoplastic medication is stopped.

Alopecia areata is fairly common and is often an autoimmune condition that results in well-demarcated areas of alopecia on the scalp or body. T-cell–mediated alopecia areata causes a chronic idiopathic inflammatory response around the hair bulb at the base of the hair.[3] The inflammation results in hair that is not well developed and, as it hits the surface, easily breaks or is shed.[3] Stress may be a contributory factor in alopecia areata, but other conditions are also associated with this type of hair loss, and include Addison disease, lupus erythematosus, and thyroid disease.[3]

Telogen Phase Disturbance

The transient shedding of telogen phase hairs is termed *telogen effluvium*. In this condition, the hair prematurely enters the telogen phase, resulting in a sudden onset of hair loss.[4] Multiple factors, including high fever, certain medications, endocrine abnormalities, anemia, childbirth, and malnutrition, can cause telogen effluvium.[4] Telogen effluvium affects men, women, and even infants, and can persist for several months after the precipitating event.

CLINICAL PRESENTATION AND PHYSICAL EXAMINATION

The history is a critical part of the evaluation of a person with alopecia. The provider should inquire about the onset, duration, and rapidity of the hair loss; any acute or chronic illnesses; current and past medications; and any symptoms that may be related to trichotillomania. It is important to determine whether the patient has had this type of hair loss before. Long and insidious hair loss is more indicative of androgenetic alopecia. Alopecia areata is often recurrent. An acute illness, such as a high fever, can trigger telogen effluvium, as can hyperthyroidism or hypothyroidism. A family history of hair loss may represent a clue for androgenetic alopecia, sometimes a hereditary disorder.

It is also important to inquire about associated symptoms. Scalp itching, pain, or flaking can suggest an inflammation of the scalp from psoriasis or contact dermatitis from hair dye. These conditions inflame the scalp and can cause hair breakage with resultant alopecia. In addition, symptoms of scalp itching and flaking can indicate tinea capitis, a fungal infection of the scalp that weakens the hairs and produces alopecia.

The physical examination begins with an evaluation of the pattern of hair loss. Androgenetic alopecia in men usually is seen as recession of the hairline at the temples and thinning in the frontal areas and the vertex. Women with androgenetic alopecia usually have diffuse thinning that is most pronounced in the frontal and parietal areas. A rim of hair along the frontal hairline is usually preserved.

Alopecia areata usually is initially seen as well-demarcated patches of hair loss on the scalp, eyebrows, and eyelashes. Singular, "exclamation point" hairs are sometimes visible. These exclamation point hairs are normal distally but are thinned proximal to the scalp. The scalp is not inflamed in alopecia areata. Men may experience alopecia areata in the beard area. When the whole scalp is affected, the process is called *alopecia totalis*.[5] If the whole body is involved, the process is called *alopecia universalis*.[5,6]

Anagen effluvium tends to result in a diffuse loss of hair, as does telogen effluvium. Scarring of the scalp suggests an inflammatory process, such as lupus or lichen planus follicularis. Scaling on the scalp may suggest psoriasis or tinea capitis. Patchy hair loss with regrowing hairs of multiple lengths suggest trichotillomania, a condition in which the patient pulls or twists the hair.

DIAGNOSTICS

Findings from the history and physical examination guide diagnostic testing. If there is scaling on the scalp that is suggestive of tinea capitis, a sample of several hairs or a scalp scraping is examined after preparation with potassium hydroxide (KOH). The presence of hyphae in the KOH preparation confirms the fungal cause of the alopecia.

A hair pull test, in which a few dozen hairs are grasped (with the patient's permission) firmly at the base and pulled, can help determine a telogen or anagen effluvium. A positive test result is noted when five or more hairs that include anagen hairs (with the follicle sheath) are pulled.[7] The hair bulb from these pulled hairs is examined with a magnifying glass or under a microscope to identify the characteristic appearance of anagen and telogen hairs.

If telogen effluvium is suspected and there is no obvious cause, an underlying illness should be considered (e.g., a thyroid disorder or iron deficiency anemia). If anemia is considered, iron studies should include serum iron, iron-binding capacity, and ferritin, in addition to a complete blood count (CBC).[4] A scalp biopsy and trichogram may also be of benefit.[4]

A hormonal evaluation of a woman with androgenetic alopecia is not necessary unless she has other signs of a hormonal imbalance, such as irregular menses, infertility, hirsutism, cystic acne, virilization, or galactorrhea. In these women, evaluation for alopecia may include testosterone or dehydroepiandrosterone-5 (DHEA-5) levels, in addition to the other hormonal tests indicated by their symptoms.

Secondary syphilis is a cause of patchy alopecia. Patients suspected of having secondary syphilis should have a Venereal Disease Research Laboratory (VDRL) test performed. Finally, a scalp biopsy is sometimes helpful when the cause of the alopecia is not clear.

INITIAL DIAGNOSTICS

Alopecia

LABORATORY
- Hair pull test and microscopy
- TSH
- Complete blood count differential

ADDITIONAL DIAGNOSTICS
- Serum iron[a]
- Iron binding capacity[a]

- Ferritin[a]
- Scalp biopsy[a]
- Trichogram[a]
- Dehydroepiandrosterone-5[a]
- Venereal Disease Research Laboratory[a]

[a]If indicated.

DIFFERENTIAL DIAGNOSIS

The differential diagnosis of hair loss is extensive. Table 40.1 can be used to differentiate among these conditions. The cause can usually be isolated with a careful history, physical examination, and some diagnostic tests. Some commonly seen causes include: systemic illness, childbirth, certain medications (heparin, propranolol, vitamin A, warfarin, propylthiouracil, isotretinoin, lithium, beta blockers, amphetamines, acitretin), metabolic abnormalities, chemotherapy and radiation, scalp infection, folliculitis, burns, Traction alopecia or Trichotillomania.

INTERPROFESSIONAL COLLABORATIVE MANAGEMENT

- The role of the primary care provider is to distinguish normal hair loss from hair loss associated with illness or another disorder.[5] When an external factor is found with anagen or telogen effluvium, the key to the management of alopecia is removal of this causative factor. Anagen effluvium as a result of chemotherapy will be reversed when the medication is stopped and the hair matrix is allowed to mature again. Telogen effluvium will also be reversed when the causative factor or event is over or corrected and the hair cycle is allowed to return to normal.

TABLE 40.1 Diagnosis of Alopecia

Disease	Duration (Year)	Scalp	Pattern	Pull Test
Alopecia areata	<1	Normal	Patchy; "exclamation point" hairs[a]	±
Anagen effluvium	Duration of chemotherapy	Normal	Diffuse	Hair breakage
Tinea capitis	<1	Scale, crust	Patchy	Hair breakage
Trichotillomania	>1	Normal to scarring	Patchy with stubble	—
Telogen effluvium	<1	Normal	Diffuse	Telogen
Androgenetic alopecia	>1	Normal	Pattern baldness	—
Systemic disease	<1	Normal	Diffuse	Normal/↑ telogen
Hair breakage	<1	Normal	Patchy	Age appropriate

[a]Short, stubby, straight hairs.

- Consultation with dermatologist is indicated if the cause of the patient's alopecia is unclear or if standard management within a reasonable time frame is not effective.
- Patients should be referred to a dermatologist or surgeon for consideration of hair transplantation.
- Patients with suspected trichotillomania may benefit from treatment with a selective serotonin reuptake inhibitor (SSRI) and a mental health referral.

Pharmacologic Management

Two medications, minoxidil (Rogaine) and finasteride (Propecia), are currently approved by the US Food and Drug Administration (FDA) to treat androgenetic alopecia.[4] Finasteride is Pregnancy Category X, so Minoxidil is the only medication approved by the FDA for use by women.[4] Applied twice a day to the dry scalp, minoxidil side effects include dryness and irritation of the scalp. Finasteride, an oral medication, inhibits the change of testosterone to DHT, the hormone responsible for causing the miniaturization of hairs in androgenetic alopecia. Both minoxidil and finasteride should be used for 8 to 12 months to determine efficacy, and require continued treatment to maintain hair growth.[5]

Alopecia areata can spontaneously resolve, but if it does not, treatment options are available (although not FDA approved). Therapies include ultraviolet B light, cyclosporine, and topical and intralesional corticosteroids.[4] Anthralin, an antipsoriatic agent, and minoxidil are two topical agents that can be effective treatments.[4] Topical immunotherapy, or contact sensitization, is also very effective.[4]

COMPLICATIONS

Some types of hair loss are the result of systemic illness. Complications can result from these illnesses. In addition, complications can occur as a result of the psychological effects that patients may experience with hair loss.

PATIENT AND FAMILY EDUCATION

Patients with androgenetic alopecia may be reassured to know that this is a common disorder. They should be reminded that there are no restrictions on the types of grooming products that they use. In addition, the frequency of hair washing will not affect the hair loss process.[5]

Patients with alopecia areata should know that spontaneous remissions and recurrences are common. They should also know that vitiligo, atopy (eczema, asthma, and hay fever), and thyroid disease are more common in people with alopecia areata.[8,9]

REFERENCES

1. Wolff, K., Johnson, R., & Saavedra, A. P. (2017). Disorders of hair follicles and related disorders. In K. Wolff, R. A. Johnson, A. P. Saavedra, & E. K. Roh (Eds.), *Fitzpatrick's color atlas and synopsis of clinical dermatology* (8th ed.). New York, NY: McGraw-Hill.
2. Bolognia, J. L., & Braverman, I. M. (2015). Skin manifestations of internal disease. In D. Kasper, A. Fauci, S. Hauser, D. Longo, J. Jameson, & J. Loscalzo (Eds.), *Harrison's principles of internal medicine* (19th ed.). New York, NY: McGraw-Hill.
3. McCann, S. A., & Huether, S. E. (2018). Structure, function, and disorders of the integument. In K. L. McCance & S. E. Huether (Eds.), *Pathophysiology: The biologic basis for disease in adults and children* (8th ed.). Philadelphia, PA: Elsevier.
4. Malkud, S. (2015). Telogen effluvium: A review. *Journal of Clinical and Diagnostic Research: JCDR, 9*(9), WE1–WE3.
5. Habif, T. P., Dinulos, J. G., Chapman, M. S., et al. (2018). *Skin disease diagnosis and treatment* (4th ed.). Edinburgh: Elsevier.
6. Alkhalifah, A. (2013). Alopecia areata update. *Dermatologic Clinics, 31*(1), 93–108.
7. Jackson, A. J., & Price, V. H. (2013). How to diagnose hair loss. *Dermatologic Clinics, 31*(1), 21–28.
8. Mohan, G. C., & Silverberg, J. I. (2015). Association of vitiligo and alopecia areata with atopic dermatitis. *JAMA Dermatology, 151*(5), 522–528.
9. Patel, D., Li, P., & Bauer, A. J. (2017). Screening guidelines for thyroid function in children with alopecia areata. *JAMA Dermatology, 153*(12), 1307–1310.

CHAPTER **41**

ANIMAL AND HUMAN BITES

Elizabeth A. Talbot

 Immediate surgical consultation and hospitalization indicated for crush injury, fractures, disfigurement, hand cellulitis, and hemorrhage.

DEFINITION AND EPIDEMIOLOGY

Every year millions of people throughout the world sustain bite wounds. Although many of these bites are minor, there is a significant risk of injury and infection. In the United States, there are millions of occurrences; dog bites alone account for 800,000 medical visits yearly, 366,000 of which are emergency room visits.[1] Animal and human bites incur large health care costs, with dog bites in the United States estimated to cost one billion dollars per year.[1]

Domestic animals inflict the majority of bite wounds. Dog bites account for most of the domestic animal bites that require medical care, yet dog bites have had the lowest incidence of wound infection (2% to 13%).[2,3] Even though most dog bites are relatively minor, severe injuries can occur. These can include crush injuries, destructive soft tissue injuries, neurovascular injuries, orthopedic injuries, and death.[4] Severe dog bite wounds most commonly affect the extremities, are seen more often in children and young adults, and can occur when the animal is provoked. Cat bites are the second most common type of mammalian bite, accounting for up to 15% of bite wound cases per year—mostly in the hand, forearm, and arm, and occurring more commonly in older women.[1] Six percent of cat bite victims require hospitalization, because the infection rate is much higher—the result of the deep puncture wounds from the cat's sharp teeth.[1]

Human bites can occur during physical altercations (i.e., fights), and these include the special circumstance of closed-fist injuries (CFIs). CFIs are injuries of the skin overlying the knuckles, incurred when a person strikes another person's tooth (often in the setting of alcohol ingestion). Human bites have overall infection rates of around 10%,[5] can be inflicted by a young child, occur accidentally during sexual activity, or be self-inflicted (e.g., nail biting). Bites not located on the hand have an infection rate similar to that of routine lacerations, but the CFI, or "fight bite," has a much higher complication rate because of the high penetrating force that causes local tissue destruction and the contamination of oral flora which then may cause cellulitis, osteomyelitis, tendinitis, tenosynovitis, and/or septic arthritis.

Patients may also present to primary care following a bite by other pets, a wild rodent, reptile, fish, bird, or larger animal. Often these presentations arise out of concern regarding any need for postexposure prophylaxis or, less commonly, because of subsequent infection.

PATHOPHYSIOLOGY

The morbidity and mortality associated with mammalian bites are mostly related to immediate tissue injury or subsequent mono- or polymicrobial infection at the bite site. The pathogens of these infections may include the oral flora of the biter, the skin flora of the victim, and the environment in which the bite took place. Infections involving aerobes alone (24% to 44%) or mixed aerobes and anaerobes (54% to 66%) are the most common.[2] The risk factors for infection are listed in Box 41.1.

Animal bite infections arising from the animal's oral flora may be caused by a variety of pathogens, which are usually bacterial. The most common aerobic bacteria are *Pasteurella multocida* and other *Pasteurella* species, *Streptococci*, *Staphylococci*, and *Corynebacterium* species.[1–3,5] Common anaerobic isolates include *Bacteroides*, *Actinomyces*, *Porphyromonas*, and *Fusobacterium* species.[1–3,5] A rare but serious bacterial pathogen notoriously present in dogs' mouths (but also in cats') is *Capnocytophaga canimorsus*, which can cause a devastating sepsis, especially in patients who are immunocompromised.[6]

The primary care clinician seeing a patient with an animal bite must also consider viral pathogens. Among viral pathogens associated with animal bites, rabies is the most feared. Bats, raccoons, skunks, and foxes are the most common carriers in the United States, whereas dogs and cats are the most predominant carriers in other countries.

Rarer pathogens transmitted through animal bites include *Francisella tularensis* (which causes tularemia), *Leptospira interrogans* (the spirochete that causes leptospirosis), *Bartonella henselae* (also known as cat-scratch disease), *Yersinia pestis* (the bacteria that causes plague and is endemic among ground rodents in the western United States), and rat-bite fever (caused by either *Streptobacillus moniliformis* in North America or *Spirillum minus* in Asia).

Beside the animal mouth pathogens that are introduced by a bite, environmental pathogens can be inoculated by the bite, including *Clostridium, tetani* (the cause of tetanus), and certain dirt fungi such as *Sporothrix schenckii* (sporotrichosis, or rose gardener's disease) and blastomycosis.

Like animal bites, human bites are also often polymicrobial, with some overlap of pathogens—but there are some important differences. *Pasteurella* and *Capnocytophaga* species are not transmitted through human bites, but *Eikenella corrodens* is often present in infected human bite injuries (particularly clenched-fist injuries).[6] *E. corrodens* must be appreciated as a possible cause of post-human bite infection because it may be resistant to empirically chosen antibiotics and can produce β-lactamases. It also grows fastidiously, and can lead to serious indolent infections including subacute endocarditis.[2] Hospitalization is usually recommended, because human bites—especially of the hands—are polymicrobial (e.g., *E. corrodens, streptococci,* and *Staphylococcus aureus*).[6] Methicillin-resistant *Staphylococcus aureus* (MRSA) is an increasingly recognized pathogen from human bite wounds.[7] *Streptococcus pyogenes* is also found in human bites.[8] Rarer organisms from human bites include herpes simplex virus types 1 and 2, and hepatitis B and C viruses. Human immunodeficiency virus (HIV) has a biologic possibility of transmission through a bite wound, but the risk of transmission is extremely low.[9]

CLINICAL PRESENTATION AND PHYSICAL EXAMINATION

A careful history from the bite victim is necessary and needs to include the location and time of the bite (patients may present several days after the bite occurrence); the species and behavior of the animal; the domestication and rabies vaccine status of the animal; and whether the animal was provoked. Elicit and document the victim's drug allergies; current immunization status for tetanus and rabies; alcohol use; current medications; and past medical history with an emphasis on immunocompetence, history of splenectomy, venous or lymphatic insufficiency, or liver disease. If the injury is related to a human bite, the presence of infectious diseases in the biter should be investigated. Sometimes patients are reluctant to admit to human bite wounds, particularly when associated with a clenched-fist or sexually incurred injury, but human bites can transmit blood-borne pathogens such as hepatitis B, hepatitis C, or HIV.

It is also important to determine if an animal bite is rabies prone. Both animal and human bites should be considered tetanus prone and managed for potential exposure.

The physical examination should document the location, extent, and depth of the wound; type of wound (puncture, scratch, tear, or avulsion); and tenderness and other signs of infection (e.g., fever, erythema, edema, streaking, warmth, fluctuation, adenopathy, purulent discharge). There should be careful testing for involvement of underlying tendons (e.g., tendon laceration), joints (joint space penetration, range of motion), and nerves, and for signs of compartment syndrome (disproportionate pain, paresthesia, pallor, paralysis).[6]

BOX 41.1

Risk Factors for Bite Wound Infection

Age older than 50 years

Advanced liver disease, alcoholism, asplenia, diabetes mellitus

Crush injury, puncture wound, penetrating injury of the periosteum or joint capsule

Location on the hand or foot

Failure to irrigate and to debride wound during initial management

Treatment delay of more than 12 h

Preexisting or resulting edema at the bite site

Peripheral vascular disease

INITIAL DIAGNOSTICS

ANIMAL AND HUMAN BITES

- For infected wounds: CBC; erythrocyte sedimentation rate; CRP, aerobic, and anaerobic wound cultures; blood cultures if febrile
- For deep or complex wounds: X-ray studies for any bone or joint involvement or foreign body
- For human bites: Human immunodeficiency virus, hepatitis B, and hepatitis C testing of biter

---

Additional Diagnostics

C-reactive protein level and erythrocyte sedimentation rate (ESR) can be used to monitor response to treatment.[10] For bites that occur near joints, or those that look severely infected, radiographs should be obtained to look for fractures, the presence of foreign bodies, soft tissue injury, subcutaneous gas, and osteomyelitis.[8]

INTERPROFESSIONAL COLLABORATIVE MANAGEMENT

Nonpharmacologic Management

After assessing for and treating life-threatening injuries, the provider should irrigate the wound and treat the patient in accordance with the following management principles:

- Irrigate the wound vigilantly with at least 150 mL (more is recommended) of sterile saline solution (tap water is acceptable if sterile saline is not available).[8,11] Devitalized tissue, foreign bodies, and clots are cautiously debrided. Aggressive drainage, irrigation, and wound packing are necessary if cultures reveal an established wound infection. Most wounds do not develop signs of infection until 24 to 72 hours after the bite.[2]
- Bites to the face, whether of animal or human origin, should be managed with extensive irrigation, cautious debridement, preemptive antibiotics, and primary closure, and are most often (depending on the bite) referred to emergency room or plastic surgery immediately.[12]
- It is generally accepted that most cat and human bites, deep puncture wounds, clinically infected wounds, wounds more than 6 to 12 hours old, and bites to the hand should be left open because of the high risk of infection.[1–5,11] These wounds can be closed by delayed primary closure or by secondary intention.
- Wounds involving the hand or foot should be immobilized and elevated for 1 to 3 days.[11]
- Close outpatient follow-up monitoring (usually every 24 hours) is recommended to track complications or treatment failures.

Pharmacologic Management

Antimicrobial therapy is obviously indicated in infected wounds, but treatment of fresh, uninfected wounds is still controversial. Prophylaxis is indicated for high-risk bites and for high-risk patients. Patients who present with a cat bite or hand bite, whether related to human or animal bite, require 5- to 7-days prophylaxis.[6,11] Some recommend that antibiotic prophylaxis be given for all bite wounds except for patients who are seen 72 hours after injury with no signs of infection.[2]

The selection of antibiotics is based on knowledge of the most common microorganisms encountered and on susceptibility testing of cultured microorganisms from infected wounds. Principles include:

- For fresh bites, prophylactic therapy is most effective with amoxicillin–clavulanic acid, 500 mg/125 mg every 8 hours daily for 5 to 7 days. Clindamycin in combination with doxycycline or TMP-SMZ is appropriate for patients with a penicillin allergy and necessary because clindamycin alone is not efficacious against *Pasteurella*. Levofloxacin or ciprofloxacin are additional treatment choices.[6,12] Macrolides should be reserved for pregnant patients allergic to β-lactamase.[13]
- Older infected bites require 7 to 14 days of hospitalization and intravenous targeted antibiotic therapy when soft tissue is involved. In bone or joint infections, longer courses of antibiotics are needed and referral to an infectious diseases specialist is indicated.[12]

The incidence of MRSA colonization in domestic animals is possible.[7] Empiric coverage can be considered in regions in which the incidence of community-acquired MRSA incidence is high. Choice of MRSA therapy should be guided by local antibiograms until cultures are available, but trimethoprim-sulfamethoxazole, doxycycline, or clindamycin can be used, although resistance to clindamycin is increasing. Oral linezolid can be used in more severe cases that do not require hospitalization. Parenteral vancomycin, daptomycin, linezolid, ceftaroline, or tigecycline can be considered in more complicated or systemic infections for MRSA coverage.[7]

Agents such as dicloxacillin, cephalexin, erythromycin, and clindamycin should not be used empirically as sole agents for infected bites because they lack activity against *Pasteurella* and *Eikenella* species (common in animal and human bites, respectively).[11]

If the bite victim has completed a full primary tetanus immunization series (usually at childhood) but has not had a Td booster within the past 5 years, vaccination with tetanus toxoid and diphtheria (Td) or tetanus, diphtheria toxoid, and acellular pertussis (Tdap) should be administered.[14] Patients who have not completed a full primary series or whose vaccination status is unknown will require tetanus immune globulin, 250 to 500 units intramuscularly, with the first of three monthly doses of tetanus toxoid.[4] For more information, see Chapter 51.

RABIES

The decision to provide rabies postexposure prophylaxis should be based on the guidelines of local, city, or state public health departments, the Centers for Disease Control and Prevention, and the Advisory Committee on Immunization Practices (ACIP).[14] The most common animal reservoirs of rabies in the United States are bats, with cases found in every state except Hawaii, but the bite of many mammals might be considered rabies-prone and warrant prophylaxis. Lagomorphs (e.g., rabbits) and rodents (e.g., hamsters, guinea pigs, gerbils, mice, rats, and squirrels) are almost never found to have rabies, and have not been found to transmit rabies to humans, so bites from these animals are not generally considered rabies-prone.

When a patient reports a bite by an animal that may have had rabies, the wound must be immediately washed with soap and water or 1% povidone-iodine solution, which significantly lowers rabies transmission rates.[4] The public health authorities can aid decisions about and implementation of appropriate quarantine (isolation and observation) or sacrifice of the biting animal for pathologic brain examination. Dogs and cats that can be quarantined should be watched for 10 days, because studies have shown that animals with rabies present in the saliva will sicken and die within this time frame.[15] If the animal becomes sick, prophylaxis should be started for the victim.

An exception to the watchful waiting of quarantine is when the bite is to the head or neck because the incubation period can be shorter.[16] In that scenario, postexposure prophylaxis should always be started immediately. If the quarantined animal is healthy after 10 days of quarantine, the rabies prophylaxis can be stopped.

Postexposure prophylaxis should be considered in high-risk bites even when the bite happened in the distant past. A previous case report describes a patient who developed rabies 8 years after having been bitten.[17]

Postexposure prophylaxis consists of passive immunization with 20 IU/kg of human rabies immune globulin (HRIG) or purified chick embryo cell vaccine (PCECV) per kilogram, with half the dose injected around the wound and half given intramuscularly (gluteal or deltoid).[18] In addition, active immunization with 1 mL of human diploid cell vaccine (HDCV) or PCECV given intramuscularly (deltoid) on days 0, 3, 7, and 14 is indicated. Individuals with a history of pre-exposure immunization with HDCV should receive an HDCV booster on days 0 and 3 but do not require HRIG.[18]

INDICATIONS FOR REFERRAL AND HOSPITALIZATION

Other indications include:

- Involvement of a joint, nerve, bone, or tendon or compartment syndrome (orthopedic referral)
- Possible compartment syndrome
- Significant hand bites (hand surgery referral)
- Extensive wounds requiring reconstructive surgery (plastic surgery referral)
- Head injuries (otolaryngologic or neurosurgery referral)[2,4]

Infection is the most serious delayed complication of bite wounds, resulting in cellulitis, lymphangitis, tenosynovitis, septic arthritis, and osteomyelitis, which may benefit from infectious diseases consultation and/or admission for evaluation and intravenous antibiotics. Common triggers for referral include:

- Patients with systemic manifestations of infection (fever, rigors, hypotension)
- Severe cellulitis
- Infected bites refractory to oral or outpatient therapy

Decisions around rabies postexposure prophylaxis are often made collaboratively with the public health department, as is an evaluation for blood-borne pathogen transmission due to human bites.

Emotional trauma, especially occurring in children victims of bites, may evolve into posttraumatic stress disorder (PTSD). Psychosupportive referral may prevent or expedite recovery from PTSD.

PATIENT EDUCATION AND HEALTH PROMOTION

All patients should be encouraged not to provoke domestic animals or to handle wild animals, especially raccoons, skunks, foxes, and bats. A rabies vaccine for pets (both dogs and cats) is mandatory in the United States but not in many foreign countries, including Mexico. Nervousness, aggressiveness, excessive drooling or foaming at the mouth, or fearlessness should raise the suspicion of rabid animals and prompt notification of the animal warden or health authorities.

Preventive measures include teaching children about safe play with pets. Parents can also be educated about supervisory practices while their children play with pets and selection factors in choosing pets. In addition, they can be taught the benefits of spaying or neutering their pets to help control feral animal populations.[19] On a broader level, legislative efforts such as control of high-risk breeds can also help in bite prevention. A review done in Canadian municipalities showed decreased bite rates in areas with higher ticketing rates by animal control.[20]

Pre-exposure immunization with HDCV should be considered for high-risk groups, such as animal handlers, veterinarians, certain laboratory workers, and persons living in or visiting countries with a significant rabies risk. The regimen would be 1 mL intramuscularly on days 0, 7, and 21 or 28, and a booster every 2 years.[6]

Td or Tdap boosters should be given every 10 years routinely in all patients. Instructions to clean all bite wounds and to seek medical care immediately should be given, especially for fight bites to the hand.

RESOURCES

Helpful resources include your local or state health department and the CDC (https://www.cdc.gov/rabies/exposure/index.html).

REFERENCES

1. Aziz, H., Rhee, P., Pandit, V., Tang, A., Gries, L., & Joseph, B. (2015). The current concepts in management of animal (dog, cat, snake, scorpion) and human bite wounds. *The Journal of Trauma and Acute Care Surgery, 78*(3), 641–648.
2. Brook, I. (2009). Management of human and animal bite wounds: An overview. *Current Infectious Disease Reports, 11*(5), 389–395.
3. Cavalcanti, A., Porto, E., Ferreira dos Santos, B., et al. (2017). Facial dog bite injuries in children: A case report. *International Journal of Surgery Case Reports, 41,* 57–60.
4. Benfield, R., Plurad, D. S., Lam, L., et al. (2010). The epidemiology of dog attacks in an urban environment and the risk of vascular injury. *The American Surgeon, 76*(2), 203–205.
5. McBrien, B. (2016). Fight bite injury: Emergency department assessment and management. *Emergency nurse: the journal of the RCN Accident and Emergency Nursing Association, 24*(7), 34–37.
6. Collins, N., & Rose, J. (2017). Hand trauma. In C. Stone & R. L. Humphries (Eds.), *Current diagnosis & treatment: Emergency medicine, 8e.* New York, NY: McGraw-Hill. Retrieved from http://accessmedicine.mhmedical.com.ezproxy.simmons.edu/content.aspx?bookid=2172&sectionid=165062479. (Accessed 07 May 2018).
7. Gustavsson, O., Johansson, A. V., Monstein, H. J., et al. (2016). *European Journal of Clinical Microbiology & Infectious Diseases: Official Publication of the European Society of Clinical Microbiology, 35,* 1315. https://doi.org/10.1007/s10096-016-2667-z.
8. Rothe, K., Tsokos, M., & Handrick, W. (2015). Animal and human bite wounds. *Deutsches Arzteblatt International, 112*(25), 433–443. doi:10.3238/arztebl.2015.0433.
9. Pettitt, D. A., et al. (2012). A human bite. *British Medical Journal, 345,* e4798.
10. Pääkkönen, M., et al. (2010). Sensitivity of erythrocyte sedimentation rate and C-reactive protein in childhood bone and joint infections. *Clinical Orthopaedics and Related Research, 468*(3), 861–866.
11. Chin-Hong, P. V., & Guglielmo, B. (2018). Common problems in infectious diseases & antimicrobial therapy. In M. A. Papadakis, S. J. McPhee, & M. W. Rabow (Eds.), *Current medical diagnosis & treatment.* New York, NY: McGraw-Hill.
12. Stevens, D. L., et al. (2014). Practice guidelines for the diagnosis and management of skin and soft tissue infections: 2014 Update by the Infectious Diseases Society of America. *Clinical Infectious Diseases: An Official Publication of the Infectious Diseases Society of America, 59*(2), e10–e52.
13. Murase, J. E., Heller, M. M., & Butler, D. C. (2014). Safety of dermatologic medications in pregnancy and lactation: Part I. Pregnancy. *Journal of the American Academy of Dermatology, 70*(3), 401.e1–401.e14.
14. Centers for Disease Control and Prevention. (April 27, 2018). Morbidity and mortality weekly report. Prevention of pertussis, tetanus, and diphtheria with vaccines in the United States: Recommendations of the Advisory Committee on Immunization Practices (ACIP). Retrieved from https://www.cdc.gov/mmwr/volumes/67/rr/rr6702a1.htm. (Accessed 6 May 2018).
15. Dyer, J. L., et al. (2013). Rabies surveillance in the United States during 2012. *Journal of the American Veterinary Medical Association, 243*(6), 805–815.
16. Garg, S. R. (2014). Rabies manifestations and diagnosis. In *Rabies in man and animals* (pp. 37–49). Delhi, India: Springer.
17. Boland, et al. (2014). Phylogenetic and epidemiologic evidence of multiyear incubation in human rabies. *Annals of Neurology, 75,* 155.
18. Rupprecht, C. E., et al. (2010). Use of a reduced (4-dose) vaccine schedule for postexposure prophylaxis to prevent human rabies. *MMWR. Recommendations and Reports: Morbidity and Mortality Weekly Report. Recommendations and Reports, 59*(RR-2), 1–9.

19. Gielen, A., et al. (2012). Dog bites: An opportunity for parent education in the pediatric emergency department. *Pediatric Emergency Care, 28*(10), 966.

20. Clarke, et al. (2013). Animal control measures and their relationship to the reported incidence of dog bites in urban Canadian municipalities. *The Canadian Veterinary Journal. La Revue Vétérinaire Canadienne, 54*(2), 145.

CHAPTER **42**

BENIGN SKIN LESIONS
Glen Blair

 Specialist referral is indicated for lesions that are not readily identifiable as benign or suspected of being malignant and should be biopsied or evaluated at the earliest possible time.

INTRODUCTION

Dermatologic issues are common complaints in the primary care arena and it is incumbent on the primary care provider to have a basic understanding of common cutaneous lesions, whether they be malignant or benign. Lesions that are not readily identifiable as benign or suspected of being malignant (irregularity in color, shape, or surface texture, or change in size, color, or morphology) should be biopsied or evaluated by a dermatology specialist at the earliest possible time. However there are numerous benign skin lesions that are easily recognizable and may require no dermatologic evaluation at all. Diagnosis of a benign lesion may spare the patient significant anxiety and possibly the additional expense associated with a dermatologic referral. Additionally, patients wishing to have benign lesions removed need to understand that the procedures used to remove benign lesions are often expenses not covered by insurance. We will discuss five benign lesions that are commonly found on the skin exam: acrochordon, angioma, dermatofibroma, sebaceous hyperplasia, and seborrheic keratosis (SK).

ACROCHORDON
Definition

Acrochordons or *skin tags* (Fig. 42.1) are small fibrovascular papules that commonly develop on and in the skin folds of the neck, axillae, inframammary and inguinal regions, and the eyelids. They create discomfort in the patient due to their appearance, but also because of their propensity to cause local inflammation and discomfort.

They vary in color from flesh-toned to hyperpigmented and range in size from 1 to 8 mm. While they are benign lesions, they are sometimes associated with obesity and metabolic disorders such as diabetes.[1] These lesions have no inherent malignant potential, but should be evaluated if there is a change in size, color, or shape.

Management

Treatment, again, may be fee-for-service, and includes scissor excision; electrocautery, which may cause scarring; and local application of cryotherapy (liquid nitrogen), which may cause local hypo- or hyperpigmentation.

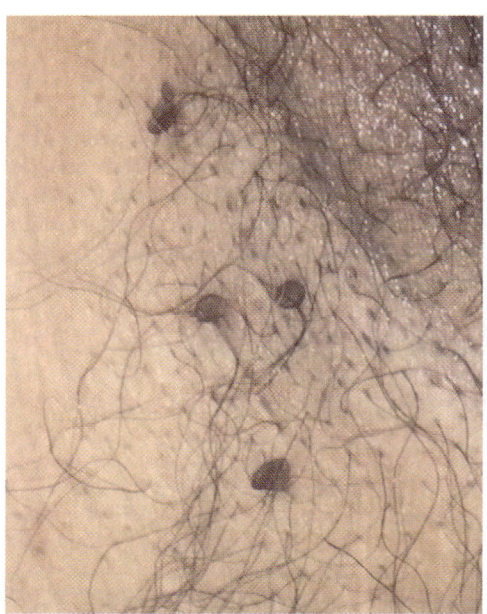

FIG. 42.1 Skin tags.

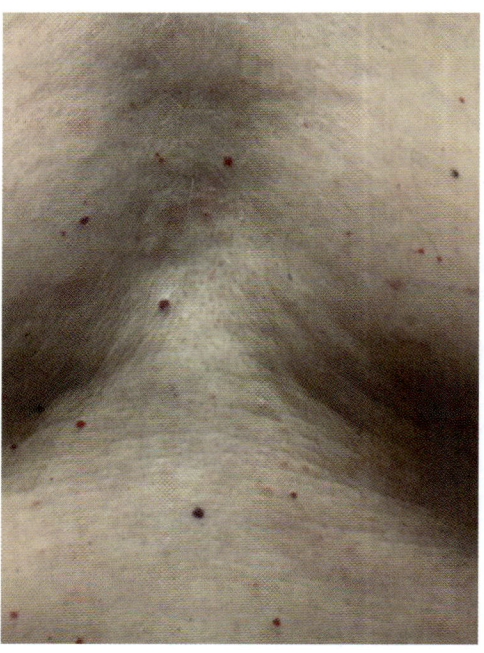

FIG. 42.2 Cherry angiomas.

ANGIOMA
Definition and Epidemiology

Angiomas, sometimes called *cherry angiomas* (Fig. 42.2), are common vascular lesions that develop on the trunk and extremities after the third of fourth decade of life and increase in number with age. They are red or violaceous non-blanching macules or papules arising from capillaries, and they range in size from 3 to 5 mm in diameter.[2] When present on the vulva or scrotum, they are referred to as *Fordyce*.[1]

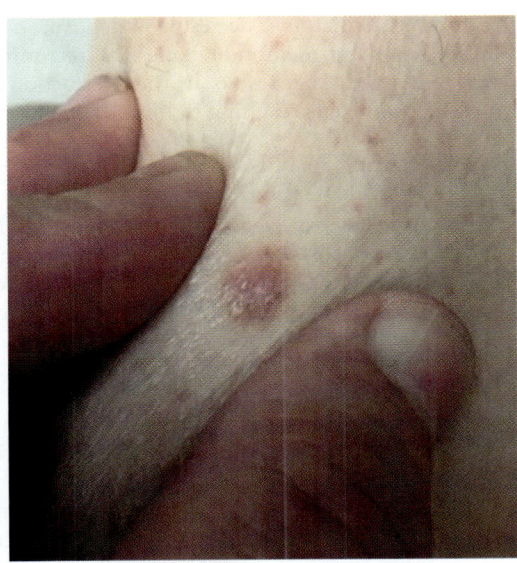

FIG. **42.3** Dermtofibromas.

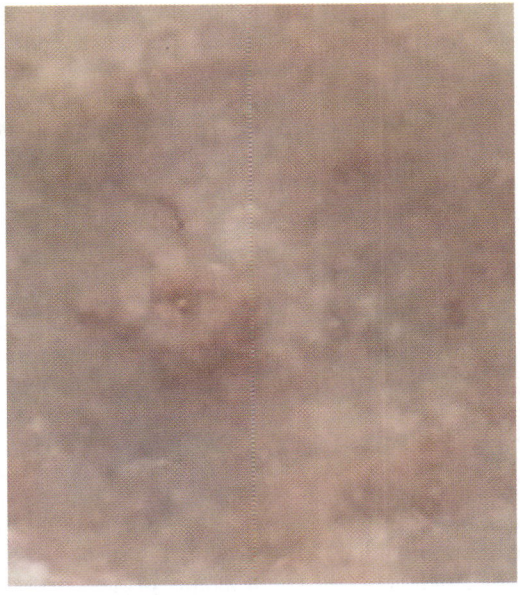

FIG. **42.4** Sebaceous hyperplasia.

Management

Angiomas are not associated with any disease and treatment is cosmetic, consisting of electrodessication, curettage, or laser.

DERMATOFIBROMA
Definition

Dermatofibromas (Fig. 42.3) are firm, intradermal nodules in the skin, found more commonly in women and on the legs, although they can be found in men and on other parts of the body. They may be caused by local trauma such as from body hair removal or insect bites. They tend to be asymptomatic but may be occasionally pruritic or tender. They can by flesh-colored, tan, hyperpigmented, or violaceous. Diagnosis can often be established by identifying the *dimple* or *Fitzpatrick* sign, by squeezing the lesion with the thumb and forefinger, causing the lesion surface to dimple.

Management

Treatment for lesions because of discomfort or for cosmetic reasons is a deep excision, taking care to remove the deepest part of the lesion to prevent recurrence.[2] Patients should be informed that the scar from excision may be less appealing in appearance than the presenting lesion.

SEBACEOUS HYPERPLASIA
Definition and Epidemiology

Sebaceous hyperplasia (Fig. 42.4) is characterized by the enlargement of sebaceous glands beneath the skin associated with a pore or follicle.[1] The lesion tends to be yellow and have a raised outer area with a central dell, similar to a basal cell carcinoma (BCC). They also have "crown vessels," which are different from the "arborizing vessels" associated with BCC in that the vessels occupy the periphery of the lesion, not the central dell as occurs in BCC.[1] Sebaceous hyperplasia lesions present primarily on the face, mostly the forehead, cheeks, and nose. These lesions are associated with aging and pregnancy and are more common in transplant patients.

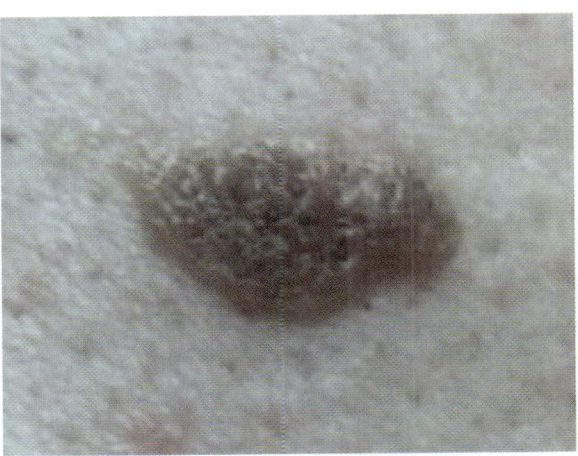

FIG. **42.5** Seborrheic keratosis.

Management

If diagnosis of BCC cannot be ruled out, these patients should be referred for biopsy. If the diagnosis is clear, treatment is optional and includes electrodessication, phototherapy, and laser therapy. Scarring is common.

SEBORRHEIC KERATOSIS
Definition and Epidemiology

SK (Fig. 42.5) are the most common benign non-melanocytic skin lesion on the body, typically presenting as waxy or verrucous appearing papules or plaques that have a "stuck-on" appearance on the skin.[3] They vary in color from flesh-toned to tan, brown, or black and are found anywhere on the body, frequently on the trunk, and sparing the palms and soles. They can vary in size from 2 mm to 3 cm. Some lesions are peppered with small keratinized cysts called *horned cysts.* SK lesions are usually easily identified by their appearance, but can vary such that they must be distinguished from malignant melanomas.[2]

Lesion biopsy or referral to dermatology for atypical lesions may be appropriate. *Dermatosis papulosa nigra* is a variant found more commonly in people of color characterized by small dark papules on the face. *Stucco keratosis* is a variant of light brown or white keratosis on the feet, ankles, and lower tibia.[1] Patients often feel disfigured by these lesions because they can present conspicuously and treatment therefore is often for cosmetic reasons.

Management

While removal of uncomplicated SK may not be covered by insurance, the treatment of inflamed or irritated SK's typically is. Treatment is often accomplished by cryotherapy, but curettage or shave biopsy are also reasonable options.[2]

CONCLUSION

Primary care providers need a basic understanding of common cutaneous lesions, both malignant and benign, as dermatologic issues are common complaints in primary care. Lesions that are not readily identifiable as benign or suspected of being malignant (irregularity in color, shape, or surface texture or change in size, color, or morphology) should be biopsied or evaluated by a dermatology specialist as soon as possible.

REFERENCES

1. Bobonich, M. A., & Nolen, M. E. (2015). *Dermatology for advanced practice clinicians* (pp. 169–178, 167, 165). China: Wolters Kluwer.
2. Higgins, J. C., Maher, M. A., & Douglas, M. S. (2015). Diagnosing common benign skin tumors. *American Family Physician, 92*(7), 601–607.
3. Habif, T. B. (2010). *Clinical dermatology* (5th ed., p. 776). Mosby Elsevier.

CHAPTER **43**

BULLOUS PEMPHIGOID

Ellen M. McCafferty O'Connell

DEFINITION AND EPIDEMIOLOGY

Bullous pemphigoid (BP) is an autoimmune disorder characterized by large, tense, subepidermal blisters that occur on normal or erythematous skin. It belongs to the group of pemphigoid diseases characterized by the presence of circulating immunoglobulin G (IgG) autoantibodies against structural proteins of the dermal-epidermal junction leading to tissue damage and blister formation.[1] Incidence increases in older adults, with the majority of patients diagnosed older than 60 years.[2,3] Males and females are equally affected, and there is no apparent racial predilection. Childhood-onset BP has been reported in the literature; however, is it generally self-limited.[4]

PATHOPHYSIOLOGY

The typical lesions of BP are subepidermal blisters. A blister is a fluid-filled cavity formed within or beneath the epidermis. Blisters are characterized by size: a vesicle is less than 10 mm, a bullae greater than or equal to 10 mm. Blisters may be clear or blood-tinged if there is disruption in blood vessels. The hallmark of BP is the presence of circulating and tissue-bound IgG autoantibodies specific for the hemidesmosomal BP antigens BP230 and BP180.[1,5,6] These autoantibodies target the hemidesmosomes (BP 180 and 230), triggering complement activation

and inflammatory mediators. The result is deposition of IgG and C3 in the basement membrane zone. The recruitment of neutrophils and eosinophils results in the destruction of the basement membrane zone, resulting in blister formation.[2,3]

CLINICAL PRESENTATION AND PHYSICAL EXAMINATION

Patients with BP often experience a nonbullous prodromal phase characterized by mild to severe pruritus accompanied by erythematous, eczematous papules, and/or urticarial lesions. These nonspecific skin eruptions last several weeks to months and may be the only early signs of the disease, often delaying the diagnosis of BP.[1,6] Constitutional symptoms are absent except in severe widespread disease.

The bullous phase may appear suddenly with intense pruritus and widespread blister formation symmetrically distributed primarily on the lower abdomen and the flexor aspects of the upper and lower extremities including the axillae and medial aspects of groin and thighs. The tense oval or round blisters are filled with either clear or hemorrhagic exudate erupting on either normal or erythematous skin accompanied by urticarial plaques and papules. Blisters may persist for several days, either rupturing or collapsing, resulting in oozing erosions and crusts.[5] This disruption in skin integrity may result in post-inflammatory hyper- or hypopigmentation. Oral lesions develop in 20% of patients; however, eyes, nose, esophagus, and anogenital areas are rarely affected.[2] Triggers that have been reported to precipitate the onset of BP include traumatic, pharmacologic, or infectious agents. Trauma to the skin such as burns, radiotherapy, and ultraviolet radiation can trigger BP. Drugs associated with the onset of BP include furosemide, phenacetin, enalapril, ibuprofen, and several antibiotics (penicillamine, ampicillin, penicillin, and cephalexin).[1,5,6] Infections such as human herpesvirus (HHV), Epstein-Barr virus, cytomegalovirus, and hepatitis B and C may contribute to the induction of BP.[5] New studies are examining an association between BP and neurological diseases such as Parkinson's and cerebrovascular accident (CVA).[3]

Physical examination begins with general appearance and vital signs, observing for signs of discomfort or toxicity. A full body exam should be done focusing on the axillae, groin, and flexor aspects of the extremities and lower legs for papular or urticarial lesions, excoriations, hemorrhagic crusts, vesicles, and erosions. Mucous membranes must be inspected for blisters or erosions in the oropharynx, conjunctiva, and genitalia. Nikolsky sign, the ability to split or dislodge the epidermis from the dermis by applying lateral pressure with a finger resulting in an erosion, is negative in patients with BP.[7–9]

DIAGNOSTICS
Essential Diagnostics

The diagnosis of BP relies on both evaluation of clinical features and immunopathologic findings. Direct immunofluorescence (DIF) microscopy of a skin biopsy specimen obtained from perilesional skin remains the gold standard for the diagnosis of BP, demonstrating the presence of IgG and/or C3 deposits along the dermal-epidermal border.[1,6]

Indirect immunofluorescence microscopy studies can be used to document the presence of IgG autoantibodies in the serum that target the skin basement membrane. Circulating autoantibodies that bind to the split skin can be found in 80% to 85% of patients with BP.[1,6] Indirect immunofluorescence can help differentiate similar microscopic findings that are seen in other blistering disorders.

Emerging procedures are now available including enzyme-linked immunosorbent assay (ELISA), which analyzes the BP antigen–specific IgG autoantibodies in the patient's serum.[1,6]

Immunoblotting or Western blotting shows varying sensitivity in the diagnosis of BP. In 75% of patients a reaction occurs with BP 230 antigen, and in 50% of patients a reaction occurs with BP 180 antigen.[1,6,10] Peripheral blood smear eosinophilia occurs in 50% of patients.[2] Remission is paralleled by decreased serum levels of IgE and decreased IgG of BP 180.[2]

INITIAL DIAGNOSTICS

LABORATORY
- CBC and differential
- Immunofluorescence, both direct and indirect
- ELISA for bullous pemphigoid antigen-specific immunoglobulin G autoantibodies
- Immunoblot or Western Blot for bullous pemphigoid antigens

DIFFERENTIAL DIAGNOSIS

 Priority differentials are (1) drug reactions (which can be difficult in older adults who may be taking multiple medications), (2) arthropod bite, (3) dermatitis herpetiformis (an autoimmune blistering disorder often associated with gluten sensitivity), and (4) epidermolysis bullosa (an inherited disorder diagnosed in childhood, although it may be undetected in mild cases).

BP often imitates other conditions. In the nonbullous prodromal stage, it is often confused with a variety of inflammatory dermatoses including contact dermatitis, urticaria, or arthropod reactions. To distinguish BP from these other disorders, a detailed history, clinical evaluation, histopathologic features, and direct immunology immunofluorescence microscopy are essential. It is also helpful to recognize the type of blister, tense vs. flaccid; size, vesicle vs. bullae; arrangement and location of the blisters. A flaccid blister indicates that the separation is occurring within the epidermis, common to trauma from friction, i.e., new shoes. Linear grouping of vesicles is common in contact dermatitis. Zosteriform grouping along dermatomes can indicate shingles.

INTERPROFESSIONAL COLLABORATIVE MANAGEMENT
Pharmacologic Management
The goal of treatment for BP is to reduce the formation of blisters, promote the healing of erosions, decrease itching, and prevent secondary infection. The focus of pharmacological intervention is to reduce inflammation, control pruritus, and suppress the immune system. Topical steroids (class 1) are effective in treating limited or regional disease and are applied twice daily until lesions are healed.[1,10] Systemic oral corticosteroids remain the treatment of choice and should be initiated and continued until the skin is clear. Prednisone doses in the range of 0.5 to 0.75 mg/kg/day have proven to be as effective as higher doses.[1,10] Most patients will obtain control within 28 immunosuppressive drugs such as azathioprine can be combined with systemic prednisone to induce remission.[2] Azathioprine should be avoided in younger patients due to the

increased risk of malignancy. General response is within 3 to 6 months. Once remission is achieved, therapy should be discontinued and restarted for flares.[2] Low-dose oral pulse methotrexate may be an effective alternative in patients with generalized BP. Starting dose of 10 mg weekly increasing by 2.5 mg/week if the patient is continuing to develop more blisters. It may be overlapped with clobetasol to treat pruritus. Once there is a positive response, the dose should be tapered by 2.5 mg/week every 2 months.[2] Treatment with an anti-CD20 antibody (rituximab) and IV immunoglobulins should be considered in difficult-to-control cases.[11]

Indications for Referral
Patients should be referred to dermatology for biopsy confirmation, unless the provider is skilled in obtaining dermatology biopsies. Two specimens should be taken: one near the edge of a blister is to be sent for histology in formalin; the other perilesional, about 2 to 3 mm away from the blister edge, is to be sent for DIF in Michel's media.[3] Biopsies should be obtained prior to initiating systemic corticosteroids. Gentle skin care advice should be discussed. The management of BP requires a team approach with a dermatologist, the patient's primary care provider, and in-home nursing services if indicated. Patients should be referred to dermatology for confirmation of the diagnosis and guidance with therapeutic regimes. A consultation with a dentist and/or otolaryngologist is required for patients with oropharyngeal lesions.

LIFE-SPAN CONSIDERATIONS
BP is a disease that primarily affects older adults and has been associated with significant morbidity. Living with chronic BP can lead to isolation, anxiety, and depression. Special consideration needs to address coping strategies for older adults with BP. Generalized BP and high levels of autoantibody BP is associated with higher mortality within the first year of therapy. Other risk factors include higher doses of glucocorticosteroids and low albumin levels.[2] Involvement of family members and caregivers in the management plan will help to ensure adherence to the treatment regimen and prevention of complications.

COMPLICATIONS
Secondary infections can occur as a result of the presence of skin erosions and the use of immunosuppressive medications to treat the disease process. Infections may be localized or systemic, resulting in sepsis. Prolonged use of corticosteroids can lead to osteoporosis, bone fractures, and potentially to adrenal insufficiency. Immunosuppressive medications may result in bone marrow suppression and malignancy.

PATIENT AND FAMILY EDUCATION AND HEALTH PROMOTION
- Education about the disease process and safe use of medications, especially topical steroids, is important.
- Avoiding scratching and trauma to already fragile skin should be encouraged.
- Patients and families need to know when and how to best alert their health care provider about adverse effects of therapy.
- Health promotion activities include education on protective skin care practices to avoid trauma to the skin and treatment to prevent further skin breakdown and secondary

infection. Patients are encouraged to eat a balanced diet and wear loose clothing.

- Careful attention to wound care of nonintact skin is recommended to avoid complications.

REFERENCES

1. Schmidt, E., & Zillikens, D. (2013). Pemphigoid disease. *Lancet, 381,* 320–332.
2. Habif, T. P., Campbell, J. L., Chapman, M. S., et al. (2011). *Skin disease diagnosis and treatment* (3rd ed.). St Louis: Saunders.
3. Bobonich, M. A., & Nolen, M. E. (2015). *Dermatology for advanced practice clinicians.* Philadelphia: Wolter Kluwer.
4. Heelan, K. (2013). Cutaneous drug reactions in children: An update. *Paediatric Drugs, 15*(6), 493–503.
5. Lo Schiavo, A. (2013). Bullous pemphigoid: Etiology, pathogenesis, and inducing factors: Facts and controversies. *Clinics in Dermatology, 31*(4), 391–399.
6. Bernard, P., & Antonicelli, F. (2017). *American Journal of Clinical Dermatology, 18,* 513. https://doi.org/10.1007/s40257-017-0264-2.
7. Shah, A., Roberts, E., Engelina, S., & Carras, E. (2018). The Nikolsky sign. *British Journal of Hospital Medicine, 79*(9), C142–C144.
8. Wolff, K., Johnson, R., & Saavedra, A. (2013). Genetic and acquired bullous diseases. In *Fitzpatrick's color atlas and synopsis of clinical dermatology* (7th ed., pp. 107–108). New York: McGraw Hill.
9. Kershenovich, R. (2014). Diagnosis and classification of pemphigus and bullous pemphigoid. *Autoimmunity Reviews, 13*(4–5), 477–481.
10. Kasperkiewicz, M., Zillikens, D., & Schmidt, E. (2012). Pemphigoid diseases: Pathogenesis, diagnosis, and treatment. *Autoimmunity, 45*(1), 55–70.
11. Ahmed, A., Shetty, S., Kaveri, S., et al. (2016). Treatment of recalcitrant bullous pemphigoid(BP) with a novel protocol: A retrospective study with a 6-year follow up. *Journal of the American Academy of Dermatology, 74*(4), 700–708.

CHAPTER **44**

BURNS (MINOR)
Randy Michael Gordon

 Immediate emergency department referral or specialist referral is indicated for burns that cause respiratory injury (inhalation or facial burns); burns of the hands, feet, genitals, or perianal area; full-thickness burns of more than 2% of the total body surface area (TBSA); minor burns of more than 10% TBSA in patients older than 50 years; or burns of more than 15% TBSA in patients 10 to 50 years of age.

DEFINITION AND EPIDEMIOLOGY

The skin is the largest organ of the body and functions as an excellent barrier against external injury. A burn can disturb this barrier function as a result of trauma from electrical, thermal, or chemical agents. Thermal burns constitute a large majority of these injuries.[1]

Burn injuries are among the most devastating of all injuries and a major global public health crisis. Burns are the fourth most common type of trauma worldwide, following traffic accidents, falls, and interpersonal violence. According to the American Burn Association, approximately 450,000 patients receive hospital and emergency room treatment for burns each year.[2] Over 60% of the estimated US acute hospitalizations related to burn injury involve patients who are admitted to 127 burn centers.[1] Such centers now average over 200 annual admissions for burn injury and skin disorders requiring similar treatment. This percentage has increased steadily in recent decades as emergency care and transportation have improved. The most common burns occur in the home secondary to fire or flame and scalding or hot object contact; industrial accidents occur more often than electrical and chemical injuries.[1] Nearly 70% of burn victims are male, and risk is highest between the ages of 18 and 35.[2] Seventy-seven percent of all injuries are accounted for by fire or scalding; 43% of scald injuries occur in children less than 5 years of age.[2] Although overall survival exceeds 96%, fire, burn, and smoke inhalation still account for approximately 3400 deaths each year in the United States. Older adult patients understandably have a disproportionately higher death rate.[2] The risk of death from a major burn increases with larger burn size, older age, the presence of inhalation injury, and female sex. Statistically, Caucasians account for more injuries than patients of African-American, Hispanic, and other races combined.

PATHOPHYSIOLOGY

Skin consists of two layers: the epidermis and the dermis. Skin thickness varies both by age and anatomic location: it is relatively thinner at extremes of age, whereas it is thicker on the palms, soles, and upper back. Thus, the depth and severity of thermal injury varies by both the age of the victim and the anatomic location exposed.[2] The temperature or heat content of the burning agent and the duration of exposure determine the extent of burn injury. A burn wound is best described by the following three zones of injury: the zone of coagulation, in which tissue is irreversibly destroyed with thrombosis of blood vessels; the zone of stasis, in which there is stagnation of the microcirculation; and the zone of hyperemia, in which there is increased blood flow. The zone of stasis can become progressively more hypoxemic and ischemic if resuscitation is not adequate. In the zone of hyperemia, there is minimal damage to the cells and spontaneous recovery is likely.[2]

Although many factors may influence prognosis, the severity of the burn, the presence of inhalation injury, associated injuries, the patient's age, comorbid conditions, and acute organ system failure are most important. Thermal injury results in a spectrum of local and systemic homeostatic disorders that contribute to burn shock. These include disruption of normal cell membrane function, hormonal alterations, acid-base disturbance, hemodynamic changes, and hematologic derangement.[2] The fluid and electrolyte abnormalities seen in burn shock are largely the result of alterations of cell membrane potential causing intracellular influx of water and sodium, and extracellular migration of potassium, secondary to dysfunction of the sodium pump. In patients with burns greater than 60% of total body surface area (TBSA), depression of cardiac output results in a lack of response to aggressive volume resuscitation.[2]

CLINICAL PRESENTATION AND PHYSICAL EXAMINATION

The health care provider must obtain a full history of the mechanism of injury. The type of thermal or chemical exposure, the duration of exposure, and the time since the injury are important details. This history will help determine any risk for associated traumatic, pulmonary, or ocular injury. In assessing a patient with even a minor burn, any preexisting health condition is noted; some, such as diabetes or an immunocompromised status, affect the prognosis and disposition.[2]

The size of a burn injury is quantified as the percentage of body surface area involved. The Rule of Nines is a simple and commonly used method to calculate burn size. It divides the body into segments that are approximately 9% or multiples of 9%, with the perineum forming the remaining 1%. Because of the proportionately larger heads and smaller legs of infants and children, this method must be modified in pediatric burn injury.

A burn wound is defined by the size and depth of the wound. The size of the burn is quantified by the percentage of the TBSA burned. This percentage can be estimated in several ways. A quick method assumes that the back of the *patient's* hand is approximately 1% of the patient's TBSA. Therefore, the percentage of TBSA burned is the number of "hands" equal to the size of the burn.[2]

The depth of a burn is measured by the skin layers injured, and nonprofessionals still refer to depth of injury as first, second, or third degree. Clinicians more commonly define burns by partial-thickness or full-thickness depth of injury. First-degree (superficial or partial-thickness) burns involve only the epidermis, which with the injury becomes glossy, red, and painful (e.g., a sunburn). Second-degree (partial-thickness) burns involve the dermis, which may present as dull or glossy with pink, red, or white pigmentation. The area may blister and be severely painful. Third-degree burns are full-thickness burns that extend to the subcutaneous fat. The area appears matte and may be white, brown, red, or black. The hallmark of the third-degree burn is that the burn site is insensate (See Box 51.2 in Chapter 51).

The physical examination of the burn victim should be methodic and thorough. Initial general patient assessment should include evaluation for adequacy of airway, breathing, and circulation. The clinician should be alert for circumferential burns on a limb because the injury may compromise perfusion to the involved appendage. The depth, extent (percentage of TBSA burned), and location of the burn must be accurately determined and recorded. The examination should also include evaluation for any associated injuries.[3]

DIAGNOSTICS

The skin is a significant protective physiologic barrier; infection and metabolic abnormalities can result when this barrier is disrupted. Simple thermal burns do not require diagnostic testing. For more serious injuries, a complete blood count (CBC), glucose, electrolytes, blood urea nitrogen (BUN), creatinine, and urinalysis may be necessary. Amino acid catabolism and fluid or protein loss through burn wound exudate may create increased metabolic needs and thus require laboratory evaluation for adequacy of hydration and protein stores.[3]

A chest X-ray study is indicated for a suspected inhalation injury. Wound sites with delayed healing may require cultures to determine if infection is a factor. If wounds are not healing, wound biopsy may also be indicated to facilitate detection of any underlying comorbidities or malignant neoplasms.

In the case of a chemical burn, the local poison control center can assist in determining toxicity of and antidote for the chemical. If possible, the patient should provide the chemical container or a complete description of the substance to aid in identification.[3,4]

DIFFERENTIAL DIAGNOSIS

 Priority differentials include (1) chemical burns, (2) electrical burns, (3) thermal burns, and (4) Ritter disease.

The differential diagnosis is determined primarily by history. Certain skin conditions (e.g., staphylococcal scaled skin

---

syndrome [SSSS]) and toxic epidermal necrolysis can resemble a generalized burn.

Interprofessional Collaborative Management

The severity, extent, and location of the burn guides the clinician's decisions for patient management. The American Burn Association classifies burn risk levels as major/high, moderate, and minor/low. Low-risk patients are those aged 10 to 50 years. High-risk patients are those younger than 10 years and older than 50 years or those with underlying medical conditions, such as heart disease, diabetes, or pulmonary problems. Minor burns involve less than 15% of TBSA in the 10- to 50-year age group or less than 10% of TBSA in patients younger than 10 years or older than 50 years. Minor full-thickness burns are less than 2% of TBSA in all age groups.[1]

NONPHARMACOLOGICAL MANAGEMENT

Minor burns without associated injuries can be managed in the clinician's office or outpatient setting. The goal of initial treatment for a partial-thickness thermal burn is to reduce heat and tissue injury by irrigation with cool tap water. Similarly, initial therapy for a chemical burn is to remove the offending chemical and garments, and then begin aggressive irrigation. In rare cases involving certain industrial chemicals (e.g., metal sodium), water should not be used because it can actually worsen the burn; it is important to identify the source of the chemical burn when treatment is initiated. Information as to appropriate management of a topical chemical exposure may be found in the industrial facility's Material Safety Data Sheet (MSDS) manual.

Intact blisters in burn injuries should not be ruptured because they maintain a physiologic protection function while underlying tissues begin the healing process.[3] The burn wound needs to be cleaned with mild soap and water or saline; unroofed blisters and devitalized tissue should be debrided. Finally, a dressing must be applied.

Pharmacological Management

There are several ways to dress minor burns. First, the burn is covered with a thin layer of antimicrobial cream or ointment; the most common topical therapy used is silver sulfadiazine cream (Silvadene).[3] Silvadene cannot be used on patients with sulfa allergy and should be used cautiously on patients with significant pain. This product may cause tattooing or staining and may not be appropriate for use on facial burns. When

Silvadene is used, the wound should be washed and redressed twice daily. A non-adherent secondary dressing is used to protect the burn from contamination until the site is healed. Advances in wound technology now provide silver in various delivery forms, including gels, hydrocolloids, and non-adherent dressing sheets; the slow release of silver in these formulations lengthens the time between dressing changes from 2 to 7 days, thus promoting patient comfort and decreasing trauma to the healing wound.

Some burns may require open dressings, in which a topical agent is applied without a covering. The most common sites for open dressings are the face, neck, and perineum. The wound should be thoroughly washed two or three times a day and the topical agent reapplied. Aloe vera in a gel, cream, or ointment formulation may promote healing and soothe painful areas.

Minor burns are painful, and treatment should include analgesics as needed. Ibuprofen and naproxen have antiprostaglandin properties and are effective anti-inflammatory and analgesic medications. Acetaminophen and narcotic agents, used over a short time period, are also appropriate analgesics though patient age and comorbidities are a consideration. Tetanus prophylaxis should be given as indicated.

INDICATIONS FOR REFERRAL OR HOSPITALIZATION

The American Burn Association provides guidelines for referral to a burn center, in addition to indications based on burn depth.[1] Any burn injury larger than the American Burn Association's criteria for minor burns should be referred to the nearest emergency department for further evaluation and hospitalization as necessary. Minor burns typically qualify for ambulatory care. Minor burns should be isolated, should not cross joints or be circumferential, and should not meet criteria for burn center care. Consider the patient's social situation and medical comorbidities when electing ambulatory care. Burns that may result in functional or cosmetic impairment, have an associated injury, or involve high-risk patients require a referral for emergency evaluation.

Burns that fail to heal within 2 to 3 weeks require further evaluation with a wound specialist. Consultation with a physiatrist or physical or occupational therapist should be considered when appropriate to initiate gentle range-of-motion exercises and to prevent localized contractures. Most partial-thickness burns heal within several days to a week without complications. Some swelling may occur in extremities affected by burns, which can be diminished by elevation of the limb above heart level. Some minor burns may become infected. Infections may require systemic antibiotic therapy or a change in topical therapy to manage bioburden or bacteria in the wound. Burns occurring over a joint may require a splint to promote comfort and wound healing.

Life-Span Considerations

Older adult patients exhibit varying degrees of immunosuppression. They are more at risk for complications such as infection and delayed healing with minor burns. Since there can be some systemic absorption of topical sulfa products (e.g., Silvadene), consider consultation with the patient's obstetrician or pediatrician with pregnant and nursing mothers.

PATIENT AND FAMILY EDUCATION

- All burn patients should be seen as soon as possible after injury for a clinical assessment of the depth and extent of the burn along with evaluation for additional injuries.
- Patients should be given clear discharge instructions that explain topical wound care.
- Patients should be given clear instructions about detecting any signs and symptoms of infection or vascular compromise and need to seek medical attention.
- If an extremity is involved, it should be elevated for control of pain and swelling.
- Pain medications may be required; if one is prescribed, an explanation of how to use the analgesic and of the potential side effects is also necessary.

HEALTH PROMOTION

Home and work safety is the cornerstone of burn prevention. Manufacturer recommendations for protective equipment such as gloves, protective eyewear, and ventilation with certain household cleaning products and at the work site can prevent chemical and inhalation burns. To prevent electrical burns, the electrical current must be turned off before any electrical repairs are attempted, electrical outlets should have covers, and frayed electrical cords should be repaired or the fixture discarded. A listing of chemicals used in the workplace, including product ingredients and treatment indicated for accidental exposures, should be accessible to all employees.

In the home, a working smoke alarm and fire extinguisher are essential for early fire detection and intervention. Lowering of hot water temperatures will reduce the risk of scald injuries, the most common source of burn injury in children. Pot and pan handles should be turned over the cooktop, away from the reach of children. Loose clothing should be restricted when cooking or when around open flames. Everyone should be familiar with the "stop, drop, and roll" technique to control or to extinguish fire if their clothes ignite, and children should be taught about the hazards of matches and fireworks. Similarly, education should be provided about the importance of wearing sunscreen and the damaging effects of the sun's rays.

REFERENCES

1. American Burn Association. Burn incidence and treatment in the United States—2016 fact sheet. Retrieved from http://ameriburn.org/who-we-are/media/burn-incidence-fact-sheet. (Accessed 29 November 2017).
2. DeKoning, E. (2016). Thermal burns. In J. E. Tintinalli, J. Stapczynski, O. Ma, D. M. Yealy, G. D. Meckler, & D. M. Cline (Eds.), *Tintinalli's emergency medicine: A comprehensive study guide, 8e.* New York, NY: McGraw-Hill. Retrieved from http://accessmedicine.mhmedical.com.chamberlainuniversity.idm.oclc.org/content.aspx?bookid=1658&sectionid=109438787. (Accessed 29 November 2017).
3. Benedetto, P. X., Taylor, J. S., & Sood, A. (2012). Occupational noneczematous skin diseases due to biologic, physical, and chemical agents: Introduction. In L. A. Goldsmith, S. I. Katz, B. A. Gilchrest, A. S. Paller, D. J. Leffell, & K. Wolff (Eds.), *Fitzpatrick's dermatology in general medicine, 8e.* New York, NY: McGraw-Hill. Chapter 212. Retrieved from http://accessmedicine.mhmedical.com.chamberlainuniversity.idm.oclc.org/content.aspx?bookid=392&sectionid=41138945. (Accessed 29 November 2017).
4. Chiang, A., Bruze, M., Fregas, S., & Gruvberger, B. (2018). Chemical Burns. In S. M. John, et al. (Eds.), *Kanerva's occupational dermatology.* Springer International Publishing AG, part of Springer Nature. https://doi.org/10.1007/978-3-319-40221-5_13-2. (Retrieved 1 August 2019).

CUTANEOUS ADVERSE DRUG REACTIONS

Glen Blair

 Immediate medical attention indicated for erythroderma, facial edema, mucositis, skin tenderness, and blistering, which may signify a more serious drug reaction.

Cutaneous drug reactions occur in 2% to 3% of patients taking oral, transcutaneous, and parenteral medications.[1] Given the number of prescriptions provided by primary care providers, it is incumbent on the provider to anticipate and respond quickly to any cutaneous eruption as possibly being medication mediated. Any time a dermatosis presents in a symmetrical manner, the provider should consider an adverse drug reaction (ADR) as the possible initiator of the dermatosis.[2]

Cutaneous ADRs can vary from relatively benign exanthematous eruptions to life-threatening eruptions such as toxic epidermal necrolysis (TEN). Being able to quickly identify the type of eruption and the possible causative agent are imperative for expedient patient care. Discontinuation of the suspect drug is necessary for dermatitis resolution and dermatology referral for diagnostic biopsy and treatment is often required for generalized cutaneous ADRs.

Acute exanthematous generalized pustulosis (AGEP), exanthematous drug reactions, fixed drug eruptions (FDE), drug reaction with eosinophilia and systemic symptoms (DRESS), and the continuum of Stevens-Johnson syndrome (SJS)/ TEN will be discussed in this chapter. Box 45.1 lists the most common medications associated with each cutaneous eruption, but the list is by no means exhaustive.

ACUTE GENERALIZED EXANTHEMATOUS PUSTULOSIS
Definition and Epidemiology

AGEP is an acute pustular eruption characterized by dozens to hundreds of pinhead sized pustules on a background of edematous erythema, with accentuation at flexural areas of the body.[3] Facial edema may be present.[4] This syndrome is caused by drugs in 90% of the cases, the most common medicines being aminopenicillin and macrolide antibiotics, antifungals, the calcium channel blocker diltiazem and antimalarials. Symptoms appear hours to days after the introduction of the offending drug.

Diagnostics

Patients may present with fever, leukocytosis, and mild eosinophilia. Transient elevation in serum creatinine and transaminases are rare but may occur in the older patient.[5]

Management

Healing begins as soon as the offending drug is identified and discontinued and may be characterized by generalized desquamation. Hospitalization may be required for severe cases and the patient may be monitored for liver toxicity.[4] Topical antibacterial soaps and petrolatum-based emollients may be used during the recovery phase to prevent secondary bacterial infection and to promote skin healing.[5]

BOX **45.1**

Common Medications Associated With Cutaneous Eruption

ACUTE EXANTHEMATOUS GENERALIZED PUSTULOSIS
Aminopenicillins
Anticonvulsants
Calcium channel blockers
Enalapril
Griseofulvin
Itraconazole
Macrolides
Nonsteroidal antiinflammatory drugs (NSAIDs)
Quinolones

EXANTHEMATOUS
Acetaminophen
Aminopenicillins
Carbamazepine
Cephalosporins
Macrolides
NSAIDs
Phenytoin
Quinolones
Trimethoprim-sulfamethoxazole (TMP-SMX)
Tuberculostatic agents

FIXED DRUG ERUPTION
Acetaminophen
Antimalarials
Barbiturate
Dapsone
NSAIDs
Penicillins
Quinolones
Tetracyclines
TMP-SMX
Drug reaction with eosinophilia and systemic symptoms allopurinol
Carbamazepine
Dapsone
Lamotrigine
Minocycline
Phenytoin
Sulfonamide antibiotics
Vancomycin

STEVENS-JOHNSON SYNDROME-TOXIC EPIDERMAL NECROLYSIS
Allopurinol
Carbamazepine
Chloramphenicol
Lamotrigine
Macrolide antibiotics
NSAIDs
Penicillin antibiotics
Phenobarbital
Phenytoin
Quinolones
Sulfonamides
Valproic acid

EXANTHEMATOUS DRUG ERUPTIONS
Definition and Epidemiology

Also known as *morbilliform* drug eruptions, exanthematous drug eruptions are the most common form of ADR, accounting for 95% of all cases and characterized by diffuse and symmetric distribution of erythematous macules and papules.[6] In more severe forms, mucous membranes and the face may be involved and the syndrome must be distinguished from AGEP, DRESS, or SJS/TEN.[7] It is thought to be a delayed, Type IV, T-cell mediated immune reaction where the drugs act as haptens to become full antigens. Offending medications include aminopenicillins, cephalosporins, macrolides, quinolones, sulfonamides like trimethoprim-sulfamethoxazole (TMP-SMX), anticonvulsants like carbamazepine and phenytoin, and some non-steroidal antiinflammatory drugs (NSAIDs). Patients with underlying immunodeficiency or concomitant viral infection may be more susceptible to these outbreaks.[8]

The eruption develops days to 2 weeks after starting medicine but may be sooner in previously sensitized individuals. Drugs implicated in the development of AGEP include aminopenicillins, macrolide antibiotics, calcium channel blockers, and NSAIDs.

Clinical Presentation

Systemic symptoms may include pruritus, low-grade fever, and mild eosinophilia. Progression to erythroderma, facial edema, mucositis, skin tenderness, and blistering may signify a more serious drug reaction and patients should be directed to seek immediate medical attention.[8]

Management

Recovery is typically uneventful, occurring within 2 weeks of drug identification and discontinuation and may be characterized by desquamation. Treatment is aimed at identifying the causative medication and discontinuing it, followed by topical steroids and antihistamines for symptomatic relief.

FIXED DRUG ERUPTION
Definition and Epidemiology

FDEs are characterized by the development of single or multiple red, brown, or black macules or plaques that present at the same sites upon re-exposure to the causative agent. Drugs known to cause an FDE are many and include antibiotics, NSAIDs, acetaminophen, barbiturates, and antimalarials.[9]

Lesions can develop within hours or weeks after exposure. Systemic symptoms are typically absent, but lesions themselves may burn or itch. Common sites affected include the lips, genitalia, perianal area, hands, and feet although FDEs may occur on any body surface area (BSA). Oral lesions may be erosive. FDE will occasionally present with atypical features and needs to be distinguished from Stevens-Johnson syndrome-toxic epidermal necrolysis (SJS/TEN), cellulitis, or large plaque parapsoriasis.[10]

Management

Lesions resolve in 7 to 10 days after discontinuance of the offending drug and may heal with postinflammatory hyperpigmentation. Treatment is largely symptomatic with the aim of reducing itch through the use of topical corticosteroids and oral antihistamines.

DRUG REACTION WITH EOSINOPHILIA AND SYSTEMIC SYSTEMS
Definition and Epidemiology

DRESS is a rare but potentially fatal drug reaction that includes both dermatologic and systemic manifestations, developing 2 to 8 weeks after exposure to the offending agent. It is often associated with the reactivation of the human herpes virus-6. Drugs implicated in the development of DRESS include several anticonvulsants, allopurinol, dapsone, and sulfonamides (see Box 45.1).

Clinical Presentation

A morbilliform eruption develops on the face and upper body that becomes edematous and may be accompanied be vesicles, bullae, and follicular or non-follicular pustules.

Facial edema is a hallmark of the eruption and occurs in 75% of patients.[11] Systemic symptoms may be present and include fever, malaise, lymphadenopathy, and arthralgia. Eosinophilia and leukocytosis are usually present. Acute hepatitis, myocarditis, interstitial pneumonitis, interstitial nephritis, and thyroiditis are complications that may require hospitalization and serial monitoring. Severe hepatitis is responsible for the largest share of DRESS-related deaths.[12]

Management

Hospitalization is often required for stabilization and monitoring.[13] Identification and discontinuance of the offending agent is necessary for recovery which may take weeks to months and may be complicated by relapse without re-exposure. In addition to support of affected organ systems, acute management may include topical and systemic corticosteroids for dermatologic symptoms.

Differential Diagnosis

Differential diagnosis includes AGEP, bacterial or viral skin infections, SJS/TEN, lymphoma, and acute cutaneous lupus erythematosus.

STEVENS-JOHNSON SYNDROME/TOXIC EPIDERMAL NECROLYSIS
Definition and Epidemiology

SJS/TEN represents a spectrum of mucocutaneous eruptions of varying severity that are potentially life threatening. The majority of cases are drug mediated, but a small percentage of cases occur with infection with Mycoplasma pneumonia. Medicines known to trigger SJS/TEN include macrolide and penicillin antibiotics, sulfonamides, NSAIDs, and several anticonvulsants.

Clinical Presentation

SJS/TEN is characterized by detachment of the epidermis from the dermis and manifests on the skin as blisters and erosions. Characterization of the dermatitis as SJS or TEN is determined by the percentage of BSA affected; SJS is characterized by BSA of less than 10%, TEN by BSA of greater than 30%. The space between 10% and 30% is referred to as the SJS/TEN overlap. Involvement of mucous membranes of the buccal, ocular, and genital mucosa is present in over 90% of SJS/TEN patients.[14] Patients with certain HLA phenotypes and patients with HIV infection may be at significantly higher risk.[15]

SJS/TEN develops within the first 8 weeks of drug initiation. Fever, oral, and ocular symptoms sometimes precede the cutaneous reaction by several days.

Constitutional symptoms of malaise, sore throat, arthralgias, and stinging eyes may be present. A central and facial dermatitis begins and spreads peripherally. Lesions develop as erythematous, flat macules, some with vesicles, that develop a hazy appearance after a few days.[16] The skin is tender to the touch and shears easily to touch (the *Nikolsky sign*). As the syndrome progresses, cardiovascular and metabolic disturbances occur, as do ocular, gastrointestinal, pulmonary, renal, and neurologic symptoms.[17] Mortality runs to 30% depending on the degree of skin involvement.

Diagnosis

Diagnosis is based on clinical presentation and recognition of the skin manifestation, as well as a skin punch biopsy which shows dermal inflammation and epidermal necrosis.

Management

Laboratory testing is not specific, but may highlight organ and metabolic sequelae and should be monitored closely. Treatment in a burn unit is optimal where appropriate skin care and hemodynamic support can be provided.

Differential Diagnosis

Differential diagnosis includes exanthematous drug eruption, DRESS, AGEP, FDE, and erythema multiforme.

REFERENCES

1. Kooken, A. K., & Tomecki, K. J. (2012). Drug eruptions. Retrieved from Clevelandclinicmeded.com/medicalpubs/diseasemanagement/dermatology/drug-eruptions. April.
2. Blume, J. E. (2017). Drug eruptions. Retrieved from Emedicine.medscape.com/article/1049474-overview#a5. July 11.
3. Speeckaert, M. M., Speeckaert, R., Lambert, J., & Brochez, L. (2010). Acute generalized exanthematous pustulosis: An overview of the clinical, immunological and diagnostic concepts. *European Journal of Dermatology: EJD, 20,* 425.
4. Blair, G., Griffin, V., Bobonich, M. A., & Nolen, M. E. (2015). Cutaneous drug eruptions. In M. A. Bobonich & M. E. Nolen (Eds.), *Dermatology for advanced practice clinicians* (pp. 276–277). China: Wolters Kluwer.
5. Sidoroff, A., & Chia-Yu, C. (2017). Acute generalized exanthematous pustulosis (AGEP). Retrieved from www.uptodate.com/contents/acute-generalized-exanthematous-pustulosis-agep. July 6.
6. Blair, et al. (2015). 274.
7. Ukoha, U. T., Pandya, A. G., & Dominguez, A. R. (2015). Morbilliform drug eruptions. In J. Hall & B. Hall (Eds.), *Cutaneous drug eruptions*. London: Springer.
8. Tohyama, M., & Hashimoto, K. (2011). New aspects of drug-induced hypersensitivity syndrome. *The Journal of Dermatology, 38,* 222.
9. Hall, A. (2019). Fixed drug eruption (reaction). In *Atlas of male genital dermatology*. Cham: Springer.
10. Paulmann, M., & Mockenhaupt, M. (2015). Severe drug-induced skin reactions: Clinical features, diagnosis, etiology and therapy. *Journal of the German Society of Dermatology, 13*(7), 625–643.
11. Skowron, F., Bensaid, B., & Balme, B. (2015). Drug reaction with eosinophilia and systemic symptoms (DRESS): Clinicopathological study of 45 cases. *Journal of the European Academy of Dermatology and Venereology, 29,* 2199–2205. doi:10.1111/jdv.13212.
12. Ichai, P., Laurent-Bellue, A., Saliba, F., et al. (2017). Acute liver failure/injury related to drug reaction with eosinphilia and systemic symptoms: Outcomes and prognostic factors. *Transplantation, 101*(8), 1830–1837.
13. Blair, et al. (2015). 277.
14. Stern, R. S., & Divito, S. J. (2017). Stevens-Johnson syndrome and toxic epidermal necrolysis: Associations, outcomes, and pathobiology—Thirty years of progress but still much to be done. *The Journal of Investigative Dermatology, 137*(5), 1004–1008. doi:10.1016/j.jid.2017.01.003.
15. Stewart, A., Lehloenya, R., Boulle, A., Waal, R., Maartens, G., & Cohen, K. (2016). Severe antiretroviral-associated skin reactions in South African patients: A case series and case–control analysis. *Pharmacoepidemiology and Drug Safety, 25,* 1313–1319. doi:10.1002/pds.4067.
16. High, W. Stevens-Johnson Syndrome and toxic epidermal necrolysis: pathogenesis, clinical manifestations and diagnosis. Up to Date, https://www.uptodate.com/contents/stevens-johnson-syndrome-and-toxic-epidermal-necrolysis-pathogenesis-clinical-manifestations-and-diagnosis, site update March, 2019. (Accessed 1 August 2019).
17. Blair, et al. (2015). 280.

CHAPTER 46

ECZEMATOUS DERMATITIS

Alex Bahadori

DEFINITION AND EPIDEMIOLOGY

Eczematous dermatitis (eczema) is a pruritic inflammatory skin disorder characterized by exacerbations and remissions of dry and itchy red skin. There are many different types of eczema including atopic dermatitis (AD), asteatotic eczema, contact dermatitis, nummular eczema, dyshidrotic eczema, stasis dermatitis, and id reaction (interface reaction). The most common type of eczema is AD. Onset of AD is most common at 3 to 6 months of age, affecting 1 in 10 children and 1 in 10 to 14 adults in the United States.[1] AD is also associated with other atopic (immunoglobulin E [IgE]) diseases (e.g., asthma, allergic rhinitis, urticaria, or acute reactions to foods).[1-3] AD affects persons of all races, with the international prevalence on the rise.[4] Patients with a tendency to develop these conditions are referred to as atopics. Many atopic patients also have a family history of atopy.

Eczema is often called "the itch that rashes." Patients initially are bothered by incessant itching, scratch an area, and then develop a rash at the site of scratching. Eventually, lichenification may develop at the site if it remains untreated.

PATHOPHYSIOLOGY

The primary cause of eczema continues to be poorly understood. Primary immune dysfunction resulting in IgE sensitization and/or a primary defect in the epithelial barrier with resultant secondary immunologic dysregulation have been proposed as potential underlying causes of most types of eczema.[4]

CLINICAL PRESENTATION AND PHYSICAL EXAMINATION

Eczema is characterized by pruritic, erythematous, dry patches of skin, often with scale. Linear excoriations may be seen as a secondary change (Fig. 46.1). The borders of eczematous lesions are not initially well defined. Crusting and oozing are common. Thickened skin with well-defined skin markings (lichenification) may develop in long-standing lesions as the result of scratching. In infants, eruption may involve the cheeks, scalp, forehead, and extensor extremities.[1] In adults, eczema may be generalized, with a tendency to develop lesions on the face, neck, flexural folds, wrists, and dorsa of the feet. Nummular eczema is typically round or coin shaped, and commonly appears on the upper and lower extremities. Dyshidrotic eczema may appear as dryness, patches, and/or fissures on the palms of the hands and the soles of the feet. Id reactions manifest as an acute onset of a pruritic, erythematous, and papulovesicular eruption commonly occurring on the upper and lower extremities. Id reactions occur as the result of an infection elsewhere in the body, particularly fungal infections such as tinea pedis (see Chapter 47).[5] Asteatotic dermatitis is characterized

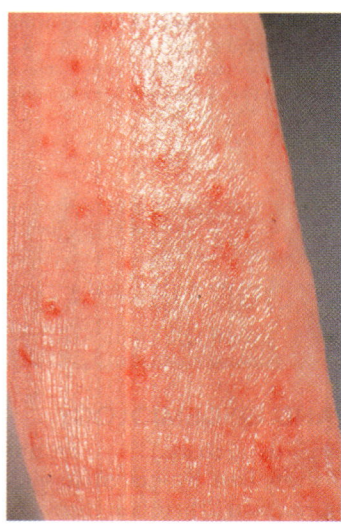

FIG. 46.1 Atopic dermatitis. Note the erythema, excoriation, and lichenification. (From Goldman, L., & Scafer, A. I. [2012]. *Goldman's cecil medicine* [24th ed.]. Philadelphia: Saunders.)

by pruritic, dry, and cracked skin with irregular scaling. It most commonly occurs on the shins of older adult patients, but it may also occur on the hands and the trunk. Stasis dermatitis occurs on the lower extremities and is usually an early cutaneous sign of chronic venous insufficiency. It typically manifests with erythematous inflamed skin in areas of edema on the lower legs. Eventually, these areas typically become hyperpigmented in appearance. Contact dermatitis (both allergic and irritant types) causes a rash on the surface of the skin that was exposed. The provider may gain clues as to the offending agent based on the location and distribution of the rash (Table 46.1). In irritant contact dermatitis, symptoms may develop minutes to hours after exposure, or they may develop months after chronic exposure. A well-demarcated area of erythema, scaling, or crusting will occur at the site of the exposure. The hands are the most common area affected, followed by wrists and forearms. Patch testing is a non invasive way of testing for multiple allergens at the same time. There are essentially no risks. The patches containing a small amount of potential allergens, are placed on the back and results are read on Day 2 of testing.[6]

DIAGNOSTICS
Essential Diagnostics

Eczematous dermatitis is a clinical diagnosis that is based on a careful history and physical examination. There are no routine imaging or serological lab tests required for diagnosis.

Additional Diagnostics

KOH preparation, skin biopsy, and skin patch testing (mainly for contact dermatitis)

Differential Diagnosis

 Priority differentials include (1) mycosis fungoides, which typically manifests as hypopigmentation with dermatitis, (2) immunodeficiency, which should be considered with severe itching in the setting of recurrent infection, and (3) scabies, which can be confirmed by scraping a burrow and microscopic identification of mites, eggs, or feces.

TABLE 46.1	Contact Dermatitis: Distribution Diagnosis
Location	**Material**
Scalp and ears	Shampoo, hair dyes, topical medicines, metal earrings, eyeglasses
Eyelid	Nail polish (transferred by rubbing), cosmetics, contact lens solution, metal eyelash curlers
Face	Airborne allergens (poison ivy from burning leaves, ragweed), cosmetics, sunscreens, acne medications (e.g., benzoyl peroxide), aftershave lotion
Neck	Necklaces, airborne allergens (ragweed), perfumes, aftershave lotion
Trunk	Topical medication, sunscreens, poison ivy, plants (phototoxic reactions), clothing, undergarments (e.g., spandex bra, elastic waistband), metal belt buckles
Axillae	Deodorant (axillary vault), clothing (axillary folds)
Arms	Same as hand; watch and watchband
Hands	Soaps and detergents, foods, poison ivy, industrial solvents and oils, cement, metal (pots, rings), topical medications, rubber gloves in surgeons
Genitals	Poison ivy (transferred by hand), rubber condoms
Anal region	Hemorrhoid preparations (benzocaine, dibucaine [nupercaine]), nystatin and triamcinolone (Mycolog II) cream
Lower legs	Topical medication (benzocaine, lanolin, neomycin), dye in socks
Feet	Shoes (rubber or leather), cement spilling into boots

From Habif, T. P. (2015). *Clinical dermatology* (6th ed.). Philadelphia: Elsevier.

Psoriasis is characterized by well-demarcated, intensely erythematous plaques with characteristic overlying silvery scale, usually located on the scalp, elbows, and knees.

Seborrheic dermatitis can be differentiated from eczema by its presentation and distribution. Seborrheic dermatitis typically manifests as nonpruritic, mildly erythematous plaques with waxy, yellow scale on the face, postauricular area, and scalp.

Tinea (or superficial fungal infection) lesions have a sharply demarcated border with scale at the edge and central clearing. They are usually limited in number and sometimes form an arciform array. A scraping of the border of the lesion and treatment of the removed sample with potassium hydroxide (KOH) reveal hyphae on microscopic evaluation. The diagnosis of eczema is differentiated on the basis of the presence of xerosis, age at presentation, history of atopic diseases, early onset, and a chronic relapsing course.[4]

INTERPROFESSIONAL COLLABORATIVE MANAGEMENT
Nonpharmacologic Management

Patient education is the cornerstone of eczema treatment. Patients must be encouraged to avoid rubbing and scratching the involved areas because this exacerbates the condition. The goals of treatment are management of pruritus to prevent scratching, continual moisturization for dryness, and control of inflammation of the eczematous lesions to maintain a healthy skin barrier.[2,3] Patients should also be encouraged to avoid any known aggravating factors or triggers. This is particularly important in cases with contact and AD. Phototherapy with narrow-band ultraviolet B light, and photochemotherapy with psoralen plus ultraviolet A light, may be helpful for some types of eczema when standard therapies have failed.

Pharmacologic Management

Antihistamines can control itching, allay anxiety, and induce sleep. Diphenhydramine (Benadryl) and hydroxyzine (Atarax) are the drugs of choice, but should be used cautiously in older adults. Nonsedating antihistamines such as levocetirizine (Xyzal) and loratadine (Claritin) may be preferred for daytime use and prolonged control of itching.

Hydration with a tepid water bath can be soothing during an acute flare of many types of eczema. The bath should be immediately followed by the application of a bland emollient such as hydrated petrolatum or Aquaphor. Other measures that may improve symptoms include wearing soft cotton clothing, maintaining cool temperatures, using a cool mist humidifier, and washing with mild detergents.[4,7]

Topical corticosteroid creams, ointments, and lotions are usually necessary to alleviate inflammation during an acute flare. Hydrocortisone 1%, a mild topical steroid, can be applied sparingly to affected areas two or three times daily for both adult and pediatric patients.[7] Acute and persistent flares of eczema may require stronger topical steroid medications such as triamcinolone 0.1% cream. Typically these medications are applied twice daily for 2 weeks, and then every 3 days as needed for control. Stronger topical steroids should not be used on the face, groin, breasts, or axillae. Use of topical steroids is limited by the wide distribution of steroid-responsive elements found in various cells and tissues. Long-term use may lead to skin atrophy such as striae, telangiectasia, and systemic side effects including growth restriction in children and glaucoma.[4] Topical corticosteroids should be discontinued when the inflammation has subsided, whereas the use of lubricants and emollients should be continued.

The nonsteroidal calcineurin inhibitor topical medications such as tacrolimus (Protopic) and pimecrolimus (Elidel) can be helpful for managing chronic moderate to severe eczema. Other newer classes of nonsteroidal medications such as Eucrisa, a phosphodiesterase 4 (PDE4) inhibitor, have been approved to target the inflammatory component. These medications are not indicated for patients younger than 2 years. They are considered safe to use on delicate skin areas such as the face, groin (external skin only), axillae, and breasts.

Newer classes of drugs recently developed and approved include the topical immunomodulatory tacrolimus and the targeted biologic dupilumab (Dupixet) which when combined with topical steroids can significantly improve clinical outcomes.[8]

Eczema patients are predisposed to skin infections. Only overt secondary bacterial, fungal, or viral infections should be treated with appropriate topical and systemic antibiotics.[7] *Staphylococcus aureus* is a common colonizer of the skin in AD and is thought to trigger multiple inflammatory cascades.[4] Additionally, those patients with id reactions may need the underlying cause also treated. Often times tinea pedis is the offending fungus, and an antifungal may need to be prescribed.

Systemic corticosteroids are seldom used in the treatment of AD and should be reserved for extreme cases that are not controlled with topical treatments.

Indications for Referral or Hospitalization

Failure to respond to topical treatments requires referral to a dermatology nurse practitioner or dermatologist for management. An eruption that is recalcitrant to treatment may resemble eczema, but actually be another disorder. For example, mycosis fungoides can sometimes resemble eczema in its early stages.

In addition, evaluation and management by an allergy nurse practitioner or allergist may be needed for optimum care of a patient with known allergies or when an allergic role is suspected in the disease.

Hospitalization may be required for intensive topical or systemic treatments. Hospitalization is also indicated for patients with secondary infection who are unresponsive to outpatient therapies.

LIFE-SPAN CONSIDERATIONS

Use of high-potency topical corticosteroids should be minimized with the very young and very old. Long-term use of topical corticosteroids should be avoided, if possible, for all age groups.

COMPLICATIONS

Secondary microbial infections are common from chronic excoriations and defects in innate immunity.

Group A β-hemolytic streptococci and staphylococci are the most common bacterial organisms. Bacterial secondary infection should be suspected, cultured when indicated, and treated in patients with purulent or weepy lesions and in cases of eczema that are slow to respond to standard therapies. Cephalexin (Keflex) is effective and well tolerated. It has been found that dilute bleach baths consisting of quarter to half cup regular strength bleach per 1 full bathtub of water (except on face and neck) twice weekly and intranasal mupirocin (Bactroban) for 3 months led to reduction in bacterial superinfections of the skin.[7]

Patients with eczema have a higher incidence of herpes simplex virus infection, molluscum contagiosum, and warts. These infections can be more frequent and widespread in patients with AD. Increases in cutaneous viral infections are related to defective cell-mediated immunity in the skin as well as to the use of topical steroids.

A particularly serious viral complication of eczematous dermatitis is eczema herpeticum. A patient with this condition has an underlying skin disorder (usually AD) and develops a widespread eruption of vesicles and erosions when experiencing a primary herpes infection or herpes infection reactivation. A Giemsa-stained scraping of the base of a vesicle will reveal multinucleated giant cells. Eczema herpeticum should be treated with oral antiviral medications (e.g., valacyclovir [Valtrex]) and supportive care.

PATIENT AND FAMILY EDUCATION

- Patients with eczema should understand that the goal is diligent avoidance of known triggers, heavy skin moisturization, and if a flare occurs, timely management of symptoms.
- Teach patients that weeks or months of control may be followed by sudden exacerbations.

- Patients should understand the proper use of antihistamines to control itching.
- Patients and caretakers require careful education on proper bathing and moisturizing, and their role in decreasing the need for topical corticosteroids.
- Patients should use a humidifier year-round to avoid dryness induced by winter dry air and air conditioning.
- People with AD should be aware of the drying effect of soaps. Mild unscented soaps can be used to wash the body folds and genital area but should be avoided on other body parts. Laundry detergents (e.g., All Free and Clear) should also be mild to prevent irritation.

HEALTH PROMOTION

Identification of individually specific aggravating factors, such as stress, infections, perspiration, weather change, dry skin, obesity, and contact sensitivity, will aid in management of all types of eczematous dermatitis.

REFERENCES

1. Silverberg, J. I. (2014). Atopic dermatitis. *Journal of the American Medical Association dermatology, 150*(12), 1380.
2. Eichenfield, L. F., Tom, W. L., Berger, T. G., et al. (2014). Guidelines of care for the management of atopic dermatitis—Section 1. Diagnosis and assessment of atopic dermatitis. *Journal of the American Academy of Dermatology, 70,* 338–351.
3. Habif, T. P. (2015). *Clinical dermatology* (6th ed.). Philadelphia: Elsevier.
4. Wollenberg, A., Oranje, A., Deleuran, M., et al. (2016). ETFAD/EADV Eczema task force 2015 position paper on diagnosis and treatment of atopic dermatitis in adult and paediatric patients. *Journal of the European Academy of Dermatology and Venereology: JEADV, 30*(5), 729–747.
5. Likit, M., Durdu, M., & Karakas, M. (2012). Cutaneous id reactions: A comprehensive review of clinical manifestations, epidemiology, etiology, and management. *Critical Reviews in Microbiology, 38*(3), 191–202.
6. Johnston, G. A., Exton, L. S., Mohd Mustapa, M. F., et al. (2017). British Association of Dermatologists'guidelines for the management of contact dermatitis 2017. *British Journal of Dermatology, 176*(2), 317–329.
7. Lio, P. A., Lee, M., LeBouidge, J., et al. (2014). Clinical management of atopic dermatitis: Practice highlights and updates from the atopic dermatitis practice parameter 2012. *The Journal of Allergy and Clinical Immunology. In Practice, 2*(4), 361–369.
8. Gooderham, M. J., et al. (2018). Dupilumab: A review of its use in the treatment of atopic dermatitis. *Journal of the American Academy of Dermatology, 78*(3), 3, S28-S36.

CHAPTER **47**

INFECTIONS AND INFESTATIONS

Duellyn Pandis

Infections and infestations are common dermatologic disorders in primary care practices. The correct diagnosis and management is critical to treatment success and patient comfort.

BACTERIAL

CELLULITIS

 Immediate referral is indicated for patients presenting with necrotizing fasciitis, immunocompromised patients, and those with severe refractory to oral antibiotics, refractory to incision and drainage, hemodynamic instability, signs and symptoms of systemic involvement, and considered high risk.

Definition and Epidemiology

Skin and soft tissue infections (SSTIs) are among the most common reasons for which patients seek outpatient care and require antibiotics. Such visits have increased over the last several years and are ranked as the 27th most common hospital discharge diagnosis, now exceeding 6.3 million annually.[1] Health care providers who know the clinical presentation of SSTIs, their causative pathogens and local antibiotic susceptibility patterns will maximize treatment efficacy and avoid inducing resistance to the limited armamentarium of antimicrobial therapies available. Cellulitis is characterized by superficial localized swelling, erythema, pain, and warmth to the area involved and frequently produce pus. Cellulitis is divided into two categories of purulent and non-purulent types.

Pathophysiology

Cellulitis can involve the deeper dermis and subcutaneous fat, spreading rapidly and extending deep from the dermis to the subcutaneous tissue. When it is left untreated, cellulitis may progress to more severe soft tissue infection and osteomyelitis and may even become limb- or life-threatening.[2-4] Cellulitis typically begins when pathogens find a portal of entry through the nonintact skin, as is seen after traumatic laceration; at sites of diabetic, vascular, or other types of skin ulceration; in chronic dermatoses with skin breakdown, such as eczema or macerated tinea pedis; surgical wound infections; or even at sites of insect bites. Cellulitis may, however, develop with no recognized trauma in the otherwise normal-appearing skin. Predisposing risk factors for cellulitis include venous or lymphatic compromise from previous episodes of cellulitis, peripheral edema, previous radiation to an affected area, history of lymph node resection, lymphedema such as occurs after a radical mastectomy and lymph node dissection in the upper extremity, and obesity.

Most cases of cellulitis in adults are caused by group A β-hemolytic streptococci. Non–group A streptococci are more likely pathogens in patients with underlying abnormalities of the lymphatic system, such as lymphedema. *Staphylococcus aureus* is less likely to be causal but should be considered in the setting of penetrating trauma, sites of injection drug use, surgical site infections, indwelling catheter skin infections, or other preexisting open wounds. Other pathogens may also be implicated in cellulitis when cellulitis occurs as a complication of animal bites, with injuries occurred in freshwater or saltwater, or in immunocompromised hosts.

Purulent SSTIs include abscesses, furuncles, and carbuncles. *Abscesses* are collections of pus that may be within the dermis or deeper layers. Typically, they are painful or tender to palpation and appear as raised lesions that may be fluctuant, red, and/or nodular. There is often a central pustule with erythematous margins, which represents inflammation rather than spreading infection (i.e., cellulitis). *Epidermoid cysts* are collections of keratinous material and usually contain skin flora; these may also become inflamed and rupture into the dermal layer. *Furuncles*, commonly known as boils, are infections that arise at the hair follicle and extend deep into the dermis, where an abscess forms. This is distinguished from folliculitis, which extends only as deep as the epidermis. A *carbuncle* forms when several adjacent furuncles coalesce, forming an inflammatory mass with pus draining from multiple follicles. These are seen more frequently in persons with diabetes. Most often, skin abscesses are polymicrobial infections, consisting of bacteria from local skin flora and the adjacent mucous membranes. Approximately 25% of the time, *S. aureus* may occur as a mono-pathogen. Furuncles and carbuncles are most commonly caused by *S. aureus*. Community-acquired (CA) methicillin-resistant *S. aureus* (MRSA) rates are dependent on local resistance patterns.

In the setting of severe immunocompromise, such as patients with neutropenic fever, human immunodeficiency virus (HIV), or acquired immunodeficiency syndrome (AIDS) with depressed CD4 count, or among patients with tropical travel, animal bites, and other exposures, the differential diagnosis of these SSTIs is extensively expanded, and consultation with an infectious disease specialist should be strongly considered.[2-4]

Clinical Presentation and Physical Examination

The Infectious Diseases Society of America classifies the severity of purulent and non-purulent SSTIs into mild, moderate, and severe.[5] Regarding purulent infection, in an immunocompetent patient who is hemodynamically stable and appears nontoxic, a mild infection could be treated on an outpatient basis with appropriate incision and drainage, and often without the need for antibiotics. Moderate infection would have purulent drainage along with systemic involvement. Patients who are considered severe are defined as those (1) refractory to oral antibiotics and if purulent, refractory to incision and drainage; (2) demonstrating hemodynamic alteration including temperature higher than 38°C, heart rate greater than 90, respiratory rate greater than 24, leukocytosis greater than 12,000 or leukopenia below 400 cells/μL; and (3) who are immunocompromised. In general, moderate and severe SSTIs require hospital admission for management.

The lower extremity is the most common site of cellulitis, although it can occur anywhere. The initial clinical presentation of cellulitis is characterized by spreading erythema, induration, warmth, and pain and may be associated with systemic symptoms such as fevers, chills, and malaise.[1,5] Bullae, abscesses, erosions, necrosis, and even focal areas of hemorrhage manifesting as ecchymosis or petechiae may develop within cellulitis. The site of entry of the bacteria may be evident as breaks in the skin or ulcerations. Careful inspection of the interdigital areas is crucial in the physical examination for lower extremity cellulitis, because macerated tinea pedis may have provided the portal of entry for bacteria. Left untreated, this predisposes to recurrent cellulitis. Regional lymph nodes may be enlarged and tender, a condition called lymphadenitis. Lymphangitic streaking may occur in the direction of a regional lymph node. Edema of the area can manifest as dimpling of the overlying skin, called peau d'orange (orange peel).[2,6]

Cellulitis may also be superimposed on concurrent skin diseases, such as stasis dermatitis, hemosiderin staining, and lipodermatosclerosis associated with venous insufficiency. The purulent skin infections, as well as purulent bursitis, may manifest with surrounding inflammatory changes clinically reminiscent of cellulitis. However, these infections are primarily purulent SSTIs, and the local erythema is more likely a result of inflammation than active infection.

For nonpurulent SSTI, diagnosis is largely by clinical recognition. The causal pathogen may be determined by culturing any existing vesicular fluid, pus, ulcer, or erosions; this is indicated to evaluate bacteriology and susceptibility patterns. If no obvious culturable source is present, empirical treatment should be pursued. Blood cultures should be obtained if there

is extensive body surface involvement, underlying comorbidities including immunodeficiencies, previous splenectomy, diabetes, lymphedema, malignancy, neutropenia, specific exposures such as animal bites or water-associated injuries, and recurrent or refractory cellulitis.

Because SSTIs have a variety of causes and corresponding management, a detailed history of exposures and comorbidities is vital for developing a pathogenic differential diagnosis. Such history includes areas of residence, detailed travel history, immune status, recent surgeries, trauma, antimicrobial therapy, hobbies, lifestyle, and animal and animal bite exposures. Mimics of purulent SSTIs (i.e., abscesses, furuncles, and carbuncles) include bursitis (infectious or inflammatory), inflamed epidermoid cyst, tophaceous gout, and other inflammatory processes.

Diagnostics

Essential Diagnostics. For mild and apparently uncomplicated infections, only Gram stain and culture of the drained purulent material need be performed. In typical cases of SSTIs, empirical treatment may also be tried without such data. Epidermoid cysts need not be cultured.

Microbiologic diagnosis should be undertaken in moderate or severe infections, for those refractory to current antibiotic treatment,[5] and in cases involving multiple sites of infection, cutaneous gangrene, or extensive surrounding cellulitis. Laboratory investigations are not warranted in otherwise healthy children and adults with cellulitis. Blood cultures have been found to be of low yield, identifying the causal organism 5% or less of the time.[4,7] The yield of skin biopsy for culture is also low in nonpurulent SSTIs (around 20%), so isolation of the causative agent is usually not attempted in otherwise healthy adults, and treatment is empirical.

In patients with longer-standing disease or in whom more deep-seated infection is suspected, radiography may be helpful to evaluate for underlying osteomyelitis and even occult abscess. Although radiographs may delineate subcutaneous emphysema in gas-producing infections, they do not have sufficient sensitivity to reliably detect necrotizing fasciitis or gas gangrene and should not delay emergent surgical management of such clinically apparent infections.

INITIAL DIAGNOSTICS

Cellulitis

LABORATORY
- CBC with differential
- Creatinine
- Bicarbonate
- Creatine phosphokinase
- Purulent focus culture
- Gram stain

IMAGING
- Radiograph to evaluate osteomyelitis
- Ultrasound[b]

ADDITIONAL DIAGNOSTICS
- Blood cultures[a]
- Needle aspirate[a]
- Punch biopsy for pathology[a]
- Culture of infection[a,1,7]

[a]Moderate to severe nonpurulent.
[b]If indicated.

Differential Diagnosis

 Priority differentials include (1) deep vein thrombosis, (2) osteomyelitis, (3) thrombophlebitis, and (4) neoplastic disease.

Other considerations should include infectious: bursitis, osteomyelitis, erythema migrans, herpes zoster (HZ); connective tissue, rheumatologic, immunologic: psoriasis, erythema nodosum, acute gout, urticaria; dermatologic: eczema, contact dermatitis, drug reactions; vascular: stasis dermatitis, deep venous thrombosis, thrombophlebitis; and other: insect bite or sting, hypersensitivity, and neoplastic.

Interprofessional Collaborative Management

Pharmacologic Management

Oral Antibiotics. For moderate or severe purulent SSTIs, systemic antibiotics that primarily target *S. aureus* are required. The decision to empirically cover MRSA (rather than methicillin-sensitive *S. aureus* [MSSA]) while awaiting culture and sensitivity results can be challenging. If the patient has failed initial non-MRSA antibiotic treatment, is critically ill, has had previous MRSA infections, or is known to be MRSA colonized, empirical antibiotics should target MRSA pending culture and susceptibility results. If the patient can take oral therapy, possible antibiotics for MRSA include trimethoprim-sulfamethoxazole (TMP-SMX) or doxycycline (or others depending on local antibiogram). If the purulent SSTI is eventually determined to be caused by MRSA, an oral cephalosporin such as cephalexin or anti-staphylococcal penicillin such as dicloxacillin is appropriate, according to the full laboratory-reported susceptibilities.

With respect to antimicrobial therapy for otherwise healthy adults with mild cellulitis, antibiotics effective against streptococci and staphylococci should be used. Penicillin, amoxicillin, amoxicillin-clavulanate, penicillinase-resistant penicillin such as dicloxacillin, a cephalosporin such as cephalexin, or clindamycin for 5 days is usually sufficient, but treatment may be extended if symptoms have not resolved within that time.[7] Care must be taken to ensure adequate doses (especially in the obese), and the dose should be appropriately adjusted for elderly patients and those with renal or hepatic impairment.

Uncomplicated cases of nonulcerative cellulitis in patients with diabetes can be treated with amoxicillin-clavulanate or quinolones. These antibiotics are chosen because they cover gram-negative organisms and anaerobes that may infect patients with diabetes. For mild cases of infected diabetic ulcers, ciprofloxacin plus either clindamycin or metronidazole may be used.[1,4,5] More severe ulcerative infections or cases of osteomyelitis require intravenous (IV) antibiotics and consultation with a surgeon for debridement.

Antiinflammatory Agents. Inflammation treated with nonsteroidal antiinflammatory agents or systemic corticosteroids accelerates the healing process. Recommendations are ibuprofen 400 mg four times a day for 5 days. Nondiabetic patients with cellulitis may be treated with systemic corticosteroids (e.g., prednisone 40 mg daily for 7 days), however the evidence is weak to moderate to support this treatment.[1,5]

Intravenous. For severe purulent SSTIs, empirical IV antimicrobial options for MRSA include vancomycin, daptomycin, linezolid, telavancin, and ceftaroline. Vancomycin is the preferred agent for severe infections in children. If the pathogen is confirmed as MSSA, therapy can be more directed using nafcillin, cefazolin, or clindamycin (depending on susceptibility pattern).[1,5]

In-Office Treatment

Incision and Drainage. In purulent SSTIs, incision and drainage is key to treatment. Small furuncles often spontaneously drain with the application of moist heat. Larger furuncles, carbuncles, and skin abscesses, however, require incision and drainage with a focus on adequate debridement of any septations or loculations.

Nonpharmacologic Management. Nonpharmacologic management of cellulitis involves postural drainage (i.e., elevation of the infected limb if possible) and compression when not contraindicated (e.g., in the setting of vascular compromise). These will allow drainage of the inflammatory milieu and help to decrease peripheral edema. Management should also address the underlying and precipitating disease(s). This may include management of systemic causes of underlying peripheral edema, venous insufficiency, peripheral vascular disease, lymphedema, tinea pedis, obesity, chronic dermatoses, and so on. In patients with cellulitis arising from ulcerative lesions, sharp debridement of necrotic or devitalized tissue should be performed to remove this nidus for infection and to reinitiate the wound-healing cascade. Daily dressing changes and use of topical solutions including nonspecific antimicrobial drugs such as povidone iodine are necessary to promote healing. Additional hyperbaric oxygen treatments may be necessary if healing is problematic.

Indications for Referral. The following patients warrant consideration for inpatient admission for management including IV antibiotics and possible consultations with infectious disease and/or dermatology specialists:

- Severely immunocompromised patients
- Patients with poor clinical response to outpatient management
- Patients with severe infections including hemodynamic compromise
- Patients in whom there is concern for necrotizing fasciitis
- Patients with diabetes mellitus
- Patients with ischemic vascular disease or other pathology of circulation affecting the ability of a wound or infection to heal
- Patients with periorbital cellulitis
- Patients with hand infections
- Patients with infections of animal or human bite wounds

Life-Span Considerations

Considerations should be made to manage medical conditions to prevent the occurrence of secondary issues as a result of poor hygiene or health maintenance. Routine physical checks are important for individuals who have the potential of developing complications associated with the disease progression.

Complications

There is some weak evidence that nonsteroidal antiinflammatory drugs (NSAIDs) or steroids hasten clinical improvement if not otherwise contraindicated. Steroids should be avoided if severe or deeper infection is possible (e.g., necrotizing fasciitis). Underlying dermatoses such as tinea pedis, stasis dermatitis, and lymphedema should be treated promptly and aggressively, particularly in patients with diabetes, so the skin does not become a portal of entry for secondary infections.

Patients with diabetes mellitus need to be monitored closely, particularly when cellulitis involves the feet or hands. As a result of decreased circulation in the extremities from microvascular compromise, persons with diabetes are at a higher risk for development of ulcerations and osteomyelitis.

Periorbital cellulitis must be distinguished from the far less frequent and more orbital severe cellulitis. Orbital cellulitis clinically manifests with exophthalmos, orbital pain, restricted eye movement, and occasionally visual disturbance. Orbital cellulitis often stems from ethmoid or maxillary sinusitis, and left untreated may lead to blindness, diplopia, brain abscess, and meningitis. Orbital cellulitis is a medical emergency and must be treated as such, including prompt evaluation with a computed tomography scan and IV antibiotics. Referral to an otolaryngologist is recommended for closer evaluation.

Periorbital cellulitis typically follows sinusitis, upper respiratory tract infection, or eye trauma and is more common in children. Symptoms typically include erythema and edema of the eyelid, conjunctivitis, and chemosis (conjunctival edema). This condition is treated with warm soaks and aggressive antibiotic therapy, such as IV nafcillin or oxacillin.[2,3,5]

Soft tissue infections of the hands must be carefully evaluated to determine whether tendon sheaths or joint or muscle spaces are involved. Necrotizing soft tissue infections are a surgical emergency. The condition starts with redness and painful swelling of the deep tissues. A black eschar rapidly develops with necrosis of the underlying tissues. If necrotizing fasciitis, cellulitis, or myonecrosis is suspected, immediate referral is indicated for prompt surgical debridement, IV antibiotics, and hyperbaric oxygen treatment if it is locally available.[2,3,5]

The causative pathogens of bite infections depend on the mouth and host skin flora, and such infections are often polymicrobial (see Chapter 41). *Pasteurella* species are classically involved in dog and cat bites, but the more familiar streptococci and staphylococci are most often identified. *Capnocytophaga, Moraxella, Corynebacterium, Neisseria,* and anaerobic bacteria are also implicated with some frequency in dog and cat bites.[1,3] *Eikenella corrodens* is a pathogen commonly associated with human bites or closed-fist injuries (CFIs). CFIs, also sometimes called clenched-fist injuries, occur when a person's closed fist strikes the teeth of another person, usually in the course of a fight. CFIs are at high risk for infection because of wound contamination with human saliva.[2,3] See Chapter 41, Human and Animal Bites for additional information.

Emerging Management Trends

Several new antibiotics are worth mentioning because of their activity against MRSA and, in the case of the lipoglycopeptides, for their remarkably convenient administration.

Ceftaroline (Teflaro). Ceftaroline is a cephalosporin with activity against gram-positive bacteria including MRSA, as well as some aerobic gram-negative bacteria, and was approved by the US Food and Drug Administration (FDA) for treatment of acute bacterial skin and skin structure infections (ABSSSIs) in May 2010. It is typically administered intravenously at 600 mg q12h and requires adjustment for renal dysfunction or severe infection.[1,5]

Dalbavancin (Dalvance). Dalbavancin is a lipoglycopeptide with activity against gram-positive organisms, including MSSA and MRSA, and *Streptococcus pyogenes*, the major pathogens in cellulitis. Dalbavancin is used for treatment of ABSSSIs. It has a long half-life, which allows once-weekly administration

at 1 g IV over 30 minutes on day 1 and 500 mg IV over 30 minutes on day 8.[1,5]

Tedizolid (Sivextro). Tedizolid is an oxazolidinone with activity against both methicillin-sensitive and methicillin-resistant strains of *S. aureus,* as well as various *Streptococcus* species and *Enterococcus faecalis*. Tedizolid was approved by the FDA in June 2014 to treat patients with ABSSSIs. It is available in both oral and IV forms.[1,5]

Oritavancin (Orbactiv). Oritavancin, another lipoglycopeptide, was approved by the FDA in August 2014 to treat patients with ABSSSIs caused by *S. aureus* (including methicillin-susceptible and methicillin-resistant strains), various *Streptococcus* species, and *E. faecalis*. Like its predecessor, dalbavancin, it is administered via IV, although the dose is 1200 mg IV once.[5]

Patient and Family Education

- Teach the patient and his or her family that cutaneous inflammation and systemic signs and symptoms often paradoxically worsen briefly after initiation of appropriate antimicrobial therapy. This may be a result of bacterial cell death, lysis, and release of proinflammatory compounds contributing to local inflammation.
- Educate patients and families about the importance of preventing skin infections by routine hygiene, use of antimicrobials, and standard first aid of any skin wounds including careful cleaning and appropriate dressings.
- In patients with diabetes, review the importance of consistently wearing well-fitted protective shoes and encourage them to make a daily visual inspection of their feet to evaluate for wounds or breaks in skin integrity.
- Outbreaks of furunculosis occur in families and within those groups in close contact (e.g., sports teams, military camps or child care centers). These outbreaks are most often caused by MSSA or MRSA. All contacts or infected persons are advised to use antibacterial soaps such as chlorhexidine and that laundering of all soiled clothing, bedsheets, towels, and so on is ensured.[4]

Health Promotion

Individuals with medical conditions such as diabetes, peripheral artery disease (PAD), eczema, or athlete's foot should pay close attention to their disease processes to ensure they maintain healthy skin. Treating the original cause of cellulitis is prevention against further development. Patients need to visit a podiatrist for nail care and callus removal and should avoiding self-treatment of these conditions with over-the-counter products.

ERYSIPELAS

 Immediate referral is indicated for rapid progression of infection, systemic involvement, worsening condition with antibiotic therapy (suspected necrotizing fasciitis), or with patients who are immunocompromised.

Definition and Epidemiology

Erysipelas is a nonpurulent SSTI infection of the upper dermis to include lymphatics. It is a superficial form of cellulitis.[5] The most commonly involved sites include the face, ears, and lower legs. It can be distinguished from cellulitis by the restriction to the superficial dermis and lymphatics. Facial erysipelas may follow a streptococcal infection of the upper respiratory tract.

Those at increased risk include children and the elderly, those with exposure to organisms, alteration in skin integrity due to trauma, atopic dermatitis, allergic contact dermatitis, skin inflammation, psoriasis, insect bites, edema, or obesity. Additional risk factors include those with altered immune systems such as kidney disease, AIDS, diabetes, preexisting skin infection, or cancer.[3,8]

Pathophysiology

Erysipelas is a distinct type of superficial cutaneous cellulitis with marked dermal lymphatic vessel involvement. Most often caused by group A Streptococcus (GAS), β-hemolytic Streptococci, *S. pyogenes*, and rarely *S. aureus*. GAS has classically been considered the predominant cause of erysipelas, but erysipelas may also be caused by *S. aureus* and group C or G Streptococcus.[4]

Clinical Presentation and Physical Examination

Very similar to cellulitis, erysipelas is characterized by erythema, edema, and pain. Patients may complain of pruritus. Classically well-demarcated borders of inflammation are present, and may have lymphatic streaking. The edema associated with erysipelas is bright red, and the skin surface is described as the skin of an orange in appearance. Erysipelas is commonly seen unilaterally and with the lower extremities as the most common location. The spaces between the toes should be carefully examined for fissures or maceration. Sudden onset of symptoms includes fever, erythema, edema, and pain at the site. Uncomplicated erysipelas is self-limiting and usually subsides over 7 to 10 days. Prompt diagnosis and treatment need to occur in individuals who are immunocompromised. Recurrence can occur especially in those who have contributing factors that are untreated.[4]

Diagnostics

Essential Diagnostics. Diagnosis is generally by physical exam. Rarely are cultures or swabs helpful in uncomplicated cases. Scrapings or swabs may prove beneficial to isolate pathogen in cases more complicated.[9]

Additional Diagnostics. Imaging may be used to rule out necrotizing fasciitis, pyomyositis, or abscess. Often what is seen on the MRI will be thickening of the subcutaneous tissue.

INITIAL DIAGNOSTICS

Erysipelas

LABORATORY
- Culture (blood or swab)[a]
- CBC[a]
- Erythrocyte Sedimentation rate (ESR)[a]
- C-reactive protein (CRP)[a]

Differential Diagnosis

The differential diagnosis must include diseases that should be considered and excluded when appropriate. These can be narrowed down with the patient history, patient's age, and any recent history of trauma.

 Priority differentials include (1) necrotizing fasciitis, (2) deep vein thrombosis, (3) contact dermatitis, and (4) insect bite.

Additional differential diagnosis considerations should include erythema migrans, acute gout, erysipeloid, HZ, stasis dermatitis, and contact dermatitis.

Interprofessional Collaborative Management

Pharmacologic Management

Antibiotics. For the uncomplicated patient, first-line treatment is oral penicillin V. 500 mg PO 4 times a day for 10 days.

If the patient is penicillin allergic, a first-generation cephalosporin or macrolide may be used.

More complicated cases need to be treated with IV antibiotics such as penicillin G 1 to 2 million units every 6 hours. Penicillin-allergic patients may be prescribed vancomycin 15 mg/kg IV q12h, additional choices include Linezolid 600 mg IV q12h, or Daptomycin 4 mg/kg IV q24h. Treatment should continue over 10 to 20 days.[5,6,9]

Pain Management

Analgesics-Antipyretics. Ibuprofen is the preferred drug for treating mild to moderate pain and also aids in fever reduction. If there is a sensitivity to NSAIDs, acetaminophen is the drug of choice.

Nonpharmacologic Management. It is important to keep the affected area elevated to reduce edema, especially with lower leg infections. The use of cool compresses can assist in pain reduction. It is important to treat the underlying cause of infection such as tinea, stasis dermatitis, or trauma.[3,4,6]

Indications for Referral. Consultation to infectious disease specialists or surgery should be made for patients who appear to have rapid progression of infection, systemic involvement, or are immunocompromised. Should condition worsen while on antibiotic therapy or necrotizing fasciitis is suspected, immediate referral to hospital is needed.[3,4,6]

Life-Span Considerations

Prognosis is excellent for those who complete appropriate therapy. Local reoccurrence is possible in patients with predisposing conditions.

Complications

The most common complications are abscess, gangrene, and thrombophlebitis. Few will develop acute glomerulonephritis, endocarditis, or septicemia. Surgical debridement may be necessary should the infection worsen.

Emerging Management Trends

Additional IV antibiotic agents recently approved by the FDA for treatment of acute bacterial skin infections include oritavancin (Orbactiv), dalbavancin (Dalvance), and tedizolid (Sivextro), see earlier discussion. These antibiotics are effective against *S. aureus*, *S. pyogenes*, *Streptococcus agalactiae*, *Streptococcus anginosus* group, and *Streptococcus intermedius* among others.

Patient and Family Education

- Outpatient setting is optimal for treatment of the noncomplicated cases. Hospitalization may be necessary for IV therapy if the disease is more extensive.
- Rest and elevation of affected area is important for the patient to have proper healing, especially with lower leg infections.
- Use cool compresses to assist in pain reduction.
- Teach patients the importance of compliance with treatment for the underlying cause of infection such as tinea, stasis dermatitis, or trauma.

• Educate patients regarding local antiseptic, wound care, and prevention with regard to predisposing conditions.[3,4,6]

IMPETIGO

 Immediate referral is indicated for Steven-Johnson syndrome, Sweet syndrome, and staphylococcal scalded skin syndrome (SSSS).

Definition and Epidemiology

Impetigo is a considered a common skin infection. It is spread rapidly by both direct and indirect contact. Climates that are hot and humid see a greater incidence of streptococcal impetigo. However, in Europe and most of the United States *S. aureus* is the contributing agent. Environmental factors, poor health, and living conditions contribute greatly to the incidence of disease. Alterations in skin integrity due to immunocompromise, insect bites, and scabies place individuals at increased risk. There are two patterns recognized: (1) bullous and (2) nonbullous. Nonbullous (small vesicle) is the most common form accounting for over 70% of all cases, which mostly occur in infants and young children but can occur in adults. Bullous impetigo is caused by *S. aureus* and occurs more often in the neonate, however, children can be affected. Nonbullous impetigo is most commonly caused by *S. aureus* in developed nations.[1,4,8]

Pathophysiology

Colonization of the nasal carriage by *S. aureus* contributes to 60% of nonbullous impetigo and 40% of bullous impetigo infections. Impetigo is a highly contagious toxin-mediated skin infection caused by *S. aureus* or group A β-hemolytic streptococcus. The common initial presentation of impetigo is vesiculopustular or bullous lesions. Nonbullous presents as small vesiculopustules; intercellular edema under the pustules with lymphadenitis is common. GAS remains a common cause of nonbullous impetigo in developing nations. Bullous impetigo does not occur as often as nonbullous. In bullous, toxins are produced causing a disturbance in desmosomal adhesion molecules, which formulate multiple blisters that coalesce together creating a larger blister. The lesions have a classic "honey-colored" yellow crust when ruptured. Lesions may occur on normal skin or an area of altered skin integrity.[4,9]

Clinical Presentation and Physical Examination

Cutaneous lesions are seen with crusts, translucent vesicle, or pustules in association with a moist erythematous weeping base when the crust is removed. Classically the crust is honey colored. Bullous lesions are more often seen in intertriginous areas, such as the face, trunk, extremities, perineal region, and buttocks. The initial presentation may begin with multiple small lesions in a single area, and by self-inoculation, the impetigo spreads. These fragile lesions enlarge rapidly and subsequently burst to form a crust. With nonbullous impetigo, lymphadenopathy is seen and patients present with constitutional symptoms.[4,6,8]

Diagnostics

Essential Diagnostics. Patient history and physical exam are commonly the only diagnostics needed.

Additional Diagnostics. For extensive or complicated cases gram stain and culture and sensitivity may be obtained

---

INITIAL DIAGNOSTICS

Impetigo

LABORATORY
• Urinalysis[a] in young children only
• ESR[a]
• Gram stain
• Culture and sensitivity[a]

ADDITIONAL DIAGNOSTICS
• Anti-DNAse B and antihyaluronidase[a] to check for previous strep infection
• Antinuclear antibodies[a] to check for the presence of chronic infection or autoimmune disease

[a]If indicated.

---

to rule out MRSA. In children ages 2 to 4 years urinalysis may be needed to reveal acute nephritis.

Differential Diagnosis

 Priority differentials include (1) ecthyma, (2) erysipelas, (3) cellulitis, and (4) herpes simplex infection.

Additional differentials that should be included are atopic dermatitis, herpes simplex infection, ecthyma, folliculitis, dermatitis herpetiformis, insect bites, scabies pediculosis, tinea corporis, varicella zoster, Steven-Johnson syndrome (fever and influenza symptoms followed by painful, blistering lesions on skin and mucous membranes), Sweet syndrome (fever, erythematous plaques and nodules, arthralgias, myalgias, fatigue), and SSSS (bullae that spread and slough).

Interprofessional Collaborative Management

Pharmacologic Management

Topical Antibiotic Therapy. Mupirocin, 2% ointment, should be applied 3 times a day for 10 days. Another choice is retapamulin 1% applied twice a day for 5 days to the affected area or until all lesions have cleared.[5]

Oral Antibiotic Therapy. Several options are available for treatment should oral antibiotics be deemed necessary. Dicloxacillin 250 mg PO 4 times a day for 7 to 10 days, cephalexin 250 mg PO 4 times a day or 25 to 50 mg/kg/day divided in to 3 to 4 doses for 7 to 10 days, azithromycin 500 mg PO on day 1, 250 mg PO on days 2 through 5, or amoxicillin/clavulanate 500 mg PO every 8 hours, or 875/125 mg twice a day.[5]

Non-Pharmacological Management. It is important to soak the crusts with wet compresses for removal of the crusts. This will allow penetration of the topical antibiotics. Additional measures include daily washing with antimicrobial cleanser chlorhexidine gluconate.

Life-Span Considerations

Impetigo can occur at any age. However, crowded living conditions or daycare facilities can prove to be an infectious environment. Individuals at additional risk are the very young and those with predisposing factors such as malnutrition or anemia.

Complications

Recurrent infection is often a sign of colonization with staphylococcal, particularly in the nasal carriage. Additional treatment should include intranasal mupirocin ointment nares twice a day for 5 days, with additional oral antibiotics such as rifampin and doxycycline.

Patient and Family Education

- Education of family and other close contacts is critical to eliminate recurrent infections.
- Close contacts may be colonized and additional sources of infection, such as shared towels, should be discussed.
- Emphasize proper hygiene, especially keeping nails short to prevent the spread of infection.
- Close contacts should also bathe in antimicrobial cleansers and possibly apply topical antibiotics to nares to reduce the colonization of pathogens.
- Infected individuals should be kept isolated to prevent spread for at least 24 hours after initiation of antibiotic therapy.[4,5,8]

Health Promotion

All individuals within close contact of the infected individual should be inspected for lesions and treated appropriately or presumptively. With neonatal impetigo, any individual that has come into contact should be evaluated or considered as asymptomatic bacterial carrier. It is important to treat any underlying skin diseases that would allow for recurrent episodes.

Erythrasma

 Immediate referral is indicated for immunocompromised patients with systemic signs/symptoms and patients with septicemia.

Definition and Epidemiology. Erythrasma is a chronic but mild bacterial infection found on the intertriginous areas of the skin. Healthy adults are not uncommonly affected. However, the diabetic, elderly, or those immunocompromised may be at increased risk. Children rarely have erythrasma. Men are more likely to have this occur in the genitocrural area and are likely to be asymptomatic, whereas women are more likely to have it occur interdigitally.[4,10]

Pathophysiology. The causative organism is most often *cornybacterium minutissimum*. It is the excessive growth of this microaerophilic, pseudodiptheroid, gram-positive rod, on the stratum corneum, the outermost layer of the epidermis. Erythrasma proliferates in tropical and sub tropical, humid, climates.[3,4]

Clinical Presentation and Physical Examination. Erythrasma appears as well-demarcated, brown-red macular patches. Fine scales appear in a wrinkled fashion. Common areas affected include the inner thighs, inguinal area, scrotum, and toe webs that appear macerated. Erythrasma presents a hyperkeratotic white macerated plaque between the fourth and fifth toes while in the other area the lesions are well demarcated, reddish-brown, wrinkled patches with central clearing commonly mistaken for tinea.[3,4,10]

Diagnostics

Essential Diagnostics. Location and character of the lesions is essential in properly diagnosing erythrasma. Confirmation comes by the demonstration from the Wood lamp illumination revealing coral-red fluorescence of lesions, resembling the burning of cigarette paper as seen in Fig. 47.1. Results may be negative if the patient bathed prior to presentation.[11,12]

Additional Diagnostics. Concurrent infection may be a factor. Therefore, it is important to perform a direct potassium hydroxide (KOH) exam to rule out dermatophytosis. Fungal

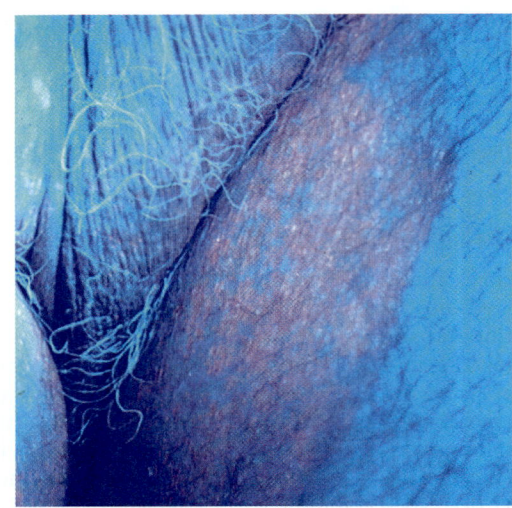

F I G . 47.1 Coral-red fluorescence upon illumination with a Wood lamp. (From Bolognia, J., Schaffer, J., & Cerroni, L. [2018]. *Dermatology* [4th ed.]. Philadelphia: Elsevier.)

spores of pityriasis versicolor and the bacterial rods of *C. minutissimum* tend to coexist. Performing a methylene blue stain will highlight both of these. By performing Wood lamp examination, KOH preparation, and Gram staining concurrently, a higher yield for positive results is likely.[13,14]

INITIAL DIAGNOSTICS
Erythrasma
LABORATORY   • Wood light examination   • Potassium hydroxide preparation   • Gram-stain   • Culture

Differential Diagnosis

 Priority differentials include (1) acanthosis nigricans, (2) allergic contact dermatitis, (3) cutaneous candidiasis, and (4) intertrigo.

Additional considerations for differentials include irritant contact dermatitis, plaque psoriasis, seborrheic dermatitis, tinea corporis, tinea cruris, and tinea pedis.

Interprofessional Collaborative Management

Pharmacologic Management

Topical Therapy. The first line of treatment for localized erythrasma can consist of different types of topical treatments. The most effective treatment between the web spaces of the toes includes benzoyl peroxide wash and 5% gel. Clindamycin 2% or azole creams twice a day for 2 weeks have been found to be effective. The fungal cell wall membrane is damaged by miconazole, allowing membrane permeability, which leaks out nutrients, ultimately resulting in cell death. If maceration is present apply the topical cream sparingly. Fusidic acid is a popular treatment but is not approved in the United States.[11]

Oral Antibiotics. With widespread erythrasma oral therapy should be initiated in combination with topical therapy.

Erythrasma is generally susceptible to penicillins, first-generation cephalosporins, erythromycin, clindamycin, ciprofloxacin, tetracycline, and vancomycin. Isolation of multiresistant strands has been found. Erythromycin is the drug of choice—500 mg PO twice a day for 14 days. Growth is inhibited by the blocking t-peptidyl t-RNA from ribosomes, which causes RNA dependent protein synthesis to stop. Appropriate prescribing may include splitting the daily doses twice a day or in more severe cases doubling the prescribing dose. Another option is clarithromycin as a single dose of 1 g PO, which disrupts growth in the same fashion as erythromycin. The third line of therapy is tetracycline. Recommended dosing is 250 mg PO 4 times daily for 14 days. Tetracycline shows Increased efficacy in treating interdigital cases, however, axillary and groin are less receptive to tetracycline.[3,13,14]

Nonpharmacologic Management. Washes to the affected area with antibacterial and/or antifungal washes are used to eliminate and decrease the numbers of *C. minutissimum* bacteria.

Life-Span Considerations. Treatment depends on the patient's medical history, the severity of disease, and tolerability of treatment. Patients intolerant to erythromycin may respond to tetracycline therapy.

Complications. Immunocompromised patients may develop septicemia; those with valvular heart disease should be closely watched for infective endocarditis. Postsurgical wound infection is possible in erythrasma patients. Medication interactions with patients' other prescribed medications may be a concern, especially with erythromycin as it is an inhibitor of the cytochrome P450 system. Metabolism by this pathway is problematic for certain concomitant medications. Tetracycline is pregnancy category D and should not be prescribed to pregnant women. It also should not be used in pediatric patients. Additional concerns with tetracycline include the risk of vestibular effects and renal toxicity, and the possibility that it may increase serum concentrations of certain medications.[11]

Emerging Trends. Red light therapy has been reported to clear erythrasma in a small sample of patients and improve overall erythrasma in others. Photodynamic therapy is not the treatment of choice; however it is an alternative adjunctive therapy in targeting and reducing erythrasma. More clinical data is needed to support the claims of this type of therapy.[11]

Patient and Family Education

- Educate the entire family in ways to reduce the risk of repeat infections by minimizing colonization. This can be accomplished with proper washing of clothing items, replacing shoes frequently, as well as the use of antibacterial washes and prophylactic application of topical therapy.
- Excessive sweating, which may make a patient more susceptible to erythrasma, can be controlled by wearing loose fitting, moisture wicking clothing and avoiding hot, humid condition whenever possible. Advocate weight loss if indicated.
- Anecdotal evidence using aluminum chloride deodorant in axilla and on feet to limit sweating has demonstrated efficacy in preventing recurrences.[4,6,11]

Health Promotion. Patients who are immunocompromised should be diligent in maintaining good hygiene and reducing exposure to moist environments. After bathing ensure areas of the body with folds or crevices are completely dry. Alternating footwear and ensuring that footwear is clean and dry prior to wearing is critical to prevent additional or worsening current erythrasma.[11]

Paronychia

Definition and Epidemiology. Paronychial infections manifest as acute or chronic inflammation of the tissues surrounding the nail, usually with an underlying bacterial or fungal infection. Other noninfectious causes are possible and include "chemical irritants, excessive moisture, systemic conditions, and medications."[3] Most commonly a microorganism penetrates the tissue after breakdown between the nail plate and nail fold. A split in the epidermis from trauma, nail-biting, a hangnail, irritation, or chronic exposure to water (such as with dishwashing) or irritants can precede the development of a paronychia.[3,15,16]

Paronychial infections may be seen more often in women than in men; this may be related to manicures or the application of acrylic nails. Patients who work with chemicals are more at risk for infections because of the irritant nature of these substances and the risk of trauma. Patients who have their hands in water are frequently at risk.[15]

Pathophysiology. There are numerous possible causative organisms for acute paronychial infections. Some organisms include *Pseudomonas*, *Proteus*, *Streptococcus*, *Staphylococcus*, *Candida albicans*, and herpes simplex virus (HSV).[16,17] A paronychial infection results when periungual tissue is inoculated by trauma, inert vehicles such as water, or soluble chemicals. The resulting infection follows the nail margin, or the infection penetrates under the nail.

If paronychial inflammation is present for longer than 6 weeks, the condition is considered a chronic paronychia. Chronic paronychia is primarily an inflammatory disorder, but *C. albicans* is also often present. It is most commonly present in workers with frequent exposure to environmental irritants (such as cooks, dishwashers, and nurses).[16]

Medications can cause chronic paronychia, increasing the risk of infection. Retinoids and protease inhibitors (e.g., lamivudine [Epivir], darunavir [Prezista], and fosamprenavir [Lexiva]) affect nail fold integrity, setting the stage for a paronychia.[10,16] An antiretroviral, indinavir (Crixivan), is associated with paronychias as a result of interference with retinoid metabolism.[16] Chemotherapeutic selective inhibition of the epidermal growth factor receptor (EGFR; e.g., cetuximab) is increasingly used to treat solid organ malignant neoplasms in patients whose standard chemotherapeutic regimens have failed. Tenderness, swelling, and pain in both fingers and toes occur after 2 weeks to months of therapy. Anatomic predisposition may increase risk in the development of paronychias.[16]

Clinical Presentation and Physical Examination. Symptoms are usually localized to one finger, and patients report throbbing pain, tenderness of the nail fold, nail, and even adjacent portions of the finger. The affected nail may display distal onycholysis, discoloration, distortion, and ridging; the affected nail folds have erythema and edema. The nail plate may have thickening and grooving longitudinally. When the examiner applies force to the affected area, there can be a release of purulent, often foul-smelling discharge.[16] Pyogenic granuloma-like lesions and granulation tissue are seen in the nail sulci in paronychias associated with indinavir and anti-EGFR agents.[12,16]

Diagnostics

Essential Diagnostics. Skin scrapings can be combined with KOH preparation on a glass slide and viewed under a microscope. Pseudohyphae and spores indicate candidal infection. Any exudate from the nail can be cultured to determine the pathogen and to guide treatment. Concerns for bone involvement or malignancy may warrant a biopsy along with imaging studies.[1]

INITIAL DIAGNOSTICS

Paronychial Infections

LABORATORY
- Potassium hydroxide preparation
- CBC and differential (if infection is suspected or if the patient is immunocompromised)
- Culture and sensitivity[a]
  Biopsy

IMAGING
- X-Ray only if bone involvement is suspected
- MRI[a]

———
[a]If indicated.

Differential Diagnosis

 Priority differentials include (1) herpetic whitlow, (2) onychomycosis, (3) psoriasis, (4) tic deformity, (5) lichen planus, (6) eczema, and (7) bacterial infection.

The differential diagnosis of paronychial infections includes trauma, bacterial origin, herpetic whitlow, onychomycosis, circulatory changes, and irritation from environmental causes (such as nail products). Malignancies of the area are possible and should be considered, especially in patients with persistent paronychia or those with a cancer history. However, paronychial infection is usually readily recognized by its appearance and absence of medication history preceding the infection. Individuals with diabetes or immunocompromised state are at a higher risk.[16]

Interprofessional Collaborative Management
Pharmacologic Management
Topical Therapy. A topical antibiotic may be added for minor cases. Topical neomycin, bacitracin, or mupirocin is indicated for pseudomonal infection.[10] Treatment of chronic paronychia includes identification and elimination of causative irritants. Topical steroids have been shown to be most often superior to topical antifungals in treating chronic paronychia. Topical triamcinolone, betamethasone, or tacrolimus 0.1% applied over 3 to 6 weeks are optional types of preparation.[1,16]

Oral Therapy. Oral antibiotic therapy is indicated for more substantial infection. The antibiotic choice depends on the suspected organism. Considerations could include TMP-SMX (good if MRSA is suspected), clindamycin, amoxicillin-clavulanate, and cephalexin. Appropriate analgesics and dosages are based on patient age and medical history. For persistent or nonresponsive cases, use of oral antifungal preparations is considered. A short course of oral corticosteroids may be considered for severe cases with multiple fingers involved. Oral antibiotic therapy should be used in conjunction with topical treatment.[1,16]

Nonpharmacologic Management. Initial treatment of minor acute paronychial infection includes warm water soaks or warm compresses four times a day, which may resolve the paronychia. Ensure the area is kept dry because moisture may prolong healing and cause further irritation.

Consultations: Specialist. Incision and drainage should be considered if the infection is not responding to noninvasive therapy or abscess is suspected. If the nail plate has separated from the underlying tissue removal of the nail may be necessary. Suspected infection of the tendons or tendon sheaths requires immediate referral to a physician or surgeon. Hospitalization may be required for surgical intervention. The surgical methods used for recalcitrant cases give better results when the nail plate is also removed simultaneously. A new surgical technique, the Swiss roll technique, has been described, which has the advantage of retaining the nail plate and allowing rapid healing without creating a defect in the skin.[16]

Life-Span Considerations. Postmenopausal women may be at greater risk for chronic candidal paronychial infections. Diminished estrogen levels are a predisposing factor for chronic candidal paronychial infections.

Complications. Patients are referred to a physician if there is continued infection after 2 weeks of treatment. Serious complications of paronychia include loss of the nail or spread of the infection into the bloodstream, deeper tissue, or bone. If it is untreated or in patients with immunosuppression or diabetes, the paronychial infection can invade deep into the digit, infecting the tendon and tendon sheaths. Infection along the tendon sheath requires immediate surgical intervention. Chronic mucocutaneous candidiasis can cause hyperkeratosis of the entire nail plate. These chronically infected nails can become distorted and may require excision. Incision and drainage is reserved for severe persistent cases.

Emerging Management Trends. The topical povidone-iodine, a broad-spectrum, resistance-free biocidal agent, and dimethylsulfoxide (DMSO) solution has proven effective in improving the signs and symptoms of paronychia. This was studied in association with chemotherapy. Penetration of the nail structure reducing inflammation and pain was seen with the use of the combination povidone–iodine in combination with DMSO. It additionally has the ability to destroy both fungal and bacterial organisms. Povidone–iodine additionally has the ability to suppress the inflammatory component of paronychia. DMSO also has the ability to deliver povidone–iodine through keratinized epithelial surfaces, thereby penetrating the nail structure, which has the ability to eradicate fungal and bacterial organisms.[18]

Patient and Family Education
- Address the individual patient's causative factors including their environmental and work exposures.
- Patients who have manicures or who wear acrylic nails should be advised to rest their nails and hands for 1 week every month.[17]
- Patients who deal with caustic chemicals and irritants should be advised to wear protective gloves.
- Patients should be instructed to wear waterproof gloves when washing dishes or clothing by hand and to keep the nails trimmed and dry to prevent further infections.

Health Promotion. It is imperative that patients understand the importance of keeping hands and nails as clean and dry as possible. Protect hands from water and wear gloves to prevent contact with irritating solutions. If surgery was performed, change bandages as directed. Contact the provider if the fingers have increased erythema, edema, or any problems with the mobility of the digit.

INTERTRIGO

 Immediate referral is indicated for rapidly progressing infections or suspicion of serious systemic involvement.

Definition and Epidemiology

Intertrigo is a superficial inflammatory bacterial or fungal skin disorder that occurs in the setting of persistent skin-to-skin contact, friction, moisture, warmth, and inadequate ventilation. It is usually characterized by varying degrees of erythema, peripheral scaling, and macerated erythematous plaques. Common intertriginous sites include inframammary and abdominal folds, inner thighs, and axillary, interdigital, and perianal areas. Sweat retention, incontinence, immobility, alterations in systemic immunity, systemic antibiotic therapy, and overgrowth of resident microorganisms are related factors. If intertrigo is not treated, affected areas with impaired skin integrity can become secondarily infected with *Candida* (most common), *S. aureus*, *Pseudomonas aeruginosa*, group A β-hemolytic streptococci, or *C. minutissimum*.[1,19]

Patients are susceptible to intertrigo at any age, but it is more common in the young and in older adults. Women with vulvovaginitis, men with balanitis, individuals infected with HIV, and prolonged steroid users are particularly susceptible.[1] Other predisposing conditions and factors include diaper use, psoriasis, eczema, diabetes, obesity, pregnancy, oral contraceptive use, chemotherapy, and living in hot and humid climates. Obesity is associated with larger skinfolds with thick layers of subcutaneous brown fat, increasing the risk of overheating, friction, and moisture.[19]

Pathophysiology. Intertrigo originates from the Latin term *inter*, meaning between, and *trigo*, which means rubbing.[17] It is a skin disorder resulting in altered barrier function, which allows opportunistic infections such as yeast, bacteria, or fungi to infiltrate the skin. Most common bacterial infections are β-hemolytic streptococci, *S. aureus*, *P. aeruginosa*, *C. minutissimum*, *K. sedentarius*. Moisture and friction are present, causing maceration in the stratum corneum, leading to erosion and skin breakdown and thus creating an opportunity for primary and secondary infections.[17] Skin in elders and in diabetic and obese individuals has a higher skin surface pH than in other individuals. The skin's barrier function may be more easily compromised in this situation, making it more vulnerable to organisms such as yeasts, bacteria, and other pathogens.[19]

Clinical Presentation and Physical Examination

Intertrigo is initially seen as mildly erythematous, moist, glistening plaques, patches, papules, and/or pustules. The borders are well defined, with areas of epidermal erosion and scaling. See Fig. 47.2 for an example of inframammary intertrigo without fungal or bacterial infection. Pinpoint pustules outside the border are diagnostically important in candidal infections. Initial symptoms usually include itching, burning, and stinging.[20] Odor, copious discharge, severe erythema, acute discomfort, fever, and abscesses may signal secondary infection.[19]

Diagnostics

Essential Diagnostics. Diagnosis is typically based on clinical appearance. Scrapings from the lesion may be examined via KOH wet mount and/or Gram stain.[5] A KOH preparation that is positive for pseudohyphae and budding spores confirms the diagnosis of *Candida* infection. Bacterial or

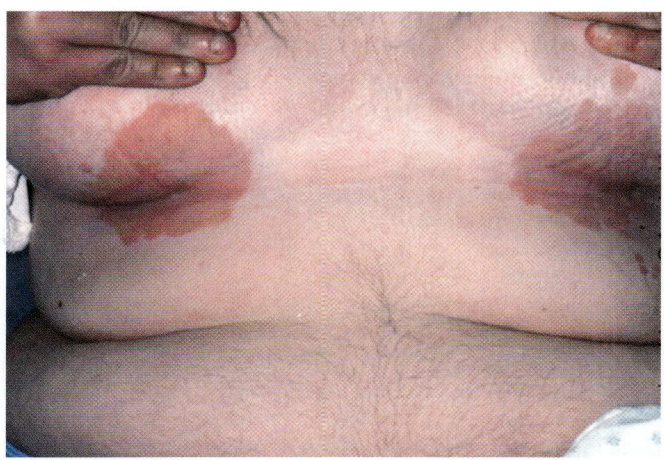

FIG. 47.2 Candida intertrigo. Notice the fringe of scale in the intertriginous area. Intertrigo in inframammary folds without evidence of bacterial infection. (Copyright © Logical Images, Inc.)

fungal superinfection (e.g., *Staphylococcus*, group A β-hemolytic streptococci, *P. aeruginosa*, *Proteus mirabilis*) may be identified by culture. Examination with a Wood lamp may indicate erythrasma (coral-red fluorescence) or *Pseudomonas* infection (yellow-green fluorescence).[1,3]

Additional Diagnostics. A biopsy may be required if intertrigo is refractory to treatment.

INITIAL DIAGNOSTICS

Intertrigo

LABORATORY
- Potassium hydroxide wet mount
- Gram stain
- Culture
- Wood lamp examination
- Additional diagnostics
- Biopsy[a]

[a]If indicated.

Differential Diagnosis

It is important to determine the underlying cause(s) of the skin eruption, because treatment options vary accordingly.

 Priority differentials include (1) candidiasis, (2) dermatophytosis, (3) erythrasma, and (4) pyoderma.

Additional diagnoses may be made as related to body site or history of chronic disease. Considerations should include:

Infectious diseases: scabies, seborrheic dermatitis, syphilis, cellulitis, granuloma inguinale, lymphogranuloma venereum

Noninfectious inflammatory diseases: atopic dermatitis, contact dermatitis (allergic, irritant), pemphigus vulgaris, familial benign pemphigus (Hailey-Haley disease), granuloma gluteale infantum, psoriasis, acrodermatitis enteropathica, keratosis follicularis

Noninflammatory diseases: acanthosis nigricans, hidradenitis suppurativa, intertrigo, lichen sclerosis

Neoplasms: Bowen disease, Paget disease, superficial basal cell carcinoma

Interprofessional Collaborative Management

Pharmacologic Management

Topical Therapy. Compresses with Burow solution may be soothing. Use of drying agents containing zinc oxide, aluminum sulfate, and calcium acetate solution is recommended. For intertrigo associated with fungal infections (including *Candida* and tinea), clotrimazole, ketoconazole, oxiconazole, or econazole may be applied 2 times daily until the rash resolves. Nystatin is effective only for candidal intertrigo. For Pseudomonas intertrigo, acetic acid 1% to 2.5%, a bactericidal, should be used. Low-potency topical corticosteroids can be used initially to gain control of inflammation.[19-21]

Oral Therapy. If an oral agent is required, the lesions should be cultured, and the results used to determine the selection of an antibiotic. secondary infections with *S. aureus*, group A β-hemolytic streptococci, *P. aeruginosa*, *P. mirabilis*, or *Proteus vulgaris* is possible Topical treatment with mupirocin, erythromycin, or clindamycin should be used. Cephalexin, ceftriaxone, cefazolin, clindamycin, erythromycin, and sulfamethoxazole-trimethoprim are typically used for oral therapy.[20,21]

In cases of recalcitrant or recurrent fungal infections, systemic antifungal therapy with agents such as oral fluconazole, itraconazole, or ketoconazole is indicated. Terbinafine is not effective in treating candidiasis. Careful monitoring of the patient for drug interactions or hepatic impairment while taking antifungals is necessary. The suggested dosage of fluconazole is 100 to 200 mg PO daily for 7 days, but obese individuals may need an increased dose.[20,21]

Nonpharmacologic Management.

The treatment of uninfected intertrigo involves keeping the skinfolds cool and dry so healing can occur. Principles of management include minimizing skin-to-skin friction, removing irritants, wicking moisture away, minimizing the source of moisture, and preventing secondary infection. The skin should be cleansed with pH balanced, no-rinse cleanser, then patted dry. Clothing should be made of either lightweight natural fibers or wicking material; textiles made with a moisture-wicking silver compound have been found to be effective. Women should wear brassieres to reduce skin-to-skin friction.[17,19]

Indications for Referral.

Referral is indicated for symptoms including fever, systemic involvement, or significant evidence of nonhealing or worsening erosions. Any patient who does not experience a resolution of symptoms within 2 weeks should be referred to a dermatologist. Immunocompromised patients require consultation with the appropriate specialist.

Life-Span Considerations

Women of childbearing age should be informed of the risk of *Candida* infections while taking oral contraceptives and during pregnancy. The growing population of older adults presents significant challenges to the provider regarding skin disorders including intertrigo. Physiologic changes of aging skin include the thinning of dermis and epidermis, which increases the risk of mechanical trauma, and an impaired immune response that increases the risk of infection. The development of incontinence and immobility increases the risk for skin breakdown. A thorough skin examination performed routinely could reveal early stages of intertrigo, thus reducing the risk for infection.[20]

Complications

A secondary bacterial infection may develop if intertrigo is left untreated or if behaviors such as scratching impair skin integrity. Aggressive infections such as with β-hemolytic streptococci may lead to considerable complications; systemic involvement must also be considered. Patients with frequent candidal infections should be evaluated for HIV infection, diabetes mellitus, or other immunocompromised states. Complications could occur if Lotrisone is used for treatment as the component betamethasone is too strong for intertriginous sites. Cornstarch is ineffective and may result in fungal growth.[21]

Emerging Management Trends

Immunocompromised individuals are at greater risk for intertrigo. It is important to closely monitor and manage the conditions of the patient at risk. Intertrigo has been documented as a primary sign of HIV. An additional scenario to be aware of is symmetrical drug-related intertriginous and flexural exanthema (SDRIFE). An erythematous rash, contact dermatitis, emerges in the skin folds after exposure to drug or food trigger. A past detailed review should be done to examine any recent changes in diet or medications.[21]

Patient and Family Education

- Intertrigo in itself is not contagious, but infections resulting from impaired skin integrity may be transferable.
- Cornstarch-containing powders should be avoided.
- Patients will benefit from the use of a balanced pH, no-rinse cleanser and a handheld hair dryer with a cool setting to dry the area.
- Women should wear bras with good support to reduce skin friction.
- Implementing measures for prevention along with therapy will lead to excellent results, however, recurrence is common.
- With comorbid health conditions, intertrigo is considered a complication resulting in secondary infections.[19,21]

Health Promotion

Weight reduction is the best way to help combat reoccurrence of intertrigo. The monitoring of comorbid conditions, exercise, and weight control will need additional social support to be effective. The provider should encourage weight loss and disease management support groups. Those who use topical steroids will need to watch for signs of skin atrophy striae or telangiectasia. When the area has healed, reinforce the importance to keep folded skin areas clean and dry. Once the affected epidermis has healed, patients should be encouraged to keep susceptible areas clean and dry. Wearing of lightweight, natural-fiber clothing or clothing made of wicking material will reduce recurrence rates.[19-21]

VIRAL

HERPES SIMPLEX

 Immediate referral to physician or obstetrician for consultation is indicated for women who are pregnant. Additionally, those with HIV and those who are co-infected should be referred to a specialist.

Definition and Epidemiology

Cutaneous infections caused by the HSV can be of two serologic types: HSV-1, primarily oral lesions; and HSV-2, mainly genital infections. However, either virus can cause infection at either site. Oral HSV-1 infection recurs more frequently and earlier than oral HSV-2 infection; likewise, genital HSV-2 infection recurs more frequently than genital HSV-1 infection.[3,22] Both HSV-1 and HSV-2 are DNA viruses. Clinically, the lesions produced by each strain of the virus are indistinguishable.

There is a high prevalence of HSV-1 and HSV-2 throughout the world. Infection with the virus shows no seasonal variation, and there are no known animal vectors. By the fifth decade of life, 90% of adults have antibodies to HSV-1. In the United States alone, at least 50 million people have genital HSV infection. Anogenital herpetic infections are on the rise among young women and MSM and are attributed to HSV-1.[22] One-third to one-half of infected individuals lack clinical manifestations of infection and can shed the virus in the absence of symptoms. HSV-2 antibodies start to develop during puberty and correlate with the onset of sexual activity.[3]

Women have a higher seroprevalence than men and seroprevalence is higher among black people than white.[3]

Pathophysiology

Transmission of HSV occurs by direct contact with active lesions or with secretions containing the virus. HSV is a double-stranded DNA virus that may enter the host through a skin disruption (e.g., small crack in the skin) or intact mucous membranes (e.g., oropharynx, cervix, conjunctiva). The virus attaches itself to epithelial cells, enters, and replicates, exploiting cellular components. Once infected, cells die and release clear fluid, causing the formation of vesicles, which can fuse to form multinucleated giant cells. During the infection process, the virus gains access to and infects regional, sensory, or autonomic nerves. The virus travels through the nerve axon to the ganglion, where it establishes a latent infection. Subsequently, the virus can reactivate and travel down the axon, where it causes a recurrent infection in the cutaneous area innervated by the affected root.[3,22]

Clinical Presentation and Physical Examination

HSV infection has three distinct phases: primary, latent, and recurrent infection. An outbreak is considered to be a primary occurrence if the patient was found to be both HSV-1 and HSV-2 seronegative before the outbreak of genital lesions.[6] A person's first occurrence of HSV infection is usually the most severe and may start after an incubation period of 2 to 14 days; however, the incubation period may range anywhere from 1 to 26 days after initial exposure.[3] Genital lesions are often painful, with an average duration of symptoms of 22 to 28 days. Persons with a different HSV type may have milder symptoms. Patients frequently report a prodrome of burning or tenderness at the site. Multiple painful round vesicles then appear at the site of infection and may be accompanied by tender lymphadenopathy in regional nodes. Fever, dysuria, vaginal discharge, or malaise may accompany the primary infection. Ulceration subsequently occurs, and lesions crust over and heal in immunocompetent patients within 2 to 3 weeks.

During the latent phase, the virus remains dormant in the ganglion of the nerve that serves the affected dermatome. The recurrent phase is characterized by virus reactivation

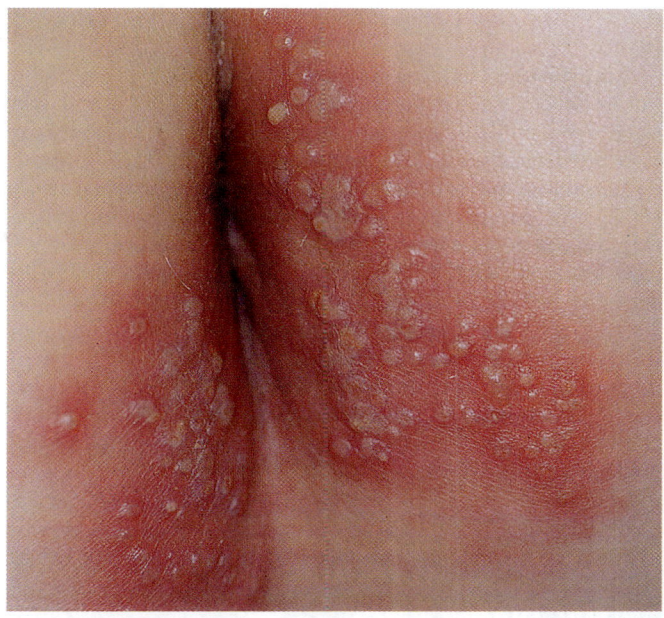

FIG. 47.3 Primary herpes simplex on the perineum and buttocks with groups of vesicles on a red base. (From Fisher, B. K., & Margesson, L. J. [1998]. *Genital skin disorders: Diagnosis and treatment.* St Louis: Mosby.)

and the reappearance of lesions in the dermatome affected during the primary infection. The outbreak may not occur at exactly the same site. Reactivation of either HSV type can be caused by local or systemic stimuli, such as immunodeficiency, trauma to mucosa, stress, depression, chronic anxiety, and poor sleep. HSV-1–specific triggers include ultraviolet light, cold weather, hot foods, lip biting, food allergy, and fever. HSV-2–specific triggers are noted to be food allergy and menses (usually 5 to 12 days before onset).[3,5,22] The primary infection may last 10 to 14 days, whereas recurrent infections are shorter and usually less severe, with markedly fewer lesions. The lesions of HSV infection are distinct. Grouped round vesicles on an erythematous base appear on the lips, facial area, throat, or genital area as seen in Fig. 47.3. The fluid contained in the vesicles turns cloudy. Vesicles rupture, leaving erosions that subsequently crust over. Often these can be confused as warts or molluscum contagiosum. Regional lymphadenopathy may be associated with primary or recurrent infections but is more common with primary infections. The various stages of lesions can often make diagnosis challenging.[4,22]

Diagnostics

Essential Diagnostics. Diagnosis of HSV infection can be made clinically with a thorough history and physical examination. However, laboratory confirmation should be considered in patients with a newly diagnosed primary infection. In addition, it is important to elicit any history of HSV infection, HIV infection, or pregnancy. The definitive test for the diagnosis of cutaneous herpes simplex infections remains viral culture. Viral cultures can take 2 to 7 days to achieve maximum sensitivity. Diagnosis may also be made with the use of fluid obtained from a freshly unroofed vesicle for Tzanck preparation or by a direct fluorescent antibody (DFA) test. Both tests have lower sensitivity rates than culture. Cultures are most likely to be positive for virus when fresh, moist lesions exist; however, the DFA test result may still be positive in crusted, healing lesions.[1,22]

Additional Diagnostics. Serologic testing is available but often does not differentiate HSV-1 from HSV-2 and may only reveal previous exposure. Antigen detection tests are also of limited usefulness in primary infections because antibody development may be delayed.[1,22] Polymerase chain reaction (PCR) tests are extremely sensitive and specific but are expensive and are not indicated for mucocutaneous infections. Serologic tests assessing for the specific immunoglobulin to HSV are available and are much more sensitive than viral cultures, PCR testing, and Tzanck smears. If ordering specific HSV serologic assay the provider should request glycoprotein G (gG-based) serologic assays. The most common test used is HerpeSelect HSV-2 enzyme-linked immunosorbent assays (ELISA), which show false positive at low index levels. Low levels should be confirmed using Biokit or the Western Blot. United States Preventive Services Task Force (USPSTF) gives a recommendation of D for routine serological screening for genital HSV in asymptomatic, pregnant adolescents and adults.[22,23]

INITIAL DIAGNOSTICS

Herpes Simplex

LABORATORY
- Viral cultures (90% sensitivity on vesicular lesion)
- Polymerase chain reaction (not approved by the FDA for genital swabs)
- Tzanck smear (not effectively sensitive)
- Serologic tests (sensitive and specific)

Differential Diagnosis

The differential diagnosis of suspected HSV infections is varied. A thorough health history, the appearance of lesions, and the results of appropriate laboratory testing help with the differentiation among these diagnoses.

 Priority differentials include (1) erythema multiforme, (2) impetigo, (3) varicella, and (4) HZ.

Varicella, herpangina, aphthous stomatitis, erythema multiforme, impetigo, Vincent angina, infectious mononucleosis, coxsackievirus infection, and Stevens-Johnson syndrome should be considered. Primary genital herpes can mimic Behçet syndrome, syphilis, candidiasis, infectious ulcerative balanitis, erosive lichen planus, atopic dermatitis, and urethritis.[3,6,9]

Interprofessional Collaborative Management

Pharmacologic Management

Topical Therapy. Evidence suggests that most cases of mild herpes labialis are self-limiting and do not require treatment. Topical medications have been shown to reduce the duration of pain; however, they may not affect the healing time. Combining topical acyclovir with hydrocortisone in medications such as topical Xerese and Denavir has been shown to be more efficient at reducing the progression of ulcerative lesions in up to 35% of patients.[1,22] Penciclovir cream (Denavir) is applied at the first sign of symptoms (e.g., tingling, itching, burning, swelling) and thereafter every 2 hours (while awake) for 4 days. Xerese (acyclovir/hydrocortisone topical) is applied 5 times a day for 5 days. Patients should avoid products with salicylic acid, which can erode the compromised skin.

Additional therapies may include the use of Sitavig (acyclovir oropharyngeal) or Acyclovir Lauriad, a muco-adhesive buccal tablet. This delivers a high concentration of acyclovir at the mucosal site. This has proven effective as a topical agent for recurrent labialis. It should be applied at the onset of prodromal symptoms. Erosion that is extensive may be treated with a compress comprised of cool water, silver nitrate 0.5%, or Burow solution applied for 20 minutes several times a day.[3]

Oral Therapy. Depending on the history and presentation of HSV multiple treatment options exists. The treatment of choice for first clinical episodes of genital HSV infections is acyclovir (Zovirax), 400 mg, given orally 3 times a day for 7 to 10 days; acyclovir, 200 mg, given orally 5 times a day for 7 to 10 days; famciclovir (Famvir), 250 mg, given orally 3 times a day for 7 days; or valacyclovir, 1 g, given orally twice daily for 7 to 10 days and with dosage, frequency, or duration reduced with renal impairment. It is also recommended that therapy is extended longer if indicated by incomplete healing despite treatment (Table 47.1).

With primary herpes labialis, acyclovir, 400 mg orally 5 times daily for 5 days, may reduce pain with eating and drinking; however, the healing period may not be reduced. On the other hand, valacyclovir—2000 mg 2 times a day for day 1, repeated with 1000 mg 2 times a day for day 2—may shorten the period

TABLE 47.1	Medication Schedule for Herpes Simplex Virus Infections
Drug	**Dosage**
INITIAL EPISODE	
Acyclovir	400 mg PO 3 times daily for 7–10 days
Acyclovir	200 mg PO 5 times daily for 7–10 days
Famciclovir	250 mg PO 3 times daily for 7–10 days
Valacyclovir	1 g PO twice daily for 7–10 days
	2000 mg PO every 12 h for 1 day for herpes labialis (cold sore); begin treatment within 48 h of symptom onset
RECURRENT EPISODES	
Acyclovir	400 mg PO twice daily for 5 days
	800 mg PO twice daily for 5 days
	800 mg PO 3 times daily for 2 days
Valacyclovir	500 mg PO twice daily for 3 days; or 1 g PO per day for 5 days
Famciclovir	125 mg PO twice daily for 5 days
	1000 mg PO twice daily for 1 day
	500 mg once, followed by 250 mg twice daily for 2 days
SUPPRESSION	
Acyclovir	400 mg PO twice daily
Valacyclovir	500 or 1000 mg PO per day (higher dose for those with more than 10 recurrences per year)
	For cold sores, reassess treatment need at 4 months
	For genital herpes simplex virus (HSV) suppression, reassess treatment need at 6 months
Famciclovir	250 mg PO twice daily

to healing and reduce pain (monitor and dose according to creatinine clearance levels with renal impairment).[3]

With primary genital herpes acyclovir, valacyclovir, and famciclovir have been shown to treat effectively. Antiviral therapy should be initiated within the first 6 days. Patients may be treated with one of the following regimens: (1) acyclovir 400 mg orally 3 times daily for 7 to 10 days; or (2) 200 mg orally 5 times daily for 7 to 10 days. Valacyclovir 500 mg 2 times daily, or famciclovir, 250 mg 3 times a day, can also be used. The duration of therapy should be extended if new lesions develop or systemic symptoms are present. Although valacyclovir and famciclovir may also be used, there is no evidence to suggest that they are any more effective clinically, and they cost considerably more. They do offer the benefit of easier administration if compliance or ease of dosage schedule is an important consideration.[22]

Recurrent episodes of orofacial herpes tend to be milder and shorter in duration than the primary infection.[3] Persons without a prodromal period with multiple painful or disfiguring lesions or more than four episodes should consider suppressive therapy. Most immunocompetent individuals with recurrent herpes labialis do not require treatment other than over-the-counter topical anesthetics for pain control. Also to be considered is the patient's ability to cope with the outbreaks. Both acyclovir and valacyclovir (Valtrex) may prevent recurrent episodes.[3,22]

Recurrent outbreaks of genital herpes that are mild and infrequent may not need to be treated. However, this will depend on the patient's desire, tolerance, and other presenting symptoms. Acyclovir, valacyclovir, and famciclovir can be chosen as oral treatment regimens for recurrent outbreaks to assist in aborting the development of lesions, reducing viral shedding, and limiting the extent of the outbreak while speeding the healing of lesions.[3] Therapy for recurrences should be initiated within the first 24 to 48 hours of the repeat episode. Treatment with acyclovir, 400 mg orally 3 times daily for 5 days, 800 mg orally twice daily for 5 days, or 200 mg orally 5 times daily for 5 days is appropriate.[3,22]

Suppressive therapy is needed for individuals with recurrent outbreaks more than 6 times per year. Patients may be treated with one of the following long-term suppressive therapy regimens: (1) acyclovir, 400 mg orally twice daily; (2) valacyclovir, 500 to 1000 mg orally every day; or (3) famciclovir, 250 mg orally twice daily. This reduces the number of recurrences and the frequency of asymptomatic shedding and may be protective for sex partners.It is important to understand that famciclovir and valacyclovir are no more effective than acyclovir for treatment of recurrent HSV infections and are costlier. Valacyclovir and famciclovir find the greatest usefulness when compliance or convenience of administration is an issue.[3,9]

Nonpharmacologic Management. The only over-the-counter treatment approved by the FDA is docosanol (Abreva). Pain and discomfort can be treated with applications of over-the-counter analgesics or anesthetics such as camphor, benzyl alcohol, pramoxine, phenol, menthol, tetracaine, or benzocaine. Protectants including petroleum jelly, lip balms, calamine, zinc oxide, allantoin, and cocoa butter may also be used.[3,4,6]

Prevention is key in the management of HSV infections. Examples of prevention strategies include widespread public education about the nature of the disease and its spread, urging the use of barrier methods for prevention of sexually transmitted infections with all sexual contact, and prophylactic antiviral therapy.[3] According to the 2015 Centers for Disease Control and Prevention (CDC) guidelines for the treatment of sexually transmitted diseases, the recommendation is to treat all patients who are experiencing initial genital herpes infections, regardless of severity, presentation, timing, or duration of symptoms, to reduce complications and possibly recurrences.[22]

 Indications for Referral Patients for whom a diagnosis of HSV is in question, who have superimposed HIV infection, who are receiving long-term suppressive therapy, or in whom conventional therapy fails should be referred to a physician or specialist. Pregnant women also represent a special population and should be referred for evaluation by their obstetrician or family physician immediately.[9]

Patients requiring large amounts of pain medication or patients who have severe disseminated infections, severe superimposed bacterial infections, inability to void, or inability to take anything by mouth should be considered for hospitalization.

Life-Span Considerations

Patients should understand that infection with HSV is lifelong and that there is no cure. There is currently no vaccination available; however, many vaccines are currently in different stages of development. These include vaccines made from proteins, peptides, or chains of amino acids and the DNA virus itself.[4,24] In most individuals, the frequency and severity of attacks diminish with time.[3] However, some evidence indicates that patients with frequently recurring HSV infections (more than six per year) can benefit from suppression with acyclovir, famciclovir, or valacyclovir.[22]

Complications

Complications of HSV infection are rare and typically occur in those who are already immunocompromised. Possible complications include aseptic meningitis, urinary retention, cutaneous dissemination, bacterial superinfection, erythema multiforme, and spontaneous abortion.[15] A cesarean section is usually performed if the mother has active herpes lesions at or around the time of delivery. Women who contract genital HSV-1 or HSV-2 infection in their third trimester of pregnancy are at high risk of infecting their newborns (30% to 50%).[15,22] Routine screening during pregnancy is not recommended by the USPSTF.[23]

Patient and Family Education

- Patients must be made aware of their ability to transmit HSV even when they have no apparent lesions or when using suppressive therapy.[22] Encouraging safe sexual practices, including the use of latex condoms and dental dams, is essential.[4,6]
- Explain the risk of neonatal transmission during pregnancy to both male and female patients.
- Encourage patients to use lip balm with sunscreen when exposed to ultraviolet light to avoid precipitation of an outbreak.
- Consider what counseling patients may need and refer appropriately. Two types of counseling are required for those newly diagnosed with genital herpes: (1) medical counseling, dealing with clinical issues; and (2) emotional counseling concerning the impact of herpes on self-esteem, sexuality, and social interactions.[3,6] Patients may experience

shame or depression because of their infection with HSV and should be referred to the American Sexual Health Association (http://www.ashasexualhealth.org/stdsstis/herpes/) for available resources.[6] The National Herpes Hotline is operated by the American Social Health Association as part of the Herpes Resource Center. The hotline, which receives more than 60,000 calls a year, provides accurate information and appropriate referrals to anyone concerned about herpes.[22] Additional support and information can be found at https://www.cdc.gov/std/herpes/default.htm on Health Promotion.

Patients can reduce their risk of acquiring genital herpes by limiting their lifetime number of sexual partners, by using condoms, and by becoming educated about transmission and shedding so they can avoid high-risk situations.[22] The risk of orolabial herpes infection can also be reduced by limiting sexual partners, incorporating the use of a dental dam, and avoiding direct contact with individuals with cold sores. Patients with orolabial and genital herpes must be counseled not to excoriate or to rub the herpes lesions because of the risk for autoinoculation of other parts of the body.

HERPES ZOSTER (SHINGLES)

 Immediate referral is indicated for herpes zoster lesions on the tip of the nose, around the eyes, and on the forehead. Hospitalization may be necessary for disseminated herpes zoster, as well as evaluation and treatment of complications.

Definition and Epidemiology

Varicella-zoster virus (VZV) disease is known worldwide by many names. VZV infections are specific to humans and are known by the following names: chickenpox virus, varicella virus, zoster virus, and human herpesvirus type 3 (HHV-3). HZ (shingles) is a dermatologic eruption caused by reactivation of the VZV that follows, sometimes by decades, a primary varicella-zoster (chickenpox) infection. A prodrome of pain or dysesthesia may precede by several days a vesicular eruption that typically occurs in a unilateral dermatomal distribution. Vesicular lesions appear during several days and may last for 7 to 10 days or more, although they can last for more than 4 weeks on rare occasions. The eruption can be extremely painful, and 5% to 20% of patients go on to develop a protracted pain syndrome called postherpetic neuralgia (PHN).[25]

The incidence of HZ increases with age. For adults aged 50 to 59, 5 out of 1000 will develop HZ, with an increase to 11 cases/1000 in those over age 80. In a single person's lifetime approximately 1 of every 3 will develop HZ, which is roughly 1 million Americans per year.[26,27]

After primary infection, VZV lies dormant in the sensory root ganglion, kept in check by the host's acquired cell-mediated immunity. The zoster eruption results from reactivation of the latent varicella infection in the dorsal root or cranial nerve ganglion cells, a process that is thought to be caused by the waning of the T-cell mediated immunity.[3,17] Zoster incidence is seen to increase with age and immune suppression, however, all ages are affected. The younger person who is affected by HZ will typically have milder symptoms. The more serious complication tends to increase with advancing age.[28] There is no pattern to who is affected based on gender or geography. Zoster is common and usually self-limited in adults, but serious complications can occur that may require consultation. HZ is

a painful cutaneous eruption that follows a single or double dermatome that does not cross the midline. Involvement of the ophthalmic branch of the trigeminal nerve can result in ocular keratitis, scarring, and loss of vision. Patients who are immunocompromised may have a disseminated infection that can result in a diffuse varicella-like eruption, neurologic complications, or visceral involvement that can cause death, most commonly from pneumonia.[28]

Pathophysiology

After initial varicella infection, the virus lies dormant in the dorsal root ganglia. Once it is reactivated, the virus replicates and travels through the axons, spreading from cell to cell until it penetrates the epidermis. Reactivation is likely to be multifactorial, with age being the most important risk factor. Immunosuppressed individuals of all types are at increased risk, as are some populations with chronic comorbid diseases, such as rheumatoid arthritis and inflammatory bowel disease. Trauma, surgery, and a recent cancer diagnosis have also been linked to zoster reactivation.[3]

HZ lesions contain high concentrations of virus that can be spread by contact and by air but are less contagious than primary infection. VZV can survive in external environments for a few hours, even a day or two. Contagion is possible once the rash has appeared and continues until the lesions have crusted.

Clinical Presentation and Physical Examination

Zoster classically is seen as a unilateral eruption within one dermatome, however, 20% of the time, an adjacent dermatome will be involved. The eruption is often preceded by a prodrome of pain, dysesthesia, or pruritus in the affected dermatome. Pain can be described as stabbing, burning, aching, or excruciating. The eruption is initially erythematous and maculopapular and becomes clusters of clear vesicles during the course of several hours to several days (Fig. 47.4). Low-grade fever and lymphadenopathy may be present. The most common areas of involvement are the thoracic, cranial (especially the trigeminal), and lumbar nerves. On the rare occasion that there is no visible eruption, a condition called zoster sine herpete, the pain is sometimes attributed to other causes (e.g., angina, renal colic, pleural pain, sciatica, or migraine), depending on

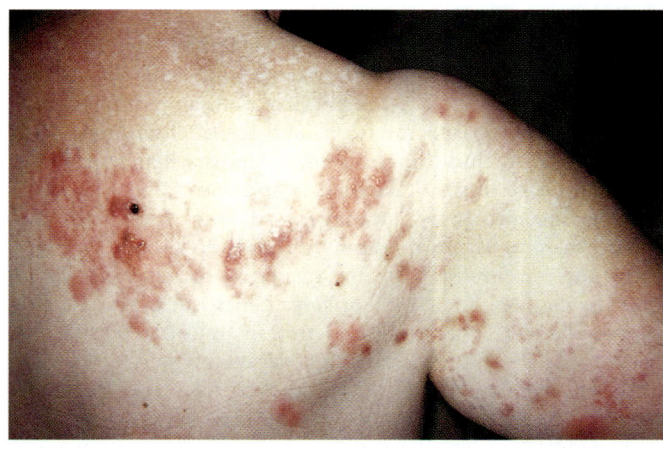

F I G . 47.4 Herpes zoster. (From Ignatavicius, D. D., & Workman, M. L. [2016]. *Medical-surgical nursing: Patient centered collaborative care* [8th ed]. St. Louis: Mosby.)

the dermatome affected. Any pain after the rash heals or any pain after 1 month, 3 months, 4 months, or 6 months can be defined as PHN. Regardless, pain can exist in varying degrees for many years.[4]

Diagnostics

Essential Diagnostics. Diagnosis is based on the clinical presentation of a vesicular eruption in a unilateral, dermatomal distribution. Without the skin eruption, zoster is a diagnosis of exclusion. Disseminated HZ is a generalized eruption of lesions along with the typical segmental distribution. Immunocompromised individuals are susceptible as well as those whose VZV viral loads are waning.[3]

Additional Diagnostics. A Tzanck test is a rapid way to confirm the diagnosis of zoster in the provider's office but does not distinguish between VZV and HSV. The DFA test is another rapid test that is available in some settings. PCR analysis is the most rapid and sensitive, although it is not available in all settings due to the expense. All of these tests are preferred to viral culture because they are more rapid and often more sensitive. Confirmation via laboratory testing may be necessary based on location of lesion to differentiate between HSV and HZ.[27]

INITIAL DIAGNOSTICS

Herpes Zoster

LABORATORY
- PCR analysis
- Tzanck preparation
- DFA test

ADDITIONAL DIAGNOSTICS
- Viral culture
- Alkaline phosphatase, bilirubin, C-reactive protein, WBC[a]

---
[a]If indicated.

Differential Diagnosis

 Priority differentials include (1) allergic dermatitis, (2) dermatitis herpetiformis, (3) contact dermatitis, and (4) coxsackievirus infection.

Additional considerations for differential diagnosis include the most likely: Herpes simplex, insect bites, burns, drug eruptions, scabies, coxsackievirus infection, impetigo, and varicella. Differentials that should always be ruled out include bullous pemphigoid, pemphigus vulgaris, dermatitis herpetiformis, epidermolysis bullosa herpetiformis, and eczema herpetic. A distribution of pain involving the chest, jaw, or left arm may mimic cardiovascular pain. Pain in the trunk could also mimic cholecystitis, appendicitis, pleurisy, duodenal ulcer, renal calculi. If prodromal sensation involves the head consider otitis media, headache, ulcerative keratitis, acute closed-angle glaucoma, trigeminal neuralgia, or stroke. Zoster pain may mimic several other diagnoses during the prodromal stages. Ruling out these is critical to prevent further disease process.[27]

The pain associated with zoster can precede the eruption by 4 or 5 days. Depending on the distribution, the pain may mimic angina, renal colic, or pleuritic pain. Once the eruption is present, the cause of the pain is more apparent. The presentation of primary varicella can be similar to that of disseminated zoster, and serologic testing may be needed in the absence of a known history of chickenpox. Eczema herpeticum is an infection of HSV inoculated into a patch of eczema,

resulting in a more widely distributed HSV infection. A DFA test, PCR analysis, or viral culture will differentiate the two.[4] Any of the numerous other vesicle-producing dermatoses, such as coxsackievirus infection, impetigo, contact dermatitis, and dermatitis herpetiformis, should be considered in the differential diagnosis.[5]

Interprofessional Collaborative Management

Pharmacologic Management

Antiviral Therapy. The treatment of uncomplicated HZ is the symptomatic treatment of lesions and prevention of secondary infection. Antiviral therapy is an essential part of zoster therapy. Studies have shown that initiation of antiviral therapy (acyclovir, famciclovir, and valacyclovir) within 72 hours of rash onset reduces the duration and severity of both the rash and the pain and reduces the risk for PHN for the localized and disseminated disease. Primary therapy includes valacyclovir 1000 mg orally 3 times a day for 7 days, famciclovir 500 mg orally 3 times a day for 7 days, or acyclovir 800 mg orally 5 times daily for 7 to 10 days.[6] Each of these medications is effective; the choice is often based on cost and convenience of administration. Dosages may need to be adjusted for renal impairment.[2,5]

Pain Control. HZ pain is difficult to treat. Most of the pain is related to nerve pain. Some of the options for control include the use of NSAIDs, gabapentin, pregabalin, amitriptyline, acetaminophen, and as a last resort opioids.

The use of oral corticosteroids is used by some clinician in combination with anti viral medication. Studies have not demonstrated efficacy in preventing post herpetic neuralgia but some patients may experience pain relief with this regime. Prednisone should not be used in patients with diabetes or those who are immunosuppressed. The prednisone dosing is 60 mg/d for 7 days, 30 mg/d for 7 days, and 15 mg/day for 7 days to finish. Development of PHN may still occur, although a 3-week tapering course may modestly reduce the duration and severity of pain and could be considered on a case-by-case basis.[3,5,6,27] Analgesic and narcotic agents may be administered if necessary.

Postherpetic Neuralgia Pain Management. The long-term effects associated with PHN can be devastating to the patient. Many treatments are available to manage this type of pain. Often it may require a creative combination of several agents to help the patient experience relief. Available options for treatment include acetaminophen, NSAIDs, and opiates. Topically applied lidocaine and capsaicin have been used successfully to reduce the pain of PHN. Anticonvulsants such as gabapentin and pregabalin are effective for treatment of neuropathic pain and have a more favorable side effect profile than their older predecessors carbamazepine and valproic acid. Caution should be used with tricyclic antidepressants related to their side effects. Recalcitrant PHN may benefit from a sympathetic block or epidural.[3,6]

Topical Therapy. Cool, moist compresses and agents, such as calamine and aluminum sulfate (Domeboro) soaks, are soothing and will help dry vesicles. Other topical treatments including lidocaine patches, nonsteroidal antiinflammatory patches, and capsaicin creams can also be helpful after skin lesions have healed Patients should be instructed to keep the area clean and dry, to avoid the topical antibiotics bacitracin and neomycin because of the high incidence of allergic contact dermatitis, and, if possible, to keep the rash covered.[2,3,6]

Preventative Therapy

Vaccination. In 2006, the FDA approved Zostavax, a live, attenuated vaccine for the prevention of zoster in patients older than 60 years. In October of 2017, the FDA approved a second vaccine to prevent zoster. Shingrix, a zoster vaccine recombinant, adjuvanted with the indication for the prevention of HZ in adults ≥ 50 years. The CDC has recommended Shingrix (recombinant zoster vaccine, RZV) as preferred over Zostavax (zoster vaccine live, ZVL). If individuals over age 60 are allergic to the components of Shingrix, it is recommended they receive the Zostavax vaccine. It is important to note that Zostavax is stored in the freezer and administered subcutaneously. Shingrix is stored in the refrigerator and is administered intramuscularly.[25]

Previous recommendation by the Advisory Committee on Immunization Practices (ACIP) at the CDC for Zostavax, included that all adults 60 years of age and older, who are not immunocompromised, be vaccinated with one dose of Zostavax vaccine regardless of chickenpox history.[25] The vaccination appears to be most effective in the 60- to 69-year age group; a significant reduction in the incidence of zoster (54%) and PHN was realized (61% measured at 30 days). In patients older than 80 years, protection against zoster occurrence was not as high (18% reduction), but efficacy against PHN was better preserved (39%).[29] Studies have recently revealed a declination in the effectiveness of the live attenuated vaccine, Zostavax. After the first year of vaccination, there was a reduction in the effectiveness of 68.7%. There was a further decline in effectiveness 8 years later, resulting in effectiveness of 4.2%. This data suggests the need for subsequent dose or doses.[29,30]

Shingrix is a subunit vaccine containing recombinant glycoprotein E in combination with a novel adjuvant. The new recommendations from the ACIP state that two doses, separated by 2 to 6 months, should be administered intramuscularly to immunocompetent adults over age 50. This indication is intended for anyone, regardless of prior history of HZ or a prior dose of Zostavax. It is indicated for those with chronic medical conditions unless a previous precaution exists. Shingrix may be administered to adults on low-dose immunosuppressive therapy, planning to receive immunosuppressive therapy, or who have recovered from an immunocompromised illness. No screening for previous varicella disease is indicated.[25–31]

Clinical trial data demonstrate RZV in all age categories has a higher efficacy against HZ than those who received ZVL. The data suggests the RZV has a higher efficacy regarding PHN pain. Based on this data the ACIP recommends Shingrix administration over Zostavax. However, the patient may choose either if there are no contraindications.[26]

Indications for Referral. Immunocompromised patients or those with disseminated HZ should be referred to a specialist for IV therapy of acyclovir or vidarabine with close monitoring of renal function along with adequate hydration. Patients who have a history of organ transplant or AIDS have a potential to have an acyclovir-resistant varicella-zoster. Treatment of record should be foscarnet IV until the lesions have healed.[6] Referral to an ophthalmologist should be sought as there are increased complications with ocular zoster.[4]

Life-Span Considerations

Consideration should be given regarding age and administration of the vaccine. There is currently no wait time between an incidence of shingles in relation to receiving the vaccination. If the patient is experiencing an acute case the administration of Shingrix should be postponed until the episode is resolved.[25]

Complications

HZ lesions on the tip of the nose, around the eyes, and on the forehead require immediate ophthalmology consultation and evaluation. These findings signal possible involvement of the branch of the trigeminal nerve that innervates the cornea, which may cause ulceration on the cornea and result in permanent damage. Motor paralysis and facial palsy (Ramsay Hunt syndrome) may follow HZ. Immunosuppressed individuals may develop dissemination, pneumonia, hepatitis, meningoencephalitis, and purpura fulminans. Patients with disseminated zoster should be evaluated for malignant disease, immunodeficiency, or AIDS.[3,4] One of the most common complications of HZ is PHN, which can last weeks to years. Management of PHN is difficult. However, many treatment options are available that may minimize the neuralgia. PHN can last anywhere from 3 months to over 10 years. Individuals with advanced age are more prone to have these long-term effects. The ACIP report noted intense pain, the changes in quality of life, and physical and emotional disabilities resulted in patients committing suicide as a way to end the pain.[3,26,31]

Emerging Management Trends

Brivudin is an antiviral that inhibits the replication of the zoster virus. It is currently available in several European countries; however, it is not available in the United States. Clinacanthus nutans is a plant from Malaysia, Indonesia, Thailand, and China used in traditional herbal medicines for the relief of inflammation and infection. Scientific data are lacking but anectodal reports of efficacy against Zoster are interestingThe recently approved vaccination Shingrix is promising for all and currently recommended for all adults ages 50 and up.[31]

Patient and Family Education

- Use moist dressings, pain management, and bedrest to relieve the discomfort of HZ lesions.
- Explain that lesions of HZ may contain VZV, enabling transmission to susceptible individuals (including infants and women of childbearing age who have not had the varicella vaccine or previous varicella infection). HZ itself is not transmissible, but VZV-naive patients are at risk for primary varicella (chickenpox) infection. Patients should avoid direct contact with susceptible persons and cover active lesions until they have crusted over, indicating that the lesions are no longer contagious.
- Alert patients and family to the possibility of PHN and be advised to seek appropriate medical attention if pain persists after the rash has cleared.[17]
- Teach patients to protect themselves from the sun, as the heat and ultraviolet rays will intensify and exacerbate the lesions.[27]

Health Promotion

Infection should be reduced by keeping the rash area clean and dry. Educate the patient regarding proper care of the rash, including avoidance of topical antibiotics, dressings with adhesive, and clothing that may be irritating or delay the healing process. Patients should be aware of postherpetic pain involvement and ways to alleviate the pain. If medication, relaxation techniques, and counseling are not beneficial with pain relief, referral to a pain management specialist should be given.[3] Consider VZ vaccination for anyone older than 50 years during routine health maintenance visits. Individual consideration must be used in this population.[25]

MOLLUSCUM CONTAGIOSUM
Definition and Epidemiology
Molluscum contagiosum virus (MCV) is a benign viral infection of the poxvirus family affecting the skin and mucous membranes. In healthy individuals MCV is self-limiting and harmless. It is seen mostly in children and adolescents and rarely affects adults. Climates that are more tropical or sub tropical have an increased incidence of MCV. It is transmitted by close contact, by fomite, or by autoinoculation (Koebner phenomenon).[2,4,32]

Individuals who are immunocompromised (HIV and low CD4 counts) will have a more severe response with lesions that are generalized over the entire body, severe replication in one location, or a longer disease course. Sexually transmitted forms of MCV occur in oral, genital, perineal, pubic, and surrounding areas.[4,15] An 11-fold increase in the incidence has been documented over the past 20 years according to a review of a recent study. This number coincides with an increase in the number of sexually transmitted diseases.[32]

Pathophysiology
MCV is in the same family as orthopox viruses (variola, vaccinia, and monkeypox). However, it differs by genus with all having similar but not exact; therefore, the disease response is quite different. The replication occurs in the cytoplasm of cells in which the proteins are responsible for the defense mechanisms that inhibit the inflammatory and immune response to occur. An epidermal tumor formation is seen with MCV while the other types of human poxviruses result in a necrotic lesion. Four subtypes of MCV exist with genotype 1 being the primary cause in children and genotype 2 as the main cause in adults and immunocompromised individuals. Sexual contact among this group tends to be the most common mode of transmission. MCVs' only known hosts are human beings.[2] The incubation period is usually 2 weeks to 6 months with lesions slowly appearing over time. Most MCV cases resolve within 9 months, however, may last as long as 4 years.[32]

Clinical Presentation and Physical Examination
MCV causes localized lesions consisting of painless, slightly itchy, flesh-colored, shiny, pearly white, or waxy dome-shaped papules with a central dimple. Their size may vary from 1 mm to 1 cm or larger nodules appearing singly or in clusters. The lesions may be found in multiple locations on the body often in intertriginous sites, such as the genital, perianal region. Lesions can also appear around the eyelid and perioral areas of the face. MCV is not seen on the palms and soles of the individual.[2,4] If the lesion ruptures or is expressed a white curd-like substance will be seen. Immune response to the lesion may appear as an erythematous patch. In the immunocompromised individual, the presentation is much more severe requiring therapy to accelerate the recovery process. Treatment should occur in the non-immunocompromised patient if the patient is having discomfort or suffering from social stigma resulting from visible lesions, or to prevent secondary infection or increased risk for trauma or bleeding based on location of lesion.[32]

Diagnostics
Essential Diagnostics. Diagnostics are generally based on clinical findings. If the disease is disseminated and there is no documentation the patient is immunocompromised, further testing should occur. If HIV disease is known, testing may be done to determine the level of invasiveness.[1]

Additional Diagnostics. A specimen may be obtained for microscopy, staining, or histopathology evaluation. Obtain the specimen by crushing or expressing the central contents of the papule. The characteristic brick-shaped viral particles inside the Henderson-Paterson inclusion bodies will be viewed upon examination of the specimen.[3,33]

INITIAL DIAGNOSTICS

Molluscum Contagiosum

LABORATORY
- Needle aspiration microscopy
- Curettage biopsy[a]
- Giemsa staining[a]
- Tzanck stain[a]
- HIV screening[a]

[a]If indicated.

Differential Diagnosis

 Priority differentials include (1) verrucae, (2) pyogenic granuloma, (3) acne, and (4) squamous cell or basal cell carcinoma.

Other differentials that should be considered include folliculitis, condylomata acuminate, syringoma, sebaceous hyperplasia, and epidermal inclusion cyst. It is important always to rule out carcinoma, melanoma, and appendageal tumors. If multiple disseminated or facial mollusca are present consider HIV disease.[9,17]

Interprofessional Collaborative Management
Nonpharmacologic Management. Watchful waiting is the most common and most conservative prescribed treatment method. MCV in immunocompetent individuals typically resolves spontaneously.[2,32]

Pharmacologic Management
Topical Destruction of Lesion. Several options are available for the destruction of the lesions. Most often curettage or liquid nitrogen (LN2) is applied. Laser surgery may be used to target and destroy the lesions. This can be an effective treatment for those who have a weakened immune system. Electrosurgery with a fine needle is a comparable method. Topical cantharidin may be applied and washed off in 4 hours or 10% KOH applied twice daily until cleared. Other topical therapies include retinoid creams, salicylic acid, silver nitrate paste, and liquefied phenol. Painful irritation and blistering are common side effects of this aggressive topical therapy. Neither Imiquimod nor podophyllotoxin have shown effectiveness with lesion destruction.[2,32]

Systemic Therapies. Oral therapies are reserved for immunocompromised individuals. Cimetidine 40 mg/kg/day has been used with minimal success. However, it does have some response as an immunomodulatory effect increasing lymphocyte proliferation. Additionally, cidofovir is also recommended as an alternative.[2]

Indications for Referral. Individuals who experience multiple, large, or a rapid onset of MCV should be tested for HIV and referred for treatment with dermatologist.[6]

Life-Span Considerations

MCV among children is spread very easily. Parents and schools should be notified to prevent risk or transmission particularly in youth who participate in contact sports. MCV in children located in the genital area may be indicative of sexual abuse.[6,9] For adults who have MCV the method of transmission is usually sexual. These lesions usually number fewer than 20 and appear on the penile shaft, upper thighs, and lower abdomen. Spread is increased with shaving, clipping, or waxing of hair.[2,3,15]

Patient and Family Education

- Education on how transmission occurs is important.
- Clean bath towels properly and do not share.
- Avoid public swimming pools or spas that may be reported as a source.
- Teach youth who play contact sports that they are at increased risk.
- Explain that self-inoculation also contributes to the spread of the lesions.[32]

Health Promotion

Individuals who have MCV located in the genital regions should practice abstinence and avoidance until the lesions have cleared. Avoid spreading the lesions by sharing of towels or shaving affected area involved.[4]

VIRAL EXANTHEMS
Definition and Epidemiology

Viral Exanthems. An exanthem rash is eruptive and usually associated with a systemic disorder. Morbilliform is a common term that means a grouping of erythematous macules. Frequently viral infections are associated with these type of skin eruptions. Often exanthems pose a challenge in diagnosing as they may have nondistinctive features. The difficulty lies with distinguishing if the exanthem is from a virus or related to drug eruption. Many classic viral diseases do present in a widely recognized pattern.[10]

Most viral exanthem (VE) rashes are seen in early and late childhood. However, when seen in adults this rash may be confused with a drug reaction. Many VE due to respiratory virus appear during winter months while enteroviruses are seen in summer and fall. Enterovirus infections usually appear within a 3- to 6-day incubation period. Attack rates are highest in children and lower socioeconomic groups. VE are more prevalent in warm, humid climates during summer and fall.[10]

The majority of viruses are highly contagious and spread by droplets. This includes measles, rubella, Gianotti-Crosti syndrome (GCS), primary human herpesvirus 6 (HHV-6), human herpesvirus 7 (HHV-7) also known as exanthema subitum or roseola infantum, pityriasis rosea, and Parvovirus B19, which is also known as erythema infectiosum, Sticker's, or fifth disease. VE spread by mosquitos are dengue, chikungunya, and Zika.[17,34,35] Approximately 110,000 people died worldwide in 2017 from measles. An outbreak of measles in 2019 resulted in 700+ cases in the United States primarily centered

in populations where the number of unvaccinated children was high. HHV-6 will affect more than 90 percent of children by adulthood. Adults can be affected by the coxsackievirus A6, which is seen more often during the winter. Many people are asymptomatic carriers of these viruses.[10,34,35]

Classically exanthems were given number names as they were named in the series. The first disease is measles, the second disease is scarlet fever (which is not viral), the third disease is rubella, the fourth disease is dukes (which is no longer accepted as a disorder), the fifth disease is erythema infectiosum, and the sixth disease is roseola.[2]

Pathophysiology

Most VEs are spread via respiratory transmission (with the exception of those that are spread by mosquitos). The proliferation of the virus in the pharynx and upper respiratory tract begins the process of virus replication. The rate of the incubation periods and thus the appearance of the rash depend on which virus is replicating. Many incubation periods vary from a few days to 2 to 3 weeks. See Table 47.2 for distinctive VE clinical description regarding transmission incubation.

The stimulation of the antibody and humoral system leads to the inflammatory reaction, which develops into flu-like symptoms and a rash. Many of the viral infections will have positive antibody titers for many years after the disease occurred. For HHV-6 and HHV-7 a herpes virus will induce a lifelong latent infection in humans.[6,10,34]

Clinical Presentation and Physical Examination

A thorough physical exam is critical for proper diagnosis. Manifestation on the skin may be the chief clue to determine the type of infection or disease. In order to determine differentials with VE a systematic approach to the physical exam should include time of year, travel history, recent exposures (individuals, animals, insects), medication changes, immune status, and most importantly health history of the individual to include childhood diseases and current immune status. During the physical exam documentation of the exanthem's initial onset of rash, morphology and change, distribution, progression, and associated symptoms will be essential in identifying the type of VE. For complete descriptions of VE transmission, infectivity, incubation, and clinical presentation, see Table 47.2. Common exanthem presentations are morbilliform-type macular and maculopapular, which include erythema infectiosum, measles, rubella, roseola, dengue, Zika, and chikungunya.[35] See Fig. 47.5 for the some of the other dermatological manifestations of Zika including facial edema and conjunctivitis. Vesicular and pustular lesions may be identified as varicella or HZ, or hand-foot-mouth disease. Papular exanthem presentations include parvovirus B19 (Fig. 47.6) and pityriasis rosea (Fig. 47.7). Physical signs and symptoms may include a combination of any of the following: rash, headache, rhinorrhea, low-grade fever, myalgias, or gastrointestinal issues.[10] The arboviral diseases of chikungunya and Zika (see Chapter 215) are very similar in presentation with more than 50% of patients presenting with a maculopapular rash of the trunk and extremities. Many will also complain of petechiae or urticaria. Zika exanthem will be seen in 98% of the patients presenting in combination with conjunctivitis and with edema of the face, hands and feet (Fig. 47.5). It is important to ask of any recent travels to areas endemic for these diseases.[36]

TABLE 47.2   Viral Exanthems Clinical Description

Virus	Transmission Method	Infectivity Period	Incubation Period	Features	Exanthem
Measles- (rubeola)	Respiratory droplets	5 days before the appearance of rash to 4 days afterward	7–14 days	Prodrome consists of fever, myalgias, cough, coryza, and conjunctivitis. The Koplik spots predates the exanthem by 1–2 days and lasts 2–4 days.	Onset 2–4 days after fever; erythematous, maculopapular, blanching rash (in later stages the rash does not blanch). Initially presents in the hairline, forehead, and behind the ears spreading cephalocaudally and moves centrifugally to involve the neck, upper trunk, lower trunk, and extremities. Day 5 rash fades in the same order it appeared.
Parvovirus B19 (erythema infectiosum, fifth disease)	Respiratory droplets	Contagious until 1–2 days after fever subsides. Active viral replication and viral shedding, which occurs approximately 5–10 days after exposure and usually lasts approximately 5 days. By the time symptoms of rash and/or arthropathy emerge, infected individuals are no longer infectious.	4–14 days	Adults may present with arthritis in hands, wrists, knees, and ankles, along with papular purpuric gloves and socks syndrome.	May appear 7–10 days after prodrome period. Bright red erythema appears abruptly over the cheeks at 1–4 days, an erythematous morbilliform rash presents on the extremities. In 4–9 days it fades reticulate lacy pattern. Exanthem may take up to 3 weeks to completely fade.
P tyriasis rosea				Prodrome may include headache, malaise, and pharyngitis, itching but generally asymptomatic.	Initial herald patch, a single oval, sharp, pink or salmon-colored lesion on the chest, neck, or back; 2–5 cm with more eruptions up to 1–2 weeks later, appearing on the trunk and proximal areas of the extremities eventually morphing into a Christmas tree appearance.
Roseola (exanthem subitem) human herpesvirus 6 and HHV-7	Respiratory droplets presumed	From onset of exposure until 3 days after fever abates.	HHV-6 is 5–15 days HHV-7 is unknown	Primarily seen in infants. Abrupt high fever 3–7 days that abates followed by abrupt onset of rash from the trunk to the extremities but spares the face. May have seizures associated with high fever as well as periorbital edema.	Rose-pink maculopapular rash
Rubella (German measles) RNA virus of the Togaviridae family	Respiratory droplets	Potentially 1–2 weeks before and during the eruption of the rash.	14–21 days	Prodrome is more prominent in adults: malaise, low-grade fever, coryza, mild conjunctivitis, and upper respiratory symptoms. Suboccipital and post auricular glands lymphadenopathy, precedes rash. Forschheimer spots appear.	Pink macules and papules on the face that spread to the trunk and extremities lasting 1–3 days fading in the same order as it appeared.
Varicella chickenpox	Respiratory droplets	Incubation 10–20 days		Malaise with low-grade fever	Tear-drop vesicles (dew on a rose petal) Presenting with multiple stages at the same time.

Continued

TABLE 47.2	Viral Exanthems Clinical Description—cont'd				
Virus	Transmission Method	Infectivity Period	Incubation Period	Features	Exanthem
Chikungunya (belongs to the same group of viruses as rubella)	Mosquito bite	Not contagious	3–7 days	Abrupt fever, headache, polyarthralgia 2–5 days after onset of fever, bilateral arthralgia, photophobia, vomiting More common in tropical climates	Maculopapular rash 3 days after onset lasting ~7 days, starts on the limbs and trunk is patchy or diffuse on extremities and trunk
Dengue	Mosquito bite	Not contagious	3–5 days	Fever, chills, headache, vomiting, myalgia/arthralgia, leukopenia and positive tourniquet test. Presumptive diagnosis based on positive symptoms.	Maculopapular eruption with islands of sparing; possible petechiae and purpura
Zika	Mosquito bite	May be spread via semen and mother to baby		Fever, headache, fatigue, aphthous ulcers arthralgias	Maculopapular rash on trunk
Hand-foot-mouth disease (HFMD) Coxsackie A16 and enterovirus 71	Spread via fecal oral possible respiratory	Incubation 4–6 days	After crusting healing in 7 days. Viral shedding up to 6 weeks.	Mild low-grade fever, sore throat, malaise for 1–2 days with submandibular and cervical lymphadenopathy. Oral lesions are the presenting sign followed by cutaneous lesion appearing within 24 h.	Red macules 3–7 mm turns pale, white oval vesicles with a red areola appear on the palms, soles, dorsal aspects of the fingers and toes and occasionally on the face, buttocks, and legs.

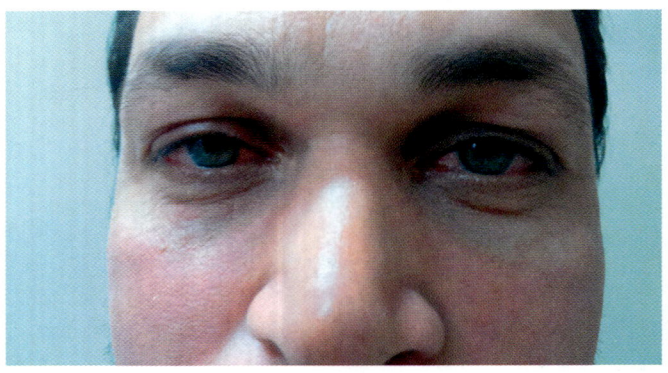

FIG. **47.5** Dengue fever: Petechia with islands of sparing on erythematous leg. (From Brasil, P., Calvet, G. A., Souza, R. V., & Siqueira, A. M. [2016]. Exanthema associated with Zika virus infection. *Lancet Infectious Diseases, 16*[7], 866.)

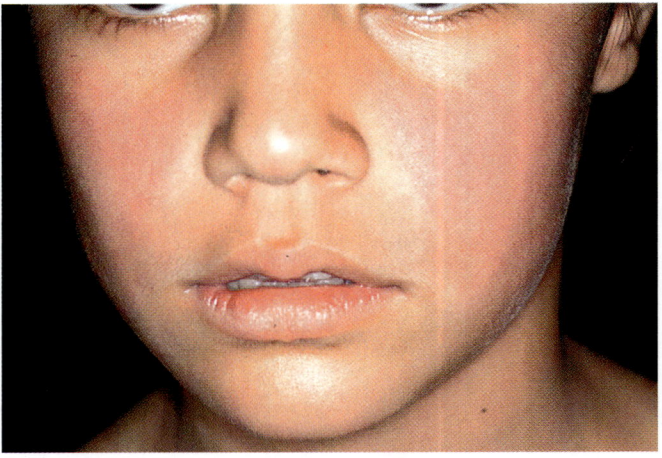

FIG. **47.6** Erythema infectiosum Parvo B19. Bright red macular lacy reticulated erythema on the cheeks. (Courtesy of Louis A. Fragola, Jr, MD; Bolognia, J., Schaffer, J., & Cerroni, L. [2018]. *Dermatology* [4th ed.]. Philadelphia: Elsevier.)

INITIAL DIAGNOSTICS

Viral Exanthem

LABORATORY
- DNA assay—polymerase chain reaction throat swab[a]
- Virus-specific IgG[a]
- Nucleic acid amplification testing[a]
- Reticulocyte count[a]
- CBC and differential[a]

[a]If indicated by the presence of more systemic features or immunocompromised status.

Diagnostics

Essential Diagnostics. Most presentation of VEs are based on clinical presentation and patient history. See Table 47.3 for more specific laboratory considerations.[3]

Differential Diagnosis

 Priority differentials include (1) all other viral exanthems, (2) mononucleosis, (3) adenovirus, (4) West Nile virus, (see Chapter 215), and (5) syphilis.

TABLE 47.3 **Viral Exanthem Laboratory Confirmation**

Virus	Diagnostic	Differential
Measles (rubeola)	Confirmation 4× or Measles-specific IgG antibody concentration, IFA, and NAT	Other VE: Roseola, rubella, measles, enteroviral infections Drug eruption, mononucleosis, Zika
Parvovirus B19 (erythema infectiosum, fifth disease)	If necessary concurrent analyses for both IgM and IgG antibodies from a single blood sample.	Other VE: Roseola, rubella, measles, enteroviral infections Group A streptococcal, HIV, mononucleosis
P tyriasis rosea	None recommended. Order: Rule VDRL: Syphilis KOH: tinea corporis Biopsy: Nummular Dermatitis Drug History: Guttate psoriasis	Secondary syphilis, Tinea corporis Nummular dermatitis, Guttate psoriasis
Roseola (exanthem subitem) Human Herpesvirus 6 and HHV-7	Polymerase chain reaction (PCR), NAT: qualitative and quantitative assays in blood	Drug eruption, acute mononucleosis (especially in adults) Enterovirus (including coxsackie, echovirus), rubella (German measles) Measles/rubeola, adenovirus, Epstein–Barr virus Fifth disease (erythema infectiosum, parvovirus) Scarlet fever, Kawasaki disease
Rubella (German measles) Togaviridae family	Rubella-specific IgM, antibodies using an enzyme immunoassay, and NAT	Other VE: Roseola, rubella, measles, enteroviral infections Drug eruption, mononucleosis, toxoplasmosis
Varicella	If necessary PCR. Acute and convalescent IgM and IgG antibody titers confirmatory	Viral exanthems, disseminated herpes simplex virus infection, atypical herpes zoster, rickettsial disease, impetigo, insect bites, syphilis
Dengue	Can be made based on positive findings on clinical exam. If during the first week PCR and Anti-DENV IgM ELISA if after 8 days Anti-DENV IgM ELISA	Chikungunya, Zika, malaria, typhoid, as well as the other viral exanthems.
Chikungunya	Anti-CHIKV IgM ELISA or IFA	Dengue, Zika, parvovirus, rubella, measles and other exanthems
Zika	Blood and urine ribonucleic acid (RNA) nucleic acid testing (NAT) and Zika virus and/or dengue virus IgM testing of serum	Chikungunya, dengue, malaria, typhoid, as well as the other viral exanthems
Hand-foot-mouth disease (HFMD) Coxsackie A16, 71	Not necessary for diagnosis. PCT may be obtained for serotyping	Herpangina, varicella, aphthous stomatitis Drug eruption, erythema multiforme, herpes

ELISA, Enzyme-linked immunosorbent assays; *HHV*, human herpesvirus type 3; *HIV*, human immunodeficiency virus; *IFA*, indirect fluorescent testing; *KOH*, potassium hydroxide; *NAT*, nucleic acid testing; *PCT*, procalcitonin; *VDRL*, venereal disease research laboratory; *VE*, viral exanthema.

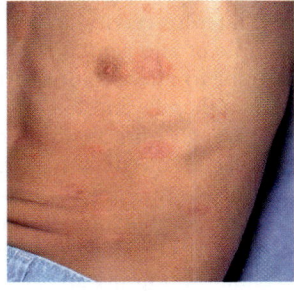

F I G . 47.7 Pityriasis rosea, classic salmon-pink. (From Ferri, F. F. [2019]. *Ferri's fast facts in dermatology: A practical guide to skin disease and disorders* [2nd ed.]. Philadelphia: Elsevier.)

Additional differentials will be based on clinical presentation, symptoms, and exam. Additional considerations include streptococcal or staphylococcal toxic shock syndrome, leptospirosis, drug eruptions, and Kawasaki disease. Please see Table 47.3 for more specific differential diagnoses.

Interprofessional Collaborative Management

Pharmacologic Management

Acetaminophen (APAP) and Nonsteroidal Antiinflammatory Drugs. The general treatment course of VE is supportive. NSAIDs may be used for symptomatic arthropathy. During the febrile phases, APAP or NSAID may be used to help control high fevers. Dosing should be as directed based on age. Careful consideration with special populations in which contraindications with medications or health issues exist.

Vitamin A. lLow serum vitamin A levels are a risk factor for measles. In the younger child, prescribing vitamin A can reduce measles-related ocular morbidity and mortality. The World Health Organization recommends prescribing a once-daily dose of Vitamin A, especially in regions where Vitamin A deficiency is common, for two days. Supplement should be given regardless of nutritional status.[3,10,37]

Antibiotic Treatment for Secondary Infections

Individuals with VE secondary infections should be treated as appropriate for the area of infection. Measles may have increased incidence of ear infections as well as kerato conjunctivitis. For all the different VEs secondary infections must be considered as part of the treatment plan.[3]

Other Helpful Medications. In hand-foot-mouth disease (HFMD) using a cyclic phosphodiesterase inhibitor, milrinone, early in the course has the ability to reduce mortality in the management of the enterovirus 71-induced illness.[4] Antiviral therapy may help improve the disease process. Depending on the severity of HHS-6 and HHS-7, for Varicella infections consider prescribing foscarnet, valacyclovir, penciclovir, famciclovir, or ganciclovir, which can lead to improvement. If the pruritis is present calamine lotion may help alleviate and calm the itch.

Nonpharmacologic Management. Management of most VEs to include dengue, Zika, and chikungunya is supportive and includes maintaining adequate hydration, general symptomatic support to alleviate malaise, and pain and fever.

Life-Span Considerations

Identification of VE is pivotal based on the patient at the time of disease presentation. Most viral infections have a typical set of features that are self-limiting, many without lifelong sequelae. Confident diagnosing will be beneficial for patient management later in life. Many strategies aimed at preventing viral infection have proven successful. Vaccinations are a key to the prevention of many of the VE diseases.

Complications

Diarrhea as the most commonly reported complication of measles however, complications from respiratory tract involvement, ocular involvement or encephalitis may lead to death. Otitis media occurs in approximately 10% of cases. Those at greatest risk include the immunocompromised individual, babies younger than 6 months and pregnant women.[1,3] Roseola has been reported in immunocompromised patients; there may be a link to suggest graft versus host as a complication of HHV-6. Cutaneous manifestations have been associated with HHV-6, which present as papular-purpuric "gloves and socks" syndrome, erythema elevatum diutinum, an infectious mononucleosis-like syndrome, the GCS, and pityriasis rosea.[10]

Primary viral infection may occur with only fever and no rash, or rash without fever. Additional secondary findings include otitis media and diarrhea. Rare complications may be seen and include febrile seizures, meningitis, encephalitis, pneumonitis, and hepatitis.[34,38] In adult patients who are unvaccinated against measles, rubella, or varicella a more severe disease course may present. For adults who have been vaccinated for measles, rubella, and varicella the vaccination may wane over time resulting in an increased risk of disease. If the disease occurred naturally, there are no latent effects with measles or rubella, however, with varicella the virus lies dormant in the nervous system and may reemerge as HZ.

Parvovirus 1B9 may interfere with erythropoiesis causing aplastic sickle cell crisis. Women who are pregnant with diagnosed B19 infection should undergo serial fetal ultrasonography during the first two trimesters to determine if the fetus is affected and to manage the treatment further. B19 infection during pregnancy can result in fetal complications including miscarriage, intrauterine fetal death, and/or non-immune hydrops fetalis.[4,38]

Patients with dengue, chikungunya, or Zika have similar complaints of severe low back pain and debilitating arthralgias, which are characteristic, and the latter may last for weeks to months. The recovery period can be lengthy.

Patient and Family Education

- Treatment of many of the VEs are self-limited; uncomplicated cases need no treatment.
- Direct patient education to the VE causative agent.
- Reassurance about the nature and course of VE are warranted in all cases.
- Mild potency topical corticosteroids may be used for symptomatic relief of pruritus.

Health Promotion

Prevention is one of the primary keys. The VEs that have a vaccine for prevention include measles, rubella, varicella, and dengue. Measles, rubella, and varicella are routine vaccinations given in childhood. However, for measles and rubella, if someone was born prior to 1957, they are considered immune as evidenced by exposure. Anyone born after 1957 should have two documented doses of the vaccine at least 28 days apart or laboratory evidence of immunity for adequate protection. Varicella vaccine administration began in 1995. Many older adults today will have natural varicella.[39] With any of these VE to decrease the risk of exposure know your environment and maintain proper handwashing techniques. Arbovirus diseases can be prevented by following precautions to avoid mosquito infection, including appropriate mosquito repellant, long sleeves, and long pants in areas at risk (see Chapter 215). A dengue vaccine was approved in 2015, but has recently been found to increase the risk of severe dengue if administered to patients who were seronegative at the time of vaccination. Pre vaccination serotesting is recommended.[40]

VERRUCA
Definition and Epidemiology

Verruca, or warts, are benign epidermal neoplasms caused by various types of the human papillomavirus (HPV), a group of double-stranded DNA viruses of the family Papillomaviridae.

More than 150 subtypes of HPV have been identified.[2] Roughly 40 of these types affect mucosal surfaces, such as the vulva, vagina, penis, anus, and oral cavity; of these, 16 have been identified as high-risk oncogenic viruses implicated in the development of numerous cervical and anogenital cancers. See Fig. 47.8 for example of ano-genital condyloma. The other virus phenotypes are apt to affect the nonmucosal cutaneous surfaces, such as the face, hands, and feet.[2]

Transmission is through direct skin contact, although contact with viral particles on inanimate objects has been known to cause infection. Genital infection is usually acquired through sexual contact. Wart subtypes with an affinity for the hands and feet typically do not affect the genitalia. Individuals with decreased cellular immunity are at risk for more resistant HPV infection. In these patients, warts can be larger and involve a greater surface area.[1,2]

Environmental and occupational factors increase the risk for development of warts. Periungual warts, for example, are much more common in butchers and in patients whose hands are exposed to chronic wet conditions. Recurrence is not unusual for warts of all types.[3]

Anogenital HPV infection is believed to be the most common sexually transmitted disease in the United States. Studies have shown that 76% of HIV–seropositive women and 42% of seronegative women are at high risk for anogenital HPV infection, and the rates for HIV-seropositive men who have receptive anal intercourse approach 100%.[40] Low-risk types 6 and 11 accounts for 90% of anogenital warts. The high-risk genotypes are responsible for 99% of the cases of cervical cancer and are emerging as the leading causes of oropharyngeal, vulvar, vaginal, and penile cancers as well.[41] Of these, type 16 is the most common, and type 18 accounts for 70% of all cervical cancers. HPV types 31, 33, 45, 52, and 58 are believed to be responsible for an additional 19% of invasive cervical cancers.

There is only one HPV vaccine, Gardasil 9, available in the United States. Cervarix was discontinued in 2016, and Gardasil 4 is no longer produced. Gardasil 9 is a nine-valent vaccine targeting HPV types 6, 11, 16, 18, 31, 33, 45, 52, and 58.[41] Gardasil has been shown to induce a significant antibody response and is the reduces the incidence of HPV-related cancers of all types. Vaccination for males and females can begin as early as age 9 but typically begins at age 11 or 12 and up to age 26. The vaccine is especially encouraged in high-risk individuals such as those with immunocompromising conditions to include gay, bisexual, men who have sex with men, and transgender individuals infected with HIV. If the series is started at age 26, the recommendation is to continue until series is complete.[41]

PATHOPHYSIOLOGY

Infection occurs when the virus comes in contact with skin that is broken or has been traumatized. The virus enters the host's epidermal epithelial cells and begins to use the host's resources to replicate. Infection remains contained within the epidermis, although the wart can become hypertrophic and behave as if it were a deep lesion, as it commonly does on the plantar surface.[15] Warts may present as projections (filiform), round domes (common), or flat (plantar). They can occur singly or in groups and can coalesce to form plaques called mosaic warts. The dermis is not penetrated therefore there is no root to the wart. However, the wart may protrude and shift the dermis. The mosaic pattern is a useful diagnostic sign. When scored with a surgical blade black dots (thrombosed black vessels) are seen.[10,15]

Autoinoculation can occur with cutaneous trauma, such as from shaving or scratching. Vertical transmission of the virus from infected mother to the fetus during passage through the birth canal can cause anogenital warts and recurrent respiratory papillomatosis in the infant. Infection by the wart virus depends on the number of viral particles, the extent of contact, and the host's cellular immunity. The virus spreads laterally for a considerable distance beyond the line that demarcates the wart from the normal skin. HPV may be actively replicating or may lie in a dormant, latent state. Spontaneous remission may occur in as many as two of three patients within 2 years. Lesions recur when the host's cell-mediated immunity can no longer hold the virus in check. Incubation periods range from 1 to 8 months.[10]

Clinical Presentation and Physical Examination

HPV infection is often asymptomatic. When it becomes apparent, it manifests in several different morphologic characteristics. Verruca vulgaris, the common wart, is a skin-colored, hyperkeratotic papule that may occur on the backs of the hands, in periungual areas, and on the knees. Filiform warts are a variant of common warts that are distinguished by their fine, finger-like projections; they typically occur on the face and may be tender. Verruca plana, the flat wart, is commonly seen on the face and extremities in crops of 1- to 2-mm papules that are smooth, flat, and skin-colored to brown. Verruca plantaris, the plantar wart, is a skin-colored papule or plaque on the weight-bearing plantar surfaces of the foot and digits; it is often studded with black pinpoint-sized areas that represent thrombosed capillaries. These warts may be extremely tender and interfere with weight bearing. The thickness of plantar warts makes them particularly resistant to multiple treatment modalities. Condylomata acuminata, or anogenital warts, are sexually transmitted and range from unobtrusive, small, skin-colored papules to large, cauliflower-like growths (Fig. 47.8). Warts have also been described on the oral and nasal mucous membranes, conjunctivae, and larynx.

The physical examination is generally by careful visual inspection. When warts are discovered on the perineum or perianal area, a vaginal examination, digital rectal examination, or anoscopy should be performed.

Diagnostics

Diagnosis of most warts can be confirmed by clinical observation. Debridement of the thickened hypertrophic epidermis on the foot with a scalpel or curette will reveal pinpoint capillaries that may bleed. This can help differentiate it from a callus (or clavus), a different type of lesion that is commonly mistaken for a wart. When it is pared, the callus will have a punctate depression and no thrombosed capillaries. The absence of skin lines within the lesion is also considered a reliable diagnostic indicator for a wart.[1,2,15]

The American College of Obstetricians and Gynecologists and the American Cancer Society recommend yearly or biennial Pap tests for women younger than 30 years and, with three consecutive normal Pap test results, every 2 to 3 years thereafter. Vaccination does not prevent the need for regular Pap

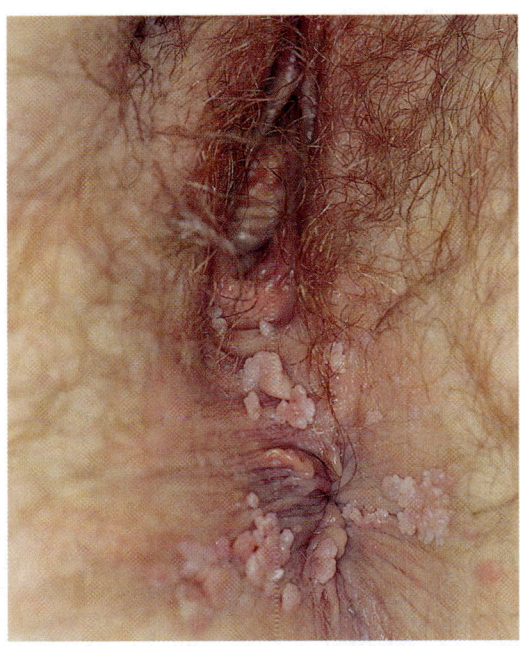

FIG. 47.8 Multiple condylomata in the perineum and perianal area. (From Fisher, B. K., & Margesson, L. J. [1998]. *Genital skin disorders: Diagnosis and treatment.* St Louis: Mosby.)

tests.[41] According to the CDC's guidelines for sexually transmitted diseases there is insufficient evidence to recommend a routine anal cancer screening. However, there is a growing body of evidence supporting the regular use of cytology-based (Pap) testing of the anus for patients at high risk, including men who have sex with men, HIV-infected patients, immunocompromised patients, and women who participate in receptive anal intercourse.[22]

INITIAL DIAGNOSTICS

Verruca

LABORATORY
- None

ADDITIONAL DIAGNOSTICS
- Lesion biopsy[a]
- Cytology[a]
- Immunoperoxidase stain[a]
- Lesion culture[a]

―――――
[a]If indicated.

Differential Diagnosis

 Priority differentials include (1) seborrheic keratosis, (2) callus, (3) lichen planus, (4) squamous cell carcinoma, (5) molluscum contagiosum, (6) amelanotic melanoma, and (7) foreign body.

Warts can appear in varied forms that mimic other common dermatologic lesions. Consideration of the differential diagnosis should be made based on the type of presenting wart. The presence of genital flat or papular warts or pearly penile papules mandate ruling out erythroplasia and condylomata lata of secondary syphilis. With genital nodular lesions, consider Nevi, angiokeratoma or skin tags. Melanoma should still be ruled out. Plane warts located on the face may be confused with perioral dermatitis, syringomas, flat seborrheic keratosis (SK), or actinic keratosis. If located on the hand, they may be mistaken for Lichen planus, stucco keratosis, or SK. Presentation on the trunk or extremities may be confused with pityriasis versicolor or guttate psoriasis.[4] Any warty lesions presenting on the palms and soles include verruca vulgaris, corn or callus, and epidermal cysts. Always rule out carcinoma and melanoma. If located on the dorsum of hands and feet periungual warts and actinic keratosis should be considered. Squamous cell carcinoma and fish tank granuloma need to be ruled out as well. For multiple lesions psoriasis, pyogenic granuloma, and actinic keratosis should be included in the differentials. Always rule out secondary syphilis with lesions on the palms and soles. Additional considerations include molluscum contagiosum, amelanotic melanoma, and foreign body.[4]

Interprofessional Collaborative Management

Most warts are benign and asymptomatic. In general, they will regress spontaneously over time. There is, however, no cure for warts. Treatment decisions are influenced by a number of factors, including the degree of discomfort or disfigurement, the motivation of the patient to undergo treatment that may be painful and protracted, and the commitment to continuing treatment at home. Patients with anogenital infection need to be evaluated for anogenital cancer and other sexually transmitted diseases and screened appropriately.

Pharmacologic Management

Topical Application. Patient-applied treatment is considered the primary option. Many of these treatments apply to both common warts and genital warts. Topical therapies need to extend at least 2 mm outside the visible confines of the wart to ensure that all infected cells are treated. Chemical destruction is done with a liquid agent or transdermal patches. Liquid preparations of salicylic acid and dichloroacetic or trichloroacetic acid (TCA) are used on common, flat, periungual, and plantar warts. Application once or twice a day along with paring or filing of the lesion has resulted in cure rates that can exceed 60%. Petrolatum ointment can be applied to the surrounding skin to protect it from a chemical burn. Treatment may take up to 12 weeks or more.[1,4,15]

For common warts destruction the first line of treatment is with salicylic acid, which may include the application of duct tape along with cryotherapy. Daily application of the salicylic acid is recommended until resolved. Flat warts are more difficult to treat, and tretinoin cream may be applied at bedtime. It may take several weeks before improvement is seen.[3,6]

Imiquimod 3.75% or 5% cream (Aldara) is topically applied by the patient. It is an immunomodulator approved for the treatment of anogenital warts but is commonly used for nongenital warts as well. It is useful in areas where scarring is of concern, such as the face, and for recalcitrant lesions in combination with regular lesion debridement. For the patient with anal intraepithelial neoplasia (AIN) and vaginal intraepithelial neoplasia (VIN) imiquimod cream may be incorporated into suppositories or applied via anal tampons for treatment.[1,5,6,10]

Patient-applied podofilox, 0.5% solution or gel, will cause necrosis of the wart. Apply 2 times a day for 3 days, no therapy for 4 days. May repeat cycle four times as necessary.

Sinecatechins 15% is a product made from green tea extract. The ointment should be applied by the patient 3 times a day until cleared, but no longer than 16 weeks. This product should not be used with an individual who is immunocompromised or has genital herpes. Mild to moderate pain and local irritation is expected.[25]

TCA or bichloroacetic acid (BCA) 80% to 90% solution is a treatment that must be performed by the health care provider as they are caustic agents. TCA/BCA treatment can be repeated weekly if necessary. More data needs to be collected on this type of treatment.

Cantharidin is an extract of a beetle that produces blistering of the skin hours after contact. It has the advantage of painless application but can be excruciating hours later. It is not currently approved by the FDA, nor is its use sanctioned when it is compounded, as with podophyllin or salicylic acid. It is often unavailable and its use is waning. Other medications include topically applied 5-fluorouracil and tretinoin and oral cimetidine.[3]

Cryotherapy. Cryotherapy with LN2 is commonly used alone or in conjunction with other modalities to treat warts. For genital warts, flat warts, and filiform warts, a single freeze-thaw application with minimal involvement of surrounding skin is usually sufficient for each wart. For warts on the palmar or plantar surfaces, individual lesions and their bases are treated for two or three freeze-thaw cycles. The procedure can be painful. Tissue destruction can cause local redness, swelling, and blistering and may take up to 2 weeks to heal. People with dark skin are at risk of hyperpigmentation and hypopigmentation from LN2 and are good candidates for trials of the topically applied medications before LN2 is used. All patients are at risk for scarring. Over-the-counter types are available for application by the patient. However, if unsuccessful in treating the wart a trained health care provider should be seen. Treatment may be required every 2 to 4 weeks for months at a time. Pain, blistering, and necrosis are common effects from LN2 therapy.

Laser Ablation. Laser ablation therapy is an option for very resistant cases. Cure rates for genital lesions are equal to other therapies with a low rate of recurrence. Most complaints from laser ablation include localized pain and swelling of the area treated.[2]

Surgical Therapy. The benefit of surgical removal is the elimination of most warts on one visit. As most warts are exophytic, they may be removed by tangential excision using a CO_2 laser, curettage, shave excision, fine scissors, or a scalpel. A trained health care provider must perform this technique which requires the use of anesthesia application. Some anogenital warts may be destroyed by electrocautery however scarring is common. Treating intraurethral warts with a CO_2 laser may be the best technique.[2]

Emerging Therapy. Injections of skin test antigens such as mumps, candida, and Trichophyton antigens have shown significant success in non-blinded studies, though controlled studies are lacking. Their use is suggested for facial lesions when scarring and pigmentation are of concern and for warts that have been resistant to treatment.[9]

Acyclic nucleoside phosphonate, Cidofovir, has proven successful in the treatment of herpes virus and HPV. 75% of patients treated with Cidofovir alone saw a complete resolution. Patients who had surgery in combination with cidofovir had 100% resolution. It has also shown promise in the treatment of refractory genital warts. The treatment is expensive and may be cost prohibitive.[1]

Indications for Referral. Referral to a dermatology specialist is advised for large warts, warts on cosmetically sensitive areas, and treatment failures or when the diagnosis is in question. Podiatry referral may be appropriate for resistant plantar warts. Obstetric-gynecologic evaluation is appropriate for pregnant women, women with intravaginal lesions or abnormal Pap test results. Urology referrals may be appropriate for lesions that are affecting normal urination or sexual performance. Gastroenterology for sigmoidoscopy may be indicated for patients with abnormal anal cytology or clinical findings suggesting rectal HPV infection.

Life-Span Considerations

Some warts have been linked to the development of cervical, genital, and mucosal carcinomas, and there are now vaccines available to protect against cancers and warts related to HPV infection. Treatment with podofilox is contraindicated in pregnancy.

Complications

The treatment of warts can be painful. Chemical destruction can leave the skin with chemical burns. Blistering and hemorrhagic bullae can develop from typical doses of cryotherapy on the frail skin. Plantar warts can be particularly painful and if left untreated may result in altered activity, abnormal gait, or foot deformities. Bacterial infections are rare. Autoinoculation from one area to another is possible.

Genital warts (condylomata acuminata) are particularly contagious and increase the risk for anogenital carcinomas in both men and women. Genital warts can be transmitted from mother to infant during childbirth.

Treatment of periungual warts can result in damage to the nail matrix and subsequent nail deformity. Nerve damage can occur if treatment is too vigorous in areas where the nerves are superficial, such as the lateral phalanges. Cryotherapy should be performed cautiously or not at all in patients with Raynaud phenomenon.

Hypopigmentation and hyperpigmentation are frequently seen with many of the ablative type therapies. Patients should be informed of this complication with the treatment by means of cryotherapy, TCA, BCA, CO_2 laser ablation, or electrodessication.[1,2,5]

Special consideration should be made for patients who are immunocompromised. Those with organ transplants or HIV-affected patients may have warts that are resistant to standard treatment. A more aggressive approach should be the initial mode of therapy.

Genital warts can increase in size with pregnancy. Many procedures may be contraindicated during pregnancy. The most appropriate treatments include surgery, cryotherapy, TCA application, and laser for removal. This would decrease the risk of transfer to the neonate during delivery.[10]

Patient and Family Education

- For common warts, patients and families should understand that most warts are benign, viral lesions that can spread from person to person in places such as showers or locker rooms. Common warts often resolve spontaneously, although that may be only after many years. Education should include self-treatment options and the side effects of medications.
- Patients should be instructed to pare hyperkeratotic warts regularly, especially those on the feet, with an instrument that is not used on any other skin surface. Soaking the area in warm water makes physical debridement more comfortable, as does the use of an exfoliating cream or lotion, such as ammonium lactate or urea.[6]

Health Promotion

Patients, parents, teens, and young adults need to be educated about the health implications of HPV infection, offered the appropriate screening, educated about prevention by barrier methods, and advised of the availability of the vaccine. This is especially relevant information to be shared before a patient becomes sexually active and during routine health maintenance visits. Routine Pap tests are still recommended regularly for sexually active women. Rectal Pap smears should become routine care for select patient populations.

FUNGAL

TINEA INFECTIONS OF THE SKIN
Definition and Epidemiology

Superficial fungal infections are common problems. Greater exposure to fungal pathogens is occurring in the health and fitness–minded population, in debilitated patients using systemic antibiotics, in diabetics, and in patients who are immunocompromised. These fungal infections can cause primary or secondary infection of the skin that complicates an accurate diagnosis of the precipitating condition. Fungal infections are not normal components of the skin flora. The fungal infection lives within the keratinized structures of the skin.[2] Fungal infections are caused typically by dermatophytes or yeast organisms. The term tinea is derived from Latin meaning worm, as a descriptive term of the serpentine flow of the lesion. The corresponding Latin term for the body region is used in conjunction with the full name.[10]

Clinically, dermatophyte infections have traditionally been classified by body region. Tinea (T.) means fungus infection. Specific body regions by definition include capitis meaning scalp. This infection can involve the eyebrows, eyelashes, or scalp and is predominantly seen in children up to age 10 and more widespread internationally. Boys tend to have a greater occurrence of T. capitis than girls prior to puberty; the reverse is true after puberty.[4]

T. corporis involves the trunk, extremities, feet, groin, face, or hand. T. pedis involves the soles of the feet and spaces between the toes. There may be a relationship based on immunity status of the individual and type of fungus. There is an increase of *Trichophyton tonsurans* among young athletes involved in close contact sports such as wrestling.[10]

T. pedis typically affects males more than females. Rates of infection increase after puberty. It is estimated that more than 70% of the population will have T. pedis during their lifetime. T. manuum indicates the involvement of the palms and spaces between the fingers. T. manuum and pedis may coexist especially if both feet are affected. This is known as the "two-feet, one-hand syndrome."[1,10]

T. cruris is seen in the inguinal region. Men frequently have more infections than women. Superficial infection increases the likelihood of having tinea. Tinea prefers moist warm areas of the skin. Living in warm tropical climates as well as summer temperatures accelerate the occurrence.[10]

Onychomycosis (or *tinea unguium*) refers to any infection of the nails caused by a dermatophyte, yeast, or sometimes mold.[10] Onychomycosis is the most common nail condition, most frequently occurs in the toenails (great toe is often first), is classified based on nail bed location of the infection, and has a reputation for being quite difficult to resolve. These infections cause nail discoloration, thickening, roughness, the splitting of the nail, and sometimes onycholysis (a painful separation of the nail from the nail bed). Onychomycosis is common in patients of advancing age as a result of a reduction in blood flow.[1,10] Other risk factors include swimming, nail trauma, diabetes, tinea pedis, psoriasis, and immunodeficiency.[10,17] Onycholysis has a significant incidence of pain and can affect patients' lives physically and psychologically, interfering with walking, exercise, and social interaction.[10]

Pathophysiology

Fungal infections are usually acquired through inhalation of endemic fungi in the environment, with soil being the natural reservoir.[10] Three major sources are typically responsible for the transmission of dermatophytes. The first is anthropophilic (human to human), the second is zoophilic (animal to human), and the third is geophilic, (soil to human or soil to animal).[10] The incubation period can take up to 3 weeks to appear. The pattern of infection is seen as growth directed outward from the center located in the stratum corneum. Fungal antigens elicit an inflammatory reaction. Males are

more prone to have Tinea infections than females as progesterone inhibits dermatophyte growth.[10] Indirect contact with fomites (infected towels, hats, upholstery, and hairbrushes) may also cause dermatophyte infections.[4]

Tinea capitis occurs most frequently during childhood. The most common in the United States is black dot, caused by *T. tonsurans*. There are three types of tinea capitis. The first is gray patch or ectothrix, which is when the cuticle of the hair is destroyed by the development of arthroconidia on the exterior of the hair shaft. Black dot or endothrix is the second, where hair invasion is seen broken off close to the surface causing the effect of a black dot. The third type is favus, which creates crusts and hair loss. T. capitis is commonly seen among children of African descent. However, it can also be seen in families living in confined quarters with animals. Zoophilic and anthropophilic are common causes.[4]

T. corporis is usually caused by *Trichophyton rubrum (T. rubrum)*, but may also be caused by *Trichophyton mentagrophytes (T. mentagrophytes)*. This is classically seen in moist warm climates and among individuals who have close physical contact, such as wrestlers, or have large amounts of facial hair.[10]

The organisms that cause T. manuus are the same as for T. pedis and T. cruris, which are *T. rubrum*, *Trichophyton interdigitale*, *Epidermophyton floccosum*, and *T. tonsurans*. Areas with less sebum production are at increased risk of developing an infection. The feet and hand have no sebaceous glands.[10]

The most common pathogens associated with tinea unguium are *T. rubrum* and *T. interdigitale*.[4,10] *Candida* organisms are rarer and may be associated with immunosuppression. A nail can be infected by multiple organisms. The infection is located inside the nail. Distal subungual onychomycosis, the most common presentation, begins with discoloration in the distal portion of the nail partially caused by the accumulation of keratinous debris under the nail.[10,15,17] Proximal subungual onychomycosis, the rarest presentation, begins deeper near the cuticle and occurs mostly in immunocompromised patients. White superficial onychomycosis has a flaky white appearance and affects the nail surface.[4,10]

Clinical Presentation and Physical Examination

Dermatophyte infections are characterized and named according to their location. Lesions appear as arcuate, oval, and annular with or without scale that has central clearing. The border of the lesion may have small pustules that can include burning or itching.

- Tinea capitis (head or scalp) can be seen initially as patchy, scaly, nonscarring areas of hair loss (Fig. 47.9). Depending on the infectious organism, the lesions may become inflamed, boggy, and pustular.[1,10]
- Tinea corporis (body) appears on the skin as erythematous plaques and papules in an annular or arciform pattern. Lesions often have slightly elevated borders with central clearing.
- Tinea manuus (hand) is often a dry, diffuse, scaly eruption of the palms, with sharply marginated plaques on the dorsum of the hands. Often if one hand is affected both feet will be affected.
- Tinea pedis (athlete's foot) can occur as interdigital scaling, maceration, and fissuring. It can also appear as a mild erythematous scaling eruption or maceration that involves the spaces between the toes and the sole and sides of the foot (moccasin distribution). Clinical types of T. pedis include

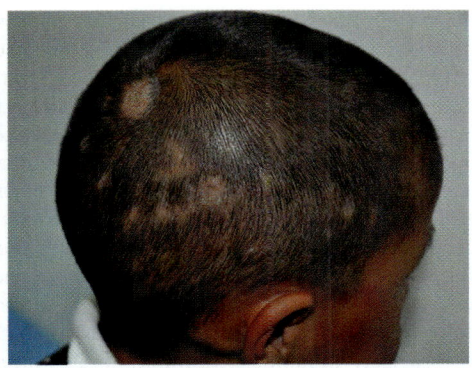

FIG. 47.9 Capitis tinea capitis. sporadic alopecia patches with scales on the scalp. (From Tang, J., Ran, X., & Ran, Y. [2017]. Ultraviolet dermoscopy for the diagnosis of tinea capitis. *Journal of the American Academy of Dermatology, 76*[2], S28–S30.)

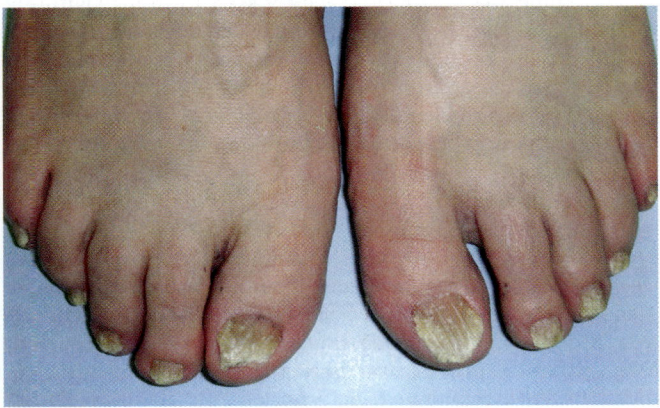

FIG. 47.10 Onychomycosis, onychclysis, yellowing, crumbling and thickening of the nails. (From Bolognia, J., Schaffer, J., & Cerroni, L. [2018]. *Dermatology* [4th ed.]. Philadelphia: Elsevier.)

the following four: moccasin, interdigital, inflammatory, and ulcerative. These are more common when the feet are enclosed creating a moist environment. Maceration is frequently seen interdigitally, and moccasin has a sharply marginated scale that is laterally distributed along the borders of the heels and soles. Coincides with onychomycosis.[10]

- Tinea cruris (jock itch) appears on the groin and upper inner thigh and extends to the gluteal folds as erythematous scaling patches with raised borders. The scrotum is often spared.
- Tinea unguium (nail), also called *onychomycosis,* (Fig. 47.10) most commonly manifests as the distal subungual type. The infection begins in the distal nail bed and spreads to infect the nail plate, causing the nail to appear thickened and yellowed or brown, with a powdery or thickened nail texture along with subungual keratinous debris. The nail surface typically has a greenish tinge with bacterial infections. Assess for onycholysis (disassociation of the nail from the nail bed). The condition of the subungual nail bed should be noted—that is, the degree of elevation and separation of the nail from the nail bed and surrounding tissue.[10] Table 47.4 describes the physical presentation of onychomycosis nail dystrophies. Pain rating and any interference with daily activities should be assessed.

TABLE 47.4 Nail Dystrophies

Nail Disorder	Clinical Presentation	Manifestations
Distal or lateral subungual onychomycosis	White to brownish-yellow discoloration of nail	Subungual hyperkeratosis; separation of nail plate and nail bed lineal channels
White superficial onychomycosis	White, sharply outlined area on nail plate; nail surface soft, dry, and friable	Common in fingernails and toenails of HIV-infected patients Nail plate not thick; no separation of nail plate and nail bed
Proximal subungual onychomycosis (rare), candidal infections	Leukonychia on proximal aspect of nail plate Thickening of nail plate Yellowish-brown discoloration	Patient may be immunosuppressed Chronic mucocutaneous candidiasis Involves all nails Eventual disintegration of nail

HIV, Human immunodeficiency virus.

Diagnostics

Essential Diagnostics. The easiest method of exam is using KOH microscopy to diagnose hair, nail, and skin. It will easily identify inflammation from moccasin types. The best sample will be collected at the erythematous active border. Translucent hyphae are observed under the microscope. Histologic tests and periodic acid–Schiff staining are reliable for an accurate diagnosis to identify organisms susceptible to specific therapeutic agents.[15]

Additional Diagnostics. A Wood lamp may be used to identify *Microsporum canis* or *Microsporum audouinii* on the hair strand. However, the most common dermatophytes that infect hair will not fluoresce. Using the Wood lamp may help to identify t.versicolor as it fluoresces a pale white yellow color or erythrasma, which produces a bright coral red fluorescence.[15]

INITIAL DIAGNOSTICS

Tinea

LABORATORY
- Potassium hydroxide
- Wood lamp[a]
- Liver function test[a]

[a]If indicated.

Differential Diagnosis

 Priority differentials include (1) atopic dermatitis, (2) contact dermatitis, (3) folliculitis, and (4) psoriasis.

Many lesions have similar appearance occurring on skin, hair, or nail areas. Patients with comorbid conditions have increased risk for many types of dermatological disorders and distinguishing the differentials is critical for expediting treatment. Inflammatory response must be considered during the physical exam. Dermatophytosis that has a central clearing can be distinguished from papulosquamous presentation such as psoriasis in which there is a uniform inflammatory response throughout the skin lesion. Onychomycosis accounts for about 50% of nail abnormalities, so consideration should be given to other causes. Psoriasis, not a fungal infection, causes pitting of

TABLE 47.5	Differential Diagnosis of Tinea	
Tinea Location	**Common**	**Consider**
Capitis	Seborrheic dermatitis Atopic dermatitis Bacterial folliculitis Pityriasis amiantacea Plaque psoriasis Primary cicatricial alopecia	Traction alopecia Alopecia areata Trichotillomania
Corporis	Erythema multiforme Nummular eczema Psoriasis Tinea versicolor Subacute cutaneous lupus 　erythematosus Cutaneous candidiasis Fixed drug eruption Lupus erythematosus	Contact dermatitis Atopic dermatitis Pityriasis rosea Seborrheic dermatitis Mycosis fungoides Parapsoriasis Secondary syphilis
Manuus, Pedis	Erythrasma Dyshidrosis Foot eczema Psoriasis, pustular psoriasis Contact dermatitis atopic dermatitis Bacterial pyodermas scabies	Bacterial coinfection Pityriasis ruba pilaris Reactive arthritis
Cruris	Erythrasma Cutaneous candidiasis Intertrigo Contact dermatitis Inverse psoriasis Seborrheic dermatitis Folliculitis	Lichen simplex chronicus Familial benign pemphigus Darier-White disease Histiocytosis
Onychomycosis	Psoriasis Lichen planus Trauma Onychogryphosis Herpetic whitlow Black nail paronychia	Pachyonychia congenita Trophic changes Yellow nail syndrome Melanoma Darier disease

the nail surface. Onychomycosis should not be confused with onychogryphosis, which is nail hypertrophy sometimes caused by trauma but more often caused by neglecting to trim the nails for an extended period. Subungual malignant melanoma can manifest as a dark stripe discoloration and requires urgent referral for evaluation. For specific differentials based on location involved, see Table 47.5, Differential Diagnosis of Tinea.

Interprofessional Collaborative Management

Pharmacologic Management

Topical Application. The treatment of tinea infections consists of removal of the infecting organisms. Acute, exudative lesions are treated with drying agents such as aluminum sulfate (Domeboro) soaks. Topical antifungal solutions and creams reduce superficial scaling and organisms; keratolytic agents remove the thick scales on the hands and feet, allowing topical antifungal agents to penetrate better. Topical applications are available to treat dermatophyte infections (Table 47.6); these medications include terbinafine (Lamisil), naftifine (Naftin), butenafine (Mentax), clotrimazole (Lotrimin), clotrimazole/

betamethasone (Lotrisone), econazole (Ecoza), ketoconazole (Nizoral), luliconazole (Luzu), miconazole OTC, oxiconazole (Oxistat), sertaconazole (Ertaczo), ciclopirox (Penlac), and tolnaftate (Tinactin). The products should be continued 1 week after clearing of the lesions to discourage recurrence; however, recurrence of tinea infections is common.[1,4,10] Tinea pedis can be treated successfully with over-the-counter terbinafine.[4]

Medicated Shampoo. For topical treatment of tinea capitis adjunct therapy of medicated shampoo should be used along with oral medications. Selenium sulfide should be used twice a week for 2 weeks. Alternatively, ketoconazole shampoo could be used twice weekly for 4 weeks.[1]

Oral Medications. Systemic antifungal medications are used for widespread tinea or infections that involve the nails or scalp. A long-standing treatment of tinea capitis is griseofulvin for 2 to 4 months or for 2 weeks after negative KOH or culture results are obtained. Griseofulvin needs to be taken with high-fat food for complete absorption. Antifungal agents such as terbinafine and fluconazole (Diflucan) are effective within 2 to 4 weeks of therapy.[1,42] The use of oral medications requires careful dosage calculation and monitoring for potential side effects. Oral ketoconazole (Nizoral) should be avoided because of risks of hepatotoxicity and serious drug interactions.[1] Treatment should not be considered complete until a follow-up negative fungal culture is obtained.[10]

Onychomycosis may be treated with oral terbinafine or with oral itraconazole (Sporanox). The oral dose of terbinafine is 250 mg daily, 6 weeks for fingernail onychomycosis and 12 weeks for toenail involvement.[1,10] Terbinafine is not recommended for patients with a history of renal or liver dysfunction. Monitoring of liver function is required every 6 weeks or if the patient experiences nausea, anorexia, or fatigue during therapy. Neutropenia has been reported as a side effect of terbinafine therapy; therefore, a complete blood count should be performed every 6 weeks or if there are symptoms suggestive of neutropenia.[10]

Varied dosage regimens are used with oral itraconazole. One regimen is 200 mg daily for 12 weeks for toenail involvement and 200 mg twice daily for 1 week, then 3 weeks off, and then 200 mg daily for 1 additional week for fingernail involvement.[42] The provider should monitor the patient for any hepatic dysfunction. A careful and complete drug history should be taken before therapy is initiated with itraconazole; itraconazole is metabolized by the cytochrome P-450 3A4 (CYP3A4) system and affects the cytochrome P-450 enzyme system, creating many drug interactions.[1] Note that topical therapy for onychomycosis is relatively ineffective. Neither the oral nor the topical form of oral terbinafine or oral itraconazole is recommended for pregnant or nursing women. Unfortunately, the recurrence of onychomycosis is high, even with compliant therapy.[10]

Complementary Approaches

Herbs and Dietary Supplements. Herbal therapies for onychomycosis have little evidence of effectiveness. Oral herbal therapies may also cause unknown drug interactions or side effects. A few natural antifungals include Mycozil, olive leaf oil, pau d'arco oregano oil, garlic, horopito, lemongrass, and Bacillus *laterosporus*.[1] For the treatment of onychomycosis, Vicks VapoRub applied once daily for 48 weeks has shown a cure rate of 22% while tea tree oil (TTO) 100% solution applied twice daily for 6 months had a cure rate of 18%. There

TABLE 47.6 Examples of Treatments for Tinea

Recommended Application to Affected Areas		Indicated for		
		Tinea (Pedis Cruris, or Corporis)	Tinea Unguium	Tinea Capitis
Clotrimazole (Lotrimin)	Twice daily	X[a]		
Miconazole (Monistat-Derm)	Once to twice daily	X[a]		
Ketoconazole (Nizoral)	Once daily	X[a]		X
Oxiconazole (Oxistat)	Once daily	X		
Ciclopirox (Loprox) (Penlac) 48w	Twice daily	X[a]	X[a]	X
Butenafine (Mentax)	Once daily	X[b]		
Econazole (Ecoza) (Spectazole)	Once to twice daily	X[a]		
Luliconazole (Luzu)	Once daily	X[a]		
Terbinafine 1% (Lamisil)[b]	Once to twice daily	X[b]	X[b] 6 months	X
Fluconazole (Diflucan) 150 mg	Oral Weekly	X 6 weeks	X[a] ×6 weeks– 9 months	X[a] 6 mg/kg/week 6 weeks
Griseofulvin 500–750 mg/day	Oral Once daily	X 6 weeks		X[b] 6 weeks
Itraconazole (Sporanox) 200–400 mg	Oral	X weekly dose	X[a] daily 12 weeks	X[a] 5 mg/kg/day × 1 week (400 mg max)
Terbinafine (Lamisil) 250 mg daily	Oral Once daily	X 2 weeks	X[b] 12 weeks	X[b] 3–6 weeks

GENERAL CONSIDERATIONS

Clinical improvement may be seen fairly soon after initiation of treatment. Twice-daily applications, when indicated, should be done morning and evening. In general, all infections should be treated for 2 weeks after infection has resolved to reduce the possibility of recurrence. Tinea pedis, tinea unguium, and tinea capitis require 6 weeks or more of treatment. Dermatophyte infections respond well to all topical therapy except areas of the body and scalp with deep, inflammatory lesions. Topicals no effect on tinea of the nail.[3]

[a]Secondary.
[b]Primary
Data from Topical antifungal agents for tinea infection, *Pharmacist's Letter/Prescriber's Letter* 30(5), 2014.

is insufficient data to provide complete recommendation for these complementary therapies.

Indications for Referral. Patients with nail stripe discolorations or persistent subungual discolorations should be referred to rule out subungual malignant melanoma. Discussion with the physician regarding recurrence and surgical or nonsurgical avulsion of nail dystrophy is also a consideration for a referral. Severe infections, combined infection with underlying disease, or infections that do not respond to treatment require a referral to a dermatologist.

Life-Span Considerations

Griseofulvin should not be prescribed to pregnant women. It is also contraindicated in lupus erythematosus, porphyria, and severe liver disease. Dosage adjustment is required for the pediatric population. Watch for drug interactions with warfarin, cyclosporine, and oral contraceptives. If prescribing itraconazole watch for enhanced toxicity of certain medications as well as reduced efficacy with H_2 blockers. Liver enzymes should be monitored for long-term use of fluconazole.[1,42]

Complications

An uncommon complication of tinea capitis is the formation of a kerion, a boggy, exudative area on the scalp, caused by a hypersensitive reaction to the fungus. Kerion formations (tinea capitis) may result in permanent hair loss and scarring.[5] Fungal infections can also be complicated by bacterial superinfections. Individuals with comorbid conditions (venous hypertension, harvested saphenous veins, chronic edema, and diabetics, etc.) can exhibit complications such as cellulitis and osteomyelitis. Other complications are associated with side effects and drug interactions with oral antifungal medications. Topical steroid use may worsen an infection, which is dermatophytic. Chronic inflammation and infection may cause nail bed cornification, causing permanent separation of the nail plate from the underlying supporting structures (onycholysis).[10,15] Patients with diabetes or peripheral neuropathy may be at higher risk for complications and need aggressive diagnosis and treatment of onychomycosis and tinea unguium.[1,15]

Patient and Family Education

- Caution patients about the use of over-the-counter steroid creams for tinea infections because prolonged use of topical steroids may cause thinning of the skin or striae.[10]
- Absorbent powders help reduce moisture and prevent reinfection.
- Encourage patients to take antifungals for the duration as directed to prevent recurrence.[10]

• With T. capitis: shave the head before treatment to decrease treatment time. Keep school-aged children with T. capitis at home until systemic treatment has begun. Family members and others should be screened for infection. Objects the head may have touched should be cleaned thoroughly as the spores may remain viable on the contaminated object.[10]

With onycholysis: review information concerning medication administration and instructions regarding signs of liver toxicity. In many cases, nails do not appear clear after the recommended course of treatment, and it may take 12 to 18 months after treatment for the patient to visually see improvement.[10] Patients should be assured that the medication remains in the nail plate for months and will continue to kill the fungus. These infections can be recalcitrant to treatment; it may take months or even years for complete resolution of the pathogens. To prevent recurrences, the patient can apply ciclopirox 2 or 3 times a week, apply terbinafine cream in the nail area weekly, and avoid trauma to the tip of the nails from tight-fitting shoes. Also, place a small strand of lamb's wool between the spaces of the toes, and keep the area dry by applying powder to the feet and keeping socks dry.[1]

Health Promotion

It is imperative that patients keep problem areas as dry as possible and avoid recurrence of tinea infestation. With regard to T. pedis, footwear should be evaluated annually for size and suitability. Patients should powder toe webs and soles, not shoes; avoid going barefoot in communal showers; wear sweat-wicking socks; and alternate several pairs of shoes for daily wear that maintain a dry, roomy environment for the feet. Using an antifungal spray in shoes may be helpful.[1,4]

TINEA VERSICOLOR
Definition and Epidemiology

Tinea versicolor (T. versicolor) is also known as Pityriasis versicolor. T. versicolor is a chronic, asymptomatic, and superficial fungal infection. Tinea versicolor is more common during the years of high sebaceous gland activity, which is usually seen in teens and young adults. The occurrence is seen worldwide with 1% in dry climates and 50% or more prevalence in the hot humid environment. Individuals with oily skin have a higher incidence of disease.[43] There is no preference in regard to skin color or sex as to whom it affects.[4] T. versicolor is difficult to cure, as relapse following treatment can be as high as 80% within 2 years.[44]

Pathophysiology

The causative organism of tinea versicolor is *Malassezia furfur*. *Pityrosporum orbiculare* is the yeast form of the organism. The fungus is found on normal skin, and the infection is caused by a change in the host's resistance to this organism. Tinea versicolor causes lesions in some individuals as a result of genetic predisposition, immunosuppression, malnutrition, pregnancy, and Cushing disease. It also occurs during periods of high heat and humidity. Thus, the condition is more prevalent during the summer and in hot, humid regions. Exposure to sunlight often initiates an episode. Resolution of hyperpigmented lesions will be seen before resolution of hypopigmented ones.[1,4,42]

Clinical Presentation and Physical Examination

Lesions vary in color and are either white or light pink in the hypopigmented version or tan or brown in the hyperpigmented version. They are slightly scaly and are round or oval coalescing papules and plaques. The usual sites for these lesions are the sternal region; the sides of the chest, abdomen, or back; the pubis; and the intertriginous areas. Hypopigmented lesions are more noticeable in the darkly pigmented skin. Patients should be reassured that repigmentation will occur after treatment and with exposure to natural sunlight. However, this process can take several months. Relapse may occur.[10]

Diagnostics

Essential Diagnostics. Diagnosis is by KOH examination, which reveals numerous short, straight hyphae and clusters of round, budding yeast; this configuration is commonly referred to as "spaghetti and meatballs." A KOH examination may be falsely negative if the patient has just showered. Wood light examination may show irregular, light, white, yellow fluorescence that fades as it improves. If the diagnosis is still in question, skin scrapings may be obtained for fungal culture on lipid-containing medium.[1,2]

> **INITIAL DIAGNOSTICS**
>
> **Tinea Versicolor**
>
> **LABORATORY**
> • Potassium hydroxide preparation
> • Wood lamp
> • Skin culture*
> • LFTs[a]
>
> ———
> [a]If indicated.

Differential Diagnosis

Vitiligo, pityriasis alba, pityriasis rosea, and small plaque parapsoriasis should be considered in the differential diagnosis. These can be narrowed down based on clinical presentation, patient history, and patient's age.

 Priority differentials include (1) vitiligo, (2) pityriasis rosea, (3) small plaque parapsoriasis, and (4) seborrheic dermatitis.

Differentials should also include VEs. Lesions may resemble seborrheic dermatitis, but tinea versicolor most commonly affects the trunk, neck, and upper extremities, whereas seborrheic dermatitis affects hairy body areas. Although it is uncommon, secondary syphilis should be considered in the differential diagnosis.[10]

Interprofessional Collaborative Management
Pharmacologic Management

Topical Treatment. Topical antifungal is the first line of treatment along with medicated shampoo. Common antifungal creams, such as the imidazoles, are useful in treating tinea versicolor (Table 47.7). Medication is applied to the entire torso during active infections to eliminate subclinical lesions. Topical shampoos or suspensions containing selenium sulfide or pyrithione zinc are affordable and effective in treatment or prophylaxis. These contain fungistatic and bacteriostatic properties that inhibit bacterial cell division. Shampoos are applied to affected areas, allowed to dry, and rinsed away after remaining in place approximately 10 minutes. This treatment is repeated for 7 to 14 consecutive days during active infections, followed by periodic use of these shampoos or soaps if the patient is prone to frequent infections. Specific instructions should be reviewed with patients with every product or drug. Perspiration may improve the distribution of oral medications on the skin surface, and refraining from bathing for at least 12 hours is recommended.[10]

TABLE 47.7 **Treatment for Candidiasis and Tinea Versicolor**

Recommended Application to Affected Areas		Candidiasis	Tinea Versicolor
Clotrimazole (Lotrimin)	Twice daily	X	X
Miconazole (Monistat-Derm)	Once to twice daily	X	X
Ketoconazole (Nizoral)	Once daily	X	X
Oxiconazole (Oxistat)	Once daily	X	
Ciclopirox (Loprox)	Twice daily	X	X
Nystatin (Mycostatin)	Twice daily	X	
Butenafine (Mentax)	Once daily		X
Econazole (Spectazole)	Once to twice daily	X	X
Terbinafine 1% (Lamisil) Over the counter	Once to twice daily		X
Fluconazole (Diflucan) 150 mg	Oral single dose	X	X 300 mg
Ketoconazole (Nizoral) 200–400 mg	Oral daily	X 5 days	X single dose
Itraconazole (Sporanox) 200 mg	Oral daily	X 3–5 days	X 7 days
Ketoconazole shampoo	Once daily × 3 days		X[a]
Selenium sulfide suspension	Once daily × 7 days		X[a]

GENERAL CONSIDERATIONS

Clinical improvement may be seen fairly soon after initiation of treatment. Twice-daily applications, when indicated, should be done morning and evening. In general, all infections should be treated for 2 weeks after infection has resolved to reduce the possibility of recurrence.

[a]Primary; [b]secondary.

HHV, Human herpesvirus type 3; *HIV*, human immunodeficiency virus; *HSV*, herpes simplex virus; *KOH*, potassium hydroxide; *VE*, viral exanthema.
References from 1, 3, 10, 41.

Ketoconazole is now available in a foam treatment which may be more favorable and increase patient adherence. The recommendation is to apply once or twice daily for 14 days along with a once weekly shampoo of ketoconazole for the most effective treatment.[44]

Oral Therapy. Systemic antifungals are the second line of treatment for patients with extensive or unresponsive disease.[42] Therapy may include itraconazole dosage, 200 mg itraconazole daily for 5 or 7 days but may vary based on prophylactic or maintenance therapy. Fluconazole may be taken at 300 mg weekly for 2 to 4 weeks. Oral ketoconazole is no longer approved for the treatment of tinea versicolor due to hepatotoxicity but topical preparations may be helpful for some patients. Caution should be taken when prescribing to special populations and those with medication contraindication. Fewer side effects and drug reactions are seen with fluconazole which is the preferred azole to be prescribed.[1,10,44]

Indications for Referral. A referral is not usually necessary. However, for rashes recalcitrant to treatment refer to dermatology for reconsideration of diagnosis.

Complications

Complications are unusual, although drug-drug interactions are possible with the systemic antifungal medications.[1,42] Careful review of the patient's current medications is essential, particularly if fluconazole or ketoconazole will be prescribed. Oral ketoconazole is no longer approved as a treatment due

to hepato-toxicity. Some patients may develop *Malassezia* folliculitis, although this disorder usually resolves with topical therapy.[1,42,44]

Emerging Management Trends

Pramiconazole is a new triazole antifungal that has been studied for the treatment of T. versicolor. When prescribed 200 mg for 3 days the cure rates were seen at 92% and 96%. This drug is currently not available in the United States.[42]

Patient and Family Education

- Teach patients to understand that tinea versicolor commonly recurs but is not a serious disorder. It is more common in warmer climates and often flares during summer months.
- To reduce recurrences, have the patient wash affected areas with selenium sulfide shampoo for 10 minutes each day for a week followed by consistent biweekly treatments.

Health Promotion

It is imperative that patients keep their hands and nails as dry as possible and avoid recurrence of tinea pedis. Nails should be trimmed and chewing or picking at nails avoided. Footwear should be evaluated annually for size and suitability. Patients should powder toe webs and soles, not shoes; avoid going barefoot in communal showers; wear sweat-wicking socks; and alternate several pairs of shoes for daily wear that maintain a dry, roomy environment for the feet. Using an antifungal spray in shoes may be helpful.

CANDIDIASIS

 Immediate referral is indicated for critically ill patients without waiting for culture confirmation if systemic infection is suspected.

Definition and Epidemiology

Candidiasis is a fungal infection caused by Candida. There are more than 150 species of Candida, which include *C. albicans*, *Candida glabrata*, *Candida tropicalis*, *Candida parapsilosis*, and *Candida krusei*.[2,45] It can normally be found on mucous membranes, in the gastrointestinal tract, in the vagina, and on the skin.[3]

Pathophysiology

Candida has a commensal relationship with diseased skin and the mucosal membranes of the intestinal tract, genitourinary, and lungs. Infection occurs when the normal host flora is interrupted, and an overgrowth occurs. Candida is usually an opportunistic organism. It is able to behave like a pathogen usually only in the presence of immunosuppression or in intertriginous areas. Predisposing factors to candidal infection include obesity, medications such as antibiotics and corticosteroids, malnutrition, diabetes and other endocrine diseases, and immunosuppressed conditions including HIV and AIDS. A local environment that is warm, moist, macerated, or occluded favors the growth of this organism.[3]

Clinical Presentation and Physical Examination

The clinical appearance of candidiasis depends on its location. Candidiasis of the mucous membranes is called *thrush*. The patient may complain of dysphagia, tender mouth, or a burning tongue. Thrush appears as white or gray membranous plaques, resembling cottage cheese, that is adherent to the buccal mucosa. If the plaques are scraped away, the base is macerated and brightly erythematous. The lesions can extend down the esophagus and to the lips and corners of the mouth. Perlèche, or angular cheilitis, is a fissuring and maceration of the corners of the mouth. The common causes of perlèche include candidal infection, bacterial infection, and irritant dermatitis.[5]

Common sites of skin infection with *Candida* organisms are axillary, gluteal, interdigital, perianal or diaper region, beneath pendulous breasts and panniculus folds, shaved areas (e.g., folliculitis of the beard), vagina, and glans penis. These intertriginous candidiasis lesions are usually pink or red moist patches bordered by a thin fringe or collarette of scale. They are sometimes surrounded by characteristic satellite pustules.[15] Vaginal thrush presents with skin maceration, intense itching, and often a "cheesy" vaginal discharge. Candid balanitis present with small papules that develop into pustules on the glans penis (Fig. 47.11).[6] If a foreskin is present pasty macerated debris from under it may lead to circular shaped erosions.[15] Candidal paronychia, or nail fold infection, is an inflammation of the nail fold. Pain may be described around and under the nail and nail bed.[6] There is rounding and lifting of the nail fold, sometimes with a pus discharge. The nail can become thickened and discolored over time. Untreated severe candidiasis in any location has the potential to cause fungal septicemia in an immunocompromised patient.[1,15] Older persons are especially susceptible to fungal infection including vulvovaginal

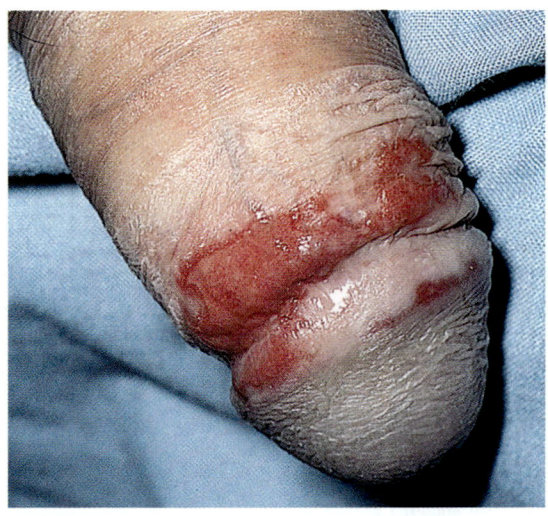

FIG. 47.11 Candida balanitis. The shaft of the penis and the glans display red round erosions. (From Swartz, M. [2014]. *Textbook of physical diagnosis: History and examination* [7th ed.]. Philadelphia: Saunders.)

infection, cutaneous candidiasis, and balanitis.[10,15] Elderly persons experience a higher risk of morbidity, including systemic fungal infections. Systemic candidiasis in the elderly may cause vague symptomology and progress to multisystem organ failure, making diagnosis vital yet challenging.[6]

Diagnostics

INITIAL DIAGNOSTICS
Candidiasis
LABORATORY • Potassium hydroxide preparation • Skin culture[a] • Skin biopsy[a]
—— [a]If indicated.

Essential Diagnostics. The diagnosis of candidiasis is based on clinical appearance, microscopic evaluation with a KOH preparation to look for budding yeast with or without hyphae, or fungal culture. Positive skin or mucous membrane cultures are not diagnostic if not confirmed by microscopic evaluation.[10]

Additional Diagnostics. None.

Differential Diagnosis

Priority differentials will differ based on location of infection.[10]

 Priority differentials include (1) bacterial infection, (2) atopic dermatitis, (3) dermatophytosis, and (4) seborrheic dermatitis.

Several areas can be affected by candidal infections. As such, each area will have a distinct differential diagnosis. The oral pharynx should include aphthous ulcers, geographic tongue, pernicious anemia, and leukoplakia. Intertriginous area differentials include miliaria, bacterial infection (erysipelas or cellulitis), erythrasma, seborrheic dermatitis, atopic dermatitis, dermatophytosis, inverse psoriasis, mycosis fungoides, and scabies. The female perianal area includes bacterial vaginosis, trichomoniasis, allergic contact dermatitis, and pediculosis pubis. The male genital area includes bacterial infection, psoriasis, and tinea. Consideration for nail differentials are bacterial infection and tinea.[4]

Interprofessional Collaborative Management

Pharmacologic Management

Topical Therapy. The treatment of candidiasis is aimed at the elimination of both the predisposing factors and the organism. In the older adult or diabetic patient, avoiding hyperglycemia and maintaining skin integrity is important for prevention. A variety of agents—powders, intravaginal agents, oral suspensions, creams, and tablets—are commonly used for the treatment of candidal infections (see Table 47.7). Oral thrush can be treated with nystatin swish and swallow, Mycostatin pastilles or clotrimazole troches.[17] Superficial infections should usually be treated with topical therapy.[1,4,6,15]

Oral Therapy. If the infection is so widespread that the use of topical agents is impractical or too expensive, oral fluconazole is appropriate and has received a high level of support from evidence-based research.[45] Table 47.7 has treatment options listed.

Probiotics and Supplements. Eating yogurt with live cultures, may help prevent vaginal or oral yeast infections.[17] Probiotics are often used to prevent yeast infections, but the evidence is mostly lacking. A small reduction is seen with the use of Lactobac orally or Femilac vaginal pessary. Intravaginal suppositories show initial evidence of improvement of symptoms with the use of 1 billion live Lactobacillus GG (Culturelle) twice daily for 7 days. Florajen is used to maintain the normal floral balance of the vagina. Eating yogurt, 150 mL, containing *Lactobacillus acidophilus* is a preventative method for recurrent vaginal candidiasis.[7,45]

Indications for Referral. Treatment is usually effective and a referral is not indicated. The differential diagnosis of candidal infection is large, however. Therefore, infections recalcitrant to treatment require a physician or dermatologist referral to look for other causes of the eruption. Patients with yeast septicemia or other systemic manifestations of infection also require a physician consultation.

Life-Span Considerations

Many conditions predispose the individual to candidiasis. These include obesity, immunodeficiency due to the disease process or medication regime, hot, humid weather, ill-fitting clothing, and a hot temperate climate.[10,15]

Complications

The most serious complication of candidiasis is fungal septicemia, which may be seen in immunocompromised patients. Candidal esophagitis is a potential complication of antibiotic therapy and may be noted in patients who are severely immunocompromised, particularly patients with AIDS.[2,10]

Patient and Family Education

- Apply simple talc powder or an antifungal powder (tolnaftate or miconazole) to intertriginous or interdigital areas twice daily during active infections or to prevent recurrence.
- Use aluminum sulfate (Domeboro solution), an over-the-counter product, to help dry excessively moist areas.
- Teach patients who are prone to fungal infections to avoid cornstarch-containing products because this substance encourages fungal growth.
- Patients using oral steroid inhalers should understand the importance of rinsing the oral cavity after use of these inhalers to prevent fungal infections.[1,6]

Health Promotion

Methods for reducing environmental factors that encourage heat, moisture, maceration, and trauma should be emphasized: drying thoroughly after bathing (especially in the axillae and toe webs and between and under the breasts), wearing absorbent materials such as cotton underwear and socks, changing socks frequently, avoiding constrictive clothing, not wearing the same shoes each day, and wearing sandals in warm weather to promote air exposure to the affected skin.[17]

INFESTATIONS

LICE

Definition and Epidemiology

Lice, ectoparasites, are wingless insects that survive by feeding on human blood. They have six legs and strong claws that they use to adhere to the shaft of the hair as well as fibers from clothing items (Fig. 47.12). Three areas of the body host different species of lice. The head louse is known as Pediculus humanus var. capitis. The body measures 2.1 to 3.3 mm in length and is elongated and narrow. They lay their eggs on the shaft of the hair. Pediculus humanus var. humanus, the body louse, is the largest in size measuring 2.3 to 3.6 mm in length. The body louse lay their eggs on fibers, and it looks very similar to the Pediculus capitis. Finally, the smallest is the pubic louse, Phthirus pubis. This louse measures 1.1 to 1.8 mm in length and has a crab-shaped body.[46] These are commonly found in the pubic hair but may also reside in thicker shafted hair such as beards, eyelashes, and eyebrows. Eggs are firmly attached and are approximately 0.8 mm in size. Lice affect all individuals worldwide regardless of socioeconomic status. Black children tend to be less affected than white and males less than females. Most common age group affected is elementary and middle school ages. Common methods of transmission include close personal contact; sharing of toys, clothes, hats, and bed linens; and sexual encounters.[4,46] Head lice are not known to be vectors of disease. However, the body louse is known to transmit epidemic typhus, trench fever, and epidemic relapsing fever. Pubic louse infection is not known to be a vector however it can be associated with other sexually transmitted diseases.[4,46]

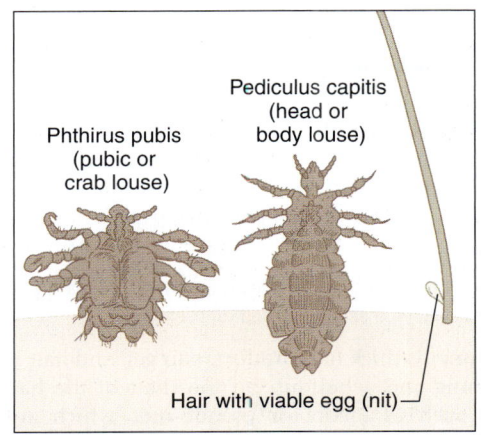

Phthirus pubis (pubic or crab louse)

Pediculus capitis (head or body louse)

Hair with viable egg (nit)

FIG. **47.12** Pediculosis. (From Buttaravoli, P., & Leffler, S. M. [2012]. *Minor emergencies* [3rd ed.]. Philadelphia: Saunders.)

Pathophysiology

Lice belong to the Anoplura family, who are dependent on their hosts. Lice feed several times per day and cannot survive more than 2 days without a blood meal. The majority of their life cycle occurs in their specific body area. During a 30-day life cycle, the female will lay between 5 to 10 eggs per day. The larvae hatch approximately 10 days later and reach maturity in 14 days.

Feeding occurs as the louse pierces the skin and injects its saliva to ingest human blood.[1,4,46]

Clinical Presentation and Physical Examination

Chief complaint regardless of location is itching and sensation that something is crawling. Pruritus with excoriation may be caused by a hypersensitivity reaction, inflammation from saliva, and fecal material from the lice. A physical exam will reveal nits and louse on the clothing or body of the individual. Head lice are commonly found at the back of the head, neck, and behind the ears.

P. corporis may be identified as linear excoriations on the main body of the individual. Hyperpigmentation with lichenification may occur with a post-inflammatory response along the trunk and neck areas. Concentrated areas of response tend to be around the waist and ancillary folds. Pubic lice may be identified by the presence of small, 3 mm in diameter, pale blue macules in the lower abdomen, thighs, buttocks, and genital area. This tends to occur as a result of prolonged infestation.[3,6,15]

Diagnostics

Essential Diagnostics. Examination of the affected area to identify louse or nits is the main way of identifying an infestation. Head and pubic lice are the easiest to identify. The body louse runs and hides and may be identified by nits on articles of clothing. If lice are not seen with the naked eye, it is important to comb the hair with a fine-toothed comb. This will detect and remove any live lice and nits. They may be viewed under a magnifying lens or by using a microscope. Using a Wood lamp to look at a nit will detect unborn louse by fluorescing white, while born louse or empty nits fluoresce gray.[6,15,46]

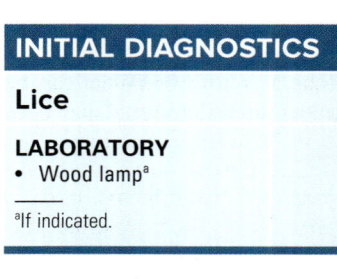

INITIAL DIAGNOSTICS

Lice

LABORATORY
- Wood lamp[a]

[a]If indicated.

Differential Diagnosis

The differential diagnosis must include diseases that should be considered and excluded when appropriate. These can be narrowed down with the patient history, patient's age, and any recent exposures.

 Priority differentials include (1) seborrheic dermatitis, (2) scabies, (3) eczema, (4) insect bites, and (5) psoriasis.

Additionally, thick hair product, hair gel, and hair spray may cause itching and a buildup on the shaft of the hair. Fungal infection such as Piedra or pseudo-nits, which are tubular casings that encircle hair shafts may also be a differential. The individual may have a psychological issue and have delusions of parasitosis.[1,4,15]

Interprofessional Collaborative Management

Pharmacologic Management

First Line Therapy. For children under the age of 2 months to 2 years Permethrin is the first line of treatment as recommended by the CDC. However, there is some resistance to many over-the-counter permethrin treatments including Nix, lindane, and some pyrethrins. Lindane is generally not recommended due to its risk of neurotoxicity and low efficacy.[6] Prescription treatments include permethrin 5%. It can be applied to dry hair and rinsed after 10 minutes. For those over age 2, malathion (Ovide) is available and is one of the more suitable forms of treatment. Precaution is given as it has a long application time, has a strong odor, and is flammable. Ivermectin lotion, 0.5% (Sklice) is approved by the FDA for those over age 6 months; it is a single application.[6,15,46]

Second Line Therapy. If needed to repeat treatment 1% permethrin cream rinse can be used with a prescription of TMP-SMX. This is an off-label indication for this medication that can be associated with many side effects and should not be used in sulfa allergic individuals. It is especially effective against eyelash infestations.[6]

Petroleum jelly and mayonnaise are thought to suffocate the louse but do not kill nits.. This is massaged over the entire surface of the hair and scalp and left on overnight. The residue is the thououghly washed from the hair and lice and nits are then carefully combed out. This method is less toxic but also less effective than chemical treatments.[1]

Spinosad (Natroba) was approved by the FDA in 2011. It kills live lice, nymphs, and nits. It is safe for ages 6 months and older, and can be repeated if live lice are seen after day 7.[46]

Complementary Approaches

Combing. After treatment, it is important to use a "nit" comb with teeth 0.2 to 0.3 mm apart, combing through the entire head at least 2 times checking for lice after each stroke. This will trap the lice. Combing is not necessary after using Sklice application.[46]

Emerging Therapy. Oral ivermectin has been used safely in many foreign countries to treat worm infections. It is not approved by the FDA for treatment of lice. However, it is effective. Ivermectin tablets are prescribed as a single oral dose based on weight and repeated in 10 days. It is contraindicated in pregnant women and children weighing less than 15 kg.[46]

Life-Span Considerations

Support to parents and infested children reassuring them that infestation is not an indication of poor hygiene. Elderly in assisted living are at increased risk. Any person who has an infestation regardless of location should notify anyone who could have potentially been in close contact with them, especially if they shared clothes or linens or were sexually active in the past 30 days.[6]

Complications

Sleep disturbances may be an annoying complication due to itching. This is especially true with young children. Antihistamines may be beneficial in alleviating the histamine response. Impetigo may occur as a secondary infection due to scratching areas bitten.[1,6]

Patient and Family Education

- Teach patients to pay close attention to detail when applying the topical treatment.
- Address patient hygiene practices, if needed.
- Teach patients to monitor for evidence of lice in members of the household and close contacts.
- Have patients discard any infested clothing or linens. For personal grooming items that are being kept, they should be soaked in hot water for 15 to 30 minutes. Clothing and linens should be laundered using hot water (at least 130°F) and machine dried using the hot cycle.[6,46]

Health Promotion

Continue to launder clothes once weekly, and do not share any clothing items or bed linens used by a person with lice. If there is a concern for the spread of disease fumigation with chemical insecticides may be necessary. If exposure occurred in the past 30 days at school or a slumber party the parent or guardian should actively look for live lice using nit comb on a weekly basis.[1,6,15,46]

SCABIES
Definition and Epidemiology

Scabies typically is a poorly defined pruritic eruption, often with linear burrows in the web spaces of the fingers. The breasts and genital areas are also often involved. The condition is commonly complicated by eczematous changes from nocturnal scratching and rubbing. The diagnosis is confirmed by scraping of a burrow and microscopic identification of mites, eggs, or feces.[10,17]

Scabies is a contagious infection caused by an infestation of the classic *Sarcoptes scabiei* mite, sometimes referred to as the *human itch mite* or *the 7-year itch*. This form is the more common and less virulent type, often affecting the young and old. Crusted scabies is caused by scabies crustosa (alternately known as Norwegian scabies, Boeck scabies, or keratotic scabies), is highly contagious, and typically tends to affect those who are immunocompromised, older, or living in poor conditions.[10,47]

Scabies can affect people of all ages and is more common in crowded living conditions and institutional facilities such as nursing homes, prisons, long-term care facilities, and day care centers. Worldwide cases number an estimated 150 million at any time, especially affecting the young and elderly in resource-poor countries. Scabies is more prevalent in hot, humid environments as well as in poor, overcrowded areas.[10,47] Scabies is usually transmitted by direct, prolonged skin-to-skin contact with an infested person, commonly through sexual contact or sharing a bed with an infected individual.[48] Animals can host scabies (var. canis, dog, and var. suis, pig) however, it is it is considered non-transmissible from animal to human.[46]

Pathophysiology

The scabies mite is not visible to the unaided eye. The female mite is responsible for the infestations. The mite is oval and has four pairs of legs (Fig. 47.13). It burrows no deeper than the stratum corneum and lays two to three eggs per day for 1 to 2 months before dying. The eggs and mites reach maturity in 28 to 30 days, starting a new cycle.[10,47] The intense pruritus experienced with scabies infestation is a hypersensitivity reaction to the mites. It usually begins 2 to 4 weeks after infection in a person who was not previously sensitized. Pruritus may

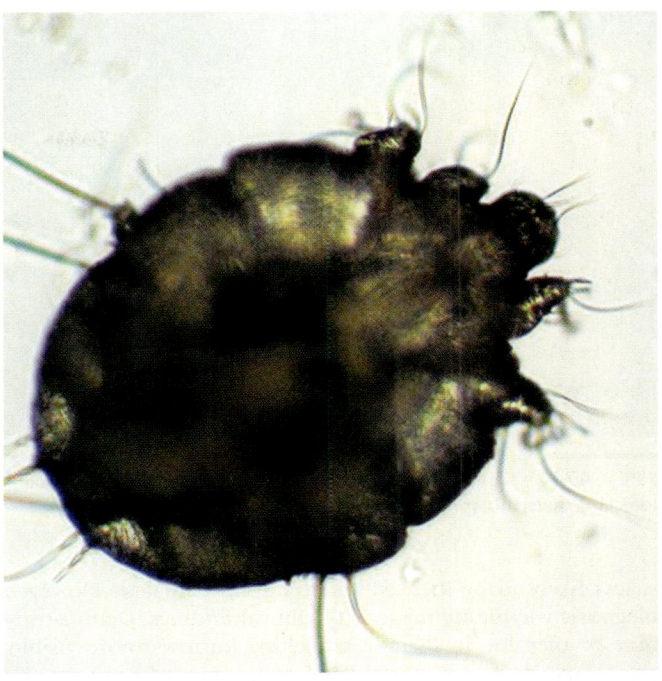

FIG. **47.13**   Scabies mite, highly magnified. (Courtesy New Zealand Dermatological Society Incorporated.)

begin within a day of reinfestation in a previously sensitized person. Scabies is usually acquired through close personal contact, although the mite can survive off the human host for up to 3 days.

Clinical Presentation and Physical Examination

The clinical presentation of scabies is variable. Most commonly, there are minimal findings in the setting of intractable pruritus, especially at night. The skin lesions of scabies can be classified into two categories: lesions at the site of infestation and lesions secondary to hypersensitivity to the mite. Small papules on an erythematous base form a disseminated tract near the waist, genitalia, breasts, buttocks, axillary folds, interdigital spaces, and wrists. The head, palms, and soles are usually spared in adults. Intraepidermal burrows are linear or serpiginous ridges that are produced by the infesting female mite. Common burrow sites are the interdigital spaces of the hands, flexures of the wrists and arms, genitals, feet, buttocks, and axillae (Fig. 47.14). A hypersensitivity reaction to the mites can manifest as urticaria, eczematous dermatitis, and scabetic nodules. Excoriations, lichen simplex chronicus, and secondary infection may result from scratching. Crusted scabies (Norwegian or hyperkeratotic) is found in severely immunocompromised or debilitated patients, or those with reduced sensation and/or immobility to scratch the itch. Itching may be mild or absent. This form of scabies is highly contagious and should be treated immediately. https://www.cdc.gov/parasites/scabies/gen_info/faqs.html Commonly found on bony prominences such as the elbows or iliac crest they present with a brownish yellow thick warty appearance.[47,48]

Diagnostics

Essential Diagnostics. The classic burrow, a straight or S-shaped ridge 2 to 10 mm long, is not always present and

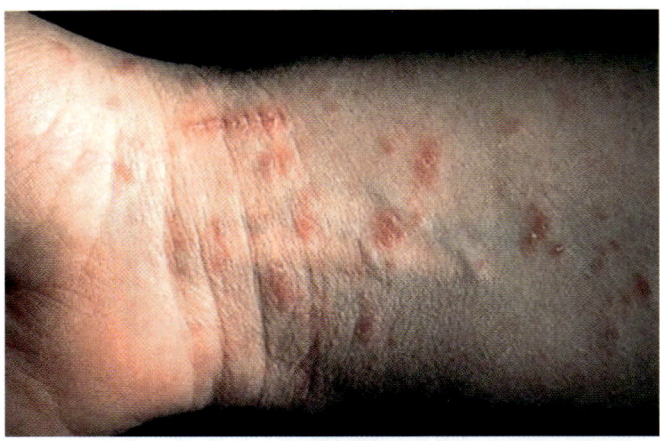

FIG. **47.14** Scabies on the wrist. (Courtesy New Zealand Dermatological Society Incorporated.)

is less likely to be seen in warm, humid climates.[3] However, diagnosis is typically made with clinical findings. Dermoscopy may be of value in diagnosis, making burrows more visible, and the ability to see a "jet-plane" appearance of a mite at one end of a burrow.[4] The "adhesive tape test" is another method of clinically diagnosing scabies. Adhesive tape is adhered to the affected area, then rapidly removed. The tape is then applied to a slide and examined under a microscope.[5]

Additional Diagnostics. Definitive confirmation is made with a "scabies prep." A drop of mineral oil is placed on a burrow, and the lesion is scraped or shaved. The sample is viewed under a microscope and examined for mites, eggs, fragments, or feces. The lack of positive findings on a scraping does not rule out the diagnosis of scabies, as the total number of mites present on any host may be fewer than 10 to 15.[48]

INITIAL DIAGNOSTICS

Scabies

LABORATORY
- Microscopic examination for mites or eggs
- Screening for sexually transmitted diseases

ADDITIONAL DIAGNOSTICS
- Biopsy to rule out other conditions if scabies is ruled out

Differential Diagnosis

The differential diagnosis must include diseases that have a similar presentation. These can be narrowed down with the patient history, patient's age, and any recent exposure or trips.

 Priority differentials include (1) seborrheic dermatitis, (2) insect bite, (3) impetigo, and (4) pediculosis.

Additional considerations include atopic dermatitis, pityriasis rosea, contact dermatitis, folliculitis, VE, psoriatic drug reaction, chickenpox, dermatitis herpetiformis, and syphilis.

Interprofessional Collaborative Management

Pharmacologic Management

Primary Treatment. Treatment is initiated with topical application of 5% permethrin cream (Elimite), applied from the neck down, giving attention to the interdigital webs, axillae, umbilicus, gluteal cleft, genitals, areas under the nails, and soles of the feet. The medication should be left on for 8 to 12 hours and then washed off. The treatment must be repeated after 7 to 14 days. Scabies can infest the hairline of older adults; massage the permethrin cream into the skin from head to toe in these patients. Also, benzyl benzoate lotion (10% to 25%) can be applied each night for 2 days in a row with reapplication at 7 days.[47] Crotamiton cream is not first-line topical treatment; this product has been associated with resistance issues.[6]

Oral ivermectin is used off-label to treat crusted scabies or if topical treatments are not effective. The dose of ivermectin is 200 mcg/kg, taken once only, but the dose may be repeated in 14 days.[6,22]

Lubrication and topical corticosteroids are used to treat persistent pruritic papules and eczematous dermatitis resulting from infestation and treatment. Antihistamines may be used to treat pruritus.[6] After 1 week, if there are no manifestations of active scabies, the infestation is considered cleared. Unfortunately, the itch after treatment may last up to 4 weeks.

Secondary Treatment. Sulfur ointment or lotion is an older treatment; it must be applied for 3 consecutive days. These sulfur preparations are not popular with patients owing to the strong odor and messiness associated with the application. Ivermectin 1% lotion is as effective as 5% cream and has a Grade A recommendation. Malathion 0.5% as well as foam preparation of synergized pyrethrins have proven effective.[47]

Crusted Scabies. Crusted scabies are difficult to treat. They have a very high mite burden and are extremely infectious. Treatment requires a prolonged course of combination therapy in which all scales and crusts are gone. Topical permethrin 5% cream should be applied from the neck down to the soles of feet and washed off after 8 to 14 hours, or benzyl benzoate lotion 25% should be applied from the neck down to the soles of feet and washed off after 8 to 14 hours. This process must repeat every 2 to 3 days for 1 to 2 weeks to help penetrate the crusted scabies. Urea cream should be applied twice-daily; this will help to decrease the hyperkeratosis.[1,47]

Other Medications for Recalcitrant Scabies. As a last resort, Lindane (Kwell) may be considered. It is no longer recommended as a first-line treatment of scabies because of toxicity concerns and side effects. However, it is considered an alternative regimen by the CDC to be used if other treatments are unavailable or have failed. One ounce of lotion (or 30 g of cream) is applied sparingly from the neck down and washed off in 8 hours.[22] Lindane is absorbed through the skin at a rate of 10%. It accumulates in the fat and binds to the brain tissue.[10]

Indications for Referral

Deaths have been associated with the use of ivermectin for scabies in older adults; thus it should be used with caution. Dermatology referral is indicated with treatment failure. Recalcitrant infestation or persistent pruritus requires physician consultation.

Life-Span Considerations

If scabies is present during pregnancy or lactation, permethrin is safe to use.[46] It can also be used in children age 2 months and up. Pregnant and lactating women may be treated with Benzyl benzoate permethrin or sulfur preparations. Malathion was not studied in pregnant women. Ivermectin is not safe to be used during pregnancy or in children weighing less than 15 kg.[46]

Complications

Ivermectin and lindane are pregnancy risk factor C; neither is recommended in breastfeeding women. The severe itching and skin abrasion can lead to breaks in the epidermis ultimately serving as an entry point for streptococci or staphylococci to enter and create a superinfection.[46] Pustules, impetigo, and ecthyma should be treated with appropriate antibiotics. Acute glomerulonephritis has been associated with streptococcal superinfection.[15] Additional caution is advised in treating individuals with secondary eczematization, erosions, or ulcers. Using standard treatment options could result in cutaneous and systemic side effects.[48]

Emerging Management Trends

Studies have been performed that have demonstrated TTO as an effective method (in vitro) of treatment against scabies mites. It was used as a topical adjuvant treatment for recalcitrant scabies. It is also effective as a bactericidal. It was shown to have superior scabicidal activity compared against the standard treatments such as permethrin 5% cream and ivermectin. It is currently being used at the Royal Darwin Hospital as a combination therapy for the management of complicated crusted scabies. Because TTO is openly licensed there is little interest by pharmaceutical companies to pursue this inexpensive option as there are no patent rights. TTO containing formulation of greater than 5% is found to be useful in the management of scabies.[48]

Patient and Family Education

- Identify and treat all household contacts.
- Wash all clothing and bedding in hot water and dry on the hot cycle; vacuum stuffed sofas and chairs. Materials that cannot be washed should be placed in a plastic bag for 1 week or dry cleaned.
- Give patients written and verbal instructions about how to use medication and how to eliminate mites in bedding and on furniture.
- Patients should be warned that symptoms may continue to be present for 2 weeks after treatment.
- Have patients compile a list of personal or household contacts from the past 30 days for evaluation and treatment, if indicated.[1,10,46]

Health Promotion

Individuals who are undergoing treatment should avoid close contact until everyone exposed has completed treatment.[46] Risks can be reduced by limiting the number of sex partners and maintaining strict personal hygiene. Maintain clean linens, clothes, and towels. Condom use does not prevent the spread of scabies.[47]

REFERENCES

1. Pouakou, G., Lagou, S., & Tsiodras, S. (2019). What's new in the epidemiology of skin and soft tissue infections in 2018. *Current Opinion in Infectious Diseases, 32*(2), 77–86.
2. Kasper, D., Fauci, A., Hauser, S., Longo, D., Jameson, J., & Loscalzo, J. (Eds.), (2014). *Harrison's principles of internal medicine* (19th ed.). New York, NY: McGraw-Hill. Retrieved from http://accessmedicine.mhmedical.com.ezproxy.hsc.usf.edu/content.aspx?bookid=1130&sectionid=79733782. (Accessed 17 January 2018).
3. Habif, T. P. (2016). *Clinical dermatology: A color guide to diagnosis and therapy* (6th ed.). Edinburgh: Elsevier.
4. Goldsmith, L. A., Katz, S. I., Gilchrest, B. A., Paller, A. S., Leffell, D. J., & Wolff, K. (Eds.). (2012). *Fitzpatrick's dermatology in general medicine* (8th ed.). New York, NY: McGraw-Hill. Retrieved from http://accessmedicine.mhmedical.com.ezproxy.hsc.usf.edu/content.aspx?bookid=392&sectionid=41138903. (Accessed January 22, 2018).
5. Stevens, D. L., Bisno, A. L., Chambers, H. F., et al. (2014). Practice guidelines for the diagnosis and management of skin and soft tissue infections: 2014 update by the Infectious Diseases Society of America. *Clinical Infectious Diseases: an Official Publication of the Infectious Diseases Society of America, 59*(2), e10–e52. doi:10.1093/cid/ciu296. (Accessed on January 17, 2018).
6. Ferri, F. F. (2018). *2018 Ferri's clinical advisor: 5 books in 1*. Philadelphia: Elsevier.
7. Torres, J., Avalos, N., Echols, L., et al. (2017). Low yield of blood and wound cultures in patients with skin and soft-tissue infections. *The American Journal of Emergency Medicine, 35*, 1159.
8. McCann, S. A., & Huether, W. E. (2014). Structure, function, and disorders of the integument. In K. L. McCance & S. E. Huether (Eds.), *Pathophysiology: The biologic basis for disease in adults and children* (7th ed.). St. Louis: Elsevier. Ch 46.
9. Prawer, S., & Bart, B. (2013). Bacterial infections. In C. Soutor & M. K. Hordinsky (Eds.), *Clinical dermatology*. New York, NY: McGraw-Hill. Retrieved from http://accessmedicine.mhmedical.com.ezproxy.hsc.usf.edu/content.aspx?bookid=2184&sectionid=165459573. (Accessed 17 January 2018).
10. Bologni, J., Schaffer, J., & Cerroni, L. (Eds.), (2017). *Dermatology: 2-volume set* (4th ed.). Philadelphia: Elsevier.
11. Erythrasma. (2016). *Clinical Advisor*. Retrieved from http://www.clinicaladvisor.com/dermatology/erythrasma/article/595282/. (Accessed 24 January 2018).
12. Blasco-Morente, G., Arias-Santiago, S., Pérez-López, I., & Martínez-López, A. (2016). Coral-red fluorescence of erythrasma plaque. *Sultan Qaboos University Medical Journal, 16*(3), e381–e382. doi:10.18295/squmj.2016.16.03.023. Retrieved from https://www.ncbi.nlm.nih.gov/pmc/articles/PMC4996308/. (Accessed 25 January 2018).
13. James, W. D., Berger, T. G., Elston, D. M., & Andrews, G. C. (2016). *Andrews' diseases of the skin: Clinical dermatology*. Philadelphia: Elsevier.
14. Polat, M., & İlhan, M. N. (2015). The prevalence of interdigital erythrasma: A prospective study from an outpatient clinic in Turkey. *Journal of the American Podiatric Medical Association, 105*(2), 121–124.
15. Habif, T. P., Campbell, J. L., Chapman, M. S., et al. (2017). *Skin disease: Diagnosis and treatment* (4th ed.). St Louis: Elsevier.
16. Relhan, V., Goel, K., Bansal, S., & Garg, V. K. (2014). Management of chronic paronychia. *Indian Journal of Dermatology, 59*(1), 15–20. doi:10.4103/0019-5154.123482.
17. Wolff, K., Johnson, R., Saavedra, A. P., & Roh, E. K. (Eds.), (2017). *Fitzpatrick's color atlas and synopsis of clinical dermatology* (8th ed.). New York, NY: McGraw-Hill. Retrieved from http://accessmedicine.mhmedical.com.ezproxy.hsc.usf.edu/content.aspx?bookid=2043&sectionid=154893879. (Accessed 25 January 2018).
18. Capriotti, K., Capriotti, J., Pelletier, J., & Stewart, K. (2017). Chemotherapy-associated paronychia treated with 2% povidone–iodine: A series of cases. *Cancer Management and Research, 9*, 225–228. doi:10.2147/CMAR.S139301.
19. Paras, V. (2018). Intertrigo: Practice essentials, background, pathophysiology. Retrieved from http://www.Emedicine.medscape.com. (Accessed 25 January 2018).
20. Kalra, M. G., Higgins, K. E., & Kinney, B. S. (2014). Intertrigo and secondary skin infections. *American Family Physician, 89*(7), 569–573.
21. Intertrigo (Intertrigo Candidiasis). (2016). *Clinical Advisor*. Retrieved from https://www.clinicaladvisor.com/dermatology/intertrigo-intertrigo-candidiasis/article/588594/. (Accessed 26 January 2018).
22. Centers for Disease Control and Prevention. (2015). Sexually transmitted diseases treatment guidelines, 2015. *MMWR. Recommendations and Reports: Morbidity and Mortality Weekly Report. Recommendations and Reports, 64*(3), 27–32. Retrieved from https://www.cdc.gov/mmwr/pdf/rr/rr6403.pdf. (Accessed 23 February 2018).
23. Bibbins-Domingo, K., Grossman, D. C., Curry, S. J., et al. (2016). Serologic screening for genital herpes infection: US preventive services task force recommendation statement. *JAMA: The Journal of the American Medical Association, 316*(23), 2525–2530. doi:10.1001/jama.2016.16776.
24. Gottlieb, S. L., et al. (2017). Modelling efforts needed to advance herpes simplex virus (HSV) vaccine development: Key findings from the World Health Organization consultation on HSV vaccine impact modeling. *Vaccine, 35*(29), 3615–3690. doi:10.1016/j.vaccine.2017.03.074.
25. Centers for Disease Control and Prevention (CDC). (2017). Shingles: Clinical overview: Varicella vaccine: Herpes zoster. Retrieved from https://

www.cdc.gov/shingles/hcp/clinical-overview.html#reference. (Accessed 29 January 2018).

26. Dooling, K. L., et al. (2018). Recommendations of the advisory committee on immunization practices for use of herpes zoster vaccines. *MMWR. Morbidity and Mortality Weekly Report, 67*(3), 103–108. Web. 30 Jan. 2018.

27. Capriotti, T. Shingles: A complete guide for clinicians; Tyring, S. Peranteau, A. (2017). Herpes Zoster (shingles, zoster, zona). *Clinical Advisor*. Web. 30 Jan. 2018.

28. Neuzil, K. M., & Griffin, M. R. (2016). Preventing shingles and its complications in older persons. *The New England Journal of Medicine, 375,* 1079–1080. doi:10.1056/NEJMe1610652.

29. Marin, M., Yawn, B., Hales, C., et al. (2015). Herpes zoster vaccine effectiveness and manifestations of herpes zoster and associated pain by vaccination status. *Human Vaccines and Immunotherapeutics, 11*(5), 1157–1164.

30. Declining effectiveness of herpes zoster vaccine in adults aged ≥60 years. (2016). *The Journal of Infectious Diseases, 213,* 1872–1875.

31. Le, P., Sabella, C., & Rothberg, M. B. (2017). Preventing herpes zoster through vaccination: New developments. *Cleveland Clinic Journal of Medicine, 84*(5), 359–366. doi:10.3949/ccjm.84a.16020.

32. van der Wouden, J. C., van der Sande, R., Kruithof, E. J., Sollie, A., van Suijlekom-Smit, L. W. A., & Koning, S. (2017). Interventions for cutaneous molluscum contagiosum. *The Cochrane Database of Systematic Reviews, (5),* CD004767, doi:10.1002/14651858.CD004767.pub4.

33. Molluscum Contagiosum (Molluscipoxvirus). (2016). *Clinical Advisor.* Retrieved from https://www.clinicaladvisor.com/dermatology/molluscum-contagiosum-molluscipoxvirus/article/589573/. (Accessed 2 February 2018).

34. Korman, A. M., Alikhan, A., & Kaffenberger, B. H. (2017). Viral exanthems: An update on laboratory testing of the adult patient. *Journal of the American Academy of Dermatology, 76*(3), 538–550.

35. Kadambari, S., & Segal, S. (2017). Acute viral exanthems. *Medicine, 45*(12), 788–793.

36. Brasil, P., Calvet, G. A., et al. (2016). Exanthema associated with Zika virus infection. *Lancet Infectious Diseases, 16*(7), 866. (Accessed December 27, 2018).

37. Drago, F., Ciccarese, G., Gasparini, G., et al. (2017). Contemporary infectious exanthems: An update. *Future Microbiology, 12,* 171–193. doi:10.2217/fmb-2016-0147.

38. Ferri, F. F. (2017). *Ferri's fast facts in dermatology: A practical guide to skin disease and disorders* (2nd ed.). Philadelphia: Elsevier.

39. Centers for Disease Control and Prevention. (2017). Epidemiology and prevention of vaccine-preventable diseases. In J. Hamborsky, A. Kroger, & S. Wolfe (Eds.), *The Pink Book, 2015* (13th ed.). Washington, DC: Public Health Foundation.

40. Durbin, A., & Gubler, D. (2019). What is the prospect of a safe and effective dengue vaccine for travelers? *Journal of Travel Medicine.* Retrieved from https://academic.oup.com/jtm/advance-article-abstract/doi/10.1093/jtm/tay5292564. (Accessed 5 May 2019).

41. Professional resource, Gardasil 9 and HPV vaccination FAQs. Pharmacist's Letter/Prescriber's Letter. December 2016. Detail-Document, Comparison of Therapies for Onychomycosis (2013). Topical Antifungal Agents for Tinea Infections (2014). Comparison of Common Probiotic Products. Pharmacist's Letter/Prescriber's Letter. July 2015. Retrieved from https://prescriber.therapeuticresearch.com. (Accessed 21 February 2018).

42. Revankar, S. Antifungal drugs. Retrieved from https://www.merckmanuals.com/professional/infectious-diseases/fungi/antifungal-drugs. (Accessed 5 May 2019).

43. Acharya, R., & Gyawalee, M. (2017). Uncommon presentation of Pityriasis Versicolor: Hyper and hypopigmentation in a same patient with variable treatment response. *Our Dermatol Online, 8*(1), 43–45. doi:10.7241/ourd.20171.11.

44. Gupta, A. K., & Foley, K. A. (2015). Antifungal treatment for pityriasis versicolor. *Journal of Fungi, 1,* 13–29. doi:10.3390/jof1010013. PMCID: PMC5770013.

45. Pappas, P. G., et al. (2016). Executive summary: Clinical practice guideline for the management of candidiasis: 2016 update by the Infectious Diseases Society of America. *Clinical Infectious Diseases: an Official Publication of the Infectious Diseases Society of America, 62*(4), 409–417.

46. CDC.gov. (2018). CDC—Global Health: Division of Parasitic disease. Parasites: Lice. Retrieved from https://www.cdc.gov/parasites/lice/index.html. (Accessed 23 February 2018).

47. Salavastru, C. M., Chosidow, O., Boffa, M. J., Janier, M., & Tiplica, G. S. (2017). European guideline for the management of scabies. *Journal of the European Academy of Dermatology and Venereology, 31,* 1248–1253. doi:10.1111/jdv.14351.

48. CDC.gov. (2018). CDC—Global Health: Division of Parasitic disease. Parasites: Scabies. Retrieved from https://www.cdc.gov/parasites/scabies/index.html.

CHAPTER **48**

NAIL DISORDERS
Kathryn D. Swartwout

Nail disorders are a common complaint in any primary care practice. Primary care providers should be familiar with the diagnosis, management, and referral points for common nail disorders such as herpetic whitlow, paronychial infections, and onychomycosis.

HERPETIC WHITLOW

 Immediate referral is indicated for patients with possible tenosynovitis who present with severe redness, swelling, pain, and stiffness in the finger. Immediate surgical intervention may be required.

DEFINITION AND EPIDEMIOLOGY

Herpetic whitlow is a self-limited viral infection of the area between the fascial planes of the distal finger, usually surrounding the nail. This infection is most often seen in patients with gingivostomatitis caused by herpes simplex, in patients with genital herpes, and in health care workers.[1,2] Symptoms develop 2 to 14 days after exposure and generally resolve in about 3 weeks. The patient is infectious until lesions are healed.[2] Auto-infection from nail biting[1] and recurrences can occur.[2]

PATHOPHYSIOLOGY

The infecting pathogen is herpes simplex virus (HSV-1 or HSV-2). Transmission may occur from a primary herpetic lesion or infected body fluids. The virus remains dormant in the nerve ganglia; secondary eruptions may be related to stress, certain foods, sun exposure, and unknown precipitants.

CLINICAL PRESENTATION AND PHYSICAL EXAMINATION

Herpetiform vesicles or blisters erupt on the distal phalanx, sometimes after a short prodromal period of flulike symptoms (particularly in the primary infection) and throbbing, tingling, numbness, or pruritus in the area of the eruption. Painful vesicles can be singular or coalescent, resemble a group of warts or a bacterial infection, and persist for 8 to 12 days; lesions then begin to dry, forming crusted fissures.[3] The course of the eruptions can persist for 21 days until resolution; healing may take longer in areas that remain moist. In addition to the vesicles, the fingertip may be edematous, erythematous streaking may be evident on the forearm, and the axillary lymph nodes may become enlarged.

The physical examination includes nail inspection for shape, configuration, texture, and herpetiform vesicles. Axillary and epitrochlear nodes should be examined for lymphadenopathy. Examination for genital herpes should be considered if there are genital symptoms.

DIAGNOSTICS
Essential Diagnostics

Diagnosis is typically established based on history and physical examination findings. If warranted, viral culture of vesicular fluid,

Tzanck smear, or serum titer may be used to confirm the diagnosis.[2]

Additional Diagnostics

If secondary bacterial infection is suspected, bacterial culture may be indicated.

DIFFERENTIAL DIAGNOSIS

Priority differentials include (1) tenosynovitis (tendon sheath infection), (2) bacterial infection, (3) candidal infection, (4) felon (painful abscess in the digital pulp), (5) paronychia, and (6) warts.

 Priority differentials include tenosynovitis and cellulitic bacterial infections that are or could become systemic.

INTERPROFESSIONAL COLLABORATIVE MANAGEMENT

Nonpharmacologic Management

Use of incision and drainage (I&D) is avoided because it may lead to superinfection[2] or longer duration of healing.[1] Cool compresses can be used to decrease erythema and to debride crusts, thus promoting healing.[3] The area should be covered with gauze to prevent transmission. The area is kept dry because moisture may prolong healing and promote superinfection.

Pharmacologic Management

Analgesics are used at doses appropriate for the patient's age and medical history. Oral antivirals (acyclovir, famciclovir, valacyclovir) may be considered for severe cases, management of recurrences, during the prodromal period, and in patients with acquired immunodeficiency syndrome (AIDS).[2] Creatinine clearance should be checked and the dose adjusted according to the creatinine clearance values if they are abnormal. L-Lysine is ineffective.[3]

INDICATIONS FOR REFERRAL AND HOSPITALIZATION

Physician referral is necessary if the virus is recalcitrant to treatment. Hospitalization should not be required.

LIFE-SPAN CONSIDERATIONS

Herpetic whitlow is generally more common in young children and young adults. Atypical presentations and more severe infection can occur in immunocompromised individuals.

COMPLICATIONS

Secondary bacterial infection in conjunction with the viral syndrome is possible. Transmission to others during viral shedding is possible. Infection can be spread to the eye and cause a serious corneal infection.

PATIENT AND FAMILY EDUCATION AND HEALTH PROMOTION

- Patients require education about the risk of infecting others and medication administration. If used in recurrences, antivirals should be administered within 48 hours of the first prodromal signs.

- Patients should be advised to keep their infected digits away from the mouth and eyes to prevent inoculation of these surfaces with the virus.
- If patients work in occupations in which they could infect other persons (e.g., health care providers, dental providers, manicurists), they should be advised to wear gloves when working.
- The provider should carefully explain signs and symptoms of infection and encourage the patient to call if complications develop.

PARONYCHIAL INFECTIONS

 Immediate emergency department or surgical referral is indicated for patients with possible tenosynovitis who present with severe redness, swelling, pain, and stiffness in the finger. Immediate surgical intervention may be required.

DEFINITION AND EPIDEMIOLOGY

Paronychial infections manifest as acute or chronic inflammation of the tissues surrounding the nail, usually with an underlying bacterial or fungal infection. Other noninfectious causes are possible and include "chemical irritants, excessive moisture, systemic conditions, and medications."[4] Most commonly a microorganism penetrates the tissue after breakdown between the nail plate and nail fold. A split in the epidermis from trauma, nail biting, a hangnail, irritation, or chronic exposure to water (such as with dishwashing) or irritants can precede the development of a paronychia. Symptoms typically develop 2 to 5 days after trauma.[4] Paronychial infections may be seen more often in women than in men; this may be related to manicures or the application of acrylic nails. Patients who work with chemicals are more at risk for infections because of the irritant nature of these substances and the risk of trauma. Other risk factors include psoriasis, diabetes mellitus, and immunosuppression.[5] Patients who have their hands in water frequently are also at risk.

PATHOPHYSIOLOGY

There are numerous possible causative organisms for acute paronychial infections. Some organisms include *Pseudomonas*, *Proteus*, *Streptococcus*, *Staphylococcus*, *Candida albicans*, and HSV. A paronychial infection results when periungual tissue is inoculated by trauma, inert vehicles such as water, or soluble chemicals. The resulting infection follows the nail margin or the infection penetrates under the nail.

If paronychial inflammation is present for longer than 6 weeks, the condition is considered a chronic paronychia. Chronic paronychia is primarily an inflammatory disorder, but *C. albicans* is also often present. It is most commonly present in workers with frequent exposure to environmental irritants (such as cooks, dishwashers, and nurses).[4] Diabetes mellitus and certain medications can cause chronic paronychia, increasing the risk for infection. Retinoids, protease inhibitors, and cetuximab have all been associated with paronychia.[6] Indinavir (a protease inhibitor used in HIV treatment) is a common cause of chronic paronychia in persons infected with HIV.[6]

CLINICAL PRESENTATION AND PHYSICAL EXAMINATION

Symptoms are usually localized to one finger, and patients report throbbing pain of the nail fold, nail, and even adjacent portions of the finger. The affected nail may display distal onycholysis, discoloration, distortion, and ridging; the affected nail folds have erythema and edema. When the examiner presses the affected area, there can be a release of purulent discharge. Greenish nail discoloration may be associated with *Pseudomonas* infection.[5]

DIAGNOSTICS
Essential Diagnostics

Diagnosis is often established based on history and physical examination findings. If exudate from the nail area is present, a bacterial culture will help determine the pathogen and guide antibiotic treatment based on sensitivities and resistances.

Additional Diagnostics

Skin scrapings can be combined with potassium hydroxide (KOH) preparation on a glass slide and viewed under a microscope. Pseudohyphae and spores indicate candidal infection. A complete blood count with differential (CBC with diff) could be indicated if systemic bacterial infection is suspected.

DIFFERENTIAL DIAGNOSIS

Priority differentials include (1) tenosynovitis (tendon sheath infection), (2) bacterial infection (especially *Staph, Strep,* or *Pseudomonas*), (3) herpetic whitlow, (4) onychomycosis, (5) psoriasis, and (6) malignancy.

 Priority differentials include tenosynovitis (surgical emergency) and cellulitic bacterial infections that are or could become systemic.

Circulatory changes and irritation from environmental causes (such as nail products) are additional considerations.[7] Malignancies of the area are possible and should be considered, especially in patients with persistent paronychia or those with a cancer history.[4] Underlying conditions such as diabetes mellitus or immunocompromised state should be considered especially with recurrences. Paronychial infection is usually readily recognized by its appearance and absence of medication history preceding the infection.

INITIAL DIAGNOSTICS

Paronychial Infections

LABORATORY
- Bacterial culture and sensitivities
- Potassium hydroxide preparation
- Complete blood count and differential (if infection complication is suspected or if the patient is immunocompromised)

INTERPROFESSIONAL COLLABORATIVE MANAGEMENT
Acute Paronychia

Nonpharmacologic Management. Treatment of minor acute paronychial infection includes warm water soaks or warm compresses four times a day. The area is kept dry because moisture may prolong healing and cause further irritation. I&D is considered if abscess is suspected or infection is not responding to noninvasive care.

Pharmacologic Management. A topical antibiotic may be added for minor cases. Topical neomycin is indicated for pseudomonal infection.[8] Oral antibiotic therapy is indicated for more substantial infection. Antibiotic choice depends on the suspected organism. Considerations could include trimethoprim-sulfamethoxazole (good if methicillin-resistant *Staphylococcus aureus* [MRSA] is suspected), clindamycin, amoxicillin-clavulanate, and cephalexin.[4] Appropriate analgesics and dosages are based on patient age and medical history. Oral antibiotics may be used in conjunction with I&D.

INDICATIONS FOR REFERRAL AND HOSPITALIZATION

Patients are referred to a physician if there is continued infection after 2 weeks of treatment. Specialist consultation is indicated if a provider skilled in I&D is not available. Complete removal of the nail plate is sometimes necessary in situations in which the nail plate has separated from the underlying tissue. Suspected infection of the tendons or tendon sheaths requires immediate referral to a physician or surgeon in the emergency department. Hospitalization may be required for surgical intervention.

CHRONIC PARONYCHIA
Nonpharmacologic Management

Treatment of chronic paronychia includes identification and elimination of causative irritants. I&D is reserved for severe persistent cases.

Pharmacologic Management

Topical steroids have been shown to be most often superior to topical antifungals in treating chronic paronychia. Topical betamethasone is the recommended preparation.[4] For persistent or nonresponsive cases, use of oral antifungal preparations is considered. A short course of oral corticosteroids may be considered for severe cases with multiple fingers involved.[4]

COMPLICATIONS

Serious complications of paronychia include loss of the nail or spread of the infection into the bloodstream, deeper tissue, or bone. If it is untreated or in patients with immunosuppression or diabetes, the paronychial infection can invade deep into the digit, infecting the tendon and tendon sheaths. Infection along the tendon sheath requires immediate surgical intervention. Chronic mucocutaneous candidiasis can cause hyperkeratosis of the entire nail plate. These chronically infected nails can become distorted and may require excision.

PATIENT AND FAMILY EDUCATION

- It is imperative that patients understand the importance of keeping hands and nails as clean and dry as possible.
- Address the individual patient's causative factors including their environmental and work exposures.
- Patients who have manicures or who wear acrylic nails should be advised of the risk of paronychia infections.
- Patients who deal with caustic chemicals and irritants should be advised to wear protective gloves.
- Instruct patients to wear waterproof gloves when washing dishes or clothing by hand and to keep the nails trimmed and dry to prevent further infections.

ONYCHOMYCOSIS

DEFINITION AND EPIDEMIOLOGY

Onychomycosis (or *tinea unguium*) refers to any infection of the nails caused by a dermatophyte, yeast, or sometimes mold.[7]

Onychomycosis is the most common nail condition, most frequently occurs in the toenails (great toe is often first), is classified based on nail bed location of the infection, and has a reputation for being quite difficult to resolve. These infections cause nail discoloration, thickening, roughness, splitting of the nail, and sometimes onycholysis (a separation of the nail from the nail bed). Onychomycosis is common in patients of advancing age, possibly from a result of a reduction in blood flow to the area. Other risk factors include swimming, nail trauma, diabetes, tinea pedis, psoriasis, and immunodeficiency.[8,9] Onycholysis has a significant incidence of pain and can affect patients' lives physically and psychologically, interfering with walking, exercise, and social interaction.

PATHOPHYSIOLOGY

The most common pathogens associated with tinea unguium are *Trichophyton rubrum* and *Trichophyton interdigitale*.[9] *Candida* organisms are rarer and may be associated with immunosuppression. Molds are also causative. A nail can be infected by multiple organisms.[3] Infection is located inside the nail. Distal subungual onychomycosis, the most common presentation, begins with discoloration in the distal portion of the nail partially caused by the accumulation of keratinous debris under the nail.[9] Proximal subungual onychomycosis, the rarest presentation, begins deeper near the cuticle and occurs mostly in immunocompromised patients. White superficial onychomycosis has a flaky white appearance and affects the nail surface.[8,9]

CLINICAL PRESENTATION AND PHYSICAL EXAMINATION

Table 48.1 describes the physical presentation of onychomycosis nail dystrophies. Pain rating and any interference with daily activities should be assessed.

Careful physical examination of the toes and fingers is essential. Typically, the nail is white or yellowed, with a powdery or thickened nail texture. The nail surface typically has a greenish tinge with bacterial infections. The examiner should assess for onycholysis (disassociation of the nail from the nail bed). The condition of the subungual nail bed should be noted—that is, the degree of elevation and separation of the nail from the nail bed and surrounding tissue (see figure 47.10).

DIAGNOSTICS
Essential Diagnostics

Accurate diagnosis is essential along with the correct identification of the causative organism due to the lengthy period and cost of the treatment.[10] Confirmation of the diagnosis may be made by microscopic examination of nail scrapings with a KOH preparation in the primary care office. However, the presence of a dermatophyte will not confirm the causative agent.[10] Thus, a fungal culture of nail debris is required and considered "gold standard."[10] It is essential to identify the invading organism as a dermatophyte or *Candida* to guide treatment. Histologic tests and periodic acid–Schiff staining are reliable for an accurate diagnosis to identify organisms susceptible to specific therapeutic agents.[3]

Additional Diagnostics

There are a number of newer and often expensive molecular assay tests available that may be useful in identifying the causative organism.[10] A CBC, creatinine clearance, and liver function tests (LFTs) may be required before initiating systemic medications.

INITIAL DIAGNOSTICS

Onychomycosis and Tinea Unguium

LABORATORY
- Potassium hydroxide smear and culture

DIFFERENTIAL DIAGNOSIS

Priority differentials include malignancy and assess for liver disease (contraindication to antifungal systemic meds).

Priority differentials include (1) malignancy, (2) psoriasis, and (3) trauma. Onychomycosis accounts for about 50% of nail abnormalities, so consideration should be given to other causes. Psoriasis, not fungal infection, causes pitting of the nail surface. Psoriasis is often mistaken for dermatophyte and fungal infections, but the two may coexist (Fig. 48.1).[3] Leukonychia, white spots or bands that appear proximally, is most likely caused by minor trauma and may be mistaken for proximal subungual onychomycosis.[11] Other conditions that cause nail findings similar to onychomycosis include eczema, trauma, lichen planus, and leukonychia.[3] Onychomycosis should not be confused with onychogryphosis, which is a nail hypertrophy sometimes caused by trauma but more often caused by neglecting to trim the nails for a long period. Subungual malignant melanoma is a nail cancer. Subungual malignant melanoma can manifest as a dark stripe discoloration and requires urgent referral for evaluation.

INTERPROFESSIONAL COLLABORATIVE MANAGEMENT
Pharmacologic Management

Confirmed onychomycosis is most effectively treated systemically. Ciclopirox, a nail lacquer applied to the nail over an extended period of time, may be considered in a patient for

TABLE 48.1	Nail Dystrophies Caused by Onychomycosis	
Nail Disorder	**Clinical Presentation**	**Manifestations**
Distal or lateral subungual onychomycosis	White to brownish-yellow discoloration of nail	Subungual hyperkeratosis; separation of nail plate and nail bed lineal channels
White superficial onychomycosis	White, sharply outlined area on nail plate; nail surface soft, dry, and friable	Common in fingernails and toenails of HIV-infected patients. Nail plate not thick; no separation of nail plate and nail bed
Proximal subungual onychomycosis (rare), candidal infections	Leukonychia on proximal aspect of nail plate. Thickening of nail plate. Yellowish-brown discoloration	Patient may be immunosuppressed. Chronic mucocutaneous candidiasis. Involves all nails. Eventual disintegration of nail

HIV, Human immunodeficiency virus.

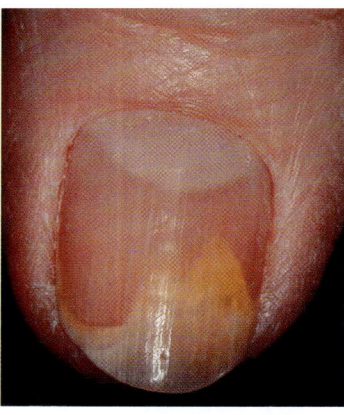

F I G . **48.1** Psoriasis of nails. (From Bolognia, J. L., Schaffer, J. V., Duncan, K. O., & Ko, C. J. [2015]. *Dermatology essentials* [1st ed.]. St Louis: Saunders.)

whom oral therapy is contraindicated or infection is limited and does not involve the nail matrix.[5] Topical antifungal creams rarely penetrate deeply enough to be effective. Onychomycosis may be treated with terbinafine (Lamisil) orally and daily for 12 weeks for toenails, 6 weeks for fingernails. This medication has a low incidence of side effects. Liver function tests should be performed at baseline and 6 weeks after starting terbinafine. The drug should not be used in patients with abnormal creatinine clearance and is Pregnancy Category B. Other oral medications that may be used are fluconazole and itraconazole.[5] *Candida* onychomycosis is preferably treated with fluconazole.[5] Indications and contraindications for all oral antifungal medications should be reviewed carefully before prescribing. Consistent, prolonged application of a topical antifungal agent after clinical response to an oral agent may prevent nail reinfection.

Indications for Referral or Hospitalization

Patients with combinations of infection and underlying disease (e.g., psoriasis) would benefit from a dermatology referral. Patients with nail stripe discolorations or persistent subungual discolorations should be referred to rule out subungual malignant melanoma. Discussion with the physician regarding recurrence and surgical or nonsurgical avulsion of nail dystrophy is also a consideration for a referral. Removal of the infected nail affords better cure rates and longer remissions.[3] Trials of various phototherapy methods for treatment of *T. rubrum* infection are promising and ongoing.

COMPLICATIONS

Chronic inflammation can cause onycholysis, a separation of the nail from the nail bed. Any patient with an underlying condition (e.g., diabetes mellitus or peripheral neuropathy) making them more susceptible to infection or delayed healing is at higher risk for onycholysis.

PATIENT AND FAMILY EDUCATION

- Review information concerning medication administration and instructions regarding signs of liver toxicity.
- In many cases, nails do not appear clear after the recommended course of treatment, and it may take 12 to 18 months after treatment for the patient to visually see improvement.[8]
- Patients should be assured that the medication remains in the nail plate for months and will continue to kill fungus.[3] These infections can be recalcitrant to treatment; it may take months or even years for complete resolution of the pathogens.
- To prevent recurrences, the patient can apply ciclopirox two or three times a week, apply terbinafine cream in the nail area weekly, and avoid trauma to the tip of the nails from tight-fitting shoes.
- It is imperative that patients keep their hands and nails as dry as possible and avoid recurrence of tinea pedis. Nails should be trimmed, and chewing or picking at nails avoided.
- Footwear should be evaluated annually for size and suitability.
- Patients should powder toe webs and soles, not shoes; avoid going barefoot in communal showers; wear sweat-wicking socks; and alternate several pairs of shoes for daily wear that maintain a dry, roomy environment for the feet. Using an antifungal spray in shoes may be helpful.

REFERENCES

1. Sanders, J. E., & Garcia, S. E. (2014). Pediatric herpes simplex virus infections: An evidence-based approach to treatment. *Pediatric Emergency Medicine Practice, 11*(1), 1–20.
2. Franko, O. I., & Abrams, R. A. (2013). Hand infections. *The Orthopedic Clinics of North America, 44*(4), 625–634.
3. Habif, T. P., Campbell, J. L., Chapman, M. S., et al. (2011). *Skin disease: Diagnosis and treatment* (3rd ed.). St Louis: Elsevier.
4. Shafritz, A. B., & Coppage, J. M. (2014). Acute and chronic paronychia of the hand. *The Journal of the American Academy of Orthopaedic Surgeons, 22*(3), 165–174.
5. Wollina, U., Nenoff, P., Haroske, G., & Haenssle, H. A. (2016). The diagnosis and treatment of nail disorders. *Deutsches Ärzteblatt International, 113,* 509–518.
6. Rigopoulos, D., Larios, G., Gregoriou, S., et al. (2008). Acute and chronic paronychia. *American Family Physician, 77*(3), 339–346.
7. Borfitz, J. (2009). Commonly missed dermatologic conditions. *The Nurse Practitioner, 34*(10), 35–45.
8. Tully, A. S., Trayes, K. P., & Studdiford, J. S. (2012). Evaluation of nail abnormalities. *American Family Physician, 85*(8), 779–787.
9. Erwin, B. L., Styke, L. T., & Kyle, J. A. (2013). Fungus of the feet and nails. *US Pharm, 36*(6), 51–54.
10. Ghannoum, M., Mukherjee, P., Isham, N., Markinson, B., Del Rosso, J., & Leal, L. (2017). Examining the importance of laboratory and diagnostic testing when treating and diagnosing onychomycosis. *International Journal of Dermatology.*
11. Habif, T. (2015). *Clinical dermatology: A color guide to diagnosis and therapy* (6th ed.). Philadelphia: Elsevier.

CHAPTER **49**

MACULOPAPULAR SKIN DISORDERS

Richard Matthew Prior

Maculopapular disorders are common conditions in patients in primary care practices. This chapter will cover the following maculopapular disorders: seborrheic dermatitis, psoriasis, pityriasis rosacea, and lichen planus.

SEBORRHEIC DERMATITIS

DEFINITION AND EPIDEMIOLOGY

Seborrheic dermatitis is a chronic, common dermatosis that occurs across the life span. It is characterized by greasy, slightly erythematous scaling that occurs in areas with the highest concentration of sweat glands or sebaceous glands, including the scalp, face, and postauricular and intertriginous areas.[1,2] The disorder affects 1% to 3% of immunocompetent adults. Men tend to be affected more than women. In adults, seborrheic dermatitis is most common in patients who are immunocompromised, such as those with human immunodeficiency virus, those who have had lymphoma, and patients who have had organ transplants. It is also common in patients who suffer from neurologic diseases such as Parkinson disease and stroke. It is much more common in infants, affecting 40% of those who are younger than 3 months of age.[2]

PATHOPHYSIOLOGY

The cause of seborrheic dermatitis is unknown. Sebaceous gland secretion, the presence of *Malassezia* yeast, and the host immune response are thought to contribute to the condition.[2]

CLINICAL PRESENTATION AND PHYSICAL EXAMINATION

Seborrheic dermatitis is seen in both young and old patients. In infants, the most common presentation is yellow or white scaling lesions on the scalp, which is called cradle cap. In adolescents and adults, the common presentation is dry, flaky scales on the scalp. This disorder is known commonly as dandruff.

On the face and auricular area, seborrheic dermatitis is seen as greasy, erythematous, sharply marginated plaques. Plaques that wax and wane are commonly seen on the sternal area. In the axillae and groin, the eruption manifests as more confluent plaques with fine scales and less well-defined borders. Lesions are usually asymptomatic, although pruritus is may be present.[2,3]

DIAGNOSTICS

Essential Diagnostics

Initial diagnostics include a wet prep with potassium hydroxide (KOH) to identify any fungal elements, guiding therapeutic choices and aiding the exact diagnosis.

Additional Diagnostics

The appearance of seborrheic dermatitis is similar to multiple skin conditions. Skin biopsy and immunofluorescence studies may be indicated to establish the exact diagnosis.

DIFFERENTIAL DIAGNOSIS

 Priority differentials are (1) eczema, (2) psoriasis, (3) tinea capitis, (4) rosacea, and (5) systemic lupus erythematous.

There are many differential diagnoses. More common diseases that can resemble seborrheic dermatitis include eczema, psoriasis, tinea capitis, rosacea, and systemic lupus erythematous. Psoriasis is often described with more circumscribed, thicker plaques with a bright silvery hue. Seborrheic dermatitis can often overlap with psoriasis in a condition known as *sebopsoriasis*. Atopic or contact dermatitis generally is accompanied by pruritus and occurs in areas of flexion. If the diagnosis is uncertain, a skin biopsy and immunofluorescence studies should be completed.[2,3]

Less common diseases that can resemble seborrheic dermatitis include Langerhans cell histiocytosis, acrodermatitis enteropathica, pemphigus foliaceus, and glucagonoma syndrome. If these disorders are considered, there should be consultation with a dermatologist.

INITIAL DIAGNOSTICS

Seborrheic Dermatitis

INITIAL	OTHER
• Potassium hydroxide wet preparation	• Skin biopsy[a]
	• Immunofluorescence studies[a]

———
[a]If indicated.

INTERPROFESSIONAL COLLABORATIVE MANAGEMENT

In general, when patients have symptoms suggestive of seborrheic dermatitis on the face or eyebrows, the scalp should be carefully examined because this is usually a "top-down" disorder, requiring treatment in that order as well. There is no cure. Treatment is targeted at controlling acute flares and maintaining remission.

Pharmacologic Management

Topical Therapies. First line therapy is topical antifungals or topical corticosteroids. Topical antifungals reduce *Malassezia* proliferation, thereby reducing the inflammatory response; topical corticosteroids serve to reduce inflammation. Topical antifungals are safe for all skin types.

For scalp lesions, ketoconazole shampoo is the most well-studied antifungal therapy and is a reasonable first option because it may be as effective as steroids but with fewer side effects. Other shampoo possibilities include ciclopirox 1% or selenium products. A Cochrane review investigated the use of short-term topical steroids and found that low-potency steroids were as effective as high-potency steroids in the short term and may actually result in better long-term clearance of symptoms than high-potency steroids. Calcineurin inhibitors (such as pimecrolimus 1% cream) may be an acceptable alternative to steroids but tend to have more side effects, such as burning and itching.[4,5]

Mainstay therapy for face and body lesions is similarly centered on topical antifungals, such as ketoconazole 2%. Face lesions often additionally require mild-potency steroids. Scales in the eyelids may cause blepharitis, which can be managed using baby shampoo and warm water to remove the scales. Lesions on the body often respond well to low- to mid-potency steroids. Calcineurin inhibitors are also effective as a short-term solution, but have a US Food and Drug Administration (FDA) "black box" warning against long-term use due to a theoretical association with skin cancer and lymphoma.

Topical steroids should not be used as maintenance therapy. Once lesions are well controlled, tar shampoos should be used for maintenance. Periodic flares of the disorder can be treated with steroids again until well controlled.

Oral Antifungal Agents. Those with severe seborrheic dermatitis may benefit from treatment with oral antifungal medication. For severe seborrheic dermatitis, prescribe oral itraconazole 200 mg/day for a week followed by a single dose of 200 mg every 2 weeks.[3,6]

Complications

Secondary candidal and bacterial infections may occur, especially around the eyes and in intertriginous areas. These should be treated with appropriate antifungal or antibiotic medications. Secondary changes such as flexural intertrigo, lichenification, otitis externa, and widespread disease may occur.[2] Periorificial dermatitis is a papular eruption that can occur around the eyes, nose, and mouth as a result of topical steroid overuse on the face. If this eruption occurs, topical steroids should be tapered off.

Indications for Referral

Patients with unresponsive seborrheic dermatitis or secondary changes with therapy should be referred to a dermatologist for further work-up. As indicated previously, several dermatoses can resemble seborrheic dermatitis but will not respond to standard therapies.[3]

PATIENT AND FAMILY EDUCATION

Explain to patients that seborrheic dermatitis is chronic and recurrent.
- Proper use of antiseborrheic preparations and monitoring for early flares will usually control the disorder.

PSORIASIS

DEFINITION AND EPIDEMIOLOGY

Psoriasis is an inflammatory papulosquamous eruption characterized by well-circumscribed erythematous macular and papular lesions with loosely adherent silvery white scale. It is a chronic, unpredictable disorder that is characterized by remissions and exacerbations throughout the life span. Approximately 3% of the population is affected by psoriasis, or approximately 7 million Americans. Psoriasis is a complex systemic disorder that may potentially result in significant morbidity. Stress, anxiety, and illness constraints on families mandate effective and convenient treatments. Symptoms can be treated; however, as yet there is no cure. Remissions are common and can last for short periods or years, with progression to arthritis in approximately 30% of cases. A genetic component appears to exist in this disorder; thus a familial tendency can increase risk.[6,7]

Patients with psoriasis score poorly on quality-of-life (QOL) measures. Patients are troubled by the appearance of the lesions and pruritus associated with the disease. Those with psoriatic arthritis (see Chapter 198) often have disability and pain. More than 80% of those with the disorder report that psoriasis often affects their emotional state and decreases their satisfaction with life. Psoriasis and psoriatic arthritis can have negative economic effects on those with the disorder; more than 92% of unemployed patients attribute their lack of a job solely to their disease.[8]

Psoriasis should be viewed as a systemic disorder that causes additional morbidity in those affected. Patients with psoriasis are more prone to inflammatory bowel disease and cardiovascular disease. They are likely to be overweight, hypertensive, diabetic, and dyslipidemic when psoriasis symptoms are present. In addition, these patients are more likely to experience sleep problems, alcohol dependence, and depression.[9]

PATHOPHYSIOLOGY

Psoriasis is a chronic, inflammatory, autoimmune disorder characterized by dermal hyperproliferation that develops in response to T cell infiltration into the skin and overexpression of multiple cytokines, including interferon, tumor necrosis factor (TNF), and interleukin-23 (IL-23). T cells are activated and produce an inflammatory response that results in the hyperproliferation of keratinocytes. Psoriasis lesions often contain 30 times the number of keratinocytes as normal skin.[6,10,11]

Psoriasis is known to have strong genetic associations. Those who have first-degree family members with the disorder are often affected as well. There is an increased incidence of psoriasis in monozygotic twins.[11]

CLINICAL PRESENTATION AND PHYSICAL EXAMINATION

In psoriasis, scaly papules and plaques form and collect on skin surfaces in well-demarcated lesions. The lesions have an erythematous base with silvery white plaques that are adherent (Fig. 49.1). The dermis is highly vascular, and tiny bleeding points are revealed if the scales are removed (Auspitz sign). Common sites for these lesions include the elbows, knees, scalp, genitals, and intergluteal cleft. In contrast to adult psoriasis, childhood psoriasis often involves the face. Many patients exhibit concomitant nail dystrophies, including pitting, yellowing of the distal portion (oil drop sign), separation of the nail plate (onycholysis), and thickening of the entire nail (hyperkeratosis).[1,6] (See Fig. 48.1).

Cutaneous trauma can induce psoriasis 1 to 3 weeks after injury. This isomorphic response, also known as the Koebner phenomenon, occurs in a linear fashion along the lines of a scratch, abrasion, sunburn, or pressure.

Discrete, scaly, "raindrop" plaques that are smaller than 1 cm, begin on the trunk, and spread to the extremities, sparing the palms and soles, are indicative of guttate psoriasis. Guttate psoriasis is occasionally seen after a streptococcal infection and is most common in adolescents. These patients are likely to develop psoriasis vulgaris (common, plaquelike psoriasis) later in life.[6,7]

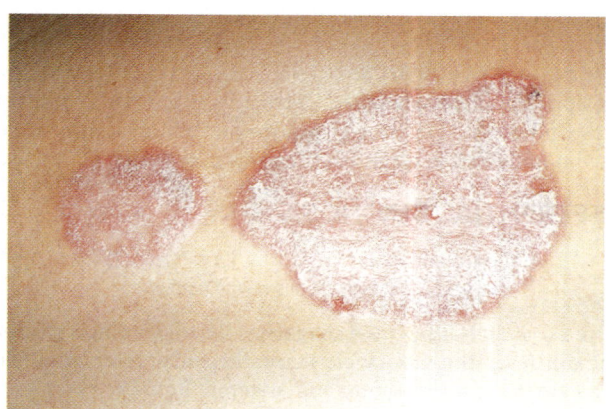

FIG. 49.1 Psoriasis. Thick, red plaques have a sharply defined border and adherent silvery scale. (From Ignatavicius, D. D., & Workman, M. L. [2016]. *Medical-surgical nursing: Patient centered collaborative care* [8th ed.]. St. Louis: Mosby.)

Erythroderma and pustular psoriasis are more serious forms of the disease. They are most common in patients older than 50 years and may be precipitated by infection, withdrawal of systemic steroids, emotional stress, or severe illness. Erythrodermic forms generally appear over a large portion of the body and can be precipitated by various treatments themselves.[6,7]

Although most psoriatic lesions are asymptomatic, itching is variable. However, picking and scratching of the lesions can produce the Koebner response, and the lesions worsen. Skinfold lesions tend to itch more than common plaquelike lesions. The axilla, intramammary folds, groin, buttocks, and genitals are common sites for intense itching, or inverse psoriasis. The bright red appearance of the lesions and affinity for dark, moist folds can make distinguishing inverse psoriasis from *Candida* infections difficult based on appearance alone.

Psoriatic arthritis is a seronegative spondyloarthropathy that affects approximately as many as 30% of the population with psoriasis. It is characterized by monoarthritis, often causing joint effusions; pain at the insertion point of tendons to bone (enthesitis); swelling of the fingers and toes (dactylitis); and changes to the nails (including pitting and splitting). In a small percentage of patients, psoriatic arthritis precedes the appearance of skin symptoms. Because as many as 16% of patients with psoriasis have undiagnosed psoriatic arthritis,[12] those who have musculoskeletal complaints should be carefully evaluated. (see Chapter 198).

DIAGNOSTICS
Essential Diagnostics

The presence of silvery scales on red, erythematous plaques is characteristic; therefore the diagnosis is usually based on presentation. However, biopsy is useful in pustular or difficult cases, and nail cultures differentiate fungal disease. Uric acid levels may be elevated in psoriasis and in gout.

Psoriatic arthritis is diagnosed clinically based on symptom scoring models, as there is no diagnostic laboratory test. As many as half of those with psoriatic arthritis may be HLA-B27 positive. Almost all patients with psoriatic arthritis are rheumatoid factor negative. Many patients who develop erosive arthritis have radiographic findings in advanced stages of the disease.

DIFFERENTIAL DIAGNOSIS

 Priority differentials include: (1) seborrhea, (2) atopic dermatitis, (3) pityriasis rosea, and (4) gout

In children, the plaques of psoriasis are thinner and less scaly than in adults with psoriasis and are often confused with seborrhea, atopic dermatitis, and diaper dermatitis. Seborrhea on the scalp tends to be patchy, red, and a bit oilier in appearance. Psoriasis is more plaquelike, with thick scales. Psoriasis typically appears on extensor surfaces, whereas atopic dermatitis is found on most flexor surfaces. Lichen planus papules have more of a purple hue, and patients exhibit Wickham striae (lacy, reticular, crisscrossed whitish lines) on many lesions. Flat warts do not have scale on the surface. Guttate psoriasis is often confused with pityriasis rosea; however, it lacks the characteristic herald patch, and the scale is thicker and more diffuse in psoriasis. Changes in the nails are often confused with onychomycosis. Culture for the presence of fungus will help to establish the diagnosis. Yellow discoloration is common in both fungal and psoriatic changes, as is nail separation. The nails in psoriasis are not well formed because debris collects underneath, again because of rapid shedding of the skin layers. This debris leads to failure in the integrity of the nail and onycholysis.

Additional diagnoses to be considered are gout, pseudogout, reactive arthritis, syphilis, squamous cell carcinoma, nummular eczema, and lichen simplex chronicus.

INTERPROFESSIONAL COLLABORATIVE MANAGEMENT
Pharmacologic

Topical Therapy. The goal of treatment is the restoration and maintenance of the barrier function of the skin. Good control can be achieved; however, it requires meticulous and consistent home care. Present therapy is aimed at reducing epidermal proliferation and decreasing inflammation. Primary care providers can reasonably manage patients whose needs are limited to topical therapy (<3% of total body surface area) and have minimal comorbidities. Patients with moderate to severe skin disease that occupies larger surface areas that cannot be realistically managed with topical steroids and/or with concerns over decreased quality of life may require systemic therapy and comanagement by a dermatologist.[7]

Topical corticosteroids produce rapid resolution of mild to moderate plaques. High-potency topical glucocorticosteroids applied ideally twice (but at least once) per day produce maximum benefit in 2 to 3 weeks. However, facial and intertriginous psoriasis should be treated with low-potency steroids. Vitamin D analogues can be used as either monotherapy or in combination with topical steroids. Calcineurin inhibitors may also be effective, particularly for facial and intertriginous areas.[6,7]

Ointments are the preferred vehicle because of better medicine penetration and support of the skin moisture barrier; however, ointments are not easily tolerated by the patient, especially if large skin surface areas are involved. Creams can be prescribed for patients who cannot tolerate ointments. Newer foam-based delivery systems provide advantages for some skin surfaces, such as the scalp, but they are expensive and often nonformulary. Solutions are available that are good vehicles for delivery of medicine to the scalp. Tolerance to steroid preparations rarely develops with plaque psoriasis, which can tolerate chronic application of high doses of steroids, but atrophy can occur with use on thinner lesions, as with inverse psoriasis. Occlusion with clear plastic wrap can increase the efficacy of therapy on large or thick plaques. Scalp psoriasis is often characterized by thick scale, which not only produces embarrassing dandruff but interferes with the steroid's ability to penetrate the dermis. Scalp lesions also respond best to topical high-potency steroids. Vitamin D analogues such as calcipotriene are also helpful for the treatment of scalp lesions and are an acceptable long-term form of therapy. Combination products of calcipotriene and betamethasone are available and can be used for 4 to 8 weeks.[6]

Research suggests that coal tar preparations may not be any more effective than placebo in treating scalp lesions. Shampoos containing the exfoliant salicylic acid are available to reduce scale buildup and to improve medication penetration. Use of topically applied mineral oil or vegetable oil and a bathing cap at bedtime is sometimes very effective at loosening and removing scale.

Intralesional Injection. For severe, recalcitrant cases, intralesional injections with a corticosteroid suspension produce satisfactory results after one or two injections; this treatment requires a dermatology referral. Limitations of this therapy include atrophy and obvious discomfort from injections.

Systemic Medications. Oral retinoids are used occasionally for psoriasis—particularly for pustular and erythrodermic psoriasis. However, they have side effects similar to those of isotretinoin and should be used with caution in women of childbearing age because they are teratogenic. Retinoids are less effective than methotrexate and cyclosporine but are safe in patients who are immunocompromised. Retinoids are not effective in patients with psoriatic arthritis.

Methotrexate, a folic acid antagonist, is highly effective in treating severe, recalcitrant psoriasis involving a large body area, acute pustular psoriasis, and psoriatic arthritis. Cell division is reduced, and the drug may also affect the inflammation. It should not be used in patients with liver or kidney disease, pregnancy, anemia, colitis, or debility. It should be reserved for patients unresponsive to other therapies and for those with psoriatic arthritis. Patients who take methotrexate are at risk for pancytopenia and should be monitored frequently with complete blood counts. Methotrexate should be avoided in pregnancy and in those who wish to become pregnant. Methotrexate and retinoid therapy should be comanaged with a dermatologist.

Cyclosporine (Neoral) is efficacious; however, it is also limited in use because of its potential nephrotoxicity. Blood pressure and serum creatinine concentration should be monitored. Relapse is also common once therapy is stopped. A dermatologist should manage patients who require cyclosporine therapy.

Biologic Agents. Biologic agents target the immune-mediated inflammation that is responsible for the psoriasis presentation. Currently, three TNF antagonists (etanercept, infliximab, and adalimumab), one monoclonal antibody that targets IL-12 and IL-23 (ustekinumab), and three IL-17A inhibitors (secukinumab, ixekizumab, and brodalumab) have been approved for the treatment of moderate to severe psoriasis. Several other biologic agents are approved for use in patients with psoriatic arthritis. Their use is increasing owing to their high degree of efficacy, low side effect profile, and improvement in QOL measures. They are given as self-administered subcutaneous or intramuscular injections or as intravenous infusions. In part because of the expense of the agents (as much as $25,000 per year), use is restricted to patients with moderate to severe disease. Insurance companies often require that other treatment modalities have been attempted and have failed before patients are approved for the biologics.[13]

Safety data are available from the use of biologics in other disease states, such as rheumatoid arthritis. Several agents come with an FDA-mandated black box warning for safety concerns relative to increased susceptibility to infection from fungi, viruses, bacteria, and mycobacteria and a possible connection to lymphoma, hematologic diseases such as aplastic anemia, melanoma, nonmelanoma skin cancers, and other solid organ cancers. There have been conflicting data about whether or not there is increased risk of infection or malignancy in patients with psoriasis who use biologics. Each medication has its own particular safety profile; thus it is good practice that patients be screened for tuberculosis and hepatitis B before initiation of therapy, to avoid latent disease activation. Histories of multiple sclerosis or other demyelinating disease and congestive heart failure are relative contraindications. Monitoring parameters include psoriasis lesion and surface area reduction, QOL

assessments, periodic liver function tests and complete blood counts, and assessment for evidence of infectious disease.[6,7]

Patients who receive biologics are essentially considered to be immunocompromised. It is therefore a good time to prior to starting biologics to check titers and to update the patient's vaccination status because live vaccines are contraindicated during treatment. However, they can be administered 2 weeks to 1 month before treatment. It is important that inactivated influenza vaccines are received yearly. Pneumococcal vaccines should be considered, even in those patients younger than 65 years of age.[14]

Phototherapy

Phototherapy in the form of ultraviolet B (UVB) light therapy has been shown to be effective for the treatment of psoriasis. The most common delivery method for the therapy is via a laser at a dermatologist's office. Targeted therapy is well tolerated, with some side effects such as blistering and erythema. The use of phototherapy requires multiple office visits, making it impractical or too expensive for some patients. Patients can be reassured that there is no evidence that narrowband therapies increase the risk of skin cancer.[7]

Combination Therapy

Combination therapy using several different treatment modalities is common, especially with particularly difficult-to-treat cases or when the treatment is poorly tolerated. Patients who have fairly significant but incomplete improvement on biologics will often still benefit from topicals. Even in patients maintained with topical treatments alone, it is useful to use multiple agents simultaneously for their synergistic effects. For smaller flares or chronicity, early treatment with combination therapies centered on topical treatments can manage the disease and minimize risk.

Selected Therapy Considerations

Guttate psoriasis should clue the provider to the need to screen for *Streptococcus*. Treatment is guided by the results of the culture.

Oral steroids should be used with caution because they can induce a pustular flare. They may be useful in controlling persistent erythroderma; however, they are not indicated in the treatment of psoriasis.

Many patients are interested in the question of whether or not diet can positively influence the severity of psoriasis. Research suggests that weight loss reduces the severity of psoriasis without therapy and that weight loss in addition to therapy significantly increases the likelihood of meeting treatment goals.[15]

Complications

Complications are usually related to infection. Scratching can introduce bacteria from beneath fingernails into lesions. Guttate psoriasis, erythrodermic psoriasis, and pustular psoriasis are also potential complications. Both erythrodermic psoriasis and pustular psoriasis are rare; however, serious sequelae, including congestive heart failure and sepsis, are potential hazards. Additional complications include psoriatic arthritis and cardiovascular disease, atrophy of skin with corticosteroid use, risk of skin cancer and cataracts with phototherapy if the eyes are not protected, and risk of effects on the metabolic profile with use of strong antimetabolites or retinoids.

Indications for Referral

A patient with recalcitrant or unresponsive psoriasis should be referred to a dermatologist for management with phototherapy, oral therapies, and biologics. If a dermatology referral is not possible, an internist may be appropriate for oral therapy.

Psoriatic arthritis often follows psoriasis by approximately 10 years. Early referral, close monitoring, and comanagement with a rheumatologist or dermatologist can help to identify appropriate patients to prevent the further debilitation to psoriatic arthritis in susceptible individuals.

PATIENT AND FAMILY EDUCATION AND HEALTH PROMOTION

- It is crucial for the patient and family to understand the chronic nature of psoriasis and the genetic and environmental factors.
- Adherence to the prescribed regimen is necessary for effective treatment; however, this requires meticulous and consistent home care.
- Patients should understand the use of moisturizers and lubricants to maintain control.
- Patients should avoid injury to skin (i.e., sunburn and other physical trauma), triggering the Koebner phenomenon.
- If possible, avoid certain medications (β-blockers, lithium, and antimalarials) that are known to worsen psoriasis
- Educate patients and families about treatment modalities and emotional support services. The National Psoriasis Foundation (www.psoriasis.org) is a not-for-profit organization dedicated to research, education, and support.

PITYRIASIS ROSEA

DEFINITION AND EPIDEMIOLOGY

Pityriasis rosea is a mild and self-limiting disorder that is frequently experienced in primary care. It most commonly affects young people, with an estimated 75% of patients being between the ages of 10 and 30 years of age. It will affect an estimated 1.3% of the population. It is a skin disorder primarily of adolescents, who comprise as many as 50% of affected patients. It can be seen in clusters, particularly in areas where individuals live in close quarters, such as military installations and college dormitories. Although mildly symptomatic, most patients and/or parents seek care due to the generalized rash, the appearance of which can be alarming.[1,6,16,17]

PATHOPHYSIOLOGY

It is thought that the disorder is caused by human herpesviruses 6 and 7, which researchers have isolated in examination of skin lesions. A pityriasis-like rash can be caused by common medications such as antibiotics, antidepressants, antihypertensives, vaccines, and other drugs. Most people who experience the disorder will confer immunity and will not experience another course of the disorder in their lifetimes.

CLINICAL PRESENTATION AND PHYSICAL EXAMINATION

Pityriasis rosea often begins with a single erythematous, scaly plaque that is 2 to 10 cm in diameter that is found on the trunk and is commonly referred to as a "herald patch." The herald patch usually precedes the widespread eruption of the rash by 1 to 2 weeks. When asked, the patient may or may not be able to identify that the herald patch. Occasionally, patients can recall experiencing a typical viral prodrome of headaches, fever, anorexia, and arthralgias/myalgias. Other than the rash, patients are often asymptomatic other than mild pruritis.

The erupting lesions are usually 5 to 10 mm in size, mildly erythematous with grayish scaling, and occur on the trunk, upper arms, and back. The lesions favor the Langer lines, which are tension lines or "cleavage" lines in the skin that are usually are not visible except in the hands. When the lesions occupy the Langer lines of the back, some providers see a pattern in the shape of a Christmas tree, which is considered characteristic of the rash. The rash will last anywhere from 6 to 8 weeks.[16–18] There may be lingering hypopigmentation, which will be more noticeable in darker skinned individuals.

The rash is known to have occasional atypical presentations. It can present with lesions on the flexural areas in adults and spare the trunk. It can be completely confined to the extremities. It occasionally presents as oral lesions on the palate. It is known at times to be persistent, lasting beyond 3 months.[19]

DIAGNOSTICS

Diagnosis is clinical. If there is any question that syphilis is a possibility, providers should order a rapid plasma reagin test. A biopsy can be helpful in atypical presentations.[6,16,17]

DIFFERENTIAL DIAGNOSIS

 Priority differentials include (1) nummular eczema, (2) tinea corporis, (3) guttate psoriasis, and (4) secondary syphilis

There are several lesions have a similar appearance to pityriasis rosea. The differentials include nummular eczema, tinea corporis, guttate psoriasis, and secondary syphilis.

INTERPROFESSIONAL COLLABORATIVE MANAGEMENT
General Treatment Measures

Pruritis can be treated with calamine or nighttime antihistamines. Systemic steroids should be avoided because they may cause the rash to flare. In adolescents and adults whose quality of life is severely affected, providers can consider oral acyclovir 400 mg three to five times per day for 1 week. The use of acyclovir for pityriasis rosea is off-label and should include a conversation on adverse effects (potential nausea and headache).[20]

Indications for Referral

A primary care provider should be able to manage pityriasis rosea. Referral to dermatology is warranted for confusing or atypical presentations and patients with significantly decreased quality of life.

PATIENT AND FAMILY EDUCATION

- Patients will benefit from reassurance that the rash is self-limiting.
- The expected resolution is within a month or two.

LICHEN PLANUS

DEFINITION AND EPIDEMIOLOGY

Lichen planus is a chronic, maculopapular skin disorder that primarily affects adults who are usually in their fourth decade of life. It consists of a characteristic papular lesion that is very pruritic and can be found a variety of body areas. Treatment consists of managing symptoms and limiting the amount of time the patient is subjected to the disorder.[6,21]

PATHOPHYSIOLOGY

The pathophysiology of lichen planus is unknown. It is thought to be autoimmune and involves activated cytokines and T cells at the dermoepidermal junction. There is a questionable relationship between lichen planus and the hepatitis C virus that is poorly understood. A very similar rash can manifest as a drug reaction, caused by common medications such as antimalarials, thiazide diuretics, and nonsteroidal antiinflammatories.[6,22]

CLINICAL PRESENTATION AND PHYSICAL EXAMINATION

The lesions of lichen planus can be remembered in that they exhibit the characteristics of the "four Ps": planar (flat), purple, polyangular, and pruritic. The lesions consist of purple papules that are 2 to 10 mm in diameter and have irregular and angular border. Close examination of the lesions reveals lacy, white lines called *Wickham striae* (Fig. 49.2). It is not unusual for the lesions to cluster and coalesce. The lesions are commonly located on the legs above the ankles, on the lower back, and flexor surfaces of the forearms and wrists. As seen in psoriasis, lesions can originate as a result of the Kobler phenomenon with damage to the skin. Lesions can last up to a year and leave a stained macule upon healing.[6,21,22]

An oral variant of the disorder is a chronic condition that affects the oral mucosa. It can be caused by oral trauma or irritation, silver amalgam fillings, and the previously mentioned medications. It results in either papular or ulcerative lesions on the tongue and buccal mucosa that also present with Wickham striae.[23]

Lichen planus can also present in the perineum. In women, it can accompany the classic lesions on the flexor surfaces with lesions with Wickham striae located on the labia minora and papules on the labia majora. It can also present in the remainder of the perineum. Erosive lesions are common and can cause pain, discharge, and dyspareunia.[21,24] In men, lichen planus lesions can present on the penis with a white, lacy lesion that is very similar in appearance to oral lesions.[6]

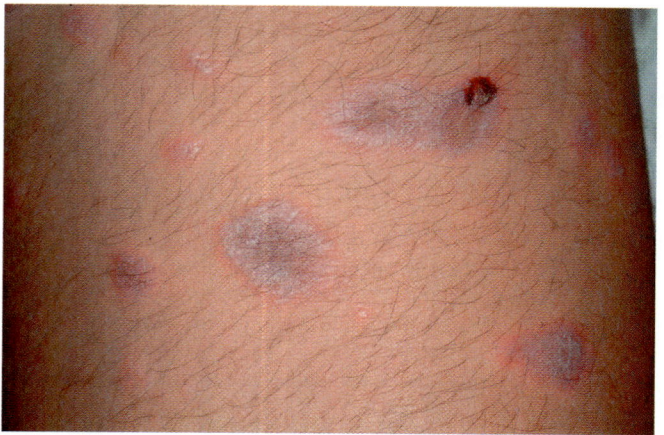

FIG. 49.2 Lichen Planus with Wickham striae. (From Paller, A. S., & Mancini, A. J. [2016]. *Hurwitz clinical pediatric dermatology* [5th ed.]. St. Louis: Elsevier.)

DIAGNOSTICS
Essential Diagnostics

The diagnosis for lichen planus is clinical.

Additional Diagnostics

If there is any doubt, a skin biopsy will confirm the diagnosis. Given the association of lichen planus with hepatitis C, providers may consider serologic testing for hepatitis C. In women with erosive lesions in the perineum, it is preferable to identify and biopsy cutaneous lesions located elsewhere, because an erosive vulvovaginal lesion may demonstrate only nonspecific changes.

DIFFERENTIAL DIAGNOSIS

 Priority differentials include (1) drug reactions, (2) tinea corporis, and (3) secondary syphilis

There are conditions that present with lesions with similar appearances. Differential diagnoses for lichen planus include drug reactions, psoriasis, tinea corporis, nummular eczema, seborrheic dermatitis, and secondary syphilis. The differential for erosive perineal lesions includes genital herpes.[6,22,24]

INTERPROFESSIONAL COLLABORATIVE MANAGEMENT
General Treatment Guidance

Antihistamines are useful at nighttime for treating the itch. Large, coalesced lesions on the wrists and legs may respond to interlesional Kenalog injections. High-potency and super-high-potency topical corticosteroids are frequently used as first line therapy for treating cutaneous lichen planus lesions. On patients with lesions covering large surface areas that are not practical for topical steroid use, primary care providers can prescribe oral prednisone 20 mg to 40 mgs once a day for 2 to 4 weeks with a subsequent 3-week taper. If the disorder does not improve, referral to a dermatologist is indicated. The disorder often responds well to systemic treatment with acitretin, sulfasalazine, and griseofulvin.[6,22,25]

Patients with oral lesions may benefit from a visit with their dentist to determine if a change to dental work or fillings are causing the problem—particularly if they have had recent dental work done. Oral mid- and high-potency topical steroids such as Orabase are generally effective. Steroid mouth rinses may be helpful for patients who have widespread involvement of the oral mucosa.[23]

Patients with asymptomatic genital lesions do not require treatment. Erosive perineal lesions respond well to high-potency topical steroids such as clobetasol 0.05% twice a day for 3 months. An alternative recommended method for prescribing topical steroids for vulvovaginal lesions is to apply a fingertip amount of steroid directly to the lesion once a day for a month, then every other day for a month and then twice a week for a month. For severe lesions, a course of oral steroids similar to that of cutaneous lesions can be considered.[6,24]

Indications for Referral

Lichen planus should be referred to dermatology when the patient has not responded to topical steroids, when the clinical picture is confusing, or when quality of life is significantly affected. Women with vulvovaginal concerns may benefit from a referral to gynecology.

PATIENT AND FAMILY EDUCATION

- Teach patients about the nature of lichen planus and the association with autoimmune responses, and explain that the lesions can persist for up to a year.
- Review that treatment is directed at resolution of symptoms and reduction of lesions

REFERENCES

1. Paller, A. S., & Mancini, A. J. (2016). *Hurwitz's clinical pediatric dermatology* (5th ed.). New York: Elsevier.
2. Borda, L. J., & Wikramanayake, T. C. (2015). Seborrheic dermatitis and dandruff: A comprehensive review. *Journal of Clinical Investigative Dermatology*, 3(2), 1–22.
3. Clark, G. W., Pope, S. M., & Jaboori, K. A. (2015). Diagnosis and treatment of seborrheic dermatitis. *American Family Physician*, 91(3), 186–190.
4. Okokon, E. O., Verbeek, J. H., Rutosalainen, J. H., Ojo, O. A., & Bakhoya, V. N. (2015). Topical antifungals for seborrhoeic dermatitis. *The Cochrane Database of Systematic Reviews*, 4, 1–130.
5. Kastarinen, H., Oksanen, T., Okokon, E. O., Kiviniemi, V. V., Airola, K., Jykka, J., et al. (2014). Topical anti-inflammatory agents for seborrheic dermatitis of the face or scalp (Review). *The Cochrane Database of Systematic Reviews*, 5, 1–105.
6. Habif, T. P. (2016). *Clinical dermatology* (6th ed.). New York: Elsevier.
7. Kim, W., Jerome, D., & Yeung, J. (2017). Diagnosis and management of psoriasis. *Canadian Family Physician*, 63, 278–285.
8. Armstrong, A. A., Schupp, C., Wu, J., & Bebo, B. (2012). Quality of life and work productivity impairment among psoriasis patients: Findings from the National Psoriasis Foundation Survey Data 2003–2011. *PLoS ONE*, 7(12), 1–6.
9. Oliveria, M. F. S. P., Rocha, B. O., & Duarte, G. V. (2015). Psoriasis: Classical and emerging comorbidities. *Anais Brasileiros de Dermatologia*, 90(1), 9–20.
10. Warren, R., & Menter, A. (2016). *Handbook of psoriasis and psoriatic arthritis*. Switzerland: Springer.
11. Meier, M. M., & McCalmont, T. H. (2013). Diseases of the skin. In G. D. Hammer & S. J. McPhee (Eds.), *Pathophysiology of disease: An introduction to clinical medicine* (Seventh ed.). New York, NY: McGraw-Hill.
12. Villani, A. P., Rouzaud, M., Sevrain, M., Barnetche, T., Paul, C., Richard, M. A., et al. (2015). Prevalence of undiagnosed psoriatic arthritis among psoriasis patients: Systematic review and meta-analysis. *Journal of the American Academy of Dermatology*, 73(2), 243–248.
13. Ronholt, K., & Iversen, L. (2017). Old and new biological therapies for psoriasis. *International Journal of Molecular Sciences*, 18, 1–23.
14. Ferreira, I., & Isenberg, D. (2014). Vaccines and biologics. *Annals of the Rheumatic Diseases*, 73, 1446–1454.
15. Upala, S., & Sanguankeo, A. (2015). Effect of lifestyle weight loss intervention on disease severity in patients with psoriasis: A systematic review and meta-analysis. *International Journal of Obesity*, 39, 1197–1202.
16. Eisman, S., & Sinclair, R. (2015). Pityriasis rosea. *British Medical Journal*, 351, h5233.
17. VanRavenstein, K., & Edlund, B. J. (2017). Diagnosis and management of pityriasis rosea. *The Nurse Practitioner*, 42(1), 8–11.
18. Drago, F., Ciccarese, G., Rebora, A., Broccolo, F., & Parodi, A. (2016). Pityriasis rosea: A comprehensive classification. *Dermatology (Basel, Switzerland)*, 232, 431–437.
19. Urbina, F., Das, A., & Sudy, E. (2017). Clinical variants of pityriasis rosea. *World Journal of Clinical Cases*, 5(6), 203–210.
20. Chuh, A., Zawar, V., Sciallis, G., & Kempf, W. (2016). A position statement on the management of patients with pityriasis rosea. *Journal of the European Academy of Dermatology and Venereology*, 30(10), 1670–1681.
21. Weston, G., & Payette, M. (2015). Update on lichen planus and its clinical variants. *International Journal of Women's Dermatology*, 1(3), 140–149.
22. Weller, R., Hunter, H., & Mann, M. (2015). *Clinical dermatology* (5th ed.). Hoboken: Wiley-Blackwell.
23. Alrashdan, M. S., Cirillo, N., & McCullough, M. (2016). Oral lichen planus: A literature review and update. *Archives of Dermatological Research*, 308, 539–551.
24. Lewis, F. M., & Bogliattol, F. (2013). Erosive vulvar lichen planus—a diagnosis not to be missed: A clinical review. *European Journal of Obestetrics & Gynecology and Reproductive Biology*, 171, 214–219.
25. Atzmony, L., Reiter, O., Hodak, E., Gdalevich, M., & Mimouni, D. (2016). Treatments for cutaneous lichen planus: A systematic review and meta-analysis. *American Journal of Clinical Dermatology*, 17, 11–22.

PIGMENTATION CHANGES

Duellyn Pandis

Pigmentation changes occur in all individuals. Many are caused by regeneration of skin after injury or trauma. This chapter covers information about two commonly occurring pigmentation disorders, vitiligo (a disease of hypopigmentation) and melasma (a disease of hyperpigmentation).

VITILIGO

 Immediate referral is indicated to rule out malignant melanoma for patients with skin macules with an irregular border and localized increased pigmentation or thickened skin in the macule.

DEFINITION AND EPIDEMIOLOGY

Vitiligo is a skin disorder characterized by either a lifelong or a rapid disappearance of pigment-producing melanocytes in the epidermis and hair follicle. Lack of melanin leads to the appearance of progressive, symmetrically patterned, milky-white macules that merge to form larger depigmented areas. The macules give a variegated appearance to the skin that is similar to the white patches on a Holstein calf, hence the origin of the word from the Greek *vitellius*, which means "calf." The disease is psychologically troublesome, affecting the patient's self-esteem and interpersonal relationships. Although the disease shows no increased prevalence among dark-skinned racial groups, the variegated appearance of the skin proves to be especially traumatic for dark-pigmented patients. The appearance of vitiligo resembles leprosy, but the lesions of vitiligo do not have the anesthetic property of leprosy. However, the similarity in appearance to leprosy presents a social stigma for those patients with vitiligo living in leprosy-affected areas of the world.[1,2] The disease manifests in two forms: type A, generalized, nondermatomal or nonsegmental distribution; and type B, a segmental or dermatomal distribution (zosteriform), characterized by rapid spread that does not cross the midline. See Figs. 50.1 and 50.2 for examples of type A and type B.[1–3]

Vitiligo is seen in 1% to 2% of the general population without regard to race, ethnic origin, or gender.[2,4] Although some patients have no vitiligo in their family history, the condition has an inherited tendency; in 30% of cases, a family history of vitiligo in parents, offspring, or siblings is reported.[2] Familial cases of vitiligo have been associated with autoimmune endocrine disorders, and a possible pathogenic connection between vitiligo and oxidative stress damage (inability of the body to remove free radicals, resulting in damage to cellular DNA, lipids, and proteins) exists.[2,4] Patients with a family history of thyroid disease, pernicious anemia, systemic lupus erythematosus, inflammatory bowel disease, and vitiligo are at risk for development of vitiligo.[2] Disease onset occurs between 10 and 30 years of age; 50% of the cases occur before the age of 20 years, and fewer cases are reported in infancy and old age.[1,2,4,5]

PATHOPHYSIOLOGY

Except for the absence of melanocytes, skin function is normal. There is a progressive destruction of pigment-producing cells at

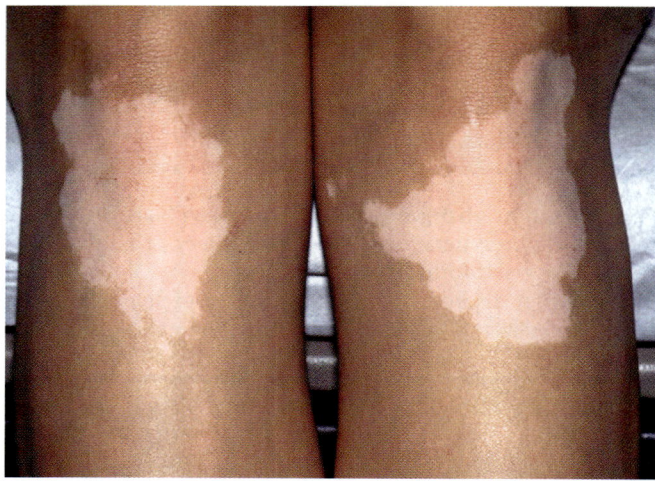

FIG. **50.1** Type A vitiligo. Sharp demarcation on the knees. (From Ferri, F. F. [2019]. *Ferri's fast facts in dermatology: A practical guide to skin disease and disorders* [2nd ed.]. Philadelphia: Saunders.)

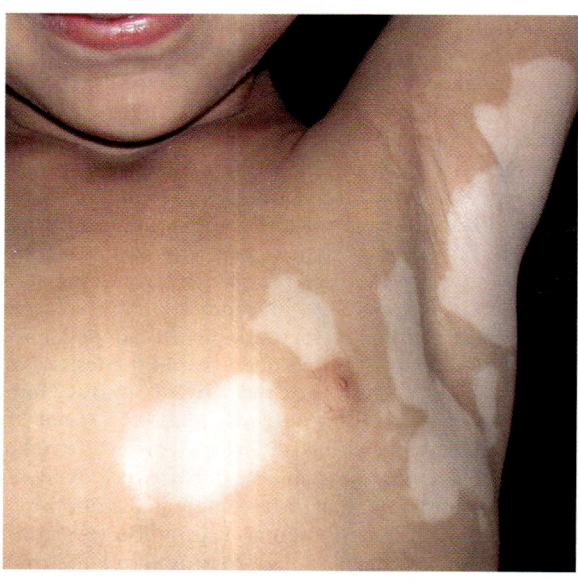

FIG. **50.2** Type B vitiligo. Segmental on chest wall and arm. (From Ferri, F. F. [2019]. *Ferri's fast facts in dermatology: A practical guide to skin disease and disorders* [2nd ed.]. Philadelphia: Elsevier.)

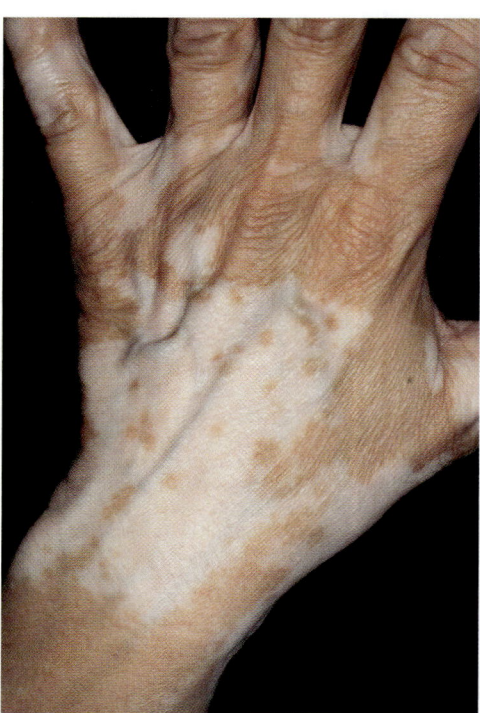

FIG. **50.3** Vitiligo. The back of the hand. (From Habif, T. P. [2016]. *Clinical dermatology: A color guide to diagnosis and therapy* [6th ed.]. Edinburgh: Elsevier.)

the border of the dermis and epidermis. While the exact cause of vitiligo is not known, multiple pathogenic theories exist and are under investigation, including autoimmune involvement, viral causes, decreased melanocyte survival, genetic defects in the structure of melanocytes, and neurochemical destruction of melanocytes.[2,4]

Several theories exist to explain the phenomenon of vitiligo. The autoimmune theory proposes that there is a destruction of the cutaneous melanocytes with loss of the melanin-producing pigment. Histologic examination indicates that lymphocytes build up within the dermis and are involved in the destruction of the melanocytes. The nonsegmental (nondermatomal) variety of vitiligo is associated with a small risk of autoimmune-related disorders, such as type 1 diabetes mellitus and thyroid disease.[1,3] Coexisting diseases such as alopecia

areata, autoimmune thyroid disorders, Addison disease, atrophic gastritis, pernicious anemia, and type 1 diabetes underscore the relationship of dermatomal vitiligo to autoimmunity. In patients with dermatomal vitiligo, serum autoimmune antibodies against melanocytes, thyroid and adrenal tissue, islet cells, gastric parietal cells, and intrinsic factors have been demonstrated.[5]

A second explanation, the neurogenic theory, supposes that a toxic substance is released by the peripheral nerve endings and interferes with the production of melanin. A third theory suggests a defect in the natural protective mechanism of melanin synthesis by melanocytes. Toxic substances accumulate during normal melanin production and later precipitate the destruction of the melanocytes.[5,6] The variation in presentation and progression of the two types of vitiligo (nonsegmental and dermatomal) indicates that the underlying pathologic condition for the two forms of disease may be distinctly different.

CLINICAL PRESENTATION AND PHYSICAL EXAMINATION

Vitiligo is characterized by a progressive and invasive hypopigmentation of the skin that is found on sun-exposed areas and extensor surfaces of the upper body. Most patients have no other clinical findings.[1,4] In general, vitiligo may follow stress; an injury to the skin, such as a burn, bruise, or contusion (Koebner phenomenon); and sunburn.[7] Chemicals, including phenols and catechols, may cause depigmentation of the skin; therefore any history of a patient with vitiligo should include questions about chemical exposure. In fair-skinned individuals, the disease may go undetected until summer, when the sun-exposed areas tan and the melanin-free areas appear a contrasting chalky white.[5] Fig. 50.3 shows several examples of

Common Locations for Hypopigmented Vitiligo Lesions

Bony surfaces: back of hands and fingers, elbows and knees
Body orifices: around the eyes, mouth, and nose
Body folds: armpits and groin
Other areas: legs, wrists, nipples, and genitals
Hair: area within the affected path turning white

vitiligo. Box 50.1 indicates the usual locations of the hypopigmented lesions of vitiligo.

Vitiligo can best be described as a white, flat macule within the epidermis that varies in size from 5 mm to 5 cm ($\frac{1}{5}$ to $1\frac{1}{5}$ inches) with a convex outer edge. Vitiligo manifesting with well-defined areas of white hair is referred to as poliosis.[8] Vitiligo should not be confused with postinflammatory hypopigmentation, in which the skin has a faded pigment appearance rather than an absence of pigment. In the common, nonsegmental or nondermatomal variety, the lesion is initially seen in a symmetrical distribution on the body parts. The segmental or dermatomal variety occurs in a band-type distribution on one side of the body. In children, the depigmentation follows a dermatomal distribution that progresses more rapidly. The border of areas in segmental or dermatomal vitiligo is not sharply demarcated but instead exhibits a tricolored, uneven appearance.[5]

Macules may eventually merge to cover the entire body in a condition termed vitiligo universalis. Variations of the disease presentation include markers of active, progressive disease. These include inflammatory lesions, confetti-type presentation, and Koebner phenomenon. Erythema, scale, and pruritus are seen with inflammatory vitiligo. Although inflammatory vitiligo has a short duration, it can cause rapid skin depigmentation. Rapidly progressive vitiligo is associated with confetti-like depigmentation.[5,6] Since melanocytes are located in the eyes, ocular changes, such as uveitis and pigmentary changes in the fundus, can occur; other findings may include healed chorioretinitis and iritis.[2]

DIAGNOSTICS
Essential Diagnostics

The clinical presentation and physical examination are generally sufficient for a diagnosis to be made. In lighter-skinned individuals and when the hypopigmentation is in underarm and genital regions, Wood light examination is necessary for diagnosis. The Wood light will illuminate depigmented areas as chalky white. In vitiligo, skin scraping and potassium hydroxide (KOH) examination fails to demonstrate the hyphae or spores that are found in tinea versicolor (Chapter 47), another common depigmenting lesion. Although it is not usually necessary, a skin biopsy will show an absence of melanocytes and melanin in the epidermis.

Additional Diagnostics

Vitiligo patients show an increased frequency of autoimmune disorders, such as thyroid disease, type 1 diabetes, and pernicious anemia.[1,2] The patient should be assessed for signs and symptoms of thyroid disease; screening for thyroid-stimulating hormone (TSH) and thyroxine (T_4) is recommended. However,

the treatment of thyroid disease has no impact on the progression of vitiligo because vitiligo does not occur as a result of an increase or reduction of thyroid hormone but instead exists as one of several components of autoimmune polyendocrine syndromes.[2,3] A fasting blood glucose is included in the initial diagnostic evaluation. A complete blood count (CBC) with indexes is performed to detect the presence of macrocytosis, followed by an evaluation for vitamin B_{12} deficiency if indicated.[1]

INITIAL DIAGNOSTICS

Vitiligo

LABORATORY
- Wood lamp examination
- Potassium hydroxide preparation

ADDITIONAL DIAGNOSTICS
- Thyroid-stimulating hormone and thyroxine
- Fasting blood glucose
- Complete blood count and differential
- Vitamin B_{12}
  Skin biopsy[a]

[a]If indicated.

DIFFERENTIAL DIAGNOSIS

 Priority differentials include (1) tinea versicolor, (2) piebaldism, (3) post-inflammatory hypopigmentation, and (4) pityriasis alba.

Additional considerations include albinism, tuberous sclerosis, leprosy, lichen sclerosus, nevus anemicus, psoriasis, chemical leukoderma, eczema, halo nevus, idiopathic guttate hypomelanosis, Leukoderma associated with melanoma and Vogt-Koyanagi syndrome, vitiligo, uveitis, and deafness.

Early or atypical lesions often require the exclusion of other hypopigmented conditions, including albinism, piebaldism, tuberous sclerosis, nevus anemicus, tinea, pityriasis alba, chemical skin exposure, and lichen sclerosus. Some of these disorders are associated with patchy depigmentation with inflammation and scaling or atrophy induration. A biopsy may be indicated to differentiate the underlying cause of depigmentation associated with these disorders.[1,2,5]

INTERPROFESSIONAL COLLABORATIVE MANAGEMENT
Pharmacologic Management

Prescribed Topical Treatments. Recent lesions and those of the facial and neck areas are the most responsive to topical steroid treatment.[4] Patients must be monitored every 2 months for evidence of skin atrophy. Positive response to treatment is indicated by the development of follicular pigmented spots that widen with time and persist. Remember that areas with minimum hair follicles are slower to repigment. Options for treatment include high-potency topical corticosteroids (betamethasone 0.1% or fluocinonide 0.05% ointment) and topical calcineurin inhibitors; tacrolimus (Protopic) and pimecrolimus (Elidel) are the usual choices.[4,5] Steroid treatment failure is seen in nearly 20% of cases; failure is likely if no response is seen by the end of 2 months.[2,5] Adhere to the rule of fingertip units when prescribing topical steroids and monitoring patients. One fingertip unit weighs 0.5 g and is the amount expressed from a tube applied to the fingertip. One half of a fingertip unit will cover the dorsum of the hand, and 2.5 fingertip units will cover the face. For lesions affecting the face, a 30-g tube should last for 10 days.[9] Oral corticosteroids have shown promise in patients with more aggressive forms of the disease; referral to a dermatologist is recommended.

Another technique is chemical depigmentation to produce an artificially induced vitiligo universalis if more than 50% to 80% of the body is affected. Studies indicate that depigmentation treatments using a combination therapy of topical mequinol, a Q-switched ruby laser, and cryotherapy show promising results.[6] Monobenzone hydroquinone (MEH) 20% cream applied twice daily produces an irreversible depigmentation that takes up to 2 to 3 months to begin and up to 9 to 18 months for a complete response. The depigmentation with MEH leads to the chalk-white coloration of the skin like that of vitiligo macules.[10] Depigmentation therapy should be initiated by a dermatologist skilled with this technique. The primary care provider may monitor the results of this therapy in conjunction with the dermatologist. Patients are generally pleased with the outcome of this treatment.

Some patients desire no treatment aside from cosmetic cover products and prefer to allow the disease to progress until all body parts are depigmented. However, it is difficult to judge how long this will take, which limits the usefulness of this approach in the treatment regimen. They may choose to use a fading cream such as monobenzone (Benoquin cream).[1,3,5]

Importance of Sun Protection and Cosmetic Coverup Preparations. Care of the patient with vitiligo involves the use of sunscreens (sun protection factor [SPF] 15 to 30) to protect the depigmented skin from burning and reduce the tanning of melanin-producing areas of the adjacent skin. Extensive sunburn can produce a response similar to Koebner phenomenon (trauma to the skin) and stimulate the depigmentation process to extend farther.

Cosmetic cover-ups assist the patient in managing the psychological aspects of the disease and improve body image and coping mechanisms. A variety of cosmetic substances are commercially available, marketed under the names Covermark (Lydia O'Leary), Dermablend (Flori Roberts), Dermage, C-ESTA Make-Up for Vitiligo, and Elizabeth Arden Concealing Cream. These products can be customized to match individual skin tones and are used by both sexes. Although these products do not come off in water, they do rub off and therefore may not be sustained for long periods of wear. Tanning creams containing dihydroxyacetone may be applied to induce the tanning of affected areas; these substances can be used for eyelids.

Photo Light Therapy. Phototherapy may include psoralen plus UVA, narrow-band UVB, an excimer or exciplex laser. Therapy is directed toward either repigmentation therapy of the affected areas or depigmentation therapy of the unaffected areas. Repigmentation involving the use of high- to mid-potency class 3 and class 4 steroid creams applied twice a day to the affected areas is usually the first approach for patients with depigmentation involving less than 10% of the body and not involving the face. Another treatment approach with proven efficacy for patients with lesser involvement or more generalized vitiligo is treatment with narrow-band ultraviolet B (UVB) light; this approach, which involves the use of psoralens, has been found to be just as effective as psoralens plus ultraviolet A (PUVA) light.[11] If treatment failure should occur, the patient

should be referred to the specialist for further evaluation and for treatment with a combination treatment which can consist of psoralens (P) and then exposing the skin to UVA (long wave ultraviolet radiation) (PUVA). PUVA treatments should be performed only by a qualified specialist. Close monitoring of the patient for response to treatment is necessary. Prevention of eye exposure to UV light must be strictly enforced by making sure that the patient wears glasses that filter all UV light. Up to 2 years of treatment may be necessary before repigmentation occurs.[1]

Surgical. Autologous skin transfer may be used when medical and phototherapy fail. The type of surgical procedures include grafts by suction-blistered epidermis, minigrafts, and transplanting in vitro–cultured epidermis-bearing melanocytes.[1]

Nonpharmacologic Management

The patient may choose not to treat their vitiligo. In these cases, the disease process follows its normal course of depigmentation.

Indications for Referral

After coexistent autoimmune disorders have been excluded, patients with vitiligo are referred to a dermatologist for treatment options. Health care providers can assist with monitoring of therapy, with a dermatology consultation for treatment questions, depigmentation therapy, oral corticosteroid therapy, or phototherapy. The involvement of eye pigment mandates a referral to an ophthalmologist for evaluation. Referral for mental health counseling may be indicated because this disorder can be psychologically stressful. In progressive forms of the disease, the patient should be referred to a specialist for evaluation for depigmentation therapy.

LIFE SPAN CONSIDERATIONS

Vitiligo can be devastating psychologically. It is important to assess for impairment or adjustment issues. Using the Dermatology Life Quality Index (DLQI), a simple 10-item questionnaire, will help to measure how much the disease impacts the life of the patient. Based on these findings referral to counseling may be indicated.

COMPLICATIONS

Treatment with steroids may involve atrophy and striae formation, which increases the risk for easy bruising and infection. Steroid-induced glaucoma and cataracts are complications of steroid application around the eyes. Complications of PUVA treatment include a phototoxic reaction and ocular damage if appropriate UV-protective sunglasses are not used. Consultation with the specialist is necessary if evidence of skin atrophy, adrenal axis suppression, or steroid-induced glaucoma is seen.[2,6]

EMERGING MANAGEMENT TRENDS

Needling as a therapy to induce pigmentation is continuing to be evaluated. A 20-gauge needle is inserted into the pigmented skin and then moved gradually to the depigmented area. Multiple insertions are performed until pinpoint bleeding occurs. After 3 sessions at 2-week intervals, repigmentation in the overall area of depigmentation was seen. This technique may prove promising for those who have failed other treatment modalities.[7]

PATIENT AND FAMILY EDUCATION

- Teach patients and their families about the nature of the pigmentation changes and the lack of scientific knowledge concerning the true cause of the disease.
- Explain that a positive treatment response is repigmentation occurring first in areas with residual melanocytes.
- Vitiligo with late-life onset or long-standing lesions is less likely to respond to treatment.
- Risk factors associated with topical steroids include easy bruising, infection, and decreased vision.
- Educate patients to observe the skin closely for the development of skin lesions suggestive of melanoma.
- Patients should avoid using more steroid cream than directed and should avoid applying steroids around the eyes and moist genital areas, where thin skin enhances systemic absorption.
- Patients should avoid sunlight for 48 hours after each PUVA treatment.
- Support for patients and families can be found at the website for The National Vitiligo Foundation (www.nvfi.org).[1]

Health Promotion

Assessment of the patient's psychological response to vitiligo includes body image adjustment, use of cosmetic coverings, and knowledge concerning the noncontagious nature of vitiligo. Family members should be included in the office visit for support and explanation concerning the benign nature of the disorder and the expected response to treatment. Instruction concerning the use of sunscreens to protect depigmented areas is critical.[1,5]

MELASMA

DEFINITION AND EPIDEMIOLOGY

Melasma or chloasma is a condition of hypermelanosis or brown hyperpigmentation due to increased melanin in the skin. This brown hyperpigmentation is located on the neck and face (Fig. 50.4). The hyperpigmentation occurs over time and can have a psychosocial impact on the patient. Individuals with darker skin tone are the most affected, however it is seen in many men and Caucasians as well.[1] When the condition occurs in pregnancy, melasma or chloasma is known as the mask of pregnancy. Melasma can be a side effect of taking oral contraceptives as well.[3]

PATHOPHYSIOLOGY

The pathology of melasma is uncertain. Contributing factors found to be associated with melasma are increased hormonal activity, increased sun exposure, and darker skin color.[2] Genetic factors, pregnancy, oral contraception use, thyroid dysfunction, and taking phototoxic medications can increase melanin production, causing melasma. Fading of the hyperpigmented areas may not occur after the contributing factors have resolved.[12]

CLINICAL PRESENTATION AND PHYSICAL EXAMINATION

Often the patient will present with concerns of discoloration or darkening on the face or neck. The color may range from light brown to dark brown to ash blue. If the epidermis is involved (epidermal melasma), the coloring of the hyperpigmentation

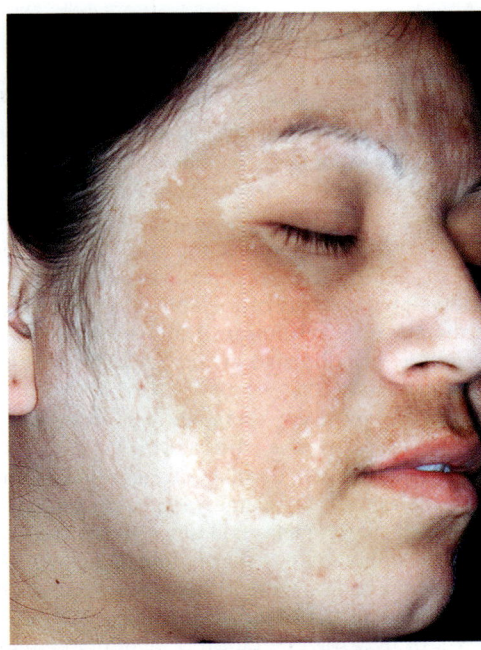

FIG. 50.4 Melasma of the cheek, temple, forehead, and upper lip. (From Habif, T. P. [2016]. *Clinical dermatology: A color guide to diagnosis and therapy* [6th ed.]. Edinburgh: Elsevier.)

will be a browner tone as opposed to the deeper dermal involvement (dermal melisma) which presents as a grey/blue hue. Melasma is classified into one of four types, based on the location of increased melanin: epidermal, dermal, mixed, or indeterminate.[12]

The hyperpigmented areas of melisma are seen classically in one of three patterns of distribution: centrofacial, malar, and mandibular. The centrofacial distribution is the most common, with hyperpigmented areas with irregular borders on a patient's forehead, cheeks, nose, upper lip, and chin. Patients with the malar pattern have hyperpigmented areas on the cheeks and nose; areas along the jawline are affected with the mandibular pattern. Other areas of the body, such as forearm extensor surfaces and mid upper chest can exhibit melasma.[12] In pregnancy, melasma is more pronounced during the second to third trimester; it may fade after delivery but darken again with additional pregnancies.[12]

DIAGNOSTICS
Essential Diagnostics

Most cases of melasma are based on the clinical findings and history of the patient. The patient may be examined with a Wood light to determine the type of melasma. Dermal melasma is not enhanced under the Wood light while epidermal is enhanced.

INITIAL DIAGNOSTICS
Melasma
LABORATORY
• Wood light

DIFFERENTIAL DIAGNOSIS

 Priority differentials include (1) post-inflammatory hyperpigmentation, (2) drug-induced pigmentation, (3) actinic lichen planus, and (4) solar lentigines.

INTERPROFESSIONAL COLLABORATIVE MANAGEMENT

Pharmacologic Management

Topical Therapy. The first line of treatment should begin with sunscreen. Lightening agents are included with the triple combination of hydroquinone 4% daily plus retinoid and corticosteroid (Tri-Luma). Common complaints include erythema, burning, dryness, and pruritus at the site of application. The second line of therapy includes glycolic or salicylic acid peels.[13] This promotes phagocytosis of melanin. It is essential to continue the therapy after resolution. Daily sunscreen, as well as topical retinoids, glycolic acid cream azelaic acid, should be used on a regular basis.[4,5]

Invasive Therapy. New therapies are emerging to treat melasma. The least invasive and newest is micro needling. The objective is to increase dermal collagen; this promotes the reduction of melasma.[14] Cryosurgery is useful in light complexions on localized spots. Fractional lasers are approved for resurfacing to create small areas of thermal damage. Intense pulsed light has moderate to poor results as lesions that are deep may not be penetrated by the laser. As with any type of therapy, there is a risk of hyperpigmentation or hypopigmentation.[1]

LIFE SPAN CONSIDERATIONS

Melasma is associated with hormonal changes as well as exposure to the sun. It is important to remember that as the aging process continues, UV protection is the mainstay of prevention.

COMPLICATIONS

There is a potential worsening of melasma after the use of Q-switched lasers as the epidermal response reacts with an inflammatory process and makes the problem worse or even darker pigmentation. Additionally, the patient could experience scaling, dryness, stinging, or burning as a result of laser therapy.[2,4,5]

PATIENT AND FAMILY EDUCATION

Patients should be aware that melasma is a long-term chronic disease.

- If resolution occurs and maintenance treatment is discontinued, the melasma will most likely return.
- Melasma that occurs during pregnancy typically resolves after delivery.
- Camouflage technique with cosmetic preparations may be an effective method to hide the discoloration. Mineral makeup is used to blend in the skin tones.[2]
- Patients should avoid sun exposure and tanning beds and understand the importance of sun-protective hats and clothing.[12]

HEALTH PROMOTION

The greatest prevention method is protection from the sun by using sunblock and a hat that provides full coverage of the face and neck. Sunblock should include titanium dioxide, as well as zinc oxide of 30% or more, which will prevent UVA and UVB from penetrating the skin.[2]

REFERENCES

1. Habif, T. P. (2016). *Clinical dermatology: A color guide to diagnosis and therapy* (6th ed.). Edinburgh: Elsevier. Chapter 19.
2. Grimes, P. E., Tsao, H. T., & Corona, R. (2018). Vitiligo: Pathogenesis, clinical features and diagnosis. In T. W. Post, P. Rutgeerts, & S. Grover (Eds.). Retrieved from https://www.UptoDate.com. (Accessed February 1, 2018).
3. Habif, T. P., Campbell, J. L., Chapman, M. S., et al. (2017). *Skin disease: Diagnosis and treatment* (4th ed.). St Louis: Elsevier.
4. Plensdorf, S., Livieratos, M., & Dada, N. (2017). Pigmentation disorders: Diagnosis and management. *America Family Physician, 96*(12), 97–804.
5. Ferri, F. F. (2019). Diseases and disorders. In *Ferri's Fast Facts in Dermatology: A practical guide to skin disease and disorders* (2nd ed.). Philadelphia: Elsevier. Chapter 3.
6. Wolff, K., Johnson, R., Saavedra, A. P., & Roh, E. K. (Eds.). (2017). *Fitzpatrick's color atlas and synopsis of clinical dermatology, 8e.* New York, NY: McGraw-Hill. Retrieved from http://accessmedicine.mhmedical.com.ezproxy.hsc.usf.edu/content.aspx?bookid=2043&sectionid=154893879. (Accessed 25 January 2018).
7. Zawar, V. J., & Karad, G. M. (2016). Needling in unresponsive stable vitiligo. *Journal of the American Academy of Dermatology, 75*, e199–e200. http://dx.doi.org/10.1016/j.jaad.2016.05.033.
8. Oakley, A. Poliosis. Retrieved from www.dermnetNZ.org/topics/poliosis. (Accessed 4 May 2019).
9. Henderson, R., & Huins, H. Fingertip Units for topical steroids. Retrieved from https://patient.info/treatment-medication/steroids/fingertip-units-for-topical-steroids. (Accessed 2 May 2019).
10. Rordam, O. M., Lenouvel, E. W., & Maalo, M. (2012). Successful treatment of extensive vitiligo with monobenzone. *The Journal of Clinical and Aesthetic Dermatology, 5*(12), 36–39.
11. Rodriques, M., Ezzedine, K., Hamzavi, I., et al. (2017). New discoveries in the pathogenesis and classification of vitiligo. *Journal of the American Academy of Dermatology, 77*(1), 17–29.
12. Chang, M. W. (2017). Diseases of hyperpigmentation. In J. Bolognia, J. Schaffer, & L. Cerroni (Eds.), *Dermatology 4e.* Philadelphia: Elsievier.
13. Sarkar, R., Arsiwala, S., & Neha, N. (2017). Chemical peels in melasma: A review with consensus recommendations by Indian pigmentary expert group. *Indian Journal of Dermatology, 62*(6), 579–584. doi:10.4103/ijd.IJD_490_17. PMC5724304.
14. Alster, T., & Graham, P. (2017). Microneedling: A review and practical guide. *Dermatologic Surgery Dermatol Surg, 0*, 1–8. doi:10.1097/DSS.0000000000001248.

CHAPTER **51**

WOUND MANAGEMENT

Tracy McClinton

DEFINITION AND EPIDEMIOLOGY

Tissue trauma accounts for significant morbidity and financial concern. Medicare expenditure in treatment of wounds in the US health care system ranges from $28.1 to $96.8 billion, with hospital outpatient services accounting for the highest cost.[1] The incidence and prevalence of acute and chronic wounds vary with populations, geographic and demographic status, and general medical conditions. Acute wounds consist of lacerations, abrasions, avulsions, crush injuries, puncture wounds, insect or mammalian bites, traumatic or surgical wounds, burns, and skin tears. Chronic wounds include pressure ulcers, venous and arterial ulcers, diabetic foot ulcers, and nonhealing surgical or traumatic wounds.

Pressure and Venous Ulcers

An estimated 2.5 million pressure ulcers are treated each year in US acute care facilities alone, and the cost of treating them ranges from $9.1 billion to $11.6 billion per year.[2] Development of a pressure ulcer increases the length of stay for hospitalized patients, and increases the mortality rate significantly.[2,3]

Venous ulcers account for 80% of ulcers found on the lower leg, and up to 60% of those patients have history of a deep vein thrombosis, a risk factor of venous ulcers. Other risk factors include but are not limited to: heredity, inadequate treatment of chronic venous insufficiency, age (peak prevalence between 60 and 80 years), female gender (1.6 female: 1 male), obesity, history of varicose vein surgery, leg injury, phlebitis, venous valve or wall degeneration, arteriovenous shunts, and congenital absence of valves. Pregnancy is also a risk factor, along with prolonged standing.[4] The estimated economic burden of health care costs of individuals with venous leg ulcers is $14.9 billion.[5] This economic burden takes into account hospitalization days, emergency department visits, outpatient/provider office visits, home health care, work-loss days, advanced therapies (such as skin substitutes), and durable medical equipment.[5] The recurrence rates of venous ulcers range from approximately 6% to 27%.[4] With such a significant impact and economic burden on society, education and prevention are key in decreasing the incidence of venous leg ulcers.

Diabetic Foot Ulcers

There are more than 20 million people in the United States with diabetes (see Chapter 186), of whom approximately 15% are at risk for ulceration making them susceptible to amputation and death.[6] Of all nontraumatic lower limb amputations in the United States, 84% are diabetes related.[6] Amputation and foot ulceration are the most common consequences of diabetic neuropathy and major causes of morbidity and disability in people with diabetes. People with diabetes are at higher risk for development of peripheral artery disease, which significantly increases the risk of amputation. The risk of ulcers or amputations also increases in people with diabetes who have poor glycemic control, visual impairment, preulcerative callus or corn, or renal complications.[7] Diabetic patients post-amputation have a mortality rate of 11% to 41% within the first year and a mortality rate of 39% to 68% within 5 years.[6]

Surgical Wounds

Surgical wounds are often treated in the outpatient setting secondary to the rising costs of acute care management and reimbursement concerns. Common complications such as wound dehiscence, blistering of the peri-wound area, or infection can delay healing in surgical wounds.[8] Signs and symptoms of infection include increased pain, purulent exudate, edema, hematoma, seroma, separation of wound edges, prolonged erythema, odor, and fever.[8,9] Dehiscence can occur as a result of many reasons, such as: impaired blood flow, hematoma, and inadequate nutrition.[9] Dehiscence can also be caused by mechanical failure such as inappropriate closure technique, excessive mobility, friction, and sheer.[9] A broad understanding of wound healing physiology and general management principles will assist the provider in facilitating maximum wound repair. Collaboration among the providers, inpatient and outpatient, as well as interdisciplinary teams, is crucial in the healing process of surgical wounds.

CLASSIFICATION OF WOUNDS

Classification of wounds is unique to wound type, and reference to established classification systems is recommended.

Wounds involving only the epidermal layer are classified as superficial or partial thickness. Examples include simple lacerations, skin tears, first-degree burns, abrasions, and shallow ulcerations. These wounds usually heal quickly and require the least intervention. Full-thickness wounds involve the epidermis and dermis, and may extend through subcutaneous tissue into muscle and bone. Examples include deep lacerations, second- and third-degree burns, various types of ulcers, and surgical or traumatic wounds.

A pressure ulcer is a localized injury to the skin or underlying tissue. The National Pressure Ulcer Advisory Panel provides staging definitions for pressure ulcers and suggested in 2016 that the term *pressure ulcer* be replaced with the term *pressure injury*. Pressure ulcer staging includes deep tissue injury, stages I to IV, and unstageable (Box 51.1). Burns are classified as first, second, or third degree (Box 51.2), and require a unique approach that often requires referral to a burn specialist (Box 51.3).

Skin tears are common in frail older adults, often occurring during routine daily activities such as washing and dressing. The shearing and friction forces against frail skin cause the tear, separating the epidermis from the dermis (partial thickness) or the dermis from underlying structures (full thickness).

Arterial and venous ulcers are classified as partial or full thickness; the diabetic foot ulcer is typically graded by one of two classification systems, the Meggitt-Wagner and the University of Texas classifications. The Meggitt-Wagner system uses grades 0 to 5 to assess wound depth (Table 51.1). The University of Texas system uses a matrix of grades and scales to assess the wound's depth and presence of infection or ischemia (Table 51.2).[10]

PATHOPHYSIOLOGY

Wound healing begins at the time of injury and often proceeds over a period of several months through the stages of hemostasis, inflammation, proliferation, and remodeling or maturation. Inflammation, which begins at the time of injury and lasts approximately seven days, is an essential first step in wound healing. The stages of inflammation and hemostasis overlap providing local vasospasm and initiation of the clotting process.[11] During the inflammation stage phagocytic cells such as macrophages and neutrophils are active. Neutrophils, oxygen, and nutrients are transported to the wound site, and proliferation begins. In this phase, epithelial cells migrate over the surface of the wound and collagen synthesis begins. Remodeling occurs during the next several months, reaching a strength approaching 80% of normal.[11,12]

Wound healing is affected by many internal and external factors. Internal factors include advanced age, preexisting comorbidities (e.g., diabetes mellitus, cardiovascular disease, autoimmune disorders, obesity, cancer), anemia, hypoperfusion, oxygenation, nutrition, hydration, and some medications (especially steroids, immunosuppressants, and chemotherapeutic drugs).[13] External factors include pressure, friction, shear, contamination (with bacteria, debris, or necrotic tissue), and wound environment (pH, moisture).[13,14]

Stages of wound healing may be interrupted by changes in the internal and external wound healing factors. Two common examples are the occurrence of anemia during wound healing, which slows the healing response as a result of decreased oxygenation, and pressure exerted over the site, which decreases perfusion and prolongs or delays wound healing.[13,14]

Surgical wounds heal by primary, secondary, or tertiary intention. Primary intention implies that the wound edges are approximated and sutured, stapled, taped, or glued. Secondary intention implies that the wound edges are not approximated, usually because of failed primary intention (dehiscence) or infection. Secondary intention healing is prolonged and results

BOX 51.1

Pressure Ulcer Staging (NPUAP/EPUAP Guidelines)

DEFINITION

A pressure ulcer is localized injury to the skin and/or underlying tissue, usually over a bony prominence, as a result of pressure or pressure in combination with shear and/or friction. A number of contributing or confounding factors are also associated with pressure ulcers; the significance of these factors is yet to be elucidated.

STAGES

Suspected Deep Tissue Injury

Purple or maroon localized area of discolored intact skin or blood-filled blister caused by damage of underlying soft tissue from pressure and/or shear. The area may be preceded by tissue that is painful, firm, mushy, boggy, warmer, or cooler as compared with adjacent tissue.

Further description: Deep tissue injury may be difficult to detect in individuals with dark skin tones. Evolution may include a thin blister over a dark wound bed. The wound may further evolve and become covered by thin eschar. Evolution may be rapid, exposing additional layers of tissue even with optimal treatment.

Stage I

Intact skin with nonblanchable redness of a localized area, usually over a bony prominence. Darkly pigmented skin may not have visible blanching; its color may differ from the surrounding area.

Further description: The area may be painful, firm, soft, warmer, or cooler as compared with adjacent tissue. Stage I wounds may be difficult to detect in individuals with dark skin tones. May indicate "at-risk" persons (a heralding sign of risk).

Stage II

Partial-thickness loss of dermis manifesting as a shallow open ulcer with a red or pink wound bed, without slough. May also manifest as an intact or open or ruptured serum-filled blister.

Further description: Shiny or dry shallow ulcer without slough or bruising.[a] This stage should not be used to describe skin tears, tape burns, perineal dermatitis, maceration, or excoriation.

Stage III

Full-thickness tissue loss. Subcutaneous fat may be visible, but bone, tendon, or muscle is not exposed. Slough may be present but does not obscure the depth of tissue loss. May include undermining and tunneling.

Further description: The depth of a stage III pressure ulcer varies by anatomic location. The bridge of the nose, ear, occiput, and malleolus do not have subcutaneous tissue, and stage III ulcers can be shallow. In contrast, areas of significant adiposity can develop extremely deep stage III pressure ulcers. Bone or tendon is not visible or directly palpable.

Stage IV

Full-thickness tissue loss with exposed bone, tendon, or muscle. Slough or eschar may be present on some parts of the wound bed. Often includes undermining and tunneling.

Further description: The depth of a stage IV pressure ulcer varies by anatomic location. The bridge of the nose, ear, occiput, and malleolus do not have subcutaneous tissue, and these ulcers can be shallow. Stage IV ulcers can extend into muscle and/or supporting structures (e.g., fascia, tendon, or joint capsule), making osteomyelitis possible. Exposed bone or tendon is visible or directly palpable.

Unstageable

Full-thickness tissue loss in which the base of the ulcer is covered by slough (yellow, tan, gray, green, or brown) and/or eschar (tan, brown, or black) in the wound bed.

Further description: Until enough slough and/or eschar is removed to expose the base of the wound, the true depth, and therefore stage, cannot be determined. Stable (dry, adherent, intact without erythema or fluctuance) eschar on the heels serves as "the body's natural (biologic) cover" and should not be removed.

Suspected Deep Tissue Injury—Depth Unknown

Purple or maroon localized area of discolored intact skin or blood-filled blister due to damage of underlying soft tissue from pressure and/or shear.

Further description: The area may be preceded by tissue that is painful, firm, mushy, boggy, warmer, or cooler as compared to adjacent tissue. Deep tissue injury may be difficult to detect in individuals with dark skin tones. Evolution may include a thin blister over a dark wound bed. The wound may further evolve and become covered by thin eschar. Evolution may be rapid exposing additional layers of tissue even with optimal treatment.

[a]Bruising indicates suspected deep tissue injury.
From National Pressure Ulcer Advisory Panel (NPUAP), European Pressure Ulcer Advisory Panel (EPUAP), and Pan Pacific Pressure Injury Alliance (PPPIA). *Prevention and treatment of pressure ulcers: quick reference guide.* Osborne Park, Western Australia.

in significant scarring. Delayed primary intention, or tertiary intention, refers to wounds that were not initially closed (usually because of infection, contamination, or wound stress) and are closed after some secondary intention healing has occurred.

CLINICAL PRESENTATION

Any break in skin integrity in the immunocompromised or diabetic patient warrants timely and complete evaluation. Early evaluation and intervention in this population of patients may prevent complications of healing, including infection.

Acute wounds are most often caused by accidental injury and include lacerations, abrasions, burns, bites, and puncture wounds. Patients with comorbidities, especially diabetes

mellitus and peripheral vascular disease, may be seen with lower extremity ulcers related to neuropathy and poor perfusion. Patients with decreased functioning resulting from brain injury, neurologic disease, or spinal cord injury often see their providers with complaints of pressure ulcers. Prevention, early identification, and appropriate management are of primary importance to avoid costly and irreversible tissue damage, especially in the medically compromised patient.

The patient's medication history is important to evaluate and guides management decisions. Immunosuppressive drugs, including chemotherapeutics and steroids, adversely affect wound healing by interrupting the inflammatory process, an important first step in mounting a healing response. Critical factors to be elicited include the patient's age, allergies,

BOX **51.2**

Burn Classification

FIRST-DEGREE (SUPERFICIAL OR EPIDERMAL) BURNS

These burns involve only the epidermis. They do not blister, but are red and quite painful. Over 2–3 days the erythema and the pain subside. By about day four, the injured epithelium peels away from the newly healed epidermis underneath, a process that is commonly seen after sunburn.

SECOND-DEGREE (PARTIAL-THICKNESS) BURNS

Partial-thickness burns involve the epidermis and portions of the dermis and can be clinically categorized as either *superficial* partial-thickness or *deep* partial-thickness burns. Superficial partial-thickness burns characteristically form blisters between the epidermis and dermis. Because blistering may not occur for some hours after injury, burns that initially appear to be only epidermal in depth (first degree) may be determined to be partial-thickness burns 12–24 h later. Most superficial partial-thickness burns heal spontaneously in less than three weeks, and do so typically without functional impairment or hypertrophic scarring. Second-degree burns often accumulate a layer of fibrinous exudate and necrotic debris on the surface, which may predispose the wound to heavy bacterial colonization and delayed wound healing, in addition to making more difficult the determination of wound depth by visual inspection.

Deep partial-thickness burns extend into the lower layers of the dermis. They possess characteristics that are distinctly different from superficial or mid-dermal partial-thickness burns. If infection is prevented and spontaneous healing is allowed to progress, these burns will heal in three to nine weeks. However, they invariably cause considerable scar formation. Even with active physical therapy throughout the healing process, hypertrophic scarring is common and joint function is usually impaired. These burns are best treated by excision and grafting. For the patient, a partial-thickness burn that fails to heal within 3 weeks is functionally and cosmetically equivalent to a full-thickness injury.

THIRD-DEGREE (FULL-THICKNESS) BURNS

Full-thickness burns involve all layers of the dermis and often injure underlying subcutaneous adipose tissue as well. Burn eschar is structurally intact but dead and denatured dermis. Over days and weeks, if left in situ, eschar separates from the underlying viable tissue, leaving an open, unhealed bed of granulation tissue. Without surgery, these burns can heal only by wound contracture with epithelialization from the wound margins. Some full-thickness burns involve not only all layers of the skin, but also deeper structures such as muscle, tendon, ligament, and bone, and are classified as deep full-thickness or fourth-degree burns. Grafting may use autologous skin grafts or biologic dressings and skin substitutes or both. (Excision and grafting using biologic dressings or skin substitutes permits closure of extensive burns in stages, with autografting done at a later date; see detailed discussion elsewhere in this chapter.) Deep full-thickness burns may require amputation or closure with alternative techniques (such as adjacent tissue transfer or microvascular procedures).

From Kagan, R. J., Peck, M. D., Ahrenholz, D. H., Hickerson, W. L., Holmes, J., 4th, Korentager, R., et al. (2013). Surgical management of the burn wound and use of skin substitutes: An expert panel white paper. *Journal of Burn Care and Research, 34*(2), e60–e79.

BOX **51.3**

Burn Center Referral Criteria

A burn center may treat adults, children, or both. Burn injuries that should be referred to a burn center include the following:
1. Partial-thickness burns of greater than 10% of the total body surface area.
2. Burns that involve the face, hands, feet, genitalia, perineum, or major joints.
3. Third-degree burns in any age group.
4. Electrical burns, including lightning injury.
5. Chemical burns.
6. Inhalation injury.
7. Burn injury in patients with preexisting medical disorders that could complicate management, prolong recovery, or affect mortality.
8. Any patients with burns and concomitant trauma (such as fractures) in which the burn injury poses the greatest risk of morbidity or mortality. In such cases, if the trauma poses the greater immediate risk, the patient's condition may be stabilized initially in a trauma center before transfer to a burn center. Physician judgment will be necessary in such situations and should be in concert with the regional medical control plan and triage protocols.
9. Burned children in hospitals without qualified personnel or equipment for the care of children.
10. Burn injury in patients who will require special social, emotional, or rehabilitative intervention.

From Bolenbaucher, R., Cotner-Pouncy, T., Edwards, C., Jackson, B., McNabb, W., Mann-Salinas, C. E. A., et al. (2016) *Burn clinical practice guideline*. Texas EMS Trauma & Acute Care Foundation Trauma Division. Retrieved from http://tetaf.org/wp-content/uploads/2016/01/Burn-Practice-Guideline.pdf. (Accessed 14 July 2018).

TABLE **51.1** **Meggitt-Wagner Classification System**

Grade	Lesion
0	Healed or preulcerative wound
1	Superficial ulcer without penetrating to deeper layers
2	Deep ulcer reaches to tendon, bone, or joint capsule
3	Deep tissues are involved and there is abscess formation, osteomyelitis, or tendinitis
4	Limited gangrene (part of the foot)
5	Extensive gangrene (entire foot)

From Santema, T. B., Lenselink, E. A., Balm, R., & Ubbink, D. T. (2016). Comparing the Meggitt-Wagner and the University of Texas wound classification systems for diabetic foot ulcers: Inter-observer analyses. *International Wound Journal, 13*(6), 1137–1141. Doi:10.1111/iwj.12429.

TABLE 51.2	Diabetic Foot Ulcer Grades (University of Texas Classification System)			
		Wound Depth		
	0	**1**	**2**	**3**
Presence of infection or ischemia	A	Preulcerative or postulcerative lesion completely epithelialized	Superficial; not involving tendon, joint capsule, or bone	Penetrating to tendon or joint capsule	Penetrating to bone or joint capsule
	B	With infection	With infection	With infection	With infection
	C	With ischemia	With ischemia	With ischemia	With ischemia
	D	With infection and ischemia	With infection and ischemia	With infection and ischemia	With infection and ischemia

Modified from Santema, T. B., Lenselink, E. A., Balm, R., & Ubbink, D. T. (2016). Comparing the Meggitt-Wagner and the University of Texas wound classification systems for diabetic foot ulcers: Inter-observer analyses. *International Wound Journal, 13*(6), 1137–1141. Doi:10.1111/iwj.12429.

occupation, nutritional status, drug or alcohol use, smoking history, and immune status, including the last tetanus booster. Moreover, the health care provider must identify conditions that adversely affect wound healing, including diabetes mellitus, autoimmune disorders, malnutrition, positive smoking history, chronic respiratory disease, and peripheral vascular disease; these affect management plans.[13,14]

PHYSICAL EXAMINATION

Assessment of the wound must follow a thorough history. The nature and age of the wound along with the patient's medical history determine management strategies. Wound location, type, depth, previous treatments, and surrounding tissue assessment guide treatment decisions.

In addition to a thorough wound evaluation (including observation for tunneling, the presence and odor of exudate, and the appearance of all tissue in and around the wound bed), a focused physical examination is important. In lower extremity wounds, perfusion is determined by pulse assessment and noninvasive diagnostic testing, such as baseline ankle-brachial indices (ABIs), if necessary. It is essential to determine the absence or presence of peripheral perfusion and associated changes of edema, tissue color and warmth, and neurovascular status.[11]

Wounds that are healing or have the potential to heal will demonstrate pink or red tissue and the absence of excessive exudate, infection, and debris. The size of the wound, measured weekly, should slowly decrease. Healing wounds are pink to red, robust, and bumpy (granulation tissue), with pink healing edges that demonstrate migration by contact with the wound bed. Tissue is not healing if it is pale or smooth, and it may have raised hard edges.

DIAGNOSTICS

X-ray studies may be necessary in acute injuries to identify bone involvement. They are also helpful in evaluating infection, foreign bodies, and deformity in the diabetic foot, although they may lag behind the clinical presentation of osteomyelitis by as long as 2 weeks.[11] Separation, fracture, or dislocation usually requires referral to a specialist. Compound fractures, especially in hand injuries, require diligent management and antibiotic administration.

Noninvasive vascular studies such as ABI or transcutaneous partial oxygen pressure are useful to determine arterial flow in patients with lower extremity ulceration.[15] Magnetic resonance imaging (MRI) is the most specific and sensitive noninvasive test for evaluation of osteomyelitis. A positive bone-to-probe test, in the presence or absence of symptoms of infection, is

a high predictor of osteomyelitis.[11] Technetium bone scintigraphy may also be abnormal in osteomyelitis.[6] The complete blood count (CBC) is useful in detecting anemia, which can slow wound healing progression by decreasing perfusion and oxygenation. A slightly elevated WBC count may indicate the inflammatory response, whereas a WBC count that continues to rise may indicate an infection. Immunosuppressive disorders delay wound healing and may be first detected on CBC. A total lymphocyte count of less than 1500 cells/mm^3 coupled with an albumin level of less than 3.5 g/dL is indicative of malnutrition, which delays wound healing.[16] Patients with diabetes who have elevated hemoglobin A$_{1c}$ levels are at increased risk of failed wound healing as a result of hyperglycemia.[15]

INITIAL DIAGNOSTICS

Wound Management

LABORATORY
- Complete blood count and differential[a]
- Hemoglobin A$_{1c}$[a]
- Albumin level[a]
- Wound culture[a]

IMAGING
- X-ray examination[a]
- Bone scan[a]

- Magnetic resonance imaging[a]
- Noninvasive vascular studies[a]

ADDITIONAL DIAGNOSTICS
- Biopsy[a]

[a]If indicated.

DIFFERENTIAL DIAGNOSIS

The nature of the injury and the location of the wound determine diagnosis as well as treatment. Diagnosis and treatment of chronic wounds are determined by history of the patient, presence of medical conditions, and location and appearance of the wound.

Ulcers: Venous and Arterial

Ulcers are chronic wounds that can be caused by several different underlying medical conditions. The diagnosis of the underlying cause is essential because treatment of this condition affects ulcer recurrence rates. Most pressure ulcers occur over bony prominences, including the sacrum, greater trochanter, ischial tuberosity, heel, and lateral malleolus.

Venous ulcers are typically located on the medial lower leg, above the medial malleolus. The wound is often large with irregular wound edges; the wound bed usually has granulation tissue or fibrinous material over the surface, with moderate to heavy exudate and minimal pain. Associated skin changes include a hemosiderin pigmentation, edema, and lipodermatosclerosis.

Arterial ulcers occur most often on the lower extremity distal to the area of impaired perfusion. They are painful and dry, have well-demarcated edges, and can be very deep with exposed support structures. The limb is traditionally thin, cool, pale or hyperemic, hairless, and shiny as a result of decreased perfusion. Diabetic foot ulcers appear most commonly on the plantar surface of the foot, often over the head of the metatarsal joint bearing the greatest pressure. They are often painless secondary to neuropathy. The borders are often punched out with surrounding callus; the ulcer base varies on the basis of arterial perfusion. With good perfusion, they have red granulation; poorly perfused ulcers are often drier, with flattened pale granulation or black eschar, warranting further vascular evaluation.

Thermal Wounds

Thermal wounds are the most common type of burn (see Chapter 44). Many patients initially are seen in the outpatient setting but may require the attention of a burn specialist. Burn center referral is based on the criteria of the American Burn Association and the American College of Surgeons (see Box 51.3).[17]

MANAGEMENT

 Immediate specialist referral is indicated for hand injuries and for deep lacerations especially if a tendon injury or fracture is suspected.[18]

 Consultation with a plastic surgeon is recommended for patients with facial or hand wounds to minimize scarring and promote a return to normal motor function.[18,19]

 Specialist referral is indicated for deep puncture wounds of the head, hand, chest, abdomen, and foot as well as wounds with continuous bleeding or requiring significant debridement.

General Principles

The use of universal precautions is essential in wound assessment and treatment. Establishing the type and nature of injury guides wound management decisions. Documentation must include the nature of the injury; wound type, location, and size in centimeters (length, width, depth); integrity of supporting structures (bone, wound, vasculature); appearance of the peri-wound; and characteristics of the exudate (Box 51.4). Normal saline 0.9% is the cleansing and irrigating product of choice in most wounds because it is isotonic, readily available, and inexpensive. Gentle surfactants, or dermal wound cleansers, may also be used and often come in a delivery system to provide adequate pressure per square inch needed for irrigation. The use of cytotoxic products, including undiluted povidone-iodine (Betadine) and hydrogen peroxide, previously thought to be beneficial, are not currently recommended.[4] Acetic acid and sodium hypochlorite should be avoided; although they are toxic to bacteria, they are also toxic to healthy tissue.[4]

Regardless of wound type, the principles of moist wound healing guide management. However, chronic wounds require specific intervention based on cause. It is imperative to ensure wound bed moisture, nutrition, perfusion, pH balance,

BOX **51.4**

Documentation of Wounds

Wound
- Location
- Width
- Depth
- Edges
- Exudate

Presence of foreign bodies
Accompanying injuries
- Fractures
- Dislocations
- Tendon or ligament injuries
- Neurologic and cardiovascular findings

Diagnostic findings, radiologic conclusions
Treatments
Follow-up

freedom from infection and debris, and protection. Antibiotic creams and ointments, including silver sulfadiazine (SSD), can be appropriate for short periods in infected wounds and may be accompanied by debridement.[20] Management of comorbid conditions and reduction of risk factors, including careful blood glucose monitoring and control, smoking cessation, correction of malnutrition, and enhancement of perfusion, are important strategies. Ensuring intake of adequate protein and essential vitamins and minerals such as vitamin C, zinc, vitamin D, vitamin B12 (cobalamin), copper, magnesium, and arginine may also enhance wound healing. All water-soluble vitamins and many minerals are necessary cofactors for the metabolic reactions in the body.[21]

Debridement. Debridement of necrotic tissue can be accomplished by surgical, mechanical, autolytic hydrogels and hydrocolloid dressings, biodebridement (larval), or enzymatic methods. Surgical debridement is used to remove hyperkeratotic or necrotic tissue and should cause only minimum healthy tissue trauma and bleeding.[4,11] Mechanical debridement involves the use of hydrotherapy and high-pressure water sprays.[4] Whirlpool treatments are not recommended by some sources because these treatments have a risk for skin burning and maceration in a population of patients in whom there are impaired healing mechanisms (the diabetic and older adult population).[22] Standard wet-to-dry dressings are considered a form of mechanical debridement but should be avoided because of the nonselectivity and potential damage to healthy tissue. Clinicians may find the need to use topical analgesics due to pain that may occur during mechanical debridement. A common topical analgesic is lidocaine/prilocaine, marketed as Eutectic Mixture of Local Anesthetics or EMLA.[4] Autolytic debridement with film, hydrocolloid, or hydrogel dressings allows leukocytes on the ulcer surface to degrade and release lysosomal enzymes that break down protein and mucopolysaccharide components of ulcer eschar; however, dressings that retain moisture are contraindicated in the presence of infection.[4,11] Biodebridement—also called maggot debridement therapy (MDT)—is approved by the FDA and occurs by application of sterilized medicinal maggots topically to the wound. Maggots have a unique capability of digesting bacteria and produce enzymes that break down necrotic tissue. Studies

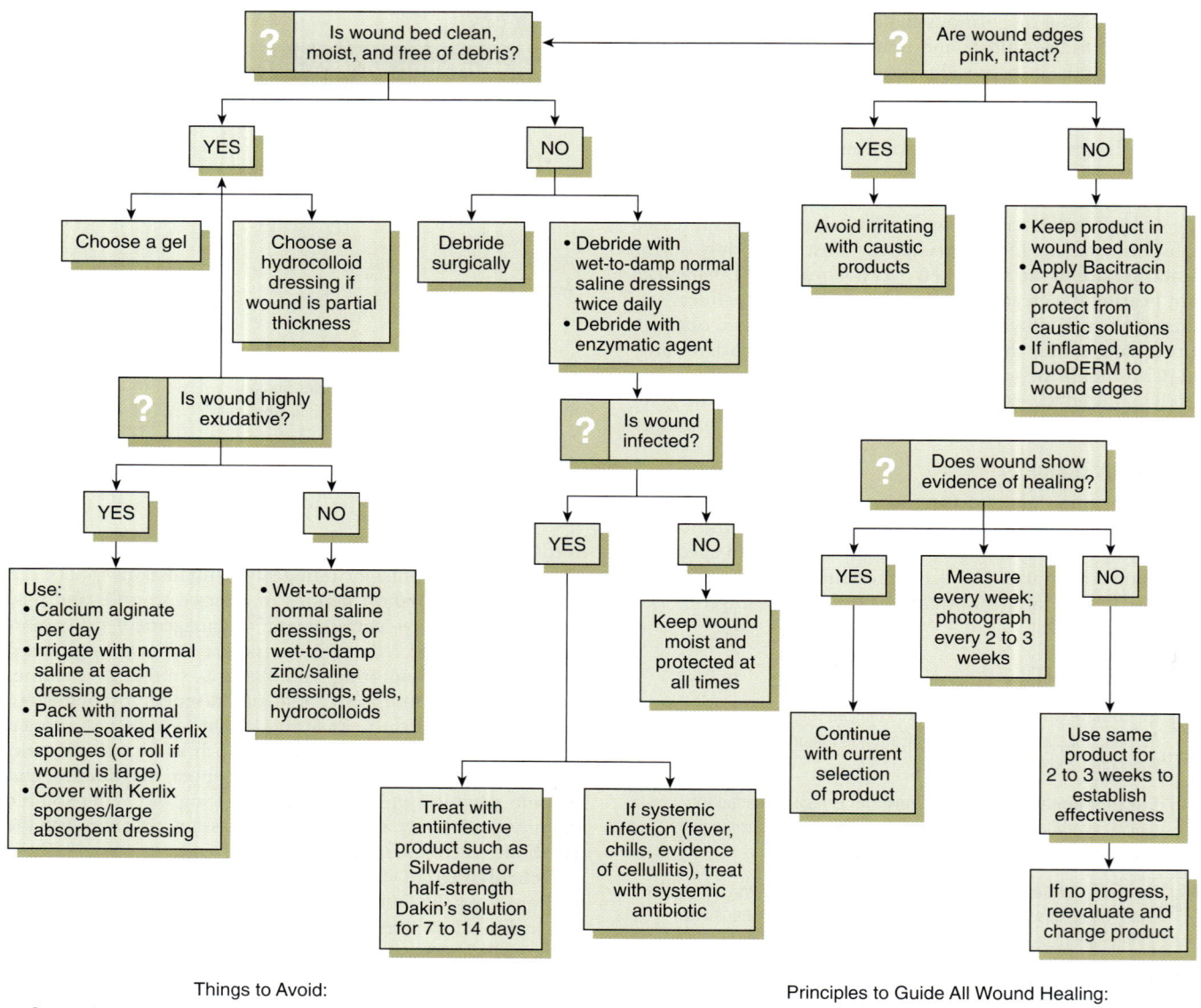

Things to Avoid:

1. Cytotoxic products such as Betadine, full-strength Dakin's solution
2. Any antibiotic product for > 14 to 21 days
3. Changing products frequently (use for 2 to 3 weeks to evaluate effectiveness)
4. Overuse of any single product, if no wound healing progress

Principles to Guide All Wound Healing:

1. Perfusion/freedom from external pressure
2. Freedom from infection
3. Freedom from debris
4. Moist environment, low pH, noncaustic/nonpainful products

F I G . 51.1   Algorithm for wound care product selection.

suggest that MDT may be more effective than standard treatment, decreasing wound healing time. However, studies do not show a decreased risk in infection compared to standard treatment.[23] Enzymatic debridement can be achieved by the use of collagenase, which has been shown to expedite debridement by the degradation of denatured collagen and is more effective than hydrogel.[4,23] Dilute Dakin solution, used at 0.05% to 0.025% concentration, has also been proven to cleanse, irrigate, and debride wounds by the degradation of collagen as well.[24] When used for a debriding agent, it should be applied by moist gauze and used no more than five days to prevent damage to healthy tissue.[25]

Dressings. A dressing is applied after wound exploration, irrigation, cleansing, debridement (when appropriate), and closure (when appropriate). Dressings serve as important components of wound management. Dressings serve various purposes, including protection, drainage absorption, insulation, maintenance of moisture and cleanliness, bacterial barriers, and as soothing components to minimize pain.[4,26] They should be easily removed without traumatizing tissue and are often multilayered. No single dressing may afford all these properties; multiple wound care products are available to choose from.[4,26]

Selection of dressing may be based on various factors, including functionality, availability, cost, and comfort. Topical wound treatment may include alginates, antimicrobial hydrofibers, hydrocolloids, foams, or gels, depending on the level of exudate the wound produces.[4,26] The wound care product selection algorithm (Fig. 51.1) can guide the selection of a dressing based on the appearance of the wound.

TABLE **51.3** Recommendations for Suturing		
Location	**Suggested Suture Size**	**Suggested Suture Removal**
Scalp	3-0 or 4-0	5–7 days
Trunk	3-0 or 4-0	7–10 days
Arms	3-0 or 4-0 3-0 or 4-0	7–10+
Legs	3-0 or 4-0	7–10+
Hands: referral indicated, although simple lacerations may be repaired	3-0 or 4-0	Palms: 7–10 days Extensor surfaces: 10–14 days
Feet (soles): referral indicated for tendon or nerve injury	3-0 or 4-0	7–14 days
Facial (including eyelids, lips, ears): pressure dressing; referral indicated	5-0 or 6-0	3–5 days
Penis, scrotum: referral indicated		
Dog bites: bites more than 6 h old and puncture wounds should not be sutured; consultation suggested for wounds less than 6 h old. Puncture wounds should be probed gently with forceps to check for foreign bodies and use 1% lidocaine to control pain as needed.		
Cat bites: puncture wounds should not be sutured		
Human bites: wounds should not be sutured		

From Jones, T. R. (2017). Wound care. In C. K. Stone & R. L. Humphries (Eds.), *CURRENT diagnosis & treatment: emergency medicine* (8th ed.). New York, NY: McGraw-Hill.

Dressings may be secured with tape, roll gauze, stockinet, binders, or adhesive films. Being mindful of minimizing tissue trauma can guide the choice of dressing security. For example, wounds that are large and highly exudative and require frequent changes should be secured with a nonadhesive bandage when possible. This will decrease skin tearing and trauma from frequent tape removal. Dressing change intervals vary and depend on the patient, wound characteristics, and type of dressing along with specific manufacturer guidelines.[26,27]

Acute Wounds

Lacerations, Abrasions, Avulsions, Crush Injuries, Bites, Puncture Wounds, and Other Traumatic or Surgical Wounds. The primary management goals for all acute wounds are to control major hemorrhage, to protect the patient and the wound, and to promote comfort by providing appropriate pain medication.[28]

It is essential to assess vascular, neurologic, and musculoskeletal (i.e., muscle, tendon, joint) function and potential injury to supportive tissues and structures.[28] After examining the wound, the health care provider must clean and debride it to remove dirt, debris, and foreign bodies.[28]

Contaminated wounds should be irrigated with normal saline solution (0.9%) or tap water. A 19-gauge needle or plastic cannula and a 35-mL syringe held 2 inches from the wound is used for high-pressure irrigation. A low-pressure bulb syringe alone does not create enough pressure for adequate irrigation.[29] Hydrogen peroxide and concentrated povidone-iodine should be avoided because of cytotoxicity to healthy tissue.[30]

Decisions about wound closure depend on the wound type, location, and depth and tension of the wound edges. A wound with smooth edges that is not grossly contaminated (e.g., a laceration from a knife or razor) may be closed by approximation of the wound edges and application of various wound adhesives

or suturing with appropriate material. Staples are an efficient closure medium but are usually used when closure must be quick and the wound is not located in an area where scarring is of concern. Wounds easily closed include small lacerations not over a joint; wounds with clean, even edges approximated without inversion or eversion; and lacerations in areas with no redundant tissue.[31] Suturing guidelines are reviewed in Table 51.3. Abrasions, avulsions, crush injuries, bites, and puncture wounds are not usually closed.

Tissue adhesive, or glue, can be an excellent substitute for stitches or staples to close simple cuts; glue causes less pain, is quicker, and needs no follow-up removal. Glue should not be used for lacerations longer than 4 cm or wounds under tension, such as over joints.[32]

Tissue approximation, when appropriate, and the application of a sterile nonadherent dressing are standard practice. Follow-up care involves observing for signs and symptoms of infection (such as increased pain, erythema, or pus) and applying a dressing to keep the wound moist, clean, and free from physical trauma.[26,33]

Tetanus immunization status should be reviewed for all patients after any type of tissue trauma. Tetanus and diphtheria toxoid and tetanus immune globulin should be administered if immunization status is unknown, if the patient has received fewer than three lifetime doses, or if the booster has not been received in 10 years. All age groups are currently recommended to receive one dose of Tdap booster immunization (tetanus, diphtheria toxoids combined with acellular pertussis vaccine). Once an adult has received one dose of Tdap, immunization with tetanus diphtheria (Td) toxoid is recommended for all patients with tetanus-prone wounds (including all contaminated wounds) if the previous immunization was more than 5 years ago[34] (see Table 51.4 and Box 51.5).

Skin Tears. Skin tears should be gently cleansed with clean water, normal saline, or a gentle, nonionic surfactant, and the

T A B L E **51.4**	**Tetanus Immunization**	
Wound Type	**Unknown Primary Immunization or Fewer than Three Doses**	**Three or More Doses**
Tetanus-prone wounds	Tetanus and diphtheria toxoid (Td) and tetanus immune globulin (TIG)	Td if > 5 years since booster
Non–tetanus-prone wounds	Td	Td if > 10 years since booster

Adult patients should receive 1 dose of Tdap (tetanus and diphtheria toxoids combined with acellular pertussis vaccine) as a replacement for Td (diphtheria and tetanus toxoids).
Doses (for age 7 years or older): TIG, 250 units IM, in separates sites.
From Jones, T. R. (2017). Wound care. In C. K. Stone & R. L. Humphries (Eds.), *CURRENT diagnosis & treatment: emergency medicine* (8th ed.). New York, NY: McGraw-Hill.

BOX **51.5**

Tetanus-Prone Versus Non–Tetanus-Prone Wounds

TETANUS-PRONE WOUNDS
- Wounds or burns that require surgical intervention that is delayed for more than 6 h
- Wounds or burns that show a significant degree of devitalized tissue or a puncture-type injury, including animal bites, particularly where there has been contact with soil or manure
- Wound containing foreign bodies
- Compound fractures
- Wounds or burns in patients who have systemic sepsis

NON–TETANUS-PRONE WOUNDS
- Wounds less than 6 h old
- Wounds with clean margins
- Wounds without devitalized tissue
- Wounds without organic contamination
- Wounds with clearly defined edges

Revised from Collins, S., White, J., Ramsay, M., & Amirthalingam, G. (2015). The importance of tetanus risk assessment during wound management. *IDCases*, *2*(1), 3–5.

---

skin flap should be as closely approximated as possible.[35] The flap should not be removed unless it is necrotic. A viable flap should not be manipulated for a minimum of 5 days. This allows the viable tissue time for adherence.[35]

An appropriate dressing should be selected based on moist wound healing principles. Dressings considered may include hydrogels, silicone foams, alginate, or nonadherent gauze mesh.[35]

Burns (see Chapter 44). Burns are described according to depth (see Box 51.2 for burn classification). Immediate action should be taken to stop the burning process by removal of the patient from the burn source, and the burn should be emergently treated with rapid and copious irrigation with cool, not cold or ice water.[36] If the patient is being transported to a burn center within 24 hours, no wound care is necessary.[36] If less than 10% of the patient's total body surface area (TBSA) is burned, dressings moistened with normal saline may be applied; for more than 10% of the patient's TBSA, covering with a clean, dry sheet is indicated; and more than 20% of the patient's TBSA suffering from burns indicates covering

the patient with a clean dry sheet and keeping the patient warm.[36] Before dressing, burn wounds should be cleansed with normal saline or a gentle surfactant and an appropriate dressing should be applied. Studies have shown that leaving blisters intact promotes faster healing. Therefore minimal debridement is warranted.[37] SSD has been the standard of care for topical treatment of burns.[37] Topical antimicrobials may also be used but will necessitate dressing changes at least twice a day.[37]

Chronic Wounds

Pressure Ulcers. Pressure ulcers are treated by removing pressure and avoiding friction, shear, and moisture.[38]

Pressure can be reduced by the use of specialty mattresses such as gel or foam overlays, alternating air pads, or low–air-loss mattresses. For immobile patients who are bed-bound or wheelchair-bound, the use of pressure-reducing foams and chair cushions are beneficial.[38] Topical treatment is based on wound size, depth, exudate, presence of necrosis, and bacterial contamination.[33]

Ulcers are cleaned after each incontinent episode or bowel movement.[39] Stage I and stage II pressure ulcers with light or no exudate can be managed with a transparent film. Hydrogel can be used on stages II, III, and IV deep wounds and with necrosis or slough. Stage III and stage IV ulcers with heavy exudates can be managed by calcium alginate or biologic products. Foam dressings can be used for a primary dressing or as a secondary dressing for wounds that require packing and stage II or stage IV ulcers with drainage.[33,40]

Venous Ulcers. Treatment of venous ulcers involves reducing edema with leg elevation and graded compression.

Ulcerations should be treated with moist wound healing along with compression therapy.[27]

Compression can be applied as an Unna paste boot or a multilayer compression wrap. Intermittent pneumatic devices can be used for patients who cannot tolerate sustained compression.[27] Some patients may have arterial insufficiency along with venous disease. Measurement of the ankle-brachial pressure index to exclude the presence of peripheral vascular disease before the application of compression is necessary.[11,27]

Arterial Ulcers. Management of arterial ulcers involves improving perfusion. Perfusion can be improved surgically and by the use of pharmacologic agents, lifestyle changes, and adjunctive therapies (such as hyperbaric oxygen therapy and arterial flow augmentation with intermittent pneumatic compression devices). The intervention selected would depend on the severity of the patient's ischemia.[27] Providing warmth to the lower extremities with cotton stockings and protecting from injury with well-fitting shoes can aid in prevention.

Topical therapy depends on the vascular supply. If there is adequate blood supply to support healing or if the patient has been successfully revascularized, debridement and a moist wound healing environment are recommended.[27,33] Arterial ulcers characterized by dry stable eschar should be left intact and treated by painting with Betadine daily to prevent infection.[27,33]

Standard compression therapy such as an Unna boot is inappropriate in the care of arterial ulcers because it dries an already dry wound bed and provides compression in a poorly perfused limb. Modified compression can be used in patients with an ABI less than 0.8, which supports a component of an arterial ulcer, with mandatory exclusion of significant arterial disease.[41]

Diabetic Foot Ulcers. Management of blood glucose concentration is an essential component for foot ulcer prevention and healing.[42,43] Off-loading areas of pressure at risk for ulceration with appropriate shoes can be effective in preventing initial or recurrent ulceration and can aide in healing of current ulcers.[43] Specific ulcer management techniques include debridement to a clean ulcer base, treatment of any infection in the ulcer, and use of modalities to promote wound healing. Once the ulcer is debrided, prevention of infection is imperative to reduce risk of amputation; however, detection of infection is often difficult secondary to neuropathy and decreased inflammatory response. Prolonged hyperglycemia may be the first indication of infection. Systemic antibiotics and assessment for osteomyelitis are essential to prevent amputation.[11,43] There is evidence showing benefit for other treatment modalities, such as bilayered living cell therapy, tissue factors, electrical stimulation, total contact casting, and hyperbaric oxygen therapy.[11,27,43] Once ulcers are healed, patients require close, continuous monitoring to minimize recurrences. Pressure-relieving modalities, including therapeutic footwear, should be used.[43]

Nonhealing Surgical or Traumatic Wounds

Wounds healing by secondary intention often have significant amount of devitalized tissue and bacterial loads.[27] Wound packing with a hydrogel (not indicated for highly exudative wounds) or calcium alginate to absorb exudate is often effective. Both of these items are now formulated with silver for antimicrobial coverage.[27]

The use of new technologic advances to enhance healing, such as negative pressure wound therapy, has promoted wound healing in large, open wounds.[43] Adjunctive therapies are useful in chronic wounds; hyperbaric oxygen therapy is an evidence-based therapy being used to treat diabetic foot ulcers with success. Negative pressure wound therapy is useful to promote healing in chronic stage III or stage IV pressure ulcers as well as nonhealing surgical wounds and some lower extremity ulcers. Ultrasound, biologic therapy, growth factors, and electrical stimulation may also be beneficial in certain wounds.[43]

COMPLICATIONS

Complications of wound healing include infection, dehiscence, delayed wound healing, extensive scarring, and sepsis. Serious infection of the face or hands and cellulitis that has not responded to oral antibiotic treatment require intravenous antibiotics or hospitalization.

INDICATIONS FOR REFERRAL OR HOSPITALIZATION

Referral decisions are guided by the location and nature of the wound; injury to bone, tendon, or vasculature; and the experience of the health care provider. Referral to a specialist is required for fractures, deep tissue injury, vascular or organ damage, facial and hand injuries, or severely contaminated wounds. Large, open wounds or deep puncture wounds most likely require referral for a surgical intervention. Chronic wounds, such as ulcers, are best managed by referral to a wound care specialist who is part of an interdisciplinary team. Facial or hand wounds that are infected may require hospitalization and intravenous antibiotics.

LIFE-SPAN CONSIDERATIONS

Older patients tend to heal more slowly, and their wounds tend to lose tensile strength, which correlates with reduced collagen.[44,45] Impaired skin integrity is common in older adults as a result of age-related skin changes, immobility, malnutrition, incontinence, immunocompromised status, polypharmacy, sensory deficits, and comorbidities. Thinning of the epidermis, dermis, and subcutaneous tissue coupled with decreased tensile strength and elasticity and poor epidermal-dermal adhesion contributes to easy skin tears, pressure ulcers, and lower extremity ulcers.[45]

In addition, wound healing time is prolonged in older adults because of decreased oxygenation and perfusion and a decreased inflammatory response. Although the same principles of wound management apply in all populations, special diligence is recommended in caring for older adults. Consideration of the diminished ability to provide self-care and to travel easily to and from medical facilities should prompt the provider to select appropriate dressings and to consider a referral to home health agencies for wound evaluation and care in the patient's setting. The risk of delayed wound healing contributes to infection, pain, and a decreased quality of life in patients who may already be compromised.[45]

EDUCATION AND HEALTH PROMOTION

Signs and symptoms of wound infection should be reviewed with the patient and family both verbally and in writing. Infection of the wound can greatly affect outcome and may impede wound healing and return of function. Demonstrating wound dressing techniques with the patient and family and observing a return demonstration when possible are helpful in ascertaining the patient's and family's understanding. A patient teaching pamphlet or video with specific directions for wound cleansing and care reinforces teaching, especially if available in the patient's primary language.

Reevaluation and follow-up evaluation for suture removal should be scheduled before discharge. Sutures are removed according to the location of the wound and the type of suture used. Referral for a home health nurse may be important for dressing changes, support in managing medications (especially antibiotics), and wound evaluation in the home. Follow-up monitoring of most wounds should occur within 7 to 10 days.

Prevention of lower extremity ulcers and diligent foot care in patients with diabetes mellitus and peripheral vascular disease will prevent amputations, decrease the cost of multiple hospitalizations, and prolong and improve the overall quality of life. Pressure-relieving interventions such as callus removal, padded hosiery to reduce callous buildup, extra-depth shoes, and insoles to redistribute foot pressure have demonstrated some benefit in ulcer prevention. Emollient moisturizers can help prevent fissures and breaks in the skin of those with diabetes and venous insufficiency. Patients at risk for pressure ulcers should be instructed in proper positioning and pressure reduction techniques.

Promotion of healthy behaviors is an essential intervention in the prevention of traumatic wounds. Health care providers should encourage home safety and reinforce child safety practices including automobile safety, helmet use, gun safety, and safe behavior around animals.

REFERENCES

1. Naussbaum, S. R., Carter, M. J., Fife, C. E., et al. (2018). An economic evaluation of the impact, cost, and medicare policy implication of chronic nonhealing wounds. *Value in Health, 21,* 27–32. Retrieved from https://www.clinicalkey.com/service/content/pdf/watermarked/1-s2.0-S1098301517303297.pdf?locale=en_US. (Accessed 19 June 2018).
2. Agency for Healthcare Research and Quality. Preventing pressure ulcers in hospitals. Retrieved from https://www.ahrq.gov/professionals/systems/hospital/pressureulcertoolkit/putool1.html. (Accessed 20 June 2018).
3. American Hospital Association. Health Research & Educational Trust. Pressure ulcers. Health Improvement Innovation Network. Retrieved from http://www.hret-hiin.org/topics/pressure-ulcers.shtml. (Accessed 24 June 2018).
4. Alavi, A., Brown, K. L., & Phillips, J. T. (2017). Venous ulcers. In S. C. McKean, J. J. Ross, D. D. Dressler, & D. B. Scheurer (Eds.), *Principles and Practice of Hospital Medicine* (2nd ed.). New York, NY: McGraw-Hill. Retrieved from http://accessmedicine.mhmedical.com.ezproxy.uthsc.edu/content.aspx?bookid=1872&sectionid=146981102. (Accessed 24 June 2018).
5. Rice, J. B., Desai, U., Cummings, A. K., et al. (2014). Burden of venous leg ulcers in the United States. *Journal of Medical Economics, 17*(5), 347–356. doi:10.3111/13696998.2014.903258. Retrieved from https://www.tandfonline.com/doi/full/10.3111/13696998.2014.903258. (Accessed 25 June 2018).
6. Embil, J. M., Trepman, E., Embil, J. M., Trepman, E., Embil, J. M., & Trepman, E. (2017). Diabetic foot infections. In S. C. McKean, J. J. Ross, D. D. Dressler, D. B. Scheurer, S. C. McKean, J. J. Ross, et al. (Eds.), *Principles and Practice of Hospital Medicine* (2nd ed.). New York, NY: McGraw-Hill.
7. American Diabetes Association. (2018). Standards of medical care in diabetes-2018. *The Journal of Clinical and Applied Research and Education, 42*(1), S113–S114. Retrieved from care.diabetesjournals.org/content/diacare/suppl/2017/12/08/41.Supplement_1.DC1/DC_41_S1_Combined.pdf. (Accessed 26 June 2018).
8. Milne, J. (2016). Managing surgical wound care: Review of leukomed control dressings. *British Journal of Nursing, 25*(6), S36–S43.
9. Yao, K., Bae, L., & Yew, W. P. (2013). Post-operative wound management. *Reprinted from Australian family physician, 42*(12), 867–870.
10. Santema, T. B., Lenselink, E. A., Balm, R., & Ubbink, D. T. (2016). Comparing the Meggitt-Wagner and the University of Texas wound classification systems for diabetic foot ulcers: Inter-observer analyses. *Int Wound Journal, 13*(6), 1137–1141. doi:10.1111/iwj.12429.
11. Frykberg, R. G., & Banks, J. (2015). Challenges in the treatment of chronic wounds. *Wound Healing Society.* Retrieved from https://www.ncbi.nlm.nih.gov/pmc/articles/PMC4528992/pdf/wound.2015.0635.pdf. (Accessed 25 June 2018).
12. LeBlond, R. F., Brown, D. D., Suneja, M., & Szot, J. F. (2014). *The skin and nails: DeGowin's diagnostic examination* (10th ed.). New York: McGrqw-Hill.
13. Barbul, A., Efron, D. T., & Kavalukas, S. L. (2015). Wound healing. In F. Brunicardi, D. K. Andersen, T. R. Billiar, D. L. Dunn, J. G. Hunter, J. B. Matthews, et al. (Eds.), *Schwartz's principles of surgery* (10th ed.). New York, NY: McGraw-Hill.
14. Karahan, A., Abbasoglu, A., Isik, S. A., Cevik, B., Saltan, C., Elbas, N. O., et al. (2018). Factors affecting wound healing in individuals with pressure ulcers: A retrospective study. *Ostomy/Wound Management, 64*(2), 32–39. doi:10.25270/owm.2018.2.3239.
15. DiPreta, J. A. (2014). Outpatient assessment and management of the diabetic foot. *The Medical Clinics of North America, 98*(2), 353–373.
16. Rocha, N. P., & Fortes, R. C. (2015). Total lymphocyte count and serum albumin as predictors of nutritional risk in surgical patients. *ABCD Arq Bras Cir Dig., 28*(3), 193–196. doi:10.1590/S0102-67202015000300012. Retrieved from http://www.scielo.br/pdf/abcd/v28n3/0102-6720-abcd-28-03-00193.pdf. (Accessed 9 July 2018).
17. Ortiz-Pujols, S. M., Thompson, K., Sheldon, G. F., Fraher, E. P., Ricketts, T. C., & Cairns, B. A. (2011). *Burn care: Are there sufficient providers and facilities?* Chapel Hill, North Carolina: American College of Surgeons Health Policy Research Institute.
18. Young, D. M., & Hansen, S. L. (2015). Hand surgery. In G. M. Doherty (Ed.), *Current diagnosis & treatment: Surgery* (14th ed.). New York, NY: McGraw-Hill.
19. Vasconez, H. C., & Buseman, J. (2014). Plastic & reconstructive surgery. In G. M. Doherty (Ed.), *Current diagnosis & treatment: Surgery* (14th ed.). New York, NY: McGraw-Hill.
20. Harper, G., Johnston, C., & Landefeld, C. (2018). Geriatric disorders. In M. A. Papadakis, S. J. McPhee, & M. W. Rabow (Eds.), *Current medical diagnosis & treatment.* New York, NY: McGraw-Hill.
21. Molnar, J. A., Underdown, M. J., & Clark, W. A. (2014). Nutrition and chronic wounds. Wound Healing Society. *Advances in Wound Care, 3*(11), 663–681. doi:10.1089/wound.2014.0530. Retrieved from https://www.ncbi.nlm.nih.gov/pmc/articles/PMC4217039/pdf/wound.2014.0530.pdf. (Accessed 9 July 2018).
22. Tao, H., Butler, J. P., & Luttrell, T. (2013). The role of whirlpool in wound care. *Journal of the American College of Clinical Wound Specialists, 4*(1), 7–12. doi.org/10.1016/j.jccw.2013.01.002. Retrieved from https://www.ncbi.nlm.nih.gov/pmc/articles/PMC3921238/pdf/main.pdf. (Accessed 12 July 2018).
23. Munro, S., et al. (2017). Maggots in the management of ulcer care. BMJ Case Reports. Retrieved from https://casereports.bmj.com/content/casereports/2017/bcr-2017-220462.full.pdf. (Accessed 1 May 2019).
24. Anthony, P. C., Sanchez, C. J., Hardy, S. K., Romano, D. R., Hurtgen, B. J., Wenke, J. C., et al. (2014). Dakin solution alters macrophage viability and function. *Journal of Surgical research., 192*(2), 692–699. Retrieved from doi.org/10.1016/j.jss.2014.07.019, https://www.sciencedirect.com/science/article/pii/S0022480414006568?via%3Dihub. (Accessed 12 July 2018).
25. Shah, S. K., & Belkin, M. (2017). Acute and chronic lower limb ischemia. In S. C. McKean, J. J. Ross, D. D. Dressler, & D. B. Scheurer (Eds.), *Principles and Practice of Hospital Medicine* (2nd ed.). New York, NY: McGraw-Hill. Retrieved from http://accessmedicine.mhmedical.com/content.aspx?bookid=1872&sectionid=146991108. (Accessed 12 July 2018).
26. Ban, K., Minei, J., Laronga, C., et al. (2017). American College of Surgeons and Surgical Infection Society: Surgical site infection guidelines, 2016 update. *Journal of the American College of Surgeons, 224*(1), 59–74.
27. Powers, J. G., Higham, C., Broussard, K., & Phillips, T. J. (2016). Wound healing and treating wounds: Chronic wound care and management. *Journal of the American Academy of Dermatology, 74*(4), 607–625. doi.org/10.1016/j.jaad.2015.08.070.
28. Singer, A. J., & Hollander, J. E. (2016). Wound evaluation. In J. E. Tintinalli, J. Stapczynski, O. Ma, D. M. Yealy, G. D. Meckler, & D. M. Cline (Eds.), *Tintinalli's emergency medicine: A comprehensive study guide* (8th ed.). New York, NY: McGraw-Hill.
29. Rapp, J., Plackett, T., Crane, J., Lu, J., Hardin, D., Loos, P., et al. (2017). Acute traumatic wound management in the prolonged field care setting. *Joint Trauma System Clinical Practice Guideline.* Retrieved from https://prolongedfieldcare.files.wordpress.com/2017/07/wound_mgmnt_pfc_24jul2017.pdf. (Accessed 13 July 2018).
30. Urban, M. V., Rath, T., & Radtke, C. (2017). Hydrogen peroxide (H2O2): A review of its use in surgery. *Wien Med Wochenschr.* doi:10.1007/s10354-017-0610-2.
31. Singer, A. J., & Hollander, J. E. (2016). Wound closure. In J. E. Tintinalli, J. Stapczynski, O. Ma, D. M. Yealy, G. D. Meckler, & D. M. Cline (Eds.), *Tintinalli's emergency medicine: A comprehensive study guide* (8th ed.). New York, NY: McGraw-Hill.
32. Brock, G. (2016). The practitioner: The occasional wound "gluing." *Canadian Journal of Rural Medicine, 21*(4), 113–116. Retrieved from https://srpc.ca/resources/Documents/CJRM/vol21n4/pg113.pdf. (Accessed 13 July 2018).
33. Dabiri, G., Damstetter, E., & Phillips, T. (2016). Wound Healing Society: Choosing a wound dressing based on common wound characteristics. *Advances in Wound Care, 5*(1), 32–41. doi:10.1089/wound.2014.0586.
34. Jones, T. R. (2017). Wound care. In C. K. Stone & R. L. Humphries (Eds.), *Current diagnosis & treatment: Emergency medicine.* New York, NY: McGraw-Hill.
35. LeBlanc, K., Baranoski, S., Christensen, D., Langemo, D., Edwards, K., Holloway, S., et al. (2016). The art of dressing selection: A consensus statement on skin tears and best practice. *Advances in Skin & Wound Care., 29*(1), 32–46. doi:10.1097/01.ASW.0000475308.06130.df. Retrieved from https://journals.lww.com/aswcjournal/Fulltext/2016/01000/The_Art_of_Dressing_Selection__A_Consensus.10.aspx. (Accessed 14 July 2018).
36. Bolenbaucher, R., Cotner-Pouncy, T., et al. (2016). Texas EMS Trauma & Acute Care Foundation Trauma Division: Burn clinical practice guideline. Retrieved from http://tetaf.org/wp-content/uploads/2016/01/Burn-Practice-Guideline.pdf. (Accessed 14 July 2018).
37. Drigalla, D., & Barth, B. (2017). Burns & smoke inhalation. In C. Stone & R. L. Humphries (Eds.), *Current diagnosis & treatment: Emergency medicine* (8th ed.). New York, NY: McGraw-Hill.
38. Palfreyman, S. J., & Stone, P. W. (2014). A systematic review of economic evaluations assessing interventions aimed at preventing or treating pressure ulcers. *International Journal of Nursing Studies, 52*(3), 769–788. Retrieved from doi.org/10.1016/j.ijnurstu.2014.06.004, https://www.journalofnursingstudies.com/article/S0020-7489(14)00161-8/fulltext. (Accessed 14 July 2018).
39. Kottner, J., & Beeckman, D. (2015). Incontinence-associated dermatitis and pressure ulcers in geriatric patients. *Giornale Italiano Di Dermatologia E Venereologia: Organo Ufficiale, Societa Italiana Di Dermatologia E Sifilografia, 150*(6), 717–729.

40. Kane, R. L., Ouslander, J. G., Resnick, B., & Malone, M. L. (Eds.), (2018). Immobility. In *Essentials of clinical geriatrics* (8th ed.). New York, NY: McGraw-Hill.

41. Alavi, A., Brown, K. L., & Phillips, J. T. (2017). Venous ulcers. In S. C. McKean, J. J. Ross, D. D. Dressler, & D. B. Scheurer (Eds.), *Principles and Practice of Hospital Medicine* (2nd ed.). New York, NY: McGraw-Hill.

42. Brownrigg, J. R. W., Apelqvist, J., Bakker, K., Schaper, N. C., & Hinchliffe, R. J. (2013). Evidence-based management of PAD & the diabetic foot. *European Society for Vascular Surgery*. dx.doi.org/10.1016/j.ejvs.2013.02.014.

43. Yazdanpanah, L., Nasiri, M., & Adarvishi, S. (2015). Literature review on the management of diabetic foot ulcer. *World J Diabetes.*, 6(1), 37–53.

44. Ulma, R. M., Aghaloo, T. L., & Freymiller, E. G. (2013). Wound healing. In R. J. Fonseca, R. V. Walker, H. D. Berber, M. P. Powers, & D. E. Frost (Eds.), *Oral & maxillofacial trauma* (4th ed.). St. Louis, Missouri.

45. Sgonc, R., & Gruber, J. (2013). Age-related aspects of cutaneous wound healing: A mini-review. *Gerontology*, 59(2), 159–164. doi:10.1159/000342344. Retrieved from https://www.ncbi.nlm.nih.gov/pubmed/23108154. (Accessed 14 July 2018).

CHAPTER 52

EVALUATION OF THE EYES

Kenneth C. Fan • James T. Banta

A complete ophthalmic examination is vital not only for routine patient care but for the diagnosis of critical local and systemic abnormalities. Whereas some problems may require a formal evaluation by an ophthalmologist, the primary care provider should be well versed in the basics of the eye examination. By achieving a better understanding of the eye examination, a primary care provider can assist patients with common complaints and refer them to a specialist when it is indicated. This chapter discusses basic eye anatomy, the components of a complete ocular evaluation, and the differential diagnosis of common presenting ophthalmic complaints.

SCREENING RECOMMENDATIONS

Because of the significant public health implications and vision's impact on quality of life, regular eye examinations are recommended at various intervals, depending on a patient's age and risk factors. Even in an otherwise healthy adult, the risk of visual impairment increases with age. Vision of 20/50 or less has been demonstrated in 9% of adults older than 60 years.

The American Academy of Ophthalmology (AAO) recommends that patients 65 years of age and older without risk factors for eye disease should have a comprehensive eye examination every 1 to 2 years. Several other academies, including the American Congress of Obstetricians and Gynecologists and the American Academy of Family Physicians, suggest similar recommendations for screening of older patients.[1,2]

In addition to more general screening guidelines, certain disease entities carry specific screening guidelines that are highly applicable to primary care providers. The AAO recommends that patients with diabetes receive eye screening—type 1 diabetics 3 to 5 years after the diagnosis, and type 2 diabetics at the time of diagnosis—to assess for diabetic retinopathy. In addition, these patients should continue to undergo screening on an annual basis. With regard to pregnancy, patients with diabetes should receive a screening examination before conception, early in the first trimester, and for 1 year postpartum.[3,4] The US Preventive Services Task Force (USPSTF) has also looked at screening for primary open-angle glaucoma (POAG) in adults but thus far has found insufficient evidence to justify routine screening.[5] The AAO has determined that population screening of POAG is not cost-effective; however, it may be more useful when it is targeted at populations at high risk for glaucoma, such as older adults, those with a family history of glaucoma, African Americans over 50 years of age, and Hispanics over 65 years of age.[6] It should be noted that in 2002, the Center for Medicare and Medicaid Services initiated coverage of glaucoma screening in the aforementioned populations.

HISTORY

The basis of a good eye examination is a thorough history. As with any medical examination, details about the history of the present illness can help hone the physical examination and give clues about an aberrant process. For patients with a new eye complaint, such as pain or vision loss, it is important to determine the quality and nature of the presenting problem. The onset of the complaint is of particular importance in ophthalmology. For instance, although a patient with a gradual worsening of vision may simply need glasses or evaluation for cataracts, a complaint of acute vision loss should be referred for immediate evaluation by an ophthalmologist. Other details should be explored, such as the location (left eye, right eye, or both), duration, character, associated factors (pain, redness, discharge, headache, nausea, or neurologic changes), aggravating and alleviating factors (pain with eye movements or with bright lights), radiation, temporal association (worse in morning or night), and severity. In addition to acute vision loss, any patient with painful vision loss or trauma should be referred to an ophthalmologist. Similarly, a patient with acute vision loss associated with neurologic signs should be emergently evaluated to rule out a cerebrovascular accident or other central nervous system processes.

A patient's past medical and ocular history can also give insight into a new problem. Information should be gathered about any previous eye disease, trauma, and surgery (both medically necessary and cosmetic or refractive). In addition, many systemic medical problems have associated ophthalmic manifestations, as discussed in more detail later in this chapter. Medication reconciliation is equally important because systemic and topical medications can be associated with both systemic effects and changes in the eye. For instance, medications commonly prescribed for erectile dysfunction (e.g., sildenafil) are sometimes associated with cyanopsia, or blue-tinted vision. The beta blocker timolol is frequently prescribed for glaucoma, and can exacerbate bradycardia and asthma in susceptible patients.

A thorough family history that includes ocular disease should be obtained because several ocular conditions are associated with a familial pattern of inheritance and can represent a threat to a patient's vision or life. Patients with a family history of glaucoma, color blindness, cataracts, macular degeneration, retinal degeneration, corneal dystrophy, and retinoblastoma have increased risks for these processes, which should be considered when obtaining the general family history. These patients should be referred to an ophthalmologist if care has not already been established.

Social and occupational factors are elucidated to better identify behaviors that increase risk for eye-related trauma or disease. Leisure or occupational activities associated with trauma to the eyes, such as construction work (particularly hammering or grinding), chemical work, and high-impact sports, should direct the physician to ask about the use of eye protection. Similarly, injection drug use or high-risk sexual behavior generates a higher risk for human immunodeficiency virus (HIV) and acquired immunodeficiency syndrome (AIDS), and can be important in correct identification of ocular diseases specific to immunocompromised states.

PHYSICAL EXAMINATION

An evaluation of the structure and function of the eyes should be approached systematically and incorporate a sound understanding of ocular and periocular anatomy. The primary measurements to determine the basic health and function of the eyes are visual acuity, pupil responses, intraocular pressure, visual fields, and extraocular movements. These metrics are analogous to vital signs for a systemic examination and are integral to every ophthalmic examination. After the assessment of these ocular vital signs, an evaluation of ocular structures should proceed from external and anterior segment structures inward to the posterior segment.

Visual Acuity

Visual acuity refers to the spatial resolving power of the eye. As the primary functional measure of the eye, it is important to measure vision accurately. Vision is typically measured at the beginning of the examination before any other test or intervention has been performed. Spurious results can otherwise be found as a result of dilating drops or corneal irritation from intraocular pressure measurements. Vision should be tested in each eye with use of the patient's refractive aids (e.g., glasses, contact lenses) or a pinhole (a technique of looking through a hole in a card to diminish refractive error). In patients with refractive error—especially high myopia—failing to test vision with the use of refractive aids or a pinhole can lead a provider to incorrectly suspect acute pathology, causing undue concern to the patient and provider.

There are many valid means of measuring vision, such as the Snellen chart, tumbling *E*s, and other instruments used for pediatric populations. Of these, the most commonly used and referenced is the Snellen chart. This chart consists of 11 lines of precisely sized block letters, or optotypes. By convention in the United States, the patient is directed to stand 20 feet away from the wall chart. With each eye, the chart is read down until the patient is unable to make out the letters. The patient's vision is recorded as a fractional value, such as 20/80, based on the last line that was successfully seen. This value indicates the equivalent distance that a person with normal vision could stand away from the chart and still read the indicated letters. In this example, a patient with normal vision could be 80 feet away from the chart and still read the letters that the patient in question can read at 20 feet. The tumbling *E* chart uses variously sized letter *E*s in different orientations for patients who have difficulty identifying letters or are illiterate.

If a patient is unable to read any letters on the Snellen chart (visual acuity <20/400), the vision can be tested by other means. The first alternative means of testing vision is to use a card of a 20/200 Snellen E. This card can be held starting directly in front of the patient's eye and slowly moved back until the patient is no longer able to identify it. This value is recorded as the number of feet the patient is able to see the letter over 200; for example, if a patient can read the card at 6 feet, the vision is recorded as 6/200. If this proves unsuccessful, finger counting can be employed. Similar to testing vision with the 20/200 card, any number of fingers are held at gradually increasing distances from the patient's eye. Vision is recorded as the maximum distance a patient can count fingers (e.g., CF at 6 feet). If a patient cannot count fingers, the patient is asked to identify the examiner's hand waving slowly in front of the eyes; a patient able to see the movement of a hand has vision recorded as HM for hand motions. If the patient fails the aforementioned tests, the final check of visual acuity is the patient's ability to perceive light. For this test, a light is shined into a patient's eye in a darkened room, and the patient is asked if any light can be seen. Care must be taken to fully cover the eye that is not being tested, as light may enter the unintended eye and lead to a false-positive result. A positive response is recorded as LP (light perception); a negative response is recorded as NLP (no light perception).

Near vision can be tested separately, as some pathologic processes yield good near vision with poor far vision and vice versa. Near vision can be tested with a Rosenbaum near card held at 14 inches. Again, each eye is tested independently, and the patient is asked to read the smallest line possible. Unlike distance vision, near vision is recorded on the Jaeger scale. This scale ranges from J16 (approximately 20/200) to J1+, which equates to 20/20 on the Snellen chart. On this scale, standard newspaper font is J5. All adults will begin to exhibit difficulties with near vision around the age of 42 or 43 years. This is because of a decrease in the flexibility of the human lens, a natural aging process known as *presbyopia*. Although this condition can cause significant patient distress, a trial of over-the-counter reading glasses generally produces a satisfactory improvement in the patient's near vision and therefore in the quality of life.

Pupil Response

Impaired pupil responses can give vital information about the function of a patient's visual system. Under standard fluorescent lighting conditions, the average adult pupil ranges from 2.6 to 5.0 mm and is round and symmetric.[7] Any variance in the size of the pupils between the eyes is defined as anisocoria. This finding can be benign, as physiologic anisocoria exists in 20% of the population,[8] and demonstrates a difference of no more than 1 mm between two normally functioning pupils. However, anisocoria can also suggest a neurologic, pharmacologic, or anatomic abnormality. In addition, previous episodes of trauma or intraocular surgery can result in an anatomically abnormal pupil; thus a detailed history is vital.

Pupil function can be assessed with a standard penlight. On initial inspection, the examiner should test each pupil independently, shining the light from a slightly oblique angle to avoid a false response from accommodation. The pupil should respond briskly to the light and hold in its constricted position. A normal pupil should not redilate in direct light, but it might demonstrate a slight fluctuation in diameter. This phenomenon is referred to as *hippus* and is of no pathologic significance. When the examiner has established the independent functioning of each pupil, he or she must next verify symmetric pupil responses with the swinging flashlight test. To perform this technique, the patient is first asked to focus straight ahead on a distant object. It is important that the patient's fixation is at distance to prevent accommodation from causing pupillary constriction and confounding the swinging flashing test. A flashlight is then directed at one eye until the pupil constricts. The flashlight is then swung quickly to the opposite eye, and the response is observed. In a normally functioning eye, equal signal is received from each eye and transmitted across synaptic pathways to achieve consensual constriction. If the pathway or the input is damaged—usually through a defect in the optic nerve—the signal is disrupted and the eyes will respond asymmetrically. For instance, if a significant injury has occurred to the left optic nerve, a flashlight shined into the right eye will produce a normal constriction in both eyes from appropriate consensual response. However, when the flashlight is swung to the left, the pupils will paradoxically dilate because of the disruption of the afferent signal from the damaged nerve. This phenomenon is known as a *relative afferent pupillary defect* (RAPD) or *Marcus-Gunn pupil*. It is important to use the swinging flashlight test to identify this condition because both pupils may respond to light, and therefore it is the relative response that is essential. An RAPD indicates significant ocular dysfunction, and if it is present for an unknown reason, the patient should be referred for further evaluation by an ophthalmologist.

Intraocular Pressure

Normal intraocular pressure is generally considered to range from 10 to 20 mm Hg. Many methods exist to measure intraocular pressure. These include the air-puff tonometer, Tono-Pen, and Goldmann applanation tonometry. Of these options, the Tono-Pen is most accessible to non-ophthalmologic offices. It consists of a pen-like device that is tapped against the center of the patient's cornea after instillation of an ocular anesthetic such as proparacaine. The Tono-Pen provides an easy-to-use, quick estimation of intraocular pressure. Unfortunately, at higher pressures the Tono-Pen is not as accurate as other methods. The gold standard of measurement is Goldmann applanation tonometry, which requires the use of a slit lamp and is something that is not typically available in non-ophthalmologic offices.

Although accurate measurement of intraocular pressure is essential to a complete eye examination, not all primary care settings have access to a measurement tool. In these cases, the physician can gather a rough estimation of the intraocular pressure by gently palpating the globes through closed lids. Under normal circumstances, the eyes should feel of a consistency similar to a grape and should be roughly symmetric. Any eye that feels rock-hard is abnormal, and should be further evaluated. In addition, a firm, painful eye that is inflamed and associated with a cloudy cornea is indicative of an acute rise in intraocular pressure. This represents an ophthalmic emergency with a strong potential for irreversible vision loss; emergent referral is indicated.

Ocular Alignment and Extraocular Movements

Ocular movements are controlled by six extraocular muscles: the four rectus muscles (superior, inferior, medial, and lateral), as well as the two oblique muscles (superior and inferior). These muscles are controlled by cranial nerves III, IV, and VI. Under normal conditions, the eyes should be symmetric and

aligned when the patient is looking forward and should move equally in all directions. Movements can be affected by a neurologic dysfunction (from trauma, compression of a cranial nerve, or ischemia), by a muscle dysfunction (such as a restrictive or inflammatory process), or by congenital abnormalities.

The examination of ocular alignment consists of three general components: the Hirschberg test, the cover-uncover test, and the alternate-cover test. These maneuvers allow the examiner to determine the presence of strabismus, a condition that may influence visual prognosis in children or cause diplopia in adults. The Hirschberg test is performed with the patient looking in primary gaze, or directly at the observer. The examiner, standing in front of the patient, then shines a bright penlight directly at the patient's eyes. The light from the penlight is seen reflecting on the patient's corneas, prompting what is referred to as the *light reflex*. In a patient with normal alignment, these reflections should be symmetrically located within the pupils. If a reflection is deviated medially (nasally) or laterally (temporally), this indicates an exotropia or esotropia, respectively.

When a disorder of ocular alignment is suspected, the cover-uncover test and alternate-cover test can be used to further evaluate the nature of the disorder. The cover-uncover test involves having a patient fixate on a distant object. The examiner then places an occluder in front of one eye to disrupt binocular vision. The occluder is removed and the newly uncovered eye is observed. Movement of the newly uncovered eye suggests underlying strabismus. Similarly, in the alternate-cover test, the patient looks at a distant object and an occluder is passed from one eye to the other. Any resulting movement in the unobstructed eye is abnormal and represents a dysfunction of ocular motility. Ophthalmologists use prisms to quantify any noted deviations.

Once the ocular alignment has been evaluated, one must examine the patient's ocular motility. The examiner asks the patient to track an object such as a pen or the examiner's index finger without moving the head (the index finger should be moved slowly to avoid making the patient dizzy). Any gross deficit in motility should be noted. There are nine diagnostic positions of gaze: straight, right, upper right, up, upper left, left, lower left, down, and lower right. Of these gazes, six (right, upper right, upper left, left, lower left, and lower right) are considered the cardinal directions of gaze. With these six, one can localize a movement deficiency of one of the extraocular muscles. Dysfunctional extraocular movement with a paretic cause can often be identified by this examination technique.

Because the oculomotor nerve (cranial nerve III) innervates the majority of extraocular muscles as well as levator palpebrae and autonomic muscles, its injury or dysfunction can have diverse presentations. In a complete cranial nerve III palsy, the patient classically has a "down-and-out" position of the affected eye and is unable to adduct the eye or move it up or down. The eyelid may demonstrate complete or partial ptosis, and a third nerve palsy can also be associated with a nonresponsive pupil in the same eye. Multiple causes of third-nerve palsy are possible, ranging from the microvascular effects of hypertension and diabetes to compressive lesions such as tumors or aneurysms. Pupil function can give a clue to the cause of a third-nerve palsy and should be checked before the instillation of dilating drops. If a nonresponsive pupil is present, this is suggestive of a compressive lesion (often an aneurysm) and necessitates referral for emergent neuroimaging and evaluation.

A trochlear nerve (cranial nerve IV) palsy can be difficult to detect; the motility examination findings can appear grossly normal. However, some patients will exhibit a decreased ability to look down in the adducted position. A head tilt away from the affected side is often present and diminishes diplopia. A patient with an abducens nerve (cranial nerve VI) abnormality will be unable to abduct the involved eye. A head turn away from the affected side will diminish diplopia. Both cranial nerve IV and VI palsies are often ischemic or traumatic in nature. However, despite this, a very thorough and comprehensive history is of utmost importance as a recent study in the AAO has demonstrated that 10% of patients with isolated cranial nerve palsies (III, IV, and VI) with at least 1 vasculopathic risk factor without other medical comorbidities were found to have other underlying causes including infarctions and neoplasms.[9]

Another important examination when evaluating the motility and position of the eyes is to check for protuberance of one or both eyes (exophthalmos or proptosis). This is especially important in a patient who reports pain or double vision or is suspected of having thyroid disease. The best way to check for proptosis is to have the patient lift up his or her chin while the provider looks at the prominence of the eyes from below. If proptosis is suspected, a referral to an ophthalmologist is recommended and should be done urgently if the patient is experiencing other ocular symptoms such as pain, headache, or double vision. Lastly, if the patient has noticed that one eye is becoming progressively proptotic, this is an indication for an urgent referral and potentially facial and head imaging.

Visual Fields

Visual field defects can result from any abnormality that affects the eye, optic nerve, optic radiations, or visual cortex. Several methods exist to precisely determine a patient's field of vision, but only confrontation visual field testing is used routinely during a standard ophthalmic examination. Confrontation field testing is performed with the examiner approximately 1 m away from the patient. The patient has one eye covered at a time, and the patient is instructed to look at the examiner's nose. The physician then presents fingers (usually one, two, or five fingers, because they are easily distinguishable and yield more accurate results) to the patient in each quadrant of vision. It is important for the provider to ensure that the patient has not changed his or her focus from the provider's nose to another area, which can dramatically alter results. If the patient is unable to count fingers, a stronger stimulus such as hand motions or light can be presented in the deficient areas. In patients capable of good cooperation, the physician can present different numbers of fingers at once in multiple quadrants. The patient is then asked for the total sum of the fingers shown. This method can confirm a suspected visual field deficit. If a field defect with an unknown cause is identified on confrontational examination, the patient should be referred to an ophthalmologist for a formal visual field test. If a visual field abnormality is present with other symptoms of concern for cerebrovascular accident or transient ischemic attack, the patient should be referred immediately to the nearest emergency room.

External Structures. The periorbital structures are composed of the eyelids, eyelashes, and lacrimal system. The eyelids are vital to maintaining ocular lubrication and are tightly opposed to the globe under normal circumstances. Both the upper and lower eyelids contain oil-secreting glands necessary for maintaining the tear film. The eyelid margin contains a continuous row of lashes that serve to protect the eye from debris. Lash loss is most frequently a sign of chronic inflammation but can be associated with a neoplastic process. Whitening (poliosis) or loss (madarosis) of lashes should be evaluated by an ophthalmologist. The medial aspect of the eyelid contains the punctum, the opening of the canalicular drainage system. During the blink cycle, the lids work as a pump to move tears from the ocular surface into the lacrimal sac. Lid abnormalities can result in pathologic changes ranging from dryness and exposure to excessive tearing. Accordingly, the lids must be examined carefully for signs of irregularity, improper positioning such as ectropion (turning outward) or entropion (turning inward), punctal patency, inflammation, and swelling. The eyelids should completely cover the ocular surface when they are closed. Any lack of closure, or lagophthalmos, suggests an underlying anatomic or functional abnormality and should be investigated.

Anterior Segment

The sclera is the firm outer wall of the globe and is composed of dense connective tissue. Typically, it has a white appearance on examination, but several local and systemic conditions can cause color variations. For instance, in conditions of hepatic dysfunction associated with jaundice, the sclera assumes a yellowish hue known as *icterus*. Similarly, in the genetic condition osteogenesis imperfecta or after local inflammation of the sclera, the sclera can be thinned and appear blue.

The conjunctiva is composed of two parts: the bulbar portion, which overlies the sclera, and the palpebral portion lining the eyelids. The bulbar conjunctiva is a moist, shiny tissue that is typically devoid of large or significant blood vessels. For the conjunctiva to be appropriately assessed, the patient is instructed to look in all directions as the lids are retracted for full exposure. The presence of prominent vessels with redness, known as *injection*, is indicative of inflammation. Although injection is commonly seen in infectious, allergic, or chemical conjunctivitis, injection is also noted with many other inflammatory conditions. The presence of a mucopurulent or watery discharge would suggest bacterial or viral conjunctivitis, respectively. In cases of conjunctival injection, the palpebral conjunctiva should be examined with a penlight. Under normal circumstances, the palpebral conjunctiva should appear pink and smooth. In the setting of conjunctivitis, it assumes a bumpy appearance (e.g., conjunctival papillae or follicles), and the conjunctival vasculature is less defined.[10] Conjunctival injection associated with severe photophobia or layered inflammatory debris in the anterior chamber (hypopyon) suggests intraocular inflammation or infection.

After trauma or Valsalva maneuvers (e.g., lifting, sneezing), conjunctival vessels can become compromised and bleed. Blood becomes trapped between the sclera and conjunctiva and results in a deep confluent red appearance that can be focal or diffuse (Fig. 52.1). This is known as a *subconjunctival hemorrhage*. Despite an often impressive appearance, it causes no ophthalmic problems and resolves without treatment, usually within 2 weeks.

A clear balloon-like swelling of the conjunctiva is known as *chemosis*. Chemosis can be associated with allergies, mechanical ventilators, trauma, and local inflammation. It is important to identify the source of chemosis. Severe chemosis can prevent

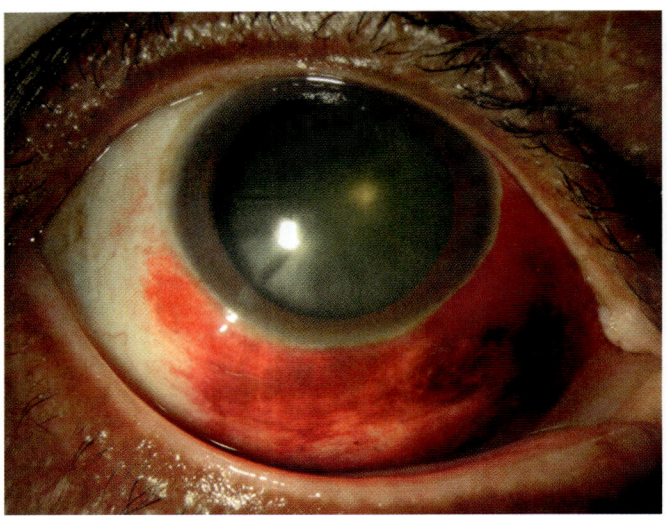

FIG. 52.1 Despite the dramatic appearance, isolated subconjunctival hemorrhage is a benign condition that does not require treatment.

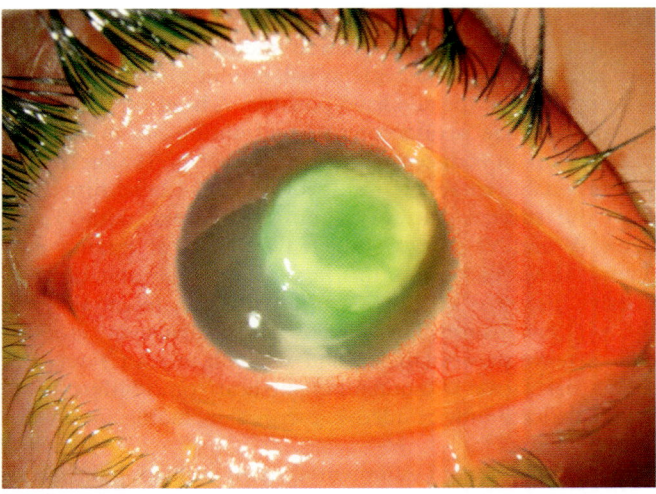

FIG. 52.2 Inappropriate contact lens use is frequently associated with severe bacterial keratitis, as illustrated in this photograph. Note the hypopyon collecting in the inferior aspect of the anterior chamber.

proper closure of the eyelids. When it is present, aggressive lubrication with ophthalmic lubricating drops and ointments is required to prevent ocular exposure.

The cornea is a curved structure composed of collagen fibers precisely arranged to achieve optical clarity. It is composed grossly of an epithelial surface, stroma, and endothelium. Damage or irritation of the epithelium can produce significant pain and irritation. The corneal epithelium is best evaluated with fluorescein dye. Under a cobalt blue light, any abrasions or irregularities in the epithelium will glow bright green. Pain associated with epithelial abnormalities will resolve completely after the use of topical anesthetic. Under no circumstances should a patient be given a bottle of topical ophthalmic anesthetic for personal use because prolonged use can result in a corneal melting and eventual perforation. Abuse of topical anesthetics is often seen among health care workers, given their relatively easy access to the drops.

It is important to note any irregularities in the clarity of the cornea, which can signify infection (typically a focal white plaque) or edema (from decomposition of corneal function or elevated intraocular pressure). The evaluation of a corneal opacity is especially important in patients who wear contact lenses and have eye pain or redness. These patients must be carefully examined for suppurative, feathery, or ring-shaped white infiltrates on the cornea (Fig. 52.2). Contact lens–related ulcers are common in patients who exhibit poor contact lens hygiene (e.g., sleeping or swimming in contact lenses, prolonged use, and poor handwashing) and can evolve rapidly. Untreated, corneal ulcers may result in permanent and severe visual loss. Any patient with an acute change in corneal clarity should be referred to an ophthalmologist for further evaluation.

The anterior chamber is defined as the space between the iris and the cornea. Aqueous humor fills the anterior chamber and is produced by the ciliary body and drains through the trabecular meshwork. This space should be deep and clear. In the setting of trauma, a shallow anterior chamber can signify a violation of the globe (open globe injury). An open globe injury is sometimes associated with expulsion of intraocular tissue or a peaked pupil. An open globe is an ophthalmic emergency and must be emergently referred. In the case of a suspected open globe, it is important not to probe or touch the eye any further and to place a hard shield over the eye to protect it from further serious damage until an ophthalmologist can evaluate and treat the patient. Typically, an open globe injury will require emergent surgery, so the patient should be restricted from eating and drinking in preparation for the operating room as soon as the diagnosis is suspected. This topic is addressed in greater detail in Chapter 61.

Numerous other severe conditions can lead to blood or inflammatory debris in the anterior chamber. Layering of blood (hyphema) or inflammatory debris (hypopyon) in the anterior chamber should prompt an immediate ophthalmic referral. In these cases, placing a hard shield over the eye is again advisable until an ophthalmologist can evaluate the eye.

The iris is the pigmented structure that forms the posterior aspect of the anterior chamber and acts as a shutter for the eye by controlling the amount of light through the pupil. The sphincter and dilator pupillae muscles produce constriction and dilation of the pupil in response to exogenous and endogenous stimuli. The iris is easily examined with a penlight with the aid of a magnifying glass, if one is available. The color of the iris can vary greatly, but it should be of a uniform color and bilaterally symmetric. Inconsistencies in the color of an iris can represent nevi, neoplasms (melanoma), hamartomas (Lisch nodules), genetic abnormalities (Waardenburg syndrome), or inflammatory nodules (sarcoidosis). Blood vessels are typically not seen on the surface of the iris. The presence of abnormal blood vessels (iris neovascularization) suggests ocular ischemia, a condition most commonly seen in association with proliferative diabetic retinopathy or central retinal vein occlusion. Patients with iris neovascularization often develop severe, recalcitrant glaucoma and require urgent ophthalmologic consultation.

The crystalline lens is a transparent, biconcave structure aligned at the center of the pupil. The lens refracts light to achieve fine focus on the retina at various distances. A penlight can be used to assess the lens, although this is difficult through a nondilated pupil. Cataracts can appear as focal opacities or a more diffuse yellow to brown discoloration. Cataractous changes are most easily assessed in the primary care setting by use of a direct ophthalmoscope to observe irregularities in a patient's red reflex. Cataracts occur naturally with age, but they can also be a sign of trauma or certain systemic conditions (e.g., diabetes, myotonic dystrophy, Fabry disease, corticosteroid exposure). Although cataracts almost never represent an ophthalmic emergency, they can cause significant visual impairment and can be removed surgically to improve a patient's quality of life.

Posterior Segment

The posterior segment is composed of vital eye structures including the vitreous, retina, and optic nerve. Examination of the posterior segment requires the assistance of an ophthalmoscope. A complete assessment of the posterior segment requires a formal evaluation by an ophthalmologist; however, the primary care provider can use a direct ophthalmoscope to identify some important, visually significant abnormalities. The direct ophthalmoscope produces a highly magnified image of the retina and optic nerve (approximately 15×). The examination should be performed in a dark room with the examiner at approximately the same height as the patient. While the examiner is standing several feet from the patient, the light from the direct ophthalmoscope is used to assess the red reflex. Any asymmetry or opacity suggests ocular disease, which should be further investigated. The examiner then takes the ophthalmoscope, held to the same eye that is being evaluated, and approaches the pupil slowly. The ophthalmoscope should be aimed slightly nasally to identify the optic disk. As the retina becomes visible, the Rekoss disk (the dial on the side of the ophthalmoscope) is turned to correct for the combined refractive errors of the examiner and patient to bring the retinal features into focus.

The vitreous humor is the gelatinous material that fills the posterior segment and attaches to the retina at several points. Under normal circumstances, it should be optically clear, allowing a crisp view of the retinal structures. With normal aging, the vitreous undergoes degenerative changes and eventually detaches from the retina (posterior vitreous detachment), causing dark floating spots (floaters). Multiple pathologic conditions can cause an abrupt increase in floaters, including vitreous hemorrhage (e.g., trauma, diabetes, retinal tears), inflammatory conditions (e.g., uveitis, endophthalmitis), and retinal detachments. Floaters associated with flashing lights, a black curtain covering part of the visual field, or decreased vision could represent serious disease, such as a retinal detachment, and should be urgently evaluated by an ophthalmologist.

The optic disk is the coalescence of the retinal nerve fiber layer as it leaves the globe to form the optic nerve. In the normal eye, it can be seen as a slightly oval pink-yellow disk with a small white depression at its center (optic cup). The cup normally encompasses 10% to 30% of the area of the optic nerve. A larger cup often represents a normal physiologic change but can be worrisome for glaucoma-related damage. With use of a direct ophthalmoscope, the optic disk should appear flat with distinct margins. A blurring of the margins suggests optic disk elevation, which can be seen with a multitude of conditions, including ocular inflammatory disorders or increased intracranial pressure. A flat, pale disk suggests optic atrophy associated with chronic ocular or neurologic disease.

The central retinal vein and artery travel along the center of the optic nerve and enter the globe through the optic disk. The vessels separate to form two main branches temporally, known as the *arcades*, and two smaller branches nasally. At the disk margin, the vessels can be identified by their size. Veins are approximately 1.5 times the size of arteries. In addition, the vessels should follow a smooth course with no significant tortuosity. The examiner should note the crossing of the arteries and veins. In a hypertensive patient, arteriovenous nicking is sometimes visible. The area between the temporal arcades is the macula. The fovea—responsible for central high-acuity vision—is located at the center of the macula. This region should be flat and regular and devoid of hemorrhages or exudates.

The peripheral retina, or the regions beyond the arcades, is difficult to evaluate with a direct ophthalmoscope. However, by having a well-dilated patient look in various cardinal directions, it is possible to view some extramacular retinal detail. If the decision is made to dilate the patient's pupils, the provider should always ensure that the anterior chamber appears grossly deep and ask the patient if there has ever been a negative reaction to dilation. If a pupil is dilated in a shallow chamber, there is a risk of causing acute angle-closure glaucoma—one of the most feared complications of dilating drops. Also, if the provider believes the patient requires urgent ophthalmic examination, it is best to leave the pupils undilated so that the ophthalmologist can make a formal assessment of the pupils. If the pupils are dilated, the peripheral retina should appear uniformly pink-orange. As with the macula, any elevation, hemorrhage, or exudates are abnormal and should be evaluated further by an ophthalmologist.

SIGNS AND SYMPTOMS OF OCULAR DISEASE
Red Eye

Red eye is one of the most common ocular concerns in the primary care setting. Often the underlying disorder is self-limited with minimum visual consequences, but it is important to recognize serious, vision-threatening conditions. The term *red eye* denotes hyperemia of the conjunctiva or sclera. It is also sometimes used to denote redness of the adnexal structures or periocular area.

The most common cause of red eye is conjunctivitis, which may be allergic, bacterial, or viral. Conjunctivitis is covered in great detail in Chapter 55. Patients may also be seen with a red eye from episcleritis or scleritis. These are inflammatory conditions, although scleritis may rarely have a microbial cause. Episcleritis is almost always self-limited and rarely requires topical anti-inflammatory therapy. This condition typically manifests with sectoral inflammation and is associated with foreign body sensation. Scleritis is a more serious condition that can be vision threatening and is often related to an underlying autoimmune disorder. Scleritis produces a boring sensation of pain and the eye is exquisitely tender to palpation. Patients with possible scleritis should be promptly referred to an ophthalmologist.

The uveal tract of the eye consists of the iris, ciliary body, and choroid. Any or all of these structures may become inflamed, causing red eye. Uveitis is an inflammation of any of these layers, including the posterior uveal structures. Iritis is an inflammation of the anterior uveal structure, the iris. These inflammatory conditions are often associated with systemic disorders, many with an autoimmune component.

Patients with uveitis should be referred to an ophthalmologist. Table 52.1 presents these and other ocular disorders that must be considered in the differential diagnosis of a patient with red eye.

Accurate diagnosis is critical in determining the appropriate therapy for red eye. For example, treatment of bacterial conjunctivitis with steroids may exacerbate the infection, and steroid use with a corneal abrasion or ulcer may lead to corneal melting and serious visual consequences. Similarly, treatment of herpetic keratitis with an antibacterial may delay appropriate therapy and lead to potentially serious consequences. Many ocular disorders can be difficult to diagnose accurately without a slit lamp. The health care provider should not hesitate to refer patients to an ophthalmologist when treatment does not produce the expected result or when the diagnosis remains obscure.

Vision Loss and Other Visual Disturbances

Visual disturbances can include decreased central or peripheral vision, metamorphopsia (distorted images), photopsia (light flashes), or vitreous opacities (floaters). Visual loss may be unilateral or bilateral, may be transient or permanent, may occur suddenly or gradually, and may involve central or peripheral vision. Complaints of decreased peripheral vision are not common in the primary care setting because patients usually perceive only significant scotomas. "Sudden" vision loss must be distinguished from "suddenly noticed." A gradual vision loss in one eye may be suddenly noticed when the better eye is inadvertently occluded by a hand or some other object. The differential diagnosis box lists common causes of sudden and gradual vision loss. Table 52.2 presents the signs, symptoms, and management of sudden vision loss.

TABLE 52.1	Red Eye: Differential Diagnosis and Management Guidelines		
Disorder	**Signs and Symptoms**	**Pain**	**Management**
DISORDERS ASSOCIATED WITH OCULAR ADNEXA REDNESS			
Blepharitis	Ocular burning; eyelid margins red with scaling or crusting	Yes	Warm compresses; daily lid scrubs; erythromycin or bacitracin ophthalmic ointment for anterior blepharitis; see Chapter 54
Cellulitis			
Orbital	Vision frequently affected; localized tenderness, erythema, edema; fever; proptosis	Yes	Referral to ophthalmologist for hospitalization, intravenous antibiotics; see Chapter 59
Preseptal	Vision usually not affected; localized tenderness, erythema, edema; fever sometimes present	Yes	Systemic, broad-spectrum antibiotics; office follow-up visit in 12–24 h; see Chapter 59
Dacryocystitis	Chronic tearing; eyelash crusting; localized tenderness; circumscribed erythema, edema in the inferior medial canthal area; may be able to express purulent material from the nasolacrimal duct	Yes	Warm compresses; gentle massage; topical and/or systemic antibiotics; see Chapter 58
Eyelid Lesions			
Chalazion	Nontender in chronic lesions; localized erythema, edema of eyelids	No	Warm compresses; daily lid scrubs; lid massage; see Chapter 54
Hordeolum	Localized tenderness, erythema, edema of eyelids; internal lesions pointing to external or internal eyelid surface; external lesions pointing to eyelid margin	Yes	Warm compresses; lid scrubs for recurrent lesions; see Chapter 54
Soft tissue hemorrhage	Localized tenderness sometimes present; erythema, ecchymosis, edema of affected area	±	Cold compresses; if orbital floor fracture suspected, computed tomography scan
DISORDERS ASSOCIATED WITH OCULAR SURFACE REDNESS			
Angle-closure glaucoma	Severe pain; nausea, vomiting; halos around lights; photophobia; cornea cloudy with variable decrease in vision; conjunctival hyperemia; pupil mid-dilated and fixed; firm globe; shallow anterior chamber	Yes	Emergent referral to ophthalmologist; with physician consultation, consider acetazolamide, 500 mg IV or PO, topical beta blocker
Chemical exposure	Pain; conjunctival hyperemia, chemosis; corneal haze; decreased visual acuity	Yes	Immediate copious irrigation essential; emergent referral to ophthalmologist; see Chapter 61
Conjunctivitis			
Allergic	Pruritus; conjunctival hyperemia, chemosis; watery or stringy discharge	No	Avoidance of allergens; cold compresses; topical and/or systemic medication; see Chapter 55
Bacterial	Photophobia with blepharospasm; mucopurulent discharge with eyelash mattering; edema, hyperemia; preauricular adenopathy only with hyperacute disorder	±	Topical antibiotic drops; systemic antibiotics necessary for gonococcal or chlamydial cause; see Chapter 55
Viral	Acute onset often associated with systemic illness; photophobia or foreign body sensation; preauricular adenopathy; hyperemia; chemosis; watery discharge; classic dendritic corneal lesion present with herpes simplex; periocular lesions present with herpes zoster ophthalmicus	±	Supportive treatment, including cool compresses, topical artificial tears; referral to ophthalmologist for herpetic conjunctivitis; see Chapter 55

TABLE 52.1   Red Eye: Differential Diagnosis and Management Guidelines—cont'd

Disorder	Signs and Symptoms	Pain	Management
Corneal foreign body, abrasion, or ulcer	Foreign body sensation with intense pain; photophobia; conjunctival hyperemia; may have decreased visual acuity; ulcers usually seen as white or opaque corneal lesion; immediate prior history of trauma common with abrasion but not erosion	Yes	Topical antibiotics (for prophylaxis) and systemic pain relievers in abrasions and after foreign body removal; no patching generally, never with ulcers or contact lens–related problems; urgent referral to ophthalmologist for erosions, emergent referral for ulcers; see Chapter 56
Dry eye	Sandy, gritty, foreign body sensation; burning; pruritus; conjunctival hyperemia; decreased visual acuity	±	Topical artificial tears; lubricating ointments at night; warm compresses; gentle eyelid massage; evaluation for systemic disorders; see Chapter 57
Episcleritis or scleritis	Mild to severe pain; circumscribed erythema of affected sclera; vision unaffected	Yes	Episcleritis usually self-limited; with possible scleritis, referral to ophthalmologist
Hyphema	Microscopic or visible blood layering in anterior chamber usually after blunt trauma; often associated with other ocular symptoms	Yes	Urgent referral to ophthalmologist
Iritis or uveitis	Pain; photophobia; conjunctival hyperemia; pupil constriction; may have epiphora but no mucopurulent discharge	Yes	Urgent referral to ophthalmologist
Keratitis	Pain, photophobia; conjunctival hyperemia; corneal cloudiness with stromal involvement	Yes	Urgent referral to ophthalmologist
Pinguecula and pterygium	Ocular irritation or pain when inflamed; dry eye symptoms; fleshy lesion medial on conjunctiva; with pterygium, lesion extending onto cornea	Yes	Ocular lubricants; topical NSAIDs; with pterygium, routine referral to ophthalmologist; see Chapter 60
Subconjunctival hemorrhage	No subjective symptoms; bright red spot of blood visible under overlying conjunctiva; remainder of conjunctiva white	No	Reassurance; no treatment necessary

NSAIDs, Nonsteroidal anti-inflammatory drugs.

TABLE 52.2   Sudden Vision Loss: Management Guidelines

Disorder	Signs and Symptoms	Management
Acute angle-closure glaucoma	See Table 52.1	See Table 52.1
Central retinal vessel occlusion	Arterial occlusion: vision loss typically more profound; cherry red macula seen against paleness of surrounding retina Venous occlusion: metamorphopsia; flame hemorrhages and dilated tortuous veins in ocular fundus	Urgent referral to ophthalmologist; with arterial occlusion, permanent vision loss possible in <2 h; physician consultation to determine underlying cause
Hyphema or other trauma	See Table 52.1	See Table 52.1
Endophthalmitis	May or may not be associated with pain; lid edema; conjunctival injection; retinal hemorrhage	Emergent referral to ophthalmologist; visual prognosis dependent on immediate treatment
Iritis or uveitis	See Table 52.1	See Table 52.1
Meningitis	Systemic presentation of meningitis; see Chapter 178	See Chapter 178
Migraine	Scintillating scotomas; photopsia; headache; photophobia; phonophobia; see Chapter 177	See Chapter 177
Optic neuritis	Variable vision loss; papilledema (present in one-third of patients); pain on eye movement; sore globe	Referral to ophthalmologist within 24–48 h
Retinal hemorrhage (macular area)	Central vision loss with no associated pain	Ophthalmologist or physician consultation; management dependent on cause
Stroke	Visual field defects; amaurosis fugax; hemianopia; see Chapter 173	Immediate emergency department referral for all patients with suspected cerebrovascular accident
Vitreous hemorrhage	Ocular fundus possibly obscured in severe cases; if retina visible, examination may reveal signs of the underlying causative disorder (diabetic retinopathy, retinopathy of prematurity, retinal tear or detachment, vitreous detachment, trauma)	Ophthalmologist or physician consultation; management dependent on cause

DIFFERENTIAL DIAGNOSIS

Vision Loss

SUDDEN
- Acute angle-closure glaucoma
- Central retinal vessel occlusion
- Hyphema or other trauma
- Endophthalmitis
- Iritis or uveitis
- Migraine
- Optic neuritis
- Retinal hemorrhage (macular area)
- Stroke
- Vitreous hemorrhage
- Corneal ulcer
- Giant cell arteritis (temporal arteritis)

GRADUAL
- Amblyopia
- Cataracts
- Corneal opacities
- Primary open-angle glaucoma
- Iritis or uveitis[a]
- Macular degeneration[a]
- Pituitary tumor[a]
- Retinal detachment[a]
- Vitreous opacities

[a]May manifest with sudden-onset vision loss depending severity of disease or complications.

Amaurosis fugax is a transient, unilateral episode of vision loss. This condition is typically caused by small embolic plaques that transiently occlude retinal circulation. Patients will initially notice a focal pattern of visual field loss that progresses to diffuse or total loss of vision that can last seconds to minutes. According to recent reviews, altitudinal patterns of visual field loss at the onset of symptoms, in contrast to diffuse patterns, are more indicative of cardiac etiologies.[11] In these cases, an embolic workup and cardiovascular evaluation are warranted.

Transient visual loss, photopsia, floaters, photophobia, metamorphopsia, or scintillating scotomas may accompany migraine headaches. Such ocular symptoms can occur without an associated headache. However, unless the patient has a clear past history of ocular migraine, these patients should be referred to an ophthalmologist to rule out other potential problems, such as retinal or vitreous detachment.

Metamorphopsia (warped or distorted central vision) is commonly seen with macular degeneration as well as a host of other ocular conditions. Any patient reporting new-onset visual distortion or a change in previously noted metamorphopsia should be referred to an ophthalmologist. Effective treatments are available for certain types of age-related macular degeneration.

Photopsia (flashes or flickers of light) may result from a retinal problem or cortical stimulation. Photopsia may be an indication of a retinal tear or a posterior vitreous detachment with retinal traction. Cortically induced photopsia may indicate migraine headache or occipital epilepsy. Retinal detachment may also produce a persistent symptom described as a curtain, shadow, or veil falling over part of the visual field.

The vitreous degenerates and liquefies with aging. When this occurs, aggregates form vitreous floaters, which are perceived by the patient as gray or black shapes floating within the visual field. Depending on the size and number, floaters may be simply annoying or may cause visual disability. If floaters occur suddenly or increase in frequency or quantity, urgent referral to an ophthalmologist is necessary. These symptoms may indicate the presence of a posterior vitreous detachment, primary vitreous hemorrhage, retinal tear, or retinal detachment.

Ocular and Periocular Pain

Ocular or periocular pain can include any discomfort in or around the eye and may be described as burning, aching, throbbing, boring, stabbing, or irritating, as with a foreign body sensation. Any condition that stimulates the numerous pain receptors in the eyelids, cornea, conjunctiva, and uveal tract will cause ocular or periocular pain. Any inflammatory disorder of the conjunctiva, superficial layers of the cornea, or uveal tract can cause ocular irritation, burning, discomfort, or frank pain. Symptoms may be related to exposure to environmental irritants such as tobacco smoke or chemical fumes. Pain may also be referred from adjacent structures innervated by the ophthalmic division of cranial nerve V (trigeminal nerve). Noninflammatory conditions affecting the optic nerve, retina, or vitreous do not usually result in pain.

Pain may occur coincidentally with other ocular symptoms, including decreased visual acuity, photophobia, ocular discharge, eyelid edema or erythema, ptosis, proptosis, or corneal cloudiness. Important history includes decrease in visual acuity, suddenness of onset, associated symptoms (including systemic symptoms such as nausea or vomiting), contact lens use, exposure to ultraviolet light (such as during outdoor activities or arc welding), neurologic or systemic disorders, and trauma.

A complete ocular assessment should be performed in any patient with ocular pain. It is also important to examine the structures of the head and neck in any patient with a history of trauma. However, the eye should never be manipulated if there is any possibility of laceration or rupture of the ocular tissues. A shallow anterior chamber or abnormally shaped pupil may indicate a loss of aqueous humor secondary to a penetrating injury. Acute glaucoma should be excluded by measuring the intraocular pressure with a Tono-Pen or similar device or by palpating the globes and comparing the affected eye with the unaffected eye. Patients with a painful eye from acute glaucoma usually have associated redness, nausea, and vomiting. The cornea and conjunctiva may be assessed to identify abrasions or ulcers by applying fluorescein dye and examining the external eye under fluorescent light. Application of a topical anesthetic such as proparacaine hydrochloride 0.5% (Ophthaine) or tetracaine hydrochloride 0.5% (Pontocaine) will help differentiate the superficial pain caused by corneal surface disorders from pain resulting from problems with the deeper structures.[12]

It may be useful to approach the differential diagnosis of ocular pain by grouping possible causes according to accompanying symptoms. This approach is summarized in Table 52.3.

Other Ocular Signs and Symptoms

Epiphora is excessive tearing. There are many different causes of epiphora including dry eye syndrome, conjunctivitis, and obstruction of the normal tear drainage system. The patient

TABLE 52.3	Symptoms Associated With Ocular Pain and Possible Causes
Associated Symptom	**Possible Causes**
Photophobia	Acute glaucoma, migraine, corneal trauma, keratoconjunctivitis, iritis, uveitis, scleritis
Nausea and vomiting	Acute glaucoma, endophthalmitis
Itching	Chemical injury, severe dry eye, allergy
Pain on eye movement	Orbital pseudotumor, myositis, posterior scleritis, optic neuritis, trauma, orbital cellulitis
Foreign body sensation	Corneal ulcer or abrasion, conjunctivitis, overexposure to ultraviolet light, entropion, trichiasis, conjunctival or eyelid lesion (rule out actual corneal or conjunctival foreign body)

San Francisco, Ca: American Academy of Ophthalmology. Retrieved from www.aao.org/ppp.

4. American Diabetes Association. (2010). *Diabetes Care, 33*(Suppl. 1), S1–S2. Retrieved from https://doi.org/10.2337/dc10-S001.
5. Moyer, V. A., U.S. Preventive Services Task Force. (2013). Screening for glaucoma: U.S. Preventive services task force recommendation statement. *Annals of Internal Medicine, 159*(7), 484–489.
6. American Academy of Ophthalmology Preferred Practice Patterns Committee. (2010). Preferred practice pattern guidelines: Primary open-angle glaucoma. San Francisco, Ca: American Academy of Ophthalmology. Retrieved from www.aao.org/ppp.
7. Witting, M. D., & Goyal, D. (2003). Normal pupillary size in fluorescent and bright light. *Annals of Emergency Medicine, 41*, 247–250.
8. Blaustein, B. H. (1994). *Ocular manifestations of systemic disease.* New York: Churchill Livingstone.
9. Tamhankar, M. A., Biousse, V., Ying, G. S., et al. (2013). Isolated third, fourth, and sixth cranial nerve palsies from presumed microvascular versus other causes: A prospective study. *Ophthalmology, 120*(11), 2264–2269.
10. Bowling, B. (2016). *Kanski's clinical ophthalmology a systematic approach, 8th edition.* Sydney, Australia: Elsevier.
11. Pula, J. H., Kwan, K., Yuen, C., & Kattah, J. (2016). Update on the evaluation of transient vision loss. *Clinical Ophthalmology, 10*, 297–303.
12. Dargin, J. M., & Lowenstein, R. A. (2008). The painful eye. *Emergency Medicine Clinics of North America, 26*, 199–216.

should be referred to an ophthalmologist when no underlying cause is apparent or if the epiphora worsens.

Ocular discharge may be clear, watery, purulent or mucopurulent, stringy, or ropy. The differential diagnosis of an ocular disorder may be aided by observing the nature of abnormal ocular secretions. Pus in the conjunctival sac causes the eyelashes to stick together and is most common in mucopurulent conjunctivitis. A profuse watery discharge with a burning or gritty sensation and pain may be present in viral conjunctivitis. Pruritus associated with a discharge varying from watery to a stringy, mucus-like consistency may indicate allergic conjunctivitis.

Photophobia may occur for no known reason. However, almost any condition resulting in ocular irritation or inflammation may cause photophobia. Conditions to consider include uveitis, conjunctivitis, conjunctival or corneal foreign bodies, corneal abrasion, keratitis, congenital glaucoma in infants, and acute glaucoma in adults. Photophobia may also result from toxic exposures, as seen in arc welders, swimmers, or skiers who do not use lenses for protection from excessive direct or reflected ultraviolet light exposure.

Pruritus is the most common complaint in allergic conditions, including allergic conjunctivitis. The symptom is usually bilateral and may be seasonal with associated hay fever symptoms. Unilateral pruritus associated with erythema and chemosis may be iatrogenic or caused by an allergic reaction to topical ophthalmic preparations or, commonly, the preservative in the preparation. Patients with other forms of non-allergic conjunctivitis, severe dry eye, or a chemical injury may also experience pruritus.

REFERENCES

1. American Academy of Ophthalmology Preferred Practice Patterns Committee. (2005). Preferred practice pattern guidelines: Comprehensive adult medical eye evaluation. San Francisco, Ca: American Academy of Ophthalmology. Retrieved from www.aao.org/ppp.
2. U.S. Preventive Services Task Force. (2009). Screening for impaired visual acuity in older adults: U.S. Preventive Services Task Force Recommendation Statement. *Annals of Internal Medicine, 151*(1), 37–43.
3. American Academy of Ophthalmology Preferred Practice Patterns Committee. (2012). Preferred practice pattern guidelines: Diabetic retinopathy.

CHAPTER **53**

CATARACTS
Zubair Ansari • James T. Banta

Priority differentials include age-related macular degeneration and diabetic retinopathy.

DEFINITION AND EPIDEMIOLOGY

Ancient physicians thought that a crystalloid structure (lens) rested in the center of the eye and was responsible for vision. People lost vision when an abnormal humor developed and flowed in front of the lens. They called this a *cataract* (Latin for waterfall).[1] Today, the term *cataract* refers to the opacification of the crystalline lens of the eye. The most recent World Health Organization estimate lists cataract as the leading cause of blindness worldwide, accounting for 48% of world blindness affecting 18 million people. Cataract causes some degree of visual impairment in nearly 20.5 million Americans or one in six Americans aged 40 years and older, and this rate is expected to rise in the foreseeable future.[2]

The most common form of cataract is associated with increasing age and progressive oxidative damage to the crystalline lens. Every person who lives long enough will develop some degree of cataract. As life expectancy increases and the population ages, visual loss from cataract will have an even greater medical and economic impact. In the United States, prevalence estimates of visually significant cataract increase with age for both men and women, from 4% and 10% for men and women aged 55 to 64 years to 39% and 46% for those older than 75 years.[2]

PATHOPHYSIOLOGY

The anatomic function of the crystalline lens is to focus incident light on the retina. Opacification of this lens, a cataract, prevents light from focusing on the retina, causing loss of vision. The natural aging process of the crystalline lens involves an increase in mass, thickness, and the development of a yellow hue with an associated loss of accommodative capacity. Initially these changes cause minimal visual impairment, but with time the lens becomes more opaque, eventually leading to a progressive decline in vision. Cataracts develop in everyone with increasing age, but their formation is hastened by trauma, exposure to certain medications (e.g., corticosteroids), metabolic disorders such as diabetes, oxidative stress from smoking or ultraviolet light, and radiation. Congenital cataracts can also form; these can be idiopathic in nature or can be caused by an underlying infection or metabolic disease.[2]

CLINICAL PRESENTATION AND PHYSICAL EXAMINATION

The classic presentation of age-related cataract is non-painful, progressive loss of visual acuity. Patients often describe blurred or hazy vision and haloes or significant glare with bright lights. A common complaint is glare from headlights while driving at night. Frequent changes in a patient's eyeglass prescription (typically increasing myopia) are common in older adults as a result of cataract progression.

There are several cataract types, each associated with particular clinical complaints. Nuclear sclerotic cataracts tend to affect distance vision more than reading vision, whereas cortical cataracts result in more symptoms of glare in dim illumination. Posterior subcapsular cataracts tend to progress more rapidly and occur in younger patients than do nuclear sclerotic and cortical cataracts. Posterior subcapsular cataracts can cause glare symptoms and difficulty reading in bright illumination.[2] Cataracts may progress during the course of months to years. Patients may occasionally report a sudden decrease in vision. In most patients the cataract has progressed slowly but is not noted because of good vision in the fellow eye. Traumatic cataracts can sometimes rapidly form in the setting of severe ocular trauma. Nontraumatic cataracts are usually bilateral but may be asymmetric.[2]

PHYSICAL EXAMINATION

Cataracts are often an isolated finding, but a full ophthalmic examination is indicated to determine if other causes of visual loss may be present. A cataract will not cause redness of the conjunctiva, corneal haze, or pain—except in rare instances of traumatic or hypermature cataracts. The pupils should constrict normally to light. Direct ophthalmoscopy may reveal hazy visualization of the optic nerve and retina as a result of the lens opacity. Cataractous lens changes are best appreciated with use of a direct ophthalmoscope with a dilated pupil, focusing on the red reflex. Nuclear sclerotic changes may cause the reflex to appear dull or asymmetric. Cortical lens changes may cause focal, segmental, or spoke-like dark areas in the reflex (Fig. 53.1); posterior subcapsular changes typically appear as a central, dark plaque (Fig. 53.2).

DIAGNOSTICS

No diagnostic tests are recommended.

DIFFERENTIAL DIAGNOSIS

 Rule out age-related macular degeneration and diabetic retinopathy. A full ophthalmologic examination may be necessary to distinguish these entities in some patients.

Many conditions can cause progressive loss of vision.

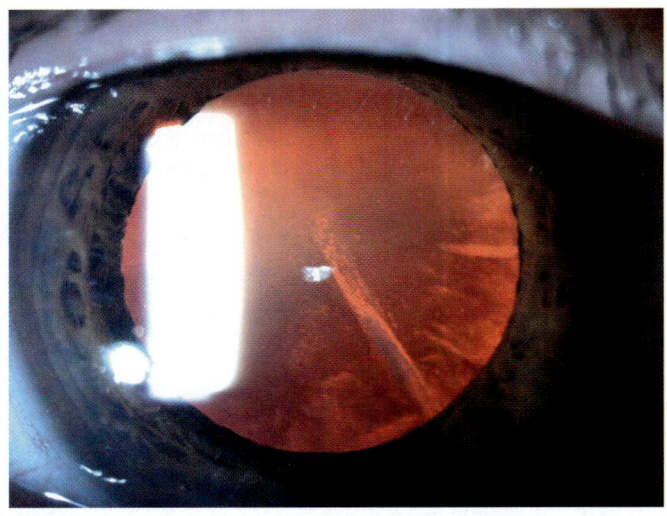

FIG. 53.1 Retroillumination photo demonstrating cortical "spokes," a finding frequently seen in people with diabetes.

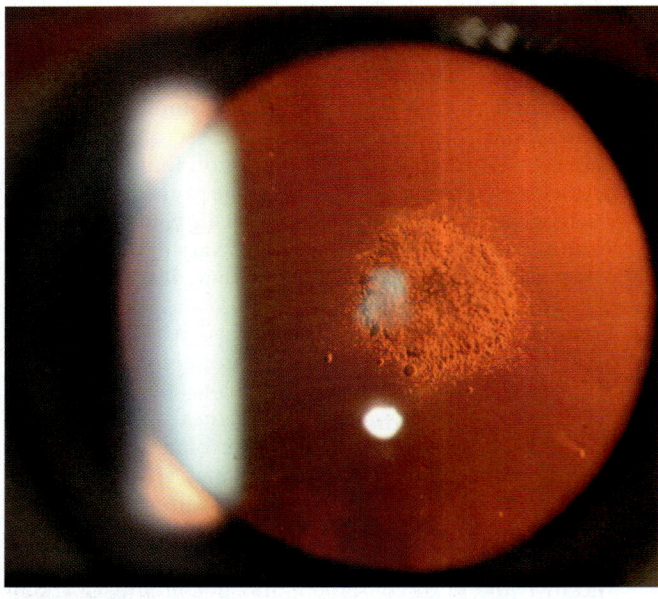

FIG. 53.2 Retroillumination photo demonstrating a small paracentral posterior subcapsular cataract.

INTERPROFESSIONAL COLLABORATIVE MANAGEMENT

Nonpharmacologic Management

Early lens changes can often be handled conservatively with a change in eyeglass prescription that may improve the patient's visual acuity. Cessation of certain tasks made difficult by the cataract, such as driving at night, may be necessary. Magnifiers, increased font size, and other visual aids may temporarily ameliorate the visual acuity loss.

Pharmacologic Management

No medical treatments or topical drops are available to reverse lens opacification.

Indication for Referral and Hospitalization

Referral for surgical treatment of cataracts is indicated when the cataract has caused visual decline to the point at which the patient's vision no longer meets his or her needs. This level will vary from patient to patient according to the patient's daily activities and warrants a discussion with the ophthalmologist on the risks and benefits of surgery.

Surgical cataract extraction is the most frequently performed surgery in the United States, and is highly successful and safe. The procedure consists of using an ultrasound device to "emulsify" the lens into microscopic fragments that are vacuumed out of the eye and replaced with an artificial lens.

LIFE-SPAN CONSIDERATIONS

In older individuals, cataracts have been associated with decreased quality of life by causing functional loss and decreased independence. Impaired vision has been shown to cause cognitive impairment that is improved by cataract surgery.[4] Impaired vision is also a safety risk. Drivers with cataracts are more likely to be involved in an at-fault automobile accident compared with those without cataracts.[5] Surgical treatment of cataract was also found to reduce the risk of falls and hip fracture.[6] Improved cataract surgical techniques, such as topical anesthesia and suture-less, clear corneal incisions, allow patients with significant medical comorbidities to be considered for cataract extraction.[7]

COMPLICATIONS

Complications of a cataract are very rare, but a hypermature cataract can cause intraocular inflammation and glaucoma, both of which are cured with surgical removal of the cataract.[2] To prevent surgical complications, it is vital for the patient to provide the ophthalmologist with a current medication list; of particular importance is the use of any systemic alpha$_1$-adrenergic antagonists, such as tamsulosin (Flomax). The current or prior use of such medications can cause intraoperative floppy iris syndrome (IFIS), which can complicate cataract surgery and result in longer postoperative recovery and poorer outcomes.[3] IFIS is most frequently associated with the selective alpha$_{1A}$ antagonist tamsulosin, but it has also been reported with other nonselective alpha$_1$ antagonists, such as terazosin (Hytrin) and doxazosin (Cardura). IFIS has been reported to occur several years after the discontinuation of tamsulosin. Studies have shown that when the surgeon is forewarned about the use of tamsulosin, the risks associated with IFIS are greatly reduced.[3]

PATIENT AND FAMILY EDUCATION

- Patients should be educated that all crystalline lenses will eventually opacify; the rate varies from person to person.
- Medical management, visual aids, and alterations of activities may ameliorate the effect of early cataract formation.
- Cataract progression will continue. Surgery may eventually be required when the patient determines the cataract has become visually significant to the point that it affects activities of daily living.

HEALTH PROMOTION

Cigarette smoking, ultraviolet light, and glycemic control in diabetics are modifiable risk factors of cataract formation.[2] Patients at risk for contusive or penetrating ocular trauma and chemical exposure should be encouraged to use appropriate eye protection.

REFERENCES

1. Aulus Cornelius Celsus. G. F. Collier (transl.) De Medicinae. OL 52211W 1831.
2. American Academy of Ophthalmology. Basic and clinical science course: lens and cataract, San Francisco. 2013.
3. Haridas, A., Syrimi, M., Al-Ahmar, B., & Hingorani, M. (2013). Intraoperative floppy iris syndrome (IFIS) in patients receiving tamsulosin or doxazosin—a UK-based comparison of incidence and complication rates. *Graefe's Archive for Clinical and Experimental Ophthalmology*, 251(6), 1541–1545.
4. Elyashiv, S. M., Shabtai, E. L., & Belkin, M. (2014). Correlation between visual acuity and cognitive functions. *The British Journal of Ophthalmology*, 98(1), 129–132.
5. Mennemeyer, S. T., Owsley, C., & McGwin, G., Jr. (2013). Reducing older driver motor vehicle collisions via earlier cataract surgery. *Accident Analysis and Prevention*, 61, 203–211.
6. Keay, L., Palagyi, A., McCluskey, P., Lamoureux, E., Pesudovs, K., Lo, S., et al. (2014). Falls in older people with cataract, a longitudinal evaluation of impact and risk: The FOCUS study protocol. *Injury Prevention: Journal of the International Society for Child and Adolescent Injury Prevention*, 20(4), e7.
7. Lai, F. H., Lok, J. Y., Chow, P. P., & Young, A. L. (2014). Clinical outcomes of cataract surgery in very elderly adults. *Journal of the American Geriatrics Society*, 62(1), 165–170.

CHAPTER **54**

BLEPHARITIS, HORDEOLUM, AND CHALAZION

Swarup S. Swaminathan • James T. Banta

 Ophthalmologist referral for any patient with chronic lid swelling, erythema, notching of the lid margin, or an atypical lid lesion associated with loss of lashes for biopsy to rule out sebaceous carcinoma, basal cell carcinoma, squamous cell carcinoma, or other malignant or benign tumors.

DEFINITION AND EPIDEMIOLOGY

Inflammation of the eyelids, also known as *blepharitis,* is one of the most frequently encountered ocular diseases. Blepharitis may be of infectious or inflammatory etiology. The disease can be divided into two basic categories anatomically: anterior and posterior blepharitis.[1,2] Anterior blepharitis involves the anterior lid margin surrounding the eyelashes and is usually associated with staphylococcal infection or seborrhea. Staphylococcal blepharitis is a disorder that predominantly affects young to middle-aged women, with exacerbations and remissions of disease. Seborrheic blepharitis is seen in a somewhat older age group, with an equal incidence in men and women.[3] Posterior blepharitis involves the posterior lid margin and is characterized by meibomian gland dysfunction, sometimes associated with rosacea. Meibomian glands are enlarged sebaceous glands aligned in a row posterior to the eyelashes. They produce a clear lipid secretion that makes up the outer layer of the tear film. All forms of blepharitis may result in a disruption of the ocular surface, dry eye syndrome, and possibly the development of hordeola or chalazia. A hordeolum is an acute infection and inflammation of one of the glands in the eyelid, whereas a chalazion is a chronic, sterile, nontender lipogranulomatous inflammatory lesion of the meibomian gland. The term "stye," used in common parlance, can refer to either of

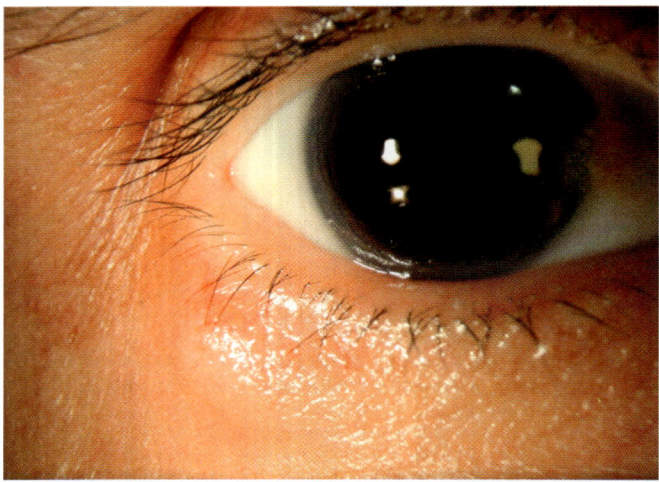

F I G . **54.1**   Unlike a hordeolum, a chalazion typically is a lid nodule with minimal erythema or pain, as illustrated in this photograph.

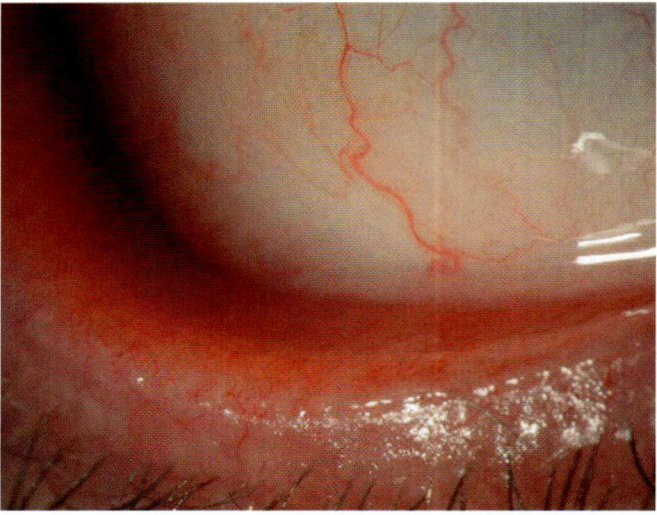

F I G . **54.2**   Lid margin telangiectasis and erythema, as demonstrated in this photograph, often accompany meibomian gland dysfunction in posterior forms of blepharitis.

these conditions. Without treatment, a hordeolum can lead to the formation of a chalazion.

PATHOPHYSIOLOGY

Anterior staphylococcal blepharitis is thought to be caused by an abnormal cell-mediated response to *Staphylococcus aureus*, ultimately resulting in lid margin inflammation. Anterior seborrheic blepharitis is associated with generalized seborrhea that may involve the scalp, nasolabial folds, skin behind the ears, and sternum. Posterior blepharitis is caused by meibomian gland dysfunction and alterations in meibomian gland secretions. Bacterial lipases may result in formation of free fatty acids, increasing the melting point of the meibum and preventing its expression from the glands, possibly enabling growth of *S. aureus* and the development of a hordeolum.[4] Certain persons may be predisposed to this condition, and hormones may play a role in creating an environment that promotes lipase-producing bacteria that alter glandular secretion.[5]

Once the meibomian gland is obstructed from excessive meibomian oil secretions or solidification of the meibum, a hordeolum may then develop.

CLINICAL PRESENTATION AND PHYSICAL EXAMINATION

Symptoms of blepharitis are often caused by ocular tear film instability and dry eye. Patients complain of burning, foreign body sensation, tearing, photophobia, itching, redness, discharge, and swollen erythematous eyelids, often worse in the morning.[6] Remissions and exacerbations are characteristic. A hordeolum or chalazion may occur at any age as a gradually enlarging localized nodule (Fig. 54.1). A hordeolum is usually painful, characterized by erythema and edema. On the other hand, a chalazion is painless and often characterized by patients as a "lump" along the eyelid. Both may cause cosmetic disfigurement and mechanical ptosis. If large, the lesion may mechanically press on the corneal surface and induce astigmatism and blurred vision.[7]

PHYSICAL EXAMINATION

The patient's face, ocular adnexa, and eye should be carefully inspected. Patients with staphylococcal blepharitis may have

lid margin erythema with fine ulceration at the base of the lashes and collarettes of fibrin along the lash. Lashes may be absent, broken, or misdirected. Patients with seborrheic blepharitis may have greasy scales along the lid margin and lashes with excess oily meibomian secretion and foamy tears. These patients may also have diffuse seborrhea with dandruff of the scalp and scaling of the brows, behind the ears, and at the base of the nose. *Demodex* blepharitis, caused by the eyelash mite, is characterized by cylindrical debris (collarette formation) encasing the base of eyelash follicles. Patients with posterior blepharitis may have hyperemia and telangiectasis of the lid margin (Fig. 54.2) and an oily and frothy tear film. Pressure on the lid margin results in expression of thick inspissated secretions. Rosacea is commonly associated with meibomian gland dysfunction, so these patients should be inspected for erythema with telangiectasis over the cheeks and nose, pustular skin eruption, and sebaceous gland hypertrophy typified by rhinophyma.[3] All types of blepharitis may also cause conjunctival injection, corneal infiltrates, excess tearing, lid crusting, discharge, and inflammation of the lid margin (see Fig. 54.2).

When a patient with a hordeolum or chalazion is examined, the lid should be palpated for swelling and masses, and the eyelid should be everted. Hordeola and chalazia are sometimes clinically indistinguishable. However, as previously mentioned, a hordeolum is often acute, tender, warm, and erythematous, whereas a chalazion is more chronic and nontender.

DIAGNOSTICS

No diagnostic tests are indicated.

DIFFERENTIAL DIAGNOSIS

 Priority differentials include dry eye syndrome, conjunctivitis (viral, bacterial, or allergic), and sebaceous carcinoma.

Chronic lid swelling and ulceration may rarely be caused by sebaceous carcinoma, which is a potentially life-threatening disease.[8] Any patient with chronic lid swelling, erythema, notching of the lid margin, or an atypical lid lesion associated with loss of lashes should be referred to the ophthalmologist for biopsy to rule out sebaceous carcinoma, basal cell carcinoma, squamous cell carcinoma, or other malignant or benign tumors.

INTERPROFESSIONAL COLLABORATIVE MANAGEMENT

Nonpharmacologic Management

Lid hygiene is the mainstay of all blepharitis treatments. Warm compresses over both eyelid margins for 5 to 10 minutes loosen lid margin debris and remove secretions. After use of the compresses, patients may use commercially available lid scrub kits or warm water with diluted baby shampoo on a cotton tip applicator at the lid margin to decrease bacterial colonization.

Pharmacologic Management

After lid scrubs, a thin strip of antibiotic ointment, such as erythromycin or bacitracin, may be applied to the eyelid margins. Artificial tears may also be beneficial. Patients with a prominent conjunctivitis component can be treated with an antibiotic solution four times a day. An antimicrobial agent effective against the majority of staphylococci, such as tobramycin 0.3% (Tobrex ophthalmic solution), is a good choice for initial therapy. In severe cases, patients may benefit from oral doxycycline 50 mg by mouth twice daily.[9,10] Treatments for both anterior and posterior blepharitis often need to be maintained for months to years and occasionally indefinitely, given its chronicity. *Demodex* blepharitis is treated with the use of tea tree oil application to the eyelashes. A relatively new treatment option is the application of hypochlorous acid 0.01% (Avenova commercially) to the eyelid margins as a spray. This has been shown to significantly decrease the bacterial load present on skin surfaces, especially staphylococci.[11] It has been advocated as an efficacious therapy for blepharitis.

Hordeola are usually self-limited, spontaneously improving in 1 to 2 weeks with conservative treatment alone. Lesions may be treated with frequent application of warm, moist compresses with light massage over the lesion. Daily lid hygiene with lid scrubs is also beneficial. Topical antibiotics are generally not effective or indicated unless an accompanying infectious blepharoconjunctivitis is present. Systemic antibiotics are generally indicated only in rare cases of secondary eyelid cellulitis.

INDICATIONS FOR REFERRAL OR HOSPITALIZATION

Any patient for whom conservative treatment fails or who develops a secondary infection, such as conjunctivitis or cellulitis, should be referred to an ophthalmologist. Patients with recurrent, atypical lesions or unexplained vision loss should also be referred. Large persistent lesions may require incision and drainage by an ophthalmologist. Cultures are not indicated for isolated, uncomplicated cases of hordeolum.

Chalazia may be self-limited in 25% to 50% of cases and can be cured or improved with conservative treatment within 1 to 3 months.[12] Chronic chalazia may require steroid injection.[13] If this is not effective, lesions can be surgically incised and removed by an ophthalmologist. Table 54.1 summarizes the specific management of hordeola, chalazia, and the different forms of blepharitis.

LIFE-SPAN CONSIDERATIONS

Hordeola can affect individuals of all ages but are more common in children and adolescents. Chalazia can affect individuals of all ages but are more common in adults. Anterior staphylococcal blepharitis is more common in younger patients, and posterior blepharitis is more common in older patients.[14]

TABLE 54.1 Management of Lid Disorders

Disorder	Compresses	Antibiotic	Steroid	Other
HORDEOLUM *Internal:* Zeis or Moll gland infection *External:* meibomian gland infection	Frequent warm, moist compresses to hasten drainage	Not indicated	None	Lid scrubs, especially if lesions recur
CHALAZION Meibomian gland inflammation	Frequent warm compresses to liquefy glandular secretions	Not indicated	Intralesional corticosteroid injection is often effective	Lid scrubs with gentle massage to help express impacted secretions
BLEPHARITIS Anterior staphylococcal	Daily warm compresses to loosen crusts	Topical ophthalmic erythromycin or bacitracin ointment	None	Daily lid scrubs to reduce sebaceous secretions
Anterior seborrheic	Daily warm compresses to loosen crusts	None	Occasional topical steroid if inflammation prominent	Daily lid scrubs to help remove oily secretions
Anterior *Demodex*	Daily warm compresses	None	Occasional topical steroid if inflammation prominent	Tea tree oil application
Posterior	Daily warm, moist compresses	Oral doxycycline in severe cases	None	Daily lid scrubs and lid massage

COMPLICATIONS

In rare cases, a hordeolum may progress to preseptal cellulitis or abscess and require systemic antibiotics. Large lesions can induce corneal astigmatism and mechanical ptosis and may restrict the superior visual field. Chronic blepharitis may result in scarring and the loss of protective eyelashes.

PATIENT AND FAMILY EDUCATION

- Patient education should emphasize daily eyelid hygiene and lid scrubs.
- Scrub lid margins at the base of the lashes with a moistened cotton-tipped applicator or a small, soft face cloth moistened with a dilute concentration of baby shampoo. After the scrub, the patient should thoroughly rinse the area and pat it dry. Alternatively, patients may prefer to perform lid scrubs with dilute baby shampoo while in the shower using a cotton-tipped applicator or the tip of the finger.
- Replace mascara and eye makeup on a regular basis to reduce the likelihood of reinoculating lids with contaminated cosmetics.[15]

HEALTH PROMOTION

Daily eyelid hygiene helps reduce bacterial colonization and accumulation of sebaceous secretions, thereby modulating the symptoms of chronic blepharitis and preventing the formation of chalazia and hordeola.

REFERENCES

1. Matoba, A. Y., Harris, D. J., Meisler, D. M., et al. (2003). *Preferred practice pattern: Blepharitis.* San Francisco: American Academy of Ophthalmology.
2. Pasternak, A., & Irish, B. (2004). Ophthalmologic infections in primary care. *Clinics in Family Practice, 6*(1), 19–33.
3. Chandler, J. W., Sugar, J., & Edelhauser, H. F. (1994). External diseases: Cornea, conjunctiva, sclera, eyelids, lacrimal system. In *Textbook of ophthalmology* (8th ed.). St Louis, MO: Mosby.
4. Kanski, J. J. (2007). *Clinical ophthalmology: A systematic approach* (6th ed.). St Louis: Elsevier.
5. Dougherty, J. M., & McCulley, J. P. (1986). Bacterial lipases and chronic blepharitis. *Investigative Ophthalmology & Visual Science, 27,* 484.
6. Sethuraman, U., & Kamat, D. (2009). The red eye: Evaluation and management. *Clinical Pediatrics, 48*(6), 588–600.
7. Cosar, C. B., Rapuano, C. J., Cohen, E. J., et al. (2001). Chalazion as a cause of decreased vision after LASIK. *Cornea, 20,* 890–892.
8. Kass, L., & Hornblass, A. (1989). Sebaceous carcinoma of the ocular adnexa. *Survey of Ophthalmology, 33*(6), 477–490.
9. Dougherty, J. M., McCully, J. P., Silvany, R. E., et al. (1991). The role of tetracycline in chronic blepharitis. *Investigative Ophthalmology & Visual Science, 32,* 2970–2975.
10. Paranjpe, D. R., & Foulks, G. N. (2003). Therapy for meibomian gland disease. *Ophthalmology Clinics of North America, 16,* 37–42.
11. Stroman, D. W., Mintun, K., Epstein, A. B., et al. (2017). Reduction in bacterial load using hypochlorous acid hygiene solution on ocular skin. *Clinical Ophthalmology, 11,* 707–714.
12. Dua, H. S., & Nilawar, D. V. (1982). Nonsurgical therapy of chalazion. *American Journal of Ophthalmology, 94*(3), 424–425.
13. Ben Simon, G. J., Huang, L., Nakra, T., et al. (2005). Intralesional triamcinolone acetonide injection for primary and recurrent chalazia: Is it really effective? *Ophthalmology, 112*(5), 913–917.
14. Sutphin, J. E. (2005). *Basic and clinical science course: External disease and cornea.* San Francisco: American Academy of Ophthalmology.
15. Wilson, L. A., Julian, A. J., & Ahearn, D. G. (1975). The survival and growth of microorganisms in mascara during use. *American Journal of Ophthalmology, 79*(4), 596–601.

CHAPTER **55**

CONJUNCTIVITIS

Jacob Starr Duker • James T. Banta

 Ophthalmologist evaluation required for patients with conjunctivitis who experience any of the following[1]: Vision loss, pain, severe, purulent discharge, corneal involvement, recurrent episodes of conjunctivitis, or no response or worsening symptoms despite treatment.

DEFINITION AND EPIDEMIOLOGY

Conjunctivitis is inflammation of the bulbar or palpebral conjunctiva, the transparent mucosal tissue that lines the eye and inner surface of the eyelids.[2] About 1% of all primary care office visits are related to conjunctivitis.[3] Approximately 70% of patients with acute conjunctivitis initially visit a primary care provider for diagnosis and management.[2,4] Commonly referred to as *pink eye*, conjunctivitis actually consists of many different disorders. Infectious causes include viruses and bacteria. Noninfectious conjunctivitis is commonly caused by allergy, atopy, or exposure to toxins.[4]

Up to 70% of all infectious conjunctivitis is viral.[2] The most common causative organism is adenovirus, the same virus implicated in the common cold.[5] Bacterial conjunctivitis is the second most common cause of infectious conjunctivitis and the most common cause in the pediatric population.[6] Other infectious causes include virus infections such as herpes and molluscum contagiosum.

The most common cause of noninfectious conjunctivitis is allergic conjunctivitis, a condition seen most frequently in the spring and summer.[7] Approximately 15% of all eye-related complaints to a primary care provider are secondary to allergic conjunctivitis.[8] Other noninfectious causes include primary ocular diseases such as toxic or cicatricial conjunctivitis and systemic diseases such as graft-versus-host disease, systemic inflammatory disorders, or neoplastic processes.[1]

PATHOPHYSIOLOGY

Viral conjunctivitis is spread by direct contact or by proximity to an infected patient.[9] Because of its highly contagious nature, viral conjunctivitis is often seen in areas of overcrowding such as schools, nursing homes, and summer camps.[2,10] About 46% of people infected with viral conjunctivitis had positive viral cultures from swabs of their hands.[11] Similarly, bacterial overgrowth in the conjunctiva occurs directly from hand-eye contact with an infected individual or from the transfer of organisms in one's own nasal and sinus mucosa.[2]

Commonly known as *hay fever*, seasonal allergic conjunctivitis is typically secondary to environmental allergens, with ragweed being the most common (75%).[8,12] Perennial allergic conjunctivitis is caused by common household allergens such as household chemicals or pet dander. In both conditions, an inflammatory response occurs once the airborne allergen contacts the ocular surface.[10] Acute allergic conjunctivitis is characterized by an immunoglobulin E mast cell–mediated hypersensitivity.[8]

Vernal conjunctivitis and atopic conjunctivitis are chronic, mast cell, and lymphocyte-mediated immune processes.

Both are considered to be more severe and chronic forms of allergic conjunctivitis.[12] Environmental allergens can trigger exacerbations.[1,12]

Conjunctivitis from a medication typically occurs with long-term use (>1 month) of an eye drop.[10] Any eye drop can be causative, but conjunctivitis is most commonly encountered with eye drops containing the preservative benzalkonium chloride (listed as an inactive ingredient). Excessive use of vasoconstrictor drops (e.g., naphazoline, tetrahydrozoline) is also common. Although vasoconstrictors are effective at acutely clearing conjunctival injection, if used for longer than 3 to 5 days, rebound vasodilation is frequently encountered and may take as long as 4 weeks to resolve.[10] The use of vasoconstrictor drops should be uniformly discouraged except for infrequent, intermittent use. Other common causes of medication-related conjunctivitis include topical antibiotics, especially aminoglycosides, and glaucoma medications.[10]

CLINICAL PRESENTATION AND PHYSICAL EXAMINATION
Viral Conjunctivitis

Evaluation of a patient with conjunctivitis should begin with a careful history. A recent upper-respiratory infection or exposure to sick individuals can point to a diagnosis of adenoviral conjunctivitis.[2,13] Ocular symptoms include acute onset of a red eye with excessive watery discharge.[4] Classically, it begins in one eye and then involves the fellow eye within days due to the phenomenon of autoinnoculation.[13] Approximately half of patients will have bilateral involvement at the time of presentation.[13]

Adenoviral conjunctivitis can occur in three different forms: adenoviral conjunctivitis, pharyngoconjunctival fever, and epidemic keratoconjunctivitis.[4,10] For examination, the lower eyelid is pulled down and the palpebral conjunctiva evaluated. There will be follicles, clear bumps ranging in size from pinpoint to 2 mm, and overlying injected conjunctival vessels (Fig. 55.1).[1,10] The second form is pharyngoconjunctival fever. The ocular examination findings are similar. However, the patient will have systemic disease: fever, headache, and sore throat.[4] Epidemic keratoconjunctivitis is clinically striking

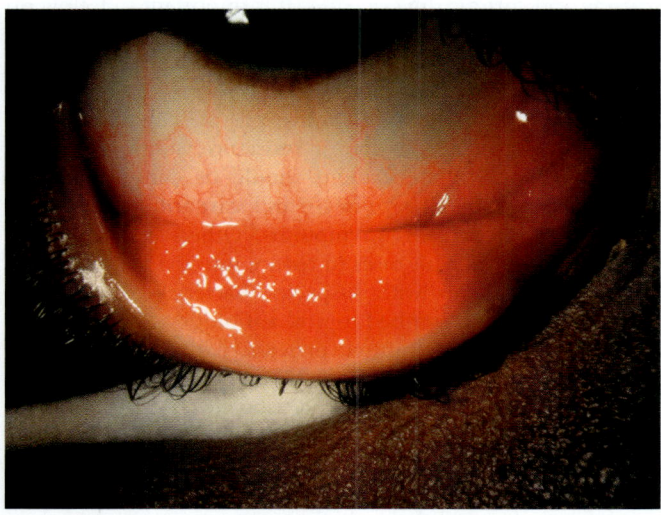

F G . 55.1 Follicles are typical of viral conjunctivitis and can frequently be appreciated without magnification.

with significant, bilateral conjunctival hyperemia and chemosis. Petechial and larger subconjunctival hemorrhages may be present in this form.[2,10] Up to one-third of patients with epidemic keratoconjunctivitis have corneal involvement, and it is appropriate to refer these patients to an ophthalmologist.[14]

When a patient with suspected adenoviral conjunctivitis is examined, it is important to palpate the anterior cervical chain of lymph nodes. At least 50% of patients have a tender preauricular lymph node (this node is located just inferior and medial to the tragus of the ear).[4] Of note, certain types of bacterial conjunctivitis can also manifest with other lymphadenopathy (specifically, *Neisseria*- and methicillin-resistant *Staphylococcus aureus* [MRSA]–associated bacterial conjunctivitis).[2]

Herpes simplex virus (HSV) infection accounts for 1.3% to 4.8% of acute conjunctivitis.[4] It can be spread by direct contact but is more commonly spread by asymptomatic shedding of viral particles. Children with primary HSV infection will often have an antecedent respiratory infection. The disease is almost always unilateral and can cause concurrent vesicular skin lesions.[4] Recurrent HSV infection can manifest similarly but often involves other ocular structures. Patients with a history of prior cold sores and presumed herpetic eye disease should be referred to an ophthalmologist.[2,10]

Molluscum contagiosum is spread by direct contact. Because it typically occurs in children, human immunodeficiency virus (HIV) infection should be considered if it is seen in adults.[2,10] Patients have a chronic follicular reaction. On examination of the eyelid margin, an umbilicated nodule is characteristic. Refer these patients to an ophthalmologist for evaluation and potential excision.[10]

Bacterial Conjunctivitis

Bacterial conjunctivitis is typically accompanied by thick, purulent discharge.[13] Patients will often report that both eyes are sticky or glued shut. These symptoms persist throughout the day but are worse in the morning.[15] Bacterial conjunctivitis can result from the overproliferation of native ocular flora or from direct spread from an infected individual.[4]

Acute conjunctivitis is the most common form of bacterial conjunctivitis. Symptoms manifest over days. In children, the causative agents include *Haemophilus influenzae* and *Streptococcus pneumoniae*. *S. aureus* is more commonly seen in adults.[9,15] Symptoms typically last for 7 to 10 days.[4]

Hyperacute onset (12 to 24 hours) of symptoms with severe purulent discharge is highly consistent with *Neisseria gonorrhoeae*.[10,15] Gonococcal conjunctivitis is typically seen in sexually active adults but can also occur in neonates via maternal-neonate transmission.[10,15] If it is seen in a child, child abuse should be suspected. Rapid progression is the hallmark of this disease. The cornea can become involved in less than 2 days and lead to permanent vision loss (Fig. 55.2).[10]

Chronic bacterial conjunctivitis is used to describe symptoms lasting longer than 4 weeks.[4] Chlamydial conjunctivitis should be suspected in sexually active adults with a nonresponsive conjunctivitis.[9] Patients typically have a concurrent genital infection.[4] Mild symptoms may be present for weeks to months, with exacerbations and remissions.[10]

Acute Allergic Conjunctivitis

Allergic conjunctivitis affects up to 40% of the US population, yet only about 10% of individuals affected will seek medical attention.[7,16] Seventy-five percent of patients with allergic

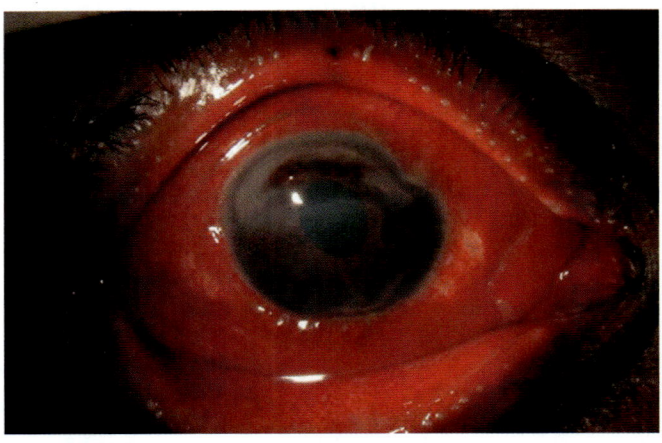

FIG. **55.2** Gonococcal conjunctivitis can progress to severe corneal thinning and even corneal perforation if left untreated. Severe corneal thinning can be seen superiorly and inferonasally in this photograph.

rhinitis will have associated conjunctivitis. Patients will often have an associated headache and fatigue. Often, patients will also have a positive family history of hay fever or atopy.[8] Unlike conjunctivitis from infectious causes, allergic conjunctivitis typically occurs simultaneously in both eyes. Its predominant feature is itching.[7,8] If discharge is present, it will be clear or stringy and white. The conjunctiva has a boggy appearance. Examination of the periocular skin shows lid discoloration, thickening, and erythema.[8] In addition, periorbital venous congestion can manifest as dark circles under the eyes (i.e., allergic shiners).[10]

Vernal and Atopic Conjunctivitis

Vernal conjunctivitis occurs in childhood, typically in the spring. It primarily affects males and resolves by the third decade.[2,10] Atopic conjunctivitis occurs in adults (>50 years) with a history of asthma, allergic rhinitis, and atopic dermatitis.[10] Twenty-five percent of older adult patients with eczema will develop atopic conjunctivitis.[2] Compared with acute allergic conjunctivitis, atopic conjunctivitis and vernal conjunctivitis are associated with more severe symptoms of severe itching, burning, and tearing. Other symptoms include blepharospasm and photophobia. Discharge is often white, thick, and ropy.[1,10] Ninety-eight percent of cases are bilateral.[17]

Giant papillary conjunctivitis is a hallmark of vernal conjunctivitis. Eversion of the upper lid will reveal a cobblestone pattern of large (>1 mm), geometric bumps.[10,17] These giant papillae can cause a droopy eyelid. In addition, corneal involvement is more common than in acute allergic conjunctivitis. Patients with vernal disease will often have a shield ulcer (an oval corneal epithelial defect of the superior cornea) in addition to the conjunctivitis.[17] This can be identified by a decrease in vision or by fluorescein staining. If it is present, the patient needs close monitoring by an ophthalmologist.[13,14]

MEDICATION TOXICITY

A variety of topical medications can induce an allergic response in the conjunctiva.[4] In addition to conjunctivitis, a contact dermatitis of the lower lids with thickening and scaling of the skin is sometimes seen.[1] Discontinuation of the offending medication leads to resolution of symptoms.[1]

DIAGNOSTICS
Essential Diagnostics

Physical examination and medical history allow for differentiation of most forms of conjunctivitis. For bacterial conjunctivitis, rapidity of onset, severity, and age at presentation often suggest the causative organism. Gram-stained smears and cultures are necessary in the immunocompromised (including neonates) and in severe or unresponsive cases.[10] For confirmation of a diagnosis of chlamydial conjunctivitis, polymerase chain reaction testing of the conjunctiva is frequently used.[10]

DIFFERENTIAL DIAGNOSIS

 Priority differentials include herpetic eye disease, gonococcal or chlamydia-related conjunctivitis, subconjunctival hemorrhage, blepharitis, foreign body, or uveitis.

Not all patients with a red eye have conjunctivitis.[5,13] Conjunctival inflammation can result from other ocular diseases. Effective treatment of the red eye depends on appropriate targeting of the underlying disease.[1]

INTERPROFESSIONAL COLLABORATIVE MANAGEMENT
Pharmacologic Management

Viral Conjunctivitis. Viral conjunctivitis is self-limited and typically lasts 5 to 14 days. Treatment is supportive with artificial tears and cool compresses. Patients should be advised that they are contagious as long as they are still tearing (i.e., shedding viral particles), or for at least 1 week.[13] Prior practice patterns recommended treatment of viral conjunctivitis with an antibiotic to prevent a bacterial superinfection. However, the occurrence of this is rare, and topical antibiotics are typically unnecessary. There is emerging evidence that a combination steroid and povidone eye drop can reduce the duration of symptoms, however, infectivity may be prolonged.[9,18]

The majority of patients with viral conjunctivitis do not have long-term sequelae. Two potentially sight-threatening consequences are corneal involvement, which can cause decreased vision, and conjunctival pseudomembranes, which can lead to scarring and chronic dry eye. Thus, it is important to follow up in 1 to 4 weeks if symptoms have not fully resolved.[2,10,13]

Bacterial Conjunctivitis. Topical treatment with antibiotics is not always necessary. Evidence shows that outcomes with topical antibiotics are equivalent to placebo at 1 week.[19] To minimize cost and antibiotic resistance, some advocate a delayed treatment plan. Patients should be educated on the self-limited nature of their disease and start antibiotics only if there is no improvement in symptoms.[9] Others advocate use of topical antibiotics in all cases to reduce infectivity rates.[1]

High-risk patients with suspected bacterial conjunctivitis should always be prescribed topical antibiotics. These patients include immunocompromised patients, patients with uncontrolled diabetes, health care workers, and patients with any history of glaucoma surgery.[1,19,20] Reasonable initial choices for a topical antibiotic include trimethoprim–polymyxin B or fluoroquinolone drops, four times a day for 1 week. Corticosteroids are rarely indicated and should not be used without the supervision of an ophthalmologist.[13]

The following types of bacterial conjunctivitis require systemic treatment:

- *H. influenzae:* treat with oral amoxicillin-clavulanate (if not allergic) because of the potential for extraocular involvement (otitis media, pneumonia, and meningitis).[21]
- Gonococcal: ceftriaxone, 250 mg intramuscularly, one dose (or ciprofloxacin, 500 mg orally, if the patient has a penicillin allergy) AND one dose of azithromycin, 1 g orally—requires same-day referral to an ophthalmologist.[21,22]
- Chlamydial: azithromycin, 1 g orally, one dose (or doxycycline, 100 mg twice daily for 7 days).[14,22]

One-third of patients with gonococcal disease have concurrent chlamydial infection, and treatment for both diseases is recommended.[13] Remember to treat the sexual partners of patients with gonococcal or chlamydial conjunctivitis to prevent reinfection.[10]

MRSA accounts for 3% to 64% of ocular staphylococcal infections and MRSA conjunctivitis is becoming increasingly more common. These organisms are resistant to many antibiotics. Patients with suspected cases of MRSA should be referred to an ophthalmologist.[23]

Acute Allergic Conjunctivitis. A stepwise approach should be used. First, any allergens should be identified and eliminated. Typically, symptoms resolve quickly once the inciting allergen is removed.[8] Because allergic conjunctivitis is typically associated with systemic allergies, an oral antihistamine can be helpful in controlling ocular symptoms. Agents to consider include fexofenadine and loratadine.[21]

Treatment should start topically with supportive care: preservative-free artificial tears, cool compresses, and removal of contact lenses. If symptoms persist, an antihistamine-vasoconstrictor (e.g., naphazoline-pheniramine) can be added with caution.[7] With use for longer than 3 to 7 days, rebound vasodilation can occur, resulting in a medication-induced conjunctivitis. Mast cell stabilizers can be used as prophylaxis for recurrent or persistent allergic conjunctivitis. The patient should keep in mind that results take several weeks with a mast cell stabilizer. Topical cetirizine has been shown to provide rapid relief of itching.[24] If the patient has any systemic allergies, an oral antihistamine can also be helpful in controlling ocular symptoms. Topical nonsteroidal antiinflammatory drugs, immunomodulators such as cyclosporine and tacrolimus, and steroids may be beneficial, but should be used only under the supervision of an ophthalmologist.[1,7,21,25]

Vernal and Atopic Conjunctivitis. The treatment approach is similar to that for allergic conjunctivitis. However, because agents are nonspecific, simple avoidance of triggers is a difficult remedy. The provider should initiate mast cell stabilizers (e.g., cromolyn sodium, lodoxamide tromethamine) 2 weeks before the usual time of presentation for relief in vernal conjunctivitis.[10] Symptoms tend to be more refractory and severe. Ophthalmology referral is indicated in all cases.

Medication Toxicity. Treatment is twofold. First, the toxic medication must be eliminated. Second, symptomatic relief with preservative-free artificial tears should be provided.[1] A short course of topical steroids is sometimes used to reduce the duration of symptoms, particularly in more severe cases.[10,21]

INDICATIONS FOR REFERRAL AND HOSPITALIZATION

On initial evaluation, if there is any concern for a sight-threatening disease, the patient should be immediately referred to an ophthalmologist. History can provide important clues. For example, patients with recent trauma, ocular surgery, or use of contact lenses need to be referred. In addition, physical examination is important. A decrease in vision or severe ocular pain is not consistent with conjunctivitis and warrants an ophthalmology consultation. Non-ocular symptoms and signs, such as nausea and vomiting, should raise concern for acute glaucoma and prompt referral.[9,13,15]

Conjunctivitis in immunocompromised patients[1] or suspected herpetic infection (either by history of prior HSV infections or by presentation with a vesicular rash in the V1 dermatome) warrants ophthalmological referral and evaluation.[1,9]

In addition, patients with conjunctivitis who experience any of the following require evaluation by an ophthalmologist[1]: Corneal involvement, pain, severe purulent discharge, vision loss, recurrent episodes or no response, or worsening symptoms despite symptoms.

PATIENT AND FAMILY EDUCATION

Education is a key component of treatment.

Patients with noninfectious conjunctivitis need to understand the underlying cause of their disease and the chronic nature of their condition.

- Infectious conjunctivitis: The health care provider has a valuable role in interrupting the cycle of transmission. Patients should avoid touching their eyes, shaking hands with others, sharing towels or bedclothes, and swimming in public pools.[9,13,21] Teach patients and their families recommended hand washing techniques.
- Because infectious outbreaks have been linked to health care facilities, health care providers must take care to wash hands with antimicrobial soap after examination of a patient with conjunctivitis. In addition, all exposed surfaces in the examination room should be decontaminated with sodium hypochlorite (a 1 : 10 dilution of household bleach) or other disinfectants.[1]

REFERENCES

1. Ophthalmology, A. A. O. (2008). *Cornea/External disease panel.* San Francisco, Ca: American Academy of Ophthalmology. Retrieved from www.aao.org/ppp.
2. O'Brien, T. P., Jeng, B. H., McDonald, M., & Raizman, M. B. (2009). Acute conjunctivitis: Truth and misconceptions. *Current Medical Research and Opinion, 25,* 1953–1961.
3. Shields, T., & Sloane, P. D. (1991). A comparison of eye problems in primary care and ophthalmology practices. *Family Medicine, 23*(7), 544–546.
4. Azari, A. A., & Barney, N. P. (2013). Conjunctivitis: A systematic review of diagnosis and treatment. *JAMA: The Journal of the American Medical Association, 310,* 1721–1729.
5. Leibowitz, H. M. (2000). The red eye. *The New England Journal of Medicine, 343,* 345–351.
6. Hovding, G. (2008). Acute bacterial conjunctivitis. *Acta Ophthalmologica, 86,* 5–17.
7. Bielory, B. P., O'Brien, T. P., & Bielory, L. (2012). Management of seasonal allergic conjunctivitis: Guide to therapy. *Acta Ophthalmologica, 90,* 399–407.
8. Bielory, L. (2008). Ocular allergy overview. *Immunology and Allergy Clinics of North America, 28,* 1–23, v.
9. Cronau, H., Kankanala, R. R., & Mauger, T. (2010). Diagnosis and management of red eye in primary care. *American Family Physician, 81,* 137–144.
10. (2007). *Basic and clinical science course: External diseases and cornea.* San Francisco, Ca: American Academy of Ophthalmology.
11. Azar, M. J., Dhaliwal, D. K., Bower, K. S., Kowalski, R. P., & Gordon, Y. J. (1996). Possible consequences of shaking hands with your patients with epidemic keratoconjunctivitis. *American Journal of Ophthalmology, 121*(6), 711–712.
12. Gomes, P. J. (2014). Trends in prevalence and treatment of ocular allergy. *Current Opinion in Allergy and Clinical Immunology, 14,* 451–456.
13. Galor, A., & Jeng, B. H. (2008). Red eye for the internist: When to treat, when to refer. *Cleveland Clinic Journal of Medicine, 75,* 137–144.

14. Sethuraman, U., & Kamat, D. (2009). The red eye: Evaluation and management. *Clinical Pediatrics, 48,* 588–600.

15. Tarabishy, A. B., & Jeng, B. H. (2008). Bacterial conjunctivitis: A review for internists. *Cleveland Clinic Journal of Medicine, 75,* 507–512.

16. Rosario, N., & Bielory, L. (2011). Epidemiology of allergic conjunctivitis. *Current Opinion in Allergy and Clinical Immunology, 11*(5), 471–476.

17. Kumar, S. (2009). Vernal keratoconjunctivitis: A major review. *Acta Ophthalmologica, 87,* 133–147.

18. Pinto, R. D., Lira, R. P., Abe, R. Y., Zacchia, R. S., Felix, J. P., Pereira, A. V., et al. (2015). Dexamethasone/Povidone eye drops versus artificial tears for treatment of presumed viral conjunctivitis: A randomized clinical trial. *Current Eye Research, 40*(9), 870–877.

19. Visscher, K. L., Hutnik, C. M., & Thomas, M. (2009). Evidence-based treatment of acute infective conjunctivitis: Breaking the cycle of antibiotic prescribing. *Canadian Family Physician, 55,* 1071–1075.

20. Everitt, H. A., Little, P. S., & Smith, P. W. (2006). A randomised controlled trial of management strategies for acute infective conjunctivitis in general practice. *British Medical Journal, 333,* 321.

21. Kunimoto, D. Y. K. K., & Makar, M. S. (2004). *The Wills eye manual: Office and emergency room diagnosis and treatment of eye disease* (4th ed.). Philadelphia: Lippincott Williams & Wilkins.

22. 2015 Sexually Transmitted Disease Guidelines, CDC. Retrieved from http://www.cdc.gov/std/tg2015/gonorrhea.htm; (Accessed June 28, 2015).

23. Freidlin, J., Acharya, N., Lietman, T. M., Cevallos, V., Whitcher, J. P., & Margolis, T. P. (2007). Spectrum of eye disease caused by methicillin-resistant Staphylococcus aureus. *American Journal of Ophthalmology, 144*(2), 313–315.

24. Krader, C. G. (2017). Topical cetirizine latest therapy to treat allergic conjunctivitis. *Ophthalmology Times,* 30.

25. Mishra, G. P., Tamboli, V., Jwala, J., & Mitra, A. K. (2011). Recent patents and emerging therapeutics in the treatment of allergic conjunctivitis. *Recent Patents on Inflammation & Allergy Drug Discovery, 5*(1), 26–36.

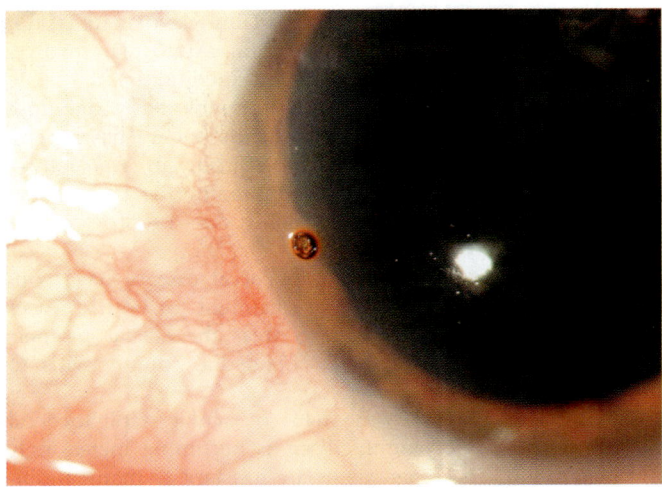

FIG. 56.1 A metallic corneal foreign body is a common presentation in young male workers, often occurring while grinding or hammering metal on metal.

Corneal surface defects must be distinguished from other serious conditions, most notably corneal inflammatory conditions, lacerations, and infections. Full-thickness lacerations can occur with ocular trauma and sometimes appear clinically similar to epithelial defects. Infectious keratitis, or corneal ulcers, are common in contact lens users. An ulcer is an epithelial defect with an infiltrate, or white area in the cornea. Other common conditions with similar presentations include herpetic keratitis, staphylococcal marginal disease, and phlyctenulosis, the last two frequently manifesting as peripheral corneal opacities with associated epithelial defects.

PATHOPHYSIOLOGY

An abrasion of the corneal epithelium may be caused by chemical or mechanical debridement resulting from trauma, chemicals, or ultraviolet radiation exposure. Corneal erosions occur if an abrasion disrupts the Bowman layer (smooth, acellular layer of tissue just beneath the corneal surface epithelium). Decreased evaporation during sleep results in the formation of a fluid layer above the incompletely healed Bowman layer and below the epithelium. This can lead to repeated sloughing of the overlying epithelium when the patient awakens and opens the lid, given the relative lack of epithelial adherence. Epithelial defects, whether abrasions or erosions, may allow bacterial, viral, or fungal organisms to invade the corneal stroma, resulting in an ulcer. Sterile corneal ulcers may also occur.

CLINICAL PRESENTATION AND PHYSICAL EXAMINATION

The most common symptom of a corneal abrasion or foreign body is sudden onset of severe eye pain in the affected eye. This pain typically resolves after application of a topical anesthetic eye drop.[3] Some patients may report a foreign body sensation instead of severe pain. Other symptoms include blurred vision, redness, tearing, light sensitivity, eyelid swelling, and blepharospasm.[4]

On physical examination, vision may be limited if the epithelial defect or foreign body falls within the visual axis. The pupils should react normally to light, and eye pressure is typically not affected. The eyelids may appear swollen in

---

CHAPTER 56

CORNEAL SURFACE DEFECTS AND OCULAR SURFACE FOREIGN BODIES

Diana M. Laura • James T. Banta

 Immediate evaluation by an ophthalmologist is indicated for hypopyon (inflammatory debris in the inferior anterior chamber); ocular contents that are extruded; a pupil that is peaked, nonreactive, or irregular (suggests a penetrating injury); nonhealing epithelial defects; metallic foreign bodies; chemical injuries (after prompt irrigation); infectious keratitis; full-thickness corneal laceration; or elevated eye pressure (>30) on tonometry.

DEFINITION AND EPIDEMIOLOGY

A corneal surface defect occurs when the corneal epithelium is interrupted. Direct trauma from foreign objects (e.g., fingers, tree branches, makeup applicators) typically causes these injuries. Airbags from motor vehicle accidents are another common source of injury. Contact lens wearers are particularly susceptible to corneal problems because prolonged use of lenses can result in injury and corneal epithelial breaks.[1] In most cases, the patient can recall a specific moment when trauma occurred.

Corneal surface foreign bodies are particularly common in workers exposed to small particles, dust, or metal grinding (e.g., construction workers, mechanics, and landscapers [Fig. 56.1]).[2] Chemicals, either splashed or inadvertently placed in the eye, can also cause surface defects. These injuries are almost universally preventable with the appropriate type of eye protection.

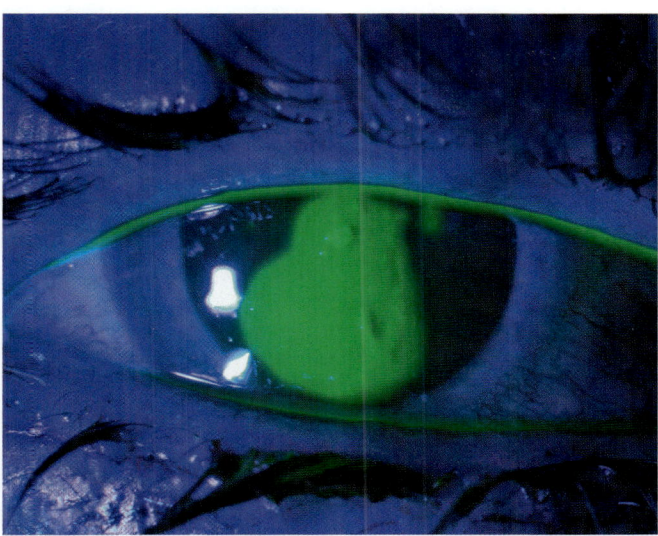

F I G . **56.2** Corneal abrasion stained with fluorescein under a cobalt blue light. The patient was inadvertently poked in the eye and complained of severe pain, decreased vision, and lid swelling.

the affected eye, and the conjunctiva is typically injected. The cornea may have some mild haze but should not be focally opacified. If there is a significant corneal opacity, an alternative diagnosis such as infectious keratitis should be considered. A foreign body may be visible on the corneal or conjunctival surface. The anterior chamber should have normal depth, and the iris should have a normal, round appearance. Presence of a hypopyon (inflammatory debris layering in the inferior portion of the anterior chamber) suggests a more serious diagnosis, and immediate referral should be made to an ophthalmologist. If the anterior chamber appears flattened, ocular contents are extruded, or the pupil is peaked, nonreactive, or irregular, this suggests a penetrating injury, and immediate referral should be made to an ophthalmologist.[5]

DIAGNOSTICS

Use of topical fluorescein dye can assist in the diagnosis of a corneal surface defect. One drop of fluorescein can be applied and viewed under a cobalt blue light or Wood lamp. A corneal abrasion should appear as a bright green area, often polygonal (Fig. 56.2). Linear, vertically oriented epithelial defects are typically caused by subtarsal (trapped under the upper eyelid) foreign bodies and should prompt eversion of the upper eyelids to check for foreign material.[6] Fluorescein staining of true surface defects should not change with the patient's blinking. If the defect appears to have a branching or dendritic pattern, a herpetic cause should be entertained.[6] An irregular iris and a shallow anterior chamber associated with an area of fluorescein staining raise the specter of a full-thickness corneal laceration and should prompt emergent ophthalmology referral.

DIFFERENTIAL DIAGNOSIS

 Priority differentials include corneal ulcer, herpetic keratitis, and dry eye syndrome.

Numerous other conditions are possible and include episcleritis, iritis, acute angle closure glaucoma, conjunctivitis,

Corneal Surface Defects and Foreign Bodies

INITIAL (CORNEAL ABRASION OR ULCER)
- Fluorescein stain

LABORATORY (CORNEAL ULCER)
- Culture and sensitivity (if immediate ophthalmology consultation is not available)

INITIAL (FOREIGN BODY)
- Fluorescein stain
- Evert eyelids and examine fornices if appropriate

full-thickness corneal laceration, staphylococcal marginal disease, phlyctenulosis, and contact lens overuse, among others.

INTERPROFESSIONAL COLLABORATIVE MANAGEMENT
Pharmacologic Management

Most patients with corneal abrasions or surface defects can be managed with supportive care, with the goals of pain relief and prevention of bacteria superinfection.[7] Treatment typically consists of topical antibiotic prophylaxis and lubricating drops and/or ointments.[5] An ophthalmic antibiotic ointment, such as erythromycin or polymyxin B–bacitracin (Polysporin), may help with pain control by providing a physical barrier between the cornea and eyelid,[1] and it is often prescribed in lieu of antibiotic eye drops. Ophthalmic ointment can be applied on the ocular surface by pulling the lower lid away from the eye while having the patient look up. Ointment is then applied into the pocket that is opened. Pressure patching, although helpful in relieving pain, may encourage infection, does not promote healing, and should be avoided.[8,9] Oral analgesics are the first-line agents for pain control, but patients should be encouraged to use ointment and artificial tears frequently because this often provides more relief than oral analgesics. Steroids are contraindicated because they inhibit healing and may encourage infection. Topical anesthetics such as proparacaine should *never* be used or prescribed for pain control. Although they provide immediate pain relief by creating a loss of feeling in the cornea, they have toxic effects in frequent and long-term use.[10] Prolonged use may lead to corneal melting. Care should be taken to inform patients of this risk, and providers should avoid leaving patients in examination rooms with topical anesthetics within reach. Cycloplegic drops are occasionally used for pain control in severe cases, particularly if the injury is severe enough to produce intraocular inflammation as is sometimes seen with trauma. However, care should be taken to avoid cycloplegic drops (because of their vasoconstrictive effect) in severe chemical burns.

A healthy corneal epithelium will repopulate rapidly, from just a few hours for a small, uncomplicated defect to 3 to 5 days with larger defects. Symptoms typically abate once the epithelium is reestablished. Patients should be informed of the typical time course and should be reassured that their pain should improve gradually over a few days. They should be advised to seek urgent ophthalmology evaluation if they develop sudden worsening of symptoms including redness, sensitivity to light, vision changes, or pain. The mnemonic *RSVP* (sudden *redness, sensitivity to light or secretion, decreased*

BOX **56.1**

Irrigation After Chemical Injuries

- Position patient comfortably at an angle.
- Place basin to collect excess fluid.
- Apply 1 drop of topical anesthetic.
- Retract lids with lid retractor.
- Deliver 1 L of normal saline through standard intravenous tubing to affected eyes.
- Flush entire area for 1 h, including fornices (areas between globe and eyelids).
- Test pH. If result is not 7.0–7.5, repeat irrigation.

BOX **56.2**

Indications for Immediate Ophthalmology Referral

- Nonhealing epithelial defects
- Metallic foreign bodies
- Chemical injuries (after prompt irrigation)
- Infectious keratitis
- Hypopyon (evidence of a fluid line in the anterior chamber near the bottom caused by inflammatory cells)
- Full-thickness corneal laceration
- Elevated eye pressure (>30) on tonometry

vision, and/or pain) can be given to help patients remember these precautions.

If a visible foreign body is present on the cornea, it must be removed. If it is not easily removed with a cotton-tipped applicator, an ophthalmology referral should be made so that the foreign body can be visualized with a slit lamp for removal. Even when a metallic foreign body is dislodged, a rust ring may persist on the cornea and cause further inflammation if it is not completely removed. Patients, especially metal or machine workers, should be asked if a high velocity injury occurred, because this can cause a penetrating eye injury.[7]

If chemical injury is suspected, *immediate* irrigation of the affected eye should be performed (before referral). A full history, including the type of chemical, should be obtained; alkali injuries in particular can lead to rapid damage. Irrigation should be performed as described in Box 56.1.[11] After irrigation, pH should measure 7.0 to 7.5.[2] If the pH is not in this range after irrigation, further irrigation should be performed. After irrigation, immediately refer the patient to an ophthalmologist.

Chemical injuries can be broadly categorized into acid or alkali. Identification of the causative chemical agent is important, and referred patients should be provided with a bottle of the chemical or at the very least specific information about the offending agent. Acid injuries tend to be less harmful; these materials cause corneal surface proteins to coagulate and create a barrier that prevents deeper penetration. On the other hand, alkaline materials (e.g., ammonia, bleach) lead to rapid damage because of saponification of fats and denaturation of collagen. Within *minutes,* alkaline materials can penetrate the anterior chamber and cause damage to intraocular structures.

INDICATIONS FOR REFERRAL AND HOSPITALIZATION

After initial management of symptoms, patients with corneal surface defects, history of metallic foreign body removal, and persistent foreign bodies should be referred to an ophthalmologist. Chemical injuries should be irrigated before referral because of the risk of rapid progression. See Box 56.2 for additional situations requiring immediate referral.

COMPLICATIONS

The most concerning complication of a corneal epithelial defect or corneal foreign body is infection. Although rare, infection is often preventable with appropriate therapy and use of topical antibiotics. Trauma with vegetable matter (e.g., tree branch) should increase suspicion and concern for infection

(often by atypical organisms, frequently fungus). Misdiagnosis of a corneal ulcer as a corneal epithelial defect can lead to scarring of the cornea and worsening of infection, resulting in further vision loss. Corneal foreign bodies may leave behind rust that can cause future inflammation or vision loss. Patients who have previously sustained surface defects may occasionally develop recurrent corneal erosion syndrome, in which spontaneous erosion occurs at the site of a previous injury weeks to months after the initial injury. If a chemical injury is not promptly treated or irrigated, severe visual impairment and ocular damage may occur.

PATIENT AND FAMILY EDUCATION

- Many workplace injuries are caused by foreign bodies, chemicals, or direct trauma, and can be easily prevented with appropriate eyewear. The Occupational Safety and Health Administration (OSHA) recommends use of safety glasses with side protection in situations such as hammering and metal grinding.[2] Safety glasses may be insufficient for workers who are performing tasks with high-velocity particles that can potentially reach the eye around the glasses. Polycarbonate safety goggles that fit snugly to the face are more appropriate in these settings.
- Welders can also develop painful corneal injuries and should wear appropriate safety equipment. Standards for eye protection are set in the American National Standards Institute (ANSI) guidelines Z78.1 and Z49.1.[12]
- Chemical injuries require prompt therapy. Work environments with hazardous chemicals should have easily accessible eyewash stations for rapid treatment.[13] ANSI standard Z358.1 provides requirements for water temperature, flow rate, distance, and functioning of eyewash stations.

HEALTH PROMOTION

Nearly all eye injuries in the workplace are preventable. Further education and awareness can reduce potentially sight-threatening accidents and the financial burden of these injuries.

REFERENCES

1. Dargin, J. M., & Lowenstein, R. A. (2007). The painful eye. *Emergency Medicine Clinics of North America, 26,* 199–216.
2. Peate, W. F. (2007). Work-related eye injuries and illnesses. *American Family Physician, 75,* 1017–1022.
3. Wirbelauer, C. (2006). Management of the red eye for the primary care physician. *The American Journal of Medicine, 119,* 302–306.
4. Cronau, H., Kankanala, R. R., & Mauger, T. (2010). Diagnosis and management of red eye in primary care. *American Family Physician, 81,* 137–145.

5 Ahmed, F., House, R. J., & Feldman, B. H. (2015). Corneal abrasions and corneal foreign bodies. *Primary Care, 42*, 363–375.

6 Pflipsen, M., Massaquoi, M., & Wolf, S. (2016). Evaluation of the painful eye. *American Family Physician, 93*, 991–998.

7 Wipperman, J. L., & Dorsch, J. N. (2013). Evaluation and management of corneal abrasions. *American Family Physician, 87*, 114–120.

8 Saccomano, S. J., & Ferrara, L. R. (2014). Managing corneal abrasions in primary care. *The Nurse Practitioner, 39*, 1–6.

9 Turner, A., & Rabiu, M. (2006). Patching for corneal abrasion. *The Cochrane Database of Systematic Reviews*, (2), CD004764.

10 Erdem, E., Undar, I. H., Esen, E., Yar, K., Yagmur, M., & Ersoz, R. (2013). Topical anesthetic eye drops abuse: Are we aware of the danger? *Cutaneous and Ocular Toxicology, 32*, 189–193.

11 Hartley, K. L., Mason, B. L., & Banta, J. T. (2007). Ocular surface (conjunctiva, cornea, and sclera). In J. T. Banta (Ed.), *Ocular trauma*. Philadelphia: Saunders Elsevier.

12 Gallogly, P. M., Vanderveldt, S. L., & Banta, J. T. (2007). Prevention of eye injuries. In J. T. Banta (Ed.), *Ocular trauma*. Philadelphia: Saunders Elsevier.

13 Khodabukus, R., & Tallouzi, M. (2009). Chemical eye injuries 1: Presentation, clinical features, treatment and prognosis. *Nursing Times, 105*, 22.

CHAPTER **57**

DRY EYE SYNDROME

Nandini Venkateswaran • James T. Banta

 Immediate consultation with the on-call ophthalmologist is required for visual loss, severe eye pain, or corneal ulceration.

DEFINITION AND EPIDEMIOLOGY

Dry eye syndrome is a multifactorial disorder characterized by abnormalities in the tear film. Tear film instability can damage the ocular surface and patients can consequently experience a wide range of dysesthesias and visual disturbances.[1] The disorder is known by many names including *dry eye syndrome, ocular surface disease, keratoconjunctivitis sicca, aqueous tear film deficiency,* and *dysfunctional tear syndrome.*

Dry eye is one of the most common reasons that adults consult an eye care professional. It is also treated frequently by primary care physicians, and perhaps most commonly, by patients themselves. Prevalence estimates for dry eye have varied widely, ranging from as low as 0.6% to as high as 57% based on the population studied and the stringency of the definition of the disease.[2] Several large cross-sectional studies have estimated that 5 million Americans have moderate to severe dry eye disease, and up to 20% of the population report occasional dry eye symptoms.[3]

Most published estimates of dry eye disease have focused on older age groups in which this disorder is thought to be more prevalent; however, there is increasing evidence that the condition is occurring increasingly at younger ages.[4]

PATHOPHYSIOLOGY

Dry eye is a surprisingly complex condition. The tear film is responsible for nourishing and lubricating the ocular surface, and providing immune protection. In addition, the tear film functions as the anterior refracting surface of the eye and, as such, plays a pivotal role in maintaining optical clarity.

A healthy tear film is created by complex interactions of the lacrimal glands and ducts, cornea and conjunctiva, eyelids, and meibomian glands, and it is maintained by autonomic and reflexive functions of the peripheral somatosensory and motor nervous system.[1] The tear film itself is formed with each blink and is composed of three layers: an inner mucin layer, an intermediate aqueous layer, and an outer lipid layer. The outer lipid layer, produced largely by secretions of the meibomian glands in the upper and lower eyelids, limits evaporative loss of the underlying aqueous layer between blinks.

A deficiency in any layer of the tear film or in any component of the lacrimal functional unit can lead to dry eye. Broadly speaking, dry eye can be classified into two mechanistic categories: *aqueous-deficient* and *evaporative* dry eye. Aqueous-deficient dry eye typically localizes to the lacrimal gland, and lacrimal gland insufficiency may be caused by Sjögren disease (a primary or secondary autoimmune infiltration of the lacrimal and salivary glands leading to dry eye and dry mouth), other infiltrative diseases of the lacrimal, or primary hyposecretion. Evaporative dry eye similarly has many causes, although the most common is meibomian gland dysfunction, in which the lipid-producing meibomian glands in the eyelids are obstructed at their openings (Fig. 57.1). Other causes of evaporative dry eye include poor eyelid closure (lagophthalmos), inadequate blinking, and ocular rosacea.

Despite the apparent simplicity of this classification scheme, most patients with dry eye will have components of both mechanisms contributing to their disease. Regardless of the cause, inflammation plays a central role in exacerbating and perpetuating dry eye disease. Inflammatory cytokines affect tear film osmolarity, leading to increased tear film instability and evaporative loss, which in turn leads to further inflammation.[5] Breaking this inflammatory cycle is critical in the management of dry eye disease.[6]

There are several similarities between dry eye disease symptoms and pain complaints elsewhere in the body. There is growing evidence that a significant number of patients with chronic dry eye describe features of neuropathic ocular pain,

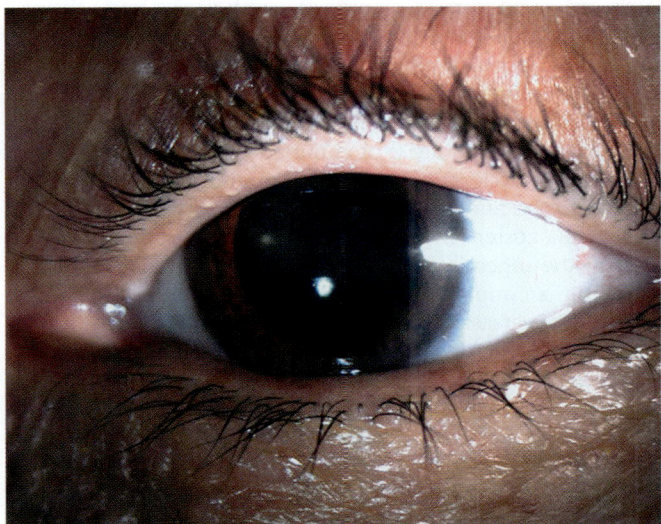

FIG. **57.1** Meibomian gland dysfunction. Meibomian glands are situated in the upper and lower eyelids, posterior to the eyelashes, and secrete the outer lipid layer of the tear film. Clogged meibomian glands are visible along the nasal portion of the upper lid in the photograph. Blockage of the meibomian glands leads to decreased tear film lipids, increased evaporation of the underlying aqueous layer, and tear film instability.

pain that is transmitted by an altered or sensitized neuronal system.[7] Dysfunctional adaptation of the corneal pain apparatus, including changes in corneal nerve morphology and neurotransmission,[8,9] can occur as a result of ocular surface inflammation, ocular trauma, or genetic predispositions, and may contribute to the development of a more persistently symptomatic disease phenotype.[10,11]

CLINICAL PRESENTATION AND PHYSICAL EXAMINATION

The symptoms of dry eye may be vague and nonspecific, and the clinician must carefully distinguish dry eye from other conditions that affect the ocular surface. Patients with dry eye most often have a chief concern of dryness, foreign body sensation (a scratchy or gritty feeling in the eyes), burning or stinging pain, itching, or ocular fatigue. They may also secondarily complain of redness or light sensitivity or note transient blurred vision that is relieved by blinking. Often, their symptoms are worsened by activities that require visual concentration (e.g., reading or computer use) or by low-humidity environments (e.g., airplane travel). Paradoxically, some patients may demonstrate excessive tearing, a reflexive hypersecretion of tears caused by corneal irritation. Many contact lens users report increasing intolerance to their lenses.

A careful medical history, including current medications and a complete review of systems should be obtained, because many systemic diseases and treatments can cause or exacerbate the symptoms of dry eyes. For example, many commonly prescribed anticholinergic drugs (including antihistamines and tricyclic antidepressants), alpha blockers (e.g., tamsulosin), antihypertensives (including diuretics and beta blockers), oral corticosteroids, and even vitamins have been associated with dry eye symptoms.[12] Autoimmune diseases including lupus and rheumatoid arthritis can cause a secondary Sjögren syndrome, leading to aqueous-deficient dry eye. Similarly, infiltrative processes affecting the lacrimal gland, such as lymphoma, sarcoidosis, graft-versus-host disease, orbital inflammatory pseudotumor, or IgG4-related disease can cause lacrimal gland insufficiency. Thyrotoxicosis and thyroid eye disease can cause exophthalmos, eyelid retraction, and incomplete eyelid closure.[13] Cranial nerve VII palsies (e.g., Bell palsy) causing partial or complete paralysis of the orbicularis oculi muscle may also lead to eyelid malposition, poor eyelid closure, and exposure of the ocular surface. Reactivation of varicella zoster virus (shingles) within the ophthalmic division of the trigeminal nerve may lead to diminished corneal sensation, an impaired blink reflex, and exposure of the ocular surface.[14] Decreased corneal sensitivity and lower rates of spontaneous blinking are also seen in patients with Parkinson disease.[15]

Physical examination by the primary care provider should include measurement of visual acuity (in each eye separately) and an external inspection of the ocular adnexa, including the skin, eyelids, conjunctiva, and cornea. If available, fluorescein dye can be used in conjunction with a cobalt blue–filtered light source to highlight pathology on the corneal surface. Attention should be given to eyelid and cranial nerve (especially V and VII) function, because incomplete eyelid closure (lagophthalmos) can cause corneal exposure and evaporative dry eye. The health care provider should evaluate for eyelid retraction and proptosis (hallmarks of thyroid eye disease) and consider screening for thyroid dysfunction. In addition, a complete physical examination—with close attention to the skin and joints—should be completed to screen for an associated autoimmune condition.

Although examination of the ocular surface by an ophthalmologist can help establish a diagnosis of dry eye syndrome, there is often a poor correlation between signs and symptoms in dry eye syndrome.[16] Some patients will report severe symptoms with little objective evidence of ocular surface disease; others will note only mild symptoms despite dramatic findings clinically. This discrepancy between signs and symptoms can complicate the diagnosis and management of patients with dry eye.

DIAGNOSTICS

The diagnosis of dry eye is based on a combination of patient history, subjective patient symptoms, objective testing, and clinical examination.

Two basic tests help distinguish aqueous-deficient from evaporative dry eye.

- A Schirmer test can be performed to assess aqueous production (Fig. 57.2). A narrow piece of filter paper is placed in the inferior cul-de-sac, and tear production is measured by how wet the paper is after 5 minutes. The test can be performed with topical anesthesia (to measure basal tearing) or without anesthesia (to measure basal plus reflex tearing). A cutoff of less than 5 mm (with anesthesia) or less than 10 mm (without anesthesia) is considered abnormal.[17] An abnormal Schirmer test result suggests aqueous-deficient dry eye.
  - For patients with aqueous-deficient dry eye suspected of having Sjögren syndrome, a serologic evaluation including SS-A (anti-Ro), SS-B (anti-La), rheumatoid factor, and antinuclear antibodies should be obtained.[17]
- Tear breakup time can be recorded with the aid of a slit-lamp biomicroscope. Fluorescein dye is instilled and the tear film is visualized with a cobalt blue filter. The amount of time between the last blink and the first discontinuity in the tear film is recorded as the tear breakup time, and a recording of less than 10 seconds is considered abnormal.[17] An abnormal tear breakup time suggests evaporative dry eye.

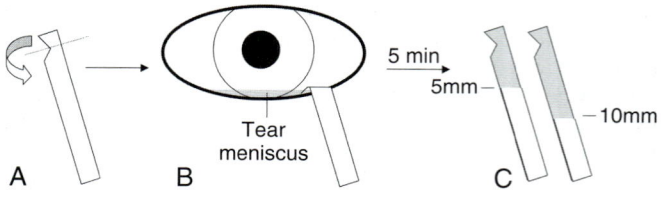

FIG. 57.2 Schirmer test. A narrow strip of filter paper is used to measure the production of tears. The Schirmer strip is folded at the notch (A) and placed over the lower eyelid margin with the short end resting in the tear meniscus of the inferior fornix (B). The strips are removed after 5 minutes, and the amount of moisture is measured (C). If the test is performed with topical anesthesia, then only basal tear secretion is measured, and less than 5 mm of wetting is considered diagnostic of aqueous tear deficiency. If the test is performed without topical anesthesia, then basal plus reflex tear secretion is measured, and less than 10 mm of wetting is considered diagnostic of aqueous tear deficiency.

Patient symptom questionnaires are important adjuncts for the diagnosis and management of dry eye syndrome; however, they vary by areas of focus and utility as screening tools versus monitoring of disease progression. The Ocular Surface Disease Index (OSDI) is a simple, reliable, and reproducible way to assess dry eye severity and to monitor patients' response to treatment.[18] There are several other validated questionnaires in addition to the OSDI that are employed for the assessment of dry eye disease. These include the Dry Eye Questionnaire-5 (DEQ-5), McMonnies Questionnaire (MQ), Impact of Dry Eye on Everyday Life (IDEEL) Questionnaire, National Eye Institute Visual Functioning Questionnaire-25 (NEI-VFQ 25), Symptom Assessment in Dry Eye (SANDE) Questionnaire, and Standard Patient Evaluation of Eye Dryness (SPEED) Questionnaire. Health care providers can employ one or more questionnaires that they feel are best suited for their patient population.[19]

DIFFERENTIAL DIAGNOSIS

 Priority differentials include trichiasis, conjunctivitis, and corneal abrasion.

A diagnosis of dry eye syndrome requires the exclusion of other more serious diseases of the ocular surface. There is a broad range of possible causes of ocular surface irritation. It is important to localize the problem and distinguish among these conditions because each is managed differently.

INTERPROFESSIONAL COLLABORATIVE MANAGEMENT

Nonpharmacologic Management

Management of dry eye should be approached in a stepwise fashion according to the severity of disease and a review of treatment guidelines was most recently authored in 2017.[20] Most patients will require a systematic escalation of treatment combining several different behavioral, pharmacologic, and nonpharmacologic approaches. Lifestyle or workplace modifications can help alleviate the symptoms of dry eye, and patients should be advised to avoid windy, smoky, or low-humidity environments. Patients should be counseled to avoid direct exposure to the drying effects of air conditioning and fans and to limit the uninterrupted time spent reading or working on the computer without a break.

Eyelid inflammation (blepharitis) and meibomian gland dysfunction (see Fig. 57.1) can often be treated with lid hygiene measures. These measures include frequent warm compresses and gentle lid scrubs with nontearing baby shampoo.

The primary care provider can help to alleviate symptoms of dry eye by reviewing the patient's systemic medications and making dietary recommendations. Exacerbating medications, including anticholinergics, beta blockers, and diuretics, should be avoided (or substituted with medications in other drug classes) whenever possible. Many of the dietary modifications and supplements that primary care providers routinely recommend for cardiovascular health (e.g., Mediterranean diet,

fish oil, omega-6 fatty acids, vitamin D) may have a beneficial effect on patients' dry eye symptoms.[21,22]

Pharmacologic Management

Artificial tears are usually the first line of treatment of dry eye disease and can be used by the patient as needed. A wide variety of artificial tear drops are available over the counter. Patients should be encouraged to try a variety of commercially available drops to find the artificial tear formulation(s) that work best for them. High-viscosity gels and ointments provide better tear retention time and protection of the ocular surface but tend to cause visual blurring; therefore, they are recommended for nighttime use or in patients with more severe dry eye. The preservatives in topical eye drops can also irritate the ocular surface, so preservative-free formulations are often beneficial for patients requiring drops more than four to six times per day (including their other topical ophthalmic drops, such as those for the treatment of glaucoma).

As a general rule, use of eye drops that contain vasoconstrictive agents such as tetrahydrozoline (e.g., Visine) should be discouraged, because these drops can produce a rebound vasodilation and worsening conjunctival injection without addressing the underlying causes. Occasionally, patients may report the illicit use of topical anesthetic drops obtained from a doctor's office. These should be confiscated from the patient because their abuse may lead to severe complications including corneal opacities, ulceration, and even perforation. When ocular lubricants and behavioral changes fail to alleviate the symptoms of dry eye, it is important to consult an ophthalmologist for consideration of pharmacologic treatment options.

Ophthalmologists may prescribe a short course of topical corticosteroids, which can help to quiet the inflammatory component of dry eye disease. However, this therapy should not be used chronically or without close follow-up, given the increased risk of glaucoma, cataract formation, and infection. Treatment with cyclosporine ophthalmic emulsion 0.05% (Restasis) or with small-molecule integrin antagonist lifitegrast 5% (Xiidra) can be recommended by an ophthalmologist. Both Restasis and Xiidra are options approved by the Food and Drug Administration for the long-term treatment of dry eye.[20] Low-dose oral doxycycline is also gaining popularity in the management of aqueous-deficient dry eye secondary to meibomian gland dysfunction and/or ocular rosacea.[22] The ophthalmologist may also consider punctal occlusion, moisture goggles, or therapeutic contact lenses to improve tear retention. In extreme cases refractory to conventional therapies, some experts recommend autologous serum tears to lubricate the eyes and to reduce inflammation, although robust efficacy data from clinical trials are lacking.[23]

INDICATIONS FOR REFERRAL OR HOSPITALIZATION

Patients should be referred promptly to the ophthalmologist on call for visual loss, severe pain, or corneal ulceration.[17] Straightforward cases of dry eye with mild, intermittent symptoms can be self-managed by the patient—with lifestyle modifications, artificial tears, and eyelid hygiene—under the guidance of a primary care provider.

Patients should be referred to an ophthalmologist for dry eye symptoms that are moderate to severe, symptoms that are persistent or poorly controlled despite use of artificial tears four to six times daily, or are associated with any known or suspected ocular or systemic diseases.

Patients should be referred to an ophthalmologist before initiating any pharmacologic therapy for dry eye. A non–eye specialist provider should never initiate the use of ocular corticosteroids because of the risk of glaucoma, cataract formation, and infection.[6]

Hospitalization is rarely required, except in the case of patients with severe sight-threatening complications (e.g., corneal ulceration) who are unable to provide adequate care for themselves on an outpatient basis.

LIFE-SPAN CONSIDERATIONS

Dry eye is a chronic condition that frequently requires long-term therapy. It is more common in older adults and particularly common in postmenopausal women.[24]

COMPLICATIONS

Failure to treat dry eye early in the course of disease can lead to chronic changes in corneal nerve morphology and neurotransmission[8,9] and cause chronic neuropathic ocular pain,[10,11] making the disease more difficult to treat later. Severe dry eye can cause conjunctival adhesions, death of limbal stem cells leading to scarring and neovascularization of the cornea, or exposure of the ocular surface leading to corneal thinning, ulceration, and infection.

PATIENT AND FAMILY EDUCATION

- Patients should be advised that dry eye is a chronic condition that usually requires long-term management and treatment. The most effective treatment plan involves the patient, the ophthalmologist, and the primary care provider in a collaborative, ongoing, and stepwise approach to management. Many behavioral, nonpharmacologic, and pharmacologic treatment options are available to patients, and most report good control of their symptoms with appropriate therapy.
- Patients with dry eye symptoms should avoid low-humidity, smoky, or windy environments.
- Patients should take frequent breaks during activities that require close visual attention, such as reading and computer work.
- Regular eyelid hygiene is important, including frequent warm compresses and gentle lid scrubs with baby shampoo.
- Over-the-counter artificial tears are readily available as a first-line therapy for dry eye, although eye drops with preservatives should be limited to 4 to 6 times per day.
- Severe disease can be managed with more powerful antiinflammatory topical medications, but only under the supervision of a trained eye care professional.

REFERENCES

1. Lemp, M. A., & Foulks, G. N. (2007). The definition and classification of dry eye disease: Report of the Definition and Classification Subcommittee of the International Dry Eye Workshop (2007). *The Ocular Surface*, 5(2), 75–92.
2. Tomlinson, A. (2006). Epidemiology of dry eye disease. In P. A. Asbell & M. A. Lemp (Eds.), *Dry eye disease: The clinician's guide to diagnosis and treatment* (p. 1). New York: Thieme.
3. Lemp, M. A. (2008). Advances in understanding and managing dry eye disease. *American Journal of Ophthalmology*, 146(3), 350–356.
4. Farrand, K. F., Fridman, M., Stillman, I. O., et al. (2017). Prevalence of diagnosed dry eye disease in the United States among adults aged 18 years and older. *American Journal of Ophthalmology*, 182, 90–98.
5. Stern, M. E., Schaumburg, C. S., & Pflugfelder, S. C. (2013). Dry eye as a mucosal autoimmune disease. *International Reviews of Immunology*, 32(1), 19–41.
6. Pflugfelder, S. C. (2004). Antiinflammatory therapy for dry eye. *American Journal of Ophthalmology*, 137(2), 337–342.
7. Rosenthal, P., & Borsook, D. (2012). The corneal pain system. Part I: The missing piece of the dry eye puzzle. *The Ocular Surface*, 10, 2–14.
8. Benitez del Castillo, J. M., Acosta, M. C., Wassfi, M. A., et al. (2007). Relation between corneal innervation with confocal microscopy and corneal sensitivity with noncontact esthesiometry in patients with dry eye. *Investigative Ophthalmology & Visual Science*, 48, 173–181.
9. Bourcier, T., Acosta, M. C., Borderie, V., et al. (2005). Decreased corneal sensitivity in patients with dry eye. *Investigative Ophthalmology & Visual Science*, 46, 2341–2345.
10. Galor, A., Zlotcavitch, L., Walter, S. D., et al. (2015). Dry eye symptom severity and persistence are associated with features of neuropathic pain. *The British Journal of Ophthalmology*, 99(5), 665–668.
11. Galor, A., Levitt, R. C., Felix, E. R., et al. (2015). Neuropathic ocular pain: An important yet underevaluated feature of dry eye. *Eye (Lond)*, 29(3), 301–312.
12. Fraunfelder, F. T., Sciubba, J. J., & Mathers, W. D. (2012). The role of medications in causing dry eye. *Journal of Ophthalmology*, 2012, 285851.
13. Ismailova, D. S., Fedorov, A. A., & Grusha, Y. O. (2013). Ocular surface changes in thyroid eye disease. *Orbit (Amsterdam, Netherlands)*, 32(2), 87–90.
14. Kaufman, S. C. (2008). Anterior segment complications of herpes zoster ophthalmicus. *Ophthalmology*, 115, S24–S32.
15. Reddy, V. C., Patel, S. V., Hodge, D. O., & Leavitt, J. A. (2013). Corneal sensitivity, blink rate, and corneal nerve density in progressive supranuclear palsy and Parkinson disease. *Cornea*, 32(5), 631–635.
16. Schein, O. D., Tielsch, J. M., Munoz, B., et al. (1997). Relation between signs and symptoms of dry eye in the elderly. A population-based perspective. *Ophthalmology*, 104(9), 1395–1401.
17. American Academy of Ophthalmology Cornea/External Disease Panel. (2013). *Dry eye syndrome preferred practice pattern*. San Francisco: American Academy of Ophthalmology. Retrieved from http://one.aao.org/preferred -practice-pattern/dry-eye-syndrome-ppp-2013. (Accessed 12 August 2014).
18. Schiffman, R. M., Christianson, M. D., Jacobsen, G., Hirsch, J. D., & Reis, B. L. (2000). Reliability and validity of the Ocular Surface Disease Index. *Archives of Ophthalmology*, 118(5), 615–621.
19. Grubbs, J. R., Jr., Tolleson-Rinehart, S., Huynh, K., & Davis, R. M. (2014). A review of quality of life measures in dry eye questionnaires. *Cornea*, 33(2), 215–218.
20. Jones, L., Downie, L. E., Korb, D., et al. (2017). TFOS DEWS II Management and Therapy Report. *The Ocular Surface*, 15(3), 575–628.
21. Jalbert, I. (2013). Diet, nutraceuticals and the tear film. *Experimental Eye Research*, 117, 138–146.
22. Galor, A., Gardner, H., Pouyeh, B., Feuer, W., & Florez, H. (2014). Effect of a Mediterranean dietary pattern and vitamin D levels on dry eye syndrome. *Cornea*, 33(5), 437–441.
23. Pan, Q., Angelina, A., Zambrano, A., et al. (2013). Autologous serum eye drops for dry eye. *The Cochrane Database of Systematic Reviews*, (8), CD009327.
24. Gayton, J. L. (2009). Etiology, prevalence, and treatment of dry eye disease. *Clin Ophthalmol.*, 3, 405–412.

CHAPTER **58**

NASOLACRIMAL DUCT OBSTRUCTION AND DACRYOCYSTITIS

Andrew J. Rong • James T. Banta

 Red Flags include older adults or frail patients with acute dacryocystitis, patients with signs and symptoms of sepsis, preseptal or orbital cellulitis

DEFINITION AND EPIDEMIOLOGY

The *nasolacrimal duct*, commonly known as the *tear duct*, is a tubular structure that drains excess tears from the eyes into the nose. A complete or partial obstruction at any point along this structure is called a *nasolacrimal duct obstruction* (NLDO).[1] There are two types of acquired NLDO: primary and secondary. Primary acquired NLDO is the most common clinical syndrome of acquired NLDO in adults and is typically caused by inflammation or fibrosis without any precipitating cause.[2] Secondary acquired NLDO is caused by a myriad of precipitating factors, including infection, inflammation, neoplasm, and trauma. Patients affected by NLDO have disruption of normal tear drainage, causing problems that range from the annoyance of constant tearing to more serious conditions such as *dacryocystitis*, an inflammation of the lacrimal sac.

ANATOMY AND PATHOPHYSIOLOGY

The lacrimal drainage system consists of the *superior and inferior canaliculus*, the *lacrimal sac*, and the *nasolacrimal duct*. Tear drainage begins with contraction of the palpebral orbicularis oculi, a muscle that encircles the lids and tear ducts. Fluid enters openings in the upper and lower lid margin (*the puncta*), before being pumped through the canaliculi, into the lacrimal sac, and finally through the nasolacrimal duct. The tears exit into the nasal cavity through a valve (*the valve of Hasner*) and an opening (*the inferior meatus*) under the inferior turbinate.[3] In normal development, the nasolacrimal duct becomes patent to the inferior meatus of the nose during the first few weeks of life and before the onset of tear production. In 5% of newborns, the valve persists beyond this period, and parents may notice the clinical symptoms of a congenital NLDO.[4,5]

Acquired inflammation originating at the eye, lacrimal system, nose, or sinuses can induce swelling and scarring of the lacrimal system's mucous membranes, resulting in acquired NLDO. Congenital or acquired forms of NLDO can lead to stasis of tear flow and the development of secondary infections such as canaliculitis, dacryocystitis, and abscess formation. Obstruction that is not congenital may result from involutional stenosis, trauma, neoplasia, or anatomic obstructions (e.g., a deviated septum, polyps, or hypertrophied inferior turbinates).

CLINICAL PRESENTATION AND PHYSICAL EXAMINATION

Adults with partial or complete obstruction of the nasolacrimal duct often have chronic tearing, ocular discharge, and eyelash crusting.[1] More serious cases may also cause painful swelling below the medial canthus and a mucopurulent discharge from the punctum. The clinical history helps differentiate an excess accumulation of tears caused by a drainage obstruction versus excess tear production. *Epiphora*, the accumulation of tears in the palpebral fissure with eventual overflow down the cheeks, denotes lacrimal outflow deficiency (Fig. 58.1). A history of chronic allergies, sinusitis, previous nasal or sinus surgery, prior midfacial fractures, or radiation therapy may predispose patients to NLDO.[6] Systemic inflammatory diseases such as granulomatosis with polyangiitis, sarcoidosis, Crohn disease, and ulcerative colitis are other known associations.[7–9]

Physical examination includes careful observation of the ocular adnexa and surface structures for signs of inflammation. Gross examination findings may include overflow of tears, mucoid or purulent discharge, conjunctival injection, and erythema over the lacrimal sac. Pressure over the lacrimal sac may produce a mucoid reflux from the punctum, indicative of lower system obstruction. The medial canthus should be carefully examined for focal swelling, fluctuance, erythema, or

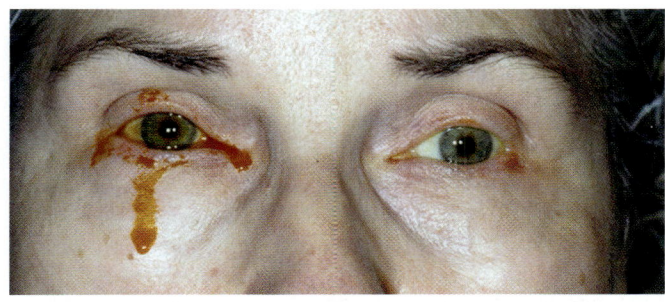

F I G .   **58.1**   After the application of fluorescein in both eyes, normal clearance of tears is seen on the left side. Pooling of tears and frank tearing are seen on the right side, indicative of nasolacrimal duct obstruction.

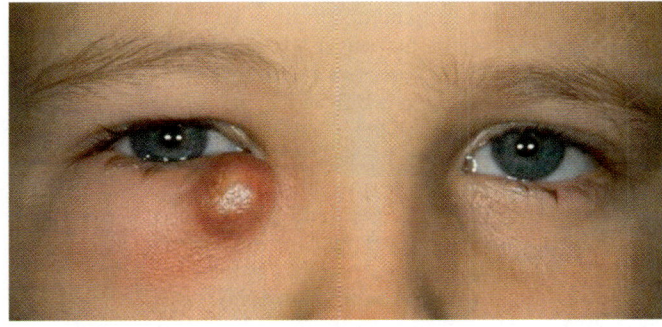

F I G .   **58.2**   Dacryocystitis commonly manifests as erythematous, fluctuant swelling just inferior to the medial canthus.

tenderness overlying the lacrimal sac, suggestive of dacryocystitis (Fig. 58.2). Fever and leukocytosis may also be present in acute dacryocystitis. Finally, a nasal speculum may be used to examine the nares for any mucosal swelling, tumors, or other anatomic abnormality that could narrow the distal opening of the nasolacrimal duct in the vicinity of the inferior turbinate.

DIAGNOSTICS

Diagnostic tests are usually unnecessary. In some cases, the ophthalmologist will test the lacrimal drainage system by directly cannulating the canaliculus and injecting sterile water or saline to check for patency of the system. In select cases of suspected trauma, tumors, or anatomic abnormalities, computed tomography or magnetic resonance imaging of the lacrimal system can be useful in the evaluation of patients with epiphora. In cases of dacryocystitis or purulent discharge, culture and sensitivity testing may help guide antibiotic therapy. If fever is present, a complete blood count (CBC) may be considered to evaluate for leukocytosis.

INITIAL DIAGNOSTICS

Nasolacrimal Duct Obstruction

LABORATORY
- Culture and sensitivity (if purulent discharge is present)
- CBC and differential (if fever is present)

IMAGING
- CT with contrast/MRI[a]

[a]If indicated.

DIFFERENTIAL DIAGNOSIS

 Priority differentials include orbital cellulitis, conjunctivitis, neoplastic process, punctual stenosis, blepharitis, and chronic dry eyes.

Chronic tearing and ocular irritation in an adult may also indicate punctal stenosis or eyelid malpositions. In patients with blood-tinged tears or a suspected mechanical obstruction, a neoplastic process must be ruled out. Preseptal or orbital cellulitis must also be considered in patients with severe swelling, mucopurulent discharge, and pain.[10]

INTERPROFESSIONAL COLLABORATIVE Management

Nonpharmacologic Management. About 96% of all congenital NLDO will resolve over a period of 12 months, and most clinicians recommend observation up to this time point.[11] The Crigler massage, a maneuver where downward pressure is applied on the lacrimal sac, can be performed by clinicians in an attempt to force open a blocked valve of Hasner by hydrostatic pressures. This maneuver has been estimated to resolve NLDO by 56% during the first 2 months of life and may prevent the patient from further interventions.[11]

Pharmacologic Management. Temporizing conservative management consists of warm compresses and topical antibiotics if an infection is suspected. In cases of dacryocystitis, the initial treatment for adults includes warm compresses, topical broad-spectrum antibiotic eye drops, and oral penicillinase-resistant antibiotics. Antibiotic choice is further guided by Gram stain and cultures. Topical antibiotics include trimethoprim sulfate and polymyxin B sulfate (Polytrim), tobramycin (AKTob, Tobrex), ciprofloxacin 0.3% (Ciloxan), and ofloxacin 0.3% (Ocuflox), one drop every 1 to 6 hours.[12] Systemic therapy may include cephalexin (Keflex), amoxicillin and clavulanate (Augmentin), or erythromycin (Erythrocin).[6] In the absence of mucopurulent drainage, prolonged use of topical antibiotics is not necessary.

INDICATIONS FOR REFERRAL OF HOSPITALIZATION

Any child with NLDO that does not resolve by the first year of life, any patient with a prolonged history of excess tearing, or any case of dacryocystitis should be referred for evaluation by an ophthalmologist. Children with congenital NLDO often require lacrimal duct probing by an ophthalmologist to relieve the anatomical obstruction. Further symptoms of tearing and intermittent conjunctivitis require repeat probing and/or stent placement.

Acquired NLDO does not benefit from nasolacrimal duct probing, and definitive treatment usually requires surgery.

As a general rule, acute dacryocystitis is managed medically. However, if a painful lacrimal sac abscess is pointing to a head, incision and drainage of the abscess may be beneficial. Once the episode of acute dacryocystitis has resolved, definitive treatment is through a *dacryocystorhinostomy* (DCR), a surgery that bypasses the lacrimal drainage system and is successful in up to 90% of cases.[13]

COMPLICATIONS

Acquired NLDO may progress to secondary infection, dacryocystitis, mucocele, pyocele, chronic conjunctivitis, preseptal and orbital cellulitis, or abscess formation. Oral antibiotics are necessary in cases of abscess formation, ineffective topical antibiotic therapy, orbital cellulitis, or recurrent dacryocystitis. The presence of dacryocystitis or an abscess with systemic signs of fever, malaise, or leukocytosis may require hospitalization with intravenous antibiotic therapy in seriously ill patients. Older adults or frail patients may develop sepsis as a result of acute dacryocystitis.

Patient and Family Education

- Adult patients should be informed about the signs and symptoms of dacryocystitis in the setting of NLDO, including mucopurulent discharge, pain, redness, and fever.
- Patients should also understand that the definitive treatment of acquired NLDO and dacryocystitis is surgery and that antibiotics are used to treat the infection, but will not resolve the obstruction.
- Children may be conservatively managed with nasolacrimal duct massage until 12 months of age, after which probing of the nasolacrimal duct should be performed.

REFERENCES

1. Dantas, R. R. (2010). Lacrimal drainage system obstruction. *Seminars in Ophthalmology, 25*(3), 98–103.
2. Linberg, J. V., & McCormick, S. A. (1986). Primary acquired nasolacrimal duct obstruction: A clinicopathologic report and biopsy technique. *Ophthalmology, 93*(8), 1055–1063.
3. Wobig, J. L., & Dailey, R. A. (2004). *Oculofacial plastic surgery: Face, lacrimal system, and orbit.* New York: Thieme.
4. Schaeffer, J. P. (1912). The genesis and development of the nasolacrimal passages in man. *The American Journal of Anatomy, 13,* 1–23.
5. Cassady, J. V. (1952). Developmental anatomy of the nasolacrimal duct. *Archives of Ophthalmology, 47,* 141–158.
6. Mills, D. M., & Meyer, D. R. (2006). Acquired nasolacrimal duct obstruction. *Otolaryngologic Clinics of North America, 39*(5), 979–999, vii.
7. Bartley, G. B. (1992). Acquired lacrimal drainage obstruction: An etiologic classification system, case reports, and a review of the literature. Part 2. *Ophthalmic Plastic and Reconstructive Surgery, 8,* 243–249.
8. Mauriello, J. A., Jr., & Mostafavi, R. (1994). Bilateral nasolacrimal duct obstruction associated with Crohn's disease successfully treated with dacryocystorhinostomy. *Ophthalmic Plastic and Reconstructive Surgery, 10,* 260–261.
9. Satchi, K., & McNab, A. A. (2009). Lacrimal obstruction in inflammatory bowel disease. *Ophthalmic Plastic and Reconstructive Surgery, 25*(5), 346–349.
10. Sullivan, J. H., Shetlar, D. J., & Whitcher, J. P. (2007). Lids, lacrimal apparatus, and tears. In P. Riordan-Eva & J. P. Whitcher (Eds.), *Vaughan and Asbury's general ophthalmology* (17th ed.). New York: McGraw-Hill.
11. Stolovitch, C., & Michaeli, A. (2006). Hydrostatic pressure as an office procedure for congenital nasolacrimal duct obstruction. *Journal of AAPOS, 10*(3), 269–272.
12. Usha, K., Smitha, S., Shah, N., et al. (2006). Spectrum and the susceptibilities of microbial isolates in cases of congenital nasolacrimal duct obstruction. *Journal of AAPOS, 10*(5), 469–472.
13. Dolman, P. J. (2003). Comparison of external dacryocystorhinostomy with nonlaser endonasal dacryocystorhinostomy. *Ophthalmology, 110*(1), 78–84.

CHAPTER **59**

PRESEPTAL AND ORBITAL CELLULITIS

Ann Q. Tran • James T. Banta

 Immediate evaluation and treatment is required for visual impairment, proptosis, increased orbital swelling, afferent pupil defects, boring pain, or suspected fungal etiology in diabetic or immunocompromised patients.

DEFINITION AND EPIDEMIOLOGY

Periorbital infections are classically divided anatomically into whether the findings are isolated anterior to the orbital septum (preseptal cellulitis) or posterior to the orbital septum (orbital cellulitis). The distinction is critical, as orbital cellulitis can extend to the orbital apex and beyond, leading to rapid blindness and potentially fatal consequences. Both disease entities are more common in children, with preseptal infection occurring much more frequently than orbital infection, but individuals of all ages can be affected.[1,2] Males are disproportionately affected compared with females at a ratio of 2:1, and the mean age is 7 years in both boys and girls.[3]

PATHOPHYSIOLOGY

Infection arises from three principle sources: local spread from adjacent structures such as the sinuses and lacrimal system, inoculation after skin trauma from lacerations or bug bites, or bacteremic spread from the upper respiratory system or the heart. Younger patients under the age of five with comorbidities or a history of trauma more commonly present with preseptal cellulitis. Children over the age of five with a clinical diagnosis of acute cellulitis and fever more commonly present with orbital cellulitis.[4]

Several anatomic factors predispose the orbit to infection. The orbital septum acts as a natural barrier to the passage of microorganisms; however, an initial preseptal cellulitis may spread to involve the orbit. Veins in the midface are valveless, permitting the direct posterior spread of infectious organisms into structures such as sinus cavities. The paranasal sinuses surround the orbit inferiorly, medially, and superiorly. The ethmoid sinus is separated from the medial orbit by the lamina papyracea, meaning "of paper" because the bone is paper-thin. Unsurprisingly, local spread from ethmoid sinusitis is the most common cause of orbital cellulitis in all age groups, and more than 90% of all cases of orbital cellulitis occur as a secondary extension of acute or chronic bacterial sinusitis.[1,5]

Given the pathogenesis of the disease, the most common organisms are those found in upper respiratory infections. In the pediatric population *Staphylococcus*, *Streptococcus* and *Haemophilus species* are the most causative organisms. There is a growing rise of methicillin-resistant *Staphylococcus aureus* (MRSA), but a prominent decrease in *Haemophilus influenza* type b due to vaccination.[6] Patients over the age of 15 are more likely to have polymicrobial infections. In immunocompromised or diabetic patients, a fungal cause such as *Aspergillus* or *Mucor* should be considered. Early signs in these patients, including apical boring pain, increased cellulitis, proptosis, and abrupt visual failure, should be evaluated promptly.[1]

CLINICAL PRESENTATION AND PHYSICAL EXAMINATION

Careful physical examination will elucidate key information regarding the location and the severity of the infection. Preseptal cellulitis typically manifests with eyelid edema, warmth, and erythema that may be severe (Fig. 59.1). The eye is typically spared, without conjunctival injection or chemosis. In contrast, orbital cellulitis causes axial proptosis, lid swelling, conjunctival chemosis and injection, elevated intraocular pressure, and pain or restriction with eye movement (Fig. 59.2).[5] The patient may report decreased visual acuity and diplopia. Decreased visual acuity and an afferent pupillary defect are

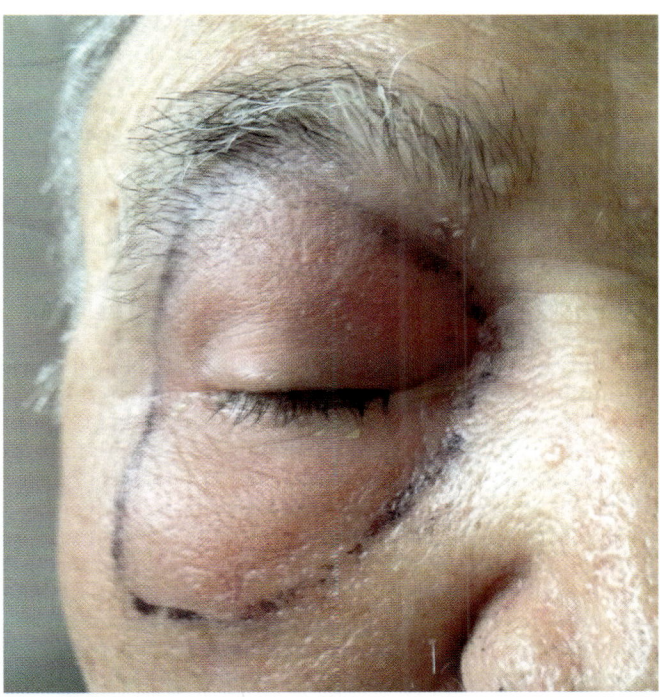

FIG. 59.1 Warm, erythematous skin with sparing of the eye is typical of preseptal cellulitis. A skin marker can be used to outline the area of erythema and monitor the response to treatment.

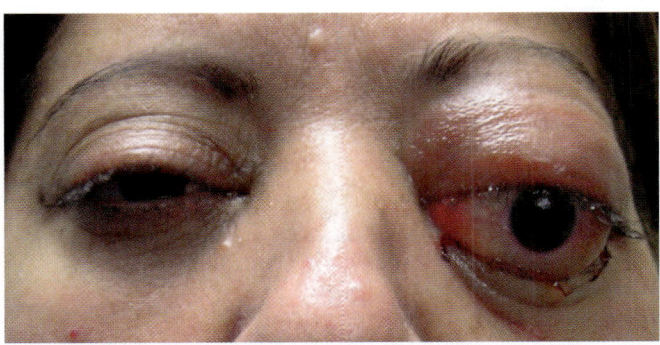

FIG. 59.2 Orbital cellulitis often presents with a dramatic appearance of axial proptosis, chemosis, and restricted ocular motility. This is an emergency and requires immediate ophthalmic care.

suggestive of optic nerve compromise, one of the most feared complications of orbital cellulitis. Patients with both preseptal and postseptal infections may be febrile, but systemic malaise is typically associated with postseptal disease. A history of neck stiffness or mental status change is worrisome for underlying meningitis. If trauma is implicated, the patient usually is seen 48 to 72 hours after the inciting event. However, in the presence of a retained foreign body, the clinical presentation of cellulitis can occur weeks to months after the injury.[6]

A thorough examination should include an evaluation of the patient's vital signs, mental status, neck flexibility, visual acuity (including color vision), pupillary response, extraocular muscle function (cranial nerves III, IV, XI), and pain with extraocular movements. Intraocular pressure may be elevated due to venous congestion from orbital inflammation. The globe and ocular adnexa should be inspected for swelling, redness, focal tenderness, hypoesthesia, and fluctuance or drainage. Close inspection should be undertaken to rule out foreign bodies or a focal source of infection such as dacryocystitis or eyelid abscess. In diabetic or immunocompromised patients, a black eschar located in the nasal cavity or hard palate may herald underlying fungal infection.

DIAGNOSTICS

An accurate history and physical examination will provide most of the information required to reach a diagnosis. All patients with suspected orbital cellulitis should undergo a computed tomography (CT) scan of the orbits and paranasal sinuses with contrast if possible. Radiographic findings of sinusitis (mucosal wall thickening, opacification, air-fluid levels), a foreign body, orbital fat stranding, signs of periosteal abscess (a heterogeneous or homogeneous collection in the subperiosteal space surrounded by an enhancing border suggestive of pus or fluid), and displacement of extraconal fat or muscle as well as diffuse enhancement of the orbit may be seen.[7] Given that approximately 75% of patients with orbital cellulitis develop leukocytosis, a complete blood count (CBC) with differential is indicated. Blood cultures may be helpful when bacteremia is suspected, and culture specimens should be taken from any drainage or abscess that is directly accessible. However, imaging should not be delayed to perform any of the aforementioned ancillary tests.

INITIAL DIAGNOSTICS

Preseptal and Orbital Cellulitis

LABORATORY
- CBC with differential
- Specimen samples for Gram stain, culture with sensitivity
- Blood cultures

IMAGING
- CT scan of the orbits and sinuses (with contrast if possible)

DIFFERENTIAL DIAGNOSIS

 Priority differentials include thyroid eye disease, idiopathic orbital inflammatory syndrome, and severe conjunctivitis.

Both infectious and noninfectious orbital disease may cause eyelid swelling, bulging of one or both eyes, and double vision. Broadly speaking, orbital disease may be grouped into five general categories, including inflammatory, infectious, neoplastic (both benign and malignant), traumatic, and related to malformation (e.g., congenital or vascular).

INTERPROFESSIONAL COLLABORATIVE MANAGEMENT
Pharmacologic Management

Appropriate oral therapy for preseptal cellulitis includes broad-spectrum antibiotics, such as a third-generation cephalosporin or amoxicillin-clavulanate. In suspected MRSA infections, drugs such as clindamycin, doxycycline, and double-strength trimethoprim-sulfamethoxazole are effective. A follow-up evaluation should be scheduled within 12 to 24 hours to monitor for signs of progression or lack of response to antibiotic therapy. Regardless of age, patients with significant systemic symptoms, cellulitis that fails to respond to oral antibiotics, or

possible orbital cellulitis should be referred to an ophthalmologist or otolaryngologist for hospitalization, urgent imaging, and intravenous antibiotic therapy. Patients are monitored closely during the first 24 to 48 hours of hospitalization for any clinical deterioration, which could suggest abscess formation or intracranial extension that may necessitate surgical intervention.[1,8] Patients with subperiosteal abscesses larger than 2 cm may have improved treatment outcomes with prompt drainage.[9]

Given the likelihood of the primary care provider to care for patients who are diabetic (or, less commonly, immunocompromised), it is imperative to identify a possible fungal cause. The most feared complication, rhino-orbital mucormycosis, can progress rapidly. Early tissue biopsy and radical excision with both local antifungal irrigation and systemic antifungal administration may be both sight saving and lifesaving, underscoring the importance of aggressive treatment and prompt referral to an ophthalmologist.[8]

INDICATIONS FOR REFERRAL OR HOSPITALIZATION

Patients with decreased visual acuity, proptosis, diplopia, restricted ocular movement, globe involvement, systemic symptoms, or neurologic signs should be referred to an ophthalmologist emergently or hospitalized for emergent imaging. Patients with preseptal cellulitis treated with oral antibiotics that do not improve within 24 hours should also be referred to an ophthalmologist. Patients with documented orbital cellulitis require hospitalization for initiation of intravenous antibiotics, imaging, and other supportive therapy as indicated.

LIFE-SPAN CONSIDERATIONS

Older adults and immunocompromised individuals may not demonstrate the same degree of inflammatory signs and may not be febrile in spite of a severe underlying infection; a heightened degree of suspicion is necessary to appropriately manage these individuals.[1]

COMPLICATIONS

Orbital cellulitis is a potentially fatal condition and blindness may occur in up to 11% of patients, necessitating prompt clinical identification of this disorder. Other complications include cavernous sinus thrombosis; central retinal artery or vein thrombosis; subperiosteal, orbital, epidural, subdural, or brain abscess; and optic neuropathy.[1,2,5]

PATIENT AND FAMILY EDUCATION

- When oral antibiotic therapy is prescribed, instruct patients to return before their scheduled follow-up visit (in 12 to 24 hours) if their symptoms increase in severity.
- Remind patients to complete the full course of antibiotic therapy and to return before the end of therapy if signs and symptoms do not continue to improve or if there is any worsening of the condition.
- Inform patients and their families that fever, lethargy, and irritability are signs of possible sepsis or meningitis, and require immediate evaluation and treatment.

HEALTH PROMOTION

Address risk factors for frequent sinus infections, such as smoking and untreated allergic rhinitis. Discuss the importance of diabetes control (normalizing blood sugar and A1C measurements; diabetes is a risk factor for the development of more serious fungal infections.

REFERENCES

1. Holds, J. (2013). Orbital inflammatory and infectious disorders. In *Basic and clinical science course, 2013–2014, Section 7*. San Francisco: American Academy of Ophthalmology.
2. Kanski, J. J. (2007). Orbit. In *Clinical ophthalmology: A systematic approach* (6th ed.). Edinburgh: Butterworth-Heinemann/Elsevier.
3. Nageswaran, S., Woods, C. R., Benjamin, D. K., Jr., Givner, L. B., & Shetty, A. K. (2006). Orbital cellulitis in children. *The Pediatric Infectious Disease Journal*, 25(8), 695–699.
4. Albert, D. M. (2008). Infectious processes of the orbit. In *Albert and Jakobiec's principles and practice of ophthalmology* (3rd ed.). Philadelphia: Saunders/Elsevier.
5. Botting, A. M., McIntosh, D., & Mahadevan, M. (2008). Paediatric pre- and post-septal peri-orbital infections are different diseases. A retrospective review of 262 cases. *International Journal of Pediatric Otorhinolaryngology*, 72(3), 377–383.
6. Kennerdell, J. S. (2001). *Practical diagnosis and management of orbital disease*. Boston: Butterworth-Heinemann.
7. Rutar, T., Chambers, H. F., Crawford, J. B., Perdreau-Remington, F., Zwick, O. M., Karr, M., et al. (2006). Ophthalmic manifestations of infections caused by the USA300 clone of community-associated methicillin-resistant *Staphylococcus aureus*. *Ophthalmology*, 113(8), 1455–1462.
8. Sridhara, S. R., Paragache, G., Panda, N. K., & Chakrabarti, A. (2005). Mucormycosis in immunocompetent individuals: An increasing trend. *The Journal of Otolaryngology*, 34(6), 402–406.
9. Dewan, M. A., Meyer, D. R., & Wladis, E. J. (2011). Orbital cellulitis with subperiosteal abscess: Demographics and management outcomes. *Ophthalmic Plastic and Reconstructive Surgery*, 27(5), 330–332.

CHAPTER 60

PINGUECULAE AND PTERYGIA

John W. Hinkle • James T. Banta

DEFINITION AND EPIDEMIOLOGY

Pingueculae and pterygia are two of the most common ocular surface abnormalities encountered by primary care providers. A pinguecula is a benign, yellow-white nodule on the bulbar conjunctiva, most often located nasal to the cornea. A pterygium is a similarly benign growth of fibrovascular conjunctival tissue that extends onto the surface of the cornea. The word *pterygium* is derived from the diminutive of the Greek word *pterygion*, meaning "wing"—an apt name given the winged shape of the lesion. Both pingueculae and pterygia usually grow slowly and commonly manifest in patients 20 to 50 years of age. A meta-analysis estimated the prevalence of pterygium to be 10.2%,[1] and both pterygium and pingueculae are more common in men than women and in lower latitudes with greater sun exposure.[2]

PATHOPHYSIOLOGY

Both pingueculae and pterygia have degenerative components. Histologic analysis reveals elastotic degeneration of stromal collagen and disruption of the basement membrane of the conjunctival epithelium. Tissue stains show that pterygia have more pronounced fibrovascular proliferation. It has been hypothesized that the barrier created by corneal limbal cells must be violated in order for this proliferation to involve the superficial cornea.[3] Corneal involvement in pterygia includes infiltration of the Bowman layer, a strong layer of collagen

directly beneath the corneal epithelium. Disruption of this layer can lead to scarring and focal opacification of cornea.

Although the pathogenesis of these entities is multifactorial and incompletely understood, exposure to ultraviolet (UV) light, particularly UV-B, has been associated with development of pterygia.[4,5] Heredity, chronic conjunctival inflammation, and viral infections have also been implicated.[6-8] As they are degenerative processes, development before the age of 20 years is very unusual. Pingueculae and pterygia have no common systemic associations, although they may occur more frequently in conditions that confer a proclivity for skin neoplasms, such as xeroderma pigmentosum. However, despite this association and the link to UV light exposure, pterygia and pingueculae themselves carry no significant malignant potential.

CLINICAL PRESENTATION AND PHYSICAL EXAMINATION

Both pingueculae and pterygia arise and grow slowly over the course of years. Common patient complaints include dryness, irritation, foreign body sensation, itching, redness, and a bothersome cosmetic appearance. Severe dryness from tear film irregularity induced by the lesion may cause intermittent blurry vision. In more advanced stages of disease, a pterygium may cause persistently decreased vision. By physically deforming the cornea, a pterygium can induce astigmatism—irregularity of the corneal shape—and cause blurred vision. Furthermore, with time a pterygium may also impair vision by extending from the periphery into the central cornea, obstructing the visual axis.

Pingueculae and pterygia can be diagnosed clinically. Most lesions are identifiable with the naked eye. The overwhelming majority of lesions appear on the horizontal meridian at either the 3-o'clock or 9-o'clock position, more frequently nasally than temporally. A single eye may have two pinguecula, two pterygium, or a combination of both.

Pingueculae appear as elevated, yellowish-white lesions immediately adjacent to but not encroaching onto the cornea. They typically do not have abnormal vasculature, large feeder vessels, or bleed spontaneously. Pingueculitis, or localized inflammation of a pinguecula, may occur, in which case the lesion will appear pinkish with dilated blood vessels (Fig. 60.1). In this scenario, patients classically report increased redness and irritation in the area.

Some believe a pterygium arises from preexisting pinguecula, though they are commonly observed without any known precursor. Like pingueculae, pterygia are almost exclusively seen on the horizontal meridian. The base of the pterygium, the wider aspect of the "wing," is on the conjunctiva and tapers to the head overlying the cornea (Fig. 60.2). Pterygia commonly involve only a millimeter or two of the cornea. However, in advanced stages they can extend to obscure the central visual axis. The corneal aspect of a pterygium can be whitish or clear and may be detectable only by changes in corneal contour and blood vessels that track from the conjunctival base. Analogous to pingueculitis, an inflamed pterygium will have prominently dilated blood vessels and a pink or reddish hue.

DIAGNOSTICS

Slit-lamp examination provides the best view of the ocular surface details. If a slit lamp is unavailable, careful examination with the naked eye under adequate lighting is usually sufficient to diagnose these two external lesions. Orienting the lighting

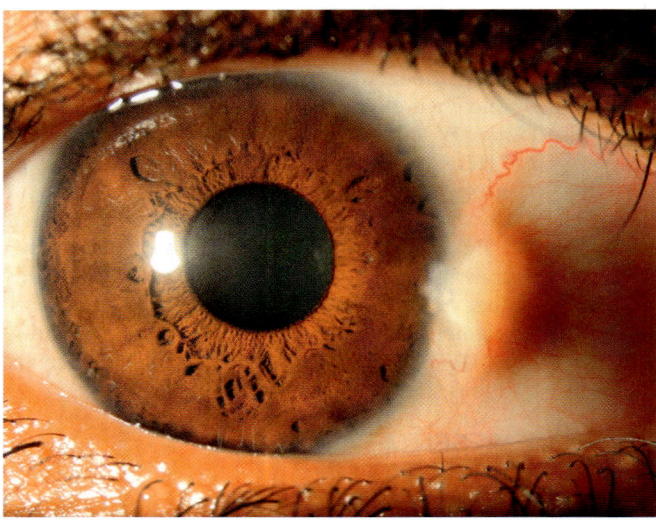

FIG. 60.1 An elevated, inflamed pinguecula can cause foreign body sensation and chronic redness.

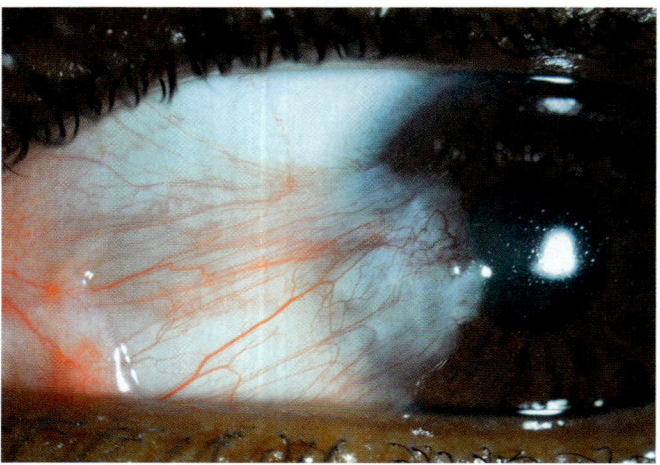

FIG. 60.2 Typical appearance of a medium-sized pterygium.

obliquely may reveal subtle differences in elevation and coloration suggesting the diagnosis of a pterygium or pinguecula.

In differentiating pingueculae and pterygia from other ocular surface abnormalities, examination of the cornea under a cobalt blue light after fluorescein staining can be helpful. Fluorescein highlights defects of the corneal or conjunctival epithelium. Neither pingueculae nor pterygia involve epithelial breakdown, so they do not stain strongly with fluorescein. In addition, pathology associated with corneal epithelial defects often cause more acute pain and photophobia.

INITIAL DIAGNOSTICS

Pinguecula and Pterygium

- Clinical examination
- Fluorescein stain (if indicated)

DIFFERENTIAL DIAGNOSIS

 Priority differentials include episcleritis, corneal ulcers, and squamous neoplasia.

Episcleritis can present with localized irritation and a slightly raised conjunctival area, but does not involve the cornea. The hyperemia of episcleritis should blanche after instilling phenylephrine 2.5% drops. Corneal ulcers can present with pain and decreased vision alongside an opacity of the cornea, but these lesions progress much more rapidly than either pterygium or pinguecula, will likely stain with fluorescein testing, and can produce purulent discharge. Squamous neoplasia can mimic pterygium or pinguecula in appearance and time course. However, cancer should be suspected if the lesion is not at the usual 3 o'clock or 9 o'clock position; has extremely prominent, tortuous blood vessels; or is found in an immunosuppressed patient.

INTERPROFESSIONAL COLLABORATIVE MANAGEMENT

Nonpharmacologic Management

Treatment should initially be directed toward symptomatic improvement. Dry eye, foreign body sensation, itchiness, and redness typically respond well to preservative free artificial tear drops, which may be purchased over the counter and are very well tolerated. These may be used as frequently as is needed and may be used indefinitely as they do not interfere with other medications. Other over-the-counter eye drops, such as tetrahydrozoline (Visine) and naphazoline (Clear Eyes), induce vasoconstriction in the conjunctiva and should be avoided because their chronic use can cause rebound inflammation and worsening redness. UV protection in the form of wide-brimmed hats and sunglasses with UVB protection should be advised to prevent progression and the development of new lesions in patients with pterygium or pinguecula.

Pharmacologic Management

Inflamed pterygia or pingueculae respond well to a short course of lower potency topical steroid drops, such as loteprednol (Lotemax) or fluorometholone (FML). These particular topical steroids are preferred because of the lower risk of complications such as elevation of intraocular pressure compared to other steroid formulations. Corneal ulcers and epithelial defects should be ruled out definitively before anti-inflammatory treatment is started, and the treatment should not extend beyond 4 to 7 days without ophthalmic consultation. A general dosage guideline for these topical medications is four times daily for 4 to 7 days.

INDICATIONS FOR REFERRAL AND HOSPITALIZATION

An inflamed eye that does not responded to treatment within a few days should prompt a nonurgent ophthalmic examination. On occasion, pterygia require excisional surgery and should be referred for evaluation. The primary indications for surgery are (1) chronic pain and redness refractory to conservative therapy, and (2) visual compromise as a result of astigmatism or visual axis obstruction. Recurrence of the pterygium and excessive scarring are the most common complications of excision. The recurrence rate is reduced by placement of a conjunctival autograft (typically harvested from the same eye) or topical application of an antimetabolite intraoperatively (e.g., mitomycin

C). Novel adjuvant management strategies targeting inflammation and angiogenesis (antivascular endothelial growth factor injections) are being developed and incorporated in efforts to reduce recurrence—a frustrating and not infrequent complication.[9]

As previously mentioned, other pathology can masquerade as pterygium or occur simultaneously. The prevalence of ocular surface squamous neoplasia in specimens from excised pterygia ranges from 0% to 10%.[10] Given this association, all excised pterygia should undergo histological examination so that further treatment can be initiated if necessary.

PATIENT EDUCATION

Patients who spend a lot of time outdoors or those with preexisting pterygia and pingueculae should be encouraged to wear sunglasses with UV filters and wide-brimmed hats to reduce exposure to UV light. They can also be counseled about the low-risk and often times effective treatment of symptoms with preservative-free artificial tears.

REFERENCES

1. Liu, L., Wu, J., Geng, J., Yuan, Z., & Huang, D. (2013). Geographical prevalence and risk factors for pterygium: A systematic review and meta-analysis. *BMJ Open, 3*(11), 1–8.
2. BCSC External Disease and Cornea, 2016–2017, pp. 316–317.
3. Raizada, I. N., & Bhatnagar, N. K. (1976). Pinguecula and pterygium (a histopathologic study). *Indian Journal of Ophthalmology, 24*(2), 8–16.
4. Detorakis, E. T., & Spandidos, D. A. (2009). Pathogenetic mechanisms and treatment options for ophthalmic pterygium: Trends and perspectives. *International Journal of Molecular Medicine, 23*(4), 439–447.
5. Chui, J., Di Girolamo, N., Wakefield, D., et al. (2008). The pathogenesis of pterygium: Current concepts and their therapeutic implications. *The Ocular Surface, 6*(1), 24–43.
6. Bradley, J. C., Yang, W., Bradley, R. H., Reid, T. W., & Schwab, I. R. (2010). The science of pterygia. *The British Journal of Ophthalmology, 94*, 815–820.
7. Foster, C. S., & Mauro, J. (2009). Pterygia: Pathogenesis and the role of subconjunctival bevacizumab in treatment. *Seminars in Ophthalmology, 24*(3), 130–134.
8. Chui, J., et al. (2008). The pathogenesis of pterygium: Current concepts and their therapeutic implications. *The Ocular Surface, 6*(1), 24–43.
9. Ang, L. P., Chua, J. L., & Tan, D. T. (2007). Current concepts and techniques in pterygium treatment. *Current Opinion in Ophthalmology, 18*(4), 308–313.
10. Oellers, P., Karp, C., Sheth, A., et al. (2013). Prevalence, treatment and outcomes of coexistent ocular surface squamous neoplasia and pterygium. *Ophthalmology, 120*(3), 445–450.

TRAUMATIC OCULAR DISORDERS

Nimesh A. Patel • James T. Banta

 Red flags include ocular trauma with visual loss, retrobulbar hemorrhage (history of contusive trauma, decrease in vision, inability to open the eye, 360 degrees of subconjunctival hemorrhage), retinal detachment, open globe injury (e.g., full-thickness laceration), ruptured globe, chemical injuries, penetrating and perforating injuries, corneal and intraocular foreign bodies, and orbital fractures.

DEFINITION AND EPIDEMIOLOGY

Ocular trauma encompasses a number of physical injuries, both mechanical and chemical, sustained by the eye (globe) and ocular adnexa. These tissues can sustain a number of different injuries. For nonophthalmologists, these injuries may seem complex and foreign. To facilitate classification and communication among health care professionals, a terminology system was devised to allow a standardized description and classification of ocular trauma.[1,2] Table 61.1 lists the standard definitions that are used to describe traumatic ocular injuries.[3]

The most vital distinction is between open and closed globe injuries. This information is crucial because it determines the clinical management of the patient and provides important prognostic information.[4] If the patient has not sustained a full-thickness injury, then the patient has a *closed* globe injury. If there is a full-thickness wound, it is an *open* globe injury. Closed globe trauma is further divided into contusions and lamellar lacerations. Contusions are the most common form of ocular injury, and occur when the eye is impacted but the wall of the eye remains intact. The sequelae of an ocular contusion are vast and include corneal abrasion, hyphema, traumatic iritis, iridodialysis, lens dislocation, vitreous hemorrhage, retinal hemorrhage, and retinal detachment. A *lamellar laceration* refers to a partial-thickness wound of the eye wall but the integrity of the globe is maintained.

Full-thickness injuries are often inappropriately described and lead to confusion between a referring provider and the ophthalmologist. Too often, both primary care providers and ophthalmologists describe a patient who has sustained a full-thickness injury to the globe as having a "ruptured globe." This is correct only if the person has sustained an ocular contusion (typically with a blunt object) resulting in a *rupture* of the eye wall. Common mechanisms for a ruptured globe include high-velocity projectiles (e.g., racquetball, bungee cord) and assault (e.g., fist, bat, paintball). These injuries are highly destructive to intraocular contents and have a guarded prognosis. By contrast, if a sharp object creates a full-thickness eye wall injury, it is classified as a laceration. Common mechanisms of lacerations include work-related activities (e.g., cutting tile, landscaping) and accidents (e.g., children playing with scissors). Lacerations can be further divided into penetrating injuries, perforating injuries, and intraocular foreign bodies. *Penetrating* injuries are caused by an object entering and exiting the eye wall through the same wound. *Perforating* injuries have a separate entry and exit wound. An *intraocular foreign body* is present when a portion of the insulting object enters and remains in the eye.

The annual number of eye injuries treated by medical personnel was estimated at nearly 2 million by a large national survey.[5] The Baltimore Eye Survey reported a cumulative lifetime prevalence of eye injury of 14.4% in the general population of an urban area.[6] McGwin and colleagues estimated the rate of injury to be 6.98 injuries per 1000 persons. Of those injuries, 50.7% were treated in emergency departments, 38.7% in private offices of physicians, 8.1% in outpatient facilities, and 2.5% within inpatient facilities. Most injuries were sustained by men younger than 30 years.[5,7] The most commonly encountered injuries were superficial injuries of the eye and adnexa and foreign bodies on the ocular surface.[5]

Ocular trauma is recurrent in nature. In the Beaver Dam Eye Study, Wong et al. noted that an initial episode of ocular trauma increased the likelihood of recurrent trauma in the next 5 years by a factor of 3.27.[8] The rates of injury were also higher among blue-collar and farm workers compared with white-collar workers, with odds ratios of 1.58 and 1.32, respectively. Epidemiologic studies such as these assist in identifying at-risk

TABLE 61.1　Birmingham Eye Trauma Terminology

Term	Definition	Explanation
Eye wall	Sclera and cornea	Although the eye wall technically has three coats posterior to the limbus, for clinical and practical purposes, violation of only the most external structure is taken into consideration.
Closed globe injury	No full-thickness wound of the eye wall	
Open globe injury	Full-thickness wound of the eye wall	
Contusion	No (full-thickness) wound of the eye wall	The injury results from direct energy delivery by the object or from the changes in the shape of the globe.
Lamellar laceration	Partial-thickness wound of the eye wall	The wound of the eye wall is not "through" but "into."
Rupture	Full-thickness wound of the eye wall caused by a blunt object	Because the eye is filled with incompressible liquid, the impact results in momentary increase of the intraocular pressure. The eye wall yields at its weakest point (at the impact site or elsewhere; e.g., an old cataract wound dehisces even though the impact occurred elsewhere). The actual wound is caused by an inside-out mechanism.
Laceration	Full-thickness wound of the eye wall caused by a sharp object	The wound occurs at the impact site by an outside-in mechanism.
Penetrating injury	Entrance wound	If more than one wound is present, each must have been caused by a different agent.
Intraocular foreign body	Retained foreign object(s)	This is technically a penetrating injury but grouped separately because of different clinical implications.
Perforating injury	Entrance and exit wounds	Both wounds are caused by the same agent.

Modified from Kuhn, F., Morris, R., & Witherspoon, C. D. (2002). Birmingham Eye Trauma Terminology (BETT): terminology and classification of mechanical eye injuries. *Ophthalmology Clinics of North America, 15*, 139–143.

populations and creating appropriate prevention strategies. For example, Dannenberg and associates found in their study of penetrating ocular trauma in the workplace that only 6% of the injured were wearing protective eyewear at the time of their injury,[9] clearly highlighting the need for protective eyewear in high-risk settings.

Haring et al. performed a review on all sports-related ocular trauma between 2000 and 2013. They found that out of 120,847 injuries, 81% were male and the most frequent causes were basketball (22.6%), baseball or softball (14.3%), and air gun or paintball (11.8%).[10]

Children are not immune to ocular trauma. One study has shown that up to 43% of open globe injuries are sustained in patients younger than 18 years.[11] A large study of pediatric globe injuries in Los Angeles demonstrated that sharp objects cause the majority of injuries (67%), and that most injuries occur at home (72%).[12]

PATHOPHYSIOLOGY
Mechanical Injuries

When mechanical energy is imparted to the eye, the manner in which it is delivered and the amount imparted largely determine the type and degree of injury.[13] Minor trauma may cause only limited injuries, such as subconjunctival hemorrhage, superficial abrasions of the periocular skin, painful abrasions of the cornea, or lacerations of the conjunctiva.

Ocular trauma associated with a higher level of mechanical energy is often mitigated by the size of the object. Large objects will often not fit in the confines of the orbital rim within which the globe rests. Thus a large blunt object with high mechanical energy may create a blowout fracture of the thin orbital walls as a result of the pressure on the orbital rim and contents. The thin orbital bones act as a "crumple zone," allowing most of the energy to be absorbed by the orbit while sparing the eye. However, a similar amount of energy imparted by a smaller blunt object that fits in the confines of the orbital rim can cause more severe injuries such as hyphema (caused by shearing of iris blood vessels), iridodialysis (disinsertion of the iris root), lens dislocation, vitreous hemorrhage, retinal detachment, or globe rupture.

A globe rupture results when the eye is bluntly impacted and cannot sustain the forces imparted. Because the eye contains incompressible fluids, the sudden increase in pressure from a mechanical trauma can cause an enormous transfer of energy to the eye wall. The eye wall may rupture if the pressure is high enough at weak points, such as previous surgical sites, the insertions of the extraocular muscles, or the limbus (junction of the cornea and sclera). Ruptures often cause devastating visual loss secondary to retinal detachments, massive hemorrhage, loss of intraocular contents, intraocular infections, and a number of other complications.

Mechanical energy imparted from sharp objects typically results in lacerations of the eye wall. In contrast to ruptures, these injuries are sustained at the site of impact and mechanically disrupt the eye wall at that location. These injuries can be equally devastating but often have a better prognosis, especially if the injury is confined to the anterior segment of the eye.

Chemical Injuries

Ocular injury due to chemical exposure varies depending on the nature of the chemical, the duration of exposure, and the degree of ocular penetration. While acids can be quite destructive to the ocular surface because the dissociated anions of the acid lead to denaturation and coagulation of the ocular proteins, the eye proteins act as an acid buffer to limit ocular penetration. By contrast, alkaline substances release hydroxyl ions that saponify cell membranes and cations that interact with the structural proteins of the eye wall. This allows for deeper ocular penetration of alkaline substances and more extensive ocular injuries.

Retrobulbar Hemorrhage

Retrobulbar hemorrhage occurs in cases of contusive trauma and is a true ophthalmic emergency. There is bleeding posterior to the globe, usually from the infraorbital artery, into the closed orbital space, resulting in a compartment syndrome. With the increase in posterior pressure, the optic nerve becomes stretched and compressed. This leads to blockage of venous drainage and central retinal artery occlusion if untreated.

CLINICAL PRESENTATION

The clinical presentation of eye trauma is highly variable. Given this variability, patients may have multiple presenting symptoms including pain, redness, decreased vision, diplopia, and photophobia. The most commonly encountered traumatic injuries are superficial injury of the adnexa and external eye (e.g., corneal abrasion, subconjunctival hemorrhage) and a foreign body on the ocular surface.[5] These typically present with an abrupt onset of redness, foreign body sensation, tearing, and photophobia. A complaint of pain with blinking is common with a corneal or conjunctival foreign body. This pain is usually improved with topical anesthetic drops such as tetracaine.

Contusive trauma may affect the orbit or the globe itself. Patients who sustain orbital fractures may acutely report diplopia, pain with eye movement, hypoesthesia of the cheek and upper lip, and subcutaneous or conjunctival emphysema. Retrobulbar hemorrhage can present with decrease in vision, inability to open the eye, and 360 degrees of subconjunctival hemorrhage.

A hyphema is a layered collection of blood in the anterior chamber of the eye (Fig. 61.1) and is a common manifestation of contusive ocular injury. Patients report blurred vision and pain. Elevated intraocular pressure is the most feared complication and can lead to permanent loss of vision. Vitreous hemorrhage or retinal detachment may present with marked decrease in vision.

Open globe trauma usually is associated with a history of projectile injury or severe contusion of the eye (Fig. 61.2). The clinical presentation of an open globe can be subtle. A very high index of suspicion should be maintained, particularly in patients with a high-risk profile (e.g., construction, landscaping, mechanic). Signs of a potential open globe injury include 360 degrees subconjunctival hemorrhage, pupil irregularity, low intraocular pressure, poor vision, and abnormal contour of the globe on computed tomography (CT) scan.

PHYSICAL EXAMINATION

Although intraocular pressure measurement and slit lamp microscopy may not always be available, the other elements of the examination should be possible in most clinic or emergency departments, and the information gathered will be invaluable to the accepting physician should the patient require referral.

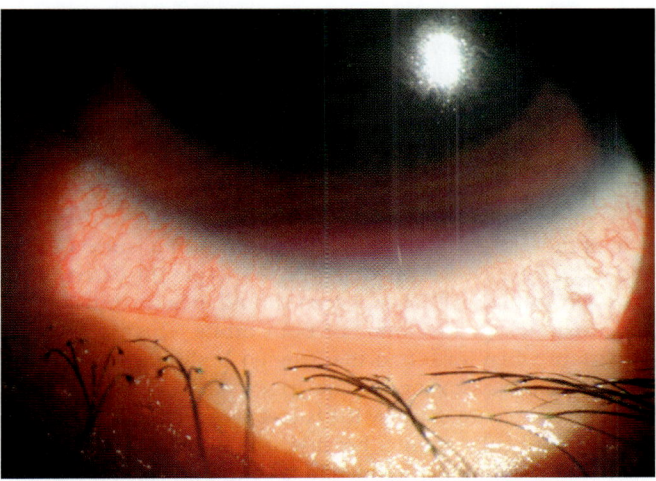

FIG. **61.1** A small layered hyphema after an ocular contusion.

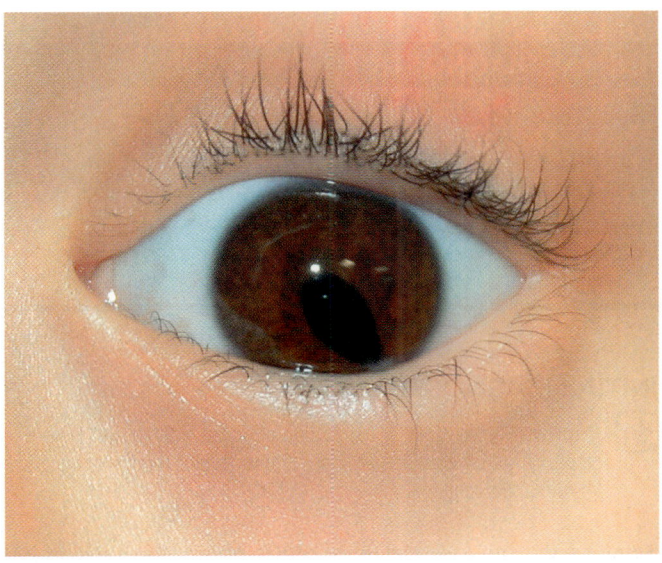

FIG. **61.2** Peaking of the pupil after ocular trauma is indicative of an open globe injury and should lead to immediate referral to an ophthalmologist.

Measurement of the intraocular pressure is contraindicated if there is a possibility of an open globe injury.

The most important assessment is the visual acuity. If no eye charts are available, there are smartphone applications or web-based charts that can be downloaded and printed. Eternal exam includes assessing extraocular movements and palpation of the orbital rim to look for fractures. With use of a bright light source (e.g., flashlight, penlight), the ocular surface and anterior chamber can be visualized to check the integrity of anterior segment structures and to assess the pupil. Periorbital lacerations should be explored to rule out foreign bodies or potential penetration sites.

DIAGNOSTICS

Once an adequate examination has been performed, there are several tools that can aid in establishing a diagnosis. If a laceration of the cornea is suspected, a Seidel test can be performed.

A moistened fluorescein strip is liberally applied to the ocular surface. When it is viewed with a cobalt blue light source, a full-thickness laceration is confirmed if a stream of aqueous disrupts the thick layer of fluorescein. Imaging studies are often very helpful and should be considered in eye injuries. Ultrasound can be used to assess for retinal detachment and intraocular foreign body but is typically useful only if technicians trained specifically in ocular ultrasound are available. CT scan is the "gold standard" for eye injuries. In a study, CT was shown to be 73% sensitive and 95% specific for detection of open globe injuries.[14] The CT scan should include thin coronal and axial cuts (1 to 2 mm) of both orbits. This is especially important when an intraocular foreign body is suspected. CT is also vital in assessing the integrity of the bony orbit. Magnetic resonance imaging (MRI) is less useful in the acute management of ocular trauma because it is inferior to CT scan in defining orbital bone trauma and is contraindicated if a metallic foreign body is suspected. If a retrobulbar hemorrhage with compartment syndrome is highly suspected, treatment should not be delayed with further imaging studies.

INITIAL DIAGNOSTICS

Eye Trauma

LABORATORY
- Seidel test in any patient suspected of having an open globe

IMAGING
- Ultrasound or computed tomography (CT) scan in any patient suspected of having an intraorbital or intraocular foreign body

INITIAL DIAGNOSIS

 Priority differentials in the setting of ocular trauma are (1) open globe, (2) retrobulbar hemorrhage, (3) intraocular foreign body, and (4) retinal detachment.

Some of the other sequelae of ocular trauma include orbital fracture, eyelid laceration, subconjunctival hemorrhage, corneal foreign body, chemical keratoconjunctivitis, corneal abrasion, hyphema, traumatic iritis, and vitreous hemorrhage.

The manifestations of ocular trauma are numerous and varied (Box 61.1). They range from mildly uncomfortable, self-limited issues to potentially blinding and even systemically threatening conditions. One of the key elements to formation of a differential diagnosis is an attempt to determine which structures in the eye have been traumatized.

INTERPROFESSIONAL COLLABORATIVE MANAGEMENT
Pharmacologic Management

Small corneal abrasions and subconjunctival hemorrhages are generally self-limited and do not require referral if further injury can be ruled out. Corneal abrasions can be treated with artificial tears and topical antibiotics. Chemical injury is initially managed with copious irrigation. Hyphema and traumatic iritis are treated with cycloplegic drops and topical steroids. Topical anesthetic drops should never be prescribed or given to the patient to take home as this can lead to melting of the cornea.

BOX 61.1

Manifestations of Ocular Trauma

ADNEXA AND ORBIT
- Eyelid laceration
- Orbital fracture
- Retrobulbar hemorrhage
- Traumatic optic neuropathy
- Orbital foreign body

CORNEA AND ANTERIOR SEGMENT
- Chemical burn
- Corneal abrasion
- Corneal or conjunctival foreign body
- Conjunctival laceration
- Subconjunctival hemorrhage
- Corneal laceration
- Traumatic iritis
- Hyphema
- Iridodialysis and cyclodialysis
- Traumatic glaucoma

POSTERIOR SEGMENT
- Vitreous hemorrhage
- Commotio retinae
- Traumatic choroidal rupture
- Chorioretinitis sclopetaria
- Purtscher retinopathy
- Shaken baby syndrome

COMBINED OR MIXED
- Globe laceration or rupture
- Intraocular foreign body

Indications for Referral and Hospitalization

In general, ocular trauma with vision loss requires ophthalmology consultation to discuss or examine the patient. Patients with corneal foreign bodies should also be referred to ophthalmology, even if the foreign body is partially removed, because residual material (e.g., rust ring) needs to be completely removed. If open globe is suspected, a shield is placed over the eye and topical and systemic antibiotics are initiated. Retrobulbar hemorrhage is a sight threatening condition and lateral canthotomy with cantholysis should be performed as soon as possible.

LIFE-SPAN CONSIDERATIONS

Ocular trauma occurs across the life span and can have a debilitating effect on those who sustain it. It is estimated by the U.S. Eye Injury Registry that 500,000 years of eyesight are lost annually as a result of ocular trauma.[15] In addition, a total of approximately 4 billion dollars annually in direct costs has been attributed to workplace eye injuries alone.[15] The lifetime prevalence of sustaining an eye injury regardless of severity is approximately 20%.[6,8] This number of injuries highlights the importance of instituting preventive measures.

Complications

Infections can sometimes complicate chemical injuries, lacerations of the periocular adnexa, and partial-thickness or full-thickness lacerations of the globe. A particularly hazardous complication is the development of posttraumatic endophthalmitis (intraocular infection) after open globe injury. Several large studies have shown that endophthalmitis can complicate open globe injuries with an incidence ranging from 6.8% to 11.9%.[16,17] Another serious complication is the development of retinal detachment in open and closed globe injuries. Chemical injuries are often complicated by the destruction of the normal ocular surface and intraocular structures, leading to corneal opacification and severe glaucoma. Hyphema can be complicated by glaucoma and corneal blood staining.

PATIENT AND FAMILY
Education

Extensive collection of epidemiologic data by researchers and organizations such as the U.S. Eye Injury Registry and Prevent Blindness has led to a better understanding of when and where eye injuries occur. It behooves clinicians and employers to educate their patients and workers to implement the consistent use of protective devices.

- Stress the importance of eye protective devices at work and in recreation activities.
- Educate patients and their families to seek immediate medical attention for increased symptoms or decrease in vision.

HEALTH PROMOTION

Protective eyewear has been shown to be an effective deterrent to ocular injury on the battlefield, in the workplace, in the sports arena, and at numerous other locations.[18,19] At a minimum, 2-mm polycarbonate safety glasses with side shields should be used for all high-risk activities (e.g., landscaping, construction, impact sports). For even higher-risk activities, such as hammering metal on metal or grinding, polycarbonate goggles should be used because foreign bodies can still reach the eye around spectacle lenses. Eyewash stations should be available in all workplaces in which splash injuries or chemical exposures are possible.

REFERENCES

1. Kuhn, F., Morris, R., Witherspoon, C. D., et al. (1996). A standardized classification of ocular trauma. *Ophthalmology*, *103*(2), 240–243.
2. Kuhn, F., Morris, R., Witherspoon, C. D., et al. (1996). A standardized classification of ocular trauma. *Graefe's Archive for Clinical and Experimental Ophthalmology*, *234*(6), 399–403.
3. Kuhn, F., Morris, R., & Witherspoon, C. D. (2002). Birmingham Eye Trauma Terminology (BETT): Terminology and classification of mechanical eye injuries. *Ophthalmology Clinics of North America*, *15*(2), 139–143, v.
4. Kuhn, F., Maisiak, R., Mann, L., et al. (2002). The ocular trauma score (OTS). *Ophthalmology Clinics of North America*, *15*(2), 163–165, vi.
5. McGwin, G., Jr., Xie, A., & Owsley, C. (2005). Rate of eye injury in the United States. *Archives of Ophthalmology*, *123*(7), 970–976.
6. Katz, J., & Tielsch, J. M. (1993). Lifetime prevalence of ocular injuries from the Baltimore eye survey. *Archives of Ophthalmology*, *111*, 1564–1568.
7. May, D. R., Kuhn, F. P., & Morris, R. E. (2000). The epidemiology of serious eye injuries from the United States Eye Injury Registry. *Graefe's Archive for Clinical and Experimental Ophthalmology*, *238*, 153–157.
8. Wong, T. Y., Klein, B. E., & Klein, R. (2000). The prevalence and 5-year incidence of ocular trauma. The Beaver Dam Eye Study. *Ophthalmology*, *107*(12), 2196–2202.
9. Dannenberg, A. L., Parver, L. M., Brechner, R. J., et al. (1992). Penetration eye injuries in the workplace. The National Eye Trauma System Registry. *Archives of Ophthalmology*, *110*(6), 843–848.
10. Haring, R. S., Sheffield, I. D., Canner, J. K., & Schneider, E. B. (2016). Epidemiology of Sports-Related eye injuries in the United States. *JAMA Ophthalmology*, *134*(12), 1382–1390. doi:10.1001/jamaophthalmol.2016.425.
11. De Juan, E., Sternberg, P., & Michels, R. G. (1983). Penetrating ocular injuries. Types of injuries and visual results. *Ophthalmology*, *90*(11), 1318–1322.
12. Rostomian, K., Thach, A. B., Isfahani, A., et al. (1998). Open globe injuries in children. *Journal of AAPOS*, *2*(4), 234–238.
13. Duma, S. M., Ng, T. P., Kennedy, E. A., et al. (2005). Determination of significant parameters for eye injury risk from projectiles. *The Journal of Trauma*, *59*(4), 960–964.
14. Joseph, D. P., Pieramici, D. J., & Beauchamp, N. J., Jr. (2000). Computed tomography in the diagnosis and prognosis of open-globe injuries. *Ophthalmology*, *107*(10), 1899–1906.
15. Kuhn, F., & Pieramici, D. (Eds.). (2002). *Ocular trauma: Principles and practice* (p. 468). New York: Thieme.
16. Essex, R. W., Yi, Q., Charles, P. G., et al. (2004). Post-traumatic endophthalmitis. *Ophthalmology*, *111*(11), 2015–2022.
17. Zhang, Y., Zhang, M. N., Jiang, C. H., et al. (2010). Endophthalmitis following open globe injury. *The British Journal of Ophthalmology*, *94*(1), 111–114.
18. Ari, A. B. (2006). Eye injuries on the battlefields of Iraq and Afghanistan: Public health implications. *Optometry (St. Louis, Mo.)*, *77*(7), 329–339.
19. Taban, M., & Sears, J. E. (2008). Ocular findings following trauma from paintball sports. *Eye (London, England)*, *22*(7), 930–934.

CHAPTER 62

AURICULAR DISORDERS

Terry Mahan Buttaro • Teresa Denk Smajda

 Immediate referral to a physician or hospital admission is indicated for severe cases of cellulitis or malignant otitis externa which require intravenous antibiotics and possibly surgical debridement.

DEFINITION AND EPIDEMIOLOGY

Auricular disorders are conditions that affect the external ear. The incidence and prevalence of the individual conditions vary. The auricular disorder may be a secondary issue or may be discovered during the physical examination. Auricular disorders may be benign conditions associated with other disease processes, may be related to cultural practices such as body piercing, or may be a symptom of a serious illness that requires immediate referral and treatment.

Certain disease processes are associated with specific abnormalities of the auricle. Patients with Addison disease may have calcification of the cartilage. The nodules of Hansen disease (leprosy) may appear on the earlobe and initially be noticed as multiple nodules on the ear and face. Patients with chronic arthritis may have hard nodules develop in the auricle. These rheumatoid nodules are usually accompanied by similar nodules on the hands, elbows, knees, or heels. Auricular pain, erythema, and edema can be associated with cellulitis, relapsing polychondritis, a rheumatologic disorder that affects the cartilage of the ears, nose, and laryngobronchial system.[1,2] Relapsing polychondritis is often related to other disorders (e.g., systemic vasculitis or systemic lupus erythematosus), but can be related to nonrheumatologic disorders also (e.g., primary biliary cirrhosis, Hashimoto thyroiditis, or myelodysplasia).[2] Hearing loss, cardiac abnormalities, and glomerulonephritis are associated with relapsing polychondritis, which, although not common, can affect people of all ages.[2]

A more common auricular disorder is tophi: painless, hard or gritty, and irregular uric acid crystal deposits in the auricle. They form in relation to high uric acid levels. Pressure exerted on tophi may result in the expulsion of a white crystalline substance.

Injuries and infections are the more common auricular disorders seen in primary care offices. A hematoma of the auricle occurs in response to blood disorders or trauma. A bluish-tinged hematoma can develop in the pinna after an injury. This type of lesion may be accompanied by laceration and require incision and drainage by an ear, nose, and throat surgeon. If the lesion is not drained, the resultant deformity is commonly referred to as *cauliflower ear.*[3]

Other common auricular problems include infections and tears related to earlobe and helix piercing. Keloids, hypertrophic scar tissue that is not cosmetically acceptable, but is otherwise benign, can also occur at the pierced site.[4] Keloids occur more often in dark-skinned people.[4] Multiple helix piercing can cause a perforation-like appearance.

Chondrodermatitis nodularis helicis is a benign, chronically inflamed lesion—usually found on the helix or antihelix.[5] The lesion most often affects elders, men more often than women, and is painful and possibly crusting. A shave biopsy is necessary to distinguish the lesion from carcinoma.[5] Photodynamic therapy (PDT), cryotherapy, intralesional steroid injection, electrodessication, and nodular excision are potentially successful treatment modalities.[5]

Malignant otitis externa is a severe form of otitis externa. It results in a severely edematous, erythematous, and tender auricle. It can quickly dissect through fascial planes and lead to a life-threatening infection of the head and face. It is most likely to occur in patients with diabetes and in those who have compromised immune systems. Causative organisms include fungal infections and *Pseudomonas aeruginosa*, especially in people with diabetes, and in more recent years, methicillin-resistant *Staphylococcus aureus*.[6]

Skin cancer is probably the most common significant auricular disorder seen in primary care. Basal cell carcinoma (BCC) is the most frequent form of skin cancer found on the auricle and the least likely to become malignant. It is a slowly growing cancer often found in sun-exposed areas, such as the top of the auricle.[7] BCC is found more often in older persons, in fair-skinned patients, and in patients who have a history of sun exposure. A shiny, irregular, painless lesion, this form of cancer rarely metastasizes, but in some cases BCC can be invasive and thus concerning.[7] Squamous cell carcinoma (SCC) is also commonly found on the auricle, usually in fair-skinned patients and in patients with a history of sun exposure. The typical lesion has a raised, crusted border around a center ulcer. SCC is a more serious form of skin cancer, although still relatively benign compared with melanoma. SCC can potentially metastasize to regional lymph nodes and cause death.[7]

PATHOPHYSIOLOGY

The auricle is the external ear structure that is composed chiefly of cartilage covered by skin. It is firm and elastic. It is divided into three parts: the top portion is the helix, the midsection is the antihelix, and the lower portion is the lobe. The function of the outer ear is to aid in receiving sound waves from the environment.

CLINICAL PRESENTATION AND PHYSICAL EXAMINATION

The presentation of auricular disorders is myriad and depends on the underlying cause of the disorder. Often, the patient is being seen for a general examination or follow-up. The complaint related to an auricular disorder is usually a minor issue, but the parameters of the disorder should be noted and include the onset, duration, and intensity of any symptoms. Any medications, treatments, or remedies that have been used on the auricle or systemically should also be documented, as should all related symptoms and past history of treatments and outcomes. For tears and infection, the patient may be seen after a specific episode of trauma or with an erythematous, tender earlobe. Malignant otitis externa may manifest as a sequela to an infection or a respiratory illness, and most often occurs in immunosuppressed or diabetic patients.[6] A detailed history and physical examination aid the diagnosis.

The physical exam includes a complete inspection and palpation of the auricle. The top of the auricle crosses a line drawn from the occiput to the corner of the eye. The ears of neonates are usually flat; however, in older infants, this may indicate persistent side lying. Protruding ears should be examined to exclude edema from insect bites or infection. Normal earlobes are similar in size and placement and should move freely and painlessly. Infected pierced earlobes will be warm, tender, and erythematous, and may have exudates. The lobes of older patients may be more prominent or pendulous. Dry or scaly skin of the external ear may indicate psoriasis, seborrhea, or eczema, which can occur on and be limited to the ear. The external ear may also have skin breakdowns or erosions from prolonged pressure from eyeglasses or oxygen tubing. Cancerous or precancerous lesions are most often found on the top of the auricle. They may appear as shiny, irregular, painless lesions (BCC), or as raised, crusted lesions around a center ulcer (SCC).[7] Painless lesions can sometimes be better palpated than observed.

DIAGNOSTICS

The diagnostic tests depend on the underlying disease process. A biopsy should be performed on any small, crusted, ulcerated, or indurated lesion that does not heal properly. If the biopsy findings are positive, a complete cancer screening should be ordered. Rheumatoid factor should be obtained in patients with rheumatoid nodules. If tophi are present, a uric acid chemistry profile is indicated. Calcification nodules indicate the need for endocrine studies and further assessment for Addison disease. A CBC/differential is indicated if malignant otitis externa or other infectious process is suspected.

INITIAL DIAGNOSTICS

Auricular Disorders

LABORATORY
- Culture and sensitivity[a]
- CBC/differential[a]
- Uric acid[a]
- Rheumatoid factor[a]
- Endocrine studies[a]

OTHER DIAGNOSTICS
- Biopsy[a]

---
[a]If indicated.

DIFFERENTIAL DIAGNOSIS

 Priority differentials include malignant otitis externa, an infectious process, or cancerous lesion.

The more common differential diagnoses include a cancerous lesion, gout, infection, injury, malignant otitis externa, or rheumatoid nodule. Addison disease, Hansen disease, and relapsing polychondritis are additional considerations.

INTERPROFESSIONAL COLLABORATIVE MANAGEMENT

Nonpharmacologic and Pharmacologic Management

Mild infections of the earlobe or pinna that are a result of piercing can be treated with topical alcohol and antibiotic ointment. However, more concerning infections may require pharmacological treatment with an oral cephalosporin or penicillin.[8] Patients with a severe infection may require hospitalization and usually treatment with an intravenous cephalosporin (cefazolin) or penicillin (nafcillin).[8]

Indications for Referral or Hospitalization

Patients with perichondritis, malignant otitis externa, or signs of mastoiditis require immediate referral to a physician or an otolaryngologist, admission to a hospital, and aggressive antimicrobial therapy usually aimed against *Pseudomonas* and/or *Staphylococcus aureus*.[8] Patients with very early malignant otitis externa disease can be treated with an oral fluoroquinolone, with frequent follow-up. However, a culture obtained from the affected auditory canal is recommended as other infectious processes may be the cause and often a cephalosporin or antipseudomonal penicillin in combination with a fluoroquinolone is necessary.[8] A biopsy should be performed on any chronically inflamed lesion, as well as any cancerous or suspicious lesion, to determine if it is malignant.

Auricle lacerations require immediate consultation with a plastic surgeon or skilled emergency physician. Antibiotic therapy is usually also recommended.

LIFE-SPAN CONSIDERATIONS

Life-span considerations are related to the specific disease disorder. Complications from piercing are more likely in the young. Skin cancers are most likely to occur in middle-aged and older patients.

COMPLICATIONS

Complications are unusual but do occur. Trauma, if untreated, may result in painful nodules or a distorted cauliflower ear. Painless pinnal nodules may be a complication of Addison disease, and any painless nodule may represent a carcinoma. Infections, if untreated, may spread systemically. Recurring pinnal infections should prompt concern for relapsing polychondritis, a degenerative cartilage disease that can cause tinnitus or deafness.[2]

PATIENT AND FAMILY EDUCATION

Understanding of the importance of sunscreen protection for the ears is essential. In addition, the signs of skin cancer—asymmetry, borders (irregular, ragged, notched, or blurred), color (irregular), and diameter (a lesion that is 6 mm [¼ inch] or growing)—should be carefully explained. The provider should stress the importance and correct way of cleaning and caring for the external ear canal and auricle. When selecting ear-piercing facilities, patients should look for facilities that employ licensed personnel and are inspected or approved by public health authorities. In addition, caution is advised if wearing heavy or dangling earrings, because the earring might be torn from the ear.

HEALTH PROMOTION

Health promotion is primarily related to the specific disease. Sunscreens and protective clothing are the best choices for the prevention of skin cancer.

REFERENCES

1. Lustig, L. R., & Schindler, J. S. (2019). Ear, nose, and throat disorders. In M. A. Papadakis, S. J. Mcphee, & M. W. Rabow (Eds.), *Current medical diagnosis and treatment*. New York: McGraw-Hill. http://accessmedicine.mhmedical.com .ezproxy.simmons.edu/content.aspx?bookid=2449&sectionid=194433886. (Accessed 04 May 2019).
2. Langford, C. A. (2018). Relapsing polychondritis. In J. Jameson, A. S. Fauci, D. L. Kasper, S. L. Hauser, D. L. Longo, & J. Loscalzo (Eds.), *Harrison's principles of internal medicine, 20e*. New York: McGraw-Hill. http://accessmedicine .mhmedical.com.ezproxy.simmons.edu/content.aspx?bookid=2129&sectionid =192285778. (Accessed 04 May 2019).
3. Munter, D. W., & McGuirk, T. D. (2010). Head and facial trauma. In K. J. Knoop, L. B. Stack, A. B. Storrow, & R. Thurman (Eds.), *The atlas of emergency medicine* (3rd ed.). New York: McGraw-Hill.
4. Ko, C. J. (2012). Dermal hypertrophies and benign fibroblastic/myofibroblastic tumors. In L. A. Goldsmith, S. I. Katz, B. A. Gilchrest, A. S. Paller, D. J. Leffell, & K. Wolff (Eds.), *Fitzpatrick's dermatology in general medicine* (8th ed.). New York: McGraw-Hill. (Accessed 4 May 2019).
5. Usatine, R. P., Smith, M. A., Chumley, H. S., & Mayeaux, E. J., Jr. (2013). Chondrodermatitis nodularis helicis and preauricular tags. In R. P. Usatine, M. A. Smith, H. S. Chumley, & E. J. Mayeaux Jr. (Eds.), *The color atlas of family medicine* (2nd ed.). New York: McGraw-Hill.
6. Hosmer, K. (2016). Ear disorders. In J. E. Tintinalli, J. Stapczynski, O. Ma, D. M. Yealy, G. D. Meckler, & D. M. Cline (Eds.), *Tintinalli's emergency medicine: A comprehensive study guide, 8e*. New York: McGraw-Hill. http://accessmedicine .mhmedical.com.ezproxy.simmons.edu/content.aspx?bookid=1658&sectionid =109387021. (Accessed 04 May 2019).
7. Curti, B. D., Leachman, S., & Urba, W. J. (2018). Cancer of the skin. In J. Jameson, A. S. Fauci, D. L. Kasper, S. L. Hauser, D. L. Longo, & J. Loscalzo (Eds.), *Harrison's principles of internal medicine, 20e*. New York: McGraw-Hill. http:// accessmedicine.mhmedical.com.ezproxy.simmons.edu/content.aspx?bookid =2129&sectionid=192015390. (Accessed 04 May 2019).
8. Rubin, M. A., Ford, L. C., & Gonzales, R. (2018). Sore throat, earache, and upper respiratory symptoms. In J. Jameson, A. S. Fauci, D. L. Kasper, S. L. Hauser, D. L. Longo, & J. Loscalzo (Eds.), *Harrison's principles of internal medicine, 20e*. New York: McGraw-Hill. http://accessmedicine.mhmedical.com.ezproxy.simmons.edu/ content.aspx?bookid=2129&sectionid=192012234. (Accessed 04 May 2019).

CHAPTER **63**

CERUMEN IMPACTION
Ani Sinanyan

DEFINITION AND EPIDEMIOLOGY

Cerumen impaction occurs when increased amounts of hard cerumen either partially or completely occlude the external ear canal. Cerumen is a natural substance that can become dry and immobile and occlude the canal. Although cerumen is an important defense against infection, many think a buildup of earwax is a sign of uncleanliness and make efforts to remove the wax. This can compromise the integrity of the ear's defenses against infection and actually contribute to cerumen impaction. Ear plugs, hearing aids, earbuds used to listen to music and talk on the phone, and probes such as cotton-tipped swabs

used to clean the ear can cause cerumen impaction. The presence of cerumen can also decrease efficacy of hearing aids.[1]

Clinicians should diagnose cerumen impaction only when an accumulation of cerumen is associated with either or both of the following conditions: patient symptoms and prevention of needed assessment of the ear. An exception is if the patient is a young child, an older adult, or is cognitively impaired and not able to express symptoms. These individuals are at higher risk for cerumen impaction because they are often unaware of or unable to express any symptoms associated with it. Hearing loss associated with cerumen impaction may further impair cognitive function.[1]

PATHOPHYSIOLOGY

Cerumen is a soft, yellow, waxy protective substance that is secreted by glands in the external ear canal. It is part of the mechanism that protects the ear canal and tympanic membrane (TM) from dirt and debris. When cerumen is formed relatively close to the TM, it is soft and fluid, colorless, and odorless. As the cerumen moves toward the distal part of the ear canal through the process of mandibular movement, it becomes drier and darker and develops its characteristic odor. If an individual uses a swab to clean the ear canal or another item that obstructs normal movement of the cerumen, the harder cerumen that is not removed or allowed to naturally progress to the outer ear is pushed against the TM. Cotton-tipped swabs can leave fibers from the swab, which then hold the cerumen in a mass. Excessive cerumen production, a narrow ear canal, or obstruction may also predispose a patient to impaction.[2]

CLINICAL PRESENTATION AND PHYSICAL EXAMINATION

Patients with cerumen impaction typically complain of unilateral or bilateral fullness or hearing loss; otalgia, itching, discomfort, tinnitus, cough, vertigo, and dizziness are also common complaints. Because hearing changes thought to be from cerumen impaction can also be from other causes (e.g., TM rupture), an expanded history to identify such problems should be obtained.[1-3]

The physical examination requires that the outer ear be inspected for size, shape, color, and placement; the lobe, helix, and preauricular and postauricular lymph nodes should be bilaterally palpated. The body temperature and lymph nodes are usually normal. The ear should be inspected by having the patient tip his or her head toward the opposite shoulder. In adults, the pinna is pulled gently up and backward; for young children and infants, the ear is pulled downward. The largest speculum that fits into the ear canal is gently inserted. Cerumen impaction may prevent the speculum from being fully inserted.

An impaction appears as a light yellow to dark brown mass that prevents or partially blocks visualization of the TM. Blood in the external ear canal appears as bright red to black and may be liquid or a solid mass. Sanguineous drainage often appears as honey-colored fluid. Whenever a cerumen impaction is noted in one ear, the other ear should be examined as well.

DIAGNOSTICS

No diagnostics are indicated.

DIFFERENTIAL DIAGNOSIS

The primary differential diagnosis is a foreign body in the external ear canal. Perforation of the TM, otitis, middle ear disease, and dysfunction of the eustachian tube can also cause symptoms similar to cerumen impaction.

INTERPROFESSIONAL COLLABORATIVE MANAGEMENT

When cerumen removal is needed, first verify if patients have a history of a ruptured TM, tympanostomy tubes, or recent ear surgery. When such history is present, some modes of cerumen removal are contraindicated. Foreign objects such as beans or other vegetable matter tend to swell with the irrigating solution, complicating removal.[1,3]

- If there is a contraindication to instilling fluid into the ear canal, removal with a cerumen spoon or curette is appropriate. If direct visualization is possible, the cerumen is in the lateral third of the external ear canal, and the patient is able to remain still during removal.
- If there is no contraindication to instilling fluid into the ear canal, a commercial ceruminolytic agent (e.g., any brand of carbamide peroxide) or two or three drops of baby oil or mineral oil, liquid docusate sodium, or hydrogen peroxide can be inserted in the affected ear daily for 3 to 5 days. This may resolve the impaction.
  - If a patient is known to have dry skin in the ear canal, ceruminolytics containing hydrogen peroxide should be avoided because the peroxide can further dry the skin.[4]
  - Although any ceruminolytic agent seems to be better than no treatment at all, there is no evidence that any one particular ceruminolytic is superior to any other.[1,5] However, only carbamide peroxide has been approved by the U.S. Food and Drug Administration (FDA) for this use.[2]
- If the ceruminolytic agent does not cause resolution of the impaction, removal with a cerumen spoon or curette can be performed.
- If the cerumen is deeper in the canal or is not cleared with the ceruminolytic agent and/or curette, irrigation with water or normal saline at body temperature using an ear syringe, a device specifically designed for ear irrigation, or a regular syringe with a flexible catheter can be performed.
  - If not already used, a ceruminolytic agent may be instilled in the canal for 15 to 20 minutes before the irrigation to soften the cerumen and aid in its removal.
  - The auricle should be straightened as much as possible and the irrigant directed upward in the canal to minimize the pressure against the TM.
  - The canal should be irrigated until clear unless the patient experiences pain or dizziness.
  - If the patient is immunocompromised, a sterile solution should be used.[1,2]
- Pain, injury to the skin of the ear canal with hemorrhage, and acute otitis externa are possible complications after cerumen removal. Patients on anticoagulants are at higher risk for bleeding.[1]

The clinical indication for use of antibiotics and topical steroids after removal of a cerumen impaction is determined by the amount of excoriation and other conditions, such as diabetes or an immunocompromised status. When warranted, hydrocortisone–neomycin sulfate–polymyxin B sulfate (Cortisporin otic solution) or a mixture of white vinegar and rubbing alcohol in the canal every day for 2 or 3 days after the procedure can reduce the risk of otitis externa.[1]

- Reassess the patient at the conclusion of in-office treatment for cerumen impaction and document resolution of the impaction.[1] If the impaction is not resolved, additional treatment should be prescribed. If full or partial symptoms persist despite resolution of impaction, clinicians should consider alternative diagnoses and referral to an otolaryngology specialist.[1]

LIFE-SPAN CONSIDERATIONS

In older adults, the glands that produce cerumen may become less productive, which can result in cerumen that is drier and more likely to collect in the canal and become impacted. Those with cognitive or communication deficits may also be unable to express symptoms of cerumen impaction.

Adults who work in noisy industries and are required to wear hearing protection may have an increased risk of cerumen impaction. Individuals requiring use of hearing aids, earplugs, or swim molds, and those who insert foreign bodies into the external auditory canal, can increase the incidence of impaction by pushing the cerumen into the canal. Clinical practice guidelines recommend examination of such patients for cerumen impaction during health care encounters, although no more frequently than every 3 months.[1]

COMPLICATIONS

Cerumen accumulation can decrease auditory acuity and cause pressure on and perforation of the TM. Removal of cerumen that has adhered to the wall of the external ear canal may leave an abraded or irritated area that can develop into otitis externa. Hearing loss and injury to the TM are other potential complications. In addition, if the impaction is not completely removed, water retention behind the impaction can occur, predisposing the patient to infection.

INDICATIONS FOR REFERRAL OR HOSPITALIZATION

Patients with suspected perforation, chronic cerumen impaction, tympanostomy tubes, recent ear surgery, or pus or necrotic tissue in the ear canal should be referred to an otolaryngologist, as should patients who experience acute pain, dizziness, hearing loss, or damage to the external ear canal or TM during the ear lavage.

PATIENT EDUCATION AND HEALTH PROMOTION

Patients should be educated that cerumen (earwax) is normal and that the external ear canal does not require cleaning. Gentle cleaning of the outer ear and canal with a cloth is all that is usually needed to remove wax and any dirt extruded from the canal. Avoidance of use of ear swabs and inserting other items into the ear will both prevent cerumen impaction and help prevent injury to the ear canal and TM. The American Academy of Otolaryngology–Head and Neck Surgery has a useful patient handout on earwax and care. This can be found at www.entnet.org/content/earwax-and-care.

Because patients who wear hearing aids or other ear-occluding items are more at risk for the development of cerumen impaction, they should try to decrease or to eliminate wearing of these items when not needed and while sleeping.

If not contraindicated, one or two drops of commercial ceruminolytic (carbamide peroxide) once or twice a week will help prevent cerumen from becoming hard and embedded. Ear syringes can also be used to gently direct clean warm water to the roof of the ear canal. Patients should be cautioned about the need to follow directions related to use and cleaning of ear syringes. Patients should be advised not to use any other home removal technique or device for cerumen removal. Although mentioned as an option for providers in the otolaryngology clinical practice guideline on cerumen impaction, oral irrigation tools should not be used by patients because they may rupture the TM even at low pressures.[1,2]

Patients should also be cautioned not to use cotton-tipped swabs or other implements to clean the ear canal. These items can push the cerumen farther into the ear and cause perforation of the TM. Soft cloths and soap and water should be used to clean the auricle. Patients must understand the importance of a medical evaluation if pain or discharge is noted.[1,6]

Patients should be cautioned to never use ear candling (also called *ear coning* or *thermal-auricular therapy*) for cerumen removal. This has no observable positive effects and is associated with considerable risks of burns to the tissues within the ear canal, perforation of the TM, external otitis, and temporary hearing loss. The FDA concluded that there is no validated scientific evidence to support the efficacy of ear candles and warns against their use.[1,2,6]

REFERENCES

1. Michaudet, C., & Malaty, J. (2018). Cerumen impaction and management. *American Family Physician, 98*(8), 525–529.
2. Pray, W. S., & Pray, J. J. (2012). Treating minor ear problems. *U. S. Pharmacist, 37*(5), 16–23.
3. Kessler, B. External ear obstructions. The Merck Manual Online Medical Library. Retrieved from https://www.merckmanuals.com/professional/ear,-nose,-and-throat-disorders/external-ear-disorders/external-ear-obstructions. (Accessed 4 May 2019).
4. McCarter, D. F., Courtney, A. U., & Pollart, S. M. (2007). Cerumen impaction. *American Family Physician, 75*(10), 1523–1528.
5. Burton, M. J., & Doree, C. (2009). Ear drops for the removal of ear wax (review). *The Cochrane Database of Systematic Reviews*, (1), CD004326.
6. American Academy of Otolaryngology (2017). Retrieved from https://www.entnet.org/content/experts-update-best-practices-diagnosis-and-treatment-earwax-cerumen-impaction-important. (Accessed 4 May 2019).

CHAPTER **64**

CHOLESTEATOMA

Sharon Smart

DEFINITION AND EPIDEMIOLOGY

Cholesteatoma is an abnormal collection of epithelial cells in the middle ear or mastoid process that cause the formation of a benign tumor. It can occur as a congenital abnormality during fetal development of the temporal bone, but may also be acquired and occur as a complication of a ruptured tympanic membrane (TM; primary cholesteatoma), chronic otitis media, surgical procedure, or chronic inflammatory process of the middle ear (secondary cholesteatoma).[1]

PATHOPHYSIOLOGY

Congenital cholesteatomas occur during fetal development when squamous epithelium cells collect in the inner ear, causing keratinaceous debris to collect behind the TM. The exact cause of this is unclear.[2] Primary cholesteatomas occur after injury to the TM, often related to middle ear infection

or eustachian tube dysfunction. Secondary cholesteatomas are the result of epithelial cell deposits that occur after a TM perforation or TM surgery (such as tympanoplasty). The epithelial debris serves as a rich medium for bacterial growth, resulting in chronic otorrhea and inflammation. The tumor can cause erosion of surrounding bone causing hearing loss, dizziness, and, if left untreated, facial nerve injury, meningitis, or brain abscess.[2]

Common bacteria associated with cholesteatomas include *Staphylococcus aureus, Streptococcus, Pseudomonas aeruginosa, Escherichia coli, Proteus mirabilis, Klebsiella pneumoniae,* and anaerobes, which are generally the source of the malodor of the otorrhea.[3]

CLINICAL PRESENTATION AND PHYSICAL EXAMINATION

Cholesteatomas can develop over years. Malodorous otorrhea and hearing loss are common presenting symptoms. Some patients will complain of tinnitus or vertigo (the result of labyrinth erosion which can cause a fistula).

The physical examination should include the entire ear, as well as evaluation of cranial nerve VII, the facial nerve. The otoscopic examination requires adequate brightness to provide sufficient illumination of the inner ear. Visualization of the entire TM (including the posterosuperior and anterosuperior quadrants) is necessary both for patency (e.g., a small TM perforation is possible) and the appearance of white colored debris and/or pearl-colored lesions behind the TM.[4] Removal of cerumen or debris from infection may be necessary for adequate exposure of the entire TM, but cholesteatomas can be small and easily missed by an inexperienced provider, especially if the TM is scarred or obscured.

Congenital cholesteatomas are typically identified as a pale whitish discoloration or spherical white cyst behind an intact TM. In primary acquired cholesteatoma, findings include retraction of the pars flaccida and, less commonly, the pars tensa. Retraction pockets are identified by careful inspection of the TM and can be shallow or deep. Shallow pockets may be seen with otoscopy; deep pockets can contain debris and not be visible. Other common findings include a whitish keratin mass, purulent otorrhea, polyps, granulation tissue on the surface of the TM, and ossicular erosion.

In secondary acquired cholesteatoma, the findings depend on the cause. Routine examination techniques for nystagmus and balance function may be warranted for patients with vestibular dysfunction.

ESSENTIAL DIAGNOSTICS

An audiogram can reveal conductive hearing loss and is an important diagnostic tool, though hearing can be unaffected if there is no damage to the ossicular chain. A computed tomography (CT) scan can aid in determining the location of a cholesteatoma and any affected surrounding structures. Tympanostomy tube placement may improve the quality of the CT scan.

ADDITIONAL DIAGNOSTICS

Magnetic resonance imaging (MRI) is useful if findings suggest a neoplasm or an encephalocele, but MRI technology is unable to determine tissue characteristics (e.g., inflammation) because of the small diameter of the ear and mastoid and the common presence of an inflammatory process.

DIFFERENTIAL DIAGNOSES

Primary differential diagnoses include squamous cell carcinoma, adenocarcinoma, and acoustic neuroma.

Other considerations should include otitis externa, chronic otitis media without cholesteatoma, a foreign body or grafted material in a surgically repaired ear, ossicular dysfunction, or otosclerosis causing hearing loss.

INTERPROFESSIONAL COLLABORATIVE MANAGEMENT

Nonpharmacological

- Removal of debris from the ear canal, as well as avoidance of water entering the external auditory canal, is crucial.

Pharmacological

Treatment with an antibacterial agent (e.g., ofloxacin) for coverage of the common bacterial organisms associated with otitis media or otitis externa is indicated to reduce the inflammation and bacterial infection in the involved ear.[5] Aminoglycosides and other ototoxic gents should be avoided if the TM is not intact. Follow-up evaluation is necessary to ensure full healing, because in many cases, the infection does not completely subside. Patients with a recurrent infection should be referred to otolaryngology or a CT scan of the affected ear considered.

INDICATION FOR REFERRAL OR HOSPITALIZATION

- All patients with cholesteatoma should be referred to otolaryngology for confirmation of diagnosis.
- Referral to audiology is necessary for audiogram and determination of hearing loss.
- Surgical referral is the definitive treatment for cholesteatoma.[4,5] If surgery is not performed, the cholesteatoma can increase in size and cause significant complications.

COMPLICATIONS

Cholesteatomas can reoccur. Chronic inflammation and otorrhea, disequilibrium, meningitis, brain injury, hearing loss, tinnitus, and/or vertigo are possible sequelae. Nerve compression, a possible surgical complication, can occur and result in facial twitching or paralysis.[2]

PATIENT AND FAMILY EDUCATION

It is important that patients and families understand that recurrent and residual cholesteatoma disease after primary surgical intervention can be common. Postoperatively, regular follow-up (e.g., annually or as indicated) monitoring for recurrence is recommended.[1,5]

REFERENCES

1. Lustig, L. R., & Schindler, J. S. (2019). Ear, nose, & throat disorders. In M. A. Papadakis, S. J. McPhee, & M. W. Rabow (Eds.), *Current medical diagnosis & treatment*. New York, NY: McGraw-Hill. http://accessmedicine.mhmedical.com.ezproxy.simmons.edu/content.aspx?bookid=2449&sectionid=194433886. (Accessed 4 May 2019).
2. Haddad, J., & Keesecker, S. (2015). Congenital malformation. In *Nelson textbook of pediatrics* (20th ed., pp. 3081–3083.e1). Elsevier.
3. Chole, R. (2015). Chronic otitis media, mastoiditis and petrositis. In *Cummings otolaryngology* (6th ed., pp. 2139–2155.c4). Saunders, an imprint of Elsevier.
4. Swartz, J., & Hagiwara, M. (2011). Inflammatory Disease of the Temporal Bone. In *Head and neck imaging* (5th ed., pp. 1183–1229). Mosby.
5. Chang, C. (2012). Cholesteatoma. In A. K. Lalwani (Ed.), *CURRENT diagnosis & treatment in Otolaryngology—Head & Neck Surgery* (3rd ed.). New York, NY: McGraw-Hill. (Accessed 4 May 2019).

CHAPTER **65**

IMPAIRED HEARING

Susan Sanner

 Immediate specialist referral to an otolaryngologist or neurologist is indicated for patients with sudden or rapidly progressive hearing loss.

DEFINITION AND EPIDEMIOLOGY

Impaired hearing is a defect in the detection and/or processing of sound waves. Impaired hearing affects both communication ability and personal safety, and can be a socially isolating experience. Hearing loss occurs at all ages, although its prevalence increases with advancing age. A complaint of hearing loss can reflect a wide variety of abnormalities and requires different considerations in children than in adults.

PATHOPHYSIOLOGY

The ear is the peripheral mechanism that converts sound waves into electrical impulses that are processed by the central auditory pathways. It is divided into three segments: the outer ear, middle ear, and inner ear. Each section must function properly for hearing to occur normally. The outer ear includes the auricle and ear canal. Its function is to collect sound waves and funnel them to the middle ear. The middle ear includes the tympanic membrane (TM) and the ossicles and the middle ear space that contains them. It transfers the sound waves to the inner ear, amplifying these vibrations as it does. Finally, the inner ear consists of the cochlea, the organ of hearing, and the semicircular canals, which functions as a primary balance system. The cochlea converts the vibratory energy into electrical impulses that are then processed by the auditory nerve pathways in the brainstem, midbrain, and cerebrum.

Hearing losses are classified into three types. The first is conductive loss, which results from sound waves being attenuated at the external auditory canal or the middle ear. The second type is sensorineural loss, resulting from malfunction in the cochlea or central auditory pathways. Sensorineural losses can be subdivided into a peripheral (cochlear) loss or a central (nerve) loss. Finally, a mixed hearing loss has both conductive and sensorineural components. The vast majority of hearing losses are peripheral, and differential diagnosis is generally focused on the peripheral mechanism. It should never be forgotten, however, that the central auditory pathways are crucial to hearing and central losses will be encountered occasionally. A number of abnormalities may lead to hearing loss of each type.

In conductive hearing loss, any component of the anatomic structures of the outer or middle ear can be involved. In the outer ear, impacted cerumen, bacterial or fungal infection (swimmer's ear), overgrowth of the bony wall (exostoses), tumors, congenital atresia, and fibrotic stenosis from recurrent infection may attenuate the sound reaching the middle ear and cochlea. In the middle ear, perforation of the TM, scar tissue, negative pressure from eustachian tube dysfunction, barotraumas, cholesteatoma, glomus tumor, otosclerosis, or any other condition that impairs the mobility of the TM or ossicles can reduce hearing sensitivity. Causes of conductive loss from middle ear disease include acute otitis media, serous otitis media, and chronic serous otitis. While otitis media is primarily associated with early childhood, it may occur at any age. Otosclerosis, which is fusion of the stapes over the oval window, is a common cause of hearing loss in adults, usually appearing between the ages of 20 and 40.[1,2] Other conditions that interfere with the mechanical transmission of sound in the middle ear are trauma that damages the ossicles and congenital malformations.

Sensorineural hearing loss usually occurs from disorders of the cochlea. Less prevalent are disorders of the central auditory nervous system (CANS)—that is, cranial nerve VIII (acoustic), the internal auditory canal, or the brain. Congenital sensorineural hearing loss may result from noninherited factors such as maternal infections (toxoplasmosis, other, rubella, CMV, HSV [TORCH complex]), medications, or from inherited autosomal abnormalities. Adventitious sensorineural hearing loss can result from such factors as infections of the inner ear, Meniere disease, inner ear barotraumas, trauma, and tumors.

Presbycusis is a gradual degeneration within the cochlea that accompanies aging. Multiple factors may be at play in any given individual, including hair cell loss, metabolic changes, and circulatory insufficiency. Multiple factors influence the rate at which hearing loss occurs: genetics, medications, infections, and exposure to noise. High blood pressure, smoking, and diabetes may hasten presbycusis. There may also be degeneration of the mechanical structures and the central auditory connections.[3]

Noise trauma is a common cause of cochlear damage and may be a factor in presbycusis.[3] Persistent or repeated exposure to excessive noise causes stress and mechanical damage to the delicate hair cells of the inner ear. High frequencies are affected initially, and over time the loss spreads to middle and lower frequencies. A loud, explosive noise may cause severe or profound damage to these structures and result in immediate hearing loss. In the United States, the Occupational Safety and Health Administration (OSHA) has set standards and guidelines for noise exposure to protect workers. The OSHA standards limit the noise level exposure and require that hearing protection be worn at certain levels and that the hearing of those working in noise be monitored annually.[4]

Sensorineural hearing loss can also be caused by diseases that involve the endocrine or metabolic systems, autoimmune disorders, and neurogenic disorders. Ototoxic medications can also cause sensorineural hearing loss. The prime suspects in ototoxicity include antineoplastics, salicylates, aminoglycosides, furosemide, and quinine-related drugs. Audiologic evaluation before inception of treatment and regular monitoring of hearing during treatment is recommended for patients receiving a course of antineoplastics or aminoglycosides.

Central sensorineural hearing losses may be caused by acoustic tumors (vestibular schwannomas), stroke, and meningiomas.

Mixed hearing loss is a combination of both conductive and sensorineural loss. Usually, the presence of a mixed hearing loss is the result of two unrelated disease processes. Occasionally, however, injury to the ear, infection, and congenital disorders may affect the outer and/or middle ear and the inner ear.

CLINICAL PRESENTATION AND PHYSICAL EXAMINATION

Hearing loss may be sudden, progressive, or fluctuating in nature. It is important to determine whether the problem is unilateral or bilateral. Associated symptoms of otalgia, ear fullness, vertigo, tinnitus, or cranial neuropathies should be documented. The medical history should incorporate current and past treatments with oral and intravenous medications or nonprescription drugs, particularly aminoglycosides, diuretics, antineoplastics, or large doses of aspirin. Chronic illnesses, hospitalizations, head injuries, and surgeries should be included in the history. A family history of hearing loss, neoplasms, renal disease, and balance disorders should be investigated. Finally, exposures to trauma and noise should also be noted.

A complete examination of the head, neck, and throat, and an evaluation of cranial nerves and the auditory and vestibular system are essential. The pinna and external auditory canal should be inspected for malformations, lesions, exudates, and obstruction. Examination of the TM should assess for mobility (via pneumoscopy) and determine whether effusion, infection, perforation, or cholesteatoma is present.

DIAGNOSTICS

The purpose of evaluating a patient with hearing loss is to determine the type of hearing loss (conductive vs. sensorineural), the severity of the impairment—whether mild, moderate, severe, or profound—and the anatomy of the impairment (external, middle, inner ear, and external auditory pathway).

Essential Diagnostics

- Weber and Rinne tests, performed in conjunction, are used to differentiate conductive and sensorineural hearing loss.
  - The Weber test is performed by placing a vibrating tuning fork at the midline of the forehead. With normal hearing or symmetric sensorineural hearing loss, the sound is heard equally in both ears. With asymmetric sensorineural loss, the sound is heard in the better ear. With an asymmetric conductive loss, the sound is heard in the poorer (greater conductive loss) ear.
  - The Rinne test compares air conduction (AC) and bone conduction (BC). A vibrating tuning fork is held next to the ear and the patient reports when he or she can no longer hear the sound. The still-vibrating fork is then placed on the mastoid process behind the ear. In normal hearing, AC is better than BC (AC > BC)—that is, the patient does not hear the tuning fork when it is placed on the mastoid. With a conductive hearing loss, BC is better than AC—that is, the patient hears the tuning fork when it is placed on the mastoid. In the presence of a sensorineural hearing loss, AC remains better than BC but the patient does not hear it at as soft a level as a normal hearing person.[5]

    A screening audiogram is optimal as it is more sensitive and specific than a tuning fork examination.[6,7] The audiogram depicts AC and BC graphically across the hearing frequencies.
  - A recent noise exposure history should be taken before administering a hearing test for more accurate results. Exposure to loud noises over the weekend, for example, may decrease hearing if tested on a Monday morning.

If the individual works in a noisy environment, a test in the morning, before the patient has been to work, is preferred.

- Tympanometry is used to determine middle ear function by measuring the impendence of the middle ear to sound.
- A formal audiogram, performed by an audiologist in a sound-treated environment, is recommended if hearing is impaired on clinical examination. Formal testing should include the following:
  - Pure tone tests by AC—to determine hearing thresholds for selected frequencies through earphones, and hence for the entire auditory system.
  - Pure tone tests by BC—to establish the thresholds for the same frequencies with a bone oscillator placed on the mastoid. This bypasses the outer and middle ear and determines the sensorineural component of the loss. Analogous to the Rinne tuning fork test, better response on this test than on the AC test indicates a conductive component to the loss.
  - Speech reception test under phones—to determine the softest level at which the patient can identify two-syllable words chosen from a closed set and to provide confirming evidence that the pure tone AC results are accurate.
  - Speech recognition testing—to evaluate the patient's ability to understand single-syllable words at a given presentation level.
  - Impedance audiometry—to evaluate middle ear function. The tympanogram determines whether the TM is intact, how well it moves, and what the air pressure is in the middle ear. Acoustic reflexes evaluate the movement of the stapedius muscle and are particularly sensitive to the presence of otosclerosis.

Additional Diagnostics

Evaluate outer hair cell function (otoacoustic emissions [OAEs]) in the inner ear and integrity of the auditory nerve and brainstem auditory pathways (auditory brainstem response [ABR]). The tests are done when indicated by the results of conventional audiometry.

- Pediatric audiologists can evaluate hearing at any age. Behavioral tests provide good estimates of hearing thresholds, and objective tests such as OAEs and threshold ABR can provide reliable information about hearing in those patients too young to respond reliably to behavioral testing.
- Laboratory tests should also be done to evaluate the patient for systemic or metabolic causes for the hearing loss. For example, CBC/differential if anemia or infection is suspected; VDRL or RPR to exclude syphilis; ESR, antinuclear antibodies, rheumatoid factor, if autoimmune disorder is a consideration; and TSH to exclude thyroid disorder.
- Magnetic resonance imaging (MRI) or computed tomography (CT) scans are useful in ruling out tumors; gauging the extent of chronic inflammatory middle ear disease and cholesteatomas; evaluating otosclerosis, erosion, or displacement of the ossicles; and identifying cochlear atresias or enlarged vestibular aqueducts,[7] which may cause sensorineural hearing loss.[8]

DIFFERENTIAL DIAGNOSIS

Once the site of lesion (outer, middle, or inner ear) is established, the differential diagnosis of hearing loss focuses on the nature of the presenting complaint: whether the loss was sudden, gradual, fluctuating, or progressive.

Causes of sudden hearing loss in adults can include sudden idiopathic sensorineural hearing loss, infections, perilymphatic fistula, ischemia of the inner ear or retrocochlear structures, multiple sclerosis, autoimmune diseases, trauma, chronic renal failure, and sickle cell anemia. Gradual hearing loss can be related to presbycusis, noise exposure, familial factors, retrocochlear neoplasm, chronic otitis media, cholesteatoma, otosclerosis, hypothyroidism, diabetes, and chronic renal failure. Differential diagnosis for fluctuating hearing loss includes otitis media, perilymphatic fistula, Meniere disease, multiple sclerosis, migraine headache, syphilis, autoimmune disorders, and sarcoidosis. Hearing loss that is rapidly progressive may result from causes that include autoimmune inner ear disease, meningeal carcinoma, vasculitis, Lyme disease, and ototoxic exposures.

DIFFERENTIAL DIAGNOSIS

 Primary differentials to consider include: (1) Congenital deformities may be accompanied by undeveloped or underdeveloped middle ear ossicles, and orthodontic/mandible structures that require reconstructive surgery. (2) Traumatic deformity associated with a blow to the head or a slap on the ear may produce bleeding, swelling, discoloration, bone fracture, or perforation. In these cases, referral may be necessary. (3) A history of active draining from the ear within the past 90 days may signify allergies or infection requiring treatment. (4) Acute or chronic dizziness may signify trauma or ototoxicity.[7]

Impaired Hearing

Sudden hearing loss is associated with autoimmune diseases, chronic renal failure, infections, ischemia of the inner ear or retrocochlear structures, multiple sclerosis, sickle cell anemia, sudden idiopathic sensoneural hearing loss, and trauma.

Factors associated with gradual hearing loss include cholesteatoma, chronic renal failure, chronic otitis media, diabetes hypothyroidism, noise exposure, otosclerosis, presbycusis, and retrocochlear neoplasm.

Fluctuating hearing loss causes include autoimmune disorders, Meniere disease, migraine headache, multiple sclerosis, otitis media perilymphatic fistula, sarcoidosis, and syphilis.

INTERPROFESSIONAL COLLABORATIVE MANAGEMENT

Conductive hearing loss associated with cerumen impaction usually resolves with removal of the impaction. Conductive loss caused by infection usually responds to resolution of the infection, although improvement in hearing loss typically lags behind clinical improvement of the infection. Otolaryngology referral is indicated for patients with hearing deficit associated with trauma, congenital hearing loss, tumors, obstructions of the external auditory canal, nonhealing TM rupture, and otosclerosis. Treatment for otosclerosis may be stapedectomy or sound amplification. TM perforation may heal spontaneously or require a surgical patch or graft. Presbycusis and some other hearing impairments can be treated with hearing aids. Parents of children with congenital or progressive hearing loss or possible syndromic loss should be referred for genetic counseling.

INDICATIONS FOR REFERRAL OR HOSPITALIZATION

 Immediate specialist referral (usually a otolaryngologist or a neurologist) is indicated for sudden or rapidly progressive hearing loss associated with trauma, infection, or unilateral symptoms.

- Referral to an otolaryngologist is appropriate when the diagnosis is unclear, when preliminary assessment indicates a serious condition, or when surgical intervention is an option.
- Referral to an audiologist is always appropriate for definitive testing and rehabilitative intervention.

LIFE-SPAN CONSIDERATIONS

Hearing loss is most often associated with aging, but hearing loss may occur at any age. Hearing loss in infancy, either congenital or adventitious, can cause delays in speech, language, and cognitive development. Early identification and intervention can prevent speech and language delays, and the consequent negative effects on cognitive development and educational attainment. In recent years, there has been a movement to institute universal neonatal screening of hearing, and 44 states have requirements for universal screening.[8] The negative effects of hearing loss are not restricted to deafness or severe impairment. Even mild losses and unilateral losses have been shown to be educationally significant.

COMPLICATIONS

Hearing impairment can result in frustration and anger when there are difficulties understanding speech; it is possible to avoid situations in which communication is difficult. The resulting social isolation can lead to depressive symptoms and cause increased strain in a marriage or other intimate relationships. In addition, a failure to hear warning signals can lead to accidents, middle-age hearing loss can cause restricted economic opportunities, and early hearing loss resulting in reduced educational attainment can result in a lifelong reduction in earning ability.

Missed diagnoses may result in significant health consequences. An untreated ear infection or cholesteatoma may result in erosion of the lamina between the middle ear space and the brain resulting in meningitis. Untreated acoustic neuromas can result in facial paralysis as the tumor impinges on other cranial nerves and ultimately death as the brainstem is displaced laterally. A number of syndromic hearing losses, such as branchio-oto-renal (BOR) syndrome and velocardiofacial (Shprintzen) syndrome, are associated with significant, even life-threatening, dysfunction of the heart, kidneys, and neurologic and other systems.[9]

PATIENT AND FAMILY EDUCATION

Patients should be aware that sudden hearing loss, difficulty understanding what people are saying, or a constant ringing in the ear requires further evaluation. A careful explanation about their particular type of hearing loss, as well as how medications (e.g., aspirin, nonsteroidal antiinflammatory drugs [NSAIDs], antibiotics, and diuretics) can cause hearing loss, is necessary.

Information about referral resources and options for management should also be discussed with patients and their families. For patients considering hearing aids, establishing realistic expectations for amplification is paramount. It should be clear that hearing cannot be completely restored and that the patient will have to relearn how to use auditory information that they have not been hearing. Family members who live with a hearing-impaired person should understand the importance of decreasing background noise, facing the person when speaking so that the face and mouth are visible, and involving the hearing-impaired person in conversations.[10]

HEALTH PROMOTION

Employees at risk for hearing loss from trauma or prolonged and elevated noise exposure are mandated by OSHA to limit their exposure and to wear protective equipment. Earplugs or protective equipment to reduce home, occupational, and recreational noise exposure should be encouraged to prevent hearing loss. Parents and children need to be informed of the risks of prolonged exposure to loud music from listening to music ear buds.

Preschoolers should be monitored for recurrent otitis media, and periodic hearing screening of school-age children should be encouraged.

Ototoxic medications should be monitored or, if possible, eliminated. Adults should be questioned periodically about hearing impairment. Questions should focus on specific areas of possible difficulty, such as difficulty hearing in noisy environments, difficulty hearing on the telephone, and difficulty understanding when the speaker's face is not visible. Ears should also be checked for ceruminosis and excess cerumen removed, if indicated.[11]

REFERENCES

1. O'Connor, A. F. (1998). Otosclerosis. In H. Ludman & T. Wright (Eds.), *Diseases of the ear* (6th ed.). London: Arnold.
2. Walling, A. D., & Dickson, G. (2012). Hearing loss in older adults. *American Family Physician, 82*(12), 1150–1156.
3. Weinstein, B. E. (2013). The aging auditory system. In *Geriatric audiology* (2nd ed., pp. 65–90). New York: Thieme.
4. Occupational Safety and Health Administration. Occupational noise exposure standard. Retrieved from www.osha.gov/pls/oshaweb/owadisp.show _document?p_table=STANDARDS&p_id=9735. (Accessed January 10, 2015).
5. Isaacson, J., & Vora, N. (2003). Differential diagnosis and treatment of hearing loss. *American Family Physician, 68*(6), 1125–1132.
6. Koike, K. J. (2013). *Everyday audiology: A practical guide for health care professionals* (2nd ed., pp. 18–19). San Diego: Plural Publishing.
7. American Academy of Otolaryngology-Head and Neck Surgery. Position statement: Red flags warning of ear disease (2014). Retrieved from http://www.entnet.org/content/position-statement-red-flags-warning-of-ear-disease; (Accessed May 4, 2019).
8. National Institute on Deafness and Other Communication Disorders. Enlarged vestibular aqueducts and childhood hearing loss. Retrieved from www.nidcd.nih.gov/health/hearing/pages/eva.aspx. (Accessed May 4, 2019).
9. McKay, S. (2013). Managing children with mild and unilateral hearing loss. In J. R. Madell & C. Flexer (Eds.), *Pediatric audiology* (2nd ed.). New York: Thieme.
10. American Speech Language Hearing Association. Patient information handouts. Retrieved from https://www.asha.org/aud/pei/. (Accessed May 4, 2019).
11. Toriello, H. V., Reardon, W., & Gorlin, R. J. (2013). *Hereditary hearing loss and its syndromes* (3rd ed.). Oxford, NY: Oxford University Press.

INNER EAR DISTURBANCES

Magen M. Price

 Immediate neurologic examination indicated for an abnormal finding which suggests a central cause.

Nearly 3% of all emergency department visits result from dizziness.[1] This complaint, as well as that of hearing loss or tinnitus, may indicate an inner ear disturbance. Vestibular neuritis, Meniere disease, and tinnitus are three of the most common inner ear disturbances.

VESTIBULAR NEURITIS
Definition and Epidemiology

Vestibular neuritis is an acute unilateral labyrinthine dysfunction, also called acute peripheral vestibulopathy or labyrinthitis. The condition is characterized by brief severe vertigo, nausea, vomiting, and imbalance following unilateral loss of peripheral vestibular function.[2] Typically, symptoms last a few days or weeks, but up to 50% of patients will develop chronic vertigo, unsteadiness, and spatial disorientation.[2,3]

Pathophysiology

Vestibular neuritis is most commonly caused by viral inflammation of the vestibular nerve, but otitis media is another possible cause. Increasing evidence suggests an association with latent herpes simplex virus type 1 (HSV-1) infection of the vestibular ganglia.[4] Inflammation of the eighth cranial nerve causes the sensation of vertigo. Research also suggests autoimmune and microvascular ischemic insults to the vestibular labyrinth as possible mechanisms of injury.[5] In addition, vestibular neuritis may also be caused by irritation from chemical products associated with acute or chronic otitis media.

Clinical Presentation and Physical Examination

Patients with vestibular neuritis complain of severe vertigo, nausea, and vomiting aggravated by head movement. Tinnitus may be present, but hearing remains intact.[4] The most severe symptoms of vertigo usually subside within 48 to 72 hours, but they can last 4 or 5 days. Although most episodes resolve spontaneously, up to half of patients will continue to experience dizziness and disequilibrium for many months.[2,3] Albeit not life-threatening, these symptoms can cause significant emotional and social stress for patients.

The history should include current medication use; history of head trauma; and duration, episodic nature, and severity of the vertigo. Past medical history and recent infection, particularly in the respiratory tract, should be elicited. Precipitating or aggravating factors, including cough, sneeze, or change in head position, and associated symptoms should be ascertained to help determine the cause of the vertigo.

A thorough ear, nose, and throat examination and a careful neurologic evaluation, including balance testing (Romberg test), are recommended. A hearing screen reveals normal hearing.[4] Spontaneous nystagmus, horizontal or rotary, is often present with fast phases directed away from the affected ear. The nystagmus may need to be evaluated by use of Frenzel lenses for greater magnification.[4] Any abnormal finding on neurologic examination suggests a central cause and should be referred for immediate neurologic evaluation.[5]

Diagnostics

Essential Diagnostics. There are no confirmatory diagnostic tests available for vestibular neuritis. Diagnosis is made upon the exclusion of differential diagnoses and assessment of clinical findings.

Additional Diagnostics. More definitive examinations to test hearing and to assess vertigo may be warranted. If a bacterial cause is suspected, a **complete blood count (CBC) with differential** may be helpful. If a tumor is suspected, **magnetic resonance imaging (MRI)** or a **computed tomography (CT) scan** is indicated.

Differential Diagnosis

Additional causes of peripheral vertigo and central vertigo must be considered.

 Priority differentials include (1) central causes of vertigo such as cerebellar disorders, (2) head trauma, and (3) multiple sclerosis.

Computed tomography (CT) (see Chapter 175) is associated with changes in head position, especially when the patient is recumbent. Meniere disease is associated with recurrent episodic vertigo, fluctuating hearing loss, and tinnitus.[4] Migrainous vertigo may occur in patients with a history of migraines.[6] Ramsay Hunt syndrome, caused by herpes zoster, includes hearing loss, facial palsy, and vertigo.[7] Cerebellar disorders are less common but potentially life-threatening.[5] Multiple sclerosis, head trauma, barotrauma, and toxins such as drugs and alcohol can also cause similar symptoms. Additional information about vertigo can be found in Chapter 175.

Interprofessional Collaborative Management

Pharmacologic Management. Treatment focuses on three goals: (1) alleviating vertigo, nausea, and vomiting; (2) treating the cause of infection; and (3) improving ventral compensation through vestibular exercises.[4] Symptomatic relief can be achieved with anticholinergics, antihistamines, long-acting benzodiazepines, or antiemetics. Anticholinergics and antihistamines are first-line agents; benzodiazepines are reserved for patients who cannot take drugs with anticholinergic effects. Meclizine, 25 to 50 mg every 6 hours, is commonly used and acceptable in pregnancy. Antiemetics may be added during an acute episode to relieve vomiting.[8] These medications should be stopped after 3 days because continuing them may hamper vestibular recovery.[8] The use of antivirals as monotherapy has not proven effective and is typically not recommended.[4] Some studies report improvement of symptoms with corticosteroids; however, more recent studies have shown little benefit. Despite conflicting evidence, it is reasonable to begin steroid therapy during the acute phase of vertigo.[4] Methylprednisolone can be given once daily for 22 days beginning with diagnosis, beginning with a 100-mg dose and gradually tapering down every 3 days.

Nonpharmacologic Management. Once the severe symptoms have passed, patients may benefit from vestibular enhancement exercises, which can be obtained through physical therapy services.[4,8]

Indications for Referral or Hospitalization

Consultation with an otolaryngologist is indicated if the diagnosis is unclear, the bacterial infection is severe, or symptoms do not resolve within 4 to 6 weeks. Associated suppurative otitis media or meningitis also necessitates referral. Severe dehydration indicates a need for intravenous rehydration and possible hospitalization.

Life-Span Considerations

Medications for symptomatic relief of vestibular neuritis can cause drowsiness and sedation. In older adults, lower doses of medications (e.g., 12.5 mg of meclizine or less) should be considered for control of sedation.

Complications

Sensorineural hearing loss can occur after resolution of inner ear inflammation. In older adults, especially, vertigo may increase the risk of falls.

Patient and Family Education

The provision of information about the disorder and reassurances will be helpful to patients and families. The importance of slowly changing positions should be discussed. In addition, adequate hydration and safety should be stressed. Patients, particularly older adults, may require assistance with activities of daily living or a walker or cane during the acute phase of the illness. Patients should avoid driving and operating heavy equipment while taking sedatives or antihistamines.

Because the disorder usually resolves within 4 to 6 weeks, patients should understand the importance of notifying the health care provider if the symptoms continue or increase in severity. Follow-up evaluation should be scheduled to reassess the patient and to ensure that the vertigo is resolving.

MENIERE DISEASE
Definition and Epidemiology

Meniere disease is a chronic condition of the inner ear characterized by recurrent vertigo and hearing loss. It is a complex of four symptoms that may or may not occur simultaneously: dizziness described as spinning vertigo, low-frequency sensorineural hearing loss, tinnitus, and a feeling of fullness in the affected ear. In the United States, estimated prevalence ranges from 9/100,000 in patients less than 18 years of age up to 440/100,000 in patients over the age of 65.[9] The majority of patients develop disease in the fourth and fifth decades of life, while approximately 10% of patients have disease onset after age 65.[9]

Pathophysiology

Meniere disease involves excess fluid (endolymphatic hydrops) and pressure in the labyrinth of the inner ear that episodically distends the structures of the labyrinth and damages the vestibular system (involved in balance) and cochlear hair cells (involved in hearing).[9] The exact cause remains unknown; however, the majority of cases are likely caused by viral infections or immune system–mediated mechanisms.[9] Up to one-third of all cases seem to originate from an autoimmune process. Less common potential causes include tumors and trauma.

Clinical Presentation and Physical Examination

Along with eliciting a careful symptom analysis, the health care provider should ask patients about a history of recurrent symptoms. Early in the disease process, patients have intermittent attacks of vertigo that last from minutes to hours, often associated with nausea and vomiting. These episodes are commonly accompanied by pressure in the ear, low-pitched tinnitus fluctuating in intensity, and unilateral hearing loss; however, only one-third of patients will present with the full triad of symptoms (vertigo, tinnitus, and hearing loss).[10] Bilateral hearing loss should not rule out Meniere disease, as up to 30% of patients often complain of bilateral involvement.[10] There can be long periods of remission. During later stages, the attacks of vertigo may occur frequently, and the hearing loss is constant.

Diagnosis of Meniere disease is based on clinical criteria and/or response to treatment; however, it is important to differentiate Meniere disease from other causes of vertigo and hearing loss.[9] A thorough head and neck examination to exclude acute otitis media or another infectious process and a comprehensive neurologic examination are important. On physical examination, sound will lateralize to the unaffected ear in the Weber test; in the Rinne test, air conduction will be greater than bone conduction. Spontaneous nystagmus occurs during attacks and may not be present between attacks.

Diagnostics

Essential Diagnostics. Diagnostic criteria for Meniere disease include two episodes of spontaneous vertigo lasting at least 20 minutes each, audiometrically documented hearing loss, tinnitus or aural fullness, and the exclusion of other causes.[11] Basic testing for Meniere disease includes an audiogram and MRI to rule out central nervous system (CNS) lesions. Laboratory testing should include thyroid-stimulating hormone (TSH), rapid plasma reagin (RPR) testing for syphilis, serum glucose, and Lyme serologies.

Additional Diagnostics. Additional testing, done by an otolaryngologist, may include vestibular testing; glycerol urea, or sorbitol "stress" tests; electrocochleography; electronystagmography; and auditory brain stem testing.[11]

INITIAL DIAGNOSTICS

Meniere Disease

- Audiogram

LABORATORY
- Thyroid-stimulating hormone
- Serum glucose
- Rapid plasma reagin
- Lyme serologies

IMAGING
- Magnetic resonance imaging (to rule out neuroma)

DIFFERENTIAL DIAGNOSIS

Meniere disease is in large part diagnosed by excluding other disorders and is classified as idiopathic. Meniere disease can be seen with only hearing loss or vertigo, symptoms seen in many disorders.

 Priority differentials include (1) transient ischemic attack, (2) acoustic neuroma, (3) cerebellar tumors, and (4) tertiary syphilis.

Other differential diagnoses include BPPV, vestibular neuritis, head trauma, vertebrobasilar insufficiency, multiple sclerosis, transient ischemic attack, migraine headache, anemia, and Cogan syndrome.[11]

Interprofessional Collaborative Management

Pharmacologic Management. If Meniere disease is suspected, patients should be referred to an otolaryngologist for testing and management. There is no cure for the disease, and treatment can be challenging. The goals of therapy include managing the episodes of vertigo and arresting the disease process. The antiviral approach has almost eliminated the need for surgical intervention.[12] If an autoimmune process is suspected, diagnosis is typically confirmed after a positive response to steroid therapy.[9] A brief oral steroid course may provide temporary relief from vertigo for several weeks; however, longer-term efficacy has not been shown. Intratympanic steroid injection into the affected ear may produce somewhat longer relief for several months.[9]

For symptomatic relief, meclizine and antiemetics such as promethazine (Phenergan) may be beneficial for some patients. Centrally acting antihistamines with anticholinergic effects can suppress the vestibular system while also providing antiemetic relief. Options include dimenhydrinate, meclizine, and promethazine. Meclizine is the least sedating option and therefore the most common therapy.[9] Benzodiazepines are often prescribed for their GABA agonist effect; however, daily use is not recommended, due to high risk for addiction and withdrawal symptoms. Lorazepam has a quick onset with a duration typical of most vertigo attacks, and may be appropriate for infrequent use.[9]

Studies suggest that betahistine may be effective for alleviating vertigo symptoms; however, it is unlikely to alleviate tinnitus in patients with Meniere disease.[13] In the United States, oral betahistine is not available, although it may be possible to obtain it by prescription from a compounding pharmacist.

Approximately 6% of patients with Meniere disease will go on to develop drop, or "Tumarkin," attacks, a potentially life-threatening condition that typically requires surgical removal of the labyrinth of the affected ear.[14] Fortunately, intratympanic gentamicin has recently proven to be a long-lasting and effective treatment against drop attacks.[14]

Nonpharmacologic Management. Salt restriction has been suggested to reduce osmotic buildup of pressure in the endolymphatic compartment; however, long-term efficacy is not proven.[9] Other dietary recommendations such as reduced caffeine and alcohol are common among Meniere disease support groups; however, the benefit remains unproven.[15]

Rehabilitation is important to promote acclimation to audiovestibular loss. Hearing aids should be prescribed as required, and vestibular rehabilitation therapy is recommended.[9] The Meniett device is a benign, noninvasive treatment that has been helpful in Meniere disease; it generates low-pressure pulses that may displace inner ear fluids, thereby relieving symptoms.[16]

Indications for Referral or Hospitalization

Referral to an otolaryngologist or a neuro-otologist is indicated for diagnostic evaluation and management. Hospitalization is rarely indicated, unless the patient becomes dehydrated or injured as a result of a fall. Hospitalization is necessary for surgical intervention.

Life-Span Considerations

Although Meniere disease is more commonly diagnosed in middle-aged adults, older adults and children can also be affected.[9] The disorder can be particularly difficult to treat in pregnancy because medications are toxic to the fetus.

Complications

Hearing loss may be permanent. If the patient develops drop attacks, injury from falls is a possible complication; proper safety education should be provided and evaluation should be performed.

Patient and Family Education

Patient education should include information about the disease, expected course, and treatment choices. Reassurance will help allay anxiety. Patient safety during acute episodes of vertigo and the sedative side effects of prescribed medications should be emphasized.

TINNITUS
Definition and Epidemiology

Tinnitus is defined as the perception of a sound when there is no sound in the environment.[17] It is usually a chronic, benign, but annoying ringing, buzzing, hissing, high-pitched screeching, whistling, or other noise in one or both ears that can be constant or intermittent. It can, however, herald a more serious disorder. It is estimated that 10% to 25% of the general population are affected. Prevalence increases with age (9% of those older than 60 years vs. 5% of those aged 18 to 44 years).[17]

Pathophysiology

The pathophysiology of tinnitus is not well understood but includes activity within the nervous system without any corresponding mechanical or vibratory activity within the cochlea.[17] Vestibular schwannoma, somatic sounds, otosclerosis, presbycusis, toxins, noise trauma, barotrauma, eustachian tube dysfunction, acoustic neuroma, vascular abnormalities, and neuromuscular conditions can all be potential causes of tinnitus.

Clinical Presentation and Physical Examination

Patients with tinnitus have varying degrees of symptoms and levels of debilitation, depending on the type and level of perceived sound. The history should include onset, duration, frequency, characteristics, and location of the sound, as well as past ear disease or injury, allergy history, noise exposure, hearing status, and all medications. A description of tinnitus can be helpful. High-pitched, continuous sounds are usually associated with sensorineural loss, and low-pitched sounds are associated with idiopathic tinnitus or Meniere disease. Tinnitus described as pulsing or rushing is usually vascular in origin. Sounds similar to the ocean may result from eustachian tube dysfunction. Clicking sounds are usually somatic and may be caused by temporomandibular joint (TMJ) dysfunction or spasms of the muscular or middle ear structures. The spasms of ear structures may be symptomatic of an underlying neurologic disorder and warrant a thorough neurologic history, complete physical examination, and consultation. If the tinnitus is associated with hearing loss, any dizziness, vertigo, ear pressure, pain, or discharge should be noted. Tinnitus can either accompany or cause insomnia and depression, so it is important to inquire about both of these conditions.[18]

The physical examination should include a complete ear, nose, throat, head, neck, and TMJ examination. If vascular tinnitus is suspected, the health care provider should include bilateral auscultation of preauricular areas, temples, orbits, mastoids, and jugular veins in various positions. Hearing tests and a complete neurologic examination (including cranial nerves) are also indicated.

Diagnostics

Essential Diagnostics. Questionnaires are available to determine the degree of tinnitus severity (e.g., the Tinnitus Handicap Questionnaire). All patients with tinnitus thought to originate in the auditory system should receive a complete audiologic evaluation performed by an audiologist. Tests may include pure tone audiogram, tympanometry, auditory reflex testing, determination of speech discrimination abilities, and otoacoustic emissions testing. An otolaryngologist or neurologist should evaluate any patient in whom vascular tinnitus is a concern.

Additional Diagnostics. There is little evidence to support routine laboratory testing for the evaluation of tinnitus, and therefore diagnosis must be guided by clinical impression.[19] Patients with unilateral sensorineural hearing loss and tinnitus should be tested for syphilis and Lyme disease.[19] Alternative laboratory testing may include a CBC and differential to rule out anemia and infection, erythrocyte sedimentation rate (ESR) to rule out autoimmune disease, serum glucose concentration, and thyroid function. If indicated, additional diagnostics include MRI and CT scan to exclude a CNS lesion.[19]

INITIAL DIAGNOSTICS
Tinnitus
• Audiology evaluation

Differential Diagnosis

The differential diagnosis should include those conditions that distinguish benign tinnitus from tinnitus caused by serious pathologic conditions.

 Priority differentials include (1) vascular disorder, (2) CNS disorder such as multiple sclerosis, and (3) vestibular schwannoma.

Excessive noise exposure and presbycusis are common causes of hearing loss and tinnitus. Medications such as aspirin can cause permanent or reversible tinnitus. Tinnitus of short duration is often caused by an acute process such as otitis, labyrinthitis, or noise exposure. Vascular disorders can cause pulsatile tinnitus and require in-depth evaluation by an otolaryngologist or neurologist. Spasm in the muscles of the ear or palate can be heard as an intermittent tapping sound. Eustachian tube dysfunction causes a sound like the ocean. Vestibular schwannoma, a benign tumor of the acoustic nerve, is usually associated with unilateral tinnitus.[19] Meniere disease is characterized by fluctuating tinnitus, hearing loss, aural fullness, or vertigo.

Interprofessional Collaborative Management

Pharmacologic Management. Most patients with mild to moderate tinnitus adjust to the condition; although it is annoying, they do not find it debilitating. Patient education and reassurance are often all that can be offered.

All ototoxic medications and excessive noise exposure need to be eliminated. Various antidepressants have been used to treat both tinnitus and the depressive symptoms associated with tinnitus, but no one medication has as yet shown significant efficacy.

Because some patients also experience insomnia, a sleeping medication or melatonin may be helpful.[18] However, all sleeping medications should be used judiciously in older adults.

Nonpharmacologic Management. Obvious local pathologic conditions should be treated (e.g., TMJ treatment or administration of antibiotics for infection). If a sensorineural hearing loss is associated, referral for the application of other treatment modalities, such as hearing aids, sound masking, and cognitive behavioral therapy, may be indicated.[19] If no hearing loss is present, sound maskers alone, such as electronic noise-generating devices, mood tapes, and radio static, may diminish the intrusiveness of tinnitus.

The evidence of benefit is unclear for alternative therapies, including vitamins, herbal remedies, biofeedback, acupuncture, and electrical stimulation, but they may help individual patients.

Indications for Referral or Hospitalization

Consultation with the primary care physician is necessary when referral to an otolaryngologist or a neurologist is indicated. If there is a suspicion that the tinnitus is not benign or if pulsatile or unilateral tinnitus is present, the patient should be seen by the appropriate specialist.

Complications

No complications are associated with chronic, benign tinnitus. Missed diagnosis of tinnitus that is caused by a serious underlying pathologic condition may lead to untreated disease and major complications.

Patient and Family Education

Information on the causes of tinnitus and hearing loss increases understanding for most patients. A discussion of treatment options and resources for treatment is beneficial. Reassurance about the benign and common experiences of tinnitus is also helpful. Resources about tinnitus can be obtained from the American Tinnitus Association (www.ata.org).

REFERENCES

1. Navi, B., Kamel, H., Shah, M., Poisson, A., Whetstone, W., Josephson, S. A., et al. (2013). The use of neuroimaging studies and neurological consultation to evaluate dizzy patients in the emergency department. *The Neurohospitalist,* 3(1), 7–14.
2. Patel, M., Arshad, Q., Roberts, R., Ahmad, H., & Bronstein, A. (2016). Chronic symptoms after vestibular neuritis and the high velocity vestibulo-ocular reflex. *Otology & Neurotology,* 37(2), 179–184.
3. Cousins, S., Cutfield, N., Kaski, D., Palla, A., Seemungal, B., Golding, J., et al. (2014). Visual dependency and dizziness after vestibular neuritis. *PLoS ONE,* 9(9), e105426.
4. Strupp, M., & Brandt, T. (2013). Peripheral vestibular disorders. *Current Opinion in Neurology,* 26(1), 81–89.
5. Jeong, S., Kim, H., & Kim, J. (2013). Vestibular neuritis. *Seminars in Neurology,* 33(03), 185–194.
6. Radtke, A. (2014). Epidemiology of vestibular migraine and related syndromes. *Vestibular Migraine and Related Syndromes,* 1, 65–72.
7. Lee, D., Yoon, T., Lee, J., Joo, Y., & Lim, S. (2013). Herpes zoster laryngitis accompanied by Ramsay Hunt Syndrome. *The Journal of Craniofacial Surgery,* 24(5), e496–e498.
8. Greco, A., Macri, G., Gallo, A., Fusconi, M., De Virgilio, A., Pagliuca, G., et al. (2014). Is vestibular neuritis an immune related vestibular neuropathy inducing vertigo? *Journal of Immunology Research,* 2014, 459048.
9. Nakashima, T., Pyykko, I., Arroll, M., Casselbrant, M., Foster, C., Manzoor, N., et al. (2016). Meniere's disease. *Nature Reviews. Disease Primers,* 2, 16028.
10. Harcourt, J., Barraclough, K., & Bronstein, A. (2014). Meniere's disease. *British Medical Journal,* 349, g6544.
11. American Academy of Otolaryngology–Head and Neck Foundation. (1995). Committee on Hearing and Equilibrium guidelines for the diagnosis and

evaluation of therapy in Meniere's disease. *Otolaryngology–Head and Neck Surgery: Official Journal of American Academy of Otolaryngology-Head and Neck Surgery, 113*(3), 181–185.

12. Gacek, R. (2015). Recovery of hearing in Meniere's disease after antiviral treatment. *American Journal of Otolaryngology, 36*(3), 315–323.

13. Azadarmaki, R., & Prasad, S. (2014). Betahistine effects on tinnitus in patients with Meniere's disease. *Otolaryngology–Head and Neck Surgery: Official Journal of American Academy of Otolaryngology–Head and Neck Surgery, 151,* P196.

14. Viana, L., Bahmad, F., & Rauch, S. (2014). Intratympanic gentamicin as a treatment for drop attacks in patients with Meniere's disease. *The Laryngoscope, 124*(9), 2151–2154.

15. Tyrrell, J., Whinney, D., Ukoumunne, O., Fleming, L., & Osborne, N. (2014). Prevalence, associated factors, and comorbid conditions for Meniere's disease. *Ear and Hearing, 35*(4), e162–e169.

16. Ahsan, S., Standring, R., & Wang, Y. (2015). Systematic review and meta-analysis of Meniett therapy for Meniere's disease. *The Laryngoscope, 125*(1), 203–208.

17. Tunkel, D., Bauer, C., Sun, G., Rosenfeld, R., Chandrasekhar, S., Cunningdam, E., et al. (2014). Clinical practice guidelines: Tinnitus. *Otolaryngology–Head and Neck Surgery: Official Journal of American Academy of Otolaryngology–Head and Neck Surgery, 151*(2S), S1–S40.

18. Baguley, D., McFerran, D., & Hall, D. (2013). Tinnitus. *Lancet, 382,* 1600–1607.

19. Yew, K. S. (2014). Diagnostic approach to patients with tinnitus. *American Family Physician, 89*(2), 106–113.

CHAPTER **67**

OTITIS EXTERNA

Jacqueline Rosenjack Burchum

Immediate referral is indicated for evidence of malignant otitis externa (Fig. 67.1).

DEFINITION AND EPIDEMIOLOGY

Otitis externa is a cellulitis of the external auditory canal that may extend to the auricle (pinna).[1] The condition is often referred to as *swimmer's ear,* although the causes are varied.

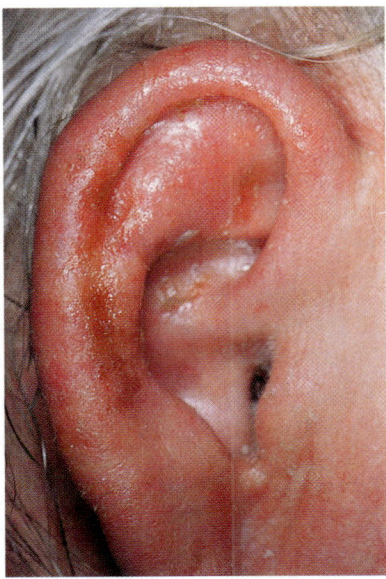

FIG. 67.1 Malignant otitis externa. (From Habif, T. P. [2016]. *Clinical dermatology: A color guide to diagnosis and therapy* [6th ed.]. St. Louis: Elsevier Saunders.)

Approximately 1 in 125 people develop acute otitis externa annually, with occurrence primarily in the warmer months and in regions with high humidity.[2] Chronic otitis externa affects 3% to 5% of the U.S. population.[2] A smaller percentage of patients with otitis externa will progress to malignant (necrotizing) otitis externa, which is a complication that is most often seen in people who are immunocompromised or who have comorbid conditions such as diabetes mellitus.[1,3–5]

PATHOPHYSIOLOGY

Risk factors for development of external otitis are typically those that compromise the integrity of the inherent defense mechanism against infection. These include removal of protective cerumen with damage to fragile skin that results from vigorous cleaning of the canal, maceration of skin that results from accumulation of moisture within the canal from swimming,[1,3–5] and alterations to the tissues that result from wearing of devices such as headphones and ear plugs.[1]

In the United States, more than 90% of cases have a bacterial cause. The most common causative organisms are *Pseudomonas aeruginosa* and *Staphylococcus aureus.*[1,5] Fungi such as *Candida* and *Aspergillus* organisms are uncommon causes of acute otitis externa, but may be present in chronic otitis externa or after antibiotic treatment of acute otitis externa.[1] Patients with recurrent otitis externa should be evaluated to determine whether the episode represents a fungal infection, treatment failure, or recurrence.

CLINICAL PRESENTATION AND PHYSICAL EXAMINATION

The usual presentation of acute otitis externa is pain of the affected ear and auricle developing over the course of 48 hours or less. The pain is often accompanied by a feeling of fullness or itching. Other signs and symptoms that may be present include drainage from the affected ear and hearing loss.[2,4] Presentation of chronic otitis externa is primarily one of intense pruritus.[5]

The classic finding in acute otitis externa is pain and tenderness on palpation of the tragus and on repositioning of the auricle to allow inspection of the canal.[1,3–5] The canal may be erythematous and edematous. Often the canal is filled with debris and sloughed tissue. The tympanic membrane may be erythematous; alternately, it may be poorly visualized because of edema or cerumen and exudate in the canal. Advanced cases of acute otitis externa are often accompanied by complete obstruction of the canal. The cellulitis may extend to the external ear with enlargement of periauricular lymph nodes.[1,4] Hearing deficits may occur in advanced cases.[1]

Chronic otitis externa has a very different presentation. The canal is often dry, and cerumen may be absent. Excoriations may be present secondary to use of objects inserted to relieve the itching that accompanies this condition. Discharge may be present. The canal may be narrowed, but this is secondary to thickened canal walls that occur over time rather than to the edema that is responsible for narrowed canals in acute otitis externa.[5]

DIAGNOSTICS

Essential Diagnostics

Diagnostic testing is usually unnecessary. A culture of canal drainage with antibiotic sensitivities is indicated if there is no improvement after 14 days of antibiotic therapy.[3] Microscopic analysis of drainage using potassium hydroxide (KOH) can identify a fungal cause.

Additional Diagnostics

If the condition progresses to malignant otitis externa, osteomyelitis can occur. With malignant otitis externa, a complete blood count will demonstrate an increased leukocyte count and an erythrocyte sedimentation rate will also be elevated.[5] If osteomyelitis is suspected, magnetic resonance imaging (MRI) is the most sensitive diagnostic test to detect this complication, while gallium scans are the most specific.[3,5]

INITIAL DIAGNOSTICS

Otitis Externa

LABORATORY
- Culture and sensitivity[a]
- Potassium hydroxide preparation of drainage[a]

[a]If indicated.

DIFFERENTIAL DIAGNOSIS

It is important to distinguish otitis externa from other conditions that cause ear pain, drainage, inflammation, or hearing loss. Patients with recurrent otitis externa should be evaluated to determine whether the episode represents a treatment failure rather than a recurrence.

 Priority differentials include (1) acute otitis media, (2) malignant otitis externa, and (3) chronic suppurative otitis media.

INTERPROFESSIONAL COLLABORATIVE MANAGEMENT

Management of otitis externa focuses on clearing debris from the canal, managing the pain, and treating the infection and inflammation. This is accomplished through both pharmacologic and nonpharmacologic therapy.

Pharmacologic Management

Nonsteroidal Antiinflammatory Drugs or Acetaminophen. For mild to moderate pain, nonsteroidal antiinflammatory drugs (NSAIDs) offer the benefit of both analgesia and control of inflammation; however, acetaminophen may be substituted if NSAIDs are not well tolerated.[1,3,5]

Opioids. Opioids may need to be given during the initial 48 to 72 hours if the pain is severe.[1,3,5] These should not be prescribed routinely, however.

Topical Anesthetics. Topical anesthetics such as benzocaine otic solution were once frequently prescribed for pain management; hence patients who had a previous episodes of otitis externa may request ear drops for pain. However, citing a lack of safety and efficacy concerns, the US Food and Drug Administration required that these medications be removed from the U.S. market in 2015.[6]

Topical Antibiotics. Topical antibiotics are indicated for uncomplicated conditions in which inflammation is confined to the ear canal.[1] If the ear canal is severely swollen, insertion of a wick into the affected ear may be necessary to allow the medication to access the deeper recesses of the canal.

In the absence of culture and sensitivity results, it is important to choose medications that are effective against both *P. aeruginosa* and *S. aureus.* This ensures coverage against the most common causes.

Fluoroquinolone antibiotics are effective against *P. aeruginosa* and *S. aureus.*[1,3,5,7] Examples include ofloxacin (Floxin otic) and ciprofloxacin (Cetraxal, Ciloxan). These are also available as antibiotic-corticosteroid combinations such as ciprofloxacin with hydrocortisone (Cipro HC) to promote resolution of both infection and inflammation. Fluoroquinolones are safe to use in patients with nonintact tympanic membranes or tympanostomy tubes.[1,3]

Aminoglycoside antibiotics such as neomycin are another option for treating acute otitis externa.[1,3,5,7] Neomycin is effective against *S. aureus* but not *P. aeruginosa,* so it is commonly combined with polymyxin B for *P. aeruginosa* coverage in products such as Cortisporin. Ototoxicity is a potential complication of aminoglycoside therapy, and it is important to not use this category of antibiotics if the tympanic membrane is not intact.[1]

For fungal infections that commonly cause chronic otitis externa, acidification with 5% acetic acid (white vinegar) or a 1:1[1] or 1:2[7] solution of vinegar and alcohol is often effective, though it may cause a stinging sensation. Antifungal solutions such as clotrimazole otic are effective against common causative fungi. Fungal infections may also be treated with fluconazole (Diflucan) if there are no contraindications because of potential drug-drug interactions (e.g., warfarin).[7]

Nonpharmacologic Management

Because debris in the canal can interfere with healing and prevent penetration by topical medications, it should be gently removed.[1] If the tympanic membrane is intact, aural lavage with hydrogen peroxide, saline, or even water may be helpful. These should be warmed to room temperature.[1] Cleansing may also be accomplished by gently suctioning or using cotton-tipped swabs under direct observation via otoscope.[1]

LIFE-SPAN CONSIDERATIONS

Otitis externa is most common in young people.[1,2,4] Malignant otitis externa primarily affects older patients.[2–4]

Complications

Malignant otitis externa is an invasive osteomyelitis of the ear that occurs when the bacterial infection extends into cartilage and bone.[1,3,4] This condition can become life threatening. It is usually caused by *P. aeruginosa* and is most commonly seen in patients who are older, who have diabetes, or who are immunocompromised.[1,4] It is associated with severe pain, necrotic ulcerations, and fever. Facial paralysis and other cranial nerve abnormalities may also occur.[2,4]

 Immediate otolaryngologist consultation is indicated for patients with malignant otitis externa (see Fig. 67.1).

PATIENT AND FAMILY EDUCATION

Patients with otitis externa need to be educated about causes, management, and prevention of their condition. Many patients will not know how to administer topical otic medications, so it will be important to review medication administration in addition to teaching about medication schedules and potential adverse effects.

Patients need to know that improvement should occur within 48 to 72 hours. If the condition should worsen rather than improve, they should be promptly reevaluated for complications. Resolution typically occurs in 7 to 10 days. If symptoms continue beyond this time, patients should be evaluated for treatment failure.

HEALTH PROMOTION

Prevention should center on avoidance of conditions that contribute to the development of otitis externa. Cerumen provides lubrication, as well as a protective barrier against water and bacteria, so patients should be instructed to avoid use of cotton-tipped swabs and similar objects to clean the ears. Swimming allows prolonged exposure of the canal to water, so explaining to patients and families that it will be helpful to use a blow dryer to dry out the ear after swimming is important.[1,3] A 1:1 or 1:2 mixture of white vinegar and rubbing alcohol drops in each ear after swimming will restore an acidic environment and promote drying.[1,3,5] Ear plugs may also be used when swimming; however, these have also been identified as a risk factor for otitis externa.[1]

REFERENCES

1. Rosenfeld, R. M., Schwartz, S. R., Cannon, C. R., et al. (2014). Clinical practice guideline: Acute otitis externa. *Otolaryngology–Head and Neck Surgery: Official Journal of American Academy of Otolaryngology–Head and Neck Surgery, 150*(IS), S1–S24.
2. Centers for Disease Control and Prevention (CDC). (2011). Estimated burden of acute otitis externa. *MMWR. Morbidity and Mortality Weekly Report, 60*(19), 605–609.
3. Goldman, L., & Schaffer, A. (2016). *Goldman-Cecil medicine* (25th ed.). St. Louis: Elsevier Saunders.
4. Dains, J. E., Baumann, L. C., & Scheibel, P. (2015). *Advanced health assessment and clinical diagnosis in primary care* (5th ed.). St Louis: Elsevier Mosby.
5. Ferri, F. F. (2018). *Ferri's clinical advisor 2018.* St Louis: Elsevier Mosby.
6. Unapproved and misbranded otic prescription drug products; Enforcement action dates. (2015). 80 Fed. Reg. 38212.
7. Kesser, B. W. (2018). External otitis (Acute). https://www.merckmanuals.com/professional/ear,-nose,-and-throat-disorders/external-ear-disorders/external-otitis-acute. (Accessed 4 May 2019).

CHAPTER 68

OTITIS MEDIA
Margaret Thorman Hartig • Sharon Little

Immediate referral is indicated for acute otitis media (AOM) in children 6 months or younger, and in children who appear lethargic or toxic, to determine the need for hospitalization and sepsis workup. Referral is also indicated for AOM in children with cochlear implants, tympanostomy tubes, and anatomic or craniofacial abnormalities.

DEFINITION AND EPIDEMIOLOGY

Otitis media (OM), characterized by fluid in the middle ear, is associated with varied inflammatory or infective processes that may be bacterial, fungal, or viral in origin, and is most often associated with upper respiratory tract infections or allergies. This disorder accounts for a significant number of all antimicrobial prescriptions in primary care.[1,2] OM is the most frequent childhood infectious illness, with the peak incidence at 6 to 15 months of age, but adults and elders are also affected

and is seen in all age groups.[2] Severity and presentation vary. Symptoms and findings often are part of a continuum, despite the common practice of identifying discrete diagnoses. This continuum and its subtypes complicate diagnosis, as one condition often evolves into another.

AOM, a bacterial or viral infection of the middle ear fluid, has a rapid onset and short duration. Otitis media with effusion (OME) describes accumulation of serous fluid in the middle ear without acute inflammation. OME can precede or follow AOM, but barotrauma or allergy also can precipitate an occurrence. Middle ear effusion (MEE) signifies an accumulation of serous fluid in the middle ear and can be associated with AOM, often persisting for weeks or months after an episode of AOM.

Chronic effusion (known also as serous OM or "glue ear") is characterized by hearing impairment and may persist for several months, with or without signs of infection.[1] Children aged 3 to 7 years old are most commonly affected. Recurrent OM is defined as three or more distinct episodes in 6 months or four or more episodes in the preceding 12 months with at least one episode in the past 6 months.[1]

PATHOPHYSIOLOGY

OM is a dysfunction of the middle ear and middle ear mucosa.[1,2] The actual cause is multifactorial, related to anatomy, pathophysiology, and cell biology.[1,2] Antecedent events may be viral, bacterial, or allergic. Viral upper respiratory tract infections or allergies often precede otitis and result in edema of the eustachian tube and nasopharynx.[1,2] Narrow eustachian tubes, common in infants and young children, may predispose patients to episodes of OM. Exposure to cigarette smoke acts in several ways to increase an individual's risk for OM. In general, smoking increases the risk for upper respiratory tract infections. In addition, smoke may decrease the mucociliary functioning in the eustachian tube. When middle ear secretions accumulate in the eustachian tube, the opportunity for pathogen growth, both bacterial and viral, also increases. The most common bacterial causative agents are *Streptococcus pneumoniae* and *Haemophilus influenzae*. Group A β-hemolytic *Streptococcus*, *Staphylococcus aureus*, and *Moraxella catarrhalis* also cause infections, but on a less frequent basis.[1,2]

Bacteria are the most frequent cause of otitis infections; however, in one study, two-thirds of the infections were caused by a combination of bacteria and viruses.[1,2] This combination complicates recovery because viruses may increase inflammation, decrease neutrophil function, and interfere with antibiotic penetration.

CLINICAL PRESENTATION AND PHYSICAL EXAMINATION

Clinical findings and severity of symptoms (i.e., otalgia and fever) experienced are aligned with criteria for categorizing the types of AOM, distinguishing it from OME and determining treatment. Three 2013 clinical practice guidelines presented by the American Academy of Pediatrics consider age, severity of symptoms, otorrhea, and laterality in diagnosing and treating AOM.[2] These criteria require thoroughness in the physical examination that may not be well received by the child in pain.

Presence of rapid-onset otalgia, worse in a prone position, remains the common initial complaint of patients with AOM. Infants and younger children often have nonspecific symptoms, such as ear rubbing, rhinorrhea, vomiting, diarrhea, and fever.

Specific symptoms and signs are linked with causative bacteria. Patients with OME or serous otitis may be asymptomatic or have mild pain with no symptoms of acute infection.[3] Conductive hearing loss is most common. Other symptoms include imbalance or vertigo, mild stuffiness, and a fullness or popping sensation in the ear.

The history should include incidents (especially recent) of ear infections, upper respiratory tract infections, allergies, smoke exposure, and any treatments and their effectiveness. Health care providers also should note the development of the current illness, including the onset and duration of symptoms, ear pain or drainage, fever, irritability, hearing loss, tinnitus, and dizziness. Associated symptoms, including headache, eye drainage, nasal congestion, sore throat, and mouth pain, require investigation. Knowledge of activities that involve barometric pressure changes, such as scuba diving and flying, is helpful because these may affect equilibrium and cause discomfort from air in the middle ear. As with any infectious process, the patient's immune status must be considered.

The physical exam can be challenging in young children, but the ear pain can also be significant in adults—especially if bullous myringitis (bullae on the tympanic membrane [TM]) is present. A significant change in status should be noted. For example, a lethargic child barely talks or moves, indicating severe illness and possibly dehydration or sepsis. Temperature should be checked for presence of fever (above or below 39°C or 102.2°F), though body temperature and other vital signs may be within normal range (especially in older adults).

The findings on examination of the mouth, eyes, and nose may also be normal, or the patient may show signs and symptoms of upper respiratory tract infection. The frontal and maxillary sinuses often are tender on palpation and do not transilluminate. Mild to significant lymphadenopathy may be present with warm, tender, and enlarged posterior auricular and cervical lymph nodes. The ears should be examined for edema, possible drainage, posterior pinna erythema, and mastoid tenderness.

A thorough otoscopic examination is indicated to accurately determine the presence of OM. Diagnosis of AOM requires a thorough assessment with pneumatic otoscopy and adherence to defined diagnostic criteria. The American Academy of Pediatrics guidelines[2] address and discourage the not uncommon practice of deferring aggressive visualization of the TM and relying on symptomatology. The presence or absence of TM bulging is considered critical to accurate diagnosis and discrimination between AOM and OME.[2,3]

Cerumen removal may be necessary to obtain a clear view of the TM. The operating head of an otoscope provides direct visualization of the canal and access to remove the cerumen with a small plastic disposable ear curette.[1,2] Hard or flaky cerumen can be softened with a variety of products at room temperature (e.g., sodium docusate solution, hydrogen peroxide, mineral oil) in the absence of TM perforation. Removal of softened cerumen can be accomplished with a curette, irrigation with soft bulb syringe, or use of a low-pressure water stream (Waterpik is a common choice).

Ideally, the otoscope uses a bright light source and airtight seal, usually achieved with the proper-size speculum. Nondisposable speculums are recommended for best seal and light conduction, as well as less painful examinations.[2] The importance and challenge of differentiating AOM from OME with and without effusion is commonly acknowledged.[2,3] Other

findings include fluid behind the TM, which often affects the color. Fluid levels may be visible behind the membrane. Discharge in the canal without acute otitis externa suggests perforation. Purulent discharge in the ear canal may be sampled for culture and used as a basis for antibiotic selection. Bullae between the TM layers are most often associated with *Mycoplasma pneumoniae*.

Diagnosis of AOM requires bulging of the TM with obscured landmarks *or* new onset of otorrhea not caused by acute otitis externa.[2] Findings of moderate to severe bulging without other signs *or* mild bulging *and* recent (less than 48 hours) onset of ear pain *or* intense erythema of TM also qualify for AOM diagnosis. Presence of MEE also is necessary for diagnosis of AOM. Fluid levels or air bubbles may be seen behind the TM, indicating accompanying effusion, though definitive diagnosis relies on pneumatic otoscopy and/or tympanometry.[2]

Pain assessment is necessary for both determining the presence of AOM and the need for pain relief. Throbbing, painful earache with impaired hearing is a common characteristic of AOM. The Acute Otitis Media Severity of Symptom Scale (AOM-SOS) provides a seven-item, parent-reported symptom score when it is a child that is being seen.[4] The AOM-SOS is a sensitive option for evaluation.[4] Symptoms evaluated are ear tugging, rubbing, and holding; excessive crying; irritability; difficulty sleeping; decreased activity; decreased appetite; and fever. The validated scale correlates with both the diagnosis and symptoms over time. Fever is often present, and the patient may have nausea or dizziness. Cold or influenza symptoms often accompany the condition.[1,2]

In OME, fluid is present in the middle ear without signs or symptoms of acute infection. The TM often is dull gray, although it may appear injected.[2,3] Ear pain may still be present in infants, although it tends to be milder and often intermittent. Older children may report ear fullness and/or an ear-popping sensation. Balance problems or hearing loss also may be noted and can be common in adults. School performance may be affected. In chronic serous otitis, the TM may appear retracted and amber or bluish in color with a diffuse light reflex. TMs usually have limited movement and bubbles, or a fluid line is seen behind the membrane.

DIAGNOSTICS
Essential Diagnostics

Acute Otitis Media Is Primarily a Clinical Diagnosis. Determine TM position or contour, color, translucency, and mobility.[2,3] Positions other than the usual neutral include retracted, full, and bulging. Moderate to severe bulging is the most important characteristic for the diagnosis of AOM.[2] Otorrhea may indicate MEE, especially if accompanied by abrupt relief of pain. Retraction is a common finding in OME.[3]

The color of the TM may range from gray to red. Erythema of the TM often occurs in AOM, though in young children, it may be related to crying or fever. A very white TM may be the result of scarring from previous infections or purulence behind the TM. Translucency may be obscured and cloudy or opaque with illness. Decreased or absent mobility, determined by pneumatic otoscopy, indicates the presence of MEE and is one of the necessary criteria for accurate diagnosis of AOM.[2]

Tympanometry may help with diagnosis if otoscopic examination cannot determine whether there is fluid in the middle ear.[3] Acoustic reflectometry, the use of sound waves to determine TM mobility, may also be helpful for diagnosis, although it is rarely used.

Examination of the ear canal for otorrhea in the absence of external OM is necessary for classification of AOM.

Weber and Rinne tests may be indicated to determine whether conduction and sensorineural hearing have been affected.

Additional Diagnostics

Laboratory or further diagnostic testing is not indicated for most patients with OM. There are special considerations for some patients, however.[2]

- A sinus X-ray study or a computed tomography (CT) scan of the sinuses may be indicated for patients who have recurrent or chronic OM, especially if intratemporal or intracranial complications are suspected. A contrast-enhanced CT scan of the temporal bones is the imaging study of choice.
- Allergy testing should be considered in patients who have recurrent or chronic otitis symptoms and a history of allergies or allergic rhinitis. Immune status should be considered in patients with atypical OM or those who do not respond to therapy.
- A complete blood count (CBC) with differential should be ordered in immunocompromised patients.
- Tympanocentesis may be indicated for recurrent OM to identify causative organisms.

INITIAL DIAGNOSTICS

Otitis Media

LABORATORY
- Complete blood count and differential[a]
- Serum glucose, electrolytes, BUN, creatinine, liver function tests[a]

IMAGING
- Sinus X-ray study or computed tomography (CT) scan of sinuses[a]
- Contrast-enhanced CT scan of the temporal bone[a]

OTHER DIAGNOSTICS
- Pneumatic otoscopy (position, color, translucency, mobility)[a]
- Tympanometry[a]
- Acoustic reflectometry[a]
- Weber and Rinne tests[a]
- Tympanocentesis[a]
- Culture and sensitivity[a]

[a]If indicated.

DIFFERENTIAL DIAGNOSIS

The primary challenge with differential diagnosis is distinguishing AOM from OME. The type of AOM also influences the management course.

Priority differentials include sepsis, otitis externa, OME, mastoiditis, cholesteatoma, and myringitis.

INTERPROFESSIONAL COLLABORATIVE MANAGEMENT

Professional organization guidelines define each of the AOM types and recommended treatments.[1-3]

The type of AOM determines the most appropriate treatment for individual patients. The need for antibiotic therapy is based on each person's medical history, physical examination, and presentation. Initial observation includes a plan for treatment of associated symptoms, especially pain management, and planned provider contact within 24 hours for follow-up assessment.[4,5]

Increased incidence of antibiotic resistance, awareness of overprescribing for noninfectious OME, and recognition of antibiotic side effects are not without consequence. Current recommendations are for "watchful waiting" with close follow-up within 48 to 72 hours for nonsevere AOM.[2,6] Studies support the potential benefit of waiting 48 to 72 hours to administer antibiotics with minimal risk. Parental or caregiver preference is to be considered in these decisions.

Some providers find it effective to give parents/patients a written prescription at the time of appointment, with the proviso they will wait up to 72 hours to determine the need for antibiotic therapy.[2]

PHARMACOLOGIC MANAGEMENT
Pain Management

Pain treatment should be provided for otalgia, whether or not antibiotics are prescribed. For adults with AOM, nonsteroidal antiinflammatory (NSAIDs) medications are most commonly used for pain control in adults, but for some patients (e.g., an adult on warfarin), a low dose opioid may be necessary especially if acetaminophen is not effective.

For children, acetaminophen or ibuprofen, with dose calculated according to weight, is effective for mild to moderate pain.[5] Narcotic analgesia with codeine was used in the past, but there were definite concerns about the potential for significant side effects and even death for children who were prescribed codeine. In 2018, the Federal Drug Administration changed the age range recommendation for codeine to be used only in patients 18 years or older.[7] Codeine and hydrocodone are now not recommended for children under the age of 18. The risks of prescribing any opioid for a child necessitates serious consideration and physician consultation.[7] Topical agents may provide brief relief, but evidence is limited as to extended benefits.[2] Antihistamines, decongestants, and steroids are not beneficial for treatment of AOM or OME.[2,3,6]

Antibiotics

Antibiotic recommendations are similar for both adults and children. If not penicillin allergic, amoxicillin 500 mg po every 8 to 12 hours was in the past recommended for an adult with AOM.[8] However, now amoxicillin–clavulanate 875/125 mg po every 12 hours for 7 to 10 days is indicated for adults with fever and if obvious significant discomfort is apparent. If an adult is allergic to penicillin (type 1 reaction), azithromycin or doxycycline are options, depending on the patient's medical history and potential drug-drug interactions.[8,9] Providers are encouraged, however, to check antibiotic recommendations frequently because of the increasing resistance to commonly used antibiotics.

If the patient is a child, consideration is given to age of the child and severity of the condition (including associated signs and symptoms).

Amoxicillin, 80 to 90 mg/kg/day, is the recommended first-line antibiotic for children who are not allergic and have not received it in the last 30 days *or* do not have purulent conjunctivitis.[2] Amoxicillin with β-lactamase is preferred for children not allergic *and* who have received amoxicillin in the last 30 days *or* have purulent conjunctivitis.[2] A third generation cephalosporin (e.g., cefdinir) or azithromycin is considered safe for children allergic to penicillin.[10] For children, unresponsive to initial treatment (e.g., after 48 to 72 hours), amoxicillin-clavulanate, 90 mg amoxicillin per kilogram each day with 6.4 mg clavulanate per kilogram each day or in penicillin allergic children, clindamycin 20 to 40 mg/kg/day (can be in combination with a third generation cephalosporin) in three divided doses or ceftriaxone 50 mg/kg/day IM or IV is indicated.[6]

Treatment recommendations for children with AOM include:

- AOM with otorrhea in children 6 months or older: antibiotic therapy is recommended.
- Severe AOM (bilateral or unilateral) in children 6 months or older with moderate to severe otalgia *or* fever of 39°C or higher: antibiotic therapy is recommended.
- Nonsevere AOM (bilateral) in children younger than 24 months with mild otalgia for less than 48 hours and fever less than 39°C: antibiotic therapy is recommended.
- Nonsevere AOM (unilateral) in children aged 6 to 23 months with mild otalgia and fever below 39°C: may receive either antibiotics or observation with close follow-up.[2]
- Nonsevere AOM (bilateral or unilateral) in children 24 months or older with mild otalgia for less than 48 hours and fever below 39°C may receive either antibiotics or observation with close follow-up.[2,5]

Length of antibiotic treatment varies by AOM severity and child age.[2]

- Severe AOM in children younger than 2 is treated for 10 days.
- Mild or moderate AOM in children 2 to 5 years of age is treated for 7 days.
- Mild to moderate symptoms of AOM in children 6 years or older are treated adequately at 5 to 7 days.
- Prophylactic antibiotic use for the treatment and prevention of chronic or recurrent OM in children is no longer recommended unless unusual circumstances exist.[2]
- Consultation with an otolaryngologist for tympanocentesis or drainage is necessary if no improvement with antibiotic therapy. If the tympanocentesis reveals multidrug-resistant bacteria, consultation with an infectious disease specialist is indicated.

COMPLICATIONS

Treatment decisions should be reconsidered if symptoms worsen or fail to respond to initial antibiotic treatment within 48 to 72 hours.[2,3,6]

The most common short-term consequence is decreased conductive hearing loss. MEE and chronic OME may last for months and can be a barrier to learning and language development in young children.[1-3]

Eardrum perforation is a common sequela of both AOM and OME. Hearing loss, perforation of the eardrum, cholesteatoma, acute mastoiditis, meningitis, and epidermal abscess are less common complications of OM, especially in developed countries. As noted, an additional concern is the consequence of antibiotic resistance. Antibiotic treatment of OME in the absence of bacterial infection is linked with growing drug resistance.[2,3]

INDICATIONS FOR REFERRAL OR HOSPITALIZATION

The patient with AOM who does not respond to therapy in 48 to 72 hours should be switched to an alternative therapy.

 Special referral is indicated for tympanocentesis for culture to determine antibiotic sensitivity for AOM that fails to resolve within 3 days of treatment with a second-line agent.[3] OME should be evaluated monthly for superimposed AOM with referral to ear, nose, and throat (ENT) specialist.[3]

 Speech and audiology evaluation for speech delay is indicated in younger children at 3 months for OME that fails to resolve and the potential need for ventilating tubes with or without adenoidectomy.[3]

 ENT referral for tympanostomy tubes is indicated for recurrent AOM (three episodes in 6 months or four or more episodes in 1 year with one episode in preceding 6 months).[2]

LIFE-SPAN CONSIDERATIONS

AOM is primarily a disease of young children. The incidence decreases quickly after age 7 years, when the Eustachian tube matures. In adults, AOM most often occurs in smokers and in adults who are exposed to second-hand smoke.[1]

PATIENT AND FAMILY EDUCATION

Education regarding OM risk reduction and treatment is focused most appropriately toward parents and caregivers when patients are younger.

- Treatment decisions should include the preferences of parents and caregivers regarding the prescription of antibiotics. The proposal of "watchful waiting" requires providers educate parents and caregivers about expected course of the condition. Parents need to be aware of both supportive management, such as pain management, and situations requiring upgrading to more aggressive intervention.
- Parental comfort with delaying antibiotic administration may be increased with provision of a written antibiotic prescription to be held while the child is under initial observation. Follow-up consultation initiated by the provider is critical to the decision to observe before antibiotic use. In addition, caregivers often require careful explanation about symptomatic treatment of OME and MEE, rather than antibiotic treatment in the absence of AOM.
- Parents also need to understand that antibiotic treatment alone does not necessarily relieve pain and sleeplessness. Pain relief measures are necessary whether or not the provider is waiting to initiate antibiotics.
- OM, including AOM and OME, is not contagious, allow children to return to day care or school once acute symptoms have resolved. All caregivers need to understand proper administration of antibiotics and management of pain and other symptoms. Teachers need to be aware of impaired hearing, which may continue for weeks or months after the acute infection stage.

Health Promotion

- For both children and adults: The risk of OM can be decreased by not smoking and by minimizing exposure to smoke. Smoking cessation should be encouraged in patients who smoke and in parents of children.
- For children: Breastfeeding for 3 months or more is associated with reduced incidence of AOM during the first year of life. Recurrent AOM in infants may increase with pacifier use after 6 months of age.

- In children, recent research indicates that the pneumococcal conjugate vaccine (PCV7) and influenza vaccine may have a protective effect.[1-3]

REFERENCES

1. Schilder, A. G. M., Arom, T., Bhutta, M. F., Casselbrant, M. L., Coates, H., Gisselsson-Solen, M., et al. (2017). Panel 7: Otitis media: treatment and complications. *Otolaryngology–Head and Neck Surgery: Official Journal of American Academy of Otolaryngology–Head and Neck Surgery, 156*(4S), S88–S105.
2. Lieberthal, A. S., Carroll, A. E., Chonmaitree, T., Ganiats, T. G., Hoberman, A., Jackson, M. A., et al. (2013). Clinical practice guideline. The diagnosis and management of acute otitis media. *Pediatrics, 131*, e964.
3. Rosenfeld, R. M., Shin, J. J., Schwartz, S. R., Coggins, R., Gagnon, L., Hackell, J. M., et al. (2016). Clinical practice guideline: Otitis media with effusion (update). *Otolaryngology–Head and Neck Surgery: Official Journal of American Academy of Otolaryngology–Head and Neck Surgery, 154*(1S), S1–S4. Retrieved from http://journals.sagepub.com/doi/pdf/10.1177/0194599815623467.
4. Shaikh, N., Hoberman, A., Paradise, J. L., Rockette, H. E., Kurs-Lasky, M., Colborn, D. K., et al. (2009). Responsiveness and construct validity of a symptom scale for acute otitis media. *The Pediatric Infectious Disease Journal, 28*(1), 9–12.
5. Sun, D., McCarthy, T. J., & Liberman, D. B. (2017). Cost effectiveness in watchful waiting in acute otitis media. *Pediatrics, 139.*
6. Lieberthal, A. S., Carroll, A. E., Chonmaitree, T., et al. (2014). Erratum. Clinical guideline: The diagnosis and management of acute otitis media. *Pediatrics, 133*(2), 346–347.
7. FDA Drug Safety Communication. FDA requires labeling changes for prescription opioid cough and cold medicines to limit their use to adults 18 years and older. Retrieved from https://www.fda.gov/Drugs/DrugSafety/ucm590435.htm. (Accessed 12 May 2018).
8. Limb, C. J., Sooy, F. A., Lustig, L. R., & Klein, J. O. (2018). Acute otitis media in adults. In D.G. Deschler (Ed.). UpToDate. Retrieved from https://www.uptodate.com/contents/acute-otitis-media-in-adults. (Accessed 11 May 2018).
9. Danishyar, A., & Ashurst, J. V. (2018). Otitis, media, acute. In *StatPearls [internet].* Treasure Island (FL): StatPearls Publishing. Retrieved from https://www.ncbi.nlm.nih.gov/books/NBK470332/. [Updated 2017 Nov 21]. Dosing for adults.
10. Klein, J. O., & Pelton, S. P. (2018). Acute otitis media in children. In M.S. Edwards & G.C. Isaacson (Ed.). UpToDate. Retrieved from https://www.uptodate.com/contents/search?search=otitis%20media%20children. (Accessed 12 May 2018).

CHAPTER **69**

TYMPANIC MEMBRANE PERFORATION

Leigh Dobbs

 Otolaryngologist referral is indicated for patients with significant vertigo, large or trauma-related perforations, subjective hearing loss after resolution of tympanic membrane (TM) perforation, or for TM ruptures with delayed healing.

DEFINITION AND EPIDEMIOLOGY

The tympanic membrane (TM) acts as a mechanical component in hearing process and separates the external and middle ear. A TM perforation is an opening in this otherwise intact membrane. TM perforations occur in all age groups, can be caused by a variety of conditions, and can result in conductive hearing loss.

PATHOPHYSIOLOGY

Perforation can be caused by a variety of traumatic, infectious, or neoplastic processes. The TM can be lacerated or perforated by foreign objects in the external canal (e.g., cotton swabs). Barotrauma, physical trauma, blast injury, or a fracture of the temporal skull can tear or perforate the TM. Occasionally the TM perforates with the pressure and inflammation of acute otitis media. Perforations often precede the development of a cholesteatoma.[1-4]

CLINICAL PRESENTATION AND PHYSICAL EXAMINATION

Hearing loss, a sensation of fullness or popping in the effected ear, tinnitus, and vertigo are common symptoms associated with tympanic perforation. If related to trauma, bleeding, hearing loss, and pain can be the chief complaints.[5] Frequently, TM perforations are discovered at the time of trauma, during the evaluation for middle ear infection, or associated with a cholesteatoma. Most patients with a traumatic perforation experience pain and some degree of hearing loss. In the case of infection, patients may report suppurative drainage or bleeding with or without a preceding history of pain.

The physical examination requires a thorough ear examination and an evaluation of hearing status. Patients with trauma-associated presentations should be assessed for possible skull fracture, facial nerve injury, and evidence of cerebrospinal fluid leakage from ear or nose.

DIAGNOSTICS

Infection-related tympanic membrane perforations often easily heal and specific diagnostics are not indicated. Diagnostic pneumatic otoscopy is indicated for a patient with large or trauma-related TM perforations and require referral to a healthcare provider (i.e., otolaryngologist) skilled in this procedure. Hearing loss assessment can be assessed in primary care with Weber and Rinne tests. An audiogram is helpful in evaluating the presence of extent of hearing impairment.

DIFFERENTIAL DIAGNOSIS

Primary differentials to consider are trauma, infection, or neoplasm.

INTERPROFESSIONAL COLLABORATIVE MANAGEMENT
Nonpharmacologic Management

Most TM perforations heal quickly and spontaneously unless they become secondarily infected or are very large. Some TM perforations will require surgical repair with a patch or graft. Patients should keep water out of the affected ear until the perforation has healed.

Pharmacologic Management

Antibiotic drops with low ototoxicity or systemic antibiotics are often necessary when infection is evident.[1] However, special consideration must be given to the individual with a known or suspected perforation of the TM or a history of tympanostomy tube placement, because topical antibiotics placed into the middle ear can cross the round window membrane and reach the inner ear. In animal studies, ototoxic antibiotics delivered into the middle ear space can consistently cause severe hearing loss and ototoxic injury to the organ of Corti. Although clinical experience suggests that hearing loss does not occur after a single short course of therapy in humans, prolonged or repetitive administration of topical drops has resulted in severe hearing loss.[3]

INDICATIONS FOR REFERRAL AND HOSPITALIZATION

A referral to an otolaryngologist is appropriate for large or trauma related perforations, patients reporting subjective hearing loss following the resolution of perforation, or for TM ruptures with delayed healing (i.e., 6 weeks or longer). Blast injuries have been shown to a cause inner ear trauma, as well as the obvious TM perforation, which can lead to profound hearing loss also requiring otolaryngology referral.[6] Patients with skull fractures should be evaluated in the emergency department and by an otolaryngologist to assess damage to inner ear structures.

COMPLICATIONS

A middle ear infection, cholesteatoma, and impaired hearing are potential complications of a TM perforation. The TM should heal quickly; thus routine follow-up should allow for evaluation and management of any complications, as well as timely referral to specialists when indicated.

PATIENT AND FAMILY EDUCATION

- Protect the TM while it heals.
- Prevent water from entering ear.
- Determine cause of perforation to avoid repeat TM injury.
- Stress importance of not inserting objects (e.g., cotton-tipped applicators) into ear canal.

REFERENCES

1. Lou, Z., Wang, Y., & Su, K. (2014). Comparison of the healing mechanisms of human dry and endogenous wet traumatic eardrum perforations. *European Archives of Oto-Rhino-Laryngology, 271*, 2153–2157.
2. Wohlgelernter, J., Gross, M., & Eliashar, R. (2007). Traumatic perforation of tympanic membrane by cotton tipped applicator. *The Journal of Trauma, 62*, 1061.
3. Rosenfeld, R. M., Schwartz, S. R., Cannon, C. R., Roland, P. S., Simon, G. R., Kumar, K. A., et al. (2014). Clinical practice guideline: Acute otitis externa. *Otolaryngology–Head and Neck Surgery: Official Journal of American Academy of Otolaryngology–Head and Neck Surgery, 150*(1S), S1–S24.
4. Hellstrom, S., et al. (2004). Tympanic membrane perforation. In C. Alper, C. Bluestone, & J. Dohar (Eds.), *Advanced therapy of otitis media*. Lewiston NY: BC Decker.
5. Hempel, J. M., Becker, A., Muller, J., Krause, E., Berghaus, A., & Braun, T. (2012). Traumatic tympanic membrane perforations: Clinical and audiometric findings in 198 patients. *Otology and Neurotology, 33*(8), 1357–1362.
6. Dougherty, A. L., MacGregor, A. J., Han, P. P., Viiree, E., Heltemes, K. H., & Galarneau, M. R. (2013). Blast-related ear injuries among U.S. military personnel. *Journal of Rehabilitation Research and Development, 50*(6), 893–904.

CHAPTER 70

CHRONIC NASAL CONGESTION AND DISCHARGE

Terry Mahan Buttaro

 Urgent otolaryngology consultation is indicated for patients with periorbital edema, diplopia, displaced globe, ophthalmoplegia, proptosis, reduced visual acuity, high fever, severe epistaxis, headache, or meningeal signs.

DEFINITION AND EPIDEMIOLOGY

Nasal congestion is often acute and related to an infectious process. Pregnant women, patients who overuse decongestants, and others will also present to primary care complaining of chronic nasal congestion and other dismaying symptoms that affect their quality of life. For some patients, however, symptoms of nasal congestion and discharge can be persistent and result in chronic rhinosinusitis (CRS). Affecting 1 out of 8 adults in this country, the costs of this disorder are significant, not only in terms of patient comfort, but when combined with the management costs of acute sinusitis, approach 11 billion dollars annually.[1] Rhinosinusitis differs from sinusitis in that sinusitis is most often associated with inflammation of the adjacent nasal mucosa while the characteristics that define rhinosinusitis are related to nasal cavity and paranasal sinus inflammation.[1]

Criteria for CRS diagnosis requires that patient symptoms are present 12 weeks or more and that two of the following symptoms are present: a diminished sense of smell, facial pain, nasal congestion, and mucopurulent drainage. Additional requirements for diagnosis of CRS include (1) confirmation of presence of edema or purulent mucous discharge in anterior ethmoid region or middle meatus, (2) nasal cavity or middle meatus polyps, and/or (3) radiographic documentation of paranasal sinuses inflammation.[1]

PATHOPHYSIOLOGY

There are main three variants of CRS: CRS with nasal polyposis, CRS without nasal polyposis, and allergic fungal rhinosinusitis. However, it is important to be aware that other serious inflammatory conditions (e.g., Churg-Straus vasculitis, granulomatosis with polyangiitis [GPA], or sarcoidosis) can affect the upper and lower respiratory tracts (in addition to patient organs, small arteries, and veins), and the illness presentation for these disorders can also be paranasal sinus pain and nasal discharge.

The complaint of nasal congestion is primarily the result of vascular changes and chronic inflammation in the nasal mucosa induced by a combination of immunologic, infectious, and/or environmental factors. Possible predisposing and associated factors for CRS include dysfunctional cilia as seen in smokers and those with cystic fibrosis, allergy, asthma, aspirin sensitivity, genetic factors, immunodeficiency, infection, and pregnancy. The pathophysiology and associated pathogens of the three variants differs, however. (For example, allergic fungal rhinosinusitis, a subcategory associated with CRS with nasal polyposis, is characterized by polyps, a type 1 sensitivity to fungi, and eosinophilic mucin.)[2]

CLINICAL PRESENTATION AND PHYSICAL EXAMINATION

CRS affects people of all ages, but those who are immunosuppressed are more at risk. The clinical presentation of CRS varies from patient to patient. Common complaints include cough, dental pain, facial discomfort, fatigue, fever, halitosis, headache, nasal blockage or discharge (anterior or posterior nasal drip), and reduction in or loss of smell. The symptoms can be chronic, worsening over time, and associated with asthma, allergic rhinitis, tonsillar hypertrophy, and recurrent otitis media.[3,4]

A detailed history is critical to the diagnosis. It is important to ask the patient about the onset and timing of symptoms, location of congestion on one side or both, and associated symptoms (e.g., rhinorrhea, sneezing, eye symptoms, itchiness, changes in smell, fever, purulent discharge, facial pressure, and snoring). Triggers such as pollutants, allergens, and occupational chemicals should be discerned as well as a history of allergies, asthma, aspirin sensitivity, acute sinusitis, nasal trauma, nasal surgery, nasal polyps, or a family history of seasonal or environmental allergies. A detailed medication history, smoking history, exposure to passive smoke, pollutants (recreational or workplace), and recreational drug use should also be elicited.

The physical examination in primary care is important but accurate diagnosis requires specialist consultation and diagnostic evaluation. The primary care examination should include observation for any asymmetry or deformity of the nasal structure. The patient should be asked to press on each nostril individually and breathe in to test for obstruction. Each nostril should be carefully inspected with an otoscope and wide speculum while applying gentle pressure to the tip of the nose with the examiner's thumb to widen the nostrils, and then inserting the lighted otoscope. The nasal mucous membranes are inspected for erythema, pallor, atrophy, edema, crusting, and discharge. The mucosa of the turbinates is often more erythematous in patients with chronic nasal congestion compared with the pale bluish hue or pallor seen in patients with allergic rhinitis. Any abnormalities, such as polyps, erosions, and septal deviations or perforations, should be noted and documented. A unilateral nasal polyp, especially if bleeding, heightens the suspicion for malignancy. The frontal and maxillary sinuses should also be palpated for pain.

DIAGNOSTICS
Initial Diagnostics

The clinical practice guideline for diagnosis of CRS indicates (1) the necessity of specialist consultation in diagnosing CRS, (2) the importance of distinguishing recurrent acute rhinosinusitis from CRS, and (3) aids in preventing over diagnosis and inappropriate treatment. Recommended diagnostics are concerned with objective confirmation of CRS via nasal endoscopy by an otolaryngology specialist (guideline recommendation), as well as possible surgery or sinus CT scan.[1] Anterior rhinoscopy is an additional option though also less specific.[1]

Additional Diagnostics

- Concerns for an acute infectious process warrant a complete blood count. A CRP and ESR suggest inflammation, though are not diagnostic. A chemistry profile can be beneficial in determining other organ involvement that could suggest more systemic disease.
- Skin and in vitro tests for allergen-specific immunoglobulin E may be helpful in determining whether the symptoms are related to allergic or nonallergic disease.
- For suspected immunodeficiency disorders, serum IgA, IgM, and IgG are indicated.
- Antineutrophil cytoplasmic antibodies (ANCA) with immunofluorescence and ELISA are recommended if a vasculitis or granulomatous disorder is suspected.
- Serum angiotensin converting enzyme (ACE) aids in determining the possibility of sarcoidosis, though ACE levels are elevated in other diseases (e.g., amyloidosis) as well.
- An MRI maybe indicated if CT scan suggests malignancy.

INITIAL DIAGNOSTICS
Chronic Rhinosinusitis
• Nasal endoscopy by otolaryngologist (Clinical Practice Guideline)[1]
• Sinus CT
• Anterior rhinoscopy[a]
ADDITIONAL
• CBC/differential[a]
• Chemistry profile[a]
• ESR,[a] CRP[a]
• MRI[a]
• Antineutrophil cytoplasmic antibodies[a]
• Angiotensin converting enzyme[a]

[a]If indicated.

DIFFERENTIAL DIAGNOSIS

 Primary differentials include vasculitides (e.g., GPA [Wegener], eosinophilic GPA [Churg-Strauss]), sinonasal sarcoidosis, allergic fungal rhinosinusitis, and suspected malignancy.[5]

Additional differential diagnoses for CRS include allergic, nonallergic, eosinophilic nonallergic, and vasomotor rhinitis,

as well as nonrhinogenic causes of facial discomfort. Mechanical obstruction (e.g., nasal septal deformity, polyps, or tumor), infection, pregnancy, rhinitis medicamentosa, sinusitis, and substance use disorder (e.g., cocaine) are further considerations. Headaches or other causes of facial pain are also possible causes of the patient's symptoms.

INTERPROFESSIONAL COLLABORATIVE MANAGEMENT

 Urgent otolaryngology consultation is indicated for patients with allergic fungal rhinosinusitis, GPA or microscopic polyangiitis (MPA), suspected malignancy, red flags, warning signs of complications, and severe illness.

- Referral to an otolaryngology specialist is indicated for nasal endoscopy to determine diagnosis and appropriate treatment and in the following instances:
  - Patients with severe congestion refractory to treatment after 4 weeks of intranasal corticosteroids and saline lavage
  - Foreign body removal or suspected nasal polyp or tumor

Pharmacologic Management

The goal of management for CRS is symptom control of inflammation and reduction of infectious exacerbations.

- Saline irrigations and intranasal corticosteroids can be helpful for patients who complain of nasal congestion.
- Daily saline irrigations and intranasal corticosteroids are the mainstay of treatment to minimize and control inflammation in CRS with and without nasal polyps; however, topical steroids may be less effective in patients who have CRS without nasal polyps.[4,6]
- For patients who present with nasal congestion associated with acute bacterial rhinosinusitis *without* complications, "watchful waiting" before treating with antibiotic therapy is advised, as symptoms can resolve within a few days.[1] Treatment does depend on the patient presentation, however.
- Allergic fungal rhinosinusitis is primarily treated surgically and with steroids by the otolaryngology specialists. In general, topical or systemic antifungal therapy for patients with CRS should not be prescribed, as efficacy is undetermined.[1] Immunotherapy and leukotriene modulators are possible considerations, though more research is needed to assess benefit.[2] Oral steroids are used in some situations, but long-term use is concerning because of the associated risks.
- For CRP with nasal polyps, sinus surgery to remove polyps can be helpful for some patients, but recurrent polyps are possible. Newer therapies (e.g., biodegradable eluting stents and anti-IgE anti monoclonal antibodies) are under investigation.[4]
- Antibiotics may be a consideration if an exacerbation of CRS results in acute rhinosinusitis.[6-8]
- Referral to an otolaryngologist is necessary for patients with severe congestion refractory to treatment.[7]
- Nasal congestion associated with pregnancy will resolve after delivery. Use of saline lavage for symptomatic relief is recommended. Intranasal corticosteroid use during pregnancy is labeled Category C.
- Patients with rebound nasal congestion related to topical decongestant use will have resolution 2 to 3 weeks after the offending medication is stopped.

LIFE-SPAN CONSIDERATIONS

CRS affects patients of all ages and is often overlooked in primary care practice. Symptoms may lead to chronic cough, malodorous breath, poor appetite, interrupted sleep, and a diminished quality of life.

COMPLICATIONS

Complications depend on the cause: ulcerations, infections, septal perforation, and diminished quality of life may occur if the underlying etiology of the patient's symptoms is not identified and correctly treated. Nasal inhalation of cocaine is associated with nasal bleeding, nasal congestion, rhinitis, and deviated or perforated septum.

PATIENT AND FAMILY EDUCATION AND HEALTH PROMOTION

All patients should be educated about the risks associated with decongestant use, cocaine, and chronic exposure to irritants and allergens. In addition, patients should be instructed in the proper use of saline irrigations and nasal sprays and advised that the effect of nasal corticosteroids may not be noticed for several days to weeks. Counseling should include information that this may be a lifelong condition that will require chronic management.

Pregnant patients with rhinosinusitis should be counseled in symptom management and offered reassurance that the condition will most likely resolve after delivery.

REFERENCES

1. Rosenfeld, R. M., Piccirillo, J. F., Sujana, S., Chandrasehar, M. D., et al. (2015). Clinical practice guideline (update): Adult sinusitis. *Otolaryngology–Head and Neck Surgery: Official Journal of American Academy of Otolaryngology–Head and Neck Surgery, 152*(2), S1–S39.
2. Gan, E. C., Thamboo, A., Rudmik, L., Hwang, P. H., Ferguson, B. J., & Javer, A. R. (2014). Medical management of allergic fungal rhinosinusitis following endoscopic sinus surgery: An evidence-based review and recommendations. *International Forum of Allergy & Rhinology, 4,* 702–715.
3. Cho, S. H., Kim, D. W., & Gevaert, P. (2016). Chronic rhinosinusitis without nasal polyps. *The Journal of Allergy and Clinical Immunology. In Practice, 4*(4), 575–582. http://doi.org/10.1016/j.jaip.2016.04.015///.
4. Stevens, W. W., Schleimer, R. P., & Kern, R. C. (2016). Chronic rhinosinusitis with nasal polyps. *The Journal of Allergy and Clinical Immunology. In Practice, 4*(4), 565–572. http://doi.org/10.1016/j.jaip.2016.04.012.
5. Kirsten, A. M., Watz, H., & Kirsten, D. (2013). Sarcoidosis with involvement of the paranasal sinuses—a retrospective analysis of 12 biopsy-proven cases. *BMC Pulmonary Medicine, 13,* 59. http://doi.org/10.1186/1471-2466-13-59.
6. Wei, C. C., Adappa, N. D., & Cohen, N. A. (2013). Use of topical nasal therapies in the management of chronic rhinosinusitis. *The Laryngoscope, 123*(10), 2347–2359. http://dx.doi.org/10.1002/lary.24066.
7. Sedaghat, A. M. (2017). Chronic rhinosinusitis. *American Family Physician, 95*(8), 500–506.
8. Barshak, M. B., & Durand, M. L. (2017). The role of infection and antibiotics in chronic rhinosinusitis. *Laryngoscope Investigative Otolaryngology, 2*(1), 36–42. doi:10.1002/lio2.61.

CHAPTER **71**

EPISTAXIS

Emily Karwacki Sheff • Sara Smoller • Catherine Franklin • Jason R. Lucey • Patrice K. Nicholas • Linda Evans

 Immediate referral is indicated for patients if there is extensive bleeding or for a posterior epistaxis.

DEFINITION AND EPIDEMIOLOGY

Epistaxis (nosebleed) is a common problem experienced by most individuals at some time in their lives. Epistaxis occurs in 60% of the population and is the second most common reason for emergency admission to otolaryngology services.[1] The incidence is highest in individuals younger than 10 years of age and in individuals over the age of 40. Most nosebleeds are idiopathic.[2] Some individuals are more prone to nosebleeds because of fragile mucous membranes. Local predisposing factors include nasal trauma, rhinitis, drying of the nasal mucosa from low humidity, nasal septum deviation, alcohol use, and chemical irritants (e.g., cocaine). Systemic conditions from either genetic or acquired coagulation disorders, hematologic cancers, and anticoagulation medication can cause epistaxis.[1] Herbal supplements can inhibit platelet aggregation, causing adverse effects with other prescribed medications.

PATHOPHYSIOLOGY

Bleeding can occur from the anterior or posterior naris. Between 90% and 95% of nosebleeds occur within the Kiesselbach plexus, a vascular plexus on the anterior nasal septum, and are associated with irritated mucous membranes or trauma.[2] This plexus is particularly vulnerable and easily injured. Posterior nosebleeds occur within the posterior branches of the sphenopalatine artery and account for approximately 5% of cases. In general, these nosebleeds are idiopathic or associated with vascular disease and can be difficult to control.[1] Studies have not found an association between hypertension and epistaxis, although there may be an elevated risk with potentially greater difficulty to control due to vascular changes.[3-5]

CLINICAL PRESENTATION AND PHYSICAL EXAMINATION

Patients with epistaxis initially are seen with scant to copious amounts of blood emerging from the nares. Anterior nosebleeds are usually unilateral with continuous moderate bleeding. Depending on the amount of bleeding, small clots may also emerge. Patients may report that the bleeding began spontaneously or that nasal trauma preceded the bleeding. Posterior nosebleeds can occur bilaterally, are associated with severe bleeding, and are difficult to treat. Bleeding into the pharynx is indicative of a posterior epistaxis. If the patient's condition is stable, the provider should obtain a thorough health history regarding frequency, duration, trauma, nasal obstruction, and prior treatments. It is important to inquire about other systemic conditions, prescribed and complementary alternative medications, intranasal substances, and clotting disorders in order to establish the causative factors and initiate care.[1]

Vital signs and airway safety should first be determined, and the patient should be instructed to sit up straight, tilt the head forward, and apply firm, continuous pressure for 15 minutes to the anterior aspect of the affected nostril.[1] The provider should assess for blood loss and risk for hemodynamic instability. If the epistaxis is the result of trauma, the nose should be checked for fractures. An internal examination may be deferred until the blood flow has subsided, but if the bleeding does not readily subside or nasal compression causes postnasal bleeding, the nose should be examined with a nasal speculum. The blood is cleared with suction or nose blowing to identify the site of bleeding. Topical vasoconstrictive agents such as 1 : 1000 epinephrine or 4% cocaine, applied either as a spray or on a cotton pledget, serves as both an anesthetic and a vasoconstricting agent. If this preparation is not available, a topical decongestant (e.g., oxymetazoline) can be used in conjunction with a topical anesthetic (e.g., lidocaine) to examine the nose.[1,6] The nose should be inspected to identify the bleeding site before further treatment is initiated. If the site cannot be identified, the posterior pharynx is inspected for any bleeding. Rinsing the oropharynx first with water will clear the area to permit identification of any new bleeding.[6]

DIAGNOSTICS
Essential Diagnostics

A complete blood count (CBC) with a type and screen/crossmatch should be obtained if severe bleeding has occurred. A prothrombin time (PT) and international normalized ratio (INR) should be obtained if the patient is taking an anticoagulant. Additional laboratory studies should be performed if the patient is hemodynamically unstable.[1]

Additional Diagnostics

It is important to consider any underlying condition that may have caused the epistaxis. Laboratory assessment of bleeding parameters may be necessary to exclude underlying disease, especially if the bleeding recurs without a clinical explanation.

INITIAL DIAGNOSTICS

Epistaxis

LABORATORY
- CBC and differential (if infection or extensive blood loss is present)
- Coagulation studies (in patients who are on anticoagulation medications)[a]
- Type and screen/crossmatch (with extensive blood loss)[a]
- Basic metabolic panel (if hemodynamically unstable)

---

[a]If indicated.

DIFFERENTIAL DIAGNOSIS

 Priority differentials include: (1) hypertension, (2) use of anticoagulants or antiplatelets such as warfarin or aspirin,[4] (3) use of nasal steroids and/or allergic rhinitis, (4) cocaine use, and (5) the presence of a neoplasm.[2]

Sudden epistaxis demands conscientious consideration. Although nasal trauma is the most common cause of nasal bleeding, it is critical to recognize other conditions that may result in bleeding from the nose. Other causes of recurrent epistaxis, such as systemic factors (e.g., hemophilia, von Willebrand disease, hereditary hemorrhagic telangiectasia [Osler-Weber-Rendu disease], thrombocytopenia, or tumor), chemical irritants, or warfarin toxicity should be considered.[1]

INTERPROFESSIONAL COLLABORATIVE MANAGEMENT
Anterior Epistaxis

Nonpharmacologic Management. Most cases of epistaxis can be successfully treated with the application of direct pressure to the anterior portion of the nose for 15 minutes. This technique is often successful because the most common source of epistaxis is the anterior part of the septum, where the Kiesselbach plexus is located. The patient should also be encouraged to sit upright because venous pressure is reduced in this position. The patient should also lean forward to decrease the swallowing of blood.[6]

If the bleeding continues, nasal packing may be used.[4] It is important to insert the packing properly in the nares to reduce bleeding. Two types of packing are commonly used. Merocel is a nasal polyhydroxylated polyvinyl tampon that expands when moistened.[4] Rapid Rhino uses a coated inflatable balloon to increase the pressure and is effective as a platelet aggregator.[3,6] There should be minimal packing visible at the nares if placed appropriately. The packing strings or balloon should be taped to the face to avoid displacement.[3] Once it is in place, the pack is not removed for 24 to 48 hours.[1] If the bleeding continues, the opposite nostril should be packed in a similar fashion to increase nasal pressure. After insertion of the nasal pack, the patient must be observed for 30 minutes to determine that there is no posterior bleeding. Once there is evidence of no bleeding, the patient may be discharged home.

Pharmacologic Management

Vasoconstrictors. Depending on the amount of bleeding, short-acting topical nasal decongestants (e.g., phenylephrine 0.125% to 1% solution, one or two sprays), which act as vasoconstrictors, may help stop the blood flow. One retrospective study reported that 65% of patients seen in the emergency department with epistaxis were successfully treated with oxymetazoline and nasal pressure.[1] Of note, topical phenylephrine is NOT recommended for use.[7]

Cautery. Once the bleeding site has been identified, the area can be treated with chemical cautery (silver nitrate) or electrocautery.[1,4,6] After the bleeding has stopped, a small amount of petroleum is applied in the nares and the patient is observed for 30 minutes.

Antibiotics. It is important to note that there are not any studies to support the use of antibiotics to prevent infection and many providers opt not to treat anterior nasal bleeds with a prophylactic antibiotic. However, individualized patient care is key, as patients with an increased risk of infection (e.g., older adults or those who are immunocompromised) may benefit from an antibiotic being prescribed.[8] In some cases, prophylactic antibiotics such as cephalexin (250 mg) 4 times daily or amoxicillin-clavulanate (875 mg/125 mg every 12 hours) may be indicated when nasal packing is used, to prevent infection.[1]

Consultations: Emergency Department (Posterior Epistaxis). Continued bleeding suggests that there is a posterior bleed and requires specialist consultation and possible hospitalization. Depending on the ability to access the site or control the bleeding, extensive packing may be required and not all healthcare providers or office settings are equipped to manage acute epistasis. If the bleeding cannot be managed within 15 minutes, patients should be transferred to an emergency department. The packing should be done in an emergency department, operating room or specialist's office because of discomfort and risk of hypoxia.

Surgical intervention may be necessary if medical measures are not sufficient to eliminate epistaxis. In this case, posterior packs with a balloon catheter (Epistat) provide bidirectional pressure to control the bleeding until the patient can be brought to surgery.[6] Nasal endoscopy is performed to visualize the bleeding site.[1] Surgical techniques such as arterial ligation or vascular embolization may be considered by an otolaryngologist. This technique is certainly necessary when the bleeding becomes life-threatening and other treatments have failed.

Epistaxis management is variable, but one study found that chemical cautery was most effective for initial treatment whereas direct vascular control (e.g., ligation, embolization) managed recurrent epistaxis.[1]

Consultation: Otolaryngologist. A nasal obstruction may require endoscopy or imaging studies by an otolaryngologist.

COMPLICATIONS

Complications are rare because most nosebleeds are easily controlled. However, respiratory function can be compromised, and patients may become hypotensive or anemic if bleeding is severe. Other complications are usually related to treatment and include necrosis, abscess formation, septal perforation, and sinus infection.[1] Toxic shock syndrome has also been reported as a complication of nasal packing; thus, appropriate antibiotic therapy may be prescribed at the discretion of the provider while the packing is in place.[1] Posterior packing can cause a vagal response resulting in hypotension and bradycardia.[1] One study showed that patients who undergo embolization are at higher risk for a stroke compared with a nasal packing procedure.[2] This may be related to comorbid conditions rather than to complications from the procedure.

EMERGING MANAGEMENT TRENDS

Treatment for epistaxis remains highly variable.[4] Topical tranexamic acid, an antifibrinolytic agent, has been increasingly studied for its use and outcomes in uncomplicated epistaxis patients, and research has shown promising results.[9,10] However, more studies must be done to fully evaluate its role in treatment plans.

PATIENT AND FAMILY EDUCATION AND HEALTH PROMOTION

Once the bleeding has stopped, the patient is advised to avoid vigorous exercise and aspirin-containing medications for several days or weeks. The patient and family should also understand the importance of calling the health care provider if the bleeding recurs (particularly while packing is in place) and recognize the necessity of follow-up evaluation within 48 to 72 hours to ensure healing of the lesion.

Avoidance of tobacco and hot, spicy foods is also advisable because they may cause vasodilation. Avoidance of nasal trauma, including digital self-trauma, is an obvious necessity. Lubrication of the mucous membranes with petroleum jelly, nasal saline, or bacitracin ointment may relieve nasal discomfort and reduce the need to manipulate the nasal passages.[1] Home humidification may also prevent the nasal irritation that results from a dry environment. Patients should also understand how to treat nosebleeds at home by applying firm pressure to the nostrils for 10 to 30 minutes.

REFERENCES

1. Simmen, D. B., et al. (2015). Epistaxis. In P. W. Flint, et al. (Eds.), *Cummings otolaryngology* (6th ed., pp. 678–690). Philadelphia, PA: Sunders.
2. Pinder, & Epistaxis, D. (2019). BMJ Best Practice. Retrieved from http://bestpractice.bmj.com/topics/en-gb/421.
3. Kao, H. (2016). Control of facial hemmorhage. In D. Kademani & P. S. Tiwana (Eds.), *Atlas of Oral and Maxillofacial Surgery* (pp. 654–661). St.Louis: Saunders.
4. Newton, E., Lasso, A., Petrcich, W., & Kilty, S. J. (2016). An outcomes analysis of anterior epistaxis management in the emergency department. *Journal of Otolaryngology-Head and Neck Surgery. 45*, 24.
5. Sarhan, N. A., & Algamal, A. M. (2015). Relationship between epistaxis and hypertension: A cause and effect or coincidence? *Journal of the Saudi Heart Association, 27*, 79–84.
6. Kumar, S. (2015). Ears, nose and throat emergencies. In P. Cameron, et al. (Eds.), *Textbook of adult emergency medicine* (4th ed., Vol. 18, pp. 620–625). Philadelphia: Elsevier.
7. Groudine, S. B., Hollinger, I., Jones, J., & DeBouno, B. A. (2000). New York State guidelines on the topical use of phenylephrine in the operating room. The Phenylephrine Advisory Committee. *Anesthesiology, 92*, 859.
8. Lange, J. L., Peeden, E. H., & Stringer, S. P. (2017). Are prophylactic systemic antibiotics necessary with nasal packing? A systematic review. *American Journal of Rhinology & Allergy, 31*(4), 240–247. https://doi.org/10.2500/ajra.2017.31.4454.
9. Logan, J. K., & Pantle, H. (2016). Role of tranexamic acid in the management of idiopathic anterior epistaxis in adult patients in the emergency department. *American Journal of Health-System Pharmacy, 73*(21), 1755–1759.
10. Kamhieh, Y., & Fox, H. (2016). Transexamic acid in epistaxis: A systematic review. *Clinical Otolaryngology, 41*(6), 771–776.

CHAPTER 72

NASAL TRAUMA

Sara Smoller • Jason R. Lucey • Catherine Franklin • Emily Karwacki Sheff • Patrice K. Nicholas • Linda Evans

 Immediate emergency department referral is indicated for nasal trauma associated with airway compromise, evidence of intracranial injury, uncontrollable bleeding, leaking cerebrospinal fluid (CSF), or suspicion for cervical spine injury.

DEFINITION AND EPIDEMIOLOGY

Nasal injuries are important not only because they may be associated with critical life-threatening complications, but also because of the potential for long-term cosmetic disfigurement, which can lead to poor social and psychological outcomes for patients.[1] Nasal trauma occurs with high frequency owing to the prominence of the nose on the face and the relative fragility of the nasal bones compared with other facial bone structures.[1] The nasal bones are fractured more often than other facial bones, and these injuries occur more than twice as often in men as in women.[2]

PATHOPHYSIOLOGY

Nasal trauma is the result of a severe blow to the face. In adults, most facial blows are related to automobile accidents, sports injuries, falls, or altercations.[2,3] Because facial anatomy is complex, injuries to the nose and face can involve damage to skin, mucous membranes, muscle, nerve, bone, cartilage, and vascular structures, thus often requiring emergency room evaluation.[1,2]

CLINICAL PRESENTATION AND PHYSICAL EXAMINATION

The mechanism of injury and the patient's past medical history, allergies, and current medications should be discerned. Distinguishing between an isolated nasal injury and one that is associated with other conditions such as concussion, facial or orbital injury, or cervical spine injury is of utmost importance. Questions about loss of consciousness, headache, nausea and vomiting, diplopia, visual changes, facial numbness, prior nasal injury or surgery, and malocclusion or other dental injury should be asked.[2,3] Interviewing a witness to the injury other than the patient may be helpful to describe the patient's behavior and appearance immediately after the injury occurred. Specific history questions related to nasal injuries might include the following: Can you breathe through both of your nostrils? Did you have any bleeding from the nostrils (one or both), and how long did it last? Have you ever had a broken nose or nasal surgery before? Have you noticed any change in your sense of smell?[2]

The physical examination requires that the health care provider determine the presence of periorbital ecchymosis, edema, abrasions or lacerations, epistaxis, or CSF leakage (clear or blood-tinged liquid); trauma to the teeth, neck, or chest; and any obvious deformity. Inspection from multiple perspectives (e.g., frontal, worm's eye, and bird's eye views) can help identify subtle abnormalities.[2,3] Respiratory and cervical spine stability and vital signs should be assessed. Assessing patency of airflow through the nostrils can help determine the presence of potential obstruction caused by deviation of a fractured septum, soft tissue edema, or a potential septal hematoma.[1]

The dorsum (bridge) of the nose should be gently palpated for deformity, instability, crepitus, and point tenderness. It is also important to assess for a palpable step-off of the infraorbital rim; this indicates a zygomatic complex fracture.[1] If orbital involvement is suspected, a detailed examination should include assessment of extraocular muscle (EOM) function looking for diplopia on upward gaze caused by entrapment of the inferior rectus muscle, as well as investigation for facial anesthesia secondary to infraorbital nerve injury.[1] Stability of the teeth and palate should also be evaluated.

Intranasal examination with adequate lighting and use of a nasal speculum (if available) is conducted to visualize the internal nasal structures including the mucosa, septum, and turbinates, and to rule out septal hematoma and CSF leakage.[2,5] Septal fracture, displacement or deviation, or laceration should also be noted.[2] Septal hematomas will appear as a rounded bluish or purplish mass against the nasal septum and requires urgent drainage to prevent cosmetic long-term complications.[1] Presence of clear fluid in the nasal cavity is concerning for CSF leakage and requires immediate emergency referral.[5] If bleeding is active, a combination of direct pressure, topical vasoconstrictors, or nasal packing should be used as needed to aide in visualization and to help control bleeding.[1,2]

DIAGNOSTICS
Essential Diagnostics

Choice of imaging techniques for a nasal injury is influenced by the associated findings and mechanism of injury. For injuries in which there is suspicion of intracranial involvement or facial skull fracture (e.g., CSF rhinorrhea; orbital or facial or

sinus step-off; EOM palsy; or high-speed mechanism), computed tomography (CT) scan is the preferred modality.[1,3] For isolated nasal bone injuries, plain X-ray examination may confirm the findings from the physical examination; however, X-ray studies of the nasal bones seldom provide additional information and are not recommended unless there is suspicion of extensive trauma that extends beyond a simple nasal fracture.[1,2] Deferring initial X-ray examination of nasal bones is appropriate and will not influence the plan of care if tenderness and swelling are isolated to the nasal bridge; if both nares are patent; if there is no significant deformity or angulation seen; and if no septal hematoma is present.[1]

INITIAL DIAGNOSTICS

Nasal Trauma

IMAGING
- Computed tomography scan
- X-ray study
- High-resolution ultrasound

Additional Diagnostics

Another less widely available imaging option for nasal and facial injuries is high-resolution ultrasonography, which has been shown to be both sensitive and specific in identifying nasal fractures.[2]

DIFFERENTIAL DIAGNOSIS

 Priority differentials include (1) concussion, (2) septal hematomas, (3) zygomatic arch fractures, (4) maxillary sinus fractures, and (5) orbital fractures.

The differential diagnosis of nasal trauma is based on the force of the trauma, with higher-speed mechanisms being more concerning for potentially life-threatening or disfiguring injury. Frontal sinus fractures result from trauma to the forehead and, because of the location, may initially be seen as a nasal fracture. Brisk hemorrhage from the nasal cavity accompanies these fractures. Fractures of the posterior wall of the frontal sinus may cause dural tears and leakage of CSF into the nasal cavity.

INTERPROFESSIONAL COLLABORATIVE MANAGEMENT

Initial treatment consists of cool, local pressure to the affected areas to decrease edema and bleeding. A nasal fracture without deformity or septal hematoma may be treated with ice, head elevation, and analgesia (e.g., acetaminophen), with close otolaryngology follow-up in 3 to 5 days for reevaluation once swelling has subsided.[1] Ideally, a displaced fracture would be manually reduced under general or local anesthesia in the initial postinjury hours by a trained provider or otolaryngologist, but many specialists prefer to allow initial swelling to subside in the first 3 to 5 days after injury before manipulation.[1,3] Closed nasal fracture reduction in children should be performed within the first several days after injury given children's tendency to heal more quickly than adults. Open reduction is not recommended in children and, if required, is delayed until nasal growth is complete.[5]

Recommendations vary around the use of antibiotics for patients undergoing open or closed fracture repair or for injuries in which nasal packing is used (e.g., incision and drainage of septal hematoma).[1,4,8] Patients with severe facial/nasal trauma or open fractures warrant antibiotic prophylaxis.[1] Assessment of tetanus vaccination status and appropriate prophylaxis are indicated for any nasal injury with a wound.[1]

CONSULTATIONS

In primary care practice, nasal injuries are frequently referred to otolaryngology for follow-up within the first week of the injury. After swelling has subsided (usually after 3 to 5 days), a more detailed examination for airflow obstruction deformity can be performed, and, if necessary, reduction and manipulation of the fracture can be done with the appropriate anesthesia. Again, any suspicion of leaking CSF or other more complex skull or facial fractures mandates more immediate referral to the emergency department or specialist.

LIFE-SPAN CONSIDERATIONS

Pediatric

Fractures of the nasal bones in infants and very young children are not as common as in older children and adolescents.[3] Nasal skeletal structure in early childhood is mostly composed of cartilage and, in general, infants and younger children are engaged in activities with lower risk of high-impact trauma compared with older children and teens. As with any injury in pediatric patients, the clinician should include abuse in the differential diagnosis and involve social services or legal authorities as mandated by reporting laws if the situation warrants it.[3]

Geriatric

Falls and associated trauma are a significant, common, and potentially life-threatening problem in older adults.[6] The clinician should include a general assessment of fall risk in the evaluation of any older adult patient with nasal trauma. The cause of a fall should be investigated and other comorbid conditions leading to the fall should be considered. Risk factors for falls include, but are not limited to, neurologic diseases, syncope, polypharmacy, and visual imparment.[6]

Severe complications of head trauma (even with fairly minor mechanisms such as a fall from a standing position) in older patients, such as intracranial bleeding, may occur without overt neurologic deficits on initial examination.[7] The clinician should have a low threshold for referring older adult patients who have fallen to the emergency department for further evaluation, appropriate imaging, and access to specialty care.[7]

COMPLICATIONS

Nasal trauma may result in a nasal septal hematoma that separates the septal cartilage from the adherent mucoperichondrium, which supplies the septum with nutrition.[8] A hematoma that remains untreated can result in septal cartilage necrosis due to an inadequate blood supply.[8] This loss of nasal cartilage can result in many complications, including: saddle nose deformity, septal perforation, and septal abscess.[2,8] Treatment of a septal hematoma requires urgent surgical incision, drainage, and packing by a trained provider (emergency department or otolaryngologist).[2]

Nasal septum deviations and fractures are often a complication of nasal trauma.[8] The deviation may cause varying degrees of nasal obstruction and predispose the patient to sinusitis and epistaxis.[2] This is a result of the blockage of mucociliary clearance.[2] Septal ulcers and perforations may occur after repeated trauma and even constant nose picking. In addition, nasal foreign bodies may mimic nasal trauma or fracture; this may occur as a result of trauma to the face in adults or introduction of a foreign body in the nasal cavity in the pediatric population.[9]

PATIENT AND FAMILY EDUCATION

The patient should understand the signs and symptoms of complications and who to call if problems develop. In particular, the patient should return for evaluation if the pain becomes intense, if bleeding is profuse, and if nasal discharge becomes purulent with a foul odor.[8] Signs and symptoms of worsening intracranial injury (e.g., headache, confusion, vomiting, vision changes) should be reviewed, and the patient instructed to seek emergency care if they develop.[3] If nasal packing (for epistaxis or septal hematoma drainage) has been placed, the patient should understand the importance of prompt scheduled follow-up for its removal.[3] Routine risks and benefits of any analgesics or antibiotics should be reviewed. Ice application and elevation of the head of the bed for sleeping may provide comfort and control soft-tissue swelling. The patient should avoid any nose touching or picking, increase the degree of humidified air at home, and increase fluid intake. The dressings should not get wet, and swimming is not allowed until dressings are removed and wounds adequately healed.[2] Nose blowing should be avoided during the recovery period.[2] Lastly, prevention of sports-related nasal injuries should be encouraged through counseling on the use of protective headgear, including face shields available for many sports.[4]

REFERENCES

1. Mayersak, R. J. (2018). Facial trauma In R. M. Walls, R. S. Hockberger, & M. Gausche-Hill (Eds.), *Rosen's emergency medicine* (9th ed., pp. 330–334). Philadelphia: Saunders/Elsevier.
2. Chegar, B. E., & Tatum, S. A. (2015). Nasal fractures. In P. W. Flint, B. H. Haughey, K. T. Robbins, J. R. Thomas, J. K. Niparko, V. J. Lund, et al. (Eds.), *Cummings otolaryngology-head and neck surgery* (6th ed., pp. 493–505). Philadelphia: Saunders/Elsevier.
3. Aronovich, S., & Costello, B. J. (2013). Nasal fractures. In R. J. Fonseca (Ed.), *Oral and maxillofacial trauma* (4th ed., pp. 491–505). St. Louis: Saunders/Elsevier.
4. Rodriguez, K. D. (2018). Nasal fracture. In E. N. Meyers & C. H. Snyderman (Eds.), *Operative otolarynology head and neck surgery* (3rd ed., pp. 1287–1291). Elsevier.
5. O'Handley, J. G., Tobin, E. J., & Shah, A. R. (2016). Otorhinolaryngology. In R. E. Rakel & D. Rakel (Eds.), *Textbook of family medicine* (9th ed., p. 311). Philadelphia: Elsevier.
6. Berry, S. D., & Kiel, D. P. (2016). Falls. In B. Resnick (Ed.), *Geriatric nursing review syllabus: A core curriculum in advanced practice geriatric nursing* (5th ed., pp. 259–267). New York: American Geriatric Society.
7. Hogan, T. M., & Rios-Alba, T. (2014). Emergency care. In R. J. Ham, P. D. Sloane, G. A. Warshaw, J. F. Potter, & E. Flaherty (Eds.), *Ham's primary care geriatrics* (6th ed., pp. 177–192). Philadelphia: Saunders/Elsevier.
8. Marston, A. P., O'Brien, E. K., & Hamilton, G. S. (2017). Nasal injuries in sports. *Clinics in Sports Medicine, 36*(2), 337–353.
9. Simmen, D. B., et al. (2015). Epistaxis. In P. W. Flint, et al. (Eds.), *Cummings otolaryngology* (6th ed., pp. 678–690). Philadelphia, PA: Saunders.

CHAPTER **73**

RHINITIS

Pamela Sue Porter

 Red flags include recurrent epistaxis or sinusitis, pulmonary involvement, visual changes, unilateral symptoms, hilar adenopathy.[1]

Rhinitis, an inflammation of the sinus nasal cavity, can be caused by various exposures that trigger the body's response to remove the foreign material from the nasal cavity. Exposure to viruses, outdoor and indoor allergens, and occupational irritants can cause irritation to the epithelial lining of the nasal cavity. The result is increased congestion and nasal secretion related to mucosal and membrane swelling.

DEFINITION AND EPIDEMIOLOGY

Allergic rhinitis (also known as allergic rhinosinusitis or AR) is a heterogeneous, inflammatory response affecting the paranasal and sinus mucosa. AR is characterized by sneezing, rhinorrhea, mucosal swelling, obstruction, conjunctivitis, and nasal-ocular and pharyngeal itching in response to an allergen exposure.[2] The membranes typically have a pale, violaceous color and are edematous (boggy). In more severe cases, systemic symptoms of fatigue, headache, and cognitive impairment may be present. This disorder is caused by an immunoglobulin E (IgE)–mediated[1] mast cell hypersensitivity response to foreign allergens and can affect individuals in any age group; patients with atopy are particularly susceptible.[2] The symptoms are reversible with avoidance of the specific allergens, pharmacotherapy, targeted treatment, and immunotherapy. Symptoms may also spontaneously resolve as the body adapts or is desensitized.

The hallmark of AR is the temporal correlation of symptoms with exposure to indoor or outdoor allergens, and time of year. Seasonal allergies occur in relation to seasonal exposures (e.g., pollens, trees and flowers in the spring, grasses in the summer, ragweed in the fall). Perennial AR is associated with indoor exposures to environmental antigens (e.g., animal dander, dust mites, foods, insect stings, cockroach droppings, mold spores, and chemicals) in the patient's living area and possibly from new medications.

The prevalence of AR varies by location and depends on the type and quantity of airborne allergens. Recent estimates state that up to 14% of adult Americans experience AR, although that number may in fact be higher.[3]

PATHOPHYSIOLOGY

The nose and paranasal sinuses contain a large epithelium mucosal membrane surface that covers the passageway, the nasal bones, and turbinates that filter and humidify the air as it passes over the nasal mucosa. This is where inhaled particles/allergens are trapped before they can flow into the lower respiratory structures. Most allergens are large and become trapped in the mucous membranes of the nasal tissue. In the mucous membranes, there is an initial reaction between the allergen and intraepithelial mast cells, which proceeds deeper to the perivascular mast cells, both of which are sensitized with specific IgE. In addition to IgE, the mucosal surface in the nose also contains IgA. The IgE attaches to the mucosal and submucosal mast cells, and the intensity of the symptoms is directly related to the allergen dose. When an allergen is inhaled, the IgE attached to the mast cells within the mucosa and submucosa stimulates the release of histamine and leukotrienes, causing local tissue edema and increased drainage (Fig. 73.1).

CLINICAL PRESENTATION AND PHYSICAL EXAMINATION

AR should be suspected with seasonal or recurrent sneezing, disturbances of taste or smell, nasal congestion, dry mouth, postnasal discharge, and fatigue. Nasal discharge is usually thin and clear, and the patient may complain of nasal obstruction, and teeth and facial discomfort. Watery, itchy, and puffy eyes

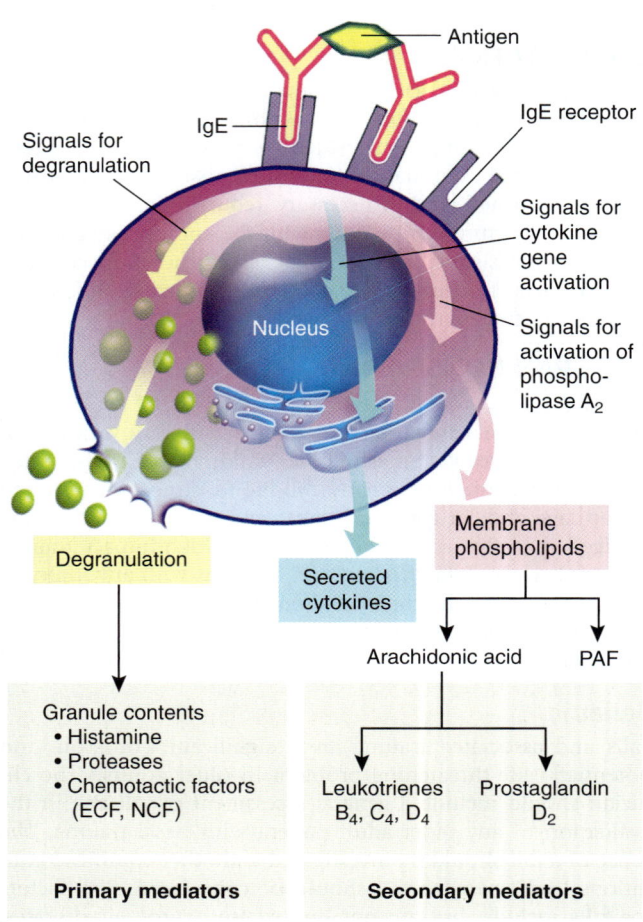

FIG. 73.1 Activation of mast cells leading to degranulation of preformed mediators (primary mediators) and synthesis of newly formed (de novo) mediators (secondary mediators). *IgE*, Immunoglobulin E. (From McCance, K. L., & Huether, S. E. [2019]. *Pathophysiology: The biologic basis for disease in adults and children* [8th ed.]. St. Louis: Elsevier.)

commonly occur, but fever and chills are unusual. Often, the patient has a personal or family history of asthma, eczema, or other atopic disease.

A detailed environmental exposure history is essential. Dust mites, animal dander, and indoor allergens should be suspected when winter symptoms predominate because heating systems disseminate dust particles and aggravate symptoms during the winter months. Patients with seasonal symptoms are typically allergic to outdoor allergens such as pollen and ragweed. Symptoms that occur during late spring and early summer are generally triggered by grass pollens, whereas symptoms during late summer and early fall tend to be linked to weed pollens. Tree pollens tend to be associated with symptoms in late winter or early spring. These generalizations vary with geographic changes and daily fluctuations in allergen counts.

Because symptoms related to AR cause itching in the nose and throughout the upper respiratory tract, the pattern of symptoms is important.[3] How frequently do these symptoms occur? How do the symptoms impact daily life? When is the patient asymptomatic? What medications has the patient been using? Where and when do symptoms occur? Is there associated itching, and if so, where?

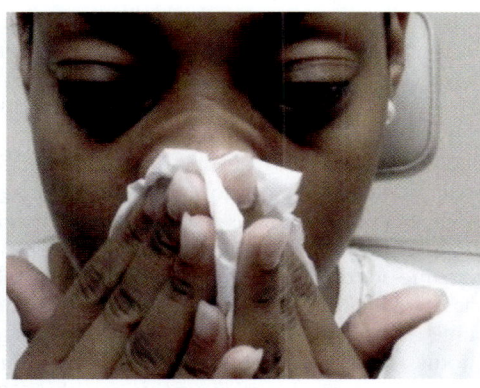

F I G . 73.2 Patient with nasal drip and modified "allergic salute" leading to the creation of a nasal crease. (From Woodbury, K., & Ferguson, B. J. [2011]. Physical findings in allergy. *Otolaryngologic Clinics of North America, 44*[3], 603–610.)

The exact anatomic location of congestion should also be determined. Anatomic obstructions tend to cause unilateral nostril blockage, whereas nasal polyps generally cause bilateral obstruction.

A thorough medication review is also necessary because often medications are associated with rhinitis.[2] Common culprits include reserpine, methyldopa, nonsteroidal antiinflammatory drugs (NSAIDs), oral contraceptives, β blockers, and snorting or sniffing street drugs (e.g., cocaine, heroin).

The physical examination can be performed with either a nasal speculum or an otoscope with an attached speculum. The nasal mucosa is typically pale (in contrast to viral or bacterial disease) because of chronic venous engorgement from the histamine and leukotrienes. The upper airway examination will also reveal swollen nasal turbinates with bleeding, mucus, crusting, and other signs of inflammation. Other common findings can include enlarged tonsils, postnasal drip, the well-recognized "allergic salute" (a crease across the nose from manipulating the tip of the nose), and conjunctival irritation (Fig. 73.2).

ESSENTIAL DIAGNOSTICS

Diagnosis of AR is primarily clinically based; patients report the hallmark symptoms of sneezing, rhinorrhea, and nasal and pharyngeal itching in the absence of infection. If there is a question about the cause of the symptoms, nasal cytologic studies (Wright stain) can demonstrate neutrophils or eosinophils and determine whether the symptoms are related to an infection or AR. If further diagnostic tests are desired, the patient should be referred to an allergist for testing. Additional tests can include scratch or patch tests, used to test for skin response to suspected allergens. Radioallergosorbent tests (RASTs) determine serum levels of allergen-specific IgE titers, but skin testing is more sensitive and is the preferred diagnostic. However, RASTs are helpful in diagnosis of food-related allergies and can be used in patients with dermatographism or equivocal skin test results, or in patients

INITIAL DIAGNOSTICS

Allergic Rhinitis

LABORATORY
- Nasal cytology–Wright stain
- Radioallergosorbent tests

OTHER
- Allergic scratch tests

who cannot discontinue antihistamines. Enzyme-linked immunosorbent assay (ELISA) is also used to identify common allergens and has high specificity.[2] Nasal cytology samples can be collected via nasal swab or collected with anterior rhinoscopy which enables direct visualization of the middle meatus, sphenoethmoidal recesses, and nasopharynx with a rigid or flexible nasal endoscope after the area is anesthetized with a topical anesthetic.

DIFFERENTIAL DIAGNOSIS

 Primary differentials include nasal-septal trauma, substance use (e.g., cocaine, heroin), granulomatosis with polyangiitis (i.e., Wegener granulomatosis), sarcoidosis, polyposis, and intranasal masses or tumors.

Health care providers should exclude structural abnormalities within the nasopharynx, irritant exposure, pregnancy, hypothyroidism, idiopathic rhinitis, rhinitis medicamentosa, or prolonged use of topical α-adrenergic agents before considering a diagnosis of AR. Fever, facial pain, and purulent sinus drainage suggest infectious sinusitis.

INTERPROFESSIONAL COLLABORATIVE MANAGEMENT

- Specialist referral is indicated for patients who do not respond to recommended therapies and for patients with recurrent epistaxis or sinusitis, pulmonary involvement, visual changes, unilateral symptoms, or hilar adenopathy.
- Referral for allergen immunotherapy. Subcutaneous or sublingual immunotherapy can be effective treatment for patients with severe AR symptoms or for those who have not responded to traditional treatments,[3-5] or if allergens cannot be avoided. Immunotherapy is generally considered if symptoms are present for more than 6 months, if symptoms are not relieved by environmental control and pharmacologic agents, and if the cost of immunotherapy is less than that of pharmacologic therapy. Subcutaneous injections are given every week in progressively increasing doses until a maintenance dose has been achieved; after that, injections are given monthly. Sublingual preparations are also available and involve the patient taking a tablet under the tongue and allowing it to absorb for up to 2 minutes before swallowing.
- There is a risk of immediate and delayed reactions with immunotherapy. Generalized reactions tend to occur within 20 to 30 minutes, but more systemic reactions can be delayed. Although the risk of a severe reaction is small, the response can be fatal. Therefore, patients should wait in the office for 30 minutes after the injection and carry an EpiPen, if appropriate. The proper resuscitative equipment should be accessible in the office if immunotherapy is offered, and a physician should be readily available.

Nonpharmacologic Management

Environmental Control. The most important treatment for AR is environmental control.[3] Because the patient is typically allergic to several allergens, control of the indoor and outdoor environment is crucial. Nonspecific irritants (e.g., smoke) and indirect contact (e.g., secondary contact with animal dander) can cause symptoms that are indistinguishable from those of allergies. Although techniques to control environmental allergens are arduous, time-consuming, and sometimes expensive, they are often essential for symptom control. In general, it tends to be the time commitment involved, not the cost, that makes environmental control difficult for patients.

If the allergen is outdoors, minimizing both direct and indirect exposure is recommended. Long-sleeved clothing and a mask may also be necessary to minimize direct contact. However, it is often the indirect contact—when the allergen is brought into the house—that proves to be most bothersome. Keeping the windows closed, especially between 10 p.m. and 5 a.m., and when windy outside, and then bathing and changing clothes immediately after entering the home aids in minimizing exposure.

Indoor allergens can also be the cause of complaints. House dust contains the waste products of dust mites that live in furniture, carpets, bedding, and mattresses. Stuffed animals are a significant problem for some patients. Pets, particularly cats and dogs, are also a major cause of allergic symptoms. Removal of the pet is not an effective means of environmental control because many people are not willing to give up their animal. Effective strategies include keeping the pet out of the bedroom at all times; keeping the pet outdoors as much as possible; washing the pet and pet bedding weekly; ventilating the home frequently to promote air exchange; having someone who is not allergic clean regularly with a high-efficiency particulate air (HEPA) or double-bag vacuum; and minimizing carpeting, drapes, and upholstered furniture. Attempts to eliminate cockroach proteins include storing foods in tightly sealed containers and having the pest eliminated. When possible, carpets should be eliminated, but if that is not an option, carpeting should be made of synthetic and short-napped fibers. Rugs should be washable; all loose or old rugs should be removed. Curtains (which should be cotton and, preferably, washable) and furniture should be cleaned and wiped regularly; dust-catching blinds should be avoided.

Other recommendations include keeping closet doors shut; covering machine-washable polyester pillows, mattresses, and comforters with allergy-free and zippered plastic covers; wet dusting; washing stuffed animals, sheets, and comforters in hot water (>54°C [130°F]) at least weekly; removing house plants and books; trimming bushes from the house; cleaning central heating and air-conditioning units; cleaning walls; using mold inhibitors when painting; reducing mold growth and humidity; and using a frost-free refrigerator. HEPA furnace filters and room cleaners may also decrease allergen exposure.

Controlling environmental exposures is important in controlling symptoms, but the provider-patient relationship is also crucial. Environmental recommendations should be reasonable and made with compassion and clarity.

Pharmacologic Management

Pharmacologic interventions are appropriate if strict environmental control has not worked sufficiently, but they should be used only when allergies significantly affect quality of life. Because pharmacologic agents may be used for extended periods, the safety, side effect profile, and cost-effectiveness of each agent must be considered carefully. Pharmacologic therapy often combines several different medications to provide patients with optimum symptom relief.

Treatment of AR is multifaceted and includes a combination of medical therapies and behavior modifications. Nasal irrigation using normal saline 100 to 150 mL and positive pressure to wash the allergens from the nasal passage is very effective

in removing allergens, mucus, inflammatory mediators, and mast cells to decrease symptoms.[3] A recent study revealed that solutions containing magnesium and potassium promote cellular repair, limit inflammation, and reduce apoptosis of respiratory cells.[6]

Intranasal steroids should be first-line treatment for AR[3,7] because systemic treatments do not target the nasal mucosa as effectively. The benefit of intranasal steroids is that they provide a targeted dose of steroids, allowing maximal efficacy and sparing systemic steroid doses and side effects. Steroids exert their effects by reducing the inflammatory response and inhibiting cytokine release;[7,8] patients can note effectiveness as soon as 6 to 8 hours after the dose and side effects are minimal. For older adults, inhaled nasal corticosteroids are likely the safest because they have minimal side effects when used correctly.[3] Patients should be instructed on the correct use of intranasal sprays to minimize irritations, prevent epistaxis, and increase medication effectiveness by placing the medication on the most reactive membranes. Specific recommendations for corticosteroid nasal spray application are to: (1) gently blow nose or use saline irrigation to remove excess secretions; (2) have patient lean head forward and look at the floor with the nasal spray aiming nearly vertical; (3) then using the hand opposite the nostril being treated, aim the nozzle slightly up and outward (lateral and cephalad) away from the septum; (4) and spray without sniffing or while sniffing very gently, keeping the medication in the nares, to prevent sucking the medication back into the throat. The medication will not help if in the throat so the patient should understand to gargle and rinse the mouth and throat if that occurs. Patients also need to understand that 2 to 4 weeks of continued use is necessary to see maximum benefit.[7] Several intranasal steroids are available for use, and there is no demonstrable difference among the different steroids, so patients may start with any of the available preparations. When treating pregnant patients, budesonide, an intranasal steroid, is U.S. Food and Drug Administration (FDA) Pregnancy Risk Factor B.

Intranasal steroids have a good safety profile with few systemic side effects. The most common reported side effects are nasal burning, stinging, and dryness.[7] Patients may also report headaches, epistaxis, and pharyngitis.[7]

Oral antihistamines are an additional treatment option in AR because histamine is the primary mediator of the nasal allergic reaction and increases nasal secretion; blocking histamine can potentially interrupt the damaging chemical mediator cascade, producing symptoms from both the allergic and viral pathologic processes.[3,7] Oral antihistamines can be effective in reducing sneezing, pruritus, and rhinorrhea, but overall are less effective than intranasal steroids in reducing the congestion associated with the allergic response.[7] The second-generation antihistamines are preferable because they have far fewer central nervous system side effects, require only once-daily administration, and offer quick relief with a 1- to 2-hour onset of action.[8] The second-generation antihistamines are effective throughout the allergic cycle. With the exception of cetirizine, the second-generation antihistamines do not produce significant sedation. These should therefore be considered a first-line treatment of AR before use of first-generation antihistamines and for those who cannot tolerate inhaled nasal steroids or those patients with narrow-angle glaucoma or benign prostatic hyperplasia.[7] Initially more expensive than the first-generation agents, second-generation antihistamines, such as loratadine, cetirizine, and fexofenadine, are now available in generic formulations, and can provide improved quality of life and work performance.

Although the second-generation antihistamines are very effective, they tend not to alleviate nasal congestion. Therefore combination formulations with decongestants, such as fexofenadine and pseudoephedrine (Allegra-D) or loratadine and pseudoephedrine (Claritin-D), are useful. Unfortunately, the decongestant component can cause sleeplessness, tachycardia, tremors, and other side effects. Antihistamines and decongestants are contraindicated for patients with hypertension, prostate enlargement, or narrow-angle glaucoma.

First-generation antihistamines can also be considered as a treatment option for AR, but they are much more sedating than their newer counterparts. In addition to their sedating side effects, the first-generation antihistamines have poor selectivity for the H_1 receptors, and often have an effect on the muscarinic receptors as well, causing constipation, blurred vision, and urinary retention. Several options are available over the counter, including diphenhydramine and chlorpheniramine, and there are also prescription agents (e.g., hydroxyzine or promethazine). Compliance with the first-generation antihistamines can be low because they often need to be administered several times per day. In general, the first-generation antihistamines should be reserved for nighttime symptoms when patients may desire the sedating side effects of these medications.

Other intranasal agents that can be helpful in controlling AR include azelastine, cromolyn, and ipratropium bromide.[3] Azelastine is an antihistamine spray, but it is expensive and can cause an unpleasant taste if it is not used correctly.[3] Intranasal cromolyn affects the inhibition of mast cell degranulation, thus it affects local cytokine release. The major problem is the administration regimen, which is four times daily. Nevertheless its safety profile makes intranasal cromolyn an appealing choice for some patients, and it is available over the counter.

Montelukast, a leukotriene receptor antagonist, is an oral treatment option for patients who are unwilling to use a nasal inhaler and for those who need multimodal therapy or have asthma.[3] A once-a-day oral medication, Montelukast has been used for many years and is associated with few side effects.[3]

Intranasal ipratropium bromide, an anticholinergic agent, is most effective for rhinorrhea and sneezing, but is less useful for nasal congestion. It is the treatment of choice for gustatory and vasomotor rhinitis and is often used to treat symptoms of the common cold. It is generally safe and well tolerated. The most common drug-related problems are dryness and epistaxis.

For pregnant and breastfeeding women, it is important that all medications should be discussed with the obstetrician/gynecologist and pediatrician before taking any medicine. Oral decongestants should be avoided during the first trimester and in breastfeeding mothers.

One nonpharmacologic intervention that has shown efficacy in AR is nasal saline irrigation. Patients can use a variety of devices, including a neti pot or plastic bottle to rinse the nares and potentially sinus cavities with isotonic saline. Plastic squeeze bottles have a more thorough lavage than the neti pots or nasal sprays, so may have better results.

COMPLICATIONS

Complications of AR are rare but potentially serious. Increased asthma and other pulmonary disease exacerbations are related to rhinitis, and sleep apnea can be a problem in untreated rhinitis. Thus treatment with medications and strict environmental control can be beneficial.

INDICATIONS FOR REFERRAL OR HOSPITALIZATION

- Older adults with new-onset rhinitis may need a physician evaluation to exclude anatomic obstruction.
- However, most patients with new-onset rhinitis have been recently exposed to a new and offending agent and can be managed effectively without a referral. Some patients require a referral to an otolaryngologist.
- Any patient who sees a health care provider because of new nasal congestion should undergo a nasal examination for assessment of anatomic problems. Although nasopharyngeal neoplasms are rare, nasal polyps are common and often require surgical intervention. These patients can also have aspirin sensitivity and allergic asthma. A deviated septum can also produce symptoms that mimic classic rhinitis.
- A second careful review of the patient's history, medication use, exposure to cigarette smoke and perfumes, and occupational exposures is indicated before any referral is made. In addition, a home visit and review of inhaler technique are invaluable. Medications and medical problems that may be contributing to the symptoms should be investigated. T-cell deficiencies (e.g., with acquired immunodeficiency syndrome [AIDS]), cystic fibrosis, hypothyroidism, and humoral deficiencies should be considered. A referral to an allergist is indicated if the signs and symptoms continue and anatomic problems have been excluded.
- AR does not usually require hospitalization. Rare circumstances include anaphylaxis, a life-threatening hypersensitivity immune response, or the need for a surgical procedure (e.g., nasal polypectomy). Hospitalization is typically required for treatment and continued observation.

PATIENT AND FAMILY EDUCATION

- Once the environmental allergens have been identified, recommendations can be made and a therapeutic regimen agreed on. Education is crucial in the management of AR. A dramatic improvement in symptoms is often noted when patients become experts on the triggers that activate symptoms. An allergy diary is therefore often useful. Reducing exposure to dust mites, animal dander, molds, cockroaches, pollens, smoke, and other irritants is essential.
- Patients should also understand how to use nasal inhalers correctly and the importance of using inhalers regularly to promote their effectiveness. The side effect profile of these medications and of over-the-counter and prescription antihistamines and decongestants should also be discussed.

IDIOPATHIC, OR VASOMOTOR, RHINITIS
Definition and Epidemiology

Vasomotor rhinitis, which is now known as *idiopathic* or *nonallergic* rhinitis, is an important, often overlooked, nonallergic, noninfectious cause of perennial nasal congestion and rhinorrhea. Idiopathic rhinitis is not associated with itchiness of the eyes and nose or sneezing. It occurs in response to environmental triggers, such as cold air, strong smells, irritants, changes in weather, some medications (angiotensin-converting enzyme [ACE] inhibitors, β blockers), stress, exercise, and certain foods as well as increased estrogen levels (e.g., pregnancy and use of oral contraceptive pills). In contrast to the symptoms of AR, which tend to be seasonal and periodic, nonallergic symptoms tend to occur year-round and to be chronic.

Pathophysiology

Nonallergic rhinitis is not immune related; the symptoms of nonallergic rhinitis are provoked by environmental stimuli. It is distinguished from other types of rhinitis by its lack of purulent discharge. It has been postulated that the cause of nonallergic rhinitis is neurogenic, involving an abnormal balance that favors parasympathetic control over sympathetic control of the nasal mucosa,[2] leading to intermittent vascular engorgement of the nasal mucous membranes. The underlying cause of this imbalance is unknown.

Clinical Presentation and Physical Examination

With nonallergic rhinitis, patients often report perennial nasal congestion but little discharge. Any discharge is generally described as watery. There are few if any symptoms on arising, but nasal congestion can begin shortly after getting out of bed. Exposure to cold, stress, odors, spicy foods, alcohol, sunlight, and other environmental factors are often cited as causes.[9] These irritants appear to be nonspecific triggers for exaggerated physiologic responses.

One characteristic that distinguishes idiopathic rhinitis from AR is that itching, sneezing, and other irritative symptoms tend to occur with AR, whereas obstructive symptoms and rhinorrhea tend to occur with nonallergic rhinitis. Tearing and itching of the eyes and sneezing are common in AR but uncommon with nonallergic rhinitis. Sneezing can occur at times with idiopathic rhinitis, usually in response to temperature changes.

Physical Examination. The physical appearance of the nasal mucosa often differs in AR and nonallergic rhinitis. The nasal mucosa is typically pale in AR, but it is often erythematous in idiopathic rhinitis.

INITIAL DIAGNOSTICS

Idiopathic Rhinitis

LABORATORY
- Nasal eosinophils

OTHER
- Skin testing

Differential Diagnosis

 Primary differentials should include obstruction caused by trauma or tumor, cancer, foreign bodies, and bacterial infections.

The patient history helps distinguish idiopathic rhinitis from AR. There is no definitive test, but certain diagnostic procedures can be useful. Skin testing results are often positive in AR but not in idiopathic rhinitis. If positive, the skin test response to a seasonal allergen in a patient with perennial symptoms is not necessarily clinically significant. Medication side effects, hypothyroidism, pregnancy, rhinitis medicamentosa, AR, aspirin sensitivity, infections, and nasal obstructions should also be considered in patients with symptoms of idiopathic rhinitis.

Interprofessional Collaborative Management
- Referral to allergist or immunologist is recommended.

Nonpharmacologic Management

As with AR, environmental avoidance is the best treatment; immunotherapy is often not effective. Idiopathic rhinitis is chronic, and avoidance of stimuli is important. Smoking, perfumes or colognes, spicy foods, and other stimuli should be discouraged.

Pharmacologic Management

Unlike AR, idiopathic rhinitis does not usually respond to antihistamines. Oral decongestants are often effective, as are saline irrigations and intranasal steroids. Environmental avoidance is the best treatment; immunotherapy is often not effective.

Complications

Although little information is available on the long-term complications of idiopathic rhinitis, chronic problems can occur. Patients can experience sleep deprivation and a diminished quality of life.

Indications for Referral or Hospitalization

Most patients can be managed effectively. A referral may be indicated if the diagnosis remains elusive, if treatments have not been effective, or if anatomic causes are a consideration.

Patient and Family Education

It is important for the patient to understand that idiopathic rhinitis is a chronic condition and that the effectiveness of symptomatic treatment is limited. A detailed environmental history with minimization of potential exposures is most beneficial. Many of the measures that are effective for patients with AR will be effective for patients with idiopathic rhinitis. Regular use of topical decongestants should be avoided because of the potential for development of a tolerance to these agents.

OTHER CAUSES OF RHINITIS
Infectious

Upper respiratory tract infections typically are associated with rhinitis. A coexistent infection is present, and relatively prompt relief of symptoms occurs with resolution of the infection. Purulent discharge is common but not always present. Viral rhinitis is usually caused by a rhinovirus or coronavirus and has a specific incubation period and duration. Rhinoviruses are responsible for the majority of viral rhinitis cases (or the "common cold," as most patients term the illness).[10] Infection with the rhinovirus occurs through direct contact with infected secretions, usually hand-to-hand contact with an infected patient. Once the virus is contracted, infection proceeds as the virus attaches to a variety of cellular receptors. The virus then replicates and causes an infiltration of neutrophils, lymphocytes, and other inflammatory cells, which cause the mucus-secreting glands within the submucosa to become hyperactive. The turbinates become engorged, and several mediators, including prostaglandins, histamine, interleukins, and tumor necrosis factor, are released and are responsible for the rhinorrhea patient's experience during acute viral rhinitis.[10] Coronaviruses are similar, but they specifically infect the ciliated epithelial cells in the nasopharynx through either aminopeptidase N (a receptor) or sialic acid receptors, and damage the ciliated cells when the virus replicates, releasing the same cascade of mediators.[10] There are some coronaviruses that do cause the common cold but some coronaviruses tend to be more serious (e.g., SARS or MERS) and fortunately are not as common.[10]

Bacterial rhinitis, or infectious rhinitis, often originates from allergic or viral swelling of the nasal mucosa, affecting the drainage from the sinuses and trapping microorganisms within the warm, dark, moist environments of the sinuses. Signs and symptoms of a primary bacterial or primary viral rhinitis are indistinguishable, and a bacterial cause is recognized only after a secondary infection, such as sinusitis, develops.

Anatomic

Anatomic causes of rhinitis include a deviated nasal septum, nasal polyps, and nasal tumors.

In particular, neoplasms should be suspected in older adults. The most common cause of anatomic problems is nasal polyps, which can cause impressive obstructive symptoms. These are often found incidentally in patients with asthma who also have aspirin sensitivity. Symptoms can be perennial and difficult to differentiate from AR or idiopathic rhinitis. Treatment options include intranasal steroids and surgery.

Rhinitis Medicamentosa

Symptoms of nasal congestion may result from the chronic administration of sympatholytic drugs, NSAIDs, or topical decongestants. This most commonly develops with tolerance to topical decongestants. After the patient uses topical decongestants for approximately 1 or 2 weeks, the nasal mucosa develops rebound engorgement through increased blood flow. Although these symptoms tend to continue for days or weeks, discontinuation of the offending drug is curative. A 1- to 2-week course of nasal steroids or, rarely, systemic steroids can be helpful during the withdrawal period.

Pharmacologic Causes

Various medications, including β blockers, ACE inhibitors, chlorpromazine, estrogen, and oral contraceptives, can cause symptoms that mimic those of AR.

Nonpharmacologic Management

Treatment involves discontinuation of the medication.

Food- or Drink-Related Rhinitis

Symptoms of rhinitis may occur after ingestion of food or alcohol. The exact cause is unknown, but it may be a cholinergic reaction or other mechanism. If the rhinitis is caused by a food allergy, gastrointestinal, dermatologic, or systemic manifestations are usually present. Treatment involves avoidance of the trigger food or drink.

Other Medical Causes

Pregnancy and hypothyroidism are other common causes of rhinitis. Other causes also include cocaine use and atrophic changes. Treatment is directed at the underlying medical problem.

REFERENCES

1. Lakhani, N., North, M., & Ellis, A. K. (2012). Clinical manifestations of allergic rhinitis. *Journal of Allergy & Therapy* https://www.omicsonline.org/clinical-manifestations-of-allergic-rhinitis-2155-6121.S5-007.php?aid=6951. (Accessed 25 February 2018).
2. Boyce, A., & Austen, K. (2014). Allergies, anaphylaxis, and systemic mastocytosis. In D. Kasper, A. Fauci, S. Hauser, D. Longo, J. Jameson, & J. Loscalzo (Eds.), *Harrison's principles of internal medicine* (19e). New York, NY: McGraw-Hill.
3. Dykewicz, M. S., Wallace, D. V., Baroody, F., Bernstein, J., et al. (2017). Treatment of seasonal allergic rhinitis. https://www.aaaai.org/Aaaai/media/../2017-Rhinitis-Guideline-Updates.pdf. (Accessed 5 May 2019).
4. Durham, S. R., & Penagos, M. (2016). Sublingual or subcutaneous immunotherapy for allergic rhinitis? *The Journal of Allergy and Clinical Immunology, 137*(2), 339–349, e10. doi:10.1016/j.jaci.2015.12.1298.
5. Walker, S. M., Durham, S. R., Till, S. J., et al. (2011). Immunotherapy for allergic rhinitis. *Clinical and Experimental Allergy: Journal of the British Society for Allergy and Clinical Immunology, 41*(9), 1177–1200.
6. Principi, N., & Esposito, S. (2017). Nasal irrigation: An imprecisely defined medical procedure. *International Journal of Environmental Research and Public Health, 14*(5), 516. http://doi.org/10.3390/ijerph14050516.
7. Sur, D. K., & Scandale, S. (2015). Treatment of allergic rhinitis. *American Family Physician, 92*(11), 985–992.
8. Minor, S. (2013). Allergic rhinitis: What's best for your patient. *The Journal of Family Practice, 62*(3), E1–E10.
9. Shah, S. B., & Emanuel, I. A. (2012). Nonallergic & allergic rhinitis. In A. K. Lalwani (Ed.), *CURRENT diagnosis & treatment in Otolaryngology—Head & neck surgery* (3e, Chapter 14). New York, NY: McGraw-Hill.
10. Dolin, R. (2014). Common viral respiratory infections. In D. Kasper, A. Fauci, S. Hauser, D. Longo, J. Jameson, & J. Loscalzo (Eds.), *Harrison's principles of internal medicine* (19e). New York, NY: McGraw-Hill.

CHAPTER **74**

SINUSITIS

Jessica Helen Fortunak

 Physician consultation is recommended when there is evidence of visual changes, periorbital cellulitis, mental status changes, high fever, or acute focal pain.

DEFINITION AND EPIDEMIOLOGY

Rhinosinusitis is a symptomatic inflammation of the mucosal surface of the paranasal sinuses. This common disorder develops in over 30 million Americans per year or about 1 in 8 adult Americans, resulting in over $11 billion in direct health care costs and even greater expense when lost productivity and decreased quality of life is included.[1] Rhinosinusitis is differentiated into subclassifications including acute, subacute, and chronic rhinosinusitis (CRS) based on the patient's duration of symptoms. Acute rhinosinusitis (ARS) resolves in less than 4 weeks; subacute rhinosinusitis resolves within 4 to 12 weeks; and CRS continues beyond 12 weeks. This important distinction dictates treatment guidelines.

ARS is an inflammatory process of the paranasal sinuses caused by viral, bacterial, allergic, or fungal infections. Rhinosinusitis is usually precipitated by an acute viral respiratory tract infection which extends into the paranasal sinus cavities. In the vast number of cases the infection remains viral with only 0.5% to 2% being complicated by bacterial infections.[1] Acute bacterial rhinosinusitis (ABRS) is generally caused by *Streptococcus pneumoniae*, *Haemophilus influenzae*, or *Moraxella catarrhalis*, while *S. pneumoniae* is the most common pathogen in all age groups. Less common pathogens include *Chlamydia pneumoniae*, *Streptococcus pyogenes*, viruses, and fungi.[2]

The symptoms of ARS are often confused with those of an upper respiratory tract infection. The presenting signs and symptoms include nasal congestion, purulent nasal discharge, and a headache that becomes more intense when the patient bends forward. Fever, fatigue, and other constitutional symptoms are common. The onset is abrupt, with infection in one or more paranasal sinuses.[3] The benefits versus risks of antibiotic therapy in decreasing the symptoms and duration of illness have been documented.[4]

There is an association between sinusitis and asthma. The incidence of sinusitis in patients with asthma ranges from 40% to 75%. Treatment of the sinus infection results in improvement of asthma symptoms.[5]

Chronic sinusitis occurs with episodes of prolonged sinus infection (more than 12 weeks) that resist treatment, or with recurrent acute infections that are inadequately treated and never resolve. The presentation of this disease is the frequent exacerbation of sinus infections that are caused by gram-negative or anaerobic microorganisms.

Approximately 10% to 12% of cases of chronic maxillary sinusitis are secondary to dental infection.[6] Identification of an anaerobic infection that can result in an anaerobic brain abscess is vital to prevent hematogenous spread from the sinuses.

Gram-negative bacilli may cause sinusitis in patients who are intubated through the nares or who have a nasogastric tube placed in the nares. The trauma and obstruction caused by these invasive devices can lead to a sinus infection.[7]

PATHOPHYSIOLOGY

Most sinus disease involves the maxillary and anterior ethmoidal sinuses. The maxillary sinus is the largest of the paranasal sinuses, and its ostium into the nose is superiorly placed, thereby failing to take advantage of gravity. These anatomic characteristics cause it to be the most commonly infected sinus. In addition, during a viral infection such as influenza or the common cold, infected secretions are forced into the sinus cavity likely with nose blowing causing inflammation of the sinus cavity. Furthermore, the viral infection causes decreased ciliary clearance leading to increased sinus and nasal obstruction which prolongs the infection.

Bacterial sinusitis is most often a complication of viral rhinosinusitis but is also associated with allergies, dental infection, or fluid introduced into the sinuses by diving and swimming. Sinusitis may also develop when fluid is trapped in the sinuses by anatomic abnormalities, such as a deviated septum, adenoidal hypertrophy, neoplasms, foreign body, or ciliary dysfunction as seen in patients with cystic fibrosis.

CRS is thought to result from an ARS infection that has not completely resolved due to continued inflammation and impaired sinus drainage. Patients with chronic sinusitis typically have an anatomic abnormality that inhibits normal ciliary mucus clearance, are immunocompromised, have continued allergen or irritant exposure, or an incompletely treated bacterial or fungal infection.

CLINICAL PRESENTATION AND PHYSICAL EXAMINATION

ARS is characterized by nasal congestion, dental pain, postnasal drip, halitosis, headache, fever, ear fullness, otalgia, fatigue, and decreased or lack of smell. Sensations of pain in the teeth and forehead are worse in the morning and when the patient bends forward from the waist. Pain may be referred to the upper incisor and canine teeth through the branches of the trigeminal nerve, which traverse the floor of the sinus.[6] Although facial and dental pain are seen in ABRS, research has not demonstrated a link between these symptoms and their correlation with the specifically infected sinus cavity.[1] Thus pain at the frontal sinus area is not sensitive for frontal rhinosinusitis and the same is true for ethmoid and maxillary symptoms. A sore throat, cough, frequent throat clearing, and upset stomach are common due to persistent postnasal drainage.

ABRS is characterized by three cardinal symptoms of mucopurulent discharge, nasal obstruction, and facial pain or pressure that demonstrate high sensitivity and relatively high specificity for this diagnosis.[1] Patients with ABRS typically present with persistent ARS symptoms for greater than 10 days without improvement or have a period of initial improvement followed by worsening of symptoms (double worsening), or a sudden onset of severe symptoms for 3 to 4 days (i.e., fever >102°F and purulent discharge or facial pain).[1]

The four cardinal symptoms seen in CRS include purulent nasal drainage, nasal obstruction, facial pain or pressure, and decrease or loss of smell lasting more than 12 weeks.[8] Frequent throat clearing and cough are also common. Nasal obstruction is most commonly bilateral and if unilateral raises concerns about neoplasm, foreign body, or anatomic abnormality. Worsening of asthma is not unusual and may be a result of the sinobronchial reflex, mouth breathing, and postnasal drip containing inflammatory chemicals from the sinuses.[5] The patient with chronic sinusitis may also experience an increase in allergic symptoms, including nocturnal asthma, allergic rhinitis, and eczema.[5] When a patient is in a prone position, sinusitis symptoms worsen, especially at night.

The physical exam should determine the presence of fever, vital signs, and associated concerning patient symptoms. General inspection for facial asymmetry, periorbital edema, or cellulitis should be performed while the patient's history is obtained. Assessment of speech for hyponasal quality may indicate nasal obstruction. Anterior rhinoscopic evaluation of the nasal tract should assess for nasal turbinate edema, erythema, discharge, patency of nares, septal deviation, and polyps. However, examination of the nose with a nasal speculum is often inadequate in evaluating sinusitis. Transillumination of the sinuses can, in some instances, provide helpful information, although this does not differentiate between a viral and a bacterial cause of the sinus inflammation. If the sinuses can be transilluminated, they are not likely to contain fluid. The inability to transilluminate the sinuses suggests the presence of fluid in the sinuses. However, this test must be done with care because improper technique can result in a false reading.[9] Examination of the eyes, noting periorbital swelling, "allergic shiners" (dark circles under the eyes), and erythema should precede palpation and percussion of the frontal and maxillary sinuses for tenderness. The pharynx should be examined for postnasal drip, erythema, and lymphoid hypertrophy. As otitis media commonly occurs with sinusitis, an otic examination is prudent. The sinuses drain into the nasopharynx, and bacteria found in this discharge is easily transported through the eustachian tube to the middle ear, creating a middle ear infection. In patients with fever and headaches, assessment and documentation for meningeal irritation (absence of Kernig and Brudzinski signs) are important for both children and adults.[10]

The teeth should be examined for caries and the gingivae should be examined for inflammation. Approximately 10% to 12% of patients with maxillary sinus infections have dental root infection, and therefore the maxillary teeth should be tapped to determine if the teeth are infected.[6]

DIAGNOSTICS
Essential Diagnostics

ARS and ABRS are diagnosed empirically based on history and physical exam as diagnostics cannot differentiate between viral, bacterial, or fungal CRS. Diagnosis is confirmed with nasal endoscopy (first line allows for aspiration of mucus and culture, and identification of polyps and anatomical defects) and computed tomography (CT) without contrast (gold standard for diagnostic certainty in patients with prolonged or complicated course, such as recurrent ABRS, patients who have orbital, intracranial, soft tissue involvement, or in patients with comorbidities such as immunodeficiency, diabetes, or a history of facial trauma or surgery).[1]

ADDITIONAL DIAGNOSTICS

MRI

INITIAL DIAGNOSTICS

LABORATORY
- None indicated

IMAGING
- Acute rhinosinusitis and ABS–none
- Chronic rhinosinusitis–Nasal Endoscopy, computed tomography without contrast

DIFFERENTIAL DIAGNOSIS

 Priority differentials include (1) foreign body or malignancy in patients with unilateral nasal discharge, (2) dental abscess in patients with poor dentition and fever, (3) trigeminal neuralgia in patients with unilateral facial pain without nasal symptoms, (4) meningitis in patients with headache and fever, (5) orbital cellulitis in patients with eye pain and edema, (6) head injury in patients with history of trauma associated with cerebrospinal fluid (CSF) draining from the nose, and (7) fungal rhinosinusitis in immunocompromised patients or those with diabetes mellitus.

The more common differential diagnoses include viral upper respiratory infection, allergic rhinitis, and migraine.

INTERPROFESSIONAL COLLABORATIVE MANAGEMENT

Nonpharmacologic Management

Watchful waiting can be used as initial management in patients with diagnosed uncomplicated ABRS who have planned follow-up with their provider in the event symptoms worsen or last beyond 7 days, at which time antibiotic treatment would be initiated.[1]

Pharmacologic Management

There are no known treatments to shorten the course of ARS. Antibiotics are not recommended since they are not effective in treatment of viral illness. Symptomatic treatment is recommended. Recommended treatment of ARS includes analgesics and NSAIDs for pain control, nasal saline and/or oral or topical decongestants to decrease nasal congestion, and topical nasal steroids to improve nasal congestion and facial pain (off-label use).[1] For a patient diagnosed with ABRS, analgesics or NSAIDs are indicated for pain control. One study found that patients who used topical nasal steroids demonstrated a 7% increase in symptom resolution compared to patients who did not use nasal steroids.[1] Nasal saline, either isotonic or hypertonic, has been shown both when used alone and in combination with other treatments to decrease nasal symptoms, improve

quality of life, and decrease adjunct medication use in patients with ABRS.[1]

In patients who fail to improve during the watchful waiting period or who do not qualify for watchful waiting due to inability to follow up, antibiotics are initiated. Antibiotic classes are chosen to cover the most common pathogens (*S. pneumonia, M. catarrhalis,* and *H. influenzae*) and include amoxicillin-clavulanate as first line treatment.[11] In patients with a penicillin allergy, doxycycline is recommended, but the choice of specific antibiotic should be individualized based on each patient's risk factors and comorbid conditions, as well as focused on geographic regional resistance patterns.[11] Similar improvement rates are seen among 5- and 10-day treatment courses, however patients treated for 10 days demonstrate increased adverse events.[1] Treatment failure is seen in patients who do not have symptom improvement and the provider has re-confirmed the diagnosis of ABRS and assessed for complications. In these patients, the choice of antibiotic treatment is based on likely resistant organisms.

Treatment for CRS is guided by the absence or presence of polyps. The next step in treatment includes identification and management of comorbidities that contribute to CRS symptoms, including allergies, asthma, cystic fibrosis, ciliary dysfunction, and immune deficiency.[1] Nasal steroids are the cornerstone treatment used to combat inflammation, the primary cause of CRS, and should be used for at least 8 to 12 weeks.[1] Saline irrigation with at least 200 mL of warmed sterile saline helps to improve quality of life through increased mucus clearance, removal of allergens, improved ciliary action, and protection of the nasal mucosa.[1] Evidence is lacking to support antibiotic treatment of CRS for patients with or without polyps. However, expert opinion suggests treatment with antibiotics in patients who have a confirmed bacterial infection through nasal endoscopy with culture.[8] For patients with nasal polyps, research demonstrates that use of short-term corticosteroids (<3 weeks) decreased symptoms, and improved quality of life and endoscopy findings, but these were not long-term benefits.[8]

INDICATIONS FOR REFERRAL AND HOSPITALIZATION

The patient who is not symptom-free after the second treatment with antibiotics should be referred to an otolaryngologist. A referral to an allergist may also be indicated as 20% to 60% of patients with CRS, especially those with nasal polyps, have allergic rhinitis.[12] If the patient with chronic recurrent sinusitis has allergies, immunotherapy as indicated by skin testing may be necessary. Surgery may be indicated if the symptoms of sinusitis do not respond to medical therapy. Goals of endoscopic nasal surgery include removing nasal obstruction, improving sinus drainage, and increasing access to use of topical medications and treatments to improve the patient's quality of life.[8] Medical treatments after surgery are continued as the surgery is not considered curative.

Immediate referral is indicated for immunocompromised patients with suspected fungal sinusitis and for patients with suspected acute bacterial sinusitis associated with visual changes, mental status changes, or periorbital edema.[13] Hospitalization for intravenous therapy and surgical consultation for biopsy or debridement are imperative.[13,14]

Scuba divers with chronic sinusitis can experience sinus barotraumas. This condition is not usually serious, but these patients can be at risk for neurologic compromise. For this reason, scuba divers with chronic sinusitis should be evaluated by an otolaryngologist.[14]

COMPLICATIONS

In the antibiotic era, it is uncommon for sinusitis to become life-threatening. However, a chronic infection may interfere with quality of life because chronic sinusitis can continue for extended periods, possibly years. The cost in time, pain, expense, and emotional stress is significant.

Osteomyelitis of the frontal bone is a potential complication of sinusitis that has been increasing in the pediatric population.[15] If osteomyelitis develops, fever, pain, and edema over the involved bone will be present. The edema is called Pott's puffy tumor.[16]

An orbital infection is another possible complication of sinus infection because the orbit is surrounded on three sides by the paranasal sinuses. This complication occurs more often when the ethmoid sinuses are infected, and the bacteria can extend through the lamina papyracea. The orbital infection may cause so much edema that the patient has difficulty with vision. Visual loss can also result from pressure on the optic nerve, which can cause a permanent loss of vision. In addition, if the optic nerve becomes infected, the infection can spread to the intracranial vault. Intracranial suppuration can develop, creating a brain abscess or meningitis. Patients with this condition are usually acutely ill and have an elevated temperature, severe headache, and symptoms of increased intracranial pressure.[17]

Invasive fungal sinusitis is a rare but potentially fatal complication of chronic sinusitis in patients with a comorbid immunologic disorder, such as malignant neoplasm, human immunodeficiency virus (HIV) infection, diabetes, or drug-induced neutropenia. Prompt recognition of the serious signs and symptoms (fever, facial pain, epistaxis, and cognitive or visual changes in an immunocompromised patient) associated with invasive fungal sinusitis is essential to prevent proliferation of the infection.[13] Invasive fungal sinusitis should not be confused with allergic fungal sinusitis, a benign but unremitting sinus infection more common in young people with asthma.[13]

PATIENT AND FAMILY EDUCATION

In patients with CRS an important educational priority is correct use of nasal steroids to gain the most benefit from this treatment. Instructions include shaking the bottle, bending the neck forward slightly, using the right hand to spray the medicine into the left nare by pointing the nozzle away from the septum, and then switching hands and repeating treatment on the opposite nare. Patients should also be reminded to avoid hard sniffing. Patients should be aware that although the symptoms of an upper respiratory tract infection and sinusitis are similar, antibiotic therapy is not beneficial in viral rhinosinusitis.[4] However, upper respiratory tract infections that increase in severity, do not resolve after 10 to 14 days, and are accompanied by symptoms suggestive of bacterial sinusitis, may require treatment. The patient treated for sinusitis should be instructed to return for further evaluation if the symptoms have not improved in 48 to 72 hours. In addition, the patient must be able to recognize complications such as periorbital swelling and know to contact the health care provider immediately.

Patients with upper respiratory tract infections should understand the importance of blowing the nose gently to prevent the introduction of nasal fluid into the sinuses.[18] Patients should also know the signs and symptoms of viral respiratory infections and be warned against the side effects of first-generation antihistamines, NSAIDs, decongestants, and cough suppressants.[4]

HEALTH PROMOTION

If allergic rhinitis is a precursor to sinusitis, environmental control should be stressed. Humidified air and increased fluid intake are important to relieve nasal discomfort and to liquefy secretions. Warm, moist air in the form of steam inhalation or warm compresses may relieve the feeling of pressure and headache, and any activity that might introduce fluid into the sinuses, such as swimming or diving, should be avoided. Smoking cessation and frequent handwashing are also strongly encouraged.

REFERENCES

1. Rosenfeld, R. M., Picarillo, J. F., Chandrasekhar, S. S., Brook, I., Kaparaboyna, A. K., Kramper, M., et al. (2015). Clinical practice guideline (update): Adult sinusitis. *Otolaryngology–Head and Neck Surgery: Official Journal of American Academy of Otolaryngology–Head and Neck Surgery, 152*(2S), S1–S39.
2. Grossman, S. C. (2014). Respiratory tract infections, neoplasms, and childhood disorders. In *Porth's pathophysiology* (9th ed.). Philadelphia: Lippincott Williams & Wilkins.
3. Southwick, F. S. (2014). Eye, ear, nose, and throat infections. In *Infectious diseases: A clinical short course* (3rd ed.). New York: McGraw Hill.
4. IDSA clinical practice guideline for acute bacterial rhinosinusitis in children and adults. Retrieved from https://www.idsociety.org/practice-guideline/rhinosinusitis/. (Accessed 5 May 2019).
5. Mahmoud, G. (2013). How closely related are allergic rhinitis, asthma, and chronic sinusitis? *Ear, Nose, and Throat Journal, 92*(9), 410–413.
6. Pokorny, A., & Tataryn, R. (2013). Clinical and radiologic findings in a case series of maxillary sinusitis of dental origin. *International Forum of Allergy & Rhinology, 3*(12), 973–979.
7. Agrafiotis, M., Vardakas, K. Z., Gkegkes, I. D., Kapaskelis, A., & Falagas, M. E. (2012). Ventilator-associated sinusitis in adults: Systematic review and meta-analysis. *Respiratory Medicine, 106*, 1082–1095.
8. Sedaghat, A. R. (2017). Chronic rhinosinusitis. *American Family Physician, 96*(8), 500–506.
9. Bickley, L. S., & Szilagyi, P. G. (2013). *Bates' guide to physical examination and history taking* (11th ed.). Philadelphia: Lippincott Williams & Wilkins.
10. Kennedy, D., & Lee, J. (2012). Paranasal sinuses: Embryology, anatomy, endoscopic diagnosis, and treatment. In K. J. Lee's (Ed.), *Essential otolaryngology: Head & neck surgery* (10th ed.). New York: McGraw-Hill.
11. Lustig, L. R., & Schindler, J. S. (2018). Ear, nose, & throat disorders. In M. A. Papadakis, S. J. McPhee, & M. W. Rabow (Eds.), *Current medical diagnosis & treatment* New York, NY. McGraw-Hill.
12. Rudmik, L., & Soler, Z. M. (2015). Medical therapies for adult chronic sinusitis: A systematic review. *Journal of the American Medical Association, 314*(9), 926–939.
13. Chandrasekharan, R., Thomas, M., & Rupa, V. (2012). Comparison study of orbital involvement in invasive and noninvasive fungal sinusitis. *The Journal of Laryngology and Otology, 126*(2), 152–158.
14. Jeong, J. H., Kim, K., Seok, H., & Kim, K. R. (2012). Sphenoid sinus barotraumas after scuba diving. *American Journal of Otolaryngology, 33*(4), 477–480.
15. Severino, M., Livonage, S., Novelli, V., Cheesborough, B., Saunders, D., Gunny, R., et al. (2012). Skull base osteomyelitis and potential cerebral vascular complications in children. *Pediatric Radiology, 42*, 867–874.
16. Domville-Lewis, C., Friedland, P. L., & Santa Maria, P. L. (2013). Pott's puffy tumour and intracranial complications of frontal sinusitis in pregnancy. *The Journal of Laryngology and Otology, 27*, S35–S38.
17. Calik, M., Iscan, A., Abuhandan, M., Yetkin, I., Bozkus, F., & Torun, M. F. (2012). Masked subdural empyema secondary to frontal sinusitis. *The American Journal of Emergency Medicine, 30*, 1657e1–1657e4.
18. Medline Plus. Sinusitis. U.S. National Library of Medicine National Institute of Health. Retrieved from www.nlm.nih.gov/medlineplus/sinusitis.html. (Accessed 5 May 2019).

SMELL AND TASTE DISTURBANCES

Emily Karwacki Sheff • Jason R. Lucey • Catherine Franklin • Linda Evans • Patrice K. Nicholas

 Emergency department referral for brain imaging (computed tomography and/or magnetic resonance imaging) and/or immediate neurologist evaluation is indicated for patients whose symptoms are suspicious for an acute life-threatening intracranial process (e.g., intracranial hemorrhage related to significant head trauma or stroke, suspicion of malignancy based on history and examination findings).

DEFINITION AND EPIDEMIOLOGY

Disorders of smell and taste can be seriously debilitating to patients and are often diagnostic dilemmas for health care providers. Olfactory dysfunction can be described as loss of the sense of smell (anosmia), smell distortion (parosmia), or diminished sense of smell (hyposmia).[1,2] These dysfunctions can result from aging, tobacco, toxins, medications, malignant neoplasms, nasal inflammation, infection, malnutrition, head or facial trauma, Parkinson disease, Alzheimer disease, multiple sclerosis, diabetes, or inflammatory autoimmune conditions.[3–6]

Taste disorders include diminished taste (hypogeusia), unpleasant taste (aliageusia), and any persistent taste (dysgeusia). Ageusia, or absent taste, does occur but is less common.[7] Taste disorders are often caused by conditions similar to those causing smell disorders, but can also be associated with endocrine dysfunction, anesthesia, malignant neoplasms, head and neck irradiation, procedures, iatrogenic causes, kidney or gastric dysfunction, metabolic or hepatic disorders, environmental exposure, substance use disorder, or psychiatric disorders.[8–11]

PATHOPHYSIOLOGY

During the process of smelling, odorant molecules are taken in through the nose; these molecules must pass through the nasal cavity to reach the cribriform area and become soluble in the mucus that lies over the dendrites of the olfactory receptor cells.[12] The inability of odorant molecules to reach the receptor cells of the olfactory nerve (cranial nerve [CN] I) is the most common cause of olfactory dysfunction. Therefore, anosmia or hyposmia can be caused by any disease process that prevents the odorant molecules from reaching these receptor cells. The dysfunction may occur in reception or transmission. Barriers to reception may include physical barriers—polyps, septal deformities, rhinitis, and nasal tumors—or epithelial cell changes that occur with aging, trauma, and chemical or iatrogenic exposure.[3–6] Transmission may be affected by neurodegenerative diseases.[13,14]

Similar to the impact that damaged nasal mucosa receptors have on smell, damaged taste receptors (buds) can impair taste. This is especially prevalent with aging, which results in the loss of taste buds.[15,16] Other factors that can impair taste include heavy smoking, viruses, medications, chemical exposure, environmental exposure, iatrogenic exposure, and radiotherapy of the head and neck.[7,17,18] Ageusia also may result from disease of the chorda tympani or the gustatory fibers, but is rare. Lesions involving sensory pathways to the taste centers of the brain, or diseases of the taste centers of the brain itself, can also interfere with the sense of taste.[15]

CLINICAL PRESENTATION AND PHYSICAL EXAMINATION

Problems with taste and smell may or may not be associated with symptoms related to disorders that cause ageusia and anosmia. Most often, the presenting complaint is loss of taste or smell after an upper respiratory tract infection. In young adults, the loss of smell often results from head trauma. If a patient has lost or experienced a decreased sense of smell, a thorough evaluation for intranasal and intracranial disease is required. A complete medical, social (including substance use disorder and occupation), and medication history is essential to diagnosis. Onset of symptoms (gradual versus acute) and associated symptoms should also be determined since a large number of cognitively well-functioning adults with olfactory dysfunction are unaware of the condition.[19]

The physical examination should confirm the patient's subjective complaint. Assessment for the loss of taste and smell focuses on the CNs that provide information about taste and smell. CN I is a sensory nerve. Testing of this nerve begins with asking the patient to identify odors that are nonirritating and aromatic, such as coffee, isopropyl alcohol, and toothpaste. After testing of CN I, the provider should inspect the nasopharynx for abnormalities (e.g., polyps), crusting, amount of mucus present, and any signs of upper respiratory tract problems. The pharyngeal examination should determine the presence of lesions, inflammation, or exudate.[1,3,6,11,20]

The glossopharyngeal nerve (CN IX) is a mixed sensory-motor nerve. The sensory portion controls the taste sensation for the posterior third of the tongue. CN IX is tested along with the facial nerve (CN VII), which is also a mixed sensory-motor nerve. The sensory part of CN VII controls taste sensation for the anterior two thirds of the tongue. Each side of the tongue should be tested with sweet, salty, sour, and bitter flavors. The patient should protrude the tongue while identifying the taste and rinse the mouth before testing the other side. This process should be repeated with the posterior portion of the tongue.[1,3,6,11,20]

After determining whether the complaint is related to olfactory or taste dysfunction, a more comprehensive examination, including weight, vital signs, and a conscientious ear, nose, throat, and neurologic evaluation, is necessary.

ESSENTIAL DIAGNOSTICS

Assessment of odor and taste identification is an essential component of diagnostic testing for the loss of taste and smell. Two tests that are appropriate for the primary care office are the University of Pennsylvania Smell Identification Test and the Sniffin' Sticks.[20] If these tests are unavailable, the patient should be referred to a specialist for specific assessment of smell and taste dysfunction and associated causes.[21]

ADDITIONAL DIAGNOSTICS

Laboratory testing should include a complete blood count (CBC), electrolytes, blood urea nitrogen (BUN), creatinine, liver function tests (LFTs), thyroid-stimulating hormone (TSH), antinuclear antibodies, and erythrocyte sedimentation rate (ESR). If Sjögren syndrome is suspected, antibodies to Ro/SSA and La/SSB should be assessed.[22] Levels of vitamin and metal concentrations may be indicated, depending on social history. Magnetic resonance imaging (MRI) is used to evaluate soft tissues and mucosal edema; computed tomography (CT) is useful to assess the skull base and sinuses.[3] Further testing should be based on clinical presentation and physical findings.[21]

DIFFERENTIAL DIAGNOSIS

 Priority differentials include allergic and bacterial rhinitis, viral infections, head trauma, sinusitis, nasal polyps, and benign neoplasms.

The differential diagnosis for the loss of taste or smell includes disease processes that can affect the upper respiratory tract. Anosmia can also be congenital or related to a meningioma, glioma, dementia, or aneurysm. Depression can be a cause of dysosmia.[23] Aging, olfactory dysfunction, infection, radiotherapy, medications, malnutrition, Sjögren syndrome, gastroesophageal reflux, endocrine disorders, trauma, benign neoplasms, Turner syndrome, degenerative disorders (e.g., Alzheimer or Parkinson disease), occupational or environmental exposure to chemicals and metals, cancer, and cancer therapy should be considered in the differential diagnosis of taste disorders.[3,4,6,7,13]

INTERPROFESSIONAL COLLABORATIVE MANAGEMENT

Treatment will vary according to the cause of a disrupted sense of taste or smell. It is particularly important to distinguish between olfactory and taste disturbance. Treatment of rhinitis, sinusitis, infection, gastroesophageal reflux disease (GERD), or anemia may restore the lost function. If possible, medications that may be associated with this disorder should be discontinued or changed.

If the cause of the change in smell sensation seems to stem from blockage of sinuses, oral or intranasal glucocorticoid steroid treatment is effective in most cases. Other adjunct treatments may include antihistamines and leukotriene inhibitors. Referral to a specialist may be indicated if these interventions are ineffective, in which case surgery is often performed with variable effects on restoration of smell and taste.[21]

Dysgeusia, in conditions other than aging, is treated with elimination of the offending agent. The diet should be reviewed and the overuse of condiments eliminated. Treatment of GERD with a proton pump inhibitor or H_2 receptor antagonist is often effective. Tricyclic antidepressants (TCAs), because of their analgesic proprieties, may be helpful for complaints of burning mouth.[24]

CONSULTATIONS

If these measures are unsuccessful, the patient should be referred to an otolaryngologist for a comprehensive nose and throat examination. Patients with suspected central nervous system disorders or conditions that cause destruction of the neuroepithelium or its central pathway require referral to a neurologist. Patients whose symptoms are related to allergies may benefit from consultation with an allergist, whereas those with dental disorders require referral to a dentist.

- Otolaryngology referral: if suspected nasal pathway obstruction (e.g., polyps or deviated septum) and symptoms not abated with first-line primary care treatments (e.g., inhaled nasal corticosteroid). Also for persistent dysgeusia after controlling for GERD or persistent burning mouth syndrome despite first-line TCA therapy or elimination of potential medication cause.
- Neurology referral: for patients whose symptoms are suspicious for systemic central nervous system disorders (e.g., multiple sclerosis, Parkinson disease, Alzheimer disease, other neurodegenerative processes).
- Allergy referral: for poorly controlled allergic rhinitis or sinusitis despite first-line primary care interventions.
- Dental referral: if suspected dental disorder cause (if indicated by examination findings).
- Rheumatology referral: for suspected Sjögren disease (if indicated by initial laboratory test results).
- Endocrinology referral: for suspected endocrine disorders (if indicated by initial laboratory test results).
- Referral to smell and taste specialist—for any patient whose quality of life is significantly impaired or who has no easily treatable cause.[3,21]

COMPLICATIONS

Complications of smell and taste disorders include a permanent loss of smell or taste. The loss of taste and smell can indicate a serious problem, such as a brain tumor or degenerative nerve disease. The loss of these senses profoundly affects quality of life, and depression is a potential problem.[3] Patients may lose their appetite and lose weight. Olfactory and taste dysfunction can also compromise safety, with decreased sensitivity to avoid harmful substances.[1,3]

LIFE-SPAN CONSIDERATIONS
Pediatrics

- Because sinonasal disorders (allergic rhinitis, rhinosinusitis, nasal polyps, upper respiratory infections) account for the most common reasons for smell and taste disturbances, special attention to the ear, nose, and throat history and examination is called for with younger patients.[25]
- Head trauma history (e.g., sports injuries, use of helmets for recreational activities) and concussion history may help elucidate cause in pediatric patients.

Senior Adult

- Loss of taste in geriatric patients is largely related to decreased olfaction, which declines significantly with age.[4]
- Decreased smell and taste sensation may lead to potentially dangerous situations (e.g., inability to detect smell of spoiled food or gas stove that is left on; decreased appetite and food intake, malnutrition).
- Smell and taste disturbances may be early signs of neurodegenerative diseases such as Alzheimer disease or Parkinson disease.[4,7,10]
- Medications and polypharmacy should be considered in older patients as a potential cause.
- Nutritional deficiencies (e.g., zinc, copper, vitamin B_{12} or B_3) may play a role.[4]

PATIENT AND FAMILY EDUCATION AND HEALTH PROMOTION

If the sensory loss is permanent, the patient should be instructed to take extra care in avoiding harmful substances, both in environmental chemicals and in food. Patients who have lost the sense of smell should be counseled to install smoke detectors and to use electrical rather than gas appliances. Food in the refrigerator may need to be dated or handled with extra care. Personal hygiene should be based on routine and physical inspection.

REFERENCES

1. Scangas, G. A., & Bleier, B. S. (2017). Anosmia: Differential diagnosis, evaluation, and management. *American Journal of Rhinology & Allergy, 31*(1), 3–7. doi:10.4140/TCP.n.2016.624.
2. Boesveldt, S., Postma, E. M., Boak, C., Welge-Luessen, A., Schöpf, V., Mainland, J. D., et al. (2017). Anosmia—A clinical review. *Chemical Senses, 42*(7), 513–523. doi:10.1093/chemse/bjx025.
3. Devere, R. (2017). Disorders of taste and smell. *Continuum, 23*(2), 421–446. doi:10.1212/CON.0000000000000463.
4. Syed, Q., Hendler, K. T., & Koncilja, K. (2016). The impact of aging and medical status on dysgeusia. *The American Journal of Medicine, 129*(7), 753.e1–753.e6. doi:10.1016/j.amjmed.2016.02.003.
5. Li, Y., Kang, W., Zhang, L., Zhou, L., Niu, M., & Liu, J. (2017). Hyposmia is associated with RBD for PD patients with variants of SNCA. *Frontiers in Aging Neuroscience, 9,* 303. doi:10.3389/fnagi.2017.00303.
6. Ruggiero, G. F., & Wick, J. Y. (2016). Olfaction: New understandings, diagnostic applications. *The Consultant Pharmacist: The Journal of the American Society of Consultant Pharmacists, 31*(11), 624–632. doi:10.4140/TCP.n.2016.624.
7. Tarakad, A., & Jankovic, J. (2017). Anosmia and ageusia in Parkinson's disease. *International Review of Neurobiology,* doi:10.1016/bs.irn.2017.05.028. In Press, corrected proof.
8. Alvarez-Camacho, M., Gonella, S., Campbell, S., Scrimger, R. A., & Wismer, W. V. (2017). A systematic review of smell alterations after radiotherapy for head and neck cancer. *Cancer Treatment Reviews, 54,* 110–121. doi:10.1016/j.ctrv.2017.02.003.
9. Kazour, F., Richa, S., Desmidt, T., Lemaire, M., Atanosova, B., & El Hage, W. (2017). Olfactory and gustatory functions in bipolar disorders: A systematic review. *Neuroscience and Biobehavioral Reviews, 80,* 69–79. doi:10.1016/j.neubiorev.2017.05.009.
10. Doty, R. L. (2017). Olfactory dysfuncation in neurodengerative diseases: Is there a common pathological substrate? *The Lancet. Neurology, 16*(6), 478–488. doi:10.1016/S1474-4422(17)30123-0.
11. Murtaza, B., Hichami, A., Khan, A., Ghiringhelli, F., & Khan, N. (2017). Alteration in taste perception in cancer: Causes and strategies of treatment. *Frontiers in Physiology, 8,* 134.
12. Fleischer, J., Pregitzer, P., & Krieger, J. (2017). Access to the odor world: Olfactory receptors and their role for signal transduction in insects. *Cellular and Molecular Life Sciences,* doi:10.1007/s00018-017-2627-5. [Epub ahead of print].
13. Doty, R. L. (2017). Olfactory dysfunction in neurodegenerative diseases: Is there a common pathological substrate? *The Lancet. Neurology, 16*(5), 478–488. doi:10.1016/S1474-4422(17)30123-0.
14. Xydakis, M. S., & Belluscio, L. (2017). Detection of neruodegernative disease using olfaction. *The Lancet. Neurology, 16*(6), 415–416. doi:10.1016/S1474-4422(17)30125-4.
15. Iannilli, E., Broy, F., Kunz, S., & Hummel, T. (2017). Age-related changes of gustatory function depend on alteration of neuronal circuits. *Journal of Neuroscience Research, 95*(10), 1927–1936. doi:10.1002/jnr.24071.
16. Somekawa, S., Mine, T., Ono, K., Hayashi, N., Obuchi, S., Yoshida, H., et al. (2017). Relationship between sensory perception and frailty in a community-dwelling elderly population. *The Journal of Nutrition, Health and Aging, 21*(6), 710–714. doi:10.1007/s12603-016-0836-5.
17. Eaker, J. J., Öberg, S., & Rosenberg, J. (2017). Loss of smell and taste after general anesthesia: A case report. *Anesthesia and Analgesia Case Reports,* doi:10.1213/XAA.0000000000000612.
18. Skiba-Tatarska, M., Kusa-Podkańska, M., Surtel, A., & Wysokińska-Miszczuk, J. (2016). The side-effects of head and neck tumors radiotherapy. *Polski Merkuriusz Lekarski: Organ Polskiego Towarzystwa Lekarskiego, 41*(241), 47049.
19. Wehling, E., Lundervold, A. J., Espeset, T., Reinvang, I., Bramerson, A., & Nordin, S. (2015). Even cognitively well-functioning adults are unaware of their olfactory dysfunction: Implications for ENT clinicians and researchers. *Rhinology, 53*(1), 89–94. doi:10.4193/Rhin14.081.
20. Poupon, D., Hummel, T., Haehner, A., Welge-Luessen, A., & Frasnelli, J. (2017). Nostril differences in the olfactory performance in health and disease. *Chemical Senses, 42*(8), 625–634. doi:10.1093/chemse/bjx041.
21. Bhattacharyya, N., & Kepnes, L. J. (2015). Contemporary assessment of the prevalence of smell and taste problems in adults. *The Laryngoscope, 125,* 1102–1106.
22. Sefanski, A. L., Tomiak, C., Pleyer, U., Dietrich, T., Burmester, G. R., & Dörner, T. (2017). The diagnosis and treatment of Sjögren's Syndrome. *Deutsches Ärzteblatt International, 114*(20), 354–361.
23. Taalman, H., Wallace, C., & Miley, R. (2017). Olfactory functioning and depression: A systematic review. *Frontiers in Psychiatry, 8,* 190. doi:10.3389/fpsyt.2017.00190.
24. Breessan, V., Stevanin, S., Bianchi, M., Aleo, G., Bagnasco, A., & Sasso, L. (2016). The effects of swallowing disorders, dysgeusia, oral mucositis and xerostomia on nutritional status, oral intake and weigh lossi in head and neck cancer patients: A systematic review. *Cancer Treatment Reviews, 45,* 105–119.
25. Boesveldt, A., Postma, E. M., Boak, C., Welge-Luessen, A., Schöpf, V., Mainland, J. D., et al. (2017). Anosmia—A clinical review. *Chemical Senses, 42*(7), 513–523. doi:10.1093/chemse/bjx025.

CHAPTER 76

TUMORS AND POLYPS OF THE NOSE

Emily Karwacki Sheff • Jason R. Lucey • Sara Smoller • Catherine Franklin • Patrice K. Nicholas • Linda Evans

NASAL TUMORS AND POLYPS

 Immediate referral to the emergency department is indicated for any physical examination findings suggestive of airway compromise or acute neurologic changes caused by a facial mass.

Definition and Epidemiology

Primary sites for malignant tumors can occur in the nose, nasopharynx, and paranasal sinuses. The broad spectrum of malignant lesions that occur in the nose and paranasal sinuses includes carcinomas, lymphomas, sarcomas, and melanomas. The most common, however, is squamous cell carcinoma.

The most common type of benign tumor is an inverted papilloma, which arises from the common wall between the nose and maxillary sinuses. A highly vascular benign tumor, the juvenile angiofibroma, is common in adolescent boys, bleeds easily, and can cause nasal obstruction. These tumors are nonmalignant, but they can cause considerable problems as they spread through the nasopharynx.[1]

Nasal polyps represent an inflammatory disorder of the nose and paranasal sinuses that can result in chronic nasal obstruction and a diminished sense of smell. The cause of these pale, edematous masses is unknown, but the lesions are commonly seen in patients with allergic rhinitis, which predisposes them to polyp formation, asthma, and, in some patients, with acute or chronic infections.[2] Nasal polyps occur in up to one-third of patients and children with cystic fibrosis, and a majority of cystic fibrosis patients have some form of sinus disease.[3,4]

Pathophysiology

The pathophysiology of benign and malignant tumors of the nasopharynx is varied and makes diagnosis difficult. However, a basic understanding of the different pathologic conditions can assist in diagnosis. Squamous cell carcinomas arise from the keratinocytes of the epithelium. This cancer develops in normal skin, in preexisting actinic keratosis, or in a patch of leukoplakia. The incidence is higher in men and can be associated with smoking, alcohol consumption, and sunlight exposure.[5] The inverted cell papillomas develop from the squamous cells in which the epithelium is invaginated into the vascular connective tissue stroma. They are invasive and behave in a locally malignant manner. Potentially serious complications involve invasion of the orbit or cranial vault.[5] Juvenile or nasopharyngeal angiofibromas are vascular and may actually hemorrhage. These tumors may be associated with familial adenomatous polyps and almost exclusively occur in adolescent males who often have red hair and fair skin.[5] They also typically act in a locally malignant manner, spreading from the nasopharynx to the nasal cavity, the sphenoid, and the parasinuses, and may extend extradurally.

Nasal polyps originate mostly from the mucous membrane linings of the maxillary sinuses and prolapse into the nasal cavity. Polyps may be classified into four types: *antrochoanal* (non-eosinophilic, unilateral masses), *idiopathic* (unilateral or bilateral eosinophilic without lower airway involvement), *eosinophilic* (associated with asthma or aspirin sensitivity), and *polyps with underlying systemic disease* (e.g., cystic fibrosis, Churg-Strauss syndrome, Kartagener syndrome).[2]

Clinical Presentation and Physical Examination

Malignant tumors can occur in the nose, nasopharynx, and paranasal sinuses. In general, these malignant neoplasms remain asymptomatic until late in their course. Early symptoms are nonspecific, mimicking those of rhinitis or sinusitis. Unilateral nasal obstruction and discharge accompanied by pain, recurrent hemorrhage, headache, or visual or olfactory changes suggest the presence of cancer. For this reason, any patient with unilateral or persistent nasal symptoms requires thorough evaluation.

Benign nasal tumors are associated with nasal obstruction, discharge, or facial swelling. These tumors can bleed easily and cause recurrent epistaxis. The tumor is usually easily visualized because of its growth and spread.

Symptoms of nasal polyps include nasal obstruction, hyposmia or anosmia, recurrent sinusitis, headache, and postnasal drip. In some patients, nasal polyps are accompanied by intrinsic asthma and intolerance to acetylsalicylic acid.[1] A developing polyp is teardrop shaped; when mature, it resembles a peeled seedless grape.

A complete examination of the head and nasopharynx is essential. The vestibules should be inspected with a penlight while the patient's head is tipped back. The use of a nasal speculum and/or a topical vasoconstrictor spray such as phenylephrine (if available) can improve visualization of intranasal structures.[6] Each naris should be inspected for erythema, edema, discharge, bleeding, or tumor. In most cases, nasal polyps are seen bilaterally. If unilateral polyps are seen, further workup should be done to rule out a neoplasm.[2] Further examination includes pharyngeal inspection, sinus palpation, and determination of lymph node involvement.

Diagnostics

Essential Diagnostics. Endoscopic evaluation and biopsy are the gold standard for definitive diagnosis and treatment of suspected tumors.[6] Complete blood studies are necessary to determine the presence of anemia or other hematologic disease.

Additional Diagnostics. Other diagnostic testing for benign tumors and nasal polyps can include sinus X-ray studies for information about fluid levels and bone involvement, but computed tomography (CT) scan or magnetic resonance imaging (MRI) is usually indicated if tumor is suspected.

INITIAL DIAGNOSTICS

Nasal Tumors and Polyps

LABORATORY
- CBC and differential

IMAGING
- Sinus X-ray studies
- Computed tomography scan or magnetic resonance imaging[a]

———
[a]If indicated.

Differential Diagnosis

Priority differentials include: (1) benign or malignant polyps, (2) granulomatosis with polyangiitis (GPA) (Wegener granulomatosis), (3) mucoceles, and (4) granulomas without systemic involvement.

GPA, previously known as Wegener granulomatosis, is a systemic vasculitis of unknown cause characterized by glomerulonephritis plus granulomas of the nose and lung.[7] The most destructive lesions of bone, cartilage, and soft tissue of the nose and paranasal sinuses are ultimately found on biopsy to be malignant neoplasms, such as lymphomas or carcinomas. The cause of this rare disorder is unknown. Without treatment, GPA is invariably fatal; most patients survive less than a year after diagnosis.[8,9] However, the prognosis is good if the disease is diagnosed and treated early. The disease usually occurs in those older than 40 years, with equal frequency in men and women. It can also affect the skin, eyes, heart, gastrointestinal system, nervous system, and musculoskeletal system.[7]

Most patients with this condition initially complain of respiratory tract symptoms, such as nasal congestion, nasal ulcerations, rhinitis, and sinusitis. Otitis media, otorrhea, hearing loss, gingival hypertrophy, cough, dyspnea, or hemoptysis also frequently occur, and fever, weakness, malaise, weight loss, conjunctivitis, rashes or skin lesions, and polyarthralgias are other common complaints.[9] The lungs are affected in 40% of newly diagnosed patients.[9] As the disease progresses, the percentage of lung involvement progresses, eventually reaching 80%, but patients with pulmonary involvement can be asymptomatic.[9] Renal disease is rarely apparent on initial presentation, although hematuria, red blood cell casts, and impaired renal function suggest renal involvement.[10]

Physical exam findings may be absent initially despite numerous subjective complaints. If physical signs are present, they are usually associated with the upper respiratory tract and include nasal congestion and crusting, rhinorrhea, ulceration of the nasal septum, and epistaxis. The destruction of the nasal septum that results in saddle nose deformity, a characteristic sign of GPA, occurs late in the disease process. Infrequently, there may be erosions through the skin that cover the nose and sinuses.[9] If there is pulmonary involvement, localized rales, rhonchi, and wheezing can be heard during auscultation. Other physical findings include unilateral proptosis, red eye, otitis media, symmetric polyarticular arthritis, and purpura.

Interprofessional Collaborative Management

The main goal of treatment is to reduce the size of the nasal polyps thus improving the patient's symptoms. This can be achieved primarily through pharmacologic measures.

Pharmacologic Management

Glucocorticoids. The successful treatment of small polyps involves the use of nasal topical steroids. If the use of topical nasal steroids is not helpful, a 2016 Cochrane review suggested that short course of an oral corticosteroid may benefit some adults with small polyps, but more research is necessary.[11]

Antihistamines may also be used for symptom management, but have little to no effect on the polyp itself.[2]

Complementary Therapy. Research has shown that the use of topical intranasal capsaicin may be effective in treating nasal polyps. However, more studies and larger sample sizes are needed to show if a true benefit exists.[2]

Consultations: Surgical. When medical management is unsuccessful, evaluation by an otorhinolaryngologist is necessary.

Surgical removal is an option, however nasal polyps frequently return so this mainly provides symptomatic relief related to polyp size or location. Malignant tumors should be surgically excised and therefore necessitate referral to a specialist; benign tumors can be removed endoscopically.[2] If the tumor is malignant, chemotherapy or radiotherapy may be indicated.

Consultations: Rheumatologist. A patient suspected of having GPA should be referred to a specialist as soon as the disease is suspected (usually rheumatology, but nephrology or pulmonology consultation often will also be required). In general, most patients will be hospitalized for diagnosis and the initiation of treatment.

Consultations: Ear, Nose, and Throat Specialist. Nasal polyps/obstructive symptoms unrelieved by first-line primary care measures (i.e., nasal corticosteroids) merit an ear, nose, and throat (ENT) consultation. Additionally, all suspected tumors (benign or malignant) require ENT evaluation.

Life Span Considerations

Pediatric.

- Juvenile angiofibroma should be considered in the differential diagnosis of obstructive nasal symptoms, especially in adolescent males (in particular those with a fair complexion and red hair).[10]
- Cystic fibrosis patients (often children) frequently have nasal polyps or other sinus obstructive symptoms.[3]

Geriatric. Age is a risk factor for malignancy in general, and epidemiologic surveys have found that most malignant nasal cavity tumors are diagnosed when a patient is older than 60 years.[12]

Complications

Complications of benign tumors and polyps include chronic nasal obstruction and olfactory dysfunction. Patients may have frequent recurrence of the tumors or polyps, necessitating frequent surgical procedures.[2] A cancerous tumor may carry a terminal prognosis despite extensive therapy.

The complication for GPA is the inability to create a remission. If the patient does not receive early treatment, the disease is typically fatal.[9] Once proteinuria or hematuria develops, progression to renal failure can be rapid.[8] Morbidity may result from the disease or be related to toxicity from the treatment.

Emerging Management Trends

The mainstay of treatment for benign nasal polyps remains intranasal glucocorticoids with the overarching goal to reduce their size, and eliminate them if possible. With regard to nasal tumors, an increasing body of research has looked at the presence of the human papilloma virus (HPV) in nasal malignancies, including nasal tumors, and although it is still rare, management of nasal tumors has evolved to consider HPV.[12]

Patient and Family Education

Patients with benign or malignant tumors need to understand the importance of therapy. The patient should be aware of the signs and symptoms of complications or disease recurrence and the importance of continued follow-up monitoring. Patients need to understand the necessity of adherence to therapy and frequent follow-up evaluation. Medication and side effects must be explained and understood.

It is important that patients with GPA are able to recognize the signs of renal, pulmonary, and other complications. In particular, they should be alert for the recurrence of nasal discharge, sinusitis, fever, and pulmonary changes.

REFERENCES

1. Lustig, L. R., & Schindler, J. S. (2013). Ear, nose and throat disorders. In M. A. Papadakis, et al. (Eds.), *Current medical diagnosis and treatment 2018* (57th ed.). New York: McGraw-Hill.
2. Insalaco, L. (2018). Nasal polyps. In F. F. Ferri (Ed.), *Ferri's clinical advisor 2018 e-book: 5 books in 1*. Elsevier.
3. Beer, H., Southern, K. W., & Swift, A. C. (2015). Topical nasal steroids for treating nasal polyposis in people with cystic fibrosis. *The Cochrane Database of Systematic Reviews*, (6), CD008253, doi:10.1002/14651858.CD008253.pub4.
4. Haddad, J., & Keesecker, S. (2016). Nasal polyps. In R. M. Kliegman, et al. (Eds.), *Nelson textbook of pediatrics* (20th ed.). Philadelphia: Elsevier.
5. Kumar, V., Abbas, A. K., & Aster, J. C. (2015). Head and neck. In *Robbins and Cotran pathologic basis of disease* (9th ed.). Philadelphia: Elsevier.
6. Murr, A. H. (2016). Approach to the patient with nose, sinus, and ear disorders. In L. Goldman & A. I. Schafer (Eds.), *Goldman-Cecil medicine* (25th ed.). Philadelphia: Saunders.
7. Hellmann, D. B., & Imboden, J. B., Jr. (2018). Rheumatologic, immunologic and allergic disorders. In M. A. Papadakis, et al. (Eds.), *Current medical diagnosis and treatment 2018* (57th ed.). New York: McGraw-Hill.
8. Stone, J. H. (2016). The systemic vasculitides. In L. Goldman & A. I. Schafer (Eds.), *Goldman-Cecil medicine* (25th ed., p. 270, 1793–1801). Phildelphia: Saunders.
9. Reginato, A. M., & Yang, N. B. (2018). Granulomatosis with polyangitis. In F. F. Ferri (Ed.), *Ferri's clinical advisor 2018 e-book: 5 books in 1*. Elsevier.
10. Langford, C. A., Fauci, A. S., Langford, C. A., et al. (2015). The vasculitis syndromes. In D. Kasper, A. Fauci, S. Hauser, et al. (Eds.), *Harrison's principles of internal medicine* (19th ed.). New York: McGraw-Hill.
11. Head, K., Chong, L., Hopkins, C., Philpott, C., Schilder, A. G. M., & Burton, M. J. (2016). Short-course oral steroids as an adjunct therapy for chronic rhinosinusitis. *The Cochrane Database of Systematic Reviews*, (4), CD011992, doi:10.1002/14651858.CD011992.pub2.
12. American Cancer Society. (2019). Nasal cavity and paranasal sinus cancer. Retrieved from https://www.cancer.org/cancer/nasal-cavity-and-paranasal-sinus-cancer/about/key-statistics.html (Accessed May 5, 2019).

Evaluation and Management of Oropharynx Disorders

CHAPTER **77**

DENTAL ABSCESS

Erin A. Lyden

 Immediate referral is indicated for airway obstruction, trismus, unable to swallow secretions, infection spread, and systemic symptoms.

DEFINITION AND EPIDEMIOLOGY

The term *dental abscess* refers to any abscess found in tissues around the tooth. The most common type of dental abscess is an acute infection of the apical tissue.[1] These infections are often encountered in members of the general population who have untreated dental caries.[1] This type of dental abscess along with toothaches comprise more than half of all nontraumatic dental emergencies.[2] Proper evaluation and treatment of these infections are important in the prevention of life-threatening complications.[3]

PATHOPHYSIOLOGY

Poor dental hygiene resulting in dental caries, trauma, or an unsuccessful root canal can all lead to acute dental abscesses.[1] Dental abscesses arise as a result of infection by normal oral flora in a carious tooth or as a result of traumatized gingival mucosa.[2] Dental or apical abscesses begin with necrosis of the tooth pulp, leading to bacterial invasion of the pulp chamber and deeper tissues (root canals). Necrosis of these areas can occur with or without pain. However, once the bacteria are able to enter the root canal, bacteria with their toxic materials enter the periodical space, creating an inflammatory response and pus formation. This response causes acute inflammation, which initiates a cascade of signs and symptoms. The abscess in the periapical tissue, if not handled appropriately, can enter deeper fascial spaces, leading to severe infections and mortality.[1,2]

Multiple organisms are common in acute dental abcesses.[1,2] These infections are usually a blend of both facultative anaerobes and strict anaerobes. Most of the facultative anaerobes found are *Streptococcus anginosus* or viridans streptococci. The strict anaerobes most frequently identified are species including *Prevotella* and *Fusobacterium*.[1,2]

CLINICAL PRESENTATION AND PHYSICAL EXAMINATION

Abscesses usually occur in the setting of carious teeth or poor dental hygiene and cause localized pain, edema, erythema, and purulent discharge from the affected site.[1,2,4] The site may be heat sensitive and friable.[1] The tooth may be partially elevated

out of the socket and the pain responds poorly to analgesic agents. If the abscess is minor, systemic signs may not be evident. More advanced infections may be associated with fever and lymphadenitis.[4] Although pain is a common sign with this type of infection, take special note in patients who have been on glucocorticoids, have diabetes mellitus, and are of an advanced age, because they may deny pain or report only mild pain.[5]

A detailed history of the pain, symptoms, and previous dental care and procedures should be taken, followed by a thorough oral examination. Inspection of the gingiva surrounding the area of pain will reveal edema and erythema of the soft tissues and possibly a purulent discharge from a draining sinus tract.[1,3,6] The tooth may be mobile and painful to manipulation. The abscess should be visualized and palpated by the practitioner.[3] If the infection has progressed beyond the local area, orbital cellulitis, retropharyngeal space invasion, fascial plane invasion, or cavernous sinus thrombosis can occur. Signs of severe infection include trismus, airway compromise, and dysphagia. A patient unable to handle his or her own secretions or with involvement of the fascial spaces of the head and neck needs emergent care. Any patient whose outpatient therapy fails should receive inpatient treatment.[3,4]

ESSENTIAL DIAGNOSTICS

Physical examination remains the standard of diagnosis for an acute dental abscess. Routine radiologic screening is not recommended because thickening of the periodontal membrane is the only finding visible before abscess formation, and abscesses develop rapidly. Chronic abscesses may reveal a radiolucent area at the tooth apex.[2] A complete blood count (CBC) may be indicated if cellulitis is suspected. Other diagnostics depend on potential complications.

DIFFERENTIAL DIAGNOSIS

All oral lesions must be evaluated for potential malignancy. If there is doubt about the lesion, a biopsy is necessary to exclude malignant disease, especially in populations predisposed to oral cavity cancer. Individuals at high risk for oral cancers include those with a history of heavy tobacco and/or heavy alcohol use and individuals infected with human papillomavirus (HPV). Of all cancers diagnosed annually, oral cavity and pharyngeal cancer comprise approximately 3%, but a missed diagnosis significantly affects morbidity.[7]

INTERPROFESSIONAL COLLABORATIVE MANAGEMENT

Nonpharmacological Management

Management of a periapical abscess is primarily by incision and drainage (I&D).[1,2] However, definitive treatment may involve dental extraction, allowing the release of pressure and drainage of the abscess, or root canal of the involved tooth or teeth.[3,6] Emergent surgery is indicated if there is a question of airway compromise or when the patient decompensates.[8]

Pharmacologic Management

Antibiotics. Antibiotic coverage is controversial in uncomplicated abscesses and not necessarily indicated, although commonly prescribed, despite increasing concerns about antibiotic resistance.[8] If there are signs of infection in adjacent tissues, antibiotics should be used without any delay to prevent further complications. With oral antibiotic therapy, penicillin or clindamycin are first-line recommendations. Macrolide antibiotics are acceptable alternatives. If there is a known resistance in the geographic area, then amoxicillin-clavulanate should be used.[2,3] Culture of the purulent discharge can result in a more specific bacterial diagnosis, and appropriate therapy can then be implemented. Analgesics are used to provide comfort to the patient as needed.

Hydration. Hydration of the patient is necessary to ensure appropriate delivery of the antibiotic therapy chosen.[3]

CONSULTATIONS: DENTIST

Patients should be given follow-up instructions for dental consultation within 2 to 3 days of I&D.[3]

COMPLICATIONS

Complications arising from dental abscesses can range from minor to life-threatening. Minor complications include the need for antibiotic therapy, dental extraction, or endodontic work (i.e., root canal). Major complications can include orbital cellulitis, fascial plane infections, osteomyelitis, dentocutaneous fistula, cavernous sinus thrombosis, and bacteremia with sepsis.[2,5] Up to 57% of deep neck-space infections may be caused by dental abscesses.[3] In addition, the life-threatening complication of Ludwig angina is a possibility. This infection of the deep mandibular space is manifested with trismus, drooling, induration of the tongue and submandibular area, tachypnea, and dyspnea. Airway compromise can occur. Ludwig angina is rare in children.[1,2,5]

INDICATIONS FOR REFERRAL OR HOSPITALIZATION

Dental abscesses are comanaged with dentists or endodontists to ensure adequate resolution of the initial infection, to prevent complications, and to institute preventive treatment. When signs and symptoms of periodontal abscess, periodontitis, bacteremia, orbital cellulitis, cavernous sinus thrombosis, or fascial plane involvement are present, prompt hospitalization and team management with a dentist or endodontist and an infectious disease consultant are indicated.[9] Other indications for hospitalization include edema and erythema of the eyelids, exophthalmos, and conjunctival edema. Deep neck-space infection is also an indication for hospitalization.[1,2]

PATIENT AND FAMILY EDUCATION AND HEALTH PROMOTION

Early and proper dental care prevents most dental infections. Ninety-one percent of adult Americans have dental caries. It is important that primary care providers stress the importance of regular care and proper dental checkups.[9] Twice-daily brushing, flossing, and appropriate dental hygiene should be stressed. Early care of carious teeth can prevent future dental infections.

Fluoride treatment of the local water supply and dietary fluoride supplements are excellent preventive measures.[10,11]

REFERENCES

1. Ogle, O. E. (2017). Odontogenic infections. *Dental Clinics of North America*, 61 http://dx.doi.org/10.1016/j.cden.2016.11.004.
2. Siqueira, J. F., & Rocas, I. N. (2013). Microbiology and treatment of acute apical abscesses. *Clinical Microbiology Reviews*, 26(2), 255–273.
3. Hodgdon, A. (2013). Dental and related infections. *Emergency Medicine Clinics of North America*, 31, 465–480.
4. Laudenbach, J. M., & Simon, Z. (2014). Common dental and periodontal diseases, evaluation and management. *The Medical Clinics of North America*, 98(2014), 1239–1260.
5. Durso, S. C. (2011). *Oral manifestations of disease. Harrison's principles of internal medicine* (18th ed.). New York: McGraw Hill.
6. Wadia, R., & Ide, M. (2017). Periodontal emergencies in general practice. *Primary Dental Journal*, 6(2).
7. National Cancer Institute. SEER stat fact sheets: oral cavity and pharynx cancer. Retrieved from http://seer.cancer.gov/statfacts/html/oralcav.html; (Accessed May 15, 2018).
8. Cope, A., Francis, N., Wood, F., Mann, M. K., & Chestnutt, I. G. (2014). Systemic antibiotics for symptomatic apical periodontitis and acute apical abscess in adults. *The Cochrane Database of Systematic Reviews*, (6), CD010136.
9. American Dental Association. Six ways to prevent adult cavities. Infographic. https://www.mouthhealthy.org/en/~/media/MouthHealthy/Files/Infographics/ADA_MH_6ways_Flyer. (Accessed May 15, 2018).
10. Hathaway, B., Grandis, J. R., & Johnson, J. T. (2015). Dental infection and its consequences. In D. Schlossberg (Ed.), *Clinical infectious disease*. New York: Cambridge University Press. ch 8.
11. American Dental Association. ADA applauds USPHS final recommendation on optimal fluoride level in drinking water. Retrieved from www.ada.org/en/public-programs/advocating-for-the-public/fluoride-and-fluoridation/ada-applauds-hhs-final-recommendation-on-optimal-fluoride-level-in-drinking-water; (Accessed May 15, 2018).

CHAPTER **78**

DISEASES OF THE SALIVARY GLAND

Lisa M. O'Neal

 Immediate referral is indicated for patients with suspected salivary gland malignancies.

DEFINITION AND EPIDEMIOLOGY

The salivary glands include the paired parotid glands, the submandibular and sublingual glands, and numerous minor salivary glands found in the upper aerodigestive tract; these glands produce saliva to aid in the breakdown of food. Diseases that affect the salivary glands are divided into neoplastic and nonneoplastic categories.[1] The nonneoplastic category is further divided into infectious and noninfectious origins; neoplastic diseases are either benign or malignant. Acute suppurative sialadenitis (bacterial parotitis) is covered in Chapter 81.

Salivary gland infections are found in all age groups and populations and can be encountered in the primary care setting. However, malfunction of the salivary gland is most common in adults and typically involves a decrease in the production of saliva.[1] Malignant neoplasms involving the salivary glands account for less than 5% of all head and neck tumors, not including skin cancers.[2] The distribution of salivary tumors is more common among men than women.[3] Salivary tumors can occur at any age, and the risk of developing a salivary gland cancer increases with age. The average age at time of diagnosis is 64 years.[3]

Salivary tumors in older adults most commonly affect the parotid glands.[1] Radiation treatment to the head and neck and work-related exposure to certain radioactive substances may increase one's risk of developing a salivary gland cancer.[3] Work-related exposure is also a concern for those working with silica or nickel dust, asbestos mining, manufacture of rubber products, and some types of woodworking.[3] There does not appear to be any increased incidence of salivary gland cancer from inheritance or in individuals with a history of family members with salivary gland cancer.[3] A diet low in vegetables and high in animal fat may increase one's risk for developing salivary gland cancer.[3] Cell phone use was shown in a singular study to increase the risk of developing benign parotid gland tumors. However, other studies have shown no relation; research is still ongoing.[3]

PATHOPHYSIOLOGY

Recurrent parotitis, sialolithiasis (salivary gland stones), branchial cleft anomalies, Sjögren syndrome (SS), xerostomia, ptyalism (hypersalivation), sialosis, and benign lymphoepithelial lesion of Godwin are classified as noninfectious salivary gland disorders. Sialectasis (dilation of a salivary duct, either acquired or congenital) can lead to recurrent parotitis. Dilation of the duct and gland can be produced by either stone formation or strictures. Sialolithiasis, which mainly affects the submandibular glands, refers to the formation of stones or calculi in the glands. The stones are predominantly hydroxyapatite, and there may be more than one.[4] The higher mucin content of the saliva produced in the submandibular glands, combined with an antigravity flow of saliva, contributes to stone formation.[5] The stagnant saliva in the gland also leads to the formation of stones. Elevated serum levels of calcium and phosphorus are not associated with stone formation.[5] First branchial cleft anomalies affect the salivary glands, primarily the paired parotid glands. Infected cysts and sinus tracks associated with these anomalies usually are initially seen in the preauricular area and can affect the facial nerve.[4]

SS is an autoimmune disorder that affects the salivary glands. On pathologic evaluation, a lymphocytic infiltrate with acinar atrophy, ductal epithelial hyperplasia, and metaplasia can be found. Benign lymphoepithelial lesion of Godwin is an inflammatory condition often found in association with human immunodeficiency virus (HIV) infection. It can be confused pathologically with malignant lymphoma, metastatic carcinoma, sarcoidosis, or chronic sialadenitis.[6]

Xerostomia means dry mouth. Several diseases, as well as radiotherapy (RT) and drug therapy, cause these symptoms. The production of excess saliva is called ptyalism; drug treatments (atropine) and other medical conditions are usually the underlying causes.[1] Sialosis refers to bilaterally recurring salivary gland edema. Acinar cell hypertrophy, interstitial edema, and striated duct atrophy may be present on pathologic examination. Alcoholism, metabolic disorders such as diabetes and various vitamin deficiencies, obesity, and malnutrition also initiate enlargement of the salivary glands. Certain drugs, including the phenothiazines, heavy metals, thiourea, and iodide-containing substances, cause salivary gland enlargement as a result of their cholinergic effects.[7]

Infectious diseases that affect the salivary glands include mumps parotitis (which is the most common cause of

suppurative acute siladenitis, with 85% of cases occurring in children younger than 15 years)[8] and other viral infections, syphilis, HIV infection, and granulomatous diseases. Granulomatous diseases affecting the salivary glands include tuberculosis, sarcoidosis, cat-scratch disease, uveoparotid fever (Heerfordt syndrome), and actinomycosis.[4]

Neoplastic changes also affect the salivary glands. Studies have shown that 2% to 4% of all head and neck neoplasms are salivary gland tumors.[4] The majority of salivary gland tumors involve the paired parotid glands, whereas 8% of salivary gland tumors are found in the submandibular glands and 22% in the minor glands.[4]

Benign tumors that involve the salivary glands have been classified by the World Health Organization (WHO) into 13 subtypes. Because of the epithelial and myoepithelial tissue components of the salivary glands, the tumors are defined by their dominant tissue type.[4] Of the benign tumors, pleomorphic adenoma (PA) is the most common and is most frequently found in the parotid gland. Warthin tumor, also known as adenolymphoma, is the second most common benign neoplasm of the salivary glands; this tumor is cystic and is found solely in the parotid glands.[4] Studies have questioned whether or not Warthin tumors are truly parotid neoplasms but rather a disease of the parotid lymph nodes.[4]

The remaining subtypes of benign epithelial tumors make up approximately 15% of all tumors.[4] Diagnosis is dependent on definitive histology of the benign neoplasm.[4]

Malignant tumors of the salivary glands have been classified by WHO into 24 subtypes. The parotid gland is the most common site for metastatic disease. The majority (60% to 70%) of patients will have mucoepidermoid carcinoma (MEC), adenoid cystic carcinoma, acinic cell carcinoma, or polymorphous low-grade adenocarcinoma.[4,9]

MECs are the most common cancers of the major and minor salivary glands and are most commonly seen in the parotid gland. Furthermore, MEC has been found to have a strong predilection for the lower lip.[8] The majority of MECs are low or intermediate grade and can be surgically treated. However, if the MEC is high grade, there is greater potential for metastasis.[4]

Adenoid cystic carcinoma accounts for approximately 10% of the malignant salivary gland tumors overall, but 30% of the minor salivary gland tumors.[4] These types of tumors often manifest with a nerve palsy because of their predilection for perineural spread. Prognosis after 10 to 15 years is poor (mortality 80% to 90%) because of metastases to other organs.[4]

Acinic cell carcinomas are found predominantly (80%) in the parotid gland and are slow growing and can be a cause of facial weakness. They can occur in both parotids and can metastasize to the cervical lymph nodes and can reoccur.[4]

CLINICAL PRESENTATION AND PHYSICAL EXAMINATION

Presentation of salivary gland inflammation and infection can vary greatly, because some patients will be completely asymptomatic whereas others will have pain, fever, chills, and other concerns. The noninfectious entities that cause enlargement of the salivary gland usually manifest with painless swelling of the salivary gland. One exception is sialolithiasis, evidenced by painful edema of the affected gland and increased symptoms with meals, "meal-time syndrome."[4] Patients with sialolithiasis oftentimes have a history of recurrent acute suppurative siladenitis.[8] SS, commonly seen in women aged 40 to 60 years, is associated with connective tissue diseases such as rheumatoid arthritis, polyarteritis nodosa, and systemic lupus erythematosus. SS symptoms are associated with the classic xerostomia, abnormal taste, keratoconjunctivitis sicca, dry tongue, and intermittent unilateral or bilateral swelling of the salivary gland.[4,10] Bilateral salivary gland cysts characterize the benign lymphoepithelial lesion of Godwin, whereas a lack of saliva is associated with xerostomia; excess saliva production results in ptyalism. Other conditions associated with ptyalism include epilepsy, cerebral palsy, rabies, and stomatitis.

Infectious diseases of the salivary glands usually cause a rapid onset of colicky pain with meals, edema, induration of the affected gland, malaise, and chills.[6] Additional exam findings in an infectious process include a tender, swollen gland and tender lymphadenopathy. With HIV infection, generalized parotid gland enlargement and xerostomia can be presenting features.[4]

Benign and malignant processes of the salivary gland are seen initially as painless, slow-growing, unilateral masses. These may be cystic, as in Warthin tumor. A prior history of radiation therapy may be elicited. A small number of patients complain of pain, and a few have facial nerve paralysis or palsy.[4] Squamous cell carcinoma and malignant mixed tumors have a history of rapid growth and may manifest with facial pain and fixation of underlying structures. The salivary glands may also be the sites of metastatic spread of other malignant neoplasms of the head and neck, most commonly squamous cell carcinoma and malignant melanoma; the primary sites are found above the clavicles.[5] Primary malignant lymphomas have been reported but are rare. Firm lymphadenopathy is associated with malignancy. In general, all salivary tumors should be surgically excised to confirm diagnosis and decrease morbidity and mortality.[8]

The superficial location of the salivary glands allows the practitioner to thoroughly inspect and palpate the glands during physical examination. Inspection includes visual observation of the head, mouth, and neck. Both the major and minor salivary gland regions are inspected for enlargement.[4,8] Salivary gland swelling is more discrete, larger, and smoother than swelling of lymphatic origin. Any facial nerve paralysis is noted, because this type of paralysis can be indicative of a malignant parotid neoplasm.[4] Intraoral inspection includes visualization of the duct orifices to identify obstruction.[4]

Nonneoplastic, noninfectious diseases of the salivary glands manifest as unilateral or bilateral swelling of the affected gland. In the case of sialolithiasis, a stone may be palpated in the submandibular duct, or parotid stones may be noted at the orifice of the Stensen duct.[5] SS, xerostomia, and keratoconjunctivitis accompany unilateral or bilateral swelling of the salivary gland. Dry papillae on the tongue may be present. Bilateral cystic masses may be palpated with a benign lymphoepithelial lesion of Godwin. Sialosis manifests as a bilateral, recurrent swelling of the affected glands.

Infectious diseases of the salivary gland result in inflammation, edema, and bilateral or unilateral involvement of the gland. Purulent discharge is present in acute bacterial infections. With a localized parotid abscess, pitting edema may be found. In viral infections such as mumps parotitis, which is highly contagious and can be spread via airborne droplets of salivary, nasal, and urinary secretions, a bilaterally and painfully enlarged gland and difficulty in opening the jaws (trismus) may be encountered.[5,8]

Neoplastic diseases are usually distinguished by painless, firm masses that may be fast or slow growing. Patients seen late in the course of their disease may exhibit paralysis of the facial nerve, fixation of underlying structures, palpable neck lymphadenopathy, and possible skin involvement.[4,8] If a patient presents with nonacute facial weakness, examination of the parotid gland is indicated, and if a mass is found upon palpation, immediate referral to an otolaryngologist is indicated.[8]

DIAGNOSTICS

Essential Diagnostics

Evaluation of salivary gland disease relies heavily on the patient's history and physical examination. It is important for the health care practitioner to determine chronicity and whether there is a history of chronic inflammatory disorders.[4] Patients often have vague complaints of pain and/or swelling with few or no other symptoms; therefore diagnosis can be difficult. Radiographic diagnostic studies (i.e., sialography, plain-film radiography, computed tomography [CT], and magnetic resonance imaging [MRI]) are extremely useful in clarifying the cause of vague symptoms.[9] In patients with known salivary gland disease, radiographic diagnostic studies can aid in planning and treatment of the disease.[4] Ultrasound combined with fine-needle aspiration cytology (FNAC) or core biopsy examination is useful, economical, and accurate in the diagnosis of major salivary gland disease and differentiation of malignant from benign disease in 90% of cases.[10] Ultrasound with FNAC is able to distinguish between salivary stones and cystic and noncystic disease.[10] Diagnostic examination of the deep parotid salivary gland lobes with ultrasound and FNAC is limited owing to location of these lobes near the mandible.[4]

Fine-needle aspiration is indicated for patients with chronic parotid lesions to exclude tuberculous parotitis, an uncommon disorder.[6]

A culture of purulent discharge from the affected ducts is performed if one suspects infectious entities. Anaerobic cultures diagnose actinomycosis. Systemic evaluation of blood serum establishes a diagnosis of HIV infection, mycobacterial disease, toxoplasmosis, and tularemia.[6]

Additional Diagnostics

Depending on the etiology of the salivary gland disorder, further diagnostic studies can be used to identify the underlying pathology and subsequent treatment can be prescribed. For example, identification of acid-fast bacilli on microscopy and culture, via drainage of pus or aspiration, gives a definitive diagnosis of *Mycobacterium tuberculosis*.[4] Cat-scratch disease is indicated with the presence of serum immunoglobulin G (IgG) and IgM.[4]

Viral titers are requested if viral infectious agents such as mumps paramyxovirus are suspected. Antibodies to the S and V antigen at levels greater than 1:192 are expected with mumps. Mumps virus can be isolated in urine samples. CT scans or ultrasonographic evaluations of the glands are used to exclude neoplastic disease. Sialography in conjunction with conventional radiographic films is used to diagnose sialolithiasis.[4] Conventional radiography is used to diagnose submandibular gland stones because 65% of these are radiopaque. SS is diagnosed by minor salivary gland biopsy, usually performed on the mucosal surface of the lip, and by measurement of salivary flow and autoantibodies (anti-Ro and anti-La).[4] Lidocaine with epinephrine is not used for this biopsy procedure because the epinephrine interferes with the pathologic diagnosis. Most recent studies have determined that salivary gland ultrasonography (SGUS) has good sensitivity and high specificity in differentiating SS from undifferentiated connective tissue diseases that have common symptoms of SS.[10] Rheumatoid factors and antinuclear factor levels should be measured, serum protein electrophoresis performed, autoantibodies SSA and SSB assessed, and other autoimmune study results obtained, if indicated by the history and examination.

INITIAL DIAGNOSTICS

Diseases of the Salivary Glands

LABORATORY
- Culture of discharge[a]
- Viral titers[a]

IMAGING
- Computed tomography scan[a]
- Ultrasound of salivary gland[a]

OTHER
- Fine-needle aspiration biopsy with cytology[a]
- Oral mucosa biopsy (lip)[a]
- Sialography[a]
- Skin testing[a]

———
[a]If indicated.

DIFFERENTIAL DIAGNOSIS

 Priority differentials include malignant tumors affecting the salivary glands: (1) mucoepidermoid carcinoma, (2) acinic cell carcinoma, (3) adenocarcinoma, (4) adenoid cystic carcinoma, (5) malignant mixed tumors, and (6) squamous cell carcinoma.[4]

The differential diagnosis of noninfectious, nonneoplastic salivary gland disease includes drug therapy, sialolithiasis, branchial cleft anomalies, SS, xerostomia, ptyalism, and metabolic disorders such as diabetes. Infectious conditions that can affect the salivary gland are numerous and include HIV infection; viral infections caused by mumps paramyxovirus, cytomegalovirus, and Epstein-Barr virus; bacterial infections, including *Staphylococcus aureus* and streptococci, tuberculosis, tularemia, actinomycosis, and cat-scratch disease; and parasitic diseases such as toxoplasmosis.[6]

Neoplastic involvement of the salivary glands includes both benign and malignant disease. Included in the differential diagnosis for benign lesions are PA, Warthin tumor, monomorphic adenoma, and oncocytoma.

The salivary glands can also be the site of metastatic disease to the head and neck. Included in these metastatic tumors are malignant melanoma, squamous cell carcinoma, and lymphoma. Primary malignant lymphoma of the salivary glands has been reported but is rare.[4]

INTERPROFESSIONAL COLLABORATIVE MANAGEMENT

- Indications for referral include recurrent or chronic symptoms, suspected neoplasm or salivary stone, or infection or swelling that is unresponsive to treatment and complications from infection.

- Management of many noninfectious diseases of the salivary glands is conservative and is conducted by a team of qualified health care providers. This includes pain management and hydration. Many noninfectious, nonmalignant salivary gland problems are caused by lack of adequate hydration. Recurrent parotitis may be treated with surgical removal of the affected gland if the patient remains symptomatic. Sialolithiasis is managed with warm compresses, analgesics, and sialagogues. Sialagogues are agents that stimulate the production and flow of saliva, such as lemon balls and chewing gum. Fluid and electrolyte replacement should be addressed. Surgical removal of the offending stone may be required, as well as a consultation with an otolaryngologist. Branchial cleft anomalies are treated with surgical excision. SS is treated symptomatically with local and systemic therapy to address the xerostomia and xerophthalmia.[11] Ptyalism may require surgical intervention, intraparotid injections of botulinum toxin A, or neodymium:yttrium-aluminum-garnet (Nd:YAG) laser treatment.[10] Furthermore, a specialist in autoimmune disease should be consulted.[3]

- Management of infectious diseases of the salivary glands depends on the cause of the disease. Management of acute suppurative parotitis is discussed in Chapter 81. Viral infection of the salivary glands, most commonly caused by the mumps paramyxovirus, requires conservative therapy that consists of adequate hydration, rest, and possibly diet modification. Hospitalization and consultation with infectious disease specialists is necessary if infection progresses to involve other organs or structures.[4] Infections that are suspected to be HIV infection should be evaluated by an HIV specialist. Granulomatous infection of the salivary glands should be treated with the appropriate agents. Tubercular infections and nontubercular mycobacterial infections may require surgical removal because these infections may not respond to traditional therapies. Actinomycosis is treated with intravenous penicillin G, followed by oral clindamycin (PNC) for several months.[12] Doxycycline or sulfamethoxazole can be substituted if the patient is allergic to penicillin.[11] Surgical removal may be required. Cat-scratch disease can be treated symptomatically without antibiotic therapy. Toxoplasmosis can be treated with combination therapy that consists of pyrimethamine and trisulfapyrimidines, although in most cases this regimen is reserved for those who have systemic disease, are immunocompromised, or are pregnant.[6] Parenteral antibiotics, such as the aminoglycosides streptomycin and gentamicin, can be used for tularemia. Tetracycline has also been used for tularemia but with mixed results.

- Suspected benign or malignant salivary gland masses are managed surgically. With surgery involving the parotid gland, preservation of the facial nerve is critical unless the nerve is already nonfunctional or has tumor involvement. A superficial parotidectomy is the surgical procedure of choice. Some surgeons propose that both the deep and superficial lobes of the parotid gland be treated with a total parotidectomy. Tumors of the minor salivary glands are treated with surgical excision. The extent of the procedure is dictated by the tumor site and the disease.[4]

- Neck dissection performed at the time of the surgical procedure may be indicated for tumors larger than 4 cm (1⅗ inches), cancers that originate in the submandibular gland, and primary squamous cell carcinoma. If there is undifferentiated carcinoma or high-grade MEC, a neck dissection is performed at the time of the initial surgery.[4]

- RT as a primary treatment modality is no longer recommended, although postoperative RT may be necessary for certain tissue types.[10] A recent analysis comparing the effectiveness of adjuvant chemoradiotherapy (CRT) versus RT alone for patients older than 66 years with locally advanced salivary gland carcinoma was conducted. The results showed that adjuvant CRT was associated with an increased risk of mortality and hospitalization with treatment-related toxicity compared with adjuvant RT alone.[12]

COMPLICATIONS

Complications of diseases of the salivary glands include recurrent bouts of salivary gland swelling, pain, and stone formation, which may necessitate surgical intervention. Xerostomia produces serious dental caries because of the lack of saliva. Saliva has properties that aid in the prevention of caries. Dry mouth seriously affects the patient's quality of life, necessitating dietary changes and frequent sips of water. Infectious causes of salivary gland disease have a potential for sepsis. Encephalitis, orchitis, meningitis, and cochleitis are serious consequences of mumps paramyxovirus infection. On occasion, development of islet cell antibodies leading to acute onset of type 1 diabetes can occur. Bacterial infections and granulomatous diseases can be serious in patients who are immunocompromised. Patients diagnosed with SS have a significantly increased risk of developing mucosa-associated lymphoid tissue lymphoma (MALT).[4]

Benign tumors of the salivary gland rarely cause complications unless they are neglected and invade the facial nerve, underlying structures, or overlying skin. The recurrence rate is low for tumors excised appropriately and properly. However, malignant tumors of the salivary glands can be difficult to treat. Tumors such as adenoid cystic carcinoma, squamous cell carcinoma, and adenocarcinoma may metastasize to other local and regional sites. To ensure a good outcome, it is important to initiate appropriate surgical consultation if a tumor is suspected.[4]

PATIENT AND FAMILY EDUCATION

Patients should be encouraged to examine themselves for signs of salivary gland disease. Painful or painless swelling of the salivary glands, xerostomia, ptyalism, and purulent discharge from salivary gland ducts are important conditions to investigate. Patients undergoing prolonged surgical procedures, especially gastrointestinal procedures, should maintain adequate hydration to avoid acute suppurative sialadenitis.

HEALTH PROMOTION

Important topics for health promotion include adequate hydration, attention to oral hygiene, and immunizations. In addition, it is important that the patient be instructed to avoid risk factors such as radiation exposure, tobacco smoking, and exposure to animals that may be vectors of disease.

REFERENCES

1. Schiff, B. A. (2016). Salivary gland disorders, The Merck Manual. Retrieved from https://www.merckmanuals.com/professional/ear,-nose,-and-throat-disorders/tumors-of-the-head-and-neck/salivary-gland-tumors.html. (Accessed 6 April 2018).
2. Chernichenko, N., Linkov, G., Li, E., Bakst, R. L., Chen, C., He, S., et al. (2013). Oncoloytic vaccinia virus therapy of salivary gland carcinoma. *JAMA Otolaryngology–Head & Neck Surgery*, *139*(2), 173–182.
3. American Cancer Society. (2017). Salivary gland cancer. Retrieved from https://www.cancer.org/cancer/salivary-gland-cancer/about/what-is-key-statistics.html. (Accessed 6 April 2018).
4. Bradley, P., & O'Hara, J. (2012). Diseases of the salivary glands. *Surgery*, *30*(11), 611–616.
5. Jackson, N. M., Mitchell, J. L., Walvekar, R. R., et al. (2010). Inflammatory disorders of the salivary glands. In C. W. Cummings, P. W. Flint, & B. H. Haughey (Eds.), *Otolaryngology: Head and neck surgery* (5th ed.). Philadelphia, PA: Elsevier.
6. Cummings, C. W., Haughey, B. H., Thomas, J. R., et al. (2010). *Otolaryngology: Head and neck surgery* (5th ed.). Philadelphia: Elsevier.
7. Miranda-Rius, J., Brunet-Llobet, L., Lahor-Soler, E., & Farré, M. (2015). Salivary secretory disorders, inducing drugs, and clinical management. *International Journal of Medical Sciences*, *12*(10), 811–824. http://doi.org/10.7150/ijms.12912.
8. Wilson, K. F., Meier, J. D., & Ward, P. D. (2014). Salivary gland disorders. *American Family Physician*, *89*(11), 882–888.
9. Durso, S. C. (2014). Oral manifestations of disease. In D. Kasper, A. Fauci, S. Hauser, D. Longo, J. Jameson, & J. Loscalzo (Eds.), *Harrison's principles of internal medicine, 19e*. New York, NY: McGraw-Hill. http://accessmedicine.mhmedical.com.ezproxy.simmons.edu/content.aspx?bookid=1130&sectionid=79725733. (Accessed April 06, 2018).
10. O'Connor, R., Mitchell, D. A., & Brennan, P. A. (2014). Focused review of investigation, management and outcomes of salivary gland disease in specialty-specific journals. *The British Journal of Oral and Maxillofacial Surgery*, *52*, 483–490.
11. Papadakis, M. A., & McPhee, S. J. (Eds.), (2017). Actinomycosis. In *Quick medical diagnosis & treatment*. New York, NY: McGraw-Hill. http://accessmedicine.mhmedical.com.ezproxy.simmons.edu/content.aspx?bookid=2033&sectionid=152400803. (Accessed April 08, 2018).
12. Tanvetyanon, T., Fisher, K., Padhya, T., Otto, K. J., Caudell, J. J., & Trotti, A. (2015). Adjuvant chemo-radiotherapy (CRT) versus radiotherapy (RT) alone for locally advanced salivary gland carcinoma among older population: SEER-Medicare analysis. *Journal of Clinical Oncology*, *33*(15_suppl), 6028.

CHAPTER 79

EPIGLOTTITIS
Lisa M. O'Neal

 Immediate emergency department referral or physician consultation is indicated for patients with suspected epiglottitis as it can lead to sudden respiratory obstruction and death.

DEFINITION AND EPIDEMIOLOGY

Epiglottitis (supraglottitis) is an acute inflammation of the supraglottic region of the oropharynx characterized by inflammation and edema of the epiglottis, vallecular, arytenoids, and aryepiglottic folds.[1] Owing to the high vascularity and loose mucosa of the epiglottic region, sudden airway obstruction and possible death can result.[1] Epiglottitis is typically caused by a bacterial infection and less commonly results from a viral illness or caustic and thermal injury to the epiglottis. Thermal epiglottitis is a rare and potentially life-threatening disease caused by direct thermal injury or inhalation of steam or aspiration of heated liquids.[2,3] Crack cocaine use in teens and young adults has also been associated with thermal injury to the hypopharynx.[4]

Epiglottitis is a rare but serious life-threatening condition because of the potential for laryngospasm and irrevocable loss of the airway.[2] From the 1950s to the early 1990s, epiglottitis typically occurred more often in children than in adults. The most common bacterial pathogen responsible for epiglottitis in children was *Haemophilus influenzae* type B (Hib). More recently, however, the incidence of epiglottitis in adults has shown a steady increase and is approximately 2.5 times greater than that in children.[5,6] In the United States, epiglottitis in adults is estimated to be 1 to 4 in 100,000 per year.[7] The dramatic decline in childhood epiglottitis is due to the advent of the vaccination for *Haemophilus* organisms.[1] Overall, the incidence is now decreasing in all age groups, possibly as a result of a general decrease of Hib disease in the general population. It should be noted, however, that a recent case report found *H. influenzae* type A as the responsible pathogen for severe invasive disease in countries with a Hib vaccination program.[8] Other pathogens associated with epiglottitis include groups A, B, and C streptococci; *Streptococcus pneumoniae*; *Klebsiella pneumoniae*; *Candida albicans*; *Staphylococcus aureus*; *Haemophilus parainfluenzae*; *Neisseria meningitidis*; varicella-zoster virus; and various other viral pathogens.[9]

Male predominance is reported with epiglottitis; however, male/female ratios have varied. The mean age of adults with epiglottitis is 44.94 years.[10] There is no seasonal predilection for epiglottitis; however, two studies have shown an increase in cases during the summer months.[5]

Epiglottitis among adults may follow an unpredictable clinical course, ranging from relatively benign disease to rapidly progressive disease with acute airway obstruction and possibly death. Recent studies have noted the increased incidence of adult epiglottitis without identifying a causative pathogen.[6] The mortality rate for children is less than 1%, but the mortality rate for the adult population is in the range of 6% to 7%.[6]

PATHOPHYSIOLOGY

Various microorganisms can cause epiglottitis. In the postvaccine era for children younger than age 5, Hib continues to be an important cause of epiglottitis.[8] In patients with underlying disease, *Aspergillus, Klebsiella,* and *Candida* organisms have been identified. A viral cause has been postulated for some cases of adult epiglottitis, especially the milder cases. Traditionally, epiglottitis is associated with an infectious organism, bacteria, combined viral-bacterial infections, and fungi.[6] Investigators have identified noninfectious causes of epiglottitis, which can include inflammation in association with thermal injury (crack cocaine and marijuana smoking), ingestion of caustic substances (automatic dishwashing detergent), systemic disease (diabetes mellitus, hypertension, obstructive pulmonary disease, seizure disorder, alcohol and drug abuse, tobacco smoking), chemotherapy for head and neck cancer, trauma by foreign objects, and burns associated with bottle-fed infant formula.[5,11,12]

CLINICAL PRESENTATION AND PHYSICAL EXAMINATION

Patients with epiglottitis are initially seen with an acute occurrence of severe odynophagia, dysphagia, fever, and shortness of breath with sitting up and leaning forward in an effort to enhance air flow.[9,12] Other complaints include the inability to swallow their own secretions, neck tenderness, lymphadenopathy, cough, drooling, stridor, respiratory distress, and hoarseness. The patient may adopt the tripod position (leaning forward with hands braced on the knees), using accessory muscles for respiration.[5] Dyspnea and stridor are common signs of epiglottitis in children, whereas odynophagia, dysphagia, and voice change are common presenting symptoms in adults.[12] The onset and duration of symptoms before the patient's initial contact with the health care provider vary. Depending on the severity of symptoms, patients may seek treatment after having symptoms for less than 8 hours, or they may have had them for more than 4 days.

The physical exam of patients requires precautions. If epiglottitis is suspected, the pharynx should not be examined with a tongue depressor, because this may precipitate an airway emergency. Any inspection of the oral cavity requires that emergency airway management equipment be immediately available in case of laryngospasm; laryngospasm can cause sudden airway occlusion.

Patients with epiglottitis may or may not have fever and a toxic appearance, depending on the severity of the infection or the cause of the inflammation. Generalized toxemia is a result of acute epiglottitis.[12] If assessment of the adult patient reveals the presence of anterior neck tenderness with severe sore throat, epiglottitis should be suspected.[5] Patients experiencing respiratory distress, posturing in the upright "sniff" or tripod position, dysphagia, and refusal to swallow are all reliable signs of epiglottitis.[5] Indirect laryngoscopy may reveal an erythematous, edematous epiglottis with a narrow glottic opening. Substernal and supraclavicular retractions, tachycardia, tachypnea, and inspiratory stridor are common. With severe respiratory distress, changes in mental status, anxiety, pallor, cyanosis, and other signs of hypoxia may be present.

DIAGNOSTICS
Essential Diagnostics

The gold standard for a definitive diagnosis of epiglottitis is made by direct visualization via laryngoscopy with a flexible fiberoptic scope or a laryngeal mirror.[13] It provides accurate visualization of the epiglottis and it shows the extent of epiglottic swelling.[5] Examination via fiberoptic laryngoscope should be done with caution as it can precipitate airway obstruction.[14] Indirect laryngoscopy is considered a safe diagnostic tool in the adult population but not in children.[15] A recent study showed that sonography is an accurate, noninvasive, and rapid diagnostic tool for epiglottitis in the emergency setting.[16] A positive diagnosis of epiglottitis is achieved by evaluating the diameter of the anteroposterior diameter of the epiglottis.[16]

A lateral neck film can be useful but is not always diagnostic in the adult population.[14] Findings on the lateral neck film suggestive of epiglottitis include a swollen epiglottis manifesting as a "thumbprint" sign (Fig. 79.1).[17,18] Because they have a low sensitivity rate (true positives), lateral neck films are not a true diagnostic tool and are being replaced with direct visualization of the epiglottis with fiberoptic nasopharyngoscopy.[17] It should be noted that if the thumbprint sign is present, it is a significant predictor for imminent airway compromise and rapid clinical deterioration.[12] Prophylactic airway management is not indicated for an adult with epiglottitis; however, securing the airway should take precedence over the performance of laboratory examinations or radiologic studies.[3] Computed tomography (CT) and magnetic resonance imaging (MRI) are not commonly used for the diagnosis of epiglottitis; however, they are useful in the evaluation of complications (infection and abscess formation) of epiglottitis.[14]

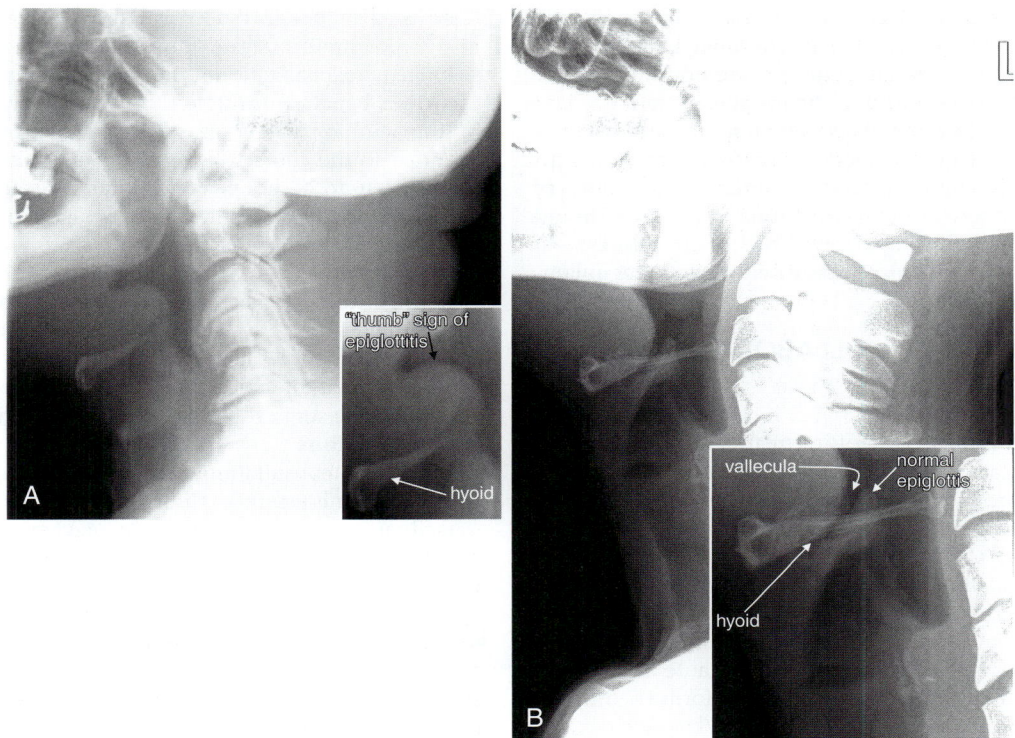

FIG. 79.1 Epiglottitis in an adult. (A) Lateral cervical soft-tissue X-ray showing epiglottitis in a 64-year-old man. The epiglottis is thickened, showing a classic "thumb sign." (B) Normal soft-tissue X-ray for comparison. The brightness and contrast have been increased to point out the normal thin epiglottis, which is partially hidden behind the hyoid bone. The vallecula is seen as a narrow space anterior to the epiglottis. An anterior-posterior (AP) X-ray is not shown for this case, because the AP view is not usually diagnostic in cases of epiglottitis. (From Broder, J. [2011]. *Diagnostic imaging for the emergency physician.* Philadelphia: Saunders.)

Additional Diagnostics

A complete blood count (CBC) often reveals leukocytosis with a shift to the left and bandemia.[15] Blood cultures may be obtained to guide antibiotic therapy and exclude septicemia. Recent literature indicates that microbiologic studies are not very helpful, because no definite organism is identified in the majority of cases of epiglottitis in adults.[5] The low percentage of positive pharyngeal and blood cultures is presumed to be related to anaerobic bacterial causes or cases of partially treated disease.[5] Analysis of arterial blood gases (ABGs) may also be indicated.

DIFFERENTIAL DIAGNOSIS

 Priority differentials include conditions causing airway obstruction: (1) foreign body aspiration, (2) caustic ingestion, (3) angioedema, (4) anaphylaxis, (5) diphtheria, and (6) peritonsillar and retropharyngeal abcess.[10]

Multiple conditions have a similar presentation. The differentials that should be considered are Ludwig angina, retropharyngeal and peritonsillar infections, tumor, caustic ingestions, allergic drug reactions, laryngeal trauma, uvulitis, bacterial tracheitis, angioedema, foreign body aspiration, and thermal injury.

Signs and symptoms of Ludwig angina, retropharyngeal abscess, and peritonsillar cellulitis or abscess are similar to those of epiglottitis because all are associated with an infectious process. Ludwig angina is a severe diffuse form of cellulitis with an acute onset affecting the submental, sublingual, or submandibular spaces. Clinical presentation of Ludwig angina includes clinical signs of fever, dysphagia, inability to swallow, and stridor.[19] Ludwig angina typically results from a dental infection and can be easily diagnosed by CT scan.[19] Retropharyngeal abscess can also be identified by CT scan and can be excluded by negative findings on physical examination.[20] Peritonsillar cellulitis or abscess can be excluded by negative physical examination findings.

INITIAL DIAGNOSTICS

Epiglottitis

- Airway stabilization mandatory before further diagnostic evaluation
- Pulse oximetry

LABORATORY
- CBC and differential
- Blood cultures with sensitivities
- ABGs

IMAGING
- Sonography (Ultrasound)
- Lateral neck X-ray examination, chest X-ray examination

OTHER DIAGNOSTICS
- Fiberoptic nasopharyngoscopy in the emergency room or surgical suite[a]

[a]Primary recommended imaging diagnostic.

A tumor, gastroesophageal reflux disease, trauma to the larynx, allergic drug reaction, or angioedema may manifest with signs similar to those of epiglottitis. A tumor or trauma to the larynx may cause sore throat, hoarseness, dysphagia, and respiratory distress; however, infectious findings are negative. Allergic drug reactions or angioedema typically manifest with respiratory distress and dermatologic findings.[5] A history of illicit drug use or thermal injury or trauma to the neck should be elicited. Crack cocaine vaporizes at high temperatures, and the extreme heat of the inhaled vapors may incite acute inflammation of the epiglottis.[3]

INTERPROFESSIONAL COLLABORATIVE MANAGEMENT

Airway Management

- Immediate mainstay of epiglottitis treatment is airway management. Patients should be allowed to sit upright in a quiet environment with humidified oxygen. Treatment of epiglottitis consists of close observation for airway management, antibiotics if indicated, and in some cases, steroids. The patient should be hospitalized in the intensive care unit for aggressive airway monitoring. Sedation, racemic epinephrine, and inhaled medications should be avoided. The patient is considered to have an unstable airway, and equipment should be at the bedside to perform cricothyrotomy or emergent intubation if necessary.[10,21]
- Isolation is sometimes recommended for the first 24 hours after the initiation of antibiotic therapy. Patients with an increased risk of airway obstruction (those with respiratory distress, tachycardia, tachypnea, or increased white blood cell count) may require an artificial airway by intubation or tracheotomy; an anesthesia provider should be immediately available. Intubation is preferred, if indicated, over tracheostomy because of the ease of removal of the endotracheal tube a couple of days after edema has subsided, the absence of surgical complications, and lower or equal mortality and complication rates.[15] Continuous oxygen therapy and monitoring of oxygen saturation are necessary.[12]

Pharmacologic Management

Intravenous Broad-Spectrum Antibiotics

- Intravenous broad-spectrum antibiotics should be initiated as soon as possible.[22] In the past, the usual treatment for epiglottitis was ampicillin and chloramphenicol; however, because of ampicillin-resistant *H. influenzae*, this regimen is no longer recommended.[23] Chloramphenicol is considered a second-line treatment,[23] but is not often used because of the increased risk of aplastic anemia.
- Until culture and sensitivity results are available, second- and third-generation cephalosporins (e.g., ceftriaxone given intravenously; cefotaxime), ampicillin-sulbactam, clindamycin, or levofloxacin is the recommended treatment.[5,23] Adult doses are as follows: ceftriaxone 50 to 75 mg/kg IV once/day (max 2 g/day),[1] cefotaxime 2 g every 4 to 8 hours, or ampicillin-sulbactam 1.5 to 3 g every 6 hours.[15] Antibiotic treatment is for 10 to 14 days.[15] Vancomycin is a consideration if methicillin-resistant *Staphylococcus aureus* (MRSA) or sepsis is a concern.
- Although many experts advocate the use of steroids, it is not a universal standard of treatment.[24,25] However, in the absence of any specific contraindications, a short course of steroids (i.e., dexamethasone or budesonide aerosols) can

be used to possibly decrease airway inflammatory edema and potentially negate the need for intubation and prolonged hospitalization. Randomized controlled trials that prove a benefit from steroid use are not available.[5,12]

- If anaerobic bacteria are suspected, metronidazole may be added to the course of therapy.[5] Epiglottitis should resolve within 36 to 48 hours after initiation of treatment; this can be confirmed via flexible laryngoscopy. If not, other diagnoses should be considered.[5]

Vaccination

- If epiglottitis has been found to be caused by *H. influenza* type B, it can be effectively prevented with the HiB vaccine.[1]

Surgery

- Management of epiglottitis caused by abscess formation will require surgical debridement by a specialist.[14]

Consultations

- Immediate consultation with otolaryngology and an anesthesiologist is essential. Consultation of the aforementioned facilitates initial safe airway management. An infectious disease specialist should be consulted if the patient does not respond to empiric antibiotics.

LIFESPAN CONSIDERATIONS

With the changes in the ages of those affected by Hib infection, careful evaluation of all age groups is suggested. As noted, epiglottitis is becoming a commonly found condition in adults as compared to children.[24] However, if epiglottitis is suspected in a child with stridor, examination of the pharynx or larynx should be avoided because it can precipitate complete airway obstruction.[1] Instead, the child's airway must first be secured via nasotracheal intubation prior to subsequent interventions.[1] Furthermore, a recent study found that adults with diabetes mellitus and other comorbidities such as respiratory problems or compromised immunity, are at an increased risk for developing acute epiglottitis.[24] Additionally, it was found that diabetic patients with acute epiglottitis have a higher incidence of developing total airway obstruction in a shorter amount of time.[24] Patients of older age (50+),[25] a body mass index greater than 25.0, epiglottic cyst, or pneumonia upon admission had a significant increase in developing severe epiglottitis.[24,26] A suspicion of epiglottitis should prompt an immediate referral to an emergency department capable of airway support. A careful history, including illicit drug use, should be documented.[8]

COMPLICATIONS

Epiglottitis is a serious and potentially fatal condition. Death from airway obstruction may result. Rapid and careful intervention is required in an effort to avoid life-threatening complications. Other potentially fatal complications include septicemia and meningitis, resulting from the spread of infection. Other complications, such as pulmonary edema, epiglottic abscess, vocal cord granuloma, and pneumomediastinum, have been reported.

EMERGING MANAGEMENT TRENDS

Patients with acute epiglottitis necessitate immediate intervention because it is a true airway emergency. Furthermore, studies have shown that airway management is not only the immediate priority in treatment of acute epiglottitis, but also determines the initial prognosis.[21]

Spontaneous respiration using intravenous anesthesia and high-flow nasal oxygen (STRIVE Hi) is a new and upcoming airway management technique that combines the benefit of high-flow nasal oxygen (HFNO) and spontaneous ventilation. This new technique has proven to preserve airway patency, carbon dioxide levels, and oxygenation in patients with severe airway obstruction or respiratory compromise. Use of STRIVE Hi in the management of acute epiglottitis can increase patient safety during intubation because it provides continuous positive airway pressure, reduces airway resistance, and improves airway patency.[21] This technique has also been found to facilitate a controlled tracheostomy, which in some cases of airway obstruction is required.

PATIENT AND FAMILY EDUCATION

Explanation of all procedures is necessary to allay patient and family anxiety. The importance of the medical regimen should be stressed to enhance adherence. If steroids are prescribed, information on steroids and tapering of doses must be reviewed. If illicit drug use is documented, education and referral for counseling should be attempted. The causes of thermal epiglottitis should be discussed with patients who are at risk for the injury (parents of children, illicit drug users).[2]

HEALTH PROMOTION

Health promotion should include an age-appropriate immunization status review. Cases of thermal inhalation injuries resulting in epiglottitis have been documented in crack cocaine users. Caustic ingestions, foreign bodies, and other thermal inhalations have also resulted in signs and symptoms of epiglottitis.[2]

REFERENCES

1. Saski, C. T. (2016). Epiglottitis (Supraglottitis). The Merck Manual. Retrieved from https://www.merckmanuals.com/professional/ear,-nose,-and-throat-disorders/oral-and-pharyngeal-disorders/epiglottitis. (Accessed 4 April 2018).
2. Kudchadkar, S. R., Hamrick, J. T., Mai, C. L., Berkowitz, I., & Tunkel, D. (2014). The heat is on … thermal epiglottitis as a late presentation of airway steam injury. The Journal of Emergency Medicine, 46(2), e43–e46.
3. Rajeshwari, S. (2011). Acute upper airway obstruction in children and adults. Trends Anaesth Crit Care, 1(2), 67–73.
4. Singh, A., Thawani, R., & Kshitij, T. (2017). Crack cocaine–induced laryngeal injury. The American Journal of Emergency Medicine, 35(2), 381.e5–381.e7.
5. Al-Qudah, M., Shetty, S., Alomari, M., & Alqdah, M. (2010). Acute adult supraglottitis: Current management and treatment. Southern Medical Journal, 103(8), 800–804.
6. Pourmortez, M., Chaudhari, D., Litchfield, J., & Young, M. (2016). Acute epiglottitis in immunized adults. Tennessee Medicine E-Journal, 2(1), Article 3. Retrieved from http://ejournal.tnmed.org/home/vol2/iss1/3 WAS 9.
7. Pang, C., & Mohammed, R. (2017). Acute epiglottitis in an older person. Age and Ageing, 46(3), 531.
8. Cerqueira, A. M., Tsang, R. S. W., Jamieson, F. B., & Ulanova, M. (2014). A case of acute epiglottitis caused by Haemophilus influenza type a in an adult. JMM Case Rep, 1(3), 1–6.
9. Harris, C., Sharkey, L., Koshy, G., Simler, N., & Karas, J. A. (2012). A rare case of acute epiglottitis due to Staphylococcus aureus in an adult. Infect Dis Rep, 4(1), e3.
10. Lindquist, B., Zachariah, S., & Kulkarni, A. (2017). Adult epiglottitis: A case series. The Permanente Journal, 21, 16–89. PMC.
11. Shah, R. K., & Stocks, C. S. (2010). Epiglottitis in the United States: National trends, variances, prognosis and management. The Laryngoscope, 120, 1256–1262.
12. Abdallah, C. (2012). Acute epiglottitis: Trends, diagnosis and management. Saudi J Anaesth, 6(3), 279–281.
13. Westerhuis, B., Bietz, M. G., & Lindemann, J. (2013). Acute epiglottitis in adults: An under-recognized and life-threatening condition. South Dakota Medicine: The Journal of the South Dakota State Medical Association, 66(8), 309–311, 313.
14. Chen, C., Natarajan, M., Bianchi, D., Aue, G., & Powers, J. H. (2018). Acute Epiglottitis in the immunocompromised host: Case report and review of the literature. Open Forum Infectious Diseases, 5(3), ofy038. doi:10.1093/ ofy038.
15. Behlau, I. (2015). Croup, supraglottitis, and laryngitis. In D. Schlossberg (Ed.), Clinical infectious disease (2nd ed.). Cambridge, UK: Cambridge University Press.
16. Ko, D. R., Chung, Y. E., Park, I., Lee, H. J., Park, J. W., You, J. S., et al. (2012). Use of bedside sonography for diagnosing acute epiglottitis in the emergency department: A preliminary study. Journal Ultrasound Med, 31(1), 19–22.
17. Takata, M., Fujikawa, T., & Goto, R. (2016). Thumb sign: Acute epiglottitis. BMJ Case Reports.
18. Angirekula, V., & Multani, A. (2015). Images in clinical medicine. Epiglottitis in an adult. The New England Journal of Medicine, 372(5), e20.
19. Candamourty, R., Venkatachalam, S., Ramesh Babu, M. R., & Suresh Kumar, G. (2012). Ludwig's angina—an emergency: A case report with literature review. J Nat Sci Biol Med, 3(2), 206–208.
20. Bellis, M., Herath, J., & Pollanen, M. S. (2016). Sudden death due to acute epiglottitis in adults: A retrospective review of 11 postmortem cases. The American Journal of Forensic Medicine and Pathology, 37(4), 275–278.
21. Lee, P. K.-G., Booth, A. W. G., & Vidhani, K. (2018). Spontaneous respiration using intravenous anesthesia and high-flow nasal oxygen (STRIVE hi) management of acute adult epiglottitis: A case report. A&A Practice, 10(4), 73–75.
22. Kjaerulff, A. M., Rusan, M., & Klug, T. E. (2017). Clinical evaluation of intravenous ampicillin as empirical antimicrobial treatment of acute epiglottitis. Acta Oto-Laryngologica, 138(1), 60–65.
23. Barker, B., & Brightling, C. (2017). Pharmacological treatment of bacterial infections of the respiratory tract. Anaesthesia & Intensive Care Medicine, 12(11), 522–525.
24. Ma, J. G., & An, J. X. (2018). Acute epiglottitis in a diabetic adult patient. Chinese Medical Journal, 131(1), 109–110.
25. Chroboczek, T., Cour, M., Hernu, R., Baudry, T., Bohé, J., Piriou, V., et al. (2015). Long-term outcome of critically ill adult patients with acute epiglottitis. PLoS ONE, 10(5), e0125736. https://doi.org/10.1371/journal.pone.0125736.
26. Suzuki, S., Yasunaga, H., Matsui, H., Fushimi, K., & Yamasoba, T. (2015). Factors associated with severe epiglottitis in adults: Analysis of a Japanese inpatient database. The Laryngoscope, 125(9), 2072–2078.

CHAPTER 80

ORAL INFECTIONS

Erin A. Lyden • Lisa M. O'Neal

Immediate referral is indicated for any known or obvious oral infection with systemic symptoms and no other obvious cause.

DEFINITION AND EPIDEMIOLOGY

The American Academy of Periodontology has emphasized the direct connection between oral health and general health; accordingly, it is imperative for providers to treat oral infections and to promote oral hygiene.[1] The most common oral infectious lesions are candidiasis, herpes labialis, and recurrent aphthous stomatitis.[2,3] Other oral lesions are also discussed in this chapter because their recognition is important in the differential diagnosis of systemic disease or oral cavity cancer.

Viral infections of the mouth include those caused by the common herpes simplex virus types 1 and 2 (HSV-1 and HSV-2). HSV-1 is the type most associated with oral lesions, believed to infect up to 90% of the population.[3] However, it is estimated that only 40% have symptomatic outbreaks.[3] Human papillomavirus (HPV) is also found in the oral cavity, manifesting with papillomatous soft tissue lesions. HPV can be transmitted by direct contact, including sexual contact. HPV-associated cancers are estimated to make up 30% of cancers in the United States.[3]

ons of the mouth frequently cause periodon-
Oral bacterial infections are under intense
use they have been linked to systemic dis-
liovascular disease and diabetes.[1]

ns is the most common fungus to infect
the oral cavity. ungal infections of the mouth are encountered across the spectrum of patient age. Thrush, or candidal
infection of the oral mucosa, is caused by the overgrowth
of *C. albicans*, fungi that are normally found in the flora of
the gastrointestinal tract. Reports state that as many as 50%
of adults may have *Candida* as part of their normal oral flora.
Immunocompromised hosts and patients who wear dentures
are susceptible to these oral mucosal lesions, as are patients
with diabetes, ulcerative colitis, Crohn disease, gluten sensitivity, or poor oral hygiene, and others with poor general health.
These lesions may occur from infancy through maturity and
can be a recurrent source of irritation. Inhaled steroids are also
a risk factor for candidiasis.[3]

Aphthous ulcers (recurrent aphthous ulceration, canker
sores) are defined as shallow, painful, and often recurrent
lesions of the oral mucosa. These are the most common oral
mucosal lesions in North America.[3,4] Prevalence is estimated
at 5% to 50%.[4] Aphthous ulcers typically affect adolescents
and young adults, with more females than males affected. Incidence has been noted to be 20% to 40% in the general population.[3] Patients with known ulcerative colitis, Crohn disease,
or gluten-sensitive enteropathy may have aphthous ulcers as a
feature of these conditions.[3,4]

Stomatitis is a general term that refers to the inflammation of
the soft tissues of the oral cavity. Chemical or heat injuries can
initiate stomatitis; aspirin can cause an ulcerative lesion when
it is used as a topical anesthetic on the oral mucosa. Burns
sustained from hot food or liquids can also cause mucosal
irritations. Certain food substances, chewing gum, oral mouth
rinses, and dental products can induce painful lesions.[3]

Aphthous ulcers and stomatitis are often encountered in
primary care practice. Other entities are associated with oral
lesions and may include mechanical irritation, drug reactions,
local trauma (broken teeth, cheek gnawing), nutritional deficiencies, and stress. These forces irritate and inflame the sensitive oral mucosa. Conditions may be localized to the oral
mucosa or associated with systemic disease; therefore, it is
important to accurately diagnose and appropriately care for
oral lesions.[3,4]

PATHOPHYSIOLOGY

Herpes labialis occurs when HSV-1 is introduced to the oral
mucosa through oral secretions. After the initial outbreak, the
virus typically remains in the trigeminal ganglion (HSV-1)
and is commonly reactivated at a later time.[3,5] HPV invades
the mucosal epithelium and the basal layer, where the viral
DNA infects the host DNA. Over 150 HPV types have been
identified, of which only nine are known to cause cancer and
another six are being investigated. HPV type 16 is mostly associated with oral cavity malignancy.[6]

Gingivitis is most commonly associated with bacterial overgrowth in persons with poor oral hygiene. As few as 4 or 5
days without oral care can initiate the infectious process, and
continued inattention to dental health can eventually lead to
tooth and bone loss.[7] Research has now proven the significant
role that oral health and gingivitis have in the development of
coronary heart disease, atherosclerosis, and stroke.[8]

Overgrowth of *C. albicans* (thrush) occurs when the normal
oral flora is out of balance or when the host immunity is
somehow compromised.[9]

Aphthous ulcers are a common presenting problem for all
age groups. Although the exact cause of these ulcers is unknown,
it is thought to be autoimmune in nature.[2] Other proposed
etiologic factors include physical or emotional stress; trauma
associated with physical, chemical, or local agents; deficiencies
of vitamin B_{12}, folic acid, or iron; familial or genetic predisposition; microbial agents; and hypersensitivity states such
as gluten-sensitive enteropathy.[4] Generalized stomatitis may
be caused by poor oral hygiene, ill-fitting dentures, and nicotine abuse. Mechanical trauma, chemical trauma from caustic
substances, or hot foods may also traumatize the mucosa.[3]
Thrush more typically occurs with underlying diabetes or with
immunocompromised states. Parenteral antibiotic and steroid
use have been implicated as precursors to oral candidiasis.[2,3]

CLINICAL PRESENTATION AND PHYSICAL EXAMINATION

Patients with herpes simplex typically report a prodromal set
of symptoms that include localized pain, tingling, and burning
with erythema.[2,3] These symptoms are followed by the eruption of vesicles that evolve into painful ulcerative lesions.[3] The
patient may experience an incubation period of 4 to 7 days
after exposure.[2]

The lesions of HSV are vesicular with an erythematous base.
The vesicles may coalesce and ulcerate before healing. Recurrent lesions may be triggered by fever, stress, and exposure to
sunlight.[3] Rarely, can this infection be severe and result in secondary bacterial infections or affect visceral organs.[5]

HPV infections manifest as white, verrucous lesions individually or in clusters. The lesions can be found on the lips, hard
palate, or gingiva. They are painless but may become ulcerative
in response to local trauma.[6] The Pap smear is currently the
screening tool for genital HPV, but there is currently no screening examination for oral HPV.[5]

The candidal infection, thrush, usually appears as white,
cottage cheese–like lesions that are easily removed with a swab.
The underlying tissue may bleed after manipulation. Children
with thrush may have a white coating in the mouth, and they
often have difficulty feeding.[2,3] Patients with xerostomia may
have thrush more often, because saliva is an oral protectant
against overgrowth of this yeast.[2,3]

Gingivitis manifests as an inflammation of the gingiva,
possibly with areas of ulceration with or without purulent discharge from the affected areas.[7] Patients typically report bleeding with eating (hard food such as chips and crusty breads) or
tooth care. Chronic gingivitis may cause only minimal findings.[1,3] However, even minor manipulation of the gingiva may
cause local bleeding.[9]

Aphthous ulcers are painful, shallow ulcerations of the
nonkeratinized oral mucosa and occur as solitary or multiple
lesions. A prodrome of burning or pricking of the oral mucosa
has been reported.[4] The lesions may be recurrent but are not
typically found on the anterior hard palate or gingiva.[3] Ranging
in size from 2 mm to several centimeters, aphthous ulcers may
have a gray-yellow, pseudomembranous base surrounded by
erythema. The disease itself is self-limited, usually lasting 10 to
14 days depending upon the offending cause.[4]

There are three categories of aphthous ulcers. Minor aphthous ulcers are the most common and range in size from 2 to

10 mm (0.08 to 0.4 inch); healing occurs during 7 to 14 days. Many people attribute these minor ulcers to stress, trauma, or even menses. Major aphthous ulcers may be seen as painful lesions that are larger than 1 cm in diameter and are often in a state of cyclic eruption. Scarring is associated with these lesions. The third category is the herpetiform ulceration, which is often mistaken for lesions of HSV. These lesions are small (2 to 3 mm [0.08 to 0.12 inch]), are widely scattered or closely grouped, and may be recurrent. Cultures of these lesions are negative for virus.[2,3]

DIAGNOSTICS

Essential Diagnostics

Herpes simplex infection can be diagnosed based on clinical presentation. However, several laboratory methods exist to verify diagnosis, including Tzanck smear, viral culture of specimens taken from an active lesion, and serum antibody titers.[2,3]

HPV lesions may be tentatively diagnosed based on physical examination; excisional biopsy and pathologic evaluation provide definitive diagnosis. Specific typing of the virus is accomplished with immunohistochemical evaluation.[3]

Candidal infections can also be diagnosed based on the physical examination and presentation, but a microscopic examination of oral scrapings will reveal the classic findings of hyphae. Cultures on a mycologic medium (Sabouraud dextrose agar, Pagano-Levin) may be obtained for confirmation.[2,3]

Gingivitis is diagnosed by physical examination; no diagnostic studies are required. If a specific cause is suspected (systemic disease, medication), the appropriate laboratory test may be requested.[1,3,8]

Aphthous ulcerations and lesions of nicotinic and traumatic stomatitis are diagnosed based on clinical presentation and physical examination.[2-4]

Additional Diagnostics

Laboratory examination may be performed to assess the patient's state of health or confirm diagnosis. This may include complete blood count (CBC); serum glucose; erythrocyte sedimentation rate; serum iron, folate, and vitamin B_{12} levels; potassium hydroxide (KOH) examination; and Tzanck smear.[2-4]

DIFFERENTIAL DIAGNOSIS

 Priority differentials include: (1) oral carcinoma, (2) aphthous ulcers, (3) drug reactions, (4) nutritional deficiencies, (5) systemic disease (diabetes, Crohn disease, Behçet syndrome, hand-foot-and-mouth disease), (6) immune dysfunction, and (7) infectious causes (bacterial, viral, fungal).

Carcinoma of the oral cavity should be suspected with oral erosive lesions that are slow to heal (longer than 2 weeks without resolution) or with thickened white patches that adhere to the oral mucosa.[6] Although similar in appearance to aphthous ulcers, herpetic lesions originate from vesicles and are usually found only on the oral mucosa attached to bone structures. Additional causes of mucosal ulceration that are indicative of systemic disease include bullous pemphigoid,[2] Behçet syndrome, Crohn disease, ulcerative colitis, immune dysfunction, and hand-foot-and-mouth disease.[3,4]

Bullous pemphigoid is a cutaneous disorder in which lesions commence as fixed urticarial plaques followed by clear bullae that appear on both normal and urticarial areas. This chronic eruption primarily affects flexor surfaces but may be generalized. The lesions occur in crops and transiently affect the oral mucosa.[2]

Behçet syndrome produces ulcerative lesions on oral and genital areas, with associated symptoms of uveitis and arthritis. Involvement of the central nervous system is less common; the ocular effects of Behçet syndrome include retinal vasculitis and necrosis. Loss of vision can occur, even with aggressive treatment.[3,4]

The lesions of Crohn disease affect the mucosal surfaces of the gastrointestinal tract, including the oral cavity. Extensive or recurrent oral lesions necessitate careful evaluation for gastrointestinal symptoms, investigation of immune status, and screening for diabetes or other systemic disorders.[2,4]

Hand-foot-and-mouth disease less commonly affects the buttocks and proximal extremities. This viral disease produces a mild, self-limited illness. Inquiry concerning the sudden onset of gastrointestinal symptoms is helpful when clear vesicular lesions that ulcerate are found in the mouth and on the hands and feet.[2,3]

INTERPROFESSIONAL COLLABORATIVE
Management

Management of Herpes Simplex Virus Infection

- Management of localized oral manifestations of HSV infection in immunocompetent patients may include the topical applications (e.g., zinc oxide, zinc sulphate), antiviral ointments or oral antiviral medications such as acyclovir and valacyclovir. Anesthetic creams can also be implemented to ease symptomatic pain.[5] These agents may be most effective if they are taken when the patient is in the prodromal phase.[2] Recent meta-analysis has shown that use of a topical corticosteroid with an antiviral shortened healing time and had a significantly lower recurrence rate.[5]
- Symptomatic treatment of acute and recurrent herpes labialis should always include hydration, analgesia, antipyretics, and nutritional support. Recurrent episodes of herpes labialis may benefit from oral suppressive therapy with antiviral agents.[2,3]

Management of Oral Papillomas

- Oral papillomas are currently treated by surgical excision. There are HPV vaccines currently targeting genital HPV; in the recent past, these vaccines were not approved for prevention of oral papillomas. However, new study results have shown that the HPV vaccination significantly reduces oral HPV infection, which is a considerable risk factor for developing oropharyngeal cancer.

Management of Candidal Infections

- Candidal infections may be treated in several ways because antifungal agents are now supplied in many forms. A nystatin oral suspension, 4 to 6 mL, four times daily for 7 to 14 days, and troches are commonly prescribed.[9] For patients with dentures, nystatin powder is applied to the dentures three or four times daily. Oral clotrimazole troches, 10 mg, five times daily, or miconazole mucoadhesive buccal 50-mg tablet applied to the mucosal surface once daily for 7 to 14 days, are also widely prescribed.[9] Antifungal creams may be applied under dental appliances. Some infections, considered moderate to severe, may respond only to systemic therapy with fluconazole, 100 to 200 mg/day for 14 days (reduce dose for creatinine clearance <50 mL/min).[9] Patients with recurrent candida infections should be checked for diabetes.

- In patients with diabetes, maintenance of proper glucose levels is an important therapeutic component.[2,3]

  Management of Gingivitis
- Gingivitis is commonly treated with attention to oral hygiene. Brushing twice daily, with greater importance on brushing before bedtime, and flossing at least once daily is recommended.[1] When gingivitis inflammation is present, interdental cleaning with an interdental brush (IDB) is preferred for effective plaque removal.[7] Management of gingivitis is considered to be both a primary and secondary prevention strategy with regard to periodontitis and secondary periodontitis, respectively.[7]

  Management of Aphthous Stomatitis (Aphthae, Canker Sores)
- Aphthous stomatitis can be a vexing problem because recurrence is common. Treatment is directed at symptomatic relief. Methods of symptomatic relief with unclear benefit include the application of topical steroids (e.g., triamcinolone in Orabase, a dental paste) or a steroid mouth rinse with betamethasone syrup.[4] Dexamethasone elixir, 0.5 mg/mL, 5-mL swish and spit four times daily, has been used in adults for severe or recurrent episodes.
- Current treatments that are likely to reduce the severity and duration of episodes but are not likely to affect recurrence rates include (1) carbamide peroxide (Gly-Oxide) rinse, or bismuth subsalicylate (Kaopectate) and diphenhydramine (Benadryl) mixed in equal measures and applied to the irritated surfaces as a mouth rinse six times a day, and (2) avoidance of irritating, acidic, hot, or spicy foods.
- Other treatments with likely benefit are varied mouth rinse preparations. Viscous lidocaine is also used as a rinse, but careful observation is needed because this treatment may affect the swallowing and gag reflexes.
- Amlexanox oral paste, $\frac{1}{4}$ inch of paste four times daily after oral care, is also indicated. Several preparations or "mouthwash" recipes have been developed to assist in the relief of patients with aphthous stomatitis. One such compounded suspension consists of 30 mL of diphenhydramine elixir and 60 mL of Mylanta (aluminum and magnesium hydroxide), taken as a 5-mL swish and swallow three times daily and at bedtime.[4] Another compound is 60 mL of Maalox and 4 g of sucralfate used in the same manner.[4]
- Other treatments include a combination of diphenhydramine liquid, dexamethasone, nystatin suspension, and tetracycline (from capsules), swished and swallowed, 1 tsp six times a day (after and between meals and at bedtime).[4] Advice from a pharmacist should be obtained concerning this formulation.
- Acemannan oral gel or rinse, as needed, can be used to soothe irritated tissue. For children and those in whom tetracycline is prohibited, amoxicillin-clavulanate can be substituted for the tetracycline.[4] However, severe eruptions may respond only to systemic steroids.
- A recent study found that using a desiccating agent may accelerate the healing process. More specifically, HybenXTM (Epien Medical s.r.l.), which is a concentrated mixture of sulfates, and a desiccating agent consisting of 50% sulfuric acid and 28% sulfonated phenolics.[4]

CONSULTATIONS

Severe cases of aphthous ulcers may need referral for assessment of the patient's immune status and need for systemic therapy.[2]

A physician or subspecialist in infectious diseases should be consulted if questions arise concerning possible carcinoma or if the patient is immunocompromised. Patients with routine eruptions are not candidates for hospitalization, but severely immunocompromised patients or patients with diabetes may need hospitalization for treatment of the underlying disease.[2,3] Alcohol or tobacco use and HPV infection increase the risk for oral cancers, and patients with ulcers or nonhealing lesions present for more than 2 weeks without resolution or improvement should be referred for evaluation.[6] Patients with obvious poor dental hygiene should be referred to a dentist.

LIFE-SPAN CONSIDERATIONS

HPV infection is the most common sexually transmitted disease in the United States. Infection by the specific HPV 16 virus is the precursor to about 70% of oropharyngeal cancers.[6] Oropharyngeal cancers are also more prevalent in young white men.[6] One current vaccine, Gardasil, protects against HPV 16. Consequently, if vaccinated with Gardasil, the likelihood of contracting HPV infection and subsequent sequalae, can be significantly reduced or possibly eliminated.[6] "The National Advisory Committee on Immunization Practices recommends routine HPV vaccination for girls and boys ages 11 and 12, as well as individuals ages 13 to 26 if they haven't received the vaccine already."[6] Most recently, Gardasil has been approved for use in boys and men (9 to 26 years of age). Practitioners should stress the importance of getting vaccinated before the patient reaches sexual age, as it provides the best protection.

COMPLICATIONS

Complications associated with HSV oral infections are uncommon in immunocompetent individuals. In immunosuppressed patients, these infections may lead to widespread systemic infections.[2,3,5]

Candidal infections of the oral cavity can be managed without complication in most instances. However, care should be taken to identify patients who may be immunocompromised or nutritionally at risk so that their needs can be adequately assessed.[2]

Gingivitis is not considered to cause acute complications, but long-term inattention to oral hygiene can lead to painful and costly periodontitis and tooth loss. Investigators are researching the role of periodontal disease in the development of heart disease and have most recently implicated oral infections, specifically periodontitis, as a risk factor for development of atherosclerotic cardiovascular disease (CVD).[1,7,8]

Aphthous stomatitis is usually a short-lived entity with few if any complications. In patients with major aphthous ulcers, oral intake should be monitored.[2]

Oral HPV infection is often a silent disorder until the patient becomes symptomatic or an oral lesion is identified by a health care provider. HPV has been implicated in some oropharyngeal cancers, particularly cancer of the tonsils.[9]

PATIENT EDUCATION AND HEALTH PROMOTION

HSV infections are spread by contact with the virus, and this can include sharing of lip balms or other materials with a viral carrier. Kissing and sharing of drinking utensils should be avoided to prevent the spread of the virus. Asymptomatic viral shedding occurs frequently, and avoidance of contact only when lesions are present does not offer protection.[2,3,5] These same precautions should be offered to individuals with manifestations of HPV infection. Orogenital contact is a common method of transmission of HPV, and this information should be shared with the individual and his or her partner. Education about the risk of HPV-related oral cancer is essential.[3,6]

Practitioners should inform and educate patients about HPV vaccination. Recent studies show that HPV vaccination is correlated with cancer prevention. Furthermore, the HPV vaccine may also provide further protection against oral HPV infections that are linked to oropharyngeal cancers.[9] Alcohol and tobacco cessation should also be discussed with patients, and appropriate cessation programs or medications should be referred.

Candidal infections can be anticipated in patients who are taking long courses of steroids and antibiotics; treatment of these patients should be started as soon as symptoms occur. Patients who are known to be immunocompromised should be monitored regularly for the signs and symptoms of developing candidal infections and treated accordingly. Patients with diabetes should be instructed in proper glycemic control measures and routine surveillance of skin and mucosal surfaces.[2]

Careful, daily attention to dental hygiene is the key to prevention of gingivitis and periodontitis. Dental health care providers recommend a routine daily brushing and flossing regimen.[1,3]

Aphthous stomatitis is usually a recurrent eruption. Treatment of the underlying causes, if known, may alleviate future outbreaks. Crohn disease, ulcerative colitis, stresses, deficiencies of vitamin B_{12} and folic acid, iron deficiency, and estrogen sensitivity have been implicated in outbreaks. Avoidance of irritating food, beverages, and chemicals may alleviate some of the symptoms and decrease the number of recurrences.[4]

REFERENCES

1. American Academy of Periodontology. (2015). More than a quarter of U.S. adults are dishonest with dentists about how often they floss their teeth. *American Academy of Periodontology*, Retrieved from www.perio.org/consumer/quarter-of-adults-dishonest-with-dentists#.VdfVmxEihHQ.mailto. (Accessed August 22, 2015).
2. Lyons, F., & Ously, L. (2015). *Dermatology for the advanced practice nurse*. New York: Springer.
3. Flint, P. W., Haughty, B. H., Thomas, J. R., et al. (2015). *Cummings otolaryngology: Head and neck surgery* (6th ed.). St Louis: Mosby.
4. Lauritano, D., Petruzzi, M., Nardi, G. M., Carinci, F., Minervini, G., Stasio, D., et al. (2015). Single application of a dessicating agent in the treatment of recurrent aphthous stomatitis. *Journal of Biological Regulators and Homeostatic Agents*, 29(3), 77s–84s.
5. Arain, N., Paravastu, S. C. V., & Arain, M. A. (2015). Effectiveness of topical corticosteroids in addition to antiviral therapy in the management of recurrent herpes labialis: A systemic review and meta-analysis. *BMC Infectious Diseases*, 15(82).
6. Oral Cancer Foundation: HPV/Oral Cancer Facts. (last updated March 2016). Retrieved from https://oralcancerfoundation.org/understanding/hpv/hpv-oral-cancer-facts/. (Accessed 24 April 2018).
7. Chapple, I. L. C., Van der Weijden, F., Doerfer, C., Herrera, D., Shapira, L., Polak, D., et al. (2015). Primary prevention of periodontitis: Managing gingivitis. *Journal of Clinical Periodontology*, 42(Suppl. 16), S71–S76.
8. Eholy, K. E., Genco, R. J., & Van Dyke, T. E. (2015). Oral infections and cardiovascular disease. *Trends in Endocrinology and Metabolism*, 26(6), 315–321.
9. National Cancer Institute at the National Institutes of Health. HPV Vaccination linked to Decreased Oral HPV Infections. Retrieved from https://www.cancer.gov/news-events/cancer-currents-blog/2017/hpv-vaccine-oral-infection. (Accessed 24 April 2018).

CHAPTER **81**

PAROTITIS
Lisa M. O'Neal

Immediate referral is indicated for any patient suspected to have a parotid abscess, and first-line antibiotics and surgical decompression is needed.

DEFINITION AND EPIDEMIOLOGY

The parotid gland is the largest of the three major salivary glands in the body. An inflammatory reaction of the parotid gland is defined as parotitis. This is not to be confused with sialadenitis, which is defined as the inflammation or infection of a salivary gland.[1] Parotitis may be caused by bacterial, viral, fungal, or mycobacterial invasion. The parotid gland is most commonly affected by an inflammatory process, and infections can range from acute to severe. Assessment of the disease process should differentiate between local primary infections of the parotid gland, such as bacterial sialadenitis, and systemic infection, in which the gland is inflamed from a generalized inflammatory process caused by a virus. Viruses most commonly associated with parotitis are the paramyxovirus (cause of mumps) and the human immunodeficiency virus (HIV).[2]

Inflammatory conditions of the parotid gland include acute viral inflammation, commonly caused by mumps, and acute suppurative sialadenitis, often caused by *Staphylococcus aureus*. Chronic inflammatory conditions of the parotid are caused by infection with *Mycobacterium tuberculosis* (tuberculosis [TB]) and HIV.[3] Noninfective causes of parotitis can be related to Sjögren syndrome (SS) and sarcoidosis.[3]

Acute suppurative parotitis is more likely to be encountered in the sixth to seventh decade of life, with a higher incidence in men, and with the right side involved more frequently than the left.[2] Older adults are at a higher risk of development of acute suppurative parotitis because of a medication-induced (e.g., anticholinergics and antihistamines) decrease in salivary flow.[2] Other factors that are associated with acute suppurative parotitis include chronic illness (e.g., diabetes mellitus, hypothyroidism, renal failure, rheumatoid arthritis), an immunocompromised host, poor oral hygiene, salivary duct obstruction, autoimmune disease (SS), recent surgical procedure, radiotherapy, and hypovolemia.[2] Acute suppurative parotitis has been identified as a common postoperative occurrence in patients undergoing major abdominal and hip repair surgery; this has been attributed to postoperative dehydration and is usually identified within the first 2 weeks after surgery.[2] Acute suppurative parotitis is rarer now because antibiotic use in the perioperative setting is more common, and there is increased attention to perioperative hydration, nutrition, and oral hygiene.[1]

PATHOPHYSIOLOGY

The parotid gland is most susceptible to infection because it secretes serous saliva versus mucinous saliva.[2] Serous saliva lacks lysosomes, immunoglobulin A antibodies, and sialic acid, all with bacteriostatic properties, thus predisposing the parotid gland to a greater risk of infection compared with its counterparts.[2] Multiple factors contribute to the development of parotitis. Most commonly, the infection begins with retrograde migration of oral cavity flora through the Stensen duct, stasis of saliva, ductal obstruction, decreased stimulation of saliva, decreased mastication, and poor oral hygiene contributes to retrograde migration.[2,3] Ill patients, recent surgical patients, and those with acute or chronic hypovolemia can develop stasis and retrograde migration. Although most of these infections occur in adults, they can occur in children also. Presentation of parotitis in the pediatric population is usually an isolated occurrence and associated with a viral or bacterial infection.[4] Parotitis is also the classic symptom of infection with paramyxovirus (mumps).[5]

CLINICAL PRESENTATION AND PHYSICAL EXAMINATION

The onset of parotitis is usually rapid and associated with localized pain, edema, and induration of the infected gland.[3] Systemic symptoms include fever, chills, anorexia, and malaise.[6] Viral inflammatory reactions are most often seen with edema (usually bilateral) and pain, which is exacerbated by mastication.[3] Parotitis associated with a bacterial infection (acute suppurative sialadenitis) often occurs in a hypovolemic elder and consists of unilateral parotid enlargement and cellulitis.[3] Intraorally, pus can be visualized with manual pressure on the parotid duct orifice.[3] Chronic inflammatory conditions of the parotid caused by the infective agent *M. tuberculosis* appear much like a malignant neoplasm, with enlargement of and pain in the affected gland.[3] The mass is usually unilateral and associated with matted lymph nodes.[3] Infection with HIV may produce bilaterally enlarged, painless parotid glands that gradually produce smaller amounts of saliva, resulting in complaints of xerostomia.[6]

The physical examination for parotitis requires bimanual palpation of the gland with attention to the Stensen duct. In bacterial parotitis, palpation of the gland elicits a suppurative discharge from the Stensen duct.[2] Bilateral edema is suggestive of viral infection, and a clear discharge is found on palpation of the duct. Suppurative discharge should be cultured. If the process has been present for several days, fluctuance of suppurative sialadenitis may not be palpable because of the anatomic septations in the parotid.

DIAGNOSTICS
Essential Diagnostics

The diagnosis of parotitis is based on the clinical presentation and physical examination. A complete blood count (CBC) with differential may reveal leukocytosis with neutrophilia in suppurative cases.[1] Appropriate cultures and sensitivities should be performed and fungal and mycobacterial studies requested when indicated. Caution should be taken when evaluating cultured pus from the Stensen duct, because it is often contaminated by the normal oral flora.[1]

Radiographs or oblique soft tissue films of the mouth and jaw should be obtained if obstruction caused by a sialolith (calculus) is suspected.[1] Computed tomography (CT) scan with contrast medium is an excellent study because it may delineate ductal stones or a suppurative process.[1] Ultrasonography is the most cost-effective and safest diagnostic tool for identifying sialoliths and diagnosing inflammatory parotid disease.[1]

Additional Diagnostics

Magnetic resonance imaging (MRI) is most useful in identifying parenchymal changes of the parotid gland and possibly identifying atrophy, which is commonly associated with SS,[1] or if neoplasms or abscesses are suspected.[2] If a neoplasm is suspected, a biopsy is indicated.[7]

INITIAL DIAGNOSTICS	
Parotitis	
LABORATORY	**IMAGING**
• CBC and differential	• X-ray studies[a]
• Culture and sensitivity	• CT scan with contrast[a]
	• Ultrasound[a]
	• MRI[a]

————
[a]If indicated.

DIFFERENTIAL DIAGNOSIS

 Further investigation of painless enlargement of the parotid gland is indicated and requires further investigation to exclude a malignant process. Fine-needle biopsy or surgical excision is indicated.

 Priority differentials for parotitis include the following: (1) SS, (2) sarcoidosis, (3) immunoglobulin G4 (IgG4)-related disease.[6]

The differential diagnosis of parotitis should include bacterial, viral, mycobacterial, and fungal infections. In addition to paramyxovirus, identified agents of infection include cytomegalovirus, Coxsackie A virus, Epstein-Barr virus, influenza A, parainfluenza virus type 3, lymphocytic choriomeningitis, human herpesvirus type 6, echovirus, and HIV.[1] Mechanical or extrinsic factors, such as radiotherapy or drug-induced parotitis, should also be included in the differential diagnosis. In addition, anticholinergic medications can initiate parotitis. Such medications include antiparkinsonian agents, atropine, dicyclomine hydrochloride, glycopyrrolate, scopolamine, and hyoscyamine sulfate. Many psychotropic medications have an atropine-like effect and can cause parotid swelling.[2,8]

INTERPROFESSIONAL COLLABORATIVE MANAGEMENT
Nonsurgical Management

- Nonsurgical treatments include parenteral antibiotics and possibly hospitalization for parenteral antibiotic therapy.
- Culture and sensitivity testing are important because multidrug-resistant organisms are common.[9]

Pharmacologic Management

- Recommended antibiotic therapy is initially empirical and includes amoxicillin with clavulanate, dicloxacillin, clindamycin, or a cephalosporin in addition to metronidazole.[5,9]
- Culture results will further direct antimicrobial therapy and identify if methicillin-resistant *S. aureus* is present, thus requiring vancomycin or linezolid.[2] Response to antimicrobial therapy should be identified within 48 to 72 hours of initiation of therapy and should be continued for 1 week after symptoms have ceased.[2]
- Fluid and electrolyte replacement are necessary.[2]
- Attention to proper oral hygiene and the use of sialagogues (agents that stimulate the production and flow of saliva, such as sugar-free hard candy and chewing gum) are also recommended.[5]

- There is a questionable role for the use of steroids.
- Analgesics and local heat for relief of pain are beneficial. External bimanual massage (from distal to proximal) of the duct is also recommended.[2]

INDICATIONS FOR CONSULTATIONS: SURGERY

- Surgical consultation is necessary if the infection is refractory for more than 3 or 4 days; therefore, requiring possible surgical drainage.[3]
- Radiology consult should occur to obtain a CT scan or ultrasound examination of the parotid and neck. This is indicated if abscess formation has occurred after 3 or 4 days while the patient is taking aggressive parenteral antibiotics. Because of the usually debilitated states of patients predisposed to parotitis, a poor prognosis is associated with postoperative patients who develop parotitis. A 20% mortality rate is associated with the development of this infection.[2]

Consultation with an otolaryngologist, a head and neck surgeon, is highly recommended. Patients who develop parotitis often require hospitalization for fluid replacement, careful monitoring, and intravenous antibiotics.

LIFESPAN CONSIDERATIONS

Parotitis can occur in the pediatric population and is referred to as juvenile recurrent parotitis (JRP). JRP often occurs in children between the ages of 4 months and 15 years of age.[10] The etiology is unknown, but usually resolves by puberty.[10] JRP is characterized by recurrent inflammation of the parotid gland, either unilateral or bilateral, and is accompanied by pain, decreased function of the gland, erythema, and sometimes fever.[10] Though JRP is self-limiting, occasionally it can progress to chronic parotitis, thus necessitating a parotidectomy.[11] Recent literature indicates that ductal corticosteroid infusion (DCI) is an effective, low-risk procedure in the treatment of JRP. Sialendoscopy and sialography have a therapeutic role in the treatment of JRP and continue to be used as a treatment modality, but should be reserved for patients for whom conservative management fails (i.e., DCI).[10,11]

Elder patients and patients on certain antipsychotic medications should be monitored closely. A recent review showed that there is an association between sialorrhea (hypersalivation) and clozapine-induced parotitis (clozapine is an atypical antipsychotic). Patients in psychiatric care and the elder population do not undergo routine head and neck examinations with parotid gland assessment. Furthermore, a study found that elder patients who are not on clozapine, have a predisposition for root caries, dental avulsion, and periodontal disease. As such, routine dental examination should also be performed.[8]

COMPLICATIONS

Complications include abscess formation and the need for surgical drainage.[2,4,5,12] The discomfort associated with this disorder may prevent the patient from eating and drinking, increasing the risk of hypovolemia and further compromising the patient. Suppurative parotitis is a rare occurrence postoperatively because of the routine use of preoperative and intraoperative antibiotic therapy. However, if it is left untreated, severe complications can arise (Box 81.1).[1] Chronic parotitis may develop as a result of an acute episode of suppurative

---

BOX 81.1

Severe Complications of Parotitis

Sepsis with or without shock
Soft tissue infection extending into the neck, face, mediastinum
Osteomyelitis of the mandible
Lemierre syndrome
Airway obstruction
Invasion of the external auditory canal
Facial nerve palsy (common with parotid malignancy)

---

parotitis.[6] Complications of viral parotitis include orchitis, pancreatitis, meningoencephalitis, and deafness.[3]

PATIENT AND FAMILY EDUCATION AND HEALTH PROMOTION

Preoperative attention to hydration and overall health status should be addressed if the patient is not a candidate for emergent surgery. After diagnosis, attention to hydration, parenteral antibiotics, oral hygiene, and sialagogue use should be addressed. Patients should be instructed in proper oral hygiene, which includes brushing and flossing the teeth and proper care of dentures and dental appliances. The side effects of medications should be discussed with the patient to determine whether medication is causing decreased salivary secretions.[1]

REFERENCES

1. Rhodes, M., & Benson, B. J. (2015). Acute suppurative parotitis. *Hospital Medicine Clinic, 4*(2), 191–204.
2. Jackson, N. M., Mitchell, J. L., Walvekar, R. R., et al. (2010). Inflammatory disorders of the salivary glands. In C. W. Cummings, P. W. Flint, & B. H. Haughey (Eds.), *Otolaryngology: Head and neck surgery* (5th ed.). Philadelphia, PA: Elsevier.
3. Bag, A. K., Cure, J. K., Chapman, P. R., Singhal, A., & Mohamed, A. W. H. (2018). Imaging of inflammatory disorders of salivary glands. *Neuroimaging Clinics of North America, 28*, 255–272.
4. Faizal, B., Abraham, S. M., & Krishnakumar, T. (2017). Study of evaluation of symptoms of juvenile recurrent parotitis prior to and after sialendoscopy. *The Open Pain Journal, 10*, 29–36.
5. Family Practice Notebook. Acute suppurative sialoadenitis. Retrieved from www.fpnotebook.com/ent/Salivary/ActSprtvSldnts.htm. (Accessed 7 June 2015).
6. Ugga, L., Ravanelli, M., Pallottino, A. A., Farina, D., & Maroldi, R. (2017). Diagnostic work-up in obstructive and inflammatory salivary gland disorders. *Acta Otorhinolaryngologica Italica, 37*(2), 83–93.
7. Wilson, K. F., Meier, J. D., & Ward, P. D. (2014). Salivary gland disorders. *American Family Physician, 89*(11), 882–888.
8. Glass, M., Muzyka, B. C., Hermida, A. P., Glass, O. M., & Zalewska, A. (2018). Clozapine induced parotitis in Elderly—A cause for sialorrhea. *American Journal of Geriatric Psychiatry, 26*(3), s77–s78. Poster session presented at the AAGP Annual Meeting, Supplement 1.
9. Steehler, M., Agnew, A. W., & Anon, J. B. (2015). Current bacteriology and antibiotic management of acute suppurative parotitis in the hospitalized patient: A retrospective study and literature review. *Journal of Otology and Rhinology, 4*, 2.
10. Premnath, K. P. B., Thomas, J., Ray, B., & Jayakrishnan, V. (2016). Multimodality diagnostic features and treatment by sialography of juvenile recurrent parotitis: A case report. *International Journal of Scientific Study, 4*(9), 176–178.
11. Roby, B. B., Mattingly, J., Jensen, E. L., Gao, D., & Chan, K. H. (2015). Treatment of juvinile recurrent parotitis of childhood: An analysis of effectiveness. *JAMA Otolaryngology Head and Neck Surgery, 141*(2), 126–129.
12. Franklyn, J., Gaikwad, P., Lazarus, E., Thomas, A., & Muthusami, J. (2017). Parotid abscess: A clinical analysis of 40 cases in a tertiary care hospital in India. *Journal of Oral and Maxillofacial Surgery, Medicine, and Pathology, 29*, 189–192.

CHAPTER **82**

PERITONSILLAR ABSCESS

Erin A. Lyden

 Immediate referral is indicated for patients with peritonsillar abscess, respiratory compromise, or unable to swallow secretions

DEFINITION AND EPIDEMIOLOGY

A peritonsillar abscess (PTA) is an accumulation of pus within the peritonsillar tissues between the tonsil and the pharyngeal constrictor muscle.[1] PTA is a common deep infection of the head and neck.[1,2] The abscess frequently occurs in patients with a history of recurrent, chronic, or improperly treated tonsillitis.[1]

Peritonsillar cellulitis and abscess formation commonly occur between the ages of 20 and 40.[2] The incidence rate for PTA varies internationally.[3] The incidence of PTAs reported in the United States has remained virtually the same in children despite a major decline in the number of tonsillectomies performed.[3] The risk of recurrence is higher if the patient is younger than 30 years and for patients who smoke.[4]

PATHOPHYSIOLOGY

PTAs were previously believed to be a direct result of inadequately treated tonsillitis. The tonsillitis progresses to cellulitis, and eventually pus formation occurs in the peritonsillar tissue. However, now there are two theories regarding the pathogenesis of PTAs.[5] One study found that 79% of patients reported symptoms of a sore throat before PTA, whereas another study reported that 68% of patients denied such symptoms before the PTA diagnosis.[5] In addition to the theory that PTA is a complication of acute tonsillitis is the theory of blocked Weber glands.[5] These are salivary glands located on the upper soft palate. It has been suggested that infection secondary to poor oral hygiene or other sources (e.g., infections and smoking) could cause scarring that leads to an eventual blockage of the ducts of the Weber glands.[5] These glands are reported to assist in the removal of debris in the tonsil area. If these glands are obstructed by debris, inflammation, or pus, their function is impaired, which contributes to the development of PTA.[5]

These infections tend to have multiple bacteria in them. However, the primary bacteria is most often Group A *Streptococcus*.[6]

CLINICAL PRESENTATION AND PHYSICAL EXAM

The presentation typically consists of fever, chills, fatigue, malaise, halitosis, dysphagia, severe sore throat, and otalgia.[6] The patient may appear acutely ill and often reports pain radiating to the ear of the affected side. Trismus (spasms of the masticator muscles) is often noted. Drooling is typically present because of the inability to handle secretions. A "hot potato" (hoarse) voice is commonly noted.[2]

Clinical examination will reveal marked edema and erythema of the peritonsillar tissue and soft palate; this tissue is often fluctuant and covered with exudate.[7] The findings are almost always unilateral, with the tonsil typically displaced downward and medially. The uvula is edematous and displaced to the opposite side.[2] Other findings include trismus, tender cervical adenopathy, tachycardia, pooling of saliva or drooling, and signs of dehydration.[7]

DIAGNOSTICS
Essential Diagnostics

PTAs are easily diagnosed on the basis of physical findings. A computed tomography (CT) scan with contrast will confirm abscess formation and the presence of gas. Ultrasonography, either oral or cutaneous, in a cooperative, nonemergent patient also can be a useful diagnostic tool.[1] Ultrasonography is being used more often at the bedside for confirmation and guidance in draining the abscess.[8]

A complete blood count (CBC) should be performed, which will often reveal leukocytosis.[8]

Additional Diagnostics

The monospot heterophile antibody test may be performed to exclude infectious mononucleosis.[9] Culture and sensitivity testing of aspirate from the abscess typically reveals both aerobic and anaerobic bacteria.[7,10] Serum electrolytes may be ordered if the patient reports decreased oral intake. As with any other suspected infectious process, Gram stain, culture, and sensitivity should be performed on any aspirated purulent material.[1]

Differential Diagnosis

When considering a diagnosis of PTA, the health care provider must exclude other conditions that manifest with similar signs and symptoms.

Priority differentials include infectious mononucleosis, tumors, and peritonsillar cellulitis. Other differentials include epiglottitis, retromolar or retropharyngeal abscesses, and lymphoma.[6,7,10]

Infectious mononucleosis can be excluded on the basis of clinical presentation, physical examination, and serologic findings. With mononucleosis, headache, malaise, fatigue, and anorexia are typically present before the sore throat. A tumor in the peritonsillar region is eliminated from diagnostic consideration by a lack of the physical findings usually present in an infectious process. A CT scan and—possibly—a biopsy is indicated if a tumor is suspected.[6,10]

The signs and symptoms of PTAs are similar to those of epiglottitis, which is a potentially fatal condition if not diagnosed. Epiglottitis is less likely when there is peritonsillar swelling with preserved ability to swallow and no stridor auscultated over the larynx on physical examination. Indirect visualization of the epiglottis is a reliable method in the adult and may be necessary to exclude epiglottitis as a cause of symptoms.[11]

Retropharyngeal abscesses may be similar in their presentation. Both conditions reveal an ill or toxic patient, with signs of infection and neck pain. A retropharyngeal abscess can be identified with a CT scan.[7]

INTERPROFESSIONAL COLLABORATIVE MANAGEMENT
Pharmacologic Management

Antibiotics. As an adjunct to surgical intervention, the antibiotic regimen appears to vary based on otolaryngologist preference and geographic location. Clindamycin is widely used antibiotic for PTA. In some cases, it is preferred by the provider, and in others it is used if the patient has a known penicillin allergy.[12] One review stated that the use of combined penicillin and metronidazole was effective in at least 98% of cases.[13]

Steroids. Steroid medication is used to aid in the relief of fever, pain, trismus, and dysphagia.[2,12]

Hydration. Helping the patient with the oral intake of nutrients is also essential.[2]

Optimum hydration of the patient must be maintained, either orally or intravenously. The importance of hydration cannot be stressed enough. These patients have difficulty swallowing, and dehydration can lead to other complications.[2]

Nonpharmacologic Management

Surgical Intervention. Antibiotic therapy is not sufficient for the effective treatment of a PTA. Surgical intervention is required with needle aspiration, incision and drainage, or tonsillectomy. The majority of PTAs can be treated effectively with needle aspiration, antibiotics, pain medication, and the maintenance of hydration.[4] A tonsillectomy may be indicated in certain situations, such as recurrent tonsillitis or history of PTA.[11] Careful attention to analgesia is required, along with adequate hydration. The use of intravenous antibiotics plus a single high dose of intravenous steroids versus intravenous antibiotics alone in PTA patients has been shown to be superior.[12]

INDICATIONS FOR CONSULTATION: OTOLARYNGOLOGIST

After the diagnosis of a PTA has been made, patients should be referred immediately to an otolaryngologist for an evaluation concerning surgical intervention and antibiotic therapy. Hospitalization may not be necessary, although the patient is usually hospitalized after aspiration and started on intravenous antibiotics. Patients may be discharged in 24 hours or less if symptoms subside and the abscess does not reappear. Follow-up should occur after 24 to 36 hours. Referral to an otolaryngologist is necessary if tonsillectomy is indicated.[5]

LIFE-SPAN CONSIDERATIONS

Although PTA is usually seen in people from the late teens to 40 years of age, a high index of suspicion must be maintained in all age groups.[5] Early detection and treatment can prevent life-threatening complications.[12]

COMPLICATIONS

Serious and potentially fatal complications may result from a PTA. The abscess can result in airway obstruction from spread of the infection. Rupture of the abscess with aspiration of the infected material can cause severe and serious sequelae. If untreated, the infection may spread to involve the superior constrictor muscle, other deep spaces of the neck, and the mediastinum. Necrosis of the muscle may result. Internal jugular vein thrombosis with septic pulmonary embolism can also occur.[12]

Other complications of PTA include thrombophlebitis, chronic PTA, glottic edema, epiglottitis, septicemia, endocarditis, myocarditis, and hemorrhage. Poststreptococcal complications, such as rheumatic fever and glomerulonephritis, may result if the infected material consists of group A β-hemolytic streptococci. Thrombosis of the internal jugular vein (Lemierre syndrome) is a rare sequela, which is usually the result of infection with *Fusobacterium necrophorum*. Intravenous antibiotic therapy and surgical treatment of the abscess are required. Ligation or excision of the internal jugular vein is mandatory if septic emboli are noted. Extension of the abscess

into the carotid artery sheath is a complication of extending infection.[7,12]

PATIENT AND FAMILY EDUCATION

Education concerning PTA as a complication of tonsillitis is important. PTA can recur, and therefore the signs and symptoms should be described to the patient and family. These include fever, chills, malaise, odynophagia, ear pain, inability to open the mouth, dysphagia, drooling, and a "hot potato" voice.[6,7] The provider should also discuss the possible side effects of antibiotic therapy. These side effects may include nausea, vomiting, diarrhea, abdominal pain, lethargy, vaginitis, or a secondary yeast infection. Signs and symptoms of an allergic reaction, including urticaria, shortness of breath, wheezing, or tightness in the chest, indicate the necessity for immediate emergency treatment.

HEALTH PROMOTION

Patients with histories of recurrent tonsillitis, chronic tonsillitis, and inadequately treated tonsillitis should be monitored closely for signs of PTA. Consultation with an otolaryngologist is a must for these patients.[13] PTA is increased in individuals with poor oral hygiene and in smokers. For this reason, the importance of good oral health and smoking cessation should be discussed with patients.[4,5,9]

REFERENCES

1. Blair, A. B., Booth, R., & Baugh, R. (2015). Unifying theory of tonsillitis, intratonsillar abscess and peritonsillar abscess. *American Journal of Otolaryngology, 36.*
2. Kocak, H. E., Acipayam, H., Elbistanli, M. S., Yigider, A. P., Alakhras, W., Kiral, M. N., et al. (2018). Is corticosteroid a treatment choice for the management of peritonsillar abscess? *Auris, Nasus, Larynx, 45,* http://dx.doi.org/10.1016/j.anl.2017.04.008.
3. Qureshi, H., Ference, E., Novis, S., Pritchett, C. V., Smith, S. S., & Schroeder, J. W. (2015). Trends in the management of pediatric peritonsillar abscess infections in the U.S., 2000–2009. *International Journal of Pediatric Otorhinolaryngology, 79,* http://dx.doi.org/10.1016/j.ijporl.2015.01.021.
4. Liu, Y., Su, H., Tsai, Y., Chang, K., Chi, C., Lin, M., et al. (2017). Initial factors influencing duration of hospital stay in adult patients with peritonsillar abscess. *Clinical and Experimental Otorhinolaryngology, 10*(1), https://doi.org/10.21053/ceo.2015.01718.
5. Powell, E. L., Powell, J., Samuel, J. R., & Wilson, J. A. (2013). A review of the pathogenesis of adult peritonsillar abscess: Time for re-evaluation. *The Journal of Antimicrobial Chemotherapy, 68*(9).
6. Bacon, E., & Tabbut, M. (2016). When a peritonsillar abscess is not a peritonsillar abscess: Using bedside emergency ultrasound to change the diagnosis. *The American Journal of Emergency Medicine, 34,* http://dx.doi.org/10.1016/j.ajem.2015.11.031.
7. Gottlieb, M., Long, B., & Koyfman, A. (2018). Clinical Mimics: An emergency medicine-focused review of streptococcal pharyngitis mimics. *The Journal of Emergency Medicine,* https://doi.org/10.1016/j.jemermed.2018.01.031.
8. Gekle, R., Raio, C., Falkoff, M., & Neufeldt, J. (2014). Technology advancements in the diagnosis and treatment of peritonsillar abscess. *The American Journal of Emergency Medicine, 32,* http://dx.doi.org/10.1016/j.ajem.2014.03.017.
9. Klug, T. E., Rusan, M., Clemmensen, K. K., et al. (2013). Smoking promotes peritonsillar abscess. *European Archives of Oto-Rhino-Laryngology, 270*(12), 3163–3167.
10. Chen, Y., Yang, Q., Wang, T., et al. (2014). Application of enhanced CT in the differential diagnosis of peritonsillar abscess and intratonsillar abscess. *Zhonghua Er Bi Yan Hou Tou Jing Wai Ke Za Zhi, 49*(2), 131–135.
11. Page, C., Chassery, G., Boute, P., et al. (2010). Immediate tonsillectomy: Indications for use as first-line surgical management of peritonsillar abscess (quinsy) and parapharyngeal abscess. *The Journal of Laryngology and Otology, 124,* 1085–1090.
12. Flint, P. W., Haughty, B. H., Thomas, J. R., et al. (2015). *Cummings otolaryngology: Head and neck surgery* (6th ed.). St. Louis: Mosby.
13. Powell, J., & Wilson, J. A. (2012). An evidence-based review of peritonsillar abscess. *Clinical Otolaryngology, 37*(2), 136–145.

CHAPTER 83

PHARYNGITIS AND TONSILLITIS

Erin A. Lyden

 Immediate emergency department referral is indicated for pharyngeal abscess, signs of airway obstruction, dysphagia, drooling, trismus, voice changes, and unilateral pharyngeal pain.

DEFINITION AND EPIDEMIOLOGY

Pharyngitis is a condition that encompasses inflammation of the pharynx from either infection or irritation.[1] An illness affecting both children and adults, pharyngitis is a common reason for people to seek health care and accounts for around 6% of visits to health care providers.[2] Pharyngitis can manifest as an acute illness or a chronic condition. The causes are numerous and include both infectious and noninfectious agents.[1]

Noninfectious causes of pharyngitis include referred pain, allergies, trauma from foreign bodies or burns, cancer, and irritation. Irritation of the pharynx may result from dust, smoke, dryness, or toxins, either inhaled or swallowed.[1,2]

Infectious agents responsible for pharyngitis include viruses, bacteria, and, uncommonly, fungi or parasites. Viral infection is the most common cause of pharyngitis in all age groups and can occur during any season.[1,2] Viruses are responsible for 30% to 60% of cases in adults. In these cases the most common cause is the rhinovirus.[1] Other possible responsible agents include Epstein-Barr virus (EBV; the cause of mononucleosis), herpes simplex virus, influenza virus, parainfluenza virus, and coronavirus.[1–4]

Bacterial pharyngitis is more common in children (30% to 40%), peaking at ages 5 to 15, than in adults (5% to 10%).[1–3] *Streptococcus pyogenes* is the etiologic agent for an estimated 15% to 30% of acute pharyngitis cases.[4] *S. pyogenes* includes groups A, C, and G β-hemolytic streptococci. Group A β-hemolytic *Streptococcus* (GAS) is the most important to identify because it is responsible for acute rheumatic fever (ARF) and poststreptococcal glomerulonephritis. Infection with GAS typically peaks in the late winter and early spring, but it can be seen year-round.[1,2,5] Group C disease is more common among college students and adolescents. Community-wide and food-borne causes of pharyngitis have been connected to group G organisms.[1] Other offending agents include mycoplasmas, *Arcanobacterium haemolyticum*, chlamydiae, *Neisseria gonorrhoeae*, corynebacteria, and anaerobic bacteria.[1,4]

Tonsillitis and pharyngitis are similar in clinical presentation, physical findings, diagnosis, and management (Fig. 83.1). Tonsillitis is an acute or chronic inflammation of the tonsil and results from the same offending microorganisms as the previously termed pharyngitis. Most often the pharyngeal tonsils are affected which the term pharyngitis encompasses.[6]

PATHOPHYSIOLOGY

The normal flora of the oral pharynx region consists of various and numerous microorganisms. These microorganisms are not harmful unless the immune system is weakened, resulting in increased susceptibility to illness.[1] Pharyngitis or tonsillitis develops from exposure to a viral or bacterial agent that is not part of the normal flora, although some people can harbor

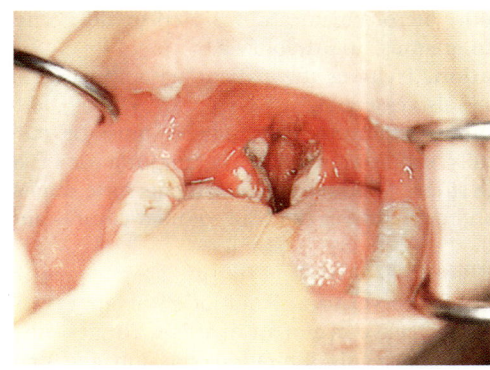

F I G . 83.1 Pharyngitis and tonsillitis. (From Barkauskas, V. H., Stoltenberg-Allen, K., Baumann, L. C., & Darling-Fisher, C. [1998]. *Health and physical assessment* [2nd ed.]. St Louis: Mosby.)

or be colonized with pathogenic bacteria and remain free of infection (carrier state).[1] When these microorganisms attack the pharyngeal cells, an inflammatory response occurs.[3] The extent of the local or systemic response depends on the particular agent.[1–4,7]

CLINICAL PRESENTATION AND PHYSICAL EXAMINATION

The clinical presentation of pharyngitis or tonsillitis varies according to the offending agent. Noninfectious pharyngitis has an initial appearance somewhat different from that of infectious pharyngitis. Typically, with noninfectious pharyngitis the patient reports a sore throat and dryness; if environmental allergens are the cause, symptoms often include rhinorrhea, watery eyes, and postnasal drip.[1,2,5] Patients receiving radiation therapy or chemotherapy may report pain, dryness, and dysphagia. Oropharyngeal candidiasis (thrush) may be present in these patients secondary to the immunosuppression.[8]

The infectious causes of pharyngitis or tonsillitis are bacterial and viral. The presentation of symptoms can be similar. Viral causes are more common and usually self-limiting (about 1 week).[2–4] Patients typically report the sudden onset of a sore throat, fever, malaise, cough, headache, myalgias, and fatigue. Patients may also report rhinitis, conjunctivitis (adenovirus), congestion, and a cough with sputum production.[2,4,6]

In viral pharyngitis, clinical findings may include mild erythema with little or no pharyngeal exudate, although the pharynx may appear swollen, boggy, or pale. Painful or tender lymphadenopathy is not typically present.[1,3,5] Infectious mononucleosis, is an exception, typically it produces headache, fatigue, high fever, pharyngeal erythema, tonsillar hypertrophy, white to gray-green exudate, petechiae at the junction of the hard and soft palate, and posterior cervical adenopathy. Hepatomegaly and splenomegaly may be identified in less than 50% of patients. Jaundice may be present in severe cases.[1,4]

One of the most common causes of bacterial pharyngitis or tonsillitis is GAS. In the winter months, it is estimated that 15% to 25% of pharyngitis cases in children are caused by GAS.[4,6] This disease is most prevalent in children younger than 15 years.[5] The transmission of GAS is by direct contact with respiratory secretions or large droplets, and the incubation period can be 2 to 5 days. It is often spread in the classroom setting.[9]

Patients may report a sudden onset of sore throat, painful swallowing, fever (temperature higher than 38.5°C [101.3°F]), chills, headache, nausea, vomiting, and abdominal pain.[1,4,6] With bacterial pharyngitis, rhinitis, cough, conjunctivitis, and myalgias are not typically present.[2,4]

Other bacterium may be causative and should be investigated if indicated. These include group C and G streptococci, *N. gonorrhoeae, Fusobacterium necrophorum,* and *A. haemolyticum.*[4]

In GAS infection, the physical examination reveals marked erythema of the throat and tonsils; patchy, discrete, white or yellowish exudate; pharyngeal petechiae; and tender anterior cervical adenopathy (see Fig. 83.1). Patients with previous exposure to GAS may exhibit the typical diffuse exanthem of scarlet fever, a sandpaper-type rash, and erythematous (strawberry) tongue.[1,4] Pressure on the tonsillar pillars may produce purulent drainage. The uvula may also be edematous, and a temperature higher than 38.3°C (101°F) is typical. On occasion, GAS infection may be seen with an erythematous, persistent sore throat with little fever and no exudate.[1]

DIAGNOSTICS

Although it is sometimes difficult to differentiate between viral and bacterial pharyngitis and tonsillitis, clinical presentation and exclusion criteria may indicate the diagnosis. No specific diagnostic test exists for viral pharyngitis.[1]

Diagnostic studies used to detect GAS infection include a throat culture, a rapid antigen detection test (RADT), and sometimes an antistreptolysin O (ASO) titer. The ASO titer is not used during initial diagnostic screening but is obtained to identify or to confirm a diagnosis of GAS infection weeks to months later.[2,4] The RADT is often used versus the traditional throat culture because it is rapid and convenient. If the diagnosis of GAS infection is suspected and the RADT result is negative, a throat culture is performed for confirmation in children.[10] The guidelines put out by the Infectious Disease Society of America recommends that anyone with pharyngitis be swabbed with either a throat culture or RADT unless viral-related symptoms are obvious (i.e., cough or rhinorrhea). However, in the chance that the RADT result is negative, a back-up throat culture should be performed only in children.[10]

Numerous studies have evaluated the efficacy of a clinical scoring system in the diagnosis of GAS pharyngitis. Medical societies have recommended various clinical indicators in an attempt to standardize diagnosis. The Centor criteria—tonsillar exudates, swollen and tender anterior cervical lymph nodes, lack of cough, and history of fever—have proved to be predictive of a positive diagnosis in adult patients.[2] To calculate a Centor score for an individual patient, 1 point is added for each of the following findings: absence of cough, tonsils with exudates or swelling, tender and swollen anterior cervical nodes, and temperature higher than 38°C (100.4°F); thus the score can range from 1 to 4. Some sources use age to modify the score, subtracting 1 point if the patient is over 45.[2]

There remains disagreement concerning the precise use of the Centor score to guide diagnosis and testing. The differences in recommendations arise from concern regarding potential sequelae of rheumatic fever.[2] US guidelines from the Infectious Diseases Society of America recommend culture and RADT testing based on the patient's history of exposure to streptococci, a previous history of rheumatic fever or post-streptococcal glomerulonephritis, or clinical signs and symptoms suggestive of streptococcal infection.[10]

An investigation conducted in a large retail health system found that the use of local biosurveillance data on the recent local proportion of positive streptococci results on throat culture or a DNA probe test to modify the Centor score improved the score's ability to predict GAS infection.[11] A complete blood count (CBC) can be helpful in some situations (e.g., infectious mononucleosis or deep neck infection such as peritonsillar abscess).

DIFFERENTIAL DIAGNOSIS

The presence of an inflamed pharynx requires further investigation. The differential diagnosis includes infectious mononucleosis, allergies, thrush, peritonsillar cellulitis or abscess, pharyngeal abscess, epiglottitis, leukoplakia, upper respiratory tract infection (URI) sexually transmitted disease, and possibly even HIV.

Infectious mononucleosis differs from pharyngitis or tonsillitis in clinical presentation, physical examination, and serologic findings. This diagnosis is seen more commonly in adolescents and young adults.[2] These patients usually present with headache, malaise, fatigue, and anorexia before the sore throat occurs. Hepatosplenomegaly may be noted during the physical examination.[2,4] A CBC often reveals leukocytosis with a right shift of atypical lymphocytes.[4] A positive Monospot test result reveals heterophil antibodies.[1,2,5] The Monospot test is highly specific and sensitive, but it may take 2 to 3 weeks of illness to produce a positive result. Therefore an initial false-negative finding may occur.[5] Symptoms of teary eyes and watery discharge from the eyes, pruritus, rhinitis, postnasal drip, pale and boggy nasal mucosa, and erythematous pharynx with mucus are commonly seen with seasonal allergies.

Thrush, a white, thick, cheese-like material that can be scraped off, is identified with a positive potassium hydroxide test result. Peritonsillar cellulitis differs from pharyngitis by the physical examination findings and the absence of pus on aspiration. A peritonsillar abscess can be diagnosed by presenting signs and symptoms, and the aspiration of pus. Tonsillitis may be present with pharyngitis.[1]

Although presenting signs and symptoms of a URI are similar to those of mild viral pharyngitis, a URI usually has associated symptoms such as cough, congestion, rhinitis, sneezing, injected conjunctiva, erythematous and edematous nasal mucosa, and erythematous pharynx.[1,2] Epiglottitis must be excluded by radiographic imaging or by direct laryngoscopy once it is suspected; however, patients with epiglottitis typically cannot effectively swallow their own saliva.[1]

Severe exudative pharyngitis or tonsillitis is usually present in mononucleosis. A thick, gray membrane over the tonsils and pharynx is indicative of diphtheria. Leukoplakia, a white patch, is a premalignant change that may arise anywhere on the oral mucosa. Leukoplakia lesions cannot be removed with a tongue depressor as is seen with oral thrush (Fig. 83.2). If it is suspected, a thorough history is warranted. If the lesion remains for more than 2 weeks, a biopsy is indicated.

INTERPROFESSIONAL COLLABORATIVE MANAGEMENT

Indications for Referral or Hospitalization

An evaluation by an otolaryngologist should be sought for recurrent GAS infections or for complications that may result from pharyngitis. In addition, potential airway obstruction from pharyngitis or abscess requires immediate referral to an

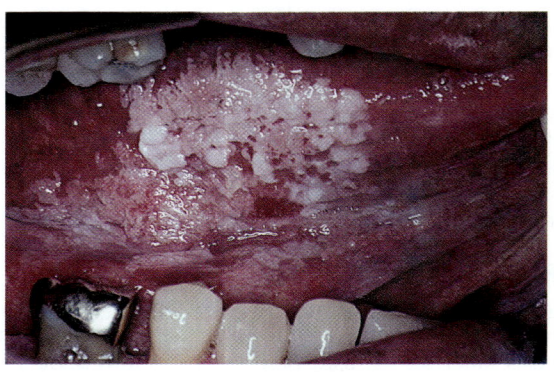

F I G. **83.2** Leukoplakia on the ventral aspect of the tongue. (From Eisen, D., & Lynch, D. P. [1998]. *The mouth: Diagnosis and treatment.* St Louis: Mosby.)

otolaryngologist and hospitalization. Peritonsillar abscess and retropharyngeal abscess require hospitalization for observation and intravenous antibiotics. Abscesses usually require incision and drainage. Patients with acute renal failure (ARF) and post-streptococcal glomerulonephritis may require hospitalization, depending on symptoms. Patients diagnosed with ARF require antibiotic prophylaxis, although debate exists about the duration of prophylaxis.[1]

Pharmacologic Management

Viral Pharyngitis and Tonsillitis

Analgesic/Antipyretics. Acetaminophen or nonsteroidal antiinflammatory drugs should be used for sore throat, fever, and general malaise. Anesthetic throat lozenges may be used but should be avoided in young children or anyone at risk of choking.[1,2] Aspirin also should be avoided because of the risk of Reyes syndrome.[2] Fluids, humidification, voice rest, and warm saline gargles are used to ease discomfort in both viral and bacterial pharyngitis.[2]

Bacterial Pharyngitis and Tonsillitis. As with viral pharyngitis, symptomatic treatment is initiated along with appropriate antibiotic therapy.

Antibiotics. Antibiotic therapy with penicillin or amoxicillin for 10 days is indicated in GAS pharyngitis primarily to prevent complications and sequela, such as suppurative tonsillitis, glomerulonephritis, and rheumatic fever.[2,5,10] Penicillin is often prescribed because of its low cost, safety, and efficacy. For those allergic to penicillin, clindamycin or clarithromycin for 10 days is appropriate. Another option is azithromycin for 5 days.[10]

Treatment of non–group A streptococcal infection is given for symptomatic relief because the organisms are not linked to serious sequelae and do not produce a major antibody response.[2]

Nonpharmacologic Management

Surgery. The management of chronic pharyngitis or tonsillitis with GAS infection may require tonsillectomy. Tonsillectomy is not performed as often as in the past due to retrospective studies that suggest there is little benefit and a chance of significant post-surgical complications.[12]

LIFE SPAN CONSIDERATIONS

More than 11 million visits occur annually for pharyngitis in the United States. Pharyngitis is an entity that affects all age groups and populations. The highest numbers of bacterial infections occur in those under 15.[2] EBV is most often found in patients aged between 15 and 24 years.[5] A comprehensive head and neck examination and history are required for accurate assessment of the situation and for appropriate treatment to be prescribed. Pharyngitis that lasts more than 2 weeks in an adult smoker should be considered a cancer unless proven otherwise.[8] Prompt and proper diagnosis of patients who truly have *S. pyogenes* infections can have a significant effect on the morbidity of the disease.[3]

COMPLICATIONS

Complications from chronic tonsillitis include upper airway obstruction, sleep apnea, and sleep disturbances. Complications from acute streptococcal infections can be divided into suppurative and nonsuppurative entities. Suppurative complications include streptococcal pharyngitis, otitis media, sinusitis, impetigo, pneumonia, and necrotizing fasciitis. Nonsuppurative complications associated with GAS infection include ARF and poststreptococcal glomerulonephritis.[1,3]

Unfortunately, glomerulonephritis may result even with proper treatment. ARF can be prevented by prompt antibiotic therapy for the prescribed time. Because the diagnosis of GAS pharyngitis is difficult on the basis of clinical findings alone, the practitioner should use recommended guidelines in the assessment of the patient thought to have GAS pharyngitis.[5,10]

PATIENT AND FAMILY EDUCATION

Education is extremely important, and adherence to antibiotic therapy must be stressed. Patients should understand that they are infectious until 24 hours after the start of antibiotic therapy and that a full course of antibiotics is required to prevent reinfection or complications.[2]

In general, patients should start to feel better 24 to 48 hours after the start of antibiotic therapy. Patients should be encouraged to use a new toothbrush 48 hours after antibiotic therapy is started to decrease the possibility of a recurrent infection. The old toothbrush should be discarded.[2]

Education for the patient with viral pharyngitis is important. Supportive measures should be encouraged. Patients can expect symptom resolution of the pharyngitis during a 1- to 3-week period.[1] Antibiotics are inappropriate in viral infections, but patients and families may require considerable teaching to understand the importance of avoiding antibiotic therapy when appropriate.[1,2,13] Patients and families need to understand to return for evaluation if there is a return of fever and symptoms.

HEALTH PROMOTION

Health promotion involving pharyngitis covers many areas. Proper oral hygiene should be addressed with all age groups at all visits. Education regarding the misuse of antibiotic therapy for viral entities should also be stressed.[2,10] Of importance is teaching patients, families, and health care workers about the need for an appropriate handwashing technique. Limiting exposure to individuals with pharyngitis also must be included in patient teaching.[3,13]

REFERENCES

1. Flint, P. W., Haughty, B. H., Thomas, J. R., et al. (2015). *Cummings otolaryngology: Head and neck surgery* (6th ed.). St Louis, MO: Mosby.

2. Ruppert, S. D., & Vaunette, P. F. (2015). Pharyngitis: Soothing the sore throat. *The Nurse Practitioner, 40*(7), 18–25.

3. Pham, L. L., Bourayou, R., Maghraoui-Slim, V., & Kone'-Paut, I. (2017). Laryngitis, epiglottitis, and pharyngitis. In J. Cohen (Ed.), *Infectious disease* (4th ed., pp. 229–235). China: Elsevier.

4. Arnold, J. C., & Nizet, V. (2018). Pharyngitis. In S. S. Long (Ed.), *Principals and practice of pediatric infectious disease* (5th ed., pp. 202–208). Philadelphia, PA: Elsevier.

5. Singer, S. F. (2018). Ear, nose and throat. In R. Olympia, R. O'Neill, & M. Silvis (Eds.), *Urgent care medicine: Secrets* (pp. 8–15). Philadelphia, PA: Elsevier.

6. Farooqi, I. A., Akram, T., & Zaka, M. (2017). Incidence and empiric use of antibiotics therapy for tonsillitis in children. *International Journal of Applied Research, 3*(12).

7. Pizzorno, J. E., Murray, M. T., & Joiner-Bey, H. (2016). Streptococcal phyaryngitis. In *The clininian's handbook of natural medicine* (pp. 911–913). St. Louis, MO: Elsevier.

8. National Cancer Institute. (2016). Oral complications of chemotherapy and head/neck radiation (PDQ) Health Professional Version. Retrieved from https://www.cancer.gov/about-cancer/treatment/side-effects/mouth-throat/oral-complications-hp-pdq.

9. Martin, J. M. (2010). Pharyngitis and streptococcal throat infections. *Pediatric Annals, 39*(1).

10. Infectious Disease Society of America. (2012). Recommendations. *Clinical Infectious Diseases: an Official Publication of the Infectious Diseases Society of America, 55.* Retrieved from https://academic.oup.com/cid/article/55/10/e86/321183.

11. Fine, A. M., Nizet, V., & Mandl, K. D. (2011). Improved diagnostic accuracy of group A streptococcal pharyngitis with use of real-time biosurveillance. *Annals of Internal Medicine, 155*(6).

12. Burton, M. J., Glasziou, P. P., Chong, L. Y., & Venekamp, R. P. (2014). Tonsillectomy or adenotonsillectomy versus non-surgical treatment for chronic/recurrent acute tonsillitis (Review). *The Cochrane Database of Systematic Reviews,* (11), CD001802.

13. Mayo Clinic Staff. (2018). Sore throat, Mayo Clinic. Retrieved from www.mayoclinic.org/diseases-conditions/sore-throat/basics/definition/CON-20027360?p=1.

CHAPTER 84

ACUTE BRONCHITIS
Patricia Polgar-Bailey

DEFINITION AND EPIDEMIOLOGY

Acute bronchitis is an acute and self-limited inflammation of the trachea and major bronchi, generally characterized by cough lasting 1 to 3 weeks without evidence of bronchial consolidation (as seen in pneumonia) or underlying cardiopulmonary disease.[1] Clinically, it is diagnosed on the basis of acute cough, with or without phlegm, and occasionally dyspnea and wheezing. It is typically viral in origin[2] and is considered part of the spectrum of upper respiratory infections (URIs), which also includes acute otitis, pharyngitis, tonsillitis, and acute sinusitis, but by definition bronchitis is an inflammation of the lower respiratory tract.[3]

Cough is the most frequent illness-related reason for visits to primary care physicians, accounting for approximately 8% of all visits.[4] The most common causes of acute cough are URIs and acute bronchitis, which together account for approximately 60% of diagnosed cases.[3] In the United States, acute bronchitis affects approximately 5% of the population annually and is the most common cause of acute cough.[5] Symptom relief is the primary reason for seeking medical attention, and of those who seek care, most do so within the first week of illness.[6] Each episode of acute bronchitis results in approximately 2 to 3 missed work days.[7] A higher incidence of acute bronchitis has been noted during the autumn and winter months, when other URIs occur with frequency.[4] Environmental factors such as living in substandard housing also predispose individuals, particularly children, to higher rates of acute bronchitis.[8]

Viruses account for an estimated 90% or more of cases of acute bronchitis and include most commonly influenza A and B viruses, parainfluenza virus, and respiratory syncytial virus (RSV), and less commonly coronavirus, adenovirus, rhinovirus, and human metapneumovirus.[9] Influenza occurs in distinct outbreaks and can result in significant morbidity because of its rapid spread.[6] The incidence of RSV is high in households with small children and in areas where older adults predominate, such as geriatric wards, senior day care settings, and nursing homes, and it can be a significant cause of morbidity in older adults.[6] Severe acute respiratory syndrome (SARS), first defined by the World Health Organization in 2003, is caused by a novel coronavirus.[6]

Less than 10% of cases of acute bronchitis are bacterial in origin, and these are more common in patients with chronic health problems.[5] These less common nonviral causes of acute bronchitis include atypical bacteria that also cause community-acquired pneumonia (CAP), such as *Bordetella pertussis*, *Mycoplasma pneumoniae*, *Moraxella catarrhalis*, and *Chlamydia pneumoniae* (as distinguished from *Chlamydia trachomatis*, which causes pneumonia in neonates). Common upper respiratory flora such as *Haemophilus influenzae* and *Streptococcus pneumoniae* are often found in sputum samples of patients with acute bronchitis, but it is unclear if their presence contributes to disease development.[3]

PATHOPHYSIOLOGY

Acute bronchitis is generally a viral infection and the role of bacteria in this infection remains controversial since bronchial samples rarely show bacterial etiology. Although the causative pathogen for acute bronchitis is rarely identified, the cause of cough in uncomplicated acute bronchitis tends to be multifactorial. It is the result of edematous changes in the mucous membrane of the tracheobronchial tree, epithelial cell damage, the release of proinflammatory mediators, and an increase in secretions. Destruction of the bronchial epithelium and loss of ciliary function are usually minimal with the common cold viruses but may be more extensive with *M. pneumoniae* and influenza viruses. Transient airflow obstruction and bronchial hyperresponsiveness occur in approximately 40% of previously healthy adults without concomitant conditions and usually resolve within 6 weeks.[6]

Acute bronchitis may be associated with a variety of symptoms, depending on anatomic distribution of the pathogen involved. For example, rhinovirus, a pathogen generally presumed to cause URI, has been found in a significant percentage of bronchoalveolar lavage specimens. Viral infection of lower airways may help explain the association between viral infection, such as that caused by rhinovirus, and asthma exacerbations.[4] Cigarette smoking and chemical irritants may increase the severity of the infection. Undiagnosed asthma may be a factor, but this can be difficult to establish because of the transient bronchial hyperresponsiveness and abnormal spirometry results that often accompany acute bronchitis.

CLINICAL PRESENTATION AND PHYSICAL EXAMINATION

A cough with or without sputum production is the most common symptom reported with acute bronchitis. It is because the cough is so bothersome and slow to resolve that patients tend to seek treatment.[9] Characteristics of the cough may vary. It is often described as dry and nonproductive, but it commonly progresses to a productive cough as the illness evolves. The sputum may be clear at the onset of the infection and become mucoid. Approximately 50% of patients with acute bronchitis report a cough productive of purulent sputum.[3] A common but inaccurate belief is that a productive cough or purulent sputum is indicative of a bacterial infection and requires antibiotic therapy. In fact, in otherwise healthy individuals, the production of purulent sputum is the often the result of sloughing of the tracheal bronchial epithelium and inflammatory cells.[3] The cough may also produce a burning substernal pain with inspiration. Nasal and pharyngeal symptoms subside after 3 or 4 days, but the cough usually remains prominent and progressive, typically lasting for 10 to 20 days (though it may occasionally persist for up to 5 or 6 weeks).[4] A low-grade fever, wheezes, rhonchi, and coarse rales may be present. However, substantial abnormalities in vital signs are infrequent, especially in older adults, even when symptoms have been present for a week or more.[4] Approximately 40% to 60% of patients may have significant reductions (a value below 80% of predicted) in forced expiratory volume in 1 second (FEV_1), with gradual improvement during the ensuing 5 to 6 weeks.[4,7] Individuals with *M. pneumoniae* or *C. pneumoniae* infections often have lower FEV_1 values and demonstrate a greater degree of reversibility than do those with viral causes.[6]

DIAGNOSTICS
Essential Diagnostics

Diagnostic tests are generally not necessary in the diagnosis of acute bronchitis. Cough and normal vital signs, in the absence of tachypnea, tachycardia, rales, and egophony, are strongly suggestive of acute bronchitis and minimize the likelihood of pneumonia.

Additional Diagnostics

Laboratory testing is not usually indicated in the evaluation of acute bronchitis but if done, a significant leukocytosis is more likely with a bacterial infection than with a viral illness. Elevated C-reactive protein levels were associated with an increased likelihood of pneumonia in a large primary care trial. Similarly pneumonia can generally be ruled out in patients with C-reactive protein levels of less than 10 mcg/dL and no dyspnea or fever.[9] Routine sputum cultures are not helpful because they are often contaminated by bacterial flora that normally colonize the nasopharyngeal area. Viral cultures and serologic assays should not be routinely performed because they are rarely helpful in identifying the causative agent and as a result are not useful in guiding treatment.[3,6] Rapid diagnostic tests exist for several of the pathogens that cause acute bronchitis. However, not all of these tests are widely available, and routine use in outpatient settings is not cost-effective or necessary. Their use is indicated when there is suspicion of a treatable organism or an infectious outbreak in the community, there are specific signs and symptoms that are identifiable and suggestive of the illness, and diagnosis and treatment would impact the care of the patient. Multiplex polymerase chain reaction testing of nasopharyngeal swabs or aspirates is being developed for diagnosis of infections resulting from *B. pertussis*, *M. pneumoniae*, or *C. pneumoniae*.[4]

A chest radiograph may be useful if the history and physical examination suggest the possibility of CAP. A heightened suspicion of CAP is reasonable in older adults because they may be seen initially with more subtle symptoms of lower respiratory tract infections or cough without any other distinctive signs and symptoms. Data suggest that only one-third of individuals 75 years of age and older who had CAP had temperatures higher than 38°C and heart rates above 100 beats per minute.[4] According to the American College of Chest Physicians (ACCP) 2006 clinical practice guidelines, the absence of the following findings reduces the likelihood of pneumonia sufficiently eliminate the need for a chest radiograph: heart rate above 100 beats per minute; respiratory rate above 24 breaths per minute; oral body temperature higher than 38°C; and chest examination findings of focal consolidation, egophony, or fremitus.[6]

DIFFERENTIAL DIAGNOSIS

 Immediate emergency department referral should be considered for dyspnea, high fever, tachycardia and evidence of consolidation or presence of symptoms for 2 weeks or more.

Distinguishing between acute bronchitis and a simple URI within the first several days of illness is difficult, but a cough that persists for longer than 7 days is suggestive of acute bronchitis.[5] Because acute bronchitis is a clinical diagnosis, how providers assign the diagnosis varies. For example, some providers diagnose acute bronchitis only if a productive cough is present, whereas others make the determination based on the presence of purulent sputum. Discolored sputum is commonly but mistakenly interpreted by both patients and health care providers as clinical evidence of bacterial infection. There has been no evidence to indicate correlation between discolored sputum and a bacterial cause of acute bronchitis.[10] A cough that lasts for longer than 3 weeks should prompt consideration of another diagnosis.

Other causes of cough, with or without phlegm production, include the common cold, reflux esophagitis, acute asthma, chronic obstructive pulmonary disease (COPD), and pneumonia. The symptoms of the common cold or URI, such as nasal stuffiness, discharge, sneezing, sore throat, and cough, can also be present in acute and chronic bronchitis.[5] Acute sinusitis in the context of a cold may stimulate cough receptors.[5]

Because pneumonia is the third most common cause of cough (following asthma), usually not self-limited, often bacterial in origin, and associated with considerable morbidity and mortality when it is not treated with antimicrobial therapy, distinguishing between acute bronchitis and pneumonia is of primary importance.[11] This is particularly true in elders, because older adults are less likely to have respiratory or nonrespiratory symptoms.[6]

Acute bronchitis is an inflammation of the trachea and bronchi and should be differentiated from asthma and bronchiolitis, which are acute inflammations of the small airway and generally characterized by wheezing, tachypnea, respiratory distress, and hypoxemia. Acute bronchitis should also be distinguished from bronchiectasis, which is associated with bronchial dilation and chronic cough.[4]

Infection with *B. pertussis* should also be considered in adults who have a paroxysmal cough lasting longer than 2 weeks, especially in the context of a community outbreak. Fever is less common with pertussis infection than with viral bronchitis.[4] Although infection with *B. pertussis* is rarely life-threatening in adults, its diagnosis is important because of the complications it can cause in older adults or in infants who have not been vaccinated against the disease.

Epidemiologic data may be helpful in the diagnosis of acute bronchitis. For example, contact with a confirmed case of pertussis and paroxysmal cough or post-tussive vomiting strongly suggest *B. pertussis* infection. Outbreaks in specific populations, such as military personnel or college students, may suggest *M. pneumoniae* or *C. pneumoniae* infection.[6] Nursing homes and long-term care facilities tend to harbor a wide range of viral

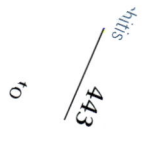

,ens, including influenza and parainfluenza coronaviruses, some of which are difficult .andard viral cultures.[12] Residents of these increased risk for the nosocomial spread of ..es.

...sis of chronic bronchitis should be considered only for ... e patients who have had cough and sputum production on most days of the month for at least 3 months of the year during 2 consecutive years. During influenza outbreaks, the presence of both cough and fever is highly predictive of influenza.[4] Other differential diagnoses include rhinitis, sinusitis, foreign body aspiration, tuberculosis, tumors, and other chronic lung diseases.

There is considerable clinical overlap in the symptoms of acute bronchitis, other respiratory symptoms, and asthma. Data suggest that many patients are misdiagnosed with acute bronchitis and their cough is more likely caused by asthma, an acute exacerbation of chronic bronchitis, or a mild URI such as the common cold.[4]

INTERPROFESSIONAL COLLABORATIVE MANAGEMENT

Nonpharmacologic Management

The mainstay of treatment in acute bronchitis is directed toward symptom reduction and supportive care. Data suggest that 85% of patients diagnosed with acute bronchitis will improve without specific treatment.[7]

Pharmacologic Management

Despite evidence that only 5% to 10% of acute bronchitis cases have a bacterial cause, data indicate that antibiotics continue to be prescribed for approximately two-thirds (approximately 71% to 73%) of patients in the United States.[13,14] Despite current Agency for Healthcare Research and Quality guidelines[15] that discourage the routine use of antibiotics for acute bronchitis, the percentage of patients receiving antibiotics for acute bronchitis has increased, and patient expectations for antibiotic therapy are largely responsible for this trend.[1] More than half of the antibiotic prescriptions are for extended-spectrum antibiotics.[6] Certain populations are more likely to receive unnecessary antibiotics, including elders and cigarette smokers. There is no evidence that cigarette smokers with acute bronchitis, in the absence of underlying COPD, are in need of antibiotics any more than nonsmokers are.[6] Studies of uncomplicated acute bronchitis in the general population demonstrate little benefit from antibiotic use when a treatable pathogen is not identified, even with smokers. Any benefit demonstrated has been of questionable clinical significance (i.e., decrease in symptoms by only a fraction of a day with the use of the three most commonly prescribed antibiotics[15]), which is offset by the risks of antibiotic use, including serious adverse effects (e.g., *Clostridium difficile* diarrhea, anaphylaxis), drug-drug interactions, financial burden, and the possibility of future antibiotic resistance.[6] In addition, antibiotic therapy for acute bronchitis has not been shown to have any impact on activity limitations.[16] The problem of antimicrobial resistance has become a serious public health threat, and rates of resistance to penicillin and macrolide antibiotics are particularly high. Decreasing the inappropriate use of antibiotics is the first step in decreasing antibiotic resistance.

Antitussive therapy is commonly prescribed, but the evidence for its effectiveness is weak.[6,7] According to the ACCP

2006 evidence-based guidelines for the diagnosis and management of acute bronchitis, antitussive agents are occasionally useful and can be offered for short-term symptomatic relief of coughing.[6] A dextromethorphan cough preparation or benzonatate may help alleviate the cough. Codeine or hydrocodone may be useful at bedtime if the cough is severe. Antipyretics, bed rest, and increased fluid consumption to thin the secretions are also beneficial treatments. In trials involving the use of β-adrenergic bronchodilators for uncomplicated acute bronchitis in adults, there was no demonstrated reduction in symptoms, including cough. Subgroups of patients with airflow obstruction and wheezing at the onset of illness did experience some benefit from the bronchodilators.[6] Based on these studies, the ACCP guidelines and other recommendations state that β-adrenergic bronchodilators should not be routinely used to alleviate cough, but in those patients with acute bronchitis and wheezing associated with the cough, bronchodilators may be useful.[6,17] According to the ACCP guidelines, there is no consistent favorable evidence for the use of mucokinetic agents for cough, and they are not recommended.[6]

Antibiotic therapy is recommended if pertussis is suspected. Pertussis is an acute bacterial infection of the respiratory tract caused by *B. pertussis*, a gram-negative bacterium. *B. pertussis* is transmitted primarily through aerosolized droplets of respiratory secretions or by direct contact with an infected person.[18] Studies indicate that pertussis may be present in 10% to 20% of patients with cough lasting longer than 2 weeks. Unfortunately, distinguishing pertussis from other sources of acute cough is difficult because pertussis in adults with previous immunity does not lead to the classic features of whooping cough that are seen in children. Suspicion of pertussis should be limited to individuals with a high probability of exposure, such as in community outbreaks. Patients with confirmed and probable pertussis should receive antimicrobial antibiotic therapy and be isolated for 5 days from the start of treatment.[6] Early treatment of pertussis is very important. If treatment is started early in the course of illness, during the first 2 weeks before coughing paroxysms occur, symptoms may be reduced. Treatment before receipt of confirmatory test results should be considered if clinical history is strongly suggestive of pertussis or if the patient is at risk for severe or complicated disease.[18] If diagnosis is late and antimicrobial therapy is not started within the first 5 to 7 days of symptom onset, therapy is less likely to alter the course of the illness. However, antimicrobial therapy may still decrease shedding of the bacteria and in that way limit spread of the disease.[18] Persons with pertussis are infectious from the beginning of the catarrhal stage (runny nose, low-grade fever, common cold symptoms) through the third week after the onset of paroxysmal cough or until 5 days after the onset of antibiotic therapy.[18]

Macrolides are used as first-line therapy for the treatment of pertussis. Trimethoprim-sulfamethoxazole can also be used if macrolides are not an option.

On March 12, 2013, the Food and Drug Administration (FDA) issued a warning that azithromycin can cause abnormal changes in the electrical activity of the heart that may lead to a potentially fatal irregular heart rhythm in some patients. An alternative to azithromycin should be considered in persons with known cardiovascular disease, including (1) those with known prolongation of the QT interval, a history of torsades de pointes, congenital long QT syndrome, bradyarrhythmias, or uncompensated heart failure; (2) those on drugs known to prolong the QT interval; and (3) those with ongoing proarrhythmic conditions such as uncorrected hypokalemia or hypomagnesemia or clinically significant bradycardia and patients receiving class IA (quinidine, procainamide) or class III (dofetilide, amiodarone, sotalol) antiarrhythmic agents.[18]

The most common pathogen isolated in acute bronchitis is influenza; therefore, anti-influenza agents may be effective if influenza is diagnosed and treatment initiated within 48 hours after onset of symptoms (see Chapter 93).[4] Because pneumonia is the third most common cause of cough illness, the presence of pneumonia should be excluded.

Even though older adults may not always manifest the typical features of pneumonia, such as fever and other vital sign abnormalities, the predictive value of these simple clinical tools remains high and should not be neglected. For atypical manifestations of pneumonia in older adults, such as diminished appetite, increased falls, and altered mental status, see Chapter 93.

Studies suggest that several factors contribute to and influence the decision to prescribe an antibiotic, including patient beliefs, desires, and expectations and provider perceptions about what is indicated clinically and what is necessary to ensure patient satisfaction.[19] Patients frequently expect to receive antibiotics for acute bronchitis, perhaps because they received antibiotics for similar symptoms in the past. In one study, less than 50% of the general public accurately identified antibiotics as being effective against bacterial infections and not against viral infections.[4] Nonetheless, patient expectations are among the strongest predictors of a provider's decision to prescribe an antibiotic, even though providers' perceptions of patient expectations are unclear or inaccurate up to 50% of the time.[9,19] Some providers also erroneously believe that if they do not prescribe antibiotics, the patient is more likely to return for another visit and take up more time. A study by Li and colleagues found that patients who received antibiotics during the index visit did not have a decreased rate of return visits.[19] In fact, the results suggested that patients who received antibiotics may have had higher expectations for a rapid resolution of their symptoms compared with those who, in lieu of obtaining an antibiotic prescription, received more education and counseling about the natural history of viral infections.[18] Providers also perceive that visits in which an antibiotic prescription is given take significantly less time and result in higher patient satisfaction than do visits in which no antibiotic prescription is given. Neither of these perceptions has been supported by research. Patient satisfaction with an office visit for acute bronchitis does not depend on receiving antimicrobial therapy but rather is centered on the nature of the provider-patient relationship as experienced during that visit. Even though acute bronchitis is a common diagnosis that resolves on its own, patients' satisfaction is primarily related to how much time was spent explaining the illness and answering their questions.

Indications for Referral or Hospitalization

Acute bronchitis that does not respond to symptomatic treatment and lingers longer than 2 weeks may require physician referral. Patients with progressive dyspnea, oxygen saturation less than 90%, and signs of sepsis require hospitalization for intravenous therapy, enhanced pulmonary therapy, and intravenous antibiotics.

COMPLICATIONS

Although acute bronchitis is often viral and self-limited, complications do occur. The development of a chronic cough, usually the result of postbronchitis reactive airway disease, can cause discomfort and sleep loss. Pneumonia results from bacterial superinfection and can cause dyspnea, chest pain, and anxiety in addition to other symptoms. If the cough lasts 3 weeks or longer, a chest X-ray study is indicated in the absence of other known causes. Acute respiratory failure, although uncommon, is a potential sequela. Individuals with chronic bronchitis are more susceptible to superinfection and can develop exercise intolerance and hypoxia.

PATIENT AND FAMILY EDUCATION

Reassurance and education are probably the most important modalities for treatment of acute bronchitis. Education should include a realistic expectation of the duration of the cough (generally 10 to 14 days) and the general ineffectiveness of antibiotic therapy for this diagnosis. Rest, increased fluids, and breathing of moist air from a clean humidifier or warm shower should be encouraged. Patients should be counseled about smoking cessation and the need to avoid air pollution and irritants. An appropriate face mask can be helpful if work involves chemicals, dust, or other irritants. Patients should be encouraged to call their health care provider if the symptoms continue or increase in severity.

The Centers for Disease Control and Prevention (CDC) recommends that providers refer to acute bronchitis as a "chest cold" to minimize expectations that antibiotics are appropriate therapy. In addition, the CDC offers the following suggestions to decrease antibiotic prescribing and use:

- Explain that antibiotic use increases the risk of antibiotic-resistant infections, and provide educational materials on antibiotic resistance.
- Identify and validate patient concerns.
- Recommend specific symptomatic therapy.
- Spend time answering questions, and offer an alternative plan if symptoms worsen.[17]

Additional patient education information can be obtained from the American Lung Association, 61 Broadway, 6th floor, New York, NY 10006; 800-586-4872; www.lungusa.org.

REFERENCES

1. Dempsey, P., Businger, A., Whaley, L., et al. (2014). Primary care clinicians perceptions about antibiotics prescribing for acute bronchitis: A qualitative study. *BMC Family Practice, 15,* 194.
2. Smith, S., Smucny, J., & Fahey, T. (2014). Antibiotics for acute bronchitis. *JAMA: The Journal of the American Medical Association, 312*(24), 2678–2679.
3. Blush, R. (2013). Acute bronchitis: Evaluation and management. *The Nurse Practitioner, 38*(1), 14–20.
4. Wenzel, R., & Fowler, A. (2010). Acute bronchitis. *The New England Journal of Medicine, 355*(20), 2125–2130.
5. Tackett, K., & Atkins, A. (2012). Evidence-based acute bronchitis therapy. *Journal of Pharmacy Practice, 25*(6), 586–590.
6. Braman, S. (2006). Chronic cough due to acute bronchitis: ACCP evidence-based clinical practice guidelines. *Chest, 129,* 95S–103S.
7. Worrall, G. (2008). Acute bronchitis. *Canadian Family Physician, 54,* 238–239.
8. Chenoweth, D., Estes, C., & Lee, C. (2009). The economic cost of environmental factors among North Carolina children living in substandard housing. *American Journal of Public Health, 99,* S666–S2674.
9. Kinkade, S., & Long, N. (2016). Acute bronchitis. *American Family Physician, 94*(7), 560–565.
10. Altiner, A., Wilm, S., Däubener, W., et al. (2009). Sputum colour for diagnosis of a bacterial infection in patients with acute cough. *Scandinavian Journal of Primary Health Care, 27,* 70–73.

11. Evertsen, J., Baumgardner, D., Regnery, A., et al. (2010). Diagnosis and management of pneumonia and bronchitis in outpatient primary care practices. *Primary Care Respiratory Journal: Journal of the General Practice Airways Group, 19*(3), 237–241.

12. Falsey, A., Dallal, G., Formica, M., et al. (2008). Long-term care facilities: A cornucopia of viral pathogens. *Journal of the American Geriatrics Society, 56,* 1281–1285.

13. Singh, M., & Koyfman, A. (2015). Are antibiotics effective in the treatment of acute bronchitis? *Annals of Emergency Medicine, 65*(5), 566–567.

14. Dallas, A., Magin, P., Morgan, S., et al. (2014). Antibiotic prescribing for respiratory infections: A cross-sectional analysis of the ReCEnt study exploring the habits of early-career doctors in primary care. *Family Practice, 32*(1), 49–55.

15. National Guideline Clearinghouse. Management of uncomplicated bronchitis in adults. Retrieved from www.guideline.gove/content.aspx?id=38668. (Accessed 7 May 2015).

16. Benninger, M., & Segreti, J. (2008). Is it bacterial or viral? Criteria for distinguishing bacterial and viral infections. *The Journal of Family Practice, 57*(Suppl. 2), S5–S11.

17. Kolinsky, D., & Schwarz, E. (2016). Do β-2 agonists for acute bronchitis provide any benefit? *Annals of Emergency Medicine, 67*(6), 702–703.

18. Centers for Disease Control and Prevention. Pertussis treatment. Retrieved from www.cdc.gov/pertussis/clinical/treatment.html. (Accessed 4 June 2015).

19. Li, J., De, A., Ketchum, K., et al. (2009). Antimicrobial prescribing for upper respiratory infections and its effect on return visits. *Family Medicine, 41*(3), 182–187.

CHAPTER **85**

ASTHMA

Patricia Polgar-Bailey

DEFINITION AND EPIDEMIOLOGY

 Emergency evaluation/treatment is indicated for persons with signs and symptoms suggestive of respiratory compromise, including respiratory rate >30/min, pulse rate >120 beats per minute, O_2 saturation (on room air) <90%, peak expiratory flow (PEF) <50% predicted or best, drowsiness, confusion, or silent chest.

Asthma is a chronic inflammatory disorder of the airways characterized by increased responsiveness of the tracheobronchial tree to various stimuli, resulting in episodic reversible narrowing and inflammation of the airways.[1,2] In susceptible individuals, this bronchial inflammation causes recurrent episodes of wheezing, shortness of breath, chest tightness, and cough. These episodes are usually associated with widespread but variable airflow obstruction that is often reversible, either spontaneously or with treatment. The inflammation also causes an associated increase in the existing bronchial hyperresponsiveness to a variety of stimuli.[1,2]

Asthma attacks can vary from mild to life threatening and can be triggered by many factors, including allergens, infections, exercise, abrupt changes in weather, and exposure to airway irritants such as tobacco smoke.[2] The concept of asthma as a chronic and inflammatory process represented a significant change in the previous understanding of the disease. During the past decade, there have been substantial advances in the understanding of the genetics, pathogenesis, and natural course of the disease, which have had important implications for its management, particularly the development of new, targeted therapies, especially for severe asthma.[1]

Asthma is the most common chronic respiratory disorder among all age groups and affects 4.3% to 27% of people worldwide.[3] Although the global prevalence of asthma increased markedly during the latter half of the of the 20th century, it appears to have plateaued since then, especially in countries with the highest asthma rates such as the United Kingdom.[1] An exception to this is the United States, where the prevalence of asthma increased from 7.3% (20.3 million persons) in 2001 to 8.4% (25.7 million persons) in 2010. In 2016, prevalence among children (persons younger than 18 years) was 8.3% and was highest among poor children (13.5%) and among non-Hispanic black children (11.6%). Prevalence among adults was 8.3%. The poor are disproportionately affect by asthma; 11.8% of those at 100% of the federal poverty level (FPL) or less are affected, as compared with 7.1% of those at 450% of the FPL or greater.[4] These statistics, as striking as they are, may still underestimate the actual prevalence of asthma, especially in communities where access to care, including emergency care, is limited.[5] Persons of black (10.2%) and American Indian or Alaska Native (9.4%) races had higher asthma prevalence compared with white persons (8.2%). Among Hispanic groups, asthma prevalence was higher among persons of Puerto Rican (14.3%) than Mexican (5.7%) descent.[6]

Asthma attack prevalence refers to the number of people who had at least one asthma attack during the previous year; it is a crude indicator of how many people have uncontrolled asthma or are at risk for a poor outcome, such as hospitalization.[6] In 2016, at least half (46.9%) of those diagnosed with asthma reported having an asthma attack within the past year.[7] Asthma attack prevalence decreases with age; a greater proportion of children than adults (57.2% vs. 50.7%) were reported to have had an asthma attack within the preceding 12 months. Women have a 35% higher asthma attack prevalence than men, but this pattern is reversed among children, in whom the attack prevalence for boys was 3.4% compared with a prevalence of 2.2% for girls.[6] A greater proportion of persons who had an asthma attack reported being in fair or poor health (24.8%) than of those who did not have an asthma attack (17.9%).[7]

Asthma interferes with daily activities, including attending school and going to work. On average each year, children miss approximately 4 days of school and adults miss 5 days of work because of asthma.[7] Occupational asthma is currently the most common occupational ailment. Widespread exposure in the workplace environment to airborne dusts, gases, vapors, or fumes contributes to both the development of asthma and the worsening of asthma for those already affected. An estimated 1.9 million cases of asthma among adults are work related, accounting for 15.7% of current adult asthma cases. Work-related asthma significantly differs by age; the incidence is highest among persons aged 45 to 64 years (20.7%).[7] Asthma accounts for 10.1 million lost work days annually and a total annual economic cost of $19.7 billion—$14.7 billion in direct costs, and another $5 billion in lost productivity.[7]

Asthma is one of the most common reasons for visits in ambulatory settings; in 2016 there were 8.9 million office visits related to asthma and a disproportionate number for ED visits and hospitalizations are due to asthma. Asthma is a condition that can be treated effectively in primary care, resulting in fewer ED visits, improved continuity of care, and decreased health care costs based on Centers for Disease Control and Prevention (CDC) 2017 health statistics for US adults.[8]

Although the asthma prevalence is higher among children, asthma deaths in children are relatively rare, at 2.8 per million compared with 10 per million for adults.[6] Women have an asthma death rate higher than that of men.[6] High mortality rates are associated with high rates of hospitalization in impoverished urban areas. Most of those hospitalized or seen in the ED had been there before, reflecting the fact that inadequate health care results in increased costs.

Asthma hospitalization rates have been highest among African Americans, women, and children; likewise, death rates have consistently been disproportionately higher among African Americans, especially those aged 15 to 24 years.[6] Although prevalence is higher among racial and ethnic minorities, a more valid relationship may exist between socioeconomic status and increased asthma prevalence, morbidity, and mortality than between race and asthma prevalence. Asthma mortality has also been associated with poverty, urban living conditions, exposure to oxidant pollutants, and passive smoking. Allergic asthmatic children exposed to high levels of indoor allergens, such as those associated with cockroaches, rodents, and mold, have more severe and more frequent episodes of asthma.

The financial impact of asthma is considerable. At least 1% of all US health care costs are spent on asthma—an estimated $3300 per person with asthma annually.[7] Direct and indirect asthma-related costs are estimated to be $56 billion per year, with ED visits and hospitalizations responsible for the majority of the cost.

Worldwide, an estimated 300 million people are affected by asthma, and the prevalence of asthma ranges from 1% to 18% of the population, depending on the country.[2] It is estimated that the number of people with asthma will grow by more than 100 million by 2025.[7] Workplace conditions, such as exposure to fumes, gases, or dust, are responsible for 11% of asthma cases worldwide. Prevalence rates vary widely depending on the country, which reflects a true difference in prevalence as well as different diagnostic standards. The prevalence has been increasing in low- and middle-income countries and plateauing in high-income countries. Deaths from asthma worldwide have been estimated at 250,000 per year, but mortality does not appear to correlate well with prevalence.[9] Although the cost to control asthma on a global scale is high, the cost of not treating asthma is even higher.

PATHOPHYSIOLOGY

It is currently believed that the primary event in asthma is airway inflammation and that airway hyperresponsiveness and airflow obstruction are secondary and symptomatic features of the disease. Underlying airway inflammation (which involves cellular infiltration, edema, nerve irritation, and vasodilation) results in constriction of airway smooth muscle, increased production of mucus, and airway hyperresponsiveness. The airflow limitation associated with asthma is caused by a variety of changes in the airway, all of which are influenced by airway inflammation. These changes include bronchoconstriction (bronchial smooth muscle contraction that quickly narrows the airways in response to a variety of stimuli, including allergens and irritants), airway hyperresponsiveness (an exaggerated bronchoconstrictor response to stimuli), and airway edema (hypersecretion of mucus and mucous plugs as the disease becomes more persistent, which further limit flow). With time, remodeling of airways may occur, and reversibility of airway obstruction may be incomplete in some persons. Possible changes in airway structure include subbasement fibrosis, hypersecretion of mucus, epithelial cell injury, smooth muscle hypertrophy, and angiogenesis (the growth of new blood vessels from existing blood vessels).

The development of asthma appears to involve an interplay among host factors, particularly genetics, and environmental factors that occur at a crucial time in the development of the immune system, although a definitive cause of the inflammatory process has not been established.

Different immune responses influence the development of asthma, including the Th1-type and Th2-type cytokine responses. Numerous factors affect the balance between these responses early in life and increase the likelihood that the Th1 immune response—which fights infection—will be downregulated, and that the Th2 immune response—which contributes to the development of allergic diseases and asthma—will dominate. This is known as the hygiene hypothesis, which postulates that early in life, exposure to other children (e.g., presence of older siblings and early enrollment in childcare, which increase the likelihood of exposure to respiratory infection), less frequent use of antibiotics, and "country living" are associated with a Th1 response and a lower incidence of asthma, whereas the absence of these factors is associated with a persistent Th2 response and higher rates of asthma.

Asthma also has an inheritable component, but the genetic factors involved remain complex.[1] One factor involved is atopy, which is the genetic tendency for development of immunoglobulin E (IgE)–mediated hypersensitivity reactions in response to environmental antigens and allergens; it is considered one of the strongest predisposing factors for the development of asthma. Certain stimuli induce asthma by causing or increasing airway inflammation, whereas other stimuli provoke bronchoconstriction in individuals who already have asthma or airway hyperresponsiveness. Inducers, stimuli that are known to increase inflammation, include inhaled allergens, low-molecular-weight sensitizers, viral or mycoplasmal respiratory infections, and high concentrations of noxious gases. Stimuli that trigger or cause bronchoconstriction include exercise, cold air, laughter, emotional upset, and inhaled irritants. Triggers of sudden severe bronchoconstriction include acetylsalicylic acid or nonsteroidal antiinflammatory drugs (NSAIDs), β-adrenergic blockers, food allergens, certain food additives, stings, bites, injections (e.g., allergy shots), and inhaled allergens.

These stimuli set the stage for a cascade of cellular activation, which includes subsequent cytokine release and neurologic excitation. The antigenic response is limited by certain cellular processes such as mast cell activation through cytokines and infiltration by inflammatory cells, including neutrophils, eosinophils, and lymphocytes. The inflammatory cells are also the source of mediators that induce bronchoconstriction, excess production of mucus, airway edema, and further influx of inflammatory cells, all of which lead to bronchial obstruction. The late-phase reaction, which generally occurs 3 to 8 hours after antigen exposure, is the result of new cellular infiltration and activation. Nocturnal and early morning bronchospasm, which occurs with relative frequency in persons with asthma, may be related to circadian variations in cortisol and epinephrine levels, vagal tone, and inflammatory mediators.

One common, often overlooked, exacerbating factor of asthma is esophageal reflux of gastric contents. The incidence of gastroesophageal reflux in adults with asthma ranges from 25% to 80%.[10] Gastroesophageal reflux resulting in distal esophageal stimulation with acid may cause bronchoconstriction or may increase bronchial reactivity through vagal mechanisms. Although the potential mechanism exists for gastroesophageal reflux disease (GERD) to cause asthma symptoms and it is fairly well accepted that GERD may be an exacerbating factor, particularly in difficult-to-control asthma, it remains unclear whether there is a true causal relationship between reflux episodes and asthma symptoms.

In addition to the aforementioned factors, environmental factors appear to play a role in the development of asthma, although the nature of specific environmental contributions is not clearly defined. Exposure in utero to tobacco smoke is associated with an increased risk of wheezing, but it is not clear whether this is linked to subsequent development of asthma. Air pollution (ozone and particular matter) and diet (obesity or low intake of omega-3 fatty acids) have been associated with asthma, although the contribution of these factors to the development of asthma has not been clearly defined.

As mentioned, asthma has a strong genetic component. However, for this to manifest, interaction with environmental factors must occur. At least some of the difference in asthma prevalence between white and minority populations may be a result of differences in genetic susceptibility. Most of the evidence to date suggests that the explanation for these differences is most likely the disparity in socioeconomic, environmental, behavioral, and cultural factors and in access to routine health care.[10]

Asthma is a disease that varies within and among individuals, but inflammation of the airways is a persistent feature, even in persons with mild asthma. Although asthma is considered to be a disease of reversible airflow obstruction, chronic airway inflammation can lead to progressive airway remodeling and airflow obstruction, eventually resulting in an irreversible deterioration of airway function.[1] At present, asthma has no cure, but effective management can reduce its impact on quality of life and morbidity.

CLINICAL PRESENTATION AND PHYSICAL EXAMINATION

The clinical hallmarks of asthma include episodic wheezing associated with dyspnea, cough, and sputum production. Between episodes, symptoms may improve or completely resolve. Symptoms vary from mild to severe, with varying effects on activity. An increased index of suspicion for asthma is essential when respiratory symptoms, including cough, wheeze, shortness of breath, chest tightness, and soreness, persist or recur often. Refer to Box 85.1 for a guide to the assessment of asthma and recommended education.

Although wheezing is probably the symptom most typically associated with asthma, the most common symptom of asthma and often the most troublesome is cough. However, cough is also the third most common presenting symptom in the ambulatory setting, with a corresponding long list of potential causes. Coughing is the only asthma symptom 7% to 57% of the time; this type of asthma is referred to as cough-variant asthma. Cough can be the principal or only manifestation of

---

BOX **85.1**

Management of an Asthma Attack: Home Treatment

ASSESS SEVERITY

- Patients at high risk for a fatal attack require immediate medical attention after initial treatment.
- Symptoms and signs suggestive of a more serious exacerbation such as marked breathlessness, inability to speak more than short phrases, use of accessory muscles, or drowsiness should result in initial treatment while immediately consulting with a clinician.
- Less severe signs and symptoms can be treated initially with assessment of response to therapy and further steps as listed below.
- If available, measure PEF; values of 50%-79% predicted or personal best indicate the need for quick-relief medication. Depending on the response to treatment, contact with a clinician may also be indicated. Values below 50% indicate the need for immediate medical care.

INITIAL TREATMENT

- Inhaled SABA: up to 2 treatments 20 min apart of 2-6 puffs by MDI or nebulizer treatments.
- Exacerbations of lesser severity may need fewer puffs than suggested above.

RESPONSE TO INITIAL TREATMENT

Good Response	Incomplete Response	Poor Response
No wheezing or dyspnea (assess tachypnea in young children).	Persistent wheezing and dyspnea (tachypnea).	Marked wheezing and dyspnea.
PEF is ≥80% predicted or personal best.	PEF is 50%–79% predicted or personal best.	PEF is <50% predicted or personal best.
Actions	**Actions**	**Actions**
Contact clinician for follow-up instructions and further management.	Add oral systemic corticosteroid.	Add oral systemic corticosteroid.
May continue inhaled SABA every 3–4 h for 24–48 h.	Continue inhaled SABA.	Repeat inhaled SABA immediately.
Consider short course of oral systemic corticosteroids.	Consult clinician urgently (this day) for further instruction.	If distress is severe and nonresponsive to initial treatment: • Call your doctor **and** • **Proceed to ED** • Consider calling 911

MDI, Metered dose inhaler; *SABA,* short-acting beta₂ agonist (quick-relief inhaler).
From National Asthma Education and Prevention Program (NAEPP): *Expert panel report 3: guidelines for the diagnosis and management of asthma,* National Institutes of Health (NIH) Publication No. 08-4051, Bethesda, Md, 2007, U.S. Department of Health and Human Services, NIH, National Heart, Lung, and Blood Institute (NHLBI). Available at www.nhlbi.nih.gov/guidelines/asthma/asthgdln.htm.

asthma, especially in young children. Cough is often treated symptomatically, which can easily result in a delayed or missed diagnosis of asthma. Asthma should be considered in the differential diagnosis of all patients with a cough because it is such a common cause. Most persons with a cough do not have associated variable airflow obstruction; if obstruction is present and reversible with bronchodilator medication, the diagnosis of asthma is confirmed.

In addition to chronic cough, asthma has several common clinical presentations. An acute asthmatic episode is characterized by airway obstruction, manifesting with symptoms of breathlessness and anxiety and often accompanied by wheezing and sometimes coughing. These symptoms may resolve within several hours if treatment is given or within 1 to 3 days even without specific intervention, or they may progress to more severe airway obstruction and respiratory compromise if no therapy is provided. Between acute asthmatic episodes, airflow is normal and symptoms are absent. Several specific conditions are associated with acute asthma exacerbations.

Exercise-induced asthma refers to the development of airway obstruction in an individual after the cessation of exercise, even after brief periods of exercise. Symptoms usually begin 5 to 10 minutes after the completion of exercise and resolve within 1 to 4 hours. Certain forms of exercise, including skiing, ice hockey, and running in the cold, more commonly precipitate airway obstruction; other forms of exercise, such as swimming, less commonly precipitate airway obstruction, probably because of the warmer and more humid air being inspired. Cold or dry air often predisposes an asthmatic individual to airway obstruction, such as occurs when a person enters a dry, air-conditioned environment (such as an indoor mall) from the warmer, more humid outside air.

Common allergens that precipitate asthma include cat allergen (dander), house dust mite allergen, cockroach allergen, and tree and grass pollen. Viral illnesses can also induce airway obstruction in asthmatic individuals; symptoms may persist for weeks to months if therapy is not initiated. Occupational exposures are common asthma triggers. Early responses may occur within several hours; however, late responses may not occur for 8 to 12 hours after exposure. Often, occupation-induced asthma symptoms may persist long after the individual has left the workplace, an important consideration in the differential diagnosis.

Approximately 1% to 10% of individuals with moderate to severe asthma have aspirin-exacerbated respiratory disease (AERD) (aspirin-induced asthma), which is characterized by symptoms of moderately severe airway obstruction, rhinorrhea, sneezing, tearing, dermal changes, and, in some cases, gastrointestinal symptoms (nausea, vomiting, cramping) on exposure to aspirin or other prostaglandin (H synthase type 1) inhibitors. The onset of AERD occurs most often when patients are in their 20s and 30s.[11] The diagnosis of aspirin-induced asthma is important for two reasons: aspirin-containing drugs should be avoided because these drugs may induce life-threatening asthma attacks, and effective treatment is available specifically for this type of asthma. In trials in which patients with AERD were challenged with selective NSAIDs, there was a small risk of respiratory symptoms with selective NSAIDs. However, cyclooxygenase-2 (COX-2) inhibitors with etoricoxib did not appear to exacerbate airway inflammatory or obstruction in persons with AERD.[11]

There is substantial evidence that persons affected by problems of socioeconomic deprivation and psychosocial issues such as anxiety, depression, and stress are at increased risk for asthma exacerbations. Adverse events, especially when accompanied by chronic stressors such as poverty and mental illness, have been shown to increase the risk of asthma exacerbations.[12,13]

The physical examination of the patient with asthma or suspected asthma can be divided into four objectives: (1) diagnosis and differential diagnosis, (2) assessment of asthma severity, (3) identification of adverse effects of medications, and (4) identification of concomitant medical problems. A complete physical examination is necessary if assessment of respiratory exertion or compromise is needed, coexisting medical conditions must be identified or evaluated, or the presentation is complex.

The diagnosis of asthma is based on the history, physical examination, and certain diagnostic tests, particularly spirometry. The physical examination, although an essential part of the evaluation, may correlate poorly with objective measures of airway obstruction, such as pulmonary function tests (PFTs). In the asymptomatic patient, the physical examination findings may be entirely normal. Nonetheless, assessment of the severity of asthma and airway obstruction is the most important objective in evaluating a person with asthma. Wheezing may be detectable or elicited during forced expiration. In general, mild bronchospasm is associated with expiratory wheezing. As obstruction becomes more significant, wheezing is heard during both the inspiratory and expiratory phases, with a prolongation of the latter. With profound obstruction, wheezing may be heard only during the inspiratory phase or may be entirely absent. With severe obstruction, the intensity of the breath sounds diminishes. As obstruction increases, accessory muscles of respiration are used; with significant obstruction, there may be evidence of hyperinflation with a low diaphragm and an increased anteroposterior diameter.

Severe asthma exacerbations are characterized by labored respirations, diaphoresis, anxiety, and breathlessness (inability to finish a complete sentence). A respiratory rate of 30 breaths per minute or more and a heart rate of 120 beats per minute or more suggest severe bronchospasm. Other signs and symptoms that often herald impending respiratory failure include agitation, confusion, somnolence, and cyanosis. Unilateral loss of breath sounds may reflect mucous plugging and secondary atelectasis, but pneumothorax must also be considered in this situation. However, even a careful physical examination provides only a crude estimate of airway obstruction, and significant airway obstruction is possible even when the physical examination findings are entirely normal. Assessment of respiratory status is best accomplished through measurement of lung function with spirometry or peak flow meters. Classification of asthma severity and recommended step for initial treatment is presented in Table 85.1. The physical examination is also important in identifying adverse effects of asthma medications. Side effects of β_2-adrenergic medications and theophylline include tachycardia and tremors. Inhaled corticosteroids (ICSs) can cause oral thrush and dysphonia. Adverse effects of oral (systemic) corticosteroids include central adiposity, hypertension, ecchymoses, cataracts, kyphosis, muscle weakness, and alterations in mental status.

Coexisting medical problems can be conceptualized in two ways. Certain comorbid conditions, such as nasal polyps,

TABLE 85.1 Classification of Asthma Severity and Recommended Step for Initial Treatment

	Intermittent Asthma	Persistent Asthma		
		Mild	Moderate	Severe
CURRENT IMPAIRMENT				
Symptoms	≤2 days/week	>2 days/week, but not daily	Daily	Throughout the day
Nighttime awakenings	≤2 times/month	3–4 times/month	>Once a week, but not nightly	Often 7 times/week
SABA used to control symptoms (but not to prevent EIB)	≤2 days/week	>2 days/week, but not daily, and not more than once on any day	Daily	Several times a day
Effect on normal activity	None	Minor limitation	Some limitation	Severe limitation
Lung function tests	Normal FEV_1 between exacerbations FEV_1 >80% of predicted FEV_1/FVC normal[a]	FEV_1 >80% of predicted FEV_1/FVC normal[a]	FEV_1 >60% but <80% of predicted FEV_1/FVC reduced 5%[a]	FEV_1 <60% of predicted FEV_1/FVC reduced > 5%[a]
FUTURE RISK				
Exacerbations requiring oral glucocorticoids	0–1/year	≥2/year	≥2/year	≥2/year
Recommended step for initial treatment	Step 1	Step 2	Step 3	Step 4 or 5

[a]Normal values for FEV_1/FVC by age group: 8 to 19 years, 85%; 20–39 years, 80%; 40–59 years, 75%; 60–80 years, 70%.
EIB, Exercise-induced bronchospasm; *FEV_1,* forced expiratory volume in 1 second; *FVC,* forced vital capacity; *SABA,* short-acting β₂ agonist.
From Burchum, J., & Rosenthal, L. (2019). *Lehne's pharmacology for nursing care* (10th ed.). St. Louis: Elsevier.

allergic rhinitis, sinusitis, and eczema, are commonly associated with asthma. In addition, some coexisting medical problems may be unrelated to asthma, but their identification and management have important implications for asthma therapy and control. Such possible comorbidities include glaucoma, hypertension, gastroesophageal reflux, diabetes mellitus, arthritis, and current malignant neoplasms.

DIAGNOSTICS

A diagnosis of asthma is based on three components: (1) demonstration of episodic symptoms of airflow obstruction (e.g., wheeze, cough, shortness of breath), (2) evidence that airflow obstruction is at least partially reversible, and (3) exclusion of other conditions from the differential diagnosis.[14] A thorough history and physical examination are essential to making the diagnosis of asthma. Physical findings can be helpful in identifying significant obstruction as it occurs but at best provide only a crude estimate of the degree of obstruction. However, significant obstruction may not manifest as an abnormal physical finding; in addition, findings are likely to be completely normal between episodes. In fact, reduced expiratory flow rates (forced expiratory volume at 1 second [FEV_1]) and increased airway resistance may not be recognized as dyspnea until a 30% to 40% decline in FEV_1 has occurred.

Initial Diagnostics

Objective measures of pulmonary function, such as spirometry and peak flow meters, are essential in establishing the diagnosis of asthma and assessing its severity. Spirometry is currently recommended at the time of initial assessment to confirm the diagnosis of asthma, after treatment is initiated and symptoms and PEF have been stabilized, and at least every 1 to 2 years.[14]

Although spirometry provides many measures, the most useful for evaluation of asthma are the peak expiratory flow rate (PEFR), FEV_1, maximum midexpiratory flow rate (MMEFR), and forced vital capacity (FVC). Results are compared with expected values, derived from a population of healthy, nonsmoking adults, and are expressed as a percentage of the expected value.

The most common pulmonary function abnormality in mild asthma is the decreased rate of airflow throughout the vital capacity as reflected by abnormalities in the PEFR, FEV_1, and MMEFR (forced expiratory flow [FEF_{25-75}]). During bronchospasm, spirometry reveals obstruction with decreases in FEV_1 and MMEFR. The FEV_1/FVC ratio is also reduced. As obstruction increases, an increased residual volume and functional residual are noted. One of the diagnostic hallmarks of asthma is reversal of obstruction after the administration of a bronchodilator, which corresponds with both clinical improvement and improved spirometric values. In addition to helping establish the diagnosis of asthma, spirometry helps to assess the adequacy of therapy, the need for further therapy and evaluation during emergencies, and the need for hospital admission. The severity of asthma attacks must be assessed by accurate and reproducible measures of airflow. Health care providers tend to underestimate the degree of airway obstruction in individuals with acute asthma, and knowledge of a person's pulmonary function has potentially important implications for treatment. For this reason, the NAEPP guidelines recommend the use of PFTs as part of the assessment and monitoring during the treatment of acute asthma. During a severe asthma attack, recording of the entire spirogram may be difficult, but the FEV_1 can still be measured. As the asthma attack resolves, both the PEFR and the FEV_1 increase, whereas the MMEFR usually remains significantly diminished.

Most patients with controlled asthma will not exhibit reversibility in FEV_1 at each visit, particularly those who are being treated for asthma, and therefore the test lacks sensitivity. Repeated testing at different visits may be helpful.[2]

PEF measurements with use of a peak flow meter may also be helpful in the diagnosis and management of asthma, but measurements of PEF are not interchangeable with other measurements of lung function such as FEV_1 because values obtained with different peak flow meters vary and the range of predicted values is too wide.[2] In addition, PEF measurements are effort dependent and may not be an accurate reflection of a person's pulmonary function. PEF measurements done in the office should always be compared with the patient's previous "personal best" using his or her own peak flow meter.

The terms reversibility and variability refer to changes in symptoms accompanied by changes in airflow limitation that occur spontaneously or in response to treatment. Reversibility refers to rapid improvements in FEV_1 or PEF minutes after use of a quick-relief medication such as a bronchodilator or sustained improvement during days or weeks after the introduction of a long-term control medication such as an ICS.[2] In contrast, variability refers to the change (improvement or deterioration) in asthma symptoms and lung function occurring during a longer time. Variability may be experienced in the course of a day (diurnal variability), from day to day, from month to month, or seasonally. Obtaining a history of variability is an integral aspect of asthma diagnosis and management.

Additional Diagnostics

Other laboratory tests that may be used to diagnose asthma or be included as part of the evaluation are airway responsiveness testing, arterial blood and other serum analysis, radiography, electrocardiography (ECG), and sputum cultures. Airway responsiveness testing measures the bronchoconstrictor response elicited by a standard stimulus. The FEV_1 is measured after inhalation of an aerosol containing graded amounts of a bronchoconstrictor agonist. The most commonly used bronchoconstrictor is methacholine, but histamine, exercise, eucapnic voluntary hyperventilation, or inhaled mannitol can also be used for bronchial provocation. These tests are moderately sensitive for a diagnosis of asthma but have limited sensitivity. For example, airway hyperresponsiveness to inhaled methacholine can also occur in patients with allergic rhinitis.[2] Individuals with asthma often have atopy, which is often reflected in blood eosinophilia. Total serum IgE levels are elevated in persons with asthma and associated with disease severity, but IgE levels cannot predict response to treatment.[15] The data from studies in pediatric populations unambiguously suggest a positive relationship between atopy and asthma severity, but studies in adults show an inconsistent relationship between the two.[15]

In general, the chest radiographs of individuals with asthma are normal. Therefore chest radiography is not indicated in the routine evaluation of patients with asthma unless physical examination findings are suggestive of infectious illness or respiratory complications such as pneumomediastinum or pneumothorax. If an asthma exacerbation is severe enough to warrant hospital admission, a chest X-ray film should be taken. The X-ray film may show hyperinflation (indicated by diaphragmatic depression) and abnormally translucent lung fields.

Between asthma attacks, in the absence of respiratory infection, the sputum is usually clear. During an asthma attack, even in the absence of infection, the sputum may be yellow to green. This does not necessarily indicate infection; the color change may be from eosinophil peroxidase. Sputum culture specimens are generally not obtained unless there is suspicion of an acute contagious respiratory infection.

ECG is not part of the routine evaluation of a patient with asthma. If it is performed during an asthma exacerbation, ECG in the absence of cardiac disease is usually significant only for sinus tachycardia. In severe attacks, right-axis deviation, right-bundle branch block, cor pulmonale, or even ST-T wave abnormalities may occur. If these abnormalities resolve as the asthma attack abates, no further cardiac evaluation is necessary. Electrocardiographic findings should be monitored during asthma attacks for patients with significant cardiac disease to monitor for myocardial infarction, which can result from attack-induced stress.

DIFFERENTIAL DIAGNOSIS

The medical conditions most likely to be confused with asthma involve the upper respiratory system (e.g., croup, vocal cord dysfunction [VCD]) and lower respiratory system (e.g., pneumonia, chronic obstructive pulmonary disease [COPD]), the cardiovascular system (e.g., valvular disease and cardiomyopathy), and the gastrointestinal system (e.g., GERD).

Not all wheezing is caused by asthma, and other causes should be excluded before a diagnosis of asthma is made. Spirometry can be used to help differentiate asthma from other possible conditions in the differential diagnosis. An FEV_1 of 80% of predicted or less with a reduced FEV_1/FVC ratio that normalizes or significantly improves with bronchodilator therapy raises the suspicion of asthma. Other causes of wheezing and upper airway obstruction include tracheomalacia, tracheal or bronchial masses, and laryngeal (vocal cord) dysfunction. The presence of stridor or focal wheezing on physical examination and with flow limitation on a flow-volume loop is characteristic of tracheomalacia and tracheobronchial masses. VCD can mimic asthma and may coexist with asthma, but it is a distinct disorder. VCD is caused by abnormal apposition of the vocal cords during the respiratory cycle and can generally be treated effectively by speech therapy. Laryngoscopy is needed to confirm VCD. VCD is often initially misdiagnosed as asthma and often inappropriately and ineffectively treated with high-dose systemic steroids. VCD should be considered in atypical asthma patients who do not respond well to asthma medications and in athletes who have exercise-related breathlessness unresponsive to asthma medication. COPD is characterized by airflow limitation that is not fully reversible, is usually progressive, and is associated with an abnormal inflammatory response of the lungs to noxious substances. Persons with COPD, including emphysema and chronic bronchitis, may have acute episodes of airway obstruction and wheezing, especially during exacerbations of their disease. COPD is often accompanied by a history of smoking, reduced response to bronchodilator therapy, and irreversible PFT changes over time. In addition, COPD may be distinguished from asthma by signs of hyperinflation, such as diminished breath sounds, decreased heart sounds, and a flattened diaphragm. Chest wall deformities are suggestive of restrictive lung diseases. Dullness to percussion may indicate pneumonia or a pleural effusion. Foreign body aspiration should be considered if lateralizing wheezes are heard. Although asthma can usually be distinguished from COPD, in some individuals who develop chronic respiratory symptoms, it may be difficult to differentiate between the two. It may be helpful for primary care providers to use symptom-based questionnaires to assist in differentiating COPD from asthma.

α_1-Antitrypsin (AAT) deficiency is an inherited disorder caused by an inborn error in the liver's production of AAT, which is the dominant protease in the lung and protects alveoli from the destructive effects of serine proteases. AAT deficiency causes a syndrome of abnormalities, including neonatal jaundice, airflow obstruction, premature emphysema, and cirrhosis of the liver. The primary respiratory effect of AAT deficiency is degradation of the protein elastin, a protein that is essential for the elastic recoil required for pulmonary expiratory function. As a result, chronic persistent airflow obstruction develops. AAT deficiency is a well-established cause of panacinar emphysema, but its role in the pathophysiologic process of asthma is less well understood. The prevalence of AAT deficiency is approximately 0.01% to 0.02% in those with emphysema; the prevalence of AAT deficiency among patients with asthma is not known.[16] Individuals with AAT deficiency often have symptoms similar to those of bronchial asthma; pulmonary function may be normal, especially among those who do not smoke. Hence a diagnosis of AAT deficiency is often missed or delayed. However, bronchopulmonary infections are common in persons with AAT deficiency, and their family history almost always includes lung disease. Asthmatic patients with AAT deficiency usually have more severe disease and often respond less to bronchodilators than do those without the disorder. Health care providers should have a high level of suspicion for AAT deficiency in young persons whose symptoms do not respond to appropriate asthma therapy, especially in the absence of smoking. Diagnosis of AAT deficiency is based on AAT serum levels but may also involve other diagnostic measurements, including PFTs, chest radiography, serum electrophoresis, and genotyping. Although management of AAT deficiency has some similarities to that of asthma, it also has important differences; diagnosis of AAT deficiency has critical implications for an individual's prognosis and quality of life.

INTERPROFESSIONAL COLLABORATIVE MANAGEMENT

Although the role of inflammation in the pathogenesis of asthma was recognized in the 1991 National Heart, Lung, and Blood Institute (NHLBI) guidelines on asthma management, asthma was not defined as a chronic inflammatory disorder of the airways until years later. Inflammation is currently understood to be one of the preeminent problems in asthma, which has shifted the focus of treatment from symptomatic to preventive therapy, including the need for antiinflammatory medications, environmental controls, and patient education. The Global Initiative for Asthma (GINA) was created to increase awareness among health professionals, public health authorities, and the general public to improve the prevention and management of asthma through a concerted worldwide effort. GINA and the CDC have identified asthma control as consisting of strategies to: (1) reducing impairment/symptom control and (2) risk reduction. Symptom control refers to preventing asthma symptoms, reducing rescue medication use, maintaining lung function, and maintaining normal activity. Risk reduction includes minimizing the need for ED visits and hospitalizations and preventing asthma exacerbations.[2]

Nonpharmacologic Management

Risk reduction includes treating modifiable risk factors and comorbidities and incorporating nonpharmacologic therapies and strategies.

Smokers with asthma should be strongly encouraged at every visit to quit, and access to resources and counseling should be provided. Minimizing exposure to tobacco smoke should also be encouraged. Physical activity should be encouraged to promote overall health, including advice about exercise-induced bronchoconstriction. Occupational sensitizers should be removed as soon as possible.

Pharmacologic Management

Asthma symptom control refers to the extent to which the effects of asthma are evident or have been reduced or removed by treatment. GINA refers to asthma as being "well controlled," "partly controlled," or "uncontrolled" based on as assessment of current symptoms and activity limitations (Box 85.2). Risk factors for future risk and poor asthma outcomes are also identified in Box 85.2. Classification of asthma by severity of symptoms is helpful in guiding disease management at the initial assessment of a patient. However, as emphasized by GINA, it is important to recognize that asthma severity involves both the severity of the underlying disease process and its responsiveness to treatment.[2] Severity should not be considered an invariable or static feature of a person's asthma; rather, it is a factor that may change over time.

Asthma treatment is adjusted in a continuous cycle that includes assessment of symptoms, adjusting treatment, and reviewing the response to the treatment (see Table 85.1). The long-term goals of asthma management include controlling symptoms and risk reduction, including reducing the risk of exacerbations, airway damage, and medication side effects.[2]

There are two main classes of asthma medications: controller medications and reliever medications. Every patient should have a "reliever medication" (i.e., bronchodilator inhaler), and most adults and adolescents with asthma will need a "controller medication" to reduce serious exacerbations, even those individuals who have relatively infrequent exacerbations.[2] Controller medications include ICSs and long-acting β agonist bronchodilator combinations (ICS/LABA). Add-on controller medications include long-acting anticholinergic, Anti-IgE, Anti-IL5 and systemic corticosteroids. Reliever medications include short-acting β_2 agonist bronchodilators (SABAs), low-dose ICS/formoterol, and short-acting anticholinergics.

For pharmacologic therapy, a stepwise approach is recommended, in which drug dosages and classes of medications are "stepped up" as needed to control symptoms and stepped down when possible. This stepwise approach to asthma management is summarized in Table 85.2.

Step 1: As Needed

Reliever Medication: as needed SABA for relief of symptoms.
Regular use of a daily controller medication should be considered as soon as possible after the diagnosis of asthma has been made, because early treatment with low-dose ICS leads to better lung function than if it is delayed and patients not using ICS, who experience severe exacerbations, have lower long-term lung function than those who have started on an ICS.[2] In addition, regular low-dose ICS is recommended for all patients with asthma who have symptoms more often than twice a month, waking

BOX **85.2**

Assessment of Symptom Control and Future Risk

A. LEVEL OF ASTHMA SYMPTOM CONTROL

In the past 4 weeks, has the patient had:

	Yes/No	Well Controlled	Partly Controlled	Uncontrolled
		None of these	1–2 of these	3–4 of these
Daytime symptoms more than twice/week?				
Any night waking due to asthma?				
Reliever med needed more than twice/week?				
Any activity limitation due to asthma?				

B. RISK FACTORS FOR POOR ASTHMA OUTCOMES

Risk factors should be assessed at diagnosis and periodically every 1–2 years, particularly for patients experiencing asthma exacerbations.

Measure FEV_1 at start of treatment, after 3–6 months of controller treatment to record "personal best" lung function, and then periodically for ongoing assessment.

Having uncontrolled asthma symptoms is an important risk factor for exacerbations.

The following risk factors increase the risk of exacerbations, even if the patient is experiencing few asthma symptoms:

- ICS not prescribed; poor ICS adherence; incorrect inhaler technique
- High SABA use (with increased mortality if >1 × 200-dose canister/month)
- Low FEV_1 especially if <60% predicted
- Higher bronchodilator reversibility
- Major psychological or socioeconomic problems
- Exposures: smoking; allergen exposure if sensitized
- Comorbidities: obesity; chronic rhinosinusitis; confirmed food allergy
- Sputum or blood eosinophilia; elevated FENO in allergic adults taking ICS
- Pregnancy
  Other major independent risk factors for exacerbations include:
- Ever being intubated or in intensive care for asthma
- Having one or more asthma exacerbations in the last 12 months
  Risk factors for medication side effects include:
- *Systemic*: frequent OCS; long-term, high-dose, and/or potent ICS; also taking P450 inhibitors
- *Local*: high-dose or potent ICS; poor inhaler technique

FEV_1, Forced expiratory volume in 1 second; *ICS*, inhaled corticosteroids.
Adapted from Global Initiative for Asthma (GINA). (2018). *Pocket guide for asthma management and prevention: A pocket guide for health professionals.* Retrieved from www.ginasthma.org.

due to asthma more than once a month, and any asthma symptoms plus risk factors for exacerbations.[2]

Step 2

Reliever medication: As-need SABA

Preferred controlled choice: Low-dose ICS

Other controller options include leukotriene receptor antagonist (LTRA).

For purely seasonal allergic asthma, start ICS immediately upon onset of symptoms and discontinue using 4 weeks after exposure ends.

Step 3

Reliever medication: As-needed SABA or low-dose ICS/formoterol

Preferred controller choice: Low-dose ICS/LABA

Other controller options include medium/high-dose ICS + LTRA (or + theophylline).

Step 4

Reliever medication: As needed SABA or low-dose ICS/formoterol

Preferred controller choice: Medium/high-dose ICS/LABA

Other controller options include tiotropium by mist inhaler for patients 12 years of age or older with a history of exacerbations, or high-dose ICS/LABA or slow-release theophylline (adults).

Step 5: Consultation Recommended

For a complete guide to managing asthma and when to review response and adjust treatment, refer to the *GINA Pocket Guide for Asthma Management and Prevention, 2018.*[2]

For a list of asthma medication classes, specific medications, their actions, indications, and side effects, refer to Tables 85.3–85.8.

Despite the fact that this approach to asthma therapy has been recommended for more than 2 decades, studies indicate that asthma control, as defined by the asthma management guidelines, is not being achieved in the majority of patients.[8] There remains an overreliance on short-acting bronchodilators and underuse of antiinflammatory medications on the part of both practitioners and persons with asthma. This suggests that the underlying pathophysiologic mechanism of asthma and its implications for therapy are still not widely understood. As emphasized in the EPR stepwise approach, all patients except those with mild, intermittent asthma benefit from maintenance antiinflammatory medication. The use of antiinflammatory medications for maintenance (long-term control) of mild to moderate asthma results in fewer asthma exacerbations, fewer ED visits, decreased cost of care, fewer school or work days missed, and improved quality of life.[14] Despite the guidelines, research suggests that asthma is often undertreated because of inappropriate prescribing or under prescribing and poor adherence of patients to therapy.[12]

Once treatment for asthma has been initiating, decisions to "step up" treatment are based on assessment of symptoms, adjusting treatment, and reviewing the response. Guidelines for this stepwise approach can be found in Table 85.2. Observing

TABLE 85.2   Stepwise Approach to Managing Asthma in Patients 12 Years and Older

| | Long-Term Control Drugs (Taken Daily) | | Quick-Relief Drugs (Taken PRN) |
	Preferred	Alternative	
Step 1	No daily medication needed		SABA
Step 2	Low-dose IGC	Cromolyn, LTRA, or theophylline	SABA
Step 3	Low-dose IGC + LABA or Medium-dose IGC	Low-dose IGC + either LTRA, theophylline, or zileuton	SABA
Step 4	Medium-dose IGC + LABA	Medium-dose IGC + either LTRA, theophylline, or zileuton	SABA
Step 5	High-dose IGC + LABA		SABA
Step 6	High-dose IGC + LABA + oral glucocorticoid		SABA

IGC, Inhaled glucocorticoid; *LABA,* long-acting β₂ agonist; *LTRA,* leukotriene receptor antagonist; *SABA,* short-acting β₂ agonist.
From Burchum, J., & Rosenthal, L. (2019). *Lehne's pharmacology for nursing care* (10th ed.). St. Louis: Elsevier.

inhaler technique and discussing adherence and barriers to use is essential. Removing risk factors, such as smoking, β-blockers, NSAIDs, and allergen exposure, is also important.

Another integral component of asthma management is the treatment of coexisting diseases, including rhinitis, sinusitis, and GERD. Evidence from clinical trials suggests no benefit from antibiotic therapy for asthma exacerbations, whether it is administered routinely or when the suspicion of bacterial infection is low. The NAEPP EPR recommendation is that antibiotics not be used in the treatment of acute asthma exacerbation except for the treatment of certain comorbid conditions, such as fever and purulent sputum, evidence of pneumonia, and bacterial sinusitis.[14] Intranasal glucocorticoids may be helpful in the management of chronic rhinitis, whereas antibiotics are indicated for bacterial sinus infections.[14] Annual influenza vaccination is recommended for all persons with persistent asthma. For persons with GERD, acid-suppressive therapy may decrease asthma symptoms. Individuals with GERD often do not describe symptoms suggestive of GERD; approximately 25% to 30% of patients with asthma have clinically silent reflux.[17]

Given the known role of environmental triggers in the pathophysiologic process of asthma, it is essential that environmental interventions be implemented along with clinical approaches in the management of asthma. Interventions at the household level must include efforts to eliminate cockroaches, rodents, and mold. Individual efforts to sustain pest-free environments, especially in apartment complexes, will be effective only if efforts at the building, neighborhood, and city level are in place to bolster those efforts. Common asthma risk factors and actions to reduce exposure to them are listed in Table 85.9.

MONITORING THERAPY AND ASTHMA SEVERITY

Asthma management guidelines stress the importance of assessment of pulmonary function with use of PEFR meters rather than basing assessment on the individual's perception of dyspnea (POD). There is often no correlation between POD

TABLE 85.3   Inhaled Glucocorticoids: Formulations and Dosages

| Drug | Formulation | Dosage | |
		Adults	Children
Beclomethasone dipropionate (QVAR)	MDI: 40 or 80 mcg/inhalation	40–320 mcg twice daily	40–80 mcg twice daily (5–11 years)
Budesonide (Pulmicort Flexhaler) (Pulmicort Respules)	DPI: 90 or 180 mcg/inhalation Suspension for nebulization	360–720 mcg twice daily 250–500 mcg once or twice daily *or* 1000 mcg once daily	180–360 mcg twice daily (6–17 years) 500–1000 mcg/day (1–8 years)
Ciclesonide (Alvesco)	MDI: 80 or 160 mcg/inhalation	80–320 mcg twice daily	80–320 mcg twice daily (12 years and up)
Flunisolide (AeroBid)	MDI: 80 mcg/inhalation	160–320 mcg twice daily	80–320 mcg twice daily (6–11 years)
Fluticasone propionate (Flovent HFA) (Flovent Diskus)	MDI: 44, 110, or 220 mcg/inhalation DPI: 50, 100, or 250 mcg/inhalation	88–440 mcg twice daily 100–1000 mcg twice daily	88 mcg twice daily (4–11 years) 50–100 mcg twice daily (4–11 years)
Mometasone furoate (Asmanex Twisthaler)	DPI: 110 or 220 mcg/inhalation	220–440 mcg once or twice daily	110 mcg once daily (4–11 years)

DPI, Dry-powder inhaler; *MDI,* metered-dose inhaler.
From Burchum, J., & Rosenthal, L. (2019). *Lehne's pharmacology for nursing care* (10th ed.). St. Louis: Elsevier.

TABLE 85.4 Leukotriene Modifiers: Preparations and Dosages

Drug (Brand Name)	Preparation	Dosage
Montelukast (Singulair)	Granules: 4 mg/pkt Chewable tablets: 4, 5 mg Tablets: 10 mg	12–23 months: one pkt of 4-mg granules daily 2–5 years: one pkt of 4-mg granules or one 4-mg tablet every evening 6–14 years: one 5-mg chewable tablet every evening 15 years and older: one 10-mg tablet every evening *EIB prophylaxis: one 10-mg tablet at least 2 hr before exercising**
Zafirlukast (Accolate)	Tablets 10, 20 mg	5–11 years: 10-mg tablet twice daily 12 years and older: 20-mg twice daily
Zileuton (Zyflo, Zyflo CR)	IR tablet: 600 mg ER tablet: 600 mg	12 years and older: • IR tablet: one 600-mg tablet 4 times daily • ER tablet: two 600-mg tablets twice daily

*No additional dose should be taken for at least 24 h. Patients already taking montelukast daily should not take any more to prevent EIB.
EIB, Exercise-induced bronchospasm; *ER,* extended release; *IR,* immediate release; *pkt,* packet.
From Burchum, J., & Rosenthal, L. (2019). *Lehne's pharmacology for nursing care* (10th ed). St. Louis: Elsevier.

TABLE 85.5 β_2-Adrenergic Agonists

Drug (Brand Name)	Formulation	Initial Dosage	
		Adults	**Children**
INHALED AGENTS: SHORT ACTING			
Albuterol (ProAir HFA, ProAir RespiClick, Proventil HFA, Ventolin HFA)	MDI (90 mcg/inhalation)	2 inhalations every 4–6 h PRN	2 inhalations every 4–6 h PRN
(Proventil)	Solution for nebulization	1.25–5 mg every 4–8 h PRN	0.63–2.5 mg/kg every 4–6 h PRN
Levalbuterol (Xopenex HFA)	MDI (45 mcg/inhalation)	2 inhalations every 4–6 h PRN	2 inhalations every 4–6 h PRN
(Xopenex)	Solution for nebulization	0.63 mg every 6–8 h PRN	0.31–1.25 mg every 4–6 h PRN
INHALED AGENTS: LONG ACTING[a]			
Aclidinium bromide[b] (Tudorza Pressair)	DPI (400 mcg/inhalation)	1 inhalation every 12 h	Safety and efficacy not established
Arformoterol[a,b] (Brovana)	Solution for nebulization	15 mcg every 12 h	Safety and efficacy not established
Formoterol (Foradil Aerolizer)	DPI (12 mcg/inhalation)	1 inhalation every 12 h	1 inhalation every 12 h
(Perforomist)[b]	Solution for nebulization	20 mcg every 12 h	Safety and efficacy not established
Indacaterol[b] (Arcapta Neohaler)	DPI (75 mcg/inhalation)	1 inhalation every 24 h	N/A
Olodaterol (Striverdi Respimat)[b]	Respimat (2.5 mcg/inhalation)	2 inhalations every 24 h	N/A
Salmeterol[a] (Serevent Diskus)	DPI (50 mcg/inhalation)	1 inhalation every 12 h	1 inhalation every 12 h
ORAL AGENTS			
Albuterol Generic	Tablets, syrup	2 or 4 mg 3–4 times/day	2 mg 3–4 times/day
(VoSpire ER)	Tablets (extended release)	8 mg every 12 h	4 mg every 12 h
Terbutaline (generic only)	Tablets	5 mg 3 times/day	2.5 mg 3 times/day

[a]When used to treat asthma, must always be combined with an inhaled glucocorticoid.
[b]Approved only for chronic obstructive pulmonary disease, not asthma.
DPI, Dry-powder inhaler; *HFA,* hydrofluoroalkane propellant; *MDI,* metered-dose inhaler.
From Burchum, J., & Rosenthal, L. (2019). *Lehne's pharmacology for nursing care* (10th ed.). St. Louis: Elsevier.

and simultaneous peak flow measurements and that the majority of individuals have a blunted POD (i.e., an underestimation of respiratory compromise), resulting in undertreatment of asthma, a delay in treatment changes, and perhaps even a predisposition to fatal asthma attacks. Therefore it is recommended that all individuals with moderate to severe asthma learn how to monitor PEF and have a flow meter at home. PEF monitoring during exacerbations should be encouraged for all those with moderate to severe, persistent asthma, and PEF should guide management. In addition, long-term daily peak flow monitoring is recommended for individuals with

Text continued on p. 461

TABLE 85.6   Anticholinergics: Preparations and Dosages

Drug (Brand Name)	Preparation	Formulation	Dosage
Aclidinium (Tudorza Pressair)	DPI	400 mcg per actuation	400 mcg twice daily
Ipratropium (Atrovent HFA)	Solution MDI	500 mcg/vial 17 mcg per actuation	500 mcg 3–4 times daily by nebulizer 2 inhalations 4 times daily (maximum dosage 12 inhalations/24 h)
Tiotropium (Spiriva)	HandiHaler DPI	18 mcg capsules[a]	18 mcg once daily
Umeclidinium (Incruse Ellipta)	DPI	62.5 mcg per actuation	62.5 mcg once daily

[a]Capsules are for insertion into DPI device and must not be swallowed.
DPI, Dry-powder inhaler; *HFA*, hydrofluoroalkane propellant; *MDI*, metered-dose inhaler.
From Burchum, J., & Rosenthal, L. (2019). *Lehne's pharmacology for nursing care* (10th ed). St. Louis: Elsevier.

TABLE 85.7   Glucocorticoids and Long-Acting β_2 Agonists: Formulations and Dosages

Drug (Brand Name)	Inhaler	Formulation	Dosage[a]
Budesonide/formoterol (Symbicort)	HFA	80 mcg/4.5 mcg 160 mcg/4.5 mcg	2 inhalations twice daily 2 inhalations twice daily
Fluticasone/vilanterol (Breo Ellipta)	DPI	100 mcg/25 mcg 200 mcg/25 mcg	1 inhalation once daily 1 inhalation once daily
Fluticasone/salmeterol (Advair Diskus)	DPI	100 mcg/50 mcg 250 mcg/50 mcg 500 mcg/50 mcg	1 inhalation twice daily 1 inhalation twice daily 1 inhalation twice daily
Fluticasone/salmeterol (Advair HFA)	HFA	45 mcg/21 mcg 115 mcg/21 mcg 230 mcg/21 mcg	2 inhalations twice daily 2 inhalations twice daily 2 inhalations twice daily
Mometasone/formoterol (Dulera)	HFA	100 mcg/5 mcg 200 mcg/5 mcg	2 inhalations twice daily 2 inhalations twice daily

[a]Dosing is the same for children and adults when prescribed as recommended for age. These drugs are not approved for children younger than 12 years. Fluticasone/vilanterol is not approved for children younger than 18 years.
DPI, Dry-powder inhaler; *HFA*, hydrofluoroalkane propellant.
From Burchum, J., & Rosenthal, L. (2019). *Lehne's pharmacology for nursing care* (10th ed). St. Louis: Elsevier.

TABLE 85.8 β_2 Agonists and Anticholinergics: Formulations and Dosages

Drug (Classification)	Brand Name	Preparation	Formulation Per Inhalation	Dosage
Ipratropium/albuterol (anticholinergic + SABA)	DuoNeb Combivent Respimat	Solution Inhaler	500 mcg ipratropium/2500 mcg of albuterol 20 mcg ipratropium/100 mcg albuterol	3 mL 4 times daily using a nebulizer 1 inhalation 4 times daily (maximum 6 inhalations in 24 h)
Indacaterol/glycopyrronium (LABA + anticholinergic)	Utibron Neohaler	Inhaler	27.5 mcg indacaterol/15 mcg glycopyrronium (glycopyrrolate)	1 inhalation twice daily
Olodaterol/tiotropium (LABA + anticholinergic)	Stiolto Respimat	Inhaler	2.5 mcg of olodaterol/2.5 mcg tiotropium	2 inhalations once daily
Umeclidinium/vilanterol (anticholinergic + LABA)	Anoro Ellipta	Inhaler	62.5 mcg umeclidinium/25 mcg vilanterol	1 inhalation once daily

Parameter	Mild	Moderate	Severe	Respiratory Arrest Imminent
Breathless	Walking Can lie down	Talking Infant: softer, shorter cry; difficulty feeding Prefer sitting	At rest Infant stops feeding Hunched forward	
Talks in …	Sentences	Phrases	Words	
Alertness	May be agitated	Usually agitated	Usually agitated	Drowsy or confused
Respiratory rate	Increased	Increased	Often >30/min	Paradoxical

TABLE 85.8 β₂ Agonists and Anticholinergics: Formulations and Dosages—cont'd

Normal Rates of Breathing in Awake Children				
Age			**Normal Rate (Breaths Per Minute)**	
<2 months			<60	
2–12 months			<50	
1–5 years			<40	
6–8 years			<30	
Accessory muscles and suprasternal retractions	Usually not	Usually	Usually	Paradoxical thoracoabdominal movement
Wheeze	Moderate, often only end-expiratory	Loud	Usually loud	Absence of wheeze
Pulse (beats per minute)	<100	100–120	>120	Bradycardia

Guide to Limits of Normal Pulse Rate in Children				
Age			**Normal Rate (Beats Per Minute)**	
Infants, 2–12 months			<160	
Preschool, 1–2 years			<120	
School age, 2–8 years			<110	
Pulsus paradoxus	Absent <10 mm Hg	May be present 10–25 mm Hg	Often present <25 mm Hg (adult) 20–40 mm Hg (child)	Absence suggests respiratory muscle fatigue
FEF after initial bronchodilator (% predicted or % personal best)	>80%	Approximately 60%–80%	<60% predicted or personal best (100 L/min adults) or response lasts <2 h	
Fa_{O_2} (on air)	Normal (test not usually necessary)	>60 mm Hg	<60 mm Hg; possible cyanosis	
and/or				
Pa_{CO_2}	<45 mm Hg	<45 mm Hg	>45 mm Hg; possible respiratory failure	
Sa_{O_2}% (on air)	>95%	91%–95%	<90%	

Drug	Low Daily Dose ≥12 Years of Age and Adults	Medium Daily Dose ≥12 Years of Age and Adults	High Daily Dose ≥12 Years of Age and Adults
INHALED CORTICOSTEROIDS			
Beclomethasone HFA 40 or 80 mcg/puff	80–240 mcg	>240–480 mcg	>480 mcg
Budesonide DPI 90, 180, or 200 mcg/inhalation	180–600 mcg	>600–1200 mcg	>1200 mcg
Flunisolide 250 mcg/puff	500–1000 mcg	>1000–2000 mcg	>2000 mcg
Flunisolide HFA 80 mcg/puff	320 mcg	>320–640 mcg	>640 mcg
Fluticasone HFA/MDI 44, 110, or 220 mcg/puff	88–264 mcg	>264–440 mcg	>440 mcg
Fluticasone DPI 50, 100, or 250 mcg/inhalation	100–300 mcg	>300–500 mcg	>500 mcg
Mometasone DPI 200 mcg/inhalation	200 mcg	400 mcg	>400 mcg
Triamcinolone acetonide 100 mcg/puff	300–750 mcg	>750–1500 mcg	>1500 mcg

Continued

| TABLE 85.8 | β_2 Agonists and Anticholinergics: Formulations and Dosages—cont'd | | |

Medication	≥12 Years of Age and Adults	Potential Adverse Effects	Comments (Not All-Inclusive)
ORAL SYSTEMIC CORTICOSTEROIDS			
Methylprednisolone 2-, 4-, 8-, 16-, 32-mg tablets Prednisolone 5-mg tablets, 5 mg/5 mL, 15 mg/5 mL Prednisone 1-, 2.5-, 5-, 10-, 20-, 50-mg tablets; 5 mg/mL, 5 mg/5 mL	7.5–60 mg daily in a single dose in AM or every other day as needed for control Short-course "burst": to achieve control, 40–60 mg/day as single or 2 divided doses for 3–10 days	Short-term use: reversible abnormalities in glucose metabolism, increased appetite, fluid retention, weight gain, mood alteration, hypertension, peptic ulcer, and rarely aseptic necrosis. Long-term use: adrenal axis suppression, growth suppression, dermal thinning, hypertension, diabetes, Cushing syndrome, cataracts, muscle weakness, and—in rare instances—impaired immune function. Consideration should be given to coexisting conditions that could be worsened by systemic corticosteroids, such as herpes virus infections, varicella, tuberculosis, hypertension, peptic ulcer, diabetes mellitus, osteoporosis, and *Strongyloides* infection.	For long-term treatment of severe persistent asthma, administer single dose in AM either daily or on alternate days (alternate-day therapy may produce less adrenal suppression). Short courses or bursts are effective for establishing control when initiating therapy or during a period of gradual deterioration. There is no evidence that tapering the dose after improvement in symptom control and pulmonary function prevents relapse. For patients unable to tolerate the liquid preparations, dexamethasone syrup at 0.4 mg/kg/day may be an alternative. However, studies are limited, and the longer duration of activity increases the risk of adrenal suppression.
INHALED LONG-ACTING β_2 AGONISTS			
Salmeterol DPI: 50 mcg/blister Formoterol DPI: 12 mcg/single-use capsule	1 blister every 12 h 1 capsule every 12 h	Tachycardia, skeletal muscle tremor, hypokalemia, prolongation of QTc interval in overdose. A diminished bronchoprotective effect may occur within 1 week of chronic therapy. Clinical significance has not been established. Potential risk of uncommon, severe, life-threatening, or fatal exacerbation; see text for additional discussion regarding safety of LABAs.	Should not be used for acute symptom relief or exacerbations. Use only with ICS. Decreased duration of protection against EIB may occur with regular use. Do not blow into inhaler after dose is activated. Each capsule is for single use only; additional doses should not be administered for at least 12 h. Capsules should be used only with the inhaler and should not be taken orally.
COMBINED MEDICATIONS			
Fluticasone/salmeterol DPI: 100 mcg/50 mcg, 250 mcg/50 mcg, or 500 mcg/50 mcg HFA: 45 mcg/21 mcg, 115 mcg/21 mcg, 230 mcg/21 mcg	1 inhalation twice daily; dose depends on level of severity or control	See notes for ICSs and LABAs.	Do not blow into inhaler after dose is activated. 100/50 DPI or 45/21 HFA for patients who have asthma not controlled on low- to medium-dose ICS. 250/50 DPI or 115/21 HFA for patients who have asthma not controlled on medium- to high-dose ICS.
Budesonide/formoterol HFA MDI: 80 mcg/4.5 mcg, 160 mcg/4.5 mcg	2 puffs twice daily; dose depends on level of severity or control	See notes for ICSs and LABAs.	There have been no clinical trials in children <4 years of age. Currently approved for use in youths ≥12 years of age. Dose for children 5–12 years of age based on clinical trials using DPI with slightly different delivery characteristics. 80/4.5 for patients who have asthma not controlled on low- to medium-dose ICS 160/4.5 for patients who have asthma not controlled on medium- to high-dose ICS

TABLE 85.8 β₂ Agonists and Anticholinergics: Formulations and Dosages—cont'd

Medication	≥12 Years of Age and Adults	Potential Adverse Effects	Comments (Not All-Inclusive)
CROMOLYN/NEDOCROMIL			
Cromolyn MDI: 0.8 mg/puff Nebulizer: 20 mg/ampule Nedocromil MDI: 1.75 mg/puff	2 puffs 4 times a day 1 ampule 4 times a day 2 puffs 4 times a day	Cough and irritation; 15%–20% of patients complain of an unpleasant taste from nedocromil.	One dose of cromolyn before exercise or allergen exposure provides effective prophylaxis for 1–2 h. Not as effective for EIB as SABAs. 4- to 6-week trial of cromolyn or nedocromil may be needed to determine maximum benefit. Dose by MDI may be inadequate to affect hyperresponsiveness. Once control is achieved, the frequency of administration may be reduced. Safety is the primary advantage of these agents.
IMMUNOMODULATORS			
Omalizumab (anti-IgE) Subcutaneous injection, 150 mg/1.2 mL following reconstitution with 1.4 mL sterile water for injection	150–375 mg SC every 2–4 weeks, depending on body weight and pretreatment serum IgE level	Pain and bruising of injection sites in 5%–20% of patients Anaphylaxis has been reported in 0.2% of treated patients. Malignant neoplasms were reported in 0.5% of patients compared with 0.2% receiving placebo; relationship to drug is unclear.	Do not administer more than 150 mg per injection site. Monitor patients after injections; be prepared and equipped to identify and treat anaphylaxis that may occur. Whether patients will develop significant antibody titers to the drug with long-term administration is unknown.
LEUKOTRIENE MODIFIERS ***Leukotriene Receptor Antagonists***			
Montelukast 4- or 5-mg chewable tablet 4-mg granule packets 10-mg tablet	10 mg every bedtime	No specific adverse effects have been identified. Rare cases of Churg-Strauss have occurred, but the association is unclear.	Montelukast exhibits a flat dose-response curve. Doses >10 mg will not produce a greater response in adults. No more efficacious than placebo in infants ages 6–24 months. As long-term therapy may attenuate exercise-induced bronchospasm in some patients, but less effective than ICS therapy.
Zafirlukast 10-mg tablet 20-mg tablet	40 mg daily (20-mg tablet twice daily)	Postmarketing surveillance has reported cases of reversible hepatitis and, rarely, irreversible hepatic failure resulting in death and liver transplantation.	For zafirlukast, administration with meals decreases bioavailability; take at least 1 h before or 2 h after meals. Zafirlukast is a microsomal P450 enzyme inhibitor that can inhibit the metabolism of warfarin. INRs should be monitored during coadministration. Monitor hepatic enzymes (ALT). Warn patients to discontinue use if they experience signs and symptoms of liver dysfunction.
5-Lipoxygenase Inhibitor Zileuton 600-mg tablet	2400 mg daily (give tablets 4 times a day)	Elevation of liver enzymes has been reported. Limited case reports of reversible hepatitis and hyperbilirubinemia.	For zileuton, monitor hepatic enzymes (ALT). Zileuton is a microsomal P450 enzyme inhibitor that can inhibit the metabolism of warfarin and theophylline. Doses of these drugs should be monitored accordingly.

Continued

TABLE 85.8 β₂ Agonists and Anticholinergics: Formulations and Dosages—cont'd

Medication	≥12 Years of Age and Adults	Potential Adverse Effects	Comments (Not All-Inclusive)
METHYLXANTHINES			
Theophylline Liquids, sustained-release tablets, and capsules	Starting dose: 10 mg/kg/day up to 300 mg maximum; usual maximum: 800 mg/day	Dose-related acute toxicities include tachycardia, nausea and vomiting, tachyarrhythmias (supraventricular tachycardia), central nervous system stimulation, headache, seizures, hematemesis, hyperglycemia, and hypokalemia. Adverse effects at usual therapeutic doses include insomnia, gastric upset, aggravation of ulcer or reflux, increase in hyperactivity in some children, difficulty in urination in elderly men who have prostatism.	Adjust dosage to achieve serum concentration of 5–15 mcg/mL at steady state (at least 48 h on same dosage). Because of wide interpatient variability in theophylline metabolic clearance, routine serum theophylline level monitoring is essential. Patients should be told to discontinue if they experience toxicity. Various factors (diet, food, febrile illness, age, smoking, and other medications) can affect serum concentrations.
INHALED SHORT-ACTING β₂ AGONISTS			
Albuterol CFC MDI: 90 mcg/puff, 200 puffs/canister Albuterol HFA MDI: 90 mcg/puff, 200 puffs/canister Levalbuterol HFA MDI: 45 mcg/puff, 200 puffs/canister Pirbuterol CFC MDI Autohaler: 200 mcg/puff, 400 puffs/canister	*Doses apply to all four SABAs.* 2 puffs 5 min before exercise 2 puffs every 4–6 h, as needed for symptoms	Tachycardia, skeletal muscle tremor, hypokalemia, increased lactic acid, headache, hyperglycemia Inhaled route, in general, causes few systemic adverse effects. Patients with preexisting cardiovascular disease, especially the elderly, may have adverse cardiovascular reactions with inhaled therapy.	*Comments apply to all four SABAs.* Drugs of choice for acute bronchospasm Differences in potencies exist, but all products are essentially comparable on a per-puff basis. An increasing use or lack of expected effect indicates diminished control of asthma. Not recommended for long-term daily treatment. Regular use exceeding 2 days/week for symptom control (not prevention of EIB) indicates the need for additional long-term control therapy. May double usual dose for mild exacerbations. For levalbuterol, prime the inhaler by releasing 4 actuations before use. For HFA: periodically clean HFA actuator, because drug may plug orifice. Nonselective agents (i.e., epinephrine, isoproterenol, metaproterenol) are not recommended because of their potential for excessive cardiac stimulation, especially at high doses.
Albuterol Nebulizer solution: 0.63 mg/3 mL, 1.25 mg/3 mL, 2.5 mg/3 mL, 5 mg/mL (0.5%)	1.25–5 mg in 3 mL of saline every 4–8 h, as needed	Same as with MDI.	May mix with cromolyn solution, budesonide inhalant suspension, or ipratropium solution for nebulization. May double dose for severe exacerbations.
Levalbuterol (R-albuterol) Nebulizer solution: 0.31 mg/3 mL, 0.63 mg/3 mL, 1.25 mg/0.5 mL, 1.25 mg/3 mL	0.63–1.25 mg every 8 h, as needed for symptoms	Same as with MDI.	Compatible with budesonide inhalant suspension. The product is a sterile-filled preservative-free unit-dose vial.

TABLE 85.8 β₂ Agonists and Anticholinergics: Formulations and Dosages—cont'd

Medication	≥12 Years of Age and Adults	Potential Adverse Effects	Comments (Not All-Inclusive)
ANTICHOLINERGICS			
Ipratropium HFA MDI: 17 mcg/puff, 200 puffs/canister Nebulizer solution: 0.25 mg/ mL (0.025%) Ipratropium with albuterol MDI: 18 mcg/puff of ipratropium bromide and 90 mcg/puff of albuterol, 200 puffs/canister Nebulizer solution: 0.5 mg/3 mL ipratropium bromide and 2.5 mg/3 mL albuterol	2–3 puffs every 6 h 0.25 mg every 6 h 2–3 puffs every 6 h 3 mL every 4–6 h	Drying of mouth and respiratory secretions, increased wheezing in some individuals, blurred vision if sprayed in eyes. If used in the ED, produces less cardiac stimulation than SABAs.	Multiple doses in the ED (not hospital) setting provide additive benefit to SABA. Treatment of choice for bronchospasm caused by β-blocker medication. Does not block EIB. Reverses only cholinergically mediated bronchospasm; does not modify reaction to antigen. May be an alternative for patients who do not tolerate SABAs. Has not proven to be efficacious as long-term control therapy for asthma. Ipratropium with albuterol nebulizer solution contains EDTA to prevent discoloration of the solution. This additive does not induce bronchospasm.
SYSTEMIC CORTICOSTEROIDS			
Methylprednisolone 2-, 4-, 6-, 8-, 16-, 32-mg tablets Prednisolone 5-mg tablets, 5 mg/5 mL, 15 mg/5 mL Prednisone 1-, 2.5-, 5-, 10-, 20-, 50-mg tablets; 5 mg/mL, 5 mg/5 mL	Short course "burst": 40–60 mg/ day as single or 2 divided doses for 3–10 days	Short-term use: reversible abnormalities in glucose metabolism, increased appetite, fluid retention, weight gain, facial flushing, mood alteration, hypertension, peptic ulcer, and rarely aseptic necrosis. Consideration should be given to coexisting conditions that could be worsened by systemic corticosteroids, such as herpes virus infections, varicella, tuberculosis, hypertension, peptic ulcer, diabetes mellitus, osteoporosis, and *Strongyloides* infection.	Short courses or bursts are effective for establishing control when initiating therapy or during a period of gradual deterioration. Action may begin within an hour. The burst should be continued until patient achieves 80% PEF personal best or symptoms resolve. This usually requires 3–10 days, but may require longer. There is no evidence that tapering the dose after improvement prevents relapse in asthma exacerbations. Other systemic corticosteroids such as hydrocortisone and dexamethasone given in equipotent daily doses are likely to be as effective as prednisolone.
Methylprednisolone acetate Repository injection: 40 mg/ mL, 80 mg/mL	240 mg IM once		May be used in place of a short burst of oral steroids in patients who are vomiting or if adherence is a problem.

DPI, Dry-powder inhaler; *EIB*, exercise-induced bronchospasm; *HFA*, hydrofluoroalkane propellant; *ICS*, inhaled corticosteroids; *LABA*, long-acting β₂ agonist; *NSAID*, nonsteroidal antiinflammatory drug; *PEF*, peak expiratory flow.
From Burchum, J., & Rosenthal, L. (2019). *Lehne's pharmacology for nursing care* (10th ed.). St. Louis: Elsevier.

moderate to severe asthma to help maintain control of symptoms; however, if long-term monitoring is not done, periodic short-term monitoring is recommended for evaluating responses to therapy or assessing the effect of environmental exposures. All individuals with asthma who experience periodic severe asthma exacerbations may benefit from peak flow monitoring.[14]

Peak flow monitoring helps individuals to follow the course of their disease, predict exacerbations, identify triggers, and assess their response to treatment. PEF values, specifically the individual's personal best PEF, should be used as the basis for an action plan. An individual's personal best PEF can be estimated after a 2- to 3-week period, during which the PEF is recorded at least once a day in the early afternoon. Additional measurements should be made after β₂-adrenergic inhalers are used for symptomatic relief. The personal best is usually achieved in the early afternoon after maximum effect of any

therapy has stabilized or resolved the symptoms. The personal best should be reassessed periodically to account for progression of disease. A PEF value that is significantly higher than all the other measurements should be interpreted with caution; rather than reflecting a personal best, an outlying value may occur because of spitting or coughing into the peak flow meter.[1]

A zone system similar to a traffic light has been successfully used to help patients interpret their symptoms and PEFR results. The use of this system is particularly helpful for asthmatic patients who are unable to recognize the severity of their asthma on the basis of symptoms, which is estimated to be the case for more than 50% of patients. In addition, many studies have shown that asthma symptoms correlate poorly with the level of airway obstruction as determined by spirometry (FEV₁ and PEF). After treatment, subjective improvement in asthma symptoms may occur without a corresponding improvement in the degree of airway obstruction. For this reason, current

TABLE 85.9	Risk Factors and Actions to Reduce Exposures
Risk Factor	**Actions**
Domestic dust mite allergens (so small they are not visible to the naked eye)	Wash bed linens and blankets weekly in hot water and dry in a hot dryer or the sun. Encase pillows and mattresses in air-tight covers. Replace carpets with linoleum or wood flooring, especially in sleeping rooms. Use vinyl, leather, or plain wooden furniture instead of fabric-upholstered furniture. If possible, use vacuum cleaner with filters.
Tobacco smoke (whether the patient smokes or breathes in the smoke from others)	Stay away from tobacco smoke. Patients and parents should not smoke.
Allergens from animals with fur	Remove animals from the home, or at least from the sleeping area.
Cockroach allergen	Clean the home thoroughly and often. Use pesticide spray—but make sure the patient is not at home when spraying occurs.
Outdoor pollens and mold	Close windows and doors and remain indoors when pollen and mold counts are highest.
Indoor mold	Reduce dampness in the home; clean any damp areas frequently.
Physical activity	Do not avoid physical activity. Symptoms can be prevented by taking a rapid-acting inhaled β_2 agonist, a chromone, or a leukotriene modifier before strenuous exercise.
Drugs	Do not take β-blockers or aspirin or nonsteroidal antiinflammatory drugs if these medicines cause asthma symptoms.

Modified from Global Initiative for Asthma (GINA). *Pocket guide for asthma management and prevention: A pocket guide for physicians and nurses* (updated 2015). Retrieved from www.ginasthma.org.

guidelines recommend that airway obstruction be measured objectively in assessing patients with chronic asthma.[14]

The zone system consists of green, yellow, and red zones (or lights if the traffic light analogy is used). The green zone (or light) corresponds to a PEF measurement that is at least 80% of an individual's personal best or optimum control. For patients with irritable airways who decompensate quickly, the cutoff may be adjusted to 90%. A measurement in the green zone reflects good asthma control and that it is safe to proceed. The yellow zone means caution and refers to a PEF measurement that is within 50% to 80% of the individual's personal best or optimum control. Some guidelines use a range of 60% to 80% for the yellow zone; the more conservative value of 60% promotes earlier intervention as the patient's condition begins to deteriorate. Symptoms that interfere with daily activities may be present; typical symptoms include cough, wheeze, chest tightness, shortness of breath, and nocturnal awakening. A measurement in the yellow zone indicates the need for a temporary increase in medication dose or frequency. The specific medication change is tailored to each individual and may include increased bronchodilator therapy, increased or added corticosteroid therapy, and a short course of oral corticosteroids.

In many ways, the yellow zone is the key to the entire asthma action plan (AAP) because a measurement in this zone reflects worsening airway obstruction, which will usually continue to worsen if action is not taken. The written AAP should identify at what point the provider should be contacted; in general, patients should be instructed to contact their health care provider for mild to moderate symptoms that do not respond to treatment or for PEFs that remain within the yellow zone (50% to 80% of personal best). The presence of a PEF value or symptoms in the red zone means danger and indicates the need for emergency treatment. A reduction in the PEF of 50% (or 40%) and dyspnea are the general criteria for the red zone. Other associated symptoms may include inability to blow into the peak flow meter, accessory respiratory muscle use, difficulty walking or talking because of asthma, and cyanosis. Immediate

use of inhaled rescue bronchodilator therapy and initiating or increasing oral corticosteroid therapy are necessary. If the PEFR does not improve after emergency treatment, the individual should be instructed to call 911 (or an emergency number) or to proceed to the ED (or to his or her health care provider). The AAP should clearly state in the red zone portion when patients need to seek emergency care.

It has been well established that improving asthma adherence can lead to better control. However, despite growing awareness of the importance of asthma education, adherence to asthma treatment, including medications, the use of peak flow meters, and avoidance of environmental irritants, is still poor. The provider-patient relationship is central to improving adherence; all specific strategies aimed at improving adherence (such as simplifying medication regimens or using AAPs) must be developed in a therapeutic, trusting provider-patient relationship to be effective. Studies have shown that asthma therapy based on influencing behavior and self-management of acute exacerbations results in improved control and decreased asthma morbidity.[17]

Current practice guidelines recommend a follow-up visit 1 to 3 months after starting treatment and every 3 to 12 months after that, except in pregnancy when visits as often as every 4 to 6 weeks may be indicated.[2]

A wide range of risk factors contribute to poor asthma control, and these may be related to genetics, patient characteristics, variability of disease pathogenesis and severity, medication use, and environmental factors. Comorbidities such as GERD, sleep apnea, rhinitis, or rhinosinusitis may complicate disease management.[18] In addition, the association between obesity and asthma has become increasingly recognized during the past decade. A positive correlation between the risk of developing asthma and increased body mass index (in a dose-response manner) has been demonstrated.[19] There is an increased risk of morbidity from asthma among those who are morbidly obese. Treatment of obesity and other comorbidities can improve asthma control and enhance efficacy of medications.

INDICATIONS FOR REFERRAL AND HOSPITALIZATION

The current NIH guidelines state that all patients who have had an asthma-related hospitalization (and thus, by definition, have chronic severe asthma) be evaluated by an asthma specialist. In addition, general reasons for consultation with a specialist include poorly controlled asthma, asthma that is unresponsive to appropriate therapy, the desire to obtain a second opinion, and periodic patient evaluation. Specific reasons for specialist consultation may include classification of asthma type and severity, interpretation of PFT results, assessment of possible occupational asthma, allergy skin testing, and advice about pharmacotherapy. Evidence of poorly controlled asthma, including frequent missed days of work or school, dissatisfaction with the quality of life, and frequent ED visits and hospitalizations, may reflect lack of recognition of the disease severity by the patient or health care provider or treatment plans that are too simplistic. In such cases, referral to an asthma specialist is warranted and will likely improve control and the quality of life and decrease asthma-related morbidity and mortality.

LIFE-SPAN CONSIDERATIONS

The preparation for pregnancy in women with asthma should, if possible, begin well in advance to achieve good asthma control before and during the pregnancy. In approximately equal proportions of women, the control of asthma will improve, worsen, or remain unchanged during pregnancy. Just as with any individual, unmanaged asthma in a pregnant woman may result in ED visits, hospitalizations, respiratory failure, and even death. In addition, poorly managed asthma has been associated with certain complications of pregnancy, including an increased incidence of preeclampsia, eclampsia, low birth weight, premature delivery, and infant death.[1] Given the potential for and possible consequences of asthma complications during pregnancy, it is vitally important that pulmonary function (minimally peak flow monitoring) be monitored throughout pregnancy. Because a 20% drop in peak flow often precedes the onset of symptoms, pregnant women need to be able to recognize when they decrease to less than 80% of their baseline. In addition, an appreciation of ability to improve or lack of improvement is essential so that appropriate prompt treatment can be initiated.

The basic management of asthma during pregnancy is similar to that in nonpregnant individuals. To minimize the need for medications, environmental and lifestyle controls assume an even more important role. No asthma therapy has been proven to be absolutely safe during pregnancy. For women who require only β_2-adrenergic agonists, albuterol is usually the drug of choice. For women requiring antiinflammatory medication, the use of budesonide or cromolyn is considered relatively safe. For more long-acting asthma treatment control, salmeterol is pregnancy category C. Tapered regimens of oral prednisone are used for pregnant women with an acute asthma exacerbation, because the risks of anoxia to the fetus outweigh the possible risks of oral corticosteroid therapy.[1] Another asthma medications that can be considered is zafirlukast (pregnancy risk factor B), a leukotriene modifier. Conversations with the pregnant woman's obstetrician should be ongoing for a pregnant woman with an acute asthma exacerbation.

Asthma tends to be less well recognized among older adults because symptoms are often attributed to other respiratory ailments, such as COPD, congestive heart failure, pulmonary aspiration, pulmonary embolism, and bronchogenic carcinoma.[12] However, the tools usually used to diagnose asthma are still helpful in the differential diagnoses in this population.

If the clinical picture is indistinguishable from either COPD or asthma, it is often useful to consider age at onset; asthmatics have generally experienced symptoms at an earlier age and had a clearer history during their younger years.

In addition, subjective awareness and perception of symptoms tend to be poorer among older adults. For these reasons, asthma remains underdiagnosed and suboptimally treated in this population. In older adults, chronic bronchitis may coexist with asthma, which may affect management. Asthma medications may aggravate coexisting medical conditions, such as cardiac disease and osteoporosis; adjustments in the pharmacotherapy may need to be made. Certain drugs commonly used in older people, including aspirin and β-blockers, may adversely affect asthma. Finally, older adults may have particular difficulty with inhaler administration; their technique should be carefully reviewed, and devices such as spacers may be especially helpful in improving drug delivery in this population. Overall, asthma in older adults tends to be associated with poor overall health and reduced mobility, despite adjustment for living conditions, depression, cognition, visual or auditory impairment, and joint pain.

Nonetheless, appropriate care in older individuals is achievable. Most adverse reactions to asthma drugs may require dose adjustment but are typically not significant enough to warrant discontinuation of the drug. The use of a large-volume spacer improves the inhalation technique, and most older individuals prefer this device to the metered dose inhaler alone.

COMPLICATIONS

Complications of asthma include status asthmaticus and fatal asthma. Status asthmaticus is present when symptoms do not improve or remit with initial treatment of an acute exacerbation. During status asthmaticus, despite maximum therapy, respiratory failure may develop. Signs and symptoms of respiratory failure include paradoxical thoracoabdominal movement, absence of wheeze, bradycardia, and deterioration in mental status. If an exacerbation is severe enough that respiratory failure seems possible, intubation should be performed sooner rather than later.

The increasing rates of asthma morbidity and mortality are disturbing. The reasons for these increasing rates are unclear; however, certain risk factors for fatal asthma have been identified. Comorbidity (such as from cardiovascular disease or COPD) and serious psychiatric disease or psychosocial problems increase the risk of fatal or near-fatal asthma. Difficulty perceiving airflow obstruction or its severity and a history of sudden severe exacerbations also increase the risk of fatal asthma. However, a period of 2 to 7 days of worsening asthma symptoms rather than a sudden deterioration often precedes hospitalizations, providing a window of opportunity to implement more aggressive therapy in an effort to prevent fatal or near-fatal events. Additional risk factors include hospitalization or emergency care for asthma within the past month, prior asthma-related intensive care unit admission, three or more ED visits or two or more hospitalizations for asthma during the past year, and prior intubation for asthma. Other risk factors include current use or withdrawal from systemic glucocorticoids and the use of three or more canisters of inhaled SABAs per month. Urban residence, low socioeconomic status, and illicit drug use also increase the risk for fatal asthma.[14] These risk factors affirm the need for interventions designed to prevent and to control asthma, as well as therapy that includes the self-management of asthma symptoms during periods of exacerbation, especially for those at high risk.

Research has demonstrated that, in comparison with other patient groups, adults with asthma who have lower socioeconomic status and less education are likely to receive care that has less continuity and is less intensive after hospital or ED discharge. In addition, a minority of these patients tend to have AAPs or adequate communication with their health care providers during the acute stages of the exacerbation. In addition, those most at risk for fatal asthma are more likely to depend primarily on the ED for management of exacerbations. In other words, those individuals who are at highest risk for complications of asthma are likely to receive the type of care that increases rather than mitigates the risk of future complications.

PATIENT EDUCATION

Patient education is both one of the most important and one of the most challenging aspects of asthma management (Table 85.10). Asthma is a chronic disease and, like other chronic diseases, requires ongoing maintenance and prevention. Asthma that is treated only episodically when exacerbations occur will result in symptomatic relief at best. To achieve the other goals of asthma treatment (such as preventing symptoms, maintaining near-normal pulmonary function, minimizing the adverse effects of pharmacotherapy, and minimizing the need for ED visits and hospitalizations), patients and their families need to be well educated about:

- The disease, its basis, and their role in monitoring symptoms and preventing exacerbations
- The role of environmental triggers and strategies for minimizing them
- The importance of an individualized asthma management plan
- The use of peak flow measure
- Proper inhaler technique

TABLE 85.10 **Delivery of Asthma Education by Clinicians During Patient Care Visits**

Assessment Questions	Information	Skills
RECOMMENDATIONS FOR INITIAL VISIT		
Focus on: Expectations of visit, Asthma control, Patient's goals for treatment, Medications, Quality of life *Ask relevant questions:* What worries you most about your asthma? What do you want to accomplish at this visit? What do you want to be able to do that you can't do now because of your asthma? What do you expect from treatment? What medicines have you tried? What other questions do you have for me today? Are there things in your environment that make your asthma worse?	*Teach in simple language:* What is asthma? Asthma is a chronic lung disease. The airways are very sensitive. They become inflamed and narrow; breathing becomes difficult. The definition of asthma control: few daytime symptoms, no nighttime awakenings because of asthma, able to engage in normal activities, normal lung function. Asthma treatments: two types of medicines are needed: *Long-term control:* medications that prevent symptoms, often by reducing inflammation *Quick relief:* short-acting bronchodilator relaxes muscles around airways Bring all medications to every appointment. When to seek medical advice. Provide appropriate telephone number.	*Teach or review and demonstrate:* Inhaler and spacer or VHC use. Check performance. Self-monitoring skills that are tied to an action plan: Recognize intensity and frequency of asthma symptoms. Review the signs of deterioration and the need to reevaluate therapy: Waking at night with asthma Increased medication use Decreased activity tolerance Use of a written AAP that includes instructions for daily management and for recognizing and handling worsening asthma.
RECOMMENDATIONS FOR FIRST FOLLOW-UP VISIT (2–4 WEEKS OR SOONER AS NEEDED)		
Focus on: Expectations of visit, Asthma control, Patient's goals for treatment, Medications, Quality of life *Ask relevant questions from previous visit and also ask:* What medications are you taking? How and when are you taking them? What problems have you had using your medications? Please show me how you use your inhaled medications.	*Teach in simple language:* Use of two types of medications. Remind patient to bring all medications and the peak flow meter, if using, to every appointment for review. Self-assessment of asthma control using symptoms and/or peak flow as a guide.	*Teach or review and demonstrate:* Use of a written AAP. Review and adjust as needed. Peak flow monitoring if indicated. Correct inhaler and spacer or VHC technique.

TABLE 85.10	Delivery of Asthma Education by Clinicians During Patient Care Visits—cont'd	
Assessment Questions	**Information**	**Skills**

RECOMMENDATIONS FOR SECOND FOLLOW-UP VISIT

Focus on:	*Teach in simple language:*	*Teach or review and demonstrate:*
Expectations of visit	Self-assessment of asthma control, using symptoms and/or peak flow as a guide.	Inhaler/spacer or VHC technique.
Asthma control		Peak flow monitoring technique.
Patient's goals for treatment	Relevant environmental control and avoidance strategies:	Use of written AAP. Review and adjust as needed.
Medications		
Quality of life	How to identify home, work, or school exposures that can cause or worsen asthma	Confirm that patient knows what to do if asthma gets worse.
Ask relevant questions from previous visits and also ask:		
Have you noticed anything in your home, work, or school that makes your asthma worse?	How to control house-dust mites, animal exposures if applicable	
Describe for me how you know when to call your doctor or go to the hospital for asthma care.	How to avoid cigarette smoke (active and passive)	
What questions do you have about the AAP? Can we make it easier?	Review all medications.	
Are your medications causing you any problems?		
Have you noticed anything in your environment that makes your asthma worse?		
Have you missed any of your medications?		

RECOMMENDATIONS FOR SUBSEQUENT VISITS

Focus on:	*Teach in simple language:*	*Teach or review and demonstrate:*
Expectations of visit	Review and reinforce all:	Inhaler/spacer or VHC technique.
Asthma control	Educational messages	Peak flow monitoring technique, if appropriate.
Patients' goals of treatment	Environmental control strategies at home, work, or school	Use of written asthma action plan. Review and adjust as needed.
Medications	Medications	
Quality of life	Self-assessment of asthma control, using symptoms and/or peak flow as a guide	Confirm that patient knows what to do if asthma gets worse.
Ask relevant questions from previous visits and also ask:		
How have you tried to control things that make your asthma worse?		
Please show me how you use your inhaled medication.		

VHC, Valved holding chamber.
From Burchum, J., & Rosenthal, L. (2019). *Lehne's pharmacology for nursing care* (10th ed.). St. Louis: Elsevier.

REFERENCES

1. Martinez, F. D., & Vercelli, D. (2013). Asthma. *Lancet, 382,* 1360–1372.
2. Global Initiative for Asthma (GINA). Pocket guide for asthma management and prevention: A pocket guide for health pofessionals, updated 2018. Retrieved from www.ginasthma.org. (Accessed 8 December 2018).
3. To, T., Stanojevic, S., Moores, G., et al. Global asthma prevalence in adults: Findings from the cross-sectional world health survey. Retrieved from https://bmcpublichealth.biomedcentral.com/articles/10.1186/1471-2458-12-204. (Accessed 8 December 2018).
4. Centers for Disease Control and Prevention (CDC). Asthma prevalence in the U.S. Retrieved from www.cdc.gov/asthma/asthmadata.htm. (Accessed 8 December 2018).
5. Keet, C. A., McCormack, M. C., Pollack, C. E., Peng, R. D., McGowan, E., & Matusi, E. C. (2015). Neighborhood poverty, urban residence, race/ethnicity, and asthma: Rethinking the inner-city asthma epidemic. *The Journal of Allergy and Clinical Immunology, 135,* 655–662.
6. Centers for Disease Control and Prevention (CDC). Most recent asthma data. Retrieved from cdc.gov/asthma/most_recent_data.htm. (Accessed 8 December 2018).
7. American Academy of Allergy, Asthma and Immunology. (2015). Asthma statistics. Retrieved from www.aaaai.org/media/statistics/asthma-statistics.asp; (Accessed 18 September 2015).
8. Centers for Disease Control and Prevention (CDC). (2017). Asthma faststats. Retrieved from www.cdc.gov/nchs/fastats/asthma.htm. (Accessed 19 January 2019).
9. Asthma and Allergy Foundation of America and the National Pharmaceutical Council. Ethnic disparities in the burden and treatment of asthma. Retrieved from www.aafa.org. (Accessed 3 February 2019).
10. Mastronarde, J. G. (2012). Is there a relationship between GERD and asthma? *Gastroenterol Hepatology, 8*(6), 401–403.
11. Varghese, M., & Lockley, R. F. (2008). Aspirin-exacerbated asthma. *Allergy, Asthma, and Clinical Immunology: Official Journal of the Canadian Society of Allergy and Clinical Immunology,* 75–83.
12. Roberts, S. E., Button, L. A., Hopkins, J. M., et al. (2012). Influence of social deprivation and air pollutants on serious asthma. *European Respiratory Journal, 40,* 785–788.
13. Mendes, N. A., Santa Anna, C. C., & de Fatima Bazhuni Pombo March, M. (2013). Stress in children and adolescents with asthma. *Journal of Human Growth and Development, 23*(1), 80–83.
14. National Asthma Education and Prevention Program (NAEPP). (2007). Expert panel report 3: Guidelines for the diagnosis and management of asthma, NIH Publication NO. 08-5846. Bethesda, MD: U.S.Department of Health and Human Services, National Institutes of Health (NIH), National Health, Lung and Blood Institute (NHLBI).

15. Fatemi, F., Sadroddiny, E., Gheib, A., Mohammadi Farsani, T., & Kardar, G. A. (2014). Biomolecular markers in the assessment and treatment of asthma. *Respirology (Carlton, Vic.)*, *19*, 514–523.

16. Mathur, S. K., & Viswanathan, R. K. (2014). Relevance of allergy in adult asthma. *Current Allergy and Asthma Reports*, *14*, 437–452.

17. Hsu, J., Sircar, K., Herman, E., et al. (2018). EXHALE: A technical package to control asthma. National Center for Environmental Health. Centers for Disease Control and Prevention.

18. Currie, G., & Lee, K. (2005). Beneficial anti-inflammatory effects of leukotriene receptor antagonists in asthma. *Chest*, *127*, 1458.

19. Wechsler, M. E. (2014). Getting control of uncontrolled asthma. *The American Journal of Medicine*, *127*(11), 1049–1059.

CHAPTER **86**

CHEST PAIN (NONCARDIAC)

David Patrick Murphy • Bethany Meyers Bartlett

 Immediate referral is indicated for hemodynamic instability, concern for acute coronary syndrome based on symptoms or electrocardiogram (ECG) changes, and concern for life-threatening etiologies such as pulmonary embolism, pneumothorax, esophageal rupture, or aortic dissection.

DEFINITION AND EPIDEMIOLOGY

Noncardiac chest pain is a recurrent substernal chest pressure or other chest discomfort believed to be unrelated to the heart after a reasonable cardiac evaluation. Because heart disease is the leading cause of death in the United States, and because patients are commonly initially seen with chest pain in the primary care setting, it is important to be able to distinguish the cardiac from the noncardiac causes of chest pain.[1] Research indicates that it is possible to accurately differentiate between the two in most cases. In a study of all patients initially diagnosed with noncardiac chest pain, 93.6% had no evidence of adverse cardiac events, 3.5% had possible evidence of adverse cardiac events, and only 2.8% had a definite cardiac event.[2]

Nevertheless, the symptoms of chest pain are frightening to patients, but reassuringly, most episodes seen in the primary care setting are not of cardiac origin. According to one report, 67% of chest pain diagnoses were the result of musculoskeletal, gastrointestinal, psychiatric, or pulmonary disorders. Only 16% were secondary to cardiac causes of all types, and another 16% were idiopathic (Table 86.1).[3]

Interestingly, even when patients have risk factors or indications for invasive diagnostic workups, data consistently show that a large percentage of these patients still do not have a cardiac cause of their pain. For example, one study found that more than 40% of patients recommended to undergo cardiac catheterization had normal or insignificantly diseased coronary arteries.[4] In another study, 81% of moderate-risk women with chest pain syndrome were prospectively demonstrated to be experiencing noncardiac discomfort. Of the remainder, only 2.5% of women actually experienced cardiac events.[5]

The correct diagnosis for chest pain is most often obtained with a detailed history, supporting physical examination findings, and an ECG or chest radiograph if indicated. Ruling out cardiac causes of chest pain or other noncardiac life-threatening conditions is an essential first step. The evaluation of cardiac chest pain is discussed separately in Chapter 102.

TABLE 86.1 Causes of Chest Pain in the Primary Care Setting

Final Diagnosis	Percentage of Episodes[a]
Musculoskeletal conditions and chest-wall pain	36.2
Gastrointestinal conditions	18.9
Nonspecific chest pain	16.1
Stable angina	10.5
Psychogenic pain	7.5
Respiratory condition	5.1
Nonischemic cardiac condition	3.8
Acute cardiac ischemia	1.5

[a]Study included 399 patients in 12 family practice clinics in Michigan.[3]

BOX 86.1

Sample Questions for Patients With Chest Pain

- Where is the pain?
- How long have you had the pain?
- Do you have recurrent episodes of pain?
- How long does each episode last?
- What makes the pain better or worse? (breathing? lying flat? moving your arms, neck?)
- How would you describe the pain? (burning? crushing? throbbing? stabbing? knifelike?)
- When does the pain occur? (with exertion? after eating? when moving your arms?)
- Is the pain associated with shortness of breath? (cough? palpitations? nausea and vomiting? fever? leg pain? coughing up blood?)

Modified from Swartz, M. B. (Ed.). (2006). The heart. In *Textbook of physical diagnosis: History and examination* (5th ed.). Philadelphia: Elsevier.

PATHOPHYSIOLOGY

The sympathetic chain, vagus, and phrenic nerves are responsible for carrying pain impulses in the thoracic cage. All the structures in the chest, including the chest wall, esophagus, lungs, heart, and diaphragm, have overlapping innervation. Thus, pain from different organs, including those in the abdomen that abut the diaphragm (i.e., liver, spleen, stomach), may have similar referral patterns. In addition, patients may have a difficult time localizing pain from deep structures, whereas diseases involving more superficial structures, such as the chest wall and pleura, are more easily localized. Because there is no sensory innervation in the lung parenchyma, disease involving the alveoli or interstitium does not cause chest pain unless the pulmonary vasculature, bronchi, or pleura is involved.[6]

CLINICAL PRESENTATION AND PHYSICAL EXAMINATION

The history is crucial in determining the differential diagnosis and appropriate management in individuals complaining of chest pain. Careful questioning usually clarifies the cause. Some examples of questions are listed in Box 86.1. The following descriptions should be pursued when the patient is questioned[7]:

Quality: "Can you describe your pain?" Myocardial ischemia typically manifests as a tightness or vise-like, constricting, or heavy pressure sensation. On the other hand, pleuritic pain or pain that is positional, sharp, or reproducible with palpation is often not cardiac.

Location: "Where is your pain?" Pain that localizes to a small area of the chest suggests pleural or chest wall involvement. However, ischemic pain is often difficult to localize. In fact, in an observational study in patients admitted with chest pain, patients who vocalized larger areas of discomfort were more likely to be experiencing a cardiac event than patients who complained of smaller areas.[8]

Intensity: "How severe is your pain?" Pain from an aortic dissection, pneumothorax, or pulmonary embolism all tend to have an abrupt start with the greatest intensity at the beginning. Ischemic chest pain is more gradual, and psychogenic causes of chest pain have a vaguer onset.

Duration: "How long does your pain last?" If the chest pain lasts only seconds or has been constant for weeks, it is unlikely cardiac. Ischemic cardiac pain typically lasts for a few minutes.

Aggravation: "What provokes your pain or makes it worse?" Symptoms related to eating, such as dysphagia, odynophagia, and heartburn, are more suggestive of an upper gastrointestinal cause, whereas chest pain that worsens with physical exertion is usually more reflective of cardiac ischemia. Aggravation of the pain with position changes, deep breathing, or cough is often indicative of a musculoskeletal or pleural disorder.

Alleviation: "What makes your pain better?" Repeated palliation with antacids or food suggests a gastrointestinal source. Esophageal and cardiac causes are generally attenuated with sublingual nitroglycerin. Pain that lessens with rest and the cessation of physical activity strongly suggests an ischemic cause.

Associated symptoms are also helpful in distinguishing chest pain etiologies. For example, acid regurgitation, cough, difficult or painful swallowing, and belching would be suggestive of gastroesophageal reflux disease (GERD) or other esophageal disease. Although cough and dyspnea can be of cardiac origin, they are also suggestive of pulmonary etiology. Fever, weight loss, fatigue, or other constitutional symptoms can be associated with malignancy, whereas rash and arthralgias with constitutional symptoms may suggest an autoimmune etiology. Other information to be elicited includes whether the patient has engaged in any recent unusual or strenuous physical activity, has had recent upper respiratory viral illness, has a history of melena, or has signs or symptoms of anemia. It is important to determine the patient's medical history, including whether the patient has a history of similar symptoms; if the patient has a history of heart disease, risk factors for heart disease, such as hypertension, hyperlipidemia or diabetes; or a history of musculoskeletal, gastrointestinal, pulmonary, or psychiatric disorders. A thorough review of current medications, including over-the-counter, herbal, and illicit substances, should be obtained. A family history of heart disease or other illnesses may also help determine risk for certain chest pain etiologies. Finally, a social history should be obtained and include daily caffeine intake, the use of tobacco or alcohol, and if the patient has experienced recent significant psychosocial

stressors. All this information may contribute to the decision-making process.

The diagnosis of chest pain in the clinical setting has classically been based on some of the factors listed earlier, including location, description, and precipitants of the pain. This has led to a widely accepted classic angina syndrome, which has been shown to correlate well with underlying coronary artery disease (CAD) in both men and women. However, research indicates that women, older individuals, and patients with diabetes and CAD often experience less typical symptoms, which can result in a missed diagnosis and improper treatment.[5]

The physical examination of a patient with chest pain starts with an assessment of his or her general appearance and vital signs. The evaluation must begin with an exclusion of cardiac disease. The general appearance suggests the severity and possibly the seriousness of the symptoms. Abnormalities in vital signs suggest an infectious, pulmonary, cardiac, or malignant process. Hemodynamic instability should prompt immediate referral to the emergency department. The majority of patients with noncardiac chest pain should have normal vital signs.

The neck examination should focus on the presence of lymphadenopathy in the cervical chains or supraclavicular fossa. Elevation of the neck veins indicates volume overload and possible heart failure. Tracheal deviation points to a possible pneumothorax.

A general inspection of the chest may reveal a rash, such as the unilateral rash of herpes zoster in a thoracic dermatome. Evidence of trauma may confirm a history of domestic violence or indicate its existence, even if the patient did not discuss it.

Palpation of the chest and range of motion of the upper body may cause chest pain in the presence of costochondritis, musculoskeletal disease, fibromyalgia, rib fracture, or trauma. Dullness to percussion over a portion of the posterior chest indicates either a pleural effusion or a consolidative pulmonary process such as pneumonia.

Auscultation of the lungs may elicit asymmetric breath sounds, pleural friction rub, wheezing, crackles, or absent or decreased breath sounds, all of which should prompt additional investigation with a chest radiograph. The cardiac examination should evaluate for the presence of murmurs, extra heart sounds (S_3 or S_4), displaced point of maximal impulse or friction rubs.

Examination of the abdomen may reveal tenderness in the epigastric area or the right or left upper quadrants, causing irritation of the diaphragm and resultant referred chest pain. Finally, many patients with noncardiac chest pain will actually have completely normal physical examination findings.

DIAGNOSTICS
Essential Diagnostics

The diagnostic testing options for chest pain are often limited in the primary care setting. Pulse oximetry should be used to determine the oxygen saturation. If the patient's chest pain seems cardiac in origin, a 12-lead ECG may demonstrate characteristic abnormalities. Although a normal ECG reduces the likelihood of an acute coronary syndrome by 70% to 90%, it does not completely rule out cardiac ischemia. An ECG should always be interpreted in the context of the patient's history and risk factors for heart disease.[9]

A chest X-ray (postero-anterior and lateral) study is a useful diagnostic tool for detecting cardiac and pulmonary abnormalities.

For typical GERD symptoms, the empirical response to a proton pump inhibitor (PPI) trial has been shown to be a reasonable first-line means to diagnose GERD as a source of chest pain.[10]

Additional Diagnostics

A complete blood count (CBC) with differential, an arterial blood gas (ABG), D-Dimer, BNP, or ESR may also be indicated.[11] In individuals younger than 40 years, a normal ECG may be sufficient to rule out cardiac disease. However, in older patients or in those with risk factors (e.g., smoking, obesity, diabetes, hyperlipidemia, stress), cardiac enzymes, echocardiogram, stress testing, or coronary angiography also may be necessary.[2] However, in many cases, a detailed history, physical examination, and possibly an ECG or chest radiograph should reveal enough information to form a hypothesis regarding the cause of the patient's symptoms.

DIFFERENTIAL DIAGNOSIS

 The differential diagnosis of noncardiac chest pain can be considered if the primary differentials of cardiac ischemia, pulmonary embolism, pneumothorax, aortic dissection, esophageal rupture, and other life-threatening conditions have been excluded or determined unlikely based on the initial history, physical exam, and diagnostic evaluation.

The differential diagnosis should include musculoskeletal, gastrointestinal, pulmonary, and psychiatric disorders.

Musculoskeletal conditions are the most common cause of noncardiac chest pain in the primary care setting, accounting for one-third to one-half of primary care visits with the chief complaint of chest pain.[12] Chest pain related to musculoskeletal conditions is often nagging and persistent, lasting anywhere from hours to weeks. Patients usually complain of superficial chest pain localized in a small area. The symptoms are aggravated by position, deep breathing, turning, or arm movement. Causes of musculoskeletal chest-wall pain include isolated musculoskeletal disorders such as costochondritis, lower rib pain syndromes, and routine muscle strains; systemic rheumatologic diseases such as rheumatoid arthritis, ankylosing spondylitis, fibromyalgia; and other systemic nonrheumatologic diseases such as trauma, stress fractures, and neoplasms.

Fibromyalgia is a common rheumatologic cause of chest pain. It is a complex widespread pain syndrome, often with visceral and somatic pain components. It is often part of a larger spectrum of central sensitization that includes depression, chronic headaches, posttraumatic stress disorder, functional gastrointestinal disorders, and chronic fatigue. Complaints such as fatigue, nonrestorative sleep, chronic headache, gastrointestinal complaints, or cognitive disturbance may indicate fibromyalgia as the cause of chest pain. Specific tender points on the second rib lateral to the costochondral junction and the midpoint of the upper border of the trapezius, although not specific, are of importance in making the diagnosis.[13]

Herpes zoster, a dermatologic condition, can cause acute chest pain, which is usually described as a burning sensation, usually in a unilateral dermatomal distribution. Pain often occurs before the onset of vesicular lesions, so physical examination findings may not be present at the time of the initial complaint, making diagnosis difficult.[1] A history of zoster or varicella may be helpful in making this diagnosis.

Gastrointestinal conditions account for approximately 10% to 20% of noncardiac chest pain in the primary care

setting.[12] In one study, gastroesophageal disease was the most common cause in persons for whom myocardial infarction (MI) was ruled out.[1] The gastroesophageal causes of chest pain include most commonly GERD, and less commonly esophageal rupture or perforation (Boerhaave syndrome), esophageal spasm, pill-induced esophagitis, peptic ulcer, pancreatitis, and cholecystitis. Symptoms highly suggestive of an esophageal disorder, especially reflux disease, include dysphagia, odynophagia, regurgitation, heartburn, and cough.[1,14] Clinical history alone cannot reliably differentiate between cardiac and esophageal chest pain. For example, chest pain associated with GERD also may be triggered by exertion or have other characteristics similar to angina, such as relief with nitroglycerin.[15] However, pain related to an esophageal disorder is more likely to last for hours, to occur retrosternally without radiation, to interrupt sleep, and to be related to meals more often than cardiac chest pain. It is also more often related to other esophageal symptoms, such as dysphagia and heartburn. One important point to consider is that cardiac and gastrointestinal diagnoses can coexist, and the management of one should not eliminate consideration of therapy for the other. In fact, one publication interestingly revealed that over 30% of patients sent to cardiology had concurrent gastrointestinal disease and that patients with true CAD might still benefit from PPI therapy, because of decreased chest pain and fewer emergency department visits with the addition of gastroesophageal medical management.[16]

With regard to esophageal perforation, this is usually caused by instrument-induced damage, foreign body impaction, forceful straining or vomiting, and diseases of the esophagus, such as esophagitis or neoplasm. The classic history for esophageal perforation is profound, sudden, severe, and constant pain from the neck to the epigastrium that is worsened by swallowing. Pain may occur after severe retching and vomiting.

Recent use of prescriptions such as doxycycline, nonsteroidal antiinflammatory drugs (NSAIDs), or alendronate may suggest pill-induced esophagitis. Although any pill, if it is not swallowed properly and with enough fluid, may cause esophagitis, alendronate has received much attention for this side effect, earning specific recommendations to swallow the pill with at least 6 to 8 ounces of water and to remain upright for at least 30 minutes after swallowing. In one study, 65.8% of cases of pill esophagitis were related to the use of antibiotics, especially in the tetracycline group.[17] Accidental ingestion of caustic substances can also cause chemical esophagitis.

Chest pain can be caused by a pulmonary source if the pulmonary vasculature, parenchyma, or pleural tissue is affected; the associated pain is frequently described as pleuritic in nature, such as pain worsened with breathing, coughing, chest movement, sneezing, or talking. Pleuritic pain also may be described as stabbing or shooting chest pain or, if mild pain, as "a stitch in the side." Pleuritic pain can be caused by pulmonary embolism or pneumonia with inflammation extending to the pleural surface; autoimmune disorders such as lupus; viral infection is a common cause of pleuritic pain in otherwise healthy individuals; and medications such as procainamide, hydralazine, and isoniazid can cause pleuritic chest pain.[6]

Pulmonary embolism is a common and often missed diagnosis and is suggested by the onset of dyspnea, pleuritic chest pain, severe hypoxia, and the presence of risk factors such as recent surgery, underlying malignant disease, and a sedentary lifestyle.[1] These symptoms are obviously nonspecific and require a high degree of clinical suspicion with special attention to known risk factors of pulmonary embolism, such as immobilization, history of previous venous thromboembolism, recent surgery, pregnancy, or malignant disease.

Patients who have pneumonia as the underlying cause of their chest pain are usually easily diagnosed on the basis of the cough, fever, sputum production, and findings on physical examination and chest X-ray study.

A diagnosis that should be considered in patients with the sudden onset of sharp, stabbing chest pain is pneumothorax. Patients with primary spontaneous pneumothorax are typically young, tall, thin men who smoke and have no history of lung disease.[6] Secondary spontaneous pneumothoraces occur in patients with cystic fibrosis, chronic obstructive pulmonary disease, human immunodeficiency virus (HIV), and *Pneumocystis* pneumonia.

Psychiatric diseases may underlie symptoms of chest pain in some primary care patients. In one study, patients with noncardiac chest pain and no abnormalities on upper endoscopy or other explanation for their symptoms had a higher prevalence of panic disorder, obsessive-compulsive disorder, and major depressive episodes.[12] These patients tend to be younger and female, and have atypical symptoms and other diagnosed psychiatric illnesses. In patients, especially older women, with acute life stressors and symptoms of a panic attack, Takotsubo stress cardiomyopathy should be considered whether or not the patient's ECG shows changes, especially if there are vital sign changes present such as bradycardia or hypotension.[18]

Vascular causes of chest pain outside of pulmonary embolism should also be considered. Important items to explore in a patient's history are a family history of sickle cell anemia, which would prompt evaluation of sickle crisis, or acute chest syndrome. Aortic dissection is an unlikely cause of chest pain in the primary care setting but must be considered. Aortic dissection typically presents with acute onset chest and back pain that is severe, sharp, and may have a ripping or tearing quality.

Finally, brief consideration should be given to chest pain caused by nonischemic cardiac sources such as pericarditis, mitral valve prolapse, or Takotsubo cardiomyopathy as mentioned above. Pericarditis is inflammation of the pericardial sac; patients often complain of pleuritic pain that is improved by sitting up or leaning forward. It can be diagnosed based on history, cardiac friction rub on physical exam, and ECG findings (typically diffuse ST segment elevation). Mitral valve prolapse also may cause chest discomfort without ECG changes. Patients may have a personal or family history of an associated connective tissue disorder, and the characteristic mid-systolic click on examination.

INTERPROFESSIONAL COLLABORATIVE MANAGEMENT

Management of patients with chest pain depends on the cause of the disease process. The following management section will focus on the most common noncardiac causes of chest pain.

For musculoskeletal chest pain, reassurance is an important component of management as chest pain is a distressing experience for patients. Other components of nonpharmacologic management include temporary avoidance of provoking activities, heat if muscle spasm is present, or ice to help reduce pain and/or swelling. Home stretches and physical therapy may likewise be appropriate for some causes of musculoskeletal chest pain.

For GERD, evidence-based behavioral and lifestyle modifications include weight loss for patients who are overweight or have had recent weight gain, avoidance of eating meals 2 to 3 hours before bed, elevating the head of the bed, avoidance of dietary triggers in patients who have noted specific triggers and improvement of symptoms with elimination, and tobacco cessation. Also, there is some new but limited evidence that dietary fiber improves GERD symptoms.[19]

Psychiatric disease as a cause of noncardiac chest pain is common; however, it should always be a diagnosis of exclusion. For suspected psychiatric causes including panic disorder, depression, or generalized anxiety disorder, patients have been shown to benefit from cognitive behavioral therapy.[20]

Pharmacologic Management

Pharmacologic treatment of mild to moderate musculoskeletal chest pain includes topical agents, such as diclofenac or capsaicin creams, and lidocaine patch or gel; and oral analgesics such as acetaminophen and NSAIDs. For severe, acute pain, such as in trauma or fracture, prescription-strength NSAIDs, parenteral ketorolac, or a short course of opioid analgesics can be considered. If muscle spasm is involved, muscle relaxants, such as cyclobenzaprine and methocarbamol, can be considered, although there are no strong data to support their use. For neuropathic pain, chronic pain, and fibromyalgia, antidepressants (e.g., TCAs, selective serotonin reuptake inhibitors [SSRIs], SNRIs) can be beneficial. Anticonvulsants, such as gabapentin and pregabalin, also have been used for these indications.

For mild or infrequent GERD symptoms, consider initial treatment with H_2 receptor antagonists with or without additional antacids, or initiate a PPI. For severe or frequent GERD symptoms, initiating PPI therapy is generally recommended as PPIs are more effective for controlling GERD symptoms than H_2 receptor antagonists.[21]

If a pulmonary disorder is suspected and confirmed by a chest radiograph, treatment will be self-evident. In the case of pneumonia, first-line treatment with antibiotics is indicated (see Chapter 93).

If a diagnosis of panic disorder, depression, or generalized anxiety disorder is suspected, SSRIs are effective.

Even in patients who did not meet *Diagnostic and Statistical Manual of Mental Disorders*, Fourth Edition (DSM-IV), criteria for these disorders but who did not otherwise have an explanation for their symptoms, use of SSRIs demonstrated a benefit of reducing daily noncardiac chest pain by 50%.[22]

INDICATIONS FOR REFERRAL OR HOSPITALIZATION

Emergency department referral or specialist referral is necessary when a cardiac origin of chest pain or a life-threatening noncardiac cause cannot be excluded. See Box 86.2 for a list of common red flags that warrant escalation of care. This list is by no means all-inclusive, and a practitioner's clinical judgement is the ultimate reason to refer.

Referral to a pain management specialist should be considered for musculoskeletal chest pain that is not responding to the above management strategies. These patients may benefit from local injection of corticosteroids and local anesthetics.

Referral to a rheumatologist should be considered for the diagnosis of new rheumatologic conditions.

In patients with suspected reflux causing chest pain, a lack of response to high-dose PPI therapy should prompt a referral to a gastroenterologist for endoscopy and further evaluation.

For all patients older than age 50 diagnosed with pneumonia, a follow-up chest X-ray study should be done 6 to 8

BOX **86.2**

Clinical Signs Warranting Immediate Transfer to Higher Level of Care

- Respiratory distress (breathlessness, tachypnea, hypoxia, hypoxemia)
- Significant hypotension or hypertension
- Signs of abnormal perfusion—cyanosis, altered mental status
- Asymmetric breath sounds
- New heart murmurs, rubs, or gallops
- Pulsus paradoxus >10 mm Hg
- Abnormal electrocardiogram findings or cardiac enzymes if done in clinic
- Widened mediastinum on chest X-ray examination
- Significant hematemesis
- Pleuritic chest pain
- Sharp chest pain radiating through to the back
- Subcutaneous crepitus

weeks after treatment to document resolution of the infiltrate and to assess for an underlying cause of the process, such as a malignant neoplasm or another structural defect. A pulmonologist should be consulted for any mass on chest X-ray film or for patients with recurring or nonresolving pneumonia. An intraparenchymal or pleura-based mass causing chest pain deserves additional workup with chest computed tomography (CT), pain management with analgesics, and a referral to a pulmonologist.

Referral to a mental health professional should be considered for all patients with a psychiatric cause of chest pain.

Referral to cardiology should be considered for chest pain that is of unclear etiology or if the patient has significant risk factors warranting further cardiac evaluation.

LIFE-SPAN CONSIDERATIONS

Patient age is often an important factor in determining the diagnosis. Younger patients' chest pain is generally caused by more benign underlying conditions, whereas older patients with more risk factors and comorbid conditions are more likely to have serious causes of their chest pain.

In patients who have been diagnosed with noncardiac chest pain, although data are limited, most studies show no significant increase in mortality. However, patients with chronic noncardiac chest pain may have debilitating symptoms, impaired functional status, chronic use of drugs, repeated admissions to the hospital, and repeated cardiac and noncardiac procedures.[23]

COMPLICATIONS

Pulmonary embolism can be life-threatening if diagnosis and treatment are delayed. Thus, clinical suspicion of pulmonary embolism is important in all patients who are seen with respiratory or cardiac complaints. A pneumothorax can develop into a tension pneumothorax if it is not treated appropriately. With a tension pneumothorax, there is a mediastinal and tracheal shift to the contralateral side, hypotension, and an increase in respiratory distress. This condition can be rapidly fatal if it is not diagnosed and treated. Pneumonia can proceed to respiratory failure even in young and otherwise healthy patients. Esophageal perforation leads to mediastinitis. Finally, acute aortic dissection can result in cardiac valvular insufficiency,

rapid hemodynamic collapse, and death if it is not addressed promptly.

PATIENT AND FAMILY EDUCATION AND HEALTH PROMOTION

- Ensure that patients are well informed about their diagnosis, its natural history, and possible complications to improve the probability of a positive outcome.
- Emphasize how to distinguish between the current cause of chest pain and cardiac or life-threatening chest pain and what to do if these conditions are recognized, including when to call 911 (or universal emergency number).
- If any medications are prescribed, instructions should incorporate the correct administration of the drugs and their possible side effects.

Chest pain can be an understandably distressing condition for patients given concern for serious underlying cardiac pathology. If noncardiac chest pain is the diagnosis, reassurance is an important aspect of the clinical visit. However, the encounter can be used to promote lifestyle changes to minimize cardiac risk including exercise, weight loss, and a healthy, well-balanced diet. If the patient smokes, he or she should receive counseling on the importance of tobacco cessation at every visit.

REFERENCES

1. Karnath, B., Holden, M., & Hussain, N. (2004). Chest pain: Differentiating cardiac from noncardiac causes. *Hospital Physician, 38*, 24–27, 38.
2. Miller, C., Lindsell, C., Khandelwai, S., et al. (2004). Is the initial diagnostic impression of "noncardiac chest pain" adequate to exclude cardiac disease? *Annals of Emergency Medicine, 44*(6), 565–574.
3. Klinkman, M. S., Stevens, D., & Gorenflo, D. W. (1994). Episodes of care for chest pain: A preliminary report from MIRNET: Michigan Research Network. *The Journal of Family Practice, 38*, 345–352.
4. Patel, M. R., Dai, D., Hernandez, A. F., et al. (2014). Prevalence and predictors of nonobstructive coronary artery disease identified with coronary angiography in contemporary clinical practice. *American Heart Journal, 167*(6), 846–852.
5. Sanfilippo, A., Abdollah, H., Knott, C., et al. (2005). Defining low risk for coronary heart disease among women with chest pain syndrome. *Journal of Women's Health (2002), 14*(3), 240–247.
6. Weinberger, S. E., & Cockrill, B. A. (2008). Presentation of the patient with pulmonary disease: Pleural disease. In *Principles of pulmonary medicine*. Philadelphia: Elsevier.
7. Fang, J., & Bjorkman, D. (2001). A critical approach to non-cardiac chest pain: Pathophysiology, diagnosis, and treatment. *The American Journal of Gastroenterology, 96*, 958–968.
8. Marcus, G. M., Cohen, J., Varosy, P. D., et al. (2007). The utility of gestures in patients with chest discomfort. *The American Journal of Medicine, 120*, 83.
9. Panju, A. A., Hemmelgarn, B. R., Guyatt, G. H., et al. (1998). The rational clinical examination: Is this patient having a myocardial infarction? *JAMA: The Journal of the American Medical Association, 280*, 1256–1263.
10. Badillo, R., & Francis, D. (2014). Diagnosis and treatment of gastroesophageal reflux disease. *World Journal of Gastrointestinal Pharmacology and Therapeutics, 5*(3), 105–112.
11. Cayley, E. W. (2005). Diagnosing the cause of chest pain. *American Family Physician, 72*(10), 2012–2021.
12. Ebell, M. H. (2011). Evaluation of chest pain in primary care patients. *American Family Physician, 83*(5), 603–605.
13. Almansa, C., Wang, B., & Achem, S. R. (2010). Noncardiac chest pain and fibromyalgia. *The Medical Clinics of North America, 94*, 275–289.
14. Ho, K. Y., Kang, J. Y., Yeo, B., et al. (1998). Non-cardiac, non-esophageal chest pain: The relevance of psychological factors. *Gut, 43*, 105–110.
15. Henrikson, C. A., Howell, E. E., Bush, D. E., Miles, J. S., Meininger, G. R., Friedlander, T., et al. (2003). Chest pain relief by nitroglycerin does not predict active coronary artery disease. *Annals of Internal Medicine, 139*(12), 979.
16. Liuzzo, J. P., Ambrose, J. A., & Diggs, P. (2005). Proton pump inhibitors for patients with coronary artery disease associated with reduced chest pain,

emergency department visits, and hospitalizations. *Clinical Cardiology*, *28*(8), 369.

17. Zografos, G. N., Georgiadou, D., Thomas, D., Kaltsas, G., & Digalakis, M. (2009). Drug-induced esophagitis. *Diseases of the Esophagus*, *22*(8), 633–637.

18. Prasad, A., Dangas, G., Srinivasan, M., Yu, J., Gersh, B. J., Mehran, R., et al. (2014). Incidence and angiographic characteristics of patients With apical ballooning syndrome (Takotsubo/stress cardiomyopathy) in the HORIZONS-AMI trial: An analysis from a multicenter, international study of ST-elevation myocardial infarction. *Catheterization and Cardiovascular Interventions*, *83*(3), 343–348.

19. Ness-Jensen, E., Hveem, K., El-Serag, H., et al. (2016). Lifestyle intervention in gastroesophageal reflux disease. *Clinical Gastroenterology and Hepatology*, *14*(2), 175–182.

20. Van Peski-Oosterbaan, A. S., Spinhoven, P., van Rood, Y., et al. (1999). Cognitive-behavioral therapy for non-cardiac chest pain: A randomized trial. *The American Journal of Medicine*, *106*, 424–429.

21. Sigterman, K. E., Van Pinxteren, B., Bonis, P. A., et al. (2013). Short-term treatment with medications for heartburn symptoms. Cochrane Review.

22. Varia, I., Logue, E., O'Connor, C., et al. (2000). Randomized trial of sertraline in patients with unexplained chest pain of non-cardiac origin. *American Heart Journal*, *140*, 367–372.

23. Fass, R., & Achem, S. R. (2011). Noncardiac chest pain: Epidemiology, natural course and pathogenesis. *Journal of Neurogastroenterology and Motility*, *17*(2), 110–123.

CHAPTER **87**

CHRONIC COUGH

Patricia Polgar-Bailey

DEFINITION AND EPIDEMIOLOGY

Cough is a common symptom in persons with a wide range of respiratory and nonrespiratory diseases, as well as individuals who are not ill. Cough, an important reflex action and respiratory defense mechanism, is designed to prevent the aspiration of foreign material into the lower respiratory tract and to clear excessive secretions, mucus, fluids, foreign matter, and infectious organisms from the larynx, trachea, and large bronchi. Cough has a protective role, which is illustrated by the possible complications resulting from cough suppression, such as infections. However, cough can also transmit disease through airborne droplets and the contamination of objects, and it can be associated with complications, particularly when it is chronic. Excessive and chronic cough can result in numerous complications, including headache, anorexia, vomiting, throat pain, subconjunctival hemorrhages, fatigue, insomnia, myalgia, dysphonia, perspiration, urinary incontinence, syncope, rib pain and rib fractures, inguinal or abdominal wall herniations, diaphragmatic rupture, anxiety, and depression.[1] Chronic cough can have a profound psychological and emotional impact. Many adults with chronic cough report feeling self-conscious about their cough and can become socially isolated owing to the associated complications, such as incontinence. In addition, older adults with chronic cough often feel anxious that "something's wrong"; in studies, a significant percentage have expressed a specific fear of cancer.[1] Chronic cough may be a symptom of underlying disease. For these reasons, a persistent chronic cough is a cause for concern for both the patient and the health care provider.

Coughs may be classified as acute (lasting <3 weeks), subacute (lasting 3 to 8 weeks), and chronic (persisting beyond 8 weeks).[1] Most coughs are acute and self-limited; 90% are caused by viral upper respiratory tract infections, two-thirds of which clear within 2 weeks.[2] Nonviral causes of acute cough include exacerbations of asthma and exposure to environmental pollutants.

A cough that persists for more than 3 weeks and for which initial treatment has failed should be investigated. Subacute cough is generally caused by bacterial sinusitis or asthma, but it can also be caused by upper respiratory infections. The cough that follows a viral or virus-like infection (e.g., *Mycoplasma pneumoniae* or *Bordetella pertussis*) is sometimes referred to as a postinfectious cough. A postinfectious cough, by definition, lasts no longer than 8 weeks; chest radiograph findings are normal, and the cough eventually resolves, generally without intervention. Thus, subacute postinfectious cough can be distinguished from chronic cough by the duration of symptoms; the chronic cough lasts for 8 weeks or more, and usually much longer.[1] The American College of Chest Physicians (ACCP) has developed evidence-based clinical practice guidelines for the management of postinfectious cough, which can be found at https://www.ncbi.nlm.nih.gov/pubmed/16428703/.[3]

Cough is reportedly the most frequent reason for visits to primary care providers and accounts for approximately 8% of all encounters.[4] In the United States and Europe, cough is estimated to affect 9% to 33% of the population, and its prevalence may be increasing as a result of worsening environmental pollution.[2] Chronic cough is often related to cigarette smoking, and the prevalence of chronic cough is three times higher in smokers than in nonsmokers or ex-smokers.[2] Chronic bronchitis (primarily from cigarette smoking) is another common cause of chronic cough. Exposure to secondhand smoke and other irritants also increases the risk for development of a chronic cough.

Chronic cough can have many causes in addition to exposure to cigarette smoke, but only a few diseases account for most cases. In adults, the three most common causes of chronic cough with normal chest radiography include the corticosteroid-responsive eosinophilic airway diseases (asthma, cough variant asthma, and eosinophilic bronchitis), upper airway cough syndrome (previously referred to as postnasal drip syndrome), and gastroesophageal reflux disease (GERD). These have been referred to as the pathogenic triad of chronic cough, accounting for almost all cases of cough in immunocompetent, nonsmoking adults who have normal chest radiographs and are not taking angiotensin-converting enzyme (ACE) inhibitors. The incidence of ACE inhibitor–induced cough has been estimated at 10%, but there is geographic variation and in certain countries, such as China, the prevalence is estimated to be as high as 44%.[1]

PATHOPHYSIOLOGY

When a neural receptor along the respiratory tree is stimulated, an afferent signal is transmitted to the "cough center" of the brain, which is located in the medulla. From this center, through a complex reflex arc, the impulse is passed down the efferent pathway to the expiratory musculature.

The receptors of the afferent limb can be found anywhere along the respiratory tree. These include the vagus from the ears, larynx, trachea, bronchi, pleurae, and gastrointestinal tract; the trigeminal from the nose and the sinuses; the glossopharyngeal from the pharynx; and the phrenic from the diaphragm.

The efferent limb consists primarily of the phrenic and spinal nerves. After the stimulus reaches the cough center, the cough begins with a deep inspiration to approximately 50% of the vital capacity. This allows maximum expiratory flow by increasing the lung elastic recoil and by decreasing airway frictional resistance. During this phase, the glottis opens widely to allow rapid entry of large amounts of air into the lung. The glottis rapidly closes and the abdominal and intercostal muscles contract, increasing the intrapleural pressures to 100 to 200 mm Hg. In a fraction of a second, the glottis reopens, causing an explosive release of air. During this phase, the tracheobronchial tree narrows, resulting in forces sufficient to strip mucus off the walls, creating sputum.

CLINICAL PRESENTATION AND PHYSICAL EXAMINATION

A careful and detailed history will provide the diagnosis in the majority of cases of cough. A cough that lasts for 3 consecutive months for more than 2 consecutive years is indicative of chronic bronchitis. A sudden onset of cough in the supine position with an associated sour taste in the mouth suggests esophageal reflux. A cough associated with constant throat clearing and thick mucus production, especially on rising from bed, is consistent with upper airway cough and sinusitis. A cough associated with rhinorrhea or sneezing may be a viral syndrome or the common cold. If it recurs annually at the same time of year, allergic rhinitis is possible. Intermittent productive cough associated with wheezing is most probably asthma. A loud hacking cough during the daytime that is nonproductive, leads to exhaustion, and is associated with emotional stress may suggest psychogenic cough. In addition, some authors have attributed certain sputum characteristics to a particular disease process (Box 87.1). Evaluation of these attributes may also aid in diagnosis.

ACE inhibitors can cause a nonproductive cough more commonly in women, nonsmokers, and persons of Chinese ethnicity.[1] The onset of cough may occur within hours of the first dose or can be delayed for weeks to months after the initiation of ACE inhibitor therapy. The cough is not dose related and usually resolves within 1 to 4 weeks after cessation of therapy; however, in a small percentage of patients, the cough may linger for up to 3 months after termination of therapy.[3]

The history and physical examination can help establish the cause of cough in the majority of cases. Obvious physical examination findings include the following:

- Pharyngeal erythema with or without cobblestoning of the mucosa and purulent secretions, as seen in sinusitis, upper airway cough, or allergic disease
- Diffuse inspiratory crackles characteristic of pulmonary edema or fibrosis

---

BOX **87.1**

Sputum Characteristics of Various Pulmonary Disorders

- Hemoptysis: bronchogenic cancer, pulmonary embolus, tuberculosis
- Yellow-green, purulent: bronchitis
- Pink frothy: pulmonary edema
- Fetid purulent: anaerobic infections
- Rust colored: pneumococcal pneumonia
- Foam, serous, mucopurulent layers: bronchiectasis

- Expiratory wheezes as in asthma or chronic obstructive pulmonary disease (COPD)
- Occasional hair rubbing against the eardrum or cerumen impaction in the canal resulting in the irritation of the auricular branch of the vagus nerve, and triggering the cough[2]

If the cause of the cough remains elusive after a thorough history and physical examination, a chest radiograph should be obtained, even though radiographic findings are diagnostic in only a minority of cases. A normal chest radiograph usually excludes malignant disease, bronchiectasis, persistent pneumonia, sarcoidosis, and tuberculosis. The next step is to reconsider the most likely remaining causes of chronic cough, keeping in mind that chronic cough may fail to resolve because of inaccurate diagnosis or incorrect or insufficient therapy.

DIAGNOSTICS
Essential Diagnostics

A chest radiograph will reveal the presence of a lung mass or parenchymal abnormalities, such as sarcoidosis, fibrosis, emphysema, and congestive heart failure. If chest films reveal abnormalities, further diagnostic studies may be indicated, possibly including computed tomography (of the chest which can reveal atypical infections or lung masses). Pulmonary function testing (PFT) and oxygen saturation levels may suggest a diagnosis of COPD, asthma, or restrictive lung disease.[1] Cardiac studies are indicated if heart failure is suspected. Bronchoscopy should be planned only for a specific diagnosis, keeping in mind that bronchoscopy has been shown to be of little diagnostic benefit when chest radiograph or computed tomography (CT) findings are normal or nonlocalizing.[4] If the diagnosis is still not found, routine PFTs are indicated, and if these results are negative, a methacholine challenge test is necessary to rule out asthma. At this point, more than 50% of coughs will have been diagnosed.

Additional Diagnostics

If the cause is still undetermined, a gastrointestinal evaluation with a barium swallow study and 24-hour pH esophageal monitoring should be considered. Further diagnostic tests include a CT scan of the sinuses and otolaryngologic evaluation. The majority of patients should now have a definitive diagnosis. Undiagnosed cases of cough may include psychogenic cough. There is a select group of patients who have a syndrome referred to as chronic idiopathic cough, for which the cause remains elusive. In some cases, the precipitating cause of the cough may have disappeared, but its effect on the cough reflex may be more prolonged. An example of this might be a transient upper respiratory tract viral infection or an exposure to respiratory toxins, which can cause inflammatory neuropathic changes in the sensory nerves, thereby inducing more prolonged damage to the respiratory mucosa. Approximately 25% to 50% of patients have multiple causes of cough.[5]

Individuals with a compromised immune system require additional diagnostic testing as part of the initial workup. If a patient is immunocompromised, especially because of human immunodeficiency virus (HIV) infection, a chest radiograph and oxygen saturation level should be obtained earlier in the assessment. Chronic comorbid conditions and acute critical illnesses can cause further depression of the immune system, thereby increasing the risk of infection.

DIFFERENTIAL DIAGNOSIS

 Red flags include signs and symptoms suggestive of cardiac disease (particularly left ventricular failure), interstitial lung disease, bronchogenic carcinoma, sarcoidosis, foreign body aspiration, postradiation pneumonitis, and metastatic lung carcinoma, all of which may have a cough as the sole presenting symptom.

The causes of cough are plentiful and diverse. In adults of all ages and in children older than 1 year, corticosteroid-responsive eosinophilic airway diseases (asthma and eosinophilic bronchitis), upper airway cough syndrome (postnasal drip syndrome), and GERD are the three most common causes of chronic cough.[1] Upper airway cough syndrome is believed to be the most common cause of chronic cough and should be one of the first conditions considered. In general, it occurs after viral upper respiratory tract infections. Other causes of upper airway cough syndrome include perennial rhinitis (e.g., rhinitis caused by seasonal allergens), irritants, drugs, vasomotor responses, chronic sinusitis, and medications (e.g., ACE inhibitors). There are no signs and symptoms specific to the cough caused by upper airway cough syndrome; therefore it can be difficult to make the diagnosis based on the history and physical examination findings alone. Postnasal drip, often associated with rhinorrhea and nasal congestion, is characterized by a sensation of nasal secretions or a "drip" at the back of the throat, often accompanied by the need to clear the throat. Throat clearing and a cobblestone appearance on the posterior pharynx are features suggestive of, but not definitive for, upper airway cough because they can occur in other conditions, and these signs and symptoms often correlate poorly with cough.[1] The diagnosis of upper airway cough syndrome is often based on response to a trial of therapy. Upper airway cough syndrome may occur in association with some other chronic condition, so it is important to consider other possible causes of the cough, particularly if the cough does not resolve after therapy.

Early asthma and other related eosinophilic conditions may manifest as chronic cough. Bronchial asthma is the second most common cause of chronic cough in immunocompetent adults. Cough can be one of the first signs of worsening asthma (cough-variant asthma), as well as the symptom most reported by patients with chronic asthma, irrespective of having achieved good asthma control with inhaled bronchodilators. The cough may precede audible wheezes, dyspnea, or airflow obstruction. A subset of asthmatics will have cough-variant asthma, in which cough is the only symptom with an otherwise normal physical examination.[1] In particular, older persons with asthma may have a history of chronic cough with no wheezing. Cough-variant asthma is often characterized by a dry, nocturnal cough and is associated with a drop in early morning peak flows.[2] Given the high and increasing prevalence of asthma, it should always be considered a possible cause of chronic cough, especially when persistent cough is exacerbated by cold or exercise or when the cough worsens at night. Airway hyperresponsiveness, cough hypersensitivity, and normal pulmonary function are also suggestive of cough-variant asthma.[2] The degree and reversibility of obstruction are most accurately assessed by spirometry, which measures forced expiratory volume in 1 second (FEV_1). An FEV_1 of less than 80% predicted value that is strongly responsive to inhaled beta$_2$ agonist bronchodilators (an increase of at least 12% in the measured FEV_1) is strongly suggestive of asthma.

If the PFT results are normal, an attempt to induce bronchospasm with use of a bronchoconstrictor, such as methacholine, should be tried. This is known as the methacholine challenge test—the negative predictive value of which is close to 100, so a negative test essentially rules out asthma.[1] A nebulized solution of methacholine is administered in a stepwise fashion, incrementally increasing the dose and repeating the spirometry after each dose. A 20% drop in FEV_1 from baseline is considered a positive result. Other substances used as bronchoconstrictors include histamine, cold air exposure, and ultrasonic water mists.

Cough is reported by 70% of patients with COPD; 46% report daily cough.[2] Cigarette smoking is the most important risk factor for cough and sputum production in patients with COPD. Patients with COPD cough very frequently while awake, with a frequency of coughs ranging from 10 to 59 coughs per hour and a mean of 21 coughs per hour.[2]

Chronic bronchitis, from exposure to cigarette smoke and other irritants, is another common cause of chronic cough, although it accounts for a much smaller percentage of those who seek treatment, probably because many persons with "smoker's cough" do not seek medical care. Spirometry reveals an airflow obstruction that does not respond significantly to inhaled bronchodilators (or improvement in FEV_1 of >12%). Smoking cessation is the most effective therapeutic intervention because the majority of patients will have resolution or improvement of cough within 8 weeks. Unfortunately, the cough of persistent smokers is usually resistant to most if not all forms of therapeutic interventions, other than the elimination of tobacco smoke or other environmental irritants.

Cough is a common symptom of occupational exposure; common causative agents include dust, organic materials, and low-molecular-weight irritants, such as hydrochloric acid and organic oils.[2] The relationship between occupational exposures and cough should be suspected if there is an improvement in symptoms over the weekend or at other times when the patient is not at work.

Bronchiectasis, another major airway disease, also may cause chronic cough. Bronchiectasis is associated with an overproduction of secretions, combined with a reduced clearance of secretions, resulting in excessive airway secretions. As much as 30 mL of mucoid or mucopurulent sputum may be produced daily and may be accompanied by fever, hemoptysis, and weight loss.[2] The cough is functional; it helps clear secretions. Bronchiectasis may be associated with some of the other common causes of chronic cough, such as postnasal drip, asthma, chronic bronchitis, and GERD. Purulent sputum, when left standing in a cup, may separate into three layers—frothy top, serous middle, and purulent bottom—and cultures are often positive for *Haemophilus influenzae*, *Staphylococcus aureus*, and *Pseudomonas aeruginosa*. Chest radiography can show increased thickening of the bronchial wall, particularly in the lower lobes in advanced disease.[2] The most efficient diagnostic modality is a high-resolution CT scan; characteristic findings include intrapulmonary thickening of the airway wall, enlargement and distortion of the peripheral airways, mucous plugging, and evidence of bronchiolitis.[2]

Gastroesophageal reflux has been estimated to be a causative factor in up to 73% of chronic coughs and one of the three most common causes of cough in nonsmoking, immunocompetent adults who have normal chest X-ray films.[3] This cough can occur at any age, although it occurs most often in the middle to late 60s, and occurs slightly more often in women. Gastric reflux to the larynx can cause reflux laryngitis with associated thickening, redness, and edema of the posterior larynx.[2] Patients may report abdominal complaints, such as dyspepsia or heartburn, but may also have throat clearing, persistent cough, and hoarseness. It is also not unusual for patients to have no symptoms at all. The reflux material does not necessarily need to be aspirated or even to reach the glottis to cause cough or bronchospasm. Studies commonly used for diagnosis include barium swallow, esophagoscopy, manometry, and pH probe monitoring. Although the most sensitive and specific test for GERD is 24-hour esophageal pH monitoring, it is generally not recommended in the routine evaluation of GERD because of the inconvenience of this test. An alternative approach is to treat patients diagnosed with GERD empirically with antireflux medications such as proton pump inhibitors or H_2 histamines. If individuals do not respond well to medical therapy, additional diagnostic testing or surgery may be indicated. Patients with GERD may continue to cough despite the use of antireflux medications, supporting the evidence that other substances such as bile, pepsin, and other gastric enzymes may be causing the cough.[2]

Infectious causes such as mycoplasma, pertussis, and tuberculosis are becoming more prevalent and need to be considered as important differentials of chronic cough. The cough that follows a viral or virus-like infection has been referred to as a postinfectious cough and is a relatively common complaint in the primary care setting. An upper respiratory infection may result in a subacute postinfectious cough, lasting less than 8 weeks, or it may result in a cough lasting much longer.[4] The pathogenesis of postinfectious cough is not clearly understood, but it is thought to result from widespread disruption of the epithelial integrity and inflammation of the upper or lower airways, with or without airway transient hyperresponsiveness.[4] Persistent inflammation of the upper airways, especially the nose and paranasal sinuses, can cause or contribute to postinfectious cough. Despite the presence of bronchial hyperresponsiveness and transient inflammation of the lower airways, eosinophilic inflammation, which is typical of asthma, is absent.[4]

Ear canal irritation is a cause of cough in approximately 3% of healthy people.[2] Cerumen, foreign bodies, or any irritation of the auditory meatus can irritate the auricular branch of the vagus nerve and trigger a cough.

Chronic cough is a result of more than one cause in up to 20% of patients.[6] Although many health care providers are concerned about missing lung carcinoma, isolated chronic cough is a rare presentation of lung cancer. Other rare causes of cough include esophageal diverticulitis, stomach ulcer, and pericardial effusion.

The literature suggests that psychogenic cough is generally a loud, barking cough, which is associated with high stress and typically does not occur at night. However, a cough that is not psychogenic can also be barking or honking, and most persons with chronic cough usually do not wake up during the night once they have fallen asleep. In addition to not coughing at night, patients with psychogenic cough are not awakened by cough and generally do not cough during enjoyable distractions. Because a psychogenic cough has no distinguishing features or diagnostic tests, it should remain a diagnosis of exclusion after all other possibilities have been eliminated. In a small percentage of cases, the cause will be undetermined.

There are innumerable other causes of chronic cough that should be considered if the more common causes of chronic cough are excluded. These include obstructive sleep apnea, idiopathic pulmonary fibrosis, recurrent aspiration (common in older adults), chronic tonsillar enlargement, a foreign body or retained suture, hyperthyroidism or retrosternal goiter, tracheobronchial collapse, Hodgkin disease, Zenker diverticulum, endemic fungi, and a "tic" cough.

INTERPROFESSIONAL COLLABORATIVE MANAGEMENT

Therapy is either antitussive (to prevent, control, or eliminate cough) or protussive (to make cough more effective and productive). Antitussive treatment is indicated when the cough serves no useful purpose, such as clearing the airway, and it can be specific or nonspecific. Specific treatment is directed at the aggravating factors or mechanism directly responsible, such as smoking cessation. Nonspecific therapy is directed at the symptom and is meant to control the cough when specific therapy has failed or is not possible (e.g., inoperable lung cancer). Protussive treatment is indicated for patients for whom coughing serves a useful function, as with cystic fibrosis.

Nonpharmacologic Management

Exposure to cigarette smoke and ACE inhibitor therapy are the most important potential aggravating factors of cough.[6] Removal of either of these factors often results in a substantial improvement in the cough. Persistence of cough after discontinuation of the ACE inhibitor is suggestive of another cause of cough. Treatment with ACE inhibitors may sensitize the cough reflex, which can exacerbate other causes of cough, such as asthma—the onset of which has been associated with the use of ACE inhibitors.[6] In general, there is a temporal association between the onset of ACE inhibitor therapy and cough, but lack of such an association does not exclude ACE inhibitor therapy as a cause of the cough. According to the ACCP evidence-based clinical practice guidelines for ACE inhibitor–induced cough, therapy with ACE inhibitors should be discontinued "regardless of the temporal relationship between the onset of cough and the initiation of ACE inhibitor therapy."[3] If the ACE inhibitor is the causative agent, the cough usually resolves within 1 to 4 weeks after the cessation of therapy; however, in some patients, resolution of the cough may be delayed for up to 3 months after discontinuation of therapy. According to the ACCP guidelines, in patients for whom cough resolves after cessation of ACE inhibitor therapy and for whom there is a compelling reason to treat with this class of drugs, a repeated trial of ACE inhibitor therapy may be attempted. If cessation of ACE inhibitor therapy is not an option, pharmacologic therapy (including sodium cromoglycate, theophylline, sulindac, indomethacin, amlodipine, nifedipine, ferrous sulfate, and picotamide) should be attempted. The ACCP guidelines recommend that in patients with persistent or intolerable ACE inhibitor–induced cough, the patient's therapy be changed to an angiotensin receptor blocker, which does not appear to cause cough in patients with a history of ACE inhibitor–induced cough.[3]

PHARMACOLOGIC THERAPY

Specific therapy is encouraged for the causative agent if a definitive diagnosis is found. Empirical therapy is appropriate when there is a reasonable suspicion of a specific diagnosis. Asthmatic patients should be treated with inhaled beta$_2$ agonists, inhaled corticosteroids, or inhaled nonsteroidal antiinflammatory medications (such as cromolyn sodium or nedocromil sodium), and occasionally oral steroids.

Upper airway cough caused by sinusitis is treated with oral decongestants, nasal steroids, and possibly—but not necessarily—antibiotics. When upper airway cough is related to allergic or nonallergic rhinitis, an H$_1$ antihistamine is an appropriate alternative to antibiotic therapy. Antibiotics are indicated when there is purulent nasal drainage and sinus tenderness.

Chronic bronchitis is best treated with smoking cessation, an ipratropium bromide inhaler, and a beta$_2$ agonist inhaler. When purulent sputum is present, a 7- to 10-day course of antibiotics is indicated.

Management of GERD involves a trial of antireflux therapy. A trial of acid suppression therapy, such as with a proton pump inhibitor, is reasonable if GERD is thought to be a contributing factor, even in the absence of specific gastrointestinal symptoms.[6] However, it may take several months before the full benefit of therapy is realized. In addition, preventive lifestyle changes, such as losing weight, stopping smoking, eating a diet low in acidic foods, and raising the head of the bed, may help to reduce the tone of the lower esophageal sphincter, thus mitigating symptoms.

Demulcents are agents high in sugar content and are believed to coat the sensory receptors in the upper airways. They also promote swallowing, which may help suppress the cough reflex. Expectorants, such as guaifenesin, are believed to change the consistency of the sputum, thus making it easier to expectorate.

Opiates increase the latency threshold of the cough center. Codeine, oxycodone, and nonopiate dextromethorphan are standard therapy for severe nonproductive coughs. All are central nervous system depressants and, except for dextromethorphan, are addictive. Local anesthetics, such as nebulized lidocaine, are extremely effective and directly suppress the sensory nerve; however, these agents are difficult to administer.

INDICATIONS FOR REFERRAL OR HOSPITALIZATION

All patients with coughs that do not respond to or resolve with treatment require physician consultation. Patients with coughs related to cardiac disease, carcinoma, foreign body aspiration, or other suspected pathologic conditions require referral to the appropriate specialist with documentation of diagnostic evaluation, treatment, and treatment evaluation. Hospitalization may be indicated for wheezing and hypoxia, as well as for bronchoscopy or other therapeutic interventions (Box 87.2).

BOX **87.2**

Indications for Referral

POTENTIALLY SERIOUS CAUSES OF CHRONIC COUGH

Condition	Suggestive History of Clinical Features
Asthma	Wheezing, triggers such as exercise, cold air
Tuberculosis	Fever, weight loss, night sweats, hemoptysis, from an endemic area
Carcinoma (primary or metastatic)	Weight loss, hemoptysis, smoking history, older age, history of cancer
Chronic aspiration	History of cerebrovascular accident
Heart failure	History of cardiac disease, dyspnea, orthopnea, dependent edema
COPD	Smoking history, chronic sputum production
Interstitial lung disease	Dyspnea, possible environmental exposures, inspiratory crackles

ABNORMALITIES REQUIRING SPECIALIST INTERVENTION

- Gastroesophageal reflux disease requiring 24-h pH monitoring
- Any suspicion of allergy requiring bronchoprovocation testing
- Occupational exposure requiring legal intervention
- Suspicion of sarcoid, carcinoma, bronchiectasis, carcinoid, Zenker diverticulum requiring bronchoscopy
- Retrosternal goiter requiring surgery
- COPD patients requiring home oxygen supplementation
- Chest X-ray film suggestive of empyema

COPD, Chronic obstructive pulmonary disease.

COMPLICATIONS

Patients often develop costochondritis or hemoptysis as a result of strenuous coughing. Although usually not serious, these developments can be frightening for patients and families. Another recognized complication of cough is rib fracture, which occurs more commonly with chronic cough than with acute cough. Cough-induced rib fractures occur most often in ribs five through nine and along the lateral aspect of the rib cage (similar to the anatomic distribution of rib fractures seen in rowers), and are likely related to the repetitive mechanical stress to the ribs caused by coughing. Reduced bone density is a risk factor for cough-related rib fractures, although such fractures also occur in individuals with normal bone density. Chest radiography has a relatively low sensitivity for detecting cough-induced rib fractures. Other complications of chronic cough include ruptures, emphysematous blebs, syncope, wheezing, dyspnea, and sleep interruption.

PATIENT AND FAMILY EDUCATION AND HEALTH PROMOTION

- Elimination of aggravating or contributing factors such as cigarette smoke or other environmental triggers.
- Education regarding the viral origin of most coughs, and that it may take 4 to 8 weeks before the cough resolves.
- The importance of taking antibiotics only when indicated.
- Education regarding the signs and symptoms of serious cough-related illness.

REFERENCES

1. Terasaki, G., & Paauw, D. S. (2014). Evaluation and treatment of chronic cough. *The Medical Clinics of North America, 98,* 391–403.
2. Chung, K. F., & Pavord, I. D. (2008). Prevalence, pathogenesis and causes of chronic cough. *Lancet, 371,* 1364–1374.
3. Braman, S. S. (2006). Post-infectious cough: ACCP evidence-based clinical practice guidelines. *Chest, 129*(Suppl. 138), 138S–146S.
4. Holzinger, F., Beck, S., Dini, L., Stöter, C., & Heintze, C. (2014). The diagnosis and treatment of acute cough in adults. *Deutsches Arzteblatt International, 111,* 356–363.
5. Barnes, T., Afessa, B., Swanson, K., et al. (2004). The clinical utility of flexible bronchoscopy in the evaluation of chronic cough. *Chest, 126,* 268–272.
6. Pavord, I. D., & Chung, K. F. (2008). Management of chronic cough. *Lancet, 371,* 1375–1384.

CHAPTER **88**

CHRONIC OBSTRUCTIVE PULMONARY DISEASE

Maureen Bell Boardman

 Immediate referral is indicated for concerns of congestive heart failure, interstitial lung disease, and lung cancer.

DEFINITION AND EPIDEMIOLOGY

Chronic obstructive pulmonary disease (COPD) is a preventable and treatable disease characterized by airflow limitation; it is usually progressive, not fully reversible, and associated with an abnormal inflammatory response of the lungs. The chronic airflow limitations of COPD are caused by a combination of both small airway disease and parenchymal destruction. These changes do not always occur together, but can occur at different rates over time.[1]

Chronic inflammation causes structural changes and a narrowing of the small airways and destruction of the lung parenchyma that leads to the loss of alveolar attachments to the small airways and decreases lung elastic recoil. These changes diminish the ability of the airways to remain open during expiration. The loss of small airways is felt to contribute to airflow limitation and mucociliary dysfunction, which are characteristic features of the disease.[1]

COPD does not include other obstructive lung diseases such as asthma, even though asthma shares the same pathophysiologic common denominator as obstructive bronchiolitis and emphysema, which is a slowing of the expiratory flow rate.[2] Asthma involves inflammation of the small airways. Although it is generally reversible, asthma can result in progressive airflow obstruction that over time becomes less and less reversible and resembles the obstruction seen with COPD.

COPD is the third leading cause of death in the United States and the fourth leading cause of death worldwide.[1] Centers for Disease Control and Prevention statistics show that COPD has advanced from being the fourth to being the third leading cause in 2014.[3,4] According to Social Security disability statistics, it is second only to coronary heart disease in causing disability. This shows a marked increase in the numbers of COPD cases worldwide since 1990, when it was ranked sixth. In the United States, where mortality from multiple chronic conditions declined from 1970 to 2002, COPD mortality rates increased.[1] Approximately 15.7 million adults in the United States have been diagnosed with COPD.[4] However, almost 24 million US adults have evidence of impaired lung function, indicating that the true prevalence of COPD is likely to be greatly underdiagnosed.[5]

COPD is predominantly a smoker's disease that clusters in families and worsens with age. Approximately 80% to 90% of COPD deaths are caused by smoking.[5] A hereditary pattern caused by α_1-antitrypsin deficiency contributes to the pure emphysematous form of this disease.

The risks for COPD include genetic, behavioral, socioeconomic, and environmental factors. Cigarette smoke and an occupation that involves regular exposure to a dusty environment are the two major external factors. Because smoking cessation slows the decline in the expiratory airflow, it is clear that smoking is a powerful factor in determining outcome. When the disease is advanced, however, degeneration of lung function will probably continue even with smoking cessation. COPD is more common among individuals who are poor or undereducated. Cigarette smoking is also more common in these groups, but indigent populations still have worse lung function even with adjustment for smoking status. Other contributing factors include crowded living conditions with exposure to frequent viral infections, poorly ventilated homes, inadequate nutrition, exposure to passive cigarette smoke, and suboptimum care for childhood respiratory infections. Air pollution from the burning of wood and other biomass fuels has also been identified as a risk factor for COPD.[1]

Morbidity and mortality rates from COPD are higher in Caucasians than in African Americans or any other racial group in the United States.[6] Mortality has always been higher in men than in women. However, data from the past three decades have demonstrated a gender shift in the number of smoking-related COPD cases being diagnosed each year.[5] Some studies have suggested that women are more susceptible to the effects of smoking than men[1]; 2014 marked the eleventh consecutive year in which more women than men died as a result of COPD.[5]

PATHOPHYSIOLOGY

The cause of obstructive lung disease is not well understood, but chronic inflammation, anatomical changes, and airway hyper reactivity play important roles, as does the underlying pathophysiologic disorder (e.g., chronic bronchitis, emphysema, asthma, α_1 antitrypsin, and other disorders). The inflammatory process continues unabated even after withdrawal of prolonged exposure to bronchial irritants such as smoke, dust, and fumes. The result is airway edema, airway wall thickening, excess production of mucus, and loss of ciliary function. Airflow is obstructed during both inspiration and expiration. Widespread bronchial narrowing with mucous plugging produces hypoxemia because of the mismatching of ventilation and perfusion. Hypercapnia results from the lack of ventilation. Chronic hypoxia and hypercapnia increase pulmonary arterial resistance and may lead to the development of pulmonary hypertension and, eventually, cor pulmonale. A sudden worsening of symptoms in severe obstructive bronchitis can precipitate acute right-sided heart failure. Obstructive bronchiolitis causes much less parenchymal damage than emphysema does; therefore, diffusing capacity, lung volumes, and compliance of lung tissue are not greatly altered.[7]

Enlargement of air spaces in emphysema is the result of alveolar wall destruction. This process is not completely understood but probably results from increased numbers of activated neutrophils that produce elastases, enzymes that destroy the elastin elements in the alveolar walls. Neutrophil-derived elastase is one of a group of destructive proteases contained in alveolar tissue. Usually, a small amount of neutrophil elastase is inactivated by anti-elastases (also known as antiproteases), which are found in the serum and lung lining layer. The prime anti-elastase, which is present in the largest quantities, is α_1-antitrypsin.

Even though they account for less than 3% of cases, patients with a hereditary deficiency of α_1-antitrypsin have less inhibition of elastase and a much higher risk for development of emphysema.[7] The primary role of α_1-antitrypsin is to inhibit the function of several proteases, most notably human neutrophil elastase. Human neutrophil elastase degrades the protein elastin, which is key to the elastic recoil mechanism necessary for the lung's expiratory function. The lack of α_1-antitrypsin can lead to panacinar emphysema. Because the alveoli have lost their recoil mechanism, the driving force during respiration decreases and causes a chronic persistent airflow obstruction. In addition to inhibiting proteases, α_1-antitrypsin inhibits the function of lymphocytes, macrophages, and neutrophils.[8] Patients with a hereditary deficiency of α_1-antitrypsin have less inhibition of elastase and a much higher risk for development of emphysema.

Cigarette smoking also increases elastase activity by causing an influx of elastase-rich neutrophils into the alveoli and by causing the oxidative inactivation of antitrypsin. These processes result in a 30-fold increase in the risk for COPD.

Regardless of the mechanism, the end result of COPD is the destruction of alveolar architecture and the capillary bed lying within the alveolar wall. Initially, the reduction in size of the vascular bed parallels the fall in alveolar surface area. Ventilation still roughly matches perfusion, and significant hypoxemia does not ensue. As the disease progresses, the elastic recoil of the airways is lost, and the poorly supported non-cartilaginous airways collapse during expiration. Expiratory flow rates fall as a result, causing decreased airflow. Because this airflow obstruction is not uniform throughout the lung, there is uneven distribution of ventilation and blood perfusion. This uneven distribution cause's arterial hypoxemia (decreased PaO_2); decreased ventilation causes hypercapnia (increased $PaCO_2$).

CLINICAL PRESENTATION AND PHYSICAL EXAMINATION

Diagnosis of COPD requires a thorough patient history, physical examination, and diagnostic testing. The most common presenting complaints are dyspnea, cough, and/or sputum production. These symptoms are not necessarily noticed by patients until late in the course of this disease, when irreversible changes may have already occurred.

COPD must be considered as a diagnosis in every patient who smokes, even in the absence of respiratory symptoms. Discussing smoking habits at every visit is an important strategy in the prevention of irreversible disease. Documentation should include onset of smoking, the average number of packs per day, and whether the patient has made any successful cessation attempts. Information about other respiratory symptoms, such as cough, sputum production, and exertional dyspnea, should be elicited and quantified.

The important medical history includes any recurrent or prolonged respiratory tract infections that have required antibiotic treatment. A childhood history of frequent respiratory tract infections and bronchitis and any history of asthma, recurrent sinus infections, or nasal polyps should be documented because such conditions are common in patients with COPD.

The family history, including allergies, tuberculosis, cystic fibrosis, COPD, and other chronic lung conditions, should be elicited. A detailed occupational history with special attention to exposure to noxious inhalants such as fumes and mineral and biologic dust is essential.[1]

The physical examination findings in early disease are often normal. Even without the findings of advanced COPD, it is impossible to exclude the diagnosis in the person at risk. However, if COPD is suspected based on the history and examination, it can be confirmed physiologically with simple spirometry.[1] In the late stages of COPD, the general physical findings include those resulting from hyperinflation. Inspection of the skin may show tobacco stains on the fingers and, occasionally, clubbing of the fingernails (convex nail plates). Chest inspection reveals an increase in the anteroposterior diameter, an increase in the intercostal spaces, and, in severe cases, abnormal retraction of the interspaces during inspiration. With inspiration, there is diminished movement of the rib cage and increased movement of the abdominal wall. Abdominal and sternocleidomastoid muscles may be well developed but accompanied by diminished muscle mass in the thighs and legs. A forward-sitting posture with both hands on the knees to fix the shoulders, thereby permitting more effective use of the accessory cervical muscles, may be noted. Pursed-lip breathing with prolonged expirations is also characteristic of COPD.[1]

There is increased resonance on chest percussion. The diaphragm seems low and moves poorly with deep inspiration and expiration. Diminished transmission of breath sounds on auscultation is the most reliable finding; this indicates chronic airflow limitation. Early inspiratory crackles are commonly found. Wheezing may be elicited with forced expiration, but it is a nonspecific symptom and is more characteristic of asthma.[1]

Lung disease causes hypertrophy of the right ventricle of the heart, resulting in cor pulmonale. Therefore, chronic cor pulmonale may be present in the advanced stage of COPD. The physical examination may reveal neck vein distention, peripheral edema, and hepatomegaly from an elevated right atrial pressure. Pulmonary hypertension and distention of the right ventricle cause a pronounced cardiac impulse in the epigastrium.

DIAGNOSTICS

Early detection of COPD is important for decreasing the associated morbidity and mortality. Symptoms of COPD do not usually occur until a significant amount of lung damage has occurred. A clinical diagnosis of COPD should be considered in any patient who has dyspnea, chronic cough, sputum production, and a history of exposure to risk factors for the disease, such as smoking or occupational exposures to dust and chemicals.[1] A simple office maneuver called forced expiratory time may help determine if further testing is needed. The patient is asked to take a deep breath in and then to breathe out as quickly and completely as possible with the mouth open. The practitioner auscultates the trachea with the diaphragm of the stethoscope and times the audible expiration. A forced expiratory time of 6 seconds or more suggests obstructive pulmonary disease.[9] The diagnosis should be confirmed by spirometry. Spirometry is considered the gold standard of diagnosis and assessment of COPD because it is the most reproducible, standardized, and objective way of measuring airflow limitation. Forced vital capacity (FVC), forced expiratory volume in

BOX **88.1**

Classification of COPD by Severity

STAGE I: MILD COPD
Mild airflow limitation (FEV_1/FVC < 70%; $FEV_1 \geq$ 80% predicted) and usually, but not always, chronic cough and sputum production. At this stage, the individual may not be aware that his or her lung function is abnormal.

STAGE II: MODERATE COPD
Worsening airflow limitation (50% $\leq FEV_1$ < 80% predicted) and usually a progression of symptoms, with shortness of breath developing with exertion.

STAGE III: SEVERE COPD
Further worsening of airflow limitation (30% $\leq FEV_1$ < 50% predicted), increased shortness of breath, and repeated exacerbations. Exacerbations that have an impact on a patient's quality of life and prognosis are seen in patients with FEV_1 < 50% predicted.

STAGE IV: VERY SEVERE COPD
Severe airflow limitation (FEV_1 < 30% predicted) or FEV_1 < 50% predicted plus chronic respiratory failure. At this stage, quality of life is very impaired, and exacerbations may be life-threatening.

COPD, Chronic obstructive pulmonary disease.
Modified from Global Initiative for Chronic Obstructive Lung Disease. (2014). *Pocket guide to COPD diagnosis, management, and prevention of chronic obstructive pulmonary disease: A guide for healthcare professionals.* NHLBI/WHO Workshop Report, Washington, DC. Retrieved from http://goldcopd.org/wp-content/uploads/2018/02/WMS-GOLD-2018-Feb-Final-to-print-v2.pdf.

BOX **88.2**

Combined COPD Assessment

PATIENT GROUP A—LOW RISK, FEWER SYMPTOMS
Typically GOLD 1 or GOLD 2 and/or no or one exacerbation per year and no hospitalization for exacerbation; and CAT score below 10.

PATIENT GROUP B—LOW RISK, MORE SYMPTOMS
Typically GOLD 1 or GOLD 2 and/or no or one exacerbation per year and no hospitalizations for exacerbation; and CAT score above 10.

PATIENT GROUP C—HIGH RISK, FEWER SYMPTOMS
Typically GOLD 3 or GOLD 4 and/or more than two exacerbations per year or more than one with hospitalization for exacerbation; and CAT score below 10.

PATIENT GROUP D—HIGH RISK, MORE SYMPTOMS
Typically GOLD 3 or GOLD 4 and/or more than two exacerbations per year or more than one with hospitalization for exacerbation; and CAT score above 10.

COPD, Chronic obstructive pulmonary disease.
Modified from Global Initiative for Chronic Obstructive Lung Disease. (2014). *Global strategies for the diagnosis, management, and prevention of chronic obstructive pulmonary disease.* NHLBI/WHO Workshop Report. Washington, DC: U.S. Government Printing Office.

1 second (FEV_1), and the ratio of the two (FEV_1/FVC) are the primary spirometric measurements used for diagnosis. The presence of a post bronchodilator FEV_1/FVC of less than 0.70 and FEV_1 of less than 80% predicted confirms airflow limitation that is not fully reversible.[1] COPD is usually a progressive disease; the general patterns of symptom development are well established, and lung function usually worsens over time despite medical intervention (Box 88.1).

The concept of staging COPD based on FEV_1 alone is now thought to be inadequate. Newer research indicates the management of stable COPD should be based on a combination of factors including a symptomatic assessment, spirometric classification, and future risk of disease progression, with the focus on exacerbations.[1]

The COPD Assessment Test (CAT) is a short but comprehensive eight-item measure of health status impairment in patients with COPD.[1] It has been validated and can be easily used in a routine practice setting. It is scored from 0 to 40, with scores greater than 10 indicating more severe symptoms.

There is a large body of accumulated data in patients classified according to the Global Initiative for Chronic Obstructive Lung Disease (GOLD) spirometry grading system. The data show an increased risk of exacerbations, hospitalization, and death with worsening airflow limitations. The assessment of exacerbation risk is seen as a risk of poor outcomes overall (Box 88.2).[1]

A posteroanterior and lateral chest X-ray study is rarely diagnostic in COPD unless significant bullous disease is present. However, X-ray examination is useful in detection of COPD complications, such as pneumonia, pulmonary hypertension,

and pneumothorax, as well as in establishing the presence of comorbidities, such as cardiac failure. Radiographic changes in COPD include flattening of the diaphragm and blunting of the costophrenic angle on the posteroanterior view, enlargement of the retrosternal space on the lateral view, flattening or concavity of the diaphragmatic contour on the lateral view, and irregularity of lung field lucency.[1]

Pulse oximetry to estimate oxygen saturation can be helpful, but arterial blood gas measurements are necessary to assess and to manage patients during exacerbations and when oxygen therapy is indicated. Elevations of hematocrit and hemoglobin provide a measure of the severity of hypoxemia. Phlebotomy may become necessary if the elevation is severe. An electrocardiogram can indicate the severity of the lung disease and the presence of cor pulmonale. Significant findings include sinus tachycardia, multifocal atrial tachycardia, signs of right atrial enlargement (peaked P waves in leads II, III, and aVF), signs of right ventricular hypertrophy (a tall R wave in lead V_1 and a deep S wave in lead V_6), and right-axis deviation.[8]

Sputum is not routinely examined, but its inspection can help differentiate between a pulmonary infection and an

INITIAL DIAGNOSTICS

Chronic Obstructive Pulmonary Disease

INITIAL
- Spirometry (FVC and FEV_1)
- Pulse oximetry

LABORATORY
- CBC and differential[a]
- ABGs[a]
- α_1-Antitrypsin

IMAGING
- Chest X-ray study (posteroanterior and lateral views)[a]

OTHER
- ABGs, arterial blood gases

[a]If indicated.

exacerbation of reactive airways. The detection of neutrophils or eosinophil in the sputum will guide treatment between antibiotics and corticosteroids. An α_1-antitrypsin level is recommended by the World Health Organization for all patients who develop COPD.[10] Testing is also indicated for symptomatic adults with airflow obstruction, in patients with bronchiectasis when the cause is unclear, and in those patients with liver disease.[11]

DIFFERENTIAL DIAGNOSIS

Distinguishing COPD from other causes of chronic cough or dyspnea is important for initial diagnosis and in acute exacerbations.

Certain features may help distinguish COPD from some of the most common pulmonary diseases that share similar signs and symptoms. The onset of COPD is more likely to be in midlife and associated with a long history of smoking and slowly progressing symptoms. The onset of asthma is usually earlier in life, with varying symptoms occurring during the night and early morning. The patient often has a family history of asthma and may also have allergies, rhinitis, or eczema. The airflow limitations associated with asthma are largely reversible, but it is important to note that some patients with asthma will develop COPD and some patients will have both asthma and COPD (Asthma-COPD Overlap Syndrome).[10,12]

Features suggestive of congestive heart failure include fine basilar crackles on auscultation and volume restriction versus airflow limitation on pulmonary function tests. A dilated heart and pulmonary edema may be noted on chest radiography. Bronchiectasis is associated with large volumes of purulent sputum and is commonly associated with bacterial infection. Coarse crackles may be noted on auscultation, and bronchial dilation and bronchial wall thickening may be seen on chest radiography or computed tomography.[1] Interstitial lung disease and lung cancer also are evident on chest radiography or computed tomography.

Other respiratory disorders should also be considered in the differential diagnosis. These include bronchiectasis, tuberculosis, nontuberculous mycobacterial lung disease, and cancer.

INTERPROFESSIONAL COLLABORATIVE MANAGEMENT

Certain therapeutic interventions for symptomatic COPD improve survival, and some improve symptoms. In the presence of hypoxemia, smoking cessation and oxygen therapy improve survival. Interventions that improve symptoms include pharmacotherapy, education, exercise, psychological support, nutrition, and surgery.

The goals of treatment are to reverse or reduce airflow obstruction; to control cough and secretions; to prevent and eliminate infection; and to control complications, including polycythemia, hypoxemia, and right-sided heart failure. It is important to relieve underlying depression and anxiety, to maximize exercise tolerance, and to educate patients about avoidance of aggravating factors such as bronchial irritants.[1]

Nonpharmacologic Management

Smoking cessation is the single most important intervention to reduce the rapid decline of lung function in patients who smoke.[1] Treatment of tobacco use and dependence should be regarded as a primary and specific intervention. Smoking should be part of the routine evaluation of every health care visit, and every patient should be offered smoking cessation programs that involve multiple interventions that address the multifactorial causes of tobacco use.[1] In addition, providers should always express strong interest in helping their patients quit. Patients may be more inclined to stop smoking if they know their providers care that they stop smoking and if they understand that their smoking cessation is critical to prevention of premature loss of lung function. The most comprehensive smoking cessation guidelines are available at www.surgeongeneral.gov/tobacco.

Home oxygen is used in later stages of COPD because unlike some pharmacotherapeutics, it improves survival in hypoxemic COPD. The long-term administration of oxygen for more than 15 hours per day has been shown to increase survival in patients with chronic respiratory failure.[1] Other benefits of long-term oxygen include reduced polycythemia, reduced pulmonary artery pressures, reduced dyspnea, and improvement in neuropsychiatric test results. Another benefit may be the reduction of nocturnal arrhythmias, but it is unclear whether this translates into reduced mortality.

The Medicare criteria for 24-hour supplemental oxygen are PaO_2 of 55 mm Hg or less and an oxygen saturation of 88% or less while breathing room air. Patients with cor pulmonale or erythrocytosis (hematocrit >55%) and a PaO_2 of 56 to 59 mm Hg also qualify.[1] Patients with exercise-induced desaturation below 88% should use oxygen during exercise to reduce dyspnea and to prevent hypoxemia. A number of studies have shown that use of oxygen during exercise can increase the duration of exercise and reduce the severity of end-exercise breathlessness.[1] In the presence of daytime hypoxemia ($PaO_2 < 55$ mm Hg), a hematocrit greater than 50% to 55%, morning headaches, daytime sleepiness, and poor exercise tolerance are indications of oxygen desaturation during sleep.[13] Monitoring of oxygen saturation during the night may be indicated for these patients because sleep can cause hypoventilation and nocturnal hypoxemia. Oxygen therapy at night will reduce the incidence of nocturnal hypoxemia.[13]

The need for long-term oxygen therapy should be reassessed 30 to 90 days after an acute exacerbation if that was the situation for which oxygen was prescribed. Oxygen therapy may be discontinued if the patient no longer meets the blood gas criteria. The development of simpler and more portable oxygen tanks and devices has helped improve the quality of life and increase mobility for persons requiring long-term oxygen therapy.

Pulmonary Rehabilitation

The principal goals of pulmonary rehabilitation are to reduce symptoms, to improve quality of life, and to increase physical and emotional participation in everyday activities.[1] The benefits of pulmonary rehabilitation are well documented in a large number of clinical trials. Pulmonary rehabilitation is a multidisciplinary team approach to care. It is designed to be highly individualized to meet the needs of each patient. The team makeup may vary from program to program but usually consists of a physician, respiratory therapist, exercise therapist or physical therapist, occupational therapist, psychosocial staff, and dietitian-nutritionist. Instruction on nutrition, exercise, upper body weight training, and breathing techniques and guidance for maximizing energy reserves are critical components of any rehabilitation program. Pulmonary rehabilitation programs are also an excellent source of support for both patients and family members.

Exercise Training

Patients at all stages of COPD appear to benefit from exercise programs, which have improved both patients' exercise tolerance and symptoms of dyspnea and fatigue.[1] Programs emphasize lower extremity training, upper extremity training, and strength training. Most pulmonary rehabilitation exercise programs consist of 10- to 45-minute sessions, daily to weekly, for 4 to 10 weeks, depending on resources.[1] Participants are also taught breathing strategies such as pursed-lip breathing and controlled coughing to improve their ability to perform activities of daily living.

Psychological Support

Patients with COPD may feel anxious, depressed, and fatigued. Counseling is recommended for those patients exhibiting signs and symptoms of major depression. COPD and associated dyspnea often result in immobility, which contributes to social isolation and depression. Pulmonary rehabilitation programs can be helpful in interrupting this vicious circle. In addition, antidepressants can be beneficial in COPD patients with depression. Depression and anxiety often improve when airflow obstruction is improved.

Nutrition

COPD often precipitates weight loss because the increased work of breathing can double resting energy expenditures. This, along with decreased physical activity, tends to diminish fat and muscle stores. Weight loss is also aggravated by disease exacerbations or anorexia from medications or emotional issues. Severe dyspnea, coughing, and sputum production can interfere with eating. A reduction in body mass index is an independent risk factor for mortality in COPD patients.[1] Patients should be encouraged to eat frequent, small meals instead of a large meal; large meals cause abdominal distention, which impairs diaphragmatic function. Vitamin supplementation and commercially prepared drinks are convenient, easily digested, and high in protein, calories, and vitamins. Nutritional counseling is a recommended component of pulmonary rehabilitation programs.

Surgery

Endoscopic bronchial valve treatment and lung volume reduction surgery (LVRS). The proposed benefit of LVRS is improved elastic recoil and diaphragmatic function, which is accomplished by reducing the volume of the lung and thereby decreasing hyperinflation. In addition, LVRS increases the elastic recoil pressure of the lung and thereby improves expiratory flow rates.[1] In a randomized control trial that compared LVRS with medical treatment in patients with upper lobe emphysema and low exercise capacity, LVRS in this small subset of patients resulted in significant improvement. However, in patients who had other emphysema distribution or high exercise capacity before treatment, the advantage of surgery over medical treatment was less significant. In patients with severe emphysema patients with an FEV_1 of less than 20% predicted and homogeneous emphysema on CT LVRS resulted in higher mortality than medical management.[1] A more recent therapy, endobronchial valve therapy, involves the placement of a one-way valve in the bronchus of the more severe emphysematous lobe. The result prevents air from entering the area on inspiration but allows expiration of air, thereby causing volume reduction

in that lobe. Despite its beneficial results in a select group of patients, these procedures are appropriate for a select number of patients who meet the criteria.[14]

Bullectomy is an older surgical procedure for bullous emphysema that involves removal of a large bulla that does not contribute to gas exchange and is or has caused previous complications. Bullectomy in a selected group of patients with preserved underlying lung is associated with decreased dyspnea, improved lung function, and exercise tolerance.[1]

Lung transplantation in appropriately selected patients with advanced COPD has been shown to improve both quality of life and functional capacity. However, lung transplantation is limited by the shortage of donor organs and its cost. Costs remain elevated for years after the surgery because of the high cost of both complications and the immunosuppressive regimens that must be used long term. Lung transplantation has also failed to show a survival benefit in patients with end-stage emphysema after 2 years.[1]

PALLIATIVE CARE AND HOSPICE

COPD is a chronic disease that consists of a gradual decline in health and increasing symptoms as well as episodes of acute exacerbation. Therefore, palliative care should be an essential component in the treatment of all patients with advanced COPD. Palliative care offers COPD patients a focus on quality of life, optimized function, and assistance with decision-making about end-of-life care, as well as providing emotional and spiritual support to both patients and their families. Unfortunately, patients with COPD are less likely to receive these services then patients with lung cancer.[1]

The National Hospice and Palliative Care Organization provides guidance for referring patients with noncancerous diseases such as COPD for services.[15] These guidelines recognize the appropriateness of providing hospice services for patients with advanced COPD.

Pharmacotherapy

There is currently no pharmacologic treatment that mitigates the rate of decline of lung function or reduces or abolishes symptoms, but pharmacotherapy can improve exercise tolerance, reduce the number and severity of exacerbations, and improve lung function (Table 88.1). Pharmacotherapy should be based on the severity of disease and the patient's tolerance for certain drugs. In addition, a stepwise approach may be helpful.

Inhaled bronchodilators relieve bronchospasm and corticosteroids reduce inflammation. Though not commonly used, theophylline and other methylxanthines can enhance bronchodilation, albeit within a narrow therapeutic range. Antibiotics will not mitigate a COPD exacerbation unless an infection precipitates the infection. Even though few patients with COPD actually have α_1-antitrypsin deficiency and the long-term efficacy of replacement therapy is unclear, its identification and treatment are important. Diuretics may also be useful in patients with cor pulmonale.

Bronchodilators. Bronchodilators can alleviate the symptoms of COPD, improve exercise tolerance, decrease the frequency of exacerbations, and improve the quality of life. With most bronchodilators, the preferred route is inhalation of long-acting agents, but for older adults effective use of a metered dose inhaler (MDI) can be challenging. The use of a spacer may facilitate inhalation.

TABLE 88.1   Pharmacologic Agents for Chronic Obstructive Pulmonary Disease Therapy

Agent	Recommended Dose Range	Notes
ANTICHOLINERGICS		
Short Acting		
Ipratropium bromide		
MDI, 20, 40 mcg/inhalation	2–4 puffs 4–6 times/day	Poorly absorbed systemically; few side effects; should be used regularly (not prn)
Solution for nebulization, 500 mcg/2.5 mL	3–4 times/day, separate doses by 6–8 h	Precautions with narrow-angle glaucoma
Long Acting		
Aclidinium bromide, DPI, 400 mcg/inhalation	1 inhalation twice a day	Same as ipratropium bromide
Tiotropium DPI, 18 mcg/inhalation	1 inhalation daily	Same as ipratropium bromide
β_2-ADRENERGIC AGONISTS		
Short Acting		
Albuterol sulfate		
MDI, 90 mcg/inhalation	1–2 puffs every 4–6 h	Use on prn basis preferable to a fixed-use schedule
Solution for nebulization, 0.5 mL of 0.5% solution	3–4 times/day	No more than 12 inhalations daily
		Relatively short-acting drug; avoid excessive use
		Caution with cardiac disease, hyperthyroidism, diabetes, seizure disorders
Bitolterol mesylate		
MDI, 370 mcg/inhalation	2 puffs at 1- to 3-min intervals every 8 h followed by a third puff if needed	
	Maximum dose: 3 puffs every 6 h	Same as albuterol
Solution for nebulization, 2 mg/mL; dilute to 2–4 mL	2–4 times/day	
Levalbuterol		
MDI, 45 mcg/inhalation	2 puffs every 4–6 h	Same as albuterol
Solution for nebulization		
0.31 mg/3 mL of NS	3–4 times/day	
0.63 mg/3 mL of NS	3–4 times/day	
1.25 mg/3 mL of NS	3–4 times/day	
Metaproterenol sulfate		
MDI, 650 mcg/inhalation	2–3 puffs every 3–4 h	Same as albuterol
Solution for nebulization, 5.0% solution	0.2–0.3 mL of 5.0% solution in 2.5 mL of normal saline, 3–4 times/day	
Pirbuterol acetate, MDI, 200 mcg/inhalation	2 puffs every 4–6 h	Same as albuterol
Terbutaline sulfate, MDI, 200 mcg/inhalation	2 puffs every 4–6 h	Same as albuterol
Long Acting		
Salmeterol xinafoate		
DPI, 50 mcg	1 puff every 12 h	
MDI, 21 mcg/inhalation	Maximum 2 doses/day	Not for treatment of acute attacks
		May be helpful for nocturnal symptoms in COPD because it is a long-acting preparation
Formoterol		
MDI, DPI, 4.5 mcg, 12 mcg	Maximum 2 doses/day	Same as salmeterol
Indacaterol		
MDI, 75 mcg	1 inhalation daily	Same as salmeterol
Arformoterol		
Solution for nebulizer, 15 mcg/2 mL	Maximum two treatments a day	Same as salmeterol

Continued

TABLE 88.1	Pharmacologic Agents for Chronic Obstructive Pulmonary Disease Therapy—cont'd	
Agent	**Recommended Dose Range**	**Notes**
METHYLXANTHINE		
Theophylline		
Immediate-release tablets	10 mg/kg/day in four divided doses	Follow serum levels to regulate dose between 8 and 13 mg/day; reduce dose in patients with liver disease, cardiac disease, or seizures
Sustained-release tablets	10 mg/kg/day in 1–3 doses	Check for drug-drug interactions
ORAL CORTICOSTEROIDS		
Methylprednisolone	40–48 mg/day in d vided doses for 3–4 days	Used to treat acute exacerbations
Prednisone	40 mg po daily × 5 days	Used to treat acute exacerbations
		Used for patients not responding to optimum doses of other drugs
		Steroid therapy associated with many side effects: osteoporosis, cataracts, hypertension, diabetes, peptic ulcers, psychic disorders, aseptic necrosis of hip, masking of infections, increased appetite, weight gain, and cushingoid effects
		Replace this form of steroid with inhaled form as soon as possible
INHALED CORTICOSTEROIDS		
Beclomethasone dipropionate, MDI, 40 mcg/inhalation, 80 mcg/inhalation	2 puffs 2 times a cay	Teach patients that inhaled corticosteroids are not bronchodilators. Must be used regularly to be effective; mouth should be rinsed after use. Side effects: hoarseness, dry mouth, oral fungal infections
Budesonide, DPI, 90 mcg/inhalation, 180 mcg/inhalation	1–2 inhalations bid	Same as beclomethasone dipropionate
Ciclesonide, MDI, 80 mcg/inhalation, 160 mcg/inhalation	1–2 inhalations bid	Same as beclomethasone dipropionate
Mometasone furoate, MDI, 110 mcg/inhalation, 220 mcg/inhalation	1–2 inhalations daily to bid	Same as beclomethasone dipropionate
Fluticasone propionate, MDI, 44, 110, or 220 mcg/puff	2–4 puffs bid; initial 88 mcg bid; maximum 440 mcg bid	Same as beclomethasone dipropionate
COMBINATION LONG-ACTING β_2 AGONIST PLUS GLUCOCORTICOSTEROID IN ONE INHALER		
Formoterol/budesonide, MDI, 80/4.5, 160/4.5 mcg/inhalation	2 inhalations bid	Same as beclomethasone dipropionate
Fluticasone furoate, DPI, 100/25 mcg/inhalation	1 inhalation daily	Same as beclomethasone dipropionate
Mometasone/formoterol, MDI, 100 mcg/inhalation, 200 mcg/inhalation	2 inhalations bid	Same as beclomethasone dipropionate
Salmeterol/fluticasone		Same as beclomethasone dipropionate
DPI 50/100, 50/250, 50/500 mcg/inhalation	1 inhalation bid	
MDI 45/21, 115/21, 230/21 mcg/inhalation	2 inhalations bid	
ANTICHOLINERGIC PLUS β_2 AGONIST		
Ipratropium bromide/albuterol, MDI, 20/100 mcg 0.5 mg/2.5 mg/3 mL	1 inhalation qid 1 vial nebulizer 4–6 times a day	Same as ipratropium bromide and albuterol
ANTICHOLINERGIC PLUS LONG-ACTING β_2 AGONIST		
Umeclidinium/vilanterol, 62.5/25 mcg/inhalation	1 inhalation daily	Severe hypersensitivity to milk proteins
PHOSPHODIESTERASE-4 INHIBITOR		
Roflumilast, 500 mcg	1 tablet daily	Contraindicated in moderate to severe liver disease

COPD, Chronic obstructive pulmonary disease; *DPI*, dry powder inhaler; *MDI*, metered dose inhaler; *NS*, normal saline.

Bronchodilators include β_2-adrenergic agonists and anticholinergics. Anticholinergics are a more effective first choice in patients with nonasthmatic COPD but are less effective than β_2-adrenergic agonists in patients with asthmatic COPD. The American Thoracic Society recommends anticholinergics as the first line of maintenance therapy for patients with daily COPD symptoms. In patients who have intermittent symptoms, a short-acting β_2-adrenergic agonist should be the first choice.[16]

Anticholinergic Therapy. Anticholinergics are effective first-line therapy for patients with COPD. Stimulation of the cholinergic nerves to the bronchial smooth muscle causes bronchoconstriction. Decreased cholinergic stimulation lessens bronchoconstriction. The cholinergic receptors are plentiful in the proximal airways, and these are the ones that influence COPD. Adrenergic receptors are more plentiful in the distal airways, which play a larger role in asthma.

The effects of anticholinergics are slower in onset but are more prolonged and intense, making them more useful for patients with sustained symptoms. Anticholinergics are subcategorized into short-acting and long-acting preparations. The short acting preparation has relatively few systemic side effects because of its poor systemic absorption and needs to be used on a regular basis, not as needed. There have been reports of an unexpected small increase in cardiovascular events in COPD patients treated regularly with some short-acting anticholinergics, so careful monitoring is indicated.[17] Long-acting anticholinergics are used once a day and have 24-hour duration of action.

β_2-Adrenergic Agonist Therapy. β_2-Adrenergic agonists (bronchodilators) cause bronchial smooth muscle dilation and can also improve mucociliary clearance. The major side effects include tachycardia and tremor from stimulation of β_1 receptors in muscle.

Short-acting agents in this class have a 4- to 6-hour duration. The dose should not exceed 4 to 12 inhalations per day for the shorter-acting preparations or twice daily for the longer-acting preparations. The longer-acting inhaled preparations or the oral form of these medications may be more helpful in patients with nocturnal symptoms. Although there are continuing concerns about the safety profile of these medications in patients with cardiovascular disease, the Summit study results suggest these medications are effective and safe at least in patients with moderate pulmonary dysfunction.[18]

Still toxicity and drug-drug interactions must be avoided in older adults requiring careful monitoring.

Inhaled Corticosteroids

The World Health Organization's GOLD guidelines suggest that inhaled corticosteroid use in addition to a (long-acting β-adrenergic (LABA) is appropriate and reduces exacerbations for symptomatic COPD patients especially those with stage III and stage IV COPD) with an FEV_1 of less than 60% predicted and repeated exacerbations. However, the GOLD guidelines also reveal that for most patients with COPD, inhaled glucocorticosteroids alone do not modify FEV_1 decline.[1]

There is a place for inhaled corticosteroids in the stepwise approach to the treatment of symptomatic COPD. The FEV_1 should be rechecked after 3 to 4 months of therapy with inhaled corticosteroids. If the FEV_1 improves or stays the same, the same dose should be continued. If the FEV_1 declines, discontinuation of the inhaled steroid should be considered. The side effects of inhaled corticosteroids are minimal and include dysphonia and oral candidiasis. Oral candidiasis can

be minimized by rinsing the mouth with water or mouthwash after every use or by using a spacer.

Combination Therapies. There are currently three different combinations of inhaled medications (i.e., short-acting β_2 agonist and anticholinergic, long-acting β_2 agonist and long-acting anticholinergic, and long-acting β_2 agonist and inhaled glucosteroid) available in one device with several options in each classification.

The pairing of an anticholinergic and a short-acting β_2 agonist in one MDI has been shown in multiple studies to be superior in the treatment of COPD than either drug alone. The combination has also been shown to reduce exacerbations, to lower cost, and to improve lung function and quality of life.[1]

The combination long-acting anticholinergic agent and long-acting β_2 agonist improves lung function compared to placebo and has also been shown to be more effective than long-acting bronchodilator monotherapy for preventing exacerbations.[1]

The combination of a long-acting β_2 agonist plus corticosteroid in patients with moderate to very severe COPD and exacerbations is more effective than either component alone in improving lung function and health status and reducing exacerbations. In patients with an FEV_1 of less than 60%, the combination therapy decreased the decline of lung function. However, combination therapy increased the likelihood of pneumonia and failed to demonstrate statistically significant effects on mortality in a large clinical trial.[1]

Issues Related to Inhaled Delivery Systems

When any treatment is prescribed to be given by the inhaled route the importance of education and training in inhaler device technique can't be stressed enough. There is a wide variety of devices available for inhalation and each works slightly differently. On average, studies have shown more than two-thirds of patients make at least one error in using an inhalation device. There been a significant relationship identified between incorrect inhaler use and symptom control in patients with COPD in observational studies.[1] Therefore the "teach-back" approach method is recommended using either placebo devices or requesting the patient bring their own devices to visits. Additionally, patients who use more than one inhaler each day may do better when prescribed inhalers requiring a similar inhalation technique (e.g., prescribing two MDIs vs. prescribing an MDI and a dry powder inhaler).[19]

Methylxanthine Therapy. Methylxanthine therapy is considered a third-line agent because the bronchodilatory effect is limited and its therapeutic range is narrow. Low-dose methylxanthine therapy reduces exacerbations in patients with COPD but does not increase post bronchodilator lung function, and because of the significant risk for toxicity, inhaled bronchodilators are preferred.[1] Newer slow-release preparations have improved the problems related to its narrow therapeutic index and complex pharmacokinetics, leading to more stable plasma levels. If levels rise, the risk of toxicity increases with little therapeutic gain. Methylxanthine therapy is not recommended for patients receiving H_2 receptor blockers and fluoroquinolone or macrolide antibiotics because it is metabolized by cytochrome P-450 mixed function oxidases, and there is a likelihood of reduced methylxanthine clearance and an increased risk of toxicity.

Corticosteroids. Oral corticosteroids do provide some improved airflow and gas exchange in acute exacerbations of COPD.[1] The current recommended outpatient treatment for an acute exacerbation is prednisone 40 mg po daily for 5 days only.[10,20] For some patients, longer therapy may be necessary, but long-term therapy with oral corticosteroids is problematic; complications include skin damage, cataracts, diabetes, obesity, peptic ulcer disease, osteoporosis, and secondary infection.

Phosphodiesterase-4 Inhibitors. A phosphodiesterase-4 enzyme inhibitor was approved for the treatment of patients with bronchitis-associated COPD.[1] This medication breaks down intracellular cyclic adenosine monophosphate (cAMP) and reduces inflammation.[1] A once-a-day oral medication, it can be used with glucocorticoid therapy, but cannot be used as monotherapy. It is contraindicated in patients with moderate or severe liver dysfunction.[1]

Mucoactive Agents. Some patients with COPD form increased quantities of abnormal mucus. The value of muco-active agents that decrease sputum viscosity and adhesiveness, which facilitates expectoration, has not been established in patients with COPD, although a few patients with viscous sputum may benefit from mucoactive agents. Increasing hydration by the intravenous route, aerosolized route, or oral route does not decrease the thickness of secretions.

Antibiotics. The infectious agents in COPD exacerbations can be viral or bacterial. Several randomized placebo-controlled studies of antibiotic treatment in COPD exacerbations have demonstrated a small beneficial effect of antibiotics on lung function. The patients who showed significant beneficial effects were the ones with an increase in all three of the following cardinal symptoms: dyspnea, sputum volume, and sputum purulence. There was also some benefit in those patients with an increase in two of these cardinal symptoms if increased purulence of sputum was one of the two. Another study in patients with severe exacerbations that required mechanical ventilation indicated that not giving antibiotics was associated with increased mortality and an increased incidence of nosocomial pneumonia.[1] With bacterial infections, the most common pathogens include *Streptococcus pneumoniae, Haemophilus influenzae, Chlamydia pneumoniae,* and *Moraxella catarrhalis.*[1]

The antibiotic choice depends on patient risk factors (i.e., age, severity of exacerbation, cardiovascular health, local resistance patterns, and the cost of treatment). The mainstay antibiotics are broad-spectrum oral agents. Typical antibiotic choices for the common bacteria associated with severe exacerbations infections macrolides, doxycycline, and trimethoprim-sulfamethoxazole for mild exacerbations.[21] Augmentin or levofloxacin are indicated for more serious exacerbations. If the patient is moderately ill or needs to be hospitalized, the antibiotic choice needs to be supported by sputum culture and sensitivity testing.[1]

Immunizations. There is evidence that persons with COPD benefit from immunization against respiratory pathogens. A yearly immunization with the influenza vaccine is essential to decrease morbidity and mortality from influenza epidemics and has been shown to reduce serious illness and death in COPD patients by about 50%.

Updated recommendations for the pneumococcal vaccine recommend not only that all patients with a diagnosis of COPD receive a pneumococcal vaccine regardless of age, but also that all smokers receive a pneumococcal vaccine.[21,22] Patients 65 or older when they receive the pneumococcal vaccine should receive only a single dose.[22] Patients aged 19 to 64 who have COPD or are smokers should receive another dose of the vaccine at age 65 or if at least 5 years have passed since their previous dose.[21,22] Current guidelines do not recommend multiple revaccinations secondary to uncertainty regarding clinical benefit and safety. Additionally, all adults 65 years or older are advised to receive Prevnar 13 once, and Prevnar 13 is recommended for patients with COPD.[21] The recommended intervals between administration of PCV13 and PPSV23 and the order in which the two vaccines are given differ based on age and risk group.[21] However, in most adults the current recommendation is a year between the two vaccines, regardless of the order in which the two vaccines are given. The recommendations are based on an improved immune response against serotypes in both vaccines compared to a single dose of either vaccine.[21,22]

INDICATIONS FOR REFERRAL OR HOSPITALIZATION

Consultation is appropriate when the disease progresses, the need for oral corticosteroids is evident, when presentation includes escalation of symptoms and fever, when hospitalization is indicated, when continuous or nocturnal oxygen is required, and when there is evidence of right-sided heart failure and cor pulmonale is present.

Indications for consultation with a pulmonary specialist include:

1. Severe disease evidenced by persistent dyspnea with activities of daily living and frequent recurrent exacerbations despite therapy.
2. Evaluation for and maintenance of oxygen therapy, including consideration of nocturnal oxygen therapy or transtracheal oxygen therapy.
3. Preoperative assessment for any surgery placing the patient at high risk for pulmonary complications
4. Failure to respond to treatment for an acute exacerbation
5. Consideration of long-term intermittent antibiotic therapy
6. Persistent pulmonary infiltrates on chest radiograph with no response to antibiotic therapy
7. Evaluation of sleep disturbances, including obstructive sleep apnea
8. Management of acute respiratory failure, or if mechanical ventilation is a consideration
9. Cor pulmonale with clinical right-sided heart failure unresponsive to usual therapy
10. Consideration of α_1-antitrypsin augmentation therapy[23]

Hospitalization is based on the severity of the underlying respiratory dysfunction, the progression of symptoms, new or worsening cor pulmonale, or the existence of other comorbidities. Hypoxemia and hypercapnia are probably increasing if a patient does not respond adequately to treatment or is confused or unable to walk, eat, or sleep without aid. Hospitalization is warranted in these cases.

Some patients require admission to a specialized respiratory care unit. Issues that require admission include severe dyspnea that does not respond to initial emergency therapy; changes in mental status including confusion, lethargy, and coma; persistent or worsening hypoxemia or severe respiratory acidosis despite supplemental oxygen; the need for invasive mechanical ventilation; and hemodynamic instability and the need for vasopressors.[1]

COMPLICATIONS

Complications may be caused not only by the condition of COPD but also by the treatment. Drug effects should always be considered if there is a change in clinical condition.

Corticosteroids are associated with hyperglycemia and frequent use increases the risk for osteoporosis and compression fractures. Some of these complications can be prevented by keeping the corticosteroid dose as low as possible, encouraging calcium supplementation, and prescribing bisphosphonate therapy for patients who are unable to reduce their prednisone dose to less than 20 mg every other day.[8]

Theophylline toxicity should be considered in the presence of gastrointestinal symptoms, tremors, headache, or tachycardia. Other medications may affect the metabolism of theophylline. Corticosteroid or diuretic therapy may be responsible for hyperglycemia, hypokalemia, or azotemia.

Depression or marked anxiety often accompanies COPD. Patients with stable COPD tolerate antidepressant therapy, but depression most often improves when airflow obstruction improves.

Anti-inflammatory therapy needs to be maximized during acute infections. Atypical mycobacterial disease should always be considered if chest radiographs show cavitary apical disease. Placement of an intermediate-strength purified protein derivative (PPD) skin test and a sputum examination for acid-fast bacilli are indicated.

Fungal infections are important in the differential diagnosis of certain infiltrates in patients with COPD. Histoplasmosis is endemic in the Ohio and Mississippi river valleys. In the southwestern United States, coccidioidomycosis is endemic and can be seen in epidemic proportions after a dust storm. *Aspergillus* organisms are fungi that can be particularly dangerous in patients with COPD. Consultation is recommended before specific antifungal therapy is initiated.[15]

Three other complications occur as a result of the COPD disease process: sleep disorders, acute respiratory failure, and cor pulmonale. Although it is not always recognized, nocturnal oxygen desaturation in patients with COPD is fairly common and is often observed throughout rapid eye movement (REM) sleep. Patients who are not obese develop coexisting upper airway obstruction. However, in some individuals who are obese, there is an added obstructive component to the usual mechanisms of transient hypoxemia. Sleep-related hypoxemia is suggested by an increased hematocrit in a patient with morning headaches and daytime somnolence. Often, the patient's sleep partner reports intense snoring. Overnight home monitoring with pulse oximetry establishes the diagnosis. It is appropriate to prescribe home oxygen for nocturnal use if home monitoring with a pulse oximeter identifies an oxygen saturation of less than 88% and if symptoms of headache, fatigue, and poor exercise tolerance are present. Continuous positive airway pressure (CPAP) through a well-fitting nasal mask is helpful for patients with an obstructive component. If nocturnal oxygen desaturation is suspected, a referral should be made to a pulmonologist or sleep disorder specialist.[16]

Acute respiratory failure is the most severe complication of COPD. Acute worsening of arterial blood gases necessitates consultation and possible hospitalization.

Cor pulmonale is a severe complication of COPD and is an indication for consultation. Its pathologic definition is right ventricular enlargement, hypertrophy, or dilation secondary to lung disease.[15] Peripheral edema, elevation of the neck veins, and a congested liver reflect right-sided heart failure. In the presence of a significant degree of COPD and an elevated hematocrit with hypoxemia, the diagnosis of cor pulmonale as a complication of COPD can be made without further expensive tests other than electrocardiography. Standard therapy for cor pulmonale is to treat the underlying airflow obstruction and improve oxygenation. Restriction of salt intake to 2 g/day and a 24-hour diuretic can benefit those with mild heart failure. If decompensation continues, the addition of supplemental oxygen is indicated to achieve arterial oxygen saturation in the 90% to 95% range 24 hours a day. Hematocrit or hemoglobin levels should be monitored at 4- to 8-week intervals. If the patient is adequately oxygenated, the elevated hematocrit will resolve within that period. Persistent erythrocytosis reflects insufficient oxygen administration or the presence of desaturation during sleep despite the oxygen. A sleep study at this point may help determine whether additional therapy, such as CPAP, is needed during the night.

PATIENT AND FAMILY EDUCATION AND HEALTH PROMOTION

1. Smoking cessation education should be offered at every visit for a COPD patient who continues to smoke.
2. Pulmonary rehabilitation is a structured program, specifically designed for patients with COPD who have demonstrated that self-management and behavior modification can be achieved, resulting in a substantial decrease in morbidity.
3. Advanced care planning includes the need for patients and families to understand that acute exacerbations of COPD may cause respiratory failure, a need for ventilator support, and the possibility of death. Providers should help patients and their family members make decisions about advance planning and their preferences for end-of-life care during stable periods of health. These discussions can help prepare patients with advanced COPD for a life-threatening exacerbation of the disease.

REFERENCES

1. Global Initiative for Chronic Obstructive Lung Disease. Global strategies for the diagnosis, management, and prevention of chronic obstructive pulmonary disease. NHLBI/WHO Workshop Report, 2017. Retrieved from www.goldcopd.org/uploads/users/files/GOLD_Report_2017_Apr2.pdf. (Accessed 1 December 2017).
2. Parmet, S. (2006). Chronic obstructive pulmonary disease. *JAMA: The Journal of the American Medical Association, 290*(17), 2362.
3. Murphy, S. L., Xu, J., & Kochanek, K. D. (2013). Deaths: Final data for 2010. *National Vital Statistics Reports: From the Centers for Disease Control and Prevention, National Center for Health Statistics, National Vital Statistics System, 61*(4), 1–117.
4. Centers for Disease Control and Prevention. (2017). Chronic obstructive pulmonary disease (COPD). Retrieved from https://www.cdc.gov/copd/index.html. (Accessed 19 May 2018).
5. American Lung Association. Chronic obstructive pulmonary disease (COPD) fact sheet, 2017. Retrieved from www.lung.usa.org/lung-disease/copd/resources/facts-figures/COPD-Fact-Sheet.html. (Accessed 1 December 2017).
6. Wheaton, A. G., Cunningham, T. J., Ford, E. S., & Croft, J. B. (2015). Employment and activity limitations among adults with chronic obstructive pulmonary disease—United States, 2013. *MMWR. Morbidity and Mortality Weekly Report, 64*(11), 289–295.
7. Celli, B. R. (1995). Pathophysiology of chronic obstructive pulmonary disease. *Chest Surgery Clinics of North America, 5*(4), 623–633.
8. Goroll, A. H. (2014). Management of chronic obstructive pulmonary disease. In A. H. Goroll, L. A. May, & A. G. Mulley (Eds.), *Primary care medicine: Office evaluation and management of the adult patient* (7th ed.). Philadelphia: Lippincott.
9. Bickley, L. A. (2016). The thorax and lungs. In L. A. Bickley (Ed.), *Bates guide to physical examination and history taking* (12Th ed.). Philadelphia: Lippincott Williams & Wilkins.
10. Global strategy for the diagnosis, management and prevention of chronic obstructive pulmonary disease (2018 Report). Retrieved from http://goldcopd.org/wp-content/uploads/2017/11/GOLD-2018-v6.0-FINAL-revised-20-Nov_WMS.pdf. (Accessed 19 May 2018).

11. Sandhaus, R. A., Turino, G., Brantly, M. L., Campos, M., Cross, C. E., Goodman, K., et al. (2016). The diagnosis and management of alpha-1 antitrypsin deficiency in the adult. *Chronic Obstructive Pulmonary Diseases*, 3(3), 668–682. http://doi.org/10.15326/jcopdf.3.3.2015.0182.

12. American Academy of Family Physicians (2016). COPD and asthma: Differential diagnosis. Retrieved from https://www.aafp.org/dam/AAFP/documents/journals/fpm/COPD-Asthma.pdf. (Accessed 19 May 2018).

13. Bhullar, S., & Phillips, B. (2005). Sleep in COPD patients. *COPD*, 2(3), 355–361.

14. Eberhardt, R., Gompelmann, D., Herth, F. J., & Schuhmann, M. (2015). Endoscopic bronchial valve treatment: Patient selection and special considerations. *International Journal of Chronic Obstructive Pulmonary Disease*, 10, 2147–2157. http://doi.org/10.2147/COPD.S63473.

15. National Consensus Project for Quality Palliative Care: Clinical practice guidelines for quality palliative care—2013. Retrieved from www.national consensusproject.org. (Accessed 1 December 2017).

16. Celli, B. R., Decramer, M., Wedzicha, J. A., Wiksin, K. C., Agusti, A. A., Criner, G. J., et al. (2015). An official American Thoracic Society/European Respiratory Society statement: Research questions in COPD. *European Respiratory Review*, 24, 159–172.

17. Sharafkhaneh, A., Majid, H., & Gross, N. J. (2013). Safety and tolerability of inhalational anticholinergics in COPD. *Drug, Healthcare and Patient Safety*, 5, 49–55. http://doi.org/10.2147/DHPS.S7771.

18. Brook, R. D., Anderson, J. A., Calverley, P. M., Celli, B. R., Crim, C., Denvir, M. A., et al. (2017). Cardiovascular outcomes with an inhaled beta2-agonist/corticosteroid in patients with COPD at high cardiovascular risk. *Heart (British Cardiac Society)*, 103(19), 1536–1542. http://doi.org/10.1136/heartjnl-2016-310897.

19. Bosnic-Anticevich, S., Chrystyn, H., Costello, R. W., Dolovich, M. B., Fletcher, M. J., Lavorini, F., et al. (2017). The use of multiple respiratory inhalers requiring different inhalation techniques has an adverse effect on COPD outcomes. *International Journal of Chronic Obstructive Pulmonary Disease*, 12, 59–71. http://doi.org/10.2147/COPD.S117196.

20. Institute for Clinical Systems Improvement. (2016). Health Care Guideline: Diagnosis and Management of Chronic Obstructive Pulmonary Disease (COPD). Retrieved from https://www.icsi.org. (Accessed 19 May 2018).

21. Centers for Disease Control and Prevention (CDC). (2015). Intervals between PCV13 and PPSV23 vaccines: Recommendations of the Advisory Committee on Immunization Practices. *MMWR. Morbidity and Mortality Weekly Report*, 64(34), 944–947.

22. Centers for Disease Control. Recommended adult immunizations schedule 2017. Retrieved from www.cdc.gov/vaccines/schedules/downloads/adult/adult-combined-schedule.pdf. (Accessed 13 December 2017).

23. Petty, T. L. (2001). *Frontline treatment of COPD*. Denver: Snowdrift Pulmonary Foundation.

CHAPTER **89**

DYSPNEA

David Patrick Murphy • John David Wagner

 Immediate referral is indicated for myocardial ischemia/infarction, heart failure exacerbation requiring inpatient treatment, and significant pneumothorax, or pulmonary embolism.

DEFINITION AND EPIDEMIOLOGY

Dyspnea encompasses a broad array of discrete unpleasant sensations, such as air hunger, increased work of breathing, chest tightness, feelings of suffocation, and respiratory fatigue.[1] Although breathlessness is expected after vigorous exercise, dyspnea is a cardinal manifestation of cardiopulmonary disease that warrants appropriate evaluation and treatment. It is also a common and disabling symptom of chronic lung disease, and measures of dyspnea are commonly used in evaluating outcomes in these diseases.[2] Dyspnea is a very common complaint in the United States and accounts for 3 to 4 million emergency department visits annually. It was noted to be among the top

three reasons for adults aged 65 and older to visit the emergency department. Its overall prevalence is about 9%, and this figure increases significantly with increasing age to about 17% of patients older than age 65.[3,4]

PATHOPHYSIOLOGY

The mechanisms that trigger dyspnea are complex and vary by disease. This is further complicated by a respiratory system that is unique in that respiratory motor drive has both autonomic (brainstem) and voluntary (cortical) sources of command. It has been suggested that dyspnea occurs whenever sensory input from receptors in the airways, lungs, and chest wall does not match up with respiratory drive.[5] These sensory receptors may respond to chemicals, stretch, irritation, or passive distention. For example, there appears to be a dissociation between sensory input and motor output in conditions that impose a mechanical load on the respiratory system by decreasing compliance of either the lung (e.g., pneumonia, pulmonary edema, fibrosis) or the chest wall (e.g., kyphoscoliosis, rib fractures, circumferential thorax burns), or by inhibiting airflow (e.g., asthma, chronic bronchitis, emphysema).[6] In addition, neuromuscular weakness or fatigue may cause dyspnea symptoms because of the inability of weakened muscles to generate an expected level of ventilation. Hypoxemia and hypercapnia stimulate chemoreceptors that may cause dyspnea through increased respiratory motor drive. Surprisingly, there is a poor correlation between dyspnea and blood gas abnormalities. Dyspneic patients are often perplexed to learn that they have adequate oxygen saturation or that supplemental oxygen administration does not relieve symptoms. Blood gases are of value in monitoring severity of illness, but many clinicians overestimate their value as measures of dyspnea.[1] Increased carbon dioxide production, lower pH, and to a lesser degree, hypoxemia, stimulate the efferent motor drive for ventilation; however, their importance physiologically in monitoring the adequacy of ventilatory response is less clear. What the physiologic mechanisms of dyspnea have in common is that some combination of stimuli triggers an awareness of a threat to the ability to breathe or a threat to self.[7]

CLINICAL PRESENTATION AND PHYSICAL EXAMINATION

Dyspnea is a common complaint, and the following dimensions are useful in elucidating the disease process that causes dyspnea: quality, timing, intensity, associated symptoms, and environmental exposures. These factors provide indications as to what the mechanism of the cause may be. A good history of the complaint is essential because dyspnea, like pain, is primarily dependent on a patient's perception and self-report of the symptom.

Quality

Dyspnea is typically described as the unpleasant sensation of tightness, increased work or effort, and air hunger or unsatisfied inspiration. The descriptors patients use for dyspnea sensations may be diagnostically useful.[8-10] For example, patients with obstructive lung disease such as asthma or chronic obstructive pulmonary disease (COPD) tend to complain of "chest tightness" or "constriction." Diseases associated with an increased mechanical load (resulting from decreased compliance or increased airway resistance), such as interstitial lung disease or cystic fibrosis, are often associated with feelings of excessive "work" or "effort." Patients with an increased drive to breathe (e.g., resulting from hypoxemia or hypercapnia) experience air hunger and may complain that they "can't get enough air in." This can also be related to decreased oxygen-carrying capacity—for example, in severe anemia or carbon monoxide poisoning. It is important to note that causes of dyspnea probably activate multiple dyspnea mechanisms, leading to a composite of sensations that defy easy classification. For example, asthma that is mild may manifest as chest tightness only, whereas common later signs of more acute or severe disease include increased work of breathing or severe air hunger (Table 89.1).

Timing

Although it is often impossible to pinpoint the precise onset of dyspnea, it is important to distinguish between acute and chronic symptoms. Sudden onset of dyspnea often heralds serious cardiopulmonary disease that requires immediate evaluation and treatment (e.g., pulmonary embolism, pneumothorax, myocardial infarction). Relative stability, intermittent exacerbations, or progressive debilitating symptoms may characterize chronic dyspnea. Patients who experience increasing symptoms or intermittent exacerbations should be carefully reevaluated for worsening disease or a new problem.

TABLE 89.1 Respiratory Descriptions and Causes

Quality or Description	Common Causes
Tightness, constriction	Asthma, COPD, bronchiectasis, foreign body, bronchitis
Increased work or effort	Severe kyphoscoliosis, obesity, pleural effusion, myasthenia gravis, Guillain-Barré syndrome, spinal cord injury, myopathy
Air hunger, unsatisfied inspiration	Pulmonary embolism, pneumonia, CHF, altitude, metabolic acidosis, anemia, interstitial lung disease, cystic fibrosis

CHF, Congestive heart failure; *COPD*, chronic obstructive pulmonary disease.

Intensity

Dyspnea severity is difficult to quantify and there are many proposed methods of trying to quantify it. This is an area of study that is still under development.[11] Activity limitation is commonly used as a surrogate marker because it is a more objective form of measure. Dyspnea is almost always first noticed with physical exertion and may progress to symptoms at rest. The degree of activity necessary to elicit symptoms may be quantified by asking questions such as "How many flights of stairs can you climb?" or "How far can you walk on level ground?" One commonly used scale for classifying the severity of dyspnea was proposed and published by the Medical Research Council (Table 89.2). Other measures that have been proposed include the Baseline Dyspnea Index. These measures may be repeated on subsequent visits to assess patient improvement with treatment. Another method for measuring intensity is use of quality-of-life measures such as the Chronic Respiratory Disease Questionnaire. There is no single broadly accepted form of measurement; the most important thing is to find the one that fits best in one's individual practice and use it consistently. Practitioners should be cautious, however, and not rely too heavily on a patient's grading of symptoms or ignore other clinical signs and symptoms.[12,13]

Associated Symptoms

In addition to dyspnea, cardinal symptoms of pulmonary disease are chest pain, cough, hemoptysis, and wheezing. Chest pain is one manifestation of ischemic heart disease but may also result from pneumothorax, pulmonary embolism, or rib trauma. A patient reporting leg or hip pain preceding or concurrent with onset of dyspnea should raise suspicion for pulmonary embolism. Hemoptysis is a distressing symptom that may accompany dyspnea. Expectorated blood can originate from the nose, airways, or lung parenchyma. Cough is a common symptom of acute and chronic pulmonary disease. Persistent cough is most often caused by upper airway cough syndrome (previously referred to as postnasal drip syndrome), gastroesophageal reflux, or asthma. Wheezing signifies airway disease, such as asthma or COPD), or focal obstruction by a

TABLE 89.2 The Modified Medical Research Council Scale

Grade	Degree	Description of Breathlessness
0	None	I only get breathless with strenuous exercise.
1	Slight	I get short of breath when hurrying on level ground or walking up a slight hill.
2	Moderate	On level ground, I walk slower than people of the same age because of breathlessness, or I have to stop for breath when walking at my own pace on the level.
3	Severe	I stop for breath after walking about 100 yards or after a few minutes on level ground.
4	Very severe	I am too breathless to leave the house, or I am breathless when dressing.
Grade	**Degree**	**Defining Clinical Characteristics**
0	None	Not troubled with breathlessness except with strenuous exercise
1	Slight	Troubled by shortness of breath when hurrying on level ground or walking up a slight hill
2	Moderate	Walks more slowly than people of the same age when on level ground because of breathlessness or has to stop for breath when walking at own pace on level ground
3	Severe	Stops for breath after walking about 100 yards or after a few minutes on level ground
4	Very severe	Too breathless to leave the house or breathless when dressing or undressing

tumor, such as a carcinoid lesion, or aspirated foreign body. Patients who are initially seen with fever, chills, or night sweats should be evaluated for acute or chronic lung infections, including pneumonia, tuberculosis, and chronic bronchitis.

Dyspnea is often accompanied by fear and anxiety. A dyspnea-panic cycle has been described in which the sensation of breathlessness leads to anxiety, which creates muscle tension, which in turn leads to increased dyspnea and panic. Thus the anxiety associated with dyspnea can become a vicious circle leading to future attacks of dyspnea.[14,15]

Exposures

The lungs are uniquely susceptible to various environmental hazards, including air pollution, dust, smoke, carbon monoxide, and an array of occupational exposures (e.g., silica, asbestos, chemical exposure). A careful history of current and past tobacco use is essential in the evaluation of tobacco-related diseases such as asthma, chronic bronchitis, emphysema, spontaneous pneumothorax secondary to bullous disease, ischemic heart disease, respiratory bronchiolitis, and eosinophilic granuloma. In addition, many medications and therapeutic radiation are known to damage the lungs. Table 89.3 lists the steps to take in the assessment of dyspnea.[7]

The physical examination begins with careful assessment of the patient's vital signs. Normal respiratory rate in adults ranges from 12 to 20 breaths per minute, and a rapid or labored breathing pattern is often but not always evident in dyspneic patients. Many practitioners consider pulse oximetry a "vital sign" because it usually provides a reliable measure of arterial oxygen saturation. A normal oxygen saturation level, however, does not rule out carbon dioxide retention and ventilatory insufficiency; carbon dioxide levels must be directly measured with an arterial blood gas sample. Expiratory peak flow measurement may also be included in the initial assessment of patients with known airway disease or wheezing.

Breathing pattern and body position provide important clues to disease severity. The acutely dyspneic patient often sits upright and leans forward to optimize breathing mechanics. The inability to speak in full sentences, and accessory respiratory muscle use, indicate increased work of breathing. Patients with COPD often adopt a characteristic "pursed-lip" appearance. Shallow, rapid breathing or panting is characteristic of interstitial lung disease in patients with poor or decreased lung compliance. The skin may be diaphoretic, and the patient may appear anxious. Bluish discoloration of the skin and mucous membranes (cyanosis) results from increased amounts of deoxygenated hemoglobin. Central cyanosis, detected in the tongue and mucous membranes, is a more reliable indicator of oxygenation than peripheral cyanosis, which can also result from intense vasoconstriction of vessels in the extremities. Mental status may be depressed by either severe hypoxemia or hypercapnia. Digital or finger clubbing is an important finding often attributed to various lung diseases, but it is also seen in other disorders, such as inflammatory bowel disease and congenital heart disease.

The lung examination includes careful inspection of the thorax and abdomen. Chest wall deformities may limit lung expansion and contribute to dyspnea. During normal inspiration, the chest rises and the abdomen moves outward due to contraction of the downward moving diaphragm. Conversely, during inspiration in a patient with inspiratory muscle fatigue, the chest rises due to accessory muscle contraction and the abdomen paradoxically moves inward because of upward movement of the weakened diaphragm. This pattern of breathing is said to be paradoxical and indicates diaphragmatic weakness or fatigue. Palpation of the chest wall is useful in assessing tracheal position, symmetry of chest movement, areas of tenderness, and crepitus (subcutaneous air from pneumothorax or pneumomediastinum). Airless lung transmits sounds more efficiently than air-filled lung and is the basis for auscultatory consolidative findings, including bronchial breath sounds, egophony (E to A changes), and whispered pectoriloquy. The classic example of a disease that causes lung consolidation is pneumonia, although any process that fills (pus, water, blood, protein, or cells) or collapses alveoli yields these findings. Abnormal, or adventitious, lung sounds are distinguished by whether they are continuous (high-pitched sounds are wheezing, low-pitched sounds are rhonchi) or discontinuous (crackles). Wheezing signifies bronchoconstriction or airway obstruction from secretions, tumor, or foreign body. Crackles are heard in a number of disease processes, including congestive heart failure (CHF) and interstitial lung disease. Pleural friction rubs are grating sounds that may occur on inspiration or expiration as inflamed pleural surfaces rub against each other.

A detailed discussion of the cardiac examination is beyond the scope of this chapter, but it is an important component of the evaluation of dyspneic patients. The pulse should be carefully analyzed for rate and rhythm. Atrial fibrillation is a common arrhythmia that can usually be diagnosed at the bedside by its "irregularly irregular" character. Left ventricular dysfunction and valvular heart disease also lend themselves to bedside diagnosis through palpation and auscultation. The extremities should also be assessed for pulse and edema.[16,17]

TABLE 89.3	Assessment of Dyspnea: Dos and Don'ts
Do	**Don't**
Ask about the qualitative experience of dyspnea (such as chest tightness, work of breathing).	Rely on blood gases for assessing the severity of dyspnea.
Ask about associated affective states (anxiety, panic, depression).	Rely on orders such as "Call physician for O_2 sat <90%" as a trigger for the reevaluation of dyspnea. Consider an order such as "Assess dyspnea intensity q shift. Call physician for dyspnea >6 (0–10 scale)."
Try to quantify the intensity of dyspnea and associated suffering (e.g., use a 0–10 scale).	
Ask how dyspnea is affecting the patient's life (e.g., reduced activity, sleep disorder).	
Ask about concerns for the future (fear of suffocation, greater disability).	

From Hallenbeck, J. (2009). Pathophysiology and treatment of dyspnea. *Pulmonary, Critical Care, Sleep Update*. Northbrook, IL: American College of Chest Physicians.

In summary, the physical examination is an essential part of the workup of dyspneic patients and should be used to help direct the diagnostic evaluation. The absence of specific physical examination findings can be of greater diagnostic usefulness than positive findings in patients with chronic dyspnea. For example, interstitial lung disease and CHF are unlikely causes of dyspnea in a patient without crackles on lung examination.

DIAGNOSTICS

Further diagnostic workup is guided by the history and physical examination findings, and the studies required depend on whether dyspnea is acute or chronic.

Essential Diagnostics

A plain chest radiograph is helpful in elucidating many causes of dyspnea. Pneumothorax and pleural effusion are usually easily detected on a plain chest radiograph, although small effusions may require decubitus views for confirmation. Parenchymal infiltrates occur in many different disease processes, but in the context of an acute infectious syndrome imply pneumonia. CHF is recognized by cephalization of vessels, Kerley B lines, and enlarged cardiac silhouette. Frank pulmonary edema manifests with bilateral perihilar air space filling (batwing appearance) and pleural effusions. Radiographic findings of hyperinflation, flattened hemidiaphragms, increased anterior clear space, and bullae support a diagnosis of COPD. The chest radiograph is usually normal or reveals only subtle abnormalities in asthma and pulmonary embolism.

The workup for pulmonary thromboembolic disease can be complicated and is often driven by the availability and expertise of local medical resources. An appropriate evaluation may initially include D-dimer, a ventilation/perfusion ($\dot{V}/\dot{Q}$) scan, or computed tomographic angiography. Symptomatic lower extremity clots (the source of most pulmonary emboli) are usually detected by lower extremity doppler ultrasound. Pulmonary angiography remains the definitive test for the diagnosis of pulmonary embolism.

If there is any suspicion for myocardial ischemia or infarction, electrocardiography (ECG) and measurement of cardiac enzymes are likely indicated. Likewise, if history and physical suggest heart failure exacerbation, B-type natriuretic peptide (BNP) or its N-terminal prohormone precursor (NTproBNP) might be in order. Keep in mind that BNP/NTproBNP testing has substantially higher sensitivity than specificity. This is why it is much better suited for ruling out heart failure in patients with a low to intermediate pretest probability of CHF.

Additional Diagnostics

Spirometry is essential to the diagnosis and management of asthma and COPD. A decrease in the ratio of forced expiratory volume in 1 second to forced vital capacity (FEV_1/FVC) is the spirometric hallmark of obstruction. Bronchoprovocation testing with either methacholine or exercise may be necessary to diagnose asthma in patients with normal baseline spirometry. Proportionately reduced FEV and FVC suggest restriction (a useful mnemonic for restrictive lung processes is *PAINT*: pleural disease, alveolar filling process, interstitial lung disease, neuromuscular disease, or thoracic cage abnormalities), which should be confirmed with lung volume measurements. Diaphragmatic and respiratory muscle weakness may be detected with maximum inspiratory pressure and maximum expiratory

pressure maneuvers, although these tests are neither sensitive nor specific.

Cardiac rhythm disturbances and hypertrophy may be noted on routine ECG, although intermittent arrhythmias may be detected only by long-term monitoring (e.g., telemetry, Holter, or event monitoring). Echocardiography is extremely useful in assessing left ventricular function, cardiac valve status, pericardial effusions, and, in some cases, pulmonary hypertension.

Other routine studies with usefulness in the evaluation of patients with dyspnea include hemoglobin level to exclude anemia, and thyroid function tests to exclude hyperthyroidism. More sophisticated testing, such as formal cardiopulmonary exercise testing and cardiac catheterization, obviously requires referral to specialists.[17]

INITIAL DIAGNOSTICS

Dyspnea

LABORATORY
- Cardiac enzymes[a]
- D-dimer[a]
- B-type natriuretic peptide/N-terminal prohormone precursor[a]

IMAGING
- Chest X-ray studies (posteroanterior and lateral)[a]
- Computed tomography scan[a]
- $\dot{V}/\dot{Q}$ scan or pulmonary angiography[a]
- Lower extremity Doppler ultrasound[a]

OTHER DIAGNOSTICS
- Electrocardiography[a]

[a]If indicated.

DIFFERENTIAL DIAGNOSIS

Dyspnea is most commonly caused by cardiopulmonary disease, although anemia, neuromuscular weakness, gastroesophageal reflux, deconditioning, and psychogenic causes must be considered. The most common causes of acute dyspnea are asthma, bronchitis, pneumothorax, pneumonia, pulmonary embolism, chest trauma with rib fractures or pulmonary contusions, ischemic heart failure, psychogenic causes, and acute blood loss. Less commonly, acute dyspnea can be due to airway obstruction, foreign body aspiration, carbon monoxide poisoning, neuromuscular weakness, or pleural effusion. The majority of patients with long-standing dyspnea have one of four causes: asthma, COPD, interstitial lung disease, or cardiomyopathy. Other causes of chronic dyspnea to consider include anemia, cystic fibrosis, gastroesophageal reflux disease, obesity, pectus excavatum, pleural effusion, pulmonary hypertension, sarcoidosis, severe kyphoscoliosis, and spondylitis.

INTERPROFESSIONAL COLLABORATIVE MANAGEMENT
Nonpharmacologic Management

The treatment of dyspnea entails treatment of the underlying disease process and symptomatic relief. Supplemental oxygen should be administered initially to all acutely dyspneic patients and to chronically dyspneic patients who are hypoxemic. The standard Medicare criteria for supplemental oxygen are as follows: PaO_2 at rest of less than 55 mm Hg, or oxygen saturation of 88% or less. Patients with a PaO_2 of 56 to 59 mm Hg or an oxygen saturation of 89% or less warrant supplemental oxygen if they have underlying CHF or pulmonary hypertension. These criteria are based on two large studies that demonstrated improved survival in hypoxemic COPD patients treated with supplemental oxygen.[18-22] Patients who undergo desaturation during sleep or exercise also qualify for supplemental oxygen, although the data supporting these indications are not as strong. Administration of supplemental oxygen may worsen carbon dioxide retention in some patients with COPD. These patients require an arterial blood gas assessment to ensure adequate carbon dioxide elimination. Energy conservation strategies (e.g., walking slowly; periodically using resting positions, such as leaning forward while sitting in a chair; avoiding fatigue; and spacing chores at times of feeling well) and specific breathing techniques are often effective in patients with obstructive lung disease. Patients with difficulty mobilizing secretions (e.g., those with chronic bronchitis, bronchiectasis, cystic fibrosis) benefit from chest physiotherapy and airway clearance adjuncts, such as the flutter device or vest airway clearance system.

Formal pulmonary rehabilitation programs effectively incorporate dyspnea management for patients with long-term disease such as COPD. Therapies include exercise training, education, nutrition intervention, and psychosocial support. These programs have been shown to improve quality of life as well as reduce health care utilization and psychosocial issues.[23-26]

Pharmacologic Management

Anxiolytics and narcotics are sometimes effective in relieving dyspnea but must be used cautiously because of inherent respiratory depressant properties. Opioid medications are among the most studied medications for the relief of dyspnea, and there can be significant relief of dyspneic symptoms; however, no improvement in oxygenation occurs. Typically these medications are used in palliative medicine at the smallest effective dose that does not cause significant side effects.

Indications for Referral or Hospitalization

Patients with chronic dyspnea should be referred to a pulmonary specialist when the cause is not obvious from the history, physical examination, and screening studies, including complete blood count (CBC), chest radiography, and spirometry. Echocardiography and treadmill stress testing may help differentiate between cardiac and pulmonary disease before the consultation.

The decision to hospitalize a patient depends initially on identifying the likely cause of respiratory distress. Conditions that need to be readily identified and mandate hospital admission include pulmonary embolism and myocardial infarction. Criteria for hospitalization of patients with other conditions such as pneumothorax, pleural effusion, CHF exacerbation, asthma, and COPD depend on the severity of the illness, response to treatment, and presence of comorbid conditions.

COMPLICATIONS

Dyspnea limits a patient's activities of daily living. The consequences of uncontrolled dyspnea symptoms may include anxiety, depression, loss of job, and social isolation. Physical deconditioning results from decreased exercise and leads to a downward spiral of ever-decreasing activity.

PATIENT AND FAMILY EDUCATION AND HEALTH PROMOTION

Patients with chronic dyspnea need to be taught techniques that control symptoms and warning signs of the need for medical assistance. Pulmonary rehabilitation programs provide intense education for patients with severe pulmonary disease but are expensive and not always available. All patients who use inhaled bronchodilators and corticosteroids should be regularly instructed in proper inhaler techniques, including the use of spacer devices. Asthmatic patients may benefit from home peak flow monitoring to detect worsening airflow obstruction, which offers an opportunity for early intervention. Smoking cessation is critical in the management of any cardiopulmonary disease, and providers play a pivotal role in educating their patients about the adverse effects of tobacco use and strategies to stop smoking.

REFERENCES

1. Beach, D., & Schwartzstein, R. (2006). The genesis of breathlessness: What do we understand? In S. Booth & D. Dudgeon (Eds.), *Dyspnea in advanced disease*. Oxford, England: Oxford University Press.
2. Kaplan, R. M., & Ries, A. L. (2005). Quality of life as outcome measures in pulmonary diseases. *Journal of Cardiopulmonary Rehabilitation, 25*, 321–331.
3. Niska, R., Bhuiya, F., & Xu, J. (2010). National hospital ambulatory medical care survey: 2007 emergency department summary. *National Health Statistics Reports*, 1–31.
4. Currow, D. C., Plummer, J. L., Crocket, A., & Abernathy, A. P. (2009). A community population survey prevalence and severity of dyspnea in adults. *Journal of Pain and Symptom Management, 38*, 533–545.
5. Schwartzstein, R. M., Simon, P. M., Weiss, J. W., et al. (1989). Breathlessness induced by dissociation between ventilation and chemical drive. *The American Review of Respiratory Disease, 139*, 1231–1237.
6. Pratter, M. R., Curley, F. J., Dubois, J., et al. (1989). Cause and evaluation of chronic dyspnea in a pulmonary disease clinic. *Archives of Internal Medicine, 149*, 2277–2282.
7. Hallenbeck, J. (June 1, 2009). The pathophysiology and treatment of dyspnea. *Pulm Crit Care Sleep Update*.
8. Moy, M. L., Woodrow Weiss, J., Sparrow, D., et al. (2000). Quality of dyspnea in bronchoconstriction differs from external resistive loads. *American Journal of Respiratory and Critical Care Medicine, 162*(1 2pt), 451–455.
9. O'Donnell, D. E., Chau, L. K., & Webb, K. A. (1998). Qualitative aspects of exertional dyspnea in patients with interstitial lung disease. *Journal of Applied Physiology, 84*(6), 2000–2009.
10. Mahler, D. A., Harver, A., Lentine, T., et al. (1996). Descriptors of breathlessness in cardiorespiratory diseases. *American Journal of Respiratory and Critical Care Medicine, 154*, 1357–1363.
11. Murray, R. J., & Nadel, J. A. (2010). Dyspnea. In *Murray and Nadel's textbook of respiratory medicine* (4th ed.). Elsevier.
12. Parshall, M., Schwartzstein, R., & Adams, A. (2012). An official American Thoracic Society statement: Update on the mechanisms, assessment, and management of dyspnea. *American Journal of Respiratory and Critical Care Medicine, 185*(4), 435–452.
13. Worster, A., Balion, C. M., Hill, S. A., Santaguida, P., Ismaila, A., McKelvie, R., et al. (2008). Diagnostic accuracy of BNP and NT-proBNP in patients presenting to acute care settings with dyspnea: A systematic review. *Clinical Biochemistry, 41*, 250–259.
14. Bailey, P. H. (2004). The dyspnea-anxiety-dyspnea cycle—COPD patients' stories of breathlessness: "It's scary when you can't breathe." *Qualitative Health Research, 14*, 760–778.
15. Periyakoil, V. S., Skultety, K., & Sheikh, J. (2005). Panic, anxiety and chronic dyspnea. *Journal of Palliative Medicine, 8*, 453–459.
16. Guo, L., et al. (2014). Diagnostic utility of N-terminal-proBNP in differentiating acute pulmonary embolism from heart failure in patients with acute dyspnea. *Chinese Medical Journal, 127*(16), 2888–2893.
17. Mahler, D. A., Selecky, P. A., Harrod, C. G., Benditt, J. O., Carrieri-Kohlman, V., Curtis, J. R., et al. (2010). American College of Chest Physicians consensus statement on the management of dyspnea in patients with advanced lung or heart disease. *Chest, 137*, 674–691.

18. (1980). Continuous or nocturnal oxygen therapy in hypoxemic chronic obstructive lung disease: A clinical trial. Nocturnal Oxygen Therapy Trial Group. *Annals of Internal Medicine, 93,* 391–398.

19. (1981). Long-term domiciliary oxygen therapy in chronic hypoxic cor pulmonale complicating chronic bronchitis and emphysema. Report of the Medical Research Council Working Party. *Lancet, 1,* 681–686.

20. Ries, A. L., Bauldoff, G. S., Carlin, B. W., Casaburi, R., Emery, C. F., Mahler, D. A., et al. (2007). Pulmonary re- habilitation: Joint ACCP/AACVPR evidence-based clinical practice guidelines. *Chest, 131,* 4S–42S.

21. Department of Health and Human Services. (December 2011). Centers for Medicare and Medicaid Services oxygen therapy supplies: complying with documentation and coverage requirements. ICN 904883. https://www.scanhealthplan.com/media/1483/medicare-coverage-of-oxygen-therapy.pdf.

22. Moore, R. P., Berlowitz, D. J., Denehy, L., Pretto, J. J., Brazzale, D. J., Sharpe, K., et al. (2011). A randomised trial of domiciliary, ambulatory oxygen in patients with COPD and dyspnea but without resting hypoxaemia. *Thorax, 66,* 32–37.

23. Fishman, A. P. (1994). Pulmonary rehabilitation research: NIH workshop summary. *The American Review of Respiratory Disease, 149,* 825–833.

24. Ries, A. L. (1990). Position paper of the American Association of Cardiovascular and Pulmonary Rehabilitation: Scientific basis of pulmonary rehabilitation. *Journal of Cardiopulmonary Rehabilitation, 10,* 418–441.

25. 1997). Pulmonary rehabilitation: Joint ACCP/AACVPR evidence-based guidelines. *Chest, 112,* 1363–1396.

26. Oh, E. G. (2003). The effects of home-based pulmonary rehabilitation in patients with chronic lung disease. *International Journal of Nursing Studies, 40,* 873–879.

CHAPTER **90**

HEMOPTYSIS

Patricia Polgar-Bailey

DEFINITION AND EPIDEMIOLOGY

Hemoptysis refers to the expectoration of blood from the lung parenchyma or tracheobronchial tree. It can range from a small amount of blood-streaked sputum, which is commonly seen in bronchitis, to a massive hemorrhage, which is a medical emergency because it rapidly causes death by asphyxiation. The classifications—nonmassive and massive—are based on the volume of blood loss; however, there are no uniform definitions for these categories. Hemoptysis is generally classified as nonmassive if the blood loss is less than 100 to 200 mL/day, whereas massive hemoptysis refers to more than this amount in 24 hours.[1] Massive hemoptysis is uncommon, occurring in less than 5% of patients with hemoptysis. However, the associated mortality rate ranges from 7% to 30% to as high as 58%, which demonstrates the need for urgent evaluation and management.[1,2] Even slight bleeding may signify a serious condition, such as bronchogenic carcinoma, tuberculosis, or erosion of the thoracic aneurysm. Therefore blood loss volume is more helpful in directing management than in making a diagnosis.

The most common causes of hemoptysis in the United States are, in descending order, acute and chronic bronchitis, lung cancer, pneumonia, and tuberculosis. Similarly, these are the most common causes of hemoptysis seen in the primary care setting. However, tuberculosis is a leading cause of hemoptysis in developing countries and should be high on the list of differential diagnoses for patients who are from countries with a high prevalence of the disease or who have traveled to countries where tuberculosis is endemic.[1] Less common causes of hemoptysis include influenza viruses, malignant carcinomas,

and pulmonary barotrauma secondary to diving.[3,4] Hemoptysis can also be a sign of an underlying hereditary disorder, such as Osler-Weber-Rendu syndrome, also known as hereditary hemorrhagic telangiectasia (HHT). HHT is an autosomal dominant disorder that is typically characterized by a triad of telangiectasia (including pulmonary), recurrent epistaxis, and a family history of the disorder.[5]

PATHOPHYSIOLOGY

For hemoptysis to occur, there must be some communication between the airways and the blood vessels of the lungs. The lungs receive blood from two relatively independent circulations: pulmonary and bronchial. The pulmonary circulation is characterized by lower pressures and higher volumes and is supplied with mixed venous blood through the pulmonary arteries. In contrast, the bronchial circulation supplies oxygenated blood in a high-pressure, low-volume circuit.

The bronchial arteries can become enlarged and more numerous in association with a variety of inflammatory or neoplastic diseases. Chronic inflammation, often associated with infectious processes, can lead to destruction of the connective tissue of blood vessels or result in erosion through the vessel wall. Angiographic studies have revealed that hemoptysis typically originates from disruptions of the branches of the bronchial arterial tree. This is presumably related to the connection of these arteries to the proliferative nests of small vessels often found in areas of inflammation and tumors.

CLINICAL PRESENTATION AND PHYSICAL EXAMINATION

It is common for patients to confuse hemoptysis with hematemesis or epistaxis. Patient history, including factors such as age, nutritional status, occupational and environmental exposures, and comorbid conditions, can be useful in differentiating among the three conditions and can help to narrow the differential diagnosis. Taking a thorough travel history is important because tuberculosis and bronchiectasis appear to be decreasing as causes of hemoptysis in the United States, whereas they are still frequent causes of hemoptysis in other parts of the world. Recent travel may have also increased the risk of parasitic infections, which can cause hemoptysis.

In addition, a description of the blood and accompanying symptoms can be helpful in differentiating between hemoptysis and hematemesis. Blood from the airways is usually bright red or pink, liquid or clotted in appearance, and frothy because of the presence of surfactant. The pH is alkaline, and it tends to be mixed with macrophages and neutrophils. Blood originating in the gastrointestinal tract is usually dark red, brown, or black; it has a coffee-ground appearance and is rarely frothy. It is acidic and may be intermixed with food particles. Absence of nausea and vomiting and a history of lung disease raise the suspicion of hemoptysis, whereas the presence of nausea and vomiting and coexisting gastric or hepatic disease suggest hematemesis.[1]

It is important to carefully determine the chronology and volume of hemoptysis. Quantifying blood loss may be difficult, even in patients who are clinically stable, because they are often anxious and, as a result, usually overestimate the amount of blood loss. However, every effort should be made to determine the rate and volume of blood loss, which can include observing as the patient coughs and using a graduated container. Urgent evaluation and possible hospitalization are indicated if more than 50 mL of blood has been expectorated in the previous 24 hours. For smaller amounts of blood loss, a thorough diagnostic evaluation can be initiated in the primary care setting.

Mild hemoptysis, recurring sporadically over a few years, is common in smokers, who may have chronic bronchitis with intermittent flares of acute bronchitis. However, abrupt hemoptysis associated with cigarette smoking can also be seen with bronchogenic carcinoma. A long history of small-volume, recurrent hemoptysis with little or no sputum production is suggestive of processes such as bronchogenic carcinoma, bronchial adenoma, and vascular malformation. A history of chronic sputum production suggests an infectious cause, such as bronchitis, bronchiectasis, lung abscess, or tuberculosis. Hemoptysis associated with bacterial pneumonia is suggested by an acute onset of fever, sputum production, and, commonly, pleuritic chest pain. Hemoptysis is commonly a late symptom of bronchogenic carcinoma and is preceded by a chronic cough, fatigue, and constitutional symptoms. Environmental exposure to asbestos, arsenic, chromium, nickel, and certain ethers can increase the risk for hemoptysis.[1] Occupational history may be helpful in elucidating the cause of hemoptysis. For example, after repetitive deep dives, breath-hold divers are often affected by a common syndrome characterized by typical symptoms such as cough, sensation of chest constriction, blood-striated expectorate (hemoptysis), and, rarely, an overt acute pulmonary edema syndrome, often together with various degrees of dyspnea. Similar clinical features had been previously observed in scuba divers, swimmers, and athletes engaged in strenuous efforts during terrestrial sport activities.[4] A travel history may be helpful. Tuberculosis is endemic in many parts of the world, and parasitic causes should be considered.[1]

PHYSICAL EXAMINATION

The presence of a fever suggests infection. A thorough examination of the ears, nose, and throat can detect upper airway sources of bleeding, such as laryngeal carcinoma lesions. Cervical, supraclavicular, or axillary adenopathy raises the suspicion of an intrathoracic malignant neoplasm. The presence of stridor or findings suggestive of chronic obstructive pulmonary disease, congestive heart failure, or pneumonia can be determined by auscultation of the chest.

Localized wheezing may indicate a local obstruction, foreign body, or bronchogenic carcinoma. A pleural friction rub may be the only sign of pulmonary infarction associated with a pulmonary embolism. Isolated crackles are nonspecific for the location of the primary disease because they may represent an inflammatory reaction to blood aspirated from another site.

Digital clubbing is suggestive of chronic lung disease, such as bronchiectasis or malignant neoplasm. Cardiac examination may help determine the presence of mitral stenosis. Localized adenopathy, especially a supraclavicular node, may be indicative of a lung malignant neoplasm. A bleeding disorder is suggested by the presence of petechiae or ecchymoses.

DIAGNOSTICS
Essential Diagnostics

Chest radiography should be performed as part of the initial evaluation because it may help localize the bleeding and identify the cause. It can also provide images for later comparison to evaluate resolution of disease. Important diagnostic findings include an air-fluid level of a lung abscess, the "crescent sign" of a mycetoma, a nodule that suggests a neoplasm, evidence of volume loss, or consolidation distal to an airway obstruction.

Computed tomography (CT) is suggested for initial evaluation of patients at high risk of malignancy who have suspicious findings on chest radiography. CT should be considered in patients with risk factors (e.g., 40 years or older, smoking history of at least 30 pack-years) who demonstrate negative or nonlocalizing findings. CT and fiberoptic bronchoscopy have complementary roles in the evaluation of patients with hemoptysis, and the combination of these two tests has been shown to give a higher yield of specific diagnoses than either test alone. Fiberoptic bronchoscopy allows direct visualization of the airways and localization of the bleeding source. Biopsy specimens and lavage samples from the airways and alveolar spaces can be sent for cytologic and microbial studies. This procedure is relatively safe, is well tolerated, and can be performed on an outpatient basis. The proper timing for fiberoptic bronchoscopy is somewhat controversial. Most thoracic specialists prefer to perform bronchoscopy early in the course of hemoptysis. However, some believe that bronchoscopy is indicated primarily if hemoptysis has been present for longer than 1 week or if the likelihood of cancer is greater because of systemic symptoms or risk factors.

A complete blood count (CBC) is reasonable to obtain in all patients with hemoptysis to rule out thrombocytopenia and to evaluate for anemia and/or microcytosis indicative of chronic blood loss or malignancy. Blood typing and crossmatch may be obtained for patients with hemodynamic instability from blood loss or those in whom a CBC reveals anemia that warrants transfusion.

Additional Diagnostics

Coagulation studies may be reasonable to obtain in patients with a history of coagulopathy or current anticoagulant use. Renal function tests should be performed before imaging with contrast media and in patients with suspected vasculitis. Sputum testing (Gram stain, acid-fast bacilli smear, fungal cultures, cytology) should be obtained if massive hemoptysis or an infectious cause is suspected. If a pulmonary embolus is suspected, especially if there are risk factors for deep venous thrombosis and pulmonary thromboembolism, a ventilation/perfusion lung scan should be obtained.

DIFFERENTIAL DIAGNOSIS

 Immediate emergency management is indicated for massive hemoptysis (a rate of more than 200 mL/day) which can be life threatening. Hemoptysis and pleuritic chest pain, especially in the context of malignancy, are suggestive of pulmonary embolism.

Minor hemoptysis is generally not life threatening. Despite a thorough evaluation, many patients who are seen with hemoptysis do not receive a specific diagnosis, at least not initially. The goals of further evaluation are to determine the cause, to provide specific treatment (if available), and to rule out underlying disease. The differential diagnosis is extensive and includes airway diseases, neoplasms, pulmonary vascular diseases, cardiovascular disease, and miscellaneous causes such as the use of anticoagulants or fibrinolytics. The most common cause of acute mild hemoptysis is bronchitis or infections such as pneumonia. Other common causes include lung cancer and lung abscesses, tuberculosis, bronchiectasis, and pulmonary thromboembolism. A history of recurrent pneumonia or hemoptysis with onset during adolescence suggests possible intralobular pulmonary sequestration or hereditary syndromes such as HHT, although the presentation may be mistaken for other causes such as bronchiectasis or lung abscess.[5,6] Pulmonary embolism is an important diagnosis to consider when the presentation includes hemoptysis and pleuritic chest pain or when the patient's history is significant for malignant disease, especially adenocarcinoma, which can contribute to hypercoagulation, thus increasing the risk for a pulmonary embolism.[1,7]

DIFFERENTIAL DIAGNOSIS

Hemoptysis

PULMONARY
- Bronchial adenoma
- Bronchiectasis[a]
- Bronchitis[a]
- Bronchogenic carcinoma
- Bronchopulmonary sequestration
- Cystic fibrosis
- Foreign body
- Fungal infections
- Lung abscess[a]
- Lung cancer[a]
- Metastatic tumor
- Mycetoma (aspergilloma or fungus ball)
- Noninvasive aspergillosis or mucormycosis
- Nontubercular mycobacteria
- Parasitic infection
- Pneumonia[a]
- Pulmonary contusion or trauma
- Pulmonary embolism[a]
- Pulmonary-renal syndromes (Goodpasture syndrome, systemic lupus erythematosus, Wegener granulomatosis)
- Tuberculosis[a]

CARDIOVASCULAR
- Arteriovenous malformation
- Bleeding diathesis
- Congestive heart failure[a]
- Mitral valve prolapse and mitral stenosis

MISCELLANEOUS
- Medications (anticoagulants, fibrinolytics, amiodarone)
- Pulmonary artery rupture caused by pulmonary arterial (Swan-Ganz) catheterization[a]

[a]Common causes.

INTERPROFESSIONAL COLLABORATIVE MANAGEMENT

The overall goals of management include bleeding cessation, aspiration prevention, and treatment of the underlying cause.

The most common presentation in primary care is acute mild hemoptysis caused by bronchitis. Low-risk patients with normal chest films can be treated on an outpatient basis with close monitoring and appropriate oral antibiotics, if clinically warranted. Outpatient evaluation by a pulmonologist should be considered if hemoptysis persists or if the cause remains unclear.

An abnormal mass on a chest radiograph necessitates outpatient bronchoscopy.

For patients with a normal chest radiograph and risk factors for lung cancer or recurrent hemoptysis, outpatient fiberoptic bronchoscopy is indicated to evaluate for neoplasm. High-resolution CT scan is indicated when clinical suspicion for malignancy exists, when sputum and bronchoscopy do not offer a cause, or when chest radiography demonstrates peripheral or other parenchymal disease.

Patients with negative findings on chest radiography, CT, and bronchoscopy have a low risk of malignancy and can be observed for 3 years. No specific recommendations can be made regarding chest CT or radiography during that interval, but imaging should be based on risk factors. If hemoptysis recurs, multidimensional CT angiography should be considered. Bronchoscopy may also complement imaging during the observation period.

Patients with massive hemoptysis require rapid and decisive care; diagnosis and treatment must occur simultaneously. Patients with massive hemoptysis require intensive care and early consultation with a pulmonologist. As with any potentially serious condition, evaluation of airway, breathing, and circulation is the initial step in treatment because asphyxiation is the primary cause of death. Supplemental oxygen and fluid resuscitation are crucial.

Assistance from a cardiothoracic surgeon should be considered because emergency surgical intervention may be necessary. Emergency lung resection is feasible in appropriately selected patients with radiologically localized disease and massive hemoptysis.[8]

Bronchial artery embolization is an effective immediate treatment for massive hemoptysis. Because the bleeding recurrence rate is high in patients with lung cancer or idiopathic bronchiectasis, surgery should be considered in these patients after initial stabilization by bronchial artery embolization.[9] Bronchial artery embolization may be best used as a temporizing measure in patients unsuitable for emergency lung resection.[8] Other treatments modalities for massive hemoptysis include cold saline lavage, epinephrine, and endobronchial stent tamponade.[10]

Indications for Referral or Hospitalization

The following criteria warrant referral or hospitalization:
- Causes of hemoptysis with high risk of bleeding (e.g., lesions with pulmonary artery involvement or aspergillosis)
  - Abnormal gas exchange (respiratory rate >30 breaths per minute, oxygen saturation <88% in room air, or need for high-flow oxygen [>8 L/min] or mechanical ventilation)
  - Hemodynamic instability (hemoglobin <8 g/dL [80 g/L] and/or a decrease of more than 2 g/dL [20 g/L] from patient's baseline, consumptive coagulopathy, or hypotension requiring fluid bolus or vasopressors)
  - Massive hemoptysis (>200 mL/48 hours or >50 mL per episode in patients with chronic pulmonary disease)
- Respiratory comorbidities (e.g., chronic obstructive pulmonary disease, previous pneumonectomy, cystic fibrosis
- Other comorbidities (e.g., ischemic heart disease) or medical conditions requiring anticoagulation (e.g., atrial fibrillation, artificial heart valves).[1]

COMPLICATIONS

Patients with hemoptysis resulting from noninfectious causes are at risk for frequent recurrences. Massive hemoptysis often recurs, both suddenly and without warning, and may be fatal. The most obvious complication is asphyxiation, which accounts for the majority of deaths from hemoptysis.

PATIENT AND FAMILY EDUCATION

Hemoptysis is frightening for patients and their families, and may be a symptom of serious underlying disease. Education should include:

- Information about the diagnostic evaluation
- Management is tailored to the underlying cause
- The importance of adherence to the prescribed treatment.
- Smoking cessation, given that rate of recurrence in patients who smoke is high

Because hemoptysis can be particularly disconcerting, emotional support for the patient and family is especially important.

REFERENCES

1. Earwood, J. S., & Thompson, T. D. (2015). Hemoptysis: Evaluation and management. *American Family Physician, 91*(4), 243–249.
2. Wong, B. K. Hemoptysis—massive or not. Proceedings of UCLA Healthcare, vol 18. 2014 (no page numbers).
3. Jovanovic, M., Jain, V., Galiveeti, S., & Ramasamy, V. (2014). A case of necrotising pneumonia in the setting of influenza infection. *Journal of Pulmonary & Respiratory Medicine, 4*, 201.
4. Cialoni, D., Sponsiello, N., Marabotti, C., Marroni, A., Pieri, M. Maggiorelli, F., et al. (2012). Prevalence of acute respiratory symptoms in breath-hold divers. *Undersea and Hyperbaric Medicine: Journal of the Undersea and Hyperbaric Medical Society, Inc, 39*(4), 837.
5. Sarkar, M., Dasgupta, C. S., & Goswami, A. (2015). Hereditary hemorrhagic telangiectasia: Presenting with epistaxis. *Journal of Universal Surgery, 3*(1), 9.
6. Ojha, V., Samui, P. P., & Dakshit, D. (2015). Role of endovascular embolisation in improving the quality of life in a patient suffering from complicated intralobar pulmonary sequestration—a case report. *Respiratory Medicine Case Reports.*
7. Kamouh, A., Nelson, A., Vats, S., Powell, R., & Missov, E. (2014). Pulmonary tumor thrombotic microangiopathy associated with right ventricular rupture and hemopericardium: A case report. *Journal of Cardiology Cases, 9*(6), 230–232.
8. Alexander, G. R. (2014). A retrospective review comparing the treatment outcomes of emergency lung resection for massive haemoptysis with and without preoperative bronchial artery embolization. *European Journal of Cardio-Thoracic Surgery, 45*(2), 251–255.
9. Fruchter, O., Schneer, S., Rusanov, V., Belenky, A., & Kramer, M. R. (2015). Bronchial artery embolization for massive hemoptysis: Long-term follow-up. *Asian Cardiovascular and Thoracic Annals, 23*(1), 55–60.
10. Ho, H. J., Cheng, C. Y., & Wang, B. Y. (2013). Massive hemoptysis controlled with transection of a pulmonary vein and bronchus-a case report. *Journal of Cardiothoracic Surgery, 8*(1), 1–4.

CHAPTER **91**

LUNG CANCER
Melissa C. Storms

 Red flags in patients without a diagnosis of lung cancer:

- Changes in a chronic cough should prompt consideration of malignancy.
- Weight loss of more than 10 pounds, focal skeletal pain (from bone metastases), or neurologic complaints such as headache or extremity weakness (from brain metastases) are the symptoms that most commonly indicate the presence of metastatic disease.

DEFINITION AND EPIDEMIOLOGY

Lung cancer, also referred to as *bronchogenic carcinoma*, encompasses multiple malignancies involving the lung or airways.

The vast majority of lung cancers are categorized as non–small cell lung cancer (NSCLC) or small–cell lung cancer (SCLC) based on the histologic characteristics.

Although lung cancer was notably uncommon near the turn of the 20th century, increased exposure to tobacco smoke has caused a global epidemic of lung cancer.[1] In 2017 there were projected to be an estimated 222,500 new cases of lung cancer and 155,870 deaths in the United States.[2] Although recently there has been a slight decline in the incidence of lung cancer within the United States, lung cancer remains the leading cause of cancer death among both males and females in this country. The 5-year survival rate for lung cancer as a whole is less than 20%.[3] The primary risk factor for lung cancer is cigarette smoking, which accounts for 80% to 90% of cases. Other risk factors include secondhand smoke, pipe and cigar smoking, air pollution, radiation (including radon gas), and occupational exposures such as asbestos, nickel, chromium, and arsenic.[4]

NSCLC represents approximately 80% to 85% of lung malignancies. The primary subtypes of NSCLC are adenocarcinoma (40%) and squamous cell carcinoma (25% to 30%), with the remainder consisting of large cell carcinomas and other less common variants.[5] Historically, these histologic subtypes have been grouped together as NSCLC and managed in a similar fashion, although there are some treatment considerations based on histology. SCLC comprises approximately 10% to 15% of lung cancers. Although smoking is linked with all forms of lung cancer, it is most strongly associated with SCLC and squamous cell carcinoma. Adenocarcinoma is the most common type of lung cancer in nonsmokers.

PATHOPHYSIOLOGY

The precise path that causes the malignant transformation of bronchoepithelial cells is not fully understood. Smoking tobacco is the primary cause in the vast majority of lung cancers. Yet, only approximately 10% of smokers will develop lung cancer, which points to significant host factors that may control an individual's susceptibility to cancer.[6] Carcinogens such as tobacco smoke, radon, and asbestos fibers induce tissue injury with resultant genetic and epigenetic changes. Over time these changes cause various pathways that control cellular proliferation to become dysregulated, which ultimately leads to tumor formation, invasion, and metastasis.[7] Individuals have varying inherent genetic susceptibility to these carcinogens, and epidemiologic studies suggest there can be a familial predisposition to lung cancer independent of tobacco smoke exposure.[1]

Specific acquired genetic abnormalities in non–small cell lung tumors have been identified that have significant clinical implications. The two most important of these acquired abnormalities are the epidermal growth factor receptor (*EGFR*) gene mutations and the anaplastic lymphoma kinase (*ALK*) translocations. *EGFR* mutations are present in approximately 15% of adenocarcinomas in the United States and are more commonly seen in nonsmokers, females, and individuals of Asian descent. *EGFR* mutations are found in 30% to 50% of lung cancers in Asia. *ALK* translocations are identified in approximately 4% of adenocarcinomas in the United States, most frequently in nonsmokers and younger patients. As discussed later, specific therapies targeting these molecular defects have been developed with encouraging results.[1] Tumor specimens for adenocarcinomas are now routinely being tested for these abnormalities. Other so-called driver mutations with approved target treatment include *ROS1* and *BRAF* V600E. Specific genetic abnormalities are not routinely tested in SCLC and squamous cell NSCLC.

CLINICAL PRESENTATION AND PHYSICAL EXAMINATION

The majority of patients are symptomatic at presentation, with the most common symptoms being cough (up to 75% of cases), weight loss (up to 68%), dyspnea (up to 60%), chest pain (up to 49%), and hemoptysis (up to 35%). Cough is particularly seen with squamous cell carcinomas and small cell carcinomas owing to their tendency to involve central airways, whereas adenocarcinomas are more often peripherally located. Although cough is common in a smoking population in general, changes in a chronic cough should prompt consideration of malignancy. In addition, recurrent pneumonias in a similar anatomic area may indicate a neoplasm causing postobstructive changes, and further investigation is warranted.[8]

Although lung cancer can spread to any organ, the most common sites of metastasis are the liver, bones, adrenal glands, and brain. About a third of patients will have symptoms caused by distant metastasis at presentation. Weight loss of more than 10 pounds, focal skeletal pain (from bone metastases), or neurologic complaints such as headache or extremity weakness (from brain metastases) are the symptoms that most commonly indicate the presence of metastatic disease. Nonspecific symptoms of anorexia, weight loss, and/or fatigue are also common.[8] Signs, symptoms, and associated syndromes of lung cancer are summarized in Table 91.1.

Many of the symptoms of SCLC and NSCLC are similar, but SCLC symptoms tend to progress more rapidly, typically over 8 to 12 weeks. NSCLC has a slower tempo, with tumor growth typically seen over many months.

On physical examination, the signs that most commonly indicate metastatic disease are palpable lymphadenopathy greater than 1 cm, bone tenderness, hepatomegaly, focal neurologic findings, or a soft tissue mass. Lung cancer is also a common cause of superior vena cava syndrome, with the corresponding physical exam findings of facial edema and plethora, dilated neck veins, and a prominent venous pattern on the chest.[8] In addition, as with other malignancies, lung cancer is a hypercoagulable state, and patients may have deep vein thrombosis on presentation.

DIAGNOSTICS
Essential Diagnostics

Lung cancer may initially be detected on a screening low-dose computed tomography (CT) scan. This is recommended by the U.S. Preventive Services Task Force (USPSTF) in adults aged 55 to 80 years who have a 30 pack-year smoking history and currently smoke or have quit within the past 15 years. Screening should be discontinued once a person has not smoked for 15 years, develops a life-limiting medical condition, or if the patient would not be willing or able to receive curative therapy.[9]

When lung cancer is suspected based on an abnormal screening CT scan or history and physical examination findings, laboratory evaluation and imaging are indicated as summarized in the Initial Diagnostics box. If there is no prior imaging, most patients will initially undergo a chest radiograph. If this is abnormal or the clinical suspicion remains high, a contrast-enhanced CT scan of the thorax should be

TABLE 91.1	Signs, Symptoms, and Syndromes of Lung Cancer
Extent of Disease	**Associated Signs, Symptoms, and Syndromes**
Primary tumor in the lung	Cough, dyspnea, hemoptysis, chest pain or discomfort
Tumor spread to regional nodes or intrathoracic structures	Dyspnea from airway compression as a result of bulky adenopathy Pain and dyspnea from pleural or chest wall involvement Hoarseness caused by recurrent laryngeal nerve palsy (particularly with left-sided tumors) Pancoast tumor: a superior sulcus tumor that causes shoulder and arm pain as a result of brachial plexus involvement Horner syndrome (unilateral ptosis, meiosis, and lack of facial sweating): caused by ipsilateral invasion of the sympathetic chain Superior vena cava (SVC) syndrome: tumors obstructing the SVC will cause neck and facial swelling, dilated neck veins, and dyspnea
Metastatic disease	Weight loss and generalized fatigue are more common in metastatic disease. Bone metastases may cause bone pain or pathologic fractures. Lesions are usually osteolytic. Adrenal metastases may rarely cause adrenal insufficiency. Brain metastases can cause headache, weakness, nausea and vomiting, and seizures, although they may be asymptomatic as well. Liver metastases can cause pain and hepatomegaly. Liver function tests will frequently be normal until very advanced. Pleural or pericardial effusions may cause pain or dyspnea.
Paraneoplastic syndromes	Hypercalcemia results from bony metastases or tumor secretion of parathyroid hormone–related peptide. This may cause altered mental status, constipation, nausea, polyuria, and dehydration. Syndrome of inappropriate antidiuretic hormone (SIADH) causes hyponatremia and is more commonly seen with SCLC. Paraneoplastic neurologic syndromes are most commonly associated with SCLC. These include Lambert-Eaton myasthenic syndrome, cerebellar ataxia, and limbic encephalitis.

SCLC, Small cell lung cancer.
Data from Ost, D. E., Yeung, S. C., Tanoue, L. T., & Gould, M. K. (2013). Clinical and organizational factors in the initial evaluation of patients with lung cancer: Diagnosis and management of lung cancer (3rd ed.): American College of Chest Physicians evidence-based clinical practice guidelines. *Chest, 143*(5). E121–E141.

performed that includes the liver and the adrenal glands. If the CT findings are suspicious for lung cancer, most patients will then undergo a procedure to confirm the diagnosis. Modalities for obtaining a cytologic or histologic diagnosis include sputum cytology, CT-guided needle biopsy, bronchoscopy including endobronchial ultrasound, thoracentesis with cytologic examination of pleural fluid, and surgical approaches including mediastinoscopy. Biopsy specimens determine the histology, and also provide tissue for molecular analysis (including testing for an EGFR mutation or ALK rearrangement) in adenocarcinomas. In NSCLC, tissue may also be tested for expression of the programmed death-ligand 1 (PD-L1), which may affect treatment decisions. If there is insufficient tissue for molecular analysis and/or PD-L1, then a liquid biopsy (i.e., blood draw) can be performed to garner that information.

Once a tissue diagnosis is confirmed, staging is completed with an evaluation of any sites of suspected metastatic disease, which is most often done with a positron emission tomography (PET) scan. Given the propensity for SCLC to metastasize to the brain, all patients with SCLC undergo brain imaging with magnetic resonance imaging (MRI) or CT scan. Brain imaging is also indicated in patients with NSCLC with seemingly more advanced disease, or if there are any neurologic signs or symptoms.

Regarding laboratory studies, it is appropriate to perform a complete blood count (CBC) and a comprehensive metabolic panel (CMP). Patients with lung cancer often have abnormal blood counts including anemia, leukocytosis, and/or thrombocytosis. The CMP provides insight into possible paraneoplastic electrolyte disturbances, including syndrome of inappropriate antidiuretic hormone (SIADH) and hypercalcemia, as well as abnormalities in liver function tests (in the setting of advanced liver metastases) and elevation in alkaline phosphatase (seen with bone metastases).

In general, the goal of this initial evaluation is to confirm the diagnosis and to establish the stage (i.e., the extent of disease). Staging considerations can be complex, and referral to a thoracic oncology program or a pulmonologist is indicated if the initial evaluation suggests likely lung cancer.

INITIAL DIAGNOSTICS

Lung Cancer

LABORATORY
- Complete blood count
- Comprehensive metabolic panel, including liver function tests

IMAGING
- Chest radiograph: optional
- Contrast-enhanced computed tomography (CT) scan of the thorax (including the liver and adrenals)
- Positron emission tomography/CT scan
- Magnetic resonance imaging or CT of the brain

Staging for NSCLC is based on the TNM (tumor, nodes, metastasis) system and is described in detail in the American Joint Committee on Cancer (AJCC) cancer staging manual.[10] The tumor stage (T1 to T4) is based on the size, location, and involvement of adjacent structures. The nodal stage (N1 to N3) is divided into three categories: N1 (ipsilateral peribronchial or hilar lymph nodes), N2 (ipsilateral mediastinal nodes), and N3 (contralateral or supraclavicular nodes). Metastatic (M)

spread is present or absent. A simplified schema of staging and treatment is presented in Table 91.2. Staging will help identify patients who are candidates for curative therapies (surgery or definitive chemoradiation) as opposed to palliative therapies (chemotherapy and/or radiation therapy). SCLC uses a more simplified staging scheme wherein disease is determined to be either limited stage or extensive stage.

DIFFERENTIAL DIAGNOSIS

 Priority differentials include: (1) infection, (2) granuloma, and (3) metastatic lesion from another cancer.

Pulmonary nodules (<3 cm in size) can be benign (e.g., infections, granulomas) or malignant. The larger the nodule or mass (>3 cm in size), the more likely it is to be malignant. Metastases from another cancer (e.g., melanoma, renal cell carcinoma, breast cancer, or colorectal cancer) may sometimes manifest as a solitary lesion, although typically metastases have multiple foci on presentation.

INTERPROFESSIONAL COLLABORATIVE MANAGEMENT

In general, the management of lung cancer involves one or a combination of treatment modalities, including surgery, radiation therapy, chemotherapy, targeted therapy, immunotherapy, or best supportive care. As discussed later, the treatment strategy is determined by the type of lung cancer (NSCLC vs. SCLC), stage, performance status, pulmonary status, comorbidities, and patient preferences. Performance status (usually assessed by either the Karnofsky scale or ECOG [Eastern Cooperative Oncology Group] scale) is a particularly important consideration because patients with poor functional status may derive less or no benefit from certain treatments, and a supportive approach with palliative care may be the optimal course.

Pharmacologic Management

Stage I and II Non–Small Cell Lung Cancer. Surgery is the primary curative therapy for early-stage lung cancer (stages I and II). With the pathologic type of staging assessment, overall survival rates at 5 years for stage I NSCLC are approximately 70% to 80%, and 50% to 60% for stage II.[11] Unfortunately, only 25% of patients in the United States will be at these early stages on presentation.[12] Surgical resection typically involves lobectomy (removal of one lung lobe) or pneumonectomy (removal of the entire lung). At the time of the surgery, the surgeon will also perform mediastinal lymph node sampling to allow for complete pathologic staging of the tumor. For patients who have stage I NSCLC according to the final pathologic assessment, there is typically no additional therapy after surgery, though the American Cancer Society notes that adjuvant chemotherapy can be recommended in some instances, but further research is needed.

For patients with resected stage II NSCLC, adjuvant chemotherapy improves survival and is generally recommended.[12]

Some patients do not wish to undergo surgery or are not candidates because of comorbidities or poor pulmonary reserve. For patients who have stage I tumors (i.e., small tumors without apparent spread to the lymph nodes), an increasingly used treatment is stereotactic body radiation therapy (SBRT). In general, radiation therapy delivers energy to kill malignant cells. With conventional radiation therapy, a specific amount of energy called a *fraction* is delivered daily to a specific target,

TABLE 91.2 Simplified Schema for Staging and Treatment of Lung Cancer

Stage	Simplified Staging Description	Typical Treatment Strategies
NON–SMALL CELL LUNG CANCER		
I	Small tumors without any lymph node involvement	Surgical resection Stereotactic body radiation therapy (SBRT) for nonsurgical candidates
II	Medium-sized tumors that may invade adjacent structures (i.e., chest wall) OR Smaller tumors that have also spread to ipsilateral non-mediastinal (e.g., hilar) lymph nodes	Surgical resection with consideration of adjuvant chemotherapy Definitive chemotherapy or radiation for nonsurgical candidates
IIIA	All but the largest tumors that have also spread to the ipsilateral mediastinal and/or subcarinal lymph nodes OR The largest tumors (i.e., those that invade structures such as the heart, great vessels, trachea, vertebral body) but have not yet spread to the mediastinal lymph nodes	An area of ongoing debate May involve preoperative chemotherapy with or without radiation followed by surgery, *or* definitive chemotherapy and radiation therapy
IIIB	Any size tumor that has also spread to the mediastinal lymph nodes on the opposite side or to any supraclavicular lymph nodes OR The largest tumors (as earlier) that have also spread to mediastinal lymph nodes on the same side	Not considered resectable Definitive chemotherapy and radiation therapy
IV	Tumors that have spread to distant sites (e.g., bone, brain, adrenals, or contralateral lung) or that cause malignant pericardial or pleural effusions	Not curable Palliative treatment involving chemotherapy, immunotherapy, and/or targeted therapy
SMALL CELL LUNG CANCER		
Limited	Disease that can be encompassed within one radiation port and that generally corresponds to one hemithorax with the associated lymph nodes	Chemotherapy and radiation
Extensive	Disease that has spread beyond the hemithorax or to distant sites	Palliative chemotherapy

Lung cancer staging and treatment are an evolving and complex science, and this table does not represent all the nuances of current staging or treatment. It is meant to give a general practitioner a working knowledge of the basic categories. For a more accurate and in-depth depiction of current staging, please refer to Rami-Porta, R., Asamura, H., Travis, W., & Rusch, V. W. (2017). Lung cancer—major changes in the American Joint Committee on Cancer eighth edition cancer staging manual. *Cancer, 67*(2), 139–155.

and treatment may last for weeks. More recently, the technique of SBRT has allowed radiation oncologists to deliver the entire amount of energy in a single fraction or over just a few fractions to a very exact, though relatively small, targeted area. For nonsurgical candidates with stage II disease (i.e., larger tumors or those that have spread to hilar lymph nodes), a combination of chemotherapy and conventional radiation therapy is usually employed.

Stage III Non–Small Cell Lung Cancer. Most patients with stage III disease are treated with curative intent, although the 5-year overall survival is between 13% and 36%.[11] Treatment of stage III tumors is an area of controversy in lung cancer management, particularly for stage IIIA, wherein the precise role and timing of surgery remains unclear. Some patients with stage IIIA tumors will receive preoperative chemotherapy or chemoradiation therapy followed by surgical resection, others may receive definitive chemoradiation therapy without surgery, and some may have surgery followed by chemotherapy or radiation therapy. Stage IIIB tumors are considered unresectable, and the primary treatment is definitive chemoradiation therapy.[13]

Stage IV Non–Small Cell Lung Cancer. Stage IV or metastatic NSCLC is not considered curable. Treatment is palliative with the goals of reducing symptoms, improving quality of life, and prolonging survival. Systemic therapy is the mainstay of treatment. In good performance status patients, chemotherapy alone has led to 1-year survival rates of 40% and 2-year survival rates of 20%. The median overall survival for metastatic NSCLC is 10 to 12 months.[14]

Survival may be longer in patients with predictive biomarkers, including those with targetable genetic alterations or PD-L1 positivity. Patients who do not have good performance status (i.e., those who spend 50% or more of their time in bed) typically do not benefit from chemotherapy, and best supportive care is recommended.

An important advance in treatment has been the development of targeted therapies directed at specific molecular defects that have been found in nonsquamous lung cancer cells. Oral tyrosine kinase inhibitors (TKIs) exist for the *EGFR* mutation, *ALK* rearrangement, *ROS1* rearrangement, and *BRAF* V600E mutation. The targeted treatments can result in significant tumor response with fewer side effects and treatment-related deaths compared with conventional chemotherapy. For example, osimertinib, an oral third-generation EGFR-TKI has led to progression-free survival of 19 months and 80% 2-year overall survival.[15] Unfortunately, despite the often dramatic initial responses to treatment, these agents are not curative and eventually the tumors will progress.

Immunotherapy is another important treatment option for patients with metastatic NSCLC. Immune checkpoint inhibitors work by inhibiting the programmed cell death protein 1 (PD-1) receptor or PD-L1, which enhances the antitumor immune response. In first-line treatment, immunotherapy may be used as a single agent (in patients with PD-L1 positivity) or in combination with doublet chemotherapy (in nonsquamous NSCLC). If not used in the first-line setting, immunotherapy is recommended for subsequent therapy at the time of disease progression. When compared to chemotherapy, immunotherapy has improved survival, longer duration of response, and fewer severe treatment-related adverse events (AEs).[16]

In addition to systemic therapy for metastatic disease, radiation therapy is frequently employed to palliate specific symptomatic areas such as painful bone metastases, lesions that are obstructing airways, or brain metastases causing cerebral edema. Unfortunately, virtually all patients with stage IV NSCLC will die of their disease, and therefore addressing the palliative care needs of these patients is crucial.

Small Cell Lung Cancer

SCLC grows extremely rapidly, and therefore the majority of patients have metastatic disease at diagnosis. Even in patients who do not have apparent metastatic sites, the assumption is generally that they have "occult" micrometastases. Therefore, surgery does not play a significant role in the management of SCLC. The specific treatment for SCLC is based on the determination of whether the disease is limited stage or extensive stage. For limited-stage SCLC, treatment involves combined chemotherapy and radiation therapy. Although SCLC often responds very well initially to chemotherapy, the majority of patients will relapse. The median survival in limited stage disease is 30 months, with a 2-year overall survival around 50%.[17] Extensive-stage SCLC is not curable, and chemotherapy is the mainstay of treatment. Median survival is 9 to 11 months, and only 5% of patients are alive at 2 years.[18]

INDICATIONS FOR REFERRAL OR HOSPITALIZATION

When lung cancer is suspected, basic imaging and laboratory tests should be performed. When the suspicion remains high or is confirmed, referral is indicated, ideally to a full-service, multidisciplinary thoracic oncology program that has pulmonologists, thoracic surgeons, thoracic radiologists, and medical and radiation oncologists. If such a thoracic oncology program is not readily available, a pulmonologist can guide the initial staging and biopsy evaluation.

Although there is no clearly identified optimal time frame for the staging and diagnostic evaluation, a reasonable expectation would be that a prompt and efficient diagnostic evaluation take place over 2 to 4 weeks and that treatment be initiated within 1 month after diagnosis. This time frame may need to be adjusted based on patient-specific factors such as the tempo of disease, patient anxiety, and patient comorbidities.[8]

Of note, surgical outcomes in lung cancer are better when surgery is performed by board-certified thoracic surgeons with a focus on lung cancer, and thus national guidelines recommend lung cancer surgery be performed in high-volume settings.[16]

There are several presentations (potential oncologic emergencies) in patients with known or suspected lung cancer that require more urgent or emergent evaluation:

- Severe back pain, particularly if associated with neurologic deficits (weakness, bowel or bladder changes, saddle

anesthesia) may indicate spinal cord compression or cauda equina syndrome.
- Dyspnea with plethora and dilated neck veins can be seen with superior vena cava syndrome.
- Rapidly progressive or severe respiratory compromise may be the result of a large effusion, a lesion causing airway obstruction, or a pulmonary embolism.
- Seizures, focal neurologic deficits, or altered mental status may indicate brain metastases.
- Altered mental status, lethargy, and evidence of dehydration can be seen with severe hypercalcemia.
- Unilateral lower extremity edema and pain may indicate venous thrombosis.
- Severe pain from a metastatic lesion, particularly a bone metastasis, that cannot be easily controlled with oral analgesics may require parenteral narcotics.
- Fever in a patient receiving chemotherapy requires urgent evaluation and treatment, especially in the context of neutropenia.
- In patients receiving immunotherapy, immune-mediated toxicities (particularly pneumonitis and colitis) require prompt evaluation and treatment.

LIFE-SPAN CONSIDERATIONS

When making treatment decisions, age should always be considered in the context of comorbidities and performance status. The "functional age" of a patient is more important than the chronologic age. Older patients who are fit and have good performance status can be considered for similar treatment options as younger patients. However, a more individualized, case-by-case approach is likely better for patients with borderline performance status (i.e., symptomatic but out of bed more than 50% of the day) and/or who are very elderly. For patients with metastatic NSCLC who have poor performance status (i.e., in bed more than 50% of the day), treatment is unlikely to improve quality of life or survival, except in rare instances when the tumor possesses an *EGFR* mutation or *ALK* rearrangement and targeted agents can be used. For all other patients with poor performance status, best supportive care is the most appropriate treatment option.

COMPLICATIONS

With lung cancer there can be many complications associated with both the underlying malignancy and the treatments. Patients may require urgent evaluation and treatment for disease-related conditions, including epidural spinal cord compression, superior vena cava syndrome, hypercalcemia, pain crises, and venous thrombosis. Treatment with chemotherapy and/or immunotherapy also has many potential side effects, including chemotherapy-induced neutropenic fever and immune-mediated toxicities. It is important to note that because of improvements over the past 2 decades in antiemetics, notably the development of 5-hydroxytryptamine$_3$ (5-HT$_3$) receptor antagonists such as ondansetron, the burden of chemotherapy nausea and vomiting for the regimens typically used in the lung cancer treatment has been significantly reduced.

PATIENT AND FAMILY EDUCATION AND HEALTH PROMOTION

The most pressing issue in lung cancer remains preventing exposure to tobacco smoke to stop new cases from developing. A smoker has 20 times the risk of developing lung cancer compared with a person who has never smoked. For individuals who do stop smoking, the risk of lung cancer diminishes significantly over time, although in the long term it still remains at least twice that of an individual who never smoked.[1] It is never too late to stop smoking. Continued smoking after diagnosis with lung cancer is associated with second primary cancers, treatment complications, and decreased survival.[16]

Given the high prevalence and lethality of lung cancer, many studies have focused on early detection and screening. The National Lung Screening Trial (NSLT), a large, randomized controlled trial involving more than 50,000 participants, showed a 20% decrease in lung cancer mortality in heavy smokers who were screened with annual low-dose CT scans for 3 years.[19] Based on these results, multiple medical societies, including the USPSTF and the American Cancer Society, now recommend lung cancer screening for high-risk individuals. Although this is a promising development, most likely smoking-prevention and smoking-cessation efforts will have a greater ability to reduce lung cancer–associated morbidity and mortality.

For those who have been treated with curative intent for lung cancer, issues of survivorship and surveillance may fall into the domain of the primary care provider. Specific guidelines vary by stage and treatment, but the National Comprehensive Cancer Network generally recommends that patients have follow-up appointments and surveillance CT scans of the chest every 3 to 6 months for 3 years, every 6 to 12 months until year 5, and then annually. The purpose is to detect recurrences and new primaries. Smoking cessation interventions are critical, and smoking status should be assessed at each visit. In addition, patients should be encouraged to maintain a healthy weight and an active lifestyle. Alcohol consumption should be limited. Routine PET scans are not considered beneficial and are not recommended.[16]

REFERENCES

1. Niederhuber, J. E., Armitage, J. O., Doroshow, J. H., Kastan, M. B., & Tepper, J. E. (Eds.), (2014). *Abeloff's clinical oncology* (5th ed.). Philadelphia: Churchill Livingstone.
2. American Cancer Society. Key statistics for lung cancer. Retrieved from https://www.cancer.org/cancer/non-small-cell-lung-cancer/about/key-statistics.html. (Accessed 6 November 2017).
3. American Cancer Society. Cancer facts and statistics, 2017 estimates. Retrieved from https://cancerstatisticscenter.cancer.org/?_ga=2.176624032.489626778.1509987087-1610671551.1503416458#!/. (Accessed 6 November 2017).
4. Alberg, A. J., Brock, M. V., Ford, J. G., Samet, J. M., & Spivack, S. D. (2013). Epidemiology of lung cancer. In Diagnosis and management of lung cancer (3rd ed): American College of Chest Physicians evidence-based clinical practice guidelines. *Chest, 143*(5), E1–E29.
5. American Cancer Society. What is non–small cell lung cancer? Retrieved from https://www.cancer.org/cancer/non-small-cell-lung-cancer/about/what-is-non-small-cell-lung-cancer.html. (Accessed December 15, 2017).
6. Nana-Sinkam, S. P., & Powell, C. A. (2013). Molecular biology of lung cancer. In Diagnosis and management of lung cancer (3rd ed): American College of Chest Physicians evidence-based clinical practice guidelines. *Chest, 143*(5), E30–E39.
7. Herbst, R. S., Heymach, J. V., & Lippman, S. M. (2008). Lung cancer. *The New England Journal of Medicine, 359*(13), 1367–1380.
8. Ost, D. E., Yeung, S. C., Tanoue, L. T., & Gould, M. K. (2013). Clinical and organizational factors in the initial evaluation of patients with lung cancer. In Diagnosis and management of lung cancer (3rd ed): American College of Chest Physicians evidence-based clinical practice guidelines. *Chest, 143*(5), E121–E141.
9. U.S. Preventive Services Task Force. Final Update Summary: Lung Cancer: Screening. July 2015. Retrieved from https://www.uspreventiveservicestaskforce.org/Page/Document/UpdateSummaryFinal/lung-cancer-screening. (Accessed December 15, 2017).
10. Edge, S., Byrd, D., & Compton, C. (2010). *AJCC cancer staging manual* (7th ed.). Chicago: Springer.
11. Detterbeck, F., Boffa, D., Kim, A., & Tanoue, L. (2017). The eighth edition lung cancer stage classification. *Chest, 151*(1), 193–203.
12. Howington, J. A., Blum, M. G., Chang, A. C., Balekian, A. A., & Murthy, S. C. (2013). Treatment of stage I and II non–small cell lung cancer. In Diagnosis and management of lung cancer (3rd ed): American College of Chest Physicians evidence-based clinical practice guidelines. *Chest, 143*(5 Suppl.), e278S–e313S.
13. Ramnath, N., Dilling, T. J., Harris, L. J., et al. (2013). Treatment of stage III non–small cell lung cancer. In Diagnosis and management of lung cancer (3rd ed): American College of Chest Physicians evidence-based clinical practice guidelines. *Chest, 143*(Suppl. 5), e314S–e340S.
14. Reck, M., Rodriguez-Abreu, D., Robinson, A., et al. (2016). Pembrolizumab versus chemotherapy for PD-L1-positive non-small-cell lung cancer. *The New England Journal of Medicine, 375*(19), 1823–1833.
15. Soria, J., Ohe, Y., Vansteenkiste, J., et al. (2018). Osimertinib in untreated *EGFR*-mutated advanced non-small-cell lung cancer. *The New England Journal of Medicine, 378*(2), 113–125.
16. National Comprehensive Cancer Network (NCCN). Clinical practice guidelines in oncology. Non–small cell lung cancer. Retrieved from www.nccn.org/professionals/physician_gls/pdf/nscl.pdf. (Accessed Dec 29, 2017).
17. Faivre-Finn, C., Snee, M., Ashcroft, L., et al. (2017). Concurrent once-daily versus twice-daily chemoradiotherapy in patients with limited-stage small-cell lung cancer (CONVERT): An open-label, phase 3, randomized, superiority trial. *The Lancet Oncology, 18*, 1116–1125.
18. National Comprehensive Cancer Network (NCCN). Clinical practice guidelines in oncology. Small cell lung cancer. Retrieved from https://www.nccn.org/professionals/physician_gls/pdf/sclc.pdf. (Accessed Dec 29, 2017).
19. National Lung Screening Trial Research Team, Aberle, D. R., Adams, A. M., et al. (2011). Reduced lung-cancer mortality with low-dose computed tomographic screening. *The New England Journal of Medicine, 365*(5), 395–409.

CHAPTER **92**

PLEURAL EFFUSIONS AND PLEURISY

Patricia Polgar-Bailey

PLEURAL EFFUSIONS

Definition and Epidemiology

A pleural effusion is an abnormal amount of fluid within the pleural space. The pleura, a serous, semitransparent, elastic membrane, covers the lung parenchyma, mediastinum, diaphragm, and rib cage, and is divided into the parietal and visceral pleurae. The parietal pleura lines the chest cavity, covering the chest wall, diaphragm, and mediastinum. It contains sensory nerves, and its blood supply comes from the systemic circulation and hence has hydrostatic pressure. The visceral pleura covers the entire surface of both lungs, including the interlobular fissures, and contains no pain fibers. Its blood flow is supplied by branches of the pulmonary circulation. The parietal and visceral pleurae are continuous at the hilum, where they are penetrated by both the pulmonary and bronchial vessels. The pleural space is an area approximately 10 to 20 mm in width, situated between the mesothelium of the parietal and visceral pleurae. Pleural fluid is normally produced in quantities just sufficient to lubricate the parietal and visceral surfaces. This small amount of fluid is constantly replenished and reabsorbed; absorption is principally through the lymphatic system. Approximately 0.16 to 0.36 mL of fluid per kilogram is normally contained within the pleural space, with a total volume of less than 20 mL and total fluid flow of 100 to 200 mL, unless some disease process or trauma has caused fluid or solid tissue to collect there.

More than 1.5 million persons develop pleural effusions each year in the United States.[1] A common manifestation of many pulmonary and systemic diseases, pleural effusions are frequently associated with congestive heart failure (CHF) but can result from a variety of other disorders. These include pulmonary tuberculosis, pulmonary embolus, and other lung diseases; chest injury or trauma; abdominal infections or pancreatitis; cancers, including lung, breast, and lymphoma; and connective tissue diseases, such as rheumatoid arthritis and lupus. Pregnancy and certain types of surgery (e.g., heart, lung, abdominal, and organ transplantation) also increase the risk for development of pleural effusions. Medical therapeutics, including radiotherapy and some medications (e.g., nitrofurantoin and amiodarone), are also associated with the development of pleural effusions. More than 90% of all pleural effusions in developed countries are caused by CHF, malignancy, pneumonia, and pulmonary embolism. Tuberculosis is a common cause of pleural effusions in tuberculosis endemic areas.[1] Viral infections are a common cause of pleural inflammation, which often manifests as pleural effusions. Some of the most common viruses implicated in the development of pleural effusions include influenza, coxsackievirus, respiratory syncytial virus (RSV), cytomegalovirus (CMV), adenovirus, human herpesvirus 8 (HHV-8), dengue virus, human T-lymphotropic virus 1 (HTLV-1), simian virus 40 (SV40), parvovirus B19, varicella, herpes simplex virus (HSV), and Epstein-Barr virus (EBV).[3] Although a malignant cause is always a concern with pleural effusions, at least 60 benign causes of pleural effusions have been identified and benign causes are at least twice as likely as malignant causes in most epidemiologic series.[2]

Pathophysiology

An increased amount of fluid (an effusion) accumulates in the pleural space whenever the rate of fluid formation exceeds the rate of fluid absorption. Numerous conditions may lead to pleural effusions, including viral and bacterial infections, neoplasms, thromboemboli, cardiovascular dysfunction, and immunologic dysfunction (Box 92.1). Mechanisms that contribute to increased pleural fluid accumulation include an increase in microvascular pressure (e.g., CHF), a decrease in plasma osmotic pressure (e.g., hypoalbuminemia), an increase in the permeability of microcirculation (e.g., pneumonia), a decrease in pleural pressure (e.g., atelectasis), an impaired lymphatic drainage from pleural spaces (e.g., malignant effusions), and the movement of fluid across the diaphragm from the peritoneal cavity (e.g., inflammation from acute pancreatitis). Parapneumonic effusions are the most common type of effusion and are associated with bacterial infections such as pneumonia, lung abscesses, and bronchiectasis.[4] Malignant pleural effusions are a common problem encountered in persons with advanced cancer and are generally associated with significant symptom burden and mortality. Lung cancer in men and breast cancer in women are the most common causes of malignant pleural effusions.[5] Other common causes of malignant pleural effusions include lymphomas and genitourinary tract and gastrointestinal tract tumors.[5]

Pleural effusions are often categorized as transudates and exudates on the basis of the amount of protein detected in the pleural fluid. Exudative pleural effusions result primarily from pleural and lung inflammation (e.g., pneumonia) or

---

BOX **92.1**

Potential Causes of Pleural Effusions

- Amyloidosis
- Atelectasis
- Benign asbestos-related effusions
- CHF (most common cause)
- Cirrhosis
- Drug-induced effusions
- Endocrine dysfunction
- Esophageal perforation
- Hemothorax
- Hepatic and splenic abscesses
- Immune conditions
  - Rheumatoid arthritis
  - Systemic lupus erythematosus
  - Sjögren syndrome
  - Wegner granulomatosis
  - Ankylosing spondylitis
  - Churg-Strauss syndrome
  - Sarcoidosis
- Infectious conditions (most common causes of exudative effusions)
  - Bacterial
  - Tuberculosis
  - Fungal
  - Viral (respiratory, cardiac, hepatic)
  - Parasitic
- Intra-abdominal abscesses
- Malignant disease
  - Primary lung cancer
  - Metastatic disease to pleura (most commonly in lung and breast carcinomas)
  - Mesothelioma
- Medications
  - Amiodarone
  - Bromocriptine
  - Dantrolene
  - Metronidazole
  - Nitrofurantoin
  - Procarbazine
- Nephrotic syndrome
- Pancreatic disease
- Peritoneal dialysis
- Peritonitis
- Pneumonia
- Postoperative
  - Postcardiac surgery
  - Lung transplantation
  - Abdominal surgery
- Pulmonary embolism
- Radiotherapy
- Viral illness, including human immunodeficiency virus (HIV) and acquired immunodeficiency syndrome (AIDS)

CHF, Congestive heart failure.
Modified from Quinn, T., Alam, N., Aminazad, A., Marshall, M. B., & Choong, C. K. (2013). Decision making and algorithm for the management of pleural effusions. *Thoracic Surgery Clinics, 23*, 11–16.

impaired lymphatic drainage of the pleural space (e.g., malignant disease). In fact, a variety of disease mechanisms, including pneumonia and other infections, malignant carcinomas, immunologic and lymphatic abnormalities, and iatrogenic factors, can cause exudates. Transudative effusions develop when systemic factors alter the formation or absorption of pleural fluid, rather than from pleuritic disease. They are produced by imbalances in hydrostatic and osmotic pressures across the pleural membrane and are usually bilateral. Transudates have a lower specific gravity and lower concentrations of protein and lactate dehydrogenase compared with exudative effusions. CHF is probably the most common cause of transudative pleural effusions, but other disease processes that cause movement of fluid from the peritoneal space or retroperitoneal space, such as cirrhosis, nephrosis, and glomerulonephritis, can cause transudates.

Age-related changes affecting the respiratory system play an important role in the development of pleural effusions. In addition to the expected changes related to aging, years of exposure to particulate matter, dust, occupational toxins, and episodic respiratory infections increase the risk for development of a pleural effusion.

Clinical Presentation and Physical Examination

Persons with pleural effusions often are asymptomatic when they are seen initially. When symptoms do occur, the most common presenting complaints include dyspnea, nonproductive cough, pleuritic chest pain, and activity intolerance. Dyspnea often increases with recumbent positions, and cough tends to worsen as the size of the effusion increases. Pleuritic pain is associated with inflammation of the parietal pleura and is caused by irritation of its sensory fibers. This pain is often sharp, unilateral, and localized to the affected area, although it may also be experienced in the lower chest and ipsilateral shoulder or referred to the abdomen. Exacerbating factors include deep inspiration, cough, and other movement of the upper body. Constrictive pericarditis is a relatively common cause of pleural effusions, and chest pain and dyspnea are common associated symptoms.[6]

Malignant tumors involving the parietal pleura generally cause steady, dull pain compared with the sharp, intermittent pain associated with an acute inflammatory process. Pleural effusions cause compression of adjacent lung tissue and reduce the amount of possible lung expansion, which may result in varying degrees of dyspnea, depending on the size and functional status of the underlying lung and the rate of fluid accumulation. However, dyspnea does not necessarily correlate with blood oxygen levels or the size of the pleural effusion but rather seems to be related to the increased thoracic cage size, which affects respiratory muscle function. Dyspnea is a common presenting symptom associated with malignant pleural effusions and is occasionally accompanied by chest pain and cough. Chest pain is usually related to involvement of the parietal pleura, ribs and intercostal muscles, and other structures. The nonproductive cough is generally a result of lung compression and bronchial irritation. Associated constitutional symptoms include weight loss, malaise, and anorexia.

A thorough history is important and can be helpful in discriminating between the symptoms associated with the effusion and those of the primary underlying pathophysiologic process. Information about the presence of fever, cough, sputum production, dyspnea, or abdominal pain should be elicited. Past medical history, including systemic and chronic illnesses, previous surgeries, prior exposures (such as to tuberculosis and asbestos), and previous alcohol abuse, is important.

Physical examination findings can be suggestive of a pleural effusion; however, the clinical manifestations of the effusion may be overshadowed by the underlying disease process. Common exam findings include decreased or absent breath sounds over the effusion, decreased respiratory excursion, dullness to percussion, reduced or absent tactile fremitus, and decreased or absent bronchial breath sounds, sometimes with egophony (E-to-A change) at the upper fluid borders. Pleural inflammation is often accompanied by a friction rub that is transitory and that generally disappears as fluid accumulates in the pleural space. Small effusions (<500 mL) may be associated with minimum or no findings. In situations in which effusions are greater (>1500 mL) or pulmonary compromise is more substantial, the use of accessory muscles of respiration, inspiratory lag, cyanosis, bulging intercostal margins, mediastinal shift, and jugular vein distention may be evident. In addition to assessing the respiratory status, the provider needs to perform a complete physical examination to identify signs that may be manifestations of systemic or acute illness and suggest the cause of the effusion. For example, nonthoracic signs such as jugular vein distention and an S_3 gallop are suggestive of CHF. A right ventricular heave or thrombophlebitis suggests pulmonary embolus. Lymphadenopathy or hepatosplenomegaly may be associated with hepatic disease, and ascites may be indicative of a hepatic cause.

Diagnostics

Essential Diagnostics. Once a pleural effusion is suspected, a chest radiograph should be obtained to confirm its presence and to look for other abnormalities that might help determine its cause. Normal amounts of fluid are not visible on chest radiographs; effusions of 200 mL of fluid can be detected on posteroanterior radiography and as little as 50 mL of fluid on lateral radiography.[1] Effusions that are detected appear as blunting and medial displacement of the sharp costophrenic angle, pleura-based densities, infiltrates, hilar adenopathy, or signs of CHF. A subpulmonary effusion is suspected if the diaphragm is elevated. Although chest radiographs are limited in their ability to diagnosis pleural effusions and do not attain 100% sensitivity until pleural effusions are more than 500 mL,[5] they can provide other diagnostic clues to the cause of the effusion. For example, large unilateral effusions usually shift the mediastinum to the contralateral hemithorax, and lack of such a shift with a large effusion may indicate a bronchial obstruction, lung tumor, mesothelioma, or fixed mediastinum from tumor or fibrosis.

Although most pleural effusions are seen on chest films, several conditions other than pleural effusions may produce similar findings. Chest ultrasound and computed tomography (CT) are more reliable for detection and localization of small pleural effusions.[5] Smaller effusions should be confirmed by ultrasonography, which will detect effusions of 5 to 50 mL and is 100% sensitive for effusions of more than 100 mL. Ultrasonography is also more sensitive than CT in detecting pleural fluid septations.[1] In addition to their use in detecting smaller effusions, ultrasound examinations are used to guide diagnostic thoracentesis, resulting in improved yield and decreased complication rates. One of the benefits of chest CT is that it allows imaging of the underlying lung parenchyma or mediastinum and thereby permits identification of possible causes of the pleural effusion, such as pulmonary, bronchial, or pleural malignancy. In addition, chest CT can characterize the effusion in terms of its size and location and the presence of loculations.[5]

Additional Diagnostics. Positron emission tomography (PET) scans are helpful in the evaluation of malignant pleural effusions.[5]

Once a pleural effusion has been discovered, identification of the disease process, procedure, or drug that caused the effusion is essential. Diagnostic evaluation relies heavily on examination of pleural fluid obtained by thoracentesis. Guidelines recommendations affirm that, whenever possible, thoracentesis be performed with ultrasound guidance to increase the likelihood of successful aspiration and to mitigate the risk of organ puncture. The odds ratio for pneumothorax with ultrasonography compared with without is 0.3 to 0.8 and associated with overall lower hospital costs.[1] The pleural fluid should always be sampled unless the underlying cause of the effusion has already been established. Although a definitive diagnosis, such as the finding of malignant cells, can be established in only 25% of cases, relevant information (from fluid analyses, including cellular counts, chemistry profiles, cultures, and stains) that is useful for clinical decision-making and for exclusion of certain causes of a pleural effusion is obtained in an additional 15% to 20% of cases. In certain situations, when the clinical diagnosis and cause of the effusion are relatively secure and the clinical course is uncomplicated (e.g., uncomplicated CHF, small effusions after thoracic or abdominal surgery, postpartum effusion), therapy may be initiated and a thoracentesis performed only if the response to therapy is inadequate. However, whenever the cause of a pleural effusion is unclear, a diagnostic thoracentesis is generally warranted.[6]

Thoracentesis has no absolute contraindications. However, relative contraindications include bleeding diathesis or systemic anticoagulation, small volume of pleural fluid, mechanical ventilation, patient's inability to cooperate, and cutaneous disease such as herpes zoster infection at the needle entry site. Preprocedure laboratory studies should include a complete blood count (CBC), prothrombin time, and partial thromboplastin time. Coagulation therapy should be considered if the platelet count is less than 50,000/µL or if the clotting time is prolonged.[5] The complication rate of thoracentesis is approximately 20% and includes pain at the puncture site, cutaneous and internal bleeding, pneumothorax, cough, empyema, and spleen or liver puncture; therefore it is essential to obtain informed consent before the procedure is initiated. The most common complications are vagal reactions and pneumothoraces.[5]

Other tests needed to establish a definitive diagnosis may include a CT scan of the chest, thoracoscopy, fiberoptic bronchoscopy, and pleural biopsy. A thoracotomy should be performed only if other diagnostic tests have not been helpful.[5] A chest CT scan is not obtained initially to confirm the presence of a pleural effusion; it is most useful after thoracentesis for further evaluation of suspected parenchymal or pleural abnormalities. Cytologic examination of the pleural fluid is an efficient and minimally invasive method to establish a diagnosis of cancer. Fiberoptic bronchoscopy can be useful if an endobronchial malignancy is suspected, especially if symptoms include hemoptysis and stridor, because biopsy specimens can be taken at the time of the procedure.[5] Thoracoscopy allows for direct visualization of the visceral and parietal pleura, and biopsy of the pleura can be done simultaneously. Thoracoscopy is usually performed with the patient under general anesthesia, but it can also be done using local anesthesia or sedation.[5] Open pleural biopsy is required when other procedures have failed to provide a diagnosis.[6] It can be done using local anesthesia. Multiple biopsy specimens (at least four) should be taken at one site. Pleural biopsy can help to establish a diagnosis of tuberculosis (sensitivity >85%), malignancy (sensitivity 45% to 60%), and amyloidosis.[5] Contraindications include thrombocytopenia (platelet count <50,000 µ/L), skin infections at the site of incision, small effusions (because of risk of injury to infradiaphragmatic viscera), and severe respiratory disease (because of risk of pneumothorax). Potential complications of pleural biopsy include hemothorax, pneumothorax, superficial and pleural infection, and injury to the liver or spleen.[5] In 15% of pleural effusions, the cause is not identified, despite repeated cytology and pleural biopsy.[5]

INITIAL DIAGNOSTICS

LABORATORY
- Pleural fluid analysis (protein, lactate dehydrogenase, pH, cholesterol [including in exudative effusion], white blood cells, red blood cells, cultures, cytology, acid-fast bacilli)

IMAGING
- Chest X-ray examination
- Ultrasound[a]
- Computed tomography scan[a]
- Thoracoscopy[a]
- Positron emission tomography scan[a]

OTHER DIAGNOSTICS
- Thoracentesis[a]
- Fiberoptic bronchoscopy[a]
- Pleural biopsy[a]

[a]If indicated.

Differential Diagnosis

 Immediate intervention and referral required for signs and symptoms suggestive of heart failure (hypoxia and pulmonary edema), pulmonary embolism (dyspnea, pleuritic chest pain, and recent immobilization) and malignancy (lung mass or history of cancer).

A number of diseases, including pneumothorax, pulmonary embolism, CHF, neoplasms, trauma, and tuberculosis, can cause symptoms similar to those characteristic of pleural effusions. Once a pleural effusion has been established, the differential diagnosis is based on the presence of transudative or exudative effusions, although a number of conditions can cause both. A transudative pleural effusion is generally associated with a systemic condition rather than with a pleural disease. An exudate usually suggests a pathologic condition that specifically involves the pleural space. Pleural fluid characterized by high erythrocyte counts (>100,000/mm³) is most often seen in cases of trauma, malignant disease, and pulmonary embolism. Other laboratory evaluations, such as a pleural fluid eosinophil count, glucose concentration, and pH, can be used to help distinguish among the potential causes of the effusion. A predominance of neutrophils in the pleural fluid suggests that an acute process, such as pancreatitis, may be affecting the pleura.

A pleural fluid eosinophilia of greater than 10% is most often caused by blood or air in the pleural space and is uncommon in patients with cancer or tuberculosis, unless there is a history of repeated thoracenteses. Pleural effusions with a low glucose concentration (<60 mg/dL) suggest a complicated parapneumonia or malignant effusion. Lactate dehydrogenase correlates positively with the degree of pleural inflammation. If the lactate dehydrogenase level increases with repeated thoracenteses, it suggests that the degree of inflammation is increasing, and it is important to aggressively pursue a diagnosis.

Less common causes of pleural effusions with associated clinical cues include abdominal abscess, cirrhosis, endometriosis, postpartum effusion, mesothelioma, nephrotic syndrome, and rheumatoid arthritis.[1]

Interprofessional Collaborative Management

Management. Management is based on treatment of the cause of the effusion, and a number of specialists may be needed, depending on the cause. In addition, symptomatic treatment is aimed at making the patient more comfortable, beginning when the evaluation is initiated and while the underlying cause is being treated. When an effusion is large, the removal of only 300 to 500 mL through thoracentesis may result in a marked decrease in dyspnea. Indomethacin is often used successfully to treat pleuritic pain and does not suppress respirations, as do narcotics. Malignant pleural effusions, especially in the face of advanced disease, are generally difficult to treat, and management often focuses on providing comfort measures. Some effusions are caused by viral infections and most often resolve without medical intervention.

Indications for Referral or Hospitalization

The evaluation and treatment of a pleural effusion depend on the underlying disease process, degree of respiratory distress, and other contributory factors such as coexisting health problems. Persons without evidence of respiratory compromise can often be assessed and treated on an outpatient basis. Those with substantial respiratory compromise should be admitted to the hospital for further evaluation and treatment. Referral to a specialist is necessary to establish a definitive diagnosis and management plan.

Complications

Complications depend on the cause and extent of the effusion, accompanying respiratory or systemic compromise, comorbid conditions, and treatment modalities available. Malignant pleural effusions are a major cause of morbidity in cancer patients with advanced disease. Treatment is usually palliative, although treatment of the primary malignant neoplasm and temporizing symptomatic relief (e.g., repeated thoracentesis for recurrent effusions) may be helpful.

Patient and Family Education

Education varies, depending on the cause of the pleural effusion. In all cases, teaching must include:

- An explanation of the diagnostic tests, such as thoracentesis, and the potential for chest tube placement and any additional surgical procedures
- Relief of uncomfortable symptoms, such as dyspnea and pain, and assistance with activity intolerance.

Because multiple specialists are often involved in the evaluation of a pleural effusion, the health care provider's role in coordinating care and keeping the patient well informed and at the focus of decision-making is essential.

PLEURISY
Definition and Epidemiology

Pleurisy, also known as pleuritis, is an inflammation of the pleura. The chest pain of pleurisy is caused when the pleural layers rub together and pain fibers in the parietal pleura are stimulated. Pleurisy is not a diagnosis but rather a possible symptom of numerous localized and systemic disease processes.[7] Pleuritic pain is usually described as sharp or stabbing; it is generally exacerbated by deep breathing, coughing, or sneezing, and it is usually experienced over the lower portion of the chest.

Pathophysiology

Pleurisy is caused by pleuritis, which is an inflammation of the pleural lining, with or without pleural effusion. The pleural layers are highly permeable and in close contact with microcirculation, which makes them responsive to local or systemic immunologic or inflammatory processes. Pleurisy has a variety of causes; it sometimes develops with excess fluid in the pleural cavity (wet pleurisy) and sometimes without (dry pleurisy). Secondary pleurisy is the result of some other chest disease, such as pneumonia, tuberculosis, or lung abscess, in which germs reach the pleura as well as the lungs and cause inflammation.

The most common causes of pleuritis include viral and bacterial infections, as well as tuberculosis in areas of high tuberculosis prevalence.[8] Other common causes of pleuritis include pulmonary infarction and connective tissue diseases such as lupus erythematosus. Trauma to the chest wall is a less common cause of pleurisy, as is coronary bypass or valve replacement surgery (postpericardiotomy syndrome).[9]

Pleurisy is rarely caused by malignant processes; malignant tumors that involve the pleura generally cause a steady, dull pain compared with the sharp, stabbing, intermittent pain associated with pleural inflammation. Certain drugs, including nitrofurantoin, methotrexate, and procarbazine, have been associated with pleurisy.[9]

Clinical Presentation and Physical Examination

A thorough history is instrumental in determining the differential diagnosis for any type of chest pain. Pain on breathing (which may be mild to severe, depending on the degree of inflammation) and a stabbing or shooting chest pain are characteristics of pleurisy. Pain is usually localized, but sometimes the pain may be felt in the shoulder. Milder pleurisy may be described as a "stitch in the side." Pleuritic pain is generally made worse by breathing, deep inspiration or chest movement, or forced breathing movements such as coughing, sneezing, or talking. Patients will often adopt a position that limits movement of the affected area. The most comfortable position for the patient is often lying on the affected side, which limits expansion of the chest wall.

The physical examination in pleuritic pain can reveal increased tenderness with deep palpation, usually located directly over the site of inflammation. Rapid and shallow breathing may be associated symptoms, with limited chest wall expansion on the affected side. Percussion over the affected area may be dull if there is underlying consolidation or pleural effusion. Increased or diminished fremitus may also denote the presence or absence of consolidation. A pleural friction rub, which varies in intensity from a faint scratching sound to a loud creak, confirms the diagnosis of pleurisy. However, the absence of a pleural friction rub does not negate the presence of pleurisy because the presence of pleural fluid may mitigate or even nullify the rub.

A pleural friction rub may be heard during both phases of respiration but is often most pronounced at or near the end of inspiration. It disappears when patients hold their breath. A pleural friction rub may be localized or heard over a wider area and is generally most audible over the lateral and posterior regions of the inferior thorax. It is rarely heard over the upper thorax and lung apexes because of the limited movement of the lung in these areas compared with the lung bases. In general, a rub is heard only if the person takes a deep breath; a rub, even if it is present, is not audible during splinting or shallow breathing. Crackles can sometimes sound similar to a rub, but a cough usually diminishes crackles and has no effect on a rub. A sound similar to a pleural friction rub can be produced by sliding a stethoscope over the skin; firm pressure of the stethoscope on the skin should eliminate this "false rub" and intensify the sound of a real friction rub if it is present.

Pleuritic inflammation can sometimes lead to pleural effusions. Pleural effusions often ease the pain temporarily by providing a cushion between the inflamed membranes and, as a result, give a false sense of improvement when the situation is really getting worse. Large collections of pleural fluid can compress the lungs and further compromise respiration.

Some common symptoms associated with pleurisy may also suggest the underlying disease process giving rise to the pleurisy. A cough productive of purulent sputum may indicate an underlying lung disease, such as pneumothorax, pneumonia, tuberculosis, or pulmonary embolism.[7] Fever and chills suggest an underlying infectious process. Rigors can sometimes occur with bacterial pneumonia. Joint pain or rashes raise the suspicion of an underlying connective tissue disorder.

Diagnostics

Essential Diagnostics. Several laboratory tests, although not diagnostic of pleurisy, may help elucidate the underlying cause. An elevated leukocyte count with a shift to the left suggests a bacterial infection such as pneumonia, an esophageal rupture, or an abscess. Leukopenia may reflect a viral process or lupus erythematosus. A chest X-ray examination may help diagnose bacterial pneumonia, pneumothorax, esophageal rupture, or problems below the diaphragm, such as a subphrenic abscess or effusion.

Additional Diagnostics. Thoracentesis and pleural fluid analysis can help identify the underlying cause once the existence of a pleural effusion has been established. If the cause of the pleurisy is still unclear, other studies, including CT scan of the chest, ventilation/perfusion scan, pleural biopsy, and esophageal contrast studies, may be indicated.

> **INITIAL DIAGNOSTICS**
>
> ## Pleural Effusions
>
> **LABORATORY**
> - Complete blood count/differential
> - Pleural fluid analysis[a]
>
> **IMAGING**
> - Chest X-ray examination
> - Computed tomography scan[a]
> - Ventilation/perfusion scan[a]
>
> **OTHER DIAGNOSTICS**
> - Thoracentesis[a]
>
> ---
> [a]If indicated.

Differential Diagnosis

 Immediate intervention required for cardiac pain (angina, acute myocardial infarction, dissecting aortic aneurysm) often characterized by pain radiating to the neck, jaw, or arms which worsens with exertion, which is not characteristic of pleurisy.

Problems that originate in other chest wall structures can produce pain similar to that of pleurisy; these conditions include pneumothorax, rib fractures, costochondritis, vertebral fractures, and nerve root pain from herpes zoster infection. The presence of a pleural friction rub confirms the pleuritis, but a patient history, physical examination, and pertinent diagnostic tests are still necessary to determine the most likely differential diagnosis.

Pleural effusion is a finding commonly associated with pleurisy and may be helpful in determining the diagnosis. Viral infections, rheumatic disease, and sarcoidosis often cause pleurisy in the absence of a pleural effusion. In contrast, pneumonia, *Mycobacterium tuberculosis* infection, lupus pleuritis, and postcardiac injury syndrome are typically associated with pleural effusions.

The patient's history may be helpful in narrowing the differential diagnosis. For example, a recent leg fracture with casting raises the possibility of a pulmonary embolism. Occupational asbestos exposure might suggest asbestos pleurisy. A history of lupus erythematosus or sarcoidosis increases the suspicion of systemic connective tissue disease as the underlying cause of the pleurisy.[10]

Many types of pain experienced in the chest area are not pleuritic. Cardiac chest pain is often central and diffuse and is described as a pressing or squeezing rather than a sharp and intermittent pain. Pericardial pain can be similar in character to pleuritic pain but is usually felt on the anterior side of the chest and back and is exacerbated by lying down. Chronic chest pain is not usually a result of parenchymal lung disease because the lung and visceral pleura are not innervated by pain fibers.

Interprofessional Collaborative Management

The management of pleurisy is based on treatment of the underlying disease. Comanagement with a specialist is necessary for all except the most benign causes of pleural inflammation. Drainage of the pleural space may be indicated if a pleural effusion is present. Certain systemic causes of inflammation, such as lupus erythematosus, respond well to corticosteroids. Nonsteroidal antiinflammatory drugs are used to provide symptomatic pain relief. Malignant diseases rarely cause pleurisy, and pleurisy usually resolves with appropriate and prompt treatment.

Indications for Referral or Hospitalization

A referral is often necessary to determine or to treat the underlying cause of the pleurisy. The requisite evaluation and management depend on the cause of the inflammation. Patients without evidence of respiratory compromise or acute illness can often be evaluated and treated on an outpatient basis. Patients with more significant respiratory compromise or highly contagious disease (e.g., active pulmonary tuberculosis) may need to be hospitalized for further evaluation and treatment.

Complications

The extent and complications of pleural inflammation depend on the underlying disease process. Some causes are self-limited and have no chronic sequelae or complications. If the inflammation is chronic or pleural repair processes cause fibrosis, an inelastic membrane (pleural peel) may form around the lung. This membrane causes lung entrapment and impairs respiratory function.[9]

Patient and Family Education

Patient education varies according to the cause of the pleurisy. Teaching must include:

- An explanation of and rationale for all diagnostic tests
- Symptomatic relief

As in all cases in which multiple practitioners may be involved, the role of the health care provider is important in coordinating care and in keeping the patient well informed and at the focus of decision-making.

REFERENCES

1. Saguil, A., Wyrick, K., & Hallgren, J. (2014). Diagnostic approach to pleural effusions. *American Family Physician, 90*(2), 99–104.
2. Thomas, R., & Lee, Y. C. (2013). Causes and management of common benign pleural effusions. *Thoracic Surgery Clinics, 23*, 25–42.
3. Nestor, J., Huggins, T., Kummerfeldt, C., DiVietro, M., Walters, K., & Sahn, S. (2013). Viral diseases affecting the pleura. *Journal of Clinical Virology, 58*, 367–373.
4. Davies, H. E., Davies, R. J., Davies, C. W., et al. (2010). Management of pleural infection in adults: British Thoracic Society pleural disease guideline 2010. *Thorax, 65*(Suppl. 2), ii41–ii53.
5. Quinn, T., Alam, N., Aminazad, A., Marshall, M. B., & Choong, C. K. (2013). Decision making and algorithm for the management of pleural effusions. *Thoracic Surgery Clinics, 23*, 11–16.
6. Warnick, S. J., & Morgeson, J. S. (2010). Recurrent pleural effusions and a normal cardiac CT. *The Journal of Family Practice, 59*(8), 9–12.
7. Robinson, T. (2011). Identification, assessment and management of pleurisy. *Nursing Standard, 25*(31), 43–48.
8. Jiang, J., Shi, H. Z., Liang, Q. L., et al. (2007). Diagnostic value of interferon-γ in tuberculosis pleurisy: A metaanalysis. *Chest, 131*, 1133–1141.
9. Kelly, B., Nicholas, J., Chhablani, R., et al. (2000). The postpericardiotomy syndrome as a cause of pleurisy in rehabilitation patients. *Archives of Physical Medicine and Rehabilitation, 81*, 517–518.
10. Palavutitotai, N., Buppajarntham, T., & Katchamart, W. (2014). Etiologies and outcomes of pleural effusions in patients with systemic lupus erythematosus. *Journal of Clinical Rheumatology: Practical Reports on Rheumatic and Musculoskeletal Diseases, 20*(8), 418–421.

CHAPTER 93

PNEUMONIA
Geri Cage Reeves

DEFINITION AND EPIDEMIOLOGY

Pneumonia remains one of the leading causes of morbidity and mortality in the United States, especially in older adults and in those with underlying chronic disease. In 2015, pneumonia and influenza combined were ranked as the eighth leading cause of death in the United States, with the majority of deaths attributable to pneumonia.[1] Worldwide, in children younger than 5 years, pneumonia is the second leading cause of death.[2] The number of hospitalizations for community-acquired pneumonia (CAP) is comparable with that for malignant neoplasms and exceeds hospitalizations for myocardial infarct and diabetes mellitus combined. In the United States the annual direct cost of CAP is more than 17 billion dollars.[3,4]

The Infectious Diseases Society of America (IDSA) defines CAP as an acute infection of the pulmonary parenchyma that is frequently associated with at least two symptoms of active infection, occurring in individuals who have not been hospitalized or resided in a long-term care facility for 14 days before the onset of symptoms.[5] Hospital-acquired pneumonia (HAP; aka nosocomial pneumonia) is defined as pneumonia that occurs 48 hours or more after hospital admission that did not appear to be incubating at the time of admission. Ventilator-associated pneumonia (VAP) is defined as a type of HAP that develops more than 48 hours after endotracheal intubation. Health care–associated pneumonia (HCAP), a relatively new clinical entity, is defined as pneumonia that occurs in a nonhospitalized patient with extensive health care contact, as defined by one or more of the following: intravenous therapy, wound care, or intravenous chemotherapy during the prior 30 days; residence in a nursing home or other long-term care facility; hospitalization in an acute care hospital for 2 or more days during the prior 90 days; or attendance at a hospital or hemodialysis clinic during the prior 30 days.[5]

PATHOPHYSIOLOGY

The lungs are usually a sterile environment maintained by a host of natural defenses. The airways act as a filtration and humidification system for inspired air. Epithelial cells line the entire respiratory tract and contain cilia that constantly beat upward toward the pharynx. This action is a physical means of elimination of foreign material. In addition, an intact gag reflex prevents the entry of particles, mucus, and food debris. Finally, the immune system is responsible for defense mechanisms, such as the action of phagocytes, macrophages, neutrophils, complement, and immunoglobulins, which retard advancement of pathogenic organisms that do gain access to this normally sterile environment.

In the healthy adult, these host mechanisms prevent disease much of the time. However, a number of mechanisms allow pathogens to gain entry into the lungs; these mechanisms include an altered level of consciousness from stroke, seizure, anesthesia, alcohol abuse, intoxication, and the sleep state. Epiglottic closure may be compromised in these situations and allow normal oral flora to gain entry. Certain other conditions may predispose an individual to recurrent pneumonia. These include compromised immune function, cystic fibrosis, esophageal abnormalities, bronchial obstruction, and bronchiectasis.

Pneumonia can be classified as typical and atypical, although the clinical presentation is often similar.[7] Typical pneumonia is caused by organisms such as *Streptococcus pneumoniae*, which accounts for 60% to 70% of all bacterial CAP cases. Atypical pneumonia, so called because the organisms are not detectable on Gram stain or cultivatable on standard bacteriologic media, is caused by *Mycoplasma pneumoniae*, *Chlamydophila pneumoniae*, *Legionella* species, and respiratory viruses.[5] In addition, patients are more likely to be exposed to certain types of pneumonia according to the setting. The most common causes of CAP in outpatients include *S. pneumoniae*, *M. pneumoniae*, *Haemophilus influenzae*, *C. pneumoniae*, and respiratory viruses.[5] Common pathogens in inpatient, non–intensive care unit (ICU) settings include *S. pneumoniae*, *M. pneumoniae*, *C. pneumoniae*, *H. influenzae*, *Legionella* species, and respiratory viruses. Common causes in inpatient ICU settings include *S. pneumoniae*, *Staphylococcus aureus*, *Legionella* species, gram-negative bacilli, and *H. influenzae*.

Comorbidities also influence susceptibility to different types of pneumonia. *Moraxella catarrhalis* and *Klebsiella pneumoniae* infections are more commonly diagnosed when there is coexistent alcoholism. *S. aureus* and *H. influenzae* infections often occur after a primary influenza infection. *M. catarrhalis*, a gram-negative organism not thought to be pathogenic, is most commonly found in those with chronic lung conditions such as chronic obstructive pulmonary disease (COPD). It is also found in patients with other underlying chronic lung conditions such as malignant disease, with steroid use, and with diabetes.[8]

Another organism responsible for pneumonia is *Legionella pneumophila*. This organism was first implicated in 1976 after 182 people became ill in Philadelphia while attending an American Legion convention. The organism is a gram-negative bacillus that survives in water and soil. Contamination with the organism is acquired through inhalation of aerosolized droplets, thus making air-conditioning ventilating systems an obvious reservoir.

Clues to the specific cause of the pneumonia can be found in the patient's history. The CAPs include the organisms found in Table 93.1.

The incidence of some causes of pneumonia is linked to the season of the year and the geographic area. Influenza illness in the winter increases the prevalence of secondary *S. pneumoniae*, *S. aureus*, and *H. influenzae* pneumonias. *H. influenzae* is known to have a short incubation period and moves through communities quickly. Mycoplasmal infection usually moves through communities slowly because of a longer incubation period and lower communicability. *Legionella* organisms have been known to infect a large number of people simultaneously by infecting many within a group from a single reservoir.

CLINICAL PRESENTATION AND PHYSICAL EXAMINATION

In most cases of CAP, diagnosis is made by history and physical examination; identification of the causative agent is usually not necessary. Although the list of organisms causing CAP is long and increasing, relatively few organisms are responsible for most cases of pneumonia. In primary care practice, two of the most important issues related to pneumonia are awareness of the most common infectious pathogens and their treatment and decisions about the appropriateness of outpatient treatment. The clinical presentation of pneumonia includes

---

TABLE 93.1 **Epidemiologic Characteristics Related to Specific Pathogens in Community-Acquired Pneumonia**

Condition	Commonly Encountered Pathogens
Alcoholism	*Streptococcus pneumoniae*, oral anaerobes, *Klebsiella pneumoniae*, *Acinetobacter* species, *Mycobacterium tuberculosis*
COPD or smoking	*Haemophilus influenzae*, *Pseudomonas aeruginosa*, *Legionella* species, *S. pneumoniae*, *Moraxella catarrhalis*, *Chlamydophila pneumoniae*
Aspiration	Gram-negative enteric pathogens, oral anaerobes
Lung abscess	CA-MRSA, oral anaerobes, endemic fungal pneumonia, *M. tuberculosis*, atypical mycobacteria
Exposure to bat or bird droppings	*Histoplasma capsulatum*
Exposure to birds	*Chlamydophila psittaci* (if poultry: avian influenza)
Exposure to rabbits	*Francisella tularensis*
Exposure to farm animals or parturient cats	*Coxiella burnetii* (Q fever)
HIV infection (early)	*S. pneumoniae*, *H. influenzae*, *M. tuberculosis*
HIV infection (late)	The pathogens listed for early infection plus *Pneumocystis jiroveci*, *Cryptococcus*, *Histoplasma*, *Aspergillus*, atypical mycobacteria (especially *Mycobacterium kansasii*), *P. aeruginosa*
Hotel or cruise ship stay in previous 2 weeks	*Legionella* species
Travel to or residence in southwestern United States	*Coccidioides* species, hantavirus
Travel to or residence in Southeast and East Asia	*Burkholderia pseudomallei*, avian influenza, SARS
Influenza active in community	Influenza, *S. pneumoniae*, *Staphylococcus aureus*, *H. influenzae*
Cough 12 weeks with whoop or posttussive vomiting	*Bordetella pertussis*
Structural lung disease (e.g., bronchiectasis)	*P. aeruginosa*, *Burkholderia cepacia*, *S. aureus*
Injection drug use	*S. aureus*, anaerobes, *M. tuberculosis*, *S. pneumoniae*
Endobronchial obstruction	Anaerobes, *S. pneumoniae*, *H. influenzae*, *S. aureus*
In context of bioterrorism	*Bacillus anthracis* (anthrax), *Yersinia pestis* (plague), *Francisella tularensis* (tularemia)

CA-MRSA, Community-associated methicillin-resistant *Staphylococcus aureus*; *COPD*, chronic obstructive pulmonary disease; *HIV*, human immunodeficiency virus; *SARS*, severe acute respiratory syndrome.
From Mandell, L. A., Wunderink, R., Anzueto, A. et al. (2007). Infectious Diseases Society of America/American Thoracic Society consensus guidelines on the management of community-acquired pneumonia in adults. *Clin Infect Dis, 44*(Suppl 2), S27–S72.

a history of fever, chills or rigors, malaise, and cough with or without sputum production.[9] The patient may also report hemoptysis, dyspnea, and pleuritic chest symptoms. The provider should focus on symptoms of bacterial, viral, and atypical pneumonia syndromes. Chest auscultation may reveal rales that do not clear with a cough, which may be found in both bacterial and atypical pneumonia. Consolidation, including dullness to percussion, bronchial breath sounds, and egophony (E-to-A changes), is found more commonly in the bacterial pneumonia syndromes. Chest radiographs are highly variable and may be normal in the early course of the disease. In addition, chest radiographs of patients with viral and mycoplasmal pneumonia may show large infiltrates with minimum outward symptoms. A prodrome of headache and sore throat is often associated with atypical pneumonia. Patients aged 18 to 44 years are almost twice as likely as those older than 75 years to complain of pleuritic chest pain and to have fever.

Some patients (e.g., older adults) may show none of the classic signs of pneumonia but may have atypical complaints such as fatigue, lethargy, decreased appetite, increased falls, and mental status changes (such as confusion, stupor, or coma). In addition, older adults are more likely to be seen initially with tachypnea but less likely to have a cough or fever.

Bacterial Pneumonia Syndromes

Gram-Positive Bacteria. S. pneumoniae is the leading cause of pneumonia in any adult age group with or without comorbid conditions.[7,8] Those at risk for S. pneumoniae infection characteristically have some chronic condition, such as diabetes, COPD, asplenia, advanced age, cigarette smoking, congestive heart failure, dementia, alcoholism, or immunosuppression. From 20% to 60% of all hospitalized patients are infected with pneumococci.[7]

The history may include an abrupt onset of high fever with shaking chills, productive cough with purulent sputum, and possibly pleuritic-type chest pains. Physical examination may reveal signs of consolidation (egophony, increased fremitus, dullness to percussion, rales, and rhonchi), and chest films reveal single or multiple lobar consolidation. Sputum analysis by Gram stain indicates gram-positive diplococci in pairs and short chains and large numbers of polymorphonuclear leukocytes.

S. aureus, although rarely a cause of CAP, must be considered, especially after a primary influenza infection, in older adults and in those with diabetes. Suppurative conditions, including empyema, lung abscess, and pneumothorax, are common complications. Seeding to distant sites, such as bones, joints, liver, endocardium, and the meninges, may also occur.

Group A streptococci rarely cause CAP but have been found in epidemics among close groups that live together, such as military units. Symptoms may be similar to those of S. pneumoniae infection, and Gram stain reveals clumped spherical cocci, similar in appearance to a bunch of grapes.

Gram-Negative Bacteria. H. influenzae, another causative agent of CAP, is a small, gram-negative rod with a polysaccharide capsule. There are six serotypes, of which type B is the most severe and invasive (causing meningitis and sepsis). Some strains of H. influenzae are nonencapsulated and therefore cannot be typed. These are also capable of causing disease, but the disease is usually noninvasive and therefore less severe. These nontypable strains of H. influenzae are usually found in acute bronchitis. Pneumonia caused by H. influenzae is usually

caused by an encapsulated strain. Older adults and those with underlying chronic lung conditions are most susceptible to this bacterium. The history usually includes an abrupt onset of fever, shaking chills, and cough with purulent sputum. The patient may describe pleuritic chest pain, and physical examination reveals signs of consolidation. A bronchopneumonia pattern is seen on the chest radiograph.

Aerobic gram-negative bacilli rarely colonize the upper airway in healthy individuals but are often found in people with an underlying disease such as alcoholism and in those who reside in health care facilities or nursing homes. Aspiration of the organisms is thought to be the mode of infection. Pseudomonas organisms, K. pneumoniae, and Escherichia coli may also become pulmonary pathogens. The mortality rate associated with gram-negative pneumonia is relatively high compared with other types of pneumonia. Therefore a history of recent hospitalization or nursing home residency should heighten suspicion for a gram-negative pathogenesis. Polymicrobial infection is seen more often in older adults, and increased colonization of gram-negative bacilli of the upper airway is related to recent antimicrobial use, decreased activity, diabetes, and alcohol use.

M. catarrhalis is a β-lactamase–producing gram-negative aerobic diplococcus that was recently identified as a common pathogen found in individuals with COPD.[7,8] In patients with COPD, it is often the only organism isolated from the lower respiratory tract. Other chronic conditions, such as alcoholism, steroid use, diabetes, and malignant disease, increase the risk for M. catarrhalis infection. The highest incidence of this infection tends to be in the winter months.

Atypical Pneumonia Syndromes

Atypical pneumonia syndromes largely refer to pneumonias caused by nonbacterial organisms and by bacterial organisms that do not share the expected characteristics of most bacteria. M. pneumoniae is one of the most common causes of atypical pneumonia in the United States and other parts of the world. Mycoplasma infection can occur at any age, but infection rates are highest among school-aged children, military recruits, and college students.[10] This atypical pneumonia syndrome is characterized by a prodrome of fever, headache, myalgias, and dry cough. These individuals usually appear less ill than those with bacterial pneumonia. Symptoms may last up to 6 weeks and include a dry, hacking cough that may require a narcotic cough suppressant. Because of the long incubation period, mycoplasmal infection may spread slowly among family members. It should be viewed as a systemic disease with a pulmonary component.

The physical examination usually reveals fine rales with no signs of lung consolidation. A cutaneous manifestation may be present in the form of maculopapular eruptions. Rarely, examination of the tympanic membranes shows evidence of bullous myringitis, which can be very painful. Chest radiographs reveal patchy alveolar densities or nonhomogeneous segmental infiltrates. The white blood cell count may be normal or only slightly elevated. Full recovery is expected with no residual effects in a previously healthy individual. However, the disease can be severe in those with sickle cell anemia, in older adults, and in those with immunosuppression.

C. pneumoniae (TWAR strain) has a higher incidence in older adults. Transmission of the organism is thought to be person to person and has been implicated in outbreaks of pneumonia in residents of long-term care facilities, in a prison, and among military recruits.[11-13]

Symptoms are similar to those of mycoplasmal infection. Clinical presentation may include laryngitis, a hoarse voice, and nonexudative pharyngitis in addition to the symptoms described for mycoplasmal infection. Laryngitis is not present in any other atypical pneumonia syndrome. Chest radiographs may show patchy consolidation, interstitial infiltrates, or funnel-shaped lesions. The white blood cell count is usually normal.

Multiple viruses, including adenoviruses, respiratory syncytial virus (RSV), and parainfluenza virus, may also cause pneumonia. Predilection for infection in children is most common. Cytomegalovirus and *Pneumocystis* may be the cause of pneumonia in the immunocompromised host. For years, *Pneumocystis* was referred to as *Pneumocystis carinii* pneumonia (PCP) and was known to be the most common serious acquired immunodeficiency syndrome (AIDS)-defining opportunistic infection in the United States. DNA analysis demonstrated extensive diversity within the genus *Pneumocystis*, with different host species having different DNA sequences. In recognition of its genetic and functional distinctness, the organism that causes human PCP is currently named *Pneumocystis jiroveci*. Infection with hantavirus organisms was initially recognized in the southwestern United States. Caused by exposure to infected rodents (e.g., a rodent bite, breathing air contaminated with rodent excretion, or touching rodent droppings), hantavirus pulmonary syndrome (HPS) has been identified in 34 states and in countries outside the United States. A viral-like illness, HPS causes fever, myalgias, nausea, vomiting, dizziness, and thrombocytopenia.[14] HPS resembles acute respiratory distress syndrome and quickly can cause pulmonary failure.[7]

Causative agents associated with CAP include the coronavirus (CoV) responsible for severe acute respiratory syndrome (SARS), human metapneumovirus (hMPV), and community-acquired methicillin-resistant *Staphylococcus aureus* (CA-MRSA). Although SARS-CoV was not documented in humans until 2002, it has been hypothesized that a previously unknown animal CoV may have mutated and infected humans. SARS-CoV is highly contagious, so aggressive infection control measures are necessary to prevent spread of the disease. Middle East respiratory syndrome (MERS)-CoV is a more recently identified severe CoV that causes respiratory distress and death in 27% of cases.[15] MERS-CoV initially seemed to be associated with travel to the Arabian peninsula but has been identified in other countries as well.[15] Person-to-person contact is likely, but the actual cause is not yet known.[15]

Another pathogen associated with CAP is hMPV, a paramyxovirus first isolated in 2001 in children hospitalized with acute infections. Since then, hMPV has been reported in all age groups, with varying stages of disease, from those who are asymptomatic to those with severe bronchitis and pneumonia. There is no specific treatment for hMPV.[16]

CA-MRSA, a combination of well-known health care–associated strains and newer isolates with distinctive genotypes, is a virulent and resistant pathogen and causes outbreaks of serious infections, including skin and soft tissue infections and necrotizing pneumonia.[16]

RSV is an important cause of pneumonia in older adults, particularly those living in long-term care facilities. Treatment is supportive.[17]

L. pneumophila is the pulmonary pathogen responsible for legionnaires' disease. Symptoms of infection include dry cough, fever with a temperature of 38.3°C to 38.8°C (101°F to 102°F), altered mental status, relative bradycardia, headache, and gastrointestinal symptoms including diarrhea.

ESSENTIAL DIAGNOSTICS
Chest Radiography

Chest radiography is most valuable when the results are considered in the context of the history and physical examination. According to the IDSA and American Thoracic Society (ATS) guidelines, a chest radiograph is required for the routine evaluation of patients who are likely to have pneumonia, to establish the diagnosis and to aid in differentiating CAP from other common causes of cough and fever.[5] Posteroanterior and lateral chest radiographs confirm pneumonia when new infiltrates are found on the films. In addition, chest radiography may provide clues to the type of pneumonia. Bacterial patterns on the chest radiograph include lobar consolidation, cavitation, and large pleural effusions. Lobar consolidation is more common in typical pneumonia, and bilateral, diffuse infiltrates are seen more commonly in atypical pneumonia.[7] A chest radiograph that is normal does not exclude the diagnosis of pneumonia. Chest radiographs early in the course of the disease (i.e., first 24 hours) may be normal.[18] In addition, immunosuppression, dehydration, and neutropenia may result in false-negative findings. Comparison of the current chest radiograph with old radiographs is important to assess for changes. Computed tomography (CT) scan of the pulmonary system is a diagnostic consideration.[18]

Pulse Oximetry

All patients should be screened by pulse oximetry, which may suggest both the presence of pneumonia in patients without obvious signs of pneumonia and unsuspected hypoxemia in patients with diagnosed pneumonia.

ADDITIONAL DIAGNOSTICS
Sputum Analysis

Analysis of sputum can be helpful in identifying a causative agent in pneumonia; however, ATS guidelines do not recommend this diagnostic test for outpatients diagnosed with CAP.[5] Culture and Gram stain are excellent methods of identifying the pathologic agent when needed. A good sputum sample comes from the bronchial tree; it is not the same as saliva from the mouth. Although it is not usually available during the clinic visit, sputum produced on awakening in the morning is typically a good sample because of the strong reflex to cough on rising to an upright position. Sputum that contains less than 10 squamous epithelial cells and more than 25 neutrophils is considered an adequate sample. The patient is encouraged to rinse the mouth with water several times before trying to produce a sample. Inhalation of a warmed 3% to 10% saline solution may help the patient to provide an adequate sample.

Other Tests

ATS diagnostic recommendations for CAP patients requiring hospital admission include assessment of gas exchange by either telemetry or arterial sampling, complete blood count (CBC) with differential, blood chemistry, and liver function tests. Patients with severe pneumonia should have blood cultures. Patients with chronic liver disease are likely to have bacteremia with CAP. Leukopenia is also associated with a high incidence of bacteremia, so two sets of blood cultures should be obtained. Evidence for benefit of routine bronchoscopy does not exist.[5]

INITIAL DIAGNOSTICS

Pneumonia

LABORATORY
- Sputum analysis-culture and Gram stain[a]
- CBC and differential[a]
- Blood chemistries[a]
- Blood cultures[a]
- Complement fixation[a]
- Arterial blood gases[a]
- Viral culture[a]

IMAGING
- Chest X-ray examination
- CT scan[a]

OTHER DIAGNOSTICS
- Bronchoscopy[a]

[a]If indicated

DIFFERENTIAL DIAGNOSIS

 Rule out pulmonary embolus, heart failure, inflammatory lung diseases (e.g., systemic vasculitis and sarcoidosis), foreign body aspiration (especially in young children), pulmonary tumors, and tuberculosis in patients who have immigrated within the past 5 years or in those who have a history of intravenous drug use or other risk factors for human immunodeficiency virus.

Other considerations in the differential diagnosis should include asthma or COPD exacerbation, acute or chronic bronchitis, heart failure, and lung cancer.

MANAGEMENT

Nonpharmacologic Management

The treatment of pneumonia, both CAP and nosocomial, has been standardized to some degree by the publication of consensus guidelines by the IDSA and ATS. The initial management decision after diagnosis is to determine if the patient can be treated on an outpatient basis. Patients at low risk for death and who are treated appropriately in the outpatient setting do not require hospitalization. Severity assessment tools (e.g., the pneumonia severity index [PSI], CURB-65, A-DROP, SCAP) can assist in determining patients who require hospitalization. Successful treatment of pneumonia depends on the correct empirical antibiotic selection and knowledge of its proven effectiveness in vivo. A working knowledge of the organisms that most commonly infect different age groups and the habits or characteristics that put an individual at risk for specific causative agents is essential.

Pharmacologic Management

Resistance patterns to all antibiotics are an increasing problem—currently more evident and widespread than at any other time in medical history. Careful, prudent use of antibiotics is absolutely necessary to curb this growing problem. The routine practice of trying to cover for all pathogens, especially gram-negative organisms, should be avoided to decrease increased resistance. Initiation of antibiotic treatment in patients with CAP is empirically determined because the history and physical examination will not determine a specific cause of the disease. Despite the use of sputum culture, Gram stain, and chest radiographs, providers cannot always accurately identify

the causative organism. The patient's age, competency of the host immune system, underlying chronic conditions, patterns of resistance in the community, and knowledge of the most likely pathogens must be considered to accurately determine empirical antimicrobial therapy.

The recommendations for treatment of CAP are taken from the most recent guidelines and recommendations published by the ATS and IDSA in 2007.[5] Since the first publication of recommendations in 1993, there has been a shift in focus from age groups and comorbid conditions as the basis for drug selection to the most likely pathogens combined with modifying factors and coexisting cardiopulmonary disease. Empirical antibiotic therapy is based on whether the patient is being treated in an outpatient or inpatient non-ICU or ICU setting. In outpatient settings, for previously healthy individuals with no use of antimicrobial therapy within the previous 3 months, a macrolide antibiotic is recommended. Doxycycline is a secondary recommendation. For individuals with comorbidities, such as heart disease, lung disease, liver disease, renal disease, diabetes mellitus, alcoholism, malignant disease, asplenia, and immunosuppressive conditions or use of immunosuppressive drugs, a respiratory fluoroquinolone or β-lactam plus a macrolide is recommended.[5] For inpatients in non-ICU settings, a respiratory fluoroquinolone or a β-lactam antibiotic is recommended. For inpatients in ICU settings, a β-lactam (cefotaxime, ceftriaxone, or ampicillin-sulbactam) plus either azithromycin or a respiratory fluoroquinolone is recommended. For penicillin-allergic patients, a respiratory fluoroquinolone and aztreonam are recommended. Special concerns related to the selection of empirical antibiotic therapy include the possibility of *Pseudomonas* infection. In such situations, an antipneumococcal, antipseudomonal β-lactam (piperacillin-tazobactam, cefepime, imipenem, or meropenem) plus either ciprofloxacin or levofloxacin is recommended. Additional recommendations, particularly those based on level III evidence, can be found in the IDSA/ATS consensus guidelines.

Other antibiotics are also available for treatment of CAP. Recommendations for treatment of CA-MRSA include vancomycin and linezolid.[5] Linezolid, an oxazolidinone, is active against many gram-positive pathogens, including CA-MRSA, anaerobes, vancomycin-resistant enterococci, and penicillin-resistant *S. pneumoniae*. The main concern with CA-MRSA is the necrotizing aspect of the infection. Many of the treatment options mentioned before have not yet been shown to decrease toxin production. Therefore, in some situations, linezolid may be the best choice. Risk factors for other uncommon causes of CAP are included in Table 93.1.

Early treatment with oseltamivir or zanamivir is recommended for influenza A and B.[5] Intravenous peramivir is an additional treatment option. Use of oseltamivir and zanamivir is not recommended in patients with uncomplicated influenza and symptoms present for more than 48 hours' duration, but these drugs may be used to decrease the risk of viral shedding in hospitalized patients or for influenza pneumonia.

Patients with an illness comparable to influenza and with known exposure to poultry in areas with previous H1N1 infection should be tested for H1N1 and droplet precautions, and routine infection control measures should be observed. Patients with suspected H1N1 infection should be treated with oseltamivir, zanamivir, or peramivir and antibacterial agents targeting *S. pneumoniae* and *S. aureus*, the most common causes of secondary bacterial infection in patients with influenza.[5]

Older adults and those with coexisting illness are at increased risk for development of more virulent pneumonia, have longer healing times, need more supportive treatment, and require closer follow-up monitoring, especially with delayed resolution of pneumonia.

Younger individuals without comorbid disease who are infected with pneumonia usually respond more quickly and have fewer complications. According to the IDSA/ATS guidelines, patients admitted through the emergency department (ED) should receive their first dose of antibiotic while still in the ED. It is recommended that patients be switched from intravenous to oral antibiotics once they are hemodynamically stable and improving clinically, have a functioning gastrointestinal tract, and are able to tolerate oral medications.[5]

The choice of antibiotic therapy depends on careful consideration of the consequences of failure to respond to initial outpatient treatment, the need for hospitalization, and the likelihood of adherence to the treatment regimen. Other considerations include the existence of a supportive home environment, access to ED care if needed, the presence of an involved individual to identify significant changes in this illness should they occur, and the opportunity for follow-up in 24 to 48 hours. In addition, reducing health care costs while maintaining optimal care is a growing concern. Strategies for reducing the cost of antibiotic therapy include choosing monotherapy (if adequate) instead of combination therapy and using agents with longer half-lives to allow once-daily administration, which leads to improved medication adherence and decreased costs.[7] Transitioning patients to oral therapy as soon as it is clinically appropriate can significantly decrease the length of an inpatient stay, decreasing costs. Other strategies to reduce cost include avoiding agents with serious or costly side effects and avoiding agents with known resistance. In addition, avoiding agents that require therapeutic monitoring or laboratory tests or antibiotics with poor tissue penetration can reduce the costs associated with antibiotics.[7]

INDICATIONS FOR REFERRAL OR HOSPITALIZATION

 Physician consultation is usually required for delayed resolution of pneumonia and inpatient treatment.

Severity-of-illness scores, such as the CURB-65 criteria (confusion, uremia [blood urea nitrogen >20 mg/dL], respiratory rate >30 breaths per minute, low blood pressure [<90 mm Hg systolic or 60 mm Hg diastolic], age 65 years or older), or prognostic models, such as the PSI, can be used to identify patients with CAP who may be candidates for outpatient treatment.[21,22] For patients with CURB-65 scores of 2 or higher, more intensive treatment through hospitalization or intensive in-home health services is usually warranted.[5] For the PSI, patients without a history of any of the following five coexisting conditions, neoplastic disease, heart failure, cerebrovascular disease, renal disease, liver disease, or vital sign abnormalities are assigned to class I (low risk for death within 30 days). If one or more risk factors are present, the evaluation of illness proceeds to step 2. This second step stratifies the remaining patients into risk classes II, III, IV, or V, based on the total number of points assigned to each risk factor.

The use of objective admission criteria can decrease the number of patients unnecessarily hospitalized with CAP. However, it is important to keep in mind that objective criteria do not replace the health care provider's clinical judgment. Determination of subjective factors, including the patient's ability to safely and reliably take oral medication and the availability of outpatient support resources should also be considered.[5] Certain clinical criteria observed in the patient warrant hospitalization. However, the health care provider's clinical judgment always supersedes written recommendations.

LIFE-SPAN CONSIDERATIONS

Older adults have the highest rates of CAP in the United States. Advanced age is associated with a variety of age-related declines in immune system function (immune senescence) and prevalent comorbidities. As a result, elders constitute the largest immunocompromised population in the United States, putting them at risk for new infectious agents. Pathogens that are not typical causative agents of pneumonia must be considered possible causative agents in all older adults. Both clinical features and physical examination findings may be lacking or altered in older adult patients.[5] Furthermore, older adults are more likely to have CAP caused by a resistant organism or tuberculosis and to require hospital admission.[19] Supportive treatment and closer follow-up monitoring are especially important in the elderly patient with pneumonia.

Symptoms and signs of pneumonia in children may be subtle. The combination of fever and cough is suggestive of pneumonia. Other respiratory findings, such as tachypnea or increased work of breathing, may precede cough. The longer fever, cough, and respiratory findings are present, the greater the likelihood of pneumonia.[20] Older children may complain of pleuritic chest pain, but this is an inconsistent finding. Occasionally, the predominant manifestation may be abdominal pain, caused by referred pain from the lower lobes.

COMPLICATIONS

With minimum diagnostic testing and empirical antibiotic treatment, most patients will improve and show resolution of pneumonia. In most cases, improvement is seen within 48 to 72 hours after initiation of antibiotics. Pneumonia that fails to resolve shows little clinical improvement after 4 weeks of therapy. Fever, cough, sputum production, and shortness of breath may still be present. Chest radiographs also do not show improvement within this time frame.

When there is poor response to therapy, possibly the initial antibiotic choice was not correct, there was poor adherence to the oral antibiotic therapy, or the diagnosis of pneumonia was not accurate. Considerations should include the possibility of opportunistic fungal infections, *P. jiroveci*, tuberculosis, bronchogenic carcinoma, Wegener granulomatosis, bronchiolitis obliterans with organizing pneumonia, and heart failure. Diagnostic bronchoscopy, CT scan, and transthoracic needle aspiration and biopsy may be warranted to exclude these. If the diagnosis is still undetermined and there is no resolution, an open lung biopsy may be considered, and consultation with a pulmonologist is clearly warranted. Other complications of pneumonia include abscess, empyema, pulmonary vascular congestion, and pulmonary embolism.

PATIENT AND FAMILY EDUCATION AND HEALTH PROMOTION

- Provide directions for use of the antibiotic and information on potential untoward effects of the drug.

- Follow-up in 24 to 48 hours by telephone contact or in the office. This will improve adherence to the prescribed therapy, provide an opportunity to address side effects of drug therapy, and allow progress to be monitored.
- Drink adequate fluids and to use an antipyretic to control fever and myalgias when needed.

Use of cough medicines should be avoided because the cough reflex and sputum expectoration enhance removal of thick secretions. For adult patients with a constant, nonproductive cough, a narcotic such as codeine at night allows more restorative sleep.

Patients at risk for pneumonia should receive the pneumonia vaccination and should also be encouraged to receive influenza vaccination (the flu shot) each year. Avoiding smoke and contact with persons who have a respiratory infection also decreases the risk of pneumonia. In an effort to reduce the spread of respiratory infections, respiratory hygiene measures, including the use of hand hygiene and masks or tissues for patients with cough, should be used in outpatient settings and EDs. Daily exercise and a diet of healthy foods high in vitamins, nutrients, and fiber should also be encouraged.

REFERENCES

1. Murphy, S. L., Xu, J., Kochanek, K. D., Curtin, S. C., & Arias, E. Deaths: Final data for 2015. National Vital Statistics Reports Vol 66 (6).
2. Wu, J., Yang, S., Cao, Q., Ding, C., Cui, Y., Zhou, Y., et al. (2017). Pneumonia mortality in children aged <5 years in 56 countries: A retrospective analysis of trends from 1960 to 2012. *Clinical Infectious Diseases: an Official Publication of the Infectious Diseases Society of America*, 65, 1721–1728. November 15.
3. File, T. M., & Marrie, T. J. Burden of community acquired pneumonia in North American adults. Post graduate medicine. Retrieved from http://www.tandfonline.com/loi/ipgm20. (Accessed 7 December 2017).
4. Fiore, A. E., Shay, D. K., Haber, P., et al. (2007). Prevention and control of influenza: Recommendations of the Advisory Committee on Immunization Practices (ACIP) 2007. *MMWR. Recommendations and Reports: Morbidity and Mortality Weekly Report. Recommendations and Reports*, 56(RR–6), 1–54.
5. Mandell, L. A., Wunderink, R., Anzueto, A., et al. (2007). Infectious Diseases Society of America/American Thoracic Society consensus guidelines on the management of community-acquired pneumonia in adults. *Clinical Infectious Diseases: an Official Publication of the Infectious Diseases Society of America*, 44(Suppl. 2), S27–S72.
6. File, T. M., Jr. (2010). Recommendations for treatment of hospital-acquired and ventilator-associated pneumonia: Review of recent international guidelines. *Clinical Infectious Diseases: an Official Publication of the Infectious Diseases Society of America*, 51(Suppl. 1), S42–S47.
7. Lutfiyya, N. W., Henley, E., Chang, L. F., et al. (2006). Diagnosis and treatment of community-acquired pneumonia. *American Family Physician*, 73, 442–450.
8. Ariza-Prota, M., Pando-Sandoval, A., Garcia-Clemente, M., Fole-Vasquez, D., & Casan, P. Community-acquired *Moraxella catarrhalis* bacteremic pneumonia: Two case reports and review of the literature. Case Reports in Pulmonology. Vol 2016. Retrieved from http://dx.doi.org/10.1155/2016/5134969. (Accessed 7 December 2017).
9. Marrie, T. J., et al. (2015). Acute bronchitis and community-acquired pneumonia. In M. A. Grippi, J. A. Elias, J. A Fishman, R. M. Kotloff, A. I. Pack, & R. M. Senior (Eds.), *Fishman's pulmonary diseases and disorders* (5th ed.). New York: McGraw-Hill.
10. Baum, S. G. (2010). Mycoplasma pneumonia and atypical pneumonia. In G. L. Mandell, J. E. Bennett, & R. Dolin (Eds.), *Principles and practice of infectious diseases* (7th ed., p. 2481). Philadelphia: Churchill Livingstone.
11. Janssens, J. P. (2005). Pneumonia in the elderly (geriatric) population. *Current Opinion in Pulmonary Medicine*, 11, 226.
12. Oketm, I. M., Ellidokuz, H., Sevinc, C., Kilinc, O., Aksakoglu, G., Sayiner, A., et al. (2007). PCR and serology were effective for identifying *Chlamydophila pneumoniae* in a lower respiratory infection outbreak among military recruits. *Japanese Journal of Infectious Diseases*, 60, 97.
13. Conklin, L., Adjemian, J., Loo, J., Mandal, S., Davis, C., Parks, S., et al. (2013). Investigation of a *Chlamydia pneumoniae* outbreak in a federal correctional facility in Texas. *Clinical Infectious Diseases: an Official Publication of the Infectious Diseases Society of America*, 57, 639.
14. Barlam, T. F., & Kasper, D. L. (2015). Approach to the acutely ill infected febrile patient. In D. Kasper, A. Fauci, S. Hauser, D. Longo, J. Jameson, & J. Loscalzo (Eds.), *Harrison's principles of internal medicine* (19th ed.). New York: McGraw-Hill.
15. Dolin, R. (2015). Common viral respiratory infections. In D. Kasper, A. Fauci, S. Hauser, D. Longo, J. Jameson, & J. Loscalzo (Eds.), *Harrison's principles of internal medicine* (19th ed.). New York: McGraw-Hill.
16. Edwards, K. M., et al. (2013). Burden of human metapneumovirus infection in young children. *The New England Journal of Medicine*, 368, 633.
17. Loeb, M. B. (2009). Influenza and respiratory syncytial virus. In J. B. Halter, J. G. Ouslander, M. E. Tinetti, S. Studenski, K. P. High, & S. Asthana (Eds.), *Hazzard's geriatric medicine and gerontology* (6th ed.). New York: McGraw-Hill.
18. Fishman, J. A., et al. (2015). Approach to the patient with pulmonary infection. In M. A. Grippi, J. A. Elias, J. A. Fishman, R. M. Kotloff, A. I. Pack, & R. M. Senior (Eds.), *Fishman's pulmonary diseases and disorders* (5th ed.). New York: McGraw-Hill.
19. High, K. (2005). Pneumonia in older adults. *Postgraduate Medicine*, 118(4), 18–27.
20. Murphy, C. G., van de Pol, A. C., Harper, M. B., & Bachur, R. G. (2007). Clinical predictors of occult pneumonia in the febrile child. *Academic Emergency Medicine: Official Journal of the Society for Academic Emergency Medicine*, 14, 243.
21. Lim, W. S., van der Eerden, M. M., Laing, R., et al. (2003). Defining community-acquired pneumonia severity on presentation to the hospital: An international derivation study. *Thorax*, 58, 377.
22. Fine, M. J., Auble, T. E., Yealy, D. M., Hanusa, B. H., Weissfeld, L. A., Singer, D. E., et al. (1997). A prediction rule to identify low-risk patients with community-acquired pneumonia. *The New England Journal of Medicine*, 336, 243.

CHAPTER **94**

PNEUMOTHORAX

Patricia Polgar-Bailey

DEFINITION AND EPIDEMIOLOGY

Pneumothorax is defined as the presence of air in the pleural space leading to a loss of negative intrathoracic pressure. Processes leading to a pneumothorax may be spontaneous, traumatic, or iatrogenic. A spontaneous pneumothorax occurs in the absence of thoracic trauma and can be categorized into primary or secondary. A primary spontaneous pneumothorax (PSP) develops in the otherwise healthy patient without underlying lung disease or trauma. A secondary spontaneous pneumothorax occurs in the presence of underlying lung disease but in the absence of trauma. A traumatic pneumothorax may result from penetrating or blunt force trauma to the chest wall.[1] An iatrogenic pneumothorax occurs secondary to a medical procedure such as a pleural biopsy, central venous line placement, or positive-pressure mechanical ventilation.[2] Any pneumothorax, regardless of type, may evolve into a tension pneumothorax in which there is increasing positive pressure in the pleural space caused by air being able to enter but not escape.

PSP occurs most frequently in young adults aged 20 to 30.[2] Additional risk factors include cannabis or cigarette smoking, male gender, underlying lung disease, tall stature, and thin body habitus.[2] There is also evidence to suggest that pregnancy and family history may also be risk factors.

There is notable variance in the occurrence of primary pneumothorax between genders. This is evidenced by an incidence in men of 7.4 to 18 per 100,000 per year in the United States compared with 1.2 to 6 per 100,000 women per year in the United States.[3]

A pneumothorax can be potentially life threatening. Astute assessment skills and prompt intervention are essential in the diagnosis and management of pneumothorax.

PATHOPHYSIOLOGY

The exact pathophysiology of PSP is unknown but is thought to be associated with subclinical or undiagnosed lung disease. The most common cause of PSP is spontaneous rupture of pleural apical blebs, lying in or just under the visceral pleura. The cause of these blebs in otherwise healthy individuals is unclear, although smoking has been shown to play a clear role by increasing the lifetime risk for development of a pneumothorax.

A secondary pneumothorax can result from underlying pulmonary diseases such as chronic obstructive pulmonary disease, tuberculosis, lung cancer, asthma, endometriosis, and cystic fibrosis.[2] Both penetrating and blunt force trauma can cause a traumatic pneumothorax irrespective of age, sex, or underlying lung disease. An iatrogenic pneumothorax is the complication resulting from a medical procedure, including invasive procedures such as the insertion of central lines and barotrauma related to surgery or mechanical ventilation. There does not appear to be any relationship between physical activity and pneumothorax; most episodes of PSP occur at rest. Although many distinct factors may contribute to a pneumothorax, it is the loss of negative pressure when air enters the pleural space that causes the lung or a portion of it to collapse.

CLINICAL PRESENTATION AND PHYSICAL EXAMINATION

The clinical history and physical examination findings associated with a pneumothorax vary and are primarily dependent on the size of the pneumothorax (volume of air in the pleural space).[1] The pertinent history would include history of previous pneumothorax, trauma, or smoking; current medications; allergies; history of strenuous exercise; recent medical procedures and other medical conditions.

Although some patients with pneumothorax may be asymptomatic, the most common complaints are an acute onset of breathlessness and unilateral pleuritic chest pain.[1,2] In general, the symptoms associated with a secondary pneumothorax are more severe than those associated with a primary pneumothorax.

The physical findings reflect the size and nature of the pneumothorax. A tension or large pneumothorax is a medical emergency. Acute respiratory distress, diaphoresis, tachycardia, hypoxemia, tachypnea, tracheal deviation, and cyanosis are unmistakable and associated with a large or tension pneumothorax.[1,2] A smaller pneumothorax may cause mild dyspnea and chest discomfort, or the patient may be asymptomatic.

DIAGNOSTICS
Essential Diagnostics

The diagnosis of pneumothorax can generally be established by plain chest radiography, including upright posteroanterior (PA), anteroposterior (AP), and/or lateral views, and portable chest radiography remains part of the standard work-up for a suspected traumatic pneumothorax. However, chest radiography may alone be inadequate for detection of a pneumothorax as; sensitivities approximate 50%.[4] A computed tomography (CT) scan is the "gold standard" for the identification of

pneumothorax because of its ability to differentiate between a pneumothorax and underlying bullous lung disease, such as complex cystic lung disease, or when accurate size measurements are required. However, chest CT is not widely used owing to delayed diagnosis and risk for hemodynamic compromise associated with transportation out of the clinical area and generally reliable confirmation with chest radiography.

ADDITIONAL DIAGNOSTICS

Ultrasound has emerged as a reliable method of detecting pneumothorax and is especially useful in detecting small occult pneumothoraces and traumatic pneumothoraces. Pulse oximetry and arterial blood gases (ABGs) can be used to determine level of hypoxia.

DIFFERENTIAL DIAGNOSIS

 Immediate intervention required for rapidly evolving hypotension, tachypnea, tachycardia, and cyanosis which raise suspicion of a tension pneumothorax, a medical emergency.

A contralateral shift of the mediastinum and trachea can also occur with spontaneous pneumothorax and is not, in and of itself, suggestive of tension pneumothorax.[4]

Dyspnea and chest pain are identified with a large number of clinical problems. It is important to ascertain whether there has been a history of lung disease (e.g., emphysema, cancer, or chronic obstructive pulmonary disease). Many pneumothoraces occur as a result of trauma, and therefore rib fractures, contusions, costochondral separation, and muscle strains need to be excluded. Other differential diagnoses to consider include pulmonary embolism, myocardial infarction, dissecting aortic aneurysm, pleurisy, pericarditis, and costochondritis. It is useful to remember that half of all patients with PSP have at least one recurrence, making a history of pneumothorax significant.[5] The final diagnosis of pneumothorax is made once the presence of air in the pleural space, seen as a visceral pleural line that parallels the chest wall without peripheral lung markings, is identified.[6]

Diagnosis should also include the size of the pneumothorax. Size can be expressed as the percentage of lung volume lost or measurement of distance from the outer edge of the pleural space to the most apical portion of the lung margin, or conversion tools such as the Rhea method and Collins method can be used.

INTERPROFESSIONAL COLLABORATIVE MANAGEMENT

Controversy exists regarding the management of a pneumothorax.[7] Variation is based on pneumothorax type, size, and contributing factors. Treatment of pneumothorax can involve the following options: observation, needle aspiration, small-bore catheter, chest tube, chest tube plus pleurodesis, chest tube plus thoracotomy, and, very rarely, chest tube plus sternotomy. Treatment strategies may also include methods to prevent recurrence, especially in PSP.

Traditionally, no treatment is needed if the pneumothorax is small (less than 2 to 3 cm between the lung and chest wall) and the patient is clinically stable. Observation alone is appropriate for mildly symptomatic patients with small, closed pneumothoraces as well. The risks associated with observation include expansion of pneumothorax and worsening of symptoms. The need to return for care in the event of worsening symptoms must be stressed to the patient and family before discharge.

Signs of cardiopulmonary compromise and/or worsening symptoms require intervention. Simple (needle) aspiration is considered first-line treatment for all primary pneumothoraces requiring intervention. Research suggests that needle aspiration is at least as safe and effective as tube thoracostomy for management. Simple aspiration is not routinely recommended for secondary spontaneous pneumothorax because underlying lung disease is a relative contraindication. Placement of a small-bore catheter is another less-invasive option. With the catheter-over-wire or catheter-over-needle technique, a small catheter is placed into the pleural space to allow release of the accumulated air. The catheter can also be attached to a one-way valve such as a Heimlich valve. This method is recommended for PSP as well as secondary spontaneous and recurrent pneumothorax. It is not contraindicated in the patient with underlying lung disease. Small-bore catheters are not indicated in the case of a traumatic pneumothorax. The final treatment option is placement of a tube thoracostomy, commonly known as a chest tube. Tube thoracostomy involves placing a hollow plastic tube into the pleural space; the tube is left in place until the lung reexpands and the leak seals. Tube thoracostomy is indicated for traumatic pneumothorax because of its ability to drain larger volumes of air in addition to blood and other fluids. Ventilatory support may be indicated in some cases. Options to decrease the likelihood of recurrences include the instillation of chemical sclerosing agents (such as talc, doxycycline, tetracycline, or minocycline) through a chest tube or thoracoscope, laser therapy, pleural abrasion, and thoracotomy.[2,5]

Secondary spontaneous pneumothorax usually requires more aggressive management because of the decreased reserve in patients with underlying disease. These patients should almost always be hospitalized for definitive treatment and prevention.[5]

A tension pneumothorax requires immediate intervention. The diagnosis of tension pneumothorax can be made based on the clinical presentation. The clinician should not wait for radiographic confirmation to begin treatment. Treatment should be implemented immediately to prevent cardiopulmonary compromise and/or death. A large-bore angiocatheter is inserted into the pleural space at the second anterior intercostal space on the affected side. Air is released immediately, but the angiocatheter must be left in place until a chest tube can be inserted.[5]

In cases in which there is a persistent air leak or failure of the lung to reexpand, a respiratory specialist or thoracic surgeon should be consulted. In patients with human immunodeficiency virus (HIV) infection and underlying lung disease, such as cystic fibrosis, early and aggressive intervention and specialist referral are recommended.

INDICATIONS FOR REFERRAL OR HOSPITALIZATION

Outpatient treatment is reserved for those without evidence of pulmonary and cardiovascular compromise. Traditionally, a patient with a large pneumothorax requires hospitalization for chest tube placement and close monitoring.[5] Patients with secondary spontaneous pneumothorax almost always require hospitalization, as do patients with respiratory compromise. Patients with PSP, regardless of size, should be referred to a pulmonologist because of the large incidence of recurrence and the possibility of subclinical lung disease. All patients with pneumothorax (other than simple traumatic) warrant evaluation by a pulmonologist both to rule out underlying lung disease and to define clinical management. Because of the variation in treatment recommendations, the attending physician and/or pulmonologist should be consulted regarding the patient's plan of care.

LIFE-SPAN CONSIDERATIONS

Efforts should be made to minimize and to treat all possible exacerbating and complicating factors. Patients who required no intervention should refrain from air travel until resolution of the pneumothorax is confirmed by chest radiography.[4] Diving should be permanently avoided after a pneumothorax unless the patient had bilateral surgical pleurectomy.

COMPLICATIONS

Complications resulting from a large pneumothorax may include cardiac and ventilatory compromise, which can be fatal. Chest tube placement can lead to numerous complications, including pulmonary edema, lung infarction, infection, trauma, bleeding, and subcutaneous emphysema.

PATIENT AND FAMILY EDUCATION

Patient education should center on information about the cause, prevention, and treatment of a pneumothorax. Recurrence is more likely to occur in those with preexisting lung disease.[4]

- Smoking cessation when relevant. Smoking remains the only modifiable risk factor for PSP recurrence.
- Air travel and scuba diving must be avoided until resolution of the pneumothorax has been confirmed.

HEALTH PROMOTION

The focus of health promotion is aimed at smoking cessation and the elimination of trauma. Contrary to common belief, PSP typically occur at rest so avoidance of exercise to prevent recurrence is not recommended.

REFERENCES

1. Tintinalli, J. E., Kelen, G. D., Stapczynski, J. S., Ma, O. J., & Cline, D. M. (Eds.), (2010). *Tintinalli's emergency medicine* (7th ed.). New York: McGraw-Hill.
2. Bintcliffe, O., & Maskell, N. (2014). Spontaneous pneumothorax. *British Medical Journal, 348*, g2928.
3. Light, R. W. (2013). *Pleural diseases* (6th ed.). Philadelphia: Lippincott, Williams and Wilkins.
4. Noppen, M. (2010). Spontaneous pneumothorax: Epidemiology, pathophysiology and cause. *European Respiratory Review, 19*, 217–219.
5. Fauci, A. S., Braunwalkd, E., Kasper, D. L., et al. (Eds.), (2011). *Harrison's principles of internal medicine* (18th ed.). New York: McGraw-Hill.
6. Ouellet, J. F., Ball, C. G., Panebianco, N. L., & Kirkpatrick, A. W. (2011). The sonographic diagnosis of pneumothorax. *Journal of Emergencies, Trauma, and Shock, 4*(4), 504–507.
7. Brims, F. J., & Maskell, N. A. (2013). Ambulatory treatment in the management of pneumothorax: A systematic review of literature. *Thorax, 68*, 664–669.

CHAPTER 95

PULMONARY EMBOLISM

Patricia Polgar-Bailey

DEFINITION AND EPIDEMIOLOGY

Pulmonary embolism (PE) is the blockage of one or more of the pulmonary arteries or their branches by a thrombus or other embolic material that dislodges and enters the pulmonary circulation.[1,2] Emboli may be caused by thrombi, fat, or other foreign material such as parasites. The most common cause of PE is a thrombus or blood clot that has formed in the pelvis or legs.[1] The focus of this chapter is pulmonary emboli caused by thrombi.

The true incidence of PE is unknown; more than half of all PEs go undiagnosed.[3] Estimates of PE incidence range from 300,000 to 600,000 people affected each year. It is the third most common cause of cardiovascular death, with approximately 100,000 to 200,000 deaths in the United States each year.[4] Of patients with acute PE, 8% to 10% die within the first hour.[1] Many occurrences go undiagnosed and are not identified until autopsy. It is estimated that as many as one in three cases are not identified.[2] A review of clinical studies from 1939 to 2000 found the prevalence of PE diagnosed at the time of autopsy to range from 9% to 55%.[3]

PATHOPHYSIOLOGY

PE is not a disease but a complication of an underlying issue. Most frequently, the PE is the result of a thrombus that has entered pulmonary circulation.[1] Several factors contribute to susceptibility to thrombus formation, including stasis, vascular damage, and hypercoagulability.[3] Deep venous thrombosis (DVT) poses the greatest risk for PE; the thrombus develops most commonly in the lower extremities and pelvis.[1] The deep vein thrombus dislodges from the originating vessel, travels through the venous system, enters the lung via the right ventricle, and partially or completely occludes one or more of the pulmonary arteries or its branches or one or more of the pulmonary arteries or its branches.[1] The resulting hemodynamic response is dependent on the size of the embolism, cardiopulmonary reserve, and other neurohumoral effects.[2] It is estimated that 10% of emboli will cause pulmonary infarction.[1]

Clinical Presentation and Physical Examination

The clinical presentation is nonspecific and varies greatly, making the diagnosis of PE difficult. A key piece of the clinical picture is the patient's history. Those with a recent history of surgery, trauma, long bone fracture, travel, period of immobility, malignancy, stroke, paralysis, heart failure, smoking, central venous instrumentation, pregnancy or postpartum status, estrogen therapy, or a history of previous PE are at risk for PE.[2] The clinical assessment, inclusive of history, is not diagnostic but instead should prompt the provider to include PE in the differential diagnosis.

The classic presentation includes dyspnea, tachypnea, pleuritic chest pain, and calf or thigh pain and swelling.[3] Studies suggest that tachypnea is the most sensitive clinical sign.[2] Other symptoms include hemoptysis, orthopnea, tachycardia, jugular venous distention, and abnormal lung sounds.[3] Complaints of calf or thigh leg pain and swelling are not indicative of PE but suggestive of DVT. Atypical presentations may include complaints of nonspecific malaise, weakness, dizziness, syncope, and extremity discomfort.[2]

The physical findings vary greatly and reflect the nature of the PE.[2] The occult PE may be fatal because it is not routinely suspected or diagnosed; however, it may be benign because healthy lung tissue can filter out small emboli. An embolus of any size can produce cardiopulmonary signs depending on the affected area, including acute respiratory distress, tachycardia, hypotension, abnormal heart sounds, jugular vein distention, hypoxemia, tachypnea, cyanosis, and abnormal lung sounds.[1,5] A thorough, accurate physical examination is important because abnormal physical examination findings are subsequently used as part of clinical prediction tools.[1]

DIAGNOSTICS

An appropriate diagnostic work-up varies and is patient and symptom specific. The combination of patient presentation, history, and physical examination findings should be used to guide diagnostic testing. A PE clinical prediction model can also be used to determine the risk of PE and suggest diagnostic tests. The Wells score, revised Geneva score, and pulmonary embolism rule-out criteria (PERC) score are three clinical decision rules that have been validated and can be used to determine the need for imaging.[3]

Essential Diagnostics

The electrocardiogram (ECG) is an integral part of PE evaluation. An ECG cannot diagnose PE but may demonstrate myocardial infarction, atrial fibrillation, and right ventricular dysfunction.[3] It is important to remember the ECG is neither sensitive nor specific and does not identify the cause of the ECG abnormality.

Abnormalities seen on the chest X-ray film may include pleural effusion, diaphragmatic elevation, Hampton hump, Westermark sign, or atelectasis but are not specific to PE.[2,3] In the past, the most widely used imaging modality for PE diagnosis has been the ventilation/perfusion (V/Q) scan,[5,6] which measures both the ability of air to enter the lungs and the perfusion to the lungs. A defect in perfusion coupled with abnormal ventilation can suggest a low, intermediate, or high probability of PE. Computed tomography (CT) angiography has largely replaced the V/Q scan and is currently the "gold standard" for PE diagnosis because of its rapid result and ability to directly visualize PE.[4] CT angiography is more invasive, expensive, and contraindicated in clinical scenarios in which contrast cannot be used.[3] Spiral chest CT with intravenous (IV) contrast is commonly used because of its availability and noninvasive nature. Owing to the high levels of radiation and contrast that may be involved in PE imaging, clinical decision tools were designed to provide providers with a diagnostic strategy and mitigate patient exposure and risk.

ADDITIONAL DIAGNOSTICS

Laboratory tests are nonspecific to PE and are used primarily to detect the cardiopulmonary effects of PE, as well as to exclude other differential diagnoses.[1,2,5] Arterial blood gases (ABGs) are used to evaluate oxygenation and the need for supplemental oxygenation or advanced ventilation.[3] Elevated troponin and brain natriuretic peptide (BNP) levels result in microinfarction and myocardial stretch. They are predictive of

PE complications and mortality.[6] D dimer is the product of the degradation of cross-linked fibrin.[7] This is an important measurement in the patient whose PE is caused by a thrombus, wherein the concentration increases in the presence of acute DVT.[5] Serum D-dimer assays have good negative predictive value and sensitivity but have poor positive predictive value and specificity, making them a useful tool for excluding but not confirming the diagnosis of PE.[8] D dimer is not useful in the postoperative, trauma, hospitalized, or critically ill patient because of the coagulation and fibrolysis that occur as a result of the disease process.[4]

DIFFERENTIAL DIAGNOSIS

 Immediate referral is indicated for suspected cases of pulmonary embolism because the patient's condition may deteriorate rapidly and serious long-term consequences may develop.

Diagnosis is made based on the likelihood of PE combined with the presence of an alteration in ventilation. Patients can be categorized as low risk, intermediate or moderate risk, or high risk.[2] Risk factors can be classified into one of three categories: venous stasis, endothelial or vessel wall injury, and hypercoagulability—the Virchow triad.[1] The PERC rule and Wells criteria can also be used to assign risk.[2] There is no diagnostic test capable of definitively diagnosing PE. Acute PE should be classified as massive or submassive; the term *massive* refers to a PE that causes hemodynamic instability or shock.[5] The presence of hypotension has a high correlation with acute right ventricular failure and subsequent death.

The aforementioned diagnostic tests are helpful in ruling out other possible causes of the symptoms being experienced, which include lung disease (acute or chronic), pneumothorax, pneumonia, acute respiratory distress syndrome, pericarditis, and pleurisy. Heart failure, myocardial infarction, and dissecting aortic aneurysm should also be considered in the differential diagnosis until ruled out. Nonthrombotic pulmonary emboli should also be considered: air embolism, fat emboli, or other substance possibly used by IV drug user.

INTERPROFESSIONAL COLLABORATIVE MANAGEMENT

Compared with recent advances in the treatment of cardiovascular diseases, such as myocardial infarction and stroke, the treatment and outcome for acute PE has remained relatively unchanged, prompting the development of interdisciplinary proactive approaches to the treatment of PE.[9]

Initial management is aimed at hemodynamic stabilization and ensuring adequate oxygenation.[3] Supplemental oxygen should be administered if hypoxemia is present. Pulse oximetry should be monitored, with a goal of at least 92%. Bilevel positive airway pressure ventilation or intubation with mechanical ventilation is indicated with severe hypoxemia or hemodynamic compromise. Administration of IV fluid is indicated for the initial management of hypotension. IV fluids should be cautiously administered to prevent fluid overload in patients with right-sided heart failure. Norepinephrine, dopamine, and epinephrine can be used when there has been a lack of response to IV fluids or if signs of shock are present.

Anticoagulation is the mainstay of PE management because it stops clot progression and allows endogenous fibrolysis to occur.[2] Unless contraindicated, anticoagulation should begin if PE is suspected.[9] Unfractionated heparin, low-molecular-weight heparin, fondaparinux, warfarin, and rivaroxaban are anticoagulation treatment options. The American College of Chest Physicians suggests low-molecular-weight heparin as the first line anticoagulant.[3,9] The recommended dose is 1 mg/kg given subcutaneously every 12 hours for enoxaparin, 200 U/kg once daily for dalteparin, and 175 U/kg once daily for tinzaparin.[2] Fondaparinux is given subcutaneously as a once-a-day injection at a dose based on weight categories. The advantages of low-molecular-weight heparins include standardized dosage without the need for regular monitoring and subcutaneous administration.[5] Low-molecular-weight heparins are frequently used to bridge the transition to an oral vitamin K antagonist.[2] Unfractionated heparin is administered intravenously at a bolus dose of 80 U/kg followed by an infusion starting at 18 U/kg/h, titrated based on activated partial thromboplastin time (aPTT).[3] It is the treatment of choice for patients with renal impairment. There are currently a variety of direct oral anticoagulants approved for treatment of pulmonary embolus, but warfarin, an oral vitamin K antagonist, is still the most commonly prescribed anticoagulant. The dose should be adjusted until the patient has adequate anticoagulation, exhibited by an international normalized ratio (INR) of 2.0 to 3.0 with a goal of 2.5.[2] The duration of oral anticoagulant therapy is dependent on embolism characteristics and patient risk factors.[3] The average length of treatment is 3 months. Long-term treatment—longer than 3 months—is indicated for high-risk patients.

Surgical management may include removal of the embolism (embolectomy) and the insertion of an inferior vena cava filter (IVCF). An IVCF prevents future pulmonary emboli in the patient with lower extremity DVT.[4] IVCFs are indicated in patients with recurrent PE, contraindications to anticoagulation, or significant risk for PE recurrence.[6]

Fibrinolytics may rapidly reverse right-sided heart failure and can lower the rate of death and PE recurrence.[6] Guidelines suggest fibrinolytic therapy for patients with massive PE who exhibit hypotension and have a low risk for bleeding.[3] The preferred regimen is 100 mg of recombinant tissue plasminogen activator (tPA) given intravenously over 2 hours.[6]

Current guidelines recommend the utilization of multidisciplinary PE Response Teams (PERTS) to encourage multidisciplinary decision-making. Similar to a "Code Stroke" or "Code STEMI," PE should be considered a "lung attack" and appropriate resources alongside of the development of hospitalized PERT programs and institutional collaboration should be used to improve outcomes.[9]

INDICATIONS FOR REFERRAL OR HOSPITALIZATION

Because of the increased mortality rate, all patients with suspected PE should receive an immediate evaluation.[6] The initial management of PE traditionally takes place in the hospital setting with transition to outpatient management once the patient has been properly anticoagulated. Low-risk patients with adequate support and the ability to participate in care can be managed as outpatients if they are hemodynamically stable. Patients with chronic PE and infarction should be referred to a pulmonologist for long-term monitoring.

LIFE-SPAN CONSIDERATIONS

Many patients who are diagnosed with acute PE will experience a recurrence.[5] The patient should be monitored for resolution of acute PE and associated complications. Daily use of vascular compression stockings is recommended to improve lower extremity venous blood return and to decrease the risk of deep vein thrombus formation. Indefinite anticoagulation may be indicated for high-risk patients who require lifestyle modifications because of bleeding precautions. Weight loss, smoking cessation, and control of chronic health conditions are suggested to limit the risk of recurrence.[5] In addition, avoiding extended periods of immobility and using prophylactic anticoagulation before surgical procedures should be encouraged.

COMPLICATIONS

Immediate complications resulting from PE include significant cardiopulmonary compromise leading to death. The acute PE usually resolves with few or no residual effects. For some, infarction occurs at the level of injury or the PE does not resolve and chronic thromboembolic pulmonary hypertension or postthrombotic syndrome may develop.[5] In the case of chronic thromboembolic pulmonary hypertension, the patient will exhibit a mean pulmonary artery pressure that is greater than 25 mm Hg that persists for at least 6 months after the diagnosis of PE. Postthrombotic syndrome is defined as chronic calf swelling, brownish discoloration of the lateral medial malleolus, and venous ulceration in severe cases.

PATIENT AND FAMILY EDUCATION

- Educate those being treated with anticoagulation therapy on measures to reduce risk of bleeding, including the use of a soft-bristled toothbrush, waxed floss, and an electric razor.
- Avoid contact sports and other activities that can result in blunt trauma.
- Importance of taking the prescribed anticoagulant exactly as prescribed with routine monitoring by a health care provider.

HEALTH PROMOTION

Patients should be educated regarding management of risk factors associated with PE development because of the increased incidence of recurrent PE.[7] Avoidance of smoking and immobility should be discussed. The patient should also inform the provider of his or her history of PE when surgical intervention or venous catheterization is necessary or if the patient is pregnant. Women of childbearing age should not take combined oral contraceptive pills.

REFERENCES

1. Kessenich, C. R., & Erigo-Backman, R. C. (2012). Computed tomography angiography and pulmonary embolism. *The Nurse Practitioner, 37*(10), 10–11.
2. Ouellette, D. W., & Patocka, C. (2012). Pulmonary embolism. *Emergency Medicine Clinics of North America, 30,* 329–375.
3. Morici, B. (2014). Diagnosis and management of acute pulmonary embolism. *JAAPA, 27*(4), 18–22.
4. Tarbox, A., & Swaroop, M. (2014). Pulmonary embolism. *International Journal of Critical Illness & Injury Science, 3.*
5. Goldhaber, S. Z., & Bounameaux, H. (2012). Pulmonary embolism and deep vein thrombosis. *Lancet, 379,* 1835–1846.
6. Fauci, A. S., Braunwald, E., Kasper, D. L., et al. (Eds.), (2011). *Harrison's principles of internal medicine* (18th ed.). New York: McGraw-Hill.
7. Riva, N., Dentali, F., & Ageno, W. (2014). How can we improve the diagnosis of deep vein thrombosis and pulmonary embolism at the primary level? *Clinical Practice, 11*(2), 131+.
8. Yellumahanthi, K., Waits, J. O. B., Tucker, M., & Gilmore, S. (2014). Positive predictive value of D-dimer in diagnosing pulmonary embolism in patients with no risk factors. *American Journal of Clinical Medicine, 10*(1), 8.
9. Jaber, W. A., Fong, P. P., Weisz, G., et al. (2016). Acute pulmonary embolism. *Journal of the American College of Cardiology, 67*(8), 991–1002.

CHAPTER **96**

PULMONARY HYPERTENSION

Anthony S. Gemignani

 Immediate emergency department referral is indicated for patients with suspected pulmonary embolism, acute coronary syndromes (STEMI/NSTEMI/unstable angina), or acute decompensated heart failure (with or without reduced ejection fraction).

DEFINITION AND EPIDEMIOLOGY

Pulmonary hypertension (PH) occurs as a common end point for a number of disease processes in which increased pulmonary vascular resistance results in increased right-sided heart pressure. The hemodynamic definition for this condition consists of a mean pulmonary arterial pressure (mPAP) ≥25 mm Hg at rest or 30 mm Hg with exercise.[1] The World Health Organization (WHO) divides this condition into five distinct groups based on underlying pathophysiology.[2] Proper classification of the specific type of PH is important because strategies for managing the condition focus on treatment of the respective underlying disease processes.

According to the modified WHO criteria (4th World Symposium on Pulmonary Hypertension), Group 1 Pulmonary Hypertension (also called Pulmonary Arterial Hypertension [PAH]) is caused by adverse remodeling of the small arteries within the pulmonary circulation. The underlying causes may be idiopathic (IPAH), heritable (HPAH), or associated with a wide range of conditions that increase either vascular resistance or blood flow. These conditions include several forms of congenital heart disease, connective tissue disorders, portal hypertension, human immunodeficiency virus (HIV) infection, exposure to drugs and toxins, schistosomiasis, and chronic hemolytic anemia.[2,3] PAH is generally considered a diagnosis of exclusion, made only after PH Groups 2 through 5 have been ruled out. The definition of PAH includes mPAP ≥25 mm Hg, and pulmonary capillary wedge pressure (PCWP) <15 mm Hg and/or pulmonary vascular resistance >3 Wood units.[3]

WHO Group 2 represents PH secondary to increased left-sided heart pressure. This is the end product of left-sided heart failure which may be systolic (heart failure with reduced ejection fraction [HFrEF]), diastolic (heart failure with preserved ejection fraction [HFpEF]), or valvular (e.g., severe mitral or aortic stenosis) in nature. Patients with Group 2 PH have evidence of elevated left-sided pressure (measured as elevated PCWP) and a modest transpulmonary gradient (<10 mm Hg difference between mPAP and PCWP).[1]

WHO Group 3 is associated with chronic lung disease, with obstructive sleep apnea and chronic obstructive pulmonary disease (COPD) being the most common causes of this type of PH. The presence of hypoxia is thought to play a key role in its development, although other mechanisms also contribute to the disease.

WHO Group 4 (also called chronic thromboembolic pulmonary hypertension [CTEPH]) is caused by multiple pulmonary emboli. This results in obstruction to arterial blood flow leading to increased pulmonary vascular resistance and elevated pulmonary arterial (PA) pressures.

WHO Group 5 describes PH arising from multifactorial causes and consists of a heterogeneous collection of systemic disease processes including hematologic, inflammatory, and metabolic disorders. This final group also encompasses rare processes such as tumor obstruction, fibrosing mediastinitis, and chronic renal failure on dialysis.[2]

The prevalence of PH in both the United States and the world has not been well characterized, primarily due to the fact that most PH is subclinical in nature.[4] Of the WHO subtypes, Group 1 has been by far the most studied. A multicenter registry has estimated that the prevalence of Group 1 disease (PAH) in the United States is 10.6 cases per million adults and an incidence of 2.0 cases per million adults per year. This type of PH occurs more commonly in women (4:1 female to male ratio), and the mean age at the time of diagnosis is 50 years.[5] The prognosis of PAH is poor, with an estimated median survival of 2.8 years and 1-, 3-, and 5-year survival rates of 68%, 48%, and 34%, respectively.[3] Risk factors for poor prognosis include advanced functional class (New York Heart Association [NYHA] class III or IV), poor exercise capacity, high right atrial pressure, significant right ventricular dysfunction, evidence of right ventricular failure, and the presence of underlying connective tissue diseases (e.g., systemic sclerosis).[2,3,6] The median survival is 6 years for patients with PAH and functional class I and II symptoms, compared with 2.5 years for patients with functional class III symptoms, and just 6 months for patients with functional class IV symptoms.[3]

PATHOPHYSIOLOGY

PH develops from increased resistance to blood flow through the PA circulation resulting in an elevation in right-sided heart pressure. This condition is generally present at rest but is exacerbated with exercise. During exercise, cardiac output increases three- to five-fold and there is markedly increased flow through the pulmonary vasculature. In healthy individuals, the pulmonary arteries are compliant and accommodate the increase in flow with little change in PA pressure. In the disease states associated with PH, several different pathologic processes result in the common end point of increased resistance to flow through the pulmonary circulation with an associated rise in PA pressure.[7]

In PAH (Group 1 PH) the primary pathologic feature is abnormal vascular remodeling within the small arteries, resulting in smaller-caliber vessels with increased stiffness. Several factors play a role in this process, including genetic predisposition, vascular growth factors, endothelial dysfunction, and abnormal vasomotor control.[2]

The pathologic state in Group 2 PH is related to increased pulmonary venous pressure associated with elevated left-sided heart pressures. This results in impaired blood flow through the lungs and elevation in PA pressures. This type of PH may be significantly improved with volume management (diuresis) and optimization of left heart function. Group 3 PH is closely associated with lung disease and driven by hypoxia. In this disease, increased pulmonary vascular resistance is most commonly caused by hypoxia-mediated vasoconstriction with thickening of the vascular media (vascular remodeling), although polycythemia, with increased blood viscosity, also likely plays a role.[8] Group 4 PH is a condition in which multiple, usually small, pulmonary emboli progressively obstruct the PA circulation resulting in increased PA pressures.[9] Group 5 PH arises from unknown or multifactorial mechanisms. The

---

BOX 96.1

Updated Clinical Classification of Pulmonary Hypertension

1. Pulmonary arterial hypertension (PAH)
   1.1. Idiopathic PAH
   1.2. Heritable
       1.2.1. *BMPR2*
       1.2.2. ALK1, endoglin (with or without hereditary hemorrhagic telangiectasia)
       1.2.3. Unknown
   1.3. Drug- and toxin-induced
   1.4. Associated with
       1.4.1. Connective tissue diseases
       1.4.2. HIV infection
       1.4.3. Portal hypertension
       1.4.4. Congenital heart diseases
       1.4.5. Schistosomiasis
       1.4.6. Chronic hemolytic anemia
   1.5. Persistent pulmonary hypertension of the newborn
2. Pulmonary veno-occlusive disease (PVOD) and/or pulmonary capillary hemangiomatosis (PCH)
3. Pulmonary hypertension caused by left heart disease
   3.1. Systolic dysfunction
   3.2. Diastolic dysfunction
   3.3. Valvular disease
4. Pulmonary hypertension caused by lung diseases and/or hypoxia
   4.1. Chronic obstructive pulmonary disease
   4.2. Interstitial lung disease
   4.3. Other pulmonary diseases with mixed restrictive and obstructive pattern
   4.4. Sleep-disordered breathing
   4.5. Alveolar hypoventilation disorders
   4.6. Chronic exposure to high altitude
   4.7. Developmental abnormalities
5. Chronic thromboembolic pulmonary hypertension (CTEPH)
6. Pulmonary hypertension with unclear multifactorial mechanisms
   6.1. Hematologic disorders: myeloproliferative disorders, splenectomy
   6.2. Systemic disorders: sarcoidosis, pulmonary Langerhans cell histiocytosis, lymphangioleiomyomatosis, neurofibromatosis, vasculitis
   6.3. Metabolic disorders: glycogen storage disease, Gaucher disease, thyroid disorders
   6.4. Others: tumoral obstruction, fibrosing mediastinitis, chronic renal failure on dialysis

ALK1, Activin receptor-like kinase type 1; *BMPR2*, bone morphogenetic protein receptor type 2; *HIV*, human immunodeficiency virus.
Modified from Simonneau, G., Robbins, I. M., Beghetti, M., et al. (2009). Updated clinical classification of pulmonary hypertension. *J Am Coll Cardiol, 54*:S43.

---

underlying mechanisms that result in increased pulmonary pressures share components with PH Groups 1 to 4 though are difficult to isolate given that multiple disease processes may be occurring simultaneously (Box 96.1).

As has been previously described, an increase in pulmonary vascular resistance is the primary driver of all subtypes of PH. It is important to know, however, that a number of other pathologic states may also contribute to increased pulmonary pressures. These include increased blood viscosity, increased baseline pulmonary blood flow (i.e., left-to-right intracardiac shunting), and more rare conditions such as extrinsic compression of the pulmonary vasculature by chest masses. Although an increase in PA pressures is the distinctive characteristic of PAH, it is the ability of the right ventricle to cope with the progressive increase in PA pressures (rather than the pressure itself) that determines functional capacity and survival.[10]

CLINICAL PRESENTATION AND PHYSICAL EXAMINATION

Patients with PH are frequently asymptomatic, or minimally symptomatic, until the condition becomes severe. Sixty percent of patients initially present complaining of dyspnea. Other associated symptoms include fatigue, chest discomfort, syncope, cough, edema, and decreased exercise tolerance. Symptoms are insidious, and the average time from the onset of symptoms to diagnosis is more than a year.[6] It is important to take a careful history when PH is suspected because clues to the underlying cause of the disease may be elicited through careful questioning. In addition, when diagnosing a condition commonly associated with PH (i.e., obstructive sleep apnea, mitral stenosis, autoimmune diseases), it is important to assess the patient for signs of PH because early diagnosis of this condition may result in more effective treatment.

PHYSICAL EXAMINATION

Findings suggestive of PH include a loud second heart sound (arising from an enhanced pulmonic component of the sound), murmurs of tricuspid and/or pulmonic regurgitation, evidence of right ventricular dilation (lifts or heaves, loud S_3 on inspiration, or "right-sided" S_3), and decreased carotid pulse. As right ventricular dysfunction develops, patients may begin to manifest jugular vein distention, increased liver size, ascites, and edema (all signs of volume overload associated with advanced disease). In general, lung fields are clear to auscultation. Patients with PH can also experience tachyarrhythmia, most commonly an atrial flutter.[2,3,9]

DIAGNOSTICS

When PH is suspected, the initial workup should include electrocardiogram (ECG), chest radiography (CXR), and pulmonary function tests (PFTs), because these studies may show evidence consistent with PH but can also identify alternative causes of a patient's dyspnea. In patients with PH, the ECG may show evidence of right-sided heart strain (e.g., S wave in lead I, Q wave in lead III, and an inverted T wave in lead III). Chronic right ventricular pressure overload may also result in findings consistent with right ventricular hypertrophy on the ECG tracing (right-axis deviation and an R wave–to–S wave ratio of more than 1 in lead V_1).[6] Chest X-ray examination often reveals prominent pulmonary arteries and cardiomegaly, and PFTs may show evidence of a reduction in gas transfer.[11] Normal ECG, chest X-ray studies, and PFT results do not wholly exclude the diagnosis of PH however.

Imaging modalities to evaluate for PH include echocardiography or cardiac magnetic resonance imaging (cMRI). Echocardiography using Doppler techniques may be used as a screening tool for the presence of PH by providing an estimate of PA systolic pressure. In addition, other echo findings such as the presence of septal flattening, right ventricular hypertrophy,

and right-sided chamber dilation may provide additional clues to the presence and severity of disease. A recent meta-analysis of Doppler echocardiography for the assessment of PH found a sensitivity and specificity of 88% and 56%, respectively.[12] This modality, although generally useful, is subject to technical limitations and therefore the findings must be interpreted in the context with other available data. More invasive investigation via right-sided heart catheterization may be indicated if other findings suggest the PH is more severe than estimated by the echo-based Doppler technique.

Cardiac MRI is becoming an increasingly popular tool when an accurate assessment of right ventricular size and function is necessary. The study provides information about stroke volume, cardiac output, PA distensibility and stiffness, and alterations in right ventricular morphology.[13-15] In addition, cMRI may be useful in serial assessments to follow therapeutic response in PH because of its high accuracy and low inter-observer variability.[16]

Additional workup may include arterial blood gases (ABGs) to demonstrate hypoxia and respiratory alkalosis, chest computed tomography (CT), or ventilation/perfusion ($\dot{V}/\dot{Q}$) scan to exclude pulmonary embolism, serologic studies to screen for connective tissue diseases, and brain natriuretic peptide (BNP) for patients with known PAH to aid in monitoring progress.[17] In rare cases, a **lung biopsy** may be necessary to exclude interstitial lung disease.[3,6]

Although the aforementioned studies may help evaluate for PH, right heart catheterization (RHC) is the standard for hemodynamic assessment and definitive diagnosis of PH. The purpose of RHC is to evaluate for evidence of elevated left-sided pressures and pulmonary venous hypertension (via assessment of PCWP), and to determine severity and prognosis (via evaluation of mPAP, right atrial pressure, and cardiac index). Administration of vasoactive agents during the study may be necessary to evaluate for pulmonary vasoreactivity and tailor therapeutic interventions.[16]

INITIAL DIAGNOSTICS

Pulmonary Hypertension

- Electrocardiogram: screen for evidence of severe pulmonary hypertension (i.e., RVH) and evaluate for evidence of myocardial ischemia or infarction
- Chest X-ray: imaging of chest may find evidence of PH, or alternative diagnoses
- Pulmonary function test: assess severity of underlying lung disease
- Echocardiography, including Doppler: useful in providing initial estimate of pulmonary arterial systolic pressure

---

Additional Diagnostics

- Chest CT
- Ventilation/perfusion (V/Q) scan
- cMRI
- Right heart catheterization
- Arterial blood gas analysis
- Serologic studies (ANA, RF)
- BNP level
- Lung biopsy

DIFFERENTIAL DIAGNOSIS

 Primary differentials include large (saddle, segmental) pulmonary embolism, acute coronary syndromes (STEMI/NSTEMI/unstable angina), acute decompensated heart failure (with or without reduced ejection fraction), and pneumonia.

PH frequently arises as a complication of underlying disease processes and therefore the differential for PH primarily consists of those diseases without significant superimposed PH. These include COPD, coronary artery disease (with angina), and heart failure with both preserved and reduced ejection fraction.

All three of these diagnoses commonly give patients symptoms of exertional dyspnea, the most common clinical complaint for individuals with significant PH.

Although definitive diagnosis of PH is made by measurement of PA pressure, elucidating the cause can be quite challenging because of the myriad diseases that lead to PH. The differential diagnosis of the underlying causes resulting in PH includes lung disease (restrictive, obstructive, mixed), chronic liver disease, heart disease (congenital, valvular, and myocardial), PA stenosis, pulmonary venous hypertension, thromboembolic disease, connective tissue disease (especially systemic sclerosis), sarcoidosis, and sickle cell disease. Other causes to consider include parasitic infection and intravenous drug use. Although it is rare in the United States, schistosomiasis is the leading cause of PH worldwide.[18]

INTERPROFESSIONAL COLLABORATIVE MANAGEMENT

The ultimate treatment goals for patients with PH are slowing disease progression and improving survival. Surrogate markers for this include reduction of PA pressures with normalization of cardiac output, improvement in symptoms (most commonly dyspnea), and enhancement of functional capacity (as measured by exercise endurance, usually by the 6-minute walk test). Management is directed by the causative factor and thorough diagnostic workup is of the utmost importance in order to focus management strategies. Good management of PH can require close collaboration between the primary care provider and one or multiple different specialists including a cardiologist, a pulmonologist, and/or a sleep medicine specialist.[2]

Non-Pharmacologic Management

Non-pharmacologic management for PH may be variably effective depending on the underlying cause of PH. A structured strategy targeting weight loss may be particularly effective for patients with WHO Groups 2 and 3 PH as obesity has been implicated in some forms of heart failure and is nearly always present among those with obstructive sleep apnea. Careful monitoring of dietary intake with emphasis on avoidance of excess salt can also be useful to alleviate the symptoms associated with volume overload that frequently occur in patients with significant PH. Regular exercise within the limits imposed by the underlying condition is recommended for most patients. In those with severe PH exercise may need to be conducted in a monitored setting as significant exertion in the end-stage of the disease may result in significant pre-syncopal symptoms or even frank syncope. In patients with PH associated with sleep apnea (Group 3) the use of positive pressure ventilation may be useful in blunting disease progression.[19] Treatment strategies for Group 3 PH may also include curtailing nicotine addiction (if present) and using supplemental oxygen.

Pharmacologic Management

Individuals with symptomatic PH are candidates for medical therapies aimed at reducing physical manifestations of the disease process. Diuretics are a mainstay of treatment for the volume overload associated with PH.[16] Digoxin has been shown in animal studies to offer some benefit in preserving right ventricular contractility, reducing circulating norepinephrine levels, and increasing resting cardiac output.[20] Anticoagulation is recommended to counteract thrombin deposition that occurs in the pulmonary circulation especially in those with Group 4 PH.[17,18]

Additional medical therapies aimed at specific underlying mechanisms are also available for some patients with severe PH. The majority of these medications have been developed primarily for use in patients with WHO Group 1 disease and initiation of these medications mainly occurs under the guidance of a specialist (usually a pulmonologist or cardiologist specifically trained in the management of PH). Primary care providers should have a low threshold to refer their patient to a PH specialist if workup has been consistent with severe symptomatic PH. Medical therapies for this group of patients are primarily accomplished with vasodilators (calcium channel blockers, prostanoids, endothelin receptor antagonists, or phosphodiesterase inhibitors). While fewer than 10% of patients demonstrate pulmonary vasoreactivity (reduction in mPAP greater than or equal to 10 mm Hg to an absolute mPAP less than 35 to 40 mm Hg with either no change or an increase in cardiac output after the administration of short-acting vasodilators), this subset of patients has been shown to derive significant long-term benefit from calcium channel blockers.[3] Calcium channel blockers have been shown to reduce mPAP and pulmonary vascular resistance as well as improve quality of life and survival in those who exhibit pulmonary vasoreactivity. Treatment doses of calcium channel blockers for PAH are higher than those used for treatment of systemic hypertension (see Table 96.1).[16]

Prostacyclin synthase is reduced in patients with PAH, resulting in inadequate production of prostacyclin I₂, a vasodilator with antiproliferative effects.[3] Prostanoids induce vasodilation and prevent platelet aggregation and inflammation through activation of cyclic adenosine monophosphate. The three US Food and Drug Administration (FDA)–approved prostanoids are epoprostenol, treprostinil, and iloprost. Epoprostenol, administered by continuous intravenous infusion, is the first-line treatment for functional class IV patients and also serves as a rescue therapy for patients in whom other drugs have failed. Epoprostenol improves functional class, exercise tolerance, hemodynamics, and survival of patients with idiopathic PAH. However, drawbacks to epoprostenol include its short half-life of approximately 6 minutes, instability at room temperature, and risk of infection with intravenous administration. Treprostinil (available for intravenous infusion or subcutaneous injection) has a longer half-life, minimizing the risk of cardiovascular collapse with inadvertent infusion cessation. Newer inhaled prostanoids (e.g., iloprost) were developed with the thought that intrapulmonary selectivity would decrease right-to-left shunt blood flow and minimize systemic

TABLE 96.1   Therapies for Pulmonary Arterial Hypertension

Medications	Year FDA Approved	Indications	Dose	Side Effects
CALCIUM CHANNEL BLOCKERS				
Amlodipine	1995	Responsive to vasodilator testing	2.5–20 mg PO daily	Peripheral edema, pulmonary edema, palpitations, flushing, fatigue, dizziness
Diltiazem	1995	Responsive to vasodilator testing	60–240 mg PO daily to tid	Edema, headache, AV block, bradycardia, hypotension, vasodilation, dizziness
Nifedipine	1995	Responsive to vasodilator testing	30–240 mg PO bid	Flushing, peripheral edema, dizziness, headache, nausea, heartburn
PROSTANOIDS				
Epoprostenol	1995	NYHA III-IV	2–40 ng/kg/min IV	Tachycardia, flushing, hypotension, dizziness, headache, anxiety, nausea, vomiting
Treprostinil	2002 (subcutaneous) 2004 (intravenous) 2009 (inhalation)	NYHA II-IV	0.625–40 ng/kg/min IV or SC 18–54 mcg inhaled qid	Flushing, headache, rash, diarrhea, nausea
Iloprost	2004	NYHA III-IV	2.5–5 mcg inhaled at maximum 9 doses/d	Flushing, hypotension, headache, nausea, flu-like syndrome, cough, jaw pain
ENDOTHELIN RECEPTOR ANTAGONISTS				
Bosentan	2001	NYHA II-IV	62.5–125 mg PO bid	Edema, headache, hepatotoxicity, inhibition of spermatogenesis, respiratory tract infection
Ambrisentan	2007	NYHA II-IV	5–10 mg PO daily	Peripheral edema, headache, flushing, palpitations, decrease in hemoglobin, nasal congestion
PHOSPHODIESTERASE INHIBITORS				
Sildenafil	2005	NYHA II-IV	2.5 mg or 10 mg IV daily 5 mg or 20 mg PO tid (taken 4–6 h apart)	Flushing, headache, dyspepsia, visual disturbances, epistaxis
Tadalafil	2009	NYHA II-IV	40 mg PO daily	Flushing, headache, dyspepsia, myalgia, respiratory tract infection

AV, Atrioventricular; *FDA,* US Food and Drug Administration.

side effects. However, because of the short half-life of iloprost, use of the drug requires inhalation 6 to 9 times daily, and its regular use has proved impractical for many patients.[16]

Patients with PAH are found to have increased levels of circulating plasma endothelin-1, a potent vasoconstrictor that promotes pulmonary artery smooth muscle cell proliferation.[16] Bosentan and ambrisentan are endothelin receptor antagonists that combat vasoconstriction and improve exercise capacity. Bosentan is associated with reversible hepatotoxicity in 5% to 10% of patients; therefore serial monitoring of a patient's hepatic function is necessary. Ambrisentan is often prescribed to those who cannot tolerate bosentan, given its lower risk of hepatotoxicity.

Naturally occurring nitric oxide works to increase pulmonary vascular relaxation and reduce cellular proliferation through cyclic guanosine monophosphate. Phosphodiesterase type 5 degrades nitric oxide. Two phosphodiesterase inhibitors, sildenafil and tadalafil, have been shown to improve functional capacity and reduce mPAP by inhibiting degradation of nitric oxide and may be used to improve some patients' symptoms.[11,16]

INDICATIONS FOR REFERRAL OR HOSPITALIZATION

Because accurate diagnosis is crucial, referral to an appropriate specialist is recommended. Imaging, cardiac catheterization, pulmonary function testing, medication recommendations, and lung transplantation all require specialist referral. Both cardiologists and pulmonologists have expertise in the workup and management of PH. In late-stage disease referral to a palliative care specialist may also be considered. For patients with end-stage PH, lung transplantation (or heart-lung transplantation if heart damage is extensive) may be an option, although the waiting list for organ transplants is often long. Transplantation criteria include the patient's age, medical history, and overall condition at the time of transplantation. The risk management and complications of transplantation should be thoroughly explained.

Providers caring for patients with severe PH should have a low threshold for hospitalization as patients with PH often have limited hemodynamic reserve and may decompensate rapidly.

LIFE-SPAN CONSIDERATIONS

The prognosis of PH is mainly dependent upon the severity of disease and the degree of functional impairment associated with the disease. Signs of poor prognosis include poor functional tolerance (NYHA functional class III or IV), poor exercise capacity, severely elevated PA pressure, or evidence of right heart failure. History of syncope in the setting of severe PH is of particular concern. In the presence of the findings described above, careful outlining of end-of-life goals of care may be particularly germane to the patient's care.

Complications

Complications of PH generally do not occur until the condition becomes severe but may eventually result in the development of right ventricular hypertrophy, dilation, and failure with associated symptoms of volume overload. Cardiac arrhythmias, both atrial and ventricular in origin, are also possible.[17] Other complications include acute pulmonary embolism, pulmonary hemorrhage, and pneumonia. In addition to physical symptoms associated with PH, other factors, such as anxiety, depression, adverse side-effects of therapy, functional limitations, and social isolation, may lead to significant impairment in quality of life.[10] Hospitalization may be necessary for medication adjustment, monitoring, and imaging. The most common cause of death in patients with clinically severe PH is right ventricular failure.[18]

PATIENT AND FAMILY EDUCATION

Patients with PH often require a tremendous amount of support from health care providers. Careful explanation of the disease and the need for moderation during activity is important because exercise may increase pulmonary vascular resistance and hypoxia. The side effects and adverse reactions of all medications should be carefully explained and understood by both patients and families. The importance of a low-salt diet and the avoidance of over-the-counter medications (unless approved by the health care provider) should be stressed.[18,21]

Familial PH accounts for 6% to 10% of patients with PAH.[3] Most cases occur in individuals with no known family history.[21,22] Families need education and support if a genetic workup is chosen.

HEALTH PROMOTION

Group 1 PH is a relatively rare disease process, and the exact mechanisms of the disease are still being investigated. Overall prognosis has historically been poor, and patients have had little hope for remission of this progressive disease until recently. Because PH occurs as a secondary complication to a wide range of disorders including COPD, sleep apnea, sickle cell crisis, connective tissue diseases, cardiac diseases, and thromboembolism, these disease processes must be monitored for the onset of complications suggestive of significant PH. Lung diseases are the most common causes of PH; therefore raising awareness of lung disease prevention is crucial.[23] One of the most important preventive measures for elimination of lung disease is smoking cessation.

REFERENCES

1. Ryan, J. J., Thenappan, T., Luo, N., et al. (2012). The WHO classification of pulmonary hypertension: A case based imaging compendium. *Pulmonary Circulation, 2*(1), 107–121.
2. Nazzareno, G., Marc Humbert, J. L., Vachiery, S. C., et al. (2015). 2-15 ESC/ERS Guidelines for the diagnosis and treatment of pulmonary hypertension: The Joint Task Force for the Diagnosis and Treatment of Pulmonary Hypertension of the European Society of Cardiology (ESC) and the European Respiratory Society (ERS): Endorsed by: Association for European Paediatric and Congenital Cardiology (AEPC), International Society for Heart and Lung Transplantation (ISHLT). *European Heart Journal, 37*(1), 67–119.
3. Simonneau, G., Robbins, I. M., Beghetti, M., et al. (2009). Updated clinical classification of pulmonary hypertension. *Journal of the American College of Cardiology, 54*, S43.
4. McLaughlin, V. V., Archer, S. L., Badesch, D. B., et al. (2009). ACCF/AHA 2009 expert consensus document on pulmonary hypertension: A report of the American College of Cardiology Foundation Task Force on Expert Consensus Documents and the American Heart Association: Developed in collaboration with the American College of Chest Physicians, American Thoracic Society, and the Pulmonary Hypertension Association. *Circulation, 119*, 2250–2294.
5. Neuman, J. H., & Hemnes, A. R. (2010). Pulmonary hypertension. In *Breathing in America: Diseases, progress and hope* (pp. 175–184). New York: American Thoracic Society.
6. Badesch, D. B., Raskob, G. E., Elliott, C. G., et al. (2010). Pulmonary arterial hypertension: Baseline characteristics from the REVEAL Registry. *Chest, 137*, 376–387.
7. Rounds, S., & Cutaia, M. V. (1998). Pulmonary hypertension: Pathophysiology and clinical disorders. In G. L. Baum, J. D. Crapo, B. R. Celli, et al. (Eds.), *Textbook of pulmonary medicine* (6th ed.). Philadelphia: Lippincott-Raven.
8. Rich, S., & McLaughlin, V. V. (2005). Pulmonary hypertension. In D. P. Zipes, P. Libby, R. O. Bonow, & E. Braunwald (Eds.), *Braunwald's heart disease: A textbook of cardiovascular medicine* (7th ed., pp. 1807–1842). Philadelphia: Elsevier.
9. Elwing, J., & Panos, R. J. (2008). Pulmonary hypertension associated with COPD. *International Journal of Chronic Obstructive Pulmonary Disease, 3*(1), 55–70.
10. Fedullo, P. F., Auger, W. R., Kerr, K. M., & Rubin, L. J. (2001). Chronic thromboembolic pulmonary hypertension. *The New England Journal of Medicine, 345*, 1465–1472.
11. Badano, L. P., Ginghina, C., Easaw, J., et al. (2010). Right ventricle in pulmonary arterial hypertension: Haemodynamics, structural changes, imaging, and proposal of a study protocol aimed to assess remodeling and treatment effects. *European Journal of Echocardiography: The Journal of the Working Group on Echocardiography of the European Society of Cardiology, 11*, 27–37.
12. Kiely, D. G., Elliot, C. A., Sabroe, I., et al. (2013). Pulmonary hypertension: Diagnosis and management. *British Medical Journal, 346*, 1–12.
13. Taleb, M., Khuder, S., Tinkel, J., et al. (2013). The diagnostic accuracy of Doppler echocardiography in assessment of pulmonary artery systolic pressure: A meta-analysis. *Echocardiography (Mount Kisco, N.Y.), 30*(3), 258–265.
14. Paz, R., Mohiaddin, R. H., & Longmore, D. B. (1993). Magnetic resonance assessment of the pulmonary arterial trunk anatomy, pulsatility and distensibility. *European Heart Journal, 14*, 1524–1530.
15. Tardivon, A. A., Mousseaux, E., Brenot, F., et al. (1994). Quantification of hemodynamics in primary pulmonary hypertension with magnetic resonance imaging. *American Journal of Respiratory and Critical Care Medicine, 150*, 1075–1080.
16. Blyth, K. G., Groenning, B. A., Martin, T. N., et al. (2005). Contrast enhanced-cardiovascular magnetic resonance imaging in patients with pulmonary hypertension. *European Heart Journal, 26*, 1993–1999.
17. Agarwal, R., & Gomberg-Maitland, M. (2011). Current therapeutics and practical management strategies for pulmonary arterial hypertension. *American Heart Journal, 162*(2), 201–213.
18. Fauci, A. S., Braunwald, E., Kasper, D. L., et al. (Eds.), (2008). *Harrison's principles of internal medicine* (17th ed.). New York: McGraw-Hill.
19. Friedman, S. E., & Andrus, M. W. (2012). Obesity and pulmonary hypertension: A review of pathophysiologic mechanisms. *Journal of Obesity, 2012*, 505274.
20. Humbert, M., Segal, E. S., Kiely, D. G., et al. (2007). Results of European post-marketing surveillance of bosentan in pulmonary hypertension. *The European Respiratory Journal, 30*, 338–344.
21. Humbert, M., Sitbon, O., Chaouat, A., et al. (2006). Pulmonary arterial hypertension in France: Results from a National Registry. *American Journal of Respiratory and Critical Care Medicine, 173*, 1024–1030.
22. Galiè, N., Hoeper, M. M., Humbert, M., et al. (2009). Guidelines for the diagnosis and treatment of pulmonary hypertension. *European Heart Journal, 30*, 2493–2537.
23. Badesch, D. B., Abman, S. H., Simmoneau, G., et al. (2007). Medical therapy for pulmonary arterial hypertension. *Chest, 131*, 1917–1928.

CHAPTER **97**

SARCOIDOSIS

Janet Rico

DEFINITION AND EPIDEMIOLOGY

Sarcoidosis is a multisystem, inflammatory, granulomatous process that commonly affects young and middle-aged adults. The assessment of its incidence is dependent on health care access and consistency of diagnostic criteria and screening. The disease primarily involves the lungs and intrathoracic lymph system (90%) and can impact any other organ (Table 97.1). More than 80% of patients are 20 to 45 years of age; the disease is rare in children and older adults. Individuals of Irish, German, Scandinavian, and West Indian descent are more at risk for the disease.[1] The incidence of sarcoidosis in the United States is higher in African Americans than in whites, with greater morbidity reported. It is important to consider that initial presentation of sarcoid is approximately 10 years earlier in blacks than Caucasians.[2] Reports of sarcoidosis appear to be rare in Africa, India, and Central and South America, probably because of the absence of mass screening programs and the presence of more common granulomatous diseases such as tuberculosis.[3] No clear genetic basis has been established for sarcoidosis, but genetic factors may modulate its evolution and expression. Sarcoidosis is commonly seen in families. The likelihood for development of the disease ranges from 26% to 73% in individuals with an affected first-degree relative.[4] Occupational and environmental exposures have been associated with sarcoidosis including exposures to dust and pesticides.[5] A study of more than 20,000 World Trade Center 911 responders found increased incidence of sarcoid-like granulomatous pulmonary disease, further supporting a possible link to environmental exposures.[6]

TABLE 97.1 Clinical Features of Sarcoidosis

Organ System	Symptoms or Presentation
Pulmonary	Dyspnea, cough, wheezing, chest pain
Upper airway	Dyspnea, nasal congestion, hoarseness, stridor, polyps
Dermatologic	Nodules, papules, plaques
Ocular	Photophobia, tearing, pain, decreased visual acuity, lacrimal gland enlargement, uveitis, glaucoma, blindness
Rheumatologic	Polyarthropathy, monoarthropathy, myopathy
Neurologic	Headache, hearing loss, paresthesias, seizures, cranial nerve palsy
Cardiologic	Syncope, dyspnea, arrhythmias, congestive heart failure, cardiac tamponade
Gastrointestinal	Dysphagia, abdominal pain, jaundice, hepatomegaly
Hematologic	Lymph node enlargement, hypersplenism
Renal	Kidney failure, calculi

PATHOPHYSIOLOGY

The characteristic pathologic feature of sarcoidosis is the noncaseating granuloma. The disease is notable for a heightened immune response against an unclear target with T cells playing a primary role. An unidentified antigen precipitating an exaggerated immune response has been hypothesized as the initiating event. The collection of macrophages and T cells that compose the granuloma releases various chemokines and cytokines, including tumor necrosis factor. Tumor necrosis factor is known to be critical to granuloma formation and preservation.[7]

The granuloma in pulmonary sarcoid is likely to be preceded by an alveolitis that involves the interstitium more than the alveolar spaces. Although the initial antigen is unknown, the alveolitis begins an accumulation of helper T lymphocyte (CD4) cells and macrophages. It is believed that activated macrophages may be responsible for the eventual development of fibrosis in some patients with sarcoidosis.

In the lung, granulomatous inflammation and fibrosis result in ventilation/perfusion imbalance and widening of the alveolar-arterial oxygen gradient. In the early stages, PaO_2 may be within the normal range at rest but decreases with exertion.

CLINICAL PRESENTATION AND PHYSICAL EXAMINATION

Sarcoidosis may affect almost any organ system; however, 90% of affected individuals have pulmonary involvement.[8] Sarcoidosis can occur in acute, subacute, or chronic form and is initially discovered asymptomatically with an abnormal chest radiograph in approximately 50% of patients.[4] Patients who are symptomatic with this disorder often have nonspecific pulmonary symptoms—dry cough, dyspnea, chest pain, fever, fatigue, anorexia, weight loss, and, occasionally, chills and night sweats. The nonspecificity of these symptoms can delay diagnosis.[1] The symptoms and related organ involvement consistent with sarcoidosis are listed in Table 97.1. Sarcoid of the upper respiratory tract (SURT) involves the nasopharynx, larynx, and trachea, and occurs in approximately 5% of patients with sarcoid and can cause upper airway obstruction with worsening symptoms of dyspnea.[9]

Hoarseness and nasal obstruction may occur as a result of vocal cord and nasal mucosa granulomas (polyps). Hemoptysis is rarely seen; when present, it suggests mycetoma.[10]

It is unusual for adventitious lung sounds to be detected on auscultation. Wheezing is occasionally audible in patients with advanced disease. Digital clubbing is rare. Dyspnea, dry cough, and chest pain occur commonly. Chest pain can be severe and difficult to distinguish from cardiac chest pain.[11]

Rheumatologic symptoms occur in 4% to 38% of patients with sarcoidosis.[12] These can manifest as an acute arthritis commonly involving the ankle, chronic polyarthritis, or myopathy.

Ocular lesions are seen in up to 25% of patients and the initial presentation in 5% of patients.[13] Anterior uveitis is seen frequently. Symptoms may include redness, photophobia, and decreased visual acuity.[3] Other ocular lesions seen include posterior uveitis, retinal vasculitis, keratoconjunctivitis, and conjunctival follicles.[10]

Skin lesions are seen in 20% to 30% of patients. A maculopapular rash over the face and hairline is the most common subacute lesion.[12] Erythema nodosum is seen more commonly in women; when it occurs in combination with hilar adenopathy, polyarthralgias, and fever, it is referred to as Löfgren syndrome.[11] Löfgren syndrome is a common sarcoid presentation and includes bihilar lymphadenopathy, ankle edema, fever, and erythema nodosum. This constellation of symptoms has a 95% diagnostic specificity for the disease.[1]

Clinical involvement of the central nervous system is unusual, occurring most frequently with other organ involvement. Neurological involvement alone is seen in only 1% of cases.[14] Asymptomatic granulomas can occur in any part of the female reproductive system, including the breast.

ESSENTIAL DIAGNOSTICS

There is no conclusive diagnostic pathway for sarcoid. Chest radiographs are abnormal in more than 90% of patients. In general, one of the following patterns is demonstrated: (1) bilateral hilar lymphadenopathy (BHL; 50% to 80% of cases); (2) parenchymal interstitial infiltrates (25% to 50%), with a predilection for upper and mid lung field distribution; or (3) both lymphadenopathy and interstitial disease. BHL is often the lesion that suggests the diagnosis of sarcoidosis.

Unless lymphadenopathy is present, the appearance of the chest radiograph may be indistinguishable from that of other interstitial lung disorders. Typically, radiographic lesions are bilateral and are distributed relatively symmetrically; asymmetric involvement is occasionally seen.

The Scadding staging, based on the appearance of the chest radiograph, has been in widespread use since 1957. The consensus now favors the following classification[4]:

Stage 0: Normal chest radiograph
Stage I: BHL
Stage II: BHL with pulmonary infiltrates
Stage III: Pulmonary infiltrates without BHL
Stage IV: Pulmonary fibrosis

One should note that there is large interrater variability between assessing patients in stages II and III and III and IV.[15]

Computed tomography (CT) and high-resolution computed tomography (HRCT) of the chest are superior to conventional chest radiography in defining the extent of parenchymal abnormalities in sarcoidosis. HRCT can help differentiate between reversible (mostly inflammatory) changes and irreversible (presumably fibrotic) alterations.

Labs: Hypergammaglobulinemia is seen in 30% to 80% of cases of sarcoidosis. Rheumatoid factor can be positive. The serum level of angiotensin-converting enzyme (ACE) is elevated in approximately 75% of patients with untreated sarcoidosis. Its utility in monitoring disease progression is not clear.[16] Anemia occurs in 4% to 20% of patients.[10] Leukopenia, eosinophilia, and thrombocytopenia can be seen, although not commonly. The erythrocyte sedimentation rate (ESR) is often elevated, but this can be a nonspecific finding. Hypercalcemia and hypercalciuria occasionally occur secondary to increased gastrointestinal absorption, abnormal vitamin D metabolism, and increased calcitriol production by sarcoid granulomas.

Skin testing often reveals cutaneous anergy.

Pulmonary function test (PFT) results may be normal or may reveal a restrictive pattern. This may be of most value in monitoring the course of the disease in individual cases. Radionuclide scanning reveals high uptake of gallium 67 (^{67}Ga) in pulmonary lesions of sarcoidosis. However, ^{67}Ga is also taken up by the lungs in patients with a large number of other diseases, therefore a high level of ^{67}Ga is not specific

for sarcoidosis, and determination of the level is not recommended as part of the routine evaluation.[4]

It is often reassuring to have a tissue biopsy diagnosis, and there are many techniques for this. The most specific location for biopsy is the lung. Bronchoscopy with transbronchial biopsy specimens is positive in 50% to 60% of patients who do not have radiographic evidence of parenchymal disease. This positivity increases to 85% to 90% when there are radiographic abnormalities. Bronchoalveolar lavage performed at the time of fiberoptic bronchoscopy retrieves inflammatory and immune effector cells from the lower respiratory tract that can also be diagnostic. Open lung biopsy through mediastinoscopy may yield tissue diagnosis when bronchoscopy has failed.[17] Biopsy specimens can also be taken from other organ systems suspected to have sarcoid involvement (conjunctivae, skin, lymph nodes).

DIFFERENTIAL DIAGNOSIS

 Priority differentials include laryngeal obstruction, malignancy, and tuberculosis.

Sarcoid is basically a diagnosis of exclusion. Many conditions are associated with dyspnea, diffuse pulmonary infiltration, and granulomas. Laryngeal obstruction, hypersensitivity pneumonitis, asbestosis, silicosis, drug effects, bacterial or fungal infections, vascular diseases, and malignant neoplasms should all be considered. It is most important to differentiate sarcoidosis from tuberculosis, another granulomatous disease with public health implications. Tuberculin skin testing should be included as part of the evaluation.

INTERPROFESSIONAL COLLABORATIVE MANAGEMENT
Nonpharmacologic Management

Overall primary care management focuses on the patient's needs and presenting symptoms. The patient may need oxygen support, pulmonary rehab services, psychiatric and/or social work support, and physical and occupational therapy if function has been impacted.

Pharmacological Management

The indications for treatment are not standardized, and there is no US Food and Drug Administration–approved therapeutic agent. Nearly half of all patients with sarcoid will require systemic treatment. Response to therapy is variable, and a large number of patients undergo a natural remission or follow a benign course.[4] No treatment is recommended for asymptomatic patients with stage I or stage II disease. Patients with fever, erythema nodosum, or joint pains often respond to nonsteroidal antiinflammatory drugs (NSAIDs). Prednisone, usually dosed at 20 to 40 mg/day, may occasionally be needed to control symptoms, with dose lowering over 3 to 6 months based on response and side effects.[18] If there are symptoms of dyspnea or if a cough develops, airway obstruction may be present and corticosteroid therapy is advisable. Oral corticosteroids are used cautiously with great respect for potential toxicity. In some cases, inhaled corticosteroids may be effective.[4]

Patients with stage II disease who are symptomatic are treated with corticosteroids. Only observation is suggested for patients who are asymptomatic and have only mild impairment of lung function. Treatment is needed for individuals who have progressive impairment of lung function. Patients with stage III or stage IV sarcoidosis almost always require treatment with corticosteroids or another type of immunosuppressive treatment, but this is often unsatisfying.

Alternatives to steroids are used for patients who develop severe side effects, do not respond to prednisone, or prefer not to take oral corticosteroids. Disease progression despite adequate corticosteroid therapy for longer than one year is also an indication for treatment with these agents.[11,19]

Anti-metabolites are used in patients who have failed steroid therapy or when there are contraindications. Methotrexate and azathioprine are the most commonly used. Leflunomide and mycophenolate have also been used.

When steroids or antimetabolites, or both, are ineffective, targeted TNF inhibition therapy (infliximab or adalimumab) may be considered. Other medications in trials for treatment include concurrent use of levofloxacin, ethambutol, azithromycin, and rifampin.[18] Treatment of non-inflammatory consequences of sarcoidosis also need to be considered such as treatment for related pulmonary hypertension and heart failure.

More and larger studies are required before these drugs can be recommended as part of the routine therapy for sarcoidosis.

INDICATIONS FOR REFERRAL OR HOSPITALIZATION

Sarcoidosis is a serious multisystem disease that requires physician consultation, specifically pulmonary consultation. However, other specialists may also be consulted dependent on the involved system. Lung biopsies are usually necessary for diagnosis and require referral to a pulmonary specialist. If other biopsies are indicated, the appropriate specialist should be consulted. Therapy during the acute and chronic phases should be directed by the physician or specialist to ensure proper treatment. Hospitalization may be necessary for patients with severe dyspnea and hypoxia or severe cardiac dysfunction.

LIFE-SPAN CONSIDERATIONS

Sarcoidosis does not affect pregnancy but may flare after delivery. Sarcoidosis in children younger than 15 years showed the

---

BOX **97.1**

Complications of Sarcoidosis

Lung scarring. Untreated pulmonary sarcoidosis can lead to irreversible interstitial scarring (fibrosis) and pulmonary hypertension.

Skin involvement. Skin involvement is common with hyperpigmented papules and erythema nodosum.

Eye disease. Inflammation can affect almost any part of the eye and usually causes watering, redness, and pain. In a few cases, sarcoidosis can lead to blindness or serious eye diseases, such as cataracts and glaucoma.

Nervous system problems. Cranial neuropathies are the most common manifestations. A small percentage of people with sarcoidosis develop problems related to the central nervous system when granulomas form in the brain and spinal cord. Inflammation in the facial nerves can cause facial paralysis.

Fertility problems. In men, sarcoidosis can affect the testes and possibly cause infertility. Severe sarcoidosis may make it difficult for some women to become pregnant, but many women with the disease give birth to healthy children.

Heart and liver problems. Arrhythmias or cardiomyopathy can be seen in the most severe cases. Granulomas that form in the liver can affect its ability to function.

Muscle and joint problems. Muscle and joint problems, including acute and chronic arthritis and myopathy, can occur.

Data from Mayo Clinic: *Sarcoidosis: Complications.* Retrieved from www.mayoclinic.com/health/sarcoidosis/DS00251/DSECTION=complications.

---

same organ distribution as in adults. The prognosis for children seems better than that for adults.[8] Patients older than 70 years are more likely to be seen with systemic symptoms[4] and have a higher likelihood of adverse reactions to treatment, particularly corticosteroids.

COMPLICATIONS

Many complications of sarcoidosis (Box 97.1), including osteoporosis, hypertension, hyperglycemia, and gastric ulcers, occur as a result of corticosteroid therapy. Relapses are common and are determined by the reappearance of clinical signs and symptoms, chest radiograph abnormalities, and an elevated ACE level. In this situation, a return to a previously high maintenance dose is sufficient to control recurrence.

Patients with sarcoidosis have demonstrated high levels of depression and stress as measured by health-related quality-of-life (HRQOL) assessments. This is likely because young people in the prime of their professional lives are most commonly affected by the disease or side effects of the medications. In one study, those taking corticosteroids had lower HRQOL scores, reflecting worse HRQOL, compared with unmatched historical controls not treated with corticosteroids.[20] Possible reasons for the association between corticosteroid use and poorer HRQOL include increased disease severity, medication side effects, and concomitant mental health issues, such as depression and stress. This relationship needs to be further investigated.

In a few cases, sarcoidosis can be fatal. Death is usually a result of progressive scarring of the lungs and respiratory failure or the result of an arrhythmia, which may lead to sudden death.[21]

PATIENT AND FAMILY EDUCATION

The nature of the disease, including its varied presentation, must be carefully explained to patients. Medications, if indicated, and their side effects need to be discussed. It is important that patients understand the risk for worsening lung impairment or other organ damage if compliance with therapy is poor. It is important that patients be familiar with the clinical signs suggestive of recurrence of sarcoidosis.

REFERENCES

1. O'Regan, A., & Berman, J. S. (2012). In the clinic: Sarcoidosis risk factors and clinical features. *Annals of Internal Medicine, 156*(9).
2. Judson, M. A., Boan, A. D., & Lackland, D. T. (2012). The clinical course of sarcoidosis. Presentation, diagnosis and treatment in a large white and black cohort in the U.S. *Sarcoidosis, Vasculitis, and Diffuse Lung Diseases, 29*, 119.
3. Lazarus, A. (2009). Sarcoidosis: Epidemiology, etiology, pathogenesis, and genetics. *Disease-A-Month, 55*(11), 649–660.
4. California Thoracic Society. (2008). Diagnosis and treatment of sarcoidosis. Retrieved from www.thoracic.org/statements/resources/interstitial-lung-disease/sarcoid1-20.pdf.
5. Newman, L. S., et al. (2004). A case control etiologic study of sarcoidosis: Environmental and occupational risk factors. *American Journal of Respiratory and Critical Care Medicine, 170*(12), 1324–1330.
6. Crowley, L. E., Herbert, R., Moline, J. M., Wallenstein, S., Shukla, G., Schechter, C., et al. (2011). "Sarcoid like" granulomatous pulmonary disease in World Trade Center disaster responders. *American Journal of Industrial Medicine, 54*, 175–184. doi:10.1002/ajim.20924.
7. Loke, W. S. J., Herbert, C., & Thomas, P. S. (2013). Sarcoidosis: Immunopathogenesis and immunological markers. *International Journal of Chronic Diseases*, http://dx.doi.org/10.1155/2013/928601.
8. Iannuzzi, M., & Fontana, J. (2011). Sarcoidosis. *JAMA: The Journal of the American Medical Association, 305*(4), 391–397.
9. Baughman, R. P., Lower, E., & Tami, T. (2010). Upper airway: Sarcoidosis of the upper respiratory tract (SURT). *Thorax, 65*, 181–186. doi:10.1136/thx.2008.112896.
10. Iannuzzi, M. C., Rybicki, B. A., & Teirstein, A. S. (2007). Sarcoidosis. *The New England Journal of Medicine, 357*(21), 2153–2165.
11. Baughman, R. P., Costabell, U., & du Bois, R. M. (2008). Treatment of sarcoidosis. *Clinics in Chest Medicine, 29*(3), 533–548.
12. Abril, A., & Cohen, M. (2004). Rheumatological manifestations of sarcoidosis. *Current Opinion in Rheumatology, 16*(1), 51–55.
13. Jamilloux, Y., Kodjikian, L., Broussolle, C., & Seve, P. (2014). Sarcoidosis and uveitis. *Autoimmunity Reviews, 13*(8), 840–849.
14. Hebe, R., Dubaniewicz-Wybieralska, M., & Dubaniewicz, A. (2015). Overview of neurosarcoidosis: Recent advances. *Journal of Neurology, 262*, 258–267.
15. Rutters, J. C., Drent, M., & Van den Bosch, J. M. M. (2009). European Respiratory Society Monograph. 46 (Interstitial Lung Diseases), 126–154. doi: 10.1183/1025448x.00046008.
16. Ungprasert, P., Carmona, E. M., Crowson, C. S., & Matteson, E. L. (2016). Diagnostic Utility of Angiotensin-converting enzyme in sarcoidosis: A population-based study. *Lung, 194*, 91.
17. Yanardag, H., Caner, M., Kaynak, K., et al. (2006). Clinical value of mediastinoscopy in the diagnosis of sarcoidosis: An analysis of 68 cases. *The Thoracic and Cardiovascular Surgeon, 54*(3), 198–201.
18. Baughman, R. P., & Grutters, J. C. (2015). New treatment strategies for pulmonary sarcoidosis: Antimetabolites, biological drugs, and other treatment approaches. *The Lancet. Respiratory Medicine, 3*(10), 813–822.
19. Lazar, C. A., & Culver, D. A. (2010). Treatment of sarcoidosis. *Seminars in Respiratory and Critical Care Medicine, 31*(14), 501–518.
20. Cox, C., Donahue, J., Kataria, Y., et al. (2004). Health-related quality of life of persons with sarcoidosis. *Chest, 125*, 997–1004.
21. Mayo Clinic. Sarcoidosis: Complications. Retrieved from www.mayoclinic.com/health/sarcoidosis/DS00251/DSECTION=complications.

CHAPTER 98

CARDIAC DIAGNOSTIC TESTING: NONINVASIVE ASSESSMENT OF CORONARY ARTERY DISEASE

Susan Sanner

There are numerous noninvasive ways to evaluate a patient with symptoms of cardiovascular disease (CAD). Each test has its advantages; each also has limitations (Table 98.1). The optimum assessment of CAD is a thorough history and physical examination that includes prior medical history of myocardial infarction or CAD, appropriate risk assessment, and the patient's present complaint (e.g., angina, radiating pain, tingling, or numbness) in conjunction with determining any family history of CAD.[1] In addition, immediate electrocardiographic (ECG) and laboratory biomarker testing should be considered to ensure a proper diagnosis and an adequate interventional plan.[1] Cardiac catheterization is indicated if ECG findings and biomarkers indicate an acute myocardial infarction. This chapter addresses the evaluation of suspected CAD in the absence of acute infarction.

Invasive coronary angiography (ICA) is considered the standard diagnostic test for CAD involving any obstructive lesion producing symptoms or individuals at risk of acute coronary syndrome (ACS). Due to risks and cost, however, this test may not be ideal for some patients.[1] Noninvasive tests, which are categorized as functional and anatomic tests, provide diagnostic and prognostic information that may improve risk stratification, ultimately guiding subsequent testing and intervention. Functional tests indicate whether symptoms are correlated with areas of ischemia and include exercise ECG, exercise/pharmacologic stress echocardiography, exercise/pharmacologic cardiac nuclear imaging with single-photon emission computed tomography (SPECT) or positron emission tomography (PET), pharmacologic stress magnetic resonance imaging (MRI), computed tomography (CT), and Doppler ultrasound-derived flow reserve measurement. Noninvasive anatomic tests include coronary CT angiography (CCTA) and coronary artery calcium scoring (CACS).[1]

Guided by the 2013 American College of Cardiology Foundation/American Heart Association (ACCF/AHA) Appropriate Use Criteria, providers may select which test is most beneficial in diagnosing CAD across patient presentations: (1) patients with signs and/or symptoms and/or various levels of risk for CAD; (2) patients with prior test results or coronary revascularization for follow-up evaluation; (3) patients scheduled for noncardiac surgery; and (4) patients with an exercise prescription or referral to cardiac rehabilitation. In general, some tests in the initial evaluation of patients with ischemia-related symptoms (newly diagnosed heart failure, arrhythmias, and syncope) were found to be Appropriate or May Be Appropriate. The exception are cases where low pre-test probability or low risk limited the benefit of most testing except for the exercise ECG. In addition, it is appropriate to test for the evaluation of new or worsening symptoms following a prior test. Testing in asymptomatic patients is generally considered Rarely Appropriate, except for calcium scoring and exercise testing in intermediate and high-risk individuals and rated May Be Appropriate.[2] In general, selection of the proper cardiac test (see Table 98.1) for an individual depends on the person's risk stratification, age, and tolerable level of activity.[2]

PATHOPHYSIOLOGY OF CORONARY ARTERY DISEASE

CAD exists when coronary arteries are narrowed by atherosclerotic plaque formation, plaque rupture, or spasm. This narrowing impedes coronary blood flow, resulting in hypoperfusion of the myocardium. The hypoperfusion produces first diastolic and then systolic dysfunction, with characteristic signs and symptoms, including chest pain. Typical ECG changes of ischemia result, although the ST-segment and T-wave changes that are central to demonstration of ischemia occur relatively late in the ischemic cascade.

Role of Inflammation and Atherogenesis

Inflammation has been implicated as one of the major processes that mediate the acceleration and progression of CAD and its complications. Inflammatory pathways have been very closely linked with the early development of atherosclerotic disease with plaque formation in coronary arteries, producing CAD. Inflammation and plaque composition both have an impact on the occurrence of acute plaque rupture, a cause of acute myocardial infarction.

Relation to Cardiac Stress Testing

Unlike most other circulatory beds in the body, the coronary circulation allows maximum oxygen extraction from the blood when the body is at rest. In a stress test or exercise tolerance test (ETT), patients are asked to perform incremental exercises that result in positive chronotropic (rate) and inotropic (strength of contraction) stimulation of the cardiovascular system, which in turn increases myocardial oxygen demand. Increases in oxygen demand obligate an increase in myocardial blood flow. The healthy coronary circulation can increase flow approximately five times above the baseline level. The fundamental pathophysiologic change in CAD is a limitation of the ability of the

TABLE 98.1   Exercise Testing Comparisons

Test	Benefits and Indications	Limitations
Exercise stress testing	Assesses ischemia, functional capacity, prognosis Equipment widely available Accuracy established in different populations	Lower sensitivity than other tests listed Poor specificity with women, resting ECG ST-T abnormalities, LVH does not indicate site or extent of infarct
Exercise myocardial perfusion imaging	Reproducible results Improved sensitivity and specificity higher diagnostic accuracy	Increases costs over treadmill testing Requires longer than treadmill exercise alone Modest radiation exposure Artifacts from soft tissue (breast) or in obese patients attenuate signal, decrease specificity
CMR imaging	High resolution of cardiac structure, function, and morphology No radiation exposure Stress perfusion MRI an option Three-dimensional capability Can be used with most cardiac stents	Use in claustrophobic patients can be difficult because of patient ability to stay in MRI machine Use of gadolinium-based contrast agents in patients with class 4 or 5 disease contraindicated in patients with implantable ferromagnetic objects (defibrillators)
Exercise radionuclide angiography	Well validated to identify patients with severe disease Risk stratification after MI Good images with obese patients or those with COPD Accurate information about ejection fractions	Limited availability and high expense Uses bicycle, not treadmill exercise Inaccurate when heart rate is irregular Reduced specificity with women, abnormal resting left ventricular function
Exercise echocardiography	Shorter test time, lower cost than nuclear imaging Assesses multiple parameters: global and regional ventricular function, chamber size, wall thickness, valve function Used with resting ECG abnormalities, LBBB Detects reversible ischemia (wall motion abnormalities develop with stress)	Images limited with obesity or obstructive lung disease Does not detect non–blood flow limiting blockages Reduced accuracy with resting wall motion abnormalities (prior MI, paced rhythm certain types of cardiac surgeries)
Pharmacologic stress with dipyridamole or adenosine	Accurate assessments in patients unable to complete exercise protocol Useful assessment in patients with claudication or musculoskeletal limitations Side effects rapidly reversible by ending infusion or administering aminophylline	Cannot assess functional capacity Contraindicated with hypotension, sick sinus syndrome, high-grade heart block, hyperreactive airways, caffeine or theophylline dependence, oral dipyridamole therapy Chest pain during test not indicative of CAD
Dobutamine echocardiography	Improves CAD assessments in patients unable to exercise Side effects rapidly reversible by terminating infusion or administering a beta blocker Perfusion defects represent true myocardial ischemia	Cannot assess functional capacity Contraindicated with recent MI (<1 week), unstable angina, high-grade heart block, BBB, severe aortic stenosis, hypertrophic obstructive cardiomyopathy, supraventricular dysrhythmias, ventricular tachycardia (history or current), uncontrolled hypertension, large aneurysm, severe pulmonary hypertension, beta blocker dependence

BBB, bundle branch block; *CAD*, cardiovascular disease; *CMR*, cardiac magnetic resonance; *COPD*, chronic obstructive pulmonary disease; *ECG*, electrocardiographic; *LBBB*, left bundle branch block; *LVH*, left ventricular hypertrophy; *MI*, myocardial infarction.
Risk Assessment Tools to Guide Decision-Making in the Primary Prevention of Atherosclerotic Cardiovascular Disease: A Special Report From the American Heart Association

coronary arterial circulation to vasodilate appropriately. As a result, the ability to increase coronary blood flow in the face of increased myocardial oxygen demand is limited, leading to an imbalance between oxygen supply and demand and resulting in myocardial ischemia.

OVERVIEW OF CARDIAC DIAGNOSTIC TESTING
Noninvasive Tests and Biomarkers for Coronary Artery Disease

There is evidence that supports the use of noninvasive markers for the diagnosis of subclinical CAD. C-reactive protein,

interleukin-6, and monocyte-macrophage colony-stimulating factor are markers that have shown predictive value for future adverse cardiovascular events. However, which of these noninvasive markers have a role in risk stratification for primary and secondary CAD prevention remains under investigation.[3-6]

Recent American College of Cardiology (ACC) guidelines provide some guidance about noninvasive testing and markers for asymptomatic CAD based on an individual patient's risk for CAD.

ACC guidelines have as a class 1 recommendation (suggested) based on Level B evidence (limited populations studied) that health care providers ascertain risk for CAD in asymptomatic individuals by use of a global assessment such as the Framingham score.[4] Other tools used to assess cardiovascular risk in patients include the ACC ASCVD Risk estimator available @ http://tools.acc.org/ASCVD-Risk-Estimator-Plus/#!/calculate/estimate/, or for preoperative patients, the Revised Cardiac Risk Index available@ https://qxmd.com/calculate/calculator_195/revised-cardiac-risk-index-lee-criteria. The ACC guidelines use the level of risk determined by these scores to evaluate the evidence and to classify recommendations for the use of various testing modalities in the investigation and determination of subclinical cardiovascular disease. For example, the ACC guidelines suggest that C-reactive protein can be used in asymptomatic men older than 50 years and women older than 60 years with low-density lipoprotein cholesterol below 160 mg/dL to determine if statin therapy is indicated and in asymptomatic intermediate-risk men older than 50 years and women older than 60 years to assess risk of cardiovascular disease.[4] Ankle-brachial index assessment is acceptable for intermediate-risk individuals to determine their risk for subclinical cardiovascular disease.[4]

Recent evidence suggests that the CACS may be beneficial for identifying CAD and is most likely to be useful in approaches for improving risk assessment in individuals who are at intermediate risk, although its role is not completely clear. The CACS is directly related to the plaque burden where zero constitutes a normal CACS; less than 10 is a low score and greater than 400 is a high score.[5,6] Even with a designated score, evidence does not support targeted treatment of patients with high-risk CACS to improve outcomes.[7] According to the (AACF)/AHA 2013 guidelines for assessment of cardiovascular risk, CACS may also be beneficial in asymptomatic adults with cardiovascular disease. Its primary advantage is that no patient preparation is required. However, owing to the issue of cost for a CACS determination, the exposure to radiation, and the unclear role of calcium scoring in low- to intermediate-risk patients with ACS, the ACC/AHA guidelines recommend CACS for individuals for whom, after having undergone a quantitative risk assessment, the treatment decision is unclear. CACS, in this case, may be able to help inform treatment.[4]

Overall, adequate risk assessment is the most challenging for individuals who are considered at low or intermediate risk for a cardiac event. Therefore the usefulness of inflammatory markers to predict a future cardiac event remains unclear and warrants further research.[5-8]

Exercise Tolerance Test

Exercise stress testing is generally inappropriate for detection of ischemia in asymptomatic patients with no history of revascularization.[9] The standard first-line approach to initial testing for CAD is the ETT, during which the patient (attached to a 12-lead electrocardiogram) is continuously monitored during graded exercise. It is used to detect CAD in patients with chest pain or dyspnea on exertion who are at intermediate risk of ACS as determined by ACCF/AHA guidelines for stable ischemic heart disease (SIHD).[9,10] Multiple protocols are available for the ETT (Bruce Protocol and Naughton Protocol).[10] The primary goal of the ETT is to increase workload incrementally to induce ischemia or until a predetermined workload is reached. Multiple studies are available that have validated the efficacy and safety of ETT in patients with low risk of chest pain. Studies have also reported on the safety and efficacy

of immediate exercise testing in low-risk patients who have normal ECG findings and biomarker levels and are not serially evaluated before stress testing.[11,12] The ETT also provides data on the patient's functional capacity, which has been shown to be a significant predictor of future cardiac events.[12] In an ETT, patients are asked to perform incremental exercises based on standardized protocols. These result in positive chronotropic (rate) and inotropic (strength of contraction) response of the cardiovascular system, increasing myocardial oxygen demand. The normal hemodynamic response to these stimuli is an increase in absolute coronary blood flow. However, this ability is reduced in the presence of CAD, which leads to an imbalance between oxygen supply and demand, resulting in myocardial ischemia and ischemic changes in the electrocardiogram.

The ECG response of normal hearts is maintenance of an "isoelectric" ST segment during exercise and recovery. By standard criteria, a positive test result for CAD is defined by the development of horizontal or downsloping ST-segment depression of 1 mm measured 80 msec after the J point of the QRS complex (the junction between the QRS complex and the ST segment). ECG changes such as upsloping ST segment (elevation) or isolated T-wave downsloping (depression) have not demonstrated significant predictive value.

Because the interpretation of the test is based primarily on the development of characteristic ischemic ST-segment and T-wave changes, it is not surprising that resting ECG abnormalities can lead to a reduction in test sensitivity and specificity. The specificity of the routine ETT is reduced if the patient has had a prior myocardial infarction or if the patient has a resting bundle branch block conduction abnormality, paced rhythm, preexcitation syndromes, or inability to exercise because this produces persistent ST-segment and T-wave abnormalities.[12]

A number of other factors can interfere with the sensitivity of the exercise test in detecting CAD. Because an increase in coronary blood flow is related to an increasing heart rate and systolic blood pressure, clearly the sensitivity of the test is effort dependent. The standard is the peak heart rate achieved during exercise. Specifically, a test result is considered negative for CAD only if the patient exercises to at least 85% of the age-predicted maximum heart rate without evidence of inducible ischemia (maximum heart rate = [220 − age]). If the patient fails to achieve this "target" heart rate, the test should be considered nondiagnostic or insufficient to exclude ischemia. On the other hand, if there is evidence of ischemia (typical angina, ischemic ST changes) before the patient's target heart rate is reached, the test is considered strongly predictive of significant CAD. A second important predictor of more advanced CAD is exercise-induced hypotension (i.e., a fall in systolic blood pressure of at least 20 mm Hg at any point during exercise). It is helpful to correlate the ischemic leads on exercise electrocardiography to the underlying coronary anatomy to roughly identify the culprit artery or arteries.

Medications such as beta blockers, digoxin, certain calcium channel blockers, and other antihypertensives can attenuate the heart rate, making the rest of the exercise test less diagnostic.[12] The decision to discontinue beta blockers 1 or 2 days before testing is influenced by the purpose of the exercise test. For ETTs ordered to detect angina, it is recommended that the cardiologist be consulted about withholding the medication before the test is performed. ETTs performed to assess effectiveness of pharmacologic therapy require normal daily medication regimens. Imaging studies such as nuclear cardiac scanning may be useful in patients who undergo a stress test during beta blocker therapy.[2]

Another potential contributor to the ETT's lack of sensitivity is derived from the limitations of the surface electrocardiogram related to the spatial distribution of the electrical abnormalities that occur in ischemia. This concept may be better understood if the electrocardiogram is considered an imaging tool that examines the electric forces of cardiac depolarization and repolarization. To detect ischemia, the repolarization phase of the cardiac cycle—the ST segment and T wave—is examined for abnormalities. ST-segment and T-wave changes in the surface electrocardiogram are related to both the extent and the severity of myocardial ischemia. As might be expected, the ETT is more sensitive for the detection of severe disease. Ischemia that is confined to the posterior or lateral segments of the left ventricle can be more difficult to detect.

When considering ETT, health care providers should be aware of its contraindications. For these patients, consultation with a cardiologist is recommended. Some absolute contraindications to ETT include active endocarditis, decompensated heart failure, acute myocardial infarction in previous 2 days, inability to exercise, persistent stable angina, uncontrolled cardiac arrhythmias including supraventricular ectopy and sustained ventricular arrhythmias with hemodynamic compromise, high-grade heart block, and hemodynamically significant aortic stenosis.[9,10] Relative contraindications include complete heart block, cardiomyopathy, known left main CAD, recent stroke or transient ischemia attack (TIA), severe hypertension (>200 mm Hg or diastolic > 110 mm Hg), and tachyarrhythmias with uncontrolled ventricular rate.[9,10]

Imaging Adjuncts to the Exercise Tolerance Test

In the evaluation of patients with stable chest pain syndromes and normal surface ECG recordings, the conventional ETT typically provides adequate clinical information for diagnostic purposes. Similarly, in patients with known CAD and stable coronary syndromes, the ETT is typically adequate as a means of observing disease progression for purposes of prognostication and timing of revascularization procedures. However, with respect to the delineation of damaged myocardial regions and residual myocardial viability in zones of prior injury, it has become clear that adjunctive radiopharmaceutical or cardiac ultrasound imaging substantially improves test sensitivity and specificity (Box 98.1).

B O X 98.1

Indications for Coupling of Nuclear or Ultrasound Imaging to Standard Exercise Tolerance Test

- Left ventricular hypertrophy with ST-segment and T-wave abnormalities on resting electrocardiography
- Baseline ST-segment and T-wave abnormalities on resting electrocardiography for any reason
- Recent myocardial infarction, particularly with persistent rest ST-segment abnormalities
- Clinical use of digoxin
- Wolff-Parkinson-White syndrome
  Bundle branch block
  Ventricular pacemaker

The various imaging modalities that can be used as adjuncts to the graded exercise test can be viewed in the context of the ischemic cascade. Myocardial perfusion imaging (MPI) is designed to detect the spatial distribution of myocardial blood flow (i.e., to define the regional heterogeneity of flow that characterizes regional ischemia). Cardiac ultrasound imaging (two-dimensional echocardiography [2DE]) is designed to detect the abnormalities in regional wall motion that develop as a consequence of regional myocardial ischemia.

Examining the limitations of routine exercise testing from a historical perspective yields interesting information. The limitations detailed previously were clinically acceptable when the exercise study was performed principally as a binary diagnostic test (to determine whether CAD was present or absent) in patients with chest pain. The limited sensitivity of this test in a subgroup of patients with minimum CAD did not produce significant consequences. However, even for patients with minimum CAD, the ETT did not yield significant answers about CAD status, primarily because these patients have a cardiovascular event rate of only 1% to 2% per year.

With the advent of effective coronary revascularization surgery, the ETT has assumed additional predictive clinical relevance. It is clear that powerful predictors of outcomes reside in clinical data and in ETT results independent of the ST-segment response, such as the hemodynamic response and the aerobic work capacity as reflected by exercise duration.

In contrast, the more recent expansion of interventional therapies for coronary revascularization has resulted in an important shift in the data that practitioners seek from provocative testing. For example, in patients with stable coronary syndromes, the judicious application of percutaneous coronary intervention requires that both the presence and territorial distribution of ischemia be defined. Furthermore, in patients who have sustained prior myocardial injury, decisions about revascularization require a definition of ischemia both within and remote from the site of injury as well as tissue viability within the zone of infarction.

The usefulness of these adjunctive imaging modalities depends in part on the prevalence of disease in the population of patients being studied. In general, these adjunctive modalities are most useful in populations with an intermediate pretest clinical probability of disease.[4]

Myocardial Perfusion Imaging. MPI offers a method of visualizing blood flow to the heart by injection of a radioactive cardiac-specific tracer. This improves the diagnostic accuracy of a stress test because it gives another method of detecting perfusion defects aside from measuring ST depression on the electrocardiogram. MPI also offers the additional advantage of estimating left ventricular function. The technique is also used independently of a stress test in the evaluation of patients with acute active chest pain.[13] The 2014 ACC/AHA/AATS/PCNA/SCAI/STS Focused Update Guideline for the Diagnosis and Management of Patients With SIHD indicates its usefulness in patients with presumed SIHD who have unacceptable ischemic symptoms despite medical therapy and who are candidates for coronary revascularization (class I, LOE: C) and when defining the extent and severity of CAD in patients with suspected SIHD whose clinical characteristics and results of noninvasive testing (excluding stress testing) indicate a high likelihood of severe ischemic heart disease (IHD) who are candidates for coronary revascularization (class IIa, LOE: C).[13] It is not routinely performed after adequate stress testing has been negative for ischemia.

At present, thallium chloride Tl-201 and technetium Tc 99m sestamibi are the radiopharmaceutical agents used for the detection of CAD in MPI. They appear comparable for CAD detection in patients with stable coronary syndromes. A number of sources have documented the clinical efficacy of sestamibi and thallium.

Thallium 201 was the first agent used in clinical practice. It is a cation that acts similarly to potassium and is taken into viable cardiac myocytes. It distributes in cardiac tissue roughly in proportion to regional blood flow. It has a half-life of 73 hours. Clinically, it is injected while the patient is at peak exercising or shortly after the pharmacologic stress test agent is administered. Images are taken immediately and then again in 3 to 4 hours. On the initial image, the defects may represent either regional ischemia or nonviable myocardium.[14]

The second agent that is commonly used is ^{99m}Tc sestamibi. It acts as a calcium analogue when it is taken up by the myocytes. It has a shorter half-life of about 6 hours. Once it is taken up by the myocytes, its distribution is quite different from that of thallium, and it is well suited to the imaging of patients with ACSs. When a sestamibi scan is performed, a second injection is given at the time of the delayed image. Interpretation of the scan is very similar to that of thallium imaging.[14]

Unlike thallium-based perfusion imaging, sestamibi image acquisition can be performed up to several hours after tracer injection. This allows appropriate treatment and triage of patients with acute myocardial infarction and unstable angina; the image acquired after such treatment will represent the status of myocardial perfusion at the time of tracer injection. Tracer injection can be repeated at a later time to assess myocardial salvage—residual viability in infarct patients—or to define the presence, extent, and territorial distribution of ischemia in patients with unstable angina. Sestamibi imaging provides the capacity to "simultaneously" define left ventricular systolic function and myocardial perfusion. This offers a means to assess the impact of reperfusion therapies in patients with ACSs.

Researchers have found that sestamibi imaging in the emergency department may be useful in identifying low- versus high-risk patients with suspected myocardial ischemia.[14] Furthermore, although MPI with ^{201}Tl is typically coupled with exercise or pharmacologic stress, rest-redistribution imaging may provide valuable information in patients with unstable coronary syndromes who are not suitable candidates for stress studies.

Because the diagnosis of perfusion defects requires the detection of decreased flow in one region relative to another, there will be occasional instances of false-negative scans in patients with severe three-vessel or left main CAD. These "balanced" flow disturbances (i.e., a decrease in coronary flow in more than two geographic territories) should be suspected in patients in whom clinical suspicion of severe CAD is high but whose MPI reveals uniform tracer uptake.

Because MPI increases diagnostic accuracy of stress testing, the ACC/AHA guidelines recommend its use in several patient subsets. It should be used if there is any baseline ECG abnormality that would interfere with measurement of stress-induced ST-segment changes, such as left ventricular hypertrophy, bundle branch blocks, and digoxin use. MPI is also a useful tool for use with high-risk diabetic patients.[13]

Exercise Echocardiography. The practice of exercise echocardiography has expanded dramatically in recent years. Current data suggest that adjunctive echocardiographic imaging enhances the sensitivity and specificity of CAD detection to an extent comparable to that provided by nuclear techniques.[2] The 2DE evidence for ischemia includes an abnormal left ventricular ejection fraction (LVEF) response to exercise or the development of regional wall motion abnormalities. The exercise is performed with a bicycle or treadmill, and dobutamine is the most common pharmacologic agent used simultaneously with the echocardiography imaging. The image quality may be enhanced by the injection of echogenic microbubbles.

As previously demonstrated in thallium imaging, the sensitivity of the 2DE technique for CAD detection is enhanced in patient subsets with multivessel CAD or prior myocardial infarction. In addition, the sensitivity of exercise echocardiography is decreased in patients with resting wall motion abnormalities. In practical terms, patients in whom adequate ultrasound imaging views cannot be obtained (often including obese patients and those with severe emphysematous lung disease or tachycardia) should be considered for alternative imaging modalities.

A positive exercise echocardiogram is defined by stress-induced decrease in regional wall motion, decreased wall thickening, or regional compensatory hyperkinesis. Some of the advantages of this test are that it is faster to perform than a nuclear stress test because the delayed images are obtained much sooner, there is no associated radiation exposure, it is less costly, and it can be more readily performed in an office setting. A limitation of the test is that it is dependent on the operator's experience. Test results can also be altered by obesity, lung disease, and tachycardia.

Comparison of Myocardial Perfusion Imaging With Two-Dimensional Echocardiography. Exercise 2DE with Doppler flow study is comparable to MPI for the detection of CAD. There is a greater accumulation of literature for MPI with respect to prognostication in patients with CAD. In addition, it appears that MPI may be preferable to 2DE for the recognition of incremental ischemia in myocardial regions characterized by abnormalities of resting wall motion. Furthermore, quantification of myocardial perfusion data has been more extensively validated than comparable quantification of cardiac ultrasound data; cardiac ultrasound imaging has been limited by the technical difficulties in the endocardial border recognition. The majority of studies with exercise 2DE have been limited to qualitative visual assessment. It is also clear that the early 2DE data were acquired in patient groups with a relatively high incidence of significant CAD. Finally, MPI (e.g., rest-redistribution ^{201}Tl scintigraphy and rest-injected ^{99m}Tc- sestamibi) is more amenable to the detection of ischemia in patients with unstable coronary syndromes, in whom exercise is contraindicated. Serial rest 2DE images acquired in patients with unstable coronary syndromes may occasionally be useful if new or more extensive wall motion abnormalities can be detected during recurrent ischemia.

In contrast, 2DE offers access to the incremental information about left ventricular contractile performance that is analogous to that provided by exercise radionuclide ventriculography. LVEF response to exercise provides important prognostic information in patients with CAD; such information is available only inferentially by myocardial perfusion scintigraphy (i.e., pulmonary thallium uptake). Finally, with respect to viability assessment, the detection of preserved contractile function in myocardial segments supplied by diseased coronary arteries is essential.

Three-Dimensional and Doppler Flow Echocardiography. Three-dimensional (3D) echocardiographic techniques are currently available that use MRI and computer-assisted 3D acquisition systems for 2DE. Three-dimensional technology has recently become available and provides a unique view of structure and function within the heart. Current evidence-based guideline evaluations, however, center on 2DE with Doppler flow study.[2] Doppler flow studies are used to localize and to quantify obstructions in the cardiovascular system. Primarily, the addition of a Doppler flow study to echocardiography enhances the ability to evaluate prosthetic valve function, to detect and to evaluate the blood shunting from a septal defect, and to gauge the severity of valvular stenosis or regurgitation.[2]

Cardiac Magnetic Resonance Imaging and Ultrafast Computed Tomography Cardiac Scans. Although historically it has been difficult to image the moving structures of the heart, the role of cardiac magnetic resonance (CMR) in the assessment and management of patients with CAD has increased. Advantages of using CMR include the lack of ionizing radiation and its flexible, high spatial resolution and three-dimensional functions that allow cardiac imaging in any desired plane.[15] CMR is primarily used to evaluate myocardial ischemia in individuals with chronic CAD using one of two major CMR techniques.[16] First, the Dobutamine stress functional CMR, although very accurate in the assessment of ischemia, is used less often due to the use of gadolinium. This is considered one of the disadvantages of this technique due to concerns regarding the use of gadolinium-based contrast agents in patients with chronic kidney disease as well as the inability to image most patients with pacemakers or implantable cardioverter-defibrillators due to safety concerns.[2] Despite the disadvantages, however, CMR has evolved into a gold-standard technique for the assessment of myocardial viability in patients with CAD late gadolinium enhancement (LGE). In patients with CAD prior to revascularization, evaluation of the transmural extent of LGE enables prediction of recovery of function with revascularization.

The second and most commonly used technique is vasodilator first-pass contrast-enhanced perfusion CMR. Comparisons of vasodilator stress perfusion CMR and dobutamine stress CMR suggest a higher sensitivity for contrast-enhanced perfusion imaging and higher specificity for dobutamine wall motion imaging. Based on multimodality appropriate use criteria, stress CMR is considered appropriate for patients with high pretest probability for CAD or intermediate pretest probability of CAD with an uninterpretable electrocardiogram (ECG) or inability to exercise.[3] It is also appropriate for patients with an abnormal ECG who are intermediate to high risk as well as those with an abnormal or uncertain exercise ECG or those with obstructive CAD of uncertain significance noted on CT or invasive coronary angiography.[2]

Current investigations of 3D technology also involve ultrafast electron beam computed tomography (EBCT). This emerging 3D technology performs a heart scan at a rapid rate, thus "freezing" cardiac motion. Coronary artery calcification is analyzed, and a total calcium score for a patient's coronary arteries is calculated on the basis of the areas of calcification and the maximum CT calcium density. Calcium generally does not appear in normal coronary arteries, so calcium deposits are determined to be a strong marker of atherosclerosis. However, EBCT does not define the location and extent of cardiac disease, and it does not image soft noncalcified plaque. A negative calcium score does not imply the absence of plaque. With significant CAD (50% stenosis), only 2.5% of coronary segments have no detectable calcium on EBCT.[3] However, coronary calcium scoring has recently been proved to be accurate in predicting CAD risk in apparently healthy middle-aged men in several studies.[2] EBCT scanning has also been found to be beneficial in motivating patients to adopt lifestyle changes and to implement aggressive cardiovascular risk reduction strategies. Recent ACC guidelines suggest calcium scoring for intermediate-risk individuals (class IIa, benefit outweighs cost); in individuals at low to intermediate risk, calcium scoring is considered class IIb (beneficial only in selected patients).[2]

Pharmacologic Stress Testing

The clinical usefulness of adjunctive imaging modalities has been expanded by coupling such techniques to "pharmacologic" stress, an important advantage in patients who are unable to perform conventional treadmill or ergometer exercises. Pharmacologic agents currently in use are coronary vasodilators (e.g., dipyridamole [Persantine] and adenosine) and inotropic-chronotropic drugs (e.g., dobutamine).

The vasodilator drugs are applied to assess the effective coronary flow reserve (i.e., the ratio of maximum flow to basal flow). Because the extraction of tracer is proportional to blood flow, the coupling of vasodilators with MPI allows the detection of regional flow disturbances. These regional perfusion abnormalities can be characterized as reversible (normal uptake at baseline, with decreased uptake after vasodilator) or fixed (indicative of prior infarction). The fact that vasodilators do not induce ischemia but simply unmask regional variations in flow reserve means that the ECG portion of the test will rarely demonstrate ischemic changes. However, on rare occasions, ECG changes may be observed, and up to 20% of patients may experience angina. Ischemia may be caused by "coronary steal." The effects of dipyridamole can be reversed by intravenous administration of aminophylline, and the effects of adenosine and dobutamine can be reversed by discontinuation of the infusion.

Another approach is to induce cardiac ischemia by use of a beta agonist such as dobutamine, which is administered in gradually increased doses until the goal heart rate is achieved (the provocation of ischemic chest pain or ST-segment changes may also lead to termination of the test). Dobutamine increases cardiac work, initially by an inotropic effect; a normal cardiac response to dobutamine is an increase in global left ventricular contractility. The chronotropic effects of this agent become apparent at higher infusion rates (20 to 50 mg/kg/min). Most commonly, inducible ischemia occurs at these higher infusion rates. Dobutamine is useful in patients who cannot tolerate the bronchoconstriction associated with adenosine administration.

As previously described, the development of regional wall motion abnormalities is often an early manifestation of ischemia. For this reason, dobutamine is most commonly coupled with 2DE (which is performed after each increase in dose) to determine regional abnormalities in left ventricular function or decreases in LVEF. The onset of new regional hypokinesis in a previously normally contracting segment is highly predictive of CAD in the artery supplying the dysfunctional segment. Alternatively, MPI can be coupled with dobutamine in patients with poor echocardiographic windows. The accuracies of dobutamine echocardiography and dobutamine MPI are comparable.

DIAGNOSTIC TESTING FOR CARDIOVASCULAR DISEASE IN WOMEN

CAD is the leading cause of death for women in the United States, but a considerable body of research has demonstrated that women have different patterns of CAD and different responses to cardiac testing than their male counterparts.[17] Although CAD is the leading cause of death in women, this disorder often is not diagnosed expeditiously. Unfortunately, studies investigating women and CAD are limited. Women are more likely to have nonobstructive or single-vessel disease compared with men, which decreases the diagnostic accuracy of stress testing.[18]

Single-photon emission CT imaging is technically limited in women because of breast tissue and smaller coronary artery size.[18] Recent evidence, particularly from the Women's Ischemia Syndrome Evaluation study, a multicenter study sponsored by the National Heart, Lung, and Blood Institute, has demonstrated that many women without obstructive CAD continue to have symptoms and a poor quality of life.[18] Many of these women have evidence of stress-induced ischemia, which is likely to be related to endothelial dysfunction of the microvasculature.[18]

As a result, there is limited evidence to suggest the most appropriate cardiovascular diagnostic testing for women.

All patients, even if asymptomatic, require risk stratification according to the Framingham risk score (low, intermediate, or high) to identify CAD risk equivalents.[2] At present, the ACC/AHA guidelines do not recommend stress tests for asymptomatic patients, unless the patient (men 45 years or older, women 55 years or older) is sedentary and wishes to begin exercising aggressively.[2] The exception is asymptomatic women with diabetes and peripheral arterial disease. These women are classified as high risk; diabetes and peripheral arterial disease are CAD risk equivalents. The recommendation for asymptomatic women with diabetes, peripheral vascular disease, and possible kidney disease is for secondary prevention strategies to prevent future cardiac events.[2]

For women who are symptomatic but who have a normal resting ECG recording, good exercise tolerance, and no coronary risk factors, an exercise stress test is appropriate; diagnostic imaging is not recommended for low-risk women who are asymptomatic.[2] For women who are symptomatic and have known CAD, an abnormal resting ECG recording, questionable exercise tolerance, or coronary risk factors (e.g., diabetes, peripheral arterial disease), stress test imaging is recommended.[2]

SUMMARY

Cardiologists are generally aware of the test limitations inherent in exercise testing. The use of additional testing to better diagnose CAD noninvasively has evolved in the development of numerous testing modalities that are yielding more sensitive results. Tests that provide diagnostic information of the left ventricle specifically along with status reports of the regional myocardial perfusion gradient have obviously gained widespread use as adjunct modalities to arrive at a more comprehensive cardiac diagnosis with improved treatments and outcomes.

Cardiac ultrasound and MPI are of comparable usefulness in detecting CAD. The data with respect to prognostication are most extensive for MPI techniques, but ultrasound-based data are accumulating.

Both functional studies and perfusion imaging have demonstrated clear usefulness in addressing the complex question of myocardial viability. These testing modalities are used to assess the presence of functional heart muscle in patients with IHD and regional contractile dysfunction.

MPI techniques and ultrasound-derived techniques are competitive. It is clear that these modalities may in fact be complementary in the evaluation of selected patients with CAD. The ACC/AHA Task Force on Practice Guidelines suggested that exercise MPI or exercise echocardiography may be used as the initial test for diagnosis in patients with chronic stable angina who are able to tolerate exercise.[2] The ACC/AHA Committee on Clinical Application of Echocardiography recognizes that exercise or pharmacologic stress echocardiography can be used to evaluate the presence or extent of ischemia, even when there is an underlying ECG abnormality that affects interpretation of the ECG recording, such as prior ischemia, left bundle branch block, or Wolff-Parkinson-White syndrome.[2] There is conflicting evidence on whether echocardiographic techniques are preferable when there are no resting ECG abnormalities.[2] For asymptomatic patients at risk for CAD, it is unclear whether exercise testing is beneficial because there have been no clinical trials investigating exercise testing in this population.[2]

In addition, multiple studies have documented gender-related differences associated with cardiovascular disease. In women, CAD is less frequently diagnosed, which in turn helps contribute to making it the leading cause of death in women. Women are more likely to have single-vessel or nonobstructive cardiac disease compared with men, which makes it less likely for an accurate diagnosis by use of stress exercise.

REFERENCES

1. Noninvasive testing for coronary artery disease, Executive Summary, Effective Health Care Program. Agency for Healthcare Research and Quality. Retrieved from www.ahrq.gov. (Retrieved 27 May 2018).
2. Wolk, M. J., Bailey, S. R., Doherty, J. U., et al. (2014). ACCF/AHA/ASE/ASNC/HFSA/HRS/SCAI/SCCT/SCMR/STS 2013 multimodality appropriate use criteria for the detection and risk assessment of stable ischemic heart disease: A report of the American College of Cardiology Foundation Appropriate Use Criteria Task Force, American Heart Association, American Society of Echocardiography, American Society of Nuclear Cardiology, Heart Failure Society of America, Heart Rhythm Society, Society for Cardiovascular Angiography and Interventions, Society of Cardiovascular Computed Tomography, Society for Cardiovascular Magnetic Resonance, and Society of Thoracic Surgeons. *Journal of the American College of Cardiology, 63*(4), 380–406. PMID: 24355759.
3. Krintus, M., Kozinski, M., Kubica, J., et al. (2014). Critical appraisal of inflammatory markers in cardiovascular risk stratification. *Critical Reviews in Clinical Laboratory Sciences, 51*(5), 263–279.
4. Goff, D. C., & Lloyd-Jones, D. (2014). 2013 ACC/AHA guideline on the assessment of cardiovascular risk. A report of the American College of Cardiology/American Heart Association Task Force on Practice Guidelines. *Journal of the American College of Cardiology, 63*(25 Pt. B), 2935–2959. doi:10.1161/01.cir.0000437741.48606.98.
5. Ammirati, E., Moroni, F., Norata, G., Magnon, M., & Camici, P. (2015). Markers of inflammation associated with plaque progression and instability in patients with carotid atherosclerosis. *Mediators of Inflammation, 2015,* http://dx.doi.org/10.1155/2015/718329.
6. Rusnak, J., Fastner, C., Behnes, M., Mashayekhi, K., Borggrefe, M., & Akin, I. (2017). Biomarkers in stable coronary artery disease. *Current Pharmaceutical Biotechnology, 18*(6), 456–471. doi:10.2174/1389201018666170630120805.
7. Shaw, L. J., Giambrone, A. E., Blaha, M. J., et al. (2015). Long-term prognosis after coronary artery calcification testing in asymptomatic patients: A cohort study. *Annals of Internal Medicine, 163,* 14–21.

8. Krintus, M., Kozinski, M., Kubica, J., et al. (2014). Critical appraisal of inflammatory markers in cardiovascular risk stratification. *Critical Reviews in Clinical Laboratory Sciences, 51*(5), 263–279.

9. Fletcher, G. F., Ades, P. A., Kligfield, P., et al. (2013). American Heart Association Exercise, Cardiac Rehabilitation, and Prevention Committee of the Council on Clinical Cardiology, Council on Nutrition, Physical Activity and Metabolism, Council on Cardiovascular and Stroke Nursing, and Council on Epidemiology and Prevention. Exercise standards for testing and training: A scientific statement from the American Heart Association. *Circulation, 128*(8), 876.

10. Garner, K., Pomeroy, W., & Arnold, J. (2017). Exercise stress testing: Indications and common questions. *American Family Physician, 96*(5), 293–300.

11. Yang, E. H., Kamran, S., & Ptaszny, M. (2013). Non-invasive assessment of coronary artery disease. *Hospital Medicine Clinics, 2*(3), A1–A10, e305–e336.

12. Karthik, A., Girish, D., & McArdle, B. (2013). The role of non-invasive imaging in coronary artery disease detection, prognosis, and clinical decision making. *The Canadian Journal of Cardiology, 29*, 285–289.

13. Fihn, S. D., Blankenship, J. C., & Alexander, K. P. (2015). 2014 ACC/AHA/AATS/PCNA/SCAI/STS focused update of the guideline for the diagnosis and management of patients with stable ischemic heart disease: A report of the American College of Cardiology/American Heart Association Task Force on Practice Guidelines, and the American Association for Thoracic Surgery, Preventive Cardiovascular Nurses Association, Society for Cardiovascular Angiography and Interventions, and Society of Thoracic Surgeons. *The Journal of Thoracic and Cardiovascular Surgery, 149*(3), e5–e23.

14. Crownover, B. K., & Bepko, J. L. (2013). Appropriate and safe use of diagnostic imaging. *American Family Physician, 87*(7), 494–501.

15. Kramer, C. M. (2016). The role of CMR in the assessment and prognosis of patients with stable CAD. American College of Cardiology. *Expert Opinion.* Retrieved from https://www.acc.org/latest-in-cardiology/articles/2016/02/22/08/49/role-of-cmr-in-the-assessment-and-prognosis-of-patients-with-stable-cad. (Retrieved 28 May 2018).

16. Gotschy, A., Niemann, M., & Kozerke, S. (2015). Cardiovascular magnetic resonance for the assessment of coronary artery disease. *International Journal of Cardiology, 193*, 84–92. doi:10.1016/j.ijcard.2014.11.098.

17. American College of Cardiology, ACC News Story, Women and Heart Disease: New Data Reaffirm Lack of Awareness by Women and Physicians 2017. Retrieved from http://www.acc.org/latest-in-cardiology/articles/2017/06/22/10/01/women-and-heart-disease-new-data-reaffirm-lack-of-awareness-by-women-and-physicians. (Retrieved 28 May 2018).

18. Vavas, S., Hong, S., & Rosen, S. (2012). Non-invasive diagnostic techniques for coronary artery disease in women. *Clinical Cardiology, 35*(3), 149–155.

CHAPTER **99**

ABDOMINAL AORTIC ANEURYSM

Joanne Sandberg-Cook

DEFINITION AND EPIDEMIOLOGY

An abdominal aortic aneurysm (AAA) is a progressive, permanent, localized dilation of the abdominal aorta with aortic diameter of 3.0 cm or more, or a 50% increase in diameter compared with the adjacent normal segment.[1]

The aorta is a conduit that carries blood to the body and is divided by the diaphragm into the thoracic and abdominal aorta. It is composed of three layers: the tunica intima, tunica media, and tunica adventitia. In adults, the normal diameter of the abdominal aorta varies with age, height, gender, and body habitus, but the average infrarenal aortic diameter in an adult is approximately 2.0 cm and typically less than 3.0 cm. The prevalence of an AAA located in the infrarenal section of the aorta is at least three times greater than a thoracic aortic aneurysm.

Aneurysms are described by their shape, which help identify a true aneurysm. A true aneurysm involves all three layers of the aorta. The more common, fusiform aneurysm is a symmetric weakness of the entire circumference of the aorta that produces a bulge. A saccular aneurysm is an asymmetric weakness or bleb on the side of the aorta; these defects result from trauma or an internal wall defect caused by an ulcer. A pseudoaneurysm, or false aneurysm, is an enlargement of only the outer layer of the blood vessel wall. AAAs are also described by size (a small aneurysm has a diameter <4.0 cm, a medium aneurysm has a diameter of 4.0 to 5.4 cm, a large aneurysm has a diameter ≥5.5 cm, and a very large aneurysm has a diameter ≥6.0 cm), as well as involvement of the renal or visceral vessels.

AAA is an important clinical diagnosis because it is associated with considerable risk of rupture and death as the aneurysm enlarges to a diameter of more than 5.0 cm (1.96 inches). In the United States, 15,000 deaths/year are attributed to AAAs, and it is the 10th leading cause of death in men older than 55 years.[2] Treatment is usually recommended when an AAA grows to larger than 5.5 cm in diameter. Most patients who have a ruptured AAA will die before reaching the hospital, and of those who make it to the hospital and have surgery, the outcome is dependent on their presenting clinical condition, but typically the mortality rate has been stated as anywhere from 80% to 90%.[3] The high mortality rate has not changed over the past 20 years although the incidence of aneurysm and rupture has leveled and appears to be decreasing.[3] This decrease is likely due to earlier detection, better treatment of cardiovascular risk factors including hypertension and hyperlipidemia, and lifestyle changes including fewer people smoking. There has been considerable improvement in operative technique with broader use of endovascular repair of both aneurysms and ruptures.

Aortic aneurysms are complex problems with genetic and environmental risk factors. Major risk factors for AAA include advancing age (>65), male gender, family history of an AAA, and cigarette smoking (current or past). Additional risk factors include atherosclerotic vascular disease, hypertension, hyperlipidemia, and other vascular aneurysms (e.g., iliac, femoral, popliteal aneurysms).[4] There is an association between chronic obstructive pulmonary disease (COPD) and AAA which remains poorly understood. The high prevalence of AAA in patients with COPD may be related to medications (oral steroids), smoking, and/or coexisting disease rather than to a common pathway of pathogenesis.

Individuals younger than age 60 are not as affected by AAA. Males are affected more than females at a 6:1 ratio.[2] Smoking is the greatest environmental risk factor for AAA development. An AAA is over seven times more likely to develop in a smoker than a nonsmoker, with duration of smoking being a key variable.[5] First-degree male relatives of patients with AAA have two to four times the normal risk for AAA. Female first-degree relatives appear to have similar risk, but the data are less certain.[2] Those with a decreased risk of AAA development include women, non-Caucasians, diabetics, and regular exercisers.[4] Factors associated with an increased risk of rupture include female gender, large initial aneurysm diameter, age over 80 years, current smoking, and elevated blood pressure.[6] Risk factors for aneurysm development, expansion, and rupture are listed in Table 99.1.

TABLE 99.1	Risk Factors for Aneurysm Development, Expansion, and Rupture
Symptom	**Risk Factors**
AAA development	Tobacco use Hypercholesterolemia Hypertension Male gender Family history (male predominance)
AAA expansion	Advanced age Severe cardiac disease Previous stroke Tobacco use Cardiac or renal transplant
AAA rupture	Female gender Low FEV_1 Larger initial AAA diameter Higher mean blood pressure Current tobacco use Cardiac or renal transplant Critical wall stress–wall strength relationship

AAA, Abdominal aortic aneurysm.
From Chaikof, E. L., Palmon, R. L., Eskandari, M. K., et al. (2018). The care of patients with abdominal aortic aneurysms. *J Vasc Surgery, 67*(1), 2–77.

PATHOPHYSIOLOGY

AAA is a disease of the medial wall layer of the aorta. It is characterized by degeneration of the extracellular matrix proteins and the presence of an inflammatory cell infiltrate composed predominantly of T cells. Degradation of the cell wall proteins in the medial layer occurs as a result of complex interactions among genetic factors, inflammatory cytokines, matrix metalloproteinases (MMPs), tissue inhibitors of MMPs, and others. The consequences include dissolution and fragmentation of collagen and elastin, leading to expansion of the vessel wall.[2] When the aortic wall tension exceeds the tensile strength of the wall collagen and the wall can no longer withstand the repetitive force of systolic contraction, the aneurysm ruptures.

CLINICAL PRESENTATION AND PHYSICAL EXAMINATION

Although an AAA may cause symptoms as a result of the pressure on surrounding structures, most are asymptomatic at initial diagnosis. Asymptomatic AAAs are generally detected during an incidental radiologic or surgical procedure. Alternatively, in thin patients, a supine abdominal examination may readily show a pulsatile abdominal mass.

Thromboembolic phenomena may herald the presence of an AAA. Microembolic infarcts in the lower extremity of a patient may suggest either abdominal or popliteal aneurysm. Embolization of mural thrombus from an abdominal aneurysm may be seen with acute limb ischemia caused by femoral or popliteal occlusion.[7]

The classic diagnostic triad of ruptured AAA is hypotension, pulsatile abdominal mass, and abdominal pain or back pain. The triad is encountered in less than 50% of patients with a ruptured AAA.[7] Symptoms of AAA may include a sensation of abdominal discomfort, back pain, pulsation of abdomen, or flank pain.[5,7] Less frequently, individuals may complain of pain in the legs, chest, or groin area. They may also report anorexia, nausea, vomiting, or dyspnea. In a patient with a history of aneurysm or pulsatile mass, abdominal pain must be considered to represent a rapidly expanding or ruptured aneurysm and must be treated accordingly.

Measurement of blood pressure and body mass is indicated. Palpation of the abdomen for AAA is recommended. The patient is positioned supine with knees flexed to relax the abdominal wall. The examiner places the palm over the epigastrium to detect a transmitted pulsation. The examiner then places both hands on the abdomen with palms down and an index finger on either side of the pulsating area to measure the aortic width. An aneurysm expands laterally with each systole. An AAA is suspected when the aorta is judged to be at least 3.0 cm (1⅕ inches) in maximum diameter. Auscultation may reveal a bruit over the mass, but abdominal bruits are not specific for AAA formation.

Unfortunately, only 30% to 40% of aneurysms are noted on physical examination, with detection dependent on the skill of the examiner and the size of the aneurysm. The sensitivity of abdominal palpation increases with AAA diameter, from 29% for AAAs of 3.0 to 3.9 cm to 76% for AAAs of more than 5.0 cm. The sensitivity of abdominal palpation also increases (91%) when the abdominal girth is less than 100 cm (40-inch waistline) compared with 53% when abdominal girth is 100 cm or greater. Overall, when the girth is less than 100 cm and the AAA is more than 5.0 cm, abdominal palpation is highly sensitive (100%) for detection of AAA.[7] If on examination one finds a pulsatile mass in the groin or popliteal fossa, this raises suspicion for an AAA, because multiple aneurysms often coexist.[5,7]

DIAGNOSTICS

Given the high mortality associated with emergency ruptured AAA repair, early detection and repair before rupture are the mainstay of AAA management. The American College of Cardiology (ACC) and American Heart Association (AHA) practice guidelines for management of peripheral arterial disease recommend that "Men 60 years of age or older who are either a sibling or offspring of patients with AAAs should undergo a physical examination and ultrasound screening for detection of aortic aneurysms." And "men who are 65 to 75 years of age who have ever smoked should undergo a physical examination and a 1-time ultrasound screening for detection of AAAs." The US Preventive Services Task Force (USPSTF) recommendation statement recommends "1-time screening for AAA with ultrasonography in men aged 65 to 75 years who have ever smoked." The USPSTF recommends that clinicians selectively offer screening for AAA in men aged 65 to 75 who have never smoked rather than routinely screening all men in this group.[8] The Screening Abdominal Aortic Aneurysms Very Efficiently (SAAAVE) Act was approved by the United States Congress in January 2007. The SAAAVE Act permits a single screening aortic ultrasound examination as part of the "Welcome to Medicare" package for patients with defined risk factors for AAA. Males aged 65 to 75 years who have smoked more than 100 cigarettes in their lifetime or patients of any age or either sex with a strong family history are eligible for this screening examination.[9]

Ultrasonography is the imaging study ordered most often for screening and initial confirmation of an aneurysm. It can measure anteroposterior, transverse, and longitudinal dimensions of an AAA. Ultrasonography can provide a reasonably accurate measurement of initial size and can be used for serial follow-up evaluation. This modality is widely available, is painless, does not expose the patient to ionizing radiation, and is inexpensive. It can also visualize important anatomic markers such as relation of major arterial branches and adjacent organs. Duplex ultrasound can provide additional information on aortic flow.[10]

Computed tomography angiography (CTA), often with three-dimensional imaging, is the preferred and most widely used imaging modality before aortic aneurysm repair. It accurately demonstrates dilation of the aorta and the relationship to major branch vessels, both proximally and distally. It will show the degree of calcification, presence of mural thrombus, inflammatory aneurysms, aneurysmal leakage, penetrating aortic ulcer, length of the aneurysm neck, iliac artery, and whether other organs have become displaced.[7,10] It is noninvasive but does expose the patient to ionizing radiation and contrast medium, which can be harmful, especially in patients with kidney disease.

Standard contrast aortography has limited utility as a screening tool but may be indicated in select individuals, including those with suspected suprarenal extension, suspected visceral or renal artery disease, iliofemoral occlusive disease, horseshoe kidney, prior aortic or colonic surgery, and unusual aneurysms (e.g., mycotic, aortocaval fistula).[10] The procedure uses ionizing radiation and contrast. Most institutions, however, are using CT angiography, magnetic resonance imaging (MRI), or magnetic resonance angiography (MRA) for the preoperative evaluation of AAA.

MRI and MRA may also be used to diagnose aortic disease and for preoperative planning. MRI and MRA have limitations, including inability to be used for patients with pacemakers or other metallic hardware that would affect the magnetic field. In addition, for certain patients, claustrophobia or unstable medical conditions would preclude their being in the tube during the necessary acquisition time. The advantage of MRI or MRA is its absence of iodinated contrast material and radiation exposure. The use of gadolinium is contraindicated in patients with renal failure. With pre–endovascular aneurysm repair (EVAR) planning, contrast-enhanced MRA is comparable to CTA.[10]

INITIAL DIAGNOSTICS

Abdominal Aortic Aneurysm

LABORATORY
- None

IMAGING
- Abdominal ultrasound
- CTA
- MRI or MRA

DIFFERENTIAL DIAGNOSIS

 Red flags include onset of severe abdominal or back pain with a tearing sensation and signs of hypotension including weakness, dizziness, orthostasis.

The differential diagnoses for AAA include conditions associated with abdominal pain or back pain. CT is the most readily available method to rule out alternative causes of abdominal pain. Common, concerning causes of abdominal pain include nephrolithiasis, myocardial infarction, gastric ulcer perforation, pancreatitis, diverticulitis, bowel obstruction, and appendicitis (see Chapter 109).

INTERPROFESSIONAL COLLABORATIVE MANAGEMENT

Patients with an AAA of 4.0 cm or larger should be referred to a vascular physician. Recent evidence suggests that outcomes for open and endovascular repair are better at large, urban institutions where experienced staff is trained and large numbers of procedures are performed.[5] Once an AAA has been identified, it can be managed with traditional open surgical repair, minimally invasive abdominal EVAR, or continued surveillance. The goal of AAA management is to prevent aneurysmal rupture while minimizing surgical risk. Thus the size of the aneurysm, the shape of the aneurysm, and the patient's medical status, life expectancy, and preference are critical factors in deciding the timing of elective AAA repair.[5] AAA size is the best predictor of rupture risk.[11] A fair amount of controversy persists about the best timing for and method of AAA repair (i.e., open vs. endovascular repair [EVAR]) when preoperative risk factors and postoperative complications are considered.[11]

The majority of aneurysms expand slowly at a rate of 0.2 to 0.3 cm/year, or 10% of the diameter. However, the risk of rupture increases significantly when an AAA exceeds 5.0 cm in diameter. Smoking increased the risk of rupture substantially. Recent guidelines suggest that the screening intervals decrease as the aneurysm increases with a recommendation to screen annually in patients whose aneurysms measure 4.0-4.9 cm.[12] In the United Kingdom Small Aneurysm Trial (UKSAT), the relative risk of rupture was increased in women, those with AAAs of increased diameter, smokers, and patients with COPD.[6] Another factor found to be important in rupture risk was asymmetry in the aneurysm.

Elective repair is appropriately indicated for healthy patients with AAAs measuring 5.0 to 6.0 cm.[5,12,13]

PREOPERATIVE CARDIAC RISK STRATIFICATION

Several older, large surveys have demonstrated that coronary artery disease is the most important underlying medical illness contributing to morbidity and mortality among individuals who undergo major vascular surgery, regardless of the type of peripheral vascular surgery, particularly in individuals 70 years of age or older.[14] The ACC/AHA developed guidelines to aid in cardiac risk stratification before noncardiac surgery. According to the ACC/AHA guidelines, aortic and other vascular procedures are considered high risk. Patients with an active cardiac condition such as unstable coronary syndrome, decompensated heart failure, significant arrhythmia, or severe valvular disease may require cancellation or delay of surgery until further testing, which may include coronary angiography or even cardiac bypass surgery, and/or implementation of medical management is done. Patients should proceed to surgery without further cardiac evaluation only when they have no clinical predictors or minor clinical predictors (minor clinical predictors include advanced age older than 70, electrocardiogram [ECG] with left ventricular hypertrophy, left bundle branch block, nonspecific ST-T abnormalities, cardiac rhythm other than sinus, uncontrolled hypertension) with moderate to excellent functional capacity on cardiac stress testing.

Preoperative noninvasive testing, such as a resting 12-lead ECG, is recommended for all within 30 days of the planned procedure. Pharmacologic stress testing is indicated when patients are undergoing high-risk vascular surgery and they have two or more intermediate predictors of clinical risk (mild angina pectoris, prior myocardial infarction, compensated or prior congestive heart failure, diabetes mellitus, renal insufficiency) and unknown or poor functional capacity (≤4 METs). Preoperative echocardiography is recommended for patients with dyspnea or heart failure. Results of noninvasive testing are then used to plan further perioperative management. This may include intensified medical therapy and/or further cardiac testing, and perhaps cancellation or delay of surgery.[5]

Other medical conditions may increase the mortality rate of aneurysm repair by twofold or threefold. They include chronic renal failure (serum creatinine level > 3 mg/dL or hemodialysis), COPD (forced expiratory volume [FEV]/FEV_1 < 0.70), and liver cirrhosis with portal hypertension. These conditions increase the mortality rate from between 3% and 5% to between 8% and 10%.[5] In a Canadian North American study, the most significant predictors of mortality were electrocardiographic changes indicative of ischemia, COPD, and increased creatinine concentration.

Open Surgical Repair

Open surgical repair of an AAA is the classic and generally reliable approach especially appealing in younger patients as long-term complications are rare.[15] However, it is not the preferred option now given the success of endovascular repair. The most recent (2018) Society of Vascular Surgery guidelines recommends that open repairs be done only in institutions that perform >10 open repairs a year with a <5% mortality rate.[5] The aorta is usually approached through a midline or a left flank retroperitoneal incision. A prosthetic graft is positioned in the aorta, extending from a segment of normal aorta above the aneurysm to a segment of normal aorta below the aneurysm. If the aneurysm extends to the iliac arteries, a bifurcated prosthetic graft is used. The wall of the aneurysm is closed over the newly placed graft.

Today, most patients undergoing open surgical repair of an AAA have their preoperative workups done on an outpatient basis and are admitted for same-day surgery. Hospital discharge ranges from 5 to 7 days postoperatively, and recovery ranges from 6 weeks up to 3 months depending on health status and the patient's overall medical condition. CTA should be performed within 5 years after open repair of AAA to detect aneurysmal degeneration.

Endovascular Stent Grafts

Endovascular AAA repair (EVAR) was first performed in 1991 and is now the preferred surgical repair technique for both elective repair and repair of ruptured aneurysms as recommended by the Society for Vascular Surgery.[5] A number of studies have documented the efficacy and generally satisfactory results of a variety of transluminally placed endovascular grafts and as techniques and training has improved immediate postoperative outcomes remain very positive.[5,15,16] EVAR repair is associated with reduced length of hospital stay, decreased recovery time, a smaller incision, and fewer complications, which accounts for its appeal to patients and physicians.

EVAR requires accurate preoperative imaging evaluation for appropriate patient selection based on aneurysm morphology and access vessel size and patency. The proximal aortic neck and iliofemoral arteries are important areas of imaging. Endoluminal repair of AAA is achieved through exclusion of the aneurysm from the circulation by means of a prosthetic graft that is inserted from a remote site to the desired intraluminal location, under radiologic guidance, and then secured by an expandable stent attachment system. The devices may be commercially manufactured or custom made. They include a bifurcated graft or a tube graft with a single limb (aorto–uni-iliac), uncovered, branched, and fenestrated devices. New devices have allowed EVAR to be offered to a greater number of patients.[17] The development of the superspecialty of vascular therapy and the dissemination of skills have increased the rate of endoluminal use.

The procedure time is usually less than 2 hours. Most procedures are performed with the patient under epidural anesthesia combined with conscious sedation. Only infrequently does an endovascular patient require an intensive care unit stay. Patients are sent home after computed tomography (CT) confirmation of graft placement and the absence of a leak at the attachment sites for the graft, with more than 85% of patients discharged on their first or second postoperative day.[16] Patients report a return to a sense of preoperative health status 11 days after endoluminal repair versus 47 days after open surgical repair.

The first routine follow-up visit with the vascular surgeon occurs 1 month after hospital discharge, at which time another CT scan is obtained to reaffirm the position of the graft, presence or absence of any leak, and evidence of sac shrinkage. Thereafter, CT scans are obtained at prescribed intervals, usually again at 6 months, then 12 months and yearly thereafter depending on stability of the aneurysm and prosthesis. Aortic remodeling after EVAR is a slow process that continues for several years.

Ruptured AAAs present a unique challenge to endovascular repair. Because the first indication of their presence is often the back pain and hypotension associated with acute enlargement and rupture, the primary goal is stabilization of the patient. This is accomplished by gaining control of the rupture and preventing further hemorrhage. Once the patient is stabilized, repair of the aorta can be accomplished. With increasing surgical experience, improvement in technology, and the availability of a range of graft sizes, this less invasive method of repair has been applied with success and is now the recommended method.[5]

Multiple guidelines recommend lifelong annual imaging after EVAR to identify complications such as endoleaks or residual aortic sac enlargement, and to prevent death from aneurysm rupture after EVAR.[18,19] Compliance with follow-up imaging is strongly recommended, and patients need to be educated about this before the procedure. Those having an EVAR AAA repair emergently appear to be at a higher risk of loss to follow-up imaging.[18]

LIFE SPAN CONSIDERATIONS

In general, AAA is considered a disease of older white men (≥65 years), but younger individuals with certain risk factors may be affected and need to undergo repair. Aneurysms are more commonly symptomatic in younger patients. Perioperative mortality and morbidity rates are not significantly different for young patients compared with older patients (≥65 years) with degenerative (atherosclerotic) AAAs. Technique (open vs. endovascular) is determined not by age but by the assessed risk to the patient and the size of the AAA.

COMPLICATIONS

Complications vary for surgical repair and endoluminal repair of AAAs.

In most large series, the 30-day mortality rate for open surgical repair is 3% to 5%, for EVAR 1% to 2%.[5] If electrocardiographic changes of ischemia, COPD, and elevated creatinine concentration are present, the mortality rate rises sharply. By comparison, patients with none of these factors have a perioperative mortality of less than 2%. Early surgical complications of arterial thrombosis, anastomotic rupture or bleeding, peripheral emboli, and limb loss are rare at centers with experience. Furthermore, the incidence of long-term complications is very low but includes anastomotic pseudoaneurysm, graft thrombosis, aortoenteric fistula, graft infection, anastomotic hemorrhage, colonic ischemia, and atheroembolism.

The 30-day mortality rates for stent graft repairs are less than open repair to those for standard surgical repair. The most common early complications include groin hematoma, arterial thrombosis, iliac artery rupture, and thromboemboli.

The most common long-term problem of EVAR is endoleak.[20] An endoleak involves persistent filling of the aneurysm sac from either an anastomotic site or collateral blood vessels, most commonly caused by persistent bleeding from lumbar or inferior mesenteric artery branches in the AAA sac. Endoleaks occur in 20% to 50% of patients who have undergone EVAR. Appropriate classification (types I–V) is crucial for subsequent management. Endoleaks close spontaneously in more than 50% of cases by 6 to 12 months after the procedure. Secondary catheter-based reinterventions are required to close an additional 10%. Surgical intervention has been required to treat 2% to 3% of long-term leaks.[20] Even after successful EVAR, aneurysm expansion may occur, leading to eventual rupture and open surgical repair. Other common late complications include severe graft kinking, graft migration, graft thrombosis, and renal dysfunction.

PATIENT EDUCATION

During the period of surveillance of small aneurysms, patient education addresses modification of risk factors such as hypertension and smoking to slow AAA expansion, and management of diabetes and hyperlipidemia.[5]

Physical activity is encouraged, such as walking, bike riding, or other aerobic exercise, but patients should avoid activities that include heavy lifting or exercises that involve undue strain. Also addressed are protocols for surveillance, indications for emergent evaluation, and surveillance of first-degree relatives.

During the periprocedural phase, patient education focuses on the trajectory of care, including hospital stay and post-discharge recovery. Reinforcement of the vascular surgeon's instructions including care of the incision or catheterization site, resumption of activities of daily living, and protocols for long-term monitoring are also discussed.[19]

Hypertension and cigarette smoking are critical risk factors for expansion of AAA. Although beta blockade has not demonstrated a significant difference in the rate of expansion of small AAAs or the need for surgery, treatment with beta blockers continues because of its effect on reducing coronary events.[5] Smoking cessation needs to be addressed and encouraged at every visit, along with referral to a smoking cessation counselor. However, smoking cessation does not preclude the development of AAA, nor will smoking cessation prevent expansion of an existing AAA.

The frequency of surveillance depends on the size of the aneurysm at the most recent ultrasonographic study. Patients must commit to serial ultrasonographic examinations or consider early repair of a small aneurysm with discussion of the inherent risks and benefits of open surgical vs. endovascular repair vs. ongoing monitoring.

At the initial visit with the vascular physician, the patient will be educated about both the standard open surgical procedure and the endovascular stent graft procedure. The explanation should include early and late results of both types of procedures to inform the patient and to assist in decision-making.

After the detection of an AAA, patients should be counseled to report new-onset symptoms of aneurysmal enlargement, such as abdominal or back pain, to the vascular physician. Symptoms of impending rupture requiring immediate emergency care include severe abdominal pain, flank pain, or back pain unrelieved by position change. The abdominal pain may be characterized as deep, boring, or tearing. Low back pain may be dull, radiating to the legs, similar to musculoskeletal pain. The flank pain may radiate to the groin and be associated with hematuria.

HEALTH PROMOTION

There is strong evidence to suggest a genetic predisposition to AAA.[11] First-degree male relatives of patients with AAA have two to four times the normal risk for AAA,[11] suggesting the importance of periodic ultrasonographic screening after the age of 50 years in these family members.[11]

There is also strong evidence suggesting the relationship between smoking and the development of AAA in men.[2,5] For this reason, the USPSTF recommends screening with ultrasonography for men older than 65 years with a past or current history of smoking.[15]

REFERENCES

1. Kuivaniemi, H., Reyer, E. J., Elmore, J. R., et al. (2014). Update on abdominal aortic aneurysm research: From clinical to genetic studies. *Scientifica (Cairo)*, *2014*, 564–573.
2. Persson, S.-E., Boman, K., Wanhainen, A., et al. (2017). Decreasing prevalence of abdominal aortic aneurysm and changes in cardiovascular risk factors. *J Vasc Surg*, 65(3), 651–658.
3. Soden, P. A., & Schermerhorn, M. L. (2017). The epidemiology of ruptured abdominal aortic aneurysms (RAAA). In B. Starnes, M. Mehta, & F. Verth (Eds.), *Ruptured abdominal aneurysm*. Cham: Springer.
4. Stackelberg, O., Wok, A., Eliasson, K., et al. (2017). Lifestyle and risk of screening-detected abdominal aortic aneurysm in men. *J Am Heart Association*, 6e004725.
5. Chaikof, E. L., Palmon, R. L., Eskandari, M. K., et al. (2018). The care of patients with abdominal aortic aneurysms. *J Vasc Surgery*, 67(1), 2–77.
6. Gokani, V. J., Sidloff, D., & Bath, M. J. (2015). A retrospective study: Factors associated with the risk of abdominal aortic aneurysm rupture. *Vascular Pharmacology*, 65–66.
7. Beckman, J. A., & Creager, M. A. (2013). Clinical evaluation of aortic aneurysm. In M. A. Creager, J. A. Beckman, & J. Loscalzo (Eds.), *Vascular medicine: A companion to Braunwald's heart disease* (2nd ed.). Philadelphia: Elsevier.
8. LeFevre, M. L. (2014). US preventive Services Task Force. Screening for abdominal aortic aneurysms: US Preventive Services Task Force recommendations statement. *Annals of Internal Medicine*, 161, 281–290.
9. SAAVE Act Background. http://www.vascularweb.org/healthpolicyandgovern mentrelations/Pages?saave-act-background.aspx. (Accessed 21 September 2018).
10. Reis, S., Majdalany, B., Aburahma, A., et al. (2017). ACT appropriateness criteria pulsatile abdominal mass suspected abdominal aortic aneurysm. *JACR*, 14(5), s258–s265.
11. Debus, E. S., & Grundmann, R. T. (2017). Abdominal aortic aneurysm (AAA). In *Evidenced-based therapy in vascular surgery*. Cham: Springer.
12. Gerhard-Herman, M., Gorner, H., & Barrett, C. (2017). 2016 ACC/AHA guidelines on the management of patients with lower extremity peripheral artery disease. *Journal of the American College of Cardiology*, 69(11).
13. Robertson, V., & Bown, M. (2018). Abdominal Aortic Aneurysm Screening, epidemiology and open surgical repair. *Surgery*, 36(6), 295–299.

14. Fleisher, L. A., Fleischmann, K., Auerbach, A., et al. (2014). 2014 ACC/AHA guidelines on perioperative evaluation and management of patients undergoing non-cardiac surgery. *Journal of American College of Cardiology*, 64(22), e77–e137.

15. Paravastu, S. C. V., Jayarajasingam, R., Cottam, R., Palfreyman, S. J., Michaels, J. A., & Thomas, S. M. (2014). Endovascular repair of abdominal aortic aneurysm. *The Cochrane Database of Systematic Reviews*, (1), Art. No.: CD004178, doi:10.1002/14651858.CD004178.pub2.

16. Badger, S., Forster, R., Blair, P. H., Ellis, P., Kee, F., & Harkin, D. W. (2017). Endovascular treatment for ruptured abdominal aortic aneurysm. *The Cochrane Database of Systematic Reviews*, (5), Art. No.: CD005261, doi:10.1002/14651858.CD005261.pub4.

17. Eagleton, M. J., Follansbee, M., Wolski, K., Mastracci, T., & Kuramochi, Y. (2016). Fenestrated and branched endovascular aneurysm repair outcomes for type II and III thoracoabdominal aortic aneurysms. *Journal of Vascular Surgery*, 63(4), 930–942.

18. Garg, T., Baker, L. C., & Mell, M. W. (2015). Adherence to postoperative surveillance guidelines after endovascular aortic aneurysm repair among Medicare beneficiaries. *Journal of Vascular Surgery*, 61, 23–27.

19. Troutman, D. A., Chaudry, M., Dougherty, M. J., & Calligaro, K. D. (2014). Endovascular aortic aneurysm repair may not be necessary for the first three years after an initially normal duplex postoperative study. *Journal of Vascular Surgery*, 60, 558–562.

20. Candell, L., Tucker, L. Y., Goodney, P., et al. (2014). Early and delayed rupture after endovascular abdominal aortic aneurysm repair in a 10-year multicenter registry. *Journal of Vascular Surgery*, 60, 1146–1153.

CHAPTER **100**

CARDIAC ARRHYTHMIAS

Andrea Efre

 Emergency transportation to hospital indicated for cardiac arrhythmias that cause hemodynamic instability, acute symptoms, signs of acute myocardial infarction, or myocardial ischemia

 Immediate referral to cardiology indicated for a complete cardiac evaluation with additional testing is indicated in new onset cardiac arrhythmia, when cardiac structure is suspected as the cause, or when symptoms of the arrhythmia cannot be controlled

DEFINITION AND EPIDEMIOLOGY

Cardiac arrhythmias are electrical abnormalities of the cardiac conduction system that can vary in severity from trivial to life-threatening. These may occur in the presence or absence of structural heart defects or cardiac disease, and may be divided into categories by rate or location. Rate classifies the arrhythmia by the speed of the heart rate: tachyarrhythmia (>100 beats/min) and bradyarrhythmia (<60 beats/min). Location identifies where the arrhythmia originates: atrial, atrioventricular (AV), ventricular, and supraventricular (originates from above the ventricles). Symptoms are more closely related to the ventricular rate and to the severity of underlying heart disease than to the origin of the arrhythmia. Cardiac arrhythmias may cause minor symptoms such as palpitations or dizziness but may also predispose to the development of lethal conditions such as stroke, embolism, or sudden cardiac death.[1]

Tachyarrhythmias

More than half of all cardiac arrhythmias involve the atria. Atrial fibrillation (AF), atrial flutter, and other supraventricular tachyarrhythmias are often triggered by excessive sympathetic stimulation, atrial stretch caused by ventricular overload, atrial infarction, myocardial infarction, pericarditis, electrolyte abnormalities, hypoxia, or underlying lung disease.[2] By far the most common supraventricular arrhythmia is AF and is often associated with structural heart disease or other co-occurring chronic conditions. It is slightly more common in men, and there is an increased prevalence with age (older than 60 years of age).[3] AF occurs in 8% to 22% of patients with STEMI, and new-onset AF is associated with shock, heart failure (HF), stroke, and 90-day mortality.[2] This information is important to keep in mind when identifying a new onset AF.

Ventricular tachyarrhythmias, especially in the presence of serious underlying organic cardiac disease, may predispose the patient to sudden cardiac death and increased mortality rates. Sudden cardiac death claims many lives in the United States, with the majority being older adults; approximately 80% of these deaths are caused by ventricular fibrillation (VF) in the context of ischemic heart disease. Structural cardiovascular anomalies and congenital rhythm abnormalities (such as long QT syndrome or Brugada syndrome) are thought to be the cause of unexplained deaths in the younger population.[1]

Ventricular arrhythmias such as sustained ventricular tachycardia (VT) and VF are common early after the onset of STEMI and are also the most common cause of out-of-hospital cardiac arrest with STEMI. There are multiple factors in the possible cause of these arrhythmias, which include ongoing ischemia, hemodynamic instability, electrolyte abnormalities, enhanced automaticity, and reentry mechanisms.[2] Ventricular arrhythmias such as accelerated idioventricular rhythm may follow myocardial insult and are known as reperfusion arrhythmias; they are related to the restoration of normal myocardial blood flow and may occur after myocardial infarction (MI) or revascularization procedures such as percutaneous coronary intervention.[1]

Bradyarrhythmias

Bradyarrhythmias may result from abnormalities in conduction between the sinoatrial (SA) node and atrium, within the AV node, or in the intraventricular conduction pathways. The cause of disruption in normal conduction may include coronary spasm, myocarditis, rheumatic fever, mononucleosis, Lyme disease, sarcoidosis, amyloidosis, and neoplasms. Additionally, bradycardic arrhythmias may co-occur in conditions such as hypothyroidism, advanced liver disease, hypothermia, or severe hypoxia, or related to medications such as calcium channel blockers (CCB), beta blockers, or digoxin. The cause of an intermittent bradycardia may be difficult to determine and may be related to intrinsic disease of the SA or AV node. The rhythm of sinus bradycardia may be noted as an incidental finding and considered normal in highly trained athletes. The presence of symptoms with sinus bradycardia should lead to further investigation and a possible treatment plan.

Bundle branch block (BBB) may be intermittent or chronic, and symptomatic or asymptomatic. Possible causes include structural heart disease, congenital conditions, cardiac disease, and coronary artery disease. Right bundle branch block (RBBB) is associated with right ventricular hypertrophy, ischemic heart disease, pulmonary embolus, atrial septal defect, rheumatic heart disease, myocarditis, cardiomyopathy, and Brugada syndrome. Left bundle branch block (LBBB) is associated with ischemia, MI, aortic stenosis or regurgitation, dilated cardiomyopathy, and Lyme disease. The rhythm disturbances of BBB do not always require treatment, but it is imperative to determine and manage the underlying cause as well as to treat any associated symptoms.

PATHOPHYSIOLOGY

The functional components of the cardiac conduction system subdivide into (1) impulse-generating tissue (SA and AV nodes) and (2) impulse-propagating tissue (e.g., His-Purkinje system). This intrinsic conduction system is comprised of several specialized subpopulations of cells that either spontaneously generate electrical activity (pacemaker cells) or preferentially conduct this activity throughout the chambers in a coordinated fashion.[4] SA nodal cells operate as electrically coupled oscillators that discharge synchronously and the function of the SA node as a pacemaker requires a delicate balance of intercellular electrical coupling.[5]

Electrical signaling in the heart involves the passage of ions, mainly Na+, K+, Ca2+, and Cl−, through ionic channels; creating a movement across the cell membrane and a flow of current that generates excitation and signals in cardiac myocytes.[5] The changes in cellular voltage across the cell membranes of the SA node are known as the cardiac action potential. The cardiac transmembrane action potential consists of five phases: phase 0, upstroke or rapid depolarization; phase 1, early rapid repolarization; phase 2, plateau; phase 3, final rapid repolarization; and phase 4, resting membrane potential and diastolic depolarization.[5] These phases can be affected, intentionally or unintentionally, by factors such as electrolyte imbalances, medications, and changes in the autonomic nervous system.

As the natural pacemaker of the normal heart, the SA node maintains rhythm and rate. If stimulated, suppressed, or blocked, it will induce a tachyarrhythmia or bradyarrhythmia. The pacemaker function may then be assumed by "escape" foci in the atrial tissue, the AV node, the bundle of His, the Purkinje fibers, or the ventricular myocardium. The intrinsic rates of each part of the conductive system may be influenced (increased, decreased, or blocked) by factors such as cardiac disease, ischemia, medications, electrolytes, or changes in the endocrine system.

Cardiac arrhythmias are a result of abnormal impulse formation or conduction, and can be categorized into one or more of three mechanisms: (1) abnormal automaticity, (2) triggered activity, or (3) reentry.

- *Abnormal automaticity (enhanced or suppressed):* Automaticity is a natural property of all myocytes, which may be suppressed or enhanced by factors such as electrolyte imbalance, medications, hypoxia, ischemic heart disease, scarring, or increased age, and can result in atrial or ventricular tachyarrhythmias.[6,7] Abnormal or enhanced automaticity is a deficit in the ability of the cardiac cells to depolarize spontaneously. Enhanced automaticity results in increased conduction of impulses and results in tachycardia (e.g., sinus tachycardia). Abnormal automaticity may lead to irregularity of the impulse conduction, causing erratic or ectopic rhythms of the atria or ventricles. Suppressed automaticity decreases conduction of the SA node and can result in sinus node dysfunction or sick sinus syndrome.
- *Triggered activity:* Triggered activity usually occurs after an early or delayed depolarization that precipitates multiple depolarizations and causes ventricular arrhythmias. They may be induced by electrolyte imbalances or medications, as in antiarrhythmic or digoxin toxicity.[6] An example of a triggered arrhythmia is torsades de pointes.[7]
- *Reentry:* Reentry arrhythmias require a circular movement of the impulse across the myocardium. Most tachyarrhythmias are thought to be caused by a reentry mechanism and include bidirectional conduction and unidirectional block.[6] They may start and terminate suddenly and are often paroxysmal. If a large area is involved, it is known as a macro-reentry arrhythmia and occurs through concealed accessory pathways; the best example is Wolff-Parkinson-White (WPW) syndrome, but macro-reentry arrhythmias can also cause AF and atrial flutter. Micro-reentry arrhythmias affect a small area; examples include VT or VF after MI. An example of a reentry arrhythmia is AV nodal reentry tachyarrhythmia.

The pathophysiology of arrhythmias is additionally defined in the differential diagnosis section to include the expected electrocardiographic changes.

CLINICAL PRESENTATION

Tachyarrhythmias

Tachyarrhythmias may be entirely asymptomatic or may cause symptoms that affect the patient's activities of daily living. Symptoms are mostly related to the ventricular rate, extent of underlying heart disease, ventricular function, and associated precipitating factors. Palpitations are the most common symptom of tachyarrhythmias. In patients with paroxysmal attacks, palpitations start and terminate abruptly and are usually rapid but regular. In patients with AF the palpitations are typically irregular and tend to be more sustained. Extra-systoles may also cause palpitations or an awareness of isolated extra beats, and the pause that follows may be symptomatic. Other causes of palpitations include thyrotoxicosis, hypovolemia, regurgitant valvular disease, anemia, hypoglycemia, pheochromocytoma, fever, anxiety, symptoms of menopause, stimulants such as caffeine, street drugs, and medications.

When interviewing the patient with tachyarrhythmias and/or palpitations, determine if there is a history of underlying heart disease, a family history of heart disease or a previous history of rhythm disturbance and its treatment. Evaluate for coronary risk factors, and inquire about the use of alcohol, tobacco, caffeine, sympathomimetics (commonly found in over-the-counter cold medicines or diet aids), and prescription medication use (e.g., theophylline or thyroid supplements). It is also prudent to ask about the use of street drugs, especially those known to be stimulants, such as cocaine, methamphetamines, synthetic cannabinoids (e.g., spice), and synthetic cathinones (known as bath salts).

Tachyarrhythmias tend to shorten diastole and ventricular filling may become compromised, causing a drop in blood pressure, cardiac output, and coronary perfusion. Symptoms include palpitations, lightheadedness, dizziness, syncope, dyspnea, or fatigue, with fatigue being the most common presenting symptom of AF, and are caused by irregularity in the ventricular rate control, loss of coordinated atrial contraction (e.g., AF), beat-to-beat variability in ventricular filling, and sympathetic activation.[3] A serious tachyarrhythmia may result in hemodynamic decompensation, causing significant hypotension, chest pain, HF, change in level of consciousness, or sudden cardiac death. It is important to assess both the arrhythmia and its tolerance by the patient to determine the degree of urgency and the appropriate setting for intervention.

Bradyarrhythmias

Bradycardia refers to any heart rate below 60 beats/min, may occur with or without symptoms (especially in healthy individuals), and may be discovered as an incidental finding on routine electrocardiography. In such cases it is most likely that the needs of the body are being met despite the slow heart rate. Symptoms accompanying bradycardia are largely dependent on the ventricular rate relative to metabolic demand and on the presence of underlying cardiac disease. Those with limited cardiac reserve are less tolerant of a slow rate than those with normal heart function. Subtle symptoms may include irritability, lassitude, inability to concentrate, apathy, or forgetfulness, but more significant symptoms of palpitations, fatigue, dizziness, lightheadedness, and syncope are not uncommon. Sinus node dysfunction may manifest as sinus bradycardia or prolonged sinus pauses, typically resulting in fatigue, dizziness, confusion, exertional intolerance, diminished mental acuity, syncope, and/or congestive HF.[6]

Relevant aspects of the history include a careful review of all medications and the identification of underlying cardiac disease. It is important to discern whether the symptoms occur at rest or with exertion, and if there are outstanding, aggravating, or alleviating factors. If bradycardic symptoms occur only with straining, such as with vomiting or moving the bowels, then a vagal mechanism is likely to be the cause. It is also appropriate to question additional symptoms in the review of systems such as lethargy, weight gain, constipation, changes to the skin, hair, or nails, or eyelid edema as they are subjective findings of hypothyroidism, which may be the cause of a bradyarrhythmia.

PHYSICAL EXAMINATION

The initial examination should include evaluation of blood pressure, pulse, temperature, mental status, evidence of diaphoresis, respiratory effort, and manifestations of anxiety. Alterations in rate and pulse volume and irregularity may accompany ventricular ectopic beats, depending on the timing and force of ventricular contractions, which may be observed by labile blood pressure. Orthostatic vital signs are helpful to exclude orthostatic hypotension as a cause of syncope, dehydration, or hypovolemia, which could be the root of a reflex tachycardia (requiring prompt intervention). The patient's hydration status also includes examination of skin turgor and status of mucous membranes.

Assessment of the neck should include inspection, observing the neck veins for jugular venous distention (JVD) (a sign of HF), and for the presence of a goiter (suggesting thyroid disorder). Inspection of the neck vasculature may provide information about atrial activity. The *a wave* (atrial contraction) reflects a slight rise in atrial pressure near the end of diastole, and occurs just before S_1 (the beginning of the carotid pulse). The *v wave* (venous filling) is produced by right atrial filling during right ventricular systole (when the tricuspid valve is closed) and occurs just before or coincides with S_2.[8] A prominent *a wave* can occur in increased resistance to right atrial contraction and may be seen in heart blocks, supraventricular tachycardia (SVT), and junctional rhythms, whereas an absence of the *a wave* suggests loss of atrial systole suggesting AF.[8]

The carotid pulses are palpated for amplitude, contour, timing, and presence of thrills. Auscultation of the carotid arteries should be performed initially with the diaphragm of the stethoscope to detect the higher frequency of the arterial bruits, then with the bell to detect the low-pitched sounds of higher-grade stenosis.[8] The presence of a bruit would suggest atherosclerosis and contraindicates carotid massage as a diagnostic or treatment option.

The chest is inspected and palpated for parasternal lifts, heaves, and thrills. Palpation of the point of maximum impulse (PMI) and percussion of the left side of the chest establish the size and location of the heart. Enlargement of the cardiac silhouette suggests ventricular hypertrophy or cardiomyopathies, which are triggers for some arrhythmias.

Auscultation of the heart sounds for regularity, rate, murmurs, clicks, or the presence of extra heart sounds is essential. An accentuated S_1 may be heard in some tachyarrhythmias, and a diminished S_1 may be found in AV nodal blocks. A varying S_1 may be a sign of complete heart block or AF, as the mitral valve is in varying positions before ventricular contraction. The splitting of S_2 may be heard in patients with premature ventricular contractions (PVCs) or RBBB, and paradoxical splitting of S_2 may be related to LBBB.[8] An S_3 is a significant finding of increased ventricular filling and can be a sign of fluid overload, HF, or decreased myocardial contractility, which may be end points of an arrhythmia. Note that S_3 may be a normal finding in a child, young adult, or pregnant female, who may also have the presence of a cardiac arrhythmia. An S_4 heart sound is pathologic and is caused by resistance in ventricular filling. It may be associated with AV nodal conduction delays.

The presence of an S_3 and/or S_4 in an athlete should be investigated because it may be a sign of athletic heart syndrome. Electrocardiographic findings may include sinus bradycardia, AV nodal block, or RBBB, and there may be lateral displacement of the PMI owing to the increased heart size. These patients should be referred to a cardiologist for further evaluation because the differentiation of benign findings from the ominous possibility of sudden cardiac death can be difficult to determine.

A heart murmur is most often associated with underlying valve disorders; however, a benign systolic ejection murmur may accompany tachycardia with or without valvular disease. Absence of a murmur is not necessarily a significant finding because rapid rates can often make accurate auscultation difficult. The patient should always be reexamined after the heart rate is controlled. An S_3 sound is a significant finding, as are JVD and peripheral edema—signs of fluid overload—and may warn of impending HF or be an indication that the rhythm is poorly tolerated by the patient.

As part of the complete assessment, the examiner should observe the overall appearance of the patient, and consider signs of discomfort, restlessness, dyspnea, or distress. Auscultate the lungs for rales, wheezes, or rhonchi and evaluate for signs of cyanosis. Other important findings include signs of hypothyroid or hyperthyroid, such as exophthalmos, lid lag, an enlarged or nodular thyroid gland, or skin, nail, and hair changes. When the presenting complaint is syncope, near-syncope, dizziness, confusion, or altered level of consciousness, a neurologic examination should be performed to explore the possibility of noncardiac causes.

If there is a positive history, or suspected use, of street drugs, physical manifestations will depend on the type of drug and route used. The examiner should be observant for signs of use: needle markings (e.g., intravenous use), burns to the mouth or fingers (e.g., from pipe use), sores to the nasal area, epistaxis or increased rhinorrhea (e.g., insufflation), or skin or gum abscesses or rotten teeth. Carefully placed body jewelry, tattoos, and skin branding marks may mask signs of needle use or skin popping scars.

ESSENTIAL DIAGNOSTICS
12-Lead Electrocardiogram

The 12-lead electrocardiogram (ECG) is indicated for initial evaluation of a suspected arrhythmia. This diagnostic tool has the notable limitation of providing only a 12-second view of the heart's electrical activity. Although sustained rhythms may easily be captured, paroxysmal rhythms may be elusive. However, even when the rate and rhythm are normal, the resting ECG may yield valuable information about the cause of the arrhythmia. The first priority is to identify ST- or T-wave changes that indicate MI or myocardial ischemia. Other significant findings are ventricular hypertrophy, effects of medication toxicity, and electrolyte imbalance, such as peaked T waves noted in hyperkalemia.

Indications of conduction abnormalities may also be present and include the widened QRS complex of intraventricular conduction delay, and the shortened PR interval that accompanies preexcitation syndromes such as WPW syndrome. Additionally, prolongation of the QT interval (which is often affected by medications) is linked to lethal arrhythmias such as torsades de pointes. The QTc is the abbreviation used for the QT interval that has been corrected for rate, and is a more accurate measurement. When abnormal rhythms are captured on the 12-lead ECG, it is prudent to record a rhythm strip by allowing the tracing to continue for several minutes to fully evaluate the rhythm.

Holter Monitor

Continuous ambulatory electrocardiographic rhythm monitoring with a Holter monitor is a useful tool for evaluation of a suspected arrhythmia, especially when symptoms are inconsistent or paroxysmal in nature. Ambulatory monitoring may also be useful in the definitive correlation of bradyarrhythmias when evaluating the need for a pacemaker. Use of this portable device allows continuous recording of the heart's activity during a 24- to 48-hour period, which may identify arrhythmias that are unable to be captured in a one-time setting on a 12-lead ECG in the primary care setting. The patient keeps a diary of activities and symptoms that can later be correlated with the tracing. This is worn while patients go about their usual activities. It is important to encourage the patient to continue their routine activities, as the tendency is to limit activities when the monitor is on, making reproduction of the arrhythmia phenomena less likely.

Laboratory (Serum Testing)

Based on presenting symptoms, history, and clinical findings, laboratory testing may assist in determining the underlying cause of the arrhythmia. These tests might include a complete blood count (CBC) to determine the presence of anemia or infection, and serum electrolyte values including potassium, calcium, and magnesium to evaluate disturbances such as hypokalemia, hyperkalemia, hypocalcemia, hypercalcemia, or hypomagnesemia. A blood glucose measurement is helpful if hypoglycemia is suspected, and blood urea nitrogen (BUN) and creatinine levels are beneficial in determining fluid volume status. A thyroid-stimulating hormone (TSH) level should be drawn if hyperthyroidism or hypothyroidism is suspected. Measuring a toxicity level may be useful for patients being treated with medications that might cause arrhythmia (e.g., digoxin). Toxicology screening for stimulants such as cocaine or amphetamines may be beneficial. Cardiac biomarkers should be measured if ACS or coronary ischemia is suspected as the cause of the arrhythmia (evaluate coronary risk factors for questionable ACS).

Cardiology Imaging

Two-dimensional transthoracic echocardiography with Doppler (2D Echo) should be performed during the initial workup of all arrhythmia patients to determine atrial and ventricular size, systolic function, and underlying structural heart disease. This is useful in guiding decisions for antiarrhythmic and antithrombotic therapy, particularly with regard to the patient with AF.

Radiologic Imaging

Chest radiography is useful to identify structural disease or the presence of HF, pneumonia, or an underlying pulmonary condition as the cause of the arrhythmia.

Stress Testing

Stress tests are an example of provocative testing and can be performed by exercise (usually on a treadmill) or pharmacologically. Causes of exercise-induced arrhythmias may include ischemia, increased sympathetic activity, congenital conduction disturbances, and medications. It is important to verify the absence of coronary ischemia before initiating antiarrhythmic agents. Nuclear images of the myocardium at baseline and after exercise show disruption of myocardial blood flow from ischemia. Exercise stress testing can be very useful in diagnosing causes of palpitations, as exercise can provoke electrocardiographic changes or induce arrhythmias which may remain unidentified at rest. This is especially useful if the symptoms occur with, or are worsened by, activity. Exercise testing can also be useful to evaluate the adequacy of rate control in AF.[3]

ADDITIONAL DIAGNOSTICS
Smartphone Technology

The addition of smartphone-based technology is changing the way that patients are monitored and has become a useful diagnostic tool. The fitness industry started using smartphone applications with a monitoring chest band or watch to encourage people to monitor their heart rate, steps, calories, and fitness levers, and medical companies are utilizing similar technology for ECG recording. The recordings are noninvasive, inexpensive, and the patient can record during symptoms as long as the arrhythmia lasts long enough to activate the application.

Smartphone-based ECG monitors provide surveillance for long-term intermittent monitoring with recordings from electrodes embedded in a smartphone case or a card that connects via low-energy Bluetooth technology to smartphone applications.[9] The company AliveCor (San Francisco) has produced technology that records, stores, and transmits an ECG tracing when the user places their fingers on a small electrode pad or places the two electrodes on their chest.[10] Such technologies are being used and further developed for monitoring and diagnosing arrhythmias and AF. The European Society of Cardiology guidelines for the management of AF also support the use of digital decision tools, in the form of freely accessible smartphone apps, to assist in diagnosis and management of AF.[11]

Event Monitor and Loop Recorder

For the patient with infrequent symptoms, intermittent ambulatory electrocardiography (event recording) may be more appropriate because these devices can be worn for a long time. There are two types of these recorders. One type is worn externally and is activated by the user at the onset of symptoms. Patient-activated electrocardiographic event recorders can help assess the relation to symptoms, whereas auto-triggered event recorders may detect asymptomatic episodes. These technologies may also provide valuable information to guide drug dosage for rate control or rhythm management.[3]

The second type is an implantable loop recorder for long-term monitoring, used for diagnosis in patients with recurrent unexplained episodes of palpitations or syncope. The implanted device records the ECG during activity, or symptoms can record when it is activated by the patient. The device has an automatic recording triggered by arrhythmia and has an additional feature that allows the patient to activate the recording. New devices may offer remote transmission of the data back to the cardiologist. Implantable loop recorder monitoring is useful in detecting arrhythmias and guiding treatment plans. It may be used to evaluate for lethal bradycardias and sudden cardiac death in hemodialysis patients.[12]

The implantable loop recorder may stay in place for months or several years; battery life tends to last 24 months or more. It can provide additional diagnostic value in patients with syncope or non-syncopal, real or apparent, transient loss of consciousness.[13] More recently, smartphone technology and applications have been used with implanted loop recorders and external recordings with wireless connection via the smartphone for longer-term monitoring to detect AF after ablation.[9]

Tilt-Table Test

Provocative testing in the form of a tilt-table test is used to evaluate syncope. The patient is observed as the table is angled in varying degrees. Symptoms and hemodynamic status are monitored to see if syncope is related to a vasodepressor, cardiac, or neurologic reason. Arrhythmias, usually bradyarrhythmias, may be elicited with position change and induce syncopal symptoms. An example is malignant vasovagal syndrome, which is evidenced by exaggerated vagal response to emotional or painful stimuli. Tilt-table tests are performed in a monitored setting by a specialist, usually a cardiologist or an electrophysiology (EP) cardiologist, or a neurologist if syncope is suspected to be noncardiac.

Electrophysiologic Studies

Rhythms that put the patient at high risk for adverse events warrant referral to a specialist for electrophysiologic studies to properly identify and treat the problematic rhythm. The arrhythmias are often tachycardic in nature and may include very rapid SVT, WPW syndrome, complex ventricular ectopy, and VT. EP studies have been used to identify patients who are at risk for sudden cardiac death, and may also be indicated for investigation of AV block, intraventricular conduction disturbance, sinus node dysfunction, tachycardia, and unexplained syncope or palpitations.[14] If congenital heart defects are suspected to be the source of an arrhythmia, electrophysiological studies may be useful in evaluating if the arrhythmia is related to extra electrical pathways (known as accessory pathways). The procedure will evaluate the origin and specific location of extra pathways and may lead to ablation of the offending source cells (if reachable and appropriate).

Transesophageal Echocardiography

Transesophageal echocardiography (TEE) is performed by a specialist physician and is used to determine the presence or absence intracardiac thrombus, which must be identified before cardioversion is used as a treatment. For patients with asymptomatic WPW syndrome, the TEE procedure can be very helpful in determining their risk for sudden cardiac death.[15]

Carotid Sinus Massage and Valsalva Maneuvers

Valsalva maneuvers and carotid sinus massage may be used as a diagnostic test to induce bradycardia, although it should only be considered if monitoring and resuscitation equipment are available. Transient AV block results in the slowing of ventricular response, enabling identification of the underlying rhythm. These techniques may terminate rhythms for which the AV node is part of the reentry circuit, such as in atrioventricular nodal reentry tachycardia (AVNRT), and are therefore used as therapeutic treatments. The provider should evaluate atherosclerotic risk factors, assess for carotid bruits, and ensure correct technique is used before performing carotid massage. Carotid sinus massage during simultaneous recording of the ECG is useful to provoke symptomatic bradycardia in carotid sinus syndrome, a disorder in which bradycardia occurs in response to carotid sinus hypersensitivity. Carotid sinus massage is usually performed by a specialist in a monitored setting (e.g., emergency provider, cardiology provider, or EP cardiologist).

INITIAL DIAGNOSTICS

Cardiac Arrhythmias

ESSENTIAL DIAGNOSTICS: CARDIAC MONITORING
- 12-Lead ECG
- Vital signs

LABORATORY (SERUM TESTING)
- CBC
- Serum electrolytes including calcium and magnesium, BUN, creatinine, and glucose
- TSH
- Toxicology: for street drug or medications like Digoxin (if indicated)
- Cardiac biomarkers (if appropriate)

IMAGING
- Echocardiography (to evaluate underlying structural heart disease)
- Chest x-ray examination (to identify structural disease)

Note: *Holter monitor and stress test are useful second steps in diagnostic cardiac monitoring*

DIFFERENTIAL DIAGNOSIS OF TACHYARRHYTHMIAS
Narrow Complex Tachycardia

Narrow complex tachycardia includes rhythms with a rate over 100 beats/min and QRS duration of 0.12 second or less. The rhythms in the following paragraphs are included in this group and are described as they appear on the ECG.

Sinus Tachycardia. In sinus tachycardia, there is a P wave preceding each QRS complex in a consistent 1:1 relationship.

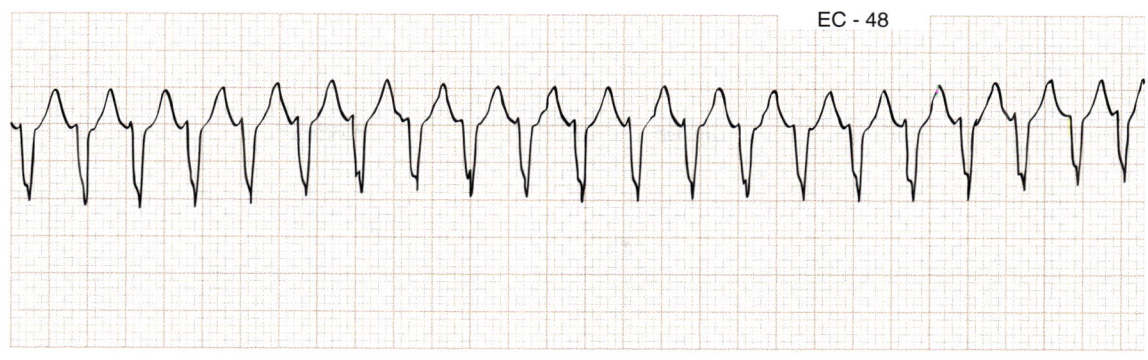

F I G . **100.1** Paroxysmal supraventricular tachycardia. Note the narrow, regular QRS complexes. (From Walls, R. M., Hockberger, R. S., & Gausche-Hill, M. [2018]. *Rosen's emergency medicine: Concepts and clinical practice* [9th ed.]. Philadelphia: Elsevier.)

The rhythm is regular, the P waves are identical, the QRS complexes are normal and narrow, and the PR and QRS intervals are within normal ranges. The rate is above 100 beats/min.

Atrial Tachycardia. Classic atrial tachycardia is defined as three or more consecutive premature atrial beats from a single atrial focus (unifocal), which may be located in the right or left atria, that have identical non-sinus P wave morphology on the ECG.[16]

Multifocal Atrial Tachycardia. Multifocal atrial tachycardia is characterized by multiple ectopic foci stimulating the atria and is defined as three of more consecutive (non-sinus) P waves of different shapes with a rate of 100 or more per minute, that originate from multiple foci.[16] The P-P interval and the PR interval may be variable, making it difficult to distinguish from AF. This rhythm is usually seen in patients with pulmonary, cardiovascular, or metabolic disturbances, or medication side effects.

Paroxysmal Supraventricular Tachycardia. Paroxysmal supraventricular tachycardia (PSVT) is a rapid (rate of 140 to 240 beats/min), generally regular rhythm that is typically initiated by a single beat and starts and stops abruptly (Fig. 100.1). The P waves may differ slightly in morphologic appearance compared with the sinus rhythm. The QRS complex is most typically narrow. P and QRS waves may exist in a 1:1 relationship, or variable AV block may alter this relationship. If the rate is very fast, P waves may not be clear, or may be buried in the previous ST or T wave making diagnosis more difficult.[16]

Atrioventricular Nodal Reentry Tachycardia. The reentry tachyarrhythmia of AVNRT is the most common mechanism for SVT. There are dual pathways within the AV node that are responsible for the reentrant circuit conduction. P waves, when they are visible, exist in a 1:1 relationship with the QRS complex. In very fast rhythms they are buried within the QRS complex and may not be visible or may be seen as a distortion at the end of the QRS complex. This distortion appears as a pseudo-S wave in leads II, III, and aVF or a pseudo-R wave in lead V_1.[16] The rate is usually 140 to 180 beats/min and regular. The QRS complex is narrow and morphologically similar to that of the sinus rhythm. It is typically paroxysmal in nature and will terminate with the Valsalva maneuver or carotid sinus massage.

Atrioventricular Reentry Tachycardia. With atrioventricular reentry tachycardia (AVRT), the reentry is the result of an accessory pathway between the atria and ventricles that bypasses the AV node. This mechanism is responsible for preexcitation syndromes, the most common being WPW syndrome.

Wolff-Parkinson-White Pattern. In WPW syndrome an AV bypass tract connects the atria and the ventricles, circumventing the AV junction and causing preexcitation of the ventricles. The directional change causes a physiologic lag through the AV junction that can be noted by the slurred upstroke of the QRS, known as the Delta wave. The classic triad of WPW is the presence of the delta wave, the shortened PR interval, and the widened QRS complex.[16]

Atrial Flutter. In atrial flutter, the atrial rate ranges from 250 to 350 beats/min, producing a sawtooth appearance of the P waves. The atrial rate of 300 beats/min usually has a 2:1 conduction to the ventricle, producing a QRS rate of 150 beats/min.

Atrial Fibrillation. The diagnosis of AF requires an ECG or rhythm strip demonstrating irregular R-R intervals, no distinct P waves on the surface ECG, and an atrial cycle length that is usually less than 200 ms.[9] The term "irregularly-irregular" is often used to identify AF; the wavy disorganized baseline and the irregular ventricular response (R to R interval) are classic signs of the arrhythmia. They occur because the normal P wave is replaced by fibrillatory *f waves*, with varying amplitude and polarity.[16] In addition, the AV node allows only a fraction of the atrial impulses to reach the ventricle, which is often in a haphazard, irregular manner. The term *AF with rapid ventricular response* is used when the ventricular rate increases over 100 beats/min. At significantly higher rates the underlying rhythm becomes difficult to distinguish from SVT (Fig. 100.2).

The diagnostic workup for AF should include a 12-lead ECG, a full cardiovascular evaluation, 2D Echo, and consideration of a TEE to identify intracardiac thrombi prior to treatment.[11] In addition, patients with concurrent signs of MI should undergo a stress test or cardiac catheterization as appropriate, and those with signs of cerebral ischemia or stroke require computerized tomography for diagnosis confirmation.[11] When initially diagnosing AF for the first time, search for the cause, as some are reversible. Common causes include MI, pericarditis, myocarditis, cardiomyopathy, rheumatic heart disease, mitral valve disease, hyperthyroidism, electrocution, cardiothoracic and noncardiac surgery, acute alcohol intoxication or withdrawal, stimulant ingestion, pneumonia, or pulmonary embolism.[3]

Wide-Complex Tachycardia

Wide-complex tachycardia involves rhythms with a rate over 100 beats/min and QRS duration of 0.12 second or greater.

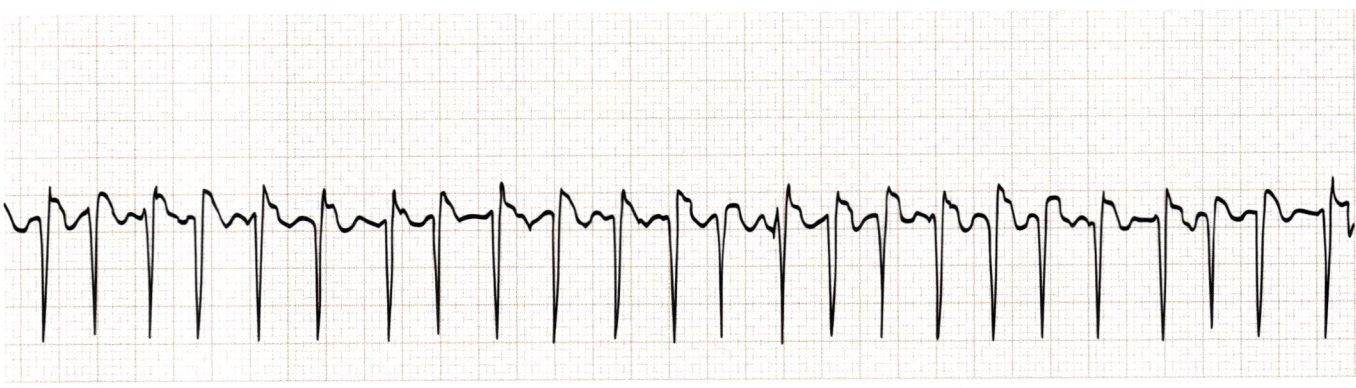

FIG. 100.2 Atrial fibrillation with rapid ventricular response. (From Walls, R. M., Hockberger, R. S., & Gausche-Hill, M. [2018]. *Rosen's emergency medicine: Concepts and clinical practice* [9th ed.]. Philadelphia: Elsevier.)

Cardiac Arrest

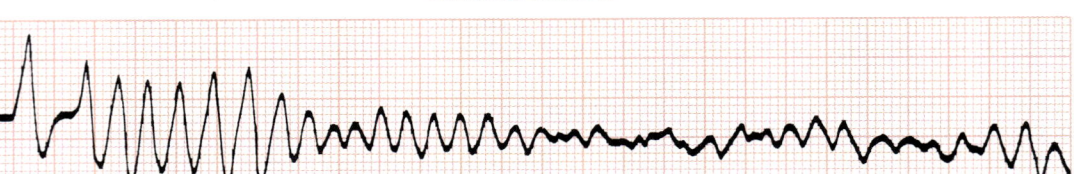

FIG. 100.3 Ventricular tachycardia *(VT)* transitioning to ventricular fibrillation *(VF)*. (From Goldberger, A. L., Goldberger, Z., & Shvilkin, A. [2018]. *Goldberger's clinical electrocardiography: A simplified approach* [9th ed.]. Philadelphia: Elsevier.)

The rhythms in the following paragraphs are included in this group and are described as they appear on the ECG.

Supraventricular Tachycardia With Aberrancy. In SVT with aberrancy the QRS duration is longer than 0.12 second but typically not more than 0.14 second. Often, a triphasic RSR right bundle branch pattern is seen in lead V_1. Because of the fast ventricular rate, the P wave may be buried in the previous beat or may present as a peaked or notched T wave in the previous beat. Carotid sinus massage may slow or even terminate the tachycardia. Differentiation between SVT with aberrant conduction VT may be challenging but is critical because treatment approaches differ significantly according to the origin of the arrhythmia. A combination of leads is superior to one lead in making this differentiation.[17]

Ventricular Tachycardia. VT is defined as three or more consecutive ventricular ectopic beats with a rate over 100 beats/min.[16] The rhythm may be sustained (>30 seconds) or non-sustained (<30 seconds). The QRS width is usually greater than 0.14 second, and may be monomorphic in nature (QRS complexes appear the same) or polymorphic (the QRS shape changes from beat to beat) (Fig. 100.3).

Differentiation of VT from SVT with aberrancy is not always possible. Usually SVT with aberrancy would have a BBB morphology, so the absence of BBB on the ECG suggests it may be VT. Another criterion is AV dissociation; P waves are independent and unrelated to the QRS complex. Other indicators that favor a diagnosis of VT are extreme right-axis deviation (northwest) between 180 and −90 degrees; concordance of the QRS pattern in all precordial leads (e.g., all have negative deflections); and a wide QRS pattern inconsistent with typical right or left bundle branch patterns.[17] Using carotid sinus massage

may assist in the differentiation of VT and SVT with aberrancy; it may slow down the rate of SVT long enough to offer an improved view of the rhythm, but VT will not respond.

Ventricular Outflow Tract Tachycardia. One of the most common causes of idiopathic VT is right ventricular outflow tract (RVOT) tachycardia, which originates from the outflow tract of the right ventricle. It is usually triggered by sympathetic stimulation (anxiety, excitement, exercise, and stimulants) and more often seen in younger patients (20 to 30 years) without underlying structural heart disease. Typical ECG findings have a wide QRS complex, a LBBB morphology and, usually, an inferior QRS axis.[18] Precordial leads that show a transition of the R wave in V_3 are more likely to be septal in the origin of the right outflow tract. These ECG changes increase with stimulation, stress, and activities, so exercise stress testing is beneficial to provoke the arrhythmia so a more definitive diagnosis may be made. It is possible for the VT to originate from the left ventricular outflow tract and manifest in a similar fashion on the ECG, making the specific diagnosis challenging; such cases should be referred to EP cardiology.

Torsades De Pointes. The most common polymorphic VT is torsades de pointes, which is characterized by polymorphic QRS complexes that change in amplitude and cycle length. It is associated with QT prolongation, which may be congenital or idiopathic or a result of electrolyte imbalances (particularly hypokalemia or hypomagnesemia). The arrhythmia may also be induced by long QT intervals produced by medications, such as quinidine, antiarrhythmic agents, antipsychotics, and some antibiotics used routinely in primary care (including azithromycin and moxifloxacin). Patient outcome will be improved if differentiation of this arrhythmia is made early, because the treatment for torsades de pointes differs markedly from standard VT treatments.

Other types of polymorphic VT may be congenital or acquired. Congenital causes include long QT syndrome (corrected QT interval >0.40 second), Brugada syndrome (ECG exhibits RBBB pattern and ST-segment elevation in the precordial leads), and the more unusual diagnosis of catecholamine-induced polymorphic VT. Acquired polymorphic VT is usually induced by drug toxicity or electrolyte abnormalities. Differential diagnosis of these types of VT can be difficult and should be referred to a cardiology specialist.

Ventricular Fibrillation. VF is a rapid, disorganized electrical activity within the ventricles with no discrete QRS complexes. The heart is unable to contract, and therefore no systole (pulse) is possible. Recognizing this arrhythmia is vital to the patient's chances of survival because defibrillation is required immediately (see Fig. 100.3).

Additional Complexes

Premature Atrial Contractions. Premature atrial contractions (PACs) are ectopic or irregular beats that occur prior to the next sinus beat. They are initiated in the left or right atrium and not by the SA node. The irregularity often causes the patient to complain of a sensation of palpitations, skipping heart rate, or extra beats, especially if they are numerous. They are typically identified on the ECG within an underlying sinus rhythm, which would be completely regular were it not for the premature beats. The PAC is a normal-looking complex (P, QRS, and T) in every way except that it occurs prematurely. The PR interval may differ slightly from that of the prevailing rhythm, although it remains within the normal range. Because the PAC depolarizes the sinus node, there is typically a partially compensatory pause before the next sinus beat.

Premature Junctional Contractions. Premature junctional contractions (PJCs) originate in the AV node and are another cause of irregularity in the heart rhythm. The impulse is carried to the ventricles along normal pathways; the resultant QRS complex is narrow and appears similar to the QRS complexes of the sinus rhythm. There may be retrograde conduction to the atria, yielding a P wave that can occur before, during, or after the QRS complex. If the P wave occurs before the QRS complex, the PR interval is less than 0.12 second. When a P wave is visible, it is typically negative in leads II, III, and aVF.[16]

Premature Ventricular Contractions. PVCs are extra premature beats that originate in the ventricle. They are characterized by wide, bizarre QRS complexes (>0.12 second) that interrupt the prevailing rhythm (Fig. 100.4) They may be unifocal (originating from one focus) or multifocal (originating from

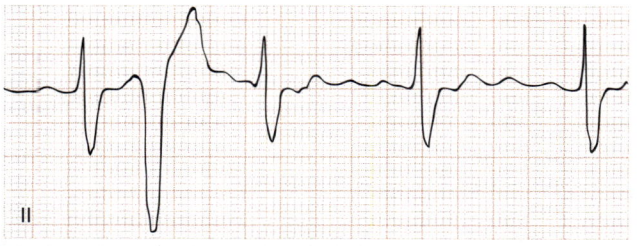

FIG. 100.4 Premature ventricular contraction. (From Walls, R. M., Hockberger, R. S., & Gausche-Hill, M. [2018]. *Rosen's emergency medicine: Concepts and clinical practice* [9th ed.]. Philadelphia: Elsevier.)

multiple points of focus). The P wave is typically absent, and the beat is most often followed by a full compensatory pause (the distance from the QRS preceding the PVC to the QRS that follows it is equal to twice the R-R interval of the prevailing sinus rhythm). Typically the T-wave deflection is in opposition to that of the QRS complex.[17] The description of PVCs is included here because of their association with ventricular tachyarrhythmias.

DIFFERENTIAL DIAGNOSIS OF BRADYARRHYTHMIAS

Sinus Bradycardia

In sinus bradycardia, the SA node fires at a rate of less than 60 beats/min with a 1:1 relationship between each P wave and QRS complex. The time that is taken for each electrical conduction is normal, the PR intervals are 0.20 second or less, and QRS intervals are 0.12 second or less.

Heart Blocks (Atrioventricular Nodal Blocks)

The electrical activity starts in the SA node and travels through the AV node to reach the ventricles. A heart block may occur at any part of this journey. SA exit block is the sudden cessation of sinus rhythm that results in long pauses that usually occur in a fixed pattern. Atrioventricular nodal blocks occur as conduction through the AV node is delayed or blocked completely. These types of blocks are separated into three groups: first-degree AV block, second-degree AV block, and third-degree AV block. The AV block may be transient, intermittent, or permanent and may be differentiated further by measuring the length of the PR interval and identifying the presence of a QRS complex. Normal conduction continues rapidly to all sections of the ventricular muscle by way of the right and left bundle branches. If disruption occurs on this part of the electrical journey it results in an intraventricular block, such as a BBB or fascicular block.

First-Degree Block. In first-degree AV block the PR intervals are equal and longer than 0.20 second, but every P wave is conducted to the ventricle, resulting in a related QRS complex.

Second-Degree Block. There are many types of second-degree AV block, but two are specifically identified in primary care: type I (sometimes referred to as Mobitz type I) and type II (Mobitz type II). The differentiating factor for second-degree AV blocks when compared with other blocks is the consistent absence of a QRS complex that is missed or "skipped" in a timed fashion (e.g., three complete complexes followed by a P wave where a QRS is missing). The atrium-ventricle conduction ratio is usually 3:2 or 4:3, and a typical pattern of complexes occurs.

Second-Degree, Type I. In second-degree AV block Mobitz type I, there is progressive prolongation of the PR interval until a P wave is not conducted to the ventricle. This rhythm is also called Wenckebach block (Fig. 100.5).

Second-Degree, Type II. In second-degree AV block Mobitz type II there is a constant PR interval until a P wave does not conduct to the ventricle and the QRS complex is skipped (missing) (Fig. 100.6). This type of second-degree AV block is less common and a little more severe than Mobitz type I and has a higher propensity to progress to complete heart block.

Third-Degree AV Block. In third-degree AV block none of the atrial impulses are conducted to the ventricle. This rhythm is often referred to as complete heart block or AV disassociation. The P waves have no relationship to the QRS complexes (they

Mobitz Type I (Wenckebach) Second-Degree AV Block

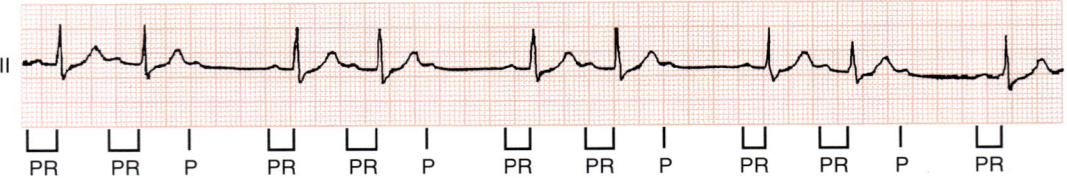

FIG. 100.5   Mobitz type 1 (Wenchebach) second-degree atrioventricular block. (From Goldberger, A. L., Goldberger, Z., & Shvilkin, A. [2018]. *Goldberger's clinical electrocardiography: A simplified approach* [9th ed.]. Philadelphia: Elsevier.)

Mobitz type II second-degree AV block

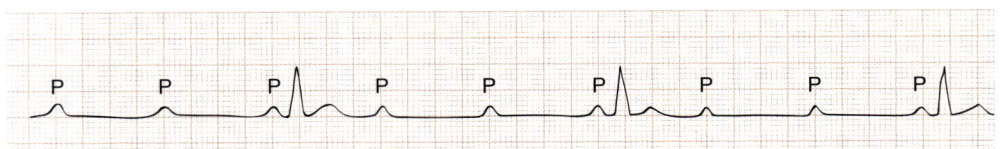

FIG. 100.6   Second-degree *AV* block Mobitz type II. (From Walls, R. M., Hockberger, R. S., & Gausche-Hill, M. [2018]. *Rosen's emergency medicine: Concepts and clinical practice* [9th ed.]. Philadelphia: Elsevier.)

Third-Degree (Complete) Heart Block

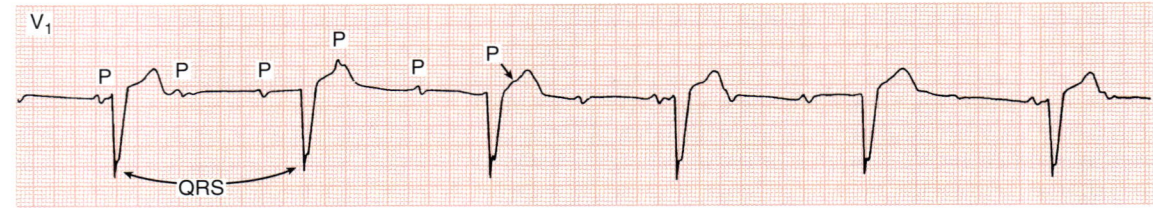

FIG. 100.7   Third-degree (complete) heart block. (From Goldberger, A. L., Goldberger, Z., & Shvilkin, A. [2018]. *Goldberger's clinical electrocardiography: A simplified approach* [9th ed.]. Philadelphia: Elsevier.)

are dissociated) (Fig. 100.7). Typically, the pacemaker function is picked up by an escape focus, resulting in either a junctional or ventricular escape rhythm. A junctional escape rhythm is characterized by a slow rate (40 to 60 beats/min) with QRS complexes of normal width that are not related to P waves. A ventricular escape rhythm typically produces a bradycardia of less than 40 beats/min and is characterized by wide QRS complexes (>0.12 second) that are also not connected to, or associated with, P waves.

Bundle Branch Blocks

In BBB the conduction is disrupted as it journeys down the bundle branches. The impulse is stopped at the blocked bundle and is forced to travel across the myocardium to depolarize the opposite ventricle. This depolarization across the ventricle takes longer than the normal bundle conduction, which causes a time lapse that increases the QRS duration. A QRS duration of 0.10 to 0.11 second results from incomplete BBB, whereas a QRS duration of 0.12 second or longer results from complete BBB. It is important to evaluate a BBB using a 12-lead ECG for multiple views of the rhythm.

Right Bundle Branch Block. The ECG shows a small R wave followed by an S wave and then a final R in lead V_1, whereas V_6 will show a deep, slurred S wave after initially normal Q and R waves.

Left Bundle Branch Block. The ECG shows a broad, slurred S wave in lead V_1 and an R in lead V_6.

Hemiblocks. The left bundle branch is further divided into the left anterior fascicle and the left posterior fascicle. When conduction is impaired in only one of the fascicles, a hemiblock occurs (which is usually related to loss of blood supply, and mostly found after MI). In addition to the LBBB, a right-axis deviation will be noticed on the ECG with left posterior hemiblock, and a left-axis deviation will occur with left anterior hemiblock.

INTERPROFESSIONAL COLLABORATIVE MANAGEMENT

The first priority with cardiac arrhythmias is to establish the presence of a pulse. Secondly, determine hemodynamic stability (blood pressure and clinical symptoms) to differentiate stable from unstable arrhythmias. Thirdly, record a 12-lead ECG to further identify the arrhythmia and to rule out MI as the cause: Identify ST elevation, depression, or T-wave changes on the 12-lead ECG, and evaluate symptoms (e.g., chest pain, dyspnea, diaphoresis, nausea, fatigue) and recognize coronary risk factors.

Management of Tachyarrhythmias

Although many of the symptoms caused by arrhythmias are the result of the heart rate and the hemodynamic response, the individual patient response is variable between episodes. The effect of an arrhythmia on hemodynamics is largely dependent on the rate rather than its cause. This may be a result of shortened ventricular filling time, the severity of underlying heart disease, the presence of AV synchrony, the ventricular activation sequence, and the autonomic balance. For patients with atrial tachyarrhythmias who are hemodynamically unstable, immediate synchronized cardioversion is to be recommended.[3] For stable patients, nonpharmacological methods or medications may be more appropriate.

Nonpharmacological Management. Nonpharmacological management starts with eliminating stimulants that could provoke the arrhythmia. Ensuring adequate hydration, oxygenation, stability of electrolyte balance, and reduction of environmental stressors is helpful. If the arrhythmia is caused by a toxin, determine if an antidote is needed or if resolution is expected over time as the toxin is cleared.

Pharmacological Management. The decision to initiate antiarrhythmic therapy depends on the severity and frequency of the arrhythmia and the hemodynamic consequences versus the risks associated with the therapy itself. Antiarrhythmic medications have significant side effects, one of which is a worsening of the arrhythmia known as proarrhythmia. The need for long-term antiarrhythmic therapy must be individualized to each patient's needs because the severity of symptoms is highly variable, based on the clinical situation and the presence or absence of underlying coronary artery disease.[19] In addition, structural heart disease has been associated with an increased risk of drug-induced proarrhythmia manifested by ventricular arrhythmias.[3]

The two general conditions for which antiarrhythmic therapy is appropriate are: a potentially life-threatening arrhythmia, and an arrhythmia that is hemodynamically significant or symptomatic, which mostly involve ventricular arrhythmias and AF. The Vaughn-Williams is the most commonly used classification system and separates antiarrhythmic medications into four classes based on their mechanism of action and target cell (excluding digoxin and adenosine).[7,19,20]

- Class I: sodium channel blockade drugs; further divided into three subgroups as follows:
  - Class Ia—quinidine, procainamide, and disopyramide
  - Class Ib—lidocaine, mexiletine, and tocainide
  - Class Ic—flecainide, propafenone, and moricizine
- Class II: beta blockers
  - Selective agents such as atenolol, bisoprolol, and metoprolol
  - Nonselective agents such as nadolol and propranolol
  - Nonselective and alpha receptor blockers such as carvedilol and labetalol
- Class III: potassium channel blocking and include sotalol, dofetilide, ibutilide, amiodarone, and bretylium
- Class IV: calcium channel blockers
  - Dihydropyridines such as amlodipine, felodipine, nicardipine, and nifedipine
  - Nondihydropyridines—SA and AV node depressants such as diltiazem and verapamil

Management of the arrhythmia is individualized and specific to each type of rhythm disturbance. The following section will discuss each tachyarrhythmia in more detail.

Sinus Tachycardia

Sinus tachycardia is typically remedied by treatment or elimination of the underlying cause (e.g., fever, hypovolemia, hyperthyroidism, anxiety). Elimination of tobacco, alcohol, caffeine, stimulants, or sympathomimetics (such as those found in over-the-counter cold medications, nasal sprays, and diet supplements) may result in a return to normal heart rate.

If the tachycardia is unresolved by removal of the underlying cause, a diagnosis of syndrome of inappropriate sinus tachycardia (IST) may be considered. It is defined as a sinus-initiated heart rate higher than 100 beats/min at rest for longer than 24 hours (mean >90 in 24 hours), usually associated with palpitations. Before managing this diagnosis, the provider should ensure that all possible underlying causes have been investigated and should eliminate possible stimulants with lifestyle modifications. Pending approval for IST in the United States, ivabradine (Corlanor) holds considerable promise for treatment, with 70% of patients reporting reduction of symptoms and increased exercise performance.[20] Beta blockers are not the primary therapy but may be useful when combined with ivabradine.[20]

Multifocal Atrial Tachycardia

Multifocal atrial tachycardia occurs primarily in older patients with comorbid disease. Sixty percent of these patients have significant pulmonary disease.[17] The diagnosis often occurs in the setting of congestive HF, exacerbation of the underlying pulmonary condition, or electrolyte imbalance. As with sinus tachycardia, therapy is directed at correction of the precipitating factor (e.g., improving oxygenation, correcting electrolyte imbalance).[17]

Paroxysmal Supraventricular Tachycardia

The use of vagal maneuvers or carotid massage may be useful in slowing the ventricular rate of PSVT. After vagal maneuvers a trial of adenosine followed by intravenous verapamil or diltiazem are reasonable treatment options to attempt before cardioversion. However, it is recommended that an external cardioverter-defibrillator be readily available, especially as AF is possible after the medications are used.[17] Adenosine is contraindicated in patients with asthma because it may precipitate AF. Narrow-complex PSVT may also be treated pharmacologically by slowing of AV conduction with digoxin, CCB, or beta blockers or by suppression of atrial automaticity with class IA, IC, or III antiarrhythmic agents.[17]

Caution is necessary when managing wide-complex PSVT; careful monitoring is required during medication administration. Pharmacologic agents that increase the refractoriness of the AV node (digoxin, CCB, and beta blockers) may decrease the refractoriness of the accessory pathway and have the potential to cause a faster ventricular rate when used alone. Class IA, IC, and III agents are preferred because they increase the refractoriness of the bypass tract.[17]

Most cases of PSVT are reentrant and amenable to radiofrequency ablation when symptoms are significant and recurrent. Ablation is most often preferable to antiarrhythmic agents because of safety and tolerability concerns.

 Caution indicated for wide-complex PSVT and should be managed in conjunction with a cardiologist and usually necessitates hospitalization.

Atrial Fibrillation or Atrial Flutter

Management of the patient with AF or atrial flutter may be challenging because the best approach is often not clear and treatment must be highly individualized and based on symptoms, underlying disease processes, and co-combined conditions.

Treatment of patients with AF traditionally consists of three main components: (1) anticoagulation for stroke prevention; (2) rate control (80 to 110 bpm); and (3) rhythm control. However, recent studies have called attention to include risk factor modification as the fourth aspect of management. These risk factors include obesity, sleep apnea, hypertension, diabetes, alcohol consumption, and physical inactivity.[9]

Anticoagulation and rate control therapies are initially used along with lifestyle modifications, but if the patient has symptoms beyond these interventions, a rhythm control therapy may be added.[11] If the patient remains significantly symptomatic (palpitations, fatigue, dyspnea, or exercise intolerance) catheter ablation has been associated with an improvement of the patients quality of life.[9] Therefore, based on symptoms, age, lifestyle, underlying disease and structure of the heart, and patient preference, an early referral to cardiology and an electrophysiologist may be considered part of the initial management of the AF patient. It is important to consider the patient's preference in their plan of care, and determine if nonpharmacological, pharmacological, or procedure/surgical approaches are most acceptable.

Prevention of Thromboembolism in Atrial Fibrillation. Although AF is not considered a lethal arrhythmia, it carries a significant risk of stroke and embolism, and increased risk of HF. Therefore prevention of thromboembolism is a therapeutic goal of long-term treatment. Stroke risk is measured using the CHA_2DS_2-VASc score. For patients with non-valvular AF with prior stroke, transient ischemic attack, or a CHA_2DS_2-VASc score of 2 or higher, oral anticoagulants are recommended.[3]

Anticoagulation may be accomplished with warfarin, a vitamin K antagonist. It is effective at multiple sites of action in the coagulation cascade, which is why it has been the mainstay oral anticoagulant treatment in the prevention of stroke for patients with AF for decades.[3] However, it is not without its drawbacks. The constant monitoring and the risk of bleeding make it a medication requiring thoughtful consideration. Warfarin dose should be titrated to maintain the international normalized ratio (INR) between 2 and 3. The INR is measured at least weekly during initiation of therapy, and monthly when stable.[3]

Use of a direct thrombin or factor Xa inhibitor is an alternative to warfarin and does not require serum monitoring. Currently there are four medications available in this category: dabigatran (a direct thrombin inhibitor) and the factor Xa inhibitors rivaroxaban, edoxaban, and apixaban.[11] Of these medications, a 2018 review of 320 articles published over an 8-year period (2000 to 2008) conducted for AHRQ demonstrated apixaban as the safest DOAC for stroke prevention in Afib, though all Factor xa inhibitors were slightly more efficacious in preventing strokes than warfarin (https://www.ncbi.nlm.nih.gov/pubmed/30480925). These medications are substrates for the efflux transporter P-glycoprotein and indicated for use in nonvalvular AF to prevent thromboembolism.[3] Dabigatran (factor IIa inhibitor) is a prodrug with the advantage that it is not metabolized by the cytochrome P-450 system; rivaroxaban, edoxaban, and apixaban are direct inhibitors of factor Xa and are partially metabolized by cytochrome P-450 enzymes, and therefore are contraindicated with drugs that are strong P-450 3A4 (CYP3A4) inducers or combined with P-glycoprotein.[3]

Severe bleeding is a side effect of both warfarin and the factor Xa inhibitors; the risks of bleeding versus the benefits of stroke prevention must be considered. Interaction with other medications may increase or decrease the potency and effectiveness of the drugs. P-glycoprotein inhibitors (ketoconazole, verapamil, amiodarone, dronedarone, quinidine, and clarithromycin) may increase plasma concentrations. In addition, P-glycoprotein inducers (phenytoin, carbamazepine, rifampin, and St. John's wort) can decrease levels to subtherapeutic levels. These medications should not be used for patients with AF and mechanical heart valves and are not recommended in patients with AF and end-stage chronic kidney disease (or dialysis) because of a lack of clinical trial evidence establishing safety and efficacy.[3] Before initiation of therapy with one of these medications, renal status should be established with serum creatinine and then periodically during use of the medication. Edoxaban is contraindicated for patients with nonvalvular AF if the patient's creatinine clearance is greater than 95 mL/min. Until recently, there was no antidote available to reverse the effects of these medications, but fortunately the limited half-life ususually lessened the need for a reversal agent. For patients with uncontrollable bleeding associated with rivaroxaban (Xarelto) or apixaban (Eliquis), the FDA has approved a factor Xa inhibitor antidote (ANDEXXA). Idarucizumab (Praxbind), a monoclonal antibody fragment is the approved antidote for patients with AF who develop uncontrollable bleeding while taking dabigatran. Research continues with this group of medications to establish better understanding of clinical variables such as the patient's age, dose and administration interval, and renal function.

Antiplatelet monotherapy is not recommended for stroke prevention in AF patients, regardless of stroke risk, and combinations of oral anticoagulants and platelet inhibitors increase bleeding risk and should be avoided unless there are other indications for platelet inhibition.[11] If the patient has an allergy to anticoagulants, clopidogrel plus aspirin is superior to aspirin alone in stroke prevention but is still significantly less effective than warfarin. Anticoagulation in low-risk patients (those younger than 60 years without heart disease) may be accomplished with this combination, although decreased stroke risk is offset by increased risk of bleeding complications.[3,11]

Older adults potentially have multiple comorbidities and a higher risk factor for stroke. (CHA_2DS_2-VASc identifies 65 to 74 years as a minor risk factor and 75 years or older as major risk factor.) Symptoms may be minimal and somewhat atypical with increased age. The risks and comorbidities must be factored into management decisions.[3]

Rate Control in Atrial Fibrillation. Rate control often relives symptoms of AF and is an acceptable goal in hemodynamically stable patients. Little robust evidence exists about the best type of treatment to control the rate, but acute or long-term rate control is achieved with beta blockers, diltiazem, verapamil, digoxin, or combination therapy.[11,21] The choice of drug and amount of rate control will depend on patient characteristics, symptoms, hemodynamics, left ventricular function, and ejection fraction. Beta blockers and nondihydropyridine CCB are the drugs of choice for rate control alone as they have a rapid onset of action and effectiveness (verapamil and diltiazem are the only CCBs to control rate).

The ideal resting rate has long been considered to be 60 to 75 beats/min,[22] but The 2010 Rate Control Efficacy in Permanent Atrial Fibrillation: a Comparison between Lenient versus Strict Rate Control II (RACE II) revealed that lenient heart rate control (< 110 bpm) was noninferior to strict rate control and did not result in increased heart failure or deaths: https://www.nejm.org/doi/full/10.1056/NEJMoa1001337. Additionally, this study was important because more lenient control may help prevent falls in older adults.

If necessary, digoxin can be added to assist in rate control, and its inotropic properties can be useful. A combination therapy with beta blockers and digoxin is useful in controlling rate for patients with EF <40%, whereas CCB should be avoided in those patients, as they can have a negative inotropic effect in patients with limitations of ventricular function.[11] However, a 2015 study by Washam et al. indicated that patients with AF have increased mortality, vascular death, and sudden death when digoxin is used.[21] Therefore periodic serum levels should be measured to establish a nontoxic therapeutic level (0.8 to 2 ng/mL for AF, and toxicity level >2 ng/mL).

A number of antiarrhythmic drugs also have rate-limiting properties (amiodarone, dronedarone, sotalol, and propafenone), in addition to being antiarrhythmic, but due to the significant side effects they should be used sparingly, and only in patients needing rhythm control therapy.[11] Ablation of the atrioventricular node/His bundle and implantation of a permanent ventricular pacemaker can control ventricular rate in a symptomatic patient when medications fail. The procedure carries a low rate of complications and low long-term mortality risk, especially when the pacemaker is implanted a few weeks before the AV nodal ablation.[11] However, AV nodal ablation is irreversible and the patient becomes pacemaker dependent, which is a different procedure to a catheter ablation used for rhythm control.

Rhythm Control in Atrial Fibrillation. One major consideration in determining treatment is the patient's tolerance of the lost atrial contraction that accompanies AF. Loss of AV synchrony and irregularity of the ventricular rhythm both lead to labile blood pressure and can cause a decline in cardiac output. If the patient is unstable, symptomatic, or it is deemed necessary, an initial attempt to restore normal sinus rhythm may be made with synchronized cardioversion and/or a pharmacologic converting agent. However, evaluation of thromboembolism risk should be made before restoration of atrial contraction. Reasons to choose restoration of sinus rhythm include symptom relief, prevention of embolism, and reduction in the risk of cardiomyopathy or HF. However, prolonged duration of the AF and left atrial enlargement can reduce the ability to be successful in maintaining normal sinus rhythm.[17,19]

Pharmacological cardioversion restores sinus rhythm in approximately 50% of patients with recent-onset AF, and can be achieved with dofetilide, flecainide, propafenone, ibutilide, or amiodarone,[11] but each medication carries side effects, and structural heart disease must be identified before administration. Long-term antiarrhythmic drug therapy may be used for symptom control, but in deciding to use a pharmacologic agent consider proarrhythmia and side effects. Each antiarrhythmic carries its own risks, and safety considerations should be made when selecting an agent. Amiodarone, dronedarone, sotalol, dofetilide, flecainide, propafenone, quinidine, and disopyramide may be used.[3,11] Dronedarone should not be used for ventricular rate control in permanent AF, HF, or left ventricular systolic dysfunction because it increases the risk of stroke, MI, systemic embolism, and cardiovascular death.[3] Administration of other antiarrhythmics with dronedarone should be avoided; there can be interactions with CCB, antiseizure medications,

and other medications metabolized by the CYP3A or CYP2D6 hepatic pathways.

Amiodarone is the most effective antiarrhythmic drug for maintenance of sinus rhythm in patients with paroxysmal or persistent AF and is more effective than dronedarone, sotalol, or propafenone.[3] Amiodarone should be initiated by a physician in the hospital with a loading dose (intravenous bolus, followed by a maintenance therapy). Proarrhythmias are a serious side effect, and lethal arrhythmias are possible with both intravenous and oral medication. Amiodarone has a very long half-life (40 to 50 days) and accumulates in the skin, liver, and cornea. Before initiation of amiodarone, baseline monitoring parameters should be attained, including liver and thyroid function tests and pulmonary function tests. Routine observation and diagnostic testing for hepatic and pulmonary toxicity is imperative, as is thyroid monitoring. Regular referrals to optometry or ophthalmology specialists for corneal monitoring are also necessary.

Finally, those with problematic or refractory AF may be candidates for electrical synchronous cardioversion, AV nodal ablation or modification, and/or pacemaker implantation. The surgical maze procedure has been shown to be useful in controlling the tachyarrhythmia that occurs with AF.[11] Electrical and pharmacologic cardioversion carry the risk of thromboembolism. When the rhythm has been sustained for longer than 48 hours, anticoagulation therapy should be uninterrupted for 4 weeks before and for at least 4 weeks after elective cardioversion. TEE may be used to evaluate or exclude the presence of left atrial thrombus before cardioversion. If an atrial thrombus is present, cardioversion is postponed for more adequate anticoagulation (usually 3 to 4 weeks) and TEE can be repeated.[3]

Premature Atrial and Junctional Contractions

In general, PACs and PJCs do not usually require treatment, but the cause should be investigated. In a non-diseased heart of normal structure these irregularities of the rhythm may be a result of increased stimulation (as previously described in the sinus tachycardia discussion). Their occurrence may diminish or disappear when these stimuli are withdrawn. More concerning causes include ischemia, hypokalemia and hypomagnesemia, hypoxia, and myocardial stretch in early congestive HF. If possible, correct the underlying cause. Symptom management may be necessary, based on individual patient situations, and possibly achieved with beta blockers.

Premature Ventricular Contractions

PVCs occur in both normal and diseased hearts, and are of no prognostic significance in the structurally normal heart. As with PACs and PJCs, management follows identifying and treating the underlying cause. In the primary care setting beta blockers are the drugs of choice and can provide symptom relief when patients feel the PVCs and complain of palpitations or the sensation of skipped beats. Complex ventricular ectopy (defined as more than 10 PVCs per minute over 24 hours or non-sustained VT) is rare in the normal heart and should provoke an evaluation for underlying cardiac disease.

Ventricular Tachycardia

Clinical management of non-sustained VT first includes identification and management of any underlying cause (e.g., myocardial ischemia, electrolyte imbalance, digoxin toxicity, hypoxia,). Patients with previous MI, structural heart disease, or low ejection fractions who have non-sustained VT are at particularly high risk for adverse events, including sudden death. Beta blockers reduce these risks, but referral for electrophysiological testing should be considered for this group as well as for those with severe symptoms.[17]

Sustained VT with a pulse including evaluation of hemodynamic status requires treatment at an acute care facility; it is not managed in the primary care setting. An emergency medical response team must be activated for immediate emergency management. Management should follow basic life support and advanced cardiac life support guidelines by the American Heart Association. Therapy to prevent recurrent sustained VT may include pharmacologic management, implantable cardioverter-defibrillator (ICD) implantation, or a combination of the two.

Antiarrhythmic therapy for VT has remained unchanged for the past decade and continues to be limited by the potential for toxicity and proarrhythmia side effects. Intravenous administration of amiodarone, lidocaine, or procainamide is used for acute termination of the arrhythmia, and amiodarone and sotalol remain the principal agents used in the chronic treatment of VT.[17,20] Sotalol has a significant adverse effect of torsades de pointes and therefore is initiated in an inpatient setting with continuous ECG monitoring. Beta blockers remain the first-line therapy for patients with systolic HF and after acute MI.

The treatment of polymorphic VT requires consultation with a cardiologist. Beta blockers may be useful in the management of congenital VT, such as long QT syndrome and catecholaminergic polymorphic ventricular tachycardia (CPVT).[20] Long QT syndrome and Brugada syndrome usually require implantation of an internal defibrillating device in patients with syncope and complex ventricular arrhythmias. Torsades de pointes is an emergency ventricular arrhythmia that requires immediate intervention and defibrillation.

Electrophysiologic studies with radiofrequency ablation are appropriate for some patients with reentrant VT, and the electrophysiologist will evaluate ventricular function before treatment. Patients may be best managed with ICD implantation. Biventricular pacing can be incorporated into a combination device with an ICD. The use of an ICD is the gold-standard therapy in patients with structural heart defects who are at risk of ventricular arrhythmias.[20]

Right Ventricular Outflow Tract

RVOT is the most common subtype of idiopathic ventricular arrhythmias.[18] Traditional detection is the Holter monitor, but more recently long-term monitoring systems are used. It is also identified when induced by activity during an exercise stress test. Beta blockers or CCB may provide symptom relief. RVOT VT is usually benign, but occasionally can induce left ventricular dysfunction, and, very rarely, VF or polymorphic VT.[18] Referral to a cardiologist or electrophysiologist for radiofrequency catheter ablation is an option, especially if symptoms remain uncontrolled with medication and lifestyle changes. The irregular heartbeats can be obliterated with ablation and is a more permanent treatment.

MANAGEMENT OF BRADYARRHYTHMIAS

The initial management of bradyarrhythmias begins with evaluating the hemodynamic stability of the patient and analysis of the underlying cause. The unstable patient with a bradyarrhythmia will require a pacemaker to stabilize the heart rate,

which may be initially external until an implantable device is placed.

Nonpharmacological Management. The nonpharmacological management of a bradyarrhythmia starts with the investigation and removal of the offending cause. Medications routinely prescribed for chronic disease processes should be reviewed for a bradyarrhythmia side effect, including beta blockers, CCB, digoxin, clonidine, and opiates. Withdrawal of the offending drug may be all that is required for restoration of adequate ventricular rate. Correction of electrolyte imbalances, in particular hyperkalemia, may also resolve the problem. Underlying conditions of hypothyroidism or Lyme disease could also be the causative factor of bradyarrhythmia and are mostly reversible with appropriate treatment of the disease. If a reversible cause of the bradyarrhythmia cannot be identified and corrected (in which sinus rhythm is restored), a referral to a cardiologist is prudent to evaluate for pacemaker and to complete a full cardiac exam with structural heart disease consideration. Patients with asymptomatic bradycardia may or may not require further intervention; this is largely determined by symptomology, stability, and the type of rhythm (detailed in the following paragraphs).

Pharmacological Management: The initial emergency medication used for bradyarrhythmia is atropine, as a temporary measure to increase the atrial rate. However, atropine will not be effective at restoring atrial rate if there is a block causing the rate to be initiated below the atria. Atropine must be used with caution in patients with coronary risk factors, as increases in the heart rate may worsen ischemia and cause MI. If the bradyarrhythmia is symptomatic or becoming unstable, atropine is used as a temporary measure along with hemodynamic support while awaiting the placement of a temporary pacemaker, which can be achieved rapidly through transcutaneous electrodes or the insertion of a transvenous pacer wire in a hospital setting. Management of each bradyarrhythmia is individualized and specific to the type of rhythm disturbance or block; the following section will discuss each bradyarrhythmia in more detail.

Sinus Bradycardia

Sinus bradycardia is treated only if the patient is symptomatic (e.g., lightheadedness or syncope associated with decreased heart rate). Withdrawal of drugs that produce an increase in vagal tone (e.g., edrophonium chloride or digitalis) or that decrease sympathetic tone (e.g., beta blockers, CCB, amiodarone, or reserpine) may result in an increase in sinus node activity. If symptomatic or decompensating, atropine can be used to increase the heart rate by blocking vagal tone, but a permanent pacemaker may be necessary for patients with chronic, symptomatic bradycardia. When symptoms cannot be proved to be caused by bradycardia, but sinus node dysfunction is suspected, pacing is discouraged in asymptomatic patients, even when resting heart rates are lower than 40 beats/min. However, pacing is supported in patients with syncope of unexplained origin when major abnormalities in sinus node function are demonstrated at electrophysiologic testing.[23]

Heart Blocks

Heart block is treated first by correction of any underlying causes. The initial priority for any type of new heart block is to identify coronary risk factors and investigate for coronary ischemia with a 12-lead ECG.

Immediate transfer to an emergency facility with interventional cardiology is indicated for a patient with coronary risk factors and observable ischemia on ECG to rapidly address reperfusion.

If the heart is free from disease and is structurally normal, the causes of heart block are usually acquired. These causes may include hyperkalemia, hypothyroidism, overactive vagus nerve, or sensitivity reaction to medications or toxicity. Pharmacologic agents such as digitalis, beta blockers, CCB, or class III agents (sotalol, amiodarone) could be responsible for the arrhythmia. Removal of the offending agent or treatment of the underlying cause should assist in the cessation of most heart blocks (including SA exit block).

Atropine reverses cholinergic-mediated reductions in AV nodal conduction and heart rate and may be useful in treating first-degree AV block in a symptomatic patient. However, it is not likely to be as effective in second- or third-degree AV block. Hemodynamic instability is more likely in third-degree AV block and usually requires intervention with a temporary pacemaker while the underlying cause is treated. Virtually all patients with third-degree AV block will require a permanent pacemaker unless the block resolves after the underlying condition is treated. An example of this type of heart block could be seen in a chronic kidney disease patient with third-degree AV block related to hyperkalemia, and digitalis toxicity after missing hemodialysis.

Bundle Branch Blocks

The sudden development of a BBB requires evaluation for coronary disease, structural defects, or medication that could have initiated a new-onset rhythm. Management focuses on treatment of the underlying cause and treatment of any specific symptoms. There are no pharmacological options for treating BBB or fascicular blocks. Once a BBB becomes chronic, it is periodically monitored and usually remains asymptomatic. A temporary pacemaker may be necessary in the initial management while the underlying cause is treated. As soon as the need for continuous pacing is determined, referral to a cardiologist or EP cardiologist will be necessary for the implantation of a permanent pacemaker. Patient follow-up and periodic checks of the pacemaker's function will be managed by the cardiologist.

INDICATIONS FOR REFERRAL OR HOSPITALIZATION

 Immediate emergency department referral and hospitalization is required if the arrhythmia produces hemodynamic decompensation such as hypotension, syncope, or chest pain, and a loss of pulse requires initiation of cardiopulmonary resuscitation.

Cardiology Referral. The treatment of serious, recurrent, or potentially life-threatening arrhythmias require referral to a cardiologist. Therapies may be initiated on an inpatient basis and managed on an outpatient basis. Patients requiring treatment of severe bradycardias and AV blocks may be referred to a cardiologist as treatment usually requires the placement of a permanent pacemaker.

Electrophysiology Cardiologist. Referral to an electrophysiologist is required if treatment of the arrhythmia warrants electrophysiologic studies or procedures such as a pacemaker, catheter radiofrequency ablation, or ICD implantation. Radiofrequency ablation is an option provided by electrophysiologists to locate the source of an arrhythmia and manipulate or eradicate it. Electrophysiologic studies are also required for guided pharmacologic therapy in the treatment of complex, potentially life-threatening arrhythmias, if the patient is refractory to standard drug therapy, or if the drug therapy itself produces life-threatening proarrhythmia.

LIFE SPAN CONSIDERATIONS

Older patients have the highest incidence of arrhythmias as well as other comorbid conditions. Renal, hepatic, and cardiovascular disease will greatly affect left ventricular function, tolerance of the arrhythmia, and ability for clearance of antiarrhythmic agents. Interactions with other agents must also be considered in treating an older patient for arrhythmias. For example, if amiodarone is prescribed for a patient who is taking warfarin or digoxin, the plasma levels of these drugs will increase.

COMPLICATIONS

An important determinant of mortality from an arrhythmia is the degree and nature of left ventricular dysfunction. Sudden cardiac death is a real and present danger with complex ventricular arrhythmias, particularly in the setting of underlying cardiac disease. Exacerbation of cardiac ischemia or infarction or HF may also occur with tachyarrhythmias or bradyarrhythmias. Reduction in cardiac output will result in decreased perfusion to other vital organs (e.g., brain, kidney). The risk of thromboembolism and stroke with AF has been previously discussed, as have the proarrhythmic effects of many of the antiarrhythmic agents. Lethal proarrhythmias are a serious adverse reaction that must be considered and monitored for in patients receiving antiarrhythmic therapy.[17,19]

PATIENT AND FAMILY EDUCATION

- Educate patients and their loved ones on the risks and benefits of all appropriate interventions before initiating them. Encourage self-management and empower patients to participate in shared decision-making to increase compliance with treatment management plans.
- Careful medication teaching, including proper scheduling of doses, potential side effects, and interactions with over-the-counter medications, is essential.
- The families of patients with arrhythmias should learn cardiopulmonary resuscitation and develop an emergency plan. Family or others who are able to act in a timely and appropriate fashion may influence the outcome and survival of the affected individual

HEALTH PROMOTION

As some arrhythmias are induced or worsened by outside stimulants or stressors, lifestyle modifications such as eliminating or reducing alcohol, caffeine, decongestant medications, cigarettes, or illicit drugs like cocaine may be utilized to reduce the chances of an arrhythmia. It has been suggested that some risk factors of AF are modifiable, such as hypertension, obesity, endurance exercise, obstructive sleep apnea, thyroid disease, and alcohol consumption.[9] For those risk factors that are not modifiable, such as age, gender, structural heart damage, or congenital causes, the best strategy may be awareness and early intervention at first onset of symptoms. The widespread implementation of automated external defibrillators has reduced mortality from lethal arrhythmias and should continue to be promoted in communities and workplaces to treat sudden cardiac death.

REFERENCES

1. Tester, D. J., & Ackerman, M. J. (2014). Genetics of cardiac arrhythmias. In D. L. Mann, D. P. Zipes, P. Libby, & R. O. Bonown (Eds.), *Braunwald's heart disease: A textbook of cardiovascular medicine* (10th ed., pp. 617–627). Philadelphia: Elsevier.

2. O'Gara, P. T., Kushner, F. G., Ascheim, D. D., et al. (2013). 2013 ACCF/AHA guideline for the management of ST-elevation myocardial infarction: A report of the American College of Cardiology Foundation/American Heart Association Task Force on Practice Guidelines. *Journal of the American College of Cardiology, 61*(4), e78–e140.

3. January, C. T., Wann, L., Alpert, J. S., et al. (2014). 2014 AHA/ACC/HRS guideline for the management of patients with atrial fibrillation: A report of the American College of Cardiology/American Heart Association Task Force on Practice Guidelines and the Heart Rhythm Society. *Journal of the American College of Cardiology, 64*(21), e1–e76.

4. Laske, T. G., Shrivastav, M., & Iaizzo, P. A. (2015). The cardiac conduction system. In P. A. Iaizzo (Ed.), *Handbook of cardiac anatomy, physiology, and devices* (3rd ed., pp. 215–233). Switzerland: Springer International Publishing.

5. Rupart, M., & Zipes, D. (2014). Electrophysiological considerations. In D. L. Mann, D. P. Zipes, P. Libby, & R. O. Bonown (Eds.), *Braunwald's heart disease: A textbook of cardiovascular medicine* (10th ed., pp. 629–661). Philadelphia: Elsevier.

6. Fu, D. G. (2015). Cardiac Arrhythmias: Diagnosis, symptoms, and treatments. *Cell Biochemistry and Biophysics, 1–6.*

7. Roukoz, H., Lü, F., & Sakaguchi, S. (2015). Catheter ablation of cardiac arrhythmias. In P. A. Iaizzo (Ed.), *Handbook of cardiac anatomy, physiology, and devices* (3rd ed., pp. 494–495). Switzerland: Springer International Publishing.

8. Bickley, L. S., Szilagyi, P. G., & Hoffman, R. M. (2017). *Guide to physical examination and history taking* (12th ed., pp. 374–399). Philadelphia: Wolters Kluwer.

9. Calkins, H., Hindricks, G., Cappato, R., Kim, Y. H., Saad, E. B., Aguinaga, L., et al. (2017). 2017 HRS/EHRA/ECAS/APHRS/SOLAECE expert consensus statement on catheter and surgical ablation of atrial fibrillation. *Heart Rhythm, 14*(10), e275–e444.

10. Nguyen, H. H., & Silva, J. N. (2016). Use of smartphone technology in cardiology. *Trends in Cardiovascular Medicine, 26*(4), 376–386.

11. Kirchhof, P., Benussi, S., Kotecha, D., Ahlsson, A., Atar, D., Casadei, B., et al. (2016). 2016 ESC Guidelines for the management of atrial fibrillation developed in collaboration with EACTS. *European Heart Journal, 37*(38), 2893–2962.

12. Koplan, B., Charytan, D., Podoll, A., et al. (2014). Implantable loop recorder monitoring detects a high incidence of bradycardia leading to pacemaker implant in hemodialysis patients: Preliminary results from the Monitoring in Dialysis (MiD) study. *Circulation, 130*(2).

13. Maggi, R., Rafanelli, M., Ceccofiglio, A., Solari, D., Brignole, M., & Ungar, A. (2014). Additional diagnostic value of implantable loop recorder in patients with initial diagnosis of real or apparent transient loss of consciousness of uncertain origin. *Europace: European Pacing, Arrhythmias, and Cardiac Electrophysiology: Journal of the Working Groups on Cardiac Pacing, Arrhythmias, and Cardiac Cellular Electrophysiology of the European Society of Cardiology, 16*(8), 1226–1230.

14. Miller, J., & Zipes, D. (2014). Diagnosis of cardiac arrhythmias. In D. L. Mann, D. P. Zipes, P. Libby, & R. O. Bonown (Eds.), *Braunwald's heart disease: A textbook of cardiovascular medicine* (10th ed., pp. 662–720). Philadelphia: Elsevier.

15. Gupta, M., Hoyt, W., & Snyder, C. S. (2014). The use of trans-esophageal electrophysiology study to identify a high risk asymptomatic Wolff Parkinson White syndrome patient. *Open J Pediatr, 4,* 231–235.

16. Goldberger, A. L., & Goldberger, Z. D. (2017). *Shvilkin A. Clinical electrocardiography: A simplified approach* (9th ed.). Philadelphia: Elsevier.

17. Olgin, J., & Zipes, D. (2014). Specific arrhythmias: Diagnosis and treatment. In D. L. Mann, D. P. Zipes, P. Libby, & R. O. Bonown (Eds.), *Braunwald's heart disease: A textbook of cardiovascular medicine* (10th ed., pp. 748–797). Philadelphia: Elsevier.

18. Fuenmayor, A. J. (2014). Treatment or cure of right ventricular outflow tract tachycardia. *Journal of Atrial Fibrillation, 7*(1).

19. Miller, J., & Zipes, D. (2014). Therapy for cardiac arrhythmias. In D. L. Mann, D. P. Zipes, P. Libby, & R. O. Bonown (Eds.), *Braunwald's heart disease: A textbook of cardiovascular medicine* (10th ed., pp. 685–720). Philadelphia: Elsevier.

20. Williams, E. S., & Viswanathan, M. N. (2013). Current and emerging anti-arrhythmic drug therapy for ventricular tachycardia. *Cardiol Ther, 2*(1), 27–46.

21. Washam, J. B., et al. (2015). Digoxin use in patients with atrial fibrillation and adverse cardiovascular outcomes: A retrospective analysis of the rivaroxaban once daily oral direct factor Xa inhibition compared with vitamin K antagonism for prevention of stroke and embolism trial in atrial fibrillation (ROCKET AF). *Lancet, 385*(9985), 2363–2370.

22. Morady, F., & Zipes, D. (2014). Atrial fibrillation: Clinical features, mechanisms, and management. In D. L. Mann, D. P. Zipes, P. Libby, & R. O. Bonown (Eds.), *Braunwald's heart disease: A textbook of cardiovascular medicine* (10th ed., pp. 798–813). Philadelphia: Elsevier.

23. Swerdlow, C. D., Wang, P. J., & Zipes, D. P. (2014). Pacemakers and implantable cardioverter-defibrillators. In D. L. Mann, D. P. Zipes, P. Libby, & R. O. Bonown (Eds.), *Braunwald's heart disease: A textbook of cardiovascular medicine* (10th ed., p. 744). Philadelphia: Elsevier.

CHAPTER 101

CAROTID ARTERY DISEASE

Virginia Curtin Capasso • Alicia Wierenga

DEFINITION AND EPIDEMIOLOGY

Carotid stenosis (CS) is defined as atherosclerotic narrowing of the extra-cranial arteries (60% to 99%)[1] most often occurring at the bifurcation of the carotid artery with involvement of the proximal internal carotid artery (ICA). Prevalence of the disease is highest among older adults and persons with hypertension and heart disease.[2] The overall estimated prevalence of carotid artery stenosis (CAS) (defined as 70% or 75% to 99% stenosis) is 0.5% to 1%.[2]

CS may be symptomatic or asymptomatic. Symptomatic CS is manifested by focal neurological dysfunction, including transient ischemic attack (TIA), ischemic stroke, or a range of other subtle but enduring neurological deficits.[3] TIA is a syndrome of acute neurological dysfunction referable to the distribution of a single brain artery and characterized by symptoms that resolve in less than 24 hours without permanent neurological deficit.[4-6] Ischemic stroke involves neurological deficit that persists longer than 24 hours.[4] Even in the presence of high-grade CS, patients may truly be asymptomatic or exhibit nonspecific symptoms that do not qualify as symptomatic ischemic events.[3]

Stroke is now the fifth leading cause of death and serious long-term disability in the United States.[1,7] Although the risk of stroke increases with age from the fifth decade onward, there has been a trend of progressively decreasing age-adjusted incidence of first stroke per 1000 persons since 1950.[8] The most important factors contributing to the decreased incidence of stroke include intensive therapy to control blood pressure, blood lipids, and diabetes in order to prevent cardiovascular disease.[9,10]

The risk of having a stroke varies by race and ethnicity.[7] The stroke rate for blacks is almost double the rate for whites.[11] Although the mortality rates associated with stroke have declined substantially over the past five decades for all races and ethnicities, blacks continue to have the highest mortality rate due to stroke.[11] In addition, the mortality rate for Hispanics has been rising since 2013.[12]

The vast majority of strokes (80% to 90%) are ischemic, 15% to 20% of which result from atheroembolization due to CS.[1,13] The risk of ischemic stroke is highest among individuals with symptomatic or asymptomatic CAS greater than 80%.

PATHOPHYSIOLOGY

Atherosclerotic CS originates near the bifurcation of the common carotid artery (CCA) in the region of the bulb.[14,15] Conditions near the bulb that contribute to the development of atherosclerotic plaque include turbulent flow due to the change in the caliber of the vessel proximal and distal to the bulb, variable shear stress, flow separation and nonlaminar flow, and increased contact time between bloodborne particles, such as lipids, and the vessel wall.[6] A fatty streak, consisting of monocytes that differentiate into lipid-laden macrophages, or foam cells, eventually develops into an atherosclerotic plaque. As the plaque enlarges, blood flow to the brain can be reduced or interrupted by severe narrowing or occlusion of the ICA. In addition, turbulence may damage the atherosclerotic plaque, resulting in intraplaque hemorrhage, loss of intimal continuity or ulceration, and thrombus formation. Fragments of a fractured plaque or thrombus may embolize to smaller distal arteries. Interruption of cerebral blood flow and cerebral infarction are the potential life-threatening sequelae.

CLINICAL PRESENTATION AND PHYSICAL EXAMINATION

Clinical presentation of ischemia in the carotid territory typically includes the following symptoms: contralateral weakness of the face, arm, or leg, or both; contralateral paresthesia of the face, arm, or leg, or both; or transient ipsilateral blindness (amaurosis fugax).[16] If the right cerebral hemisphere is involved, other manifestations may include anosognosia (lack of self-awareness of an illness or disability), asomatognosia (lack of awareness of all or part of one's body), neglect, and visual or sensory extinction. Signs of left hemispheric involvement include aphasia, alexia (severe reading problems), anomia (difficulty naming people or objects seen), and agraphesthesia (disorder of directional cutaneous kinesthesia characterized by difficulty recognizing a written number or letter traced on the skin after parietal damage).

Physical examination findings indicative of stroke include facial/eyelid drooping, motor or sensory deficits, and speech disturbances. Hollenhorst plaques may be present on ocular examination. Neck auscultation may elicit carotid bruit that has been shown to have sensitivity of 63% and a specificity of 61% (range, 70% to 99%) for high-grade CS in neurologically symptomatic patients.[17] Ratchford et al. found that only 25% of a selected high-risk subgroup of asymptomatic patients with an audible bruit had ≥ 60% stenosis.[18]

DIAGNOSTICS
Initial Diagnostics

Duplex ultrasound is now the first-line diagnostic tool for CS. This test has high sensitivity and specificity, although it yields many false positives in the general population.[10] Indications for carotid duplex ultrasound include:

- Serial surveillance of known stenosis (>20%) in asymptomatic individuals
- Vascular assessment in a patient with multiple risk factors for atherosclerosis (hypertension, hyperlipidemia, tobacco smoking, first-degree relative with atherosclerosis manifested before age 60, family history of ischemic stroke)[6]
- Stroke risk assessment in patient with symptomatic coronary artery disease (CAD) or peripheral arterial disease (PAD)
- Amaurosis fugax or Hollenhorst plaque(s) visualized on retinal examination
- Hemispheric TIA
- Stroke in a candidate for carotid revascularization
- Serial surveillance after carotid revascularization procedure (carotid endarterectomy [CEA], carotid artery stenting [CAS], or carotid-to-subclavian bypass graft)[6]
- Intraoperative monitoring during CEA

A meta-analysis of studies of color duplex ultrasound demonstrated that when the peak systolic velocity is ≥130 cm/s, the sensitivity and specificity are very high, at 98% and 88%, respectively, in detecting stenotic ICA lesions ≥50%. In the setting of a peak systolic velocity of ≥0 cm/s, the sensitivity and specificity of duplex ultrasound are 90% and 94%, respectively, in the detection of stenotic lesions ≥70%.[19] For recognizing carotid occlusion, duplex ultrasound has been shown to have a sensitivity of 96% and specificity of 100%.[20] There is also high agreement between duplex ultrasound and the gold standard, digital subtraction arteriography, in the detection of more than 45% stenosis in the carotid artery.[19,21]

Additional Diagnostics

Alternate diagnostic testing consisting of multi-planar computed tomography angiography (CTA) or contrast-enhanced magnetic resonance angiography (MRA) may be necessary under the following circumstances: (1) duplex ultrasound cannot be obtained, (2) results of duplex ultrasound are inconclusive, (3) further evaluation of the severity of stenosis and identification of intrathoracic or intracranial vascular lesions is needed prior to intervention for severe CS. CTA diameter may accurately estimate stenosis.[6] CTA also can provide imaging from the aortic arch to the Circle of Willis, defining bone and soft tissue structures surrounding the diseased carotid arteries, tracing the course of a vessel that is tortuous or has a high bifurcation, and directly imaging the vessel lumen allowing evaluation of stenosis. CTA may be preferred for patients who are not suitable candidates for MRA due to claustrophobia, implanted pacemakers, or other incompatible devices. MRA may overestimate the degree of CS. Catheter-based angiography may still be necessary to detect and characterize extracranial

---

INITIAL DIAGNOSTICS

Carotid Artery Disease

IMAGING
- Carotid ultrasound (U/S)
- Computed tomographic angiography (CTA)[a]
- Magnetic resonance angiography (MRA)[a]
- If indicated[a]

LABORATORY[a] (may vary by physician)
- Complete blood count
- Serum glucose, electrolytes, BUN creatinine
- Lipid panel
- Coagulation studies
- Type and cross for blood transfusion
- CK, CK-MB, troponin
- Electrocardiogram
- Chest x-ray

[a]for patients undergoing carotid revascularization[22]

cerebrovascular disease when noninvasive imaging is inconclusive, not feasible because of technical limitations, or noninvasive imaging studies yield discordant results.[4]

DIFFERENTIAL DIAGNOSIS

The differential diagnosis of symptomatic CS includes intracranial arterial stenosis, atheromatous disease of the aortic arch, partial seizure, radiculopathy, neuropathy, microvascular cerebral or spinal pathology, and lacunar stroke. Causes of intracranial arterial stenosis include atherosclerosis, intimal fibroplasia, vasculitis, adventitial cysts, or vascular tumors. Intracranial arterial occlusion may occur because of thrombosis or embolism arising from the aortic arch, cardiac chambers, heart valves, or a defect in the septum of the heart allowing a right-to-left shunt. Symptoms and signs of ischemia or infarction in the vertebrobasilar system include ataxia, cranial nerve deficits, visual field loss, dizziness, imbalance, and incoordination.[4] Partial seizures are associated with brief, stereotyped, repetitive behaviors and require electroencephalogram to confirm the diagnosis. Etiologies that account for purely sensory symptoms (that is, numbness, pain, or paresthesia) include radiculopathy, neuropathy, microvascular cerebral or spinal pathology, and lacunar stroke.

Symptoms not typically associated with carotid territory events include vertigo, ataxia, diplopia, visual disturbances, dysarthria, nausea, vomiting, decreased consciousness, and weakness, which may include quadriparesis.[16]

 Complaint of amaurosis fugax and a finding of Hollenhorst plaque on funduscopic examination are associated with significant stenosis at the carotid bifurcation and stroke risk comparable to transient cerebral ischemia.[16]

Interprofessional Collaborative Management

CS therapy may consist of medical management, surgical or interventional procedures, or a combination of treatments. The cornerstones of medical management include smoking cessation, statin therapy, antihypertensive treatment, and antiplatelet therapy. Surgical treatment consists of CEA. Interventional procedures include carotid angioplasty and stenting (CAS).

Medical Management

Statin Therapy. Generally, the goal of statin therapy is a low-density lipoprotein (LDL) level less than 100 mg/day, although the target LDL in the ongoing Carotid Revascularization and Medical Management for Asymptomatic Carotid Stenosis (CREST-2) trial is aggressive at less than 70 mg/dL.[4,23] Given current evidence, a statin regimen often consists of atorvastatin (80 mg daily), since, compared to placebo, it has been shown to reduce the 5-year risk of ischemic stroke by 22%.[24]

Hypertensive Therapy. The relationship between hypertension and stroke is firmly established.[25] The risk of stroke increases 30% to 45% for each 10 mm Hg increase in blood pressure. The 2017 American College of Cardiology/American Heart Association Hypertension Guideline established new criteria for stage 1 hypertension, that is, greater than 130 mm Hg/80 mm Hg.[26] First-line anti-hypertensive medications for high-risk patients with stage 1 hypertension may include thiazide diuretics, dihydropyridine calcium channel blockers (e.g., amlodipine), angiotensin-converting enzyme (ACE) inhibitors, and angiotensin-receptor blockers (ARB) (see Chapter 104).

Due to their efficacy, thiazide diuretics and calcium channel blockers are preferred for most Americans, including Black patients with diabetes, provided the Black adult does not have heart failure or chronic kidney disease.[26] For many patients, combination therapy with an ACE or ARB combined with a thiazide diuretic or CCB is recommended to achieve the goal blood pressure below 130/80 mmHg.[26]

Antiplatelet Therapy. Antiplatelet therapy is started for symptomatic CS. Based on the results of two studies, current antiplatelet therapy consists of aspirin (75 mg to 325 mg) and clopidogrel (75 mg). The studies include the Clopidogrel and Aspirin for Reduction of Emboli in Symptomatic Carotid Stenosis (CARESS) trial,[27] which demonstrated that the combination therapy was more effective than aspirin alone in reducing symptomatic embolization. The Clopidogrel in High Risk Patients with Nondisabling Cerebrovascular Events (CHANCE) trial also showed a benefit for patients receiving combination therapy for 21 days after TIA.[28]

Surgical Therapy: Carotid Endarterectomy

CEA is a surgical procedure involving incision of the CCA, extending distally through the bifurcation to the ICA beyond the offending plaque. The plaque is everted from the external carotid artery (ECA), then the ICA. The arteriotomy is closed using a patch of autogenous vein, Dacron, or bovine pericardium.[29] Completion angiogram or duplex ultrasound may be done to evaluate residual stenosis, which occurs in less than 1% of cases.

The American Heart Association 2011 collaborative guidelines[4] recommend CEA within 6 months for patients with symptomatic CS. Criteria for CEA include (1) average to low surgical risk; (2) reduction of the diameter of the lumen of the ipsilateral ICA by more than 70% as measured by noninvasive imaging, or more than 50% as measured by catheter angiography; and (3) an anticipated rate of perioperative stroke or mortality of less than 6%. When compared with CS, CEA may be preferred when arterial anatomy is unfavorable for endovascular intervention.

The effectiveness of CEA plus medical management versus medical management alone on event rates has been studied in symptomatic patients and asymptomatic patients. Studies of the effectiveness of CEA in symptomatic patients (i.e., history of TIA or mild stroke and 30% to 99% ipsilateral CS) include two large randomized trials: North American Symptomatic Carotid Endarterectomy Trial (NASCET[30]) and the European Carotid Surgery Trial (ECST).[31] In these studies, randomization was stratified by severity of stenosis, although the trials differed on method of measurement of CS and definitions of outcome events. Three studies compared the effectiveness of CEA plus medical therapy versus medical therapy alone in asymptomatic patients, including Asymptomatic Carotid Atherosclerosis Study (ACAS),[32] Asymptomatic Carotid Surgery Trial (ACST),[33] and the Veterans Affairs Cooperative Study (VACS).[34]

Carotid Endarterectomy for Symptomatic Patients. In NASCET,[30] high-grade stenosis was defined as 70% to 99% reduction of the diameter of the vessel lumen at the point of greatest stenosis. Lower-grade stenosis was defined as 30% to 69% reduction in luminal diameter. After 18 months of follow-up, NASCET stopped enrolling patients in the high-grade stenosis group (70% to 99%) because the benefit of CEA over medical therapy alone was clear. At 2 years, the cumulative risk of stroke was significantly lower for the CEA group (9%) than for the medical management group (26%). NASCET also demonstrated a benefit of CEA for patients with 50% to 69% CS. The 30-day rate of death or stroke was 6.7%. At 5 years, the rate of ipsilateral stroke was 15.7% for the CEA group versus 22% for the medical management group. No benefit was found for CEA among individuals with less than 50% CS.

In the ECST, randomization also was stratified according to severity of stenosis, which was defined as mild (10% to 29%), moderate (30% to 69%), and severe (70% to 99%).[31] ECST also showed highly significant benefit of CEA for patients with severe stenosis but no benefit for patients with lower-grade stenosis. After adjustment for primary end points and duration of follow-up, the benefit of CEA for symptomatic patients with high-grade CS was similar for men and women in NASCET and ECST.

The Very Urgent Carotid Endarterectomy Confers Increased Procedural Risk Study found that patients who sustained a neurologic event and were treated with CEA were at higher risk for mortality and stroke if the procedure was done at day 0 to 2 after event (11.5%) versus day 3 to 7 (3.6%).[35]

Carotid Endarterectomy for Asymptomatic Patients. Several studies have examined the effect of CEA in asymptomatic patients (i.e., atherosclerotic narrowing of the proximal ICA exceeding 50% to 60% in the absence of previous referable symptoms of TIA or stroke),[30] although the end points of the studies varied. VACS[34] compared the rates of TIA, stroke, and death among individuals treated with surgery plus aspirin and risk factor modification versus with medical management alone. At 30 days, the death rate was 1.9%, stroke rate was 2.4%, and combined event rate was 4.3% for patients who underwent surgery. At 5 years, the rate of adverse events was significantly lower for patients undergoing CEA (10%) versus medical therapy (20%).

In ACAS, TIA was not included as an end point.[32] The trial was stopped early, when an advantage of CEA was apparent among patients with greater than 60% CS. The 30-day death rate was 2.3%. After mean follow-up of 2.7 years, the projected 5-year rates of ipsilateral stroke, perioperative stroke, and death for patients treated surgically and medically were 5.1% and 11%, respectively. The benefit was not substantiated for women.[6]

In ACST, asymptomatic patients with hemodynamically significant CS were randomized to two groups: (1) immediate surgery plus medical therapy and (2) medical therapy alone or surgery delayed until necessary.[33] At 30 days the risk of stroke and death was 3.1% in both groups. The 5-year adverse event rate demonstrated an important advantage for the early surgery group (6.4%) over the delayed surgery group (11.4%).

When the results of ACAS and ACST are compared, the 5-year risk for any stroke or perioperative death in the nonsurgical group was lower in the ACST (11.8%) versus ACAS (17.5%), although the absolute reduction in 5-year risk with surgery in ACST (5.3%) was essentially the same as ACAS (5.1%). The 30-day risk for any stroke or perioperative death also was lower in ACAS at 1.5% versus 3.1% in ACST. Neither study showed an increased benefit from surgery for increasing degrees of stenosis (60% to 99%).[36]

Complications of Carotid Endarterectomy. Possible complications of CEA include hypertension (20%), hypotension (5%), hemorrhage, acute arterial occlusion, stroke, MI (1%), venous thromboembolism (0.1%), cranial nerve palsy,

infection, arterial restenosis, and death. The risk of stroke or death is higher among symptomatic patients (3.2%) than asymptomatic patients (1.4%), patients with hemispheric symptoms versus retinal symptoms, urgent operation versus nonurgent operation, reoperation versus primary surgery, and those with renal insufficiency.[29] Intracerebral hemorrhage may occur as a consequence of hyperperfusion syndrome, although the rate is less than 1% among patients whose blood pressure is stable preoperatively and well controlled perioperatively.

Cranial nerve injuries occur in 5% to 7% of cases that, in decreasing order of frequency and with most common clinical presentation, usually involve the hypoglossal nerve (atrophy of tongue musculature), marginal mandibular nerve (asymmetrical smile), recurrent laryngeal nerve (hoarseness), spinal accessory nerves (weakness of trapezius muscle), and Horner syndrome. Cranial nerve dysfunction is linked to a duration of surgical procedure longer than 2 hours. Approximately 25% of cranial nerve injuries resolve before discharge from the hospital.

Wound complications include infection (≤1%) and hematoma (≤5%). Factors contributing to wound complications include perioperative antiplatelet therapy, duration of surgery, and perioperative heparin and protamine therapy.

Arterial restenosis occurs at two predictable timeframes—within 18 months, but usually within 6 months after CEA, and at 5 years or more after surgery. The earlier restenosis is due to intimal hyperplasia. The later restenosis is due to progressive atherosclerotic disease. Surveillance of the extracranial carotid arteries by noninvasive imaging, to detect new ipsilateral or contralateral lesions, is recommended at 1 month, 6 months, 1 year, and annually after CEA.[8] Surveillance may be discontinued when the patient is no longer a candidate for intervention. The collaborative AHA guidelines[6] recommend repeat CEA or CAS for symptomatic patients with greater than 50% recurrent stenosis or asymptomatic patients with greater than 80% recurrent CS and periprocedural risk of stroke or death less than 6%. Revascularization by CEA or CAS is not recommended in symptomatic patients with less than 70% CS that has remained stable over time.

Interventional Procedures: Carotid Angioplasty and Stenting

Carotid angioplasty and stenting involves retrograde arterial catheterization, traditionally through a femoral approach, although iliofemoral occlusive disease may necessitate brachial or radial access and anomalies of the aortic arch may require direct cannulation of the cervical CCA. In general, the procedure involves insertion of a 5-F catheter over a 0.035-inch guidewire into the CCA; the wire is positioned in the ECA. A series of stents and catheters are deployed into the CCA within a few centimeters of the lesion, with care taken to avoid inadvertent arterial dissection. To prevent embolization and consequent neurologic complications, an embolic protection device (EPD) is positioned in the straight portion of the distal ICA. Subsequently, angioplasty is performed with a 3- to 4-mm balloon to ensure safe passage of the stent and retrieval of the stent delivery system. A self-expanding stent using a balloon that is undersized by 20% to 40% of the ICA diameter and stent length is deployed. At the end of the procedure, the EPD is removed. Completion angiogram visualizing the extracranial and intracranial circulation in two or more views is performed. Anticoagulation is discontinued. If an arterial closure device is used, the need for normalization of the ACT is eliminated.

The collaborative AHA guidelines[4] recommend CAS only for symptomatic patients who meet the following criteria: (1) average or low risk of complications associated with endovascular intervention; (2) narrowing of the arterial lumen of more than 70% as shown by noninvasive imaging, or more than 50% as demonstrated by catheter angiography; and (3) risk of periprocedural stroke or death below 6%. CS may be preferred over CEA when the neck anatomy is unfavorable for arterial surgery (e.g., previous neck surgery or radiation injury).

The findings of International Carotid Stenting Study (ICSS)[37] demonstrated a higher adverse event rate that may be attributable to the use of EPDs, especially of the distal filter type.[38] These findings have prompted several iterations of innovation in neuroprotection devices and strategies, leading to (1) direct transcervical access to the CCA, thereby avoiding the embolic risk of traversing the aortic arch and supra-aortic vasculature, and (2) a low-resistance shunt between arterial and venous circulations with high and low flow rates, thereby eliminating the need for ECA occlusion and reducing or eliminating an active aspiration step.[39] There is inferential evidence from Embolic Protection with Reverse Flow (EMPiRE)[40] trials that flow reversal is a better protection strategy than distal filters. The Silk Road Trial, which completed enrollment in 2014, was a single-arm study that enrolled 400 high-risk symptomatic and asymptomatic patients and incorporated transcarotid access with a flow reversal system.[38] The Silk Road system (Silk Road Medical) has been associated with a very low overall stroke risk, in the 1% range, which is comparable to the rate achieved with CEA.[41]

Complications of Carotid Artery Stenosis. Complications of CAS are categorized as cardiovascular, neurological, device malfunction, general medical, access-site complications, restenosis, and mortality.

Cardiovascular complications include baroreceptor reflexes, MI, arterial dissection or thrombosis, transient vasospasm, and recurrent stenosis. The rate of target-vessel perforation and MI is generally low at 1%. Baroreflex responses (that is, bradycardia, hypotension, and vasovagal reaction) occur in 5% to 10% of patients undergoing CAS. Transient vasospasm occurs in 10% to 15% of procedures as a result of instrumentation with guidewires, catheters, and protection devices. Restenosis after CAS, which ranges from 3% to 5%, can be minimized by avoiding multiple high-pressure balloon inflations, particularly in heavily calcified vessels.

In order of decreasing frequency, neurological complications include stroke (as high as 4.1%), non-disabling stroke (2.9%), disabling stroke (1.5% to 2%), TIA (1% to 2%), intracranial hemorrhage and hyperperfusion syndrome related to hypertension and anticoagulation (<1%), and seizures related to hypoperfusion (<1%).

Device malfunction can involve deployment failure of the stent, EPD, or flow reversal system. In addition, the stent may be malformed or, rarely, migrate after deployment.

General risks include access-site injury (5%), although most of these injuries involve pain or hematoma and are self-limiting. Other risks include wound infection, pseudoaneurysm, bleeding from the access site, and contrast-induced nephropathy.

Post-Procedural Care. Immediate post-procedural care focuses on prevention, assessment, and treatment of per-

procedural complications. Medical management includes dual-antiplatelet therapy with aspirin (81 mg to 325 mg daily) and, for at least 4 weeks, clopidogrel (75 mg daily). Medications for blood pressure control, hyperlipidemia, and diabetes also are resumed or initiated. The patient is usually discharged on post-procedural day one or two. If the patient has persistent hypotension, hospitalization may be extended for hydration and oral adrenergic therapy. Long-term post-procedural management includes continued antithrombotic therapy with aspirin and serial surveillance for stent patency and areas of recurrent stenosis using noninvasive imaging techniques. Serial surveillance should occur at 1 month, 6 months, 1 year, and then annually thereafter. Surveillance can be terminated when the patient is no longer a candidate for intervention.

Comparison of Outcomes: Carotid Endarterectomy and Carotid Artery Stenosis

Numerous studies have compared the outcomes of CEA and CAS. These studies include the Carotid Revascularization Using Endarterectomy or Stenting Systems (CaRESS) study,[42,43] SAPPHIRE Study,[44,45] EVA-3S,[46] ICSS,[37] SPACE trial,[47,48] and CREST.[49]

CaRESS was a nonrandomized study that compared symptomatic patients with greater than 50% CS and asymptomatic patients with greater than 75% CS who underwent CEA and CAS. Study results revealed no significant differences in event rates (i.e., MI, stroke, and death at 30 days and 1 year and restenosis and revascularization at 1 year) for patients undergoing the two types of revascularization procedures.

SAPPHIRE is the only study that has compared the outcomes of high-risk patients (i.e., age greater than 80 years, New York Heart Association Class III or IV heart failure, chronic obstructive pulmonary disease, greater than 50% contralateral CS, prior CEA or CAS, or prior coronary artery bypass graft [CABG] surgery) undergoing CEA and CAS. Rates of periprocedural MI, stroke, and death were almost twice as high for CEA as for CS at 30 days and 1 year, possibly as a consequence of determining the rate of MI only on the basis of sensitive cardiac serum biomarker data. Among symptomatic patients, the periprocedural event rate was similar following CEA (16.5%) and CAS (16.8%). Among asymptomatic patients, the rate of MI, stroke, and death after CEA (21.5%) was over twice the event rate after CAS (9.9%). At 1 year, CEA was associated with significantly higher rates of cranial nerve palsy (4.9% and 0%, respectively) and target-vessel revascularization (4% and 0.6%, respectively) than CAS. At 3 years, the rates of stroke and target-vessel revascularization were similar for CEA and CAS.

Several other studies have compared the outcomes of conventional-risk patients who underwent CEA and CAS. The Endarterectomy Versus Angioplasty in Patients with Symptomatic Severe Carotid Stenosis (EVA-3S) study was terminated early because of a significantly higher rate of stroke in the CAS group (24%) versus the CEA group (9%) (P = .01).[46] In the SPACE trial,[47,48] which randomized symptomatic patients with high-grade CS (>70% by ultrasound), TIA, or stroke, there was no significant difference between treatment groups on outcomes at 30 days. In the ICSS, a European multicenter randomized controlled trial that compared the safety and effectiveness of CEA versus CAS in symptomatic patients with greater than 50% stenosis, the 120-day composite adverse event rate for stroke, death, or MI was 5.2% in the CEA group versus 8.5% in the CAS group (P = .006).[37]

The Carotid Revascularization Versus Endarterectomy Trial (CREST)[49] compared the periprocedural risk of stroke, death, and MI and ipsilateral risk of stroke up to 4 years after CEA and CAS in conventional-risk, symptomatic patients with greater than 50% CS and asymptomatic patients with greater than 60% stenosis. Rates of 30-day MI, stroke, or death were not significantly different between CEA (4.5%) and CAS (5.2%). After mean follow-up of 2.5 years, results revealed that there also was no significant difference in the overall rate of primary events for CEA (6.8%) and CAS (7.2%). However, significant differences existed between CEA and CAS on the periprocedural rate of stroke (2.3% versus 4.1%, respectively) and MI (2.3% versus 1.1%, respectively). At 1 year, major and minor stroke was shown to have a greater impact on quality of life than MI. Furthermore, improved outcomes were observed with CEA for patients older than 70 years, whereas patients younger than 70 years had better outcomes with CAS. Similar to the SAPPHIRE study, the rate of cranial nerve palsy in CREST was higher after CEA than CAS.

Medical Versus Surgical and Interventional Management

Currently, there is controversy about whether newer aggressive medical therapy is as effective as CEA and CAS in treatment of CS. In response, there are several ongoing trials intended to clarify best practices for medical, surgical, and interventional management of patients, of both genders across the lifespan, who have varying degrees of CS greater than 50%. These include ECST-2, ACST-2, SPACE-2, and CREST-2. ECST-2 is a randomized controlled trial comparing CEA and CAS in combination with optimal medical therapy (OMT) for atherosclerotic CAS with OMT alone for symptomatic and asymptomatic stenosis greater than 50%. ACST-2 is a randomized controlled trial recruiting patients who require either medical or procedural treatment. SPACE-2 is randomizing patients with asymptomatic CS to treatment with CEA, CAS, or OMT. The CREST-2 study also will compare CEA, CAS, and OMT in patients with asymptomatic carotid artery disease.[6]

Life Span Considerations

In review, in the absence of medical therapy, CS advances with age, increasing from the fifth decade and affecting about 10% of those over age 80 years. The severity of CS is generally worse for men than women. The prevalence of TIA also increases with age, although the lifetime risk of stroke decreased significantly for both men and women between 1950 and 2004. Among women, the risk of stroke increases with age. Higher risk is associated with menopause before age 42 and postmenopausal hormonal therapy.

The CREST trial, which compared outcomes of symptomatic patients and asymptomatic patients treated with CEA and CAS, revealed that for patients younger than 70 years, CAS had more favorable outcomes while CEA yielded better outcomes for patients older than 70 years. Even octogenarians safely underwent CEA.

Patient Education/Health Promotion

Patient education focuses on the pathogenesis and consequences of CS, indications, approaches and complications of treatment approaches (that is, CEA and CAS), associated medical management, risk factor reduction to prevent recurrent CS and the plan for ongoing follow-up.

During the peri-procedural period, the patient must be able to recognize and report signs of complications of CEA or CAS. For patients in both groups, the importance of adherence with the antihypertensive and lipid reduction regimen in preventing hyperperfusion syndrome and stroke is emphasized, as is the need for the patient to report transient loss of consciousness, severe headache, and transient or persistent neurologic deficit. For patients who have undergone CEA, signs and symptoms of infection of the neck incision are stressed. Immediate treatment and reporting of bleeding, hematoma, and catheterization site complications are emphasized with patients who have undergone CAS.

Secondary prevention of recurrent CS and ischemic stroke is directed at reducing cardiovascular risk factors.[24] The target for normal blood pressure is less than 130 mm Hg/80 mm Hg, which may require a regimen of antihypertensive medications.[26] Additional lifestyle modifications include salt restriction (<1500 mg/day);[50] weight loss if necessary to achieve a body mass index less than 30 kg/m²; consumption of a diet rich in fruits, vegetables, and reduced saturated and total fat; and moderate-intensity exercise for 30 minutes three to five times per week. Glycemic control and blood pressure control are important for patients with diabetes. Statin therapy may be titrated to achieve an LDL of less than 75 mg/dL and reduce cholesterol. For adults with heterozygous hypercholesterolemia (HeFH) and clinical cardiovascular disease, injections of PCSK9 protein inhibitors may be added every 2 weeks which reduce LDL cholesterol by 36% to 59%.[51] Smoking cessation is a critical component of secondary prevention; counseling, nicotine products (excluding vaping), and smoking cessation medications have been shown to be effective at promoting successful smoking cessation. Alcohol consumption should be limited to light to moderate levels (that is, two drinks per day for men and one drink per day for women who are not pregnant.)

REFERENCES

1. LeFevre, M. L., Others. (2014). Screening for asymptomatic carotid artery stenosis: U.S. Preventive Services Task Force recommendation statement: Screening for asymptomatic carotid artery stenosis. *Annals of Internal Medicine, 161*(5), 356–362. doi:10.7326/M14-1333.
2. Jonas, E., Feltner, C., Amick, H. R., Sheridan, S., Zheng, Z. J., Watford, D. J., et al. (2014). *Screening for asymptomatic carotid artery stenosis: A systematic review and meta-analysis for the U.S. Preventive Services Task Force. Evidence synthesis no. 111.* AHRQ publication no. 13-05178-EF-1. Rockville, MD: Agency for Healthcare Research and Quality.
3. Lanzino, G., others. (2009). Treatment of carotid artery stenosis: Medical therapy, surgery, or stenting. *Mayo Clinic Proceedings. Mayo Clinic, 84,* 362–368.
4. Brott, T. G., others. (2011). Guideline on the management of patients with extracranial carotid and vertebral artery disease: A report of the American College of Cardiology Foundation/American Heart Association Task Force on Practice Guidelines, and the American Stroke Association, American Association of Neuroscience Nurses, American Association of Neurological Surgeons, American College of Radiology, American Society of Neuroradiology, Congress of Neurological Surgeons, Society of Atherosclerosis Imaging and Prevention, Society for Cardiovascular Angiography and Interventions, Society of Interventional Radiology, Society of NeuroInterventional Surgery, Society for Vascular Medicine, and Society for Vascular Surgery. Circulation. *Stroke; a Journal of Cerebral Circulation, 42,* e420–e463. Retrieved from http://stroke.ahajournals.org/content/42/8/e420.full.pdf. (Accessed 19 August 2018).
5. Easton, J. D., et al. (2009). Definition and evaluation of transient ischemic attack: A scientific statement for healthcare professionals from the American Heart Association/American Stroke Association Stroke Council; Council on Cardiovascular Surgery and Anesthesia; Council on Cardiovascular Radiology and Intervention; Council on Cardiovascular Nursing; and the Interdisciplinary Council on Peripheral Vascular Disease. *Stroke; a Journal of Cerebral Circulation, 40,* 2276–2293.

6. O'Brien, M., & Chandra, A. (2014). Carotid revascularization: Risks and benefits. *Vascular Health and Risk Management, 10,* 403–416.

7. Centers for Disease Control and Prevention. Stroke Facts. Retrieved from: https://www.cdc.gov/stroke/facts.htm. (Accessed 31 July 2018).

8. Kleindorfer, D., Panagos, P., Pancioli, A., et al. (2006). Incidence and short-term prognosis of transient ischemic attack in a population-based study. *Stroke; a Journal of Cerebral Circulation, 36,* 720–723.

9. Lackland, D. T., Roccella, E. J., Deutsch, A. F., Fornage, M., George, M. G., Howard, G., et al. American Heart Association Stroke Council, Council on Cardiovascular and Stroke Nursing, Council on Quality of Care and Outcomes Research, Council on Functional Genomics and Translational biology. (2014). Factors influencing the decline in stroke mortality; a statement from the American Heart Association / American Stroke Association. *Stroke; a Journal of Cerebral Circulation, 45,* 315–353.

10. U.S. Preventative Services Task Force. (2016). Final recommendation Statement: Carotid Artery Stenosis: Screening. Retrieved from: https://www.uspreventiveservicestaskforce.org/Page/Document/Recommendation StatementFinal/carotid-artery-stenosis-screening. (Accessed 1 August 2018).

11. Benjamin, E. J., Blaha, M. J., Chiuve, S. E., et al. on behalf of the American Heart Association Statistics Committee and Stroke Statistics Subcommittee. (2017). Heart disease and stroke statistics—2017 update: A report from the American Heart Association. *Circulation, 135,* e229–e445.

12. Vital Signs. (2017). Recent trends in stroke death rates—United States, 2000-2015. *MMWR, 66.*

13. Safian, R. D. (2017). Asymptomatic carotid artery restenosis: Revascularization. *Progress in Cardiovascular disease, 59,* 591–600.

14. Kleindorfer, D., others. (2005). Incidence and short-term prognosis of transient ischemic attack in a population-based study. *Stroke; a Journal of Cerebral Circulation, 36,* 720–723.

15. Johnston, S., Others. (2003). Prevalence and knowledge of transient ischemic attack among US adults. *Neurology, 60,* 1429–1434.

16. Ricotta, J. J., AbuRahma, A., Ascher, E., et al. (2011). Updated Society for Vascular Surgery guidelines for management of extracranial carotid disease. *Journal of Vascular Surgery, 54,* e1–e31.

17. Zhu, C. Z., & Norris, J. W. (1990). Role of carotid stenosis in ischemic stroke. *Stroke; a Journal of Cerebral Circulation, 21,* 1131–1134.

18. Ratchford, E. V., Jin, Z., Di Tullio, M. R., Salameh, M. J., Homma, S., Gan, R., et al. (2009). Carotid bruit for detection of hemodynamically significant carotid stenosis: The Northern Manhattan Study. *Neurological Research, 31*(7), 748–752.

19. Jahromi, A. S., Cinà, C. S., Liu, Y., et al. (2006). Sensitivity and specificity of color duplex ultrasound in the estimation of internal carotid artery stenosis: A systematic review and meta-analysis. *Journal of Vascular Surgery, 41,* 962–972.

20. Nederkoorn, P. J., van der Graaf, Y., & Hunink, M. G. M. (2003). Duplex ultrasound and magnetic resonance angiography compared with digital subtraction angiography in carotid artery stenosis: A systematic review. *Stroke; a Journal of Cerebral Circulation, 34,* 1324–1332.

21. Grant, E. G., Duerinckx, A. J., El Saden, S. M., et al. (2003). Carotid artery stenosis: Grayscale and Doppler ultrasound diagnosis—Society of Radiologists in Ultrasound consensus conference. *Ultrasound Quarterly, 19,* 190–198.

22. Rosenfield, K., Matsumura, J. S., Chaturvedi, S., et al. (2016). Randomized trial of stent versus surgery for asymptomatic carotid stenosis. *The New England Journal of Medicine, 374,* 1011–1020.

23. Howard, V. J., Meschia, J. F., Lal, B. K., et al. (2017). Carotid revascularization and medical management for asymptomatic carotid stenosis: Protocol of the CREST-2 clinical trials. *International Journal of Stroke: Official Journal of the International Stroke Society, 12*(7), 770–778.

24. Silleson, H., Amarenco, P., Hennerici, M. G., et al. (2008). Stroke Prevention by Aggressive Reduction in Cholesterol Investigators. Atorvastatin reduces the risk of cardiovascular events in patients with carotid atherosclerosis: A secondary analysis of Stroke Prevention by Aggressive Reduction in Cholesterol Levels (SPARCL) trial. *Stroke; a Journal of Cerebral Circulation, 39*(12), 3297–3302.

25. Lawes, C. M., Bennett, D. A., Feigin, V. L., & Rodgers, A. (2004). Blood pressure and stroke: An overview of published reviews. *Stroke; a Journal of Cerebral Circulation, 35*(4), 1024.

26. Whelton, P. K., Carey, R. M., Aronow, W. S., et al. (2018). 2017 ACC/AHA/AAPA/ABC/ACPM/AGS/APhA/ASH/ASPC/NMA/PCNA guideline for the prevention, detection, evaluation, and management of high blood pressure in adults: A report of the American College of Cardiology/American Heart Association Task Force on Clinical Practice Guidelines. *Journal of the American College of Cardiology, 71,* e127–e248.

27. Markus, H. S., Droste, D. W., Kaps, M., et al. (2013). Dual antiplatelet therapy with clopidogrel and aspirin in symptomatic carotid stenosis evaluated using Doppler embolic signal detection: The Clopidogrel and Aspirin for Reduction of Emboli in Symptomatic Carotid Stenosis. *Curr Vac Pharmacol, 11*(4), 514–523.

28. Wang, Y., Wang, Y., Zhao, X., et al. (2013). CHANCE Investigators. Clopidogrel with aspirin in acute minor stroke or transient ischemic attack. *New England Journal of Medicine, 369*(1), 11–19.

29. Hobson, R. W., Mackey, W. C., Ascher, E., et al. (2008). Management of atherosclerotic carotid artery disease: Clinical practice guidelines of the Society for Vascular Surgery. *Journal of Vascular Surgery, 48,* 480–486.

30. North American Symptomatic Carotid Endarterectomy Trial (NASCET) Investigators. (1991). Clinical alert: Benefit of carotid endarterectomy for patients with high grade stenosis of the internal carotid artery. National Institutes of Neurological Disorders and Stroke, Stroke and Trauma Division. *Stroke; a Journal of Cerebral Circulation, 22,* 816–817.

31. 1995). Randomized trial of endarterectomy for recent symptomatic carotid stenosis: Final results of the MRC Carotid Surgery Trial. *Lancet, 351*(9113), 1379–1387.

32. Walker, M. D., Marler, J. R., Goldstein, M., et al. (1995). Endarterectomy for asymptomatic carotid artery stenosis. *JAMA: The Journal of the American Medical Association, 273*(18), 1421–1428.

33. Halliday, A. W., Thomas, D., & Mansfield, A. (1994). The Asymptomatic Carotid Surgery Trial (ACST) rationale and design. *European Journal of Vascular Surgery, 8,* 703–710.

34. Hobson, R. W., Weiss, D. G., Fields, W. S., et al. (1993). Efficacy of carotid endarterectomy for asymptomatic carotid stenosis: The Veterans Affairs Cooperative Study Group. *The New England Journal of Medicine, 328,* 221–227.

35. Strömberg, S., Gelin, J., Österberg, T., et al. (2012). Very urgent carotid endarterectomy confers increased procedural risk. *Stroke; a Journal of Cerebral Circulation, 43,* 1331–1335.

36. Executive Committee for the Asymptomatic Carotid Atherosclerosis Study. (1995). Endarterectomy for asymptomatic carotid artery stenosis. *JAMA: The Journal of the American Medical Association, 273,* 1421–1428.

37. Ederle, J., Dobson, J., Featherstone, R. L., et al. (2010). Carotid artery stenting compared with endarterectomy in patients with symptomatic carotid stenosis (International Carotid Stenting Study): An interim analysis of a randomized controlled trial. *Lancet, 375,* 985–997.

38. Pinter, L., Ribo, M., Loh, C., et al. (2011). Safety and feasibility of a novel transcervical access neuroprotection system for carotid artery stenting in the PROOF Study. *Journal of Vascular Surgery, 54,* 1317–1323.

39. Ansel, G. M., Hopkins, L. N., Jaff, M. R., et al. (2010). Safety and effectiveness of the INVATEC MO.MA proximal cerebral protection device during carotid artery stenting: Results from the ARMOUR pivotal trial. *Catheterization and Cardiovascular Interventions, 76*(1), 1–8.

40. Clair, D. G., Hopkins, L. N., Mehta, M., et al. (2011). Neuroprotection during carotid artery stenting using the GORE flow reversal system: 30-day outcomes in the EMPiRE Clinical Study. *Catheterization and Cardiovascular Interventions, 7*(3), 420–429.

41. Kwolek, C. J., Jaff, M. R., Leal, J. I., et al. (2015). Results of ROADSTER multicenter trial of transcarotid stenting with dynamic flow reversal. *Journal of Vascular Surgery, 62,* 1227–1235.

42. CaRESS steering committee. (2005). Carotid revascularization using endarterectomy or stenting systems (CaRESS) phase I clinical trial: 1-year results. *Journal of Vascular Surgery, 42,* 213–219.

43. CaRESS steering committee. (2005). Carotid revascularization using endarterectomy or stenting systems (CaRESS) phase I clinical trial: 1-year results. *Journal of Vascular Surgery, 42,* 213–219.

44. Yadav, J. S., Wholey, M. H., Kuntz, R. E., et al. (2004). Protected carotid artery stenting versus endarterectomy in high risk patients. *The New England Journal of Medicine, 351,* 1493–1501.

45. Yadav, J. S., for the SAPPHIRE Investigators. (2005). Durability of carotid stenting for prevention of stroke: 3-year follow-up of the SAPPHIRE trial and the U.S. Carotid Feasibility. *Circulation, 112,* 416 abstract.

46. Mas, J. L., Chatellier, G., Beyssen, B., et al. (2006). Endarterectomy versus stenting in patients with symptomatic severe carotid stenosis. *The New England Journal of Medicine, 355,* 1660.

47. The SPACE Collaborative Group. (2006). 30 day results from the SPACE trial of stent- angioplasty versus carotid endarterectomy in symptomatic patients: A randomized non-inferiority trial. *Lancet, 368,* 1239–1247.

48. Eckstein, H. H., Ringleb, P., Allenberg, J. R., et al. (2008). Results of the Stent-Protected Angioplasty Versus Carotid Endarterectomy (SPACE) study to treat symptomatic stenosis at 2 ears; a multi-national, prospective, randomized trial. *The Lancet. Neurology, 7,* 893–902.

49. Brott, T. G., Hobson, R. W., Roubin, G. S., et al. (2010). Stenting versus endarterectomy for treatment of carotid artery stenosis. *The New England Journal of Medicine, 363,* 11–23.

50. https://www.heart.org/en/healthy-living/healthy-eating/eat-smart/sodium/how-much-sodium-should-i-eat-per-day. (Accessed 18 September 2018).

51. Curfman, G. (2015). PCKS9 Inhibitors: a major advance in cholesterol low-ering drug therapy. Retrieved from: http://www.health.harvard.edu/blog/pcsk9-inhibitors-a-major-advance-in-cholesterol-lowering-drug-therapy-201503157801. (Accessed 13 September 2018).

CHAPTER **102**

CHEST PAIN AND CORONARY ARTERY DISEASE

Sule Steve Salami • Terry Mahan Buttaro

- **Immediate transfer to the emergency department** is indicated for all patients who are thought to be having or are having an acute myocardial infarction.
- **Hospital admittance** is indicated for oatients who have unstable angina pectoris, defined as new-onset angina (angina occurring within 1 month), angina occurring at rest and with minimum exertion, or crescendo angina.

DEFINITION AND EPIDEMIOLOGY

Coronary heart disease (CHD), the primary cause of death for both men and women in the United States, includes acute myocardial infarction (MI), angina pectoris, atherosclerotic car-dicvascular disease (ASCVD), and all forms of chronic ische-mic heart disease. In 2015, 114,023 Americans died of CHD, a decline over the previous 10 years.[1] Despite the decrease in car-dicvascular deaths in this country, over 90 million people have cardiovascular or cerebrovascular disease, with associated esti-mated costs (direct and indirect) greater than $329.7 billion.[2] For African Americans, the risk of cardiovascular disease is increased, primarily because of diabetes, hypertension, and obesity, though these three co-morbidities increase the risk of coronary artery disease (CAD) for everyone.[3] Older adults also have a greater risk of developing cardiovascular disease, partly related to physiologic changes (arterial stiffening, fibrosis, left ventricular [LV] hypertrophy, alterations in endothelial cell function, and inflammation).[4]

Other causes of cardiovascular disease involve genetics, life-style, and CAD risk factors: obesity, diet, hypertension, high cholesterol, smoking, stress, and diabetes.[5] Of concern is that heart disease death rates in adults with diabetes are two to four times higher than the rates for adults without diabetes.[6]

Risk Factors for Coronary Artery Disease

Current theorization is that it is the composition, morphol-ogy, and stability of the coronary artery plaque rather than the degree of plaque stenosis that determines the risk of cardio-vascular events. To decrease the frequency of cardiovascular morbidity and mortality, modification of controllable cardiac risk factors is necessary. Historically, risk factors have been sub-divided into factors that are nonmodifiable, such as age and family history, and factors that are modifiable, such as smoking cessation, dyslipidemia, diabetes mellitus, increased waist-to-hip ratio, physical inactivity, atherogenic diet, psychosocial stress, hypertension, and even "particulate matter air pollu-tion."[7, p.1149] In addition, there are sex-specific nontraditional CAD risks in women that include pregnancy-related disor-ders (preterm delivery, gestational hypertension, preeclamp-sia. gestational diabetes mellitus, and persistent weight gain after pregnancy). Women who have a diagnosis of polycystic ovary syndrome, functional hypothalamic amenorrhea, or have incurred breast cancer therapy also have a greater than average risk for CAD.[8]

Although some cardiac risk factors are more predictive of coronary artery events than others, there are specific recom-mendations to modify risk factors for patients who have CAD (Table 102.1). Just 1 hour a day of moderate-intensity exer-cise can lessen the risk of CAD about 30%, while decreasing sodium intake by 1 g lessens the risk of cardiovascular death by 16%.[9]

Patient-Related Delays and Initial Treatment

Early reperfusion for patients with an acute MI improves LV systolic function and survival; therefore every effort must be made to minimize hospital delay. Although time is critical in the treatment of MI, it is patient delay, not transport or system inadequacy, that is often the greatest impediment to timely medical treatment. Older adults and women especially do not seek timely medical care when experiencing a STEMI or other cardiac symptoms, but many patients delay seeking care.[10,11] This despite community-wide educational efforts to increase patient awareness of concerning cardiac symptoms. The reasons for patient delay in seeking treatment include (1) inappropriate reasoning that symptoms are not serious; (2) attribution of symptoms to other causes; (3) belief it would be a "false alarm"; (4) not wanting to call a family member or friend except when "really sick"; (5) preconceived stereotypes of who is at risk for a heart attack; (6) little understanding of the importance of calling EMS or 911 and the availability of treatment (reperfusion therapies); (7) attempted self-treatment with prescription and/or nonprescription medications; and (8) possibly financial concerns.[12]

PATHOPHYSIOLOGY
Chronic Stable Angina

Chronic stable angina is chest pain precipitated by exertion and relieved by rest. A reduction in myocardial oxygen supply or increases in myocardial oxygen demand are the determinants of coronary ischemia. Although the pathologic process for unstable angina and the pathologic process for chronic stable angina both result from atherosclerotic lesions in the coronary arteries, the pathophysiologic mechanism of each varies.

Under normal circumstances, an increase in myocardial oxygen demand is balanced by an increase in myocardial oxygen supply. The three most important factors that deter-mine myocardial oxygen demand are heart rate, systemic blood pressure (peripheral vascular resistance), and LV wall tension.[13] Heart rate and the systolic blood pressure exert independent influence on myocardial oxygen requirements because both determine myocardial workload (heart rate × systolic blood pressure = myocardial workload). Therefore activities (e.g., exercise, hurrying, lifting) and increased metabolic demands (e.g., with fever, anemia, thyrotoxicosis) that increase the work-load of the heart in the presence of a fixed and limited oxygen supply will increase myocardial oxygen requirements precipi-tating ischemia and angina.

The coronary arteries exhibit changes in vascular tone that play a significant role in the development of coronary ische-mia. Under normal circumstances, the endothelial or inner-most lining of the coronary artery responds to vasoactive stimuli, such as mental stress, cold, and catecholamines, by

TABLE 102.1 AHA/ACC Secondary Prevention for Patients With Coronary Artery Disease and Other Atherosclerotic Vascular Disease

Risk Factor	Goal
Smoking	Complete cessation
Blood pressure control	<140/90 mm Hg <130/80 mm Hg if patient has heart failure or renal insufficiency
Lipids	Initial evaluation before statin initiation Fasting lipid panel Check ALT and CK level Age <75 years without contraindications, conditions, or drug-drug interactions influencing statin therapy—begin on high-intensity statin therapy Age >75 years or with conditions or drug-drug interaction or a history of statin intolerance—initiate moderate-intensity statin therapy Educate on healthy lifestyle habits Reduce saturated fats to <7% calories Triglycerides <200 mg/dL If triglycerides are ≥200 mg/dL, non-HDL-C should be <130 mg/dL Non-HDL-C = Total cholesterol − HDL-C
Physical activity	30 min, 7 days per week (minimum 5 days per week)
Weight management	Body mass index of 18.5–24.9 kg/m^2 Waist circumference: men <40 inches, women <35 inches
Diabetes mellitus	Hemoglobin A$_{1c}$ <7% is advised
MEDICATIONS	
ASA	75–162 mg PO daily; if ASA is contraindicated, use clopidogrel or warfarin. ASA is used alone or in combination with antiplatelet medications, depending on clinical situation.
β blockers	All patients who have had myocardial infarction, acute coronary syndrome, or left ventricular dysfunction with or without heart failure symptoms, unless contraindicated
ACE inhibitors	All patients with left ventricular ejection fraction ≤ 40% and those with hypertension, diabetes, or chronic kidney disease, unless contraindicated
Influenza vaccination	All patients

Includes peripheral arterial disease, atherosclerotic aortic disease, and carotid artery disease.
ACC, American College of Cardiology; *ACE*, angiotensin-converting enzyme; *AHA*, American Heart Association; *ALT*, alanine aminotransferase; *ASA*, acetylsalicylic acid; *CK*, creatine kinase; *HDL-C*, high-density lipoprotein cholesterol.
From Smith, S. C., Jr, Benjamin, E. J., Bonow, R. O., et al. (2011). AHA/ACCF secondary prevention and risk reduction therapy for patients with coronary and other atherosclerotic vascular disease: Update. *Journal of the American College of Cardiology, 58*(23):2432–2446.

releasing endothelium-derived relaxing factor (EDRF) to maintain vasodilation. In the presence of atherosclerosis, however, the endothelial function is impaired; hence the vasoconstrictive response is unopposed, leading to constriction at the site of atherosclerosis and adjacent areas. This results in a decrease in myocardial blood flow and induces coronary ischemia.

Silent Myocardial Ischemia (Asymptomatic Coronary Heart Disease)

Asymptomatic occurrences of ischemia can be more common than symptomatic episodes in patients with exertional angina symptoms.[7] Silent myocardial ischemia occurs when there is objective evidence of ischemia in the absence of symptoms. Since the advent of continuous ambulatory electrocardiographic monitoring, many patients with typical stable angina have been found to have frequent episodes of asymptomatic ischemia.[14] The clinical implications of silent ischemia are not well understood, but there can be an increased incidence of ischemia, MI, and sudden death in asymptomatic patients. Patients with a previous MI are more at risk for a coronary

event associated with asymptomatic ischemia,[14] **and** patients with diabetes have a greater risk of cardiovascular mortality compared with those without diabetes.[13,15] Ischemia can occur with or without evidence of increased myocardial oxygen demand.

The pathogenesis of silent myocardial ischemia is not clear, although several hypotheses exist. It has been suggested that some individuals have a higher endorphin level than others do, which may play a role in the perception of pain. Additionally, some patients have a higher ischemic pain threshold and greater tolerance of cold-induced ischemia. Furthermore, autonomic dysfunction, particularly in patients with diabetes, is thought to contribute to silent ischemia.

Microvascular Angina

Microvascular angina affects women (usually postmenopausal) more than men and is characterized by chest discomfort with exercise and a positive stress test.[16] Yet, angiography reveals that there is no obstruction of the coronary arteries.[16] The cause is still not fully understood, although epicardial and microvascular dysfunction as well as spasm may cause a decreased blood supply to the coronary arteries and the subsequent chest discomfort that these patients experience.[16] Unfortunately, in the past, patients with demonstrated microvascular angina were told that there was nothing wrong and yet these patients do require treatment that involves improving coronary circulation and/or decreasing myocardial oxygen demand.[16]

Vasospastic Angina (Variant Angina, Coronary Artery Spasm, Prinzmetal Angina)

In vasospastic angina, coronary artery spasm can cause chest discomfort at rest evidenced by ST elevation or depression on electrocardiogram (ECG).[17] Spasm can occur in any coronary artery and the exact cause is not certain. Impaired regulatory mechanisms effecting vasoconstriction and vasodilation in the smooth muscle cells of the coronary vessels are a possible cause. A change in balance within the sympathetic and parasympathetic systems is a possible factor affecting blood flow within the coronary arteries, but endothelial dysfunction effects on the coronary artery smooth muscle is also suspect, and other pathologies may also play a role.[17] Whatever the cause, the resulting spasm causes obstruction, angina, and if prolonged, MI.

Unstable Angina and Non–ST-Segment Elevation Myocardial Infarction

The pathophysiologic mechanisms of an MI can be divided into those that decrease myocardial oxygen supply and those that increase myocardial oxygen demand. The known reason for these changes are formation of a thrombus related to one, and possibly more than one, of the following: (1) a structure-changing event causing a vulnerable coronary plaque to erode, rupture, or calcify, resulting in a thrombus forming within the coronary artery and initiating an inflammatory response; (2) vasoconstriction of a coronary artery; (3) intraluminal narrowing over time; and (4) increased myocardial oxygen related to tachycardia, thyrotoxicosis, or illness (e.g., bacterial or viral infection) demand.[18]

When plaque rupture occurs, it stimulates chemotactic factors for circulating monocytes. Monocytes enter the vessel wall, transform into tissue macrophages, and ingest oxidized LDLs. Over time, lipid-filled macrophages (foam cells) die, creating an extracellular lipid pool with eventual formation of a fibrous cap. Proteolytic enzymes produced by activated macrophages erode the fibrous cap, producing areas that are fragile and prone to rupture. Increases in shear stress and vasomotor changes placed on this vulnerable lesion make it highly likely to rupture. Plaque rupture causes vessel damage and initiates platelet activity. Platelet aggregation and activation develop a platelet-rich "white clot" over the endothelial damage, causing partial obstruction of flow in the artery and thus unstable angina and non–ST-segment elevation myocardial infarction (NSTEMI). The role of the inflammatory response as a trigger for plaque rupture is significant and emphasizes the benefit of high-sensitivity C-reactive protein in evaluating cardiovascular risk.

Bacterial and viral infections can also make plaques more vulnerable and unstable with a predisposition to rupture and thrombose.

When plaque rupture occurs, the size of the resultant thrombus, whether it is a small mural thrombus or an occlusive thrombus, depends on several factors, including the amount of thrombogenic substrate that is exposed, the amount of local blood flow disturbance, and the actual thrombotic propensity of the vessel.

Therefore lesion disruption is a dynamic process that may lead to transient vessel occlusion and ischemia by a labile thrombus, resulting in unstable angina. These thrombotic occlusions often resolve spontaneously; however, they can recur within hours or days. In other cases, formation of a fixed thrombus and a more chronic occlusion may occur, resulting in acute MI.

Coronary artery narrowing of less than 80% typically does not induce development of collateral vessels. For this reason, smaller plaques that rupture are more likely to cause a significant clinical event during thrombotic occlusion of the vessel as a result of the absence of protective collateral flow.

Acute ST-Segment Elevation Myocardial Infarction

In most cases, MI occurs when an atherosclerotic plaque ruptures and then serves as a nidus for thrombus formation with resultant coronary artery occlusion, ischemia, myocyte necrosis, infarction, and death.[7] The atherosclerotic plaque most likely to rupture is the nonocclusive plaque, which may rupture several times before MI is produced. With each rupture, blood, fibrin, and platelet aggregates accumulate in the plaque, forming intra-intimal or intra-plaque thrombus and resulting in increases in plaque size, intraplaque pressure, and obstruction of the coronary lumen. When such a plaque ruptures, fissures, or ulcerates, MI or sudden death may occur. Plaque rupture with resulting thrombus formation is the common physiologic mechanism underlying unstable angina, MI, and sudden death. The amount of myocardial injury sustained is directly related to several factors, including the amount of thrombus present, the ability of the intrinsic lytic system to promote lysis, the impact of local vasoconstrictor substances on impeding blood flow, whether the vessel affected is partially or totally occluded, the presence or absence of collateral vessels and the quantity of blood supplied to the affected area, and the amount of myocardium supplied by the affected vessel.

The platelet is not only the smallest cell but is also the most active in thrombus formation. The platelet consists of membranes, tubules, granules, and receptors. During activation, the resting platelet undergoes a dramatic change that induces platelet–platelet interaction or aggregates. Such platelet aggregates play an important role in acute coronary syndrome (ACS) and MI. Patients who died of unstable angina, MI, and sudden cardiac death have platelet aggregation, fibrin, and microthrombi as common findings. Because platelets are important in the pathophysiologic process of acute ischemic syndrome and MI, inhibition of platelet activation should be beneficial in reducing and preventing ACS.

MINOCA: Suspected Myocardial Infarction With Nonobstructed Coronary Arteries

Myocardial infarction with nonobstructed coronary arteries (MINOCA) is described as the occurrence of an acute MI, but without an obvious cause (i.e., no obstruction).[19] Cardiac registries' prevalence measurements indicate that 10% of patients with diagnosed MI do not have obstructions in their coronary arteries.[20] In 2015, researchers used PubMed and Embase to conduct a meta-analysis of studies mentioning nonobstructed coronary arteries in the setting of MI. For this review, these researchers defined MINOCA as documented presence of MI with angiographic findings of less than 50% stenosis in any epicardial artery. Findings from this meta-analysis indicate that MINOCA is a finding in 6% of MI patients, confers a better than 12-month mortality prognosis than in documented CAD (prognosis for patients with MINOCA is still guarded), and has structural dysfunction, coronary spasm, and thrombotic disorders found in association.[20] Current recommendations are to consider MINOCA as a working diagnosis while evaluating these patients for treatable underlying causes with magnetic resonance imaging (MRI), provocative testing, and evaluation for thrombophilia.[20]

CLINICAL PRESENTATION
Chronic Stable Angina

The patient with chronic stable angina demonstrates characteristic symptoms that occur with predictable frequency, severity, duration, and provocation. These symptoms occur with exertion, are relieved by rest or no more than one nitroglycerin (NTG) tablet, and in general last for only 1 to 3 minutes. Chronic stable angina remains constant unless an acceleration of the disease process intervenes. The clinical presentation can best be evaluated by a detailed history of angina quality, location, radiation, severity, duration, and precipitating and relieving factors. Associative factors such as dyspnea, diaphoresis, nausea, vomiting, eructations, diarrhea, and fatigue should also be evaluated (Box 102.1).

William Heberden first defined the peculiar discomfort of myocardial ischemia as angina pectoris, which translated means "strangling in the chest." The majority of patients do not refer to their angina symptoms as pain; thus, questioning related to "chest pain" may prove misleading, and the diagnosis of angina pectoris may be missed. Discomfort originating in the chest may arise from many structures, including the skin, subcutaneous tissue, bone, muscle, vascular structures, nerves, pleura, lungs, pericardium, heart, esophagus, and gastrointestinal viscera.

Adjectives used to describe the quality of angina can be variable; it is often conveyed as a pressure, heaviness, aching, constriction, tightness, squeezing, numbness, or burning sensation.

BOX 102.1

History Questions for the Patient With Angina

Chest pain information
- Precipitating factors (exertion, meals, stress, cold)
- Quality (pressure, squeezing, burning, stabbing)
- Radiation (shoulders, arm, wrist, neck, jaw, back)
- Relief measures (rest, nitroglycerin [hallmark], food)
- Severity (1–10 scale)
- Timing (activity, bedtime, meals, history of occurrence, duration)

Associative factors
- Dyspnea
- Provoked by activity (chest pain first or dyspnea)
- Orthopnea (how many pillows)
- Paroxysmal nocturnal dyspnea (how soon after retiring to bed)
- Diaphoresis
- Gastrointestinal complaints (nausea, vomiting, diarrhea)
- Fatigue

Cardiac risk factors
Current medication profile

Patients may demonstrate a clenched fist over the sternal area (Levine sign) to further elucidate this feeling. The location of discomfort is predominantly behind the midsternum (retrosternal) or just to the left of the sternum, in an area approximately the size of a clenched fist. If the patient is able to localize the area of discomfort as being no larger than a fingertip, the sensation is seldom related to myocardial ischemia, and other causes should be considered. Myocardial ischemia can also encompass the territory between the epigastrium and the lower jaw, lower teeth, and hard palate, with sensations of tightness or constriction in the throat area. Atypical symptoms are more common in women, older adults, and diabetic patients.

Radiation symptoms are not uncommon and are related to involvement of the C8 to T4 spinal ganglia. These ganglia receive impulses from the heart and from peripheral dermatomes that are transmitted to the spinal cord through afferent nerve fibers. When myocardial ischemia occurs, the sharing of these ganglia can produce discomfort to the other dermatomal areas. Thus stimulation of the dermatomes affecting the brachial plexus can result in discomfort or numbness anywhere along the medial surface of the left arm, including the fourth and fifth digits. Isolated wrist discomfort has also been reported. The right arm and lateral surfaces can be affected, although with less frequency.

Stimulation of the cervical plexus can result in suprascapular and intrascapular discomfort. Precipitating factors, including increased exertion, coitus, and emotion, tend to induce myocardial ischemia by increasing circulating catecholamine levels. This increases the metabolic oxygen needs of the heart in the setting of a limited oxygen supply, thereby producing angina symptoms. Eating of a large meal may precipitate discomfort, as can the increased metabolic demands from fever, chills, thyrotoxicosis, anemia, hypoglycemia, exposure to cold air, and the nicotine from cigarette smoking.

Relief of stable angina symptoms generally occurs within 1 to 3 minutes after the discontinuation of activity or with rest. When angina is related to emotional upheaval, it may take longer for catecholamine levels to decrease, and angina symptoms may persist for a longer period. NTG administration will usually provide relief within 5 minutes and is a useful diagnostic tool. When symptoms persist for longer than 20 minutes, the patient should no longer be considered to be having chronic stable angina and should be instructed to seek prompt medical attention.

Although cessation of activity generally produces relief of pain, it has been noted that some patients who develop angina with walking are able to continue walking, with eventual alleviation of the angina. These patients are able to "walk through" the angina event. There are several proposed hypotheses for the relief of angina during exercise. These include dilation of functioning collateral blood vessels during exercise; relief of coronary arterial spasm; and vasodilation of systemic blood vessels with a corresponding decline in systemic arterial blood pressure and heart rate, which in turn reduces myocardial oxygen demand.

Anginal Equivalents

Myocardial ischemia can be experienced as dyspnea, indigestion, nausea, numbness in the upper extremities, and fatigue rather than actual chest pressure, particularly in women.

Symptoms of dyspnea are generally noted to be stable when they occur with moderate exertion and unstable when they occur with minimum exertion, with rest, or when they begin to awaken the patient during the night. The cause of stable symptoms is related to increased myocardial demand, and the cause of unstable symptoms is related to decreased myocardial supply. The dyspnea produced is caused by myocardial ischemia resulting in diastolic dysfunction, which produces increased left-sided filling pressures. Fatigue often follows an activity and resolves within several minutes. The cause is related to LV dysfunction resulting in decreased cardiac output.

Microvascular Angina

The clinical presentation for microvascular angina is chest pain, often unpredictable and occurring with rest, routine physical activity, or stressful events. Unlike chest pain from stable angina, chest discomfort from microvascular disease is generally more intense, lasts for longer periods of time, and does not go away with rest. The discomfort is generally not responsive to NTG. Although there is no apparent gender difference in the perception of angina, the syndrome of microvascular angina seems more common in women.

Vasospastic Angina

The sine qua non of vasospastic or variant angina pectoris is a history of spontaneous or unprovoked episodes of typical angina. Discomfort occurs predominantly at rest and is usually not provoked by exertion. The differential diagnosis on presentation should be unstable angina until it is proven otherwise.

Unstable Angina and Non–ST-Segment Elevation Myocardial Infarction

Diagnosis of unstable angina and NSTEMI depends predominantly on a detailed patient history. The most important factors from the initial history that enhance the likelihood of the patient experiencing an episode of ischemia are the nature of symptoms, prior history of CAD, age older than 65 years, and number of risk factors present for CAD. The Thrombolysis in Myocardial Infarction (TIMI) risk score is one of several valued tools for use in the emergency department for risk stratification and therapeutic decision-making (Table 102.2).[21] The risk score encompasses these factors and adds electrocardiographic findings and cardiac marker data as well as aspirin use in the previous 7 days. The use of aspirin and concomitant angina was found to be a powerful predictor of unstable angina or NSTEMI. In addition, several factors may suggest an acceleration of the patient's chronic angina symptoms to unstable angina or NSTEMI. These factors may include occurrence of the angina event with less provocation or at rest, prolongation of the angina symptoms, increase in the severity of symptoms, and newly associated findings with the chest discomfort. Physical examination findings of pulmonary edema, new or worsening mitral regurgitation murmur, S_3 heart sound, hypotension, bradycardia, or tachycardia suggest that the patient is at high risk. According to guidelines, a 12-lead ECG, preferably with and without chest pain, should also be obtained. It is particularly important to assess the duration of angina events and whether rest pain has been present to determine the patient's short-term risk of complications.

Acute ST-Segment Elevation Myocardial Infarction

Classically, acute MI is diagnosed as a constellation of symptoms. Chest pain described as pressure, heaviness, squeezing, crushing, and aching is often associated with nausea, vomiting, diaphoresis, or dyspnea. In general, the pain involves the sternum or epigastrium; in many cases, it may radiate to the

| TABLE 102.2 | TIMI Risk Score for Patients With Unstable Angina and NSTEMI: Predictor Variables |

Predictor Variable	Point Value of Variable	Definition
Age ≥65 years	1	
≥3 risk factors for CAD	1	Risk factors: Family history of CAD Hypertension Hypercholesterolemia Diabetes Current smoker
Aspirin use in last 7 days	1	
Recent, severe symptoms of angina	1	≥2 anginal events in last 24 h
Elevated cardiac markers	1	CK-MB or cardiac-specific troponin level
ST deviation ≥0.5 mm	1	ST depression >0.5 mm is significant; transient ST elevation ≥0.5 mm for <20 min is treated as ST-segment depression and is high-risk; ST elevation ≥1 mm for more than 20 min places these patients in the STEMI treatment category
Prior coronary artery stenosis ≥50%	1	Risk predictor remains valid even if this information is unknown

Calculated Timi Risk Score	Risk of ≥1 Primary End Point[a] in ≤14 Days	Risk Status
0 or 1	5%	Low
2	8%	Low
3	13%	Intermediate
4	20%	Intermediate
5	26%	High

[a]Primary end points: death, new or recurrent MI, or need for urgent revascularization. *CAD*, Coronary artery disease; *CK-MB*, Creatine kinase muscle-brain fraction; *MI*, myocardial infarction; *NSTEMI*, non–ST-segment elevation myocardial infarction; *STEMI*, ST-segment elevation myocardial infarction; *TIMI*, Thrombolysis in Myocardial Infarction.
From O'Connor, R. E., Brady, W., Brooks, S. C., Diercks, D., Egan, J., Ghaemmaghami, C., et al. (2010). 2010 American Heart Association guidelines for cardiopulmonary resuscitation and emergency cardiovascular care: part 10: Acute coronary syndromes. *Circulation, 122,* S787–S817.

arm, elbow, jaw, or neck. Any combination of these symptoms may occur in an individual patient. Epigastrium pain secondary to acute MI may be misdiagnosed as indigestion, and referred pain to the shoulder on deep inspiration may be misdiagnosed as being splenic in nature. In the older patient, MI may manifest as a sudden onset of dyspnea, weakness, loss of consciousness, or confusion. Although chest discomfort may be the most common presenting symptom, it may be atypical or absent in some patients with ACS (silent acute MI).

PHYSICAL EXAMINATION

Inspection of the chest may reveal the point of maximum impulse (PMI) to be downward or laterally displaced, suggestive of cardiomegaly, perhaps from hypertension. The PMI may also have a rocking quality, possibly related to a LV aneurysm from a previous MI. The thorax should be inspected to determine the presence of any rashes or vesicles, which may suggest a herpetic cause of the discomfort. Inspection of the neck veins should be performed to assess the jugular venous pulse for any elevation. The contour of the internal jugular waveforms should also be noted. A funduscopic examination may reflect hypertension or diabetic retinopathy. Xanthomas or an early arcus senilis may be indicative of elevated cholesterol levels. The peripheral circulation should be assessed for any vascular lesions suggestive of arterial or venous disease.

Palpation during cardiac assessment is confined to assessment of the upstroke of the carotid artery pulse and the PMI of the cardiac apex. The carotid upstroke should be of normal volume and intensity. A prolonged carotid upstroke may indicate aortic stenosis because ventricular emptying becomes delayed when it is ejected across a significantly stenotic valve. Conversely, a brisk carotid upstroke may indicate aortic regurgitation or hypertrophic cardiomyopathy.

Auscultation of the chest may reveal a ventricular gallop (S_3) produced just after the second heart sound, which may be either physiologic or pathologic in nature. A physiologic S_3 may be heard in children and adults up to 35 to 40 years old. It may also be noted in women during their third trimester of pregnancy. A pathologic S_3 may be related to decreased myocardial contractility and is suggestive of heart failure caused by volume overload of the ventricles. This may be related to either mitral or tricuspid regurgitation.

An atrial gallop (S_4) may be noted just before the first heart sound and is produced by an increased resistance to ventricular filling caused by ventricular stiffness after atrial contraction. LV causes of an S_4 include cardiomyopathy, hypertension, MI, and aortic stenosis. Right ventricular (RV) causes include pulmonary hypertension and pulmonary stenosis. An S_4 may also be noted in trained athletes.

A pansystolic murmur audible at the apex during an episode of chest pain is most likely consistent with mitral regurgitation. It is often secondary to papillary muscle dysfunction as a result of LV ischemia. A ventricular septal defect after MI should also be considered and further evaluated with echocardiography.

Inflammation around the pericardium may produce a pericardial friction rub, which generally has one systolic and two diastolic components. The systolic component is produced when the ventricles contract in systole, whereas the diastolic components are produced in early and late diastole. The early diastolic component is a result of rapid, passive ventricular filling, whereas the late diastolic component occurs with atrial contraction. The sound produced is very high and of a scratching or grating quality.

Adventitious breath sounds suggest heart failure. Their occurrence and the presence of any vascular bruits, indicating further vascular disease, should prompt further evaluation.

The physical examination findings are usually normal when the patient is not having episodes of variant angina; however, during episodes, the patient may develop hypertension and

---

BOX 102.2

Cardiac Physical Assessment

INSPECTION

Point of maximum impulse (PMI): displaced downward and laterally, aneurysmal

Skin and extremities: color, edema, xanthomas, lesions

Neck veins: elevated jugular venous distention, contour of internal jugular pulse

Thorax: rashes, zoster

Funduscopic examination: evaluation for risk factors—diabetes mellitus, elevated cholesterol

PALPATION

Carotid upstroke: may be prolonged with aortic stenosis

PMI: may be diffuse with cardiac enlargement

AUSCULTATION

Ventricular gallop (S_3): heart failure

Atrial gallop (S_4): hypertension, myocardial infarction; caused by resistance of ventricular filling

Systolic mitral regurgitation murmur consistent with an ischemic papillary muscle

Pericardial friction rub: inflammation around the pericardial sac; may have one systolic and two diastolic components

Adventitious breath sounds

Carotid bruits: other vascular location

---

tachycardia in response to the pain. In addition, the patient may have associated diaphoresis, nausea, and radiation of pain to the arm. Auscultation of the chest during an episode may reveal a gallop or transient systolic murmur originating from the mitral valve.

The diagnosis of an acute coronary event is primarily based on the patient history, ECGs, and laboratory data. The physical examination findings will support this diagnosis and help determine whether the patient is in heart failure or is manifesting evidence of a cardiac arrhythmia. The patient will understandably be anxious and on occasion will be diaphoretic. The pulse rate and blood pressure may be normal; however, with an extensive area of MI, the patient may have a compensatory tachycardia and be hypotensive (Box 102.2).

DIAGNOSTICS

Chronic Stable Angina

Electrocardiography. In chronic stable angina, the ECG can be useful for detection of cardiac ischemia during actual episodes of angina. During this period, ST-segment depressions with symmetric T-wave inversions in the affected leads may be noted. During pain-free intervals, however, the ECG will revert to normal limits. Other possible changes include evidence of a prior MI, LV hypertrophy, and repolarization abnormalities.

Exercise Tolerance Testing (Stress Testing). Because of the nondiagnostic potential of the ECG in patients with intermittent episodes of chest pain, for those patients in whom the diagnosis of coronary ischemia remains unclear, an exercise tolerance test within 72 hours of presentation of symptoms should be obtained. Stress testing, which may be pharmacologic or exercise based, is performed for diagnostic, prognostic, and management purposes. With an overall sensitivity of

50% and specificity of 90%, exercise stress testing can be a cost-effective strategy for evaluation of CAD.

Stress testing for patients with a history of chest pain or angina-type symptoms should always be implemented with imaging. Imaging with either thallium or sestamibi should be added for those patients with uninterpretable resting ECGs resulting from the following conditions: preexisting 1-mm ST-segment depressions, LV hypertrophy with strain, left bundle branch block (LBBB), digoxin therapy, ventricular pacing, or Wolff-Parkinson-White syndrome.

The most commonly used definition for a positive result of exercise tolerance testing is the development of electrocardiographic changes consistent with ischemia. The standard criteria for test positivity include horizontal or down-sloping ST depression of 1 mm (0.1 mV) or more at 60 to 80 msec after the J point. When modest resting ST depression is present on the upright control ECG before exercise, only additional ST depression during exercise is measured for analysis. Markedly depressed up-sloping ST-depression responses to exercise (2.0 mm at 80 ms after the J point) could identify underlying CAD and future adverse events in highly symptomatic patients with angina.

The ST-segment changes on a stress test are indicative of viable cardiac muscle being supplied by a narrowed coronary artery. The time frame in which symptoms or electrocardiographic changes appear should be noted, as should the hemodynamic response. Stress testing should not be performed in individuals with exacerbation of heart failure, uncontrolled cardiac arrhythmias, severe hypertension, unstable angina, acute evolving MI, or critical aortic stenosis.

The Duke's Treadmill Score (DTS) is a point system to predict 5-year mortality utilizing a treadmill stress test with a standard Bruce protocol. The scoring system itself is based on the duration of exercise, ST-segment deviation (depression or elevation), and the presence and severity of angina during the exercise.

$$DTS = Exercise\ time\ (minutes) - (5 \times ST\ deviation\ in\ mm)$$
$$- (4 \times angina\ index)$$

See Box 102.3.

Computed Tomography Angiography. Imaging techniques in noninvasive coronary arteriography with multidetector computed tomography (MDCT) or multislice computed

---

BOX **102.3**

Dukes Treadmill Score

$$DTS = Exercise\ time\ (minutes) - (5 \times ST\ deviation\ in\ mm)$$
$$- (4 \times angina\ index)$$

Patients are categorized as low, intermediate, or high risk.
- Low risk (score > 5) indicates a 5-year survival of 97%.
- Intermediate risk (score between 4 and −11) indicates 5-year survival of 90%.
- High risk (score < −11) indicates 5-year survival of 65%.
  In high-risk patients, 74% had three-vessel or left main occlusive coronary disease on angiography.

From Mark, D. B., Hlatky, M. A., Harrell, F. E., Lee, K.L., Califf, R. M., & Pryor, D. B. (1937). Exercise treadmill score for predicting prognosis in coronary artery disease. *Annals of Internal Medicine, 106*, 793–800.

---

tomography (MSCT) scanners permit imaging of the beating heart with no or little motion artifact. The presence and extent of coronary artery calcification serve as a marker of the extent of coronary atherosclerosis rather than the actual severity of coronary artery vessel stenosis. Coronary artery calcifications can be seen without a dye load; however, for the provider to visualize the coronary artery anatomy for stenosis, intravenous iodine containing contrast needs to be administered. With this in mind, one absolute contraindication to this type of testing is pregnancy. Relative contraindications to this testing include a contrast allergy, hyperthyroidism, and renal insufficiency. It is important to note that coronary computed tomography angiography (CTA) is highly sensitive, with a detection rate over 90%, but is not very specific. This means that a negative result will essentially rule out CAD with 90% accuracy, but if the test result is positive, this result is less conclusive and further imaging studies such as with an invasive cardiac catheterization procedure will need to be considered.

The Dilemma

Once the decision is made that a noninvasive imaging study is needed to further evaluate the patient with chest pressure, the decision then becomes whether to perform a nuclear stress test or cardiac CTA. It may be helpful to understand the benefits and concerns with each study. One fact that may not be well appreciated is the amount of radiation exposure for each test. Historically, radiation exposure had been a major concern for CTA, with some centers exposing a patient to 25 to 30 mSv (millisieverts) of radiation. However, advances in technology can now allow CTA with 1 to 3 mSv or less. (Think of a chest radiograph as exposing a patient to 0.1 mSv of radiation.) Nuclear stress testing, on the other hand, exposes the patient to approximately 13 mSv of radiation. Given the enhanced degree of temporal resolution, newer scanners can image the heart with improved accuracy without the need to slow the heart rate (hence there is not always a need to administer β blockers). Further CTA can often provide information about noncardiac findings, including pulmonary embolism, aortic dissection, and lung masses, which nuclear testing does not provide. Thus, given the low radiation exposure, higher amount of diagnostic accuracy, and additional noncardiac information that is obtained, many would argue that CTA is indeed the gold standard.

However, morbidly obese patients may have decreased penetration, which can result in poor image quality, making it difficult to visualize the mid to distal coronary arteries, although newer scanners have made improvements in this area. Reimbursement continues to be a major issue, and many insurance companies will approve a CTA only based on their "appropriateness criteria," and then only after a stress test has been performed and has yielded equivocal results. Some centers are concerned with the coronary calcium score, which is obtained first, and will not proceed to coronary artery CT scan if the value is greater than 800. Artifact from the calcium reduces the accuracy of testing; however, newer technology is able to subtract the calcium interference, so at centers with newer scanners this is no longer an issue. For patients who have had coronary artery bypass graft (CABG) surgery, CTA can be effective in evaluating the potency of the bypass grafts. Unfortunately for patients with coronary artery stents, it is challenging to image the inside of the stent to determine any evidence of in-stent restenosis, and therefore CT scanning has generally not proven helpful for this patient population.

Microvascular Angina

Diagnosing microvascular disease has been challenging, because standard testing used to diagnose CAD in the larger vessels has not proven helpful in these smaller vessels. This type of angina usually does not result in any wall motion abnormality on a cardiac echo. Stress testing may produce ST changes similar to those of CAD, but perfusion imaging will be abnormal only 30% of the time. Anemia, thought to slow the growth of cells needed to repair damaged blood vessels, should be ruled out. For those patients who undergo left heart catheterization/coronary angiography, the absence of myocardial blush could signify the presence of microvascular atherosclerotic heart disease.

Variant Angina

Electrocardiography. Transient ST-segment elevation on a 12-lead ECG during an episode of variant angina is essential to make the diagnosis. Electrocardiographic changes are usually observed in the leads related to the ventricular areas supplied by the affected vessels. On occasion, electrocardiographic changes may be dramatic but resolve readily with the use of sublingual NTG or nifedipine.

Echocardiography. An echocardiogram obtained during a period of variant angina may reveal segmental wall motion abnormality, depending on the severity of the spasm and duration of the episode.

Exercise Tolerance Testing. An exercise tolerance test should be performed to exclude atherosclerotic disease. Most patients with noncritical CAD who have variant angina have a negative exercise tolerance test result.

Coronary Angiography. Patients with unprovoked chest discomfort at rest that is typical of angina may have variant angina. An exercise tolerance test should be the initial testing modality. On occasion, the result of this test may be negative for ischemia, even though the patient is still experiencing chest discomfort. At that time, patients may undergo coronary arteriography to evaluate further for CAD. If variant angina is indeed suspected, all vasoactive medications should be discontinued at least 24 hours before coronary arteriography or any other provocative testing. Provocation of spasm with acetylcholine has been used to induce endothelial cell vasoreactivity. However, this practice has fallen out of vogue because of the potential to induce global spasm and hence lethal cardiac arrhythmias. Therefore diagnosis of variant angina is typically made from a patient history revealing nonexertional events that often are nocturnal.

Unstable Angina and Non–ST-Segment Elevation Myocardial Infarction

Electrocardiography. In patients with chest pain or other symptoms suggestive of an ACS, a 12-lead ECG should be obtained and evaluated for ischemic changes within 10 minutes of the patient's arrival at an emergency facility. Serial electrocardiography should be performed for the next 15 to 30 minutes if chest pressure persists despite the lack of initial ECG changes coupled with continuous telemetry monitoring. During an episode of angina the electrocardiographic findings depend on several factors, including location of the involved vessel, amount of myocardium involved, duration of ischemia,

and transient nature of the pathophysiologic process. During an episode of ischemia, the electrical properties of the myocardial cells within and surrounding the area of ischemia are altered, producing changes on the surface ECG. ST-segment depression, along with symmetrically inverted T waves, is generally present within minutes during an acute ischemic event. According to guidelines of the Agency for Healthcare Research and Quality, ST depressions of more than 1 mm indicate a high likelihood of an unstable angina event, whereas ST depressions of 0.5 to 1 mm indicate an intermediate likelihood. These changes generally return to baseline once the ischemic event has resolved. As a rule, Q waves do not develop, and there is no distinct change in the R wave. Persistence of ST-segment depression for longer than 48 hours usually differentiates an unstable angina event from NSTEMI. An absence of ST-segment or T-wave changes does not exclude the possibility of myocardial ischemia. In particular, ischemia affecting the left circumflex territory is not always demonstrated on the ECG.

In addition, ST-segment and T-wave changes may be seen in a variety of disease processes, including infiltrative myocardial disease (neoplasm, sarcoidosis, amyloidosis, hemochromatosis); chest deformities; muscular dystrophy; electrolyte abnormalities; cerebrovascular accidents; pharmacologic treatments (digoxin, tricyclics); hyperventilation; and anxiety.

Exercise Tolerance Testing. An exercise stress test is not performed in those individuals experiencing MI.

Laboratory Data. Laboratory blood work for the patient with a potential unstable angina pattern should consist of hemoglobin and hematocrit levels to exclude anemia as a precipitating factor. Measurements of sodium, potassium, chloride, carbon dioxide, blood urea nitrogen, and creatinine should be obtained. A fasting blood glucose level and fasting cholesterol profile should be obtained to identify potential coronary risk factors. Thyroid functions should be considered to exclude hyperthyroidism or hypothyroidism. Magnesium levels should be considered for repletion purposes. Serial cardiac troponin I or T levels (when a contemporary assay is used) should be obtained at presentation and 3 to 6 hours after symptom onset. Samples for C-reactive protein analysis may also be drawn to determine the presence of an inflammatory response. Measurement of B-type natriuretic peptide or N-terminal pro-B type natriuretic peptide may be considered to assess risk for heart failure.

Echocardiography. The echocardiogram is helpful during an acute ischemic event in several ways. Most important, it assists in detecting the location and extent of regional or global LV dysfunction. Second, it assists in risk stratification before discharge. Finally, it is helpful for future evaluation of the remodeling. Echocardiography detects ischemia by evaluating the motion and thickening of the LV walls. This becomes particularly helpful when the patient has chest pressure and nondiagnostic electrocardiographic findings.

Although there are many techniques to assess ventricular wall motion including LV myocardial stain measured by tissue Doppler imaging (TDI) or speckle tracking echocardiography (STE), the method most commonly used is two-dimensional echocardiography with M-mode echocardiography. In acute coronary ischemia, two-dimensional and M-mode echocardiography may demonstrate abnormal wall motion of the ischemic section, which occurs almost immediately. Wall motion abnormalities, however, can be influenced by any abnormalities in the adjacent muscle to which the ischemic area is attached.

Perhaps a more specific finding for ischemic cardiac muscle would be the inability of the affected myocardial muscle to thicken during systolic contraction. The nonischemic, or normal, region reveals normal motion and thickening toward the LV cavity during systole. The M-mode echocardiogram is ideal for measuring wall thickness and chamber dimensions, whereas the color Doppler study is used in conjunction with M-mode echocardiography to assess a regurgitant lesion.

ST-Elevation Acute Myocardial Infarction

STEMI is a clinical syndrome defined by characteristic symptoms of myocardial ischemia in association with persistent ST elevation in the absence of LV hypertrophy or LBBB coupled with the release of cardiac biomarkers. MI is defined as new ST elevation at the J point in at least two contiguous leads of 2 mm (0.2 mV) or more in men or 1.5 mm (0.15 mV) or more in women in leads V_2 to V_3 and/or of 1 mm (0.1 mV) or more in other contiguous chest leads or the limb leads. The majority of patients will evolve ECG evidence of Q-wave infarction. New or presumably new LBBB has been considered a STEMI equivalent but should not be considered diagnostic of acute MI in isolation. Baseline ECG abnormalities other than LBBB (e.g., paced rhythm, LV hypertrophy, Brugada syndrome) may obscure ECG interpretation. In addition, ST depression ≥ to 2 mm in the precordial leads (V_1 to V_4) may indicate transmural posterior injury; multilead ST depression with coexistent ST elevation in lead aVR has been described in patients with left main or proximal left anterior descending artery occlusion. Rarely, hyperacute T-wave changes may be observed in the very early phase of STEMI, before the development of ST elevation. Although the 12-lead ECG is useful in localizing the region of myocardial ischemia, it is limited in both the sensitivity and the specificity needed to distinguish the culprit coronary artery (Table 102.3 and Figs. 102.1–102.3).

It is important to note that other disease states can demonstrate ST-segment elevations, such as hypertrophic cardiomyopathy, variant Prinzmetal angina, pericarditis, takotsubo cardiomyopathy, spontaneous coronary artery dissection, hyperkalemia, and early LV repolarization. Early depolarization changes can be differentiated from the ST-segment elevation of an acute MI by the following: an upward concavity of the ST segment, an elevated takeoff of the ST segment at the J point (the junction of the end of the QRS complex and the beginning of the ST segment), and a distinct notching or slurring on the downstroke of the R wave. Therefore the history and presenting symptoms remain the important factors in the diagnosis of an acute or chronic coronary syndrome.

Echocardiography may provide evidence of focal wall motion abnormalities and facilitate triage in patients with ECG findings that are difficult to interpret. If doubt persists, immediate referral for invasive angiography may be necessary to guide therapy in the appropriate clinical context.

Laboratory Data

The ACC recommends the use of troponin I and troponin T as the definitive cardiac diagnostic biomarkers because of their high sensitivity and specificity (Table 102.4). Like the CK-MB levels used previously, cardiac troponin levels become elevated within 3 to 4 hours. Troponins continue to be released for up

TABLE 102.3	Twelve-Lead Electrocardiogram and Myocardial Infarction Territory
Lead	Territory
II, III, aVF	Inferior wall
II, III, aVF, V_5, V_6	Inferoapical wall
I, aVL, V_5, V_6	Inferolateral wall
V_1–V_4	Anterior wall
I, aVL, V_1–V_6	Anterolateral wall
V_1–V_3	Anteroseptal wall (ST-segment elevations)
V_5–V_6	Apical wall
I, aVL, V_5–V_6	Lateral wall
V_1–V_3	Posterior wall (ST-segment depressions; tall, upright R wave)
V_1–V_2	Septal wall (ST-segment elevations)

ECG, Electrocardiogram.

ECG Sequence With Anterior Wall Q Wave Infarction

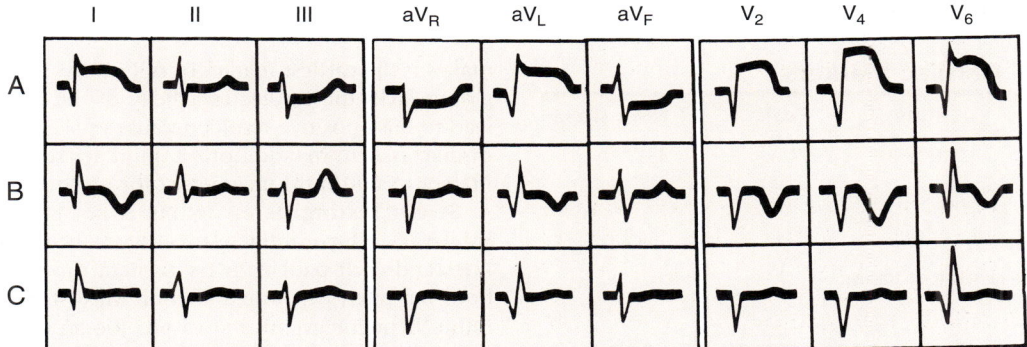

FIG. 102.1 (A) Acute phase of an anterior wall infarction: ST elevations and new Q waves. (B) Evolving phase: deep T-wave inversions. (C) Resolving phase: partial or complete regression of ST-T changes (and sometimes of Q waves). In A and B, note the reciprocal ST-T changes in the inferior leads (II, III, and *aVF*). *ECG*, Electrocardiogram. (From Goldberger, A. L. [2012]. *Goldberger clinical electrocardiography: A simplified approach.* [8th ed.]. Philadelphia: Elsevier.)

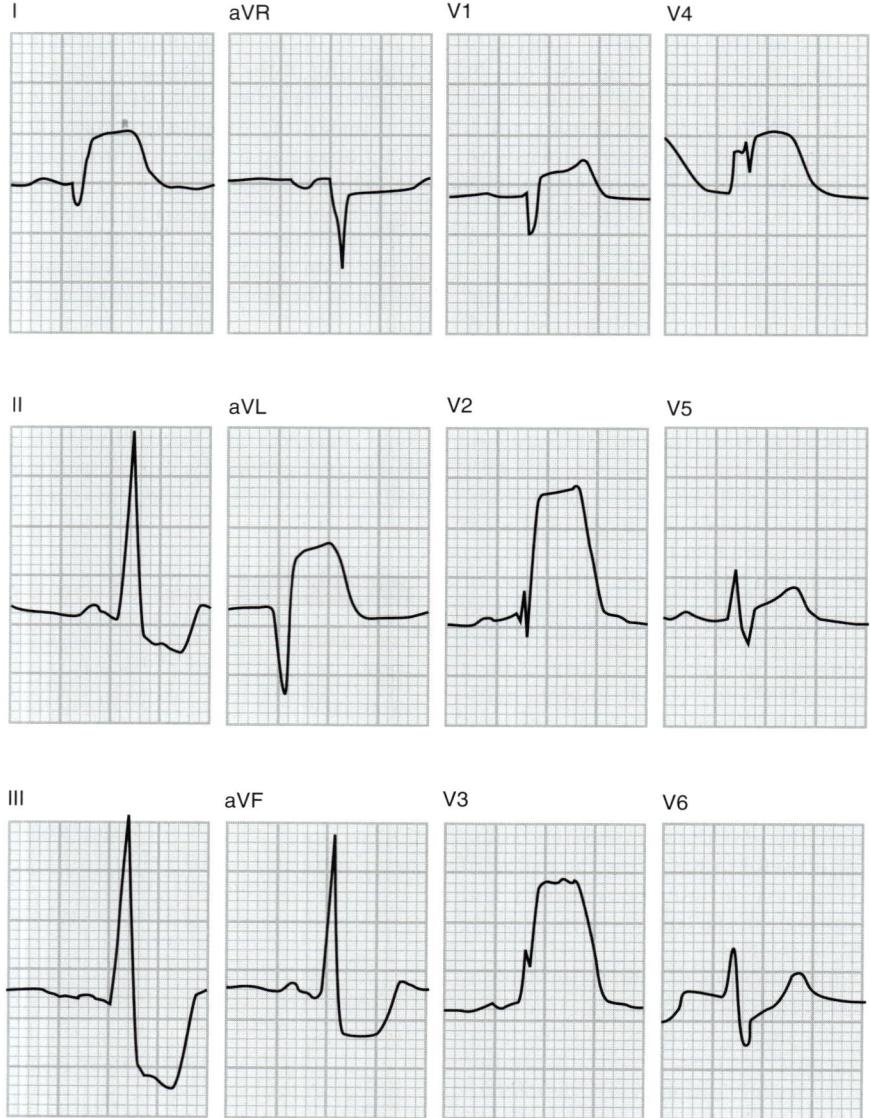

F I G. 102.2 Large anterior (or anterolateral) myocardial infarction. There is marked ST-segment elevation in leads V1 through V5 and in leads I and aVL. This infarction, caused by occlusion of the proximal left anterior descending artery, therefore covers the anterior, septal (V1 through V3/V4), and lateral (V4 to V5 and I/aVL) portions of the left ventricle. In addition, reciprocal ST-segment depression is seen in the inferior leads (II, III, aVF). A Q wave is present in aVL. (From Sidebotham, D., McKee, A., Gillham, M., et al. [2007]. *Cardiothoracic critical care*. Philadelphia: Butterworth Heinemann.)

TABLE 102.4 Cardiac Markers			
Cardiac Marker	**Rises**	**Peaks**	**Normalizes**
CK-MB isoforms	3–12 h	24 h	48–72 h
Myoglobin	1–3 h	6 h	24 h
Troponins T and I	3–12 h	3–4 h	14 days

CK-MB, Creatine kinase muscle-brain fraction.

to 11 days (7- to 14-day range) after a cardiac event. Troponin is a useful diagnostic test in predicting an acute coronary event and serving as a late cardiac marker. Myoglobin is found exclusively in both cardiac and skeletal striated muscle. It is released within 1 to 3 hours after a myocyte cell injury, which currently makes it the earliest marker of cell injury. Unfortunately, myoglobin lacks the cardiac specificity of the troponins. This can lead to false-positive results because of skeletal, renal, or other cardiac issues. In addition, a mild leukocytosis of approximately 15,000/mm³ may persist for up to 1 week.

Stress Testing. Stress testing is not performed during an ST-elevation myocardial event. Based on the ACC/AHA guidelines and each patient or risk/benefit profile, stress testing is, however, often performed after an MI to determine the risk of future ischemic events and to provide an exercise prescription for cardiac rehabilitation.

Echocardiography. Two-dimensional echocardiography can be of value in identifying wall motion abnormalities; estimating left ventricular ejection fraction (LVEF); assessing for pericardial effusion, ventricular aneurysm, and LV thrombus;

ECG Sequence With Inferior Wall Q Wave Infarction

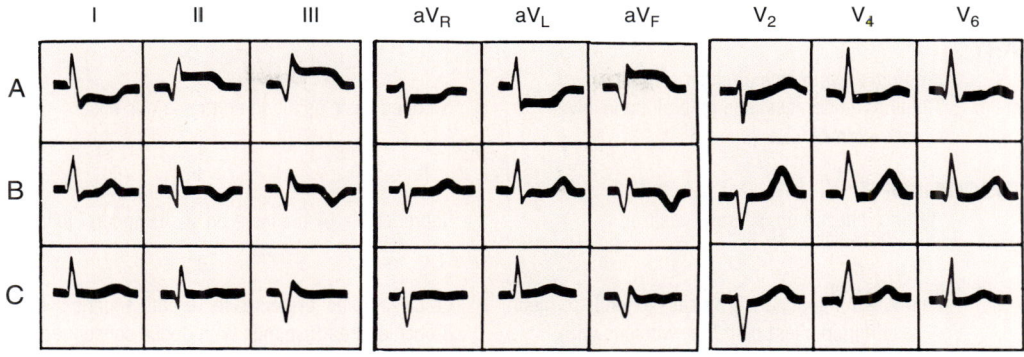

F I G . **102.3** (A) Acute phase of an inferior wall myocardial infarction: ST elevations and new Q waves. (B) Evolving phase: deep T-wave inversions. (C) Resolving phase: partial or complete regression of ST-T changes (and sometimes of Q waves). In A and B, notice the reciprocal ST-T changes in the anterior leads (I, aV_L, and V_2). *ECG*, Electrocardiogram. (From Goldberger, A. L. [2006]. *Clinical electrocardiography: A simplified approach.* [7th ed.]. Philadelphia: Mosby.)

and corroborating clinical and physical diagnosis of RV infarction. Doppler echocardiography is useful in the detection of valvular regurgitant lesions as well as ventricular and atrial septal defects. Echocardiography performed early in the course of an evolving MI is helpful in diagnosis and can aid in the decision-making process. In addition, the echocardiogram can provide prognostic information about LV function and identify patients who may be at risk for development of complications. Therefore serial echocardiograms are beneficial for future comparison.

DIFFERENTIAL DIAGNOSIS

 Aortic dissection, pulmonary embolus, MI, and spontaneous pneumothorax must be considered, expediently detected, diagnosed, and managed in the differential diagnosis of chest pain.

Other conditions in the differential diagnosis to be considered include takotsubo cardiomyopathy; spontaneous coronary artery dissection; and gastrointestinal, pulmonary, valvular, inflammatory, integumentary, and psychological disturbances (Table 102.5).

INTERPROFESSIONAL COLLABORATIVE MANAGEMENT

Chronic Stable Angina

Treatment of chronic stable angina involves many modalities. Because this is a chronic disease, it is important to have a good provider–patient relationship and a means of objectively evaluating specific therapeutic interventions. The majority of patients should initially undergo noninvasive stress testing for diagnosis and risk stratification.

The medication regimen should include acetylsalicylic acid, β blockers, lipid-lowering agents, and nitrates as needed. Nitrate tolerance is a major limitation to continuous nitrate therapy. To avoid tolerance, it is recommended that a daily nitrate-free interval of a minimum of 8 hours be provided. This interval is usually scheduled during the night when angina is less likely to occur. Calcium channel blockers are reasonable options for symptom relief if β blockers are contraindicated or poorly tolerated or as an additional agent for symptom

relief. Renin-angiotensin-aldosterone system blockers such as angiotensin-converting enzyme (ACE) inhibitors or angiotensin blockers should be implemented in patients with LVEF less than 40% and patients with diabetes, hypertension, or chronic kidney disease. Ranolazine is recommended to be used as a substitute for β blocker therapy or in addition to β blockers and/or calcium channel blockers for the treatment of chronic angina. Ranolazine is thought to inhibit the late inward sodium current during systole, which leads to reductions in intracellular calcium accumulation, LV wall tension, and oxygen consumption. It does not affect contractility or coronary blood flow, but may cause hypotension, bradycardia, and QT prolongation and is contraindicated with concurrent QT-prolonging drugs or with a preexisting prolonged QT interval. It should also be avoided with the use of CYP3A4 inhibitors and in patients with hepatic impairment. Renal function must be monitored.

Patients should be cautioned about specific angina triggers. Lifting a heavy load or performing arm exercise (isometric exercise) may precipitate angina symptoms because of an increase in myocardial oxygen demand. Walking in cold air may induce coronary vasoconstriction. It is advisable, therefore, to educate patients to cover the nose and mouth with a scarf when walking in cold weather. Finally, patients should be encouraged to exercise to a level below their anginal threshold to avoid the potential complications resulting from inactivity.

For those patients who are symptomatic despite maximal guideline medical directed therapy or for those with high-risk findings on noninvasive stress test, coronary angiography is appropriate only when the information derived from the procedure will significantly influence patient management, and the patient is agreeable to, and a candidate for, a percutaneous or surgical revascularization. As an alternative to invasive angiography many clinicians proceed to CTA, which may be a more appropriate and safer approach than routine invasive angiography.

Silent Myocardial Ischemia

Myocardial ischemia can occur without symptoms. It has been observed that asymptomatic ST segment depression during

TABLE 102.5 Differential Diagnosis: Chest Pain

Diagnosis	Symptoms	Physical Examination Findings
INTEGUMENTARY		
Herpes zoster	Prodromal symptoms of chest pressure Tingling, tenderness, and pain along involved dermatomes	Grouped vesicles along erythematous base
CHEST WALL DISCOMFORT		
Costochondritis	Anterior chest pain, sharply localized	Reproducible by pressure on costochondral junction
LUNGS		
Pneumonia	Pain when inflammatory process extends to pleura, resulting in chest pain that worsens with inspiration Fever, chills, cough, sputum production, dyspnea	Crackles, rales, or decreased breath sounds over affected area Bronchial breath sounds with dense consolidation, increased fremitus, and egophony (E-to-A changes) Dullness to percussion
Pneumothorax	Sudden-onset, severe unilateral chest pain, generally pleuritic in nature Dyspnea	Diminished breath sounds on affected side Mediastinal emphysema may be present
Pneumothorax, tension	Same as pneumothorax, yet with substernal chest pressure with throat tightness	Same as pneumothorax, but hypotension may be present Tracheal and mediastinal shift
Pulmonary embolus	Dyspnea Chest pain secondary to pulmonary infarction or inflammatory response (pleuritic)	Decreased breath sounds in affected area Hypotension with massive pulmonary embolus as a result of low cardiac output Hemoptysis, tachycardia, and hypoxia
Pulmonary hypertension	Mimics symptoms of ischemic chest pain Dyspnea	Prominent parasternal lift at lower left sternal border or xiphoid Pulmonic, tricuspid, or mitral regurgitation murmur S_4 may be audible
HEART		
Aortic stenosis	Easy fatigability, dyspnea on exertion, syncope or near-syncope, anterior chest pressure	Systolic murmur best heard over right base Delayed carotid upstrokes
Aortic dissections	Sudden onset of severe tearing, stabbing pain over anterior chest (proximal dissection) or interscapular-abdominal region (distal dissection) Diaphoresis, nausea, vomiting, near-syncope	Hypertension in 50% of patients Pulses diminished or absent Neurologic symptoms (decreased cerebral–spinal cord perfusion) Aortic regurgitation murmur may be present as a result of aortic root dissection
Mitral valve prolapse	Sharp left anterior chest pain, generally occurring in response to stress or emotional events Chest discomfort lasting seconds to days Palpitations and dyspnea	Mitral valve click may be noted in systole at left lower sternal border
Pericarditis Spontaneous coronary artery dissection (SCAD) Takotsubo cardiomyopathy	Anterior chest pain that may radiate to shoulder area if diaphragmatic surface of pericardium is involved Sharp chest pain that increases with inspiration or supine positioning (pleuritic) and lessens with forward positioning Chest pain, dyspnea Chest pain. Shoulder pain, dyspnea, diaphoresis, nausea, weakness Chest pain, dyspnea, heart failure, syncope	Fever with bacterial or viral cause Friction rub may or may not be present Possible hypotension, tachypnea, tachycardia, S_3 gallop, systolic ejection murmur (SEM) or holosystolic murmur, jugular venous distention (JVD), and/or bibasilar rales Clinical signs may be absent Exam findings similar to acute myocardial infarction (MI). SCAD is a consideration in women Hypotension, mental status change, dyspneic, systolic murmur
GASTROINTESTINAL SYMPTOMS		
Reflux (gastroesophageal reflux disease) Acute cholecystitis	Substernal burning that may radiate to neck; occurs 30–60 min after eating Nausea, vomiting, and anorexia	Right upper quadrant pain, epigastric pain Right upper quadrant tenderness plus Murphy sign Fever may be present
PAIN DISORDERS		
	Intense anxiety that may last for several days Avoidance behavior because of inability to seek a safe refuge during an attack period Chest pain that is atypical Hypertension may be noted	

ambulatory ECG monitoring occurs more often than symptomatic ST-segment depression in patients with CAD.

Management of patients with asymptomatic myocardial ischemia must be individualized. Exercise stress testing should be considered for evaluation of ischemia in asymptomatic male patients older than 45 years with one or more of the following risk factors: hypercholesteremia, hypertension, history of tobacco use, diabetes, or family history of early CAD. Diabetic patients without symptoms and with only one of the following risk factors should undergo exercise stress testing: age older than 35 years, type 2 diabetes for longer than 10 years or type 1 diabetes for longer than 15 years, any additional atherosclerotic risk factors for CAD, PVD, or presence of microvascular disease. The Asymptomatic Cardiac Ischemia Pilot Study (ACIP) enrolled patients in the 1990s and found that revascularization was better than medical therapy in reducing silent ischemic episodes and possibly cardiovascular events.[22] Asymptomatic patients with silent ischemia and significant left main CAD or three-vessel CAD and impaired LV function are appropriate candidates for CABG surgery. Among patients with recent MI, silent ischemia verified by exercise stress test imaging and followed by percutaneous coronary intervention (PCI) reduced long-term risk of major cardiac events.

Microvascular Angina

The treatment of microvascular disease is aimed to relieve pain. Varied medication categories have been studied, but β blockers may be first prescribed. They work by lowering adrenergic tone and reducing myocardial oxygen demand, as well as enhancing endothelium-dependent vasodilation. Calcium-channel blockers, ACE inhibitors, or ranolazine have also been used successfully. Sublingual nitrates may benefit symptomatic episodes, but long-acting nitrates have proven disappointing. Xanthine derivatives such as aminophylline have been shown to improve the time to exercise-induced angina, time to ST depression, and magnitude of ST depression.[25] These could be used when chronic airway disease and microvascular angina coexist. Some studies have found imipramine to possibly be beneficial in pain modulation.[24] Statin therapy and lifestyle changes are also recommended.[24] Other medications, including metformin for women without diabetes, have also been suggested to improve vascular function and decrease myocardial ischemia; however, further trials are required.[25] Lifestyle changes and risk factor modifications, including the initiation of physical activity, should also be implemented. Many patients will have resolution of symptoms but may have periods of exacerbations. It is important to note that there does not appear to be a risk for MI or sudden cardiac death despite the presence of symptoms, and therefore reassurance of the patient is an important part of therapy.

Vasospastic Angina

Acute treatment of the chest pain episode is usually sublingual NTG. Nondihydropyridine calcium channel blockers (e.g., diltiazem) are recommended for the long-term treatment of variant angina, although amlodipine had been proven useful. Continuous nitrate therapy is not recommended because of problems with tolerance, but targeted nitrates may be helpful in patients with a predictable pattern of pain.

The natural history of spasm is one of periods of symptomatic exacerbation followed by periods of relative quiescence. Once a patient who is receiving therapy has been without symptoms for 6 to 12 months, medication withdrawal can be attempted. Patients with spasm without significant fixed coronary stenosis are not candidates for mechanical intervention.

Unstable Angina and Non-ST Segment Elevation Myocardial Infarction

Early risk stratification should be performed to determine the likelihood of an acute cardiac ischemic event from NSTEMI. The immediate management of this population of patients consists of a detailed patient history, physical examination, and 12-lead ECG within 10 minutes of arrival at an emergency facility (further ECGs every 15 to 30 minutes may be indicated). Cardiac specific troponin (troponin I or T) levels should be measured at presentation and at 3 to 6 hours after symptom onset. From this information, the health care provider can usually assign the patient with chest pain to one of four categories: a noncardiac cause, a stable angina cause, a possible acute coronary artery syndrome, or a definite coronary artery syndrome. Risk analysis using the Heart Score for Major Cardiac events or the TIMI Risk Score can aid in determining the risk analysis, but all patients with unstable angina or NSTEMI should be referred to a cardiologist for further management.

Per the 2014 ACC/AHA Guideline for the management of patients with non-ST elevation ACS, a non-enteric-coated aspirin, 162 to 325 mg, to chew unless contraindicated, should be immediately given unless the patient has an aspirin allergy.[26] Oxygen is indicated only if needed. Additional treatment recommendations include daily β blocker therapy provided there are no contraindications (e.g., cocaine-associated MI), and sublingual NTG (contraindicated in patients with severe aortic stenosis) as needed. Identifiable precipitating clinical circumstances should be uncovered, as should any secondary causes (e.g., fever, anemia, hypotension, cardiomyopathy, aortic stenosis, thyrotoxicosis, or recent stressful events). Symptoms of unstable angina may resolve once the precipitating event has been treated. Low-risk patients should be seen for follow-up evaluation within a 72-hour period, at which time symptoms should be reevaluated for any further instability. Early exercise tolerance testing should also be performed. Patients should be educated about cardiac risk factors and aggressive plans for risk factor modification.

Patients in the intermediate or high-risk category should be hospitalized for careful monitoring, risk stratification, and management. If the symptoms of ACS are identified in the office setting, immediate referral to an emergency department should be undertaken. Oxygen is recommended for patients with respiratory distress or oxygen saturation less than 90%. The patient should be given sublingual NTG and chewable aspirin immediately *unless* the patient has taken a phosphodiesterase inhibitor within the past 48 hours.[26] If chewable aspirin is not available, a regular aspirin tablet should be crushed and given to the patient. Once the patient is in the emergency department setting, β blocker therapy should be initiated within 24 hours if the presenting hemodynamic profile permits, with the dose titrated to a heart rate of 50 to 60 beats/min. Contraindications to β blocker therapy include (1) signs of heart failure; (2) evidence of a low-output state; (3) increased risk for cardiogenic shock; or (4) PR interval greater than 0.24 seconds, second- or third-degree heart block without a cardiac pacemaker, active asthma, or reactive airway disease.

Transthoracic echocardiography is recommended to access LV function.[27] ACE inhibitors and angiotensin II receptor blockers have improved survival rates in patients with acute MI and are most beneficial to patients experiencing anterior wall infarction, pulmonary congestion, or LVEF less than 40%, according to AHA guidelines.

Heparin should be considered with a bolus of 80 units/kg of body weight and then infused at 14 units/kg/h. The dose is then titrated to achieve an activated partial thromboplastin time of 1.5 to 2.0 times the control value. Low-molecular-weight heparin (e.g., enoxaparin) may also be considered in lieu of intravenous heparin therapy.

Invasive therapy (PCI) for revascularization may be indicated for patients who do not respond to medical interventions.[26] Fibrinolytic therapy is not recommended.

Guidelines indicate that initiation of statins within 24 hours of acute MI or ACS has reduced major cardiac events.

High-intensity statin therapy should be initiated or continued in all patients who have no contraindications to its use. A P2Y12 inhibitor (e.g., clopidogrel, prasugrel, or ticagrelor) in addition to aspirin should be administered for up to 12 months in all patients who undergo PCI. For some patients, longer dual-antiplatelet therapy may be a consideration.[26,28]

Acute ST-Segment Elevation Myocardial Infarction

Treatment goals for the patient with an acute MI are to restore blood supply to cardiac muscle, relieve pain, and decrease the incidence of complications (such as heart failure, myocardial rupture, valvular dysfunction, and fatal and nonfatal arrhythmias). With these goals in mind, patients with an acute evolving STEMI should be transferred to a hospital with a dedicated chest pain center and interventional cardiac program within 90 minutes. Primary PCI is the recommended method of reperfusion when it can be performed in a timely fashion by experienced operators.[29] At non–PCI capable hospitals, when the anticipated time of transfer would exceed 120 minutes, fibrinolytic therapy should be administered within 30 minutes of the time of first medical contact to patients with an evolving STEMI in the absence of contraindications. Reperfusion therapy should be administered to all eligible patients who experienced the onset of symptom within the previous 12 hours because benefit can still be achieved when therapy is instituted 3 to 6 hours after the onset of infarction, and some benefit is possible when therapy is given up to 12 hours after the onset of infarction if chest pain is ongoing and ST-segment elevation is apparent in electrocardiographic leads that do not demonstrate new Q waves. Delays in reperfusion have been shown to increase mortality rates. General contraindications to lytic therapy include recent surgery or head trauma, active internal bleeding, suspected aortic dissection, pregnancy, diabetic hemorrhagic retinopathy, severe hypertension, and history of cerebrovascular accident or allergic reaction to the thrombolytic agent. Hemorrhagic stroke is the most common hemorrhagic complication. The rate increases with advancing age. Patients older than 70 years have strokes at twice the rate of younger patients; however, older patients may benefit from lytic therapy. Decisions about thrombolytic therapy must be made on a case-by-case basis in these patients.

Adjunctive antithrombotic therapy at the time of primary PCI would include aspirin in doses of 162 to 325 mg before PCI, and after PCI should be continued indefinitely. Heparin is usually administered by weight adjustment to keep the partial thromboplastin time at 1.5 to 2 times normal. Unless contraindicated, a loading dose of a P2Y12 receptor inhibitor (preferably ticagrelor, but clopidogrel or prasugrel is also appropriate) should be given as early as possible or at the time of primary PCI to patients with evolving STEMI and should be continued for at least 1 year in patients with drug-eluting stents (DESs). The Dual Antiplatelet Therapy (DAPT) Study showed that continuation of a P2Y12 receptor inhibitor and aspirin therapy for up to 30 months, when compared with the continuation of aspirin alone, in patients with drug eluding stents, resulted in a significantly reduced rate of stent thrombosis.[28] Since bleeding is a concern with DAPT, the decision to continue these treatments for patients after a year is individualized.

Oral β blocker therapy should be initiated in the first 24 hours in patients with STEMI who do not have any symptoms of heart failure, a low output state, or cardiogenic shock. Other concerns related to β blocker therapy would include a PR interval greater than 0.24 seconds, second- or third-degree heart block, active asthma, or reactive airway disease. Patients with initial contraindications should be reevaluated to determine if the prior contraindications have resolved.

The use of ACE inhibitors has improved mortality rates and prevention of heart failure and recurrent MI in patients with LVEF of 40% or less. If possible, ACE inhibitors should be started once the patient is hemodynamically stable. Renal issues should also be considered when ACE inhibitor therapy is started; renal artery stenosis is a contraindication to this therapy. Among lower-risk patients with normal LVEFs, ACE inhibitor therapy initiated early in the course of hospitalization has improved survival rates for patients with acute MI.

Calcium channel blockers are effective in acute and chronic stable angina, in lowering blood pressure and in controlling heart rate in patients with atrial fibrillation who are intolerant of β blockers. They have not been shown to have any beneficial effect on infarct size or the rate of reinfarction. They should not be given to patients with LV systolic dysfunction. The use of immediate-release nifedipine is contraindicated in patients with STEMI because of hypotension and reflex sympathetic activation with tachycardia.

Nitrates can assist with relief of symptoms by decreasing LV preload and to some extent increasing coronary blood flow. Nitrates are further useful to treat hypertension or heart failure. Nitrates should not be given to STEMI patients with hypotension, marked bradycardia, RV infarction, or phosphodiesterase type 5 inhibitor use within the previous 24 to 48 hours.

Pharmacologic Therapy for Coronary Artery Disease

Aspirin. Aspirin is effective in the treatment of CAD because of its effects on platelets and vascular endothelial cells. In platelets, aspirin irreversibly inhibits the synthesis of cyclooxygenase, preventing the formation of thromboxane A_2, which is responsible for platelet aggregation. In vascular endothelial cells, aspirin temporarily inhibits the synthesis of cyclooxygenase, which inhibits prostacyclin production and platelet aggregation. The clinical benefits of aspirin have been demonstrated at doses of 75 to 325 mg/day.

Aspirin reaches appreciable plasma levels within 20 minutes and results in platelet inhibition within 60 minutes. The antiplatelet effect of aspirin lasts for the 10-day life of the platelet; however, 10% of circulating platelets are replaced on a daily basis. Normal hemostasis can be achieved with only 20% of aspirin-free platelets. This becomes an important consideration in the timing of aspirin withdrawal for elective surgical procedures.

Aspirin therapy has proved to benefit patients in the acute phase of an evolving MI and should be routinely administered orally with an initial loading dose of 325 mg unless an anaphylactic aspirin allergy is known. Enteric-coated tablets should be chewed or crushed for more rapid absorption. For primary prophylaxis, the U.S. Preventive Services Task Force recommends daily low-dose aspirin for adult men and women who have a 10% or greater risk of CVD, are age 50 to 59 years, have a life expectancy of 10 years, do not have an increased bleeding risk, and are agreeable to take a daily low dose aspirin for at least 10 years.[30] For older patients (age 60 to 69), the recommendations are individualized, but different: the patient should not have a bleeding risk and should have a 10-year life expectancy and be willing to take a daily low-dose aspirin.[28]

The American Diabetes Association recommendation for low-dose aspirin for primary prevention for both type 1 and 2 patients, male or female, aged 50 years or more with a minimum of one additional risk factor for cardiovascular disease (albuminemia, dyslipidemia, smoking, or family history of premature atherosclerosis CVD), but without an increased risk of bleeding, is 72 to 162 mg aspirin daily.[31]

β Blockers. β blockers are a mainstay of therapy for patients with CAD. β blockers decrease myocardial oxygen consumption by decreasing the heart rate at rest and with exercise, by lowering the blood pressure, and by reducing myocardial contractility, thereby eliciting a negative inotropic effect. In contrast, these agents are not useful for vasospastic angina and may worsen the condition. β blockers have been shown to reduce total mortality, rate of nonfatal infarction, infarct size, cardiovascular mortality, and sudden cardiac death.

β blockers can be classified according to their relative cardioselectivity and lipid solubility. They may be nonselective (have an affinity for both β$_1$ and β$_2$ receptors) or selective (have an affinity for β$_1$ receptors). β$_1$ receptors are located in the myocardium, with small amounts of β$_2$ receptors in the atrium. β$_2$ receptors are primarily located in the bronchioles, peripheral vascular smooth muscles, and other specialized sites, such as pancreatic islet cells. Thus blockade of β$_2$ receptors may lead to bronchoconstriction or bronchospasm and peripheral vascular constriction, resulting in claudication. In addition, the mechanism whereby insulin-induced hypoglycemia is countered by stimulation of the liver to mobilize liver glycogen is β$_2$ receptor dependent. Thus blockade of β$_2$ receptors in a patient with diabetes may lead to an inappropriate response to hypoglycemia. This is important because patients with CAD and asthma, COPD, diabetes, or intermittent claudication may benefit from a low dose of β$_1$-selective agents administered with caution. However, as the dose of such agents is increased, selectivity is lost, and both types of receptors become blocked (Box 102.4).

Side effects of β blockers include fatigue, impotence, cold extremities, bronchospasm, worsening claudication, bradycardia, and cardiac conduction disturbances. Central nervous system side effects are based on the agent's lipid solubility property. Agents that are lipid soluble readily cross the blood–brain barrier and are more likely to cause insomnia, depression, and nightmares; this may be seen in any patient but is commonly observed in older adults. Patients should be cautioned that sudden discontinuation of β blocker therapy may precipitate angina symptoms or lead to MI as a result of rebound tachycardia. Although much has been written about the β blocker

---

BOX 102.4

β Blocker Agents

NONSELECTIVE β$_1$ AND β$_2$ BLOCKERS
Propranolol (Inderal)
Timolol (Blocadren)
Nadolol (Corgard)
Sotalol (Betapace)
Penbutolol (Levatol)

NONSELECTIVE, VASODILATORY
Labetalol (Trandate, Normodyne)
Pindolol

CARDIOSELECTIVE, β$_1$ RECEPTORS ONLY
Acebutolol (Sectral)
Atenolol (Tenormin)
Metoprolol (Lopressor, Toprol-XL)
Esmolol (Brevibloc)
Bisoprolol (Zebeta)
Nebivolol (Bystolic)

COMBINATION α$_1$ AND NONCARDIOSELECTIVE β BLOCKER
Carvedilol (Coreg)

---

withdrawal syndrome, the incidence is low. However, in discontinuing the drug, one should be prudent and taper the drug during several days. Some β blockers have the capacity to stimulate either one or both β$_1$ and β$_2$ receptors—hence the term *intrinsic sympathomimetic activity*, as seen with pindolol. This property limits the efficacy of treating patients with angina because at higher doses the heart rate is not decreased and may even be increased. These agents may be beneficial in patients who have symptomatic sinus bradycardia when they are treated with other β blockers. The major effect of β blockers with sympathomimetic activity is lowering of blood pressure. Labetalol possesses both β- and α-blocking actions. This drug can be used to treat patients with angina as well as patients with significant hypertension.

Nitrates. Nitrates are recommended for the treatment of stable and unstable angina and the management of an acute MI. The clinical effectiveness of nitrates is in their ability to promote vascular smooth muscle relaxation, resulting in arteriolar and venous dilation. In smaller doses, nitrates dilate the venous system, which causes peripheral pooling and decreased venous return to the heart (preload). This reduction in preload decreases the LV size, ventricular filling pressures, and myocardial wall tension. In larger doses, nitrates dilate the arterial vasculature, lowering systemic blood pressure (afterload) and thereby decreasing the resistance to ventricular ejection, making it easier for the heart to contract. This overall reduction in LV workload decreases myocardial oxygen consumption. The arteriolar dilating effect, however, may produce a reflex tachycardia, thereby increasing myocardial oxygen consumption. This effect may be attenuated by concurrent use of β blockade. In addition, the combination of nitrates with dihydropyridine (DHP) calcium channel blockers should be undertaken cautiously because postural hypotension may be a problem.

TABLE 102.6	Nitrate Preparations				
Preparation	**Starting Dose**	**Maximum Dose**	**Onset of Action**	**Duration of Action**	
Nitroglycerin (Nitrostat)	0.4 mg (1 tablet)	3 tablets in 15 min	1 min	<30 min	
Nitroglycerin (Nitrolingual)	0.4 mg (metered spray)	3 sprays in 15 min	1 min	<30 min	
ISDN (Isordil, Sorbitrate)	20 mg every 4–6 h	240 mg/day	60–90 min	4–6 h	
ISDN-SR (Dilatrate-SR)	40 mg every 8–12 h				
ISMN (Ismo, Monoket)	20 mg in AM and 20 mg 7 h later				
ISMN-SR (Imdur)	30–60 mg/day	120–240 mg/day			
Nitroglycerin ointment (2%) (Nitro-Bid, Nitrol)	½ inch every 4–6 h	4–5 inches every 3–4 h	30–60 min	3–6 h	
Nitroglycerin patch (Transderm-Nitro, Nitro-Dur, Nitrodisc, Deponit)	5 mg/24 h (0.1–0.4 mg/h)	2–3 patches of 15 mg in 24 h	30 min	24 h	

Regimen for nitrate preparations should include a dose-free interval each day to prevent refractory tolerance.
ISDN, Isosorbide dinitrate; *ISMN*, isosorbide mononitrate.

Coronary vasodilation is induced through the exogenous production of nitric oxide from nitrate metabolism, which is now known to be EDRF (endothelial derived relaxing factor). In the coronary circulation, damage to the endothelial layer from atherosclerosis results in decreased availability of EDRF and a decreased vasodilatory response is the result. Nitrates are endothelium-independent vasodilators and therefore do not require a functioning endothelium to deliver a vasodilating response. Nitrate administration results in the endogenous production of nitric oxide, which replaces the vasodilating effects of EDRF and promotes coronary vessel vasodilation.

Three nitrate preparations are currently available for use in the United States (Table 102.6): NTG, isosorbide dinitrate (ISDN), and isosorbide mononitrate (ISMN). Sublingual nitroglycerin tablets in doses of 0.4 mg are most useful for acute angina events because of the rapid course of action of sublingual NTG. Sublingual NTG is also recommended for prophylactic use before the patient engages in a physical activity or a stressful event that has historically precipitated an angina event. Sublingual NTG works within 3 to 5 minutes; however, anti-ischemic effects last for less than 30 minutes. Because of its short duration of action, sublingual NTG should be combined with oral nitrates for sustained effectiveness. According to the ACC/AHA 2007 guidelines for the management of patients with unstable angina or NSTEMI, "Health care providers should instruct patients with suspected ACS for whom NTG has been prescribed previously to take not more than 1 dose of NTG sublingually in response to chest discomfort/pain. If chest discomfort/pain is unimproved or is worsening 5 minutes after 1 NTG dose has been taken, it is recommended that the patient or family member/friend/caregiver call 911 immediately to access EMS before taking additional NTG. In patients with chronic stable angina, if symptoms are significantly improved by 1 dose of NTG, it is appropriate to instruct the patient or family member/friend/caregiver to repeat NTG every 5 minutes for a maximum of 3 doses and call 911 if symptoms have not resolved completely."[29]

NTG tablets retain their potency for up to 6 months after the bottle has been opened. Patients should be encouraged to keep NTG tablets in their amber-colored glass bottle, protected from moisture and extremes of temperature and light.

NTG spray is particularly useful for patients with visual or neurologic impairments, who may have difficulty handling a small tablet. The spray is delivered at a metered dose of 0.4 mg and should be applied to the surface of the tongue. Patients should be reminded not to inhale the spray. Each canister contains approximately 200 doses, and the canister will maintain its potency for up to 3 years.

Oral NTG is the nitrate of choice in the ambulatory population and can be taken as either ISDN or ISMN. ISDN is extensively metabolized in the liver, where more than half of it is converted to ISMN. Because of this bypass effect, ISDN is not effective for treatment of angina or enhancement of exercise capacity in doses of less than 20 mg every 4 hours. In 1991, the U.S. Food and Drug Administration approved ISMN, which does not undergo hepatic degradation, so that 100% of it is available after oral administration. The main advantage of the ISMNs is that they can be administered once or twice daily, whereas ISDNs must be administered three or four times per day.

Topical NTG is absorbed through the skin and can be administered either as a 2% ointment or by premeasured skin patches in doses of 5, 10, 15, or 20 mg/day. The advantage of NTG ointment over other methods of administration is that the ointment can be removed promptly if any side effects develop. However, its disadvantages seem to outweigh its advantages in the ambulatory population. The ointment is messy to apply, can soil clothing, is seldom dosed consistently each time, and may produce a localized rash. The NTG patch produces a more controlled dose and is generally favored over the ointment. Although topical NTG is initially effective, long-term use can lead to nitrate tolerance and thus a decreased therapeutic effect. It is therefore recommended that topical NTG be removed from the skin for 8 to 12 hours daily.

Nitrate tolerance results from plasma nitrate levels sustained from continued nitrate administration. It is important to identify nitrate tolerance because it leads to a reduction in anti-ischemic benefits. The cause of nitrate tolerance is a complex, multifactorial phenomenon, and the mechanism remains elusive. However, the theory that is commonly associated with nitrate tolerance involves vascular depletion of sulfhydryl groups. The metabolism of nitrates requires the use of sulfhydryl to form intracellular nitric oxide from nitrates. This is the active molecule that stimulates guanylate cyclase to produce vasodilation. Continuous use of nitrates produces excess nitric oxide formation, thus depleting sulfhydryl groups.

Calcium Channel Blockers

DIHYDROPYRIDINES

Amlodipine (Norvasc)
Isradipine (DynaCirc)
Felodipine (Plendil)
Nicardipine (Cardene)
Nifedipine (Procardia, Adalat)
Nisoldipine (Sular)

NONDIHYDROPYRIDINES

Diphenylalkylamine derivative: verapamil (Calan, Covera-HS, Isoptin, Verelan)
Benzothiazepine derivative: diltiazem (Cardizem, Dilacor, Tiazac)

A sulfhydryl donor such as acetylcysteine has been used in experiments to counteract nitrate tolerance.

To avoid the effects of nitrate tolerance, intervals free of nitrates must occur. For oral ISDN administration, an administration schedule of three times per day (8 AM, 1 PM, and 6 PM) rather than four times per day should be prescribed. With sustained-release ISDN administration, administration at 8 AM and 2 PM would support nitrate-free intervals in the evening. Topical nitrates should be removed for 8 to 12 hours daily. This schedule provides periods during the evening hours when the patient is without anti-ischemic therapy. For this reason and because of the reflex tachycardia often seen with vasodilation in response to nitrate therapy, combination therapy with β blockers or calcium channel blockers is recommended.

Calcium Channel Blockers. Calcium channel blockers are used in the treatment of hypertension and angina pectoris. They selectively inhibit the influx of calcium into the calcium L-channel in both smooth muscle and myocardial cells. All have a peripheral arteriolar and coronary vasodilating effect and a negative inotropic effect, although the latter is modest in the case of nifedipine. Two distinct classes of calcium channel antagonists have emerged on the basis of molecular structure (Box 102.5): the DHPs, with a chemical structure similar to nifedipine; and the non-DHPs, such as verapamil (papaverine derivative) and diltiazem (benzothiazepine derivative).

The DHPs are more vascular selective; thus their dominant effect is peripheral and coronary vasodilation. They have minimum or no effect on the sinus and atrioventricular nodes. The rapid vasodilatory effects of these agents may lead to reflex tachycardia, exacerbation of heart failure, and stimulation of the renin-angiotensin system. These undesirable effects are more common among the short-acting DHPs, which should be avoided in the patient with an acute MI. Extended-release non-DHPs may be considered in patients with unstable angina or NSTEMI instead of β blockers or as adjuncts to β blocker therapy in the presence of ongoing ischemia or hypertension.

Angiotensin-Converting Enzyme Inhibitors and Angiotensin II Receptor Blockers. The conical shape of the heart is designed for optimum efficiency in performance and energy use. MI induces alteration in the contour of the heart, leading to decreased LV performance and increased energy requirement for a given workload. Preservation of the contour of the heart after MI is essential for effective LV performance and prevention of the development of left-sided heart failure and valvular regurgitation. There are significant survival benefits for older patients with heart failure who are compliant with ACE inhibitor therapy.

It is clear that stimulation of the renin-angiotensin-aldosterone system plays an important pathophysiologic role in the development of heart failure and poor LV performance. ACE inhibitors can therefore inhibit or counteract the adverse hemodynamic and neurohumoral effects (increased preload, afterload, heart rate, sympathetic tone, catecholamines, and renin-angiotensin system activity) contributed by the system.

Heart failure guidelines have shown that administration of ACE inhibitors shortly after acute MI, once the patient is hemodynamically stable, has prevented the development of heart failure in patients with LV dysfunction but without clinical heart failure. In addition, ACE inhibitors reduced long-term mortality in patients with and without clinical evidence of heart failure through the ability of the inhibitors to reverse the major hemodynamic and neurohumoral abnormalities associated with poor LV performance. Angiotensin receptor blockers should be used in patients who are intolerant of ACE inhibitors and have heart failure or have had an MI with LVEF of less than 40%.

Anticoagulation. The use of anticoagulation with aspirin and heparin has significantly reduced the short-term risk of thromboembolic complications during an acute MI. Therapeutic levels may be difficult to maintain with heparin infusions, but an alternative to unfractionated heparin is the use of low-molecular-weight heparin and Factor xa inhibitors. Enoxaparin and fondaparinux have been shown to reduce mortality and reinfarction but can be administered only to patients with normal renal function.

A significant percentage of patients with ACS experience major vascular events either during or within the first few months after their hospital stay. Another recommended adjunctive therapy for ACS are P2Y12 inhibitors (e.g., clopidogrel, prasugrel, or ticagrelor), which bind to the adenosine diphosphate receptors on platelets, causing a decrease in platelet aggregation. P2Y12 has been shown to reduce cardiovascular morbidity and mortality when it is administered to patients with NSTEMI. In patients up to 75 years of age experiencing a STEMI, there is a reduction in major cardiac event mortality.

Cases in which there is a mural thrombus represent another circumstance for anticoagulation. Ventricular mural thrombi are more common in patients with a large rather than a small area of MI. Thrombi are often observed in the left ventricle, particularly in the apex, where aneurysm and pseudoaneurysm commonly form. On rare occasions, with extensive infarction, thrombus may be observed in the RV apex. Warfarin (Coumadin) therapy is indicated in patients with a mural thrombus, especially in cases in which the thrombus is mobile, has an irregular surface, and is protruding. Warfarin therapy is generally initiated for 3 to 6 months, after which time echocardiographic evaluation to assess the presence or absence of mural thrombus is performed. If the thrombus persists after warfarin therapy, it does not necessarily indicate continued embolic potential unless there is evidence of mobility. In addition, warfarin therapy is indicated in patients with severe LV dysfunction and an LVEF of less than 20%.

LIPID GUIDELINES

Lifestyle modifications, including adherence to a heart-healthy diet, regular exercise, avoidance of tobacco products, and maintenance of a healthy weight, remain an important component of health promotion and ASCVD risk reduction. Lipid lowering with the use of statins has also been supported for the primary prevention of ASCVD in high-risk individuals and for secondary prevention in all individuals. In 2013, the American College of Cardiology (ACC) and American Heart Association (AHA) released guidelines on the treatment of blood cholesterol.[32] These guidelines are available in a mobile application to assist health care providers in determining if statin therapy may be indicated in patients who do not otherwise have a compelling indication to initiate therapy. The Pooled Cohort Equation estimates the 10-year primary risk of ASVD among patients between 40 and 79 years of age without preexisting cardiovascular disease. Though there are concerns that the Pooled Cohort Equation needs updating, it has largely replaced the Framingham risk score for clinical risk assessment. Four statin benefit groups have been identified and include individuals in need of primary or secondary prevention. The first group includes those in need of secondary prevention who have demonstrated clinical ASCVD. This is defined by an ACS, history of MI, stable or unstable angina, coronary or other arterial revascularization, stroke, transient ischemic attack (TIA), or peripheral vascular disease (PVD). The other three categories involve patients in need of primary prevention. The first of these categories involves those with elevations of low-density lipoprotein cholesterol (LDL-C) above 190 mg/dL without a secondary cause such as high saturated fats or causative drugs. The next category involves those primary prevention patients with diabetes aged 40 to 75 years with LDL-C of 70 to 189 mg/dL. The last category involves those without diabetes aged 40 to 75 years with LDL-C of 70 to 189 mg/dL and an estimated 10-year ASCVD risk score higher than 7.5%. These guidelines base the intensity of statin therapy to reduce ASCVD risk according to those most likely to benefit (Table 102.7). There are no more low-density lipoprotein (LDL) treatment targets. For those individuals unable to tolerate high-intensity statin therapy, moderate-intensity statin therapy is recommended.

TABLE 102.7 **High-, Moderate-, and Low-Intensity Statin Therapy**

High-Intensity Statin Therapy	Moderate-Intensity Statin Therapy	Low-Intensity Statin Therapy
Daily dose lowers LDL-C on average by approximately >50%	Daily dose lowers LDL-C on average by approximately 30% to <50%	Daily dose lowers LDL-C on average by 30%
Atorvastatin 40–80 mg Rosuvastatin 20–40 mg	Atorvastatin 10–20 mg Rosuvastatin 5–10 mg Simvastatin 20–40 mg Pravastatin 40–80 mg Lovastatin 40 mg Fluvastatin 40 mg bid	Simvastatin 10 mg Pravastatin 10–20 mg Lovastatin 20 mg

From Stone, N., Robinson, J., Lichtenstein, A., et al. (2014). ACC/AHA guideline on the treatment of blood cholesterol to reduce atherosclerotic cardiovascular risk in adults: A report of the American College of Cardiology/American Heart Association Task Force on Practice Guidelines. *Journal of the American College of Cardiology, 63*(25 Pt B), 2889–2934; Lloyd-Jones, D. M., Morris, P. B., Ballantyne, C. M., Birtcher, K. K., Daly, D. D., DePalma, S. M., et al. (2016). 2016 ACC Expert Consensus Decision Pathway on the Role of Non-Statin Therapies for LDL-Cholesterol Lowering in the Management of Atherosclerotic Cardiovascular Disease Risk. *Journal of the American College of Cardiology, 68*(1), 92–125; DOI: 10.1016/j.jacc.2016.03.519.

Non-statin therapies are considered when patients do not tolerate statins. Ezetimibe is initially recommended; bile acid sequestrants are a second choice (though not for patients with triglycerides >300 mg/dL.).[33]

Proprotein convertase subtilisin/kexin type 9 inhibitors (PCSK9 inhibitors) are indicated for patients with statin intolerance and also for those patients who have ASCVD or familial hypercholesterolemia with elevated LDL-C levels despite treatment with a statin. The currently available PCSK9 inhibitors, alirocumab and evolocumab, are monoclonal antibodies that bind to LDL receptors and decrease LDL (Table 102.8). There can be associated hypersensitivity reactions and patients can develop antibodies to these medications.[34]

LIFE SPAN CONSIDERATIONS: WOMEN AND HEART DISEASE

Heart disease is the primary cause of death in women in the United States. Sixty-four percent of women who experienced sudden cardiac death were asymptomatic.[35]

The gender differences between men and women with respect to coronary anatomy, clinical presentation, and treatment modalities have been under investigation. Women have a lower prevalence of anatomically obstructive CAD with greater rates of myocardial ischemia than men.[8] Studies have shown microvascular dysfunction, plaque erosion, and abnormal coronary reactivity to be implicated in the greater rate of ischemia for women.[8] The clinical presentation of women often is not the typical midsternal chest tightness with shoulder and arm radiation that men often experience. Instead, women may be seen initially with indigestion, progressive fatigue, or dyspnea. Because the mortality rate from STEMI is higher in women than in men, it is important that gender bias be eliminated from the clinical decision-making and that the nuances of CAD in women be acknowledged. Current data continue to show disparity in diagnosis and management of ACS and acute MI in women.

The diagnosis of CAD in women has also proved difficult because of false-positive results of exercise tolerance testing in women. The electrocardiographic response to such testing in women has been shown to be an abnormal ischemic response, despite normal coronary arteries. Speculation in this area suggests women's lower hematocrit levels and higher circulating estrogen levels as plausible culprits. Radionuclide testing may be performed to provide greater test sensitivity and specificity. Despite the increased accuracy of this testing, a significant number of false-positive results still occur, mainly as a result of breast attenuation artifact, which may produce septal and anterior wall defects. Stress echocardiography may prove a more accurate method of noninvasive CAD testing in women.

COMPLICATIONS

The complications of ischemic heart disease and MI are potentially life-threatening. Recurrent ischemia and reinfarction can increase the area of nonfunctioning myocardial tissue, creating mechanical complications such as papillary muscle rupture, ventricular aneurysm, and ventricular septal defect. Rhythm and conduction disturbances may arise without premonitory signs. Chest pain and anxiety associated with cardiac disease can produce hypertension, increasing afterload and oxygen demand. Heart failure, hypotension, and shock impair systemic perfusion and cardiac function.

TABLE 102.8	PCSK9 Inhibitors	
Medication	**Dose**	**Common Adverse Effects**
Airocumab (Praluent) Recommended for treatment of atherosclerotic heart disease or heterozygous familial hypercholesterolemia	75 mg SQ every 2 weeks *Or* 300 mg SQ every 4 weeks	*Contraindicated if history of previous hypersensitivity reaction (vasculitis or allergic reaction requiring hospitalization).* Possible injection site or allergic reaction Increased LFTs Cough Influenza Nasopharyngitis Sinusitis Muscle spasm and pain Potential for development of anti-drug antibodies
Evolocumab (Repatha)	For homozygous familial hypercholesterolemia: 420 mg SQ once a month For primary heterozygous familial hyperlipidemia: 140 mg SQ every 2 weeks or 420 mg SQ monthly For cardiovascular disease prevention in patients with known cardiovascular disease: 140 mg SQ every 2 weeks or 420 mg SQ monthly.	*Allergic reaction including angioedema, difficulty breathing* Injection site reaction Hypertension Myalgias Cough, upper respiratory infection Nausea Dizziness Palpitations Ventricular extra systoles Angina Potential for development of anti-drug antibodies

From Chaudhary, R., Garg, J., Shah, N., & Sumner, A. (2017). PCSK9 inhibitors: A new era of lipid lowering therapy. *World Journal of Cardiology, 9*(2), 76–91. http://doi.org/10.4330/wjc.v9.i2.76.

INDICATIONS FOR REFERRAL OR HOSPITALIZATION

- The patient whose condition is complicated by multiple comorbid diseases (e.g., diabetes mellitus, hypertension, heart failure, hyperlipidemia, and PVD) should be referred to a cardiologist. Patients with chronic stable angina who develop a change in angina pattern should also be referred to a specialist. In addition, all patients with a documented history of coronary ischemic syndrome should be co-managed with a cardiologist. The patient's symptoms and comorbid diseases should determine the frequency of visits to the specialist.
- Ischemic CAD represents a spectrum of coronary insufficiency ranging from chronic stable angina, unstable angina, or non Q wave MI (subendomyocardial infarction) to transmural MI. Hospitalization is based on specific criteria.

PATIENT AND FAMILY EDUCATION

- Patients need to be educated about CAD and heart attack warning signs. Deaths from acute MI can occur within the first hour of onset. Patients and families should understand the importance of calling 911 or an ambulance if symptoms of a heart attack occur. These include chest pressure or discomfort; pain radiating to the arm, neck, or jaw; diaphoresis; nausea or vomiting; shortness of breath; dizziness; rapid or irregular pulse; and loss of consciousness. All families with a family member who has CAD should be encouraged to learn CPR.
- Discussions with patients and families should include a review of instructions for taking aspirin and NTG in response to chest pain.
- Careful management of comorbid illnesses along with a thorough understanding of the disease process and prescribed medical regimen is important for patients with CAD.

Women who are candidates for hormone replacement therapy should be educated about the risks and benefits of estrogen or hormone replacement therapy after menopause.

HEALTH PROMOTION

Adherence to guidelines for ideal cardiovascular health is paramount to decrease coronary artery morbidity and mortality. Risk factor modification includes smoking cessation; aspirin or other antithrombotic therapy; alcohol and drug use management; lipid lowering; ACE inhibitor use; β blocker therapy; and management of hypertension, weight, exercise, diabetes, and atrial fibrillation.

REFERENCES

1. AHA/ASA Heart Disease and Stroke Statistics 2018 At-a-Glance. https://healthmetrics.heart.org/wp-content/uploads/2018/02/At-A-Glance-Heart-Disease-and-Stroke-Statistics-2018.pdf. (Accessed 11 August 2018).
2. American College of Cardiology. (2018). CDC Report Shows Increased Black-White Disparities Related to CVD. https://www.acc.org/latest-in-cardiology/articles/2018/04/03/13/34/cdc-report-shows-increased-black-white-disparities-related-to-cvd. (Accessed 19 August 2018).
3. American Heart Disease. (2015). African Americans and Heart Disease. http://www.heart.org/en/health-topics/consumer-healthcare/what-is-cardiovascular-disease/african-americans-and-heart-disease-stroke. (Accessed 12 August 2018).
4. Cunningham, S. G., Brashers, V. L., & McCance, K. L. (2014). Structure and function of the cardiovascular and lymphatic systems. In *Pathophysiology: The biologic basis for disease in adults and children.* St. Louis: Elsevier.
5. National Institute of Health. Coronary heart disease risk factors. https://www.nhlbi.nih.gov/health-topics/coronary-heart-disease-risk-factors. (Accessed 11 August 2018).
6. American Heart Association/American Stroke Association. Statistical Fact Sheet 2014 Diabetes. https://www.heart.org/idc/groups/heart-public/@wcm/@sop/@smd/documents/downloadable/ucm_462019.pdf. (Accessed 12 August).

7. Brashers, V. L. (2014). Alterations of cardiovascular function. In K. L. McCance & V. L. Brashers (Eds.), *Pathophysiology: The biologic basis for disease in adults and children* (p. 1149). St. Louis: Elsevier.

8. Garcia, M., Mulvagh, S. L., Bairey Merz, C. N., Buring, J. E., & Manson, J. E. (2016). Cardiovascular disease in women; Clinical perspectives. *Circulation Research, 118*, 1273–1293.

9. World Heart Federation. (2017). Risk Factors. https://www.world-heart-federation.org/resources/risk-factors/. (Accessed 12 August 2018).

10. Sederholm, L. S., Isaksson, R.-M., Ericsson, M., Ängerud, K., & Thylén, I. (2018). Gender disparities in first medical contact and delay in ST-elevation myocardial infarction: A prospective multicentre Swedish survey study. *BMJ Open, 8*(5), e020211. http://doi.org/10.1136/bmjopen-2017-020211.

11. Ouellet, G. M., Geda, M., Murphy, T. E., Tsang, S., Tinetti, M. E., & Chaudhry, S. I. (2017). Prehospital delay in older adults with acute myocardial infarction: The ComprehenSIVe evaluation of risk factors in older patients with acute myocardial infarction study. *Journal of the American Geriatrics Society, 65*(11), 2391–2396.

12. Consumer Reports. $164 Per Mile: Surprise Ambulance Bills Are A Growing Problem & Difficult To Avoid. https://www.consumerreports.org/consumerist/164-per-mile-surprise-ambulance-bills-are-a-growing-problem-difficult-to-avoid. (Accessed 12 August).

13. Antman, E. M., & Loscalzo, J. (2018). Ischemic heart disease. In J. Jameson, A. S. Fauci, D. L. Kasper, S. L. Hauser, D. L. Longo, & J. Loscalzo (Eds.), *Harrison's principles of internal medicine* (20th ed.). New York, NY: McGraw-Hill. http://accessmedicine.mhmedical.com.ezproxy.simmons.edu/content.aspx?bookid=2129&sectionid=192029847. (Accessed 12 August 2018).

14. Conti, C. R., Bavry, A. A., & Petersen, J. W. (2012). Silent ischemia: Clinical relevance. *Journal of the American College of Cardiology, 59*(5), 435–441.

15. Aronson, D., & Edelman, E. R. (2014). Coronary artery disease and diabetes mellitus. *Cardiology Clinics, 32*(3), 439–455. http://doi.org/10.1016/j.ccl.2014.04.001. (Accessed August 15, 2018).

16. Park, J. J., Park, S.-J., & Choi, D.-J. (2015). Microvascular angina: Angina that predominantly affects women. *The Korean Journal of Internal Medicine, 30*(2), 140–147. http://doi.org/10.3904/kjim.2015.30.2.140.

17. Rodriguez Ziccardi, M., & Gossman, W. G. Angina, Prinzmetal. [Updated 2017 Jun 12]. In: StatPearls [Internet]. Treasure Island (FL): StatPearls Publishing; 2018 Jan-. Retrieved from https://www.ncbi.nlm.nih.gov/books/NBK430776/.

18. Giugliano, R. P., Cannon, C. P., & Braunwald, E. (2018). Non-ST-segment elevation acute coronary syndrome (non-ST-segment elevation myocardial infarction and unstable angina). In J. Jameson, A. S. Fauci, D. L. Kasper, S. L. Hauser, D. L. Longo, & J. Loscalzo (Eds.), *Harrison's principles of internal medicine* (20th ed.). New York, NY: McGraw-Hill. http://accessmedicine.mhmedical.com.ezproxy.simmons.edu/content.aspx?bookid=2129&sectionid=192029959. (Accessed August 13, 2018).

19. Pasupathy, S., Tavella, R., & Beltrame, J. F. (2017). Myocardial infarction with nonobstructive coronary arteries (MINOCA): the past, present, and future management. *Circulation, 135*, 1490–1493.

20. Sivabaskari, P., Tracy, A., Dreyer, R. P., et al. (2015). Systematic review of patients presenting with suspected myocardial infarction and non-obstructed coronary arteries (MINOCA). *Circulation, 132*(19), e232.

21. Jaffrey, Z., Hudson, M. P., Jacobsen, G., et al. (2007). Modified Thrombolysis in Myocardial Infarction (TIMI) risk score to risk stratify patients in the emergency department with possible acute coronary syndrome. *Journal of Thrombosis and Thrombolysis, 24*(2), 137–144.

22. Pepine, C. J., Sharaf, B., Andrews, T. C., Forman, S., Geller, N., Knatterud, G., et al. (1997). Relation between clinical, angiographic and ischemic findings at baseline and ischemia-related adverse outcomes at 1 year in the asymptomatic cardiac ischemia pilot study. *Journal of the American College of Cardiology, 29*(7), 1483–1489.

23. Ong, P., Athanasiadis, A., & Sechtem, U. (2015). Pharmacotherapy for coronary microvascular dysfunction. *European Heart Journal. Cardiovascular Pharmacotherapy, 1*(1), 65–71. https://doi.org/10.1093/ehjcvp/pvu020, https://academic.oup.com/ehjcvp/article/1/1/65/2599633. (Accessed August 21, 2018).

24. Samim, A., Nugent, L., Mehta, P. K., Shufelt, C., & Merz, C. N. B. (2010). Treatment of angina and microvascular coronary dysfunction. *Current Treatment Options in Cardiovascular Medicine, 12*(4), 355–364. http://doi.org/10.1007/s11936-010-0083-8, https://www.ncbi.nlm.nih.gov/pmc/articles/PMC3914311. (Accessed August 21, 2018).

25. Jadhav, S., Ferrell, W., Greer, I. A., et al. (2006). Effects of metformin on microvascular function and exercise tolerance in women with angina and normal coronary arteries: A randomized, double-blind, placebo-controlled study. *Journal of the American College of Cardiology, 48*(5), 956–963.

26. Amesterdam, E. A., Wenger, N. K., Brindis, R. G., Casey, D. E., et al. (2014). 2014 AHA/ACC guideline for the management of patients with non–ST-elevation acute coronary syndromes: a report of the American College of Cardiology/American Heart Association Task Force on practice guidelines. *Circulation, 130*, e 344–e426. https://www.ahajournals.org/doi/abs/10.1161/cir.0000000000000134. (Accessed August 22, 2018).

27. Jneid, H., Addison, D., Bhatt, D. L., et al. (2017). 2017 AHA/ACC clinical performance and quality measures for adults with ST-elevation and non-ST-elevation myocardial infarction: A report of the American College of Cardiology/American Heart Association Task Force on Performance Measures. *Journal of the American College of Cardiology, 70*(16), 2048–2090.

28. Mauri, L., Kereiakes, D. J., Yeh, R. W., et al. (2014). Twelve or 30 months of dual antiplatelet therapy after drug eluting stents. *The New England Journal of Medicine, 371*(23), 2155–2166.

29. O'Gara, P., Kushner, F., Ascheim, D., et al. (2013). 2013 ACCF/AHA guideline for the management of ST elevation myocardial infarction. *Circulation, 61*(4), e78–e140.

30. U.S Preventive Services Task Force. https://www.uspreventiveservicestaskforce.org/Page/Document/UpdateSummaryFinal/aspirin-to-prevent-cardiovascular-disease-and-cancer. (Accessed 21 August 2018).

31. American Diabetes Association. Cardiovascular Disease and Risk Management: Standards of Medical Care in Diabetes—2018. http://care.diabetesjournals.org/content/41/Supplement_1/S86. (Accessed 22 August 2018).

32. Stone, N. J., Robinson, J. G., Lichtenstein, A. H., Goff, D. C., Lloyd-Jones, D. M., Smith, S. C., et al. (2014). Treatment of blood cholesterol to reduce atherosclerotic cardiovascular disease risk in adults: synopsis of the 2013 American College of Cardiology/American Heart Association cholesterol guideline. *Annals of Internal Medicine, 160*, 339–343. doi:10.7326/M14-0126.

33. Lloyd-Jones, D. M., Morris, P. B., Ballantyne, C. M., Birtcher, K. K., Daly, D. D., DePalma, S. M., et al. (2016). 2016 ACC expert consensus decision pathway on the role of non-statin therapies for LDL-cholesterol lowering in the management of atherosclerotic cardiovascular disease risk. *Journal of the American College of Cardiology, 68*(1), 92–125. doi:10.1016/j.jacc.2016.03.519.

34. Rosental, L. D. (2017). Prophylaxis of atherosclerotic cardiovascular disease: Drugs that help normalize cholesterol and triglyceride levels. In L. D. Rosenthal & J. R. Burchum (Eds.), *Lehne's pharmacotherapeutics for advanced practice providers*. St. Louis: Elsevier.

35. Centers for Disease Control and Prevention. Women and heart disease fact sheet. https://www.cdc.gov/dhdsp/data_statistics/fact_sheets/fs_women_heart.htm. (Accessed 22 August 2018).

CHAPTER 103

HEART FAILURE

Barbara G. Rosato

 Immediate referral is indicated for new onset of heart failure (acute or worsening dyspnea) in patients with no previous history of heart disease or acute decompensation of heart failure.

DEFINITION AND EPIDEMIOLOGY

Heart failure (HF) is a complex syndrome characterized by the inability of the heart to meet the body's metabolic demands; it is a clinical diagnosis. It results from any structural or functional cardiac disorder that impairs the ventricle's ability to fill or to eject blood properly. While the terms have been used interchangeably, cardiomyopathy and left ventricular dysfunction contribute to the development of HF.[1] HF has been divided into two main types:

1. HFrEF: HF with reduced ejection fraction of 40% or lower, notable for a reduction in the contractility of the left ventricle. Left ventricular systolic dysfunction is often associated with clinical symptoms when the left ventricular ejection fraction (LVEF) falls below 40%, resulting in pump failure.

HFrEF has historically been associated with symptomatic HF, and is also known as systolic HF.

2. HFpEF: HF with preserved ejection fraction of 50% or higher, associated with impairment of ventricular filling and relaxation, wherein the left ventricular filling pressures are often high, resulting in a reduced stroke volume with exertion, causing HF symptoms. HFpEF now accounts for approximately 50% of all patients with HF.[2]

Given the current definitions by EF, a "gray area" exists. There is consideration of an intermediary category based on an EF between reduced and preserved EF. HF of mid-range ejection fraction (HFmrEF) is characterized by an LVEF of 40% to 49% and features of both systolic and diastolic dysfunction.[3] An understanding of this category allows for guideline-directed medical therapy.

Coronary artery disease is the most common cause of HFrEF, while hypertension, atrial fibrillation (AF), and diabetes are common antecedents of HFpEF. It has been hypothesized that HFpEF may be more than just one problem (Table 103.1).

Etiology

The etiology of HF can be divided into the following three broad categories:

1. Anatomic or functional abnormalities of the coronary vessels, myocardium, or cardiac valves, of either sudden or gradual onset affecting the contractility of the heart
2. Neurohormonal overexpression that causes activation of the adrenergic nervous system and renin-angiotensin-aldosterone system (RAAS)
3. Extracardiac factors that cause excessive demand on the cardiovascular system.[2]

The most common diseases associated with HF are coronary artery disease, hypertension, and dilated cardiomyopathies (Box 103.1). Most forms of heart disease predispose the patient to HF over time; viral, metabolic, and toxic insults to the myocardium can cause acute symptomatic HF that may become chronic if left untreated. Early diagnosis and treatment can improve quality of life and life expectancy for people who have HF.

Cardiomyopathy. Cardiomyopathy, the most common cause of HF, is a disease process of the myocardium that affects the heart's pumping ability in the absence of other cardiovascular causes, such as coronary artery disease, hypertension, valvular heart disease, or congenital heart disease.[4] A classic definition for cardiomyopathies notes the complexity of the process to include mechanical and electrical dysfunction that results in hypertrophy or dilation of the myocardium.[5] Classification of cardiomyopathies is based on structure and function of the heart muscle. Classifications include dilated cardiomyopathy (DCM), hypertrophic cardiomyopathy (HCM), restrictive cardiomyopathy (RCM), and arrhythmogenic cardiomyopathy. Further differentiation reflects the cause of the cardiomyopathy, such as systemic disorders, infection, inflammation, inherited, and idiopathic. Amyloidosis is an underdiagnosed cause of heart failure and should be a consideration especially in patients with HFpEF and low-voltage EKG, and hypertrophy on echo, but not on EKG.

Clarification is made between nonischemic versus ischemic cardiomyopathy, as in the situation of coronary artery disease, to guide treatment and prognosis.[5] Furthermore, staging cardiomyopathies based on phenotype (M), organ involvement (O), genetic transmission (G), pathogenesis (E), and disease

stage (S) aids clinical providers in identifying patients who are genetically predisposed.[4]

Incidence and Prevalence

HF is a societal epidemic in the United States because of its incidence, prevalence, and high cost. HF is a leading cause of morbidity and mortality due to the aging population and those with cardiovascular disease at risk for developing HF.[6]

TABLE 103.1   HFrEF Versus HFpEF in Heart Failure: Differences in History, Physical Examination Findings, and Diagnostic Test Results[a]

Parameter	HFrEF	HFpEF
HISTORY		
Coronary artery disease	+++	++
Hypertension	++	++++
Diabetes	++	++
Valvular heart disease	++++	+
Paroxysmal dyspnea	++	+++
PHYSICAL EXAMINATION		
Cardiomegaly	+++	+
Soft heart sounds	++++	+
S_3 gallop	+++	+
S_4 gallop	+	+++
Hypertension	++	++++
Mitral regurgitation murmur	+++	+
Rales	++	+
Edema	+++	+
Jugular venous distention	+++	+
CHEST X-RAY EXAMINATION		
Cardiomegaly	+++	+
Pulmonary congestion	+++	+++
ELECTROCARDIOGRAPHY		
Low voltage	+++	−
Left ventricular hypertrophy	++	++++
Q waves	++	+
ECHOCARDIOGRAPHY		
Left atrial enlargement	++	++
Low ejection fraction	++++	−
Left ventricular dilation	++	−
Left ventricular hypertrophy	++	++++

[a]Plus signs indicate "suggestive" (the number reflects relative weight). Minus signs indicate "not very suggestive."
Modified from Young, J. B. (2002). Assessment of heart failure. In W. S. Colucci (Ed.), *Atlas of heart failure: Cardiac function and dysfunction* (3rd ed.). Philadelphia: Current Medicine.

BOX 103.1

Causes of Heart Failure

ANATOMIC OR FUNCTIONAL ABNORMALITIES OF THE CORONARY VESSELS, MYOCARDIUM, OR CARDIAC VALVES

Ischemic heart disease
Valvular heart disease
Pericardial disease
Congenital defects
Chronic tachycardia
Idiopathic cardiomyopathies
- Dilated
- Hypertrophic
- Restricted

EXTRACARDIAC FACTORS THAT CAUSE EXCESSIVE DEMAND ON THE CARDIOVASCULAR SYSTEM

Toxic cardiomyopathy (e.g., alcohol, chemotherapeutic agents)
Hypertension
Endocrine or metabolic disorders (contractility not usually impaired; rather, metabolic demands are in excess of normal cardiac output; volume overload of the left ventricle)

NONCARDIAC DISEASE

Viral illness (parvovirus, cytomegalovirus, Epstein-Barr virus, hepatitis, Lyme disease, varicella, and others)
Thyrotoxicosis
Anemia
Iron overload disease
Pregnancy
Fever, systemic infection
Arteriovenous fistulas
Vitamin B_1 deficiency (beriberi)
Amyloidosis, sarcoidosis

CONNECTIVE TISSUE DISEASES

Systemic lupus erythematosus
Polymyositis
Progressive systemic sclerosis (scleroderma)

PULMONARY DISEASES

Cor pulmonale secondary to chronic obstructive pulmonary disease
Pulmonary hypertension

Data from Funk, M., & Winkler, C. G. (2008). Epidemiology of heart failure. In D. K. Moser, B. Riegel (Ed.), *Cardiac nursing: A companion to Braunwald's heart disease.* St Louis: Elsevier.

There are 960,000 new cases identified each year. The lifetime risk of HF for both men and women is high, between 20% and 45%, respectively, from age 45 to 95.[6] Worldwide, 1% to 2% of the population has HF in developed countries; the prevalence approaches 10% in those older than 70 years.[3] In the United States, the direct and indirect cost of HF by 2030 is estimated to be $70 billion. This total includes the cost of health care services, medications, and lost productivity.[6]

Risk Factors. Many individuals with HF have antecedent hypertension or myocardial infarction (MI). Other risk factors include amyloidosis, coronary artery disease, diabetes mellitus, HIV infection, renal disease, obesity, smoking, and increasing age. African Americans have a higher prevalence of HF than other ethnicities, with an increased prevalence of hypertension, diabetes, and lower socioeconomic status.[6]

PATHOPHYSIOLOGY

HF is a clinical syndrome characterized by signs and symptoms of volume excess. Whereas there can be several causes of the HF, common pathophysiologic mechanisms characterize this important condition. Understanding these mechanisms is critical to selection of successful therapeutic interventions.

Heart Failure With Reduced Ejection Fraction

Systolic dysfunction, which accounts for about half of all HF cases, is a decrease in both ejection fraction (40% or less) and cardiac output. In systolic dysfunction, when looking at a hemodynamic model, the three determinants of ventricular function—preload, contractility, and afterload—are usually altered. Preload is the degree of myocardial fiber stretch at the end of ventricular filling. When the heart ejects subnormally, there is an increased volume of blood left in the ventricular chambers (increased left ventricular end-systolic volume). This excess volume leads to distention of the ventricles and increased interventricular pressure at the onset of diastole. Filling must then occur at higher pressures during diastole. At small increases of volume and pressure, nonfailing myocardial fibers have the intrinsic property of increasing their force of contraction in an attempt to "revert" the subsequent volume and pressure conditions of both heart ejection and filling back to normal. This intrinsic property also enables the heart to maintain cardiac output during states of pressure or volume overload. However, in the failing heart, the failing myocardial fibers are both excessively overloaded and stretched beyond lengths commensurate with the normal reflex-increased force of contraction. This results in left ventricular remodeling, with dilation and impaired contractility, and activation of the sympathetic and RAASs. The ventricular dysfunction in HFrEF is accompanied by a decrease in myocardial contractility, a reduction in ejection fraction, and often a reduction in stroke volume and cardiac output. If HF is left untreated, symptoms develop and worsen, with declining functional capacity, recurrent acute decompensated events, life-threatening arrhythmias, and pump failure. Effective treatment of HF, primarily pharmacotherapy, depends on the interruption of left ventricular remodeling and the pathophysiologic processes that accompany it.

Afterload is the amount of left ventricular wall tension that develops during systole; it is determined by both the size of the ventricular chamber and the dynamic vascular resistance against which the heart contracts. According to Laplace's law, an increase in the radius of the ventricle results in an increase in wall tension. Because systolic blood pressure closely approximates afterload, it is a clinically important indicator of myocardial load or afterload. The LVEF is a function of afterload and an afterload-dependent measure of contractility. Chronic elevation of cardiac afterload can lead to ventricular enlargement, reduction in ejection fraction, and reduction in stroke volume and cardiac output. Several systemic mechanisms exist for the body to compensate for the reduction in cardiac output. Early on, these compensatory mechanisms serve to increase cardiac output and tissue perfusion. In the long run, however, they lead to further cardiac injury and further decompensation.[2]

Heart Failure With Preserved Ejection Fraction

The prevalence of HFpEF has increased dramatically. Controversy surrounds the true cause(s) of HFpEF. One mechanism believed responsible is increased ventricular stiffness and reduced compliance of the left ventricle, which produces a rise in cardiac filling pressures during diastole. Left ventricular distensibility is reduced during part or all of diastole, and filling pressures must increase to maintain a constant ventricular volume. Whereas filling pressures in the left ventricle are increased during rest and exercise, the failure of a normal rise in cardiac output during exertion results in characteristic symptoms of HF, particularly dyspnea. The heart attempts to initially compensate for this impaired distensibility through the "booster" effect of augmented left atrial contraction, resulting over time in left atrial dilation.

The incidence of HFpEF increases with age and is more prevalent in older adult women. Recent studies have suggested that proinflammatory conditions such as hypertension, obesity, diabetes, smoking, and COPD lead to cardiac muscle inflammation and subsequent fibrosis.[7] The most common factors associated with HFpEF are hypertension, ischemia resulting from coronary artery disease, aortic stenosis, and infiltrative or restrictive myocardial diseases.[3]

Compensatory Mechanisms

Several interrelated compensatory mechanisms attempt to maintain normal ventricular contractility, ventricular pressures, cardiac output, and blood pressure. The three primary compensatory mechanisms are increased sympathetic adrenergic activity with a resultant increase in circulating neurohormones, neuroendocrine activation of the RAAS, and ventricular remodeling. In addition, as HF progresses, neurohormonal alterations in peripheral vasculature and renal function occur. Sodium and water retention through the renal tubules results in decreased renal perfusion and rising blood urea nitrogen and creatinine concentrations, broadly called cardiorenal syndrome, which can be chronic or acute. The same compensatory mechanisms in early and acute stages gradually fail as HF progresses, and they are responsible for the eventual deterioration in cardiac function.[2]

Sympathetic Adrenergic Activity. Baroreceptors and chemoreceptors in the heart and vascular system, sensitive to stretch, pH, and CO_2, help regulate blood pressure. Cardiac reflexes regulate heart rate. Abnormalities in both baroreceptor and cardiac reflexes have been documented in HF.[2] In a healthy heart, stimulation of the baroreceptor reflex results in activation of the parasympathetic nervous system and inhibition of the sympathetic nervous system. Heart rate and systemic vascular resistance are reduced, and normal blood pressure and cardiac output are maintained.

In HF, however, a decrease in cardiac output leads to activation of the sympathetic nervous system and blunting of the baroreceptor reflex. The result is an elevation in heart rate, compensating for low cardiac output in an attempt to maintain perfusion to vital organs. As HF progresses, further depression of the baroreceptor function leads to greater sympathetic overactivity despite intense vasoconstriction and volume retention.

Increasing activation of the sympathetic nervous system stimulates release of catecholamines from cardiac adrenergic nerves and the adrenal medulla; this in turn causes vasoconstriction in less metabolically active organs (e.g., skin, kidneys). It

results in venoconstriction, which increases preload by increasing venous return. Catecholamines also affect the cardiac cells, producing an increased myocardial oxygen demand, myocyte hypertrophy, and tissue necrosis. Progressive HF occurs as cardiac cells progressively enlarge and die. As a result of sympathetic activation, plasma norepinephrine levels are elevated. The degree of plasma norepinephrine elevation correlates with the severity of HF and may be predictive of mortality.[8]

Neuroendocrine Activation. Two additional vasoconstrictor systems act as compensatory mechanisms and therefore are affected by HF: the RAAS and arginine vasopressin. The RAAS is activated by a decline in blood pressure in the renal juxtaglomerular cells, which causes an increase in the release of the enzyme renin. The release of these hormones causes maladaptive remodeling of the ventricles; blockade of these hormones has been found to be beneficial in HF treatment.[2] The natriuretic peptides, brain natriuretic peptide (BNP) and amino-terminal pro-B-type natriuretic peptide (NT-proBNP), promote vasodilation, diuresis, and regulation of cardiac remodeling. As a result of activation of RAAS and sympathetic nervous system causing increased wall stress, the natriuretic peptides are released and eventually broken down by neutral endopeptidase, neprilysin.[9]

Ventricular Remodeling. Cardiac remodeling is an alteration in both the structure and function of the heart as a response to cardiac injury or hemodynamic strain in association with neurohormonal activation. Remodeling can be physiologic (adaptive; as in the case of pregnant women and trained athletes) or pathologic (maladaptive; in disease states). Both myocardial hypertrophy and dilation occur in varying degrees as a progressive process, even in the absence of further myocardial injury, infection, or ischemic events.[10]

Dilation is a result of an increase in the ventricular end-diastolic volume and represents an early compensatory response in volume overload in an attempt to increase contractility and to preserve cardiac output. With an ischemic event, there is a loss of cardiomyocytes, leading to a thinning of the cardiac wall and decreased contractile activity. Dilation preserves stroke volume and maintains cardiac output, but it also significantly increases wall stress, which increases myocardial oxygen demand, a deleterious condition if significant coronary artery disease is present. As a result of injury and death of the cardiac cells as well as excessive wall stress, an inflammatory response is triggered creating fibrosis of cardiac tissue.[10]

The condition of ventricular hypertrophy is a direct result of attempts to compensate for the increase in wall stress.[10] With hypertrophy, the cardiac myocytes eventually enlarge leading to ventricular wall thickening and impaired contractility. Hypertrophy also increases the force of the ventricular contraction. Persistent wall stress promotes decompensation of the myocardium. An inflammatory response of increased cytokine activity is being investigated as a trigger for creating fibrosis, suggesting another component of ventricular remodeling.[10]

CLINICAL PRESENTATION

HF is associated with a constellation of symptoms, the result of heart muscle damage and the body's physiologic response mechanisms. A careful history and review of symptoms are extremely important because they yield clues to the cause of HF; HF should never be the only diagnosis (Box 103.2). Clinical presentation of HF is wide ranging, from mild, exertionally related dyspnea resulting from fluid retention to cardiogenic

BOX 103.2

Critical Components of a Patient's History That Assist With Diagnosis and Management of Heart Failure

- History of HF (American Heart Association [AHA]/American college of Cardiology [ACC] stage C)
- Known coronary artery disease
- History of high blood pressure
- History of or current arrhythmias
- History of hypertension
- Family history of cardiomyopathy, sudden cardiac death, coronary artery disease
- Recent viral illness, fevers
- Travel outside of the United States (particularly Mexico or South American countries)
- Any history of Lyme disease, tuberculosis, human immunodeficiency virus (HIV) infection, hepatitis; recent rashes
- History of substance use (e.g., heavy alcohol use, diet pills, cocaine, cigarettes)
- Any medications that could exacerbate volume status, such as nonsteroidal antiinflammatory drugs (NSAIDs), prednisone
- History of any chemotherapy or any radiation therapy to the chest
- Recent pregnancy
- History of autoimmune disease (sarcoid, amyloid, thyroid disease)
- Recent extreme stress

REVIEW OF SYSTEMS
- Presence of fatigue
- Lightheadedness or dizziness
- Syncope or presyncope
- Dyspnea on exertion
- Dyspnea at rest
- Orthopnea
- Paroxysmal nocturnal dyspnea
- Cough
- Chest pain, heaviness, or tightness
- Palpitations
- Abdominal bloating or fullness
- Loss of appetite
- Weight gain (or loss)
- Edema or swelling

CLASSIFICATION OF HEART FAILURE

Symptoms and activity limitations have been quantified to assist in classifying a patient's status and guiding therapy. The American College of Cardiology (ACC) and the American Heart Association (AHA) have devised a classification system that grades HF by stage (Table 103.3) to include patients at risk for the development of HF (stage A) and those with end-stage, advanced disease (stage D). Complementary to the ACC/AHA staging system is the New York Heart Association (NYHA) classification, which illuminates the patient's reported functional status and symptom burden. As an example, a patient with a prior history of HF who experiences shortness of breath while making the bed may be assigned to ACC/AHA stage C and NYHA class III HF.[1]

PHYSICAL EXAMINATION

The examination of a patient of HF is preceded by a careful history. Assessment of perfusion and volume status gives clues to the degree of decompensation or the management of HF. Signs of volume overload, reduced cardiac output, enlarged heart, and arrhythmia must be considered.[12] Important elements include assessing jugular venous distention, narrow pulse pressure, apical pulse displacement, heart sounds for S3 gallop and cardiac murmur, adventitious lung sounds, and edema (Table 103.4).[3]

DIAGNOSTICS

There is no single diagnostic test for HF, largely because it is a clinical spectrum that is based primarily on a careful history and examination. The diagnostic evaluation should be aimed at those studies necessary to determine the type and degree of ventricular dysfunction (primarily systolic or diastolic), to uncover correctable causes of cardiomyopathy, to determine prognosis, and to guide treatment.

INITIAL DIAGNOSTICS

DYSPNEA
Laboratory
- Brain natriuretic peptide or pro-BNP
- Serum electrolytes
- Magnesium[a]
- Renal function

Imaging
- Echocardiogram
- Chest radiograph
- Electrocardiogram

[a]If indicated

shock and lethal arrhythmias. Cardinal symptoms of HF are dyspnea and fatigue, often but not always associated with volume overload.[11]

The cardinal symptoms of dyspnea and fatigue and the typical signs of HF, such as lower extremity edema and jugular venous distention, are nonspecific and must be evaluated along with a patient's history, review of symptoms, and physical examination findings, corroborated by further cardiac investigations. Patients may describe symptoms of paroxysmal nocturnal dyspnea and orthopnea as well as shortness of breath with exertion or at rest. Some people experience abdominal fullness or bloating along with lack of appetite (Table 103.2).[1] The 2013 HF guidelines suggest the usefulness of a multivariate risk score to estimate subsequent risk of mortality in both ambulatory and hospitalized patients with HF.[1]

When HF is suspected, the diagnostic evaluation is preceded by a history and physical examination, followed by an assessment of cardiac structure and function. Patients should be evaluated for coronary disease and ischemia. In addition, important aspects in the diagnostic evaluation of each patient with HF are establishment of the risk of arrhythmia, identification of exacerbating factors (e.g., anemia, ischemia, or infection) for HF, and diagnosis of any comorbidities. Echocardiography, chest radiography, electrocardiography, cardiac catheterization, cardiac magnetic resonance imaging (MRI), positron emission tomography–computed tomography (PET/

TABLE 103.2 **Symptoms of Heart Failure**

Symptoms	Why It Happens	What Patients With Heart Failure May Describe
Shortness of breath (dyspnea)	Pressure is increased in the pulmonary veins because the heart cannot keep up with the supply. This can cause pulmonary congestion or pulmonary edema (interstitial and alveolar congestion), which leads to left ventricular overload and worsening symptoms of failure.	Breathlessness during activity, at rest, or while sleeping (called paroxysmal nocturnal dyspnea); these symptoms worsen with severity of heart failure (HF). Difficulty breathing while lying flat (orthopnea) or complaints of waking up tired or feeling anxious and restless.
Persistent coughing, bronchospasm, or wheezing	Persistent pulmonary interstitial or alveolar edema (sometimes called cardiac asthma), worsen when recumbent.	Coughing that produces white or pink blood-tinged mucus may not always be present.
Edema	As blood flow out of the heart is impeded, blood returning to the heart through the veins backs up, causing fluid to build up in the tissues. The kidneys are less able to dispose of sodium and water, also causing fluid retention. This is evidence of right-sided HF.	Swelling in the feet, ankles, legs, or abdomen or weight gain. Patients may find that their pants or shoes feel tight.
Tiredness, fatigue	The heart cannot pump enough blood to meet the needs of body tissues, resulting in decreased oxygen saturation. The body's normal vascular response to exercise is altered; blood is diverted away from less vital organs, particularly muscles in the limbs, and sent to the heart and brain. Muscle deconditioning plays a role here as well. Loss of potassium induced by increased aldosterone also leads to muscle fatigue.	Tired feeling all the time and difficulty with everyday activities, such as shopping, climbing stairs, carrying groceries, or walking.
Lack of appetite, nausea	The digestive system receives less blood, causing problems with digestion. Medications, particularly diuretics, may be poorly absorbed. Hepatic congestion may often lead to discomfort.	Feeling of being full or nauseated, or loss of appetite.
Confusion, impaired thinking, lightheadedness	Changing levels of certain substances in the blood, such as sodium, can cause confusion. Poor cardiac output with decreased perfusion to the brain may also cause these symptoms.	Memory loss and feelings of disorientation; a caregiver or relative may notice this first.
Increased heart rate	Compensatory mechanism for the loss in stroke volume; the heart beats faster.	Heart palpitations, described by patients as a sensation that the heart is racing or throbbing.
Nocturia	Nocturnal diuresis lessens the degree of fluid retention. Nocturnal diuresis results from fluid reabsorption and redistribution in the supine position as well as a reduction in renal vasoconstriction that occurs at rest.	Patient reported; diuretics confound the picture.

CT), blood hematology, serum laboratory testing, and, in selected cases, exercise tolerance testing are common diagnostic tests used in the evaluation of patients with HF.

The initial evaluation of the patient with symptoms of HF includes the hematology and serum laboratory tests listed in Table 103.5. B-type (brain) natriuretic peptide (BNP), combined with history, physical examination findings, other values such as echocardiographic indices, and cardiovascular risk factors, augments the assessment of patients with suspected HF and is recommended as a screening test in all patients with suspected HF.[1]

Essential Diagnostics

Brain Natriuretic Peptide. In the setting of dyspnea and volume overload, evidence suggests natriuretic peptide biomarkers can support the diagnosis or exclusion of HF in both the ambulatory and acute care settings.[13] B-type (brain)

natriuretic peptide (BNP) is a peptide synthesized and secreted almost exclusively by ventricular myocardial cells in response to elevations in end-diastolic pressure and volume. BNP is a substrate of neprilysin and cannot be interpreted if the patient is taking an angiotensin receptor neprilysin inhibitor (ARNI), one of the newer classes of medications to treat HFrEF.[9] Rather, the NT-proBNP should be used. BNP has higher sensitivity than specificity and thus can be helpful to rule out HF[13] and both have high negative predictive value. Evidence demonstrates, for patients at high risk for HF, a screening BNP $\geq$ 50 pg/mL can guide early identification and treatment of HF.[13] BNP levels can be increased with age, acute coronary syndrome, AF, anemia, COPD, pulmonary HTN, pneumonia, sepsis, valvular disease and renal dysfunction, but may be lower in obese patients.[3]

Laboratory Studies. Other laboratory tests search for the etiology of the presentation or exacerbation of HF. These include complete blood cell count, urinalysis, serum

TABLE 103.3 Classification of Heart Failure

NEW YORK HEART ASSOCIATION FUNCTIONAL CLASSIFICATION

Class I	No limitations. Ordinary physical activity does not cause undue fatigue, dyspnea, or palpitations.
Class II	Slight limitation of physical activity. Such patients are comfortable at rest. Ordinary physical activity results in fatigue, palpitations, dyspnea, or angina.
Class III	Marked limitation of physical activity. Although patients are comfortable at rest, less than ordinary activity will lead to symptoms.
Class IV	Inability to carry on any physical activity without discomfort. Symptoms are present even at rest. With any physical activity, discomfort is experienced or increased.

ACC/AHA HEART FAILURE STAGES

Stage A	At high risk for heart failure (HF) with no identified structural or functional abnormality; no signs or symptoms.
Stage B	With structural heart disease that is strongly associated with the development of HF but without signs or symptoms.
Stage C	Symptomatic HF associated with underlying structural abnormalities.
Stage D	Advanced structural cardiac disease and marked symptoms of HF at rest with maximal medical therapy or requiring advanced therapies.

Data from Yancy, C. W., Jessup, M., Bozkurt, B., Butler, J., Casey, D. E., Jr, Drazner, M. H., et al. (2013). 2013 ACCF/AHA guideline for the management of heart failure: a report of the American College of Cardiology Foundation/American Heart Association Task Force on Practice Guidelines. *Journal of the American College of Cardiology, 62*(13), e147–e239.

electrolytes, blood urea nitrogen, serum creatinine, glucose, fasting lipid profile, liver function tests, thyroid-stimulating hormone, and possibly HIV testing for new-onset heart failure. Other biomarkers include cardiac troponin to assess for myocardial injury related to CAD or chronic HF. Elevated troponin levels, in acute or chronic HF, are associated with increased mortality.[1] Both BNP and cardiac troponins have been useful to establish a prognosis of chronic and acute HF, respectively, though BNP can be lower in obese patients and elevated in a variety of other conditions.[13]

Echocardiography. The value of echocardiography cannot be overestimated in the diagnostic evaluation of suspected HF. It represents the single most effective tool in widespread clinical use for the assessment of HF.

Approximately 50% of patients with HF have left ventricular systolic dysfunction, defined as a LVEF of less than 40%. Transthoracic Doppler echocardiography is rapid and safe and provides information about biventricular systolic performance, wall thickness, and chamber dimensions as well as segmental or regional wall motion abnormalities and valvular function. Evaluation of the mitral, tricuspid, and aortic valves with regurgitation grading is important, as is a determination of estimated pulmonary artery pressures from secondary tricuspid

regurgitation. LVEF is determined. Diastolic function can often be detected as well; Doppler echocardiography allows the characterization of abnormal left ventricular filling in diastole. The ACC and AHA guidelines recognize echocardiography as the preferred diagnostic tool for evaluation of the cause of HF.[1]

Evaluation for myocardial ischemia should be considered in most patients who have developed new left ventricular systolic dysfunction by echocardiography. Referral to a cardiologist is recommended. The evaluation modality ultimately chosen depends on pretest probability of disease and whether the patient is a candidate for an intervention.

Electrocardiography. An electrocardiogram should be obtained as part of the assessment of patients with possible HF. It may be a useful diagnostic test in the workup of patients thought to have HF to assist in evaluation of heart rhythm, presence of wide QRS (left ventricular bundle branch block) or left ventricular hypertrophy, and evidence of MI or ongoing ischemia.

Chest Radiography. In patients with a new diagnosis of HF, a chest radiograph (posteroanterior and lateral) is recommended.[1] The size and shape of the cardiac silhouette and the presence of interstitial and alveolar edema comprise the radiologic evidence of HF. A common chest radiographic finding in HF is cardiomegaly, with a cardiothoracic ratio (the ratio of the diameter of the heart at its widest point to the maximum width of the thoracic cavity; the normal ratio is less than 1:2) that is increased more than 50%. This ratio is non-specific, and widespread use of echocardiography has rendered chest radiography less important and insensitive for the diagnosis of HF.

Additional Diagnostics

Exercise or Stress Testing for Heart Failure. The exercise test, or stress test, for functional capacity is not currently recommended as part of the routine evaluation for HF. It is sometimes done as part of a pre–cardiac transplantation workup to evaluate symptoms that are disparate from what other objective indicators would suggest or to distinguish between cardiac and pulmonary causes of symptoms. It is sometimes used in disability determinations.

Cardiac Catheterization. Clinical information gleaned from cardiac catheterization and measurement of hemodynamics is invaluable in patients with HF who have advanced symptoms or suboptimum response to medical therapy. Hemodynamic evaluation or right-sided heart catheterization provides hemodynamic measurements and assessments along with a measurement of cardiac output, which can guide medical therapy and provide data to identify the timing of valvular surgery. It is useful when patients have respiratory distress and impaired perfusion and when determination of volume status is uncertain based on clinical assessment. Left-sided heart catheterization (coronary artery angiography) is reasonable to diagnose the presence, extent, and severity of coronary artery disease when ischemia may be contributing to HF.[1]

Cardiac Magnetic Resonance Imaging

Cardiac MRI is becoming an important imaging technique for the diagnosis of myocardial infiltrative processes and scar burden. Cardiac MRI allows a reproducible and accurate evaluation of myocardial morphology, function, perfusion, and tissue damage in a noninvasive way. If there is suspicion of an infiltrative disease process or uncertainty about scar burden,

TABLE 103.4   **Signs of Heart Failure**

Sign	Indicates	Physical Examination
Jugular venous distention	An index of right atrial pressure; when elevated, it is an indicator of volume overload. (Tricuspid regurgitation may alter the examination findings.) With normal pressure, the upper level of visible jugular vein is approximately 4 cm above the sternal notch.	With the patient at a 45-degree angle, note the upper limit of visible pulse in the internal jugular. In some patients, this pressure may be normal at rest, but it rises to abnormal levels with compression of the right upper quadrant. This sign is known as the hepatojugular or abdominal jugular reflex. The internal or external jugular vein is compressed in the supraclavicular fossa, and as the examiner's finger strips the vein cephalad, blood rises in the more proximal portion of the vein; the height of this blood volume above the patient's clavicles reflects the central venous pressure. The height of the venous column normally falls during inspiration as a result of the accompanying decrease in intrathoracic pressure.
Crackles, frothy or pink sputum, pleural effusions	Pulmonary fluid transudate moves to interstitial spaces and alveoli, usually in lung bases because of gravity. Pulmonary edema. Occur with volume overload—transudative.	Lung examination. Dull or absent breath sounds.
Third heart sound	Early diastolic rapid ventricular filling associated with left ventricular systolic dysfunction.	S_3 is best heard with patient in left lateral position.
Fourth heart sound	Overdistention of ventricles during late diastole as the stiff ventricles expand further to accommodate final diastolic filling by atrial contraction (atrial "kick").	Best heard with patient in left lateral position; absence of S_3 suggests early failure or the presence of diastolic dysfunction.
Aortic stenosis	Small volume, high velocity.	Harsh murmur, usually loud.
Mitral regurgitation	Large volume, low turbulent flow.	Soft holosystolic murmur.
Tricuspid regurgitation	Large volume in right ventricle.	Hepatic congestion, edema, ascites.
Hepatomegaly, right upper quadrant tenderness	Liver enlargement or stretching of the hepatic capsule.	Right upper quadrant tenderness indicates enlarged or tender liver.
Ascites, anasarca, or edema	Caused by volume overload.	Edema of subcutaneous tissue may be found in abdomen, chest, buttocks. Ascites may be suggested by protuberant abdomen, but the examination is not reliable. Pitting or firm edema of lower extremities is common in heart failure (HF).
Altered hemodynamics	Changes in cardiac output by stroke volume and heart rate.	May appear with symptoms and signs of low output, such as lightheadedness, impaired cognition, tachycardia, cool extremities, hypotension.
Tachycardia	Changes in heart rate caused by arrhythmia or activation of baroreceptors, which in turn activate sympathetic nervous system. These compensatory mechanisms along with the renin-angiotensin-aldosterone and vasopressin release help modulate heart rate early on with a drop in pressure. Ultimately tachycardia will ensue, unless it is masked by medication (such as β blockers, digoxin, calcium channel blockers).	Heart rate measurement; evaluation of rhythm is important.
Displaced point of maximal impulse	Displacement of the palpable apical impulse away from the midclavicular line toward the anterior axillary line indicates left ventricular enlargement.	The palpable apical impulse should be a quick tap, narrow in distribution, not more than 1 to 2 cm (⅖ to ⅘ inch) in diameter. An impulse that is palpable with the palm of the hand, lasts longer, or is forceful indicates increased cardiac output or ventricular hypertrophy. Palpable impulse may be elicited with the palm placed on the sternum. This finding is a right ventricular tap or heave, indicating right ventricular enlargement and volume overload.
Hypotension, cool extremities	Caused by low cardiac output; sometimes medication related.	Blood pressure measurement.

TABLE 103.5   Laboratory Evaluation

Laboratory Test	Comments
Complete blood count	Anemia, iron deficiency, or iron overload can exacerbate heart failure (HF).
Serum electrolytes, including calcium and magnesium	Hyponatremia can be associated with volume overload and diuretic use. Potassium aberrations should be detected and corrected. Helpful before initiation of aldosterone antagonist. Abnormalities in calcium or magnesium may aggravate or induce arrhythmias.
Blood urea nitrogen and serum creatinine	Before initiation of angiotensin-converting enzyme (ACE) inhibitors. Renal function may be altered in HF because of poor renal perfusion, medications, age, or diabetes.
Lipid profile	Risk factor modification.
Fasting blood glucose concentration or glycohemoglobin level	Diabetes.
Urinalysis	Evaluate for proteinuria, evidence of kidney disease.
Liver function tests	Hepatic congestion may cause abnormalities.
Serum albumin	Low albumin level may cause edema.
Thyroid-stimulating hormone	Hypothyroidism or hyperthyroidism can lead to HF.
Brain natriuretic peptide (BNP) or pro-BNP	See Diagnostics.

MRI may be useful. Currently, use of MRI is not widespread, and it is recommended only if other imaging techniques are not diagnostically satisfactory.

Positron Emission Tomography–Computed Tomography

PET/CT is currently an accepted standard in noninvasive imaging of coronary perfusion in patients with suspected or known coronary artery disease. PET/CT allows accurate noninvasive clinical decision-making about coronary artery disease. Because of its high negative predictive value, PET/CT is playing an important role in noninvasive selection of coronary artery disease patients for revascularization. It is not mentioned in the ACCF/AHA guidelines specifically.[1]

Endomyocardial Biopsy. The role of right ventricular endomyocardial biopsy in the diagnostic evaluation is not well defined. The ACCF/AHA 2013 guidelines suggest performing it if it might be deemed useful.[1]

Differential Diagnosis

 Priority differentials include (1) acute myocardial infarction or ischemia, (2) pulmonary emboli, (3) acute decompensation heart failure, (4) tachyarrhythmia, and (5) pneumonia.

Dyspnea is a common presenting symptom in primary care. Initial evaluation of the patient with dyspnea is to determine the severity of the dyspnea; acute symptoms require immediate evaluation. Dyspnea is most commonly caused by underlying respiratory or cardiac disease but can also be associated with other conditions, such as metabolic diseases, psychogenic disorders, mechanical obstruction, and neuromuscular diseases. Therefore systematic evaluation of dyspnea is critical for proper diagnosis of the underlying disease.

Cardiac Conditions

Myocardial ischemia or infarct must be ruled out with biomarkers and electrocardiogram. Dyspnea is a known anginal equivalent in many patients who have coronary artery disease but who lack classic anginal symptoms. Women and persons with diabetes, in particular, frequently do not have classic anginal symptoms of chest pain but will have dyspnea or dyspnea on exertion. In addition, valvular disorders, pericardial disease, cardiac arrhythmias amyloid heart disease and HIV-associated cardiomyopathy can also cause dyspnea. A careful history and negative physical examination findings suggestive of HF (e.g., elevated jugular venous pressure, edema, S_3) can lead the clinician to further focused diagnostic testing or cardiology consultation for more extensive evaluation.

Pulmonary Conditions

Pulmonary Emboli. Pulmonary embolism is a common and potentially deadly medical condition that may mimic the acute dyspnea of pulmonary edema. However, the symptoms of pulmonary embolism may be subtle and range from none to mild dyspnea with pleuritic chest pain to cardiac arrest. The most common cause of a pulmonary embolus is lower extremity deep venous thrombosis, which can cause unilateral leg pain and swelling that can suggest embolus as a cause of chest pain and dyspnea. Patients at risk for pulmonary embolus include those with previous thrombosis or hereditary factors (hypercoagulable states); those with acquired factors, such as prolonged immobility, cardiac disorders (AF, prosthetic cardiac valve), obesity, hormonal therapy, and malignant neoplasms; and postoperative patients. In pulmonary embolus, arterial blood gas analysis may show hypoxemia, but this is nondiagnostic. Diagnostic tools that can be used in the evaluation of suspected pulmonary embolus include a moderately sensitive D-dimer assay, which has a high negative predictive value in low-probability patients; a ventilation/perfusion scan, which exhibits ventilation/perfusion mismatch in a pulmonary embolus; and a helical CT scan of the chest.[3]

Chronic Pulmonary Disease. The dyspnea of HF might be confused with chronic pulmonary conditions. The most common obstructive disorders are chronic obstructive pulmonary disease (COPD), chronic bronchitis, and asthma; restrictive disorders include underlying pulmonary diseases (e.g., interstitial fibrosis) and extrapulmonary causes (e.g., obesity and thoracospinal abnormalities). COPD represents a spectrum of disease severity and pathophysiologic changes and is a common comorbidity in patients with HF. Mortality and morbidity rates in patients with coexistent HF and COPD are high, and these patients present unique diagnostic and management issues.[14]

Orthopnea and paroxysmal nocturnal dyspnea may result from either COPD or HF or a combination of both. These entities may be difficult to identify on the basis of symptom analysis: past medical history, risk for HF, and physical examination findings (sudden weight gain, S_3, S_4, jugular venous distention, peripheral edema) in combination with other symptoms, such as increased fatigue, may help elucidate the cause as HF.

Pleural Effusions

A pleural effusion is an abnormal collection of fluid in the pleural space, which lies between the lung and the chest cavity. Fluid accumulation may result from excess fluid production or decreased absorption and is indicative of underlying disease from pulmonary or nonpulmonary causes. Common causes include HF, infections, malignant disease, and pulmonary embolus.

Dyspnea associated with pleural effusions is usually more chronic in nature. Symptoms may worsen with exertion, and hypoxia may occur in some patients. Pleural effusions produce dyspnea through compression of underlying lung parenchyma and reduction in ventilated lung volume.[14]

Other Diagnostic Considerations

Neuromuscular disorders, such as myasthenia gravis, amyotrophic lateral sclerosis, and Guillain-Barré syndrome, may cause dyspnea by weakness of the respiratory muscles.

Anxiety as the sole cause of dyspnea is uncommon and is always a diagnosis of exclusion. Health care providers must remember that anxiety is common with dyspnea of any cause, adds to the perceived severity, and prolongs the duration of the dyspnea. Many other medical conditions can cause dyspnea and should be included in the differential diagnosis in the evaluation of a patient who has symptoms at rest or with exertion. Anemia, obesity or deconditioning, kyphoscoliosis, and hypersensitivity reactions (allergens, medications) are a few common conditions that should be considered.

INTERPROFESSIONAL COLLABORATIVE MANAGEMENT

Chronic or acute HF requires sufficient diagnostic testing for determination of the specific cause. Coronary artery disease, valvular heart disease, and pericardial disease may be treatable either percutaneously or surgically, mandating appropriate diagnostic studies. Once a specific diagnosis has been made, the first strategy in the treatment of HF is to relieve congestion; next, specific reversible causes are treated. Once reversible causes have been treated, management of the residual HF can be initiated. HF caused by diastolic dysfunction must be differentiated from that caused by systolic dysfunction because treatment options differ; currently, there are evidence-based guidelines for HFrEF but only recommendations for the treatment of HFpEF.

In general, the primary objectives in treatment of HF are fourfold: relief of symptoms and signs, prevention of further myocardial injury, prevention of recurrence of clinical failure (congestive or low output), and improvement in prognosis.[2] Correct selection and application of pharmacologic therapy

require a careful history and physical examination as well as an understanding of the physiologic process of HF.

Use of ACC/AHA Classifications to Guide Therapy

The ACC/AHA classification stages represent a framework for management of left-sided HF (see Table 103.4). In patients assigned to stage A (at high risk, no structural abnormality or symptoms of HF), clear benefit exists for identifying and treating lipid disorders and also hypertension to attain a systolic blood pressure less than 130.[13,15] Standard therapy of angiotensin-converting enzyme (ACE) inhibitor or angiotensin receptor blocker (ARB) for patients with diabetes and other cardiovascular risk factors, as well as control of arrhythmias and tachycardic ventricular rates, can mitigate the development of HF. According to expert consensus opinion, these patients should be screened periodically for signs and symptoms of HF, and primary prevention issues should be addressed: smoking cessation, dietary salt reduction, avoidance of illicit drug use, limitation of alcohol consumption, regular exercise.[1] Recent evidence suggests a screening BNP along with echocardiography for those with risk factors and early intervention by a cardiology team may prevent HF.[13]

For patients assigned to stage B (those with structural heart disease, previous MI, left ventricular systolic dysfunction, and asymptomatic valvular disease, but without symptoms of failure), a screening BNP can be useful.[13] Clear evidence exists for the use of ACE inhibitors, or ARBs if the patient is intolerant of ACE inhibitors, and β blockers, irrespective of the ejection fraction. Valvular repair or replacement for hemodynamically significant stenosis or regurgitation is recommended according to contemporary guidelines outlined by the ACCF/AHA. The use of digoxin for patients with systolic dysfunction in sinus rhythm, in the absence of HF symptoms, is not recommended, nor is the use of calcium channel blockers or nutritional supplements. Patients with ischemic or nonischemic cardiomyopathy who have LVEF of less than 35% and are receiving maximally tolerated medical therapy should be considered for a prophylactic implantable cardioverter-defibrillator (ICD).[1]

Management of patients assigned to stage C (with known structural heart disease and with prior or current symptoms of failure) includes the health promotion measures previously mentioned in conjunction with daily weights, dietary sodium restriction, reduced exercise during periods of acute decompensation, and close monitoring for decompensation. In these patients, nonadherence to prescribed medication and dietary regimens can precipitate rapid deterioration.

Identification and treatment of sleep-disordered breathing and sleep apnea can be beneficial and improve functional status. Cardiac rehabilitation and exercise training may improve overall clinical status in clinically stable patients and may improve functional status, quality of life, and even perhaps mortality.[1]

Avoidance of medications that can adversely affect these patients, such as nonsteroidal antiinflammatory drugs (NSAIDs) and calcium channel blockers, should be stressed. Pharmacologic therapy in stage C typically involves four classes of medications: a diuretic, a renin-angiotensin system inhibitor (an ACE inhibitor, ARB, or ARNI)[13], a β blocker, and an aldosterone antagonist.[1]

In stage C, additional interventions have demonstrated value in selected patients. These include the use of digoxin for symptom control, ivabradine,[13] hydralazine and nitrates, and biventricular pacemakers and ICDs in appropriate patients. Nutritional supplements have not been recommended as part of treatment for any of the HF stages.[1]

Patients assigned to stage D with refractory HF require meticulous control of fluid balance. Clear evidence exists for benefit of ACE inhibitors or ARBs or ARNIs and β blockers. However, the increased role of neurohormonal factors in compensation of severe HF can place stage D patients at risk for hypotension and renal insufficiency with ACE inhibition, as well as at greater risk for increasing failure with β blockade. Hypotension is also common with initiation of ARNIs requiring careful monitoring. Thus these agents should be used with caution in these patients, and dose reductions may be needed. Selected stage D patients may be candidates for specialized interventions, such as circulatory support measures, cardiac transplantation, and left ventricular assist devices (LVADs); these patients need to undergo rigorous evaluation for appropriateness of these advanced therapies. In addition, palliative care measures may include inotropic support and morphine to relieve breathlessness. End-of-life care issues should be addressed early and compassionately, because symptom management becomes a main focus of care in these patients.

Nonpharmacologic Therapy

Education. Patient education regarding self-care principles has been shown to improve medication adherence and understanding of disease process, and reduce hospitalizations. The current ACCF/AHA HF treatment guidelines include self-care education as a class 1 recommendation for patients with HFpEF and HFrEF. Self-care principles, such as smoking cessation, medication compliance, immunization updates, fluid restriction, and daily weight monitoring, should be discussed with all HF patients and reinforced frequently. Patients with sleep apnea should be treated.[1,7,13]

Diet. Reduced-sodium diets have been recommended for the management of HF, although no clinical studies have as yet evaluated a specific sodium restriction. Dietary sodium restriction of 2 to 3 g is advised for HF patients, including those with preserved systolic function and patients with reduced ejection fractions. More rigid dietary sodium restriction (<2 g) may be more appropriate for patients with moderate to severe HF.[1] Most patients with HF can benefit from specific dietary instructions and guidelines on how to read the labels on all food packages. A licensed dietitian with specialized training in HF can be an invaluable asset to the HF patient and family. Involvement of family members who prepare the foods cannot be underestimated; they should be included in all dietary education.

Sudden increases in sodium intake in patients with well-compensated but relatively severe HF can lead to acute decompensation. Holidays and seasonal festivities are particularly a problem because of the alteration in food preparation, increase in daily activity levels, and increase in emotional stressors during these times. Patients with alcohol-induced cardiomyopathy should completely abstain from alcohol. Alcohol is a cardiac toxin; therefore patients with HFrEF should be advised to limit or avoid alcohol completely.[5,12]

Exercise. The benefits of a regular exercise program have been well documented for patients with HFpEF and HFrEF. Evidence suggests a structured exercise program can reduce mortality and hospitalization rates. Patients demonstrated improved exercise tolerance and reported improved health-related quality

of life.[1] It has been suggested that this benefit is a result of improved endothelial function, blunted catecholamine response, and improved peripheral oxygen uptake.

All major societies with HF treatment guidelines include an exercise training recommendation, although a program is not clearly outlined. Guidance has been based on functional capacity and activity that provokes mild to moderate exertion.[3] Thirty minutes of aerobic activity daily should be recommended to patients with stable HF.[7] In 2014, Medicare expanded its coverage to include cardiac rehabilitation programs in patients with LVEF of 35% or lower and NYHA class II to IV symptoms who are on optimal medical therapy for at least 6 weeks, but not for those patients with preserved EF.[7]

Pharmacologic Management

Overview. Pharmacotherapy for the treatment of HF can be subdivided by the pathophysiologic process (HFrEF versus HFpEF) and by the level of symptomatic presentation defined by the NYHA classification system. Whereas evidence-based therapies for the treatment of systolic dysfunction and HF are clearly defined, the treatment of HFpEF remains less clear. In patients with HF in the setting of either reduced LV function or preserved LV function as well as signs and symptoms of volume overload, initial therapy focuses on the relief of symptoms by treatment of volume excess with diuretics. In all patients with HFrEF (ejection fraction ≤40%), with or without evidence of volume overload, ACE inhibitor therapy is recommended. For patients who are intolerant of ACE inhibitors because of cough or other side effects, an ARB or ARNI should be considered. Patients started on an ARNI should be carefully monitored, as hypotension is a common side effects. β blocker therapy is beneficial in all patients with current or prior symptoms of HFrEF. Currently only three β blockers—carvedilol, metoprolol succinate, and bisoprolol—are proven to reduce mortality in patients with HF. In patients who have signs of fluid overload, such as elevated jugular venous pressure, weight gain, or pulmonary crackles, initial therapy should be a diuretic to reduce volume excess and an ACE inhibitor (or ARB). β blocker therapy should not be considered until the patient is decongested and has stabilized. Digoxin is an appropriate therapy for symptom control in patients with HFrEF and has been shown to reduce hospitalizations. Additional drug therapy includes the use of aldosterone antagonists, such as spironolactone for patients who are NYHA functional class II to IV.[1] Although not currently endorsed in the HF management guidelines, there are data to support benefit in patients with NYHA functional class I symptoms.[13] Hydralazine-isosorbide combination therapy is beneficial in the African-American population[1] and in patients intolerant of ACE inhibitors or ARBs. Renal function, potassium level, and other comorbid conditions may affect decisions for therapy.[1]

The 2013 ACCF/AHA guideline for the management of HF recommends blood pressure control (i.e., both systolic and diastolic) according to the currently published practice guidelines in patients with HFpEF. Ventricular rate control in patients with AF is recommended. Diuretic therapy in the setting of volume excess such as pulmonary congestion, peripheral edema, and abdominal bloating is recommended for relief of symptoms.[1]

Angiotensin-Converting Enzyme Inhibitors. The role of the ACE inhibitor emerged from the recognition that neurohormonal activation contributes to the pathogenesis of HF. By suppressing the production of angiotensin II, a potent vasoconstrictor, ACE inhibitors decrease systemic and pulmonary vascular resistance by preventing the release of aldosterone and norepinephrine while elevating the levels of the vasodilator hormone bradykinin. Multiple large randomized trials have shown that ACE inhibitor therapy improves mortality in symptomatic and asymptomatic patients with HFrEF, decreases HF symptoms, and improves overall clinical status. Therefore ACE inhibitor therapy remains the cornerstone of chronic medical management in patients with HFrEF and should be considered a priority in all symptomatic or asymptomatic patients, unless there is an absolute contraindication. ACE inhibitors should be used with caution in patients with prior allergy including anaphylaxis, hyperkalemia, baseline hypotension, bilateral renal artery stenosis, or serum creatinine level greater than 3 mg/dL.[1] There is no creatinine level that absolutely limits the use of ACE inhibitors, although in patients with chronic kidney disease, renal function should be monitored closely. Guidelines suggest that a 50% increase in serum creatinine or a value of 3 mg/dL or estimate glomerular filtration rate of less than 25 mL/min/1.73 m^2 is reasonable to continue. RAAS therapy should be discontinued for doubling of creatinine or a value of 3.5 mg/dL or eGFR of less than 20 mL/min/1.73 m^2.[16] Absolute contraindications also include angioedema associated with ACE inhibitors and pregnancy. Cough can occur as a side effect of ACE inhibitors in close to 20% of treated patients. Although not dangerous, this can be annoying, and alternate therapy with ARBs is often considered.[1] Patients who begin ACE inhibitors should have their blood pressure, renal function, and serum potassium level monitored within 7 to 10 days and then periodically throughout the year. Target doses should be attempted in all patients.

Angiotensin Receptor Blockers. ARBs act directly on the angiotensin-renin-aldosterone system. These agents modify the effects of angiotensin II, the substance that promotes vasoconstriction, abnormal cell growth, and the release of aldosterone, but do not interfere with kinins, resulting in fewer adverse drug reactions.[1] ACE inhibitors remain the first-line choice for inhibition of the renin-angiotensin system, but as a result of multiple trials, ARBs and ARNIs have been endorsed as an effective option for those who are ACE inhibitor intolerant.[13] Cautions, contraindications, and monitoring parameters are similar to those outlined for ACE inhibitors.

Neprilysin Inhibitor. As noted, BNP counters the detrimental effects of RAAS activation, which causes vasoconstriction, sodium and water retention, and aldosterone secretion. Neprilysin inactivates BNP, thus newer strategies include inhibition of this peptide.[9] The PARADIGM-HF trial (Prospective Comparison of ARNI with ACEI to Determine Impact on Global Mortality and Morbidity in Heart Failure) was stopped early because of the significant improvement in survival in patients with LVEF of 40% or below with class II to IV symptoms who were treated with ARB-neprilysin inhibition compared with enalapril.[9] The 2017 ACC/AHA/HFSA Heart Failure guidelines recommend that patients with chronic HF NYHA class II or III be transitioned to an ARNI, if tolerating an ACE-I or ARB, to further reduce morbidity and mortality.[13] As BNP is a substrate of neprilysin, NT-proBNP should be used for monitoring. An ANRI should not be used concurrently with an ACE-I or ARB as the risk for renal impairment, hyperkalemia, and angioedema is increased. For this reason, patients should have a 36-hour window between the last dose of ACE-I or ARB before starting an ANRI. As with other RAAS inhibitors, potassium level and renal function should be monitored frequently.[9] Recent studies have not determined the benefit of an ANRI for HF patients with a preserved EF.

Hydralazine and Oral Nitrates. The 2013 ACCF/AHA Guidelines for the Management of Heart failure state that hydralazine combined with oral nitrate is an appropriate alternative for patients who are unable to tolerate ACE inhibitors.[1] In addition, there are data to support the use of this combination in addition to standard HF treatment in the African-American population. Studies have shown a reduction in mortality and hospitalizations in this population of patients.[3]

Hydralazine is a direct arteriolar vasodilator, and isosorbide dinitrate is a venodilator. The combination of these agents results in an increase in cardiac output secondary to decreased impedance to ventricular ejection and decreased preload. Side effects include headache, palpitations, gastrointestinal (GI) issues, and nasal congestion. Compliance with this regimen has been problematic because of these side effects and the three-times-daily administration, with large number of tablets required with uptitration. Initiation of both drugs is at low doses with weekly uptitration as tolerated.[1]

Mineralocorticoid Receptor/Aldosterone Antagonists. Aldosterone contributes to the detrimental neurohormonal activation that is associated with ACE and the renin-angiotensin system. Interrupting this effect leads to improved endothelial function and reduced left ventricular remodeling as well as positive effects on heart rate variability and ventricular arrhythmias. For HFrEF, several studies suggest a benefit of a mineralocorticoid receptor antagonist (MRA), such as spironolactone or eplerenone, to reduce hospitalizations, morbidity, and morality.[17] Unfortunately, the same benefit was not realized for HF patients with preserved EF.[18] Use of these agents promotes hyperkalemia and requires careful patient selection, initiation, and monitoring. Concomitant potassium supplementation should be avoided. Interruption in therapy or discontinuation may be necessary for worsening renal function or acute kidney injury. Renal function and potassium concentration should be carefully monitored within 7 days after initiation or increase of therapy periodically thereafter to minimize the risk of hyperkalemia or renal impairment. When initiating a MRA, creatinine should be less than 2.0 mg/dL or less than 2.5 mg/dL (or eGFR > 30 mL/min) for women and men, respectively, and potassium level is less than 5.0 mEq/L.[13] Gynecomastia or breast tenderness occurs in approximately 10% of patients using spironolactone. This is less frequent with eplerenone.[1,17]

Diuretics. Diuretics are used to relieve symptoms of systemic and pulmonary congestion caused by volume overload in both systolic and diastolic HF. Many factors contribute to the sodium and water retention that causes volume overload in HF. Diuretics promote sodium and fluid excretion, thus relieving both the symptoms and the accompanying signs of volume overload.

Initial therapy with a thiazide diuretic or low-dose loop diuretic may be appropriate in mild HF. A loop diuretic, which is more potent, is more efficacious when taken on an empty stomach, and should be used for more symptomatic HF, renal insufficiency, or persistent edema. Persistent congestion despite a thiazide diuretic trial necessitates changing to a loop diuretic. Symptoms of severe HF or significant renal dysfunction will require a loop diuretic agent, either orally or intravenously. Patients may become resistant to oral diuretic therapy in increasing doses from a single class. Response may improve

TABLE 103.6   Diuretics Used in Treatment of Chronic Heart Failure*

Drug	Initial Dose	Recommended Maximum Dose	Potential Adverse Reactions
THIAZIDE DIURETICS			
Hydrochlorothiazide	12.5–25 mg/day	200 mg/day	Postural hypotension, hypokalemia, hyperuricemia
Chlorthalidone	25 mg/day	100 mg/day	
LOOP DIURETICS (increased efficacy if taken on an empty stomach)			
Furosemide	20–40 mg/day to twice daily	600 mg/day	Same as with thiazide diuretics
Bumetanide	0.5–1 mg/day	10 mg/day	
Torsemide	10–20 mg/day		
POTASSIUM-SPARING DIURETICS			
Spironolactone	12.5–25 mg/day	50 mg/day for heart failure (HF)	Hyperkalemia (especially if given with angiotensin-converting enzyme [ACE] inhibitors), gynecomastia, rash
Eplerenone	25 mg/day	50 mg/day	Less gynecomastia than with spironolactone
THIAZIDE-RELATED DIURETIC			
Metolazone (Zaroxolyn)	2.5 mg as single dose initially	5–10 mg/day	Same as with thiazide diuretics

Modified from Yancy, C. W., Jessup, M., Bozkurt, B., Butler, J., Casey, D. E., Jr, Drazner, M. H., et al. (2013). 2013 ACCF/AHA guideline for the management of heart failure: A report of the American College of Cardiology Foundation/American Heart Association Task Force on Practice Guidelines. *Journal of the American College of Cardiology, 62*(13), e147–e239.
*Patients with renal or hepatic impairment may require a lower diuretic dose.

with oral diuretics in combination from two different classes (i.e., loop diuretic and thiazide-like diuretic) or intravenous diuretic therapy. Patients unresponsive to intravenous diuretics or with anasarca from excessive volume overload may benefit from advanced therapies, such as ultrafiltration. Diuretic dosage is summarized in Table 103.6. The standing dose of a diuretic depends on the patient's body size, age, estimated glomerular filtration rate, renal function, amount of edema, and compliance with a low-sodium and fluid-restricted diet.[1] Caution is advised for patients using low-sodium seasonings as a salt replacement, as some products are high in potassium.

Use of high-dose diuretic therapy can cause electrolyte abnormalities, such as hypokalemia and hypomagnesemia, that require close monitoring and cautious repletion. An aldosterone antagonist, such as spironolactone, may minimize potassium wasting in patients with hypokalemia and can be used in these patients with close monitoring of electrolyte and renal function.[18] With disease progression, the use of intermittent intravenous diuretics to overcome the neurohormonal responses that are antecedent to the increase in sodium and fluid retention may be necessary. Eventual diuretic resistance is common in advanced HF or in long-term diuretic therapy. Metolazone, a potent oral thiazide-like agent, can be added with caution to loop diuretic therapy to enhance the effect. Metolazone may be effective in patients with reduced renal function, but it should in general not be prescribed on a daily basis.[1]

Digoxin. The cardiac glycosides, such as digoxin, have been used to treat HF for more than 200 years. Digoxin improves symptoms and reduces hospitalization rates, but it has a low therapeutic index. It modestly improves mortality in patients with NYHA class II or III HR.[1] Digoxin may be used to slow ventricular rates in patients with HF and AF. In addition, digoxin may be used as an add-on therapy in patients who are tolerating other standard HF medical therapy.[1]

Digoxin acts as a positive inotropic agent by increasing intracellular calcium concentration in myocytes by altering calcium-sodium exchange. In addition, digoxin may resensitize baroreceptors that have been suppressed by increased neurohormonal sympathetic activity.

There are numerous interactions between digoxin and other drugs, particularly amiodarone, quinidine, procainamide, diltiazem, verapamil, antibiotics, and anticholinergic agents. There are no data to support regular measurement of serum digoxin levels. Electrolyte abnormalities can exacerbate digoxin toxicity.

β Blockers. One of the most important mechanisms responsible for progression of HF is activation of the sympathetic nervous system. This observation led to the hypothesis that drugs that interfere with the actions of the sympathetic nervous system (e.g., β blockers) can be beneficial in HF. β blockers reduce heart rate and thereby reduce myocardial oxygen consumption, inhibit the release of renin, and decrease the activation of the renin-angiotensin system.[1]

In numerous trials, β blockers in selected patients with HF have been shown to improve ventricular function, hemodynamics, functional status, and exercise tolerance, reduce HF exacerbations, and improve mortality. However, this is not a β blocker class effect. Only carvedilol, metoprolol succinate, and bisoprolol have been shown to reduce morbidity and mortality.[1]

β blockers are currently recommended for all patients with LVEF of 40% or less. β blockade should be used with caution in those with HF who have bradycardia, high-degree heart block, or severe COPD. The benefits are especially well described for patients with a history of MI and most patients with left ventricular dysfunction.[3] In addition, a study showed that continuation of β blocker therapy in patients with acutely decompensated systolic HF noted a decreased risk of in-hospital mortality and short-term rehospitalization.[3] Initiation of therapy is recommended at low doses and only when patients are hemodynamically stable.

Ivabradine. Ivabradine is a hyperpolarization-activated cyclic nucleotide-gated channel blocker that inhibits sinus node activity without affecting ventricular repolarization or myocardial contractility. It has been shown to reduce HF hospitalization and death from worsening HF in patients with LVEF of 35% or less and heart rate of 70 beats per minute or more who are being treated with standard HF medical therapy. It is not indicated for patients in AF because its action is directed at the sinus node. Common adverse reactions include bradycardia, hypertension, AF, and visual brightness. Current guidelines recommend prescribing for patients who have NYHA II-III stable HF with an EF ≤ 35%, on maximally tolerated β blocker doses and have a sinus heart rate of ≥ 70 beats per minute.[3,13]

Antiplatelet and Anticoagulation. For patients with HF, there has been no evidence to support the use of antiplatelets or anticoagulation, beyond treatment for underlying or concomitant conditions, such as CAD, previous percutaneous interventions, previous thromboembolic events, or AF.[1,3]

Device Therapy

Implantable Cardioverter-Defibrillators and Cardiac Resynchronization Therapy. In patients with reduced ejection fraction, with or without prior MI, who are receiving standard HF medications, ICDs prevent sudden cardiac death. Numerous studies have shown that ICDs detect and terminate malignant ventricular arrhythmias, therefore reducing mortality. ICDs are appropriate for both primary and secondary prevention of sudden cardiac death in patients with LVEF of 35% or lower.[1,3] Patients with LVEF of 35% or lower who are on optimal HF medical therapy; are at least 40 days post-MI; or are 90 days from index diagnosis if the cause is nonischemic, have NYHA class II to III symptoms, and have life expectancy of at least 1 year may be candidates for prophylactic ICD implantation.[1]

ICD implantation is a prophylactic therapy for patients with HFrEF. Cardiac resynchronization therapy (CRT) or biventricular pacing is a therapeutic intervention indicated in patients with ventricular dyssynchrony evidenced by left bundle branch block (LBBB), QRS duration of 150 ms or less, and LVEF of 35% or less who have NYHA class II or III symptoms. This therapy has been shown to modify the disease process by improving LVEF and reducing LV size and functional mitral regurgitation as well as reversing ventricular remodeling. Only about 35% of qualifying patients show benefit from this therapy, and benefit is usually evident by 3 months after implantation, although some patients show late improvement. Although benefits can be significant, permanently implanted device therapy is not without drawbacks, including device malfunction, lead integrity issues, infection, and inappropriate shocks, which can all decrease quality of life.[1,3] Cardiac electrophysiologists are the experts in this subspecialty and can counsel patients regarding the risks and benefits of device therapy as well as guide device selection.

Revascularization

Some HF patients may benefit from revascularization. Most patients with newly diagnosed systolic dysfunction should be evaluated for cardiac ischemia by either stress testing or coronary angiography. Certain patients with reduced ejection fraction and coronary artery disease may benefit from revascularization, such as percutaneous coronary intervention or coronary artery bypass grafting, because this may improve survival as well as reduce symptoms. Decision criteria related to revascularization are beyond the scope of this chapter.

Advanced Heart Failure Therapies

Inotropic Agents. Positive inotropic agents, which are given by intravenous infusion, increase the force of myocardial contraction. Long-term parenteral administration of positive inotropic agents such as phosphodiesterase inhibitors (milrinone) and β-adrenergic agonists (dobutamine) has resulted in improved symptoms but increased rates of sudden cardiac death because of their potential proarrhythmic effect. The continuous or intermittent parenteral administration of positive inotropic agents remains largely palliative in patients with stage D HF. Inotrope infusion can be a bridge to recovery, a bridge to decisions regarding further advanced HF therapy, or a bridge to cardiac transplantation. These agents can be helpful as short-term infusions for patients with refractory volume overload or threatened end-organ dysfunction. The temporary institution of an intravenous inotropic agent can transiently improve systolic function, palliate low-output states, and improve end-organ dysfunction.[1]

Mechanical Circulatory Support. Mechanical circulatory support (MCS) can be considered for short-term management in the acutely ill hospitalized patient or for longer-term therapy. Short-term devices are placed percutaneously and used in the critical care areas of specialized centers. These devices are a bridge to recovery or a bridge to decisions regarding a longer-term therapy. LVADs are the most commonly used longer-term MCS device. LVADs have emerged as a destination or bridge to transplant therapy in patients with stage D HF. These devices are implanted and managed in specialty centers. They are designed to augment cardiac output and improve survival, functional capacity, and quality of life in selected stage D patients.[3]

Cardiac Transplantation. Cardiac transplant is the gold standard of advanced HF therapies. It is the most effective therapy for stage D HF. Five-year post-transplant survival is approximately 70%. Patients who may be considered should be referred to an advanced HF program or cardiac transplant center. Unfortunately, cardiac transplantation is an option for relatively few patients because of the limited supply of donor hearts. Life expectancy of patients who qualify for transplant is typically less than 1 year. Because of recent advances in LVAD technology, this therapy has emerged as a more viable option for patients waiting for transplant.[1]

INDICATIONS FOR REFERRAL OR HOSPITALIZATION

Patients with HF may benefit from cardiology consultation when symptoms appear to be refractory to the standard therapies of diuretics, ACE inhibitors, aldosterone antagonists, and β blockers. The onset of arrhythmias, coronary ischemia, or MI should prompt consultation. In addition, consideration of input from a cardiologist should be entertained in all young patients with either ischemic or nonischemic DCM, HCM, worsening ejection fraction over time, NYHA class III or class IV symptoms, need for device therapy (ICD) or resynchronization (RCT), or HF advanced therapies evaluation.

Even with pharmacologic advances in HF management, the 30-day hospital readmission rate among older patients remains above 20%.[19] Patient-centered care focuses on careful transitions from the inpatient setting to the community. Clear documentation of inpatient events and therapies and medication reconciliation facilitate the transition and reduce the risk of readmission.[1]

With the rapidly increasing prevalence of HF worldwide and the financial burden this is placing on the health care system, disease management programs and strategies to manage HF patients are important interventions for reducing hospital readmission rates. The fatality rates of 30 days, 1 year, and 5 years after hospitalization for HF were 10.4%, 22%, and 42.3%, respectively.[6] Several types of disease management programs have been studied, including HF clinics, home health advanced practice nurses, community-based case managers, patient telemanagement, cardiac rehabilitation, emergency department observation units, and HF subacute care. Recently hospitalized HF patients as well as those at high risk for hospital admission (renal insufficiency, multiple comorbid illnesses) should be considered for referral to a disease management program.[1]

HF clinics have provided a mechanism for patients to be seen in a clinic for physical assessment, medication instruction and frequent diuretic titration, dietary education, and exercise training. Some nurse-run clinics focus on patient education and resource finding, while advanced practice registered nurses who run HF clinics are instrumental in frequent diuretic titration, uptitration of medical therapy, and referral for appropriate advanced therapies. For patients with HF who are unable to attend clinic sessions, the home health advanced practice nurse may be an appropriate referral. The health care provider with expertise in HF can see the patient in his or her home for assessment of weight, vital signs, heart and lung sounds, and other physical examination findings to assess for HF. During the home visit, the provider can continue patient teaching about medications, diet, and activity and develop a plan with the patient and family for emergency care and when to call the health care provider.

The use of telemedicine technology as a tool in disease management is expanding rapidly to meet the needs of patients in integrated health care delivery systems. A number of innovative attempts at telemedicine with patients with HF are under way and may be potential alternatives for management of these patients at home. Specifically, patients with HF are using telephone and computer technology to transmit data on vital signs, symptoms, and weight to a central repository where the health care providers can review trends. The data are currently variable regarding the effectiveness of this intervention for improving clinical outcomes for HFrEF and HFpEF.[3]

For patients presenting to the acute care setting with acute HF symptoms, the history and physical examination allows understanding of their state of congestion and adequacy of perfusion. Four hemodynamic categories have been identified for the purpose of guiding therapy and predicting mortality outcomes. The categories, dry or wet and warm or cold, are based on assessment of filling pressures and perfusion, respectively. Defining filling pressures, patients may present with low/normal (dry) or elevated (wet) pulmonary capillary wedge pressure indicating congestion. Normal (warm) or decreased (cold) cardiac index aids in understanding cardiac perfusion.[3]

Indications for hospitalization include new-onset HF with symptoms of congestion for treatment and diagnostic evaluation, clinical or electrocardiographic evidence of acute myocardial ischemia (acute coronary syndrome), pulmonary edema or acute decompensated HF, oxygen saturation below 90%, severe medical complications (e.g., pneumonia, renal failure), anasarca, symptomatic hypotension or syncope, hemodynamically significant cardiac arrhythmias, HF refractory to maximal outpatient oral treatment program, and need to evaluate home support for safe management in the community. In addition, hospitalization may be necessary for administration of intravenous diuretics or for more advanced therapies, such as inotropic support for low-output states or initiation of antiarrhythmic medications.[1]

LIFE SPAN CONSIDERATIONS

HF with preserved systolic function is more prevalent with increasing age. All comorbidities should be treated in these patients with HF, particularly anemia, thyroid abnormalities, diabetes, and sleep apnea.[13] Recommendations include management of systolic hypertension with diuretics, ACE inhibitors, and β blockers for goal BP less than 130/80[13] and use of β blockers and nitrates to treat myocardial ischemia. NSAIDs should be avoided in older adult patients at risk for HF because of the propensity of these agents to promote fluid retention and to affect renal function.[1]

HF is a progressive and deadly disorder; 50% of HF patients are likely to die within 5 years of diagnosis. Consideration should be given to early involvement of HF patients in a palliative care program. Palliative care specialists provide decision support surrounding advanced therapies and assistance with symptom management and facilitate discussions about end-of-life decisions. The trajectory of this disease process is variable, and prognosis statistics are simply predictions. Early involvement of the palliative care team is critical for emotional support of patients and families as they negotiate their way through a progressive, chronic disease process.[1,3,12]

There are guideline-driven management and therapies for patients with HFrEF; however, patients with HFpEF continue to present a clinical challenge because treatment remains empirical.[7] Ongoing research into the underlying pathophysiologic mechanism of and treatment approaches for HFpEF will lead to improved therapies and outcomes for these patients. These are exciting developments in the understanding and management of HF. Further investigations and consultations with cardiac specialists will guide use of these in individual patients with HF.

COMPLICATIONS

Acute decompensated HF is one of the leading causes for hospitalizations in the elderly population. There are many factors that can precipitate an acute exacerbation, such as acute MI, pulmonary emboli, medications contraindicated for HF patients (ionotropic drugs, NSAIDs, or steroids), poorly controlled hypertension, AF (new onset, paroxysmal, or persistent), tachyarrhythmias, endocrine abnormalities, infectious source, medication nonadherence, and poor self-care behaviors (high salt and fluid intake, increased alcohol intake).

AF is more likely to develop in patients with HF. The symptoms of AF and HF can become a cycle of worsening cardiac function related to ventricular rate and activation of neurohormonal vasoconstrictors leading to fibrosis and remodeling. In treating HF patients with AF, rhythm control does not demonstrate better outcomes than rate control. The etiology or precipitating factors of AF, such as thyroid disease, uncontrolled hypertension, or exacerbation of COPD, should be identified and corrected.[3] Goals of therapy include reducing risk of thromboembolism and maintaining adequate LV function with the consideration of anticoagulants, β-blockers, and digoxin for pharmacologic treatment.[1]

Cardio-oncology is a rapidly growing area; both oncologists and cardiologists recognize the increasing prevalence of HF in cancer patients and screen patients more aggressively both before and after potentially cardiotoxic chemotherapy or radiation therapy or during stem cell transplant evaluation. Primary care clinicians should be aware of the potential for chemotherapy-induced cardiomyopathy and HF in patients, even years after they have completed chemotherapy, and refer appropriately.

PATIENT AND FAMILY EDUCATION

Many of the important concepts for management of HF are discussed in previous sections of this chapter. Patients and their families can take an active role in management of their disease process and develop self-care skills.[20]

- Ongoing education about the cause, symptoms, and prognosis of HF, including advanced therapies and end-of-life care discussions, and integrating culture and self-care beliefs;
- Encouraging self-care behaviors, such as diet, exercise, smoking cessation, alcohol intake in moderation, immunizations, and monitoring and managing symptoms, such as recording daily weights and elevating edematous lower extremities;
- Understanding the pharmacologic treatments for HF, including action, doses, and side effects and empowering patients and families to titrate medications based on symptoms, such as titrating dose of diuretic for weight gain greater than 5 pounds in 2 days;
- Treating concomitant disease, such as CAD, hypertension, hyperlipidemia, sleep apnea, anemia, and depression.

HEALTH PROMOTION

Prevention of HF is linked to prevention of ischemic heart disease as well as to control of hypertension in the primary care setting. Accordingly, all patients should be screened for heart disease risk and encouraged to reduce their risk by adopting a healthy lifestyle, including maintenance of normal weight, low-fat diet, tobacco avoidance, and exercise. Interventions to screen for heart disease risk include a family history, blood pressure measurement, lipid screen, and blood glucose concentration or hemoglobin A_{1c} level to screen for diabetes. Patients should be encouraged to seek medical attention promptly for any heart attack signs or symptoms, unexplained fatigue, or dyspnea. In addition, patients should be screened for familial cardiac conditions, such as HCM and sudden cardiac death, and referred to a cardiologist if family history is positive. Other cardiovascular diseases need close monitoring with timely intervention for any condition change.

REFERENCES

1. Yancy, C. W., Jessup, M., Bozkurt, B., Butler, J., Casey, D. E., Drazner, M. H., et al. (2013). 2013 ACCF/AHA guideline for the management of heart failure. *Journal of the American College of Cardiology*, 62(16), e147–e239. http://dx.doi.org/10.1016/j.jacc.2013.05.020.
2. Braunwald, E. (2013). Heart failure. *JACC. Heart Failure*, 1(1), 1–20.
3. Ponikowski, P., Voors, A. A., Anker, S. D., Bueno, H., Cleland, J. G. F., Coats, A. J. S., et al. (2016). 2016 ESC Guidelines for the diagnosis and treatment of acute and chronic heart failure. *European Heart Journal*, 37, 2129–2200.
4. Arbustini, E., Narula, N., Tavazzi, L., Serio, A., Grasso, M., Favalli, V., et al. (2014). The MOGE(S) classification of cardiomyopathy for clinicians. *Journal of the American College of Cardiology*, 64(1), 304–318. http://dx.doi.org/10.1016/j.jacc.2014.05.027.
5. Braunwald, E. (2017). Cardiomyopathies: An overview. *Circulation Research*, 121, 711–721. doi:10.1161/CIRCRESAHA.117.311812.
6. Benjamin, E. J., Blaha, M. J., Chiuve, S. E., Cushman, M., Das, S. R., Deo, R., et al. on behalf of the American Heart Association Statistics Committee and Stroke Statistics Subcommittee. (2017). Heart disease and stroke statistics-2017 update: A report from the American Heart Association. *Circulation*, 135(10), e146–e603. doi:10.1161/CIR.0000000000000485.
7. Redfield, M. M. (2016). Heart failure with preserved ejection fraction. *The New England Journal of Medicine*, 375(19), 1868–1877. doi:10.1056/NEJMcp1511175.
8. Florea, V. G., & Cohn, J. N. (2014). The autonomic nervous system and heart failure. *Circulation Research*, 114 1815–1826. doi:10.1161/CIRCRESAHA.114.302589.
9. Jhund, P. S., & McMurray, J. J. V. (2016). The Neprilysin Pathway in Heart Failure: A review and guide on the use of sacubitril/valsartan. *Heart (British Cardiac Society)*, 102(17), 1342–1347. doi:10.1136/heartjnl-2014-306775.
10. Burchfield, J. S., Xie, M., & Hill, J. A. (2013). Pathologic ventricular remodeling mechanisms: part 1 of 2. *Circulation*, 128(4), 388–400. doi:10.1161/CIRCULATIONAHA.113.001878.
11. Butler, J., Fonarow, G. C., Zile, M. R., Lam, C. S., Roessig, L., Schelbert, E. B., et al. (2014). Developing therapies for heart failure with preserved ejection fraction: Current state and future directions. *JACC. Heart Failure*, 2(2), 97–112. doi:10.1016/j.jchf.2013.10.006.
12. Lindenfeld, J., Albert, N. M., Boehmer, J. P., Collins, S. P., Ezekowitz, J. A., Givertz, M. M., et al. (2010). Executive summary: HFSA 2010 comprehensive heart failure practice guideline. *Journal of Cardiac Failure*, 16(6), 475–539. doi:10.1016/j.cardfail.2010.04.005.
13. Yancy, C. W., Jessup, M., Bozkurt, B., Butler, J., Casey, D. E., Jr., Colvin, M. M., et al. (2017). 2017 ACC/AHA/HFSA focused update of the 2013 ACCF/AHA guideline for the management of heart failure: a report of the American College of Cardiology/American Heart Association Task Force on Clinical Practice Guidelines and the Heart Failure Society of America. *Journal of the American College of Cardiology*, 70(6), 776–803. http://dx.doi.org/10.1016/j.jacc.2017.04.025.
14. Hawkins, N. M., Petrie, M. C., Jhund, P. S., Chalmers, G. W., Dunn, F. G., & McMurray, J. J. V. (2009). Heart failure and chronic obstructive pulmonary disease: Diagnostic pitfalls and epidemiology. *European Journal of Heart Failure*, 11, 130–139. doi:10.1093/eurjhf/hfn013.
15. Mitter, S. S., & Yancy, C. W. (2017). Contemporary approaches to patients with heart failure. *Cardiology Clinics*, 35, 261–271. http://dx.doi.org/10.1016/j.ccl.2016.12.008.
16. Damman, K., Wilson Tang, W. H., Felker, M., Lassus, J., Zannad, F., Krum, H., et al. (2014). Current evidence on treatment of patients with chronic systolic heart failure and renal insufficiency. *Journal of the American College of Cardiology*, 63(9), 853–871. http://dx.doi.org/10.1016/j.jacc.2013.11.031.
17. Wang, A., Elshehadeh, R., Rao, D., Yap, E., Lee, A., Mossobir, F., et al. (2016). Roles of aldosterone receptor antagonists in heart failure, hypertension, and chronic kidney disease. *The Journal of Nurse Practitioners*, 12(3), 201–206.
18. Pitt, B., Pfeffer, M. A., Assmann, S. F., Boineau, R., Anand, I. S., Claggett, B., et al. (2014). Spironolactone for heart failure with preserved ejection fraction. *The New England Journal of Medicine*, 370(15), 1383–1392.
19. McClintock, S., Mose, R., & Smith, L. F. (2014). Strategies for reducing the hospital readmission rates of heart failure patients. *The Journal of Nurse Practitioners*, 10(6), 430–433.
20. Clark, A. M., Spaling, M., Harkness, K., Spiers, J., Strachan, P. H., Thompson, D. R., et al. (2014). Determinants of Effective Heart Failure Self-care: A systematic review of patients' and caregivers' perceptions. *Heart (British Cardiac Society)*, 100, 716–721.

CHAPTER 104

HYPERTENSION

Terry Mahan Buttaro

 Hospitalization is recommended for those with a blood pressure of 180/120 mm Hg and evidence of target organ dysfunction.

DEFINITION AND EPIDEMIOLOGY

Blood pressure is the force in arterial structures created by interplay of flow, volume, and constriction. Hypertension has been defined by determining the levels of blood pressure that cause target organ damage, morbidity, and mortality as arterial flow is delivered. In the United States, an estimated 75 million people including children have hypertension, many of them unknowingly.[1] Most patients with hypertension have primary, or essential, hypertension; a smaller number have secondary hypertension. Whatever the cause, identifying and treating hypertension is necessary to prevent the complications associated with this disorder that has sometimes been referred to as the "silent killer."

INCIDENCE AND PREVALENCE

Systolic and diastolic blood pressures rise throughout childhood and early and middle adulthood; each is an independent predictor of cardiovascular and cerebrovascular disease, occurring alone or concurrently, in individuals younger than 50 years. The rate of rise in diastolic blood pressure tends to level off or to drop slightly in approximately the fifth decade of life. Systolic blood pressure continues to rise with advancing age, making isolated systolic hypertension more prevalent in the older adult. This is a concern because in adults age 85 or older with a systolic blood pressure 160 mm Hg or greater, hypertension has been associated with stroke.[2]

In some African Americans, salt sensitivity related to enhanced renal sodium reabsorption increases the likelihood of hypertension and the risk of cardiovascular disease, stroke, and renal complications. As a result, affected patients have a higher mortality rate related to hypertension than people of other ethnic backgrounds.[3]

Risk Factors

Genetics, obesity, metabolic syndrome, high dietary fat intake, excessive sodium ingestion, physical inactivity, obstructive sleep apnea, excessive alcohol intake, smoking, and stress are just some of the factors associated with hypertension.[3] Glucose intolerance and low intake of magnesium and potassium are other possible influences. In general, the risks for hypertension are significant for both systolic and diastolic measurements.

PATHOPHYSIOLOGY

Primary hypertension is theorized to be related to genetic as well as environmental factors.[4]

The sympathetic nervous system (SNS), either through response to perceived hypovolemia (baroreceptor response) or physical or psychological stressors is responsible for sustaining blood pressure. However, SNS stimulation can cause peripheral and insulin resistance, procoagulant effects, and vascular remodeling. These changes contribute to hypertension in

varied ways. For example, insulin resistance impairs endothelial function, while vascular remodeling and procoagulant effects cause vasospasm and blood vessel narrowing. These factors, when combined with overactivity of the renin-angiotensin-aldosterone system and natriuretic hormone dysfunction, cause hypertension.

Sodium intake also impacts blood pressure and may be related to excess circulating volume, but sodium may also directly affect cardiac hypertrophy, contractility, and vascular resistance. Age, African-American heritage, diabetes, low renin levels, and nonmodulating hypertension often predict salt sensitivity. Hypertension associated with salt sensitivity has been postulated to be caused by (1) inability to normally excrete sodium through the kidneys; (2) resetting of the pressure-natriuresis curve, requiring higher blood pressures to maintain normal sodium and water balance; (3) abnormal electrolyte transport, resulting in disturbances in the cytosolic sodium and calcium balance and increased vasoconstriction; or (4) low renin levels, reduced numbers of nephrons, and modified SNS activity.[5]

Additionally, epidemiologic studies generally support a link between higher salt intakes and the prevalence of hypertension.[6]

Renin is released by the juxtaglomerular apparatus of the kidney in response to a low-flow state (reduced renal perfusion pressure or low circulating intravascular volume), SNS stimulation or catecholamine release, and hypokalemia. Once released, renin acts on angiotensinogen to create angiotensin I. In the pulmonary circulation, angiotensin-converting enzymes (ACEs) change angiotensin I to angiotensin II, a potent vasoconstrictor that over time and with prolonged production causes arterial stiffening and hypertrophy. Vascular hypertrophy results in increased peripheral resistance, depression of angiogenesis, or vessel regression. Angiotensin II also causes aldosterone stimulation, which enhances sodium and water reabsorption from the renal tubules and effectively increases circulating volume. The resulting higher blood pressure should provide feedback to maintain homeostatic responses; however, feedback loops may not work properly in some individuals, allowing higher circulating levels of renin and thus higher blood pressure.

There may also be a correlation among obesity, insulin resistance, and hypertension, resulting in impaired salt excretion and enhanced sodium reabsorption, increased SNS activation, and increased angiotensin II and aldosterone production, all of which are associated with higher blood pressure readings.[5]

The Dietary Approaches to Stop Hypertension (DASH) study showed a relationship between lower potassium intake and hypertension. In this study, it was found that blood pressure also decreased in response to a universally recommended diet that contains generous servings of fruits, vegetables, and low-fat dairy products with reduced sodium and saturated and total fat and increased potassium.[6,7]

Excessive alcohol consumption (more than two drinks per day) has been associated with hypertension and other cardiovascular risks and should be suspected in individuals who have been resistant to treatment. Alcohol may raise blood pressure by causing increases in SNS activity, activation of the renin-angiotensin system, or decreases in peripheral vascular tone and impairment of baroreceptor effectiveness. Marked increases in blood pressure may occur with acute alcohol withdrawal but are unrelated to mechanisms of chronic hypertension. Overall reduction of alcohol intake results in a lowered blood pressure and cardiovascular risk in hypertensive heavy drinkers.[8]

Blood pressure rises with acute exercise and is most dramatic and serious in those with uncontrolled hypertension. However, regular exercise can be beneficial if the person can adhere to an established exercise routine and is recommend as an aid in lowering blood pressure. Regular isometric exercise has been shown to prevent the development of hypertension.[5] Regular aerobic exercise has been shown to reduce the incidence of cardiovascular events.

Secondary Hypertension

Secondary hypertension is less common and is associated with a variety of medical conditions including renal vascular disease (renal artery stenosis [RAS]), renal parenchymal disease, pheochromocytoma, hyperaldosteronism, coarctation of the aorta, acromegaly, Cushing syndrome, sleep apnea, and thyroid disease. Alcohol, nonsteroidal antiinflammatory drugs (NSAIDs), steroids, oral contraceptives, and occasionally hormone replacement therapy are exogenous causes (Table 104.1). Anxiety and pregnancy are additional considerations.

Renal Artery Stenosis. RAS results in hypertension when there is a 70% to 80% blockage of a renal artery, often activating the renin-angiotensin system. Two different mechanisms have been shown to cause RAS. In individuals younger than 30 years, fibrodysplasia or fibromuscular dysplasia causes tight fibrous bands that alternate with normal or thin tissue along the renal artery, usually the medial portion. Fibrodysplasia affects more women than men. After age 50, atherosclerosis is the more likely cause of RAS and usually manifests in the proximal artery, extending from aortic plaque. Hypertension from RAS can coexist with essential hypertension; in older adults, RAS is likely to be a frequent contributor to hypertension. Percutaneous renal angioplasty with or without stenting is the preferred treatment of fibromuscular dysplastic RAS.[9] Medical treatment of atherosclerotic RAS is common, but treatment with angioplasty, often with stenting, is also used.[10]

Pheochromocytoma. Pheochromocytoma is a catecholamine-producing tumor of the adrenal glands and is a fairly rare cause of hypertension. A small percentage of these tumors are malignant. Hypertension seen with pheochromocytoma is constant in 50% of cases and labile in the other 50%. Approximately 50% of cases involve the five *H*s: hypertension, headache, hyperhidrosis, hypermetabolic state, and hyperglycemia. Bilateral headache, hyperhidrosis, and palpitations occur in 95% of the cases.[11]

Primary Hyperaldosteronism. Primary hyperaldosteronism, a rarer cause of hypertension, is suspected in patients with unprovoked hypokalemia.[11] Adrenal adenoma (see Chapter 185) accounts for the majority of cases of primary

---

TABLE 104.1 Secondary Hypertension

	Clues			
	History and Physical	**Screening**	**Diagnostic Testing**	**Treatment**
CONDITION: ENDOGENOUS				
Renovascular condition (RAS)	Age < 30 years (fibromuscular) or > 50 years (atherosclerotic) History of atherosclerosis or risk factors Family history of RAS Abdominal bruits	Urinalysis Creatinine	Captopril flow scan Renal magnetic resonance arteriography Renal arteriography	Control hypertension: beta blockers Avoid ACE inhibitors Angioplasty Bypass surgery
Pheochromocytoma	Five *H*s (hypertension, headache, hyperhidrosis, hypermetabolic state, hyperglycemia) Hypertension after anesthetics, tricyclics Family history of endocrine disorders Hypertension after abdominal palpation Labile hypertension	Spot urine VMA 24-h urine VMA and metanephrines	Spot urine VMA 24-h urine VMA and metanephrines Plasma catecholamines (clonidine suppression test) CT scan of abdomen and pelvis Scintigraphy/MIBG imaging	Control hypertension: alpha blocker followed by beta blocker, or alpha-beta blocker Surgery (to check for extrarenal and malignant masses)
Hyperaldosteronism	Weakness Headache Fatigue Hypertension Hypokalemia	Unprovoked hypokalemia	Aldosterone levels before and after saline challenge Renin levels 24-h urinary aldosterone 17-Hydroxycorticosteroids CT scan of abdomen and pelvis Adrenal scintigraphy (if CT scan is normal) Adrenal vein catheterization (if CT scan and scintigraphy are normal)	If adrenal tumor: surgery If bilateral hyperplasia: potassium-sparing diuretics

Continued

TABLE 104.1   Secondary Hypertension—cont'd

		Clues		
	History and Physical	**Screening**	**Diagnostic Testing**	**Treatment**
Coarctation of the aorta	Young age Arm blood pressure > leg blood pressure Possible claudication Fatigue Late systolic murmur Apical heave	Chest x-ray study	Echocardiography Chest CT scan Aortography	Surgery Angioplasty Stent

Thyroid disorder	Weight change
	Fatigue
	Metabolic change
	Temperature intolerance
	Edema
	Change in bowel habits
	Thyromegaly
		Thyroid-stimulating
		    hormone
		Weakness
		Muscle spasms
		Unprovoked
		    hypokalemia
			Triiodothyronine
			Thyroxine
			Thyroid-binding hormone
				Treatment of underlying
				    disorder
				Control hypertension in
				    interim

Renal parenchymal
    disease:
Polycystic kidney disease
Glomerulonephritis
Diabetic nephropathy
Chronic renal failure
Obstruction
Creatinine
	Edema
	Nocturia
	Diabetes
	History of UTIs
	Pruritus
	Family history of polycystic kidney
	    disease
	24-h urine: protein, creatinine,
	    creatinine clearance
		Urinalysis	Renal ultrasound
			Intravenous pyelography
			Diabetes testing
				Depends on specific cause;
				    control of volume
				    intake, diuretics, and
				    additional medical
				    therapy; ACE inhibitor if
				    diabetic (otherwise use
				    with caution), control
				    of glycemia, relief of
				    obstruction

Cushing syndrome	Hirsutism
	Edema
	Buffalo hump
	Moon facies
	Truncal obesity
	Red-purple striae
		24-h urine: free
		    cortisol
			Dexamethasone suppression
			    test
			Pituitary MRI
			CT scan of thorax, abdomen
				Surgery
				Control hypertension

Other:
    Anxiety
    Pregnancy
    Sleep apnea				

CONDITION: EXOGENOUS

Alcohol	History of use			
Cocaine				Cessation of substance
NSAIDs	History of arthritis			Alternative treatment if necessary
Steroids	History of steroid-dependent conditions			

Sympathomimetics
    (over-the-counter cold
    remedies)
	History of recent URI			

Weight control remedies				
Erythropoietin				
MAOIs				

ACE, Angiotensin-converting enzymes; *CT,* computed tomography; *MAOIs,* monoamine oxidase inhibitors; *MIBG,* metaiodobenzylguanidine; *MRI,* magnetic resonance imaging; *NSAIDs,* nonsteroidal anti-inflammatory drugs; *RAS,* renal artery stenosis; *URI,* upper respiratory tract infection; *UTI,* urinary tract infection; *VMA,* vanillylmandelic acid.

hyperaldosteronism and is correctable by surgery. Bilateral adrenal hyperplasia is medically managed and is the second cause of primary hyperaldosteronism.

Coarctation of the Aorta. Coarctation of the aorta (a localized stricture of the aorta) is usually found in youth. It is typified by hypertension in the presence of claudication, delayed femoral pulses, decreased blood pressure in the lower extremities, and notching of ribs on chest x-ray films.[12] Treatment usually involves surgical repair, with angioplasty and stenting a less frequent option.[13]

Cushing Syndrome. Seventy percent to 85% of individuals with Cushing syndrome have hypertension.[12,14] Cushing syndrome is caused by hypersecretion of glucocorticoids by the adrenal cortex, the result of an adrenal tumor or overstimulation by the anterior pituitary (see Chapter 185).

Use of Certain Medications. A variety of medications, herbal supplements, and illicit drugs can cause high blood pressure. Oral corticosteroids, anabolic steroids, oral contraceptives, and NSAIDS are well-known precipitants, but some SSRIs (fluoxetine), SNRIs (venlafaxine), amitriptyline, and amphetamines may also result in hypertension. Decongestants, stimulants, energy drinks, cocaine, and other illicit substances also can increase blood pressure.

Obstructive Sleep Apnea. Obstructive sleep apnea, which affects up to 38% of the population and an even greater percentage of older adults, is associated with hypertension[15] and most likely is related to a variety of processes including a hypoxia-driven SNS discharge. It is more common in aging and in individuals with elevated body mass index,[16] but there is a possible relationship with leptin, which may be associated with the development of obesity, obstructive sleep apnea, and hypertension (see Chapter 206).[17,18] Treatment of OSA can aid hypertension management, but other treatments may also be needed.[19]

Renal Parenchymal Disease. There is a correlation between renal parenchymal disease and hypertension, but renal disease is also considered a result of hypertension.[11] Renal insufficiency is apparent when creatinine levels rise higher than 1.5 mg/dL and the glomerular filtration rate falls to less than 50 mL/min. Renal parenchymal disease encompasses glomerular diseases (e.g., chronic renal failure, systemic lupus erythematosus, nephritis, diabetic nephropathy, glomerulonephritis, renal vasculitis) and interstitial diseases (e.g., polycystic kidney disease, chronic interstitial nephritis).

Genetics. Previous studies have found a genetic link to some secondary causes of hypertension, such as hyperaldosteronism. More recently, researchers at Queen Mary University and Imperial College London identified many more genes associated with hypertension, some of which have previously been identified with other health problems.

CLINICAL PRESENTATION AND PHYSICAL EXAMINATION

Many patients with hypertension are asymptomatic, so the importance of screening cannot be overemphasized. Symptoms of high blood pressure usually occur only after the physical consequences of end organ damage arise. Stroke, CAD, heart failure symptoms, renal dysfunction, retinopathy, and aortic dissection are potential presenting conditions that result from long-standing undiagnosed hypertension. Secondary causes of hypertension are more likely to manifest with early symptoms

reflective of the underlying cause, such as diabetic nephropathy and Cushing syndrome.

The medical history, physical examination, and laboratory data obtained from a patient with high blood pressure should focus on eliciting the presence of cardiovascular risk factors, dysfunction of target organs, and evidence of possible secondary causes of hypertension.[20]

Cardiac risk factors are assessed in the medical history. The health risks associated with hypertension are compounded by tobacco use, hyperlipidemia, left ventricular hypertrophy, glucose intolerance, and positive family history. In addition, a complete cardiovascular, cerebrovascular, renovascular, endocrine, and family history should be elicited.

Any recent surgical, psychological, social, environmental, or traumatic stress should also be determined, because such events may precipitate a temporary elevation in blood pressure or suggest a secondary cause of hypertension. For example, pheochromocytoma can adversely affect hemodynamic stability during surgery.

All over-the-counter and prescribed medications (both currently and formerly used by the patient) should be listed, including nicotine, herbal treatments, steroids, oral contraceptives, NSAIDs, sedatives, sympathomimetics, amphetamines, cyclosporine, erythropoietin, tricyclic antidepressants, monoamine oxidase inhibitors, and alpha- and beta-adrenergic agonists.[20] The dosage, frequency, and duration of medications should be documented. A dietary assessment of sodium, cholesterol, fat, and alcohol intake must also be obtained.

The provider should elicit clues for potential secondary causes of hypertension, such as sleep apnea (loud snoring, erratic sleep, daytime somnolence), pheochromocytoma (severe headaches, diaphoresis, palpitations), aldosteronism (muscle cramps, weakness, polyuria, polydipsia, nocturia, rhabdomyolysis, paresthesias), mineralocorticoid alteration (licorice intake, chewing tobacco, oral steroid use), and renovascular conditions (hypokalemia).

Symptoms indicative of target organ damage must be sought. These symptoms can be neurovascular (transient weakness or blindness, loss of visual acuity, severe headache, confusion, lethargy, seizures), vascular (coarctation, impotence, claudication), cardiovascular (chest pain, dyspnea, palpitations, syncope), and renal (oliguria, hematuria, dysuria).

The physical exam first involves accurate assessment of blood pressure. The patient should be seated with feet on the floor for a total of 5 minutes. A blood pressure cuff of the appropriate size (with the bladder of the cuff encompassing at least 80% of arm circumference) is applied 1 cm ($\frac{2}{5}$ inch) above the antecubital fossa. The patient's arm is positioned with support level with the heart; the sphygmomanometer must be at the provider's eye level. The systolic value is the level at which the first Korotkoff sound appears; the diastolic value is the level at which sound disappears. An average of at least two measurements is recommended. Blood pressure and heart rate are measured in each arm while the patient is seated with feet on the floor. Measurements are repeated with the patient standing for older adults and when warranted by concerns for orthostasis.

Height, weight, and body mass index (BMI) are recorded to guide weight management decisions. Other components of the physical examination are necessary to determine evidence of end-organ impairment and secondary causes for hypertension.

Sustained hypertension produces a vascular effect. Retinal changes include arteriolar narrowing, arteriovenous nicking, exudates, hemorrhages, and, in severe cases, papilledema. The carotid arteries, aorta, and renal arteries may have bruits, and impaired cerebral circulation may manifest as deficits on neurologic testing. Evidence of cardiac dysfunction (e.g., adventitious lung sounds, cardiac gallops, or displaced apical pulse) or left ventricular enlargement indicates complications of hypertension and affects treatment decisions. Pulse changes (diminished or absent) and skin changes (thinning, loss of extremity hair) point to peripheral circulatory impairment.

It is important to note striae, neurofibroma, and pruritic areas. Radial-femoral pulse delays and differences in blood pressure between arms or between arms and legs require further evaluation. Renal artery bruits or enlarged kidneys are evidence of kidney involvement. Thyroid findings of enlargement, bruits, or nodules necessitate additional testing.

DIAGNOSTICS

A diagnosis of hypertension is based on measurements obtained at at least two office visits, usually 2 weeks apart.[20] Classification and treatment of hypertension are guided by age, ethnicity, comorbidities, and blood pressure guidelines. Treatment is always individualized and based on shared decision making, but for all patients life-style changes are discussed with the patient. These include weight loss when indicated, increased exercise, a low-salt diet, the DASH diet, and alcohol in moderation.

There are varied associations with recommendations about blood pressure goals in adults and elders. In 2014, JNC 8 classified a blood pressure of BP 120-139/<80-89 as "prehypertension, thus a normal blood pressure was deemed to be less than 120/80 mg/Hg. A diagnosis of hypertension was described as a blood pressure of 140/90 or higher in individuals younger than 60 and in individuals with Diabetes, chronic kidney disease, and cardiovascular disease.[21] A blood pressure of 150/90 or higher was considered hypertension for those 60 years of age or older.

In 2017, the results of the Systolic Blood Pressure Intervention Trial (SPRINT) revealed that lowering systolic blood pressure to less than 120 mm Hg for high-risk, nondiabetic patients with hypertension, even in older adults, resulted in cardiovascular disease and heart failure reduction as well as a decrease in all cause mortality (https://www.acc.org/latest-in-cardiology/clinical-trials/2015/09/23/10/40/sprint).

In 2017, the American Heart Association and American College of Cardiology (AHA/ACC) guidelines stated that the goal blood pressure recommendation should be less than 130/80 for older adults and for those adults younger than age 60 with an ASCVD score greater than 10%. AHA/ACC recommended the same BP goal (<130/80) for adults with diabetes, chronic kidney disease or cardiovascular disease.

The 2019, the American Diabetes Association recommends that patients with a blood pressure greater than 140/90 mm Hg be started on a medication to lower the blood pressure. Preferred medications for patients with diabetes include ACE inhibitors, ARBs, dihydropyridine calcium channel blockers and thiazide–like diuretics (http://clinical.diabetesjournals.org/content/37/1/11). More aggressive treatment (combination therapy) is recommended for patients with diabetes and a blood pressure 160/100 mm Hg or higher (http://clinical.diabetesjournals.org/content/37/1/11).

The National Kidney Foundation describes hypertension as a blood pressure of a systolic pressure of 140 or more or diastolic pressure of 90 or greater, but addresses the risks inherent when a patient's blood pressure is greater than 130/80 mm Hg (https://www.kidney.org/news/newsroom/factsheets/High-Blood-Pressure-and-CKD).

It can be challenging for healthcare providers when guidelines are conflicting, but it is important to remember that organizations release guidelines at different points in time and research is ongoing. Additionally, co-morbid disorders increase the risk of a cardiovascular event. Thus when treating a patient with hypertension or another health condition, each patient should be evaluated and treated individually, based not only on the health problem but also on patient risks for an adverse event. This is particularly important when treating frail older adults with hypertension, because the risk for falls can be greater in older adults depending on a variety of factors. For this reason, when treating patients with hypertension, target blood pressure values are established based on the patient's unique characteristics, comorbidities, risk for falls or other complications, and tolerance to medication.

Routine evaluation of a patient's hypertension should include calculation of the patient's 10 year atherosclerotic cardiovascular risk available at http://www.cvriskcalculator.com/calculated?age=72&gender=0&race=0&total-chol=181&hdl=89&sbp=124&dbp=80&treated=0&diabetes=0&smoker=0. A urinalysis and complete blood count (CBC) and determination of serum potassium, blood urea nitrogen (BUN), serum creatinine, fasting blood glucose, plasma lipoprotein, serum uric acid, and calcium concentrations should be obtained. Electrocardiography (ECG) is performed to assess evidence of ischemic heart disease or left ventricular hypertrophy. Left ventricular hypertrophy manifests on ECG with a large S wave in V_1 and a large R wave in V_5. These two deflections add up to more than 35 mm.

INITIAL DIAGNOSTICS

Hypertension

LABORATORY
- Urine albumin to creatinine ratio
- Complete blood count and differential
- Fasting blood glucose serum electrolytes, electrolytes
- Blood urea nitrogen
- Creatinine, calcium, phosphorus, uric acid
- Fasting lipid profile
- Thyroid-stimulating hormone[a]
- 24-h urine cortisol (if Cushing syndrome is suspected)

- 24-h creatinine, catecholamines, and metanephrines (if pheochromocytoma is suspected)

IMAGING
- Chest x-ray examination[a]
- Abdominal ultrasound[a]
- Renal angiography[a]

OTHER DIAGNOSTICS
- Electrocardiography
- Echocardiography[a]

[a]If indicated

DIFFERENTIAL DIAGNOSIS

The differential diagnosis of a patient with hypertension includes primary and secondary hypertension. Causes of secondary hypertension (see Secondary Hypertension above) should always be excluded, as treatment of an underlying secondary cause may ultimately resolve the hypertension. The more commonly noted secondary causes of hypertension are noted and their symptoms and diagnostic testing can be found in Table 104.1. Less common causes of secondary hypertension include acromegaly, hypercalcemia caused by hyperparathyroidism, primary aldosteronism, and central sleep apnea.

Among the other differential diagnoses is white coat hypertension, which, although somewhat controversial, is described as an elevated blood pressure related to the anticipation or anxiety associated with visiting a health care provider. When white coat hypertension is suspected, home or ambulatory blood pressure monitoring may be beneficial. If home monitoring is recommended, the patient's sphygmomanometer should be evaluated for comparative efficacy in the office and the patient should be instructed or supervised in proper technique. If ambulatory blood pressure monitoring is considered, coverage by insurance should be confirmed. Some cases of white coat hypertension are thought to be predictive of high blood pressure; in such cases, the patient's risk factors for a cardiovascular event should be assessed and both nonpharmacologic and pharmacologic treatments encouraged.

INTERPROFESSIONAL COLLABORATIVE MANAGEMENT

Indications for Referral or Hospitalization

- Hospitalization is indicated for a patient with blood pressure of 180/120 mm Hg or greater associated *with* target organ dysfunction Frequently these patients have a systolic blood pressure greater than 200 mgHg.[22] Target organ symptoms should be rapidly assessed. Retinopathy may be the first presenting sign; grade 3 or grade 4 retinopathy with exudates and hemorrhage is a significant physical finding.[23] Neurologic symptoms include altered mental status, dizziness, blurred vision or loss of vision, focal neurologic deficits, and gastrointestinal symptoms. Cardiac symptoms include chest pain (or an anginal equivalent) or dyspnea accompanied by electrocardiographic changes, rales, and an S_3 on physical examination and possibly heart failure on chest x-ray study. Vascular symptoms may include tearing or burning chest pain and interscapular pain, with a variation in bilateral arm or leg blood pressure measurements, decreased pulses in lower extremities, or widened mediastinum on the chest x-ray film. Renal signs may include oliguria, hematuria, proteinuria, and red cell casts by urinalysis.
- In patients with an elevated BP 180/120 or greater, *but evidence of acute end organ damage is not present*, blood pressure control can be managed on an outpatient basis and hospitalization is not recommended by 2017 American College of Cardiology/American Heart Association Guideline for the Prevention, Detection, Evaluation, and Management of High Blood Pressure in Adults. Discussion regarding outpatient treatment with a physician or nephrologist is necessary.
- Consultation is recommended:

  Physician consultation is necessary when hypertension is resistant to therapy (failure of three full-dose, or maximally tolerated, antihypertensive drugs, including a diuretic) and when secondary causes attributable to lifestyle considerations, habits, or nonadherence to medication recommendations have been excluded.

Patients with known secondary hypertension caused by RAS should be referred to a vascular interventionalist or surgeon.

- Primary aldosteronism may require specialized input from an endocrinologist.
- Pheochromocytoma will require collaboration with medical physician and surgeon.

Patients with autonomic failure who have orthostatic hypotension but hypertension while supine are challenging and would benefit from a consultation with a specialist in autonomic dysfunction or hypertension.[24]

Nonpharmacologic Treatment

Lifestyle modifications for patients with hypertension or prehypertension include regular exercise, the maintenance of a healthy weight, tobacco cessation, reduction of daily dietary sodium to below 2300 mg, and alcohol intake in moderation.

Exercise: Each patient's exercise prescription is dependent on their overall health. In general, for healthy adults with hypertension, moderate-intensity aerobic exercise should be done at least 30 minutes daily. In addition, 2 or 3 days each week should include dynamic resistance exercise. The total amount of exercise each week should be 150 minutes or more.[25]

Alcohol use: The maximum recommended daily amount of alcohol is one drink a day for women (no alcohol if pregnant), and two drinks a day for men, but alcohol increases blood pressure, and avoiding alcohol is recommended. A recent study suggests that for all of us, less than 100 ounces of alcohol a week is associated with the least mortality.[26]

Weight management: When indicated, weight loss is recommended, though it is not easy to lose weight and then maintain the loss. Referral to a nutritionist, Weight Watchers, or other weight loss program can be helpful for some patients. The American Heart Association also has weight loss recommendations that can be helpful; these are available at https://www.heart.org/-/media/data-import/downloadables/pe-abh-why-should-i-lose-weight-ucm_300472.pdf. A calorie calculator can also be helpful for some patients: https://www.calculator.net/calorie-calculator.html?ctype=standard&cage=72&csex=f&cheightfeet=5&cheightinch=6&cpound=130&cheightmeter=180&ckg=60&cactivity=1.2&printit=0&x=75&y=19.

Smoking cessation is advised for all patients, and providers are encouraged to always ask patients if they smoke or are exposed to smoke and use the 5 As at every patient encounter: **Ask** about a patient's tobacco use, **Advise** the patient to stop smoking, **Assess** the patient's readiness to stop, **Assist** the patient when ready to quit, and **Arrange** follow-up to help support the patient. Bupropion and varenicline are medications available to aid smoking cessation, but nicotine replacement therapy can also be helpful for some patients. Patients who are not yet ready to quit smoking can be encouraged to try and decrease smoking by eliminating only one cigarette a week, and that can be helpful for some.

Stress management: Learning to cope with stress can be helpful for us all. Walking, relaxation, yoga, biofeedback, and meditation exercises can be helpful.

Pharmacologic Treatment

Medical regimens are based on age, ethnicity, and comorbidities, as well as patient preferences. The health care provider will need to use judgment regarding the patient's safety and stability in determining the best plan with the patient. ACE inhibitors, angiotensin receptor blockers (ARBs), thiazide diuretics, and calcium channel blockers (CCBs) are the recommended treatment categories for hypertension, but other medication categories are sometimes used for resistant hypertension or because of patient allergies or medication side effects. Choosing the medication(s) involves not only judgment based on each patient's comorbidities, current medications, safety, and stability but also the patient–provider partnership. JNC 8 recommendations are to start Black patients on a dyhydropine CCB (e.g., amlodipine) and/or a thiazide diuretic. Asian patients often do better when prescribed a CCB or ARB.[27] Non-Black patients should be started on thiazide diuretic, ACE inhibitor, angiotensin blocker, CCB, or combination (e.g., lisinopril/hydrochlorothiazide).[28] ACE inhibitors (or ARBs) are recommended for all patients with diabetes, and this includes Black individuals with diabetes.

For patients with chronic kidney disease and/or diabetes, regardless of age or ethnicity, the JNC 8 target blood pressure is below 140/90.[28] Medical treatment should include an ACE inhibitor or an ARB either as initial treatment or as a second agent.

Beta blockers are not recommended for hypertension therapy but are indicated in settings of known CAD, thoracic aortic disease, and heart failure with reduced ejection fraction (HFrEF).[29] Nondihydropyridine CCBs (e.g., diltiazem, verapamil) are contraindicated in patients with HFrEF, but dihydropyridines (e.g., amlodipine) are acceptable to use for blood pressure control. Also in patients with HFrEF, loop diuretics, such as furosemide or torsemide, along with spironolactone may be used for volume management as well as blood pressure management, though careful monitoring of serum electrolytes is necessary.

Most people require two medications for adequate blood pressure control.[20] For nonorthostatic patients whose blood pressures are at or below 160 mm Hg systolic or 100 mm Hg diastolic, two-drug therapy (e.g., lisinopril/hydrochlorothiazide) has been suggested as initial pharmacologic treatment.[20] Combining two medications (in one pill) may improve adherence, plus decrease medication costs for the patient.

Follow-up should be performed in 1 to 4 weeks to assess blood pressure results and monitor the patient's serum electrolytes and renal status. If a thiazide diuretic such as chlorthalidone (the preferred diuretic because of a longer half-life) or hydrochlorothiazide or loop diuretic is initially prescribed, a chemistry profile 5 to 7 days after the medication is started is indicated because of the risk of significant electrolyte disturbance (hyponatremia or hypokalemia). For patients with renal dysfunction (GFR < 30 mL/min) or heart failure, loop diuretics are indicated and laboratory follow-up should also occur within 5 to 7 days after the drug is started.[29] When ACE inhibitors or ARBs are prescribed, potassium and renal function should also be carefully monitored.

If blood pressure is not at target, either the dose of the initial drug can be increased or a second drug can be added. The provider should continue to follow patient blood pressures until goal blood pressure is achieved and uptitrate and/or add a third drug as needed. Continuous monitoring every 3 months is recommended to determine treatment efficacy and monitor electrolytes and renal status.

Resistant hypertension occurs when blood pressure readings are not at goal despite maximal dose of three drugs, including a diuretic. Frequently, though not always, resistant hypertension is associated with poor adherence to the recommended

therapies, so discussing this issue with the patient is important. Medication side effects, costs, and polypharmacy are only some of the causes of poor adherence to treatment.

LIFE SPAN CONSIDERATIONS

In general, systolic blood pressure rises with age, whereas diastolic blood pressure reaches a peak at around 50 to 60 years of age and then may begin to decrease mildly. Isolated systolic hypertension is especially a problem for patients older than 60 years and is thought to result from aging, vascular stiffening, and diminished artery compliance. Isolated systolic hypertension responds well to most antihypertensive medications and especially to diuretics and CCBs. Advancing age does not preclude pharmacologic therapy but does require gentle initiation and advancement to prevent excessive drops in blood pressure or orthostatic hypotension, which can result in falls.

ACC 2017 guidelines recommend treatment for ambulatory adults over age 65 living in the community. The goal systolic blood pressure for these patients is <130 mm Hg. For patients with hypertension, multiple comorbidities, or a more finite life expectancy in this age group, treatment is based on the patient's wishes and clinician judgment.[29]

The JNC 8 blood pressure goal recommendation for adults less than age 60 is a blood pressure equal to or less than 140/90; for adults over age 60, the blood pressure goal is equal to or less than 150/90. For adult patients of any age with diabetes, the JNC 8 goal blood pressure is less than 140/90. For adult patients of any age with chronic kidney disease, the goal blood pressure is less than 140/90.[28]

Secondary hypertension should be considered when hypertension develops before the age of 30 years (e.g., coarctation of the aorta or fibromuscular RAS) or after the age of 65 years (e.g., atherosclerotic RAS). Hypertension during pregnancy (preeclampsia) is always a concern requiring immediate conversation with OB/GYN specialists and hospitalization.

COMPLICATIONS

Long-term complications of hypertension include left ventricular hypertrophy, heart failure, CAD, myocardial infarction, sudden death, aortic dissection, cerebrovascular disease, proteinuria, renal insufficiency, atherosclerotic conditions, retinopathy, and hypertensive urgencies and emergencies. Complications can be caused by long-term uncontrolled hypertension that assails target organs over time or by sudden surges of acute hypertension that result, for example, from acute glomerulonephritis or cocaine ingestion. A decline in cognitive functioning and a higher incidence of dementia and Alzheimer disease have been associated with hypertension in older individuals.[30]

Hypertensive Urgency and Hypertensive Crises

Hypertensive emergencies are relatively rare events, and in fact most patients with elevated blood pressures have hypertensive urgency. Earlier and more pervasive diagnosis and treatment have reduced the incidence of emergencies related to untreated high blood pressure and have reduced mortality rates. A hypertensive crisis is present when blood pressure is high enough to threaten target organs acutely and there can be a variety of presentations. The differentiation between hypertensive emergencies and hypertensive urgencies was addressed by JNC 7 and not changed in JNC 8 (Box 104.1).[31]

The initial assessment of hypertensive crises should be aimed at two primary goals: (1) determining a threat to the most commonly affected target organs (fundi, brain, heart, and kidneys) and (2) finding a cause (consider stimulant, alcohol intoxication or recent cessation of the patient's blood pressure meds). Various diagnostic options may be contaminated by drugs, therefore blood and urine samples should be collected quickly before treatment but without delaying (Box 104.2).

Parenteral antihypertensive therapy can be indicated for hypertensive urgencies, but oral therapy with labetolol or hydralazine may be appropriate and patients without end organ damage can often be treated as outpatients successfully. For hospitalized patients, intravenous clevidipine may be indicated urgently when organ damage is ongoing.[32] It may also be advisable to coordinate the treatment of the cause (e.g., relief of pain in a postoperative patient) with the adjustment or initiation of medication. Observation of the patient for several hours after treatment to determine safety and efficacy is recommended.

Hypertensive emergencies may require admission to an intensive care unit and parenteral treatment. The goal of treatment should be to reduce blood pressure slowly because rapid lowering of blood pressure can produce a shock effect in target organs, though treatment really depends on the patient presentation. The initial goal is to maintain the diastolic blood pressure at 100 mm Hg or more while lowering the mean arterial pressure 25% within the first hour, then gradually decreasing the blood pressure over the next 24 to 48 hours, though there are definite exceptions (e.g., an acute aortic dissection or neurologic emergency), thus identification of exact cause of the hypertensive emergency is essential.[33] Precipitous drops in blood pressure should be avoided. The brain maintains cerebral perfusion pressure by autoregulation, which balances perfusion by cerebral vasoconstriction or vasodilation

in response to rises and falls in blood pressure. Normal autoregulation is easily maintained with blood pressure ranges of 70/40 to 190/130 mm Hg (allowing for some individual variation). However, the autoregulation curve skews to the right and upward in patients with chronic hypertension. If blood pressure exceeds the limits of autoregulation or if blood pressure drops precipitously, signs of cerebral hypoperfusion may be present.

Initially, patients with severe hypertension may appear with headache, dizziness, altered consciousness (lethargy, slowed mentation, confusion, agitation), and nausea. Other target organs may produce profound symptoms in response to severe hypertension; pulmonary edema may occur in the setting of diastolic heart failure from excessively high afterload (peripheral resistance); retinal hemorrhage may occur. The physical examination, especially the retinal examination, should focus on target organ damage. Groups 3 and 4 Keith-Wagener-Barker funduscopic changes may be the only or the initial sign of rapid deterioration with severe hypertension. Other possible changes may include blood pressure variation between the arms resulting from coarctation or aortic dissection, electrocardiographic changes and chest pain consistent with unstable angina or myocardial infarction, and hematuria resulting from renal decompensation.

Particular caution should be exercised with older adults, patients with chronic hypertension, patients who might have hypovolemia (diuretic use, recent loss of appetite, vomiting, or diarrhea), and patients who are taking vasoactive medications. In patients of all ages, overly aggressive therapy has been associated with adverse outcomes such as blindness, coma, and death. The necessity of preventing permanent cerebral damage must be carefully achieved while lowering blood pressure enough to protect vital organs in circumstances such as acute heart failure, threatened myocardial infarction, or acute aortic dissection.

PATIENT AND FAMILY EDUCATION AND HEALTH PROMOTION

Topics that must be addressed include dietary instructions, exercise recommendations, other risk factor modifications, lifestyle issues, and side effects associated with the medication(s) prescribed. Patient comprehension is increased when handouts are given as references after the office visit.

Salt intake should be restricted to a maximum of 2.3 g/day and potentially less if possible. Measures that help with salt restriction include avoiding the addition of salt to food, cooking with herbs, using fresh fruits and vegetables instead of canned, choosing fresh meats instead of deli or processed meats (e.g., bacon, sausage), and avoiding obviously salty foods (e.g., potato chips, pretzels, salted nuts). Products with food labels showing sodium free (5 mg/serving), very low sodium (<36 mg/serving), or low sodium (<141 mg/serving) should be selected.

Exercise recommendations are geared to provision of a specific exercise prescription, with consideration of CAD screening by physician consultation or stress testing in men older than 40 years and women older than 50 years.

The goal should be an established routine of exercise that is enjoyable and maintains interest with consistent progression of activity. Factors that need emphasis include adequate hydration, stretching, and warm-up and cool-down periods with more strenuous exercise.

Self-monitoring of blood pressure is a reasonable goal. If the patient agrees, family members should be provided with information concerning therapeutic recommendations. Individual knowledge concerning the optimum level of blood pressure, the factors affecting blood pressure, the necessity of treatment for control rather than cure of high blood pressure, and the dangers of quick weight loss programs is crucial. When a patient is prescribed medication, the dose, the medication's mechanism of action, the monitoring required, and the side effects are important topics to discuss to ensure patient understanding. Involvement of patients in the decision-making process, exploration of feelings concerning treatment regimens, exit interviews, and regular follow-up visits help the patient achieve therapeutic goals.

REFERENCES

1. Centers for Disease Control and Prevention. (2018). High blood pressure. https://www.cdc.gov/bloodpressure. (Accessed 16 September 2018).
2. Lionakis, N., Mendrinos, D., Sanidas, E., Favatas, G., & Georgopoulou, M. (2012). Hypertension in the elderly. *World Journal of Cardiology*, 4(5), 135–147. http://doi.org/10.4330/wjc.v4.i5.135.
3. Mozaffarian, D., Benjamin, E. J., Go, A. S., Arnett, D. K., et al. on behalf of the American Heart Association Statistics Committee and Stroke Statistics Subcommittee. (2015). Heart disease and stroke statistics—2015 update: A report from the American Heart Association. *Circulation*, 131, e29–e322.
4. Brashers, V. L. (2014). Alterations in cardiovascular function. In K. L. McCance & S. E. Huether (Eds.), *Pathophysiology. The biologic basis for disease in adults and children* (7th ed.). St. Louis: Elsevier.
5. Frohlich, E. D. (2009). Current challenges and unresolved problems in hypertensive disease. *The Medical Clinics of North America*, 93(3), 527–540.
6. Eckel, R. H., Jakicic, J. M., Ard, J. D., et al. (2014). 2013 AHA/ACC guideline on lifestyle management to reduce cardiovascular risk: A report of the American College of Cardiology American/Heart Association Task Force on Practice Guidelines. *Journal of the American College of Cardiology*, 63(25_PA), doi:10.1016/j.jacc.2013.11.003.
7. Conlin, P. R., Chow, D., Miller, E. R., et al. (2000). The effect of dietary patterns on blood pressure control in hypertensive patients: Results from the Dietary Approaches to Stop Hypertension (DASH) trial. *American Journal of Hypertension*, 13(9), 949–955.
8. Fernandez-Sola, J. (2015). Cardiovascular risks and benefits of moderate and heavy alcohol consumption. *Nature Reviews. Cardiology*, doi:10.1038/nrcardio.2015.91.
9. Chrysant, S. G., & Chrysant, G. S. (2014). Treatment of hypertension in patients with renal artery stenosis due to fibromuscular dysplasia of the renal arteries. *Cardiovascular Diagnosis and Therapy*, 4(1), 36–43. http://doi.org/10.3978/j.issn.2223-3652.2014.02.01.
10. Aronow, W. S. (2017). Atherosclerotic renal artery stenosis. *Annals of Translational Medicine*, 5(12), 264. http://doi.org/10.21037/atm.2017.03.105.
11. Calhoun, D. A., Jones, D., Textor, S., et al. (2008). Resistant hypertension: Diagnosis, evaluation, and treatment. A scientific statement from the American Heart Association Professional Education Committee of the Council for High Blood Pressure Research. *Hypertension*, 51, 1403–1419.
12. Sukor, N. (2011). Secondary hypertension: A condition not to be missed. *Postgraduate Medical Journal*, 87, 706–713.
13. Suradi, H., & Hijazi, Z. M. (2015). Current management of coarctation of the aorta. *Global Cardiology Science & Practice*, 2015(4), 44. http://doi.org/10.5339/gcsp.2015.44.
14. Isidori, A. M., Graziadio, C., Paragliola, R. M., Cozzolino, A., Ambrogio, A. G., Colao, A., et al. on behalf of the ABC Study Group. (2015). The hypertension of Cushing's syndrome: Controversies in the pathophysiology and focus on cardiovascular complications. *Journal of Hypertension*, 33(1), 44–60.
15. Senaratna, C. V., Perret, J. L., Lodge, C. J., Lowe, A. J., et al. (2017). Prevalence of obstructive sleep apnea in the general population: A systematic review. *Sleep Medicine Reviews*, 34, 70–81. doi:10.1016/j.smrv.2016.07.002. [Epub 2016 Jul 18].
16. Konecny, T., Kara, T., & Somers, V. K. (2014). Obstructive sleep apnea and hypertension—an update. *Hypertension*, 63(2), 203–209. http://doi.org/10.1161/HYPERTENSIONAHA.113.00613.
17. Landsberg, L., Aronne, L. J., Beilin, L. J., et al. (2013). Obesity-related hypertension: Pathogenesis, cardiovascular risk, and treatment. A position paper of the Obesity Society and the American Society of Hypertension. *Journal of Clinical Hypertension (Greenwich, Conn.)*, 15, 14–33.
18. Imayama, I., & Prasad, B. (2017). Role of leptin in obstructive sleep apnea. *Annals of the American Thoracic Society*, 14(11).
19. Ahmad, M., Makati, D., & Akbar, S. (2017). Review of and Updates on Hypertension in Obstructive Sleep Apnea. *International Journal of Hypertension*, 2017, 1848375. http://doi.org/10.1155/2017/1848375.
20. Weber, M. A., et al. (2014). Clinical practice guidelines for the management of hypertension in the community. A statement by the American Society of Hypertension and the International Society of Hypertension. *Journal of Clinical Hypertension*, 16(1), 14–26.
21. American College of Cardiology Foundation. 2017 Guideline for the prevention, Detection, Evaluation and Management of High Blood Pressure in Adults. https://www.acc.org/~/media/Non-Clinical/Files-PDFs-Excel-MS-Word-etc/Guidelines/2017/Guidelines_Made_Simple_2017_HBP.pdf. (Accessed 15 September 2018).
22. Breu, A. C., & Axon, R. N. (2018). Acute treatment of hypertensive urgency. *Journal of Hospital Medicine*, 12, 860–862. doi:10.12788/jhm.3086. Published online first October 31, 2018.
23. James, P. A., et al. (2014). 2014 Evidence-based guidelines for the management of high blood pressure in adults. Report from the panel members appointed to the Eighth Joint National Committee (JNC 8). *JAMA: The Journal of the American Medical Association*, 311(5), 507–520.
24. Shibao, C., Gamboa, A., Diedrich, A., et al. (2006). Management of hypertension in the setting of autonomic failure: A pathophysiologic approach. *Hypertension*, 45, 469–476.
25. Pescatello, L. S., MacDonald, H. V., Lamberti, L., & Johnson, B. T. (2015). Exercise for hypertension: A prescription update integrating existing recommendations with emerging research. *Current Hypertension Reports*, 17(11), 87. http://doi.org/10.1007/s11906-015-0600-y.
26. Wood, A. M., et al. (2018). Risk thresholds for alcohol consumption: Combined analysis of individual-participant data for 599912 current drinkers in 83 prospective studies. *Lancet*, 391, 10129.
27. Cheung, T. T., & Cheung, B. M. Y. (2014). Managing blood pressure control in Asian patients: Safety and efficacy of losartan. *Clinical Interventions in Aging*, 9, 443–450. http://doi.org/10.2147/CIA.S39780.
28. JNC 8 Hypertension guideline algorithm. http://www.nmhs.net/documents/27JNC8HTNGuidelinesBookBooklet.pdf. (Accessed 17 September 2018).
29. ACC. 2017 Guideline for high blood pressure in adults. https://www.acc.org/latest-in-cardiology/ten-points-to-remember/2017/11/09/11/41/2017-guideline-for-high-blood-pressure-in-adults. (Accessed 16 September 2018).
30. Lorius, N., Locascio, J., Rentz, D., et al. (2015). Vascular disease and risk factors are associated with cognitive decline in the Alzheimer's disease spectrum. *Alzheimer Disease and Associated Disorders*, 29(1), 18–25.
31. National Heart, Lung, and Blood Institute. (2004). The seventh report of the Joint National Committee on Prevention, Detection, Evaluation, and Treatment of High Blood Pressure. NIH Publication No. 04–5230. Bethesda, Md: U.S. Department of Health and Human Services.
32. Tulman, D. B., Stawicki, S. P., Papadimos, T. J., et al. (2012). Advances in management of acute hypertension: A concise review. *Discovery Medicine*, 13(72), 375–383.
33. Muiesan, M. L., Salvetti, M., Amadoro, V., et al. (2015). An update on hypertensive emergencies and urgencies. *The Journal of Cardiovascular Medicine*, 16, 372–382.

CHAPTER **105**

INFECTIVE ENDOCARDITIS

Lauren Curtis

 Immediate specialist consultation and transfer to the emergency department is indicated for patients with fever and suspected endocarditis.

DEFINITION AND EPIDEMIOLOGY

Infective endocarditis (IE) refers to a microbial infection within the endothelium of the heart. Vegetations form and adhere to the endothelial structures. The heart valves are most often involved, but the disease may also occur within a septal defect, on the chordae tendineae, or on the mural endocardium.

The majority of IE cases are the result of bacterial infections. However, increasing numbers of cases of IE caused by fungal, chlamydial, and rickettsial organisms have been reported; hence the change in name from *bacterial endocarditis* to *IEs*.[1-5] Despite diagnostic and therapeutic advancements, IE remains a life-threatening disease associated with serious complications and carries a high mortality.

IE has been classified as acute or subacute according to its clinical course. Acute IE is a fulminant process; death can occur within days to less than 6 weeks. The usual culprit organisms are *Staphylococcus aureus, Streptococcus pyogenes, Streptococcus pneumoniae,* and *Neisseria gonorrhoeae*. Subacute IE (death occurring within 6 weeks to 3 months) and chronic IE (death occurring later than 3 months) are usually classified together. These two forms of IE have a more subtle course; the usual causative organisms are the *Viridans streptococci*. Although classifications based on acuity are helpful, a more descriptive system has been introduced and is of greater therapeutic and prognostic value. IE may be classified according to the evolution of the disease, the infectious pathogen, and the presence of a preexisting disease or risk factor (e.g., acute native valve endocarditis [NVE] involving *V. streptococci*).[3,6,7]

Currently more than half of patients diagnosed with IE are older than 50 years; the ratio of male-to-female patients is greater than 2 : 1.[4] IE continues to be characterized by increased morbidity and mortality and is now the fourth most common life-threatening infection syndrome.[5] Certain populations are at higher risk, including but not limited to users of injectable drugs; individuals with structural cardiac abnormalities, implantable devices, or cardiac and vascular prostheses; immunosuppressed patients; and individuals with a history of IE.[2,3] It is difficult to know the exact numbers of patients afflicted by IE, but approximately 10,000 to 15,000 new IE cases in the United States as well as an alarming 20% to 30% mortality rate have been reported.[2] *S. aureus* is the most common cause of IE in the industrialized world, mainly because of the risk associated with health care contact.[2-4,7] Successful management of IE requires a multispecialty collaborative effort.[1-4]

Native Valve Endocarditis

NVE is the most common type of IE and affects the mitral valve (28% to 45%), the aortic valve (5% to 36%), and both mitral and aortic valves (35%); the tricuspid valve is rarely affected (5% to 10%).[3,7,8]

Native Valve Endocarditis Risk Factors. Predisposition to NVE seems to be greatest when structural heart disease has created a defect, resulting in turbulent blood flow.[3,4] Any structural heart disease (e.g., rheumatic heart disease, mitral valve prolapse, congenital heart disease) or degenerative cardiac lesion (e.g., calcification of the mitral annulus, calcified nodular lesions secondary to atherosclerotic disease, post–myocardial infarction thrombus) may predispose a patient to IE.[8]

In many countries, rheumatic heart disease is still a common cause of IE; it has been implicated in 37% to 76% of infections.[3] IE has been associated with mitral valve prolapse, especially in the setting of mitral valve regurgitation. Mitral valve prolapse without mitral insufficiency is a more common abnormality and is associated with a small risk of endocarditis. Previous endocarditis is a risk factor for IE due to the valvular damage that results from the infection.[3,8]

Congenital heart disease anomalies including bicuspid aortic valve, patent ductus arteriosus, ventricular septal defect, coarctation of the aorta, bicuspid aortic valve, tetralogy of Fallot, and pulmonic stenosis account for 10% to 20% of the cases.[2] Advances in the management of structural abnormalities and surgical correction of congenital abnormalities have significantly reduced the number of individuals at risk for IE.[2,3,6,8]

IE can occur on valves that are morphologically normal; in recent years, an increasing number of patients have no detectable predisposing cardiac lesion. Other predisposing factors for NVE are advanced age, diabetes, injection drug use, long-term hemodialysis, and immunosuppression, including human immunodeficiency virus (HIV) infection.[4,9]

Native Valve Endocarditis Infectious Organisms. Streptococcal and staphylococcal species account for 80% of NVE in non–injection drug users.[2,3] Higher mortality is seen in patients with *S. aureus* infection, diabetes, advanced age, and IE complications (stroke, congestive heart failure [CHF], paravalvular abscess). *S. aureus* is the culprit organism in most cases of acute IE; it causes systemic toxicity, often with metastatic infection, and carries a 40% mortality.[3,5]

V. streptococci are normal inhabitants of the oropharynx and account for approximately 30% to 40% of all streptococcal IE.[2,3] *Streptococcus gallolyticus* (formerly bovis) is the causative organism in a small percentage of cases and is strongly associated with malignant or premalignant gastrointestinal lesions; therefore evaluation for colon cancer should be conducted in patients with *S. gallolyticus* IE.[2]

Group B streptococci are normal flora of the gastrointestinal tract, oropharynx, vagina, and urethra in 5% to 12% of the population. Group B streptococci account for less than 5% of cases, yet these organisms are capable of affecting normal valves, leading to rapid destruction of the valve and embolization of vegetative matter. Mortality rates can approach 50%.[2,3] Enterococci are indigenous to the gastrointestinal tract and urethra; the number of IE cases caused by enterococci appears to be increasing. IE caused by enterococci is usually seen in both older men and younger women who have a recent history of genitourinary surgery, trauma, or malignant disease. Albeit rarely, it may also occur in women who have undergone an obstetric procedure.[2,3]

Other potential pathogens in NVE include fastidious gram-negative organisms grouped by the acronym of *HACEK* (*Haemophilus aphrophilus; Actinobacillus actinomycetemcomitans; Cardiobacterium hominis; Eikenella corrodens;* and *Kingella kingae*). These organisms are components of the flora of the oropharynx and upper respiratory tract and account for approximately 3% to 10% of cases of IE in patients who do not use injection drugs.[2] Although the clinical course is typically subacute, these organisms are capable of producing large friable vegetations with high risk of embolization, causing CHF and often necessitating valve replacement. Although it was previously difficult to identify the HACEK organisms, they are now reliably isolated with automated blood culture systems.[2,3,5]

NVE caused by other gram-negative organisms including *Pseudomonas* species and *Escherichia coli* is rare and usually associated with central venous catheters and implantable endovascular devices. Recent health care contact is common in these patients.[3]

Fungal IE represents less than 5% of NVE cases. *Candida* and *Aspergillus* species account for the majority of fungal endocarditis, usually in patients with predisposing conditions including but not limited to central venous catheters, dialysis catheters, prosthetic valves, immunosuppression, and implanted cardiac devices. Large vegetations often develop, extension into surrounding tissue and apparatus is seen, and surgical intervention frequently is required. The prognosis remains poor, despite aggressive combined medical and surgical interventions.[2,5]

Culture-negative endocarditis occurs in 5% to 15% of cases of IE. It is usually associated with previous exposure to antibiotics or infection with extremely fastidious organisms or intracellular bacteria that cannot be routinely cultured in blood with the standard blood culture techniques, including *Bartonella* species and *Coxiella burnetii*. Close work with the microbiology and pathology laboratories can help identify organisms that may require longer incubation periods, enhanced culture mediums, special serology testing, and tissue biopsy.[2,3,7]

Prosthetic Valve Endocarditis

Prosthetic valve endocarditis (PVE) comprises 10% to 20% of all IE cases and occurs with similar frequency in both the aortic and mitral valves. The first 12 months after valve replacement surgery represent the highest risk of infection; bioprosthetic and mechanical prostheses are infected with similar frequency.[2,3,9–11] Risk factors associated include prior NVE, long cardiopulmonary bypass time during valve replacement, and male sex.

Transcatheter aortic valve replacement (TAVR), a minimally invasive catheter-based technique using bioprosthetic valves, has resulted in increasing numbers of procedures performed in the United States and globally as a consequence of widening indications. TAVR has emerged in the last decade as an alternative option for patients at inoperable, high, and intermediate risk for surgical aortic valve replacement (SAVR). PVE in TAVR patients has an incidence of 1.1% per person year. Risk factors associated with PVE in TAVR patients include younger age, male sex, diabetes mellitus, moderate to severe aortic regurgitation, chronic obstructive pulmonary disease, peripheral artery disease, chronic kidney disease Stage 3B or greater, hemodialysis, ischemic heart disease, intubation, and CoreValve use. The most common agents reported are enterococci species, *S. aureus*, and coagulase-negative staphylococci. Mortality rate is estimated between 22% and 74.5%.[6,11]

PVE is categorized as early when symptoms occur within 60 to 365 days after surgery, or late when symptoms occur more than 1 year after surgery. Early PVE is usually nosocomial, and the result of perioperative or immediate postoperative infection; it occurs either intraoperatively through direct contamination of the surgical field or postoperatively through contamination of central lines, pacemaker wires, or other indwelling sources. Despite prophylactic antibiotic therapy, the majority of early infections are the result of *S. aureus*, coagulase-negative staphylococci, or fungi.[3,7] The organisms involved in PVE are similar to those seen in NVE. Infections associated with early PVE usually result in rapid valvular dysfunction and destruction of the integrity of the suture line, thus heralding an acute and rapidly deteriorating course with a high morbidity and mortality rate. *Streptococcus* species, enterococci, gram-negative bacilli, and diphtheroids are often involved within the first year after surgery.[3,7,10]

Because late PVE is often caused by less virulent organisms, it usually has a subacute course; however, if the offending organism is virulent, late PVE may also manifest as an acute, fulminant infection. Late fungal endocarditis accounts for 10% to 15% of cases and carries a higher mortality.[2,3] Common presentations in PVE include but are not limited to CHF, conduction system abnormalities, valve dehiscence, and regurgitant murmurs.[7] Staphylococci, streptococci, and enterococci are the organisms mainly responsible for community-acquired late PVE.[3,7] PVE usually requires a combination of medical and surgical approaches.[2,5]

Endocarditis in Injection Drug Users

Those who develop endocarditis associated with injection drug use tend to be 20 to 40 years of age (80%) and are most often male (4 : 1).[3,5] The actual risk of infection among injection drug users is variable, depending on the drugs injected, the method of preparation, and the frequency of use. In this population, infection involving the tricuspid valve or in combination with another valve is most common (50% to 60%). Up to 75% of these patients may develop septic pulmonary emboli.[2,3] Right-sided endocarditis is otherwise rare; therefore injection drug use should be suspected. Involvement of the mitral valve alone is seen in 10.8% of cases, and in the aortic valve, 18.5% of cases. Involvement of both the aortic and mitral valves is seen in 12.5% of patients. The majority of individuals (66% to 75%) who develop IE have structurally normal valves before the infection; a minority have an underlying cardiac lesion from congenital heart disease or previous endocardial infection. Use of injection drugs predisposes the patients to recurrent and polymicrobial IE.[2,3]

Skin flora is the most common source of pathogenic microorganisms in users of injection drugs; contaminated drugs and drug paraphernalia are also bacterial sources. *S. aureus* is the most common offending organism; it is isolated in 50% to 60% of total cases and tends to be less virulent in IE originating from the right side. *Streptococcus* species, *Pseudomonas aeruginosa*, polymicrobial infections, and diphtheroids have also been implicated as causative pathogens.[2,3,5]

Right-sided endocarditis is associated with pneumonia and septic pulmonary emboli as a result of direct embolization in approximately 75% to 85% of patients. These patients appear ill, with high fevers and shaking chills. Patients with a clinical syndrome consistent with tricuspid valve endocarditis should also be evaluated for a potential extracardiac source of the endovascular infection, such as septic thrombophlebitis. The overall mortality rate for right-sided endocarditis is approximately 2% to 6%, whereas left-sided involvement is associated with a much higher mortality.[2,5]

Health Care–Associated Endocarditis

Health care–associated endocarditis (HCA-IE) refers to IE in patients with history of health care system contact (e.g., wound care, care in a dialysis center or specialty nursing home, or chemotherapy within the last 30 days; or hospitalization for 2 or more days within the last 90 days). Community-acquired IE is defined as diagnosis within 48 hours of admission, without extensive health care contact. Non-nosocomial IE is defined as the occurrence of symptoms within 48 hours of hospital admission, with extensive health care contact. Nosocomial IE is defined as IE that is diagnosed more than 48 hours after hospital admission.[3,7] Data suggest that most cases of nosocomial and non-nosocomial IE are caused by *S. aureus*, and at higher rates than previously reported; *Enterococcus* species were second in frequency.[3,9] Invasive interventions have increased during the recent decades, increasing the risk of nosocomial bacteremia and subsequent IE. HCA-IE represents 34% of all episodes of IE and frequently affects elderly patients with poor general condition and comorbidities.[9]

CARDIAC IMPLANTABLE ELECTRONIC DEVICE ENDOCARDITIS

Permanent pacemakers and implantable cardioverter-defibrillators are examples of cardiovascular implantable electronic devices (CIEDs). Advances in cardiovascular device technology have had a positive impact on patient outcomes with respect to quality and quantity of life. According to the American Heart Association (AHA), implantation rates for permanent pacemakers and implantable cardioverter-defibrillators increased dramatically over the study period from 1993 to 2008.[12] With the population living longer and greater numbers of devices being implanted, rates of infection have markedly increased from 0.13% to 0.19%; infection may occur in the device pocket or leads as well as in valvular or nonvalvular endocardium.[2,12] Elevated risk of infection also appears correlated to the following: advanced age; comorbid conditions (diabetes, CHF, malignancy COPD, renal failure); device revision; multiple leads; temporary pacing prior to pacemaker implant; absence of preprocedural antibiotic prophylaxis; hematoma formation; inexperienced operators; and low-volume implantation centers.[9,12,13] Early infections, within 6 months of implantation, are generally caused by skin flora organisms, mainly *Staphylococcus* species. Those organisms demonstrate the ability to form biofilm. Biofilm is an accumulation of bacteria on bacteria, adherent to the surface of the device and encased in extracellular slime; this dense formation of bacteria is more resistant to antibiotics as well as to host defenses.[12,13] Mortality rate is estimated to be 25%.[9]

PATHOPHYSIOLOGY

The development of endocarditis depends on the invasion of the bloodstream by a pathogen capable of attaching to an endothelial surface. The normal endothelium is not conducive to bacterial deposition. A high-velocity jet stream, a narrow valvular orifice, and flow from a high- to a low-pressure chamber are hemodynamic features that predispose the patient to endocarditis. The forceful flow denudes the endothelium and allows platelet and fibrin deposition. The layering of platelets and fibrin creates nonbacterial sterile vegetation (nonbacterial thrombotic endocarditis [NBTE]), which in turn provides an ideal medium for bacterial adherence and growth.[3,14] Virulent microorganisms, especially the staphylococcal species, are capable of attaching to even normal endothelium.[3,4]

Microorganisms typically attach just distal to the narrowed orifice of a turbulent jet, such as on the atrial surface of the mitral leaflets in mitral regurgitation or on the ventricular surface of the aortic cusps in the setting of aortic insufficiency. After colonization of the endothelial surface, bacteria begin the replication process. Further platelet and fibrin deposition over the bacteria provides insulation from phagocytic cellular defenses, which allows the microorganisms to thrive and to form vegetations. Proliferation of the microorganism leads to local valvular destruction, tissue invasion, and possible embolization of the vegetative material.[2–4]

Morphologic characteristics of the vegetations depend on the offending organism and the duration of the infection. Lesions range from small, flat, or granular deposits to large, pedunculated, and friable formations. During the course of effective antimicrobial therapy, leukocytes and fibroblasts penetrate vegetations. This healing process results in fibrosis, occasionally with calcification, and eventual reendothelialization of the valvular surface.[3]

Embolization of vegetative matter is not uncommon and most often involves the renal, splenic, coronary, or cerebral circulation. Pulmonary embolism is a complication associated with right-sided endocarditis or fungal infections. Embolization of septic material can lead to abscess formation. Mycotic aneurysms occur as a direct result of septic invasion into the arterial wall or septic embolization, which weakens the vessel wall and predisposes it to rupture.[3]

Persistent bacteremia triggers an immune complex response of both the humoral and cell-mediated immune systems. As seen in many chronic infections, a generalized hypergammaglobulinemia develops. Immune complexes containing immunoglobulins G, M, and A along with complement are deposited along the glomerular basement membrane of the kidney, precipitating glomerulonephritis. Peripheral manifestations of arthritic discomforts and cutaneous vasculitis may also be attributed to deposition of immune complexes in the joints and mucocutaneous vessels.[3,7]

CLINICAL PRESENTATION AND PHYSICAL EXAMINATION

The clinical history of IE is highly variable according the causative organism. IE should be suspected in a variety of different clinical situations. It may present as an acute, rapidly progressive infection, but also a subacute or chronic disease state with low-grade fevers and nonspecific symptoms. Up to 90% of IE patients present with fever, often associated with chills, poor appetite, and weight loss. Heart murmurs can be found in 85% of patients, while up to 25% of patients have embolic complications at the time of diagnosis. The virulence of the invading microorganism, underlying health of the patient, duration of infection, valvular structures involved, and presence or absence of CHF dictate the pace and severity of the disease course.[1–3]

Fever

Fever is present in the majority of patients but may be absent in older adults, immunocompromised patients, patients with CHF or renal failure, or patients previously treated with antibiotics.[2–4] The degree of fever depends on the causative microorganism; high-grade fevers are primarily associated with virulent organisms and acute infections. Most patients defervesce with 3 to 7 days of appropriate antimicrobial therapy; however, fever may be protracted in some patients, usually resolving within 2 weeks of treatment. Persistent fever may suggest secondary infection, an ineffective antimicrobial regimen, or abscess formation.[2,3,7]

Neurologic Findings

Evidence of cerebral emboli may be seen in approximately 15% to 35% of patients with IE, and is the most common clinical neurologic finding.[7] Half of the patients presenting with these events precede the diagnosis of IE. Staphylococcal IE may manifest with neurologic phenomena as the first sign. The middle cerebral artery is the most commonly involved territory. Brain abscesses, seizures, purulent meningitis, arteritis, cerebral emboli, intracerebral bleeding, subarachnoid hemorrhage, and encephalopathy have also been reported.[2,3,5,7]

Mycotic aneurysms are potentially life-threatening complications that occur in a small percentage of patients. They typically occur early in the course of the disease but can occur months or even years after a bacteriologic cure has been achieved. A severe unrelenting headache, transient neurologic changes, or signs of cranial nerve involvement suggest the possibility of an intracranial mycotic aneurysm.[2,3,5,7]

Ophthalmologic Findings

A complete funduscopic examination in those diagnosed with or suspected to have IE is recommended. Roth spots are exudative, edematous hemorrhagic lesions of the retina. They may cause changes in visual acuity. Endogenous endophthalmitis can be one of the consequences of IE; usual symptoms are decreased vision and/or eye pain. It can cause severe vision impairment and vision loss.[3]

Cardiac Findings

The signs and symptoms of IE vary according to the causative organism and the degree of systemic involvement. Valvular infection can result in the disruption of valvular integrity, including perforation of a valve leaflet, rupture of chordae tendineae or papillary muscles, and leaflet prolapse. Penetration of bacteria into the adjacent myocardium can result in myocardial or paravalvular abscesses, which may contribute to development of conduction system disturbances, heart block, and pericarditis.[7] Further penetration of infection may produce fistulas between cardiac chambers. Large vegetations associated with fungal or *Haemophilus* infections can cause obstruction of the valvular orifice. Even after a bacterial cure has been achieved, fibrosis of the valve leaflets can result in hemodynamically significant valvular stenosis or regurgitation.[3]

Heart murmurs are detectable in the majority of patients but may be absent early in the course of the illness, in patients with right-sided endocarditis, or in older adults. A new murmur of regurgitation or change in an existing murmur suggests an acute, virulent process and often heralds the development of CHF in 30% to 40% of cases. The diagnosis of IE must be entertained in any patient with a new heart murmur or a change in an existing heart murmur and fever of unknown origin.[2–4,7]

CHF predicts a grave prognosis along with poor surgical outcome. Nevertheless, substantially reduced mortality rates are seen in the individual who undergoes valve surgery, if necessary. CHF may be secondary to valvular destruction, rupture of one of the chordae, obstruction of the valve by bulky vegetations, coronary embolization resulting in myocardial infarction, myocarditis, myocardial abscess formation, or prosthetic dehiscence.[2,3,5]

Pulmonary Findings

Pulmonary embolism is most often associated with tricuspid valve endocarditis in injection drug users. It may also occur in patients with indwelling central venous catheters or in patients with left-sided endocarditis who have left-to-right shunting from a septal defect.[2,5] Patients may have clinical pulmonary signs and symptoms, pleural effusion, pneumonia, pleuritic chest pain, and cough with or without blood-streaked sputum. Pneumothorax may also be a complication of septic pulmonary emboli.[3]

Splenic and Dermatologic Findings

Splenomegaly has declined significantly, with rates reported at 11%, possibly because of increasing acute IE and/or shorter time to diagnosis. Splenic septic emboli, although common, are usually asymptomatic. Prolonged fever or localized symptoms should prompt CT scan to rule out splenic abscess.

Petechiae may be noted on the conjunctivae, palate, buccal mucosa, and extremities; they are present in 20% to 40% of patients and usually only for the first few days. Splinter hemorrhages are linear, subungual hemorrhages appearing in the proximal nail bed, and are common in subacute IE.[2,3] Janeway lesions and Osler nodes are cutaneous lesions associated with endocarditis. Janeway lesions are nontender, hemorrhagic macules (1 to 4 mm) on the palms and soles and are the result of septic embolization. Osler nodes are painful nodules on the finger and toe pads that last hours to days. They have also been noted on the forearms, ears, and dorsa of the feet and are associated with immune complex deposition. The resulting inflammatory response leads to swelling, redness, and pain that characterize these lesions. Osler nodes are rare in acute IE but are present in 10% to 25% of subacute cases; they are not specific to IE.[2,3]

Renal Findings

Renal failure is associated with severe and/or prolonged IE and is usually reversible with treatment of the infection. Uremia is often the result of glomerulonephritis secondary to immune complex deposition on the glomerular basement membrane.[3,7] It may also occur secondary to septic embolization leading to renal infarction, or in the setting of severe sepsis and/or cardiogenic shock. The urinalysis may reveal microhematuria with or without proteinuria.[7]

Musculoskeletal Findings

Musculoskeletal manifestations may be seen early in the course of IE. Complaints of arthralgias and myalgias are common. Arthralgias tend to involve the proximal joints and lower extremities and may be monoarticular. Myalgias, often localized to the thigh or calf, are commonly unilateral and have no radicular pattern. These discomforts are often described at the time of presentation and may be related to elevated circulating immune complexes.[3,7]

Findings With Cardiovascular Implantable Electronic Devices

IE in patients with CIEDs can manifest as an acute or subacute process. Infection may be indolent and ongoing for weeks, or acute and associated with symptoms such as sepsis, high fever, rigors, and organ dysfunction. Local inflammatory changes at the pocket site are often seen. Examples are exposure of the leads or device, pain, discomfort, erythema, and drainage. Malaise, anorexia, presence or absence of fever, and decreased functional capacity are also possible complaints.[3,12]

DIAGNOSTICS
Essential Diagnostics

Blood cultures are the cornerstone in diagnosing IE. Three sets of blood cultures should be obtained from different venipuncture sites *before* antimicrobial therapy is initiated. For establishment of the diagnosis of IE, every effort should be made to isolate the pathogenic microorganisms from the blood. Additional blood cultures may be useful in patients who have been recently exposed to antibiotics. Culture specimens can be obtained at any time; a febrile state at the time of culture is not critical, but the initial blood culture sets should be drawn

INITIAL DIAGNOSTICS

For Suspected Infective Endocarditis

LABORATORY TESTS

- **Blood cultures**—PRIOR to initiating antibiotic treatment, at least three sets of blood cultures (second set procured at least 1 h after the first), each set from a different site. Among patients with untreated endocarditis who ultimately have a positive blood culture, 95% of all blood cultures are positive. Negative blood cultures may be present in 10% of patients.[2,4,5,7]
- **Complete blood count**—The white cell count is usually within normal limits in less virulent infections, perhaps with a slight shift to the left. A marked leukocytosis with a shift to the left is a common finding in endocarditis caused by a virulent microorganism.[7]
- **Inflammatory markers**—CRP and erythrocyte sedimentation rate (ESR) are nonspecific, but may be elevated.
- **Serologic tests** can be used for organisms difficult to recover by blood culture: *Brucella, Bartonella, Legionella, Chlamydia psittaci,* and *C. burnetii.* Pathogens can also be identified in vegetations by culture of excised valve tissue and microscopic examination with special stains.[7,14]
- **Electrocardiogram**—Continuous electrocardiograms are necessary to monitor for perivalvular abscess involvement. https://www.kidney.org/news/newsroom/factsheets/High-Blood-Pressure-and-CKD

IMAGING

- **Transthoracic echocardiogram** (TTE) is recommended in patients with staph bacteremia and suspected IE to identify vegetations, characterize the hemodynamic severity of valvular lesions, assess ventricular function and pulmonary pressures, and detect complications.[14-15]
- **Transesophageal echocardiography** (TEE) is recommended in all patients with known or suspected IE when TTE is nondiagnostic, when complications have developed or are clinically suspected, or when intracardiac device leads are present. TEE is preferred for evaluation of suspected endocarditis in patients with valve prostheses (sensitivity for vegetations in this setting is 82%–95%).[14]
- **Cardiac CT** is reasonable to evaluate morphology/anatomy in the setting of suspected paravalvular infections when the anatomy cannot be clearly delineated by echocardiography.[14]

at least 1 hour apart.[2,3,5,7,8] Negative blood cultures may be present in 10% of patients.[2,4] Negative culture data should prompt further investigation into other possible causes of the fever and symptoms. If there is high clinical suspicion of IE in a patient with negative blood cultures, intensive efforts should be undertaken to identify fastidious microorganisms. Pathogens may potentially be isolated from embolized material or excised valve tissue.[2,11]

Laboratory tests including complete blood count should be ordered. The white cell count is usually within normal limits in less virulent infections, perhaps with a slight shift to the left. A marked leukocytosis with a shift to the left is a common finding in endocarditis caused by a virulent microorganism.[7] Serologic tests can be used for organisms difficult to recover by blood culture: *Brucella, Bartonella, Legionella, Chlamydia psittaci,* and *C. burnetii.* Pathogens can also be identified in vegetations by culture and microscopic examination with special stains.[7,14]

Echocardiography plays an important role in the evaluation of highly suspected or documented endocarditis. Vegetations appear as abnormal sessile or pedunculated echogenic masses attached to valve leaflets. Unfortunately, vegetations smaller than 2 mm can be difficult to identify with TTE; body habitus and emphysema limit the sensitivity of this study (46% to 65%).[7,8] With its greater resolution, TEE has been shown to be more sensitive in detection of abscesses (87%) and vegetations (95%).[2,3,5]

Identification of vegetations in the presence of a prosthetic valve is more difficult because the prosthesis causes acoustic shadowing of parts of the ultrasound image; in this setting, the sensitivity of TTE falls to approximately 36%.[2] TEE is capable of imaging prosthetic valves reliably; its sensitivity for vegetations in this setting is 82% to 95%. Consequently, TEE is preferred for evaluation of suspected endocarditis in patients with valve prostheses.[2,3,7,8]

In addition to documenting the presence of vegetations in patients with endocarditis, echocardiography provides additional data of prognostic importance. First, the size, location, and mobility of vegetations as determined with echocardiography may be useful predictors of subsequent embolism. Second, echocardiography reliably identifies leaflet damage or associated valvular regurgitation that arises as a consequence of endocarditis. Finally, echocardiography can detect evidence of local invasion by an aggressive infection, such as an abscess or a fistula formation, that may be an indication for surgical repair.[8,9]

ADDITIONAL DIAGNOSTICS

ESR is elevated except in patients with cardiac or renal failure. Rheumatoid factor can be detected in half of the patients who have an infection lasting longer than 3 to 6 weeks. Circulating immune complexes are present in most patients; however, these levels decline as the infection is effectively treated. The serum complement level is usually decreased, especially in patients with glomerulonephritis. The urinalysis result is most often abnormal with proteinuria, microscopic hematuria, or pyuria. Serum creatinine concentration may be elevated and reflects the degree of renal involvement secondary to glomerulonephritis or renovascular embolization. Although these laboratory findings are common, they are of limited diagnostic value in IE.[2,3,7]

DIFFERENTIAL DIAGNOSIS

 Red Flag: Fever occurs in most cases of acute rheumatic fever (ARF). However, there is no definitive test, so the diagnosis of ARF relies on the presence of a combination of typical clinical features together with evidence of the precipitating group A streptococcal infection, and the exclusion of other diagnoses.[7]

 Red Flag: Fever, hemodynamic changes, new heart murmur. Rule out: Left atrial myxoma that may obstruct left atrium (LA) emptying, causing dyspnea, a diastolic murmur, and hemodynamic changes resembling those of mitral stenosis. Patients have complaints suggestive of a systemic disease, such as weight loss, fever, anemia, systemic emboli, and elevated serum IgG and interleukin 6 (IL-6) concentrations. Auscultatory findings may change markedly with body position. The diagnosis can be established by the demonstration of a characteristic echo-producing mass in the LA with TTE.[7]

 Red Flag: Polyarthritis, neurological complaints. Rule out: Systemic lupus erythematosus (SLE). Antinuclear antibodies (ANA) are positive in > 98% of patients during the course of disease.

BOX **105.1**

Duke Criteria for Diagnosis of Infective Endocarditis

MAJOR CRITERIA

1. Positive blood cultures: one of the following:
   a. Typical organisms consistent with infective endocarditis from two separate cultures (*Viridans streptococci, Streptococcus bovis,* HACEK group, *Staphylococcus aureus,* or community-acquired enterococci in the absence of a primary focus)
   b. Microorganisms consistent with infective endocarditis from persistently positive blood cultures (two positive cultures >12 h apart; or all of three or a majority of four or more separate cultures with the first and last sample at least 1 h apart)
   c. Single positive blood culture for *Coxiella burnetii* or anti–phase I immunoglobulin G antibody titer >1:800
2. Evidence of endocardial involvement: echocardiogram demonstrating vegetation, abscess, new prosthetic valve dehiscence, or new valvular regurgitation (worsening or changing of preexisting murmur not sufficient). (Transesophageal echocardiography is recommended for prosthetic valves rated at least "possible infective endocarditis" by clinical criteria or complicated infective endocarditis, such as paravalvular abscess. Transthoracic echocardiography is the first approach in other patients.)

MINOR CRITERIA

1. Predisposition: preexisting heart conditions or injection drug use
2. Fever: temperature of 38°C (100.4°F) or higher
3. Vascular phenomena: arterial emboli, septic pulmonary emboli or infarcts, mycotic aneurysms, intracranial hemorrhage, conjunctival hemorrhage, Janeway lesions
4. Immune phenomena: nephritis, Osler nodes, Roth spots, rheumatoid factor

5. Microbiologic evidence: positive blood cultures that do not meet major criteria or serologic evidence of active infection with a microorganism consistent with endocarditis

DEFINITION OF INFECTIVE ENDOCARDITIS ACCORDING TO THE DUKE CRITERIA
Definite Infective Endocarditis
Pathologic criteria
    Microorganisms: documented by culture or histologic examination of vegetation, embolic material, or intracardiac abscess; or
    Pathologic lesions: presence of vegetation or intracardiac abscess, histologic confirmation of active endocarditis
Clinical criteria
    Two major criteria; or
    One major criterion and three minor criteria; or
    Five minor criteria

Possible Infective Endocarditis
Presentation and findings that are consistent with diagnosis but fall short of definite criteria (but not "rejected"—one major criterion and one minor criterion or three minor criteria)

Infective Endocarditis Rejected
Firm alternative diagnosis established; or
Resolution of symptoms after 4 days or fewer of antibiotic therapy; or
No pathologic evidence at surgery or autopsy after 4 days or fewer of antibiotic therapy

Modified from Nishimura, R. A., Otto, C. M., Bonow, R. O., et al. (2017). AHA/ACC Focused Update of the 2014 AHA/ACC guideline for the management of patients with valvular heart disease. *Circulation, 135*(25), e1159–e1195.

Ninety percent of patients are women of child-bearing years. Most people with SLE have intermittent polyarthritis, varying from mild to disabling, Lupus dermatitis, nephritis, cognitive dysfunction and headaches, pleuritis, anemia, abdominal discomfort, ocular manifestations, and vascular events such as TIA and stroke.[7]

The diagnosis of IE is based on careful history, physical examination, blood cultures, laboratory results, electrocardiography, chest radiography, and echocardiography. Several sets of criteria for IE have been described. The most widely accepted are the Duke criteria (Box 105.1). This diagnosis must be considered in any patient with a cardiac murmur, changes in an existing murmur, and/or a fever of unknown origin. IE should also be entertained in any febrile injection drug user, patient with a prosthetic valve and evidence of valvular dysfunction, or patient with a cerebrovascular accident.[3] Last, IE should be suspected in any patient with an implantable device (i.e., permanent pacemaker or implantable cardioverter-defibrillator) with erythema at the pocket site, cutaneous erosion of the device itself, or drainage from the pocket.[12,16] The definitive diagnosis of IE requires the isolation of a pathogenic organism from the blood, embolic material, and the demonstration of endocardial vegetations on echocardiography, or at the time of surgery or autopsy.[2,4,16] For patients with suspected device endocarditis,

additional cultures of the device pocket and hardware should be obtained on explantation.[12,16]

The diagnosis of endocarditis is rejected if an alternative diagnosis is established, if symptoms resolve and do not recur with ≤4 days of antibiotic therapy, or if surgery or autopsy yields no histologic evidence of endocarditis. Illnesses not classified as definite endocarditis or rejected as such are considered cases of possible IE.[7]

Other conditions can mimic the signs and symptoms of IE, which makes a definitive diagnosis difficult at the time of initial presentation. A comprehensive diagnostic evaluation will usually yield an accurate diagnosis in a timely manner. Disease processes such as ARF, atrial myxoma, SLE, lymphoma, tuberculosis, thrombotic thrombocytopenic purpura, connective tissue disorders, sickle cell disease, and NBTE can produce a similar constellation of symptoms. Diagnosis of IE requires a high degree of suspicion given its complexity; the Duke criteria remain the most sensitive and specific diagnostic tool available.[2,3,5,7]

INTERPROFESSIONAL COLLABORATIVE MANAGEMENT
Pharmacological Management

The identification of the infecting organism is imperative. Blood cultures should be obtained before appropriate antibiotic therapy is initiated. Consultation with an infectious disease specialist is indicated and further antibiotic changes based on antibiotic sensitivity data and infectious disease consultation.[14] Parenteral administration of antibiotics is preferred to ensure predictably high serum levels. Throughout the prolonged course of treatment, ongoing assessment of the patient's response to therapy and vigilance for the development of potential complications are crucial. Clinical improvement with reduction of fever is usually seen within 1 week of appropriate antimicrobial therapy. Blood cultures should be rechecked and should become negative after effective antimicrobial treatment. Persistent fevers and/or bacteremia should raise the suspicion of an intracardiac abscess, metastatic foci of infection, or inadequate antimicrobial therapy.[2,3,7]

The selection of antimicrobial agents and the duration of therapy vary by microorganism isolated and the duration of infection. IE caused by highly penicillin-sensitive *V. streptococci* can often be cured within 2 weeks with a dual regimen of penicillin G or ceftriaxone and an aminoglycoside. Intracardiac prostheses or infections of longer duration (which produce large vegetations) require a prolonged antibiotic course for a successful cure to be achieved.[5]

Multiple organisms are the infectious agents in NVE. The prominent infectious agents are streptococci, enterococci, staphylococci, HACEK organisms, and fungal organisms. *V. streptococci* usually infect abnormal valves and are typically highly sensitive to penicillin, although some strains are exhibiting variable penicillin resistance.[4] *S. gallolyticus* (bovis) a virulent microorganism associated with significant valvular damage and resultant hemodynamic compromise as well as a high risk of embolism. Treatment options are guided by the degree of penicillin sensitivity; concurrent use of aminoglycosides may be required.[2,4] Group B streptococci may not be eradicated by penicillin alone, and aminoglycoside adjuvant antibiotic therapy may be necessary.[3,5] Enterococci may be resistant to penicillin; the treatment of these organisms has become further complicated by β-lactamase–producing and aminoglycoside-resistant strains. Overall, enterococcal IE therapy will need to be tailored according to the antibiotic susceptibilities.[2,3,5,7]

Staphylococcal species are highly resistant to penicillin because of their ability to produce β-lactamase. Either oxacillin or vancomycin is the preferable therapy, depending on the methicillin sensitivity profile of the organism.[3,5,7] Increasing resistance to these antibiotics has complicated the treatment in recent years.[5]

Valve infection with fungal organisms represents a challenge. Historically, therapy is a combination of parenteral antifungal therapy and valve replacement surgery. The availability of new antifungal agents presents the opportunity for reevaluation of therapy principles.[3,4,6] In CIED endocarditis, antimicrobial therapy should be directed toward oxacillin-resistant staphylococcal species; vancomycin should be administered until the source of infection is known.[12]

Treatment recommendations are formulated by the AHA (Table 105.1). Although these recommendations do not include all subgroups or potential pathogens, they do provide treatment regimens for the most commonly encountered causes of IE and incorporate recommendations for antibiotic resistance. The Infectious Disease Society of America (IDSA) website is also a valuable source of information in determining appropriate treatments.

Nonpharmacological Management

Early recognition of cardiac decompensation and intensive intervention are critical. Decisions about timing of surgical intervention should be made by a multispecialty heart valve team of cardiology, cardiothoracic surgery, and infectious disease specialists.[14] Failure of antimicrobial therapy and/or the development of refractory CHF is an indication for surgical intervention. A recent study showed decreased 1-year mortality rates for patients with IE and heart failure who underwent valve surgery rather than medical treatment alone.[14] Other intracardiac complications requiring surgical intervention include valvular dehiscence, ruptured chordae tendineae, valvular destruction, persistent large vegetations, perforation of valve leaflets, and formation of an aneurysm or abscess. In these situations, surgical intervention may be lifesaving.[4] Early surgery during initial hospitalization before completion of a full therapeutic course of antibiotics is indicated in patients with left-sided IE caused by *S. aureus*, fungal, or other highly resistant organisms.[14] Early surgery in left-sided IE caused by gram-negative bacteria, recurrent emboli, early PVE, or late PVE secondary to *S. aureus* is also indicated.[5,9] CIED endocarditis warrants complete removal of all hardware including the leads and generator, regardless of location.[12,17] Local or superficial infection may not warrant complete removal of all hardware.

INDICATIONS FOR REFERRAL OR HOSPITALIZATION

- Patients with suspected IE should be referred to an emergency department ideally with cardiac surgery availability.
- Patients with IE should be evaluated and managed with consultation of a multispecialty heart valve team including an infectious disease specialist, cardiologist, and cardiac surgeon. In surgically managed patients, this team should also include a cardiac anesthesiologist.[14]
- Patients with IE who have undergone adequate in-hospital treatment may be considered for referral for outpatient parenteral antibiotic therapy (OPAT). OPAT requires scheduled home health care visits by the registered nurse and regular follow-up with the patient's primary experienced clinician.[7]

COMPLICATIONS

The acute complications associated with IE are numerous, may involve all major organ systems, and are potentially life-threatening. Death and persisting morbidity may result from cerebral or coronary artery emboli. Cardiac complications are often the result of direct pathogen invasion, such as valve dysfunction, CHF, paravalvular abscess, and major prosthesis dehiscence. Metastatic complications result from septic embolization or immune complex deposition. Splenic abscess can occur in 3% to 5% of patients with IE. Mycotic aneurysms occur in 2% to 15% of IE patients and may involve cerebral arteries and present as headaches, focal neurological deficits, or hemorrhage. Mycotic aneurysms may also be extra cerebral aneurysms which present as pain, mass, ischemia, or bleeding.[7]

Another concern is the possibility of a relapse. After completion of the antibiotic course, the following should be completed: new baseline TTE, referrals for drug rehabilitation services (if necessary), dental evaluations, prompt removal of intravenous catheter, and ongoing patient education about IE.[5]

Text continued on p. 614

TABLE 105.1   Some Suggested Antibiotic Regimens

Antibiotic[a]	Dose[b]	Duration of Treatment	Comments
NATIVE VALVE ENDOCARDITIS CAUSED BY PENICILLIN-SENSITIVE _VIRIDANS STREPTOCOCCI_ AND _STREPTOCOCCUS GALLOLYTICUS_ (BOVIS)			
Penicillin G (evidence exists for benefit)	12 18 million units/24 h IV, continuously	4 weeks	Preferred in most patients older than 65 years and in patients with impaired renal or cranial nerve VIII function.
Or			
Ceftriaxone (evidence exists for benefit)	2 g/24 h IV or IM in 1 dose	4 weeks	
Alternative treatments: Penicillin G	12–18 million units/24 h IV, either continuously or in 6 equal doses	2 weeks	
Or			
Ceftriaxone[c]	2 g/24 h IV or IM in one dose	2 weeks	
Plus			
Gentamicin (evidence exists for benefit)	3 mg/kg per 24 h IV or IM in a single dose	2 weeks	Gentamicin dosage is based on ideal body weight, not actual body weight.
Vancomycin (evidence exists for benefit)	30 mg/kg per 24 h IV in two divided doses, levels monitored not to exceed 2 g/24 h unless serum levels monitored	4 weeks	Recommended for patients allergic to penicillin or ceftriaxone. Follow recommended peak-trough levels.
PROSTHETIC VALVE OR OTHER PROSTHETIC MATERIAL ENDOCARDITIS CAUSED BY _V. STREPTOCOCCI_ AND _S. GALLOLYTICUS_ (BOVIS)			
Penicillin-Susceptible Strains			
Penicillin G (evidence exists for benefit)	24 million units/24h IV, either continuously or in 4–6 doses	6 weeks	
Or			
Ceftriaxone[c] (evidence exists for benefit) with or without:	2 g/24 h IV or IM in 1 dose	6 weeks	
Gentamicin[b]	3 mg/kg per 24 h IV or IM in 1 dose	2 weeks	The addition of gentamicin has not demonstrated higher cure rates compared with monotherapy. Not recommended with creatinine clearance <30 mL/min.
Vancomycin[c] (evidence exists for benefit)	30 mg/kg per 24 h IV in 2 divided doses, not to exceed 2 g/24 h	6 weeks	Recommended only for patients allergic to penicillin or ceftriaxone.
Penicillin-Resistant Strains			
Penicillin G (evidence exists for benefit)	24 million units/24 h IV, either continuously or in 4–6 doses	6 weeks	For relatively or fully resistant strains with MIC >0.12 mcg/mL.
Or			
Ceftriaxone (evidence exists for benefit)	2 g/24 h IV or IM in 1 dose	6 weeks	
Plus			
Gentamicin (evidence exists for benefit)	3 mg/kg per 24 h IV or IM in 1 dose	6 weeks	See above for gentamicin recommendations.
Vancomycin (evidence exists for benefit)	30 mg/kg per 24 h IV in two divided doses, not to exceed 2 g/24 h	6 weeks	Recommended only for patients allergic to penicillin or ceftriaxone.

TABLE 105.1 Some Suggested Antibiotic Regimens—cont'd

Antibiotic[a]	Dose[b]	Duration of Treatment	Comments
NATIVE VALVE ENDOCARDITIS CAUSED BY STRAINS OF *V. STREPTOCOCCI* AND *S. GALLOLYTICUS* (BOVIS) RELATIVELY RESISTANT TO PENICILLIN G			
Penicillin G	24 million units/24 h IV, either continuously or in 4–6 equal doses	4 weeks	Patients with penicillin-resistant strains (MIC > 0.5 mcg/mL) should be treated with the regimen recommended for enterococcal endocarditis (see below).
Plus			
Gentamicin (evidence exists for benefit)	3 mg/kg per 24 h IM or IV in a single dose	2 weeks	Dose should be adjusted to achieve a peak concentration of 3–4 mcg/mL.
Vancomycin (evidence exists for benefit)	30 mg/kg per 24 h IV in two equal doses, not to exceed 2 g/24 h unless serum levels monitored	4 weeks	Vancomycin is recommended for patients allergic to penicillin or ceftriaxone.
THERAPY FOR ENDOCARDITIS INVOLVING A NATIVE OR PROSTHETIC VALVE OR OTHER PROSTHETIC MATERIAL RESULTING FROM *ENTEROCOCCUS* SPECIES CAUSED BY STRAINS SUSCEPTIBLE TO PENICILLIN AND GENTAMICIN IN PATIENTS WHO CAN TOLERATE β-LACTAM THERAPY[a]			
Ampicillin (evidence exists for benefit)	12 g/24 h IV in 6 doses	4–6 weeks	4 weeks if native valve and symptoms ≤3 months in duration; 6 weeks if symptoms >3 months.
Or			
Penicillin G	18–30 million units/24 h IV, either continuously or in 6 equal doses	4–6 weeks	A minimum of 6 weeks for prosthetic valve or prosthetic cardiac material.
Plus			
Gentamicin (evidence exists for benefit)	3 mg/kg ideal body weight in 2–3 equally divided doses	4–6 weeks	
OR			
Double β-lactam Ampicillin	2 g IV every 4 h 6	6 weeks	
PLUS			
Ceftriaxone	2 g IV every 12 h	6 weeks	
THERAPY FOR ENDOCARDITIS INVOLVING A NATIVE OR PROSTHETIC VALVE OR OTHER PROSTHETIC MATERIAL RESULTING FROM *ENTEROCOCCUS* SPECIES CAUSED BY A STRAIN SUSCEPTIBLE TO PENICILLIN AND RESISTANT TO AMINOGLYCOSIDES OR STREPTOMYCIN-SUSCEPTIBLE GENTAMICIN-RESISTANT IN PATIENTS ABLE TO TOLERATE β-LACTAM THERAPY			
Double β-lactam Ampicillin Plus Ceftriaxone	12 g/24 h IV in 6 doses 2 g IV every 12 h	4–6 weeks	4 weeks if native valve and symptoms ≤3 months in duration; 6 weeks if symptoms >3 months.
Alternative for streptomycin susceptible/ gentamicin resistant			
Ampicillin sodium	2 g IV every 4 h		
Penicillin G	24 million units/24 h IV, either continuously or in 6 equal doses	4–6 weeks	Minimum of 6 weeks for prosthetic valve or prosthetic cardiac material.
Plus			
Streptomycin (evidence exists for benefit)	15 mg/kg ideal body weight per 24 h IV or IM in two equally divided doses	4–6 weeks (a minimum of 6 weeks for prosthetic valve or prosthetic cardiac material)	

Continued

TABLE 105.1   Some Suggested Antibiotic Regimens—cont'd

Antibiotic[a]	Dose[b]	Duration of Treatment	Comments
VANCOMYCIN-CONTAINING REGIMENS FOR VANCOMYCIN- AND AMINOGLYCOSIDE-SUSCEPTIBLE PENICILLIN-RESISTANT *ENTEROCOCCUS* SPECIES FOR NATIVE OR PROSTHETIC VALVE (OR OTHER PROSTHETIC MATERIAL) IE IN PATIENTS UNABLE TO TOLERATE β-LACTAM			
Unable to Tolerate β-Lactams			
Vancomycin[b]	30 mg/kg per 24 h IV in two equally divided doses	6 weeks	
Plus			
Gentamicin	3 mg/kg per 24 h IV or IM in three equally divided doses	6 weeks	
Penicillin resistance; intrinsic or β-lactamase producer			
Vancomycin	30 mg/kg per 24 h IV in two equal doses, not to exceed 2 g/24 h unless serum levels monitored	6 weeks	Vancomycin is recommended for patients allergic to penicillin.
Plus			
Gentamicin[e] (limited evidence exists for benefit)	3 mg/kg per 24 h IV or IM in three equally divided doses	6 weeks	
With Intrinsic Penicillin Resistance			
Vancomycin	30 mg/kg per 24 h IV in two equal doses, not to exceed 2 g/24 h unless serum levels monitored	6 weeks	Infectious disease consultation is recommended.
Plus			
Gentamicin	1 mg/kg IM or IV every 8 h		
THERAPY FOR ENDOCARDITIS INVOLVING A NATIVE OR PROSTHETIC VALVE OR OTHER PROSTHETIC MATERIAL RESULTING FROM *ENTEROCOCCUS* SPECIES CAUSED BY STRAINS RESISTANT TO PENICILLIN, AMINOGLYCOSIDES, AND VANCOMYCIN			
Linezolid	600 mg IV or orally every 12 h	≥6 weeks	Linezolid use may be associated with potentially severe bone marrow suppression, neuropathy, and numerous drug interactions. Patients with IE caused by these strains should be treated by a care team including specialists in infectious diseases, cardiology, cardiac surgery, clinical pharmacy, and, in children, pediatrics. Cardiac valve replacement may be necessary for cure.
Or			
Daptomycin		≥6 weeks	Use with infectious disease consultation.
STAPHYLOCOCCAL ENDOCARDITIS IN THE ABSENCE OF PROSTHETIC MATERIAL			
Oxacillin-Susceptible Strains			
Nafcillin or oxacillin (evidence exists for benefit)	12 g/24 h IV in 4–6 doses	6 weeks	For uncomplicated right-sided infective endocarditis, 2 weeks.
In Patients Who Are Penicillin Allergic (Nonanaphylactoid Type)			
Cefazolin[c] (evidence exists for benefit)	6 g/24 h IV in 3 doses	6 weeks	Avoid cephalosporins in patients with anaphylactoid-type reactions to penicillin.

TABLE 105.1 Some Suggested Antibiotic Regimens—cont'd

Antibiotic[a]	Dose[b]	Duration of Treatment	Comments
Oxacillin-Resistant Strains			
Vancomycin (evidence exists for benefit)	30 mg/kg per 24 h IV in 2 doses	6 weeks	Adjust vancomycin to a trough concentration of 10–20 mcg/mL.
STAPHYLOCOCCAL ENDOCARDITIS IN THE PRESENCE OF PROSTHETIC MATERIAL			
Oxacillin-Susceptible Strains			
Nafcillin or oxacillin	12 g/24 h IV in 6 doses	≥6 weeks	Vancomycin should be used in patients with anaphylactoid reactions to penicillin.
Plus			
Rifampin	900 mg/24 h IV or PO in 3 doses	≥6 weeks	
Plus			
Gentamicin[e] (evidence exists for benefit)	3 mg/kg per 24 h in 2–3 doses	2 weeks	
Oxacillin-Resistant Strains			
Vancomycin	30 mg/kg per 24 h in 2 doses	≤6 weeks	Adjust vancomycin to a trough concentration of 10–20 mcg/mL.
Plus			
Rifampin	900 mg/24 h IV or PO in 3 doses	≤6 weeks	
Plus			
Gentamicin[e] (evidence exists for benefit)	3 mg/kg per 24 h IV or IM in 2–3 doses	2 weeks	
ENDOCARDITIS CAUSED BY HACEK MICROORGANISMS[f]			
Ceftriaxone[c] (evidence exists for benefit)	2 g/24 h IV or IM in a single dose	4 weeks NVE 6 weeks PVE	Cefotaxime or other third- or fourth-generation cephalosporin may be substituted.
Or			
Ampicillin-sulbactam (limited evidence exists for benefit)	12 g/24 h IV in 4 doses	4 weeks	
Or			
Ciprofloxacin (limited evidence exists for benefit)	1000 mg/24 h PO or 800 mg/24 h IV in 2 doses	4 weeks	Recommended only for patients unable to tolerate cephalosporin or ampicillin therapy. In patients with prosthetic valves, treatment is recommended for 6 weeks.

[a]Desirable peak serum gentamicin level (1 h after infusion) is approximately 3–4 mcg/mL. Desirable peak serum vancomycin level (1 h after infusion) is 30–45 mcg/mL for twice-daily administration.

[b]Doses recommended are for adults with normal renal function.

[c]Cephalosporins should not be used in patients with immediate-type sensitivity reactions to penicillins (urticaria, angioedema, anaphylaxis).

[d]All enterococcal endocarditis must be tested for antimicrobial susceptibility.

[e]Gentamicin should be given close to nafcillin, oxacillin, or vancomycin doses.

[f]HACEK microorganisms include *Haemophilus parainfluenzae, Haemophilus aphrophilus, Haemophilus paraphrophilus, Actinobacillus actinomycetemcomitans, Cardiobacterium hominis, Eikenella corrodens,* and *Kingella kingae.*

IE, Infective endocarditis; *MIC,* minimal inhibitory concentration; *NVE,* native valve endocarditis; *PVE,* prosthetic valve endocarditis.

Modified from Baddour, L. M., Wilson, W. R., Bayer, A. S., et al. (2015). Infective endocarditis in adults: Diagnosis, antimicrobial therapy, and management of complications: A scientific statement for healthcare professionals from the American Heart Association. American Heart Association Committee on Rheumatic Fever, Endocarditis, and Kawasaki Disease of the Council on Cardiovascular Disease in the Young, Council on Clinical Cardiology, Council on Cardiovascular Surgery and Anesthesia, and Stroke Council. *Circulation, 132,* 1435–1486.

BOX **105.2**

Cardiac Conditions Associated With High Risk of Adverse Outcome From Infectious Endocarditis

ENDOCARDITIS PROPHYLAXIS RECOMMENDED (HIGH RISK)

Prosthetic cardiac valves, including transcatheter-implanted prostheses and homografts

Prosthetic material used for cardiac valve repair, such as annuloplasty rings and chords

Prior episode of infective endocarditis

Unrepaired cyanotic CHD

Repaired CHD with prosthetic material or device (surgical or catheter intervention within 6 months)

Repaired CHD with residual defects at or adjacent to repair site

Cardiac transplant recipients with development of valvulopathy

CHD, Congenital heart disease.
Modified from Baddour, L. M., Wilson, W. R., Bayer, A. S., et al. (2015). Infective endocarditis in adults: Diagnosis, antimicrobial therapy, and management of complications: A scientific statement for healthcare professionals from the American Heart Association. American Heart Association Committee on Rheumatic Fever, Endocarditis, and Kawasaki Disease of the Council on Cardiovascular Disease in the Young, Council on Clinical Cardiology, Council on Cardiovascular Surgery and Anesthesia, and Stroke Council. *Circulation. 132,* 1435–1486.

BOX **105.3**

High-Risk Procedures and Endocarditis Prophylaxis[a]

ENDOCARDITIS PROPHYLAXIS RECOMMENDED
Dental Procedures
Perforation of oral mucosa
Manipulation of gingival tissue (most dental procedures, such as cleanings, extractions, implant placements, periodontal procedures)
Exposure or manipulation of periapical region of tooth

Respiratory Tract Procedures
Procedures involving incision or biopsy of respiratory mucosa
- Tonsillectomy, adenoidectomy
- Bronchoscopy (only with incision of respiratory mucosa)

Infected Skin, Skin Structure, or Musculoskeletal Tissue Procedures
Surgical procedures involving infected skin or musculoskeletal structures

[a]For patients with underlying risk factors listed in Box 105.2.
Modified from Nishimura, R. A., Carabello, B. A., Faxon, D. P., et al. (2008). ACC/AHA 2008 guideline update on valvular heart disease: Focused update on infective endocarditis. *Journal of the American College of Cardiology, 52*(8), 676–685; and Baddour, L. M., Wilson, W. R., Bayer, A. S., et al. (2015). Infective endocarditis in adults: Diagnosis, antimicrobial therapy, and management of complications: A scientific statement for healthcare professionals from the American Heart Association. American Heart Association Committee on Rheumatic Fever, Endocarditis, and Kawasaki Disease of the Council on Cardiovascular Disease in the Young, Council on Clinical Cardiology, Council on Cardiovascular Surgery and Anesthesia, and Stroke Council. *Circulation, 132,* 1435–1486.

Patients with a relapse in NVE often respond to further antimicrobial treatment, but surgical intervention should be considered, especially in patients with prosthetic valves.[2,5]

On occasion, it is impossible to completely eradicate the microorganism with antimicrobial therapy, and surgery may not be an option because of the high operative risk associated with comorbid conditions. In this case, chronic suppressive therapy may be considered in an attempt to prevent the manifestations and complications of endocarditis.[14]

Life Span Considerations

Because IE is associated with significant morbidity and mortality, primary prevention for patients at risk needs to be considered. The cardiac conditions believed to predispose patients to IE are listed in Box 105.2. Identification of patients at risk is essential and is the responsibility of all providers. The AHA's current recommendations for IE prophylaxis being reserved for those at high risk are summarized in Box 105.3 and Table 105.2. The 2017 AHA/American College of Cardiology (ACC) focused update recognizes that "there is not universal agreement on which patient populations are at higher risk of developing IE than the general population. Protection from endocarditis in patients undergoing high-risk procedures is not guaranteed." Further study of dental prophylaxis for IE is needed. There is no evidence for IE prophylaxis in gastrointestinal procedures or genitourinary procedures, absent known active infection. The AHA/ACC recommendation for prophylaxis is limited to those patients at highest risk of adverse outcomes with IE. These include patients with a history of prosthetic valve replacement, patients with prior IE, select patients with congenital heart disease, and cardiac transplant recipients. IE has been reported to occur after TAVR at rates equal to or exceeding those associated with SAVR and is associated with a high 1-year

mortality rate of 75%. High-risk persons should establish and maintain the best possible oral health to reduce potential sources of bacterial seeding. Optimal oral health is maintained through regular professional dental care and the use of appropriate dental products.[14]

Aging is associated with an increased morbidity and mortality in this already potentially deadly infection. Compromised physical functions are in danger of decompensation in this fragile population. Nutritional fitness is usually compromised at baseline, and reserve is low. Prompt evaluation by the medical team should be initiated if endocarditis is in the differential diagnosis.

PATIENT EDUCATION AND HEALTH PROMOTION

Education of patients and family members is crucial. The etiology and treatment of IE as well as the diagnostic tests should be carefully explained. Patients should understand the importance of preventive therapy and current prophylaxis recommendations. Emphasis on oral health and improved access to dental care should be a primary focus, especially for those with highest risk of predisposition and adverse outcome from IE. Patients should understand the risk of relapse, the early recognition of signs and symptoms, and the importance of obtaining follow-up diagnostics; health care provider evaluations should be emphasized. Every effort should be made to actively engage the patient with prescribed treatment, because lack of patient adherence to regimens may adversely affect treatment outcomes.[14]

TABLE 105.2 Antibiotic Prophylaxis for Dental, Oral, or Respiratory Tract Procedures

Patient Situation	Antibiotic	Route	Adult Dose	Pediatric Dose
Standard prophylaxis[a]	Amoxicillin	Oral	2 g	50 mg/kg
Inability to take standard oral medication[a]	Ampicillin	IM or IV	2 g	50 mg/kg
	or			
	Cefazolin	IM or IV	1 g	50 mg/kg
	or			
	Ceftriaxone	IM or IV	1 g	50 mg/kg
Allergy to penicillin or ampicillin[a]	Cephalexin[b,c]	Oral	2 g	50 mg/kg
	or			
	Clindamycin	Oral	600 mg	20 mg/kg
	or			
	Azithromycin	Oral	500 mg	15 mg/kg
	or			
	Clarithromycin	Oral	500 mg	15 mg/kg
Allergy to penicillin or ampicillin and inability to take oral medications[a]	Cefazolin[b]	IM or IV	1 g	50 mg/kg
	or			
	Ceftriaxone[b]	IM or IV	1 g	50 mg/kg
	or			
	Clindamycin	IM or IV	600 mg	20 mg/kg

[a]All regimens: to be given in a single dose, 30–60 min before the procedure.
[b]Cephalosporins should not be used in patients with hypersensitivity reaction to penicillins.
[c]Other first- or second-generation oral cephalosporins may be used in equivalent adult dose.
Modified from Nishimura, R. A., Carabello, B. A., Faxon, D. P., et al. (2008). ACC/AHA 2008 guideline update on valvular heart disease: Focused update on infective endocarditis. *Journal of the American College of Cardiology, 52*(8), 676–685.

REFERENCES

1. Habib, G., Lancellotti, P., Antunes, M. J., et al. (2015). 2015 ESC Guidelines for the management of infective endocarditis: The Task Force for the Management of Infective Endocarditis of the European Society of Cardiology (ESC). Endorsed by: European Association for Cardio-Thoracic Surgery (EACTS), the European Association of Nuclear Medicine (EANM). *European Heart Journal, 36*(44), 3075–3128.
2. Sabe, M. A., & Griffin, B. P. (2013). Infective endocarditis. In B. P. Griffin (Ed.), *Manual of cardiovascular medicine* (4th ed.). Philadelphia: Lippincott Williams & Wilkins.
3. Fowler, V. G., Scheld, W. M., & Bayer, A. S. (2014). Endocarditis and intravascular infections. In J. E. Bennett, R. Dolin, & M. J. Blasser (Eds.), *Mandell, Douglas, and Bennett's principles and practice of infectious diseases* (8th ed., Vol. 1). Philadelphia: Elsevier.
4. Hoen, B., & Duval, X. (2013). Infective endocarditis. *The New England Journal of Medicine, 368*(15), 1425–1433.
5. Baddour, L. M., Wilson, W. R., Bayer, A. S., et al. (2015). Infective endocarditis in adults: Diagnosis, antimicrobial therapy, and management of complications: A scientific statement for healthcare professionals from the American Heart Association. American Heart Association committee on rheumatic fever, endocarditis, and Kawasaki disease of the council on cardiovascular disease in the young, council on clinical cardiology, council on cardiovascular surgery and anesthesia, and stroke council. *Circulation, 132*, 1435–1486.
6. Cahill, T. J., Baddour, L. M., Habib, G., et al. (2017). Challenges in infective endocarditis. *Journal of the American College of Cardiology, 69*(3), 325–344.
7. Karchmer, A. W. (2014). Infective endocarditis. In D. Kasper, A. Fauci, S. Hauser, D. Longo, J. Jameson, & J. Loscalzo (Eds.), *Harrison's principles of internal medicine* (19th ed.). New York, NY: McGraw-Hill.
8. Cahill, T. J., & Prendergast, B. D. (2016). Infective endocarditis. *Lancet, 387*(10021), 882–893.
9. Ambrosioni, J., Hernandez-Meneses, M., Téllez, A., et al. (2017). The changing epidemiology of infective endocarditis in the twenty-first century. *Current Infectious Disease Reports, 19*, 21.
10. Prendergast, B. D., & Tornos, P. (2010). Surgery for infective endocarditis: Who and when? *Circulation, 121*, 1141–1152.
11. Amat-Santos, I. J., Ribeiro, H. B., Urena, M., et al. (2015). Prosthetic valve endocarditis after transcatheter valve replacement: A systematic review. *JACC. Cardiovascular Interventions, 8*(2), 334–346.
12. Rusanov, A., & Spotnitz, H. M. (2010). A 15-year experience with permanent pacemaker and defibrillator lead and patch extractions. *The Annals of Thoracic Surgery, 89*, 44–50.
13. Palraj, R., Knoll, B. M., Baddour, L. M., & Wilson, W. R. (2014). Prosthetic valve endocarditis. In J. E. Bennett, R. Dolin, & M. J. Blasser (Eds.), *Mandell, Douglas, and Bennett's principles and practice of infectious diseases* (8th ed., Vol. 1). Philadelphia: Elsevier.
14. Nishimura, R. A., Otto, C. M., Bonow, R. O., et al. (2017). 2017 AHA/ACC focused update of the 2014 AHA/ACC guideline for the management of patients with valvular heart disease. *Circulation*.
15. Sekar, P., Johnson, J. R., Thurn, J. R., Drekonja, D. M., Morrison, V. A., Chandrashekhar, Y., et al. (2017). Comparative sensitivity of transthoracic and transesophageal echocardiography in diagnosis of infective endocarditis among veterans with *Staphylococcus aureus* bacteremia. *Open Forum Infectious Diseases, 4*(2), ofx035. doi:10.1093/ofid/ofx035.
16. Sohail, M. R., Wilson, W. R., & Baddour, L. M. (2014). Infections of nonvalvular cardiovascular devices. In J. E. Bennett, R. Dolin, & M. J. Blasser (Eds.), *Mandell, Douglas, and Bennett's principles and practice of infectious diseases* (8th ed., Vol. 1). Philadelphia: Elsevier.
17. Kiefer, T., Park, L., Tribouilloy, C., et al. (2011). Association between valvular surgery and mortality among patients with infective endocarditis complicated by heart failure. *JAMA: The Journal of the American Medical Association, 306*(20), 2239–2247.

CHAPTER **106**

MYOCARDITIS

Joanne Sandberg-Cook

 Emergency department referral is indicated for patients with atypical chest pain, dyspnea on exertion, fatigue, orthopnea, and paroxysmal nocturnal dyspnea. The symptoms, though nonspecific for myocarditis, may indicate left ventricular failure.

DEFINITION AND EPIDEMIOLOGY

Myocarditis, also known as inflammatory cardiomyopathy, includes any pathologic process in which inflammation involving the myocardium is identified. The basic definition given by the World Health Organization (WHO) is "an inflammatory disease of the myocardium diagnosed by established histological, immunological and immunochemical criteria."[1] There are multiple potential causes and therefore varying clinical presentations and outcomes. In addition, the currently accepted gold-standard diagnostic test, endomyocardial biopsy (EMB), is infrequently used; therefore the criteria of this very specific definition will likely not apply to the majority of patients who are ultimately diagnosed with myocarditis using less invasive techniques. To add to the confusion, the Dallas criteria,[2] defined as histologic evidence of inflammatory infiltrates within the myocardium, have been criticized as too insensitive, nonspecific, and unable to predict response to treatment, especially given newer, less invasive diagnostics approaches. The actual incidence of myocarditis is not well defined, with a wide variation of reported cases. For example, in autopsy studies of sudden cardiac death in adolescents and young adults, the prevalence of microscopic evidence of myocarditis has been variably reported to be 2% to 42%[3]; biopsy-proven myocarditis has been reported at 9% and 16% in adults diagnosed with nonischemic dilated cardiomyopathy[4] and in 46% of children with an identified cause of dilated cardiomyopathy.[5]

It is important to note the distinction between cardiomyopathy and myocarditis. *Cardiomyopathy* refers to any situation in which myocardial systolic or diastolic function is impaired and is generally categorized in three separate types; dilated, hypertrophic, or restrictive. There are multiple causes of systolic myocardial dysfunction, the most common in developed nations being ischemic in origin as a result of the presence of coronary artery disease. The most common cause of dilated cardiomyopathy is idiopathic (unexplained), whereas myocarditis is only one cause of dilated cardiomyopathy and accounts for 10% to 50% of cases.[4]

PATHOPHYSIOLOGY

Myocarditis is an underdiagnosed, heterogeneous condition that can be caused by a multitude of insults to the myocardium. The causative agent is most often infectious, such as viral (including human immunodeficiency virus [HIV]), bacterial, protozoal (Chagas disease, a major cause of dilated cardiomyopathy in Latin America), spirochetal (Lyme disease), rickettsial, or fungal. A number of toxins can cause severe myocarditis; ethanol and certain chemotherapeutic agents belonging to the anthracycline family are among the most common. Myocarditis may also be the result of drug-induced allergies (including penicillin allergy) or autoimmune diseases such as systemic lupus erythematosus. Histologic diagnosis is made by examination of tissue obtained by EMB and depends on analysis of the type of inflammation present (lymphocytic, polymorphic, eosinophilic) as well as correlation with other systemic and physical findings. Frequently the cause remains undetermined, although new molecular techniques have shown that viruses seem to be the most important cause in North America and Europe. Viruses that have been identified include enteroviruses, adenoviruses, influenza, herpesvirus, Epstein-Barr virus, cytomegalovirus, hepatitis B and C, and HIV.[4]

The myocardium is damaged by direct viral cytopathic effects as well as by damage by autoantibodies triggered by the ongoing inflammatory process. Families with a genetic predisposition for developing viral-induced autoantibodies and subsequent dilated cardiomyopathy have been identified.[6]

CLINICAL PRESENTATION AND PHYSICAL EXAMINATION

Initial presentation can be varied and ranges from mild symptoms of fever, atypical chest pain, fatigue, and palpitations with possible transient electrocardiographic (ECG) changes to potentially fatal cardiogenic shock and/or arrhythmias and sudden death. Should myocarditis progress to significant systolic dysfunction, the symptoms would be the same as seen in any cause of left ventricular dysfunction (dyspnea on exertion, fatigue, orthopnea, paroxysmal nocturnal dyspnea). In cases involving the right ventricle, either through direct involvement or because of the underlying left-sided failure, the patient may report ankle swelling, bloating, or loss of appetite as a result of the development of bowel edema. Chest pain, usually of the pleuritic kind, may be a prominent finding if there is pericardial involvement.

Myocarditis is more frequent in younger age groups, although it can occur at any age. The presentation may well be subtle, so the diagnosis should be considered in any patient with symptoms suggestive of a cardiac cause, with the understanding that other cardiac diagnoses such as coronary artery disease, endocarditis, or a noncardiac inflammatory process should always be ruled out. It must also be recognized that patients with established cardiac diagnoses, such as coronary disease or valvular heart disease, may also develop acute myocarditis, which should especially be considered if the signs and symptoms do not correlate well with the known existing condition. When this is suspected, the gold standard for diagnosis remains EMB.[7]

Resting tachycardia with an exaggerated chronotropic response to any exertion would be an expected finding on physical examination. Mild cases of myocarditis may include normal physical examination findings or just a low-grade fever and tachycardia. In cases that progress to significant systolic dysfunction, the physical findings would be the same as seen in any cause of left ventricular dysfunction (pulmonary rales, third or fourth heart sounds, or occasionally a murmur of mitral regurgitation [MR] caused by the functional MR seen in moderate to severe left ventricular dilation). There may be a pericardial friction rub in cases involving the pericardium. In cases in which right ventricular dysfunction is a prominent finding, one would see an elevation of the jugular venous pressure, evidence for hepatic congestion in the form of hepatic enlargement and possible right upper quadrant tenderness, and pedal edema, with the development of ascites and anasarca in extreme cases. The astute clinician will be aware of the fact that patients with chronic heart failure can be symptomatic but have few if any obvious physical findings.

DIAGNOSTICS

There are no accepted, specific criteria for making a diagnosis of myocarditis short of EMB. The diagnosis is most frequently made by a combination of clinical presentation coupled with the results of noninvasive testing, most frequently echocardiography. In the right clinical setting (e.g., fever, recent flulike illness), documentation of decreased left (and sometimes right) ventricular function in a more global distribution and lack of regional wall motion abnormalities (RWMAs)—which would be more suggestive of an ischemic cause—are suggestive of a diagnosis of acute myocarditis. In facilities experienced in cardiac magnetic resonance imaging (MRI), a more sensitive finding, in addition to the lack of RWMAs, would be evidence of patchy focal edema and the presence of subepicardial foci of late gadolinium enhancement (LGE), a finding typical of acute myocarditis. Because of the lack of specific criteria in making this diagnosis, it is currently recommended that patients with a suspected diagnosis be referred to a tertiary center with expertise in cardiac MRI or, if deemed necessary, EMB.[8]

As is true with all patients suspected of having a cardiac diagnosis, an ECG should be obtained initially. This is most often abnormal in patients with acute myocarditis, although there are no findings that would be specific for this diagnosis. The ECG might demonstrate all degrees of atrioventricular (AV) block, right or left bundle branch block, nonspecific ST-T wave changes or T-wave abnormalities, atrial fibrillation, or, more ominously, ventricular tachycardia. Of some possible help, the ST elevations that can be seen in acute myocarditis are more frequently concave upward, as they are in pericarditis, and more likely to be diffuse—that is, not restricted to any one specific vascular distribution.

All patients with suspected myocarditis should have an initial echocardiogram to evaluate the degree of left and right ventricular dysfunction, chamber size, and wall thickness and to rule out other potential diagnoses such as valvular or ischemic disease. Global ventricular dysfunction is the most common finding, but one might see RWMAs, although not in the expected distribution of any one vascular territory. In addition, the echocardiogram may demonstrate significant wall thickening and depression of systolic function consistent with the acute edema seen in marked inflammatory conditions. Sequential echocardiograms are very useful in following possible progression or response to therapy. At present, echocardiography is preferable to nuclear studies owing to a lack of sensitivity and specificity of the latter with present techniques. As mentioned previously, cardiac MRI can be very helpful and may be the imaging modality of choice in a facility with that expertise. Stress testing is not recommended in cases of suspected myocarditis owing to the risk of precipitating an arrhythmia in this setting (unless there is a need to rule out an ischemic cause for symptoms).

Biomarkers are helpful and confirmatory in making the diagnosis of acute myocarditis. The markers of acute inflammation, such as erythrocyte sedimentation rate (ESR) and C-reactive protein (CRP), will frequently be elevated but of course are nonspecific as to cause. Specific cardiac biomarkers are more explicit, with troponins being more sensitive than creatine phosphokinase (CPK). These tests will not necessarily, however, help differentiate myocarditis from other cardiac conditions, and the results may be normal at the time of testing. This is also true of brain natriuretic peptide (BNP).

Testing for specific viral antibodies can be unreliable because infection with these agents is frequent in most populations without causing acute myocarditis. Proof of progression from immunoglobulin M (IgM) to IgG antibodies might be helpful, as might testing for HIV when suspected or Lyme disease in areas where it is known to be endemic. Testing for cardiac autoantibodies may be useful, although these tests are not routinely available.

INITIAL DIAGNOSTICS

Myocarditis

LABORATORY	IMAGING
• Complete blood count and differential	• ECG
• ESR	• Echocardiogram
• CRP	• Cardiac MRI
• Troponins	**OTHER**
• IgM to IgG	• EMB

DIFFERENTIAL DIAGNOSIS

The differential diagnosis in patients with symptoms and signs consistent with a diagnosis of myocarditis includes those conditions associated with similar symptoms of dyspnea, fatigue, fever, chest discomfort, palpitations, and presyncope or syncope. Because acute myocarditis is a potentially dangerous condition that can rapidly progress to a life-threatening situation or fatal outcome, rapid diagnostic testing, very close follow-up, and, in general, immediate hospitalization are warranted in all cases of suspected myocarditis.

Other important diagnoses to consider and exclude are those that are more common and potentially dangerous. These include atypical presentations of acute coronary syndromes or myocardial infarction, pulmonary embolism, or other, potentially reversible cause of dilated cardiomyopathy. Other considerations would include underlying valvular disease, cardiomyopathy, endocarditis, pneumonia, or other causes of systemic inflammation not necessarily involving the heart.

INTERPROFESSIONAL COLLABORATIVE MANAGEMENT

 Immediate specialist referral is indicated for all cases of suspected myocarditis.

 Immediate emergency department referral is indicated for all cases in which immediate specialist referral is not available or there are clear symptoms or signs of congestive heart failure or persistent arrhythmia.

Nonpharmacologic Management

The fundamental principles of clinical management include bed rest and avoidance of stimulants such as alcohol, caffeine, and nicotine. Exercise is to be avoided, especially in athletes. Strenuous exercise should not be resumed for 6 months from the date of symptom onset. Competitive athletes should undergo a complete reevaluation including MRI and inflammatory biomarkers between 3 and 6 months. There is concern regarding the effect of myocardial scarring after an episode of myocarditis. If scarring is noted on repeat cardiac MRI, a shared decision-making approach regarding return to competitive sport should be undertaken.[3]

Medical therapy should be instituted in comanagement with a cardiologist or directly by the consulting cardiologist and consists of the same regimen one would use in any cause of heart failure; angiotensin-converting enzyme (ACE) inhibitors or angiotensin receptor blockers (ARBs), loop diuretics (furosemide or torsemide), and β blockers as tolerated. Caution is advised in the use of β blockers in patients with severe left ventricular dysfunction; β blockers may be held until congestive heart failure comes under control. Arrhythmias are treated as in any other situation: temporary pacing for symptomatic brady-arrhythmias or high-grade AV block, rate control or consideration of cardioversion for atrial fibrillation, and antiarrhythmic therapy as indicated for ventricular arrhythmias. Anticoagulation with heparin or warfarin may be indicated in cases of persistent atrial fibrillation or severe left ventricular dysfunction.[10]

Antiviral therapy may be helpful in specific cases depending on the viral agent. Involvement of an infectious disease specialist is recommended if antiviral therapy is being considered. High-dose intravenous immune globulin (IVIG) may be helpful in cases refractory to conventional therapy in either virally mediated or autoantibody-mediated cases. Immunosuppressive therapy using prednisone and/or azathioprine can be helpful in EMB-proven cases without viral etiology. In patients with hypereosinophilia, consideration should be given to the possibility of drug-induced hypersensitivity. The offending agent must be discontinued and should not be reintroduced.

PROGNOSIS AND LIFE-SPAN CONSIDERATIONS

The eventual outcome and prognosis of myocarditis depend on the cause, the patient's clinical status at presentation, and the severity of disease. In about 50% of cases, especially in those with preserved left ventricular function, acute myocarditis resolves in 2 to 4 weeks. Twenty-five percent of patients will progress to chronic cardiac dysfunction, and 12% to 25% can deteriorate acutely and die or progress to end-stage congestive heart failure, requiring consideration of transplantation.[4] Biventricular dysfunction at the initial presentation is a main predictor of death or the eventual need for transplantation.[1,7]

Close follow-up at appropriate intervals—depending on degree of left ventricular function, the patient's physical functionality, and his or her response to therapy for residual heart failure (or lack thereof)—is important both to track recovery as well as to monitor for possible relapse.

PATIENT AND FAMILY EDUCATION

Any visit to a caregiver is likely to be associated with some degree of trepidation or anxiety. This can be especially true of any person who is not feeling well, and any existing anxiety can be magnified when the diagnosis in question involves cardiac issues. Because myocarditis is a potentially life-threatening or disabling disease, it is important to clearly and compassionately explain the process, its effects on cardiac function, and the possible complications that might ensue. This should be done in the context of the overall good prognosis of many patients and the fact that there are advanced therapies for myocarditis, its potential complications, and heart failure. Most important, it should be made clear that the provider, as caregiver, will be there to see the patient and family through this potentially complex, intimidating, and frightening experience.

REFERENCES

1. Richardson, P., McKenna, W., Bristow, M., et al. (1996). Report of the 1995 World Health Organization/International Society and Federation of Cardiology Task Force on the Definition and Classification of Cardiomyopathies. *Circulation, 93*, 841–842.
2. Aretz, H. T., Billingham, M. E., Edwards, W. D., et al. (1985). Myocarditis: A histopathologic definition and classification. *The American Journal of Cardiovascular Pathology, 1*, 1–10.
3. Basso, C., Calabrese, F., Corrado, D., & Thiene, G. (2001). Postmortem diagnosis of sudden cardiac death victims. *Cardiovascular Research, 50*, 290–300.
4. Caforio, A. L., Oankuweit, S., Arbistini, E., et al. (2013). Current state of knowledge on aetiology, diagnosis, management and therapy of myocarditis: A position statement of the European society of Cardiology Working Group on myocardial and pericardial diseases. *European Heart Journal, 34*, 2636–2648.
5. Towbin, J. A., Lowe, A. M., Colan, S. D., et al. (2006). Incidence, causes, and outcomes of dilated cardiomyopathy in children. *JAMA: The Journal of the American Medical Association, 296*, 1867–1876.
6. Kindermann, I., Kindermann, M., Kandolf, R., et al. (2008). Predictors of outcomes in patients with suspected myocarditis. *Circulation, 118*, 639–648.
7. Kindermann, I., Barth, C., Mahfould, F., et al. (2012). Update on myocarditis. *Journal of the American College of Cardiology, 59*, 779–792.
8. Leone, O., Veinot, J. P., Angelini, A., et al. (2012). Consensus statement on endomyocardial biopsy from the association for European Cardiovascular Pathology and the Society for Cardiovascular Pathology. *Cardiovascular Pathology, 21*, 245–274.
9. Marion, B. J., Zipes, D. P., & Kovacs, R. J. (2015). Eligibility and disqualification recommendations for competitive athletes with cardiovascular abnormalities: Preamble, principles, and general considerations: A scientific statement from the American Heart Association and the American College of Cardiology. *Journal of the American College of Cardiology, 66*, 2343–2349.
10. Sinagra, G., Anzini, M., Pereira, N., et al. (2016). Myocarditis in clinical practice. *Mayo Clin Proc, 91*(9), 1256–1266.

CHAPTER 107

PERIPHERAL ARTERIAL AND VENOUS INSUFFICIENCY

Susan Sanner

 Red flags include severe claudication, resting pain, gangrene, nonhealing wounds, absent or diminished pulses, a blue, cold limb.

PERIPHERAL ARTERIAL INSUFFICIENCY

Peripheral arterial insufficiency results when there is insufficient blood flow to the extremities; it includes disease of the aortoiliac, femoropopliteal, and intrapopliteal arterial segments. It is much more likely to occur in the lower extremities, although the use of catheter interventions has made the incidence of upper extremity problems more common. In the United States it is estimated that 8.5 million people have arterial occlusive disease, which is more prevalent in those 50 years of age and older.[1] The incidence in this population is estimated to be 1 in every 20 individuals.[1] If the symptoms have been present for weeks or months, peripheral artery disease (PAD) is defined as chronic. If the symptoms develop over hours or days, it is referred to as acute.

CHRONIC ARTERIAL INSUFFICIENCY

DEFINITION AND EPIDEMIOLOGY

Chronic arterial insufficiency is a disease that has increasing prevalence as the population ages (18% for individuals between 60 and 90 years of age) and is seen more frequently in males.[2]

Because the major cause of PAD is atherosclerosis, the risk factors are the same as those for coronary artery disease (see Chapter 102). Vascular disease is among the most common complications of diabetes, but hypertension, hyperlipidemia, hyperhomocysteinemia, and tobacco use are all independent risk factors. Smokers are twice as likely to develop claudication.[2] Genetic factors have also long been recognized as playing a role in the development of PAD, and an increased level of homocysteine has been associated with atherosclerosis.[1] Even in younger patients, premature atherosclerosis is the most common cause of chronic arterial insufficiency, although rare causes also include entrapment syndromes and adventitial cystic disease of the popliteal artery. Because nontraditional risk factors such as ethnicity may also influence the prevalence of PAD, all individuals above 65 years of age, those older than 50 years with a history of smoking or diabetes, and those with suspected PAD including exertional leg symptoms and non-healing wounds should be screened.[1,3]

Numerous studies have confirmed that most patients with clinically obstructive arterial disease have underlying coronary artery disease or diabetes. These patients have a 40% increased risk of stroke and a 20% to 60% risk of myocardial infarction (MI), with a twofold to sixfold increase in the risk for cardiac death.[1,3]

In cases of severe obstructive disease and acute limb ischemia, the risk for amputation is determined not by the mere appearance of claudication but by disease severity, the sudden appearance of limb ischemia, and the timeliness and ability to restore limb circulation. The occurrence of acute limb ischemia carries with it a 30-day amputation rate of 10% to 30% regardless of whether thrombolysis has been used.[3]

PATHOPHYSIOLOGY

Atherosclerosis is an abnormality of the arteries and therefore can impact any organ in the body. The individual may be asymptomatic until a complication develops.[4] For example, extensive atherosclerosis may lead to aneurysmal dilation and rupture of the vessel; constriction of one or both renal arteries may cause renal hypertension and resultant damage; and vascular insufficiency in the legs may cause intermittent claudication. A severely compromised limb may also lead to gangrene with eventual loss of the limb. Obstruction may also occur in vasculature that supplies the intestines. Chronic arterial insufficiency results from diverse systemic conditions that can affect the arteries in various parts of the circulatory system even in the absence of clinical symptoms in more than one arterial system.[2] The disease entities that result in arterial insufficiency include degenerative diseases (collagen abnormalities found in Marfan or Ehlers-Danlos syndrome), dysplastic disorders (e.g., fibromuscular dysplasia), and vascular inflammatory processes (e.g., arteritis). Arterial insufficiency can also be a result of thrombosis, thrombotic embolism, radiation-induced arteritis, autoimmune conditions, and, the most common cause, arteriosclerosis.[4]

In patients without atherosclerosis, the pathophysiology of chronic arterial insufficiency involves loss of structural integrity of the artery wall. This loss produces arterial dilation and favors aneurysm formation, with its associated risk of rupture or occlusion as a result of aneurysmal dissection[4]; it can affect arteries in the carotid, renal, and iliac circulation most commonly but is not restricted to those circulatory beds.[4]

In patients with underlying arteriosclerosis, the atherosclerotic plaque causing leg ischemia is identical to that seen in coronary artery disease and carotid disease. The plaque is an intimal lesion that may affect any of these vessels. The blockage may build up slowly, allowing collateral vessels to develop and thereby minimizing symptom progression until such time as the flow is inadequate to support metabolic needs.

Alternatively, intraplaque hemorrhage and thrombosis may lead to sudden expansion and acute symptoms.

The infrarenal aorta and iliac arteries are classified as the inflow arteries, whereas the femoral, popliteal, and tibial vessels are classified as the outflow vessels. Obstruction of the aortoiliac and femoral arteries is often seen in smokers, whereas disease in the smaller vessels, such as that seen in tibial artery disease, is much more common in patients with diabetes. There is evidence that the presence of a reduced ankle-brachial index (ABI) and diabetes are associated with the development of rest pain and ulcerations from inadequate perfusion.

CLINICAL PRESENTATION AND PHYSICAL EXAMINATION
Risk Factors

Certain groups of patients are at risk for PAD. This includes patients who are older than 65 years of age (21% had asymptomatic or symptomatic PAD in one study),[1] those between the ages of 50 to 64 years with a history of diabetes, smoking, hyperlipidemia, hypertension, or family history of PAD; and patients younger than age 50 who have diabetes and another risk factor for atherosclerosis (e.g., smoking, dyslipidemia, hypertension, hyperhomocysteinemia). It also includes patients with known atherosclerotic disease in another vascular bed (e.g., coronary, carotid, subclavian, renal), mesenteric artery stenosis, or abdominal aortic aneurysm (AAA)[1] as well as patients with exertional leg symptoms suggestive of claudication or with ischemic rest pain and those with abnormalities of lower extremity pulses. All of these patients should undergo a comprehensive vascular review of symptoms (Box 107.1).[1,5]

It is imperative to recognize that each patient with PAD is unique; the reported discomfort associated with PAD includes "tiredness," "giving way," "soreness," or "pain." Although the classic or "textbook" symptom of peripheral arterial insufficiency is claudication, patients can report two or more symptoms in two or more locations. Primary care providers must take a careful history of each symptom, including the impact of each symptom on work, activities of daily living, and recreational activities; the symptoms should be interpreted in the context of patient comorbidities and the presence of the previously discussed PAD risk factors.[3] When present, claudication is a tightening or cramping pain that is precipitated by exercise and relieved by rest. These symptoms most frequently occur in

---

BOX 107.1

Components of a Vascular Review of Symptoms (Including Family History)

Assess for presence of
- Exertional leg symptoms (fatigue, aching, numbness, or pain; record location of symptoms such as buttock, thigh, calf, or foot)
- Impaired walking function
- Other non–joint-related exertional lower extremity symptoms (not typical of claudication)
- Poor wound healing in legs or feet
- Pain at rest in lower leg or feet; note whether this occurs when patient is recumbent or upright
- Abdominal pain that occurs after eating and is associated with weight loss
- First-degree relative with abdominal aortic aneurysm

the calf muscles but can also occur in the thighs or buttocks, depending on the location of the stenosis. Claudication occurs with exercise because of an increased demand for blood that cannot be met by the stenotic vessels. Subsequently, lactic acid and other metabolites build up in the muscle, causing discomfort. Claudication is assessed by how far a patient can walk before pain ensues. Although the distance may be reduced by an incline, cold weather, or a recent meal, it tends to be fairly consistent. Pain is always relieved immediately by stopping the activity and never occurs when the patient is at rest. The thigh or buttock muscles are sometimes affected first. This is indicative of iliac artery obstruction (Leriche syndrome).

As the obstruction becomes more severe, the patient may develop pain at rest because circulation to the feet is impaired. Characteristically the patient will go to bed and be awakened after a couple of hours by pain in the toes that is relieved only by gravity to enhance peripheral blood flow (e.g., getting out of bed or hanging the feet over the side of the bed). The patient may resort to sleeping in a chair to avoid the pain. Ischemic rest pain tends to be consistent; it occurs every night, unlike the intermittent leg cramps seen so often in older adults, which are not related to arterial insufficiency.

For effective, collaborative care of the patient with suspected vascular insufficiency, there must be a standard set of measurements. The American College of Cardiology (ACC) and American Heart Association (AHA) 2016 guidelines recommend components of the vascular physical examination supplemented by vascular testing (see the section on diagnostics, later). Components of the vascular physical examination include measurement of blood pressure in both arms at least once during the initial assessment and vascular examination that includes inspection of legs and feet, palpation of lower extremity pulses for quality and amplitude (femoral, popliteal, dorsalis pedis, and posterior tibial), assessment of abdominal aortic pulsation, and auscultation for femoral bruits (Box 107.2).[1]

Inspection of the limbs may reveal muscle wasting and loss of hair. With more severe disease, there is not enough blood to sustain viability, and tissue loss ensues, usually beginning in the toes or heels. Tissue loss may manifest as ulceration, dry gangrene, or wet gangrene. Reduced temperature in an affected limb may be noted. Careful pulse examination is important. Absent femoral pulses suggest inflow disease, whereas the absence of popliteal pulses implies isolated tibial disease.

One physical sign that can be helpful in the diagnosis of peripheral vascular disease is dependent rubor. If the ischemic leg is elevated for 30 seconds, it becomes pale, because blood is unable to travel uphill. This renders the tissue ischemic, and the capillaries vasodilate. If the leg is then made dependent, blood travels down to those dilated capillaries, and a deep red color ensues. The longer the rubor takes to develop, the worse the ischemia. A careful history and physical examination will allow a good assessment of the functional severity of the obstruction and its likely location.

The severity of the patient's peripheral arterial insufficiency can be graded based on the vascular history and physical examination findings. Fontaine's stages or Rutherford's categories are the most widely used tools to provide a standardized system of classifying the severity of peripheral disease based on symptoms, gangrene, or ulcerations.[6] The distances that define mild, moderate, and severe claudication are part of the Fontaine classification and are based on a distance of 200 m (650 ft).

BOX 107.2

Components of the Vascular Physical Examination

Measure blood pressure in both arms; record findings and note any discrepancy.

Auscultate carotid arteries bilaterally for bruits; record findings.

Palpate carotid pulses bilaterally; record upstroke and pulse amplitude.

Auscultate abdomen and flank for bruits; record findings.

Palpate abdomen; measure and record width of aortic pulsation.

Palpate, estimate, and record the intensity of the following pulses bilaterally: brachial, radial, ulnar, femoral, popliteal, dorsalis pedis, and posterior tibial.

Use the following scale for pulse intensity documentation: 0 = absent, 1 = diminished, 2 = normal, 3 = bounding.

If upper extremity insufficiency is suspected, perform an Allen test and record results.

Auscultate femoral arteries for bruits; record findings.

Assess lower extremities for indications of more severe peripheral artery disease, such as distal hair loss, trophic skin changes, or hypertrophic nails; record findings.

Remove patient's shoes and socks; assess feet for color, temperature, skin integrity, ulcerations; examine intertriginous areas for lesions or ulcerations; record findings.

Measure and record ankle-brachial index.

Data from Gerhard-Herman, M. D., Gornik, H. L., Barrett, C., Barshes, N. R., Corriere, M. A., Drachman, D. E., et al. (2017). 2016 AHA/ACC guideline on the management of patients with lower extremity peripheral artery disease: Executive summary: A report of the American College of Cardiology/American Heart Association Task Force on Clinical Practice Guidelines. *Circulation*, 135(12), e686–e725. doi:10.1161/CIR.0000000000000470.

They are not specified in the Rutherford classification of symptoms. In addition, there is a separate Rutherford scale for acute limb ischemia.[6] Any patient with intermittent claudication, leg pain at rest, or nonhealing wounds in the lower extremity that persist for 4 weeks or more warrants an evaluation for PAD.

DIAGNOSTICS

Depending on the clinical scenario and the urgency of the patient's condition, there is a role for noninvasive testing to supplement the history and physical examination. The level of testing should be limited initially to those studies that confirm the presence of arterial disease and those that will alter the course of treatment. The main reason for physiologic testing is to verify a vascular origin for the patient's complaints and to localize the level of the lesion. In addition, such testing can be used to assess the adequacy of tissue perfusion and wound-healing potential.

The initial diagnostic test for lower extremity PAD is the resting ABI. It is used in patients with one or more of the following: exertional leg symptoms, nonhealing lower extremity wounds, history consistent with PAD in patients 65 years and older, or symptoms in patients 50 years and older with a smoking history or diabetes.[1] The most useful tools in assessing peripheral arterial insufficiency in the office are a portable Doppler instrument and a sphygmomanometer cuff. With these tools, it is possible to compare the systolic pressure at the brachial artery with that in the dorsalis pedis and posterior tibial arteries. This measurement is expressed as the ABI and should be lower in the affected extremity than in the normal one. An ABI of 0.9 or less is indicative of PAD. An ABI of 0.75 to 0.5 is consistent with claudication, and an ABI below 0.5 is consistent with rest pain and/or tissue loss. An ABI higher than 1.4 is also considered abnormal and can indicate the potential for noncompressible calcified vessels. Along with low ABI, high ABI is also associated with higher cardiovascular risk.[1,3,7] The clinical significance of ABI results provide guidance on continued evaluation of PAD. An ABI greater than 1.4 is consistent with calcified arteries, warranting the use of the toe-brachial index (TBI) to determine the presence of disease. Peripheral vascular resistance (PVR) may be used to determine levels of disease. For patients with normal ABI results (1.0 to 1.4) and high clinical suspicion for PAD based on symptoms, treadmill exercise testing should be considered. Exercise testing may also be considered when the patient has a borderline ABI reading (0.91 to 0.99). PVR may be useful if there is a need to determine level of disease in cases where mild (0.71 to 0.9) and moderate disease (0.41 to 0.7) are present. Patients with mild disease may be asymptomatic but may present with claudication. Severe disease (ABI < 0.4) is usually associated with poor wound-healing potential. Angiographic imaging is appropriate for patients with nonhealing wounds or gangrene so as to determine reperfusion options.[1,4,7]

In summary, the AHA/ACC 2016 guidelines for managing patients with lower extremity PAD recommend resting ABI for patients with history or physical exam findings suggestive of PAD in order to establish the diagnosis (Level 1). In patients at increased risk of PAD but without history or physical exam findings suggestive of PAD, obtaining resting ABI is still reasonable (Level 1I). There is no benefit, however, to perform resting ABI on patients who do not have increased risk of PAD and have no history or physical exam findings suggestive of PAD (Level III).[1]

Additional physiologic testing may be indicated (exercise treadmill ABI testing, TBI, and perfusion assessment measures that include transcutaneous oxygen pressure [T$_c$PO$_2$] or skin perfusion pressure [SPP]). For example, exercise treadmill ABI testing is useful in establishing lower extremity PAD in the symptomatic patient when resting ABI results are normal or borderline. The TBI is useful in establishing the diagnosis of PAD in the setting of noncompressible arteries (ABI > 1.40).

Anatomic imaging studies such as duplex ultrasound may be conducted on the lower extremities to diagnose anatomic location and severity of stenosis when revascularization is being considered for symptomatic patients with PAD (Level I). Invasive angiography may also be considered for patients with chronic leg ischemia (CLI) when revascularization is being considered (Level I) and is also reasonable for patients with severe claudication who have had an inadequate response to guideline directory medical therapy (GDMT) and revascularization is being considered (Level IIa).[1] In patients with symptomatic PAD, noninvasive or invasive angiography should not be performed (Level III).[1]

Patients with mild claudication may have palpable pulses at rest but lose them with exercise. This is best demonstrated in the vascular laboratory with an exercise noninvasive study. During this test, the patient is placed on a treadmill and ABIs are measured at rest, while exercising, and on recovery.

Related medical conditions, such as obesity and peripheral edema, sometimes make it impossible to assess the pulse status. In these situations the pocket Doppler instrument may be invaluable. A normal pulse is triphasic but becomes increasingly monophasic with proximal obstruction. With practice, it is relatively simple to distinguish these pulses. If Doppler ultrasonography reveals good triphasic pulses in the feet, significant ischemia in that extremity is unlikely.

Patients should be referred to the vascular laboratory for formal evaluation if there is concern for arterial insufficiency or to ascertain the location and severity of occlusive lesions. The prevalence of atherosclerosis in other arterial beds (coronary, carotid and renal, and mesenteric arteries) is higher in patients with PAD. Aggressive treatment of risk factors through GDMT, rather than screening, is the major approach to prevent adverse cardiovascular ischemic events from asymptomatic disease in other arterial beds. The US Preventive Services Task Force (USPSTF) recommends one-time screening for AAA with ultrasonography in men ages 65 to 75 years who have ever smoked. The USPSTF recommends against routine screening for AAA in women who have never smoked. The only justification for screening in other arterial beds is if revascularization would result in a reduced risk of MI, stroke, or death.

INITIAL DIAGNOSTICS

Chronic Arterial Insufficiency

INITIAL
- Doppler ankle and arm indexes

LABORATORY
- Serum glucose, lipid profile, high-sensitivity C-reactive protein, and homocysteine

IMAGING
- Digital subtraction angiography
- Color-assisted duplex ultrasonography

- Magnetic resonance angiography
- Computed tomography angiography

OTHER DIAGNOSTICS
- Segmental limb pressure measurement
- Pulse volume recording
- Toe-brachial index assessment
- Velocity waveform analysis
- Treadmill testing
- Plethysmography

DIFFERENTIAL DIAGNOSIS

The presence of peripheral neuropathy in diabetes makes the diagnosis of peripheral insufficiency difficult. Damage to the peripheral nerves may mask the symptoms of arterial insufficiency. Thus if patients have no feeling in their legs, they may simply complain that their legs get tired of walking. Without sensation, there may be no rest pain, and patients may be initially seen with nonhealing ulcers and possibly painless gangrene. Other conditions that should be considered include cauda equina syndrome related to spinal stenosis and Buerger disease, an inflammatory occlusive disease of medium and smaller arteries primarily related to nicotine use, common leg cramps, and musculoskeletal disorders.

Upper Extremity Arterial Disease

It is important not to forget about the upper extremities in evaluating patients with known or suspected arterial disease. Patients with compromised flow to the upper extremities can have typical ischemic pain of one or more muscle groups but may also have atypical pain or no symptoms at all. The presentation may be only a difference in the systolic blood pressure between one arm and the other.

In other cases, patients may report dizziness during arm exertion, which can be indicative of disease in the subclavian artery. Subclavian steal syndrome implies the presence of significant symptoms caused by arterial insufficiency to the brain (vertebrobasilar insufficiency) or the upper extremity, which is also supplied by the affected subclavian artery.[8]

A review of symptoms and upper extremity vascular examination must be performed in all patients at risk for PAD or with documented PAD. Further testing would be determined based on examination findings and symptoms. This may include duplex ultrasound, transcranial Doppler studies, magnetic resonance angiography, or computed tomography (CT) angiography.[9]

INTERDISCIPLINARY COLLABORATIVE MANAGEMENT

 Referral to a vascular specialist is indicated for patients with superficial ulcers who do not improve with bed rest and treatment. More extensive ulcers require immediate vascular consultation.

Nonpharmacologic Management

Management of chronic arterial insufficiency depends on the severity of the symptoms. If the patient has stable claudication and is managing without much difficulty, it is reasonable to treat him or her conservatively. Patients with mild claudication of recent onset are likely to improve with conservative measures alone. These include lifestyle modifications as indicated, particularly tobacco cessation. Hypertension, hyperlipidemia, and diabetes must be treated aggressively to reduce long-term risk. Compression stockings may be used in selected PAD patients to treat leg swelling and reduce the risk for deep venous thrombosis (DVT) provided that the ABI is 0.8 or higher and the use of the compression stockings does not compromise circulation to the extremity or increase claudication symptoms.[1,10]

Studies comparing exercise with angioplasty have shown that a daily exercise program involving walking to the point of pain as often as possible is as effective as angioplasty in providing relief of symptoms.[1] Components of a structured exercise program to relieve claudication include (1) an initial session of treadmill or track walking of 30 minutes, with an increase of subsequent sessions to reach 1 hour per session three times a week; (2) in each session, walking at a speed and grade that produce moderate claudication pain within 3 to 5 minutes; (3) resting until claudication resolves; and (4) repeating the exercise and rest cycles until the session duration is achieved.[1,10] Because the ABI does not change, it is believed that this beneficial effect is produced by training the muscles rather than by increasing flow to the foot.

Diabetic patients with neuropathy or arterial insufficiency require regular podiatry consultation. The podiatrist will determine the frequency of visits based on callus development. With appropriate shoes and care of calluses and nails, many patients with ischemia can avoid problems for long periods. Regular podiatric visits enable early recognition of potential problems and ensure expeditious referral and treatment.

Pharmacologic Management

These patients are at high risk for coronary artery disease, so it is prudent to start them on antiplatelet therapy. Aspirin alone (81 to 325 mg/day) or clopidogrel alone (75 mg/day) is recommended to reduce the risk of MI, stroke, and vascular death in patients with symptomatic PAD (Level I).[1,11] Clopidogrel can be used as an alternative to aspirin or in combination with aspirin (reserved for high-risk patients not at risk for bleeding).[12] In asymptomatic patients with PAD with mild to moderate ABI results, antiplatelet therapy is also reasonable (Level IIa).[11,12] For asymptomatic patients with borderline ABI results (0.91 to 0.99), the use of antiplatelet therapy to reduce the risk of MI, stroke, or vascular death is uncertain (Level IIb).[1,10,11] The effectiveness of using a combination of aspirin and clopidogrel to reduce the risk for cardiovascular ischemic events in patients with symptomatic PAD is not clear (Level II b).[1,11]

Any antiplatelet regimen must be based on an individual patient's clinical characteristics (risk of PAD, risk of bleeding) and tolerance for the medications in conjunction with cost and future evidence-based guidelines.[1,12] The use of anticoagulant therapy to improve vessel patency after lower extremity bypass surgery is unclear (Level IIb). In addition, anticoagulation therapy should not be used to reduce the risk of cardiovascular ischemic events (Level III).[1]

It has been shown that statin therapy helps stabilize plaque and lowers the level of low-density lipoprotein (LDL); moreover, studies have suggested that bypasses are more durable if the patient is taking a statin. Treatment with a statin is indicated for all patients with PAD (Level IA).[1]

Antihypertensive medications should be administered to patients with hypertension and PAD to reduce the risk of MI, stroke, heart failure, and cardiovascular death (Level 1A). The use of angiotensin-converting enzyme inhibitors (ACEIs) or angiotensin-receptor blockers (ARBs) can be effective to reduce the risk of cardiovascular ischemic events in patients with PAD (Level IIa).[1]

Pentoxifylline (Trental) is no longer recommended for the treatment of claudication (Level III).[1] Cilostazol (Pletal), a phosphodiesterase type 3 inhibitor, has been shown to be an effective therapy to improve symptoms and increase walking distance in patients with claudication (Level IA).[12] The main contraindication for using cilostazol is a history of congestive heart failure.

The use of B-complex vitamin supplements to lower homocysteine levels and thus to prevent cardiac events has no benefit and therefore is not recommended (Level III).

Surgical Management

Once the extent of the severe ischemia has been identified, arteriography is indicated to demonstrate the extent and location of the obstruction. Treatment may involve angioplasty (with or without stent placement) or surgery. Magnetic resonance arteriography has been a popular alternative to arteriography, but the risk of gadolinium-induced complications has limited its use in patients with renal failure. CT angiography has become more popular, particularly in patients with aortoiliac disease, because it is less invasive. In general, neither arteriography nor CT should be ordered without consultation with a vascular medicine specialist or a vascular surgeon. The vascular specialist can perform arteriography and decide at that time whether to proceed with an angioplasty or stent or to refer the patient for surgery. Patients are often treated with a hybrid procedure in which an inflow stent is placed at the same time as an outflow surgical procedure is performed.[13]

COMPLICATIONS OF CHRONIC PERIPHERAL ARTERIAL DISEASE

Lower extremity ulcers may result from neuropathy, arterial insufficiency, infection, or a combination of these. Infections such as cellulitis or ulcers with extensive involvement may result in osteomyelitis. The presence of infection can also disturb blood glucose control, complicating diabetes management.

Peripheral neuropathy is associated with the development of calcification of the arteries. This is not directly related to the atherosclerotic lesion, which is an intimal lesion, but it does render the vessels relatively incompressible. This means that the ABI may be artificially elevated and less helpful in assessing the degree of ischemia. In these cases the pulse volume recording can be particularly helpful.

Thirty percent of patients with neuropathy also have an autonomic neuropathy, which is sometimes called an autosympathectomy. This condition results in the diversion of blood from the nutrient vessels to the skin, making the skin unnaturally warm. Thus it is possible to see a diabetic patient with a minor skin lesion but with no symptoms and a warm foot that is critically ischemic. Failure to recognize this may result in further loss of tissue.

Abdominal Aortic Aneurysm

PAD is a risk factor for AAA. Its prevalence increases with age, beginning in patients 55 years of age with the highest prevalence in patients 75 years of age and older. The prevalence is also higher in patients with symptomatic PAD and in those with atherosclerotic risk factors. Although there are no data to support AAA screening in patients with asymptomatic PAD, it is reasonable to perform a screening duplex ultrasound in patients with symptomatic PAD (Level IIa)[1] (see Chapter 99).

Renal Artery Stenosis

Atherosclerosis is the most common etiology of renal artery stenosis, causing more than 90% of cases. Fibromuscular dysplasia is the second most common cause. The result of intervention is more favorable for fibromuscular dysplasia than for renal artery atherosclerosis. Open surgical repair (OSR) via endarterectomy or bypass is less preferred than percutaneous angioplasty and stenting, although randomized trials (Angioplasty and Stenting for Renal Artery Lesions [ASTRAL] and Cardiovascular Outcomes in Renal Atherosclerotic Lesions [CORAL]) failed to demonstrate a clinical benefit of renal artery intervention compared with best medical therapy for patients with moderate stenosis and hypertension. Restenosis is common after renal artery angioplasty and surgical bypass. Recurrent stenosis is also common after reintervention. Although there are several intervention techniques for angioplasty, no one method appears to be superior over the others. CT angiography is used to detect renal artery in-stent restenosis. This test has been shown to be effective and sensitive but not specific for detecting renal artery stenosis. Diagnostic ultrasonography (DUS) is the most common test used for follow-up after renal artery intervention. Overall there is no evidence documenting the efficacy of a surveillance protocol after renal artery intervention. After renal artery angioplasty with or without stenting or renal artery bypass or endarterectomy, clinical follow-up and a baseline DUS is recommended within a month of the procedure and again at 6 and 12 months and then annually (Level II, C). Contrast-enhanced imaging is recommended for loss of renal parenchyma as determined by DUS findings (Level II, B).[14]

Diabetic Foot Ulcer

Diabetic neuropathy is a polyneuropathy and has a motor component. The paralysis of the intrinsic muscles results in clawing of the foot, and the patient tends to develop traumatic lesions over the metatarsal heads and on the tops of the toes. Healing may be impaired by relative arterial insufficiency.

Infection

Any infection requires treatment with appropriate debridement and antibiotics (see Chapter 51). Bed rest is indicated to minimize damage, which may go undetected if neuropathy is present. If the ulcer is superficial, it can be treated on an outpatient basis with non–weight bearing, dressing care, and a first-generation cephalosporin. If the ulcer is deep or has significant cellulitis, hospitalization with the institution of broad-spectrum antibiotics is advised. Failure to heal with treatment suggests arterial insufficiency and merits referral to a vascular surgeon or vascular medicine specialist for possible arteriography.

LIFE SPAN CONSIDERATIONS

Women, particularly postmenopausal women, exhibit complications associated with PAD at a higher rate than men, yet risk assessment, risk modification, and early detection and intervention do not occur at the same rate as in male patients. Complicating the picture are the nonspecific symptoms that women with PAD exhibit, including bilateral claudication, extremity fatigue, and rest discomfort. Women tend also to be more likely to be nonwhite and living alone, less likely to be married, and more likely to delay treatment because of financial concerns.

Primary care providers are well advised to consider the holistic nature of atherosclerotic disease—whether found in the coronary, peripheral, renal, or cerebral arteries—and to incorporate PAD risk screening and risk reduction for patients with CAD risk factors such as hypertension, diabetes, and hyperlipidemia.

EDUCATION AND HEALTH PROMOTION

All patients should be advised to follow a low-carbohydrate, low-fat diet; to exercise regularly; and to avoid all tobacco products. Patients should understand the importance of lifestyle modification to reduce the risk of cardiovascular disease and diabetes.

Patients with diabetes, particularly if neuropathy is present, should be instructed to visually inspect their feet daily and to seek professional help for any foot lesion. Many patients with diabetes are terrified of amputation and should be reassured that—with good podiatric care and immediate attention to any problem—amputation can possibly be avoided. All patients with arterial insufficiency should have their toenails cut by a podiatrist. In addition, patients should be given instructions about general foot protection measures, including the importance of properly fitting shoes, avoiding synthetic materials in shoes that causes them not to "breathe," and always wearing shoes or slippers to protect their feet. Direct contact with very hot or very cold substances or surfaces must be avoided. It is imperative to seek immediate medical evaluation for prolonged pain, sudden color changes, or a numb feeling in the extremities.

ACUTE ARTERIAL INSUFFICIENCY

 Acute arterial occlusion is an emergency in which treatment delay can impair limb viability or threaten life. The sudden onset of a pale, cold, pulseless limb is an acute emergency.

DEFINITION AND EPIDEMIOLOGY

Acute arterial insufficiency is the sudden onset of the symptoms of ischemia. The incidence of acute arterial occlusion seems to be increasing,[15] partly as a result of better diagnosis and recognition but also because patients with advanced heart disease are living longer and undergoing more invasive procedures. It is critical to make the diagnosis expeditiously to avoid loss of limb or life.

PATHOPHYSIOLOGY

Acute ischemia may result from an embolus (from another source) that occludes or obstructs flow to a distal vessel. The most common source of an embolus is the heart. This may be a clot that forms on the ventricular wall after an MI or a clot from the atrium in patients with atrial fibrillation. Rarely, a tumor in the heart, such as atrial myxoma, may break off and travel to the peripheral vessels.

Acute thrombosis of preexisting atherosclerotic lesions is the other major cause of acute ischemia. This type may be less severe than acute ischemia secondary to embolization because collateral circulation has had time to develop. Aneurysms of the abdominal aorta or popliteal artery may cause acute ischemia secondary to acute thrombosis of the aneurysm. Once the embolus becomes lodged, the arteries and veins distal to the occlusion go into spasm. After a few hours, vasodilation occurs, and the thrombus begins to organize. At this point, the ischemia becomes irreversible. It is generally accepted that if acute occlusion of the limb occurs and there is no collateral circulation, necrosis will begin after 6 hours unless the ischemia is relieved.

CLINICAL PRESENTATION AND PHYSICAL EXAMINATION

Classically the patient reports a sudden onset of pain in an extremity. A history of recent MI or atrial fibrillation and the presence of normal circulation in the other limb suggest an embolus as the source of acute limb ischemia. A previous history of peripheral vascular disease would suggest acute thrombosis as the cause.

On examination, the limb is usually pale and pulseless with absent or diminished capillary refill. If there is loss of sensation or immobility of the foot, tissue loss is imminent. These signs and symptoms are often referred to as the five *P*s: pain, pallor, pulselessness, paresthesias, and paralysis.

If left untreated, the limb becomes edematous, mottled, and eventually gangrenous. The sudden onset of pain with signs of acute ischemia and mottling from the waist down suggests acute aortic occlusion and demands immediate diagnosis and treatment if the patient is to survive.

DIAGNOSTICS

Diagnosis of acute limb ischemia is generally based on the clinical presentation and physical examination. Doppler studies may be necessary to confirm the presence or absence of arterial pulses. Arteriography may be indicated in some circumstances.

INITIAL DIAGNOSTICS

Acute Arterial Insufficiency

INITIAL	IMAGING
• Doppler studies	• Arteriography[a]

[a]If indicated.

DIFFERENTIAL DIAGNOSIS

The patient's history usually suggests whether the ischemia is related to an embolus or a thrombus. The most common error is misdiagnosis of acute ischemia as an acute neurologic event. The consequent delay in treatment can result in limb loss or, in the case of acute aortic occlusion, death. Careful pulse examination at the time of presentation will avoid this problem. Other causes of acute arterial insufficiency or arterial occlusion include blue-toe syndrome and aneurysms.

Blue-Toe Syndrome

Bluish discoloration or localized gangrene of the feet without evidence of ischemia, infection, or peripheral neuropathy is known as blue-toe syndrome, which results from microemboli from the heart, aorta, or peripheral arteries that are small enough to lodge in the capillaries. These emboli may be small thrombi from the heart or from an aortic or popliteal aneurysm. They may also be cholesterol emboli or atheroemboli from atherosclerotic plaques in the aorta, iliac arteries, or femoral arteries.

When blue-toe syndrome is suspected, careful physical examination for the presence of an abdominal or popliteal aneurysm is mandatory. If there is no evidence of ischemia, infection, or peripheral neuropathy, cardiac echocardiography and an abdominal ultrasound study should be obtained. If these tests are negative for a clot or abdominal aneurysm, antiplatelet therapy is initiated and the patient closely monitored. Consultation with a vascular specialist is necessary. The lesion will usually improve during the next few weeks, but if it does not or if emboli recur, transesophageal echocardiography and aortography of the thoracic aorta to the femoral arteries are indicated. If a localized lesion is discovered, it can be addressed, although diffuse atherosclerosis of the suprarenal aorta is often the source. In these cases, recurrent embolization often leads to renal failure and distal gangrene. Ligation of the iliac arteries with axillobifemoral bypass and preparation for dialysis are some of the available therapies.

Aneurysm

An aneurysm is a localized enlargement of an artery that causes symptoms by expansion, rupture, or thrombosis. A true aneurysm is said to be present when the wall of the aneurysm is an arterial wall. If the wall is compressed connective tissue, however, the rupture is a contained rupture, or false aneurysm.

Infrarenal aortic aneurysms (see Chapter 99) are a common cause of death secondary to rupture. They are often asymptomatic, although they may cause an acute onset of back or abdominal pain. If a pulsatile abdominal mass is discovered on physical examination, further evaluation with either an abdominal ultrasound study or a CT scan is indicated. If the presence of an aneurysm is confirmed, referral to a vascular surgeon is indicated.

Femoral or popliteal aneurysms are less common but may be detected on physical examination and usually cause symptoms by expansion and thrombosis. They are often associated with aortic aneurysms; an abdominal ultrasound study should also be obtained if either of these is detected.

Patients with aneurysms should be advised that this condition is often congenital and that any blood relatives older than 50 years should consult their primary care providers about having an abdominal ultrasound examination to screen for an aortic aneurysm.

INTERDISCIPLINARY COLLABORATIVE MANAGEMENT

 Hospitalization and prompt referral to a vascular specialist for evaluation and treatment are essential as soon as the diagnosis of acute arterial occlusion is made. Immediately upon diagnosis, a bolus of intravenous heparin (5000 U) should be given to prevent a clot from forming distal to the occlusion.

Treatment of the occlusion includes surgical or percutaneous embolectomy, percutaneous arterial thrombolytic delivery, or intravenous thrombolytic therapy. No matter the options available, treatment should be instituted within 6 hours of the occlusion to prevent permanent injury.

COMPLICATIONS

Complications are dependent more on the effect of the acute occlusion than on the cause. Thus patients with an embolus at the time of a massive MI will do poorly in comparison with those whose clot is from atrial fibrillation. Fortunately, invasive treatment for patients with PAD has changed dramatically over the last few decades. Endovascular repair procedures have been used more, thus reducing bypass surgery by 42% and the amputation rate by 29%.[7] Surgical bypass has become much safer over the last two decades. Other factors that have improved patient outcomes include a shift to endovascular therapy or limited open surgery to achieve revascularization in high-risk patients, better patient selection, more effective medication regimens, and improved intraoperative care and postoperative management.[7]

EDUCATION AND HEALTH PROMOTION

It is important to review the signs and symptoms of acute arterial occlusion with the patient and family members at regular intervals. For other educational points for review, see the Education and Health Promotion section under Chronic Arterial Insufficiency.

PERIPHERAL VENOUS INSUFFICIENCY

Peripheral venous insufficiency occurs whenever there is obstruction to venous return in the superficial or deep veins of the upper or lower extremities. Important clinical syndromes related to venous insufficiency include DVT, venous stasis, varicose veins, stasis dermatitis, and leg ulceration.

DEEP VENOUS THROMBOSIS OF THE LOWER EXTREMITY

DEFINITION AND EPIDEMIOLOGY

DVT is the development of a blood clot in the deep veins of the lower or occasionally upper extremity. A DVT may also involve the iliac veins and the vena cava. DVT is characterized by a relatively loose thrombotic attachment to the vein wall until the healing process starts. This loose attachment puts the patient at risk for mobilization of the clot until it stabilizes.

Although the term *phlebitis* is often used to describe DVT, the term should in fact be reserved for superficial venous thrombosis (SVT; also known as superficial phlebitis). SVT is an inflammation of the affected superficial veins as a result of local trauma, venous stasis, varicosities, or infection; chemical injury may result from an intravenous injection. Because SVT is part of an inflammatory process that involves the superficial vessel wall, there is no risk of pulmonary embolism unless the process extends to involve the deep system or the thrombus is larger than 5 cm in diameter. It is estimated that 23% of American adults have varicose veins and 6% have more advanced chronic venous disease (CVD), including skin changes due to healed or active venous ulcers.[16]

Fortunately evaluation and treatment of patients with venous disease has improved over the past two decades owing to the availability of duplex ultrasonography and the introduction of percutaneous endovenous ablation techniques (endovenous laser therapy [EVLA] and radiofrequency ablation [RFA]). Open surgical treatment techniques such as vein stripping of varicose veins performed under general anesthesia has been largely replaced by percutaneous procedures performed in the office setting.[17]

PATHOPHYSIOLOGY

The deep veins of the lower extremity are the main conduits through which the legs are emptied of blood. Blood travels back to the heart as a result of compression of the deep veins by the leg muscles. Valves in the vein prevent reflux back down the vein due to gravity. Blood runs from the superficial system to the deep veins through perforator veins, which are also protected from reflux by the presence of valves. Any condition that produces stasis or hypercoagulability is likely to result in the formation of clots in the deep veins. A major risk factor is surgery, particularly gynecologic operations and orthopedic procedures on the hip and knee. Bed rest produces stasis and thus may result in DVT. Long airplane or car rides are also risk factors.

Patients who have a tendency for hypercoagulation, particularly patients with malignant disease, may also be seen with DVT. A lesser but definite risk factor for DVT is the use of estrogen preparations (e.g., contraceptives or hormone replacement therapy); this should be considered in patients with other risk factors (see Chapter 217).

A clot may form in any part of the deep venous system and may either propagate or remain localized. It can cause symptoms in two ways. First, there is a local effect in obstruction of blood flow, which rarely is so significant that it results in venous gangrene. Second, the clot may become detached and migrate to the lungs, forming an embolus. This is a common cause of death in at-risk patients (see Chapter 95).

CLINICAL PRESENTATION AND PHYSICAL EXAMINATION

Clinical signs and symptoms are highly variable and non-specific but remain the cornerstone of diagnostic strategy. A history of previous DVT, prolonged inactivity, estrogen use, pregnancy, or recent surgery or trauma should be obtained from the patient. The classic signs of DVT are leg edema and calf tenderness. Calf pain on dorsiflexion of the foot is known as Homan's sign. All these signs are relatively nonspecific; up to 50% of patients with DVT have no symptoms at all.

The history and examination for SVT differ from those for DVT. The patient may have a localized area of edema, erythema, and tenderness over a superficial vein, with increased temperature in the surrounding skin. The primary risk factor is varicose veins.

DIAGNOSTICS

The diagnosis of SVT is based on the clinical findings; diagnostic tests are not usually needed. However, every patient with superficial phlebitis should undergo a duplex ultrasound examination to rule out a DVT as well to visualize the size of the thrombus. If a DVT is suspected on the basis of clinical signs or risk factors, the diagnosis can be made simply by duplex ultrasound examination of the legs. Test results should document clot visualization, normal blood flow, compressibility of the veins, augmentation of flow with respiration, or reflux in the deep and superficial systems. There are controversies as to whether testing is needed for the symptomatic leg only or for both.[18]

The differential diagnosis of DVT includes: SVT (also known as superficial phlebitis), ruptured Baker cyst, chronic venous stasis, or cellulitis. Any of these can cause pain, redness or swelling of the suspect extremity, usually the lower leg. A careful review of risk factors including a history of cancer or recent travel can help in deciding upon further diagnostic testing (see Chapter 217 for a more extensive review of DVT and other venous thromboembolic diseases).

INTERDISCIPLINARY COLLABORATIVE MANAGEMENT

Management of deep venous thrombosis is covered in Chapter 217. Management of superficial phlebitis consists of nonsteroidal antiinflammatories; either oral of topical, limb elevation, and compression with an elastic bandage. Low-molecular-weight heparin (LMWH) may be recommended in cases where there is thrombus extension into the deep venous system or if the thrombus is large.[19,20]

Management of DVT during pregnancy or immediately post partum should be done on an individual basis after consultation with a vascular specialist and obstetrician. Heparin is usually safe during pregnancy but warfarin is contraindicated because of serious risk to the fetus, especially in the first trimester. LMWH has made the management of DVT during pregnancy safer and easier.

A number of measures have been shown to be effective for DVT prophylaxis in surgical patients. Cuffs that provide intermittent leg pressure to reduce stasis are often combined with unfractionated heparin or LMWH until the patient is mobile. LMWH has been approved for DVT prevention in surgical patients who are at very high risk (e.g., hip replacement).

COMPLICATIONS

Pulmonary embolism is one of the major causes of postoperative morbidity and mortality. In high-risk patients the key to prevention is appropriate surveillance for DVT and the postoperative measures already described. Pulmonary embolism usually occurs within 2 weeks of a DVT. See Chapter 95 for a full discussion of pulmonary embolism, including diagnostic studies and management.

CHRONIC VENOUS STASIS

DEFINITION AND EPIDEMIOLOGY

Chronic venous stasis results from increased pressure in the deep veins. This condition produces edema, varicose veins, chronic skin changes, and potentially ulceration.

PATHOPHYSIOLOGY

Human beings are relatively poorly adapted to walking on two legs for long periods. The distribution of blood to the feet is accomplished by the heart in concert with gravity, but it is only the muscle pump and fragile venous valves that return the blood to the heart. Prolonged standing and a tall stature increase hydrostatic pressure on the valves. During pregnancy the hormone relaxin, which allows the pelvis to stretch, also causes the veins to distend and the valves to become incompetent. Resolution of this condition after pregnancy is often incomplete, resulting in increased venous stasis. Obesity and age-associated loss of tissue turgor are also factors that produce venous stasis.

Increased pressure may also result from proximal venous obstruction secondary to an old DVT or more commonly from reflux secondary to valvular incompetence. The latter may result from recanalization after a DVT or it may be primary in nature.

Even if the valves of the perforator and saphenous veins remain competent, deep venous hypertension will affect the foot and ankle. The foot tends to swell, particularly if the patient stands much of the day. The point of maximum pressure is the ankle; the skin becomes thickened and may react to the pressure with an eczematous reaction known as stasis eczema. Consequently blood cells in the tiny venules break down under high pressure and hemosiderin is deposited under the skin to produce a characteristic brown staining, which progresses with time.

CLINICAL PRESENTATION AND PHYSICAL EXAMINATION

The clinical appearance of chronic venous stasis varies according to whether the superficial or deeper veins are affected. Chronic edema and skin discoloration on the legs and ankles may be present. Varicose veins, ulceration, and even cellulitis may result.

DIAGNOSTICS AND DIFFERENTIAL DIAGNOSIS

Diagnostic tests are unnecessary because the diagnosis is based on the clinical history and physical findings. The physical findings also guide the diagnosis. However, the peripheral edema associated with chronic venous stasis may also be caused by other disease entities. DVT, SVT, medications, congestive heart failure, lymphatic obstruction, and malnutrition may all be associated with edema of the lower extremity.

INTERDISCIPLINARY COLLABORATIVE MANAGEMENT

Compression stockings or elastic bandages and periodic leg elevation are the most important ways of controlling chronic venous insufficiency and preventing skin ulcers. Careful monitoring is important when venous ulcers occur. Treatment of venous stasis ulcers is a time-consuming and chronic endeavor. Many dressing options are available (see Chapter 51 for a discussion of wound care). Infected ulcers should be treated with the appropriate antibiotic.

COMPLICATIONS

Venous ulcers are the most common complication of chronic venous stasis (see discussion below). A superimposed infection and cellulitis are additional concerns. Severe edema may result in decreased mobility and an increased risk for falls or DVT.

INDICATIONS FOR REFERRAL OR HOSPITALIZATION

Venous ulcers or peripheral edema that does not respond to conventional therapies may require a referral to a wound care specialist. Severe ulcers with extensive tissue loss may require evaluation by a plastic surgeon for possible grafting. Most patients can be successfully managed with careful outpatient follow-up visits. However, hospitalization may be indicated for severe edema, infection, or surgical valvuloplasty.

PATIENT AND FAMILY EDUCATION

The most effective treatment of leg swelling and stasis dermatitis is the use of support stockings.[17,18] Severe stasis eczema may require the use of 0.5% hydrocortisone cream in combination with compression. The hydrocortisone cream should be discontinued once the condition has resolved.

VARICOSE VEINS

PATHOPHYSIOLOGY

Varicose veins are caused by pathologic distention and proliferation of the superficial veins. Varicose veins include primary and secondary varicose veins as well as spider veins.

Primary varicose veins are usually familial. There is no previous history of DVT, and the varicosities are usually exacerbated by pregnancy. Progressive dilation of the superficial veins may be local or more extensive. Primary varicose veins result from incompetent perforators, which produce local varicosities, or from incompetence of the saphenous vein valves, which produces more generalized varicosities. Secondary varicose veins result from a previous DVT. Most commonly these are caused by incompetent valves after recanalization. When the deep venous system is totally occluded, these varicose veins may represent the main venous drainage from the leg; in this instance, removal of the veins would be harmful. Telangiectasia or spider veins may result from increased pressure in the superficial veins. It is not clear why this condition is more predominant in some patients.

CLINICAL PRESENTATION AND PHYSICAL EXAMINATION

The pooling of blood in large varicose veins tends to produce symptoms of heaviness and discomfort in the legs while standing. Large varicose veins are unsightly and may produce severe anxiety and cause major lifestyle changes. Trauma to varicose veins may result in severe bleeding, particularly in older adults, because their skin may be atrophic and thus provides less protection.

DIAGNOSTICS AND DIFFERENTIAL DIAGNOSIS

Diagnosis is based on inspection of the lower extremities when the patient is standing. The important diagnostic for varicose veins is the duplex scan to determine whether the deep system is patent and whether there is saphenofemoral reflux. Individual incompetent perforators in the leg may also be identified. If varicosities are not present, venous and arterial insufficiency, peripheral neuritis, and arthritis should be considered (for peripheral venous insufficiency, see the boxes titled Diagnostics and Differential Diagnosis).

INTERDISCIPLINARY COLLABORATIVE MANAGEMENT

Asymptomatic varicose veins do not require treatment. There is no effective way to reduce venous pressure in the lower legs except with support stockings. Treatment by a specialist may involve closing the vein, thereby shunting blood to deeper vessels. This can be done in a variety of ways, including sclerotherapy, laser therapy, endovenous ablation, or endoscopic vein surgery. Removal of the varicose veins may be indicated if more conservative measures fail. Ambulatory phlectomy or vein stripping and ligation are the most commonly performed procedures. Spider veins can be treated by either injection or laser treatment. Increasingly, obliteration of the long saphenous vein with use of a catheter and a radiofrequency generator or a laser has reduced the morbidity of saphenectomy; this can be done with the patient under local anesthesia in the office.[19]

COMPLICATIONS

A superficial varicosity will occasionally rupture, and significant bleeding may be noted. Topical compression and elevation of the extremity will usually control the bleeding. Skin ulcerations are an additional complication of varicose veins.

PATIENT AND FAMILY EDUCATION

It is important to inform patients that none of the treatments for varicose veins eradicate the problem of high venous pressure. Therefore recurrence is the rule rather than the exception. This knowledge may affect a patient's decision to proceed with surgery. Patients should also understand that compression stockings and periodic leg elevation are beneficial.

VENOUS STASIS ULCERS

DEFINITION AND EPIDEMIOLOGY

Venous stasis ulceration can occur following a DVT especially if there is permanent damage to the affected vein (s) with residual chronic swelling. However, the introduction of heparin and the prompt diagnosis and treatment of DVT has resulted in venous stasis ulceration as a consequence of DVT much less common. Ulcers that occur in the setting of chronic venous stasis (see above) are much more common.

PATHOPHYSIOLOGY

A number of factors contribute to venous ulceration. At first, peripheral edema increases as a result of incompetent valves in the venous system. This edema leads to capillary distention and the leakage of fluid and other substances into the surrounding tissue. If there is trauma to the skin of the affected extremity, oxygen and essential nutrients for healing are prevented from reaching the injured area. As a result, a superficial, irregularly shaped ulceration occurs. These ulcers can continue to erode, and cellulitis and superimposed infection can occur.

CLINICAL PRESENTATION AND PHYSICAL EXAMINATION

The patient with venous stasis ulceration is typically seen with an ulcer above the medial malleolus, and other signs of venous stasis are usually present. The ulcers have a distinctive presentation that permits differentiation from ischemic or diabetic ulcers (Box 107.3). At the time of presentation, the wound may

---

BOX **107.3**

Characteristics of Leg Ulcers by Cause[a]

VENOUS STASIS
- Occur around the ankle, particularly the medial side
- History of phlebitis
- Signs of venous stasis
- Painful when secondarily infected
- Improved by elevation

ISCHEMIC
- Occur at tips of extremities or heel
- History of claudication common
- Very painful, but much worse on elevation
- Absent pulses on physical examination
- Secondary infection likely to spread very quickly

NEUROPATHIC (DIABETIC)
- Occur at pressure points
- Painless, but coexistent neuritic pain possibly confusing
- Often present after secondary infection

[a]More than one cause may be involved.

---

be secondarily infected. Pulses may not be palpable because of local swelling or coexistent ischemia.

DIAGNOSTICS AND DIFFERENTIAL DIAGNOSIS

Diagnostic tests are usually unnecessary. A portable Doppler instrument can be used to assess pulses if they are not readily palpable. The differential diagnosis should encompass all peripheral ulcers (for peripheral venous insufficiency, see the boxes titled Diagnostics and Differential Diagnosis).

INTERDISCIPLINARY COLLABORATIVE MANAGEMENT

Management of venous stasis ulceration consists of wound debridement by an experienced practitioner and an appropriate dressing that will manage the wound exudate without causing further skin irritation or damage (see Chapter 51).[17,18] Antibiotics are appropriate if the wound is infected or cellulitis is present.[18,19]

COMPLICATIONS

Superimposed infection and cellulitis are potential concerns with venous stasis ulceration. Osteomyelitis (see Chapter 166) is an additional complication of chronically infected ulcers.

PATIENT AND FAMILY EDUCATION

Patient education is important in preventing recurring venous stasis ulcers. Patients must understand the importance of appropriately fitted compression stockings worn daily. If severe edema is present, an external pneumatic compression stocking may be necessary to control end-of-day lower extremity edema.

Many patients fail to wear their prescribed support stockings because the wrong stockings are provided and patients find them uncomfortable or difficult to put on. In general, knee-high stockings are much better tolerated than any tight support that crosses the knee. The main exceptions are for pregnant women and women with varicose veins in the thigh, who may find support pantyhose comfortable. In ordering stockings, the key factor is pressure (Table 107.1). The thick or fine-knit quality of the stockings affects only durability and patient acceptance.

TABLE **107.1** **Recommendations for Support Stockings**[a]

Pressure (mm Hg)	Recommendations
0–10	Normal socks
10–20	Over-the-counter support stockings Recommended for individuals who are on their feet all day and for prophylaxis for deep venous thrombosis when traveling
20–30	Lowest-pressure therapeutic stocking Good for individuals who are looking for more pressure than over-the-counter stockings or who cannot tolerate the higher pressures
30–40	Standard pressure for therapeutic stockings Instruct patients to shower in the evening so that these stockings can be put on before getting out of bed; otherwise, they will be difficult for many patients, particularly older adults, to put on.
40–50	Should be prescribed only for patients who do not have enough compression with 30–40 mm Hg. These are almost impossible to get on.

[a]Consult vascular specialist for use in patients with peripheral artery disease.

REFERENCES

1. Gerhard-Herman, M. D., Gornik, H. L., Barrett, C., Barshes, N. R., et al. (2017). 2016 AHA/ACC guideline on the management of patients with lower extremity peripheral artery disease: Executive summary: a report of the American College of Cardiology/American Heart Association Task Force on Clinical Practice Guidelines. *Circulation, 135*, e686–e725. doi:10.1161/CIR.0000000000000470.

2. Hikmet, H., Oruc, A. L., Ertain, V., et al. (2017). Determinants of chronic total occlusion in patients with peripheral arterial occlusive disease. *Angiology, 68*(2), 151–158. doi:10.1177/0003319716641827.

3. Carman, T. L., & Ang, S. K. (2014). Peripheral arterial disease and venous thromboembolism. In B. A. Williams, A. Chang, C. Ahalt, et al. (Eds.), *Current diagnosis and treatment: Geriatrics, 2e.* New York, NY: McGraw-Hill.

4. Mitrovic, I. (2019). Cardiovascular disorders: Vascular disease. In D. Hammer & S. McPhee (Eds.), *Pathophysiology of disease: An introduction to clinical medicine 8e.* New York, NY: McGraw-Hill.

5. Kullo, I., & Rooke, T. (2016). Peripheral artery disease. *The New England Journal of Medicine, 374*, 861–871.

6. Demirtas, S., Karahan, O., Yazici, S., et al. (2014). The relationship between complete blood count parameters and Fontaine's Stages in patient with peripheral arterial disease. *Vascular, 22*(6), 427–431. doi:10.1177/1708538114522227.

7. Fabiani, I., Calogero, E., Riccardo, N., et al. (2018). Critical limb ischemia: A practical up-to-date review. *Angiology, 69*(6), 465–474. doi:10.1177/0003319717739387.

8. Potter, B., & Pinto, D. (2014). Clinician update: Subclavian steal syndrome. *Circulation, 129*, 2320–2323. https://doi.org/10.1161/CIRCULATIONAHA.113.006653.

9. Policha, A., Baldwin, M., Lee, V., et al. (2018). Clinical Significance of reversal of flow in the vertebral artery identifies on cardiovascular duplex ultrasound. *Journal of Vascular Surgery, 67*(2), 568–572. Labropoulos, N., Nandivada, P., Bekelis, K. Prevalence and impact of the subclavian steal syndrome. Ann Surg. 2010: 252: 166.

10. Hennion, D. Y., & Siano, K. (2013). Diagnosis and treatment of peripheral arterial disease. *American Family Physician, 88*(5), 306–310.

11. Katsanos, K., Spiliopoulos, S., Saha, P., et al. (2015). Comparative efficacy and safety of different antiplatelet agents for prevention of major cardiovascular events and leg amputations in patients with peripheral arterial disease: A systematic review and network Meta-Analysis. *PLoS ONE, 10*, e0135692.

12. Agrawal, K., & Eberhardt, R. (2015). Contemporary management of peripheral artery disease. *Cardiology Clinics, 33*(1), 111–137.

13. Glaser, J., & Damrauer, S. (2017). Surgical management of peripheral artery disease. In E. Mohler & M. Jaff (Eds.), *Peripheral artery disease 2e.* Hoboken, New Jersey: John Wiley and Sons, ltd.

14. Zierler, E. R., Jorday, W. D., Lal, B. K., et al. (2018). The society of vascular surgery practice guidelines on follow-up after vascular surgery arterial procedures. *Journal of Vascular Surgery, 68*(1), 256–284.

15. Creager, M. A., Kaufman, J. A., & Conte, M. S. (2012). Clinical practice. Acute limb ischemia. *The New England Journal of Medicine, 366*, 2198.

16. Nelson, E. A., & Adderly, U. (2017). Venous leg ulcers. *American Family Physician, 95*(10), 662–663.

17. Gloviczki, P., Comerata, A., Dalsing, M., et al. (2011). The care of patients with varicose veins and associated chronic venous disease: Clinical practice guidelines of the Society for Vascular Surgery and the American Venous Forum. *Journal of Vascular Surgery, 53*(5), 2S–48S.

18. Robert-Ebadi, H., & Righini, M. (2017). Management of distal deep vein thrombosis. *Thrombosis Research, 149*.

19. Le Gal, G., Robert-Ebadi, R., Carrier, M., et al. (2015). Is it useful to also image the asymptomatic leg in patients with suspected deep vein thrombosis? *Journal of Thrombosis and Haemostasis 13*, 563–566.

20. Cosmi, B. (2017). Superficial vein thrombosis: New prospectives and observations from recent clinical trials. *Clin Adv Hem Onc.*

CHAPTER **108**

VALVULAR HEART DISEASE AND CARDIAC MURMURS

Andrea Efre • Elizabeth Remo

 Immediate Referral

Cardiology Referral: Pathologic murmurs or concerning signs that require evaluation by a cardiologist include diastolic murmurs, holosystolic murmurs, systolic murmurs grade 3 or above, a murmur with a new extra heart sound (S3, S4, or a click), or a murmur that increases in intensity when the patient stands.

Hospitalization: Acute or chronic valvular disease that becomes hemodynamically unstable or requires acute management of complications—such as heart failure, pulmonary edema, or uncontrolled angina—requires hospitalization. This is recommended for advanced diagnostic testing with cardiac catheterization, angioplasty, or treatment with percutaneous procedures or surgical intervention. Patients with acute valvular disease related to bacterial endocarditis may require hospitalization for intravenous antibiotic therapy.

DEFINITION AND EPIDEMIOLOGY

Valvular heart disease (VHD) refers to a damaged or dysfunctional heart valve, which is most often caused by calcific changes related to advanced age or inherent congenital conditions of the valve structure. Historically rheumatic fever was the primary cause of VHD, but with the advancement of primary prevention (through early detection and treatment of streptococcal throat infections), the United States and Europe currently have a very low prevalence.[1] Mortality rates remain high in other parts of the world, more predominantly in Oceania, South Asia, and central sub-Saharan Africa.[2]

The prevalence of valve disease in the US population is 2.5%, with no difference between males and females.[3] Aortic stenosis (AS) and mitral regurgitation (MR) are the most common types of degenerative valvular disease. VHD accounts for 10% to 20% of all cardiac surgical procedures in the United States, with two-thirds of valve operations being aortic valve replacement (AVR), most often for AS.[1] Many patients with mild to moderate valvular disease are able to be managed medically, but continued advancements are transforming the therapeutic approach to include newer transcatheter techniques such as transcatheter aortic valve replacement (TAVR), catheter-based mitral valve repair device closure, or closure of paravalvular leaks.[1,4]

The management of VHD is experiencing a paradigm shift toward the multidisciplinary care of a heart valve team within an institutional Heart Valve Center (HVC).[1,4] This integrated approach guides patient management toward optimal treatment strategies for the presenting valvular problem. The team usually includes cardiologists (invasive and noninvasive), cardiac surgeons, cardiac anesthesia, cardiac imaging, and nurses with expertise in VHD.[1,4–6]

PATHOPHYSIOLOGY

The structural integrity of the valves and their ability to function normally is vital to blood flow and maintenance of the cardiac cycle. Damaged, diseased, leaking, or stiff valves may disrupt flow, increasing workload, and affecting contractility, conduction, and cardiac stability. Valve stenosis (a stiffness of the valve) can decrease the ability of the valve to fully open. Valve regurgitation (incompetence or leaking of the valve) means that the valve does not close tightly or has a backflow of blood through the valve.

The aortic and pulmonic valves are semilunar (shaped like a half moon) and open during ventricular systole. The mitral and tricuspid valves are often called atrioventricular valves because they lie between the atria and ventricles. They open during diastole to allow refilling of the ventricles from the atria. As the heart valves close, heart sounds arise from vibrations of the valvular leaflets, the adjacent cardiac structures, and the flow of blood.[7]

Closure of the mitral and tricuspid valves produces the first heart sound (S_1) and begins systole. When the aortic and pulmonic valves close, the second heart sound (S_2) identifies the end of systole and the start of diastole. The second heart sound has two components: the aortic (A_2) sound is usually louder, reflecting the high pressure in the aorta; and the pulmonic (P_2) sound is relatively soft, reflecting the lower pressure of the pulmonary artery. It is not uncommon to hear a splitting of S_2 during inspiration, in which the right heart filling time, right ventricular stroke volume, and right ventricular ejection duration are all increased; this then causes delay in the closure of the pulmonic valve, splitting S_2 into two audible components. During expiration, these two components usually fuse back to a single S_2 sound.[7] The intensity of A_2 and P_2 decreases with aortic and pulmonic stenosis (PS) and a single S_2 may result.[8] VHD is primarily evidenced by a cardiac murmur, which is an audible heart sound caused by turbulent blood flow and is covered in detail throughout this chapter. However, not all murmurs indicate valvular or structural heart disease.[8]

CLINICAL PRESENTATION AND PHYSICAL EXAMINATION

The symptoms of heart valve disease are determined by the causative valve, and do not necessarily indicate the severity of the valvular dysfunction. If the activities of daily living are affected by symptom severity, further evaluation by a HVC is required. Common clinical complaints associated with valvular disorders may include but are not limited to chest pain, palpitations, dizziness, syncope or near syncope, fatigue, exercise intolerance, and dyspnea. Symptoms may be directly caused by a valvular problem, sequelae of the valvular dysfunction, or comorbidity unrelated to the valve. For example, orthopnea, paroxysmal nocturnal dyspnea, chronic cough, and wheezing may indicate mitral valve stenosis; they may also be related to left ventricular (LV) heart failure or a symptom of an unrelated chronic pulmonary condition. Further information on symptomology is detailed further on with each valvular problem.

The physical exam of a patient with VHD starts with inspection and palpation of the chest wall. Initially palpating the apical pulsation at the location of the point of maximum impulse (PMI) will help identify heart size, which may be achieved with the patient sitting upright, slightly leaning forward, or in a left lateral lying position. Displacement of the impulse laterally suggests enlargement of the heart and can be seen in ventricular enlargement, heart failure, and cardiomyopathies caused by VHD. Palpation is performed using the palm and/or finger pads obliquely against the chest wall for the presence of heaves or lifts (a rhythmic impulse that lifts

---

BOX 108.1

Grades of Murmurs

Grade 1	Very faint; heard with intent listening and may not be heard in all positions
Grade 2	Quiet, but heard immediately after placing the stethoscope on the chest
Grade 3	Moderately loud
Grade 4	Loud, with palpable thrill
Grade 5	Very loud with thrill. May be heard when the stethoscope is partly off the chest
Grade 6	Very loud with thrill. May be heard with stethoscope entirely off the chest

---

the fingers), and the ball of the hand is used for palpation of thrills (a buzzing vibratory sensation).[7] A palpable thrill over a valvular area characterizes a louder murmur of grade 4 (VI) or higher intensity (Box 108.1).[7,8]

Auscultation for heart sounds should include an evaluation of the S_1 and S_2 sounds, extra heart sounds (S_3 and S_4) and murmurs. It is important to use a systematic approach and the correct location and to utilize both the diaphragm and the bell of the stethoscope for thorough evaluation of all four valves. The diaphragm is best used for picking up the higher-pitched sounds of S_1 and S_2, such as the murmurs of aortic and MR and pericardial friction rubs. The bell is more sensitive to the lower-pitched sounds of S_3 and S_4 and the low rumbling murmur of mitral stenosis (MS).[7] Knowledge of the type of stethoscope being used (acoustic or electronic) will help ensure that gentle or quiet murmurs are identified. Overly firm pressure on the bell can stretch the underlying skin and make it function as the diaphragm, causing low-pitched sounds like S_3 and S_4 to disappear.[7]

When a murmur is identified, it is important to determine the timing, location, radiation, intensity (grade), quality, and pitch. These characteristics aid in the identification of the murmur, which is a vital part of managing VHD (Table 108.1). In addition, there are maneuvers or positions that may be used to improve the differentiation of murmurs, such as left lateral lying, squatting, or leaning forward while sitting. Using other techniques such as the Valsalva maneuver, isometric handgrip, or changing respiratory rhythm can also be helpful.

Timing

Timing distinguishes between systolic and diastolic murmurs and clarifies the relationship of the murmur to the heart sounds; it is a prerequisite to identifying the events of the cardiac cycle. As the heart rate increases, diastole shortens and systole and diastole approach similar intervals. When this occurs, differentiation between S_1 (beginning of systole) and S_2 (beginning of diastole) can be more challenging. Palpation of the carotid pulse while simultaneously auscultating the heart can help determine timing and to identify systolic murmurs that coincide with the carotid upstroke.[7]

Location and Radiation

The location where a murmur is best heard should be identified by anatomical location rather than valve area. This is done in order to accommodate variable sound transmission, radiation, or relocation of the sound due to cardiac dilation, ventricular

TABLE 108.1   Murmurs

Diagnosis	Characteristic	Location, Radiation	Physical Examination Findings	Effect of Valsalva Maneuver	Electrocardiographic Findings	Chest X-Ray Findings
COMMON SYSTOLIC MURMURS						
Aortic stenosis	Harsh, crescendo-decrescendo	Right sternal border; radiation to neck	Delayed carotid upstroke; narrowed pulse pressure; systolic thrill at second right intercostal space	Decreased murmur	Left atrial enlargement; left axis deviation; atrioventricular conduction delay; LVH	Aortic valve calcification; LVH
PS	Variable intensity, medium pitch, harsh quality; crescendo-decrescendo	Third and fourth left intercostal spaces; radiation down the left sternal border to the apex and possibly the base	Ejection sound heard best in the second and third intercostal spaces; reveals normal S1 and widely split S2	Increased murmur	Right axis deviation; increased R wave amplitude in lead V1; increased P wave amplitude associated with right atrial abnormality; Q waves may be seen in severe PS in leads V1–V3	Dilated pulmonary trunk or a main pulmonary artery may be present in congenital disease
Mitral regurgitation	Pansystolic blowing	Apex; radiation to axilla	Laterally displaced, hyperdynamic apical impulse; brisk carotid upstroke	No change	LVH	Left ventricular enlargement
Mitral valve prolapse	Midsystolic to late systolic; occasionally honking; may have midsystolic click; click and murmur can be intermittent	Lower left sternal border	May have scoliosis or pectus excavatum in connective tissue disorder	Murmur or click may move to later systole or disappear	Usually within normal limits; occasionally flat or inverted T in leads I, III, aVF	Skeletal abnormalities, if present
Tricuspid regurgitation	Early systolic, midsystolic, late systolic, or pansystolic	Lower left sternal border; radiation to right sternal border	Sustained precordial lift	Decreased murmur	Right atrial hypertrophy; right axis deviation	Usually normal
Hypertrophic cardiomyopathy	Peaks midsystole	Left sternal border	Murmur decreased with change from standing to squatting; S4 gallop may be present	Increased murmur	Left atrial enlargement; increased voltage; may have LVH	May have slight cardiac enlargement
Benign or innocent[a]	Early systolic; crescendo-decrescendo; changes intensity with rate	Variant	No underlying systemic findings; no findings of cardiac enlargement or failure; murmur disappears with breath holding	Murmur disappearing	Normal recording	Normal findings
Ventricular septal defect	Pansystolic; louder in midsystole	Left sternal border; radiation to right sternal border	May have systolic thrill at lower left sternal border	Increased murmur	May have left atrial and ventricular enlargement	
COMMON DIASTOLIC MURMURS						
Aortic regurgitation	Loud, blowing, high-pitched	Lower left sternal border	Widened pulse pressure; abrupt rise and fall in carotid upstroke	Increased murmur	LVH; sinus tachycardia	LVH; aortic valve calcification; ascending aortic dilation

Continued

TABLE 108.1 **Murmurs—cont'd**

Diagnosis	Characteristic	Location, Radiation	Physical Examination Findings	Effect of Valsalva Maneuver	Electrocardiographic Findings	Chest X-Ray Findings
PR	Soft, high-pitched decrescendo murmur during the first half of diastole; Graham-Steele murmur	Third and fourth left intercostal spaces; increased audibility when patient is sitting and leaning forward	Normal S1 and S2 (split S2); silent systole; increases in intensity during inspiration	Decreased murmur	RV hypertrophy	May show minimally thickened pulmonic valve leaflet; RV enlargement
Mitral stenosis	Low-pitched, diastolic rumble (mid)	Apex, left lateral position	Opening snap	No change or increased murmur	Left atrial enlargement; right axis deviation	Left atrial enlargement; calcified mitral valve
Tricuspid stenosis	Decrescendo, low-pitched	Fourth or fifth left intercostal space	Absent right ventricular impulse; diastolic thrill; lower left intercostal border may have opening snap at fourth left intercostal space	Decreased murmur	Height of P wave in lead II >2.5 mm; PR shortened; right atrial hypertrophy	Right atrial and vena cava shadows

[a]Whether a murmur is benign or innocent cannot be determined with 100% accuracy.
LVH, Left ventricular hypertrophy; *PR,* pulmonic regurgitation; *PS,* pulmonic stenosis; *RV,* right ventricular.
Modified from Mann, D. L., Zipes, D. P., Libby, P., & Bonown, R. O. (Eds.), (2014). *Braunwald's heart disease: A textbook of cardiovascular medicine* (10th ed.). Philadelphia: Elsevier; Bickley, L. S., Szilagyi, P. G., & Hoffman, R. M. (2017). *Bates' guide to physical examination and history taking* (12th ed.). Philadelphia: Wolters Kluwer.

hypertrophy, anomalies of the great vessels, or dextrocardia.[7] The most common areas of auscultation are as follows:

- Right upper sternal border or second intercostal space (aortic area)
- Left upper sternal border or second intercostal space (pulmonic area)
- Lower left sternal border (tricuspid area)
- Apex (mitral area)

Intensity

The intensity or loudness of the murmur is related to the velocity of blood flow but does not equate with the severity of the underlying problem. A loud murmur of a small muscular ventricular septal defect (VSD) in an adolescent that is destined to close spontaneously is a good example. Murmurs are graded by the intensity of the sound and the addition of a palpable thrill on a scale of 1 to 6 (often documented in Roman numerals I to VI) (see Box 108.1). The intensity of the murmur may be diminished in patients who are obese, very muscular, or with emphysematous lungs.[7]

Quality and Pitch

The quality of the murmur is an expression of its tone. Descriptive characteristics include terms such as *blowing, harsh, rumbling,* or *musical.* The pitch refers to the sound frequency and is categorized as a low, medium, or high.[7]

SYSTOLIC MURMURS

Murmurs are classified into where they are heard within the cardiac cycle, but the cause of the murmur is not concluded solely by the characteristics of the murmur. Systolic murmurs

are organized into *early systolic, midsystolic, late systolic,* or *pansystolic* (also known as *holosystolic*). Midsystolic murmurs are the most common, and early systolic murmurs are the least common. Additional terms used are *ejection murmurs* (systolic) and *regurgitant murmurs* (pansystolic).

Early Systolic murmurs are usually high-pitched, sharp, and associated with pathologic halting of the aortic and pulmonic valves as they open in early systole.[7] The early murmur can be caused by mitral or tricuspid regurgitation (TR) or VSD.[8]

Midsystolic murmurs are described as crescendo-decrescendo (diamond-shaped) sounds that build in intensity as velocity increases and then decrease well before S_2. This type of murmur is typically heard in aortic or PS where there is obstruction of the blood flow across the valve. It may also be associated with a hyperkinetic state, hypertrophic obstructive cardiomyopathy, or a left-to-right shunt such as an atrial septal defect.[7,8] Midsystolic ejection murmurs are the most common murmurs and may be innocent (without anatomical abnormality), or physiologic (related to anatomical changes), or pathologic (caused by a structural abnormality).[7] A Valsalva strain maneuver can increase the murmur of hypertrophic cardiomyopathy to define it from the other systolic murmurs.[7]

Late systolic murmurs usually start in mid- or late systole and continue up to S_2 in a crescendo pattern. This murmur is typically seen in mitral valve prolapse (MVP) or tricuspid valve prolapse.

Pansystolic murmurs result from blood flow transferring from a high-pressure chamber to a low-pressure chamber, which occurs in incompetent and regurgitating mitral or tricuspid valves or VSD. The pressure gradient and murmur intensity are largely unchanged throughout systole, causing a plateau-shaped murmur from S_1 to S_2.

DIASTOLIC MURMURS

Diastolic murmurs are almost always pathologic and indicate heart disease. They are identified as early diastolic, mid-diastolic, or late diastolic. There are two basic reasons for diastolic murmurs to be heard. The first is due to regurgitation flow across the incompetent aortic or pulmonic valves, which is a high-pitched early decrescendo murmur heard best with the diaphragm of the stethoscope. The second type is a low-pitched rumbling mid-diastolic or late diastolic murmur of obstructed, stenosed mitral or tricuspid valves. These are best appreciated using the bell of the stethoscope at the apical area with the patient lying slightly on the left side. The duration rather than the intensity (grade) of the murmur correlates with the severity of the obstruction.

Early diastolic murmurs start immediately after S_2 and typically have a decrescendo sound pattern that ends before S_1. These are pathologic murmurs associated with AR or pulmonic regurgitation (PR); they are high-pitched and heard best at the base with the patient sitting and leaning forward. A Graham Steell murmur is a high-pitched early diastolic murmur heard best at the left sternal edge in the second intercostal space; it is associated with pulmonary regurgitation. If the murmur is loudest at the right of the sternum, it suggests an eccentric regurgitant stream from dilation of the aortic root, which can be seen in Marfan syndrome, aortic dissection, syphilitic aortitis, or damage to a single aortic cusp, as in endocarditis.[9]

Mid-diastolic murmurs start a short time after S_2 and may fade or merge into a late diastolic murmur. They are usually low-pitched rumbles at the apex caused by mitral or tricuspid stenosis (TS), left or right atrial tumors (myxomas), or severe atrial regurgitation (AR), which may obstruct flow across the mitral valve during diastole.[8] Hyperdynamic states such as anemia, fever, the presence of an atrial septal defect, or VSD may create shunting of blood from one chamber to the other during diastole, producing a mid-diastolic murmur.

Late diastolic murmurs are also known as presystolic murmurs, as they start late in diastole and typically continues up to S1 as low-pitched rumbles heard mostly in the apex. Late diastolic murmurs are usually associated with MS (they accentuate as S1 is reached), or the mid- to late Austin Flint murmur of severe aortic AR. It is possible that patients with atrial fibrillation may lack the presystolic accentuation of the diastolic rumbles because they have no atrial contraction.

CONTINUOUS MURMURS

Continuous murmurs begin in systole and extend at least partway into diastole; they are usually associated with rapid blood flow, high- to low-pressure shunts, or localized stenosis. The classic continuous murmur of patent ductus arteriosus is characterized by a crescendo in systole and decrescendo into diastole best heard at the left upper sternal border with a thrill or hyperdynamic LV impulse. Fistulas or localized arterial obstructions may also produce continuous murmurs. The continuous murmur of a venous hum is a benign high-flow state heard in the neck of some children and adolescents; it disappears with compression of the jugular vein. Another benign continuous murmur (also referred to as a *mammary shuffle murmur*) is that of a woman in the late stages of pregnancy or lactating shortly postpartum; it can be reduced with firm pressure over the breast.

FUNCTIONAL BENIGN MURMURS (INNOCENT)

Innocent (accidental) murmurs are asymptomatic; they are found in healthy children and related to the sounds made by blood flow through an anatomically and physiologically normal heart. They are common in infants and children (prevalent in over 50% of children), with peak occurrence being in those between 3 and 6 years or 8 and 12 years of age.[10] Innocent murmurs are systolic (usually mid-systolic); they have a musical or vibratory quality and are heard between the mid-left sternal border and the apex. Some murmurs that are categorized as innocent or accidental include the Still murmur, pulmonary flow murmur, peripheral pulmonary stenosis, supraclavicular systolic murmur, systolic murmur of pulmonary flow in neonates, venous hum, and mammary souffle (rare and found in adolescents). The most common functional murmur is the Still murmur (a classic vibratory parasternal-precordial murmur), which constitutes more than 50% of all accidental murmurs.[10] Other innocent benign murmurs may be known as functional, harmless, physiological, irrelevant, evolving, benign, habitual, infantile, growth murmurs, or flow murmurs.

Differentiation of a benign functional murmur is based on the lack of symptoms and other abnormal physical findings. Murmurs that are caused by an increased cardiac output (e.g., as a result of fever, thyrotoxicosis, or anemia) may be termed functional because they are caused by excess flow across the outflow tract. Although innocent murmurs are usually associated with children, it is possible for an older adult with no underlying cardiovascular disease to have a distorted flow without a significant gradient across the valve or to have an outflow murmur from the ejection of blood into a kinked and tortuous aorta.

DIAGNOSTICS

Initial diagnostic testing should include a 12-lead electrocardiogram (ECG), a chest x-ray, and an echocardiogram. Among these, the echocardiogram is the standard diagnostic test for the initial evaluation of patients with suspected or known VHD.[5] Preliminary diagnostic testing may be managed in the primary care setting, but more specific cardiac diagnostic testing and treatments require consultation with cardiology.

Echocardiogram

Transthoracic echocardiography (TTE) with two-dimensional (2D) imaging and Doppler studies is used to evaluate hemodynamic capacity, valvular structure, and valvular function; it also serves to measure ventricular dimensions and EF. The valvular exam detects causes of regurgitation by documenting flail or prolapsing leaflets, a dilated aortic root, or evidence of a vegetation. However, the greatest effect of Doppler echocardiography is its ability to assess the severity of the regurgitation and assist in determining the optimal time for valve replacement, especially in the asymptomatic patient. Color Doppler imaging provides an assessment of the amount of regurgitation and the upstream and downstream pressures. TTE can be challenging in patients with a large body habitus. For these patients, a TEE or cardiac MRI may be a more effective diagnostic tool.

TABLE 108.2	Stages of Progression of Valvular Heart Disease	
Stage	**Definition**	**Description**
A	At risk	Patients with risk factors for development of VHD
B	Progressive	Patients with progressive VHD (mild-to-moderate severity and asymptomatic)
C	Asymptomatic severe	Asymptomatic patients who have the criteria for severe VHD: C1: Asymptomatic patients with severe VHD in whom the left or right ventricle remains compensated C2: Asymptomatic patients with severe VHD, with decompensation of the left or right ventricle
D	Symptomatic severe	Patients who have developed symptoms as a result of VHD

VHD, Valvular heart disease.
From American College of Cardiology/American Heart Association Task Force. (2014). 2014 AHA/ACC Guideline for the Management of Patients With Valvular Heart Disease: Executive Summary: A Report of the American College of Cardiology/American Heart Association Task Force on Practice Guidelines. *Journal of the American College of Cardiology, 63*(22), 2438–2488.

Echocardiography is recommended for the initial evaluation of patients with known or suspected VHD to confirm the diagnosis, establish etiology, determine severity, assess hemodynamic effects, and determine prognosis.[5] Patients with significant obstruction and modest symptoms or those who are asymptomatic but have severe obstruction may require more frequent evaluation. Significant changes in status, such as murmur changes or onset of symptoms, necessitates a TTE. In addition, periodic assessment of asymptomatic patients with known VHD is recommended so as to monitor the progression of valvular disease (Table 108.2), valvular function, change in symptoms, or physical examination findings.[5]

12-Lead Electrocardiogram

The 12-lead ECG is used to evaluate the conduction, rhythm, and performance of the heart in VHD. Although the valves are not responsible for the conduction system, the effects of valvular disease may cause atrial or ventricular conduction abnormalities discernible on the 12-lead ECG. Sequelae related to valve disorders may include atrial fibrillation, acute MI, acute coronary syndrome, and atrial or ventricular hypertrophy, all of which may be evidenced by conduction changes on the 12-lead ECG. Additional investigation using a 24-hour ambulatory ECG monitoring device (e.g., Holter monitor or Zio patch) is recommended in the presence of palpitations, lightheadedness, dizziness, syncope, ventricular arrhythmias, or prolonged QT intervals.[1]

Chest X-Ray

A chest radiograph (CXR) may appear normal in patients with valvular disease, or there may be evidence of sequelae such as atrial enlargement, ventricular hypertrophies, and a dilated aortic root. Therefore it is prudent to include a CXR in the evaluation of a patient with suspected or known VHD to assess cardiac size, features of the cardiac borders, prominence of the vasculature, presence of calcifications, and size of the aorta.

Stress Test

Exercise stress testing is reasonable in selected patients with asymptomatic severe VHD to assess the hemodynamic response to exercise, presence of symptoms, or assist in determining prognosis.[5]

Cardiac Catheterization

The severity of valvular obstruction can be determined using cardiac catheterization to record the gradient across the valve and by calculating the valve area. Additional functional assessment of the left ventricle and valvular function can confirm results obtained by Doppler echocardiography. Cardiac catheterization is recommended for hemodynamic assessment in symptomatic patients when noninvasive tests are inconclusive or the severity of the valve lesion is questionable.[5]

INITIAL DIAGNOSTICS

Valvular Heart Disease and Cardiac Murmurs

IMAGING
- TTE with 2D Doppler studies
- 12-Lead ECG
- Chest x-ray

ADDITIONAL DIAGNOSTICS[a]
- Stress test with exercise ECG
- Cardiac magnetic resonance imaging
- Cardiac catheterization

[a]If indicated.

DIFFERENTIAL DIAGNOSIS

A diagnosis of VHD is primarily based on the type of murmur and echocardiogram findings, which are covered in detail throughout the following sections. Management of patients with VHD is guided by the recommendations of the American College of Cardiology and American Heart Association. General recommendations include a thorough history and complete physical examination on all patients with suspected or known heart disease, including progression staging and treatment (see Table 108.2). Patients are expected to be active participants in the entire decision-making process.[11]

AORTIC STENOSIS

DEFINITION AND EPIDEMIOLOGY

AS is the most common type of VHD and is associated with advanced age (calcification), valve anatomy (bicuspid valves increase the risk by 50%), and clinical risk factors including hypertension, smoking, diabetes, and hyperlipidemia.[1,12,13] The etiology has shifted from rheumatic to calcific over the past three decades with the successful treatment of streptococcal pharyngitis. During the later decades of life, inflammation, fibrosis, calcification, and stenosis develop due to repetitive mechanical trauma of the blood against the valve over many years.

PATHOPHYSIOLOGY

The normal aortic valve orifice measures 3 to 4 cm². Progression of AS is measured using peak aortic valve velocity, which corresponds to the mean aortic valve gradient. Severe AS is defined as having a peak aortic valve velocity of greater than

4.0 m/s or a mean aortic valve gradient of greater than 40 mm Hg. When the aortic valve is smaller than 1.0 cm^2, the prognosis is poor.[1,5,12] A large pressure gradient across the aortic valve may be sustained for many years without a reduction in contractile function, with LV dilation generally a very late manifestation. Persistent pressure overload to the left ventricle may eventually lead to LV dilation, left atrial enlargement, and pulmonary hypertension.

CLINICAL PRESENTATION AND PHYSICAL EXAMINATION

AS leads to an imbalance in myocardial oxygen supply, which is responsible for the three classic symptoms of exertional angina, syncope, and heart failure.[12] Chest pain, exercise intolerance, and anginal symptoms can manifest despite preserved LV function, but severe AS carries a higher risk of sudden death when anginal symptoms are present. LV dysfunction leads to symptoms of fatigue, cough, progressive dyspnea on exertion, orthopnea, and paroxysmal nocturnal dyspnea. Heart failure is a late sign of AS and is associated with a poor prognosis.[12]

When a patient is being examined, the classic crescendo-decrescendo midsystolic murmur of AS is most audible at the right upper sternal border at the second intercostal space, but it can radiate significantly across the chest down the left sternal border to the apex or up to the carotid arteries. It is frequently harsh at the base but may be musical at the apex and often loud in intensity (grade 3/6 or greater) with a palpable thrill. Paradoxical splitting of the second heart sound (S$_2$) may occur as a result of delayed aortic valve closure. In severe stenosis, the A$_2$ is often inaudible; therefore no splitting of S$_2$ is appreciated. In younger patients with congenital or bicuspid AS, the murmur may be preceded by a systolic aortic ejection click that can radiate to the right upper sternal border or to the apex.

LV hypertrophy (LVH) may produce a sustained thrust or heave of the PMI, but displacement of the apical impulse does not usually occur unless LV failure is present. The carotid pulse has a slow rise with delayed peak and small volume (pulsus parvus and pulsus tardus). A notch or shudder in the upstroke (anacrotic notch) may be appreciated. AS is often accompanied by MR, caused by MVP, and it can be difficult to recognize two distinct systolic murmurs.[1] In differentiating AS from the systolic murmur of hypertrophic obstructive cardiomyopathy, the Valsalva maneuver is helpful. The Valsalva release of squatting will increase the murmur intensity of AS, which resolves on standing. However, the strain phase (or standing) of the Valsalva maneuver decreases venous return, resulting in a smaller LV outflow tract and an increase in the murmur intensity in hypertrophic cardiomyopathy.

DIAGNOSTICS

Transthoracic 2D echocardiography of the aortic valve shows the thickened, calcified, immobile leaflets of AS and evaluates for significant obstruction of flow. The Doppler portion provides measurements of the outflow gradient, enabling a reasonable calculation of the aortic valve area that closely approximates cardiac catheterization measurements. Poststenotic dilation of the aorta, LV wall thickening, dilation of the left ventricle, or reduced contractility (ejection fraction) are often seen in AS. However, if these findings are normal, severe disease is not excluded. The 12-lead ECG may demonstrate normal sinus rhythm with signs of LVH. Conduction abnormalities—such as first-degree atrioventricular block, bundle branch block, and

intraventricular conduction disturbances—are fairly common. Atrial fibrillation usually represents either end-stage disease with LV decompensation or other associated disease. The CXR may demonstrate rounding or prominence of the left ventricle as a result of concentric hypertrophy of the left ventricle, poststenotic dilation of the aorta, and calcification of the valve cusps, or the CXR findings may be completely normal.

INTERPROFESSIONAL COLLABORATIVE MANAGEMENT

Nonpharmacologic Management

Periodic monitoring for symptom development and disease progression is the usual treatment for asymptomatic AS. Patients with moderate or severe AS should not engage in competitive sports that require high dynamic and static muscular activity.[5] With severe AS, once symptoms manifest, valve obstruction must be relieved to prevent a poor outcome.

Pharmacologic Management

Medical therapy for asymptomatic patients with AS is no longer recommended by the American Heart Association unless the patient has associated high-risk medical conditions that would warrant treatment.[5] Recommended medical therapy for AS is associated with risk factor reduction and may include antihypertensives for blood pressure management and statin therapy for the prevention of coronary artery disease.[5]

INDICATIONS FOR REFERRAL AND HOSPITALIZATION

The TAVR is a percutaneous interventional procedure that repairs AS by placing a new valve within the old one (without removing the native one). TAVR is usually used for those patients who have a heightened surgical risk. It uses a transfemoral approach or a transapical approach (through the tip of the left ventricle) for a minimally invasive surgical procedure. The replacement valve has three bovine (cow) or porcine (pig) leaflets mounted in a frame that is loaded in a catheter and deployed into position within the native damaged aortic valve.[14] In comparing the bovine and porcine valves in TAVR, there is a higher incidence of AR with the porcine valve secondary to the architecture and positioning of the implant, but no difference in early mortality rates has been seen.[14] Other complications include thromboembolic stroke and other vascular complications. Significant AR, mitral valve disease and bicuspid or non calcified valve, hypertrophic cardiomyopathy, recent MI or CVA or TIA within the past 6 months are among the several contraindications to TAVR.[15]

Surgical AVR remains the most widely acceptable standard and uses a mechanical or bioprosthetic (tissue) valve. Survival after AVR is better with a mechanical than with a bioprosthetic valve.[1] However, bioprosthetic valves are indicated in patients for whom anticoagulation therapy is not preferred. Both the TAVR and surgical AVR carry risk factors, with TAVR posing a slightly higher risk of developing infective endocarditis and the surgical AVR having a higher risk of atrial fibrillation or major bleeding.[11]

Percutaneous interventions (e.g., TAVR) and/or surgical interventions (surgical AVR) are now recommended in the management of severe symptomatic AS (stage D) and asymptomatic AS (stage C) in patients with surgical risk factors who meet the indications for valve replacement.[11] In a patient undergoing other cardiac surgery, it is reasonable to consider surgical AVR for stage B or C with an aortic velocity of 3.0 to 3.9 m/s.[5]

AORTIC REGURGITATION

DEFINITION AND EPIDEMIOLOGY

AR occurs when the aortic valve fails to close completely, allowing blood to flow back into the left ventricle during ventricular diastole. This process may be either chronic or acute and may be a result of primary disease of the valve leaflets or of distortion of the wall of the aortic root. In patients with isolated AR who undergo valve replacement, more than 50% of the AR is caused by aortic root disease.[1]

PATHOPHYSIOLOGY

In chronic AR, the slow progression of the disease results in increased LV volume. The left ventricle adapts to the increased volume, which over time causes LVH.[5] Pathologic processes affecting the aortic valve that lead to chronic AR include inflammation (e.g., resulting from rheumatic fever, syphilis, rheumatoid arthritis), structural processes (e.g., unicuspid, bicuspid, aneurysm), disruptive processes (e.g., trauma, infective endocarditis, dissection), congenital conditions, and stress from hypertension. Acute AR is most commonly a result of infective endocarditis, dissecting aortic aneurysm, or acute chest trauma. There is no time for adaptation to occur, so left ventricular volume overload leads to severe pulmonary congestion and decreased cardiac output.

CLINICAL PRESENTATION AND PHYSICAL EXAMINATION

Patients with chronic AR may remain asymptomatic for many years. But when the severity of the disease increases, the clinical manifestations of LV enlargement develop. These include exertional dyspnea, orthopnea, paroxysmal nocturnal dyspnea, and fatigue. Angina pectoris and nocturnal angina may be troublesome and diaphoresis may occur when the heart rate or diastolic pressure is low.[1] Symptoms of AR that may cause distress include tachycardia, palpitations, chest discomfort, or awareness of the heartbeat when lying down.[1]

Severe AR may cause three distinct types (or stages) of murmurs, the first being in early diastole, when the murmur may occupy part or all of diastole. It is a high-pitched, blowing, decrescendo sound due to the regurgitant flow across the incompetent valves. It may be best heard along the left sternal border (the second to fourth intercostal spaces) with the patient in a seated position slightly leaning forward and with the breath held after expiration.[7,9] In addition to the diastolic murmur, the second type is caused by the progressive changes of severe AR, which increase pulse pressure and produce a short systolic aortic flow murmur near the sternum.[9] The third type of murmur in severe AR is the Austin Flint murmur, which is sometimes referred to as a mitral diastolic murmur and suggests a large regurgitant flow. There are two diastolic components (mid- and late) to the rumbling sound, which is heard at the apex; it begins immediately after S_2 and is loudest just before S_1 (presystolic).[9] The Austin Flint murmur resembles the characteristic murmur of MS (but the mitral valve is normal); it appears to be created by severe aortic reflux impinging on the anterior leaflet of the mitral valve or the free wall of the left ventricle.[1]

In patients with mild or moderate chronic AR, a diastolic regurgitant murmur is not always auscultated.[5] This makes differentiation from other diastolic murmurs difficult, as in pulmonary valve regurgitation or a VSD with a large left-to-right shunt. In aortic root enlargement or secondary AR, the murmur may radiate along the right sternal border.[8] The diastolic murmur of acute AR is both softer and of shorter duration than chronic, and additional features of acute AR include tachycardia, a soft S_1, and the absence of peripheral findings of significant diastolic runoff.[8]

An increase in pulse pressure from AR leads to strong bounding pulses with rapid rises and falls. A Corrigan pulse or water-hammer pulse result from the forceful ejection of blood in early systole and regurgitation during early diastole.[1] A bisferiens pulse (increased pulse pressure with a double systolic peak) is possible and is more readily recognized in the brachial and femoral arteries than in the carotid arteries. There may also be a slight bobbing of the head with each heartbeat (the de Musset sign).[1] Confirmatory findings of a widened pulse pressure include the Traube sign (booming sounds heard over the femoral artery), the Müller sign (pulsations of the uvula), the Duroziez sign (diastolic murmur heard over the femoral artery when proximally compressed), or the Quincke sign (capillary pulsations through the patient's fingertips).[1] If chronic severe AR has progressed, exam findings may include signs of heart failure, hepatomegaly, and ascites.

DIAGNOSTICS

TTE is used to measure the valve, aortic root, LV function, and EF; it is helpful in identifying a bicuspid valve, thickening of the valve cusps, congenital abnormalities, prolapsed valve, flail leaflet, or vegetation.[1] Doppler color imaging is the most sensitive and accurate evaluation of AR and is able to detect mild degrees of regurgitation that may be inaudible on physical examination.[1] It provides the necessary anatomical and hemodynamic measurements for the staging of AR, confirming its presence, severity, and cause.[5]

The 12-lead ECG findings in chronic AR is mostly limited to signs of LVH; they are not a strong predictor of AR severity.[1] When AR is secondary to inflammatory processes, a prolonged PR interval (first-degree atrioventricular block) may be present. An LV strain pattern may exist that correlates with the presence of ventricular dilation.[1] In acute severe AR there should be no evidence of LVH, and there is usually a normal sinus rhythm or sinus tachycardia.

As the severity of chronic AR increases, the LV contour enlarges, producing a boot-shaped heart silhouette on the CXR film. The aortic knob and ascending aorta become prominent with moderate to severe chronic AR. Patients with acute AR do not demonstrate cardiac enlargement but will exhibit increased venous redistribution to the upper lobes because of pulmonary venous and capillary hypertension secondary to an increased LV end-diastolic pressure and left atrial pressure. Any new onset of symptoms in patients diagnosed with mild to moderate AR, such as angina or dyspnea, may indicate progression and warrant further diagnostic testing.

INTERPROFESSIONAL COLLABORATIVE MANAGEMENT
Nonpharmacologic Management

Appropriate management of AR requires accurate diagnosis of the cause and staging of the disease process. Clinical staging of chronic AR is determined by symptomatic status, regurgitation severity, LV volume, and systolic function. Evaluation for surgical treatment, according to current recommendations, may be indicated in asymptomatic patients (stage C) and symptomatic patients (stage D).[1] Interdisciplinary management is considered when a patient becomes symptomatic.

Pharmacologic Management

Asymptomatic patients with mild or moderate AR and normal or minimally increased heart size do not require therapy; however, annual follow-up is recommended. The presence of systemic arterial diastolic hypertension in patients with mild to moderate AR or severe AR should be treated with a dihydropine calcium channel blocker, angiotensin-converting enzyme inhibitors (ACEIs), angiotensin receptor blockers (ARBs) or other antihypertensive that does not cause slowing of the ventricular heart rate.[1] Atrial fibrillation and bradycardia are common complications and should be prevented. In patients with tachyarrhythmia, beta blockers may be used with caution. In asymptomatic patients at high risk for surgery, pharmacologic management is preferred.[1] In most patients with AR, antibiotic prophylaxis for infective endocarditis is not needed.

INDICATIONS FOR REFERRAL AND HOSPITALIZATION

Surgical intervention is recommended for symptomatic patients (stage D) and asymptomatic patients (stage C) who have a LVEF below 50%.[1,5] AVR is also recommended for asymptomatic patients (stage C) and those with progressive AR (stage B), undergoing other cardiac surgery.[1] LVEF below 50% is an independent risk factor associated with poor outcomes. Therefore surgical recommendations should be highly considered before LV function deteriorates. The available types of surgical interventions are similar to AS and can be found in the relevant section of this chapter. On the other hand, asymptomatic patients with severe AR and normal LV function have excellent prognoses and do not require surgical intervention.[1]

MITRAL STENOSIS

DEFINITION AND EPIDEMIOLOGY

The predominant cause of MS is rheumatic fever; at the time of surgical mitral valve replacement, 99% of patients show rheumatic changes.[1] Approximately 25% of all patients with rheumatic heart disease have isolated MS, 40% have combined MS and regurgitation, and 38% have multivalve involvement with MS.[1] The marked reduction of rheumatic carditis has reduced the overall occurrence of MS. Additional causes in the older population include heavy calcification of the mitral annulus with extension into the leaflets, causing obstruction to LV inflow.[6] The obstruction of MS across the valve during diastole results in a pressure gradient between the left atrium and the left ventricle. The increased left atrial pressure is transmitted to the pulmonary veins and capillaries and eventually to the pulmonary arteries and right side of the heart. Less common causes of MS are related to obstruction across the mitral valve that prevents normal emptying of the left atrium into the left ventricle during diastole. These causes include congenital stenosis, vegetation, clots, benign tumors (atrial myxomas), and profound calcification of the mitral annulus

Damage to the mitral valve from rheumatic fever causes thickening at the leaflet edges, fusion of the commissures, and chordal shortening and fusion.[1] The thickened, scarred valve leads to a characteristic funnel-shaped valve deformity sometimes referred to as a fish-mouth appearance. The pathologic hallmarks of rheumatic disease are Aschoff bodies in the myocardium (not found in the valve tissue), which are identified in only 2% of autopsied patients with chronic valve disease.[1]

In pregnancy, mitral stenosis is a commonly diagnosed valvular abnormality due to the increase in circulating volume. For women in developing countries, MS a significant cause of maternal death usually related to rheumatic mitral stenosis.

PATHOPHYSIOLOGY

There is usually no detectable pressure gradient across the normal mitral valve even when flow is increased with exercise. As the valve area is reduced, the gradient across the valve increases. The normal mitral valve area is 4 to 5 cm^2; but if it is measured at less than 2.5 cm^2, hemodynamically significant stenosis is present.[16] However, MS usually becomes symptomatic when the mitral valve opening is reduced to 1.5 cm^2 or less.[1,16] With this degree of obstruction, the mean gradient, even at rest, is likely to be more than 20 mm Hg throughout diastole. With a further rise to 25 to 30 mm Hg, the left atrial pressure will exceed plasma oncotic pressure and episodes of orthopnea or paroxysmal nocturnal dyspnea will develop.[1] Chronic elevation of left atrial pressure produces a passive pressure load on the pulmonary vessel and causes hypertrophy and hyperplasia. This causes pulmonary hypertension to develop and may lead to right ventricular hypertrophy (although typically the left ventricle remains normal). It is common for patients with MS to have atrial fibrillation, especially with increasing age, making a greater risk for thrombus formation and systemic embolism more concerning due to left atrial enlargement and stasis of blood flow.[1]

CLINICAL PRESENTATION AND PHYSICAL EXAMINATION

The principal symptom of MS is dyspnea, which is graded according to the New York Heart Association (NYHA) classification. Patients with asymptomatic MS are assigned to functional class I. Patients with dyspnea that occurs with greater than ordinary exertion are assigned to class II; patients with dyspnea that occurs with only mild exertion (less than ordinary activity) are assigned to class III; and those with dyspnea on minimum exertion—with episodes of orthopnea, paroxysmal nocturnal dyspnea, or pulmonary edema—are assigned to class IV.

The dyspnea may be accompanied by cough or wheezing and hemoptysis may occur as a result of pulmonary hypertension; in rare instances this may be extensive.[1,16] Hoarseness (Ortner syndrome) may develop from compression of the left recurrent laryngeal nerve by a dilated left atrium.[1] A small number of patients report anginalike chest pain, which may be caused by concomitant coronary artery disease, pulmonary embolus, or pulmonary hypertension. Fatigue and weakness are symptoms of severe MS (valve size <1 cm^2) when pulmonary vascular resistance is elevated and secondary to a low cardiac output and pulmonary congestion with exercise.[1] Patient with MS who have atrial fibrillation may also complain of palpitations due to the increase in embolic events, and the clinician should investigate symptoms of thromboembolic events.

When a patient with MS is being examined, the diastolic murmur of MS is typically a low-pitched rumbling sound best heard during exhalation with the bell of the stethoscope directly over the apex and in the left lateral position or with mild exercise, like hand grips.[7] There are three additional auscultatory findings associated MS; these include a loud S1, a loud P_2, and an opening snap that initiates the diastolic murmur. The murmur has two components: the mid-diastolic (rapid ventricular filling) and the late diastolic, also called presystolic (atrial contraction). It starts after S_2 and follows a decrescendo pattern but ends with an accentuation leading up to S_1 (which is usually loud). The opening snap of the mitral valve (just after S_2) is most audible over the apex with the diaphragm. It may sound a little like an S_3, but S_3 is caused by LV volume overload, which is not usually present in MS unless MR or AR coexists.[1]

The murmur of MS can be hard to hear, making it difficult to differentiate from the diastolic murmurs of TS, the murmur of atrial tumors (myxomas) or the rumbling of the Austin Flint murmur. If pulmonary hypertension exists, the P_2 may become accentuated and loud on auscultation and the right ventricular impulse may become palpable.[1] In severe chronic MS, low cardiac output and systemic vasoconstriction may cause pinkish-purple patches to appear on the cheeks; these are known as mitral facies. In patients with atrial fibrillation, there may be an irregular pulse and signs of right-sided heart failure, and the jugular venous pulse pressure may disappear.[1]

DIAGNOSTICS

TTE quantifies the gradient and valve area affected by MS and identifies valvular lesions or causes of mitral obstruction. It shows leaflet thickening, restriction of opening, and doming of the leaflets in diastole caused by symmetric fusion of the commissures.[1] The atrial size and ventricular function, especially in the right ventricle, are evaluated. The color Doppler study is helpful to detect the presence and extent of regurgitation and to improve clarity of the valve area measurements. A transesophageal echocardiogram (TEE) is used to exclude left atrial thrombus or when TTE images are not optimal.[1] Coronary arteriography may still be required in adults to exclude coronary artery disease in patients with conflicting TTE and TEE results. Exercise Doppler echocardiography is useful to assesses exercise duration and pulmonary pressures or to clarify the cause if there is a discrepancy in diagnostic findings and symptom severity.

The characteristic findings on the 12-lead ECG are evident only as MS worsens into more severe obstruction. Typically there is an underlying normal sinus rhythm with left atrial enlargement, evidenced by widened, notched P wave in the limb leads and pronounced terminal P negativity in V1. There may also be signs of right axis deviation and right ventricular hypertrophy. However, the signs of left atrial enlargement and right heart strain disappear if the patient enters into atrial fibrillation.

CXR examination in a patient with MS may reveal left atrial enlargement, which is initially more evident on the lateral view; but as severity worsens, the frontal view reveals enlargement of the cardiac silhouette and lung fields, which should be identified. The double density sign of atrial enlargement is seen in a frontal view and occurs when the right side of the left atrium is pushed into the lung behind the right cardiac shadow and creates a double shadow or double right heart border. The left atrial enlargement also causes changes to the main bronchus, with widening of the carina angle to greater than 90 degrees. The left atrial appendage bulges and creates a discrete convex bump on the left upper heart border (this is confirmed in the lateral view). With chronic pulmonary hypertension, the pulmonary vessels become prominent and flow redistributes fluid in the upper lobes. Severe MS obstruction may result in interstitial edema, manifesting as Kerley B lines, which are dense short horizontal lines most commonly seen in the costophrenic angles. However, severe long-standing mitral obstruction may result in Kerley A lines seen as straight, dense lines up to 4 cm in length running toward the hilum as well as the findings of pulmonary hemosiderosis and rarely of parenchymal ossification.[1]

INTERPROFESSIONAL COLLABORATIVE MANAGEMENT

Nonpharmacologic Management

Management of MS is determined by identification of the cause and accurate staging of the disease process. Stages are determined by the patient's symptoms, valve anatomy, hemodynamics, and the effect of valve obstruction on the left atrial and pulmonary circulation. Stage A (risk of MS) has normal left atrial size and normal flow velocities with only doming of the valve during diastole.[5] Stage B (progressive) is characterized by rheumatic valve changes with commissural fusion, diastolic valve doming, a mitral valve area greater than 1.5 cm^2, and diastolic pressure half-time below 150 ms.[5] Stage C is severe, asymptomatic MS where valve changes are accompanied by a mitral valve area smaller than 1.5 cm^2 and diastolic pressure half-time exceeding 150 ms. In addition, left atrial enlargement and elevated pulmonary artery pressures are also present in stage C and beyond.[5] Stage D is severe symptomatic MS wherein the valve anatomy, hemodynamics, and valve obstruction sequelae are accompanied by decreased exercise tolerance and exertional dyspnea. Occupations that demand strenuous physical exertion should be avoided by patients with more than mild MS.

Pharmacologic Management

The goals of medical therapy include the prevention of rheumatic fever, prevention and treatment of complications secondary to progression of the disease, and early intervention as well as timing of treatment.[1] Recurrent episodes of rheumatic fever may be prevented by penicillin prophylaxis.[1] Anemia should also be addressed promptly because of its demand on the heart and reduced amount of circulating oxygenated blood, causing tachycardia. The use of oral diuretics and sodium restriction may help relieve symptoms of congestion (i.e., fluid overload).

Patients with MS who have atrial fibrillation associated with ventricular dysfunction can be treated with digoxin. Patients who develop symptoms with exercise can be treated with beta blockers or calcium channel blockers to slow the ventricular rate.[5,16] Use of anticoagulation is indicated for the prevention of systemic embolism, with a prior history of embolic events, and where there is a known history of left atrial thrombus in patients with MS (moderate by echocardiography) and atrial fibrillation.[1] Patients with MS in chronic atrial fibrillation are at a much higher risk of embolic events if they are not receiving anticoagulant therapy. If warfarin is used as an anticoagulant, an international normalized ratio (INR) between 2 and 3 should be maintained.[1] No benefit of anticoagulation has been shown for patients in normal sinus rhythm without a prior history of embolism.

INDICATIONS FOR REFERRAL AND HOSPITALIZATION

Interdisciplinary management is necessary in patients with moderate to severe MS. Consultation with a cardiologist is recommended to those who are symptomatic, difficult to manage, or diagnosed with severe VHD. Consultation should occur when the diagnosis is unclear or when cardioversion, surgery, or balloon valvuloplasty is being considered. Referral to an HVC is recommended to discuss treatment options for asymptomatic patients with severe VHD and those who may benefit from valve repair or replacement.[5]

There are several options of procedures that have been found to be effective in the treatment of MS. The balloon mitral valvulotomy (BMV) is an interventional procedure in which a large balloon is inflated across the mitral valve to dilate the leaflets. This procedure is an option for asymptomatic patients with severe MS (<1 cm^2), symptomatic patients high risk for surgery, or patients with mild MS with pulmonary hypertension (>25 mm Hg) during activity or of unexplained causes.[1] Degree of calcification and regurgitation, valve morphology, and presence of thrombi in the atrium are considerations in determining the type of surgical intervention needed.[5]

Surgical valve repair is recommended for patients with severe MS and significant symptoms if they are not candidates for BMV or had an unsuccessful BMV procedure, have severe MS and severe pulmonary HTN, or have moderate to severe MS with recurrent embolic events while on anticoagulation.[1] Several approaches for surgical valvotomy include a closed mitral valvotomy, an open valvotomy, and valve replacement. If possible, the preferred surgical approach is open valvotomy, especially if the mitral valves are highly distorted or calcified.[1] A closed valvotomy procedure uses a transatrial or transventricular approach to repair the mitral valve.[1] Patients who undergo an open valvotomy are connected to a cardiopulmonary bypass unit so that surgeons can achieve a direct view of the valve.[1] If the valve cannot be repaired, valve replacement is performed. Because atrial fibrillation is so common in patients with MS, a surgical ablation can be performed during surgery (Maze procedure/atrial compartment operation), thus eliminating possible thrombotic complications.[5] Normal gains of atrial function and maintenance in sinus rhythm are seen in about 80% of patients who undergo the Maze procedure in conjunction with the surgical intervention.[1] The prosthetic valve of choice is a mechanical valve, especially when atrial fibrillation is present, because of the need for chronic anticoagulation.[1]

MITRAL REGURGITATION

DEFINITION AND EPIDEMIOLOGY

Mitral valve disease is the most common of the valvular heart disorders, particularly in ageing populations, with greater than 10% prevalence in people 75 years of age and older.[6] MVP is the most common cause of MR in the United States; it is so significant that it is discussed in more detail in a specific section following that on MR. Ischemic LV dysfunction and dilated cardiomyopathy are the second leading causes of MR in the United States.[1] Approximately 30% of patients with coronary artery disease who are being considered for coronary artery bypass grafting (CABG) have some degree of MR.[1] Other causes of MR include rheumatic heart disease, annular calcification, and infective endocarditis. Less common causes of MR include collagen vascular diseases, hypereosinophilic syndrome, carcinoid, and exposure to certain drugs.[1,5] However, regurgitation from connective tissue diseases, such as Marfan syndrome, tends to progress more rapidly than chronic MR of rheumatic origin.[1] Acute rheumatic fever is a frequent cause of isolated severe MR among adolescents in developing nations, and these patients often have a rapidly progressive course.[1] Acute regurgitation may be a result of spontaneous rupture of the chordae tendineae, blunt chest trauma, or disruption of a papillary muscle as a sequela of a myocardial infarction, most often an inferior infarct. Dilation of the left ventricle from any cause is likely to result in failure of the mitral leaflets to coapt.

PATHOPHYSIOLOGY

The mitral valve is a bicuspid valve, but its anatomical structure consists of four cusps, with the anterior (aortic cusp) and posterior (mural cusp) being the two largest and two smaller commissures. There are three groups of chordae tendineae supported by two sets of papillary muscles and the mitral annulus that make up the supporting valvular apparatus. Damage, necrosis, or strain to the apparatus can result in MR, but the primary reason is abnormality of the leaflets.

Chronic MR is usually classified into primary (degenerative or structural) or secondary (functional).[6] Primary MR (degenerative) is caused by structural disease of the valve, valvular leaflets, or valvular components (leaflets, chordae tendineae, papillary muscles, or annulus) usually seen with infectious endocarditis, connective tissue disorders, cardiac disease from radiation, rheumatic heart disease, or progressive MVP.[5] The damage of rheumatic mitral valve disease (e.g., classic fish-mouth appearance) is discussed in the MS section but is the same pathophysiologic changes noted in MR.

Secondary MR is further divided into functional or ischemic types and depends on the contributing coronary artery disease. Secondary MR is usually caused by a damaged left ventricle or mitral annulus (e.g., from MI or cardiovascular disease), which causes deformation of a normal valve.[1,5,6] The burden placed on the heart as a result of MR is dependent on the amount of reflux and the ability of the ventricles and atria to compensate. Pulmonary hypertension rarely develops in the patient who has developed MR gradually over time. However, in functional MR there is long-standing LV dysfunction, which increases the atrial pressures and leads to increased pulmonary pressures and eventual failure.[5]

During systole the left ventricle simultaneously ejects blood forward through the aortic valve and backward across an incompetent valve into the left atrium. In moderate to severe MR, approximately 50% of the regurgitant volume is ejected into the left atrium before the aortic valve opens.[1] The volume of regurgitant flow depends on the size of the regurgitant orifice and the pressure gradient between the left ventricle and left atrium. The increased preload and afterload plus the depressed contractility further increase LV size and enlarge the mitral annulus, resulting in worsened regurgitance.[1] Regurgitant flow is decreased by any agent that decreases LV size (such as diuretics) or shifts the balance toward the forward output (such as afterload-reducing vasodilators). In contrast, regurgitation is increased by any factor that enlarges the left ventricle, depresses myocardial function, or increases resistance to forward flow (such as hypertension or AS). Effective (forward) cardiac output is usually depressed in severely symptomatic patients with MR, whereas total LV output is usually elevated.[1]

With chronic MR, the increased volume of blood ejected back into the left atrium causes stretching and thinning of the atrial wall. The large thin-walled atrium accommodates the large volume of blood ejected into it during ventricular systole. Although the pressure in the left atrium and pulmonary capillaries and veins is elevated during systole, the left atrial pressure decreases to nearly normal during ventricular diastole. The left ventricle dilates and becomes hypertrophied in response to the increased volume from the left atrium, so that sufficient cardiac output is maintained. Initially the additional volume to be ejected by the ventricle (increased preload) results in enhanced emptying. Therefore the EF is increased. Normal EF or other measures of cardiac systolic performance are likely to represent significantly abnormal ventricular function.

In contrast, patients with acute MR develop a rapid increase in left atrial pressure as a result of the sudden volume overload into a normal, nondilated left atrium and ventricle. This results in suddenly increased pressures in the left atria and the pulmonary vasculature and elevated LV end-diastolic pressure. Pulmonary hypertension and pulmonary congestion producing interstitial edema may ensue.

CLINICAL PRESENTATION AND PHYSICAL EXAMINATION

The patient with MR may remain asymptomatic for decades, but typical symptoms include fatigue due to reduced cardiac output; later in the course of the disease, dyspnea on exertion may occur from LV dysfunction. Cardiac arrhythmias and atrial fibrillation are associated with MR, but palpitations or tachycardia may occur with or without evidence of atrial fibrillation. The severity of symptoms and clinical outcome of chronic MR depend on the degree of regurgitation and also on associated valvular abnormalities, underlying ventricular dysfunction, and concomitant coronary artery disease.[1] Symptoms of CHF usually appear late in the course of chronic MR as a result of the gradual increase in volume overload. By the time symptoms appear, the degree of ventricular dysfunction may have progressed to such an extent as to be irreversible. In asymptomatic patients with severe MR, the rate of progression to symptoms such as LV dysfunction, pulmonary hypertension or atrial fibrillation is 30% to 40% at 5 years.[1] Acute MR symptoms develop from sudden overload of the left atrium and include congestive hepatomegaly, edema, and ascites due to right-sided heart failure along with elevated pulmonary vascular resistance and pulmonary hypertension.[1]

The hallmark murmur of MR is the harsh pansystolic (holosystolic), blowing murmur best heard at the apex and radiating to the axilla, back, or left sternal border.[7] The murmur is more likely to radiate to other locations if there is papillary muscle dysfunction, partial rupture, or damage to the supporting structures. Auscultation of the patient with chronic MR reveals a soft S_1 and often a wide split S_2 due to the shortening of LV ejection; in patients with severe pulmonary hypertension, the P_2 is louder than the A_2.[1] An audible S_3 is present when there is hemodynamically significant MR, reflecting volume overload of the left ventricle; therefore S_3 is indicative of predominant regurgitation.

Pansystolic murmurs are pathologic; therefore the murmur of MR or mitral insufficiency should be differentiated from the pansystolic murmurs of TR, VSD, or patent ductus arteriosus (rare). The murmurs may be difficult to distinguish from long systolic ejection murmurs, especially if the patient is tachycardic. The murmur of MR does not become louder with inspiration, as it does with TR.[7] Bedside maneuvers can be used to enhance or diminish the murmur to differentiate it from other causes. The murmur of MR is usually intensified by isometric exercise, such as alternating hand grasps, which increases the impedance to LV ejection and increases regurgitation.[1] Maneuvers that decrease LV volume by decreasing impedance to LV outflow or venous return (such as sudden standing) will result in a decreased murmur, as will more chronically decreasing ventricular volume with diuresis. It should be noted that it is possible to have severe MR without an audible murmur because of the equalization of LV and left atrial pressures.

The apical impulse (point of maximal impulse, or PMI) is hyperkinetic and displaces downward and to the left if volume overload is present in the left ventricle.[1,7] Arterial pulses are brisk and hyperdynamic. Palpation of the carotid arterial pulse is helpful in differentiating MR from AS; the carotid arterial upstroke is sharp and severe in MR and delayed in AS.[1]

DIAGNOSTICS

A baseline evaluation with TTE is indicated for primary MR or suspected chronic MR to evaluate LV size and function, left atrial size, right ventricular function, pulmonary artery pressure, and mechanism and severity of the MR.[5] In severe MR echocardiographic imaging is used to identify the cause of the valve dysfunction and shows enlargement of the left atrium and left ventricle, with increased systolic motion of both chambers. The addition of color Doppler echocardiography is helpful to determine the severity of the MR as it is reflected in the width of the regurgitant jet across the valve and by the size of the left atrium. Reversal of flow in the pulmonary veins during systole and a high peak mitral inflow velocity also are useful signs of severe MR.[1] Chronic MR usually produces a volume overload pattern and a large left atrium.

The hemodynamic effects of MR on the left atrium and left ventricle can be estimated using TTE. Patients with LV dysfunction may increase end-systolic and end-diastolic volumes, reduce the EF, and shorten rate. The TTE is significantly useful for patients with acute MR, as direct visualization of the valve aids in rapid and accurate diagnosis, allowing for lifesaving interventions.

The 12-lead ECG findings of chronic and severe MR are the same as those in MS; there is usually an underlying normal sinus rhythm with left atrial hypertrophy in the early stage and atrial fibrillation later. If the MR is secondary to underlying ventricular dysfunction and dilation, evidence of LVH may be noted. The CXR film demonstrates an increase in both LV and left atrial size (which is detailed in the MS radiology section).

Cardiac magnetic resonance imaging (cMRI) is indicated in patients with chronic primary MR to assess left ventricular (LV) and right ventricular (RV) volumes, function, or MR severity and when these issues are not satisfactorily addressed by TTE. Additional imaging—including stress nuclear, positron emission tomography, cMRI, stress echocardiography, cardiac CT angiography, or cardiac catheterization with coronary arteriography—is useful to establish etiology of chronic secondary MR (stages B to D) and to assess myocardial viability, which influences the management plan for functional MR.[5]

INTERPROFESSIONAL COLLABORATIVE MANAGEMENT

Nonpharmacologic Management

The management of chronic primary MR is determined by severity and presence or absence of negative prognostic features, including symptoms, LV dysfunction, size increase, and pulmonary hypertension. Patients with MR may remain asymptomatic for decades, with only a small percentage progressing to more severe MR requiring surgery.[5] The progression of MR varies with each patient, and the prognosis worsens with delayed MR correction.

Interdisciplinary management should be considered for patients with acute MR or once the patient with chronic MR becomes symptomatic and surgery is considered. The goal of treatment is to correct MR before onset of LV systolic dysfunction to prevent adverse effects on patient outcomes. Asymptomatic patients with MR and normal sinus rhythm without atrial or LV enlargement can participate in exercise without any restrictions.[5] Patients with MR associated with pulmonary hypertension, LV enlargement, or evidence of heart failure cannot engage in competitive athletic exercise.[5]

Pharmacologic Management

Medical management includes beta-adrenergic blockade, ACEIs or ARBs, and possibly aldosterone antagonists. These therapies aid in reducing the severity of MR in a failing heart. Vasodilator therapy is not indicated for normotensive asymptomatic patients with chronic primary MR.[5]

INDICATIONS FOR REFERRAL AND HOSPITALIZATION

Referral to an HVC for early repair or very careful surveillance is required.[5] Surgical therapy is aimed at improving symptoms, relieving severe pulmonary hypertension, and decreasing LV volume and mass. Surgical techniques used to treat MR are valve repair or reconstruction and valve replacement. Valve repair, the preferred treatment, repairs the disrupted functional component of the valve. Mitral valve repair retains the tethering effect of chordal attachments, which may prevent postoperative dilation of the left ventricle and decreases the chance of LV dysfunction that arises after mitral valve replacement. Surgery recommendations are based on MR stages.[5] Mitral valve surgery should be performed when the patient's left ventricle nears but does not exceed the parameters of systolic dysfunction (LVEF ≤60% or LV end systolic dimension ≥40 mm).[5] In 2013, the US Food and Drug administration approved the use of MitraClip, a percutaneous surgical approach, for asymptomatic high-risk patients with diagnosed degenerative MR.[17]

New recommendations have been made in regard to the surgical intervention of both primary and secondary MR. Mitral valve surgery is now acceptable for asymptomatic patients with preserved LV size and function, with a progressive increase in LV size, or the presence of decreased LVEF.[11] Patients with persistent chronic severe MR despite goal-directed medical therapy now have the option of choosing sparing of the MV chord versus annuloplasty with repair.[11] The updated guidelines also confirm that there still continues to be a questionable benefit in repairing the moderate MR valve in conjunction with CABG.

Antithrombotic therapy continues to be an important factor to consider with prosthetic valves.[11]

Patients with marked LV dysfunction may remain symptomatic even after surgical treatment. Such patients may show a decrease in EF and an increase in end-systolic volume immediately after surgery, essentially increasing the afterload that the ventricle faces. These patients may require vasodilator treatment in the immediate postoperative period and in fact may be difficult to wean off bypass. Such patients may benefit from only partial repair of the valve, leaving some regurgitation.

MITRAL VALVE PROLAPSE

DEFINITION AND EPIDEMIOLOGY

MVP is the most common cause of MR and mitral valve disease in developed nations and is twice as frequent in women as in men.[1,9] With a prevalence of 2% to 3%, MVP affects over 7 million individuals in the United States and more than 170 million people worldwide.[18] MVP has been given many additional names, including the floppy valve syndrome, systolic click-murmur syndrome, Barlow syndrome, billowing mitral cusp syndrome, myxomatous mitral valve syndrome, and redundant cusp syndrome.[1,19] MVP is also the most common cardiac condition predisposing patients to infective endocarditis.[1]

MVP may be classified into two groups, syndromic and nonsyndromic. Syndromic MVP is usually associated with connective tissue disorders such as Marfan syndrome and Ehler-Danlos syndrome. The familial (nonsyndromic) form of MVP appears to be inherited, and family history that includes a three-generation pedigree is a useful tool.[18] Echocardiographic findings of MVP have been reported in a large number of first-degree relatives of patients with established MVP.[1] Nonsyndromic MVP is more prevalent in young women and usually benign; if diagnosed in older men, however, it is more likely a severe disease and carries a higher risk of complications and surgical repair.[1,18] The survival and outlook for a patient with MVP is generally very good, and a large majority remain asymptomatic for many years without any change in clinical or laboratory findings.[1,19]

PATHOPHYSIOLOGY

MVP is typically described as a malcoaptation of one leaflet (SiMVP) or both (BiMVP) leaflets of the mitral valve during systole. It more commonly involves the posterior leaflet. The leaflets bulge (prolapse) upward into the left atrium, causing a regurgitation of blood back to the left atrium. Displacement of the prolapsed leaflets is measured by echocardiography at more than 2 mm above the annular high points of the valve at end systole.[1,18,19]

The most common cause of MVP is idiopathic myxomatous degeneration, which is a deterioration of the fibrous collagen layer valve that thins and is replaced by myxomatous (mucoid) matter. This causes abnormal stretching of the valve leaflets and the chordae tendineae. The valve leaflets become floppy and the chordae become longer and thinner. The billowing movement of the leaflet places stress on the chordae and papillary muscles, which may be the cause of the nonischemic chest discomfort. The floppy valve leaflets pull on the chordae, causing lengthening and rupture—cardinal features of the MVP syndrome.[1]

CLINICAL PRESENTATION AND PHYSICAL EXAMINATION

Most persons with MVP are asymptomatic and remain that way throughout their lives. When symptoms do occur, they usually involve palpitations, syncope, presyncope, and chest discomfort.[1] The latter may be difficult to distinguish from that of angina pectoris but is often atypical, with severe stabbing pain at the cardiac apex that is prolonged and not clearly related to exertion.[1] Symptoms of fatigue, palpitations, postural orthostasis, anxiety, panic attacks, and depression are commonly associated with MVP but are most likely related to an imbalance of the autonomic nervous system rather than a direct result of the valvular disease.[1] The severity of symptoms often does not match the severity of the valvular prolapse, with some patients describing severe symptoms but having limited prolapse and others showing significant prolapse with no symptoms. If MVP progressed to severe MR, one may note signs of fatigue, dyspnea, exercise intolerance, orthopnea, paroxysmal nocturnal dyspnea, or heart failure.

Palpitations or the sensation of a rapid or irregular heartbeat is a common complaint of patients with symptomatic MVP and may result from a variety of arrhythmias. It has been suggested that BiMVP is associated with sudden cardiac death but only limited data support this; therefore although BiMVP seems to be associated with an increased risk of ventricular tachycardia, it does not appear to increase the risk of death and should not raise concern if it occurs in the absence of other cardiac abnormalities.[20]

Most cases of MVP are diagnosed on routine physical examination. The murmur of MVP reveals a classically late systolic crescendo-type murmur that is usually loud and musical. It is often preceded by a midsystolic click (but not always), which is a snapping extra heart sound best heard at the lower left sternal border or at the apex and often only intermittently appreciated.[7,9]

The presence of an apical systolic murmur varies with the degree of MR. The sounds can sometimes be manipulated or enhanced with bedside maneuvers. Several positions are recommended to identify MVP, including supine, seated, squatting, and standing. Squatting uses the Valsalva release phase, which delays the systolic click and murmur due to increased venous return. This is different from the Valsalva strain of standing, in which the sounds are heard earlier and closer to S_1.[7,9]

The murmur of MVP is a late-systolic murmur characterized by a midsystolic click. This non-ejection systolic click heralds the onset of the murmur. The murmur is slightly different from the other murmur of mitral insufficiency that is heard with MR, which is pansystolic. The click in MVP can be differentiated from an aortic ejection click because it occurs after the beginning of the carotid pulse upstroke.[1]

DIAGNOSTICS

Echocardiographic imaging provides details of the integrity of the valve apparatus and shows the underlying cause of the regurgitation, such as rupture of the chordae tendineae, in MVP. The 2D echo must show the mitral leaflets billowing by at least 2 mm into the left atrium to diagnose MVP, and thickening of the leaflet by more than 5 mm supports the diagnosis.[1] TTE can provide information regarding LV size and function, evaluate the severity of MR, and evaluate flail leaflets in patients with ruptured chordae.

Patients with MVP may demonstrate inverted T waves and nonspecific ST-segment changes in the inferior and left precordial leads of the ECG; however, this is more common if the patient is symptomatic. These changes may be a manifestation of ischemia to the papillary muscles resulting from the strain placed on these muscles by the prolapsed valve leaflets. Stress ECG and thallium Tl-201 or sestamibi exercise scans should be used when there is a need to differentiate MVP from coronary artery disease. This is especially important when the patient with suspected MVP complains of chest discomfort.

Supraventricular tachycardia is not uncommon in MVP. Other ventricular and supraventricular arrhythmias and conduction disturbances may also occur. There seems to be a slightly increased incidence of sudden death, presumably as a result of ventricular fibrillation, although this finding has not been firmly established.

INTERPROFESSIONAL COLLABORATIVE MANAGEMENT

Nonpharmacologic Management

Patients with MVP are usually asymptomatic and require no intervention other than clinical and echocardiographic follow-up evaluation every 3 to 5 years.[1] The prognosis of patients with MVP is good, and many of these patients remain asymptomatic for years with no notable changes in their clinical findings.[1] However, if a long systolic murmur is present in an asymptomatic patient, frequent monitoring is highly recommended.

Pharmacologic Management

A common complication of MVP is progressive MR, wherein patients may develop an increase in left atrial and ventricular size, pulmonary hypertension, and congestive heart failure.[1] Beta-blocker therapy is often used for the management of palpitations secondary to PVCs or self-limiting SVTs as well as in the treatment of nonischemic or ischemic chest pain.[1] Aspirin therapy is recommended for those with a prior history of neurologic events. Appropriate anticoagulation therapy should be initiated in patients with a prior history of left atrial thrombus or arrhythmia, such as atrial fibrillation.[1]

INDICATIONS FOR REFERRAL AND HOSPITALIZATION

Interdisciplinary management and life span considerations for MVP are related to the severity of the MR and are similar to the previously described measures for the treatment MR. In patients with associated symptoms of syncope or near-syncope, a referral for arrhythmia evaluation is recommended. Radiofrequency ablation is recommended in patients with frequent or prolonged SVTs.[1] Serious complications such as cardiac surgery, infective endocarditis, and cerebrovascular events may occur, however rare. Surgical treatment of MVP, such as mitral reconstruction secondary to a ruptured chordae tendinae, may be necessary when the MR has been progressive and severe.[1] Refer to MR management for surgical options.

PULMONARY VALVE DISORDER

DEFINITION AND EPIDEMIOLOGY

The etiology of a pulmonic valve disorders is unknown, but there seems to be an association with other cardiac conditions, congenital anomalies or in babies born to mothers with rubella. Rheumatic heart disease is a rare manifestation of pulmonic valvular disease and associated more with regurgitation than with stenosis. Carcinoid disease may be a causative factor in both PS and PR.[21] In children with tetralogy of Fallot, the right ventricular outflow tract and pulmonic valve are commonly affected and cause insufficiency of the valve, usually requiring multiple surgical interventions before adulthood.[21] Patients diagnosed with pulmonary valve stenosis may have a thickened, immobile, or fused heart valve that is unable to open fully. The most common etiology of PS is the congenital form, responsible for approximately 8% to 10% of cardiac birth defects.[1,22]

Congenital defects are the most common explanation for PR, including tetralogy of Fallot, abnormal valve motions and Marfan syndrome. There are also acquired causes of PR such as endocarditis, primary cardiac tumors, carcinoid heart disease, rheumatic heart disease, trauma or in rare incidences pulmonary hypertension.[22] Mild PR may be found in 40% to 78% of patients who have normal anatomy of the pulmonic valve, but severe PR is rare and usually caused by congenital heart disease (such as tetralogy of Fallot), or in patients who have undergone surgical repair of congenital heart defects.[22] The presence of PR postoperatively is used as a determinant of short- or long-term adverse outcomes.[22] The amount of regurgitation is influenced by the valve size, afterload in the right ventricle, and right ventricular diastolic compliance.[21]

PATHOPHYSIOLOGY

Pulmonary valve stenosis affects the right side of the heart, causing increased pressure in the right ventricle, thus making it difficult to pump blood out of the heart. It also causes an interruption in the pulmonic blood flow out of the heart to the pulmonary arteries. Disruption of the oxygenated blood flow through the pulmonary artery into the lungs may lead to pulmonary manifestations.

The severity of pulmonic valve regurgitation is classified in stages (see Table 108.2). Hemodynamic consequences in patients with severe PR include right ventricular enlargement and an echocardiographic pattern consistent with volume overload.[5] About 20% of patients with congenital heart disease will have abnormality in the pulmonic valve and right ventricular outflow tract.[22] Valvular dilation, right sided heart failure, arrhythmia, and death are commonly seen in patients with progressive PR.[22]

CLINICAL PRESENTATION AND PHYSICAL EXAMINATION

Patients with mild to moderate pulmonary valve stenosis may remain asymptomatic. Severe valvular stenosis may cause symptoms of dyspnea and fatigue. Rarely, patients with severe stenosis have symptoms of exertional angina, syncope, or sudden death. In patients with right heart involvement, peripheral edema may be present.

Initially, patients with severe PR may be asymptomatic. Symptoms related to PR may vary depending on the cause of the regurgitation and the effect on the RV function.[5] Anatomical disruption in the valve leaflets and resulting annular dilation plays a significant role in symptomatology. Significant RV dilation and the severity of systolic dysfunction are key factors that dictate presence of symptoms.[22]

The pulmonic valvular sound is best heard over the second to third intercostal spaces, left of the sternum, and may reveal a normal S_1 and wide splitting of S_2 (most likely caused by dilatation of the pulmonary artery, pulmonary hypertension, and PS).[1,7] The murmur of PS is harsh and medium-pitched with a crescendo-decrescendo pattern.[7] Severe PS causes a prolonged duration and delayed peak of the sound. The intensity may vary from soft to loud with increasing volume, which is associated with a palpable thrill.[7] A precordial heave or palpable impulse from the right ventricle may be present in severe PS.

The murmur of PR is soft, pitched, and heard during diastole, with a normal S_1 and widely split S_2 that increases in intensity with inspiration and is heard in the absence of pulmonary hypertension.[1] If the murmur is secondary to pulmonary hypertension, a midsystolic ejection murmur in the second left intercostal space is audible.[1] An S_3 and S_4 is heard typically in the left fourth intercostal space and increased with inspiration. If the pulmonary artery pressure exceeds 55 mm Hg, a high-pitched, blowing, decrescendo murmur is auscultated in the left second to fourth intercostal spaces; this is also known as the Graham Steell murmur.[1] Although PR is primarily a diastolic murmur, the presence and severity of pulmonary hypertension plays a role in the characteristics of the auscultatory findings. Palpation of the left parasternal area is recommended to identify the systolic pulsation of PR related to the hyperdynamic right ventricle and enlarged pulmonary artery.[1]

DIAGNOSTICS

TTE may reveal an abnormal increased pressure in the right side of the heart in pulmonic valve disease, with enlargement of the atria in PS and right ventricular hypertrophy in PR. TTE is also helpful in evaluating the severity of the regurgitation and the identification of valvular pathology.[22] The gold standard in quantification of pulmonic valve regurgitation in patients with congenital heart disease is cine MRI (cMRI).[24] The right ventricular systolic end volume is a critical value in determining significant PR and is best evaluated using cMRI.

The 12-lead ECG findings are usually normal in patients with mild pulmonary stenosis. However, right axis deviation and increased R-wave amplitude in lead V1 may be noted. Greater P-wave amplitude may be seen in right atrial enlargement. In severe PS, Q waves may be present in V1 to V3. The ECG findings in PR are usually secondary to pulmonary hypertension and consistent with RVH. The configuration of rSr in the right precordial leads reflects right ventricular diastolic overload.[1] Radiologic findings are nonspecific for pulmonic valvular disease but may include a mildly thickened pulmonic valve leaflet, right atrial enlargement, right ventricular enlargement, or enlargement of the pulmonary artery.

INTERPROFESSIONAL COLLABORATIVE MANAGEMENT
Nonpharmacologic Management

Management of PS is dependent on the congenital anomaly affecting the valvular structures, such as constriction and obstruction from plaque buildup in the valvular ring and cusps. Patients with PR does not necessarily require a specific treatment unless with a diagnosis of tetralogy of Fallot.[1] Valvular disease progression must be closely monitored to avoid consequences such as heart failure, arrhythmias, and death.

Pharmacologic Management

Medical management for pulmonic valvular disorders is indicated to help alleviate symptoms; it includes the use of diuretics in patients with pulmonary edema. Treatment for PR is focused on primary conditions, such as infective endocarditis and pulmonary hypertension. Precautionary antibiotics may be prescribed to prevent bacterial endocarditis.

INDICATIONS FOR REFERRAL AND HOSPITALIZATION

Surgical intervention is rarely required for pulmonic valve disease, as the symptoms are rarely severe enough to warrant surgery. However, if necessary, transcatheter pulmonic valve replacement is the most common approach. A leaflet repair or replacement with a biological or mechanical valve may be achieved with an open heart surgical approach. The preferred treatment for PS in infants is the percutaneous balloon pulmonary valvuloplasty.[23] This method instantaneously relieves pressure in the right ventricle, allowing ease of blood flow out of the heart and into the pulmonary arteries. Other methods of treatment include transannular patches; however, this must be done within the child's first year of life.[25] There is a higher risk of surgical reintervention in children as compared with adults.

TRICUSPID VALVE DISEASE

DEFINITION AND EPIDEMIOLOGY

Tricuspid valve disease is most commonly rheumatic in origin, with TR being more common than TS, or a combination of both TS and TR may be seen.[1] Additional causes of TS include connective tissue diseases, congenital atresia, right atrial tumors, or other obstructions of right atrial emptying.[1] Valvular calcification is rare and more common in women.[1] The backflow of blood into the right atrium from tricuspid valve disease may result in right atrial enlargement. Medical conditions, such as heart failure and cardiomyopathies, may contribute to this valvular disease but may also occur as a consequence of the disease process. Ventricular dilation secondary to arterial and pulmonary hypertension as well as pulmonic conditions such as emphysema may subsequently cause TR.[26] Inflammatory disease processes—such as infective endocarditis, rheumatic heart disease, trauma, degenerative processes, carcinoid syndrome, or congenital heart disease—are also contributing factors to TR.[26] Additional conditions that may cause TR include congenital heart disease (such as PS and pulmonary hypertension secondary to Eisenmenger syndrome), primary pulmonary hypertension secondary to right ventricular infarction, associated atrial septal defect, or rarely cor pulmonale.[1]

PATHOPHYSIOLOGY

The stiff and narrowed valvular movement of TS impedes blood flow from the right atrium to the right ventricle, resulting in a diastolic pressure gradient that is augmented during inspiration or exercise and reduced when the blood flow declines during expiration.[1] Right ventricular pressure and cardiac output decrease as the blood is prevented from traveling through the stenotic valve. Regurgitation and inadequate closure of the valve cause backflow to the atrium. Atrial dilation in TS may result in severe passive congestion and hepatosplenomegaly.[1] Severity is greatly affected by conditions causing right ventricular expansion and dilation, thus increasing the size of the valvular ring.[26] Tricuspid valve prolapse caused by myxomatous

changes in the valve and chordae tendineae may result in TR and additionally occurs in approximately 20% of patients with MVP.[1]

CLINICAL PRESENTATION AND PHYSICAL EXAMINATION

The severity of tricuspid valve disease dictates symptomatology and clinical symptoms may not be present until the valvular disease becomes severe. Patients may present with symptoms of fatigue, tiredness, or lethargy due to the low cardiac output from both TS or TR. Anasarca, ascites, or discomfort is caused by hepatomegaly secondary to elevated systemic venous pressure.[1] Patients may complain of a fluttering feeling of discomfort in the neck caused by the jugular venous pulse.[1]

The presence of TR is generally well tolerated, but when pulmonary hypertension and TR coexist, the cardiac output declines and symptoms of right-sided heart failure become exaggerated. These symptoms may include ascites, painful congestive hepatomegaly, massive edema, throbbing pulsations of the neck, and systolic pulsations of the eyeballs (more common if mitral disease is also present).[1] Activities of daily living may increase in difficulty in proportion to the severity of the disease as well as reduced exercise tolerance.

Upon examination, a mild diastolic murmur of TS may be heard along the left lower parasternal border in the fourth intercostal space. This reflects the blood flowing through the stenotic valve and is usually high-pitched, soft, and short in duration.[1] The auscultatory finding of TS is often missed because it is masked by the louder and more prominent heart sounds from MS. The presence of peripheral cyanosis, peripheral edema, a jugular venous pulse, distended neck veins, hepatosplenomegaly, or hepatic pulsations are all physical findings of TS due to right atrial backflow, but the lung fields should remain clear.[1]

The typical ausculatory finding of TR is a pansystolic (holosystolic) blowing murmur, usually short in duration, heard best at the lower left sternal border; it may radiate to the right of the sternum and left midclavicular line.[1,7] In addition there is often an S_3 sound from the right ventricle (accentuated by inspiration). If TR is secondary to pulmonary hypertension, P_2 may be accentuated.[1] The murmur has similarities to MR, but the S_1 sound is not as soft as in MR; the murmur of TR is augmented during inspiration (Carvallo sign).[1,7] The murmur of TR may also increase with exercise, leg raising, and hepatic compression, known as the Mueller maneuver.[1] The amplitude of the right ventricular impulse is increased in TR and may be sustained.[7] A venous systolic thrill and murmur in the neck may be auscultated in severe TR and a prominent v wave and y descent may be noted in the jugular venous pulse.[1] Weight loss, cachexia, cyanosis, jaundice, ascites, and jugular venous distention may be present on the physical exam of a patient with severe TR.[1]

Diagnostics

Echocardiography of the tricuspid valve is used to detect valvular anatomy and to estimate the severity of TS or TR. It also serves to assess pulmonary arterial pressure, right ventricular function, and pressures of the right atria, right ventricle, and end diastole.[1] In patients with TS, findings include thickened and restricted motion of the valvular leaflets and a reduced diameter of the tricuspid orifice.[1] In patients with TR, the TTE findings may show evidence of right ventricular diastolic overload, paradoxical motion of the ventricular septum, exaggerated or delayed closure of the valve, and the presence of prolapse.[1] Doppler findings of a prolonged slope of the antegrade flow are comparable to measurements of TS and TR performed by cardiac catheterization.[1] In addition, Doppler findings in TR may detect carcinoid heart disease or reveal vegetation caused by endocarditis in patients with TR.[1]

ECG findings may be normal or nonspecific in tricuspid valve disease, especially in the absence of atrial fibrillation. Right atrial enlargement with a P wave amplitude exceeding 0.25 mV in leads II and V1 may be found in TS. There may be signs of right atrial dilation noted in TS if the QRS amplitude is reduced in V1.[1] Patients with TR may exhibit incomplete right bundle branch block, Q waves in lead V1, or atrial fibrillation.[1]

Radiographic findings for both TS and TR may reveal cardiomegaly, and the right atrium may be prominent or enlarged.[1] Angiographic findings reveal thickened and decreased mobility of leaflets, a narrowed valve orifice, and a thickened atrial wall in patients with TS.[1] cMRI may be used to evaluate the geometric relationship of the right ventricle and the valve annulus and leaflets in patients with functional TR.[1]

INTERPROFESSIONAL COLLABORATIVE MANAGEMENT
Nonpharmacologic Management
Management of tricuspid valve disease is dependent on the underlying cause and presenting symptoms. A conservative approach is preferred in patients with TR. Isolated TR is rare; it is usually secondary to rheumatic heart disease but commonly seen associated with mitral valve disease. Therefore initial management is focused on the mitral valve.

Pharmacologic Management
Medical management, such as the use of diuretics, in patients with TS is focused on reducing the accumulation of excess salt and water. Although the prevention of bacterial endocarditis is no longer indicated, immediate treatment in the presence of bacterial endocarditis is critical in preventing further valvular damage. If needed, beta-blocker therapy may be prescribed for the management of tachyarrhythmia.

INDICATIONS FOR REFERRAL AND HOSPITALIZATION
Significant damage to the valves may require valve repair or replacement with a biological or mechanical device. Surgical management is the ideal treatment of choice in patients with severe TS. However, it is not usually indicated as a sole intervention based on TS alone. Patients with TS are likely to have MS as well, and treating TS alone may only contribute to increased pulmonary congestion or edema postoperatively.[1] Indications for surgery include a mean diastolic pressure gradient greater than 5 mm Hg, a tricuspid orifice of smaller than 2.0 cm, and planned mitral valve repair or replacement.

TS is almost always accompanied by TR; therefore surgical intervention is preferred for optimal symptom improvement. Two valvular device options include a large bioprosthesis or a mechanical prosthesis. Use of a bioprosthesis is preferred because of its longer durability and lesser risk for thrombosis.[1] If a patient is not a surgical candidate, a tricuspid balloon valvuloplasty may be done in combination with the mitral balloon valvuloplasty.

MULTI-VALVULAR DISEASE
It is possible to have multi-valvular disease, the most frequent cause being rheumatic fever, degenerative calcification, or a connective tissue disorder such as Marfan syndrome.[1] The dysfunction of a valve can increase chamber pressures, affect blood flow through the heart, and therefore cause strain on other valves. For this reason it is not uncommon to have multi-VHD. An example of this is seen in the progression of mitral valve disease, which may result in pulmonary hypertension and can lead to TR due to atrial dilation.

Clinical presentation and physical exam findings will depend on the location of the valves involved and the severity of each lesion. Diagnostic testing with 2D color Doppler echo and possibly cardiac catheterization and angiography will provide a thorough evaluation of each valve and the cardiac anatomical structure. It is important to discover and measure the degree of multi-valvular involvement before surgical valve repair, as failure to correct all significant valvular disease during the same surgery increases mortality considerably.[1]

The choice between a bioprosthetic or mechanical valve for surgical replacement becomes more complicated in a multivalvular approach. The bioprosthesis does not require anticoagulation therapy, but the longevity and durability of the valve are less than those of a mechanical valve. When multiple prosthetic valves are inserted in the left side of the heart they should be of the same type, such as two bioprostheses or two mechanical prostheses. If two mechanical prostheses are selected for the mitral and AVRs, but the tricuspid valve also needs replacing, the use of a bioprosthesis in the tricuspid position is suggested.[1]

LIFE SPAN CONSIDERATIONS
Life span considerations for patients with VHD are determined based on the valve involved, the severity of the valve disease, the symptomology, and subsequent sequelae. The progression of valvular disease is staged based on symptomology and diagnostic testing, which help manage treatment options and determine prognosis. The degree of symptoms and the status of the cardiac pump, especially LV function, help determine the considerations and outcomes. All female patients planning a pregnancy should be referred to a cardiologist for evaluation, testing, and guidance prior to the pregnancy. Age may be a factor in diagnosing VHD, such as AS, a condition most often seen in the aging population. However, the severity of valvular dysfunction and effects on the cardiac cycle are more important prognostic factors than is age.

COMPLICATIONS
Complications of VHD vary based on the cause of the underlying valve disease, the location, and the obstruction of blood flow through the valve (stenosis vs. regurgitation). Increasing severity of the valvular dysfunction and the involvement of surrounding anatomical structures augment the risk of complications. Heart failure, cardiac arrhythmias, and thromboembolic events such as stroke are serious potential sequelae of valvular dysfunction.

Additional complications may arise from the pharmacologic treatment or surgical repair of the valve.

Infective endocarditis may occur in either the native or prosthetic valve, and suspicion for this should be confirmed via TEE. The presence of infective endocarditis in a prosthetic valve requires surgical intervention.[5] In native valve endocarditis, early surgical intervention may be considered if the vegetation is mobile and greater than 10 mm in length.[5]

Cardiac arrhythmias, specifically atrial fibrillation, may occur in about 10% of patients with AS and 75% of patients with MR.[1] Atrial fibrillation in AS should raise the possibility of a concomitant mitral valve disease, especially in the presence of a dilated left atrium. Progressive deterioration of ventricular function, as manifested by symptoms of dyspnea and angina, is a complication and an indication for immediate evaluation by TTE.[5] The presence of atrial fibrillation may require prompt cardioversion to prevent impairment of LV performance and systemic embolization.

Valve dysfunction increases the risk of thromboembolic events. The added danger of clot formation with atrial fibrillation increases the possibilities of pulmonary emboli or stroke. In comparison to the other heart valves, the tricuspid valve's position carries the greatest risk of increased valvular thrombus due to the lower pressures and velocity of blood flow.[1]

PATIENT AND FAMILY EDUCATION

Patients diagnosed with a valvular disorder require basic knowledge of their medical condition for early management and to prevent complications. Patients are recommended to immediately report the development of or any change in symptoms, such as fatigue, dyspnea, weight gain, rapid heartbeat, or chest discomfort. A change in current symptoms or onset of new symptoms can signify disease progression.

It is also critical for patients to have a good understanding of their management plan. The prescribed medication regimen should be clearly explained and its importance reinforced at every visit. For patients with severe VHD it is important to discuss the indications for prophylactic antibiotic therapy, such as before instrumentation procedures (e.g., dental procedures).

HEALTH PROMOTION

A global initiative to expand the focus beyond cardiovascular disease prevention is critical in addressing needs and opportunities to combat the increasing concerns of morbidity and mortality. Reduction of cardiac risk factors and lifestyle modifications can impact overall cardiovascular health and slow the progression of heart disease. Therefore health promotion should include advice on dietary adjustments, increasing physical activity, smoking cessation, alcohol reduction, and compliance with medical therapy. In addition, the early detection and initiation of medical management of VHD may prevent the development of comorbid conditions such as heart failure and hypertensive heart disease.

REFERENCES

1. Otto, C. M., & Bonow, R. O. (2014). Valvular heart disease. In D. L. Mann, P. Zipes, P. Libby, & R. O. Bonown (Eds.), *Braunwald's heart disease: A textbook of cardiovascular medicine* (10th ed., pp. 1446–1515). Philadelphia: Elsevier.
2. Søndergaard, L., Saraste, A., Christersson, C., & Vahanian, A. (2018). The year in cardiology 2017: Valvular heart disease. *European Heart Journal*.
3. Benjamin, E. J., Blaha, M. J., Chiuve, S. E., Cushman, M., Das, S. R., Deo, R., et al. (2017). Heart disease and stroke statistics—2017 update: A report from the American Heart Association. *Circulation, 135*(10), e146–e603.
4. Endicott, K., Lambdin, J., Morrisette, J., Kirkpatrick, A., Nagy, C., Mordini, F., et al. (2017). Heart valve clinic: A model for treatment of structural heart disease. *World Journal of Cardiovascular Surgery, 7*(1), 1.
5. Nishimura, R. A., Otto, C. M., & Bonow, R. O. (2014). 2014 AHA/ACC guideline for the management of patients with valvular heart disease: A report of the American College of Cardiology/American Heart Association Task Force on Practice Guidelines. *Circulation, 129*, e521–e643.
6. Nishimura, R. A., Vahanian, A., Eleid, M. F., & Mack, M. J. (2016). Mitral valve disease—current management and future challenges. *The Lancet., 387*(10025), 1324–1334.
7. Bickley, L. S., Szilagyi, P. G., & Hoffman, R. M. (2017). *Bates' guide to physical examination and history taking*. Philadelphia: Wolters Kluwer.
8. Fang, J. C., & O'Gara, P. T. (2014). The history and physical examination. In D. L. Mann, D. P. Zipes, P. Libby, & R. O. Bonown (Eds.), *Braunwald's heart disease: A textbook of cardiovascular medicine* (10th ed., pp. 95–112). Philadelphia: Elsevier.
9. McGee, S. (2018). *Evidence-based physical diagnosis e-book*. Elsevier Health Sciences.
10. Begic, E., & Begic, Z. (2017). Accidental heart murmurs. *Medical Archives., 71*(4), 284.
11. Mastiasz, R., & Rigolin, V. H. (2018). 2017 focused update for management of patients with valvular heart disease: Summary of new recommendations. *JAHA, 7*, e007596.
12. Czarny, M. J., & Resar, J. R. (2014). Diagnosis and management of valvular aortic stenosis. *Clinical Medicine Insights Cardiology, 8*(S1), 15–24.
13. Rashedi, N., & Otto, C. M. (2015). Aortic stenosis: Changing disease concepts. *Journal of Cardiovascular Ultrasound, 23*(2), 59–69.
14. Bhatheja, S., Panchal, H. B., Barry, N., Mukherjee, D., Uretsky, B. F., & Paul, T. (2016). Valvular performance and aortic regurgitation following transcatheter aortic valve replacement using Edwards valve versus CoreValve for severe aortic stenosis: A meta-analysis. *Cardiovascular Revascularization Medicine, 17*(4), 248–255.
15. Mahmaljy, H., & Young, M. (2019). Transcatheter Aortic Valve Replacement (TAVR/TAVI, percutaneous replacement) [updated 2019 Jan 11]. In *StatPearls [Internet]*. Treasure Island (FL): StatPearls Publishing. Retrieved from https://www.ncbi.nlm.nih.gov/books/NBK431075/.
16. Ray, R., & Chambers, J. (2014). Mitral valve disease. *International Journal of Clinical Practice, 68*(10), 1216–1220.
17. Feldman, T. (2015). MitraClip for degenetrative and functional mitral regurgitation in high-risk patients. ACC. Retrieved from: http://www.acc.org/latest-in-cardiology/articles/2015/03/23/13/40/mitraclip-for-degenerative-and-functional-mitral-regurgitation-in-high-risk-patients.
18. Parwani, P., Avierinos, J. F., Levine, R. A., & Delling, F. N. (2017). Mitral valve prolapse: Multimodality imaging and genetic insights. *Progress in Cardiovascular Diseases*.
19. Krishnaswamy, A., & Griffin, B. P. (2013). Myxomatous mitral valve disease. In C. M. Otto & R. O. Bonow (Eds.), *Valvular heart disease: A companion to Braunwald's heart disease* (4th ed., pp. 278–294). Philadelphia: Saunders.
20. Nordhues, B. D., Siontis, K. C., Scott, C. G., Nkomo, V. T., Ackerman, M. J., Asirvatham, S. J., et al. (2016). Bileaflet mitral valve prolapse and risk of ventricular dysrhythmias and death. *Journal of Cardiovascular Electrophysiology, 27*(4), 463–468.
21. Pignatelli, R. H., Noel, C., & Reddy, S. C. (2017). Imaging of the pulmonary valve in the adults. *Current Opinion in Cardiology, 32*(5), 529–540.
22. Shillcutt, S. K., Tavazzi, G., Shapiro, B. P., & Diaz-Gomez, J. (2017). Pulmonic regurgitation in the adult cardiac surgery patient. *Journal of Cardiothoracic and Vascular Anesthesia, 31*(1), 215–228.
23. Hong, D., Qian, M. Y., Zhang, Z. W., Wang, S. S., Li, J. J., Li, Y. F., et al. (2017). Immediate therapeutic outcomes and medium-term follow-up of percutaneous balloon pulmonary valvuloplasty in infants with pulmonary valve stenosis: A single-center retrospective study. *Chinese Medical Journal, 130*(23), 2785.
24. Zdradzinski, M. J., Elkin, R. L., Hart, S. A., Flamm, S., & Krasuski, R. A. (2015). Incremental value of cardiac magnetic resonance imaging for assessing pulmonic valve regurgitation. *Journal of Heart Valve Disease*.
25. Tasoglu, I., Atalay, A., Aksoy, O. N., & Polat, V. (2018). Pulmonary valve cusp augmentation for pulmonary regurgitation after percutaneous balloon pulmonary valvuloplasty of valvular pulmonary stenosis. *Cardiology in the Young, 1-4*.
26. Harris, C., Croce, B., & Munkholm-Larsen, S. (2017). Tricuspid valve disease. *Annals of Cardiothoracic Surgery, 6*(3), 294.

Evaluation and Management of Gastrointestinal Disorders

CHAPTER 109

ABDOMINAL PAIN AND INFECTIONS

Vicki Chandler

 Specialist referral is indicated for suspected gastrointestinal bleeding, bowel obstruction, orthostatic vital sign changes, abnormal findings, jaundice, positive pregnancy test result, severe localized or unilateral lower abdominal pain, or a history of trauma and any indication of peritoneal irritation.

DEFINITION AND EPIDEMIOLOGY

Abdominal pain is a common reason patients seek care in primary care offices, urgent care centers, and emergency rooms. Gastrointestinal discomfort is also a challenging condition to diagnose because the pain can be related to something as benign as abdominal gas or a more serious condition requiring emergency care.[1] There are many causes of abdominal pain, and the patient's description of the discomfort may be vague, but for any patient reporting abdominal discomfort, the health care provider's first priority is to determine whether the patient's pain is the result of an acute abdomen, indicating an emergency referral.[1]

PATHOPHYSIOLOGY AND CLINICAL PRESENTATION

There are several major mechanisms of abdominal pain, including pain from obstruction of a hollow viscus, capsular distention, peritoneal irritation, mucosal ulceration, vascular insufficiency, altered body motility, nerve injury, abdominal wall injury, and pain referred from an extra-abdominal site. Determination of the specific type of pain gives a provider valuable information about the possible cause of the pain. Abdominal wall pain is often described as a constant achy feeling. Visceral pain, the pain arising from a hollow viscus, is usually the result of distention or spasm of a hollow organ, as in early intestinal obstruction; it is commonly described as dull and crampy and is poorly localized. Parietal pain is a sharp, well-localized pain arising from irritation of the parietal peritoneum, such as the pain of acute appendicitis with inflammation spread to the peritoneum. Referred pain is an aching type of pain experienced away from the disease process and is perceived to be near the surface of the body. The pain referral phenomenon is a result of the shared central pathways for afferent neurons from different locations (e.g., pain from an inflamed gallbladder may be felt in the right scapula[1]).

Location of the abdominal pain is another factor that can aid in identifying the cause of the patient's discomfort. Pain localized to the right upper abdominal quadrant generally emanates from the chest cavity, liver, gallbladder, stomach, bowel, or right kidney or ureter. Left upper quadrant pain is usually associated with the heart or chest cavity, spleen, stomach, pancreas (especially acute pancreatitis), or left kidney or ureter. The source of left lower abdominal pain can include the bowel, left ureter, or pelvis and is most commonly associated with diverticulitis, particularly when the pain is protracted and severe.[2] Right lower quadrant pain is associated with the appendix, bowel, right ureter, or pelvis, with the most common diagnosis being appendicitis. Cholecystitis or peptic ulcer perforation also must be considered. Pain that migrates across several quadrants is typically associated with the bowel, whereas abdominal wall pain from trauma or inflammation can occur in any quadrant.

In some patients, abdominal pain can be subtle and the diagnosis obscure. This is particularly true in older adults, whose symptoms may be atypical and nonspecific.[3] Older adults are also more likely to be hypotensive, lethargic, or confused. Patients with dementia are especially at risk for having their symptoms dismissed as being an element of dementia rather than an underlying pathology.[4]

Lower abdominal or pelvic discomfort in females can suggest a gynecologic problem (e.g., an ovarian cyst). In women of childbearing age, even those with a history of tubal ligation, abdominal pain, or abnormal vaginal bleeding, it is imperative to perform a pregnancy test to exclude the possibility of ectopic pregnancy.[5]

An accurate diagnosis in patients complaining of acute abdominal pain is highly dependent on history, physical examination, and appropriate laboratory and radiologic procedures. Previous abdominal surgery, medication history (including over-the-counter drugs, vitamins, and supplements), allergies, social and sexual history, last menstrual period, dietary history, last food or fluid ingested, and family history of abdominal pain are important considerations that should be elicited. Causes of acute abdominal pain that should be considered include appendicitis, cholecystitis, diverticulitis, small bowel obstruction, perforated peptic ulcer, peritonitis, ruptured ectopic pregnancy, pelvic inflammatory disease, ruptured abdominal aortic aneurysm (AAA), hypercalcemia, superior mesenteric artery syndrome, and acute intermittent porphyria.[6] In female patients, it is important to obtain a sexual history and to consider pelvic inflammatory disease or ectopic pregnancy.[6] It is also essential to remember that acute diseases of the chest, including myocardial infarction, congestive heart failure, pulmonary infarction, and pneumonia, may mimic primary diseases of the abdomen.[6]

APPENDICITIS

 Immediate surgical referral is indicated for appendicitis.

DEFINITION AND EPIDEMIOLOGY

Acute appendicitis is an inflammatory disease of the wall of the appendix that may result in perforation with subsequent peritonitis. In the United States, appendicitis affects approximately 300,000 people yearly, often resulting in emergency surgery.[7,8]

PATHOPHYSIOLOGY

Appendicitis is primarily thought to be caused by the blockage of the appendiceal lumen, leading to distention of the appendix as a result of accumulated intramural fluid with secondary bacterial infection. Acute appendicitis is described as simple, gangrenous, or perforated on the basis of operative findings. In simple appendicitis, the appendix is viable and intact. Gangrenous appendicitis is characterized by necrosis of the appendiceal wall. Perforated appendicitis refers to disruption of the appendix. Acute appendicitis is thought to be secondary to obstruction of its orifice, with secondary bacterial infection.[8]

The main cause of appendiceal lumen obstruction is hyperplasia of the lymphoid tissue, which most often occurs during adolescence. Other causes of lymphoid tissue hyperplasia are bacterial, viral, parasitic, or fungal infections, inflammation such as inflammatory bowel disease, fecaliths, foreign bodies, and cancer.[8] When the appendiceal lumen becomes obstructed, the mucosa continues to secrete fluid until the intraluminal pressure exceeds venous pressure. At this point, the appendix becomes hypoxic, the mucosa ulcerates, and bacteria invade the wall. Infection causes additional swelling and ischemia as a result of thrombosis of small intramural vessels. Gangrene and perforation usually develop in 24 to 36 hours. Perforation leads to a release of the luminal contents into the peritoneal cavity.[8]

CLINICAL PRESENTATION AND PHYSICAL EXAMINATION

The most reliable historical feature in the diagnosis of acute appendicitis is the sequence of symptoms. The three signs and symptoms most predictive of acute appendicitis include pain that starts in the epigastrium or periumbilical area, migration of the pain to the right lower quadrant, and abdominal rigidity.[6] The pain can be diffuse or occur at other sites in the abdomen, including the left lower quadrant.[6] Another predictor is the duration of the pain; patients with appendicitis have been shown to have pain of a shorter duration than that of patients with other disorders.[9]

Anorexia and nausea are quite common, with the latter occurring after the pain onset; vomiting is possible.[1] Often the symptoms are subacute and nonspecific; crampy abdominal discomfort that comes and goes, some malaise, and possibly a change in bowel habits occurs initially.[1] Constipation, or rarely diarrhea accompanied by a low grade fever, follows the onset of pain. Not all patients will have every symptom; however, when the symptoms occur in any other order, the diagnosis of appendicitis should be questioned.[6,9]

A thorough physical examination (including a pelvic examination for a female patient) after obtaining a careful history is necessary. A fever is usually present. Abdominal tenderness is elicited by asking the patient to cough. Localized tenderness is a valuable physical finding, and the patient can often specify the painful spot with one finger. By systematically performing a thorough abdominal examination starting in the upper abdomen in an area without pain and ending in the area of pain, localized tenderness can be determined, usually in the right lower quadrant between the umbilicus and the anterosuperior iliac spine (McBurney point). The Rovsing sign (right lower quadrant pain) is elicited by palpating the left lower quadrant.[1] There may be signs of peritoneal irritation, including guarding, rebound tenderness, and obturator sign (elicited by passive rotation of the right leg with the patient supine and the right hip and knee flexed) and psoas sign (the supine patient raises the straightened right leg against resistance by the practitioner. The "Bump" sign is elicited when a patient notes abdominal pain when driving over a speed bump or when the stretcher a patient is lying on is "bumped" causing increased abdominal pain. Having patients jump up and down (the Markle sign) or off one step can also cause an increase in abdominal discomfort. A rectal examination is necessary and may reveal tenderness or a mass.

DIAGNOSTICS

Acute appendicitis is suggested by the history and physical examination findings. An elevated white blood cell count is present in 70% to 90% of patients with acute appendicitis, and a left shift is present 95% of the time.[1] The health care provider should immediately refer a patient with suspected appendicitis for surgical consultation. A serum beta human chorionic gonadotropin (β-hCG) level should be obtained in women of childbearing age because appendicitis is common in pregnancy and it is necessary to exclude a ruptured ectopic pregnancy. Serum amylase and lipase levels are necessary. Sickle cell disease should be excluded in patients of African, Indian, Mediterranean, or Spanish descent.[1] A C-reactive protein level is also necessary, as is a urinalysis.

Imaging studies are not required in most cases of suspected appendicitis. However, imaging modalities may be necessary if the presentation is atypical or in patients at the extremes of age. Plain abdominal radiographs show nonspecific signs and are not recommended. Ultrasonographic evidence of appendicitis includes appendiceal wall thickening, luminal distention, and lack of compressibility. Ultrasound is useful in children and in pregnant women and if the cause of the discomfort seems gynecologic, although ultrasound can generally be limited by operator skill and interpretation. A computed tomography (CT) scan is most useful for diagnosis if the cause of the abdominal pain is unclear.[1]

INITIAL DIAGNOSTICS

Appendicitis

LABORATORY
- Complete blood count (CBC) and differential
- Serum glucose, electrolytes, blood urea nitrogen (BUN), creatinine
- C-reactive protein
- Serum β-hCG
- Sickeldex test
- Urinalysis

IMAGING
- CT scan

ADDITIONAL DIAGNOSTICS
- Laparoscopy or laparotomy
- Ultrasound

DIFFERENTIAL DIAGNOSIS

Conditions that mimic acute appendicitis include gastroenteritis, mesenteric lymphadenitis, acute salpingitis, mittelschmerz, ruptured ectopic pregnancy, ruptured corpus luteum cyst, ureteral colic, Meckel diverticulitis, sigmoid diverticulitis, perforated peptic ulcer, cholecystitis, intestinal obstruction, cecal diverticulitis, intestinal ischemia, regional enteritis (Crohn disease), and perforated colonic carcinoma. Basilar pneumonia may also be confused with appendicitis.

 Primary differentials include ectopic pregnancy in women of childbearing age and sickle cell anemia in African Americans.

INTERPROFESSIONAL COLLABORATIVE MANAGEMENT
Pharmacologic Management

Abdominal discomfort in older patients should always be evaluated and appropriate treatment initiated. In patients with uncomplicated appendicitis, antibiotic therapy is a possible option, although controversial because appendicitis can recur.[10] Perioperative systemic antibiotics, such as metronidazole and ceftizoxime, have been shown to prevent wound infection in simple appendicitis. If the appendix is perforated, antibiotic therapy to cover anaerobic as well as aerobic pathogens is initially indicated until culture results are available. Antibiotics are also indicated for patients with suspected septicemia and patients scheduled for laparoscopic surgery.

Indications for Referral and Hospitalization

Immediate surgical referral or a transfer to the emergency department is indicated for suspected appendicitis or other acute abdominal pain. Treatment of appendicitis is usually a prompt appendectomy, preferably within 24 hours of symptom onset to prevent perforation and peritonitis. Hospitalization is indicated for monitoring and surgical care, if necessary.

If surgery is required, patients should have nothing by mouth and intravenous fluid and electrolyte repletion initiated as necessary. Surgery for an appendiceal abscess may spread a localized infection to other parts of the peritoneal cavity; therefore percutaneous CT-guided drainage of an abscess is used to allow the acute inflammation to resolve before elective appendectomy is performed.[11]

Lifespan Considerations

Hyperplasia of the lymphoid tissue, which can obstruct the appendiceal lumen, occurs during adolescence. Therefore adolescents who present with signs and symptoms of appendicitis should be evaluated promptly.[8]

Families of older patients should understand that pain perception may be diminished, especially if the patient takes an analgesic. Misdiagnosis at the first health care visit and using analgesics can delay treatment for appendicitis and lead to appendix perforation.[12] Any of the previously listed symptoms in older adults, even if unaccompanied by abdominal pain, should be evaluated by a medical professional.[4]

COMPLICATIONS

Complications of appendicitis include gangrene, perforation with peritonitis, and abscess formation. Pylephlebitis, which is septic thrombophlebitis of the portal venous system, should be suspected in any patient with appendicitis who has shaking chills. Septicemia, urinary retention and infection, small bowel obstruction, and mesenteric thrombophlebitis may also occur. Common complications associated with appendectomy include wound infection, pneumonia, intraperitoneal abscesses, enterocutaneous fistulas, wound or inguinal hernias, and possibly minor bleeding.

PATIENT AND FAMILY EDUCATION

- Abdominal pain may be a sign of serious illness or may be related to a chronic disorder
- Localized abdominal pain or pain that increases in severity warrants discussion with the health care provider
- Abdominal pain accompanied by fever, chills, severe vomiting or diarrhea, significant rectal bleeding, black and tarry stools, weakness, or dizziness requires a visit to the health care provider

SMALL BOWEL OBSTRUCTION
DEFINITION AND EPIDEMIOLOGY

 Immediate surgical referral is indicated for small bowel obstruction.

Small bowel obstruction, a common cause of acute diffuse abdominal pain, refers to either a partial or complete obstruction of the bowel lumen or paralysis (ileus) of the intestinal musculature. As a result, fluid and gas accumulate proximal to the obstruction, causing nausea, vomiting, abdominal distention, and pain.[13] It is essential to recognize bowel obstruction because it can cause vascular compromise, bowel ischemia, and peritonitis. Adhesions, hernias, and tumors are the most common causes of small bowel obstruction, although other conditions, such as fecal impaction, ischemia, abscesses, inflammatory bowel disease, volvulus, intussusception, strictures, gallstones, cystic fibrosis, and radiation enteritis, can also be responsible.[14] Ileus is associated with abdominal surgery; abdominal and other infectious processes (e.g., pneumonia, sepsis); electrolyte disorders; and medications (e.g., anticholinergics, calcium channel blockers, narcotics, tricyclics, and other drugs).[14]

PATHOPHYSIOLOGY

In a bowel obstruction, distention results in decreased absorption and increased secretions that cause further distention and fluid and electrolyte imbalances. Bacterial proliferation may occur as a result of stasis. Distention increases the risk of bowel perforation and diffuse peritonitis. Mechanical obstruction of the bowel lumen may occur from lesions (e.g., adhesions; congenital, inflammatory, or neoplastic lesions), femoral or indirect inguinal hernia, polypoid tumors, intussusception, volvulus, gallstone ileus, impacted feces, or bezoar formation.[13] Intussusception, often recognized as an abdominal mass on examination with a history of acute symptom onset, occurs when a bowel segment telescopes into the adjacent bowel, resulting in symptoms of intermittent bowel obstruction. Volvulus results from abnormal twisting of a bowel segment along its mesenteric axis.[14]

CLINICAL PRESENTATION AND PHYSICAL EXAMINATION

Bowel obstruction manifests with intermittent and crampy abdominal pain, vomiting, obstipation, abdominal distention, hyperactive bowel sound, and fever. The pain is usually relieved by vomiting, intestinal tube decompression, or the passage of intestinal contents through a partial obstruction. Pain that progresses in severity, localizes, or becomes constant demonstrates progression to a strangulated obstruction; this condition requires urgent surgery. The presentation of a patient with ileus differs slightly in that bowel sounds are more frequently decreased or absent.[13]

A careful history of the chronicle of the illness, the patient's medication history, the last bowel movement, and the presence of flatus is necessary. A prior history of bowel obstructions, abdominal irradiation, abdominal inflammation or cancer, or abdominal or pelvic operations should be identified because these conditions are all associated with bowel obstructions.

The physical examination for any patient with an intestinal obstruction requires provider attentiveness to the patient's general appearance and vital signs. A fever suggests an infectious process, whereas hypovolemia is associated with tachycardia and orthostatic hypotension. The physical examination should determine whether the patient's symptoms are related to a nonabdominal cause (e.g., pneumonia, myocardial infarction) or an abdominal process. A distended, tympanic abdomen accompanied by peristaltic rushes and high-pitched tinkling sounds may be present initially, but bowel sounds may be absent as the disorder progresses. Diffuse midabdominal tenderness is common; localized tenderness, abdominal guarding, rebound tenderness, and rigidity are concerning signs. The rectal examination may reveal stool, masses, tenderness, or occult blood. Particular attention needs to be placed on examination of potential hernial orifices, especially the area of the femoral ring because of its small opening and potential for bowel strangulation. Women should receive a vaginal exam to rule out any gynecologic pathology that can cause an obstruction.[13]

DIAGNOSTICS

A small bowel obstruction can be diagnosed with plain radiography or ultrasound, although an abdominal CT is often used and is indicated if an abdominal infection or mechanical obstruction is suspected and to determine the underlying cause of the obstruction.[13,14] If x-rays are appropriate, upright and supine views of the abdomen and an upright view of the chest are necessary. The upright abdominal film identifies a distended bowel proximal to the obstruction in addition to air-fluid levels. It may show free air if perforation has occurred. The supine radiograph may distinguish between ileus and obstruction. If an ileus is present, the radiograph will show distended loops in both the large and small bowel; with an obstruction, the segment proximal to the obstruction is distended, and the distal bowel loops are decreased in caliber. Diagnostic evaluation should determine the presence of intraperitoneal masses, ascites, gallstones, renal calculi, foreign bodies, and gas within the bowel wall, portal venous system, or biliary tree and may require magnetic resonance imaging (MRI).[14]

Laboratory data usually reflect a progressively increasing white blood cell count and electrolyte abnormalities. Dehydration may result in elevated hematocrit, creatinine, and BUN. Other diagnostics include a urinalysis and, if indicated, a lactate dehydrogenase test and liver panel. Serum amylase and lipase may be mildly elevated.[13] Serum β-hCG should be measured to exclude pregnancy in women of childbearing age.

INITIAL DIAGNOSTICS

Small Bowel Obstruction

LABORATORY
- CBC and differential
- Serum glucose, electrolytes, BUN, creatinine
- Liver panel[a]
- Lactate dehydrogenase[a]
- Serum β-hCG (in women of childbearing age)

IMAGING
- Abdominal x-ray studies (upright and supine)[a]
- Chest x-ray studies[a]
- CT scan[a]

ADDITIONAL DIAGNOSTICS
- MRI[a]
- Transabdominal ultrasound[a]

[a]If indicated.

DIFFERENTIAL DIAGNOSIS

The differential diagnosis of small bowel obstruction requires that other abdominal conditions be excluded. Appendicitis, constipation, gastroenteritis, pancreatitis, paralytic ileus, intestinal perforation, ischemic colitis, inflammatory bowel disease, mesenteric thrombosis, and retroperitoneal hemorrhage are all possible differentials that should be considered Addison disease, poisoning, diabetes mellitus, ovarian torsion, and tertiary syphilis (e.g., tabetic crisis) may also mimic small bowel obstruction.[13,14]

 Priority differentials include appendicitis, ileus, mesenteric thrombosis, and retroperitoneal hemorrhage.

INTERPROFESSIONAL COLLABORATIVE MANAGEMENT

Nonpharmacologic Management

Initial management of bowel obstruction includes restriction of all oral intakes, intravenous fluid therapy, electrolyte and acid-base correction, and optimization of cardiopulmonary and renal function. Nasogastric tube for decompression is often necessary.[13]

Pharmacologic Management

Antibiotic therapy is usually not indicated. However, broad-spectrum intravenous antibiotics are indicated in cases of strangulated bowel or as an adjunct to surgery.[13] An antiemetic can be administered for systemic relief.

Indications for Referral and Hospitalization

 Immediate hospitalization and consultation with a surgeon is required for suspected small bowel obstruction.

 Urgent laparotomy is required if the patient does not respond to supportive care or has advanced illness, ischemia, or perforation. Delay in surgical intervention for a strangulated small bowel obstruction can result in more postoperative complications, longer hospital stays, and a higher mortality rate.[13]

COMPLICATIONS

A bowel obstruction may progress to bowel ischemia. Physical and diagnostic signs of ischemic bowel include fever, severe and continuous pain, hematemesis, peritoneal signs, hypotension, gas in the bowel wall or portal vein, abdominal free air, and acidosis.

PERFORATED PEPTIC ULCER

 Immediate hospital referral is indicated for suspected perforated peptic ulcer.

DEFINITION AND EPIDEMIOLOGY

The prevalence of peptic ulcer disease (PUD) in the United States is decreasing, largely because of proton pump inhibitor therapy and treatment of *Helicobacter pylori* infection. However, peptic ulcer perforation still occurs and is a life-threatening complication that occurs more commonly with duodenal ulcers than with gastric ulcers.[15] Perforation may lead to a free perforation into the peritoneal cavity or perforation of an adjacent organ such as the pancreas, with resulting peritonitis or pancreatitis. Factors that predispose a patient to peptic ulcers are *H. pylori* infections, medications (e.g., aspirin, bisphosphonates, nonsteroidal antiinflammatory drugs, potassium chloride), gastric malignancy, tobacco abuse, and hypersecretory states such as Zollinger-Ellison syndrome.

PATHOPHYSIOLOGY

Most often PUD is caused by the repeated use of nonsteroidal antiinflammatory drugs or *H. pylori* infection. *H. pylori* is a gram-negative bacterium that is transmitted via the fecal-oral route in early childhood. The infection lingers for decades into adulthood and causes both peptic and duodenal ulcers. It is also a risk factor for gastric adenocarcinoma and mucosa-associated lymphoid tissue (MALT). The eroded lining of the stomach lining can lead to perforation, and the release of gastric contents into the abdominal cavity causes peritonitis. In addition, the ulcer can perforate to nearby organs such as the liver or pancreas, with resulting elevations in serum liver enzymes, amylase, and lipase.[16]

CLINICAL PRESENTATION AND PHYSICAL EXAMINATION

The most common presentation of a perforated peptic ulcer is the abrupt onset of severe abdominal pain followed rapidly by peritoneal signs. Pain begins in the epigastrium and spreads rapidly throughout the abdomen with frequent early radiation of pain to the scapular areas. Vomiting of coffee-ground emesis, hematemesis, or melena or hematochezia occurs in some patients. The abruptness, severity, and rapid progression of symptoms lead the patient to seek prompt medical attention. Clinically, patients often demonstrate signs of improvement, such as decreased pain and vomiting, 6 to 12 hours after perforation. However, peritoneal signs remain, the clinical improvement does not last long, and the patient can then become obviously ill within several hours.[15]

In some patients, especially older adults, the pain may be absent or slight. The patient may have a history of abdominal discomfort and at presentation usually complains of severe upper abdominal tenderness, especially in the epigastric region.

Physical exam findings include boardlike abdominal rigidity in peptic ulcer perforation. Tachycardia is common, as is orthostasis if vomiting or bleeding occurs. Continued spilling of gastric and intestinal contents into the peritoneum causes chemical peritonitis and subsequent hypovolemia with the development of progressive hypotension and fever.[15]

DIAGNOSTICS

Perforation is suggested by the history and physical examination. The suspected diagnosis is confirmed by the detection of pneumoperitoneum on upright abdominal or chest x-ray films. A left lateral decubitus radiograph usually demonstrates air over the liver. Perforation is also confirmed with upper gastrointestinal contrast with water-soluble contrast medium; extravasation of contrast material is evidence of perforation. When the diagnosis is suspected and the x-ray studies are normal, the diagnosis may be confirmed by endoscopy. Laboratory tests include a CBC with differential; serum electrolyte values; BUN, creatinine, and serum amylase levels; *H. pylori* testing and urea breath test; and stool specimen for occult blood. A serum β-hCG measurement is necessary for women of childbearing age.[17]

INITIAL DIAGNOSTICS

Perforated Peptic Ulcer

LABORATORY
- CBC and differential
- Serum glucose, electrolytes, BUN, creatinine
- Serum amylase
- Stool for occult blood
- *H. pylori*
- Serum β-hCG (in women of childbearing age)

IMAGING
- Abdominal x-ray studies (upright, left lateral decubitus)

ADDITIONAL DIAGNOSTICS
- Endoscopy
- Urea breath test

DIFFERENTIAL DIAGNOSIS

The differential diagnosis of a perforated peptic ulcer includes acute pancreatitis, acute cholecystitis, perforated acute appendicitis, colonic diverticulitis, intestinal obstruction, ruptured ectopic pregnancy, perforated colon, and postemetic esophageal rupture. Myocardial infarction may also mimic a perforated peptic ulcer.[15]

 Priority differentials include perforated acute appendicitis, ruptured ectopic pregnancy, and myocardial infarction.

INTERPROFESSIONAL COLLABORATIVE MANAGEMENT

Nonpharmacologic Management

Management includes intravenous fluid resuscitation, correction of electrolyte abnormalities, and continuous nasogastric suction for decompression.

Pharmacologic Management

Intravenous proton pump inhibitors and broad-spectrum antibiotics are also required. Blood transfusions may be necessary in the presence of hemorrhage.

Indications for Referral and Hospitalization

 Immediate hospitalization and consultation with a gastroenterologist and surgeon are indicated for a patient with suspected perforated ulcer.

Endoscopy is effective in some situations, but surgery may be necessary for patients in whom the bleeding is not controlled and who are hemodynamically unstable, show signs of peritonitis, or have free extravasation of contrast material on upper gastrointestinal studies. Early suspicion, recognition, and endoscopic or surgical repair are the keys to survival and decreased morbidity.[16,17]

COMPLICATIONS

Malabsorption of some vitamin and minerals can occur after a peptic ulcer perforation.[16] Despite the widespread use of H₂ blockers and proton pump inhibitors, the mortality rate of patients with perforated peptic ulcers continues to be significant, especially in older patients.[16]

PATIENT AND FAMILY EDUCATION

- Because older patients may not have as dramatic onset of pain or peritoneal findings as in younger adults, it is necessary to monitor any increase in abdominal pain in older adults.[17]
- Older adults are also at higher risk because of using high-risk medications such as aspirin, nonsteroidal antiinflammatory drugs, warfarin, selective serotonin reuptake inhibitors, and bisphosphonates.
- Long-term tobacco and alcohol use combined with the frailty of aging increases the risk of perforated peptic ulcers.[16]

PERITONITIS

 Immediate hospital referral is indicated for suspected peritonitis.

DEFINITION AND EPIDEMIOLOGY

Spontaneous bacterial peritonitis refers to an ascetic fluid infection in the absence of a clear precipitating factor, such as a perforated viscus. The most common cause of primary spontaneous bacterial peritonitis in adults is cirrhosis complicated by variceal hemorrhage and ascites.[18] Secondary peritonitis refers to spillage of gastrointestinal or genitourinary microorganisms into the peritoneal space and is most often the result of peritoneal dialysis or a perforated viscus (e.g., acute pancreatitis, appendicitis, diverticulitis, cholecystitis, perforated gastric or duodenal ulcer) or penetrating wounds of the bowel.[18] In these instances a secondary infection may occur as either generalized peritonitis or a localized abscess.

PATHOPHYSIOLOGY

Primary peritonitis is thought to result from increased pressure in the portal vein of a cirrhotic liver causing portal hypertension.[19] Fluid accumulates in the perineal cavity of the abdomen, otherwise known as ascites. Portal hypertension causes arteries to dilate, blood pressure to drop, and renal arteries to constrict.[19] Salt and water then accumulate in the body and abdomen. This fluid can migrate through the intestinal walls and cause bacteria to proliferate in the peritoneal fluid, which leads to bacterial peritonitis.[19] An uncommon cause of primary peritonitis is from prolonged proton inhibitor use.[19] Enteric microorganisms account for the majority of pathogens in patients with cirrhosis. *Escherichia coli* is the most commonly identified pathogen, but viridans streptococci, *Staphylococcus aureus*, *Klebsiella*, and enterococci have also been identified.[18]

CLINICAL PRESENTATION AND PHYSICAL EXAMINATION

Many patients have a high fever, chills, and acute abdominal pain that can be diffuse, localized, or referred. Patients with cirrhosis may not complain of pain and may run only a low-grade fever.[19] Additional complaints include diffuse abdominal pain, tenderness, nausea, vomiting, and diarrhea or constipation.

Prominent physical examination findings include abdominal distention, rigidity, decreased bowel sounds, diffuse abdominal tenderness, rebound tenderness, and guarding. Fever, tachycardia, tachypnea, and hypotension may also be present. Rectal examination may reveal tenderness if abscesses occur near this area.

DIAGNOSTICS

The diagnosis of peritonitis should be suspected on the basis of fever, abdominal pain and tenderness, and leukocytosis. Initially, a chest and abdominal x-ray study, CBC and differential, and serum electrolyte values with BUN and creatinine levels may be obtained in the primary care setting. Suspected peritonitis, especially that accompanied by decreasing bowel sounds, increasing tenderness, and rebound tenderness, warrants a laparotomy for confirmation of the diagnosis. Hospitalization and consultation with an internist, gastroenterologist, and surgeon are therefore required.

Patients with cirrhosis and spontaneous bacterial peritonitis should be diagnosed on the basis of the clinical appearance, presence of ascites, and ascitic fluid analysis. Patients with ascites require a paracentesis in the hospital setting with peritoneal fluid analysis for cell count, differential, protein concentration, and Gram stain and culture.[19] The diagnosis of primary bacterial peritonitis requires more than 250 to 500 white blood cells/mm³ in the ascitic fluid, with more than 50% of them being polymorphonuclear neutrophils.[20] The ascitic fluid analysis will typically show a neutrophil count greater than 250/mL, low protein concentration, pH of less than 7.35, and a lactate concentration of more than 25 mg/dL.[20]

INITIAL DIAGNOSTICS

Peritonitis

LABORATORY
- CBC and differential
- Serum glucose, electrolytes
- BUN, creatinine
- Ascitic fluid analysisª
- Serum β-hCG (in women of childbearing age)

IMAGING
- Chest radiograph
- Abdominal radiograph

ADDITIONAL DIAGNOSTICS
- Kidney, ureter, and bladder (KUB)
- CT scan
- Laparotomy or endoscopyª
- Ultrasound-guided aspirationª

ªIf indicated.

DIFFERENTIAL DIAGNOSIS

Diseases that may mimic peritonitis include pancreatitis, appendicitis, diverticulitis, gastroenteritis, salpingitis, ischemic colitis, or other abdominal infection. Pneumonia and secondary causes of peritonitis should also be considered, including perforated duodenal or gastric ulcer, small bowel infarction or perforation, large bowel perforation, and cholecystitis with or without perforation or pericholecystic abscess.

 Priority differentials include appendicitis, pancreatitis, and ischemic colitis.

INTERPROFESSIONAL COLLABORATIVE MANAGEMENT

Nonpharmacologic Management

Fluid resuscitation and careful monitoring of vital signs and fluid balance are critical. A nasogastric tube may be necessary.

Pharmacologic Management

With primary bacterial peritonitis, the peritoneal fluid Gram stain is often negative; therefore antibiotic therapy is usually empirical and is based on the most likely pathogens.[20] Current empirical therapy recommendations for primary bacterial peritonitis include a third- or fourth-generation cephalosporin or a quinolone until culture results are available.[19,20] Antimicrobial therapy should be continued for those patients in whom peritoneal cultures are sterile but there is a strong suspicion of primary bacterial peritonitis.[20] Clinical improvement and a decline in the ascitic fluid leukocyte count (<250/mm³) should occur after 24 to 48 hours of antimicrobial therapy; a failure to respond to therapy should prompt investigation for other pathologic conditions. Patients with secondary bacterial peritonitis may require surgical management and will require metronidazole in addition to ertapenem or another carbapenem.[20] A β-lactam/β-lactamase combination can be substituted for the carbapenem in the treatment of secondary bacterial peritonitis.[20]

Preventive treatment in patients with cirrhotic ascites is recommended to reduce the incidence of spontaneous bacterial peritonitis. Low-dose antibiotics to keep the bacteria concentration decreased should be given after the acute infection is resolved to prevent reinfection.[19] Probiotics can be used to allow beneficial bacteria to proliferate in the gastrointestinal tract. New studies reveal that probiotics decrease the transmission rate of bacteria between the intestinal wall and the peritoneum.[19]

COMPLICATIONS

Primary peritonitis is an ominous sign in the cirrhotic patient. Renal failure, recurrent gastrointestinal bleeding, and liver failure are potential concerns that increase morbidity and mortality. It is crucial that this condition be detected and diagnosed promptly. In addition, those who have bacterial peritonitis are more likely to have future episodes.[19]

PATIENT AND FAMILY EDUCATION

Patients with cirrhosis and their caretakers need to know that obvious symptoms of infection such as fever and abdominal pain may be decreased due to immunosuppression. Subtle signs of peritonitis should be evaluated early since it is associated with decreased chances of survival.

RUPTURED AORTIC ANEURYSM

 Immediate hospital and surgical referral is indicated for a ruptured aortic aneurysm.

DEFINITION AND EPIDEMIOLOGY

An AAA is an abnormal, progressive dilatation of the abdominal aorta that may rupture and cause exsanguination into the peritoneum.[1] Most aneurysms are asymptomatic until they rupture. When they do rupture, the mortality rate is as high as 85% to 90%.[21] Fortunately, screening and risk management recommendations have decreased the prevalence of this potentially fatal disorder.

Risk factors for AAA include male gender, a positive family history, advanced age, white race, smoking, hypertension, and atherosclerosis.[21]

PATHOPHYSIOLOGY

It used to be believed that aneurysms were secondary to atherosclerosis; however, it is widely accepted as a degenerative process of all vessel wall layers.[21] Four steps lead to the development of aortic aneurysms. The first is lymphocyte and macrophage invasion of the aorta wall. Next, elastic tissues and collagen in the media and adventitia are destroyed.[22] Third, smooth-muscle cells are depleted and the media wall thins. Neovascularization, or the formation of microvascular networks within the aneurysm wall, is the final step.[21] The resulting rupture typically causes significant hemorrhage and profound hemodynamic instability.

CLINICAL PRESENTATION AND PHYSICAL EXAMINATION

Although AAA is a leading cause of sudden death, patients may be asymptomatic before rupture. In some cases, rupture may be preceded by abdominal, flank, or back pain. Patients with a contained rupture can be seen several days after the rupture with abdominal, flank, or back pain.[21,22] In many cases, rupture of an AAA is accompanied by the sudden onset of severe abdominal pain that may be confined to the flank, low back, or groin with radiation to the back that brings the patients in urgently. Faintness and syncope may occur as a result of blood loss and gradually worsen until shock finally supervenes.[21,22]

Abdominal examination findings might include abdominal distention and abdominal, flank, or back pain and tenderness.[21,22] Also associated with AAAs are pulsations that are felt directly over the mass and displace the examining fingers laterally. An aortic bruit may be present. During dissection, a pulsatile, painful mass can be palpated in the abdomen between the xiphoid process and the umbilicus. Peripheral pulses may be unequal or absent but can be normal. Profound shock may rapidly ensue as a result of intraperitoneal leakage of blood and hypotension.

DIAGNOSTICS

Screening for AAA is recommended for men ages 65 to 75 with a positive history of smoking (at least 100 cigarettes smoked over a lifetime). The 2015 United States Preventative Services Task Force determined that the evidence evaluating the risk and benefit of screening women age 65 to 75 who had ever smoked was inconclusive to recommend AAA screening. The 2005 guideline also did not recommend screening for aortic aneurysm in women.[22] Additional diagnostic tests are not required if a ruptured AAA is suspected. The patient should be hospitalized immediately, with resuscitation and therapy in the operating room. If the diagnosis of rupture is in doubt and time allows, a **CT scan** is the standard for evaluation of an AAA because it can determine the extent of the aneurysmal process. **Angiography** is used preoperatively in elective repairs to demonstrate aortic and vascular anatomy and renal vessel involvement. An ultrasound examination can be a helpful screening tool in the early stages of the disease process or in the questionable emergency department patient. Abdominal plain x-ray films may show a soft tissue mass in the region of the abdominal aorta. A chest radiograph should also be obtained to evaluate the thoracic aorta. Laboratory tests should include a CBC, type and crossmatch, electrolytes, and renal function tests.[21,22]

INITIAL DIAGNOSTICS

Ruptured Aortic Aneurysm

LABORATORY
- CBC and differential
- Serum glucose, electrolytes
- BUN
- Creatinine
- Serum β-hCG (in women of childbearing age)
- Type and crossmatch

IMAGING
- Chest x-ray studies
- CT scan or MRI

- Transthoracic echocardiography
- Angiography
- Ultrasound
- Abdominal x-ray studies

ADDITIONAL DIAGNOSTICS
- Electrocardiography

DIFFERENTIAL DIAGNOSIS

 Priority differentials include myocardial infarction.

The most common misdiagnosis of ruptured AAA is myocardial infarction. Other diseases or conditions that may mimic AAA include a perforated peptic ulcer, diverticulitis, appendicitis, peritonitis, acute pancreatitis, pyelonephritis, renal colic, renal infarct, and mesenteric ischemia. Consideration of a ruptured AAA is essential in the differential diagnosis for all these disorders.

INTERPROFESSIONAL COLLABORATIVE MANAGEMENT
Indications for Referral and Hospitalization

 Immediate emergency room evaluation is necessary for a patient with suspected ruptured AAA.

A ruptured AAA is a surgical emergency with high mortality rates. The patient should be sent from the office via ambulance to the emergency room for prompt evaluation. Sometimes the triad of hypotension, shooting back or abdominal pain, and a pulsatile abdominal mass are absent. Misdiagnosis can occur in nearly 60% of cases.[22] A patient with abdominal pain and shock should have an immediate surgical consultation to determine whether the patient should be taken emergently to surgery. When a rupture is strongly suspected, resuscitation procedures should happen as testing is being done. After rupture confirmation with imaging, the decision should be made to take the patient directly to the operating room because emergency surgery is the only chance the patient has for survival. The surgeon can do either endovascular or open repair.[21,22]

COMPLICATIONS
Postoperative complications of ruptured AAA repair include colon infarction, sepsis, congestive heart failure, myocardial infarction, arrhythmias, liver dysfunction, renal failure, respiratory failure, pneumonia, and lower extremity ischemia.[21,22]

REFERENCES

1. Jacobs, D. O., & Silen, W. (2015). Abdominal pain. In D. Kasper, A. Fauci, S. Hauser, D. Longo, J. Jameson, & J. Loscalzo (Eds.), *Harrison's principles of internal medicine* (19th ed.). New York, NY: McGraw-Hill.
2. Tursi, A., et al. (2015). Moderate to severe and prolonged left lower-abdominal pain is the best symptom characterizing symptomatic uncomplicated diverticular disease of the colon: A comparison with fecal calprotectin in clinical setting. *Journal of Clinical Gastroenterology, 49*(3), 218–221.
3. Chih-Hao, L., Chien-Hsin, L., & Ying-Hsin, C. (2017). Elderly woman with fever and abdominal discomfort. *Annals of Emergency Medicine, 70*(1), 18–40.
4. Knight, C., & Dening, K. H. (2017). Management of long-term conditions and dementia: The role of the admiral nurse. *British Journal of Community Nursing, 22*(6), 295–302.
5. O'Brien, M. C., et al. (2016). Acute abdominal pain. In J. E. Tintinalli, J. Stapczynski, O. Ma, D. M. Yealy, G. D. Meckler, D. M. Cline, et al. (Eds.), *Tintinalli's emergency medicine: A comprehensive study guide* (8th ed.). New York, NY: McGraw-Hill.
6. Glass, C. A., & Malone, A. (2017). Abdominal pain. In J. C. Cash & C. A. Glass (Eds.), *Family practice guidelines*. New York: Springer Publishing Company.
7. Flum, D. R. (2015). Acute appendicitis—appendectomy or the "antibiotics first" strategy. *The New England Journal of Medicine, 372*, 1937–1943.
8. D'Souza, N., & Nugent, K. (2016). Appendicitis. *American Family Physician, 93*(2), 142–143.
9. Elniel, M., Grainger, J., Nevins, E. J., Misra, N., & Skaife, P. (2018). 72 h is the time critical point to operate in acute appendicitis. *Journal of Gastrointestinal Surgery: Official Journal of the Society for Surgery of the Alimentary Tract, 22*(2), 310–315.
10. Salminen, P., Paajanen, H., Rautio, T., et al. (2015). Antibiotic therapy vs appendectomy for treatment of uncomplicated acute appendicitis: The APPAC Randomized Clinical Trial. *JAMA: The Journal of the American Medical Association, 313*(23), 2340–2348.
11. Luo, C.-C., Cheng, K.-F., Huang, C.-S., Lo, H.-C., We, S.-M., Huang, H.-C., et al. (2016). Therapeutic effectiveness of percutaneous drainage and factors for performing an interaval appendectomy in pediatric appendiceal abscess. *BMC Surgery, 16*, 72.
12. Ozturk, A., Korkmaz, M., Ataly, T., Karakose, Y., Akinci, O. F., Bozer, M., et al. (2017). The role of doctors and patients in appendicitis perforation. *The American Surgeon, 83*(4), 390–393.
13. Price, T. G., Orthober, R. J., et al. (2016). Bowel obstruction. In J. E. Tintinalli, J. Stapczynski, O. Ma, D. M. Cline, R. K. Cudulka, & G. D. Meckler (Eds.), *Tintinalli's emergency medicine: A comprehensive study guide* (8th ed.). New York, NY: McGraw-Hill.
14. O'Malley, R. G., Al-Hawary, M. M., Kaza, R. K., Wasnik, A. P., Platt, J. F., & Francis, I. R. (2015). MDCT findings in small bowel obstruction: Implications of the cause and presence of complications on treatment decisions. *Abdominal Imaging, 40*, 2248–2262.
15. Del Valle, J. (2015). Peptic ulcer disease and related disorders. In D. Kasper, A. Fauci, S. Hauser, D. Longo, J. Jameson, & J. Loscalzo (Eds.), *Harrison's principles of internal medicine* (19th ed.). New York: McGraw-Hill.
16. Fashner, J., & Gitu, A. C. (2015). Diagnosis and treatment of peptic ulcer disease and H. pylori infection. *American Family Physician, 91*(4), 236–242.
17. Gratton, M. C., Boyle, A., et al. (2016). Peptic ulcer disease and gastritis. In J. E. Tintinalli, J. Stapczynski, O. Ma, D. M. Cline, R. K. Cudulka, & G. D. Meckler (Eds.), *Tintinalli's emergency medicine: A comprehensive study guide* (8th ed.). New York, NY: McGraw-Hill.
18. Bacon, B. R. (2015). Cirrhosis and its complications. In D. Kasper, A. Fauci, S. Hauser, D. Longo, J. Jameson, & J. Loscalzo (Eds.), *Harrison's principles of internal medicine* (19th ed.). New York: McGraw-Hill.
19. Kowdley, K. (2015). Spontaneous bacterial peritonitis. *Gastroenterologia Y Hepatologia, 11*(1), 70–73.
20. Greco, E. F., & Bohnen, J. A. (2015). The acute abdomen and intra-abdominal sepsis. In J. B. Hall, G. A. Schmidt, & J. P. Kress (Eds.), *Principles of critical care* (4th ed.). New York: McGraw-Hill.
21. Kent, K. C. (2014). Abdominal aortic aneurysms. *The New England Journal of Medicine, 371*, 2101–2108.
22. Keisler, K., & Carter, C. (2015). Abdominal aortic aneurysm. *American Family Physician, 91*(8), 538–543.

CHAPTER **110**

ANORECTAL COMPLAINTS

Priscilla Marsicovetere

Anorectal complaints stem from a variety of disorders of structure and/or function, including hemorrhoids, anal fissure, pruritus ani, and anorectal abscess and fistula. In these conditions, symptoms can range from pain and bleeding to tissue prolapse and skin irritation. Similar anorectal symptoms can be seen with other disorders, such as polyps, condyloma, malignant neoplasms, and dermatologic disorders. Most of these conditions are not life-threatening and can be treated in an outpatient setting. The correct diagnosis and treatment require a detailed patient history and thorough physical examination. The history should elicit information on at least location and duration of pain, stool consistency, constitutional symptoms, family history of colorectal issues, sexual history, abdominal pain, and current medications. Dietary history must be included because inadequate fiber intake, suboptimal fluid intake, and foods known to alter bowel habits may be revealed as contributory to benign anorectal symptoms.[1]

HEMORRHOIDS

 Urgent surgical intervention is indicated for incarcerated fourth-degree hemorrhoids.

DEFINITION AND EPIDEMIOLOGY

Hemorrhoids are nonpathologic venous cushions in the submucosal layer of the anal canal. They are suspended by the connective tissue of the internal anal sphincter. They are a normal part of human anatomy and help maintain anal closure and continence. Three main cushions are typically present in the left lateral, right posterior, and right anterior portions of the anal canal. Hemorrhoids are classified based on their location—external hemorrhoids lie below the dentate line and are covered by squamous epithelium, while internal hemorrhoids are located above the dentate line and are covered by columnar epithelium.[2] Although hemorrhoids are normal anatomic structures, they are infrequently referred to until symptoms arise. Symptomatic hemorrhoidal disease will develop in up to 75% of the population at some point in their lifetime,[2] with a peak incidence between the ages of 45 and 65 years.[3] Development of hemorrhoids before the age of 20 is rare.[4-6]

PATHOPHYSIOLOGY

The exact cause of hemorrhoids is not well understood but is thought to be multifactorial. Weakening of the anatomic structures that support hemorrhoidal cushions can occur as a person ages. Additional risk factors include pregnancy, straining, lifting, prolonged standing, and prolonged straining with bowel movements, all of which lead to increased intra-abdominal pressure. The increased pressure, over time, can lead to vascular engorgement with the overlying mucosa becoming thin and friable. Trauma to the underlying vessels—as can occur with a hard bowel movement—then leads to painless bright red blood per rectum. Symptoms can progress to

include prolapse of the hemorrhoidal tissue if the underlying cause is not corrected. Although the prolapse may reduce spontaneously initially, over time it can result in persistent leakage of mucus, blood, or fecal matter from the anus. Low-fiber diets, toileting habits (spending prolonged periods on the commode, with straining), and genetics are also thought to be possible contributing factors.[1]

CLINICAL PRESENTATION AND PHYSICAL EXAMINATION

The most common presenting symptom of hemorrhoids depends on the location of the hemorrhoid: external or internal. External hemorrhoids are located distal to the dentate line in tissue that is highly innervated by somatic nerves, and therefore sensitive to touch, temperature, and stretch. Internal hemorrhoids, however, are located proximal to the dentate line and have no somatic sensory nerves and are therefore usually painless.

External hemorrhoids are typically asymptomatic unless thrombosis develops. When this occurs, the patient will complain of an acutely painful perianal lump. The patient may also report anal irritation and pruritus. Symptoms of a thrombosed external hemorrhoid can also include edema.[7] Pain from a thrombosed external hemorrhoid will typically be severe in the first couple of days and then will gradually subside thereafter.

Internal hemorrhoids typically present with painless bright red blood per rectum with bowel movements, occasionally with intermittent, reducible prolapse. The blood may be seen on the toilet paper, in the toilet water, or coating the stool. Blood mixed within the stool or dark-colored blood often indicates more proximal disease, whereas bright red blood on the outside of the stool is more suggestive of anorectal pathology.

Internal hemorrhoids can be divided into four categories classified by the degree of prolapse. First-degree hemorrhoids cause bright red, painless bleeding and may bulge but do not prolapse through the anal orifice. Second-degree hemorrhoids prolapse during defecation but reduce spontaneously. Patients with second-degree hemorrhoids report bleeding and perineal itching from chronic moisture secreted by the anal canal mucosa. Third-degree hemorrhoids prolapse with defecation and require manual reduction. Patients with third-degree hemorrhoids have pain secondary to local ischemia and mucoid drainage.[8] Fourth-degree hemorrhoids are permanently prolapsed and are not reducible. It is important to note that the degree of prolapse does not imply incarceration, nor dictate the need for intervention. Hemorrhoidal symptomology and effect on quality of life should guide therapy.[1,7] However, incarcerated fourth-degree hemorrhoids require urgent surgical intervention.[8]

The physical examination requires that the entire perineum and perianal area be inspected with the patient in a comfortable position (prone jackknife, lithotomy, or left lateral position) while the patient is both at rest and straining.[7] Gentle spreading of the buttocks will reveal any abnormalities of the perianal skin, as well as any protrusion of tissue at the anal outlet. With Valsalva, prolapse may be reproduced. External hemorrhoids can be visualized around the anal orifice as the patient bears down. Digital rectal exam allows for palpation of any abnormal lesions within the anal canal. An internal hemorrhoid is not palpable on rectal examination unless it is thrombosed. Anoscopy allows direct visualization of the anus and lower rectum, with full view of the internal hemorrhoids.

With the anoscope fully inserted into the rectum, Valsalva will allow visualization of bulging and prolapsing internal hemorrhoids. It will also permit examination of the anus and lower rectum for other sources of bleeding.

Severe rectal pain is unusual but if present suggests a gangrenous or thrombosed hemorrhoid. Gangrenous hemorrhoids are fourth-degree internal hemorrhoids and require immediate surgical evaluation.

DIAGNOSTICS

The diagnosis of hemorrhoids is almost always a clinical one. Laboratory testing is generally not helpful, but if the history reveals heavy, prolonged bleeding, a complete blood count (CBC) should be obtained to assess for anemia. Anoscopy plays a critical role in diagnosing hemorrhoids, as it allows for direct visualization of the entire anus and distal rectum, where hemorrhoids are anatomically located. If no bleeding source is found during anoscopy, examination with rigid proctoscopy, flexible sigmoidoscopy, or colonoscopy can be performed to assess more proximal segments of the rectum and colon. If the patient is older than age 50 or has a family history of colorectal cancer, the entire colon should be visualized via colonoscopy.[7] A thrombosed external hemorrhoid can be identified on physical examination as a tender blu-ish lump at the anal outlet, and no additional workup is required.

INITIAL DIAGNOSTICS

Hemorrhoids

- Digital rectal exam
- Anoscopy

LABORATORY
- Complete blood count with differential
- Serial fecal occult blood testing

ENDOSCOPIC EVALUATION
- Rigid proctoscopy
- Flexible sigmoidoscopy
- Colonoscopy

DIFFERENTIAL DIAGNOSIS

The differential diagnosis includes other anorectal conditions that can cause bleeding, pain, or protrusion. The primary conditions that should be considered when evaluating a patient for hemorrhoids are anal cancer, colorectal cancer, and rectal prolapse. Other possible etiologies include perianal skin tags, hypertrophied anal papillae, anal or rectal polyps, anal fissure, anorectal abscess, anal papillitis, proctitis, inflammatory bowel disease, and condyloma or other sexually transmitted infection.

 Red flag symptoms include increased age, family or personal history of colorectal cancer, persistent anorectal bleeding despite treatment, weight loss, or iron deficiency anemia. These symptoms should prompt more extensive evaluation to rule out anal malignancy, colorectal malignancy, intraepithelial neoplasia, and inflammatory bowel disease.

INTERPROFESSIONAL COLLABORATIVE MANAGEMENT

Guidelines for the treatment of benign anorectal disorders such as hemorrhoids were published by the American College of Gastroenterology in 2014.[7] The treatment of hemorrhoids is usually based on the degree of the patient's symptoms and may

be categorized as medical management, in-office procedures, and surgical intervention.[1] Most hemorrhoids are managed conservatively, and some patients require little or no treatment.

Nonpharmacologic Management

A high-fiber diet and increased fluid intake are recommended for the treatment of symptomatic hemorrhoids.[7] Fiber (20 to 30 g/day) is a bulking agent that absorbs water and helps soften the stool, thus preventing constipation and straining. According to a Cochrane review, fiber is an effective treatment for symptomatic hemorrhoids, with reduction in hemorrhoidal prolapse and bleeding.[9]

If a thrombosed external hemorrhoid is identified within 3 days of onset, it can be evacuated by first infiltrating a local anesthetic into the base of the hemorrhoid. An elliptical excision is then made into the thrombus, and the clot is expressed. Relief is immediate. This procedure can usually be carried out in the clinic setting by an experienced health care provider but is not indicated in children or in patients who have bleeding disorders, are immunocompromised, or are pregnant. Post-procedure care includes a gauze pad applied to the site for 12 hours, followed by a sitz bath to remove the bandage and cleanse the area. Continued daily sitz baths and a minipad to protect clothing are recommended for several more days. If a thrombosed external hemorrhoid has been present for more than 3 days or is not very painful, no excision is required and conservative measures, including mild analgesics, sitz baths, and topical anesthetic ointments, can be used.[5,7,8]

Patients with hemorrhoid symptoms should be counseled about modification of bathroom habits to decrease the risk of symptom recurrence or progression. These include avoiding prolonged sitting on the commode and straining with bowel movements. Restrict sitting on the commode to no more than 2 minutes and consider use of a foot stool under the feet to mimic the squatting position.[10]

Pharmacologic Management

Stool softeners are sometimes used in addition to fiber therapy to keep stools soft. Laxatives have a limited role in the initial management of hemorrhoids, because the variability in stool consistency associated with chronic laxative use makes hemorrhoid management more difficult.[1] Topical analgesics or hydrocortisone creams and suppositories or foams (Table 110.1) and over-the-counter oral analgesics can help reduce inflammation and promote patient comfort.

Researchers continue to investigate newer anesthetic, analgesic, antiinflammatory, and vasoconstrictive preparations to relieve the discomfort associated with hemorrhoids. In a small study, Rectogesic (glyceryl trinitrate 0.2%) ointment relieved pain, high anal canal resting pressures, and rectal bleeding.[11] Phlebotonics, most often composed of natural plant compounds, have proven effective in the management of first- and second-degree hemorrhoids by decreasing vascular endothelial inflammation and normalizing capillary permeability.[12]

Indications for Referral and Hospitalization

Patients with first- to third-degree hemorrhoids that remain symptomatic after dietary and lifestyle modification should be referred for in-office procedures such as rubber band ligation, sclerotherapy, and infrared coagulation. The most common in-office procedure is rubber band ligation, in which a small set of rubber bands is placed at the base of enlarged hemorrhoidal

TABLE 110.1 **Topical Anorectal Antiinflammatory Preparations**

Preparation	Actions	How Supplied	Usual Dosage and Administration
ProctoCream-HC 2.5% (hydrocortisone acetate)	Antiinflammatory and antipruritic	Cream	Apply to affected area 2–4 times per day, depending on severity of condition.
Anusol-HC 2.5% (hydrocortisone)	Antiinflammatory and antipruritic	Cream	Apply to affected area 2–4 times per day, depending on severity of condition.
Analpram-HC 1% and 2.5% (hydrocortisone acetate and pramoxine)	Antiinflammatory and antipruritic, topical anesthetic	Cream	Apply to affected area 2–4 times per day, depending on severity of condition.
Anusol-HC suppositories (hydrocortisone acetate)	Antiinflammatory and antipruritic	Suppositories	Place 1 suppository in rectum in morning and 1 at night for 2 weeks.
ProctoFoam-HC (hydrocortisone acetate and pramoxine)	Antiinflammatory and antipruritic, topical anesthetic	Aerosol container and anal applicator	Apply to affected area nightly for 2 weeks; may be used up to 3–4 times a day.

Topical anal preparations containing hydrocortisone should not be used continuously for more than 2 weeks to avoid skin atrophy.

tissue. The banded tissue infarcts and sloughs off in 7 to 10 days, resulting in reduction of the enlarged tissue and fixation of the residual hemorrhoidal tissue in the upper anal canal.[13] This is a relatively painless procedure, as long as the bands are properly placed above the dentate line.

For more symptomatic hemorrhoids, or those that fail to respond to nonoperative management, referral for operative management is indicated. Only 5% to 10% of patients, typically those with third- or fourth-degree hemorrhoids, go on to require surgery.[13] Surgical options include excisional hemorrhoidectomy, stapled hemorrhoidopexy, and Doppler-assisted hemorrhoidal artery ligation.[7] Excisional hemorrhoidectomy is the most effective treatment for hemorrhoids.

LIFE SPAN CONSIDERATIONS

Symptomatic hemorrhoids are a common disease entity. Although they can occur at any age in both sexes, they are more common in adults between 45 and 65 years of age. The prevalence in the United States has been estimated to be as high as 75% of adults older than 50 years.[14]

COMPLICATIONS

Fourth-degree hemorrhoids are at risk for strangulation because they are irreducible. Strangulated hemorrhoids can become gangrenous, requiring immediate surgical intervention.[8]

Rubber band ligation is now a common treatment, occasionally associated with vasovagal response, pain and, very rarely, infection or sepsis. Urinary retention and fever onset immediately after rubber band ligation may be the initial sign of perianal sepsis, and mandates emergent patient evaluation. Hemorrhoidectomy has been associated with bleeding, urinary tract infections, urinary retention, anal stenosis, and, rarely, infection. Stapled hemorrhoidectomy has been associated with a higher recurrence of hemorrhoids and prolapse.[7,15] However, compared to excisional hemorrhoidectomy, the stapled surgery affects fewer nerve endings, which results in less postoperative pain.[16]

PATIENT AND FAMILY EDUCATION

• Patients should be instructed in how to increase dietary fiber and in the correct use of topical antiinflammatory agents—namely, that topical corticosteroids should be used judiciously to avoid thinning of the perianal skin with risk for maceration secondary to excess wiping.

• Preventive measures, including increasing fluid intake, keeping the stool soft, avoiding prolonged periods on the commode and straining during bowel movements, exercising regularly to help promote regular bowel movements, and keeping the anal area clean and dry, are important education reminders for patients.

• The importance of follow-up care, particularly if symptoms do not resolve with conservative measures, should be stressed.

ANAL FISSURE

DEFINITION AND EPIDEMIOLOGY

Anal fissures, painful linear cracks or tears in the lining of the anal canal distal to the dentate line, are a frequent cause of rectal bleeding and are common in children and middle-aged adults. In 90% of cases, the fissure occurs in the posterior midline of the anal canal; other locations (e.g., lateral positions, or in the anterior midline) within the canal are considered atypical. A fissure present for less than 6 weeks is considered acute, whereas a fissure present for longer than 6 weeks is designated chronic. An acute fissure looks like a superficial, longitudinal tear in the distal anoderm. A chronic fissure, on the other hand, is characterized by edema and fibrosis, with fibrous induration of the sides and visible fibers of the internal anal sphincter at the base. A chronic fissure will often be accompanied by a tender sentinel skin tag at the distal margin, and a hypertrophied anal papilla at the proximal margin.

PATHOPHYSIOLOGY

Most anal fissures are caused by trauma to the anal canal from passage of a large, hard stool. Pathophysiology is associated with high resting sphincter tone coupled with relative ischemia in the posterior midline of the internal anal sphinter.[17] The diminished blood flow is thought to predispose the mucosa to ischemia and tearing during bowel movements.[2] Other causes include frequent diarrhea, which can result in a chemical burn from severe alkalinity, and anal stenosis, which may predispose the patient to fissure formation. An acute fissure often resolves without intervention. However, a chronic ulcer surrounded by scar tissue may develop if the underlying sphincter goes into involuntary spasm, thereby worsening the diminished blood flow to the area.

Most anal fissures occur in the posterior midline. A fissure located in an atypical (e.g., off-posterior midline) position usually indicates a sexually transmitted disease, tuberculosis, human immunodeficiency virus (HIV) infection, ulcerative colitis, Crohn disease, malignant neoplasm, or other underlying disorder and necessitates referral to a subspecialist.[17,18]

CLINICAL PRESENTATION AND PHYSICAL EXAMINATION

Classic symptoms of an anal fissure are severe, sharp rectal pain during and after bowel movements and small amounts of bright red blood seen on the toilet paper. The patient may report a history of a tearing sensation while passing firm stool or diarrhea. Some patients avoid having a bowel movement because of the pain and thus produce even harder stools, which exacerbates the problem.[18]

The physical examination should be done gently and with reassurance because of the severe pain associated with an anal fissure. The patient should be properly positioned and a topical anesthetic applied to enable adequate visualization of the anus. The fissure is most easily visualized by gently spreading the buttocks to expose the area. An acute anal fissure appears to be a laceration, whereas a chronic anal fissure will have an indurated, fibrotic appearance and a tender sentinel skin tag.[2,17] If the fissure is touched with a cotton-tipped applicator, the symptoms will often be reproduced, helping to confirm the diagnosis. If the fissure is extremely painful, digital rectal and anoscopic examination should be deferred.

INITIAL DIAGNOSTICS

Anal Fissure

- Visual inspection

ADDITIONAL DIAGNOSTICS
- Digital rectal exam
- Anoscopy

DIFFERENTIAL DIAGNOSIS

The three primary conditions that should be considered when evaluating a patient for fissure are anal carcinoma, perianal abscess, and thrombosed external hemorrhoid.

Red flag symptoms include a personal history of anal carcinoma, persistent anorectal pain and bleeding despite treatment, bloody diarrhea, and weight loss. These symptoms should prompt more extensive evaluation to rule out anal malignancy, colorectal malignancy, intraepithelial neoplasia, and inflammatory bowel disease. Other differential diagnoses to be considered include anorectal conditions that can cause pain and bleeding. Chronic anal fissures are often misdiagnosed as hemorrhoids because of the presence of a sentinel tag. Other possible etiologies include inflammatory bowel disease, leukemia, lymphoma, tuberculosis, syphilis, and other sexually transmitted infections.

INTERPROFESSIONAL COLLABORATIVE MANAGEMENT
Nonpharmacologic Management

Most acute fissures, and over half of chronic fissures, will resolve without medical treatment.[2,7,16] The primary goals of management are to bulk and soften the stool and minimize constipation, and to relax the muscles of the anal canal. The American College of Gastroenterology recommends supportive measures such as increased fiber, stool softeners, and sitz baths as first-line treatment.[7]

Pharmacologic Management

Suppositories or foam-containing antiinflammatory agents may also be used to treat fissures (see Table 110.1). Topical anesthetic gel (lidocaine [Xylocaine] 2% jelly) applied before bowel movements can be helpful in reducing pain and spasm. Chronic anal fissures may be treated with topical nitrates or topical or oral calcium channel blockers.[7] Topical nitroglycerine ointment 0.2% administered two to three times a day for 6 to 8 weeks is efficacious. However, the rate of concomitant headache with nitroglycerine use occurs in up to 70% of patients, which often affects compliance with usage.[2] Topical 2% diltiazem applied twice daily for 6 to 8 weeks has proven effective in the healing of chronic anal fissures without the vasodilatory side effects associated with nitroglycerine.[19]

Indications for Referral and Hospitalization

Patients with chronic or recurrent anal fissures that fail to respond to conservative treatment strategies should be referred for local botulism toxin injection into the sphincters, which relaxes the muscle, breaks the spasm, and thereby allows for fissure healing. The gold standard treatment of chronic anal fissure, however, is lateral internal sphincterotomy (LIS), which reduces internal sphincter tone, allowing the fissure to heal.[20] LIS is recommended for patients in whom botulism toxin injections fail.[7]

LIFE SPAN CONSIDERATIONS

While there is very little population-based data on the incidence of anal fissures, they are commonly seen in young and middle-aged adults but can occur at any age. Both sexes seem to be equally affected. Although they are common, the exact incidence of this disease is unknown,[21] but a 2014 retrospective analysis of 1243 anal fissure patients found the average lifetime risk to be approximately 7.8%.[22]

COMPLICATIONS

Surgical procedures for anal fissure may be accompanied by significant postoperative complications, such as pain, bleeding, and recurrence. Complications of LIS also include poor wound healing and incontinence (typically only to flatus, but occasionally also to feces), though rare.[21] Botulinum toxin has a lower risk of incontinence than LIS, but a higher rate of fissure recurrence.[23]

PATIENT AND FAMILY EDUCATION

- Patients should be informed that healing can take up to 6 weeks with conservative measures.
- If topical nitrates or calcium channel blockers are prescribed, patients should understand how to use these preparations and be able to recognize associated side effects.
- Prevention includes keeping the stools soft with fiber powder, a high-fiber diet, adequate fluid intake, and avoiding straining during bowel movements.

PRURITUS ANI

 Red flag symptoms include weight loss or refractory symptoms, which should prompt more extensive evaluation to rule out malignancy, intraepithelial neoplasia, and dermatopathologic diseases such as Paget or Bowen disease.

DEFINITION AND EPIDEMIOLOGY

Pruritus ani, or itching of the anus and perianal skin, is a fairly common condition affecting up to 5% of the population.[17] It is the second most common anorectal condition after hemorrhoids. Although the true prevalence of this disorder is unknown, there is an increased prevalence in age 30 to 50, and men are affected four times more often than women.[14,21,24]

PATHOPHYSIOLOGY

There are greater than 100 different causes of pruritus ani.[2] Up to 90% of cases, however, are idiopathic and are classified as primary pruritus.[21] Secondary causes can be related to cancer, dermatologic conditions, anal disorders, hyperhidrosis, infections or infestations (e.g., scabies, pediculosis, fungus, or pinworms), medications, malignant neoplasms, and common systemic illnesses (e.g., renal insufficiency, liver disease, or diabetes). Pruritus ani may also be related to improper hygiene or to the ingestion of certain foods or beverages that may affect the function of the internal anal sphincter. Pathophysiologically, symptoms develop as a result of local irritation. An inflammatory response thereafter ensues, leading to histamine-induced itching. A self-propagating itch-scratch cycle results, with scratching exacerbating the inflammation, causing an irresistible urge to scratch even more. Chronic pathologic changes can result in the perianal area becoming lichenified, appearing whitened with fine fissuring of the skin.[17]

CLINICAL PRESENTATION AND PHYSICAL EXAMINATION

The patient often reports an uncontrollable urge to scratch the anus. The symptoms tend to be worse at night or after a bowel movement. Sometimes the itching will involve the perianal area, buttocks, and vulva or scrotum. Scratching provides only transient relief and can exacerbate the itch-scratch cycle.[2]

Diagnosis is made by a careful history and physical examination. If the pruritus is chronic, the perianal skin may appear moist, excoriated, and macerated. A digital rectal examination is indicated to assess for any mass or lesion. Anoscopy should be performed to assess for anorectal, infectious, or dermatologic disease.

DIAGNOSTICS

The diagnosis of pruritus ani is primarily a clinical one, made by history and physical examination. History should seek to uncover potentially reversible causes, including dietary and lifestyle contributors. The ITCH acronym has been used to help identify potential causes: I-infection, T-topical irritants, C-cutaneous and cancer, H-hypersensitivity.[2] Some cases of pruritus ani are related to an infectious process (e.g., β-hemolytic streptococci, *Staphylococcus aureus*, and *Corynebacterium minutissimum*).[21] Thus, cultures may be useful. If the pruritus is primarily nocturnal, cellophane tape can be applied to the perianal skin in the early morning. The tape is then placed on a glass slide and examined under a microscope for pinworm eggs. Suspected sexually transmitted disease requires the appropriate workup to exclude chlamydia, gonorrhea, syphilis, and other diseases. For refractory symptoms, a perianal skin biopsy may be warranted to exclude malignancy or other dermatopathology.

INITIAL DIAGNOSTICS

Pruritus Ani

- Visual inspection
- Digital rectal exam
- Anoscopy

ADDITIONAL DIAGNOSTICS

- Cultures
- Microscopic examination for pinworm eggs
- Biopsy of perianal skin for refractory symptoms

DIFFERENTIAL DIAGNOSIS

Anorectal disorders, diarrhea, and constipation are common causes of pruritus ani.[21] The ITCH acronym is helpful in the initial evaluation and exploration of differential diagnoses associated with pruritus ani:

Infections—Infections such as Candida albicans, herpes, HIV, pinworms, and other bacterial infections should be considered.

Topical irritants—Soaps, detergents, and restrictive clothing are all topical irritants that should be considered.

Cutaneous causes—Cutaneous causes such as cancer should be considered.

Hypersensitivities—Hypersensitivities to foods and medication should be determined.[2]

INTERPROFESSIONAL COLLABORATIVE MANAGEMENT

Nonpharmacologic Management

Once pathologic causes of pruritus ani have been excluded, patient education should be aimed at perianal hygiene and breaking the itch-scratch cycle that leads to the chronicity of the condition.[2]

A psyllium product can be used to bulk the stool to prevent fecal soilage if loose stools are a problem. Medications and foods that cause loose stools should be avoided if at all possible. The anal area should be kept clean and dry, and overly vigorous wiping or scratching should be avoided. According to Markell and Billingham, a hair dryer on the cool setting can help dry the anal area more thoroughly.[21] Perfumed toilet paper, soaps, and hygiene products should not be used, but cornstarch applied sparingly can be helpful.[21] Tight-fitting clothing should also be avoided, and constipation prevented.[21]

Pharmacologic Management

Any identified infectious or dermatologic disease should be treated. A 1% hydrocortisone cream can be used initially, but should be discontinued after 2 weeks to avoid skin atrophy.[21] If severe nocturnal itching is a problem, an antihistamine with antipruritic properties, such as hydroxyzine (Atarax), can help the patient sleep and assist in breaking the itch-scratch cycle.[21] Relief of symptoms usually occurs in 4 to 6 weeks. Witch hazel has also been used as an anti-pruritic. Barrier creams containing zinc oxide help protect the skin from moisture while promoting healing. For patients who do not respond to these therapies, intradermal methylene blue injections have relieved the disorder for some patients.[21]

Indications for Referral and Hospitalization

Patients with persistent symptoms after 2 weeks of appropriate therapy should be referred to dermatology for further evaluation.[2] Suspicious lesions require biopsy, and any signs or symptoms suggesting pathology of the bowel require colonoscopy to exclude malignant disease. If medical treatment has failed, referral to a gastroenterologist or colorectal specialist is indicated.

LIFE SPAN CONSIDERATIONS

Pruritus ani is most common in the fourth, fifth, and sixth decades. However, this disorder can occur at any age.[21]

COMPLICATIONS

Scratching associated with pruritus ani can cause excoriations and dermatologic changes. These can become infected and require antibiotic therapy. Vaginal infections are also potential complications. Pruritus ani related to pinworm infestation can be easily spread to others, and reinfection is common.

PATIENT AND FAMILY EDUCATION

- To help identify offending foods, the patient can be taught an elimination diet.
- The patient should be instructed about proper anal hygiene habits and to avoid scratching the area.
- Sitz baths several times a day can provide comfort and hygiene; be sure to thoroughly dry the perianal area afterwards. Pat dry or use a blow dryer on the cool cycle.
- Avoid tight-fitting clothing, as well as undergarments made from moisture-trapping fabrics such as nylon.

ANORECTAL ABSCESS OR FISTULA

DEFINITION AND EPIDEMIOLOGY

An anorectal abscess is an infection that occurs from obstruction of the duct of an anal gland at the level of the dentate line. The abscess may form, then spread to adjacent pelvic tissue or the perianal skin. An anorectal fistula is the abnormal communication between the abscess and the perianal skin. An abscess is the acute manifestation of the infection, and a fistula is the chronic manifestation. The incidence is two times higher in men than in women,[25] with the most common ages being the third and fourth decades of life.[14] Up to 35% of patients with Crohn disease are affected by at least one instance of perianal fistula formation.[26] In Crohn disease, however, the abscess-fistula complex appears to arise from penetrating inflammation rather than infection of an anal gland.[27]

PATHOPHYSIOLOGY

The most common cause of anorectal abscesses and fistulas is bacterial infection of the anal crypt glands. These glands may become infected if obstruction with resulting stasis occurs from trauma, hard stools, foreign bodies, or diarrhea. The suppurative process then tracks through the planes of the anorectal tissue, and typically presents as a purulent collection at the anal verge. Other possible causes of anorectal abscesses or fistulas include neoplasms, ruptured diverticula, and inflammatory bowel disorders (e.g., Crohn disease).[28] Abnormal communication between the anorectal canal and the perianal skin results in fistula formation with resultant drainage of purulent material.

CLINICAL PRESENTATION AND PHYSICAL EXAMINATION

The most common complaints of patients with an anorectal abscess are anal or perianal pain and swelling. The pain increases with movement, sitting, or bowel movements. Malaise and fever may also be present. The most common complaint of patients with an anorectal fistula is persistent purulent drainage with a history of abscess that has either been drained surgically or spontaneously. A careful history is necessary to determine whether the patient has a history of immunocompromise, diabetes, Crohn disease, or anorectal abscess or fistula, as these conditions can alter the expected course and treatment of the abscess and fistula.

Physical examination of the perineum may reveal erythema, heat, swelling, and tenderness. If the abscess is located higher in the anorectum, the perineum may be unrevealing and the abscess may manifest as localized fluctuance and tenderness on digital rectal examination. On anoscopy, pus may be seen exuding from the internal opening of the fistula tract into the anal canal. A fistula may be seen with purulent drainage oozing from a sinus or opening in the perineal skin, as well. If the abscess has resolved, and induration is no longer present, a palpable linear cord may be felt between the anal outlet and the site of prior abscess on the perianal skin. Inguinal lymph nodes may be enlarged.

DIAGNOSTICS

Most abscesses and fistulae do not require any laboratory workup or imaging. In the presence of systemic symptoms, however, a CBC may reveal leukocytosis. Several imaging modalities are available to evaluate abscess and fistula, if indicated. Ultrasound, computed tomography (CT), or magnetic resonance imaging (MRI) is indicated in cases of recurrent and complex cases (e.g., those involving inflammatory bowel disease).[25] These studies can provide valuable information on the location and extension of the abscess and fistula tracts. In patients with Crohn disease and perianal pathology, CT has proven useful in delineating abscesses and fistulae from isolated rectal inflammation.[29] MRI has reported accuracy rates of greater than 90% for mapping fistulous tracts and identifying the internal opening.[29]

INITIAL DIAGNOSTICS

Anorectal Abscess or Fistula

- Visual inspection
- Digital rectal exam
- Anoscopy

ADDITIONAL DIAGNOSTICS

- Complete blood count with differential: if fever, serious underlying medical issues, or an unclear diagnosis.
- Computed tomography scan
- Magnetic resonance imaging Pelvis
- Colonoscopy
- Small bowel examination to assess for evidence of Crohn disease

Differential Diagnosis

The differential diagnosis of anorectal abscess primarily includes fissure, thrombosed hemorrhoids, and pilonidal disease. Also included in the differential diagnosis are hidradenitis suppurativa, anorectal malignant neoplasm, actinomycosis, sexually transmitted diseases, and lymphoma. With recurrent fistulas, Crohn disease should be considered.

Red flag symptoms are refractory anal pain, back pain, weight loss, and a change in bowel habits. These symptoms should prompt more extensive evaluation to rule out malignancy, intraepithelial neoplasia, and inflammatory bowel disease.

INTERPROFESSIONAL COLLABORATIVE MANAGEMENT

Nonpharmacologic Management

The first-line treatment of anorectal abscess is incision and drainage. The severity and location of the abscess dictate the treatment setting. Perianal and ischiorectal abscesses may be treated in an outpatient setting, whereas more complex abscess presentations require management in the operating room.[25]

Pharmacologic Management

In general, antibiotic use with incision and drainage of a simple perianal abscess does not improve healing or reduce recurrence rate, and so is therefore not routinely recommended. Antibiotics are indicated in patients with anorectal abscess complicated by cellulitis, systemic signs of infection, or underlying immunosuppression.[29] Management of perianal abscess and fistula can include treatment with ciprofloxacin and/or metronidazole.[30] Consultation regarding appropriate re-treatment should be obtained; it is dictated by patient comorbidities and path of the fistula tract.

Indications for Referral or Hospitalization

Early referral to a surgeon for operative incision and drainage is essential for complex abscess-fistula complexes, as delayed or inadequate treatment can lead to extensive or life-threatening suppuration with massive tissue necrosis and possible sepsis.[16]

Surgical options for the management of chronic anal fistulas include fistulotomy, fistulectomy, debridement with seton placement, fibrin glue, fistula plug, ligation of the intersphincteric fistula tract (LIFT), and sphincter-sparing advancement flaps.[25]

COMPLICATIONS

Anal sphincter injury is the most serious complication after surgical management of anal fistulae, resulting in impaired continence. A 2010 Cochrane Review with 479 patients demonstrated that sphincter division with primary fistulotomy or fistulectomy was associated with a significant decrease in abscess or fistula persistence, but an increased risk of continence disturbance at 1-year follow-up.[27] Anal fistulae in Crohn patients is associated with poor and delayed wound healing and a high risk of incontinence.[16]

PATIENT AND FAMILY EDUCATION

- Postoperatively, the patient should be instructed to keep the stools soft with bulk-forming agents, a high-fiber diet, and stool softeners.

- Warm sitz baths can help with hygiene, promote healing, and provide comfort until healing is complete.
- The importance of follow-up visits to effectively manage conditions contributing to anorectal abscess and subsequent fistula formation should be emphasized.

REFERENCES

1. Rakinic, J., & Poola, V. P. (2014). Hemorrhoids and fistulas: New solutions to old problems. *Current Problems in Surgery, 51,* 98–137.
2. Henderson, P. K., & Cash, B. D. (2014). Common anorectal conditions: Evaluation and treatment. *Current Gastroenterology Reports, 16*(10), 408.
3. Mounsey, A. L., Halladay, J., & Sadiq, T. S. (2011). *American Family Physician, 84*(2), 204–210. Copyright © 2011 American Academy of Family Physicians.
4. Jonahson, J. F., & Sonnenberg, A. (1990). The prevalence of hemorrhoids and chronic constipation. *Gastroenterology, 98,* 380–386.
5. Hulme-Moir, M., & Bartolo, D. C. (2001). Hemorrhoids. *Gastroenterology Clinics of North America, 30,* 183–197.
6. Ohning, G. V., Machicado, G. A., & Jensen, D. M. (2009). Definitive therapy for internal hemorrhoids; new opportunities and options. *Reviews in Gastroenterological Disorders, 9,* 16–26.
7. Wald, A., Bharucha, A. E., Cosman, B. C., & Whitehead, W. E. (2014). American College of Gastroenterology (ACG) clinical guideline: Management of benign anorectal disorders. *The American Journal of Gastroenterology, 109,* 1141–1157.
8. Hall, J. F. (2013). Modern management of hemorrhoidal disease. *Gastroenterology Clinics of North America, 42,* 759–772.
9. Alonso-Coello, P., Mills, E., Heels-Ansdell, D., et al. (2006). Fiber for the treatment of hemorrhoids complications: A systematic review and meta-analysis. *The American Journal of Gastroenterology, 101,* 181–188.
10. Chang, J., McLemore, E., & Tejirian, T. (2016). Anal health care basics. *The Permanente Journal, 20*(4), 15–22.
11. Tjandra, J. J., Tan, J. J., Murray-Green, C., et al. (2006). Rectogesic (glyceryl trinitrate 0.2%) ointment relieves symptoms of hemorrhoids associated with high resting anal canal pressures. *Colorectal Disease: The Official Journal of the Association of Coloproctology of Great Britain and Ireland, 9*(5), 457–463.
12. Perera, N., Liolitsa, D., Iype, S., et al. (2012). Phlebotonics for haemorrhoids. *The Cochrane Database of Systematic Reviews,* (8), CD004322.
13. Rivadeneira, D., Steele, S., Ternent, C., et al. (2011). *Diseases of the Colon and Rectum, 54,* 1059–1064.
14. Delashaw, M., & Foley, K. (2006). Managing anorectal complaints. *Emergency Medicine, 38*(5), 44–50.
15. Giordano, P., Gravante, G., Sorge, R., et al. (2009). Long-term outcomes of stapled hemorrhoidopexy vs conventional hemorrhoidectomy: A meta-analysis of randomized controlled trials. *Archives of Surgery (Chicago, Ill.: 1960), 144*(3), 266–272.
16. Schubert, M. C., Sridhar, S., Schade, R. R., & Wexner, S. D. (2009). What every gastroenterologist needs to know about common anorectal disorders. *World Journal of Gastroenterology, 15*(26), 3201–3209.
17. Fargo, M. V., & Latimer, K. M. (2012). Evaluation and management of common anorectal conditions. *American Family Physician, 85*(6), 624–630.
18. Herzig, D. O., & Lu, K. C. (2010). Anal fissure. *The Surgical Clinics of North America, 90*(1), 33–44.
19. Nelson, R. L., Thomas, K., Morgan, J., et al. (2012). Nonsurgical therapy for anal fissure. *The Cochrane Database of Systematic Reviews,* (2), CD003431.
20. Stewart, D., Gaertner, W., Glasgow, S., et al. (2017). Clinical practice guideline for the management of anal fissures. *Diseases of the Colon and Rectum, 60,* 7–14.
21. Markell, K. W., & Billingham, R. P. (2010). Pruritus ani: Etiology and management. *The Surgical Clinics of North America, 90*(1), 125–135.
22. Maple, D., Schum, M., & Von Worley, A. (2014). The epidemiology and treatment of anal fissures in a population-based cohort. *BMC Gastroenterology, 14,* 129.
23. Chen, H. L., Woo, X. B., Wang, H. S., et al. (2014). Botulinum toxin injection versus lateral internal sphincterotomy for chronic anal fissure: A meta-analysis of randomized control trials. *Techniques in Coloproctology, 18,* 693–698.
24. Ansari, P. (2016). Pruritus ani. *Clinics in Colon and Rectal Surgery, 29,* 38–42.
25. Sneider, E. B., & Maykel, J. A. (2013). Anal abscess and fistula. *Gastroenterology Clinics of North America, 42,* 773–784.
26. Scharl, M., & Rogler, G. (2014). Pathophysiology of fistula formation in Crohn's disease. *World Journal of Gastrointestinal Pathophysiology, 5*(3), 2015–2212.

27. Vogel, J., Johnson, E., Morris, A., et al. (2016). Clinical practice guideline for the management of anorectal abscess, fistula-in-ano, and rectovaginal fistula. *Diseases of the Colon and Rectum, 59*, 1117–1133.

28. Rizzo, J. A., Naig, A. L., & Johnson, E. K. (2010). Anorectal abscess and fistula-in-ano: Evidence-based management. *The Surgical Clinics of North America, 90*(1), 45–68.

29. Lohsiriwat, V. (2016). Anorectal emergencies. *World Journal of Gastroenterology, 22*(26), 5867–5878.

30. Marzo, M., Felice, C., Pugliese, D., Andrisani, G., Mocci, G., Armuzzi, A., et al. (2015). Management of perianal fistulas in Crohn's disease: An up-to-date review. *World Journal of Gastroenterology: WJG, 21*(5), 1394–1403. http://doi.org/10.3748/wjg.v21.i5.1394.

CHAPTER **111**

CHOLELITHIASIS AND CHOLECYSTITIS

Meghan Glynn

 Immediate referral is indicated for acute cholecystitis

DEFINITION AND EPIDEMIOLOGY

Cholelithiasis and cholecystitis are worldwide disorders that result from inflammatory, infectious, neoplastic, metabolic, and congenital conditions. Gallbladder disease affects all cultures and is prevalent in most Western countries.[1] The highest incidence of acute cholecystitis occurs in adults of middle age and older. Although gallbladder disease also occurs in adolescents, it is seen at increased rates after the age of 40 years. Acalculous cholecystitis is less common but is associated with more severe morbidity. Risk factors for gallbladder disease include ethnicity, with Native Americans having an increased incidence in North America. Moreover, gallbladder disease is more common in females and during pregnancy. Other risk factors include family history, diet, medications (e.g., estrogen, oral contraceptives, thiazide diuretics), obesity, rapid weight loss, history of gastric bypass surgery, and hyperalimentation, as well as comorbid disorders such as diabetes, Crohn disease, alcoholic and biliary cirrhosis, and hyperparathyroidism.

PATHOPHYSIOLOGY

Gallstones are formed from bile constituent crystals and are divided into three primary types of stones: cholesterol, pigmented, and mixed. Small gallstones pass uneventfully through the common bile duct and do not cause distress. Larger stones may obstruct the cystic or common bile duct, causing increased pressure to the ductal system that results in pain, nausea, and vomiting as a result of the contractile spasms of the smooth muscle. Because of the blockage, bile is prevented from entering the duodenum, reducing the body's ability to digest fat. The undigested fat passes from the small intestine into the large intestine, where bacteria convert the excess undigested fat into fatty acid derivatives. The fatty acid derivatives alter water absorption from the colon, which results in diarrhea and excess fluid loss. The obstruction prevents bile secretion into the small intestine, causing jaundice.

The gallbladder becomes inflamed as a result of various processes, including continued blockage of the cystic or common bile duct. This inflammation causes the release of prostaglandins and other chemicals that further inflame

gallbladder tissue. In most cases, bacterial infections contribute to the inflammatory response in acute cholecystitis.[2] Human immunodeficiency virus (HIV) disease may lead to opportunistic infections of the biliary tract. The most common bacteria involved in biliary tract infections are *Escherichia coli*, *Klebsiella* organisms, *Enterobacter*, and enterococci.[3] Gangrene of the gallbladder and possible perforation can result if the process is not stopped.

Cholecystitis can also occur in the absence of stones; this condition is labeled *acute* or *chronic acalculous cholecystitis*. Acalculous cholecystitis is classified as acute if the duration of symptoms is less than 1 month and as chronic if the symptoms have been present longer than 3 months. The pathophysiology of this condition is poorly understood. The inflammatory process resembles that of cholecystitis except that gallstones are not present. A common cause of chronic acalculous cholecystitis is hypokinetic biliary dyskinesia, but decreased gall bladder emptying is another possible cause. Severe weight loss, sepsis, trauma, or other serious illness in a hospitalized patient is associated with acute acalculous cholecystitis and can be life-threatening.[4]

CLINICAL PRESENTATION AND PHYSICAL EXAMINATION

Most patients with gallstones are asymptomatic.[5] Classically, symptomatic cholelithiasis manifests as biliary colic with intermittent or steady, right upper quadrant abdominal pain that radiates to the right posterior shoulder within an hour of eating any type of large meal, specifically a meal with a high fat content. The pain may be constant or intermittent and tapering, sometimes without complete relief. It is described as mild to severe and lasts 1 to 6 hours. The biliary colic is accompanied by nausea and vomiting. There can be a history of these episodes, which increase in frequency.

Acute cholecystitis develops in a manner similar to symptomatic cholelithiasis, but biliary colic lasts longer than 4 to 6 hours. There usually is a history of intermittent colic consistent with chronic cholecystitis, and the patient may have anorexia, fever, and chills with the nausea and vomiting observed in symptomatic cholelithiasis. As the gallbladder becomes progressively inflamed, the pain in the right upper quadrant becomes sharp. The Charcot triad of right upper quadrant abdominal pain, fever, and jaundice can be observed if a stone is lodged in the common bile duct.

Patients with chronic cholecystitis often describe a recurrent, mild to moderate right upper quadrant and epigastric abdominal pain accompanied by nausea and vomiting. The pain may radiate to the region of the posterior right shoulder and scapula and is often associated with consuming fatty foods.

Traditionally, patients with acute acalculous cholecystitis are critically ill and require hospitalization. Presentation includes generalized complaints, fever, nausea, vomiting, and loss of appetite. The patient often has no significant medical history, although surgery, trauma, burns, and other disorders have been associated with acalculous cholecystitis. This condition should be considered in all patients who are seen with right upper quadrant pain in the absence of gallstones.

The physical examination in symptomatic cholelithiasis and chronic cholecystitis may be unremarkable, depending on the severity of the condition. Right upper quadrant abdominal pain may be accompanied by tenderness. The diagnosis is based on the history, the exclusion of other disorders, and the results of the gallbladder ultrasound examination.

With acute cholecystitis, patients may have moderate distress from systemic toxicity, including tachycardia and fever. The right upper quadrant abdominal pain is associated with tenderness and muscle guarding or rigidity. The gallbladder is not commonly palpable, but a distended tender gallbladder confirms the diagnosis. Hypoactive bowel sounds and presence of Murphy sign (an inability to take a deep breath because of the discomfort during palpation beneath the right costal margin) may be noted. Dehydration is not uncommon. Jaundice is present in some patients and is the result of biliary obstruction or chronic hemolysis.

The physical findings in acalculous cholecystitis resemble those of symptomatic gallstones: right upper quadrant pain, vomiting, fever, jaundice, and presence of Murphy sign.

DIAGNOSTICS

Essential Diagnostics

Laboratory testing should be individualized, but a complete blood count (CBC) with differential, urinalysis, liver function tests (LFTs), and serum pancreatic enzymes are usually indicated. Serum electrolyte values and blood urea nitrogen (BUN) and creatinine concentrations are necessary to determine fluid and electrolyte status as well as renal function. Blood cultures are indicated if sepsis is suspected. A test for human chorionic gonadotropin (hCG) is essential in women of childbearing age if potentially teratogenic clinical imaging studies are considered. Electrocardiography is necessary if cardiac risk factors are present or if cardiac involvement is suspected.

INITIAL DIAGNOSTICS

Cholelithiasis and Cholecystitis

LABORATORY
- Complete blood count and differential
- Liver function tests (bilirubin, alkaline phosphatase)
- Serum electrolytes, blood urea nitrogen, and creatinine[a]
- Serum pregnancy test, human chorionic gonadotropin[a]

IMAGING
- Ultrasound
- Biliary scintigraphy
- Endoscopic retrograde cholangiopancreatography[a]

[a]If indicated.

Although history and physical examination findings help to support diagnosis of cholecystitis, an ultrasound is ordered to help confirm diagnosis. Ultrasound is the most practical imaging study for evaluation of the gallbladder and is not contraindicated in pregnancy. In addition to detecting the gallstones, ultrasound may show gallbladder thickening and "sonographic Murphy sign"; the examination is similar to the physical examination techniques, except that when performed during the ultrasound examination, there is confirmation that the gallbladder is being pressed when the patient responds.

Additional Diagnostics

Follow-up diagnostics are based on ultrasound findings and include computed tomography (CT), preferably with contrast; cholescintigraphy (hepatobiliary iminodiacetic acid [HIDA] scan); or magnetic resonance imaging (MRI).[5,6] Plain abdominal radiographs will demonstrate biliary air, marked hepatomegaly, and, in some cases, gallstones. A chest x-ray study will exclude right lower lobe pneumonia. An abdominal CT scan may be indicated in some instances if other imaging tests are not conclusive.

DIFFERENTIAL DIAGNOSIS

 Priority differentials include (1) bowel obstruction, (2) chronic cholecystitis, (3) diverticulitis, (4) gastritis, and (5) hepatitis. However, the differential diagnoses for cholecystitis are extensive. The physical examination, laboratory results, and imaging aid in narrowing the differentials.

INTERPROFESSIONAL COLLABORATIVE MANAGEMENT

In general, asymptomatic gallstones do not require surgical intervention. However, there is a chance that the patient will become symptomatic. Thus, gastroenterologists and surgeons would consider the benefit of a prophylactic cholecystectomy in some instances.[7]

Pharmacologic Management

The initial management of symptomatic gallbladder disease begins with isotonic intravenous rehydration and correction of electrolyte abnormalities. Oral hydration is contraindicated during this time. Antispasmodic and antiemetic medications are used for uncomplicated cholelithiasis. In addition to an antiemetic, a nasogastric tube should be used for protracted vomiting to decompress the stomach. Although meperidine was frequently used in the past to manage pain, an injectable nonsteroidal antiinflammatory prostaglandin inhibitor (e.g., ketorolac tromethamine) is also an effective pain reliever in nonbacterial gallbladder distention.[7]

Ursodeoxycholic acid used either alone or in combination with chenodeoxycholic acid can decrease the pain associated with biliary disease and aid in gallstone dissolution.[8,9] This treatment is an option for patients with mild symptoms, stone size less than 0.5 to 1 cm, and normal gallbladder function. However, side effects such as diarrhea can make this treatment intolerable for patients. Moreover, the addition of a 3-hydroxy-3-methylglutaryl-coenzyme A (HMG-CoA) inhibitor may help to reduce the cholesterol saturation index. Studies disagree as to whether or not the addition of statin will assist with the dissolution and prevention of gallstones. Ezetimibe has also been considered because it inhibits cholesterol absorption; however, its ability to prevent or dissolve gallstones needs further studying.[10] These treatments take time, but they may be appropriate for patients who are not surgical candidates.

With uncomplicated symptomatic cholelithiasis, discharge is appropriate once the condition has stabilized and oral hydration is maintained. Surgical consultation before discharge is advised because many patients will have recurrent symptoms.

Acute cholecystitis should be suspected if the symptoms do not resolve within 4 to 6 hours; in this case, timely surgical referral for laparoscopic cholecystectomy is essential.[11] Prophylactic antibiotics may be indicated for patients with acute complicated cholecystitis.[12]

Consultations: Surgery

Medical dissolution, biliary lithotripsy, or surgical intervention requires further consultation to ensure optimum health care.

Patients who have diabetes or asymptomatic disease or who are not candidates for surgery should have a consultation with a gastroenterologist or surgeon to determine whether further management is required.

After initial stabilization of the patient, treatment options for uncomplicated symptomatic cholelithiasis include medical dissolution therapy (oral or direct gallbladder irrigation), biliary lithotripsy, cholecystostomy (as an alternative surgical procedure), and open or laparoscopic cholecystectomy.

Although recently less common, biliary lithotripsy can be considered in some patients with gallstones. The relatively painless shock waves fracture the stones into smaller pieces that are then passed into the small intestine. The criteria for biliary lithotripsy are specific; eligibility may include stone size or calcification and gallbladder function.

Cholecystostomy is an alternative surgical procedure to open or laparoscopic cholecystectomy and is used if the patient has too much inflammation or is too ill for cholecystectomy. Either operatively or percutaneously, stones and bile are removed through the gallbladder fundus, and a tube is placed as an external drain.

In some instances, an open cholecystectomy may be indicated. The open surgical approach is necessary when the laparoscopic method is contraindicated. Contraindications include coagulopathy, cirrhosis, portal hypertension, pregnancy, peritonitis, severe cardiopulmonary disease, and prior surgical adhesions. Cholecystostomy is the treatment of choice with severe disease or extensive inflammation.[9]

Because of its safety, convenience, reduced postoperative pain, and shorter hospitalization (outpatient surgery at some facilities) leading to reduced costs, laparoscopic cholecystectomy is the standard treatment of symptomatic gallbladder disease. Surgical drainage or removal of the gallbladder is indicated with laparoscopic cholecystectomy or ultrasound-guided percutaneous cholecystostomy. Choledocholithiasis, or stones in the common bile duct, can also be managed through the laparoscopic approach, although this will be too difficult in some instances to manage safely. Some laparoscopic approaches require a conversion to the open cholecystectomy procedure.

In addition to the initial treatment of gallstone disease, antibiotics may be indicated. Bacteria associated with acute cholecystitis include *E. coli*, *Klebsiella pneumoniae*, *Clostridium welchii*, *Clostridium perfringens*, and *Streptococcus faecalis*. Therapeutic antibiotics are used for preoperative prophylaxis, acute cholecystitis, and cholangitis. In acalculous cholecystitis, broad-spectrum antibiotics with gram-negative coverage (e.g., piperacillin) are necessary.[5,9]

COMPLICATIONS

Potential organ damage depends on the location of the gallstone obstruction in the biliary system. The most common complication is choledocholithiasis. In general, symptomatic gallstones require surgical intervention. If it is left untreated, the disease has potential complications, including a pus-filled gallbladder, which can lead to perforation. Local perforation can occur within 1 week after the onset of acute cholecystitis and can lead to the formation of a pericholecystic abscess and potential mortality. Should a large gallstone pass into the intestinal lumen, a small bowel obstruction (also known as a *gallstone ileus*) can occur. Gas-forming bacteria (*Clostridium* and coliform organisms) can lead to an emphysematous cholecystitis that also can result in gallbladder perforation. The

gallbladder may become gangrenous if extensive inflammation occurs and causes necrosis and thrombosis of the cystic artery. Gangrenous cholecystitis is more common in older patients who have comorbidities or who delay treatment. These patients not only will have the symptoms of cholecystitis, but they also will have sepsis.[5] Stones lodged in the ampulla of Vater can cause gallstone pancreatitis. The porcelain gallbladder, an uncommon condition associated with cancer, is observed on plain radiographs. The porcelain appearance of the gallbladder rim is caused by calcification of the gallbladder.

The complication rate of gallstone disease varies and depends on the procedure chosen to manage the disease, the size of the gallstone, the patient's age, and comorbid issues.

PATIENT AND FAMILY EDUCATION

Patients who are obese should be counseled about the increased risk of gallstone formation and understand the importance of lifestyle and dietary changes.[1] Some risk factors have been implicated in but not clearly demonstrated for cholelithiasis; still, physical exercise and weight control are beneficial for all patients.

If gallstones are incidentally noted on x-ray, ultrasound, or other clinical imaging studies of the abdomen, reassurance that asymptomatic stones do not require surgery is needed. Patients with symptomatic gallbladder disease need an explanation of laboratory and imaging tests, referral, and management.

Many patients who are anticipating laparoscopic cholecystectomies underrate or have unrealistic expectations about postoperative pain and activity. Preparatory guidance in this area may be efficacious to ensure a more realistic understanding of the postoperative course. Older patients can expect to spend additional time in the hospital or in rehabilitation after cholecystectomy.

REFERENCES

1. Gaby, A. R. (2009). Nutritional approaches to the prevention and treatment of gallstones. *Alternative Medicine Review: A Journal of Clinical Therapeutic*, 4(3), 258–267.
2. Neal, D. D., Moritz, M. J., & Jarrell, B. E. (1996). Liver, portal hypertension, and biliary tract. In B. E. Jarrell & R. A. Carabasi (Eds.), *Surgery* (3rd ed.). Baltimore, MD: Williams & Wilkins.
3. Barie, P. S., & Eachempati, S. R. (2010). Acute acalculous cholecystitis. *Gastroenterology Clinics of North America*, 39, 343. (Accessed 18 September 2019).
4. Jones, M. W., & Ferguson, T. (2019). Acalculous cholecystitis. [updated 2019 Apr 6]. In *StatPearls [internet]*. Treasure Island (FL): StatPearls Publishing. Retrieved from https://www.ncbi.nlm.nih.gov/books/NBK459182/.
5. Yusoff, I. E., Barkun, J. S., & Barkun, A. N. (2003). Diagnosis and management of cholecystitis and cholangitis. *Gastroenterology Clinics of North America*, 32, 1145–1168.
6. Yarmish, G. M., Smith, M. P., Rosen, M. P., et al. (2013). Expert panel on gastrointestinal imaging. Appropriateness criteria right upper quadrant pain (online publication). Reston, VA: American College of Radiology. Retrieved from http://guidelines.gov/content.aspx?id=23817. (Accessed 4 January 2018).
7. Olsen, J. C., McGrath, N. A., Schwarz, D. G., et al. (2008). A double-blind randomized clinical trial evaluating the analgesic efficacy of ketorolac versus butorphanol for patients with suspected biliary colic in the emergency department. *Academic Emergency Medicine: Official Journal of the Society for Academic Emergency Medicine*, 15, 718.
8. Petroni, M. L., Jazrawi, R., Pazzi, P., et al. (2001). Ursodeoxycholic acid alone or with chenodeoxycholic acid for dissolution of cholesterol gallstones: A randomized multicentre trial. *Alimentary Pharmacology and Therapeutics*, 15(1), 123–128.
9. Greenberger, N. J., & Paumgartner, G. (2015). Diseases of the gallbladder and bile ducts. In D. Kasper, A. Fauci, S. Hauser, D. Longo, J. Jameson, & J. Loscalzo (Eds.), *Harrison's principles of internal medicine* (19th ed.). New York: McGraw-Hill. Retrieved from http://accessmedicine

.mhmedical.com.ezproxy.simmons.edu:2048/content.aspx?bookid=1130&Sectionid=79749108. (Accessed 18 May 2019).

10. Bodmer, M., Brauchli, Y. B., Krahenbuhl, S., et al. (2009). Statin use and risk of gallstone disease followed by cholecystectomy. *JAMA: The Journal of the American Medical Association, 302*, 2001.

11. Stevens, K. A., Chi, A., Lucas, L. C., et al. (2006). Immediate laparoscopic cholecystectomy for acute cholecystitis: No need to wait. *American Journal of Surgery, 192*(6), 756–761.

12. Darkahi, B., Videhult, P., Sandblom, G., et al. (2012). Effectiveness of antibiotic prophylaxis in cholecystectomy: A prospective population-based study of 1171 cholecystectomies. *Scandinavian Journal of Gastroenterology, 47*, 1242.

CHAPTER **112**

CIRRHOSIS

Donna M. Glynn

 Immediate referral to a hepatologist should be considered for a diagnosis of cirrhosis

DEFINITION AND EPIDEMIOLOGY

Cirrhosis is the end-stage consequence of progressive hepatic fibrosis affecting normal liver function. It is a serious, irreversible disease—the result of exposure to persistent toxins and resulting in liver failure and death.

The most common causes of cirrhosis in the United States are chronic hepatitis B and C virus (HBV and HCV), alcoholic liver disease, nonalcoholic fatty liver disease (NAFLD), and nonalcoholic steatohepatitis (NASH).[1] Various pharmacotherapeutics including acetaminophen, amiodarone, methotrexate, isoniazid, varied antibiotics, and carbon tetrachloride are also associated with cirrhosis. The cause can be inherited or idiopathic, but primary and secondary biliary cirrhosis, infections, viruses, hemochromatosis, polycystic liver disease, right-sided heart failure, autoimmune hepatitis, and other disorders play a key role in the development of cirrhosis.

Fibrosis, the replacement of normally functioning liver tissue by injured scar tissue, results in varied-size nodules that impair function. In advanced stages, the impaired hepatic vasculature results in a shunting of the portal and arterial blood supply, causing portal hypertension, obstructive biliary channels, destruction of liver cells, hepatocellular carcinoma, and eventual liver failure.[2]

Liver biopsy is an important diagnostic tool in the diagnosis of cirrhosis to stage the severity of the fibrosis and to establish a plan of care, though newer tests (Fibrotest/Fibroscan) can also be helpful. Cirrhosis is typically classified as micronodular, macronodular, or mixed.[3] Micronodular cirrhosis, often associated with alcoholic liver disease, occurs when the repeated presence of an offending agent prevents the regeneration of normal tissue. As a result, the regenerating tissue produces small nodules that have limited functional abilities. As the disease progresses, the liver becomes smaller in size and the nodules become larger with diffuse fat accumulation. Macronodular cirrhosis is seen in chronic viral hepatitis and hepatocellular carcinoma and is distinguished by larger nodules (2 to 3 cm [⅘ to 1⅕ inches] in diameter) that may contain their own blood supply. The larger nodules resemble scar tissue and also have limited functional abilities. Mixed-form cirrhosis, a combination of both macronodules and micronodules, has mixed characteristics, and liver functions are also varied.[3]

Data regarding the prevalence and progression of cirrhosis are limited and variable, likely because of undiagnosed cirrhosis in the adult population. In the United States, 40,545 deaths were attributed to cirrhosis in 2016, and cirrhosis is now considered the 8th leading cause of death in this country.[3,4] The Model for End-Stage Liver Disease (MELD) is a prognostic tool for cirrhosis. Based on the underlying cause of the cirrhosis and the serum creatinine, bilirubin, and international normalized ratio (INR), the MELD tool is used as a prediction tool for patients with cirrhosis and for prioritizing candidates for liver transplantation (www.mdcalc.com/meld-score-model-for-end-stage-liver-disease-12-and-older).[2,5,6]

The prognosis of cirrhosis depends on the cause and classification of the disease. If the cirrhosis is related to alcohol or hepatotoxic drugs, the major factor that determines survival is the patient's ability to stop drinking alcohol or taking hepatotoxic drugs.

PATHOPHYSIOLOGY

Primary biliary cirrhosis (PBC) is the autoimmune destruction of the intrahepatic bile ducts and eventual development of cirrhosis and liver failure. Hepatocellular injury occurs when the liver is continually exposed to toxins (e.g., alcohol, elevated triglycerides) or diseases (e.g., hepatitis) that produce toxemia, inflammation, ischemia, and necrosis of the hepatic tissue. The persistent inflammation and necrosis stimulate hepatocellular regeneration, causing the development of fibrous (scar) tissue such as collagen by fibroblasts. As the regeneration process progresses, rigid nodules form, distorting the normal surrounding hepatic tissue. This deformation produces increased resistance to normal blood circulation, decreased blood flow, and even obstruction of normal portal venous flow, resulting in decreased liver function abilities.[2,6]

Portal hypertension develops when increased hydrostatic pressure within the portal venous circulation occurs, the result of inflammation and obstruction of blood flow. As cirrhosis progresses, the rising pressure in the portal circulation will increase resistance to portal venous flow. Collateral circulation develops new vascular channels and shunts that bypass areas of obstruction to maintain adequate blood flow.[2,6] The collateral path to portal circulation occurs most commonly in the peritoneum, retroperitoneum, and thoracic cavities, but also in the rectum, esophagus, and gastric areas. The complications of the collateral circulation include ascites, splenomegaly, and esophageal varices. These collateral vessels contain varicosities susceptible to spontaneous rupture, hemorrhage, and subsequent death.

CLINICAL PRESENTATION AND PHYSICAL EXAMINATION

The onset of symptoms can be insidious, and patients with cirrhosis can be asymptomatic. In PBC, the earliest reported symptoms include pruritus, weight loss, and fatigue.[5] Other concerns associated with cirrhosis are nonspecific and include weakness, malaise, dark urine, or pale stools. As the patient's condition worsens, anorexia is present and is often associated with nausea and vomiting. Hematemesis can also be a common presenting concern. Abdominal pain, if present, is related to ascites and the stretching of the muscles around the enlarged liver. Chest pain caused by cardiomegaly has also been reported. Menstrual abnormalities, impotence, and sterility are other concerns. Neuropsychiatric symptoms such as difficulty concentrating, irritability, and confusion are associated with liver function failure. Jaundice is a late-stage presenting symptom. The initial clinical presentation of patients with advanced cirrhosis is common.

A careful history, particularly a personal history of alcohol, toxic drug, or substance use, and a specific review of the patient's social and work history, can identify high-risk behaviors such as intravenous drug use. Additional necessary information includes a thorough review of all medications, including herbal and over-the-counter products; allergies; past medical history; and family history. A history of recent blood transfusion or residence in an area of high hepatitis virus incidence also can suggest the diagnosis of cirrhosis.

Jaundice, spider angiomata, gynecomastia, ascites, splenomegaly, palmar erythema, digital clubbing, and asterixis may be the presenting signs of cirrhosis. Low-grade fever, anorexia, and right upper quadrant pain can be present. As the cirrhosis progresses, patients may experience a decrease in mean arterial pressure. The liver may be nodular, firm, enlarged, or shrunken (seen in late stages of cirrhosis), and the spleen may be enlarged. A fluid wave and increased abdominal girth will be evident if ascites is present. The presence of high pressures in the portal circulation often leads to the development of a venous hum (best heard over the epigastrium) and rectal and esophageal varices. As a result of the fluid shifts, peripheral edema is found in the feet, legs, and hands. Delirium, lethargy, and coma occur in the later stages of cirrhosis.[5]

Other physical signs associated with cirrhosis include weight loss; tremors; cheilosis or glossitis; spider angiomata on the face, chest, and abdomen; palmar erythema; Dupuytren contracture; horizontal white bands on nail beds (Muehrcke nails); whitening of the proximal two thirds of the nails and reddening of the remainder (Terry nails); digital clubbing; gynecomastia and testicular atrophy in men; and changes in body hair distribution in women. A sweet breath odor may be discernable in patients, referred to as *fetor hepaticus*. Asterixis, or liver flap, can be elicited with severe cases of liver failure.[3]

In patients with portal hypertension, a Cruveilhier-Baumgarten murmur may be heard. This murmur is described as a venous hum, is best auscultated over the epigastrium, and may be augmented by the Valsalva maneuver.[5]

DIAGNOSTICS

In the early stages of cirrhosis, there are often no significant diagnostic findings. It is with the presence of laboratory abnormalities that the potential for liver dysfunction is questioned. No single diagnostic biochemical marker is available regarding cirrhosis.

Essential Diagnostics

Although not found in all patients, hypoalbuminemia, elevated serum protein, hyperbilirubinemia, and elevated liver enzymes (aspartate transaminase [AST] and alanine aminotransferase [ALT]) all indicate hepatocellular inflammation or injury. ALT is used to evaluate acute versus chronic liver injury. The alkaline phosphatase and γ-glutamyl transpeptidase levels are also often elevated. The evaluation of liver function test results and the decision to proceed with further testing and possible biopsy are based on the history and physical examination findings.[3]

Prothrombin time (PT), partial thromboplastin time (PPT), and serum albumin should be evaluated to determine hepatic synthesis and clotting function[2]; such measurements are a useful tool in the MELD score. Albumin synthesis is directly correlated to liver function, and levels of albumin will decrease as the cirrhosis advances. In addition, decreased levels of platelets are common in patients with chronic liver disease, placing the patient at increased risk for bleeding.[2,7]

The Lok index is an online calculator that uses blood chemistries to determine the likelihood of cirrhosis in patients with HCV. The index uses the platelet count, AST, ALT, and INR to assess that probability.[8]

Additional Diagnostics

Additional diagnostics depend on the patient presentation, but it is important to determine the exact cause of the cirrhosis in newly diagnosed patients. Initial serologic workups may include a screen for antimitochondrial antibodies (a marker of PBC that distinguishes PBC from secondary biliary cirrhosis), antinuclear antibodies, anti-smooth muscle antibodies, antibodies to hepatitis C, hepatitis B surface antigen, and antibodies to hepatitis B core antigen and surface antigen. Fasting serum ferritin, transferrin saturation, and total iron-binding capacity should be obtained to exclude hereditary hemochromatosis.[2] If the transferrin saturation is significantly elevated (>45%), genetic testing for hereditary hemochromatosis (C282Y and H63D) is indicated. FibroTest (FT) is a serum marker that combines the quantitative results of five serum markers (α_2-macroglobulin, haptoglobin, γ-glutamyl transpeptidase, total bilirubin, and apolipoprotein A-I) with the patient age and gender and provides a measure of the degree of fibrosis in the liver.[9]

Other abnormalities in laboratory results are common. Pancytopenia, anemia (frequently macrocytic), thrombocytopenia, abnormal clotting mechanisms, and prolongation of PT all contribute to an increased potential for gastrointestinal bleeding.[7] Hyponatremia can indicate advanced illness, but other electrolyte abnormalities and renal insufficiency are also common. Ultrasound is used to assess liver size, portal circulation, and the presence of occult ascites or tumor. The imaging will also detect portal hypertension, ascites, and portal vein thrombosis. Fibroscan, another way to determine the extent of liver fibrosis, is a pulse echo ultrasound that calculates liver stiffness in a noninvasive way.[10] Computed tomography (CT) is not used to diagnose cirrhosis, and the benefits of magnetic resonance imaging (MRI) in the diagnosis and management of cirrhosis are still unclear.

In the past, liver biopsy, unless contraindicated, was necessary for the diagnosis of cirrhosis and staging of fibrosis.[9] A biopsy specimen would be obtained by a radiographically guided percutaneous procedure or via the transjugular or laparoscopic route. Bleeding was always a concern because of the risk of platelet abnormalities. The Fibroscan, also known as transient elastography, and Fibrotest are now more frequently used to diagnose fibrosis and cirrhosis because they are less invasive and present less risk to the patient.[11] However, liver biopsy can be beneficial in determining the cause of the patient's cirrhosis and in the end remains the gold standard.

Magnetic resonance elastography (MRE) estimates liver stiffness resulting from fibrosis. MRE is an additional safe, effective method of evaluating fibrosis in patients with chronic hepatitis C and for some patients may be more accurate.[12,13]

INITIAL DIAGNOSTICS

Cirrhosis

LABORATORY
- Complete blood count and differential
- Serum glucose, electrolytes, blood urea nitrogen, creatinine
- Liver function tests

IMAGING
- Ultrasound

ADDITIONAL DIAGNOSTICS
- Alpha fetoprotein[a]
- Hepatitis screen
- Fasting serum ferritin

- Transferrin saturation
- Total iron-binding capacity
- Serum protein electrophoresis[a]
- Serum ceruloplasmin[a]
- Fibrotest[a]

Imaging
- Doppler ultrasound
- Fibroscan
- MRE[a]

Other Diagnostics
- Esophagogastroscopy
- Liver Biopsy
- Liver biopsy

[a]If indicated.

DIFFERENTIAL DIAGNOSIS

Priority differentials include primary biliary cholangitis (PBC), secondary biliary cirrhosis, thrombosis, tumor, and hemochromatosis. Hepatocellular injury has varied causes, but it can be idiopathic. PBC is a chronic, progressive cholestatic disease of unknown cause. Nonsuppurative, granulomatous inflammatory destruction of the small interlobular bile ducts occurs within the liver and results in the development of cholestasis, liver failure, and cirrhosis.

Secondary biliary cirrhosis occurs when the disease is related to extrahepatic disease, as seen with cardiac failure, hemochromatosis, or Wilson disease. Patients with neuropsychiatric symptoms should be evaluated for Wilson disease. Uremia, nephrotic syndrome, metabolic disorders, pericarditis, various blood dyscrasias, biliary disease, and hepatitis are conditions that impair liver function and mimic cirrhosis. Thrombosis resulting from cardiac or hematologic manifestations can obstruct blood flow and alter liver function. The presence of a tumor (hepatocellular carcinoma or metastatic tumors) can be detected by imaging and is suspected if the serum alpha-fetoprotein concentration is elevated. The presence of diabetes and endocrine disturbances in an older patient may suggest hemochromatosis. NASH, primary sclerosing cholangitis, or a parasitic infection such as *Schistosoma mansoni* should also be considered as a possible cause of hepatocellular injury.

INTERPROFESSIONAL COLLABORATIVE MANAGEMENT

Cirrhosis is considered an irreversible disease process, but recent advances provide hope that early identification and future therapies will permit reversibility. Currently, progression is dependent on the cause, treatment, and patient adherence to treatment recommendations. The main focus of treatment involves the prevention of further liver dysfunction and the treatment of complications. The MELD classification tool can also be used for 3-month predication of survival with cirrhosis regardless of cause.

Primary care providers must focus on the elimination of causative factors and the promotion of a healthy lifestyle to delay the long-term consequences of cirrhosis. Patients should be immunized with polyvalent pneumococcal vaccine, yearly influenza vaccine, and, unless already immune, both hepatitis A and B vaccines.[3] Reversible causes of cirrhosis such as alcohol or hepatotoxic medications such as nonsteroidal antiinflammatory drugs (NSAIDs) must be eliminated because continued use will result in a limited life expectancy.

Pharmacologic Management

Patients who have ongoing viral hepatitis B or C infection can have increased life expectancy with antiviral therapy.[14] Polymerase inhibitors and protease inhibitors used in the treatment of hepatitis C have been shown to be effective in eradication and therefore prevention of cirrhosis.[15]

Esophageal varices and the risk of bleeding is a serious complication of decompensated cirrhosis. Management is directed to both control and prevent bleeding. The use of nonselective β-blocker therapy has been proven to reduce the risk of bleeds by 40%. Patients should undergo esophagogastroduodenoscopy routinely to evaluate for varicies.[16] When β-blocker therapy is contraindicated or the patient is unable to tolerate it, endoscopic variceal ligation is considered. The combination of β-blocker therapy and endoscopic variceal ligation has been proven effective in recurrent variceal bleeding.[16]

To identify the cause of ascites and develop an effective treatment plan, diagnostic paracentesis is necessary. Management of ascites includes dietary sodium restriction to 1 to 2 g/day. Spironolactone is also a consideration to improve fluid diuresis; furosemide may be added to augment diuresis and prevent hyperkalemia. Monitoring of electrolytes, blood urea nitrogen (BUN), and creatinine is required. If ascites is refractory to diet and pharmacologic intervention, placement of peritoneovenous shunts, or repeated large-volume paracentesis may be required.

Spontaneous bacterial peritonitis (SBP) is an infection of the ascitic fluid in patients with cirrhosis, necessitating careful monitoring for patients at risk. The presentation includes abdominal pain, fever, and altered mental status. Hospitalization is required, and patients are treated with cephalosporin or fluoroquinolone therapy.[16] For patients with recurrent bacterial peritonitis, antibiotic prophylaxis is required.[16]

Hepatorenal syndrome (HRS) results from renal vasoconstriction and progressive renal failure. Treatment is difficult because diuretic therapy needs to be discontinued and dehydration needs to be corrected. Fluid overload is a common complication, and hemodialysis is a necessary consideration.[16]

Hepatic encephalopathy is associated with severe liver disease. Symptoms of hepatic encephalopathy include changes in cognition, mood disturbance, and disorientation. Numerous factors, including infections, medications, gastrointestinal bleeding, and constipation, are associated with the development of hepatic encephalopathy requiring careful management. The serum ammonia level may or may not be elevated. Lactulose 30 to 45 mL by mouth three times per day (tid) or four times per day (qid) to produce two or three daily soft stools helps treat and prevent hepatic encephalopathy, but the underlying cause should also be corrected. If the patient develops diarrhea, the dose should be decreased to prevent fluid and electrolyte imbalance. Rifaximin is used in addition to lactulose to treat hepatic encephalopathy. Neomycin is also used to treat hepatic encephalopathy. Because the nutritional state of the patient is compromised, close oversight of all systems is necessary to ensure management of iron deficiency, fluid and electrolyte balance, and protein-calorie malnutrition. The health care provider and nutritionist can design a patient-centered plan that will focus on consumption of a low-sodium diet, combined with protein 1.2 to 1.5 g/kg/day and adequate fiber (25 to 45 g daily), with foods that meet the patient's physical, emotional, and cultural needs. Multivitamin supplementation each day is also advised. Patients with Wernicke encephalopathy also require thiamine supplementation.[16]

Co-Management With Specialists

Management of the patient with cirrhosis is complex and requires coordinated effort with a gastroenterologist and other specialists.[17] For patients with drug or alcohol abuse, the initial priority is to assist in eliminating the offending agent from use. Drug and alcohol treatment programs can help both the patient and the family. Collaboration with mental health specialists provides information about the patient's progress with alcohol or drug abuse and determines safe medication choices for patients if pharmacologic support for detoxification is needed.

The availability of social services is helpful in acquiring financial, physical, or psychologic assistance; attaining therapeutic home aides and home health nursing care; recommending support groups; or arranging transportation. If long-term care is needed, the social worker can provide information about available facilities that will meet the patient's and family's needs.

COMPLICATIONS

The complications that occur in cirrhosis are discussed in the management of the disease and the disease process. Individuals with a diagnosis of cirrhosis will undergo many complications during the course of the disease, and early identification and treatment are critical to improve their quality of life.

PATIENT AND FAMILY EDUCATION

The patient and family should understand the benefits of the treatment plan. Dietary discipline, avoidance of hepatotoxic drugs (including NSAIDs), and support group activities are ways to achieve a successful outcome.[18] The importance of reducing the risk of gastrointestinal bleeding, recognizing the signs of variceal bleeding, and taking the appropriate course of action if bleeding occurs should be discussed.

Patients with cirrhosis may be depressed. However, the use of antidepressant drugs is not usually indicated because of the high risk of over-sedation and toxicity. Consultation with a psychopharmacologist can assist in designing a treatment regimen that could help the patient through this depression. Signs and complications of depression, as well as indications for immediate intervention, should be reviewed with the patient and family.

RESOURCES

MELD Score: www.mdcalc.com/meld-score-model-for-end-stage-liver-disease-12-and-older

Lok index: medcalc3000.com/LokIndex.htm

REFERENCES

1. National Institute of Diabetes and Digestive and Kidney Disease. Cirrhosis. Retrieved from http://www.niddk.nih.gov/health-information/health-topics/liver-disease/cirrhosis/Pages/facts.aspx. (Accessed May 18, 2019).
2. Bacon, B. R. (2015). Cirrhosis and its complications. In D. Kasper, A. Fauci, S. Hauser, D. Longo, J. Jameson, & J. Loscalzo (Eds.), *Harrison's principles of internal medicine* (19th ed.). New York, NY: McGraw-Hill.
3. Friedman, L. S. (2019). Liver, biliary tract, & pancreas disorders. In M. A. Papadakis, S. J. McPhee, & M. W. Rabow (Eds.), *Current medical diagnosis & treatment*. New York, NY: McGraw-Hill. http://accessmedicine.mhmedical.com.ezproxy.simmons.edu/content.aspx?bookid=2449&sectionid=194440813. (Accessed May 18, 2019).
4. Centers for Disease Control and Prevention. Chronic liver disease and cirrhosis. www.cdc.gov/nchs/data_access/Vitalstatsonline.htm. (Accessed on May 18, 2019).
5. Andersen, D. K., Billiar, T. R., Dunn, D. L., Hunter, J. G., Matthews, J. B., & Pollock, R. E. (Eds.). (2014). *Schwartz's principles of surgery* (10th ed.). New York, NY: McGraw-Hill.
6. Heuman, D. M., Abou-Assi, S. G., Habib, A., et al. (2004). Persistent ascites and low serum sodium identify patients with cirrhosis and low MELD scores who are at high risk for early death. *Hepatology (Baltimore, Md.)*, 40(4), 802–810.
7. Afdhal, N., McHutchinson, J., Brown, R., et al. (2008). Thrombocytopenia associated with chronic liver disease. *Journal of Hepatology*, 48, 1000–1007.
8. Chou, R., & Wasson, N. (2013). Blood tests to diagnose fibrosis or cirrhosis in patients with chronic hepatitis C virus infection. *Annals of Internal Medicine*, 158(11), 807–820.
9. Sharma, S., Khalili, K., & Nguyen, G. C. (2014). Non-invasive diagnosis of advanced fibrosis and cirrhosis. *World Journal of Gastroenterology*, 20(45), 16820–16830. doi:10.3748/wjg.v20.i45.16820.
10. Grace, N. D., & Minor, M. A. Portal hypertension & esophageal variceal hemorrhage. In N. J. Greenberger, R. S. Blumberg, & R. Burakoff (Eds.), *CURRENT diagnosis & treatment: Gastroenterology, hepatology, & endoscopy* (3rd ed.). New York, NY: McGraw-Hill. http://accessmedicine.mhmedical.com.ezproxy.simmons.edu/content.aspx?bookid=1621&sectionid=105187152. (Accessed May 18, 2019).
11. Avila, P., & Grace, N. D. Cirrhosis and its complications. In S. C. McKean, J. J. Ross, D. D. Dressler, & D. B. Scheurer (Eds.), *Principles and practice of hospital medicine* (2nd ed.). New York, NY: McGraw-Hill. http://accessmedicine.mhmedical.com.ezproxy.simmons.edu/content.aspx?bookid=1872&sectionid=146982218. (Accessed May 18, 2019).
12. Crespo, S., Bridges, M., Nakhleh, R., et al. (2013). Non-invasive assessment of liver fibrosis using magnetic resonance elastography in liver transplant recipients with hepatitis C. *Clinical Transplantation*, 27(5), 652–658.
13. Xiao, H., Shi, M., Xie, Y., & Chi, X. (2017). Comparison of diagnostic accuracy of magnetic resonance elastography and Fibroscan for detecting liver fibrosis in chronic hepatitis B patients: A systematic review and meta-analysis. *PLoS ONE*, 12(11), doi:10.1371/journal.pone.0186660. e0186660.
14. Bruno, S., Stroffolini, T., & Colombo, M. (2007). Sustained virological response to interferon-alpha is associated with improved outcome in HCV-related cirrhosis; a retrospective study. *Hepatology (Baltimore, Md.)*, 45, 579–587.
15. Jack, K. (2014). Hepatitis C: From discovery to eradication. *Gastrointest Nurs*, 7, 26–35.
16. Fowler, C. (2013). Management of patients with complications of cirrhosis. *Nursing Practice (Edinburgh, Scotland)*, 38(4), 14–22.
17. Grattagliano, I., Ubaldi, E., Bonfrate, L., & Portincasa, P. (2011). Management of liver cirrhosis between primary care and specialists. *World Journal of Gastroenterology*, 17(18), 2273–2282. doi:10.3748/wjg.v17.i18.2273.
18. Amodio, P., et al. (2013). The nutritional management of hepatic encephalopathy in patients with cirrhosis: International Society for Hepatic Encephalopathy and Nitrogen Metabolism consensus. *Hepatology (Baltimore, Md.)*, 58, 325. Retrieved from http://www.jwatch.org/na31703/2013/07/19/nutritional-management-patients-with-cirrhosis-and-hepatic#sthash.vFgCHJvg.dpuf.

CHAPTER **113**

CONSTIPATION
Courtney L. Betts

 Immediate referral is indicated for sudden change in bowel habits after the age of 50, weight loss, blood in the stool, anemia, family history of colon cancer or inflammatory bowel disease, acute constipation in the elderly.[1,2]

DEFINITION AND EPIDEMIOLOGY

Constipation, one of the most common gastrointestinal complaints in the United States, affects approximately 20% of the general population with 235 million dollars spent annually in medical costs and more than 820 million dollars spent on laxatives.[1-4] This chronic disorder disproportionately affects women, children, older adults, people of low socioeconomic status, obese patients, non-white individuals and people with low-fiber diet.[2,5] Up to 50% of nursing home residents have constipation and 74% of the residents use daily laxatives.[6] Constipation in older adults can be secondary to diminished vitality, decreased fluid intake, diets high in fat and protein and low in fiber, decreased activity, and the consequences of many illnesses and medications (Box 113.1).[6] Although it is not usually considered life-threatening, constipation can be disconcerting and disabling and can cause a decrease in quality of life.[1,5,7] It can also be associated with hemorrhoids, anal fissures, rectal prolapse, impaction, and ileus.[5,8]

Constipation is usually defined by practitioners as a decrease in the frequency of bowel movements to fewer than three per week,[6,8] and patients usually describe symptoms of passing hard stools, straining, and incomplete defecation.[6] For Rome IV criteria to be fulfilled (a consensus on gastrointestinal [GI] disorders compiled by leading experts), two or more of the following must have been present for at least 3 months with onset 6 months before diagnosis: fewer than three bowel movements per week, the passage of hard or lumpy stools (Bristol stool chart types 1 and 2, Fig. 113.1), a sensation of straining with more than 25% of defecations, a feeling of incomplete evacuation or anorectal obstruction in more than 25% of defecations, or use of manual maneuvers to aid defecation in more than 25% of defecations.[1,9] In addition, soft, easily passed stools are not present without the use of medication such as laxatives, and there is insufficient criteria for irritable bowel syndrome.[1] The Rome criteria were most recently updated in 2016.[10] Compared to early versions of Rome criteria, Rome IV is moving away from the terminology of "functional" GI disorders to "Disorders of Brain-Gut Interaction."[10] There is developing understanding regarding gut bacteria, gut permeability, and altered immune function (among others) and how these affect GI disorders.[10] In addition, new with the Rome IV is the category of opioid-induced constipation related to the change in bowels when taking opioids.[10] True clinical diagnosis of constipation is the finding of a large amount of feces in the rectal ampulla on digital examination or excessive feces in the colon, rectum, or both on the abdominal radiograph.

PATHOPHYSIOLOGY

The primary function of the large intestine is to store and to concentrate fecal material before defecation. If the fecal contents remain in the large intestine for long periods, almost all

---

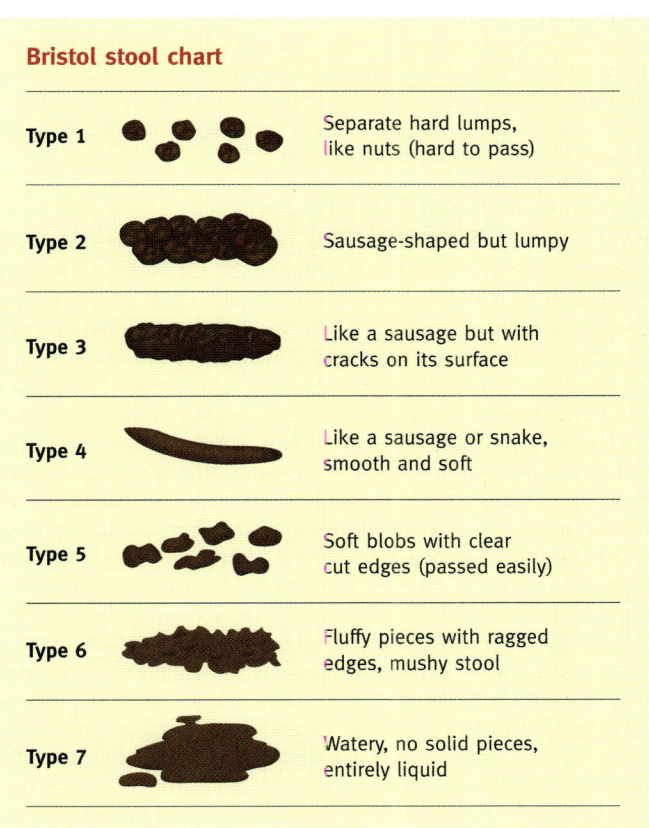

Bristol stool chart

Type 1		Separate hard lumps, like nuts (hard to pass)
Type 2		Sausage-shaped but lumpy
Type 3		Like a sausage but with cracks on its surface
Type 4		Like a sausage or snake, smooth and soft
Type 5		Soft blobs with clear cut edges (passed easily)
Type 6		Fluffy pieces with ragged edges, mushy stool
Type 7		Watery, no solid pieces, entirely liquid

FIG. 113.1 Bristol stool chart. (Data from Emmanuel, A., & Butt, S. [2015]. Small intestine and colon motility. *Medicine, 43*[5], 271–275.)

water is absorbed, resulting in hard stools. Normal colonic motility depends on the integrity of the central nervous system, autonomic nervous system, gut wall innervation and receptors, circular smooth muscle, gastrointestinal neurotransmitters, and hormones. Healthy adults have normal gut transit time, whereas total gut transit time is prolonged in patients with constipation.

Causes of constipation can be classified as either acute or chronic. Acute constipation can be indicative of another pathologic condition (see differential diagnosis) and requires immediate attention.[2] However, acute constipation usually occurs with dietary changes, travel, or stress and often resolves on its own or with minimal intervention.[1] Chronic constipation is further differentiated between primary (idiopathic) or secondary. Primary causes include: irritable bowel syndrome (constipation predominant), disordered colonic transit (normal or slow transit), and evacuation disorders (a failure to adequately empty the rectal contents) such as dyssynergic defecation.[1,5] Dyssynergic defecation is the inability of the abdominal and pelvic floor muscles to coordinate correctly and empty stool; this problem can affect half of patients with chronic constipation.[11] Identifying if the patient has dyssynergic defecation is important because different treatments will be more effective.[9]

Secondary causes of constipation are related to medical and psychogenic conditions, medications, structural abnormalities, and lifestyle.[5,8] These include ignoring the urge to defecate; inadequate fiber or fluid intake; medications; pregnancy; hypothyroidism; hypoparathyroidism; diabetes; hypokalemia; hypercalcemia; motility disorders; psychological disturbances; and neurologic disorders, such as Parkinson disease, multiple sclerosis, and disorders of the peripheral or central nervous system.[2,5,8] Fistulas, hemorrhoids, rectoceles, abscesses, neoplasms, and other functional abnormalities are also associated with constipation, but the cause can be idiopathic or even related to irritable bowel syndrome.[1,2,6,12]

CLINICAL PRESENTATION AND PHYSICAL EXAMINATION

Constipation is a subjective complaint and varies from one individual to another. Patients may have daily bowel movements but still feel constipated.[8] Patients may complain of constipation and describe a feeling of nausea, bloating, straining, cramping, and difficulty passing stools. A stool diary for 7 days can be helpful and should include when the change in bowel pattern occurred; the number of stools per day and week; the last bowel movement; the need to strain during defecation; the sensation of incomplete evacuation; the need to self-disimpact or the need for vaginal splinting; and any episodes of fecal incontinence, diarrhea, abdominal pain, or blood or pain with defecation.[1,5,8] Patients can use the Bristol stool chart (see Fig. 113.1) to assess bowel transit time.[5] Patients who indicate that their main concerns are incomplete evacuation, feeling of obstruction, and manual disimpaction may have a defecatory disorder.[8] Possible systemic, neurologic, or other related symptoms should be elicited in addition to a past history of associated illnesses, a 24-hour dietary and fluid review, and a complete medication review (including laxative and over-the-counter medication use). Alarm symptoms and factors include sudden change in bowel habits after the age of 50, weight loss, blood in the stool, anemia, and family history of colon cancer or inflammatory bowel disease.[1,5]

The physical examination is performed to exclude or to verify the symptoms of constipation, though it is not uncommon to have normal findings. Orthostatic hypotension or tachycardia implies dehydration; weight loss suggests anorexia or carcinoma. The oral examination may suggest poor dentition, ill-fitting dentures, lesions, or dehydration. Abdominal scars indicate a surgical history. Peristalsis and bowel sounds may be increased or decreased, suggesting a threatened obstruction or ileus. There may be increased dullness over areas of stool, and masses may be palpated. Rebound tenderness suggests a peritoneal inflammation. A gynecologic examination may demonstrate a rectocele. A digital rectal examination should determine anal abnormalities, sphincter tone and function, pain, lesions, rectal prolapse, impaction, hemorrhoids, or fissures. The neurologic examination may elicit autonomic dysfunction or neuropathy. Perineal descent is assessed by having the patient bear down while lying in the left lateral position (normal perineal descent while straining is 1 to 4 cm).[13]

DIAGNOSTICS
Essential Diagnostics

If abdominal discomfort, nausea, or vomiting is present, abdominal x-ray studies or abdominal computed tomography (CT) scan and complete blood count (CBC) with differential are necessary to exclude obstruction, ileus, megacolon, and volvulus.[14] Alarm symptoms mandate an evaluation for an obstructing neoplasm with colonoscopy.[8] CBC, thyroid-stimulating hormone (TSH), and a chemistry profile, including calcium and blood glucose concentrations, are indicated in chronic constipation if metabolic diseases are suspected.[5] Urinalysis and culture may reveal chronic cystitis, which is often related to constipation. If alarm symptoms are not present, it is reasonable to start with a trial of laxatives before additional diagnostic tests.[2]

Additional Diagnostics

Anorectal manometry, balloon expulsion test, colonic transit assessment (wireless motility capsule or radiopaque marker test), barium and magnetic resonance defecography, and colonic manometry can also be considered depending on patient presentation and physical exam.[5] Rectal balloon expulsion testing and anorectal manometry are important diagnostics when considering dyssynergic defecation.[1,2,5]

INITIAL DIAGNOSTICS

Constipation

LABORATORY
- Complete blood count with differential
- Urinalysis[a]
- Stool for occult blood
- Thyroid-stimulating hormone
- Serum glucose, serum electrolytes including calcium, blood urea nitrogen, creatinine

IMAGING
- Abdominal radiography (kidneys, ureters and urinary bladder [KUB], flat plate, and upright)[a]
- Abdominal ultrasound[a]

OTHER DIAGNOSTICS
- Colonoscopy[a]

[a]If indicated.

DIFFERENTIAL DIAGNOSIS

It is critical to recognize the pathologic conditions that first manifest as constipation. Acute-onset constipation requires emergent evaluation to identify ileus, intra-abdominal infection (e.g., appendicitis, diverticulitis), toxic megacolon, or an obstructing lesion.[14,15] Causes of chronic constipation that must be considered include anxiety or other psychogenic disorder, colorectal carcinoma, colonic obstruction, ovarian cancer, hypothyroidism, hypopituitary disorder, diabetes, hypokalemia, hypercalcemia, motility disorder, rectal fissure, scleroderma, multiple sclerosis, Parkinson disorder, amyotrophic lateral sclerosis (ALS), and irritable bowel syndrome.[5,7]

 Priority differentials include (1) intra-abdominal infection (2) ileus (3) toxic megacolon (4) obstructive lesion.

INTERPROFESSIONAL COLLABORATIVE MANAGEMENT

Nonpharmacologic Management

The initial approach should include management of secondary causes such as medical and psychogenic conditions, medications, structural abnormalities, and lifestyle changes including dietary measures, periodic exercise, and bowel training.[16] See Box 113.1 for a list of medications.

Stool Diary. Advise patient to keep a stool diary (note frequency of stooling, types of stools using Bristol stool chart [see Fig. 113.1], and any associated symptoms), both to substantiate the constipation and to aid in determining the effectiveness of interventions.[16]

Fiber. Increase fiber to 25 to 30 g/day over a period of weeks.[16] It is important to increase fiber slowly because it can cause bloating, gas, and abdominal discomfort.[5] Six prunes twice a day have been shown to increase stool frequency.[16] Fiber increases the stool's water absorbency, which in turn increases bulk and weight of the stool, making it easier to pass.[3] It should be noted that fiber is unlikely to help constipation in patients with slow transit constipation or outlet dysfunction.[3,16] Fiber supplements combined with increased fluids are recommended if a patient is unable to consume the required diet.

Bowel Habits. Instruct patients to allow enough time for satisfactory bowel elimination and to attempt to defecate during a specific time period each day. Encourage the patient to toilet 30 minutes after eating a meal because eating stimulates the gastrocolic response. Suggest placing feet on a foot stool while on the toilet, or using a toilet that is low to the ground may also be helpful.[16]

Pharmacologic Management

Pharmacologic treatment is appropriate if there is no response to conservative measures.

Stool Softeners or Emollients. Stool softeners, such as docusate sodium, may be added to soften the stool if bulk-forming agents are ineffective; however, there is little evidence suggesting the effectiveness of stool softeners for treatment of chronic constipation.[6,13] Mineral oil, an emollient, will soften stool, but it has been associated with aspiration and lipoid pneumonia, prevents absorption of fat-soluble vitamins, and can cause fecal incontinence; it is not generally recommended.[14]

Probiotics. Changes can occur in gut microbes from diet, toxins, lifestyle, and/or antibiotics; probiotics may return immunologic balance to the gut.[17] Probiotics, such as *Lactobacillus*, *Bifidobacterium*, and *Saccharomyces*, may help increase stool frequency.[16–18]

Osmotic Laxatives. Osmotic laxatives (magnesium hydroxide, polyethylene glycol (PEG), lactulose, sorbitol) are hypertonic medications that cause secretion of water through osmosis into the intestinal wall, resulting in diarrhea.[6] Osmotic laxatives, such as PEG, are first-line treatment compared with stimulant laxatives, because there is more research showing efficacy of PEG.[1] PEG is also more effective than lactulose.[1,16] Lactulose should be used cautiously in patients with diabetes. PEG or milk of magnesia should be used judiciously in patients with a history of congestive heart failure or renal insufficiency to avoid fluid and electrolyte abnormalities.[16]

Simulant Laxatives. Stimulant laxatives (senna, bisacodyl) increase intestinal motility by stimulating colonic mucosa and decreasing water absorption.[16] The chronic use of senna or bisacodyl was previously contraindicated, but new studies show no evidence of injury to the enteric nervous system with long-term use.[6]

Enemas. Enemas are useful when there are mobility issues and fecal impaction is a concern.[3] Tap water enemas are safer if frequent use is needed, as electrolyte imbalances can occur with phosphate enemas.[3]

Secretagogues. Lubiprostone, linaclotide, and plecanatide are newer drugs that increase fluid secretion into the lumen and improve colonic transit.[1,5] Lubiprostone, a chloride channel activator, does not cause electrolyte imbalances; nausea is a common side effect.[5] Women who may potentially be pregnant should have a negative pregnancy test before starting lubiprostone and should use contraceptives while taking lubiprostone.[1] Linaclotide, a guanylate cyclase-C receptor agonist, is generally safe and effective; a common side effect is diarrhea.[1] Plecantaide is a guanylate cyclase-C agonist that was approved for the market in 2017; a common side effect is diarrhea.[1]

Serotonergic Agents. 5-Hydroxytryptamine receptor 4 (serotonin) agonists (tegaserod maleate, prucalopride) have either been taken off the U.S. market because of adverse cardiovascular events reported in some uses or are only approved in Canada and Europe.[5]

Opioid Antagonists. PAMORA (peripherally acting mu-opioid receptor antagonists), such as naloxegol and methylnaltrexone, are useful in treating opioid-induced constipation; however, the goal is to reduce the opioids as the first step to improving constipation.[1]

Other Treatments. Patients with constipation related to pelvic floor dysfunction or neurologic injury may benefit from biofeedback training.[11] Surgical evaluation is necessary for patients with rectal prolapse and for those who require surgical intervention.[2] Sacral nerve stimulation is used for some patients with intractable constipation; however, it is not approved in the United States and studies are inconclusive.[2] Acupuncture may also be considered.[19]

The phases of constipation management are listed in Box 113.2.

INDICATIONS FOR REFERRAL OR HOSPITALIZATION

Nausea, vomiting, fever, and abdominal pain may indicate an ileus or ischemia and must be managed accordingly.[15] Treatment is usually supportive and requires physician consultation when hospitalization is necessary to provide parenteral fluids

BOX **113.2**

Constipation Management

PHASE 1
Make lifestyle changes.
- Exercise regularly.
- Develop regular bowel habits.

Make dietary changes.
- Increase dietary fiber to 25–30 g/day (prunes, bananas, bran, beans, broccoli, spinach, carrots, corn, potato, apple, and pears with skin).
- Decrease fats, particularly cheese.
- Increase fluids to 1.5–2 L/day.

PHASE 2
Use bulk-forming laxatives.
- Psyllium (Metamucil) 2.5–30 g daily in divided doses
- Methylcellulose (Citrucel) 2 g daily in divided doses
- Calcium polycarbophil (FiberCon), 1 tablet with 8 oz of water 1–4 times daily, followed by a second glass of water

PHASE 3
Use stool softeners.
- Docusate sodium: 100 mg PO twice daily followed by 8 oz of water

PHASE 4
Use osmotic laxatives.
- MiraLax: 17 g in 8 oz of water prn daily[a]
- Milk of magnesia: 30 mL PO prn at bedtime
- Lactulose: 15–30 mL PO daily to twice a day, up to 60 mL/day in divided doses[a]

PHASE 5
Use stimulant laxatives.
- Bisacodyl: 5–15 mg PO daily prn
- Senna (Senokot): 2 tablets PO prn at bedtime
- Bisacodyl (Dulcolax) suppository: 1 per rectum every 3 days prn

PHASE 6
Use intestinal secretagogues.
- Lubiprostone 24 mcg twice a day[a] for chronic constipation
- Linaclotide 145 mcg daily[a] for chronic constipation
- Plecanatide 3 mg PO daily[a]

PHASE 7
Severely constipated patients may require both oral laxatives and enemas or a suppository to alleviate constipation.

---

[a]These products may be expensive.
Data from Rao, S. Chronic constipation: Assessment and treatment options. http://www.gastroendonews.com/Review-Articles/Article/08-17/Chronic-Constipation-Assessment-and-Treatment-Options/42171/ses=ogst?enl=true; National Institute of Diabetes and Digestive and Kidney Diseases. (2018). Eating, diet, & nutrition for constipation in children.[21] https://www.niddk.nih.gov/health-information/digestive-diseases/constipation-children/eating-diet-nutrition; Feldman, M., Friedman, L., & Brandt, L. (2010). *Sleisenger and Fordtran's Gastrointestinal and Liver Disease* (9th ed.). Philadelphia: Saunders; and Greenberger, N. (2018). Constipation. https://www.merckmanuals.com/professional/gastrointestinal-disorders/symptoms-of-gi-disorders/constipation.

and pain management. Referral to a gastroenterologist is indicated if a pathologic condition is suspected or if therapies are unsuccessful.

LIFE SPAN CONSIDERATIONS
Older adults are more prone to constipation.[20] Common causes include medications, disease, diet, and lack of physical activity.[3] Studies show constipation in older adults can be related to physiological changes (e.g., altered colonic motility, decreased inhibitory nerves in the smooth muscle membrane, and altered rectal sensitivity).[3,20]

COMPLICATIONS
Complications of constipation include the development of ileus, ischemic bowel, megacolon, hernia, hemorrhoids, fecal impaction, or rectal or uterine prolapse.

PATIENT AND FAMILY EDUCATION
It is imperative that lifestyle changes be reinforced to establish consistent bowel habits. Patients should not delay in responding to the call to defecate and should be encouraged to sit on the toilet, with feet placed on a stool, at the same time each day for approximately 10 minutes; this should occur preferably after meals or the ingestion of a warm liquid to stimulate the gastrocolic reflex. The promotion of a low-fat, high-fiber diet and 2 L of fluid per day are recommended. However, dietary fiber should be gradually introduced to avoid severe cramping and bloating. It is important that patients receive a careful explanation of medication side effects and understand the importance of avoiding laxatives during pregnancy or unless necessary. Patients should also contact the health care provider for any change in bowel habits or if the constipation is associated with fever, bleeding, weight loss, and abdominal pain.

REFERENCES
1. Rao, S. Chronic constipation: assessment and treatment options. Retrieved from http://www.gastroendonews.com/Review-Articles/Article/08-17/Chronic-Constipation-Assessment-and-Treatment-Options/42171/ses=ogst?enl=true. (Accessed 16 December 2017).
2. Rao, S., Rattanakovit, K., & Patcharatrakul, T. (2016). Diagnosis and management of chronic constipation in adults. *Gastroenterology & Hepatology*, 13, 295–305.
3. Vazuez Roque, M., & Bouras, E. (2015). Epidemiology and management of chronic constipation in elderly patients. *Clinical Interventions in Aging*, 10, 919–930.
4. Rao, S. Health-care burden and cost of constipation and fecal incontinence: the silent afflictions. Retrieved from http://www.gastro.org/news_items/2015/5/6/health-care-burden-and-costs-of-constipation-and-fecal-incontinence-the-silent-afflictions. (Accessed 16 December 2017).
5. Brenner, D., & Shah, M. (2016). Chronic constipation. *Gastroenterology Clinics of North America*, 45, 205–216.
6. De Giorgio, R., Ruggeri, E., Stanghellini, V., Eusebi, L., Bazzoli, F., & Chiarioni, G. (2015). Chronic constipation in the elderly: A primer for the gastroenterologist. *BMC Gastroenterology*, 15, 130.
7. Bharucha, A. E., Pemberton, J. H., & Locke, G. R. (2013). American Gastroenterological Association technical review on constipation. *Gastroenterology*, 144, 218–238.
8. Bharucha, A. E., Dorn, S. D., Lembo, A., & Pressman, A. (2013). American Gastroenterological Association medical position statement on constipation. *Gastroenterology*, 144, 211–217.
9. Lacy, B., Mearin, F., Chang, L., Chey, W., Lembo, A., Simren, M., et al. (2016). Bowel disorders. *Gastroenterology*, 150, 1393–1407.
10. Simren, M., Palsson, O. S., & Whitehead, W. E. (2017). Update on Rome IV criteria for colorectal disorders: Implications for clinical practice. *Current Gastroenterology Reports*, 19, 15.
11. Rao, S. (2016). Diagnosis and treatment of dyssynergic defecation. *Journal of Neurogastroenterology and Motility*, 22(3), 423–435.

12. Anal fistula. Cleveland Clinic. Retrieved from https://my.clevelandclinic.org/health/diseases/14466-anal-fistula. (Accessed 20 December 2017).

13. Lembo, A. Constipation. *Sleisenger and Fordtran's Gastrointestinal and Liver Disease*, Chapter 19, 270–296.e9.

14. Greenberger, N. Constipation. Retrieved from https://www.merckmanuals.com/professional/gastrointestinal-disorders/symptoms-of-gi-disorders/constipation. (Accessed 18 May 2019).

15. Ansari, P. Intestinal obstruction. Retrieved from https://www.merckmanuals.com/professional/gastrointestinal-disorders/acute-abdomen-and-surgical-gastroenterology/intestinal-obstruction. (Accessed 18 May 2019).

16. Lacy, B., Mearin, F., Chang, L., Chey, W., Lembo, A., Simren, M., et al. (2016). Bowel disorders. *Gastroenterology, 150*(6), 1393–1407.

17. Wilkins, T., & Sequoia, J. (2017). Probiotics for gastrointestinal conditions: A summary of the evidence. *American Family Physician, 96*(3), 170–178A.

18. Martinez-Martinez, M., Calabuig-Tolsa, R., & Cauli, O. (2017). The effect of probiotics as a treatment for constipation in elderly people: A systematic review. *Archives of Gerontology and Geriatrics, 71*, 142–149.

19. Emmanuel, A., & Butt, S. (2015). Small intestine and colon motility. *Medicine, 43*(5), 271–275.

20. Schuster, B., Kosar, L., & Kamrul, R. (2015). Constipation in older adults: Stepwise approach to keep things moving. *Canadian Family Physician, 61*, 152–158.

21. Eating, diet, & nutrition for constipation in children. National Institute of Diabetes and Digestive and Kidney Diseases. Retrieved from https://www.niddk.nih.gov/health-information/digestive-diseases/constipation-children/eating-diet-nutrition. (Accessed 18 May 2019).

CHAPTER **114**

DIARRHEA, NONINFECTIOUS

Michelle Freshman

DEFINITION AND EPIDEMIOLOGY

Diarrhea is generally appreciated as an increase in stool frequency of more than three unformed stools per day, typically appearing loose or liquid, often characterized by urgency, and consistent with a daily stool weight greater than 250 g.[1,2] By contrast, hyperdefecation, or pseudodiarrhea, is an increase in stool frequency without a concomitant change in stool consistency.[2] Diarrhea can range from a mild, self-limited episode to a severe, life-threatening illness. Acute diarrhea, lasting less than 2 weeks, whether it is infectious or noninfectious, usually improves without intervention. Persistent diarrhea over 2 to 4 weeks may be associated with a protozoal or other endemic infection.[3] When diarrhea continues for a month without improvement, it is considered chronic. Along with diarrhea, fecal incontinence may occur, although they can be distinct.

Among inhabitants of industrialized countries with adequate sanitation, chronic diarrhea may account for 1% to 5% of cases annually.[2,4] Congregate-dwelling, immunocompromised, and hospitalized elderly patients are at increased risk.[5]

Although the majority of acute and persistent cases of diarrhea are infectious, a much smaller percentage of cases are noninfectious,[3] being caused by trauma, medications, toxins, transient ischemia, diverticulitis, or flares of irritable bowel syndrome (IBS) or inflammatory bowel disease (IBD). In fact, reports of IBS alone may be as high as 11% worldwide[6] and an estimated 10% to 20% in the United States, with as many as one-third of these cases featuring diarrhea as the predominant type (IBS-D).[5] Yet more recent surveillance data in English-speaking countries, using new criteria for IBS citing abdominal pain as integral to the diagnosis, supports

a prevalence of IBS-D closer to 6%.[7–9] Criteria for characterizing IBS-D can overlap with other organic entities such as celiac disease and microscopic colitis, which would require microscopic evidence for definitive diagnosis.[2] Aside from protracted episodes of functional bowel disease (including IBS-D), chronic diarrhea is usually related to a host of malabsorptive, autoimmune, endocrine, malignant, and surgical conditions. It can be intermittent or continuous, with or without extraintestinal complications.

 Prompt medical evaluation is indicated if diarrhea is associated with fever, significant abdominal pain, bloody stool, dehydration, significant unintentional weight loss, or family history of colorectal cancer in first degree relative under age 50, as this raises the risk of colorectal cancer ninefold.[6,10]

PATHOPHYSIOLOGY

Approximately 9 to 10 L of fluid enters the small intestine daily, yet only a fraction leaves the body within stool.[1,11] In 95% of individuals, 200 mL of fluid or less is excreted—more with higher dietary fiber. The colon recovers up to four times its usual volume but is dependent on a tempered flow rate, allowing enough time for the maximal reabsorption of 800 mL to occur. The small intestine absorbs 7.5 L and the large intestine absorbs 1.3 L[1]; this volume accounts for nearly all of the excess reabsorption of water. A key mechanism in water regulation is epithelial transport—that is, sodium and chloride regulation across the membrane surface by cholinergic, adrenergic, and serotonergic mediators.[8] A second critical factor is the integrity of the mucosal barrier through intracellular junctions, which supports these ion exchanges. However, disruption of the barrier alone does not lead to profuse diarrhea.[11] The complexity involved in solute transport and barrier permeability as well as motility (such as the influence of 5-HT on transit time), in addition to inflammatory mechanisms (such as microflora alterations in short-chain fatty acids produced by fermentation of carbohydrates)[12] has given way to evolving research into immune dysfunction, including the role of reduced microbiome diversity as well as the brain-gut axis.[8,11,13,14] The acronym ALPINE (autocrine, luminal, paracrine, immune, neural, and endocrine) has been proposed to explain the multiple concurrent mechanisms at work in watery diarrhea; these influence the paracellular pathway, epithelium, muscle, and blood flow, affecting permeability, transport, and motility.[11]

Although some focus on three presentation categories—watery (secretory and osmotic diarrhea), fatty, and inflammatory diarrhea—others separately account for osmotic, secretory, fatty, and inflammatory disorders (including noninvasive infections) as well as motility and functional irregularities. In fact, these entities can overlap in some conditions.

Osmotic diarrhea includes malabsorptive disorders and results from ingested, solute-rich molecules (e.g., sugar-free gum, alpha glucosidase, ampicillin, clindamycin, polyethylene glycol, methyldopa, quinidines, hydralazine, angiotensin-converting enzyme inhibitors (ACEIs), procainamide, propranolol, enteral feeds, laxatives with magnesium, phosphates)[1] leaving the vascular space and entering the colon. This, in turn, draws more water and salt into the intestinal lumen or may prevent water from entering the vascular space. Stool osmolality differentiates osmotic from secretory sources. Diarrhea starts postprandially and typically ends with fasting or discontinuation of the identified ingredient.

Secretory diarrhea is the most common type. It is more likely to result in very watery stools as the absorptive function of the gut is compromised. The net secretion of anions (sodium, chloride, bicarbonate, and potassium) and solute (mainly glucose) transporters at the level of the mucosal barrier (facing the apical lumen and basolateral circulation) as well as changes in the activation of cyclic nucleotide and calcium signaling pathways favor secretion over absorption.[5] Along the intestinal epithelium are intestinal crypts, promoting secretion, and intestinal villi, promoting absorption by enterocytes.[5] Secretory diarrhea typically involves chemical (bacterial enterotoxins, viruses, parasites, drugs), mechanical (surgery, radiation), or functional disruptions (congenital diseases like cystic fibrosis, bacterial overgrowth, bile acid malabsorption) that produce an excess of electrolyte, nutrient, and water content in the colon. Adequate surface area and contact time to absorb intestinal nutrients and water is critical and may vary with the segmental length or type of diseased or resected intestinal tissue.[2] HIV enteropathy is thought to involve loss of adequate crypt and villous function, leading to inflammation, further membrane damage, and autonomic nerve impairment.[15] Nonosmotic medications, endocrine disorders, and cancers also contribute. Large-volume isotonic or hypertonic fluid enters the colon, and the resulting watery diarrhea does not typically resolve with fasting. Large-volume secretory diarrhea is more likely to present without white or red blood cell exudate, fever, or systemic complaints. Nocturnal diarrhea can be a defining feature. Medications contributing to secretory diarrhea include amoxicillin-clavulanate, caffeine, cholinesterase inhibitors, cholestyramine, secretory laxatives (senna, bisacodyl), levodopa benaserazide, metformin, misoprostol, nonsteroidal antiinflammatory drugs (NSAIDs), and simvastatin.[1]

Steatorrhea, a subset of secretory diarrhea known as *fatty diarrhea*, is usually associated with malabsorption or maldigestion involving mucosal changes, ileal disease or surgery, bile acid deficiency, or pancreatic exocrine insufficiency. For example, loss of intrinsic factor from surgery or a damaged ileum will result in unconjugated bile salts that spill into the colon, pulling additional water into the lumen. Bile acid malabsorption is associated with cases involving disease or surgery in up to 100 cm of the ileum and can lead to diarrhea; resection or disease involving more than 100 cm of the ileum is more likely to cause steatorrhea.[16] Up to 20% of ingested carbohydrates may elude small bowel absorption in well adults, contributing to an increase in bacterially activated short-chain fatty acids, which in turn stimulates 5-HT before becoming absorbed in the colon.[8,11]

Overlapping conditions exist. A significant number of patients with chronic IBS with diarrhea predominance (IBS-D) and microscopic colitis (diagnosed in 10% to 15% of chronic diarrhea patients)[17] also have diarrhea that responds to bile acid binders in the absence of structural change.[16] Pale, sticky, foul-smelling stool can also be the result of celiac disease caused by malabsorption of gluten and in some patients; this condition overlaps with microscopic colitis possibly due to human leukocyte antigen patterns similar to those that characterize subtypes of celiac disease.[18] Malabsorption of bile acids resulting from the use of biguanides by diabetics may cause vitamin B_{12} malabsorption with diarrhea.[1,16] Diabetic diarrhea results from nerve damage.[19] Long-term use of neomycin/polymyxin/bacitracin as well as antiretrovirals, colchicine,

L-thyroxine, methyldopa, octreotide, and orlistat specifically contribute to steatorrhea.[1] Likewise, small intestinal bacterial overgrowth syndrome (e.g., after cholecystectomy) is associated with malabsorption. Maldigestion results from decreased bile salts due to congestion (e.g., cirrhosis, bile duct obstruction) and pancreatic dysfunction (e.g., chronic pancreatitis, cystic fibrosis).[2]

The inflammatory type of diarrhea results from injury to the absorptive mechanism of the epithelium. Tight junctions (zona occludens) prevent extracellular fluid absorption. The expression of claudins, which affects permeability at tight junctions, has been implicated in IBD.[11] Without an intact epithelium, serum and blood can pass into the lumen and water cannot be absorbed adequately. NSAIDs can contribute to this type of injury.[1] Vascular injury, whether mechanical or drug-induced due to vasoconstriction (ergotamine, cocaine),[1] can also cause inflammatory diarrhea. Exudative or inflammatory conditions resulting in febrile illness or blood and pus in the stool are typically associated with pain. Tumor necrosis factor (TNF) and interleukin-6 production as a result of T-cell and neutrophil activation during inflammation are linked to chloride secretion; moreover, the inhibition of sodium absorption and further chloride excretion has links to other inflammatory pathways.[5] Thus water absorption is compromised. Diverticulitis, ischemic colitis, IBD, pseudomembranous colitis from *Clostridium difficile* invasion after antibiotic exposure, and a range of other viral, bacterial, and parasitic infections contribute to inflammatory diarrhea (cytomegalovirus, *Entamoeba histolytica*, tuberculosis).[2] Cancer treatment–induced diarrhea may be considered a subcategory of the exudative or even secretory type, inclusive of radiation enteritis.

Motility or dysregulation due to motor complex malfunction can drive gastrointestinal contents along the tract more quickly, resulting in inadequate absorption of fluid from the colon.[1] Some of these transit dysfunctions may also be considered secretory-type diarrheal disorders but include such a variety of conditions as to warrant separate mention.[11] Postsurgical complications may result in diarrhea. Surgeries with a high likelihood of causing this adverse effect include cholecystectomy, vagotomy, the Whipple procedure (pancreaticoduodenectomy), the Billroth II procedure (gastrojejunostomy), gastric bypass (Roux-en-Y), ileocolonic resection, and ileocecal valve removal or compromise. Bile salt malabsorption features largely in significantly resected or diseased ileum, causing an overflow into the colon and an osmotic gradient (with secretory and osmotic features in the barrier crossing). Erythromycin and metoclopramide shorten colonic transit time.

Motility disorders also include diarrhea-predominant IBS. Defined by commonly accepted Rome IV diagnostic criteria for functional gastrointestinal disorders, IBS-D is thought to result from the impact of many altered pathways, including that of opioid receptors (μ, κ, and δ).[13,20,21] Regulatory enzymes affecting ion secretion are more readily seen in the colorectal mucosa of IBS-D patients.[11] Postinfectious IBS-D occurs in about 10% of patients with intestinal gastroenteritis, especially in older patients, women, and those with severe symptoms; it may resolve in months or years, although data conflict.[14] There is some effort to move away from the term *functional*; however, these disorders are thought to represent a spectrum of presentations. Symptoms in any one patient can vary over time. Lately there has been more focus on the biopsychosocial influences on nonorganic diarrhea—such as dietary influences on gut flora, abnormal motility, increased perception of visceral sensations, immune dysregulation–mucosal membrane permeability through leaky tight junctions, intraluminal antigens causing inflammation of the submucosa—as well as recognition of the premorbid psychological, social stressors, and comorbid responses (gut-brain axis) as contributing factors.[11,13]

One treatment focus has been on the hormone serotonin, with more receptors in the gut than the brain. The serotonin reuptake transporter has a critical effect on the increase or decrease of gastrointestinal motility through the 5-HT$_3$ and 5-HT$_4$ receptors, which have been harnessed in medical therapy directed against diarrhea-predominant IBS.

A subset of patients with functional bowel disease have significant psychological disorders that are more likely to respond to psychiatric comanagement, including those with factitious diarrhea, who might tamper with stool samples or simulate or perpetuate symptoms for secondary gain or out of emotional distress.

CLINICAL PRESENTATION AND PHYSICAL EXAMINATION

The initial history should include the patient's normal stool pattern as compared with the new-onset diarrhea. Charting of when the diarrhea began—whether the onset was abrupt or gradual, the course's duration, and daily stool consistency and frequency (discrete or continuous) as well as when diarrhea occurs with respect to mealtime and sleep—will help frame the clinical picture. Any improvement or worsening of the condition or associated symptoms should be elicited as part of the history.

Attention should be given to new-onset urgency; lower abdominal spasms, whether across the abdomen or localized to one side; relief of spasms after a movement; rectal discomfort or tenesmus; a sense of incomplete evacuation; or fecal incontinence. Bloody or mucopurulent exudates in the stool might reveal an inflammatory source. Greasy, bulky, rancid-smelling stools that are difficult to flush suggest fat or carbohydrate malabsorption related to small bowel or pancreatic dysfunction. Whether the stool is mostly watery or unformed is also helpful in sorting out a potential secretory source. Alternating patterns of diarrhea and constipation, diarrhea that awakens the patient from sleep, and any history of hemorrhoids will help to determine the diagnosis. A previous history of manual disimpaction and chronic constipation or recent narcotic use might suggest overflow diarrhea in the setting of fecal impaction.

It is important to gauge symptom relief achieved in relation to diet and over-the-counter or prescription medication. Associated signs and symptoms (e.g., nausea, vomiting, dehydration, abdominal cramping, pain, fever, chills, and rash) must be gleaned. Recent history of illness may point to postinfectious IBS-D. Foreign travel may contribute, particularly if a lingering viral, protozoal, helminthic, or mycobacterial source might be at root.[22] Likewise, an opportunistic infection can arise in an immunocompromised host. Other pertinent information includes increased thirst, dark or concentrated urine, oliguria, dizziness, and urinary tenesmus in consideration of renal insufficiency or undiagnosed diabetes or dehydration.

Determination of whether unintentional weight loss (gradual or acute) has occurred is critical; this may prompt a diagnosis of IBD, Addison disease, hyperthyroidism, or malignant disease (such as medullary thyroid cancer) in the absence of other findings, especially in older adults. Growth retardation or delayed onset of puberty can suggest celiac disease, juvenile-onset diabetes, or cystic fibrosis.

Medications are also commonly associated with diarrhea. This occurs as often as 7% of the time,[1] particularly involving magnesium, antihypertensives, NSAIDs (3% to 9% of those treated can have diarrhea, with an association in microscopic colitis and possibly IBD[18]), proton pump inhibitors, serotonin-receptor reuptake inhibitors and other antidepressants,[1] antibiotics, theophyllines, and chemotherapy agents.[4] The risk of developing microscopic colitis increases in association with proton pump inhibitors, antiplatelet agents, and statins, among others.[18] Chronic prednisone use can result in hypercortisolism with symptomatic diarrhea. Finally, over-the-counter and complementary products warrant further investigation for possible adverse effects or toxicity.

Allergic reactions to prescription medications and environmental exposures as well as food-related reactions are important. A dietary history should include any nutritional or dietary supplements or diet aids, especially sugar-free products that contain xylitol, sorbitol, or mannitol, which are poorly absorbed. Patients whose food sources lack niacin (vitamin B3 from tryptophan) secondary to alcoholism or food deprivation may develop pellagra, which is associated with diarrhea, dementia, and dermatitis.

The history should elicit previous medical conditions, in particular Addison disease, Behçet disease, vasculitis, common variable immunodeficiency (CVID) disease, cystic fibrosis, celiac disease with signs of dermatitis herpetiformis or osteoporosis, autoimmune enteropathy, diabetes mellitus type 1 or acquired diabetes mellitus, human immunodeficiency virus (HIV) infection or AIDS, hyperthyroidism or potentially over-medicated hypothyroidism, sarcoidosis, scleroderma, ischemia or renal blood flow difficulties, pancreatic insufficiency or other pancreatic conditions, appendectomy (associated with Crohn disease), protein-losing enteropathies, short bowel syndrome, gastrin excretion symptoms of Zollinger-Ellison syndrome, or pancreatic tumor.[22] A personal history of intestinal lymphoma, carcinoid, or other gastrointestinal tumors or prior radiation therapy to the abdomen or pelvis is important because radiation enteritis can result in diarrhea many years later. Gastric bypass or a Billroth II or Whipple procedure and associated complications—such as fistulas, blind loops, and strictures—may contribute to bacterial overgrowth and chronic mucosal surface changes, leading to diarrhea. Obstetric injury to the anal sphincter may be especially pertinent if there is fecal incontinence. A family medical history of the same or other chronic gastrointestinal conditions or cancers would be clinically relevant.

A social history of tobacco use, alcohol abuse, or illicit drug or recently unsupervised narcotic use may contribute to diarrhea. Smoking has been shown to increase the risk and earlier presentation of lymphocytic and collagenous colitis.[18] Diarrhea can be associated with weight-loss medications, amphetamines, and caffeinated products, including stimulating energy drinks and tea preparations. Finally, laxative abuse and other disturbed eating patterns, such as bulimia, might raise concern for self-injurious behavior. Munchausen syndrome, factitious diarrhea for secondary gain, malingering, and hypochondriasis are also seen. Situational stress, heightened anxiety, and panic attacks, which can be seen in association with depression, might contribute to a change in bowel pattern.

The physical examination includes temperature and orthostatic vital signs (blood pressure and heart rate [lying, sitting, and standing]) to assess volume depletion, rare autonomic neuropathy of diabetes, or amyloidosis.[11] The patient's mental status should be noted along with other signs or symptoms of wasting, including weight loss.

Dry mucous membranes, decreased skin turgor, and absent jugular venous pulsation would suggest significant dehydration. A close assessment should be done for skin pallor or hair thinning in patients with anemia; adrenocorticotropic hormone (ACTH)–related darkening of palmar creases and other sites, as in Addison disease; dermatographia (mast cell disease); icteric conjunctiva in advanced liver disease; evidence of exophthalmos and eyebrow thinning (hyperthyroidism); eye redness and pain of uveitis, episcleritis, or dry eyes (Whipple disease, IBD, lid lag in hyperthyroidism); subcutaneous bleeding resulting from lack of vitamin K or prolonged prothrombin time (cirrhosis); and erythema nodosum (ulcerative colitis). The head and neck should be assessed for evidence of immunocompromise, such as lymphadenopathy or oral leukoplakia in those undergoing cancer treatment or in AIDS patients, macroglossia (in rare cases of amyloidosis), or mouth ulcers in IBD, as well as thyromegaly or thyroid nodules. Carotid bruits may indicate arterial flow disease. Flushing might relate to carcinoid syndrome or mastocytosis.

A cardiovascular examination is indicated to exclude the cardiac complications associated with some illnesses, such as tachycardia in hyperthyroidism. Chest findings would be unusual except in suggesting systemic or metastasized diseases. Wheezing or a right-sided heart murmur might signify a carcinoid tumor. During the abdominal examination, care should be taken in noting abdominal scars, visible distention, and audible activity of the bowel including a succussion splash, which may provide evidence of delayed gastric emptying. In addition, an indication of impaired arterial flow would be seen in bounding abdominal pulses and heard as bruits. For completion of the examination, palpation should be performed for tenderness, rigidity, rebound, guarding, masses, organomegaly (enlarged liver from neuroendocrine tumor, amyloidosis, alcoholic fatty liver), or ascites. Gauging anorectal sphincter tone as well as performing a digital rectal examination for masses, fecal impaction or incontinence, or bleeding would be included. In the female patient with lower abdominal symptoms, a pelvic examination is imperative.

Tremor may be a sign of hyperthyroidism. Joint pain might point to IBD, reactive arthritis after enteritis such as Reiter syndrome, or a vitamin D and calcium deficiency resulting from malabsorption. Distal extremity edema suggests interstitial fluid shift, possibly from extravascular fluid leak or protein malabsorption as a result of chronic malnutrition or protein-losing enteropathy (PLE).

DIAGNOSTICS
Acute Diarrhea

Essential Diagnostics. For the patient who has mild, afebrile, acute diarrhea, diagnostic evaluation is not usually indicated. These brief episodes are typically viral or food-borne illnesses, are self-resolving, and require little or no intervention. If an infectious source is suspected, stool should be tested for occult blood, fecal leukocytes, ova, and parasites; a stool culture may reveal common pathogens; and sensitivity testing will also be necessary (see Chapter 211). In patients

with a temperature above 38.8°C (102°F), bloody diarrhea, abdominal pain, more than six unformed stools in a 24-hour period, profuse watery diarrhea, and dehydration or in the case of patients who are frail or older, immunocompromised, or toxic-appearing, a stool sample should be sent for C. difficile toxin A or B analysis with secondary consideration of IBD.

The patient's weight is a key factor, especially in persistent or chronic cases.

A complete blood count (CBC) with differential revealing an elevated white blood cell count may indicate general inflammation or infection; low hematocrit and hemoglobin would indicate anemia or acute blood loss, which may corroborate a positive stool guaiac test result over time. A complete metabolic panel including liver function would reveal electrolyte or enzyme abnormalities. A compromise in kidney function would suggest dehydration or concomitant illness, contributing to a source of albumin wasting.[23] A fecal calprotectin can help determine if the cause of the patient's diarrhea is inflammatory or noninflammatory.

Additional Diagnostics. In the absence of an infectious cause, plain abdominal x-ray examination of the kidneys, ureters, and bladder (KUB), flat and upright, is necessary if a small bowel obstruction or stool impaction with overflow incontinence is suspected. Emergent indications for upper endoscopy with small bowel follow-through include small bowel torsion causing partial or full obstruction, possibly resulting from colitis-related strictures, bowel perforation, toxic megacolon, or ileus with fecal leaking.

If diarrhea continues after 2 weeks and the suspected cause is noninfectious, then colitis, diverticulitis, pancreatitis, irritable bowel, and IBD would lead the list of differential diagnoses.

INITIAL DIAGNOSTICS

Acute Diarrhea

LABORATORY
- Complete blood count with differential[a]
- Serum glucose, electrolytes, blood urea nitrogen, creatinine[a]
- Stool for fat, osmolality, laxative screen[a]
- Stool for occult blood and fecal leukocytes[a]
- Stool for fecal calprotectin[a]
- Stool for ova and parasites, culture, C. difficile A & B toxins[a]

IMAGING
- X-ray of kidneys, ureters, bladder[a]
- Computed tomography of abdomen[a]
- Sigmoidoscopy or colonoscopy[a]
- Upper endoscopy with small bowel follow-through and biopsy[a]

[a]If indicated

Chronic Diarrhea

Essential Diagnostics. The cornerstone of diagnosis in chronic diarrhea is stool analysis. Diarrhea in the setting of blood in stool and pus should prompt a Wright stain for white blood cells in cases of bacterial bowel disease or IBD. Also, HIV infection, recent surgery, chemotherapy, transplantation, and antibiotic or antiretroviral use would suggest an infectious cause (see Chapter 211).

Aside from a complete metabolic panel and CBC, a 24-hour stool pH, electrolyte panel, osmotic gap, weight, fecal elastase, and qualitative and quantitative fecal fat along with a stool screen for laxatives, if indicated, should help in the diagnosis of malabsorption (small bowel mucosal transport dysfunction), maldigestion (inability to hydrolyze triglycerides), or laxative abuse. A small osmotic gap (<50 mOsm/kg) points to a low electrolyte concentration, secretory type; a large gap (>125 mOsm/kg) points to a hypertonic gradient, osmotic type, where ingested ions are poorly absorbed, as in carbohydrate malabsorption due to celiac disease.

Additional Diagnostics. Although stool weight can confirm excess output, a more precise indicator is fecal liquidity, which in cases of diarrhea refers to the marked inability of the stool to absorb excess water. The quantitative 72-hour screening, which is performed after the patient's intake of a high-fat regimen (>100 g/day), can help quantify excess fat in stool. Although a stool weight over 1000 g/day is more ominous for a neuroendocrine tumor, up to 25% of diarrhea patients may have a normal stool weight value.[11] Multi-day collections can also be evaluated for excess bile salts in some research centers. Coincident IBS-D or chronic functional diarrhea can present with bile acid malabsorption in 33% to 60% of cases[11] and on pooled analysis closer to 22.5%.[11] Qualitative fecal fat or Sudan III stain will be misleading if the condition results from the ingestion of Olestra or use of the diabetic medication acarbose. Otherwise the spot Sudan stain identifies cases of fatty diarrhea with 76% sensitivity and 99% specificity, achieving a higher sensitivity with more specific characterization of the sample.[11] A fecal elastase below 200 mcg/g points to chronic pancreatitis with exocrine insufficiency. Steatorrhea can also point to small bowel disturbances. In maldigestion, small bowel bacterial overgrowth syndrome might also show up as an acidic sample due to fermented short-chain fatty acids from bacterial digestion or as a significantly elevated serum folate level in the setting of gastrointestinal bloating, flatulence, and diarrhea.

Serum eosinophilia may reflect eosinophilic gastroenteritis, eosinophilic colitis, or mastocytosis, which could be confirmed by a serum tryptase level, especially if there is a significant association with the use of various medications—penicillin, NSAIDs, or narcotics—or mast cells on skin biopsy.

In cases of watery diarrhea, poorly absorbed carbohydrates or magnesium overload should be considered. A hydrogen breath test using lactose, D-xylose (if available), or similar sugar molecules may help make the diagnosis of lactose intolerance, small bowel bacterial overgrowth syndrome, or carbohydrate malabsorption as in sucrase or fructase enzyme deficiencies, especially if fecal pH is acidic. A separate stool magnesium level in excess of 45 μmol/L (90 mEq/L) might raise suspicion of factitious tampering through laxative overuse.

A wider investigation of secretory diarrheal causes might include a cosyntropin stimulation test for Addison disease if fatigue, weight loss, and malaise persist in the absence of other signs, even absent electrolyte shifts. Low albumin and abnormal liver function test results might point to cirrhosis or a chronic illness state. Hypokalemia with or without hypoalbuminemia in IBD is associated with poor outcome in toxic megacolon.[24] The relationship between C-reactive protein (CRP) and hypoalbuminemia (CRP/albumin) in acute severe ulcerative colitis has been associated with a higher probability of colectomy and may warrant earlier use of monoclonal infliximab therapy by day 3 of hospital admission in steroid-refractory patients.[25] The rapid loss of blood proteins into the gut with or without

erosions of the membrane or increased lymphatic pressure is called PLE and is thought to relate to an underappreciated but critical, possibly subclinical loss of albumin, for which earlier detection of this loss of plasma protein might reduce mortality.[23] In patients with a low albumin level but normal kidney and liver function, PLE can be associated with as many as 60 gastrointestinal illnesses, including Crohn disease, Whipple disease (*Tropheryma whippeli* infection), and celiac disease.[23] Although the calculation of α1-antitrypsin clearance, which helps determine existence of PLE in feces, may be no better than a CRP or ESR in predicting a Crohn relapse, a low albumin state can possibly be associated with a reduced duration of concentration of TNF alpha-blocker therapy when $alpha_1$-antitrypsin clearance is high.[23]

An elevated hemoglobin A_{1c} level would help to establish diabetes mellitus, as would signs of neuropathy and acanthosis nigricans in patients with insulin resistance if not associated with Cushing disease or polycystic ovary syndrome. An abnormally low thyroid-stimulating hormone concentration (with confirmatory T3 and free T4) obtained as a result of evident tachycardia and weight loss should prompt consideration of hyperthyroidism.

Other laboratory tests may include immunoglobulin A (IgA) with anti–tissue transglutaminase, which may be used alone given its high positive predictive value, and antiendomysial antibodies for celiac disease in the absence of IgA deficiency. IgA or IgM deficiency in the setting of an already low IgG level may lead to the diagnosis of CVID or common variable hypogammaglobulinemia, with its constellation of infectious, pulmonary, gastrointestinal, and potentially malignant manifestations.

Various pancreatic conditions can lead to secretory diarrhea. Plain abdominal radiography and computed tomography (CT) scan will help to differentiate pancreatitis from a pancreatic mass. Magnetic resonance imaging (MRI) is best in cases of suspected pancreatic insufficiency if anatomic landmarks can be seen. Radiopaque markers found in the colon by x-ray imaging after 5 days is a sign of slow transit and/or stool impaction, possibly contributing to overflow seepage. A secretin stimulation test, which would follow a positive stool chymotrypsin level, may be performed when a pancreatic exocrine disorder or a tumor is suspected, although these are difficult to perform and have low sensitivity and specificity. In practice, pancreatic enzyme replacement often precedes if not replaces this test as a more cost-effective approach. Other rare neuroendocrine disorders may be implicated in situations of low potassium concentration or fatigue. Urine excretion of 5-hydroxyindoleacetic acid in the setting of facial flushing or wheezing might lead to a diagnosis of carcinoid, gastrin in consideration of Zollinger-Ellison syndrome, calcitonin for medullary thyroid adenocarcinoma or bone metastases, and vasoactive intestinal polypeptide (VIP) for VIPoma; however, these tests are usually of low yield given a high false-positive rate in the absence of leading clinical indicators.

Fecal leukocytes on Wright stain with microscopy or a fecal calprotectin or lactoferrin level can lead the investigation for bacterial infection or IBD, although it is limited by variable sensitivity. Often a CRP and erythrocyte sedimentation rate (ESR) is drawn if IBD is suspected. Fecal marker tests are thought to be better than CRP levels in determining an organic versus a functional cause; a normal ESR is more likely to point to functional bowel disease, as is the case with normal fecal and inflammatory markers.[11] Thiopurine methyl-transferase (TPMT) and the metabolite panel are sometimes ordered if there is clinical suspicion of IBD and the anticipated use of azathioprine. A serum albumin concentration should be checked in IBD flares.

Further diagnostic tools include magnetic resonance angiography for ischemic colitis, sigmoidoscopy, colonoscopy, and abdominal and pelvic CT. Colonoscopy can be helpful in diagnosing 15% to 31% of the causes of chronic diarrhea[2] and in particular for establishing microscopic colitis, both collagenous and lymphocytic colitis, followed by IBD (revealed as the source much less often) because this may be the etiology for chronic watery diarrhea 2% to 15% of the time.[1] Congo red staining is used on biopsy for amyloidosis. Although IBD can be appreciated in some cases on upper endoscopy with small bowel follow-through as well as on colonoscopy with microscopic analysis of the gastrointestinal mucosa, the yield of upper endoscopy for unspecified diarrhea is considered low.[2] Ulcers, fistulas, and strictures would favor a diagnosis of IBD. Both sigmoidoscopy (for left-sided symptoms) and colonoscopy are useful to diagnose carcinoma and chronic laxative use.

Another consideration is that an infection may overlie pre-existing colitis, such as pseudomembranous colitis.

A small bowel biopsy, when narrowing in on a diagnosis, will distinguish amyloidosis, bacterial overgrowth (by aspirate analysis in research centers), Behçet disease (a vasculitis more prominent in the Middle East), celiac disease, Crohn disease or ulcerative colitis, eosinophilic gastroenteritis, jejunal diverticulitis, intestinal lymphangiectasia (congenital as well), lymphoma, mastocytosis, and small bowel carcinoma. Wireless capsule endoscopy, increasingly preferred over small bowel follow-through, might be necessary for an enhanced three-dimensional visualization and biopsy of the distal ileum if the lesions are very small. A [75]SeHCAT (radiation) retention study (available in Europe and Canada) provides evidence of bile salt malabsorption, although a trial of bile salt resin replacement is typically prescribed in the United States before further testing would be ordered. It may be that fibroblast growth factor 19 (FGF-19) ileal hormone deficiency arising from a failure of the liver to make it or from ileal disease, may serve as a marker for bile acid diarrhea or a bile salt synthesis precursor such as serum C4, but neither is commonly available.[2,11]

 Gastroenterologist consultation is warranted if the initial workup does not suggest a cause. Further endoscopic visualization through endoscopic ultrasound or capsule endoscopy, as well as endoscopic biopsy or serum testing with CT and octreotide scan for rare endocrine tumors are likely to be necessary.

DIFFERENTIAL DIAGNOSIS
Acute Noninfectious Diarrhea
Once the commonly occurring infectious causes are no longer under consideration, medications rise to the top of the differential list. Magnesium-containing antacids and laxatives lead the list in contributing to acute noninfectious diarrhea. Antibiotics are commonly implicated as well. In fact, over 700 medications have been associated with diarrhea after initiation.[1] Toxins such as organophosphate insecticides (typically found in migrant farm workers), unpasteurized milk, mushrooms, lead, mercury, arsenic, food additives such as monosodium

---

glutamate (MSG), and ciguatera and scombroid (environmental toxins found in fish) also cause diarrhea. Abrupt-onset, large-volume diarrhea with bleeding, pain, or fever may result from mesenteric vascular insufficiency or intestinal angina (an emergency that may lead to bowel necrosis and death without revascularization or stenting), ischemic colitis involving low flow to the inferior mesenteric artery of the left lower quadrant, diverticulitis, or obstruction.

Chronic Noninfectious Diarrhea
Toxins from bacterial processes are the most likely cause of chronic diarrhea; however, many noninfectious causes are possible (e.g., HIV-associated noninfectious diarrhea or tube feedings and pseudomembranous colitis associated with *C. difficile*) (Box 114.1). There is also a graft-versus-host disease phenomenon that results in chronic diarrhea.

Chronic noninfectious diarrheas represent a multitude of disease entities, some with overlapping features. Celiac disease, which produces secretory diarrhea, involves mucosal changes of the duodenojejunal brush border, malabsorption of gluten, and fatty stool. Diabetes, an endocrine disorder with pancreatic effects, is a secretory cause of diarrhea featuring a glucose malabsorption component, which can eventually lead to PLE

Differential Diagnosis: Chronic Noninfectious Diarrhea

- Medication or toxin exposure
- Irritable bowel syndrome, diarrhea predominant
- Carbohydrate malabsorption, celiac disease
- Microscopic colitis (collagenous and lymphocytic)
- Inflammatory disease (Crohn disease, ulcerative colitis)

and dysmotility. Therefore categorical delineations may not be as well circumscribed as suggested.

Excess magnesium, sulfate, and phosphate ingestion, most often associated with antacids and laxatives, can cause osmotic diarrhea. Cathartics or saline purgatives likewise draw water into the gut. Other highly osmotic molecules include sugar alcohols such as sorbitol and mannitol found in sugar-free (diabetic) candy or chewing gum and undigested lactulose. Sucrase-isomaltase malabsorption can be controlled through avoidance diets. Other carbohydrate malabsorption (maltose, glucose-galactose, fructose) may result from disaccharide insufficiency, although excess fructose can cause diarrhea in healthy individuals.

Cow's milk or soy milk protein intolerance as well as lactose intolerance may be discovered early in life. Whereas the majority of individuals have lactase enzyme activity until they are weaned in early childhood, a minority of those of northern European descent appear to have lactase enzyme activity continuing into adulthood, which is considered the result of a genetic mutation. Typically, no diagnostics are indicated other than a trial of abstinence from foods or liquids that contain lactose, although some prefer to conduct hydrogen breath tests. After a hiatus, a retrial of lactose-containing foods in smaller quantities throughout the day will sometimes allow some tolerance, particularly if calcium supplementation cannot be achieved otherwise. Adults rarely have food allergies (1% to 2%); of note, kiwi, banana, avocado, and walnut allergy complex has been associated with latex allergy.[11] An infectious source that may persist for several years is Brainerd diarrhea from unpasteurized milk or untreated water.[3]

Watery diarrhea that persists despite efforts to eliminate potential sources can result from a secretory disorder. There is usually no blood or white blood cell debris, and no constitutional symptoms are seen. Causes of secretory diarrhea include primary gastrointestinal disorders, nongastrointestinal inflammatory diseases, and endocrine disorders such as unusual neuroendocrine tumors. Although celiac disease might be considered a gluten malabsorption or mucosal disorder, it is treated as a secretory one. Heavy alcohol use associated with malnutrition and atrophic gastritis both may result in low vitamin B_{12} absorption into the small intestine, causing pernicious anemia along with secretory diarrhea. Chronic alcohol consumption has been linked with diarrhea possibly due to an altered mucosal surface, causing hemorrhage, inflammation, increased permeability, a change in intestinal motility possibly due to nitric oxide overproduction, as well as carbohydrate and nutrient malabsorption, even colorectal cancer.[26]

Chronic diarrhea can also be inflammatory and accompanied by pain, fever, pus, and bleeding. Examples include lymphogenous or collagenous colitis, Crohn disease and ulcerative colitis (including ulcerative jejunoileitis), ischemic colitis, diverticulitis, Behçet syndrome, pseudomembranous colitis, primary or secondary immunodeficiency, eosinophilic gastroenteritis, diarrhea after cancer treatment, and radiation colitis. Malabsorption disorders that cause PLE, such as autoimmune enteropathy and gluten malabsorption, are similar.

When changes in the intestinal mucosa occur, whether or not they are caused by an autoimmune disease or inflammation, muscle innervation and, in turn, peristalsis can be affected. This causes malabsorption of fluid and nutrients and rapid transit in a state of overactive motility or IBDs, such as ulcerative colitis and Crohn disease. Crohn disease may strike anywhere along the whole gut (mouth to anus) and affects the full thickness of the bowel wall. Ulcerative colitis usually affects the mucosal layer in the distal sigmoid but has been known to arise occultly in the left side of the colon or distal ileocecal valve, causing high-volume stool with pus and bloody exudates, significant cramps, and even fever in severe cases. Mucosal changes associated with inflammation as a result of IBD, collagenous and lymphocytic colitis (10% to 15% of diarrhea cases),[17] diverticulitis, or Behçet disease cause secretory diarrhea. Small intestinal ischemic colitis is often associated with poor vascular flow. Other than infectious and neoplastic sources, further inflammation of the intestinal wall and ulceration of the mucosa can result from diverticulitis and radiation enteritis.

Another cause of chronic secretory diarrhea is the disruption of fat absorption. Pancreatic insufficiency can produce a malabsorption of fats, causing fatty stool, bloating, and malodorous gas. Small bowel surface loss as a result of bacterial overgrowth can cause malabsorption, as is the case in cystic fibrosis. An example of small intestinal malabsorption is gluten-sensitive enteropathy, or celiac disease, which causes an inflammatory reaction with loss of mucosal surface area resulting in steatorrhea and malnutrition. Gluten-sensitive enteropathy is a complex disorder composed of impaired absorption, increased intestinal permeability, and, in 10% of patients, pancreatic insufficiency. Chronic pancreatitis is the most common, but it develops into permanent scarring and progressive dysfunction. Bile acid malabsorption may be more closely linked to IBS-D, microscopic colitis, and perhaps functional diarrhea, accounting for one-third of the 1% of people in Western countries experiencing chronic diarrhea.[16] Diarrhea resulting from motility dysfunction is highly prevalent, whether it is caused by the use of stimulant laxatives or NSAIDs, diabetic enteropathy, hyperthyroidism, scleroderma, strictures or adhesions from surgery, radiation enteritis, or prokinetic agents.

Although functional disorders are typically grouped separately, both affect transit time. The Rome IV consensus statement defines IBS as recurrent abdominal pain on average 1 day/week during the preceding 3 months associated with at least two or more of the following: (a) an increase related to defecation, (b) a change in stool frequency, (c) a change in the form (appearance) of stool, with greater than 25% of stools being loose/watery. Criteria must be fulfilled for the preceding 3 months with symptom onset at least 6 months prior to diagnosis (see Chapter 121).[7] The new criteria focus on the number of days an individual has a change from her or his baseline stool consistency with increasing recognition of the complexity of brain-gut axis processes; functional diarrhea, by contrast, is loose or watery stool without pain.[13] An empirical management approach serves both entities unless there are persistent symptoms, which might warrant more workup.[2]

Stress or psychiatric disease may play a role in functional bowel disease. Self-neglect or substance use (e.g., alcoholism) may result in malabsorption, a cofactor or prevailing cause of diarrhea. Unsupervised narcotic withdrawal causes rapid transit in the gut. Other severe malnutrition states as a result of socioeconomic or behavioral neglect may set the stage for further illness or infectious complications. Last, factitious diarrhea includes those cases caused by deception or self-injury. The motivation is often secondary gain, as for sympathy, treatment with controlled medications, or relief from responsibilities. Factitious causes may account for up to 15% of otherwise unexplained cases, which are made more difficult on occasion by patient tampering with samples. In some cases of severe psychological illness the behavior may perpetuate without insight.

Toxic megacolon, ischemic colitis, acute severe ulcerative colitis with hypoalbuminemia, or colon cancer must be ruled out in patients who present with fever, dehydration, severe abdominal pain, bloody stool, unintentional weight loss, or history of colon cancer in first-degree family members diagnosed at age 50 or younger.

INTERPROFESSIONAL COLLABORATIVE MANAGEMENT
Nonpharmacologic Management
For overflow incontinence, manual disimpaction and subsequent low-volume tap water or solute-filled enemas, along with the side-lying position and turning back and forth, may help to move the bowels. For fecal incontinence unresponsive to bulking agents or loperamide, anorectal biofeedback guided by a specialized physical therapist can be remarkably effective in the setting of anorectal dysfunction diagnosed by MR defecography and anorectal manometry.

Celiac disease is managed by a gluten-free diet (i.e., strictly avoiding wheat, buckwheat, oats, rye, barley, and malt). A mere one-third of an average-sized piece of bread is enough to lead to symptoms. Church wafers or inert ingredients in medications have been known to be unexpected culprits. Because there is some correlation between celiac disease and microscopic colitis, strict gluten avoidance may also help. But if diarrhea persists, further testing might reveal this second source.

One popularly adopted, evidence-based approach to IBS-D symptom management is to adhere to a low-FODMAP diet (consisting of low levels of fermentable oligo-di-monosaccharides and polyols), although this may be less effective on the diarrhea component of the syndrome.[11,27] Another entity that has been seen to respond to a low-FODMAP diet is runner's diarrhea, a multifactorial phenomenon more pronounced in long-distance runners than other athletes, which responds to a well-hydrated low-fiber/protein/fat regimen excluding NSAIDs, bicarbonate, and caffeine.[12]

Patients living with chronic disease may benefit from psychological counseling. Depression or despondency is not unusual in the face of ongoing medical surveillance, treatment, and uncertainty. The associated toll on financial and emotional resources alone can be daunting. Acknowledging these stressors can help patients express their concerns and seek appropriate support. Patients with IBS have been shown to benefit from relaxation therapy and psychological support, although their traction is harder to gauge from short-term studies; stress

is thought to predispose IBD patients to flares, and relaxation techniques have shown improvement in multiple domains.[28] For example, within guidelines established by the American College of Gastroenterology, 19% of patients were reported anxious and 21% depressed without respect to disease activity; depression also correlated with a risk for medication nonadherence.[29]

Pharmacologic Management
Fluid and electrolyte replacement is essential in the treatment of acute diarrhea. Oral fluid replacement should be initiated at home or in the office to manage a mild, uncomplicated episode of diarrhea. A hyperosmolar solution containing glucose and electrolytes is advised to prevent future intestinal intraluminal fluid overload. Zinc has been seen to play a role in shortening illness duration.[5] If the patient's condition fails to respond to oral rehydration, intravenous hydration may be indicated. Solid food products should be reintroduced as symptoms resolve and stools become more formed.

Medications can be used for symptomatic relief of nausea and vomiting, abdominal cramping, and diarrhea. If nausea is the main complaint, treatment with promethazine (Phenergan) or prochlorperazine maleate (Compazine), both having anticholinergic effects, or ondansetron, a serotonin 5-HT$_3$ antagonist, can be effective. Absorbents such as attapulgite (Kaopectate), 30 mL by mouth every 30 minutes as needed to a maximum of eight doses a day, and bismuth subsalicylate (Pepto-Bismol), 30 mL by mouth every 30 minutes if needed to a maximum of eight doses per day, typically serve to control diarrhea (as do activated charcoal, kaolin-pectin, attapulgite, and smectite).[4] The tablet form of bismuth subsalicylate, one or two tablets every 4 to 6 hours to a maximum 8 tablets in 24 hours, and antispasmodic-anticholinergic sedatives such as atropine-scopolamine-hyoscyamine-phenobarbital (Donnatal, immediate release), one or two tablets up to three times a day, are used to decrease abdominal cramping. Because these products may cause aspirin intoxication, they should be used cautiously. Patients taking warfarin should be warned as well, because anticoagulation will be affected. Also, bismuth subsalicylate should not be given to HIV-positive or immunocompromised patients, who are at risk for encephalopathy. Secretory diarrhea related to neuroendocrine tumors (VIPomas, carcinoids) is treated with octreotide, 50 to 150 mcg subcutaneously three times a day. This agent is a somatostatin analogue that stimulates intestinal fluid and electrolyte absorption and stops intestinal fluid secretions. Octreotide is also used off label to treat AIDS-related chronic, noninfectious diarrhea. A newer agent, crofelemer 125 mg twice daily, is a Food and Drug Administration (FDA)–approved botanical for HIV/AIDS-related patients with diarrhea on antiretroviral therapy.[2,15]

Depending on the cause of chronic diarrhea, treatment may be curative, suppressive, or empirical. If the cause of the diarrhea is not known but is not thought to be worrisome, treatment commonly includes the antimotility agent loperamide, available over the counter, once or twice initially followed by one tablet after each loose stool (to a maximum of eight tablets daily). This mu-receptor agonist does not cause dependency and can be used daily in a low dosage to fend off motility-related frequency. Likewise, diphenoxylate with atropine, a controlled substance requiring an opioid-monitoring attestation in some states due to its central effects, may be helpful in more difficult cases, although there is no effect on anorectal sphincter tone. Other far less common opiate options include codeine, 15 to 60 mg up to four times daily (the maximum daily dose is 320 mg); deodorized tincture of opium, initially two or three drops four times daily, which is rarely used; and morphine, 2 to 20 mg up to four times daily in appropriate settings. These intestinal transit inhibitors aid in slowing motility, decreasing secretions, increasing fluid absorption, and increasing blood flow. Because narcotic agents are potentially habit forming, they should be reserved for patients with chronic, intractable diarrhea and prescribed in consultation with the physician. Clonidine, 0.1 mg to 0.3 mg three times daily, is an α_2-adrenergic agonist that inhibits intestinal electrolyte secretion but also lowers blood pressure. Octreotide (natural somatostatin or its analogues) provides further antisecretory support for short-bowel syndrome, gastrointestinal endocrine tumors, chemotherapy side effects, and carcinoid syndrome.[2,4] Clonidine and octreotide are both potential agents for the treatment of diarrhea due to nocturnal diabetic autonomic neuropathy.[19] Other investigative antisecretories have been tested with mixed results.[5]

For IBS-D in women with refractory diarrhea, alosetron hydrochloride, 0.5 to 2 mg daily, is available with an education requirement in the Prescribing Program for Lotronex (see Chapter 121) to recognize the risk for ischemic colitis, intestinal ileus, obstruction, and perforation. In addition, eluxadoline 100 mg twice daily, a mixed peripherally acting μ- and κ-receptor opioid agonist/δ-opioid antagonist, has been FDA-approved for IBS-D.[21] There is also a new indication in IBS-D for rifaximin 550 mg taken three times daily, for up to 14 days.[6]

Collagenous colitis responds best to budesonide 9 mg daily initially and 6 mg daily for maintenance. Bismuth subsalicylate (two tablets four times a day for 8 weeks), mesalamine, and prednisone are second-line treatments and not as effective in lymphocytic colitis. Alternatively, colesevelam (1875 mg daily, up to twice daily), or cholestyramine (4 g daily, up to four times a day) can be helpful. Use of NSAIDs, weight loss, and age 50 or greater (as opposed to abdominal pain or PPI use) are associated with the development of microscopic colitis.[17]

Empirical treatment with antibiotics should be considered in cases of small intestinal bacterial overgrowth syndrome if it is likely that excessive dyspepsia with flatulence and watery diarrhea might be associated with an elevated folate level. Rifaximin, 550 mg twice daily for a week, is currently recommended; an alternative is metronidazole, 250 mg three times daily, or ciprofloxacin, 500 mg twice daily for a week, with the caveat that its use may cause tendon injury. Ideally, if there are likely to be repeated courses, any antibiotic used for this purpose would be alternated with a second in order to prevent antibiotic resistance. Probiotics that stimulate the bowel to colonize increased levels of advantageous bacteria continue to prompt research and may be used as an adjunct.[5]

If *C. difficile* colitis is diagnosed, metronidazole, 500 mg three times a day for 10 to 14 days, or vancomycin, 125 mg orally four times a day for 10 to 14 days, may be used. Unfortunately some resistant strains have arisen, and a small subset of patients can have a difficult time surmounting this secondary infection. Rifaximin, 200 to 400 mg twice a day to three times a day, is another treatment option, as is, in limited use, fecal transplant.[30]

For diarrhea caused by bile salt malabsorption from intestinal resection or terminal ileal disease, colesevelam hydrochloride (Welchol), 1875 g twice daily, although not approved by the FDA for this indication, is a preferred agent in practice. It is common to start with cholestyramine (Questran), 4 g one or two times a day up to 24 g daily, to gauge response.

Anti-inflammatory treatments are appropriate for inflammatory causes such as Crohn disease and ulcerative colitis. Antimotility agents should not be used with IBD. Depending on severity of presentation, location and history of the course of IBD, sulfasalazine or mesalamine would be advised in addition to a steroid course or ongoing treatment. In more severe cases, azathioprine or 6-mercaptopurine, with or without mesalamine suppositories or enemas, with ongoing steroid suppression or weaning, might lead to a remission. Some patients cannot tolerate 6-mercaptopurine or azathioprine treatment if their TPMT enzyme level is too low (see Chapter 120). Monoclonal antibodies are now in common use for moderate to severe cases of Crohn disease: these include infliximab (Remicaide), adalimumab (Humira), certolizumab pegol (Cimzia), natalizumab (Tysabri), vedolizumab (Entyvio), and ustekinumab (Stelara) and ulcerative colitis: golimumab (Simponi), adalimumab, infliximab, and vedolizumab. Monoclonal therapy may be used as an independent approach or as an add-on treatment.

Finally, some clinicians will resort to a trial of codeine, which has been used in variable immunodeficiency disease but may lead to tolerance, heightened nausea, and sedation. Following a low-fat diet is no longer recommended because fat-soluble vitamins must be absorbed; if therapy is successful, weight should also be maintained.

Indications for Referral or Hospitalization

In patients with severe dehydration or protracted vomiting, intravenous fluids should be initiated in a medical setting. If the illness persists beyond 3 weeks despite treatment measures, malignant neoplasms and disease states such as diabetes, thyrotoxicosis, lupus, HIV infection, and IBD should be further considered. IBD can manifest as a bowel obstruction or severe anorectal fistula beyond pouchitis. Surgery, potentially colectomy, in severe, protracted cases might be a primary consideration. Renal and cardiac comorbidity would be a factor in ischemic colitis, which is considered to be a gastrointestinal emergency. Older adults are more likely to be hospitalized with diarrheal illness and have a higher mortality. Urgent physician or hospital-based consultation with surgical staff is imperative in these cases. Acute insult to the bowel, as through trauma or ischemic attack, necessitates hospitalization because significant complications may arise. Diverticular disease may also necessitate hospitalization and treatment if it is unresponsive to past outpatient therapy (see Chapter 115).

LIFE-SPAN CONSIDERATIONS

In young adults IBS may occur as a postviral complication. In general IBS has a bimodal distribution, appearing in young adults or older adults for the first time, with a female and constipation predominance. Crohn disease and ulcerative disease are split roughly equally by sex and disease type and are considered to have a bimodal distribution by age at onset, although these groupings are clustered closely in time. These two peaks in symptom onset occur between the ages of 15 and 40 years and the ages of 50 and 80 years, and both entities have a genetic and ethnically Jewish predisposition, although new-onset diarrhea late in the seventh decade (median age at onset) is more likely to be microscopic colitis. Microscopic colitis typically affects women in the fifth to seventh decades of life. Detection of celiac disease is on the rise because of more sensitive and specific testing assays; it can first manifest in children, sometimes in pregnancy, or as late as the sixth decade as diarrhea. A history of small birth size, childhood illnesses, Irish or Scottish descent, and concomitant diabetes are risk factors. Diabetic complications such as diabetic enteropathy are more likely to affect patients with long-standing disease.

Older adults are more likely to have a worse case of *C. difficile* colitis, with a higher risk of relapses and death. Medications have a multitude of side effects. The majority of patients older than 65 years have diverticula. Tube feeding in elders can be a cause of iatrogenic diarrhea, causing a dumping syndrome from the high solute content when it is infused directly into the small bowel. In the geriatric patient, fecal impaction must be ruled out.

COMPLICATIONS

Complications from diarrhea are usually a result of dehydration. Regardless of the cause, attention should be directed toward fluid and electrolyte replacement. Electrolyte disorders—particularly hypocalcemia, hypomagnesemia, and hypokalemia—are common in persistent diarrhea. Continuous diarrhea can necessitate hospitalization for fluid and electrolyte replacement if the patient is unable to maintain hydration with oral fluid replacement. Sepsis and cardiovascular collapse are potential complications, and infants, older adults, and immunosuppressed patients are more susceptible to these complications. Refractory diarrhea is usually a symptom of a more serious illness and requires diagnostic evaluation and immediate physician consultation.

Surgery is sometimes necessary to address recurrent IBD due to bowel perforation, stricture or blockage, obstruction, or sepsis. Duration of IBD (especially at a younger age), extent of disease (e.g., strictures, pseudopolyps), family history of sporadic colorectal cancer (nine times greater risk if a first-degree relative was diagnosed before age 50), and primary biliary cholangitis correlate with a greater the risk of colon cancer.[10] Colonoscopies are recommended after 8 years of disease and frequently every 1 to 2 years thereafter depending on extent of disease; proctitis and ulcerative proctosigmoiditis do not confer increased risk, although a baseline should be established.[10] Extraintestinal manifestations can include eye-related inflammatory changes including chronic dry eyes (keratoconjunctivitis sicca), primary biliary cholangitis, osteopenia or osteoporosis, arthritis, pyoderma gangrenosum, ulcerating erythema nodosum, anemia, and melanoma as well as a variety of corticosteroid-related effects.[22]

For some patients, postoperative diarrhea can persist for years. In patients who have dumping syndrome after vagotomy or gastric surgery affecting transit, concentrated carbohydrates can be a trigger. Avoidance of liquids with meals and lying down afterward can help relieve a common reaction of sweating, dizziness, and flushing. Some gastrointestinal surgeries will lead to motility disorders stemming from stagnation in the small intestine.

Relapses of *C. difficile* colitis are common in older adults and are more likely in cases of extended fever, stool incontinence, immunosuppression, and use of H_2 receptor antagonist acid-suppression therapy. Fecal microbiota transplant has been approved, with requirements for investigational therapy usage by the FDA. Enteral feedings or comorbidities may further complicate the condition.

In celiac disease, patients may first notice a persistent erythematous rash called *dermatitis herpetiformis*. In addition to the abdominal bloating and steatorrhea coupled with foul-smelling stool, there is a potential for weight loss caused by anorexia and resulting stunted growth. Untreated or recalcitrant celiac disease can lead to other endocrine (osteopenia or osteoporosis), hematologic (vitamin B12 deficiency anemia due to small intestinal damage), neurological (ataxia), and oncological (T-cell lymphoma) conditions as well as infertility.

For those diagnosed with IBS, there is a phenomenon in which the entity is associated with interstitial cystitis and endometriosis, which may mean that a patient will seek specialty management from three specialists instead of one. Complications of CVID can lead to significant dehydration, bowel blockage, and anemia. The effects of a surgically shortened ileum can range from anemia resulting from lack of intrinsic factor to dumping syndrome. Gastric bypass surgery has a host of complications necessitating adequate vitamin and electrolyte replacement and nutrient supplementation.

Amyloidosis is a multi-organ syndrome in which damage may manifest in the heart, kidneys, liver, intestines, and nervous system. Recalcitrant high-volume diarrhea may lead to dangerous levels of potassium loss, and hypokalemia has cardiac implications. Laxative abuse may lead to metabolic acidosis if there is a severe decrease in sodium bicarbonate, which may affect the heart.

PATIENT AND FAMILY EDUCATION

Diseases of malabsorption or complications of intestinal surgery that have led to malabsorption offer an opportunity to promote healthful choices in nutrient and vitamin supplementation with periodic laboratory surveillance. For those with celiac disease, multiple societies provide online resources to find food alternatives, medical information, and support. Regular exercise programs in many instances are thought to be of benefit to the patient with chronic noninfectious diarrhea.

If infectious, toxin- or medication-related, autoimmune, endocrine, surgical, and other gastroenterological causes have been excluded, the clinician is left with a host of functional diseases for which symptom management is key. Functional bowel disease, including IBS-D as well as mixed IBS (involving alternating diarrhea and constipation predominance at baseline), is thought to be influenced by diet and stress, with further insults from caffeine, nicotine, and alcohol.

HEALTH PROMOTION

Therapeutic support or referral for psychological counseling is paramount for those with a significant psychological component to their illness. Community, hospital- and office-based support groups can be very helpful, as can online authoritative disease education and referral sites. Research has pointed to the positive impact of the relaxation response as a mind-body intervention on IBS and IBD in deregulating the common genetic expression of natural killer cells, among many others, as demonstrated by peripheral blood transcriptome analysis.[28]

REFERENCES

1. Philip, N. A., Ahmed, N., & Pitchumoni, C. S. (2017). Spectrum of drug-induced chronic diarrhea. *Journal of Clinical Gastroenterology, 51*(2), 111–117.

2. Schiller, L. R., Pardi, D. S., & Sellin, J. H. (2017). Perspectives in clinical gastroenterology and hepatology. Chronic diarrhea: Diagnosis and management. *Clinical Gastroenterology and Hepatology: the Official Clinical Practice Journal of the American Gastroenterological Association, 15,* 182–193.

3. DuPont, H. L. (2016). Persistent diarrhea: A clinical review. *JAMA: The Journal of the American Medical Association, 315*(24), 2712–2723.

4. Abdullah, M., & Firmansyah, M. A. (2013). Clinical approach and management of chronic diarrhea. *Acta Medica Indonesiana, 45*(2), 157–165.

5. Thiagarajahgarajah, J. R., Donowitz, M., & Verkman, A. S. (2015). Secretory diarrhea: Mechanisms and emerging therapies. *Nat Rev Gastroenterol Hepatol, 12,* 446–457.

6. Chang, L., Lembo, A., & Sultan, S. (2014). American Gastroenterological Association Institute technical review on the pharmacological management of irritable bowel syndrome. *Gastroenterology, 147,* 1149–1172.

7. Schmulson, M. J., & Drossman, D. (2017). What is new in Rome IV. *Journal of Neurogastroenterology and Motility, 23*(2), 151–163.

8. Bharucha, A. E., Chakraborty, S., & Sletten, C. D. (2016). Common functional gastroenterologic disorders associated with abdominal pain. *Mayo Clinic Proceedings Mayo Clinic, 91*(8), 1118–1132.

9. Simren, A., Palsson, O. S., & Whitehead, W. E. (2017). Update on Rome IV criteria for colorectal disorders: Implications for clinical practice. *Current Gastroenterology Reports, 19,* 15.

10. 2010). AGA Medical position statement on the diagnosis and management of colorectal neoplasia in inflammatory bowel disease. *Gastroenterology, 138,* 738–745.

11. Camilleri, M., Sellin, J. H., & Barrett, K. E. (2017). Reviews in basic and clinical gastroenterology and hepatology. Pathophysiology, evaluation, and management of chronic watery diarrhea. *Gastroenterology, 152,* 515–532.

12 de Oliveira, E. P. (2017). Runner's diarrhea: What is it, what causes it, and how can it be prevented? *Current Opinion in Gastroenterology, 33,* 41–46.

13 Drossman, D. A., & Hasler, W. L. (2016). Rome IV-functional GI disorders: Disorders of the gut-brain interaction. *Gastroenterology, 150*(6), 1257–1261.

14 Downs, I. A., Aroniadis, O. C., Kelly, L., et al. (2017). Postinfection irritable bowel syndrome. The links between gastroenteritis, inflammation, the microbiome, and functional disease. *Journal of Clinical Gastroenterology, 51*(10), 869–877.

15. Clay, P. G., & Crutchley, R. D. (2014). Noninfectious diarrhea in HIV seropositive individuals: A review of prevalence rates, etiology, and management in the era of combination antiretroviral therapy. *Infectious Diseases and Therapy, 3*(2), 103–122.

16. Camilleri, M. (2014). Advances in understanding of bile acid diarrhea. *Expert Review of Gastroenterology & Hepatology, 8*(1), 49–61.

17. Cotter, T. G., Binder, M., Harper, E., et al. (2017). Optimization of a scoring system to predict microscopic colitis in a cohort of patients with chronic diarrhea. *Journal of Clinical Gastroenterology, 51,* 228–234.

18. Pisani, L. F., Tontini, G. E., Vecchi, M., et al. (2016). Microscopic colitis: What do we know about pathogenesis? *Inflammatory Bowel Diseases, 22*(2), 450–458.

19. Kaur, N., Kishore, L., & Singh, R. (2014). Diabetic autonomic neuropathy: Pathogenesis to pharmacological management. *Journal of Diabetes & Metabolism, 5*(7), 402. doi:10.4172/2155-6156.1000402.

20. Schiller, L. R., Pardi, D. S., Spiller, R., et al. (2013). Gastro 2013 APDW/WCOG Shanghai Working Party report: Chronic diarrhea: definition, classification, diagnosis. *Journal of Gastroenterology and Hepatology, 29,* 6–25.

21. Lembo, A. J., Lacy, B. E., Zuckerman, M. J., et al. (2016). Eluxadoline for irritable bowel syndrome with diarrhea. *The New England Journal of Medicine, 374,* 242–253.

22. Chachu, K. A., & Osterman, M. T. (2016). How to diagnose and treat IBD mimics in the refractory IBD patient who does not have IBD. *Inflammatory Bowel Diseases, 22*(5), 1262–1274.

23. Levitt, D. G., & Levitt, M. D. (2017). Protein losing enteropathy: Comprehensive review of the mechanistic association with clinical and subclinical disease states. *Clin and Exper Gastroenterol, 10,* 147–168.

24. Woodhouse, E. (2016). Toxic megacolon: A review for emergency department clinicians. *Journal of Emergency Nursing, 42,* 481–486.

25. Gibson, D. J., Harley, K., Doherty, J., et al. (2017). CRP/Albumin ratio. An early predictor of steroid responsiveness in acute severe ulcerative colitis. *Journal of Clinical Gastroenterology, 1–5.*

26. Grad, S., Abenavoli, L., & Dumitrascu, D. L. (2016). The effect of alcohol on gastrointestinal motility. *Reviews on Recent Clinical Trials, 11,* 191–195.

27. De Roest, R. H., Dobbs, B. R., Chapman, B. A., et al. (2013). The low FODMAP diet improves gastrointestinal symptoms in patients with irritable bowel syndrome: A prospective study. *International Journal of Clinical Practice, 67*(9), 895–903.

28. Kuo, B., Bhasin, M., Jacquart, J., et al. (2015). Genomic and clinical effects associated with a Relaxation Response Mind-Body Intervention in patients with irritable bowel syndrome and inflammatory bowel disease. *PLoS ONE, 10*(4), e0123861. doi:10.1371/journal.

29. Davis, S. C., Robinson, B. L., Vess, J., et al. (2018). Primary care management of ulcerative colitis. *The Nurse Practitioner, 43*(1), 11–19.

30. Shayto, R. H., Abou Mrad, R., & Sharara, A. I. (2016). Use of rifaximin in gastrointestinal and liver diseases. *World Journal of Gastroenterology, 22*(29), 6638–6651.

CHAPTER **115**

DIVERTICULAR DISEASE
Priscilla Marsicovetere

Diverticular disease is one of the most common conditions in the Western world. It is the eighth most common outpatient diagnosis in the United States[1] and accounted for more than 216,000 hospital admissions in 2012 at an aggregate cost of $2.2 billion in health care and $100 million in medication costs.[1] The considerable costs are predominantly driven by hospital bed days, but they also include intensive care unit costs, endoscopy, computed tomography (CT), ultrasound, and clinic and emergency visits.[2] The exact pathogenesis of the disease is unknown but is thought to include environmental, genetic, and dietary factors.[1] Diverticular disease occurs more often with increasing age and as dietary practices include more refined foods. The disease manifests in a variety of clinical spectrums, including diverticulosis, segmental colitis associated with diverticular disease (segmental colitis associated with diverticulosis [SCAD]), symptomatic uncomplicated diverticular disease (SUDD), diverticulitis, and diverticular bleeding or hemorrhage. Clinical presentation depends greatly on the severity of the inflammatory process and the presence or absence of complications.[3] Among patients with diverticula, 80% to 85% will remain asymptomatic, whereas 10% to 25% will experience diverticulitis at some point in their lives.[2,4]

DIVERTICULOSIS

DEFINITION AND EPIDEMIOLOGY

The basic unit of diverticular disease is the diverticulum, which is an outpouching of mucosa through the colon wall. Clinically diverticulosis is defined by the presence of numerous diverticula and presents as an uncomplicated asymptomatic or symptomatic process without inflammation or bleeding. Asymptomatic diverticulosis is typically an incidental finding on imaging performed for other indications.[1]

The prevalence of colonic diverticulosis varies greatly in different geographic areas of the world. It is most common in the Western Hemisphere and is rare in Africa, Asia, and many parts of South America. This distinction was noted in a landmark 1971 article by Painter and Burkitt, who found that the greatest difference in the diets of these populations was the amount of fiber consumed.[5] In studying the colonic transit times and stool weights of more than 1000 people in the United Kingdom and sub-Saharan Africa, the authors found statistically significant longer transit times and lower stool weights in the UK population than in the African population. The amount of dietary fiber was thought to be the contributing factor to these findings—higher fiber content resulted in faster colonic transit time, larger stool volumes, and more frequent bowel movements.

The rising incidence of diverticular disease seemed to coincide with the Industrial Revolution, the advent of roller milling, and the process of refining sugar, which removed a large source of fiber from Western diets. Interestingly, the first reports of increasing diverticular disease appeared in the literature at about the same time as the first cohort of children raised on refined sugar and white flour reached the age where diverticular disease begins to occur, or about 40 years after the start of the Industrial Revolution.[6]

Whereas the prevalence of diverticulosis in Western society has been estimated as high as 60% in people older than 60 years,[7] studies from less industrialized regions (e.g., Africa and Asia) document prevalence rates of less than 0.2%.[8] Diverticulitis in Africa and Asia commonly involves the right colon, as compared with left colon involvement in Western countries.[9] The worldwide prevalence of diverticular disease is not precisely known, but in the United States and other developed countries its prevalence approaches 1% to 2% of people under 30 years of age, about 10% of people greater than 40 years of age, more than 60% of people greater than 70 years of age, and approximately 80% of those greater than 85 years of age.[4,6,10,11] It affects men and women equally.[11] Patients younger than age 40, however, are more commonly male.[8] A familial pattern has been noted from twin studies.[12]

A possible genetic connective tissue defect has also been posited because of reports of diverticula in young patients with Marfan syndrome or Ehlers-Danlos syndrome.[6]

PATHOPHYSIOLOGY

Colonic diverticula are defects of the bowel wall, especially the sigmoid, that develop with advancing age. They are saclike herniations of the mucosa through the muscularis propria and are actually pseudodiverticular because they do not contain the muscle layer.

The pathophysiologic changes common to diverticulosis of the colon are not entirely clear. Diverticula tend to arise in areas of weakness of the colonic wall, generally between the mesenteric and antimesenteric teniae, where the vasa recta penetrate the muscle.[10] Herniation of the mucosa is thought to result from two factors: (1) an increased pressure gradient between the colonic lumen and the serosa and (2) areas of relative weakness in the colonic wall.[13] Indeed, microscopic studies have shown muscular atrophy at the site of diverticula, which makes them particularly susceptible to herniation of the mucosa in the setting of increased intraluminal pressure.[6,10]

A commonly accepted hypothesis of diverticulum formation is that low-fiber diets decrease the amount of intraluminal bulk in the colon, causing muscle hypertrophy as the colon tries to move the fecal matter along.[13] Lack of fecal bulk is thought to produce uncoordinated and irregular colonic peristalsis, which creates sacculations in the colon wall. There is increased pressure within these sacs, which results in diverticular outpouchings at weak points, or natural breaks, in the muscle layer of the colon where the nutrient vessels, the vasa recta, pass through the muscularis propria into the submucosa.[6,10]

Another possible contributing factor of diverticular formation is that the colon wall, which is covered by connective tissue, loses its flexibility and tensile strength with age. The role of collagen and the tensile strength of the colonic wall was studied by Wess et al. in 1995 to determine whether lack

of collagen was responsible for weakness of the muscular wall of the colon.[14] Researchers found that because the collagen content does not change with age, the changes seen in diverticulosis were more likely due to qualitative, not quantitative, changes in the collagen. With advancing age past 40 years, collagen in the colonic mucosa, the layer primarily responsible for tensile strength, becomes stiffer and less resistant to stretching. This was thought to make the wall more susceptible to tears in the setting of higher intraluminal pressures, thus leading to small herniations and the formation of diverticular disease.

Additional risk factors for diverticular disease include the consumption of aspirin and nonsteroidal antiinflammatory drugs (NSAIDs), lack of exercise, obesity, the consumption of red or processed meats, and smoking.[4,8]

A genetic component has also been identified, because monozygotic twins are twice as likely as dizygotic twins to develop diverticulosis.[4]

In terms of size and distribution, diverticula range from 1 or 2 mm to giant diverticula. In Western societies, diverticula occur predominantly in the sigmoid colon. In Asian countries, right-sided diverticula are more common.[9]

CLINICAL PRESENTATION AND PHYSICAL EXAMINATION

Patients with uncomplicated colonic diverticula, or diverticulosis, are often asymptomatic and rarely seek medical attention; approximately 75% of these individuals are never seen with a clinical problem.[13,15] Asymptomatic diverticula are typically an incidental finding when the colon is studied for another reason with a barium enema, colonoscopy, CT scan, or ultrasound examination. The clinical significance of asymptomatic diverticula is unclear, and they do not indicate a need for treatment or further follow-up.[1]

Symptomatic patients may complain of intermittent abdominal pain, bloating, excessive flatulence, or irregular defecation. In general there is a change in stool caliber, with descriptors that can range from flattened or ribbonlike to hard pellets. Associated complaints include urinary dysfunction, anorexia, nausea, vomiting, and heartburn. Older individuals often report recurrent bouts of steady or crampy pain (mostly in the left lower quadrant) in combination with constipation or alternating periods of diarrhea and constipation. They may also have abdominal distention that is relieved by the passage of flatus or stool. These symptoms are often classified as SUDD, and often mimic irritable bowel syndrome (IBS).[1] SUDD and IBS share an underlying pathophysiology that includes visceral hypersensitivity and slowed colonic motility. However, it is unclear whether SUDD and IBS are on a continuum in terms of their pathophysiology, and whether IBS patients are more likely to have diverticulosis.

Another variety of uncomplicated diverticulosis occurs when there is nonspecific segmental inflammation in the interdiverticular mucosa without involvement of the diverticular orifice; that condition is termed SCAD.[1] The pathophysiology of SCAD is not well understood, but is thought to be multifactorial, related to fecal stasis or localized ischemia.[16] As with SUDD, the presentation can include abdominal pain, altered bowel habits or diarrhea, and rectal bleeding.

Physical examination findings (including the pelvic and rectal examinations) for patients with uncomplicated symptoms are usually normal. The vital signs are often within normal limits. In case of SUDD or SCAD, physical findings may reveal mild left-lower-quadrant tenderness with a thickened palpable sigmoid colon. Rectal bleeding is infrequent, but painless bright red bleeding or maroon-colored stools suggest a diverticular bleed.[17]

DIAGNOSTICS

Asymptomatic diverticulosis requires no diagnostic workup. For symptomatic diverticulosis, a complete blood count (CBC) should be obtained in the setting of rectal bleeding. Microcytic anemia can be present in patients with chronic bleeding from diverticular disease. Mean corpuscular volume (MCV) may be elevated in acute bleeding secondary to reticulocytosis. Plain abdominal x-ray films will be normal and are unnecessary, although they are sometimes ordered to exclude the presence of free air in the abdomen. The diagnosis of diverticulosis or segmental colitis (as with SCAD) can be established by direct view on colonoscopy or flexible sigmoidoscopy. A barium or water-soluble enema can be utilized to diagnose the extent of diverticulosis. A CT scan of the abdomen can also diagnose diverticulosis.

INITIAL DIAGNOSTICS

Symptomatic Diverticulosis

- Flexible sigmoidoscopy or colonoscopy[a]

LABORATORY
- Complete blood count and differential[a]
- Stool for occult blood

IMAGING
- Barium enema
- Water-soluble enema
- X-ray of the kidneys, ureters, and bladder[a]
- Computed tomography scan

[a]If indicated

DIFFERENTIAL DIAGNOSIS

 Red flag symptoms include increased age, family or personal history of colorectal cancer, persistent symptoms despite treatment, and weight loss. These symptoms should prompt more extensive evaluation to rule out malignancy or infectious disease.

The hallmark of symptomatic diverticulosis is colicky abdominal pain in the absence of an inflammatory process. The cause of this pain is not fully understood but may be related to spasms in the sigmoid colon or an element of obstruction related to the spasms. This clinical entity must be differentiated from diverticulitis and any disease that causes abnormal intestinal motility.

The challenge is to distinguish patients who have symptomatic diverticular disease from those who have diverticula plus other lesions that may be responsible for the symptoms. IBS and colorectal cancer should be considered in the differential diagnosis. In patients with localized right-sided abdominal pain, appendicitis must be considered.[13]

The top three differentials are diverticulitis, colorectal malignancy, and IBS. The differential also includes inflammatory bowel disease, radiation-induced colitis, gynecologic inflammatory or neoplastic diseases, endometriosis, ectopic pregnancy, obstruction of the small or large bowel, gastroparesis, lactose intolerance, celiac disease, chronic constipation, infections (pseudomembranous colitis, cystitis, pyelonephritis), and anorectal disease.

INTERPROFESSIONAL COLLABORATIVE MANAGEMENT

Nonpharmacologic Management

A strong inverse relationship has been found between dietary fiber intake, which reduces the risk of constipation, and symptomatic diverticular disease.[11] In the United States, adults consume approximately 11 to 23 g of fiber per day, half of the 27 to 40 g of daily fiber recommended by the World Health Organization and less than the 20 to 35 g proposed by the American Dietetic Association.[18] Increased fiber intake can be achieved through the consumption of whole grains and cereals, fruits, vegetables, and legumes. These foods should be introduced gradually over a period of weeks to months to avoid excessive bloating and flatulence. Bran, a concentrated form of fiber, can be used as an adjunct to fiber consumption but should not be a replacement for other high-fiber foods. Fiber can also be consumed as commercially available high-fiber supplements or bulk formers such as psyllium hydrophilic mucilloid, methylcellulose, and calcium polycarbophil. These products must be taken with several glasses of fluid to be effective and produce a softer, more frequent stool.

To help alleviate symptoms, increased exercise is recommended to improve bowel function.

Pharmacologic Management

Anticholinergic and antispasmodic agents have been used without substantiated evidence of their effectiveness in treating diverticular symptoms. They may be used to relieve spasms.

Indications for Referral and Hospitalization

Surgical resection for pain relief in the absence of documented inflammatory complications is associated with a high rate of symptom recurrence and is therefore not recommended.[13]

Uncomplicated diverticular disease can be managed in the primary care setting. Refractory or worsening symptoms or questionable radiographic findings necessitate referral to a gastroenterologist for further evaluation. Patients with suspected diverticular abscess or rectal bleeding warrant further evaluation, and a referral for lower endoscopy is indicated. Although the health care provider assumes responsibility for patient education, a referral to a dietitian may be beneficial for patients with recurrent, painful disease.

LIFE-SPAN CONSIDERATIONS

Diverticular disease is usually observed in adults above 40 years of age, and the incidence increases with age. Younger adults, however, can also develop diverticular disease and associated complications such as diverticulitis and diverticular bleeding.[13]

COMPLICATIONS

The most common complication of diverticular disease is acute diverticulitis.[19] Hemorrhage from diverticula is also a common complication. Other less common complications include abscess, bowel perforation, peritonitis, strictures, fistulas, and small bowel obstructions.[8]

PATIENT AND FAMILY EDUCATION AND HEALTH PROMOTION

The patient's diet and symptoms should be reviewed at every session for prevention and health promotion.

The goal of 30 to 35 g of fiber per day should be encouraged. It is important that patients be advised to increase their fiber intake gradually to prevent flatulence and abdominal discomfort. Patients can often tolerate 5 to 10 g increments every couple weeks on the basis of symptoms. Bloating or flatulence resulting from increased fiber intake usually resolves with continued use. Maintenance of ideal body weight, daily exercise, reduced consumption of red and processed meats, and avoidance of tobacco and alcohol as well as the routine use of NSAIDs may also reduce the risk of developing diverticula.

DIVERTICULITIS

 Hospitalization is indicated for patients with fever above 101.3°F, signs of peritonitis, suspected abscess, intestinal obstruction, sepsis, and hypovolemia. Hospitalization should also be considered for diabetic or immunosuppressed patients, older adults, and patients with chronic renal failure.

DEFINITION AND EPIDEMIOLOGY

Diverticulitis is the most common complication of diverticulosis and affects 10% to 25% of patients at some time during their lives.[19-21] It is characterized by the inflammation of one or more colonic diverticula. The severity of diverticulitis can range from mild, self-limiting uncomplicated disease to a life-threatening condition complicated by perforation, abscess, fistula, or bleeding.[20,22] Complicated diverticulitis occurs in up to 25% of cases, and the majority of these patients have no prior knowledge of the disease. Perforation can be a patient's first symptom and is the most significant cause of morbidity and mortality.[13]

PATHOPHYSIOLOGY

The inflammation associated with diverticulitis is thought to result from the stagnation of fecal material in a single diverticulum.[1] This produces a fecalith that leads to pressure necrosis of the mucosa and subsequent inflammation. As the inflammatory process progresses, perforation can occur. A *micro*perforation is easily contained by the pericolic tissues and becomes a localized phlegmon. A *macro*perforation may result in a walled-off pericolic abscess whose erosion may produce fistulas into adjacent structures, such as the urinary bladder, vagina, small bowel, and anterior abdominal wall. If there is free perforation in the abdominal cavity, fecal peritonitis may occur.[23]

CLINICAL PRESENTATION AND PHYSICAL EXAMINATION

The diagnosis of diverticulitis is often clinical, especially in a patient with known diverticula. Most patients with infection or localized inflammation have mild to moderate aching abdominal pain usually present in the left lower quadrant (93% to 100%) accompanied by fever (57% to 100%) and leukocytosis (69% to 83%).[13] Diffuse abdominal pain is possible, indicating possible macroperforation.[24] The pain can be constant or intermittent, with associated nausea and vomiting in up to one-third of patients. A change in bowel habits, such as constipation or loose stools, may or may not be present. Hematochezia is uncommon in diverticulitis and is more suggestive of other diagnoses. In some instances the patient is initially seen with complications of diverticulitis, such as recurrent urinary tract infections or a feculent vaginal discharge resulting from

fistulization. In other cases a patient may exhibit few or no symptoms and therefore may not seek medical attention for several days. Older patients or those who are immunocompromised may have minimal abdominal pain, no fever, and relatively benign findings on physical examination but still have sepsis.[13]

The physical examination of patients with diverticulitis may reveal tenderness in the left lower quadrant with localized guarding and rigidity. Mild distention may be present. Very rarely, a mass may be palpated in the left iliac fossa.[24] The presence of a rigid board-like abdomen indicates severe disease associated with peritonitis, as do rebound tenderness and the absence of peristalsis.[4] Rectal examination may be normal but might reveal tenderness or a mass if a pelvic abscess is present.[4] Fever may or may not be present depending on the severity of the infection and the age and immune status of the patient.[13] If present, fever (typically below 102°F), tachycardia, and hypotension should raise suspicion for complicated disease. Stools are not usually positive for occult blood, but hematochezia is possible. In female patients, a pelvic examination is a necessary component of the physical examination to assess for a gynecologic etiology of symptoms.

DIAGNOSTICS

In mild cases, the diagnosis of acute diverticulitis can be made clinically based on history and physical examination alone. For more symptomatic cases, however, diagnostic testing and clinical management are guided by symptom severity, signs of peritonitis, and the patient's ability to tolerate oral intake. Leukocytosis has been found in nearly 55% of patients with acute diverticulitis; therefore a CBC should be obtained.[4] C-reactive protein (CRP) can also be ordered, as it has been found to be an indicator of the presence of complicated disease when values are greater than 170 to 200 mg/L.[25-27] Urinalysis may reveal white blood cells if the inflammatory process is adjacent to the bladder or ureter. The presence of bacteria in the urine sample consistent with urinary tract infection is suggestive of a fistula. A pregnancy test is indicated for premenopausal and perimenopausal women, particularly if antibiotic treatment, imaging, or surgery is being considered.

A CT scan of the abdomen is the test of choice in patients with symptomatic diverticulitis, particularly if complications are suspected. The use of intravenous contrast is recommended. Typical findings include bowel wall thickening, pericolic fat stranding, and pericolic fluid.[4,28] Abscess, free air, and fistula formation can also be visualized. In addition, CT gives a more accurate estimate of the degree of inflammation than other studies[29] and has the advantage of delineating the extent of an extraluminal disease process; it can also direct therapeutic intervention in case of complicated disease (e.g., percutaneous drainage of an intra-abdominal abscess).[21] A disadvantage of CT is the potentially harmful effects of ionizing radiation.

Ultrasound and MRI are possible alternative imaging modalities. Ultrasonography is used to reveal extracolic fluid collections and to guide percutaneous drainage of pelvic and paracolic abscesses; however, ultrasonography is more operator-dependent than CT.[29] Patients may not be able to tolerate the external pressure, and imaging is limited in an obese patient. MRI can reveal excellent soft tissue detail and does not involve ionizing radiation. However, MRI takes significantly longer than CT and has not been shown to have similar sensitivity or specificity. In addition, patients with certain types of surgical clips, metallic fragments, or cardiac pacemakers cannot undergo MRI.[4] Supine and upright plain x-ray films can be obtained to assess for a small or large bowel obstruction or free abdominal air (which indicates perforation). A barium enema is not recommended with acute diverticulitis because of the risk of barium peritonitis.[29] Colonoscopy should be avoided in acute diverticulitis due to risk of perforation[4,21] but is useful after the inflammatory process subsides to rule out a malignant etiology of symptoms.[23]

INITIAL DIAGNOSTICS

Diverticulitis

- Complete blood count and differential
- C-reactive protein
- Urinalysis
- Blood urea nitrogen, creatinine (before computed tomography scan in older adults or in patients with renal insufficiency)
- Colonoscopy (4–6 weeks after the acute episode has resolved)

IMAGING
- Computed tomography scan
- Ultrasound
- Magnetic resonance imaging[a]
- Water-soluble contrast enema
- Angiography (if the patient is bleeding)
- Endoscopy
- Flexible sigmoidoscopy

[a]If indicated.

DIFFERENTIAL DIAGNOSIS

 Priority differentials include acute appendicitis, gastroenteritis, cystitis, colitis, ectopic pregnancy, testicular torsion, and malignancy.

The differential diagnoses are considerable. Red flag symptoms include increased age, family or personal history of colorectal cancer, persistent symptoms despite treatment, and weight loss. These symptoms especially should prompt more extensive evaluation to rule out malignancy.

Further differentials to consider include mechanical and inflammatory disorders of the gastrointestinal tract, urologic and gynecologic disorders, functional disorders, and malignancy.[4,13] Other possible diagnoses include acute appendicitis, gastroenteritis, cystitis, ischemic or radiation colitis, infectious colitis, pelvic inflammatory disease, endometriosis, ovarian cyst, ectopic pregnancy, and testicular torsion.

INTERPROFESSIONAL COLLABORATIVE MANAGEMENT

NONPHARMACOLOGIC MANAGEMENT

For decades antibiotics have been the cornerstone of treatment for acute diverticulitis, owing in large part to the belief that symptoms were due to the obstruction of a diverticulum leading to microperforation and the translocation of bacteria.[1] In recent years, however, studies have challenged this view. Several studies have shown no benefit in the use of antibiotics in the management of some patients with uncomplicated diverticulitis. In 2012, Chabok et al. investigated the need for antibiotic therapy to treat acute uncomplicated diverticulitis and found no statistically significant difference in outcome in patients treated with antibiotics and those managed conservatively.[30] In

2014, Isacson et al. performed a retrospective-based population cohort study to assess the applicability of a selective "no antibiotic" policy and its consequences in terms of complications and recurrence and found that withholding antibiotics was safe and did not result in higher complication or recurrence rates.[31] Further, in a 2016 multicenter study, Daniels et al. performed a randomized controlled trial of observation versus antibiotic treatment for a first episode of uncomplicated acute diverticulitis in 528 patients and found that there was no prolongation of recovery time in those treated without antibiotics.[32] These studies may herald a shifting paradigm in the treatment of uncomplicated diverticular disease. For patients with acute diverticulitis, antibiotic therapy is necessary to avoid sepsis and other complications.[33]

After an attack of diverticulitis, a short-term, low-fiber diet consisting of 15 g or less of dietary fiber is prescribed to reduce the volume of fecal material in the lower bowel and to prevent irritation of the colon. Once the patient is asymptomatic, a gradual modification to a diet high in fiber may help to reduce pressure inside the colon, thus reducing the chances of future attacks. A colonoscopy is recommended 4 to 6 weeks after symptoms resolve in order to exclude malignancy.[13]

PHARMACOLOGIC MANAGEMENT

Spontaneous resolution is common for many patients with low-grade fever, mild leukocytosis, and minimum abdominal tenderness. In cases where antibiotics continue to be utilized in the treatment of uncomplicated diverticulitis, outpatient management typically consists of conservative treatment with bowel rest (e.g., clear liquids and follow-up in 48 to 72 hours), increased fluid intake, and oral antibiotics to cover colonic flora. The most common antibiotic regimens in the United States include trimethoprim-sulfamethoxazole (Bactrim DS, 160/800 mg twice daily) plus metronidazole (500 mg three times daily), amoxicillin-clavulanate potassium (Augmentin, 875/125 mg), or ciprofloxacin (500 mg twice daily) plus metronidazole (500 mg three times daily) for 7 to 14 days.[13,28] The success rate with such outpatient management has been estimated at 94% to 97%.[28] These patients do not require hospitalization. Pain medication is discouraged; symptomatic relief may be achieved with warm packs. Nonopiate analgesics may be used if necessary. Rifaximin, as well as anti-inflammatories including mesalamine and probiotics, are newer therapies that have been used in the treatment of diverticulitis, especially SUDD.[33] However, these agents have not been shown to decrease the risk of diverticulitis complications or recurrence.[1]

Indications for Referral and Hospitalization

With complicated diverticulitis, patients can be acutely ill with systemic peritonitis, sepsis, and hypovolemia. Any patient with a temperature of 38.5°C (101.3°F) or higher and with marked tenderness, signs of localized peritonitis, intestinal obstruction, or suspected intra-abdominal or pelvic abscess should be admitted to the hospital. Hospitalization is also recommended for diabetic or immunosuppressed patients, older adults, and patients with chronic renal failure in whom diverticulitis is suspected in the absence of the previously listed criteria.[13] Older adults are especially prone to complications from diverticular disease, including risk of diverticular rupture and peritonitis.[34] Hospital management includes assessment of fluid status and intravenous replacement, nasogastric suction if there is an obstruction or ileus, blood cultures, and broad-spectrum intravenous antibiotics that cover gram-negative anaerobes and gram-negative aerobes. Treatment time depends on symptom resolution and is usually maintained for 7 to 10 days. Further evaluation and management depend on patient assessment and response to initial treatment. If fever, abdominal signs, and leukocytosis have mostly resolved and bowel function has returned with the passage of flatus, a liquid diet can be started and slowly advanced to a low-fiber diet. When the patient is asymptomatic, a high-fiber diet can gradually be introduced. The patient is discharged with a regimen of oral antibiotics, such as metronidazole, 500 mg three times daily for 7 to 10 days. Studies such as a barium enema or colonoscopy should be performed 4 to 6 weeks after hospital discharge. A CT scan with contrast enhancement is required if the patient's condition does not improve after 2 to 4 days of medical treatment; if the diagnosis is in doubt; or if a pelvic or abdominal abscess, fistula, or obstruction is suspected.[13]

Most patients with uncomplicated diverticulitis recover with medical treatment and do not have escalation of acute symptoms even if they have additional attacks in the future. Standard convention has been to refer these patients for surgical consultation after a second episode, but the most recent American Gastroenterological Association (AGA) and American Society of Colon and Rectal Surgeons (ASCRS) guidelines both suggest against elective colonic resection in patients with uncomplicated diverticulitis and recommend that an individualized approach to symptoms—rather than a numerical threshold—should guide management.[35,36] For complicated disease, the decision regarding surgical intervention is based on factors including the patient's age, comorbidities, frequency and severity of attacks, and CT-graded severity of attacks. Elective surgical management typically consists of a single-stage procedure to decrease morbidity and mortality. A laparoscopic approach has been used for sigmoid resection. This approach decreases hospitalization time and shortens recovery.[23]

COMPLICATIONS

Complications of diverticulitis include free perforation with fecal peritonitis, suppurative peritonitis secondary to ruptured abscess, abdominal or pelvic abscess, fistula, and obstruction. It is estimated that 30% of patients will have recurrent diverticulitis. The chance of recurrence after the first episode is 90% within 5 years. Patients who experience a second episode have more than a 50% chance of having a third episode.[9] Fiber can reduce the risk of recurrence in up to 70% of patients.[37]

Historically, patients between 40 and 50 years of age were thought to be at increased risk for the development of complications,[13] with less response to medical management, leading to increased risk of recurrences with complications. Aggressive treatment with early surgery was thus deemed appropriate. However, more recent studies have found that young patients do not experience a more virulent or recurrent disease course compared with older patients and do not require more aggressive treatment, particularly surgical intervention, for the prevention of complications or recurrence.[38]

Immunosuppressed patients are at especially high risk for complications because they may not experience a normal inflammatory response and subsequently can develop spontaneous colon perforation and perforated diverticula.[13] Aggressive management of these patients includes emergency surgical intervention.

PATIENT AND FAMILY EDUCATION

During the convalescent period, patients benefit from a low-fiber diet (<15 g/day) and careful diet instruction. Whole-grain breads and cereals, raw fruits and vegetables, and legumes should be avoided.

Patients need not avoid nuts, seeds, or popcorn as no relationship has been found between consumption of those foods and the development of diverticulitis.[24]

A low-fiber diet can be liberalized as the patient's condition improves. Once stable and pain-free, patients can reintroduce a high-fiber diet slowly, during several weeks, to avoid any abdominal distention or excessive flatulence.

It is important that patients establish a regular bowel movement pattern that avoids constipation. A high-fiber diet will keep stools soft and easy to pass.

Patients should be aware of the importance of reporting recurrent pain promptly, especially if the pain is associated with chills or fever. Urgent hospitalization may be necessary.

DIVERTICULAR BLEEDING

Massive bleeding is an urgent situation that requires referral to a gastroenterologist. In older patients with bleeding, transient hypovolemia can be a serious problem for major organs, and immediate hospitalization must be considered.

DEFINITION AND EPIDEMIOLOGY

Diverticular bleeding is the most common cause of lower gastrointestinal bleeding, accounting for 3% to 15% of episodes of mild hematochezia and approximately 40% of episodes of severe hematochezia.[13,39,40] Diverticular hemorrhage resolves spontaneously in 70% to 90% of cases.[39-41] However, rebleeding occurs in 25% to 47% of patients.[42] Persistent bleeding or acute and massive bleeding presenting with hemodynamic instability requires intervention. Hemorrhage from a colonic diverticulum generally begins without warning in an older individual with otherwise asymptomatic diverticulosis.

PATHOPHYSIOLOGY

Bleeding arises from the rupture of one of the branches of the vasa recta adjacent to a diverticulum. The most significant risk factor for diverticular bleeding is the use of NSAIDs, because they inhibit prostaglandin synthesis and platelet aggregation, leading to bleeding if diverticular disease is present.[39,43] Cerebrovascular disease and hyperuricemia are also significant predictors of diverticular bleeding.[39] The most common site of massive bleeding is the right colon, particularly in older adults.[13,34] Diverticular bleeding is neither chronic nor occult. Iron deficiency anemia associated with occult blood in the stool should not be attributed to diverticulosis without an appropriate diagnostic evaluation.

CLINICAL PRESENTATION AND PHYSICAL EXAMINATION

The typical presentation of a diverticular bleed is painless hematochezia. Diverticular bleeding usually occurs in an older patient with diverticulosis who has previously been asymptomatic or undiagnosed. The patient will most likely not experience abdominal cramping, which is a reflection of the noninflammatory pathogenesis of the bleeding. The patient may pass a large volume of bright red to dark maroon blood with or without signs of hypovolemia. The patient may have an additional one or two such movements and then no more, or the bleeding may continue for several days. There are no distinctive features by which to distinguish diverticular bleeding from other causes of lower gastrointestinal bleeding.

Physical examination findings are typically normal, although the digital rectal examination can reveal anorectal lesions (e.g., hemorrhoids) as the source of bleeding. The oropharynx, nasopharynx, abdomen, and perineum should all be examined to exclude other sources of bleeding. If the bleeding has stopped, the patient may be normotensive. If the bleeding is ongoing, however, the patient may be tachycardic and hypotensive. If blood loss is excessive, signs of hypovolemia with postural vital signs or shock may be present.[13]

DIAGNOSTICS

A CBC will help to determine not only the extent of blood loss (anemia), but also whether the bleeding has been ongoing. Upper gastrointestinal bleeding can be excluded by esophagogastroduodenoscopy and aspiration of gastric contents. Once an upper gastrointestinal source of the bleeding has been excluded, colonoscopy is the diagnostic tool of choice to evaluate for a source of the bleeding even when it is aggressive.[39,40] Colonoscopy can be used to both identify the source of the bleeding and apply endoscopic therapy. If no bleeding source is found during colonoscopy, nuclear scintigraphy (tagged red blood cell scan) followed by angiography can be performed to localize the bleeding site. Mesenteric angiography can be used as a diagnostic tool to localize the bleeding site and as a therapeutic intervention whereby vasoconstrictive drugs or an artificial blood clot can be infused to control the hemorrhage. A barium enema study should never be the initial test in patients with diverticular bleeding because angiography or colonoscopy will be precluded until the contrast material has been evacuated, thereby resulting in a delayed examination.

INITIAL DIAGNOSTICS

Diverticular Bleeding

- Complete blood count and differential and manual platelet count
- Esophagogastroduodenoscopy
- Colonoscopy

LABORATORY
- Stool for occult blood
- Coagulation studies including liver function tests

IMAGING
- Nuclear scintigraphy
- Angiography
- Red blood cell nuclear bleeding scan

DIFFERENTIAL DIAGNOSIS

 Priority differentials include colorectal malignancy, ischemic colitis, and inflammatory bowel disease. Red flag symptoms include profound anemia, increased age, family or personal history of colorectal cancer, persistent symptoms despite treatment, and weight loss. These symptoms should prompt more extensive evaluation to rule out malignancy.

Diverticular bleeding is a diagnosis of exclusion. The differential diagnosis is broad and includes upper gastrointestinal sources, malignancy, inflammatory diseases, and anorectal conditions. Any gastrointestinal lesion that has the potential for massive hemorrhage (e.g., a duodenal ulcer or Meckel diverticulum) can manifest in a manner similar to diverticular bleeding and must be excluded.[44] The differential also includes colonic polyps, infectious colitis, duodenal ulcer, Meckel diverticulum, vascular ectasia, hemorrhoids, anorectal lesion, angiodysplasia, and foreign body.

INTERPROFESSIONAL COLLABORATIVE MANAGEMENT

Although massive gastrointestinal bleeding is a life-threatening condition, the prognosis for diverticular bleeding is generally favorable. Most bleeding stops spontaneously and does not recur. The exception for recurrence includes use of NSAIDs, advanced age, documented diverticulitis, cerebrovascular disease, or a history of chronic renal failure. Any of these factors increases the risk for a repeat bleed.[45] Treatment of diverticular bleeding should begin with conservative medical management. Most patients can be observed as inpatients without the need for urgent diagnostic or invasive therapeutic maneuvers.

NONPHARMACOLOGIC MANAGEMENT

The primary interventions for diverticular bleeding are hemodynamic stabilization and resuscitation. Anal or rectal bleeding should be excluded with a digital rectal examination and anoscopy. Most cases of mild to moderate hemorrhage stop spontaneously with medical management that includes establishment of intravenous access and insertion of a nasogastric tube to exclude an upper gastrointestinal source of bleeding. Laboratory tests should include a CBC, electrolytes, coagulation studies, and blood type with cross-match. Patients with suspected lower gastrointestinal bleeding should undergo colonoscopy to identify the source; if a source is found, endoscopic therapy such as clipping, endoscopic band ligation, and injection therapy can be applied.[40] The patient with persistent diverticular bleeding also has several therapeutic options, including selective intra-arterial infusion of vasopressin, angiographic embolization, and surgical resection.[15]

INDICATIONS FOR REFERRAL AND HOSPITALIZATION

Surgical intervention is required for massive and persistent bleeding that does not respond to medical treatment and interventional radiology. Surgery may also be recommended on an elective basis for patients with recurrent hemorrhages.[44]

COMPLICATIONS

The complications of diverticular hemorrhage are related to hypovolemia and circulatory collapse. Older patients tolerate the hemorrhage poorly because of the ischemic risk to major organs with each bleeding episode.

PATIENT AND FAMILY EDUCATION

Explicit patient education is essential because of the risk for recurrent bleeding after the first episode. It is important to advise patients to report symptoms immediately in order to avoid complications such as hypovolemia and circulatory collapse.

REFERENCES

1. Rezapour, M., Ali, S., & Stollman, N. (2017). Diverticular disease: An update on pathogenesis and management. *Gut and Liver* (online publication).

2. Mayl, J., Marchenko, M., & Frierson, E. (2017). Management of acute uncomplicated diverticulitis may exclude antibiotic therapy. *Cureus*, 9(5), e1250.

3. Horesh, N., Wasserberg, N., Zbar, A. P., et al. (2016). Changing paradigms in the management of diverticulitis. *International Journal of Surgery*, 33(Pt. A), 146–150.

4. Wilkins, T., Embry, K., & George, R. (2013). Diagnosis and management of acute diverticulitis. *American Family Physician*, 87(9), 612–620.

5. Painter, N. S., & Burkitt, D. P. (1971). Diverticular disease of the colon: A deficiency disease of Western civilization. *British Medical Journal*, 2(5759), 450–454.

6. Hobson, K. G., & Roberts, P. L. (2004). Etiology and pathophysiology of diverticular disease. *Clinics in Colon and Rectal Surgery*, 17(3), 147–153.

7. Weizman, A., & Nguyen, G. (2011). Diverticular disease: Epidemiology and management. *Canadian Journal of Gastroenterology*, 25(7), 385–389.

8. World Gastroenterology Organisation Practice Guidelines. Diverticular disease. Retrieved from: www.worldgastroenterology.org/assets/downloads/en/pdf/guidelines/07_diverticular_disease.pdf. (Accessed 30 June 2014).

9. Fong, S. S., Tan, E. Y., Foo, A., Sim, R., & Sheong, D. M. (2011). The changing trend of diverticular disease in a developing nation. *Colorectal Disease: The Official Journal of the Association of Coloproctology of Great Britain and Ireland*, 13(3), 312–316.

10. Deery, S. E., & Hodin, R. A. (2017). Management of diverticulitis in 2017. *Journal of Gastrointestinal Surgery: Official Journal of the Society for Surgery of the Alimentary Tract*, 21(10), 1732–1741.

11. McSweeney, W., & Srinath, H. (2017). Diverticular disease practice points. *Australian Family Physician*, 46(11), 829–832.

12. Strate, L. L., et al. (2013). Heritability and familial aggregation of diverticular disease: A population-based study of twins and siblings. *Gastroenterology*, 144(736).

13. Prather, C. (2012). Inflammatory and anatomic disease of the intestine, peritoneum, mesentery, and omentum. In L. Goldman & A. I. Schafer (Eds.), *Goldman's Cecil Medicine* (24th ed.). Philadelphia: Elsevier.

14. Wess, L., Eastwood, M. A., Wess, T. J., Busuttil, A., & Miller, A. (1995). Cross-linking of collagen is increased in colonic diverticulosis. *Gut*, 37, 91–94.

15. Tursi, A., & Papagrigoriadis, S. (2009). The current and evolving treatment of colonic diverticular disease. *Alimentary Pharmacology and Therapeutics*, 30(6), 532–546.

16. Ludeman, L., & Shepherd, N. A. (2002). What is diverticular colitis? *Pathology*, 34, 568.

17. Bickley, L. S., & Szilagyi, P. G. (2013). *Bates' Guide to Physical Examination and History Taking* (11th ed.). Philadelphia: Lippincott Williams & Wilkins.

18. Cordain, L., Eaton, S. B., Sebastian, A., et al. (2005). Origins and evolution of the Western diet: Health implications for the 21st century. *The American Journal of Clinical Nutrition*, 81(2), 341–354.

19. Jackson, J. D., & Hammond, T. (2014). Systematic review: Outpatient management of acute uncomplicated diverticulitis. *International Journal of Colorectal Disease*, 29(7), 775–781.

20. Tan, J. P., Barazanchi, A. W., Singh, P. P., et al. (2016). Predictors of acute diverticulitis severity: A systematic review. *International Journal of Surgery*, 26, 43–52.

21. Moubax, K., & Urbain, D. (2015). Diverticulitis: New insights on the traditional point of view. *Acta Gastro-Enterologica Belgica*, 78(1), 38–48.

22. Isacson, D., Thorisson, A., Andreasson, K., et al. (2015). Outpatient, non-antibiotic management in acute uncomplicated diverticulitis: A prospective study. *International Journal of Colorectal Disease*, 30(9), 1229–1234.

23. Watkins, T., Embry, K., & George, R. (2013). Diagnosis and management of acute diverticulitis. *American Family Physician*, 87(9), 612–620.

24. Humes, D. J., & Spiller, R. C. (2014). Review article: The pathogenesis and management of acute colonic diverticulitis. *Alimentary Pharmacology and Therapeutics*, 39(4), 359–370.

25. Bolkenstein, H. E., van de Wall, B. J. M., Consten, E. C. J., et al. (2017). Risk factors for complicated diverticulitis: Systematic review and meta-analysis. *International Journal of Colorectal Disease*, 32(10), 1375–1383.

26. Kechagias, A., Rautio, T., Kechagias, G., et al. (2014). The role of C-reactive protein in the prediction of the clinical severity of acute diverticulitis. *The American Surgeon*, 80(4), 391–395.

27. van de Wall, B. J., Draaisma, W. A., van der Kaaij, R. T., et al. (2013). The value of inflammation markers and body temperature in acute diverticulitis. *Colorectal Disease: The Official Journal of the Association of Coloproctology of Great Britain and Ireland*, 15(5), 621–626.

28. Linzay, C. D., & Pandit, S. (2017). Diverticulitis, acute. In *StatPearls [Internet]*. Treasure Island (FL): StatPearls Publishing. Retrieved from https://www-ncbi-nlm-nih-gov.dartmouth.idm.oclc.org/books/NBK459316/. Jun [Updated 2017 Nov 12].

29. American College of Radiology (ACR) Appropriateness criteria. Left lower quadrant pain—suspected diverticulitis. Retrieved from www.acr.org/~/media/ACR/Documents/AppCriteria/Diagnostic/LeftLowerQuadrantPainSuspectedDiverticulitis.pdf. (Accessed 28 June 2015).

30. Chabok, A., Påhlman, L., Hjern, F., et al. (2012). AVOD Study Group. Randomized clinical trial of antibiotics in acute uncomplicated diverticulitis. *The British Journal of Surgery*, 99, 532–539.

31. Isacson, D., Andreasson, K., Nikberg, M., Smedh, K., & Chabok, A. (2014). No antibiotics in acute uncomplicated diverticulitis: Does it work? *Scandinavian Journal of Gastroenterology*, 49, 1441–1446.

32. Daniels, L., Ünlü, Ç., de Korte, N., et al. (2017). Randomized clinical trial of observational versus antibiotic treatment for a first episode of CT-proven uncomplicated acute diverticulitis. *The British Journal of Surgery*, 104, 52–61.

33. Carabotti, M., & Annibale, B. (2018). Treatment of diverticular disease: An update on latest evidence and clinical implications. *Drugs in Context*, 7, 212526.

34. Lutwak, N. (2013). Mild to moderate diverticulitis: What's new in diagnostic approach, treatment, and prevention of reoccurrence? *American Family Physician*, 21(7).

35. Feingold, D., Steele, S. R., Lee, S., et al. (2014). Practice parameters for the treatment of sigmoid diverticulitis. *Diseases of the Colon and Rectum*, 57, 284–294.

36. Stollman, N., Smalley, W., Hirano, I., & AGA Institute Clinical Guidelines Committee. (2015). American Gastroenterological Association Institute guideline on the management of acute diverticulitis. *Gastroenterology*, 149, 1944–1949.

37. Reinhard, T. (2014). Diverticular disease. *Todays Dietician*, 16(3), 46–50.

38. van Dijk, S. T., Rottier, S. J., van Geloven, A. A. W., et al. (2017). Conservative treatment of acute colonic diverticulitis. *Current Infectious Disease Reports*, 19(11), 44.

39. Cirocchi, R., Grassi, V., Cavaliere, D., et al. (2015). New trends in acute management of colonic diverticular bleeding: A systematic review. *Medicine*, 94(44), e1710.

40. Yamada, A., Niikura, R., Yoshida, S., et al. (2015). Endoscopic management of colonic diverticular bleeding. *Digestive Endoscopy: Official Journal of the Japan Gastroenterological Endoscopy Society*, 27(7), 720–725.

41. Reddy, V., & Longo, W. E. (2013). The burden of diverticular disease on patients and healthcare systems. *Gastroenterologia Y Hepatologia*, 9(1), 21–27.

42. Akutsu, D., et al. (2015). Endoscopic detachable snare ligation: A new treatment method for colonic diverticular hemorrhage. *Endoscopy*, 47(11), 1039–1042.

43. Taki, M., Oshima, T., Tozawa, K., et al. (2017). Analysis of risk factors for colonic diverticular bleeding and recurrence. *Medicine*, 96, 38.

44. Triadafilopoulos, G. (2012). Management of lower GI bleeding in older adults. *Drugs and Aging*, 29(9), 707–715.

45. Aytac, E., Stocchi, L., Gorgun, E., & Ozuner, G. (2014). Risk of recurrence and longterm outcomes after colonic diverticular bleeding. *International Journal of Colorectal Disease*, 29(3), 373–378.

CHAPTER **116**

OROPHARYNGEAL DYSPHAGIA IN ADULTS

Talli McCormick

 Emergency room evaluation is indicated for patients with new-onset inability to swallow and for those who have experienced an acute choking episode requiring the Heimlich maneuver.[1]

DEFINITION AND EPIDEMIOLOGY

Oropharyngeal dysphagia is a swallowing disorder that involves dysfunction of one or more stages in the sequence of swallowing. This type of dysphagia differs from upper gastrointestinal disorders in that the dysfunction involves oral, pharyngeal, and laryngeal structures. The dysphagia may be mild or severe,

BOX 116.1

Potential Causes of Oropharyngeal Dysphagia

IATROGENIC
- Medication side effects (e.g., xerostomia, chemotherapy, neuroleptics)
- Postsurgical muscular or neurogenic disorders (e.g., head and neck cancers, stroke)
- Radiation therapy
- Corrosive (pill injury, intentional)

INFECTIOUS
- Botulism, diphtheria, Lyme disease, syphilis
- Mucositis (e.g., herpes, cytomegalovirus, *Candida* organisms)

METABOLIC
- Amyloidosis
- Cushing syndrome
- Thyrotoxicosis
- Wilson disease

MYOPATHIC
- Connective tissue disease
- Myasthenia gravis
- Myotonic dystrophy
- Oculopharyngeal dystrophy
- Polymyositis
- Sarcoidosis
- Paraneoplastic syndromes

NEUROLOGIC
- Amyotrophic lateral sclerosis
- Brain-stem tumors
- Cerebral palsy
- Dementia

- Guillain-Barré syndrome
- Head trauma
- Huntington disease
- Multiple sclerosis
- Parkinson disease

POLIOMYELITIS
- Postpolio syndrome
- Stroke
- Tardive dyskinesia

STRUCTURAL
- Cervical webs
- Congenital disorders (cleft palate, diverticula, pouches)
- Cricopharyngeal bar

OROPHARYNGEAL TUMORS
- Osteophytes and skeletal abnormalities
- Zenker diverticulum

PSYCHIATRIC
- Anxiety or stress causing globus sensation
- Depression or grief

ENVIRONMENTAL
- Poor positioning
- Eating or being fed too quickly or too large a bolus
- Inappropriate consistency
- Poor oral health or hygiene
- Distractibility

Modified from Cook, I. J., & Kahrilas, P. J. (1999). AGA technical review on management of oropharyngeal dysphagia. *Gastroenterology, 116*(2):455–478; and Blackington, E., McCormick, T., Willson, B., et al. (2001). Oropharyngeal dysphagia in the elderly. *Advance Nurse Practice, 9*(7):45.

resulting in malnutrition, dehydration, choking, aspiration, impaired healing, pneumonia, and even death. Estimates of incidence and prevalence vary, but Rofes and colleagues report that over 16 million people in the United States and over 40 million in Europe are affected.[2] Dysphagia results in a reduced quality of life in those affected and their caregivers.

Dysphagia is most commonly associated with stroke (70%),[3] Parkinson disease (and other neurodegenerative diseases, including dementia),[4,5] and traumatic brain injuries.[3–5] "Stroke is the second most common cause of death and of adult disability worldwide,"[6] but estimates suggest that perhaps 90% of people with community-acquired pneumonia may have dysphagia.[7]

Recently, chronic obstructive pulmonary disease (COPD) has been considered in dysphagia research. It is the third-leading cause of death worldwide and a leading cause of hospitalization. As breathing and swallowing share space and neurons, potentially competing activities occur here. To swallow safely, breathing must briefly stop. It is thought that altered breathing may contribute to dysphagia and that dysphagia may contribute to exacerbations of COPD.[8] Screening for swallowing is frequently done in new stroke patients[9] but not commonly performed for patients with COPD.[8]

PATHOPHYSIOLOGY

Dysphagia may be either oropharyngeal or esophageal. The cause can be neurologic, neuromuscular, metabolic, pharmacologic, infectious, psychiatric, environmental, or structural. Identification of the causative agent or disease is paramount in the assessment and treatment of dysphagia. Structural causes are more common in esophageal dysphagia, and functional causes are more likely in oropharyngeal dysphagia (Box 116.1). Structural causes include trauma or surgery, tumor, webs, strictures or stenoses, diverticula, infection, and, in some cases, cervical osteophytes or cricopharyngeal bars.[10]

To more fully understand dysphagia, it is essential to appreciate the anatomy and physiology of normal swallowing. Swallowing has three commonly described phases: oral, pharyngeal, and esophageal. In addition to these three phases, there are preparatory phases to the act of eating. Most of us decide when we are hungry and what and how much we would like to eat. We prepare food or go to a restaurant. We decide with whom we will eat. These decisions involve autonomy, fairly intact cognition, and normal neuromuscular function. Nursing home residents and homebound older adults may have significant limitations or restrictions in this preparatory phase.[11]

During the oral phase, much sensory information is gathered about the food and the involved structures. Quantity, shape, consistency, and moisture content are determined along with the temperature, taste, and location of the food. The touch and pressure exerted on the oral structures, especially the tongue and hard and soft palates and pillars, are transmitted to the brain stem for further action and distribution. This continuous assessment by the sensory system allows precise communication with the muscles of mastication.

Chewing (mastication) involves cranial nerves (CNs) V (trigeminal), VII (facial), IX (glossopharyngeal), and XII (hypoglossal) in addition to the muscles of the jaw, cheeks, tongue, and palate. The lips remain closed during chewing, while the tongue and teeth prepare the food into a bolus of the proper size and consistency. The soft palate descends to help hold the food within the mouth during chewing. The teeth close, the tongue places the bolus in its central groove, and the bolus is then rapidly pushed, or transferred, through the pillars (fauces) into the pharynx.

At this point the bolus passes a ring of sensory receptors at the base of the tongue, pillars, soft palate, and posterior pharyngeal wall. Sensory impulses indicating the presence of a bolus are sent by CN IX to the swallowing center in the brain stem, which then initiates the involuntary phase of the swallow.[11] Sensory input is also crucial to the pharyngeal stage. As the tongue pushes the bolus to the posterior pharynx, the soft palate flattens upward and backward (CN V), sealing off the nasopharynx. Simultaneously, the hyoid and larynx begin to move upward and forward (CN X [vagus]), tipping back the epiglottis and widening the esophageal opening. The pillars lower, and the tongue presses against the posterior pharyngeal wall (CN IX) to block retrograde movement of the bolus into the oral cavity. Sensory fibers of CN X transmit information to the swallowing center in the brain stem. The impulse returns by the motor component of the vagus nerve and initiates peristalsis of the pharyngeal constrictors to propel the bolus toward the esophagus, passing the valleculae and piriform sinuses. The soft palate descends, the larynx continues to rise, and the epiglottis descends. As the epiglottis descends to block the laryngeal opening, the upper esophageal sphincter (UES) or cricopharyngeal sphincter opens to allow the bolus to pass into the esophagus.[11]

As the food bolus enters the esophagus, these processes begin in reverse. Once the food bolus is in the esophagus, the UES closes and peristalsis and gravity propel the bolus toward the stomach. The lower esophageal sphincter (LES) opens, and the bolus enters the stomach. Normal transit time depends on bolus consistency but is generally 2 to 4 seconds.[11] The cerebellum is thought to play a significant role in the modulation and choreography of the swallowing process, but further research is needed.[12]

CLINICAL PRESENTATION AND PHYSICAL EXAMINATION

Dysphagic patients can be initially seen with malnutrition, weight loss, dehydration, coughing or choking with eating, impaired healing, or even pneumonia. Problems in the oral stage include poor bolus control, spillage either from the lips or into the pharynx, dry oral membranes, pocketing or oral residue, and difficulty with chewing. Pharyngeal dysphagia often results from weakness or poor coordination of the pharyngeal muscles. This can cause delayed swallowing, failure of airway protection, nasal or oral regurgitation, or it can leave residue in the pharynx after swallow, manifesting as coughing, choking, or gurgling.

Xerostomia (dry mouth), either intrinsic or extrinsic, can be a contributing factor in dysphagia. Independently of impaired function, patients with xerostomia often perceive difficulty in swallowing and a change in sensation or motion with or without actual difficulties.[13] Globus, the sensation of a lump in the throat, can occur alone or may coexist with esophageal dysphagia, particularly when it is accompanied by chest pain or heartburn.[14] Globus alone is merely a sensory experience; swallowing itself is unimpaired.

A detailed history is the most important step in differential diagnosis. Because dysphagia can be associated with neurologic disease, a thorough neuromuscular history is important. Obtaining an accurate history can be complicated by a patient's reduced alertness and possible cognitive and speech impairments, which can also affect the patient's ability to participate in examinations, diagnostics, and treatment strategies. Assessment of the impact of dysphagia on patient function and quality of life as well as social interactions is paramount. A geriatric depression scale or other measure of anxiety and depression may be of value.

Onset, progression, location, and duration of symptoms and preferred food consistency aid in diagnosis. A short duration associated with weight loss can indicate malignant disease.[10] Abrupt onset associated with neurologic impairment suggests a cerebrovascular accident. Studies have estimated that 8% to 80% of new stroke patients will have dysphagia, and in 10% to 30% of these, the dysphagia will persist beyond 1 month.[2] Swallowing of thin liquids is often a problem after a stroke. Gradual progressive onset is more likely to be associated with Parkinson disease, amyotrophic lateral sclerosis, sarcoidosis, myasthenia gravis, Alzheimer disease, or other chronic diseases. Parkinson disease is the most common movement disorder in older adults and leads to tongue rigidity and tremor, making bolus formation and transfer into the pharynx difficult. Difficulty in swallowing of only solids suggests a structural cause but not necessarily the location of the impairment. Ability to point to where the food "sticks" is useful for oropharyngeal obstructions and correlates well with radiographic studies.

Eating or being fed too rapidly may result in either oral or nasal regurgitation and choking. Coughing up food after meals can indicate a pharyngeal diverticulum.[10] Frequent swallowing can indicate oral or pharyngeal residue. Positioning of the patient, degree of distraction, companions or assistants, utensils used, food consistency, and likes and dislikes can all provide information useful not only in the differential diagnosis but also in deciding on treatment strategies.

A complete review of all medications is necessary because some medications are thought to cause or contribute to swallowing dysfunction. Further study of the interactions of medications and swallowing is indicated. Medications such as alendronate sodium (Fosamax), nonsteroidal antiinflammatory drugs (NSAIDs), and potassium can cause direct damage to the esophageal mucosa (Box 116.2). Xerostomia, altered esophageal sphincter pressure, and reduced alertness are other medication side effects that can affect swallowing.[11]

The first step in identifying dysphagia is asking patients or families whether there is a problem. Heijnen and colleagues[15] compared asking "What about swallowing?" with the EAT-10

Medication-Related Conditions That Cause Oropharyngeal Dysphagia

XEROSTOMIA
- Antidepressants
- Antispasmodics
- Antihypertensives
- Anticholinergics
- Antihistamines
- Bronchodilators
- Sedatives

CENTRAL NERVOUS SYSTEM DEPRESSION
- Anticonvulsants
- Antianxiety agents (alprazolam, diazepam, chlordiazepoxide)
- Antispasmodics (dantrolene, baclofen)
- Antidepressants (trazodone, amitriptyline, desipramine)
- Neuroleptics (haloperidol, chlorpromazine, thioridazine)
- Sedatives

IMMUNOSUPPRESSION
- Antibiotics
- Cytotoxic agents

INCREASED SALIVATION
- Anticholinesterase
- Clonazepam
- Clozapine

NEUROMUSCULAR JUNCTION BLOCKADE
- Aminoglycoside antibiotics
- Botulinum toxin (Botox)

MYOPATHY
- Corticosteroids
- Lipid-lowering agents
- Colchicine
- L-Tryptophan

MUCOSAL INJURY
- Alendronate (Fosamax)
- Tetracycline
- Nonsteroidal antiinflammatory drugs
- Potassium
- Ferrous sulfate

LOWER ESOPHAGEAL SPHINCTER PRESSURE
- Theophylline
- Nitrates
- Calcium channel blockers
- Beta blockers
- Hormone replacement therapy
- Anticholinergics

tool. This single question was 75% consistent with the results of the EAT-10, which has been shown to be reliable and valid in identifying swallowing dysfunction.[16] Just asking a patient whether he or she has trouble swallowing is a sensible initial step in assessing for dysphagia.

A thorough physical examination aids in the differential diagnosis, establishes the existence of deficits and impairments, and determines whether malnutrition or pneumonia is present.[10] A complete oral examination will reveal oral health and hygiene, including dentition, oral sensation, tongue strength, mobility, coordination, and specific cranial nerve function. Altered speech or voice, particularly nasal speech or a gurgling voice, should be noted. Nasal speech can indicate soft palate dysfunction, whereas a gurgling or wet voice is more indicative of weak pharyngeal constrictors. The presence or absence of the gag reflex is not predictive of swallowing dysfunction or risk of aspiration because the gag reflex may be absent in 20% to 40% of healthy adults.[17] Trial sips of water or spoonfuls of applesauce or pudding can reveal specific deficits. Observation and palpation of laryngeal elevation can detect delayed swallowing. The pharyngeal swallow should occur within approximately 1 second.

The complete neuromuscular examination includes CN function (particularly CN V, VII, IX, X, and XII) and assessment of muscle strength or weakness, muscle atrophy, or altered coordination. Involuntary movements, tremor, or gait disturbance should also be determined. A mental status assessment with particular emphasis on level of alertness and ability to concentrate and cooperate is important. Head injuries, deformities, or past operations on the head, neck, or trunk may affect dysphagia or the ability to participate in diagnostic studies. Despite skillful and comprehensive physical examination, the risk for aspiration may not be fully appreciated without the use of radiographic studies.[18]

Numerous "bedside evaluations" of swallowing are in use around the world. It is difficult to compare studies using differing methods of swallowing evaluation. Timely assessment after an acute event is important to properly identify swallowing disfunction and determine appropriate interventions.[9] Guidelines recommending screening for dysphagia in acute stroke exist in the United Kingdom, Europe, Canada, the United States, and Australia but are imperfectly implemented.

There is some support for the idea that the respiratory system may have a role in optimal swallowing. Gross and colleagues found that pharyngeal swallowing time was longer in subjects at residual lung volume than in those at total lung capacity or functional residual capacity.[19] This implies a possible regulatory role of subglottic air pressure in optimum swallowing.

Careful assessment of oral health and hygiene habits is also important in dysphagia. Poor oral health and hygiene are risk factors for aspiration pneumonia and subsequent death.[20] Sjögren and colleagues have suggested that 1 in 10 deaths from pneumonia among elderly nursing home patients may be prevented by improved oral hygiene.[21] Intensive oral care and hygiene are recommended as a means of reducing pathogen load in aspirators.

DIAGNOSTICS

Videofluoroscopy (VFS), also called videofluoroscopic examination of swallowing (VFES) or modified barium swallow (MBS), is the "gold standard" and is a commonly used imaging procedure. This is a study that visualizes and records imaging of the actual swallow. The primary purpose of the MBS is to determine if and to what degree aspiration occurs. Patients must be able to sit upright, hold still, and follow commands during the examination. With the use of contrast material, this radiographic study is designed to assess functional impairment of swallowing in four categories: delay in swallowing initiation, nasopharyngeal regurgitation, aspiration, and pharyngeal residue. A variety of consistencies and bolus volumes are usually assessed during the MBS. This study not only aids in diagnosis but also helps determine the effectiveness of various positions, consistencies, or maneuvers used in treatment.

The fiberoptic endoscopic examination of swallowing (FEES), plus or minus video, is another widely used visualization of the swallowing structures and function.

If a structural rather than functional cause is suspected, nasoendoscopy could be considered. This procedure permits direct visualization of the oral cavity, nasopharynx, pharynx, and larynx. Lesion biopsy samples can simultaneously be obtained.

If muscle weakness or problems with sphincter relaxation are suspected, manometry can measure intraluminal pressures during the swallow. Manometry can be synchronized with VFS (manofluorography) to distinguish more subtle findings.

Ultrasound examination, electromyography, and electroglottography are other diagnostic procedures that can be appropriate, although these tests are more limited. Computed tomography (CT) or magnetic resonance imaging (MRI) of the head and neck can aid in diagnosis but does not describe the actual swallow mechanism.

INITIAL DIAGNOSTICS

Oropharyngeal Dysphagia

IMAGING
- Modified barium swallow
- Computed tomography or magnetic resonance imaging[a]

OTHER DIAGNOSTICS
- Fiberoptic endoscopic examination of swallow

[a]If indicated.

DIFFERENTIAL DIAGNOSIS

Priority differentials include pharyngeal abscess associated with fever, sore throat, neck stiffness and swelling; obstruction related to a pill, foreign body, tissue injury, pharyngeal carcinoma, or metastasis; or inflammation or ulceration.

Barium is contraindicated if there is any risk of perforation.[1]

The tragedy of oropharyngeal dysphagia is not recognizing that it is there. Health care providers must have an index of suspicion in conditions where swallowing difficulties are known to occur. Stroke, pneumonia and COPD, dementia, as well as Parkinson and Huntington diseases are some of the conditions more frequently associated with dysphagia, and such patients should be screened (see Box 116.1). In patients with unexplained weight loss, weakness or muscle wasting, avoidance of foods or fluids, or significant depression, providers should consider swallowing difficulty as a part of the differential. See Box 116.3 for more differential diagnoses.

INTERPROFESSIONAL COLLABORATIVE MANAGEMENT
Indications for Referral or Hospitalization

Physician Consultation. A gastroenterologist should be consulted for a suspected gastroesophageal problem. Structural causes of dysphagia—such as tumors, strictures, webs, and diverticula—are usually treated with surgery or dilation and will require consultation with the appropriate specialist.

Cricopharyngeal myotomy is the most common surgical treatment for oropharyngeal dysphagia of structural origin, and consistent evidence of its benefit is available.[22] Referral to a neurologist is warranted if the cause of the dysphagia is neurogenic. Studies exploring the use of myotomy for dysphagia of neurogenic origin are very different. Data conflict and are often methodologically and sometimes qualitatively weak. Nonetheless, myotomy may offer benefit to 50% of patients with neurogenic dysphagia.[10] It is suggested that patients who benefit may be those with a higher preoperative hypopharyngeal intrabolus pressure related to resistance of flow across the UES.[22] In patients who have difficulty in coordinating the UES or cricopharyngeal muscle and the pharynx, improvement and patient satisfaction in swallowing has been shown with botulinum toxin (Botox) injections into the UES.[23]

Chemotherapy or radiation therapy may be indicated for tumors requiring consultation with an oncologist. If oral health and hygiene are of concern, referral to a dentist for evaluation and treatment is indicated. Counseling or psychiatric consultation is necessary for patients experiencing grief or depression associated with the dysphagia.

 Consultation with speech/language therapists and dieticians is indicated for dysphagic patients and their families. Other referrals will be dictated by the cause of the dysphagia. Moderate to severe cases of oropharyngeal dysphagia require referral to a speech therapist, particularly if therapeutic swallowing techniques are needed.

Medications and Sensory Stimulation

According to Miarons and colleagues, the limited information regarding medication influence on swallowing is based on small studies and case reports.[24] Nearly 1000 patients who were old, frail, and poorly functional, with multiple illnesses and medications, were studied and no medications that "altered swallowing after adjustment for confounding variables" (p. 697) were identified. Nonetheless, more dysphagia was seen in patients taking antidepressants, antipsychotics, and antidementia medicines and less in patients on angiotensin converting enzyme inhibitors (ACEIs) and β blockers. The researchers noted other studies showing improved swallowing safety and speed with agents that increase the concentration of substance P, such as capsaicin and piperine, and ACEIs.[24] This may be a mechanism of action in the Japanese studies noted further on. In addition, Asian populations may have an altered ACE gene compared with Europeans, perhaps explaining differences in responses to ACEIs.[25] ACEIs may also help in muscle wasting conditions.

Antipsychotics inhibit dopamine and thereby may affect swallowing, and sedatives may reduce the level of consciousness; both may increase the risk of aspiration. Avoidance of these medications in dysphagic patients may reduce the risk of aspiration pneumonia.[26]

In patients using multiple medications who have associated diagnoses of frailty, poor function and dependence, depression, dementia, and others, it is important to recognize the risk of swallowing dysfunction and to look for it.

The knowledge that cough can be stimulated by ACEIs has been of interest to researchers in dysphagia. Takahashi and colleagues used ACEIs in older adult Japanese patients and found a decrease in aspiration pneumonia.[27] On the other hand Lee, in China,[28] studying lisinopril in dysphagia patients with

BOX **116.3**

Differential Diagnosis: Oropharyngeal Dysphagia

MECHANICAL PROBLEMS
Acute inflammations
- Herpes simplex
- Tonsillitis, epiglottitis, pharyngitis, esophagitis
- Infectious and inflammatory bone and mucosal disorders

Chemical agents (aspirin, lozenges, gargles, alcohol)
Medications (see Box 116.2)
Skeletal or muscle anomalies
Macroglossia
Pharyngoesophageal diverticulum
Carcinoma
Surgery
- Oral or palatal resections
- Glossectomy
- Supralaryngectomy; partial or total laryngectomy
- Tracheoesophageal puncture
- Chest surgery (coronary artery bypass graft)
- Endarterectomy
- Anterior cervical spine surgery

Irradiation
Cervical spine disease
Nasoenteric tubes
Tracheostomy tubes
Esophageal stenosis, webs, rings, stricture

NEUROGENIC PROBLEMS
Riley-Day syndrome
Acquired central nervous system disorders
- Stroke syndromes and vascular disorders
- Capsular infarct
- Pseudobulbar palsy
- Apraxias and agnosias
- Lacunar disease

Movement disorders
- Parkinson disease
- Dystonias and dyskinesias
- Huntington disease
- Palatal myoclonus

Poliomyelitis and other systemic infections
- Diphtheria
- Botulism
- Rabies
- Tetanus

Amyotrophic lateral sclerosis
Acquired peripheral nervous system disorders
Recurrent laryngeal neuropathies
Central nervous system neuropathies
- Guillain-Barré syndrome
- Diabetes
- Leukemia
- Lymphoma
- Carcinoma
- Other neuropathies

Neurodevelopmental disorders
- Cerebral palsy
- Abnormal oral and pharyngeal reflexes
- Abnormal salivation
- Others

MYOGENIC PROBLEMS
Myasthenia gravis
Neuromuscular esophageal disorders
- Scleroderma
- Achalasia
- Diffuse spasm
- Others

OTHER CONDITIONS
Dementias
Multiple sclerosis
Tuberculosis
Syphilis
Neoplasms
Degenerative disorders
Psychopathology
Feeding phobias
Atypical parent-child interactions
Sensory deficits

---

cerebrovascular disease, found an increase in mortality and no change in incidence of pneumonia and stopped the study.

The relationship of pharyngeal sensation, silent aspiration, and cough reflex has been explored in many Japanese studies. Ebihara and colleagues[29] found that oral stimulation and awareness were key in addressing swallowing delay. They found that capsaicin stimulated warm receptors whereas menthol stimulated cold receptors and that both improved a delayed swallowing reflex. In addition, black pepper oil was effective in reducing latent time to swallow in patients with diminished consciousness.[29] Ice massage is widely used in Japan to trigger swallowing in stroke patients.[30]

A variety of chemicals and temperatures applied in the oral cavity, especially to the faucial pillars, have shown some efficacy. A published review of stimulation reports that sour (lemon juice, citric acid); cold (menthol or a metal probe); warm, pungent (capsaicin, piperine); and carbonation all improving the onset of swallow.[31,32] The combination of more than one therapy may be more effective than a single method.

Pownall and others reviewed the literature regarding the use of electrical stimulation.[33] Electrotherapies may be peripheral or cortical; applied to the neck, palate, or pharynx; or used noninvasively over the brain. Pownall uses the acronym NMES to apply to all transcutaneous neuromuscular electrical stimulations. A number of these treatments, particularly in conjunction with more traditional treatments, have shown improvement in swallowing and quality of life in small samples. Mechanisms may involve improving sensory signals, muscle strength, coordination, and feedback with the swallowing areas of the brain.

TABLE 116.1	Swallowing Therapy Techniques, Rationales, and Indications	
Technique	**Execution (Rationale)**	**Indication**
DIETARY MODIFICATION		
Thickened liquids	Reduce tendency to spill over tongue base	Disordered tongue function Pre-swallow spill or aspiration Impaired laryngeal closure
Thin liquids	Offer less resistance to flow	Weak pharyngeal contraction Reduced cricopharyngeal opening
MANEUVERS		
Supraglottic swallow	Breath hold, double swallow, forceful expiration (closes vocal folds before swallowing)	Aspiration: reduced or late vocal fold closures
Supersupraglottic swallow	Effortful breath hold (closes vocal folds before and during swallow) Increase anterior tilting of arytenoids	Aspiration (poor closure of laryngeal introitus)
Effortful swallow	Effortful tongue action (increases posterior motion of tongue base)	Poor posterior tongue base motion
Mendelsohn maneuver	Prolong hyoid excursion guided by manual palpation (prolongs opening of upper esophageal sphincter)	Poor pharyngeal clearance and laryngeal movement
POSTURAL ADJUSTMENTS		
Head tilt	Tilt posteriorly at swallow initiation (gravity clears oral cavity) Tilt laterally to unaffected side (directs bolus down stronger side)	Poor tongue control Unilateral pharyngeal weakness
Chin tuck; positive improvement in swallowing scores	Chin down (widens valleculae, displaces tongue base and epiglottis posteriorly)	Aspiration, delayed pharyngeal response, reduced posterior tongue base motion
Head rotation	Rotate head to affected side (isolates damaged side from bolus path, reduces lower esophageal sphincter pressure) Rotate head to affected side with extrinsic pressure on thyroid cartilage (increases adduction)	Unilateral pharyngeal weakness Unilateral laryngeal dysfunction Unilateral pharyngeal dysfunction
Lying on side, elevation	Right or left lateral (bypass laryngeal introitus)	Aspiration, bilateral pharyngeal impairment, or reduced laryngeal elevation
FACILITATORY TECHNIQUES		
Strengthening exercises	Various	Nonprogressive disease
Biofeedback	Augment volitional component	Poor pharyngeal clearance
Thermal stimulation; reduces transition and swallow duration	Cold, tactile stimulation to anterior faucial pillar	Delayed or absent swallow response
Surface electrical stimulation; increases swallowing improvement	Electrical stimulation of pharyngeal and laryngeal musculature	
Gustatory stimulation	Sour bolus (facilitates swallow response)	Huntington chorea, stroke

From Cook, I. J., & Kahrilas, P. J. (1999). AGA technical review on management of oropharyngeal dysphagia. *Gastroenterology, 116*(2):470; and Speyer, R., Baijens, L., Heijnen, M., & Zwijnenberg, I. (2010). Effects of therapy in oropharyngeal therapy by speech and language therapists: a systematic review. *Dysphagia, 25*(1):40–65.

Swallowing Strategies and Therapies

Head positioning, swallowing maneuvers, and dietary textural modifications seem to demonstrate evidence of benefit in the treatment of functional dysphagia.[10] Newer interventional techniques also show promise, although studies regarding efficacy are small and some swallowing improvement may be related to normal recovery.[34] Table 116.1 provides data on swallowing therapy techniques, rationales, and indications. Many therapeutic measures require autonomy and fairly intact cognitive function for memory and learning. For patients with certain strokes, Alzheimer disease, and some other neurologic diseases, this requirement may limit the usefulness of these techniques. Dietary modifications may be the best choice for many of these patients.

Aspiration and Nonoral Feeding in Dysphagia of Functional Origin

Previous practice standards were that patients found to have severe aspiration not treatable with dietary or positional modifications should receive nonoral feeding to prevent aspiration. It is clear that aspiration is evidence of severe swallowing dysfunction and that death is associated with aspiration pneumonia.[10] However, the relationship between aspiration and risk for the development of pneumonia is not as obvious. DiBardino and Wunderink found that aspiration did not predict a risk of respiratory morbidity.[35] Similarly, Falsetti and coworkers discovered that 6 of 49 dysphagic patients had normal VFS findings.[36] A study by Terpenning and others suggested an increased risk of aspiration pneumonia in patients who have COPD or diabetes mellitus or who require assistance with feeding.[37] Aspiration pneumonia was also more common in subjects with oral *Porphyromonas gingivalis*, decayed teeth, and visible dental plaque. Although these authors hypothesized that poor healing associated with diabetes and poor pulmonary clearance could contribute to the development of pneumonia, they did not find an association with stroke.[37] Harvey and colleagues proposed that patients with compromised functional capacity may be fed too quickly or with boluses that were too large.[38] In summary, it appears that aspiration probably contributes to the risk of pneumonia but may not be the only important contributor; nonoral feeding may not reduce this risk in all patients and may increase this risk in some patients.

COMPLICATIONS

Because complications associated with dysphagia include impaired quality of life, coughing, choking, aspiration, malnutrition, dehydration, pneumonia, and death, gastrostomy tube placement may be necessary and appropriate for some patients with progressive neurological disease or the inability to swallow. Other comorbid illnesses or conditions may affect dysphagia or contribute to the development of pneumonia. Pulmonary rehabilitation may be indicated for patients with concurrent lung disease. Suspected pneumonia should usually be evaluated at the hospital, especially if gastric fluid is thought to be the aspirate. Malnutrition, dehydration, or acute dysphagia may require hospital admission.

PATIENT AND FAMILY EDUCATION

The most important aspects of education include patient feeding, positioning, maneuvers, and dietary textural modifications. Speech therapists can teach patients and families positioning and maneuvers to improve swallowing efficacy. The Silver Spoons program, a volunteer program, was designed to facilitate safe feeding and can also assist family members or institutional staff.[38] Paying careful attention to bolus size and consistency—including taste, texture and visual appeal—allowing plenty of time for meals, and ensuring proper positioning of the patient for meals will improve safety and satisfaction.

Discussion concerning the risks and benefits of feeding tubes in specific disease entities is important for patients, families, and often staff. Feeding tubes may not be appropriate for patients with severe dementia.[39] Cultural and religious preferences must be respected. Other concurrent illnesses may also be important considerations. More research is needed, but for any given patient, the decision to place a feeding tube must remain individualized and be carefully considered.

HEALTH PROMOTION

Regular health screenings and recommendations for diet, exercise, and smoking cessation can prevent or delay the onset of disease, particularly in those with a strong family history of

stroke. Once dysphagia is established, good oral hygiene, dental care, careful attention to positioning and swallowing techniques, and management of comorbid illnesses—particularly respiratory illnesses and diabetes—can help prevent pneumonia. Counseling can be beneficial for patients with a family history of hereditary neurologic or myopathic disorders associated with dysphagia. Support for families caring for dysphagic members may also help reduce caregiver stress.

REFERENCES

1. Charous, S. J. (June 2018). Evaluation of dysphagia. *BMJ Best Practice*. http://bestpractice.bmj.com/topics/en-us/226. (Accessed 3 September 2018).
2. Rofes, L., Arreola, V., Almirall, J., Cabré, M., Campins, L., García-Peris, P., et al. (2011). Diagnosis and management of oropharyngeal dysphagia and its nutritional and respiratory complications in the elderly. *Gastroenterology Research and Practice*.
3. Martino, R., Foley, N., Bhogal, S., Diamant, N., Speechley, M., & Teasell, R. (2005). Dysphagia after stroke: Incidence, diagnosis, and pulmonary complications. *Stroke; a Journal of Cerebral Circulation*, 36(12), 2756–2763.
4. Hartelius, L., & Svensson, P. (1994). Speech and swallowing symptoms associated with Parkinson's disease and multiple sclerosis: A survey. *Folia Phoniatrica et Logopaedica: Official Organ of the International Association of Logopedics and Phoniatrics (IALP)*, 46(1), 9–17.
5. Steele, C. M., Greenwood, C., Ens, I., et al. (1997). Mealtime difficulties in a home for the aged; not just dysphagia. *Dysphagia*, 12, 43–50, Discussion 51.
6. Murray, C. J., Vos, T., Lozano, R., Naghavi, M., Flaxman, A. D., Michaud, C., et al. (2013). Disability-adjusted life years (DALYs) for 291 diseases and injuries in 21 regions, 1990-2010: A systematic analysis for the global burden of disease study 2010. *Lancet*, 15(380), 2197–2223.
7. Clavé, P., Arreola, V., Romea, M., Medina, L., Palomera, E., & Serra-Prat, M. (2008). Accuracy of the volume-viscosity swallow test for clinical screening of oropharyngeal dysphagia and aspiration. *Clinical Nutrition: Official Journal of the European Society of Parenteral and Enteral Nutrition*, 27, 806–815.
8. Gross, R. D., Atwood, C. W., Ross, S. B., Olszewski, J. W., & Eichhorn, K. A. (2009). The coordination of breathing and swallowing in chronic obstructive pulmonary disease. *American Journal of Respiratory and Critical Care Medicine*, 179, 559–565.
9. Boaden, E., Doran, D., Burnell, J., Clegg, A., Dey, P., Hurley, M., et al. (2017). Screening for aspiration risk associated with dysphagia in acute stroke. *The Cochrane Database of Systematic Reviews*, (6), CD012679, doi:10.1002/14651858.CD012679.
10. Cook, I. J., & Kahrilas, P. J. (1999). AGA technical review on management of oropharyngeal dysphagia. *Gastroenterology*, 116(2), 455–478.
11. Blackington, E., McCormick, T., Willson, B., et al. (2001). Oropharyngeal dysphagia in the elderly. *Advance for Nurse Practitioners*, 9(7), 42–49.
12. Mihai, P. G., Otto, M., Domin, M., Platz, T., Hamdy, S., & Lotze, M. (2016). Brain imaging correlates of recovered swallowing after dysphagic stroke: A fMRI and DWI study. *Neuroimage Clinical*, 12, 1013–1021.
13. Logemann, J. A., Curro, F. A., Pauloski, B., & Gensler, G. (2013). Aging effects on oropharyngeal swallow and the role of dental care in oropharyngeal dysphagia. *Oral Diseases*, 19, 733–737. doi:10.1111/odi.12104.
14. Kwiatek, M. A., Mirza, F., Kahrilas, P. J., et al. (2009). Hyperdynamic upper esophageal sphincter pressure: A manometric observation in patients reporting globus sensation. *The American Journal of Gastroenterology*, 104, 289–298.
15. Heijnen, B. J., Speyer, R., Bülow, M., & Kuijpers, L. M. F. (2016). 'What about swallowing?' Diagnostic performance of daily clinical practice compared with the Eating Assessment Tool-10. *Dysphagia*, 31, 214–222.
16. Belafsky, P. C., Mouadeb, D. A., Rees, C. J., Pryor, J. C., Postma, G. N., Allen, J., et al. (2008). Validity and reliability of the Eating Assessment Tool (EAT-10). *The Annals of Otology, Rhinology, and Laryngology*, 117(12), 919–924.
17. Lim, K., Hew, Y., Lau, H., Lim, T., & Tan, C. (2009). Bulbar signs in normal population. *The Canadian Journal of Neurological Sciences*, 36(1), 60–64.
18. Smith Hammond, C. A., & Goldstein, L. B. (2006). Cough and aspiration of food and liquids due to oral-pharyngeal dysphagia: ACCP evidence-based clinical practice guidelines. *Chest*, 129, 154S–168S.
19. Gross, R. D., Atwood, C. W., Grayhack, J. P., et al. (2003). Lung volume effects on pharyngeal swallowing physiology. *Journal of Applied Physiology*, 95(6), 2211–2217.
20. Terpenning, M. (2005). Geriatric oral health and pneumonia risk. *Clinical Infectious Diseases: an Official Publication of the Infectious Diseases Society of America*, 40, 1807–1810.

21. Sjögren, P., Nilsson, E., Forsell, M., Johansson, O., & Hoogstraate, J. (2008). A systematic review of the preventive effect of oral hygiene on pneumonia and respiratory tract infection in elderly people in hospitals and nursing homes: Effect estimates and methodological quality of randomized controlled trials. *Journal of the American Geriatrics Society, 56*(11), 2124–2130.

22. Allen, J., White, C. J., Leonard, R., et al. (2010). Effect of oropharyngeal muscle surgery on the pharynx. *The Laryngoscope, 120*(8), 1498–1503.

23. Terré, R., Panadés, A., & Mearin, F. (2013). Botulinum toxin treatment for oropharyngeal dysphagia in patients with stroke. *Neurogastroenterology and Motility, 25*(11), 896–904.

24. Miarons, M., Campins, L., Palomera, E., Serra-Prat, M., Cabré, M., & Rofes, L. (2016). Drugs related to oropharyngeal dysphagia in older people. *Dysphagia, 31*, 697–705. doi:10.1007/s00455-016-9735-5.

25. Ohkubo, T., Chapman, N., Neal, B., Woodward, M., Omae, T., & Chalmers, J. (2004). Effects of an angiotensin-converting enzyme inhibitor-based regimen on pneumonia risk. *American Journal of Respiratory and Critical Care Medicine, 169*(9), 1041–1045.

26. Knol, W., van Marum, R. J., Jansen, P. A., Souverein, P. C., Schobben, A. F., & Egberts, A. C. (2008). Antipsychotic drug use and risk of pneumonia in elderly people. *Journal of the American Geriatrics Society, 56*, 661–666.

27. Takahashi, T., Morimoto, S., Okaishi, K., Kanda, T., Nakahashi, T., Okuro, M., et al. (2005). Reduction of pneumonia risk by an angiotensin I-converting enzyme inhibitor in elderly Japanese inpatients according to insertion/deletion polymorphism of the angiotensin I-converting enzyme gene. *American Journal of Hypertension, 18*, 1353–1359.

28. Lee, J., Chui, P. Y., Ma, H. M., Auyeung, T. W., Kng, C., Law, T., et al. (2015). Does low dose angiotensin converting enzyme inhibitor prevent pneumonia in older people with neurologic dysphagia—A randomized placebo-controlled trial. *Journal of the American Medical Directors Association, 16*(8), 702–707. doi:10.1016/j.jamda.2015.05.009. [Epub 2015 Jun 27].

29. Ebihara, S., Kohzuki, M., Sumi, Y., & Ebihara, T. (2011). Sensory stimulation to improve swallowing reflex and prevent aspiration pneumonia in elderly dysphagic people. *Journal of Pharmacological Sciences, 115*(2), 99–104.

30. Nakamura, T., & Fujishima, I. (2013). Usefulness of ice massage in triggering the swallow reflex. *Journal of Stroke and Cerebrovascular Diseases, 22*, 378–382.

31. Rofes, L., Cola, P. C., & Clavé, P. (2014). The effects of sensory stimulation on neurogenic oropharyngeal dysphagia. *Journal of Gastroenterology and Hepatology Research, 3*(5), 1066–1072.

32. Malik, S. N., Khan, M. S. G., Ehsaan, F., et al. (2017). Effectiveness of swallow maneuvers, thermal stimulations and combination of both in treatment of patients with dysphagia using functional outcome swallowing scale. *Biomedical Research, 28*(4), 1479–1482.

33. Pownall, S., Enderby, P., & Sproson, L. (2017). Electrical stimulation for the treatment of dysphagia. In A. Majid (Ed.), *Electroceuticals.* Cham.: Springer. https://doi.org/10.1007/978-3-319-28612-9_6.

34. Speyer, R., Baijens, L., Heijen, M., & Zwijnenberg, I. (2010). Effects of therapy in oropharyngeal therapy by speech and language therapists: A systematic review. *Dysphagia, 25*(1), 40–65.

35. DiBardino, D., & Wunderink, R. (2015). Aspiration pneumonia: A review of modern trends. *Journal of Critical Care, 30*(1), 40–48.

36. Falsetti, P., Acciai, C., Palilla, R., Bosi, M., Carpinteri, F., Zingarelli, A., et al. (2009). Oropharyngeal dysphagia after stroke: Incidence, diagnosis, and clinical predictors in patients admitted to a neurorehabilitation unit. *Journal of Stroke and Cerebrovascular Diseases, 18*(5), 329–335.

37. Terpenning, M. S., Taylor, G. W., Lopatin, D. E., et al. (2001). Aspiration pneumonia: Dental and oral risk factors in an older veteran population. *Journal of the American Geriatrics Society, 49*, 557–563.

38. Harvey, T., Coulter, S., Zublena, L., & Woodard, E. (2013). Silver spoons: Volunteers and patient-centered meals. *Nursing Management, 44*(4), 8–10.

39. Campbell, M., Dove-Medows, E., Walch, J., Sanna-Gouin, K., & Colomba, S. (2011). The impact of a multidisciplinary educational intervention to reduce PEG tube placement in patients with terminal-stage dementia: A translation of research into practice. *Journal of Palliative Medicine, 14*(9), 1017–1021.

CHAPTER **117**

GASTROESOPHAGEAL REFLUX DISEASE
Michelle Freshman

 Prompt medical evaluation by a gastroenterologist is indicated if the patient has unintentional weight loss, dysphagia for solids or liquids, odynophagia, unexplained anemia, or chronic tobacco and alcohol exposure.

 Alarm symptoms include gastrointestinal bleeding, anemia, dysphagia, odynophagia, unintentional weight loss, early satiety, age older than 55 at presentation, recurrent vomiting, and epigastric mass.

DEFINITION AND EPIDEMIOLOGY

Gastroesophageal reflux refers to the retrograde movement of gastric contents from the stomach to the esophagus. This occurs multiple times daily in the general population followed by rapid clearance of refluxed material from the distal esophagus, without injury. Swallowing initiates primary peristalsis; distention of the esophagus or acidification promotes secondary peristalsis. When the capacity of the esophageal mucosa to tolerate caustic refluxate is overwhelmed, this normal physiologic process can produce pathologic signs and symptoms in the oropharynx, larynx, esophagus, and respiratory tract. Symptoms may be directly attributable to the degree and time of acid exposure, but the correlation is weak.[1] An individual is said to have *gastroesophageal reflux disease* (GERD) in the setting of chronic symptom distress with or without mucosal damage.

GERD is one of the most prevalent clinical conditions of the gastrointestinal tract,[2] affecting between 8% and 33% worldwide,[3] and 10% to 20% of adults at least weekly in Western countries, although these accounts are subjective.[4] Prevalence among American (15% to 20%), British (10% to 15%), Swedish (5% to 10%), and Chinese citizens (0.1% to 5.0%) is variable depending on the source, and many populations have yet to be quantified: Africa, Brazil, India, and Russia.[2,5] Estimates of US expenditure range from $9.3 billion to $12.3 billion per year, largely due to proton pump inhibitor (PPI) therapy.[1,6] Although body mass index (BMI) may be a factor, sex and older age appear to be less so.[5] Some 4% to 7% of patients with GERD experience progressive disease associated with aspiration (most often related to age, comorbidities, or large hiatal hernia).[4] A serious complication of GERD is Barrett esophagus (BE) seen in 5% to 15% of chronic GERD patients,[1,7] from which a much smaller percentage develop esophageal adenocarcinoma (EAC).

The most common symptoms of GERD are heartburn (retrosternal area pain) and acidic regurgitation. Aside from typical symptoms, atypical and extraesophageal symptoms (EESs) are frequently reported.[8] Atypical symptoms include epigastric fullness, epigastric pressure, epigastric pain, dyspepsia, nausea, bloating, and belching, which may suggest GERD, but actually represent microaspirations and overlap with other entities.[8] Moreover, atypical symptoms respond much less well to PPI therapy.[1] Symptomatic GERD affects quality of life, may contribute to tissue injury, and is associated with EESs such as dental erosions, sore throat, laryngitis, hoarseness, chronic cough, wheezing, asthma, and broncho-spasm, to which some add burning of mouth and tongue, globus sensation, or shortness of breath.[5] As proposed with atypical symptoms of GERD, in cases of EESs, microaspirations or a vagally mediated response triggered by the distal esophagus has been theorized, although GERD may not be involved at all.[3,8]

Nevertheless, severity of symptoms is not a reliable indicator of mucosal damage or prognosis. There are two types of reflux disease: nonerosive reflux disease (NERD) and erosive reflux disease (ERD). The nonerosive, endoscopically negative type is more prevalent, and is characterized by symptoms that correlate with abnormal durations of acid exposure time (AET) and/or response to PPIs.[9] In fact, 50% to 85% of patients have NERD[5] and less than 60% respond to standard therapy.[10] By contrast, ERD is established by identifying inflammatory changes in the mucosa showing high-grade esophagitis (LA classification grades C or D), which correlates with higher nocturnal acid exposure,[11] peptic structuring, or BE on esophago-gastroduodenoscopy (EGD).[1]

Beyond GERD are two functional disorders in the absence of EGD findings, but positive ambulatory pH or pH-impedance monitoring: reflux hypersensitivity (RH), where symptoms correlate with physiologic reflux, and functional heartburn (FH), where symptoms do *not* correlate with physiologic reflux. The number of patients diagnosed with these entities is higher when considering those who do not respond to twice-daily PPI therapy.[3] A significant proportion of individuals with endoscopically negative GERD have been shown to have pH testing abnormalities on impedance testing. Although esophageal damage is marked by erosions, ulcers, or strictures in the esophagus, exclusive of malignant disease, a small percentage of endoscopically negative, symptomatic GERD will progress to erosive GERD.[12] However, conversion from NERD to ERD or the probability of misdiagnosis between entities is low, favoring stability of disease in NERD despite symptom distress.[2] Several other Rome IV-defined functional conditions exist: e.g., functional chest pain, which excludes all esophageal and cardiac disease despite symptoms more than once per week; globus sensation; and functional dysphagia in the absence of structural (including congenital), motor, or histological abnormalities.[13]

In patients with no findings on EGD or pH monitoring, functional GERD is suspected and may still be responsive to standard GERD therapy. In fact, up to 47% of patients with RH or FH respond to PPI therapy.[3]

Alarm symptoms include gastrointestinal bleeding, anemia, dysphagia, odynophagia, unintentional weight loss, early satiety, age older than 55 at presentation, recurrent vomiting, and epigastric mass.[5,11,14]

PATHOPHYSIOLOGY

No single mechanism explains all cases of symptomatic GERD; however, multiple factors are thought to be involved in the pathogenesis of reflux[4]:

- Transient lower esophageal sphincter (LES) relaxations (TLESRs)
- Low resting LES pressure
- Poor esophageal acid clearance, with increased volume and causticity
- Defects in esophagogastric motility or peristalsis
- Impaired mucosal resistance and other protective defenses

- Altered hiatal and gastroesophageal anatomy (involving hiatal crura, phrenoesophageal ligament, esophageal shortening)
- Hypersensitivity to gastric acid

TLESRs, the first factor, have been shown to be the cause of most reflux events. Intervals of LES relaxation, which allow the gastric contents to reflux into the esophagus, result in esophageal damage. TLESRs account for most reflux events. Anatomic variations such as hiatal hernia, shortened abdominal length, or obesity can contribute.[5]

LES pressure is maintained or increased by acetylcholine; relaxation of the LES occurs in response to nitric oxide, as seen in response to swallowing, often augmented by the crural diaphragm and phrenoesophageal ligament[12] when intra-abdominal pressure increases. Patients with chronic symptoms usually have a hiatal hernia, which reflects movement of the proximal stomach upward through the diaphragm into the chest, where the crural diaphragm becomes separated from the LES. This separation is highly correlated with severe esophagitis, especially in the setting of esophageal stricture or BE. However, the presence of a hiatal hernia alone does not confirm the presence of reflux esophagitis because the majority of patients with hiatal hernias do not have any symptoms. Other conditions increase intra-abdominal pressure and cause retrograde movement of refluxate. In pregnancy there is an increased prevalence of reflux, especially in the final trimester, which results from the relaxant effects of circulating estrogen and progesterone on the LES.

A third factor is intensity of acid exposure. The proton pump ultimately drives the production of acid in the stomach. This acidification pathway results from gastric parietal cells in response to histamine, acetylcholine, and gastrin,[5] using hydrogen-potassium adenosine triphosphate molecules in the secretory canaliculi to dislodge hydrogen ions, which in turn acidifies the stomach pH to 1.5 to 3.5, typically tested as a pH less than 4.[5,9] Once acid reflux has occurred, impaired acid clearance prolongs exposure of the mucosa to the damaging effects of the reflux. Evidence suggests that the acid component of the refluxate is the primary cause of heartburn and subsequent erosion. Other factors include the duration of the acid reflux event on the esophageal mucosa and the extent and composition of refluxate. Secondary causes of GERD involving heightened acid exposure include rare hypersecretory disorders. The most common of these disorders, Zollinger-Ellison syndrome, is caused by gastrin-producing tumors of the duodenum, pancreas, or both. In this disease, an overproduction of gastrin-driven acid output refluxes upward, causing severe GERD pain or peptic stricture. In addition, the role of bile refluxate (bile, bicarbonate, pancreatic enzymes), in the context of epidemic obesity and bariatric surgery, has been seen to contribute to duodenogastroesophageal mucosal injury.[15]

A fourth pathogenic factor is the inability of the esophagus to clear itself of reflux material, resulting in longer exposure to gastric contents. Abnormalities in peristalsis increase the risk for esophagitis. This includes delayed gastric emptying when gastric contents wash back into the esophagus as a result of their increased time in the stomach. Connective tissue disorders, gastric outlet obstruction caused by ulceration and stricture, and delayed gastric emptying from a variety of causes (such as postviral infections, gastric stasis, neuromuscular disease, vagal nerve disorders, idiopathic gastroparesis, pyloric dysfunction, duodenal dysmotility, duodenogastroesophageal bile reflux, and functional disorders of the gut) also result from inadequate refluxate clearance. A decrease in esophageal peristalsis can be more pronounced in patients with scleroderma, diabetes mellitus, hypothyroidism, amyloidosis, and eating disorders.

A fifth factor is the integrity of the protective barrier of the mucosal lining. The inability of the mucosa to resist breakdown in the face of excessive refluxed gastric acid, along with pepsin, bile, trypsin, and pancreatic enzymes of the small intestine, may lead to erosive esophagitis in the majority of patients with ulcers and strictures. In fact, recent focus on the volume of refluxate cleared during secondary peristalsis (usually around 90%) and the nature of the chemical clearance (salivary bicarbonate and epidermal growth factor), which contributes to mucosal repair, has led to establishing a mean nocturnal baseline impedance (MNBI) and postreflux swallow-induced peristaltic wave (PSPW) testing in research settings, which is considered superior to pH monitoring or ambulatory impedance-based calculations of AET for NERD versus FH or hypersensitive esophagitis disorders.[9] Saliva, along with alkaline secretion from the esophageal glands, serves as a potent buffer in neutralizing acid. Salivation decreases during sleep, which in turn prolongs acid clearance and may correlate with increased symptom severity at night. Reduced salivary secretion, such as in Sjögren disease or sicca syndrome, can lead to esophagitis. Eosinophilic esophagitis (EoE), both PPI responsive and non–PPI responsive, is an allergy-mediated disease. Altered structural anatomy is also a factor in establishing an accurate diagnosis.

Finally, there is evidence to support the prevalence of GERD in individuals evaluated for excessive acid exposure despite normal findings on 24-hour pH monitoring studies. Of 128 patients in one study, 55% had confirmed normal acid exposure, but within 4 to 6 years 87% of these subjects continued to complain of GERD, leading to the suspicion that hypersensitivity plays a significant role.[5] The Rome IV criteria for RH describes normal acid reflux on standard pH testing, but allows for a variety of potential histologic changes of the esophageal mucosa (dilated intracellular spaces, basal cell thickness, papillary elongation), which FH patients lack.[13]

CLINICAL PRESENTATION AND PHYSICAL EXAMINATION

The most common symptom of GERD is heartburn, which is usually described as a burning, retrosternal discomfort. Other terms for heartburn include *indigestion, acid regurgitation, sour stomach,* and *bitter belching.* A hot sensation usually begins inferiorly and radiates up the entire retrosternal area to the neck, occasionally to the back, and rarely into the arms. The sensation may become so intense that it is described as pain. Heartburn is usually relieved with antacids, baking soda, or milk, but these remedies are often short-lived.

Heartburn is frequently precipitated by food intake and occurs within 1 hour of eating, particularly after a large fatty meal. Other foods that precipitate heartburn are sugar, peppermint, chocolate, coffee, garlic, and onions because they lower pressure in the LES. Alcohol effects lower LES pressure, decrease lower esophageal smooth muscle contractility, reduce gastric acid production, and can cause mucosal inflammation and hemorrhage, but it has not independently been associated with BE; in fact, red wine may be protective.[7,16] In chronic

alcoholics, LES pressure is increased with reduced clearance in the setting of autonomic neuropathy, but can reverse when alcohol is withdrawn.[16] Tobacco smoking may have a dual role in causing by promoting bile movement from the intestine to the stomach while prolonging effective neutralization by delaying saliva secretion. Other foods that commonly cause heartburn are citrus products, tomato-based foods, and spicy foods. These foods do not affect LES pressure but are instead direct mucosal irritants. Other direct irritants include aspirin, nonsteroidal antiinflammatory drugs (NSAIDs), potassium, and even swallowing of large tablets. The prevalence of GERD is higher in patients on benzodiazepines, calcium antagonists, and aspirin, but GERD is less often seen in patients on oral contraceptives and hormone replacement therapy.[5] Patients may also report heartburn or acid regurgitation that increases after going to bed, especially after eating late in the evening. This pain usually occurs within 1 to 2 hours of bedtime and may awaken a patient from sleep. Several other maneuvers, including bending over, lifting, straining, and exercising, or even the sleeping position may also precipitate heartburn because of increased intra-abdominal pressure. Weight gain is associated with an increase in GERD symptoms, erosive esophagitis, and BE.[3]

Other symptoms of GERD, outside of esophageal burning and regurgitation, are termed EESs, involve the respiratory and oropharyngeal tracts, and may also be associated with other entities. A subset, extraesophageal reflux (EER), involves the respiratory tract.[4] Another subset is laryngopharyngeal reflux (LPR).[6] Because these conditions may relate to GERD, they are included in the workup and treatment. Some variations of cough, sore throat, hoarseness, postnasal drainage, globus sensation, asthma, water brash, dysphagia, odynophagia, chest pain, sleep disturbance, nausea, and vomiting are described as EESs. Recent recharacterizations of these symptoms as functional disorders has helped frame alternative diagnoses.[13]

Acid regurgitation, bitter acidic fluid in the mouth, usually occurs at night or when bending over. Acid regurgitation may be associated with extraesophageal complications should the refluxate extend beyond the esophagus to the lungs, larynx, pharynx, or oral cavity. This symptom should be differentiated from vomiting. Water brash is the appearance of salty-tasting fluid in the mouth because of stimulated saliva secretion. If delayed gastric emptying is the cause of GERD, abdominal fullness, nausea, and early satiety may be present.

Dysphagia, in patients with GERD, and odynophagia are more predictive of severe disease and should be considered alarm symptoms. More than one alarm symptom increases the sensitivity to 67% of complicated cases, particularly advanced age older than 55 years and alarm symptoms for EAC.[11] Dysphagia, an impairment of swallowing food into the stomach, is experienced immediately after swallowing. Patients may say that the food "sticks," "hangs up," or "stops." This may be stemming from the oropharynx in the upper esophageal area or lower in the esophagus and reflects peristaltic dysfunction, inflammation, peptic stricture, or a Schatzki ring. Esophageal strictures are highly correlated with hiatal hernia.[17] Dysphagia and food impaction are hallmarks of EoE, which may be driven by reflux as a precursor and is thought to depend on the role of impaired esophageal mucosa and immune activation.[18] Alternatively, GERD may be associated with a globus sensation, which is a heightened perception of something stuck, like a "lump" in the throat, despite the lack of a diagnosable artifact. A recent onset of severe dysphagia might reflect esophageal cancer (see Chapter 116).[19] Odynophagia is sharp pain on swallowing and usually occurs under the sternum. Odynophagia is more commonly associated with infectious esophagitis (fungal, viral, or bacterial) or pill ulceration.

Chest pain can mimic angina, which may be explained by shared neural pathways. Esophageal disorders are considered the most common cause of noncardiac chest pain. Symptoms that are more suggestive of esophageal problems include pain that continues for hours, interrupts sleep, or is retrosternal without lateral radiation and pain that is meal related or relieved with antacids. Some association of GERD symptoms with obstructive sleep apnea has been observed, but causal direction with respect to reflux and apnea has yet to be determined. Obesity may be a confounder in both. Pain that is not exercise induced is also suggestive of an esophageal disorder.

When GERD is overlooked as a factor, many of these atypical GERD symptoms can be refractory to treatment. As described earlier, some conditions, such as dyspepsia, may overlap with GERD; erosive esophagitis and nonerosive esophagitis are said to be present in 20% of patients with dyspepsia, the most common finding, followed by peptic ulcer.[12] However, symptom control in response to standard GERD treatment, including surgery, may serve to uncover reflux as a factor. Comanagement, especially in respiratory illnesses such as asthma, pulmonary fibrosis, and aspiration pneumonia, is increasingly standard practice.

Medications may contribute to GERD by decreasing salivation, esophageal motility, LES tone, or a combination of these factors. Decreased LES pressure results from the administration of nitrates, tricyclic antidepressants, benzodiazepines among other sedatives, anticholinergics, bronchodilators, and methylxanthine derivatives (such as caffeine, aminophylline, and theophylline) as well as a wide assortment of cardiac medications including α-adrenergic blockers, β blockers, and calcium channel blockers.[5]

The physical findings are not likely to be quite as important as a careful history. Because there is an association between dental erosions and GERD, an oral examination may suggest GERD in a patient with extensive loss of enamel and exposed dentin. Halitosis might also be a sign. Cutaneous evidence of smoking can be associated with GERD, as well as scleroderma, evidenced as thickened, tight, shiny skin, or sclerodactyly and facial telangiectasia. Weight loss is a concern, particularly in patients who have dysphagia; by contrast, obesity can lead to symptoms. Respiratory wheezes and cough may be seen if there is associated asthma. Epigastric tenderness or hemoccult-positive stool may be the result of esophageal erosions, ulcerations, or even severe inflammation. Any abdominal mass would suggest malignant neoplasia.

DIAGNOSTICS

Further diagnostic testing should be considered in patients with a failed empirical trial suggesting an alternative diagnosis, with sudden onset of symptoms in a patient aged 50 years or older, with alarm symptoms suggesting complicated disease (anemia, dysphagia, bleeding, odynophagia), and with long-standing symptoms of sufficient duration to put patients at risk for BE. The purpose of evaluating patients with long-term symptoms is to exclude complications of GERD.

Essential Diagnostics

A basic complete blood count (CBC), fecal *Helicobacter pylori* antigen, and fecal hemoccult may indicate anemia and its potential source, although intestinal bleeding does not register as anemia early on. As for upper intestinal imaging, a barium radiography will help characterize mechanical obstructions such as strictures, hiatal hernia, and esophageal shortening to inform surgical approach, but it has poor sensitivity and specificity and should not be used as a screening test. The more commonly ordered diagnostic, EGD, has good sensitivity in cases of erosive disease with typical symptoms (95%) but is best used with those with risk factors for BE or EAC, particularly one or more alarm symptoms.[11] In refractory GERD (medically unresponsive) high-definition, high-resolution, flexible video EGD with mucosal biopsy is the gold standard.

Additional Diagnostics

EGD is appropriate for patients with long-standing or poorly controlled GERD or in the presence of alarm features. Because EGD is notoriously problematic as a screening tool in those with reflux symptoms, it is better used (1) to examine patients who have breakthrough symptoms despite 4 to 8 weeks of twice-daily PPI therapy; (2) to monitor severe erosive esophagitis after 2 months of PPI therapy to assess healing or rule out BE; (3) to monitor patients with a history of esophageal stricture who have recurrent dysphagia; (4) to screen high-risk individuals with chronic GERD or to survey high-risk individuals with GERD and BE with or without dysplasia; and (5) to screen atypical or extraesophageal presentations as part of a presurgical evaluation or to perform stricture dilation.[5,17,19]

Because heartburn and regurgitation lead the clinician to diagnose GERD above other diagnoses, patients are commonly treated with PPI therapy without EGD. This risks missing a potential case of BE, EoE (defined as more than 15 eosinophils per high-powered field), and PPI-responsive eosinophilia.[14,18] BE is an important diagnosis to be made; it represents a change in typically observed esophageal mucosa and may develop into EAC within a rare, unfortunate subgroup of patients with GERD. The incidence of BE has risen significantly within the past 30 years.[20] Los Angeles criteria for the extent and severity of inflammatory findings (grades A to D) at initial EGD of higher grade (C/D) indicates a heightened risk for progression to BE.[2] The Montreal consensus definition for classification of BE includes all three types of columnar metaplasia (specialized intestinal, characterized by goblet cells; gastric junctional type, also known as cardiac type; and gastric fundic type), but the presence of metaplasia (goblet cells) in the columnar epithelial lining of the distal esophagus is the only type of esophageal columnar epithelium known to predispose to malignancy, so it is a preferred diagnosis.[4]

In cases of dysphagia, EGD is always indicated initially because dilation of a possible stricture can occur at the same time as the diagnostic procedure. Biopsy specimens of the gastric mucosa obtained during EGD may reveal gram-negative *H. pylori*, which affects 20% to 50% of the industrialized world's population and 80% of the developing world's population.[21] Opinion is divided as to whether patients should be tested and treated for *H. pylori* before long-term PPI therapy. There is some association with the location of *H. pylori* and gastric and duodenal ulcers (in 1% to 10%), gastric carcinoma

(0.1% to 3%, a sixfold increased risk), and gastric mucosa–associated lymphoid tissue lymphoma (rare); the majority will develop symptoms.[21] It is also linked to vitamin B_{12} and iron deficiency. In general, patients treated for *H. pylori* have a decrease in GERD symptoms.[5] Although *H. pylori* is associated with some protective effects with respect to developing GERD, esophageal carcinoma, pediatric allergies, and asthma, on the whole it is thought better eradicated in cases of peptic ulcer disease, carcinoma of the stomach, and functional dyspepsia, given that its cost-effectiveness is not established in broad testing and treatment.[11,21]

Gastric emptying scans are useful for early satiety, nausea, and vomiting symptoms. Dynamic barium videography is useful to examine swallowing irregularities and look for structural defects. Endoscopic ultrasound can assist in excluding mechanical obstruction.[13]

Ambulatory pH testing (24-hour catheter based or greater than 48-hour wireless) and high-resolution esophageal manometry are of benefit to patients with refractory symptoms and before reflux surgery by classifying the acidity, volume, and percentage duration of reflux in relationship to esophageal contractions. Esophageal pH testing can be performed with or without PPI and H_2 receptor antagonist acid suppression therapy. Typically, those with refractory, proven GERD should be tested on therapy. Esophageal pH testing with a single- or dual-sensor pH probe positioned above the LES (and below the upper esophageal sphincter, if the second sensor is used) for 24 hours contributes to the composite DeMeester score (greater than 14.72 indicates pathologic reflux).[10]

INITIAL DIAGNOSTICS

Gastroesophageal Reflux Disease (GERD)

LABORATORY
- Complete blood count and differential[a]
- Stool for occult blood × 3[a]
- *H. pylori* serum antibody or fecal antigen[a]
- Iron and vitamin B12 studies (if *H. pylori* is positive)

ADDITIONAL DIAGNOSTICS
- Esophagogastroduodenoscopy with biopsy specimens[a]
- 24-h ambulatory pH monitoring by transnasal catheter[a]
- 48-h ambulatory pH monitoring by radiotelemetry capsule[a]
- Multichannel intraluminal impedance testing[a]
- Endoscopic ultrasound[a]
- High-resolution manometry[a]
- Barium esophagram (for complications of GERD)[a]
- Gastric emptying scan[a]

[a]If indicated.

Esophageal manometry measures LES sphincter compliance and is especially useful in fundoplication surgeries in clarifying presurgical cofactors; it is sometimes repeated postsurgically if there are significant, persistent symptoms that medication cannot relieve. Although these studies can be useful, the most common manometric finding in patients with GERD is a normal LES pressure with normal esophageal motility.

New advances in technology using a radiotelemetry capsule, such as the Bravo (Medtronic) capsule, allow remote-controlled testing without the discomfort of a nasogastric tube to capture esophageal pH during a 48-hour period. Also, in some settings,

multichannel intraluminal impedance pH technology is used to look at acidic and nonacidic volume in the distal esophagus. Esophageal impedance detects retrograde bolus movement, pH, and location of reflux whether on or off of suppressive therapy. This test is especially important in identifying potential surgical candidates. If the amount of AET on ambulatory reflux monitoring is normal, the compliance of the esophagus is tested. Combined impedance-pH monitoring is considered standard testing in refractory cases,[9] and is particularly useful for those on PPIs.[10]

High-resolution manometry excludes motor disorders by closely measuring the esophagus during swallowing with reproducible pressure gradient measurements to mark severity of LES incompetence and to plan the surgical approach. In the face of atypical symptoms, proof of reflux is essential.[4]

The Lyon Consensus published in 2018 comprises several tests to more precisely affirm, negate, or sway inconclusive evidence to or away from a GERD diagnosis: the number of reflux episodes, AET (as a percentage), and the perception of symptoms associated with reflux episodes, whether by ambulatory reflux monitoring (on or off-PPI) or with (the preferred but costly) impedance-pH monitoring, in addition to a conclusive EGD. An AET of less than 4% is normal; AET greater than 6% is abnormal; reflux episodes of fewer than 40 in 24 hours is normal and more than 80 in 24 hours is abnormal.[1] For indeterminate findings, there are many more detailed analytics with respect to anatomic landmarks and motor function that can be assessed through high-resolution manometry. However, controversy exists with respect to the use of symptom association probability (SAP) and symptom index (SI) are considered less reliable than postreflux, swallow-induced perstaltic wave index and MNBI, especially for those with normal AET, who may otherwise be considered non-GERD, but who may yet benefit from PPI therapy as hypersensitive reflux patients.[9] Another academic measure, bolus exposure time (BET), the sum of all pH refluxate in the distal esophagus divided by time upright, is thought to separate ERD and NERD from FH and RH.[10]

Because empiric treatment can be helpful and cost-effective, patients more often receive a prescription for heartburn than an EGD. However, a response to PPIs is not necessarily an indication of GERD. A report found that those with erosive esophagitis responded to PPIs 69% of the time; those with NERD, 49%; and those with neither EGD nor pH findings, 35%.[1] Others argue that more stringent testing, such as multichannel intraluminal impedance-pH monitoring (MII-pH) and esophageal manometry to include detection of nonacid reflux and peristaltic abnormalities, are the best discriminators.[9] Much of the focus of establishing a GERD diagnosis is the correlation between symptoms and symptomatic pH monitoring, evidence of excess acid (even weakly acidic refluxate without mucosal changes), or responsivity to proton pump inhibition therapy.[2] Mucosal evidence on EGD can clinch the diagnosis, but becomes harder to confirm when the histopathology is less clear or the LA esophagitis score is at a lower grade, which may or may not correlate with symptoms.[1]

DIFFERENTIAL DIAGNOSIS

The symptoms of GERD can be similar to those of cholelithiasis, peptic ulcer disease, gastritis, angina, esophageal motility disturbances, and gastrointestinal malignant neoplasms. These disorders can be distinguished from GERD through the use of ultrasonography, upper gastrointestinal x-ray studies, endoscopy, esophageal manometry, electrocardiography, or coronary angiography, depending on the degree of clinical suspicion, particularly if the patient has a poor response to empirical GERD treatment.

Because symptoms and tests do not offer satisfactory correlations, different phenotypes have emerged. There are patients who respond to PPI therapy who have evidence of abnormal AET (greater than 6%) on ambulatory pH reflux testing and LA high-grade esophagitis, BE (ERD), or no esophagitis (NERD), and patients who report a positive symptom reflux correlation without an abnormal distal esophageal acid exposure attributable to RH. Both situations are thought more likely to respond to PPIs.[14] Patients with a third phenotype cannot stop their PPI treatment, and are proven to have improvement on some PPI treatment, but are no better with more aggressive PPI regimens, suggesting they have an additional factor.[1] A fourth phenotype includes FH patients for whom symptoms do not correlate with acid exposure. These are patients who do not need PPIs, but rather alternative strategies for acid suppression and reflux mitigation.[14] Patients who do not respond to twice-daily PPIs have either refractory GERD (refluxed acid contents with heartburn or regurgitation, without or without a functional component) or refractory heartburn (due to other physiologic mechanisms with or without a functional component).[1]

Of note, coincident depression is widely associated with heartburn symptoms.[22] More specifically, some early evidence points to major depression as being more likely associated with FH, whereas anxiety was more likely associated with hypersensitive and erosive esophagitis patients, which underscores the need to weigh the factor of comorbid psychological illnesses, their potential impact, and mitigation through cotreatment.[22]

Another consideration is EoE, particularly PPI-responsive EoE, which is seen more often in young men with a history of atopy in the setting of reflux, dysphagia, odynophagia, and even stricture. It is a uniquely managed entity that is captured on histology since diagnosis has become more standardized. Prompt treatment is recommended with steroid inhaler solutions, such as fluticasone propionate, 220 mcg, used twice daily. Leukotriene modifiers and other antihistamines or oral steroids may be used, depending on the severity.

GERD may be the most common cause of esophagitis, but there are other causes, including cytomegalovirus, herpes, or *Candida* infections in patients who are immunocompromised. Medications such as tetracycline and potassium chloride, if dissolved in the esophagus, result in "pill esophagitis." In unexplained cases of chest pain, cough, hoarseness, or asthma, GERD should be considered.

Finally, there are many extraesophageal manifestations of GERD. These atypical symptoms of GERD may come to the attention of otolaryngologists, cardiologists, or pulmonologists initially and include odynophagia, tooth decay, gingivitis, sour or brackish water taste, halitosis, dysphagia or globus sensation, cough, hoarseness, laryngitis, earache, sinus pain, hiccups, noncardiac chest pain, asthma, bronchiectasis, aspiration pneumonia, idiopathic pulmonary fibrosis, and sleep disturbances, as discussed earlier. GERD is also associated with irritable bowel syndrome and peptic ulcer disease.[5] Moreover, newer entities proposed by the Montreal consensus meeting incorporate GERD in their classification: reflux cough syndrome, reflux laryngitis syndrome, reflux asthma syndrome, reflux dental erosion syndrome, and associated possibilities—pharyngitis, sinusitis, idiopathic pulmonary fibrosis, and otitis.[4]

DIFFERENTIAL DIAGNOSIS

 Priority differential diagnoses include cardiac ischemia, aspiration pneumonia, esophageal cancer, gastric obstructing tumor, pyloric stenosis, peptic stricture, BE, peptic ulcer disease, Zollinger-Ellison syndrome, and achalasia.

Other considerations for GERD should be BE, erosive esophagitis, NERD, EoE/eosinophilic gastritis, and FH.

INTERPROFESSIONAL COLLABORATIVE MANAGEMENT

Goals of therapy are prompt and sustained symptom control; healing of the injured esophageal mucosa; and prevention of complications, including stricture formation, BE, and adenocarcinoma (Fig. 117.1).

Nonpharmacologic Management

Lifestyle modifications may benefit patients with GERD, although these changes alone are unlikely to control symptoms (Box 117.1). Modifications include elevating the head of the bed, sleeping on the right side of the body,[3] lowering fat intake, ceasing smoking, loosening restrictive clothing, and avoiding recumbency for 2 to 3 hours after a meal. Avoidance of chocolate, alcohol (especially excessive, although data conflict on the effects with respect to amount and type of alcohol consumed),[16] carbonated drinks, peppermint, coffee, citrus, onion, and garlic can guard against chemically reduced LES pressure. Some research has shown a higher association of functional dyspepsia and irritable bowel disease with refractory symptoms in those with documented abnormal reflux and higher baseline anxiety contributes to persistent symptoms.[10] For patients with functional esophageal reflux unresponsive to once-daily PPI, there is a role for complementary and alternative medical therapies including acupuncture and diaphragmatic breathing techniques.[3]

Pharmacologic Management

Many heartburn patients do not seek medical care but rather choose antacids and over-the-counter acid suppressants. Antacids are helpful but have a shorter duration of effect. Alginate-based antacids provide effective relief but are less effective in nonacid reflux and regurgitation management.[4]

All four of the histamine$_2$ receptor antagonists (H$_2$RAs) approved for use in the United States are available over the counter and decrease gastric acid, particularly after a meal. They include cimetidine, famotidine, nizatidine, and ranitidine. H$_2$RAs in divided doses may be effective in a patient with

BOX **117.1**

Lifestyle Changes for Management of Gastroesophageal Reflux Disease

- Decreased meal size
- Raised head of bed
- Reduced alcohol consumption
- Reduced carbonated drinks
- Reduced dietary fat, acidic and spicy foods, garlic, onion, mint, and caffeinated products
- Smoking cessation
- Weight loss

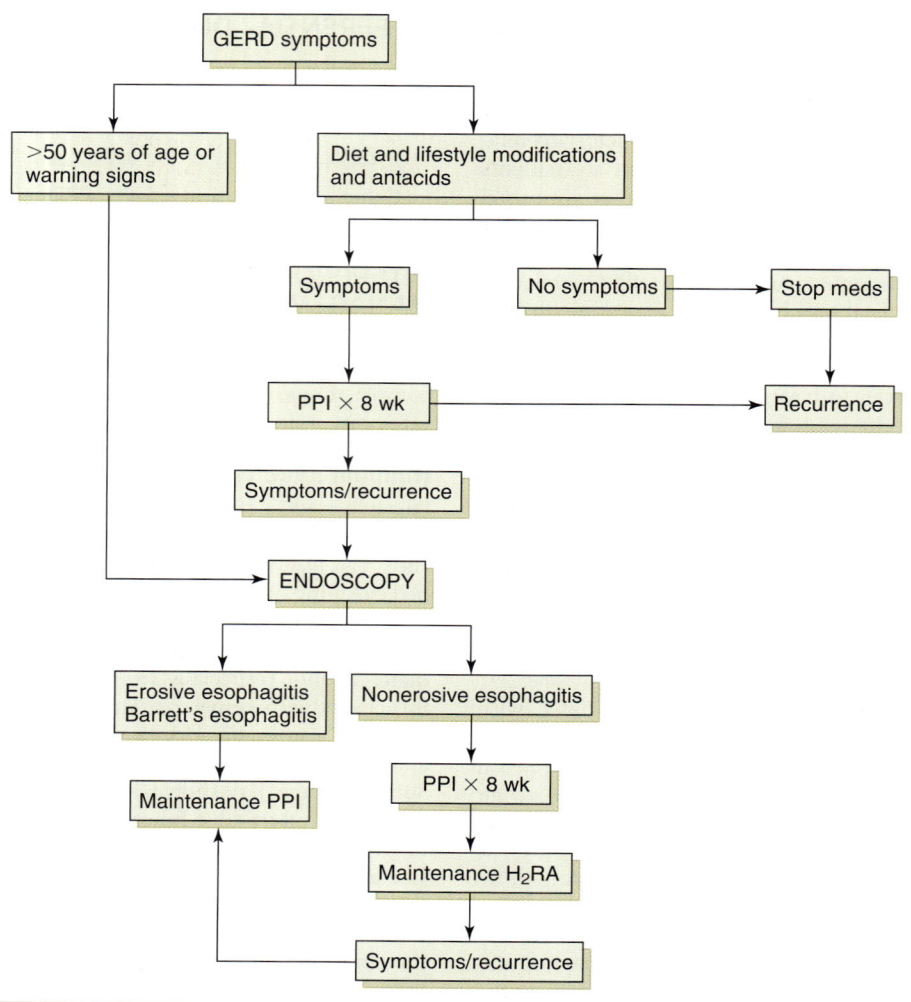

FIG. 117.1 Gastroesophageal reflux disease *(GERD)* algorithm. *H₂RA,* H₂ receptor antagonist; *PPI,* proton pump inhibitor.

mild GERD and are considered equivalent in equipotent doses. Unfortunately, there is a risk of tolerance.[4] Over-the-counter PPIs have disclaimers that patients seek medical advice if treatment for more than 14 days is required. In fact, a trial dose of 7 days' duration was shown as long enough to establish sensitivity in 71% of erosive esophagitis patients and 78% in those with ambulatory pH-positive results, although specificity was 41% and 54% respectively, leading the authors to conclude that there was a mixture of GERD and non-GERD etiologies.[3] Prescription treatment for 2 to 3 months is sufficient to determine efficacy and to promote esophageal healing, as necessary (see Fig. 117.1).

The use of prescription-dose PPIs for acid suppression and maintenance therapy is well documented as the treatment of choice for GERD. PPIs prevent acid (H^+ as well as K^+)[3] production at the final juncture of the histamine, gastrin, and acetylcholine pathways, and thus outperform histamine-blocking H₂RAs. Six PPIs are available: dexlansoprazole, esomeprazole, lansoprazole, omeprazole, pantoprazole, and rabeprazole. PPIs provide slow-onset and time-limited suppression. The medication has to concentrate in the acidic secretory canaliculi of the parietal cell before rendering the resulting refluxate weakly acidic or alkaline.[3] Because of interaction and reduced efficacy when taken together, PPIs and H₂RAs can be used together

if administered at different times of day to offer an alternative to high-dose PPIs. Twice-daily administration is seen as more effective than a single higher dose initially (especially for nighttime control), and three-times-a-day dosing is rarely advantageous.[3]

PPIs are superior to H₂RAs (even in high doses multiple times a day) in controlling symptoms, healing esophagitis, and improving quality of life. PPIs should ideally be given one-half hour to 45 minutes before breakfast. Administration can be increased to twice daily. The second dose should be given 1 hour before the evening meal. In the face of persistent symptoms, confirmation of correct timing of PPI administration and compliance with daily or twice-daily administration should be sought, along with lifestyle modifications, before considering the trial an inadequate response, because adherence to this regimen has been seen to hover around 50%.[14] Despite daily use of PPIs, 10% to 40% of patients still have GERD, although compliance is variable.[3,5] The thought is that some may have weakly acidic or weakly alkaline refluxate associated with regurgitation or atypical GERD symptoms, even bile salt exposure in a nonacidic esophageal environment, but this is still not well established.[15] Specifically, regurgitation as a symptom of GERD does not respond as well to PPI therapy: risk ratio 1.4 over placebo, number needed to treat (NNT) nearly 6, which is only slightly better than noncardiac chest pain with negative GERD testing (NNT 22) or laryngeal symptoms alone (NNT 79).[3]

Sometimes a step-down approach with successful PPI use can allow reduction in use, particularly if there is no erosive esophagitis or BE. Patients with NERD can use PPIs on demand. With PPIs, a reduction in dose should happen slowly to avoid producing a rebound of GERD symptoms. Another concern has been increased risk of PPI-associated *Clostridium difficile* infection, although it is modest.[23] This has been borne out by the US Food and Drug Administration (FDA), which has led to the recommendation of testing for this pathogen in cases of unremitting diarrhea after recent start of PPI therapy.[5] The most salient concern with PPIs is reduced gastric acid associated with increased risk of gastric cancer, gastric carcinoids, or colorectal cancer possibly due to the promotion of *H. pylori* colonies under conditions of hypergastrinemia, but this has yet to be established, even when cases of colorectal cancer were restricted to more than 7 years of PPI use.[5,23] With the exception of small intestinal bacterial overgrowth, it seems that prolonged exposure to PPIs does not result in excess fracture risk in men and women, myocardial infarction, kidney, spontaneous bacterial peritonitis, dementia, salmonella, campylobacter, pneumonia, vitamin B_{12}, no-heme iron, or calcium or magnesium deficiencies.[23] No routine monitoring, including nutrient levels, or stepped-up cancer screening recommendations have yet been made.[1,23] Despite the step-down approach, it has been reported that 42% have to return to PPIs.[1] A newer acid blocker, vonoprazan fumarate, a potassium-competitive acid blocker that inhibits the attachment of potassium ions to the proton pump in the final step of gastric acid secretion in gastric parietal cells, has not yet been approved by the FDA because of excess gastrin concerns.[13]

Another strategy in GERD management is to promote gastric emptying and to increase LES pressure. Promotility agents (e.g., metoclopramide, domperidone) may be used in selected patients as an adjunct to acid suppression, particularly if there is an element of delayed gastric emptying. The currently available agents are not ideal for monotherapy because they may produce undesirable side effects. Another consideration is the use of neuromodulators, which exert mostly centrally mitigating effects on pain sensation.[3] Classes involved include tricyclic antidepressants (amitriptyline, nortriptyline) in significantly reduced doses for pain receptor modulation, and trazadone, selective serotonin reuptake inhibitors, and serotonin-norepinephrine reuptake inhibitors, although evidence points to marginal responses and more research is needed.[3]

TLSER reducers and pain modulators for weakly acidic refluxate might better address the perception of pain experienced by the patient. Medication strategies using γ-aminobutyric acid type B (GABA$_B$) agonists such as baclofen (especially at nighttime) have been useful. Sucralfate has been used in healing of peptic ulcers but may not be appropriate in NERD.[3]

Endoscopic Therapies

Endoscopic techniques for GERD have been developed. These techniques are less invasive than the standard surgical approach, laparoscopic fundoplication, but have narrow application.

Radiofrequency using a delivery catheter to remodel the esophageal junction and LES has evolved over the past 15 years. The catheter is positioned, and needles are deployed into the muscles of the gastroesophageal junction. Energy is delivered to create a series of thermal lesions, which are thought to thicken the sphincter for more resistance. It may be used in a stepwise progression before antireflux surgery or in addition to other techniques. To this end, three other techniques have been used with some durability of positive impact in very select cases: transoral incisionless fundoplication, which uses T-fasteners to sutures to form a mechanical barrier between the esophagus and stomach; a stapling device used in anterior fundoplication; and electrical stimulation to increase resting LES.[3]

Surgery

In patients who are responsive to PPI treatment, and have documented reflux and LES incompetence with inadequate control, surgery can improve symptom control and quality of life.[3] There are minimally invasive endoscopic techniques and more involved laparoscopic, rarely open, antireflux surgeries. One technique that is used to address LES compliance is endoscopically implanting titanium-enclosed magnets into the relatively intact esophageal junction, especially if regurgitation is the prominent feature of proven GERD.[3]

Antireflux surgery includes conventional (open) Nissen fundoplication and laparoscopic partial and total fundoplication for patients with well-documented, chronic, symptomatic GERD (including ambulatory reflux monitoring usually off their acid suppressive medication), although enthusiasm for antireflux surgery has waned since its peak in 2009, because outcomes are similar to long-term PPI use in proven GERD.[3] The longer the distal esophagus is exposed to acid, the absence of esophageal outflow obstruction on manometry, having a response to acid blockers with typical symptoms and a hiatal hernia correlates with a good response to surgical intervention. In addition, bariatric Roux-en-Y surgery to address morbid obesity provides effective reflux reduction. By contrast, the gastric-sleeve approach worsens reflux.[3] Finally, there is a role for selected surgery in cases of BE to prevent EAC.[7]

Patients with atypical symptoms and EESs, and those whose symptoms are refractory, respond less effectively to surgery, although patients with respiratory symptoms, NERD, hypersensitive esophagus, or LPR may be candidates, depending on symptom correlation with acid or nonacid reflux.[4] Inappropriate patients include those with achalasia, diffuse esophageal spasm, nutcracker esophagus, eosinophilic esophagus, or scleroderma.[4]

Complications include a high rate of postoperative dysphagia, bloating, and flatulence. To address this, there are several variations on approach, particularly the anterior partial fundoplication and reoperative procedures if necessary. The posterior partial fundoplication is indicated for qualifying normal-weight patients with GERD. In contrast, gastric bypass surgery would be a good choice for patients with a BMI greater than 40. With all surgeries, repair of hiatal hernia is obligatory and correlated with improvement; still, there is an antireflux failure rate of 10% to 15%, wherein symptoms persist or new symptoms develop. In fact, since the introduction of Nissen fundoplication in 2001, a small cohort of patients demonstrated that 42% (laparoscopic approach) and 49% (conventional approach) reported using daily PPI.[24]

Indications for Referral or Hospitalization

It is important to identify patients who might benefit from maximum long-term medical therapy or experience complications. Patients who initially receive 2 months of empirical treatment without success or whose symptoms recur when medications are stopped should undergo EGD to determine whether esophagitis is present (see Fig. 117.1).

A gastroenterology referral is indicated if the patient is older than 50 years or has the warning signs of dysphagia (both solid and liquid), odynophagia, unexplained iron deficiency anemia, weight loss, fecal occult bleeding, new-onset motility disorder, or anorexia.[25]

Patients who have refractory symptoms, including EER symptoms, will need further consultation and management, ideally within a multidisciplinary framework. Newer techniques, such as 180- or 360-degree circumferential mucosal impedance testing, may help establish multiple distances above the squamocolumnar junction.[26] When otolaryngologists, allergists, cardiologists, pulmonologists, surgeons, psychopharmocologists, speech language pathologists, and nutritionists are consulted for diagnosis and management, the challenge is to continue to provide cross-disciplinary communication to optimize the patient's outcome.

LIFE SPAN CONSIDERATIONS

GERD can affect patients of any age, including infants. Both age and nutritional status affect esophageal mucosal resistance, which is less robust than that of the stomach because it is not designed to resist prolonged acid exposure.

Patients with pregnancy-related reflux can use antacids, sucralfate, and H2RAs. As women enter perimenopause and postmenopause, the use of exogenous hormone replacement, including estrogen, progesterone, tamoxifen, selective estrogen receptor modulators, and over-the-counter hormone preparations, rises. Each of these medication classes has been shown to raise the risk of GERD in women.

Increased age is associated with more neuromuscular, hormonal, renal, cardiac, and pulmonary function decreases, whereas there is less impact on the gastrointestinal tract.[27] Some disturbances are associated with age: dysphagia, more common in patients over 80, has a higher associated mortality rate and achalasia has an early and late age presentation, the latter peaking after age 60.[27] Delayed gastric emptying and small intestinal bacterial overgrowth are among the more common entities in advanced age; GERD itself may be unreported because it may not be perceived as distinctly at a younger age, whereas at an older age the higher risk for polypharmacy may contribute to GERD symptoms rather than physiologic decline.[27] With advanced age, arthritic pain and bone health in the prevention and management of osteopenia and osteoporosis may result in the use of bisphosphonates and NSAIDs, which can exacerbate mild GERD symptoms. PPIs are recommended to prevent risk of ulcer-related bleeding with long-term NSAID use.

Although symptom severity in patients aged 60 years and older may be similar to that in younger patients, evidence suggests that the proportion of patients with heartburn alone may decrease in an older cohort, whereas the incidence of erosive esophagitis and BE may increase.[8] Older patients on H2-receptor antagonists may experience drowsiness or falls, and there is a caveat in use in this population due to increased risk of delirium or renal clearance concern.[5] Low-dose tricyclic antidepressants used to address functional reflux symptoms may exert anticholinergic effects particularly in older patients leading to urinary retention, constipation, headache, dizziness, and somnolence.

Long-term results of antireflux surgery appear to show a benefit in patients achieving their best control of symptoms with PPIs, whereas those who are refractory to intensive therapy have more variable responses postoperatively. If surgery is indicated for a patient older than 65 years, outcomes are thought to be comparable to those of younger patients, although postoperative stay is potentially longer because of comorbidities.

COMPLICATIONS

Complications of GERD include hemorrhage and perforation, esophageal ulcers, peptic strictures, BE, and adenocarcinoma. Dental erosions, pharyngeal ulcerations, laryngeal damage, and sleep derangements can also occur.[5] Strictures, which form from mucosal scarring, may impede the progress of food from the mouth to the stomach. These inflamed bands develop over time and are characterized by dysphagia and a possible reduction in heartburn because the stricture may block some of the reflux. Dilation may be necessary if symptoms are persistent despite PPI therapy and may need to be repeated months to years later.

BE, an infrequent premalignant condition, is associated with chronic (more than 5 years) esophageal injury resulting from reflux. It is estimated that 5% to 15% of patients with chronic GERD develop BE, defined as a length of metaplastic columnar epithelium greater than 1 cm located in the distal esophagus (above the esophagogastric junction), which has replaced squamous epithelium.[2,7] It is diagnosed histologically, when patches of normal gray-white, stratified squamous cell mucosa of the esophagus change into the light pink columnar epithelium. Biopsy specimens of the gastroesophageal junction with careful landmarking are critical for accurate diagnosis and staging (Prague criteria).[20]

In half of BE cases, patients have undergone endoscopy in the absence of prior reflux symptoms. In fact, a history of erosive esophagitis has not been established as a clear risk factor for BE in patients with GERD symptoms. In the general population 1% to 2% of subjects in studies have been shown to have BE; in one study of EAC, 40% reported no prior GERD symptoms.[7] However, those with GERD and BE tend to develop symptoms at an earlier age and have more complications. BE is associated with the following risk factors: white race, male sex, tobacco use or past use, central obesity, age older than 50, and family history of BE or EAC in a first-degree relative, and would warrant EGD screening in all cases of GERD with two or more risk factors.[7] Those with dysplasia or BE are at further risk for developing EAC in the absence of NSAIDs, PPIs, or statin use.[7] Patients with BE, particularly those with high-grade dysplasia (this is a significant risk factor for EAC), which has a median survival of less than 1 year,[25] have a 5-year survival of less than 20%.[7] A distinction between BE and intestinal metaplasia cardia suggests that the latter finding, which is associated with H. pylori, is far less likely to develop into EAC; on the other hand, any suspicious lesions in BE require careful biopsy, separate from surveillance biopsies, because they are more likely to contain advanced dysplasia or early neoplasia.[20]

The risk for EAC (with a survival rate of less than 3% at 5 years in symptomatic patients) is 10 times higher in individuals with BE.[20] Early work with genetic and molecular markers, indicating a likelihood of progression to dysplasia, have not been validated yet by larger studies; alternatively, broad EGD surveillance along current risk stratifications are not cost-effective, including in women with GERD but no significant risk factors.[7,25] *H. pylori* infection may be a protective factor.[7] If BE is present, periodic high-definition/high-resolution white light (if available) EGDs with biopsies of raised nodules or depressed lesions, excluding erosive esophagitis LA grade C or D, are recommended to assess and to grade the development of dysplasia or malignant transformation, ideally confirmed by a gastroenterology pathologist with audit documentation to check on progression.[25] Surveillance endoscopy every 3 to 5 years in patients without dysplasia, with four-quadrant mucosal biopsies of every 1 to 2 cm of involved mucosa, is generally recommended: at 6 months and 12 months to confirm low-grade dysplasia (which affects 15% to 40% of BE patients)[25] with consideration of endoscopic eradication, and then annually (as diagnosed with white-light endoscopy under maximal acid suppression)[25]; and every 3 months if high-grade dysplasia has been identified, with consideration of endoablative therapy.[7,17,20] If there is complete eradication of BE-related low-grade dysplasia (LGD), patients should be under surveillance every year for 2 years and then every 3 years thereafter or more frequently if eradication is not achieved.[25] Advanced imaging techniques, such as electronic or virtual chromoendoscopy, have been associated with increased yield of dysplasia detection.[17]

For those with complete eradication of intestinal metaplasia, whether by medication, an endoluminal procedure, or surgery (preferred in younger patients with hiatal hernia and LES incompetence),[4] surveillance for high-grade dysplasia or T1a EAC should continue at 3, 6, 12, 18, and 24 months, and then yearly.[20]

Unfortunately, there are disparities in the classification of BE low-, high-grade, and neoplasia, and the tendency is to overcall low-grade dysplasia rather than nondysplasia.[25] Regardless, the risk of cancer progression is as great as 7% a year in patients with high-grade dysplasia (or as low as 0.2% to 0.5% in BE patients with nondysplastic neoplasia); however, more than 90% of patients with BE succumb to causes other than EAC.[7]

As for other complications arising from antireflux surgery, a proportion of antireflux postoperative patients continue acid-blocking medication despite negative results of 24-hour pH monitoring.[6] Laparoscopic fundoplication complications include dysphagia, flatulence, and the inability to belch, among other bowel complaints. Furthermore, the surgical wrap around the LES is known to weaken over time.

PATIENT AND FAMILY EDUCATION

Education is essential for patients with GERD and their families. Patients should avoid fatty foods, caffeinated and carbonated drinks, acidic and spicy foods, chocolate, peppermint, and excessive alcohol consumption. Foods that may elicit symptoms for one person may not necessarily produce symptoms in another; therefore, selective avoidance of foods that precipitate symptoms is necessary. Raising the head of the bed or using wedge pillows can offer modest improvement and help avoid nighttime symptoms. Sleeping on the right side of the body apparently offers an advantage over the left.[3] Ultimately, a screening upper endoscopy is recommended in cases of chronic GERD or difficult-to-treat symptoms to determine if there is an erosive component or if complications are present. Medication adherence presents its own challenge and accounts for reduced efficacy in a substantial proportion of patients.

HEALTH PROMOTION

Lifestyle modifications include optimizing BMI through proper diet and exercise and controlling comorbidities such as chronic allergy, asthma, and obstructive sleep apnea by adhering to medical and mechanical therapy can help promote immune health and mitigate the impact of and each entity's independent contribution to reflux.[3] Patients with psychological symptoms have higher reports of reflux; moreover, more severe GERD symptoms are associated with increased psychological distress.[22] To this end, therapeutic counseling and stress management strategies are ever more necessary components of heartburn relief and, ideally, heartburn prevention.

REFERENCES

1. Gyawali, C. P., Kahrilas, P. J., Savarino, E., et al. (2018). Modern diagnosis of GERD: The Lyon consensus. *Gut*, 1–12.
2. Savarino, E., de Bortoli, N., De Cassan, C., et al. (2017). The natural history of gastro-esophageal reflux disease: A comprehensive review. *Diseases of the Esophagus: Official Journal of the International Society for Diseases of the Esophagus / I.S.D.E.*, 30, 1–9.
3. Gyawali, C. P., & Fass, R. (2018). Management of gastroesophageal reflux disease. *Gastroenterology*, 154, 302–318.
4. Fuchs, K. H., Babic, B., Breithaupt, W., et al. (2014). EAES recommendations for the management of gastroesophageal reflux disease. Consensus statement. *Surgical Endoscopy*, 28, 1753–1773.
5. Hert, A. M. (2013). Evidence-based recommendations for GERD treatment. *The Nurse Practitioner*, 38(8), 27–34.
6. Francis, D. O., Rymer, J. A., Slaughter, J. C., et al. (2013). High economic burden of caring for patients with suspected extraesophageal reflux. *The American Journal of Gastroenterology*, 108, 905–911.
7. Shaheen, N. J., Falk, G. W., Iyer, P. G., et al. (2015). ACG Clinical Guideline: Diagnosis and management of Barrett's esophagus. Practice guidelines. *The American Journal of Gastroenterology*, 1–21.
8. Badillo, R., & Francis, D. (2014). Diagnosis and treatment of gastroesophageal reflux disease. *World Journal of Gastrointestinal Pharmacology and Therapeutics*, 5(3), 105–112.
9. Frazzoni, L., Frazzoni, M., de Bortoli, N., et al. (2018). Critical appraisal of Rome IV criteria: Hypersensitive esophagus does belong to gastroesophageal reflux disease spectrum. *Ann of Gastro*, 31, 1–7.
10. Wang, F., Li, P., Ji, G.-Z., et al. (2017). An analysis of 342 patients with refractory gastroesophageal reflux disease symptoms using questionnaires, high-resolution manometry, and impedance—pH monitoring. *Medicine*, 96(5), 1–6.
11. Taylan, K. (2017). To whom and when the upper gastrointestinal endoscopy is indicated in gastroesophageal reflux disease? What is the role of routine esophageal biopsy? Which endoscopic esophagitis classification should be used? *The Turkish Journal of Gastroenterology*, 28(Suppl. 1), S22–S25.
12. Subramanian, C. R., & Triadafilopoulos, G. (2014). Refractory gastroesophageal reflux disease. *Gastroenterology Report*, 1013.
13. Suzuki, H. (2017). The application of the Rome IV criteria to functional esophagogastroduodenal disorders in Asia. *Journal of Neurogastroenterology and Motility*, 23(3), 325–333.
14. Gawron, A. J., & Pandolfino, J. E. (2013). Ambulatory reflux monitoring in GERD—which test should be performed and should therapy be stopped? *Current Gastroenterology Reports*, 15(4), 316.
15. Eldredge, T. A., Myers, J. C., Kiroff, G. K., et al. (2018). Detecting bile reflux—the enigma of bariatric surgery. *Obesity Surgery*, 28, 559–566.
16. Grad, S., Abenavoli, L., & Dumitrascu, D. L. (2016). The effect of alcohol on gastrointestinal motility. *Reviews on Recent Clinival Trials*, 11, 191–195.
17. van Rhinj, B. D., Weijenborg, P. W., Verheij, J., et al. (2014). Proton pump inhibitors partially restore mucosal integrity in patients with proton pump inhibitor–responsive esophageal eosinophilia but not eosinophilic esophagitis. *Clinical Gastroenterology and Hepatology*, 12, 1815–1823.
18. Sharma, V. K. (2014). Role of endoscopy in GERD. *Gastroenterology Clinics of North America*, 43, 39–46.
19. Johnson, D. A., Katz, P. O., Armstrong, D., et al. (2017). The safety of appropriate use of over-the-counter proton pump inhibitors: An evidence-based review and Delphi consensus. *Drugs*, 77, 547–561.
20. Sharma, P., Katzka, D. A., Gupta, N., et al. (2015). Quality indicators for the management of Barrett's esophagus dysplasia, and esophageal

adenocarcinoma: International consensus recommendations from the American Gastroenterological Association Symposium. *Gastro, 149,* 1599–1606.

21. Malnick, S. D., Melzer, E., Attali, E., et al. (2014). *Helicobacter pylori:* Friend or foe? *World Journal of Gastroenterology, 21*(27), 8979–8985.

22. Fass, R., & Fass, S. (2017). Psychological comorbidity and chronic heartburn: Which is the chicken and which is the egg? *Digestive Diseases and Sciences, 62,* 823–825.

23. Freedberg, D. E., Kim, L. S., & Yang, Y.-X. (2017). The risks and benefits of long-term use of proton pump inhibitors: Expert review and best practice advice from the American Gastroenterological Association. AGA Clinical Practice Update: Expert Reviews. *Gastro, 152,* 706–715.

24. Oor, J. E., Roks, D. J., Broeders, J. A., et al. (2017). Seventeen-year outcome of a randomized clinical trial comparing laparoscopic and conventional Nissen fundoplication. A plea for patient counseling and clarification. *Annals of Surgery, 266*(1), 23–28.

25. Wani, S., Rubenstein, J. H., Vieth, A. M., et al. (2016). Diagnosis and management of low-grade dysplasia in Barret's esophagus: Expert review from the clinical practice updates committee of the American Gastroenterological Association. AGA clinical practice update: Expert review. *Gastro, 151,* 822–835.

26. Kavitt, R. T., Lal, P., Yuksel, E. S., et al. (2017). Esophageal mucosal impedance pattern is distinct in patients with extraesophageal reflux symptoms and pathologic acid reflux. *Journal of Voice: Official Journal of the Voice Foundation, 31*(3), 347–351.

27. Gidwaney, N. G., Bajpai, M., & Chokhavatia, S. S. (2016). Gastrointestinal dysmotility in the elderly. *Journal of Clinical Gastroenterology, 50*(10), 819–827.

CHAPTER **118**

GASTROINTESTINAL HEMORRHAGE

Tracia L. O'Shana

 Immediate emergency room evaluation/urgent consultation with a gastroenterologist is indicated for patients with acute GI bleeding.

DEFINITION AND EPIDEMIOLOGY

Gastrointestinal (GI) bleeding is a common finding in the ambulatory care setting. Patients may report the symptoms as black tarry stools (melena), bright red stools (hematochezia), and even bright red vomitus (hematemesis) or coffee ground emesis.[1] GI hemorrhage can occur anywhere in the GI tract from the mouth to the anus and can be overt or occult (Box 118.1).[2] Overt GI bleeding is considered major when it is accompanied by hemodynamic instability and minor when it is not. Occult bleeding is nonvisible bleeding that can be detected by stool testing or indirectly suggested by iron deficiency anemia.[3]

GI bleeding may be related to ulceration, inflammation, erosion of a blood vessel, or neoplasm. Management of GI bleeding has remained constant for several decades. Hemodynamic stabilization of the patient, cessation of active bleeding, and prevention of recurrent bleeding have long remained the goals of medical management for this disorder. Upper GI bleeding occurs in up to 150 individuals per 100,000 per year, and the incidence of lower GI bleeding appears to be similar.[4] Many of these patients require emergency treatment, hospitalization, and intensive care monitoring.

Upper and lower GI tract bleeding are differentiated according to anatomic source. Patients with upper gastrointestinal bleeding (UGIB) from a source proximal to the ligament of

---

B O X **118.1**

Bleeding Definitions

Overt: Visible bright red or maroon blood in feces or emesis
Occult: No visible blood in feces or emesis
Obscure: Patient may be seen with iron deficiency anemia (IDA) or may have a positive fecal occult blood test (FOBT) result
Obscure/Occult: IDA recurrent or persistent; positive FOBT result; may or may not have visible bleeding; no bleeding source found at time of original endoscopy
Obscure/Overt:
- IDA recurrent or persistent; positive FOBT result; no visible blood in feces; no source identified
- Blood visible in feces and emesis; bleeding recurrent or persistent; no source found at original endoscopy

Modified from Zuckerman, G. R., Prakash, C., Askin, M. P., & Lewis, B. S. (2000). AGA technical review on the evaluation and management of occult and obscure gastrointestinal bleeding. *Gastroenterology, 118*(1):201–221.

Treitz may be asymptomatic, have subtle signs of anemia and hypovolemia, or have a dramatic presentation with hematemesis, melena, or hematochezia.[5] Causes of UGIB are classified as variceal and nonvariceal bleeding. The most common cause of nonvariceal bleeding is peptic ulcer disease (i.e., duodenal and gastric ulcers).[6] Nonspecific mucosal abnormalities, such as erosions, are also a significant cause of nonvariceal bleeding.[6] Low-dose aspirin and other nonsteroidal antiinflammatory drugs (NSAIDs) are frequently implicated in UGIB and are associated with morbidity and mortality.[5,7,8] Other causes of UGIB include anticoagulants, antiplatelets such as clopidogrel, esophagitis, and gastroesophageal varices. Lower gastrointestinal bleeding (LGIB) from a source distal to the ligament of Treitz can cause occult blood loss or massive hematochezia and shock.[9] Lower GI bleeding causes include cancer, diverticulosis, polyps, colitis, ulcers, angiodysplasia, postpolypectomy bleeding, aortocolonic fistula, stercoral ulcer, anastomotic bleeding, anorectal hemorrhoids, fissures, and rectal ulcers.

PATHOPHYSIOLOGY

GI bleeding can be associated with various GI disorders including esophagitis, peptic ulcer disease, gastritis, *Helicobacter pylori*, esophageal or gastric varices, colitis, diverticulosis, inflammatory bowel disease, gastric and colonic cancers, gastric and colonic polyps, hemorrhoids, proctitis, and angiodysplasia.[2] Peptic ulcers are defects in the mucosa of the duodenum or stomach caused by a breakdown in normal mucosal defenses and ulcer erosion into a blood vessel. Contributing factors include smoking, NSAIDs, excess stomach acid production, and *H. pylori*.

Bleeding caused by gastritis is related to diffuse superficial lesions in the gastric mucosa that are usually associated with local irritants or *H. pylori*. Gastritis can also be caused by major physiologic stressors, including burns, sepsis, trauma, and long-distance running, secondary to decreased splanchnic blood flow and the resultant decrease in mucus production, bicarbonate secretion, and prostaglandin synthesis, all leading to a breakdown in the normal mucosal defenses. NSAIDs inhibit cyclooxygenase, decreasing the synthesis of protective prostaglandins, and may have direct effects on the gastric mucosa, causing both irritation and superficial lesions. Alcohol ingestion causes gastric mucosa production of leukotrienes, which may be responsible for vascular stasis, engorgement, and increased vascular permeability, resulting in hemorrhage.[10]

H. pylori, a gram-negative spiral bacterium has adaptive mechanisms to survive in the human stomach, including the conversion of urea, water, and acid to ammonia and bicarbonate. It is the secretions of toxins, disruption of the mucous layer, and direct adherence to the gastroduodenal surface epithelium that render the underlying mucosa vulnerable to peptic acid damage. Improved hygiene and eradication have caused the prevalence of *H. pylori* in peptic ulcer disease to markedly decrease.[11] Treatment of this organism has been shown to cure ulcer disease and to decrease the incidence of ulcer recurrence and rebleeding (see Chapter 126).[12-14]

Esophageal varices are dilated submucosal veins arising as a consequence of portal hypertension.[15] The most common cause of portal hypertension in the United States is cirrhosis from alcohol, hepatitis, and nonalcoholic fatty liver disease, but schistosomiasis and other parasitic diseases are common causes worldwide.[12-18]

Colitis can be infectious or ischemic. Bloody diarrhea is associated with *Campylobacter*, *Salmonella*, and *Shigella* infection (see Chapter 211), but ischemic colitis, which has varied causes, is also a cause of rectal bleeding, as is inflammatory bowel disease (see Chapter 120) and anorectal pathology (see Chapter 110).

Diverticulosis, a common cause of acute LGIB, can occur at the penetration site of colonic arteries. A rupture into the diverticular sac results in LGIB.[10]

Angiodysplasias, small vascular tufts formed by capillaries, veins, and venules, representing an acquired arteriovenous malformation[14,15] are vascular lesions found in the GI tract.[1] Although massive bleeding is occasionally associated with these lesions, bleeding is more often slow, chronic, and occult.

CLINICAL PRESENTATION AND PHYSICAL EXAMINATION

Overt blood loss from the GI tract can manifest in numerous ways. Hematemesis is bloody vomitus that appears fresh and bright red or is older and like coffee grounds in appearance. Melena is stool that is black, shiny, and foul smelling as a result of blood degradation. These clinical signs generally originate from an upper GI source. The presence or history of black or red hematemesis confirms an upper GI source after bleeding from the nose and oropharynx has been excluded.

Hematochezia is the passage of bright red to mahogany-colored blood from the rectum as pure blood, blood mixed with stool, blood clots, or bloody diarrhea. These manifestations are more overt or obvious, but occult blood loss is often more subtle. In general, patients with a lower GI source of bleeding have hematochezia, a clear nasogastric (NG) aspirate,[9] and a normal blood urea nitrogen (BUN)/creatinine ratio. In addition, patients can have symptoms associated with blood loss, such as presyncope, dyspnea, angina, postural hypotension, and shock, with no overt bleeding source. Occult blood loss can manifest as iron deficiency anemia or as a positive result of a routine fecal occult blood test (FOBT).

Patient history should include the amount, duration, and source of any signs of bleeding along with any associated symptoms, including dizziness, abdominal pain, chest pain, shortness of breath, diaphoresis, and weakness. The patient should be questioned about prior episodes of bleeding and about other illnesses that can result in bleeding, such as cirrhosis, cancer, coagulopathies, and connective tissue disease. All significant past medical and surgical conditions, and any allergies and medication use, including alendronate, potassium chloride, anticoagulants, and over-the-counter preparations (especially aspirin and NSAIDs), should be elicited and documented. A careful history of alcohol, tobacco, and illicit drug use is also necessary.

The physical examination is brief and focused. The initial general appearance and mental status of the patient should be noted. Vital signs are the most important factor in considering initial triage and should be obtained early and frequently. The earliest sign of hypovolemia is tachycardia; hypotension does not occur unless the fluid loss is greater than 10% of extracellular fluid (ECF) volume.[19] Blood loss of 1000 mL or more over a short period of time causes tachycardia and hypotension. With losses greater than 1000 mL, the heart rate is usually greater than 100 beats per minute and the systolic blood pressure is usually less than 100 mg Hg.[20] The skin should be examined for color, temperature, turgor, moisture, and capillary refill. Cutaneous lesions on upper extremities, lips, and oral mucosa may reveal hereditary hemorrhagic telangiectasia or blue rubber bleb nevus syndrome. These can be related to a family history of GI bleeding. Other cutaneous manifestations that should be noted on the physical examination include signs of cirrhosis such as spider nevi, palmar erythema, and scleral icterus.

The cardiovascular examination should focus on the heart rate and the character of the peripheral pulses. In the stage of early blood loss, peripheral arteries constrict and blood is shunted to vital organs.[20] Postural change in blood pressure should be immediately noted. If the systolic blood pressure falls more than 20 mm Hg, the diastolic blood pressure decreases more than 10 mm Hg, or the heart rate increases by more than 20 beats/min when an adult patient stands from a supine position, intravascular fluid loss is likely and hospital admission should be considered (level of evidence: moderate).[19-21] If blood loss continues, hypovolemic shock occurs. The diminished blood flow to the kidneys results in oliguria, tubular necrosis, and possibly renal failure. A deficiency in blood flow to the brain and in the coronary arteries can result in irreversible anoxia and death.

The abdomen should be inspected, auscultated, percussed, and palpated to identify a mass, tenderness, guarding, Cullen's sign, or rigidity. Abdominal pain, particularly cramping in the periumbilical area and abdominal distention, may indicate rapid intestinal transit of blood and a major bleed. A careful rectal examination can detect hemorrhoids, fissures, or rectal carcinoma. The stool should be examined for gross blood or melena, indicating acute bleeding that may require urgent intervention. If bleeding is not obvious, the stool should be tested for occult blood.[21] However, it is important to be cognizant of the highly variable specificity and sensitivity in stool occult blood testing. After the patient is stabilized, a thorough physical examination should be performed in search of non-GI sources of bleeding, such as increased or menstrual bleeding in the presence of iron deficiency anemia.[22]

DIAGNOSTICS

Laboratory evaluation of all patients with GI bleeding should include a complete blood count, with a focus on red blood cells, hemoglobin, hematocrit, and platelet count to assess baseline blood loss and platelet adequacy. The patient's blood should be typed and cross matched for 4 to 6 units of packed red blood cells. Laboratory studies include serum glucose, electrolytes, BUN, creatinine, glomerular filtration rate; liver function tests (LFTs); and prothrombin time (PT) and activated partial thromboplastin time (aPTT). An increased BUN level with normal creatinine concentration is suggestive of an upper GI source.[12] Arterial blood gases (ABGs) may be helpful in assessing oxygenation and clarifying the patient's acid-base status. Electrocardiography (ECG) should be performed for all patients with chest or abdominal pain or a history of cardiac or pulmonary disease. Radiographic studies may include an acute abdominal series if there is suggestion of a perforated viscus or intestinal obstruction accompanying bleeding.

NG tube lavage that reveals blood or coffee ground–like material confirms the diagnosis of UGIB and may suggest that the bleeding is caused by a high-risk lesion.[23] It is worth noting that 16% of patients with actively bleeding lesions at endoscopy may not demonstrate blood in the NG tube aspirate and therefore have a low sensitivity for UGIB.[23] The gastric lavage may not be positive for blood if the bleeding has ceased or if the bleeding is occurring beyond a closed pylorus in cases such as duodenal ulcers. Bilious fluid return on NG lavage indicates an open pylorus, thus increasing the sensitivity for detection of postpyloric bleeding. NG tube lavage has also been used to clear the stomach for improved visualization before endoscopic evaluation.

Further diagnostic studies, such as endoscopy, barium studies, bleeding scans, and angiography, should be performed at the discretion of the consulting gastroenterologist or surgeon.[21,22] Early consultation should be prompted if an acute bleed is suspected.

INITIAL DIAGNOSTICS

Gastrointestinal Bleeding

LABORATORY
- Stool for occult bleeding
- Complete blood count with differential
- Serum glucose, electrolytes, blood urea nitrogen, creatinine, calcium
- Liver function tests
- Prothrombin time/activated partial thromboplastin time
- Arterial blood gases[a]
- *H. pylori*
- Type and crossmatch

IMAGING
- Abdominal x-ray studies
- Bleeding scans or angiography[a]
- Upright chest x-ray study (for severe abdominal pain)
- Computed tomography (CT) of abdomen and surgical

consultation (if all other test results remain negative and the patient continues to have severe abdominal pain with intestinal bleeding)

OTHER DIAGNOSTICS
- Blood pressure tilts for orthostatic hypotension
- Electrocardiography
- Endoscopy[a]
- Barium studies[a]
- Air-contrast enema[a]
- Nuclear scintigraphy[a,b]
- Selective mesenteric angiography[a,b]
- Enteroscopy[a]
- Anoscopy[b]
- Sigmoidoscopy[b]
- Colonoscopy[b]

[a]If indicated.
[b]For evaluation of lower gastrointestinal bleeding.

DIFFERENTIAL DIAGNOSIS

The sources of GI bleeding may be categorized as inflammatory, mechanical, vascular, neoplastic, systemic, or anomalous. Vomiting, coughing, retching, or blunt abdominal trauma before bleeding suggests a Mallory-Weiss tear, the majority of which occur in the upper stomach. Painful UGIB is suggestive of peptic ulcer disease, gastritis, esophagitis, or duodenitis; severe pain and peritoneal signs suggest a perforated viscus. The bleeding of esophageal varices is suggested by a history of cirrhosis and painless bleeding.

Bleeding from colonic diverticula is the most common cause of acute LGIB. The bleeding is an arterial bleed at the neck or dome of the diverticulum but spontaneously ceases in most cases. Ischemic colitis, a common cause of LGIB, is usually associated with acute, temporary reduction in mesenteric blood flow in the "watershed" areas of the colon at the splenic flexure and the rectosigmoid junction. This transient ischemic event causes necrosis of the colonic mucosa and, as a result, diarrhea, abdominal pain, and bleeding. Postprandial abdominal pain or pain that is disproportionate to the physical findings is also suggestive of ischemic colitis. Other lower GI sources of bleeding associated with abdominal pain include inflammatory bowel disease and infectious colitis. Infectious diarrhea should not be overlooked in a patient with bloody diarrhea.[24] Enterohemorrhagic *Escherichia coli* (especially *E. coli* O157:H7) is responsible for numerous infections worldwide[25] and is commonly associated with the ingestion of undercooked ground meat, contaminated water, or unpasteurized milk.

Painless bleeding may be related to diverticulosis, angiodysplasia, or hemorrhoids. Rectal pain may be associated with bleeding from anal fissures or anal or rectal carcinoma. Constipation may suggest malignant disease or hemorrhoids (Box 118.2).

MANAGEMENT

The most important concept in the management of acute GI bleeding is that resuscitation and stabilization must precede diagnostic and therapeutic interventions. The initial priorities are the establishment of an adequate airway, ensuring oxygenation and ventilation, followed by restoration of the circulatory status to normal. All patients with hemodynamic instability (shock, orthostatic hypotension, decrease in hematocrit of at least 6%, or active bleeding) should be admitted to the intensive care unit (ICU) for resuscitation and close monitoring.

Any patient thought to have significant bleeding should immediately have two large-bore intravenous lines or a central line placed. Fluid resuscitation should be vigorous and should consist of crystalloid infusions of normal saline or lactated Ringer solution at rates as rapid as the patients cardiopulmonary system will allow to correct the volume deficit. Consideration of a central venous pressure line or a Swan-Ganz catheter should be given for patients with underlying cardiac, pulmonary, renal, or hepatic disease to prevent fluid overload. A Foley catheter should be placed to assist with determination of volume status, with a minimum urinary output of 30 to 50 mL/h in the adult.

The blood product of choice is initially packed red blood cells for patients continuing to bleed, patients in shock, patients with very low hemoglobin and hematocrit values, or patients who have symptoms related to poor tissue oxygenation (e.g., angina).[22] High-risk patients, such as older adults and those

Differential Diagnosis: Gastrointestinal Bleeding

UGIB (ORIGINATING ABOVE THE LIGAMENT OF TREITZ)

- Oral or pharyngeal lesions: swallowed blood from nose or oropharynx
- Swallowed hemoptysis
- Esophageal: varices, ulceration, esophagitis, Mallory-Weiss tear, carcinoma, trauma
- Gastric: peptic ulcer (including Cushing and Curling ulcers), gastritis, angiodysplasia, gastric neoplasms, hiatal hernia, gastric diverticulum, pseudoxanthoma elasticum, hereditary hemorrhagic telangiectasia (Rendu-Osler-Weber syndrome)
- Duodenal: peptic ulcer, duodenitis, angiodysplasia, aortoduodenal fistula, duodenal diverticulum, duodenal tumors, carcinoma of ampulla of Vater, parasites (e.g., hookworm), Crohn disease
- Biliary: hematobilia (e.g., penetrating injury to liver, hepatobiliary malignant neoplasm, endoscopic papillotomy)

LGIB (ORIGINATING BELOW THE LIGAMENT OF TREITZ)

Small Intestine

- Ischemic bowel disease (mesenteric thrombosis, embolism, vasculitis, trauma)
- Small bowel neoplasm: leiomyomas, carcinoids
- Hereditary hemorrhagic telangiectasia
- Meckel diverticulum and other small intestine diverticula
- Aortoenteric fistula
- Intestinal hemangiomas: blue rubber bleb nevi, intestinal hemangiomas, cutaneous vascular nevi
- Hamartomatous polyps: Peutz-Jeghers syndrome (intestinal polyps, mucocutaneous pigmentation)

- Infections of the small bowel: tuberculous enteritis, enteritis necroticans
- Volvulus
- Intussusception
- Lymphoma of the small bowel, sarcoma, Kaposi sarcoma
- Irradiation ileitis
- Arteriovenous malformation of the small intestine
- Inflammatory bowel disease
- Polyarteritis nodosa
- Other: pancreatoenteric fistulas, Henoch-Schönlein purpura, Ehlers-Danlos syndrome, systemic lupus erythematosus, amyloidosis, metastatic melanoma

Colon

- Carcinoma (particularly left colon)
- Diverticular disease
- Inflammatory bowel disease
- Ischemic colitis
- Colonic polyps
- Vascular abnormalities: angiodysplasia, vascular ectasia
- Radiation colitis
- Infectious colitis
- Uremic colitis
- Aortoenteric fistula
- Lymphoma of large bowel
- Hemorrhoids
- Anal fissure
- Trauma, foreign body
- Solitary rectal or cecal ulcers

LGIB, Lower gastrointestinal bleeding; *UGIB*, upper gastrointestinal bleeding.

with severe comorbid conditions such as coronary artery disease, should maintain hemoglobin above 7 g/dL.[21,26] Indications for transfusions have become more restrictive, with recent data suggesting more judicious use of blood products. Animal studies suggest that overtransfusion in cirrhotic patients may actually increase bleeding related to portal hypertension.[26–28] Randomized trials with cirrhotic patients have shown that transfusions should be used to maintain a hemoglobin at or above 7 g/dL. Furthermore, this threshold has been shown to improve outcomes for noncirrhotic patients with UGIB as well.[29] For patients with massive blood loss, whole blood may be used. Close monitoring of coagulation parameters and serum calcium concentration must accompany every five units of packed red blood cell transfusions because dilutional coagulopathy is a risk in major bleeding for patients receiving multiple blood transfusions. Specific ratios of fresh frozen plasma, platelets, packed red blood cells and, in some cases, cryoprecipitate are necessary. Fresh frozen plasma (FFP) is used to correct coagulopathy (international normalized ratio [INR] >1.5),[29] while patients with platelet counts of less than 500,000 should be transfused with platelets. Prothrombin complex concentrate can be used in place of FFP, if necessary. Tranexamic acid (TXA) injection is an additional treatment consideration for patients with serious GI bleeding.[30]

Many patients, especially older adults, will often take medications that may exacerbate bleeding. Aspirin or other antiplatelet medications such as Plavix are frequently used in patients with prior history of coronary artery disease or stroke. Coumadin, low-molecular-weight heparin, and new antithrombin inhibitors such as dabigatran or rivaroxaban may be used in patients with a history of atrial fibrillation, pulmonary embolism, deep vein thrombus, or mechanical valves. Some of the anticoagulation can be reversed with medication. Vitamin K and FFP can reverse the coagulopathy from Coumadin.[31] Antiplatelet agents in general bind irreversibly, and transfusion of platelets may be necessary to counter the antiplatelet effects. Reversal agents for dabigatran, a direct thrombin inhibitor, and the direct Factor Xa inhibitors (e.g., apixaban) are now available for use in hospitalized patients with bleeding associated with these medications.[32] The risks and benefits of the anticoagulation should be weighed and individualized with every patient before reversal of the anticoagulation.

In most cases of suspected acute UGIB, acid suppressive therapy with proton pump inhibitors (PPIs) can be started empirically because the majority of upper GI lesions are acid responsive. Metaanalysis of randomized controlled trials in patients with UGIB suggests that PPI therapy is associated with reduced rebleeding and reduced need for surgery.[33] In addition, high-dose bolus and continuous infusion intravenous PPI (80 mg intravenous push followed by 8 mg/h for 24 hours) has been shown to reduce the proportion of UGIB patients with bleeding sources that need to be treated with specific endoscopic therapy.[34] Patients can then be transitioned to once or twice daily oral PPI therapy.[35] Given the broad efficacy of PPI in UGIB, patients with symptoms of UGIB should be started empirically on PPI therapy.[36] H_2 receptor antagonists (e.g., ranitidine, famotidine) should not be routinely used for patients with acute ulcer bleeding.[33]

Preendoscopy risk in UGIB can be assessed several different ways. Two models, the Glasgow Blatchford score and its modified version, are validated systems for calculating a given patient's risk for requiring endoscopic intervention.[37,38] The modified Glasgow Blatchford score is simplified with fewer clinical parameters.[37]

The diagnostic test of choice in UGIB is endoscopy. Endoscopy has the advantage of identifying patients with continued bleeding or high-risk lesions who will benefit from endoscopic therapy. Therapeutic endoscopy can achieve hemostasis once a bleeding lesion has been identified. High-risk endoscopic findings include arterial bleeding, adherent clot, visible vessels, and varices. Endoscopy is also helpful in stratifying those patients found to have lesions with low risk of rebleeding to early discharge. Those at risk for rebleeding, resulting in increased morbidity and mortality, are patients older than 60 years, those with coagulopathies and other concurrent illnesses, and anyone hospitalized at the time of bleeding.

All patients who are diagnosed with gastric or duodenal ulcers should be screened for *H. pylori* infection by biopsy or noninvasive methods, including urea breath tests and fecal *H. pylori* antigen and treated appropriately.[39] In addition, treatment with PPIs is recommended for patients with peptic ulcer disease. Intravenous PPI drip should be reserved for patients with high risk of rebleeding or those who are unable to tolerate oral intake.

Esophageal varices are related to increased portal hypertension causing variceal rupture and bleeding. Intravenous octreotide, a long-acting analogue of somatostatin, aids in controlling acute upper GI bleeding. Octreotide decreases splanchnic and hepatic blood flow and decreases transhepatic and variceal pressures, thus reducing portal pressures.[40] In patients with GI bleeding and cirrhosis, prophylactic broad-spectrum antibiotics (typically third-generation cephalosporins) should also be given for 7 days from the time of bleeding presentation to prevent the risk of infectious complications.[40-42]

The most common definitive therapy for gastroesophageal varices is endoscopic sclerotherapy or band ligation. According to Sarin and colleagues,[43] endoscopic variceal ligation is as effective as propranolol for the prophylactic treatment of high-risk varices. Endoscopic sclerotherapy involves intravariceal injection of a sclerosing agent. It has proven to be as effective as somatostatin alone for actively bleeding varices. However, a combination of medical and endoscopic therapy is superior to either treatment alone. For patients who rebled despite endoscopic therapies, alternative therapies include balloon tamponade, surgical operations, and transjugular intrahepatic portosystemic shunt (TIPS). Balloon tamponade with a Sengstaken-Blakemore tube may cause severe complications, including aspiration, ulceration, and perforation if it is used improperly. Surgical operations include shunt procedures to decompress the portovenous system, esophageal transection,

and devascularization of the gastroesophageal junction. A TIPS procedure is performed by interventional radiologists and involves creation of a shunt between the portal and hepatic vein to decompress the portal system and to achieve hemostasis. An additional benefit of a TIPS procedure as salvage therapy is that in certain high-risk patients it has been shown to significantly decrease overall mortality if used early.[43,44]

Diagnostic modalities available for the evaluation of overt LGIB include sigmoidoscopy, colonoscopy, nuclear scintigraphy, selective mesenteric angiography (with vasopressin infusion or selective embolization), enteroscopy, and operative therapy. The evaluation of the patient with LGIB depends on the severity of the bleeding.[14] Vigorous fluid resuscitation should precede any diagnostic evaluation. Patients who are hemodynamically stable should first undergo colonoscopy. Colonoscopy in this setting is the diagnostic procedure of choice because of its accuracy and therapeutic capability. In addition, urgent colonoscopy has been associated with a decreased hospital length of stay.[45] Preparation facilitates endoscopic evaluation and increases safety, visualization, and diagnostic yield.[46]

Radionuclide evaluation or a bleeding scan (red blood cell scan) can detect a hemorrhage as slow as 0.1 mL/min.[47] Technetium 99 m–labeled red cells are injected, and scans are taken shortly thereafter to look for extravasation. Because technetium has a short half-life in the intravascular space, detection of abnormality requires the patient to be actively bleeding at the time of the evaluation. Unfortunately, red blood cell scans have a low diagnostic yield but may have a role in localizing an active bleed before more invasive imaging. Mesenteric angiography is useful in patients with continuous active bleeding who have had a normal finding on endoscopic evaluation or a positive nuclear medicine scan or who are too unstable for conventional endoscopic evaluation. Angiography also offers therapeutic interventions for bleeding cessation, including vasopressin infusion and targeted embolization.

A small number of patients with evidence of overt bleeding will have normal endoscopic evaluation findings and are classified as having overt, obscure GI hemorrhage. Evaluation should then focus on looking for small bowel sources of bleeding through either wireless capsule endoscopy (WCE) or enteroscopy. WCE involves ingestion of a capsule that records images throughout the intestine, which are transmitted to a recorder given to the patient. The images are then reviewed by a gastroenterologist; if small bowel bleeding is seen, further action can be taken with small bowel enteroscopy. Enteroscopy involves the passage of either a colonoscope or special enteroscopes beyond the ligament of Treitz to directly examine the small bowel.[48] Methods of enteroscopy include push, intraoperative, spiral, and balloon enteroscopy, all of which differ in their ability to examine the distal small bowel. Causes of small bowel bleeding that can be detected by enteroscopy or WCE include angioectasias, small bowel tumors, and ulcerations from inflammatory bowel disease or NSAID enteropathy.[3] WCE should be performed first because it has been shown to have a higher diagnostic yield than push enteroscopy, but it does have the disadvantage of not having any therapeutic capabilities. In patients who have clinical evidence of small bowel obstruction, WCE should be used with caution. Prior to considering the WCE, a patency capsule study could be performed.

Indications for consideration of LGIB surgical management include transfusion of 4 units or more in 24 hours or more than 10 units overall, and significant rebleeding that occurs within 1 week of initial cessation and in the presence of comorbid disease. Emergency surgery can be lifesaving but associated with high morbidity and mortality if the location of the lesion is not identified before the surgical procedure. Surgical resection can be associated with rebleeding in up to 30% of cases.[2]

Interdisciplinary Management

Asymptomatic patients in whom GI bleeding is suggested during routine screening or hemodynamically stable patients with minor bleeding may be appropriately evaluated on an outpatient basis with specialty referral for endoscopy or radiologic studies.[22] For cases of chronic GI loss, management should be based on whether the patient has anemia. A patient with a positive FOBT result should undergo colonoscopy to exclude malignancy. If the study findings are negative or there are upper GI symptoms or concomitant anemia, evaluation with upper endoscopy should be considered as well, given that up to 40% of patients with a positive FOBT result can have peptic ulcer disease or esophagitis.[49]

For intermittent scant hematochezia, examination of the full colon versus a focused examination with sigmoidoscopy and anoscopy can be tailored based on the age of the patient. Healthy patients younger than 40 years most likely have a distal lesion such as hemorrhoids and fissures and may not need to undergo full colonoscopic evaluation. Anyone older than age 50 or having worrisome symptoms such as weight loss or change in bowel habits should undergo a full colonoscopic evaluation.[46]

LIFE SPAN CONSIDERATIONS

Mortality associated with GI bleeding is higher in older adults, primarily a result of comorbid disease.[49] Variceal bleeding occurs in more than 70% of patients with chronic liver disease; 20% or more of patients die of a variceal bleeding episode.[50] The patient with LGIB tends to be older than the patient with UGIB and hence has more comorbid illness.[49] The incidence of LGIB is unclear. Overall mortality for hospitalization for LGIB has been reported to be approximately 3.5%; positive predictors of mortality include intestinal ischemia, comorbid illness, male gender, and age older than 70 years.[49] This increase in age may be related to the increased incidence of diverticulosis, angiodysplasia, and neoplasms in older adults.

COMPLICATIONS

Many of the complications of GI bleeding are associated with the diagnostic or therapeutic modalities used in its treatment. Serious complications of angiography include bowel ischemia and infarction, dye allergy, and potential renal failure. Complications of upper or lower endoscopy include perforation, bleeding, aspiration, and adverse reactions to conscious sedation.

INDICATIONS FOR REFERRAL OR HOSPITALIZATION

All patients with acute UGIB require urgent consultation with a gastroenterologist. Patients with hematochezia or signs of ongoing bleeding should also be immediately referred. A surgical consultation should be obtained for any patient who is hemodynamically unstable, has an abdominal aortic aneurysm or graft, has high risk of rebleeding despite endoscopic therapy, or has a suspected perforation.[5,51]

Admission to the ICU is recommended for all high-risk patients with hemodynamically unstable GI bleeding or rebleeding and for patients who have red hematemesis or grossly bloody gastric aspirate, an abdominal aortic aneurysm or a graft, any bleeding with severe anemia, a large drop in hematocrit, or unstable comorbid disease.[5,51]

Hospitalization is recommended for patients with melena who are hemodynamically unstable or who have had recent bleeding with significant but stable comorbid disease.[5] A select group of patients may be discharged home after urgent endoscopy, provided they are hemodynamically stable, have no comorbid disease, and have no high-risk endoscopic findings.[5]

PATIENT AND FAMILY EDUCATION

Patients should understand that NSAIDs, aspirin products, alcohol, tobacco, and stress can affect peptic ulcer disease. NSAIDs and aspirin products need to be avoided in newly diagnosed ulcer disease to promote healing. If these medications cannot be stopped, concurrent use of a PPI is paramount to prevent recurrence; however, the risk of rebleed can be significant. In addition, older adults may be particularly susceptible to GI bleeding and should understand the risks associated with aspirin and NSAIDs and the importance of taking these medications with food.

Substance use should be identified and patients actively encouraged to participate in alcohol or tobacco cessation programs. Stress management classes can be indicated for those patients whose lifestyles indicate that behavioral change in this area could be beneficial. All patients should have thorough education and demonstrate an understanding of all medication use, interactions, and possible side effects.

HEALTH PROMOTION

In 2018, the American Cancer Society Guidelines recommended a screening colonoscopy or sensitive stool-based test (e.g., fecal immunochemical test [FIT] or Cologuard, a home-based stool test) for men and women of average risk to begin at age 45. The rationale for this change is the increase in colon cancers before age 50. The current recommendation from the United States Preventive Services Task Force is that all men and women of average risk have the first screening colonoscopy at age 50 years. The American College of Gastroenterology Screening Guidelines recommend screening at age 50 years for patients who have an average risk, but recommend that screening for African Americans should begin at age 45.

For those with a strong family history of colon cancer in a first-degree relative diagnosed before the age of 60 years, screening should begin at the age of 40 years or 10 years before the age at diagnosis of the youngest affected relative.[49] Esophagogastroduodenoscopy for variceal screening is recommended for all newly diagnosed patients with cirrhosis.[43]

REFERENCES

1. Reyes, S. M., & Bronner, J. (2017). Gastrointestinal bleeding. In C. Stone & R. L. Humphries (Eds.), *CURRENT diagnosis & treatment: Emergency medicine* (8th ed.). New York, NY: McGraw-Hill. http://accessmedicine.mhmedical.com.ezproxy.simmons.edu/content.aspx?bookid=2172&sectionid=165059683. (Accessed 29 May 2018).
2. Bull-Henry, K., & Al-Kawas, F. H. (2013). Evaluation of occult gastrointestinal bleeding. *American Family Physician, 87*(6), 430–436.
3. American Society for Gastrointestinal Endoscopy Standards of Practice Committee. (2010). The role of endoscopy in the management of obscure gastrointestinal bleeding. *Gastrointestinal Endoscopy, 72*(3), 471–479.

4. Antunes, C., & Copelin, E. L., II. (2018 Jan.). Gastrointestinal Bleeding, Upper. [Updated 2017 Nov 19]. In: StatPearls [Internet]. Treasure Island (FL): StatPearls Publishing. Retrieved from: https://www.ncbi.nlm.nih.gov/books/NBK470300/.

5. Wilkins, T., Khan, N., Nabh, A., & Schade, R. R. (2012). Diagnosis and management of upper gastrointestinal bleeding. *American Family Physician, 85,* 469–476, 1.

6. Saltzman, J. R. (2015). Acute upper gastrointestinal bleeding. In N. J. Greenberger, R. S. Blumberg, & R. Burakoff (Eds.), *CURRENT diagnosis & treatment: Gastroenterology, hepatology, & endoscopy* (3rd ed.). New York, NY: McGraw-Hill. http://accessmedicine.mhmedical.com.ezproxy.simmons.edu/content.aspx?bookid=1621&sectionid=105185120. (Accessed 30 May 2018).

7. Jutabha, R., Jensen, D. M., Martin, P., Savides, T., Han, S. H., & Gornbein, J. (2005). Randomized study comparing banding and propranolol to prevent initial variceal hemorrhage in cirrhotics with high-risk esophageal varices. *Gastroenterology, 128*(4), 870–881.

8. Lanas, A., Ping, W., Medin, J., & Millis, E. J. (2011). Low doses of acetylsalicylic acid increase risk of gastrointestinal bleeding in a meta-analysis. *Clinical Gastroenterology and Hepatology, 9*(9), 762–768, e6.

9. Strate, L. L., & Gralnek, I. M. (2016). Management of patients with acute lower gastrointestinal bleeding. *The American Journal of Gastroenterology, 111*(4), 459–474. http://doi.org/10.1038/ajg.2016.41.

10. Yardley, J. H., & Hendrix, T. R. (1999). Gastritis, duodenitis, and associated ulcerative lesions. In T. Yamada, D. H. Alpers, L. Laine, et al. (Eds.), *Textbook of gastroenterology* (3rd ed.). Philadelphia: Lippincott.

11. Perez-Aisa, M. A., Del Pino, D., Siles, M., et al. (2005). Clinical trends in ulcer diagnosis in a population with high prevalence of *Helicobacter pylori* infection. *Alimentary Pharmacology and Therapeutics, 21*(1), 65–72.

12. Soll, A. H. (1996). Consensus conference: Medical treatment of peptic ulcer disease: practice guidelines: Practice Parameters Committee of the American College of Gastroenterology. *JAMA: The Journal of the American Medical Association, 275,* 622–629.

13. Hopkins, R. J., Girardi, L. S., & Turney, E. A. (1996). Relationship between *Helicobacter pylori* eradication and reduced duodenal and gastric ulcer recurrence: A review. *Gastroenterology, 110,* 1244–1252.

14. Gunnlaugsson, O. (1985). Angiodysplasia of the stomach and duodenum. *Gastrointestinal Endoscopy, 31,* 251–254.

15. Kazushige, B., Inokuchi, K., Koyanagi, N., Nakayama, S., Sakata, H., Kitano, S., et al. (1981). Prediction of variceal hemorrhage by esophageal endoscopy. *Gastrointestinal Endoscopy, 27*(4), 213–218.

16. Brewer, T. G. (1993). Treatment of acute gastroesophageal variceal hemorrhage. *The Medical Clinics of North America, 77*(5), 993–1009.

17. Bacon, B. R. (2016). Cirrhosis and its complications. In D. Kasper, A. Fauci, S. Hauser, D. Longo, J. Jameson, & J. Loscalzo (Eds.), *Harrison's principles of internal medicine* (19th ed.). New York, NY: McGraw-Hill.

18. King, C. H., & Mahmoud, A. F. (2014). Schistosomiasis and other trematode infections. In D. Kasper, A. Fauci, S. Hauser, D. Longo, J. Jameson, & J. Loscalzo (Eds.), *Harrison's principles of internal medicine* (19th ed.). New York, NY: McGraw-Hill. http://accessmedicine.mhmedical.com.ezproxy.simmons.edu/content.aspx?bookid=1130&sectionid=79741082. (Accessed 30 May 2018).

19. Lewis, J. L. (2016). Volume depletion. https://www.merckmanuals.com/professional/endocrine-and-metabolic-disorders/fluid-metabolism/volume-depletion. (Accessed 1 June 2018).

20. Doig, A. K., & Huether, S. E. (2014). Alterations of digestive function. In K. L. McCance & S. E. Huether (Eds.), *Pathophysiology: The Biologic Basis for Disease in adults and Children* (7th ed., pp. 1426–1428).

21. Laine, L., & Jensen, D. M. (2012). Management of patients with ulcer bleeding. *The American Journal of Gastroenterology, 107,* 345–360.

22. Ferri, F. F. (2002). Gastrointestinal bleeding. In F. F. Ferri (Ed.), *Ferri's clinical advisor 2002.* St Louis: Mosby.

23. Aljebreen, A. M., Fallone, C. A., & Barkun, A. N. (2004). Nasogastric aspirate predicts high-risk endoscopic lesions in patients with acute upper-GI bleeding. *Gastrointestinal Endoscopy, 59*(2), 172–178.

24. Oldfield, E. C., & Wallace, M. R. (2001). The role of antibiotics in the treatment of infectious diarrhea. *Gastroenterology Clinics of North America, 30*(3), 817–835.

25. Page, A. V., & Liles, W. C. (2013). Enterohemorrhagic *Escherichia coli* infections and the hemolytic-uremic syndrome. *The Medical Clinics of North America, 97*(4), 681–695.

26. Colomo, A., Hernandez-Gea, V., Muniz-Diaz, E., et al. (2008). Transfusions strategies in patients with cirrhosis and acute gastrointestinal bleeding. *Hepatology (Baltimore, Md.), 48,* 413A.

27. Castaneda, B., Morales, J., Lionetti, R., et al. (2001). Effects of blood volume restitution following a portal hypertensive-related bleeding in anesthetized cirrhotic rats. *Hepatology (Baltimore, Md.), 33,* 821–825.

28. Hebert, P. C., Wells, G., Blajchman, M. A., et al. (1999). A multicenter, randomized, controlled clinical trial of transfusion requirements in critical care. Transfusion Requirements in Critical Care Investigators, Canadian Critical Care Trials Group. *The New England Journal of Medicine, 340,* 409–417.

29. Barkun, A. N., Bardou, M., Kuipers, E. J., et al. International Consensus Upper Gastrointestinal Bleeding Conference Group. (2010). International consensus recommendations on the management of patients with nonvariceal upper gastrointestinal bleeding. *Annals of Internal Medicine, 152*(2), 101–113.

30. Chertoff, J., Lowther, G., Alnuaimat, H., & Ataya, A. (2017). The use of tranexamic acid for upper gastrointestinal bleeding by medical and surgical intensivists: A single center experience. *Gastroenterology Research, 10*(4), 235–237.

31. Anderson, M. A., Ben-Menachem, T., et al. (2009). ASGE guideline: Management of antithrombotic agents for endoscopic procedures. *Gastrointestinal Endoscopy, 70*(6), 1060–1070.

32. Almegren, M. (2017). Reversal of direct oral anticoagulants. *Vascular Health and Risk Management, 13,* 287–292. http://doi.org/10.2147/VHRM.S138890.

33. Leontiadis, G. I., Sharma, V. K., & Howden, C. W. (2007). Proton pump inhibitor therapy for peptic ulcer bleeding: Cochrane collaboration meta-analysis of randomized controlled trials. *Mayo Clinic Proceedings. Mayo Clinic, 82,* 286–296.

34. Sachar, H., Vaidya, K., & Laine, L. (2014). Intermittent vs continuous proton pump inhibitor therapy for high-risk bleeding ulcers: A systematic review and meta-analysis. *JAMA Internal Medicine, 174*(11), 1755–1762.

35. Ayoub, F., Khullar, V., Banerjee, D., et al. (2018). Once versus twice-daily oral proton pump inhibitor therapy for prevention of peptic ulcer rebleeding: A propensity score-matched analysis. *Gastroenterology Research, 11*(3), 200–206.

36. Lau, J. Y., Leung, W. K., Wu, J. C. Y., et al. (2007). Omeprazole before endoscopy in patients with gastrointestinal bleeding. *The New England Journal of Medicine, 356,* 1631–1640.

37. Cheng, D. W., Lu, Y. W., Teller, T., et al. (2012). A modified Glasgow Blatchford Score improves risk stratification in upper gastrointestinal bleed: A prospective comparison of scoring systems. *Alimentary Pharmacology and Therapeutics, 36,* 782.

38. Blatchford, O., Murray, W. R., & Blatchford, M. (2000). A risk score to predict need for treatment for upper-gastrointestinal haemorrhage. *Lancet, 356,* 1318.

39. Gisbert, J. P., Esteban, C., Jimenez, I., et al. (2007). 13C-urea breath test during hospitalization for the diagnosis of *Helicobacter pylori* infection in peptic ulcer bleeding. *Helicobacter, 12*(3), 231–237.

40. Laine, L. (2014). Gastrointestinal bleeding. In D. Kasper, A. Fauci, S. Hauser, D. Longo, J. Jameson, & J. Loscalzo (Eds.), *Harrison's principles of internal medicine* (19th ed.). New York, NY: McGraw-Hill. http://accessmedicine.mhmedical.com.ezproxy.simmons.edu/content.aspx?bookid=1130&sectionid=79726350. (Accessed 1 June 2018).

41. Velayos, F. (2003). Upper and lower gastrointestinal bleeding in the critically ill patient. In P. E. Parsons & J. P. Wiener-Kronish (Eds.), *Critical care secrets* (3rd ed.). Philadelphia: Hanley & Belfus.

42. Garcia-Tsao, G., Sanyal, A. J., Grace, N. D., & Carey, W. (2009). Prevention and management of gastroesophageal varices and variceal hemorrhage in cirrhosis. AASLD practice guidelines. *Hepatology (Baltimore, Md.), 46*(3), 922–938.

43. Sarin, S. K., Wadhawan, M., Agarwal, S., et al. (2005). Endoscopic variceal ligation plus propranolol versus endoscopic variceal ligation alone in primary prophylaxis of variceal bleeding. *The American Journal of Gastroenterology, 100*(4), 797–804.

44. Garcia-Tsao, G., Sanyal, A. J., Grace, N. D., et al. (2007). Prevention and management of gastroesophageal varices and variceal hemorrhage in cirrhosis. *Hepatology (Baltimore, Md.), 46,* 922–938, 34.

45. Strate, L. L., & Syngal, S. (2003). Timing of colonoscopy: Impact on length of hospital stay in patients with acute lower intestinal bleeding. *The American Journal of Gastroenterology, 98*(2), 317–322.

46. Davila, R. E., Rajan, E., Adler, D. G., et al. (2004). ASGE guideline: The role of endoscopy in the patient with lower-GI bleeding. *Gastrointestinal Endoscopy, 60*(4), 497–504.

47. Eisen, G. M., Dominitz, J. A., Faigel, D. O., et al. (2001). An annotated algorithmic approach to acute lower gastrointestinal bleeding. *Gastrointestinal Endoscopy, 53*(7), 859–863.

48. Kee Song, L., & Topazian, M. (2014). Gastrointestinal endoscopy. In D. Kasper, A. Fauci, S. Hauser, D. Longo, J. Jameson, & J. Loscalzo (Eds.), *Harrison's principles of internal medicine* (19th ed.). New York, NY: McGraw-Hill. http://accessmedicine.mhmedical.com.ezproxy.simmons.edu/content.aspx?bookid=1130&sectionid=79747298. (Accessed 1 June 2018).

49. Strate, L. L., Ayanian, J. Z., Kotler, G., et al. (2008). Risk factors for mortality in lower intestinal bleeding. *Clinical Gastroenterology and Hepatology, 6*(9), 1004–1010.

50. Mallet, M., Rudler, M., & Thabut, D. (2017). Variceal bleeding in cirrhotic patients, *Gastroenterology Report, 5*(3), 185–192, https://doi.org/10.1093/gastro/gox024. (Accessed 1 June 2018).

51. Rex, D. K., Boland, C. R., Dominitz, J. A., Giardiello, F. M., et al. (2017). Cancer Screening: Recommendations for Physicians and Patients from the U.S. Multi-Society Task Force on Colorectal Cancer. http://gi.org/wp-content/uploads/2018/04/Multi-Society-Task-Force-Colorectal-Cancer-Screening-Recommendations-Guideline-Summary.pdf. (Accessed 1 June 2018).

CHAPTER **119**

HEPATITIS

Terry Mahan Buttaro

 Emergent admission to the hospital and gastroenterology and hepatology consultation are indicated for patients with signs of increasing liver failure or decompensation of cirrhosis. Physician specialist consultation/referral should be considered for patients with newly diagnosed hepatitis.

DEFINITION AND EPIDEMIOLOGY

Hepatitis, an inflammation of the liver, has many causes: alcohol, autoimmune disease, malnutrition, metabolic defects, medications, nonalcoholic fatty liver disease, and viruses. If the inflammation continues, the result is chronic liver disease (CLD), cirrhosis, end-stage liver disease, and possibly liver cancer.[1] Unfortunately the death rates associated with cirrhosis and CLD seem to be increasing in some populations; 31% in patients 45 to 64 years of age from CLD and cirrhosis, 3% in patients 65 years of age or older.[2]

Viral Hepatitis

Six hepatitis viruses are responsible for causing acute hepatitis (A, B, C, D, E, and G). Only three of the six cause chronic hepatitis (B, C, and D). Most viral hepatitis is attributed to five main groups of viruses that attack the liver: hepatitis A virus (HAV), hepatitis B virus (HBV), hepatitis C virus (HCV), hepatitis D virus (HDV; also known as hepatitis delta virus and occurring only as a coinfection with HBV), and hepatitis E virus (HEV). Other viruses may cause a secondary hepatitis that never becomes chronic and resolves with the viral infection. Acute viral hepatitis can last up to 6 months and can range in severity from a clinically asymptomatic infection to fulminant hepatic failure and death. Chronic viral hepatitis is considered to be the presence of virus at least 6 months after initial exposure and can range in severity from mild disease with minimum inflammation to cirrhosis, hepatocellular carcinoma (HCC), liver failure, and need for transplantation.

Worldwide, the number of deaths associated with hepatitis infections is increasing, mostly related to the cirrhosis or liver cancer sequelae associated with hepatitis.[3] In the United States, the incidence of both HBV and HCV infections has also increased, and the prevalence of these two infections is greater than that of human immunodeficiency virus (HIV).[4–6] There are many risk factors, including intravenous drug use, high-risk sexual behavior, and incarceration. Viral hepatitis is common among inmates of correctional facilities, emphasizing the importance of immunizations and other risk reduction

programs such as needle exchanges, not only in prisons but also in our communities.[7,8] HAV, HBV, and HCV all cause inflammation by affecting the hepatocytes, leading to acute disease with similar symptoms but differing levels of pathogenicity.[9]

HAV, an RNA virus identified over 20 years ago, is a common cause of acute viral hepatitis in the United States and worldwide. The highest incidence occurs in areas of low socioeconomic status, poor sanitation, and poor access to clean drinking water, including Africa, Asia, and Central America. There have been intermittent outbreaks in the United States, causing approximately 3000 cases annually. Although the incidence of HAV infection was decreasing in the U.S because of the recommendation and use of vaccination, more recently there has been an increased number of outbreaks.[10] HAV is transmitted by the fecal-oral route, through blood, person-to-person contact, and the ingestion of contaminated food (e.g., shellfish) or water. The virus can survive for months in both fresh and salt water. HAV can be found in liver cells, bile, stool, and blood and has an incubation period of 2 to 6 weeks. All strains of this virus belong to the same serotype; as a result, HAV immune globulin provides worldwide protection. The vaccination involves an injection followed by a booster (6 to 12 months later), which can provide immunity for 20 years. The virus can be inactivated by boiling for 1 minute or by exposure to formaldehyde, chlorine, or ultraviolet radiation.

Patients are most infectious in the late incubation period because the virus excretes a large amount of virus 11 days before the antibodies appear in the blood. Clinical symptoms appear approximately 4 weeks after exposure, but the majority of adults and children younger than 6 years are asymptomatic. This contributes to the easy spread of the virus, which can be found in the stool 2 to 3 weeks before and up to 1 week after the development of clinical jaundice. Despite the presence of HAV in the liver, viral shedding in feces, viremia, and infectivity rapidly decrease once jaundice has appeared. Patients are contagious when they are asymptomatic, after jaundice occurs, and about a week more. An important exception involves neonates, who can be infectious for months. HAV infection is an acute disease; rarely, relapses can occur 30 to 90 days after the primary illness. There are rare cases when extrahepatic manifestations—including vasculitis, nephritis, myocarditis, encephalitis, and others—occur. HAV infection does not progress to chronic hepatitis.

HBV infection is endemic worldwide. Many patients are asymptomatic, but some will present and be quite ill. In North America and Europe, HBV infection is more common among adolescents and young adults and is spread by sexual contact and intravenous drug use. In Asia and Africa, HBV infection is seen mostly among newborns and young children and is spread by vertical transmission from mother to child. People with chronic HBV have an increased lifetime risk of cirrhosis and HCC infection. It is recommended that individuals in high-risk groups (Box 119.1), including all who were born in Asia or have direct family members born in Asia, be screened for hepatitis B surface antigen (HBsAg) for HBV. Risk factors are listed in Box 119.1.

A safe and effective vaccine against HBV is available. Recommendations to prevent transmission of HBV include universal vaccination of weight-appropriate (2000 g or greater) infants at birth with a second dose in 1 to 2 months and a third dose at 12 months; screening of all pregnant women to prevent perinatal infection; vaccination of all patients with CLD (including

BOX 119.1

High-Risk Groups for Hepatitis Screening

BORN IN AREAS OF HIGH-PREVALENCE HEPATITIS B VIRUS

- Asia and Pacific Islands
- Middle East
- Mediterranean: Italy, Greece, Malta, Portugal, Spain
- Indigenous to the Arctic region
- South America
- Eastern Europe
- Caribbean

OTHER RISK FACTORS

- Household or sexual contact
- Injection drug use
- Multiple sexual partners, male same-sex partners
- Inmates of correctional facilities
- Chronically elevated alanine aminotransferase or aspartate aminotransferase
- Human immunodeficiency virus or hepatitis C virus infection
- Hemodialysis
- Pregnancy

Modified from Keefe, E. B., Dieterich, D. T., Han, S. H., Jacobson, I. M., Martin, P., Schiff, E. R., et al. (2008). A treatment algorithm for the management of chronic hepatitis B virus infection in the United States: 2008 update. *Clinical Gastroenterology and Hepatology 6*, 1314–1340.

autoimmune, alcoholic, and nonalcoholic fatty liver disease and immunoprophylaxis of infants born to HBsAg-positive women, which indicates infection).[11,12] All children and adolescents not vaccinated must be immunized, as must unvaccinated adults at risk of infection.[11,12]

HBV infection can present a clinical picture similar to that of the other subtypes, with a severity that can range from asymptomatic to fulminant and fatal liver failure. Progression to CLD, cirrhosis, and hepatocellular cancer (HCC) is possible. HBV can be found in blood, tears, cerebrospinal fluid, breast milk, saliva, vaginal secretions, and seminal fluid. Transmission of HBV also occurs parenterally, sexually, and perinatally. Heterosexual contact with a person infected with HBV is the most common mode of transmission, followed by injection drug use, homosexual activity, and vertical transmission from mother to child at the time of birth. Babies who acquire HBV infection at birth often go through an immune tolerant phase where ALT is normal despite high viral titer and positive HBeAG.

Transmission from blood transfusions is rare in the United States because of extensive blood screening processes. HBV is not transmitted through the fecal-oral route or by arthropod vectors. Compared with the general population, health care workers—especially surgeons, phlebotomists, and dialysis nurses—and the spouses of infected persons—are at an increased risk for contracting HBV infection.[13]

HCV infection—a significant cause of cirrhosis, hepatocellular carcinoma (HCC), and liver transplantation—has reached epidemic proportions in the United States, with an estimated 2.7 million to 3.9 million people chronically infected.[14] HCV is a blood borne infection that has increased exponentially with the increase in intravenous drug use.[14] This disorder has also

reached epidemic proportions throughout the world, with a suspected 71 million people infected.[15]

HCV is a single-stranded RNA genome with a high rate of replication (10^{12} virions per day) and mutation. These characteristics lead to chronic infection, which is difficult to treat. At least six strains and multiple subtypes of the virus have been identified. Once a person is infected with HCV, the body initiates humoral and cellular mechanisms. Although it is uncommon to see fulminant hepatic failure with acute HCV infection, up to 85% of such patients develop chronic infection.[16] Some people clear the virus, possibly because they have a strong cellular immune response to HCV. Ineffective cellular immune responses lead to inflammation and damage to the liver. Extrahepatic manifestations of chronic HCV infection occur when humoral immune responses are continually stimulated. These can involve the skin, kidneys, and nerves. An increased risk of cirrhosis after HCV seroconversion is older age, alcohol use, hypertension, white race, and anemia.[17]

Other causes of HCV include blood transfusions received before July 1992, receipt of clotting factor concentrates produced before 1987, chronic hemodialysis, injection of illegal drugs, and intranasal drug use (sharing needles or straws). There is no evidence that arthropod vectors transmit HCV. Other possible transmission issues include tattoos, manicures or pedicures, and body piercings. These practices are not regulated and are possible risk factors, especially if there are multiple exposures or the work is done in questionable environments. Health care workers and emergency medical personnel are at risk from needle sticks, sharps, or mucosal exposure to HCV-positive blood. Sexual transmission is uncommon, although bleeding, sexually transmitted disease, not using protection (condoms, dental dams), presence of sores (oral, penile, vaginal), or having multiple partners increases the risk of acquiring HCV infection through sexual contact. Long-term partners of chronically infected persons should be tested at least once.[18] The rate of vertical transmission from mother to child during delivery is presently 2.5% in the United States, indicating the importance of screening women for HCV infection before pregnancy.[19] Coinfection with HCV and HIV (see Chapter 209) is becoming more prevalent, now estimated to be about 25% and creating unique challenges in management.[20]

HDV is a defective RNA virus that requires coinfection with HBV for replication and is considered to be a severe form of viral hepatitis. Worldwide, 15 million people are infected with HDV.[21] Several genotypes are known. It can be transmitted with HBV or may superinfect an individual who is already infected with HBV. It is transmitted parenterally through injection drug use, blood transfusions, and rarely through sexual contact. Perinatal transmission is uncommon and can be prevented through HBV prophylaxis. During the past two decades, HDV circulation has decreased because of the use of HBV vaccine; however, the challenge of migration of infected persons from endemic areas continues to be a concern.

HEV is another RNA virus with four known human genotypes that have been responsible for large outbreaks in developing countries. This virus has a short incubation period (15 to 60 days) and usually results in a self-limited disease in an immune-competent host. There are groups that are at risk for severe disease and possible chronicity. Similar to HAV, HEV is most commonly spread by the ingestion of contaminated water. Areas endemic for HEV infection are Asia, northeast Africa, the Middle East, and Mexico. In the United States, the seroprevalence is low (6%).[22] Infection during pregnancy can lead to liver failure and death, especially during the third trimester.

HGV is another single-stranded RNA virus classified in the Flaviviridae family. It shares a similar structure with HCV and is actually two independent viruses, but it does not seem to cause or worsen CLD, even in patients with HBV or HCV. Little is actually known about HGV, although it is transmitted sexually and through blood. It is also possible that HGV infection can be transmitted from the mother to the fetus via the placenta. As yet there is no test or treatment for HCG, although it has been identified throughout the world in patients with HBV and HCV.[23]

Alcoholic hepatitis is a common, life-threatening cause of liver failure. This toxic liver injury is associated with chronic, excessive alcohol consumption, usually for 10 years or longer. In the United States, alcoholism is one of the most common causes of cirrhosis and cirrhosis-related deaths.[24] Factors that increase the risk of alcoholic hepatitis include the consumption of more alcohol daily than recommended, genetic predisposition, environment, age when the person started consuming alcohol, and a body mass index higher than 25 in women and 27 in men. It has been suggested that the drinking pattern may play a role and that daily drinking increases the risk compared with drinking less frequently. It has also been proposed that recent alcohol intake and not lifetime consumption could be a strong predictor of alcoholic cirrhosis, as excessive alcohol can lead to a fatty and inflamed liver, which in turn can lead to cirrhosis.[25]

Nonalcoholic Fatty Liver Disease

Nonalcoholic fatty liver disease (NAFLD) and nonalcoholic steatohepatitis (NASH), a spectrum of chronic disorders associated with the metabolic syndrome (see Chapter 192), are now the most common CLDs in the United States.[26] The prevalence of NAFLD, affecting approximately 60 million people in the United States, has increased steadily and corresponds with increases in obesity, visceral obesity, type 2 diabetes, insulin resistance, and hypertension.[27,28] There is a 20% to 40% incidence of NASH in those who have NAFLD.[26,29] NASH, a subcategory of NAFLD, is more serious because it is characterized by inflammation (steatohepatitis) and scarring of the liver, which can progress to cirrhosis, end-stage liver disease, and liver failure. NASH is now the most frequent cause of cirrhosis and, in the near future, is expected to be the most common reason for liver transplantation. NASH may be a part of the metabolic syndrome, as abdominal obesity, hyperlipidemia, and diabetes are associated with increases in the content of liver fat, and insulin resistance is proposed to be the cause of too much fat storage in the liver. Hispanics seem to have a higher risk of NAFLD, whereas African Americans seem to have less risk.[30]

Drug-induced liver injury (DILI) is a rare reaction associated with common medications, including nonsteroidal antiinflammatory drugs (NSAIDs) and antimicrobial agents. Half of all cases of acute liver failure are caused by drug hepatotoxicity, and it is thought that there may be a genetic predisposition to DILI. Some drugs, such as acetaminophen, produce a predictable, dose-related injury, but most reactions are unpredictable. These reactions usually occur in one of two patterns: (1) an allergic reaction that occurs within 6 weeks of initiation of the drug (e.g., phenytoin) or (2) a metabolic reaction that occurs with up to 1 year of continuous use, as noted with isoniazid. Hundreds of therapeutic agents—including prescription drugs, over-the-counter medications, nutritional supplements, and herbal remedies—have been implicated in DILI, but there will likely be more as newer medications are approved. The National Institute of Diabetes and Digestive and Kidney Diseases together with other agencies created the DILI Network and LiverTox website (https://livertox.nih.gov/intro.html) to provide information about medications, herbals, and liver injury. Offending drugs include the commonly prescribed amoxicillin–clavulanic acid, nitrofurantoin, sulfamethoxazole-trimethoprim, and minocycline.[31] Health care providers should always consider DILI and obtain a thorough drug history, including information about recent and past exposure to therapeutic agents, supplements, and herbal products. Details of the patient's occupation and work environment as well as the use of herbal preparations and "traditional" medications should also be determined.

Autoimmune hepatitis is a rare condition that can occur in anyone, young or old. Although it is often associated with other autoimmune processes in the patient or family members, medications (hydralazine, methyldopa, minocycline, nitrofurantoin) are also a possible cause. The clinical spectrum varies and there are two variations (types 1 and 2) identified by serology testing. Patients can be asymptomatic or have mild to severe symptoms with acute or fulminant liver failure. Often newly diagnosed patients have already developed cirrhosis. Treatment is usually with corticosteroids, but azathioprine can be added or used alone. Fulminant disease may require liver transplantation.[32]

PATHOPHYSIOLOGY
Process of Inflammation and Development of Cirrhosis

The process of inflammation and development of scarring and cirrhosis is similar for all causes of hepatitis. The pathologic process of hepatitis involves inflammation and damage to the hepatocytes. Fibrosis and scarring with isolated hepatocyte injury and focal necrosis can develop. Mononuclear infiltration, which consists mostly of lymphocytes, invades the tissue, particularly around the portal triads. Cellular edema and death can occur. There may be a minor degree of periportal necrosis of hepatocytes around these triads, which gives the liver an appearance of piecemeal necrosis on microscopic examination. After the hepatocyte degenerates, its cytoplasm shrinks and condenses to form an acidophil body. The available space is then temporarily filled by monocytes. Although characteristic of acute viral hepatitis, these cytologic changes are not specific to this disease and can also be found with drug-induced injuries and other disease processes.

The inflammatory and scarring processes can cause "bridging" fibrosis between portal triads. This level of fibrosis and moderate inflammation is a sign that cirrhosis will develop if the damage continues. Increased numbers of liver cells begin to die, which may lead to more collapse and condensation of the liver stroma. This may occur over months in a severe acute injury but is more commonly seen in chronic infection. Bridging and confluent necrosis can resolve, enabling complete regeneration and histological recovery in acute hepatitis. Chronic hepatitis, however, can remain mild, with little or no scarring developing. If scarring does develop, it is unlikely to improve without treatment. Over time, cirrhosis can lead to liver failure, HCC infection, and death.

Pathogenesis of Hepatitis

HAV infection is a self-limiting acute disease spread from person to person. The replication cycle is slow and has not been shown to cause chronic infection. The virus is thought to be transported across the intestinal epithelium after oral inoculation and is taken up by hepatocytes. Although HAV can be transmitted via a transfusion if the blood is infected, it is shed in the feces, which continues the fecal-oral transmission.[33] Viral loads peak at 2 weeks postexposure and are undetectable by 6 to 8 weeks. Symptoms usually develop at week 4, at the same time as the beginning of the humoral response to the viral proteins. Immunity to HAV occurs after the illness and is evidenced by serum IgG.

Hepatitis E is primarily transmitted by the fecal-oral route, but transmission varies with genotype and can occur through blood transfusion as well as food and water contamination. It is primarily problematic in developing countries rather than in the United States and may also be transmitted perinatally. It does not cause CLD, cirrhosis, or liver cancer[34] but is associated with mortality in pregnancy.[33] After oral ingestion, it is taken up in the portal circulation and produces viremia. It is excreted in the feces, and it is not known whether it replicates in the small bowel.

HBV is a DNA virus in the Hepadnaviridae family. Transmitted through blood and body fluids, the virus enters the hepatocyte nucleus and begins replication. The viral load peaks at 7 to 8 weeks after exposure. HBV initiates a type I interferon (IFN) response, and it is thought that viral clearance occurs in part with CD4 and CD8 T cells.[35] The infection has separate phases that reflect disease progression: immune tolerance (minimal activity in the liver), immune clearance (active with chronic inflammation in the liver), inactive carrier of HBsAg (minimal fibrosis), resolution (scant fibrosis), and reactivation (active, moderate fibrosis). Progressive fibrosis leads to cirrhosis. Each phase has serologic markers that helps determine the phase. Ongoing viral replication leads to cirrhosis, HCC, or both.[33]

HDV spread through parenteral exposure infects hepatocytes, causing inflammation, destruction, and hepatocellular injury. It occurs only when a person is infected with HBV and is HbsAg-positive; this is required for transmission. The infection can be associated with a severe course of hepatitis, fibrosis, decompensation, and cancer, although some patients will have a milder disease burden. It is an immune-mediated disease process, but the level of viremia is not directly associated with the stage of liver disease. The degree of control of infection may be associated with cellular immune responses.[36]

HCV is a parenterally transmitted RNA virus from the Flaviviridae family and has a remarkable ability to persist within a host by evading the adaptive and innate components of the immune system. The life cycle and survival mechanisms of HCV are increasing. HCV enters the host cell, uncoats the viral genome, translates viral proteins, replicates the genome, and assembles and releases virions. HCV infection impairs all parts of the adaptive immune system with multiple viral factors that allow it to evade detection and elimination. HCV is unique compared with HAV and HBV. The viral cycle has rapid turnover and elicits a strong type I IFN response. Multiple factors affect the course of the infection, including age, sex, the patient's symptoms, antiviral T-cell response, and immunogenetic polymorphisms.[37]

There are six HCV genotypes and multiple subtypes that aid in determining treatment. Most people infected will develop chronic HCV, but treatment can eliminate HCV RNA and decrease the sequelae associated with HCV infection.

Alcoholic Hepatitis. It is possible that just one alcoholic drink a day for a woman or 2 a day for a man will cause steatosis (fatty liver) by promoting fat deposition in the liver.[33] Steatosis is the first change to occur, followed by steatohepatitis, an inflammatory degenerative process that results in hepatocyte death, immunologic changes, and lipid peroxidation. The ethanol is oxidized in the mitochondria, producing toxins that have harmful effects on lipid and carbohydrate metabolism. Acetaldehyde is increased, causing hypoxia at the terminal veins in the liver, and oxygen-derived free radicals may cause damage and dysfunction of the liver cells.[33] Proinflammatory cytokines are expressed, stimulating cells to produce collagen, which leads to fibrosis, cellular damage within the liver, cirrhosis, and a greater risk of acquiring HCC infection.[33]

Drug-Related Hepatotoxicity. Liver damage from hepatotoxins—such as chlorpromazine, rifampin, and estrogens—is variable, depending on the drug, dose, and individual hypersensitivity. Damage can appear quickly or may take weeks to months to appear after the medication is begun. Proposed mechanisms include alteration of the membranes, interference with the hepatic uptake process, and free radicals causing lipid peroxidation.

Autoimmune hepatitis is an uncommon disorder associated with elevated transaminases, human leukocyte antigens, and hypergammaglobulinemia. The pathophysiology is not clear. A genetic predisposition combined with an environmental trigger may stimulate autoallergens that create autoantibodies such as antinuclear antibodies, smooth muscle antibodies, and others. The resultant inflammatory response in the liver is likely T cell–mediated, possibly also involving B cells and stimulating liver injury.[33,38]

CLINICAL PRESENTATION

Patients with liver failure may present acutely, but often liver disease is quiescent and determined through routine laboratory screening. For all patients, symptom onset should be elicited, especially if jaundice or other symptoms are present, and a thorough medication (including herbal, over-the-counter, illicit, and recreational drugs) list should be determined. Alcohol use and amount, as well as family history and all risk factors (occupations, sexual contacts, travel, transfusions, toxins), must be explored.

Acute Hepatitis

Most people are not aware when they develop acute hepatitis because the symptoms are similar to those of any other mild viral illness. Symptoms can include anorexia, fatigue, myalgias, nausea, fever, headaches, arthralgias, vomiting, and abdominal pain. Jaundice can occur, especially with HBV, but it is rare in other viral hepatitis illnesses. Acute viral hepatitis occurs after an incubation period of varying length based on the specific virus. HBV and HDV infections are clinically indistinguishable from one another. Suspicion of HEV infection should be increased in patients with clinical symptoms of hepatitis and a recent travel history to an underdeveloped country.

Alcoholic hepatitis can have a widely variable presentation, and patients can be asymptomatic or have nonspecific symptoms—such as fatigue, weight loss, or anorexia, nausea, vomiting, and abdominal discomfort—suggesting advanced liver disease; patients can appear ill, be malnourished, and can be feverish.[33] There may be signs of cirrhosis such as jaundice, ascites, encephalopathy, and upper gastrointestinal bleeding.[33]

Severe cases can mirror the presentation of sepsis or biliary obstruction.

Drug-induced liver disease can present similarly to a non-specific febrile, or viral-like illness. The diagnosis of chronic hepatitis can be challenging because patients are often not symptomatic until liver damage has progressed.

Autoimmune hepatitis may manifest as an acute illness with liver failure or with complaints of vague symptoms that include fatigue, right-upper-quadrant abdominal discomfort, polymyalgia, and arthralgia of small joints. Often, though, patients are asymptomatic.

NAFLD is rarely an acute presentation and therefore, unfortunately, often not diagnosed. Some patients can have right-upper-quadrant pain, especially if there is a large amount of fat in the liver and the liver is slightly enlarged.

PHYSICAL EXAMINATION

The physical examination of all patients includes vital signs, mental status, and evidence of cardiac, pulmonary, abdominal, and other systemic complications. A low-grade fever with acute hepatitis is far more common with HAV and HEV infections, although patients with HBV can develop a serum sickness–like syndrome that can include fever, arthralgias, and rash. Dark-colored urine and clay-colored stools may precede the onset of clinical jaundice by 1 to 5 days. With the onset of jaundice, these constitutional symptoms usually diminish, but patients with jaundice often have both hepatomegaly and splenomegaly. The onset of jaundice or the icteric phase can be observed when the serum bilirubin concentration is higher than 4 mg/dL; this is most easily observed in the sclerae or under the tongue. Symptomatic hepatitis is difficult to miss, but half the patients with acute hepatitis do not develop jaundice.

In alcoholic hepatitis, the physical findings may be consistent with cholestasis. Fever, jaundice, and leukocytosis may be present. Rashes are common, and patients can have tender hepatomegaly, ascites, or encephalopathy (ranging from asterixis to coma), but splenomegaly is uncommon. There may be findings of malnutrition as well as a hepatic bruit. Physical signs of alcoholic and nonalcoholic cirrhosis are similar, but spider telangiectasia (especially on the trunk and upper extremities), parotid enlargement, gynecomastia, palmar erythema, and hepatomegaly may be more common with alcoholic cirrhosis.[39]

Drug-induced hepatitis is suggested by the presence of extrahepatic manifestations. Fever, rash, and eosinophilia suggest drug hypersensitivity but are relatively nonspecific findings. Presenting signs may include pseudomononucleosis syndrome (phenytoin), systemic vasculitis (allopurinol and sulfonamides), and bone marrow suppression (NSAIDs).

DIAGNOSTICS

Initial testing should include a complete blood count (CBC) and liver function tests (LFTs). The first sign of hepatitis may be the elevation of the serum aminotransferases aspartate aminotransferase (AST) and alanine transaminase (ALT). These enzymes increase proportionately during the prodromal phase

of hepatitis and can reach 20 times normal (in acute hepatitis). The levels in chronic hepatitis can be normal but may be mildly elevated or two or three times normal. The total bilirubin level can be elevated with acute hepatitis, and it can continue to increase as the ASTs decline; it may reach 20 mg/dL. In alcoholic hepatitis a bilirubin greater than 20 mg/dL is not uncommon and may be elevated for several weeks. There are equal proportions of direct and indirect bilirubin in patients with hepatitis, and bilirubin will also be present in the urine. The prothrombin time (PT) is usually normal in patients with acute hepatitis but may become prolonged in those with severe hepatitis; thus PT can be used as a marker of prognosis. If the PT is more than three times normal (international normalized ratio [INR] 1.5), the patient should be evaluated for fulminant hepatic failure. The white blood cell count, hemoglobin level, and hematocrit are usually within normal limits. The platelet count may be normal or may be decreased in fulminant hepatic failure. An elevation in α-fetoprotein is not unusual in cirrhosis, HCC, or CLD and is sometimes used as a marker or monitor of liver function.

Other laboratory tests that may indicate advancing liver damage are platelet and albumin levels, which will be lower than normal with the progression to cirrhosis. Anemia may be present. Alkaline phosphatase levels are usually normal or mildly elevated. Alkaline phosphatase is not specific to the liver. An elevated alkaline phosphatase level can indicate a fatty liver, obstruction, or disease in the bile ducts. If an elevated alkaline phosphatase level is documented, it is useful to determine how much of it is from the liver. Fractionation will show the percentages from the liver, bone, and intestines. The elevation of AST levels does not seem to correlate with the histologic severity of the disease.

Testing for Hepatitis

- HAV infection should be suspected if hepatitis infection occurs after the ingestion of contaminated food or shellfish, after natural disasters, in institutionalized adults or children, in patients returning from travel to an endemic area, or in children or families of children in day care facilities. Diagnosis can be confirmed by the presence of immunoglobulin M (IgM) anti-HAV during the acute illness. Eventually the IgM anti-HAV decreases over several months and IgG anti-HAV rises and persists indefinitely.
- Initial testing for HBV and HCV infection can be done and will aid in determining acute, chronic, or previous infection that has resolved.
  - Chronic HBV infection: HBsAg-positive, anti-HBc–positive IgM, anti-HBc–negative, and anti-HBs-negative.
  - Further sub-categorization of chronic HBV infection can also be further sub-categorized. For example, serology results in a chronic inactive carrier will reflected by a positive HBsAg, negative anti HBs, negative anti-HBc IgM, negative HBeAG, and positive anti-HBe, and viral load <20k. This indicates the possibility for reactivation but poses a lower risk of liver disease.
  - Chronic HBeAG positive (immune active) or chronic HBeAG negative (immune escape): are both characterized by positive HBsAg, negative anti HBs, and anti-HBc IgM, but differentiated by HBeAg or anti HBeAg.[40]
  - Acute hepatitis infection: HbsAg-positive, anti-HBc–positive IgM, anti-HBc–positive, but anti-IgM–HBs negative.

- HBV immunity: Hepatitis B surface antibody (HBsAg)–negative
  - If immunized from natural infection, patient will be HbsAg-negative but anti-HBc– and anti-HBs–positive.
  - If immunized from vaccine, patient will be HbsAg-negative but anti-HBc–negative and anti-HBs–positive.
  - Patients who are positive for HBsAg and HBcAb (hepatitis B core antibody) should be referred for more detailed testing because interpretation can be difficult.
  - HBV antigen (HBeAg) and antibody testing: for patients with recurrent HbsAg-positive results, testing for HBeAg is indicated. A patient with negative HBeAg and low HBV DNA can be a carrier.
- If HCV antibody is present, the viral load should be tested by polymerase chain reaction (PCR) **(HCV RNA)**. Some patients who are infected with HCV do clear the virus on their own and no viral load will be detected with HCV RNA testing. Repeat HCV RNA testing in 6 months is recommended for these patients. For others, the level of virus load detected can range from a few to more than several million international units per milliliter. If the viral load is detectable, the patient is considered to have chronic HCV. Testing of the genotype for HCV can help with decisions about treatment. Genotype 1 is most often seen in patients who live in the United States, but worldwide travel mandates specific testing.
- HDV infection should be considered in patients with acute HBV infection who develop fulminant hepatic failure or in those with chronic HBV infection who show evidence of deterioration. Anti-HDV can be detected to confirm the diagnosis of HDV infection.
- HEV infection should be considered in patients returning from travel to endemic areas. Diagnosis can be made by testing IgM antibody to HEV, but the results can be variable. Further testing with HEV RNA (serum or stool) can aid diagnosis, and PCR testing sites are available through the Centers for Disease Control (CDC).[41]
- Alcoholic hepatitis typically manifests as a cholestasis type of liver disease, with abnormalities seen as elevations in bilirubin, alkaline phosphatase, and γ-glutamyl transferase levels. The ratio of AST to ALT is often greater than 2.0, which is considered diagnostic of this disease. Anemia and leukocytosis are present in a significant number of patients with alcoholic hepatitis. In more severe disease, PT and INR may be prolonged, and the albumin concentration is often low.
- Laboratory testing for drug-induced liver disease is helpful in excluding other causes of liver disease. Liver biopsy is indicated when the diagnosis remains unclear. Diagnosis depends on the history of exposure; consistent clinical, laboratory, and liver biopsy findings in select cases; and the resolution of liver injury after the presumed toxin has been removed.
- Diagnosis of autoimmune hepatitis usually requires the expertise of a hepatologist. Type 1 autoimmune hepatitis is associated with + ANA antibodies and/or anti–smooth muscle antibodies, anti–soluble liver/liver pancreatic antigen, antiactin antibodies, or atypical perinuclear antineutrophil cytoplasmic antibodies. Laboratory identification of type 2 autoimmune hepatitis is suggested by anti–liver/kidney microsomal (LKM) antibody type 1 and/or anti–liver cytosol antibody type 1 or anti–soluble liver/liver pancreatic antigen.

- Liver biopsy is the most accurate test that can determine the amount of inflammation and scarring and is also necessary when the diagnosis is uncertain or if certain conditions, such as autoimmune hepatitis, are suspected. Scoring mechanisms can be used to provide a fairly standardized measure of the severity of liver disease.
- Ultrasonography and computed tomography (CT) are equally useful in documenting tumors, fatty tissue, and size of the liver. The ultrasound examination is more cost-effective, providing screening information. There are noninvasive liver fibrosis tests (e.g., ultrasound-based transient elastography, a reasonable alternative to liver biopsy) that are currently implemented. The tests can provide an estimate of the severity of steatosis, fibrosis, and inflammation.
- The tests specific for NASH and hepatitis HCV infection are improving and can be used as an adjunct to the management of these conditions when indicated.[32] Fibro*Spect* testing for fibrosis and inflammation in NASH may be helpful and aid in staging the degree of fibrosis.

DIFFERENTIAL DIAGNOSIS

- Viral causes, alcoholic liver disease, autoimmune hepatitis, NAFLD, NASH, and medications and toxins should be initial considerations. However, it is always important that patients be evaluated for other causes of liver disease. For instance, chronically elevated results of LFTs may be caused by alcoholic liver disease, drug- or toxin-induced hepatitis, hepatic steatosis, cholestatic conditions, metabolic diseases, granulomatous hepatitis, pericholangitis associated with inflammatory bowel disease, celiac sprue, or biliary or pancreatic disease. The most common cause of chronically elevated LFTs is NAFLD
- Chronic hep B can present as membranous glomerulonephritis, Polyarteritis Nodosa (PAN) or cryoglobulinemia and can be associated with other immune-mediated extrahepatic manifestations.[42-43]
- Medications associated with hepatitis include acetaminophen (especially when associated with alcohol use), isoniazid, methotrexate, amoxicillin–clavulanic acid, minocycline, methyldopa, nitrofurantoin, rifampin, and the cholesterol-lowering statins. However, numerous medications can cause a change in liver function requiring a careful review if LFTs are abnormal. Regular monitoring of LFTs is necessary because elevations can indicate the presence of liver inflammation.
- A secondary hepatitis can be caused by other viruses, such as Epstein-Barr virus, cytomegalovirus, HIV, herpes simplex virus, varicella zoster virus, adenovirus, and coxsackie virus. Secondary hepatitis usually resolves along with the viral illness.
- Hemochromatosis, or iron overload, is the most common inherited disorder in the United States. Testing of iron saturation and ferritin is used for screening. If elevated levels of iron are found, a genetic test for hemochromatosis is available.
- Autoimmune hepatitis can be screened with antinuclear and smooth muscle antibody. Further testing may be necessary to distinguish type 1 from type 2 autoimmune hepatitis.
- Wilson disease, an autosomal recessive condition that results in toxic copper accumulation in the liver and other organs, must also be considered. Low levels of serum ceruloplasmin,

elevated levels of urinary copper, and Kayser-Fleischer rings in the eyes can establish a diagnosis of Wilson disease.

- Sarcoidosis can affect the liver and is often noted in African Americans. Obtaining an angiotensin-converting enzyme level may be used to screen for sarcoid, although it is not specific for sarcoid and can be elevated for various reasons.
- Celiac sprue has been known to elevate LFTs, which may be the only clinical sign of the disease. A celiac antibody panel plus, if positive, a small bowel (duodenal) biopsy by endoscopy can confirm the diagnosis.
- Other possible causes include alpha$_1$-antitrypsin deficiency and cholestatic conditions (primary sclerosing cholangitis, primary biliary cirrhosis).

INTERPROFESSIONAL COLLABORATIVE MANAGEMENT

Referral to a hepatologist is indicated for patients with chronic HBV infection associated with abnormal AST levels, positive HBV DNA findings, and positive or negative HBV e antigen (HBeAg) (especially with elevated alanine AST or HBV DNA), cirrhosis, and coinfection with HDV or HCV.

- Chronic hepatitis B treatment is individualized and best managed by the hepatologist. Currently used medications recommended for chronic hepatitis B by the American Association for the Study of Liver Diseases include the interferon alpha preparations (peginterferon 2a and interferon alpha 2b), and the nucleoside analogues (lamivudine, entecavir, tenofovir, adenovir, and telbivudine).[44–45] Adherence to therapy is very important.[5] Missing doses, decreasing doses, and poor compliance affect treatment response. All patients with chronic HBV infection should be screened for HDV and HIV infection as well as fibrosis and HCC. Biopsy may also be indicated. Generally patients with chronic HBV infection and fibrosis receive antiviral therapy if the alanine AST is greater than normal and the HBV DNA level is greater than 2000 IU/mL.[46] The HBV e antigen status is no longer a consideration for these patients, and fibrosis does not have to be present for these patients to be treated with antiviral therapy. It is important to note that these treatments are individualized for each patient depending on patient status and comorbidities.[46]
- Patients with both HBV and HIV infection require specialist coordination. Some HBV meds will interact with HIV antiretroviral treatment. In some instances long-term treatment may be needed if there is no seroconversion. Resistance can be an issue, and medications can be added or changed as needed.
- Acute management of HAV and HBV infection consists primarily of treating the acute symptoms and providing supportive care. Most patients do well and experience no concerning sequelae. HAV infection does not develop chronicity, but some carriers of HBV in the United States develop chronic HBV infection. In the acute uncomplicated course of HBV infection, the majority of patients do not require hospitalization and symptomatic care is all that is needed. LFTs should be monitored every 2 weeks until normalization.
- HCV infection can be acute or chronic. Patients with the acute illness are not treated but are monitored, and not all of these will develop chronic hepatitis C.[47] Unfortunately patients are often not even aware that they have been infected, nor are they aware of the risk of developing

cirrhosis or liver cancer and of infecting others. This points to the importance of the primary care screening of patients for HCV and is why the United States Preventive Services Task Force (USPSTF) recommends offering one-time screening for HCV infection to adults born between 1945 and 1965. There are currently a variety of treatments for chronic infection based on HCV genotypes, treatment status (naive or previously treated unsuccessfully), and current liver function. So that primary care providers will feel more comfortable treating affected patients, the American Association for the Study of Liver Diseases (AASLD) and the Infection Diseases Society of America have delineated the specific testing and treatments for chronic HCV infection by genotype, previous history of treatment or treatment-naive status, and the presence or absence of cirrhosis.[48] Often, however, patients with chronic HCV infection are treated by specialists, because monitoring is necessary and drug-drug interactions are possible. The newer direct-acting antiviral drug combinations (e.g., Ledipasvir/Sofosbuvir [Harvoni] or sofosbuvir/velpatasvir [Epclusa]) indicated for genotype 1a treatment-naive patients without cirrhosis and currently used to treat chronic HCV can be better tolerated than interferon and ribavirin, although these medications are still used for some patients.[48] The improvement in treatments has increased the cure rate and many patients do well. One barrier to treatment is cost; insurance coverage can be a significant factor, and adherence to therapy is vital to cure the infection.

- The treatment of alcoholic hepatitis is abstinence from alcohol. The involvement of family, friends, counseling, and support groups may be helpful. Patients experiencing an acute episode should be hospitalized because acute alcoholic hepatitis can be life-threatening. Discharge is considered when the patient is stable and the bilirubin level decreases. Malnutrition is a strong contributor to the morbidity and mortality associated with alcoholic hepatitis; therefore assessment by a dietitian, adequate diet therapy, and vitamin replacement for deficiencies are essential. Parenteral administration of vitamin B is preferred to oral therapy for better absorption in alcoholic patients. Multi-vitamin preparations that include folic acid, thiamine, vitamins A and D, and essential minerals are also important. In the absence of hepatic encephalopathy, a high-protein diet is recommended. Corticosteroid therapy in the treatment of alcoholic liver disease has been equivocal and poses significant risk. The use of pentoxifylline is considered off label and controversial in the treatment of severe alcoholic hepatitis, but it has been used to help prevent hepatorenal syndrome, a complication that is a major cause of mortality. Transplantation is considered in patients with proven long-term abstinence, but recidivism is a concern. For successful treatment, a focus on reducing recidivism rates with early and frequent outpatient visits is important. Several other medications suggested for patients with alcohol use disorder include naltrexone, nalmefene, acamprosate, disulfiram, topiramate, and baclofen, but studies of efficacy and safety are needed.[49] Carbohydrate-deficient transferrin testing may be used to identify heavy alcohol use and is not detectable after 2 weeks of abstinence. It may be useful for monitoring on an outpatient basis.[50]
- Drug-induced liver disease is best managed by removal of the suspected drug or offending agent. In the case of severe

drug-induced liver failure, urgent liver transplantation can be lifesaving. Currently, the only specific treatment available is the administration of N-acetylcysteine for acetaminophen overdose. In general, corticosteroids have no value in the treatment of drug-induced liver disease.

- NAFLD is a significant health concern. Diagnosis and monitoring are important. Although there is currently no treatment for NAFLD, weight loss, diet, and exercise are recommended. Vitamin E, 400 to 800 IU daily in combination with weight loss, can decrease ALT levels to within normal parameters and aid in the resolution of NASH.[26] Treatment of hyperlipidemia with diet and medication is also important because it plays a role in the development of NAFLD. Patients with diabetes should be on a low-carbohydrate diet and medication as appropriate to control blood glucose levels.[26] Lowering saturated fats and polyunsaturated fats in the diet should be a goal. The Mediterranean diet is recommended. There is no effective pharmacological treatment at this time.

LIFE-SPAN CONSIDERATIONS

The liver is a remarkable organ that is capable of regeneration. The treatment of hepatitis has been shown to halt progression and improve liver histology if the causative agent is removed. If hepatitis is treated and cirrhosis does not develop, patients can lead normal lives and their life spans will be unaffected. If cirrhosis develops, the life span can be greatly reduced because cirrhosis is a leading cause of death.

Hepatitis is often insidious, and liver damage can be ongoing without the patient's knowledge. Signs or symptoms often do not appear for many years. Lifestyle becomes an important factor, but it is not the sole issue in deteriorating liver disease. Some patients have aggressive disease, and treatment is difficult. Thus, it is imperative that health care providers screen for risk factors and routinely monitor LFT results. Abnormal LFT results should never be ignored. The sooner identification and treatment can begin, the better the prognosis.

COMPLICATIONS

- The most significant complications of hepatitis are cirrhosis, liver failure, and HCC.
- The greatest risk with chronic HBV is HCC, which can occur without the development of cirrhosis. All patients with chronic HBV need HCC surveillance with imaging and laboratory tests every 3 to 6 months.
- Fulminant hepatic failure occurs in a small percentage of patients with acute HAV and HBV infection. Rapid elevation of PT (more than three times normal), hyperbilirubinemia, and hepatic encephalopathy indicate fulminant hepatic failure. Hospitalization with rapid organ transplantation is the only treatment option; without transplantation, the mortality rate is very high.
- Hepatic encephalopathy, which can result in coma and death, occurs with the development of cirrhosis and accumulation of ammonia in the brain. Treatment is with rifaximin and lactulose. Rifaximin is a poorly absorbed antibiotic that has its effect in the intestinal tract and has a wide antibacterial spectrum. It helps to reduce blood ammonia and has been effective in treating hepatic encephalopathy. Rifaximin is used in combination with lactulose, which requires a large enough dose to produce three loose stools a day.

But adhering to these recommendations can be an issue for patients.

- Alcohol is a factor in the progression of liver damage. Regular alcohol use increases the risk of cirrhosis, liver failure, and cancer, especially if alcohol ingestion continues. Physical and psychosocial problems and malnutrition are other complications associated with alcoholism.
- NAFLD, a silent disorder associated with obesity and the metabolic syndrome, is becoming a leading cause of cirrhosis and liver transplantation. Once diagnosed, patients need regular monitoring of their liver function at least every 6 months.
- The prognosis of drug-induced liver disease is highly variable and depends on the clinical circumstances and causative agent involved. There is a much poorer prognosis with some agents because they induce acute hepatic necrosis or cause progressive CLD and cirrhosis.

PATIENT AND FAMILY EDUCATION

- Screening for NAFLD is important and should be done in patients who are obese, diabetic, who have the metabolic syndrome, and those with any transaminase elevations
- HCC surveillance should be undertaken in anyone with cirrhosis. Follow-up appointments with laboratory studies (CBC, INR, and liver and renal status) and MELD-Na score calculation (https://www.mdcalc.com/meldna-meld-na-score-liver-cirrhosis) every 3 months is indicated for patients with chronic HCV infection.
- The diagnosis of HCV infection has a profound effect on patients and families and their quality of life. Patients with all forms of hepatitis require careful education about the cause, prevention, transmission, treatment options, and complications. The benefit of rest, diet, avoidance of hepatotoxic substances (especially alcohol), and medications should be emphasized.
- HAV can be prevented. Contact with obviously contaminated food or water should be avoided, and infected individuals should not handle or prepare food. In addition, personal objects should not be shared, and hands should be washed thoroughly after patient contact. Health care workers should wear gloves when handling blood or body fluids. Travelers to underdeveloped countries should avoid eating uncooked shellfish, fruits, or vegetables or drinking water that could be contaminated. Currently the CDC recommends immune globulin for all travelers to developing countries where HAV infection is endemic. Hepatitis A immune globulin should be considered for travel that is going to be longer than 6 months. Prophylaxis against hepatitis A should be given as soon as possible after exposure (0.02 mL/kg intramuscularly), although it is of no benefit if it is not given within 2 weeks of exposure. Immunization with immune globulin lasts for 6 months. A hepatitis A vaccine is currently available.
- The prevention of HBV infection involves the routine screening of pregnant women, prophylaxis of infants born to infected women, and routine infant immunization. The hepatitis B vaccine should also be offered to persons at risk. The vaccine is given in a series of three injections; the first two doses are given 1 month apart and the third dose is given 6 months after the second dose. Antibodies to HBV develop in approximately 90% to 95% of vaccinated individuals but

may be as low as 50% to 70% among individuals who are immunocompromised. A positive HBsAb indicates immunity. To prevent transmission, therapy should be initiated immediately after exposure to HBV. The recommendations for prophylaxis after sexual exposure to HBV include hepatitis B immune globulin (0.06 mL/kg IM) within 14 days of exposure and simultaneous hepatitis B vaccination, with the second and third injections at 1 and 6 months, respectively. HBV and HCV infections are transmitted by blood; therefore patients must understand the importance of not sharing razor blades, toothbrushes, or nail clippers. Partners of infected patients must be tested as well because sexual transmission is possible. Barrier protection should be used, and partners should be told about the patient's hepatitis infection. Long-term monogamous partners can use their discretion if the partner is hepatitis-negative, but all partners should be tested every few years to detect any seroconversion. Household contacts have an extremely low risk of infection. Patients with chronic hepatitis should clean up their blood spills with bleach and bag any bloodstained material before placing it in the trash.

- All patients with liver disease should understand the significant risk for the development of cirrhosis, liver failure, and cancer with alcohol ingestion. Patients should be counseled and resources provided to help them stop drinking. Referral to psychotherapy, substance use counselors, Alcoholics Anonymous, and support groups can be helpful. Family members and significant others must be included in counseling and therapy.
- Patients with chronic hepatitis should be vaccinated for both HAV and HBV as appropriate. Education regarding their disease, possible complications, the importance of adhering to the treatment regimen, and contributing factors to the disease must be addressed. Patient education can be a valuable tool that can improve patient adherence.[38]

HEALTH PROMOTION

The prevention of hepatitis is possible with healthy lifestyles and the avoidance of situations that increase risk. A healthy lifestyle includes alcohol and substance use avoidance, safe sexual practices, vaccinations, and regular checkups that include the monitoring of LFT results.

Once hepatitis has been diagnosed, complications and disease progression can be deterred by abstaining from alcohol and substance use, obtaining vaccinations, becoming knowledgeable about the disease, and maintaining regular follow-up appointments with the health care provider.

All patients with liver disease should understand the significant risk for development of cirrhosis, liver failure, and cancer with alcohol ingestion. Patients should be counseled and resources provided to help them stop drinking. Referral to psychotherapy, substance use counselors, Alcoholics Anonymous, and support groups can be helpful. Family members and significant others should be included in counseling and therapy.

Patients with chronic hepatitis should be vaccinated for both HAV and HBV as appropriate. Education regarding their disease, possible complications, the importance of adhering to the treatment regimen, and contributing factors to the disease must be addressed. Patient education can be a valuable tool that can improve patient adherence.[38]

REFERENCES

1. American Liver Foundation. The progression of liver disease. Retrieved from https://liverfoundation.org/for-patients/about-the-liver/the-progression-of-liver-disease/#1503433005041-1b714e18-b29f).
2. QuickStats. (2017). Death rates for chronic liver disease and cirrhosis, by sex and age group—national vital statistics system, United States, 2000 and 2015. *MMWR. Morbidity and Mortality Weekly Report*, 66, 1031–DOI. http://dx.doi.org/10.15585/mmwr.mm6638a9.
3. WHO global hepatitis report. Retrieved from http://apps.who.int/iris/bitstream/handle/10665/255016/9789241565455-eng.pdf;jsessionid=E2EBBC452F3B0CC26D625D0E4627E64B?sequence=1.
4. U.S. Department of Health and Human Services. Hepatitis B basic information. Retrieved from https://www.hhs.gov/hepatitis/learn-about-viral-hepatitis/hepatitis-b-basics/index.html.
5. Centers for Disease Control and Prevention. Viral hepatitis. Retrieved from https://www.cdc.gov/hepatitis/statistics/2016surveillance/commentary.htm.
6. Burchum, J. R. (2018). Antiviral agents I: Drugs for non-viral HIV viral infections. In L. D. Rosenthal & J. R. Burchum (Eds.), *Lehne's pharmacotherapeutics for advanced practice providers*. St. Louis: Elsevier.
7. Sequera, V.-G., Valencia, S., García-Basteiro, A. L., Marco, A., & Bayas, J. M. (2015). Vaccinations in prisons: A shot in the arm for community health. *Human Vaccines & Immunotherapeutics*, 11(11), 2615–2626. doi:10.1080/21645515.2015.1051269.
8. Hunt, D. R., & Saab, S. (2009). Viral hepatitis in incarcerated adults: A medical and public health concern. *The American Journal of Gastroenterology*, 104, 1024–1031.
9. Duffy, D., Mamdouh, R., Laird, M., et al. (2014). The ABCs of viral hepatitis that define biomarker signatures of acute viral hepatitis. *Hepatology (Baltimore, Md.)*, 59, 1273–1282.
10. Centers for Disease Control and Prevention. Hepatitis fact sheet. Retrieved from https://www.cdc.gov/hepatitis/hav/pdfs/hepageneralfactsheet.pdf. (Accessed 29 May 2019).
11. Centers for Disease Control and Prevention. (2019). Recommended immunization schedule for children and adolescents aged 18 years or younger. United States. Retrieved from https://www.cdc.gov/vaccines/schedules/hcp/imz/child-adolescent.html. (Accessed 29 May 2019).
12. Centers for Disease Control and Prevention. Prevention of hepatitis B virus infection in the United States: Recommendations of the Advisory Committee on Immunization Practices. Retrieved from https://www.cdc.gov/mmwr/volumes/67/rr/rr6701a1.htm.
13. Keefe, E. B., Dieterich, D. T., Han, S. H., et al. (2008). A treatment algorithm for the management of chronic hepatitis B virus infection in the United States: 2008 update. *Clinical Gastroenterology and Hepatology*, 6, 1314–1340.
14. Hepatitis C online. HCV epidemiology in the United States. Retrieved from https://www.hepatitisc.uw.edu/pdf/screening-diagnosis/epidemiology-us/core-concept/allThis. (Accessed 1 August 2018).
15. World Health Organization. Hepatitis. Retrieved from http://www.who.int/news-room/fact-sheets/detail/hepatitis-c. (Accessed 1 August 2018).
16. Pietrangelo, A. (2018).Hepatitis C by the numbers: Facts, statitistics, and you. Retrieved from https://www.healthline.com/health/hepatitis-c/facts-statistics-infographic#prevalence. (Accessed 1 August 2018).
17. Butt, A. A., Yan, P., Lo Re, V., et al. (2015). Liver fibrosis progression in hepatitis C virus infection after seroconversion. *JAMA Internal Medicine*, 175 (2), 178–185. doi:10.1001/jamainternmed.2014.6502. https://jamanetwork.com/journals/jamainternalmedicine/fullarticle/1984248. (Accessed 1 August 2018).
18. U.S. Department of Veterans Affairs. Viral hepatitis. Sex and sexuality: Entire lesson. Retrieved from https://www.hepatitis.va.gov/patient/daily/sex/single-page.asp. (Accessed 1 August 2018).
19. Hughes, B. L., Page, C. M., & Kuller, J. A. (2017). Hepatitis C in pregnancy: Screening, treatment, and management. Retrieved from https://www.ajog.org/article/S0002-9378(17)30930-4/pdf. (Accessed 1 August 2018).
20. Centers for Disease Control and Prevention. HIV/AIDS and viral hepatitis. Retrieved from https://www.cdc.gov/hepatitis/populations/hiv.htm. (Accessed 1 August 2018).
21. Romeo, R. Hepatitis delta: Natural history and outcome. Retrieved from http://onlinelibrary.wiley.com/enhanced/doi/10.1002/cld.250. (Accessed 1 August 2018).
22. Ditah, I. 1., Ditah, F., Devaki, P., Ditah, C., Kamath, P. S., & Charlton, M. (2014). Current epidemiology of hepatitis E virus infection in the United States: Low seroprevalence in the National Health and Nutrition Evaluation Survey. *Hepatology (Baltimore, Md.)*, 60(3), 815–822. doi:10.1002/hep.27219. [Epub 2014 Jul 17].

23. Centers for Disease Control and Prevention. Guidelines for viral hepatitis surveillance and case management. Retrieved from https://www.cdc.gov/hepatitis/statistics/surveillanceguidelines.htm. (Accessed 3 August 2018).

24. Singal, A. K., Battaler, R., Ahn, J., Kamath, P. S., & Shaw, V. J. (2018). ACG clinical guideline: Alcoholic liver disease. Retrieved from www.cdc.gov/vaccines/schedules/hcp/imz/child-adolescent.html. (Accessed 3 August 2018).

25. Askgaard, G., Gronbaek, M., Kjaer, M. S., et al. (2015). Alcohol drinking pattern and risk of alcoholic liver cirrhosis: A prospective cohort study. *Journal of Hepatology*, 62(5), 1061–1067.

26. Banini, B. A., & Sanyal, A. J. (2016). Nonalcoholic fatty liver disease: Epidemiology, pathogenesis, natural history, diagnosis, and current treatment options. Clinical medicine insights. *Therapeutics*, 8, 75–84.

27. Arrese, M., & Feldstein, A. E. (2017). NASH-related cirrhosis: An occult liver disease burden. Retrieved from https://aasldpubs.onlinelibrary.wiley.com/doi/full/10.1002/hep4.1033. (Accessed 29 May 2019).

28. Calzadilla Bertot, L., & Adams, L. A. (2016). The natural course of non-alcoholic fatty liver disease. *International Journal of Molecular Sciences*, 17(5), 774. http://doi.org/10.3390/ijms17050774.

29. National Institute of Diabetes and Digestive and Kidney Diseases. Definition & facts of NAFLD & NASH. Retrieved from https://www.niddk.nih.gov/health-information/liver-disease/nafld-nash/definition-facts. (Accessed 29 May 2019).

30. Lorbec, G., Urlep, Z., & Rozman, D. Pharmacogenomic and personalized approaches to tackle nonalcoholic fatty liver disease. Retrieved from https://www.futuremedicine.com/doi/full/10.2217/pgs-2016-0047. (Accessed 29 May 2019).

31. Chalasani, N., Bonkovsky, H. L., Fontana, R., et al. (2015). Features and outcomes of 899 patients with drug-induced liver injury: The DILIN Prospective Study. *Gastroenterology*, 148(7), 1340–1352, e7.

32. Mann, N. P., Czaja, A. J., Dorham, J. D., Krawitt, E. L., Mieli-Vergani, G., Vergani, D., et al. (2010). Diagnosis and management of autoimmune hepatitis. Retrieved from https://www.aasld.org/sites/default/files/guideline_documents/autoimmunehepatitis2010.pdf. (Accessed 29 May 2019).

33. Doig, A. K., & Huether, S. E. (2014). Alterations of digestive functions. In K. L. McCance & S. E. Huether (Eds.), *Pathophysiology; the biologic basis for disease in adults and children* (7th ed.). The incubation period is 4 to 6 weeks. St. Louis: Elsevier.

34. Levinson, W., Chin-Hong, P., Joyce, E. A., Nussbaum, J., & Schwartz, B. (Eds.), (2018). Brief summaries of medically important organisms: Introduction. In *Review of medical microbiology & immunology: A guide to clinical infectious diseases* (15th ed.). New York, NY: McGraw-Hill. http://accessmedicine.mhmedical.com.ezproxy.simmons.edu/content.aspx?bookid=2381&sectionid=187698504. (Accessed 25 July 2018).

35. Duffy, D., Mamdouh, R., Laird, M., et al. (2014). The ABCs of viral hepatitis that define biomarker signatures of acute viral hepatitis. *Hepatology (Baltimore, Md.)*, 59, 1273–1282.

36. Abbas, Z., & Afzal, R. (2013). Life cycle and pathogenesis of hepatitis D virus: A review. *World Journal of Hepatology*, 5(12), 666–675. http://doi.org/10.4254/wjh.v5.i12.666.

37. Bunchorntavakul, C., Jones, L. M., Kikuchi, M., et al. (2015). Distinct features in natural history and outcomes of acute hepatitis C. *Journal of Clinical Gastroenterology*, 49(4), e31–e40.

38. Than, N. N. (2016). Autoimmune hepatitis progress form immunosuppression to personalized regulatory T cell therapy. *Canadian Journal of Gastroenterology and Hepatology*.

39. Amini, M., & Runyon, B. A. (2010). Alcoholic hepatitis 2010: A clinician's guide to diagnosis and therapy. *World Journal of Gastroenterology*, 16, 4905–4912.

40. Hyun, C. S., Lee, S., & Ventura, W. R. (2019). The prevalence and significance of isolated hepatitis B core antibody (anti-HBc) in endemic population. *BMC Research Notes*, 12(1), 251. doi:10.1186/s13104-019-4287-z.

41. Centers for Disease Control and Prevention. Hepatitis E questions and answers for health professionals. Retrieved from https://www.cdc.gov/hepatitis/hev/hevfaq.htm. (Accessed 3 August 2018).

42. Kappus, M. R., & Sterling, R. K. (2013). Extrahepatic manifestations of acute hepatitis B virus infection. *Gastroenterology and Hepatology*, 9(2), 123–126.

43. Kupin, W. L. (2017). Viral-associated GN: Hepatitis B and other viral infections. *Clinical Journal of American Society of Nephrology*, 12(9), 1529–1533. https://doi.org/10.2215/CJN.09180816.

44. Dienstag, J. L. (2008). Chronic hepatitis. In J. Jameson, A. S. Fauci, D. L. Kasper, S. L. Hauser, D. L. Longo, & J. Loscalzo (Eds.), *Harrison's principles of internal medicine* (20th ed.). New York, NY: McGraw-Hill.

45. Terrault, N. A., Bzowej, N. H., Chang, K. M., Hwang, J., Jonas, M. M., & Murad, M. H. (2016). AASLD guidelines for treatment of chronic hepatitis B. *Heapatology*, 63(1), 261.

46. Martin, P., et al. (2015). A treatment algorithm for the management of chronic hepatitis B virus infection in the United States: 2015 update. *Clinical Gastroenterology and Hepatology*, 13(12), 2071–2087, e16.

47. Centers for Disease Control and Prevention. Hepatitis C questions and answers for health professionals. Retrieved from https://www.cdc.gov/hepatitis/hcv/cfaq.htm#C1. (Accessed 3 August 2018).

48. American Association for the Study of Liver Diseases and The Infectious Diseases Society of America. (2018). HCV Guidance: Recommendations for testing, managing, and treating hepatitis C. Retrieved from https://www.hcvguidelines.org/.

49. Liu, J., & Wang, L. (2017). Baclofen for alcohol withdrawal. *The Cochrane Database of Systematic Reviews*, (8), Art. No.: CD008502, doi:10.1002/14651858.CD008502.pub5.

50. Solomons, H. D. (2012). Carbohydrate deficient transferrin and alcoholism. *Germs*, 2(2), 75–78. http://doi.org/10.11599/germs.2012.1015. (Accessed 3 August 2018).

CHAPTER **120**

INFLAMMATORY BOWEL DISEASE

Terry Mahan Buttaro

 Immediate physician consultation is indicated for patients who develop weight loss, nausea, vomiting, severe abdominal pain, significant blood loss, and malnutrition and other systemic symptoms.

DEFINITION AND EPIDEMIOLOGY

Ulcerative colitis (UC) and Crohn disease (CD) are chronic inflammatory bowel diseases (IBDs) thought to comprise diverse disorders of the intestinal tract and affecting about 3 million people in the United States.[1] Both disorders typically have periods of remission and exacerbation, and although they have many similarities, there are also significant differences. A third category, known as IBD–unclassified, can account for up to 15% of all patients with IBD.[2] The unclassified disease involves the colon but the distinction between UC and CD cannot be made.[3] Later, as UC or CD symptoms and features manifest, a diagnosis may be determined. The diagnosis of indeterminate colitis should be used only after colectomy and histopathology of the colon have failed to distinguish between UC and CD.

UC is a chronic inflammation of the lining of the colonic mucosa and, to some extent, the submucosal layer. Beginning in the rectum, the inflammation is diffuse, continuous, and may involve the entire colon (pancolitis) or only part of it (left-sided colitis). The worst of the disease is seen in the rectum and this may be indicative of the disease above, but it is not usually found worse higher in the colon compared with the rectal involvement. The disease can involve only the rectum (proctitis) or the rectosigmoid colon, but some patients have disease extending proximally to the splenic flexure (left-sided UC). Many patients experience a major impact on their quality of life, and approximately 50% do not experience a stable period of remission for any significant amount of time.[4,5]

CD also is associated with chronic inflammation, but all layers of the intestinal tract wall (transmural inflammation) and any portion of the intestinal tract from the mouth to the anus can be affected. CD is also heterogeneous, with a variable presentation and response to treatment. The presentation is affected by site involvement and whether the disease is only inflammatory or also complicated by fibrostenosis or penetration of the bowel wall, creating fistulous tracts. CD can affect any area of the digestive system from the mouth to the anus. The majority of patients with CD have disease in the small intestine (ileitis or regional enteritis), but some will have inflammation that involves both the ileum and colon and a small number will have disease only in the colon (Crohn colitis, not to be confused with UC).[6]

The transmural involvement in CD is responsible for many of the complications that occur. Although the inflammation can be patchy (unlike UC, which is nearly always continuous), the involvement of all layers of the bowel wall creates many problems. Fibrostenosis occurs from the inflammation and can partially or completely obstruct the lumen of the intestinal wall (stricturing). Intestinal wall weakening, caused by the inflammation, results in sinus tracts or fistulas (penetrating disease), abscesses, and perforation. Fistulas can develop from bowel to bowel (enteroenteric), bowel to skin (enterocutaneous), bowel to bladder (enterovesical), or bowel to vagina (enterovaginal). The fistulas frequently occur perianally; other complications include abscesses, large tender skin tags, and the need for surgically placed drains and repair.[3]

The annual incidences of UC and CD are similar in both age at onset and worldwide distribution. IBD occurs more frequently in colder climates and industrial-urbanized societies with a Westernized lifestyle, but the incidence is rising in developing countries and in Asia. IBD affects men and women equally, but there may be some regional differences. The peak age at onset is frequently in the second or third decade and a second peak in the 6th decade but IBD can occur at any time across the life span. The incidence in the pediatric population is increasing, especially for CD.

The cause of IBD is unknown, though there appears to be an abnormal immune response to intestinal microbial flora, shifting the composition of the flora in the affected individual. Altered interactions between the intestinal flora and the immune system in the mucosa of the intestines may be contributing to the inflammatory response. Environmental factors also play a role. These include long-term dietary patterns and age, both of which affect the gut microbiota.[7]

Genetics are also proposed to be a cause of IBD and may be linked with the microbiome as well. Several genes have been identified that increase the individual's susceptibility to IBD, with different genetic patterns for UC and CD. Mutations of these genes have an impact on the microbiome, which increases the inflammatory response.[7] In affected individuals, the immune system is dysregulated and triggered by environmental factors. These factors may include luminal bacteria, infection, or tobacco. For some persons with IBD, there seems to be a familial tendency in that these individuals have a first-degree relative with IBD. This occurs more often in CD and more frequently in children.[6] Ethnicity may be implicated in IBD (e.g., patient has ancestors from northern Europe or of central and eastern [Ashkenazi] Jewish descent).[6]

Cigarette smoking is also a strong environmental factor affecting IBD. Smoking may affect the course of UC, demonstrating a protective role, whereas in CD current smoking is a strong independent risk factor for the early development of structuring and fistulizing, postoperative recurrence of ileal CD, and disease requiring maintenance therapy. A higher level of tobacco pack-years will increase risk, as smokers are twice as likely as nonsmokers to develop CD. Smoking cessation can improve the disease course, and individuals who can stop smoking may have fewer IBD problems than those who continue to smoke.[8]

PATHOPHYSIOLOGY

Several factors are associated with IBD. A proposed mechanism of inflammation is an infection or other toxin releasing cell wall products that upregulate macrophages and granulocytes. The latter activate circulating cells that migrate into the mucosa, releasing a variety of inflammatory factors such as cytokines, proteases, and oxygen-derived free radicals. These factors all promote inflammation, and the patient has no means of downregulating the system to inhibit the inflammation. Either the tissue responds by resolving with scarring or other secondary immune reactions continue to create irreversible damage.[8]

The pathophysiology involves the role of the microbiome plus the impact of genetic profiles and environmental factors linked together to explain the development of IBD.[9,10] More than 70 genes associated with IBD (UC, CD, or both) have been identified.[11] *NOD2* (CD susceptibility gene) mutations are associated with an altered structure of the gut microbiota.[12] Anti–*Saccharomyces cerevisiae* antibodies (ASCAs) are associated with CD, and antineutrophil cytoplasmic antibodies (ANCAs) are associated with UC. Other studies have examined associations among genotype, phenotype, disease course, and response to treatment. This knowledge contributes to the understanding of the clinical manifestations of IBD, such as disease location, behavior, natural history, and response to medications as well as their side effects.[11]

There are differences between UC and CD even though clinically they may seem similar. UC is identified by continuous lesions of the intestinal mucosa, noted first in the large intestine, most often the left colon extending to the rectum. The inflammation can be mild (edematous and hyperemic) or more acute, with obvious ulcerations, hemorrhagic areas, abscesses, and even necrosis.[13]

CD is primarily located in the ileocolon and is associated with skip lesions. Fissures, both longitudinal and transverse, expand not only to other parts of the colon but also to lymphoid tissue. The mucosal structure in CD has a cobblestone appearance with granulomas and fissured lesions between the intestinal loops.[13]

CLINICAL PRESENTATION

UC and CD can have similar presentations and can be difficult to distinguish. People may complain of symptoms for varying lengths of time, and it is not unusual to have someone report abdominal pain or diarrhea intermittently for years before other symptoms develop. In most cases the symptoms of abdominal pain and diarrhea are present in both diseases, although abdominal pain may be the only presenting complaint. The abdominal pain may be diffuse (generalized lower pain) or localized to the right or left lower quadrant. The pain is usually a cramping sensation and can be intermittent or constant.[1,10]

Tenesmus, spasms in the rectum, urgency, and fecal incontinence may be reported with active rectal inflammation. Stools are often loose or watery and may include blood if the colon is involved. Rectal bleeding is usually present with colitis, either UC or CD (if the lower colon is involved). Patients may report blood seen only on the toilet paper after wiping, blood in the stool, clots, or large amounts of blood.[14] With proctitis, rectal bleeding may be the only complaint, or constipation may be reported rather than diarrhea.

Other complaints may include fatigue, weight loss, anorexia, fever, chills, nausea, vomiting, joint pain, and mouth sores. CD may manifest with only vague complaints of fatigue and abdominal cramping but is also associated with intestinal obstruction, symptoms of vomiting, bloating, and no stool as well as perianal disease (anal fissures, perirectal abscess, or fistula). Some patients, especially in late adolescence and early adulthood, have obstruction, abscesses, or fistulas and are diagnosed at surgery.

Extraintestinal signs and symptom are possible in both these disorders. These can include oral ulcerations, lesions such as erythema nodosum, episcleritis, primary sclerosing cholangitis, osteopenia, osteoporosis, polyarthritis, and sacroiliitis.[13]

Pertinent history includes recent antibiotic use or travel, the health of other household members, family history of IBD, previous history of abdominal pain or diarrhea, and a thorough medication review.

PHYSICAL EXAMINATION

The presentation can vary from minimal or no distress to severe illness. Fever and accompanying tachycardia can be present but often are not. All weight ranges are seen, from underweight to obese. People, especially the young and older adults, can demonstrate significant weight loss and failure to thrive. Conjunctival inflammation or oral aphthous ulcers may be present. Abdominal examination can reveal hyperactive bowel sounds. Palpation of loops of bowel may be noted as "fullness" in the lower abdomen and can reveal tenderness there, which may be more prominent on one side or the other, although the abdomen can be diffusely tender. A mass, especially in the lower right quadrant, can signify ileocecal inflammation. Rectal examination for occult blood may be positive, with frank blood and tenderness. Perianal lesions—such as skin tags, anal fissure, and perianal fistulas—are more suggestive of CD but can be present in UC. Anal stenosis, abscess, or purulent drainage from a fistulous tract may be seen on rectal examination. Perianal disease is suggestive of IBD but can also be seen in healthy people. Joints do not usually appear red or edematous. Skin lesions (e.g., erythema nodosum, pyoderma gangrenosum, papulonecrotic skin lesions, or rashes) may also be noted.

DIAGNOSTICS
Blood Tests

A complete blood count (CBC) is useful to determine the presence of anemia. The platelet count will often be elevated in the presence of active inflammation or infection. C-reactive protein (CRP) and erythrocyte sedimentation rate (ESR) can be elevated but are nonspecific markers of inflammation. CRP can be useful as a monitor of disease activity if it is elevated with active disease, but not everyone will have an increase in CRP response to active inflammation. These tests may not be useful for diagnosis but may have value in following a patient's progress. CD may result in malabsorption, especially after a small bowel resection, thus glucose, electrolyte values, blood urea nitrogen, creatinine, liver function, vitamin D, vitamin B_{12}, and folate levels should be monitored to determine status.

Genetic testing may be helpful in identifying IBD, distinguishing CD from UC, and demonstrating the likelihood of more aggressive CD (prognostic test).[15] The serogenetic markers include ANCAs and perinuclear antineutrophil cytoplasmic antibodies (pANCAs); ASCA immunoglobulin A (IgA) and IgG; outer membrane protein C (anti-OmpC) IgA; and flagellin (anti-Fla2, anti-FlaX, and anti-CBir1).[16,17] Other markers can be tested in an IBD panel. *NOD2/CARD15* genetic testing is prognostic for CD and can indicate the likelihood of more aggressive disease over time.

A recent study reported sensitivity and specificity of biomarker testing in patients younger than 18 years of age (sensitivity for IBD 86%, CD 91%, UC 82%; specificity for IBD 86%, CD 76%, UC 91%).[15] A positive test result can be helpful for diagnosis but does not obviate the need for other diagnostic testing. False-negative test results do occur and clinical judgment should override the test results.

Stool Tests

Initial presentation of diarrhea and subsequent flares should be evaluated for infection. Stool testing for ova and parasites should be performed two times to eliminate the most common pathogens. Testing may be done for *Giardia* stool antigen, *Entamoeba histolytica*, and, for patients experiencing a flare, *Clostridium difficile*; the latter is especially important if the patient has recently used antibiotics. Special cultures for other organisms can be requested (*Bacillus*, *Escherichia coli* O157:H7, *Campylobacter*, *Salmonella*, *Shigella*, *Vibrio cholerae*, *Yersinia*). Patients (male and female) with rectal symptoms should be tested for sexually transmitted disease. Fecal leukocytes, a marker of inflammation, can be tested in the stool specimen. Fecal calprotectin is also used to determine inflammation in the bowels.[16]

Radiography

Enterography by computed tomography (CT) or magnetic resonance imaging (MRI) is a diagnostic and monitoring tool in the management of CD. A more accurate test for small bowel disease, CT can detect bowel wall inflammation, perforation, and abscess and is used selectively when appropriate. There is growing concern about exposure to excessive radiation that occurs especially with CT scans. Responsible practitioners must carefully weigh the benefits of the scan versus the increasing radiation risk. This is especially important in IBD, which, as a chronic, lifelong illness, will potentially require multiple radiologic tests. MR enterography is safer because there is no radiation and it is an alternative procedure for viewing the small bowel.

Small bowel series are used infrequently to determine small bowel involvement and can demonstrate an abnormal terminal ileum and fistulas, but they are not as sensitive as other testing. There are moderate false-positive and false-negative rates with barium studies. As a result, the barium enema is of limited use in the diagnosis of IBD and is most useful in detecting colonic distention, obstruction, fistulas, strictures, or tumors. If a barium enema is used, a laxative should be taken by the patients after barium studies because they can become extremely constipated and the barium can remain for weeks in the intestines. A barium enema *should not* be used in patients with moderate to severe colitis because there is perforation risk when the colon is weakened from inflammation. MRI may be helpful in detecting fistulas and abscesses in patients with perianal CD.

Endoscopy

Flexible sigmoidoscopy examines the lower 76 cm (30 inches) of the colon and is useful to determine the source of bright red rectal bleeding. Colonoscopy can be useful in differentiating UC and CD. Bowel cleansing is necessary for colonoscopy, and several preparations are available. Split-dose preparations are used for a morning colonoscopy; single doses are used for colonoscopies done in the afternoon. Polyethylene glycol electrolyte lavage solution is commonly used, although the colonoscopy preparation often depends on the gastroenterologist's preference. Hydration during the preparation is extremely important and must be emphasized to the patient. Caution must be exercised for patients with a history of congestive heart failure or decreased kidney function (serum creatinine >1.5).

Both UC and CD may have distinguishing features endoscopically that, if found, may help to differentiate one from the other. On endoscopy, UC mucosal inflammation will be continuous with disease in the rectum up to the point where the inflammation stops. CD can have "skip areas," patchy sections of normal mucosa intermixed with inflamed mucosa, giving a cobblestone appearance to the mucosa. However, these distinguishing features are not always present, making diagnosis difficult. A useful endoscopic finding in CD is an inflamed or abnormal terminal ileum.

Capsule endoscopy (a swallowed capsule with a camera inside) takes pictures of the small intestine and transmits them to a box worn by the patient. Many lesions and abnormalities missed by small bowel radiology can then be visualized. This test is covered by insurance but requires specific indications and other testing to be completed first. It can be valuable in the diagnosis and monitoring of CD, but caution should be exercised to ensure that there is no stricture or narrowing of the small bowel because the capsule may then become lodged. Small bowel enteroscopy (e.g., single or double balloon enteroscopy or spiral enteroscopy) can be used to evaluate CD or bleeding in the small bowel.

Mucosal biopsy samples, usually 3 to 4 mm in size, are especially helpful in the diagnosis and monitoring of IBD. On microscopic examination, acute and chronic inflammation can be seen. It may be difficult to distinguish UC from CD; in these patients, the disease may be labeled "indeterminate colitis" until a clear diagnosis can be made. UC can have cryptitis and crypt abscesses, whereas CD can show aphthous ulcers and granulomas.

DIFFERENTIAL DIAGNOSIS

 Further evaluation is needed for rectal bleeding; rectal bleeding should never be ignored or assumed to be benign.

When a patient presents with the common symptoms of IBD, several issues should be excluded: abdominal pain, rectal bleeding, and diarrhea. Bleeding may be related to hemorrhoids, ischemia, diverticular disease, a fissure, drugs (e.g., by aspirin, nonsteroidal anti-inflammatory drugs [NSAIDs], anticoagulation), infection, or a colonic polyp or cancer. Abdominal pain can be due to diverticulitis and, in women, endometriosis or pelvic inflammatory disease. Abdominal pain and diarrhea without bleeding may signify appendicitis, lactose intolerance,

irritable bowel syndrome, or diarrhea predominant (IBS-D), a chronic benign functional disorder associated with altered loose bowel habits, bloating, and abdominal pain relieved by defecation. (See Chapter 121.)

Infectious causes of diarrhea (with or without bleeding) must be excluded. The most common pathogenic organisms to consider are *Giardia*, *Campylobacter jejuni*, *C. difficile* (especially with a history of recent antibiotic use), *E. coli*, *Salmonella*, and *Shigella*. Other causes include viral infection, celiac disease, lactase deficiency, bacterial overgrowth, bile acids (after cholecystectomy), hyperthyroidism, and diabetes (enteropathy). If a host is immunocompromised, infections with such organisms as cytomegalovirus, *Cryptosporidium*, and *Mycobacterium avium-intracellulare* should be excluded.

Noninfectious causes include acute self-limited colitis, ischemic colitis (especially in patients older than 60 years), radiation enteritis or colitis (history of radiation to abdomen or pelvis; may be a late sequela), Behçet syndrome, lymphoma, and systemic vasculitis. A rare cause of diarrhea (usually with excessive watery stools and flushing) is neuroendocrine tumors and carcinoid syndrome.

Over-the-counter medications that can be a source of diarrhea include antacids with magnesium, mints with sorbitol, and laxatives. Other medications that can cause diarrhea include metformin and proton pump inhibitors. Medications associated with microscopic (lymphocytic, collagenous) colitis include antibiotics, chemotherapeutic agents, colchicine, magnesium-containing antacids, metformin, misoprostol, NSAIDs, proton pump inhibitors, and gold.

INTERPROFESSIONAL COLLABORATIVE MANAGEMENT

Indications for Referral or Hospitalization

- The diagnosis of IBD can be challenging and requires physician consultation. Referral for diagnostic and follow-up endoscopy procedures as well as for management is the best approach. Once a patient has a treatment regimen, health care providers may be able to comanage the IBD, but continual close consultation with a gastroenterologist is necessary for optimal management and various treatment options.
- Hospitalization is sometimes necessary for bowel rest, hydration, and parenteral medication.

Pharmacotherapy

The American Gastroenterology Association provides guidance for the treatment of UC, CD, and other gastrointestinal issues (https://www.gastro.org/guidelines/ibd-and-bowel-disorders). There are varied treatment categories (including treatment for CD patients after surgical resection), and it is important to note that commonly used medications for IBD are not approved by the US Food and Drug Administration (FDA) but are considered to be used "off label," despite having been employed for many years.[17] In general UC and CD are treated with the same medications, although severity scores guide clinical treatment and are based on each patient's disease course, inflammatory burden, complications, impact of disease on the patient's activities, and prognosis. Some patients with mild disease can be treated in primary care, but greater disease severity will require referral and collaboration with a gastroenterologist. Five medication categories are used to treat IBD: antibiotics,

TABLE 120.1 Therapeutic Options for Inflammatory Bowel Disease

Disease Intensity	Disease Form	
	Ulcerative Colitis	**Crohn Disease**
Mild	5-Aminosalicylate: PO or rectal	Mesalamine: PO Metronidazole: PO Budesonide: PO Ciprofloxacin: PO
Moderate	5-Aminosalicylate: PO or PR Infliximab: IV	Glucocorticoid: PO Azathioprine: PO Mercaptopurine: PO Infliximab: IV
Severe	Glucocorticoid: PO or IV Cyclosporine: IV Infliximab: IV	Glucocorticoid: PO or IV Methotrexate: IV or SubQ Infliximab: IV
Refractory	Glucocorticoid: PO or IV Azathioprine: PO Mercaptopurine: PO	Infliximab: IV
In remission	5-Aminosalicylate: PO Azathioprine: PO Mercaptopurine: PO	Mesalamine: PO Azathioprine: PO Metronidazole: PO Mercaptopurine: PO Infliximab: IV

IV, Intravenous; *PO*, oral or by mouth; *PR*, rectal or per rectum; *SubQ*, subcutaneous. From Rosenthal, L. D., & Burchum, J. R. (2018). *Lehne's pharmacotherapeutics for advanced practice providers* (1st ed.). St. Louis: Elsevier.

5-aminosalicylates, glucocorticoids, immunosuppressants, and immunomodulators (Table 120.1).

5-Aminosalicylates. Patients with mild to moderate inflammatory bowel disease are usually initially treated with one of the 5-aminosalicylates, or 5-ASAs (i.e., sulfasalazine [Azulfidine], mesalamine [5-ASA], olsalazine [Dipentum], or balsalazide [Colazal]).[17] Mesalamine is recommended for mild CD, but otherwise the 5-ASAs have a limited role in CD.[17] First-line treatments for UC do include 5-ASA mesalamine products. Sulfasalazine is a sulfapyridine and a 5-ASA product connected by a bond. 5-ASA has been shown to be the active ingredient, and the sulfapyridine is responsible for most of the side effects. Several 5-ASA topical and oral products are available and effective in establishing remission in UC. Topical mesalamine medications are recommended and effective for proctitis. The rectal suspension of mesalamine is effective at inducing and maintaining remission in UC, especially left-sided UC. The combination of rectal and oral therapy can be effective for pancolitis.

Rarely, a patient may be allergic to 5-ASA; if so, the drug should be stopped. Patients will have had a worsening of their colitis symptoms, which will improve with discontinuation of the medication.

Corticosteroids. Oral and parenteral steroids can be useful in treating moderate to severe disease in both UC and CD patients but are avoided (or limited) if possible because of potential long-term side effects, including the development of diabetes, osteoporosis, and/or cataracts. Steroids are currently used to treat moderate to severe UC that is not responding to mesalamine; they have been shown to induce remission in mild to moderately active CD. Budesonide, recommended for

mild CD, is an enteric-coated synthetic steroid subject to high first-pass metabolism, potentially decreasing the risk of side effects.[17] It has similar (or slightly less) efficacy to corticosteroids and releases more in the distal ileum and right colon (useful for CD). However, there is a once-a-day oral preparation (Uceris) that is designed to be released throughout the colon and is indicated for both mild to moderate CD or UC. Once remission is achieved, corticosteroids are tapered off as soon as possible, although long, slow tapers (over 2–3 months) may be necessary to prevent a flare.

Topical rectal steroids in the form of a retention enema or foam can provide relief of urgency and spasm in the rectum in addition to healing the inflamed mucosa. Rectal steroids are used for a few weeks, usually until there is an improvement of rectal symptoms. There is some absorption of the steroid systemically; thus, long-term use (more than a few months) is not routinely recommended.

Immunosuppressants

 Immediate referral/consultation with a gastroenterologist is indicated for patients taking azathioprine who develop elevated liver enzymes twice normal or higher. Leukopenia, thrombocytopenia, or pancreatitis developing during treatment with azathioprine warrant immediate discontinuation of the drug and referral to the gastroenterologist for further evaluation.

Both azathioprine (Imuran), a prodrug that becomes mercaptopurine when metabolized, and 6-mercaptopurine (Purinethol) are used for the treatment of UC and CD, allowing the patient to avoid steroids and prevent steroid dependency. These medications must be taken for up to 6 months before disease remission occurs and cannot be used in isolation (i.e., monotherapy).[17] Phenotype and metabolite testing of 6-mercaptopurine can determine those in whom the drug is likely to become toxic and who should not take it.[18] Laboratory monitoring (CBC, LFTs, amylase and lipase levels) at baseline, weekly for 4 weeks, monthly for 3 months, and then every 3 months is necessary because of the potential adverse effects.

If an elevated liver enzyme level is found, the test should be repeated in 1 to 2 weeks. If the levels remain elevated or continue to rise, the drug should be discontinued and the patient referred to the gastroenterologist for further evaluation. Levels that are twice normal or higher are especially concerning and should prompt immediate referral to a gastroenterologist.

Other immunosuppressants used to treat IBD include cyclosporine and methotrexate, both with concerning side effects. Cyclosporine is primarily used for patients with severe CD and UC.[17] Concerns with cyclosporine include immunosuppression, an expected side effect, but also neurotoxicity and renal dysfunction.[17] Methotrexate has been shown to be effective in CD, but serious side effects are decreased if a lower weekly dose is used.[17]

Immunomodulators. Monoclonal antibodies have made a significant difference in the treatment of IBD, especially for patients with CD. Although immunomodulators are suggested for severe and refractory inflammatory bowel disease, it is not uncommon for patients with severe, new-onset IBD to be given these medications earlier.[17,19] The trend is to start a biologic earlier in the course and to taper off other medications for IBD. After surgery in CD patients with a risk factor for recurrence, antitumor necrosis factor (anti-TNF) prophylaxis is often prescribed to aid in preventing progression.[19] Several immune modulators are available for treatment: infliximab (Remicade,

Inflectra), adalimumab (Humira), certolizumab (Cimzia), and golimumab (Simponi). These are considered anti-TNF monoclonal antibodies.[19] Infliximab, an anti-TNF monoclonal antibody, is indicated for induction and maintenance of remission in CD. It is effective in treating fistulas, allowing patients to avoid or taper off steroids (steroid sparing), and is also indicated for UC. It is administered intravenously every 2 months, but some patients need to have the interval shortened to every 6 weeks for efficacy. The standard treatment regimen is to give a dose at 0, 2, and 6 weeks and then a maintenance dose every 8 weeks. Infusion reactions and a serum sickness–like reaction can occur because of the development of autoantibodies with infliximab, which is 25% mouse antibody and 75% human. Given alone or in combination with other immunomodulators, infliximab has induced remission and improvement in patients with refractory CD. Infusion reactions may be avoided by not extending the interval beyond 2 to 3 months and pretreating with corticosteroids and antihistamines.[5]

Adalimumab (fully human anti-TNF monoclonal antibody) is indicated for induction and maintenance of remission in moderate to severe CD that has not responded to conventional therapy. It is a subcutaneous injection given every 2 weeks after an induction dose.

Certolizumab is a pegylated monoclonal antibody (10% mouse antibody, 90% human) that is given by subcutaneous injection every 4 weeks. The response and remission rates are similar for all three medications for CD.[5]

Golimumab (Simponi) is used to treat UC and is given subcutaneously. The patient receives 200 mg initially and then 100 mg a week later. Thereafter 50 mg maintenance therapy is given every 4 weeks.[20]

Vedolizumab (Entyvio) is also a monoclonal antibody, but is a selective adhesion molecule inhibitor (as is natalizumab, [Tysabri]), not a TNF blocking agent. Both are indicated for CD and are sometimes used in combination with steroids or immunosuppressants, as are the anti-TNF medications. Vedolizumab specifically targets the gastrointestinal tract, causing an interruption in the inflammatory cascade. Patients with UC or CD who do not respond to other treatments are potential candidates for vedolizumab or natalizumab therapy. Vedolizumab does not cause progressive multifocal leukoencephalopathy (PML), but PML is a risk with natalizumab.

There are serious risks associated with all the immunomodulators, thus requiring vigilant follow-up, laboratory studies at least every 3 to 6 months, and patient education including information about the adverse effects of these medications: demyelinating disorders, serious infections, lymphoma and malignant neoplasms, activation of tuberculosis and other viruses, heart failure, pancytopenia, and a lupus-like syndrome. All patients must have a negative tuberculin test response (purified protein derivative [PPD]) before beginning therapy and repeat the PPD test yearly as long as they are receiving a biologic. It is recommended that patients be tested for hepatitis B and C as well as testing for other viruses that may be dormant. Patients should be up to date on vaccines including tetanus, Pneumovax, and influenza. A documented vaccination history is important, and guidelines have been developed for IBD patients.[21] Patients must report any sign of infection or new symptoms, and the biologic must be stopped until the infection is treated.

Adherence to therapy is important for the greatest efficacy to be maintained. Usually, patients who are doing well are continued on a biologic indefinitely. Newer therapies are being developed and extensive research is ongoing.

Antibiotics. Metronidazole can be effective in treating perianal disease and in healing fistulas associated with CD (not UC), but long-term treatment is necessary.[17] Ciprofloxacin is also helpful for CD but not effective for patients with UC.[17] Antibiotics are primarily used for infection because *C. difficile* is common with IBD. Probiotics may have some limited use but more studies are needed.[22]

Combination Therapy

There may be some benefit to combination therapy with these drugs. Immunomodulators have been used in combination with anti-TNF agents, but more research is needed to determine correct combinations, dosing, and treatment guidelines.[19]

Nonpharmacologic Management

Surgery. Some patients with UC and CD will require surgery for refractory disease. Patients with intractable disease generally do not respond to high doses of medications and may be systemically sick, with weight loss, anemia, nausea, and vomiting. Surgery is also indicated when dysplasia or cancer is confirmed on biopsy.

In UC, a total colectomy is often necessary. After surgery, patients no longer have the colonic disease and all IBD medications can be discontinued. Complications such as liver disease and ankylosing spondylitis may still be present, and treatment of these and other complications must be continued. Options for surgical treatment include an ileostomy and an ileal pouch–anal anastomosis (IPAA). With an IPAA, the colon is removed except for some rectal tissue, the small intestine is anastomosed to the rectum, and an internal pouch is created to store stool. Patients have no external bag but have several loose stools a day and can develop complications, including pouchitis.[10]

In CD, the average time from diagnosis to surgery is about 3 years. Surgery is indicated for a lack of response to medical therapy, small bowel obstruction, fistulas, and abscesses. A small bowel or colonic resection is the most common surgical procedure, although colectomy may be necessary in some patients. Many patients do well after surgery, but recurrence is possible. Approximately one-third of patients who have had a resection will require a second procedure, and a smaller number of patients will require additional surgical procedures.

Many novel surgical techniques are being tried at various centers, constantly seeking better ways to help patients. Variations on ileoanal pouch procedures, stricture plasties, and a multitude of other procedures continue to be advanced with the goals of preserving continence and repairing fistulas. Laparoscopic surgery for CD of the small bowel or terminal ileum and total colectomy for UC or CD is possible.

LIFE SPAN CONSIDERATIONS

IBD does not decrease the life span unless complications develop or the patient is not managed properly. Issues of malnutrition, malignant disease, and infection are factors that can have an impact. Compliance with treatment regimens, surveillance for colorectal cancer, and attention to complications will maximize patients' health.

COMPLICATIONS

There is an increased risk of colorectal cancer in patients with IBD. The risk is related to the extent of colonic involvement in both UC and CD. Patients with proctitis do not have increased risk over that of the general population. The risk in UC begins to increase after 8 years of disease and continually rises. Initial colorectal cancer screening for those with pancolitis or left-sided colitis should begin at 8 years after disease onset and then be performed every 1 to 3 years.[10]

A number of extraintestinal manifestations can occur with IBD. These primarily involve the eyes, mouth, peripheral joints, skin, and blood vessels. Some are related to the inflammatory activity of the bowel and can occur with active inflammation, improving when the IBD improves. These manifestations include aphthous stomatitis, iritis, uveitis, episcleritis, arthritis, and skin lesions (i.e., pyoderma gangrenosum, erythema nodosum).

Peripheral arthritis occurs in patients with UC and CD: knees, ankles, and shoulders are most often affected. A small number of patients with CD develop ankylosing spondylitis. Treatment of the underlying IBD is the best management approach for the arthritis, although symptomatic treatment can be used. Caution should be used in treating patients with NSAIDs, because these medications can trigger a flare of IBD.

Anemia is the most frequently seen extraintestinal complication in IBD; iron deficiency is the most common cause. Indices that should be monitored include iron saturation, ferritin, and reticulocyte count. Depending on the small bowel involvement of IBD and adverse gastrointestinal effects of oral iron supplements, patients may need parenteral iron supplementation. A hematology consultation would be appropriate for iron deficiency refractory to oral supplementation. There are also some data to suggest that oral iron may exacerbate disease.[23]

Other complications include liver disease (primary sclerosing cholangitis), gallstones, malabsorption (CD of the small bowel), and adrenal stones. Both men and women with IBD are at risk for osteoporosis independent of steroid use. All patients should have a bone density scan at baseline and every 2 years.

PATIENT AND FAMILY EDUCATION

- IBD has a significant impact on the quality of life of patients and their families. The stigma of a chronic bowel disease creates a unique set of problems. Patients may be afraid or unwilling to discuss their disease with loved ones, friends, and coworkers. Embarrassment about the symptoms and the need to be near a bathroom can prevent patients from participating in activities and outings. Fear of pain and diarrhea may keep them from eating, and they may become malnourished. Frequent visits and embarrassing, uncomfortable procedures may prevent them from seeking medical care when needed. There is a tendency for patients to accept their symptoms and not expect to be in remission; they should be reminded that the goal is remission, not just improvement.
- Patients receiving a biologic or immunomodulator should seek medical attention for any signs of infection or new symptom.
- Better education for better disease management is essential. A clear understanding of the disease process, potential complications, medication side effects, and risks (such as cancer) is imperative. The need for regular health care visits and the importance of treatments and scheduled procedures

should be emphasized. The patient should understand the importance of a well-balanced diet and be informed that there is no specific diet to follow for IBD. Written materials, videos, and educational meetings are available. The Crohn's and Colitis Foundation of America is a national patient organization that can provide information and support. Many local support groups can also provide a forum enabling learning and support for patients and their families.

- Health care providers should remember that these patients will be overwhelmed. Repetition is necessary to ensure that they understand. Visual aids are available that can help patients understand the disease and the necessary procedures and tests. In addition, because patients can obtain a great deal of misinformation from the media and well-meaning friends, relatives, and others, correction of misinformation and misconceptions will help. Above all, establishing a trusting, comfortable relationship and listening carefully to patients are vital to the long-term management of IBD.

HEALTH PROMOTION

IBD is a disease of remission and exacerbation. Cigarette smoking exacerbates CD, and patients should be encouraged to stop smoking because the risks of smoking far outweigh any benefit.

A healthy lifestyle and stress management should be encouraged.

Adherence with the prescribed treatment regimen and regular follow-up are the two most important strategies patients can implement to maximize their health. Maintaining regular follow-up with their health care providers and contacting their providers with early signs of a flare-up will minimize problems.

Patients with IBD are at higher risk for colon cancer and need regular colon cancer surveillance. Patients and family members must understand the medication regimen, the importance of not self-adjusting doses, and what monitoring is necessary.

RESOURCES

American College of Gastroenterology: www.acg.gi.org

Centers for Disease Control and Prevention: www.cdc.gov/ibd

Crohn's and Colitis Foundation of America: www.ccfa.org; info@ccfa.org; 800-932-2423

National Diabetes, Digestive Diseases and Kidney Diseases (NIDDK) Information Clearinghouse: www.niddk.nih.gov/health-information/health-topics/digestive-diseases

REFERENCES

1. Centers for Disease Control and Prevention. Inflammatory Bowel Disease. https://www.cdc.gov/ibd/data-statistics.htm. (Accessed 30 May 2019).
2. Bharadwaj, S., Narula, N., Tandon, P., & Yaghoobi, M. (2018). Role of endoscopy in inflammatory bowel disease. *Gastroenterology Report, 6*(2), 75–82, https://doi.org/10.1093/gastro/goy006.
3. Tremaine, W. J. (2011). Diagnosis and treatment of indeterminate colitis. *Gastroenterology & Hepatology, 7*(12), 826–828.
4. M'Koma, A. E. (2013). Inflammatory bowel disease: An expanding global health problem. *Clin Med Insights Gastroenterol, 6*, 33–47.
5. Furfaro, F., Bezzio, C., Ardizzone, S., et al. (2015). Overview of biological therapy in ulcerative colitis; current and future directions. *Journal of Gastrointestinal and Liver Diseases, 24*(2), 203–213.
6. U.S. National Library of Medicine. (2018).Crohn Disease. https://ghr.nlm.nih.gov/condition/crohn-disease. (Accessed 30 May 2019).

7. Kostic, A. D., Xavier, R. J., & Gvers, D. (2014). The microbiome in inflammatory bowel diseases: Current status and the future ahead. *Gastroenterology*, 146(6), 1489–1499.

8. Nguyen, G. C., Devlin, S. M., Afif, W., et al. (2014). Defining quality indicators for best-practice management of inflammatory bowel disease in Canada. *Can J Gastroenterol Hepatol*, 28(5), 275–285.

9. Thompson, A. I., & Lees, C. W. (2011). Genetics of ulcerative colitis. *Inflammatory Bowel Diseases*, 17(3), 831–848.

10. Sands, B. E. (2004). From symptom to diagnosis: Clinical distinctions among various forms of intestinal inflammation. *Gastroenterology*, 126, 1518–1532.

11. Thompson, A. I., & Lees, C. W. (2011). Genetics of ulcerative colitis. *Inflammatory Bowel Diseases*, 17(3), 831–848.

12. Taleban, S. (2015). Challenges in the diagnosis and management of inflammatory bowel disease in the elderly. *Current Treatment Options in Gastroenterology*, 13(3), 275–286.

13. Doig, A. K., & Huether, S. E. (2014). Alterations of digestive function. In *Pathophysiology: The biologic basis for disease in adults and children*. St Louis: Elsevier.

14. Devlen, J., Beusterien, K., Yen, L., et al. (2014). The burden of inflammatory bowel disease: A patient-reported qualitative analysis and development of a conceptual model. *Inflammatory Bowel Diseases*, 20(3), 545–552.

15. Lockton, S., Princen, F., & Singh, S. (2014). Classification of non-IBD, Crohns' disease and ulcerative colitis in a young patient population using a multi-marker diagnostic panel. *Gastroenterologia Y Hepatologia*, 10(7 Suppl. 4), 7–8.

16. Sandborn, W. J. (2014). Highlights in anti-tumor necrosis factor monitoring and antibody monitoring from the 2014 DDW Meeting: Commentary. *Gastroenterologia Y Hepatologia*, 10(7 Suppl. 4), 17–19.

17. Rosenthal, L. D. (2017). Other gastrointestinal drugs. In L. D. Rosenthal & J. R. Burchum (Eds.), *Lehne's pharmacotherapeutics for advanced practice providers*. St. Louis: Elsevier.

18. Dean, L. (2012). Mercaptopurine therapy and TPMT genotype. 2012 sep 20 [updated 2016 May 3]. In V. Pratt, H. McLeod, W. Rubinstein, et al. (Eds.), *Medical genetics summaries [internet]*. Bethesda (MD): National Center for Biotechnology Information (US). Retrieved from https://www.ncbi.nlm.nih.gov/books/NBK100660/.

19. Cohen Benjamin, L., & Sachar David, B. (2017). Update on anti-tumor necrosis factor agents and other new drugs for inflammatory bowel disease. *British Medical Journal*, 357, j2505.

20. Löwenberg, M., de Boer, N. K., & Hoentjen, F. (2014). Golimumab for the treatment of ulcerative colitis. *Clinical and Experimental Gastroenterology*, 7, 53–59. http://doi.org/10.2147/CEG.S48741.

21. Wasan, S. K., Baker, S. E., Skolnik, P. R., et al. (2010). A practical guide to vaccinating the inflammatory bowel disease patient. *The American Journal of Gastroenterology*, 105, 1231–1238.

22. Abraham, B. P., & Quigley, E. M. M. (2017). Probiotics in inflammatory bowel disease. *Gastroenterology Clinics of North America*, 46(4), 769–782. Published online 2017 Oct 3. doi:10.1016/j.gtc.2017.08.003.

23. Stein, J., Hartmann, F., & Dignass, A. U. (2010). Diagnosis and management of iron deficiency anemia in patients with IBD. *Gastroenterologia Y Hepatologia*, 7, 599–610.

CHAPTER **121**

IRRITABLE BOWEL SYNDROME

Terry Mahan Buttaro

 Consultation with a gastroenterologist is indicated for patients with a change in bowel habits after age 50; a family history of celiac disease, colon cancer or inflammatory bowel disease; evidence of gastrointestinal bleeding; weight loss; fever; nocturnal symptoms; recent antibiotic therapy; or continuing symptoms.[1]

DEFINITION AND EPIDEMIOLOGY

Irritable bowel syndrome (IBS) is a common gastrointestinal (GI) complaint seen in primary care. In the past, IBS was classified as a "functional" GI disorder; the ROME IV criteria now describes IBS as a "gut-brain" disorder characterized by a variety of GI syndromes in varied combinations (i.e., IBS associated with predominant constipation [IBS-C], predominant diarrhea [IBS-D], mixed bowel habits [IBS-M], or unsubtyped IBS) that can be related to alterations in central nervous system processing, gut microbiota, and mucosal and immune function as well as visceral hypersensitivity and motility disturbance.[1,2] Chronic abdominal pain, bloating, distention, flatulence, and bowel changes (e.g., constipation or diarrhea that alter with each other or with normal bowel movements) are the common presenting symptoms.

The worldwide prevalence of IBS is estimated to be 7% to 16%; females are more commonly affected than males, and the age of onset is usually between 25 and 54 years.[3–5]

Young adults are most affected, although the symptoms can occur at any age. Estimated costs associated with IBS in the United States are $1.6 billion per year.[6]

PATHOPHYSIOLOGY

A complex, multifactorial disorder involving a number of physiologic processes, IBS is associated with altered GI motility, increased GI (visceral) sensitivity, microscopic inflammation, postinfectious processes (e.g., gastroenteritis or increased gut sensitivity, brain-gut signal problems, and possibly a genetic linkage. Previous studies have demonstrated that patients with IBS process sensory information from the gut differently than do persons without IBS.[7] It is possible that IBS is related to changes in the central nervous system's processing of sensory information; exaggerated normal intestinal motility patterns; or sensory abnormalities in the colon, rectum, or small intestine.[8] A number of theories of the mechanisms for altered intestinal motility and sensitivity have been evolving.

Altered Motility

Although altered motility is often mentioned as a cause of IBS, controversy remains as to the exact electrical and contractile activity of the colon in IBS. Normal bowel motility predominantly consists of segmenting contractions that function to inhibit the transit of bowel contents. Any increase in segmenting contractions with decreased transit time results in constipation, whereas a decrease in contractions with increased transit time results in more frequent stools. In patients who have IBS, the colon delays the movement of feces, allowing an increase in their absorption.[8,9] This altered motility leads to changes in stool consistency. The increase in intestinal peristalsis and motility that usually follows the ingestion of a meal is thought to be increased in patients with IBS. More consistently demonstrated in IBS is an exaggeration of normal colonic motility in response to external and enteric stimuli, such as psychological stress, anxiety, anger, various drugs, acute intestinal infection, and (more recently discovered) small bowel bacterial overgrowth.[9,10] Postinfectious IBS has also been the topic of research; a few studies have demonstrated that as many as 10% to 30% of post–acute gastroenteritis patients with previously normal bowel function develop long-term symptoms suggestive of IBS.[8,10] The exact cause of postinfectious IBS is unknown but could involve injury to the enteric nervous system, immune hypersensitivity, or chronic mucosal inflammation that results in an alteration of gut motility.[9,11] Proponents of the postinfectious theory have speculated that IBS patients are postinfectious and that efforts should be directed toward measures to prevent and treat severe cases of acute gastroenteritis.[9] Research has also shown that the use of antibiotics in acute gastroenteritis for the purpose of preventing IBS may reduce symptoms.[8,9] Another factor possibly affecting the development of IBS is the role of small bowel bacterial overgrowth. Intestinal flora provides nutrition to the host, keeps the mucosal immune system in check, and regulates epithelial growth and function. However, it has been reported that a large portion of patients with IBS have small bowel bacterial overgrowth. Therefore, the treatment of IBS symptoms may be improved with the use of probiotics.[8,9]

Enhanced Visceral Sensation

Balloon distention studies used to determine the pathogenesis of IBS in the sigmoid, ileum, and colorectum demonstrate that painful symptoms at significantly lower pressures and higher pain frequency and severity are often seen in persons with IBS compared with healthy individuals. This concept, known as *hyperalgesia*, suggests that altered visceral sensation plays a role in the pathogenesis of IBS. Other diagnostic tests include endoscopy, radiology, stool samples (fecal calprotectin measurements, fecal ova and parasites, fecal occult blood), thyroid function tests, flexible sigmoidoscopy, and colonoscopy. However, there are no biochemical and histopathological diagnostic tests that can determine all causes of IBS.

Research suggests that with IBS there is increased sensitivity to mechanical stimulation in the small bowel and colon, increased or unusual somatic referral of visceral pain, and increased sensitivity to normal intestinal functions. Several possible mechanisms of visceral afferent dysfunction have been suggested to explain the increased visceral sensitivity in IBS. These mechanisms include altered receptor sensitivity at the viscus, increased excitability of neurons in the spinal cord, and altered central modulation of sensation.

Role of Enteric Neurotransmitters

Evidence suggests that abnormalities in extrinsic autonomic innervation of the viscera occur with functional bowel disorders and that neuroimmune interactions may mediate stress-induced GI responses.[12] Research has focused on the role of enteric nervous system neurotransmitters, such as serotonin, in controlling intestinal motility and visceral afferent (sensory) responses to normal stimuli (gas, sugars, bile acids, fatty acids) and noxious stimuli (allergens, infectious agents, balloon distention). Eighty percent of the body's serotonin is located in the gut, manufactured and released from enterochromaffin cells located in the mucosa. Increases in intraluminal pressures result in the release of serotonin. These neurotransmitters stimulate afferent fibers in the mucosa and initiate a peristaltic reflex, enhancing GI motility and mediating visceral pain. Serotonin, along with corticotropin-releasing hormone (CRH), may also play a role in mediating psychological stress-induced GI responses through the brain-gut axis.[12,13] Although defecating often relieves pain, stress and food increase it.[10]

Psychosocial Factors

Studies of the relationship between psychosocial factors and IBS suggest that there is a connection between the two and that patients with IBS have a greater incidence of psychosocial stressors and abuse than healthy individuals.[14] Quality of life is affected, and patients with IBS can miss work more frequently and have an increased incidence of depression and anxiety.[9,13–15] In addition, patients with IBS often believe that stress triggers their symptoms[5]; however, many physicians are reluctant to refer patients for psychological treatment.[16]

CLINICAL PRESENTATION AND PHYSICAL EXAMINATION

Abdominal pain must be present for an IBS diagnosis.[17] The pain associated with IBS is often described as nonradiating, intermittent, and crampy; pain can occur anywhere but is usually located in the left lower abdominal quadrant.[10,15,16] Symptoms frequently occur after food or alcohol consumption.[9] Because IBS is a functional chronic disorder in which symptoms fluctuate over time, it is critical to establish the absence of nocturnal symptoms to diagnosis IBS.[10,12]

Diarrhea, constipation, or a pattern of alternating diarrhea and constipation may be reported in conjunction with abdominal pain. It is necessary to clarify what is meant by these complaints because normal patterns of defecation can range from three bowel movements per week to three bowel movements per day, so this needs to be defined by the individual patient's norm. Mucus in the stool is sometimes reported. Complaints of abdominal distention, bloating, nausea, lethargy, and backache are common[10] and most likely reflect increased sensitivity to normal amounts of intestinal gas rather than an actual increase in gas.

The likelihood of organic disease is indicated by an acute onset of GI symptoms or an onset of symptoms in patients older than 50 years. Nocturnal symptoms, bloody or greasy stool, weight loss, malnutrition, evidence of GI bleeding, anemia, recurrent nausea, vomiting, and fever are incompatible with a diagnosis of IBS and require immediate diagnostic evaluation or referral.[10] Although bleeding is not associated with IBS, it may occur secondary to an anal fissure or hemorrhoids aggravated by an alteration in bowel habits associated with IBS. However, careful diagnostic evaluation is required before rectal bleeding can be ascribed to distal benign causes.

A complete health history should be elicited in the presence of abdominal pain with an alteration in bowel habits. The history should include a thorough investigation of the presenting symptoms, the associated symptoms, and the presence of nocturnal symptoms. The patient should be questioned about the exact onset of symptoms and stool consistency based on the Bristol Stool Form Scale (available @ https://americannursetoday.com/wp-content/uploads/2015/01/Bristol-Stool-Chart-PDF.pdf), number of stools daily, and previous diagnostic evaluations for similar symptoms. A past medical and surgical history plus family history of GI problems—such as colon cancer, inflammatory bowel disease, and celiac disease—should be obtained. These are often associated with other disease processes and need further evaluation. Additionally, patients with IBS can have symptoms consistent with other comorbidities or disorders, including other functional gastrointestinal disorders (FGIDs); gastroesophageal reflux disease (GERD); psychiatric disorders such as depression, anxiety, and obsessive-compulsive disorders; chronic fatigue syndrome; fibromyalgia; gynecological disorders; and asthma.[12]

The patient should be asked about recent travel, GI infections, and the use of all prescription or over-the-counter medications that could cause diarrhea or constipation. A thorough review of diet, with particular emphasis on any food allergies or sensitivities such as lactose or fructose intolerance, should be undertaken.[10] The review of symptoms should focus on the differential diagnoses for abdominal pain with an alteration in bowel habits. A menstrual history and gynecologic review of symptoms are essential in women to exclude urogenital sources of abdominal pain, such as pelvic inflammatory disease (PID), ovarian cysts, uterine fibroids, or endometriosis. A sensitive psychosocial history should be elicited to determine sources of stress, coping mechanisms, support systems, reactions to stress in the past, and the use of psychological counseling services to cope with past stressors. A history of physical or sexual abuse as a child or an adult should also be explored at some point.

A thorough physical examination should be performed to exclude organic disease and to reassure the patient. With IBS, the physical examination findings are often unremarkable. An abdominal, pelvic, and rectal examination should be performed. Increased tympany to percussion, a palpable and tender cordlike sigmoid colon, and tenderness on rectal examination have been reported. Significant abdominal tenderness or rectal tenderness, masses, or blood in the stool warrants further investigation.

DIAGNOSTICS

The diagnostic goals for patients with suspected IBS are to establish an early diagnosis, exclude the presence of alternative or coexisting diagnoses, and avoid unnecessary diagnostic testing. When planning a diagnostic strategy for the patient with an alteration in bowel habits, the provider should consider several factors, including the duration and severity of symptoms, current medications, the demographic features, any family history of colon cancer, the nature and extent of psychosocial issues, and previous diagnostic evaluations for similar symptoms.[9,10] An initial approach should be based on the Rome IV criteria (Box 121.1), a thorough history and physical examination, and a limited diagnostic screen to exclude organic disease. Few if any diagnostic tests are required in young healthy patients who meet the symptom-based criteria for IBS and do not have "red flags" suggestive of organic disease. A diagnosis of IBS with adequate initial evaluation is rarely associated with a need for additional diagnostics in the future; however, providers should always be aware of "red flags" suggesting that there has been a concerning change.

Although the diagnosis of IBS is based on the patient's symptoms, a limited screen for organic disease should be completed. For patients with persistent pain, diarrhea, and weight loss, serological testing (i.e., tissue transglutaminase antibodies [tTG-IgA]) for celiac disease is indicated, but the patient must be on a diet that includes gluten.[10,18] Fecal calprotectin should be considered in patients with chronic diarrhea, especially if the differential diagnosis suggests inflammatory bowel disease.[19]

For patients with complaints of excess gas and bloating or constipation-predominant symptoms a kidney, ureter, and bladder (KUB) scan of the abdomen, which will aid in determining the amount of stool in the bowel, should be obtained. Other diagnostics include a complete blood count (CBC) with differential; serum glucose, electrolytes, blood urea nitrogen (BUN), and creatinine; erythrocyte sedimentation rate (ESR) or C-reactive protein; thyroid-stimulating hormone (TSH) level; and stool specimen for occult blood and fecal leukocytes. If fecal leukocytes are present, stool culture specimens for enteric pathogens, ova and parasites, and *Clostridium difficile* should be obtained. If the result for occult blood is positive, the patient should be referred to a gastroenterologist for evaluation. A colonoscopy is typically recommended for young (<40 years) healthy patients with an acute change in bowel habits or rectal discomfort. A colonoscopy should also be performed for patients older than 50 years (45 years per the 2018 American Cancer Society recommendations) or those with weight loss, anemia, occult blood, or risk factors for colorectal cancer.[20]

Many patients with IBS are also lactose-intolerant. Any patient with bloating, gas, distention, and diarrhea who cannot be diagnosed as having IBS on symptoms alone should undergo a 2-week trial of a lactose-free diet or a hydrogen breath test to exclude lactase deficiency.[21] An alternative is to have patients drink a quart of milk. If the patient does not experience symptoms, lactose intolerance is unlikely.

Liver function tests (LFTs) and an abdominal ultrasound to exclude gallstones may be required, depending on the constellation of symptoms. Patients with suspected urogenital causes of abdominal pain require further diagnostic testing or referral to a gynecologist.

BOX 121.1

Rome IV Diagnostic Criteria for Irritable Bowel Syndrome

For diagnosis, the criteria required is that the patient symptoms must be present at least 3 months and the initial symptom onset must have occurred at least 6 months prior to the diagnosis of IBS. Additional principles for diagnosis include the following:

Abdominal pain that occurred a minimum of once each week for the previous 3 months, in combination with two or more of the following features:

- Defecation-related pain
- Pain related to change in stool frequency
- Pain associated with change in appearance of stool (lumpy and hard or loose and watery)

The patient's abnormal stools should be quantified on the Bristol Stool Form Scale quantification of stool consistency on days when at least one abnormal bowel movement occurs. For example, abnormal stool types per the Bristol Stool Scale would be considered constipated if the patient describes # 1, separate hard lumps, like nuts that are described as hard to pass or # 2, sausage-shaped, but lumpy. Diarrhea on the Bristol Stool Scale would be described as a mushy stool with fluffy, ragged edges (#6), or watery without solid pieces and entirely liquid (#7).

Modified from Lacy, B. E., & Patel, N. K. (2017). Rome criteria and a diagnostic approach to irritable bowel syndrome. *Journal of Clinical Medicine, 6*(11), 99.[28]

INITIAL DIAGNOSTICS

Irritable Bowel Syndrome

LABORATORY
- CBC with differential
- ESR, C-reactive protein
- Serum glucose, electrolytes, BUN, creatinine
- TSH
- Stool for occult blood and fecal leukocytes (if fecal leukocytes are present, test for enteric pathogens, ova and parasites, and *C. difficile*)
- LFTs[a]
- Serum immunoglobulin A tissue transglutaminase antibody (if celiac disease is a consideration)[a]
- Hydrogen breath test[a]
- Fecal calprotectin[a]

IMAGING
- KUB study (flat plate and upright)[a]
- Barium enema[a]
- Abdominal ultrasound[a]

OTHER DIAGNOSTICS
- Flexible sigmoidoscopy or colonoscopy[a]

[a]If indicated.

If the initial diagnostic screen is negative, treatment of symptoms should be initiated and reevaluated in 3 to 6 weeks. This diagnostic strategy allows a more conservative and cost-effective evaluation. If the initial treatment fails, additional diagnostic studies or a referral to a gastroenterologist should be considered. IBS patients older than 50 years with new or changed symptoms require repeated evaluation.

DIFFERENTIAL DIAGNOSIS

A number of organic diseases have presentations similar to those of IBS. It is essential that they be considered in the diagnostic reasoning process. Colon cancer, inflammatory bowel disease, cholecystitis, pancreatic insufficiency, intestinal ischemia, intestinal parasites, lactase deficiency, fructose intolerance, malabsorption syndromes such as celiac disease, and viral gastroenteritis can cause abdominal pain or a change in bowel habits. Medications can cause constipation or diarrhea. Hypothyroidism can cause constipation, whereas hyperthyroidism and diabetes can cause diarrhea. Psychiatric conditions—including anxiety disorders, depression, and somatization—are also a consideration in the evaluation of the patient with a change in bowel habits.[10] Urogenital causes—such as PID, endometriosis, ovarian cyst, and uterine fibroid—are possible causes of lower abdominal pain and gynecologic symptoms in women.

INTERPROFESSIONAL COLLABORATIVE MANAGEMENT

Nonpharmacologic Management

The focus of IBS treatment is symptomatic and includes dietary modifications, medications, supportive and behavioral therapy, education, and reassurance. One important factor in the successful management of IBS appears is the establishment of a therapeutic relationship. A nonjudgmental attentive approach is essential to help patients shift their focus from finding the cause of their symptoms to finding a way to cope with them. Health care providers must make the correct diagnosis as early as possible, initiate appropriate treatment, and avoid expensive or unnecessary tests.

Because both physiologic and psychosocial factors appear to play a role in the severity of symptoms and the expression of illness, both must be considered in the development of a management plan.[9,22] Diagnosis and treatment of any underlying psychological disorders, such as anxiety and depression, are essential.[9] Most patients with IBS have mild symptoms and can be managed in a primary care setting. They usually respond to education, reassurance, and dietary and lifestyle modifications. A smaller number have moderate symptoms that can be intermittent and disabling. Patients may have psychological distress from their symptoms, but their symptoms correlate with gut physiology.[7] Cognitive behavioral therapy can be effective for patients with IBS, depression, and anxiety. In some cases psychological counseling may be indicated (quality of evidence: low).[22] A small number of patients have severe and refractory symptoms associated with psychosocial difficulties and require antidepressant medication, mental health referral, and possibly a pain management evaluation.[9] These patients require a team approach that includes co-management with a gastroenterologist. In the future, biofeedback may play an important role in the treatment of IBS as protocols are now being explored.[23]

Dietary Modification

Although true food allergies are an uncommon cause, many patients with IBS report food intolerances. Although there is no evidence that food allergy testing and food elimination diets are effective, many patients (e.g., those with nonceliac gluten sensitivity) recognize these triggers and may choose to avoid these foods.[8,10,24] These patients may also benefit from a referral to a dietician for a trial of low FODMAPs (fermentable oligo-di-monosaccharides and polyols) diet for 1 to 2 months.[24] In some cases, it is not what the patient eats but rather the act of eating that precipitates symptoms; large meals can cause cramping and diarrhea.[9] Gas, bloating, distention, and a change in bowel habits are often attributed to the intake of certain foods. Dairy products and gas-forming foods are common offenders, but foods artificially sweetened with fructose or sorbitol, carbonated beverages, caffeine, and alcohol are also possible causes.[9,18]

Although care should be taken to avoid unnecessary dietary restrictions because evidence of benefit is unclear, the initial recommendations should focus on elimination of foods suspected of causing or aggravating individual symptoms. Use of a diary to record food intake and symptoms can help to identify offending foods. Lactose intolerance should be excluded in all patients who are initially seen with symptoms of IBS.

Fiber is likely to decrease constipation, but its role in relieving abdominal pain and diarrhea is less clear. Soluble fiber therapy (i.e., oats) in IBS is recommended (quality of evidence: moderate) for patients with constipation-dominant symptoms.[19] Insoluble fiber, such as that found in wheat bran and corn, often increases symptoms of bloating and abdominal pain because of colonic distention and should therefore be provided in incremental steps of 2 to 3 g each day. Clinical experience has demonstrated that many patients benefit from fiber after an initial period of bloating and abdominal discomfort. A trial of a minimum of 20 g of fiber per day, which should be added gradually, seems reasonable for the treatment of IBS.[10]

An alternative to synthetic fiber is a diet high in whole grains and natural fiber, a daily fluid intake of 64 ounces, and a set time each day to use the bathroom. Exercise has been shown to improve many health problems; however, no data provide support for routine exercise and the improvement of symptoms.

Pharmacologic Management

Fiber. Synthetic fiber supplements are more soluble than natural fiber and may be better tolerated by some patients.[9] Slow introduction of the fiber load helps to reduce gas and bloating. Use of psyllium (Metamucil or Benefiber), calcium polycarbophil (FiberCon), or methylcellulose (Citrucel) taken daily with food or 8 oz of liquid is a pharmacologic consideration (quality of evidence: moderate).[25]

Antispasmodics. Despite a lack of clinical evidence to support benefit, antispasmodics seem to slow bowel contractions, decreasing symptoms of diarrhea and abdominal discomfort (quality of evidence: low).[25] Anticholinergics act to reduce sigmoid motility in response to a fatty meal. Medications such as dicyclomine (Bentyl), 10 to 40 mg four times daily as needed, may be tried by patients who experience postprandial abdominal pain, gas, and bloating. For maximum effectiveness, the medication should be taken 30 to 60 minutes before meals. Hyoscyamine sulfate, the active ingredient in Levsin and Donnatal, is also an effective antispasmodic but has several side effects, including urinary retention, tachycardia, and dry mouth. Clidinium, the active ingredient in Librax, is another antispasmodic but is combined with a benzodiazepine and has confusion and fatigue as common side effects. Dicyclomine acts more selectively on the smooth muscle of the GI tract and may produce fewer side effects than the nonselective anticholinergics. Analgesic medications, particularly narcotics, should be avoided if at all possible. Librax is listed in the Beers criteria as a medication that should be avoided in older adults (i.e., patients older than age 65).

Antidiarrheal Agents. Loperamide (Imodium), 2 to 4 mg 45 minutes before eating as needed (up to four times a day), decreases intestinal transit time, enhances intestinal water absorption, and strengthens rectal sphincter tone, thereby improving the diarrhea, urgency, and fecal soiling in IBS patients with diarrhea (quality of evidence: low).[25] Patients may take a maximum of 16 mg/day as needed to control symptoms. Polycarbophil can be added to help increase stool bulk. Pepto-Bismol, Kaopectate, and bile acid–sequestering agents, such as cholestyramine (Questran, Prevalite), can also be considered in the treatment of diarrhea-predominant IBS. Rifaximin (Xifaxan) 550 mg, a miscellaneous antibiotic taken three times a day for 2 weeks, has also been used successfully in the treatment of diarrhea-associated IBS (quality of evidence: moderate).[25] Usually prescribed for patients who have continued diarrhea and pain despite after trying other treatments, rifaximin can be repeated twice if necessary. Eluxadoline (Viberzi), 75 to 100 mg PO twice daily, is a more recent medication being used successfully for patients with IBS-D.[26] However, it is important to note that there are many contraindications to eluxadoline, including alcohol use, history of constipation (chronic or severe), pancreatitis, Child-Pugh class C liver impairment, cholecystectomy, and GI or biliary obstruction.

Alosetron (Lotronex), a 5-HT$_3$ receptor antagonist, is used for the treatment of abdominal pain, diarrhea, and bloating in women with severe chronic diarrhea-associated IBS who have not responded to other therapies (quality of evidence: moderate).[25] However, alosetron should be prescribed only by physicians participating in a prescribing program for this medication.

Anticonstipation Agents. Synthetic fiber is beneficial in treating constipation associated with IBS. In addition to fiber therapy, increased fluids, and regular exercise, patients with constipation may benefit from stool softeners and osmotic laxatives such as lactulose and polyethylene glycol (MiraLax), though evidence is lacking to support its use (quality of evidence: very low).[25] Stimulant laxatives should be avoided whenever possible. Lubiprostone (Amitiza), 8 mcg PO twice daily, was approved by the US Food and Drug Administration (FDA) for chronic constipation and IBS associated with constipation (quality of evidence: moderate).[25] Linaclotide (Linzess), 290 mcg PO daily, works on the guanylate cyclase-C receptor to decrease the absorption of sodium ions, which allows the secretion of water to assist in defecation; the drug is also approved for IBS associated with constipation (quality of evidence: high).[5,27]

Psychotropic Agents. Antidepressants, including tricyclic agents and selective serotonin reuptake inhibitors (SSRIs), are often used to treat IBS, particularly in patients with severe or refractory pain and symptoms, impaired daily function, and associated depression or panic attacks (quality of evidence: high).[9,25] The anticholinergic properties of the tricyclic antidepressants (amitriptyline, nortriptyline, desipramine) are believed to contribute to their effectiveness in treating the pain, gas, bloating, and frequent stools associated with IBS. Small clinical trials have shown benefit in alleviating abdominal pain. Because of their tendency to decrease transit times, which in turn causes constipation, the use of tricyclic agents should be avoided in IBS patients with constipation.

Because of the lower side effect profile of SSRIs, these should be considered instead of tricyclic agents in patients with constipation.[8] These medications reduce depression, anxiety, and somatization rather than relieving abdominal pain per se. A common side effect of SSRIs is diarrhea; therefore these drugs may prove most beneficial in treating IBS patients with constipation. There is no clinical research to support the use of benzodiazepines in IBS; their use should be avoided because of their addictive potential.

Alternative Therapies

Several alternative therapies have been studied in IBS, including probiotics, cognitive behavioral therapy, hypnosis, guided imagery, relaxation techniques, and stress management.[5] Acupuncture decreased symptoms in some studies but not all.[25,27] Alternative therapies seem to have some value in reducing GI symptoms, anxiety, and other psychological symptoms. Patients with underlying psychological issues may benefit from a referral to a psychologist, mental health clinical nurse specialist, or psychiatric nurse practitioner. For patients with severe, refractory pain, referral to a pain management program can be beneficial.

Probiotics are live microorganisms similar to the normal bacterial flora of the GI tract. Probiotics reduce inflammation or alter gut flora and seem to decrease flatulence and relieve bloating; however, the use of probiotics remains controversial (quality of evidence: low).[19,25]

Peppermint oil is a natural antispasmodic. Its GI effects are similar to those of calcium channel blockers, causing smooth muscle relaxation and aiding postprandial pain and bloating (quality of evidence: moderate).[25]

LIFE-SPAN CONSIDERATIONS

IBS is a chronic recurrent disorder that frequently develops in late adolescence to early adulthood and continues throughout life. Exacerbations are common and often correlate with life stressors. Once thought to be a disease of young women, IBS is also increasingly being recognized in men and older adults. An IBS diagnosis in an older person must be made cautiously and in consultation with a gastroenterologist to avoid missing a more serious diagnosis.

COMPLICATIONS

It is important to recognize that IBS is a chronic recurrent GI disorder in the majority of cases; serious complications from IBS are extremely rare. In some patients, the chronic nature of symptoms leads to a reduced quality of life and clinical depression. Chronic constipation may also result in hemorrhoids, anal fissures, fecal impaction, and, rarely, intestinal obstruction.

INDICATIONS FOR REFERRAL OR HOSPITALIZATION

Nocturnal symptoms, abnormal physical findings such as lymphadenopathy or an abdominal or rectal mass, anemia, bloody stools, fever, recurrent nausea and/or vomiting, weight loss, or elevated CA125 are incompatible with a diagnosis of IBS and require immediate further diagnostic evaluation or referral. Additionally, patients with a first-degree relative with GI malignant disease, IBS, or ovarian cancer require immediate evaluation and appropriate referral.

 Physician consultation and referral to a gastroenterologist are indicated if initial treatment of IBS fails, if organic disease is suspected or found, or if the patient is older than 50 years or has an established diagnosis of IBS and is reporting a change in the usual pattern of symptoms. Gastroenterology specialists are also helpful in the comanagement of patients with complex IBS.

PATIENT AND FAMILY EDUCATION

Dietary and lifestyle modifications—such as avoiding foods that trigger symptoms, increasing fluids and fiber, getting regular exercise, and using alternative therapies—should be discussed with patients. Information about what constitutes "normal" bowel habits should be provided. Bowel retraining should be encouraged by recommending sitting on the toilet (without straining) for 15 to 20 minutes each morning after breakfast. Medications for symptom control should be reviewed, including a conversation about laxative abuse.

Patients should be informed that the symptoms of IBS are very real and are caused by increased sensitivity and reactivity of the gut to stimuli, resulting in pain or abnormal motility. They should be reassured that IBS is a chronic condition characterized by periods of remission and exacerbation that often correlate with physical and psychological stressors but that IBS usually does not lead to cancer or inflammatory bowel disease. Patients should understand that although there is no cure, there is help, and that most patients learn to cope with their symptoms and lead productive lives.

HEALTH PROMOTION

The chronic nature of IBS symptoms may cause a patient with IBS to ignore a change in bowel habits resulting from an organic condition. Patients must be told that although IBS does not increase their risk for colorectal cancer, a change in bowel habits that is atypical of their usual pattern of symptoms should be reported to the health care provider. In addition, screening for colorectal cancer per current guidelines is important for all patients.

REFERENCES

1. Sultan, S., & Malhotra, A. (2017). Irritable bowel syndrome. *Annals of Internal Medicine, 166*(11), ITC81–ITC96. doi:10.7326/AITC201706060.
2. Drossman, D. A. (2016). Functional gastrointestinal disorders: History, pathophysiology, clinical features and Rome IV. *Gastroenterology, 150,* 1262–1279.
3. Ford, A. F., Lacy, B. E., & Talley, N. J. (2017). Irritable bowel syndrome. *The New England Journal of Medicine, 376,* 2566–2578.
4. Canavan, C., West, J., & Card, T. (2014). The epidemiology of irritable bowel syndrome. *Clinical Epidemiology, 6,* 71–80.
5. Schmick, M., & Hornecker, J. (2017). Irritable bowel syndrome: A review of treatment options, gastroenterology. *U. S. Pharmacist, 42*(12), 20–26.
6. Sayuk, G. S., & Gyawali, C. P. (2015). Irritable bowel syndrome: Modern concepts and management options. *The American Journal of Medicine, 128,* 817–827.
7. Faresjo, A., Grodzinsky, E., Hallert, C., & Timpka, T. (2013). Patients with irritable bowel syndrome are more burdened by co-morbidity and worry about serious diseases than healthy controls—eight years follow-up of IBS patients in primary care. *BMC Public Health, 13,* 832.
8. Forte, F., Pizzoferrato, M., Lopetuso, L., & Scaldaferri, F. (2012). The use of anti-spasmodics in the treatment of irritable bowel syndrome: Focus on otilonium bromide. *European Review for Medical and Pharmacological Sciences, 16,* 25–37.
9. National Institute of Diabetes and Digestive and Kidney Diseases. Irritable bowel syndrome. Retrieved from http://digestive.niddk.nih.gov/ddiseases/pubs/ibs/index.aspx. (Retrieved 28 June 2018).
10. Martin, S. (2014). Irritable bowel syndrome evidence-based treatment. *Clinician Reviews, 24*(1), 44–51.
11. Khanbhai, A., & Sura, D. S. (2013). Irritable bowel syndrome for primary care physicians. *British Journal of Medical Practitioners, 6*(1), 34–37.
12. Berrill, J. W., Green, J. T., Hood, K., & Campbell, A. K. (2013). Symptoms of irritable bowel syndrome in patients with inflammatory bowel disease: Examining the role of sub-clinical inflammation and the impact on clinical assessment of disease activity. *Alimentary Pharmacology and Therapeutics, 38,* 44–51.
13. Hayes, P. A., Fraher, M. H., & Quigley, E. M. (2014). Irritable bowel syndrome: The role of food in pathogenesis and management. *Gastroenterologia Y Hepatologia, 10*(3), 164–174.
14. Farhadi, A., Banton, D., & Keefer, L. (2018). Connecting our gut feeling and how our gut feels: The role of well-being attributes in irritable bowel syndrome. *Journal of Neurogastroenterology and Motility, 24*(2), 289–298. http://doi.org/10.5056/jnm17117.
15. Halpin, S. J., & Ford, A. C. (2012). Prevalence of symptoms meeting criteria for irritable bowel syndrome in inflammatory bowel disease: Systematic review and meta-analysis. *The American Journal of Gastroenterology, 107,* 1474–1482.
16. Harkness, E. F., Harrington, V., Hinder, S., O'Brien, S. J., Thompson, D. G., Beech, P., et al. (2013). GP perspectives of irritable bowel syndrome—an accepted illness, but management deviates from guidelines: A qualitative study. *BMC Family Practice, 14,* 92–99.
17. Pimentel, M. (2018). Evidenced based management of irritable bowel syndrome with diarrhea. American Institute for Value Based Medicine. https://www.ajmc.com/journals/supplement/2018/evidence-based-management-of-ibsd/evidencebased-management-of-irritable-bowel-syndrome-with-diarrhea?p=1. (Accessed 1 June 2018).
18. Celiac Disease Foundation. Screening. https://celiac.org/celiac-disease/understanding-celiac-disease-2/diagnosing-celiac-disease/screening/. (Accessed 30 June 2018).
19. Chandar, A. K. (2017). Diagnosis and treatment of irritable bowel syndrome with predominant constipation in the primary-care setting: Focus on linaclotide. *International Journal of General Medicine, 10,* 385–393. http://doi.org/10.2147/IJGM.S126581.
20. American Cancer Society. (2018). American Cancer Society updates colorectal cancer screening guideline. https://www.cancer.org/latest-news/american-cancer-society-updates-colorectal-cancer-screening-guideline.html. (Accessed 30 June 2018).
21. Rana, S. V., & Malik, A. (2014). Hydrogen breath tests in gastrointestinal diseases. *Indian Journal of Clinical Biochemistry, 29*(4), 398–405. doi:10.1007/s12291-014-0426-4.
22. Li, L., Xiong, L., Zhang, S., Yu, Q., & Chen, M. (2014). Cognitive-behavioral therapy for irritable bowel syndrome: A meta-analysis. *Journal of Psychosomatic Research, 77,* 1–2.
23. Goldenberg, J. Z., Brignall, M., Hamilton, M., Beardsley, J., & Lichtenstein, B. (2017). Biofeedback for treatment of irritable bowel syndrome. *The Cochrane Database of Systematic Reviews,* (1), Art. No.: CD012530, doi:10.1002/14651858.CD012530.
24. Losurdo, G., Principi, M., Iannone, A., Amoruso, A., Ierardi, E., Di Leo, A., et al. (2018). Extra-intestinal manifestations of non-celiac gluten sensitivity: An expanding paradigm. *World Journal of Gastroenterology, 24*(14), 1521–1530. doi:10.3748/wjg.v24.i14.1521.
25. Ford, A. C., Moayyedi, P., Lacy, B. E., Lembo, A. J., Saito, Y. A., Schiller, L. R., et al. (2014). American College of Gastroenterology monograph on the management of irritable bowel syndrome and chronic idiopathic constipation. *The American Journal of Gastroenterology, 109,* S2–S26, quiz S27.
26. Lembo, A. J., Lacy, B. E., Zuckerman, M. J., Schey, R., Dove, L. S., Andrae, D. A., et al. (2016). Eluxadoline for irritable bowel syndrome with diarrhea. *The New England Journal of Medicine, 374,* 242–253. doi:10.1056/NEJMoa1505180.

27. Love, B. L., Johnson, A., & Smith, L. (2014). Linaclotide: A novel agent for chronic constipation and irritable bowel syndrome. *American Journal of Health-System Pharmacy, 71,* 1081–1091.

28. Lacy, B. E., & Patel, N. K. (2017). Rome criteria and a diagnostic approach to irritable bowel syndrome. *Journal of Clinical Medicine, 6*(11), 99. http://doi.org/10.3390/jcm6110099.

CHAPTER **122**

JAUNDICE

Terry Mahan Buttaro

 Physician consultation is indicated for patients with new-onset jaundice.

DEFINITION AND EPIDEMIOLOGY

Jaundice, or icterus, is a yellow or greenish discoloration of the skin, sclerae, and mucous membranes caused by bile pigments of conjugated or unconjugated bilirubin.[1] There are many causes of jaundice, necessitating determination of the underlying disorder.

Jaundice can be divided into three categories: prehepatic, hepatic, and posthepatic. Prehepatic jaundice is caused by conditions that produce excessive bilirubin. Examples include any condition that causes hemolysis. Hepatic jaundice is a result of hepatic injury, including infections, toxins, autoimmune disorders, and tumors. Posthepatic jaundice, also called *obstructive jaundice,* is a result of complete or partial obstruction of the bile ducts. Pancreatic tumors and gallstones are the most common causes of posthepatic jaundice.[2]

The causes of jaundice are categorized according to (1) symptoms (acute or chronic), (2) evidence of bile duct dilation, and (3) jaundice of the conjugated or unconjugated varieties.[1] Jaundice is common in newborns and occurs in 60% to 80% of term infants 4 to 14 days after birth.[2] In older children and young adults, common causes include viral hepatitis, Gilbert syndrome, drug-induced hepatitis, pregnancy, cirrhosis, and alcoholic hepatitis. In older patients, the most common causes are cirrhosis, pancreatic cancer, metastatic cancer to the liver, sepsis, common bile duct stone, and medication-induced hepatitis.[3,4] Alcoholic liver disease, associated with loneliness and depression, is a common cause in older adults.[3] Common causes of jaundice are presented in Box 122.1.

PATHOPHYSIOLOGY

The liver plays a major role in the metabolism of bile pigments. This process is divided into three distinct phases: (1) hepatic uptake, (2) conjugation, and (3) excretion.[1] A byproduct of hemolysis is bilirubin, which is produced through the breakdown of hemoglobin in red blood cells (RBCs). There are two forms of bilirubin: indirect, or unconjugated, bilirubin (which is protein-bound) and direct, or conjugated, bilirubin. The direct form circulates freely in the blood until it reaches the liver, where it is conjugated with glucuronide transferase and excreted into the bile.[1] An increase in unconjugated bilirubin is often associated with an increase in the destruction of RBCs. An increase in conjugated bilirubin is more likely seen with liver dysfunction or obstruction.[1] Disturbance in the passage of conjugated bilirubin from the liver to the intestine is a common cause of jaundice in patients older than 60

BOX **122.1**

Classification and Causes of Jaundice

UNCONJUGATED HYPERBILIRUBINEMIA (PREDOMINANTLY INDIRECT-ACTING BILIRUBIN)
- Increased bilirubin production
- Hemolytic anemias (thalassemias, sideroblastic anemias, some pernicious anemias), hematoma, infarction
- Decreased hepatic uptake
- Posthepatitis, drug reactions, sepsis, prolonged fasting
- Decreased bilirubin conjugation (decreased hepatic glucuronosyltransferase)
- Hereditary transferase deficiency (Gilbert syndrome, Crigler-Najjar syndrome)
- Acquired transferase deficiency: drug inhibition (e.g., chloramphenicol), breast milk, hepatocellular disease
- Neonatal jaundice
- Ineffective erythropoiesis (megaloblastic anemias)
- Hematomas
- Pulmonary emboli
- Chronic hepatitis

CONJUGATED HYPERBILIRUBINEMIA (PREDOMINANTLY DIRECT-ACTING BILIRUBIN)
- Impaired excretion: intrahepatic defects
- Familial defects (Dubin-Johnson syndrome, Rotor syndrome), recurrent intrahepatic cholestasis, cholestatic jaundice of pregnancy
- Acquired disorders: viral or drug-induced hepatitis, cirrhosis, sepsis, postoperative complications, androgens. chlorpromazine, acetaminophen, sulfonamides, NSAIDs, aspirin, industrial poisons
- Impaired excretion: extrahepatic defects
- Gallstones, biliary malformation or strictures, infection, biliary or pancreatic tumors, chronic pancreatitis, pancreatic pseudocyst, metastasis to the hepatic hilum, primary bile duct lymphoma

NSAIDs, Non-steroidal antiinflammatory drugs.

years. With bile duct obstruction, bilirubin is conjugated by the hepatocytes but cannot flow into the duodenum.[1] Therefore bilirubin accumulates in the liver and enters the bloodstream, causing hyperbilirubinemia.

Extrahepatic obstructive jaundice (cholestasis) develops if the common bile duct is occluded. Frequently the cause is gallstones (choledocholithiasis), tumors (especially pancreatic carcinoma), or strictures, but there are rarer causes (e.g., parasites, pancreatic pseudocysts).[1,2,5,6] Because conjugated bilirubin is water soluble, it is excreted in the urine. This produces the characteristic orange urine with elevated conjugated bilirubin produced by inflammation.

Intrahepatic obstructive jaundice involves disturbances in hepatocyte function or obstruction of bile canaliculi. The uptake, conjugation, and excretion of bilirubin are affected, resulting in increased levels of conjugated and unconjugated bilirubin.[1]

Failure of liver cells to conjugate bilirubin causes hepatocellular damage, resulting in increased plasma concentrations of unconjugated bilirubin. In addition, bilirubin cannot pass from the liver to the intestine.[1] The causes of hepatocellular damage include infections, medications, toxins, and genetic defects leading to decreased enzyme production.

Hemolytic jaundice is caused by excessive hemolysis of RBCs. An increased amount of unconjugated bilirubin is formed through metabolism of the heme component of destroyed RBCs and exceeds the conjugation ability of the liver.[1] This causes the blood levels of unconjugated bilirubin to rise. Hemolysis can occur with blood transfusion reactions, after cardiopulmonary bypass, with sickle cell anemia, and with marrow or splenic destruction of RBCs. In sickle cell anemia, abnormal hemoglobin and a fragile cell membrane lead to hemolysis and an increase in the amount of free unconjugated bilirubin.[1] Bone marrow development problems and defective erythropoiesis are conditions in which poorly manufactured erythrocytes are fragile and have a short life span. The result is an excess of unconjugated bilirubin that reaches the liver for conjugation.[1] The most common causes of jaundice are hepatocellular destruction and mechanical obstruction of the biliary tracts.[1,2]

Jaundice can also be associated with bilirubin disorders. Crigler-Najjar, Gilbert, Dubin-Johnson, and Rotor syndromes are examples of inherited hyperbilirubinemia disorders.

CLINICAL PRESENTATION AND PHYSICAL EXAMINATION

Appropriate history includes determining whether the jaundice is acute or chronic and ascertaining associated symptoms (e.g., fever, weight loss, anorexia, rash, pruritus, abdominal pain, or musculoskeletal aches and pains). In acute jaundice, inquiry focuses on hepatitis risks: recent travel; transfusions; tattoos; intravenous drug use; alcohol intake; medications (prescription drugs, herbals, or over-the-counter preparations); food, toxin, animal, or infected person exposures; unsafe sexual practices; and symptoms of biliary tract disease.[2] Chronic jaundice may suggest hepatitis (B, C, D, or autoimmune), biliary tract disease, pancreatitis, or chronic alcohol intake. Weight loss, anorexia, malaise, and other symptoms of cancer are noted.[6] In addition, a list of medications (including over-the-counter medications) and a complete family history—including cancer, Wilson disease, G6PD deficiency, Gilbert syndrome, hemochromatosis, and hereditary hemolytic anemias—provide vital information for an appropriate diagnosis. Exposure to toxins, including use of herbal products, and a surgical history should also be elicited.[2,7]

Jaundice is most commonly observed in the face, trunk, and sclerae. Bilirubin is distributed uniformly in the sclerae and is differentiated from the normal occurrence of the yellow subscleral fat that collects in the periphery. In African Americans, the hard palate or ventral surface of the tongue helps clinical jaundice to be observed. Jaundice caused by carotene does not stain the sclerae but rather is seen in the forehead, around the alae nasi, and in the palms and soles. The patient with jaundice may have pruritus, which often accompanies obstructive jaundice. The pruritus is caused by nerve injury in the skin by the bile pigments. Cutaneous xanthomas may be seen in patients with jaundice from chronic cholestasis and suggest hypercholesterolemia. The presence of spider angiomas, palmar erythema, and ascites combined with malaise, anorexia, and right-upper-quadrant discomfort suggests chronic hepatocellular disease or cirrhosis. Colicky right-upper-quadrant pain, weight loss, and light-colored stools may be present in obstructive jaundice. Intermittent colicky right-upper-quadrant pain before the onset of jaundice suggests choledocholithiasis. Fever and chills may accompany biliary obstruction and virus- or drug-induced hepatitis. Occult blood in the stools suggests cancer as a cause of jaundice.[6]

A complete physical examination is required to determine the underlying cause of acute jaundice. Essential components are determination of vital signs (including temperature); evaluation of the skin (including the palms and soles), sclerae, and mucous membranes; assessment of the cardiovascular system for congestive heart failure; and evaluation of the abdomen for ascites, organomegaly, guarding, and tenderness.[1,3] Fever and right-upper-quadrant tenderness are most often associated with choledocholithiasis, cholangitis, or cholecystitis. An enlarged, tender liver suggests acute hepatic inflammation or a rapidly growing hepatic tumor.[2] Splenomegaly suggests portal hypertension from acute or active chronic hepatitis as well as cirrhosis.

Chronic jaundice mandates evaluation for chronic liver disease. Gynecomastia, testicular atrophy, and splenomegaly are strongly associated with cirrhosis. In addition, palmar erythema, facial telangiectasia, and Dupuytren contractures are associated with cirrhosis from chronic ethanol ingestion. Lymphadenopathy suggests malignant disease and can be related to a pancreatic tumor obstructing the splenic vein or to a metastatic lymphoma. When malignant disease is suspected, the investigation should concentrate on determining the location of the primary tumor as indicated by heme-positive stool, abdominal masses, breast masses, thyroid nodules, or supraclavicular lymphadenopathy.[6] Physical findings associated with specific liver diseases include distended neck veins and hepatojugular reflux (right-sided heart failure), xanthomas (primary biliary cirrhosis), and Kayser-Fleischer rings (Wilson disease).

DIAGNOSTICS

Liver function tests (LFTs)—including albumin, aspartate aminotransferase (AST), and alanine aminotransferase (ALT); total and direct serum bilirubin; serum alkaline phosphatase; stool guaiac; and urinalysis—are performed in addition to a complete blood count (CBC) with platelet count and a prothrombin time (PT) and International Normalized Ratio (INR). Urinalysis for bilirubin aids diagnosis because only conjugated bilirubin is associated with bilirubinuria.[8] Elevated ALT and AST levels result from hepatocellular necrosis or inflammation.[1] An AST level that is more than twice the ALT level is typical with alcoholic liver injury, although an AST greater than ALT can be present in nonalcoholic steatohepatitis (NASH) or Wilson disease. Elevated alkaline phosphatase levels can have varied causes, but those that are associated with liver problems include cholestasis, primary biliary cirrhosis, or infiltrative liver disease (e.g., tumor, abscess, granulomas).[7] A GGT level and fasting alkaline phosphatase isoenzymes should be obtained to correlate an elevated alk phos level. In obstructive liver disease, the alkaline phosphatase may be more than three times the normal level.

When the jaundice is not related to a biliary disorder or hepatic injury, the liver enzymes will be normal. A normal serum albumin concentration suggests a more acute disease process than the chronic disease associated with low serum albumin levels.[8]

Unconjugated (indirect) hyperbilirubinemia suggests a hemolytic disorder, such as an autoimmune or microangiopathic hemolytic anemia. The most common cause of mild elevations of unconjugated bilirubin is Gilbert syndrome, which, with a male predominance, affects up to 7% of the population.[1]

Direct hyperbilirubinemia results from hepatocellular inflammation, cholestatic liver disease, or extrahepatic biliary obstruction. The presence of direct hyperbilirubinemia without liver enzyme abnormalities is uncommon but is seen in pregnancy, in sepsis, or after recent surgery.[8–10] Patients with elevated conjugated bilirubin should be evaluated for evidence of viral hepatitis, drug toxicity, or hepatic congestion. Serologic studies are used to diagnose hepatitis A, B, C, and D.[2] Common causes of toxic hepatitis include acetaminophen, allopurinol, androgenic steroids, aspirin and other salicylates, nitrofurantoin, azathioprine, contraceptive steroids, chlorpromazine, erythromycin, glucocorticoids, mercaptopurine, methotrexate, plicamycin, nonsteroidal antiinflammatory drugs (NSAIDs), sulfonamides, and HIV medications (e.g., protease inhibitors).[11,12]

In patients with chronic liver disease lacking a defined cause, serum iron, transferrin saturation, and ferritin should be measured to screen for hemochromatosis. In hemochromatosis, the serum ferritin concentration is substantially elevated. Plasma iron levels may exceed 200 mcg/dL, and transferrin saturation exceeds 70%.[13] In patients younger than 30 years with abnormal LFT results or in those with hepatitis who test negative for viruses A, B, C, and D and neurological dysfunction, measurements of serum ceruloplasmin and urine copper levels are recommended to screen for Wilson disease.[2] Other laboratory diagnostics to consider include antimitochondrial antibodies (for primary biliary cirrhosis), antinuclear anti–smooth muscle and liver-kidney microsomal antibodies (for autoimmune hepatitis), and α_1-antitrypsin activity (for α_1-antitrypsin deficiency). Because chronic liver disease is associated with HIV, testing for HIV should also be done.[2,14]

Hepatobiliary imaging is recommended if the liver chemistry profile suggests cholestasis or extrahepatic obstruction. Ultrasonography is more than 90% specific and close to 90% sensitive in detecting obstruction. A computed tomography (CT) scan with and without the administration of contrast material is indicated in cases where ultrasound examination was unsatisfactory.[15] However, ultrasonography is an effective means of detecting stones in the gallbladder and is somewhat more sensitive than a CT scan.[15] Endoscopic retrograde cholangiopancreatography (ERCP) or percutaneous transhepatic cholangiography is indicated if extrahepatic obstruction is strongly suspected.[15] ERCP may relieve the obstruction in the majority of cases. Newer imaging techniques to evaluate biliary obstruction and suspected malignant neoplasms include magnetic resonance cholangiopancreatography and endoscopic ultrasonography.[8,15] Percutaneous liver biopsy is the definitive study for determination of the cause and extent of hepatocellular dysfunction or infiltrative liver disease, particularly if metastatic disease or a hepatic mass is suspected.[2]

DIFFERENTIAL DIAGNOSIS

The etiology of jaundice is multifactorial; consequently the presence of coexisting disease is an important aspect of the evaluation. The finding of unconjugated hyperbilirubinemia can be related to increased bilirubin production (hemolytic anemia) or impaired bilirubin uptake and storage (hepatitis sequelae, posthepatitis conditions, Gilbert syndrome, drug reactions). Hereditary syndromes such as Crigler-Najjar and Gilbert syndromes (resulting from impaired glucuronosyltransferase activity) and Dubin-Johnson and Rotor syndromes (resulting from faulty excretion of bilirubin) are examples of causes of unconjugated bilirubin.[1] Conjugated hyperbilirubinemia can be caused by infectious or autoimmune hepatitis, cirrhosis, cholestasis, postoperative jaundice, spirochetal infections, infectious mononucleosis, sarcoidosis, lymphomas, and industrial toxins. Fever and chills suggest cholangitis. Causes of biliary obstructions can be intrahepatic (e.g., cirrhosis, hepatitis, NASH, obstruction of bile capillaries, malignancy, the intrahepatic cholestasis of pregnancy, and a variety of other disorders) or extrahepatic (e.g., common bile duct obstruction related to pancreatic edema, gallstones, or tumor).[16] Jaundice during pregnancy is most often related to viral hepatitis, whereas newborn jaundice, which is usually transient and not concerning, can be serious and associated with erythroblastosis fetalis, hemolysis, hepatic dysfunction or excretion, and immaturity of conjugating mechanisms within the liver.[9,16] Other differentials to consider include cirrhosis, choledochal cysts, cholangitis, cholestasis, choledocholithiasis, hepatobiliary tuberculosis, hemolytic anemia, lymphoma, pancreatitis (possibly autoimmune), primary sclerosing cholangitis, sarcoidosis, tumor, drug reactions including over-the-counter and herbal products, and toxins.

INTERPROFESSIONAL COLLABORATIVE MANAGEMENT

The treatment of jaundice relates to the underlying disease process. Most patients with viral hepatitis can be treated symptomatically on an outpatient basis (see Chapter 119), although this depends on the type of hepatitis and presence of associated liver dysfunction.[17] When liver enzymes fail to return to normal levels within 6 months, liver biopsy, unless contraindicated, is indicated.[2] Cholangitis requires antibiotic therapy and surgical consultation. For patients with cholangitis, nonoperative biliary drainage can be performed through ERCP with transhepatically placed stents.[18] Surgical therapy is usually required for extrahepatic biliary obstruction. Gilbert disease, Dubin-Johnson syndrome, and Rotor syndrome beyond the neonatal period rarely require treatment to lower the bilirubin level.[19] However, treatment of the primary disease process may be indicated if the presentation of these diseases is complicated by hemolytic anemia.

The treatment of uncomplicated cirrhosis consists of voluntary restriction of activity if the patient has weakness and fatigue. The diet should be high in protein but low in sodium, and alcohol should be avoided. This regimen almost invariably results in improvement of hepatocellular function in patients with alcohol-induced cirrhosis.[20] Multivitamins and folic acid (1 mg/day) are given if the patient's diet is inadequate. Tranquilizers and sedatives should be avoided. When serum potassium concentration falls below 3.5 mEq/L, the deficit will have to be appropriately repleted with oral potassium chloride. Protein is currently not commonly restricted in patients with cirrhosis, although it may be indicated in some instances. Lactulose is used to treat encephalopathy by decreasing blood ammonia. Dosed at 20 to 30 g three or four times daily, the goal is soft stools two to four times a day.[21] Rifaximin, 550 mg every 12 hours, can be added if encephalopathy is not improving with lactulose alone.[22] Rifaximin reduces encephalopathy risk by killing ammonia-producing bacteria in the gut.[22] Liver transplantation may be an option for patients who are no longer drinking alcohol but have severe cirrhosis. For patients with cirrhosis-associated bleeding risks, vitamin K (oral, subcutaneous, or intramuscular) is also commonly used, although the benefit is not completely clear.[23]

Pruritus, which is commonly associated with jaundice, may be disabling to some patients, resulting in depression. Early treatment with agents such as cholestyramine three times per day and antihistamines three or four times daily can be helpful, as can fragrance-free soaps, fewer baths or showers, and emollient use.

Ultrasound to monitor for hepatocellular carcinoma and continued monitoring of LFTs (at least twice a year), as well as serologic values, and the results of hematologic studies (blood counts, platelets, and PT) are recommended for all patients with jaundice to determine the presence of complications.

COMPLICATIONS

The complications of jaundice are directly related to the underlying disease process. In cirrhosis, infection and gastrointestinal bleeding often precipitate decompensation. Ascites, coagulation defects, electrolyte disorders, esophageal varices, hepatic failure, hepatorenal syndrome, hyperestrinism, portal hypertension, and portal-systemic encephalopathy are among the common difficulties patients with cirrhosis can experience.

Patients with hepatitis may experience one or two relapses during their recovery period. Complications of other underlying diseases associated with jaundice range from anemia to gastrointestinal infection, hepatocellular damage, encephalopathy, and postsurgical complications. The most serious postsurgical complication of stenting is recurrent jaundice from stent occlusion and recurrent cholangitis.[18]

INDICATIONS FOR REFERRAL OR HOSPITALIZATION

The management of patients with jaundice is complex because of the myriad underlying disease processes and potential complications. The primary care physician is always consulted to determine the diagnosis and initial management plans. Consultation with a gastroenterologist, hepatologist, or surgeon is also often indicated. For patients with hepatitis B or C infection, referral to a gastroenterologist is necessary to ensure appropriate serologic testing and treatment.

PATIENT AND FAMILY EDUCATION

It is imperative that patients understand the underlying disease process and preventive regimens. The Centers for Disease Control and Prevention (CDC) recommend that all high-risk individuals be screened for hepatitis B and C and that all individuals born in the years 1945 to 1965 be offered hepatitis C screening once.[23] The CDC also has recommendations for immunization against hepatitis A and B for all age groups.[24] The appropriate levels of activity and rest, the importance of medication adherence, the need for avoidance of over-the-counter medications that interfere with hepatic function, and the avoidance of any liver-toxic chemicals including alcohol should be emphasized. Appropriate dietary instruction is essential for patients with hepatic disease, and referral to a dietitian for instruction in specific diets is desirable.

REFERENCES

1. Grossman, S. C., & Porth, C. M. (2014). *Disorders of the skin integrity and function. Porth's pathophysiology* (9th ed.). Philadelphia: Lippincott Williams & Wilkins.
2. Berk, P., & Korenblat, K. (2012). Approach to the patient with jaundice or abnormal liver tests. In L. Goldman & A. I. Schafer (Eds.), *Goldman's cecil medicine* (24th ed.). Philadelphia: Elsevier.
3. Neki, N. S. (2013). Jaundice in elders. *JK Sci J Med Educ Res, 15*(3), 113–116.
4. Casey, G. (2013). Jaundice: An excess of bilirubin. *Nursing New Zealand, 19*(1), 20–24.
5. Schulman, A. R., & Jajoo, K. Jaundice, obstruction, and acute cholangitis. In S. C. McKean, J. J. Ross, D. D. Dressler, & D. B. Scheurer (Eds.), *Principles and practice of hospital medicine* (2nd ed.). New York, NY: McGraw-Hill. http://accessmedicine.mhmedical.com.ezproxy.simmons.edu/content.aspx?bookid=1872&sectionid=146982009. (Accessed July 04, 2018).
6. Bunzo, N., Ryosuke, A., Kenjiro, K., & Kosei, H. (2013). Comparison of prognosis between patients of pancreatic head cancer with and without obstructive jaundice at diagnosis. *International Journal of Surgery, 11*(4), 344–349.
7. Langrand, J., Regnault, H., Cachet, X., Bouzidi, C., Villa, A. F., Serfaty, L., et al. (2014). Toxic hepatitis induced by herbal medicine: *Tinospora crispa. Phytomedicine: International Journal of Phytotherapy and Phytopharmacology, 21*(8–9), 1120–1123.
8. Herrine, S. K. 2018. Jaundice. *The Merck manuals online medical library for healthcare professionals.*
9. Walker, I., Chappell, L. C., & Williamson, C. (2013). Abnormal liver function tests in pregnancy. *British Medical Journal, 347*(7931), 33–35.
10. Bauer, M., Press, A. T., & Trauner, M. (2013). The liver in sepsis: Patterns of response to injury. *Current Opinion in Critical Care, 19*(2), 123–127.
11. U.S. Department of Health and Human Services. 2018. AIDS Info Fact Sheets. (Accessed July 6, 2018)@https://aidsinfo.nih.gov/understanding-hiv-aids/fact-sheets.
12. Lopez, A. M., & Hendrickson, R. G. (2014). Toxin-induced hepatic injury. *Emergency Medicine Clinics of North America, 32*(1), 103–125.
13. Cherfane, C. E., Hollenbeck, R. D., Go, J., & Brown, K. E. (2013). Hereditary hemochromatosis: Missed diagnosis or misdiagnosis? *The American Journal of Medicine, 32*(1), 1010–1015.
14. U.S. Department of Veterans Affairs, HIV/AIDS. (Accessed July 3, 2018)@ https://www.hiv.va.gov/provider/manual-primary-care/liver-disease.asp.
15. American College of Radiology. Right upper quadrant pain. American College of Radiology ACR Appropriateness Criteria. Retrieved from https://acsearch.acr.org/docs/69474/Narrative. (Accessed July 6, 2018).
16. Doig, A. K., & Huether, S. E. (2014). Alterations of digestive function. In K. L. McCance & S. E. Huether (Eds.), *In pathophysiology: The biologic basis for disease in adults and children* (7th ed.). St. Louis: Elsevier.
17. Kiser, J. J., & Flexner, C. W. Treatment of viral hepatitis (HBV/HCV). In L. L. Brunton, R. Hilal-Dandan, & B. C. Knollmann (Eds.), *Goodman & Gilman's: The pharmacological basis of therapeutics* (13th ed.). New York, NY: McGraw-Hill.
18. Gwon, D., Ko, G., Heung, K., Yoon, H., & Sung, K. (2013). Percutaneous transhepatic treatment using retrievable covered stents in patients with benign biliary strictures: Mid-term outcomes in 68 patients. *Digestive Diseases and Sciences, 58*(11), 3270–3279.
19. Viveksandeep, T. C., & Savio, J. Gilbert syndrome. (Accessed June 4, 2019)@ https://www.ncbi.nlm.nih.gov/books/NBK470200/.
20. Kline-Simon, A. H., Weisner, C. M., Parthasarathy, S., Faulk, D. E., Litten, R. Z., & Mertens, J. R. (2013). Five year healthcare utilization and costs among lower-risks drinkers following alcoholism treatment. *Alcoholism, Clinical and Experimental Research, 38*(2), 579–586.
21. American Liver Foundation (2018). H.E. 123. (Accessed June 2, 2019)@ https://he123.liverfoundation.org/treatment-basics/treatment-medications/lactulose/.
22. Iadevaia, M. D., Prete, A. D., Cesaro, C., Gaeta, L., Zulli, C., & Loguercio, C. (2011). Rifaximin in the treatment of hepatic encephalopathy. *Alcoholism, Clinical and Experimental Research, 3*, 109–117. http://doi.org/10.2147/HMER.S11988.
23. Centers for Disease Control. The ABCs of Hepatitis Fact Sheet. (Accessed July 6, 2018)@ https://www.cdc.gov/hepatitis/Resources/Professionals/PDFs/ABCTable_BW.pdf.
24. Centers for Disease Control and Prevention. Vaccination immunization schedules. Retrieved from www.cdc.gov/vaccines/schedules/hcp/imz/adult.html. (Accessed June 25, 2019).

NAUSEA AND VOMITING

Brad E. Franklin

 Red flags include nausea and vomiting accompanied by pain, severe dehydration, acute abdomen, fever, neurologic changes, anemia, hematemesis, metabolic imbalance, or a greater than 5% unintended weight loss.

DEFINITION AND EPIDEMIOLOGY

Nausea and vomiting are common presenting complaints in primary care and significantly affect quality of life.[1] One study of primary practice reported that nausea and vomiting ranked second to upper respiratory infections as presenting problems in primary care.[2] Gastroenteritis alone accounts for 10% of inpatient admissions and more than 1.5 million visits to primary care.[3] Nausea and vomiting present a diagnostic challenge to health care providers because of the varied causes such as infection, chronic medical conditions, and even treatment modalities. Often, history and physical exam help identify the underlying cause in the majority of cases.[4] Once the cause is identified, the health care provider is better able to control the symptoms and to prevent complications.[2,5]

Nausea is defined as an unpleasant or queasy, but painless, sensation that one is about to vomit. Actual vomiting may or may not occur.[1,6] Nausea usually lasts longer than vomiting and is generally relieved by vomiting. Vomiting, the forceful expulsion of liquid or food from the stomach through the mouth, should be differentiated from other symptoms that are often described by patients as vomiting, such as retching (rhythmic contractions of the respiratory and abdominal muscles without expulsion of gastric contents) or regurgitation (an effortless backward flow of food and liquids from the stomach to the mouth).[6,7] Vomiting is a protective mechanism from harmful ingested substances, but it can result from underlying disease affecting the gastrointestinal tract or surrounding structures, metabolic or endocrine function, or the central nervous system, or it can be an adverse effect of disease interventions (e.g., chemotherapy).[1,2]

PATHOPHYSIOLOGY

Vomiting is a reflex action controlled by two major central nervous system centers: the vomiting center (VC) and the chemoreceptor trigger zone (CTZ).[2,4,7,8] The VC, a collection of neurons within the medulla, is stimulated by input from multiple mechanisms, including pharyngeal, vagal, and midbrain afferents and the limbic system. Mechanical irritation can stimulate the pharyngeal afferents, leading to retching and then vomiting. The presence of noxious substances in the stomach and duodenum and the mechanical distention and contraction can sensitize chemoreceptors, and mechanical receptors can stimulate the vagal afferent pathways, which in turn stimulate the VC, leading to vomiting.[4,7,9]

The CTZ, located on the floor of the fourth ventricle, is directly sensitive to chemical agents with known emetogenic potential. It is sensitive to stimulation from serotonin, dopamine, histamine, cholinergic, adrenergic, and opiate receptors. The pharmacologic basis of most antiemetics is to block these neurotransmitters. The CTZ identifies harmful substances and transmits the information to the VC, which then initiates the vomiting reflex. Neurotransmitters, vagal afferents, or noxious agents can stimulate the CTZ, resulting in the stimulation of the VC.[4,7,9]

THE VOMITING REFLEX

Regardless of the cause of the stimulation of the VC, once stimulated it initiates a sequence of events that end with vomiting. There are three phases of vomiting: pre-ejection, ejection, and postejection. During pre-ejection, there is an increase in salivation and swallowing and a decrease in gastric tone; tachycardia, pallor, and diaphoresis occur. Relaxation of the proximal stomach and contraction of the small intestine ensue, leading to regurgitation of contents into the stomach. Pre-ejection is mediated by acetylcholine and the vagus nerve. In the ejection phase, abdominal muscles and the diaphragm contract and the lower esophageal sphincter relaxes, allowing contents into the esophagus and then into the mouth. The palate is elevated, thereby preventing propulsion of contents through the nasopharynx. Postejection is the period after expulsion of the stomach contents, usually resulting in some relief of the nausea.[9]

CLINICAL PRESENTATION AND PHYSICAL EXAMINATION

Nausea and vomiting are common presenting symptoms in primary care and can be associated with a variety of clinical presentations. The vomiting act varies very little regardless of cause.[2] The symptoms can be mild and self-limited or severe and prolonged, which can result in anorexia, weight loss, dehydration, and malnutrition. Nausea and vomiting might dominate the presentation or may be only a part of a symptom complex.[2]

When obtaining the patient's history, the clinician must have a clear determination of the patient's symptoms because a detailed history can provide clues to the diagnosis. The presentation of nausea and vomiting can vary from the gradual onset of symptoms noted with medication side effects, middle ear, gastric retention, or early pregnancy to the abrupt episodes caused by viral gastroenteritis, food poisoning, increased intracranial pressure, or acute abdominal emergency.[1,4,6] Associated symptoms can include pain, headache, dizziness, tinnitus, diarrhea, fever, mental status changes, anxiety, and other symptoms associated with pregnancy.[1,2]

A thorough history should include such details as the timing of the symptoms and their relation to meals, characteristics of the emesis, and any associated complaints. For example, early morning vomiting is associated with metabolic disturbances, alcoholic bingeing, and pregnancy. Vomiting that is triggered by meals is suggestive of pyloric channel ulcer, gastritis, or possibly a psychogenic problem. Learning the appearance of the vomitus is helpful (e.g., coffee-ground emesis suggests gastritis or ulcer disease, vomiting of gastric juice is suggestive of peptic ulcer disease and Zollinger-Ellison syndrome, and vomiting of feculent material is a sign of distal small bowel obstruction). Learning the onset, duration, and severity of symptoms is important.

The clinician should also ask about associated symptoms, past medical history, and psychosocial history. Inquiry should be made about the presence of abdominal pain, fever, jaundice, weight loss, dizziness, headache, visual disturbances, or abdominal surgery; a history of diabetes, cancer, irritable bowel syndrome, or heart disease is ascertained; and current medications and therapies, including cannabinoid use, radiation therapy, or chemotherapy, are reviewed. Gentle questioning about eating habits (binge eating), self-image, and self-induced emesis should also be conducted. A woman of childbearing age needs to be asked about the last menstrual period and whether she is sexually active, with or without contraception. Essential epidemiologic data include a history of recent foreign travel,[2] any recent exposure to commonly contaminated foods, and any recent exposure to sick contacts. It is also necessary to determine the relationship of nausea and vomiting to food (Does it occur before, during, or after eating? Is it predictable?); the force of vomiting (projectile vs. retching); and the quality of the emesis (bile, undigested food, coffee-ground emesis). Acute nausea and vomiting without warning signs can be indicative of infectious or iatrogenic causes. A 24-hour dietary review, with bowel symptoms (diarrhea versus constipation) and the time of the last void, should also be determined.[1,2]

Acute episodes of nausea and vomiting may be caused by viruses, bacterial food poisoning, cannabinoid hyperemesis and cyclic vomiting syndrome, or medication overdose.[10] Acute emergencies, such as pancreatitis, appendicitis, bowel obstruction, peritonitis, or cholecystitis, may be accompanied by fever or pain. These symptoms can also occur in acute episodes of Crohn disease, colitis, and diverticulitis. Chronic or recurrent nausea and vomiting may be psychogenic or the result of radiation therapy or chemotherapy, gastric disorders, migraine headache, diabetic gastroparesis, or a metabolic or endocrine abnormality.[1,2]

The physical examination should be directed toward searching for complications of nausea and vomiting and identifying any signs that might suggest the cause. Each area of the abdomen assessed should help narrow the possible differential diagnoses specific to that region.[11] The examination should focus on signs of dehydration, including evaluation of skin turgor, mucous membranes, and orthostatic vital signs (positional blood pressure, pulse). The general examination should include assessment of the skin for jaundice, moisture, rashes, or hyperpigmentation. Fingers should be assessed for calluses on dorsal surfaces suggesting self-induced vomiting. If self-induced vomiting is suspected, the clinician should examine the parotid gland for enlargement and check for the presence of lanugo hair and loss of tooth enamel; the patient should also be evaluated for signs of depression and anxiety. The head and neck should be assessed for evidence of dehydration, acute infection, lymphadenopathy, rigidity, or signs of thyrotoxicosis. A cardiovascular examination is necessary to determine the patient's response to the illness or other signs of infection. The abdomen should be observed for distention, visible peristalsis, abdominal or inguinal hernias, and surgical scars; auscultated for bowel sounds (presence or absence, increased or sluggish) and succussion; then palpated for rigidity, tenderness or masses, and flank tenderness. When palpating, the provider begins in areas where no discomfort is reported. Abdominal wall rigidity is indicative of an acute surgical abdomen. A rectal examination, if indicated, is helpful to determine if a fecal impaction or bleeding is present. A neurologic examination including mental status, gait, muscle weakness, asterixis, and cranial nerve function is also an essential component of the evaluation, if neurologic involvement is suspected.[1,2,6]

DIAGNOSTICS

There are currently no randomized controlled studies to guide the diagnostic evaluation; most recommendations are based on expert opinion.[1] The presentation of nausea and vomiting and the physical findings should guide diagnostic testing.[5]

Essential Diagnostics

Even though there are no specific tests to determine the cause of nausea and vomiting, laboratory tests can be useful to evaluate for the complications as well as to determine the underlying causes. The laboratory tests may include urinalysis for specific gravity; erythrocyte sedimentation rate; serum glucose concentration; electrolyte values; serum levels of ketones; blood urea nitrogen (BUN), creatinine, and amylase concentrations; liver function tests (LFTs); and drug levels (if indicated). A serum level of human chorionic gonadotropin should be obtained in women of childbearing age.

Additional Diagnostics

Urinalysis with culture and sensitivity, complete blood count (CBC), thyroid-stimulating hormone, or further endocrine studies may be indicated in some cases.[1,4,6]

Abdominal upright and plain x-ray films are necessary if an obstruction is suspected. An ultrasound examination, barium swallow study, computed tomography (CT) scan, or endoscopic examination may be indicated for masses, dysphagia, or suspected cannabinoid hyperemesis syndrome (CHS) and the cyclic vomiting syndrome in adults, gastrointestinal bleeding, or ulceration. If a cerebral hemorrhage or mass is suspected, the patient should be urgently referred to the nearest hospital where a head CT scan can be performed. Severe indigestion, epigastric pain, and vomiting could indicate myocardial infarction.[11] Electrocardiography is indicated if myocardial infarction is suspected.

INITIAL DIAGNOSTICS

Nausea and Vomiting

LABORATORY
- Urinalysis[a]
- Serum glucose, electrolytes, blood urea nitrogen, creatinine[a]
- Serum ketones[a]
- Amylase[a]
- Liver function tests[a]
- Drug levels[a]
- Human chorionic gonadotropin[a]
- Complete blood count and differential[a]

IMAGING
- Abdominal x-ray studies[a]
- Ultrasound[a]
- Barium swallow[a]
- Endoscopic examination[a]
- Head computed tomography scan[a]

OTHER DIAGNOSTICS
- Electrocardiography[a]

[a]If indicated.

DIFFERENTIAL DIAGNOSIS

Nausea and vomiting may be caused by an acute or chronic process. Differentiation of the cause will assist in treatment of the underlying disease and in patient education efforts.

Priority differentials include vomiting associated with an infectious source, chest or abdominal pain, medications or

Differential Diagnosis

ACUTE NAUSEA AND VOMITING

- Cardiac
  - Myocardial infarction
- Gastrointestinal
  - Acute abdomen (appendicitis, ischemic bowel, peritonitis, abdominal aortic aneurysm, volvulus)
  - Cholecystitis
  - Constipation
  - Infection (viral, bacterial, or parasitic)
  - Intestinal obstruction
  - Medication (chemotherapy, toxic level of some medications, anesthesia, or side effect of medications)
  - Metabolic disturbances (diabetic ketoacidosis, adrenal crisis)
- Neurologic
  - Acute labyrinthitis, Meniere disease
  - Increased intracranial pressure
  - Migraine headache
  - Motion sickness
- Pain
- Pregnancy
- Renal conditions
- Uremia

CHRONIC NAUSEA AND VOMITING

- Cancer
- Drug or alcohol use or withdrawal
- Gastrointestinal
  - Achalasia
  - Cirrhosis
  - Crohn disease
- Cyclic vomiting syndrome
  - Diabetic gastroparesis
  - Diverticular disease
  - Hepatitis
- *Helicobacter pylori* infection
  - Irritable bowel syndrome
  - Pancreatitis
  - Peptic ulcer disease
- Psychological
  - Anorexia nervosa or bulimia
  - Psychogenic

other toxic substances (e.g., alcohol), or increased intracranial pressure (Box 123.1). The possibility of cannabinoid hyperemesis syndrome (CHS) and the cyclic vomiting syndrome in teens and adults should be explored especially if there are recurrent episodes of vomiting. In women of childbearing age, pregnancy should always be a consideration.

INTERPROFESSIONAL COLLABORATIVE MANAGEMENT

Before initiating a treatment protocol, the clinician must identify the warning signs and consult with a specialist as warranted. In managing nausea and vomiting, priority should be given to recognition and correction of complications, followed by identification and treatment of underlying causes and finally, if necessary, treatment to suppress or to alleviate

symptoms.[1,5,7,9] The possibility of intestinal obstruction or acute abdomen should be eliminated before other treatment options are initiated. How nausea and vomiting are managed should be individualized to patient-specific variables, including presence of comorbidities, current medications, success of previous therapies, severity of symptoms, age of the patient, and the likely cause of the symptoms.[1,4,6]

Nonpharmacologic Management

Uncomplicated viral gastroenteritis (without metabolic imbalance or dehydration) can be managed with nonpharmacologic interventions including increased fluid intake and diet restrictions. A clear liquid diet should be followed for 24 hours, followed by 24 hours of the BRAT (banana, rice, applesauce, and toast) diet. This regimen will provide the bowel with sufficient rest. A bland diet may be necessary the following week if the patient is still symptomatic.

Pharmacologic Management

Control of vomiting is important for the comfort of the patient and prevention of complications. The use of antiemetics may be indicated. Unfortunately, only a few high-quality studies have compared the efficacy of the different antiemetic drugs on the market.[12] Antiemetic medications should be selected on the basis of the patient's medical history and the suspected cause of the nausea and vomiting. In practice, the choice of an antiemetic is also influenced by provider experience, safety, and cost.[13] Adequate fluid intake must be maintained to prevent dehydration, especially if the illness is prolonged or severe. Intake should exceed output by at least 500 mL in a 24-hour period. Assessment for hydration status should include postural vital signs along with the patient's ability to void every 2 to 3 hours. Oral hydration should be attempted in the office if the patient has postural hypotension and is able to tolerate fluid intake. If the patient is too nauseated or does not respond to oral fluid intake, intravenous hydration should be started. In general, 1 to 2 L of intravenous normal saline or lactated Ringer solution over a few hours is well tolerated. Slower rates are recommended for older adults or patients with significant comorbidities. Emergency provider consultation is recommended if postural hypotension is not corrected or if metabolic alkalosis or severe dehydration is present.

Antiemetic medications are administered to treat or to prevent nausea and vomiting (Box 123.2). These medications can be given alone or in combination with other agents. Presently, the 5-hydroxytryptamine$_3$ (5-HT$_3$ [serotonin]) receptor antagonists are the cornerstone of antiemetic therapy and are used to treat postoperative emesis and chemotherapy-induced emesis. However, there are concerns about QT prolongation with ondansetron and dolasetron.[3]

The phenothiazines were initially used to prevent chemotherapy-induced emesis. The 5-HT$_3$ receptor antagonists are also used for the prevention of nausea and vomiting associated with chemotherapy.[9] These agents used in combination with corticosteroids may offer the greatest antiemetic treatment.[9] For the refractory nausea and vomiting associated with chemotherapy, the cannabinoids may be useful.[8]

For the prevention of motion sickness, vertigo, and migraines, antihistamines and anticholinergics are excellent choices. These include diphenhydramine (Benadryl), meclizine (Antivert), dimenhydrinate (Dramamine), transdermal scopolamine, promethazine (Phenergan), and cyclizine (Marezine).[3,8]

BOX **123.2**

Antiemetic Medications

FOR GENERALIZED NAUSEA AND VOMITING
Bismuth Subsalicylate
For nausea with or without diarrhea
- Pepto-Bismol: 30 mL PO every 30–60 min; maximum 8 doses/24 h; available over the counter

Benzamides
Metoclopramide Hydrochloride
For nausea related to diabetic gastroparesis: 10 mg PO 30 min before meals and at bedtime for 2–8 weeks, depending on response

For gastroesophageal reflux: 10–15 mg PO 4 times daily prn 30 min before meals and at bedtime; do not use for more than 12 weeks

For nausea and vomiting associated with chemotherapy: 1–2 mg/kg IV slowly during 1–2 min or infused over 15 min after diluting in 50 mL of D5W, D5½NS, normal saline, Ringer solution, or lactated Ringer solution; give first dose 30 min before chemotherapy, then every 2 h prn; do not exceed 5 doses/day; may produce dystonic reaction when given IV; premedicate with diphenhydramine.

****Can cause extrapyramidal symptoms (i.e., tardive dyskinesia). Increased risk in geriatric population.[3]

Phenothiazines
Prochlorperazine (Compazine)
For severe nausea and vomiting: 5–10 mg PO 3 or 4 times daily, 5–10 mg IM every 3–4 h prn (maximum 40 mg/day), or 25 mg rectal suppository every 12 h prn; may give 2.5–10 mg IV at a rate not to exceed 5 mg/min; give IM injections in the upper outer quadrant of the gluteal muscle; use this drug when only a few doses are required for treatment. Monitor patients for hypotension.

Promethazine Hydrochloride (Phenergan)
For nausea: 12.5–25 mg PO, IM, or rectally every 4–6 h prn; use cautiously in ambulatory patients because of possible pronounced sedative effects

Trimethobenzamide Hydrochloride (Tigan)
For mild to moderate nausea and vomiting: 300 mg PO 3 or 4 times daily, 200 mg IM 3 or 4 times daily; give IM injections in the upper outer quadrant of the gluteal muscle; for short-term treatment

FOR NAUSEA AND VOMITING ASSOCIATED WITH CHEMOTHERAPY
5-HT (Serotonin) Receptor Antagonists (Also Used for Postoperative Emesis)
For prevention of postoperative and chemotherapy-induced emesis in adults
- Granisetron (Kytril): 1 mg or 0.01 mg/kg once daily IV before chemotherapy. If necessary, a repeat dose can be given in 12 h.
- Ondansetron (Zofran): 4–8 mg or 0.15 mg/kg once daily IV, or 4–8 mg 3 times daily PO
- Palonosetron (Aloxi): 0.25 mg IV ½ h before chemotherapy is initiated

Dopamine Receptor Antagonists
Phenothiazines
For prevention of chemotherapy-induced events
- Prochlorperazine (Compazine): 5–10 mg PO every 6–8 h, 5–10 mg IM, 2.5–10 mg IV every 3–4 h, or 25 mg suppository every 12 h
- Chlorpromazine (Thorazine): 10–25 mg PO every 4–6 h, 25 mg IV every 3–4 h, or 100 mg suppository every 6–8 h

Butyrophenones
For postoperative nausea
- Droperidol (Inapsine): 0.625–1.25 mg IV at time of surgical completion; 1.25–5 mg IM

Benzamides
For nausea caused by cytotoxic drugs
- Metoclopramide (Reglan): 0.5 mg–1.0 mg/kg IV every 6–8 h or 10–20 mg PO every 6–8 h
- Trimethobenzamide (Tigan): 300 mg PO every 6–8 h or 200 mg IM or suppository every 6–8 h

Cannabinoids
For chemotherapy-induced nausea and vomiting, anorexia associated with weight loss in adult AIDS patients
- Dronabinol (Marinol): 5 mg/m^2 PO 1–3 h before chemotherapy; repeated every 2–4 h prn to maximum 6 doses daily.[6] For anorexia patients, start 2.5 mg once daily and titrate up to BID; available in 2.5, 5, and 10 mg capsules.[12]

Substance P/Neurokinin₁ Antagonists
For acute and delayed nausea and vomiting associated with chemotherapy
- Aprepitant (Emend): 125 mg PO 1 h before chemotherapy, then 80 mg/day for 2 days; may be given with other agents (e.g., steroids, Zofran)

Benzodiazepines
For adjunct therapy to decrease anxiety and anticipatory emesis
- Alprazolam (Xanax): 0.5–1 mg once daily PO up to 3–6 mg/day
- Lorazepam (Ativan): 0.5–2 mg PO or IV every 4–6 h

Antihistamines and Anticholinergic Agents
For motion sickness, vertigo, and migraines
- Diphenhydramine (Benadryl): 25–50 mg PO every 6 h or 10–50 mg IV or IM
- Dimenhydrinate (Dramamine): 50 mg PO every 4 h
- Meclizine (Antivert): 12.5–50 mg PO every 24 h
- Promethazine (Phenergan): 12.5–25 mg every 4–6 h PO, IM, or IV
- Transdermal scopolamine (Transderm-Scop): 1 patch 4 h before travel, remove after 72 h; for surgery, apply 1 patch the evening before surgery, remove 24 h after surgery

Medication doses above are indicated for adults. A decrease in dosing may be necessary for older adults or for patients with impaired renal function.

Hospitalization is usually necessary for the adult treatment of cannabinoid hyperemesis syndrome (CHS) and the cyclic vomiting syndrome. Intravenous fluid resuscitation with 0.9 % sodium chloride, in addition to IV alprazolam or lorazepam, and IV proton pump inhibitor therapy are recommended in the acute phase of this disorder. Cannabis cessation is the long-term treatment goal.[14]

CONSULTATIONS

- An urgent referral for hospital admission and consultation with a specialist is indicated for patients when nausea and vomiting are accompanied by pain, severe dehydration, hematemesis, acute abdominal findings, neurologic changes, or a metabolic or electrolyte imbalance. Hospitalization may also be indicated if the patient is unable to maintain hydration status at home.
- Referral to an appropriate specialist may be necessary if the nausea or vomiting is not controlled by supportive measures such as hydration, diet change, and antiemetics; the patient's condition worsens or does not respond to treatment; a psychological component is present; the acuity of the patient's condition exceeds the experience and comfort level of the treating provider; or adequate resources are not readily available. Metabolic disturbances; pregnancy; and altered medication, drug, or alcohol levels should be managed in consultation with an interdisciplinary team.
- Consultation is required for emergencies such as acute myocardial infarction or for patients with neurologic changes.
- Prolonged or recurrent nausea or vomiting may indicate gastric paresis, irritable bowel, or pancreatitis, and requires consultation with a gastroenterologist or appropriate specialist.

COMPLICATIONS

The complications of nausea and vomiting must be identified and treated. The severity of complications is associated with the underlying condition. Untreated, nausea and vomiting can cause dehydration, hypokalemia, and metabolic acidosis. Although it is uncommon in alert patients, aspiration pneumonitis is a possibility in patients with decreased levels of consciousness.[7] Continual vomiting may result in malnutrition and dental erosion. Forceful vomiting has been the cause of Mallory-Weiss syndrome and esophageal ruptures.[1,6]

PATIENT AND FAMILY EDUCATION

Patients should be educated about adequate fluid intake, with special attention given to the types of fluid ingested. Oral rehydration solutions and broths are especially helpful in maintaining electrolyte balance. Dairy products and carbonated fluids should be avoided. A minimum of 96 to 120 ounces of fluid should be consumed each hour. An oral rehydration solution may be prepared by mixing 1 cup of orange juice, three-fourth teaspoon of salt, 1 teaspoon of baking soda, 4 tablespoons of sugar, and 1 L of water.

Because dehydration can occur easily in the presence of persistent vomiting, patients should be instructed to notify the health care provider if the following occur:

- Vomiting persists despite antiemetic use.
- Vomiting is accompanied by fever, severe abdominal pain, severe headache, neck pain, or lethargy.
- Urinary output becomes dark, or the patient does not void at least every 2 hours during the day.

- Dizziness or lightheadedness occurs with or without position change.
- Patient is vomiting blood or fluid that has the appearance of coffee grounds.

HEALTH PROMOTION

Patients should be instructed in the proper handling and storage of food products to prevent contamination and possible food poisoning. Patients traveling abroad should receive the necessary vaccinations and treatments appropriate for the country visited. Guidelines are available from the Centers for Disease Control and Prevention or through local travel clinics.

REFERENCES

1. Scorza, K., Williams, A., Phillips, D., et al. (2007). Evaluation of nausea and vomiting. *American Family Physician*, 76(1), 76–84.
2. Goroll, A. H., & Mulley, A. (2009). Evaluation of nausea and vomiting. In *Primary care medicine: Office evaluation and management of the adult patient* (6th ed.). Philadelphia: Lippincott Williams & Wilkins.
3. Flake, Z. A., Linn, B. S., & Hornecker, J. R. (2015). Practical selection of antiemetics in the ambulatory setting. *American Family Physicians*, 91(5), 293–296.
4. Harbord, M., & Pomfret, S. (2013). Nausea and vomiting. *Medicine*, 41(2), 87–91.
5. American Gastroenterological Association. (2001). American Gastroenterological Association medical position statement: Nausea and vomiting. *Gastroenterology*, 120, 261–262.
6. Mertz, A., & Hebbard, G. (2007). Nausea and vomiting in adults: A diagnostic approach. *Australian Family Physician*, 36(9), 688–692.
7. Steele, A., & Carlson, K. K. (2007). Nausea and vomiting: Applying research to bedside practice. *AACN Advanced Critical Care*, 18(1), 61–75.
8. Pasricha, P. J. (2006). Treatment of disorders of bowel motility and water flux; antiemetics; agents used in biliary and pancreatic disease. In L. L. Brunton, J. S. Lazo, & K. L. Parker (Eds.), *Goodman & Gilman's the pharmacological basis of therapeutics* (11th ed.). New York: McGraw-Hill.
9. Baker, P. D., Morzorati, S. L., & Ellett, M. L. (2005). The pathophysiology of chemotherapy-induced nausea and vomiting. *Gastroenterology Nursing*, 28(6), 469–480.
10. Blumentrath, C. G., Dohrmann, B., & Ewald, N. (2017). Cannabinoid hyperemesis and the cyclic vomiting syndrome in adults: Recognition, diagnosis, acute and long-term treatment. *German Medical Science: GMS e-journal*, 15, doi:10.3205/000247. Doc06.
11. Brown, H. F., & Kelso, L. (2014). Abdominal pain: An approach to a challenging diagnosis. *AACN Critical Care*, 25(3), 266–278.
12. Egerton-Warburton, D., Meek, R., Mee, M. J., et al. (2014). Antiemetic use for nausea and vomiting in adult emergency department patients: Randomized controlled trial comparing ondansetron, metoclopramide, and placebo. *Annals of Emergency Medicine*, 64(5), 526–532.
13. Flake, Z. A., Scalley, R. D., Bailey, A. G. (2004). Practical selection of antiemetics. *American Family Physician*, 69(5), 1169–1174.
14. Khattar, N., & Routsolias, J.C. (2018). Emergency department treatment of cannabinoid hyperemesis syndrome: A review. *American Journal of Therapeutics*, 25(3), e357–e361. doi:10.1097/MJT.0000000000000655.

CHAPTER **124**

PANCREATITIS

Kevin Dholaria • Henrique J. Fernandez • Jodie A. Barkin

 Gastrointestinal consultation and hospitalization for pain and fluid and electrolyte management is required for patients with acute pancreatitis.

ACUTE PANCREATITIS

DEFINITION AND EPIDEMIOLOGY

Acute pancreatitis is an inflammatory condition of the pancreas that may range in severity from mild to severe. The patient with acute pancreatitis typically has abdominal pain and an elevation of pancreatic enzymes. The clinical course can range from mild disease to life-threatening multiorgan failure, sepsis, and possibly death. The Atlanta symposium classified acute pancreatitis into mild (no organ dysfunction and no local or systemic complications), moderately severe (transient organ failure or local or systemic complications in absence of persistent organ failure), and severe (persistent organ failure).[1-3] The major stratifying criteria thus is the presence of organ failure, which generally encompasses pulmonary, cardiovascular, and renal organ systems. Persistent organ failure is organ dysfunction for greater than 48 hours, and transient organ failure is less than 48 hours. Local complications of acute pancreatitis include peripancreatic fluid collections, acute necrotic collections, and other less common conditions. These complications will be described further as follows. It is important to define the condition by severity for a number of reasons. It assists in triaging patients for hospitalization and level of care, as well as potentially identifying who may require early aggressive treatment. Furthermore, it may identify which patients may benefit from care in a tertiary center.

Acute pancreatitis can also be further divided into two types: interstitial edematous pancreatitis and necrotizing pancreatitis.[3] In acute interstitial pancreatitis, computed tomography (CT) when performed primarily shows homogenous enhancement of the pancreas. This comprises the majority of cases of acute pancreatitis, and has an associated mortality rate as low as 1%, with no or minimal necrosis present. Symptoms of interstitial pancreatitis usually resolve within one week.[3] Conversely, acute necrotizing pancreatitis shows areas of nonenhancement on CT with intravenous contrast, with necrosis in the pancreas, peripancreatic tissue, or a combination thereof, with the most common presentation being the combination. Necrotizing pancreatitis is graded by CT as involvement of the gland of less than 30% or 30% or more, with the latter being more severe. Severe necrotizing pancreatitis may manifest with organ failure; when present, it has a mortality rate of 10% with aseptic necrosis and up to 30% with infected necrosis.[2,4]

The causes of pancreatitis are varied. A number of factors have been implicated as precipitants and can easily be identified using the ABCs of causes of acute pancreatitis (Boxes 124.1–124.3). The most common cause of pancreatitis is gallstones, which are responsible for 45% of all cases of pancreatitis in the United States.[5] Toxins are another leading cause of acute pancreatitis, with ethyl alcohol as the precipitant in the majority of cases.[5] Standardized by gender, ethyl alcohol is the most common cause in males, with a worldwide incidence of 7.9 cases per 100,000 people per year. Gallstones are the most common cause in women, with a worldwide incidence of 4.8 per 100,000 people per year.[2,6] Other causes of pancreatitis include trauma from injury and surgery, which may disrupt the ductal system or damage the pancreas.[5] Endoscopic retrograde cholangiopancreatography (ERCP) is an important iatrogenic cause of pancreatitis and can occur in up to 5% of cases.[7] Conditions that cause hypercalcemia, such as

BOX **124.1**

The ABCs of Causes of Acute Pancreatitis

A: Alcohol, autoimmune disorders, arteritis
B: Biliary, blunt trauma
C: Congenital—pancreas divisum
D: Drugs or medications
E: ERCP, eosinophilia
F: Formations—primary and metastatic tumors
G: Genetic—*CFTR, SPINK, PRSS1*
H: Hyperlipidemia, hypercalcemia
I: Idiopathic, infectious—human immunodeficiency virus (HIV), inflammatory bowel disease

ERCP, Endoscopic retrograde cholangiopancreatography.
Courtesy Jamie S. Barkin, MD, University of Miami, Leonard M. Miller School of Medicine, Department of Medicine, Division of Gastroenterology, Miami, Florida.

hyperparathyroidism, are also implicated in the development of pancreatitis. However, the reasons for this are not clearly understood. Hyperlipidemia associated with triglyceride levels of more than 1000 mg/dL is known to increase the risk of pancreatitis.[5] Parasites and viral infections, such as human immunodeficiency virus (HIV) infection, have been implicated in the development of pancreatitis. Some medications are associated with pancreatitis (e.g., thiazide diuretics and furosemide); the exact relationship is unknown but may be related to a hypersensitivity reaction that results in pancreatic injury. Thiopurines, often used in autoimmune and chronic inflammatory disorders, carry up to a 3% risk of development of pancreatitis that is independent of dose.[8] Other toxic substances including cannabis can lead to acute pancreatitis.[9]

Anatomic variations are a possible cause of acute or chronic idiopathic pancreatitis (pancreas divisum, ansa pancreatica, and vertical course of the pancreatic duct).[10] Lesions that result in pancreatic ductal obstruction, such as tumors, also may cause pancreatitis.

PATHOPHYSIOLOGY

The exact mechanism of pancreatitis is not well understood, but the most common explanation is related to autodigestion of the pancreas. For reasons unknown, pancreatic enzymes become activated in the pancreas rather than in the intestine. Trypsinogen, an inactive enzyme produced by the pancreas, is normally released into the intestines through the pancreatic ducts and activated by trypsin. In pancreatitis, trypsin is present in the pancreas and not only digests the pancreas but also activates other enzymes, such as elastase and phospholipase A. Elastase and phospholipase A are also involved in the autodigestion of the pancreas. Elastase causes hemorrhage through breakdown of the elastic fibers of the blood vessels. Phospholipase A has been implicated in fat necrosis.[11]

Although most patients typically experience minimum organ dysfunction as a result of pancreatitis, approximately 10% to 20% develop systemic inflammatory response syndrome (SIRS). SIRS is defined by the presence of at least two of the following features: temperature below 36°C or above 38°C; heart rate above 90 beats/min; respiratory rate above 20 breaths/min or $PaCO_2$ below 32 torr; white blood cell count above 12,000 cells/mm³, below 4000 cells/mm³, or above 10% immature cells (bands).[12] Pancreatic inflammation can lead to

BOX 124.2

Extended List of Factors Associated With Acute Pancreatitis

MOST FREQUENT CAUSES

- Gallstones
- Alcoholism
- Idiopathic (may be related to diverse causes)

FREQUENT CAUSES

- Toxins
- Ethyl alcohol
- Methyl alcohol
- Cannabis
- Hereditary/Genetic
- Medications
  - Acetaminophen
  - Aminosalicylates
  - Angiotensin-converting enzyme inhibitors
  - Asparaginase (Elspar)
  - Azathioprine (Imuran) or 6-mercaptopurine
  - Chlorthalidone
  - Cimetidine
  - Corticosteroids
  - ddl (2',3'-dideoxyinosine; associated with concurrent pentamidine treatment)
  - Erythromycin
  - Estrogens (identified with type IV or V hyperlipidemia)
  - Ethacrynic acid
  - Furosemide (rare)
  - Iatrogenic hypercalcemia
  - Intravenous lipids
  - L-Asparaginase
  - Methyldopa (rare)
  - Metronidazole (rare)
  - Nitrofurantoin
  - Nonsteroidals
  - Olsalazine, 5-ASA (rare)
  - Pentamidine (rare)
  - Phenformin (rare)
  - Ranitidine
  - Sulfonamides (rare)
  - Sulindac
  - Tetracycline (rare)

- Thiazide diuretics
- Valproic acid
- Blunt abdominal trauma
- Crohn disease of the duodenum
- End-stage renal disease with chronic dialysis
- Iatrogenic trauma: cardiopulmonary bypass, endoscopic retrograde cholangiopancreatography, endoscopic sphincterotomy, manometry of the sphincter of Oddi, organ transplantation, postoperative pancreatitis after abdominal or thoracic surgery
- Hyperparathyroidism associated with hypercalcemia
- Infection
  - Parasitic: *Ascaris* worms, clonorchiasis
  - Viral: coxsackievirus, cytomegalovirus, mumps, and fulminant viral hepatitis
  - Bacterial: *Campylobacter jejuni, Mycoplasma pneumoniae, Salmonella* organisms, microlithiasis
- Lipid abnormalities (hypertriglyceridemia)
- Metabolic abnormalities: hypercalcemia associated with excessive doses of vitamin D, parathyroid adenoma, familial hypocalciuric hypercalcemia, hypercalcemia associated with total parenteral nutrition
- Pancreatic divisum
- Pancreatic outflow obstruction: afferent loop obstruction, annular pancreatitis
- Penetrating peptic ulcer
- Pregnancy
- Surgery (endoscopic retrograde cholangiopancreatography)
- Trauma
- Tumor: primary and metastatic

LESS FREQUENT CAUSES

- Organophosphorus insecticides
- Scorpion venom
- Pancreatic cancer
- Periampullary duodenal diverticulum
- Refeeding after fasting
- Rheumatologic disorders: systemic lupus erythematosus, mixed connective tissue disorders, scleroderma
- Thrombotic thrombocytopenic purpura
- Vasculitis

BOX 124.3

Factors Associated With Acute Pancreatitis in HIV-Positive Patients

INFECTION

- Cytomegalovirus
- *Cryptococcus*
- Cryptosporidia
- *Mycobacterium avium* and *Mycobacterium tuberculosis*
- *Toxoplasma gondii*

MEDICATIONS

- Didanosine
- Pentamidine
- Trimethoprim-sulfamethoxazole

SIRS by the activation of an inflammatory cascade mediated by cytokines, immunocytes, and the complement system. The inflammatory cytokines cause macrophages to migrate to the lungs, kidneys, and other tissues distant from the pancreas. SIRS can lead to a fulminant course with multiorgan failure and the development of local or systemic complications, which as aforementioned is used to classify patients as having mild, moderately severe, or severe disease.[3,13,14]

CLINICAL PRESENTATION AND PHYSICAL EXAMINATION

The main presentation of acute pancreatitis is the sudden onset of constant, sharp, poorly localized abdominal pain that radiates to the back in about 50% of patients. The pain usually persists for several hours to days. The pancreas is in a retroperitoneal location, and signs of peritoneal irritation, such as rebound tenderness, are frequently absent. Pain that is characterized as dull, colicky, or located in the lower abdomen is generally not typical of pancreatitis, and other etiologies should be considered. About 90% of patients have associated nausea and vomiting.[3]

Early recognition of pancreatitis in clinical practice is of utmost importance. Given the nonspecific nature of symptomatology, acute pancreatitis may be misdiagnosed by physical examination alone. The most common presentation is intense abdominal pain so severe that the patient is reluctant to take a deep breath. This results in hypoventilation and contributes to the increased incidence of respiratory complications, such as atelectasis; therefore crackles may be present in lungs on examination. The pain is worse in the supine position and often increases in severity with time. Many patients are initially seen with symptoms of dehydration caused by nausea and vomiting, which may result in tachycardia, orthostatic hypotension, and shock. Abdominal distention caused by the leakage of fluid into the retroperitoneum is common and results in protrusion of abdominal contents forward. Direct and rebound tenderness secondary to peritonitis are late signs associated with severe acute pancreatitis, which is associated with a grave prognosis.[15] Upper abdominal palpation of a mass may suggest the presence of a pancreatic pseudocyst. Evidence of retroperitoneal hemorrhage, although rare, may be observed. Cullen sign (bruising of the periumbilicus) or Grey Turner sign (bruising of the flank) is consistent with retroperitoneal bleeding that can develop in acute severe pancreatitis. The occurrence of Cullen and Grey Turner signs is rare and associated with increased mortality. Jaundice, an uncommon finding, also may occur and is related to compression of the common bile duct by edema or a mass of the head of the pancreas.

DIAGNOSTICS
Essential Diagnostics
Serum amylase and lipase are the most common laboratory tests used to diagnose acute pancreatitis. Rising 6 to 12 hours after the onset of symptoms, serum amylase levels usually return to normal within 3 to 5 days in uncomplicated cases. This elevation is not always seen in alcoholic pancreatitis, especially in patients with chronic alcoholic pancreatitis, or in hypertriglyceridemia-associated pancreatitis because of laboratory delineation. Serum amylase elevation is considered a nonspecific finding because serum amylase may be elevated in other conditions with an extrapancreatic cause, such as diseases of the salivary glands, which also produce amylase. Further, mild elevations in amylase or lipase in the setting of multiorgan failure and shock may be incidental findings of systemic hypoperfusion and not true acute pancreatitis. A threefold elevation of serum lipase level is more diagnostic, especially in patients seen several days after the acute attack, and serum lipase is elevated in both alcoholic and nonalcoholic pancreatitis.[16] Trending of amylase and lipase levels in an acute episode is not indicated, and management should be driven only by symptomatology.

Hemoconcentration, hyperglycemia, and electrolyte abnormalities are commonly found as a result of intravascular volume depletion. Hyperbilirubinemia and transient hypocalcemia may also be present. Elevated bilirubin and alkaline phosphatase, with or without the presence of elevated aminotransferases, should raise the suspicion for biliary obstruction—a common presentation of biliary pancreatitis.

Abdominal radiographs are useful in the exclusion of other causes of abdominal pain, such as bowel obstruction, ileus, or perforated bowel, but are not diagnostic for acute pancreatitis. Chest x-ray studies may show infiltration, left lower lobe atelectasis, or effusion. Abdominal ultrasonography offers a sensitivity as high as 95% in diagnosing uncomplicated cholelithiasis, though its sensitivity decreases in setting of biliary pancreatitis due to concurrent bowel distention.[17] Nonetheless, abdominal ultrasonography is recommended to be performed in all patients with acute pancreatitis to evaluate for biliary etiologies and gallstones.[14] Additional imaging should be used only when the diagnosis is not conclusive from the history, physical examination, and laboratory findings or when the medical practitioner suspects a complicated course.

Additional Diagnostics
CT imaging is not routinely indicated as the diagnosis is obvious in many cases and most will have a mild, uncomplicated course. Intravenous contrast-enhanced CT scanning, however, is the most useful imaging technique, not only for diagnosis of acute pancreatitis but also for detection of local complications of pancreatitis. This should be delayed until the patient is rehydrated if there is uncertainty of diagnosis because impairment of pancreatic perfusion and signs of pancreatic necrosis can take several days.[18] If a patient is not improving clinically after 72 hours, CT with contrast or magnetic resonance imaging (MRI) is recommended to assess for the presence of local complications.[14] MRI and magnetic resonance cholangiopancreatography (MRCP) are used in the diagnosis of acute pancreatitis. MRI is considered more useful in the effort to categorize acute fluid collections and assess main pancreatic duct anatomy and is more sensitive in diagnosis of milder forms of pancreatitis. MRCP is better able to delineate the pancreatic and bile ducts.

The diagnosis of acute pancreatitis can only be made if the patient meets at least 2 of the 3 Revised Atlanta Classification criteria: clinical symptomology characteristic of acute pancreatitis, serum amylase or lipase at least three times greater than the upper limit of normal, and/or radiographic findings consistent with pancreatitis.[14] Thus, if the patient meets only clinical symptoms suggestive of pancreatitis or biochemical evidence, then a radiologic study such as CT imaging can be considered in the right clinical scenario for further evaluation.

In 20% of patients diagnosed with pancreatitis, the cause is unknown. The majority of these patients will have no further episodes. Patients with recurrent acute pancreatitis may benefit from endoscopic ultrasound (EUS) for further evaluation of pancreatic parenchyma and ducts, or ERCP as a therapeutic modality to remove common bile duct stones or debris.[19] Patients with unexplained pancreatitis who are older than 40 years are at increased risk of pancreatic malignancy and should have further imaging with CT or EUS. ERCP should be used only as a therapeutic modality because it can exacerbate biliary pancreatitis with manipulation of the pancreatic duct. In cases of idiopathic pancreatitis, patients should be referred to centers of expertise.

There have been multiple scoring systems used over time including Apache II criteria, Bedside Index of Severity in Acute Pancreatitis (BISAP), Ranson Criteria, and so on. All of these scoring systems have fallen out of favor and have been replaced by evaluating for the presence and persistence of organ failure with presence of SIRS criteria as a surrogate marker for this as predictors of increased morbidity and mortality.

INITIAL DIAGNOSTICS

Acute Pancreatitis

LABORATORY
- CHEM-12 (electrolytes, blood urea nitrogen, creatinine, hepatic function panel)
- Fasting lipid profile for triglycerides[a]
- Complete blood count
- Serum human chorionic gonadotropin (in women of childbearing age)
- Urine toxicology screen and serum ethanol level
- Amylase/Lipase level—once only

IMAGING
- Kidney, ureter, bladder
- Abdominal ultrasound
- Chest x-ray study
- MRI/MRCP[a]
- Endoscopic ultrasound[a]
- Computed tomography scan if no improvement after 72 h[a]

OTHER DIAGNOSTICS
- Electrocardiogram
- Endoscopic retrograde cholangiopancreatograph (only as a therapeutic modality)[a]

[a]If indicated.
MRCP, Magnetic resonance cholangiopancreatography; *MRI*, magnetic resonance imaging.

DIFFERENTIAL DIAGNOSIS

 Primary differentials include myocardial infarction, bowel obstruction, or acute cholecystitis.

Any patient who presents with abdominal pain requires meticulous assessment, because many disease processes may have symptomatic overlap. A thorough history of the pain, including location, time of onset, severity, and quality, in addition to associated symptoms will assist in determining the diagnosis. Questions about gastrointestinal function, such as appetite, nausea, vomiting, and the presence of blood in the stool, will be useful. The possibility of gynecologic conditions also must be considered in women with abdominal pain.[20]

INTERPROFESSIONAL COLLABORATIVE MANAGEMENT

Nonpharmacologic Management

Recognition of underlying abdominal emergencies and the need for quick surgical intervention for extrapancreatic processes is essential. Treatment of pancreatitis is generally aimed at decreasing pancreatic inflammation with rehydration and correcting any predisposing factors, such as removal of gallstones in gallstone pancreatitis. Hospitalization is generally indicated for analgesia and intravenous rehydration, as well as for monitoring of vital signs, volume status, and electrolytes. Level of treatment should be based on severity criteria previously mentioned, and one should have a low threshold for intensive care unit monitoring. Patients should be treated as if they have a burn injury because third spacing of fluids is commonly seen. Monitoring of fluid status is critical; these patients require large amounts of fluids for correction of intravascular volume depletion. The foundation of therapy is early intravenous hydration. This should be administered with at least 1 L initially and then continued at 150 to 250 mL/h during the initial 24 hours of hospitalization depending on the comorbidities of the patient. This has been shown to decrease morbidity and mortality of

acute pancreatitis. Lactated Ringer solution has shown to be the preferred solution for rehydration in acute pancreatitis because it has a more neutral pH and better electrolyte balance.[21] This is particularly true in both the prevention of and treatment for post-ERCP pancreatitis.[22] Strict monitoring of intake and output should be used to follow overall fluid balance. BUN and hematocrit should be followed every 6 to 12 hours, and should decrease with rehydration and help dictate further fluid administration.[23]

Pharmacologic Management

There is no medication that has been shown to be effective in treating acute pancreatitis. Pain is typically treated with opioid analgesics. Meperidine is used cautiously because of the propensity of its metabolites to accumulate and to cause neuromuscular irritation and possibly seizures. Morphine has been shown in human studies to cause an increase in pressure of the sphincter of Oddi; however, there is no evidence that this has a negative effect on the condition of the pancreas. Fentanyl is sometimes used, but, like all opioids, it can cause respiratory depression.

Antibiotic therapy for acute pancreatitis is not appropriate when the patient is admitted; it has not been shown to prevent pancreatic infection.[24,25] If the patient later in the course develops a secondary infection or suspected infected pancreatic necrosis, antibiotics can be used. In the setting of a suspected infected fluid collection, fluid aspiration via interventional radiology or EUS guidance can be obtained for culture and sensitivities if there is no clinical response to an initial empiric course of antibiotics. Antibiotic prophylaxis is contraindicated in acute pancreatitis because of the potential development of resistant bacterial or fungal pancreatitis and has not been associated with any statistically significant differences in subsequent morbidity or mortality. Probiotics have also been examined and have not been shown to have any benefit for preventing complications and may lead to increased mortality.[26]

There are no specific guidelines for the treatment of hypertriglyceridemia-induced pancreatitis, though IV insulin drip therapy used concurrently with intravenous hydration (or a dextrose solution if necessary) is being used to decrease the elevated triglycerides more quickly. Once stabilized, initiating fibrate therapy, and possibly a statin as well, is suggested. Apheresis is also in some situations, though controversial as consistent evidence of efficacy is lacking.[27,28] In the past, patients with pancreatitis were kept NPO (nothing by mouth) until resolution of pain or normalization of pancreatic enzymes. As previously mentioned, there is no role for trending pancreatic enzymes. The paradigm regarding nutrition in acute pancreatitis has changed where early feeding is encouraged. In cases of mild pancreatitis, immediate oral feeding appears to be safe.[29,30] In moderately severe or severe pancreatitis, enteral feedings are encouraged when able to be tolerated. The recurrence of pain indicates the need to restrict oral intake and also to look for complications, such as fluid collections, necrosis, or development of pseudocysts. Enteral feeding has been shown to be superior to parenteral nutrition for overall decreased morbidity and mortality.[31] Initiation of enteral feeding within 48 hours of onset of pancreatitis is associated with fewer complications and may decrease severity of the episode of pancreatitis. A nasogastric or nasojejunal feeding tube can be used to support enteral feeding if indicated.[30,31,32]

Intravenous contrast-enhanced CT scanning to determine the presence of necrosis or other complications is indicated for patients who do not respond to supportive measures. CT scanning should be performed no earlier than 72 hours after the start of the episode to enable appropriate estimation of the extent of pancreatic necrosis. ERCP with or without EUS may be necessary for management of common bile duct stones causing biliary pancreatitis. Pancreatic necrosis should be managed conservatively with a step-up approach focusing on supportive care measures, followed by catheter drainage if there are ongoing symptoms and need for drainage of infected necrosis. Intervention with EUS or a minimally invasive surgical approach should be considered for those patients with walled-off infected necrosis who are not clinically improving despite treatment with antibiotics.[33] The advent of EUS-guided placement of lumen apposing metal stents has enabled cyst-gastrostomy of fluid collections with immediate drainage, and endoscopic necrosectomy for walled-off necrosis (WON).[34] Timing of the intervention is of utmost importance, and treatment should be delayed for at least 3 to 4 weeks after the initial episode of acute pancreatitis to allow for maturation of fluid collection walls and to enable delineation of tissue planes. Open necrosectomy should be reserved for severe refractory cases in which minimally invasive approaches fail; this procedure is associated with poor prognosis.[35,36]

INDICATIONS FOR REFERRAL OR HOSPITALIZATION

The treatment of acute pancreatitis is primarily supportive and requires gastroenterology consultation. Hospitalization is indicated for all patients for early large-volume intravenous fluid replacement, careful observation, frequent assessment of vital signs, laboratory analyses including electrolytes and glucose concentration, and parenteral analgesia. Nutritional and surgical consultations may also be recommended. The only exception to the need for hospitalization may be the setting of mild acute pancreatitis post-ERCP if the patient is able to maintain oral hydration and oral analgesia at home.

COMPLICATIONS

Patients who have recovered from acute pancreatitis are at significant risk for recurrence if the initial cause has not been elucidated and corrected. Continued pain, malabsorption, or new-onset diabetes mellitus warrants immediate investigation. The majority of patients will recover with supportive therapy, although approximately 25% of patients will have complications. These complications include hypocalcemia and other metabolic abnormalities, blindness (Purtscher retinopathy), pseudocysts, necrosis, hemorrhage, and multisystem organ failure. The majority of deaths are caused by multiorgan system failure mediated by the SIRS. Long term, if there is disruption with disconnection of the pancreatic duct due to an episode of acute pancreatitis, this may lead to recurrent complications including fluid collections, as well as pancreatic exocrine insufficiency.

PATIENT AND FAMILY EDUCATION AND HEALTH PROMOTION

Patients should understand that severe abdominal pain with or without radiation, nausea, vomiting, or diaphoresis requires immediate evaluation. It is also important that patients understand the risk of repeated attacks of pancreatitis, the need to avoid possible precipitants, and the importance of adherence to prescribed therapy. Patient education about contributing factors, such as alcohol use, must be discussed. Because the mortality rate from alcoholic pancreatitis is high, alcohol should be avoided. A low-fat diet, weight loss, exercise, and normalization of triglyceride levels, with medications if needed, should be the goal for patients with pancreatitis associated with hypertriglyceridemia. Medications that may have caused the pancreatitis should also be avoided.

CHRONIC PANCREATITIS

DEFINITION AND EPIDEMIOLOGY

Chronic pancreatitis, an inflammatory condition of the pancreas, is characterized by morphologic and histologic changes in the pancreas that result in exocrine and endocrine insufficiency. Chronic pancreatitis differs from acute pancreatitis in that acute pancreatitis usually does not result in long-term pancreatic insufficiency, whereas the inflammatory changes in chronic pancreatitis permanently impair the exocrine and endocrine function of the gland. There are, however, reports of chronic pancreatic insufficiency in patients with acute pancreatitis with severe necrosis, especially in the head of the pancreas. The prevailing opinion regarding the parenchymal injury in acute pancreatitis, such as that induced by passage of a gallstone, is that it is both pathologically and morphologically different from the injury that occurs in chronic pancreatitis.

Chronic pancreatitis is a disease of multiple causes including chronic alcoholism, duct obstruction from tumors, strictures, hypercalcemia, hyperlipidemia, genetic mutations, congenital anatomic abnormalities such as pancreas divisum, and autoimmune and possibly dietary or environmental causes (Box 124.4). The TIGAR-O system can be used to identify major predisposing risk factors for chronic pancreatitis: (1) toxic-metabolic, (2) idiopathic, (3) genetic, (4) autoimmune, (5) recurrent and severe acute pancreatitis, and (6)

BOX **124.4**

Causes of Chronic Pancreatitis

- Alcohol abuse
- Hereditary pancreatitis
- Ductal obstruction
- Congenital anatomic abnormalities
- Tropical pancreatitis
- Autoimmune disease
- Cystic fibrosis
- Hyperparathyroidism
- Hypertriglyceridemia
- Hereditary pancreatitis (mutation of trypsinogen gene)
- Idiopathic pancreatitis (associated with atherosclerotic disease)
- Nutritional deficiencies (of antioxidants, such as selenium or vitamin C or E)

Data from Freedman, S. D., & Lewis, M. D. *Etiology and pathogenesis of chronic pancreatitis in adults.* www.uptodate.com/contents/etiology-and-pathogenesis-of-chronic-pancreatitis-in-adults?source=search_result&search=chronic+pancreatitis&selectedTitle=3~93.

obstructive.[37] In a substantial number of cases (approximately 10% to 20%), no identifiable cause can be found.

Alcohol is a major factor in both acute and chronic pancreatitis. Alcohol abuse accounts for 50% to 70% of cases of chronic pancreatitis.[38] Although the exact pathogenesis is not clearly understood, the risk appears related to the duration and amount of alcohol consumed rather than to the type of alcohol or the pattern of consumption.[38] A small group of patients may have hereditary causes for chronic pancreatitis, including genetic mutations in PRSS-1, SPINK, and CFTR. Genetic testing should be considered in recurrent acute pancreatitis or chronic pancreatitis. Pancreatic duct obstruction from trauma, calcific stones, or tumors can result in chronic pancreatitis also. Tropical pancreatitis is a common cause of pancreatitis in parts of India and the tropics. Systemic diseases, such as lupus erythematosus and cystic fibrosis, have been linked to chronic pancreatitis as well. Malnutrition or consumption of sorghum may play a role in the development of chronic pancreatitis in southern India, Indonesia, and central Africa and South Africa. Uncommon causes of chronic pancreatitis include severe malnutrition, hemochromatosis, trauma, sicca syndrome, radiation injury, gastric surgery, and tuberculosis.

In patients older than 40 years, the finding of pancreatic exocrine dysfunction or new onset endocrine dysfunction with diabetes mandates an evaluation for pancreatic cancer. Pancreatic exocrine dysfunction in adults aged 20 to 40 years should trigger an investigation for cystic fibrosis because 85% of patients with cystic fibrosis have some pancreatic insufficiency and may have a delayed presentation of their underlying cystic fibrosis. Fifty percent of patients with chronic pancreatitis die within 25 years of diagnosis; up to 49% of those deaths are related to complications including pancreatic cancer.[39]

The most widely used classification for chronic pancreatitis is the Marseilles-Rome classification system modified by Sarles. It divides the condition into categories based on morphology, epidemiology, and molecular biology.[2,40]

PATHOPHYSIOLOGY

The pathophysiologic mechanism of chronic pancreatitis is multifactorial and not completely understood. It is postulated that increased pancreatic secretion causes proteinaceous plugs to form within the interlobular and intralobular ducts, with obstruction of the ducts and subsequent scarring and damage because of inflammatory changes, resulting from autodigestion.[41] Patients with recurrent episodes of acute pancreatitis may go on to develop chronic pancreatitis.

CLINICAL PRESENTATION AND PHYSICAL EXAMINATION

Chronic pancreatitis most commonly manifests with abdominal pain, and signs and symptoms related to pancreatic exocrine or endocrine insufficiency. Abdominal pain may be severe, recurrent, or constant and is typically epigastric, with potential referral to the upper back, anterior chest, or flank. Nausea and vomiting may accompany the pain. Usually the discomfort is not relieved by food or antacids and intensifies with alcohol or fatty food. Pain often occurs 15 to 20 minutes after eating. Weight loss, diarrhea, and steatorrhea with oily stools may be reported as a result of fat malabsorption; however, malnutrition and micronutrient deficiencies may be present long before the development of gross steatorrhea. When the destruction of pancreatic function results in diabetes, the typical symptoms

of polyuria, polydipsia, and polyphagia may be observed. Glucose intolerance occurs frequently, typically requiring insulin administration as the disease progresses. Patients with severe pancreatic dysfunction have difficulty digesting complex foods or absorbing products of digestion. Significant protein and fat deficiencies occur when more than 90% of pancreatic exocrine function is lost.[41,42]

The physical examination, even in the presence of severe pain, may reveal few overt findings. Weight loss or abdominal tenderness may be present. Jaundice, signifying common bile duct obstruction, is less common. If pancreatic dysfunction results in severe malabsorption, signs of malnutrition will be evident.[42]

DIAGNOSTICS

Laboratory data are useful to exclude other causes of abdominal pain and to determine whether pancreatic insufficiency exists. In contrast to acute pancreatitis, elevated serum amylase and lipase levels are not typically present. There is a minimal if any increase in pancreatic enzymes in the blood because of significant fibrosis, which results in decreased concentration of these enzymes within the pancreas. Complete blood count (CBC) and liver chemistry results are typically normal. Increased bilirubin and alkaline phosphatase levels can indicate compression of bile ducts and should prompt investigation for fibrosis, edema, or tumor. The presence of pancreatic insufficiency is indicated by elevated blood glucose concentration or steatorrhea. Steatorrhea can be diagnosed with Sudan stain of the feces and examination for fecal fat. The patient should eat a minimum of 100 g of fat daily, and stool is collected during a 72-hour period. A fecal fat level of more than 7 g is diagnostic of malassimilation.[42] This is cumbersome for patients and has therefore been replaced by other markers such as fecal elastase. Fecal elastase has a high negative predictive value for pancreatic insufficiency and high sensitivity in patients with moderate and severe pancreatic failure.[43]

When the diagnosis is not clear clinically, the next step is pancreatic imaging. Imaging studies visualizing structure and pancreatic function tests complement one another. Abdominal radiography, EUS, CT scan, MRI, ERCP, and MRCP are diagnostic imaging studies that are useful in chronic pancreatitis. In one-third of patients, abdominal radiographs (kidney, ureter, bladder [KUB]) may demonstrate pancreatic calcifications, thereby supporting the diagnosis. Abdominal ultrasonography may expedite early diagnosis because pancreatic enlargement and calcifications can be seen earlier than on abdominal radiography. The sensitivity of CT and MRI approaches 90% for diagnosis of advanced chronic pancreatitis. Evidence of ductal dilation with focal enlargement, fluid collections, or calcifications on CT or MRI indicates chronic pancreatitis. EUS is an increasingly common diagnostic and therapeutic modality in the management of chronic pancreatitis. It is now the gold standard because one can visualize the pancreatic parenchyma and examine the features of the ductal system with much less risk for complications compared with ERCP. Stone formation in the pancreatic duct seen on EUS is a largely predictive feature of chronic pancreatitis. Other EUS findings include visible side branches, cysts, lobularity, irregularity or dilation of a main duct, hyperechoic foci, hyperechoic strands, and a main duct with hyperechoic margins. The severity of chronic pancreatitis correlates with the number of EUS findings observed. The Rosemont classification system has been proposed as a means to diagnose chronic pancreatitis using EUS, and takes into account a hyperechoic or echogenic appearance of the pancreas as well as measurements and appearance of the pancreatic ducts, side branches, and presence of strictures.[44,45] MRCP is useful in assessing the pancreatic ducts as a noninvasive method. ERCP should not be used as a primary diagnostic modality for chronic pancreatitis, and should be used only for therapeutic interventions.

The secretin stimulation test is considered the definitive test in assessing pancreatic function. This diagnostic test involves measurement of the bicarbonate concentration originating from the pancreas in the duodenal fluid after the administration of secretin. Secretin causes the secretion of bicarbonate-rich fluid from the pancreas. A peak bicarbonate concentration of less than 80 mEq/L is consistent with chronic pancreatitis. The test can be done either with fluoroscopic placement of a double lumen tube or endoscopically. This test is not widely utilized due to availability.

Laboratory tests may be used to diagnose autoimmune chronic pancreatitis, including erythrocyte sedimentation rate, immunoglobulin G4, rheumatoid factor, antinuclear antibodies, and anti–smooth muscle antibody.[42]

INITIAL DIAGNOSTICS

Chronic Pancreatitis

LABORATORY
- Complete blood count and differential
- Serum amylase
- Serum lipase
- Serum bilirubin
- Serum glucose
- Serum alkaline phosphatase
- Stool for steatorrhea (fecal fat)/fecal elastase

IMAGING
- Kidney, ureter, bladder, abdominal ultrasound

- Computed tomography scan, magnetic resonance imaging, magnetic resonance cholangiopancreatography
- Endoscopic ultrasound

OTHER DIAGNOSTICS
- Endoscopic retrograde cholangiopancreatography[a]
- Secretin stimulation test[a]

---

[a]If indicated.

DIFFERENTIAL DIAGNOSIS

 The primary priority differential is pancreatic cancer, but mesenteric vascular disease and autoimmune disorders are also possible causes that should be considered.

A strong history of alcoholism suggests the diagnosis of chronic pancreatitis in the patient with abdominal pain. However, pancreatic cancer, peptic ulcer disease, cholelithiasis, biliary tract obstruction, irritable bowel syndrome, and pancreatic stones should be excluded when the diagnosis of chronic pancreatitis is being considered.

In addition, because pancreatic cancer may manifest with signs and symptoms similar to those of chronic pancreatitis, patients may require MRCP or EUS for diagnosis. *Pancreatic cancer should be suspected as a cause of chronic pancreatitis when a patient is older than 50 years or has any of the following: (1) new-onset diabetes mellitus; (2) change in bowel habits;*

(3) negative history of alcohol use; (4) recent weight loss; (5) a short duration of symptoms and/or the presence of other constitutional signs and symptoms (e.g., fatigue, insomnia, anorexia). These symptoms can originate from pancreatic cancer and should be considered a "red flag," prompting additional workup with EUS and tumor markers, given a high suspicion for malignancy. Tumor markers (carcinoembryonic antigen, CA 19-9) may be normal with early pancreatic cancer as CA 19-9 level should be viewed as a marker of ductal obstruction.[42]

Further imaging with ultrasound or angiography can be used to exclude mesenteric vascular disease as the origin of chronic abdominal pain. Finally, the health care provider must recognize that chronic pancreatitis can occur in the setting of autoimmune diseases such as Sjögren syndrome, systemic lupus erythematosus, and primary biliary cirrhosis, and use appropriate testing to exclude associated conditions as warranted by the patient's history and presentation.

INTERPROFESSIONAL COLLABORATIVE MANAGEMENT

The aims of treatment of chronic pancreatitis include treatment of pancreatic exocrine and endocrine dysfunction, pain control, and correction of symptomatic pancreatic structural abnormalities. Pain management can be challenging, but there are now pain management guidelines to guide practitioners caring for patients with chronic pancreatitis. Initially, current guidelines recommend the stepwise escalation of analgesic drugs with increasing until the patient's pain pain relief is obtained. Alcohol and smoking cessation is also important, not only for immediate pain relief but also in avoiding future episodes. Pancreatic enzyme therapy, antioxidants, and endoscopy are further considerations that may be helpful.[48,49] These management goals require medical and possibly surgical intervention.[48]

Pharmacologic Management

In chronic pancreatitis, patients experience nutritional deficiencies and chronic pain. The intense pain of chronic pancreatitis coupled with inconsistent pain relief is a risk factor for narcotic addiction. A short course of opiates with low-dose amitriptyline and nonsteroidal medication may break the pain cycle. Nerve blocks have not been found to provide long-term pain relief in the treatment of chronic pancreatitis, and results are widely variable. Studies have found that the celiac nerve block provides relief of pain for 2 to 4 months, if at all, and poses a risk for irreversible nerve damage.[42] Early involvement of a pain management team may provide additional benefit to patients and potentially minimize addiction sequelae. Uncoated pancreatic enzymes combined with acid suppression to allow for maximal absorption are thought to be useful for pain control to suppress the production of pancreatic enzymes.

Nutritional deficiencies result from malassimilation of ingested food from exocrine pancreatic insufficiency and endocrine insufficiency resulting in diabetes mellitus with loss of calories. Steatorrhea and diarrhea are produced by exocrine dysfunction and may be compounded by potential small intestinal bacterial overgrowth due to malassimilated food contents remaining in the intestinal lumen. Malassimilation is managed by pancreatic enzyme replacement. The starting dose of pancreatic enzyme replacement in patients with severe chronic pancreatitis may be as high as 90,000 United States Pharmacopeia (USP) units of lipase with each meal and 45,000 USP units with snacks.[46,47] Pancreatic enzyme function may be increased by intake of acid-suppressing medications. Enzyme supplementation is recommended for all patients with chronic pancreatitis and may have a role to decrease pain that has not responded to other conservative measures. Pancreatic enzyme replacement therapy comes in coated and uncoated forms; the uncoated form requires acid suppression, because an acidic environment will neutralize the pancreatic enzymes. The coated form of enzymes is usually used to correct pancreatic exocrine insufficiency. Normalization of the patient's diarrhea and/or steatorrhea and improvement of nutritional parameters are indicative of efficacy of enzyme replacement, and stool frequency and consistency have been shown to improve and correlate with improvements in fecal elastase with pancreatic enzyme replacement therapy. Additional nutritional support with supplementation of fat-soluble vitamins (A, D, E, and K) may be necessary.

Nonpharmacologic Management

When a patient has pain nonresponsive to medical therapies, surgical interventions may be necessary. Extracorporeal shock wave lithotripsy of calcified pancreatic stones can be helpful in relieving the obstruction of pancreatic ducts, blocking secretions in the 22% to 60% of patients with chronic pancreatitis who have pancreatic duct stones. Endoscopic therapy may provide pain relief in some patients by decompressing an obstructed pancreatic duct with placement of a stent or pancreatic duct sphincterotomy and stone extraction. However, studies have shown that the presence or absence of stones does not correlate with the existence of pain.[42] A randomized controlled trial examining patients with chronic pancreatitis and a dilated duct showed that surgical drainage resulted in better pain scores than for those patients undergoing endoscopic drainage.[47]

Surgical options for chronic pancreatitis include denervation procedures, which involve interruption of the nerve fibers passing through the celiac ganglion and splanchnic nerves from the pancreas. Another surgical intervention for patients with a dilated duct involves decompression and drainage of the pancreatic duct. Gastric and biliary drainage may be necessary as well because of obstruction or strictures of the bile duct or duodenum. Resection of a portion of the pancreas may be an option for those patients with ongoing pain who are not considered candidates for drainage procedures. Resection of the pancreatic head may provide pain relief in up to 85% of patients. Patients who have undergone pancreatectomy may have exocrine and endocrine dysfunction. Pancreatic insufficiency can result with extensive resection, and severe diabetes can ensue, which can be very difficult to treat given the absence of counter-regulatory hormones. Autologous islet cell transplantation after entire gland resection is becoming increasingly common especially for those with episodes of recurrent acute pancreatitis, as reimplantation of islets into the portal vein minimizes the risk of development of brittle diabetes, and a subset of these patients may remain insulin independent. Total pancreatectomy is a last resort in patients who have not responded to all other treatments. Despite the availability of these techniques, the criteria for surgical intervention are controversial. Consultation with a gastroenterologist is advised for diagnostic verification and collaborative management. Invasive studies may be indicated as the patient's condition changes or as complications follow.[41]

INDICATIONS FOR REFERRAL OR HOSPITALIZATION

The primary care or collaborating physician is consulted for the initial diagnosis and management. Subsequent deterioration or complications in the patient's status warrant continued physician guidance. Initial testing for stable, uncomplicated patients can be accomplished in the outpatient setting. Patients with chronic pancreatitis may have superimposed episodes of acute pancreatitis, which should be appropriately managed as described in the acute pancreatitis section. Hospitalization is required for the management of serious complications and for surgical drainage or resection procedures. Given the complications and risk of progression to pancreatic cancer, patients with chronic pancreatitis should be referred to a gastroenterologist to tailor long-term management plans and ensure close follow-up. Incidentally found suspicious lesions or changes in imaging of the pancreas in a patient with known chronic pancreatitis should also prompt immediate referral to a gastroenterologist for further evaluation.

LIFE-SPAN CONSIDERATIONS

Steatorrhea, diabetes, and pancreatic calcifications are complications commonly experienced by older adults with long-standing chronic pancreatitis. Other causes of malabsorption in older adults with steatorrhea should be considered. Celiac disease, small bowel bacterial overgrowth, and pancreatic cancer must be excluded.

COMPLICATIONS

Chronic pancreatitis can be associated with a variety of complications. The most common complications are pseudocyst formation and mechanical obstruction of the duodenum and common bile duct.[50] Diabetes, exocrine insufficiency, malnutrition, pancreatic ascites, pleural effusion, splenic vein thrombosis, gastric varices due to splenic vein thrombosis with left-sided portal hypertension, and pain are other complications associated with chronic pancreatitis.[50] The most feared complication of chronic pancreatitis is development of pancreatic cancer. The development of extrahepatic biliary obstruction is signified by serum alkaline phosphatase levels that are twice the normal level for longer than 2 months. Portal hypertension may occur as a result of thrombosis in the splenic or portal veins, pancreatic abscess, common bile duct obstruction, peptic ulcer, pseudoaneurysm of adjacent arteries, gastrointestinal bleeding, ascites from a leaking pseudocyst or damaged duct, and pancreatic cancer.

PATIENT AND FAMILY EDUCATION

It is vital that patients and families understand the recurrent, chronic character of the disease. Careful explanation of each individual's etiologic factors and the need for alcohol abstinence is necessary. Patients with pancreatic endocrine insufficiency should receive diabetic education, because they are susceptible to macrovascular and microvascular complications. Patients with pancreatic exocrine insufficiency must understand the origin of steatorrhea, the purpose and dosage of dietary supplements and pancreatic enzyme replacement when appropriate, and supplementation with fat-soluble vitamins and calcium. It is important to clarify and to update guidelines for follow-up care, pain management, and symptoms requiring immediate attention.

PANCREATIC PSEUDOCYST

DEFINITION AND EPIDEMIOLOGY

Pseudocysts develop in approximately 10% of patients with chronic pancreatitis. They are the result of an encapsulation by fibrous tissue of an acute fluid collection. A pancreatic pseudocyst is an acute fluid collection persistent longer than 4 weeks, occurring after an episode of acute pancreatitis. Pseudocysts do not contain necrotic debris. Conversely, necrotic collections lasting longer than 4 weeks after an episode of acute pancreatitis is defined as WON.[3] The prefix *pseudo-* is used because this localized collection of material does not have an epithelial lining, a hallmark of a true cyst.

Pseudocysts form as sequelae of acute pancreatitis or in association with chronic pancreatitis. Other, less common causes include gallbladder disease causing pancreatitis, and surgery or trauma to the pancreas. Pseudocysts, occurring singularly or as multiple lesions, develop primarily in the body or tail of the pancreas but are found outside the pancreas.

PATHOPHYSIOLOGY

Pseudocysts develop as a result of ductal disruptions and contain a large concentration of pancreatic enzymes. Pseudocysts may be single or multiple, small or large, and located in or outside of the pancreas. An absence of epithelial tissue distinguishes pseudocysts from pancreatic cysts.

CLINICAL PRESENTATION

Most pancreatic pseudocysts are asymptomatic. When symptoms occur, the presenting symptoms are typically related to the location and extent of the fluid collection, or its complications—that is, leakage, infection, or erosion into adjacent organs such as the splenic vein. Abdominal pain may be a presenting symptom related to expansion of the pseudocyst. Other symptoms associated with pseudocyst formation include low-grade fever, jaundice, diaphragm inflammation, pleural effusion, and ascites. Pseudocyst expansion may also contribute to duodenal or biliary obstruction, vascular occlusion, and fistula formation into adjacent viscera. Gastrointestinal bleeding can result when a pseudoaneurysm forms from adjacent vessel necrosis and bleeds into a pancreatic duct.[51] Secondary infection of pseudocysts is uncommon compared with WON.

DIAGNOSTICS

Diagnostics include pancreatic imaging by CT, MRI, or ultrasonography. If pleural effusion or ascites is present along with the pseudocyst, the thoracentesis or paracentesis fluid has amylase levels above 1000 international units (IU)/L when the origin is pancreatic.[52] Biopsy and carcinoembryonic antigen levels of cystic fluid from suspicious cystic lesions exclude premalignant growths and malignant neoplasms.[52,53] This is accomplished by CT-guided percutaneous needle aspiration or via EUS with fine-needle aspiration. MRCP, EUS, or ERCP before surgery is indicated to determine ductal and pseudocyst anatomy. Serologic analysis includes amylase, glucose, alkaline phosphatase, and bilirubin concentrations. Elevations of blood glucose and amylase levels are common. Increased serum alkaline phosphatase or bilirubin levels indicate compression of the common bile duct as it passes through the pancreas from extrahepatic biliary obstruction.

DIFFERENTIAL DIAGNOSIS

 The important priority differential is a pancreatic neoplasm. Additional concerns include pseudoaneurysm as well as an infected or ruptured pseudocyst.

The presence of pancreatic fluid masses requires investigation. Pseudocysts can be confused with and should be distinguished from pancreatic cystic tumors including cystadenomas, cystadenocarcinomas, intraductal papillary mucinous neoplasms (IPMNs), and other pancreatic cysts including retention cysts, and congenital conditions. Concerns that a fluid collection is not a pseudocyst are prompted by a patient's history of no prior episodes of acute pancreatitis, signs or symptoms of chronic pancreatitis, or pancreatic trauma, and by the absence of inflammatory changes on CT scan. The cyst on imaging may have features that suggest it is not a pseudocyst—for example, thick walls or septations.[51] EUS with fine-needle aspiration is used to exclude malignancy in cystic lesions because pancreatic neoplasms may be cystic.

INTERPROFESSIONAL COLLABORATIVE MANAGEMENT

The decision process for pseudocyst management contains several steps. First, alternative diagnoses, particularly the possibility that the cyst may represent a neoplasm, must be excluded. Next, the provider considers whether a complication of pseudocyst (e.g., biliary or duodenal obstruction) is present. If the pseudocyst is increasing rapidly in size and/or the hemoglobin is decreasing, consideration should be given to a pseudoaneurysm, which occurs in approximately 10% of patients with a pancreatic pseudocyst.[51] Complication rates rise dramatically after the presence of the pseudocyst for longer than 13 weeks. In patients without discomfort, neoplasm, or complications, conservative management may be possible and the pancreatic pseudocyst safely monitored.[51] Currently, there are several drainage options for pseudocysts that are based on the cyst's location and the patient's symptoms. These options are multiple internal drainage procedures that can be performed endoscopically and percutaneously guided by CT. Indications for drainage include rapid enlargement, compression of surrounding structures, pain, gastric outlet obstruction with associated symptoms of pain/nausea/vomiting, and signs of infection. One should allow maturation of the pseudocyst wall for at least 4 weeks before arranging for drainage.

Initial evaluation, laboratory tests, and imaging studies can be performed in the primary care setting. Complications, invasive diagnostics, and evaluation for surgery require collaboration with specialists in radiology, surgery, and gastroenterology.

INDICATIONS FOR REFERRAL OR HOSPITALIZATION

If a pseudocyst or another complication is suspected, the collaborating physician is consulted during the initial visit. Long-term management requires careful and continued collaboration with the primary care physician.

COMPLICATIONS

Infected pseudocysts may cause severe pain, high fever, chills, and leukocytosis. If infection is clinically suspected, an empiric course of antibiotics should be initiated. If there is no clinical response, then guided needle aspiration is indicated for culture and sensitivity. Without clinical response to antibiotics or with continued enlargement of the pseudocyst and symptoms as above, then CT or EUS guided drainage is indicated. Furthermore, pseudocysts may erode and perforate structures, resulting in rupture into the peritoneal cavity or gastrointestinal tract. Stomach perforation can manifest with few symptoms and require no treatment; acute peritoneal perforation necessitates surgical intervention and can be fatal, as opposed to gradual leakage, which results in pancreatic ascites. Colon perforation is seen with abdominal pain and self-limited bloody diarrhea. Pseudocysts can also erode blood vessels, creating a pseudoaneurysm and producing hemorrhage and shock. Three clinical findings are associated with pseudoaneurysm formation: gastrointestinal bleeding, sudden pseudocyst enlargement, and unexplained decrease in hematocrit.[52] Elevated serum amylase levels and ascitic fluid containing amylase and protein suggest a leaking pseudocyst.

PATIENT AND FAMILY EDUCATION

Patients at risk for pseudocyst formation should be educated about the symptoms of a pseudocyst and the necessity to contact their health care provider for increased or persistent pain. Patients with known pseudocysts should receive instruction concerning the cause of their condition, complications, symptoms, and indications to seek medical attention.

ACKNOWLEDGMENTS

The authors wish to extend their thanks to Jamie S. Barkin, MD, for reviewing this chapter.

REFERENCES

1. Bradley, E. L., 3rd. (1993). A clinically based classification system for acute pancreatitis. Summary of the International Symposium on Acute Pancreatitis, Atlanta, Ga, September 11 through 13, 1992. *Archives of Surgery (Chicago, Ill.: 1960), 128*(5), 586–590.

2. Fernandez, H., & Barkin, J. (2010). Acute pancreatitis. In P. R. McNally (Ed.), *GI/liver secrets* (4th ed.). Philadelphia: Elsevier.

3. Banks, P. A., Bollen, T. L., Dervenis, C., et al. (2013). Classification of acute pancreatitis—2012: Revision of the Atlanta Classification and definitions by international consensus. *Gut, 62*(1), 102–111.

4. Forsmark, C. E., & Baillie, J. (2007). AGA institute technical review on acute pancreatitis. *Gastroenterology, 132*(5), 2022–2044.

5. Parsons, P., & Wiener-Kronish, J. (Eds.), (2003). *Critical care secrets* (3rd ed.). Philadelphia: Hanley & Belfus.

6. Lankisch, P. G., Karimi, M., Bruns, A., et al. Time trends in incidence of acute pancreatitis in Luneburg: A population-based study. Abstracts of papers submitted to the 38th annual meeting of the American Pancreatic Association, Chicago, Ill, November 1–3, 2007.

7. Testoni, P. A., Mariani, A., Giussani, A., et al. (2010). Risk factors for post-ERCP pancreatitis in high- and low-volume centers and among expert and non-expert operators: A prospective multicenter study. *The American Journal of Gastroenterology, 105*(8), 1753–1761.

8. van Geenen, E. J., de Boer, N. K., Stassen, P., et al. (2010). Azathioprine or mercaptopurine-induced acute pancreatitis is not a disease specific phenomenon. *Alimentary Pharmacology and Therapeutics, 31*(12), 1322–1329.

9. Barkin, J. A., Nemeth, Z., Saluja, A. K., et al. (2017). Cannabis-induced acute pancreatitis: A systematic review. *Europe PubMed Central, 46*(8), 1035–1038.

10. Adibelli, Z. H., Adatepe, M., Imamoglu, C., Esen, O. S., Erkan, N., & Yildirim, M. (2016). Anatomic variations of the pancreatic duct and their relevance with the Cambridge classification system: MRCP findings of 1158 consecutive patients. *Radiology and Oncology, 50*(4), 370–377. doi:10.1515/raon-2016-0041.

11. Cole, L. (2001). Unraveling the mystery of acute pancreatitis. *Nursing, 31*(12), 58–63.

12. American College of Chest Physicians/Society of Critical Care Medicine Consensus Conference. (1992). Definitions for sepsis and organ failure and guidelines for the use of innovative therapies in sepsis. *Critical Care Medicine, 20*(6), 864–874.

13. Mitchell, R. M., Byrne, M. F., & Baillie, J. (2003). Pancreatitis. *Lancet, 361*(9367), 1447–1455.

14. Tenner, S., Baillie, J., DeWitt, J., & Vege, S. (2013). American College of Gastroenterology Guideline: Management of acute pancreatitis. *The American Journal of Gastroenterology.*

15. Young, S., & Thomson, J. (2008). Severe acute pancreatitis. *Continuing Education in Anaesthesia Critical Care & Pain, 8*(4), 125–129.

16. Baillie, J. (2001). Acute pancreatitis. *Emergency Medicine, 33*(8), 12–19.

17. Surlin, V., Saftoiu, A., & Dumitrescu, D. (2014). Imaging tests for accurate diagnosis of acute biliary pancreatitis. *The American Journal of Gastroenterology, 20*(44), 16544–16549.

18. Shea, Y., Furlan, A., Almusa, O., et al. (2012). The Revised Atlanta Classification for acute pancreatitis: A CT imaging guide for radiologists. *Emergency Radiology, 19*(3), 237–243.

19. van Santvoort, H. C., Besselink, M. G., deVries, A. C., et al. (2009). Early endoscopic retrograde cholangiopancreatography in predicted severe acute biliary pancreatitis: A prospective multicenter study. *Annals of Surgery, 250*(1), 68–75.

20. Rhoads, K., & Varma, M. (2003). The acute abdomen. In P. Parsons & J. Wiener-Kronish (Eds.), *Critical care secrets* (3rd ed.). Philadelphia: Hanley & Belfus.

21. Wu, B. U., Hwang, J. Q., Gardner, T. H., et al. (2011). Lactated Ringer's solution reduces systemic inflammation compared with saline in patients with acute pancreatitis. *Clinical Gastroenterology and Hepatology: the Official Clinical Practice Journal of the American Gastroenterological Association, 9*, 710–717.

22. Barkin, J. A., & Barkin, J. S. (2017). Periprocedural intravenous fluid administration for the prevention of post-endoscopic retrograde cholangiopancreatography pancreatitis. *Pancreas, 46*(7), e57–e58.

23. Working Group IAP/APA Acute Pancreatitis Guidelines. (2013). IAP/APA evidence-based guidelines for the management of acute pancreatitis. *Pancreatology, 13*(4 Suppl. 2), e1–e15.

24. Wittau, M., Mayer, B., Scheele, J., et al. (2011). Systematic review and meta-analysis of antibiotic prophylaxis in severe acute pancreatitis. *Scandinavian Journal of Gastroenterology, 46*(3), 261–270.

25. Crockett, S. D., Crockett, S., et al. (2018). American Gastroenterological Association Institute Guideline on initial management of acute pancreatitis. *Gastroenterology, 154*(4), 1096–1101.

26. Besselink, M. G., van Santvoort, H. C., Buskens, E., et al. (2008). Probiotic prophylaxis in predicted severe acute pancreatitis: A randomized, double-blind, placebo-controlled trial. *Lancet, 371*(9613), 651–659.

27. Chaudhary, A., Iqbal, U., Anwar, H., & Siddiqui, H. U. (2017). Acute pancreatitis secondary to Severe hypertriglyceridemia: Management of severe hypertriglyceridemia in emergency setting. *Gastroenterology Research, 10*(3), 190–192. doi:10.14740/gr762e. Epub 2017 Jun 30.

28. Rawla, P., Sunkara, T., Thandra, K. C., & Gaduputi, V. (2018). Hypertriglyceridemia-induced pancreatitis: Updated review of current treatment and preventive strategies. *Clinical Journal of Gastroenterology, 11*(6), 441–448. doi:10.1007/s12328-018-0881-1. Epub 2018 Jun 19.

29. Echerwall, G. E., Tingstedt, B. B., Bergenzaun, P. E., et al. (2007). Immediate oral feeding in patients with acute pancreatitis is safe and may accelerate recovery—a randomized clinical study. *Clinical Nutrition: Official Journal of the European Society of Parenteral and Enteral Nutrition, 26*, 758–763.

30. Crockett, S. D., Crockett, S., et al. (2018). Gastroenterological Association Institute Guideline on initial management of acute pancreatitis. *Gastroenterology, 154*(4), 1096–1101.

31. Al-Omran, M., Albalawi, Z. H., Tashkandi, M. F., et al. (2010). Enteral versus parenteral nutrition for acute pancreatitis. *The Cochrane Database of Systematic Reviews*, (1), CD002837.

32. Petrov, M. S., van Santvoort, H. C., Besselink, M. G., et al. (2008). Enteral nutrition and the risk of mortality and infectious complications in patients

with severe acute pancreatitis. *Archives of Surgery (Chicago, Ill.: 1960), 143*(11), 1111–1117.

33. McClave, S. A. (2013). Nutrition in pancreatitis. *World Review of Nutrition and Dietetics, 105,* 160–168.

34. Walter, D., Will, U., Sanchez-Yague, A., et al. (2015). A novel lumen-apposing metal stent for endoscopic ultrasound-guided drainage of pancreatic fluid collections: A prospective cohort study. *Endoscopy, 47*(1), 63–67.

35. van Santvoort, H. C., Besselink, M. G., Bakker, O. J., et al. (2010). A step-up approach or open necrosectomy for necrotizing pancreatitis. *The New England Journal of Medicine, 362*(16), 1491–1502.

36. Besselink, M. G., Verwer, T. J., Schoenmaeckers, E. J., et al. (2007). Timing of surgical intervention in necrotizing pancreatitis. *Archives of Surgery (Chicago, Ill.: 1960), 142*(12), 1194–1201.

37. Etemad, B., & Whitcomb, D. C. (2001). Chronic pancreatitis: Diagnosis, classification, and new genetic developments. *Gastroenterology, 120*(3), 682–707.

38. Cote, G. A., Yadav, D., Slivka, A., et al. (2011). Alcohol and smoking as risk factors in an epidemiology study of patients with chronic pancreatitis. *Clinical Gastroenterology and Hepatology, 9*(3), 266–273.

39. Otsuki, M. (2003). Chronic pancreatitis in Japan: Epidemiology, prognosis, diagnostic criteria and future problems. *Journal of Gastroenterology, 38*(4), 315–326.

40. Sarles, H. (1989). Classification and definition of pancreatitis. Marseilles-Rome 1988. *Gastroentérologie Clinique et Biologique, 13*(11), 857–859.

41. Puylaert, M., Kapural, L., Van Zundert, J., et al. (2011). Pain in chronic pancreatitis. *Pain Practice, 11*(5), 492–505.

42. Nair, R. J., Lawler, L., & Miller, M. R. (2007). Chronic pancreatitis. *American Family Physician, 76*(11), 1679–1688.

43. Gullo, L., Ventrucci, M., Tomassetti, P., et al. (1999). Fecal elastase 1 determination in chronic pancreatitis. *Digestive Diseases and Sciences, 44,* 210–213.

44. Stevens, T., & Parsi, M. A. (2013). Endoscopic ultrasound for the diagnosis of chronic pancreatitis. *World Journal of Gastroenterology, 16*(23), 2841–2850.

45. Catalano, M. F., Sahai, A., Levy, M., et al. (2009). EUS-based criteria for the diagnosis of chronic pancreatitis: The Rosemont classification. *Gastrointestinal Endoscopy, 69*(7), 1251–1261.

46. DiMagno, M. J., & DiMagno, E. P. (2013). Chronic pancreatitis. *Current Opinion in Gastroenterology, 29*(5), 531–536.

47. Thorat, V., Reddy, N., Bhatia, S., et al. (2012). Randomised clinical trial: The efficacy and safety of pancreatin enteric-coated minimicrospheres (Creon 40000 MMS) in patients with pancreatic exocrine insufficiency due to chronic pancreatitis—a double-blind, placebo-controlled study. *Alimentary Pharmacology and Therapeutics, 36*(5), 426–436.

48. Cahen, D. L., Gouma, D. J., Nio, Y., et al. (2007). Endoscopic versus surgical drainage of the pancreatic duct in chronic pancreatitis. *The New England Journal of Medicine, 356*(7), 676–684.

49. Drewes, A. M., Bouwense, S. A. W., Campbell, C. M., et al. (2017). Guidelines for the understanding and management of pain in chronic pancreatitis. *Pancreatology, 17*(5), 720–731. doi:10.1016/j.pan.2017.07.006. https://mission-cure.org/blog/new-guidelines-for-managing-the-pain-of-chronic-pancreatitis/. Epub 2017 Jul 13.

50. Braganzo, J. M., Lee, S. H., McCloy, R. F., et al. (2011). Chronic pancreatitis. *Lancet, 377*(9772), 1184–1187.

51. Turner, B. G., & Brugge, W. R. (2010). Pancreatic cystic lesions: When to watch, when to operate, when to ignore. *Current Gastroenterology Reports, 12*(2), 98–105.

52. Cannon, J. W., Callery, M. P., & Vollmer, C. M., Jr. (2009). Diagnosis and management of pancreatic pseudocysts: What is the evidence? *Journal of the American College of Surgeons, 209*(3), 385–393.

53. Lim, S. J., Alasadi, R., Wayne, J. D., et al. (2005). Preoperative evaluation of pancreatic cystic lesions: Cost-benefit analysis and proposed management algorithm. *Surgery, 138*(4), 672–679.

CHAPTER **125**

TUMORS OF THE GASTROINTESTINAL TRACT

Lauren Jean Welton

Tumors of the gastrointestinal tract may be benign or malignant. It is essential that malignant tumors be identified as

early as possible and treated appropriately. This chapter focuses on the common malignant neoplasms of the esophagus, stomach, small intestine, and colon; common benign tumors of the gastrointestinal tract are also discussed.

TUMORS OF THE ESOPHAGUS

DEFINITION AND EPIDEMIOLOGY

Esophageal carcinoma is a malignant neoplasm of the esophagus. In 2015, esophageal carcinoma accounted for 16,890 new cancer cases and 15,590 cancer deaths in the United States alone.[1] Esophageal cancers are often not identified until in advanced stages, and morbidity and mortality are very high due to their aggressive nature.[2] Esophageal cancer is the sixth leading cause of death from cancer and the eighth most common cancer in the word.[2] The 5-year survival rate is about 15% to 25%.[2] Esophageal cancer is identified as adenocarcinoma or squamous cell carcinoma during histologic exam of the tissue. Esophageal squamous cell carcinoma is the most common histologic type worldwide; however, adenocarcinoma is most prevalent in Western countries.[2] There are known risks factors with each histologic type. Adenocarcinoma of the esophagus is eight times more common in males than in females and five times more common in Caucasians than in African Americans in the United States.[2] Squamous cell carcinoma remains that most common subtype in African Americans.[2] The prevalence of esophageal cancer is higher in Turkey, Iran, Kazakhstan, and northern and central China, which make up the "Asian Esophageal Cancer Belt."[2] In areas where incidence is high, early diagnosis is more frequent. In some areas of China, screening endoscopy in the general population has proven to be cost effective due to the high prevalence of squamous cell carcinoma.[2]

Other risk factors for squamous cell esophageal carcinoma include smoking, alcohol consumption, and Tylosis, which is an autosomal dominant disease.[2] About 6% to 14% of patients with gastroesophageal reflux disease (GERD) will develop Barrett esophagus, which is a premalignant lesion; 0.5% to 1% of these patients will develop adenocarcinoma.[2] Observational studies have indicated that the use of nonsteroidal antiinflammatory drugs, proton pump inhibitors, and statins are linked with low rates of progression to adenocarcinoma.[2] Endoscopic screening for adenocarcinoma in patients with Barrett esophagus remains the standard of care worldwide but has not proven to be cost-effective.[2] Obesity is also emerging as a significant risk factor for the development of esophageal adenocarcinoma.[2]

PATHOPHYSIOLOGY

Squamous cell carcinomas develop from cells in the proximal portion of the esophagus, and adenocarcinomas develop from glandular cells in the distal portion of the esophagus.

Esophageal adenocarcinomas associated with Barrett esophagus arise from metaplasia of the distal esophagus occurring in association with long-term gastroesophageal reflux.[2]

CLINICAL PRESENTATION AND PHYSICAL EXAMINATION

Dysphagia and weight loss are classic presenting symptoms of esophageal carcinoma. More than 90% of patients will have solid food dysphagia which progressively worsens.[3]

Odynophagia can also be present. Tumors can extend into the tracheobronchial tree, which can result in fistula formation; these patients may present with coughing on swallowing or pneumonia.[3] Back or chest pain may suggest extension into the mediastinum.[3] Hoarseness can occur when the recurrent laryngeal nerve is involved.[3] **The physical exam** of the patient is often unremarkable. However, supraclavicular and cervical lymphadenopathy can suggest metastatic disease.[3]

DIAGNOSTICS
Essential Diagnostics
Upper gastrointestinal endoscopy with biopsy remains the gold standard for screening and diagnosis.[2]

Additional Diagnostics
New-onset dysphagia should prompt an evaluation for an esophageal tumor. Workup may begin with a barium esophagogram followed by upper gastrointestinal endoscopy if indicated.[3] After confirmation of the diagnosis, computed tomography (CT) of the chest and abdomen is commonly used to evaluate for evidence of metastatic disease.[3] Endoscopic ultrasound, fine needle aspiration lymph node biopsy, positron emission tomography, and bronchoscopy can also be utilized when indicated for further staging of the disease.[3]

INITIAL DIAGNOSTICS

Esophageal Tumors

LABORATORY
- Complete blood count
- Comprehensive metabolic panel

IMAGING
- Contrast radiography
- Chest x-ray examination[a]
- Computed tomography (CT) scan[a]
- PET/CT scan

- Radionuclide bone scans[a]
- Ultrasound[a]

OTHER DIAGNOSTICS
- Upper gastrointestinal endoscopy with biopsy and cytologic tests
- Barium esophagography
- Bronchoscopy[a]

[a]If indicated.

DIFFERENTIAL DIAGNOSIS
The priority differentials in an adult patient with new onset progressive dysphagia differentials should include (1) esophageal squamous cell carcinoma, (2) esophageal adenocarcinoma, (3) adenocarcinoma of the gastric cardia, (4) achalasia, and (5) peptic stricture. Other differentials to consider include corrosive stricture and other esophageal motility disorders.[3] Symptoms of dysphagia, especially in a patient older than 45 years, mandate a complete evaluation to exclude esophageal carcinoma.[3]

INTERPROFESSIONAL COLLABORATIVE MANAGEMENT
Gastroenterologic, oncologic, and surgical consultations are critical for the evaluation of esophageal tumors. Cancer of the esophagus is usually treated with surgery, radiotherapy, chemotherapy, or a combination of these therapies.[1] Treatment and overall survival after diagnosis depend upon the stage of the disease. Staging of the disease uses the American Joint Committee on Cancer (AJCC) staging system, which factors in the involvement of tissue layers (T), lymph node involvement (N), and metastases (M).[4]

Primary Surgical Management
Surgery is the treatment of choice and recommended for patients with localized esophageal cancer.[5] In early stage disease (T1N0), surgery alone is appropriate.[1] In more advanced disease, chemotherapy or chemoradiotherapy may be used in conjunction with surgical management and is discussed further below.

Chemotherapy and Chemoradiotherapy
Definitive chemoradiotherapy is only recommended for patients with localized cancer of the esophagus who are unfit for surgery.[4] Chemotherapy may be consider in palliation of metastatic disease.

Chemoradiotherapy and chemotherapy agents such as Cisplatin can be used before surgery in attempt to shrink the tumor in turn making the operation easier and diminishing the risk of spread.[5] Chemoradiotherapy in conjunction with surgical intervention is recommended for all people with node-positive adenocarcinoma, adenocarcinoma that extends beyond muscularis propria, and for patients with squamous cell carcinoma who have undergone incomplete surgical resection.[4] In locally advanced squamous cell carcinoma of the esophagus, the addition of esophagectomy to chemoradiotherapy offers little to no benefit to overall survival.[5] In patients with medically operable squamous cell carcinoma, concurrent chemoradiotherapy improved overall survival significantly when compared with radiotherapy alone.[1]

COMPLICATIONS
Because of the distensibility of the esophagus, esophageal carcinoma tends to be silent until late in its course. Complications are usually related to mediastinal extension or esophageal narrowing and may include obstruction, hemorrhage, perforation, and fistula formation. Because the esophagus lacks a true serosa, cancer is often not contained at the time of diagnosis. The lungs and liver are the most common sites of hematogenous metastasis. Complications of esophageal resection include torsion or gangrene of the gastric, colonic, or jejunal pull-up; anastomotic leak; anastomotic stricture; subphrenic abscess; chylothorax; hemorrhage; wound infection and dehiscence; sepsis; dumping syndrome; vocal cord paralysis; and reflux esophagitis.

PATIENT AND FAMILY EDUCATION
Patients should be educated on the disease process and potential next steps to anticipate including referral to gastroenterology, oncology, and possibly surgery. Smoking cessation, alcohol moderation, and weight management counseling should be emphasized. If dysphagia is present, dietary restrictions should be imposed depending upon the degree.

HEALTH PROMOTION
Patients should be screened for risk factors of esophageal cancer, as previously discussed including age, race, gender, country of origin, GERD, smoking, alcohol use, and obesity, so that appropriate screening diagnostics can be initiated. Primary prevention of esophageal cancer includes smoke cessation, avoidance of heavy alcohol consumption, and weight management.

TUMORS OF THE STOMACH

DEFINITION AND EPIDEMIOLOGY

Gastric cancer is the fourth most common cancer in the world after lung, breast, and colorectal cancers.[6] Gastric cancer is also the third most common cause of cancer-related deaths worldwide, resulting in 750,000 deaths every year.[7] In high-income countries such as the United States, the incidence of gastric cancer is falling; however, the increased age of the world's population has led to a rise in the total number of deaths from gastric cancer.[7] Decreased incidence of gastric cancer is associated with improvements in food conservation and diet, as well as eradication of *Helicobacter pylori* in the last 50 years.[8] More than 90% of gastric malignancies are histologically classified as adenocarcinoma.[8] Gastric lymphoma, gastric carcinoid tumors, and gastrointestinal mesenchymal tumors can also occur.

Helicobacter pylori is noted as the primary risk factor for gastric cancer.[7] Atrophic gastritis, intestinal metaplasia, and dysplasia have also been recognized in the pathogenesis of gastric cancer.[8] Dietary risk factors include decreased consumption of fruits and vegetables and increased intake of salt, nitrates and nitrites, and smoked and poorly preserved foods.[9] Genetic factors linked to gastric carcinoma include hereditary nonpolyposis colorectal cancer, familial polyposis, and first-degree relatives of patients with gastric cancer. A partial gastrectomy for peptic ulcer disease is also associated with an increased risk of gastric carcinoma.[9]

PATHOPHYSIOLOGY

Gastric cancer can be divided into two histologic types—intestinal and diffuse. The World Health Organization differentiates histologic types further in five major subtypes: papillary, tubular, mucinous adenocarcinoma, poorly cohesive, and mixed carcinoma.[8] The first three subtypes correspond with intestinal type, and the diffuse type corresponds to the poorly cohesive type.[8] The intestinal type is more common in males, older age groups, and in high-risk geographic regions, while the diffuse type is more frequent in younger individuals with a more uniform geographic distribution.[8] Ninety percent of gastric cancers are considered sporadic.[8] Gastric carcinomas spread by direct extension, lymphatic spread, hematogenous metastasis, and peritoneal seeding.

CLINICAL PRESENTATION AND PHYSICAL EXAMINATION

Symptoms may not present until the disease is advanced and can be nonspecific. Possible symptoms include unexplained weight loss, upper abdominal pain, anorexia, nausea, and early satiety. Other symptoms include a change in bowel habits, dysphagia, melena, anemic symptoms, and hemorrhage.[9]

The physical exam is typically unremarkable. A small portion of patients may have a palpate gastric mass. Metastases may also manifest as an enlarged left supraclavicular lymph node (Virchow node), an enlarged periumbilical lymph node (Sister Mary Joseph node), an enlarged ovary (Krukenberg tumor), or a mass on the Blumer shelf on rectal examination.[3]

DIAGNOSTICS

Essential Diagnostics

Diagnosis of a primary gastric tumor is made with upper endoscopy, which allows for direct visualization of the tumor and biopsy. Pathologic evaluation of tumor biopsy should then be performed. Staging of malignant gastric tumors is then assessed preoperatively using endoscopic ultrasound and CT scans of the abdomen and chest.[6]

Additional Diagnostics

Blood studies may reveal hypochromic, microcytic anemia secondary to iron deficiency. Liver function tests may be abnormal if liver metastasis is present.[3] The stool is often positive for occult blood.

INITIAL DIAGNOSTICS

Gastric Tumors

LABORATORY
- Liver function tests
- Complete blood count and differential
- Stool for occult blood

IMAGING
- Computed tomography (CT) scan of abdomen
- PET/CT scan

OTHER DIAGNOSTICS
- Upper gastrointestinal endoscopy and biopsy
- Endoscopic ultrasound
- Barium upper gastrointestinal series
- Diagnostic laparoscopy

DIFFERENTIAL DIAGNOSIS

Priority differentials include (1) gastric lymphoma, (2) leiomyosarcoma, (3) carcinoid tumors, (4) gastric metastasis from lung, breast, and melanoma, and (5) gastrointestinal stromal tumor (GIST). Kaposi sarcoma of the stomach, which may be present in patients with acquired immunodeficiency syndrome (AIDS), and hypertrophic gastropathy (Meniere disease) are also included in the differential diagnosis.

INTERPROFESSIONAL COLLABORATIVE MANAGEMENT

Gastroenterologic, surgical, and oncologic consultations are essential for a patient with gastric cancer.

Endoscopic Mucosal Resection

Endoscopic mucosal resection is a newly proposed approach for patients with early gastric carcinoma and favorable prognostic features (histologically well-differentiated carcinoma limited to mucosa, <2 cm, absence of ulceration) as an alternative to surgical resection.[6]

Surgical Management

Radical surgery is the standard for curative treatment of gastric carcinoma.[6] Nearly half of gastric cancers are inoperable due to advanced staging by the time they are diagnosed, leading to a 5-year survival rate of almost zero.[7] Those who are candidates for surgical resection often require extensive surgery with a 5-year survival rate of 20% to 30%.[7] Relapse rates after "curative" gastrectomy remain in the range of 40% to 60%.[8]

Chemotherapy

In combination with surgical resection, adjuvant chemotherapy with or without radiotherapy has been shown to provide significant survival advantage in patients with advanced gastric cancer.[6]

In patients with inoperable advanced gastric cancer, systemic chemotherapy is the mainstay of treatment. Patients with inoperable, recurrent, or metastatic tumors have a median survival of 3 to 5 months without chemotherapy, while palliative treatment with chemotherapy has been shown to extend overall survival by 6.7 months in comparison to supportive care alone.[8]

COMPLICATIONS

Gastric carcinomas are detected at an advanced stage, and the prognosis of this neoplasm remains poor. Intraperitoneal dissemination of the tumor may occur with involvement of the omentum, peritoneum, and serosa of the intestine. Other complications include gastric outlet obstruction, gastrointestinal bleeding, distensibility, malnutrition, and ascites.

PATIENT AND FAMILY EDUCATION

Although gastric tumors and small colon tumors may be associated with aging, cancer can affect younger patients. Weight loss, anorexia, difficulty swallowing, abdominal pain, change in bowel habits, and blood in the stool are signs of gastrointestinal cancers. Patients should be reminded to notify their health care provider if any of these symptoms occurs. In addition, patients should routinely be asked about a family history of gastrointestinal or other cancers.

HEALTH PROMOTION

A well-balanced diet rich in fruits and vegetables is important for overall good health. Such a diet will provide sufficient vitamins and antioxidants to maintain health. Consumption of smoked and highly salted, nitrated food should be avoided or severely limited.[9] Only food that is refrigerated and kept under safe conditions should be consumed. Avoidance of all tobacco products is strongly recommended. Because infectious agents have been associated with gastric cancer, it is important to practice good hygiene. Diagnosis of *H. pylori* infection and subsequent treatment also contribute to a reduction in the incidence of gastric cancer.[9]

TUMORS OF THE SMALL INTESTINE

DEFINITION AND EPIDEMIOLOGY

The small bowel accounts for 75% of the gut length, but small bowel tumors are relatively uncommon, only accounting for 1% to 3% of malignant gastrointestinal tumors.[10] Adenocarcinoma accounts for about one-third of small bowel tumors; other common malignant tumors include carcinoid tumors, stromal tumors, leiomyosarcomas, and lymphoma.[11] The average diagnostic age ranges between 50 and 70 years of age, and there is a slight male predominance.[11]

The four most common benign tumors of the small intestine are fibromas, neurofibromas, leiomyomas, and lipomas.[12] Hamartomatous polyps occur throughout the gastrointestinal system but are most predominantly in the small intestine in Peutz-Jeghers syndrome and are considered benign; however, 40% to 60% of these patients develop cancer.[3]

Patients with Crohn disease have an increased risk for development of carcinoma of the small bowel, and adenocarcinoma develops years earlier than expected for this malignant neoplasm.

PATHOPHYSIOLOGY

Adenocarcinomas of the small intestine are aggressive tumors that most commonly occur at the ampulla of Vater. It is thought that these arise in a similar manner to colorectal adenocarcinomas in which a polyp becomes malignant.[3,9] Small

bowel lymphoma accounts for 5% of lymphoma cases occurring more often in patients with AIDS, immunosuppressive therapy, and Crohn disease.[3] Carcinoid tumors are neuroendocrine tumors that most commonly occur in the small bowel. All carcinoid tumors should be considered malignant. Metastasis often occur with carcinoid tumors larger than 2 cm.[13] Carcinoid syndrome may occur as a result of hormone secretion from these tumors which results in facial flushing, diarrhea, asthma-type wheezing, skin lesions, and cardiac manifestations.[3] The vast majority of patients with carcinoid syndrome also have hepatic metastases.[3]

CLINICAL PRESENTATION AND PHYSICAL EXAMINATION

Abdominal pain is the most common symptom expressed by patients with either benign or malignant small bowel tumors. Large lesions of the small intestine may produce partial or intermittent obstruction, bleeding, intussusception, and volvulus.[3] Symptoms could include nausea, vomiting, cramping, abdominal distention aggravated by eating, weakness, fatigue, and weight loss.[9] Anemia may be present. Unless patients manifest carcinoid syndrome as previously discussed in pathophysiology, there are no definitive signs or symptoms which suggest cancer of the small bowel.

The physical exam is often benign. Duodenal adenocarcinomas that involve the Vater ampulla may cause obstructive jaundice or pancreatitis.[3] Hepatomegaly, ascites, and jaundice may indicate advanced metastatic disease.[3] Pulmonic stenosis may cause a systolic murmur in patients with carcinoid syndrome.[3]

DIAGNOSTICS
Essential Diagnostics

Standard diagnostic methods include gastroscopy, colonoscopy, and CT. Video capsule endoscopy (VCE), enteroscopy, and octreotide scans may also be pursued.[10] VCE is thought to be superior to small bowel barium radiography.[14] Data regarding computed tomography-enterography/enteroclysis and magnetic resonance-enterography/enteroclysis is limited, although MRE does have a high sensitivity and specificity for small bowel tumors.[14]

Additional Diagnostics

Diagnostic laparoscopy/laparotomy may be pursued if other diagnostic tests are negative.[10] Complete blood count (CBC) with differential may reveal anemia. Although nonspecific, stool may also be tested for occult blood.

INITIAL DIAGNOSTICS

Small Intestine Tumors

LABORATORY
- Complete blood count and differential
- Stool for occult blood
- Serotonin and metabolites
- Urinary 5-HIAA[a]

IMAGING
- Small Bowel Follow-though (SBFT)

- Enteroclysis
- Endoscopy[a]
- Capsule endoscopy[a]
- Arteriography[a]
- Scintigraphy[a]
- Computed tomography scan[a]

OTHER DIAGNOSTICS
- Laparotomy[a]

[a]If indicated.

DIFFERENTIAL DIAGNOSIS

Priority differentials include (1) small bowel adenocarcinoma, (2) carcinoid tumor, (3) stromal tumor, (4) leiomyosarcoma, and (5) lymphoma.

Small bowel tumors may be considered one of the less common causes of intestinal obstruction, occult gastrointestinal blood loss, weight loss, and unexplained abdominal pain. In addition to the priority differentials, other differential diagnoses to consider include adhesions, hernias, intussusception, volvulus, intra-abdominal abscesses and hematomas, endometriosis, pelvic inflammatory disease, Crohn disease, ischemia, hematoma associated with oral anticoagulant therapy, radiation enteritis, amyloidosis, ingested foreign bodies, gallstones, bezoars, and intestinal parasites.

INTERPROFESSIONAL COLLABORATIVE MANAGEMENT

Gastroenterologic, oncologic, and surgical consultations are essential to provide optimum care for patients with small bowel tumors.

Surgical Management

Early diagnosis and surgical resection provide the only possibility for curative management of small bowel adenocarcinoma. Five-year survival reaches 65% with stage 1 disease versus 4% in stage 4 disease.[11] Adenocarcinomas and neuroendocrine tumors should be treated with surgical resection and radical lymphadenectomy.[11] Patients with GIST should undergo resection, but lymphadenectomy is not required.[11] Palliative resections may be considered.[11]

Chemotherapy and Chemoradiotherapy

Data regarding adjuvant chemotherapy and radiotherapy in operative small bowel cancers is limited.[11] Although lacking standardized protocols, adjuvant chemotherapy is often based on studies regarding adjuvant chemotherapy in colorectal cancers.[11]

PATIENT AND FAMILY EDUCATION

Patient and family education for tumors of the small intestine is the same as that for tumors of the stomach.

HEALTH PROMOTION

See the Health Promotion section under Tumors of the Colon and Rectum.

TUMORS OF THE COLON AND RECTUM

DEFINITION AND EPIDEMIOLOGY

Colorectal cancer is the third most common cancer and cancer-related cause of death in the United States. In 2014 approximately 137,000 people were diagnosed with colorectal cancer, which also accounted for approximately 50,000 deaths.[15] Adenocarcinomas account for the majority of all malignant tumors of the colon and rectum.[3] Approximately one-third of these cancers are located in the rectum, including the anus, and two-thirds in the colon.[16] Rectal cancers are classified as lesions located 3 to 12 cm from the anal verge.[16] There is a slightly higher proportion of left-sided colon cancers than right-sided colon cancers.[17] Risk factors for the development of colorectal cancer include age greater than age 50, prior colorectal cancer, ulcerative colitis, hereditary and genetic factors, familial polyposis syndromes, long-term cigarette smoking, and a high-fat high-caloric diet.[3,17,18]

PATHOPHYSIOLOGY

Genetic and environmental factors contribute to the development of colorectal cancer. Colon cancer develops from mucosal polyps. Adenomatous and hyperplastic are the most common types. The majority of colon cancers arise from adenomas. Colorectal adenocarcinomas may be polypoid, ulcerating, or infiltrative. Adenocarcinomas arise from a varied progression of events that can be genetic in origin and involve a series of mutations that result in a malignant neoplasm. Colorectal adenocarcinoma can spread intraluminally or by direct extension, hematogenous spread, lymphatic dissemination, or transperitoneal seeding. More than 80% of colorectal cancers are a result of malfunction of tumor suppressor genes *p53*, *APC*, and *DCC*.[3]

CLINICAL PRESENTATION AND PHYSICAL EXAMINATION

The symptoms of colon adenocarcinoma depend on the location of the tumor. Cancers of the proximal colon usually attain a larger size before becoming symptomatic compared with cancers of the left side of the colon and rectum. Fatigue, shortness of breath, angina caused by hypochromic microcytic anemia, and melenic liquid stool may be the principal means of presentation of right-sided colonic masses. Abdominal discomfort may be present as the tumor increases in size. Obstruction is uncommon because of the large diameters of the cecum and ascending colon. The left side of the colon has a smaller lumen than the proximal colon, and therefore obstructive symptoms may occur. Left-sided symptoms include cramps, gas pain, and decrease in the caliber of the stool. Adenocarcinomas of the descending and sigmoid colon are often circumferential and may also cause obstruction.

Patients with colon adenocarcinoma may experience colicky abdominal pain, especially after meals, and a change in bowel habits. Constipation may alternate with an increased frequency of defecation. Hematochezia may be present with distal rather than proximal lesions, and bright red blood passed through the rectum may be seen with cancers that involve the left side of the colon and rectum. Approximately half of patients with colon cancer experience anorexia and weight loss.

The physical exam is typically benign. Patients with advanced disease may initially be seen with a palpable abdominal mass and signs of distention or intestinal obstruction. Inguinal nodes may be enlarged with left-sided cancer, and the liver may be enlarged because of metastasis.[3]

DIAGNOSTICS
Essential Diagnostics

Colonoscopy is the gold standard for tumor visualization and biopsy. Visual inspection and digital rectal examination should also be performed.

Additional Diagnostics

The air-contrast barium enema can diagnose many colon cancers but does not permit biopsy. Carcinoembryonic antigen (CEA) is not useful for screening but may be a valuable marker for recurring cancer.[19] The metastatic evaluation includes a CT scan, a chest x-ray study, CEA, and liver function tests (LFTs).[3]

DIFFERENTIAL DIAGNOSIS

Priority differentials include (1) adenocarcinoma, (2) diverticulitis, (3) ulcerative colitis, and (4) Crohn disease. Other differential diagnoses of colorectal tumors to consider include benign tumors, tuberculosis, amebiasis, fungal masses, schistosomiasis, viral lesions such as cytomegalovirus, feces, lymphoid polyps and lymphoma, carcinoid tumors, metastatic lesions, and Kaposi sarcoma. Obstructing lesions may include strictures from inflammation, radiation and ischemic colitis, and volvulus. In addition, extrinsic compression may occur from endometriosis and pancreatitis.

INTERPROFESSIONAL COLLABORATIVE MANAGEMENT

Gastroenterologic, oncologic, and surgical consultations are necessary to provide optimum care for patients with colorectal tumors.

Surgical Management

Surgical resection of colorectal cancer remains the standard of treatment. Regional lymph node excision at time of resection is standard of care and will assist with final staging of the neoplasia. Rectal cancer resections should include total mesorectal excision, which has been shown to decrease the rate of local recurrences.[3,16,17]

Chemotherapy and Chemoradiotherapy

Combination chemotherapy has been shown to improve the prognosis of patients with rectal cancer.[16] The addition of radiotherapy has also been shown to decrease local recurrence to 50% to 60% compared to surgery alone.[16] It is generally accepted that chemoradiation therapy should be initiated prior to surgery.[16] Postoperative chemotherapy is recommended for patients with node-positive colon cancer and may be recommended in select patients with node negative disease.[3] For patients with metastatic disease, chemotherapy may be utilized to slow tumor progression.[3]

COMPLICATIONS

Colorectal cancer may cause large bowel obstruction or perforation in cancers that reach an advanced stage. Rate of recurrence within the abdominal cavity, including liver metastasis, is high. Distant metastases, which are thought to be disseminated by hematogenous spread, may occur to the lungs, adrenal glands, bones, and brain. Weight loss, fatigue, rectal bleeding, abdominal and pelvic pain, coughing, change in bowel habits, and bone pain may signal recurrent disease.

PATIENT AND FAMILY EDUCATION

Only approximately 34% to 59% of Americans undergo recommended colorectal cancer screening.[15] Screening can reduce mortality and help identify colorectal cancers at an earlier stage, resulting in more favorable outcomes. The United States Preventive Services Task Force currently recommends routine screening for patients 50 years of age through 75 years of age.[15] According to the American Cancer Society, acceptable means of surveillance for average-risk adults include annual fecal occult blood testing using high sensitivity tests, annual fecal immunochemical test, fecal DNA test, flexible sigmoidoscopy every 5 years, colonoscopy every 10 years, or CT colonography every 5 years.[3] Patients who have a first-degree relative with history of colorectal cancer require screening colonoscopy starting age 40 or 10 years younger than the relative's age at diagnosis.[3] If the first-degree relative was older than age 60 at time of diagnosis, repeat colonoscopy can be done every 10 years; if the relative was younger than age 60 at time of diagnosis, screening should be repeated every 5 years.[3] It should be noted that colonoscopy is the only test that allows for examination of the entire colon and is the most sensitive test for detecting adenomas and cancer.[3]

HEALTH PROMOTION

Promotion of a healthy lifestyle is essential in the prevention of colorectal cancer. Weight management and regular exercise should be emphasized. Patients should be encouraged to increase intake of whole grains, fruits, and vegetables while decreasing intake of processed and red meats.[9] Avoidance of tobacco products should be discussed, and counseling regarding responsible alcohol intake should also be provided.[9]

REFERENCES

1. Vellayappan, B. A., Soon, Y. Y., Ku, G. Y., Leong, C. N., Lu, J. J., & Tey, J. C. S. (2017). Chemoradiotherapy versus chemoradiotherapy plus surgery for esophageal cancer. *The Cochrane Database of Systematic Reviews*, (8), Art. No.: CD010511, doi:10.1002/14651858.CD010511.pub2.
2. Domper Arnal, M. J., Ferrández Arenas, Á., & Lanas Arbeloa, Á. (2015). Esophageal cancer: Risk factors, screening and endoscopic treatment in Western and Eastern countries. *World Journal of Gastroenterology: WJG*, 21(26), 7933–7943. doi:10.3748/wjg.v21.i26.7933.
3. Papadakis, M. A., McPhee, S. J., & Rabow, M. W. (2017). *Current medical diagnosis and treatment* (56th ed.). New York: McGraw-Hill.
4. Best, L. M. J., Mughal, M., & Gurusamy, K. S. (2016). Non-surgical versus surgical treatment for oesophageal cancer. *The Cochrane Database of Systematic Reviews*, (3), Art. No.: CD011498, doi:10.1002/14651858.CD011498.pub2.
5. Kidane, B., Coughlin, S., Vogt, K., & Malthaner, R. (2015). Preoperative chemotherapy for resectable thoracic esophageal cancer. *The Cochrane Database of Systematic Reviews*, (5), Art. No.: CD001556, doi:10.1002/14651858.CD001556.pub3.
6. Mocellin, S., & Pasquali, S. (2015). Diagnostic accuracy of endoscopic ultrasonography (EUS) for the preoperative locoregional staging of primary gastric cancer. *The Cochrane Database of Systematic Reviews*, (2), Art. No.: CD009944, doi:10.1002/14651858.CD009944.pub2.
7. Ford, A. C., Forman, D., Hunt, R., Yuan, Y., & Moayyedi, P. (2015). *Helicobacter pylori* eradication for the prevention of gastric neoplasia. *The Cochrane Database of Systematic Reviews*, (7), Art. No.: CD005583, doi:10.1002/14651858.CD005583.pub2.
8. Wagner, A. D., Syn, N. L. X., Moehler, M., Grothe, W., Yong, W. P., Tai, B. C., et al. (2017). Chemotherapy for advanced gastric cancer. *The Cochrane Database of Systematic Reviews*, (8), Art. No.: CD004064, doi:10.1002/14651858.CD004064.pub4.
9. Information and Resources about for Cancer: Breast, Colon, Lung, Prostate, Skin. American Cancer Society. http://www.cancer.org/. Accessed June 3, 2019.
10. Rozhledy v Chirurgii: Mesicnik Ceskoslovenske Chirurgicke Spolecnosti [01 Jan 2016, 95(9):344-349].

11. Minardi, A. J., Jr., Zibari, G. B., Aultman, D. F., McMillan, R. W., & McDonald, J. C. (2017). Evaluation of prognostic factors and adjuvant chemotherapy in patients with small bowel adenocarcinoma who underwent curative resection. *Journal of the American College of Surgeons.*

12. Tumors of the digestive system. The Merck Manuals—Trusted Medical and Veterinary Information. http://www.merckmanuals.com/. Accessed June 3, 2019.

13. Walsh, J. C., Schaeffer, D. F., Kirsch, R., et al. (2016). Ileal "carcinoid" tumors—small size belies deadly intent: High rate of nodal metastasis in tumors ≤1 cm in size. *Human Pathology*, 56, 123–127. doi:10.1016/j.humpath.2016.05.023.

14. Pennazio, M., Spada, C., Eliakim, R., Keuchel, M., May, A., Mulder, C. J., et al. (2015). Small-bowel capsule endoscopy and device-assisted enteroscopy for diagnosis and treatment of small-bowel disorders: European Society of Gastrointestinal Endoscopy (ESGE) Clinical Guideline. *Endoscopy*, 47(04), 352–386. doi:10.1055/s-0034-1391855.

15. Moreno, C. C., Mittal, P. K., Sullivan, P. S., Rutherford, R., Staley, C. A., Cardona, K., et al. (2016). Colorectal cancer initial diagnosis: Screening colonoscopy, diagnostic colonoscopy, or emergent surgery, and tumor stage and size at initial presentation. *Clinical Colorectal Cancer*, 15(1), 67–73. https://doi.org/10.1016/j.clcc.2015.07.004.

16. Resende, H. M., Jacob, L. F. P., Quinellato, L. V., Matos, D., & da Silva, E. M. K. (2015). Combination chemotherapy versus single-agent chemotherapy during preoperative chemoradiation for resectable rectal cancer. *The Cochrane Database of Systematic Reviews*, (10), Art. No.: CD008531, doi:10.1002/14651858.CD008531.pub2.

17. Lee, G. H., Malietzis, G., Askari, A., Bernardo, D., Al-Hassi, H. O., & Clark, S. K. (2015). Is right-sided colon cancer different to left-sided colorectal cancer?—A systematic review. *European Journal of Surgical Oncology (EJSO)*, 41(3), 300–308. https://doi.org/10.1016/j.ejso.2014.11.001.

18. Erdrich, J., Zhang, X., Giovannucci, E., et al. (2015). Proportion of colon cancer attributable to lifestyle in a cohort of US women. *Cancer Causes and Control*, 26, 1271. https://doi.org/10.1007/s10552-015-0619-z.

19. Nicholson, B. D., Shinkins, B., Pathiraja, I., Roberts, N. W., James, T. J., Mallett, S., et al. (2015). Blood CEA levels for detecting recurrent colorectal cancer. *The Cochrane Database of Systematic Reviews*, (12), Art. No.: CD011134, doi:10.1002/14651858.CD011134.pub2.

CHAPTER **126**

PEPTIC ULCER DISEASE

Donna M. Glynn

 Immediate referral is indicated for gastrointestinal bleeding, gastric outlet obstruction, and perforation.

DEFINITION AND EPIDEMIOLOGY

Peptic ulcer disease (PUD) is a pathologic, destructive, chronic disorder characterized by ulceration of the gastric and duodenal mucosa. The two common causes of peptic ulcers in the United States are *Helicobacter* infections (*Helicobacter pylori*) and the use of nonsteroidal antiinflammatory drugs (NSAIDs). During the last decades of the 20th century, the incidence of PUD declined dramatically. This decline is attributed to the discovery and effective use of acid suppressants and the treatment of *H. pylori* infections. However, gastric and duodenal ulcers continue to have a serious impact on the economics of health care and society because of recurrence rates, increased office visits, medication costs, diagnostic costs, and patient quality-of-life concerns. Therefore, it is essential to obtain a thorough health history, to identify potential risk factors, and to provide a cost-effective diagnosis and treatment plan.

PUD may be defined as a full-thickness defect in the mucosa of the stomach or duodenum caused by an imbalance both in the amount of acid and pepsin production and in the ability of the gastric and duodenal lining to protect itself. It is estimated that approximately 4.5 million people in the United States are affected annually, and the hospitalization rate for PUD is approximately 30 patients per 100,000 cases. Lifetime prevalence is estimated at 11% to 14% in males and 8% to 11% in females.[1] *H. pylori*, a spiral, flagellated, gram-negative, rod-shaped bacterium, was first identified and linked to gastritis in the 1980s and is a major causative organism in the development of ulcer disease. With the discovery of the bacterium, the treatment of PUD has changed from acid suppression to eradication of the bacterium. Excluding individuals who are using NSAID therapy, 61% of duodenal ulcers and 63% of gastric ulcers have been found to test positive for *H. pylori*.[1]

The second most common cause of PUD is the use of NSAIDs and low-dose aspirin. NSAIDs are commonly prescribed medications and available over the counter. As many as 30% of individuals taking NSAIDs will have adverse gastrointestinal (GI) events. Factors that increase the risk of an adverse event in individuals using NSAID therapy include a previous history of PUD, advanced age, long-term NSAID use, comorbidities, and concurrent use of anticoagulants.[1] Because of advancing age and the increased prevalence of osteoarthritis, the risk of PUD is significant in older patient populations. The discovery of cyclooxygenase 1 (COX-1) and COX-2 led to the development of COX-2–selective NSAIDs as an alternative therapy. COX-2 inhibitors are generally considered safer for the GI tract; however, this class of medication, which is commonly prescribed for arthritis pain, can also cause gastric or duodenal ulcer formation and has been linked to adverse cardiovascular events.[2]

Other risk factors for the development of PUD include family history, cigarette smoking, chronic obstructive pulmonary disease, major trauma, oral steroids, bisphosphonate therapy, caffeine ingestion, alcohol, cirrhosis, and physiologic stress. Certain conditions and genetic factors have also been identified as risk factors for the development of PUD. Zollinger-Ellison syndrome, antral G cell hyperplasia, cystic fibrosis, short bowel syndrome, hyperparathyroidism, and noncompliance with an *H. pylori* treatment regimen are documented in the development of PUD.[1]

PATHOPHYSIOLOGY

The function of the GI tract is the digestion of food and absorption of nutrients. This process is achieved by high concentrations of acid and pepsin that are secreted from the parietal cells of the stomach. The surface of the mucosa secretes alkaline mucus that protects the mucosa from self-digestion. Under normal conditions, a balance is present between gastric acid secretion and gastroduodenal mucosal defense. However, when this system is interrupted, the protective tissue is damaged, and erosion or ulcer formation occurs. A peptic ulcer can affect one or all layers of the gastric lining or duodenum. Gastric ulcers are commonly found distal to the junction between the antrum and the acid secretory mucosa. Duodenal ulcers are primarily located in the duodenal bulb or at the pyloric duodenal junction. Most patients with duodenal ulcers have impaired bicarbonate secretion, which is associated with *H. pylori*.[3] Reduction of the production of acid and pepsin is key to the promotion of healing and prevention of recurrence. Spontaneous remissions and exacerbations are commonly associated with PUD.

H. pylori, a spiral, flagellated organism, is acquired through the orofecal route. Once it is ingested, *H. pylori* attaches to the gastric mucosa, colonizes the entire gastric epithelium, and produces local tissue injury that results in the release of cytotoxins and proteases. NSAID therapy has been shown to damage the gastric mucosa by suppression of gastric prostaglandin synthesis. Acid suppression continues to be the key component in the management of NSAID-associated PUD.

CLINICAL PRESENTATION AND PHYSICAL EXAMINATION

Although some patients are asymptomatic, the most common presenting chief complaint is epigastric pain or dyspepsia. Upper abdominal pain or discomfort is the most common presentation, with pain centered in the epigastrium. This discomfort is often described as a sharp, burning, aching, gnawing pain occurring 2 to 5 hours after meals or in the middle of the night. The patient will report that the pain is usually relieved with the ingestion of food or antacids; however, the symptoms are recurrent, with episodes lasting from hours to days to months. Peptic ulcers may be associated with food provoking symptoms. Patients may report pain with eating, postprandial belching, fullness, fatty food intolerance, nausea, and vomiting. Changes in the intensity, duration, or location of the pain may indicate penetration or perforation of an ulcer.[4]

Inspection, auscultation, and percussion generally yield negative findings. In rare presentations, auscultation may reveal a succussion splash 4 hours or longer after meals, which would indicate a duodenal or pyloric channel ulcer, causing gastric outlet obstruction. Palpation may produce epigastric tenderness midline between the umbilicus and xiphoid process. If a perforation has occurred, the patient will have a rigid abdomen and generalized rebound tenderness. Rectal examination should be included with testing for melena.

DIAGNOSTICS
Essential Diagnostics

There is no reliable blood testing that can accurately confirm PUD. A complete blood count (CBC) will exclude anemia. Blood chemistries will assess liver function and calcium levels. Serologic antibody testing and stool monoclonal antigen tests are available for *H. pylori*; however, it is better if the patient is not taking a PPI for 14 days before doing the stool antigen test. The serologic antibody test for *H. pylori* is not impacted by PPIs, but this test is unable to determine if the patient has a previous or active *H. pylori* infection.

Endoscopy will provide the most accurate diagnosis of PUD and allows for multiple biopsies to exclude malignancy and confirm *H. pylori*.[5] Barium radiography is still performed, but only in patients who are not eligible or who are unwilling to undergo endoscopy.[5]

INITIAL DIAGNOSTICS

Endoscopy

LABORATORY
- Complete blood count and differential
- *Helicobacter pylori* testing (serum)
- Serum chemistries
- Stool for occult blood

DIAGNOSTICS
- Barium radiography

ADDITIONAL DIAGNOSTICS
- *H. pylori* testing (breath, fecal)

DIFFERENTIAL DIAGNOSIS

Differential diagnosis for PUD is based on the symptoms reported and the location of the pain.

Priority differentials include cholecystitis, gastroesophageal reflux disease (GERD), irritable bowel disease, or nonulcer dyspepsia. Cholecystitis causes right upper quadrant abdominal discomfort. Vague abdominal pain with reports of diarrhea or constipation may be associated with diverticulosis, irritable bowel syndrome, or nonulcer dyspepsia. GERD, pancreatitis, and malignant disease should also be considered. Zollinger-Ellison syndrome is a condition of excessive acid production. This should be considered if the individual does not respond to the traditional diet, smoking cessation, and pharmacologic therapy.

INTERPROFESSIONAL COLLABORATIVE MANAGEMENT
Pharmacologic Management

First-line treatment of PUD is antisecretory therapy. If NSAID or COX-2 inhibitor use is documented, the medications should be discontinued. If objective findings include anemia, GI bleeding, rigid abdomen, weight loss, or new-onset dyspepsia in an individual older than 50 years, an immediate physician consultation is indicated. If symptoms persist after a limited course of antisecretory therapy, referral to a gastroenterologist for endoscopy is appropriate.

Treatment options for PUD include histamine$_2$ receptor antagonists (H$_2$RAs), proton pump inhibitors (PPIs), and prostaglandin therapy. The H$_2$RAs include cimetidine, famotidine, nizatidine, and ranitidine. These preparations inhibit gastric acid secretion by blocking the H$_2$ receptors of the parietal cells. H$_2$RA therapy is associated with 75% to 98% healing during a 4- to 6-week period in documented PUD. Therapy needs to be continued with maintenance administration at bedtime for 1 year to prevent recurrence. H$_2$RA therapy is available over the counter, which presents new challenges for the primary care providers. Again, an in-depth history that includes over-the-counter medication use is extremely important in contemplating treatment options.

PPIs are the most potent and most expensive treatment option for PUD. Omeprazole, lansoprazole, rabeprazole, and esomeprazole effectively block the production of acid secretion. Daily administration eliminates acid production and also improves patient compliance. Investigation of over-the-counter medication use is once again required because PPI therapy is available for purchase without prescription.

Prostaglandin therapy protects the gastric and duodenal mucosa and should be considered for individuals with documented PUD who are unable to discontinue NSAID use. Misoprostol is the only available agent for the prevention of NSAID-induced gastric ulcers; it inhibits acid production and prevents duodenal damage. The therapeutic dose has been shown to produce transient side effects of cramping and diarrhea, which can be eliminated with a lower dose. Sucralfate is also indicated for treatment of active duodenal ulcer and maintenance of healed duodenal ulcers.

Treatment options for *H. pylori* eradication continue to be closely evaluated for efficacy and compliance. Treatment for *H. pylori*–associated ulcer disease is achieved with a combination of acid-inhibiting therapy and antibiotics, though there are concerns about antibiotic resistance and patient adherence to *H. pylori* treatment.[6] The current American College of Gastroenterology (ACG) guideline recommendations include a PPI plus clarithromycin 500 mg po twice a day and amoxicillin 1 g po twice for 7 to 14 days *or* a PPI plus clarithromycin 500 mg po twice a day and metronidazole 500 mg po twice a day for up to 14 days.[5,6] The patient should not have taken a macrolide in the past to be prescribed this regimen.[6] A total of 10 to 14 days of treatment with metronidazole, tetracycline, a PPI, and bismuth is an additional option.[6] Patients should be queried about previous antibiotic therapy and the ACG guidelines reviewed for other recommended therapies, if these treatments are contraindicated for any reason (e.g., allergy).[6]

Nonpharmacologic Management

Smoking cessation and decreasing psychological stressors have been associated with a significant decrease in PUD and *H. pylori*–associated ulcers.

COMPLICATIONS

Perforation of gastric or duodenal ulcers is a life-threatening complication of chronic ulcer disease. This is most common in older patients and requires emergency care. Other complications include hemorrhage, gastric outlet obstruction, and ulcers refractory to treatment.[5]

PATIENT AND FAMILY EDUCATION

Patient education involves the identification and modification of risk factors, specifically cigarette smoking, alcohol abuse, stress, and NSAID and aspirin use. Once a diagnosis of ulcer disease has been established, education should also include the signs and symptoms of hemorrhage, perforation, GI bleeding, and anemia. In addition, the consequences of lack of adherence to the medication regimen related to the treatment of PUD and *H. pylori* infection should be carefully reviewed.

REFERENCES

1. Anand, B. S., Katz, J., et al. (2017). Peptic ulcer disease. Retrieved from http://emedicine.medscape.com/article/181753-overview. 2017 January 29.
2. Rosenthal, L. D. (2018). *Cyclooxygenase inhibitors: Nonsteroidal anti-inflammatory drugs and acetaminophen. Lehne's Pharmacotherapeutics for Advanced Practice Providers.* Missouri: Elsevier.
3. Sung, J., Tsoi, K., Ma, T., Yung, M., Lau, J., & Chiu, P. (2010). Causes of mortality in patients with peptic ulcer bleeding: A prospective cohort study of 10,428 cases. *The American Journal of Gastroenterology, 105*(1), 84–89.
4. Vakil, N. Clinical manifestation of peptic ulcer disease. Retrieved from www.uptodate.com. June 3, 2019.
5. Fashner, J., & Gitu, A. C. (2015). Diagnosis and treatment of peptic ulcer disease and *H. pylori* infection. *American Academy of Family Physicians, 91*(4), 236–242. https://www.aafp.org/afp/2015/0215/p236.html. (Accessed 28 March 2018).
6. Chey, W. D., Leontiadis, G. I., Howden, C. W., & Moss, S. F. (2017). ACG Clinical Guideline: Treatment of *Heliobacter pylori* infection. *The American Journal of Gastroenterology, 112*(2), 212–239.

Evaluation and Management of Genitourinary Disorders

CHAPTER 127

INCONTINENCE
Leslie Neal-Boylan

DEFINITION AND EPIDEMIOLOGY

Urinary incontinence is the involuntary transient or persistent loss of urine (Box 127.1). It is experienced by 30% to 50% of women and 17% of men older than 60 years, as well as up to 50% of elderly nursing home residents.[1] Incontinence is one of the major causes of institutionalization in the geriatric population, but incontinence is not limited to the elderly. Twenty percent to 30% of young community dwellers are also affected by this disorder.[1] Urinary incontinence should not be considered normal at any age and is not an expected outcome of aging. Impaired mobility, pelvic floor weakness, race and ethnicity, weight, other comorbidities (asthma, depression, heart disease, or a history of frequent urinary tract infection [UTI]), benign prostatic hyperplasia (BPH), medications, and bowel status may all contribute to incontinence.[2]

The annual cost of managing incontinence for all age groups in the United States was nearly $66 billion in 2007 with much of the cost associated with nursing home placement.[3] However, despite its financial impact on society, incontinence is rarely addressed by patients with their health care providers. Thus it behooves health care providers to identify patients who could benefit from therapeutic regimens to minimize the overall impact of incontinence.

PATHOPHYSIOLOGY

Urinary incontinence is usually the symptom of an underlying bladder or sphincter condition, but it may also be related to an extrinsic problem that can be easily treated. There are five main types of urinary incontinence: stress incontinence, urge incontinence, mixed incontinence, overflow incontinence, and functional or transient incontinence.

Stress Incontinence

Stress urinary incontinence (SUI) is leakage of urine with any maneuvers that increase intra-abdominal pressure (coughing, sneezing). The increase in intra-abdominal pressure is transmitted to the bladder, which then overcomes the sphincteric and urethral pressure, resulting in an open urethra and urinary leakage. Stress incontinence is seen in those who have either or both of the following issues.

Anatomic Stress Urinary Incontinence. Previously termed "genuine stress incontinence," anatomic incontinence refers to hypermobility of the bladder neck (vesicourethral junction). In general, the sphincter is competent at rest, and an increase in abdominal pressure leads to increased closure pressure. When the bladder neck is mobile, a rise in intra-abdominal pressure results in rotation of the bladder neck and urethra below the pelvic floor muscles so that intra-abdominal pressure is no longer transmitted to the bladder neck and urethra. The sphincter is overcome by the increase in abdominal pressure, which is transmitted to the bladder, and leakage occurs.[4]

Intrinsic Sphincter Deficiency. Intrinsic sphincter deficiency (ISD) indicates an open bladder neck at rest. Even a mild increase in intra-abdominal pressure in individuals with ISD can result in leakage.[4] Although ISD can occur naturally, patients who have had radical pelvic surgery may also experience a compromise of their intrinsic sphincter, predisposing them to incontinence. Contemporary theories suggest that all patients with sphincteric incontinence have some degree of ISD.[4]

Urinary Urge Incontinence

Urge is the most common cause of incontinence in older adults and manifests as the sudden, often uncontrollable sensation to void.[5] This urge can then lead to urinary urge incontinence (UUI). However, in patients with severe urge, incontinence may not be realized until actual leakage occurs. Overactive bladder (OAB) is a newer term used to describe the phenomenon of urgency and frequency with or without UUI.[5] Urge and urge incontinence occur because of a rise in detrusor pressure that may be a phasic contraction, detrusor overactivity (DO), or poor bladder compliance.

Detrusor Overactivity. DO is instability of the detrusor muscle during bladder filling because of idiopathic or neurogenic causes. In both idiopathic and neurogenic DO, bladder pressures surpass sphincter and urethral pressures, causing the bladder neck to open and incontinence to occur.

Idiopathic Causes. When no defined neurologic contributor can be identified, DO is idiopathic. Prominent theories for

BOX **127.1**

Incontinence Definitions

Stress incontinence: Loss of urine associated with activities that increase intra-abdominal pressure

Urge incontinence: Involuntary loss of urine usually preceded by a strong, unexpected urge to void

Mixed incontinence: Urge and stress incontinence together

Overflow incontinence: An involuntary loss of urine associated with incomplete emptying

DO include increased stimulation of alpha$_1$ receptors in the bladder, disruption of somatic and autonomic nervous systems that help regulate voiding, disruption of afferent and efferent pathways, and increased activation of muscarinic (M_2/M_3) receptors in the bladder.[4]

Neurogenic Causes. Patients who have spinal cord injuries below T11 to L1,[2] or neurologic conditions, such as multiple sclerosis, diabetes mellitus, and spina bifida, can have a disruption in voluntary micturition control. Reflex micturition often results, leading to detrusor hyperactivity and urge incontinence.[4]

Poor Bladder Compliance. Normal bladder compliance allows large amounts of urine to be stored with minimum changes in bladder pressure.[6] With poor compliance, large bladder pressures are seen with small increases in volumes.[6] This can be a result of the loss of viscoelasticity in detrusor muscle or changes in neuroregulatory activity.

Mixed Incontinence

A combination of SUI and UUI is referred to as mixed incontinence.

Overflow Incontinence

Incomplete emptying of urine often results in passive loss of small amounts of urine when bladder pressures elevate, either episodically or continuously, as the bladder fills beyond capacity. The rise in bladder pressure may occur because of either transmitted abdominal pressure or an increase in detrusor pressure. Overflow incontinence is seen in patients with either bladder outlet obstruction or poor detrusor contractility. Bladder pressure surpasses sphincter and urethral pressure, which allows "overflow" of urine to occur. This is more commonly seen in men than in women, and causes include benign prostatic hypertrophy (BPH), radical pelvic surgery, detrusor inactivity, neurologic issues, and certain medications.

Functional or Transient Incontinence. Pathologic conditions external to the urinary tract can also cause incontinence. Such factors are indicated in Resnick's DIAPPERS mnemonic (Box 127.2). Reversal of these conditions may improve the urinary incontinence.

Clinical Presentation and Physical Examination

The presentation of incontinence can vary depending on the cause. A careful history and physical examination should exclude causes of transient incontinence that can be easily

---

BOX **127.2**

Resnick's Diappers Mnemonic

*D*elirium or confusional state
*I*nfection—urinary (only symptomatic)
*A*trophic urethritis, vaginitis
*P*harmaceuticals
*P*sychological, especially severe depression (rare)
*E*xcess urinary output (e.g., congestive heart failure, hyperglycemia)
*R*estricted mobility
*S*tool impaction

From Resnick, N. M. (1997). Urinary incontinence. In: C. K. Cassel, H. J. Cohen, E. R. Larson, et al., (Eds.), *Geriatric medicine* (3rd ed.). New York: Springer.

---

treated. SUI, UUI, mixed incontinence, and overflow incontinence can manifest similarly, so careful history taking may help delineate the type of incontinence experienced. A history should include a detailed review of symptoms related to incontinence; bowel habits; medications; medical, surgical, and genitourinary histories; history of pelvic trauma; and neurologic issues.[5] Onset, precipitants, duration, characteristics (frequency, timing, and amount), alleviating factors, and treatments tried should all be documented. Alterations in bowel or bladder habits, number of pads used, and response to previous treatments should be noted as well.

Incontinence can contribute to medical morbidities, including perineal candida infections, pressure ulcers, UTIs, urosepsis, falls, and sleep interruption. At the same time, incontinence can contribute to poor self-esteem, social withdrawal, depression, and sexual dysfunction secondary to embarrassment. Because of this, patients in the home environment may try to limit fluid intake to control incontinence. By minimizing fluid intake, patients may put themselves at risk for dehydration and its sequelae.

The physical examination for incontinence includes abdominal, genitourinary, pelvic, and rectal components. A neurologic and functional assessment, as well as an assessment of the extremities for edema, should also be made. Medication history (especially that of diuretic use), mental status, mobility, and social evaluations should be performed, especially in older adults, because impairment in any of these realms may contribute to functional incontinence.

Examination findings in men including phimosis, balanitis or infection, rectal masses, prostate nodules or asymmetry, and fecal impaction suggest underlying causes of the incontinence. In women, an assessment of urethral mobility is performed by examining the bladder neck and urethra with the patient supine while she strains. A stress test is also performed by observing for urine loss when the patient performs a Valsalva maneuver or by having the patient cough. If incontinence is not seen when the patient is examined supine, the examination should be repeated with the patient standing.

Bladder neck hypermobility can also be determined with the Q-tip test. If the Q-tip moves more than 30 degrees from a horizontal plane when it is inserted superficially into the urethra, lack of urethral support is delineated.[7] Furthermore, pelvic organ prolapse and effectiveness of the patient's ability to perform Kegel exercises (contraction of the pelvic floor) should be noted. General observation of pelvic anatomy should be made, and any abnormalities, including atrophy, should be documented. The relationship between estrogen and incontinence in perimenopausal and menopausal women has not been well defined. However, studies have noted that the risk of urinary incontinence for women taking estrogen only or estrogen-progestin formulations increases.[8] Lack of estrogen and subsequent vaginal atrophy may contribute to symptoms of stress incontinence.[9]

UUI may not be detectable on physical examination. Subjective complaints may be most beneficial in detecting urge incontinence and UUI. However, examination of pelvic anatomy and pelvic floor strength may reveal contributors to bladder symptoms, such as constipation and vaginal atrophy. Mixed incontinence requires a physical examination to assess for SUI and UUI. This should be performed as previously discussed.

Finally, overflow incontinence can often be determined through abdominal and vaginal examinations. Bladder distention may be easily palpated abdominally or vaginally. Evaluation of general pelvic anatomy should also occur.

DIAGNOSTICS
Essential Diagnostics

A urinalysis is performed to exclude hematuria, pyuria, glucosuria, or proteinuria. Hematuria, defined as more than three red blood cells per high-power field on urinalysis with a negative urine culture,[10] warrants further workup with cytology, upper tract imaging, and bladder cystoscopy. Urine cytologic studies should also be performed in patients with gross or persistent microhematuria, risk factors for bladder cancer, or irritative symptoms.[10] A urine culture is necessary to exclude a UTI in patients with pyuria or irritative symptoms, including urge and urge incontinence.[5] Blood urea nitrogen (BUN) and creatinine levels should be obtained if compromised renal function is suspected, especially with overflow incontinence. If polyuria is suspected, serum glucose and calcium tests are also recommended.

A postvoid residual (PVR) is helpful to exclude incomplete emptying and can be obtained through either pelvic ultrasound or catheterization.[5] In general, a PVR of less than 50 mL is considered normal, whereas residuals of more than 100 mL are considered abnormal and require further evaluation.[11]

Additional Diagnostics

Pad testing via the measurement of the loss of urine over a designated period (typically 1 hour or 24 hours) may be useful in combination with other tests to diagnose but may be more useful in measuring change resulting from treatment. Negative tests should be repeated.[12]

Additional testing is usually not needed for the basic evaluation of urinary incontinence unless onset is sudden, symptoms are severe, or suprapubic pain or hematuria is present. The patient should be referred to a urologist if further diagnostic testing (e.g., cystoscopy, urodynamics) is necessary or if the diagnosis is uncertain.[5] Urodynamic testing may lead to drug treatment, and healthy people may have abnormal results.[11] Ultrasound and/or MRI may be used to determine if anatomical or functional abnormalities exist.[11]

DIFFERENTIAL DIAGNOSIS

 Referral to a specialist should be expedited for patients with incontinence and an abnormal postvoid residual, prostate examination that suggests prostate cancer, a neurologic condition, symptomatic pelvic prolapse, or persistent symptoms of difficult or incomplete bladder emptying. Patients with hematuria without infection should be referred for immediate testing.

Consultation with a urologic specialist is important when there is difficulty determining the type of incontinence or when traditional treatment regimens provide inadequate relief of symptoms. Incontinence that does not respond adequately to initial treatment may be managed more effectively in collaboration with a physical therapist (PT), continence nurse, urologist, urogynecologist, or specialized nurse practitioner.

Also, consider referring the patient to a specialist if there are recurrent symptomatic UTI, a history of radical pelvic or incontinence surgery, when the diagnosis is uncertain, when

surgical intervention is being considered, or when therapy of reasonable duration has failed.

The differential diagnosis includes all the types of urinary incontinence: stress, urge, mixed, overflow, and functional (transient). Factors contributing to urinary incontinence include (1) lower urinary tract conditions (bladder cancer, stricture, prolapse), (2) intrinsic sphincteric deficiency, (3) anatomic SUI, (4) DO (idiopathic or neurogenic), (5) poor bladder compliance, (6) medication, and (7) increased urinary production.

INTERPROFESSIONAL COLLABORATIVE MANAGEMENT

If incontinence is believed to be functional, the first step in treatment is to manage the underlying condition. This may be as simple as moving a commode to the bedside of a newly immobile patient recovering from orthopedic surgery. Medical conditions that may exacerbate incontinence should be treated, and conditions that contribute to incontinence should be minimized or discontinued, if possible. A careful review of all medications is important to determine if side effects are contributing to incontinence. When all non-urologic causes of incontinence have been ruled out, the type of incontinence—based on history, physical examination, and diagnostic data—can be determined. Once it has been identified, a management plan for the type of incontinence can be initiated.

Nonpharmacologic Management

The treatment of incontinence varies per cause, but behavioral and pharmacologic therapies are generally first-line therapies in the treatment of urinary incontinence. Surgical therapies may be indicated in some individuals (Box 127.3). Education, particularly around food and fluid regulation and weight loss, can be effective for all the most common types of urinary incontinence.[13] Voiding diaries are also important in the assessment and treatment of UI. It is important to review and evaluate the patient's medications to determine if they may be causing the incontinence. However, it may be difficult to distinguish if medications are the cause and unwise to stop the medications. Constipation is associated with UI and OAB, so successful resolution of constipation may relieve incontinence.[11] Reduction in caffeine intake may reduce urgency but not have any effect on UI.[11] It is unclear whether exercise impacts UI, although people may experience UI more often during physical activity than when not exercising.

Stress Incontinence. Behavioral therapies for SUI include timed voiding, double voiding, weight loss, pelvic muscle exercises, pessary placement, and bowel management.[14] Timed voiding—voiding every 2 hours during the day—allows adequate time for the patient's bladder to fill but not overdistend. This minimizes the amount of urine in the bladder to leak when a stress maneuver does occur.[14] Use of a voiding diary may be beneficial to map voiding occurrences so the patient and health care provider can identify problematic bladder habits.

Double voiding is used for patients who empty incompletely with urination. It consists of having the patient change positions on the toilet, get up and sit back down, or just allow a few extra minutes for the bladder to contract and fully empty. In a patient with stress incontinence and incomplete emptying, improved emptying may allow improved control. Evidence

BOX **127.3**

Management of Incontinence

STRESS INCONTINENCE
- Behavioral therapies: timed or double voiding, smoking cessation, weight loss, pelvic muscle exercises with or without a physical therapist, pessary, bowel management
- Medical therapies: alpha-adrenergic agonists, tricyclic antidepressants, estrogen
- Surgical therapies: injectables, bladder neck suspensions, slings, artificial sphincters

URGE INCONTINENCE
- Behavioral therapies: as above with bladder training, scheduled voiding, bladder irritant minimization, and urge suppression
- Medical therapies: anticholinergic-antimuscarinics, vaginal estrogen
- Surgical therapies: neurosacral modulation, bladder augmentation, botulinum toxin injections

MIXED INCONTINENCE
- Combination of therapies for stress and urge incontinence

OVERFLOW INCONTINENCE
- Behavioral therapies: timed or double voiding, clean intermittent catheterization, pessary
- Medical therapies: alpha$_1$ blockers, 5α-reductase inhibitors
- Surgery to relieve urethral obstruction or stricture or to reduce prolapse

FUNCTIONAL OR TRANSIENT INCONTINENCE
- Treatment of underlying cause

suggests that bladder training with timed or double voiding does not have benefit over the long term unless the patient continues the practice.[11]

Smoking cessation helps minimize events that increase intra-abdominal pressure; smokers are often more likely to cough because of respiratory side effects and infections. Tobacco is also a bladder irritant and can increase the sense of urgency.[5] Recent research indicates, however, that smoking cessation does not necessarily improve UI symptoms.[11] Weight loss can help minimize SUI because increased abdominal girth may apply more pressure to the bladder when stress maneuvers occur.[15]

Pelvic muscle exercises, or Kegel exercises, strengthen the pelvic floor and are considered initial treatment for stress incontinence. Evidence indicates that a combination of pelvic floor exercises by digital palpation, vaginal cones, or weights and biofeedback is the most effective treatment.[16]

The exercises are beneficial because when they are performed correctly, pelvic floor contraction can help minimize stress incontinence by preventing rotation and descent of the urethra and bladder neck during physical activities that may cause symptoms.[14] They may also improve resting pressure in the urethra and increase bulk around the urethra, which may prevent stress and urge incontinence. However, patients do not always stick with the protocol or perform the exercise incorrectly.[11] Kegel exercises are performed by tightening only the pelvic floor muscles as if controlling defecation or urination.

Contraction of abdominal, thigh, and gluteal muscles should be avoided. Appropriate technique is best assessed by placing a finger in the vagina so the appropriate muscles can be isolated. Contractions should be held for up to 5 seconds followed by a period of relaxation. Exercises should be performed as three sets of 10, three times a day, for 6 months, even though benefit may not be seen for 4 to 8 weeks.[17] Referral to a PT is often beneficial for patients who are unable to appropriately isolate the pelvic floor muscles or are unsure if they are performing Kegel exercises correctly. The PT may use adjuncts such as biofeedback and electrical stimulation—for instance, with a transcutaneous electrical nerve stimulation (TENS) unit or similar device—to further improve the patient's ability to contract the pelvic floor. However, the evidence is inconsistent regarding the effectiveness of electrical stimulation.[11]

Biofeedback is used to increase awareness of pelvic floor function and help change responses to improve urination.[18] One of the simplest forms of biofeedback is the use of vaginal weights.[18] Patients are instructed to insert a weight intravaginally and to retain it during ambulation by contraction of the pelvic floor muscles.[18] Exercises should start with light vaginal weights (20 g) and gradually increase to use of heavier weights. If electrical stimulation is used, training must be performed by a professional skilled in this procedure.[5]

Pessary placement may be helpful in patients with stress incontinence or bladder or pelvic organ prolapse. There are pessaries specifically designed for incontinence that work by elevating the bladder neck. Referral to a skilled pessary fitter for appropriate fitting and management is important because patients may need to try a variety of types and sizes before obtaining a good fit.

Bowel management is important in minimizing incontinence.[11] Stool impaction can increase the likelihood of bladder irritability by an increase in external pressure on the bladder and from increased activity in the sacral nerves. Excessive straining with defecation may also contribute to denervation of the external anal sphincter and pelvic floor muscles.[19,20] This denervation is thought to result in bladder symptoms.[19] Ideally, the goal is moderation of the gastrointestinal tract so that one large, soft bowel movement per day or every other day is achieved.

Urge Incontinence. Behavioral methods for treatment of UUI also include timed and double voiding, use of a voiding diary, pelvic floor exercises with or without the assistance of a PT, weight reduction, smoking cessation, and bowel management, as indicated. However, bladder training, scheduled voiding, urge suppression techniques, and overall minimization of bladder irritants can also be recommended.

With UUI, a voiding diary documenting time and amount of each void and the time of any incontinent episode will help illustrate which treatments could be most beneficial. The patient with urge incontinence on the way to the toilet after waiting 4 to 5 hours to void may need to incorporate timed voiding every 2 hours into his or her daily routine.

Bladder training is of benefit to the patient who voids frequently (every 30 minutes to 1 hour) during the day but can sleep through the night and void 300 mL in the morning. Bladder training requires the patient to postpone voiding, to resist the sense of urgency, and to void on a predetermined schedule. Intervals of 10 to 15 minutes should be added to the current voiding pattern and then gradually increased so the patient can reach a goal of voiding every 2 to 3 hours. The bladder should be emptied at the scheduled intervals, and voiding should be delayed if urge occurs. Four or five quick Kegel exercises ("quick flicks") may alleviate bladder spasms, allowing the patient to get to the bathroom without rushing or leaking.[17]

Scheduled or prompted voiding by a caregiver may be effective when a patient cannot use the toilet independently.[11,14] Assistance with toileting should be provided every 2 to 4 hours during the day and night to minimize incontinence. Habit training, another method for decreasing incontinence in dependent patients, occurs when a toileting schedule is developed in accordance with the patient's past voiding habits. Based on a record of incontinence, a schedule can be developed to minimize episodes of incontinence.

Regulation of bladder irritants can help decrease urgency and UUI. Spicy, acidic, and caffeinated foods tend to irritate the bladder and increase the sense of urgency.[21] Chocolate, tomatoes, citrus fruits or juices, most nuts, coffee, tea, dark sodas, alcohol, and tobacco can contribute to irritative symptoms. Furthermore, moderation of overall fluid intake to 48 to 64 ounces per day can help maintain hydration while mitigating the frequency of voiding. A voiding diary may be helpful in assessing this. Posterior tibial nerve stimulation (PTNS) involves stimulation to the sacral micturition center and can benefit women with urge incontinence who have not had any relief from or cannot tolerate antimuscarinic treatment.[11]

Mixed Incontinence. After careful diagnostic evaluation, the patient may be found to have mixed incontinence. Treatment with a combination of previously described behavioral or medical therapies is warranted. Evidence suggests that pelvic floor training is not as effective as in stress UI and that electrical simulation is equally effective in mixed and stress UI conditions.[11]

Overflow Incontinence. Overflow incontinence can be managed with timed and double voiding but also with clean intermittent catheterization (CIC), a pessary, medical therapies, or surgical options. CIC is recommended for patients who have poor emptying secondary to poor detrusor function or for patients with urethral obstruction who are poor surgical candidates. This should be done often enough that CIC amounts, if the patient does not void volitionally, or total void plus CIC amounts remain less than 500 mL with each catheterization-void event.

A pessary may be helpful for prolapse that causes partial urethral obstruction. A pessary provides support to the vaginal canal so the bladder can empty more completely. However, when it is placed, stress incontinence may become more prevalent once the bladder is in proper anatomic position.

Pharmacologic Management

Stress Incontinence. α-adrenergic agonists, such as pseudoephedrine (Sudafed), increase urethral pressure, and outlet resistance to decrease incontinence. Although not curative or approved for this indication, alpha-adrenergics may improve symptoms without significant side effects.

Estrogen replacement may be helpful in treating postmenopausal stress incontinence in women who have signs of vaginal atrophy, although oral estrogen therapy does not provide any benefit.[11] Local applications of estrogen cream can provide a measurable reduction in urinary incontinence and are generally safe for most women but do not cure stress incontinence.[9,11] Periurethral estrogen creams have very low systemic levels and

can be administered daily for 2 weeks, and then twice weekly thereafter with excellent results.

Given the results of the Women's Health Initiative and other studies, women must be counseled about the risks versus benefits of hormone replacement therapy, and therapy must be used for the shortest possible time.[9]

Imipramine or other tricyclic antidepressants may be recommended, especially in younger patients, if other therapies have proved ineffective. At doses of 10 to 25 mg orally one to three times daily, imipramine has both alpha-agonist and anticholinergic effects, which make it useful for patients with SUI or mixed incontinence.[21]

In general, these drugs should be used carefully in older adults because of potential adverse effects, mostly cardiac and anticholinergic. Orthostatic hypotension with an increased risk of falls may be more likely in the elderly.

Other possible anticholinergic side effects include dizziness, fatigue, dry mouth, and constipation. If a patient decides to stop the tricyclic antidepressant, a gradual taper should be used. Duloxetine, commonly used in Europe for stress incontinence and not approved for use in the United States, should be used with caution if it is prescribed, because worsening of depression may occur initially before benefit is seen. Desmopressin can reduce UI symptoms for a 4-hour duration but does not provide relief beyond 4 hours. A few studies have tested urethral injection therapy and have so far found that urinary retention and infection were common complications from the treatment. This treatment requires further testing.[22]

Urge Incontinence. Medications are generally helpful in moderating urge incontinence. Anticholinergic-antimuscarinic agents are the cornerstone of medical therapy because they work to block impulses to muscarinic acetylcholine receptors (M_2/M_3) found in the bladder.[19] In turn, the number and strength of involuntary bladder contractions decrease, and urinary frequency is moderated. Anticholinergic agents can have side effects of dry mouth, confusion, constipation, dizziness, blurred vision, and tachycardia.

Tolterodine tartrate (Detrol) and oxybutynin chloride (Ditropan) are examples of antimuscarinic agents.[23] Oxybutynin has greater anticholinergic side effects than other anticholinergics and may be reserved for younger patients. Ditropan XL (an extended-release formulation of oxybutynin), Oxytrol (transdermal oxybutynin in a patch), and Gelnique (transdermal oxybutynin in a gel) have been shown to produce fewer anticholinergic side effects than regular oxybutynin.[23] Newer anticholinergics, such as fesoterodine (Toviaz), continue to be developed in an effort to increase efficacy while reducing side effects. Trospium (Sanctura) is a quaternary amine and, in theory, has less ability to cross the blood–brain barrier. Darifenacin (Enablex), solifenacin (VESIcare), and mirabegron (Myrbetriq) are selective for M_3 receptors, which may increase efficacy and decrease M_2-mediated side effects.[24] However, because all these drugs have the potential to cause side effects in the frail geriatric patient, they should be started at low doses and gradually titrated until either symptoms improve or non-tolerability indicates further medication trials. The long-term effects of mirabegron are so far unknown.[11] Vaginal estrogen treatments may cure urge incontinence in postmenopausal women.[11]

Tricyclics may be helpful for certain patients with UUI. Again, low doses of these drugs should be used in older adults because of the potential for adverse effects.

Mixed Incontinence. Duloxetine can improve mixed UI, particularly in patients who are unresponsive to other treatments.[11]

Overflow Incontinence. Medications are used to relieve overflow incontinence in relation to BPH. The alpha₁ blockers tamsulosin hydrochloride (Flomax) and terazosin (Hytrin), as well as the 5α-reductase inhibitors finasteride (Proscar) and dutasteride (Avodart) can be used. There is no role for these medications in women.

Complementary Approaches

A study by Jackson et al.[25] explored the use of complementary and alternative therapies in diverse patients with urinary incontinence. The remedies most frequently used included vitamins, green tea, Cranberry juice and flaxseed. Other CAM remedies used included moabi, cinnamon, ginseng, saw palmetto, aloe, yarrow, other herbs, and herbal teas.[25] Acupuncture is frequently discussed in the medical and nursing literature with mixed results.[26,27] In addition, a variety of Chinese[28-30] and other herbs[31] have been tested to treat incontinence. Further research is needed, and the clinician is advised to carefully review evidence-based literature and guidelines before attempting to use any of these remedies.

Emerging Treatments

Emerging trends in the treatment of SUI include cell-based therapy, slings, and vaginal laser treatment.[32] For the treatment of lower urinary tract symptoms in men, intraprostatic injections, prostate urethral lifts, ablative techniques, and prostatic artery embolization are showing some success.[33]

Surgical Consultation

Surgery should be considered if treatment regimens are ineffective or if patients are not able to adhere to other treatment plans. Stress incontinence is the most common type of incontinence treated with surgery. Surgery is done either to lift or to provide support to the urethra or bladder neck. Choices include retropubic suspensions, a variety of sling procedures, urethral bulking agents, and artificial urinary sphincters. Referral to a urologist or urogynecologist is recommended if surgery is being considered. The type of surgery performed depends on patient anatomy, urodynamic findings, and patient expectations.

Surgical therapies may be indicated in some patients with severe urge incontinence. Surgical therapies, done to counteract bladder contractions or to increase bladder capacity, include botulinum toxin injections, neurosacral modulation, and bladder augmentation. Botulinum injections are now licensed by the Food and Drug Administration for the treatment of OAB and neurogenic DO and can be helpful for these conditions.[25] Referral to a urologist is indicated if botulinum injections or surgical therapy are being considered. Surgery is often indicated to relieve urethral obstruction caused by BPH, stricture, or a nonreducible prolapse.

LIFE SPAN CONSIDERATIONS

Incontinence can occur at any age but is more prevalent in the older adult. Changes in the urinary tract that occur with aging can contribute to the development of incontinence. Bladder capacity, contractility, and the ability to postpone voiding are thought to decline with age. Prostate size, urethral obstruction, involuntary bladder contractions, and PVRs, on the other

hand, may increase.[34] These changes, as well as increased chronic health conditions and medications that affect the urinary tract, explain why incontinence is so prevalent in the geriatric population. Evidence is largely inconclusive regarding the effect of antimuscarinic medications on cognition in the elderly; however, Oxybutynin appears to contribute to cognitive decline. Solifenacin, Tolterodine, and Darifenacin do not appear to increase cognitive dysfunction. To date, there have been no studies comparing the use of Fesoterodine in elderly and young patients. Nor have there been any trials testing Mirabegron in the elderly.[11] Side effects from anticholinergic medications that impact cognition are cumulative.[11] It is important to conduct a thorough cognitive assessment prior to starting therapy and to monitor cognitive function throughout treatment.

PATIENT AND FAMILY EDUCATION

Effectiveness of behavioral strategies in the treatment of incontinence depends on the education and adherence of patients, families, and caregivers to the treatment plan agreed on. Plans for behavioral interventions should be realistic and meet the needs of patients and caregivers. Regular follow-up visits will help reinforce therapeutic options, support efforts to obtain treatment goals, and allow care plan modification so optimum outcomes can be obtained.

HEALTH PROMOTION

Weight management, tobacco cessation, exercise and food, and fluid adjustments can significantly impact or prevent urinary incontinence. Patient education is key to assisting patients to prevent and manage UI, regardless of the type.

REFERENCES

1. Yelina, G. (2014). Prevalence of incontinence among older Americans. *Vital and Health Statistics. Series 3, Analytical Studies, 36*(1).
2. Mathews, C. A., Whitehead, W. E., Townsend, M. K., & Gordstein, F. (2013). Risk factors for urinary, fecal or dual incontinence in the Nurses' Health Study. *Obstetrics and Gynecology, 122*(3), 539.
3. Milson, I., Coyne, K., Nicholson, S., et al. (2014). Global prevalence and economic burden of urgency incontinence: A systematic review. *European Urology, 65*(1), 96–98.
4. Wein, A. J. (2011). Pathophysiology and classification of lower urinary tract dysfunction: Overview. In A. J. Wein (Ed.), *Campbell-Walsh urology* (10th ed.). Philadelphia: Elsevier.
5. Bettez, M., Tu, L., Carlson, K., et al. (2012). 2101 update: Guidelines for adult urinary incontinence. Collaborative consensus document for the Canadian Urological Association. *Canadian Urological Association Journal = Journal de l'Association des urologues du Canada, 6*(5), 354–363.
6. Phe, V., Chartell-Kastler, E., Soler, J. M., & Denys, P. (2015). Pathophysiology of the low compliant bladder. In J. Corcos & D. Ginsberg (Eds.), *Textbook of the neurogenic bladder* (3rd ed.). Boca Raton, Florida: CRC press.
7. Chen, Y., Wen, J. G., Shen, H., et al. (2014). Valsalva leak point pressure associated O-tip angle and simple female stress urinary incontinence symptoms. *International Urology and Nephrology, 46*(11), 2103–2108.
8. Gartlehner, G., Patel, S. V., Viswanathan, M., et al. (2017). Menopausal hormone therapy for the primary prevention of chronic conditions: An evidence review for the U. S. Preventive Task Force. AHRQ Publication No. 15-05227-EF-1.
9. Cody, J. D., Jacobs, M. L., Richardson, K., et al. (2012). Oestrogens for urinary incontinence in women. *The Cochrane Database of Systematic Reviews,* (10), CD001405.
10. Davis, R., Jones, S., Baricas, D., et al. (2012). Diagnosis, evaluation and follow-up of asymptomatic microhematuria (AMH) in adults: AUA guidelines. *The Journal of Urology, 188*(6), s2473–s2481.
11. Espuña-Pons, M., Cardozo, L., Chapple, C., et al. (2012). Overactive bladder symptoms and voiding dysfunction in neurologically normal women. *Neurourology and Urodynamics, 31*(4), 422–428.

12. Lucas, M. G., Bedretdinova, D., et al. (2015). Guidelines on urinary incontinence. *European Association of Urology*, 1–90.

13. Cameron, A. P., Jimbo, M., & Heidelbaugh, J. J. (2013). Diagnosis and office-based treatment of urinary incontinence in adults. Part two: Treatment. *Therapeutic Advances in Urology*, 5(4), 189–200.

14. Salzman, H. B. (2013). Clinical management of urinary incontinence in women. *American Family Physician*, 87(9), 634–640.

15. Osburn, D., Strain, M., Gomelsky, A., et al. (2013). Obesity and female stress urinary incontinence. *Urology*, 82(4), 759–763.

16. Ferreira, M., Azevedo, M. J., Firmino-Machado, J., & Santos, P. C. (2017). Pelvic floor muscle training protocol for stress urinary incontinence in women: A systematic review. *Revista Da Associacao Medica Brasileira*, 63(7), http://dx.doi.org/10.1590/1806-9282.63.07.642.

17. Mayo Clinic Staff. Kegel exercises: a how-to guide for women. Retrieved from www.mayoclinic.org/healthy/lifestyle/womens-health.in-depth/kegel-exercises/art 20045283. (Accessed 31 August 2015).

18. Burgio, K. L. (2013). Update on behavioral and physical therapies for incontinence and overactive bladder: The role of pelvic floor muscle training. *Current Urology Reports*, 14(5), 457–464.

19. Cipullo, L., Zullo, F., Cosimato, C., et al. (2014). Pharmacological treatment of urinary incontinence. *Female Pelvic Medicine and Reconstructive Surgery*, 20(4), 185–202.

20. Lucas, M. G., Bedretdinova, D., Bosch, J. L., et al. (2012). EAU guidelines on assessment and non-surgical management of urinary incontinence. *Urology*, 62(6), 1130–1142.

21. Qaseem, A., Dallas, P., Forcien, M. A., et al. (2014). Non-surgical management of urinary incontinence in women: A clinical practice guideline from the American College of Physicians. *Annals of Internal Medicine*, 161(16), 429–440.

22. Matsuoka, P. K., Locali, R. F., Pacetta, A. M., et al. (2016). The efficacy and safety of urethral injection therapy for urinary incontinence in women: A systematic review. *Clinics (Sao Paulo, Brazil)*, 71(2), 94 100.

23. Abraham, N., & Goldman, H. B. (2015). An update on the pharmacological therapy for lower urinary tract dysfunction. *Expert Opinion on Pharmacotherapy*, 16(1), 79–93.

24. Adhuvrata, P., Cody, J. D., Ellis, G., et al. (2012). Which anticholinergic drug for overactive bladder symptoms in adults? *Cochrane Database of Systematic Review*, (1), CD005429.

25. Jackson, C. B., Taubenberger, S. P., Botelho, E., et al. (2012). Complementary and Alternative Therapies for Urinary Symptoms: Use in a diverse population sample qualitative study. *Urologic Nursing*, 32(3), 149–157.

26. Wang, M. (2017). Acupuncture for stress urinary incontinence. *JAMA: The Journal of the American Medical Association*, 318(15), 1500.

27. Rosenberg, K. (2017). Electroacupuncture is Beneficial in Women with Stress Incontinence. *The American Journal of Nursing*, 117(10), 61–62.

28. Xiao, D. D., LV, J. W., Xie, X., et al. (2016). The combination of herbal medicine Weng-li-tong with Tolterodine may be better than Tolterodine alone in the treatment of overactive bladder in women: A randomized placebo-controlled prospective trial. *BMC Urology*, 16(1), 49.

29. Chen, Y. H., Lin, Y. N., Chen, W. C., et al. (2014). Treatment of stress urinary incontinence by ginsenoside Rh2. *The American Journal of Chinese Medicine*, 42(4), 817–831.

30. Chen, Y. H., Lin, Y. N., Chen, W. C., et al. (2014). Treatment of stress urinary incontinence by cinnamaldehyde, the major constituent of the Chinese medicinal herb ramulus cinnamomi. *Evidence-Based Complementary and Alternative Medicine*, 280204. doi:10.1155/2014/280204.

31. Rangaswamy, A., & Sultana, A. (2014). Nagapattinam S. Efficacy of Boswellia serrata L. and Cyperus scariosus L. plus pelvic floor muscle training in stress incontinence in women of reproductive age. *Complementary Therapies in Clinical Practice*, 20(4), 230–236. doi:10.1016/j.ctcp.2014.08.003.

32. Samer, S., & Campeau, L. (2017). Stress urinary incontinence in women: Current and emerging therapeutic options. *Canadian Urological Association Journal = Journal de l'Association des urologues du Canada*, 11(6Suppl2), S155–S158.

33. Magistro, G., Chapple, C. R., Elhilali, M., et al. (2017). Emerging minimally invasive treatment options for male lower urinary tract symptoms. *European Urology*, 72(6), 986–997.

34. Testa, A. (2015). Understanding urinary incontinence in adults. *Urologic Nursing*, 35(2), 86–96.

CHAPTER **128**

PROSTATE CANCER

Meaghan O'Leary

 Suspected spinal cord compression is an emergency requiring early intervention for neurologc recovery.

DEFINITION AND EPIDEMIOLOGY

Other than skin cancer, cancer of the prostate is the most common malignant neoplasm in men in the United States and the second leading cause of cancer death in men of all races and Hispanic origin populations.[1] The National Cancer Institute estimated that in 2017, the United States had 161,360 new cases diagnosed and 26,730 deaths from prostate cancer.[2] One in nine men in the United States will be diagnosed with prostate cancer in his lifetime, and more than 3 million American men are living with prostate cancer.[3] Risk factors for prostate cancer include advancing age, African-American race, and a positive family history of prostate cancer. Geography is considered a risk factor; prostate cancer is more common in Caribbean men of African ancestry and men living in North America, northwestern Europe, and Australia. The majority of cases are diagnosed in men older than 65 years, with incidence rates higher in African-American men than in white men.[2] The mortality rate of African-American men is estimated to be twice that of white men.[2] As a result of early, effective screening and the aging of the U.S. population, the number of prostate cancer cases diagnosed has increased; however, deaths from prostate cancer have decreased significantly in recent years, and the majority of men diagnosed with prostate cancer do not die of the disease.[2,3]

PATHOPHYSIOLOGY

The most common type of prostate cancer is adenocarcinoma. It develops in the acinar glands located in the posterior peripheral zone of the prostate (Fig. 128.1). Histologic grading is an important predictor of prognosis. The Gleason system incorporates pathologic parameters for grading of the malignant neoplasm.[4] Tumors can arise in one or both lobes of the prostate and can spread within the prostate, through the prostatic capsule, and through the seminal vesicles or the base of the bladder, with metastasis occurring through the lymphatic and circulatory systems. The most common sites of metastasis are to the lymph nodes and bone.

CLINICAL PRESENTATION AND PHYSICAL EXAMINATION

Presenting symptoms of prostate cancer may include urinary hesitancy, urgency, nocturia, frequency, and hematuria, although the patient is usually asymptomatic in early stages of the disease. Symptoms tend to increase in intensity during a 1- to 2-month period, which is different from the slow, gradual progression in symptoms that occurs in benign prostatic hyperplasia (BPH). In more advanced disease, presenting symptoms may include back pain, impotence, and other bone pain that suggests metastasis. Other symptoms of metastasis include weight loss, constipation, malaise, hematuria, and rectal pain or symptoms related to nerve root compression, such as paresthesias or extremity weakness.

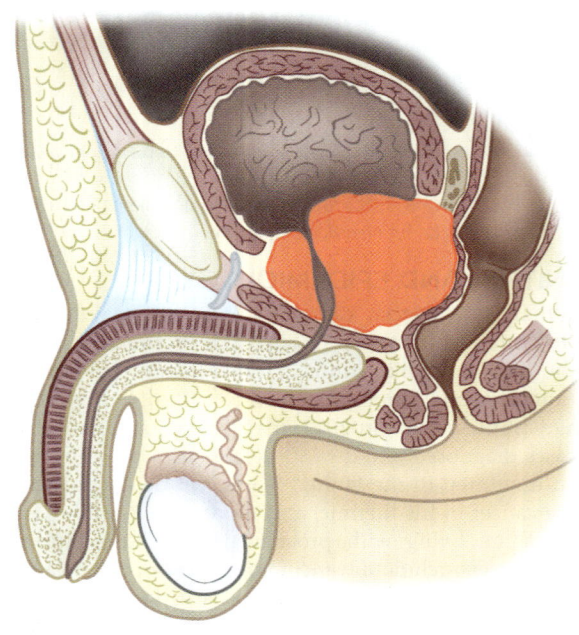

FIG. 128.1 Cancer of prostate. (From Ball, J. H., Dains, J. E., Flynn, J. A., Solomon, B. S., & Stewart, R. W. [2019]. *Seidel's guide to physical examination: An interprofessional approach* [9th ed.]. St. Louis: Elsevier.)

The most common factor in identifying prostate cancer is an elevated prostate-specific antigen (PSA). Rarely, prostate cancer can be non–PSA producing, and tumor burden will not correlate with PSA values. These patients will have the same presentation as others, with symptoms of bone pain or obstruction, and will likely have abnormal digital rectal examination (DRE) findings but a low PSA level. Patients with signs and symptoms of prostate cancer should be referred to a urologist for evaluation, even in the presence of a normal PSA level.

The DRE is used to detect initial physical abnormalities of the prostate gland. A firm nodule on rectal examination, induration, or a stony, asymmetric prostate is suggestive of prostate cancer. In early-stage disease, the findings on prostate examination will generally be normal.

DIAGNOSTICS

Measurement of the PSA level combined with DRE if elevated is considered the most sensitive and specific screening method for prostate cancer. Some controversy exists regarding initial PSA screening and interval testing. The American Urological Association (AUA) recommends that men who are considering prostate screening should discuss the benefits and risks of testing with their health care providers. The American Cancer Society recommends that men have the opportunity to make an informed decision with their health care provider about prostate cancer screening.[5] The U.S. Preventive Services Task Force continues to support the recommendation against PSA-based screening for prostate cancer. The recommendation applies to all men in the general U.S. population regardless of age.[6]

PSA is a protease enzyme secreted by the prostate gland, and levels may be elevated in both benign and malignant conditions of the prostate. A prostate level below 4 ng/mL is considered normal, although a prostate tumor may be present with a PSA level below 4 ng/mL. Algorithms exist to adjust normal values for age and race. In addition, some medications (e.g., finasteride, dutasteride) can decrease PSA values, thus requiring adjustment. Values of 4 to 10 ng/mL may be seen in early prostate cancer and other benign conditions; values above 10 ng/mL suggest prostate cancer. The use of the free PSA test and determination of PSA velocity (rate of rise) may increase specificity for prostate cancer, especially if the PSA level is elevated. A rate of rise of more than 0.75 ng/mL per year is considered highly sensitive for prostate cancer, but subsequent clinical trials have shown PSA velocity to add little predictive information to the total PSA.[7,8] Different age-specific reference ranges are sometimes considered, especially in African-American men, because cases in this population might be missed with use of the traditional reference ranges.

Similar to decisions about when PSA screening should occur, the decision regarding when to perform tissue biopsies for prostate cancer diagnosis confirmation remains controversial. In men older than 60 years, if the PSA level is higher than 4.0 ng/mL or findings on DRE are abnormal, transrectal ultrasound (TRUS) of the prostate with TRUS-guided biopsy is recommended. TRUS allows guided biopsy of suspicious hypoechoic areas. Transperineal biopsy may also be performed under general anesthesia and is associated with a lower risk of infection. Magnetic resonance imaging (MRI)–targeted biopsy is being evaluated to improve the accuracy of TRUS biopsy, especially in the setting of men with prior negative biopsies. MRI of the prostate may be performed prior to TRUS-guided biopsy to help identify areas for biopsy, but TRUS is still currently the standard of care for initial biopsy.[9] In younger men, biopsy is considered if the PSA level is above 2.6 ng/mL.

In cases with a positive finding on biopsy of the prostate and a PSA level above 10 ng/mL or a Gleason score greater than 7, a radionuclide bone scan may be necessary to determine the presence of bone metastases. Computed tomography (CT) scan of the abdomen and pelvis is important to assess the regional lymph nodes and metastasis. A CT scan of the chest can exclude metastasis to the lungs but is not routinely performed if the CT scan of the abdomen and pelvis is negative. An elevated alkaline phosphatase level suggests bone metastasis, and an elevated acid phosphatase level suggests prostatic metastasis.

INITIAL DIAGNOSTICS

Prostate Cancer

LABORATORY
- Prostate-specific antigen
- Complete blood count and differential

OTHER DIAGNOSTICS
- Needle biopsy
- Pelvic computed tomography scan
- Pelvic magnetic resonance imaging
- Bone scan

DIFFERENTIAL DIAGNOSIS

 Priority differentials include BPH and prostatitis.

In both BPH and prastatitis, there may be an abnormal DRE finding and/or PSA test result. In BPH, the prostate typically feels rubbery with no palpable nodules on DRE. In prostatitis, the DRE will usually reveal a tender, boggy prostate. Other potential differential diagnoses include bladder cancer, urinary tract infection, and urethral stricture.

- Bone pain, hematospermia, macroscopic hematuria, and renal failure are possible symptoms of advanced prostate cancer and should alert the health care provider to further investigate their etiology.[10]
- Acute neurologic symptoms, i.e., weakness, numbness, urinary retention, urinary incontinence, or fecal incontinence, could represent spinal cord compression from tumor. This is an emergency, and early intervention is crucial to neurologic recovery.

INTERPROFESSIONAL COLLABORATIVE MANAGEMENT

Treatment options are based on the stage or extent to which the cancer has spread. There are several different staging systems for prostate cancer, but the most widely used is the American Joint Committee on Cancer (AJCC) TNM system. The TNM system describes the following:

- Extent of the primary tumor (T category)
- Whether the cancer has spread to nearby lymph nodes (N category)
- Absence or presence of distant metastases (M category)

Localized disease (T1 and T2) has the most options: active surveillance (monitoring with PSA, DRE, and follow-up prostate biopsies), radiation therapy (brachytherapy or external beam radiation therapy), and surgery. Patients with disease that has gone beyond the prostatic capsule but without evidence of metastatic spread (T3) may be offered radiation therapy, hormonal therapy, or a combination of radiation and hormonal therapy as well as surgery in select situations. Patients with either local or distant metastatic disease will generally be offered hormonal therapy; however, palliative radiation therapy (beam therapy aimed at bone lesions) or palliative chemotherapy as well as salvage chemotherapy may be offered.

Treatment decisions are based on the stage at diagnosis; prognostic features of the tumor; and the patient's age, medical condition, and treatment preference. Prostate cancer has been categorized as very low-risk, low-risk, intermediate-risk, high-risk, and very high-risk to assist in developing a treatment plan. Decisions about therapy are complex and controversial. The current therapy with disease classified as intermediate-risk, high-risk, or very high-risk (histologic grade group 2 or above) is radical prostatectomy or radiation therapy with or without hormonal therapy or androgen deprivation therapy (ADT). Cryotherapy is being considered in localized prostate cancer, as well.

ADT has been used for symptomatic patients with advanced disease or for patients who do not want surgery, but evidence is mixed as to whether androgen suppression improves long-term outcomes.[9] Hormone treatments include oral estrogens, orchiectomy, luteinizing hormone–releasing hormone (LHRH) agonists, antiandrogens, and progestational agents. LHRH agonists act by initially stimulating pituitary gonadotropin production and later inhibiting it. Therapy to prevent osteoporosis may be necessary in men receiving hormonal therapy. The National Cancer Institute provides a very helpful treatment by stage section for patients on their prostate cancer treatment (PDQ) site.

Pain management is often an important treatment issue in more advanced disease. Palliative treatment with chemotherapy or radiation therapy and medication may help relieve the pain.

INDICATIONS FOR REFERRAL OR HOSPITALIZATION

A referral should be made to a urologist when an abnormality is found on DRE or the PSA level is elevated (some patients may decline referral after options and implications for treatment have been discussed). After treatment, the health care provider can offer follow-up care that includes monitoring of the PSA levels. After radical prostatectomy, the PSA level should fall to less than 0.2 ng/mL. PSA levels also fall after radiation therapy and continue to decrease for 12 months after completion of therapy. PSA levels should be tested at 6 and 12 months after treatment and annually thereafter. An increase in PSA should be evaluated with TRUS and biopsy in individuals that have had radiation therapy. Hospitalization may also be necessary in the case of advanced metastatic disease for pain control.

LIFE SPAN CONSIDERATIONS

The early detection of prostate cancer remains the key consideration in caring for male patients. In addressing this concern for men, primary care providers must demonstrate an evidence-based shared decision-making approach to care. Providers should be prepared to discuss screening recommendations and all related aspects of prostate health with adult males of all ages.

The AUA offers the following prostate cancer screening recommendation in its recent early detection of prostate cancer guideline.[11] PSA screening is not recommended for men younger than age 40 years. Routine screening is not recommended for men aged 40 to 54 years who have average risk. For patients younger than 55 years with higher risk, providers should individualize decisions for prostate screening. A shared decision-making approach to prostate cancer screening for men 55 to 69 years should be implemented. The greatest benefit of PSA screening is evidenced for men 55 to 69 years. For those men who have made the decision to screen, a screening interval of 2 years is preferred over annual screening. Evidence supporting the AUA guideline suggests that a 2-year screening interval may reduce harm and improve benefits, including a reduction in overdiagnosis and false positives.[11] PSA screening is not recommended for men older than 70 years or men with less than a 10- to 15-year life expectancy. The AUA guideline suggests that PSA screening may be of value to healthy males older than 70 years.[11]

COMPLICATIONS

The major complication of prostate cancer is metastatic disease. Risks of surgery include hemorrhage and injury to the obturator nerve, ureter, or rectum. Incontinence and impotence are also potential complications. Problems associated with radiation therapy include urinary problems, intestinal sequelae, impotence, and transient edema. Intestinal problems include diarrhea, fecal incontinence, rectal bleeding, intestinal obstruction, rectal strictures, mucous discharge, and tenesmus. Potential urologic problems include cystitis, hematuria, frequency, dysuria, and urethral stricture. The main complications of cryotherapy include urethral stricture, irritative symptoms, urinary incontinence, impotence, rectourethral fistula, bladder neck contracture, and urinary retention.

PATIENT AND FAMILY EDUCATION

Prostate health education that incorporates shared decision-making approaches is more likely to produce successful outcomes that align with patient and family preferences and values. The use of shared decision-making in health care can improve care quality and reduce costs.[12] Providers should emphasize education that incorporates best evidence of prostate cancer screening and treatment recommendations. Patients should receive individualized, well-informed treatment options.[13] Primary care providers should collaborate with urologic specialty providers and remain fully engaged and responsive to the patients' and families' needs.

HEALTH PROMOTION

As with most cancers, the exact cause of prostate cancer is not certain. Mutations in the genetic structure and a cadre of risk factors related to age, race, location, and diet are considered causes. Evidence to support significant benefits including reduction in morbidity and mortality related to prostate health is limited. There is limited evidence supporting specific nutritional recommendations to prevent prostate cancer. Despite these limitations, health promotion strategies to address modifiable lifestyle factors such as diet, stress management, and overall health are the current approaches considered. Primary care providers should promote health through lifestyle interventions that encourage overall health and wellness.

REFERENCES

1. U.S. Cancer Statistics Working Group. (2017). United States Cancer Statistics: 1999–2014 Incidence and Mortality Web-based Report. Atlanta (GA): Department of Health and Human Services, Centers for Disease Control and Prevention, and National Cancer Institute.
2. National Cancer Institute, National Institute for Health. Surveillance, Epidemiology and End Results Program: Cancer of the prostate. http://seer.cancer.gov/statfacts/html/prost.html. (Accessed 7 November 2017).
3. American Cancer Society. www.cancer.org/cancer/prostatecancer/detailedguide/prostate-cancer-key-statistics. (Accessed 11 December 2017).
4. Epstein, J. I., Zelefsky, M. J., Sjoberg, D. D., et al. (2016). A contemporary prostate cancer grading system: A validated alternative to the Gleason score. *European Urology, 69*, 428.
5. American Cancer Association. (2016). American Cancer Society guidelines for the early detection of cancer. www.cancer.org/cancer/prostatecancer/moreinformation/prostatecancerearlydetection/prostate-cancer-early-detection-acs-recommendations. (Accessed 11 December 2017).
6. Moyer, V. (2012). Screening for prostate cancer: U.S. Preventive Services Task Force Recommendation Statement. *Annals of Internal Medicine, 157*(2), 120–134.
7. Scher, H. I. (2015). Benign and malignant diseases of the prostate. In D. L. Kasper, et al. (Eds.), *Harrison's Principles of Internal Medicine* (19th ed.). New York: McGraw-Hill.
8. Vickers, A. J., Till, C., Tangen, C. M., et al. (2011). An empirical evaluation of guidelines on prostate-specific antigen velocity in prostate cancer detection. *Journal of the National Cancer Institute, 103*, 462.
9. NCCN Clinical Practice Guidelines in Oncology. (2017). Prostate cancer version 2.2017. https://www.nccn.org/professionals/physician_gls/pdf/prostate.pdf. (Accessed 29 November 2017).
10. Prostate Cancer Working Group and Ministry of Health. (2015). Prostate cancer management and referral guidance. http://www.prostate.org.nz/documents/prostate-cancer-management-referral-guidance-sept15.pdf. (Accessed 11 December 2017).
11. American Urological Association (AUA). (2013). Early detection of prostate cancer: AUA guideline. http://www.auanet.org/guidelines/early-detection-of-prostate-cancer-(2013-reviewed-and-validity-confirmed-2015). (Accessed 11 December 2017).
12. Lee, E., & Emanuel, E. (2013). Shared decision making to improve care and reduce costs. *The New England Journal of Medicine, 368*, 6–8.
13. Irvine, J., & Chung, S. F. (2014). Treatment decision-making for early prostate cancer patients—what can nurses do? *Nursing and Health, 2*, 23–29.

CHAPTER 129

PROSTATIC HYPERPLASIA (BENIGN)

Patricia Polgar-Bailey

 Immediate referral indicated for acute urinary retention, recurrent prostatic and results of DRE suggestive of prostate cancer.

DEFINITION AND EPIDEMIOLOGY

Benign prostatic hyperplasia (BPH), an almost ubiquitous phenomenon among older men, is a noncancerous enlargement of the prostate gland. Although the exact prevalence of BPH is unknown, it ranges from 50% to 70% among men 50 years of age and older and up to 80% among men 70 years of age and older.[1]

PATHOPHYSIOLOGY

The prostate gland undergoes its first growth spurt during puberty and attains an average size of 20 g ($\frac{7}{10}$ ounce) by the age of 20 years. The gland then undergoes a second growth spurt during the fifth decade of life.

The development of the prostate gland depends on androgen secretion, and both the presence of testes and advancing age are necessary for the development of BPH. Dihydrotestosterone (DHT) is the main mediator of the growth and secretory function of the prostate and is the active metabolite that results from testosterone conversion.[2] BPH seems to be related to a complex interaction between androgen and estrogen secretion; abnormal serum elevations of androgen and estrogen stimulate prostatic growth. Other factors that contribute to prostatic enlargement appear to be related to the elaboration of certain growth factors, the formation and maintenance of DHT levels, and the functioning of androgen receptors.[2]

CLINICAL PRESENTATION AND PHYSICAL EXAMINATION

Men with BPH can also have bladder outlet obstruction (BOO), lower urinary tract symptoms (LUTS), or a combination of these problems.[3] Thus the symptoms of BPH are either obstructive or irritative in character, depending on the particular BPH components involved. Obstructive symptoms include urinary hesitancy, decreased caliber and force of the stream, and postvoid dribbling. These symptoms are related to BOO. Irritative symptoms include frequency, urgency, and nocturia and occur as a result of decreased functional bladder capacity and instability or infection. In men, the term *LUTS* was originally used to describe the irritative symptoms primarily associated with BPH but has been expanded to include symptoms related to bladder storage and/or voiding disturbances; the term used now is *male LUTS* or *MLUTS*.[3] On occasion, hematuria accompanies BPH. Episodic symptoms may be present during many years with a gradual increase in the intensity of symptoms over time.

A thorough history is important and should include questions related to general health, history of type 2 diabetes, and sexual health. A family history of BPH or prostate cancer should be explored as well as any past history of urethral trauma,

TABLE 129.1	American Urological Association Symptom Index for Benign Prostatic Hyperplasia					
Questions to be Answered	**Not at All**	**Less Than One Time in Five**	**Less Than Half the Time**	**About Half the Time**	**More Than Half the Time**	**Almost Always**
Over the past month, how often have you had a sensation of not emptying your bladder completely after you finish urinating?	0	1	2	3	4	5
Over the past month, how often have you had to urinate less than 2 hours after you finished urinating?	0	1	2	3	4	5
Over the past month, how often have you found you stopped and started again several times while urinating?	0	1	2	3	4	5
Over the past month, how often have you found it difficult to postpone urination?	0	1	2	3	4	5
Over the past month, how often have you had a weak urinary stream?	0	1	2	3	4	5
Over the past month, how often have you had to push or strain to begin urination?	0	1	2	3	4	5
Over the past month, how many times did you typically get up to urinate from the time you went to bed at night until the time you got up in the morning?	0 (None)	1 (1 time)	2 (2 times)	3 (3 times)	4 (4 times)	5 (5 times)

A score of 0–7 indicates mild symptoms; 8–19, moderate symptoms; and 20–35, severe symptoms.
From Holtgrewe, H. L., Mebust, W. K., Dowd, J. B., et al. (2002). The American Urological Association symptom index for benign prostatic hyperplasia (abstract 1042). *The Journal of Urology, 167*(2), 265.

urethritis, or urethral instrumentation. Current over-the-counter and prescription medication use should be explored to determine the use of anticholinergics (including diphenhydramine and those in cold preparations), which can impair bladder contractility, or sympathomimetics such as pseudoephedrine, which increase outflow resistance. Diuretics, which can cause an increased output of urine, may lead to urinary retention, especially in the presence of a partially decompensated detrusor muscle. Frequency volume charts or voiding diaries can be used to evaluate nocturia.[3]

BPH symptoms may be quantified by a symptom index developed by the American Urological Association (AUA) to aid in classifying symptom severity and in developing a treatment plan (Table 129.1).[4] Symptoms are rated according to frequency of occurrence and aid health care providers in determining the severity of patient symptoms.[4] The AUA is working on improving the symptom index so future modifications are possible. Additional information regarding the BPH symptom index is available at https://www.jurology.com/article/S0022-5347(16)31615-9/pdf.

The physical examination requires a digital rectal examination (DRE) to evaluate the prostate gland for size, consistency, shape, symmetry, and abnormalities as well as to evaluate anal sphincter tone. Prostatic nodules or induration should be noted on rectal examination because these findings suggest prostate cancer. The normal prostate is heart shaped and measures approximately $4 \times 3 \times 2$ cm ($1\frac{3}{5} \times 1\frac{1}{5} \times \frac{4}{5}$ inches). With BPH, there may be uniform or focal enlargement of the prostate. The size of the prostate does not always correlate with symptom severity, however, and should not direct therapy. The median sulcus is often obliterated in BPH, and it is often difficult to palpate over the base of the prostate because of the gland's enlarged size in advanced stages. With BPH, the gland is nontender and should be rubbery and smooth in consistency. A focused neurologic examination is done to assess sacral nerve roots to identify neurologic problems that could be contributing to bladder symptoms. A lower abdominal examination is necessary to ascertain bladder distention from urinary retention.[3]

DIAGNOSTICS
Essential Diagnostics
A urinalysis should be performed to exclude a urinary tract infection or hematuria. Office-based bladder ultrasound examination to determine postvoid residual can be helpful in the diagnosis and treatment of BPH.

Additional Diagnostics
According to AUA guidelines, measurement of serum prostate-specific antigen (PSA) is appropriate for men with a life expectancy of more than 10 years in the presence of physical findings suggestive of prostate cancer (abnormal DRE findings) and if 5α-reductase inhibitor therapy is planned.[5]

The routine measurement of serum creatinine levels is not indicated in the initial evaluation of men with LUTS secondary to BPH because baseline renal insufficiency appears to be no more common in men with BPH than in a comparable cohort of men without BPH.[6]

Men with BPH should be advised that data from the Prostate Cancer Prevention Trial revealed that BPH is not a risk factor for prostate cancer.[7] Assessment of free PSA and PSA velocity (the rate of rise per year) may help increase specificity for prostate cancer. Noncancerous prostate growth rarely results in a PSA velocity of more than 0.75 ng/mL/year.[8]

DIFFERENTIAL DIAGNOSIS

Symptoms of BOO mandate evaluation for bladder calculi, urethral stricture, cancer of the prostate, and bladder neck contracture. Bladder cancer (as well as renal cancer) should be a consideration in a male patient with unexplained hematuria. Urinary tract infection must be excluded if there are complaints of irritative voiding symptoms. If abnormalities are found on neurologic examination and problems with urinary retention are present, neurologic disease must be considered. Prostate cancer should be considered when an asymmetric enlargement, nodule, or induration is palpated on rectal examination.

MANAGEMENT

Nonpharmacologic Management

The traditional management goal for treatment of BPH has been relief of symptoms to improve quality of life. Treatment focuses on balancing the severity of the patient's symptoms with potential side effects of therapy. For men with BPH who have mild symptoms and no complications, behavioral modifications including limiting fluids before bedtime, limiting use of caffeine and alcohol, and double voiding can be helpful.

Pharmacologic Management

In addition to watchful waiting and lifestyle modifications, treatments include α_1-adrenergic antagonist therapy, 5α-reductase enzyme inhibitor therapy, antimuscarinics, β-3 agonists and phosphodiesterase type 5 inhibitors or combination drug therapy, phytotherapeutics, balloon dilation, and surgery.[9] The benefits and risks associated with each treatment should be explained. It is important to advise the patient that if he chooses watchful waiting, other treatment approaches can be considered at any time if symptoms increase.

α-adrenergic antagonists have long been the main treatment of BPH. They work by relaxing smooth muscle in the bladder neck, prostate capsule, and prostatic urethra. Doses can be titrated up while monitoring for side effects. Terazosin and doxazosin need to be initiated at bedtime to reduce dizziness and postural effects. If patients cannot tolerate this class of medications, 5α-reductase inhibitor therapy (e.g., dutasteride and finasteride) can be initiated as monotherapy. These drugs work by shrinking prostatic glandular hyperplasia by decreasing tissue DHT levels, but it may take up to 6 to 12 months to see improvement in symptoms based on reduced prostate size. Phosphodiesterase-5 (PDE5) inhibitors such as sildenafil or tadalafil can be used for men with mild to moderate BPH symptoms and erectile dysfunction. Antimuscarinics help relax the bladder muscle, which can reduce urinary frequency, urgency, nocturia, and incontinence. Combination therapy with alpha-adrenergic antagonists and 5α-reductase inhibitors can also be used for men with large prostates and severe symptoms.[6]

Use of herbal preparations such as *Serenoa repens* (saw palmetto), rye-grass pollen extract (Cernilton), and *Pygeum africanum* (African prune tree extract) may be increasing, but there is limited evidence regarding their safety and efficacy. Saw palmetto may contribute to increased risk of bleeding, and patients need to notify their providers so that it can be stopped before invasive procedures. Balloon dilation reduces symptoms in the short term, but long-term follow-up after the procedure has not been adequately studied. Transurethral resection of the prostate (TURP), transurethral incision of the prostate, and open prostatectomy are surgical procedures that are effective for severe BPH. TURP has long been considered the gold standard treatment of BOO, but it is limited to prostates weighing less than 100 g and is associated with significant complications and mortality.[10]

INDICATIONS FOR REFERRAL OR HOSPITALIZATION

If the initial evaluation demonstrates the presence of LUTS associated with results of a DRE suggesting prostate cancer, hematuria, abnormal PSA levels, recurrent infection, palpable bladder, history/risk of urethral stricture, and/or a neurologic disease raising the likelihood of a primary bladder disorder, the patient should be referred to a urologist for appropriate evaluation before advising or beginning any treatment.[6]

Filling cystometry, uroflowmetry, urethrocystoscopy, pressure-flow studies, and measurement of postvoid residuals may be helpful in individual situations, and their need can best be determined by a urologist. Surgery may be indicated for patients who do not tolerate medical management.

COMPLICATIONS

Urinary tract infection and urinary retention are common sequelae of BPH. In addition, urinary retention can result in renal problems if it is not detected early.

PATIENT AND FAMILY EDUCATION

- Education regarding the advantages and risks of each treatment option is necessary to enhance patient understanding of symptom relief.
- Importance of monitoring symptom progression and reporting any abrupt change in symptom pattern, indicating possible complications or another pathologic process, should be stressed.

PROSTATITIS

DEFINITION AND EPIDEMIOLOGY

The prostate gland is an organ located adjacent to and inferior to the bladder. The urethra passes through the prostate gland. Prostatitis, or inflammation of the prostate gland, is a common problem in the adult male population. Bacterial prostatitis (both acute and chronic) is caused by bacterial inflammation. Recently, the National Institutes of Health (NIH) changed the classification of prostatitis. According to this new classification systems, the criteria for acute and chronic bacterial prostatitis remain the same as previously. Both types of prostate inflammation are caused by bacterial infection, but chronic prostatitis is characterized by a slower development of inflammation and duration of symptoms for 3 months. There is a third group called chronic nonbacterial prostatitis/chronic pelvic pain syndrome (CNP/CPPS), which combines the previous categories of CNP and prostadynia prostatitis. The fourth and final category is asymptomatic prostatitis.[11]

Inflammatory CP/CPPS is characterized by chronic pelvic pain and possibly voiding symptoms, in the absence of bacterial infection, although leukocytes may be present in expressed prostatic secretions or semen. In asymptomatic inflammatory prostatitis, there is evidence of inflammation without symptoms of prostatitis or urinary tract infection.

It is estimated that nearly half of all men suffer from symptoms of prostatitis at some point in their lives. It is the third most common urinary tract disease in men, after BPH and prostate cancer.[11] The prevalence of acute prostatitis is estimated to be about 10% of all prostatitis diagnoses. The prevalence of CBP is much lower, accounting for only 5% to 10% of all prostatitis cases due to this condition. In contrast, the prevalence of nonbacterial prostatitis accounts for more than 90% of all cases of prostatitis.[11]

PATHOPHYSIOLOGY

The organisms responsible for acute prostatitis are usually gram-negative organisms—those responsible for most of the lower urologic tract infections. *Escherichia coli* or *Proteus* species and *Klebsiella, Enterobacter,* and *Serratia* are the most common causative bacteria. *Pseudomonas aeruginosa* is also implicated as an infective organism. Some gram-positive cocci are considered responsible for prostatitis, including *Staphylococcus aureus,* streptococci, and enterococci. *Neisseria gonorrhoeae* and *Chlamydia trachomatis* are important organisms to consider in relation to infections in men at higher risk for sexually transmitted infection.

Acute bacterial prostatitis results from the ascent of organized, colonized bacteria from the lower urethra to the prostate. The urethral bacteria may be a result of infection or normal fecal flora. Increases in intraurethral pressure as a result of intercourse can result in bacterial deposition into the prostate. Challenges associated with bacterial eradication increase the risk of chronic infection. The use of instruments during urologic procedures is another common cause of acute bacterial prostatitis.

The most common causative pathogens of chronic bacterial prostatitis include gram-negative and gram-positive bacteria. Animal studies have demonstrated that the formation of a biofilm in the acini of the prostate contribute to an environment that favors the growth of pathogens, which include *Chlamydia trachomatis, Enterococci* species, *Klebsiella pneumonia, Proteus mirabilis, Enterobacter cloacae, Staphylococcus aureus, Trichomonas vaginalis, Ureaplasma urealyticum, Mycoplasma hominis, Serratia marcescens,* and *Pseudomonas aeruginosa.*

The cause of nonbacterial prostatitis is less clear. Causative factors contributing to the development of nonbacterial prostatitis include prior bacterial infection with organisms such as *Ureaplasma urealyticum, Chlamydia, Gardnerella,* and *Mycoplasma;* irritation from urine flow problems, chemical irritants, lower urinary tract nerve disorders and pelvic muscle abnormalities; sexual abuse; and viruses.

The cause of asymptomatic inflammatory prostatitis (category IV) is also unknown although studies suggest that men with this type of prostatitis are more likely to have bacteria in their semen. Because men with this type of prostatitis are asymptomatic, they generally learn of their diagnosis when they undergo a prostate biopsy or are being tested for infertility.

CLINICAL PRESENTATION AND PHYSICAL EXAMINATION

Fever, chills, malaise, myalgias, and arthralgias are common with acute bacterial prostatitis. Genitourinary symptoms include hesitancy, frequency, urgency, nocturia, dysuria, and a sensation of incomplete bladder emptying. Accompanying complaints may be low back pain, perineal pain, or suprapubic pain. PSA levels are often markedly elevated and should not be checked in the acute stages of prostatitis because they are not reliable indicators of either infection or cure.

The presentation of chronic prostatitis tends to be more varied than that of acute prostatitis and may include a history of recurrent urinary tract infection (usually with the same organism) and complaints of urinary frequency, urgency, and burning on urination. Perineal, inguinal, or suprapubic pain may be present.

Inflammatory prostatitis (CP/CPPS), or category III prostatitis, is characterized by prostatic pain or vague discomfort of the suprapubic, scrotal, inguinal, lower back, or perineal areas. Pain on ejaculation may also occur. Urinary symptoms, such as hesitancy, a decrease in the urinary stream, frequency, urgency, and burning on urination, may also be present.

Symptoms suggestive of nonbacterial prostatitis include pain and discomfort in the pelvic area and problems related to urinary flow, such as hesitancy, interrupted flow, postvoid dribbling, and decreased flow. Frequency, urgency, and nocturia may be present. Penile and urethral pain as well as discomfort in the lower back, suprapubic area, testicles, groin, and perineum are often reported. The patient usually has no history of urinary tract infection but may have a lifetime history of voiding difficulty.

Abdominal and rectal examinations are important components of the physical examination for symptoms related to the prostate. The abdominal examination should exclude bladder distention, and the prostate gland should be examined for size, consistency, and tenderness. Normally, the prostate is heart shaped and measures approximately $4 \times 3 \times 2$ cm ($1\frac{3}{5} \times 1\frac{1}{5} \times \frac{4}{5}$ inches). In acute bacterial prostatitis, the prostate is typically enlarged, with tenderness and induration. The prostate examination should be performed gently without excessive manipulation to avoid inducing bacteremia. Urinary retention and fever may be present.

The prostate examination in chronic bacterial prostatitis may be nonspecific or may reveal a tender or boggy prostate. In nonbacterial prostatitis, the prostate examination findings are usually normal, but a soft, boggy prostate with tenderness may occasionally be present. Physical examination in nonbacterial prostatitis is unremarkable with the exception that increased anal sphincter tone and paraprostatic tenderness may be present.

DIAGNOSTICS
Essential Diagnostics

The history and physical examination are often adequate for diagnosis of prostatitis. Physical examination should include the external genitalia, abdomen, perineum, and prostate. It is not recommended to perform a prostate massage during the DRE.

Urine analysis and culture are important in the evaluation of acute bacterial prostatitis. In acute bacterial prostatitis, the urinalysis results may reveal pyuria, bacteriuria, and varying degrees of hematuria; urine culture is necessary for organism identification. A complete blood count (CBC) is significant for increased numbers of leukocytes with a left shift. In chronic bacterial prostatitis, the urinalysis is usually normal unless there is coexistent cystitis.

Urine cultures are negative with nonbacterial prostatitis, but increased numbers of leukocytes are often seen in the specimen.

Additional Diagnostics

Postvoid residual can be helpful if the bladder is palpable or there are symptoms of incomplete emptying. Computed tomography (CT) scan or transrectal prostatic ultrasonography (TRUS) may be useful in cases of acute bacterial prostatitis if there is concern for prostate abscess.

DIFFERENTIAL DIAGNOSIS

 Immediate referral indicated for signs and symptoms suggestive of septicemia and urosepsis which can be life-threatening.

The diagnosis of acute prostatitis is usually made on the basis of the clinical presentation and the markedly tender prostate on physical examination. It can be distinguished from a urinary tract infection, acute pyelonephritis, acute epididymitis, and acute diverticulosis by a careful history, physical examination, and urinalysis. Prostatic enlargement from BPH or prostate cancer–causing urinary retention can usually be distinguished from acute bacterial prostatitis on rectal examination.

Chronic bacterial prostatitis can be differentiated from chronic urethritis and cystitis with segmented urine cultures. Common causes of urinary outflow problems, such as BPH, urethral stricture, and prostate cancer, should be considered in the differential diagnosis. Bladder carcinoma, sphincter dyssynergia, and neurogenic bladder also can cause lower urinary tract irritative symptoms. Chronic pelvic pain may be related to obstructive stones in the prostatic ducts. Rectal examination should help exclude anal disease, such as tumors, which may manifest similarly to chronic prostatitis.

The primary condition to be considered in the differential diagnosis of nonbacterial prostatitis is chronic bacterial prostatitis. The absence of positive cultures and a negative history of urinary tract infection support the diagnosis of nonbacterial prostatitis. A urinary cytologic examination and cystoscopy are indicated to exclude bladder cancer in the older man with irritative voiding symptoms and negative cultures. Interstitial cystitis and carcinoma *in situ* of the bladder may be seen with similar symptoms in the younger man.

MANAGEMENT
Pharmacologic Management

Many patients with acute prostatitis are severely ill and require broad-spectrum antibiotic therapy. Initial empirical therapy should be based on the presumed infecting organism and severity of illness. Depending on the severity of the illness, hospitalization and intravenous antibiotic therapy may be indicated. Patients who are febrile should be considered for hospitalization. Intravenous fluoroquinolones such as levofloxacin or ciprofloxacin may be selected for treatment. Intravenous therapy is changed to oral therapy when the patient is afebrile for 24 to 48 hours and able to tolerate oral intake.

Those who are less acutely ill may be treated on an outpatient basis with oral antibiotics. Trimethoprim-sulfamethoxazole (TMP/SMX) and fluoroquinolones are effective and usually considered first-line treatment choices.[11] TMP/SMX should not be used as first-line empirical therapy in areas where TMP/SMX resistance for *E. coli*, the most frequent pathogen, is greater than 10% to 20%. A 2- to 4-week course of treatment is recommended.[11] Penicillins and cephalosporins do not penetrate the prostatic epithelium and are not considered desirable options

for treatment. In general, acute bacterial prostatitis requires antibiotic therapy for a minimum of 3 weeks to prevent the development of chronic bacterial prostatitis. Local measures may be helpful in reducing discomfort. Sitz baths, three times per day, may reduce perineal pain. Analgesics, antipyretics, stool softeners, and bed rest may also be beneficial.

The treatment of chronic bacterial prostatitis is more complex because of the difficulty in attaining therapeutic intraprostatic antibiotic levels in a noninflamed prostate. The antibiotics that have demonstrated the highest effectiveness for penetration into prostatic tissue include fluoroquinolones, sulfonamides, tetracyclines, and macrolides. Fluoroquinolones have emerged as the agents of choice with overall response rates of 70% to 90% at the end of therapy, but a decline in response to 60% after 6 months.[11] In cases of resistance to fluoroquinolones, TMP/SMX can be used, but duration of treatment should be 7 to 12 weeks.[11] In addition to these therapeutic regimens, other antibiotics shown to be helpful include piperacillin, cephalosporins, aztreonam, erythromycin, imipenem, and some aminoglycosides. The combination of antibiotic therapy and alpha-blockers have been shown to provide symptom relief and reduce high recurrence rates

It may be difficult to cure chronic bacterial prostatitis. If a relapse occurs, a longer course of antibiotic therapy is necessary. If a cure is not achieved, a low dose of antibiotics may be prescribed to prevent symptomatic infection.

Supportive measures, such as warm water baths, may be helpful in the treatment of chronic bacterial prostatitis. Beverages that produce rapid bladder expansion, such as coffee, tea, and alcohol, should be avoided. The use of medications that impair bladder function (e.g., anticholinergics, sedatives, antidepressants) should be assessed.

The treatment of nonbacterial prostatitis is controversial because of the inability to isolate a causative organism. Research indicates that approximately 50% of patients with CP/CPPS (category III) prostatitis can be improved with fluoroquinolone therapy. In addition, alpha adrenergic blockers together with antibiotics have demonstrated better outcomes than antimicrobial therapy alone. Nonsteroidal antiinflammatory drugs (NSAIDs) reduce the synthesis of prostaglandin, which can reduce prostatic inflammation, and may be particularly helpful for the relief of pain. Recently some herbal-based therapies, including *Serenoa repens* and Cernilton have been shown to be beneficial compared with placebos but more research is necessary before recommendations can be made regarding their use. Supportive measures as described previously may be helpful, including warm tub baths. Normal sexual activity is not contraindicated. If patients complain of irritative voiding problems, a trial of anticholinergic medications, such as oxybutynin chloride, may be effective. If spicy foods, alcohol, and caffeine aggravate symptoms, they should be avoided.

INDICATIONS FOR REFERRAL
OR HOSPITALIZATION

Because of the severity of the illness associated with acute bacterial prostatitis and the potential chronicity of bacterial and nonbacterial prostatitis, co-management with a urologist is often indicated. Urologic referral is indicated for severe cases of acute bacterial prostatitis, when comorbidity increases the risk of sequelae, or when signs of urinary retention are present. Refractory chronic prostatitis in the presence of prostatic stones also requires urologic referral. If symptoms do not resolve after the treatment of nonbacterial prostatitis or prostatodynia, a urologic referral is necessary to exclude cystitis or bladder cancer and to confirm the original diagnosis.

Hospitalization is indicated for acute illness. If prostate enlargement results in urinary retention, urinary catheterization is contraindicated, and a percutaneous suprapubic tube is necessary until the prostatic enlargement subsides.

LIFE SPAN CONSIDERATIONS

In the older man, the possibility of coexistent BPH or prostate cancer, which can potentiate the signs and symptoms of prostatitis, should be considered.

COMPLICATIONS

A prostatic abscess rarely occurs as a complication of acute bacterial prostatitis except in immunocompromised patients. The symptoms are similar to those of acute bacterial prostatitis, but on rectal examination there is a fluctuance of the affected lobe. Diagnosis can be confirmed with TRUS. The treatment usually includes surgical drainage and antibiotics. Other complications of acute bacterial prostatitis may include pyelonephritis, epididymitis, seminal vesiculitis, and bacteremia. Chronic prostatitis/chronic pain syndrome may occur and includes LUTS, sexual dysfunction, and reduced quality of life. The syndrome is diagnosed on the basis of symptoms, particularly pain or discomfort in the pelvic region.

PATIENT AND FAMILY EDUCATION

Education should include the following information:
- Cause of the patient's symptoms and the treatment
- Rationale for the possibility of a long duration of treatment and the need to maintain adequate therapeutic levels
- Importance of follow-up care
- Use of condoms to prevent the reintroduction of bacteria into the urethra.
- Avoidance of anal intercourse with acute bacterial prostatitis.

REFERENCES

1. Egan, K. B. (2016). The epidemiology of benign prostatic hyperplasia associated with lower urinary tract symptoms. *The Urologic Clinics of North America*, 43(3), 289–297.
2. Fode, M., Sønksen, J., McPhee, S. J., & Ohl, D. A. (2013). Disorders of the male reproductive tract. In G. D. Hammer & S. J. McPhee (Eds.), *Pathophysiology of disease: An introduction to clinical medicine* (7th ed.). New York: McGraw-Hill.
3. Abrams, P., Chapple, C., Khoury, S., et al. (2009). Evaluation and treatment of lower urinary tract symptoms in older men. *The Journal of Urology*, 181(14), 1779–1787.
4. Holtgrewe, H. L., Mebust, W. K., Dowd, J. B., et al. (2002). The American Urological Association symptom index for benign prostatic hyperplasia (abstract 1042). *The Journal of Urology*, 167(2), 265.
5. American Urological Association Guideline: Management of benign prostatic hyperplasia. www.auanet.org/education/guidelines/benign-prostatic-hyperplasia.cfm. (Accessed 11 June 2015).
6. McVary, K. T., Roehrborn, C. G., Avins, A. L., et al. (2010). Management of Benign prostatic hyperplasia (Guidelines). American Urological Association. https://www.auanet.org/benign-prostatic-hyperplasia-(2010-reviewed-and-validity-confirmed-2014)#x2466. (Accessed 10 November 2018).
7. Schenk, J. M., Kristal, A. R., Arnold, K. B., et al. (2011). Association of symptomatic benign prostatic hyperplasia and prostate cancer: Results from the Prostate Cancer Prevention Trial. *American Journal of Epidemiology*, 173(12), 1419–1428.
8. Scher, H. I. (2008). Benign and malignant disease of the prostate. In A. S. Fauci, et al. (Eds.), *Harrison's principles of internal medicine* (18th ed.). New York: McGraw-Hill.
9. Presicce, F., De Nunzio, C., & Tubaro, A. (2017). Re: Is early benign prostatic hyperplasia (BPH) treatment worthwhile? *Urologia*, 84, 142–147.
10. Zhao, Z., Zeng, G., Zhong, W., et al. (2010). A prospective, randomised trial comparing plasmakinetic enucleation to standard transurethral resection of the prostate for symptomatic benign prostatic hyperplasia: Three year follow-up results. *European Urology*, 58, 752–758.
11. Khan, F. U., Ihsan, A. U., Khan, H. U., et al. (2017). Comprehensive overview of prostatitis. *Biomedicine & Pharmacotherapy = Biomédecine & Pharmacothérapie*, 94, 1064–1076.

CHAPTER 130

PROTEINURIA AND HEMATURIA
Yvette T. Wilson

 Specialist referral is indicated for signs and symptoms suggestive of nephrotic syndrome, acute renal failure, and renal failure of unknown origin. New-onset proteinuria in pregnant women requires urgent referral to exclude eclampsia.

 Proteinuria and hematuria can be signs of serious disease or neoplasm and thus require a systematic and thorough evaluation.

DEFINITION AND EPIDEMIOLOGY

Proteinuria and hematuria are not unusual findings on routine urinalysis. However, research demonstrates that there is a positive linear association between the magnitude of proteinuria and an increase in the risk of cardiovascular disease and end-stage renal disease (ESRD).[1] Current research also demonstrates that acute kidney injury (AKI) and chronic kidney disease (CKD) have a direct correlation with increased health care costs and a reduced quality of life resulting in depression and mortality.[2] Hematuria is concerning because it is the most common sign of bladder cancer. The decision to evaluate and diagnose the underpinnings of hematuria has been studied by a variety of governing bodies for medical research including the American Urological Association (AUA), which advocates the importance of implementing diagnostic protocols to maximize the detection of occult malignancies. Delays in the treatment of genitourinary (GU) cancer can result in a decreased quality of life, increased anxiety, and overall poor outcomes.[3]

Approximately 15 kg of protein is filtered through the adult kidney each day, with normally less than 150 mg excreted.[4] Proteinuria, generally defined as urinary protein excretion of more than 150 mg/day (10 to 20 mg/dL), is the hallmark of renal disease. Microalbuminuria is defined as the excretion of 30 to 150 mg of protein per day and is a sign of early renal disease, particularly in patients with diabetes.[5] Macroalbuminuria is occasionally used to describe rates of more than 300 mg/day.

Proteinuria can be classified as transient or persistent. Transient proteinuria is caused by a temporary change in glomerular hemodynamics, which causes the excess of protein. These conditions are usually of a benign or self-limited nature and include orthostatic (postural) proteinuria, dehydration, fever, exercise, and emotional stress. Congestive heart failure and seizures can also cause transient proteinuria.[6] Persistent proteinuria is defined as 1+ protein on a standard dipstick (which corresponds to approximately 30 mg/dL) two or more times during a 3-month period.[6] Persistent proteinuria indicates a pathologic process, and the etiology must be investigated. Some common causes of persistent proteinuria are listed in Box 130.1.

Common Causes of Proteinuria

DRUG INDUCED
- Lithium
- Cyclosporine
- Cisplatin
- Nonsteroidal antiinflammatory drugs

HEREDITARY
- Medullary or polycystic kidney disease

IMMUNE
- Drug allergies
- Collagen vascular disorders (lupus, vasculitis)
- Immunoglobulin A nephropathy (Berger disease)
- Sarcoidosis

INFECTIOUS
- Bacterial, fungal, or parasitic infection
- Tuberculosis

METABOLIC
- Hyperuricemia
- Hypercalcemia
- Amyloidosis

VASCULAR
- Diabetes mellitus
- Hypertension
- Sickle cell disease
- Radiation nephritis

INCREASED PRODUCTION
- Multiple causes

Although isolated proteinuria is not necessarily associated with excess morbidity and mortality, it can be a sign of serious systemic disease. Evidence suggests that changes in low levels of proteinuria are predictive of the annual decline in glomerular filtration rate and the development of ESRD in persons with nondiabetic kidney disease.[1] Even a slight increase in proteinuria has been shown to be an independent risk factor for ESRD. Therefore asymptomatic proteinuria warrants further evaluation.

In the United States, diabetes is the leading cause of ESRD, and in both type 1 and type 2 diabetes, microalbuminuria is the first sign of deteriorating renal function. As kidney function declines, microalbuminuria becomes full-fledged proteinuria. Hypertension is the second leading cause of ESRD and a significant cause of mortality worldwide.

Urinary albumin excretion has been shown to predict blood pressure progression in nondiabetic, nonhypertensive individuals and appears to precede progression to higher blood pressure stages.[7] Therefore proteinuria may be a useful biomarker for identification of individuals at risk for development of hypertension. In addition, persistent proteinuria in excess of 1 g/day has been associated with increased cardiac morbidity and mortality, especially heart failure.[8]

Certain population groups, including African Americans, Native Americans, Hispanic Americans, and Pacific Islanders, are at increased risk for development of proteinuria. Aging and obesity are also risk factors.[9] Although recent studies demonstrate an improvement in CKD prevalence, it is not consistent across all populations. There is a continued rise in prevalence among non-Hispanic black persons (most notable in persons older than 65 years), despite the decline across all other ethnic groups. The racial disparities are closely linked to awareness, evaluation, and treatment.[10]

PATHOPHYSIOLOGY OF PROTEINURIA

Proteinuria has varied causes, and protein excretion is affected by three factors: (1) prevention of excretion by the glomerular capillary wall, (2) reabsorption and catabolism by the proximal tubule cells, and (3) production of low-molecular-weight proteins.[5] Therefore proteinuria is most often classified as glomerular, tubular, overflow in origin. Inflammation can also cause proteinuria, is classified as postrenal proteinuria, and can be present in patients with a urinary tract infection (UTI) or other renal conditions associated with inflammation. Glomerular proteinuria is the most common type of persistent proteinuria, and albumin is the primary urinary protein.[5] Tubular proteinuria results when malfunctioning tubule cells no longer metabolize or reabsorb the protein that has been normally filtered. In this condition, low-molecular-weight proteins are the predominant type of protein, and the amount rarely exceeds 2 g/day. Overflow proteinuria occurs when low-molecular-weight proteins overwhelm the ability of the tubules to reabsorb filtered proteins.[4]

CLINICAL PRESENTATION AND PHYSICAL EXAMINATION

The clinical presentation of the patient with proteinuria can vary from healthy young adults with functional proteinuria related to prolonged exercise to seriously ill diabetic patients with nephrotic syndrome. All individuals should therefore be screened for proteinuria by routine dipstick testing. Especially important is the routine screening of pregnant women. Proteinuria before 24 weeks' gestation indicates likely glomerulonephritis, whereas proteinuria after 24 weeks' gestation is usually a sign of preeclampsia.[11]

Persistent proteinuria in patients with diabetes is usually a result of diabetic nephropathy. However, uncontrolled diabetes mellitus may cause transient proteinuria, most likely as a result of hyperfiltration and decreased tubular reabsorption.[12]

When proteinuria is identified, a complete and thorough history is essential. Specific areas of focus should include recent acute or chronic illness, surgery, diagnostic procedures (especially those requiring contrast media), urinary frequency or symptoms suggesting infection, risk factors for human immunodeficiency virus (HIV) infection, medications taken (including over-the-counter and herbal medications), family history of renal disease or diabetes, and recent physical activity (especially exercise or cold weather activities).

The physical examination should be comprehensive and thorough; in the case of coexistent diabetes, the severity of the diabetes should be assessed to determine whether it correlates with the severity of proteinuria. Diabetic retinopathy is often present in patients with diabetic renal disease.[13]

Essential Diagnostics

Proteinuria is usually detected on routine dipstick testing, and any value of 1+ or greater on two or more occasions should be investigated. Limitations of dipstick testing include false-negative results caused by dilution, inability to detect microalbuminuria (although ultrasensitive dipstick tests are now available that can measure low rates of microalbuminuria), false-positive results caused by certain medications, and inability of dipstick reagents to detect light-chain proteins.[6]

Once proteinuria has been identified, unless the cause is readily apparent (e.g., preeclampsia or diabetes), a 24-hour urine measurement for protein and creatinine (or spot urinary protein/creatinine ratio) is recommended, along with microscopic examination of urinary sediment, urinary protein electrophoresis, and additional assessment of renal function.[6]

A urine protein amount greater than 150 mg in 24 hours is significant, but glomerular kidney disease is usually associated with greater than a gram of proteinuria in 24 hours. Urine should be tested for Bence Jones proteins with urine protein electrophoresis (UPEP) or urine protein immunoelectrophoresis (IEP), the presence of which suggests multiple myeloma. In addition, a full blood chemistry panel with fasting blood glucose concentration, hemoglobin A_{1c} (HbA_{1c}), lipid profile, urine culture and sensitivity, and complete blood count (CBC) with differential are indicated.

Other diagnostic tests depend on presentation and differential diagnosis. Collagen disease, glomerulonephritis, hepatitis-induced vasculitis, urate-related renal disease, diabetes, and other systemic disease or structural abnormalities should be considered in the evaluation of proteinuria.

DIFFERENTIAL DIAGNOSIS

It is important to determine whether the proteinuria is persistent or transient. Transient proteinuria in an otherwise healthy patient that is secondary to an identifiable cause (e.g., exercise, fever, congestive heart failure) may be classified as functional proteinuria and does not require further diagnostic testing or evaluation.

Persistent proteinuria that cannot be classified as functional proteinuria does require further investigation. Investigation should begin with a 24-hour measurement of urine protein and creatinine clearance to determine the urinary protein excretion and the protein/creatinine ratio.[14] Although this has been the gold standard, it can be complicated for patients, and errors are common; thus, a spot urine test for a urinary protein/creatinine ratio is recommended. If the excretion rate is 3.5 g/day or more, the patient by definition has nephrotic syndrome,[14] which is usually accompanied by hypoalbuminemia, hyperlipidemia, and edema. Nephrotic syndrome mandates a nephrologist's evaluation. Diabetes is the leading cause of nephrotic syndrome and accounts for 75% of all cases.[14]

Renal function is classified as normal or abnormal if the 24-hour urinary protein excretion rate is less than 3.5 g/day. Proteinuria in the presence of normal renal function is defined as "isolated" proteinuria; in these patients, the next step is to

---

DIAGNOSTIC

INITIAL DIAGNOSTICS
- 24-hour urine measurement for protein and creatinine *or spot urinary protein creatinine ratio*
- Urine culture and sensitivity
- Laboratory evaluation of urinary sediment
- Complete blood count and differential
- Fasting blood sugar and HgbA1c
- Complete chemistry profile (kidney and liver function)
- Lipid profile

ADDITIONAL DIAGNOSTICS
- See Fig. 130.1.

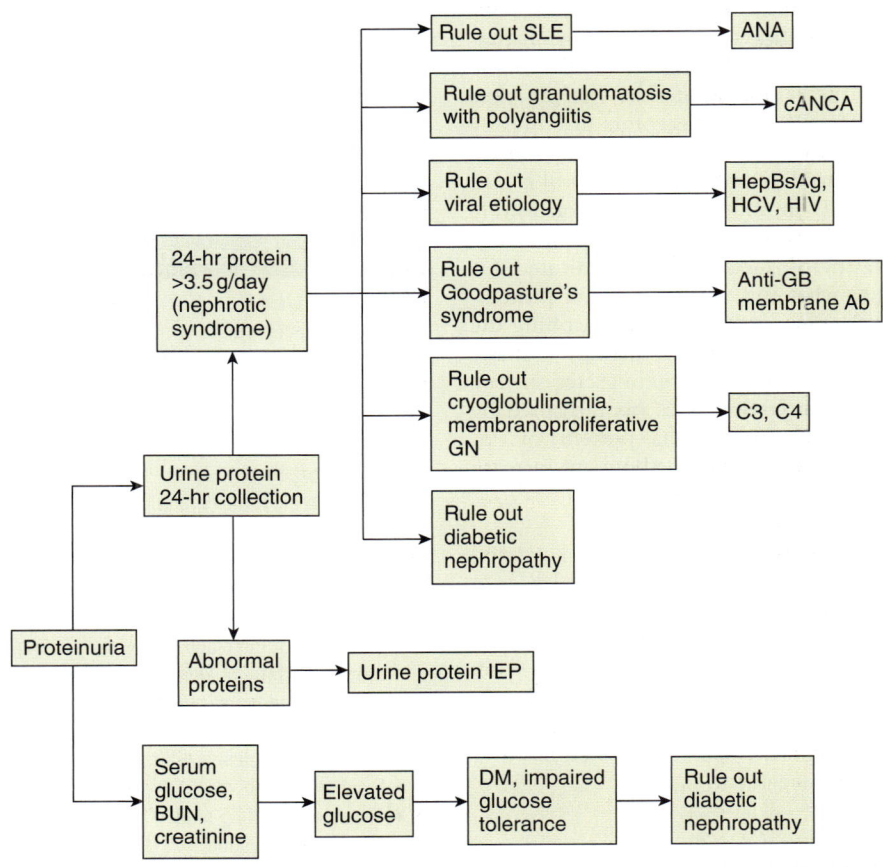

FIG. 130.1 Proteinuria. *BUN,* Blood urea nitrogen; *HIV,* Human immunodeficiency virus. (From Ferri, F. F. [2019]. *Ferri's best test: A practical guide to laboratory medicine and diagnostic imaging* [4th ed.]. Philadelphia: Elsevier.)

determine whether the proteinuria is orthostatic or nonorthostatic.[14] Urinary protein excretion can increase after prolonged standing, and therefore three early-morning voids should be checked for protein. If all the results are negative, a diagnosis of orthostatic proteinuria can be made, and no further diagnostic tests are necessary.[14] However, referral to a renal specialist is also appropriate because this is a poorly understood, although generally benign and self-limited, condition.

An alternative to 24-hour urine testing for total protein is the measurement of the urine protein/creatinine ratio using a single urine specimen and a single blood draw. The ratio is the same as the amount of grams excreted daily, so a ratio of 3.5 is equal to 3.5 g of protein per day excreted.

Patients with nonorthostatic proteinuria and normal renal function and without an elevation in Bence Jones proteins should be referred to a renal specialist. A renal biopsy may be needed to determine the cause of the proteinuria. The presence of Bence Jones proteins warrants serum protein electrophoresis and a referral for further evaluation to exclude multiple myeloma.

INTERPROFESSIONAL COLLABORATIVE MANAGEMENT

Management of proteinuria depends on the underlying cause, but some general principles apply. A careful medication review should be performed, and any medications implicated in proteinuria should be discontinued. Both angiotensin-converting enzyme (ACE) inhibitors and angiotensin receptor blockers (ARBs) inhibit the renin-angiotensin system and reduce proteinuria by decreasing the systemic arterial pressure and the intraglomerular filtration pressure.[11] ACE inhibitors incompletely block the formation of angiotensin II, which is the main effector peptide of the renin-angiotensin system. ARBs do not block all angiotensin II type 1 receptors at clinically recommended doses. Diabetes and hyperlipidemia, if present, should be aggressively managed; blood pressure control is also important. Patients with CKD should be managed aggressively to help prevent or delay the onset of ESRD (see Chapter 131). Sodium- and protein-restricted diets may be indicated for some patients. No matter what the cause, persistent proteinuria should be aggressively managed, both by controlling the underlying disease and by directing specific therapy (usually ACE inhibitors or ARBs) at reduction of protein excretion. The goal for treatment is protein excretion rates (as measured by collection of a 24-hour urine sample for total protein) of 1 g/day or less; rates higher than this have been shown to increase cardiovascular disease.

INDICATIONS FOR REFERRAL OR HOSPITALIZATION

- All patients with renal disease or abnormal renal function should be referred to a renal specialist for consultation and management guidance.
- Referrals for patients with isolated orthostatic proteinuria should be based on a thorough risk assessment and evaluation of their general health, life span considerations, and concerns for aggressive management.

COMPLICATIONS

Nephrotic syndrome with associated edema, hypoalbuminemia, and extrarenal complications is a potential consequence of proteinuria. Cardiovascular morbidity and mortality,

immobilization, hyperlipidemia, hypercoagulability, and electrolyte disturbances are additional complications.

PATIENT AND FAMILY EDUCATION AND HEALTH PROMOTION

Patient education depends on the cause of proteinuria, but diet education, diabetic teaching for patients with diabetes, and education concerning blood pressure management are usually necessary. Especially critical is that the patient and family understand the importance of diagnostic testing and regular follow-up care.

HEMATURIA

 Specialist referral and/or hospitalization is indicated for patients with large amounts of frank hematuria, severe flank pain suggestive of renal calculi, unstable vital signs, signs of urologic obstruction, or acute renal failure.

DEFINITION AND EPIDEMIOLOGY

Hematuria is generally defined as three or more red blood cells (RBCs) per high-power field.[15] Transient hematuria is defined as hematuria that occurs on one occasion, whereas persistent hematuria is defined as hematuria that occurs on two or more consecutive occasions.[6,15] Exercise-induced hematuria in healthy young adults is not associated with any known morbidity or mortality, but both transient and persistent hematuria can be signs of serious disease. Common causes of hematuria are listed in Box 130.2.

The rates for asymptomatic microscopic hematuria (AMH) in the general population range from 2.4% to 31% and vary with gender and age.[15] In older men, who are at higher risk for urologic disease, the prevalence of AMH is high. Ten percent

---

BOX 130.2

Common Causes of Hematuria

GLOMERULAR
- Glomerulonephritis
- Lupus nephritis
- Interstitial nephritis
- Pyelonephritis
- Vasculitis
- Alport syndrome
- Thin basement membrane disease

NONGLOMERULAR
- Infection
- Neoplasm of the bladder, ureter, prostate, or kidney
- Renal or bladder calculi
- Polycystic kidney disease
- Sickle cell (disease or trait)
- Trauma
- Increased bleeding time
- Hemorrhagic cystitis
- Schistosomiasis
- Nutcracker phenomenon

MISCELLANEOUS
- Drug induced
  - Warfarin, heparin
- Exercise induced
- Endometriosis

PSEUDOHEMATURIA
- Menstrual contamination
- Hemoglobinuria
- Myoglobinuria
- Porphyrins
- Red food dyes, red foods (e.g., beets)
- Drugs
  - Dilantin
  - Quinine
  - Phenothiazines
  - Rifampin
  - Pyridium
  - Sulfonamides
  - Cascara, Ex-Lax

of men older than 50 years have AMH on presentation. Gross hematuria in older men denotes a significant risk of malignant disease.[16] The likelihood of developing the disease is three to four times higher for men than for women.[17]

PATHOPHYSIOLOGY

Normal urinary excretion of RBCs is 2 million/day, which results in two or three RBCs per high-power field.[6] Isolated hematuria (hematuria unaccompanied by any other abnormal urine components) can result from bleeding anywhere from the renal pelvis to the urethra but is rarely caused by systemic disease. Hematuria related to renal disease enters the tubular field along the nephron and produces RBC casts that are indicative of the renal origin.[5,6] Bacterial infections are a common cause of hematuria, and the presence of bacteria on urinalysis is suggestive of an infectious cause. Acute cystitis or urethritis can cause gross hematuria and is more common in women than in men. The presence of proteinuria and hematuria is suggestive of glomerular or interstitial nephritis.[5]

CLINICAL PRESENTATION AND PHYSICAL EXAMINATION

Hematuria is often accompanied by clinically significant symptoms or by abnormalities in the urinalysis that can aid in identifying the source of bleeding. The patient's age, gender, and level of physical activity should always be considered (long-distance runners have been documented to have rates of hematuria as high as 13%).[18] Hematuria associated with pyuria suggests an infectious process, whereas colicky flank pain suggests pain originating from a ureter. A prostatic or urethral source is likely when bleeding occurs only at the beginning or end of micturition. The presence of hemoptysis, acute renal failure, and hematuria is highly suggestive of Goodpasture syndrome. Postinfection glomerulonephritis is signified by

hematuria and proteinuria accompanied by edema, hypertension, and a history of sore throat or skin infection, although patients often may not report any recent signs or symptoms of infection. This form of glomerulonephritis results in transient reduction of renal function in most cases.[19]

A thorough patient history should be obtained, including urinary patterns, urine color, timing of hematuria (beginning, end, or throughout micturition; transient or persistent), flank pain, history of renal calculi, UTIs, hemoptysis or bloody nasal secretions, recent acute or chronic illness, medications (including over-the-counter and illicit drugs), history of sexually transmitted disease, risk behaviors for HIV infection, and history of travel to areas with endemic schistosomiasis, a common cause of hematuria in Asia and Africa. A complete family history specifically related to renal disease, sickle cell disease or traits, and congenital deafness (indicating Alport syndrome) is also necessary.

A comprehensive physical examination, including a pelvic examination in women and a prostate examination in men, is warranted. In women, urethral and vaginal examinations are indicated to determine if there are any local causes of microscopic hematuria.[15] In uncircumcised men, the foreskin should be retracted to expose the glans penis. In both men and women, a catheterized urinary specimen is indicated if a clean-catch specimen cannot be reliably obtained.

Essential Diagnostics

Laboratory analysis of hematuria begins with a comprehensive examination of the urine and urinary sediment. Further indicated testing is systematic and based on patient symptoms (pain or painless hematuria) on presentation (Fig. 130.2).[15] A urinalysis with RBC casts indicates hematuria originating from the renal parenchyma.[4] Further evidence of a renal source is significant proteinuria (>1 g/24 hours), dysmorphic RBCs,

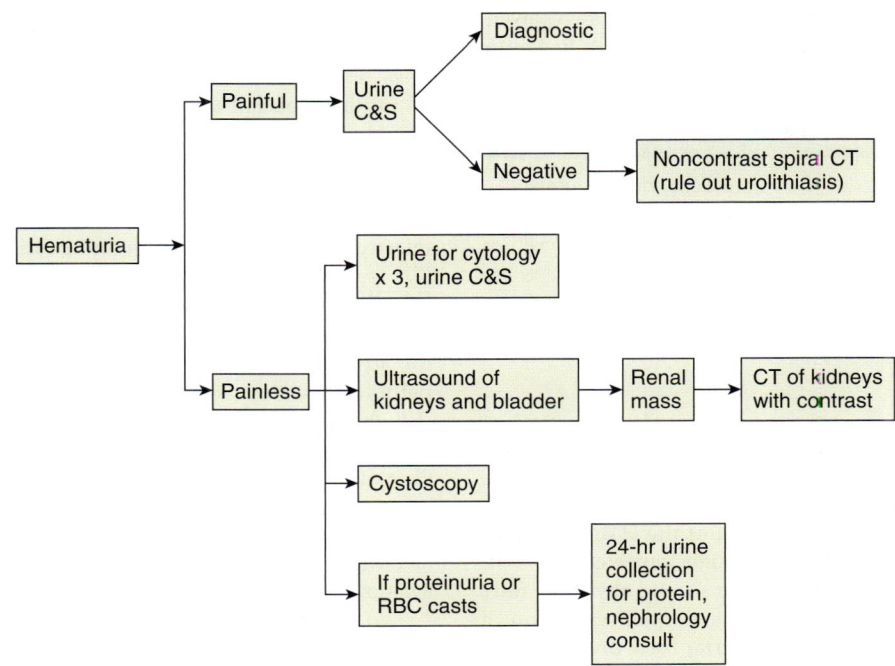

FIG. 130.2   Hematuria. *CT,* Computed tomography; *RBC,* red blood cell. (From Ferri, F. F. [2019]. *Ferri's best test: A practical guide to laboratory medicine and diagnostic imaging* [4th ed.]. Philadelphia: Elsevier.)

cola-colored urine, or renal insufficiency.[5,6] One major limitation of dipstick testing is that it detects the peroxidase activity of erythrocytes, not RBCs, in the urine. However, myoglobin and hemoglobin will also catalyze this reaction, so a positive test result may indicate hematuria, myoglobinuria, or hemoglobinuria. If the dipstick is positive for heme but no increased numbers of RBCs are seen on microscopic examination, the urine should be tested for myoglobinuria and hemoglobinuria.

Hematuria can be divided into glomerular, renal (i.e., nonglomerular), and urologic causes. Glomerular hematuria is typically associated with significant proteinuria, erythrocyte casts, and dysmorphic RBCs. However, 20% of patients with biopsy-proven glomerulonephritis are seen with hematuria alone. Berger disease (immunoglobulin A nephropathy), Alport syndrome, and thin basement membrane disease are three common causes of glomerular hematuria.[20] Nonglomerular or renal hematuria is caused by tubulointerstitial, renovascular, or metabolic disorders. As with glomerular hematuria, there is often coexisting proteinuria but no dysmorphic RBCs or erythrocyte casts. The evaluation of glomerular and nonglomerular hematuria requires an assessment of renal function and 24-hour urine or spot urinary protein/creatinine ratio. Urologic causes of nonglomerular hematuria include tumors, calculi, and infections. It is distinguished from other types of hematuria by the absence of proteinuria, dysmorphic RBCs, and erythrocyte casts. Up to 23% of patients with gross hematuria have a urinary tract malignant neoplasm, so a full workup, including cystoscopy and imaging of the upper urinary tract, needs to be done.[21]

When hematuria originates from the lower urinary tract, intact and uniform RBCs should be present.[21] The presence of intact RBCs, white blood cells, and bacteria suggests hematuria resulting from a UTI. The decision to obtain a urine culture and sensitivity should be guided by the patient's age and gender and the presence of resistant organisms in the local population. After treatment has been completed, repeated urinalysis is necessary to ensure that the hematuria has resolved. Failure to follow hematuria to resolution may result in failure to diagnose a serious condition.

INITIAL DIAGNOSTICS

HEMATURIA
- Urinalysis
- Urine culture and sensitivity[a]
- Urine for cytology[a]
- CBD and differential[a]
- Blood urea nitrogen, creatinine
- PT/PTT[a]

- Ultrasound, kidneys, ureters, bladder[a]
- Computed tomography scan abdomen/pelvis[a]
- Cystoscopy[a]
- IVP
- Renal biopsy[a]

[a]If indicated.

DIFFERENTIAL DIAGNOSIS

If the hematuria resolves after treatment of the UTI, no further diagnostic testing is indicated, although repeated UTIs in low-risk populations such as young men should always be fully investigated. If hematuria fails to resolve despite resolution of the UTI, or if it is of renal origin, a referral for a urologic evaluation is required.

In the absence of RBC casts or bacteria and white blood cells, a urologic evaluation should be performed. There are limited

data on the impact of intravenous urography (IVU), ultrasonography, computed tomography (CT), or magnetic resonance imaging (MRI) on the management of patients with microscopic hematuria. Although IVU has been the long-standing initial imaging study, CT scanning is now recommended.[15] The advantage of CT over IVU is that CT has the highest efficacy rate for the range of possible underlying pathologic processes, especially of the upper tract. If the CT scan shows a solid mass or is nondiagnostic, referral to a urologic surgeon for excision and pathologic testing is advised. The presence of renal or bladder calculi generally requires GU referral for definitive treatment. If the CT scan is nondiagnostic, the next step in the evaluation is cystoscopy, which includes inspection, biopsy, and culture of the bladder tissue. Cystoscopy is highly diagnostic for uroepithelial neoplasms. If the cystoscopy is nondiagnostic, the urologist may request a renal biopsy (see Fig. 130.2). The AUA recommends utilizing the CT for evaluating AMH because of the accuracy of detecting smaller tumors. However, there is strong support for the recommendation of utilizing the combination of renal ultrasound and cystoscopy for the first-line approach to AMH evaluation due to the lower costs.[22]

INTERPROFESSIONAL COLLABORATIVE MANAGEMENT

Management of hematuria consists mainly of identification, diagnosis, and referral. Further management considerations are based on the underlying pathologic condition, not on the presence of the hematuria itself.

COMPLICATIONS

Complications of hematuria depend on the underlying pathologic condition. Urinary obstruction, renal failure, anemia, infections, and hydronephrosis are potential complications.

INDICATIONS FOR REFERRAL OR HOSPITALIZATION

Isolated, transient hematuria or hematuria related to a UTI does not require a urology consultation. Referral to a renal or urology specialist is indicated to evaluate other causes of hematuria, given the high incidence of malignancy associated with this sign. Patients with large amounts of frank hematuria, severe flank pain suggestive of renal calculi, unstable vital signs, signs of urologic obstruction, or acute renal failure should be referred for urgent evaluation and possible hospitalization.

PATIENT AND FAMILY EDUCATION

Patient education largely depends on the cause of the hematuria; advice and educational material specific to the underlying pathologic process are appropriate. Because smoking is a major risk factor for bladder cancer, smoking cessation assistance should be offered to all smokers at every medical encounter. One of the major goals of education in asymptomatic hematuria is to reinforce the importance of the diagnostic evaluation. Other guidance should focus on the explanation of tests, medications, untoward effects, and the need for careful follow-up evaluation when indicated.

REFERENCES

1. Cravedi, P., Ruggenenti, P., & Remuzzi, G. (2012). Proteinuria should be used as a surrogate in chronic kidney disease. *Nature Reviews. Nephrology, 8,* 301–306.

2   Bello, A. K., Levin, A., Tonelli, M., Okpechi, I. G., Feehally, J., Harris, D., et al. (2017). Assessment of global Kidney Health Care Status. *JAMA: The Journal of the American Medical Association, 317*(18), 1864–1881.

3   Halpern, J. A., Chughtai, B., & Ghomrawi, H. (2017). Cost-effectiveness of Common Diagnostic Approaches for Evaluation of Asymptomatic Microscopic Hematuria. *JAMA Internal Medicine, 177*(6), 800–807.

4   Hall, J. T. (Ed.), (2011). *Guyton and Hall textbook of medical physiology* (10th ed.). Philadelphia: Saunders.

5   McPherson, R., & Pincus, M. (2011). *Henry's clinical diagnosis and management by laboratory methods* (22nd ed.). Philadelphia: Elsevier.

6   Strasinger, S., & DiLorenzo, M. (2014). *Urinalysis and body fluids* (6th ed.). Philadelphia: FA Davis.

7   National Institute of Diabetes and Digestive and Kidney Diseases. Proteinuria. www.niddk.nih.gov/health-information/health-topics/kidney-disease/proteinuria/document/proteinuria_508.pdf. (Accessed 4 September 2015).

8   Xu, H., Huang, X., Risérus, U., et al. (2014). Urinary albumin excretion, blood pressure changes and hypertension incidence in the community: Effect modification by kidney function. *Nephrology, Dialysis, Transplantation, 29*(8), 1538–1545.

9   Bhall, V., Zhao, B., Kristen, M. J., et al. (2012). Racial/ethnic differences in the prevalence of proteinuric and non-proteinuric diabetic kidney disease. *Diabetes Care, 36.*

10   Fried, L. F., & Palevsky, P. M. (2016). Decreasing prevalence of chronic kidney disease in the United States: A cause for optimism. *Annals of Internal Medicine, 165*(7), 521–522.

11   Airoldi, J., & Weinstein, L. (2007). Clinical significance of proteinuria in pregnancy. *Obstetrical and Gynecological Survey, 62*(2), 117–124.

12   Parving, H. H., Persson, F., & Rossing, P. (2015). Microalbuminuria: A parameter that has changed diabetes care. *Diabetes Research and Clinical Practice, 107*(1), 1–8.

13   He, F., Xia, X., & Wu, X. F. (2013). Diabetic retinopathy in predicting diabetic nephropathy in patients with type 2 diabetes and renal disease: A meta-analysis. *Diabetologia, 56*(3), 457–466.

14   Snyder, S., & Jones, S. J. (2014). Work-up for proteinuria. *Primary Care, 41*(4), 719–735.

15   Davis, R., Jones, S. J., Barocas, D., et al. (2012). Diagnosis, evaluation, and follow-up of asymptomatic microhematuria (AMH) in adults: AUA guideline. www.auanet.org/education/guidelines/asymptomatic-microhematuria.cfm. (Accessed 4 September 2015).

16   Tullika, G., Pinheiro, L., Atoria, C., et al. (2014). Gender disparities in hematuria evaluation and bladder cancer diagnosis: A population based analysis. *The Journal of Urology, 192*(4), 1072–1077.

17   DeGeorge, K. C., Holt, H. R., & Hodges, S. C. (2017). Bladder cancer: Diagnosis and treatment. *American Family Physician, 96*(8), 507–514.

18   Varma, P. P., Sengupta, P., & Nair, R. K. (2014). Post exertional hematuria. *Renal Failure, 36*(5), 701–703.

19   Sethi, S., Fervenza, F., Zhang, Y., et al. (2013). Atypical post-infectious glomerulonephritis is associated with abnormalities in the alternative pathway of complement. *Kidney International, 83,* 293–299.

20   Moreno, J. A., Martin-Cleary, C., Gutierrez, E., et al. (2012). AKI associated with macroscopic glomerular hematuria: Clinical and pathophysiologic consequences. *Clinical Journal of the American Society of Nephrology: CJASN, 7*(1), 175–184.

21   Saclarides, T. J., Myers, J. A., & Millikan, K. W. (Eds.), (2015). *Common surgical diseases: An algorithmic approach to problem solving.* New York: Springer.

22   Subak, L. L., & Grady, D. (2017). Asymptomatic microscopic hematuria-rethinking the diagnostic algorithm. *JAMA Internal Medicine, 177*(6), 808–809.

CHAPTER **131**

RENAL FAILURE

Chris Winkelman • Evelyn Duffy

➕ **Immediate hospitalization** is indicated for acute kidney injury (oliguria, anuria) associated with elevated serum creatinine; acute fluid and electrolyte derangement; hypotensive/hypertensive emergency; symptoms of systemic inflammatory response or sepsis; metabolic acidosis/large anion gap; acute heart failure, pericarditis

compromising mean arterial pressure, systolic blood pressure, or ventilation; or pulmonary edema or pleural effusion resulting in peripheral oxygenation (SpO_2) <92% or, if chronically hypoxemic, <88%, particularly if there is a change in mental status not improved with oxygen at less than 5 L by nasal cannula.

DEFINITION AND EPIDEMIOLOGY

Kidney damage causes loss of filtration and the retention of waste products in blood. Patients with kidney damage experience a complex and common health condition that demands the involvement of both the primary care provider and specialists. The loss of kidney filtration has two patterns of damage: chronic kidney disease (CKD) and acute kidney injury (AKI). The resultant damage is impaired kidney function. Although AKI is considered potentially reversible, both AKI and CKD can progress to kidney failure (the absence of kidney function) and is also known as end-stage renal disease (ESRD) and stage 5 CKD, replacing previously used terms such as *renal insufficiency, acute renal failure,* and *acute-on-chronic kidney disease.*[1,2]

The Kidney Disease: Improving Global Outcomes (KDIGO) group defines CKD as "abnormalities in kidney structure or function for greater than 3 months with implications for health," and this definition includes measures of kidney damage detailed in Table 131.1.[3] The international guideline recommendations (reviewed for its usefulness in the United States and accepted by the NKF) are that CKD be categorized based on the cause, glomerular filtration rate (GFR), and amount of albuminuria; these categories are illustrated in Tables 131.2 and 131.3.[3]

The Centers for Disease Control and Prevention estimates that more than 30 million Americans, 15% of the population, have CKD.[4] It is reported that 48% of patients with advanced kidney function but not on dialysis are undiagnosed.[4] Studies of provider and patient awareness of CKD have consistently found that the majority of cases are not recognized by providers and that patients themselves are unaware of their damaged kidneys.[5,6] Although CKD is more prevalent in adults aged 65 years and older, approximately one-third of older adults do not experience progressive disease.[6,7]

The current KDIGO documents related to AKI are also recognized nationally and internationally as the most sensitive and current.[2] AKI is defined as an increase in serum creatinine of 0.3 mg/dL over 48 hours or an increase of serum creatinine to 1.5 times baseline over the prior seven days; or a urine volume

TABLE **131.1**	Guidelines: Diagnosing Chronic Kidney Disease
Markers of kidney damage (one or more)	Albuminuria (albumin excretion rate. ≥30 mg/24 h; albumin/creatinine ratio ≥30 mg/g [≥3 mg/mmol])
	Urine sediment abnormalities
	Electrolyte and other abnormalities resulting from tubular disorders
	Abnormalities detected by histology
	Structure abnormalities detected by imaging
	History of kidney transplantation
Decreased GFR	GFR <60 mL/min/1.73 m² (GFR categories G3a–G5)

GFR, Glomerular filtration rate.
From Kidney Disease: Improving Global Outcomes (KDIGO). (2013). KDIGO 2012 clinical practice guideline for the evaluation and management of chronic kidney disease. *Kidney International Supplements, 3*(1), 1–150.

TABLE 131.2 Categories of Chronic Kidney Disease

GFR Categories (G)	GFR (mL/min/1.73 m²)	Terms
G1	≥90	Normal or high
G2	60–89	Mildly decreased[a]
G3a	45–59	Mildly to moderately decreased
G3b	30–44	Moderately to severely decreased
G4	15–29	Severely decreased
G5	<15	Kidney failure

[a]Relative to young adult level.
GFR, Glomerular filtration rate.
From Kidney Disease: Improving Global Outcomes (KDIGO). (2013). KDIGO 2012 clinical practice guideline for the evaluation and management of chronic kidney disease. *Kidney International Supplements, 3*(1), 1–150.

TABLE 131.3 Albuminuria Categories in Chronic Kidney Disease

	ACR (Approximate Equivalent)			
Category	AER (mg/24 h)	(mg/mmol)	(mg/g)	Terms
A1	<30	<3	<30	Normal to mildly increased
A2	30–300	3–30	30–300	Moderately increased[a]
A3	>300	>30	>300	Severely increased[b]

[a]Relative to young adult level.
[b]Including nephrotic syndrome (albumin excretion usually >2200 mg/24 h [ACR >2220 mg/g; >220 mg/mmol]).
ACR, Albumin/creatinine ratio; *AER,* albumin excretion rate.
From Kidney Disease: Improving Global Outcomes (KDIGO). (2013). KDIGO 2012 clinical practice guideline for the evaluation and management of chronic kidney disease. *Kidney International Supplements, 3*(1), 1–150.

TABLE 131.4 Staging of Acute Kidney Injury

Stage	Serum Creatinine	Urine Output
1	1.5–1.9 times baseline *or* >0.3 mg/dL (>26 µmol/L) increase	<0.5 mL/kg/h for 6–12 h
2	2.0–2.9 times baseline	<0.5 mL/kg/h for >12 h
3	3.0 times baseline *or* Increase in serum creatinine to >4.0 mg/dL (>353.6 µmol/L) *or* Initiation of renal replacement therapy *or* In patients <18 years, decrease in estimated glomerular filtration rate to <35 mL/min/1.73 m²	<0.3 mL/kg/h for >24 h *or* Anuria for >12 h

Data from Kidney Disease: Improving Global Outcomes (KDIGO) Work Group for Acute Kidney Injury. (2012). KDIGO clinical practice guideline for acute kidney injury. *Kidney International Supplements, 2*(Suppl), 1–138.

PATHOPHYSIOLOGY

The basic pathophysiologic process of kidney disease is loss of functioning nephrons. As filtration capacity falls to less than 50%, the remaining healthy nephrons exhibit hyperfiltration and hypertrophy. This process is hypothesized to contribute to increased glomerular capillary pressure, leading to secondary nephron damage and progressive disease.[9] The results are a decrease in GFR; an increase in circulating biomarkers of kidney disease, including creatinine and blood urea nitrogen (BUN); and albuminuria. Fig. 131.1 illustrates the risk for progression of CKD.

The pathophysiology of AKI is any process that interferes with perfusion, filtration, or excretion.[4] Disruption to perfusion is categorized as prerenal. Filtration abnormalities are intrinsic causes of AKI and refer to the pathology of vessels, glomeruli, or tubules and interstitium.[5] Postrenal causes of AKI include obstruction to the renal pelvis, ureters, bladder, or urethra. However, AKI can also result from combined pathologic processes. For example, poor perfusion and subsequent ischemic damage to the nephron comprise a combined prerenal and intrinsic cause of AKI. Consider the hospitalized patient with prolonged poor renal perfusion (i.e., prerenal) from a hypotensive shock state (e.g., cardiogenic, septic, or hemorrhagic shock) with concurrent acute tubular necrosis (related to endotoxin exposure or ischemic necrosis of the nephron tubules), an intrinsic cause of AKI. As a second example of combined pathology, consider the patient with untreated kidney stones leading to urinary tract obstruction—postrenal AKI—leading to fibrosis and atrophy of the obstructed kidneys—an intrinsic pathology.

Risk factors of comorbidities, age, and drugs can also contribute to prerenal, intrinsic, and postrenal AKI.[6,7] For example, comorbidities that reduce blood flow to the kidneys such as chronic heart failure (HF) or cirrhosis increase the risk for AKI. Hypovolemic states from acute blood loss, diarrhea, or dehydration lead to prerenal injury. Contrast from imaging studies may contribute to intrinsic AKI, particularly when the patient is

output of less than 0.5 mL/kg/h for 6 hours. According to this guideline, AKI severity is classed from 1 to 3, with 1 being the least severe, as illustrated in Table 131.4.[2] AKI is an abrupt loss of kidney function that occurs over 7 days or less, although damage is most often recognized within 48 hours of admission to an acute or critical care setting.[8] Annually, AKI has been reported in 0.3% to 0.5% of community-dwelling adults, 5% to 10% of all hospitalized patients, and 25% to 70% of critically ill patients.[8]

Both AKI and CKD can progress to kidney failure in a small but significant percentage of people.[3] Kidney failure (ESRD) is characterized by anuria and the need for renal replacement therapy or kidney transplant. The kidneys and the urinary tract system no longer filter blood, create filtrate, or excrete urine in amounts sufficient to clear waste and balance fluid intake with output. In addition to being a clinical diagnosis, ESRD has policy and administrative implications because patients who receive dialysis or a kidney transplant are eligible for health insurance through Medicare regardless of their age.

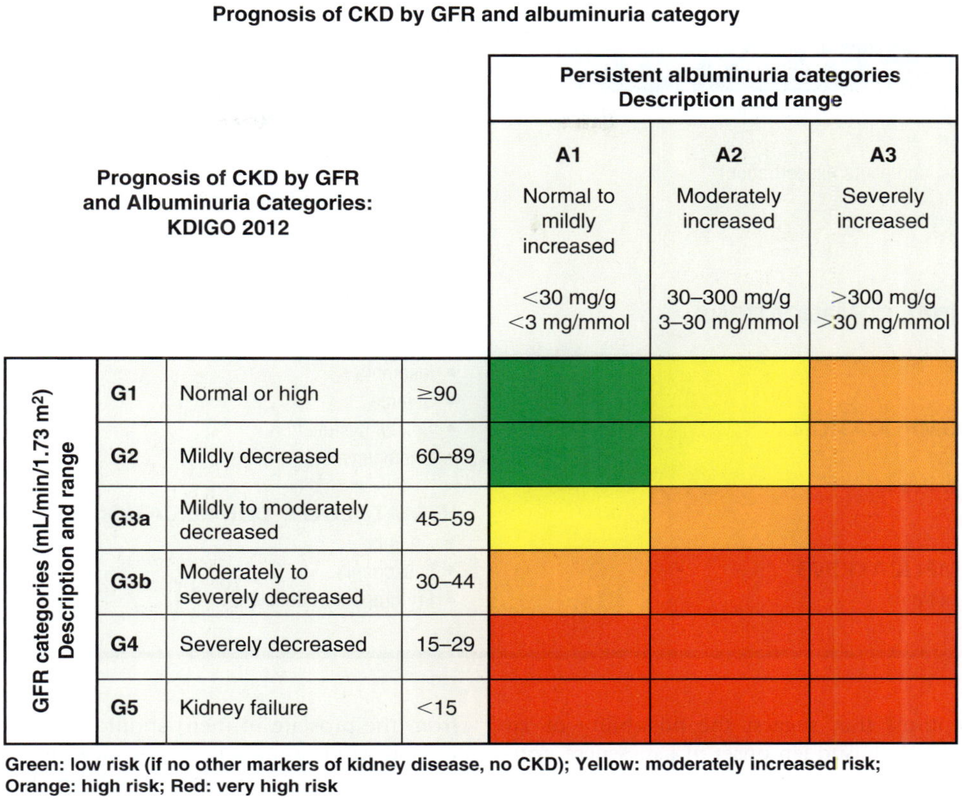

Prognosis of CKD by GFR and albuminuria category

Prognosis of CKD by GFR and Albuminuria Categories: KDIGO 2012				Persistent albuminuria categories Description and range		
				A1 Normal to mildly increased <30 mg/g <3 mg/mmol	A2 Moderately increased 30–300 mg/g 3–30 mg/mmol	A3 Severely increased >300 mg/g >30 mg/mmol
GFR categories (mL/min/1.73 m²) Description and range	G1	Normal or high	≥90	Green	Yellow	Orange
	G2	Mildly decreased	60–89	Green	Yellow	Orange
	G3a	Mildly to moderately decreased	45–59	Yellow	Orange	Red
	G3b	Moderately to severely decreased	30–44	Orange	Red	Red
	G4	Severely decreased	15–29	Red	Red	Red
	G5	Kidney failure	<15	Red	Red	Red

Green: low risk (if no other markers of kidney disease, no CKD); Yellow: moderately increased risk; Orange: high risk; Red: very high risk

FIG. 131.1 Risk for progression of kidney damage. *CKD*, Chronic kidney disease; *GFR*, glomerular filtration rate; *KDIGO*, Kidney Disease: Improving Global Outcomes. (From Kidney Disease: Improving Global Outcomes [KDIGO]. [2013]. KDIGO 2012 clinical practice guideline for the evaluation and management of chronic kidney disease. *Kidney International Supplements, 3*[1], 1–150.)

dehydrated or presents with CKD.[10,11] Inflammatory conditions, sepsis, kidney infection, toxins including drugs, and malignancies damage tubules and the interstitium, resulting in intrinsic causes of AKI.[5] Postrenal (obstructive) AKI may be caused by neoplasm, prostatic enlargement, neurogenic bladder, strictures, nephrolithiasis, and severe constipation. Combinations of prerenal and intrinsic etiologies can increase the early onset or severity of AKI. To illustrate, small vessel vascular pathology from diabetes, clotting disorders, and hypertension can combine with drug-induced nephritis to cause AKI during hospitalization or following surgery.[4]

CLINICAL PRESENTATION AND PHYSICAL EXAMINATION

CKD and AKI have few symptoms in the early stages. Ongoing progression of CKD and destruction of nephrons result in a variety of symptoms, complications, and a steady and predictable decline in functional health. ESRD and its management (dialysis or kidney transplantation) have significant complications that need to be comanaged with nephrologists and other experts.

The hallmark clinical signs of CKD and AKI are a decreased GFR, an increased serum creatinine, and albumin in the urine. The clinical symptoms are subtle and uncommon, with a GFR above 35 mL/min/1.73 m². Therefore suspicion for kidney disease should be based on recognition of the risk for kidney damage, particularly in patients with diabetes mellitus and hypertension. Diabetes is the most common cause of kidney

failure in the United States. Thirty percent of type I and 10% to 40% of type II diabetics develop kidney failure.[12] Because diabetes and hypertension are highly associated with CKD, clinical guidelines for management of both diabetes and hypertension recommend regular urinalysis with a calculation of the urinary albumin/creatinine ratio (ACR) to allow for early detection of kidney damage.[9,13] Early detection of renal disease—for both CKD and AKI—is advocated to slow progression or kidney damage and decrease complications from uremia and disrupted metabolism.

The most common cause of AKI is hospitalization with concomitant reduced renal perfusion and exposure to nephrotoxins.[3] Most patients who develop AKI have identifiable risk factors, such as CKD, advanced age, liver disease, diabetes, or vascular disease. Therefore it is essential to identify those at high risk before AKI develops. It is equally important to follow up with monitoring after a diagnosis of AKI because patients with AKI are at risk for developing CKD in the future and may be discharged with early-stage CKD.[14]

Once the GFR falls below 35 mL/min/1.73 m², a variety of cardiovascular, gastrointestinal, neurologic, metabolic, hematologic, and psychosocial problems occur. These complications are listed in Box 131.1. Clinical presentation at this point depends on the particular complication and on the underlying cause of kidney failure. All individuals with CKD should undergo screening for the complications of kidney disease to prevent morbidity and to establish a credible baseline for the individual.

BOX **131.1**

Major Complications of Stages 4 and 5 Chronic Kidney Disease

CARDIOVASCULAR COMPLICATIONS
- Atherosclerosis
- Heart failure (chronic and acute exacerbation)
- Hypertension
- Pulmonary edema
- Pericarditis

GASTROINTESTINAL COMPLICATIONS
- Nausea, vomiting
- Anorexia

NEUROLOGIC COMPLICATIONS
- Peripheral neuropathy
- Muscle cramps or twitching
- Pruritus

METABOLIC COMPLICATIONS
- Electrolyte abnormalities
- Metabolic acidosis

- Alterations in vitamin D, calcium, and phosphorus metabolism and absorption
- Mineral and bone disorders
- Hyperparathyroidism
- Hyperlipidemia

PSYCHOSOCIAL COMPLICATIONS
- Depression
- Fatigue
- Insomnia
- Suicide
- Sexual dysfunction
- Unemployment

HEMATOLOGIC COMPLICATIONS
- Anemia
- Leukopenia
- Erythropoietin deficiency

Concerning symptoms that suggest the possibility of an acute renal problem include sudden onset of listlessness, confusion, anorexia, nausea/vomiting, edema, and weight gain.

Oliguria (i.e., urine output <400 mL/day or anuria [i.e., urine output <100 mL/day]) in adults, when associated with an elevated serum creatinine, indicates a change in fluid volume status requiring diagnostic testing.

The physical examination should include both a focused examination to identify primary diseases that contribute to kidney damage (e.g., diabetes mellitus or hypertension) and a broader examination that evaluates the effects of kidney disease. Staging or categorizing kidney damage (i.e., AKI stage 1 to 3; CKD category 1 to 5) can guide the primary care provider in determining the frequency of monitoring and providing anticipatory guidance about self-management.

Common symptoms and signs result directly from diminished kidney function such as edema, hypertension, and decreased urine output. CKD may be asymptomatic until it is in the advanced stages. In older adults, there may never be clear symptoms related to declining renal function.

The provider should assess for hypotension and hypertension: take vital signs (including measurement of bilateral arm and orthostatic blood pressure); perform funduscopic evaluation for signs of arteriovenous nicking, diabetic retinopathy, and papilledema; and evaluate peripheral pulse characteristics. Volume overload from kidney damage can cause adventitious lung sounds jugular vein distention; peripheral and central edema; and a third heart sound. Pericarditis (heart "rub" sound) and pleural effusions (pleuritic chest pain; pleuritic "rub") can be a complication of CKD. A focused abdominal examination includes auscultation for renal artery bruits, palpation of the kidneys, inspection for distention that may be caused by ascites, and percussion of the suprapubic area to determine bladder distention. The skin is examined for ecchymosis, rashes (especially those suggesting collagen vascular disorders), or uremic frost and the patient should be asked about pruritus. A rectal examination to exclude obstruction (e.g.,

from the prostate in men) should be performed. A thorough mental status examination is included to screen for depression, anxiety, substance use, and cognitive dysfunction associated with kidney dysfunction.

DIAGNOSTICS
Essential Diagnostics

The most important diagnostic tool in monitoring both patients at risk for and those with diagnosed CKD is a serum creatinine test with an estimated GFR (eGFR) and a first morning or random urine sample to assess for the presence of albuminuria.[1]

Serum creatinine is a product of muscle metabolism. In patients with very high muscle mass, such as weight lifters, or very low muscle mass as a result of sarcopenia or cachexia, the eGFR will be inaccurate. The eGFR is not accurate in non–steady states, such as conditions of disease exacerbation or critical illness. The eGFR may be limited as a screening and diagnostic tool among older adults, who may have lower muscle mass that leads to reduced creatinine production or reduced kidney mass that is associated with elevated creatinine but without concerning progression.

Most laboratories now report eGFR along with serum creatinine, but if that is not available, there are recommended eGFR calculators. The preferred method is the CKD Epidemiology Collaboration (CKD-EPI) 2009 creatinine equation. Other methods include (in order of preference) the Modification of Diet in Renal Disease (MDRD) equation, the CKD-EPI 2012 creatinine equation, and the Crockhoff-Gault formula.[1] These calculators are available at www.kidney.org/professionals/KDOQI/gfr.

Serum creatinine remains the most common test for kidney function even though it can be affected by muscle mass, gender, race, and diet. Serum cystatin C–based estimates of eGFR are recommended as a diagnostic biomarker to confirm or exclude the diagnoses of kidney disease in people with GFR less than 60 mL/min/1.73 m[2].[1,2] However, the serum cystatin C test is not available at all laboratories and is expensive. Its utility in primary care settings as a diagnostic marker for CKD or AKI has not been supported in some settings.[15]

The preferred screening strategy for albuminuria is measurement of the urine ACR in an untimed urinary sample.[1,3] If the ACR is greater than 30 mg/g, a confirmatory test is done on the first morning urine. In the absence of available ACR determination, the KDIGO guidelines recommend alternatives in the following order:

- Urine protein/creatinine ratio (PCR)
- Reagent strip analysis for urine total protein with automated reading
- Reagent strip analysis for urine total protein with manual reading

An additional method for determining kidney damage is urinalysis. Examination of urine sediment or dipstick for red blood cells (RBCs) or white blood cells is recommended.[16,17]

Urine sodium can be helpful in determining the cause of the patient's symptoms. A low urine sodium may suggest hypovolemia, but low urine sodium can occur in patients on low salt diets, diuretic therapy, and some other renal disorders and thus is not highly specific.

If AKI or CKD is identified, a more comprehensive assessment of causative factors and possible complications is recommended. Not all patients require all of the evaluation; the primary care provider can individualize diagnostics based on history, established previous diagnoses or comorbidities, and an estimate of cost-effectiveness.

Additional Diagnostics

Patients with known CKD will need monitoring for metabolic acidosis, hyperphosphatemia, elevated parathyroid hormone (PTH), and decreased $1,25(OH)_2D_3$.

INITIAL DIAGNOSTICS

Renal Disease

LABORATORY
- Complete serum metabolic panel with attention to creatinine and estimation of glomerular filtration rate
- Urine albumin; urine ACR
- Urine creatinine
- Urine volume (for AKI; hourly for 3 or more hours)
- Urine sodium[a] to differentiate ATN and prerenal disease.
- Liver enzyme tests[a]
- Serum lipid profile[a]
- Glycosylated hemoglobin (HbA1C)[a] or fasting blood sugar[a]
- Serology for glomerulonephritis[a]

IMAGING
- Renal ultrasound to evaluate presence of obstruction
- Bladder ultrasound to estimate postvoid residual
- Renal biopsy for glomerular disease diagnosis

---

[a]If indicated by the presence of systemic conditions such as diabetes, high blood pressure, heart disease, liver disease, or infection and inflammatory disorders.

DIFFERENTIAL DIAGNOSIS

 Priority differentials include determining the etiology of AKI as (1) prerenal (decreased renal perfusion); (2) intrinsic renal (pathology of the renal blood vessels, glomeruli or tubules); (3) postrenal (obstructive); or (4) combinations such as prerenal and intrinsic etiologies.

For CKD, priority differentials include consideration of (1) drug or lead toxicity; (2) chronic inflammatory, cardiovascular, or cancer conditions (e.g., rheumatoid arthritis, scleroderma, hypertension, HF, sickle cell disease, multiple myeloma); and (3) diabetes as contributing to the onset and severity of kidney pathology.

Differential diagnoses related to AKI and CKD include conditions that contribute to renal damage. Vigilance is necessary to determine any underlying correctable pathologic process that may be causing kidney damage. Identifying and reversing disorders that occur acutely can mitigate the severity or progression of kidney damage. In general, a mean arterial pressure of 65 mm Hg is recommended to avoid hypoperfusion to kidneys and subsequent damage.[3] Nephrotoxin exposure, including drugs, heavy metals, and by-products of infection, should be avoided or eliminated.[18] Recognition and treatment of inflammatory conditions that contribute to AKI can mitigate intrinsic causes of AKI.

The most common type of AKI seen in primary care is prerenal AKI related to volume depletion or hypotension. Common drugs and toxins that contribute to intrinsic AKI include nonsteroidal antiinflammatory drugs (NSAIDs) used chronically, renin-angiotensin-aldosterone system (RAAS) antagonists (i.e., angiotensin-converting enzyme [ACE] inhibitors and angiotensin receptor blockers [ARBs]), many antibiotics (including aminoglycosides, quinolones, cephalosporins active against β-lactamase, sulfonamides), illicit drugs (amphetamines, heroin), antineoplastic agents, immunosuppressants, the human immunodeficiency virus (HIV) drugs indinavir and ritonavir, heavy metals, industrial chemicals, organic solvents, pesticides, and bacterial exotoxins and endotoxins.[19] Radiation can also cause AKI. Contrast used in radiographic imaging has undergone signification reformulation in recent years, with a reduced profile in terms of causing direct kidney damage, particularly when patients are well hydrated before testing.[20] Inflammatory conditions that contribute to AKI include systemic lupus erythematous, renal artery stenosis, Wegener granulomatosis, Alport syndrome, polycystic kidney disease, diabetic nephropathy, Goodpasture syndrome, multiple myeloma, nephrolithiasis, and rapidly progressive glomerulonephritis; these conditions need to be recognized.[5] In general, acute inflammatory conditions are cotreated with corticosteroids; early and appropriate administration is essential to good patient outcomes.[3,5]

Often, patients who experience AKI have preexisting conditions, such as advanced age, liver disease, diabetes, and cardiovascular disease.[19] It is not uncommon to see a patient with early-stage CKD experience AKI while hospitalized and then progress to a more serious stage of CKD; this is known as AKI on CKD. The astute primary care provider will assess the presurgical patient for CKD and risk for AKI. Recently hospitalized patients should be tested for renal function in the first 2 to 3 months after discharge to determine if kidney damage remains present, is improving, or if it is progressing.[21]

INTERPROFESSIONAL COLLABORATIVE MANAGEMENT

 Referral to a nephrologist is indicated for patients with a new diagnosis of stage 4 CKD (see Table 131.2) to discuss options and preferences for renal replacement therapy (dialysis).

Pharmacologic Management

- The management of AKI includes removing sources of nephrotoxins (contrast, drugs) and managing fluid to avoid overhydration and underhydration.[22]
- Early recognition and treatment of electrolyte imbalances, especially hyperkalemia, is essential for patient safety in both AKI and CKD.
- The management of CKD includes blood pressure control and reducing proteinuria with diet. The use of angiotensin inhibitors (ACE inhibitors) are specifically recommended to slow the progression of CKD.
- Treating metabolic acidosis with supplemental bicarbonate and attaining glycemic control are also associated with a slowed progression of CKD.

Nonpharmacologic Management

- Protein restriction through diet and smoking cessation are advised to slow the progression of CKD.
- Primary care providers need to consider the timing of referral to a nephrologist. In one study, it was noted that 64% of patients did not receive referral until the late stage of their disease.[23] The 2012 KDIGO guidelines[1,3] provide suggestions for timely referral. These include:
  - AKI or abrupt sustained decrease in GFR
  - GFR less than 30 mL/min/1.73 m^2 or CKD stage 4 or 5
  - Significant albuminuria (ACR >300 mg/g)
  - Progression of CKD defined as a decrease in any GFR category and a 25% or greater drop in GFR from baseline
  - Urine RBCs greater than 20 per high-power field (hpf)
  - Hypertension refractory to treatment with four or more agents
  - Persistent abnormalities of serum potassium or low serum albumin
  - Recurrent or extensive nephrolithiasis
  - Hereditary kidney disease

Kidney failure will require interdisciplinary management with a nephrologist. Complications for late-stage CKD or ESRD may also require an urgent referral for interdisciplinary management. For example, symptomatic hyperkalemia discovered in primary care may require an urgent request for dialysis, managed by the nephrologist. New-onset or acute exacerbation of HF may require referral to a cardiologist.

When a patient has a diagnosis of severe AKI, an emergent referral is made to a nephrologist for initiation of dialysis (see Table 131.2) to manage the following life-threatening conditions: metabolic acidosis with a pH <7.1; refractory hyperkalemia >6.5 mEq/L; volume overload unresponsive to diuretic use (particularly when hypervolemia impairs perfusion or ventilation); uremic encephalopathy; and removal of toxins or drugs that can be removed with dialysis.[3,19] The goals of management of a patient with AKI are to reverse the causes of AKI and stop progression of kidney damage.[2]

Multiple resources are available for clinicals and patients on NKF website, www.kidney.org, including educational resources, nutritional information, and clinical trials. The goal of management for a patient with stages 1 to 4 CKD is to slow progression of disease. The following management steps reflect best practices in primary care.

Consensus hypertension management guidelines currently recommend a blood pressure target of 130/80.[24] Lifestyle modifications are essential to management and include sodium restriction and weight loss. The use of RAAS antagonists (ACE inhibitors or ARBs) is recommended for treatment of hypertension in any patient with CKD and albuminuria. These drugs should not be used concurrently, nor should they be used in patients with bilateral renal artery stenosis. Their use in CKD increases the risk of hyperkalemia. Serum potassium, BUN, and creatinine measurements are repeated 1 week after initiation of ACE inhibitor or ARB therapy.

A small increase in creatinine is not a reason to discontinue the ACE inhibitor or ARB. However, a 30% increase it is usually considered to be clinically significant, although recent data suggest that adverse outcomes were noted even at levels below that threshold.[25] Of more concern is the serum potassium level that should be monitored to attain a goal of 5 mEq/L or lower. The addition of a thiazide diuretic may be useful for improved management of hypertension and to manage hyperkalemia. NSAIDs increase the risk of hyperkalemia, and patients should be advised to avoid these over-the-counter medications. If an ACE inhibitor or ARB is not tolerated, nondihydropyridine calcium channel blockers may be used an alternative.[26]

Partnering with the patient who has diabetes is essential to manage both CKD and diabetes. The HbA1c must be monitored; guidelines recommend maintaining a level below 7%. Guidelines for older adults are more generous: HbA1c for healthy older adults is < 7.5%, for frail older adults with multiple chronic conditions, < 8%; and frail with poor health or in long-term care, < 8.5%.[27] These guidelines were developed owing to reduce harm from hypoglycemia.[19,23] Certain diabetic medications may need to be adjusted or eliminated in patients with CKD. In 2016, changes were made to the guidelines for appropriate use of metformin. It is currently contraindicated in patients with an eGFR <30 mL/min/1.73 m^2, and initiation of treatment in patients with an eGFR between 30 and 45 mL/min/1.73 m^2 should be done with caution. If the eGFR falls below 45 mL/min/1.73 m^2 in a patient already taking metformin, the benefits and risks of continuing treatment should be assessed.[28]

Dietary management is essential to the overall management of CKD. Referral to a registered dietitian for medical nutritional therapy (MNT) is beneficial for optimum care, especially in patients with comorbidities such as diabetes and those who are under or over ideal body weight. Medicare provides an MNT benefit for patients with CKD or diabetes at no cost and may be provided yearly. Although protein restriction is widely recommended at 0.6 to 0.8 g/kg/day, the issue of how much to restrict protein remains controversial.[1,3] To help prevent hyperkalemia, patients should be instructed to avoid potassium-containing salt substitutes. Diets low in phosphorus (0.8 to 1 g/day) have been shown to delay the progression of kidney failure, probably as a result of the prevention of deposition of phosphate and calcium in the interstitium of the kidney.[29]

Patients with CKD are at risk for the development of mineral bone disorder (CKD-MBD), a syndrome previously called renal osteodystrophy.[26] The kidneys are critical in the maintenance of serum calcium and normal bone metabolism. These changes affect PTH and both activated and inactive forms of vitamin D. Beginning in CKD stage 3, excretion of phosphate is decreased, resulting in a need to decrease dietary phosphate. Hyperphosphatemia and hyperparathyroidism contribute to calcium removal from bones. The bone demineralization is associated with an increased incidence of atraumatic and traumatic fractures. When calcium levels are low, the patient develops osteoporosis, and, with elevated levels, vascular calcification and cardiovascular disease can develop. The recommendation is for meeting the recommended daily calcium requirements, 1000-mg/day for adults and 1200 mg/day for older adults. Preferably these goals will be met with calcium-containing foods. Meeting calcium requirements through dietary intake provides other essential nutrients and micronutrients as well. Calcium supplements vary in amount of elemental calcium and in absorption. Calcium carbonate provides 40% elemental calcium but requires stomach acid for absorption. It must be taken with meals. Calcium citrate provides 21% elemental calcium, and it may be taken without regard for food. Calcium acetate, recommended for patients with later stages of CKD, provides 25% elemental calcium and helps remove phosphate. Use of aluminum or magnesium antacids as replacement for calcium should be avoided because these can cause aluminum or magnesium toxicity. It is important to monitor serum calcium levels. Serum calcium levels need to be corrected if the patient has a concomitant low serum albumin. Calcium is bound to protein, and when albumin is decreased for any reason, the serum value will be lower than the actual calcium level. Tools are available to perform this calculation. If the corrected calcium level is high or low, an ionized calcium measurement should be ordered to confirm the result.

Vitamin D insufficiency is identified by measurement of 25-hydroxyvitamin D levels. Vitamin D replacement should be initiated when levels are below 30 ng/mL. Replacement can follow recommendations established for the general population; either ergocalciferol (D_2) or cholecalciferol (D_3) may be prescribed.[29]

Lipids must be controlled. Hyperlipidemia is both a complication of CKD and a potential factor in the progression of the disease.[1,19] Patency of vessels anywhere in the body is compromised by hyperlipidemia. Lowering of low-density lipoprotein (LDL) cholesterol in patients with coronary artery disease is recommended.[30] Many statins have limitations based on renal function; atorvastatin does not require renal dosing, and fluvastatin dosing is only a consideration in patients with severe renal dysfunction.

Anemia is a frequent complication of CKD but may have other causes. Management of anemia may help delay the progression of CKD. All potential causes of anemia should be explored to establish optimal treatment; iron deficiency, B_{12} or folate deficiency, and thalassemia screening tests should be completed before concluding that anemia is exclusively a result of CKD. The CBC with differential is monitored at least annually in patients with stage 3 CKD without anemia and twice yearly in patients with stage 4 or 5 CKD. Additional tests for anemia evaluation conducted annually are an absolute reticulocyte count, serum ferritin level, serum transferrin saturation, and serum B_{12} and folate levels. Iron replacement therapy is often required in patients with anemia related to CKD. Replacement with iron should precede initiation of erythropoiesis-stimulating agents (ESAs) because RBC production is dependent on adequate iron and iron stores. Although treatment with ESAs may be necessary in patients with CKD, all correctable causes of anemia should be treated first. Treatment with ESAs should be considered only if hemoglobin concentrations fall below 10 g/dL and must be stopped before normal values are achieved. Judicious use of ESAs helps avoid the need for RBC transfusion and improves quality of life. Decisions regarding the use of intravenous iron or ESAs should be made in conjunction with a nephrologist

For a patient with ESRD, the goal is to maximize patient survival with the use of dialysis or through kidney transplantation. Optimizing function and a sense of well-being are also important goals shared by the primary care provider, and achieving these goals can occur even when the patient does not elect to manage kidney failure with dialysis or transplant. Patients with ESRD are often older adults who have multiple comorbid conditions. The presence of a high symptom burden and the potential for early mortality among patients with ESRD suggests that primary care providers have a significant role in ensuring education about options for dialysis, establishing advance directives, and using structured shared communication with the nephrologist and other specialists to avoid or reduce complications that occur during ESRD and its treatment. Co-management with an expert in symptom management (i.e., a specialist in palliative care) may increase quality of life and function among patients with ESRD.

LIFE SPAN CONSIDERATIONS

Age increases the risk for AKI and CKD. GFR declines by approximately 5% each decade after age 40 years. Note that a decline in GFR alone is not diagnostic of CKD without the presence of other markers, particularly in older adults. All individuals with CKD should undergo screening for the complications of renal disease to prevent morbidity and to establish a credible baseline for the individual.

Critically ill pediatric patients have an incidence of stage 2 or 3 AKI of 11.6% following admission.[23] Critically ill adults experience severe AKI at a 38.9% incidence and older adults at 52.8%.[23,29] A diagnosis of AKI during hospitalization increases length of stay across the lifespan.[23] Long-term consequences of AKI in all groups include cardiovascular events, progression to CKD and ESRD, and increased mortality at 30 days following discharge, as well as over the next 1 to 10 years.[30]

COMPLICATIONS

When CKD or AKI results in ESRD, complications are systemic and require significant collaboration and intervention for maintenance of health. For example, because it takes approximately 4 to 6 weeks for a fistula to mature sufficiently for intermittent hemodialysis, this surgical procedure, completed by a vascular surgeon, needs to be planned in advance of starting hemodialysis. Box 131.1 details major complications from ESRD.

Understanding patient preferences and values can help the primary care provider communicate options for treatment, such as discussing the advantages of peritoneal dialysis or the strategies that promote adherence to a complicated medical regimen. Coaching for self-management and ongoing communication between the primary care and specialist provider (e.g., nephrologist, cardiologist, or vascular surgeon) are also valuable to achieving goals of care. The current mortality rate for US patients with ESRD is more than 20% per year, and the primary care provider can lead a discussion about end-of-life care after a diagnosis of ESRD.

Cardiovascular Management and Complications

Cardiovascular complications are the leading cause of death among patients with kidney failure (ESRD), accounting for more than 50% of deaths in the first year of dialysis.[1] Prevention of cardiovascular complications is therefore of the utmost priority in primary care, and management or co-management of cardiovascular disease falls within the primary care provider's scope of practice. Hypertension and hyperlipidemia should be aggressively managed.[26] Unfortunately, 70% of patients who begin dialysis treatment already have left ventricular hypertrophy and 40% have chronic HF.[17] Pulmonary edema and acute exacerbation of HF are major concerns in ESRD. If the patient is unstable, hospitalization and urgent dialysis may be necessary. All episodes of HF and pulmonary edema should be reported to the renal specialist so that adjustments can be made in the dialysate fluid to compensate for fluid overload.

Dietary Management and Metabolic Complications

Dietary management should be aimed at balancing electrolytes (including calcium, phosphorus, and potassium), preventing malnutrition, and maintaining fluid volume balance.[24] Daily dietary requirements for patients with ESRD depend on the type of dialysis chosen (continuous ambulatory peritoneal dialysis [CAPD] vs. hemodialysis). All patients with ESRD should be referred to a dietitian for optimization of nutritional status.

Hematologic Management and Complications

The anemia of CKD, if untreated, leads to significant functional decline, including cardiac damage and cognitive impairment. The options to treat CKD-related anemia are transfusion of RBCs, and ESAs. ESAs given subcutaneously are more effectively absorbed than ESAs given intravenously or into extracorporeal blood during hemodialysis. Bleeding risk increases with uremia from impaired platelet function. In the presence of concerning hemorrhage, administration of coagulation factors (e.g., cryoprecipitate) may help, and emergent dialysis will reduce uremia. Patients with CKD are at increased risk for infection, and careful attention should be paid to preventive measures, including vaccination with influenza, pneumococcal, and hepatitis B vaccines.

Psychosocial Management and Complications

The stress of dealing with severe chronic illness can be psychologically devastating. Patients with ESRD, especially patients on hemodialysis, are known to have high rates of depression, insomnia, and anxiety. Often ignored, sexual dysfunction occurs at high rates in both male and female patients with ESRD. The treatment of these and other psychosocial complications should begin before the onset of ESRD.

PATIENT AND FAMILY EDUCATION AND HEALTH PROMOTION

- Patient education related to a diagnosis of AKI, CKD, or ESRD is highly complex and requires carefully coordinated care.
- Numerous resources to support patient and family education along the trajectory of kidney disease are available at www.kidney.org or via phone at 1-855-NKF-CARES (1-855-653-2273). At this site, patients can access a food coach and receive help with insurance coverage and medication costs, as well as information about clinical trials, transplant, and dialysis.
  - There is a special link on the site for older adults with information specific to their unique needs.
- Guiding patients and family members to appropriate internet and social media sites is part of essential patient and family education.
- Gradually introduce different educational materials and prompt self-management to help control the course of the kidney disease to help restore a sense of independence and confidence in the patient.

The goal of care for AKI is to identify and manage reversible causes of kidney damage. Patients with AKI are at risk for early mortality and for progression to CKD; transitions from acute to primary care should include a recommendation to the primary care provider to test serum and urine to detect early CKD and slow progression of this chronic condition. CKD is associated with cardiovascular disease risk, infection, malignancy, and mortality. Early and ongoing screening will identify AKI and CKD and mitigate the life-limiting nature of multiple comorbidities. Patients with CKD should receive counseling about advance-care planning and be referred to a nephrologist before eGFR falls to <30 mL/min/1.73 m^2.

REFERENCES

1. KDIGO. (2012). KDIGO clinical practice guideline for the evaluation and management of chronic kidney disease. *Kidney International*, 3, Suppl1–Suppl150.
2. KDIGO. (2012). KDIGO clinical practice guideline for acute kidney injury. *Kidney International*, 2(Suppl. 1–138).
3. Sharfuddin, A., Weisbord, S. D., Palvesky, P. M., & Moltoris, B. A. (2016). Acute kidney injury. In K. Skorecki, G. M. Chertow, P. A. Marsden, A. S. L. Yu, & M. W. Taal (Eds.), *Brenner and Rector's the kidney* (Vol. 1, pp. 958–1011). Philadelphia, PA: Elsevier.
4. Emmett, M., & Fenves, A. Z. (2016). J.C. S. Approach to the patient with kidney disease. In K. Skorecki, G. M. Chertow, P. A. Marsden, A. S. L. Yu, & M. W. Taal (Eds.), *Brenner and Tector's the kidney* (Vol. 1, pp. 754–779). Philadephia, PA: Elsevier.
5. Raghavan, R., & Eknoyan, G. (2014). Acute interstitial nephritis—a reappraisal and update. *Clinical Nephrology*, 82(3), 149–162.
6. Pakula, A. M., & Skinner, R. A. (2016). Acute kidney injury in the critically ill patient: A current review of the literature. *Journal of Intensive Care Medicine*, 31(5), 319–324.
7. Kane-Gill, S. L., Sileanu, F. E., Murugan, R., Trietley, G. S., Handler, S. M., & Kellum, J. A. (2015). Risk factors for acute kidney injury in older adults with critical illness: A retrospective cohort study. *American Journal of Kidney Diseases: The Official Journal of the National Kidney Foundation*, 65(6), 860–869.
8. Chawla, L. S., Bellomo, R., Bihorac, A., Goldstein, S. L., Siew, E. D., Bagshaw, S. M., et al. (2017). Acute kidney disease and renal recovery: Consensus report of the Acute Disease Quality Initiative (ADQI) 16 Workgroup. *Nature Reviews. Nephrology*, 13(4), 241–257.
9. KDIGO. (2012). Clinical practice guideline for the management of blood pressure in chronic kidney disease. *Kidney International*, 2, Suppl 405–Suppl 414.
10. Ozkok, S., & Ozkok, A. (2017). Contrast-induced acute kidney injury: A review of practical points. *World Journal of Nephrology*, 6(3), 86–99.
11. Davenport, M. S., Cohan, R. H., & Ellis, J. H. (2015). Contrast media controversies in 2015: Imaging patients with renal impairment or risk of contrast reaction. *American Journal of Roentgenology*, 204(6), 1174–1181. PubMed PMID: 25730301.
12. About Chronic Kideny Disease: National Kidney Foundation; 2017 [cited 2 January 2018]. Retrieved from https://www.kidney.org/atoz/content/about-chronic-kidney-disease.
13. Farmer, A. J., Stevens, R., Hirst, J., Lung, T., Oke, J., Clarke, P., et al. (2014). Optimal strategies for identifying kidney disease in diabetes: Properties of screening tests, progression of renal dysfunction and impact of treatment—systematic review and modelling of progression and cost-effectiveness. *Health Technology Assessment*, 18(14), 1–128.
14. Bellomo, R., Ronco, C., Mehta, R. L., Asfar, P., Boisrame-Helms, J., Darmon, M., et al. (2017). Acute kidney injury in the ICU: From injury to recovery: reports from the 5th Paris International Conference. *Annals of Intensive Care*, 7(1), 49.
15. Shardlow, A., McIntyre, N. J., Fraser, S. D. S., Roderick, P., Raftery, J., Fluck, R. J., et al. (2017). The clinical utility and cost impact of cystatin C

measurement in the diagnosis and management of chronic kidney disease: A primary care cohort study. *PLoS Medicine, 14*(10), e1002400.

16. CDC (Centers for Disease Control and Prevention). National chronic kidney disase fact sheet: General information and national estimates on chronic kidney disease in the United Stated. Atlanta Georgia: U.S. Department of Health and Human Services, Centers for Diases Control and Prevention; 2014 [accessed 2 January 2018]. Retrieved from http://www.cdc.gov/diabetes/pubs/pdf/kidney_factsheet.pdf.

17. Identify & Evaluate Patients with Chronic Kidney Disease Bethesda, Maryland: National Institutes of Health: National Institute of Diabetes and Digestive and Kidney Diseases 2017 [cited 2 January 2018]. Retrieved from https://www.niddk.nih.gov/health-information/communication-programs/nkdep/identify-manage-patients/evaluate-ckd.

18. Alobaidi, R., Basu, R. K., Goldstein, S. L., & Bagshaw, S. M. (2015). Sepsis-associated acute kidney injury. *Seminars in Nephrology, 35*(1), 2–11.

19. Fatehi, P., & Hsu, C.-Y. Evaluation of acute kidney injury among hospitalized adult patients. UpToDate [Internet]. 2017. Retrieved from https://www.uptodate.com/contents/evaluation-of-acute-kidney-injury-among-hospitalized-adult-patients?source=search_result&search=acute%20kidney%20injury&selectedTitle=2~150.

20. Mamoulakis, C., Tsarouhas, K., Fragkiadoulaki, I., Heretis, I., Wilks, M. F., Spandidos, D. A., et al. (2017). Contrast-induced nephropathy: Basic concepts, pathophysiological implications and prevention strategies. *Pharmacology & Therapeutics*, PubMed PMID: 28642116.

21. Washinger, K. (2017). Acute kidney injury in adults: An underdiagnosed condtion. *The Journal for Nurse Practitioners—JNP, 13*(10), 667–746.

22. Martensson, J., & Bellomo, R. (2017). Does fluid management affect the occurrence of acute kidney injury? *Current Opinion in Anaesthesiology, 30*(1), 84–91.

23. Lameire, N., Vanmassenhove, J., & Lewington, A. (2017). Did KDIGO guidelines on acute kidney injury improve patient outcome? *Intensive Care Medicine, 43*(6), 921–923.

24. Whelton, P. K., Carey, R. M., Aronow, W. S., Casey, D. E., Jr., Collins, K. J., Dennison Himmelfarb, C., et al. (2017). 2017 ACC/AHA/AAPA/ABC/ACPM/AGS/APhA/ASH/ASPC/NMA/PCNA Guideline for the prevention, detection, evaluation, and management of high blood pressure in adults: A report of the American College of Cardiology/American Heart Association Task Force on Clinical Practice Guidelines. *Journal of the American College of Cardiology.*

25. Schmidt, M., Mansfield, K. E., Bhaskaran, K., Nitsch, D., Sorensen, H. T., Smeeth, L., et al. (2017). Serum creatinine elevation after renin-angiotensin system blockade and long term cardiorenal risks: Cohort study. *British Medical Journal, 356*, j791.

26. Hill Gallant, K. M., & Spiegel, D. M. (2017). Calcium balance in chronic kidney disease. *Current Osteoporosis Reports, 15*(3), 214–221.

27. Bansal, N., Dhaliwal, R., & Weinstock, R. S. (2015). Management of diabetes in the elderly. *The Medical Clinics of North America, 99*(2), 351–377.

28. (2016). New recommendations for use of metformin in renal impairment. *The Medical Letter on Drugs and Therapeutics, 58*(1493), 51–52.

29. Chao, C.-T., Tsai, H.-B., Lin, Y.-F., & Ko, W.-J. (2014). Acute kidney injury in the elderly: Only the tip of the iceberg. *Journal of Clinical Gerontolgoy and Geriatrics, 5*(1), 7–12.

30. Singh, M. F., Karakala, N., & Shah, S. V. (2017). Long-term adverse events associated with acute kidney injury. *Journal of Renal Nutrition, 27*(6), 462–464.

CHAPTER **132**

SEXUAL DYSFUNCTION (MALE)
Patricia Polgar-Bailey

DEFINITION AND EPIDEMIOLOGY

Sexuality is a fundamental aspect of human identity and an important determinant of one's quality of life. Sexual dysfunction can lead to sexual frustration, guilt, loss of self-esteem, and interpersonal problems. It often results in a change in partner relationships and dynamics, decreased sexual intimacy, and reduced quality of life. Despite the high prevalence of male sexual dysfunction worldwide, and an even higher incidence among certain populations—such as those with neurologic, endocrine, and other comorbidities; those with combat-related mental health disorders; and cancer survivors.[1-4] Concerns about sexual health are often not elicited by providers owing to a lack of appreciation of the impact of sexual dysfunction or fear of patient embarrassment.

Men with sexual dysfunction are often embarrassed about discussing their problem openly with health care providers. Many men associate declining sexual function with aging and do not appreciate that this is a problem for which there is treatment. In addition, men are generally less likely to seek medical care than women, and men's heath as a concept and discipline is not nearly as well developed as women's health. Men are more inclined to see a provider for problems that specifically affect men most such as baldness, sports injuries, and erectile dysfunction (ED).[5] ED, the most common sexual problem in men, often causes serious distress and prompts men to seek care when they otherwise might not. In addition, the aging population, the increase in available therapies, and the publicity regarding pharmacologic agents for the treatment of ED have increased the awareness of the scope of this problem and resulted in an increased number of men seeking treatment. Incorporation of an understanding of male sexual health and available treatment options can have a tremendous impact on the sexual health and quality of life of men affected by sexual dysfunction.

Sexual dysfunction is broadly defined as the difficulty or inability to fully enjoy sexual intercourse and more specifically includes disorders that interfere with a full sexual response cycle. The human sexual response can be described as a cycle with four phases: desire, excitement, orgasm, and resolution. Sexual dysfunction affects one or more of the first three phases. Resolution is simply the relaxation and reduction in arousal after orgasm. Resolution to the preexcitement phase occurs more rapidly with age, although this is most noticeable in older men. The amount of time that must pass before a man is capable of another ejaculation increases as men age.

The desire phase of the cycle consists of an urge to have sex, sexual fantasies, and sexual attraction to others. Hypoactive sexual desire is a lack of interest in sex or sexual activity, although the actual sexual experience may be normal. The perception or stereotype of men in Western culture is that they want sex as often as they can get it; however, hypoactive sexual desire affects as many as 16% of men, and the number of men seeking treatment for it has increased during the past decade.[6] There is an important distinction between people who have normal sexual desires but choose as part of their lifestyle not to engage in sexual relations and people with hypoactive sexual desire. Hypoactive sexual desire is also different from sexual aversion, which refers to people who find sex distinctly unpleasant or repulsive.

The excitement phase of the sexual response cycle is marked by physical changes of arousal: increases in heart rate, blood pressure, rate of breathing, and muscle tension. ED affects the excitement phase and is the persistent inability to achieve and to maintain an erection sufficient to permit satisfactory sexual performance. Since the National Institutes of Health Consensus Conference in 1988, the term *erectile dysfunction* has replaced the term *impotence*. ED is currently recognized as a medical problem with potential psychological consequences that may interfere with a man's quality of life, self-esteem, and interpersonal relationships.

Based on data from the National Health and Social Life Survey (NHSLS), the prevalence of sexual dysfunction in males is approximately 31%. Some degree of ED, the most common male sexual problem,[7] was reported by 52% of respondents in the Massachusetts Male Aging Study (MMAS[5]); a large epidemiologic study, by as many as 65.6% in a Brazilian study, and almost 60% in a Ghanaian study.[1] After adjustment for age, men with certain comorbidities, including diabetes, heart disease, and hypertension, have significantly higher probabilities for ED than men as a whole.

During the orgasmic phase of the sexual response cycle, an individual's sexual pleasure peaks, sexual tension is released, and the man's semen is ejaculated. Male sexual dysfunctions during this phase include premature ejaculation (PE) and male orgasmic disorder. In 2013, the International Society for Sexual Medicine (ISSM) developed the first evidence-based definition for PE: "a male sexual dysfunction characterized by: (1) ejaculation that always or nearly always occurs prior to or within about 1 minute of vaginal penetration (lifelong PE) or a clinically significant and bothersome reduction in latency time, often to about 3 minutes or less (acquired PE); (2) the inability to delay ejaculation on all or nearly all vaginal penetrations; and (3) negative personal consequences, such as distress, bother, frustration, and/or avoidance of sexual intimacy."[8] Data suggest that the prevalence of acquired PE in the community is approximately 4% among sexually active adults and that men with acquired PE are more likely to seek treatment than men with lifelong PE.[8] The reasons for this difference are unclear, but it has been hypothesized that men with lifelong PE may have accommodated to their rapid ejaculation, whereas those with acquired PE may be bothered to the point of seeking treatment.[8] It is estimated that approximately 30% to 50% of men with PE have concurrent ED, which typically results in early ejaculation with an incomplete erection.[9,10] Men with ED may require higher levels of stimulation to achieve an erection or may intentionally "rush" intercourse to prevent the early detumescence of a partial erection, resulting in PE.[8]

The cause of PE is not completely understood, but PE appears most commonly to result from performance anxiety, inexperience, hurried masturbation experiences, relationship factors, or psychological issues. Although less frequent, it may also be caused by prostatitis, hyperthyroidism, and withdrawal or detoxification from prescribed or recreational drugs.[8] Men with acquired PE have a higher incidence of concomitant ED and other comorbidities, including hypertension, diabetes mellitus, and chronic prostatitis, than men with lifelong PE.[8]

Men are often hesitant to discuss sexual problems with their providers and generally consult them for health-related problems less frequently than women do. In addition, the emphasis in health care visits, particularly for men, tends to be on cardiovascular diseases and other common chronic illnesses, such as hypertension and diabetes, whereas conditions that may be of a more sensitive nature are ignored, thereby reducing the opportunity for the recognition and treatment of problems that substantially affect the quality of life. Research shows that health care providers do not regularly ask about sexual dysfunction with men who are at risk, citing as reasons a lack

of time and the belief that the patient will initiate the discussion.[11] Reluctance to discuss ED on the part of both the patient and the health care provider results in underdiagnosis and lack of treatment. The partner in a relationship significantly influences a man's health-seeking behavior. Men who do not have a supportive partner or who feel particularly vulnerable or fearful or are in denial are less likely to seek help for issues related to sexual dysfunction.

Although sexual dysfunction affects a sizable portion of the male population, a lack of discussion of the condition prevents a significant number of affected men from receiving treatment. Health care providers have become well versed in asking questions about patients' sexual practices in screening for sexually transmitted diseases (STDs) and human immunodeficiency virus (HIV) infection but are less experienced and more uncomfortable when it comes to investigating sexual satisfaction among patients and their partners.[11] It is important for health care providers to include sexual assessment as a component of routine health care surveillance and to become comfortable in eliciting the information that will help identify sexual dysfunction, give insight into its cause, and guide further intervention. It is also important to remember that ED is often a sentinel or early marker for concomitant cardiovascular disease, as well as a risk factor for metabolic comorbidities. Research indicates that men with ED are at significantly greater risk of having a cardiovascular event—angina, myocardial infarction (MI), or stroke—than those without ED.[5] In addition, the relationship between "incident ED" (the first report of ED of any grade) and cardiovascular disease is comparable with that associated with current smoking, family history of MI, and hyperlipidemia.[5] The meaning of this relationship appears to vary depending on age. When ED occurs in a younger man (younger than 60 years), it is associated with a marked increase in future cardiovascular events, whereas in older men it appears to be less of a prognostic indicator.[5]

Eliciting information about sexual health is essential for a thorough assessment of health. In particular, ED can be viewed as a "barometer" of cardiovascular health, and its identification can provide an opportunity to identify and treat modifiable risk factors.[5] Health care providers are in a unique position to address sexual and relationship issues that exist between their patients and their partners. In addition to representing more holistic care, discussing and addressing sexual health concerns may uncover underlying comorbid conditions, improve quality of life and self-esteem, foster a better patient–provider relationship, and increase patient satisfaction.

PATHOPHYSIOLOGY
Disorders of Desire

The etiology of disorders of desire or reduced libido is multifactorial and involves a combination of biologic, psychological, and sociocultural factors. Several hormones combine to produce sexual desire, and lower levels of them can lower the sex drive. In men and women, sexual desire is linked to levels of androgen, testosterone, and dehydroepiandrosterone (DHEA). In men, testosterone levels peak at 19 years of age and demonstrate a linear decline of 1% per year thereafter. DHEA levels begin to decline in the 30s and continue to decline steadily until a low is reached by the age of 60 years. Because a decrease in male hormones begins early, it is suggested that screening for hypogonadism should begin at 50 years of age. Chronic physical illness, as well as stress, pain, or depression related to the illness, directly affects the desire to have sex. The sex drive can also be lowered by some pain medications, certain psychotropic drugs, and a number of illegal drugs, such as cocaine, marijuana, and amphetamines. In addition, low levels of alcohol can enhance the sex drive by reducing inhibitions, but at high levels, alcohol can reduce sex drive. Circumstances and social pressures such as job stress, marital discord and divorce, death in the family, and infertility difficulties can affect one's desire to have sex.

Disorders of Excitement

Erectile function is a neurovascular event initiated by cognitive or tactile stimulation that is processed in the brain. Chemical mediators cause the essential relaxation of tissue and perfusion of the corpora cavernosa and corpus spongiosum. Nitric oxide and cyclic guanosine monophosphate (cGMP) are the primary noncholinergic and cholinergic mediators responsible for the neurogenic aspect of erection. Engorgement of the corpora cavernosa and corpus spongiosum, in turn, compresses the veins to prevent the venous outflow of blood. This is how the erection is maintained and accounts for the vascular component of erection. Any factor that interferes with this process may lead to ED.

The cause of ED may be clearly identified (e.g., a radical prostatectomy) or may be multifactorial, requiring comprehensive assessment. Although ED was believed in the past to be psychogenic, it is currently understood to result from organic causes (e.g., vascular, neurogenic, hormonal, anatomic, or drug induced), psychological causes, or a combination of the two. A normal sexual erectile response is a complex interaction among neurotransmitter, biochemical, and vascular smooth muscle responses initiated by parasympathetic and sympathetic neuronal triggers that integrate physiologic stimuli and sexual desire. Alterations in vascular supply, hormonal changes, neurologic dysfunction, or medications and associated systemic disease may contribute to or exacerbate ED. A list of common organic and psychological risk factors for ED can be found in Box 132.1.

Psychogenic. Psychological factors that may be of etiologic significance include performance anxiety, guilt, and strict religious constraints. Life events, such as a business failure, loss of health, or deterioration in the partner relationship, may also contribute to ED because of their impact on mood, anxiety, self-esteem, and depression. Developmental vulnerabilities, such as a history of child abuse, may have a profound effect on sexual function. Psychological issues, when combined with physiologic problems, can result in significant erectile difficulties.

Hormonal Risk Factors. Testosterone deficiency may be caused by hypothalamic or pituitary tumors or treatment aimed at suppression of testosterone, such as hormonal therapy for prostate cancer. Although the primary effect of testosterone deficiency is decreased libido, ED may result as well. Other conditions that may precipitate decreased libido or ED because of their hormonal effects include hyperprolactinemia, hyperthyroidism, hypothyroidism, Cushing syndrome, and Addison disease.

Cardiovascular Risk Factors. Cardiovascular disorders that affect the penile vasculature can affect different stages of erection, including a failure to initiate erection, a failure to achieve erection, and a failure to sustain erection.

BOX **132.1**

Common Risk Factors for Erectile Dysfunction

NEUROLOGIC CONDITIONS
- Multiple sclerosis
- Peripheral neuropathy
- Radical prostatectomy
- Spinal cord injury
- Stroke
- Parkinson disease

CARDIOVASCULAR CONDITIONS
- Cardiovascular or peripheral vascular disease
- Congestive heart failure
- Hypertension
- Hyperlipidemia
- Cigarette smoking

TRAUMATIC INJURY OR PENILE ABNORMALITIES
- Trauma to perineum, pelvis, penis
- Peyronie disease (penile curvature)
- History of priapism
- History of penile fracture

RADIATION THERAPY
- Pelvic irradiation for malignant conditions

HORMONAL CAUSES
- Decreased testosterone
- Increased prolactin
- Increased luteinizing hormone
- Increased prostate-specific antigen

ENDOCRINE DISORDERS
- Diabetes mellitus
- Hypothyroidism
- Hyperthyroidism
- Pituitary adenoma
- Hypogonadism
- Obesity

PSYCHOGENIC FACTORS
- Performance anxiety
- Depression
- Psychological stress
- Relationship problems

MEDICAL CONDITIONS
- Chronic disease states
- Multiple sclerosis
- Renal failure
- Diabetes mellitus
- Sleep apnea

MEDICATIONS
- See Box 132.2

Pharmacologic Risk Factors. The major classes of drugs that affect erectile function include antihypertensives, antidepressants, and major tranquilizers. ED may result from pharmacologic effects on the central nervous system, vascular system, hormone levels, and libido (Box 132.2). Other medications that have been associated with ED include hormonal agents (e.g., antiandrogens), protease inhibitors, antihistamines, benzodiazepines, selective serotonin reuptake inhibitors (SSRIs), and cytotoxic agents.

Surgical Risk Factors. ED may occur after major surgery that potentially alters either the innervation of or the blood flow to the penis. These procedures may also affect a man's body image and self-perception of masculinity. Examples of such procedures are the radical prostatectomy, radical cystectomy, and abdominal-perineal resection. Nerve-sparing surgical techniques minimize this risk and may result in the preservation of erectile function.

Alcohol and Opioid Use. There are a limited number of studies that have evaluated sexual dysfunction (SD) in men with alcohol or opioid use. However, data indicate that men with heroin addiction or who are on methadone maintenance treatment (MMT) or buprenorphine maintenance treatment (BMT) show a higher rate of SD compared with the general population, ranging from 34% to 85% (heroin addiction), 14% to 81% (MMT), 36% to 83% (BMT), and 90% for naltrexone

BOX **132.2**

Pharmacologic Agents Implicated in the Development of Erectile Dysfunction

CARDIOVASCULAR AGENTS
- Angiotensin-converting enzyme inhibitors
- β-Blockers
- Calcium antagonists
- Centrally acting agents
- Antiarrhythmics

PSYCHOGENIC AGENTS
- Anxiolytics
- Hypnotics
- Selective serotonin reuptake inhibitors
- Serotonin-norepinephrine reuptake inhibitors
- Tricyclic antidepressants
- Antipsychotics, mood stabilizers

NEUROLOGIC AGENTS
- Anticonvulsants (phenytoin [Dilantin], phenobarbital)
- Antiparkinson agents (bromocriptine [Parlodel], levodopa, trihexyphenidyl)

OTHER PHARMACOLOGIC AGENTS
- Analgesics (e.g., opiates)
- Anticholinergics
- Antihistamines (diphenhydramine [Benadryl], hydroxyzine [Vistaril], meclizine [Antivert], promethazine [Phenergan])
- Cytotoxic agents (methotrexate)
- Diuretics (spironolactone, thiazides)
- Immunomodulators (interferon-α)
- Miscellaneous: clofibrate, dichlorphenamide, fenfluramine, ketoconazole, methadone, metoclopramide, methazolamide, norethindrone, thiabendazole
- Recreational and illicit drugs (opioids, amphetamines, cocaine, marijuana, heroin), alcohol, nicotine

maintenance.[12] Rates of SD in men with alcohol dependence are similarly higher (40% to 93%) than in men who do not drink or only drink socially.[12] The most common types of SD reported among men with opioid use or excessive alcohol use include ED, PE, retardant ejaculation, and decreased sexual desire.[12]

Other Factors. Pelvic radiotherapy (e.g., to treat prostate cancer) may damage nerves and blood vessels, potentially resulting in ED.

Disorders of Orgasm

Male orgasmic disorders (i.e., problems with ejaculation) can be caused by low testosterone levels, certain neurologic diseases, and some head and spinal cord injuries. Certain drugs, including hypertensive medications, antidepressants, anxiolytics, antipsychotics, and alcohol, can slow down the sympathetic nervous system and can also affect ejaculation. An important psychological cause of male orgasmic disorder seems to be performance anxiety and the spectator role. If a man focuses on reaching orgasm, he stops being an aroused participant and instead has a tendency to be a self-critical and fearful observer.

CLINICAL PRESENTATION AND PHYSICAL EXAMINATION

Men may not readily offer information about sexual dysfunction, even though it may be the reason for the visit. Because men often avoid routine visits and are known to underuse primary care in general, the provider could suspect that a man with vague somatic complaints might actually be in the office because of concerns about sexual dysfunction. The interactions between the provider and patient are vital in establishing rapport, and the patient's anticipation of the discussion or concern about bringing up the issue may be the source of considerable anxiety or stress. Thus sensitively introducing the subject of sexual health may help create a more comfortable atmosphere and facilitate discussion.

Providers should obtain a broad history, which includes not only sexual concerns but also relationships and life events. Open-ended questions help elucidate the onset of concerns, course over time, and factors that may improve or worsen symptoms. It is helpful to start by asking general questions about sexual activity and interest and then relate this to healthy "masculine" intimacy, rather than by directly asking questions about sexual function. It is important to keep in mind the impact that physical, psychological, and relationship issues can have on sexual health. Compassionate and normalizing statements can be helpful, such as "It is common for men who have had prostate cancer to notice changes in their interest in sexual activity."

In obtaining a history from the patient or partner, the provider may find it useful to identify three types of factors that can contribute to sexual dysfunction: predisposing factors (e.g., restrictive upbringing, disturbed relationships, traumatic sexual experiences), which might make a man more susceptible to sexual dysfunction; precipitating factors (e.g., dysfunction in the partner, discord in the relationship, depression or anxiety, comorbid medical conditions), which may have triggered the onset of the problem; and maintaining factors (e.g., performance anxiety, relationship issues, impaired self-image, poor communication), which sustain the problem.

Specific inquiries about ED should include questions that address the onset of ED (gradual or abrupt), whether there is difficulty in achieving or maintaining an erection, and the presence and quality of nocturnal erections. In addition, the onset of ED, particularly if it is associated with a specific event (e.g., stress), should be determined. Additional information to elicit includes quality and timing of the orgasm, volume and appearance of the ejaculate, presence of sexually induced genital pain or penile curvature (Peyronie disease), and partner sexual function. A brief urologic questionnaire, such as the five-item version of the International Index of Erectile Function Questionnaire, is a validated survey instrument that can be used to assess the nature and severity of ED.[13] The clinical history should include current health problems, a review of systems, and current medications including nonprescription drugs and herbal formulations. Cardiovascular risk stratification is an essential component of the evaluation of ED because of the increased incidence of cardiovascular disease. Questions about exercise tolerance, history of cardiovascular disease, and past and current medication use are important. Men with risk factors for cardiovascular disease should undergo further evaluation and management before treatment of ED is initiated.

In eliciting information about sexual health, the provider also must consider generational issues. The sexual behaviors and interests of aging "baby boomers" are now beginning to emerge through surveys, such as those conducted by AARP. For example, baby boomers appear to hold traditional values about extramarital relationships but are more willing than former generations to experiment with new activities, such as watching pornography with their partners and trying new sexual positions. Another issue to consider is the growing population of divorced and single adults who engage in sexual relationships and may be at risk for STDs, including HIV infection. Relationship issues are a major factor in the decline of sexual activity among older adults.

Relatively little research has been done on the needs and interests of sexual minority patients, but it is important to consider that homosexual men may be reluctant to disclose their sexual orientation or to discuss sexuality because of the negative associations with being gay. Transgender health and the use of cross-sex hormones (estrogens in male-bodied people and androgens in female-bodied people) is increasing around the world, and health care providers must educate themselves to adequately care for these individuals in the primary care setting. Maintaining a nonjudgmental and accepting attitude can increase the comfort level of a patient who finds it difficult to discuss issues related to sexual identity.

Patient history will guide the physical examination, which, if indicated, also focuses on detecting signs of endocrine, vascular, or neurologic deficits and penile abnormality. Testicular atrophy, gynecomastia, or signs of hypothyroidism or hyperthyroidism may indicate hormonal abnormalities. Vascular assessment includes checking pulses in the lower extremities and observing for vascular skin changes in the lower extremities (e.g., hair loss). The presence of a femoral bruit may indicate possible pelvic blood occlusion. Neurologic assessment is focused on testing for genital reflexes (bulbocavernosus, cremasteric, scrotal, sphincter tone) and light touch discrimination. During the genital examination, it is important to palpate for penile plaques, which may indicate Peyronie disease. Plaques in the tunica albuginea limit penile distensibility, causing a bend in the penis with erection. This may interfere with sexual activity by making penetration difficult.

Although approximately 75% of patients with ED have an organic cause (resulting from vascular, neuronal, or endocrine factors), psychosocial, cognitive, and interpersonal variables, often related to illness or disease, play a role in exacerbating or maintaining ED. Assessment of these issues is essential in the evaluation of ED and other types of sexual dysfunction.

DIAGNOSTICS
Essential Diagnostics

The history and physical examination will determine which diagnostic and laboratory tests are indicated. Detection of underlying medical problems is essential in the evaluation of sexual dysfunction, and appropriate diagnostic testing is indicated. There is no preferred first-line diagnostic test for ED, and routine screening is not recommended. History and physical examination are sufficient to make an accurate diagnosis in most cases.[5]

Additional Diagnostics

The American Urological Association (AUA) and the World Health Organization (WHO) recommend limited diagnostic testing for men with ED.[5] Initially, nocturnal penile tumescence is evaluated to determine whether ED is attributable to a psychogenic or organic condition. The snap gauge, a Velcro band with three colored films arranged parallel to one another, is fitted around the penis. Each film ruptures to correspond with the intracavernosal pressures found in erection. Response is gauged by the number of films broken, with none or one indicating absent rigidity and two or three indicating rigid erection. The accuracy of snap gauge results is variable.

The RigiScan (Dacomed Corporation, Minneapolis) is a more sophisticated device that provides continuous tumescence monitoring and can distinguish functional from inadequate erections in the majority of cases.[1]

Studies to evaluate penile vasculature include the intracavernosal injection of a vasoactive drug, duplex Doppler study of the penis, dynamic infusion cavernosometry and cavernosography (DICC), and internal pudendal arteriography. These tests can evaluate for anatomic abnormalities such as Peyronie disease and measure both penile inflow and outflow.[1] Neurologic studies include bulbocavernous reflex latency and nerve conduction studies.

In the absence of a reliable test, the clinician must rely on the patient's history, physical examination, and laboratory testing to determine the cause of ED. Laboratory tests include thyroid-stimulating hormone (TSH) and luteinizing hormone concentrations; serum electrolyte values; serum glucose, blood urea nitrogen (BUN), creatinine, serum testosterone, and prolactin levels; and lipid panel. Serum testosterone to detect hypogonadism maybe useful, especially in older men because the disorder is common in this population.

DIFFERENTIAL DIAGNOSIS

 Emergency treatment indicated for priapism, which may occur after intracavernous drug treatments for ED, if the erection lasts longer than 4 hours.

Incident ED is often a marker of cardiovascular disease; signs and symptoms suggestive of acute coronary artery disease warrant further evaluation.

Sexual dysfunction is considered a symptom of an underlying issue and not a disease. Causes may be organic (including vascular, neurologic, or endocrine dysfunction) or psychogenic (such as mood disorders, relational issues, or performance anxiety). Underlying causes of SD must be evaluated to determine appropriate treatment.

INTERPROFESSIONAL COLLABORATIVE MANAGEMENT

Research supports a multidisciplinary approach to the treatment of sexual dysfunction. Health care providers need to determine their own comfort level with discussions about sexuality and sexual dysfunction. In addition, health care providers need to determine whether the patient's major issues are psychogenic, relational, or organic (often all three are involved) and whether referral to a psychologist, marriage counselor, or sex therapist might be helpful. Relationship counseling (or referral) may be appropriate to help the patient and partner with any emotional and communication barriers to sexual success. Effective communication is essential, and the provider can recommend some excellent self-help books and videos.

Nonpharmacologic Therapy

Anxiety reduction techniques have been a prominent part of psychological approaches for sexual dysfunction. These techniques are based on the principle that, by removal of the source of the anxiety (e.g., by forbidding intercourse and permitting only nondemand caressing), men can overcome performance anxiety and inhibitions. Providers can help alleviate the anxiety by encouraging sensuality, extended foreplay, and a focus on pleasure rather than arousal. It is important to remind the persons involved that treatment often takes time to be fully effective and to be comfortably integrated into their sex lives.

Cognitive restructuring techniques can be used to overcome sexual ignorance and to challenge unrealistic expectations that couples may have about sexuality. Sexual dysfunction, such as ED, and associated anxiety can sometimes lead to the cessation of all sexual activity. In these situations, couples can be coached to give and to receive pleasure in other ways, such as manual or oral stimulation. Increased stimulation may also be necessary for the male partner to achieve an erection and thus can augment pharmacologic therapy.

The primary goal in the management of ED is to determine its cause and treat it when possible, rather than treating the symptom alone. ED may be associated with modifiable and reversible risk factors, including lifestyle and drug-related issues. Addressing these factors can be done before or concurrently with other specific therapies.[1] As a rule, ED can be treated successfully with current treatment options but cannot be cured. The exceptions to this are psychogenic ED, post-traumatic arteriogenic ED in young men, and ED from hormonal causes, which may resolve with specific treatment.[1] Most ED therapy is not cause specific but rather follows a structured treatment strategy that depends on a number of factors including efficacy, safety, invasiveness, cost, and patient preference.[1]

For ED with concomitant risk factors, lifestyle changes and risk factor modification should precede or accompany any pharmacologic therapy. The potential benefits of lifestyle modification are particularly apparent in men with specific comorbidities, such as cardiovascular or metabolic disorders (e.g., diabetes and hypertension). In such situations, lifestyle changes have the potential to improve not just ED and cardiovascular and metabolic health but also overall health.[1]

Psychotherapy is the preferred treatment for psychogenic ED. Sexual counseling can enhance communication, ease some of the stress associated with ED, and dispel myths. For instance, men may not realize that they do not have to have an erection to have an orgasm and may believe intercourse to be their only means of sexual expression. In mixed psychogenic and organic ED, psychotherapy may relieve anxieties and increase the success of medical or surgical intervention.

Group or individual cognitive behavioral therapy, psychosexual therapy, and relationship or couples therapy may improve sexual dysfunction. Research suggests that men who have received psychosocial interventions in addition to pharmacotherapy may have had more successful intercourse compared with those receiving medications alone. In addition, psychoeducation about the medical and psychosocial causes of ED in conjunction with reassurance and support may be adequate to restore normal sexual function.

Pharmacologic Therapy

Oral phosphodiesterase type 5 (PDE5) inhibitors facilitate erection by enhancing the effects of nitric oxide and blocking the degradation of cGMP. Inhibition of PDE5 results in smooth muscle relaxation with associated increased arterial flow, which leads to compression of the subtunical venous plexus and penile erection.[1] These medications do not initiate an erection, and sexual stimulation is required for an erection to occur. They are the first-line pharmacotherapy for ED in patients with no contraindications to their use. Currently, four PDE5 inhibitors are available in the United States: sildenafil (Viagra), vardenafil (Levitra), tadalafil (Cialis), and avanafil (Stendra).[14] They are similar in their action and efficacy. Common to all four drugs is the need for sexual stimulation to affect the release of nitric oxide. Evidence has shown the PDE5 inhibitors to be effective in a wide range of patients with ED. They are not the preferred option for men with neurogenic ED and are absolutely contraindicated in patients who are taking nitrates secondary to increased vasodilation with concomitant use (Table 132.1).

Although PDE5 inhibitors have a similar mechanism of action, there are significant differences among the agents in terms of pharmacokinetics; the ones that most directly affect patient preference are onset and duration of action. Sildenafil, vardenafil, and avanafil have a rapid onset of action and remain effective for a short time. In addition, sildenafil and vardenafil are more effective if they are taken on an empty stomach; eating of a high-fat meal before either drug is taken reduces the peak plasma concentration. Avanafil is rapidly absorbed (within 30 to 45 minutes), and food does not appear to delay or decrease drug absorption.

By facilitating a sexual response, PDE5 inhibitors may help couples return to a more satisfying sexual lifestyle. However, even with these agents, other underlying or unresolved issues may require counseling or other types of psychological interventions.

Second-line therapies for the treatment of ED include intraurethral suppositories, intracavernous injections, and vacuum pump devices. Alprostadil (prostaglandin E_1) is indicated for the treatment of ED related to angiogenic, neurogenic, psychogenic, or mixed causes. Alprostadil is available as a urethral suppository (Muse) or as a solution for intracavernosal injection (Caverject, Edex).[1] The dose is highly individualized, which requires the patient to receive a test dose in the clinical setting. For this reason, patients wishing to pursue this option are usually referred to a urologist. Efficacy rates for intracavernous alprostadil in the treatment of ED overall appear to be greater than 70%, with similar rates in certain patient subgroups such as those with diabetes or cardiovascular disease.[1] Reported satisfaction rates appear to be quite high for both patients (87.5% to 93%) and partners (86% to 90%). Complications of intracavernous alprostadil include penile pain, prolonged erections (5%), priapism (1%), and fibrosis (2%). Pain is usually self-limited after prolonged use and can be alleviated by the addition of sodium bicarbonate or local anesthesia. Contraindications to its use include men with a hypersensitivity to alprostadil, those at risk for priapism, and those with a history of bleeding disorders.[1]

For men whose only difficulty is maintaining an erection, a constriction band (e.g., Actis venous flow controller) applied

TABLE 132.1   Phosphodiesterase Type 5 Inhibitors

Drug	Sildenafil (Viagra)	Vardenafil (Levitra)	Tadalafil (Cialis)	Avanafil (Stendra)
Dose	25–100 mg on an empty stomach Starting dose is 50 mg	5–20 mg	5–20 mg 2.5 or 5 mg for once-daily use	100–200 mg approximately 30 min before sexual intercourse
Peak time	1 h	42–54 min	2 h	30–45 min
Excretion	8–12 h	8–12 h	36 h	5 h
Contraindications	Nitrates Resting blood pressure <90/50 or >170/110 mm Hg Cardiac failure Unstable angina Retinitis pigmentosa (applies to all phosphodiesterase type 5 inhibitors) Caution with α-blockers	Nitrates Same as sildenafil Associated with minor QT interval prolongation Those taking class I or class II antiarrhythmics Caution with α-blockers	Nitrates Same as sildenafil Caution with α-blockers other than tamsulosin (Flomax)	Nitrates Same as sildenafil Caution with α-blockers Caution with concomitant use of CYP3A4 inhibitors
Adverse side effects	Headache Flushing Nasal congestion Abnormal vision Dyspepsia Hearing loss	Headache Flushing Nasal congestion Abnormal vision Dyspepsia Hearing loss	Headache Flushing Nasal congestion Abnormal vision Dyspepsia Back pain Myalgias	Headache Flushing Nasal congestion Sore throat Abnormal vision Dyspepsia Back pain

at the base of the penis after erection is achieved may be all that is needed. Vacuum devices are associated with an 80% to 90% success rate and are among the least invasive and least expensive of the current treatment options. They produce an erection by creating a vacuum around the penis that triggers passive blood flow into the corpora cavernosa. Erection is then maintained by a constriction band applied at the base of the penis. A certain amount of manual dexterity is required to use these devices, but once men become comfortable with their use, many men can create an erection sufficient for vaginal penetration and intercourse.

Sexual dysfunction is a common side effect of some antidepressant medications, particularly SSRIs, serotonin-norepinephrine reuptake inhibitors (SNRIs), and some tricyclics, and are a common reason for discontinuation.

Hormonal imbalance, such as low levels of testosterone or high levels of prolactin, is a less common cause of ED. Testosterone replacement therapy (TRT) has been shown to improve libido in older men with low testosterone levels; however, the role of testosterone in the physiology of erections is unclear. Thus TRT for the treatment of ED and androgen deficiency is controversial. There is a US Food and Drug Administration (FDA) warning regarding the potential for cardiovascular or cerebrovascular events related to TRT.[15] TRT may increase prostate size and cause lower urinary tract symptoms, but a causal relationship between testosterone supplementation and prostate cancer has not been demonstrated.

Surgical management includes vascular surgery or implantation of a penile prosthesis. The goal of vascular surgery is to increase arterial inflow to the corpora cavernosa and to increase venous outflow resistance. Candidates are selected only after careful vascular examination, measurement of intracavernous pressures, and observation of the patient's response to certain pharmacologic agents. Younger men with discrete lesions, usually sustained from pelvic or perineal trauma, seem to be the best candidates for vascular surgery.

Placement of a penile prosthesis remains the third-line treatment of ED and is a therapeutic option for individuals in whom first- and second-line therapies have failed and those who cannot tolerate these therapies. Penile prostheses may be malleable, mechanical, or inflatable devices and provide girth and rigidity; they do not increase length. The decision to proceed with implant therapy often comes after treatment with the less invasive options has been unsuccessful. Complications of penile implants are infection, erosion, and component failure, and patients must be counseled regarding the risks, benefits, expectations, and possible complications of these procedures. Because of improvements in design and more durable materials, the complication rate has significantly decreased during the past few years, and patient–partner satisfaction has increased.

INDICATIONS FOR REFERRAL

Underlying or refractory medical problems should be referred to the appropriate specialist. Persistent sexual dysfunction requires consultation with a urologist who has a subspecialty in sexual dysfunction. Patients with hormonal abnormalities should be referred to an endocrinologist or urologist. Referral for sexual counseling or psychotherapy should be considered when appropriate. Modern sex therapy is short term and instructive, typically lasting 15 to 20 sessions. It centers on specific sexual problems and includes assessment and conceptualization of the problem, education about sexuality, recognition of mutual responsibility and attitude change if necessary, elimination of performance anxiety, and help with improving sexual and general communication skills to change destructive lifestyle or marital interactions. Sex therapy does not deal with broad personality issues, and if these are contributing factors, psychotherapy is indicated.

COMPLICATIONS

Unfulfilled or even destroyed relationships, lack of self-esteem, and depression are common complications of sexual dysfunction. Difficulties related to sexual health often cause the cessation of all sexual activity. This withdrawal of affection can lead to diminished sexual desire and can exacerbate whatever distance or conflict already exists in the relationship.

LIFE SPAN CONSIDERATIONS

Physical, social, and sexual maturation can be a source of satisfaction as well as confusion and anxiety for adolescents, who would like to talk with their health care provider about sexual issues, particularly those they are curious about. Masturbation is a normal and healthy activity at all ages and may serve as a substitute for partnered sexual behavior during adolescence. Creation of a trusting environment for discussion around issues of consensual or forced sexual experiences, sexual orientation, risk factors for unprotected intercourse (e.g., alcohol and drug use), and family planning will assist the adolescent in developing healthy sexual behaviors as an adult.

Reduction in sexual functioning in the later years may be associated with hormonal changes and concurrent physiologic illnesses, such as vascular and coronary artery disease, stroke, diabetes, hypertension, and hyperlipidemia. Complications from medical or surgical treatments (e.g., genitourinary and prostate surgeries) can also play a role in sexual dysfunction. Older adults are at higher risk for sexual dysfunction related to pharmacologic agent side effects and effects of prolonged cigarette smoking. The normal physical changes that accompany the aging process are inevitable, but health care providers can be helpful in preventing loss of sexual activity as a result of preventable conditions. Physical intimacy and sexual activity are integral to an individual's overall quality of life, and health care providers should assist patients of all ages in achieving and maintaining healthy sexual function.

PATIENT AND PARTNER EDUCATION

Patient education is essential to the success of treatment for sexual dysfunction. The health care provider must take the necessary time to counsel patients about the available options appropriate to their individual needs. It is important to remember that sexual dysfunction is a couple's problem and to include the partner whenever possible.

- Provide clear instructions and realistic expectations of treatment and educate regarding the couples' role in its success.
- For couples using penile injection therapy, provide emergency contact information if needed.

Follow-up is important to determine whether further intervention is needed. Patients appreciate knowing that their providers are concerned about their sexual health and are open to discussing these issues with them.

HEALTH PROMOTION

Early detection and screening for patients at high risk for sexual dysfunction should be considered in the primary care setting. Such patients include those with a history of heavy cigarette use, obesity, sleep apnea, chronic medical problems (such as hypertension, diabetes, or cardiovascular disease), psychological issues, and unresolved life stressors. Sexual dysfunction may be the first indication of underlying cardiovascular disease or serious comorbidity. Health promotion behaviors, such as smoking cessation, daily exercise, low-fat diet, and stress reduction, can minimize risk for sexual dysfunction.

REFERENCES

1. Hatzimouratidis, K., Eardley, I., Giuliano, F., Hatzichristou, D., Moncada, I., Salonia, A., et al. (2014). Guidelines on male sexual dysfunction: Erectile dysfunction and premature ejaculation. *European Association of Urology*. Retrieved from http://uroweb.org/wp-content/uploads/14-Male-Sexual-Dysfunction_LR.pdf. (Accessed 26 December 2015).
2. Fode, M., Krogh-Jespersen, S., Brackett, N. L., Ohl, D. A., Lynne, C. M., & Sønksen, J. (2014). Male sexual dysfunction and infertility associated with neurological disorders. *Asian Journal of Andrology*, 14, 61–68.
3. Breyer, B. N., Cohen, B. E., Bertenthal, D., Rosen, R. C., Neylan, T. C., & Seal, K. H. (2014). Sexual dysfunction in male Iraq and Afghanistan war veterans: Association with posttraumatic stress disorder and other combat-related mental health disorders: a population-based cohort study. *The Journal of Sexual Medicine*, 11, 75–83.
4. Chung, E., & Brock, G. (2013). Sexual rehabilitation and cancer survivorship: A state of art review of current literature and management strategies in male sexual dysfunction among prostate cancer survivors. *The Journal of Sexual Medicine*, 10(Suppl. 1), 102–111.
5. Miner, M. M. (2012). Men's health in primary care: An emerging paradigm of sexual function and cardiometabolic risk. *The Urologic Clinics of North America*, 39, 1–23.
6. Heiman, J. (2002). Sexual dysfunction: Overview of prevalence, etiological factors and treatments. *Journal of Sex Research*, 39(1), 73–78.
7. Kyle, J. A., Brown, D. A., & Hill, J. K. (2013). Avanafil for erectile dysfunction. *The Annals of Pharmacotherapy*, 47(10), 1312–1320.
8. Serefoglu, E. C., McMahon, C. G., Waldinger, M. C., et al. (2014). An evidence-based unified definition of lifelong and acquired premature ejaculation: Report of the Second International Society for Sexual Medicine Ad Hoc Committee for the Definition of Premature Ejaculation. *The Journal of Sexual Medicine*, 11, 1423–1441.
9. Rosen, R. C., MCMahon, C. G., Niederberger, C., et al. (2007). Correlates to the clinical diagnosis of premature ejaculation: Results from a large observational study of men and their partners. *The Journal of Urology*, 177, 1059.
10. Porst, H., Montorsi, F., Rosen, R. C., Gaynor, L., Grupe, S., & Alexander, J. (2007). The Premature Ejaculation Prevalence and Attitudes (PEPA) survey: prevalence, comorbidities, and professional help-seeking. *European Urology*, 51, 816–823.
11. Kirby, C. N., Piterman, L., & Giles, C. (2009). GP management of erectile dysfunction: The impact of clinical audit and guidelines. *Australian Family Physician*, 38(8), 637–641.
12. Grover, S., Mattoo, S. K., Pendharkar, S., et al. (2014). Sexual dysfunction in patients with alcohol and opioid dependence. *Indian Journal of Psychological Medicine*, 36(4), 355–365.
13. Rosen, R. C., Cappelleri, J. C., Smith, M. D., Lipsky, J., & Peña, B. M. (1999). Development and evaluation of an abridged, 5-item version of the International Index of Erectile Dysfunction (IIEF-5) as a diagnostic tool for erection dysfunction. *International Journal of Impotence Research*, 11(6), 319–326.
14. Huang, S. A., & Lie, J. D. (2013). Phosphodiesterase-5 (PDE) inhibitors in the management of erectile dysfunction. *Pharmacy & Therapeutics*, 38(7), 407, 414–419.
15. FDA Drug Safety Communication. FDA cautions about using testosterone products for low testosterone due to aging; requires labeling change to inform of possible increased risk of heart attack and stroke with use. Retrieved from: http://www.fda.gov/Drugs/DrugSafety/ucm436259.htm.

CHAPTER **133**

TESTICULAR DISORDERS
Daniel A. Blaz

 Immediate referral is warranted for sudden onset of severe pain in or swelling of the scrotum, elevation or abnormally positioning of a testicular, scrotal, or testicular erythema, tender scrotal masses, evidence of increasing hematoma, absent cremasteric reflex, and testicular or scrotal trauma. Associated but nonspecific symptoms of testicular torsion include dysuria, abdominal pain, nausea, and fever.

DEFINITION AND EPIDEMIOLOGY

Scrotal pain may be a symptom of an underlying pathologic condition of the scrotum or testis. The pain may be described as sharp, dull, aching, uncomfortable, or tender, and it is characterized as mild, moderate, or severe. The pain may be sudden in onset, remitting, or progressively escalating in severity. Scrotal pain may be the chief complaint or an incidental finding during the history and physical examination. It is necessary to determine the cause of the pain to evaluate the need for emergent referral or intervention and to exclude potentially life-threatening or fertility-threatening conditions.

Scrotal masses may be nodules or cystic changes on the skin of the scrotum; may involve intrascrotal contents, such as the testis, epididymis, spermatic cord, and tunica vaginalis; or may be the result of herniation of abdominal structures into the scrotal sac. Palpation may reveal single or multiple nodules of varying sizes with consistencies that range from soft to firm. The mass may be freely movable or fixed and may range from nontender to extremely painful to touch or manipulation. Masses may be found during testicular self-examination (TSE) or are discovered during examination and palpation of the scrotum by a health care provider. The mass may go undetected if it is small, if enlargement is gradual, or if discomfort is minimum or absent.

Scrotal swelling, or edema, may involve only one side of the scrotum (left or right hemiscrotal edema) or both sides (bilateral scrotal edema) and may indicate an underlying pathologic condition. Edema caused by a hydrocele may be benign, whereas swelling related to testicular torsion or a malignant tumor of the testis may be potentially life threatening. The clinical presentation of testicular cysts and dysplasia is enlarged testes, and both are clinically interpreted as neoplasms until otherwise evaluated. Testicular malignancy has doubled over the past 40 years and accounts for approximately 1% of all malignant neoplasms in men in the United States.[1,2]

The epidemiology of scrotal pain, masses, and swelling depends on the cause of the disorders that manifest these symptoms. Specific disorders may occur more often in certain age groups. The causes of scrotal pain, masses, or swelling discussed in this chapter are limited to those most commonly encountered in primary care: varicocele, epididymitis, epididymo-orchitis, spermatocele, hydrocele, hematocele, testicular torsion and torsion of the appendix testis, trauma, scrotal hernia, and testicular tumors.

PATHOPHYSIOLOGY

A varicocele is an abnormal dilation of the pampiniform plexus and spermatic veins in the spermatic cord.[3-5] The cause of a varicocele has been determined to be a multifactorial process that involves anatomic variations (the left gonadal vein is longer than the right, and the left testicular vein inserts at an angle into the left renal vein) and incompetent valves within the pampiniform venous plexus, which results in a backflow of blood and venous pooling.[3,4] Varicoceles usually develop slowly, are often symptomatic, and can lead to testicular damage or dysfunction and male infertility.[5] They occur in less than 1% of boys younger than 10, but this gradually increases to 15% in the young adult male age range.[4,6] Varicoceles are commonly identified in men with primary infertility, with approximately 35% to 40% of infertile males being diagnosed with a left-sided varicocele.[3,5,6] In addition, the prevalence of varicocele increases as men age, with 42% of the geriatric population having an identified varicocele.[4] Although the majority of varicoceles are left sided, bilateral varicoceles occur in approximately 30% to 80% of males.[5] A right-sided varicocele is a rare occurrence and should raise concern for a secondary cause of the varicocele, specifically an abdominal, pelvic, or retroperitoneal mass.[4,5]

Epididymitis is an acute or chronic inflammation of the epididymis and is the most common cause of acute scrotal pain in men, with the majority of cases occurring at ages 14 to 35.[7] The cause may be bacterial, viral, parasitic, chemically induced, or related to trauma, and it is further categorized as a nonspecific or specific infection or traumatic injury. Nonspecific infections are caused by gram-negative rods, gram-positive cocci, or anaerobic bacteria associated with a group of diseases with similar symptoms. Inflammation of the epididymis is occasionally caused by trauma or urinary reflux from the urethra through the vas deferens.[7,8] The two most common causes, especially in younger men, are *Chlamydia trachomatis* and *Neisseria gonorrhoeae*.[7,9] Other causative agents include *Escherichia coli*, *Haemophilus influenzae*, tuberculosis, cryptococci, and *Brucella* organisms in men who engage in unprotected anal intercourse.[7,10] Epididymitis has several nonsexually transmitted causes, including Enterobacteriaceae and *Pseudomonas aeruginosa*, which are associated with urinary tract infections and prostatitis.[10] In men older than 35 years, epididymitis is most often associated with urinary tract pathogens, structural abnormalities, and urologic procedures or instrumentation, such as transurethral resection of the prostate and urethral catheterization.[10,11] Epididymitis can also spread to the entire testicle (epididymo-orchitis) as a result of many of the same pathogens (*C. trachomatis*, *N. gonorrhoeae*, and *E. coli*) that cause epididymitis or from reflux of urine from straining, although the exact cause is unclear.[12,13]

Orchitis is a systemic, blood-borne infection that results in an acute inflammation of one or both testicles. It may coexist with infections of the prostate and epididymis; be a consequence of systemic viral infections, such as mumps; or be a complication of syphilis, mycobacterial infections, or fungal infections.[9] Orchitis is commonly caused by *C. trachomatis* and *N. gonorrhoeae* in adolescents and urinary tract pathogens such as *E. coli* in men older than 35.[12,14] When orchitis is a complication of mumps, it is seen in 25% of postpubertal males and may be accompanied by a hydrocele and scrotal wall thickening.[12,14]

A spermatocele is a benign, painless sperm-filled cyst of the epididymis located between the head of the epididymis and the testes and arising from the tubules that connect the rete testis to the head of the epididymis.[15,16] Spermatoceles typically form from the obstruction of the efferent duct and contain a milky fluid that consist of spermatozoa, lymphocytes, and debris.[15,17,18] Spermatoceles have been reported to commonly occur after vasectomies and may be present in 30% of males.[16,18]

A hydrocele is an accumulation of fluid within the tunica vaginalis surrounding the testicle; it may also result from a patent processus vaginalis at birth and sometimes closes spontaneously within the first 1 to 2 years of life.[16,19] Hydroceles are the most common cause of painless scrotal swelling; in adults they are often the result of trauma, a hernia, testicular tumor, or torsion or a complication of epididymitis.[13,15,18]

Similar to a hydrocele, a hematocele is a collection of fluid in the tunica vaginalis of the testes and manifests as a mass.[18]

However, a hematocele is a collection of blood (rather than serous fluid) and usually is precipitated by trauma and can be painful and tender on palpation.[13,18,20]

Testicular torsion is an obstruction of blood flow to the testes because of a twisting of the arteries and veins in the spermatic cord.[21-23] Testicular torsion has an overall incidence of 1 in 4000, with the majority of cases occurring from 12 to 18 years of age.[22] Testicular torsion is most often unilateral (commonly involving the left testis). There are two different types of torsion: extravaginal and intravaginal.[22] Extravaginal torsion occurs with the twisting of the spermatic cord, testis, and process vaginalis; intravaginal torsion is failure of the testis to adhere to the scrotal wall, creating a "bell clapper deformity."[14,22] Extravaginal torsion is rare and is more commonly seen in neonates; intravaginal torsion is mostly seen in adolescents.[14,22] An appendage (appendix testis) on the testicles that is vestigial tissue may twist, making it difficult to distinguish from a testicular torsion.[21] The appendix testis is located at the superior pole of the testicle and is the most common cause of acute scrotal pain in children.[14]

Trauma to the scrotum and testicles results in 4% to 8% of testicular torsions.[20] This condition results in congestion of venous blood flow and concomitant edema of the testis. Trauma to the scrotum can be caused by burns, blunt force, or penetrating injury or may be sports related; it can involve the testicle.[20] The majority of blunt force testicular trauma is isolated, but approximately half of such injuries occur during sporting activities.[20] Therefore no matter what the mechanism is for testicular torsion, it should be included within the differential diagnosis for any scrotal trauma.[20]

A scrotal-inguinal hernia results when a segment of the bowel slips through the internal inguinal ring, where it may remain in the inguinal canal or pass into the scrotal sac. An inguinal hernia may occur as a result of a defect in the anterior abdominal wall or because of a patent process vaginalis.[8] Inguinal hernias predominantly affect men (9:1) and have the highest incidence in men aged 40 to 59 years.[24] A hernia may move freely between the abdomen and the scrotum or can be spontaneously reduced by digital manipulation.[8] When a hernia becomes strangulated or is unreducible, this compromises the blood supply and requires emergent surgical reduction.[8] Strangulation should be suspected when a tender mass is palpated in the scrotum in addition to redness, nausea, and vomiting.[24]

The origin of testicular tumors can be divided into two primary categories: germ cell and stromal tumors.[1] On the basis of the histologic and genetic origin of the tumor, neoplasms of germ cell origin may be further divided into seminomas and nonseminomas.[1]

Testicular malignant neoplasms are relatively uncommon in the general population and account for only 1% of all cancers in men in the United States.[2] Testicular cancer occurs most often at ages 20 to 39 years and is the most common form of cancer in men aged 15 to 34 years, although these tumors have also been reported in infants and in older men.[2,17,25] The risk for testicular cancer in white men is more than five times that of African-American men and more than double that of Asian men.[17] Although the exact cause of testicular tumors is unknown, tumors have been associated with scrotal trauma, atrophy, undescended testicles (cryptorchidism), exogenous estrogen exposure, and family history of testicular cancer.[2,17] Males who have an undescended testicle (cryptorchidism)

have an approximately 17% higher incidence of developing testicular cancer than the general population.[2] Germ cell tumors (GCTs) are the most common type of testicular tumor and account for 90% to 95% of all primary malignant neoplasms.[1,17,25] Stromal tumors are rare and usually consist of Leydig and Sertoli cell tumor types.[17] GCTs are associated with serum tumor marker products alpha fetoprotein (AFP), human chorionic gonadotropin (hCG), and lactate dehydrogenase (LDH) and are critical to diagnosing, prognosing, staging, and monitoring treatment response of testicular cancer.[1,25] Metastasis from testicular tumors occurs primarily through the lymphatic system, usually to the retroperitoneal lymph nodes.[1,17]

Elephantiasis is caused by a filariasis (parasitic disease) that affects the scrotum, causing massive scrotal lymphedema.[26,27] Filariasis is caused by threadlike roundworms, called filariae, that are transmitted by various mosquitoes, flies, and biting midges and is most often caused by *Wuchereria bancrofti*.[27] Although this is a rare cause of testicular problems in the United States, it should be considered in the differential diagnosis in persons who have recently traveled to Africa or Asia or in health care workers involved in humanitarian missions in those areas.[27]

CLINICAL PRESENTATION

With testicular disorders, the history and presenting symptoms often suggest the underlying pathologic condition. However, because some disorders may not cause significant discomfort, all male patients should be queried about changes in testicular size or the presence of nodules or masses, pain, or penile discharge. The following disorders may be identified by the presenting complaint.

Varicocele

There are usually no visible outward signs other than a blue color through light-colored scrotal skin. The patient may be asymptomatic or complain of a dull pain, ache, or heaviness in the affected hemiscrotum that worsens with activity or straining.[4,15] Male patients may report enlargement in a testicle that decreases in the supine position; however, the mass may not be seen or palpable on lying down.[5]

Epididymitis

The patient may have a low-grade fever, chills, and a heavy sensation.[22] The history includes a sudden onset of severe pain that may be partially relieved by elevating the scrotum (Prehn sign).[10,22] Additional signs and symptoms include blood in semen, penile discharge, lower abdominal discomfort, groin pain, lump in the testicle, and pain with intercourse or ejaculation. Symptoms may also include dysuria, flank pain, and testicular pain that is made worse by a bowel movement or straining.[17]

Orchitis

The patient may report a gradual onset of acute or moderate pain, testicular swelling, and fever; he may have a concomitant hydrocele and scrotal wall thickening.[14,22]

Spermatocele

A spermatocele typically is a painless, cystic mass that is separate from the testis and located superior or inferior to it.[16] It is in general movable, firm, and painless, with distinct borders, and it is easily visible on transillumination.[15,16]

Hydrocele

Hydroceles are usually painless and may be present for long periods, partially resolve, and recur before the patient seeks medical attention.[15] Gradual enlargement of the scrotum occurs with marked edema, which may be uncomfortable because of the added weight. A hydrocele may occur secondary to a tumor when excess serous fluid accumulates in the scrotal sac.[15]

Hematocele

The patient may report a painful scrotum that is tender to palpation. The hematocele is not visible on transillumination. It may have begun after recent surgery, trauma, or a sports-related injury.[18,20]

Testicular Torsion

Testicular torsion, which involves twisting of the spermatic cord and resultant occlusion of the blood flow, is sudden in onset, is extremely painful, and may awaken the patient from sleep or be trauma induced.[20,23] In addition to testicular pain, the patient may experience abdominal pain, nausea, and vomiting; 25% of patients have a fever.[20] Two clinical signs that are suggestive of testicular torsion are a testicle that rides high in the scrotum and an absent cremasteric reflex on examination.[20]

Torsion of the Appendix Testis

The classic presentation is a gradual onset of unilateral testicular pain, edema, and tenderness over the head of the testicle.[8,21] The "blue dot sign" is often present, in which a blue discoloration is noted on transillumination, usually indicating an infarcted or ischemic appendage.[10,22]

Trauma

There may be a history of blunt or penetrating injury to the scrotum that may involve the scrotal contents, leading to severe pain, bruising, edema, nausea, vomiting, or syncope.[20] Depending on the type and extent of the injury, the patient may be in excruciating pain, have minimal pain, have a noted hematocele, or have loss of normal testicular shape because of testis rupture.

Scrotal-Inguinal Hernia

Scrotal swelling, mild to moderate pain on straining, scrotal heaviness, and the possible presence of a bulge are common complaints.[28] The edema is increased after standing in an erect position but decreases when the patient is recumbent.[29]

Testicular Tumor

The patient usually seeks medical care for evaluation of an abnormal mass found during self-examination or has symptoms similar to those of epididymitis, orchitis, or hydrocele.[25] The most common symptom or finding associated with a testicular tumor is a palpable mass that is often accompanied by edema or a sensation of fullness or heaviness in the scrotum.[2,25] Complaints, such as back or abdominal pain, nausea, anorexia, or bowel and bladder symptoms, may occur with retroperitoneal lymph node involvement and suggest metastatic disease.[1]

Elephantiasis

Elephantiasis leads to massive scrotal lymphedema, thickened scrotal skin, and, in severe cases, skin ulcerations.[27]

PHYSICAL EXAMINATION

Examination begins with inspection of the scrotum. Scrotal size can change with temperature variations because of the cremaster muscle response. Asymmetry is expected because the left hemiscrotum is normally positioned lower than the right.[30] The skin of each hemiscrotum should be inspected carefully, spreading the rugae between the fingers. Care should be taken to inspect both the anterior and posterior surfaces to detect any lesions. Each hemiscrotum should be palpated with the thumb and first two fingers of both hands. The scrotal contents should be easily movable in a sliding fashion. The testes should be smooth, equal, firm but rubbery, and the shape is round in the newborn transitioning to ovoid during puberty.[14] The size of a testicle after puberty is on average 4 to 5 cm in length, 2 to 4 cm in width, and 3 cm anteroposteriorly.[30] The normal epididymis is divided into the head, body, and tail and is located in the superior, posterior portion of the testis.[14,30] It is softer than the testis, nontender, and smooth. To palpate the spermatic cord, the provider should slide the fingers and thumb up from the epididymis. The cord should feel smooth and nontender. Documentation should include any tenderness or pain, discoloration, edema, or abnormal findings, such as those seen in the conditions discussed in the following sections.

Varicocele

Bluish color shows through the scrotal skin; when the patient stands, palpation of the soft mass reveals a "bag of worms" on the proximal spermatic cord, more frequently encountered on the left side.[4,5] Varicoceles become smaller when the patient is supine and are better seen when the patient is upright or performs a Valsalva maneuver.[4] If a right varicocele is identified, it is noted to be rare and may indicate venous obstruction, a retroperitoneal process, or abdominal or renal neoplasm.[5,31]

Epididymitis

The scrotum is red, enlarged, and extremely tender and may be difficult to distinguish from the testis.[10] The position of the testicle should be noted; it should be located in its normal anatomic position.[22] The examination should include evaluation for strong predictors of epididymitis, which include an intact cremasteric reflex, a positive Prehn sign (pain relief with the elevation of the affected testicle), and pain along the upper pole of the testicle.[10] Other elements that may be noted during the examination are fever, tachycardia, urinary tract infection symptoms (dysuria, urgency, frequency), and inflammation of the testis (orchitis).[13,22]

Orchitis

As with epididymitis, testicular edema may be so pronounced that it is difficult to distinguish the testes from the epididymis. Palpation may reveal swollen, very tense testes that are painful, and the patient may be febrile. Inflammation of the testis usually involves systemic viral infections (commonly mumps) and includes unilateral or bilateral erythema, edema, and scrotal tenderness, which occurs 4 to 7 days after initial fever.[9,11]

Spermatocele

The spermatocele is palpated as a small, nontender, freely movable mass above and behind the testis.[15,16] The mass may arise from the vasa efferentia (tubules that connect the rete testis to the epididymis), the epididymis, or cystic structures on the upper pole of the testis.[16] Transillumination of the mass in a darkened room may help visualize the mass.[15]

Hydrocele

Palpation reveals a painless mass that appears easily on transillumination.[15,17] The hydrocele may fluctuate in size and is identified by a smooth, tense scrotal mass.[15] A hydrocele that is noted in men older than 30 years can be secondary to a testicular tumor.[15,32]

Hematocele

Palpation reveals scrotal swelling that does not transilluminate and may be tender to palpation.[18,20]

Testicular Torsion

Torsion is more common in the left hemiscrotum. The scrotum may be edematous and erythematous, and the affected side may have a higher position as a result of rotation.[20,33] The spermatic cord is swollen and extremely tender, the epididymis may be felt anteriorly, and the majority of patients will have an absent cremasteric reflex.[20,33] In some instances a small area of cyanosis (blue dot sign) may be present on the scrotal skin and indicates torsion of the appendix testis.[20]

Torsion of the Appendix Testis

Torsion of the appendage testis commonly occurs in children and frequently is seen at ages 7 to 12 years.[14] On examination, the testicle will be tender along the superior pole of the testis, with scrotal edema and enlargement of the epididymis, and often the blue dot sign is identified.[14,21] Occasionally, nausea and vomiting occur but are less frequent than with a testicular torsion.[8]

Trauma

Bruising, bleeding, edema, and severe pain may be present and are highly suspicious for scrotal trauma.[18,20] Inspection should include careful comparison of coloration to determine the extent of bruising or expanding hematoma. A ruptured testis should be suspected if there is evidence of increasing hematoma or hematocele; edema; and pain.[20] Palpation should include external skin and scrotal contents. Documentation includes the time and date of injury, type of trauma, and any change in signs or symptoms since the time of injury.

Scrotal-Inguinal Hernia. Inspection reveals an enlarged hemiscrotum or a bulge in the groin area that may spontaneously reduce when the patient is supine or with manual reduction.[24] The provider will not be able to move the fingers above the mass, which should be soft and mushy but painless unless it is incarcerated and ischemic. Scrotal hernias do not transilluminate. Auscultation of bowel sounds over the mass is significant for the diagnosis of bowel in the scrotal sac.

Testicular Tumor

Inquiry should focus on previous trauma to the scrotum or perineal area and the history or presence of cryptorchidism, pain, swelling, or sensations in the scrotum. The physical examination should include inspection and palpation of the abdomen, perineal area, scrotal sac, testes, and surrounding lymph nodes. Palpation should be performed with both hands to assist in differentiating between a mass located on the body of the testicle and a mass located on or within the epididymis. The location, size, mobility, and degree of tenderness of normal structures, as well as any abnormal findings, should be noted.[17] Any solid, firm mass within the body of the testicle should be considered a tumor unless proven otherwise.[18] Additional examination of the abdomen and chest should be completed while also evaluating for gynecomastia (a sign of elevated β-hCG).[22] One in three patients is misdiagnosed with epididymitis, orchitis, or a hydrocele on initial presentation.[1] Evaluation of lymph nodes in the abdomen and groin should be performed, because bulky lymphadenopathy is noted in metastatic disease.[1] Scrotal transillumination performed in a darkened room may be used to visualize abnormalities and to detect solid versus fluid-filled masses.[7,22]

Elephantiasis

Obstruction of the lymphatic vessels leads to swelling in the torso, genitals, and lower extremities and is classically characterized by massive scrotal lymphedema.[27]

ESSENTIAL DIAGNOSTICS

Many testicular disorders are readily recognized at the time of presentation and do not require further evaluation. In general, clinical presentation and physical examination guide the choice of appropriate diagnostics.

Varicocele

Varicoceles have a grading system from 1 to 3. Grade 1 is considered small and palpable only with the patient standing while performing a Valsalva maneuver. Grade 2 is moderate and palpable with the patient standing and no Valsalva maneuver. Grade 3 is large and palpable with the patient standing and can been seen through the scrotal skin.[5]
- Semen analysis may reveal oligospermia or azoospermia, but findings can be normal.[5]
- Measurement of serum testosterone levels may be considered; varicoceles have been shown to have a negative impact on Leydig cell function.[5]
- Ultrasound examination will reveal a dilated pampiniform plexus vessel larger than 2 to 3 mm.[18]

Epididymitis
- Doppler ultrasound examination shows heterogeneous hypoechoic epididymis with hyperemia and increased intratesticular blood flow.[18,30]
- Urinalysis and complete blood count (CBC) may reveal white blood cells and bacteriuria.
- A nucleic acid amplification test (NAAT) will assist with diagnosing chlamydia and gonorrhea.[12]

Orchitis
- Doppler ultrasound examination shows heterogeneous hypoechoicity.[18]

Spermatocele
- A mass is located at the proximal aspect of the spermatic cord and can be transilluminated.[15]

Hydrocele
- A hydrocele will transilluminate and be anechoic on ultrasound examination.[18]

Hematocele

- Ultrasound examination is used to evaluate blood flow and will show echogenic debris.[18] Surgical exploration may be necessary to rule out cancer.

Testicular Torsion

- Ultrasound examination will demonstrate an enlarged testicle with diffuse hypoechogenicity, usually associated with a reactive hydrocele and edema of the epididymis and scrotum.[14] Absent blood flow seen on color flow Doppler ultrasound is both sensitive and specific for testicular torsion.[14]

Torsion of the Appendix Testis

- Transillumination may reveal a blue dot sign, and ultrasound examination of the appendage will demonstrate an oval nodule in the superior pole of the testis. If the appendage has infarcted, it can calcify and may later appear as a "scrotal pearl" during imaging.[14]

Trauma

- Ultrasound examination of the scrotum after trauma may reveal a hematocele or hematoma, which can become quite large.[14] If there is testicular rupture, a testicular fracture line may appear on ultrasound images and should be considered an emergency; prompt surgical repair should be considered.[14]

Scrotal-Inguinal Hernia

- A scrotal hernia does not transilluminate and is easily identified on ultrasound examination, showing the bowel mass within the scrotum.[18]

Testicular Tumor

- To assist practitioners in assessing the extent of testicular disease, the staging system commonly used is the American Joint Committee on Cancer staging system, which is based on surgical findings and histologic examination of retroperitoneal lymph nodes: stage I, tumor confined to testis; stage II, tumor spread to retroperitoneal nodal involvement; stage III, tumor spread beyond retroperitoneal nodes.[1]
- The diagnosis of testicular cancer is usually confirmed through direct surgical exploration of the testes and serum tumor markers (hCG, AFP, and LDH) along with chest, abdominal, and pelvic imaging.[1]

- Tumor markers are drawn before and after orchiectomy to obtain information on staging, prognosis, and treatment outcome.[1,25] A negative marker does not necessarily exclude disease, but an elevated marker is considered clinically significant.[1]
- High levels of hCG are seen in both seminomatous and nonseminomatous tumors, whereas AFP levels are elevated only in nonseminomas.[25]
- Ultrasonography is useful in evaluating testicular masses and in confirming the size and location of palpable tumors.[1] Abdominopelvic and chest computed tomography (CT) along with other imaging studies may be necessary to determine the extent and location of metastases.[1]

Elephantiasis

- The only definitive way to make the diagnosis of lymphatic filariasis is by detecting the parasite itself, either the adult worms or the microfilariae.[27]
- The microfilariae can sometimes be detected by microscopic examination of a blood sample, but people with chronic infection often do not have the microfilariae in their blood. In such cases, the urine, hydrocele fluid, or other clinical tests are necessary.
- Blood samples should be obtained during the night, when microfilariae are more numerous in the bloodstream.
- A CBC and ultrasound examination are additional diagnostics that can be considered.[27]

DIFFERENTIAL DIAGNOSIS

The differential diagnosis for any testicular disorder or acute scrotal mass or pain should first exclude the possibility of a testicular tumor. The differential diagnosis for testicular tumors includes cysts, testicular torsion, epididymitis, and epididymo-orchitis (Table 133.1).[7] A hydrocele, hernia, hematoma, or spermatocele may also mimic a testicular tumor.[32] The presence of a testicular mass is suggestive of a tumor and indicates the need for immediate referral. It is often difficult to differentiate between epididymitis and orchitis because the symptoms are similar and at times may coexist. A varicocele is more discernible than other scrotal masses because this mass classically resembles a bag of worms on palpation.[4] However, many other testicular conditions (specifically, testicular cancer in men older than 30 years) may have hydrocele development as a symptom.[15] A detailed history, a thorough physical examination, and key diagnostics (urinalysis, urine culture, ultrasound, CT, tumor markers) all aid in clarity for determining the precise diagnosis.

TABLE 133.1	Differential Diagnosis of Testicular Disorders		
Diagnosis	Symptoms	Signs	Evaluation
Appendage torsion (appendix testis)	Typically a more indolent onset of symptoms compared with testicular torsion; less likely to present with nausea or vomiting	Tender nodule typically at head of testicle or epididymis; "blue dot sign" pathognomonic	Ultrasound examination may demonstrate infarcted appendage.
Epididymitis	Typically a more indolent onset of symptoms compared with testicular torsion; less likely to present with nausea or vomiting	*Early:* firmness and nodularity isolated to epididymis *Late:* with progression, inflammation may become contiguous with testicle (termed epididymo-orchitis)	Ultrasound examination may reveal increased intratesticular blood flow, although this is a nonspecific finding.

Continued

TABLE 133.1	Differential Diagnosis of Testicular Disorders—cont'd		
Diagnosis	Symptoms	Signs	Evaluation
Epididymo-orchitis	More likely to present with systemic findings, including nausea, vomiting, fever	Large, swollen scrotal mass typically with indistinct border between testicle and epididymis	Ultrasound examination may reveal increased intratesticular blood flow, although this is a nonspecific finding.
Fournier disease	Perineal swelling, redness; fever, vomiting, lethargy	May present with an absence of visible local findings on skin inspection in early stages (pain out of proportion to examination); ecchymosis, crepitus, necrotic eschar may be present in more advanced disease	Emergent surgical consultation for debridement, broad-spectrum antimicrobials.
Hematocele	Large, painful scrotal mass; often antecedent history of trauma	Ecchymosis of scrotal skin; testicular tenderness or firmness	Ultrasound examination may reveal fluid-filled tunica vaginalis.
Hernia	Unilateral inguinal or scrotal swelling and pain	Reducible, incarcerated, and strangulated forms; incarcerated or strangulated hernia may be particularly tender on examination	Emergent surgical consultation when incarcerated or strangulated; outpatient surgical referral reasonable if readily reducible.
Hydrocele	Typically a gradual progression of swelling	Scrotal transillumination may be helpful	Ultrasound examination may reveal fluid-filled tunica vaginalis.
Idiopathic scrotal edema	Typically unilateral scrotal swelling and edema; primarily seen in boys younger than 10 years	Scrotal, perineal, inguinal erythema and edema; may be difficult to distinguish from an acute skin or soft tissue infection	Ultrasound examination.
Orchitis	Typically gradual onset of unilateral (or bilateral) testicular swelling and pain	Swelling and tenderness isolated to testis or testes, without epididymal involvement	Ultrasound examination; often seen in conjunction with other systemic diseases (viral, other); treatment is disease specific.
Scrotal skin infection	Variable depending on cause	Must distinguish between lesions localized to scrotal wall and those contiguous with deeper scrotal structures	Ultrasound or CT imaging may be helpful in determining the depth and extent of involvement if invasive process suspected.
Spermatocele or epididymal cyst	Typically a painless well-defined nodule Spermatocele is present on the head of the epididymis; epididymal cysts arise throughout the epididymis	Spermatocele will have proteinaceous fluid and spermatozoa. Epididymal cysts contain clear serous fluid	Ultrasound examination. Spermatoceles and epididymal cysts are indistinguishable.
Testicular torsion	Typically a sudden and severe onset of pain; more likely to be associated with nausea or emesis	Classic findings include an elevated testis with a transverse lie	Emergent surgery consultation in high probability cases.
Trauma	History of blunt or penetrating mechanism of injury	Variable depending on mechanism	Ultrasound examination; low threshold for surgical consultation in all but the most minor injuries.
Tumor	Typically a gradually progressive testicular mass; may be painless or painful	May palpate testicular mass, firmness, or induration	Ultrasound examination.
Varicocele	Typically a gradual onset of unilateral swelling, often painless	Abnormally enlarged spermatic cord (pampiniform) venous plexus (often described as a "bag of worms")	Ultrasound examination.
Vasculitis (e.g., Henoch-Schönlein purpura)	Testicular swelling and pain	Associated vasculitis findings (such as buttock or lower extremity purpura and renal involvement in HSP)	Ultrasound examination, other diagnostic testing guided by suspected cause (e.g., CBC, serum electrolytes with renal function in HSP).

CBC, Complete blood count; CT, computed tomography.
Modified from Davis, J. E., & Silverman, M. (2011). Scrotal emergencies. *Emergency Medicine Clinics of North America, 29*(3), 469–484.

INTERPROFESSIONAL COLLABORATIVE MANAGEMENT

Management of testicular disorders depends on the specific type of disorder.

Varicocele

- A volume discrepancy of more than 20%, along with an abnormal semen analysis, usually prompts surgical intervention. Surgical treatment by ligation of the spermatic vein (varicocelectomy) is often the treatment of choice, and there are several different surgical approaches.[4] The microsurgical subinguinal technique appears to have the highest spontaneous pregnancy rate in previously infertile couples.[4]
- Alternative treatment options include vascular ablation or embolization, and percutaneous sclerotherapy.[4]

Epididymitis and Orchitis

- Antiinfective therapy is recommended, with guidance by local sensitivity reports. The following antibiotic regimens are effective against the most common causes of epididymitis: single-dose ceftriaxone given intramuscularly (IM), 250 to 500 mg, and doxycycline, 100 mg twice daily for 10 days for men younger than 35 years; in men older than 35 years, levofloxacin (given intravenously [IV] or orally [PO]), 500 to 750 mg/day, or ciprofloxacin, 500 mg (IV or PO), for 10 to 14 days.[11,12] In severe cases, it may be necessary to use intravenous antibiotics.
- Antipyretics should be used to reduce discomfort and fever, and an antiinflammatory agent should be prescribed.[10] An antiemetic can also be prescribed for nausea and vomiting.
- Bed rest and scrotal elevation are also recommended for epididymitis.[10] Hot or cold compresses may be helpful for orchitis.

Spermatocele

- No treatment if asymptomatic or scrotal support.
- If significant discomfort is present or there is concern because of the increasing size of the mass, excision is recommended.[15]

Hydrocele

- Congenital hydroceles that occur in newborns usually resolve themselves within the first year of life; if not, surgical correction can be completed.[15,29]
- Treatment of asymptomatic hydroceles can consist of watchful waiting.[15]
- Symptomatic hydroceles can be treated with surgical aspiration, resection, or sclerotherapy.[15]

Testicular Torsion

- Treatment is prompt surgical consultation with surgical exploration with the intent to prevent ischemia and restore blood flow.[21] It is critical to restore vascularity as soon as possible because salvage rates are greater than 90% within 6 hours, greater than 50% within 12 hours, and less than 10% in 24 hours.[21]

Torsion of the Appendix Testis

- Treatment of an appendix testis with torsion often is self-limiting, but management revolves around conservative measures of antiinflammatories, rest, ice, and scrotal

support.[10] If pain persists and conservative management does not provide relief, surgical referral is appropriate.

Trauma or Hematocele

- If all scrotal contents are intact, trauma injuries can be treated symptomatically with ice, elevation, scrotal support, and bed rest.[20] However, if there is concern that the testicle has been ruptured or penetrated, or if other contents are not palpated as intact, immediate surgical exploration and intervention should be undertaken.[8,20]

Scrotal-Inguinal Hernia

- If the herniated bowel is reducible, surgical referral for possible future repair is indicated. Difficulty in reducing a hernia is cause for urgent surgical intervention. However, pain may indicate incarceration of the bowel or complete inability to reduce the hernia, which is cause for immediate emergency department referral and surgical exploration.[29]

Testicular Tumor

- Prompt evaluation is essential. The mainstays of testicular cancer treatment are surgery, chemotherapy, and radiation.[2]
- Primary treatment for seminomas involves radical orchiectomy followed by irradiation of the retroperitoneal lymph for low-stage seminomas and chemotherapy for more advanced stage seminomas.[2,25]
- Nonseminomas are also treated with radical orchiectomy followed by retroperitoneal lymphadenectomy and chemotherapy because they are more responsive to chemotherapy.[2]
- Additional management is monitoring of tumor markers hCG, AFP, and LDH.[25] Follow-up visits should include a thorough physical examination, chest imaging, and measurement of serum tumor markers monthly for the first year, every 2 months for the second year, and every 3 to 6 months for up to 5 years. Regardless of the disease stage, more than 90% of all newly diagnosed cases of testicular cancer will be cured.[25]

Elephantiasis

- The recommended treatment for *W. bancrofti* infection is diethylcarbamazine, but some research has shown response to doxycycline.[34] Diethylcarbamazine is no longer sold in the United States or approved by the US Food and Drug Administration (FDA), but it can be obtained from the Centers for Disease Control and Prevention (CDC) with positive laboratory confirmation.[34]

COMPLICATIONS

Varicoceles are associated with infertility and produce abnormal semen parameters, testicular atrophy, and Leydig cell dysfunction.[4] The condition can be reversed if the varicocele is surgically corrected, and this has been shown to improve spontaneous pregnancy rates by almost 40%.[4] Infertility is also the most serious complication of epididymitis, orchitis, and spermatocele.[9]

Testicular torsion is a medical emergency and should be surgically explored and relieved as quickly as possible to prevent the development of gangrene. A delay in treatment could result in testicular infarction and loss of the affected testicle. Manual detorsion can be attempted in certain situations with the standard medial-to-lateral rotation method (as in opening a book), but residual torsion may still remain.[8] Torsion of the appendix testis is frequently seen in adolescents and is a self-limiting condition that is treated with pain relief and limited activity.[8] In some instances, torsion of the appendix testis can recur.[8] In scrotal trauma the most pressing concern is whether the testis has been ruptured or the blood supply compromised from trauma-induced torsion of the spermatic cord.[20] A referral to a urologist or surgical consultation is required to verify that the testis and other scrotal contents are intact.[20]

Scrotal-inguinal hernia repair can have complications associated with the procedure, the most common being hematomas, scrotal ecchymosis, seromas, and infection.[24] Testicular cancer is the most common malignancy in males aged 15 to 35 years.[2] The mainstays of testicular cancer treatment are surgery (inguinal orchiectomy), chemotherapy, and radiation therapy; with these treatments, complications may occur.[2] Potential complications that may occur as a result of testicular cancer treatment are infertility, recurrent or secondary malignancy (lymphoma and myeloid dysfunctions), cardiac disease, ventral hernia, and bowel obstruction.[2,7]

INDICATIONS FOR REFERRAL OR HOSPITALIZATION

- Patients suspected of having a testicular mass, testicular torsion, or an incarcerated scrotal hernia require immediate referral to a urologist or surgeon.
- Epididymitis and minor scrotal trauma can be managed by the health care provider unless complications are present or the testis is involved in a traumatic injury. Any suspicion of testicular rupture, torsion, epididymal injury, hematocele, or other testicular defect warrants evaluation by a surgeon.[20]
- Any patient with a hydrocele that is expanding, is causing pain, or potentially was caused by a scrotal tumor should be referred to a urologist.
- Patients with varicoceles that do not respond to conservative treatment (scrotal support and antiinflammatory medications) should be referred to a urologist for more definitive treatment. Patients with an identified varicocele in addition to an abnormal semen analysis, known infertility, and testicular atrophy should be referred to a urologist.[5]

Hospitalization should be considered for any unremitting testicular or scrotal pain, if a testicular mass is suspected, or if edema from testicular involvement cannot be excluded.

PATIENT AND FAMILY EDUCATION AND HEALTH PROMOTION

Diagnosis, treatment options, potential outcomes, and the need for follow-up care should be carefully explained to patients. All patients should be encouraged to discuss their concerns or fears about the diagnosis and treatment or treatment options. These concerns and fears about potential complications and the severity of the condition should be addressed truthfully.

Patients with testicular masses require ongoing education and support from the time of diagnosis through all phases of treatment. Whenever possible, the spouse or significant other should be educated about the disease process, prognosis, treatment, and effects of treatment on relationships and sexuality. The patient and family should be encouraged to verbalize feelings and to support one another throughout the process.

Male patients, from adolescence to older age, should be instructed in the correct method of TSE and the importance of the examination for other men in their family (including teenagers, because this is the beginning of the age range for testicular cancer). The TSE should be performed monthly and is best performed after a warm bath or shower when the skin of the scrotum is relaxed.[2] Patients should see their health care providers if any abnormalities are detected in the scrotum or testes.

Although the patient's age may influence concerns about fertility, the potential loss of testicular function should not be disregarded in men of advanced age. Surgical intervention for testicular tumors may result in body image disturbances and altered sexuality in adolescence and later life. After an orchiectomy, counseling may be indicated to assist in coping with loss related to alterations in the genitals and reproductive system. For children, adolescents, or young men with a single testicle, it is recommended that protective equipment be used during athletic participation.[20]

REFERENCES

1. Kreydin, E. I., Barrisford, G. W., Feldman, A. S., & Preston, M. A. (2013). Testicular cancer: What the radiologist needs to know. *AJR. American Journal of Roentgenology, 200*(6), 1215–1225.
2. Russell, S. S. (2014). Testicular cancer: Overview and implications for health care providers. *Urologic Nursing, 34*(4), 172–176.
3. Dabaja, A., Wosnitzer, M., & Goldstein, M. (2013). Varicocele and hypogonadism. *Current Urology Reports, 14*(4), 309–314.
4. Kwak, N., & Siegel, D. (2014). Imaging and interventional therapy for varicoceles. *Current Urology Reports, 15*(4), 1–6.
5. Masson, P., & Brannigan, R. E. (2014). The varicocele. *The Urologic Clinics of North America, 41*(1), 129–144.
6. Korets, R., Woldu, S. L., Nees, S. N., Spencer, B. A., & Glassberg, K. I. (2011). Testicular symmetry and adolescent varicocele—does it need followup? *The Journal of Urology, 186*(Suppl. 4), 1614–1619.
7. Wampler, S. M., & Llanes, M. (2010). Common scrotal and testicular problems. *Primary Care, 37*(3), 613–626, x.
8. Davis, J. E., & Silverman, M. (2011). Scrotal emergencies. *Emergency Medicine Clinics of North America, 29*(3), 469–484.
9. Bachir, B. G., & Jarvi, K. (2014). Infectious, inflammatory, and immunologic conditions resulting in male infertility. *The Urologic Clinics of North America, 41*(1), 67–81.
10. Srinath, H. (2013). Acute scrotal pain. *Australian Family Physician, 42*(11), 790–792.
11. Walker, N. A. F., & Challacombe, B. (2013). Managing epididymo-orchitis in general practice. *The Practitioner, 257*(1760), 21–25, 22–23.
12. Street, E. J., & Wilson, J. D. (2014). Acute epididymo-orchitis. *Medicine, 42*(6), 338–340.
13. Crawford, P., & Crop, J. A. (2014). Evaluation of scrotal masses. *American Family Physician, 89*(9), 723–727.
14. Delaney, L. R., & Karmazyn, B. (2013). Ultrasound of the pediatric scrotum. *Seminars in Ultrasound, CT, and MR, 34*(3), 248–256.
15. Kessenich, C. R., & Bacher, K. (2014). Evaluation of a scrotal mass. *The Nurse Practitioner, 39*(5), 13–14.
16. Rioja, J., Sánchez-Margallo, F. M., Usón, J., & Rioja, L. A. (2011). Adult hydrocele and spermatocele. *BJU International, 107*(11), 1852–1864.
17. Montgomery, J. S., & Bloom, D. A. (2011). The diagnosis and management of scrotal masses. *The Medical Clinics of North America, 95*(1), 235–244.
18. Sommers, D., & Winter, T. (2014). Ultrasonography evaluation of scrotal masses. *Radiologic Clinics of North America, 52*(6), 1265–1281.
19. Lewis, M. L. (2014). A comprehensive newborn exam: Part II. Skin, trunk, extremities, neurologic. *American Family Physician, 90*(5), 297–302.
20. Hunter, S. R., Lishnak, T. S., Powers, A. M., & Lisle, D. K. (2013). Male genital trauma in sports. *Clinics in Sports Medicine, 32*(2), 247–254.
21. Sharp, V. J., Kieran, K., & Arlen, A. M. (2013). Testicular torsion: Diagnosis, evaluation, and management. *American Family Physician, 88*(12), 835–840.
22. Sandella, B., Hartmann, B., Berkson, D., & Hong, E. (2012). Testicular conditions in athletes: Torsion, tumors, and epididymitis. *Current Sports Medicine Reports, 11*(2), 92–95.
23. Karaguzel, E., Kadihasanoglu, M., & Kutlu, O. (2014). Mechanisms of testicular torsion and potential protective agents. *Nature Reviews. Urology, 11*(7), 391–399.
24. LeBlanc, K. E., LeBlanc, L. L., & LeBlanc, K. A. (2013). Inguinal hernias: Diagnosis and management. *American Family Physician, 87*(12), 844–848.
25. Motzer, R. J., Agarwal, N., Beard, C., et al. (2012). Testicular cancer. *Journal of the National Comprehensive Cancer Network, 10*(4), 502–535.

26 Brotherhood, H. L., Metcalfe, M., Goldenberg, L., Pommerville, P., Bowman, C., & Naysmith, D. (2014). A surgical challenge: Idiopathic scrotal elephantiasis. *Canadian Urological Association Journal = Journal de l'Association des urologues du Canada, 8*, E500.

27 Parmar, H. D. (2013). The surgical approach in huge scrotal lymphedema. *International Journal of Medical Science and Public Health, 2*(1), 153.

28 Ramanan, B., Maloley, B. J., & Fitzgibbons, R. J., Jr. (2014). Inguinal hernia: Follow or repair? *Advances in Surgery, 48*, 1–11.

29 Palmer, L. S. (2013). Hernias and hydroceles. *Pediatrics in Review, 34*(10), 457–464.

30 Cokkinos, D. D., Antypa, E., Tserotas, P., et al. (2011). Emergency ultrasound of the scrotum: A review of the commonest pathologic conditions. *Current Problems in Diagnostic Radiology, 40*(1), 1–14.

31 Appelbaum, L., Gaitini, D., & Dogra, V. S. (2013). Scrotal ultrasound in adults. *Seminars in Ultrasound, CT, and MR, 34*(3), 257–273.

32 Bromby, A., & Cresswell, J. (2014). Differential diagnosis of a scrotal mass. *Trends in Urology & Men's Health, 5*(1), 15–18.

33 Drlík, M., & Kočvara, R. (2013). Torsion of spermatic cord in children: A review. *Journal of Pediatric Urology, 9*(3), 259–266.

34 Centers for Disease Control and Prevention (CDC). (2018). Parasites—lymphatic filariasis. Retrieved from www.cdc.gov/parasites/lymphaticfilariasis/treatment.html. (Accessed 6 February 2019).

CHAPTER **134**

URINARY CALCULI

Daniel A. Blaz

 Immediate referral is warranted for testicular torsion, ovarian torsion, appendicitis, ectopic pregnancy, small bowel obstruction, renal infarction, and abdominal aortic aneurysm with or without aortic dissection.

DEFINITION AND EPIDEMIOLOGY

Renal and urinary calculi are calcifications or "stones" that can form anywhere within the urinary tract, specifically the kidneys (nephrolithiasis), urinary system (urolithiasis), or ureters (ureterolithiasis), or they may migrate to the lower urinary tract (bladder or urethra).[1-3] The majority of stones are found within the kidney, but stone formation may also occur in the ureter or bladder or in the presence of congenital urogenital abnormalities.[1] Renal stone formation and disease revolve around a multifactorial process that involves environmental and genetic factors and a delicate balance of metabolic substances within the urine.[1,4] In the United States, stone disease is associated with nearly $5 billion in health care costs, accounting for nearly 1.2 million emergency room visits each year and 41,000 surgical procedures annually.[5,6] Understanding the epidemiology of stone formation may help elucidate and define approaches to reduce the risk of stone formation and mitigate the health care costs related to stone disease.

The prevalence of kidney stones in adults in the United States was most recently reported from the National Health and Nutrition Examination Survey (NHANES 2007–10) at 8.8%, with men having a higher prevalence (10.6%) than women (7.1%).[7] Kidney stones are most common in men, specifically white males, and development of stones is most prevalent in males age 40 to 70 years and ages 50 to 60 for females.[3,8] The lifetime risk for kidney stone disease in Americans is 9%, and over the past several decades the risk of kidney stone development between men and women has closed, with the ratio currently 2:1.[4,8] This is thought to be related to the

rise in obesity rates among individuals, specifically in women.[7] In children, stone disease is not very common, although 40% of children who develop stones have a positive family history, suggesting a probable genetic metabolic cause.[9] The recurrence rate for stone formation is approximately 15% in the first year, with a 50% chance of experiencing another stone within the next 10 years.[4,7] The incidence of stone formation has several ethnic (age, gender, heredity) and geographic (geography, climate, season) implications that affect the development of renal stones; the highest frequency occurs in the Middle East regions of the world and the Southeast region of the United States.[6,8] Living in a hot tropical or desert climate has been shown to increase the risk of forming stones.[8]

The genetic predisposition to stone development is becoming clearer to health care providers when diagnosing hereditary stone disease.[9] Certain metabolic and genetic disorders have been shown to occur most frequently in inherited cases, with cystinuria (in adults) and primary hyperoxaluria (PH) (in children) being the two most common.[9] A positive family history of kidney stones has been documented to occur in 20% to 50% of familial cases and is a risk factor for stone development.[9,10] In addition, certain lifestyle factors have shown increased stone risk. These include obesity, low socioeconomic status, low fluid intake, high dietary salt intake, and low dietary calcium intake.[3] Other risk factors include insulin-resistant states, hypertension, gout, metabolic syndrome, primary hyperparathyroidism, chronic metabolic acidosis, and coronary artery disease.[5,7,10] Obesity is associated with insulin resistance and compensatory hyperinsulinemia, both of which can contribute to stone formation. In addition, body mass index and waist circumference have been positively associated with kidney stone formation in both men and women. Obese individuals who form stones excrete higher amounts of sodium, calcium, uric acid, and citrate, with uric acid stones found most commonly in this population.[11] Diet-related factors such as a diet that is high in salt and animal protein and excessive ingestion of substances that produce stones, such as purines (e.g., seafood, organ meats), oxalates (e.g., colas, chocolate), and phosphate, increase the incidence of stone formation.[3,4,7] Other predisposing factors include sedentary occupations (pilots and teachers), sedentary activity level, risk of dehydration, and medications (e.g., acyclovir, acetazolamide, antacids, ascorbic acid in doses of 2 g or more daily, sulfa drugs, triamterene, topiramate, methotrexate, and indinavir [Crixivan]).[3,4,8] Environmental factors, such as exposure to drinking water high in minerals, may contribute to stone formation, but it has been widely accepted that the role of increased water intake can reduce risk of stone formation.

PATHOPHYSIOLOGY

The formation of kidney stones is a multifaceted process that incorporates a delicate balance between elevated levels of stone-forming salts and inadequate inhibitory proteins.[4,6] Renal and urinary calculi are mineral deposits that develop from microscopic crystals in the loop of Henle, the distal tubule, or the collecting ducts, and they aggregate to form lithogenic structures.[4] The cause of renal and urinary calculi formation has traditionally narrowed on two agreed-on theories. The first theory involves the process of the supersaturation of urine with calcium, oxalate, and uric acid, whereby microscopic crystals form on these substances and adhere to the urothelium, creating the nidus for stone formation.[3] The second theory primarily involves the formation of calcium oxalate stones whereby deposits (Randall plaques) of subepithelial interstitial calcium act as nuclei for the formation of a stone.[3,4] In addition, more recent theories centralize on the aspect of surface molecules that promote or inhibit the formation of crystals.[4] These molecules are further influenced by the urothelial injury and repair cycle after a stone has formed, which increases the expression of the molecules and promotes enhanced crystal adhesion.[4]

One of the most common risk factors for stone formation is reduced urinary flow, and any factor that reduces urinary flow or urinary volume (e.g., dehydration or inadequate fluid intake) allows stone constituents to supersaturate and increases the risk of kidney stones.[4] Other risk factors for the formation of urinary calculi include excess dietary intake of oxalate and sodium, which promotes hyperoxaluria and hypercalciuria, respectively; gout, which promotes hyperuricosuria; and primary hyperparathyroidism, which can result in persistent hypercalciuria.[4-6] Excess dietary animal protein (meat, poultry, and fish) creates an acidic urinary milieu, resulting in citrate depletion and hyperuricosuria.[3,7,8,10] Obesity may contribute to hypercalciuria and uric acid stone formation, owing to an increase in refined sugars, low fluid intake, high calcium and oxalate, and excess dietary ingestion of meat.[3,7] Short bowel syndrome can contribute to low urine volume, acidic urine (which depletes available citrate), and hyperoxaluria.[6,7] Insulin resistance can result in an alteration in urinary pH, and gout increases the risk of hyperuricosuria, both of which increase the risk of stone formation.[1,8] In addition, stone formation is encouraged by anatomic abnormalities that reduce urine flow or cause stasis, including horseshoe kidney, genitourinary diverticula, obstructive disorders, and medullary sponge kidney. The entire process of stone formation is influenced by multiple chemical, physical, physical-chemical, biochemical, and physiologic events.

Calculi can be broadly classified as calcareous (i.e., calcium containing) stones, which are visible on imaging, and noncalcareous stones, which are often radiolucent or poorly visible on plain film radiography.[12,13] Renal and urinary calculi can be more specifically classified into five types based on their composition, with calcium-based stones being the most common, representing up to 80% of all calculi (Table 134.1).

Calcium oxalate stones are the most common type of urinary calculi and are often visible on plain radiography

---

TABLE 134.1   Types of Kidney Stones, Prevalence, and Radiopacity

Type of Stone	Prevalence (%)	Radiopacity
Calcium oxalate	75–80	Radiopaque
Calcium phosphate	5–10	Radiopaque
Struvite	5–15	Poor radiopacity
Uric acid	5–10	Radiolucent
Cystine	1–2	Poor radiopacity

Data from Pfau, A., & Knauf, F. (2016). Update on nephrolithiasis: Core curriculum 2016. *American Journal of Kidney Diseases, 68*(6), 973–985; Hornberger, B., & Bollner, M. R. (2018). Kidney stones. *Physician Assistant Clinics, 3*(1), 37–54; Türk, C., Petřík, A., Sarica, K., Seitz, C., Skolarikos, A., Straub, M., et al. (2016). EAU Guidelines on diagnosis and conservative management of urolithiasis. *European Urology, 69*(3), 468–474.

---

or unenhanced computed tomography (CT).[8,13] Hypercalciuria (>250 mg/24 h in women and >300 mg in men/24 h) is the most common metabolic abnormality associated with calcium oxalate stones.[4] The next most common cause is hypocitraturia (<325 mg/24 h), which involves a generally idiopathic deficiency of citrate (a naturally occurring stone inhibitor).[4] High acid loads (e.g., excess intake of meat, and dehydration) can contribute to or exacerbate hypocitraturia.[4,8] Urine levels of oxalate, normally a metabolic by-product, may increase as a result of the ingestion of foods high in oxalate, such as rhubarb, nuts, cocoa, tea, beans, lime peel, and green leafy vegetables; this condition is termed hyperoxaluria.[4] The most common causes of hyperoxaluria are bowel resection and intestinal disease such as malabsorptive small bowel disorders, including Crohn disease, biliary obstruction, celiac sprue, chronic pancreatitis, and bariatric surgical procedures.[4,6,7]

Calculi that consist predominantly of calcium phosphate occur more often in women, specifically pregnant women.[8] They are most often associated with acidification disorders such as renal tubular acidosis (RTA), which results in metabolic acidosis, defective urinary acidification, hypokalemia, and reduced urinary citrate concentrations.[4] Less common causes of defective urinary acidification include primary hyperparathyroidism, excessive alkalinization, and autoimmune disease.[4] Favorable conditions for calcium phosphate stone formation are high urine pH, reduced citrate excretion, and increased urinary concentration of calcium and phosphate.[4,7]

Uric acid stones account for approximately 5% to 10% of all stones and are more prevalent in patients with diabetes, gout, and metabolic syndrome.[4,8] Uric acid is an end product of purine metabolism; increased uricosuria is often a result of dehydration and excessive purine intake.[7,8] Other risk factors include a consistently low urine pH, gout, myeloproliferative disorders, insulin-resistant states, cytotoxic drugs, end ileostomies, and conditions that predispose a patient to concentrated urine.[4,6,8]

Struvite stones are composed of magnesium phosphate, ammonium phosphate, and calcium phosphate and are referred to as triple phosphate stones.[4,8] Struvite stones account for approximately 5% to 15% of all stones, are more prevalent in women, and are the leading cause of staghorn calculi.[8] Struvite stones grow rapidly, recur frequently, and occurs from urea splitting by urease, which results in high ammonium concentration and alkaline urine.[4,14] Struvite stones are an index of a urinary tract infection (UTI) usually from urea-splitting microorganisms and are often implicated in staghorn kidney stones.[8] Neurogenic bladders, foreign bodies in the urinary tract, and recurrent UTIs with urea-splitting microorganisms (e.g., *Proteus mirabilis, Ureaplasma urealyticum, Klebsiella pneumoniae*) increase the risk of struvite calculi.[4,14]

Cystinuria is an autosomal recessive disorder in which there is excessive urinary excretion of the amino acids cystine, ornithine, lysine, and arginine.[4,14] The low solubility of cystine results in stone formation, accounting for approximately 1% to 2% of all stones.[4] Cystine stones are more common in males than females, commonly appear in the second decade of life, and ultimately can lead to kidney failure.[4] Lastly, stone formation is stimulated by anatomic abnormalities that reduce urine flow or cause stasis, including horseshoe kidney, genitourinary diverticula, obstructive disorders, and medullary sponge kidney.

CLINICAL PRESENTATION AND PHYSICAL EXAMINATION

Symptoms vary and depend on the size and anatomic location of the stones. In general, symptoms include acute renal or ureteral colic (with pain radiating to the ipsilateral abdomen or groin), nausea and vomiting, hematuria (microscopic or occult blood in the urine), fever and chills, dysuria, increased urinary frequency, and vague abdominal, flank, or groin pain.[3,4,8,14] Individuals with calculi most commonly have hematuria and renal colic or severe flank pain that may migrate anteriorly and into the groin as the stone moves from the kidney toward the bladder.[4,6,12] Renal or ureteral colic is a result of obstruction of the urinary tract by the stone. This obstruction is usually in one or more of five locations: (1) the calyx; (2) the ureteropelvic junction; (3) at or near the pelvic brim, where the ureter begins to arch over the iliac vessels; (4) the posterior pelvis, where the ureter is crossed anteriorly by the pelvic blood vessels and the broad ligament; and (5) the ureterovesical junction, which is the most constricted area.[2,6] Renal or ureteral colic is often associated with nausea and vomiting, gross hematuria, and dysuria, while fever and chills may be present if infection occurs with the stone.[6] Individuals with renal or ureteral colic classically present with an acute onset of pain that climaxes and are often extremely restless as they attempt to find a comfortable position (Box 134.1).[6,10] Less often, there may be persistent microhematuria or intermittent dull pain that lasts for weeks or months. Once a stone enters the bladder, dysuria, frequency, and urgency may be the only symptoms, but upon the stone exiting the bladder, symptoms typically resolve.[3,6]

A careful medical history should be obtained and should include personal stone history, medical problems and conditions (diabetes, gout, hyperparathyroidism, recurrent UTIs, immunosuppression, and solitary functioning kidney), surgical history (kidney transplant), medications (specifically ones that are associated with kidney stone formation: allopurinol, laxatives, topiramate, sulfonamides, quinolones, triamterene, sulfonylureas, and potassium channel blockers), family history (to include kidney stone disease), occupation, dietary habits and history, and fluid intake.[6,8]

The physical examination should include assessment of systemic symptoms and meticulous abdominal examination to exclude other sources of pain, including intra-abdominal pathology (abdominal aortic aneurysm, diverticulitis, appendicitis, and gynecologic pathology). The abdominal examination typically lacks signs of peritoneal irritation and results in a soft, nontender, and nondistended abdomen.[6] Continued physical examination findings include fever, tachycardia, elevated blood pressure, severe costovertebral angle tenderness, diaphoresis, and pale, cool, and clammy skin.[6,8] Individuals who have previous documented nonobstructing stone burden or disease are often asymptomatic.[8]

DIAGNOSTICS

The cornerstones of diagnostics are a detailed history and physical examination, after which the appropriate urinalysis, laboratory studies, and imaging can be ordered.

Essential Diagnostics

Urinalysis and urine culture and sensitivity are essential to determine pH and to identify the presence of bacteria, crystals, and red blood cells.[8] Hematuria may be microscopic or gross and may occur with or without infection.[4,6] An increase in the urine pH and the presence of crystals may give clues as to the stone's composition and whether the stone is alkaline or acidic.[7] In addition, the urine should be strained, and if a stone is made available, stone analysis should be completed.[7] Urine pH above 7.0 suggests urea-splitting microorganisms, and a urine culture should be obtained to evaluate for a UTI.[7] Urine pH below 5.4 associated with metabolic acidosis is seen in the presence of distal RTA, whereas the presence of hexagonal cystine crystals is diagnostic of cystinuria.[8,9] As part of the screening evaluation, a basic (at a minimum) or complete serum metabolic panel should be performed.[8] The serum metabolic panel will aid in evaluating underlying medical conditions (e.g., gout, hyperparathyroid) and should include sodium, potassium, chloride, bicarbonate, calcium, creatinine, and uric acid.[7] A complete blood count (CBC) should be obtained in patients with a fever or with an acute stone event and will assist in ruling out an infectious cause or stone.[8] Further metabolic testing of the urine can be completed through the use of a 24-hour urine test. Currently there is conflicting evidence regarding whether a single 24-hour urine sample should be collected with the first stone event.[7] Current evidence recommends either one or two 24-hour urine samples with the patient on his or her usual diet should be obtained and measured for calcium, oxalate, citrate, magnesium, sodium, and sulfate, but two samples are preferred.[7] In the presence of elevated serum calcium, primary hyperparathyroidism should be suspected and parathyroid hormone (PTH) levels should be measured; vitamin D levels should be assessed because low vitamin D can mask primary or secondary hyperparathyroidism.[7] An abdominal x-ray study (plain film) of the kidneys, ureter, and bladder (KUB) is often the fastest imaging study to identify renal stones that are radiopaque.[12] Frequently, stones that are only larger than 5 mm are visible on plain film,

---

B O X 134.1

Signs and Symptoms of Renal Colic

- Sudden onset—brought by sudden obstruction to outflow
- Intermittent versus constant
  - Intermittent suggestive of incomplete obstruction
  - Constant suggestive complete obstruction
  - If chronically obstructed, may become painless
- Location of pain
  - Flank, lower abdomen, genitalia, groin
- Nausea vomiting
  - Present in approximately 50% of cases
- Hematuria
  - Present in 64% of cases
- Fever
  - Sign of a confined, nondraining upper tract infection. Must be surgically drained.
- Costovertebral angle tenderness to percussion
- Abdominal and genitalia examination findings often benign
- Laboratory values most often normal. Elevated creatinine and microscopic hematuria common.
- Significantly elevated white count should raise concern of nondraining urinary tract infection

From Ingimarsson, J. P., Krambeck, A. E., & Pais, V. M. (2016). Diagnosis and management of nephrolithiasis. *Surgical Clinics of North America, 96*(3), 528.

but a KUB is helpful in documenting the number, size, and location of the stones in the urinary tract.[3] A plain film is also helpful in identifying nephrocalcinosis, hyperparathyroidism, primary hyperparathyroidism, PH, RTA, or sarcoidosis.[7] The low-dose noncontrast computed tomography (NCCT) scan is considered the "gold standard" radiographic tool for diagnostic imaging of renal and urinary calculi.[3,6,10,15,16] NCCT findings indicative of an acute urinary obstruction due to a stone include renal enlargement, hydronephrosis, ureteral dilation, perinephric stranding, and periureteral edema.[15] In the event that a stone is not visualized with an NCCT scan, secondary signs of a stone can be identified (nephromegaly, hydronephrosis, hydroureter) or an alternate diagnosis can be made from the NCCT findings (testicular or ovarian torsion, ectopic pregnancy, appendicitis, renal infarction).[12] Renal ultrasound is the imaging modality of choice for pregnant women, children, and individuals in whom radiation is contraindicated.[4,6,16] A renal ultrasound examination will aid in diagnosis and can be used as a screening tool for hydronephrosis, detecting the absence of expulsed urine (ureteral jets), and identifying stones within the ureters, kidney, or renal pelvis.[10,12] Calculi that are visible on ultrasound will show up as hyperechoic with a posterior acoustic shadow, but ultrasound does have its limitations, because calculi <5 mm are difficult to see.[12] Calculi that are more distal in the urinary tract have a 75% to 79% of passing spontaneously, but as the stone increases in size, it has less chance of passing spontaneously (Table 134.2).[6] Stones that do pass should be submitted for a complete stone analysis.[16]

INITIAL DIAGNOSTICS

Urinary Calculi

LABORATORY
- CBC
- Complete metabolic panel including uric acid
- PTH
- Vitamin D
- Urinalysis, urine culture, and sensitivity
- 24-h urine for calcium, oxalate, citrate, magnesium, sodium, sulfate
- Complete stone analysis

IMAGING
- KUB
- NCCT scan
- Renal ultrasound: pregnant women, children, and if radiation is contraindicated

TABLE 134.2 Spontaneous Stone Passage Rates

Stone Size (mm)	Spontaneous Stone Passage Rates (%)
1	87
2–4	76
5–7	60
8–9	48
>10	25

Data from Ingimarsson, J. P., Krambeck, A. E., & Pais, V. M. (2016). Diagnosis and management of nephrolithiasis. *Surgical Clinics of North America, 96*(3), 517–532.

Additional Diagnostics

C-reactive protein, coagulation studies, phosphorus, uric acid, intravenous pyelogram (IVP), magnetic resonance imaging (MRI), nuclear function renal scan, and cystoscopy.

DIFFERENTIAL DIAGNOSIS

Nephrolithiasis and urolithiasis can mimic other causes of visceral pain. Therefore in persons with abdominal symptoms, it is essential to consider other common causes of abdominal and flank pain; pyelonephritis, UTI, and acute pancreatitis.[3,12]

INTERPROFESSIONAL COLLABORATIVE MANAGEMENT
Nonpharmacologic Management

Most of acute renal and urinary calculi can be managed conservatively through oral hydration, pain management, and expectant stone passage.[3,10] Stone management guidelines depend on the size and location of the stone, the presence or absence of associated infection, the presence of one or two kidneys, and the severity of symptoms (Fig. 134.1). Fluid therapy is an integral part of acute stone management. Current evidence supports fluid volume replacement for those who are dehydrated or have increased creatinine levels. It is recommended that individuals with a current stone or with previous stones increase urine volumes to >2 L/day.[3] Adequate water intake that produces large urine volumes has been shown to reduce the supersaturation of the urine with stone-forming substances.[3] In stone formers, calcium restriction is not recommended and individuals should maintain a moderate calcium intake.[8]

Calcium Stones

Calcium stones (calcium oxalate and phosphate) are the most complex of all stones in their causes and treatments. The accepted theory regarding their cause is an imbalance between urinary excretion of insoluble salts and water, which results in an environment of supersaturation.[4] Therefore nonpharmacologic treatment is aimed at raising the urine flow rate and reducing excretion of stone-forming salts. The two main causes of calcium oxalate stone formation are a diet rich in oxalate foods (which creates a state of hyperoxaluria) and endogenous autosomal recessive disorders that cause oxalate overproduction. Management of oxalate stone formers should be focused on omitting foods high in oxalate, such as colas, vitamin C, chocolate, and peanuts.[4] Management of hyperoxaluria related to bowel disease and malabsorption syndromes is multifaceted and may include a low-fat diet, restrictive oxalate intake, and administration of calcium.[7] Hyperuricosuria, which is also associated with calcium oxalate stones, is most simply managed by reducing the intake of high-purine foods that cause elevated uric acid excretion.[7,14]

Uric Acid Stones

Management of uric acid stones should include maintaining an optimal urinary output of 2.5 to 3 L/day to prevent supersaturation.[6,17] Urine alkalization is an important intervention to prevent uric acid stone formation and a diet that is low in high-purine foods and rich in fruits and vegetables aids in the prevention of uric acid stone formation.[4,17]

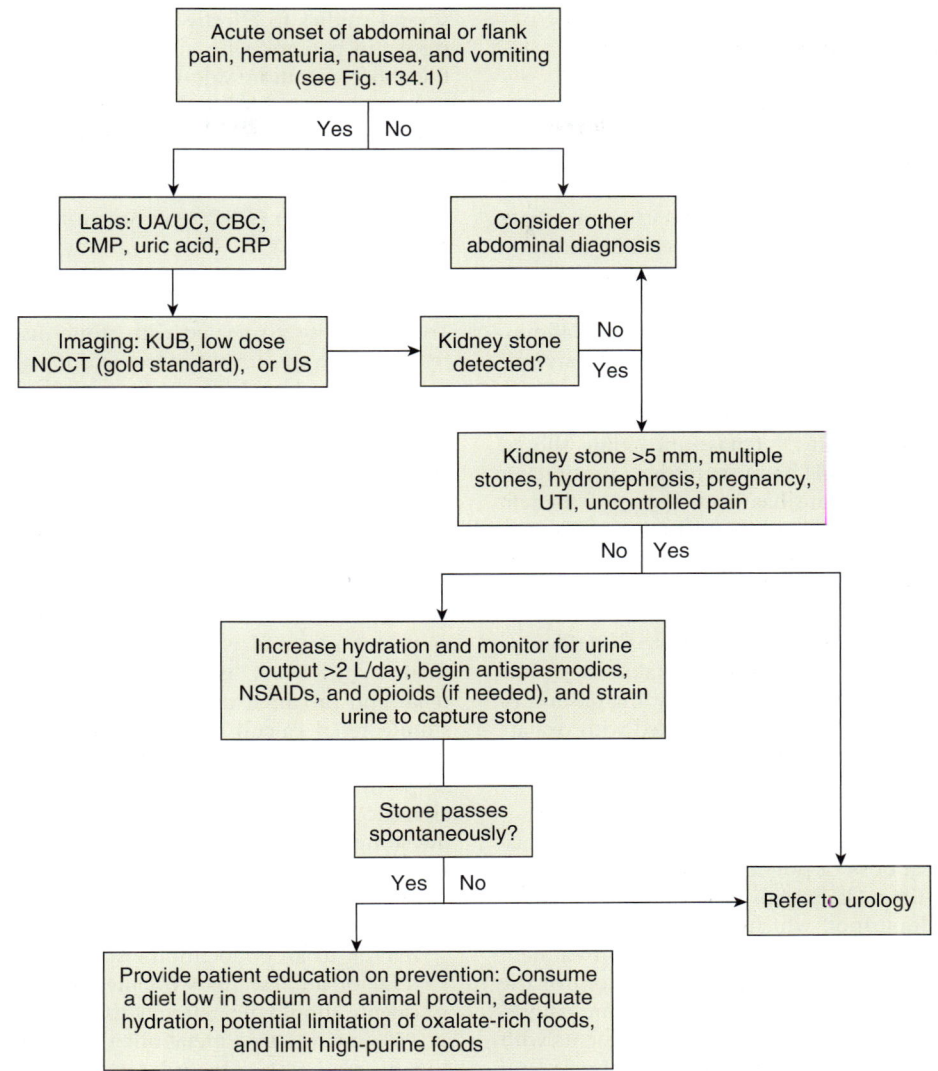

FIG. **134.1** Acute kidney stone management. *CBC,* Complete blood count; *KUB,* kidneys, ureter, and bladder; *NCCT,* noncontrast computed tomography; *NSAID,* nonsteroidal anti-inflammatory drug; *US,* ultrasound; *UTI,* urinary tract infection.

Struvite Stones

Struvite stones require early medical and surgical intervention, and therefore nonpharmacologic interventions have minimal impact, as complete stone removal is considered a definitive treatment.[3]

Cystine Stones

Prevention of cystine stones includes reduced intake of protein-rich foods, low sodium intake (≤2300 mg daily), and high intake of fluids (4 L/day).[3,7]

Pharmacologic Management

The acute management of renal colic symptoms and kidney stones should initially focus on pain relief through the use of narcotics or nonsteroidal antiinflammatory drugs (NSAIDs).[3,10,13] As kidney stones pass into the ureter, pain intensifies owing to the increasing pressure on the collecting system, ureteral spasm, and renal capsular distention.[6] NSAIDs provide relief through prostaglandin inhibition and decrease in renal blood flow, and recent literature has suggested that NSAIDs have similar efficacy as narcotics for renal colic pain.[2,3] Special issues need to be considered in prescribing NSAIDs, specifically in older adult patients who have preexisting renal disease, severe dehydration, and other comorbidities that can lead to acute kidney injury.[10] In conjunction with pain relief and adequate fluid hydration, several medical expulsion therapy (MET) medications are known to aid in the passage of kidney stones. The two most frequently used types of medications are calcium channel blockers and α-blockers, which aid in relaxing smooth muscle and widen channels to allow stone passage.[10] Nifedipine and tamsulosin are the best-studied MET medications, and with MET, stone passage rates are as high as 44% to 66%.[6] Corticosteroids have also been used as part of MET, but there is no significant evidence that supports their efficacy and therefore routine use is not recommended.[13]

PHARMACOLOGIC MANAGEMENT (STONE SPECIFIC)

Calcium Stones

The use of thiazides (hydrochlorothiazide, 25 mg orally twice daily or 50 mg orally once daily; chlorthalidone, 25 mg orally once daily; indapamide, 2.5 mg orally once daily) has been shown to be beneficial in preventing renal calcium stones because thiazide diuretics decrease urinary calcium excretion by augmenting tubular reabsorption of calcium but do not decrease intestinal absorption in absorptive hypercalciuria.[7,18] Persistent calcium stone formation may be treated with allopurinol to inhibit uric acid synthesis and to decrease urinary uric acid excretion.[18] Allopurinol has been shown to reduce the risk of recurrent calcium oxalate stones with the commonly used dose being 100 to 300 mg daily.[4,7] Potassium citrate should also be given to increase urine pH because uric acid precipitates in acidic urine; potassium citrate has been shown to benefit calcium phosphate stone formers with hypocitraturia.[7] The recommended dosing of potassium citrate is 20 to 80 mEq/day with a maximum daily dose of 100 mEq/day.[3,4] A secondary choice of alkalinizing agent is sodium citrate or bicarbonate for those who do not tolerate potassium citrate.[19] Pyridoxine (vitamin B_6) may reduce the production of oxalate by reducing enzyme activity; in one epidemiologic study, high intake of vitamin B_6 (>40 mg/day) was inversely associated with oxalate stone formation in women.[18]

Uric Acid Stones

First-line therapy is aimed at alkalinizing the urine with potassium citrate.[7] The initial dose of potassium citrate is 60 meEq/day or 20 mEq three times daily with a maximum daily dose of 100 mEq/day.[3,4] Allopurinol, which inhibits the formation of uric acid, is reserved for use in uric acid stone treatment when diet control and alkalinizing agents fail to control the condition; the commonly used dose is 100 to 300 mg daily.[4,7] Febuxostat is also used but should be limited to patients with a primary diagnosis of gout, high urinary uric acid levels, and a history of calcium stones.[4,17]

Struvite Stones

Management of magnesium ammonium phosphate (struvite) stones has focused on eliminating urease-producing bacteria (Proteus species are predominant) within the urine and stones that are colonized with bacteria.[14,18] Antimicrobial therapy to sterilize the urine is necessary to treat the infection, and, if needed, surgical intervention is required to remove the colonized stone.[18] Urease inhibitors may be used to prevent struvite formation or to slow the growth of existing calculi. The most commonly used urease inhibitor is acetohydroxamic acid (AHA).[18] It is an irreversible inhibitor of urease and can prevent the crystallization of struvite stones. However, because of its associated risk of deep venous thrombosis, it is generally reserved for patients who cannot tolerate surgical interventions.[7,18] To adequately sterilize the urine, it is paramount that surgical intervention be performed to remove the offending stone.

Cystine Stones

The mainstay of cystic stone treatment is the combination of urinary alkalization and thiol-binding medications.[4] D-Penicillamine and tiopronin (Thiola) have been shown in several studies to effectively decrease the number of recurrent stones in patients who are cystinuric stone formers.[18] Among the more common side effects of long-term D-penicillamine therapy is vitamin B_{12} deficiency. Tiopronin has fewer side effects but still poses some risk for hematologic changes, fever, proteinuria, and rash.[18] For patients who are taking these medications, specific laboratory testing should be completed at least twice a year (CBC, liver function tests, and urine protein/creatinine ratios).[18]

Indications for Referral and Hospitalization

The morbidity associated with stone disease has been greatly reduced with the advent of extracorporeal techniques for stone treatment and with the refinement of endoscopic surgery. Kidney stones 10 mm or larger usually require surgical management because they only spontaneously pass approximately 25% of the time.[6] The three major endourologic procedures are shock wave lithotripsy (SWL), percutaneous nephrolithotomy (PCNL), and ureteroscopy (URS).[6,8] It is indicated for stones that cannot be passed spontaneously, can be visualized on x-ray film, are located in the renal pelvis or upper ureter, and are smaller than 2 cm.[8] SWL is the least invasive treatment and is the treatment of choice for stones less than 1 cm.[8] PCNL is the treatment of choice for complex renal and proximal ureteral calculi larger than 2 cm or when simple renal calculi do not respond to SWL.[8] URS is used mainly in the ureter and involves the use of a fiberoptic scope through the urethra to relieve obstruction, allow basket extraction of stones, or use a laser or lithotripsy to break apart the stone.[16]

- There are several considerations for hospitalization or referral for individuals who present with a kidney stone. A stone associated with hyperparathyroidism requires a referral to an endocrinologist for further evalutaion.[7] Children or adolescents who present with a renal or urinary calculi should be referred to an urologist because up to 75% are due to a metabolic or genetic cause.[14] All patients who are being managed conservatively for a kidney stone should be instructed to return to the emergency room for any unbearable pain or symptoms of a UTI.[2] Individuals that have uncontrolled nausea and vomiting and unable to tolerate oral fluids and pain medications should be considered for hospitalization.[3] Stones larger than 5 mm and more proximal in the urinary tract are less likely to pass spontaneously and should be referred to urology for intervention.[2,3] Urinary obstruction and/or infection by a stone are considered emergent conditions and should be considered for hospitalization and referred to urology.[3]
- The development of kidney stones during pregnancy is increased owing to urinary stasis, elevated progesterone levels, and decreased bladder capacity.[8,20] Calcium phosphate stones occur more frequently in women than any other type of kidney stone, and stones occur more often in the second and third trimesters. The majority of kidney stones will pass spontaneously, but pregnant women have an increased risk of UTIs, and those who are symptomatic have double the risk for preterm labor.[20] If surgical intervention is indicated, ureteroscopic stone removal (URS) is the primary treatment with similar safety outcomes as in nonpregnant women, but PCNL and SWL have high complication rates and are generally contraindicated.[20]

COMPLICATIONS

Renal calculi are associated with an increased risk of UTIs with the potential for progression to pyelonephritis, sepsis, or chronic kidney disease.[4] Hydronephrosis, which is associated with partial or complete obstruction of the renal pelvis or ureter, is another possible complication.[12] Additional potential sequelae include renal tissue damage, scarring, and renal failure because of obstruction or stone movement, and nephrocalcinosis because of deposition of calcium phosphate in the renal parenchyma.[4]

PATIENT AND FAMILY EDUCATION AND HEALTH PROMOTION

- Patients suspected of having stones should be instructed to increase fluid intake, to strain all urine, and to use analgesics as necessary.
- Specific patient education should be based on individual risk factors, the type of stone produced by the patient, a prescribed medical regimen, and comorbidities.
- Basic approach to stone management and prevention is a delicate balance among fluid hydration, a diet low in sodium and low in animal protein, and potential limitation of oxalate-rich and high-purine foods.
- Reoccurrence of urinary calculi is 15% at 1 year, 35% to 40% at 5 years, and 50% at 10 years.[3]

An emphasis on healthy lifestyle habits, such as regular exercise, generous fluid intake (2 to 4 L/day), and a balanced diet high in fiber, is integral to stone prevention.[3,8] Effective stone prevention depends on the stone type and identification of risk factors for stone formation. Research has demonstrated that obesity is a significant factor in stone formation owing to dietary choices such as low fluid intake, high-oxalate foods, protein-rich foods, and refined sugars and overall increases the risk for uric acid stones.[8,14] Therefore the importance of exercise and weight management must be emphasized as a recommendation to reduce stone risk but also to improve renal function and insulin sensitivity. Patients should be informed that the basic approach to stone management and prevention is a delicate balance among fluid hydration, a diet low in sodium and low in animal protein, and potential limitation of oxalate-rich and high-purine foods.[3,8]

REFERENCES

1. Kirkali, Z., Rasooly, R., Star, R. A., & Rodgers, G. P. (2015). Urinary stone disease: Progress, status, and needs. *Urology, 86*(4), 651–653.
2. Sewell, J., Katz, D. J., Shoshany, O., & Love, C. (2017). Urolithiasis—ten things every general practitioner should know. *Australian Family Physician, 46*(9), 648–652.
3. Tan, J. A., & Lerma, E. V. (2015). Nephrolithiasis for the primary care physician. *Disease-A-Month, 61*(10), 434–441.
4. Pfau, A., & Knauf, F. (2016). Update on nephrolithiasis: Core curriculum 2016. *American Journal of Kidney Diseases, 68*(6), 973–985.
5. Shadman, A., & Bastani, B. (2017). Kidney calculi: Pathophysiology and as a systemic disorder. *Iranian Journal of Kidney Diseases, 11*(3), 180–191.
6. Ingimarsson, J. P., Krambeck, A. E., & Pais, V. M. (2016). Diagnosis and management of nephrolithiasis. *Surgical Clinics of North America., 96*(3), 517–532.
7. Pearle, M. S., Goldfarb, D. S., Assimos, D. G., et al. (2014). Medical management of kidney stones: AUA guideline. *The Journal of Urology, 192*(2), 316–324.
8. Hornberger, B., & Bollner, M. R. (2018). Kidney stones. *Physician Assistant Clinics, 3*(1), 37–54.
9. Manuel, F. P., D'Addessi, A., & Gambaro, G. (2013). When to suspect a genetic disorder in a patient with renal stones, and why. *Nephrology, Dialysis, Transplantation, 28*(4), 811–820.
10. Ferraro, P. M., Robertson, W., & Unwin, R. (2015). Renal stone disease. *Medicine, 43*(8), 427–430.
11. Ahmed, M. H., Ahmed, H. T., & Khalil, A. A. (2012). Renal stone disease and obesity: What is important for urologists and nephrologists? *Renal Failure, 34*(10), 1348–1354.
12. Nicolau, C., Salvador, R., & Artigas, J. M. (2015). Diagnostic management of renal colic. *Radiología (English Edition), 57*(2), 113–122.
13. Türk, C., Petřík, A., Sarica, K., et al. (2016). EAU Guidelines on Diagnosis and Conservative Management of Urolithiasis. *European Urology, 69*(3), 468–474.
14. Hoppe, B. (2014). Renal calculi in children. *Paediatrics and Child Health., 24*(7), 293–302.
15. Renard-Penna, R., Martin, A., Conort, P., Mozer, P., & Grenier, P. (2015). Kidney stones and imaging: What can your radiologist do for you? *World Journal of Urology, 33*(2), 193–202.
16. Ziemba, J. B., & Matlaga, B. R. (2015). Guideline of guidelines: Kidney stones. *BJU International, 116*(2), 184–189.
17. Heilberg, I. P. (2016). Treatment of patients with uric acid stones. *Urolithiasis, 44*(1), 57–63.
18. Eisner, B. H., Goldfarb, D. S., & Pareek, G. (2013). Pharmacologic treatment of kidney stone disease. *The Urologic Clinics of North America, 40*(1), 21–30.
19. Fattah, H., Hambaroush, Y., & Goldfarb, D. S. (2014). Cystine nephrolithiasis. *Translational Andrology and Urology, 3*(3), 228–233.
20. Pedro, R. N., Das, K., & Buchholz, N. (2016). Urolithiasis in pregnancy. *International Journal of Surgery, 36*, 688–692.

CHAPTER **135**

URINARY TRACT INFECTIONS AND SEXUALLY TRANSMITTED INFECTIONS
Patricia Polgar-Bailey

 Immediate hospitalization indicated for rigors, high fever, flank pain, nausea, vomiting, and other signs and symptoms suggestive of acute illness, including obstruction or urosepsis.

URINARY TRACT INFECTIONS

DEFINITION AND EPIDEMIOLOGY

Urinary tract infection (UTI) is a broad term describing any infection involving any part of the urinary tract, including the kidneys, ureters, bladder, and urethra. The urinary tract can be divided in the upper tract (kidneys and ureters) and the lower tract (bladder and urethra). UTIs can be classified as uncomplicated, complicated, recurrent, and asymptomatic bacteria.[1] Uncomplicated UTIs include those typically occurring in otherwise healthy, immunocompetent, nonpregnant women with no significant history of UTIs or structural abnormalities and are characterized by recent onset of mild to moderate symptoms. UTIs are considered complicated if the infection is associated with a condition, such as a structural or functional abnormality of the urinary tract, as this increases the risk of the infection being more serious than it would be in individuals without any risk factors (i.e., uncomplicated UTIs). All UTIs in males are considered complicated. Recurrent UTIs are symptomatic UTIs that occur after resolution of a previously treated UTI. They are common among young, healthy women, albeit in the absence of anatomic or physiologic abnormalities. Asymptomatic bacteriuria (ABU) refers to significant levels of bacteria in the urine with no UTI symptoms. ABU does not cause renal disease or damage.[1]

Infection of the urinary tract is one of the most common diagnoses seen in primary care and is the most frequent urologic disorder encountered.[1] These infections are responsible for more than 7 million office visits yearly in the United States, with costs exceeding $1 billion per year.[2]

UTIs are a particular problem in certain patient groups, with young, sexually active women and elderly individuals being disproportionately affected. Approximately 40% of women develop a UTI at some point in their life. There are 1000 to 4000 cases of UTI per 100,000 females annually, and fewer than 100 cases per 100,000 men.[3] Most of these infections are sporadic, with about 25% being recurrent infections. At least 20% of infections in long-term care facilities are attributed to UTIs, and the prevalence of ABU in long-term care facility (LTCF) residents can range from 20% to 50%.[4]

UTIs are unusual in men younger than 50 years with normal urologic structures but become more common with age. Common reasons for UTIs in men include prostatitis, epididymitis, orchitis, pyelonephritis, cystitis, and urethritis. Risk factors associated with UTI in men include previous UTI; enlarged prostate; history of instrumentation, catheterization, or surgery of the urinary tract; human immunodeficiency virus (HIV) infection; comorbidities; immunosuppression; abnormalities or family history of abnormalities in the urinary tract; and anal intercourse. After the age of 65 years, the incidence of UTIs in men is about 10%, whereas the incidence is 20% in similarly aged women.[5]

ABU refers to a colony count of at least 100,000/mL in the absence of symptoms. It is estimated that 8% of women have ABU.[2] It is more common in women, increases in both sexes with advancing age, and is found in as many as 43% of older women and 21% of older men, especially those living in nursing homes. In addition to advancing age and nursing home residence, ABU is also associated with pregnancy, history of indwelling catheterization, instrumentation, urinary incontinence, diabetes, multiple medical illnesses, obstructive uropathy, postmenopausal status, and impaired functional and mental status.

PATHOPHYSIOLOGY

Most UTIs in women are secondary to ascending infection from the periurethral or perianal area. Bacteria from the colon, vagina, or skin are the usual organisms causing the infection. Cystitis is more common in women than in men because of the short length of the urethra and the proximity of the urethral opening and vagina to the perianal area. Bacteria reach the bladder through the urethra and have the opportunity to ascend to the kidneys through the ureters.

A relatively narrow spectrum of microorganisms cause the majority of UTIs. The most prominent uropathogen is *Escherichia coli*. Other common uropathogens include *Staphylococcus saprophyticus* and the *Enterococcus*, *Klebsiella*, *Enterobacter*, and *Proteus genus.*[1]

Most UTIs in women are not associated with complicating conditions or serious problems. Common precipitants include sexual intercourse, use of spermicidal agents, a new sexual partner, maternal history of UTI, and history of UTI during childhood.[1] Risk factors for UTI in postmenopausal and older adult women include history of UTI before menopause, urinary incontinence, atrophic vaginitis due to estrogen

---

BOX 135.1

Risk Factors for Urinary Tract Infections

WOMEN
- Inherent anatomic risk (4-cm urethra in females versus 20-cm urethra in males)
- Fecal contamination
- History of recent urinary tract infection
- Decreased fluid intake
- Irregular bladder emptying
- Vaginal pH >4.5
- Sexual intercourse
- Failure to void within 10–15 min of coitus
- Spermicide use
- Symptomatic partner
- Pregnancy
- Menopause
- Hyperuricemia
- Neurogenic bladder
- Kidney disease

- Urologic abnormalities
- Instrumentation
- Immunosuppression
- Comorbidities (e.g., diabetes)

MEN
- Urologic abnormalities
- Neurogenic bladder
- Instrumentation
- Benign prostatic hyperplasia
- Anal intercourse
- Immunosuppression
- Comorbidities (e.g., diabetes)

CHILDREN
- Constipation
- Anatomic abnormalities
- Dysfunctional voiding
- Immunosuppression

BOX 135.2

Risks for Recurrent Urinary Tract Infections

WOMEN
Current Conditions
- Sexually active
- Immunosuppression
- Pregnancy
- Spermicide use
- New sexual partner
- Voiding problems

Past Medical History
- Post-coital UTI symptoms
- Pyelonephritis
- UTI in pregnancy

MEN
- Immunosuppression
- Voiding problems

UTI, Urinary tract infection.
Data from Al-Badr, A., & Al-Shaikh, G. (2013). Recurrent urinary tract infections, management in women: A review. *Sultan Qaboos University Medical Journal, 13*(3), 359–367.

---

deficiency, cystocele, and increased postvoid urine residual.[1] In addition, UTIs frequently occur in individuals with diabetes, obesity, urinary tract calculi, sickle cell trait, and frequent or indwelling bladder catheterization.[3] In men, the reservoirs of microorganisms are not in close proximity to the urethral opening as in women; anatomic abnormalities of the urinary tract are more likely associated with UTIs in men. Risk factors associated with UTI in men include lack of circumcision, anal intercourse, HIV infection, and prostatic hypertrophy.

Risk factors for UTIs and recurrent UTIs are listed in Boxes 135.1 and 135.2.

Urethritis is characterized by an inflammation (mechanical, chemical, viral, or bacterial) of the urethra. Nongonococcal urethritis (NGU) is most common, with *Chlamydia* being the most frequent causative organism. Other urethral pathogens include *Ureaplasma urealyticum*, *Mycoplasma hominis*, herpes simplex virus (HSV), cytomegalovirus, and, in women, *Trichomonas vaginalis* and *Gardnerella vaginalis*. Noninfectious causes include Stevens-Johnson syndrome, Wegener granulomatosis, use of spermicides, and ingestion of some acidic foods.[6] Risk factors for urethritis include being a man aged 20 to 35, being a female of reproductive age, having multiple sexual partners, engaging in high-risk sexual behavior, and having a history of a sexually transmitted infection (STI).

CLINICAL PRESENTATION AND PHYSICAL EXAMINATION

Different characteristics are associated with each type of UTI. Uncomplicated UTIs are characterized by signs and symptoms of bladder irritation: increased frequency, urgency, dysuria, suprapubic pain, odorous urine, and occasionally hematuria. The term *uncomplicated infection* implies that this is a relatively uncommon occurrence in the affected individual who is also otherwise healthy, that there are a small number of responsible pathogens susceptible to first-line narrow-spectrum antimicrobial agents, and that there are no underlying urologic or gynecologic abnormalities.

A more acute presentation, including high fever, chills, flank pain, costovertebral angle (CVA) tenderness, nausea, and vomiting, is suggestive of complicated UTI (pyelonephritis or urosepsis). A sustained bladder infection increases the risk for a complicated infection. However, kidney infection may also manifest with only bladder irritation and the absence of any of the classic signs or symptoms. Pyuria in the presence of positive urine or blood culture is indicative of a complicated UTI. Risks associated with complicated UTI include presence of urinary catheter, residual urine of 100 mL or more after voiding, obstruction in the urinary tract, azotemia resulting from kidney disease, and urinary retention.[3]

UTI is considered isolated with the first occurrence or a repeat occurrence at least 6 months from the previous episode. About 25% to 40% of infections are considered isolated. Unresolved infections persist when prescribed medications are not effective because of drug resistance or the presence of more than one organism with different drug sensitivities. UTIs are considered recurrent if they occur at least three times in 1 year or twice in 6 months. There are two basic patterns of recurrence: relapse and reinfection. Relapse refers to infection caused by bacterial persistence, i.e., infection by the previously treated pathogen, which was not completely eradicated by the course of antimicrobial therapy. Reinfection refers to recurrence of infection by introduction of a new bacterial strain or regrowth of the same organism after complete eradication with treatment. Recurrent UTIs in women are usually are a result of reinfection rather than relapse, but it can also be difficult to determine the difference.

In men, symptoms of urethritis are usually mild and gradual in onset, and include dysuria and irritative symptoms, frequency, urethral discharge, and pruritus at the distal end of the penis. Women may experience vaginal discharge or bleeding from concomitant cervicitis and lower abdominal pain. Urinalysis often demonstrates pyuria and, less commonly, hematuria. Urine cultures generally show a colony count of less than 100/mL in urethritis.

Important history to elicit from the woman with complaints of UTI symptoms includes urinary frequency, nocturia, dysuria, pruritus, fever or chills, hematuria, vaginal discomfort or discharge, pelvic discomfort, back or flank pain, date of last menstrual period, any prior history of UTIs, cervicitis, or pelvic inflammatory disease (PID). Patients should be queried about medical history, specifically immunocompromising disease or

drugs, and recent instrumentation. A recent study has shown that women with a history of UTI correctly diagnose themselves (as confirmed by urine culture) as having a UTI 61% to 90% of the time.[7]

Vaginal symptoms, external irritation on urination, and dyspareunia are helpful in sorting out vaginal causes from those referable to the urinary tract. Male patients should be asked about urethral discharge, penile lesions, history of UTIs or STIs, and prior treatment. It is important to ask all patients about sexual history and risk factors for gonorrhea or chlamydia, including new or symptomatic sex partners.

The physical examination should include assessment of vital signs, signs and symptoms of acute illness, and dehydration. A careful abdominal examination including the assessment of CVA tenderness is an important aspect of the physical examination. A pelvic examination in females should be performed if there is any indication that infection is not solely associated with the urinary tract. The vulva, vagina, cervix, periurethral area, and perianal area should be assessed for discharge, excoriations, tenderness, and ulcerations. In male patients, the penis should be checked for discharge, lesions, ulcerations, and swelling. The prostate should be checked for tenderness, swelling, masses, or nodules. A rectal examination showing a tender prostate may be indicative of acute prostatitis, and a normal or enlarged prostate indicates chronic bacterial prostatitis.

Malodorous urine is not found to be indicative of infection. The diagnosis of UTI is suggested by the history and physical examination findings and confirmed by examination of the urine.

DIAGNOSTICS
Essential Diagnostics

The urinalysis is the most important initial study and the urine dipstick is a reasonable alternative to urine culture to diagnose uncomplicated UTI. A clean-voided midstream specimen minimizes contamination from nearby sources. Leukocyte esterase reflects the presence of white blood cells (WBCs) in the urine, but not all UTIs are associated with WBCs in the urine. Evidence-based guidelines from the University of Michigan Quality Management Program report that the presence of pyuria has a sensitivity of 80% to 90% and a specificity of 50% in predicting UTI. The nitrite test is not as good at detecting UTI as not all bacteria produce nitrate reductase, and false-positive results may occur with intake of ascorbic acid.[2] However, in a more recent study of older women, these dipstick findings only resulted in 57% with a positive urine culture.[8] In addition to leukocyte esterase and urinary nitrite, the presence of blood on the dipstick is another variable that is useful in predicting the presence of a UTI.

Urine culture is the definitive test; specimens should be obtained from all patients who are pregnant, are febrile, are seriously ill, have a history of frequent UTIs, live in a community with high rates of antibiotic resistance, or have recently been hospitalized, or in whom empirical treatment has failed. Cultures should be obtained in young men because these infections are unusual and suggestive of underlying problems.

Additional Diagnostics

Urine may also be examined microscopically, which allows easier detection of red blood cells, WBCs, bacteria, and WBC casts. Correlation with subsequent culture is approximately

90%. This diagnostic is typically ordered by the provider and performed by a laboratory before culturing. Abnormalities of pH, protein, and blood are nonspecific with respect to UTIs. In the presence of symptoms but a negative dipstick result, direct demonstration by microscopy or culture should be done before the possibility of infection is excluded.

The presence of multiple bacterial species identified by culture usually suggests contamination of the specimen, except in the case of catheterization or other special circumstances. Small numbers of certain pathogens, including *Klebsiella* organisms and *E. coli*, should be regarded as suspicious. Large numbers of skin flora, such as *Staphylococcus epidermidis*, diphtheroids, and β-hemolytic streptococci, can usually be ignored. Anaerobic bacteria do not usually cause UTIs; their presence suggests communication from the bowel. *Candida* organisms usually suggest vaginal contamination.

Sterile pyuria is defined as a negative urine culture despite a positive urinalysis (e.g., positive leukocyte esterase). This condition requires further investigation because the absence of pathogens on culture does not imply the absence of infection. Renal tuberculosis, systemic illness, vaginal contamination, and kidney stones can also cause leukocytosis in the absence of a positive culture. Some infectious organisms, such as those causing NGU, do not grow on standard laboratory media. Cultures specific for these organisms should be considered if the history and physical examination findings suggest a chlamydial or nongonococcal cause. However, many patients with urethral syndrome do not have a demonstrable infectious agent even when special culture media are used. A test of cure urine culture should be obtained in men and whenever there is suspicion that an infection may not have been eradicated. Routine testing of cure cultures are not indicated unless a persistent UTI is suspected. The recurrence of a UTI within 2 weeks is suggestive of a persistent UTI.

Renal ultrasound is useful to diagnose structural abnormalities, calculi, masses, and hydronephrosis. Persistent UTIs require more extensive urologic evaluation with referral to a urologist. Indications for ultrasound evaluation of patients with UTIs include frequent recurrent UTIs in females or failure to eradicate infection despite appropriate therapy, acute pyelonephritis in males, recurrent pyelonephritis in females, and palpable bladder or renal mass. Ultrasound is recommended for children younger than 2 years with their first febrile UTI, patients of any age with recurrent febrile UTIs, patients with a family history of kidney or urologic problems, and children with high blood pressure or retarded growth.

DIFFERENTIAL DIAGNOSIS

The differential diagnosis of an acute uncomplicated UTI includes urethritis, vaginal infections, STIs that may lead to cervicitis or PID, and other STIs that may mimic symptoms of UTI but are considered distinct from UTIs. The diagnosis is usually made on the basis of the history, presenting signs and symptoms, and findings on urinalysis and culture. In the case of a negative urine dipstick result in the presence of urinary symptoms, microscopic evaluation or culture should be performed before it is decided that a UTI is not present. The combination of cervical discharge, cervical motion tenderness, and adnexal tenderness suggests cervicitis or PID. Atrophic vaginitis should be considered in a postmenopausal woman not using topical estrogen therapy. Chlamydial and gonorrheal cultures should be obtained in sexually active individuals.

Clinical syndromes in women that mimic UTIs include acute urethral syndrome (also referred to as symptomatic abacteriuria) and interstitial cystitis. Clinical presentation is characterized by bladder irritation, frequency, urgency, and dysuria. The urinalysis is often unimpressive, with few leukocytes, no bacteria, and occasionally hematuria. Urine cultures show no significant colony counts, and urethral cultures are often negative. Symptoms of interstitial cystitis also include suprapubic discomfort, especially with a full bladder, and symptoms are often relieved with voiding. No definitive therapy for interstitial cystitis has been developed.

The differential diagnoses for chronic or recurrent UTIs include structural abnormalities (such as obstructive uropathy, congenital anomalies, urinary tract fistulas), neurologic dysfunction, renal calculi and renal masses, intrarenal and perirenal abscesses, and androgenital tuberculosis. Prostate infections and STIs should be considered in all male patients with UTI.[1]

INTERPROFESSIONAL COLLABORATIVE MANAGEMENT

Uncomplicated UTIs are typically managed on an outpatient basis with oral antibiotics.

Nonpharmacologic Management

Patients should be advised to drink enough fluid to avoid dehydration. Although some lay literature suggests that cranberry juice may be helpful in preventing and treating UTIs, there is insufficient evidence to suggest that drinking cranberry juice is helpful in the management of UTIs.

Pharmacologic Management

Selection of antibiotic therapy is based on the severity of symptoms, risk of complications, previous urine culture and susceptibility results, previous antibiotic use, and local antimicrobial resistance data.

1. Recommended antimicrobial therapy for uncomplicated UTIs in nonpregnant women aged 16 years and older includes nitrofurantoin (avoid in G6PD deficiency) or trimethoprim-sulfamethoxazole (if there is a low rate of resistance). Alternatives include fosfomycin, ciprofloxacin, levofloxacin, and cephalosporins (e.g., cephalexin, cefuroxime).[1,9]
2. Treatment of lower UTIs in pregnant women during the first trimester include cephalexin, amoxicillin, amoxicillin-clavulanic acid, and ampicillin. If these agents are contraindicated (e.g., severe allergy or pathogen is not susceptible), nitrofurantoin and trimethoprim-sulfamethoxazole may be considered. During the second or third trimester, first-line therapies include cephalexin, amoxicillin, amoxicillin-clavulanic acid, and ampicillin. Trimethoprim-sulfamethoxazole and nitrofurantoin may also be considered, although both should be avoided near delivery (38 to 42 weeks). Use of nitrofurantoin near term has been associated with an increased risk of hemolytic anemia in the infant, which may be linked to mothers with G6PD deficiency.
3. Recommended antibiotics for men include trimethoprim-sulfamethoxazole, nitrofurantoin, and amoxicillin-clavulanate. Alternative choices include ciprofloxacin and cephalosporins.

4. Phenazopyridine may be prescribed along with an antibiotic as a urinary analgesic; the drug is pregnancy risk factor B.

5. Recurrent cystitis can be managed by one of several strategies: continuous prophylaxis, postcoital prophylaxis, or therapy initiated by the patient. Prophylaxis should not be initiated until the existing UTI has been eradicated, confirmed with negative culture 1 to 2 weeks after treatment.

6. Given that ABU does not cause renal disease or damage, and since studies suggest that antibiotic treatment increases the risk of subsequent symptomatic UTIs, treatment for ABU is not recommended, except in diagnostic or therapeutic procedures that involve entry to the urinary tract with a risk of mucosal damage. Screening and treatment of ABU in pregnant women has generally been recommended in order to reduce the risk of low-birth-weight infants and preterm delivery, although recent studies show mixed results in improvement in outcomes following antibiotic treatment of ABU in pregnancy.[1]

7. Postmenopausal women who experience recurrent UTIs may find symptomatic relief with topical estrogen cream.

8. Common pathogens found in a urine culture that are not considered common urinary pathogens include candida species, enterococcus, staphylococcus aureus, and Gardnerella vaginalis. In most cases, isolation of candida represents colonization and treatment of candiduria should be considered for symptomatic relief. Enterococcus also often represents colonization, but treatment is not generally necessary unless the patient is symptomatic, the urinalysis shows inflammation, or in high-risk populations. Gardnerella vaginalis is the most common cause of bacterial vaginosis, but may also cause a UTI. If there is a significant colony count and the urinalysis shows inflammation, treatment with oral metronidazole is indicated.

Indications for Referral and Hospitalization

- Indications for urology referral include presence of macroscopic hematuria, suspected malignancy, recurrent UTIs or infections that do not respond to standard antimicrobial therapy, urinary tract anomalies or obstructions, acute scrotum, and all forms of prostatitis. Hospitalization is recommended for pregnant women with pyelonephritis.

- Older adults and those with acute, severe symptoms are candidates for hospitalization and often require parenteral therapy.

- A history of diabetes mellitus, sickle cell anemia, nephrolithiasis, or excessive analgesic use increases the risk of renal papillary necrosis and subsequent obstruction and can be considered an indication for hospitalization.

Life Span Considerations

UTIs are the most common cause of bacterial infection in older adults, but are often not accompanied by the classic signs and symptoms. Symptoms are often subtle and may include a vague change in mental status, decreased appetite, lethargy, and increased falls (sustained during efforts to get to the bathroom). UTIs are also a common cause of sepsis, especially in older adults, and a risk for morbidity and mortality in nursing facilities.

Complications. The most common complication of UTI is pyelonephritis, a bacterial infection of the kidney resulting from ascending, untreated, or inadequately treated lower UTI. Uncomplicated pyelonephritis can be treated effectively on an outpatient basis, and clinical response should occur within 48 to 72 hours of starting therapy. Recommended treatment includes broad-spectrum antibiotics such as cephalosporins and fluoroquinolones. Due to increasing prevalence of resistant E. coli, TMP/SMX, ciprofloxacin, and ampicillin are generally not recommended for therapy but may be an option when susceptibilities are known. If no improvement is noted or if the patient's condition worsens, aggressive investigation for complications of renal infection or urinary obstruction should be undertaken, which generally requires hospitalization.

Complicated pyelonephritis, as characterized by complicated infections, diabetes, or other forms of immunosuppression or suspected bacteremia, requires inpatient management, including supportive care, adjustment of antibiotic regimen based on culture results, and IV volume repletion as needed. Urosepsis is a potentially life-threatening systemic complication of UTI that requires hospitalization with high-dose parenteral antimicrobial therapy.

Acute urinary infections may be associated with severe complications and even death, particularly in patients with underlying comorbidities such as diabetes and in those with indwelling urologic devices or chronic disease. Individuals with diabetes are also more likely to develop rare complications, such as emphysematous cystitis and pyelonephritis, abscess formation, and renal papillary necrosis, compared with those who do not have diabetes mellitus.

Patient and Family Education

Nonpharmacologic measures have been demonstrated to prevent episodic or recurrent UTIs.

1. Voiding 10 to 15 minutes after sexual intercourse has been shown to prevent episodic UTIs.

2. Drinking plenty of fluids (64 to 80 ounces daily), urinating frequently (at least every 4 hours), wiping from front to back, and using tampons during menstruation may also be helpful in preventing UTIs.

3. Avoiding the following may help in the prevention of UTIs: wiping more than once with the same tissue, extended soaking in a bathtub, wearing tight-fitting underwear made of nonbreathable fabric, and using spermicidal products.

4. Women who have had previous UTIs should be encouraged to seek treatment as soon as symptoms are recognized.

5. Women with recurrent UTIs should be educated about the possible benefits of antimicrobial suppression or postcoital prophylaxis, depending on the situation.

6. Intravaginal estrogen cream may be helpful for postmenopausal women with recurrent UTIs.

SEXUALLY TRANSMITTED INFECTIONS

DEFINITION AND EPIDEMIOLOGY

The terms *sexually transmitted infection* and *sexually transmitted disease* are used interchangeably. They encompass more than 25 infectious organisms that are transmitted through sexual activity along with the dozens of clinical syndromes associated with these organisms. The most common STIs in the United States are human papillomavirus (HPV), chlamydia, trichomoniasis, gonorrhea, genital herpes, syphilis, HIV, and hepatitis B.

STIs are spread by anal, oral, or vaginal sex with an infected individual. Symptoms are not always present, and knowing if sexual partners are infected can be challenging. Pregnant women infected with an STI may infect infants in utero or during birth; women may also infect infants through breastfeeding.

There are federally funded control programs for three notifiable STIs: chlamydia, gonorrhea, and syphilis. Chlamydia continues to be the most commonly reported nationally notifiable disease. Based on the latest data from the Centers for Disease Control and Prevention (CDC) surveillance report. During 2016–17, the rate of chlamydia increased 6.9%, from 494.7 to 528.8 cases per 100,000 population.[10] Rates of reported cases of chlamydia were highest among adolescents and young adults aged 15 to 24 years, and the prevalence was highest in the South, followed by the West, Midwest, and Northeast.[10]

Gonorrhea is the second most commonly reported notifiable disease in the United States. Just as with infections due to Chlamydia trachomatis, infections due to Neisseria gonorrhoeae are a major cause of PID in the United States, which can result in serious outcomes in women including tubal infertility, ectopic pregnancy, and chronic pelvic pain. In addition, evidence from epidemiologic and biologic studies indicates that gonococcal infections facilitate the transmission of HIV infection.[10] During 2016–17, the rate of reported gonorrhea cases increased 18.6%, and increased 75.2% since the lowest incidence in 2009.[10] The South has the highest prevalence of gonorrhea cases, followed by the Midwest, West, and Northeast.[10]

Syphilis is a genital ulcerative disease caused by the bacterium *Treponema pallidum*. It is associated with significant complications if left untreated and can facilitate the transmission and acquisition of HIV infection. Primary and secondary syphilis represent the earliest stages of infection and reflect symptomatic disease and provide the data for the analysis of syphilis trend data.[10] In 2017, a total of 30,644 cases of primary and secondary syphilis were reported in the United States, yielding a rate of 9.5 cases per 100,000 population. This rate represents a 10.5% increase compared with 2016 (8.6 cases per 100,000 population), and a 72.7% increase compared with 2013 (5.5 cases per 100,000 population).[10]

STIs affect males and females of all racial, cultural, and socioeconomic groups, but wide disparities are present. The CDC's data show much higher rates of reported STIs among certain racial and ethnic groups, with blacks being disproportionally affected by chlamydia, gonorrhea, and primary and secondary syphilis. Many factors contribute to this disparity, including poverty, lack of access to health care, and a relatively high prevalence of STIs in the community.[10] Based on incidence and prevalence data, it is estimated that young people aged 15 to 24 years acquire half of all new STIs and that one in four sexually active adolescent females has an STI such as chlamydia or HPV. This increased risk of acquiring STIs, compared with older adults, is due to a combination of behavioral, biological, and cultural reasons. Behavior that includes multiple partners and inconsistent use of condoms contributes to the higher risk in this age group. Adolescents may also be faced with barriers to access for STI prevention resources. Women are more vulnerable to STIs because they are more biologically susceptible than men to certain STIs such as chlamydia due to cervical ectopy, may be reluctant to insist on condom use, and are dependent on the behavior of the male partner to practice safe sex.

CLINICAL PRESENTATION AND PHYSICAL EXAMINATION

A significant number of persons with STIs have no apparent signs or symptoms. More than one site may be infected simultaneously (e.g., cervix plus urethra), and symptoms may overlap and involve more than one pathogen. Diseases are tentatively classified into syndromes to narrow the field of possible pathogens.

Because STIs do not always manifest with distinct clinical features, determination of which patients are at risk necessitates a thorough sexual history. Eliciting the history for an STI needs to be routine, standardized, and guided by the individual's age. An effective sexual history is critical for diagnosis and for counseling individuals with regard to risk reduction behaviors. The CDC suggests talking with patients about the five Ps: partners, practices, protection from STIs, past history of STIs, and prevention of pregnancy.[11] See Box 135.3 for sexual history questions and topics. With few exceptions, adolescents in the United States can be provided with confidential diagnosis and treatment of STIs without parental consent or knowledge.

The physical examination for an STI incorporates the same principles as for the history. It is routine, standardized, and sensitive to the patient's age, individual needs, and cultural heritage. Consistent examination of all areas reduces the chance of a missed diagnosis. Minimum physical examination procedures for women and men are listed in Box 135.4.

Every effort should be made to reduce anxiety. All steps of the examination should be explained before they are initiated. Female patients normally void before the examination; the necessity of obtaining a urine specimen to test for UTI, gonorrhea, or chlamydia should be kept in mind.

DIAGNOSTICS

After completing the routine screening history and examination, the health care provider may be able to assign the patient to one of several clinical syndromes. This narrows the field of possible pathogens that cause the syndrome and guides treatment. If the patient is asymptomatic, therapy is determined by the laboratory results. Partners of persons with identified STIs are evaluated and treated on the basis of their last sexual encounter and the particular STI in question. Early, specific diagnosis and treatment of symptomatic and asymptomatic persons will prevent further transmission of disease to their partners. However, appropriate diagnosis of an STI often requires multiple diagnostic tests because of the variety of STIs. Culture, nucleic acid hybridization tests, and nucleic acid amplification tests (NAATs) are critical tools used to diagnose chlamydia and gonorrhea. In most cases, urine can be used to test for gonorrhea and chlamydia; first-voided urine is preferred. Use of a urine sample for NAAT is the recommended testing method to detect gonorrhea and chlamydia.

DIFFERENTIAL DIAGNOSIS

Any signs and symptoms suggestive of acute systemic illness warrant immediate referral. Table 135.1 outlines various STIs and their associated pathogens and syndromes, appropriate diagnostics, and differential diagnoses.

BOX 135.3

Sexual History Questions

- Are you currently sexually active? (Are you having sex?)
  - If not, have you ever been sexually active?
- In the past 12 months, how many sex partners have you had?
- Are your sex partners men, women, or both? (If both, ask first two questions for each gender.)
- What kind of sexual contact do you have or have you had? Anal, vaginal, or oral?
- Do you and your partner(s) use any protection against sexually transmitted diseases?
  - If not, tell me your thoughts about this.
  - If so, what kind of protection and how often do you use this protection?
  - If sometimes, in what situations or with whom do you use protection?
- Have you ever been diagnosed with an STI?
  - When?
  - How were you treated?
  - Have you had any recurring symptoms or diagnoses?
- Have you ever been tested for human immunodeficiency virus or other STIs?
- Has your current or any former partner ever been diagnosed or treated for an STI(s)?
  - Were you tested for the same STI(s)?
  - If yes, when were you tested?
  - What was the diagnosis and how was it treated?
- Are you currently trying to conceive or father a child?
- Are you concerned about getting pregnant or getting your partner pregnant?
- Are you using contraception or practicing any form of birth control?

ADDITIONAL HISTORY
- Travel: location, date
- Dysuria, frequency, hematuria
- Adenopathy
- Fatigue, weight loss, night sweats, unexplained diarrhea, fever
- Rash, lesions, sores: location
- Pruritus: anogenital, oral, other
- Rectal bleeding, discharge, pain, constipation

ADDITIONAL HISTORY FOR WOMEN
- Vaginal discharge, bleeding, consistency, color
- Pain (abdominal, vaginal, vulvar, anal, headache, joints)
- Consistency of contraception use
- Last menstrual period, description, changes

ADDITIONAL HISTORY FOR MEN
- Penile discharge
- Pain (testes, joints, headache, anal)

STI, Sexually transmitted infection.

INTERPROFESSIONAL COLLABORATIVE MANAGEMENT

The management of STIs is often confounded by the inclusiveness of the term itself. A number of different organisms may be associated with different syndromes; for example, genital ulcers can result from herpes, chancroid, syphilis, or other infections.

BOX 135.4

Minimum Physical Examination for Sexually Transmitted Infections

- Examination of the mouth
- Examination of the lymph nodes
- Examination of the skin on the thorax, abdomen, limbs, palms, soles
- Examination of the anogenital area
- Palpation for inguinal and femoral adenopathy

ADDITIONAL EXAMINATION FOR WOMEN
- Pelvic examination, including speculum examination and bimanual examination
- Assessment for cervical motion tenderness

ADDITIONAL EXAMINATION FOR MEN
- Examination of the external genitals and anus

Because there is a broad spectrum of sources with STIs, treatment is individualized to the cause. Major curable syndromes in adults include genital ulcers, urethritis vaginitis, cervicitis, and PID. In the United States, treatments are frequently initiated against common pathogens causing these syndromes while laboratory results are pending; coinfection with more than one organism is common. Antimicrobial therapy is available for all bacterial STIs, as well as for those caused by protozoa and ectoparasites. Drugs for viral STIs are largely limited to symptom alleviation because they cannot eradicate the organism.

1. The standards published by the CDC in 2010 and updated in 2015 use the regimens listed in Box 135.5
2. For most STIs, the partners of patients should be examined.
   a. Expedited partner treatment (EPT) is considered permissible in 35 states, potentially allowable in 9 states and prohibited in 6 states.
   b. EPT is a treatment practice whereby a provider gives prescriptions or medications to the patient for treatment of an STI in his or her sexual partner.
   c. In many states, the local state or health department can assist in partner notification for selected STIs (e.g., HIV infection, syphilis, gonorrhea, hepatitis B, and chlamydia).

Indications for Referral or Hospitalization

All pregnant and HIV-positive patients should be co-managed with a specialist or collaborating physician. All treatment failures necessitate management with a specialist. Consultation or co-management with a specialist is necessary for all cases of syphilis. See Table 135.1 for further information.

LIFE SPAN CONSIDERATIONS

Prevalence rates for many STIs are highest among adolescents and young adults. Screening of asymptomatic high-risk patients, with sensitivity to age-related developmental and cultural characteristics, is required. STI prevention should be initiated before sexual activity begins, with education about healthy, safe, sexual practices and continual reinforcement throughout the life span. Additional life span considerations relate to the development of PID in women, with possible

TABLE 135.1   Summary of Sexually Transmitted Infections

Pathogen, Differential Diagnosis	Clinical Presentation	Diagnosis	Consultation, Co-Management	Complications	Management
GONORRHEA Neisseria gonorrhoeae **Differential diagnosis:** NGU, PID, candidiasis, bacterial vaginosis, endometriosis, pregnancy, salpingitis, orchitis, trichomoniasis, UTI, epididymitis	Purulent urethral discharge Dysuria Pruritus Anorectal burning Skin lesions **Female:** Frequently asymptomatic; dysuria; leukorrhea; abnormal uterine bleeding; cervical motion tenderness; vaginal discharge; pharyngeal edema or erythema	NAATs: vaginal swab, first-catch urine Culture	Treatment failure Complications	Prostatitis Epididymitis Cystitis PID Gonococcal conjunctivitis	Treat presumptively for chlamydia. Specimen testing for gonorrhea should occur before other testing. Partners are evaluated and treated. Perform syphilis serology. Offer HIV counseling and testing.
CHLAMYDIA Chlamydia trachomatis **Differential diagnosis:** PID, gonorrhea, candidiasis, bacterial vaginosis, endometriosis, pregnancy, salpingitis, orchitis, epididymitis, trichomoniasis, UTI	Often asymptomatic May infect lungs and eyes **Female:** Abnormal vaginal discharge (yellow or green), vaginal bleeding, dysuria, cervical friability or edema **Male:** Dysuria, penile discharge, itching **Those having receptive anal intercourse:** Rectal pain, discharge, bleeding	NAATs: vaginal swab, first-catch urine, pharyngeal or rectal samples Culture	Treatment failure HIV-positive patients	Reactive arthritis Chronic conjunctivitis **Female:** PID, infertility, ectopic pregnancy, chronic pelvic pain **Male:** Epididymitis, orchitis, proctocolitis **Infant:** Conjunctivitis, pneumonia	Collect specimen. Treat presumptively in patients with PID, NGU, gonococcal infection, epididymitis in men <35 years old. Perform syphilis serology. Offer HIV counseling and testing.
NONGONOCOCCAL URETHRITIS C. trachomatis (23%–55% of cases) Ureaplasma urealyticum (20%–40% of cases) Trichomonas vaginalis (25% of cases) Herpes simplex virus **Differential diagnosis:** Same as for Chlamydia	Dysuria Mucoid or purulent discharge Pruritus Hematuria Frequency Urgency Endocervical exudate, friability	Gram stain Wet mount Tests for gonorrhea and chlamydia	Treatment failure Complications	Epididymitis Penile edema Reiter syndrome Tenosynovitis	If microscopic test results are not available, treat for both gonorrhea and chlamydia.
PRIMARY SYPHILIS Treponema pallidum **Differential diagnosis:** Genital herpes; chancroid; LGV; balanitis, excoriation of nonulcerative lesions; squamous cell carcinoma	Painless, firm, round chancre(s) at site of inoculation, lasts 3–6 weeks Discrete, enlarged, painless regional lymph nodes Incubation: 10–90 days; average, 21 days	Darkfield microscopy Nontreponemal serology (RPR, VDRL) Confirm with treponemal serology (MHA-TP, FTA-ABS) Sequential serologic testing; use same testing method and laboratory	Positive diagnosis of disease All HIV-positive patients	Secondary syphilis Meningitis Cardiovascular or neurologic disease Facilitates HIV transmission Left untreated, can cause perinatal death or congenital syphilis in infants	Systemic disease: Chancre is unnoticed in 15%–39% of cases. Perform nontreponemal serology and clinical follow-up at 6 and 12 months. Note fourfold drop in titer; evaluate for HIV infection. Treatment failure: re-treatment and consultation with specialist are indicated; patients may need lumbar puncture.

SECONDARY SYPHILIS

T. pallidum

Differential diagnosis: All undiagnosed mucocutaneous skin eruptions (e.g., drug eruption, pityriasis rosea, scabies)

Clinical features	Diagnosis			Follow-up
Nonpruritic rash: rough, red, red-brown spots, sometimes very faint; may occur on mucous membranes, vagina, anus, palms, soles, trunk. Appears 2–8 weeks after chancre, may be present while chancre is resolving. Generalized adenopathy. Fever. Sore throat. Patchy alopecia. Malaise, arthralgias, weight loss. Oral mucous patches. Condylomata lata. Hepatosplenomegaly. Increased incidence is associated with crack cocaine and illicit drug use.	As for primary syphilis	As for primary syphilis	As for primary syphilis	At 6- and 12-month follow-up, assess for fourfold drop in titer. A fourfold increase in titer at any time may represent treatment failure or reinfection.

LATENT SYPHILIS (EARLY LATENT, LATE LATENT)

T. pallidum

Clinical features	Diagnosis			Follow-up
Occur after primary and secondary symptoms resolve. Difficulty coordinating muscle movements. Paralysis. Numbness. Gradual blindness. Dementia. Positive serology without evidence of clinical disease	Reactive VDRL or RPR. Reactive FTA-ABS or MHA-TP	All cases managed with specialist	Progression of disease	Latent syphilis is diagnosed as probable on the basis of documented seroconversion or a fourfold increase in titer of nontreponemal test. History of symptoms or exposure to partner during previous 12 months. Evaluate for aortitis, neurosyphilis iritis.

CHANCROID

Haemophilus ducreyi

Differential diagnosis: Genital herpes; primary syphilis; LGV; infected or traumatic lesions

Clinical features	Diagnosis			Follow-up
One or more painful genital ulcers with tender inguinal adenopathy. May have suppurative inguinal adenopathy and undermined ulcer borders	Isolation of *H. ducreyi*. Most cases diagnosed on clinical grounds. Painful ulcers 4–7 days after exposure. Usually coronal sulcus in men. Prepuce in women	Treatment failure	Successful treatment cures infection. In extensive cases, scarring despite successful therapy	Topical cleansing with gentle soaks. Symptomatic treatment to reduce swelling. Antibiotic administration to patients with nonfluctuant buboes. No need to drain lesions. Reexamine patients at 3–7 days. Larger ulcers heal more slowly. No evidence of *T. pallidum* appears on darkfield examination or by serology. Culture is negative for herpes simplex virus. Partner contact: Examine and treat within 10 days. Perform syphilis serology. Offer HIV counseling.

Continued

TABLE 135.1 Summary of Sexually Transmitted Infections—cont'd

Pathogen, Differential Diagnosis	Clinical Presentation	Diagnosis	Consultation, Co-Management	Complications	Management
GENITAL HERPES (PRIMARY, RECURRENT)					
HSV-2 and HSV-1 **Differential diagnosis:** Primary syphilis; chancroid; candidiasis; hand-foot-and-mouth disease, herpes zoster; fixed drug eruption; folliculitis	**Primary:** Vesicular lesions on erythematous base **Male:** Penis shaft, glans, urethra, rectum **Female:** Vulva, vagina, anus, cervix Painful lesions Malaise Fever Painful adenopathy Lesions ulcerative to superficial ulcers **Recurrent:** Clinical prodrome—pain, itching, burning, tingling Constitutional symptoms rare Vesicles Superficial ulcers	History and physical examination with confirmation by viral culture Moist swab of unroofed or weeping vesicle from base of ulcer Tzanck smear of scrapings from lesion looking for multinucleated giant cells Testing for HSV routine in all atypical and all undiagnosed genital ulcers	Secondary infection Ocular infection Persistent constitutional symptoms Urinary retention Primary or recurrent infection during pregnancy HIV-positive patients	Secondary infection Ocular infection Neonatal infection Premature delivery Spontaneous abortion Intrauterine growth retardation Fetal infection	Treatment is symptomatic. Infection may recur. HSV may be transmitted to sex partners even when no lesions are present. Support groups are available. Many educational resources are available.
LYMPHOGRANULOMA VENEREUM					
C. trachomatis **Differential diagnosis:** Chancroid Colitis Granuloma Inguinale Herpes simplex Syphilis	Small, nonpainful, ulcerative genital papule Painful inguinal or femoral lymph nodes follow 2–6 weeks later Proctocolitis in third stage	Based on clinical suspicion, epidemiologic information and exclusion of other etiologies.		Patients should be followed clinically until signs and symptoms have resolved. Persons who receive an LGV diagnosis should be tested for other STIs, especially HIV, gonorrhea, and syphilis.	Drainage of infected buboes. Treat with antibiotics.
GRANULOMA INGUINALE					
Klebsiella granulomatis **Differential diagnosis:** Chancroid Herpes simplex LGV Syphilis	Painless, slowly progressive ulcerative lesions on the genitals or perineum without regional lymphadenopathy; subcutaneous granulomas (pseudobuboes) also might occur. The lesions are highly vascular (i.e., beefy red appearance) and bleed.	Difficult to culture. Requires visualization of dark-staining		Relapse can occur 6–18 months after apparently effective therapy.	Treatment has been shown to halt progression of lesions, and healing typically proceeds inward from the ulcer margins; prolonged therapy is usually required to permit granulation and re-epithelialization of the ulcers.

FTA-ABS, Fluorescent treponemal antibody absorption; *HIV*, human immunodeficiency virus; *HSV*, herpes simplex virus; *LGV*, lymphogranuloma venereum; *MHA-TP*, microhemagglutination assay for antibody to *Treponema pallidum*; *NAATs*, nucleic acid amplification tests; *NGU*, nongonococcal urethritis; *PID*, pelvic inflammatory disease; *RPR*, rapid plasma reagin; *UTI*, urinary tract infection; *VDRL*, Venereal Disease Research Laboratory.

BOX **135.5**

Treatment of Sexually Transmitted Infections

UNCOMPLICATED GONOCOCCAL INFECTIONS
Recommended Regimens
Ceftriaxone 250 mg IM in a single dose
plus
Azithromycin 1 g PO in a single dose, *or*
Doxycycline 100 mg PO twice daily for 7 days *(azithromycin preferred)*

ALTERNATIVE REGIMENS
If Ceftriaxone Not Available
Cefixime 400 mg PO in a single dose
plus
Azithromycin 1 g PO in a single dose, *or*
Doxycycline 100 mg PO twice daily for 7 days *(azithromycin preferred)*
plus
Test-of-cure in 1 week

If Patient Has Severe Cephalosporin Allergy
Azithromycin 2 g PO in a single dose
plus
Test-of-cure in 1 week

Uncomplicated Gonococcal Infections of the Pharynx
Ceftriaxone 250 mg IM in a single dose
plus
Azithromycin 1 g PO in a single dose, *or*
Doxycycline 100 mg PO twice daily for 7 days *(azithromycin preferred)*

Pregnant Women
Ceftriaxone 250 mg IM in a single dose
plus
Azithromycin 1 g PO in a single dose

Alternative Regimens for Pregnant Women
Azithromycin 2 g PO in a single dose

CHLAMYDIA
Recommended Regimens
Azithromycin 1 g PO in a single dose, *or*
Doxycycline 100 mg PO twice daily for 7 days

Alternative Regimens
Erythromycin base 500 mg PO 4 times daily for 7 days, *or*
Ofloxacin 300 mg PO twice daily for 7 days, *or*
Levofloxacin 500 mg PO once daily for 7 days

Pregnant Women
Azithromycin 1 g PO in a single dose, *or*
Amoxicillin 500 mg 3 times daily for 7 days

NONGONOCOCCAL URETHRITIS
Recommended Regimens
Azithromycin 1 g PO in a single dose, *or*
Doxycycline 100 mg PO twice daily for 7 days

Alternative Regimens
Erythromycin base 500 mg PO 4 times daily for 7 days, *or*
Erythromycin ethylsuccinate 800 mg PO 4 times daily for 7 days, *or*
Ofloxacin 300 mg PO twice daily for 7 days *or*
Levofloxacin 500 mg PO once daily for 7 days

TREATMENT OF DISEASES CHARACTERIZED BY GENITAL ULCERS
Primary, Secondary, or Latent Syphilis of Less Than 1 Year's Duration
Recommended Regimens
Benzathine penicillin G 2.4 million units IM in a single dose

If Allergic to Penicillin
Doxycycline 100 mg twice a day for 14 days *or*
Tetracycline 500 mg PO 4 times a day for 14 days

EARLY LATENT SYPHILIS
Recommended Regimens
Benzathine penicillin G 2.4 million units IM in a single dose

LATE LATENT SYPHILIS OF MORE THAN 1 YEAR'S DURATION OR UNKNOWN DURATION
Recommended Regimens
Benzathine penicillin G 7.2 million units total, administered as 3 doses of 2.4 million units IM each, at 1-week intervals

GENITAL HERPES: FIRST CLINICAL EPISODE
Recommended Regimens
Acyclovir 400 mg PO 3 times daily for 7–10 days, *or*
Acyclovir 200 mg PO 5 times daily for 7–10 days *or*
Famciclovir 250 mg PO 3 times daily for 7–10 days, *or*
Valacyclovir 1 g PO twice daily for 7–10 days

GENITAL HERPES: RECURRENT EPISODES
Recommended Regimens
Acyclovir 400 mg PO 3 times daily for 5 days, *or*
Acyclovir 800 mg PO 3 times daily for 2 days, *or*
Acyclovir 800 mg PO twice daily for 5 days, *or*
Famciclovir 125 mg PO twice daily for 5 days, *or*
Famciclovir 1000 mg PO twice daily for 1 day, *or*
Famciclovir 500 mg PO once, followed by 250 mg PO twice daily × 2 days, *or*
Valacyclovir 500 mg PO twice daily for 3 days, *or*
Valacyclovir 1 g PO once daily for 5 days

CHANCROID
Recommended Regimens
Azithromycin 1 g PO in a single dose, *or*
Ceftriaxone 250 mg IM in a single dose, *or*
Ciprofloxacin 500 mg PO twice daily for 3 days, *or*
Erythromycin base 500 mg PO 3 times daily for 7 days

Continued

BOX **135.5**

Treatment of Sexually Transmitted Infections—cont'd

LYMPHOGRANULOMA VENEREUM
Recommended Regimens
Doxycycline 100 mg PO twice daily for 21 days, *or*
Erythromycin base 500 mg PO 4 times daily for 21 days

Asymptomatic Partners
Doxycycline 100 mg PO twice daily for 7 days, *or*
Azithromycin 1 g PO in a single dose

Quinolones should not be used for infections in men who have sex with men or in those with a history of recent foreign travel or who have partners with a recent history of foreign travel, infections acquired in California or Hawaii, or infections acquired in other areas with increased quinoline-resistant *Neisseria gonorrhoeae* prevalence.

From Workowski, K. A. & Bolan, G. A. (2015). Centers for Disease Control and Prevention (CDC): Sexually transmitted diseases treatment guidelines, 2015. *MMWR Recommendations and Reports,* 64(3), 1–138. Consult these guidelines for more detailed recommendations, including guidelines for treatment of pregnant patients, HIV-infected patients, allergic patients, and other specific groups.

consequences of infertility, ectopic pregnancies, and chronic pelvic pain.

Prevention of viral STIs requires the adoption of lifelong healthy sexual behaviors to help avoid acquisition and spread of infection. The prevalence of herpes increases with age because once acquired, the disease stays within the body. Factors related to the spread and acquisition of STIs often include other high-risk behaviors, such as multiple partners, use of illicit drugs, excessive alcohol use, and unsafe sexual practices, such as inconsistent or no use of condoms.

DISEASES CHARACTERIZED BY CERVICITIS AND URETHRITIS

Urethritis, or inflammation of the urethra, may be caused by an infection characterized by the discharge of mucoid or purulent material and by burning during urination. Among men, urethral infections with *Neisseria gonorrhoeae* are often symptomatic, causing them to seek treatment and to avoid serious sequelae, but this may occur after the STI has already been transmitted to others.[11] However, most presentations of chlamydia in both sexes are asymptomatic. Urethritis is classified as gonococcal if it is caused by *N. gonorrhoeae* (gonorrhea) or as NGU if *N. gonorrhoeae* is not detected. NGU in younger men is most commonly caused by *Chlamydia* but may be associated with other pathogens.

GONORRHEA
Definition and Epidemiology

Gonorrhea is an STI caused by the gram-negative diplococcus *N. gonorrhoeae*. In men, it is often characterized by a purulent urethral discharge, but it is asymptomatic in up to 80% of women.[11] Laboratory confirmation of the presence of *N. gonorrhoeae* is required for the establishment of the diagnosis.

Gonorrhea is the second most commonly reported infectious disease in the United States, with 555,608 infections reported in 2017, but this is likely an underestimate, given that all cases are not reported.[11] Populations at risk for gonorrhea include young, sexually active individuals; nonwhite urban poor; and other individuals who engage in high-risk behaviors, such as using illegal drugs or engaging in prostitution.

Pathophysiology

N. gonorrhoeae infects mucus-secreting columnar and transitional epithelium in the mucocutaneous surfaces of the genitourinary tract, pharynx, conjunctiva, and anus. Transmission occurs by sexual contact with an infected individual, by autoinoculation to the eyes, or to the neonate during childbirth via the birth canal of a pregnant woman with gonorrhea. The incubation period is usually 1 to 14 days after exposure. If untreated, gonorrhea spreads from its initial sites upward into the genital tract, prostate, and epididymis in men and into the fallopian tubes in women. Menstruation increases the risk of intraluminal ascent from the cervix and predisposes the patient to gonococcal bacteremia.

Clinical Presentation and Physical Examination

Many women and some men are asymptomatic. If symptoms develop, they usually manifest in women within 10 days of contact and in men within 2 to 5 days of infection.

Signs and symptoms of infection in females with *N. gonorrhoeae* include thin, purulent, and mildly odorous leukorrhea; dysuria; intermenstrual bleeding; dyspareunia or mild lower abdominal pain; or pharyngitis. Progression to PID may occur in 10% to 20% of females in whom symptoms are initially not present or are unrecognized. Symptoms of PID include lower abdominal pain, vaginal discharge, mucopurulent urethral discharge, dysuria, cervical motion tenderness, adnexal tenderness or mass, intermenstrual bleeding, fever, chills, nausea, and vomiting.

Gonorrhea in men usually manifests as urethritis, burning on urination, and serous penile discharge. This progresses over the next few days to copious, purulent, and sometimes blood-tinged discharge.

Infections of the pharynx, rectum, and eye may occur in men or women. Pharyngeal infection usually occurs in association with orogenital contact. The majority of pharyngeal infections are asymptomatic, but they may cause symptoms of pharyngitis with cervical lymphadenopathy. Anorectal infection may manifest with anorectal burning, mucopurulent discharge, and painful bowel movements. Ocular infections occur via autoinoculation into the eye from another infection site, such as the genitalia. Typical presentation is unilateral and purulent conjunctivitis.

Diagnostics

The CDC recommends testing for gonorrhea with US Food and Drug Administration (FDA)–approved NAATs. Vaginal swabs are preferred for detection in women, and first-catch urine in men. However, urine collection is frequently performed in women and is a less invasive method of detection. Culture should be obtained in cases of suspected treatment failure or instances of child sexual assault in boys and extragenital infections in girls.

Interprofessional Collaborative Management

Since the emergence of fluoroquinolone-resistant *N. gonorrhoeae* in 2007, the CDC no longer recommends fluroquinolones for the treatment of gonorrhea. Due to reported treatment failures in the United States and globally, the CDC no longer recommends the routine use of cefixime as a first-line treatment regimen for gonorrhea. Frequently persons with gonorrhea have a coexistent chlamydial infection. As a result, only one regimen, dual treatment with ceftriaxone and azithromycin, is recommended for the treatment of gonorrhea. Providers are urged to check the CDC and state health departments for the most current treatment recommendations

Complications

Left untreated, infection can result in a range of complications from acute salpingitis in female patients, perihepatitis (Fitz-Hugh-Curtis syndrome), and disseminated gonococcal infections to ophthalmia neonatorum in newborns. Infections caused by gonorrhea are a major cause of PID, ectopic pregnancy, and chronic pelvic pain in the United States. In untreated men, gonorrhea can cause epididymitis, a painful condition of the testicles that can result in infertility. Untreated ocular gonorrhea may result in panophthalmitis and possibly loss of the eye if not treated immediately.

EDUCATION AND HEALTH PROMOTION

Annual screening for *N. gonorrhoeae* is recommended for all sexually active women age < 25 years and for older women at increased risk of infection (e.g., those who have a new sex partner, more than one sex partner, a sex partner who is not monogamous, or a sex partner who has an STI). Additional risk factors for gonorrhea include inconsistent condom use among persons who are not in mutually monogamous relationships, previous or coexisting STIs, and exchanging sex for money.

CHLAMYDIA
Definition and Epidemiology

Chlamydia is an STI caused by an intracellular parasitic organism, *Chlamydia trachomatis*, and organisms of the genus *Chlamydophila*. Clinical syndromes associated with *C. trachomatis* include NGU, mucopurulent cervicitis, PID, lymphogranuloma venereum (LGV), acute urethral syndrome, ocular infections, proctocolitis, epididymitis, and reactive arthritis. *C. trachomatis* may be acquired by infants through an infected birth canal, causing pneumonia and conjunctivitis.

Chlamydia is the most commonly reported STI in the United States. In 2017, there were a total of 1,708,569 reported chlamydial infections in the United States reported to the CDC. During 2016–17, the rate increased 6.9%, from 494.7 to 528.8 cases per 100,000 population, with the highest age-specific rates of reported cases occurring among those aged 15 to 19 years. Rates of reported cases of chlamydia were highest among black,

American Indian/Alaska Native (AI/AN), and Native Hawaiian/Other Pacific Islander (NHOPI) women, as compared with other groups in the populations. The rate of reported cases of chlamydia among blacks was 5.6 times the rate among whites (1175.8 and 211.3 cases per 100,000 population, respectively).

Pathophysiology

There are 18 strains of *C. trachomatis*, with variants affecting the eyes and genital tract. It is usually spread by sexual contact. In women, the organism infects the columnar epithelial cells, most commonly at the transition zone of the endocervix, resulting in an inflammatory cascade. Each sexual encounter with an infected male has about a 25% chance of infecting a female. Infected mothers spread the disease to their newborns about 50% to 60% of the time, usually resulting in conjunctivitis but possibly pneumonia. The incubation period is typically 1 to 2 weeks. Coinfection with gonorrhea is common; 20% to 40% of men and women with chlamydia are likely to also have gonorrhea.[12]

Clinical Presentation and Physical Examination

Most chlamydial infections are asymptomatic. Symptoms may not appear for several weeks after contact with the organisms and include abnormal vaginal discharge, burning with urination, penile discharge, and discomfort and edema in testicle(s). The rectum may also show symptoms such as pain, discharge, and bleeding. Chlamydia should be suspected in female patients with cervicitis on the basis of mucopurulent discharge from the cervical os, easily induced bleeding, and edema in the area of ectopy.

Diagnostics

NAATs are the preferred method of testing for chlamydia and are used for both endocervical swabs and urine-based evaluation. Testing for chlamydia can be coupled with liquid-based Pap smears during routine well-visit examinations, similar to testing for gonorrhea. *Chlamydia* organisms are found within urethral, cervical, and rectal epithelial cells but not in exudate or pus.

Complications

Chlamydia can cause damage to the reproductive system, including PID, perihepatitis, and reactive arthritis, regardless of the presence or absence of symptoms. Pregnant women with chlamydia are at risk for preterm delivery, chlamydial conjunctivitis, and pneumonia in the newborn.

Education and Health Promotion

All sexually active women younger than 26 and all pregnant women should be screened for chlamydia. Routine screening is not currently recommended in men but should be encouraged in geographic areas with high prevalence. Men who have sex with men (MSM) who have receptive anal sex should be screened annually, and every 3 to 6 months for those who have multiple and/or anonymous partners.

DISEASES CHARACTERIZED BY GENITAL ULCERS

In the United States, most young, sexually active patients who have genital ulcers are infected with genital herpes, syphilis,

BOX **135.6**

Stages of Syphilis

- Primary syphilis
- Secondary syphilis
- Latent syphilis
  - Early latent syphilis
  - Late latent syphilis
- Latent syphilis, unknown duration
- Neurosyphilis
- Tertiary (late) syphilis
- Syphilitic stillbirth

or chancroid. Other infectious causes of genital ulcers include LGV and HIV; noninfectious causes include trauma, Behçet syndrome, neoplasms, and fixed drug eruptions. More than one of these diseases may be present concurrently.

SYPHILIS
Definition and Epidemiology

Syphilis is a complex systemic STI caused by *Treponema pallidum*. In 2017, a total of 30,644 cases of primary and secondary syphilis were reported in the United States—a rate of 9.5 cases per 100,000 population. This rate represents a 10.5% increase compared with 2016 (8.6 cases per 100,000 population) and a 72.7% increase compared with 2013 (5.5 cases per 100,000 population).[11] The primary and secondary syphilis rates are highest among blacks, Native Hawaiians/other Pacific Islanders, Hispanics, American Indians/Alaskan Natives, compared to Whites, in descending order of prevalence. The rate of infection among Asians was 0.8 times that of whites.[11] Increasing numbers of MSM represent newly diagnosed cases, accounting for 75% of primary and secondary syphilis. Blacks and Hispanics account for a majority of the remaining cases. It is interesting to note that the rate of congenital syphilis (passed from pregnant mother to infant) is about twice the rate of perinatal HIV transmission.[13]

Syphilis has been classified into a series of overlapping stages, which is used to guide treatment and follow-up (Box 135.6). Patients may initially demonstrate signs and symptoms of primary infection (ulcer or chancre at the infection site; Fig. 135.1), secondary infection (rash, mucocutaneous lesions, and adenopathy), or tertiary infection (cardiac, neurologic, ophthalmic, auditory, or gummatous lesions). Primary and secondary syphilis are the most infectious states of the disease.

Pathophysiology

Syphilis is usually spread through contact with infectious lesions called chancres; the infection usually enters the host during sexual activity through sites where the epithelium has been disrupted from minor trauma. Sexual contact with a partner who has early syphilis is associated with the highest risk for development of the disease. The mean time from exposure to the development of active infection (chancre formation) is 21 days (range, 10 to 60 days). Syphilis may also be transmitted from an infected pregnant woman to her developing child.

Clinical Presentation and Physical Examination

Chancres typically develop at the site of inoculation. Syphilitic lesions are painless and some patients may not be aware of them. Secondary syphilis causes more widespread findings, including macules and papules on the trunk, neck, palms, and soles. Condylomata lata, which are raised, flat, broad, grayish papular lesions, may occur in moist areas such as the anus,

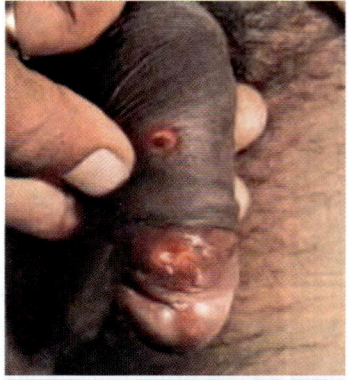
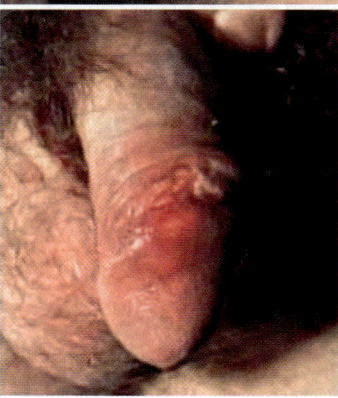

FIG. 135.1   Chancre in primary syphilis. (From Wisdom, A. [1989]. *Color atlas of sexually transmitted diseases.* Chicago: Year Book.)

scrotum, and vulva. Mucous patches (small, asymptomatic, shallow ulcerations) may develop in the oral or genital mucosa or at the angles of the mouth.[4]

The signs of primary and secondary syphilis may resolve spontaneously even without treatment. The patient then enters the latent stage of the disease, in which there are generally no clinical signs or symptoms of infection and diagnosis is made on the basis of serology. A pregnant woman with latent disease can infect her fetus.

Tertiary syphilis (late-stage syphilis) manifests after a variable period of latency in approximately one-third of patients who do not receive treatment. Late-stage syphilis may occur 10 to 20 years after initial infection. It may appear as gummatous disease (rubbery lumps or lesions found in subcutaneous tissue), cardiovascular disease, or neurosyphilis. Neurosyphilis can occur in all stages of syphilis, and the diagnosis is based on clinical findings and examination of the serum and cerebrospinal fluid.

Diagnostics

Darkfield examinations and direct fluorescent antibody tests of lesion exudate or tissue are the definitive methods for diagnosis of early syphilis. These are not typically performed in practice today owing to their complexity. Simple serologic testing with nontreponemal tests (e.g., Venereal Disease Research Laboratory [VDRL] and rapid plasma reagin [RPR]) are used for screening but are not specifically diagnostic for syphilis. These initial tests correlate with disease activity and are reported quantitatively. False positives may be associated with hepatitis, viral pneumonia, pregnancy, infectious mononucleosis, and other viral infections. Treponemal testing (e.g., fluorescent treponemal antibody absorption [FTA-ABS], *Treponema pallidum* particle agglutination [TP-PA], various enzyme immunoassays [EIAs], and chemoluminescence immunoassays) is done for diagnosis, and a positive result is usually present throughout the lifetime, regardless of treatment. Chronic false-positive treponemal findings are associated with connective tissue diseases such as systemic lupus erythematosus.

Complications

Untreated, syphilis may cause systemic disease involving neurologic and cardiovascular problems including stroke, meningitis, decreased hearing, changes in vision, and dementia.

GENITAL HERPES
Definition and Epidemiology

Genital infection with HSV infection is a condition characterized by primary involvement of the genital or anal area with visible, painful genital or anal lesions, or grouped vesicles at the site of inoculation and regional lymphadenopathy. Recurrent HSV infections are characterized by a normal course of recurring outbreaks of vesicles at the same site. Genital herpes is a chronic, lifelong viral infection caused by two types of herpes simplex virus: HSV-1 and HSV-2. Most cases of recurrent genital herpes are caused by HSV-2, and approximately 50 million people in the United States are infected with HSV-2. Oral HSV-1 infection is typically acquired in childhood. However, an increasing proportion of anogenital herpetic infections have been attributed to HSV-1 infection, which is especially prominent among young women and MSM.

Annually, 776,000 people in the United States get new genital herpes infections. In the United States, 11.9% of persons aged 14 to 49 years have HSV-2 infection. However, the prevalence of genital herpes infection is higher than that because of the increasing number of genital herpes infections are caused by HSV-1. HSV-2 infection is more common among women than among men; the percentages of those infected during 2015–16 were 15.9% versus 8.2%, respectively, among 14- to 49-year-olds. This is possibly because genital infection is more easily transmitted from men to women than from women to men during penile-vaginal sex. HSV-2 infection is more common among non-Hispanic blacks (34.6%) than among non-Hispanic whites (8.1%). A previous analysis found that these disparities exist even among persons with similar numbers of lifetime sexual partners. Most infected persons may be unaware of their infection. In the United States, an estimated 87.4% of 14- to 49-year-olds infected with HSV-2 may be asymptomatic or may be unaware that they have HSV.[14]

More women than men have herpes. Racial and ethnic distribution is similar to that of other STIs, with blacks representing 39.2% of cases, more than triple the rate in whites.

Genital herpes is spread by direct contact with lesions, mucosal membranes, or genital or oral secretions. Transmission is higher from men to women than from women to men. Shedding occurs in asymptomatic individuals about 10% of days. Most transmissions occur from an infected person with no known sores who may not be aware of harboring the infection. Most neonatal herpes is caused by HSV-2 infections transmitted during delivery. Infants of mothers who have been infected for the first time during their pregnancy, especially in the third trimester, are at high risk of serious complications. Delivery via cesarean section is recommended for all pregnant women with active lesions or early symptoms.

Pathophysiology

After an inoculation, the virus undergoes primary replication, resulting in the production of the characteristic lesion (a thin-walled vesicle on an erythematous base). Incubation ranges from 2 to 12 days, averaging 4 days. With primary infection, HSV travels along sensory nerves and establishes latency within sensory nerve fibers for life.

Reactivation may be triggered by stimuli such as fever, trauma, stress, sunlight, and menstruation. Immunocompromised individuals are likely to experience more frequent and severe reactivation. Shedding occurs in both symptomatic and asymptomatic reactivations. Recurrences for genital HSV-2 are typically more frequent than those for HSV-1.

Clinical Presentation and Physical Examination

Many people are infected with herpes but have never been symptomatic. Those experiencing symptoms usually show an outbreak of vesicles on or around the genitals, rectum, or mouth. These vesicles erode and leave painful ulcerations that may linger for 2 to 4 weeks before healing.

An initial outbreak of herpes usually lasts longer than subsequent outbreaks, has a higher rate of viral shedding, and includes symptoms such as fever, body aches, lymphadenopathy, and headache. Subsequent outbreaks are common in the first year after initial episode, with later recurrences being shorter and milder. Recurrent outbreaks may produce prodromal symptoms several hours or days before lesions appear, including tingling and shooting pains in the lower extremities and buttocks.

Diagnostics

Diagnosis of HSV infection is often a clinical decision based on the patient's history and the morphologic characteristics of the lesions. Isolation of HSV in cell culture is the preferred virologic test and requires a sample from an active lesion. Unfortunately, healing lesions affect the sensitivity of virologic testing. Several enzyme-linked immunosorbent assay (ELISA) serologic tests are available, and most are able to distinguish between HSV-1 and HSV-2. Serologic test results will not be positive at the time of the primary outbreak; seroconversion takes 2 to 12 weeks after infection. A positive serologic test result will be lifelong.

Complications

Having herpes may increase the likelihood of contracting other STIs. Infants of mothers who have been infected for the first time during their pregnancy are at high risk of serious complications.

Indications for Referral or Hospitalization

Patients for whom any suspicion of HSV in the eyes is present should be promptly referred to an ophthalmologist.

Education and Health Promotion

The CDC does not currently recommend screening for HSV.

CHANCROID
Definition and Epidemiology

Chancroid is an STI characterized by painful genital ulceration and inflammatory inguinal adenopathy. The disease is characterized by infection with *Haemophilus ducreyi*. The prevalence of chancroid has declined in the United States, and since 2013 there were no cases of chancroid occurring in the United States reported to the CDC.[10] Globally, the incidence of chancroid has also declined, although infection may still occur in some regions of Africa and the Caribbean. When cases of chancroid do occur, they are usually associated with sporadic outbreaks. As is the case with genital herpes and syphilis, chancroid increases the risk of transmission and acquisition of HIV.[10]

Pathophysiology

Chancroid is caused by a destructive toxin is produced by *H. ducreyi*, which breaks down skin and mucus membrane barriers.

Clinical Presentation and Physical Examination

Chancroid is a genital ulcer disease characterized by one or a few painful ulcers that develop after an incubation of 4 to 7 days. The most distinguishing feature is deep, raw, and painful ulcerations. Painful inguinal adenopathy, often unilateral, develops in 50% of patients 1 to 2 weeks after the primary lesion. Buboes occur and may drain spontaneously, leaving behind a nonhealing ulcer.[10]

Diagnostics

Diagnosis is often clinical. The combination of a painful genital ulcer and tender suppurative inguinal adenopathy are suggestive of chancroid. Confirmation is based on isolation via culture of *H. ducreyi* from a clinical specimen.

OTHER ULCERATIVE DISEASES

LGV and granuloma inguinale are two other causes of genital ulcers. These genital ulcers are rare in the United States but endemic to certain tropical areas.

Granuloma Inguinale

Definition and Epidemiology. Granuloma inguinale, also known as donovanosis, is caused by *Klebsiella granulomatis*. It occurs rarely in the United States, but is endemic in some tropical and developing areas, in tropical and developing areas.

Pathophysiology. Granuloma inguinale is primarily transmitted via sexual contact but may be spread fecally or to the neonate through an infected mother's birth canal. Incubation varies from 1 day to 1 year, but the median incubation is 50 days.

Clinical Presentation and Physical Examination. This infection is characterized by painless progressive ulcers and regional lymphadenopathy. The lesions bleed easily on contact. There are four types of skin lesions: nodular, ulcero-vegetative, cicatricial, and hypertrophic/verrucous. Nodular lesions (pseudobubo) are soft and may be pruritic and erythematous. They eventually erode to ulcerations. Ulcerovegetative lesions are the most common, showing painless, large, beefy-red, pus-filled ulcers, with raised borders. They are frequently found in skin folds. Cicatricial lesions appear as dry ulcers resembling scars. Hypertrophic/verrucous ulcers appear similar to genital warts.

Diagnostics. Granuloma inguinale is difficult to culture; however, it may be seen on a smear from the base of the lesion. Samples may be obtained via punch, curettage, or wedge resection and sent to pathology for review. Confirmation of diagnosis is based on the visualization of dark-staining Donovan bodies on tissue crush preparation or biopsy.[10] No FDA-cleared

molecular tests for the detection of *K. granulomatis* DNA currently exist.

Lymphogranuloma Venereum

Definition and Epidemiology. LGV is a systemic STI caused by a variety of *C. trachomatis*. It rarely occurs in the United States. Providers in the United States should be aware of this infectious disease, as rectal exposure in women or MSM can result in a proctocolitis that may mimic inflammatory bowel disease.[10]

Clinical Presentation and Physical Examination. A primary lesion that is a small, nonpainful genital papule that ulcerates after an initial 3- to 30-day incubation period characterizes LGV. Painful inguinal or femoral lymph nodes follow 2 to 6 weeks later. Proctocolitis is present in the third stage of the presentation and is more common in women. Clinical presentation may also include mucoid and/or hemorrhagic rectal discharge and pain, constipation, fever, and/or tenesmus. LGV can become a systemic infection if not treated early and proctocolitis-related LGV can lead to chronic colorectal fistulas and strictures. However, rectal LGV can also be asymptomatic. In addition, persons with genital and colorectal LGV can also develop secondary bacterial infections and have other concomitant sexually and nonsexually transmitted pathogens.[10]

DIAGNOSIS

Diagnosis is based on clinical presentation, epidemiologic information and the exclusion of other differentials for proctocolitis, inguinal lymphadenopathy, or genital and rectal ulcers. Genital lesions, rectal specimens, and lymph node specimens can be tested for *C. trachomatis* by culture, direct immunofluorescence, or nucleic acid detection. NAATs for C trachomatis are reliable on rectal specimens, but are not FDA approved for this purpose.[10]

TREATMENT

Persons with clinical syndromes consistent with LGV, including proctocolitis or genital ulcers with lymphadenopathy, should be presumptively treated for LGV. As required by state law, these cases should be reported to the health department.[10] Treatment cures infection and prevents further tissue damage, although scarring may result from the tissue damage that has already occurred. Patients diagnosed with LGV should be followed until signs and symptoms have completely resolved. In addition, persons diagnosed with LGV should be tested for other STIs, especially HIV, gonorrhea, and syphilis.

INDICATIONS FOR REFERRAL OR HOSPITALIZATION

It is not common for patients with STIs to require hospitalization. Indications include signs and symptoms of systemic disease not appropriate for outpatient treatment; ineffective outpatient treatment; and complications related to an STI, such as PID. Referral to a specialist in infectious disease is indicated for all patients with LGV, syphilis, or granuloma inguinale, as well as for all treatment failures.

PATIENT AND FAMILY EDUCATION

Patient education efforts need to focus on preventing the establishment of high-risk behaviors before sexual activity is initiated. The general public is largely unaware of the health consequences of STIs, because many infections are asymptomatic. Major health consequences, such as infertility and chronic disease, can occur years after initial infections, and the stigma associated with STIs often inhibits frank and open discussion. Population-specific educational efforts and screening for specific STIs must be established to help curb this hidden epidemic.

HEALTH PROMOTION

Efforts to prevent STIs include promotion of healthy sexual practices and targeting of high-risk behaviors often associated with the acquisition of an STI. These behaviors include excessive alcohol intake, substance use, and high-risk sexual practices such as inconsistent or no condom use and multiple sex partners. Patients who are sexually active, regardless of age, should be educated on the risk of transmitting or acquiring the different STIs and on the various transmission modes. Sensitivity to the patient's age, culture, religion, and setting are integral to successful health promotion and disease prevention activities.

Adolescents are at higher risk for STIs. Efforts targeting this age group must include an awareness of peer pressures and self-esteem, which may affect the patient's health behavior patterns. Sex education can become a controversial issue for patients, families, and schools. This age group, with few exceptions, is able to consent to confidential diagnosis and treatment of STIs. This provides the opportunity for promotion of healthy sexual practices in a nonthreatening environment.

A great deal of information is available on the Internet, for both the health care provider and the patient, from numerous reputable and informative resources. The CDC Division of STD Prevention has the current treatment guidelines and STI fact sheets with valuable links to other sites. For more information, consult the following:

- CDC, Division of STD Prevention: www.cdc.gov/STD
- CDC National STD Hotline: 800-232-4636 (24 hours/day, 7 days/week)
- American Sexual Health Association (ASHA): www.ashasexualhealth.org

REFERENCES

1. Tan, C. W., & Chlebic, M. P. (2016). Urinary tract infections in adults. *Singapore Medical Journal, 57*(9), 485–490.
2. Gradwohl, S. E., Bettcher, C. M., Chenoweth, C. E., VanHarrison, R., & Zoschnick, L. B. (2016). Urinary tract infection. University of Michigan health system quality management program, guidelines for clinical care ambulatory. p. 1–9. Retrieved from: http://www.med.umich.edu/1info/FHP/practiceguides/uti/uti.pdf. (Accessed 15 January 2019).
3. Ferri, F. F. (2014). Urinary tract infection. In *Ferri's clinical advisor 2015* (3rd ed., p. 993). Philadelphia: Elsevier.
4. Centers for Disease Control and Prevention. Healthcare-associated infection surveillance protocol for urinary tract infection events for long-term care facilities. Updated January 2019. Retrieved from: https://www.cdc.gov/nhsn/pdfs/ltc/ltcf-uti-protocol-current.pdf. (Accessed December 31, 2018).
5. Brusch, J. L. (2018). Urinary tract infection in males. Medscape. Retrieved from: http://emedicine.medscape.com/article/231574-overview#showall. (Accessed 15 January 2019).
6. Shoff, W. H. (2012). Asymptomatic bacteriuria. Medscape. Retrieved from: http://emedicine.medscape.com/article/2059290-overview#showall. (Accessed 3 August 2014).
7. Donofrio, J. C., & Weiner, S. G. (2013) Female patient self-diagnosis compared with emergency physician diagnosis of urinary tract infection. *The Journal of Emergency Medicine, 45*(6), 969–973.
8. Gordon, L. B., Waxman, M. J., Ragsdale, L., & Mermel, L. A. (2013). Overtreatment of presumed urinary tract infection in older women presenting to the emergency department. *Journal of the American Geriatrics Society, 61*(5), 788–792.
9. National Institute for Healthcare and Excellence (NICE). (2018). Lower Urinary tract infection guideline. Retrieved from: https://www.guidelines.co.uk/urology/nice-lower-urinary-tract-infection-guideline/454434.article. (Accessed 31 December 2018).
10. Centers for Disease Control and Prevention (CDC). (2017). Sexually Transmitted Disease Surveillance. Retrieved from: https://www.cdc.gov/std/stats17/default.htm. (Accessed 7 January 2019).
11. Centers for Disease Control and Prevention (CDC), Workowski, K. A., & Bolan, G. A. (2015). Sexually transmitted diseases treatment guidelines, 2015. *MMWR. Recommendations and Reports: Morbidity and Mortality Weekly Report. Recommendations and Reports, 64*(3), 1–138.
12. Struble, K. (2014). Chlamydial genitourinary infections. Medscape. Retrieved from: http://emedicine.medscape.com/article/214823-overview#showall. (Accessed 31 August 2014).
13. Centers for Disease Control and Prevention (CDC). (2017). Syphilis—CDC fact sheet, detailed version. Retrieved from: www.cdc.gov/std/syphilis/STDFact-Syphilis-detailed.htm. (Accessed 7 January 2019).
14. Centers for Disease Control and Prevention (CDC). (2017). Genital herpes—CDC fact sheet, detailed version. Retrieved from: www.cdc.gov/std/Herpes/STDFact-Herpes-detailed.htm. (Accessed 7 January 2019).

CHAPTER **136**

UROPATHIES (OBSTRUCTIVE) AND TUMORS OF THE GENITOURINARY TRACT (KIDNEYS, URETERS, AND BLADDER)

Patricia Polgar-Bailey

DEFINITION AND EPIDEMIOLOGY

Obstructive uropathy refers to structural or functional changes in the urinary tract that impair urine flow. Left untreated, obstruction can result in progressive renal damage and potential renal failure.[1] The degree, duration, and location of obstruction determine the extent of functional and pathologic alterations in the kidney. Tumors of the genitourinary tract may be benign or malignant. Benign renal tumors include adenomas, oncocytomas, and angiomyolipomas and are often incidentally found on imaging studies. Adenomas are small tumors of the renal cortex and are most often asymptomatic. Oncocytomas are adenomas of the renal collecting tubule and represent 1% to 14% of renal tumors; although considered benign, they have on rare occasions demonstrated malignant potential. Angiomyolipomas, as the name implies, contain vascular tissue, smooth muscle cells, and fatty elements. Because of the potential for hemorrhage, they may become symptomatic, manifesting with pain, hematuria, or hypertension.[2]

Obstructive uropathy is common, can occur at any age, and can be seen anywhere in the urinary tract from the urethral meatus to the renal tubules.[1] It can be classified by cause (congenital or acquired), duration (acute or chronic), degree (partial or complete), and level (upper or lower urinary tract).[1] In children, congenital disorders are seen most commonly. For adults, acquired disorders are more prevalent. Urolithiasis is the most common disorder in young adults.[3] In individuals older than 60 years, men are affected more than women, and benign prostatic hyperplasia (BPH) and prostate carcinoma are the most prevalent culprits in this age group.[4]

Renal cell carcinoma (RCC) is the most common malignant renal tumor in adults and constitutes more than 90% of all adult renal cancers.[5] Known risk factors for RCC include abdominal imaging, smoking, obesity, long-term dialysis, and a family history.[6] Occupations such as leather tanning and shoe making and exposure to asbestos, gasoline, petroleum, tar, and pitch are considered risk factors, but more data are needed to determine the amount of risk.[6] Tobacco abuse is the strongest known risk factor for RCC. There is a higher prevalence of RCC in men than in women (2 : 1); black men have the highest incidence of all ethnic groups.[2]

Wilms tumor, the most common tumor of childhood, affects approximately 1 in 10,000 children younger than 15 years. The tumor is more common in blacks than in whites, and bilateral disease is more common in females.[7,8]

Cancer of the bladder is the second most common cancer of the genitourinary tract. The male/female ratio for bladder cancer is 3 : 1, and it is more common in whites than in blacks and peaks in the sixth to seventh decade of life.[9] Known risk factors for urothelial cancers of the bladder are aging, cigarette smoking, occupational chemical exposure including iron and aluminum processing, working with metals, industrial painting, gas and tar manufacturing, transport equipment operation, and mining. Genetic abnormalities, radiotherapy, and chronic bladder irritation also increase the risk for bladder cancers.[9,10] Current tobacco smokers have a threefold increased risk for bladder cancer, and ex-smokers have a twofold increased risk.[9,11]

PATHOPHYSIOLOGY
Urinary Tract Obstruction

Obstruction of urine flow can result from intrinsic or extrinsic mechanical blockage as well as from functional defects not associated with a fixed occlusion. Lesions causing mechanical obstruction can occur at any level of the upper or lower urinary tract.[12] When the lesion is above the level of the bladder, unilateral dilation of the ureter and kidney (hydronephrosis) can occur. When the lesion is below the level of the bladder, bilateral involvement of the kidneys occurs, unless there is a solitary kidney. Forms of mechanical obstructions are listed in the differential diagnosis box.

Obstruction of urine flow causes urinary retention and increased pressure proximal to the obstruction.[1] A significant or prolonged pressure increase can lead to considerable renal tissue damage with resultant renal insufficiency or failure.[1]

Functional impairment of urine flow can also result from disorders that involve both the ureter and bladder. Neurogenic bladder dysfunction can be caused by upper neuron damage or lower spinal cord injury. Upper neuron damage may produce involuntary micturition against a closed bladder neck or external sphincter, whereas lower spinal tract injury can cause the bladder to become atonic.[13] In many cases, a significant urinary residual volume may occur, resulting in increased bladder pressure and subsequent upper tract pressures.[1,13] This may or may not be accompanied by reflux of urine into the ureters. Ischemia of the upper tracts can occur when pressures are elevated, leading to substantial renal injury and even tissue death.[1,13]

Renal Cell Carcinoma

RCC is an adenocarcinoma of the kidney that most frequently originates from the proximal tubule.[2] Evidence of metastasis is present in one-third of patients at the time of diagnosis. The most common site of metastasis is the lungs.[5] RCCs are often associated with paraneoplastic syndromes, which may produce the initial signs and symptoms (e.g., fever, anemia, cachexia, hypercalcemia, erythrocytosis, hypertension, hepatic dysfunction).[2]

RCC occurs with equal frequency in either kidney and may occur in the upper, middle, or lower poles. Tumor size at presentation varies from 1 to 10 cm or larger, and tumor size has been inversely correlated with survival.[2] Prognosis and treatment recommendations are based on the stage of disease. Two systems are commonly used for staging: the Robson staging system and the TNM (tumor, nodes, metastasis) classification of kidney cancer.[6]

Wilms Tumor

Wilms tumor is unilateral in 95% of cases and is associated with several congenital anomalies, including cryptorchidism, ureteral duplication, and hypospadias.[7] Acquired von Willebrand disease has been associated with Wilms tumor and should be considered in children with coagulation abnormalities or bleeding symptoms.[2]

Wilms tumor may be familial or sporadic in occurrence, and 15% to 20% of cases are associated with chromosomal abnormalities. The familial type is thought to be inherited by autosomal dominant transmission.[7]

Wilms tumors are usually large and multilobulated with focal areas of hemorrhage and necrosis. Metastasis (e.g., lungs, liver) is present in 10% to 15% of cases at the time of diagnosis.[7] Staging of Wilms tumor is based on the National Wilms' Tumor Study staging system and consists of five stages. The range is from stage I (tumor limited to kidney and completely excisable) to stage IV (hematogenous metastasis to lung, liver, bone, and brain) and stage V (bilateral renal involvement).[8]

Bladder Cancer

An estimated 80,470 cases of bladder cancer (about 61,700 cases in men and 18,770 cases in women) will be diagnosed in 2019; 90% of those diagnosed will be over the age of 55 with an average age of 73 at the time of diagnosis. There will be approximately 17,670 deaths due to bladder cancer in 2019.[14]

Bladder cancer develops within the urothelium, the lining of the urinary tract. The urothelium is composed of three to seven layers of transitional cells that cover the muscle layers of the bladder wall. Proliferative changes of the transitional cells may result in cancer, which may remain superficial or progress to invasive or metastatic disease.

Urothelial carcinoma (transitional cell carcinoma [TCC]) accounts for approximately 90% of all bladder cancers and may appear as papillary lesions or, less commonly, sessile or ulcerated lesions.[11] A papilloma or papillary tumor is a less aggressive transitional cell tumor. Non-TCCs include adenocarcinomas, squamous cell carcinomas, undifferentiated carcinomas, and mixed carcinomas. Squamous cell carcinomas account for 2% to 5% of bladder cancers and are more resistant to treatment.[11] They may be associated with high-grade urothelial carcinomas in which squamous differentiation has occurred or as a result of chronic infection, bladder stones, long-term indwelling urethral catheter use, or schistosomiasis.[6]

Carcinomas of the bladder are graded and staged in an effort to define the aggressiveness and extent of disease. Staging defines the depth of invasion within the bladder and progression of disease: stage 0 (mucosal changes) to stage D (lymph node involvement). The depth of invasion into muscle layers and perivesical fat increases the risk for metastasis.[11] Grading refers to the degree of cellular differentiation from normal urothelium. TCCs are graded on a numeric scale from 1 to 4, with the higher-grade tumors being more invasive and aggressive in behavior.

TCCs can progress to or initially appear as upper tract lesions. At least 90% of malignant neoplasms arising within the renal pelvis and ureter are TCCs. TCC of the upper tract is seen in nearly 5% of patients who have had bladder cancer. Conversely, at least 50% of patients first seen with upper tract urothelial carcinoma have or develop bladder cancer.[11]

CLINICAL PRESENTATION AND PHYSICAL EXAMINATION
Obstructive Uropathy

The presentation of obstructive uropathies can vary by cause. The health care provider should obtain a history with detailed review of symptoms, including onset, duration, location, aggravating and alleviating factors, characteristics of symptoms, changes in voiding or bowel patterns, and management therapies previously tried. Further inquiry should address current medications, medical and surgical histories, genitourinary history, family history (especially related to urologic issues), and history of pelvic trauma or neurologic issues.

In acute obstruction, pain is typically the most common presenting symptom.[1] Flank pain occurring in a crescendo-decrescendo pattern radiating to the lower abdomen, testes, or labia is common in acute obstruction. Flank pain that occurs only with urination is pathognomonic of vesicoureteral reflux, although reflux can also be asymptomatic.[1]

Chronic (slowly developing) obstructive lesions may be asymptomatic. Polyuria with resultant nocturia can be seen in chronic partial obstruction, whereas anuria and acute renal failure can be seen in total complete bilateral obstruction or obstruction of a solitary kidney. A pattern of oliguria or anuria alternating with polyuria or sudden onset of anuria suggests some type of obstructive uropathy.[1]

When it is incomplete, bladder outlet obstruction is often accompanied by other lower urinary tract symptoms, including frequency, nocturia, urgency, urge incontinence, hesitancy, poor stream, straining to initiate a urinary stream, postvoid dribbling, and overflow incontinence.[1,13] It is important to note changes in the pattern of urinary output, abrupt alterations versus gradual changes, and fluctuation in urinary symptoms. Recurrent urinary tract infections (UTIs) can also occur with chronic partial obstructions, so UTIs should be ruled out in patients with urologic symptoms.[1]

Clinical Presentation of Tumors

The classic triad of flank pain, hematuria, and renal mass occurs in less than 10% of patients, and consequently RCC is often not diagnosed until metastasis has occurred. Pain, hematuria, and flank mass therefore indicate advanced disease. A significant number of RCCs are found incidentally on imaging for other clinical problems.[2]

Wilms tumor affects children; the mean age at diagnosis is 3½ to 4 years. In Wilms tumor, the prevalent feature is an abdominal mass. Abdominal pain, which may suggest an acute abdomen, occurs in 30% to 40% of these patients.[7]

More than 70% of bladder cancer patients are first seen with intermittent painless gross hematuria that is often described as continuing throughout urination. Irritative voiding symptoms (e.g., urgency, frequency, dysuria) may or may not be present.[9] The presence of microhematuria also may herald a urothelial malignant neoplasm and requires further investigation.[15]

A general physical examination should be performed on all patients. Blood pressure measurement is critical because both acute and chronic hydronephrosis can be accompanied by severe hypertension.[16] Signs of azotemia (pallor, skin changes, dizziness, and lethargy) should be monitored if kidney function is thought to be disrupted.[1] A fever may indicate infection. Palpation and percussion of the abdomen can often reveal bladder distention. An enlarged, tender kidney may be noted, especially in thin patients, and it may manifest as a flank mass or increased abdominal girth. Costovertebral angle or flank tenderness can be related to urolithiasis or infection.[1] The majority of genitourinary tract tumors are not associated with specific findings on physical examination. However, approximately 80% of children with Wilms tumor will have a large, smooth, firm flank mass that often extends across the midline.[7]

In men, a digital rectal examination will help determine the size of the prostate gland and the presence of nodules posteriorly. Prostate size does not directly correlate with intensity of lower urinary tract symptoms. However, symptoms are related to the degree of obstruction caused by the prostate.[4] The penis should be inspected for evidence of meatal stricture or phimosis.

A pelvic examination should be performed for women. Careful inspection of the external genitalia, vaginal and uterine cavities, and rectum may reveal contributors to urinary obstruction. It may also yield information about anatomy, such as prolapse, that might contribute to obstruction.

DIAGNOSTICS
Essential Diagnostics

Several diagnostic studies may be helpful in diagnosing urinary obstruction. A postvoid residual provides information about the residual urine in the bladder. Catheterization provides a sterile urine specimen for analysis, and a urine culture should be done to exclude infection. Urinalysis is necessary for all patients for whom obstructive uropathy is suspected. This can detect pyuria, microscopic hematuria, and abnormalities in urine pH that can occur with calculi or infection.[1] Gross hematuria is often seen in acute obstruction and is usually caused by calculi or bladder tumor but can be a result of infection as well.[1] Uric acid crystals in the urine sediment suggest uric acid nephropathy or calculi. A hematuria workup should include cystoscopy and an imaging study of the upper tracts. Intravenous pyelography is being used less frequently in favor of the spiral CT scan (CT urography) for imaging of the kidneys, ureters, and bladder (KUB).[17]

In patients with flank pain, renal calculus must be excluded (see Chapter 134). A stone protocol non–contrast-enhanced computed tomography (CT) scan is the best test to detect a stone and obstruction without use of contrast media.[17] If stones are not suspected, a diagnostic ultrasound evaluation is the preferred procedure for visualization of the renal pelvis and diagnosis of hydronephrosis.[1] Urodynamics may be helpful in diagnosis of lower tract obstruction such as bladder outlet obstruction. Other procedures useful in determining the site of obstruction include anterograde and retrograde pyelography.

Additional Diagnostics

Routine blood studies are nonspecific. Complete blood count (CBC) and electrolyte values may be helpful in identifying anemia and alterations in fluid status. Blood urea nitrogen (BUN) and creatinine levels and glomerular filtration rate will be helpful in determining alterations in renal function if

INITIAL DIAGNOSTICS

Obstructive Uropathy and Genitourinary Tumors

OBSTRUCTIVE UROPATHY
Initial
- Postvoid residual
- Urine dip for leukocytes, nitrites, blood

Laboratory
- CBC and differential
- Serum glucose, serum electrolytes, BUN, creatinine, and glomerular filtration rate
- Microalbumin
- Urinalysis
- Urine cultures*
- Blood cultures*

Imaging
- KUB
- Intravenous pyelography
- Ultrasound (duplex Doppler ultrasonography)
- CT scan
- Anterograde and retrograde pyelography
- Diffusion-weighted magnetic resonance imaging (MRI)

Other Diagnostics
- Cystoscopy
- Urodynamics
- Diuretic renography
- Perfusion pressure-flow study

RENAL CELL CARCINOMA
Laboratory
- Urinalysis
- Urine cytology*

- CBC and differential
- Serum glucose, electrolytes (including calcium), BUN, and creatinine
- Liver function tests

Imaging
- Intravenous pyelography
- Ultrasound
- CT scans, MRI
- Renal angiography*
- Retrograde pyelography*

Other Diagnostics
- Cystoscopy

WILMS TUMOR
Laboratory
- Urinalysis
- CBC and differential
- BUN, creatinine
- Coagulation screening
- Imaging
- Ultrasound
- CT scan
- Chest x-ray studies[a]

BLADDER CANCER
Laboratory
- Urine for cytology
- Imaging
- Spiral CT (CT urography)
- Ultrasound
- Intravenous pyelography
- CT scan

Other Diagnostics
- Cystoscopy with biopsy

[a]If indicated.

BOX 136.1

Differential Diagnosis: Obstructive Uropathy and Genitourinary Tumors

OBSTRUCTIVE UROPATHY
Intrinsic (Outflow Obstruction)
Intraluminal
- Stones
- Papilla
- Clots
- Fungal balls

Structural
- Stricture
- Tumors, polyps
- Infection: granuloma
- Anatomic defects
- Valve or sphincter abnormalities

Functional
- Vesicoureteral reflux
- Adynamic ureters
- Neurogenic bladder

Extrinsic (Outflow Obstruction)
Autoimmune
- Vascular, glomerular, or tubulointerstitial disease

Abdominal
- Ileum, left colon, duodenum, gallbladder disease
- Aneurysms (aortic or renal)
- Appendicitis

Pelvic
- Prostatic hypertrophy
- Cysts, tumors of the uterus, ovaries
- Endometriosis

- Pregnancy, ectopic pregnancy
- Phimosis, meatal stenosis

Retroperitoneal
- Fibrosis
- Tumor, lymphoma

GENITOURINARY TUMORS
Renal Cell Carcinoma
Simple cyst
Angiomyolipoma
Renal abscess
Arteriovenous malformations
Renal lymphoma
Transitional cell carcinoma of renal pelvis
Adrenal cancer
Oncocytoma

Wilms Tumor
Neuroblastoma
Hepatoblastoma
Germ cell or teratoma
Hydronephrosis
Mesoblastic nephroma
Fecal mass
Renal tumor, non-Wilms tumor

Bladder Cancer
Urinary tract infections
Interstitial cystitis
Hemorrhagic cystitis
Fibrous polyp
Endometriosis
Hematoma
Bladder calculi

---

renal insufficiency is suspected.[1] Blood glucose concentration or hemoglobin A_{1c} level can help assess for diabetes. Further workup depends on results from these tests and the suspected cause of symptoms.

DIFFERENTIAL DIAGNOSIS OF URINARY TRACT OBSTRUCTION AND RENAL TUMORS

See Box 136.1.

INTERPROFESSIONAL COLLABORATIVE MANAGEMENT

 Immediate intervention required for signs and symptoms suggestive of obstruction, anuria and acute renal failure, or acute illness and may indicate advanced disease.

Treatment to relieve partial obstruction is indicated when the patient has recurrent infections, significant symptoms, urinary retention, and impaired renal function. Urinary tract obstruction complicated by infection should be relieved as soon as possible to prevent development of sepsis, to preserve

renal function, to normalize blood pressure, to correct fluid and electrolyte imbalances, and to treat pain. Acute treatment of lower tract obstruction is catheterization.[1]

Obstruction caused by BPH is not always progressive, and the patient need not be treated unless retention, recurrent infection, or unacceptable symptoms are present. Irritative symptoms often include frequency, nocturia, difficulty initiating a urinary stream, dribbling, and incontinence. Chronic urinary retention because of prostatic hypertrophy may respond to treatment with alpha$_1$ blockers.

5α-Reductase inhibitors—antitestosterone products such as finasteride (Proscar) and dutasteride (Avodart)—can also be effective for relieving symptoms of BPH by reducing prostate size, thereby increasing urinary flow (see Chapter 129).[18,19]

The decision to undertake surgical or instrumental procedures for the relief of obstruction depends on the location of obstruction, presence of infection, and status of renal function.

Relief of complete obstruction should occur as soon as possible after diagnosis. Infection in the face of an acute obstruction requires emergent treatment because relief of obstruction and antibiotics are both essential in treating the infection. Furthermore, antibiotics are given before any surgical intervention used to relieve obstruction. In cases of chronic incomplete obstruction, such as BPH, surgery is ideally done only when the urine is sterile.[1]

Renal Cell Carcinoma

The prognosis for RCC is poor unless it is diagnosed and treated before metastasis occurs. Surgical intervention for localized disease offers the only potential for cure.[2] Surgical options include a radical nephrectomy, which may be done as a laparoscopic procedure or as an open procedure. A nephron-sparing partial nephrectomy may be an option in select situations.[6]

Preoperative renal artery embolization may be used to minimize blood loss or to minimize pain or hematuria in the case of a nonresectable tumor.[2,6] For patients with disseminated disease, radiotherapy is used for palliation of metastatic lesions (e.g., to the brain, bone, or lungs). RCC has shown limited response to biologic response modifiers (e.g., interferons, interleukin).[2]

Targeted therapies for metastatic RCC have been employed for the treatment of advanced disease, with variable outcomes. Small-molecule therapy is another targeted treatment of metastatic RCC that may increase survival rates.[2]

Wilms Tumor

For the child with Wilms tumor, multimodality therapy has been successful, with cure rates currently greater than 90%.[7] Chemotherapy is recommended for bilateral disease before kidney resection. Radiation therapy is recommended in advanced cases.[8]

Bladder Cancer

Transurethral resection of the bladder tumor is usually the initial treatment of superficial bladder cancer. In cases of less aggressive cancer, follow-up surveillance may include interval urine cytologic studies and repeated cystoscopy with transurethral resection as necessary. Adjuvant intravesical therapy (e.g., bacillus Calmette-Guérin, mitomycin-C, thiotepa, doxorubicin) may be used for tumors with unfavorable prognostic features (e.g., frequent recurrence, multifocal tumors, carcinoma in situ). For muscle-invasive bladder tumors, a radical cystectomy with urinary diversion remains the standard therapy. Options for urinary diversion include ileal conduit, continent diversion, and orthotopic neobladder. Bladder conservation therapy, with combined modalities of radiation therapy and chemotherapy, may be an option for some patients.[9,11]

INDICATIONS FOR REFERRAL OR HOSPITALIZATION

Renal calculi larger than 5 to 7 mm usually do not pass spontaneously and should be treated surgically.[3] These patients as well as those with other obstructive symptoms should be referred to a urologist for consultation and initiation of an appropriate care plan. In cases of anuria and acute renal failure, a nephrology referral should be made for appropriate management because hospitalization or dialysis may be needed. In patients with a history and clinical presentation suggestive of genitourinary tumors, specialist referral and consultation should be obtained as soon as possible. Hospitalization may be indicated for cases of acute illness or advanced disease.[20]

LIFE SPAN CONSIDERATIONS

Obstructive uropathy can occur at any age. Prenatal ultrasound has made it possible to diagnose obstruction in the fetus during pregnancy. In the young adult, acute obstruction is most likely a result of calculi. In women, pelvic cancer is an important cause of obstruction, and in men, BPH and prostate cancer are common causes.[1]

Because clinical evidence of RCC occurs late in the disease and discovery is usually accidental, survival rate at 5 years with stage IIIB is 18%. If the tumor is localized to the kidney, the average 5-year survival is 96%.[2,11] Even in muscle-invasive bladder cancer, survival rates can reach 70%. Lifetime follow-up is recommended to detect recurrences and to improve survival rates for bladder cancers.[21]

Wilms tumors boast the second highest cure rates of childhood cancers, with the survival rates at 5 years being greater than 90%.[7] Prognosis is poorer with diffuse anaplasia.

COMPLICATIONS

Complications of untreated urinary tract obstruction include azotemia, life-threatening sepsis, and obstructive nephropathy that can lead to chronic renal insufficiency or renal failure. Complications of surgical procedures include infection, sepsis, bleeding, voiding difficulty, and pain.

Profound and prolonged diuresis, known as postobstructive diuresis, can follow relief of complete obstruction.[1] This diuresis—characterized by marked losses of water and solutes such as sodium, potassium, and magnesium—is usually self-limited. However, loss of solutes can often result in hypovolemia, hyponatremia, hypokalemia, and hypomagnesemia. Careful fluid replacement and monitoring of weight and serum and urine electrolyte values should be performed in these patients.[1] Box 136.2 lists complications of both obstructive uropathy and genitourinary tumors.

PATIENT AND FAMILY EDUCATION

Patients with urinary tract obstruction are frequently uncomfortable and often frightened. Every effort should be made to alleviate discomfort and to provide information and reassurance.

- All patients with obstruction should be taught the signs and symptoms of infection and how to take their temperature. If obstruction is a result of calculi, patients need to understand that the likelihood of recurrence is high.[3]
- Patients with BPH taking nonselective alpha blockers need to be advised of the potential for postural hypotension and confusion, especially if they are elderly.[22] All patients need to know how to access the health care system in an emergency situation, whether they are at home or traveling.
- Patient education for tumors of the genitourinary tract should include information about prevention, the disease process, diagnostic and staging procedures, treatment options, prognosis, and symptom management. The importance of lifelong surveillance and follow-up should be emphasized.

HEALTH PROMOTION

Adequate daily fluid intake may help prevent recurrence of urinary tract obstructions related to nephrolithiasis. Dietary

BOX **136.2**

Complications of Obstructive Uropathy and Genitourinary Tumors

URINARY TRACT OBSTRUCTIONS

- Azotemia
- Life-threatening sepsis
- Chronic renal insufficiency or renal failure
- Surgical procedures: infection, sepsis, bleeding, voiding difficulty, pain from surgical intervention
- Postobstructive diuresis

GENITOURINARY TUMORS

Renal Cell Carcinoma

- Complications of metastasis
- Anemia
- Pain
- Hypercalcemia
- Erythrocytosis

- Hypertension
- Hepatic dysfunction

Wilms Tumor

- Treatment-related morbidity including surgical complications, chemotherapy, and scoliosis from partial vertebral irradiation
- Metastasis-related morbidity
- Complications of associated congenital anomalies

Bladder Cancer

- Bladder perforation
- Hematuria
- Clot retention
- Metastasis
- Treatment-related morbidity
- Obstruction

modification, depending on the type of stone, may be indicated as well.

Unfortunately, there currently are no screening tests for cancers of the kidneys, ureters, or bladder. Urine cytologic testing may be done, but it is most sensitive and specific in high-grade urothelial cancers. Urine cytology may be falsely negative in as many of 50% to 75% of cases of low- to moderate-grade urothelial cancers.[23]

Cigarette smoking remains the greatest risk factor for bladder cancer. Health promotion that emphasizes no smoking or smoking cessation is a critical aspect of prevention.[9]

REFERENCES

1. Tanagho, E. A., & Lue, T. F. (2012). Urinary obstruction and stasis. In J. W. McAninch & T. F. Lue (Eds.), *Smith and Tanagho's general urology* (18th ed.). New York: McGraw-Hill.
2. Konety, B. R., Vaena, D. A., & Williams, R. D. (2012). Renal parenchymal neoplasms. In J. W. McAninch & T. F. Lue (Eds.), *Smith and Tanagho's general urology* (18th ed.). New York: McGraw-Hill.
3. Stoller, M. L. (2012). Urinary stone disease. In J. W. McAnich & T. F. Lue (Eds.), *Smith and Tanagho's general urology* (18th ed.). New York: McGraw-Hill.
4. Cooperberg, M. R., Presti, J. C., Shinohara, K., & Carroll, P. R. (2012). Neoplasms of the prostate gland. In J. W. McAninch & T. F. Lue (Eds.), *Smith and Tanagho's general urology* (18th ed.). New York: McGraw-Hill.
5. Patel, C., Ahmed, A., & Ellsworth, P. (2012). Renal cell carcinoma: A reappraisal. *Urologic Nursing, 32*(4), 182–191.
6. Noble, H., & Page, K. (2012). Renal cell carcinoma: Nurse's role in prevention and management. *British Journal of Nursing (Mark Allen Publishing), 21*(17), S18–S22.
7. Wang, L. L., Yustein, J., Russell, L. C., et al. (2011). Solid tumors of childhood. In V. T. DeVita, T. S. Lawrence, S. A. Rosenberg, et al. (Eds.), *Cancer: Principles and practice of oncology* (9th ed.). Philadelphia: Lippincott Williams & Wilkins.
8. Davenport, K. P., Blanco, F. C., & Sandler, A. D. (2012). Pediatric malignancies: Neuroblastoma, Wilm's tumor, hepatoblastoma, rhabdomyosarcoma, and sacrococcygeal teratoma. *The Surgical Clinics of North America, 92*(3), 745–767.
9. Turner, B., & Drudge-Coates, L. (2012). Bladder cancer: Risk factors, diagnosis, and treatment. *Cancer Nursing Practice, 11*(7), 30–36.
10. Wadhwa, N., Mathew, B. B., Jatawa, S. K., & Tiwari, A. (2013). Genetic instability in urinary bladder cancer: An evolving hallmark. *Journal of Postgraduate Medicine, 59*(4), 284–288.
11. McDougal, W. S., Shipley, W. U., Kaufman, D. S., et al. (2011). Cancers of the bladder, ureter, and renal pelvis. In V. T. DeVita, T. S. Lawrence, S. A. Rosenberg, et al. (Eds.), *Cancer: Principles and practice of oncology* (9th ed.). Philadelphia: Lippincott Williams & Wilkins.
12. Grossman, S. C., & Porth, C. M. (2014). Disorders of renal function. In *Porth's pathophysiology* (9th ed.). Philadelphia: Lippincott Williams & Wilkins.
13. Lue, T. F., & Tanagho, E. A. (2012). Neuropathic bladder disorders. In J. W. McAninch & T. F. Lue (Eds.), *Smith and Tanagho's general urology* (18th ed.). New York: McGraw-Hill.
14. American Cancer Society. About bladder cancer. Retrieved from https://www.cancer.org/content/dam/CRC/PDF/Public/8557.00.pdf. (Accessed 11 June 2019).
15. Lambert, M. (2013). AUA guidelines addressing diagnosis, evaluation, and follow up of asymptomatic microhematuria. *American Family Physician, 87*(9), 649–653.
16. Chalisey, A., & Karim, M. (2013). Hypertension and hydronephrosis: Rapid resolution of high blood pressure following relief of bilateral uretic obstructive. *Journal of General Internal Medicine, 28*(3), 478–481.
17. American College of Radiology (ACR) Appropriateness Criteria. Acute onset flank pain—suspicion of stone disease. Retrieved from www.acr.org/~/media/ACR/Documents/AppCriteria/Diagnostic/AcuteOnsetFlankPainSuspicionStoneDisease.pdf. (Accessed 23 August 2015).
18. McVary, K. T., Roehrborn, C. G., Avins, A. L., et al. (2014). American Urological Association Guideline: Management of Benign Prostatic Hyperplasia (BPH). Retrieved from https://www.auanet.orgoogle/education/guidelines/benign-prostatic-hyperplasia.cfm.
19. Shinohara, K. (2012). Disorders of the bladder, prostate, and seminal vesicles. In J. W. McAninch & T. F. Lue (Eds.), *Smith and Tanagho's general urology* (18th ed.). New York: McGraw-Hill.
20. Lee, B. K., & Vincenti, F. G. (2012). Acute kidney injury and oliguria. In J. W. McAninch & T. F. Lue (Eds.), *Smith and Tanagho's general urology* (18th ed.). New York: McGraw-Hill.
21. Chamie, K., Litwin, M. S., Bassett, J. C., Daskivich, T. J., Lai, J., Hanley, J. M., et al. (2013). Recurrence of high-risk bladder cancer: A population based analysis. *Cancer, 119*(17), 3219–3227.
22. U.S. Department of Health and Human Services. Prostate enlargement: benign prostatic hypertrophy. National Kidney and Urologic Diseases Information Clearinghouse. National Institute of Health. Retrieved from http://kidney.niddk.nih.gov/kudiseases/pubs/prostateenlargement/. (Accessed 1 July 2014).
23. U.S. Preventive Services Task Force. Screening for bladder cancer. Retrieved from www.uspreventiveservicestaskforce.org/uspstf11/bladdercancer/bladcanrs.htm. (Accessed 23 August 2015).

CHAPTER 137

AMENORRHEA

Patricia Polgar-Bailey

 Hospitalization may be necessary for women with anorexia nervosa who have lost more than 30% of their desired body weight and fail to gain weight, as well as for those with suicidal ideation.

DEFINITION AND EPIDEMIOLOGY

Amenorrhea is the absence or abnormal cessation of menstrual bleeding. It can be transient or permanent and is classified as primary or secondary depending on the absence or presence of previous menses. *Primary amenorrhea* is defined as the absence of both spontaneous uterine bleeding and secondary sexual characteristics (delayed puberty) at the age of 14 years or by 2 years after sexual maturation or the absence of menarche at the age of 16 years regardless of the presence of secondary sexual characteristics. *Secondary amenorrhea* has been variously defined and refers to the absence of menstrual bleeding in a woman with prior menstruation.[1] Although the average age for menarche in the United States is 12.7 years[1] (12.8 years for white adolescents and slightly earlier, 12.6 years, for African American adolescents), there is a range of 9 to 16 years, and factors other than race, such as nutritional status, body fat, and maternal age at menarche, are also contributory.

Primary amenorrhea has an estimated prevalence of 0.1% to 0.3%. Secondary amenorrhea is much more common, affecting 1% to 3% of women of reproductive age in the general population. Higher prevalence has been noted in specific subgroups of women, such as college students, endurance athletes (particularly runners and elite athletes in sports and activities that emphasize thinness,[2] such as ballet), and women who are obese.

Up to 25% of female athletes experience exercise-induced amenorrhea. The female athlete triad involves the combination of amenorrhea, osteoporosis, and disordered eating; it affects female athletes in all sports and at all levels of training, as well as both professional and amateur dancers.[3] Approximately 2.5% of healthy adolescents will experience pubertal delay.

PATHOPHYSIOLOGY

Aside from physiologic amenorrhea resulting from constitutional delay, pregnancy, lactation, or menopause, the pathophysiologic mechanisms for amenorrhea generally involve disorders of the sex chromosomes, hypothalamic-pituitary-ovarian axis, and related hormone production; the responsiveness of the uterine endometrium to various hormones; and the patency of the outflow tract. Because normal ovarian development depends on the presence of at least two X chromosomes, abnormalities involving X and Y chromosomes can result in gonadal failure, agonadism, gonadal dysgenesis, and androgen resistance (testicular feminization). Problems with hypothalamic synthesis or release of gonadotropin-releasing hormone (GnRH) can result in hypogonadotropic hypogonadism. Müllerian agenesis, obstruction of the vaginal outflow tract (such as with an imperforate hymen), cervical stenosis, and transverse vaginal septa are structural causes of primary amenorrhea.

Disorders of the hypothalamic-pituitary-ovarian axis can cause primary or secondary amenorrhea. Leptin, a hormone secreted by adipocytes, signals energy availability in energy-deficient states and may have a major role in the regulation, synthesis, and secretion of sex steroids, gonadotropins, and GnRH. In the face of significant energy expenditure, the body may lack a compensatory response in terms of adequate calorie intake; decreased luteinizing hormone (LH) secretion and a subsequent lack of estrogen production may result. Other pituitary hormones (triiodothyronine, growth hormone, and insulin-like growth factor 1) may also be affected. Hypothalamic causes of dysfunction have been linked to weight loss, intensive exercise, starvation, eating disorders, and psychogenic stress in nonathletic, normal-weight women and can result in pubertal delay or secondary hormonal insufficiency. Persistent amenorrhea has also been correlated with a longer duration of eating disorders and the presence of a concomitant anxiety disorder. The majority of young women with amenorrhea are estrogen deficient; a minority have normal estrogen levels that are unopposed by progesterone secondary to anovulation. Neurotransmitter abnormalities (central dopaminergic and opioid activity) may modulate the response of LH to GnRH. Amenorrhea can also be seen in obese patients; reduction of body fat can bring about return of regular menstrual flow.

Prolactinemia associated with amenorrhea after normal puberty may be caused by breastfeeding, microadenomas or macroadenomas of the pituitary, renal failure, or the use of medications (e.g., psychoactive drugs such as haloperidol, amitriptyline, benzodiazepines, cocaine). Anovulation associated with hyperprolactinemic amenorrhea is primarily caused by both impaired gonadotropin pulsatility and derangement of the estrogen-positive feedback effect on LH in the face of a continued ovarian response to gonadotropin. In polycystic ovary syndrome (PCOS), a low ratio of progesterone to estrogen is associated with menstrual irregularity and amenorrhea. Drugs (chemotherapeutic agents, thalidomide, leuprolide, heroin, gabapentin) may affect menstruation. Autoimmune disorders (systemic lupus erythematosus, Addison disease, hypothyroidism, and toxic thyroiditis) have also been associated with amenorrhea. In thalassemic patients with secondary amenorrhea, severe and progressive damage to the hypothalamic-pituitary axis has been demonstrated by gonadotropin pulse abnormalities, marked reduction in GnRH-stimulated gonadotropin levels, and even apulsatility.

CLINICAL PRESENTATION AND PHYSICAL EXAMINATION

Relevant history in the evaluation of amenorrhea includes a thorough menstrual history (age at menarche; frequency, duration, and flow of menstrual periods; last menstrual period; history of missed menses). Obtaining a complete sexual history (number of partners; date of last intercourse; method of birth control and percentage of use; number of pregnancies, abortions, miscarriages, or ectopic pregnancies; and surgical history) as well as the age at menarche and menopause for family members and any family history of infertility is also necessary.

Probable signs of past ovulatory cycles include breast tenderness, cyclic abdominal pain or bloating, and changes in the cervical mucus. The past medical history should be examined specifically for autoimmune disorders, childhood onset of type 1 diabetes mellitus, previous irradiation or chemotherapy, frequent fractures or osteoporosis, and thyroid or adrenal dysfunction. A complete medication history regarding prescribed, over-the-counter, and illicit drug use should be obtained. Nutritional and exercise factors, including disordered eating behavior, recent weight loss or gain, and athletic training, are evaluated, along with endocrinologic markers of growth and development (growth charts and the presence or absence of secondary sexual characteristics, specifically breast development and pubic hair).

A review of systems may reveal indications of systemic illness, such as thyroid dysfunction, headaches or visual disturbances (possibly indicating a cranial mass in the area of the pituitary or hypothalamus), galactorrhea, and signs of hyperandrogenism (hirsutism, truncal obesity, deepening of the voice) or hypoestrogenism (hot flashes, vaginal dryness, headaches, depression, dyspareunia, decreasing breast size). A social history may indicate substance use or stressful life events (e.g., going away to college, entering religious life or the armed forces, sudden changes in the environment, death or divorce in the family), which have been linked with amenorrhea.

The physical examination requires an evaluation of general growth and development as the presence of congenital short stature together with neck webbing and a pigeon chest suggests Turner syndrome. The exam may also reveal signs of androgen excess (hirsutism, acne, male pattern hair loss, truncal obesity, clitoromegaly >1 cm [⅖ inch]), androgen insensitivity (complete absence of axillary and pubic hair), hyperprolactinemia (galactorrhea on breast examination), decreased estrogen status (pale, dry vaginal mucosa; scant cervical mucus), or eating disorders (cachexia, hypothermia, lanugo hair, decreased blood pressure, bradycardia, dry skin, tooth decay, chipmunk cheeks, Chvostek sign). Assessment of visual acuity and a funduscopic examination are important because vision changes or retinal abnormalities may reflect an intracranial mass. The thyroid is palpated for masses or nodules. A pelvic examination assesses estrogen status by vaginal epithelium and cervical mucus; it may identify an imperforate hymen and also provides a gross evaluation of the cervix, uterus, and ovaries. Enlarged ovaries are palpable in 60% of women with PCOS and, in combination with acne, obesity, and acanthosis nigricans, suggest this diagnosis. Abdominal striae on nulliparous women may be indicative of hypercortisolism, and skin tags, fissures, and fecal occult blood may indicate inflammatory bowel disease.

DIAGNOSTICS
Essential Diagnostics

Pregnancy or lactation-induced amenorrhea must be excluded in all women of childbearing age before any other diagnostic evaluation is initiated. Next, follicle-stimulating hormone (FSH) and LH should be checked (anovulation); thyroid-stimulating hormone (TSH) concentration is determined to evaluate for hypothyroidism; and prolactin levels are obtained to check for hyperprolactinemia or possibly an early presentation of acromegaly, which produces excess prolactin and growth hormone. If prolactin levels are elevated, a magnetic resonance imaging (MRI) or computed tomography (CT) scan of the sella turcica to identify microadenomas and macroadenomas is necessary (MRI is more effective than CT in detecting empty sella syndrome). If these scans are normal, a progesterone challenge test, which classically consists of 10 mg of medroxyprogesterone administered daily for 5 to 7 days, can be used to further evaluate estrogen status. Any vaginal bleeding within 2 to 7 days after the cessation of progesterone signals a positive progesterone challenge, indicating both adequate estrogen stores and patency of the outflow tract. A negative progesterone challenge (i.e., no bleeding 2 to 7 days after cessation of progesterone) indicates either inadequate estrogen stores or an obstruction of the outflow tract. To further differentiate hypoestrogenism from obstruction, the test can be repeated after daily administration of 2.5 mg of estrogen for 21 days, followed by 10 mg of progesterone for the next 5 days. If there is still no withdrawal bleeding, investigation into structural or outflow reasons for the amenorrhea should ensue.

Additional Diagnostics

If amenorrhea is secondary to anovulation, potential causes include Cushing syndrome, adrenal or ovarian tumors, premature ovarian failure, and, more commonly, PCOS. An FSH level elevated beyond 20 IU/L after repeated measurements is indicative of ovarian failure. An elevated LH/FSH ratio (>0.2) is suggestive of PCOS; an FSH level greater than 30 IU/L indicates menopausal status.

To differentiate between pituitary and hypothalamic amenorrhea, an LH-releasing hormone test is typically performed in conjunction with imaging of the sellar region by CT or MRI. Long-term administration of pulsatile GnRH can indicate hypothalamic amenorrhea by an ovulatory response within two treatment cycles. In the absence of an ovulatory response, a pituitary cause of the amenorrhea should be suspected.

MRI has been shown to be an effective and accurate tool to evaluate the cause of primary amenorrhea and to plan for surgery, particularly when this involves congenital disorders of sexual differentiation and localization of the gonads. A hysterosalpingogram or sonohysterogram can be used to outline the uterine cavity if a bicornuate uterus or double cervix is suspected.

The clomiphene challenge test may provide information necessary for an early diagnosis to be made of waning ovarian function in hypergonadotropic amenorrhea. Increased serum dehydroepiandrosterone (DHEA; >700 mg/dL) indicates an adrenal origin for androgens in women with hirsutism, and elevated plasma testosterone levels (>90 ng/dL) suggest tumors of adrenal and ovarian origin or congenital adrenal hyperplasia;

levels above 200 ng/dL are found in the rare Sertoli-Leydig cell tumors. The level of sex hormone–binding globulin, which binds potent androgens such as testosterone and thereby controls the level of active androgens in circulation, may also provide useful clinical information.

Chemistry profiles (including serum electrolyte values and serum glucose, blood urea nitrogen [BUN], and creatinine concentrations), urinary free cortisol, thyroid antibodies, erythrocyte sedimentation rate (ESR), and hemoglobin A_{1c} can help differentiate possible causes of autoimmune-related amenorrhea[4] (Addison disease, diabetes mellitus, thyroiditis, and hypoparathyroidism), which are responsible for 20% to 40% of cases of primary ovarian insufficiency. The diagnosis of premature ovarian failure in a young woman (in general, younger than 25 or 30 years) warrants karyotyping to exclude the presence of a Y chromosome.

INITIAL DIAGNOSTICS

Amenorrhea

LABORATORY
Initial Diagnostics
- Serum human chorionic gonadotropin
- Thyroid profile
- FSH, LH
- Prolactin

Additional Testing[a]
- DHEA
- Serum glucose, electrolytes, BUN, creatinine

- Thyroid antibodies
- ESR
- Urinary free cortisol
- HbA_{1c}

IMAGING
- CT or MRI

OTHER DIAGNOSTICS
- Clomiphene challenge test
- Hysterosalpingogram

[a]If indicated.

DIFFERENTIAL DIAGNOSIS

 Co-management with the appropriate specialist mandated for evidence of anatomic or endocrinologic abnormalities. Women with eating disorders, such as anorexia nervosa, are best managed in collaboration with psychiatric or other specialized eating disorder services.

Primary Amenorrhea

Physiologic primary amenorrhea may be attributable to constitutional delay, although 97% to 99% of young women experience menarche by age 16 years and 95% by 14.5 years. Failure of the gonads to develop normally accounts for half of all cases of primary amenorrhea. Other possible causes include Turner syndrome (45, X) mosaicism; abnormal X chromosomes; the presence of an intact or fragmented Y chromosome; complex chromosomal rearrangement; chromosomal deletions; pure gonadal dysgenesis (may manifest with hyperandrogenism); steroidogenic factor 1 (SF-1) mutation; and the rare 17α-hydroxylase deficiency, which is seen with hypernatremia, hypokalemia, and hypocortisolism.
- Additional causes of primary amenorrhea include structural abnormalities (imperforate hymen, transverse septum, vaginal inversion or other trauma, congenital absence of the uterus or vagina), premature ovarian failure (may be idiopathic or secondary to radiation therapy or chemotherapeutics), malnutrition, systemic illness, tumors (ovarian,

hypothalamic, parasellar, or adrenal), and any of the disturbances in the hypothalamic-pituitary-ovarian axis that also cause secondary amenorrhea. Rare causes of primary amenorrhea include mutations in the beta subunit of FSH, vaginal inversion and uterus acollis, multiple endocrine neoplasia, progesterone-producing adrenal adenoma, increased melatonin secretion from a cystic pineal lesion, and childhood trauma.

Secondary Amenorrhea

Pregnancy is the most common cause of secondary amenorrhea; lactation and early menopause are other physiologic possibilities. Transient amenorrhea may occur in the first two postmenarchal years, after discontinuation of oral contraceptives, and in the majority of women who receive medroxyprogesterone (Depo-Provera) for contraception. Aside from these causes, secondary amenorrhea is most often linked to disordered functioning somewhere along the hypothalamic-pituitary-ovarian axis.

Other causes of secondary amenorrhea include primary ovarian insufficiency (previously referred to as *premature ovarian failure*), which may be of an autoimmune cause,[4] and chronic anovulatory disorder (PCOS, obesity-related disorder, idiopathic disorder). Less common conditions include pituitary tumors, hyperprolactinemia, Sheehan syndrome (postpartum pituitary necrosis), hypogonadotropic hypogonadism, thyroid disease, tuberculosis, and late-onset 21-hydroxylase deficiency. For the majority of women, a clinical history, physical examination, and laboratory determination of TSH, LH, FSH, and prolactin levels are sufficient for diagnosis.

Categorization of amenorrhea by cause (hyperprolactinemic, hyperandrogenic, hypergonadotropic, and hypogonadotropic) provides a helpful framework for consideration of the differential diagnosis, evaluation, and management.

Hyperprolactinemic amenorrhea can be caused by drugs (including reserpine, phenothiazines, oral contraceptives, metoclopramide, and α-methyldopa), prolactin-secreting tumors of the pituitary, or systemic illness such as acromegaly or hypothyroidism. Physiologic causes of increased prolactin levels include lactation and nipple stimulation.

Hyperandrogenic amenorrhea is seen most commonly in women with PCOS (also called *hyperandrogenic chronic anovulation* or *Stein-Leventhal syndrome*) but may also be caused by obesity, Cushing syndrome, hyperprolactinemia, thyroid disease, adrenal disease (hyperplasia, adenoma, carcinoma), androgen-secreting ovarian tumors, or drug abuse.

Hypergonadotropic amenorrhea affects about 1% of women younger than 40 years. The differential diagnosis for ovarian failure includes chromosomal (mosaicism and gonadal dysgenesis), autoimmune (Hashimoto thyroiditis, Addison disease, diabetes mellitus, hypoparathyroidism), metabolic (ovarian enzymatic defects), familial, infectious (mumps), idiopathic, and iatrogenic (irradiation, chemotherapy) causes as well as resistant ovary syndrome.

Hypogonadotropic amenorrhea, a clinical syndrome of gonadal failure caused by abnormal pituitary gonadotropin levels, can be a result of either congenital or acquired causes,[2] including functional and organic forms. Although relatively common in young women as a result of emotional or physical stress (including athletic training), depression, nutritional deficiency, weight loss, and eating disorders, it can also be caused by thyroid or adrenal dysfunction, isolated gonadotropin deficiency (Kallmann syndrome), or hypothalamic or pituitary lesions (craniopharyngiomas, germinomas, pituitary adenomas, endodermal sinus tumors, pituitary apoplexy, empty sella syndrome, postpartum ischemia, necrosis of the pituitary gland). Amenorrhea is one of the cardinal features of anorexia nervosa. Head injuries (especially head-on automobile collisions resulting in whiplash) and external irradiation can damage the hypothalamus; infections (tuberculosis, human immunodeficiency virus [HIV]) can disrupt pituitary function.

In addition to disorders of the hypothalamic-pituitary-ovarian axis, secondary amenorrhea can be caused by uterine pathologic conditions, including endometrial hyperplasia, postpartum uterine adhesions, and iatrogenic Asherman syndrome. Rare causes of secondary amenorrhea include hydrocephalus, Pendred syndrome, onchocerciasis, inhibin-secreting ovarian tumors, Sjögren syndrome, and neurosarcoidosis.

INTERPROFESSIONAL COLLABORATIVE MANAGEMENT

1. In amenorrhea caused by systemic illness or endocrinopathy, treatment of the underlying cause, such as diabetes mellitus or hypothyroidism, generally resolves the amenorrhea as a result of renewed ovarian function.

2. Spontaneous recovery of menses also occurs after diagnosis of premature ovarian failure, after prolonged irradiation-induced ovarian failure from treatment of Hodgkin disease, and in cases of chemotherapy-induced ovarian failure; there is evidence to suggest that taxane, as an adjuvant agent, may help prevent chemotherapy-related amenorrhea and that the use of oral contraceptives during chemotherapy may also decrease post-treatment amenorrhea. Gonadal function should be reassessed periodically in these women, and oral contraceptives are a good choice for hormone replacement in women not desiring pregnancy.

3. Menses generally return 6 to 14 months after a last injection of medroxyprogesterone and within 6 months after stopping of oral contraceptives in post–oral contraceptive amenorrhea. Eventual return of menstruation has been shown, after a variable interval, for less than half of women with medically refractory menorrhagia after endometrial ablation and uterine resection.

4. In perimenopausal women, amenorrheic intervals are common and do not require any treatment aside from adequate contraception when pregnancy is not desired; in these women, unplanned pregnancy is possible unless FSH levels have been consistently elevated (>30 IU/L) and the amenorrhea has been present for more than 1 year.

5. Complete recovery of gonadal function in hypothalamic amenorrhea depends on restoration of the hypothalamic-pituitary-adrenal and the hypothalamic-pituitary-thyroidal axes, and so psychological interventions[5] (such as cognitive behavioral therapy [CBT]) that focus on changing behaviors and attitudes and pharmacologic interventions that target the resultant hormonal dysfunction are often necessary; multidisciplinary approaches to treatment are generally encouraged.

6. Whereas women with anorexia or other eating disorders and endurance athletes have benefited from increased calorie intake and decreased exercise,[6] some overweight and hirsute women with hyperandrogenism may recover normal menses with control of excess body weight by calorie restriction. Menstrual return can often be predicted by a return to the weight at which previous function ceased.

7. Recombinant human leptin has been used in research settings in women with hypothalamic amenorrhea, resulting in normalization of levels of reproductive hormones, follicular development, and menstrual cyclicity.

8. Pulsatile GnRH has also been used to induce ovulation[7] in hypothalamic infertile women with PCOS. GnRH administration on alternate days has also been used to increase FSH levels, to reinstate LH pulsatility, and, in conjunction with clomiphene therapy, to induce ovulation in women with weight loss–associated amenorrhea.

9. Clomiphene has also been used alone, and naltrexone hydrochloride, an oral antiopioid, has also been studied as an agent in the management of amenorrhea resulting from hypogonadotropic syndromes.

10. Estrogen, the current standard of pharmacologic care, does not address the underlying infertility or neuroendocrine dysfunction associated with hypothalamic amenorrhea in anorexia nervosa, but early research does suggest a possible role for the administration of a weak estrogen, estriol,[8] in the spontaneous and GnRH-induced LH secretion in women with functional hypothalamic amenorrhea.

11. One review of the available literature on the use of oral contraceptives or hormone replacement therapy by these women determined that available evidence was both of low quality and mixed,[9] in terms of improving lumbar spine and total body bone mineral density. Although supplemental estrogen and progesterone (as with oral contraceptives) have been recommended for the prevention of further bone loss and subsequent fracture development in women with decreased estrogen levels, normalization of body weight is the single most important factor in regaining bone density. Irreversible bone loss can occur after 3 years of amenorrhea. Although scant direct evidence supports the use of hormone replacement therapy in amenorrheic women, there is some evidence that taking long-term triphasic oral contraceptives can increase total lumbar spine bone mineral density in women with hypothalamic amenorrhea and osteopenia and can improve both endothelial function and dyslipidemia in amenorrheic athletes.

12. Adequate calcium and, if indicated, vitamin D intake or supplementation plus weight-bearing exercise should be encouraged in women who are amenorrheic for any reason to help maintain bone density.

13. Administration of estrogen and progesterone is also necessary after hysteroscopic adhesiolysis to reestablish a functional endometrium in women with Asherman syndrome.

14. No treatment is required if women maintain normal estradiol and prolactin levels in post–oral contraceptive amenorrhea.

15. Amenorrhea caused by heroin use has been reversed with methadone maintenance.

16. Bromocriptine has been widely studied with demonstrated effectiveness for promoting menstrual bleeding and ovulation and for years has been the drug of choice for hyperprolactinemic amenorrhea and the syndrome of galactorrhea-amenorrhea. In case of relapse, this treatment should be resumed and continued.

17. An alternative, cabergoline, may be more effective and better tolerated than bromocriptine, with fewer

gastrointestinal symptoms; this drug may be a better first choice initial treatment[10] in many women. Subcutaneous pulsatile GnRH therapy combined with human chorionic gonadotropin has been proposed as a method of ovulation induction if these women should desire pregnancy.

INDICATIONS FOR REFERRAL OR HOSPITALIZATION

Suspected or confirmed genetic abnormalities that result in primary or secondary amenorrhea warrant referral to a specialist for more thorough evaluation. Young women with either Y chromosome fragments or an entire Y chromosome will need to have their gonads removed after pubertal development is complete because of the increased risk of malignant gonadoblastoma. Referral to an infertility specialist is indicated for women with ovarian reserve factors, anovulatory cycles, hyperprolactinemia, and genetic or structural factors.

Hospitalization may be necessary for women with anorexia nervosa who have lost more than 30% of their desired body weight and fail to gain weight, as well as for those with suicidal ideation. Inpatient surgical care may be indicated for women with tumors or adenomas associated with amenorrhea.

The reversible nature of most cases of hypothalamic amenorrhea resulting from stress, weight changes, or exercise as well as the temporary (6 months or less) duration of post–oral contraceptive amenorrhea can be stressed when relevant. When counseling athletes, the health care provider should remind them, as well as trainers and coaches, that amenorrhea can be an indication of overtraining and can contribute to future performance deficits, especially in light of the long-term health consequences, such as fractures and osteoporosis. Like hypoestrogenemic women, women with androgen excess are at increased risk of lipid abnormalities and coronary artery disease. Counseling may be required in an effort to reduce other contributing risk factors, such as obesity.

LIFE SPAN CONSIDERATIONS

The prognosis for present or future fertility is a major concern of many women with amenorrhea and will guide the treatment plan in most instances. For women with hypothalamic amenorrhea resulting from stress, weight loss, or exercise, reassurance about the reversible nature of the problem after requisite lifestyle modification may be all that is necessary. For other women, such as those with primary ovarian insufficiency, cryopreservation of oocytes or ovarian tissue[11] (the only option for prepubertal girls) is becoming increasingly possible. For women with structural or chromosomal abnormalities incompatible with achieving a natural pregnancy, alternatives such as adoption, egg donation, or surrogacy may need to be considered.

COMPLICATIONS

Untreated amenorrhea is associated with significant long-term morbidity, especially when it occurs in younger women. Loss of body weight is adversely related to pituitary-ovarian function, and in 20% to 30% of women with weight loss–related amenorrhea, no restoration of function is attained despite recovery of body weight.

Hypoestrogenemic amenorrhea, which includes the female athlete triad, has been associated with an increased risk of decreased bone mineral density[12] that can manifest decades later as osteoporosis and fractures. The female athlete triad has

also been linked to endothelial dysfunction,[13] with potential for cardiovascular consequences. Although some improvements in bone mineral density have been observed with appropriate treatment of amenorrhea, this recovery in bone mass has not been substantial, emphasizing the importance of early diagnosis and treatment.

The hypoestrogenemic state has also been associated with endothelial dysfunction, unfavorable lipid profiles, and a significantly increased risk of cardiovascular events. Anovulatory amenorrhea puts women at increased risk for endometrial hyperplasia and endometrial carcinoma. Women with PCOS and women with chronic hyperandrogenic anovulation have a high risk of metabolic syndrome and cardiovascular disease.[14]

PATIENT AND FAMILY EDUCATION AND HEALTH PROMOTION

Women will have varying educational needs depending on the cause of their amenorrhea, but all women should:

- receive basic nutritional counseling with an emphasis on obtaining sufficient calcium from either food sources or supplementation.
- be reminded that pregnancy can occur in the presence of amenorrhea; sexually active women not desiring pregnancy, especially adolescents, should receive appropriate contraceptive counseling.

Women with genetic or congenital abnormalities may wonder about their ability to become pregnant and need to be apprised of their reproductive potential. The necessity for gonadectomy to prevent future malignant neoplasms should be discussed with women who have Y chromosome fragments or a Y chromosome.

REFERENCES

1. Safai, A., Vasei, M., Attaranzadeh, A., Azad, F., & Tabibi, N. (2012). Chromosomal abnormality in patients with secondary amenorrhea. *Archives of Iranian Medicine, 15*(4), 232–234.
2. Bacchi, E., Spiazzi, G., Zendrini, G., Bonin, C., & Moghetti, P. (2013). Low body weight and menstrual dysfunction are common findings in both elite and amateur ballet dancers. *Journal of Endocrinological Investigation, 36*(5), 343–346.
3. Silva, C. A., Yamakami, L. Y., Aikawa, N. E., Araujo, D. B., Carvalho, J. F., & Bonfa, E. (2014). Autoimmune primary ovarian insufficiency. *Autoimmunity Reviews, 13*(4–5), 427–430.
4. Silveira, L. F., & Latronico, A. C. (2013). Approach to the patient with hypogonadotropic hypogonadism. *The Journal of Clinical Endocrinology and Metabolism, 98*(5), 1781–1788.
5. Michopoulos, V., Mancini, F., Loucks, T. L., & Berga, S. L. (2013). Neuroendocrine recovery initiated by cognitive behavioral therapy in women with functional hypothalamic amenorrhea: A randomized, controlled trial. *Fertility and Sterility, 99*(7), 2084–2091, e2081.
6. Marquez, S., & Molinero, O. (2013). Energy availability, menstrual dysfunction and bone health in sports; an overview of the female athlete triad. *Nutrición Hospitalaria, 28*(4), 1010–1017.
7. Dubourdieu, S., Fréour, T., Dessolle, L., & Barriere, P. (2013). Prospective, randomized comparison between pulsatile GnRH therapy and combined gonadotropin (FSH + LH) treatment for ovulation induction in women with hypothalamic amenorrhea and underlying polycystic ovary syndrome. *European Journal of Obstetrics, Gynecology, and Reproductive Biology, 168*(1), 45–48.
8. Genazzani, A. D., Meczekalski, B., Podfigurna-Stopa, A., et al. (2012). Estriol administration modulates luteinizing hormone secretion in women with functional hypothalamic amenorrhea. *Fertility and Sterility, 97*(2), 483–488.
9. Lebow, J., & Sim, L. (2013). The influence of estrogen therapies on bone mineral density in premenopausal women with anorexia nervosa and amenorrhea. *Vitamins and Hormones, 92*, 243–257.
10. Faje, A., & Nachtigall, L. (2013). Current treatment options for hyperprolactinemia. *Expert Opinion on Pharmacotherapy, 14*(12), 1611–1625.

11. Baker, V. L. (2013). Primary ovarian insufficiency in the adolescent. *Current Opinion in Obstetrics and Gynecology, 25*(5), 375–381.
12. Thein-Nissenbaum, J. (2013). Long term consequences of the female athlete triad. *Maturitas, 75*(2), 107–112.
13. Temme, K. E., & Hoch, A. Z. (2013). Recognition and rehabilitation of the female athlete triad/tetrad: A multidisciplinary approach. *Current Sports Medicine Reports, 12*(3), 190–199.
14. Tzeng, C. R., Chang, Y. C., Chang, Y. C., et al. (2014). Cluster analysis of cardiovascular and metabolic risk factors in women of reproductive age. *Fertility and Sterility, 101*(5), 1404–1410.

CHAPTER **138**

BARTHOLIN GLAND CYSTS AND ABSCESSES

Emily Proulx

DEFINITION AND EPIDEMIOLOGY

Bartholin glands, also known as the greater vestibular or vulvovaginal glands, were first discovered by the French anatomist Joseph-Guichard du Verney in the late 17th century[1]; their physiology was described by the Danish anatomist Gaspard Bartholin in 1677.[2] These paired glands, homologous to the male bulbourethral glands in structure, placement, and function, have narrow ducts about 2.5 cm (1 inch) long that open into the vestibule just distal to the hymenal ring at the 5-o'clock and 7-o'clock positions. The glands become active at puberty and continuously secrete mucus through their narrow ducts. This mucus lubricates the vulva, and the glands are generally not palpable unless a cyst or abscess develops. Bartholin gland cysts are usually noninfectious enlargements of the gland related to ductal obstruction, which can occur as a result of inflammation, mucus, or congenitally even narrower ducts. Bartholin gland abscesses, also called bartholinitis or Bartholin adenitis, are the result of acute infection followed by obstruction.

Bartholin gland cysts occur most often during women's reproductive years, and an individual woman's lifetime risk of developing a Bartholin cyst or abscess is approximately 2%.[3] A Korean study[4] found that the incidence increases until menopause and then declines. Another study designed to estimate the prevalence of Bartholin gland cysts in asymptomatic women serving as controls in research studies found that 3% of the participants had asymptomatic cysts of the gland that were visible on magnetic resonance imaging (MRI).[5] Half of these were on the right, nearly 43% were on the left, and the remaining 7% were bilateral. The cysts ranged in size from 0.5 to 2.7 cm, and on average the cysts were 1.3 × 1.2 × 1.3 cm. Clinicians are likely to encounter cysts of this gland approximately once per 46 pelvic examinations.[6]

PATHOPHYSIOLOGY

Cysts of the Bartholin gland are related to obstruction of the duct orifice. In the presence of an infectious process, inflammation of the gland's acinus may lead to abscess. Most cases are self-limited but can be severely discomforting.

Any opportunistic genital or genitourinary organism can be the cause of an acute inflammation, and infections can be the result of single organisms or polymicrobial in nature. Although it has long been generally held that most abscesses of the gland are caused by polymicrobial and sexually transmitted

infections, one 6-year retrospective study found that *Escherichia coli* was the single most common (47%) pathogen identified on culture,[3] and less than 8% of all cases were polymicrobial. Nevertheless, studies have also demonstrated the presence of *Chlamydia trachomatis, Neisseria sicca,* "usual genital flora,"[7] methicillin-resistant *Staphylococcus aureus,*[7] and *Brucella melitensis; Bacteroides* species have been detected in cultures from abscess formations in human immunodeficiency virus (HIV) antibody–positive women. Capnophilic bacteria, gram-negative bacteria (*Proteus* organisms), *Neisseria gonorrhoeae,* and polymicrobial flora including gram-negative and gram-positive anaerobes have also been cultured. Anaerobic and facultative aerobic organisms have also been implicated in abscess formation.

CLINICAL PRESENTATION AND PHYSICAL EXAMINATION

Bartholin gland cysts are often asymptomatic, are generally unilateral, range in size from 1 to 3 cm, and they can be chronic or recurrent. Associated pain is usually a sign of an infectious process and development of an abscess, which can often grow large and rapidly over 2 to 4 days. Women may be seen with pain (especially while walking or standing), swelling, dyspareunia, or tenderness. Specific inquiry into recent history of an infectious process may yield clues to the cause. A recent vaginal delivery or history of localized trauma should be explored.

Physical examination includes vital signs, visualization of the affected area, and assessment of accompanying inguinal node involvement. Patients usually exhibit a unilateral and edematous mass located lateral to the vestibule. If abscessed, it will also be erythematous. Cysts tend to be nontender while abscesses range from tender to extremely painful. The size may vary, and discharge from the mass is sometimes present. A speculum or bimanual examination may be too painful until the cyst or abscess has been treated.

ESSENTIAL DIAGNOSTICS

Culture of cystic contents and the cervix for sexually transmitted diseases is recommended to ensure adequate treatment of women and their sexual contacts. A complete blood count (CBC) can identify leukocytosis.

DIFFERENTIAL DIAGNOSIS

 Priority differentials include abscess with evidence of systemic infection, signs and symptoms suggestive of toxic shock syndrome, and necrotizing fasciitis.

Cysts or abscesses of the Bartholin gland represent the majority of cysts in the vulvar region and are the most common diseases of the gland. Differential diagnoses include epidermal inclusion cysts, Skene's gland cyst, hidradenoma papilliferum, and lipoma. Although solid benign tumors, adenocarcinomas, high-grade squamous intraepithelial neoplasias, carcinomas,[8] sarcomas,[9] mixed tumors, leiomyomas, adenofibromas, mucinous cystadenomas, myxoid leiomyosarcomas,[10] papillary tumors, mucocele-like changes, endometriosis,[11] and malacoplakia all can originate in (or, in the case of endometriosis, infiltrate) the Bartholin gland, these presentations are rare. Carcinoma of the Bartholin gland, which can be primary, accounts for less than 1% of all genital neoplasms in female patients. Tuberculosis of the Bartholin gland is also rare (vulval and vaginal infections account for less than 2% of genital tuberculosis) but should be considered if swelling does not resolve after excision. Primary neuroendocrine carcinoma (Merkel cell carcinoma) of the vulva can both originate in the Bartholin gland and mimic Bartholin gland abscess.

Skene's gland cysts should also be considered in the differential diagnosis. The skene's gland, also known as the lesser vestibular glands, periurethral glands, or homologous female prostate, are glands located on the anterior wall of the vagina, around the lower end of the urethra. Their presentation can be similar although typically smaller with a different location on the vulva.

INTERPROFESSIONAL COLLABORATIVE MANAGEMENT

The goal of management is to preserve the gland and its function if possible. Office procedures such as incision and drainage with or without catheter placement are the most common first-line treatments. Weekly patient follow-up is indicated after surgical incision and drainage of a Bartholin's cyst with insertion of a drain. Marsupialization of the cyst can be done if necessary. Antibiotic therapy is warranted only when cellulitis is present or concern for systemic infection is high, such as the presence of fever, chills, or changes in vital signs or mental status.

Nonpharmacologic Management

A variety of surgical options to treat Bartholin gland cysts and abscesses have been cited in the literature, ranging from simple incision and drainage techniques (with or without the insertion of a catheter) to fistulization and marsupialization (the most commonly employed surgical techniques),[12] alcohol sclerotherapy, hydrodissection procedures, and the application of silver nitrate or carbon dioxide (CO_2) lasers. Adequate pain control is an important issue for all women who have surgical intervention for Bartholin gland cysts and abscesses.

Incision and drainage is a commonly used management strategy for Bartholin gland cysts and abscesses and was once the mainstay of treatment.[13] Incision and drainage alone is not recommended as recurrence risk is high. A Word catheter is placed through the incision into the gland after I&D is performed. It allows continued drainage and reepithelialization of a tract for future drainage.

Excision of Bartholin Gland. Removal of the entire gland, once a standard procedure, is now recommended only when there is suspicion of malignancy or for recurrent abscess. Current surgical practices emphasize preservation of the gland's function.

Marsupialization and Window Operation. Both these treatments seek to create and to maintain a patent fistula for drainage of the cyst or abscess. The techniques differ significantly only in that the cyst is excised in the marsupialization procedure, whereas a "window" is cut into the cyst or abscess in the window procedure. In both marsupialization and window techniques, pudendal or local anesthesia is used, and the edges of the opened cyst cavity are sutured to the adjacent labial skin to make a permanent opening. The gland remains functional after both procedures, and the size of the fistulas created gradually decreases over time. Recurrence rates for marsupialization are 5% to 15%. Recommended follow-up care after marsupialization is 4 to 6 weeks.

Pharmacologic Management

Antibiotic treatment is reserved for Bartholin gland abscesses with surrounding cellulitis and should not be used as monotherapy. Treatment is generally initiated with broad-spectrum antibiotics since the infection is typically polymicrobial.

Carbon Dioxide Laser Therapy. With the patient under local anesthesia, the CO_2 laser is used first to create a defect from the vulvar skin to the cystic cavity as near as possible to the original duct track and then to vaporize cyst contents. The neostoma that is created permits continued drainage after the procedure without the presence of sutures or mechanical devices such as catheters or drains and allows an epithelium-lined tract to form. Glandular function is maintained, sexual function is not impaired after a 2-week healing period, and the size of the created defect is substantially reduced with complete healing (shrinking from approximately 1.5 to 0.2 cm [⅗ to 2/25 inch]). Healing typically occurs without scarring. A disadvantage of this approach is that the laser equipment is expensive to install and to maintain, but in one study the relapse-free rate exceeded 85%.[14,15]

Silver Nitrate. Insertion of silver nitrate into a scalpel-formed incision is a simple and inexpensive option for treatment; it is as effective as traditional excision techniques and has fewer complications and less scar formation[16] than marsupialization. However, chemical burning of the vulva has been observed. There is evidence to suggest that alcohol sclerotherapy to Bartholin gland cysts or abscesses is as effective as silver nitrate and is associated with fewer complications.[17]

INDICATIONS FOR REFERRAL OR HOSPITALIZATION

Health care providers not comfortable managing Bartholin gland cysts and abscesses are encouraged to refer these patients to experienced surgeons for appropriate therapy. In general, Bartholin gland cysts or abscesses are managed successfully on an outpatient basis, but systemic infection or other complications remain valid indications for hospitalization.

Women who have been treated by surgeons for Bartholin gland cysts or abscesses should have continued follow-up care with their health care providers. Providers can also check for possible sequelae to treatment, including dyspareunia, in the course of routine gynecologic or other primary care provision.

LIFE SPAN CONSIDERATIONS

Bartholin gland cysts and abscesses are most common in women of reproductive age. When adequately treated, women maintain function without reproductive or other sequelae such as dyspareunia.

COMPLICATIONS

Cyst recurrence often follows incision and drainage or aspiration alone,[18] and gland excision may be accompanied by hemorrhage, hematoma formation, trauma to surrounding tissues, rectovaginal fistula,[19] scarring, a long healing process, and subsequent dyspareunia from loss of vaginal lubrication. Toxic shock syndrome, a very rare complication, has been noted in the literature, both before and after corrective surgical procedures. True necrotizing fasciitis[20] has been noted after abscess.

PATIENT AND FAMILY EDUCATION AND HEALTH PROMOTION

Explaining to patients the basic physiology of the Bartholin gland and the pathophysiology involved in cyst or abscess may help demystify the condition and the treatment experience. Women may also benefit from an explanation of what to do and expect after a treatment strategy is used. After CO_2 therapy, for example, patients are instructed to refrain from sexual intercourse for 2 weeks; potential postoperative discomfort is managed with saltwater soaks. Women should be counseled to expect drainage of mucus for 2 or 3 days after certain procedures while the cyst or abscess resolves. Proper hygiene, sitz baths or soaks, and condom use are also helpful in the treatment and prevention of future Bartholin gland cysts and abscesses.

REFERENCES

1. Bouchet, A. (2000). [Gaspard II Bartholin and the vulvovaginal gland]. *Annales de Chirurgie, 125*(5), 483–488.
2. Pundir, J., & Auld, B. J. (2008). A review of the management of diseases of the Bartholin's gland. *Journal of Obstetrics and Gynaecology: The Journal of the Institute of Obstetrics and Gynaecology, 28*(2), 161–165.
3. Kessous, R., Aricha-Tamir, B., Sheizaf, B., Steiner, N., Moran-Gilad, J., & Weintraub, A. Y. (2013). Clinical and microbiological characteristics of Bartholin gland abscesses. *Obstetrics and Gynecology, 122*(4), 794–799.
4. Yuk, J. S., Kim, Y. J., Hur, J. Y., & Shin, J. H. (2013). Incidence of Bartholin duct cysts and abscesses in the Republic of Korea. *International Journal of Gynaecology and Obstetrics, 122*(1), 62–64.
5. Berger, M. B., Betschart, C., Khandwala, N., DeLancey, J. O., & Haefner, H. K. (2012). Incidental Bartholin gland cysts identified on pelvic magnetic resonance imaging. *Obstetrics and Gynecology, 120*(4), 798–802.
6. Patil, S., Sultan, A. H., & Thakar, R. (2007). Bartholin's cysts and abscesses. *Journal of Obstetrics and Gynaecology: The Journal of the Institute of Obstetrics and Gynaecology, 27*(3), 241–245.
7. Thurman, A. R., Satterfield, T. M., & Soper, D. E. (2008). Methicillin-resistant Staphylococcus aureus as a common cause of vulvar abscesses. *Obstetrics and Gynecology, 112*(3), 538–544.
8. Zhan, P., Li, G., Liu, B., & Mao, X. G. (2014). Bartholin gland carcinoma: A case report. *Oncology Letters, 8*(2), 849–851.
9. Kozakiewicz, B., Dmoch-Gajzlerska, E., & Roszkowska-Purska, K. (2014). Carcinomas and sarcomas of Bartholin gland. A report of nine cases and review of the literature. *European Journal of Gynaecological Oncology, 35*(3), 243–249.
10. Mowers, E. L., Shank, J. J., Frisch, N., & Reynolds, R. K. (2014). Myxoid leiomyosarcoma of the Bartholin gland. *Obstetrics and Gynecology, 124*(2 Pt. 2 suppl 1), 433–435.
11. Aydin, Y., Atis, A., & Polat, N. (2011). Bilateral endometrioma of Bartholin glands accompanying ovarian endometrioma. *Journal of Obstetrics and Gynaecology: The Journal of the Institute of Obstetrics and Gynaecology, 31*(2), 187–189.
12. Mayeaux, E. J., & Cooper, D. (2013). Vulvar procedures: Biopsy, Bartholin abscess treatment, and condyloma treatment. *Obstetrics and Gynecology Clinics of North America, 40*(4), 759–772.
13. Kroese, J., van der Velde, M., Morssink, L., Zafarmand, M., Geomini, P., van Kesteron, P., et al. (2016). Word catheter and marsupialization in women with cyst or abscess of the Bartholin gland (WoMan-trial): a randomized clinical trial. [online] www.bjog.org. Retrieved from http://dio:10.111/1471-0528.14281. (Accessed 11 December 2017).
14. Figueiredo, A. C., Duarte, P. E., Gomes, T. P., et al. (2012). Bartholin's gland cysts: Management with carbon-dioxide laser vaporization. *Revista Brasileira de Ginecologia e Obstetrícia: Revista da Federação Brasileira das Sociedades de Ginecologia e Obstetrícia, 34*(12), 550–554.
15. Di Donato, V., Bellati, F., Casorelli, A., et al. (2013). CO_2 laser treatment for Bartholin gland abscess: Ultrasound evaluation of risk recurrence. *Journal of Minimally Invasive Gynecology, 20*(3), 346–352.
16. Ozdegirmenci, O., Kayikcioglu, F., & Haberal, A. (2009). Prospective randomized study of marsupialization versus silver nitrate application in the management of Bartholin gland cysts and abscesses. *Journal of Minimally Invasive Gynecology, 16*(2), 149–152.
17. Kafali, H., Yurtseven, S., & Ozardali, I. (2004). Aspiration and alcohol sclerotherapy: A novel method for management of Bartholin's cyst or abscess. *European Journal of Obstetrics, Gynecology, and Reproductive Biology, 112*(1), 98–101.
18. Wechter, M. E., Wu, J. M., Marzano, D., & Haefner, H. (2009). Management of Bartholin duct cysts and abscesses: A systematic review. *Obstetrical and Gynecological Survey, 64*(6), 395–404.
19. Zoulek, E., Karp, D. R., & Davila, G. W. (2011). Rectovaginal fistula as a complication to a Bartholin gland excision. *Obstetrics and Gynecology, 118*(2 Pt. 2), 489–491.
20. Morris, M. W., Aru, M., Gaugler, A., Morris, R. F., & Vanderlan, W. B. (2014). Necrotizing fasciitis of the perineum associated with a bartholin abscess. *Surgical Infections, 15*(2), 131–133.

CHAPTER 139

BREAST DISORDERS
Elizabeth B. McCabe

Evaluation of breast complaints and screening for breast cancer account for a significant number of primary care visits. The most frequent breast complaints include breast pain, breast masses, and nipple discharge. Most breast masses and other breast complaints are a result of benign conditions, but some breast disease can impart actual risk for the development of breast cancer. For example, recent research suggests that women with atypical hyperplasia may have a cumulative incidence of breast cancer as high as 30% at 25 years of follow-up.[1]

For these reasons, accurate evaluation of all breast complaints and appropriate follow-up are essential. In addition, failure to adequately reassure women about their breast symptoms after a benign diagnosis heightens the need for appropriate support for women with ongoing breast symptoms.[2] Research shows that even after a benign diagnosis, up to one-third of women report that they are either unsure or not reassured about their breast symptoms. A significant percentage of women who undergo evaluation and receive a benign diagnosis for their breast symptoms remain anxious about the possibility of breast cancer or another form of breast disease.

The initial breast evaluation should be comprehensive and include a risk assessment to determine average to high-risk status, history of the present breast concern, workup to date including imaging and pathology reports of recent or past breast biopsies, past relevant medical and surgical history, and family history of both breast and ovarian cancer on both the maternal and paternal sides of the family. Education about breast health tailored to age and risk status, including screening recommendations and follow-up, should be clearly outlined for every patient regardless of the underlying breast condition.

RISK ASSESSMENT
Risk Factors

A thorough history and breast cancer risk assessment should be performed for every woman who sees her health care provider with a breast complaint. The absolute lifetime risk for development of breast cancer is approximately 12%.[3] Determination of level of risk is an important part of the risk assessment process. Several well-established risk factors associated with the development of breast cancer have been thoroughly studied and are defined by four major groups: family history or genetic factors, reproductive or hormonal factors, proliferative benign breast disease, and mammographic density.[4]

Individuals with a single first-degree relative with breast cancer have an estimated twofold risk. Individuals with two first-degree relatives have a threefold risk, and three or more impart a fourfold risk. A first-degree relative younger than 40 years at the time of diagnosis results in a threefold risk compared with a twofold risk for relatives 40 to 50 years old and a 1.5-fold risk for relatives 50 to 65 years old. Risks are also greater if relatives have bilateral breast cancer.[4] Other risks in this category include male breast cancer, ovarian cancer, and Ashkenazi Jewish ancestry.

In terms of reproductive factors, nulliparous women have the same risk as that of women who delivered their first child at the age of 30 years of age or older. Subsequent births and substantial periods of breastfeeding offer some degree of risk protection. Early menarche and late menopause result in increased duration of ovulation with the resultant hormonal effects. Women who are using hormone replacement therapy (HRT) have up to a 5% increased risk per year of use, which returns to baseline levels within a year of stopping hormone use.[4]

Certain types of benign breast disease impart significant risk for development of invasive breast cancer. Women with lobular carcinoma in situ have a 10-fold relative risk, and women with atypical ductal hyperplasia and atypical lobular hyperplasia carry a fourfold to fivefold relative risk. A doubling of risk is seen with proliferative lesions without atypia, such as intraductal papillomas. Nonproliferative lesions, such as fibroadenomas and cysts, do not increase risk.[4]

Mammographic density, estimated by the percentage of the mammogram image that is covered by opaque tissue, has been determined to be the single most important risk factor in the population of women receiving mammograms. Description of density can be found on the final mammogram report and is described as extremely dense, heterogeneously dense, scattered density, or fatty replacement of the breast tissue. Fifty percent to 75% density on a mammogram imparts a twofold to threefold risk. Approximately 14% of the population falls into this category, compared with 5% whose density is greater than 75%. Studies have shown that postmenopausal women with high breast density are at increased risk for developing breast cancer. This risk is further elevated if they are taking combined hormone therapy.[5]

It is also known that other risk factors are largely independent of one another. Efforts are ongoing at looking at all risk factors and using the information to provide individual risk status and prevention strategies.[4]

Risk Assessment Models

There are various breast cancer risk assessment tools available (www.cancer.gov/bcrisktool). Models that are used to determine a woman's risk for the development of breast cancer are the Gail model, the Claus model, the Tyrer-Cuzick Model, the BRCAPRO and the BOADICDA models. The Gail model is based on several risk factors: age, race, age at menarche, number of breast biopsies, number of biopsies with atypical hyperplasia, number of first-degree relatives with breast cancer, and age at first live birth (ww5.komen.org/BreastCancer/GailAssessmentModel.html). A 5-year score of 1.67% or greater is considered high risk. The Gail model was not designed for women younger than 35 years, with a personal history of breast cancer or ductal or lobular carcinoma in situ, or whose history suggests a possible hereditary breast cancer.[6] The Claus model predicts the cumulative probability for development of breast cancer of a woman who has a family history with both first- and second-degree relatives. This model has been most useful in assessing risk in younger women (aged 29 to 35 years) with a family history of breast cancer. There have been more validation studies performed on the Gail model, and this model tends to be more frequently used in the clinical setting.[6] The Tyrer-Cuzick Model is considered to be one of the most consistently accurate tools for predicting breast cancer risk. It determines the risk of developing both invasive and in situ cancer

and the probability of carrying a BRCA mutation. Unlike the Gail model, the Tyrer-Cuzick model incorporates detailed first- and second-degree family history.[7] The BRCAPRO and BOADICEA models are useful for identifying candidates for breast magnetic resonance imaging screening as an adjunct to mammography.

Genetic Testing

Women with a strong family history of breast cancer may be candidates for genetic testing for *BRCA* mutations. The decision to undergo genetic testing raises many psychosocial and ethical issues and should be considered after a discussion with a genetics counselor. Strong consideration to involve family members is recommended. Women who are known *BRCA1* or *BRCA2* mutation carriers have a 40% to 70% lifetime risk for development of breast cancer.[8,9] These women are considered to be at extremely high risk and require education and counseling about screening and risk reduction strategies. Screening recommendations include clinical breast examination every 6 months, annual three-dimensional (3D)/tomosynthesis mammography, and breast magnetic resonance imaging (MRI).

Risk Reduction

The best nonsurgical risk reduction strategy for *BRCA* mutation carriers is adjuvant MRI. It has been shown to be successful in detecting twice as many invasive cancers as mammography, with the majority of cancers being at an early stage at diagnosis.[10] Surgical risk reduction strategies include prophylactic mastectomy and oophorectomy. Women who undergo mastectomy reduce their breast cancer risk by 90%, and premenopausal women who undergo prophylactic oophorectomy decrease their breast cancer risk by 75%.[8] Once a woman has been identified as a mutation carrier, choices for risk reduction are typically made on the basis of age childbearing status and personal preference.

SCREENING RECOMMENDATIONS

There is ongoing debate about the appropriate age at which to initiate screening mammography in the average-risk patient, defined as a woman whose relative risk for developing breast cancer is 1.5-fold or lower and whose 5-year Gail score is below 1.7%.[8] In addition to mammography, clinical breast examination and breast self-examination have historically been recommended as routine screening practices for women.

USPSTF and the American College of Physicians screening mammography recommendations for women aged 40 to 49 continue to be individualized based on the risks and benefits of biennial screening, although the American College of Radiology (ACR), Society of Breast Imaging (SBI), and American College of Obstetricians and Gynecologists (ACOG) recommend annual mammography for women aged 40 to 74.[11] The US Preventive Services Task Force (USPSTF) and the American College of Physicians recommend biennial screening mammography for women 50 to 74 years of age and determined that the evidence to continue screening women after age 75 was inconclusive.[11] For women aged 75 or older, the USPSTF found there was insufficient evidence to recommend for or against breast cancer screening. The ACP recommends that in average-risk women aged 75 years or older or in women with a life expectancy of 10 years or less, breast cancer screening should be discontinued. The American Cancer Society and ACOG continue to recommend annual mammography.[11] Teaching breast self-examination to patients is still not recommended by the USPSTF, although women should be encouraged to discuss breast changes with their primary care provider.[11]

There is strong evidence to suggest that mammography is most useful in women aged 50 to 65 years and that mammography remains the best method for breast cancer screening among average-risk patients.[11,12] Regular breast self-examination is a very individualized decision. For those women who are interested in learning proper techniques for performing self-examination and who are interested in promoting awareness of their breast health, time needs to be allotted for providing this information.

High-risk women are those with a 5-year Gail score higher than 1.7% and whose relative risk is 1.5- to 5-fold. Screening recommendations for this group include annual clinical breast examination and mammography, consideration for chemoprevention, and discontinuation of hormonal therapy if the patient has been receiving it for more than 2 years.

Very-high-risk women include those with a personal history of invasive breast cancer, ductal carcinoma in situ, or lobular carcinoma in situ. This imparts a fourfold to fivefold risk for development of a new primary breast cancer. Other women who fall into this category are those with a prior breast biopsy showing atypical hyperplasia, known *BRCA* mutation carriers, and those with a history of mantle radiation of the chest wall for Hodgkin disease before the age of 30. Screening recommendations for this group include clinical breast examination every 6 months, annual mammography, consideration for chemoprevention, and genetic testing.[8] Screening for this population may begin as early as 25 years of age. 3D/tomosynthesis mammography and adjuvant MRI may be recommended for many of these women.[12]

Digital breast tomosynthesis (3D mammography) has been shown to have fewer false positive findings and call backs and an increase in cancer detection rate. This is particularly advantageous in younger women with dense breast tissue.[13]

In March 2019, the USPSTF drafted a recommendation that "primary care providers screen women who have family members with breast, ovarian, tubal, or peritoneal cancer or have an ethnicity or ancestry associated with BRCA1 or BRCA2 gene mutations with one of several screening tools designed to identify a family history that may be associated with an increased risk for potentially harmful mutations in breast cancer susceptibility genes (BRCA1 or BRCA2). Women with positive screening results should receive genetic counseling and, if indicated after counseling, genetic testing."[14]

Determination of average- or high-risk status for each patient is an integral step in the process of providing individualized care. Both average- and high-risk women require education about the screening tools available and how the use of these tools can be tailored to meet their individualized needs.

BREAST PAIN (MASTALGIA, MASTODYNIA)

 Urgent referral is indicated for a clinically occult mass, abscess, hematoma, seroma, or fat necrosis found on mammogram or ultrasound.

DEFINITION AND EPIDEMIOLOGY

Breast pain, often referred to as mastalgia or mastodynia, is the most common breast problem encountered in primary care and surgical practices.[15] Although increased awareness and overestimation of breast cancer risk may prompt women to be more inclined to seek medical treatment for breast concerns, mastalgia is generally underreported and up to 80% of women experience breast pain at some point in their life.[16,17] Premenstrual, or cyclic, breast pain is the most common type of mastalgia and usually occurs during the late luteal phase of the menstrual cycle, in association with the premenstrual syndrome or independently, and resolves after menses.

Noncyclic mastalgia involves constant or intermittent pain that is unrelated to the menstrual cycle.[16,17] It is less common than cyclic mastalgia and occurs most frequently in women 40 to 50 years old. It accounts for about 31% of women being seen for mastalgia.[16] Noncyclic mastalgia may result from pregnancy, mastitis, thrombophlebitis, macrocysts, benign tumors, fibrocystic breast changes, or cancer; however, these conditions explain only a minority of noncyclic mastalgia cases. Most noncyclic mastalgia occurs for unknown reasons, but it is thought to be related more often to an anatomic cause than to a hormonal one. Noncyclic breast pain usually resolves spontaneously without treatment.[16]

PATHOPHYSIOLOGY

The actual pathophysiologic mechanism of breast pain is not well understood. Cyclic mastalgia occurs during the luteal phase of the menstrual cycle and resolves with the onset of menstruation.[18] This predictable pattern of pain is likely to be hormonally mediated, despite the failure of studies to show any difference in estrogen levels among women with or without pain. It has also been shown that progesterone levels may be lower in these women and that prolactin release may be increased as a response to thyrotropin-releasing hormone.[19]

Essential fatty acids such as dietary gamma-linolenic acid have been suggested as inhibitors of prostaglandins, which possibly cause breast pain. Low plasma levels of these essential fatty acids may result in a hypersensitivity of breast tissue to circulating hormones.[18]

There is little evidence to support a relationship between breast pain and histologic findings consistent with cysts, apocrine metaplasia, and ductal hyperplasia.[19]

CLINICAL PRESENTATION AND PHYSICAL EXAMINATION

Cyclic mastalgia usually starts in the luteal phase of the menstrual cycle, increases in intensity until menses begin, and then dissipates, although pain may be present during the entire cycle with increased intensity premenstrually.[16] Cyclic mastalgia usually begins in the third or fourth decade of life. It is usually bilateral and poorly localized, although it typically involves the upper outer breast area and radiates to the upper arm and axilla. Women will describe the pain as dull, heavy, or aching. Symptoms tend to persist with intermittent relapses, but remission can occur with hormonal events such as pregnancy and menopause. Only 14% of women with cyclic mastalgia experience spontaneous resolution of symptoms, whereas 42% experience resolution at menopause.[16] In contrast, noncyclic mastalgia is often unilateral, localized, and described as a sharp, burning pain. Mastalgia is rarely the sole presenting symptom of breast cancer.[15]

There may be an association between breast pain and anxiety, depression, emotional distress, somatization, and a history of emotional abuse. Women with breast pain may experience greater cyclic fluctuations in anxiety and depression, but it remains unclear whether there is any kind of causal or consequential relationship between breast pain and psychological distress.[16]

A thorough history and breast examination is necessary for every woman who is seen with any breast problem and must be directed at identification and characterization of breast-related symptoms. The health care provider should elicit current symptoms, such as type of pain (cyclic, noncyclic, bilateral, or unilateral), presence or absence of nipple discharge with characteristics of the discharge (color, whether it is spontaneous or nonspontaneous, large or scant volume), presence of a breast mass, change in mass with the menstrual cycle, axillary masses, skin dimpling, ulceration, inflammation, and history of recent breast infections or trauma.

The history should include current medications, including hormone therapy. Prior history of any breast surgery for both cancerous and noncancerous reasons including cosmetic procedures should be obtained. In addition, age at menarche and menopause, pregnancy and lactation history, and relevant past medical and surgical history should be included. Breast cancer screening history should include the date and results of the last clinical breast examination and breast imaging. Family history of breast and ovarian cancer on both maternal and paternal sides should be obtained.

The breast examination must be methodical, and the breasts should be inspected for differences in size, skin changes, retraction or dimpling of the skin or nipple, prominent venous patterns, lesions, and signs of inflammation. The axillary, supraclavicular, and infraclavicular areas should be palpated with the woman in the sitting position. Inspection of the breasts should be performed with the woman both sitting and supine, with her hands behind her head or raised over her head. The examiner should use the flat surface of the fingertips to palpate all of the breast tissue against the chest wall. In women with a history of nipple discharge, the nipple-areola complex is compressed very gently in all directions. If this technique does not elicit discharge, firm equal pressure should be applied from the periphery toward the nipple. To distinguish discharge from multiple or single ducts, pressure must be distributed evenly over all of the ductal structures. Benign or physiologic nipple discharge is typically creamy, gray, or green. Watery, serous, or bloody fluid is considered abnormal.

Breast masses palpated on physical examination may be moveable or fixed and are typically discrete. Description of the size and location of the mass is important before obtaining any radiographic studies.

On examination of the patient with a complaint of breast pain, it is important to note if the pain is focal, regional, or diffuse. Some breast pain actually originates from the chest wall and can manifest as point tenderness.

Skin changes that may signify cancer include erythema, edema, retraction, dimpling, peau d'orange, and nipple excoriation or crustiness.

DIAGNOSTICS
Essential Diagnostics

Noncyclic breast pain is initially investigated with bilateral mammography in postmenopausal women, although the likelihood of an abnormal finding is low. A focused ultrasound examination is often performed to evaluate persistent, focal mastalgia in young women and in addition to mammography in older women.[16] Mammography is not indicated in young women with cyclic breast pain in the absence of focal pain, suspicious findings, or risk factors. However, mammography should be considered in women 30 to 35 years or older who have a family history of breast cancer or other risk factors for breast cancer.[16] Chest X-ray to rule out fractures should be considered if there is a history of breast or chest wall trauma or focal pain adjacent to the breast on the chest wall.

Additional Diagnostics

Laboratory studies are not useful in general, but a pregnancy test should be done for a woman of reproductive age if the history or physical examination findings suggest that pregnancy is possible. Other hormone levels, such as estrogen, progesterone, and prolactin, are usually within normal limits in women with breast pain and therefore are not indicated as part of the workup.[16]

INITIAL DIAGNOSTICS

Breast Pain (Mastalgia, Mastodynia)

IMAGING
- Mammography: to look for masses, asymmetry, architectural distortion, calcifications
- Ultrasound: to look for masses (solid or fluid filled) and skin thickening
- Chest x-ray: to look for rib fractures
- Use of directed US in conjunction with mammography for the evaluation of focal breast pain in women with nondense breasts may be of limited utility and contribute to unnecessary intervention because of incidental findings.[17]

DIFFERENTIAL DIAGNOSIS

The differential diagnosis of breast pain includes a normal physiologic event, chest wall or nonbreast pain, recent or past trauma with or without hematoma or fat necrosis, microcysts or macrocysts, infection, and malignant or benign tumor.

Chest wall or nonbreast pain accounts for about 7% of women seen with complaints of mastalgia. Pain that is limited to a particular area and characterized by a burning or knife-like sensation may be chest wall pain. There are several distinct types of chest wall pain, including localized or diffuse pain, radicular pain from cervical arthritis or slipping and cracking ribs, and pain from Tietze syndrome (also known as costochondritis).[16] The pain can be reproduced with pressure over the costal cartilage rather than in the more generalized pattern of mastalgia. Movement may also precipitate chest wall pain, and there is no relationship to the menstrual cycle. Chest wall syndromes can occur even in the absence of a clear precipitating event, which sometimes heightens the woman's concern that the pain has a suspicious or malignant cause.[16]

INTERPROFESSIONAL COLLABORATIVE MANAGEMENT

Nonpharmacologic Management

After a thorough history, evaluation, and risk assessment, reassurance is all that is needed for 85% of women with cyclic mastalgia. For the 15% of the women not helped with reassurance alone, use of a pain chart for at least two cycles may elucidate any patterns of mastalgia. Patients can also be reassured that breast pain has a high spontaneous remission rate (60% to 80%).[4] Providing optimal breast support is helpful. Management of cyclic mastalgia should also include reevaluation of the breast pain at a different time during the menstrual cycle, preferably soon after the menses.

A firm, supportive brassiere, low-fat diet and reduced caffeine intake may be helpful in reducing breast discomfort.

Pharmacologic Management

There is consensus that topical nonsteroidal antiinflammatory drugs (NSAIDs) may reduce breast pain and the potential benefits are thought to outweigh the risk of adverse side effects. There is insufficient evidence to evaluate the effectiveness of oral NSAIDsDanazol, tamoxifen, and gonadorelin analogues (goserelin) may reduce breast pain, but all can cause adverse effects. These agents should generally be prescribed in consultation with a specialist.[20]

Oral contraceptives may be discontinued or changed to an alternative agent with a lower estrogen and higher progesterone content.

It may be difficult to quantify breast pain because it is often variable. However, assessment of pain with a pain-rating instrument or scale can be particularly useful in evaluating cyclic breast pain and response to treatment.

INDICATIONS FOR REFERRAL OR HOSPITALIZATION

Mastalgia is infrequently associated with breast cancer. Despite this fact, any persistence in a patient's symptoms should prompt further evaluation. Failure to treat or a delay in diagnosis of an underlying problem may affect a woman's quality of life or long-term outcome.

Treatment of cyclic mastalgia with antigonadotropic agents should be managed by or in consultation with a specialist because of the severity of the side effect profile and the teratogenicity of this class of drugs.

Women with mastalgia, without evidence of disease on physical examination and imaging, whose pain is refractory to basic interventions may be considered candidates for a chronic pain referral. If the pain is severe enough and interferes with a woman's quality of life, a general surgery referral can be considered to discuss mastectomy. The benefit of this extreme intervention is not well proven.

PATIENT AND FAMILY EDUCATION AND HEALTH PROMOTION

Many women are initially seen with mild forms of mastalgia, fearful that they have cancer. Women who experience breast pain should receive a thorough clinical breast examination and reassurance that pain is an uncommon presenting symptom of breast cancer.

For most patients, a thorough evaluation without clinical or radiographic findings should provide sufficient reassurance in addition to knowing that the pain they are experiencing is typically self-limited and improves over time. A follow-up breast examination on an interval basis may be offered.

MASTITIS

 Failure to respond to appropriate antibiotic therapy is a concerning sign of a clinically occult breast abscess or a malignancy and necessitates a prompt referral.

DEFINITION AND EPIDEMIOLOGY

Mastitis refers to inflammation of the breast tissue. It can occur in both men and women. The frequency of mastitis increases with lactation, but it can occur in the nonlactating or pregnant patient. Approximately one-third of women who breastfeed develop mastitis. *Staphylococcus aureus* is the most common organism. *Haemophilus parainfluenzae, Streptococcus,* and *Escherichia coli* can be seen as well but are less common.[21] Streptococcus lactarius should be considered as a cause of lactational mastitis.[22]

Any clinical presentation of mastitis should be promptly treated. If resolution of symptoms does not occur after the initial treatment, inflammatory breast cancer should be considered, and a referral should be made for biopsy. Inflammatory breast cancer represents 1% to 3% of all breast cancer diagnoses in the United States. Almost 50% of women with inflammatory breast cancer have metastatic disease at the time of diagnosis.[23]

PATHOPHYSIOLOGY

In lactational mastitis, organisms enter the ductal system from the infant's mouth through the nipple. Infection frequently occurs in a segment of the breast where milk drainage is poor. Breast milk provides a good culture medium for these microorganisms.

Because of the increase in incidence of methicillin-resistant *S. aureus* (MRSA) soft tissue infections seen in the United States, providers who treat women with mastitis should consider MRSA as a causative organism if traditional treatment fails. MRSA mastitis in the postpartum period is more likely to result in a breast abscess.[21]

Nonpuerperal mastitis can manifest as periductal mastitis with or without periareolar abscess or whole-breast cellulitis. Periductal mastitis occurs secondary to blockage of the milk ducts by breast secretions and cellular debris.[23]

CLINICAL PRESENTATION AND PHYSICAL EXAMINATION

Puerperal mastitis is typically unilateral and may occur any time during lactation. Women with puerperal mastitis often are seen with breast engorgement and tenderness, fever, chills, anorexia, headache, and malaise. Erythema is usually confined to the area of a single breast lobule. A discrete mass is suggestive of abscess formation. The axillary lymph nodes may be tender and enlarged. Nonpuerperal mastitis is often seen in women who are immunocompromised (e.g., women with diabetes or who have undergone radiation treatment) and those with autoimmune disorders. Nonpuerperal mastitis may also be accompanied by nipple discharge. Periductal mastitis manifests with periareolar inflammation with or without an erythematous subareolar mass.[23] Mastitis is typically associated with pain, malaise, fever, and leukocytosis.

Persistent erythema involving the entire breast, accompanied by increased breast firmness and size, with or without pain, is suggestive of inflammatory breast carcinoma and necessitates immediate referral.[23]

Inflammatory breast cancer is a clinical diagnosis characterized by breast edema (peau d'orange) and erythema, with or without a palpable mass. Biopsy confirms the presence of invasive cancer.[24]

DIAGNOSTICS
Essential Diagnostics

3D/tomosynthesis mammography, if it is tolerated, should be considered when a breast infection does not respond to appropriate antibiotic therapy within 3 to 7 days. Mammography may detect a mass that may or may not be clinically evident. Findings on mammography such as architectural distortion of the tissues, asymmetry, calcifications, or subtle skin thickening are typically clinically occult. A focused ultrasound examination is indicated in any patient with symptoms of mastitis with a mass or an area of focal fullness or fluctuance. Ultrasonography may detect abscess, fluid collection, or mass. Mammography is not indicated in pregnant or lactating women with an initial presentation of mastitis.

Additional Diagnosis

Diagnosis of inflammatory breast cancer should be considered in patients who do not respond to antibiotic therapy. The diagnosis cannot be made with radiographic examination alone; pathologic examination is required for confirmation. A skin biopsy reveals dermal lymphatics congested with cancer cells, and the core biopsy of breast tissue reveals invasive breast cancer.

DIFFERENTIAL DIAGNOSIS

In lactating women, the differential diagnosis for mastitis includes breast engorgement, which is usually bilateral. Other differential diagnoses include duct ectasia, peri ductal mastitis, breast abscess, and granulomatous mastitis

In nonlactating women, inflammatory breast cancer can mimic acute mastitis or cellulitis. Failure to respond to appropriate antibiotic therapy is a concerning sign of a malignant neoplasm.

INTERPROFESSIONAL COLLABORATIVE MANAGEMENT
Nonpharmacologic Management

Methods to facilitate removal of milk from the breast include breastfeeding followed by pumping and the use of warm compresses, good support, massage of the painful areas while nursing, and analgesics.[21]

Pharmacologic Management

Most skin and soft tissue infections are due to *S. aureus* or streptococcus infections. Data suggests that approximately 68% of all nonurine isolates have been reported to be methicillin-sensitive *S. aureus* (MSSA). Treatment with a first-generation cephalosporin such as cefazolin or cephalexin is recommended. If abscess is suspected or confirmed, the preferred treatment is Bactrim (trimethoprim-sulfamethoxazole) or doxycycline after the abscess is incised and drained.[25]

Clindamycin is recommended for penicillin-sensitive patients. MRSA should be considered when women do not respond to traditional therapy. Obtaining a culture of the abscess fluid if it is present, breast milk, or nipple discharge is recommended, to confirm the diagnosis. MRSA infections may respond to treatment with oral clindamycin, trimethoprim-sulfamethoxazole, linezolid, or intravenous administration of vancomycin.[21]

Continuation of breastfeeding during treatment is encouraged, provided the infant is healthy and full term.[21] If an abscess is present, incision and drainage of the infected fluid is required. In both puerperal and nonpuerperal mastitis, acetaminophen or NSAIDs and moist heat may be beneficial.

Complications

Concerns for an underlying abscess may be present in any patient with mastitis who does not respond to a standard course of antibiotics. A focused ultrasound examination should be performed to further evaluate any area of the breast that has a mass or an area of focal prominence.

Indications for Referral

Any patient with an abscess or suspected abscess requires a referral to a surgeon or to interventional radiology once an abscess is confirmed. Surgical or radiologic intervention for drainage is indicated when a fluctuant mass, suggestive of an underlying abscess, accompanies mastitis. Intravenous antibiotics may be required to treat acute mastitis unresponsive to oral agents. Surgical referral is also indicated when inflammatory breast cancer is suspected. The diagnosis is confirmed after a skin biopsy and core needle biopsy of the concerning breast tissue is performed and shows malignancy.

PATIENT AND FAMILY EDUCATION AND HEALTH PROMOTION

Lactating women should also be reassured that mastitis is a common complication of lactation, the nutrition of the breast milk is unaffected by the infection, and a history of mastitis is not associated with an increased risk of breast cancer.

Nonpuerperal mastitis typically resolves after a course of antibiotics. Women should be instructed to monitor their breast examination after resolution of their symptoms.

In the absence of clinical concerns, the timing of the next screening mammogram should be no earlier than 3 months from the resolution of symptoms.

NIPPLE DISCHARGE AND GALACTORRHEA

 Rule out a pituitary adenoma when evaluating a patient with suspected galactorrhea. Referral to endocrinology is reasonable if suspicion remains high in the absence of an adenoma on MRI.

DEFINITION AND EPIDEMIOLOGY

Nipple discharge is commonly seen in approximately 20% to 25% of women with breast complaints.[19] It is classified as physiologic, pathologic, or galactorrhea. Nipple discharge causes significant anxiety and fear that there may be an underlying malignant neoplasm.[18]

Physiologic nipple discharge is common in premenopausal and pregnant women. It is typically bilateral and may be spontaneous or nonspontaneous. Pathologic nipple discharge is often spontaneous, bloody, serous, and involving one duct. Galactorrhea or milky discharge is associated with pituitary adenomas or hypothyroidism.[26]

PATHOPHYSIOLOGY

Most nipple discharge is physiologic in nature and is not symptomatic of any pathologic condition. It is seen in nonlactating and lactating breasts. Hormonal influences from estrogen, progesterone, and prolactin, as well as the presence of growth hormones, insulin, and adrenal hormones, may stimulate nipple discharge. When the physiologic fluid is secreted through the nipple, it is generally bilateral, arising from multiple ducts, and not spontaneous.

The most common cause of pathologic nipple discharge is intraductal papilloma, followed by duct ectasia. The presence of an associated palpable mass increases the likelihood of cancer.[14] The most common cause of bloody nipple discharge is intraductal papilloma. Approximately one-third of bloody or serous discharges are the result of a malignant neoplasm.[26]

Galactorrhea may be caused by hypothyroidism, hyperprolactinemia, and medications. Brain MRI is indicated when elevated prolactin levels are seen, to rule out prolactin-secreting pituitary tumors.[19]

CLINICAL PRESENTATION AND PHYSICAL EXAMINATION

The primary goal in evaluating nipple discharge is to determine whether it is physiologic, pathologic, or galactorrhea. Physiologic nipple discharge is characterized by discharge only with compression and by multiple duct involvement. These discharges are often bilateral, and the fluid may be clear, gray, yellow, white, or dark green.[14] Although it is not common, lactational secretions may persist for years after weaning if the breasts continue to be manually stimulated.

Nipple discharge requires further investigation if it is spontaneous, bloody, watery, large volume, or associated with a mass. Pathologic discharge is usually unilateral and involves a single duct.

Galactorrhea manifests as bilateral milky discharge and is seen with endocrine disorders such as hypothyroidism and hyperprolactinemia. Clinical signs and symptoms indicative of these complaints include lethargy, cold intolerance, constipation, dry skin, headache, amenorrhea, and defects in peripheral vision.[19]

The physical examination requires a thorough breast examination as previously described to assess for an underlying breast mass and should include gentle compression of the nipple-areola complex between the thumb and index finger. Milking of the ducts with equal pressure from various directions is required to determine the origin of the discharge from either a single duct or multiple ducts.

In the presence of galactorrhea, funduscopic examination to exclude papilledema as well as evaluation of visual acuity, visual fields by confrontation, and extraocular movements is indicated to detect a bitemporal field defect and asymmetry of field loss, which are common in parapituitary lesions. Neurologic and thyroid examinations should also be performed.

A complete medication and past medical history, including endocrine and reproductive histories, should be obtained at the time of the evaluation.

DIAGNOSTICS
Essential Diagnostics

Nipple discharge that is serous or watery should be tested for occult blood. Cytologic studies are not recommended because the absence of malignant cells does not exclude malignant disease or distinguish intraductal from invasive cancer.

Diagnostic mammography should be performed to assess for any nonpalpable masses or calcifications.[19] A focused periareolar ultrasound examination may be performed in an attempt to identify any intraductal masses or ductal abnormalities such as duct ectasia.

Pregnancy should be excluded by obtaining a human chorionic gonadotropin level in all premenopausal women experiencing amenorrhea and galactorrhea. The serum prolactin level is the single most important determination that can establish a lesion of pituitary or central nervous system (CNS) origin.

The serum prolactin level may be normal or only slightly elevated when galactorrhea is drug related. Thyroid profiles should also be obtained because primary hypothyroidism can cause elevation of serum prolactin level and galactorrhea.

Additional Diagnostics

MRI of the brain is indicated for the patient with symptoms suggestive of an intracranial mass, galactorrhea with amenorrhea, or elevated prolactin level.[19]

DIFFERENTIAL DIAGNOSIS

Duct ectasia, nonpuerperal mastitis, intraductal papilloma, and breast cancer must be considered in the presence of a nonmilky nipple discharge.

The differential diagnosis of galactorrhea includes pituitary adenomas, neurologic disorders, hypothyroidism, numerous medications, breast stimulation, chest wall irritation, and physiologic causes.

INTERPROFESSIONAL COLLABORATIVE MANAGEMENT
Pharmacologic Management

Treatment of the underlying infection, as previously described, is required if nipple discharge is related to acute mastitis. When a chemical origin for galactorrhea is suspected, discontinuation or substitution with a comparable pharmacologic agent may be attempted when possible. Restoration to the euthyroid state is indicated if hypothyroidism is present. Minimum intervention is required for galactorrhea of idiopathic, drug-related, or physiologic origin.

INDICATIONS FOR REFERRAL AND HOSPITALIZATION

Nipple discharge associated with mammary duct ectasia is not related to neoplasms. Treatment is not necessary unless there is associated periductal mastitis. With recurrent infections, surgical referral to a breast surgeon is indicated to discuss surgical excision of the involved ducts.

Spontaneous bloody or large-volume watery discharge with or without a palpable mass can be caused by intraductal papillomas. Surgical referral is recommended to determine the need for duct excision and to rule out malignant disease.

Nipple discharge that is spontaneous, unilateral, bloody, serous, or watery and arising from a single duct may be pathologic in nature and requires further investigation with a mammogram and ultrasound examination. If imaging is normal, a referral to a breast surgeon is indicated.[27]

Controversy exists about the frequency of follow-up care for pituitary microadenomas. Repeated MRI examinations are often recommended until the growth of the lesion is established, and these should be performed in conjunction with the consulting specialist. A useful resource is the American College of Radiology Appropriateness Criteria, which are evidence-based guidelines for specific clinical conditions that are reviewed annually and provide imaging and treatment procedures for specific clinical scenarios.[28]

PATIENT AND FAMILY EDUCATION AND HEALTH PROMOTION

Patients should be reassured that most causes of breast discharge are nonmalignant. In the presence of a normal prolactin level and menses, women with galactorrhea should be informed of its normal physiologic association with nipple and breast stimulation. Patients with pituitary adenoma should be reassured of the generally favorable response to treatment. Accurate and clear information, support, and close follow-up will help minimize the anxiety that many women with nipple discharge have.

PAGET DISEASE OF THE NIPPLE

 Dermatology and/or surgical referral required for biopsy of any persistent abnormality of the nipple areolar complex to rule out malignancy.

Paget disease of the nipple is a superficial manifestation of an underlying breast carcinoma, most often of ductal origin. Paget disease is believed to represent 1% to 3% of all breast cancers. It is rare in men but is associated with a poorer prognosis.[29]

PATHOPHYSIOLOGY

Controversy exists about the origin of the malignant cells seen in Paget disease. They may represent malignant breast ductal epithelial cells, which then migrate into the epidermis of the nipple.[29]

CLINICAL PRESENTATION AND PHYSICAL EXAMINATION

Paget disease manifests clinically as a unilateral, well-demarcated, erythematous, scaly plaque first appearing on the nipple and subsequently spreading to the areola. The surrounding skin is usually spared. Serous or sanguineous discharge, pain, crusting, pruritus, burning, epithelial thickening, erythema, ulceration, nipple retraction, and underlying breast mass (in up to 60% of patients) may be seen. A small vesicular lesion on the nipple, persistent soreness, pain, or pruritus of the nipple-areola complex in the absence of other clinical symptoms should be evaluated thoroughly because these may be early manifestations of Paget disease.[29]

A thorough breast examination as described previously must be conducted. Paget disease may manifest as scaling of the nipple, but it may also be accompanied by erythematous and excoriated, retracted nipples. The erosion of the areolar tissue may produce copious clear or viscous yellow exudate.

Eczema	Paget Disease of the Nipple
Usually bilateral	Unilateral
Intermittent history with rapid progression	Continuous history with slow progression
Moist initially	Moist or dry
Indistinct border	Irregular but distinct border
Areola involved, nipple may be spared	Nipple always involved and disappears in advanced cases
Itching common	Itching common

TABLE 139.1   Eczema Versus Paget Disease of the Nipple

As the disease steadily progresses, the excoriated surface of the nipple may result in a bloody discharge and associated adenopathy. There may or may not be an associated periareolar mass.

DIAGNOSTICS
Essential Diagnostics

If Paget disease is suspected, punch biopsy of the nipple may be performed as an office procedure, or the patient may be referred to a dermatologist or a general surgeon. As with all breast abnormalities, mammography is indicated but should not delay referral to a specialist.

DIFFERENTIAL DIAGNOSIS

For patients with lesions involving the nipple, Paget disease should be suspected until proven otherwise. This is true even for a lesion that has healed spontaneously, because patients have been identified with healed nipple lesions that were subsequently diagnosed as Paget disease. Paget disease is most commonly misdiagnosed as eczema (Table 139.1). Eczema involving the nipple (versus the areola) is rare and, when present, is usually bilateral. The differential diagnosis of Paget disease includes psoriasis, contact dermatitis, tinea, basal cell carcinoma, Bowen disease, and benign intraductal papilloma of the nipple. Direct spread of invasive carcinoma from the underlying breast may be considered after Paget disease has been excluded.[29]

INTERPROFESSIONAL COLLABORATIVE MANAGEMENT

Paget disease is treated with mastectomy or breast conservation surgery, which may be followed with radiation treatments.[29]

Indication for Referral

Because histologic diagnosis of Paget disease is required, surgical referral for skin biopsy or excisional biopsy of the underlying mass is indicated. Biopsy-proven Paget disease should be viewed as an invasive breast cancer, and the patient must be referred to a surgical oncologist for management.[29]

PATIENT AND FAMILY EDUCATION AND HEALTH PROMOTION

Patients undergoing evaluation for Paget disease require the same accurate information, support, and well-coordinated care that all patients anticipating a possible diagnosis of cancer are provided.

BREAST MASSES

 Surgical referral required for any clinically evident breast mass with normal breast imaging.

DEFINITION AND EPIDEMIOLOGY

Currently, one in eight women will develop breast cancer in her lifetime.[3] Up to 85% of women with newly diagnosed breast cancer do not have a family history of breast cancer.[26]

Most breast cancers are diagnosed after a biopsy of a mammographic abnormality has been performed.[30] Ninety percent of breast masses are caused by benign lesions such as cysts, fibroadenomas, and fibrocystic changes.[17] Breast masses are different entities in women who are younger than 30 years, 31 to 50 years of age, or older than 50 years. Nine of 10 new masses in premenopausal women are benign.[17]

The breast undergoes substantial morphologic changes between early adolescence and menopause, ranging from a predominance of ducts, lobules, and interlobular stroma to fibrous change and cyst formation, formerly referred to as fibrocystic disease of the breast. The term *fibrocystic changes* is now preferred because 50% to 60% of women without breast disease may have fibrocystic changes, such as breasts with nondiscrete nodules, which impart no increased risk of breast cancer and are distinguished from those that confer a small increase in relative risk.[17]

Simple cysts are the most common type of discrete mass and are characterized as a distinct entity consisting of a palpable, fluid-filled sac within the breast tissue. Although cysts may be found in younger women, they are most commonly found in women aged 35 to 50 years. Cysts are rare in postmenopausal women not receiving HRT and should be viewed as breast cancer until proven otherwise. Fibroadenomas are the most common benign solid lesion of the female breast. Characteristically, fibroadenomas are painless, well-circumscribed, freely movable masses with a rounded, lobulated, or discoid configuration. They usually have a rubbery feeling but may appear hard, especially if calcified. Fibroadenomas occur most often in women in their 20s and 30s but may occur any time after puberty and even during menopause. They are hormonally responsive and may increase in size toward the end of the menstrual cycle.

Benign phyllodes tumors are solid tumors of the breast that can manifest as a rapidly enlarging breast mass.

Focal areas of firm tissue in the breast when biopsied are often described as stromal fibrosis and represent a benign finding.

Common malignant tumors of the breast may manifest as a breast mass; these include invasive ductal carcinoma and invasive lobular carcinoma. Malignant phyllodes tumors are less often seen but often manifest as a breast mass.

Ductal carcinoma in situ may manifest as a breast mass but is frequently diagnosed due to a mammographic abnormality such as calcifications.

PATHOPHYSIOLOGY

Breast development begins at puberty under the influence of increased levels of estradiol and progesterone. These influences promote the growth of ductal structures and glandular or lobular units. During the luteal phase of the menstrual cycle, there is an increase in the rate of cell proliferation.[17]

Fibroadenomas are thought to develop in the lobules and stroma as a result of hormonal stimulation. This occurs more frequently between adolescence and the mid-20s. Women in their 30s and 40s develop adenosis or enhancement of the lobular tissue with hypertrophy, resulting in palpable fullness of the breast tissue. By their 40s and toward menopause, more patients may develop hypertrophy of the stroma.

The incidence of cysts increases with late menopause, use of HRT, and low body fat. Evidence suggests that the incidence of benign breast lesions increases in response to hormonal events. Many investigators believe that breast lesions progress in a linear fashion from usual ductal hyperplasia to atypical ductal hyperplasia to ductal carcinoma in situ and then to invasive cancer.[17]

CLINICAL PRESENTATION AND PHYSICAL EXAMINATION

Discrete masses can be solitary lesions or multiple lesions, unilateral or bilateral. Cysts, fibroadenomas, hematomas, and breast cancer can manifest as a discrete palpable mass. Cysts are fluid-filled lesions that may or may not be associated with pain. Symptomatic cysts occur in conjunction with the menstrual cycle.[26] Oil cysts may form as a result of fat necrosis associated with breast trauma.

Fibroadenomas are seen more often in adolescents and young women. They vary in size and are bilateral in approximately 10% of patients.[26] During pregnancy, fibroadenomas may enlarge. Clinically, they are discrete with well-circumscribed smooth borders. They may feel rubbery or firm and may be tender. Giant or juvenile fibroadenomas may enlarge quickly.[31]

Phyllodes tumors can be seen in young adults but more frequently occur in women in their 40s. On pathologic examination, they are benign or malignant. Clinically, they can be well circumscribed and can become very large in a short time.[31]

A palpable mass in the face of recent breast injury is often a hematoma. A mass that develops months after a traumatic injury may be caused by fat necrosis. These masses may be tender.[31]

The clinical presentation of breast cancer may include a firm, discrete mass or an area of diffuse firmness of the breast tissue, with or without skin thickening.

Physical examination should be performed as previously described. Key historical features in the evaluation of a breast lump are the length of time the mass has been present, pain, associated skin changes, presence of axillary, supra or infraclavicular adenopathy, change in size or texture over time, relationship to menstrual cycle, and nipple discharge.

The clinical breast examination of a woman with a complaint of a discrete breast mass should assess the mass, including the location, consistency or texture, mobility, size, and shape and the presence or absence of palpable lymph nodes. Nipple discharge should also be assessed if it is reported. The presence or absence of a corresponding finding in the contralateral breast should be included.

DIAGNOSTICS
Essential Diagnostics

Clinical breast examination is a method of detection, not an independent diagnostic test. Diagnostic mammography and ultrasonography are usually the initial tests for a palpable mass in women older than 25 years. Ultrasonography alone is typically done in average-risk women younger than 25 years. Use of mammography in younger women is individualized on the basis of risk status, clinical presentation, and findings on ultrasound examination. Negative imaging should not deter follow-up evaluation because 15% to 18% of mammograms appear negative in the presence of a palpable cancer.

Additional Diagnostics

Decision to perform biopsy is based on the outcome of the radiographic findings and the level of clinical suspicion. A discrete mass with normal imaging always requires surgical referral for consideration of biopsy.

DIFFERENTIAL DIAGNOSIS

The differential diagnosis of a dominant breast mass includes breast cancer, macrocyst (clinically evident cyst), fibroadenoma, and phyllodes tumors (malignant or benign). In addition, prominent areas of fibrocystic change, fibrosis or fat necrosis as a result of surgical or extraneous trauma, and a galactocele (a milk cyst in a lactating woman) may be seen as a breast mass.[15]

INTERPROFESSIONAL COLLABORATIVE MANAGEMENT

The treatment of a patient with a breast mass is governed by the patient's age, clinical history, and clinical findings. The incidence of malignant palpable masses increases after the age of 40 years. Any discrete mass requires thorough evaluation to include imaging, aspiration, or biopsy.[19]

If a cyst is detected, aspiration can be performed for both diagnosis and relief of pain. Cysts require cytologic analysis of aspirate fluid and surgical biopsy only if the aspirated fluid is bloody or if the palpable abnormality does not resolve completely after the aspiration of fluid. This approach has been supported by large studies of benign-appearing cyst fluid aspirates.[15] No cancers were ultimately identified in 6782 aspirates of low-probability samples. It is recommended that patients with a solitary breast cyst be reexamined 4 to 6 weeks after cyst aspiration to determine whether the cyst has recurred.[15]

Noncystic masses in premenopausal women that are different from the surrounding breast tissue require tissue sampling by core, needle, or excisional biopsy. Observation for one or two menstrual cycles is appropriate only for vague asymmetry or nodularity when it is unclear that a dominant breast mass is present.[15]

Any discrete, solid mass requires a tissue diagnosis to rule out malignant change.[19] Solid masses with ultrasound features consistent with a fibroadenoma can be followed clinically with serial ultrasound examinations. Core biopsy to confirm the diagnosis can be performed if there is any doubt about the ultrasound or clinical finding. Surgical excision is recommended if the mass enlarges or if the patient requests surgical removal.[19]

LIFE SPAN CONSIDERATIONS

Approximately 90% of women have some degree of fibrocystic breast changes. Hormonal status and menopause status are associated with these changes, which at times may manifest as a breast mass. Awareness of breast changes with a willingness to seek evaluation for any new finding is always recommended.

INDICATIONS FOR REFERRAL OR HOSPITALIZATION

A palpable solid mass in all women, regardless of age, necessitates both consultation with a radiologist and a breast specialist and referral for surgical evaluation. Women should be referred for mammography or ultrasound examination and a clinical breast examination. Even when fibrocystic changes are suspected, surgical evaluation of a persistent, palpable dominant mass or lump is required. Tissue diagnosis will provide a definitive diagnosis and determine the presence of high-risk lesions.

PATIENT AND FAMILY EDUCATION AND HEALTH PROMOTION

Most women are worried about developing breast cancer. Women need reassurance about the benign nature of breast lesions that wax and wane with hormonal variation as well as the rationale behind conservative versus surgical management. Education must also focus on the need for prudent breast evaluation of all breast symptoms and lesions regardless of the improbability of malignant disease. Screening recommendations should be tailored based on whether the patient is at average or high risk.

GYNECOMASTIA

 Further evaluation and/or mammography required for any palpable breast mass or concern for serious disease processes, such as endocrine disorders, other malignant neoplasms, or liver disease.

DEFINITION AND EPIDEMIOLOGY

Gynecomastia is a benign enlargement of the male breast. Unlike pseudogynecomastia or lipomastia, which refers to an excess of adipose tissue of the breast, gynecomastia is the result of proliferation of the ductular elements.[32] Gynecomastia is common in infancy, puberty, and in middle-aged-to-older men, with prevalence rates of 60%-90%, 50%-60%, and 70%, respectively.[33] Palpable breast tissue is appreciated on physical examination in 30% to 65% of men, and 50% to 70% of boys experience breast enlargement during puberty.[32] Physiologic pubertal gynecomastia typically lasts for approximately 6 months before regressing.

PATHOPHYSIOLOGY

Gynecomastia is caused by the effects of an imbalance between free estrogen and free androgens. During puberty, production of estrogen by the testes and the peripheral tissues exceeds production of testosterone, resulting in breast enlargement. As men age, the testes may secrete too little testosterone. Numerous pathways that produce androgens and estrogen can be altered. Gynecomastia is the result of an enhanced estrogen effect or a diminished androgen effect on breast tissue.[33]

Exposure to many medications and recreational drugs may cause gynecomastia. The mechanism of action for this is not well understood.[32] Gynecomastia is also associated with disease processes including Klinefelter syndrome, adrenal and testicular tumors, thyrotoxicosis, some forms of liver disease, large cell carcinoma of the lung, and some gastric and renal cell cancers.

CLINICAL PRESENTATION AND PHYSICAL EXAMINATION

Gynecomastia is often an incidental finding on physical examination. Men are often asymptomatic and can describe stable enlargement of their breast tissue. A family history to determine the presence of breast or ovarian cancer, male breast cancer, and *BRCA* mutation carriers is essential. A detailed history and review of systems should include onset and duration of symptoms, presence of pain, underlying systemic illness, medications, exposures to environmental estrogens, and recent weight gain or loss.[32]

A thorough physical examination is required to distinguish among a benign finding, a breast cancer, and a finding indicative of a serious endocrine or systemic disease.[32] The clinical findings may present unilaterally or bilaterally or as asymmetry.

The axilla should be evaluated for adenopathy. Both breasts are examined by comparing subareolar tissue with the adjacent subcutaneous fat. Tissue in gynecomastia can be soft, elastic, or firm but is not typically hard. A unilateral hard or asymmetric mass that is fixed to the skin is worrisome for a malignant neoplasm. Skin dimpling or nipple retraction may be seen with breast cancer.

In addition to a breast examination, a testicular and general physical examination should be considered to evaluate for systemic illness.

DIAGNOSTICS
Essential Diagnostics

In men with clinical findings consistent with gynecomastia, no routine imaging is recommended. If an indeterminate breast mass is identified, the initial recommended imaging study is ultrasound in men younger than age 25, and mammography or digital breast tomosynthesis in men age 25 and older. If physical examination is suspicious for a male breast cancer, mammography or digital breast tomosynthesis is recommended irrespective of patient age.[34]

Additional Diagnostics

For long-standing asymptomatic gynecomastia, laboratory tests may not be necessary. A decrease in morning testosterone and luteinizing levels reflects hypogonadism, often seen with advancing age.

Suspicion of systemic illness as a causative factor should be worked up appropriately.[32]

DIFFERENTIAL DIAGNOSIS

Adolescents with persistent gynecomastia should be further evaluated for Klinefelter syndrome, testicular or adrenal tumors, hyperthyroidism, and other hormonal causes. Further history taking to determine ongoing use of anabolic steroids, alcohol, opioids, or marijuana as a causative factor may be helpful. Persistent gynecomastia in adults should be further evaluated with hormone levels to confirm hypogonadism. A unilateral mass should suggest breast cancer until proven otherwise.

INTERPROFESSIONAL COLLABORATIVE MANAGEMENT
Pharmacologic Management

If it is thought that the gynecomastia is related to a medication, the suspected agent should be discontinued and the breast reassessed for resolution of the gynecomastia.

INDICATIONS FOR REFERRAL OR HOSPITALIZATION

Patients with gynecomastia should be referred when breast cancer is suspected or when concern exists for other serious disease processes, such as endocrine disorders, other malignant neoplasms, or liver disease.

Surgical referral is indicated when there is a discrete mass and/or a clinically abnormal nipple or nipple areolar complex, with or without a mammographic abnormality. Painful large masses or segments of breast tissue may be surgically excised.

PATIENT AND FAMILY EDUCATION AND HEALTH PROMOTION

Patients and their families can be informed that asymptomatic gynecomastia is relatively common. In adolescents, gynecomastia resolves over time, and reassurance and clinical follow-up are all that is needed. Reassurance is indicated for adults whose gynecomastia is related to an adverse reaction to a medication. Any patient whose symptoms persist and who is concerned about cosmesis may be referred for surgical removal of the affected breast tissue.

REFERENCES

1. Hartman, L. C., Degnim, A. C., Santen, R. J., et al. (2015). Atypical hyperplasia of the breast—Risk and management options. *The New England Journal of Medicine, 372,* 78–89.
2. Meechan, G., Collins, J., Moss-Morris, R., et al. (2005). Who is not reassured following benign diagnosis of breast symptoms? *Psycho-Oncology, 14,* 239–246.
3. Breast, U.S. Cancer Statistics. Retrieved from www.breastcancer.org/symptoms/understand_bc/statistics. (Accessed 12 June 2019).
4. Cuzick, J. (2008). Assessing risk for breast cancer. *Breast Cancer Research: BCR, 10*(Suppl. 4), S13.
5. Kerlikowske, K., et al. (2010). Breast cancer risk by density, menopause and post menopausal hormone therapy use. *Journal of Clinical Oncology, 28*(4), 3830–3837.
6. Barke, L. D., & Freivogel, M. E. (2017). Breast cancer risk assessment models and high-risk screening. *Radiologic Clinics of North America, 55*(3), 457–474.
7. Monticciolo, D. C., et al. (2018). Breast cancer screening in women at higher than average risk. Recommendations from the ACR. *Journal of the American College of Radiology: JACR,* In press.
8. Krontiras, H., Farmer, M., & Whatley, J. (2018). Breast cancer genetics and indications for prophylactic mastectomy. *Surgical Clinics of North America, 98*(4), 677–685.
9. Inherited Genetic Mutations. Retrieved from ww5.komen.org/BreastCancer/InheritedGeneticMutations.html. (Accessed 24 July 2018).
10. Stadler, Z. K. (2010). Weighing options for cancer risk reduction in carriers of *BRCA1* and *BRCA2* mutation. *Journal of Clinical Oncology: Official Journal of the American Society of Clinical Oncology, 28*(2), 189–191.
11. American Academy of Family Physicians. USPSTF still recommends mammography for women age 50-74. Retrieved from www.aafp.org/news/health-of-the-public/20150424mammograms.html. (Accessed 24 July 2018).
12. Qaseem, A., Lin, J. S., & Mustafa, R. A. (2019). Screening for breast cancer in average-risk women: A guidance statement from the American College of Physicians. *Annals of Internal Medicine, 170*(8), 547–560.
13. Maniero, M. B., et al. (2017). ACR appropriateness criteria breast cancer screening. Expert panel on breast imaging. *Journal of the American College of Radiology, 14*(115), 5383–5390.
14. U.S. Preventive Services Task Force. Draft Recommendation Statement BRCA-Related Cancer: Risk Assessment, Genetic Counseling, and Genetic Testing. Retrieved from https://www.uspreventiveservicestaskforce.org/Page/Document/draft-recommendation-statement/brca-related-cancer-risk-assessment-genetic-counseling-and-genetic-testing. (Accessed 11 June 2019).
15. Morrow, M. (2000). The evaluation of common breast problems. *American Family Physician, 61*(8), 2371–2378.
16. Smith, R., Pruthi, S., & Fitzpatrick, L. (2004). Evaluation and management of breast pain. *Mayo Clinic Proceedings. Mayo Clinic, 79,* 353–372.
17. Cho, M. W., Grimm, L. J., & Johnson, K. S. (2017). Focal breast pain. *Academic Radiology, 24*(1), 53–59.

18. Pruthi, S., Wahner-Roedler, D. L., Torkelson, C. J., et al. (2010). Vitamin E and evening primrose oil for the management for cyclic mastalgia: A randomized pilot study. *Alternative Medicine Review: A Journal of Clinical Therapeutic*, 15(1), 59–66.

19. Agnese, D. M., Povoski, S. P., & Souba, W. W. (2007). Benign breast disease. In W. W. Souba, M. P. Fink, G. J. Jurkovich, et al. (Eds.), *ACS surgery: Principles and practice*. New York: WebMD Professional Publishing.

20. Goyal, A. (2015). Breast pain. *Clinical Evidence Handbook*, 610–611. BMJ Publishing.

21. Rubolino-Gallego, M. L. (2010). Mastitis and MRSA. An overview of current issues. *Advance for Nurse Practitioners*, 18(3), 31–33.

22. Tena, D., Fernandez, C., & Lopez-Garrido, B. (2016). Lactational mastitis caused by Streptococcus lactarius. *Diagnostic Microbiology and Infectious Disease*, 85(4), 490–492.

23. Miller, V. G. (2010). Inflammatory breast cancer: Rare, aggressive and lethal. *The American Journal for Nurse Practitioners*, 14(3), 48–54.

24. Edge, S. B., Byrd, D. R., Compton, C. C., et al. (Eds.), (2010). *American Joint Committee on Cancer staging manual* (7th ed.). New York: Springer.

25. NH Department of Health and Human Services. NH Division of Public Health Services. 2016. State Antibiogram.

26. Meisner, A. L., Fekrazad, M. H., & Royce, M. E. (2008). Breast disease: Benign and malignant. *The Medical Clinics of North America*, 92(5), 1115–1141.

27. Onstad, M., & Stuckey, A. (2013). Benign breast disorders. *Obstetrics and Gynecology Clinics*, 40(3), 1–13.

28. Hoang, J. K., Hoffman, A. R., Gonzalez, R. G., et al. (2018). Management of incidental pituitary findings on CT, MRI, and (18)F-fluorodeoxyglucose PET: A white paper of the ACR Incidental Findings Committee. *Journal of the American College of Radiology*, 15, 966–972.

29. Whitaker-Worth, D. L., Carlone, V., Susser, W. S., et al. (2000). Dermatologic diseases of the breast and nipple. *Journal of the American Academy of Dermatology*, 43(5 Pt. 1), 733–751.

30. Barlow, W. E., Lehman, C. D., Zheng, Y., et al. (2002). Performance of diagnostic mammography for women with signs and symptoms of breast cancer. *Journal of the National Cancer Institute*, 94, 1151.

31. Miltenburg, D. M., & Speights, V. O. (2008). Benign breast disease. *Obstetrics and Gynecology Clinics of North America*, 35(2), 285–300.

32. Narula, H. S., & Carlson, H. E. (2007). Gynecomastia. *Endocrinology and Metabolism Clinics of North America*, 36(2), 497–519.

33. Thomas, P., & Stoemmer, P. (2017). Gynecomastia: Look beyond the obvious. *American Journal of Medicine*, 130(10), e439–e440.

34. Niell, B. L., Lourenco, A. P., & Moy, L. (2018). ACR Appropriateness Criteria ® Evaluation of the symptomatic male breast. *Journal of the American College of Radiology*, 15(11), S313–S320.

CHAPTER **140**

CHRONIC PELVIC PAIN

Patricia Polgar-Bailey

 Immediate referral is advised for patients with unstable vital signs and acute onset or increasing abdominal or pelvic pain.

DEFINITION AND EPIDEMIOLOGY

Chronic pelvic pain (CPP) is a continuous or episodic, nonmenstrual pain of at least 3 to 6 months duration, which may be sudden or gradual in onset, occurs at or below the umbilicus, and is severe enough to interrupt normal activities of daily life and is not related solely to menstruation, sexual activity, or bowel movements.[1] CPP may involve gastroenterologic, urologic, gynecologic, oncologic, musculoskeletal, and psychosocial systems, and its cause is often multifactorial, making it challenging for patients and providers.[2] Ideally, the cause of CPP is elucidated; however, in up to 50% to 60% of patients no clear cause is established and the absence of pathology often exacerbates the challenge of CPP.[2,3] CPP affects both men

and women. Chronic prostatitis/chronic pelvic pain (CP/CPP) is a well-established cause of pelvic pain in men[2]; however, this chapter refers to the assessment and management of CPP in women. Chronic cyclic pelvic pain (CCPP) is a subset of CPP and is generally used to describe a CPP syndrome that occurs in relation to the menstrual cycle. CCPP may also be used to describe pelvic pain that occurs in a cyclic pattern that is unrelated to the menstrual cycle.[4]

CPP is one of the most common medical problems affecting women today. In the United States CPP is estimated to affect approximately 15%–20% of women.[5] In other parts of the world the prevalence of CPP is estimated to be higher. Recent studies demonstrated prevalence rates of approximately 25% in the United Kingdom and New Zealand.[2] Data indicate that the prevalence of CPP (38 per 1000) is similar to that of migraine, back pain, and asthma.[6] CPP is considered the principal indication for 40% of gynecologic laparoscopies and 12% of all hysterectomies performed for benign disease annually in the United States.[7] Epidemiologic studies have found that women with CPP are more likely to have a history of spontaneous abortion, nongynecologic surgery, and nonpelvic complaints than women without CPP.[2] In addition, a positive correlation has been demonstrated between CPP and a history of multiple sexual partners and psychosocial trauma and abuse. Women with CPP are four times more likely to have a history of pelvic inflammatory disease (PID), as well as higher incidences of constipation, irritable bowel syndrome (IBS), depression, and anxiety than those not affected by CPP.

Potential visceral sources of CPP include the reproductive, genitourinary, and gastrointestinal tracts; potential somatic sources include the pelvic bones, ligaments, muscles, and fascia. CPP may result from psychological disorders or neurologic diseases, both central and peripheral.[8] It may be caused by one disorder, or it can be the end result of several diagnoses, with each contributing to the generation of pain and requiring management. Women with diagnoses that involve more than one organ system generally have greater pain than do women with only one system involved. The distinction between acute and chronic pain is significant. In acute pain, the pain is often a symptom of underlying tissue damage, such as anal fissure, and the diagnosis can be precise, but with CPP, the pain itself becomes the disease; CPP is itself the diagnosis.[2,9]

Populations at Increased Risk of Chronic Pelvic Pain

Physical and Sexual Abuse. A significant association exists between physical and sexual abuse and CPP. If a history of abuse is obtained, it is important to ensure that the woman is not currently being abused or in danger.

Pelvic Inflammatory Disease. Approximately 18% to 35% of all women with acute PID develop CPP.[9] The mechanisms by which CPP results from PID are not known, but the extent of adhesive disease, tubal damage, and pelvic tenderness present 30 days after treatment correlates with the likelihood of development of CPP. Whether acute PID is treated with inpatient or outpatient regimens does not appear to alter the odds for development of subsequent CPP (34% with outpatient therapy versus 30% with inpatient therapy).[9]

Endometriosis. Endometriosis is one of the leading causes of CPP in women and the most common diagnosis made at the time of gynecologic laparoscopy for the evaluation of CPP. Most often, women diagnosed with CPP in the setting of endometriosis are nulliparous, in their 20s to 30s, with symptoms associated with their menstrual cycle, including dysmenorrhea or pain.[2] Although endometriosis is diagnosed laparoscopically in approximately 33% of women with CPP, up to 40% of women with endometriosis and CPP will have no findings on laparoscopy.[2] There is often no correlation between severity of pain and pathologic findings.[2]

Interstitial Cystitis. Interstitial cystitis is a chronic inflammatory condition of the bladder. It is clinically characterized by bladder pain, urinary frequency or urgency, or nocturia in the absence of evidence of another disease that could cause the symptoms.[2] Pain is often present in the suprapubic area but may also occur in the lower back or buttock. As many as 50% of women complain of dyspareunia; fibromyalgia, vulvodynia, anxiety, and depression are often associated complaints.[2]

Irritable Bowel Syndrome. There is a strong association between CPP and IBS; an estimated 65% to 70% of people with IBS have CPP.[2] IBS is a functional gastrointestinal disorder characterized by intermittent or chronic abdominal pain that is associated with bowel symptoms such as bloating, urgency, diarrhea, and constipation. IBS is a diagnosis of exclusion and it is important to rule out other causes of bowel dysfunction such as Crohn disease, diverticulitis, sprue and lactose intolerance, and chronic appendicitis.[2] IBS is associated with certain gynecologic problems, such as endometriosis, dyspareunia, and dysmenorrhea.[10] Women with both CPP and IBS are more likely to have screening and diagnostic procedures done and are less likely to have improvement after laparoscopy compared with women with only CPP.[10]

Musculoskeletal Disorders. Faulty posture may contribute to weak and deconditioned muscles, which allow imbalances in the pelvis with formation of trigger points and hypertonicity and, as a result, pelvic pain. Other musculoskeletal disorders, such as trigger points, lumbar vertebral disorders, pelvic floor myalgia, and fibromyalgia, may cause or contribute to pelvic pain.

Postsurgical Pain. Chronic pain has been reported after several types of surgical procedures, including after cholecystectomy and groin hernia repair in less than 30% of patients and after cesarean section in 6% of patients. A study also found a 48.4% incidence of CPP in patients up to 5.6 years after surgery for pelvic fracture.[11]

PATHOPHYSIOLOGY

The pathogenesis of CPP remains poorly understood, and diagnostic studies, such as laparoscopy, reveal no obvious cause of the pain in up to 35% of cases.[2] In a US population study, 61% of women with CPP did not have a clear cause of their pain.[6] Thus chronic pain is thought to be a dynamic interaction of the combined influences of the mind and nervous system on the body. In addition to the organ system where the pain originated, other organ systems become involved and emotional changes occur with the long-term tension of CPP. For example, pain can cause muscle tension, which can in turn cause changes in the muscles of the pelvis, adjacent urinary tract (bladder, urethra), bowel, connective tissue, and even skin of the area. These secondary changes often become more significant than the original cause of the pain and also may overshadow the original disease process, making it more difficult to diagnose.

There are different theories about the development of chronic pain. According to an older theory of pain, called the Cartesian theory, neurons carry pain signals from the damaged areas through the spinal cord directly to the cortex of the brain, where the pain is perceived. This theory is now thought to be an oversimplification of the development of chronic pain.

A newer theory, the gate control theory, posits that pain signals arise from the injured or adversely affected tissues and travel through specialized nerve cells to the spinal cord, where they can be intensified, reduced, and even blocked before they are transmitted to the brain. The spinal cord acts as a functional "gate" with respect to the pain signals. This gate is influenced by local factors such as nerve inputs in the spinal cord and by descending signals from higher brain centers. Thus internal influences, other than the pain itself, and external environmental factors affect the nature of the pain's impulse transmission. If the gates are damaged by chronic pain, they may remain open even after the tissue damage has resolved or has been controlled. In other words, the pain remains despite the fact that the original cause of the pain has been treated; this type of pain is referred to as neuropathic pain, a key factor in CPP.[9]

CLINICAL PRESENTATION AND PHYSICAL EXAMINATION

The evaluation of CPP can require many office visits and become a highly frustrating experience for both patient and provider. A complete and thorough history and physical examination are crucial in developing a rational approach to women with CPP. It is important that the patient understand early on that visits are not only for evaluation and treatment but also for the formation of a continued therapeutic relationship between patient and provider.

The history should include a description of the nature, intensity, distribution, radiation, location, and daily pattern of the pain, as well as the relationship of the pain to each organ system. Associated events, including complaints of fever, sweats, fatigue, anorexia, nausea, vomiting, and constipation, should be elicited. The relationship of the pain to posture, meals, bowel movements, voiding, menstruation, intercourse, and medications as well as any factors that aggravate or alleviate the pain should be determined. Past surgeries, pelvic infections, and a history of infertility are important diagnostic clues to the origin of the pain.

It is helpful to obtain an understanding from the woman of the past and present status of her pain, the chronology, and how it developed. It can be helpful to have the woman complete a detailed pain questionnaire before her first visit. Box 140.1 includes some questions that should be included on a CPP questionnaire, but the International Pelvic Pain Society also has a Pelvic Pain Assessment Form (in English and Spanish) that is available at https://www.pelvicpain.org/IPPS/Content/Professional-Patients/Documents_and_Forms.aspx.

The physical examination should be thorough, complete, and guided by the history. It will differ from a standard gynecologic examination because it is designed to provide information beyond the condition of the female genitals. The initial part of the examination should begin with observation of the patient's general demeanor during the interview. The five major sources that contribute to pelvic pain should be completely evaluated: gynecologic, gastrointestinal, psychological, musculoskeletal, and urologic.

The abdomen should be examined to elicit a point or area of tenderness. It is important that the patient be allowed to indicate the location of the pain and the depth of palpation

EOX 140.1

Chronic Pelvic Pain Questionnaire (Sample Questions)

- How and when did the pain begin?
- What actions or activities make it better or worse?
- Does it vary based on time of day, week, or menstrual cycle?
- Does it affect your sleep?
- Has it spread beyond where it first was noted?
- Is it associated with abnormal skin sensations, muscle or joint pain, or back pain?
- Do you have any urinary pain or problems, constipation, diarrhea, or other bowel complaints?
- Has it affected your daily routine at home and at work?
- Has it led to emotional changes such as anxiety or depression?
- What have you personally done to attempt to alleviate the pain?
- What has your physician done?
- Have these methods been successful to any degree?
- What medications are you currently using?
- What do you think is causing your pain?
- What concerns you most about your pain?

Modified from the International Pelvic Pain Society. (2014). *Chronic pelvic pain, a patient education booklet.* www.pelvicpain.org, Copyright The International Pelvic Pain Society.

necessary to elicit the discomfort. If pain is experienced during palpation of the abdomen, a trigger point, hernia, endometriosis, or hematoma is likely. Costovertebral angle tenderness should also be elicited if there is tenderness with suprapubic palpation. The groin should be evaluated for inflamed lymph nodes and hernias.

The back should be examined for lordosis, scoliosis, and any tenderness over the paraspinal musculature, sacroiliac joints, or spine prominence. Range of motion should be evaluated. By having the patient lie in the lateral decubitus position, the examiner can accomplish passive thigh extension, which may reveal psoas muscle tenderness.

The pelvic examination should be performed in a gentle, stepwise manner. Attention should be given to any evidence of a vulvar pathologic condition. Pelvic relaxation should be evaluated by having the patient bear down while the practitioner separates the labia and observes for a significant cystocele, rectocele, enterocele, or cervical or uterine prolapse.

A single-digit transvaginal examination (monomanual) is necessary to elicit any tenderness or mass in the adnexa, in the cervix or posterior vagina, along the vaginal side walls, or near the base of the bladder or urethra. Special attention during palpation of the levator ani muscles, piriform muscles, and coccyx is important because all have been implicated as a cause of CPP and discomfort.

A careful speculum examination is performed to visualize the cervix and vagina and to inspect for neoplasms, prolapse, or infections. This examination may reveal vaginismus, with involuntary spasms of the vaginal musculature that make insertion of the speculum difficult.

The bimanual examination and rectovaginal examination complete the genitourinary evaluation. Particular attention should be given to areas of tenderness. Cervical motion tenderness has been associated with endometriosis, pelvic adhesive disease, inflammatory bowel disease (IBD), and ureteral colic.

A fixed retroverted uterus or an enlarged boggy uterus, the hallmark of adenomyosis, may be noted. Uterine fibroids do not classically cause pain unless they are degenerating or infarcting, but their enlargement may cause a feeling of heaviness and pressure on nerve endings in the lower abdomen and pelvis. Finally, the rectovaginal examination may reveal nodularity in the cul-de-sac that is associated with endometriosis. The examination may also help identify any rectal masses, and the piriform muscle can be evaluated for spasms and tenderness.

DIAGNOSTICS
Essential Diagnostics

Laboratory studies should be based on each patient's history and physical findings. The usual evaluation for CPP may include vaginal and cervical cultures for sexually transmitted diseases, urinalysis, urine culture, complete blood count (CBC), pregnancy test, and erythrocyte sedimentation rate (ESR).

Additional Diagnostics

A transvaginal ultrasound examination may be beneficial if the bimanual examination was difficult; if it revealed adnexal tenderness, a mass, or uterine enlargement; or if irregularity was noted.

Laparoscopy may be indicated, especially if the pelvic examination or imaging findings are abnormal. Commonly found abnormalities include endometriosis, adhesions, and chronic PID. Referral to a gynecologic surgeon should be made if abnormalities are noted.

DIFFERENTIAL DIAGNOSIS

 Red flags include weight loss, pain associated with night-waking, radiation of pain, and constitutional symptoms such as rash, arthralgia, and fever.

The differential diagnosis for CPP is extensive. From a primary care perspective, a good history and physical examination aid in the differential diagnosis. Direct questioning of the patient's view of what is wrong or of concern may be very helpful in developing a differential diagnosis.[4] IBS is believed to account for 35% to 50% of all cases of CPP.[6] IBS is a chronic functional bowel disorder that is often accompanied by gynecologic complaints and labeled as CPP. IBS consists of a constellation of symptoms, including abdominal pain or discomfort that is relieved with defecation; it is usually associated with alternating constipation and diarrhea. The pain of IBS is usually worse around the time of menstruation and may be associated with dyspareunia.

CPP and IBS are both believed to be multifactorial in origin and share some of the same psychosocial factors, including a high prevalence of depression and a history of physical or sexual abuse A diagnosis of IBS should be included in any differential diagnosis of CPP, but CPP should also remain a diagnosis of exclusion.[2] As with any other gastrointestinal complaint, more serious disease entities need to be excluded, including IBD, diverticulitis, and malignant disease.

Urinary tract problems may manifest as CPP. Because the gynecologic and urinary systems share embryologic origins, differentiation of the source of pain can be difficult. A pathologic condition of the urinary tract can demonstrate a constellation of symptoms, including pelvic pain, dysuria, urgency, hesitancy, dyspareunia, postcoital voiding difficulties, and incontinence. Urethral syndrome, chronic urethritis, interstitial cystitis, urethral diverticulum, and bladder spasms should be considered in the differential diagnosis.

Musculoskeletal diseases are also associated with CPP. These conditions include postural problems, herniated disk disease, chronic pelvic tilt, degenerative joint disease, and myofascial trigger points. Levator ani muscle spasms and piriform muscle spasms are two conditions that are easy to evaluate on physical examination and may be a source of pain and discomfort.

Levator syndrome is generally attributed to muscle spasms of the pelvic floor musculature and is associated with a wide range of musculoskeletal disorders, including piriformis and puborectalis syndromes.[2] Levator ani muscle spasms are more common in women, with an incidence of approximately 6%,[2] and are usually initially seen as sacral pain and overlooked as a possible cause of CPP. The pain is caused by contraction and spasm of the levator ani muscles. Palpation of this muscle group reveals tenderness and increasing pain with voluntary contraction. Teaching the patient to relax these muscles and the vaginal muscles will help alleviate the discomfort.

Piriform syndrome or spasms of the piriform muscle during external rotation of the leg can be reproduced by contraction of the externally rotated leg against resistance. Because the piriform muscle can be palpated transvaginally, tenderness along the muscle should be evaluated during bimanual examination. Physical therapy is usually indicated to help relieve the spasms.

An alteration in the processing of the stimuli by the spinal cord and brain in women with CPP has also been suggested as a possible cause.[6] This may be a component in other types of chronic pain, in which normal body sensations are perceived as painful.[6]

A gynecologic source of pain should always be considered. Although a pathologic condition is more likely with acute pain, certain entities are more commonly seen with CPP. Endometriosis is one of the leading causes of CPP in women.[2] Endometriosis is caused by the development of endometrial implants outside the endometrium. Because these implants can be found anywhere and are responsive to the cyclic hormonal cycle, the point source of the pain can be elusive. On physical examination, either tenderness in the cul-de-sac or along the uterosacral ligaments (early finding) or nodularity in the same locations (late finding) may be noted. The diagnosis should be confirmed by laparoscopy. In spite of laparoscopic confirmation of endometriosis, definitive criteria to determine the actual cause of the pain of endometriosis are lacking.[2]

Adhesions are scar tissue that can form between any two abdominal organs, usually after surgery or intra-abdominal infections such as PID. The pain occurs because of the stretching of usually mobile structures that are now scarred. Patients usually complain of a substantial positional component to the pain. The diagnosis can be confirmed by laparoscopy.

Other gynecologic origins of CPP include pain with ovulation, dysmenorrhea, functional ovarian cysts, ovarian torsion, chronic PID, pelvic congestion of the reproductive organ venous system, adenomyosis, and leiomyomas.

If a patient admits to depression and attributes it to the pain, management in collaboration with a psychiatrist or psychologist may be helpful.[4] Disclosure of childhood physical or emotional abuse should elicit a referral to an appropriate mental health provider but will likely not affect immediate management of the pain.[4]

If no other pathologic entity or explanation can be found for the pain, a psychiatric component such as clinical depression or somatization disorder should be considered. Screening for depression and referral to a psychiatrist can assist in this area.

INTERPROFESSIONAL COLLABORATIVE MANAGEMENT

Nonpharmacologic Management

Complementary and alternative medicine (CAM) options most commonly used for CPP include dietary supplements and herbs, acupuncture, and mind-body methods.[7] Some of these adjunctive therapies have shown promise, but more studies are necessary to demonstrate efficacy in the management of CPP.

Information for evidence-based management of CPP is not widely available, and there is little specific evidence for the role of analgesic drugs in the treatment of CPP.[4] Success in treating women with CPP is greatly facilitated by winning their trust and confidence. In general, positive reinforcement and general psychological support are important in the early diagnostic phase of CPP. Women suffer for years, and many are told the problem is psychosomatic. Consideration of depression and sleep disorders is important because treatment of these conditions enhances management of the chronic pain syndrome. If a cause of the pain is identified, appropriate management should be undertaken with the assistance of the appropriate physician specialist.

Pharmacologic Management

During the diagnostic evaluation, the pain component should be treated effectively and promptly. First-line treatment is generally nonsteroidal antiinflammatory drugs (NSAIDs) to decrease pain and inflammation.[2] Narcotics are not recommended owing to concerns for substance use and addiction potential, as well as risks of constipation or antimotility side effects, which could exacerbate the pain.

There are data to suggest that tricyclic antidepressants are effective for neuropathic pain and, for this reason, may be helpful in CPP.[4] There are limited data for the use of selective serotonin reuptake inhibitors for relief of pain in CPP and insufficient evidence for the use of any other antidepressant.

Anticonvulsants have been used for pain management for many years. Recently, gabapentin has begun to be used for chronic pain syndromes and is thought to have fewer side effects than other anticonvulsants.[4] There remains insufficient good-quality evidence for the efficacy of neuropathic medications in the context of CPP, but they may be helpful for some women.[2]

Neurostimulation has been used successfully for the treatment of neuropathic pain. It is believed that there may be a role for sacral neuromodulation in CPP syndromes.[4] Neuroablative techniques and chemical neuroablation have been used with some success in pain management. Botox has been used with some success for both pelvic floor muscle spasms and undifferentiated CPP.[2]

Laparoscopy has been used as both a diagnostic and a therapeutic tool in CPP. Adhesions are often thought to be a cause of CPP, and some women may experience improvement after laparoscopic adhesiolysis.[2] An estimated 10% of hysterectomies have been performed for CPP, but up to 40% of women will have recurrent pain after hysterectomy.[2]

Counseling and a supportive patient-provider relationship are very important, particularly because diagnostic procedures such as ultrasound and laparoscopy are used to exclude serious conditions and to provide reassurance.[6] Menstrual cycle suppression with oral, transdermal, transvaginal, or subcutaneous contraceptives (medroxyprogesterone [Depo-Provera]) may be helpful. The Mirena intrauterine device and a gonadotropin-releasing hormone agonist such as leuprolide (Lupron) may also be helpful in management of CPP.

Given the multifactorial nature of CPP, the emerging treatment models have included interdisciplinary approaches that may include standard gynecological management, as well as physical and psychological therapy. A recent 1-year prospective cohort study demonstrated the benefit of treating CPP with such an interdisciplinary approach at a single integrated center. Interventions included surgical management (e.g., excision of endometriosis or hysterectomy), medical management (e.g., hormonal and/or pain medication, trigger point injections), and/or a pain management program (including group pain workshops, individual counseling, and PT). Counseling included mindfulness-based strategies and cognitive behavioral strategies. Participants were also directed to community resources and provided with community mental health referrals as needed. The results of the study demonstrated a decrease in chronic pelvic pain severity and health care utilization and improvements in quality of life after 1 year.[1]

Given that an integrated approach within a single center may not be feasible, a strong relationship with the provider who can facilitate an interdisciplinary approach is important for patients with CPP. These visits enable discussion of the progress of the diagnostic process, reassurance and support during the evaluation period, and the development of an interdisciplinary treatment plan.

Indications for Referral or Hospitalization

The cause of CPP is often complex and multifaceted, and treatment may involve several specialists. A coordinated multidisciplinary approach has been advocated. Prompt referral to physical therapy, gastroenterology, urology, and pain management programs as indicated should be considered. Working with a consulting physician is essential to assess the need for surgical evaluation, in addition to consultation for diagnostic testing, appropriate referral to collaborating providers, and assistance with treatment planning as indicated.

LIFE SPAN CONSIDERATIONS

CPP usually occurs during a woman's late 20s and early 30s but can be seen across the reproductive life span, and the population group is varied. This can be a stressful period in a woman's life. She may be married, considering pregnancy or raising children, and involved in a career. CPP can profoundly affect a woman's personal and professional life. An open mind and the pursuit of appropriate diagnostics as well as support of the patient's fears, anxieties, and stresses can have a profound impact on the understanding of CPP and ultimate pain control.

COMPLICATIONS

Numerous pathologic conditions have been identified with CPP, and the potential for complications is incalculable. Many women suffer great frustration associated with the diagnosis and treatment of this disorder. In addition, there is often a psychogenic component to the disorder that is often not addressed.

PATIENT AND FAMILY EDUCATION

- Reassurance that the causes of CPP, although real and concerning, tend to be less urgent than the causes of acute pelvic pain can be helpful.

- Education regarding the need or lack of need for additional diagnostic testing.
- Information about the possible sources of pain and an explanation that the alleviation of pain may be best achieved by a combination of therapies, including medical, psychological, and behavioral treatments.

HEALTH PROMOTION

Helping a woman understand her body and the sources of possible pain can assist her in coping. As always, a healthy diet, regular exercise, moderation of alcohol intake, and relaxation techniques can go a long way toward improving a woman's management of the stress and anxiety associated with CPP.

REFERENCES

1. Stein, C. (2013). Chronic pelvic pain. *Gastroenterology Clinics of North America, 42,* 785–800.
2. Toye, F., Seers, K., & Barker, K. (2014). A meta-ethnograpy of patients' experience of chronic pelvic pain: Struggling to construct pelvic pain as "real". *Journal of Advanced Nursing, 70*(12), 2713–2727.
3. Fall, N. M., Baranowski, A. P., Elneil, S., et al. (2010). EAU guidelines on chronic pelvic pain. *European Urology, 57,* 35–48.
4. Stones, W., Cheong, Y. C., & Howard, F. M. (2007). Interventions for treating chronic pelvic pain in women. *The Cochrane Database of Systematic Reviews,* (4), CD000387.
5. Allaire, C., Williams, C., Bodman-Roy, S., et al. (2018). Chronic pelvic pain in an interdisciplinary setting: 1 year prospective cohort. *American Journal of Obstetrics and Gynecology, 218*(114), e1–e12.
6. Leong, F. C. (2014). Complementary and alternative medications for chronic pain. *Obstetrics and Gynecology Clinics of North America, 41,* 503–510.
7. Howard, F. (2004). Chronic pelvic pain. ACOG technical bulletin no. 51. Washington, DC: American College of Obstetricians and Gynecologists.
8. Wenof, M., & Perry, C. (2013). Chronic pelvic pain. The International Pelvic Pain Society patient education booklet. Retrieved from www.pelvicpain.org/pdf/Patient/CPP_Pt_ED_Booklet.pdf. (Accessed 15 September 2015).
9. Ness, R., Soper, D., Holley, L., et al. (2002). Effectiveness of inpatient and outpatient treatment strategies for women with pelvic inflammatory disease: Results from the Pelvic Inflammatory Disease Evaluation and Clinical Health (PEACH) Randomized Trial. *American Journal of Obstetrics and Gynecology, 186,* 929–937.
10. Williams, R., Hartman, K., Sandler, R., et al. (2005). Recognition and treatment of irritable bowel syndrome among women with chronic pelvic pain. *American Journal of Obstetrics and Gynecology, 192,* 761–767.
11. Meyhoff, C., Thomsen, C., Rasmussen, L., et al. (2006). High incidence of chronic pain following surgery for pelvic fracture. *The Clinical Journal of Pain, 22*(2), 167–172.

CHAPTER **141**

ABNORMAL UTERINE BLEEDING
Marie Elena Botte

 Immediate referral is indicated for women with acute abnormal uterine bleeding who are hemodynamically unstable require immediate access to fluid replacement and blood or platelet transfusion in an appropriate setting

DEFINITION AND EPIDEMIOLOGY

Nongestational abnormal uterine bleeding (AUB) comprises a range of clinical conditions and presentations, including timed bleeding, intermenstrual bleeding (AUB/IMB) mal heavy menstrual bleeding (AUB/HMB), that menstrual blood loss that interferes with the wom cal, emotional, social, and material quality of life.[1,2]

be either acute or chronic. Acute AUB has been defined as an episode of heavy bleeding that, in the opinion of the clinician, is of sufficient quantity to require immediate intervention to prevent further blood loss,[3] and chronic AUB has been defined as bleeding from the uterine corpus that is abnormal in duration, volume, frequency, or regularity and has been present for the majority of the past 6 months.[4,5]

The recognition of AUB, however, is contingent upon an appreciation of how normal vaginal bleeding is defined, both by women and providers. Citing worldwide confusion in the definitions and terminology used to describe the symptom of AUB in women, the International Federation of Gynecology and Obstetrics (FIGO) convened in 2005 to address the standardization, terminology, and definition of normal menstruation,[6] based on published data from the World Health Organization and records from over 6000 women. Characteristics and descriptors of "normal" menstruation were established according to FIGO's system, which aimed to develop clear, simple terminology (and to avoid ill-defined terms such as *dysfunctional uterine bleeding* as well as several terms with classical roots, such as *menorrhagia, metrorrhagia, oligomenorrhea*). The characteristics of normal menstruation that FIGO established include the four key menstrual dimensions of cycle regularity, frequency of menstruation, duration of menstrual flow, and volume of menstrual flow. Each of these dimensions is accompanied by one of three simple descriptors indicating either "normal" (between the 5th and 95th percentile for women) or terms describing beyond (more than) or below (less than) normal. Therefore normal duration of flow has been established as 4.5 to 8 days, with "prolonged" flow greater than 8 days and "shortened" flow less than 4.5 days. Similarly, normal menstrual frequency or interval has been defined as 24 to 38 days (22 to 35 in midreproductive years), and "frequent" or "infrequent" define intervals outside of these parameters. "Normal" cycle-to-cycle variation has been established as ± 2 to 20 days (over 12 months), with "irregular" cycles defined as having a variability greater than 20 days. A "normal" volume of blood loss is defined as between 5 and 80 mL, with "heavy" blood loss greater than 80 mL and "light" blood loss less than 5 mL. As a point of reference, 80 mL is equivalent to three soaked pads or six full regular-absorbency tampons per day for 3 or more days.

AUB was revisited in 2009 by the FIGO Menstrual Disorders Group, and the acronym PALM-COEIN was devised to standardize nomenclature and the underlying categories of etiology. This is a useful mnemonic that separates etiology into uterine structural abnormalities (PALM, for Polyps, Adenomyosis, Leiomyoma, Malignancy and hyperplasia) and nonstructural abnormalities (COEIN, for Coagulopathy, Ovulatory, Endometrial, Iatrogenic, and Not otherwise classified). The classification system is intentionally dynamic, with ongoing feedback and debate informing the classification and reclassification of etiologies as more is known regarding pathophysiology in areas of active inquiry. It is helpful to keep the PALM-COEIN mnemonic in mind while sorting through potential causes, symptoms, and management strategies for AUB.

AUB is a common gynecologic complaint, affecting 14% to 25% of reproductive-aged women.[5] AUB is the reason for one-third of gynecological appointments in premenopausal women[7] and greater than 70% of visits for perimenopausal and postmenopausal women.[8] The estimated worldwide prevalence of subjective, self-defined AUB has been estimated from 4% to

52%.[9] The associated direct and indirect costs of AUB can be high and have been estimated at upwards of one billion dollars in the US annually[7] related to work absence, home management, and the cost of procedures, pharmaceuticals, pads, and tampons. Age is a factor in AUB: ovulatory dysfunction is more common at the extremes of reproductive age,[10] and structural uterine alterations such as polyps and leiomyomas (also known as fibroids) are the main cause of AUB during menacme[8] (the time between menarche and menopause). Polyps, fibroids, adenomyosis, hyperplasia, and malignancy all have an increasing prevalence with age. Reproductive history is also related to risk for AUB. Increasing parity and cesarean delivery have been linked to the development of adenomyosis[11] (AUB-A), and cesarean delivery to the formation of cesarean scar defects that can cause abnormal bleeding.[12-15]

PATHOPHYSIOLOGY

Whether acute or chronic (or acute presentation in the context of a more chronic problem), the etiologies of AUB are the same. Many cases include a combination of factors, and there are certainly individuals in whom definable entities such as polyps or fibroids are identified in the workup that are not actually contributing to presenting symptoms. AUB-P (polyps) are epithelial proliferations that arise from endometrial stroma and glands; hormonal or inflammatory factors may influence their development. AUB-A (adenomyosis) is a condition where the endometrial glands and stroma are located within the myometrium, eventually causing uterine enlargement; its etiology is unclear but may involve invagination of the endometrium, metaplastic process, or altered molecular functioning of the endometriotic glands or the junctional zone of the endometrium and the myometrium.[11,16] AUB-L (leiomyomas) are very common benign monoclonal fibromuscular tumors of the myometrium that can develop in a variety of locations and are further subclassified as to whether or not they are in contact with the endometrium (submucous); submucous leiomyomas are believed to be most likely to contribute to AUB. Leiomyomas are believed to develop from normal monocytes that then transform into abnormal monocytes and then finally into clinically apparent tumors, and their growth is affected by steroid hormones, growth factors related to angiogenesis, and genetics. AUB-M (malignancy and hyperplasia, or endometrial intraepithelial neoplasia/EIN), historically occurred only rarely in premenopausal women but is now also seen in women with unopposed estrogen (obesity, metabolic syndrome) and may also be caused by uterine sarcoma (rare but increased in women >75 years and those exposed to tamoxifen or prior radiation therapy) and cervical or ovarian cancer. Premalignant proliferation is understood to be caused by monoclonal growth and mutation of tumor-suppressive genes in affected glands.[17] The majority of women with AUB-C (coagulopathy) have von Willebrand syndrome (which affects 1% of the population), and the mildest form is the most frequently diagnosed. AUB-O (ovulatory) may be caused by the effect of unopposed estrogen on the endometrium, causing marked proliferation and HMB and altered menstrual frequency, or other endocrinopathies that impact the functioning of the hypothalamic-pituitary- ovarian (HPO) axis, such as hypothyroidism, hyperprolactinemia, obesity or anorexia, extreme exercise, mental stress, and weight loss. AUB-E (endometrial) generally occurs in the context of regular cycles, normal uterine structure, and absence of coagulopathy and may involve infection, inflammation, hypoxia, primary local endometrial hemostasis, angiogenesis, aberrant prostaglandin synthesis, excessive plasminogen, and disturbances of local glucocorticoid metabolism[18] or deficiencies in the molecular mechanisms of endometrial repair.[19] AUB-I (iatrogenic) can be caused by copper intrauterine device (IUD) use, systemic or localized continuous estrogen or progesterone therapy, including contraceptive implants and IUDs,[20] gonadotropin-releasing hormone (GnRH) agonists, aromatase inhibitors, and selective estrogen receptor modulators (SERMS), through direct action on the endometrium, as well as by anticoagulant and antiplatelet therapies, endometritis from an IUD, or cesarean scar defects.[13] AUB-N (not otherwise classified) includes endometrial pseudoaneurysms, myometrial hypertrophy, and arteriovenous malformations.

CLINICAL PRESENTATION AND PHYSICAL EXAMINATION

While the upper limit of normal blood loss in menstruation has been defined as 80 mL, the average amount of blood lost during menstruation is closer to 30 to 40 mL.[21] Many women present with AUB for blood loss below this level,[22] suggesting both that abnormal bleeding in a particular woman is necessarily subjective (i.e., it is abnormal *for her*) as well as that patient distress, more than absolute blood loss per se, is a significant factor in causing women to seek care for their symptoms. Women may report difficulty leaving the home because of the amount of blood loss, limitations in social activities because of fear of soiling clothing, and decreased work productivity because of frequent pad and tampon changes.[7] While precise quantification of menstrual loss is appropriate and practical only in research settings, a pictoral blood loss assessment chart (PBAC) that visually estimates the extent of blood loss on sanitary pads and tampons[23] can be a reliable and semiobjective tool for use in clinical practice.[24]

A thorough history is essential to guide subsequent testing and treatment. Details of the current bleeding episode, related symptoms, and past medical, surgical, and gynecologic history can all guide the selection of appropriate laboratory and radiologic testing. Menstrual history, including age at menarche, typical menstrual patterns, amount of bleeding, associated pain, family history of AUB, and signs and symptoms of coagulopathy are all relevant to the determination of etiology of AUB. The initial assessment should exclude pregnancy, establish the impact of the bleeding on the woman's quality of life and functioning, and assess risk for both uterine cancer and coagulopathy. Uterine polyps (AUB-P) have been correlated with HMB, IMB, and postmenopausal bleeding (PMB) but may also be found incidentally on ultrasound or other imaging. AUB, pelvic pain, and infertility may be the presenting symptoms of adenomyosis (AUB-A). Dysmenorrhea may be a symptom of both adenomyosis and leiomyomas (AUB-L). Heavy or prolonged menstrual bleeding are the most common presenting symptoms of women with leiomyomas, but women can also present with pelvic pain, infertility, or premature birth. Depending on their location, leiomyomas may also contribute to dyspareunia. Vaginal bleeding of any amount is suspicious for malignancy (AUB-M) in postmenopausal women. Women of reproductive age, especially those with an endogenous or exogenous excess of unopposed estrogen (obesity, PCOS, hirsutism, acne, early onset diabetes) may present with amenorrhea (absence of menstrual bleeding)

or irregular bleeding[25] in endometrial malignancy. Postcoital bleeding may be a sign of surface lesions on the genital tract (such as polyps, cervicitis, vulvar atrophy or vulvar lichen planus or lichen sclerosis) but may also be caused by cervical or vaginal cancers.

A history of "flooding," (a change in pad or tampon more frequently than hourly), prolonged bleeding, clots greater than 1 inch, or a family history of bleeding problems is highly suggestive of a bleeding disorder (AUB-C). Other questions geared to identification of possible coagulopathy include a history of bleeding problems (after surgery, trauma, or childbirth), transfusion, iron-responsive anemia, epistaxis or gingival bleeding, HMB since menarche, petechiae or ecchymosis, thyroid disorders, renal disease, or hepatic dysfunction; 90% of coagulopathies can be identified by use of structured history screening criteria.[26] Ovulatory dysfunction (AUB-O) commonly presents as heavy, irregular bleeding. Iatrogenic causes (AUB-I) are suggested by careful review of current medications as well as prior medical and surgical problems and interventions.

A prompt physical examination for a woman with acute AUB is necessary to evaluate for signs of blood loss (e.g., tachycardia, hypotension, and pallor). Clinical signs of systemic disease may offer clues as to the etiology of the AUB, or to comorbid factors that may impact treatment decisions. Physical exam findings such as hirsutism, acne, PCOS, thyroid nodules or enlargement (thyroid dysfunction), petechiae, ecchymosis, hepatosplenomegaly (coagulopathy), acanthosis nigricans (insulin resistance), or obesity (unopposed estrogen) can guide further inquiry and diagnostics. A thorough pelvic examination is necessary for all complaints of AUB. The speculum exam is useful to identify vaginal or cervical lesions (infection, polyps) and to confirm the source of bleeding. A bimanual exam can assess for uterine size or irregularity (suggestive of structural causes such as leiomyoma).

DIAGNOSTICS
Essential Diagnostics

Pregnancy must be excluded in all women of reproductive age with a serum level of human chorionic gonadotropin; a complete blood count is warranted to assess for anemia. Transvaginal ultrasound (preferably) or pelvic ultrasound can identify uterine size, and structural abnormalities such as polyps or submucosal fibroids, evaluate the endometrial stripe for hyperplasia, and noninvasively suggest adenomyosis[11,27] (a diagnosis best confirmed with histology).

Endometrial sampling (after excluding pregnancy) is indicated in all women over 44 with AUB but should also be considered in women with increased risk for endometrial cancer[28] (family history, obesity, PCOS, diabetes, early menarche/late menopause, unopposed estrogen therapy, tamoxifen); postmenopausal women should be evaluated with endometrial sampling for any amount of vaginal bleeding, including spotting or staining.

Additional Diagnostics

Additional diagnostics are guided by clinical suspicion and detailed below in the diagnostics box. Thyroid-stimulating hormone and prolactin levels can evaluate for possible ovarian cause of AUB. Hysteroscopy and guided biopsy are the gold standard for diagnosis of endometrial polyps.[29] Sonohysterography, or SIS (saline infusion sonogram), is a noninvasive technique using a slow infusion of sterile saline into the uterine cavity during ultrasound imaging; this technique has been shown to be superior to ultrasound alone in the detection of polyps and fibromas.[30]

DIFFERENTIAL DIAGNOSIS

Potential causes of AUB include uterine structural abnormalities, coagulopathies, malignancy, and ovarian, hormonal, and iatrogenic factors. The classification of the etiologies of AUB is arranged according to the PALM-COEIN system of classification: AUB-P (polyp), AUB-A (adenomyosis), AUB-L (leiomyomas), AUB-M (malignancy and premalignant conditions: atypical hyperplasia/endometrial intraepithelial neoplasia (or EIN) and endometrial cancer), AUB-C (coagulopathy: von Willebrand disease, hemophilia, leukemia, liver failure), AUB-O (ovulatory disorders: PCOS, hypothyroidism, hyperprolactinemia, mental stress, obesity, anorexia or weight loss, extreme aerobic exercise), AUB-E (endometrial causes: primary disorder of local endometrial hemostasis, deficiencies in molecular mechanism of endometrial repair such as inflammation or infection), AUB-I (iatrogenic: women on therapeutic anticoagulation or chemotherapeutic agents or exogenous hormones, either systemic or local), AUB-N (not otherwise classified: arteriovenous malformation, cesarean scar defect, or isthmocele).

INTRAPROFESSIONAL COLLABORATIVE MANAGEMENT

The primary goal of treatment for women with AUB related to HMB is to control the current episode of heavy bleeding and reduce bleeding in future cycles. Selection of appropriate treatment is necessarily individualized and must consider clinical acuity and stability, the suspected etiology of the bleeding, the desire for present contraception and future fertility, as well as other potential underlying medical problems.

Pharmacologic Management

Medical management, including hormonal and nonhormonal options, is the preferred initial management strategy for women in whom pregnancy, malignancy, underlying coagulopathy, and iatrogenic causes of AUB have been excluded.[31] Intravenous administration of high-dose conjugated equine estrogen,[32] typically 25 mg every 4 hours, may be indicated (and is the only FDA approved therapy) for acute AUB.

For women with anovulation or ovulation dysfunction, combined oral contraceptives or the vaginal contraceptive ring are appropriate therapies because they prevent risks from unopposed estrogen and have been shown to decrease the number of bleeding episodes per year and HMB,[2] with continuous use (no placebo pills or week off with the ring) demonstrating a significant decrease in HMB and number of bleeding episodes per year compared to cyclic regimens.[33,34] For women who cannot tolerate or who have contraindications to estrogen, progesterone-only methods can also decrease heavy bleeding in women with AUB caused by ovulatory dysfunction. Progesterone can be given continuously and systemically (oral, IM depot medroxyprogesterone acetate), cyclically (pills on menstrual days 5 to 21), or via continuous local administration (progesterone IUD, levonorgestrel intrauterine system LNG-IUS). Women who use an IUS consecutively (i.e., the system is replaced after 5 years) continue to benefit from decreased bleeding and, in the majority of cases, cessation of bleeding.

For women who cannot take or prefer not to use hormonal therapies, hemostatic therapy with tranexamic acid[35] (an antifibrinolytic medication) and high doses of nonsteroidal anti-inflammatories have been used to reduce menstrual blood loss. There has been one randomized placebo-controlled trial of the effects of myrtle fruit syrup on HMB in Iranian women that demonstrated a decrease in the number of bleeding days and pads used, as well as quality of life improvements.[36] Metformin has also been studied and found to have an antiproliferative and antiestrogenic effect on benign abnormal endometrial proliferative disorders.[17]

Indications for Referral and Hospitalization

Surgical intervention may be necessary in acute AUB that does not respond to fluid replacement and blood transfusion, or after failed medical therapy in chronic AUB. Endometrial ablation is the targeted destruction of the endometrium for the treatment of select (benign) causes of AUB[37] and can be accomplished via laser, radiofrequency, electrical or heated fluid to coagulate or vaporize endometrial tissue. Uterine artery embolization and hysterectomy (the definitive treatment for AUB) may also be considered. Surgical therapies can result in increased quality of life but also preclude future childbearing.

Referral to gynecology is appropriate for endometrial sampling and hysteroscopy, as well as for consideration of procedures such as endometrial ablation or hysterectomy. Women with suspected coagulopathy should be evaluated and managed in consultation with a hematologist. Women with acute AUB who are hemodynamically unstable require immediate access to fluid replacement and blood or platelet transfusion in an appropriate setting.

LIFE SPAN CONSIDERATIONS

AUB affects women of all ages but decisions regarding treatment can have considerable impact on present and future reproductive potential. A woman desiring pregnancy can be informed that while IMB significantly decreases a woman's odds of conceiving in that particular cycle, it does not appear to negatively impact her immediate future reproductive potential.[38]

COMPLICATIONS

Patients with acute AUB should be promptly evaluated for signs of hypovolemia and hemodynamic instability, with an eye toward obtaining IV access and consideration of blood transfusion or clotting factor replacement.[3] AUB is a leading cause of iron deficiency anemia in women worldwide,[7] and anemia can result in fatigue, weakness, unexplained weight loss, mood swings, and impaired cognitive functioning. For women in whom initial medical management with hormonal therapies is ineffective, or those with severe bleeding or contraindications to medical management, surgical interventions including endometrial ablation, uterine artery embolization, and hysterectomy may be necessary, with implications for future childbearing. Hysterectomy is the definitive treatment for AUB but is costly and associated with potential complications such as high blood loss, infection, thromboembolic events, and injury to bowel, bladder, and ureters.

PATIENT AND FAMILY EDUCATION

Education is an important aspect of care for women with AUB, especially around choice of treatment, as many of the causes and treatments for AUB have reproductive implications.

Women with adenomyosis attempting pregnancy with or without assisted reproductive technologies (ART) should be informed that they have a higher risk of complications[11] including premature delivery (OR 1.84) and premature rupture of membranes (OR 1.98); when these women utilize IVF, there are significant reductions in pregnancy and delivery rates. Oral contraceptives and LNG-IUSs are excellent choices for women who do not currently desire pregnancy but may in the future. Women choosing endometrial ablation should expect a relatively low-risk procedure that will reduce their HMB to normal levels or less.[37] Women choosing endometrial ablation, uterine artery embolization, or hysterectomy need to understand that these choices necessarily preclude subsequent childbearing.

HEALTH PROMOTION

Although the morbidity associated with AUB varies with severity and duration of bleeding, the impact on a woman's health-related quality of life can be profound.[7] AUB can impact professional, financial, emotional, and sexual functioning.[7,24] Identifying the source of the AUB and initiating appropriate therapy can go a long way toward reinstating a woman's disrupted quality of life.

INITIAL DIAGNOSTICS

Abnormal Uterine Bleeding

LABORATORY
Initial Diagnostics
- Serum level of human chorionic gonadotropin
- Complete blood count
- Thyroid stimulating hormone
- Cervical cultures

Further Diagnostics, if Indicated
- Liver function tests
- Prolactin
- Total and free testosterone
- Dehydroepiandrosterone (DHEA-S)
- Lutenizing Hormone and Follicle-Stimulating Hormone
- Serum iron
- Total iron binding capacity
- Ferritin
- **For women >45 years or with an increased risk of endometrial cancer:**
- Endometrial sampling
- **For women with a positive coagulopathy screen:**
- Von Willebrand factor antigen
- Ristocetin cofactor assay
- Factor VIII
- **For women with acute AUB:**
- Blood type and cross match
- Platelet count
- Prothrombin time
- Partial thromboplastin time
- Fibrinogen

IMAGING
- Pelvic ultrasound, preferably transvaginal

REFERENCES

1. Hudelist, G. (2017). Heavy menstrual bleeding diagnosis and medical management. *European Journal of Obstetrics, Gynecology, and Reproductive Biology, 2*, 20.
2. Kaunitz, A. M., et al. (2009). Cycle control with a 21-day compared with a 24-day oral contraceptive pill: A randomized controlled trial. *Obstetrics and Gynecology, 114*(6), 1205–1212.
3. American College of Obstetricians and Gynecologists. (2013). ACOG committee opinion no. 557: Management of acute abnormal uterine bleeding in nonpregnant reproductive-aged women. *Obstetrics and Gynecology, 121*(4), 891–896.
4. Munro, M. G. (2017). Practical aspects of the two FIGO systems for management of abnormal uterine bleeding in the reproductive years. *Best Practice and Research. Clinical Obstetrics and Gynaecology, 40*, 3–22.
5. Whitaker, L., & Critchley, H. O. (2016). Abnormal uterine bleeding. *Best Practice and Research. Clinical Obstetrics and Gynaecology, 34*, 54–65.
6. Fraser, I. S., et al. (2007). A process designed to lead to international agreement on terminologies and definitions used to describe abnormalities of menstrual bleeding. *Fertility and Sterility, 87*(3), 466–476.
7. Liu, Z., et al. (2007). A systematic review evaluating health-related quality of life, work impairment, and health-care costs and utilization in abnormal uterine bleeding. *Value in Health, 10*(3), 183–194.
8. Lasmar, R. B., & Lasmar, B. P. (2017). The role of leiomyomas in the genesis of abnormal uterine bleeding (AUB). *Best Practice and Research. Clinical Obstetrics and Gynaecology, 40*, 82–88.
9. Surveys, O. O. P. C. A. (1995). Morbidity statistics from general practice: Fourth national morbidity study: 1991–1992. *HMSO, MB5*(3).
10. Shapley, M., et al. (2013). The epidemiology of self-reported intermenstrual and postcoital bleeding in the perimenopausal years. *BJOG: An International Journal of Obstetrics and Gynaecology, 120*(11), 1348–1355.
11. Abbott, J. A. (2017). Adenomyosis and Abnormal Uterine Bleeding (AUB-A): Pathogenesis, diagnosis, and management. *Best Practice and Research. Clinical Obstetrics and Gynaecology, 40*, 68–81.
12. Zhou, J., et al. (2016). Vaginal repair of cesarean section scar diverticula that resulted in improved postoperative menstruation. *Journal of Minimally Invasive Gynecology, 23*(6), 969–978.
13. van der Voet, L. F., et al. (2014). Long-term complications of caesarean section. The niche in the scar: A prospective cohort study on niche prevalence and its relation to abnormal uterine bleeding. *BJOG: An International Journal of Obstetrics and Gynaecology, 121*(2), 236–244.
14. Vervoort, A. J., et al. (2015). Why do niches develop in Caesarean uterine scars? Hypotheses on the aetiology of niche development. *Human Reproduction, 30*(12), 2695–2702.
15. Vervoort, A. J., et al. (2015). The HysNiche trial: Hysteroscopic resection of uterine caesarean scar defect (niche) in patients with abnormal bleeding, a randomised controlled trial. *BMC Women's Health, 15*, 103.
16. Bacon, J. L. (2017). Abnormal uterine bleeding: Current classification and clinical management. *Obstetrics and Gynecology Clinics of North America, 44*(2), 179–193.
17. Tabrizi, A. D., et al. (2014). Antiproliferative effect of metformin on the endometrium—a clinical trial. *Asian Pacific Journal of Cancer Prevention: APJCP, 15*(23), 10067–10070.
18. Critchley, H. O., & Maybin, J. A. (2011). Molecular and cellular causes of abnormal uterine bleeding of endometrial origin. *Seminars in Reproductive Medicine, 29*(5), 400–409.
19. Maybin, J. A., Critchley, H. O., & Jabbour, H. N. (2011). Inflammatory pathways in endometrial disorders. *Molecular and Cellular Endocrinology, 335*(1), 42–51.
20. Grunloh, D. S., et al. (2013). Characteristics associated with discontinuation of long-acting reversible contraception within the first 6 months of use. *Obstetrics and Gynecology, 122*(6), 1214–1221.
21. Warner, P., Critchley, H. O., Lumsden, M. A., Campbell-Brown, M., Douglas, A., & Murray, G. (2001). Referral for menstrual problems:cross sectional survey of symptoms, reasons for referral, and management. *British Medical Journal, 323*, 24–28.
22. Hale, G., Manconi, F., Luscombe, G., & Fraser, I. S. (2010). Quantitative measurements of menstrual blood loss in ovulatory and anovulatory cycles in middle and late reproductive age and the menopausal transition. *Obstetrics and Gynecology, 115*, 249–256.
23. Hingham, J., OBrien, P. M., & Shaw, R. W. (1990). Assessment of menstrual blood loss using a pictoral chart. *British Journal of Obstetrics and Gynaecology, 97*(8), 734–739.
24. Billow, M., & El-Nashar, S. A. (2016). Management of abnormal uterine bleeding with emphasis on alternatives to hysterectomy. *Obstetrics and Gynecology Clinics of North America, 43*, 415–430.
25. Adams, T., & Denny, L. (2017). Abnormal vaginal bleeding in women with gynaecological malignancies. *Best Practice and Research. Clinical Obstetrics and Gynaecology, 40*, 134–147.
26. Sriprasert, I., et al. (2017). Heavy menstrual bleeding diagnosis and medical management. *Contraception and Reproductive Medicine, 2*, 20.

27. Graziano, A., et al. (2015). Diagnostic findings in adenomyosis: A pictorial review on the major concerns. *European Review for Medical and Pharmacological Sciences, 19*(7), 1146–1154.

28. Tzur, T., Kessous, R., & Weintraub, A. Y. (2017). Current strategies in the diagnosis of endometrial cancer. *Archives of Gynecology and Obstetrics, 296*(1), 5–14.

29. Clark, T., & Stevenson, H. (2016). Endometrial polyps and abnormal uterine bleeding (AUB-P): What is the relationship, how are they diagnosed, and how are they treated? *Best Practice and Research. Clinical Obstetrics and Gynaecology, 40*, 89–104.

30. Bouzid, A., et al. (2016). [Feasibility and diagnostic value of hysterosonography performed in bleeding time in the exploration of abnormal uterine bleeding]. *Journal de Gynecologie, Obstetrique et Biologie de la Reproduction, 45*(9), 1067–1073.

31. Heikinheimo, O., et al. (2014). Bleeding pattern and user satisfaction in second consecutive levonorgestrel-releasing intrauterine system users: Results of a prospective 5-year study. *Human Reproduction, 29*(6), 1182–1188.

32. Deligeoroglou, E. Abnormal Uterine Bleeding including coagulopathies and other menstrual disorders. 2017.

33. Kaunitz, A. M., et al. (2009). Adding low-dose estrogen to the hormone-free interval: Impact on bleeding patterns in users of a 91-day extended regimen oral contraceptive. *Contraception, 79*(5), 350–355.

34. Anderson, F. D., & Hait, H. (2003). A multicenter, randomized study of an extended cycle oral contraceptive. *Contraception, 68*(2), 89–96.

35. James, A. H. (2016). Heavy menstrual bleeding: Work-up and management. *Hematology / the Education Program of the American Society of Hematology. American Society of Hematology. Education Program, 2016*(1), 236–242.

36. Qaraaty, M., et al. (2014). Effect of myrtle fruit syrup on abnormal uterine bleeding: A randomized double-blind, placebo-controlled pilot study. *Daru, 22*, 45.

37. Munro, M. G. (2017). Endometrial ablation. *Best Practice and Research. Clinical Obstetrics and Gynaecology.*

38. Crawford, N. M., et al. (2016). Prospective evaluation of the impact of intermenstrual bleeding on natural fertility. *Fertility and Sterility, 105*(5), 1294–1300.

CHAPTER **142**

DYSMENORRHEA

Elke Zschaebitz • Emily Proulx

DEFINITION AND EPIDEMIOLOGY

The term *dysmenorrhea,* from the Greek word meaning "difficult monthly flow," refers to painful menstruation. Dysmenorrhea is classified as either a primary or a secondary gynecologic disorder. Primary dysmenorrhea is defined as painful menses despite normal pelvic anatomy and ovulation occurring within 6 to 12 months after menarche, when ovulatory cycles are established.[1] However, primary dysmenorrhea can begin as late as 1 to 3 years after menarche and is characterized by cramping pelvic pain just before or with the onset of menstrual flow and typically lasting 1 to 3 days,[2] with a peak in the second and third decades of life and subsequently decreasing with advancing age. Secondary dysmenorrhea usually appears later in life, after some years of painless menstruation, and is associated with underlying pathologic processes such as endometriosis, uterine fibroids, adenomyosis, pelvic inflammatory disease, ovarian cysts, polyps, intrauterine adhesions, cervical stenosis, other pelvic pathologic conditions, or an intrauterine contraceptive device (IUD).

Dysmenorrhea is the most common gynecological symptom reported by women. Prevalence rates vary considerably based on geographical location and are widespread in diverse populations, ranging between 20% and 90%.[3] In the United States, dysmenorrhea is one of the most commonly encountered gynecologic disorders, estimated to affect 50% to 60% of reproductive-age women overall and up to 90% of adolescents. The peak incidence of dysmenorrhea is highest during adolescence, and approximately 15% of women who experience dysmenorrhea have discomfort that interferes with normal daily activity for 1 to 3 days each month, with 51% of women having missed work or school because of their symptoms.[1] It is difficult to estimate the economic burden of missed work from dysmenorrhea, but clearly it accounts for significant lost wages and diminished quality of life. Nevertheless, many women "suffer silently" and do not discuss dysmenorrhea with any health care provider. Adolescents, in particular, are unlikely to consult a health care provider about dysmenorrhea and have a tendency to self-medicate with over-the-counter medications.[1] Providers should be aware that the quality of a woman's life can be improved by reducing or relieving the discomfort of dysmenorrhea. In addition, the willingness to discuss this common but possibly sensitive issue may pave the way to a more satisfying patient-provider relationship.

PATHOPHYSIOLOGY

Primary dysmenorrhea has been attributed to ovulatory cycles and the maturation of the hypothalamic-pituitary-gonadal axis. Dysmenorrhea is caused by an excess or imbalance of prostaglandins, vasopressin, and chemical substances originating from phospholipids.[6] These chemicals cause uterine contractions, cramping, nausea, vomiting, and diarrhea. Risk factors for dysmenorrhea include adolescence, anxiety, depression, stress, body mass index below 20 or above 30 kg/m^2, menorrhagia, metrorrhagia, nulliparity, and smoking. Contractions in the menstruating uterus and pain have been attributed to the production of prostaglandins, specifically $PGF_{2\alpha}$ and PGE_2.[2] The prostaglandins also cause the nausea and diarrhea associated with dysmenorrhea. Current evidence shows that the menstrual fluid of women with primary dysmenorrhea has higher-than-normal levels of these prostaglandins.[1,7] Anovulatory cycles are associated with lower levels of prostaglandins and, as a result, usually no dysmenorrhea.[2]

Despite the supporting evidence for a link between higher prostaglandin levels and dysmenorrhea, it is likely that the explanation for menstrual pain is not as simple as the cyclic production of one hormone. Women with dysmenorrhea may have complex alterations in hormonal patterns that exist throughout the cycle and affect a number of factors, including higher basal body temperature and disrupted sleep patterns. Vasopressin may also play a role by increasing uterine contractility and causing ischemic pain as a result of vasoconstriction. Elevated vasopressin levels have been reported in women with primary dysmenorrhea.[1] In addition, women have differing perceptions of pain, and this may affect how they experience dysmenorrhea. Research suggests that many factors are related to dysmenorrhea, including younger age, low body mass index, smoking, early menarche, pelvic infections, genetic influence, and history of pelvic assault.

There is no convincing evidence that mechanical cervical obstruction or severe uterine flexion causing obstructed uterine flow is present in patients with primary dysmenorrhea, although heavy menstrual flow is associated with dysmenorrhea. Some studies have suggested that young age and nulliparity are associated with dysmenorrhea, but the correlation with age was not substantiated in other studies once parity and other factors were controlled for.[1] There is also no evidence to support an association between tubal sterilization and the prevalence of dysmenorrhea.[1]

Although dysmenorrhea is no longer considered a psychological disorder, risk factors for dysmenorrhea have been investigated, including socioeconomic, behavioral, and psychological variables. A systematic review of several studies has suggested a significant inverse relationship between age and the risk of dysmenorrhea. A concurrent family history of dysmenorrhea, perceived stress levels, and heavy or irregular menstrual cycles have also been linked to dysmenorrhea in many studies. Stress has been demonstrated to indirectly affect prostaglandin synthesis and concentrations through the release of corticotropin-releasing hormone. Prostaglandins affect uterine muscle and vascular tone, and an imbalance of prostaglandins has been linked to the occurrence of dysmenorrhea.[1] Stress inhibits the release of follicle-stimulating hormone and luteinizing hormones, leading to impaired follicular development. This pathway can alter progesterone synthesis and release, which can alter the activity of prostaglandin. Stress-related hormones also appear to influence prostaglandin synthesis and/or binding in the myometrium of the uterus. Studies have also confirmed a relationship between dysmenorrhea and psychological factors such as depression and anxiety, although the nature of these relationships are unclear.[4] Abnormal and painful menstruation in adolescent girls can also cause psychological and emotional strain and thus the relationship between dysmenorrhea and emotional distress is likely bidirectional to some extent.[5]

Fruit and vegetable intake has been found to have some benefit in the treatment of dysmenorrhea. The protective effect of oral contraceptives or other hormonal contraceptive forms such as IUDs has been evident and consistent across different study types; IUDs containing hormones were found to have a positive effect on dysmenorrhea pain. Interestingly, there was no significant association between tubal ligation and dysmenorrhea.

Conflicting results were found in studies examining sociodemographic factors such as employment, socioeconomic status, body mass index, and the effect of exercise on dysmenorrhea. No associations between alcohol consumption and dysmenorrhea were found, and the association with cigarette smoking yielded mixed results.[1] The lack of data and the conflicting data are attributed to the limited number of studies as well as the small study samples in examining variables and the biases noted in systematic reviews.

Cultural and family influences may have a profound effect on how a woman experiences dysmenorrhea. The attitudes a woman has toward menstruation are often formed early in life and may be influenced by factors that include culture, religion, family, friends, and sexual partners. Additional emotional influences may be related to perceptions of fertility, the ability to bear children, or the relationship with the sexual partner. Many women begin menstruating with little or no accurate information, and menstrual sensations and discomfort may be distressing, frightening, or viewed as punishment. A woman's beliefs about menstruation may directly affect the way she experiences it and her willingness to report any problems to her provider or to seek treatment. The variation rates examining the prevalence globally in studies are attributed to the lack of standard methods for assessing the severity of dysmenorrhea in various cultures.[1]

Secondary dysmenorrhea is associated with underlying pelvic pathology and needs to be investigated to determine the cause. Secondary dysmenorrhea is caused by a pathologic process that affects the uterus, fallopian tubes, ovaries, or pelvic peritoneum. These processes can cause pain by altering pressures in or around pelvic structures, changing or restricting blood flow, or irritating the pelvic peritoneum. They can occur with the normal physiology of menstruation or act completely independently, with symptoms appearing during specific points in the menstrual cycle. Extrauterine causes must also be considered in the differential diagnosis; associated pelvic, bladder, and abdominal structural problems as well as causes related to previous surgical history may exist with chronic pelvic pain syndromes that suggest dysmenorrhea.

CLINICAL PRESENTATION AND PHYSICAL EXAMINATION

The diagnosis of primary dysmenorrhea is based on clinical features determined with a careful and detailed history of symptoms. The history should include age at menarche, menstrual history, last menstrual period, location and severity of discomfort, associated symptoms (headache, dizziness, nausea, vomiting, diarrhea, dyschezia), amount of school or work missed, medications, method of birth control, and whether the birth control is being used correctly. Abdominal and pelvic pain not related to the menstrual cycle should also be considered in the differential diagnosis.

Pain descriptions can vary significantly from individual to individual. Young women will generally report recurrent sharp, crampy pelvic pain, spasmodic lower abdominal pain, or pain over the suprapubic area. The pain will often radiate to the back, sacrum, or inner thighs. The pain usually begins a few hours before or just after the onset of menstruation and lasts the first 1 to 3 days of menstruation; it can be associated with nausea, vomiting, diarrhea, low back pain, or headache. Some young women also have associated systemic symptoms, including nausea, vomiting, loose bowel movements, and dizziness. Consideration should be given to symptoms exacerbated by dysmenorrhea such as irritable bowel syndrome, interstitial cystitis, or migraines.[2]

Secondary dysmenorrhea is distinguished from primary dysmenorrhea by a history of pain that is inconsistent with the kind of low anterior pelvic pain described as beginning in adolescence and associated specifically with menstrual cycles. The signs and symptoms of secondary dysmenorrhea are related to an underlying pathologic process. The onset of secondary dysmenorrhea usually occurs in women 30 or 40 years of age rather than shortly after menarche. The pain is often not limited to the menses and is less related to the 48 to 72 hours of menstrual flow. There may be an array of associated symptoms in secondary dysmenorrhea, including dyspareunia, infertility, and abnormal bleeding.

Physical examination findings are normal in primary dysmenorrhea. The diagnosis is based on a careful history. It is appropriate to perform only an abdominal examination in young women with a typical history of low anterior pelvic pain beginning in adolescence and associated specifically with the menstrual cycle.

When the history or physical examination suggests secondary dysmenorrhea (i.e., an atypical history or physical findings of pelvic mass, abnormal vaginal or pelvic tenderness not limited to the menstrual cycle), the evaluation should follow accordingly and is based on the suspicion of an underlying pathologic condition. The physical examination for secondary dysmenorrhea must include a thorough abdominal, pelvic, and rectovaginal examination. Clues to diagnosis may be asymmetric enlargement of the uterus or adnexa (indicating myomas or other tumors), symmetric enlargement (indicating adenomyosis), painful nodules in the posterior cul-de-sac together with restricted motion of the uterus (indicating endometriosis), cervical stenosis (suggesting retrograde menstruation), or restricted motion of the uterus together with thickened adnexal structures (indicating pelvic scarring or adhesions).

DIAGNOSTICS

No diagnostic studies are needed for the diagnosis of primary dysmenorrhea. However, if the diagnosis of primary versus secondary dysmenorrhea is not clear or the pelvic examination suggests pelvic disease, additional diagnostic tests are indicated.

Essential Diagnostics

Pelvic ultrasonography is often a helpful initial diagnostic test to rule out anatomic abnormalities, such as ovarian cysts and endometriomas.[1] Sonovaginography (i.e., transvaginal ultrasonography with saline infusion of the uterus) may be more helpful than transvaginal ultrasonography in diagnosis of endometriosis.[1]

Additional Diagnostics

In some instances, an abdominal or pelvic computed tomography (CT) scan may be indicated. Laboratory evaluation may include a complete blood count (CBC) and differential, erythrocyte sedimentation rate (ESR), genital cultures for pathogens, serum human chorionic gonadotropin (hCG), and urinalysis and Pap test. If the final diagnosis is still unconfirmed, the patient may require a laparoscopy, hysteroscopy, or dilation and curettage.

DIFFERENTIAL DIAGNOSIS

 Red flags include unilateral dysmenorrhea, signs and symptoms suggestive of acute abdomen or STDs. Pregnancy, especially ectopic pregnancy, should always be ruled out.

The diagnosis of primary dysmenorrhea is made by a careful history and clinical presentation. Secondary dysmenorrhea is more concerning because the cause can be pathologic, requiring treatment, and difficult to determine. The causes can be broadly classified as intrauterine or extrauterine. Intrauterine causes include myomas, adenomyosis, polyps, an IUD, infection, cervical stenosis, and cervical lesions. Unilateral dysmenorrhea is relatively rare and may manifest as an acute abdomen, but it should also raise the suspicion of uterine malformation.[8] Extrauterine causes include endometriosis, tumors (myomas or malignant), inflammation, sexually transmitted infections, adhesions, psychogenic causes such as pelvic congestion syndrome, and nongynecologic causes (urologic, gastrointestinal, musculoskeletal, and psychiatric conditions). Pregnancy, especially ectopic pregnancy, should always be a consideration in a female patient of childbearing age.

Chronic cyclic pelvic pain (CCPP) is a subset of chronic pelvic pain that occurs in relation to the menstrual cycle; however, CCPP also refers to cyclically occurring pelvic pain that may not be related to the menstrual cycle. For example,

pain associated with ovulation (mittelschmerz) or pain associated with intercourse may occur with a cyclic pattern but is not related to menstruation as is dysmenorrhea.

Dysmenorrhea (primary and secondary) is also a distinct and separate entity from premenstrual syndrome (PMS), and the two should not be confused. PMS describes a predictable set of physical and affective symptoms that occur cyclically during the luteal phase and resolve quickly on or near the onset of the menstrual cycle. The ACOG define this condition as at least one symptom associated with "economic or social dysfunction; that occurs during the 5 days prior to onset of menses and is present in at least three consecutive menstrual cycles." These symptoms may be concurrent with dysmenorrhea; however, their characteristics are distinct. The cause of PMS is not known, but it is a relatively uncommon disorder during adolescence, in contrast to primary dysmenorrhea, which affects the majority of adolescent girls.

INTERPROFESSIONAL COLLABORATIVE MANAGEMENT
Nonpharmacologic Management

The role of nutrition (e.g., arachidonic acid as a precursor to prostaglandin formation) has led to an inquiry on a low-fat diet rich in fish (especially salmon, tuna, and halibut), beans, seeds (particularly pumpkin, sesame, and sunflower), whole grains, fruits, and vegetables to decrease arachidonic acid. Similarly, the impact of nutritional supplements on menstrual pain has been studied in small trials including vitamin B1 (thiamine), vitamin B3 (niacin), vitamin B6 (pyridoxine), zinc, calcium, magnesium, and omega-3 fatty acids. Patients frequently ask about herbal therapies for dysmenorrhea. The Society of Obstetricians and Gynecologists of Canada has noted that Toki-shakuyaku-san, an herbal preparation, may or may not be helpful for some patients with dysmenorrhea (Grade C, Level II: evidence is conflicting).

Other interventions include behavioral interventions such as relaxation training, biofeedback, and mind-body awareness, as well as an examination of the impact of exercise, chiropractic and osteopathic treatment, acupuncture, and transcutaneous electrical nerve stimulation (TENS). Heat therapy has been used for millennia (e.g., hot water bottles, hot baths, and heating pads). New modalities such as heat patches and wearable heating devices should not be dismissed as a treatment option.

Pharmacologic Management

A variety of therapies have been used to treat dysmenorrhea, but the standard treatments have not been well examined over the past 30 years. The mainstays for treatment of primary dysmenorrhea are nonsteroidal antiinflammatory drugs (NSAIDs), which are antiprostaglandins, and hormonal contraceptives. NSAIDs are the best-established initial therapy for dysmenorrhea. They inhibit prostaglandin synthesis and thereby provide pain relief. In addition, they decrease the volume of menstrual flow, which may mitigate the dysmenorrhea.[6] Randomized controlled trials of NSAIDs suggest that all of the NSAIDs studied are more effective in treating dysmenorrhea than acetaminophen, although no studies have clearly determined which NSAIDs are the most efficacious. NSAIDs may be the most effective when therapy is started before the onset of menstrual pain and flow, and they need not be continued for the entire menstrual cycle.[1]

Some women suffer from NSAID resistant dysmenorrhea, and therefore it is important for providers to be aware of alternative treatments.[10] Small studies have shown that cycooxygenase-2 (COX-2) inhibitors are as beneficial as NSAIDs in the treatment of dysmenorrhea.[1] The choice for any particular drug may be determined by a woman's preference based on individual experience, administration patterns, side effects, and cost.

Treatment of dysmenorrhea is a well-recognized off-label use for oral contraceptive pills,[9] although more studies need to address the efficacy of oral contraceptives in the management of dysmenorrhea. Combined oral contraceptives, and in particular monophasic contraceptives, that are in continuous use without a placebo week, therefore avoiding the withdrawal bleed, can be of benefit. Oral contraceptives suppress ovulation and creation of a cyclic pattern of serum estrogen and progesterone, resulting in diminished endometrial thickening, decreased prostaglandin release during menstruation, and consequent pain reduction. However, there are concerns that the estradiol component of OCPs could exacerbate endometriosis.[10] If the discomfort of primary dysmenorrhea is not controlled with NSAIDs or oral contraceptives, further diagnostic evaluation is indicated to exclude a pathologic pelvic condition.

There is some evidence that Mirena®, the levonorgestrel-releasing IUD, may reduce dysmenorrhea because the progestin may act directly on the endometrium to reduce endometrial proliferation, menstrual flow, and pain. This IUD has been introduced in Europe for the management of primary and secondary dysmenorrhea but is not currently labeled for this use in the United States.[1] Another option that may be available in the near future is a vasopressin receptor antagonist.

Other approaches used in the management of dysmenorrhea, including calcium channel blockers (such as nifedipine or diltiazem), tocolytic agents (such as albuterol [Salbutamol]), progestogens, acupuncture, herbal remedies, exercise, a low-fat vegetarian diet, increased dietary fiber, castor oil packs to the abdomen, vitamin E (500 IU for 2 days before and 3 days after the onset of menses or 500 IU daily during the menstrual period), fish oil supplements, psychotherapy, and hypnosis, have proven beneficial in some studies.[1] A more recent meta-analysis found moxibustion and acupoint therapy effective in treating the pain associated with dysmenorrhea, although more studies are needed. High-intensity TENS was also associated with pain improvement in dysmenorrhea in one small study (level of evidence: moderate).[10]

Narcotic analgesics should not be used for the typical level of discomfort associated with dysmenorrhea. Not only do narcotics raise issues related to prescription drug abuse, but the side effects of narcotics, such as sedation, and potential drug interactions may further affect a woman's ability to fully participate in daily life activities.

Hysterectomy is considered a viable option for the treatment of severe, refractory dysmenorrhea.[1] Presacral neurectomy and uterosacral ligament division were used in the past to treat dysmenorrhea but are rarely performed today. These treatments of primary dysmenorrhea may also assist in the treatment of secondary dysmenorrhea. However, successful treatment of secondary dysmenorrhea depends on an accurate diagnosis of the cause of the pelvic pain. In the absence of a clear diagnosis, nonacute pain can be treated empirically for a short time with some of the interventions described.

Indications for Referral or Hospitalization

Patients with recalcitrant primary dysmenorrhea and no apparent secondary causes found by physical examination, laboratory, and radiologic studies need to be referred to a gynecologist for possible surgical diagnostic evaluation and treatment. Referral is also necessary if a secondary cause requiring surgical intervention is found. In difficult cases, psychological factors must be considered, and mental health referral may be warranted.

COMPLICATIONS

Dysmenorrhea may be a difficult and frustrating condition to treat in some patients. If patients diagnosed with primary dysmenorrhea do not respond to conventional treatment, the diagnosis may need to be reassessed.

PATIENT AND FAMILY EDUCATION

- Women receiving NSAID therapy should understand the potential gastrointestinal adverse effects associated with NSAIDs.
- Modifiable risk factors, such as smoking and pelvic infections, may contribute to dysmenorrhea. Education directed toward reducing or eliminating these risk factors may be helpful.
- Stress reduction may be an effective preventive strategy for some and should be included in education about a healthy lifestyle.

HEALTH PROMOTION

Primary dysmenorrhea is a common condition throughout the world with a wide range of treatments available based on evidence and ongoing trials. The opportunity to recognize and support this condition, particularly for women who are incapacitated by their symptoms, is a need that the primary care provider can successfully fill while helping counsel healthy lifestyle choices.

REFERENCES

1. Ju, H., Jones, M., & Mishra, G. (2014). The prevalence and risk factors of dysmenorrhea. *Epidemiologic Reviews, 36*, 104–113.
2. The American College of Obstetricians and Gynecologists (2015). Dysmenorrhea: painful periods. www.acog.org/-/media/For-Patients/faq046.pdf?dmc=1&ts=20150623T1027000437.
3. Burnett, M., & Lemyre, M. (2017). No. 345—Primary dysmenorrhea consensus guideline. *Journal of Obstetrics and Gynaecology Canada, 39*(7), 585–595.
4. Payne, L., Rapkin, A., & Seidman, L. (2013). Relationships among dysmenorrhea, emotion regulation, and acute laboratory pain in healthy girls and adolescents. *Journal of Pain, 4*(1), S33.
5. Jamieson, M. A. (2015). Disorders of menstruation in adolescent girls. *Pediatric Clinics of North America, 62*(4), 943–961.
6. Majoribanks, S., Ayeleke, R. O., Farcuhar, C., et al. (2015). Nonsteroidal anti-inflammatory drugs for dysmenorrhea. *The Cochrane Database of Systematic Reviews*, (7), CD001751, http://admin.wol2.wiley.com/cochrane-database-of-systematic-reviews/table-of-contents/2015/Issue7/.
7. Wu, L., Su, C., & Liu, C. (2012). Effects of noninvasive electroacupuncture at Hegu (LI4) and Sanyinjiao (SP6) acupoints on dysmenorrhea: A randomized controlled trial. *Journal of Alternative and Complementary Medicine (New York, N.Y.), 18*(2), 137–142.
8. Borah, T., Das, A., Panda, A., et al. (2010). A case of unilateral dysmenorrhea. *Journal of Human Reproductive Sciences, 3*, 158–159.
9. Won, H., & Abbott, J. (2010). Optimal management of chronic cyclical pelvic pain: An evidence-based and pragmatic approach. *International Journal of Women's Health, 2*, 263–277.
10. Oladosu, F. A., Tu, F. F., & Hellman, K. M. (2018). Nonsteroidal antiinflammatory drug resistance in dysmenorrhea: Epidemiology, causes, and treatment. *American Journal of Obstetrics and Gynecology, 218*(4), 390–400.

DEFINITION AND EPIDEMIOLOGY

Dyspareunia is defined as recurrent or persistent genital pain with sexual activity that causes marked distress. The condition is not unique to women; men can have dyspareunia from a variety of causes, including dermatologic infections, structural abnormalities, and exposure to alloplastic materials via partners who have had pelvic floor surgery; anodyspareunia can occur in men who have receptive anal sex. However, it is much more commonly encountered in women and is therefore almost exclusively described as a women's health issue. Dyspareunia can develop secondary to other vulvar problems, including inflammatory, neoplastic, or traumatic conditions, or be associated with localized provoked vulvodynia (LPV), vaginismus, or vulvodynia. LPV, formerly known as vulvar vestibulitis, refers to severe pain on vestibular contact or with attempted vaginal entry, tenderness to pressure within the vestibule, and vulvar erythema. Vaginismus is involuntary spasm of the muscles surrounding the outer third of the vagina brought on by real, imagined, or anticipated attempts at vaginal penetration. Vulvodynia refers to idiopathic chronic vulvar pain[1] that may involve complaints of rawness, burning, stinging, or irritation; it is not necessarily related to sexual activity.

Dyspareunia is a common gynecologic complaint, which is estimated to affect around half of all women at some point in their life.[2] The problem can be thought of as either superficial (pain around the vaginal opening) or deep (pain in the lower abdomen or pelvic organs). Factors influencing dyspareunia include spontaneous and postabortive pelvic inflammatory disease, postpartum[3–5] or perimenopausal status,[6] vaginal dryness,[7] and generalized urogenital sensitivity. Women with endometriosis have a ninefold increase in risk for dyspareunia.[8,9] Psychosocial factors such as a history of childhood sexual or physical abuse, rigid religious upbringing, low physical and emotional satisfaction, decreased general happiness, or previous painful sexual experience may also be contributory. Dyspareunia has not been consistently associated with factors such as age, parity, marital status, race, income, or education, and there is no increase in prevalence among women seeking fertility treatment.[10] Hormonal and sexual history factors including oral contraception use[11] (especially before age 17 years) and first intercourse before age 15 years have been proposed as causes of LPV. Women with LPV have demonstrated lower pain threshold, higher magnitude estimation of pain, higher trait anxiety, increased somatization, poorer body image than controls, hypervigilance for coital pain, and selective attentional bias toward pain stimuli.

PATHOPHYSIOLOGY

Pain in the vulvar area can result from inflammatory conditions (endometriosis, interstitial cystitis, or inflammatory bowel disorders), atrophic dermatologic conditions, assorted pelvic pathologies including leiomyoma,[12] neoplasm, neurologic dysfunction, trauma (horseback riding, sexual abuse, traumatic childbirth,[13] and genital mutilation[14]), chemotherapy, and genital manifestations of other systemic diseases such as discoid lupus erythematosus, nonalcoholic liver disease (by decreasing vaginal lubrication), Ehlers-Danlos,[15] Charcot-Marie-Tooth,[16] and multiple sclerosis (MS).[17] Vulvar pain may be sequelae of iatrogenesis (pelvic radiation, chemotherapy, graft-vs-host reaction, pelvic surgery), an acute or chronic infectious process (human semen carries the irritating toxin ciguatera), or the result of psycho-social-sexual disturbance. Although the *Diagnostic and Statistical Manual of Mental Disorders* currently classifies dyspareunia as a sexual pain disorder, there is debate as to whether dyspareunia reflects a predominant psychopathology, a condition of sexual dysfunction, or a physical pain syndrome. However it is classified academically, there is evidence of high levels of psychological distress in some women with dyspareunia,[18–20] particularly those with PVD and vulvodynia.

Dyspareunia is often due to inadequate vaginal lubrication.[7] This can be attributable to insufficient stimulation or arousal during sexual activity or can be related to decreased estrogen, a condition noted in postmenopausal women, women taking tamoxifen for chemoprevention of breast cancer, women who breastfeed after childbirth,[4] and breast cancer survivors. Superficial dyspareunia has been associated with lichen planus and lichen sclerosis, factitious urticaria, vulvovaginal candidal infection and recurrent candidiasis, bacterial vaginosis, HSV 1 and 2 infection, HPV infection, urinary tract infections, urinary incontinence, occlusion of Bartholin's gland duct, Bowen's disease, and interstitial cystitis. Tiny mucosal tears have been implicated in focal vulvitis, and perivascular inflammation has been proposed as a mechanism causing dyspareunia in women with Sjögren syndrome. Dyspareunia after a normal pelvic examination has been linked with overexertion of the levator ani muscles and subsequent myalgia after the initiation of Kegel exercises. When the levator ani muscles are hypertonic, vaginismus can result.

In PVD, a conditioned, protective, muscle-guarding response has been proposed, leading to a pelvic floor pathologic condition. Vaginismus cannot easily be distinguished from vestibulitis/PVD by vaginal spasm and pain alone, but women with vaginismus demonstrate significantly greater vaginal and pelvic muscle tone and lower muscle strength, have a higher frequency of defensive and avoidant distress behaviors during pelvic examinations, and recall past attempts at intercourse with more affective distress.

By far the most common cause of deep dyspareunia in premenopausal women is endometriosis,[21] especially when it involves the rectovaginal area. Women with deep infiltrating endometriosis of the uterosacral ligament can have severe impairment of sexual function, and many have had deep dyspareunia for their entire sex lives. Structural abnormalities that can cause dyspareunia include glomus tumors; leiomyomas of the uterus and urethra; vaginal, urethral, and hymenal abnormalities; bladder stones; postobstetric or postoperative vulvar outlet stenosis; and stenosing lichen planus. Aortoiliac or atherosclerotic disease can diminish pelvic blood flow and lead to vaginal wall and clitoral smooth muscle fibrosis. Pelvic floor surgery can either ameliorate preexisting dyspareunia or cause it.[22,23] Episiotomies, particularly those involving the mediolateral technique and glycerol-impregnated chromic catgut, have been tied to significant increases in dyspareunia.[24] Obstetric instrumentation and perineal trauma during delivery contribute to postpartum dyspareunia.

CLINICAL PRESENTATION AND PHYSICAL EXAMINATION

Health care providers need to take an active role in inquiring specifically about discomfort during or after sexual intercourse and not simply assume that women will raise the issue if it is a problem. Women often will not voice this concern even if it is the main reason for their visit. Although some women will discuss dyspareunia with their partner, far fewer consult a health care provider for the problem.[25]

A thorough symptom analysis will guide the physical examination and should specifically include questioning about the onset of the discomfort and its relationship to particular partners, positions, times in the menstrual cycle, contraceptive devices and substances (such as latex condoms, spermicides, or lubricants), and products (such as douches, soaps, tampons, or detergents). Women may report pain with tampon use or pelvic examinations. Important information to gather includes number of pregnancies and type of delivery, surgical history, history of rape or sexual abuse, and menopausal signs and symptoms. Knowing whether the pain is on entry, postcoital, generalizable to the entire vulva, felt only with deep thrusting, or localized to a particular anatomic structure or area is helpful in determining the cause of the discomfort. Several symptom-related scales have been proposed, such as the Female Sexual Function Index, but are not widely used in clinical practice.

A thorough pelvic examination is necessary for all complaints of dyspareunia. The experience can be educational for the woman and more informative for the provider if the patient sits somewhat upright and holds a small hand mirror; this allows the woman to see what is happening and feel more in control. It is important to correlate the discomfort elicited during the pelvic examination with specific physical findings whenever possible. In addition, clarification should be sought for pain elicited to determine whether it is similar to what the woman has been experiencing during intercourse, because many women find pelvic examinations generally uncomfortable.

The external genitals should be examined for erythema, pigment changes, lesions (including herpes and condyloma), and indications of trauma or abuse. Touching of the vestibule and the hymen with a moistened cotton swab (the Q-tip test) may elicit the pain of PVD, a condition in which there is exquisite tenderness to pressure at specific sites, often accompanied by erythema.

A finger inserted gently into the introitus and gradually pressed in a posterior direction may elicit the spasms of vaginismus; conscious control of the pelvic floor musculature can be evaluated by asking the woman to squeeze and relax the muscles around the examiner's finger. Bartholin's glands, which are normally not palpable, may be tender and enlarged. A narrow, well-lubricated speculum should be used to evaluate the vagina. A bimanual examination can assess for uterine and ovarian size, fibroids, ovarian cysts, other pelvic masses, cervical motion tenderness (seen with pelvic inflammatory disease), and position of the uterus. Hemorrhoids or prolapse of the uterus, bladder, or rectum may be evident. A rectal or rectovaginal examination is generally not necessary.

DIAGNOSTICS

Wet mounts, potassium hydroxide (KOH) preparation and cultures of vaginal discharge, endocervical Pap smear, and *Chlamydia trachomatis* and *Neisseria gonorrhoeae* cultures will help rule out infection as a cause of either superficial or deep dyspareunia. The Q-tip test (assessing for localized discomfort by means of touching a swab to the vulvar or vaginal epithelium) can identify local sites of allodynia.

A complete blood count (CBC) and erythrocyte sedimentation rate (ESR) can help identify inflammation and infection; a urinalysis evaluates for urinary tract infection; and a human chorionic gonadotropin level can exclude ectopic pregnancy.

DIFFERENTIAL DIAGNOSIS

Potential causes of dyspareunia include psychological, physiological, and pathophysiologic factors, and most cases are probably multifactorial. A problem that is initially physical often has a continued and escalating psychological impact. The most likely causes of dyspareunia are endometriosis in reproductive-aged women and vaginal dryness/atrophy in postmenopausal women. Women at any phase of life can experience dyspareunia from insufficient arousal, vaginitis, vaginismus, hymenal abnormalities, dermatopathology, and postherpetic neuralgia. Dyspareunia may be focal (PVD/vulvar vestibulitis, residual scars or sutures, introital tears, herpetic lesions, urethral problems) or deep (endometriosis, fibroids, pelvic inflammatory disease, hemorrhoids, inflammatory bowel disease, retroverted uterus, uterine prolapse, pelvic adhesions or masses) and caused by irritants (contraceptive devices, spermicides, douches, feminine hygiene products, soaps, lubricants or moisturizers) or psychological factors (anxiety, previous abuse or trauma, prior painful sexual experiences).

INTERPROFESSIONAL COLLABORATIVE MANAGEMENT

Nonpharmacologic Management

Women with dyspareunia resulting from insufficient lubrication may benefit significantly from education about the physiology of female arousal and the importance of allowing adequate time before vaginal penetration for the vascular engorgement of genital tissues that results in glandular secretions. Women with mild symptoms may obtain relief from nonhormonal therapies, with or without a prescription. Vaginal lubricants should be optimally balanced in terms of pH and osmolality to be most similar to natural vaginal secretions.[7] Alternative sexual positioning (female astride to control penetration) or position changes can alleviate the pain of dyspareunia for some women, as can nonsteroidal agents, pelvic floor physical therapy,[26] or a warm bath before sex.

Some women have had a reduction in endometriosis-related dyspareunia on a gluten-free diet,[27] and others have had success with antioxidant (vitamins E and C) supplementation, suggesting a link with oxidative stress in the peritoneal cavity.[28] Psychological and behavioral treatments are first-line therapy for PVD/vulvar vestibulitis syndrome[29] and include mindfulness and cognitive behavioral therapy (CBT). PVD has been treated successfully with a low-oxalate diet and calcium citrate supplementation to neutralize urinary oxalates. Other therapeutic strategies include pelvic floor surface electromyography biofeedback, the manual techniques of pelvic floor physical therapists, and local application of capsaicin cream.

Treatment of vaginismus-related dyspareunia focuses on helping the woman regain voluntary control of the muscles of the pelvic floor,[30] and pelvic floor physical therapy is often quite helpful: therapeutic approaches most often involve pelvic floor contraction-relaxation exercises and using fingers or dilators to progressively desensitize the woman to vaginal penetration. Other approaches include biofeedback, sex and relationship counseling, psychotherapy, CBT, hypnotherapy, and lubricants.[31]

Pharmacologic Management

If the problem is estrogen-insufficient vaginal dryness, systemic estrogen or topical estrogen cream is the most effective way to build up the vascularity of the vaginal epithelium and thereby induce physiologic lubrication in moderate to severe vulvovaginal atrophy, with systemic therapies given in the lowest possible dose for the shortest possible time. For women in whom supplemental estrogen is not wanted or contraindicated, such as breast cancer survivors, ospemifene,[32-35] a selective estrogen receptor modulator, and topical aqueous lidocaine[36,37] in a compress to the vulvar vestibule have been utilized successfully. Potent topical steroids are indicated for lichen sclerosis. OnabotulinumtoxinA (Botox®) and lidocaine injections[38-40] have been used successfully in women with vaginismus. Surgical intervention is rarely required and may be detrimental to the resolution of vaginismus.

For PVD, topical amitriptyline cream (2% in sorbolene), topical estrogen cream applied twice a day for 4 to 8 weeks, and intralesional injections of interferon have been effective treatment strategies. Surgical intervention, such as a modified vestibulectomy[41] and vaginal apex repair, can be effective in cases refractory to more conservative approaches. Dyspareunia secondary to endometriosis has been treated successfully both hormonally and with surgical intervention; a combination of both may be more effective than either alone[42] and results in the lowest incidence of recurrence.

Indications for Referral

Women with dyspareunia related to severe psychological distress or anxiety may be best managed in collaboration with psychiatric or other counseling services. For severe PVD/vulvar vestibulitis unresponsive to conservative behavior-based therapies, perineoplasty or posterior vestibulectomy can be performed as a last resort and involves a crescent-shaped posterior vestibular excision followed by vaginal advancement. Surgery is less successful if there is concomitant vaginismus (unless the vaginismus is treated first), in dyspareunia present since first intercourse, and in women with associated persistent vulvar pain. Surgical referral for endomeriosis-related dyspareunia unresponsive to hormonal and nonhormonal treatment can offer women a significant improvement in symptoms.[8] For some women in whom dyspareunia is related to prior hysterectomy, surgical excision of the vaginal apex has been a successful surgical procedure.

LIFE SPAN CONSIDERATIONS

Dyspareunia affects sexually active women of all ages but may become increasingly evident at times of major transition in a woman's life, including onset of sexual activity, childbirth, and menopause.[43]

COMPLICATIONS

Dyspareunia is known to have a detrimental effect on relationships[44,45] and can affect the erectile function and sexual satisfaction of male partners.[46] The problem can continue unacknowledged and unaided for years in the absence of clinician inquiry and therapeutic involvement.[26,47-49] Although the morbidity associated with dyspareunia varies widely with its attendant cause, the impact on a woman's quality of life can be profound and should not be underestimated.

PATIENT AND FAMILY EDUCATION

Education is central in the management of dyspareunia, particularly when the cause of discomfort is attributable to insufficient sexual arousal time and lubrication, spasms of vaginismus, control of concomitant infections, or use of irritating or allergenic products. Taking the time to educate individuals about their bodies and the particular strategies necessary to attain or to resume sexual activity without discomfort is an important aspect of comprehensive, holistic primary care.

HEALTH PROMOTION

The World Health Organization (WHO) considers sexual health to be a state of physical, mental, and social well-being in relation to sexuality and also considers its quality as a health indicator. To the extent that dyspareunia has a detrimental impact on women's well-being, identification and alleviation of factors causing dyspareunia will continue to be a fruitful endeavor in the promotion of women's health.

INITIAL DIAGNOSTICS

Dyspareunia

LABORATORY
Initial Diagnostics
- Wet mount, KOH preparation
- Gonorrhea and chlamydia cultures

Further Diagnostics, if Indicated
- Pap smear
- Complete blood count and differential

- Erythrocyte sedimentation rate
- Urinalysis
- Serum level of human chorionic gonadotropin

IMAGING
- Pelvic ultrasound

REFERENCES

1. Pukall, C. (2016). Vulvodynia: Definition, prevalence, impact, and pathophysiological factors. *Sexual Medicine Reviews, 13*(3), 291–304.
2. Jamieson, D. J., & Steege, J. F. (1996). The prevalence of dysmenorrhea, dyspareunia, pelvic pain, and irritable bowel syndrome in primary care practices. *Obstetrics and Gynecology, 87*(1), 55–58.
3. Rosen, N. O., & Pukall, C. (2016). Comparing the prevalence, risk factors, and repercussions of postpartum genito-pelvic pain and dyspareunia. *Sexual Medicine Reviews, 4*(2), 126–135.
4. Trivino-Juarez, J. M., et al. (2018). Resumption of intercourse, self-reported decline in sexual intercourse and dyspareunia in women by mode of birth: A prospective follow-up study. *Journal of Advanced Nursing, 74*(3), 637–650.
5. Santoro, N. (2016). Comparing the prevalence, risk factors, and repercussions of postpartum genito-pelvic pain and dyspareunia. *Journal of Women's Health (2002), 4*(2), 126–135.
6. Santoro, N. (2016). Perimenopause: From research to practice. *Journal of Women's Health (2002), 25*(4), 332–339.
7. Edwards, D., & Panay, N. (2016). Treating vulvovaginal atrophy/genitourinary syndrome of menopause: How important is vaginal lubricant and moisturizer composition? *Climacteric: The Journal of the International Menopause Society, 19*(2), 151–161.
8. Fritzer, N., & Hudelist, G. (2017). Love is a pain? Quality of sex life after surgical resection of endometriosis: A review. *European Journal of Obstetrics, Gynecology, and Reproductive Biology, 209*, 72–76.
9. Vercellini, P., et al. (2011). Priorities for endometriosis research: A proposed focus on deep dyspareunia. *Reproductive Sciences, 18*(2), 114–118.

10. Furukawa, A. P., et al. (2012). Dyspareunia and sexual dysfunction in women seeking fertility treatment. *Fertility and Sterility, 98*(6), 1544–1548.e2.

11. Fugl-Meyer, K. S., et al. (2013). Standard operating procedures for female genital sexual pain. *The Journal of Sexual Medicine, 10*(1), 83–93.

12. Xin, J., et al. (2016). Bladder leiomyoma presenting as dyspareunia: Case report and literature review. *Medicine, 95*(28), e3971.

13. Andreucci, C. B., et al. (2015). Sexual life and dysfunction after maternal morbidity: A systematic review. *BMC Pregnancy and Childbirth, 15,* 307.

14. Berg, R. C., et al. (2014). Effects of female genital cutting on physical health outcomes: A systematic review and meta-analysis. *BMJ Open, 4*(11), e006316.

15. Hurst, B. S., et al. (2014). Obstetric and gynecologic challenges in women with Ehlers-Danlos syndrome. *Obstetrics and Gynecology, 123*(3), 506–513.

16. Gargiulo, P., et al. (2013). Sexual functioning in women with mild and severe symptoms of Charcot-Marie-Tooth disease. *The Journal of Sexual Medicine, 10*(7), 1800–1806.

17. Cordeau, D., & Courtois, F. (2014). Sexual disorders in women with MS: Assessment and management. *Annals of Physical and Rehabilitation Medicine, 57*(5), 337–347.

18. Pazmany, E., et al. (2013). Aspects of sexual self-schema in premenopausal women with dyspareunia: Associations with pain, sexual function, and sexual distress. *The Journal of Sexual Medicine, 10*(9), 2255–2264.

19. Fritzer, N., et al. (2013). More than just bad sex: Sexual dysfunction and distress in patients with endometriosis. *European Journal of Obstetrics, Gynecology, and Reproductive Biology, 169*(2), 392–396.

20. Pazmany, E., et al. (2013). Body image and genital self-image in premenopausal women with dyspareunia. *Archives of Sexual Behavior, 42*(6), 999–1010.

21. Barbara, G., et al. (2017). When love hurts. A systematic review on the effects of surgical and pharmacological treatments for endometriosis on female sexual functioning. *Acta Obstetricia et Gynecologica Scandinavica, 96*(6), 668–687.

22. Dietz, V., & Maher, C. (2013). Pelvic organ prolapse and sexual function. *International Urogynecology Journal, 24*(11), 1853–1857.

23. Crosby, E. C., et al. (2014). Symptom resolution after operative management of complications from transvaginal mesh. *Obstetrics and Gynecology, 123*(1), 134–139.

24. Islam, A., et al. (2013). Morbidity from episiotomy. *JPMA. The Journal of the Pakistan Medical Association, 63*(6), 696–701.

25. Mann, J., Shuster, J., & Moawad, N. (2013). Attributes and barriers to care of pelvic pain in university women. *Journal of Minimally Invasive Gynecology, 20*(6), 811–818.

26. Huffman, L. B., et al. (2016). Maintaining sexual health throughout gynecologic cancer survivorship: A comprehensive review and clinical guide. *Gynecologic Oncology, 140*(2), 359–368.

27. Marziali, M., et al. (2012). Gluten-free diet: A new strategy for management of painful endometriosis related symptoms? *Minerva Chirurgica, 67*(6), 499–504.

28. Santanam, N., et al. (2013). Antioxidant supplementation reduces endometriosis-related pelvic pain in humans. *Translational Research: The Journal of Laboratory and Clinical Medicine, 161*(3), 189–195.

29. Dunkley, C. R., & Brotto, L. A. (2016). Psychological treatments for provoked vestibulodynia: Integration of mindfulness-based and cognitive behavioral therapies. *Journal of Clinical Psychology, 72*(7), 637–650.

30. Reissing, E. D., Armstrong, H. L., & Allen, C. (2013). Pelvic floor physical therapy for lifelong vaginismus: A retrospective chart review and interview study. *Journal of Sex & Marital Therapy, 39*(4), 306–320.

31. Pacik, P. T. (2014). Understanding and treating vaginismus: A multimodal approach. *International Urogynecology Journal, 25*(12), 1613–1620.

32. Pinkerton, J. V., & Thomas, S. (2014). Use of SERMs for treatment in postmenopausal women. *The Journal of Steroid Biochemistry and Molecular Biology, 142,* 142–154.

33. Wurz, G. T., Kao, C. J., & DeGregorio, M. W. (2014). Safety and efficacy of ospemifene for the treatment of dyspareunia associated with vulvar and vaginal atrophy due to menopause. *Clinical Interventions in Aging, 9,* 1939–1950.

34. Shin, J. J., et al. (2017). Ospemifene: A novel option for the treatment of vulvovaginal atrophy. *Journal of Menopausal Medicine, 23*(2), 79–84.

35. Del Pup, L. (2016). Ospemifene: A safe treatment of vaginal atrophy. *European Review for Medical and Pharmacological Sciences, 20*(18), 3934–3944.

36. Goetsch, M. F., Lim, J. Y., & Caughey, A. B. (2014). Locating pain in breast cancer survivors experiencing dyspareunia: A randomized controlled trial. *Obstetrics and Gynecology, 123*(6), 1231–1236.

37. Goetsch, M. F., Lim, J. Y., & Caughey, A. B. (2015). A practical solution for dyspareunia in breast cancer survivors: A randomized controlled trial. *Journal of Clinical Oncology: Official Journal of the American Society of Clinical Oncology, 33*(30), 3394–3400.

38. Nesbitt-Hawes, E. M., et al. (2013). Improvement in pelvic pain with botulinum toxin type A: Single vs. repeat injections. *Toxicon: Official Journal of the International Society on Toxinology, 63,* 83–87.

39. Pacik, P. T., & Geletta, S. (2017). Vaginismus treatment: Clinical trials follow up 241 patients. *Sexual Medicine, 5*(2), e114–e123.

40. Pacik, P. T. (2011). Vaginismus: Review of current concepts and treatment using botox injections, bupivacaine injections, and progressive dilation with the patient under anesthesia. *Aesthetic Plastic Surgery, 35*(6), 1160–1164.

41. Swanson, C. L., et al. (2014). Localized provoked vestibulodynia: Outcomes after modified vestibulectomy. *The Journal of Reproductive Medicine, 59*(3–4), 121–126.

42. Alkatout, I., et al. (2013). Combined surgical and hormone therapy for endometriosis is the most effective treatment: Prospective, randomized, controlled trial. *Journal of Minimally Invasive Gynecology, 20*(4), 473–481.

43. Kingsberg, S. A., et al. (2013). Vulvar and vaginal atrophy in postmenopausal women: Findings from the REVIVE (REal Women's VIews of Treatment Options for Menopausal Vaginal ChangEs) survey. *The Journal of Sexual Medicine, 10*(7), 1790–1799.

44. Nappi, R. E., et al. (2013). The CLOSER (CLarifying Vaginal Atrophy's Impact On SEx and Relationships) survey: Implications of vaginal discomfort in postmenopausal women and in male partners. *The Journal of Sexual Medicine, 10*(9), 2232–2241.

45. Fritzer, N., et al. (2013). More than just bad sex: Sexual dysfunction and distress in patients with endometriosis. *European Journal of Obstetrics, Gynecology, and Reproductive Biology, 169*(2), 392–396.

46. Smith, K. B., & Pukall, C. F. (2014). Sexual function, relationship adjustment, and the relational impact of pain in male partners of women with provoked vulvar pain. *The Journal of Sexual Medicine, 11*(5), 1283–1293.

47. Sturdee, D. W., & Panay, N., International Menopause Society Writing Group. (2010). Recommendations for the management of postmenopausal vaginal atrophy. *Climacteric: The Journal of the International Menopause Society, 13*(6), 509–522.

48. Barlow, D. H., et al. (1997). Urogenital ageing and its effect on sexual health in older British women. *British Journal of Obstetrics and Gynaecology, 104*(1), 87–91.

49. Rahn, D. D., et al. (2014). Vaginal estrogen for genitourinary syndrome of menopause: A systematic review. *Obstetrics and Gynecology, 124*(6), 1147–1156.

CHAPTER **144**

ECTOPIC PREGNANCY
Patricia Polgar-Bailey

 Immediate surgical intervention is indicated for a high hCG level, abdominal pain, vaginal bleeding, hemodynamic failure, hemoperitoneum, and syncope, which are suggestive of a very active ectopic gestation.

DEFINITION AND EPIDEMIOLOGY

Ectopic pregnancy (from the Greek *ektopos*, meaning "out of place") occurs when a fertilized ovum implants anywhere outside of the uterus. Ectopic pregnancy occurs in up to 2.6% of pregnancies[1] and in 6% to 16% of women who visit the emergency department with pain or bleeding (or both) in early pregnancy.[2] The rate of ectopic pregnancy in the United States has risen dramatically in the past few decades.[3,4] Prevalence has risen sixfold since 1970, peaking in the late 1980s, perhaps because of an attendant increase in sexually transmitted diseases, increased frequency of sterilization procedures, and delayed childbearing. The incidence plateaued around the turn of the 21st century and has since increased, which in part may be related to worldwide increases in chlamydia infections.[5] The rate of ectopic pregnancy has been found to increase dramatically after the age of 30 years, especially beyond the age of 35 years.

Although the incidence of ectopic pregnancy has increased, there has been a decrease in the mortality associated with ectopic pregnancy due in part to advances in diagnostic technologies and more opportunity for conservative treatment approaches. Nevertheless, the mortality rate related to ectopic pregnancy is still high.[3] Even in developed countries, ectopic pregnancy is the second leading cause of maternal mortality and the leading cause of pregnancy-related death in the first trimester, representing approximately 6% to 9% of maternal deaths.[2,4]

Identified risk factors[6] for ectopic pregnancy are all maternal and include tubal pathologic conditions and infections (e.g., chlamydia, gonorrhea, or salpingitis), prior tubal surgery including sterilization, particularly at younger (<28) age,[7] prior ectopic gestation,[8] in vitro fertilization (embryo transfer and assisted hatching), endometriosis,[9] irritable bowel syndrome,[10] and smoking. In one Danish historical prospective controlled cohort study, daughters of mothers who experienced ectopic pregnancy had a 50% higher risk of ectopic gestation.[11] Prior medical abortion is not associated with increased risk. Risk of rupture is increased with parity and previous ectopic gestation.

Risk factors for ectopic pregnancy should be elicited for any woman when pregnancy is suspected, although identifiable factors may be absent in many women with ectopic gestation. Risk factors that interfere with fallopian tube function include past or current history of sexually transmitted infections and pelvic inflammatory disease (PID) (including recurrent chlamydial infection), pregnancy occurring while taking oral contraceptives (because of the mechanism of action of the birth control pill on the ciliary movement of the fallopian tube), previous history of ectopic pregnancy, history of infertility, in utero diethylstilbestrol (DES) exposure, documented tubal pathologic condition, prior appendectomy or pelvic operation, cesarean section, prior tubal sterilization or operation (Essure[12]), history of in vitro fertilization, and congenital malformation of the fallopian tubes. Cigarette smoking, vaginal douching, multiple sexual partners, and early age at first intercourse have weaker evidence for association. Although intrauterine devices do not increase the risk for ectopic pregnancy, pregnancies that occur with these devices in place are more likely to be ectopic. Previous induced abortion has not been associated with subsequent ectopic pregnancy.

Historically, the incidence of ectopic pregnancy and related death is higher in African American and other racial and ethnic minorities.[3] These disparities have remained despite the overall decline in ectopic pregnancy–related mortality and are attributed to delayed access to prenatal care, less social support, and different management strategies based on the treatment setting.[3] Without reliable insurance coverage and regular primary and prenatal care, women experience delays in access to health care, leading to more advanced disease at presentation and greater risk of morbidity and mortality.[13] Earlier diagnosis and treatment is important because a small, unruptured ectopic pregnancy allows for more treatment options and the possibility of avoiding salpingectomy if desired. In addition, increased incidence of chlamydia and gonorrhea infections among certain minority groups leads to more severe, underlying tubal disease and pelvic inflammatory disease, which can limit treatment options.

PATHOPHYSIOLOGY

Proposed pathophysiologic explanations for ectopic pregnancy include abnormal embryogenesis (with serious chromosomal aberration in one-third of cases), ascending *Chlamydia trachomatis* infection that scars the fallopian tubes, and luteal phase defects. History of, or current PID, and in utero DES exposure may also result in ectopic gestation. Cases have been reported that involve clear cell hyperplasia of the fallopian tube development in a cesarean section scar and occurrence after ethinyl estradiol–levonorgestrel for emergency contraception. Although implantation can occur anywhere on the cervix, in the abdomen, or on the ovary, 95% of ectopic pregnancies implant in the distal portion of the fallopian tube and on the ipsilateral side to the corpus luteal cyst.

Cervical pregnancy is the rarest form of ectopic pregnancy (accounting for <1% of all ectopic pregnancies) and has been associated with cervicouterine instrumentation. Ovarian pregnancy has been associated with ovulation induction, intrauterine insemination, and vaginal douching. Heterotopic pregnancy (simultaneous intrauterine and extrauterine gestations) is increasing in incidence, occurring in 0.3% to 0.8% of the general population and 1% to 3% of women whose pregnancies resulted from assisted reproductive technologies.[2] Persistent ectopic pregnancy involves residual trophoblastic activity and a β-human chorionic gonadotropin (β-hCG) level that rises or plateaus, whereas chronic ectopic pregnancy contains no active trophoblastic tissue and results in an hCG level that is low or absent.

CLINICAL PRESENTATION AND PHYSICAL EXAMINATION

Symptoms of unruptured ectopic pregnancy can be vague and subacute. The most common symptom of ectopic pregnancy is abdominal pain, which may manifest in isolation or in combination with vaginal bleeding or spotting, dizziness, and shoulder pain (which suggests blood irritating the diaphragm). Symptoms typically appear between 6 and 12 weeks of gestation. Amenorrhea for 1 to 2 months and the usual early signs of pregnancy (nausea, fatigue, breast heaviness) are often part of the initial presentation. Women can also be seen with generalized or unilateral pelvic or abdominal pain described as sharp, cramping, continuous, or intermittent. Less common presenting symptoms include acute urinary retention and abnormal dark, scant vaginal bleeding. Painless vaginal bleeding is the most common presentation for cervical pregnancy. Pain that radiates to the shoulder is more common in a ruptured ectopic pregnancy. Acute syncopal episodes and hypotension are possible secondary to rupture-induced peritoneal hemorrhage. Chronic ectopic pregnancy usually appears as a pelvic mass, with minimum symptoms such as intermittent pain and a low or absent hCG titer.

A thorough history and physical examination are warranted if there is any suspicion of ectopic pregnancy, although the history and physical examination, with a combined sensitivity of 50%, can neither exclude nor confirm an ectopic pregnancy. Postural vital signs and temperature are essential to indicate the presence of hypotension or infection. Speculum examination may reveal a bulging cul-de-sac (indicative of hemoperitoneum in rupture), a bluish coloration of the cervix (a normal finding in any pregnancy), and vaginal bleeding or spotting (the uterus is not able to maintain a stable endometrium at low hCG levels). Uterine enlargement occurs in roughly one-fourth of women with ectopic pregnancy, but its size may be less than expected according to dates (generally smaller than expected size at 8 weeks). Approximately 75% of women with ectopic pregnancies have abdominal tenderness, but the abdominal examination findings may be normal if the ectopic pregnancy has not ruptured; cervical motion tenderness may also be present. An adnexal mass, involuntary guarding, and peritoneal signs, although uncommon, are highly predictive of ectopic gestation.

The pelvic examination is necessary and may reveal signs that suggest a cause other than ectopic pregnancy as the source of the bleeding, such as hemorrhoids, urethral irritation, cervical lesions, or condyloma. Although tissue at the os is a sign of spontaneous abortion and an open os and heavy vaginal bleeding are predictive of an abnormal intrauterine pregnancy, absence of these signs does not differentiate ectopic from intrauterine gestation.

DIAGNOSTICS
Essential Diagnostics

Human chorionic gonadotropin (hCG) assays (pregnancy tests) have become increasingly sensitive in recent years and are the first step in the diagnosis of any suspected ectopic pregnancy. The slope of a rising hCG titer has been found to be a useful determinant of early ectopic pregnancy below the ultrasonographic discriminatory zone. In normal pregnancy, this titer doubles every 1.4 to 3.5 days, with a minimum of 66% increase suggesting viable pregnancy in clinical practice; a titer that plateaus or falls suggests either ectopic pregnancy or miscarriage, although some ectopic pregnancies (and nonviable intrauterine pregnancies) do have abnormally rising hCG levels.

One prospective study that sought to distinguish viable pregnancy from ectopic pregnancy and spontaneous miscarriage at presentation (of women to the emergency department with abdominal pain and a positive pregnancy test) with single point biomarkers,[14] found that a serum hCG level below 3736 mIU/mL was 100% sensitive, and 76% specific, for distinguishing ectopic from viable pregnancy, but that these measurements alone could not distinguish between ectopic gestation and spontaneous miscarriage. Serum CA-125 level below 41.98 U/mL, however, was 100% sensitive and 43% specific in distinguishing ectopic gestation from spontaneous miscarriage. The study suggested that the serial use of hCG and CA-125 cutoffs followed by ultrasound could detect 100% of ectopic pregnancies with 87% specificity for intrauterine gestation. Recent evidence suggests that declining hCG levels in spontaneous abortions can be distinguished from those in ectopic gestation; ectopic gestation (or retained trophoblastic tissue) has a rate of decline that is less than 21% at 2 days or 60% at 7 days. Because nearly all ectopic pregnancies have hCG titers less than 50,000 mIU/mL, a single value above this level can help rule out ectopic pregnancy.

Initial diagnostic tests also include a complete blood count (CBC) (because women with ectopic gestation are often anemic) and a blood type and Rh determination. Serum progesterone is a useful marker of viable pregnancy[15] (levels above 22 ng/mL); levels below 16 ng/mL are consistent with a failing pregnancy (whether ectopic or miscarriage), and levels below 5 ng/mL indicate nonviable pregnancies with nearly 100% sensitivity.

Ultrasonography, particularly transvaginal sonography, is the single best diagnostic tool for demonstration of viable intrauterine pregnancy, nonviable pregnancy, and ectopic gestation.[16] Ultrasound can reliably diagnose a failed pregnancy[17] in an embryo larger than 7 mm (crown rump length) in the absence of cardiac activity or the absence of an embryo when the mean sac diameter is in excess of 25 mm. Spontaneous heterotopic pregnancy was once so rare that detection of intrauterine pregnancy on ultrasound essentially ruled out ectopic gestation, but the incidence of these simultaneous intrauterine and extrauterine pregnancies has been increasing.

At low hCG levels, ultrasound is often nondiagnostic, but when hCG levels are greater than 1800 mIU/mL, sonography is helpful in establishing the location and viability of the pregnancy and is an essential investigation for all women requesting termination of pregnancy. At hCG levels of 1500 to 1800 mIU/mL, a gestational sac should be visible[4] on transvaginal ultrasound (in a singleton pregnancy); at more than 5000 mIU/mL, a yolk sac is visible. When hCG levels are 2000 mIU/mL or more and the mean sac diameter is 3 mm or more, the sensitivity for diagnosis of an intrauterine pregnancy is increased. The β-hCG discriminatory zone, the hCG level at which, if no intrauterine pregnancy is visualized on ultrasound, one can be reasonably confident that a healthy singleton intrauterine pregnancy is not present,[18] is debated at somewhere between 1000 and 2500 mIU/mL[19,20] and is a surrogate marker for gestational age. Transvaginal ultrasound has been shown to be effective at diagnosis of ectopic gestation at even lower levels for some patients. Ultrasound can detect ectopic pregnancy in one-third of women with β-hCG levels of less than 1000 mIU/mL. By 3 weeks after missed menses, virtually all viable intrauterine pregnancies, half of nonviable intrauterine and viable ectopic pregnancies, and one-fourth of nonviable ectopic pregnancies can be detected with this method. A trilaminar pattern (specific but not sensitive in ectopic pregnancy) and the thickness of the endometrium (it is thinner in ectopic gestation) as well as something called the leash sign[12] have also been studied as ways to differentiate ectopic from viable uterine gestations on ultrasound examination.

There is broad agreement regarding the combined use of transvaginal sonography and β-hCG levels in evaluating possible ectopic gestation because of an ability to detect earlier and smaller ectopic pregnancies without the attendant risks of a surgical procedure.

Additional Diagnostics

When ultrasound findings are indeterminate, diagnostic laparoscopy is considered by many to be the definitive test for diagnosis of ectopic pregnancy. However, the advent of new strategies, particularly very sensitive pregnancy tests and ultrasonography, contributes to "nearly perfect" noninvasive diagnostic acumen and permits medical management of the condition in carefully selected instances.

INITIAL DIAGNOSTICS

Ectopic Pregnancy

LABORATORY
- Serum human chorionic gonadotropin
- Complete blood count

IMAGING
- Transvaginal ultrasound

DIFFERENTIAL DIAGNOSIS

Ectopic pregnancy must be considered a likely possibility in any woman of childbearing age with abdominal pain or bleeding (or both) until it is proved otherwise. Other possible differential diagnoses include appendicitis, salpingitis, cholecystitis, PID, intrauterine pregnancy with inaccurate dates, corpus luteum cyst, gestational trophoblastic neoplasm, incomplete or missed spontaneous abortion, endometriosis, pelvic mass, ureteral calculi, and adnexal torsion. A twisted cystic teratoma or a ruptured malignant ovarian tumor may appear similar to a ruptured ectopic pregnancy.

INTERPROFESSIONAL COLLABORATIVE MANAGEMENT

 Immediate emergency department referral or physician consultation is indicated for female patients with a positive serum hCG, abdominal pain, and vaginal bleeding. Ruptured ectopic pregnancy is a surgical emergency requiring immediate admission and attention.

Nonpharmacologic Management

The major factor in determining appropriate therapy in ectopic gestation (i.e., expectant, medical, or surgical) is what is referred to as the level of activity of the ectopic gestation.[3] Less active (medically treatable) gestations are generally agreed to have lower hCG levels (typically below 5000 IU/L, but there is considerable debate as to the cutoff[3]) and no fetal cardiac activity in an asymptomatic woman who is hemodynamically stable. In very inactive ectopic gestation (low and plateauing hCG <1500), expectant management may be the most appropriate strategy.

Expectant management for appropriately selected women[21] (hCG <1500, mild clinical symptoms, small nonviable tubal ectopic pregnancy, and no significant intra-abdominal bleeding on ultrasound in a woman who is able to adhere to close follow-up) involves an intensive follow-up of the woman until she has fully recovered and includes serial hCG measurements, initially every 2 days and then weekly, until the hCG drops below 2 IU/L. Success with expectant management is inversely related to hCG level at diagnosis of ectopic pregnancy.[22] Spontaneous resolution is not uncommon, occurring in up to 80% of cases that are less vascular and less advanced (1 to 3.5 cm [⅖ to 1⅖ inches]) and in which hCG levels are initially low[22] (<1000 mIU/mL) or declining.

During the course of resolution, associated β-hCG levels become undetectable in 3 to 45 days (mean, 15.8 days). An increase in serial CA-125 levels has been explored as an aid in the early diagnosis of tubal rupture in ectopic pregnancies being managed expectantly or with medical treatment.

Pharmacologic Management

Methotrexate therapy, with or without leucovorin rescue or accompanying mifepristone, has been widely used as a nonsurgical intervention for early unruptured ectopic pregnancies[23] smaller than 3.5 cm (1⅖ inches) and with β-hCG levels below 3000 mIU/mL.[24]

A folic acid antagonist that inhibits purine and pyrimidine synthesis, methotrexate interferes with DNA synthesis and cellular multiplication. Rapidly growing tissues such as fetal and trophoblastic cells are most susceptible. Various dosage strategies have been explored,[3] with decreased occurrence and severity of side effects observed in single, low-dose intramuscular injections and increased success rates with flexible protocols and "variable dose" regimens.

Methotrexate or potassium chloride has also been used in ultrasound-guided local injections, equally successfully, in unruptured live ectopic pregnancies. Methotrexate has been used successfully to decrease the incidence of persistent ectopic pregnancy after salpingostomy, in cervical pregnancy[25] when followed by curettage, and in women eligible for expectant management. Uterine embolization with methotrexate for selected cases of early interstitial gestation may decrease the risk of hemorrhage. Appropriate candidates for methotrexate therapy should be hemodynamically stable, have no active renal or hepatic disease, and have no evidence of thrombocytopenia or leukopenia. Initial hCG levels in this population should be low, the gestational sac should be small (<3.5 cm [1⅖ inches]) or absent, and there should be no discernible fetal cardiac activity on ultrasound examination.

Methotrexate therapy has a 94% success rate as long as the woman fits the appropriate criteria. Methotrexate (1 mg/kg or 50 mg/m^2) is given intramuscularly, followed by a repeated hCG titer and symptom assessment on day 4 and another hCG titer on day 7. For women whose hCG titers do not decline significantly (by 15%), a second injection of methotrexate is indicated; this is more likely to be necessary if a yolk sac was visualized on ultrasound examination. If a woman's hCG titer declines by the seventh day, she should be monitored weekly until it is undetectable.

Side effects of treatment with methotrexate include diarrhea, nausea, perioral irritation, and transient transaminase elevations. Similar tubal patency rates have been shown after both methotrexate treatment and expectant management; subsequent fertility[23] and ovarian reserve are not affected,[26] and subsequent risk of recurrent ectopic gestation is not increased with conservative methotrexate treatment.[27]

Surgical laparoscopy[28] or laparotomy remains the only treatment choice for ruptured ectopic pregnancy, and laparoscopy is the cornerstone of treatment in most cases of ectopic gestation. Although laparoscopy is the standard treatment of all ectopic pregnancies, attendant risks include perioperative and postoperative complications, such as uncontrollable hemorrhage, adhesion formation, subcutaneous emphysema and pneumothorax, and reduced subsequent fertility.

In women with a healthy contralateral fallopian tube, salpingotomy does not confer a significant increase in future fertility over salpingectomy.[19] Regardless of treatment modality, every woman with Rh-negative blood should receive anti-D immunoglobulin (RhoGAM).

Indications for Referral or Hospitalization

Suggestive hCG levels (<1000 mIU/mL) and an indeterminate vaginal ultrasound examination necessitate further evaluation, preferably on an inpatient basis. Although transient abdominal pain is common in the second week after methotrexate administration and generally resolves within 24 hours, severe pain is an indication for hospital-based observation because it may indicate tubal rupture.

LIFE SPAN CONSIDERATIONS

All sexually active women of reproductive age are theoretically at risk for ectopic pregnancy, especially if they have one or more of the risk factors mentioned earlier. Women in their 20s are more likely to have ectopic gestation, but adolescents and perimenopausal women are also at risk. Women, including those for whom infertility is an issue, may require the provider's support in expressing and grieving the loss of the pregnancy and the baby who was expected.[29]

COMPLICATIONS

Ruptured ectopic pregnancy can result in acute, massive bleeding and poses an immediate threat to life. Rupture is more likely at higher presenting levels of hCG and with multiple ovulation or ovulation induction. Misdiagnosis, which occurs in as many as 12% of cases, can result in sudden death secondary to internal hemorrhage and infection. Nonfatal sequelae of delayed diagnosis include infection and an increased rate of salpingectomy, potentially affecting future fertility. Missed or delayed diagnoses and subsequent ruptures occur more often in women previously treated with therapeutic abortions when ectopic pregnancies were not suspected. In addition, the risk of a missed or delayed diagnosis is higher in women considered to be less at risk for an ectopic pregnancy, including those with no history of ectopic pregnancy, those with at least one child, and those who have a history of tubal ligation.

Methotrexate has adverse effects, including mucositis, abdominal cramping, and malaise. Its administration has been associated with cases of anaphylaxis, alopecia, and life-threatening neutropenia; high doses can cause bone marrow depression, hepatotoxicity, stomatitis, pulmonary fibrosis, and photosensitivity. The risk of persistent ectopic pregnancy ranges from 3% to 20% after conservative surgical therapy and is 9.8% for treatment with methotrexate. Research has shown a significantly reduced fertility rate postoperatively for some women after ectopic pregnancy and a relationship among advancing age, prior ectopic pregnancy, and declining future pregnancy rates.

PATIENT AND FAMILY EDUCATION

- All women should be apprised of their subsequent risk of reduced fertility and recurrent ectopic pregnancy.
- Condom use should be encouraged to reduce the likelihood of infection and PID because declining rates of chlamydial infection have been associated with declining rates of ectopic pregnancy.
- Women taking birth control pills should be reminded to take them as directed. Women at risk for ectopic pregnancy should alert their provider when they become pregnant.
- Women who have received methotrexate therapy for unruptured ectopic pregnancy need to refrain from sexual activity and consumption of alcohol or vitamins containing folic acid until after resolution of the ectopic pregnancy, preferably at least 3 months, because of the potential teratogenic effects of methotrexate.
- An increase in abdominal pain 5 to 10 days after methotrexate therapy warrants further clinical evaluation because of the possibility of tubal abortion or rupture.
- Good subsequent fertility rates have been demonstrated in women who received methotrexate for ectopic pregnancy (more than half conceive within 1 year of attempting pregnancy), which suggests that fertility in these cases depends more on prior medical history than on the treatment of the ectopic pregnancy.

REFERENCES

1. Stulberg, D. B., Cain, L. R., Dahlquist, I., & Lauderdale, D. S. (2013). Ectopic pregnancy rates in the Medicaid population. *American Journal of Obstetrics and Gynecology, 208*(4), 274.e271–274.e277.
2. Crochet, J. R., Bastian, L. A., & Chireau, M. V. (2013). Does this woman have an ectopic pregnancy? The rational clinical examination systematic review. *JAMA: The Journal of the American Medical Association, 309*(16), 1722–1729.
3. Papillon-Smith, J., Inam, B., & Pateraude, V. (2014). Population-based study on the effect of socioeconomic factors and race on management and outcomes of 35.535 inpatient ectopic pregnancies. *The Journal of Minimally Invasive Gynecology, 21*, 914–920.
4. Alkatout, I., Honemeyer, U., Strauss A., et al. (2013). Clinical diagnosis and treatment of ectopic pregnancy. *Obstetrical and Gynecological Survey, 68*(8), 571–581.
5. Rekart, M. L., Gilbert, M., Meza, R. et al. (2013). Chlamydia public health programs and the epidemiology of pelvic inflammatory disease and ectopic pregnancy. *The Journal of Infectious Diseases, 207*(1), 30–38.
6. Rana, P., Kazmi, I., Singh, R., et al. (2013). Ectopic pregnancy: A review. *Archives of Gynecology and Obstetrics, 288*(4), 747–757.
7. Malacova, E., Kemp, A., Hart, R., Jama-Alol, K., & Preen, D. B. (2014). Long-term risk of ectopic pregnancy varies by method of tubal sterilization: A whole-population study. *Fertility and Sterility, 101*(3), 728–734.
8. Lund Karhus, L., Egerup, P., Wesse Skovlund, C., & Lidegaard, O. (2013). Long-term reproductive outcomes in women whose first pregnancy is ectopic: A national controlled follow-up study. *Human Reproduction, 28*(1), 241–246.
9. Hjordt Hansen, M. V., Dalsgaard, T., Hartwell, D., Skovlund, C. W., & Lidegaard, O. (2014). Reproductive prognosis in endometriosis. A national cohort study. *Acta Obstetricia et Gynecologica Scandinavica, 93*(5), 483–489.
10. Khashan, A. S., Quigley, E. M. M., McNamee, R., McCarthy, F. P., Shanahan, F., & Kenny, L. C. (2012). Increased risk of miscarriage and ectopic pregnancy among women with irritable bowel syndrome. *Clinical Gastroenterology and Hepatology, 10*(8), 902–909.
11. Karhus, L. L., Egerup, P., Skovlund, C. W., & Lidegaard, O. (2014). Impact of ectopic pregnancy for reproductive prognosis in next generation. *Acta Obstetricia et Gynecologica Scandinavica, 93*(4), 416–419.
12. Al-Safi, Z. A., Shavell, V. I., Hobson, D. T., Berman, J. M., & Diamond, M. P. (2013). Analysis of adverse events with Essure hysteroscopic sterilization reported to the Manufacturer and User Facility Device Experience database. *Journal of Minimally Invasive Gynecology, 20*(6), 825–829.
13. Hsu, J. Y., Chen, L., Gummer, A. R., et al. (2017). Disparities in the management of ectopic pregnancy. *American Journal of Obstetrics and Gynecology, 217*, 49.e1–49.e10.
14. Butler, S. A., Abban, T. K., Borrelli, P. T. A., Luttoo, J. M., Kemp, B., & Iles, R. K. (2013). Single point biochemical measurement algorithm for early diagnosis of ectopic pregnancy. *Clinical Biochemistry, 46*(13–14), 1257–1263.
15. Verhaegen, J., Gallos, I. D., van Mello, N. M., et al. (2012). Accuracy of single progesterone test to predict early pregnancy outcome in women with pain or bleeding: Meta-analysis of cohort studies. *British Medical Journal, 345*, e6077.
16. Fylstra, D. L. (2014). Cervical pregnancy: 13 cases treated with suction curettage and balloon tamponade. *American Journal of Obstetrics and Gynecology, 210*(6), 581.e581–581.e585.
17. Lane, B. F., Wong-You-Cheong, J. J., Javitt, M. C., et al. (2013). ACR Appropriateness Criteria first trimester bleeding. *Ultrasound Quarterly, 29*(2), 91–96.
18. Barnhart, K. T. (2012). Early pregnancy failure: Beware of the pitfalls of modern management. *Fertility and Sterility, 98*(5), 1061–1065.
19. van Mello, N. M., Mol, F., Ankum, W. M., Mol, B. W., van der Veen, F., & Hajenius, P. J. (2012). Ectopic pregnancy: How the diagnostic and therapeutic management has changed. *Fertility and Sterility, 98*(5), 1066–1073.
20. Little, S. H., & Rockwell, P. G. (2012). Ectopic pregnancy: Zero in on these lab and imaging clues. *The Journal of Family Practice, 61*(11), 678–686.
21. Mavrelos, D., Nicks, H., Jamil, A., Hoo, W., Jauniaux, E., & Jurkovic, D. (2013). Efficacy and safety of a clinical protocol for expectant management of selected women diagnosed with a tubal ectopic pregnancy. *Ultrasound in Obstetrics and Gynecology, 42*(1), 102–107.
22. Craig, L. B., & Khan, S. (2012). Expectant management of ectopic pregnancy. *Clinical Obstetrics and Gynecology, 55*(2), 461–470.
23. Practice Committee of American Society for Reproductive Medicine. (2013). Medical treatment of ectopic pregnancy: A committee opinion. *Fertility and Sterility, 100*(3), 638–644.
24. Ustunyurt, E., Duran, M., Coskun, E., Ustunyurt, O. B., & Simsek, H. (2013). Role of initial and day 4 human chorionic gonadotropin levels in predicting

the outcome of single-dose methotrexate treatment in women with tubal ectopic pregnancy. *Archives of Gynecology and Obstetrics, 288*(5), 1149–1152.

25. Adabi, K., Nekuie, S., Rezaeei, Z., Rahimi-Sharbaf, F., Banifatemi, S., & Salimi, S. (2013). Conservative management of cervical ectopic pregnancy: Systemic methotrexate followed by curettage. *Archives of Gynecology and Obstetrics, 288*(3), 687–689.

26. Uyar, I., Yucel, O. U., Gezer, C., et al. (2013). Effect of single-dose methotrexate on ovarian reserve in women with ectopic pregnancy. *Fertility and Sterility, 100*(5), 1310–1313.

27. Wyroba, J., Krzysiek, J., Rajtar-Ciosek, A., et al. (2014). High live birth rate after conservative treatment of ectopic pregnancy with methotrexate. *Ginekologia Polska, 85*(2), 105–110.

28. Cohen, A., Almog, B., Satel, A., Lessing, J. B., Tsafrir, Z., & Levin, I. (2013). Laparoscopy versus laparotomy in the management of ectopic pregnancy with massive hemoperitoneum. *International Journal of Gynaecology and Obstetrics, 123*(2), 139–141.

29. Purandare, N., Ryan, G., Ciprike, V., Trevisan, J., Sheehan, J., & Geary, M. (2012). Grieving after early pregnancy loss—a common reality. *Irish Medical Journal, 105*(10), 326–328.

CHAPTER **145**

FERTILITY CONTROL

Richard Matthew Prior

DEFINITION AND EPIDEMIOLOGY

In the United States, 99% of sexually active women have used contraception at some time in their lives. From 2006 to 2010, 62% of women aged 15 to 44 years reported that they were currently using contraception. The most commonly used types of contraception are oral contraception, female sterilization, and condoms. Unfortunately, 47% of the women who have used more than one method of contraception decided to change or stop due to dissatisfaction.[1]

From 2006 to 2010, 37% of all births were unintended.[2] Given the high frequency of unplanned pregnancy, it is essential that health care providers educate and counsel women and their partners on the variety of feasible contraception options. It is imperative that the woman (and her partner, if desired) be involved in the care plan rather than be merely a recipient of the provider's expertise and advice. Discussion of contraceptive options should include information about the risks and benefits, potential side effects, rate of efficacy, and effects on future fertility.

The thoughtful and safe prescribing of contraception always begins with a thorough medical history. All forms of hormonal contraception carry some degree of risk, which can be partially mitigated by careful consideration of a woman's health and the contraindications for a particular method. A recent study surveyed 987 women of childbearing age and found that 13% of the sample had a contraindication to combined hormonal contraception and that 39% of those women were unfortunately taking them anyway.[3] To assist prescribers, the World Health Organization regularly publishes and updates easy-to-use eligibility criteria for contraceptive use that includes summary charts, quick reference tools, and smartphone apps for quick use in the clinic setting.

When possible emotional and health care costs are factored in, all methods of contraception have been shown to be more cost effective than unintended pregnancy.[4] Current methods of contraception are continuously improved and new contraceptives are constantly being developed, resulting in an ever-evolving variety of patient-centered, cost-effective choices.

HORMONAL CONTRACEPTION
Combined Hormonal Contraceptives

Combined hormonal contraceptives (CHC) are highly effective means of preventing pregnancy and have played an important role in contraception since the approval of the first oral contraceptive by the U.S. Food and Drug Administration (FDA) in 1960. Combined hormonal contraceptives come in the forms of oral contraceptive pills (OCPs), the contraceptive vaginal ring, and the contraceptive patch, which provide the patient with choice in deciding which delivery method is preferable. CHCs offer a quick return to fertility, with ovulation returning within a few cycles of cessation. With few exceptions, the CHC share the same indications and contraindications.

Estrogen is one of the two major hormonal components in CHCs. The role of estrogen is to promote bleeding regularity and to suppress the release of follicle-stimulating hormone.[5,6] The basic chemical structure of estrogen has been modified by pharmaceutical manufacturers to increase effectiveness, leading to the development of the two synthetic estrogens (ethinyl estradiol and, less commonly, mestranol) that are used in combined oral contraceptives today. The doses of ethinyl estradiol used in the first oral contraceptives were often in excess of 100 mcg, resulting in side effects that decreased the safety profile of the medication. Subsequent research and experience proved that doses of 50 mcg or less are sufficient to aid in the suppression of ovulation while minimizing side effects.

These estrogen compounds are delivered with a synthetic progestin, the second active hormonal compound. The progestin component provides the majority of the contraceptive effect by suppressing follicle-stimulating hormone and luteinizing hormone. This altered hormonal environment prevents ovulation, thickens cervical mucus, and promotes a uterine atmosphere that is hostile to implantation.[5,6] Several different formulations of synthetic progestins are commonly used in combined oral contraceptives in the United States.

The structural similarity of the progestins to testosterone largely determines their androgenic activity. This androgenic activity is often associated with the side effects of progestins, which may include menstrual cycle disturbances, weight gain, breast tenderness, increase in functional ovarian cysts, ectopic pregnancy, interactions with anticonvulsants, and bone density decrease.[5,7]

Newer third- and fourth-generation progestins are less adrenergic, limiting such side effects as acne, hirsutism, and hyperlipidemia.[5] The spironolactone derivative drospirenone has been combined with ethinyl estradiol to form several newer monophasic oral contraceptives. Drospirenone is a fourth-generation progestin that is a spironolactone analogue with antiandrogenic properties. It may be a good choice in women who experience significant sodium and water retention during their cycle. In one study, drospirenone was actually found to improve acne by nearly 50%. It is also known to lesson premenstrual symptoms.[8]

Dienogest is another relatively new and very potent antiandrogenic progestin that also allows for good cycle control.

Dienogest is available in both biphasic and quadriphasic preparations. Like drospirenone, it is also very effective at improving acne.[8]

Nausea, breast tenderness, and mild fluid retention resulting from the estrogen component of CHCs are common side effects. Menstrual changes, including intermenstrual (breakthrough) spotting or bleeding, occur in 25% of women during the first 3 months of CHC use and decrease significantly during subsequent prolonged use. Other estrogen-related side effects include increased breast size, weight gain, and increased skin pigmentation.[7]

Women with persistent intermenstrual bleeding after 3 months of CHC use should be evaluated for possible causes of bleeding unrelated to CHC use. Amenorrhea may also occur, especially in women who have been using CHC products for a prolonged period. Other possible side effects include fluid retention, leukorrhea, pruritus, and headaches.

Some of the "short-lived" side effects associated with CHCs tend to dissipate by the third or fourth cycle. Once the responsible hormonal component has been identified, the provider can determine whether the side effect is caused by an excess or deficiency and can present potential alternative contraceptive options that may lead to increased satisfaction.

Benefits of CHCs extend beyond that of preventing pregnancy. Lighter menses may occur and result in a decrease in the incidence or severity of iron deficiency anemia. Some women may notice a decrease in premenstrual mood symptoms and premenstrual cramping. Most combined oral contraceptives—in particular some triphasic preparations—are known to help control acne. Other advantages may include increased bone density and decreases in the incidence of pelvic inflammatory disease (PID), endometrial and ovarian cancers, and colorectal cancer.[9]

CHCs also have significant health risks and disadvantages, including a lack of protection against human immunodeficiency virus (HIV) infection, a greater threat to the health of many sexually active individuals than an unplanned pregnancy. To protect against HIV infection and other sexually transmitted infections, condoms must be used in conjunction with OCPs.

The estrogen component in CHCs has been shown to cause mild increases in both systolic and diastolic blood pressure, which may be more pronounced in some patients. Blood pressure returns to baseline after the cessation of CHCs. There is some concern that women who take CHCs are at a slightly higher risk for myocardial infarction and stroke. Current practice recommendations are that women with an untreated blood pressure lower than 140/90 mm Hg are good candidates for CHCs. Even in women with well-controlled hypertension, the risks of using a combined hormonal form of contraception likely outweigh the benefits and another method should be chosen. All women should have their blood pressure monitored at each clinic visit.[6,10,11]

Potential for venous thromboembolism is another infrequent but serious adverse effect associated with CHCs. Although the risk is quite low, thromboembolism occurs three times more frequently in women who take CHCs than in those who do not. The effect appears to be more pronounced in women who are obese, women who smoke, and in women with a history of coagulopathies. Because of the increased risk of thromboembolism, combined products should be avoided in women with a history of thromboembolism or those at risk,

such as women who experience prolonged immobility due to surgery and those with known thrombogenic mutations.[11,12]

There is a questionable relationship between CHCs and stroke. The risk is low and is likely to occur around 1.6 times more frequently in women who use contraception. There may also be an increased risk of ischemic stroke with CHC use in women with a history of migraines with aura. Some studies suggest that the risk is higher when women use preparations with greater than 50 mcg of ethinyl estradiol, which is no longer used in the United States. Although the risk is low, morbidity associated with stroke is devastating enough that current recommendations remain that migraine sufferers use a progestin-only contraceptive or nonhormonal form of contraception.[10,11]

The potential impact of CHC use on breast cancer is a concern for a great number of women interested in this form of fertility control. There continues to be debate as to the degree of effect of CHCs on the development of breast cancer. Many of the studies showing an association between CHC use and breast cancer are older and also apply to preparations that included a much higher dose of estrogen than is used today. Studies have not proved an increased risk in OCP users with a first-degree relative who has a history of breast cancer; therefore current practice guidelines do not treat family history as a contraindication. Women who have active or past breast cancer are not considered to be good candidates for any type of hormonal contraception.[11,13]

The World Health Organization's medical eligibility criteria for contraceptive use provides comprehensive guidance for the safety of use of different contraceptive methods. Combined hormonal contraception should not be prescribed for women who breastfeed and are less than 6 weeks postpartum; smoke more than 15 cigarettes per day; have a systolic blood pressure of 160 mm Hg or higher or a diastolic blood pressure of 100 mm Hg or higher; have a current or past history of deep vein thrombosis or pulmonary embolus; are immobilized for extended periods of time after surgery; have a history of coronary artery disease or stroke; or have a genetic disease that predisposes them to clotting, systemic lupus erythematosus, diabetes with end-organ damage, or severe liver diseases. The risks likely outweigh the benefits in the following categories of women: those who have blood pressure higher than 140/90 mm Hg; have adequately controlled hypertension; are less than 3 weeks postpartum; are breastfeeding and are 6 weeks to 6 months postpartum; smoke fewer than 15 cigarettes per day; have diabetes mellitus; have hyperlipidemia; have migraines without aura and are older than 35 years; or are taking anticonvulsants.[11]

The warning signs to teach CHC users can be summarized with the acronym *ACHES*:

- Abdominal pain (severe) (which may indicate liver disease)
- Chest pain (severe), cough, or shortness of breath (which may indicate angina or a pulmonary embolus)
- Headaches (severe), dizziness, weakness, or numbness (which may indicate stroke or hypertensive emergency)
- Eye problems (vision loss or blurring) or speech problems (which may indicate a stroke)
- Severe leg pain (calf or thigh) (which may indicate a deep vein thrombosis)

Women who experience any of these signs or symptoms or who develop depression, jaundice, or a breast lump should discontinue taking the pill and consult their providers. CHC users who smoke should be encouraged to quit smoking; if quitting is not possible, they should consider discontinuation of CHCs after the age of 35 years.

Oral Contraceptives

The terms *birth control pill, combined oral contraceptive,* and *oral contraceptive* generally refer to OCPs containing both estrogen and progestin. In this chapter, these terms are not used to refer to progestin-only pills, also known as *minipills.* Several different types of OCPs are available and vary according to the dose of hormones and the formulations within each cycle pack. Monophasic OCPs have a constant dose of estrogen and progestin in each of the active tablets of the cycle pack. Multiphasic OCPs have alternating doses of progestin and, in some cases, estrogen throughout the cycle. The aim of manufacturers in lowering the total monthly exogenous hormone dose while trying to simulate a woman's normal menstrual cycle is to reduce the metabolic side effects associated with OCP use.

The first oral contraceptive regimens provided 21 days of active hormone followed by 7 days of inert pills, resulting in a withdrawal bleed. The 21/7 regimen was initially adopted because the creators of the first OCP believed that women would appreciate the reassurance of a monthly period. Alternating regimens offer additional benefits of decreasing unpleasant symptoms and inconvenience associated with withdrawal bleeding. Other preparations provide a regimen of 24 active days followed by 4 days of inert pills or 24 active days followed by 2 days of decreased hormones and then 2 days of inert pills, resulting in decreased side effects caused by estrogen withdrawal, lighter menses, and decreased likelihood of ovulation.[14,15]

The FDA has approved the use of several extended OCP regimens that result in a withdrawal bleed only once a quarter. The advantages of extended regimens are that by decreasing the frequency of withdrawal bleed, women will less frequently experience the inconvenience and symptoms associated with menses such as dysmenorrhea and headaches. Common preparations use 84 days of combined hormones followed by 7 days of placebo (Seasonale); 84 days of combined hormones followed by 7 days of low-dose estrogen (Seasonique and LoSeasonique); or 84 days of a varied amount of combined hormones followed by 7 days of low-dose estrogen (Quartette).[14,15]

With perfect use, OCPs are 99.7% effective in preventing pregnancy. However, with typical use in the United States, the rate of efficacy drops to 91%.[16] At the time of prescription, the absence of pregnancy should be verified via standard laboratory tests. Traditionally, women have been instructed to begin the regimen of OCPs on either the first day of menses or on the first Sunday after menses begin, a method known as the *conventional start.* This approach ensures that the patient is not pregnant and in the case of a Sunday start aligns the days on the packaging with the actual day of the week. Another approach, known as the *quick start,* has the patient begin the regimen on the day of the visit, as the hormones in the contraceptive do not harm the fetus if the woman is pregnant at that time. Studies have shown that both methods have similar rates of effectiveness and side effects, leaving opportunity for provider and patient choice.[17]

Women should be encouraged to take OCPs at the same time every day and to associate pill taking with a certain daily habit or ritual if that facilitates compliance. Daily compliance is essential to ensuring efficacy. Women who miss one or two tablets should take two tablets for each of the missed days. Women who miss more than 2 days should continue taking the pills as prescribed but use an additional form of birth control for the remainder of the cycle. Women who often miss doses of OCPs should be encouraged to consider a form of fertility control that does not depend on daily compliance.

Secondary analysis of National Survey for Family Growth data suggests that 29% of women discontinued oral contraceptives because of dissatisfaction. Of those women, 64.6% discontinued because of side effects, and 13.1% of women discontinued OCPs because they were worried about side effects.[1] The extent and type of side effects differ slightly among individual OCPs because of variations in the amount and kind of estrogen and progestin contained within each product.

Vaginal Ring

The etonogestrel–ethinyl estradiol vaginal ring (NuvaRing) is a 54-mm-diameter vaginal contraceptive ring that delivers 15 mcg of ethinyl estradiol and 120 mcg of etonogestrel each day.[18] The flexible, circular ring is inserted in the vagina by the woman and kept in place for 3 weeks. Unlike the diaphragm, the ring does not have to be in a specific position because the hormones can be absorbed anywhere in the vagina. If for some reason the ring is out of the vagina for more than 3 hours, backup contraception should be used until the ring has been back in place for 7 days.

After 3 weeks, the ring is removed for 1 week. Withdrawal bleeding usually begins within 2 or 3 days of the ring-free week. For prevention of pregnancy, a new ring must be inserted after the ring-free week (7 days). The ring is reported to be 91% effective with typical use and 99.7% effective with perfect use.[16] The vaginal ring provides contraception with use of lower hormonal doses than in other contraceptive methods, is readily reversible, and is easy for patients to use. Side effects include vaginal complaints and headaches. It has the same contraindications as the other CHCs.[19,20]

Contraceptive Patch

Norelgestromin–ethinyl estradiol transdermal system (Ortho Evra) is the only contraceptive patch currently available in the United States. The 20-cm^2 patch delivers 35 mcg of ethinyl estradiol and 150 mcg of norelgestromin daily and is 99.7% effective with perfect use and 91% effective with typical use.[16,20] Each cycle consists of a contraceptive patch applied to the lower abdomen, buttocks, upper outer arm, or upper torso (excluding the breasts) once a week for 3 weeks. After the third week, the patch is removed for a contraceptive-free week during which withdrawal bleeding occurs.[19,20]

There remain questions about the effectiveness of the patch when prescribed to obese women. Studies exploring contraceptive patch failure in these women have demonstrated mixed results. Although obesity is not a contradiction to the patch, it would be reasonable to advise obese women that there is potential for decreased effectiveness.[20] Advantages of the contraceptive patch include ease of use, improved adherence, reversibility, and steady-state hormone levels. Spotting rates are comparable to those of OCP use. Additional side effects include breast discomfort, headache, nausea, dysmenorrhea, and skin irritation at the patch site.[19]

In November 2005 and again in 2011, the FDA issued a warning that the birth control patch could be associated with an increased risk of thromboembolism, although studies have not conclusively defined whether there is increased risk of thromboembolism compared with similarly dosed OCPs. The patch carries the same risks, warnings, and contraindications as other CHCs. All patients starting on the contraceptive patch or hormonal birth control should understand the risks of thromboembolism and the importance of stopping the medication and calling their health care providers immediately if they develop a severe headache, chest pain or pressure, shortness of breath, abdominal pain, or leg pain.[12,19]

Progestin-Only Products

Progestin-only products exist as oral contraceptives, injectable contraceptives, and implantable rods. The first progestin-only products were the progestin-only pills, which were developed in the early 1960s in response to the side effect profile associated with the estrogen component of OCPs. Progestins prevent pregnancy mainly by thickening the cervical mucus to slow sperm motility and interfering with or preventing sperm penetration. Progestins may also work by inhibiting ovulation and creating an endometrial environment inhospitable to implantation.[5]

Because of the lack of estrogen, progestin only products are not associated with some of the same potential side effects of combination oral contraceptives, such as thromboembolic disorders (e.g., myocardial infarction and cerebrovascular disease) and gallbladder disease. However, without the estrogen component to stabilize the endometrium, menstrual irregularities are a common side effect. With sustained use, however, most women will eventually experience amenorrhea.

Generally speaking, progestin-only products are safer than CHCs. The only absolute contraindication to progestin-only products is active breast cancer. The risks likely outweigh the benefits in women with an acute deep vein thrombosis or pulmonary embolism, history of heart disease, history of stroke, unexplained vaginal bleeding, history of breast cancer, or active liver disease. The oral contraceptive minipills and the contraceptive rod are particularly good progestin-only contraceptive choices for women with poorly controlled blood pressure and women with diabetes who have end-organ damage.[11]

Progestin-Only Pills (Minipills). Progestin-only pills are taken on a daily basis, with no pill-free days. Progestin-only pills have a failure rate equivalent to those of OCPs; however, they must be taken at the same time each day. Minipills are the method of choice in women who are lactating and are less than 6 weeks postpartum; the efficacy rate for these women is close to 100%.

Progestin-only pills are also useful for women who wish to use an OCP but have contraindications to combined pills.[5] Minipills are associated with a higher incidence of ectopic pregnancy compared with other contraceptive measures, but the risk is still lower than in women who do not use contraception.

Injectable Contraception

The only available injectable form of contraception available in the United States is depot medroxyprogesterone acetate (DMPA; Depo-Provera). DMPA prevents pregnancy by inhibiting ovulation. A 150-mg injection of DMPA suppresses ovulation for 14 weeks. A 104-mg preparation is generally considered to be equivalent, although the subcutaneous delivery method may be less painful and preferable to some women. With a prescribed dose given every 3 months, contraceptive efficacy is 99.8%.[16] Although DMPA has traditionally been started immediately before or during menses, new research suggests improved effectiveness if given at the time of the initial visit, as long as the provider is reasonably sure that the patient is not pregnant. DMPA injections should be administered every 12 weeks, which provides a 2-week "grace period" given the 14-week duration of action. The possibility of pregnancy should first be excluded for any woman who is more than 2 weeks late for her DMPA injection.[17,19]

A primary concern for women who take DMPA is bone loss. Studies have demonstrated that bone loss occurs primarily in the first 2 years. There is some concern that women who take DMPA may be at a slightly higher risk of fracture. For these reasons, there is an FDA "black box" warning that recommends that DMPA not be used for more than 2 years. Providers should counsel patients on the risks of bone loss. Patients should also be counseled on the risks and benefits of continuing the medication beyond the 2-year mark.

Menstrual changes occur in almost all women who use DMPA and are the most common cause for dissatisfaction and discontinued use of this form of fertility control. Irregular bleeding usually resolves within the first month of use. Amenorrhea is the most common menstrual change with persistent use of DMPA. Other side effects of DMPA include headache, abdominal or breast bloating, mood changes, decreased libido, and weight gain of 5 pounds or less.[19,21]

DMPA is a reversible form of contraception, but a return to fertility is often delayed after discontinuation of DMPA. Average return to fertility occurs in 5 to 7 months after cessation of DMPA, but fertility may not be restored for as long as 18 months in some women. DMPA is associated with certain noncontraceptive benefits, such as a reduction in or elimination of premenstrual symptoms, a reduced risk of PID, a decreased risk of endometrial cancer, and hematologic improvement in women with sickle cell disease. DMPA-induced amenorrhea may make DMPA a good contraceptive choice for women with menorrhagia, dysmenorrhea, and iron deficiency anemia as well as for women with intellectual disabilities who have menstrual hygiene problems.

DMPA is linked with certain health risks. As is the case with CHCs, DMPA provides no protection from many sexually transmitted diseases (STDs), including HIV infection. The risks of prescribing DMPA outweigh the benefits in women who are less than 6 weeks postpartum and are breastfeeding, women who are at risk for heart disease, and women with uncontrolled hypertension greater than 160 systolic or 100 mm Hg diastolic.[11]

Women should be counseled to use an additional form of contraception for the first 2 weeks after the first DMPA injection. Women who are at risk for STDs should use a barrier method of contraception, preferably condoms. Women who become concerned about their menstrual irregularities while taking DMPA or who develop signs or symptoms of infection should consult their health care providers. Women need to be informed about the likely delay in fertility after discontinuation of DMPA. DMPA is not the best choice for women who wish to become pregnant within the next 1 to 2 years; these women should be counseled about alternative contraceptive options.

Contraceptive Implants

In 1990, the contraceptive levonorgestrel (Norplant) ushered in the era of implantable progestin rods. Although Norplant is no longer being manufactured, there is currently one contraceptive implant available in the United States. A single-rod implant (Implanon) was approved by the FDA in 2006 for use by women in the United States and was then modified and reintroduced as Nexplanon. Nexplanon is a thin, flexible plastic subdermal insert, approximately 4 cm long, that delivers ethylene vinyl acetate impregnated with 68 mg of etonogestrel. The rod delivers an average of 40 mcg of etonogestrel every day, inhibiting ovulation and thickening cervical mucus.[19,21] The Nexplanon implant is reported to be 99.9% effective at preventing pregnancy.[16]

A provider trained and skilled in Nexplanon insertion can perform this procedure in the office. The implant prevents pregnancy for 3 years and does not interfere with fertility once the rod has been removed. Menstrual periods usually return to normal within a few months after removal of the rod.[19] The rod is typically inserted into the inside portion of the upper arm. If the rod is inserted within 5 days of the start of menses, a backup form of contraception is not needed during the remainder of the cycle. The most common side effect is irregular menstrual bleeding.[19,21]

Postcoital Contraception

Postcoital contraception, also referred to as *emergency contraception* (EC) or the *morning-after pill*, is intended for women who have experienced a single episode of unprotected intercourse within a given menstrual cycle. Postcoital contraception can also be used in cases of sexual assault. In the United States, three types of EC are widely accepted for use: levonorgestrel, ulipristal acetate (UA), and the copper intrauterine device (IUD).[19,22]

In 2013, the FDA approved the commercial formulation Plan B One-Step. Since marketed under a number of trade names, this EC form contains the progestin levonorgestrel as single dose 1.5 mg pill that should be taken as soon as possible within 3 days of unprotected sex. Within 72 hours of intercourse, levonorgestrel is likely to reduce the risk of pregnancy by 50%. From 72 to 120 hours after intercourse, there is a significant drop in efficacy. Perhaps the primary benefit of the levonorgestrel method is that it is available in the United States over the counter without a prescription. Common side effects include bleeding irregularities, nausea, headaches, vomiting, and abdominal pain.[19,22]

Another option includes the prescription-only selective progesterone receptor modulator UA, known by the brand name Ella. UA is prescribed as a single-dose, 30-mg tablet that is taken within 120 hours of unprotected sexual intercourse. Studies indicate that UA is as effective as levonorgestrel up to 72 hours after intercourse and may be more effective from hours 72 to 120. Side effects are similar to those of levonorgestrel.[19,22]

Perhaps the most effective method is the copper IUD, which can be used as EC as long as there is no established pregnancy and the woman has no other contraindications to IUDs. Studies have shown that up to 80% of women who received a copper IUD as a means of EC kept it as a form of long-acting contraception.[22] Providers who prescribe EC should engage the patient in a discussion about the benefits of a sustained contraception plan.

Intrauterine Devices

Intrauterine contraceptive devices are one of the safest, most effective, and most cost-effective contraception options.

Many negative perceptions of the IUD are based on the first-generation models, which were removed from the market because of side effects and morbidity. The current-generation IUDs are safer and are engineered to produce fewer side effects than their predecessors.

Two types of IUDs are currently available in the United States. The oldest is the copper T 380A (ParaGard), a T-shaped polyethylene device with a stem and cross arms partly covered by copper wire and tubing; the device can remain in place for 10 years. In addition, there are four levonorgestrel-containing IUDs: the Mirena device, which releases 20 mcg of levonorgestrel per day and can be left in place for 5 years; the Skyla device, which releases 13.5 mcg/day and can be left in 3 years; the Kyleena device, which releases 17.5 mcg per day and can be left in place for 5 years; and the Liletta device, which releases 19.5 mcg per day and can be left in place for 5 years. It should be noted that blood levels decrease over time but remain effective.[19,23]

Copper IUDs prevent fertilization primarily by creating a spermicidal environment. The IUD causes the endometrium to initiate a foreign body reaction, which results in sterile inflammation and inhibits sperm from reaching the fallopian tube. In addition, the copper ions permeate the cervical mucus and decrease sperm motility. Progesterone-releasing IUDs thicken the cervical mucus, cause atrophy of the endometrium, and perhaps inhibit ovulation. Both forms of IUD are more than 99% effective.[16,19,23]

Far fewer complications are associated with the IUDs currently in use than with the early copper-containing IUDs (including the Dalkon Shield) of the 1980s. Copper-containing IUDs can increase bleeding and dysmenorrhea—especially in the first 3 to 6 months, whereas the levonorgestrel system lessens these symptoms. Historically, one of the concerns about IUDs had been that women are at a greater risk for developing PID. This was believed to be attributed to the multifilament strings in the Dalkon Shield, which provided a convenient route for bacteria to ascend to the pelvic organs. Current IUDs possess a monofilament string that is much less likely to harbor bacteria.

Current recommendations are that women should be warned of the very small risk of PID in the 20-day postinsertion period. Only women who are symptomatic or those who are at risk for having an STD should be tested before insertion. Women who develop PID can be treated with antibiotics with an IUD in place unless they fail to improve with 72 hours of therapy.[19,23]

Of the pregnancies that do occur with IUDs in place, 50% result in spontaneous abortion. In contrast to the older-generation IUDs, neither type of IUD increases the overall risk of ectopic pregnancy compared with the risk for noncontraceptive users.[19,23]

IUDs should not be prescribed for women with known pregnancy, an active sexually transmitted infection, or active PID; in the period immediately after a septic abortion; in the presence of unexplained vaginal bleeding or untreated cervical cancer; or for women with anatomic abnormalities of the uterus (such as fibroids that disrupt the uterine cavity). IUDs are generally not recommended in women less than 4 weeks postpartum. The levonorgestrel IUDs are not recommended in women who are breastfeeding, have an acute deep vein thrombosis or pulmonary embolus, have had breast cancer within the past 5 years, or have ovarian cancer or severe liver disease.[11]

IUDs have been demonstrated to be safe for both nulliparous and parous women. Patient education should include information about checking for the IUD string as well as the signs and symptoms of possible complications, including pain, bleeding, odorous discharge, fever, and missed menses.

BARRIER METHODS

Barrier methods of fertility control are so named because they act as mechanical barriers and prevent pregnancy by blocking the passage of sperm through their surfaces. In addition, they prevent or reduce contact with genital lesions, discharges, or secretions.

Condoms

Most condoms made in the United States are manufactured from latex; approximately 3% are made from other materials. Contraception and disease prevention efficacy data are available only for latex condoms. Failure rates with condoms are as low as 2% with perfect use and as high as 18% with typical use[16] Polyurethane female condoms have the benefit of affording women direct control of contraception and disease prevention. However, failure rates for the female condom are significantly higher (5% with perfect use, 21% with typical use) than for male condoms.[16] Condoms remain the only immediately reversible method of contraception for men.

Patient education about condom use should include information about how to put on and remove a condom, the need to leave a receptacle at the tip of the condom to avoid breakage, what to do in case of condom slippage or damage, and the importance of avoiding oil-based products (e.g., petroleum jelly, cold cream) when extra lubrication is needed.

Diaphragms and Cervical Caps

Diaphragms and cervical caps are female barrier methods of contraception. Both must be individually fitted to be effective; even with correct use, failure rates are as high as 32% for nulliparous users and 16% for parous users during the first year of use.[24] Both the diaphragm and the cervical cap are used with spermicidal cream or jelly.

The diaphragm is a dome-shaped rubber cap that comes in a variety of sizes. It fits into the vagina, covering the cervix and the anterior vagina from the pubic symphysis to the posterior fornix. The diaphragm should remain in place for at least 6 hours after intercourse, but no more than 24 hours (to minimize the risk of toxic shock syndrome). Once it is in position, the diaphragm provides effective contraception for 6 hours, after which fresh spermicide must be applied if additional contraceptive protection is desired. The postpartum patient should not be fitted for a diaphragm for at least 6 weeks after childbirth.

The cervical cap is a deep, soft rubber cup that covers the surface and fits snugly around the base of the cervix. There are several sizes of cap that correspond to the woman's obstetric history. The cap provides continuous contraceptive protection during 24 hours regardless of how often intercourse occurs. Additional spermicide or jelly can be inserted vaginally without removal of the cap for repeated intercourse.[24]

Advantages of the female barrier methods include a lack of dependence on partners for contraception and none of the side effects of systemic hormones. With the exception of the female condom, all female vaginal barrier methods are used in conjunction with spermicides. Some protection against HIV infection is afforded if the spermicide contains nonoxynol-9. On the other hand, research has demonstrated that vaginal irritation caused by nonoxynol-9 may increase susceptibility to HIV infection. Reduction in the risk of other STDs, including gonorrhea and chlamydia, varies from 10% to 50%, depending on the study. Risks associated with the use of diaphragms and cervical caps include latex allergy, toxic shock syndrome, and recurrent urinary tract infections.[24]

Spermicides

A variety of over-the-counter spermicidal products are available in the United States and include foams, creams, gels, suppositories, and films. The active ingredient in all spermicides available in the United States is nonoxynol-9 or a similar agent that destroys the membrane of the sperm cell. Spermicides can be used alone but, as noted earlier, are also essential for the effective functioning of diaphragms and cervical caps.[19,24] Effectiveness varies with the type of use and compliance; failure rates vary from 29% with typical use to 18% with perfect use.[16]

One major advantage of spermicides is that they are available over-the-counter. Many women also appreciate that there is no partner involvement with this method. Side effects include allergic reactions to the active ingredient or to the particular spermicide base or vehicle, which generally manifests as vulvar pruritus or a rash. Women who are prone to yeast infections may notice an increased frequency of this problem when spermicides are used.

Cervical Sponge

The cervical sponge is available without a prescription. With perfect use, it is 91% effective for nulliparous women and 80% effective for parous women.[16] The sponge is moistened with water and inserted into the vagina. The sponge provides its contraceptive effect for up to 24 hours and must be left in place for 6 hours after intercourse, to a maximum 30-hour total. The Today Sponge available in the United States is impregnated with the spermicide nonoxynol-9.

SURGICAL STERILIZATION

Methods of surgical sterilization include tubal sterilization and vasectomy. Sterilization is the most commonly reported method of fertility control; in the United States in 2006 to 2008, it was the method used by 33% of contraceptive users aged 15 to 44 years.[1] Advantages of both male and female sterilization include its permanence, high rate of efficacy (0.5% failure rate for women and 0.15% for men), cost-effectiveness, lack of significant long-term side effects, and lack of need for partner compliance.[16] Permanence is also a disadvantage of sterilization; the procedures can sometimes be reversed, but this is difficult and expensive. In addition, sterilization provides no protection against STDs, including HIV infection.

HYSTEROSCOPIC STERILIZATION

A newer type of nonsurgical permanent sterilization has gained popularity as an alternative to tubal ligation. The Essure method involves placement of microinserts into the fallopian tubes through a hysteroscope. Over the course of 3 months, fibers in the inserts promote tissue growth and occlusion of the fallopian tubes, preventing conception. The procedure can be performed in the office setting with or without use of conscious sedation or local anesthesia. Occlusion is verified radiologically. Adverse effects are rare. This method has been shown to be slightly more effective than surgical sterilization but without the surgical risks. In 2006, Essure received an FDA "black box" warning for adverse events to include perforation of the uterus/fallopian tubes, misplacement of the inserts, pain, and allergies and hypersensitivity to the device.[25]

NATURAL FAMILY PLANNING

Natural family planning (NFP) includes any method of family planning that is based on observations of the signs of fertility rather than on interference with physiologic function. Although NFP is infrequently used,[1] it is important for health care providers to suggest NFP to those who might otherwise be unaware of its benefits or have spiritual or religious beliefs that preclude the use of barrier and hormonal contraceptives. With perfect use, NFP methods can be up to 97% effective.[16]

NFP began in the 1920s with the rhythm method, which taught couples to avoid intercourse on days when the woman was likely to be ovulating. Typically, starting at day 1 for menses, women avoided intercourse on days 12 to 19 and then altered those days depending on menstrual cycle length. Another older method, basal body temperature, relied on spikes of 0.05°F to 1°F in morning temperatures as an indicator of ovulation. Newer, more accurate methods of NFP primarily rely on identification of more sensitive physiologic indicators of fertility.

There are several methods of cervical mucus testing as a means of measuring fertility. All involve testing the quality and character of the mucus before intercourse. Mucus produced during fertile periods is clear, moist, and slippery and stretches. In contrast, mucus produced during periods of infertility is dry, cloudy, and sticky and breaks when stretched. The couple cannot adequately evaluate cervical mucus the day after intercourse and must abstain. After developing and identifying patterns, the couple can learn to identify periods of fertility and infertility. The Billings Ovulation Method and Creighton Method are formalized programs that provide the couple with education and visual aids.[26]

Another method of family planning, the symptothermal method (STM), is similar to the ovulation method but uses two other fertility signs in addition to cervical mucus: basal body temperature and the position, shape, and consistency of the cervix. STM is the most widely used method of NFP in the United States. Advocates of this method place particular emphasis on the cooperation of the man and woman in fertility regulation.[27]

With STM, the menstrual cycle is separated into three phases. The relatively infertile phase lasts from the beginning of menstruation to the onset of any mucus. The fertile phase lasts from the first sign of mucus until the beginning of the third phase. The third phase, known as the *postovulatory infertility phase* (or the *absolute infertility phase*), begins on the fourth day of a temperature elevation and the fifth day of the drying of the cervical mucus. A basal thermometer (useful for measuring subtle variations in body temperature between 35.5°C and 37.7°C [96°F and 100°F]) is used to record morning body temperatures. Typically, a biphasic curve is observed during the course of the menstrual cycle, with low temperatures recorded before ovulation and slightly higher temperatures recorded after ovulation. A typical postovulatory elevation ranges from 0.4°F to 1°F above the average of the last 6 ovulatory days. The temperature rise is caused by the presence of progesterone, which is released by the empty follicle after ovulation. At least 3 days of elevated temperatures must be recorded before the postovulatory infertile phase begins on the evening of that third day. Basal body temperature does not give any advance warning of ovulation but indicates when ovulation has passed.[27]

Palpation of the cervix is performed as an adjunct to the other signs of fertility. During the infertile period, the cervix is firm and low in the vagina, and the cervical os is closed. As ovulation approaches, the cervix softens and elevates until it is almost out of reach, and the cervical os opens. Some women find this to be a helpful sign; others do not. In some cycles, these signs provide information as to when the woman is capable of conceiving. Couples who wish to avoid pregnancy should wait to have intercourse until all signs indicate that the fertile time has passed.

REASONS FOR CONTRACEPTIVE NONUSE

In the United States, where contraception is generally widely available, it is surprising that almost 50% of pregnancies are still considered unintended. Unintended pregnancy may occur for many reasons, including nonuse of contraception, failure to use contraceptive methods consistently and correctly, and, far less frequently, method failure. Studies show that reasons for nonuse differ by event and by age at the time of the event. Common nonuse reasons include difficulty obtaining contraception, side effects, and displeasure with the current method.

Given the high rates of unintended pregnancy and the high rates of dissatisfaction with contraceptive methods, it is imperative that health care providers be skilled in prescribing contraception. This requires a well-informed, nonjudgmental approach in which the provider listens to the patient's concerns and desires, assesses risks, and sifts through that information to present a thoughtful list of contraceptive choices.

REFERENCES

1. Daniels, K., Mosher, W. D., & Jones, J. (2013). Contraceptive methods women have ever used: United States, 1982-2010. *Natl Health Stat Report.*, 62, 1–15.
2. Mosher, W. D., Jones, J., & Abma, J. C. (2012). Intended and unintended births in the United States: 1982-2010. *Natl Health Stat Report.*, 55, 1–28.
3. Lauring, J. R., Lehman, E. B., Deimling, T. A., Legro, R. S., & Chuang, C. H. (2016). Combined hormonal contraception use in women with contraindications to estrogen use. *American Journal of Obstetrics and Gynecology*, 3, E1–E7.
4. Trussel, J., Lalla, A. M., Doan, Q. V., Reyes, E., Pinto, L., & Gricar, J. (2009). Cost effectiveness of contraceptives in the United States. *Contraception*, 79, 5–14.
5. Erikkola, R., & Landgren, B. (2005). Role of progestins in contraception. *Acta Obstetricia et Gynecologica Scandinavica*, 84, 207–216.
6. Frye, C. A. (2006). An overview of oral contraceptives, mechanism of action and clinical use. *Neurology*, 66(Suppl. 3), S29–S36.
7. Chrousos, G. (2018). The gonadal hormones and inhibitors. In B. G. Katzung (Ed.), *Basic and clinical pharmacology* (14th ed.). New York: McGraw-Hill.
8. Regidor, A. P., & Schindler, A. E. (2017). Antiandrogenic and antimineralcorticoid health benefits of COC containing newer progestogens: Dienogest and drospirenone. *Oncotarget*, 8(47), 8334–83342.
9. Bahamondes, L., Bahamondes, M. V., & Shulman, L. P. (2015). Noncontraceptive benefits of hormonal and intrauterine reversible contraceptives. *Human Reproduction Update*, 21(5), 640–651.
10. Roach, R. E., Helmerhorst, F. M., Lijfering, W. M., Stijnen, T., Algra, A., & Dekkers, O. M. (2015). Combined oral contraceptives: The risk of myocardial infarction and ischemic stroke (review). *The Cochrane Database of Systematic Reviews*, (8), CD01105454.
11. World Health Organization, Department of Reproductive Health. Medical eligibility criteria for contraceptive use, 5th edition. Retrieved from http://www.who.int/reproductivehealth/publications/family_planning/Ex-Summ-MEC-5/en/. (Accessed 12 March 2018).

12. Practice Committee of the American Society for Reproductive Medicine. (2017). Combined hormonal contraception and the risk of venous thromboembolism: A guideline. *Fertility and Sterility, 107*(1), 43–51.
13. Kaminska, M., Ciszewski, T., Lopacka-Szatan, K., Miotla, P., & Staroslawska, E. (2015). Breast cancer risk factors. *Prz Menopauzalny, 14*(3), 196–202.
14. Nappi, R. E., Kaunitz, A. M., & Bitzer, J. (2016). Extended regimen combined oral contraception: A review of evolving concepts and acceptance by women and clinicians. *The European Journal of Contraception & Reproductive Health Care, 21*(2), 106–115.
15. Benson, L. S., & Micks, E. A. (2015). Why Stop Now? Extended and continuous regimens of combined oral hormonal contraceptive methods. *Obstet Gynecol Clin N Am, 42*, 669–681.
16. Hatcher, R. A., Trussell, J., Nelson, A., et al. (Eds.), (2011). *Contraceptive technology: Twentieth revised edition.* New York: Ardent Media.
17. Lopez, L. M., Newmann, S. J., Grimes, D. A., et al. (2012). Immediate start of hormonal contraceptives for contraception (review). *The Cochrane Database of Systematic Reviews,* (12), CD006260.
18. Brache, V., Payan, L. J., & Faundes, A. (2013). Current status of contraceptive vaginal rings. *Contraception, 87*, 264–272.
19. Family planning: a global handbook for providers, 2018 update. Baltimore: Johns Hopkins Bloomberg School of Public Health/Center for Communication Programs and World Health Organization, Department of Reproductive Health and Research; 2018.
20. Galzote, R. M., Rafie, S., Teal, R., & Mody, S. (2017). Transdermal delivery of combined hormonal contraception: A review of the current literature. *International Journal of Women's Health., 9*, 315–321.
21. Jacobstein, R., & Polis, C. B. (2014). Progestin-only contraception: Injectables and implants. *Best Practice and Research. Clinical Obstetrics and Gynaecology, 28*, 795–806.
22. Betur, P., Kransdorf, L. N., & Casey, P. M. (2016). Emergency contraception. *Mayo Clinic Proceedings. Mayo Clinic, 91*(6), 802–807.
23. Nelson, A. L., & Massoudi, N. (2016). New developments in intrauterine device use: Focus on the US. *Open Access Journal of Contraception, 7*, 127–141.
24. Yranski, P., & Gamache, M. L. (2008). New options for barrier contraception. *Journal of Obstetric, Gynecologic, and Neonatal Nursing, 37*, 384–389.
25. Clark, N. V., Endicott, S. P., Jorgensen, E. M., Hur, H. C., Lockrow, E. G., Kern, M. E., et al. (2017). Review of sterilization techniques and clinical updates. *Journal of Minimally Invasive Gynecology*, September 20.
26. Pallone, S. R., & Bergus, G. R. (2009). Fertility awareness-based methods: Another option for family planning. *Journal of the American Board of Family Medicine: JABFM, 22*(2), 147–157.
27. Hamilton, K. (1984). The symptothermal method of natural family planning. *Physician Assistant, 8*(11).

CHAPTER **146**

GENITAL TRACT CANCERS
Patricia Polgar-Bailey • Terry Mahan Buttaro

Gynecologic malignant neoplasms are cancers of the female genital tract; they include cancers of the endometrium, ovary, fallopian tube, vulva, vagina, and cervix. In the United States, endometrial cancer is the most commonly diagnosed gynecologic malignant neoplasm, and ovarian cancer accounts for the most deaths annually.[1,2] Although endometrial cancer is more common than ovarian cancer, it is easier to cure with surgery alone. Ovarian cancer is usually diagnosed at a later stage and therefore is difficult to cure. Fallopian tube cancers are rare and are managed like ovarian cancers.

Vulvar and vaginal cancers are also uncommon and are less familiar to patients. Few women are aware that a cancer of the vulva or vagina can develop and therefore do not seek health care at the onset of symptoms, usually burning or itching. Most vulvar or vaginal cancers are detected during a careful gynecologic examination. Of the gynecologic cancers, cervical cancer is the only one with a standardized screening tool—the Papanicolaou (Pap) test.

As a primary care provider, it is important to have a clear understanding of these six types of gynecologic cancers.

ENDOMETRIAL CANCER
DEFINITION AND EPIDEMIOLOGY
The endometrium is the inner glandular lining of the myometrium (muscle) of the uterus. This layer proliferates to prepare for implantation of a fertilized egg and sloughs on a regular cycle during the reproductive years. Once a woman reaches menopause, the endometrium remains thin because estrogen is no longer secreted from the ovaries. The proliferative characteristic of this lining is what can lead to neoplasia.

Despite being rare in females under age 45, endometrial cancer is the most common female genital tract cancer.[1] Most cases are found in older women after menopause. Three out of four cases are found in women ages 55 and older. In 2018, approximately 63,230 new cases will be diagnosed (an increase since 2015); it is estimated that 11,350 will die.[1] Although more white women are diagnosed with endometrial cancer, more African American women die of the disease, the result likely related to a variety of socioeconomic issues related to access to care and education.[3] The risk for endometrial carcinoma is primarily associated with estrogen exposure without progesterone. Estrogen that is not opposed by progesterone causes the endometrium to become thicker and hypervascular (hyperplasia). Without progesterone, the structural support needed to sustain vascularity of the thickened endometrium is not present, and spontaneous superficial random hemorrhages occur. Other risk factors include family history of ovarian, endometrial, or colon cancer; hypertension; and diabetes.

PATHOPHYSIOLOGY
Endometrial cancers are divided into two types: uterine sarcomas and varied types of endometrial carcinomas (adenocarcinomas, carcinosarcomas, squamous cell carcinomas, undifferentiated carcinomas, small cell carcinomas, and transitional carcinomas). Uterine sarcomas are uncommon and include adenosarcomas, endometrial stromal sarcomas, and leiomyosarcomas.

Adenocarcinomas are endometrioid cancers and are even further differentiated. Endometrial cancers are divided into two types, type I and type II. Type I is associated with excess estrogen that is unopposed by progesterone. Without progesterone, the structural support needed to sustain vascularity of the thickened endometrium is not present, and spontaneous superficial random hemorrhages occur. Typically occurring in women who have hyperlipidemia, hyperestrogenism, anovulatory bleeding, infertility, low parity, late menopause, and are overweight, Type I is associated with a favorable prognosis and usually is at an early stage on presentation. The excess androgen in the obese patient is converted to estrogen. Type II is not associated with these risk factors; it is most often seen in normal-weight women and has a poor prognosis.

The hyperplastic appearance of the endometrium is classified by pathologists into two categories: benign endometrial hyperplasia and endometrial intraepithelial neoplasia (EIN). This classification system is intended to stratify the patient's risk for development of malignant endometrial cells. Benign endometrial hyperplasia shows cysts, remodeled glands, vascular thrombi, and stromal microinfarcts; these are changes resulting from the duration and combination of hormonal exposures. In contrast, EIN is the premalignant state that is demonstrated microscopically as cells with altered cytologic features and crowded architecture. Patients with EIN have a 45-fold greater risk for development of an endometrial cancer, and hysterectomy is recommended.[4] According to the Collaborative Group on Epidemiological Studies on Endometrial Cancer, medium- to long-term use of oral contraceptives (i.e., for 5 years or longer) results in substantially reduced risk of endometrial cancer.[5] The reduction in risk associated with ever having used oral contraceptives differed, depending on the type of tumor, with the risk reduction being stronger for carcinomas than sarcomas. In high-income countries, use of oral contraceptives for 10 years was estimated to reduce the absolute risk of endometrial cancer arising before age 75 years from 2.3 to 1.3 per 100 women.[5]

Factors that influence the risk of endometrial cancer include factors affecting hormone levels (e.g., estrogen after menopause, birth control pills, tamoxifen), the number of menstrual cycles (over a lifetime), pregnancy, obesity, certain ovarian tumors, polycystic ovarian syndrome, use of an intrauterine device, age, diet and exercise, diabetes, a history of breast or ovarian cancer, history of endometrial hyperplasia, and a history of radiation therapy to the pelvis to treat another type of cancer.[6]

The risk of endometrial cancer is increased among first-degree relatives of patients with endometrial cancer and those with a personal history of colon and breast cancers. Patients with Lynch II syndrome, or hereditary nonpolyposis colorectal cancer (HNPCC), have about a 49% lifetime risk for development of endometrial cancer.[6,7] HNPCC is an autosomal dominant inherited cancer that is caused by a germline mutation in a DNA mismatch repair gene. These patients should be referred to an oncologist to ensure careful and frequent screening.

CLINICAL PRESENTATION AND PHYSICAL EXAMINATION

The most important sign or symptom of endometrial cancer in the postmenopausal patient is bleeding. Patients often have complaints of a single episode of postmenopausal bleeding or a fullness or pressure in the pelvis. For some women who may not bleed because of cervical stenosis, a transvaginal ultrasound examination is a helpful tool. In a postmenopausal woman, endometrial thickness (also called endometrial stripe) on transvaginal ultrasonography should not be more than 5 mm. An endometrial thickness of more than 5 mm requires assessment by a gynecologist.

The perimenopausal presentation is more challenging. These patients often have irregular menses that are heavier and more frequent than their cycle previously. This is an important sign because bleeding should become lighter and less frequent during perimenopause, not heavier and more frequent. It is important to not assume that changes in menses are related to the onset of menopause.

A detailed history of menstruation, dyspareunia, pelvic pain, fever, trauma, and intrauterine contraceptive device use should be elicited, and risk factors for endometrial cancer reviewed.

Other complaints that either premenopausal or postmenopausal women might express to the primary care provider are painful urination, dyspareunia, pelvic pain, cramping, pelvic discomfort, and postcoital bleeding.

In addition to a thorough general physical examination, the patient should undergo bimanual pelvic examination (including rectovaginal examination) and transvaginal ultrasound examination.

DIAGNOSTICS
Initial Diagnostics

If endometrial cancer is considered in the differential diagnosis, an endometrial biopsy is indicated. If there is high suspicion for cancer and the biopsy finding is normal, dilation and curettage should also be performed. If abnormalities are palpated on general or pelvic examination, a computed tomography (CT) scan with contrast enhancement of the abdomen and pelvis should be obtained to assess for spread of disease to adjacent organs or lymph nodes. Most common spread of disease is to the pelvic and para-aortic lymph nodes.

There are multiple benign causes of dysfunctional uterine bleeding; however, bleeding in the postmenopausal woman should be assumed to be cancer until proven otherwise. If a postmenopausal patient has vaginal bleeding, the priority should be tissue sampling, as a significant number of women will have cancer. If a perimenopausal patient has worsening vaginal bleeding, tissue sampling is also indicated to exclude malignant disease.

Additional Diagnostics

Once a malignant neoplasm has been ruled out, further diagnostic testing is necessary to determine the cause of the patient's symptoms. Additional diagnostics, if not previously obtained, should include serum human chorionic gonadotropic (if of reproductive age), complete blood count (CBC) with differential and platelets, vaginal wet preparations and cultures, coagulation profile, blood urea nitrogen (BUN), prothrombin/partial thromboplastin time (PT/PTT), creatinine and hormone levels.

DIFFERENTIAL DIAGNOSIS

 Immediate referral to a gynecologic oncologist is indicated if there is a high suspicion for cancer.

Differential diagnoses include endometrial cancer, atrophic vaginitis, cervicitis, cervical polyps, ovarian cysts, inflammation, infection or systemic disease, endometriosis, uterine fibroids or polyps, uterine prolapse, pelvic inflammatory disease, trauma, medications, and pregnancy.

INTERPROFESSIONAL COLLABORATIVE MANAGEMENT

Surgery is the treatment of choice for endometrial cancer. In early-stage disease, surgery can be curative. Ideally, even patients with disease that has spread outside the uterus will undergo hysterectomy to remove the bulk of the disease and the source of bleeding.

Endometrial cancer surgery includes hysterectomy, bilateral salpingo-oophorectomy, resection of gross disease, peritoneal cytology, and possibly pelvic and para-aortic lymphadenectomy, though according to Hamilton et al., the latter can be controversial.[8] The surgery should be performed in collaboration with a gynecologic oncologist who is trained to perform lymphadenectomy and lymph node sampling. Adjuvant treatment includes radiation therapy, hormonal therapy, and chemotherapy. Treatment decisions are made after surgery is complete and the staging and grading (type and morphologic features) of the disease have been assigned.

LIFE SPAN CONSIDERATIONS

The average age at diagnosis of endometrial cancer is 60 years, and the incidence increases with advancing age. When endometrial cancer occurs before the age of 40 years, it is usually associated with chronic obesity or anovulation.[9]

PATIENT AND FAMILY EDUCATION

Patients should understand that the use of estrogen plus progesterone for postmenopausal hormone replacement therapy does not increase the risk of endometrial cancer. It is also necessary that women understand the importance of evaluation for any postmenopausal bleeding even if it occurs only once or is a small amount.

OVARIAN CANCER

DEFINITION AND EPIDEMIOLOGY

Among women, ovarian cancer represents the fifth leading cause of death from cancer.[1] In 2018, the American Cancer Society estimated that there would be approximately 22,240 new cases diagnosed and 14,070 deaths from ovarian cancer with a woman's lifetime risk of getting ovarian cancer about 1 in 78, and the lifetime chance of dying from ovarian cancer about 1 in 108, slightly better than in 2016.[1,2] This cancer develops mainly in older white women, and approximately half of the women who are diagnosed with ovarian cancer are 63 years or older.[1]

During the last decade, advances have been made in the treatment of ovarian cancer; however, little advance has been made in the development of tools for early diagnosis of ovarian cancer. This disease often progresses to advanced stages with only subtle signs and symptoms. Attentiveness to patient symptoms is necessary to recognize the signs of early disease.

PATHOPHYSIOLOGY

Ovarian cancer develops in the ovary and according to the 2018 Cancer Statistics there are numerous histologic types of ovarian cancer.[2] the most common being epithelial (90%); the non-epithelial:germ cell (3%), and mesenchymal (2%) are stromal and sex cord. Although all these types are labeled ovarian cancers, it is important for the provider to understand that each histologic type is slightly different from its counterparts, and therefore oncology management of the disease may differ for each type.

The risk for development of ovarian cancer is influenced by genetic, hormonal, and environmental factors. Approximately 5% to 10% of women have a genetically acquired risk of ovarian cancer because of inherited mutations in the ERCA1 and BRCA2 tumor suppressor genes, but recent genetic research suggests that non BRCA genes may also be associated with ovarian and other cancers. The overall risk for development of ovarian cancer is 20% to 60% for those with BRCA1 mutations and 10% to 35% for those with BRCA2 mutations. Some data suggest that women with BRCA mutation-mediated ovarian cancer may have survival rates better than those of woman with sporadic ovarian cases. This may be a result of improved tumor response to platinum-based chemotherapy in those with BRCA-related cancer.[10]

Other familial genetic concerns associated with ovarian cancer include hereditary nonpolyposis colon cancer (Lynch syndrome), Peutz-Jeghers syndrome, PTEN tumor hamartoma syndrome, and MUTYH-associated polyposis.[11,12] Other risk factors are currently under investigation, but some studies suggest diet, use of talcum powder, and androgens.[12]

For patients with a family history of breast or ovarian cancer inquiring about pelvic pain, fullness, early satiety, or urinary frequency at each visit is important. Any concerns must then prompt the provider to carefully evaluate the patient and rule out malignant disease.

Other risk factors include obesity, late menopause, nulliparity, and early menarche. There is debate as to whether infertility drugs increase the risk for ovarian cancer; at this time, the data do not fully support either argument. In general, these theories are based on a theory of ovulation without stopping, in which the ovary itself is somehow disrupted and is sensitive to events of ovulation. Therefore methods to suppress ovulation, such as oral contraceptive use, multiparity, late menarche, and early menopause, would potentially decrease a patient's risk. The American Cancer Society suggests that use of oral contraceptives may offer some protection, especially for epithelial ovarian cancer.[12]

CLINICAL PRESENTATION AND PHYSICAL EXAMINATION

Goff and colleagues[13] developed a symptom index to improve early detection of ovarian cancer. These specific symptoms, if persistent, should be considered red flags for the provider: pelvic pain, abdominal pain, urinary urgency, urinary frequency, increased abdominal size, abdominal bloating, difficulty eating, and early satiety. The provider must consider all differential diagnoses and especially ovarian cancer for these symptoms and should not presume that they are related to menopause or stress.

A pelvic examination that includes a rectovaginal examination should be done but is not sensitive for detection of ovarian cancer. This examination should be done routinely on all women to adequately assess the entire pelvis for mass, fullness, or tenderness. Despite a careful examination, it is rare that an ovarian cancer is detected.

DIAGNOSTICS
Essential Diagnostics

If a pelvic mass is suspected, the initial diagnostic test that should be ordered is a transvaginal pelvic ultrasound. Once the diagnosis of a pelvic mass is established, a tumor marker, such as serum cancer antigen 125 (CA-125), OVA,1 and human epididymis protein 4 (HE4), should be ordered. CA-125 is a serum protein produced by ovarian cancer cells and elevated in most epithelial ovarian cancers, but can also be increased in many conditions, malignant and nonmalignant (Box 146.1). Unfortunately, because CA-125 is also elevated in nonmalignant conditions, it is not an adequate screening tool. OVA1 is a serum test that combines the results of five immunoassays into a single numeric result. The five assays are prealbumin (transthyretin), apolipoprotein, β_2-microglobulin, transferrin,

BOX **146.1**

Causes of Elevation of CA-125

- Acute pelvic inflammatory disease
- Endometriosis
- Functional ovarian cyst
- Meigs syndrome
- Ovarian hyperstimulation
- Uterine myoma
- Acute infection: hepatitis, pancreatitis, colitis, pericarditis, pneumonia, congestive heart failure, polyarteritis nodosa
- Renal disease
- Chronic liver disease
- Mesothelioma
- Postoperative period
- Rodent exposure (human anti-mouse antibody[HAMA] response)
- Systemic lupus erythematosus
- Autoimmune disease
- Poorly controlled diabetes

Data from DiSaia PJ, Creasman WT: *Clinical gynecologic oncology*, ed 7, St. Louis 2007, Mosby.

and CA-125. It is indicated for women who have a pelvic mass for which surgery is already planned. It is intended to aid in the assessment of the likelihood that the pelvic mass is malignant. It is particularly useful when the pelvic examination and radiographic imaging do not clearly indicate a malignant neoplasm. It is not a useful test for screening. The test result is divided into two categories, premenopausal and postmenopausal. When the probability of malignant disease is high, the test is designed to help the general gynecologist decide whether the patient's surgery should be performed by a gynecologic oncologist, who can perform a complete debulking and staging surgery.

HE4 is a more recent serum marker. Studies show that HE4 is overexpressed in 93% of serous, 100% of endometroid, and 50% of clear cell tumors, but not in mucinous ovarian carcinomas. In addition, data suggests that HE4 is elevated in more than half of ovarian cancer patients who did not have elevated CA-125 levels. The combination of markers improves sensitivity.

None of these biomarkers should be used as screening tools because they lack sensitivity and specificity and misuse can lead to unnecessary treatment. They can all be used for discrimination of pelvic masses. In addition, CA-125 and HE4 can be used for monitoring treatment and detection of recurrence.

If an ovarian cancer is suspected, the patient should undergo CT scanning to further delineate the disease process. On CT, the provider is looking for lymphadenopathy, ascites, omental caking, diaphragmatic thickening, and pleural effusion, all signs of advanced-stage disease requiring referral directly to a gynecologic oncologist for complete debulking surgery (usually includes hysterectomy, bilateral salpingo-oophorectomy, omentectomy, and node sampling). Diaphragmatic stripping, bowel resection, and splenectomy are sometimes performed as well.

Additional Diagnostics

Transvaginal ultrasonography is the gold standard assessment of the pelvis. If the ultrasound study is inconclusive, pelvic CT scan and pelvic magnetic resonance imaging (MRI) are both useful. However, if a primary care provider suspects a pelvic mass or diagnoses a mass on ultrasound examination, the patient should be referred to a gynecologist for further workup.

DIFFERENTIAL DIAGNOSIS

If a pelvic mass is suspected or diagnosed on ultrasound examination, referral should be made to a gynecologist for further evaluation.

Other conditions can manifest as a pelvic mass. These include sigmoid diverticulitis; pregnancy; a distended bladder; a low-lying distended cecum; stool in the sigmoid colon; a pelvic kidney; and a fallopian tube, uterine, or gastrointestinal tumor. Included in the differential diagnosis are fallopian tube carcinomas, which are rare, but managed and treated like ovarian cancers.

INTERPROFESSIONAL COLLABORATIVE MANAGEMENT

All patients with suspected ovarian carcinoma should be referred to a gynecologic oncologist for surgery. The standard procedure is a laparotomy to facilitate careful evaluation of the upper abdomen for evidence of disease spread that might not have been detected on radiographic imaging preoperatively.

LIFE SPAN CONSIDERATIONS

Older women are more likely to develop ovarian cancer and have worse outcomes than younger women. This is likely because of comorbidities and tolerability of aggressive treatment with surgery and chemotherapy.

PATIENT AND FAMILY EDUCATION

Patients with a familial history of ovarian cancer or known genetic abnormality associated with *BRCA1* or *BRCA2* or HNPCC should be referred to a gynecologist and possibly a gynecologic oncologist for careful surveillance. These families will benefit from referral to genetic counseling. There are many emotional challenges related to screening the relatives of the patient with ovarian cancer. The decision to undergo screening should be done in consultation with a genetic counselor.

Families and patients undergoing treatment of ovarian cancer should understand that although the disease is rare, it is generally sensitive to chemotherapy. An increasing number of medication therapies are available for ovarian cancer patients; some are novel agents that do not have the same toxicities of traditional chemotherapies. These patients generally receive chemotherapy intermittently or targeted therapy for the rest of their lives.

VULVAR CANCER

DEFINITION AND EPIDEMIOLOGY

In the United States, approximately 6020 cases of vulvar cancer were projected to be diagnosed in 2018 with an estimated 1150 deaths caused by this particular cancer.[14] The majority of these cancers will be related to human papillomavirus (HPV).[14]

PATHOPHYSIOLOGY

There are several types of vulvar cancers: squamous cell carcinoma, verrucous carcinoma, sarcoma, melanoma, basal cell carcinoma, Paget disease, and Bartholin gland adenocarcinoma. Squamous cell carcinomas arise from the skin of the vulva and consist of two subtypes. One (Bowenoid type) is associated with HPV 16, 18, and 33; the other type is associated with chronic venereal granulomatous disorders and lichen sclerosis but not HPV. Adenocarcinomas of the vulva arise from the glandular cells of the vulva, such as the Bartholin gland. Prognosis of these lesions is related to size of the lesion and lymph node involvement.

Melanoma is a rare and aggressive form of vulvar skin cancer that is often without any symptoms of burning, itching, or pain. It is thought to arise from a lesion that contains a junctional or compound nevus. It is the second most common cancer of the vulva.[15] These lesions are usually pigmented, raised, and often ulcerated. Most of these lesions occur on the labia minora and clitoris. Prognosis is related to size of the lesion and depth of invasion.

Basal cell carcinoma is usually small and occurs on the labia majora; it often has a central ulceration. It usually progresses slowly and rarely involves the lymphatics. Usually, the patient reports a repeated pattern of mild itching, slight bleeding, and then healing.

Paget disease is uncommon, usually affects postmenopausal women, and arises from glandular cells of the vulvar skin. These lesions usually are present for years before the patient seeks medical attention. Paget disease manifests with pruritus, tenderness, erythematous skin, and hyperkeratotic plaques and may be confused with candidiasis. The lesions are hyperemic, well-demarcated, thickened plaques with foci of excoriation and induration. The skin is usually smooth and thick, reminiscent of leukoplakia. The hyperemic areas are often associated with a superficial white coating that is described as "cake icing effect." These patients have an increased risk for development of an associated adenocarcinoma and concurrent adenocarcinoma somewhere else in the body. Therefore routine cancer screening with mammography, colonoscopy, and chest radiography is important. The primary treatment of Paget disease is surgical resection.

Adenocarcinoma of the Bartholin gland is rare and more often found in women in their 60s. This cancer usually presents with a mass in the deep vulvar tissues. Women often experience dyspareunia before they realize there is a problem. Although the Bartholin gland can form an abscess, enlargement of the Bartholin gland in a postmenopausal woman should be presumed to be carcinoma. Treatment involves radical pelvic surgery to extensively dissect the tissues around the gland.

Risk factors for vulvar cancers include cigarette smoking (particularly with the vulvar cancers that are caused by HPV), human immunodeficiency virus (HIV) infection or other conditions that cause immunosuppression, low socioeconomic status, vulvar intraepithelial neoplasia, other genital cancers, and lichen sclerosus.[16]

CLINICAL PRESENTATION AND PHYSICAL EXAMINATION

It is not uncommon for women to present with concerns about vulvar irritation, burning, pain, pruritus, local discomfort, excoriation, fissuring, painful irritation, bleeding, discharge, or a painful vulvar lesion that may be white, raised, hyperkeratotic, or pigmented. Many tumors are diagnosed at advanced stages because women are generally unaware of the possibility of vulvar cancer or they are embarrassed. A long-term "lump" or mass and pruritus are present in many women who are diagnosed with vulvar cancer.

Early diagnosis of vulvar cancer is important. The initial lesion may appear as a small raised area or as an ulceration that will not heal, or it may be associated with a secondary infection. The entire vulva is composed of squamous cells, and therefore lesions can arise anywhere on the vulva; the majority are usually found on the labia. The size of the tumor correlates with the risk of lymph node metastases. Careful examination of the inguinal lymph nodes is important because the cancer can metastasize easily along the inguinal lymph channels. The presence of palpable lymph nodes often represents malignant spread.[16]

DIAGNOSTICS

Definitive diagnosis requires a biopsy and further evaluation by a gynecologist. Biopsy is often done in the office with a punch biopsy procedure and local anesthetic.

DIFFERENTIAL DIAGNOSIS

If vulvar carcinoma is suspected, referral should be made to a gynecologist for further evaluation.

Vulvar carcinoma can be mistaken for other conditions, including eczema or dermatitis, ulcerative lesions such as syphilis, and granuloma inguinale. These lesions are often cultured and treated for infection before a biopsy is done, which delays diagnosis. Crohn disease can manifest as an ulcerative area on the vulva, and a lesion, on rare occasion, could be a metastasis from a distant site.

INTERPROFESSIONAL COLLABORATIVE MANAGEMENT

Treatment of vulvar cancer is usually surgery consisting of wide local excision or vulvectomy with unilateral or bilateral inguinal lymph node dissection. On occasion, the urethra or the rectum may be involved, and the oncologist will opt to treat the patient with radiation therapy or chemotherapy before resection of the tumor. Postoperatively, these patients may develop lymphedema of the lower extremity. This is managed with lymph compression stockings or compression pumps.

LIFE SPAN CONSIDERATIONS

Vulvar cancer can affect women younger than age 50, but 50% of these cancers occur in women over age 70.[16] Women age 70 are more frequently diagnosed with invasive vulvar cancer.[16]

PATIENT AND FAMILY EDUCATION

All women should understand the necessity of screening to ensure early detection of vulvar and other gynecological cancers. Primary care providers have an opportunity to educate patients and families on the possibility of development of a malignant neoplasm of the vulva as well as other cancers and the importance of seeking care as soon as symptoms arise. Screening methods include an annual pelvic examination and Pap test, monthly genital self-examination, and prompt reporting of unusual symptoms.

VAGINAL CANCER

DEFINITION AND EPIDEMIOLOGY

Vaginal cancer is an uncommon tumor that accounts for a small percentage of genital tract cancers. In the United States, there are approximately 5000 cases of vaginal cancer annually and the majority of cases are associated with HPV virus, but diethylstilbestrol (DES) exposure or previous history of cervical, vaginal, or uterine cancer are other causes.[17] Most vaginal cancers are diagnosed in women 70 years of age and older; most vaginal cancers are squamous cell carcinoma, some are adenocarcinomas, and a small number are melanomas or other rare histologic types. The survival rate is dependent on varied factors, but for squamous cell carcinomas is 54%, for adenocarcinomas of the vagina is 60%, and for melanomas is 13%.[17]

Most vaginal cancers are secondary (originating from other sites, such as the gastrointestinal tract or the breast). When the cancer involves the vagina only, it is considered a primary vaginal cancer. The grade of the tumor, the stage, and the histologic type will all affect survival.

PATHOPHYSIOLOGY

Squamous cell carcinoma and adenocarcinoma are the most common types of vaginal cancer. Squamous cell carcinomas arise from surface epithelial cells; adenocarcinomas arise from glandular cells; sarcomas arise from connective tissue; and melanomas arise from melanocytes. Non-clear cell adenocarcinoma is very rare, occurs predominantly in postmenopausal women, and has a worse prognosis than squamous cell carcinoma. Clear cell adenocarcinoma is usually associated with DES exposure in utero.

Risk factors that increase a woman's risk of vaginal cancer are young age at coitarche, greater number of lifetime sexual partners, smoking, in utero DES exposure, HPV infection, previous history of pelvic irradiation, and personal history of cervical cancer. Many vaginal cancers are caused by HPV infection. Vaginal cancers metastasize by direct extension into the surrounding tissues. The pelvic bones, bladder, rectum, and soft tissues are commonly involved.

CLINICAL PRESENTATION AND PHYSICAL EXAMINATION

Often patients with vaginal cancer are asymptomatic. The most common presenting symptom of vaginal cancer is vaginal bleeding that is not associated with discomfort.[18] Symptomatic patients may report vaginal pain, pelvic pain, dyspareunia, postcoital bleeding, dysuria, constipation, or vaginal discharge or mass. Tenesmus can be associated with posterior vaginal disease.

A thorough gynecological examination is necessary. A common site for a primary tumor is the upper third of the vagina.

DIAGNOSTICS
Essential Diagnostics

If a gross lesion is noted on vaginal examination or routine Pap testing, the provider should refer the patient for further evaluation by a gynecologist. In both cases, the patient will need to undergo colposcopic examination and biopsies of the abnormal tissue.[18]

If the patient has a history of DES exposure in utero, she should be referred to a gynecologist for surveillance because of the increased incidence of clear cell adenocarcinoma in this population. These patients should undergo Pap test of the cervix and vaginal fornix to screen for vaginal adenosis and coexisting adenocarcinoma.

Vaginal cancer is staged clinically, not surgically.[18] Careful pelvic and rectovaginal examination is essential to determine the amount of direct extension of the disease into surrounding tissues.

Additional Diagnostics

Metabolic imaging with positron emission tomography (PET) and CT scan is more sensitive than CT or MRI for the detection of metastatic disease. All patients diagnosed with a vaginal cancer should be assessed for metastatic disease.

DIFFERENTIAL DIAGNOSIS

Signs and symptoms suggestive of vaginal cancer or metastatic disease necessitate referral to a gynecologic oncologist.

The differential diagnosis of cervical lesions includes vaginal intraepithelial neoplasia, metastatic disease, or trophoblastic disease.

INTERPROFESSIONAL COLLABORATIVE MANAGEMENT

Patients with suspicious lesions require colposcopy and biopsy. The primary treatment involves surgery; wide excision or upper vaginectomy is the most common. Adjuvant treatment includes chemotherapy and radiation therapy. In rare cases, the gynecologic oncologist may perform a pelvic exenteration.

LIFE SPAN CONSIDERATIONS

Age is a risk factor for squamous cell cancer of the vagina. In the 1970s, more vaginal adenocarcinoma was seen in a younger population because of the use of DES during the first trimester in the 1950s. Because DES is no longer used, there are fewer cases of clear cell adenocarcinomas of the vagina.

PATIENT AND FAMILY EDUCATION

Patients and families should be educated about the importance of routine screening. This is especially true for women who have a history of cervical cancer or radiation therapy because vaginal cancers can be detected on routine examination with the Pap test and careful inspection.

CERVICAL CANCER

DEFINITION AND EPIDEMIOLOGY

Cervical cancer is a malignant neoplasm that develops in the squamous or glandular cells of the uterine cervix. In the United States, it is estimated that approximately 13,240 new cases of invasive cervical cancer will be diagnosed in 2018 and about 4170 women will die from this disease.[19] Cervical precancers are diagnosed far more often than invasive cervical cancer.[19]

Cervical cancer used to be one of the most common causes of cancer death for American women but has decreased because of the Pap test.

Cervical cancer generally occurs in midlife. Most cases are found in women younger than 50, but it is unusual in women younger than 20.[19] Many older women do not realize that the risk of developing cervical cancer continues as we age, yet 15% of cases of cervical cancer occur in women older than 65. However, these cancers rarely occur in women who underwent regular tests to screen for cervical cancer before they were 65.[19]

In the United States, Hispanic women seem to be the most commonly affected population to develop cervical cancer, but cervical cancer is seen in all ethnicities.[20] Unfortunately, there are still ethnic and racial disparities in the incidence of cervical cancer in the United States. The incidence of cervical cancer for African American and Hispanic women is higher than for white women and the death rate for black women related to cervical cancer is twice that of white women.[21]

Each year, millions of women undergo screening with the Pap test, invented by George Papanicolaou in the 1940s to obtain a cytologic sample of the cervix to screen for cancer or precancerous cells. It involves use of a brush or broomlike tool to sample the cells of the cervix and endocervix. The advent of the Pap test has reduced the incidence of cervical cancer in the United States by approximately 75%.[21]

Approximately 3.5 to 5.0 million of these Pap tests require some follow-up. Of these, 2 to 3 million will involve atypical cells of undetermined significance, 1.25 million will be low-grade squamous intraepithelial lesions (LSIL), and 300,000 will be high-grade squamous intraepithelial lesions.[21]

PATHOPHYSIOLOGY

Approximately three-quarters of all cervical cancers in the United States are squamous cell carcinomas; the remaining are adenocarcinomas. HPV is a precursor for the development of cervical cancer and precancer. For sexually active people in the United States, HPV infection is prevalent, but many of these infections resolve, usually within 12 months of infection. High-risk HPV types 16 and 18 account for approximately 70% of all cervical cancers; the remaining are caused by other high-risk strains of HPV (of which there are approximately 40).[22] Cervical cancers occur when high-risk HPV infection persists more than 2 years. Approximately 90% of HPV infection will become undetectable in the first 2 years after exposure to the virus. Therefore it is the remaining 10% that persists that causes cervical squamous cell and adenocarcinomas.

The transformation zone of the cervix (where the columnar cells of the endocervix are undergoing metaplasia to become squamous cells) is particularly sensitive to microtrauma and therefore to HPV infection. Most HPV-related cancers occur in this zone. As women age, the transformation zone regresses into the endocervical canal. Adolescents, who have a large transformation zone on the cervix, are at an increased risk of HPV infection; this explains why early sexual debut and multiple sex partners would increase one's risk of HPV infection and in turn one's risk for development of cervical cancer if monitoring is not done on a regular basis with Pap testing.

Important risk factors for cervical cancer that should be considered include long-term contraception use and smoking. Women who smoke have a two to three times greater risk for development of cervical cancer.[23] Immunosuppression, other cervical infections, and multiparity are other risk factors.[23]

CLINICAL PRESENTATION AND PHYSICAL EXAMINATION

Early symptoms include abnormal uterine bleeding (postmenopausal, postcoital, after douching, or intermenstrual) and foul vaginal discharge. Vaginal discharge is often described as thin and watery. Bleeding usually begins as light and serosanguineous and becomes heavier and more persistent as the

tumor enlarges. Late symptoms include pain, leg edema, and urinary and rectal symptoms.

A vaginal examination may reveal an enlarged cervix (described as a barrel cervix), friable tumor on the cervix, or ulcerative lesion that bleeds easily on contact. A Pap test will detect precancerous and cancerous lesions on the cervix or within the endocervix even if the cervix appears normal. The Pap test should include a scraping from the cervical os and a brushing from the endocervical canal. The specimen should be sent for interpretation by an experienced cytopathologist.

DIAGNOSTICS
Essential Diagnostics

The Pap test is a screening test that uses a liquid-based medium (cytology) that is spun down and plated on a slide for the pathologist. It is only a screening test and has a high false-negative rate. However, it is an effective screening tool when it is used routinely. It does not render a diagnosis; this must be obtained by tissue sampling with colposcopy (the application of acetic acid to improve visualization of abnormal cells for directed biopsy). Both the Pap test and the histologic features are described by the terminology of the Bethesda System, which was last updated in 2014.

The Bethesda System scores cervical intraepithelial neoplasia (CIN) on a grading system (1 to 3). CIN 1 is well differentiated and involves the initial third of the epithelial layer. CIN 2 is less differentiated and involves one-third to two-thirds of the epithelial layer. CIN 3 is undifferentiated in two-thirds and involves the full thickness (carcinoma in situ) up to the basal cell layer. Invasive cervical cancer involves cancerous cells that penetrate below the basal cell layer or the basement membrane.

The Bethesda System further separates cervical squamous intraepithelial lesions (CSIL) into two categories: LSIL/CIN-1 or high-grade intraepithelial lesions (HSIL/CIN 2 or 3) and also has a classification system for cervical cytology to determine specimen type and adequacy as well as interpretation of the findings. The Pap smear results can indicate that there is no evidence of intraepithelial lesions (a negative finding) or indicate atypical squamous cells of undetermined significance (ASC-US), LSIL suggesting HPV or mild dysplasia (CIN1), or HSIL indicating a moderate degree of severe dysplasia (CIN 2 or 3). Other information is available and includes vaginal infections and endometrial cells, which are concerning in females over age 45 and require further evaluation.

Additional Diagnostics

Newly diagnosed cervical cancer patients should undergo careful pelvic examination, which includes a rectovaginal examination. Cervical cancer spreads by direct extension into the adjacent tissues (bladder, rectum, parametrium, bone). It is staged clinically, not surgically. Therefore the stage is assigned at initial examination by a gynecologic oncologist. Patients should be evaluated for invasion of the tumor into the bladder and the rectum. This is done during an examination under anesthesia by cystoscopy and proctoscopy. Urine cytology can be used to detect bladder wall invasion.

DIFFERENTIAL DIAGNOSIS

 Specialist referral is indicated for signs and symptoms suggestive of cervical cancer.

Other considerations include atrophic vaginitis, cervicitis, cervical erosions, endometrial hyperplasia, and endometrial cancer, but the Pap test will aid in detection. If a cervix has an abnormal appearance on examination and the Pap test is normal, referral to a gynecologist is necessary. The liquid-based medium used for Pap tests allows the pathologist to distinguish between HPV-infected cells and inflammatory cells. In particular, this medium allows the pathologist to test the sample for the presence of HPV DNA.

INTERPROFESSIONAL COLLABORATIVE MANAGEMENT

The patient should be referred to a gynecologic oncologist for evaluation and consideration of surgery versus chemotherapy combined with radiation therapy. This determination is based on the assigned stage of the disease.

In 2006, the first HPV vaccine, Gardasil, was approved by the U.S. Food and Drug Administration (FDA). Gardasil was a quadrivalent vaccine that contains four types of HPV (16, 18, 6, 11). This was the first vaccine developed to prevent cervical cancer, precancerous cervical lesions, vulvovaginal cancer, and genital warts caused by HPV.

In 2009, a second vaccine, Cervarix, was approved by the FDA. Neither of these vaccines is currently used in the United States, as in 2015, the FDA approved Gardasil 9, a new vaccine for HPV. Gardasil 9 protects against nine types of HPV, more than the two vaccines previously marketed. In addition to providing protection against HPV 16 and 18, Gardasil also protects against two more types of HPV that cause genital warts. The vaccine is an intramuscular immunization, a three-injection series over 6 months.[24]

LIFE SPAN CONSIDERATIONS

Cervical cancer is unique in life span considerations. In most cases, women who are diagnosed with and die of cervical cancer have had HPV-related precancerous lesions for many years and have not been screened on a regular basis. In addition, this is the only cancer for which there is a preventive vaccine.[24]

PATIENT AND FAMILY EDUCATION

- Health care providers and the public need to be educated about the benefit of the HPV vaccine. Children, both females and males, can receive the 9-valent vaccine starting at age 9.[25]
- Cervical cancer is a preventable disease that can be treated successfully if it is detected early. Routine Pap testing is the key to cervical cancer prevention.

REFERENCES

1. American Cancer Society. (2018). Key statistics for endometrial cancer. https://www.cancer.org/cancer/endometrial-cancer/about/key-statistics.html. (Accessed 12 December 2018).
2. American Cancer Society. (2018). Key statistics for ovarian cancer. https://www.cancer.org/cancer/ovarian-cancer/about/key-statistics.html. (Accessed 12 December 2018).
3. Allard, J. E., & Maxwell, G. L. (2009). Race disparities between black and white women. *Cancer Control: Journal of the Moffitt Cancer Center, 16*(1), 53–56.
4. Mutter, G. L., Zaino, R. J., Baak, J. P., et al. (2007). Benign endometrial hyperplasia sequence and endometrial intraepithelial neoplasia. *International Journal of Gynecological Pathology, 26*(2), 103–114.
5. Collaborative Group on Epidemiological Studies on Endometrial Cancer. (2015). Endometrial cancer and oral contraceptives: An individual participant meta-analysis of 27276 women with endometrial cancer from 36 epidemiological studies. *The Lancet Oncology, 16*(9), 1061–1070.
6. American Cancer Society. (2018). What are the risk factors for endometrial cancer? Retrieved from https://www.cancer.org/cancer/endometrial-cancer/causes-risks-prevention/risk-factors.html. (Accessed 14 December 2018).
7. University of Texas M. D. Anderson Cancer Center. (2008). Lynch syndrome (hereditary nonpolyposis colorectal cancer syndrome or HNPCC). Retrieved from www2.mdanderson.org/app/pe/index.cfm?pageName=opendoc&docid=2133. (Accessed 17 September 2015).
8. Hamilton, C., Stany, M., Gregory, W., & Kohn, E. C. (2015). Gynecology. In F. Brunicardi, D. K. Andersen, T. R. Billiar, D. L. Dunn, J. G. Hunter, J. B. Matthews, et al. (Eds.), *Schwartz's principles of surgery* (10th ed.). New York, NY: McGraw-Hill. http://accessmedicine.mhmedical.com.ezproxy.simmons.edu/content.aspx?bookid=980&sectionid=59610883. (Accessed 14 December 2018).
9. Elliott, J. L., Hosford, S. L., Demopoulos, R. I., et al. (2001). Endometrial adenocarcinoma and polycystic ovary syndrome: Risk factors, management, and prognosis. *Southern Medical Journal, 94*(5), 529–531.
10. Karlan, B., Markman, M., & Eifel, P. (2005). Ovarian cancer, peritoneal carcinoma, and fallopian tube carcinoma. In V. DeVita, S. Hellman, & S. Rosenberg (Eds.), *Principles and practice of oncology* (7th ed.). Philadelphia: Williams & Wilkins.
11. Lu, K. H., & Daniels, M. (2013). Endometrial and ovarian cancer in women with Lynch syndrome: Update in screening and prevention. *Familial Cancer, 12*(2), 273–277.
12. American Cancer Association. Ovarian cancer risk factors. https://www.cancer.org/cancer/ovarian-cancer/causes-risks-prevention/risk-factors.html. (Accessed 17 December 2018).
13. Goff, B. A., Mandel, L. S., Drescher, C. W., et al. (2007). Development of an ovarian cancer symptom index: Possibilities for earlier detection. *Cancer, 109*(2), 221–227.
14. Cancer.Net. (2017). Vulvar cancer statistics. https://www.cancer.net/cancer-types/vulvar-cancer/statistics. (Accessed 18 December 2018).
15. Vapiwala, N., et al. (2017). https://www.oncolink.org/cancers/gynecologic/information-about-gynecologic-cancers/vulvar-cancer/all-about-vulvar-cancer. (Accessed 18 December 2018).
16. Cancer Treatment Centers of America. Vulvar cancer risk factors. https://www.cancer.org/cancer/vulvar-cancer/causes-risks-prevention/risk-factors.html. (Accessed 18 December 2018).
17. Cancer Treatment Centers of America. Types of vaginal cancer. https://www.cancer.net/cancer-types/vaginal-cancer/statistics. (Accessed 18 December 2018).
18. Ramirez, P. T. (2017). Vaginal cancer. https://www.merckmanuals.com/professional/gynecology-and-obstetrics/gynecologic-tumors/vaginal-cancer. (Accessed 18 December 2018).
19. American Cancer Association. Key statistics for cervical cancer. https://www.cancer.org/cancer/cervical-cancer/about/key-statistics.html. (Accessed 18 December 2018).
20. American Cancer Society. (2018). What are the key statistics about cervical cancer? Retrieved from www.cancer.org/cancer/cervicalcancer/detailedguide/cervical-uterine-cancer-risk-factors. (Accessed 9 December 2018).
21. Centers for Disease Control and Prevention. (2014). Human papillomavirus vaccination: Recommendations of the Advisory Committee on Immunization Practices (ACIP). *MMWR. Morbidity and Mortality Weekly Report, 63*(5).
22. Grimes, R. M., Benjamins, L. J., & Williams, B. S. (2013). Counseling about the HPV vaccine: Desexualize, educate and advocate. *Journal of Pediatric and Adolescent Gynecology, 26*, 243–248.
23. National Cancer Institute. (2015). Cervical cancer prevention. Retrieved from www.cancer.gov/cancertopics/pdq/prevention/cervical/healthprofessional. (Accessed 19 September 2015).
24. U.S. Department of Health and Human Services. HPV (Human papilloma virus). Vaccines.gov: HPV (Human papillomavirus vaccine. (Accessed 18 December 2018).
25. Centers for Disease Control and Prevention. Human Papillomavirus (HPV) ACIP Vaccine Recommendations. https://www.cdc.gov/vaccines/hcp/acip-recs/vacc-specific/hpv.html. (Accessed 18 December 2018).

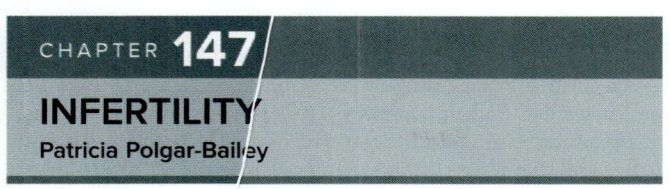

CHAPTER 147

INFERTILITY

Patricia Polgar-Bailey

DEFINITION AND EPIDEMIOLOGY

Whereas a healthy couple has approximately a chance of conceiving in a given month (natural cycle fecundity), infertility is defined as a couple's inability to conceive after 1 year of regular, timed, unprotected intercourse or therapeutic donor insemination.[1] Impaired fecundity is defined as physical difficulty in getting pregnant or the inability to carry a pregnancy to live birth. Infertility affects one couple in six, and prevalence increases dramatically with paternal and maternal age. In this chapter, infertility is contrasted with sterility, a term that applies to those members of a population for whom there is no possibility of attaining a natural pregnancy. The most recent national US data suggest that some form of infertility or subfertility was reported by 12% of men aged 25 to 44 and by 12.1% of women aged 15 to 44.[2] An estimated 15% of all couples experience infertility. The number of women in the reproductive age group who have ever received any infertility services has remained relatively constant between the 2002 and 2006-2010 surveys and corresponds to approximately 7.4 million women, or 11.9% of the population.[3]

PATHOPHYSIOLOGY

Potential causes of infertility include genetic, anatomic, endocrine, and behavioral factors. Physiologic dysfunction in men accounts for approximately 20% to 50% of all cases of infertility; ovulatory dysfunction in women contributes to up to 40% of infertility cases[4]; and tubal factors (20%), endometriosis (5%), and unexplained causes (between 10% and 25%) are other factors.

It has been difficult to estimate the true extent of male infertility is likely due to lack of evaluation of male evaluation in infertile couples.[5] Fertility treatment is often paid for out-of-pocket, and the lack of insurance data makes it difficult to quantify the problem. In addition, the empiric treatment of male infertility factor involves assisted reproductive technology (in vitro fertilization) that primarily treats the female partner and may obscure contributing male factors.[5] Male factors contribute to infertility in over 50% of cases, and 15%–20% of the most severe forms of male infertility, azoospermia, are related to genetic abnormalities.[6]

Male factor infertility can in general be attributable to chromosomal or structural defects or to endocrine abnormalities of the hypothalamic-pituitary-testicular axis. Contributing hypothalamic-pituitary disorders include congenital gonadotropin-releasing hormone (GnRH) deficiency (Kallmann syndrome); hemochromatosis; pituitary and hypothalamic tumors; infiltrative disorders (tuberculosis, sarcoidosis); hormonal disturbance (androgen, cortisol, and estrogen excess; hyperprolactinemia); and systemic disorders, such as chronic illness, obesity, and nutritional deficiencies. Structural causes include cryptorchidism, aplasia or obstruction in the male genital tract, varicoceles (usually a problem only when accompanied by other factors, such as abnormal semen analysis), congenital bilateral absence of the vas deferens (which can

indicate partial expression of a gene mutation for cystic fibrosis), and erectile or ejaculatory dysfunction. Factors influencing spermatogenesis or motility include inflammation or infection (postpubertal mumps, gonorrhea, chlamydial infection), direct injury or trauma (including postoperative), and use or abuse of substances (including alcohol, caffeine, cocaine, steroids, and marijuana).

Male factor infertility can involve a low sperm concentration (oligospermia), poor sperm motility (asthenospermia), abnormal sperm morphology (teratospermia), or, more commonly, a constellation of all three variables (oligoasthenoteratozoospermia). Poorer semen quality (reduced motility, increased DNA fragmentation, chromosomal aberrations) has been demonstrated in older men[6,7]; as men age, they produce fewer motile sperm, which are less able to travel in a straight line.[8]

Reproductive hazards for both men and women include environmental exposures,[9] possibly but not necessarily in an occupational setting, to solvents, pesticides, heavy metals, pharmaceuticals, anesthetic gases, ionizing radiation, and lead. Occupational exposures in male workers can affect the male reproductive system, leading to sperm abnormalities, hyperestrogenism, impotence, infertility, or increased spontaneous abortions in their partners. Even benzene levels at the US Occupational Safety and Health Administration (OSHA)–permissible level of 1 ppm have been associated with sperm aneuploidy[10,11]; because stem cells are affected, such exposures may have persistent reproductive effects in previously exposed workers. The websites of the National Institute for Occupational Safety and Health (www.cdc.gov/niosh/homepage.html) and OSHA (www.osha.gov) provide information on reproductive hazards and their management.

Cigarette smoking is associated with infertility in both women and men,[12–14] as is obesity.[6,15] In women, being underweight at age 20,[16] doing shift work, and having occupational exposure to chemotherapeutic drugs have also been associated with an increased subsequent risk of infertility.

Women can also have ovulatory dysfunctions that range from congenital absence of the ovaries and premature ovarian failure to various disruptions in the hypothalamic-pituitary-ovarian axis and other metabolic or endocrine conditions, such as hypothyroidism and hyperthyroidism. Uterine and fallopian pathologic conditions include current or past pelvic inflammatory disease resulting in salpingitis, endometriosis, iatrogenic Asherman syndrome after overly vigorous curettage, fibroids, bicornuate uterus, and postinfectious or operative tubal scarring and adhesions. Tubal infertility has been associated with lower family income. Pre-embryonic developmental problems and implantation problems have been postulated as possible causes of idiopathic infertility.

The pathophysiology of infertility includes theories relating to energy deficits inhibiting GnRH and luteinizing hormone (LH) secretion, interference with circadian rhythms, and the temporal pattern of endocrine functions in shift work. In addition, endogenous opioid–mediated inhibition of the hypothalamic GnRH pulse generator has been implicated in hypothalamic ovarian failure. The link between infertility and various autoimmune disorders may be related to the fact that the segment of the major histocompatibility complex that contains genes affecting reproduction also contains genes associated with various autoimmune disorders. Diabetes mellitus has been linked, at least in part, to a functional deficit of hypothalamic noradrenergic neurons, and cystic fibrosis has been connected to congenital bilateral absence of the vas deferens.

CLINICAL PRESENTATION AND PHYSICAL EXAMINATION

Ideally, both members of the couple are present for the initial interview; this is invaluable not only for the comprehensiveness of the medical history but also for providing insight into the couple's communication and decision-making style, emotional status, ability to support each other, coping strategies, and current level of functioning. Subsequent interviews with either partner alone may reveal information (e.g., previous pregnancies, abortions, or infections) that the individual is not comfortable disclosing otherwise. Essential components of relevant history to be elicited include coital frequency and timing, duration of the couple's infertility, previous pregnancy or siring of children, and age, because these factors have been consistently demonstrated to affect the prognosis.

Other needed historical information includes a thorough obstetric and gynecologic history (contraceptive use, prior pregnancy, therapeutic abortion, miscarriage, infection, pathologic conditions, or procedures). Particular attention is given to the menstrual history for cues related to ovulatory cycles, including midcycle discomfort, regular menses, premenstrual symptoms, and periods that occur every 27 to 30 days. The past medical history focuses on infections, surgeries, medications, and developmental, systemic, and autoimmune disorders. Family history is assessed for relatives with infertility or early menopause, autoimmune disorders such as lupus, and maternal diethylstilbestrol (DES) exposure. A review of systems may reveal weight changes; signs of estrogen deficiency or excess; signs of thyroid imbalance; hyperandrogenism or virilism; hyposmia (which may be related to Kallmann syndrome); or signs of galactorrhea, headaches, or visual disturbances (which are possibly suggestive of a pituitary pathologic condition).

Social history should include patterns of smoking, use of alcohol or other substances such as caffeine, exercise patterns, level of stress and coping strategies, potential eating disorders, and frequency of intercourse. Occupational history may reveal a host of potential reproductive threats, including the prolonged waiting time to pregnancy observed in female shift workers. Laboratory workers, health care workers (including anesthetists, dental assistants, and hospital personnel), farmers, painters, and construction workers may be exposed to reproductive toxins such as lead, nitrous oxide, waste anesthetic gases, and solvents. Domestic exposures include recent home renovation, contaminated air or groundwater, and domestic pesticide use. Various population-based studies have failed to find a correlation between consanguinity (uncle–niece, first cousins, and first-degree cousins once removed) and primary sterility. Infertility has also been shown not to be related to prior cervical laser surgery.

The examination of the male partner includes inspection of the genitals for abnormalities, including phimosis, varicocele (the most commonly identified genital abnormality in subfertile men), and hypospadias. The bilateral presence of the vas deferens is established, and the testes are palpated for maldescent, consistency, and size. Decreased testicular size is related to impaired spermatogenesis; the length of the testes (measured in a warm room, after the patient has been standing for several minutes) should be more than 4 cm (1⅗ inches) and the volume more than 20 mL by orchidometry.

Physical examination of the female partner includes palpation of the thyroid; breast examination to check for galactorrhea; and evaluation of signs of hypoestrogenic status (dry, pale vaginal mucosa), androgen excess (hirsutism, male-pattern hair loss, acne, obesity), or virilization (changes in body fat distribution, a lowering of the voice, or clitoromegaly). A pelvic examination also provides a gross indication of the state of the reproductive organs and may detect enlarged ovaries or other masses such as uterine fibroids. Changes in visual acuity or visual fields may be indicative of a cranial (pituitary) mass.

DIAGNOSTICS

Considerable debate surrounds the selection and interpretation of diagnostic studies in the context of a basic fertility workup because of the difficulty in establishing cutoff points for "abnormal" findings of investigations such as semen analysis and the demonstrated inability of many analyses to differentiate between fertile and infertile individuals. Complicating the issue is the likelihood that many couples have a constellation of factors, such as varicoceles and low-normal sperm count; although each may be relatively insignificant in isolation, they combine synergistically to produce clinical infertility.

Essential Diagnostics

Semen analysis should be performed early in the evaluation, usually after 2 to 7 days of abstinence. National guidelines from England and the US Institute for Clinical Systems Improvement suggest repeated semen analysis after 4 months if the first test result was normal and there has been no intervening pregnancy, though some recommendations suggest two semen samples within a much shorter period of time (weeks vs. months). All semen analysis should be conducted via the World Health Organization Laboratory Manual for Examination and Processing of Human Semen. If semen analysis indicates oligospermia, follicle-stimulating hormone (FSH), LH, and testosterone levels (drawn between 8 a.m. and 10 a.m.) should be obtained before referral to a male infertility specialist; if the serum testosterone level is low or the patient has other symptoms of hypogonadism (decreased libido or potency), a prolactin level should also be obtained. Testicular volume assessment with an orchidometer combined with basal serum FSH level can also be used to estimate future fertility in individuals who are long-term survivors of malignant disease in childhood or adolescence. The postcoital test (PCT) has received mixed reviews in the literature and is generally not recommended. It can be useful to confirm that intercourse has taken place, but it has poor sensitivity, specificity, positive predictive value, and negative predictive value. Although tests for sperm DNA fragmentation (SDF) are available and recognized as a valuable tool in the evaluation of male infertility, there remains a lack of understanding of the specific clinical scenarios where SDF test would be most helpful and the potential drawbacks of using SDF,[17] and being used in some circumstances, they are not yet recommended in best-practice guidelines from the American Society for Reproductive Medicine (ASRM) and the European Society of Human Reproduction and Embryology (ESHRE).[18,19]

Although the only definitive proof of ovulation in a particular cycle remains a subsequent pregnancy, ovulatory assessment has traditionally been done with menstrual calendars (a cycle normal in duration and frequency is suggestive of ovulation), and basal body temperature charting (biphasic curve demonstrating a consistently raised temperature in the latter half of the cycle is one of the simplest, most inexpensive, and most practical ways to assess ovulatory function, but the resultant curves can be difficult to interpret). Urinary LH can identify the LH surge that precedes ovulation by 1 or 2 days, and kits are available for home use. Such home testing, especially when done with an afternoon or evening urine sample, correlates well with peak serum LH. A plasma midluteal progesterone concentration higher than 3 ng/mL on day 21, or about 1 week before the expected onset of the next menses, is presumptive of ovulation but cannot assess the quality of the luteal phase. All female patients merit a rubella titer (if indicated), cervical cytology (Papanicolaou test [PAP] and human papilloma virus [HPV]), and nucleic acid amplification (NAAT) for *Chlamydia trachomatis* and *Neisseria gonorrhea*. Evaluation of tubal patency is most commonly done by hysterosalpingography and can even be therapeutic in that women have been known to conceive soon after this procedure. For women older than 35 years, a day-3 FSH level and an estradiol level are indicated to assess ovarian reserve (elevated day-3 FSH levels indicate a poorer outcome with assisted reproductive technologies [ARTs]).

Additional Diagnostics

Additional laboratory assessment is indicated by the patient's history and physical examination findings and is not warranted for all women concerned about their fertility, especially those with regular menstrual cycles. These tests include prolactin and thyroid assays, testosterone, and dehydroepiandrosterone (DHEA) and 17-hydroxyprogesterone tests when indicated and clomiphene challenge or day-3 FSH to evaluate ovarian reserve. Anticardiolipin antibody, antiphospholipid antibody, and antinuclear antibody assessments can be performed to exclude lupus.

INITIAL DIAGNOSTICS

Infertility

MEN
- Semen analysis X 2. If semen analysis + oligospermia, check FSH and testosterone level. If testosterone level low, check prolactin level.

WOMEN
- If semen analysis wnl, PAP smear/HPV, *Chlamydia trachomatis*, and *Neisseria gonorrhea*

IMAGING
- Hysterosalpingogram

DIFFERENTIAL DIAGNOSIS

A wide range of conditions can contribute to infertility and early pregnancy loss, including genetic, structural, and endocrine disorders; acquired infections (*Trichomonas, Chlamydia* organisms); treatment of other conditions with radiation therapy or chemotherapy; body mass index; personal behaviors such as alcohol consumption and maternal cigarette smoking; medications; sexual dysfunction; antisperm antibodies; previous genital or pelvic surgery; exposure to reproductive toxins; and other chronic medical diseases, such as thyroid dysfunction, celiac disease, inflammatory bowel disease, and hemochromatosis. Congenital causes include gonadal dysgenesis;

chromosomal mosaicism; congenital bilateral absence of the vas deferens or the uterus; Klinefelter syndrome (small hard testes, gynecomastia); Turner syndrome (short stature, pigeon chest, webbed neck); deletions in the Y chromosome genes; and isolated corticotropin deficiency, which is rare but treatable. Male factors contributing to infertility are in general determined by semen analysis.

Ovulatory dysfunction can be attributable to hyperprolactinemia; hypogonadotropic hypogonadism (these women have decreased serum estradiol levels and no withdrawal bleeding after a progesterone challenge); hypergonadotropic hypogonadism (elevated FSH levels indicating premature ovarian failure and possible presence of Y chromosome in young women); and normogonadotropic anovulatory conditions, including polycystic ovary syndrome (PCOS; a hyperandrogenic condition often seen with acne, weight gain, hirsutism, or acanthosis nigricans when hyperinsulinemia is also contributing), luteal phase defects, and multifollicular ovaries.

The term *unexplained infertility* refers to a diagnosis of exclusion, one in which the findings of standard investigations (semen analysis, tests of ovulation, tubal patency) are normal; this accounts for roughly 17% of all infertile couples.[20]

INTERPROFESSIONAL COLLABORATIVE MANAGEMENT

Although the provision of infertility services is beyond the scope of practice of most primary health care providers, they perform an important initial exploration of historical, physical examination, and selected diagnostic factors that can facilitate expedient referral to appropriate specialists when indicated. Individuals warranting an expedited workup and referral to a specialist include women without periods, with irregular periods, or with bleeding between periods as well as those who have pain with intercourse and a history of abdominal surgery, ruptured appendix, or upper genital tract infection. Men for whom similar expedited workup and referral are appropriate include those with difficulty sustaining an erection or an inability to ejaculate during intercourse and those with a history of testicular injury, infection, or maldescension.

Nonpharmacologic Management

1. Health care providers can intervene early in terms of improving modifiable lifestyle risk factors, improving coping mechanisms, providing basic preconception education and care such as updating immunization status,[21] and improving overall health for all patients who are attempting conception. General health-promoting interventions for the couple include normalizing weight, especially in overweight and obese individuals with PCOS[15]; improving nutritional status[22]; taking folate supplementation; reducing stress; and eliminating potential detrimental factors, such as cigarette smoking, caffeine, alcohol, nonsteroidal antiinflammatory drugs,[23] illicit drugs, and exposure to potential reproductive toxins. These interventions, which may increase a couple's chances of attaining successful pregnancy, might also improve their psychological health.

2. Education regarding prognosis. Of all couples diagnosed as infertile in one prospective US trial,[24] 28% of those untreated achieved pregnancy, and the rates were higher in all of the treatment modes—up to 85% in the first two cycles of medications, up to 71% in the first three intrauterine insemination (IUI) cycles, and 57% to 59% in the

first two in vitro fertilization (IVF) cycles. For all of these cycle-based treatment modalities, there was a diminishing return of efficacy as treatments continued beyond this point. In a European longitudinal multicenter cohort study, most couples (81%) diagnosed with unexplained infertility achieved an ongoing pregnancy, and the majority of these pregnancies (nearly 74%) were spontaneous.[25] Prognosis is more encouraging for shorter duration of infertility (less than 3 years), for younger women, and for those who have previously conceived a child in the same relationship. Prognosis is worse for situations involving endometriosis, male factor infertility, and tubal pathologic conditions or multiple factors.

3. It is essential from the outset to reinforce with any couple seeking treatment that appropriately directed therapy, excluding advanced reproductive technologies, is unsuccessful up to 50% of the time. Expectant management for unexplained infertility (encouraging couples to have intercourse during the "fertile window," roughly 5 days before until the day of ovulation) can be an effective strategy, especially for younger women with a shorter duration of infertility.[15] More elaborate ARTs, such as IVF and the newer intracytoplasmic sperm injection along with donor gametes and surrogacy, may provide hope for pregnancy otherwise unattainable through more conventional means. However, these approaches can be expensive[26] (upward of $10,000 for a single IVF cycle) and risky,[27] and their use often raises moral and ethical dilemmas.

4. Any treatment plan should follow a full discussion of all possible treatment options, including adoption, child-free living without intervention of any kind, and the possibility of stopping at any time in the treatment process. Discussion must address attendant benefits, risks, time required for participation, and costs along with reasonable estimations of probability for achieving pregnancy based on relevant infertility factors both with and without treatment.

5. Ongoing counseling for the couple should be offered and encouraged. Counseling may help the couple discontinue treatment when appropriate, solicit second opinions, participate in support groups, establish a (necessarily arbitrary) time limit for treatment, and take time off from treatment to give them a sense of control and balance in their lives.

Pharmacologic Management

1. When infertility is a result of hypothalamic-pituitary insufficiency in the male partner (as is the case in 1% to 2% of couples with male factor infertility), these men often respond well to gonadotropin or GnRH therapy.

2. Induction of ovulation according to a variety of protocols involving gonadotropins has been used for hypogonadotropic hypogonadism in women.

3. Chronic opiate agonist administration (naltrexone) can normalize ovarian function for women with hypothalamic ovarian failure.

4. Bromocriptine or other, newer dopamine agonists, such as cabergoline, are indicated in the treatment of hyperprolactinemia.

5. Metformin is a reasonable first-line intervention for non-obese women with anovulatory PCOS.[28]

6. Antiestrogens such as clomiphene citrate and tamoxifen are used for the induction of ovulation in women with POPS,

and Chinese herbal medicine has shown some promise in increasing the efficacy of clomiphene citrate therapy.[29]

7. Estrogen replacement for women with hypergonadotropic hypogonadism is important to prevent osteoporosis; ovulation-inducing therapies are neither useful nor indicated for these women.

8. For women with chemotherapy-induced ovarian failure, ovarian function should be reassessed periodically because spontaneous recovery has been noted.

9. Pharmacologic management of unexplained infertility[15,25] is by definition empirical; clomiphene, human menopausal gonadotropin, and various ART procedures are often used in these cases.

10. ARTs include such technologies as gamete intrafallopian transfer (GIFT). IVF, direct intraperitoneal injection of sperm, intrafollicular injection of sperm, and preimplantation genetic diagnosis. The induction of superovulation is often followed by artificial insemination of some kind; success is highly influenced by the woman's age, with cycle fecundity dropping from an average of 0.23% to 0.05% after the age of 40 years.

Women or men being managed by specialists for infertility still require basic primary care services. This enables the health care provider to assess and to intervene on behalf of the couple's functional, emotional, and psychospiritual responses to continuing therapy. Somatization is a common manifestation of the psychological stress of infertility, as are sexual problems, depressive reactions, emotional instability, relationship difficulties, and reduced self-confidence and self-esteem as well as feelings of anger, guilt, grief, isolation, and anxiety. As a result, concerns have arisen about the association between infertility treatment and perinatal depressive symptoms. According to a meta-analysis published in 2019, women who receive infertility treatment do not appear to be at increased risk of significant perinatal depressive symptoms compared with those after spontaneous conception.[30]

INDICATIONS FOR REFERRAL OR HOSPITALIZATION

Referral to a reproductive urologist is indicated for male factors identified on semen analysis. Referral to a reproductive endocrinologist or fertility specialist is indicated for an abnormal PCT result, for a basic infertility workup that does not disclose the source of the problem, or for any of the various ART procedures, should they be a couple's only hope for conception. Couples interested in exploring complementary therapeutic options may find some success with acupuncture. Pathologic conditions, including adhesiolysis and various testicular, uterine, or tubal conditions, may require surgical repair. In addition, complications from therapy (moderate to severe ovarian hyperstimulation syndrome) may necessitate hospitalization.

LIFE SPAN CONSIDERATIONS

A cultural tendency to delay childbearing combined with decreased fecundability with increasing age[31] necessitates prompt investigation into infertility in certain cases. According to the ASRM, an infertility evaluation is warranted after 1 year of coital exposure for couples in which the woman is younger than 35 years and after 6 months when she is older than 35 years. Immediate referral is reasonable for women older than age 40 or for men with suspected male factor infertility. Future fertility preservation for young men faced with a diagnosis of cancer can be assisted with sperm-banking procedures.[10]

COMPLICATIONS

In general, women with PCOS do not respond to ovulation induction as well as women with other ovulatory disorders do, and have an increased risk of ovarian hyperstimulation and spontaneous abortion when they do respond. Women with fibroids have a lower implantation rate with ART, women with endometriosis have a decreased pregnancy rate after ART procedures than do controls, and women 40 years of age or older have a higher risk for cesarean delivery after infertility treatment that is independent of other risk factors. Women who conceive with ART are more likely than their naturally conceiving counterparts to enter pregnancy with a chronic condition (such as diabetes or incompetent cervix) and to develop complications during pregnancy (pregnancy-induced hypertension, gestational diabetes mellitus, uterine bleeding), labor, and delivery.[11] Infants born after ART procedures are also at increased risk of adverse health outcomes (preterm delivery, very preterm delivery, low birth weight, infant not discharged home).[11] Other infertility treatment–related complications include a controversial association between fertility drugs and ovarian cancer and the protracted psychic anguish that can accompany successive failed treatment cycles.

The incidence and risks of multiple gestations associated with ARTs have been well documented in the literature; ART births are 18 times more likely to be twin, triplet, or higher-order births.[11] Twins that are the result of IVF also have an increased rate of preterm birth compared with spontaneously conceived twin controls.[12] (For all initial numbers of fetuses in an ART-induced multifetal pregnancy, including twins, reduction to a lower number decreases subsequent fetal loss, prematurity, and infant morbidity and mortality.[13]) Even resultant singleton pregnancies represent obstetric risks (given an increased incidence of pregnancy-induced hypertension, placenta previa, elective cesarean delivery, and preterm labor), an increased risk for major malformation, and a lower mean birth weight in ART pregnancies. Although the medical problems associated with ART-assisted multiple gestations have been widely emphasized in the medical literature, several studies note a desire among fertility patients for multiple births[14]; one study found that 67% to 90% of infertile couples expressed a desire for twins, and the majority of these couples rejected concerns about multiple gestations.[15] In another study, a significant proportion (41%) of fertility patients considered multiple birth an ideal treatment outcome.[16] This clearly indicates a need for additional education about the risks and complications associated with ARTs.

PATIENT AND FAMILY EDUCATION

Infertility and its often unsuccessful medical treatment present a conglomerate of stresses and losses with which the couple must contend, including the loss of biologic children and the experiences of pregnancy and breastfeeding. Individuals endure the stresses of complicated, expensive, and invasive treatment interventions, which can be experienced as humiliating, embarrassing, frustrating, and disappointing for women and their partners. Adjusting to infertile status is easier for individuals with positive self-esteem, an internal locus of control, and higher socioeconomic status, whereas increased anxiety and distress have been associated with advancing age, undifferentiated sex role identity, and low self-esteem. In one study, pregnant women with a history of infertility were at increased risk for alcohol abuse and were more likely to experience psychiatric disorders (phobia, generalized anxiety, bulimia, major depression, and panic disorder).[18]

Motives for medical consultation by infertile couples, in addition to the desire to have a child, include a desire for education and understanding regarding the cause of the infertility. Health care providers should be aware of a potential disparity between the medical diagnosis and the perception of the diagnosis in infertile persons, along with a tendency for patients to blame themselves for the infertility. Basic education for infertile persons includes advising them to have intercourse about twice a week and to avoid lubricants that may be spermicidal, such as K-Y Jelly, petroleum jelly, and Surgilube. In contrast, raw egg white and vegetable oil do not seem to affect sperm motility. The provider should also encourage cessation of alcohol or illicit drug use, smoking cessation, proper nutrition, normalization of body mass index (especially for women), and strategies for stress reduction. Health care providers can also provide an initial infertility workup that focuses on explaining the various diagnostic procedures and addressing couples' concerns and questions as they arise. The ASRM website (www.asrm.org) is a good source of patient information.

It is particularly important to provide couples with an accurate estimation of the success rates that are expected for various procedures and the concordant risks, discomforts, and expenses. Unfortunately, there have been fewer randomized clinical trials in the area of infertility management than in other branches of medical science, and many studies have small sample sizes, inappropriate design, and pseudorandomization. For couples able to conceive with treatment, providers of primary care can stress the normalcy of the pregnancy and help the couple through the normative developmental processes of pregnancy and parenthood.

Because the length of time that a woman has been infertile is related to her future fecundability and because fertility decreases exponentially with increasing age, many infertile individuals confront the necessity of redefining their expectations and goals related to establishing a family. Providers play an important role in facilitating the grieving process for the many losses sustained throughout the experience of diagnosis and treatment. This process is important because it constitutes the experiential prerequisite to acceptance and is essential for the couple to move on with their lives. Many providers emphasize helping couples to determine their own end point and timeline for intervention attempts, because there always seems to be some promising or potential development around the corner. Clinician support can enforce an "unsuccessful" couple's eventual realization that they have been thorough and have tried sufficient therapeutic interventions and that cessation of such interventions is reasonable and advisable. Couples can then be supported in their efforts to plan their lives in ways that may include consideration of adoption or child-free living as valid alternatives to biologic parenthood.

REFERENCES

1. Lobo, R. A. (2017). Infertility: Etiology, diagnostic evaluation, management, prognosis. In R. Lobo, D. Gershenson, G. Lentz, & F. Valea (Eds.), *Comprehensive gynecology* (7th ed., pp. 897–923). St. Louis: Elsevier.
2. National Survey of Family Growth. National Center for Health Statistics. Retrieved from https://www.cdc.gov/nchs/nsfg/index.htm. (Accessed 26 September 2019).

3. Centers for Disease Control and Prevention (CDC). (2019). Centers for Disease Control and Prevention (CDC): Infertility FAQs. Retrieved from https://www.cdc.gov/reproductivehealth/infertility/index.htm. (Accessed 15 June 2019).

4. Practice Committee of American Society for Reproductive Medicine. (2012). Diagnostic evaluation of the infertile female: A committee opinion. *Fertility and Sterility, 98*(2), 302–307.

5. Winters, B. R., & Walsh, T. J. (2014). The epidemiology of male infertility. *Urologic Clinics of North America, 41*(1), 195–204.

6. Flannigan, R., & Schlegel, P. N. (2017). Genetic diagnostics of male infertility in clinical practice. *Best Practice & Research: Clinical Obstetrics & Gynaecology, 44*, 26–37.

7. Schmid, T. E., Grant, P. G., Marchetti, F., Weldon, R. H., Eskenazi, B., & Wyrobek, A. J. (2013). Elemental composition of human semen is associated with motility and genomic sperm defects among older men. *Human Reproduction, 28*(1), 274–282.

8. Sloter, E., Schmid, T. E., Marchetti, F., Eskenazi, B., Nath, J., & Wyrobek, A. J. (2006). Quantitative effects of male age on sperm motion. *Human Reproduction, 21*(11), 2868–2875.

9. ACOG Committee Opinion No. (2013). 575: Exposure to toxic environmental agents. *Fertility and Sterility, 100*(4), 931–934.

10. Marchetti, F., Eskenazi, B., Weldon, R. H., et al. (2012). Occupational exposure to benzene and chromosomal structural aberrations in the sperm of Chinese men. *Environmental Health Perspectives, 120*(2), 229–234.

11. Xing, C., Marchetti, F., Li, G., et al. (2010). Benzene exposure near the U.S. permissible limit is associated with sperm aneuploidy. *Environmental Health Perspectives, 118*(6), 833–839.

12. Lieber, C., & Wetterauer, U. (2016). The cigarette and the sperm: A fatal liaison? *European Urology, 10*(4), 646–647.

13. Laubenthal, J., Zlobinskaya, O., Poterlowicz, K., et al. (2012). Cigarette smoke-induced transgenerational alterations in genome stability in cord blood of human F1 offspring. *FASEB Journal: Official Publication of the Federation of American Societies for Experimental Biology, 26*(10), 3946–3956.

14. Practice Committee of the American Society for Reproductive M. (2012). Smoking and infertility: A committee opinion. *Fertility and Sterility, 98*(6), 1400–1406.

15. Propst, A. M., & Bates, G. W., Jr. (2012). Evaluation and treatment of anovulatory and unexplained infertility. *Obstetrics and Gynecology Clinics of North America, 39*(4), 507–519.

16. Jacobsen, B. K., Knutsen, S. F., Oda, K., & Fraser, G. E. (2013). Body mass index at age 20 and subsequent childbearing: The Adventist Health Study-2. *Journal of Women's Health (2002), 22*(5), 460–466.

17. Majzoub, A., Agarwal, A., & Esteves, S. (2017). The clinical utility of sperm DNA fragmentation: A survey based study of fertility specialists. *Fertility and Sterility, 108*(3), e138.

18. Pacey, A. A. (2012). Assessment of male factor. *Best Practice and Research. Clinical Obstetrics and Gynaecology, 26*(6), 739–746.

19. McQueen, D. B., Zhang, J., & Robbins, J. (2019). Sperm DNA fragmentation and recurrent pregnancy loss: A systematic review and meta-analysis. *Fertility and Sterility*, American Society for Reproductive Medicine, Article in press.

20. Barbieri, R. (2019). Female infertility. In J. F. Strauss & R. L. Barbieri (Eds.), *MD Yen and Jaffe's reproductive endocrinology* (8th ed., pp. 556–558). St. Louis: Elsevier.

21. Practice Committee of American Society for Reproductive Medicine. (2018). Vaccination guidelines for female infertility patients: A committee opinion. *Fertility and Sterility, 110*(5), 838–841.

22. Schmid, T. E., Eskenazi, B., Marchetti, F., et al. (2012). Micronutrients intake is associated with improved sperm DNA quality in older men. *Fertility and Sterility, 98*(5), 1130–1137, e1131.

23. Stone, S., Khamashta, M. A., & Nelson-Piercy, C. (2002). Nonsteroidal anti-inflammatory drugs and reversible female infertility: Is there a link? *Drug Safety, 25*(8), 545–551.

24. Smith, J. F., Eisenberg, M. L., Millstein, S. G., et al. (2011). Fertility treatments and outcomes among couples seeking fertility care: Data from a prospective fertility cohort in the United States. *Fertility and Sterility, 95*(1), 79–84.

25. Brandes, M., Hamilton, C. J., van der Steen, J. O., et al. (2011). Unexplained infertility: Overall ongoing pregnancy rate and mode of conception. *Human Reproduction, 26*(2), 360–368.

26. Jain, T. (2006). Socioeconomic and racial disparities among infertility patients seeking care. *Fertility and Sterility, 85*(4), 876–881.

27. Reddy, U. M., Wapner, R. J., Rebar, R. W., & Tasca, R. J. (2007). Infertility, assisted reproductive technology, and adverse pregnancy outcomes: Executive summary of a National Institute of Child Health and Human Development workshop. *Obstetrics and Gynecology, 109*(4), 967–977.

28. Hashim, H. A. (2016). Twenty years of ovulation induction with metformin for PCOS; what is the best available evidence? *Reproductive Biomedicine Online, 32*(1), 44–53.

29. See, C. J., McCulloch, M., Smikle, C., & Gao, J. (2011). Chinese herbal medicine and clomiphene citrate for anovulation: A meta-analysis of randomized controlled trials. *Journal of Alternative and Complementary Medicine (New York, N.Y.), 17*(5), 397–405.

30. Chen, S., Wang, T., Zhang, S., et al. (2019). Association between infertility treatment and perinatal depressive symptoms: A meta-analysis of observational studies. *Journal of Psychosomatic Research, 120*, 110–117.

31. Macaluso, M., Wright-Schnapp, T. J., Chandra, A., et al. (2010). A public health focus on infertility prevention, detection, and management. *Fertility and Sterility, 93*(1), 16, e10–11.

CHAPTER **148**

MENOPAUSE

Diane C. Seibert • Diane Todd Pace

 Immediate referral is indicated for postmenopausal women, with an intact uterus, who develop abnormal uterine bleeding or signs and symptoms suggestive of breast, ovarian, lung, or colorectal cancer.

Like the onset of menarche, menopause is a normal life event that every woman will experience if she lives long enough. Unlike the onset of puberty, in many women the hormonal and physiologic changes associated with menopause are superimposed on disorders such as hypertension and osteoporosis, that commonly manifest in older adults, many of which can be traced to a complex mix of genetic predisposition, environmental exposures, access to health care, and lifestyle choices. Midlife also brings significant psychological and social change; adult children may begin their own families and aging parents may need help and support all of which may affect physical, emotional, social, and financial well-being. To optimize quality of life and health outcomes, all of these factors should be considered when developing an individualized care plan for women at or after midlife.

DEFINITION AND EPIDEMIOLOGY

Menopause is the final step in a series of reproductive events that begin in 4-week-old embryos that contain 2 X chromosomes. At 4 weeks gestation, several primordial germ cells (PGCs) begin dividing as they migrate through the embryonic gut, eventually finding their way to newly created ovaries at approximately 16 weeks gestation. Unlike somatic cells PGCs have the unique ability to divide by both mitosis (up to 5 million copies are made of the initial PGCs) and later by meiosis, where division is arrested in prophase 1 (dictyotene), until ovulation which may occur years or decades later.[1] At birth, a female infant has approximately 2 million viable oocytes; by the time of the first menstrual period, the number of viable oocytes will have dropped to around 500,000, and menopause begins when the final oocyte degrades and disappears, typically age 52.5 in North America. Atresia (cell death and degeneration) is responsible for the loss of the vast majority of oocytes during a woman's life, and although the atresia rate varies from woman to woman, the decline in oocytes number and quality is usually linear until age 37, when atresia accelerates until menopause.[2]

TABLE 148.1 **Terms Related to Menopause**

Term	Definition
Menopause	The permanent decline in gonadal hormone levels confirmed by 12 months of amenorrhea (12 months after final menstrual period [FMP]) in women with a uterus. In women without a uterus, the diagnosis can be established using other criteria including history of bilateral oophorectomy, symptoms, and/or serial measurement of endocrine markers.
Premenopause	The period of life that precedes menopause.
Premenopausal	Relating to premenopause.
Postmenopause	The period of life after menopause. The 2010 US Census Bureau reported that nearly 40 million US women were older than 55 years, past the age of natural menopause, which occurs at approximately ages 51–52 years in the United States.
Postmenopausal	Relating to postmenopause.
Menopausal transition	Begins with the onset of intermenstrual cycle irregularities and/or other menopause-related symptoms and extends through the FMP.
Perimenopause (sometimes called *climacteric*)	A clinically useful term that encompasses the most symptomatic years and means "around menopause." Perimenopause begins with the onset of intermenstrual cycle irregularities and/or other menopause-related symptoms and extends beyond menopause to include the 12 months after the FMP, thus lasting 1 year longer than the menopausal transition.
Early menopause, late menopause	Vague terms that have been used to describe menopause that occurs earlier or later than the normal range of menopause.
Premature menopause	Menopause that occurs before age 40. Approximately 1% of US women experience premature natural menopause, so of the 49 million US women who were projected to be age 15–44 years in 2015, approximately 490,000 would have experienced premature natural menopause.[5]
Primary ovarian insufficiency	Hypergonadotropic hypogonadism in a woman younger than age 40 years. Prevalence ranges from 2%–10% of women presenting with secondary amenorrhea.
Induced menopause	Cessation of menstruation after either surgical removal of both ovaries (bilateral oophorectomy/the most common cause) or iatrogenic ablation of ovarian function (by chemotherapy or pelvic radiation therapy).
Premature ovarian failure	The North American Menopause Society as well as the American Congress of Obstetricians and Gynecologists recommend that this term no longer be used.

Modified from (2014). *Menopause practice: a clinician's guide* (5th ed.). Mayfield, OH: North American Menopause Society.

As the number of functional oocytes declines, inhibin B declines and follicle-stimulating hormone (FSH) levels rise, temporarily sustaining follicular development and ovulatory function. The first clinically measurable sign of perimenopause therefore is a high serum FSH (>10 IU/L) during the early follicular phase (days 2 to 5) of the menstrual cycle. Although the elevated FHS supports the current oocyte, elevated FSH levels may contribute to the acceleration of follicular atresia because more follicles are recruited per cycle.[3] Overproduction of estradiol by this large cohort of recruited follicles may be responsible for many perimenopausal symptoms, including bloating, irritability, breast tenderness, menorrhagia, uterine fibroid growth, vasomotor symptoms (VMS), insomnia, migraines, and premenstrual syndrome (PMS) dysphoria.[4] Although rare, pregnancy is still possible late in the perimenopausal period and women are at risk for unplanned pregnancy until they have been amenorrheic for more than 1 year. Several terms associated with menopause are defined in Table 148.1.

The mean age at menarche in the United States has dropped steadily from the early 1800s and continues to decline in some populations,[6] but the age of onset of menopause has remained relatively stable for generations. The Study of Women's Health Across the Nation (SWAN) trial, which followed over 3000 women from multiple states and racial and ethnic groups, found that menopause occurred at age 52.54 years irrespective of racial or ethnic group, age of menarche, or number of lifetime pregnancies.[7] Some health and socioeconomic factors, such as self-rated health, higher body weight, lower physical activity levels, negative smoking history, prior oral contraceptive use, higher education level, and employment, were significantly associated with a later onset of menopause, suggesting that the onset of menopause is influenced by a number of factors, perhaps explaining some of the relationship between reduced morbidity and mortality in women who enter menopause later in life.[2]

The Stages of Reproductive Aging Workshop (STRAW +10) document provides definitions and descriptions of menopause (similar to Tanner staging for puberty) characterizing reproductive aging through menopause.[8] Consistent use of the STRAW +10 criteria improves clinical decision-making and supports research efforts because it offers a structure within which to compare studies conducted on women in midlife (Fig. 148.1).

The STRAW +10 criteria divide the perimenopause, menopause, and postmenopause periods into seven phases, five of which occur before the final menstrual period (FMP) and two of which occur after the FMP. As with every other developmental phase in life, individual variability is the norm, with some women moving rapidly through one or more stages, some skipping stages altogether, and some shifting back and forth between stages. In general, the transition through these 7 phases is predictable, but chronologic age does not accurately predict reproductive ability, so menopause should be included in the differential diagnosis whenever a woman reports

Stages	−5	−4	−3	−2	−1	+1	+2
Terminology	Reproductive			Menopausal Transition		Postmenopause	
	Early	Peak	Late	Perimenopause		Early	Late
Duration	Variable			Variable	1 year	4 years	Until death
Menstruation	Variable to regular	Regular		Variable >7 days different from NL	>2 skipped cycles + amenorrhea >60 days	None	
Endocrine	Normal FSH	↑ FSH		↑ FSH		↑ FSH	

Final Menstrual Period

F I G . 148.1 STRAW +10. *FSH*, follicle-stimulating hormone. (From Soules, M.R., Sherman, S., Parrott, E. Rebar, R., Santoro, N., Utian, W., Woods, N. [2001]. Executive summary: stages of reproductive aging workshop [STRAW]. *Fertility and Sterility, 76*, 874-878.)

menopausal symptoms. Because most American women will spend nearly one-third of their lives in the postmenopausal period, the implications for women, clinicians, and the health care system are extensive.

PHYSIOLOGY

Reproduction is controlled by a highly complex series of interactions among a number of different hormones. A complete discussion of all of them is beyond the scope of this chapter, but the structure and function of a few key hormones (estrogen, progestogen, androgens) are discussed here to provide a frame of reference for the management section, later.

In the early 1970s, estrogen's effects were believed to be primarily reproductive, having little effect on tissues outside the uterus and mammary glands. Over the past 40 years, however, evidence has revealed that estrogen exerts its effects on many organs. At least two distinct estrogen receptors (ER-α and ER-β) have been identified, both of which are present in ovarian and central nervous system (CNS) tissues. In other body tissues, however, one form or the other predominates. For example, ER-α is found in hepatic, uterine, and breast tissue, whereas ER-β is found in bone, blood vessels, lungs, and urogenital tissues.[9] Further complicating the estrogen picture, there are three known forms of human estrogens: estrone (E1), estradiol (E2), and estriol (E3). E1, the least abundant, is derived from stored body fat and is the primary estrogen in postmenopausal women. E2, produced by the ovarian follicle during the reproductive years, is the most potent and abundant (10% to 29%). E3, the least potent, predominates during pregnancy. Serum estradiol levels vary widely during the menstrual cycle—below 10 pg/mL early in the follicular phase, rising above 800 pg/mL at midcycle, and dropping back down to 200 to 340 pg/mL during the luteal phase. More than 95% of the circulating E2 is produced by the dominant follicle, and less than 5% is derived from peripheral conversion of E1.[9]

Progesterone, secreted during the luteal phase of the menstrual cycle, first appears right after ovulation and rises steadily for about 10 days before dropping back down to baseline if no pregnancy occurs. Normal progesterone levels range from 2 to 20 ng/mL depending on the day the level is drawn.[10]

There are five clinically important androgens in women: testosterone, dihydrotestosterone (DHT), androstenedione,

dehydroepiandrosterone (DHEA), and dehydroepiandrosterone sulfate (DHEAS). Although often referred to as androgens, androstenedione, DHEAS, and DHEA are actually prohormones that are converted to active androgens in body tissues.[11] DHEA in particular plays an important role in the production of ovarian testosterone, and recently a new DHEA-containing vaginal product (prasterone [Intrarosa]) has been FDA approved to treat vaginal symptoms associated with menopause.[12] In reproductive-age women, a slight but significant rise in serum testosterone is measurable immediately before ovulation. Evaluating serum androgen levels can be challenging for several reasons. First, only 1% to 2% of testosterone is free to circulate because two-thirds is bound to sex hormone–binding globulin (SHBG) and the remainder is bound to albumin, so changes in SHBG production or albumin levels can affect the amount of testosterone available to tissues.[13] Second, serum androgen levels do not accurately reflect the amount of androgens available to androgen-dependent or androgen-sensitive tissues such as the skin, the clitoris, or the vulva, because the ratio of plasma DHT levels to serum testosterone levels is low (0.3:1) whereas the ratio is much higher (2:1) in tissues where conversion from DHT to testosterone is actively occurring.[13]

Antimüllerian hormone (AMH) produced by the follicular granulosa cells plays an important role in follicle recruitment and selection and is a useful marker of ovarian reserve. After rising in adolescence and early adulthood, AMH levels gradually decline, becoming undetectable approximately 5 years before the FMP.[14,15] AMH levels have primarily been used in infertility settings, but as laboratory technology improves, serial AMH levels may begin to be used in primary care settings to predict the age of menopause.

The first sign that a woman is entering perimenopause (stage–3a) might be, but is not always, menstrual cycle changes. In response to declining ovarian reserve, inhibin B levels drop, and FSH levels rise to more aggressively stimulate the remaining follicles, and although the luteal phase of the cycle remains 14 days, the follicular phase shortens by 2 to 4 days, causing the overall cycle to become shorter (i.e., 25 to 26 days rather than 28 days).[10] The STRAW +10 staging illustrates this because stages−2 and −1 are characterized by significant menstrual cycle irregularity, reflecting the increasingly wide swings in hormonal levels and the increasingly frequent anovulatory cycles.

Although the FMP marks the onset of menopause, it is difficult to tell clinically when that FMP has occurred. No serum marker sensitive enough to definitively mark this transition has yet been identified, and a single assessment of several hormone levels (FSH, luteinizing hormone [LH], and estradiol, for example) is unreliable when trying to determine when the FMP has occurred. Recent large studies such as SWAN have found that using a combination of factors such as comparing E2 levels with a level drawn earlier in the perimenopausal period, race or ethnicity, and timing of the serum collection (early follicular phase) is a better predictor of the probability of a woman having had her FMP.[16] It is important to remember that although the STRAW+10 criterion of one episode of more than 60 consecutive days of amenorrhea is enough to consider a women older than 45 years in late menopausal transition, it is unreliable in women younger than 40 years who have prolonged (>120 days) episodes of amenorrhea, even when their FSH levels are in the menopausal range. These women should be evaluated for other causes of amenorrhea because once treated, many will resume regular menstruation and have had successful spontaneous pregnancies.[10]

RESEARCH AND CLINICAL TRIALS

Researchers have been studying the risks and benefits of hormone "replacement" therapy for over half a century, and although much has been learned, areas of uncertainty remain. A key thing to remember about using hormones in the postmenopausal period is the concept of "replacement." This term has fallen out of favor because current prescribing dosage levels are significantly lower than reproductive "replacement" doses of hormones would be. That said, anyone taking exogenous hormones who has not produced that dose of hormone naturally for several years may experience adverse effects ranging from minor/mild (breast tenderness) to severe (death). The risk of adding HT has to be balanced against the effects of aging in older adults. The question of risk is also more and more relevant and complex, as transgender men and women request hormone therapy to support their gender transformation.[17]

Many of the earlier case/cohort studies found that standard-dose estrogen-alone HT decreased both coronary heart disease (CHD) and reduced all-cause mortality in women younger than age 60 and within 10 years of menopause onset. The data on combined estrogen-progestogen HT were not as compelling.[18] Therefore in the late 1990s, two large randomized controlled trials, the Heart and Estrogen/Progestin Replacement Study (HERS) and the Women's Health Initiative (WHI), were launched to find answers to important questions about the impact of HT on the cardiovascular system.

HERS was designed to determine whether combined estrogen/progestin therapy (EPT) reduced the number of cardiovascular disease (CVD) events in postmenopausal women with *established CHD*. The study clearly demonstrated that HT increased risk during the first year of use, and that no long-term benefit was seen, and the authors concluded that estrogen's prothrombotic, arrhythmic, and ischemic effects during the first year counteracted any lipid improvement.[19]

The WHI was a large randomized, double-blinded, multicenter, multiyear trial designed to examine the risks and benefits of HT in healthy postmenopausal women aged 50 to 79.

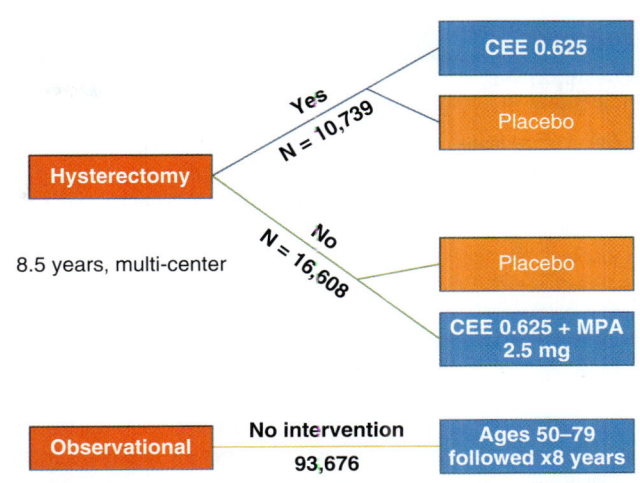

FIG. 148.2 WHI Study Design. *CEE*, conjugated equine estrogen.

There were over 100,000 women enrolled in the three arms of the trial (Fig. 148.2).

Before the trial began, two major clinical outcomes (CVD and invasive breast cancer), six minor outcomes (stroke, pulmonary embolism, endometrial cancer, CRC, hip fracture, and death from other causes), and a global index (a number reflecting the balance of risks and benefits) were identified.[20] The EPT arm was terminated 3 years early, in July 2002, because the global index rose above a predetermined risk threshold. Although the absolute risk of harm was very small and there was no difference in the number of deaths between the EPT and placebo groups, the trend toward increasing risk could not be ignored. The ET group continued to the projected end point because the global index threshold was not crossed. Overall, the trial demonstrated that the health risks and benefits of HT vary depending on the type(s) of hormones used, the woman's age when she begins taking HT, and the length of time since the last menstrual period. Although the absolute risk for harm was very low, both ET and EPT increased risk for developing venous thromboemboli and associated disorders (stroke and CVD), although the risk of ischemic stroke was rare in the 50- to 59-year age group.[21] It is important to understand that the risks and benefits for health outcomes varied by age. After 5 years or more of continuous EPT use, there was an increased risk for breast cancer, which decreased after HT was discontinued; this pattern was not seen in women taking ET only, however, so counseling women about HT risks and benefits is complex (Table 148.2). Some small studies have shown nonstatistically significant reductions in breast cancer in women using estrogen therapy.[24] Differences in risk may also be noted with different pharmacological preparations such as conjugated equine estrogen with bazedoxifene (Duavee), different types of estrogens or progestogens, and varying patient characteristics.[25]

Manson and the WHI primary investigators reported in JAMA in 2017, after 18 years of follow-up of WHI participants, that neither EPT nor ET was associated with an increased risk for CVD, cancer, or all-cause mortality. However, while HT is appropriate for managing vasomotor, genitourinary symptoms, and prevention of bone loss and fractures in menopausal women, it is not indicated and should not be prescribed for chronic disease prevention.[23–25]

TABLE 148.2   Hormone Therapy Risks and Benefits

FDA Approved Indications	Contraindications/Risks	Common Adverse Events	Benefits

• Relief of moderate to severe vasomotor symptoms (VMS)
• Prevention of bone loss and reduction of fractures in postmenopausal women (Prevention of Osteoporosis)
• Prevention/treatment of genitourinary syndrome of menopause/ vulvovaginal atrophy (GSM/VVA)
• Treatment for women with hypogonadism, POI, or premature surgical menopause for health benefits, risk reduction, and menopausal symptom treatment.
	• Unexplained vaginal bleeding
	• Severe active liver disease
	• Personal history or inherited high risk of thromboembolic disease
	• Prior estrogen-sensitive breast or endometrial cancer
	• Coronary heart disease
	• Stroke
	• Dementia
	• Hypertriglyceridemia
	• Concerns that: Endometriosis might reactivate; migraine headaches may worsen; leiomyomas may grow
	• Known hypersensitivity to active substance of therapy
	
	POTENTIAL RISKS:
	• Women > 60/> 10 years from onset of menopause who **initiate** HT have an increased risk of stroke
	• Increased risk of VTE with ET/EPT with higher risk seen in years 1 and 2 after initiation; absolute risk rare if initiated in age <60 years and <10 years from menopause onset. Transdermal use may have less effect, but meta-analysis has only been published viewing observational studies.
	• Possible risk of breast cancer with EPT
	  • Risk of effect of ET/EPT/CEE/BZA on breast cancer is complex. Types of preparation, doses, timing of initiation, duration (in some studies risk increased with longer duration), and patient characteristics effect risk outcome but should be included in discussions.
	  • Attributable risk found in WHI of CEE + MPA similar to that observed in drinking 1 daily glass of wine, with obesity, low physical activity, and other medications
	• Endometrial hyperplasia/cancer in women with uterus if estrogen is unopposed/inadequately unopposed
	• Biliary issues
	• Myocardial infarction, stroke
	• Dementia
	• Risk of gallstones, cholecystitis, and cholecystectomy increased with oral estrogen-alone and EPT
		• Nausea
		• Bloating
		• Weight gain
		• Fluid retention
		• Mood swings (progestogen-related)
		• Episodic bleeding (often related to administration type of EPT)
		• Headaches
		• Breast tenderness
			• More likely to outweigh risks for symptomatic women before age of 60 or within 10 years after FMP
			• For women who are severely symptomatic, improves health-related and menopause-specific quality of life
			• No other pharmacologic or alternative therapy found to provide more relief for VMS which is also associated with diminished sleep quality, irritability, difficulty concentrating, reduced QoL, and poorer health status
			• In women without osteoporosis prevents bone loss and reduces postmenopause osteoporotic fractures, including hip, spine, and all non-spine fractures
			• For GSM/VVA symptoms not relieved with OTC moisturizers/ lubricants and/or other nonhormonal interventions, estrogen therapy has been found to be the most effective treatment. If not needed for management of systemic symptoms (VMS), low-dose vaginal estrogen is effective/safe.
			• No link between HT and all cause or cause-specific mortality found after 18 years cumulative follow-up with WHI (including CVD or cancer) for women initiating HT at all ages.

Risks of HT differ for women promoting the need for an individualized/shared decision-making plan/not one size fits all. Risk is dependent on type of therapy, dose, duration of use, route of administration, timing of initiation, and the need for concomitant administration of a progestogen. Periodic reevaluation of risks/benefits for continuation should be a part of the shared plan of care.
Modified from *The 2017 hormone therapy position statement of The North American Menopause Society.* Accessed at: http://www.menopause.org/docs/default-source/2017/nams-2017-hormone-therapy-position-statement.pdf.

The most recent findings regarding HT risks and benefits came from the Kronos Early Estrogen Prevention Study (KEEPS). KEEPS was a 5-year, randomized, multisite, clinical trial involving over 700 women ages 42 to 58 who were within 36 months of their FMP. Participants were randomized to either placebo or treatment (CEE or transdermal estradiol in combination with cyclic oral, micronized progesterone, 200 mg 12 days each month) arms with clinical endpoints of carotid intimal medial thickness, coronary calcium levels, bone density, and mood. The authors concluded that hormone replacement started near the onset of menopause appears to be safe and relieves many menopausal symptoms of menopause.[26]

As a result of ongoing information about the HT risks and benefits, other communities are coming forward with recommendations as well. The American Association of Clinical Endocrinologists and American College of Endocrinology published a 2017 position paper stating that HT is appropriate for use in symptomatic postmenopausal women depending on their age, CVD risk factors, and time from menopause.[27] The authors also recommended transdermal estrogen and micronized progesterone (if progestins were needed) over oral estrogen and older progestins and suggested selective serotonin re-uptake inhibitors in women in which HT was inappropriate. Bioidentical hormones were not recommended, and women with diabetes should be carefully assessed for CVD prior to initiating HT.

CLINICAL PRESENTATION

The clinical presentation and symptoms of menopause vary significantly from one woman to another depending on the woman's age and underlying health status. Some manifestations such as VMS are clearly associated with menopause, but others such as sexual dysfunction are much more elusive. Management of symptoms in women at midlife must therefore be considered in the context of healthy aging, because age is a confounder for symptoms and diseases that may be associated with or directly affected by menopausal management. The primary driver for the physiologic changes associated with menopause is the dramatic decline in estrogen levels, causing a number of short- and long-term physical changes including cycle irregularity, VMS (hot flashes), urogenital atrophy (vaginal dryness, urinary incontinence, pelvic floor dysfunction), mood changes, and poor sleep and sexual functioning.

Irregular Bleeding

Abnormal uterine bleeding (AUB) is the most frequently reported perimenopausal symptom, with nearly 90% of women reporting 4 to 8 years of menstrual cycle changes before experiencing their FMP.[28] Although some women experience fewer cycles with lighter bleeding during the menopausal transition, many women seek medical assistance for prolonged or heavy menstrual bleeding, which can cause significant anemia; avoidance of activities, including sexual intercourse; and a diminished quality of life. Early in the menopausal transition, cycle irregularities are commonly caused by disruption of communication between the hypothalamus, pituitary, and ovaries, but as the FMP approaches, anovulation becomes more common, increasing the risk for unopposed estrogen exposure, endometrial hyperplasia, and cancer. Although most perimenopausal women with heavy or irregular bleeding do not have anatomic pathology, other causes of heavy menstrual bleeding such as thyroid dysfunction, pituitary adenoma, cervical polyps, uterine fibroids, endometriosis, and endometrial hyperplasia or cancer should be ruled out before attributing the cycle changes to the menopausal transition.[28]

In an effort to standardize terminology describing menstrual bleeding, in 2009 the Fédération Internationale de Gynécologie et d'Obstétrique (FIGO) Menstrual Disorders Group proposed standardizing the terms to describe menstrual bleeding (Box 148.1), and also proposed the PALM-COEIN structure (Box 148.2). By using the PALM-COEIN nomenclature, menstrual bleeding definitions and associated disorders could be organized to support clinical care but also facilitate research and evidence-based care.[29]

Depending on the clinical presentation, a comprehensive AUB workup could include laboratory tests to rule out pregnancy and sexually transmitted infections, hematologic parameters (complete blood count, liver function, coagulation profile), and serum hormone levels (thyroid, prolactin, FSH, estradiol, progesterone, testosterone, and DHEAS). Depending on these results, additional procedures might include endometrial biopsy and/or dilation and curettage, transvaginal ultrasonography, hysteroscopy, or sonohysterography.

AUB can be managed medically, hormonally, and/or surgically, and treatment should be individualized based on the severity of the AUB, the impact of the bleeding on a woman's

---

BOX 148.1

Abnormal Uterine Bleeding Terms

Old Terms	New Terms
• Menorrhagia	• Abnormal uterine bleeding (AUB)
• Hypermenorrhea	• Heavy menstrual bleeding (HMB)
• Hypomenorrhea	• Heavy and prolonged menstrual bleeding (HMPB)
• Menometrorrhagia	• Intermenstrual bleeding (IMB)
• Polymenorrhea	• Postmenopausal bleeding (PMB)
• Polymenorrhagia	
• Epimenorrhea	
• Epimenorrhagia	
• Uterine hemorrhage	
• Dysfunctional uterine bleeding	
• Functional uterine bleeding	
• Metropathia hemorrhagica	

BOX 148.2

Palm-Coein Nomenclature

PALM Structural Disorders	COEIN Nonstructural Disorders
Polyp (AUB-P)	**C**oagulopathy (AUB-C)
Adenomyosis (AUB-A)	**O**vulatory Dysfunction (AUB-O)
Leiomyoma (AUB-L)	**E**ndometrial (AUB-E)
Malignancy & Hyperplasia (AUB-M)	**I**atrogenic (AUB-I)
	Not yet classified (AUB-N)

---

quality of life, her personal preferences and contraceptive needs, and her overall health status. Often the first therapy tried is medical management, which includes nonsteroidal anti-inflammatories, tranexamic acid, and desmopressin (for women with underlying bleeding disorders). Medical management is often combined with hormonal management, which includes gonadotropin-releasing hormone (GnRH) agonists, oral progestogens and contraceptive options such as low-dose oral contraceptive pills, depot MPA, and levonorgestrel-releasing intrauterine devices (IUDs). Referral for consideration of surgical options (endometrial ablation, polypectomy, myomectomy, and/or hysterectomy) is usually reserved for women who have anatomic pathology such as fibroids, endometrial hyperplasia, and cervical disorders such as dysplasia and polyps, and procedures are tailored to treat those specific conditions.[24]

Vasomotor Symptoms

VMS, considered the hallmark of the female climacteric, are characterized by vasomotor instability, hot flashes, day sweats, and night sweats. As many as 75% of perimenopausal and postmenopausal women report experiencing VMS for 6 months to 2 years, although some women will report having hot flashes for more than 10 years. The peak incidence of hot flashes is within 2 years of the FMP[22] but the physiologic mechanisms are still not completely understood. The term *hot flash* is used to describe the sudden onset of head, neck, and chest flushing, accompanied by a feeling of intense body heat, profuse perspiration, and modest heart rate increases that lasts generally from 1 to 5 minutes. Often as skin temperatures return to normal, there are decreases in core body temperatures with significant heat loss resulting in chills for some women. Additional symptoms of diminished quality of sleep, difficulty in concentration, irritability, lower quality of life (QOL), and a reduced health status all have been associated with the presence of VMS.[30]

According to the Study of Women Across the Nation (SWAN), the prevalence of hot flashes differs across US racial and ethnic groups. Within this study of over 15,000 women, black women reported VMS most frequently with the longest duration (median 10.1 years), followed by Hispanic, White, Chinese, and Japanese women. The median overall total VMS duration reported in the study is 7.4 years.[25] Other variables for increasing VMS include obesity, low socioeconomic status, and surgically induced menopause. Factors such as depression, history of depression, anxiety, perceived stress, and poor physical health have also been associated with a higher risk. Higher education levels appear to be somewhat protective, but other factors, such as age, current smoking, alcohol use, and employment status do not appear to be significantly associated with an increased risk for developing severe VMS.[25] Conditions such as thyroid disease, infection, insulinoma, pheochromocytoma, autoimmune disorders, new-onset hypertension, diabetes, and autonomic dysfunction may also cause hot flashes and should be considered if appropriate in the differential diagnosis.[22]

Fluctuating hormone levels are associated with hot flashes. Although there have been numerous research studies and theories developed regarding the causes of hot flashes, specific mechanisms or brain areas involved in thermogenesis and heat perception are still being explored and more research is needed.[22,31]

Genitourinary Syndrome of Menopause/Vulvovaginal Atrophy

Vulvovaginal atrophy (VVA) refers to changes in the vagina and vulva that develop during the postmenopausal period as a result of declining estrogen levels in these tissues. Given that the term *VVA* does not include the anatomic areas of the urinary tract that are also affected by estrogen deficiency of menopause, a panel was convened in 2012 to discuss the need for more acceptable terminology to replace VVA. Two large societies, NAMS and the International Society for the Study of Women's Sexual Health (ISSWSH), acknowledged that a new term was needed that would be more "scientifically accurate, descriptive, inclusive, and socially acceptable." The term *genitourinary syndrome of menopause* (GSM) was adopted by both organizations and is now used by professional societies, providers, researchers, educators, and the media to improve communication, research, education, and the treatment in this area of women's health.[32]

GSM is a chronic, progressive disorder that often causes significant discomfort and worsens without treatment. The vagina may narrow and lose elasticity, become thin, pale, dry, or easily traumatized. The vaginal pH is > 5.0 and parabasal cells dominate. There is loss of rugae, fornices may become obliterated, and petechiae may be present. As a result of these changes, women with VVA often report dryness, burning, irritation, vaginal pain, and dyspareunia. These changes may be seen throughout the genitourinary tract. As many as half of midlife and older women may experience urinary symptoms such as frequency, urgency, dysuria, and recurrent urinary tract infections.[24]

Two large studies, Vaginal Health: Insights, Views and Attitudes (VIVA) and Real Women's View of Treatment Options for Menopausal Vaginal Changes (REVIVE), examined the impact of VVA on women and found that VVA negatively affects women's lives, lowers their quality of life, and has negative consequences on their sexual health.[33,34] The REVIVE survey also noted that women reported few health care practitioners had any conversations with them about VVA. These surveys and others completed in recent years continue to show that clinicians are still not evaluating for or initiating discussions with their menopausal patients about this disorder.

GSM should be evaluated and interventions individualized for each woman as appropriate based on her symptoms and how these symptoms may be creating distress. Unmet needs of women with GSM should be addressed by clinicians. It is optimal if these conversations should occur between the patient and their provider prior to symptoms developing.

Central Nervous System Effects

Mood Changes. Mood disorders, particularly depression, are nearly twice as common in women as in men. Recent randomized, controlled trials have demonstrated that the hormone shifts associated with menopause can significantly increase the risk for new-onset and recurrent depression. It does not appear to be the estrogen alone, however, because a number of menopausal symptoms are independent risk factors for depression, including VMS, insomnia, severe premenstrual or postpartum mood swings and depression, stressful life events, history of depression, high body mass index, low socioeconomic status, and hormone or antidepressant use. Estrogen helps modulate several neurotransmitter pathways, particularly serotonin and norepinephrine, helping regulate mood. Studies have also shown that transdermal estrogen and serotonergic and noradrenergic antidepressants relieve both mood and VMS.[35] If depressive symptoms appear when a woman begins taking HT, the provider should examine the type of HT being used. Estrogen, specifically 17β estradiol, has shown some antidepressant efficacy in clinical trials Progestogens have been shown to worsen mood in some women, particularly those with a history of PMS, premenstrual depressive disorder, or clinical depression. Antidepressants are the first-line intervention for depression which occurs in menopause transition/menopause. Clinicians should consider tolerability, adverse effects (sexual functioning, weight gain), positive effects on reducing menopausal symptoms such as VMS, pain, or sleep.

Insomnia. Insomnia may occur in association with or independent of hot flashes, and HT has been shown to provide substantial relief for early morning waking, even in women without significant VMS. Other causes for sleep disturbances during this period may be sleep apnea, restless legs, irritability, or depression. Age-related changes or other medical conditions may also be factors. A thorough evaluation, including consideration of an overnight sleep study, may be warranted. Treatment options vary depending on the sleep disturbance. Night awakenings due to VMS can be treated with HT. The irritability that so often accompanies insomnia also responds positively to HT. Women receiving HT have been shown to have shorter sleep latency and more frequent and prolonged rapid eye movement sleep.[24] Counseling on sleep hygiene, cognitive behavioral therapy, sleep medications, and treatments for sleep apnea all may be options to consider.

Sexual Functioning. Decline in sexual activity during the menopausal years is probably influenced more by culture and attitudes than by nature and physiology. Significant determinants of sexual activity for older women are the availability and health status of a sexual partner.[36] Data from the PRESIDE (Prevalence of Female Sexual Problems Associated with Distress and Determinants of Treatment Seeking) study point out, however, that sexual problems are reported by approximately 40% of US women and peak in women at midlife.[37] Psychological, sociocultural, interpersonal, and biologic factors occurring at midlife also contribute to sexual issues at midlife.[22] Changes in mood and well-being and untreated anxiety or depression may have an effect on sexual disorders associated with menopause. Low estrogen levels at menopause often leading to GSM also have been associated with a decline in sexual function. Due to changes in aging and the decline in endogenous androgens, most postmenopausal women will experience low levels. Although testosterone is an important factor in midlife sexual changes for women, playing a role in motivation, desire, and sexual sensation, an association between decreased androgen levels and impaired female sexual function is not clearly supported in the evidence.[22]

Sexuality is, however, important to quality of life. Factors affecting sexual function are multifactorial: medical history/illness, medications, hormones, stressors, individual's sexual self-image and behavior, partner relationships, culture, etc. Patients may be reluctant to initiate the conversation because of embarrassment, or clinicians may have discomfort in discussing the topic because of insufficient training or confidence in talking about the issues. Taking a sexual history can facilitate the discussion on sexuality and sexual health, addressing the woman's concerns and identifying any potential issues such as intimate partner violence or risk for acquiring a sexually transmitted infection. Consider introducing the conversation with "I ask all of my patients about their sexual history as a part of their exam." The online handout *Talking to Patients About Sexuality and Sexual Health* published by the Association of Reproductive Health Professionals provides a good reference guide for clinicians.[38] There are a number of instruments available to assess female sexual dysfunction in the clinical setting: Female Sexual Function Index (FSFI); Profile of Female Sexual Function (PFSF); Sexual Interest and Desire Inventory-Female (SIDI-F); Sexual Quality of Life-Female (SQoL-F); Decreased Sexual Desire Screener (HSDD).[38]

CHRONIC DISEASE

With rare exceptions, menopause occurs as women enter late midlife, when many of the disorders associated with aging begin to emerge. Estrogen has been shown to improve quality of life and reduce risk for some diseases associated with aging, but it has been shown to increase risk for adverse outcomes from some diseases in some women. The question for clinicians is how to best manage menopausal symptoms while maintaining optimal health in older women. To address these important questions, NAMS has published a series of position statements to help inform and guide clinicians in the management of midlife women.[31,39]

The disorders that are of most concern to clinicians working with menopausal women include CVD (venous thromboembolism [VTE], stroke, and CHD), osteoporosis, atrophic vaginitis, cognitive decline (Alzheimer dementia [AD]), and certain cancers (endometrial, breast, ovarian, lung, and colorectal), all of which are described here. A brief discussion of the disease is followed by what is known about the risks and benefits of HT for that particular condition.

Cardiovascular Disease

CVD is a broad term that encompasses three distinct but related disorders: CHD, stroke, and VTE. According to the American Heart Association, in 2017 nearly 800,000 Americans had a heart attack, and 114,000 deaths were due to cardiovascular disease. The classic description of myocardial infarction (MI; heart attack) often includes chest, left arm, or jaw pain or pressure, but many women are not aware that other, more atypical symptoms such as pain at rest, shortness of breath, nausea, and fatigue may be more common presenting manifestations in women. It is important to rule out MI when a woman reports chest pain, fatigue, or shortness of breath. Stroke is the second leading cause of death (behind CHD) in the world, and is the fifth leading cause of death and a leading cause of disability in the United States. In 2017 over 610,000 Americans had their first stroke and 185,000 others had a recurrent stroke.[40] CHD risk factors such as hypertension, diabetes, and hyperlipidemia are well known, but modifiable risk factors such as tobacco use, obesity, and inactivity are linked to increased risk as well, so counseling and management early in life are critical to supporting healthy aging.

A 2016 Cochrane review of randomized controlled trials is consistent with the findings of HERS and WHI, concluding that HT may be appropriate for healthy, younger menopausal women with intolerable vasomotor or genitourinary symptoms. HT is not indicated for the prevention of CVD, dementia, or osteoporosis, although it may be considered for osteoporosis prevention in women in whom non-estrogen therapies are poorly tolerated or ineffective. The authors emphasized that HT should not be prescribed for women with pre-existing CHD, thromboembolic disease, or some types of cancer. They also pointed out that the data were insufficient to evaluate the risk of long-term HT use, the use of HT in postmenopausal women younger than age 50, and that only 30% of the women participating in the trials were age 50 to 59 years when they enrolled in the study.[41]

A meta-analysis of studies related to stroke and HT found no increased risk in women less than 60 years or less than 10 years from onset of menopause. The attributable risk for stroke in the WHI was rare.[31] Looking at a meta-analysis of clinical trials of women initiating HT less than 60 years or less than 10 years from onset of menopause, evidence continues to suggest risk of VTE in the HT group compared with placebo.[23] Lower doses of oral ET, use of micronized progesterone, and transdermal HT may provide less VTE risk, but data is lacking.[31]

Osteoporosis

Osteoporosis is a serious and disabling disease that has become increasingly prevalent as the American population has aged. A study by the National Osteoporosis Foundation (NOF) estimates that 10.2 million Americans currently have osteoporosis and another 43.4 million have low bone mass (osteopenia).[42] Assuming that disease prevalence remains stable, it is estimated that within 5 years, the number of Americans affected by osteoporosis will increase from 54 million to 64.4 million, and that by 2030, 71.2 million will be affected. Osteoporosis is a major risk factor for femur, hip, spine, and forearm fracture, but is often site-specific and may not present uniformly. One woman might have osteoporosis in her spine but have normal bone density in the femoral neck, while another woman may have osteopenia in both areas. As the incidence of osteoporosis

BOX **148.3**

Prevention and Treatment Interventions for Osteoporosis

Weight-Bearing Exercise	• Early in life, promotes higher peak bone mass • Weight bearing and strength training (most beneficial for bone health) • Increases muscle mass and strength • Exercise programs for elderly to increase muscle strength and to reduce the risk of falls
Smoking Cessation	Smoking leads to lower bone mass and fractures
Nutrition	Seek out: • Dairy • Fruits and vegetables • Nutrients such as: magnesium, potassium, vitamin C, vitamin K, several B vitamins, and carotenoids • Adequate protein intake • Moderate alcohol intake Avoid: • Regular cola beverage use • Foods with low nutrient density[46]

BOX **148.4**

Risk Factors for Postmenopausal Osteoporosis

Medications	• Corticosteroids (>7.5 mg prednisone per day, or equivalent, for ≥ 6 months) • Long-term use of certain anticonvulsant medications (e.g., phenytoin) • Anticoagulant agents (e.g., heparin, warfarin) • Immunosuppressive drugs (e.g., cyclosporine) • Levothyroxine • Intramuscular medroxyprogesterone in premenopausal women • Lithium • Tamoxifen (premenopausal use)
Menstrual Status	• Early menopause without ET or HT • Premenopausal hypogonadism • Previous amenorrhea (e.g., because of anorexia nervosa or exercise-induced amenorrhea) • Hyperprolactinemia
Disease States	• Osteoporotic fracture as an adult • Primary hyperparathyroidism • Thyrotoxicosis • Cushing syndrome • Multiple myeloma • Rheumatoid arthritis • Malabsorption syndromes (e.g., celiac disease, Crohn disease) • Chronic obstructive pulmonary disease • Anorexia nervosa • Chronic liver disease • Chronic renal disease

increases, so does the incidence of pathologic fracture, but interestingly, mortality associated with osteoporotic fractures may not be all that different than mortality from other types of fractures. Melton (2014) followed 1991 adults who suffered a fracture as a result of severe (motor vehicle accident or fall from greater than standing height) trauma, moderate (fall from standing height or less) trauma, or pathologic process (i.e., metastatic cancer) for 22 years to evaluate mortality risk. The conditions most associated with the cause of death were similar across all three types of fractures and were similar to the causes of death in the general population, so osteoporotic fractures, interestingly, were not a significant risk factor for early death.[43]

Even if osteoporosis is not associated with premature death, Americans suffer over 2 million osteoporotic fractures every year resulting in pain, immobility, and the associate risk for thrombosis, nursing home placement, and isolation.[44] The cost to the individuals, families, and tax payers is high; 80% of osteoporosis-associated fractures are paid for by Medicare and femoral neck fracture is number 19 on the top 20 most expensive health conditions, which together account for almost 50% of aggregate hospital costs.[45]

The most important factors affecting osteoporosis risk are gender, age, dietary calcium intake, hormone status, genetics, medication use, and certain disease states. Additional risk factors include low vitamin D levels, excess alcohol intake, sedentary lifestyle, low lean body mass, smoking, and early onset of menopause (Box 148.3). Risk factors specifically applicable to postmenopausal women are discussed here (Box 148.4); a more in-depth discussion of osteoporosis risk factors can be found in chapter 163.

Estrogens are not approved for primary treatment of osteoporosis, but oral and transdermal estrogens and oral conjugated equine estrogen with bazedoxifene (CEE/BZA) are approved for osteoporosis prevention, decreasing bone loss, reducing fractures, and preventing height loss (Box 148.5). Studies have shown that if HT is started early, osteoporotic fractures are 20% to 50% lower, and if used for at least 5 years, the fracture risk reduction persists after HT is discontinued.[47] Overall, if HT is prescribed for osteoporosis prevention, it should be continued for at least 5 years, and alternative osteoporosis prevention and nonhormonal therapies should be reviewed with every patient.

Cognitive Decline

Multiple factors, including sleep disturbances (and attendant fatigue), hot flashes, mood changes, and midlife stressors can impact cognitive function. Women participating in the SWAN study showed a trend toward worsening memory during menopausal transition, but returned to baseline after the transition was complete.[22]

Regardless of gender, cognitive performance declines gradually with age as part of the normal aging process, but dementia, a progressive and often rapid deterioration in cognitive function, is not part of the normal aging process. More than 5 million Americans live with Alzheimer dementia (AD), the most common form of dementia, and that number of adults affected by AD doubles every 5 years after age 65.[48] US Census data estimating future AD prevalence rates indicate that unless new prevention strategies are developed, the number of older adults with AD will increase to 14 million by 2050, a nearly threefold increase over current rates.[49] Because women comprise an ever-increasing percentage of older adults, they are disproportionally affected by this disease.

The effect of estrogens on the brain varies based on the age of the woman at the time of treatment. Ovarian estradiol produced during the reproductive years and HT initiated early

Select Nonhormonal Agents Approved for Postmenopausal Osteoporosis

BISPHOSPHONATES
- Alendronate (Fosamax): prevention and treatment
  Prevention: 5 mg/day or 35 mg/week
  Treatment: 10 mg/day or 70 mg/week
- Alendronate plus cholecalciferol (Fosamax Plus D): treatment
  70 mg plus 2800 IU/week or 70 mg plus 5600 IU/week
- Risedronate (Actonel): prevention and treatment
  5 mg/day, 35 mg/week
  75 mg in 2 consecutive doses/month
  150 mg/month
- Risedronate plus calcium carbonate (Actonel with calcium): prevention
  35 mg/week (day 1) plus 1250 mg calcium for no-risedronate days (2–7) of 7-day cycle
- Ibandronate (Boniva): prevention and treatment
  Prevention and treatment: 150 mg/month (oral tablet)
  Treatment: 3 mg every 3 months (intravenous injection)
- Zoledronic acid (Reclast): treatment
  5 mg/year (intravenous infusion)

SERMS
- Raloxifene (Evista): prevention and treatment
  60 mg/day

CALCITONIN
- Calcitonin, salmon (Fortical, Miacalcin): treatment > 5 years after menopause
  200 IU/daily (nasal spray)
  100 IU every other day (subcutaneous injection)

PARATHYROID HORMONE
- Teriparatide (recombinant human parathyroid hormone [PTH]1-34; Forteo): treatment for high fracture risk
  20 mcg/day (subcutaneous injection)

Please go to http://www.menopause.org/docs/default-source/professional/nams-osteo-table-q1-2016.pdf for additional information.
Data from North American Menopause Society (NAMS). *Approved Drugs for Postmenopausal Osteoporosis in the United States and Canada*, February 2016. http://www.menopause.org/docs/default-source/professional/nams-osteo-table-q1-2016.pcf.

in the menopausal transition have been shown to be neuroprotective, but HT begun late in menopause (after age 65) has been associated with an increased risk for cognitive decline and dementia.[50] The neuroprotective effect of HT may be particularly important to discuss with women who undergo bilateral oophorectomy before the onset of menopause and with all women when they first enter menopause, but HT should not be prescribed to women already diagnosed with dementia or AD, and HT is not recommended for treatment of dementia.[50]

Cancers

Endometrial Cancer. Prolonged or unopposed exposure to estrogen in women with a uterus is a well-known risk factor for developing endometrial cancer, but other risks include early menarche, late menopause, chronic anovulation, estrogen-secreting ovarian tumors, obesity, and a history of breast or ovarian cancer.[51] The magnitude of risk varies depending on the dose and duration of exposure to estrogen. Women taking a standard dose of estrogen (0.625 mg of conjugated estrogen per day, or the equivalent) for more than 3 years incur up to a 5-fold increased risk for endometrial cancer, and the risk increases to 10-fold if unopposed estrogen is taken for more than 10 years.[22] Women in the CEE plus MPA arm of the WHI trial had a lower risk (hazard ratio [HR] 0.83, confidence interval [CI] 0.49 to 1.40) for developing endometrial cancer than women in the placebo arm.[22]

Endometrial cancer is a relatively common cancer among postmenopausal women, and because the presenting symptom is typically bleeding, it is important to remember that unexplained vaginal bleeding is cancer until proven otherwise. Unexplained vaginal bleeding must be promptly and thoroughly evaluated with either transvaginal ultrasonography or an endometrial biopsy. Endometrial thickness ≥4 mm on ultrasound or inability to adequately visualize endometrial thickness requires endometrial sampling.[22] An endometrial biopsy may not be the only test needed to evaluate uterine bleeding, because bleeding and profuse watery discharge are also associated with fallopian tube carcinoma. Therefore even if an endometrial sample is normal, if unexplained bleeding persists, additional tests and procedures, including hysteroscopy, laparoscopy, and possibly hysterectomy, may be required to diagnose the problem.[52]

When taken as prescribed, EPT can reduce the risk for endometrial cancer in postmenopausal women. Postmenopausal women with an intact uterus should be treated with adequate progestogen or with BZA to reduce the risk.[25,53] In women using cyclic HT, endometrial sampling should be considered any time bleeding occurs at other than the expected time of withdrawal bleeding. Women using continuous-combined therapy should be evaluated if irregular bleeding persists more than 6 months after HT is started.

Breast Cancer. Globally, breast cancer is the most commonly diagnosed cancer in women and the leading cause of cancer related death as well.[54] It is estimated that one in every eight American women will develop the disease during her lifetime[55] and 249,260 Americans would be diagnosed and 40,890 would die of the disease in 2016.[56] Approximately 75% of breast cancer cases are sporadic (not inherited), and 79% of cases are diagnosed in postmenopausal women over the age of 50.[57]

A number of large randomized clinical trials have explored the relationship between HT and breast cancer. The type of HT, dose, duration of use, regimen, route of administration, prior exposure of estrogen, and individual characteristics of the women may all play roles on HT effects on breast cancer risk.[22] The 18-year follow-up data from the WHI published in *JAMA* in 2017 reported no increased risk of long-term all-cause mortality or death from cancer for women initiating HT at all ages and trend toward reduced mortality in younger women (<60 years) who received HT.[58] Although hormones themselves do not appear to directly damage DNA, they do stimulate breast cell growth (including estrogen-responsive cancer cells) and influence other hormones that stimulate breast cell division.[18,59] Extended duration of HT use exerts a risk factor in some studies and different HT regimens may be associated with increased breast density which may affect mammographic interpretation. Therefore counseling woman on risks and benefits is important in the shared decision making of management options. In general, HT is contraindicated in women with breast cancer unless the decision to treat a survivor experiencing debilitating menopause-related symptoms without relief from nonhormonal alternatives follows an informed discussion and is managed with an oncology consultation. For bothersome GSM symptoms not relieved by nonhormonal options, survivors of breast cancer, in consultation with their oncologist, may use low-dose vaginal ET with experiencing only minimal systemic absorption.[22]

Ovarian Cancer. Ovarian cancer is rare (~3% of cancer diagnoses) but deadly (fifth leading cause of cancer deaths in the United States), primarily because it often remains undetected until it has reached an advanced stage.[57] If the cancer is identified and treated early (stage I), the 10-year survival rate for epithelial ovarian cancer, the most common type of ovarian cancer, can be as high as 99%; but unfortunately, up to 75% of cases are detected at stage III or IV, and survival rates are much lower than when the cancer is still localized to the ovary.[60]

The relationship between hormone use and ovarian cancer is bimodal. During the reproductive years, combined hormonal contraception (birth control pills, vaginal contraceptive ring, contraceptive patch) and bilateral tubal ligation have both been shown to decrease ovarian cancer risk by 50%.[24] Across clinical studies there have been no data to support that HT initiates or promotes the development of ovarian cancer.[22]

Lung Cancer. Lung cancer is the second most commonly diagnosed cancer (after nonmelanoma skin cancer), and more Americans die of the disease than of breast, prostate, and colon cancer combined. In 2014, 224,210 Americans were diagnosed with lung cancer and 159,000 persons died of the disease, 66% of whom were older than 65.[57] Men are at greater risk than women overall, and cigarette smokers are at higher risk in both groups; but, among nonsmokers, women are more likely than men to develop lung cancer, which raises the question of whether hormones increase the risk.

Although menopause itself has not been shown to increase the risk for developing lung cancer, studies are limited and results are inconsistent. Studies do not support any effect of HT on lung cancer incidence.[22]

Colorectal Cancer. Although its overall incidence has been declining over the past two decades, colorectal cancer (CRC) is still the third most commonly diagnosed cancer in the United States. In 2016, the latest year for which incidence data are curerntly available, 141,270 new cases of colon and rectum cancer were reported, and 52,286 deaths were due to CRC.[57] CRC risk increases with advancing age, so menopausal women are at increased risk compared with younger women.

Although menopause itself has not been associated with an increased risk for the disease, screening for CRC has been found to detect early-stage disease and improve mortality rates. According to established guidelines, women should be screened for CRC at age 50 and in general should undergo repeat testing every 10 years until age 75. A reduced incidence of CRC in women taking HT has been seen in observational studies, especially when initiated early in the menopausal period.[22]

PHYSICAL EXAMINATION

Regular physical and preventive health examinations are recommended for people of all ages, but the frequency and focus of the examination vary by the individual's age and gender and the presence of any comorbid conditions. Although few groups recommend a routine "annual" visit, all older adults should be

seen for preventive care on a regular basis. This is also the time to discuss symptoms of and examine for the presence of GSM. Several groups, including federal agencies, medical specialty societies, independent panels, and private advocacy groups, have published preventive services guidelines, including those published by the North American Menopause Society which can be found at: https://www.menopause.org/publications/clinical-care-recommendations/chapter-5-clinical-evaluation-and-counseling. Another new tool, the free mobile app from Nurse Practitioners in Women's Health called the "Well Woman Visit" (iPhone/iPad and Android), was developed to guide clinicians conducting a well-woman visit. The application compiles common clinical practice guidelines from a variety of sources (ACOG, USPSTF, CDC, NOF, ACIP, ASCCP) and has specific content on the physical exam, immunizations, CHD prevention, etc., and one of the newest features is a section dedicated to menopause management (https://www.npwh.org/pages/mobile-app).

MANAGEMENT
Lifestyle Changes

It is important to collaborate and individualize a plan of care with each woman because there is no single menopausal syndrome. For most women, menopause is a normal physiologic and developmental life event.[22] Many studies found women have mostly positive or neutral attitudes toward the transition through menopause, but for some women, symptoms do affect their QoL, and they may seek out interventions from their primary care provider. For all women, some modification of lifestyle can have a significant and positive impact on overall health regardless of age, and some lifestyle changes can improve menopausal symptoms as well.

Personal attitudes, culture, lifestyle, and even social and demographic factors may influence a woman's perception of menopause. Smoking cessation reduces the risk of lung cancer and may reduce VMS. Weight-bearing exercise improves bone density. Eating a healthy diet, limiting alcohol intake, and maintaining a normal body weight can decrease cardiovascular and breast cancer risks. Reducing stress levels can improve mental health and emotional well-being. These are all important reasons for clinicians to begin any discussion with an assessment of lifestyle behaviors and discussion on health promotion and risk reduction.

Vitamins and Minerals

A balanced diet rich in fruits and vegetables is always preferable to taking supplements. However, a woman's daily diet may not contain all the nutrients required for optimal health, and a daily multivitamin and mineral supplement may be necessary. A systematic review published in 2013 for the US Preventive Services Task Force (USPSTF) found a lack of evidence that supplements prevent either cancer or CVD.[47]

Vitamin D. Vitamin D is essential for the efficient intestinal absorption of calcium and for bone health and has been found to improve muscle strength and balance and to reduce the risk of falling. Although available in two forms—vitamin D_2 and vitamin D_3—D_3 (25-hydroxyvitamin D [25OHD]) is the naturally occurring form, is more potent, and is the one most commonly referred to when discussing this vitamin.[60] The Institute of Medicine (IOM) has published guidelines for both vitamin D serum levels (20 to 50 ng/mL [50 to 125 nmol/L]) and recommended daily allowances (RDAs) for vitamin D

TABLE 148.3   **Institute of Medicine 2011 Recommended Dietary Allowances for Vitamin D and Calcium**

Population	Recommended Daily Dose	
	Vitamin D	**Calcium**
WOMEN		
Aged 19–50 years	600 IU	1000 mg
Aged 51–70 years	600 IU	1200 mg
Aged > 70 years	800 IU	1200 mg

Data from Institute of Medicine, Food and Nutrition Board (2010). Dietary Reference Intakes for Calcium and Vitamin D. Washington, DC, National Academy Press.

supplementation in adults (Table 148.3). The USPSTF concludes that evidence is lacking to recommend greater than 400 IUs of vitamin D_3 for the primary prevention of fractures but recommends supplementation of 800 IUs to prevents falls in community-dwelling adults ≥65 years who are at increased risk of falls because of a history of falls or due to vitamin D deficiency.[61] The NOF and NAMS recommend 800 IU to 1000 IU of vitamin D_3 per day for women aged 50 years and older.[22]

Although the IOM stops short of recommending universal vitamin D screening, it does recommend routine screening in vulnerable populations (e.g., older adults or institutionalized adults; people at increased risk for micronutrient deficiency, for instance, post–bariatric surgery patients; individuals at increased risk for osteoporosis; and those taking selected medications such as oral steroids).[61]

Calcium. The importance of an adequate calcium intake for skeletal health has been well established, although its requirements fluctuate throughout a woman's life (see Table 148.3). Although results from studies are conflicting, they have suggested nonskeletal benefits of calcium, such as reduction of CRC, hypertension, and obesity, but supplements may slightly increase the risk of nephrolithiasis. If adequate calcium cannot be obtained from the diet, a separate calcium supplement may be required to reach the recommended 1200 mg of calcium per day. Women should be encouraged to divide the doses throughout the day and to take calcium with food because absorption is better when it is taken with meals.[22]

Iron. Iron may be needed during the time of menopausal transition for the woman who is having AUB and may develop iron deficiency anemia. After the FMP of menopause, iron is no longer lost through menstrual bleeding. Women can be counseled that iron is readily available in food (e.g., organ meats, beef, turkey, clams, oysters, oatmeal, beans) and fortified foods (e.g., breakfast cereals). The daily requirement of elemental iron for menstruating women is 18 mg per day; after menopause, 8 mg per day is sufficient. Postmenopausal women choosing to take a multivitamin should be advised to use an appropriate formulation. Further supplementation is not necessary unless chronic illness leads to iron deficiency anemia.[22]

Further Intervention

The next phase for developing a collaborative plan is to discuss the woman's view of menopause and her desire for intervention for symptoms affecting her QoL.

NONPHARMACOLOGICAL THERAPIES
Vasomotor Symptoms

Mild hot flashes can often be managed with lifestyle changes. Keeping the core body temperature as cool as possible or utilizing products such as a cooling pillow (e.g., Chillow Pillow) or bed fan may help. Managing other healthy lifestyles such as maintaining a healthy body weight, avoiding triggers, using relaxation techniques, and engaging in regular exercise have also been linked to minimizing VMS. Many alternative/complementary remedies such as supplements, yoga, tai chi, and acupuncture are used by 62% of Americans.[24] Herbal products including soy (with increased S-equol levels), isoflavone supplements, black cohosh (40 mg), red clover, vitamin E, and omega-3 fatty acids are popular to reduce VMS and are generally low risk, but none have been proven to be significantly more effective than placebo, and some may be harmful.[24] Clinicians should investigate use of complementary and alternative medicine (CAM) when taking a patient history and be knowledgeable when counseling women about available therapies considering: costs; time and effort involved for using CAM interventions; potential for side effects; lack of long-term clinical studies demonstrating efficacy/safety; and especially potential for drug/herb interactions.

1. Although randomized clinical trials have been few or inconsistent in validating effectiveness, some women have found the following lifestyle options to be effective in reducing VMS:
   a. Dress in layers.
   b. Lower room thermostat.
   c. Maintain healthy weight.
   d. Avoid smoking.
   e. Avoid triggers such as hot drinks, caffeine, spicy foods, alcohol.
   f. Use paced respirations (deep, slow, abdominal breathing).
2. Women who choose not to use or have contraindications to pharmacologic interventions have found some of the following OTC devices or products to be helpful in moderating VMS:
   a. Chillow Pillow©
   b. Bed fan
   c. Clothing and pajamas or gowns, bedsheets, and pillowcases made from wicking material
3. Herbal preparations. Many women purchase OTC supplements to alleviate minor menopausal symptoms. Because these products are not regulated by the FDA, there are significant concerns regarding the consistency, safety, and purity of the supplements, as well as the potential for adverse interactions with other drugs or herbal products. Women should also be aware that just because a product is labeled "natural" does not mean it is safe, and women should be counseled to discuss any new medication or OTC product with their health care provider before taking it.[22] For more information, consult the National Center for Complementary and Integrative Health (NCCIH), at https://nccih.nih.gov/. Several herbal products have been identified as options for managing VMS:
   a. Black cohosh. Study results are inconsistent compared with placebo, but this herb has been found to be at least as effective as placebo for relieving VMS in some women.[24] One OTC product, Remifemin, has been

tested in randomized, controlled trials. Long-term safety of black cohosh has not been established because most studies for managing menopausal symptoms have been conducted for only 6 months or less. Because of some complaints, however, products are required to post a warning that users should consult their provider if they have a liver disorder or discontinue use of the product if they develop symptoms of liver problems such as abdominal pain, dark urine, or jaundice.[22]

b. Relizen. Available online in the United States since 2015, this supplement has been available in Europe for more than 15 years for the treatment of vasomotor flushes. It is a pollen extract that has been shown in several small randomized clinical trials to have no estrogenic effects. The metabolic effect appears to be "serotonergic" similar to an SNRI effect. It does not have FDA approval and is considered an alternative/complementary product.[62]

4. Progesterone creams. In the United States, many brands of topical progesterone can be purchased without a prescription as lotion, gel, and cream preparations and have been used by women for treating VMS. There have been limited, small studies suggesting relief of symptoms with these products. However, because of absence of FDA oversight of these products, data regarding safety and efficacy are lacking. The effects of transdermal progesterone on endometrial protection with estrogen use are unknown, and this should not be recommended as an option for endometrial protection for women with a uterus who are taking an estrogen.[22]

5. Some studies have demonstrated value in hypnosis, yoga, acupuncture, and cognitive behavioral therapy for reducing VMS.[25]

Genital and Sexual Symptoms

Vaginal Moisturizers and Lubricants. Menopausal women may experience symptoms of vaginal dryness, irritation, and dyspareunia, although these symptoms may not become problematic until late in the postmenopausal period. Although few clinical studies have been conducted on the efficacy of these products, first-line therapies include nonhormonal OTC vaginal lubricants and moisturizers for symptoms of vaginal dryness and to reduce friction on atrophic tissue during sexual activity.[24] Products can be water-based (e.g., Astroglide, Just Like Me, K-Y Jelly, Slippery Stuff), oil-based (Elegance Women's Lubricants, olive oil), or silicone-based (Astroglide X, ID Millennium, K-Y Millennium, Pink). Some products are pH balanced (Replens, RepHresh). Some OTC products, such as Luvena, have combination benefits such as a moisturizer and lubricant. Although no OTC vaginal product treats the underlying estrogen deficiency that is causing the dryness and irritation, these products often provide significant short-term symptom relief. Women should be encouraged to experiment with products to find ones that meet their personal needs and should also be told that moisturizers may provide more relief if they are used regularly (several times a week), whereas lubricants are more helpful when used to minimize friction and irritation during sexual intercourse. Women should be discouraged from using products that contain perfumes, flavors, or warming ingredients that might cause irritation to the vaginal tissue, and douching disrupts the normal genital flora, increasing the risk for infection, and should be avoided by all women regardless of age.[22,25]

Stimulators or Vibrators. Regular sexual activity helps maintain normal vaginal lubrication and blood flow to the vagina. When sexual activity is decreased or absent, nonpenetrative sexual activity through use of oral stimulation or self-stimulation with vibrators or massage promotes blood flow to the genital area and helps maintain vaginal health and can be encouraged by self-stimulation or with partner assistance. Devices can be purchased OTC at drugstores (e.g., the Trojan Mini vibrator) or online (e.g., MiddleSexMD: www.middlesexmd.com), and more information is available on the NAMS website (www.menopause.org).

PHARMACOLOGIC THERAPY

Deciding which pharmacologic intervention to recommend to a particular woman depends on several factors, including her underlying health status, her personal preference, the cost, and the potential adverse effects of a particular medication. Many prescription therapies have been approved by the FDA to manage menopausal symptoms, including estrogens and progestogens (available in oral, transdermal, and topical formulations). Some nonhormonal therapies are FDA approved for these indications, and some FDA-approved pharmacologic options are also used off label to manage VMS symptoms. Because women may experience troublesome VMS and vaginal symptoms before reaching menopause (FMP), women should also be counseled regarding contraception options that can relieve perimenopausal symptoms while preventing an unintended pregnancy.

Contraceptive Therapy

Because there are no reliable laboratory tests to confirm definitive loss of fertility in a woman, both the American Congress of Obstetricians and Gynecologists (ACOG) and NAMS recommend that women continue contraceptive use until menopause or age 50 to 55 years.[63] Women of older reproductive age may also experience perimenopausal symptoms. Hormonal contraception offers a viable option for both symptomatic perimenopausal women and those who wish to avoid an unintended pregnancy. Low-dose combination estrogen/progestin contraceptives (pills, patch, ring) may be appropriate for healthy, lean, nonsmoking perimenopausal women but are contraindicated in women older than age 35 who smoke. Other potential contraindications include hypertension, diabetes, obesity, and other comorbidities. Progestin-only options offer potentially safer alternatives for women with these contraindications. Options for women who desire long-term contraception include long-acting reversible contraception (LARC) methods, such as the copper IUD, the two levonorgestrel-releasing intrauterine systems (LNG-IUSs), and the etonogestrel subdermal implant. The Centers for Disease Control and Prevention (CDC) has issued evidence-based guidelines, making contraceptive provision and clinical decision-making easier through publication of their "Selected Practice Recommendations" and "Medical Eligibility Criteria for Contraceptive Use." These guidelines can assist clinicians in recommending contraceptive methods according to age and medical conditions based on risks and advantages.[25,63]

Hormone Therapy

Consistent terminology is needed for discussion of pharmacologic choices for HT. In place of the old term *hormone replacement therapy* (HRT), the following terminology should be used[22]:

1. HT—hormone therapy. The FDA uses this term to distinguish therapy that includes only combination estrogen-progestogen. NAMS uses this term to encompass both types of therapy, estrogen and estrogen-progestogen therapy.
2. ET—estrogen therapy alone.
3. EPT—combined estrogen-progestogen therapy.
4. Progestogen—encompassing both natural progesterone and synthetic progestins.

HT/ET has both the primary indication and is the most effective treatment for VMS, and every systemic ET and EPT product has received regulatory agency FDA approval for vasomotor instability. Estrogen options include systemic estrogen; EPT combination products including combined estrogen-progestogen or estrogen (CEE)/bazedoxifene (BZA), a selective estrogen receptor modulator (SERM) combined with conjugated equine estrogen; or combined oral contraceptives (in women requiring contraception).[24] Estrogens are available in many prescription preparations, including as single agents in oral preparations; transdermal patch, gel, or topical emulsion preparations; and vaginal preparations for systemic or topical administration. Combination (EPT) preparations are also available in oral and transdermal preparations (Table 148.4).

Individualization of the plan of care in collaboration with the clinician is important because no consensus has been established regarding the perfect risk/benefit ratio for initiating or continuing HT.[27] A plan should be based on the woman's needs and desires after conducting a thorough history and physical examination and after a discussion with her regarding her risks and benefits for the interventions.

In October 2014, NAMS released a free app in the Apple App Store to help clinicians in prescribing HT. The Menopause Decision-Support Algorithm, discussed in an article published in Menopause: The Journal of the North American Menopause Society,[22] and the companion iPhone/iPad app, developed in collaboration with NAMS, are designed to help clinicians decide which patients are candidates for pharmacologic treatment of menopausal symptoms. The app provides clinicians with treatment options based on the woman's risk factors and her individualized choices. Within the app are links to other resources such as the Gail model breast cancer screening tool, the FRAX (Fracture Risk Assessment Tool) osteoporosis screening tool, CV screening tools, and the NAMS HT tables. This new algorithm and mobile app for menopausal symptom management incorporate current evidence-based data and research to clarify the decision-making process for clinicians; the app also includes a component for patients to seek answers to their questions about HT. Future plans include a version of the app for Android systems. An additional resource is the free app which can be downloaded to a smartphone from the National Association of Nurse Practitioners in Women's Health: NPWH: Well Woman App (menopause-specific content).

In reviewing key resources and specifically the NAMS 2017 Hormone Therapy Position Statement, the clinician can consider the following important points about prescribing HT[24,25]:

1. Estrogen and progesterone agonists share common features and effects and have potentially different properties. All HT products, including bioidentical and compounded hormones, are assumed to have similar risks until proven otherwise. Without randomized controlled trials, data for one agent should be generalized to all agents.
2. The option of HT is an individual decision in terms of quality of life and health priorities as well as personal factors such as age, time since menopause, and the risk of VTE, stroke, ischemic heart disease, and breast cancer. The type, dose and duration, route of administration, timing of initiation, and type of progestogen/or if needed, should be consistent with treatment goals and should be individualized with periodic reevaluation of benefits and risks.
3. HT is the most effective treatment for VMS, GSM, and to prevent bone loss and fracture. Benefits are more likely to outweigh risks for symptomatic women younger than 60 years or within 10 years after menopause. Absolute risks in healthy women ages 50 to 59 are low. Long-term use or HT initiation in older women, however, has greater risks, although longer duration may be more favorable for ET alone.
4. ET alone is appropriate in women after hysterectomy. Additional progestogen or BZA is required if the woman has a uterus. Administration of unopposed estrogen in a woman

TABLE 148.4	**Estrogen Products**	
Product	**Product Name(s)**	**Doses (mg/day)**
ORAL ESTROGEN PRODUCTS		
17β-estradiol	Estrace Various generics	0.5, 1.0, 2.0
CEE	Premarin	0.3, 0.45, 0.625, 0.9, 1.25
Synthetic conjugated estrogens, A	Cenestin	0.3. 0.45, 0.625, 0.9, 1.25
Synthetic conjugated estrogens, B	Enjuvia	0.3, 0.45, 0.625, 0.9, 1.25
Conjugated estrogens, CSD (synthetic)	CSD, PrC.E.S. Prpms-Conjugated estrogens	0.3, 0.625, 0.9, 1.25
Esterified estrogens	Menest Estragyn	0.3, 0.625, 1.25, 2.5 0.3, 0.625
Estropipate	Ogen Various generics	0.625 (0.75 estropipate) 1.25 (1.5), 2.5 (3.0) 0.625 (0.75), 1.5 (3.0), 5.0 (6.0)

Continued

TABLE 148.4   Estrogen Products—cont'd

Product	Product Name(s)	Doses (mg/day)
TRANSDERMAL ESTROGEN PRODUCTS		
17β-estradiol		
Patch	Alora	0.025, 0.05, 0.075, 0.1 twice/week
	Climara	0.025, 0.0375, 0.05, 0.075, 0.1 once/week
	Estradot	0.025, 0.0375, 0.05, 0.075, 0.1 twice/wk 0.014 once/week
	Estraderm	0.05, 0.1 twice/week
	Menostar	0.0375, 0.05, 0.075, 0.1 twice/week
	Minivelle	0.05, 0.1 twice/week
	Oesclim	0.025, 0.0375, 0.05, 0.075, 0.1 twice/week
	Vivelle	0.025, 0.0375, 0.05, 0.075, 0.1 twice/week
	Vivelle-Dot	0.05, 0.06, 0.025, 0.0375, 0.75, 0.1 once or twice/week
	Various generics	
Transdermal gel	Divigel	0.003, 0.009, 0.027
	EstroGel	0.75 (use lowest effective)
	Elestrin	0.0125, 0.0375 (use lowest effective)
Topical emulsion	Estrasorb	0.05 (2 packets) (use lowest effective)
Transdermal spray	Evamist	1.53 (1/day initially, adjust dose by response)
VAGINAL ESTROGEN PRODUCTS		
Creams		
17β-estradiol	Estrace	Initial: 2–4 g/day for 1–2 week
	VVA	Maintenance: 1 g 2–3 times/week (0.1 mg active ingredient per gram)
Conjugated estrogens	Premarin Vaginal Cream *Atrophic vaginitis* *Kraurosis vulvae* *United States: Moderate to severe* *dyspareunia* *Canada: Dyspareunia*	*United States:* *Atrophic vaginitis and kraurosis vulvae:* 0.5–2 g/day (0.625 mg active ingredient per gram) for 21 days then off 7 days *Moderate to severe dyspareunia:* 0.5 g/day for 21 days then off 7 days, or twice/week *Canada:* Low dose: 0.5 g intravaginal or topical twice/week Maximum recommended dose: 0.5 g/day intravaginally or topically for 21 days then off 7 days Start with 0.5 g/day; dose adjustments (0.5–2 g) may be made based on individual response
Estrone	Estragyn Vaginal Cream *Senile vaginitis* *Pruritus vulvae* *Kraurosis vulvae*	2–4 g/day (1 mg active ingredient per gram) adjusted to the lowest amount that controls symptoms; administration should be cyclic (e.g., for 21 days then off 7 days)
Rings		
17β-estradiol	Estring *United States: Moderate to severe* *urogenital symptoms caused by* *postmenopausal atrophy of the* *vagina and/or the lower urinary tract* *Canada: Atrophic vaginitis, dyspareunia,* *dysuria, and urinary urgency*	2 mg (releases 7.5 mcg/day) for 90 days
Estradiol acetate	Femring *VMS* *Severe vulvar and vaginal atrophy*	Releases 50 or 100 mcg of estradiol per day for 90 days; both doses release systemic levels and require consideration of a progestogen if the uterus is intact
Estradiol	Vagifem *Atrophic vaginitis*	Initial: 1 tablet/day for 2 week Maintenance: 1 tablet twice/week (tablet containing 10 mcg of estradiol hemihydrates, equivalent to 10 mcg estradiol)

TABLE 148.4   **Estrogen Products—cont'd**

Product	Product Name(s)	Doses (mg/day)
COMBINATION ESTROGEN-PROGESTOGEN PRODUCTS		
Oral Continuous Cyclic		
Conjugated estrogens plus MPA	Premphase	0.625 mg estrogen + 5.0 mg Progestogen 2 tablets: estrogen, and estrogen + Progestogen Estrogen alone days 1–14, estrogen + progestogen days 15–28
Oral Continuous Combined		
Conjugated estrogens plus MPA	Prempro Premplus	0.3 or 0.45 mg estrogen + 1.5 mg progestogen, 0.625 mg estrogen + 2.5 or 5.0 mg progestogen
Ethinyl estradiol plus norethindrone acetate	femhrt, FemHRT Lo femhrt, FemHRT	2.5 mcg estrogen + 0.5 mg Progestogen 5 mcg estrogen + 1 mg progestogen
17β-estradiol plus norethindrone acetate	Activella Activelle LD Activelle	0.5 mg estrogen + 0.1 mg progestogen, 1 mg estrogen + 0.5 mg Progestogen 0.5 mg estrogen + 0.1 mg Progestogen 1 mg estrogen + 0.5 mg progestogen
17β-estradiol + drospirenone	Angeliq	1 mg estrogen + 0.5 mg progestogen, 0.5 mg estrogen + 0.25 mg progestogen, 1 mg estrogen + 1 mg progestogen
Oral Intermittent-Combined		
17β-estradiol plus norgestimate	Prefest	1 mg estrogen and 1 mg estrogen + 0.09 mg Progestogen Estrogen alone for 3 days, then estrogen + progestogen for 3 days Repeated continuously
Conjugated estrogens plus MPA	Premplus Cycle	0.625 mg estrogen + 10 mg Progestogen 2 tablets: estrogen, and estrogen + Progestogen Estrogen alone for 14 days, then estrogen + progestogen for 14 days
Transdermal Intermittent-Combined		
17β-estradiol plus norethindrone acetate	CombiPatch Estalis	0.05 mg estrogen + 0.14 mg Progestogen 9 cm² patch, twice/week 0.05 mg estrogen + 0.25 mg Progestogen 16 cm² patch, twice/week
17β-estradiol plus levonorgestrel	Climara Pro	0.045 mg estrogen + 0.015 mg Progestogen 22 cm² patch, once/week
PROGESTOGENS		
MPA	Provera Provera Pak Various generics	2.5, 5, 10
Micronized progesterone	Prometrium	100, 200
OTHER ORAL PRODUCTS		
Conjugated estrogens plus bazedoxifene	Duavee *Moderate to severe VMS*	0.45 + 20 mg/day
Ospemifene	Osphena *Moderate to severe dyspareunia, a symptom of vulvar and vaginal atrophy, caused by menopause*	60 mg/day
Paroxetine	Brisdelle *Moderate to severe VMS*	7.5 mg/day

Data from North American Menopause Society, 2015. www.menopause.org/docs/default-source/2014/nams-ht-tables.pdf.

with a uterus increases the risk of endometrial cancer. Research is insufficient to recommend one regimen over another.

5. Local low-dose ET is preferred for women whose symptoms are limited to only vaginal dryness or associated dyspareunia. A progestogen is generally not indicated when ET is administered locally in a low dose for vaginal atrophy, although long-term safety data are limited.

6. Vaginal ET may help decrease recurrent urinary tract infection in postmenopausal women. Local ET may benefit some women with overactive bladder. Systemic HT may worsen or provoke stress incontinence.

7. The risk of breast cancer in women older than 50 years associated with HT is a complex issue. Current safety data do not support the use of systemic HT in breast cancer survivors, however vaginal estrogen may be used in some women with symptomatic GMS in collaboration with their oncologist.

8. The decision to continue or discontinue HT must be individualized. There is a 50% chance of VMS recurring when HT is discontinued. Symptom recurrence is similar whether the drug is tapered or abruptly discontinued. Women who initiated HT less than age 60 or less than 10 years of onset of menopause may choose to continue therapy beyond age 65 or choose to restart HT because of continuation of symptoms. To routinely discontinue systemic HT in women aged 65 years and older as recommended by Beers criteria is not supported by data.[27] Studies have shown that VMS may persist on average 7.4 years but for some women longer than 10 years. In one study 16% of women ≥ 85 years were still experiencing VMS. Additionally, some women in this older age group may be candidates for continuation of HT for prevention of osteoporosis when other choices are not acceptable.

Oral estrogen is the most widely used formulation. Because of the first-pass liver uptake, there is greater stimulation of certain proteins including a 25% increase in triglycerides, so women with hypertriglyceridemia, or who are at increased risk based on family history, should consider transdermal administration.[22,58] Oral ET also stimulates hepatic globulins, coagulation factors, and some inflammatory markers such as C-reactive protein, which have been associated with an increased risk of gallbladder disease.[22]

Transdermal and topical estrogens are not subject to first-pass liver metabolism and therefore have both known and theoretical advantages as well as disadvantages compared with oral formulations. There is no effect on increasing triglycerides. For patients with metabolic syndrome or hypertriglyceridemia, transdermal estrogen would be a better option. However, with transdermal administration and the lack of the first liver pass, there is also no improvement in high-density lipoprotein cholesterol (HDL-C) as happens with oral administration. Although there have been no large randomized controlled trials, several observational studies have suggested that transdermal ET is associated with a decreased risk of VTE.[22]

Women using topical estrogen sprays and gels should be instructed to cover areas of drug placement until it has been absorbed to avoid exposing partners, children, and pets to the medication. The most common side effect of a transdermal patch is skin irritation at the patch application site. Rotating the patch to other areas such as the buttocks, maintaining a clean site, and applying talcum powder around the patch edge to prevent formation of dirt rings may help reduce irritation.[22]

Vaginal estrogen can be administered through creams, rings, and tablets. For women who have other menopausal symptoms (VMS), all systemic ET is approved for treatment of GSM/VVA. If systemic management of symptoms is not needed, and only GSM symptoms requiring intervention for moderate to severe symptoms, including dyspareunia, is required, minimally absorbed vaginal low-dose ET is the treatment of choice for women who have no medical contraindications to its use.[25] Benefits of low-dose vaginal estrogen include restoration of vaginal blood flow, a decrease in vaginal pH, and improvement in the thickness and elasticity of the tissues. Maintenance is achieved with either twice weekly application or insertion of 17β-estradiol cream, conjugated estrogen cream, or estradiol hemihydrate 10-mcg tablets or insertion of a 17β-estradiol ring that releases hormone for 90 days. Regardless of the product used, systemic absorption is limited and progestogen therapy is usually not indicated for a woman with a uterus. (The 90-day vaginal product, estradiol acetate ring, releases estradiol at a higher dose and has FDA approval for also managing VMS symptoms; it will require a progestogen to protect the endometrium in women with a uterus.) Clinical monitoring should always be continued in women on low-dose vaginal estrogen without a progestogen because endometrial safety data do not extend beyond 1 year. Treatment can be continued for as long as distressing vaginal symptoms continue to occur.[24,25]

Product labeling for vaginal estrogen products often includes the same warnings, contraindications, and listing of adverse effects as labeling for other *systemic* estrogen products, despite the fact that low-dose vaginal ET does not typically result in significant systemic estrogen levels. A number of menopause, clinical, and scientific experts have initiated conversations with the FDA regarding changing the "boxed labeling" of topical vaginal estrogen products. Women should be counseled on this issue when given the prescription as research has shown if not given information from their provider, many will not fill the prescription after reading the product labeling and their symptoms will go untreated. Instructions to the patient prescribed the ring is that if it falls out, it can be rinsed off and reinserted, and the ring does not usually interfere with sexual intercourse but can be removed if it is uncomfortable for either partner.

Progestogen therapy can be an option to treat VMS. However, the primary role for this hormone in menopausal management is to reduce the risk of endometrial cancer associated with unopposed estrogen. Combined EPT products are available. All government-approved progestogen formulations will provide endometrial protection if the dose and duration are adequate. The progestogen product most structurally related to progesterone is an oral capsule containing micronized progesterone (Prometrium), which can be administered as an independent dose with an estrogen product. Prometrium is contraindicated for women who have an allergy to peanuts, and because of potential side effects of drowsiness and dizziness is recommended for administration at bedtime. A dose of 100 mg is usually effective for endometrial protection if administered in a continuous combined dosage schedule.[22]

EPT can be prescribed in many regimens. There is no consensus, and there is insufficient evidence to recommend any one regimen. Regimens are classified as continuous-cyclic sequential, continuous cyclic long-cycle, continuous-combined, and intermittent-combined. Each may have advantages and disadvantages, and clinicians using each regimen should be aware of any special monitoring of the endometrium that might be advised during clinical supervision of the patient. The continuous-combined regimen, which was developed to address withdrawal uterine bleeding, a major reason for discontinuation of EPT, has been the predominant regimen used in North America.[22,25] Breakthrough uterine bleeding has been observed in 40% of women on a continuous-combined regimen during the first 3 to 6 months, but most women will become amenorrheic within 12 months. Adjusting doses and evaluating for other causes of bleeding can be considered.

A tissue-selective estrogen complex (TSEC), which pairs BZA 20 mg, a novel SERM, with CEE (Duavee) 45 mg is FDA approved for the treatment of moderate to severe VMS and for prevention of osteoporosis in postmenopausal women with a uterus. This gives women another option instead of pairing estrogen with a progestogen for endometrial safety.

NAMS recommends ongoing clinical monitoring of women using HT to include at least yearly return visits, during which time the woman and her clinician should review the decision to use HT, including a discussion of any new research findings. It is recognized that more frequent visits may be required, especially for women just starting HT or for those having bothersome side effects. Although clinical guidelines and societies may differ, NAMS recommends annual mammography for women who are prescribed HT. Endometrial surveillance is not required for women using systemic ET and adequate progestogen. Data are insufficient to recommend annual endometrial surveillance in asymptomatic women using low-dose vaginal ET for the treatment of vaginal atrophy. If a woman is at high risk for endometrial cancer, is using a higher dose of vaginal ET, or is having symptoms (spotting, breakthrough bleeding), closer surveillance may be required.[22]

Estrogens are available in many prescription preparations, including as single agents in oral preparations; transdermal patch, gel, or topical emulsion preparations; vaginal preparations; and combination (EPT) preparations (see Table 148.4).

Bioidentical Hormone Therapy Products. Many well-tested FDA-approved bioidentical brand-name products are available in the United States. However, the term *bioidentical* is typically used to mean custom-made HT formulations compounded for an individual according to a provider's prescription. Custom-compounded bioidentical hormone therapy (CBHT) may provide doses, ingredients, and routes of administration not commercially available, but no formulation has been approved by any regulatory agency. CBHT agents are not tested for efficacy, safety, batch standardization, or purity and do not include package inserts like those required for FDA-approved HT products, explaining benefits and risks.[22,24,25] Often dosing on the basis of salivary testing which has not been found to be reliable because of differences in hormonal pharmacokinetics and absorption, diurnal variation, and inter/intraindividual variability, these therapies may not be safe or efficacious for patients. Third-party payers rarely reimburse prescription costs for these compounded drugs. Most of the large national organizations (NAMS, ACOG, Endocrine Society) do not support the use of CBHT unless the patient must have the hormone prescription compounded because of an allergy to an ingredient in the commercial formulation. Clinicians are encouraged, if they decide to use a compounding pharmacy for whatever reason, to check whether the company supplying the drug is accredited by the Pharmacy Compounding Accreditation Board. Also, the clinician should educate the patient on the drug's risks, benefits, safety, administration, and dosage.[22,24,25]

FOOD AND DRUG ADMINISTRATION–APPROVED NONHORMONAL PHARMACOLOGIC OPTIONS

FDA approved nonhormonal pharmacologic options are available for management of menopausal symptoms.
1. Paroxetine (Brisdelle) 7.5 mg is a nonhormone selective serotonin reuptake inhibitor (SSRI) that provides an alternative for women to manage VMS, especially women who cannot or choose not to use HT. Higher doses of paroxetine were originally approved in 1992 for treatment of psychiatric conditions that currently include depression, anxiety disorder, social anxiety disorder, panic disorder, obsessive compulsive disorder, and generalized and post-traumatic stress disorder. This lower dose of paroxetine is not approved for these indications. A potential exists for paroxetine to interact with tamoxifen owing to its potent cytochrome P-450 2D6 inhibitors.
2. Ospemifene (Osphena), a SERM, is an estrogen-like compound that acts as an estrogen agonist or antagonist. Ospemifene is an oral option for treating moderate to severe dyspareunia, a symptom of vulvar and vaginal atrophy resulting from menopause. It has not been shown to cause any increased risk of endometrial proliferation in trials up to 52 weeks. Although risks of thromboembolic stroke, hemorrhagic stroke, and VTE have been similar to those of placebo in healthy postmenopausal women studied for up to 52 weeks, concern remains about potential risk of VTE because of potential class effect.[22]
3. Prasterone (Intrarosa), the steroid DHEA, is a once-daily vaginal ovule 6.5 mg inserted HS for treatment of dyspareunia due to menopausal VVA/GSM.[32] This new option is associated with not only improvement in dyspareunia but was found to increase vaginal superficial cells, reduce parabasal cells, and reduce vaginal pH. The intracrine conversion of DHEA to estrogen and testosterone resulted in local benefits but no increase in circulating levels of androgens. Unlike the vaginal estrogens, no boxed warning was required by the FDA for prasterone. A history of breast cancer is not a contraindication; however the drug has not been studied in this population and the insert does list a warning for women who have a diagnosis of estrogen-sensitive breast cancer.[10]

NONHORMONAL PHARMACOLOGIC OPTIONS: NON–FOOD AND DRUG ADMINISTRATION–APPROVED FOR MENOPAUSAL SYMPTOMS

Although the following drugs have FDA approval for other indications, they do not have approval for menopausal symptoms. However, many of them have been studied and have been found to relieve menopausal symptoms[22,24-26]:
1. SSRIs and SNRIs:
   a. Citalopram, 10 to 20 mg/day
   b. Desvenlafaxine, 50 to 100 mg/day
   c. Escitalopram, 10 to 20 mg/day
   d. Fluoxetine, 20 mg/day
   e. Paroxetine, 12.5 to 25 mg/day
   f. Venlafaxine, 37.5 to 75 mg/day

Adverse effects of drugs in these classifications may be: dizziness; nausea; dry mouth; sweating; tiredness; insomnia; anxiety or agitation; constipation; difficulty urinating; headache; loss of appetite; reduced sexual desire, or problems with sexual arousal. Women prescribed tamoxifen for treatment of breast cancer should avoid use of paroxetine due to its metabolic inhibition of the cytochrome P450 system which may render tamoxifen less effective.

2. Clonidine: Initial oral dose for hot flash treatment is 0.05 mg twice daily, but some women may require at least 0.1 mg twice daily or the patch, 0.1 mg per day. The drug has a modest effect on symptoms. Adverse side effects include insomnia, dry mouth, constipation, and drowsiness. This may be a good choice for patients with hypertension.

3. Gabapentin may be initiated at a daily dose of 300 mg at bedtime; the dose can be increased to 300 mg twice daily and then to three times daily at 3- to 4-day intervals. Adverse side effects include dizziness, somnolence, and peripheral edema.

4. Studies have not shown that ET has any significant effect on sexual interest, arousal, or orgasmic response,[22] and no drugs are FDA approved to treat hypoactive sexual desire disorder (HSDD) in postmenopausal women. Flibanserin (Addyi), a sexual health drug, has been studied in both pre- and postmenopausal women.[64] Prescribed at 100 mg at HS, a 5-hydroxytryptophan (1A) receptor agonist and 5-hydroxytryptophan (2A) receptor antagonist that works in the brain to restore sexual desire, it is FDA approved for use in premenopausal women. Women who had a positive response to the drug had on average 2.5 to 4 additional satisfying sexual events/month compared to those in the study on placebo. Side effects of dizziness, hypotension, and somnolence were similar to other CNS drugs. These side effects can be reduced by taking the medicine at HS and avoiding alcohol intake. Clinicians who wish to prescribe flibanserin must complete a risk evaluation and mitigation strategy (REMS) program by answering 4 questions online. Pharmacists also must complete the REMS program to dispense the drug. Flibanserin may be an effective option for some women with HSDD, but clinicians need to be fully aware of prescribing requirements.

5. Testosterone: Because there are no approved testosterone products for females (specifically used clinically for treating HSDD), dosing must be compounded or clinicians may prescribe the male testosterone products (e.g., Testim) at 1/10 of the male dose. Postmenopausal women who are being prescribed testosterone therapy must be counseled on proper dosing, risks, and benefits since safety data are lacking, and they should be followed closely by their provider. Both the woman's total testosterone and SHBG levels should be evaluated to maintain the calculated free testosterone level within the physiological range for a reproductive-aged woman.[53]

IMPLICATIONS FOR PRACTICE

The perimenopausal period offers a perfect opportunity to recommend healthy lifestyle choices and to address individual health risks as women transition into late midlife. Part of this discussion should include a conversation about the risks and benefits of HT, particularly if a woman is experiencing premature or induced menopause. After a comprehensive review of the literature by an expert panel assembled by NAMS, the updated Hormone Therapy Position Statement was published in 2017. It was endorsed or supported by 33 national and international societies and suggests "that women are better served using evidenced-based information to determine the most appropriate type, dose, formulation, route of administration, and duration of use of hormone therapy."[22] The plan of care for a menopausal woman who seeks intervention from her health care provider should be individualized and developed collaboratively using a shared decision-making approach.

REFERENCES

1. De Felici, M. (2013). Origin, migration, and proliferation of human primordial germ cells. In *Oogenesis* (pp. 19–37). London: Springer.
2. Costanian, C., McCague, H., & Tamim, H. (2017). Age at natural menopause and its associated factors in Canada: Cross-sectional analyses from the Canadian Longitudinal Study on Aging. *Menopause (New York, N.Y.)*, doi:10.1097/GME.0000000000000990. [Epub ahead of print].
3. Grisendi, V., et al. (2014). Age-specific reference values for serum FSH and estradiol levels throughout the reproductive period. *Gynecological Endocrinology*, 30(6), 451–455.
4. Al-Safi, Z. A., & Santoro, N. (2014). Menopausal hormone therapy and menopausal symptoms. *Fertility and Sterility*, 101(4), 905–915.
5. U.S. Census Bureau. (2012). *Statistical Abstract of the United States*. Washington, DC: U.S. Department of Commerce.
6. Juul, F., et al. (2017). Birth weight, early life weight gain and age at menarche: A systematic review of longitudinal studies. *Obesity Reviews: An Official Journal of the International Association for the Study of Obesity*, 18(11), 1272–1288.
7. Thurston, R. C., & Joffe, H. (2011). Vasomotor symptoms and menopause: Findings from the Study of Women's Health Across the Nation. *Obstetrics and Gynecology Clinics of North America*, 38(3), 489.
8. Harlow, S. D., Gass, M., Hall, J. E., Lobo, R., Maki, P., Rebar, R. W., et al. (2012). Executive summary of the Stages of Reproductive Aging Workshop +10: Addressing the unfinished agenda of staging reproductive aging. *Climacteric: The Journal of the International Menopause Society*, 15(2), 105–114.
9. Burns, K. A., & Korach, K. S. (2012). Estrogen receptors and human disease: An update. *Archives of Toxicology*, 86(10), 1491–1504.
10. Mihm, M., Gangooly, S., & Muttukrishna, S. (2011). The normal menstrual cycle in women. *Animal Reproduction Science*, 124(3), 229–236.
11. Davis, S. R., & Worsley, R. (2014). Androgen treatment of postmenopausal women. *The Journal of Steroid Biochemistry and Molecular Biology*, 142, 107–114.
12. Key. (2016). Prasterone (Intrarosa) for dyspareunia. *Menopause*, 243–256.
13. Wierman, M. E., Arlt, W., Basson, R., Davis, S. R., Miller, K. K., Murad, M. H., et al. (2014). Androgen therapy in women: A reappraisal: An Endocrine Society Clinical Practice Guideline. *The Journal of Clinical Endocrinology and Metabolism*, 99(10), 3489–3510.
14. Broer, S. L., Broekmans, F. J., Laven, J. S., & Fauser, B. C. (2014). Anti-Müllerian hormone: Ovarian reserve testing and its potential clinical implications. *Human Reproduction Update*, 20(5), 688–701.
15. de Kat, A. C., et al. (2017). A quantitative comparison of anti-Müllerian hormone measurement and its shifting boundaries between two assays. *Maturitas*, 101, 12–16.
16. Greendale, G. A., Ishii, S., Huang, M. H., & Karlamangla, A. S. (2013). Predicting the timeline to the final menstrual period: The study of women's health across the nation. *The Journal of Clinical Endocrinology and Metabolism*, 98(4), 1483–1491.
17. Hembree, W. C., et al. (2017). Endocrine treatment of gender-dysphoric/gender-incongruent persons: An endocrine society* clinical practice guideline. *The Journal of Clinical Endocrinology and Metabolism*, 102(11), 3869–3903.
18. De Villiers, T. J., Gass, M. L., Haines, C. J., Hall, J. E., Lobo, R. A., Pierroz, D. D., et al. (2013). Global consensus statement on menopausal hormone therapy. *Climacteric: The Journal of the International Menopause Society*, 16(2), 203–204.
19. Grady, D., Herrington, D., & Bittner, V. (2002). Cardiovascular disease outcomes during 6.8 years of hormone therapy: Heart and Estrogen/progestin Replacement Study follow-up (HERS II). *JAMA: The Journal of the American Medical Association*, 288(1), 49–57.
20. Writing Group for the Women's Health Initiative Investigators. (2002). Risks and benefits of estrogen plus progestin in healthy postmenopausal women principal results from the women's health initiative randomized controlled trial. *JAMA: The Journal of the American Medical Association*, 288(3), 321–333. doi:10.1001/jama.288.3.321.

21. Manson, J. E., et al. (2017). Menopausal hormone therapy and long-term all-cause and cause-specific mortality: The Women's Health Initiative randomized trials. *JAMA: The Journal of the American Medical Association, 318*(10), 927–938.

22. NAMS-1 North American Menopause Society (NAMS). (2014). *Menopause practice: A clinician's guide* (5th ed.). Mayfield Heights, OH: NAMS.

23. Manson, J. E., Aragaki, A. K., Rossouw, J. E., et al. (2017). Menopausal hormone therapy and long-term all-cause and cause-specific mortality: The women's health initiative randomized trials. *JAMA, 318*(10), 927–938.

24. Shifren, J. L., & Gass, M. L. (2014). The North American Menopause Society recommendations for clinical care of midlife women. *Menopause (New York, N.Y.), 21*(10), 1038–1062.

25. NAMS 2 North American Menopause Society (NAMS). (2017). Retrieved from http://www.menopause.org/docs/default-source/2017/nams-2017-hormone-therapy-position-statement.pdf.

26. Harman, S. M., Brinton, E. A., Cedars, M., Lobo, R., Manson, J. E., Merriam, G. R., et al. (2005). KEEPS: The Kronos Early Estrogen Prevention Study. *Climacteric: The Journal of the International Menopause Society, 8*(1), 3–12.

27. Cobin, R. H., & Goodman, N. F. (2017). American Association of Clinical Endocrinologists and American College of endocrinology position statement on menopause - 2017 update. *Endocrine Practice*. Retrieved from http://journals.aace.com/doi/abs/10.4158/EP171828.PS. (Retrieved 23 November 2017).

28. Paramsothy, P., Harlow, S. D., Greendale, G. A., Gold, E. B., Crawford, S. L., Elliott, M. R., et al. (2014). Bleeding patterns during the menopausal transition in the multi-ethnic Study of Women's Health Across the Nation (SWAN): A prospective cohort study. *BJOG: An International Journal of Obstetrics and Gynaecology, 121*, 1564–1573.

29. Whitaker, L., & Critchley, H. O. D. (2016). Abnormal uterine bleeding. *Best Practice & Research Clinical Obstetrics & Gynaecology, 34*, 54–65. doi:10.1016/j.bpobgyn.2015.11.012.

30. North American Menopause Society. (2015). Nonhormonal management of menopause associated vasomotor symptoms: 2015 position statement of The North American Menopause Society. Retrieved from http://www.menopause.org/docs/default-source/professional/2015-nonhormonal-therapy-position-statement.pdf.

31. Freeman, E. W., Sammel, M. D., & Sanders, R. J. (2014). Risk of long-term hot flashes after natural menopause: Evidence from the Penn Ovarian Aging Study cohort. *Menopause (New York, N.Y.), 21*(9), 924–932.

32. Avis, N. E., Crawford, S. L., Greendale, G., et al. (2015). Duration of menopausal vasomotor symptoms over the menopause transition. *JAMA Internal Medicine, 175*(4), 531–539.

33. Portman, D. J., Bachmann, G. A., & Simon, J. A. (2013). Ospemifene Study Group. Ospemifene, a novel selective estrogen receptor modulator for treating dyspareunia associated with postmenopausal vulvar and vaginal atrophy. *Menopause (New York, N.Y.), 20*(6), 623–630.

34. Labrie, F., Archer, D. F., Koltun, W., et al. (2016). Efficacy of intravaginal dehydroepiandrosterone (DHEA)on moderate to severe dyspareunia and vaginal dryness, symptoms of vulvovaginal atrophy, and of the genitourinary syndrome of menopause. *Menopause (New York, N.Y.), 23*(3), 243–256.

35. Nappi, R. E., & Kokot-Kierepa, M. (2012). Vaginal Health: Insights, Views and Attitudes (VIVA)—results from an international survey. *Climacteric: The Journal of the International Menopause Society, 15*(1), 36–44.

36. Soares, C. N., Almeida, O. P., Joffe, H., & Cohen, L. S. (2001). Efficacy of estradiol for the treatment of depressive disorders in perimenopausal women: A double-blind, randomized, placebo-controlled trial. *Archives of General Psychiatry, 58*, 529–534.

37. Hayes, R., & Dennerstein, L. (2005). The impact of aging on sexual function and sexual dysfunction in women: A review of population-based studies. *The Journal of Sexual Medicine, 2*(3), 317–330.

38. Shifren, J. L., Monz, B. U., Russo, P. A., Segreti, A., & Johannes, C. B. (2008). Sexual problems and distress in United States women: Prevalence and correlates. *Obstetrics and Gynecology, 112*(5), 970–978.

39. Hebert, L. E., Weuve, J., Scherr, P. A., & Evans, D. A. (2013). Alzheimer disease in the united states (2010-2050) estimated using the 2010 census. *Neurology, 80*(19), 1778–1783.

40. American Heart Association. (2017). Heart and Stroke Statistics 2017 At-A-Glance. Retrieved from http://www.heart.org/idc/groups/ahamah-public/@wcm/@sop/@smd/documents/downloadable/ucm_491265.pdf. Retrieved 25 November 2017).

41. Marjoribanks, J., et al. (2012). Long term hormone therapy for perimenopausal and postmenopausal women. *The Cochrane Database of Systematic Reviews*, (7), CD004143, Most recent amendment: 1-16-2017.

42. Wright, N. C., et al. (2014). The recent prevalence of osteoporosis and low bone mass in the United States based on bone mineral density at the femoral neck or lumbar spine. *Journal of Bone and Mineral Research, 29*(11), 2520–2526.

43. Melton, L. J., Atkinson, E. J., St. Sauver, J. L., et al. (2014). Predictors of excess mortality following fracture: A population-based cohort study. *Journal of Bone and Mineral Research: The Official Journal of the American Society for Bone and Mineral Research, 29*(7), 1681–1590. doi:10.1002/jbmr.2193.

44. National Osteoporosis Foundation. (2014). 54 Million Americans Affected by Osteoporosis and Low Bone Mass. NOF Releases Updated Data Detailing the Prevalence of Osteoporosis and Low Bone Mass in the U.S. Retrieved from https://www.nof.org/2014/06/02/54-million-americans-affected-by-osteoporosis-and-low-bone-mass/. (Retrieved 26 November 2017).

45. Torio, C. M., & Moore, B. J. (2017). National Inpatient Hospital Costs: The Most Expensive Conditions by Payer, 2013 Healthcare Cost and Utilization Project (HCUP). Retrieved from https://www.hcup-us.ahrq.gov/reports/statbriefs/sb204-Most-Expensive-Hospital-Conditions.jsp. (Retrieved 24 November 2017).

46. Tucker, K. L. (2009). Osteoporosis prevention and nutrition. *Current Osteoporosis Reports, 7*(4), 111.

47. Fortmann, S. P., Burda, B. U., Senger, C. A., Lin, J. S., & Whitlock, E. P. (2013). Vitamin and mineral supplements in the primary prevention of cardiovascular disease and cancer: An updated systematic evidence review for the U.S. Preventive Services Task Force. *Annals of Internal Medicine, 159*(12), 824–834.

48. Centers for Disease Control and Prevention (CDC). Alzheimer's disease. Retrieved from www.cdc.gov/aging/aginginfo/alzheimers.htm. (Retrieved 28 November 2017).

49. Hebert, L. E., Weuve, J., Scherr, P. A., & Evans, D. A. (2013). Alzheimer disease in the united states (2010-2050) estimated using the 2010 census. *Neurology, 80*(19), 1778–1783.

50. Rocca, W. A., Grossardt, B. R., & Shuster, L. T. (2014). Oophorectomy, estrogen, and dementia: A 2014 update. *Molecular and Cellular Endocrinology, 389*(1), 7–12.

51. National Comprehensive Cancer Network (NCCN). (2017). Clinical Practice Guidelines in Oncology Uterine Neoplasms Version 1.2018. Retrieved from https://www.nccn.org/professionals/physician_gls/pdf/uterine.pdf. (Retrieved 28 November 2017).

52. Vyas, M. N., Rai, S., Manjeera, L., & Shetty, D. (2013). Bilateral primary fallopian tube carcinoma with the classical clinical features: A case report. *Journal of Clinical and Diagnostic Research: JCDR, 7*(4), 726–728. doi:10.7860/JCDR/2013/4518.2894.

53. Shifren, J. L., & Davis, S. R. (2017). Androgens in postmenopausal women: A review. *Menopause (New York, N.Y.), 24*, 970–979.

54. World Health Organization (WHO). (2017). Breast cancer prevention and control—breast cancer burden. Retrieved from www.who.int/cancer/detection/breastcancer/en/index1.html.

55. National Comprehensive Cancer Network (NCCN). (2017). Clinical Practice Guidelines in Oncology Breast Cancer Version 3.2017. Retrieved from https://www.nccn.org/professionals/physician_gls/pdf/uterine.pdf. (Retrieved 29 November 2017).

56. Siegel, R. L., Miller, K. D., & Jemal, A. (2016). Cancer statistics, 2016. *CA: A Cancer Journal for Clinicians, 66*(1), 7–30.

57. Centers for Disease Control. (2016). Leading Cancer Deaths, Male and Female. Retrieved from https://gis.cdc.gov/Cancer/USCS/DataViz.html. (Accessed 23 June 2019).

58. McNeil, M. (2017). Menopausal hormone therapy: Understanding long-term risks and benefits [editorial]. *JAMA: The Journal of the American Medical Association, 318*(10), 911–912.

59. The North American Menopause Society. (2014). Algorithm and mobile app for menopausal symptom management and hormonal/non-hormonal therapy decision making: A clinical decision-support tool from The North American Menopause Society. *Menopause (New York, N.Y.), 22*(3).

60. Roett, M. A., & Evans, P. (2009). Ovarian cancer: An overview. *American Family Physician, 80*(6), 609–616.

61. Singh, S., & Gambert, S. (2014). Health practitioner's guide to prescribing vitamin D and calcium. *Consultant, 54*(3), 174–180.

62. Espie, M., & Druckmann, R. How can hot flashes be managed for breast cancer patients and survivors without risk. (Poster Presentation, Annual Meeting at the North American Menopause Society, Washington, DC, October 15-18, 2014.

63. Division of Reproductive Health, National Center for Chronic Disease Prevention and Health Promotion, Centers for Disease Control and Prevention (CDC). (2013). U.S. selected practice recommendations for contraceptive use: Adapted from the World Health Organization selected practice recommendations for contraceptive use, 2nd edition. *MMWR. Recommendations and Reports: Morbidity and Mortality Weekly Report. Recommendations and Reports, 62*(RR–05), 1–60.

64. Simon, J. A., Kingsberg, S. A., Shumel, B., et al. (2014). Efficacy and safety of flibanserin in postmenopausal women with HSDD: Results of the SNOW-DROP trial. *Menopause (New York, N.Y.)*, 21(6), 633–640.

CHAPTER **149**

CERVICAL CANCER SCREENING ABNORMALITIES

Michelle Collins

DEFINITION AND EPIDEMIOLOGY

The Papanicolaou (Pap) test is a screening test for cervical cancer that involves collection of exfoliated cervical cells for cytologic staining and examination. Among the 30 million Pap tests performed annually in the United States, approximately 1.4 million (2.1%) reveal cytologic abnormalities requiring follow-up.[1] Cervical cancer affects approximately 12,200 US women annually, with 4210 women dying from cervical cancer every year. The majority of women who are diagnosed with cervical cancer have either never had cervical cancer screening prior to diagnosis, or they have not had screening in the 5 years prior to diagnosis.[2] Cervical cancer mortality has decreased by 70% since the introduction of the Pap test 75 years ago; however, health disparity research has revealed that women of lower socioeconomic status, and particularly ethnic minorities, have a higher incidence of cervical cancer mortality within the United States, with rates higher among black and Hispanic women as compared to white women. For the most recent year that data is available, 2014, Hispanic women had the highest rates of cervical cancer. Next highest rates of cervical cancer were among black, then white, then Asian/Pacific Islander (A/PI) women, and lastly American Indian/Alaska Native (AI/AN).[3] Women immigrating to the United States from countries where cervical cancer screening is not routinely conducted are a group at particularly high risk.[4]

Until the 1980s, there had not been clearly definitive evidence linking cervical cancer to any one particular cause, and certainly not to a virus. German virologist Harald zur Hausen (who went on to win the Nobel Prize in Medicine for his groundbreaking discovery) first published his work in 1983, positively identifying types of genital human papillomavirus (HPV) in cervical cancer tissue samples.[5] Though his work was not initially universally accepted, it is now common knowledge that HPV is involved in the etiology of cervical cancer. Papillomaviruses are small, double-stranded DNA viruses. Among the more than 200 types of HPV that affect humans, approximately 40 are genital subtypes, meaning that they affect the uro-ano-genital area and are spread via oral, anal, or vaginal intercourse. At least 13 of those are high-risk types, including types 16 and 18, which are the two most problematic as they are the cause of approximately 70% of all cervical cancers. HPV-16 accounts for approximately 50% of cervical cancers worldwide. Low-risk HPV subtypes, such as HPV-6 and HPV-11, are associated with genital warts and are not implicated in the etiology of malignant cervical disease.[6] Human papilloma virus is the most common sexually transmitted infection in the United States, with at least 50% of sexually active persons becoming infected with at least one type of uro-ano-genital HPV during their lifetime. By the age of 50, at least 80% of women will have been infected with a genital HPV infection.[7] Of note, transmission of the genital virus types does not require penetrative intercourse; HPV can be transmitted through direct contact of the skin and mucous membranes of infected individuals to the skin and mucous membranes of partners.

Although it is known that the presence of high-risk uro-ano-genital HPV is necessary for the development of cervical cancer, only a very small proportion of women infected with HPV actually progress to the point of developing cervical cancer, which suggests that cervical cancer is a multifactorial phenomenon. Specifically, not just the *presence* but the *persistence* of the HPV infection is thought to be the impetus for precancerous and cancerous lesions.[8] Most HPV infections resolve spontaneously, particularly in young women. What can be very confusing to both clinicians and patients is that resolution of the initial infection does not equate to virus eradication from the body. Current scientific thought is that HPV may clear the cervical cells but remain dormant in the body, showing up at a later time particularly when there is immune system compromise (as in pregnancy). The knowledge that HPV infections clear fairly easily in young women, combined with the information gleaned from tracking women with HPV for several successive years, has led to the significant revision of screening and management guidelines for women younger than age 24.

PATHOPHYSIOLOGY

The development of cervical cancer is multifactorial. Human papillomavirus infection is integral to the development of cervical dysplasia (development of abnormal cells) and oncogenic (cancerous) lesions. Identified associated risk factors for HPV infection include age at first sexual intercourse (coitarche) and number of sexual partners. Women who experience coitarche prior to the age of 16 years (noted to be 17 years in some studies, 16 in others) have shown a significantly higher association with HPV infection. They are also more at risk to have contracted the two most concerning high-risk oncogenic types, 16 and 18. Multiple studies have demonstrated that cervical HPV infections occur shortly after sexual debut. Young women who become sexually active prior to age 16 to 17 are more vulnerable to HPV infection because of the cellular changes of the cervix that occur during the pubescent period. These cellular changes leave the cervix more susceptible to the virus. The number of sexual partners (defined as more than 5) also increases the risk for HPV infection and subsequent dysplasia development.[9] Additionally, older age, vaginal pH changes, hormonal changes, cellular trauma, long-term use of combined hormonal contraception, multiparity (defined as having had three or more pregnancies), history of other sexually transmitted infections, having a sexual partner with a history of a sexually transmitted infection, younger age at first pregnancy, and cigarette smoking are all factors involved in the development of dysplasia and neoplasia.[10,11,12]

HPV contains genes that encode proteins with particular functions in the life cycle of the virus. Among high-risk HPV types, the role of E5, E6, and E7 proteins is unique, allowing high-risk types of HPV to take control of an infected host cell for its own replication and survival. A normal host cell contains two important tumor suppressor genes (*p53* and *pRb*) that act as the guardians of the cell. Among high-risk HPV types, such as HPV-16, E6 and E7 proteins interfere with the *p53* and *pRb* host cell tumor suppressor genes, disrupting the normal cell life cycle. In a normal non-replicating cell, pRb is bound to another protein, E2F, which is required for DNA replication. When HPV viral protein E7 displaces the connection between pRb and E2F, the usual control that pRb exerts over cell replication is disabled. Unbound E2F causes a normally non-replicating cell to begin the complex sequence of cell replication necessary for the survival and reproduction of HPV. Usually, if pRb is dysfunctional, the other guardian of the cell, $p53$, recognizes this dysfunction and initiates a mechanism that suspends the cell cycle processes to repair the damage. Normally, when $p53$ recognizes that the damage is not reparable, it triggers apoptosis (programmed cell death), preventing the damaged cell from future replication. However, HPV also disables $p53$, thereby allowing damaged cells to escape death and enabling HPV to thrive. This aberrant replication process increases susceptibility to gene mutation. An unstable genome gives rise to carcinogenesis.[13,14]

HPV enters the body during vaginal, anal, or oral sexual contact, or by skin-to-skin transmission through intimate sexual contact. The virus can also be transmitted via sex toys or other implements utilized during sex play.[15] HPV passes through the cervical epithelium to the basal cell layer, where it enters the normally replicating basal cell and exploits the replicating machinery of the basal cell to establish itself. The virus then begins to reproduce insidiously, eventually accompanying the host cell through natural epithelial cell maturation until it is detectable in the normally non-replicating suprabasal cells and surface epithelium.[16]

After initial infection, HPV may exist as a latent infection for a period of months. The virus then enters its productive phase, during which the virus produces a protective capsule that allows it to survive attached to superficial and exfoliated squamous cells. This protective capsule makes HPV highly infectious and sexually transmittable. Persistent HPV infection, combined with other cofactors, gives rise to cervical dysplasia, also described as cervical intraepithelial neoplasia (CIN). Low-grade lesions detected by Pap test, and confirmed by cervical biopsy, have a fairly high regression rate and frequently resolve spontaneously; the probability of regression of CIN 1 (the lowest level of CIN) is approximately 70% to 80% in adult women, and greater than 90% in adolescents and young women.[16] High-grade lesions (CIN II and III) detected by Pap tests, and confirmed by cervical biopsy, are more likely than CIN 1 lesions to progress to cervical cancer than to regress, particularly for lesions that are CIN 3 as compared with those that are CIN 2.[17] Women who are immunocompromised are at greater risk for progression of cervical disease, even with the low-grade CIN I lesion.

CLINICAL PRESENTATION AND PHYSICAL EXAMINATION

Although frank cervical cancer may appear as a visible cervical lesion on the cervix, most cervical lesions detected via cervical screening methods are not visible during routine speculum and pelvic examination.

DIAGNOSTICS: CERVICAL CANCER SCREENING

Two techniques are currently available for Pap test specimen collection. The traditional Pap test involves collection of exfoliated endocervical cells with a cytobrush or cotton swab, and collection of ectocervical cells with a wooden or plastic spatula. A cytobroom, which collects both ecto- and

endocervical cells simultaneously, is another option for cell collection. The method originally developed for Pap cell analysis still in use, albeit to a lesser extent than the liquid fixative methods, involves application of the collected exfoliated cervical cells applied directly to a glass slide in a smear-like fashion (hence the origin of the well-known term "Pap smear"; current terminology of "Pap test" is a more all-encompassing term). Fixative is then applied immediately after the specimen is smeared onto the slide. A more recent technology for Pap test specimen collection and processing uses a liquid-based medium (SurePath, ThinPrep). The examiner uses either the plastic spatula and endocervical brush, or cytobroom, for cell collection and then places the specimen in the liquid medium. The pathology laboratory then centrifuges the liquid specimen, allowing separation of the cervical cells from blood, mucus, and any cellular debris. When liquid-based medium is used for the collection and analysis of cervical cells, additional testing for gonorrhea, chlamydia, and HPV can be performed from the same specimen. Additional testing for gonorrhea, chlamydia, and HPV is not able to be performed directly from the sample placed onto the glass slide.

HPV DNA testing has been approved by the US Food and Drug Administration (FDA) as an adjunct to Pap testing when atypical squamous cells of undetermined significance (ASCUS) are detected. The FDA has also approved HPV DNA testing as a screening test for women older than 30 years as an adjunct to the Pap test. The rationale for limitation of use as a primary screen for women age 30 and older is based on the knowledge of the high prevalence of inconsequential, transient HPV infections among women younger than 30 years. To use the HPV as a primary screening tool in women younger than 30 would lead to an abundance of positive HPV results, potentially resulting in unnecessary procedures and psychosocial concerns. HPV infection among women 18 to 25 years is more commonly transient and appears to frequently resolve spontaneously or to become undetectable within a period of 2 years.[12]

The accuracy of Pap test screening depends, in large part, on proper specimen collection technique. Optimally, a Pap specimen should not be obtained during menses, or within 24 to 48 hours of having had intercourse, or having used any topical vaginal medications. Health care providers should be aware that the Pap test sample should be obtained from the transformation zone of the cervix. The normal ectocervix (external surface of the cervix) is covered by stratified squamous epithelium. The endocervix (internal surface of the cervix) contains mucus-secreting columnar epithelium. The normal physiologic process of metaplasia (cell metamorphosis from one type of cell to another) transforms columnar epithelium into squamous epithelium, with the border between the columnar and squamous epithelium known as the squamocolumnar junction. The region of the cervix where columnar epithelium transforms into modified squamous epithelium is aptly named the transformation zone. The location of the squamocolumnar junction and the transformation zone varies according to a woman's age and hormonal influences. It may be located on the ectocervix, at the cervical os, or just inside the endocervix.[14,17]

MANAGEMENT

In 2014, existing consensus guidelines for the management of women with cytologic abnormalities, based on the Bethesda system of classification for the reporting of abnormal cervical cytologic findings, were revised (Box 149.1). The three previous

The Bethesda System (Abridged)

SPECIMEN ADEQUACY
Satisfactory for evaluation
Unsatisfactory for evaluation
- Specimen rejected/not processed
- Specimen processed and examined, but unsatisfactory for evaluation of epithelial abnormality

GENERAL CATEGORIZATION
Negative for intraepithelial lesion or malignancy
Epithelial cell abnormality
Other

INTERPRETATION OF RESULT
Negative for intraepithelial lesions or malignancy
Organisms identified
- Trichomonas vaginalis
- Fungal organisms consistent with Candida species
- Shift in flora suggestive of bacterial vaginosis
- Bacteria consistent with Actinomyces species
- Cellular changes consistent with herpes simplex virus

Other non-neoplastic findings may include (optional to report; list not comprehensive):
- Reactive cellular changes associated with inflammation (includes typical repair)
- Radiation

Intrauterine Contraceptive Device
- Glandular cells status posthysterectomy
- Atrophy

Epithelial cell abnormalities
Squamous cell abnormalities
- Atypical squamous cells (ACS)
- Atypical squamous cells of undetermined significance
- Atypical squamous cells, cannot exclude high-grade squamous intraepithelial lesion (ASC-H)
- Low-grade squamous intraepithelial lesion encompassing human papillomavirus, mild dysplasia, CIN 1
- High-grade squamous intraepithelial lesion encompassing moderate and severe dysplasia, CIN, CIN 2, CIN 3
- Squamous cell carcinoma

Glandular cell abnormalities
- Atypical glandular cells (AGC)
- Atypical glandular cells, favor neoplastic (AGC)
- Endocervical adenocarcinoma in situ (AIS)
- Adenocarcinoma

Other (list not comprehensive):
- Endometrial cells in a woman ≥ 40 years of age

Modified from Verma I, Jain V, Kaur T. Application of Bethesda System for Cervical Cytology in Unhealthy Cervix. *J Clin Diagn Res.* 2014: 8(9); OC26–OC30.

levels of dysplasia and carcinoma in situ were replaced with two levels: low-grade squamous intra epithelial lesion (LSIL) and high-grade squamous intra epithelial lesion (HSIL).[18] The high-grade lesions should be noted as precursor lesions that have the *potential* to develop into invasive squamous cell carcinoma of the cervix. Atypical glandular cells, which are less frequently reported, can represent a precursor lesion for adenocarcinoma of the cervix.

Whereas the Pap test is the *screening* test for cervical cancer, the biopsy is the definitive *diagnostic* test that guides treatment decisions. If there is no evidence of biopsy-proven cervical dysplasia, or CIN, follow-up surveillance may include Pap alone or cotesting with both Pap and HPV (definitive management dependent on patient age, preceding Pap, and subsequent biopsy results). If the biopsy reveals CIN 1, patients can be managed conservatively with follow-up Pap alone or Pap plus HPV (again, dependent on patient age, preceding Pap, and subsequent biopsy results). In the case of persistent low-grade lesions (defined as present for *at least* 2 years), patients are given the option of surveillance versus treatment. If the biopsy reveals CIN II, CIN III, or more advanced abnormalities, treatment is indicated by current guidelines.[19] Women aged 21 to 24 with biopsy-confirmed CIN II may be followed with colposcopy and cytology (Pap), which is actually the *preferred* method of follow-up, with treatment being an *acceptable* option. The 2012 Consensus Guidelines for the Management of Women with Abnormal Cervical Cancer Screening Tests guide the clinician as to what is indicated after an abnormal cervical screening test result.

LIFE SPAN CONSIDERATIONS

According to current guidelines, cervical cancer screening should begin no earlier than the age of 21 years, regardless of a woman's sexual history, with the exception of women who have human immunodeficiency virus (HIV) or who are otherwise immunocompromised. Pap tests are then recommended every 3 years from the ages of 21 to 29. HPV testing (defined as testing for high-risk HPV types only) *for primary screening purposes* is not appropriate for women in this age range. Between the ages of 30 and 65, HPV testing performed *with* the Pap test *for primary screening purposes* is the preferred method of cervical surveillance, as opposed to Pap testing without HPV adjunct. Women older than 30 with a normal Pap test result and negative high-risk type HPV DNA test result can extend Pap test screening intervals to every 5 years.[12]

In 2015, the American Society for Colposcopy and Cervical Pathology (ASCCP) and the Society of Gynecologic Oncology (SGO) issued a statement of interim guidance regarding using the HPV test (approved in 2014 by the US Food and Drug Administration) as a *sole* (i.e., without the complement of the Pap test) *primary* cervical cancer screening tool. The American College of Obstetricians and Gynecologists (ACOG) initially published Practice Bulletin 157, supporting the use of the cobas® HPV Test for primary cervical cancer screening as an alternative to current cytology (Pap)-based cancer screening methods in women 25 years and older. Practice Bulletin 157 was replaced by Practice Bulletin 168 in 2016. Practice Bulletin 168 recommends that primary HPV testing (not done along with Pap, but used alone) can be considered for women 25 and over. If women have a negative primary HPV result, they do not require retesting for 3 years. If a woman's HPV test detects either of the two high-risk HPV types (16 or 18), the recommended follow-up is colposcopy. If the HPV test is negative for types 16 and 18, but positive for any other high-risk HPV types, it *should be followed* with cytology (Pap) testing. The bulletin does point out that cytology (Pap) alone or cotesting remain the principal recommendations of the chief health organizations concerned with the health care of women. The bulletin goes on to note that if screening with primary HPV testing is used, it should be done so according to the interim guidance provided in the 2015 statement from ASCCP and SGO.[20]

Cytology (Pap) alone every 3 years is an acceptable method of surveillance in the 30 to 65 age range, although Pap and HPV screening done together (cotesting) is the preferred method. For women older than 65, no screening is recommended, provided that there has been adequate negative prior screening (defined as 3 consecutive negative cytology (Pap) results or 2 consecutive negative HPV results within 10 years prior to cessation of screening, with the most recent test within the prior 5 years). Those women who have a history of CIN II or greater should continue screening past the age of 65 for a minimum of 20 years after either spontaneous regression of the CIN II or appropriate management, even if this extends screening past age 65 years. Women who have had a hysterectomy and had their cervix removed should have screening discontinued unless they have a history of CIN II or greater in the past 20 years, or have had cervical cancer.[21] Immunosuppressed women, those infected with HIV, women exposed to diethylstilbestrol in utero, and those previously treated for CIN II, III, or cancer may require more frequent screening.[22]

INDICATIONS FOR REFERRAL

Clinicians' management decisions should always be guided by the most recent screening and management guidelines.[19] Colposcopy is an office procedure conducted by a trained colposcopist in which the cervix and vagina are viewed directly under magnification, during which an ectocervical biopsy and endocervical sampling of cells may be obtained. According to most recent guidelines, patients with ASCUS lesions with a concurrent positive HPV DNA test result should be referred for colposcopy, unless they are younger than 24 years. Because HPV tends to clear the cells more impressively in younger women, those aged 21 to 24 with an ASCUS HPV-positive result do not require colposcopy—only repeat cytology (Pap) in 12 months.

A *reflex* (meaning run only *after* a Pap result is deemed as ASCUS) HPV test may be run after the initial result of ASCUS is received on a woman in the 21 to 24 age group (*acceptable* per current guidelines); it is *preferred* to repeat only cytology (Pap alone) in 12 months, without running a reflex HPV test. Women older than age 24 with an ASCUS HPV-positive result should be referred for colposcopy. For LSIL Pap results, as with ASCUS results, follow-up is age dependent. Women aged 21 to 24 with LSIL can be advised to follow up with cytology (Pap) in 12 months. Women older than 24 with LSIL should be referred for colposcopy as a next step, not just to repeat cytology (Pap). A reflex HPV DNA test is not indicated to be done after LSIL results because the vast majority of LSIL Pap results involve high-risk uro-ano-genital HPV. All patients with HSIL and ASC-H Pap results should be directed to undergo colposcopy. Women who have Pap results of "atypical glandular cells of undetermined significance" (known as AGUS or AGC) should have subsequent colposcopy with endocervical sampling. Those women with "atypical glandular cells of undetermined significance" who are 35 or older or who are at risk for endometrial cancer should also undergo endometrial sampling. Atypical glandular cells of undetermined significance Pap results can be indicative of either cervical or endometrial malignancies, or premalignant states.[19]

Additionally, if a clinician notes a visible cervical lesion, particularly an erythematous, exophytic lesion, the patient should be directed to undergo colposcopy for further evaluation regardless of the Pap test result, as some frank cervical cancers may not be detected by Pap test.

PATIENT AND FAMILY EDUCATION

HPV infection should be discussed during disclosure of an abnormal Pap test result; patient education should include information about prevalence of HPV, course of infection, risk of cervical cancer, regression rates, cofactors influencing development of cancer, and health practices that may minimize progression of dysplasia. Reassurance that cervical cancer may be prevented, when precancerous lesions are detected and treated early in the course of dysplasia, is appropriate.

In 2006, Gardasil, the first vaccine designed to prevent HPV infection, was approved by the FDA. Gardasil was developed to prevent cervical cancer, precancerous genital lesions, and genital warts caused by HPV. The vaccine is currently recommended for girls and women aged 11 to 26 years but can be given to girls as young as 9 years. The quadrivalent vaccine has been shown to be highly effective against four types of the HPV virus, including the two high-risk types (16 and 18) that cause 70% of cervical cancers. The vaccination also protected against two low-risk types of HPV (6 and 11). Cervarix, another HPV vaccine that came to market in 2009, conferred protection against the same two high-risk HPV types as Gardasil, types 16 and 18. Cervarix was recommended for females aged 10 to 25, though it is no longer available in the United States. Gardasil can be given to both males and females, while Cervarix was recommended to be given only to females. In 2015, the Advisory Committee on Immunization Practices (ACIP) recommended the addition of the 9-valent HPV vaccine Gardasil 9 to the already existing HPV vaccines. 9vHPV, approved by the FDA, contains HPV types 6, 11, 16, 18, 31, 33, 45, 52, and 58 virus-like particles (VLPs). The FDA recommended 9vHPV for use in females aged 9 through 26 years and males aged 9 through 15 years.[23]

The Centers for Disease Control (CDC) recommends routine HPV vaccination of both girls and boys at 11 or 12 years of age, though the vaccine can be given to either as young as 9. For children aged 9 through 14, Gardasil 9 can be given using either a 2-dose or 3-dose schedule. When using the 2-dose schedule, the second dose in the series is advised to be given 6 to 12 months after the initial immunization. A third dose is advised if the second dose is given less than 5 months after the first dose, with the third dose advised at least 4 months after the second dose. For the 3-dose schedule, the second dose should be given 2 months after the initial one and the third dose should be given 6 months after the initial immunization. For those aged 15 through 26, Gardasil 9 is recommended to be given using only the 3-dose schedule. The second in the series is advised to be given 2 months after the initial immunization and the third dose should be given 6 months after the initial immunization. The vaccine is given intramuscularly and is contraindicated in young women who are pregnant, or who have severe yeast allergies. Pain or erythema at the injection site can occur, as can fainting.[24]

For maximum efficacy, the best time to administer the HPV vaccine is *prior* to the onset of sexual activity, though vaccination should *not* be withheld or delayed in either males or females because of sexual debut. Individuals already infected with a type of uro-ano-genital HPV are candidates for the vaccination (if they have not yet begun the series) as they can be afforded protection from those types of HPV that they have not yet contracted. The American Academy of Pediatrics supports the vaccination age range recommendation acknowledging that the greatest patient benefit can be reached with administration prior to coitarche. Additionally, children have the most efficacious antibody responses to vaccines when they are administered at ages 9 to 15.[25]

In 2015, the ACIP announced its recommendation for the 9-valent HPV vaccine (Gardasil). 9vHPV, approved by the FDA, contains HPV types 6, 11, 16, 18, 31, 33, 45, 52, and 58 VLPs. The FDA recommended 9vHPV for use in females aged 9 through 26 years and males aged 9 through 15 years.[19]

The presence of HPV, combined with the fear of potential cervical cancer, often produces considerable psychological distress for a woman. Thus it remains imperative that the clinician offer adequate counseling and information about the nature of HPV and effect on cervical cells when giving women their abnormal Pap result. Women may express concerns about future fertility, the stigma of harboring a sexually transmitted virus, and how to approach the topic of HPV with their partners. They may be fearful of diagnostic and treatment procedures and may also have misconceptions about HPV. Women may be confused by the medical jargon associated with HPV infection discussions, abnormal test results, colposcopies, biopsies, and treatment. All providers who perform cervical cancer screening are ultimately also responsible for being able to educate and inform patients about the abnormal test results as well as further diagnosis and treatment. Excellent resources for patient education and support regarding abnormal cervical screening tests and HPV include the ASCCP (www.asccp.org), Association of Reproductive Health Professionals (www.arhp.org), American Social Health Association (www.ashastd.org), and National Women's Health Resource Center (www.healthywomen.org).

HEALTH PROMOTION

Women should be advised to have regular cervical cancer screening according to most recent consensus screening guidelines. Although condom use does not completely prevent transmission of HPV, it appears to afford modest protection against cervical HPV infection as well as to possibly slow progression of viral spread and dysplasia development after HPV infection.

Recent work in the area of nutrition and HPV has found that the ingestion of certain foods, such as nuts, fish, fruits, and vegetables, may be a protective factor against HPV infection. Foods high in vitamin A and retinol, calcium, long-chain polyunsaturated fatty acids, and antioxidants (e.g., vitamins C and E, lutein, carotene, and lycopene) have been shown to reduce the risk of cervical cancer.[21] Healthy lifestyle habits, including adequate sleep, exercise, and avoidance of smoking, should be encouraged. There is evidence that certain practices that promote good health, including good nutrition, dietary supplementation of substances such as folic acid and beta-carotene, adequate sleep, and exercise, can help the body's cells fend off HPV's effects.[22]

In addition, one of the most important steps that health care providers can take toward decreasing the incidence of cervical dysplasia is to educate women on, and recommend, vaccination for HPV protection. Vaccination continues to be under-recommended and underused, according to the CDC and Prevention 2013 National Immunization Survey–Teen (NIS-Teen). Survey results noted that only 57% of adolescent girls and 35% of adolescent boys had received one or more doses of HPV vaccine.[23]

Health care providers must be vigilant in their efforts to recognize, and then recommend vaccination for, the appropriate candidates. Cervical cancer screening, which is secondary prevention, can detect cervical dysplasia caused by HPV and help to prevent progression via treatment. However, as with any primary prevention strategy, the greatest public health benefit will be seen with widespread HPV vaccination, and ideally prior to any HPV exposure.

REFERENCES

1. Berkowitz, Z., Saraiya, M., Bernard, V., & Yabroff, K. R. (2010). Common abnormal results of Pap and human papillomavirus cotesting what physicians are recommending for management. *Obstetrics and Gynecology, 116*(6), 1332–1340.
2. National Cancer Institute. (2018). Cervical Cancer Fact Sheet. Retrieved from https://www.report.nih.gov/nihfactsheets/viewfactsheet.aspx?csid=76.
3. Centers for Disease Control and Prevention. (2018). Cervical cancer rates by race and ethnicity. Retrieved from https://www.cdc.gov/cancer/cervical/statistics/race.htm.
4. Siegel, R. L., Fedewa, S. A., Miller, K. D., Goding-Sauer, A., Pinheiro, P. S., Martinez-Tyson, D., et al. (2015). Cancer statistics for Hispanics/Latinos, 2015. *CA: A Cancer Journal for Clinicians, 65,* 457–480. doi:10.3322/caac.21314.
5. NNDB. (2018). Tracking the entire world. Retrieved from http://www.nndb.com/people/305/000176774/.
6. Shi, R., Devarakonda, S., Liu, L., Taylor, H., & Mills, G. (2014). Factors associated with genital human papillomavirus infection among adult females in the United States, NHANES 2007–2010. *BMC Research Notes, 7*(1), 544.
7. Chesson, H. W., Dunne, E. F., Hariri, S., & Markowitz, L. E. (2014). The estimated probability of acquiring human papillomavirus in the United States. *Sexually Transmitted Diseases, 41*(11), 660–664.
8. Kranjec, C., & Doorbar, J. (2016). Human papillomavirus infection and induction of neoplasia: A matter of fitness. *Current Opinion in Virology, 20,* 129–136.
9. Ribeiro, A. A., Costa, M. C., Alves, R. R. F., Villa, L. L., Saddi, V. A., dos Santos Carneiro, M. A., et al. (2015). HPV infection and cervical neoplasia: Associated risk factors. *Infectious Agents and Cancer, 10*(1), 16.
10. Yetimalar, H., Kasap, B., Cukurova, K., Yildiz, A., Keklik, A., & Soylu, F. (2012). Cofactors in human papillomavirus infection and cervical carcinogenesis. *Archives of Gynecology and Obstetrics, 285,* 805–810.
11. Schiffman, M., Wentzensen, N., Wacholder, S., Kinney, W., Gage, J. C., & Castle, P. E. (2011). Human papillomavirus testing in the prevention of cervical cancer. *Journal of the National Cancer Institute, 103,* 368–383.
12. Alliance for Cervical Cancer Prevention. (2018). Risk Factors for Cervical Cancer: Evidence to Date. https://www.gardasil9.com/about-gardasil9/schedule/?utm_source=bing&utm_medium=cpc&utm_campaign=2017%20Brand%20General%20%7C%20Exact&utm_term=gardasil&utm_content=be__group_Brand%20General_Exact&gclid=CKGhnqKqx9gCFYdegQodnnUKpA&gclsrc=ds http://screening.iarc.fr/doc/RH_fs_risk_factors.pdf.
13. Faridi, R., Zahra, A., Khan, K., & Idrees, M. (2011). Oncogenic potential of human papillomavirus (HPV) and its relation with cervical cancer. *Virology Journal, 8,* 269.
14. Hwang, S. J., & Shroyer, K. R. (2012). Biomarkers of cervical dysplasia and carcinoma. *Journal of Oncology, 2012,* 507286.
15. Anderson, T. A., Schick, V., Herbenick, D., Dodge, B., & Fortenberry, J. D. (2014). A study of human papillomavirus on vaginally inserted sex toys, before and after cleaning, among women who have sex with women and men. *Sexually Transmitted Infections,* sextrans-2014.
16. Schiffman, M., & Wentzensen, N. (2013). Human papillomavirus infection and the multistage carcinogenesis of cervical cancer. *Cancer Epidemiology, Biomarkers and Prevention: A Publication of the American Association for Cancer Research, Cosponsored by the American Society of Preventive Oncology, 22,* 553–560.
17. Stewart Massad, L., Einstein, M. H., Huh, W. K., Katki, H. A., Kinney, W. K., Schiffman, M., et al. (2013). 2012 updated consensus guidelines for the management of abnormal cervical cancer screening tests and cancer precursors. *Journal of Lower Genital Tract Disease, 17*(5 Suppl. 1), S1–S27.
18. Verma, I., Jain, V., & Kaur, T. (2014). Application of Bethesda system for cervical cytology in unhealthy cervix. *Journal of Clinical and Diagnostic Research: JCDR, 8*(9), OC26–OC30.
19. Massad, L. S., Einstein, M. H., Huh, W. K., Katki, H. A., Kinney, W. K., Schiffman, M., et al. (2013). 2012 Updated consensus guidelines for the

management of abnormal cervical cancer screening tests and cancer precursors. *Journal of Lower Genital Tract Disease*, *17*(5 Suppl. 1), S1–S27.

20. American College of Obstetricians and Gynecologists. (2016). Cervical cancer screening and prevention. Practice Bulletin No. 168. *Obstetrics and Gynecology*, *128*, e111–e130.

21. Saslow, D., Solomon, D., Lawson, H. W., Killackey, M., Kulasingam, S. L., Cain, J., et al. (2012). American Cancer Society, American Society for Colposcopy and Cervical Pathology, and American Society for Clinical Pathology screening guidelines for the prevention and early detection of cervical cancer. *Journal of Lower Genital Tract Disease*, *16*(3), 175–204.

22. American College of Obstetricians and Gynecologists. (2009). ACOG Practice Bulletin no. 109: Cervical cytology screening. *Obstetrics and Gynecology*, *114*(6), 1409–1420.

23. Petrosky, E., Bocchini, J. A., Jr., Hariri, S., et al. (2015). Use of 9-valent human papillomavirus (HPV) vaccine: Updated HPV vaccination recommendations of the Advisory Committee on Immunization Practices. *MMWR. Morbidity and Mortality Weekly Report*, *64*(11), 300–304.

24. Merck Gardasil 9. (2018). Information about Gardasil 9. Retrieved from https://www.gardasil9.com/about-gardasil9/schedule/?utm_source=bing&utm_medium=cpc&utm_campaign=2017%20Brand%20General%20%7C%20Exact&utm_term=gardasil&utm_content=be__group_Brand%20General_Exact&gclid=CKGhnqKqx9gCFYdegQodnnUKpA&gclsrc=ds.

25. Committee on Infectious Diseases. (2012). HPV vaccine recommendations. *Pediatrics*, *129*(3), 602–605.

CHAPTER 150

PELVIC INFLAMMATORY DISEASE

Sheila Ann Medina

 Immediate referral is indicated in cases of surgical emergency, failure to respond to outpatient therapy or tolerate an outpatient regimen, evidence of severe illness, and in cases of immunodeficiency.

DEFINITION AND EPIDEMIOLOGY

Pelvic inflammatory disease (PID) is a common condition that refers to a spectrum of inflammatory disorders of the upper genital tract in women. It can include any combination of endometritis, salpingitis, tubo-ovarian abscess (TOA), and pelvic peritonitis.[1] There is a wide variation in the signs and symptoms associated with PID. Acute signs and symptoms are often moderately severe, but many women have subtle or mild symptoms that go unrecognized. Nonetheless, the long-term sequelae resulting from fallopian tube damage and scarring can be serious and include ectopic pregnancy, recurrent episodes of PID, chronic pelvic pain, and infertility.[2,3]

It is estimated that each year in the United States, more than 750,000 women experience an episode of acute PID and 1 in 8 women are more likely to become infertile as a result of PID.[4,5] PID is the most common gynecologic reason for emergency department (ED) visits and hospitalizations in the United States. Women with PID account for approximately 340,000 to 410,000 cases diagnosed in the ED each year and incur health care costs exceeding $2 billion each year. PID affects more women of reproductive age, with a disproportionately higher incidence in unmarried (particularly divorced) women.[6,7] Although the number of PID-related ED visits and hospitalizations remains high, more than three-fourths of women treated for PID in the United States are now treated as outpatients, a trend that has been increasing during the past two decades.[2] Based on research looking at trends in PID from 2001 to 2013, cases of PID (based on hospitalizations and estimated ambulatory cases) have decreased significantly, but the annual estimate of acute and unspecified PID cases diagnosed in the United States for 2009 and 2010 was greater than had previously been published.[3] It is evident that PID remains an important public health concern for women and health care providers, especially those working in outpatient settings.

Direct costs for care of acute PID and its sequelae are estimated at $2.7 billion yearly, even though the majority of women receive care as outpatients.[4] The high financial and social costs related to PID are important to consider if the full impact of this disease is to be appreciated.

Risk factors for PID include being younger than 25 years, having multiple sexual partners, not currently or consistently using contraception, and living in an area with a high prevalence of sexually transmitted diseases (STDs). There is a strong correlation between the incidence of STDs and PID in any given population. Other risk factors for PID include penetration of the cervical mucus barrier during medical procedures, including the insertion of an intrauterine contraceptive device, vaginal douching, and cigarette smoking.[2] A woman's risk for PID is decreased if she uses barrier contraception, takes oral contraceptives, or has had a tubal sterilization. The risk of PID in young women is especially significant; one in five cases of PID occur in women younger than 19, and one in eight adolescent girls will develop PID compared with one in 80 women older than 24 years.[1,8] From 2001 to 2013, 46.8% of all US high school students had engaged in sexual intercourse, and 15% had had four or more partners, making STDs a major public health problem for adolescents.[9] Contact with multiple sexual partners, inconsistent use of contraception, and biologic vulnerability can account for the increased incidence of STDs in women younger than 25 years, although it does not fully account for the increased incidence of PID. Younger women with chlamydial infections of the cervix have a higher incidence of upper genital tract infection than do older women.[10]

Previous diagnosis of PID is a risk factor for subsequent episodes, with approximately 15% to 25% of all women with PID experiencing more than one episode.[10] These subsequent infections are generally new, primary attacks of PID, not flares of latent or chronic infection. Reinfection is often related to contact with untreated sexual partners. In addition, one-third of women with PID will develop chronic pelvic pain.[8]

PATHOPHYSIOLOGY

PID is usually a polymicrobial infection caused by organisms that ascend from the vagina and cervix along the mucosa of the endometrium to infect the mucosa of the fallopian tubes. The most common organisms implicated in PID (approximately 40% of cases) include *Neisseria gonorrhoeae* and *Chlamydia trachomatis*; however, microorganisms that can be part of the normal vaginal flora (e.g., anaerobes, *Gardnerella vaginalis*, *Haemophilus influenzae*, enteric gram-negative rods, and *Streptococcus agalactiae*) can contribute or possibly cause PID.[1,2,11] Newer data suggest that *Mycoplasma genitalium* may also play a role in PID and may be associated with milder symptoms.[1,11] *Mycoplasma hominis* and *Ureaplasma urealyticum* are also possible causative agents.[1] The mildest form of salpingitis involves tubal hyperemia, edema of the tubal wall, and exudate on the tubal surface and fimbriated ends.[12] If salpingitis is left untreated, further inflammatory changes of the pelvic organs occur, including tubal adhesions, pyosalpinx, and TOA.

The increased incidence of PID in young women may be explained by a larger cervical squamocolumnar junction, allowing easier colonization with *N. gonorrhoeae* or *C. trachomatis*, and by a decreased antibody response.[10] Rarely, PID can result from secondary extension of infection of adjacent organs, as in appendicitis or diverticulitis. It may also result from hematogenous dissemination of tuberculosis or as a rare complication of a tropical disease such as schistosomiasis. The following discussion refers only to ascending infections resulting in PID.

CLINICAL PRESENTATION AND PHYSICAL EXAMINATION

The clinical presentation of PID is varied. Some women are truly asymptomatic, yet diagnosis can be missed in women who have mild or nonspecific signs and symptoms. These symptoms vary based on the pathogen responsible.[13] These can include fever or chills, cramping, dysuria, low back pain, nausea and vomiting, abnormal vaginal bleeding (postcoital or intermenstrual bleeding), dyspareunia, and vaginal discharge. The most frequent presenting symptom is usually lower abdominal and pelvic pain of less than 2 weeks' duration. The pain is typically described as dull and constant, but increased by movement and sexual intercourse. The onset of symptoms often occurs in the proliferative phase of the menstrual cycle. Complaints of fever or abnormal vaginal discharge may also be present.[13]

PID caused by gonococci is usually associated with a more intense inflammatory reaction in the epithelial lining of the ovarian tube and may have a more acute presentation, often requiring hospitalization.[14] The reaction in the ovarian tube caused by chlamydia is secondary to the immune response and causes a different reaction. Approximately 5% of women will develop Fitz-Hugh–Curtis syndrome (FHCS), a perihepatitis. The initial presentation of FHCS is associated with right upper quadrant abdominal pain, but the woman will also have lower abdominal pain, pleuritic pain, and tenderness on liver palpation. These symptoms are often mistaken for hepatic disease, cholecystitis, or pneumonia.[14]

The physical examination requires assessment of abnormal vital signs (and elevated temperature is possible) and an abdominal and gynecological examination. The abdomen is assessed for presence of bowel sounds and tenderness and the gynecological exam should determine the presence of cervical motion, adnexal and uterine tenderness as well as any vaginal or endocervical discharge. Unfortunately, the clinical diagnosis of acute PID is imprecise. Lower abdominal pain may be mistakenly attributed to pregnancy (ectopic), ovarian cysts, or even appendicitis. No single history, physical, or laboratory finding is both sensitive and specific for the diagnosis of acute PID. For that reason, the Centers for Disease Control and Prevention (CDC) recommends the necessity of empirical treatment of PID for sexually active young women and other women at risk for STDs who are experiencing pelvic or lower abdominal pain, provided no other cause of the illness other than PID (e.g., diverticulitis, ectopic pregnancy, or appendicitis) is identified, and if the pelvic examination is significant for one or more of the following criteria: cervical motion tenderness, uterine tenderness, or adnexal tenderness.[1] These criteria still may not be sensitive enough to identify subtle cases of PID. The following additional criteria enhance the specificity of the aforementioned minimum criteria and support a diagnosis of PID: (1) oral temperature above 101 °F, (2) an abnormal mucopurulent

discharge from the cervix or noted in vagina, (3) positive white blood cells in vaginal secretions noted on saline microscopy, (4) erythrocyte sedimentation rate or C-reactive protein elevation, and (5) cervical infection documentation with *N. gonorrhoeae* or *C. trachomatis*.

It is not uncommon for women with PID to have a mucopurulent cervical discharge or positive WBCs when the vaginal fluid is viewed under the microscope. If the cervical discharge appears normal and there are no WBCs on the wet mount, the diagnosis of PID is unlikely; alternative causes of pain should be considered.[1]

DIAGNOSTICS

Acute PID is difficult to diagnose because of the wide variation in signs and symptoms. The clinical diagnosis of symptomatic PID has a positive predictive value for salpingitis of 65% to 90% compared with laparoscopy.[1] Diagnosis is based on the patient's risk factors, the presence of cervical motion, uterine, or adnexal tenderness on examination, and the criteria outlined above.

INITIAL DIAGNOSTICS

LABORATORY
- Serum level of HCG
- HIV Serology
- ESR[a]
- CRP[a]
- Lab documentation of cervical infection with N. Gonorrhoeae or C. Trachomatis
- Saline microscopy of vaginal fluid (determine presence of WBCs)
- HIV screening
- Syphilis screening
- CBC/differential[a]

IMAGING
- Pelvic ultrasound
- Transvaginal sonography or magnetic resonance imaging[a]
- Endometrial biopsy with histopathological evidence of endometritis[a]

OTHER
- Laparoscopy

[a]If indicated.

Essential Diagnostics

A serum pregnancy test should be performed immediately to assess for the possibility of ectopic pregnancy. Pelvic ultrasound evaluation is indicated when TOA is suspected. Additional studies to consider include the rapid plasma reagin (RPR) test for syphilis and serologic studies for human immunodeficiency virus (HIV) infection. PID can be diagnosed clinically, and empirical therapy initiated on the basis of some of the aforementioned findings. However, an evaluation that includes more extensive studies may be necessary if the diagnosis is unclear.

Additional Diagnostics

The most specific criteria for diagnosis of PID include endometrial biopsy with histopathologic evidence indicative of endometriosis; transvaginal ultrasonography, magnetic resonance imaging (MRI), or Doppler studies suggesting pelvic infection; and laparoscopic abnormalities consistent with PID.[4] However, these extensive procedures may not be warranted in all cases. Thus an accurate diagnosis of PID is difficult, given the wide variation in symptoms on presentation. However, the potential damage to the reproductive health of women with even mild or atypical PID is well documented.[1] Diagnosis and management of other causes of lower abdominal pain are unlikely to be affected by the initiation of empirical therapy for PID.

DIFFERENTIAL DIAGNOSIS

 Priority differential diagnoses include abscesses, perihepatitis, ectopic pregnancy, acute appendicitis, ovarian torsion, ovarian cyst, and tumors. Other conditions to consider include fibroids, cysts, endometriosis, corpus luteum bleeding, pelvic adhesions, benign ovarian tumor, inflammatory bowel disease (IBD), irritable bowel syndrome (IBS), diverticulitis, pyelonephritis, nephrolithiasis, and cystitis.[2]

PID can cause lower abdominal pain that is similar to the pain associated with gastrointestinal conditions, making it difficult to determine the cause of the patient's symptoms. Thus at-risk women with lower abdominal pain or pelvic pain and no other identified cause for their pain should be presumed to have PID.[5]

INTERPROFESSIONAL COLLABORATIVE MANAGEMENT

Nonpharmacological Management

The primary treatment for PID is antibiotic therapy. Nonpharmacological treatment requires identifying the patient's sex partners to assure appropriate treatment as well as education to aid in STD prevention (e.g., use of condoms).

Pharmacological Management

Treatment regimens for PID are based on CDC recommendations and include both broad-spectrum antimicrobials and anaerobic coverage, because combination therapy is necessary. Medication regimen recommendations include metronidazole for all women to provide anaerobic coverage (e.g., bacterial vaginosis) and decrease the risk of PID sequelae (i.e., recurring PID, ectopic pregnancy, chronic pelvic pain, and infertility).[1]

Oral and parenteral therapy for PID is outlined in Box 150.1.[1] Patients receiving oral therapy require follow-up

---

BOX **150.1**

CDC Oral and Parenteral Therapy for Pelvic Inflammatory Disease

PARENTERAL TREATMENT

Parenteral Regimen A

Cefotetan (Cefotan) 2 g IV every 12 h in combination with doxycycline (Vibramycin) 100 mg PO or IV[a] every 12 h

Or

Cefoxitin (Mefoxin) 2 g IV every 6 h in combination with doxycycline (Vibramycin) 100 mg PO or IV[a] every 12 h

Parenteral therapy may be discontinued 24 h after a patient improves clinically, and oral therapy with doxycycline (100 mg twice a day) should continue to complete 14 days of therapy. When tubo-ovarian abscess (TOA) is present, many health care providers use clindamycin or metronidazole with doxycycline for continued therapy rather than doxycycline alone because the combination provides more effective anaerobic coverage.

Parenteral Regimen B

Clindamycin 900 mg IV every 8 h in combination with gentamicin. The gentamycin loading dose IV or IM is 2 mg/kg of body weight followed by a maintenance dose (1.5 mg/kg) every 8 h.[b]

The parenteral therapy can be discontinued if the patient is clinically improved after 24 h, but doxycycline 100 mg PO twice a day or clindamycin 450 mg PO 4 times a day is necessary to complete a total of 14 days of therapy. When TOA is present, clindamycin may be preferable over doxycycline because clindamycin provides more anaerobic coverage.

Alternative Parenteral Regimens

Ampicillin-sulbactam 3 g IV every 6 h in combination with doxycycline (Vibramycin) 100 mg PO or IV[a] every 12 h

ORAL TREATMENT

Recommended Intramuscular and Oral Regimens

Ceftriaxone (Rocephin) 250 mg IM in a single dose in combination with

doxycycline (Vibramycin) 100 mg orally twice a day for 14 days

with or without metronidazole (Flagyl) 500 mg orally twice a day for 14 days

Or

Cefoxitin[c] 2 g IM in a single dose and probenecid 1 g orally administered concurrently in a single dose in combination with doxycycline 100 mg orally twice a day for 14 days

with or without metronidazole 500 mg orally twice per day for 14 days

Or

Other parenteral third-generation cephalosporin (e.g., ceftizoxime or cefotaxime)

in combination with doxycycline 100 mg orally twice per day for 14 days

with or without metronidazole 500 mg orally twice per day for 14 days

Alternative Oral Regimens

Azithromycin (1 g orally once a week for 2 weeks) in combination with a single ceftriaxone 250 mg IM dose is a potential alternative. Metronidazole should be considered because of the presence of anaerobic organisms. In addition, metronidazole will also treat bacterial vaginosis.

B.N.

Quinolones are no longer recommended for the treatment of pelvic inflammatory disease (PID).

Note. Ampicillin-sulbactam plus doxycycline has good coverage against *Chlamydia trachomatis, Neisseria gonorrhoeae,* and anaerobes and is effective for patients who have TOA. However, gastrointestinal side effects are common with ampicillin-sulbactam treatment.

B.N. Patients allergic to penicillin should not be treated with cephalosporins.

[a]Doxycycline should be administered orally whenever possible, because IV doxycycline is very painful. The recommendation for oral doxycycline is also indicated for hospitalized patients. The bioavailability of doxycycline is similar orally and intravenously.

[b]Once-a-day administration (3–5 mg/kg) may be substituted.

[c]Ceftriaxone has better coverage against *N. gonorrhoeae.* If Cefoxitin is used, metronidazole is necessary to treat the often-concurrent bacterial vaginosis associated with PID.

within 72 hours to assess for improvement. The repeat physical assessment should determine if direct or rebound abdominal tenderness is decreased and note if uterine, adnexal, and cervical motion tenderness is reduced. If the patient is not clinically improved within 3 days (i.e., 72 hours) after pharmacologic therapy is started, reevaluation to confirm the diagnosis and arrange parenteral therapy or surgical intervention is necessary. Test of cure for infection with *C. trachomatis* and *N. gonorrhoeae* 4 to 6 weeks after the completion of therapy is indicated.

Because of the high risk for maternal morbidity and preterm delivery, pregnant women with PID should be hospitalized and treated with parenteral antibiotics.[1] Aside from pregnancy, the CDC recommends hospitalization of women based on health care provider discretion and in certain situations (see Indications for Referral or Hospitalization). Hospitalization of adolescents with PID should be based on the same criteria used for older women.[11]

Given the significant risk of future health problems associated with PID, efforts to adhere to recommended practice guidelines and to ensure patient adherence to care are critical. Treatment of sexual partners of women with PID is imperative because of the risk for reinfection and the high incidence of urethral gonococcal or chlamydial infections in the male sexual partner. Partners who have had sexual contact with the patient during the 60 days preceding the onset of symptoms should be treated empirically with regimens effective against *C. trachomatis* and *N. gonorrhoeae*, regardless of the apparent cause of PID or pathogens isolated from the patient.[1] Sexual abstinence should be recommended until both partners have completed treatment.

Indications for Referral or Hospitalization

In certain cases hospitalization may be required to treat PID. Referral for hospitalization of the patient with PID is indicated if:
- there is a surgical emergency (e.g., inability to exclude appendicitis or ectopic pregnancy).
- the patient is pregnant, has failed to respond clinically to outpatient therapy, or is unable to follow or tolerate an outpatient regimen.
- there is evidence of severe illness, nausea and vomiting, a high fever, or patient has a pelvic abscess or TOA.
- the patient is immunodeficient (e.g., HIV positive with a low CD4 count or receiving immunosuppressive therapy).

In early observational studies, HIV-infected women with PID were more likely to require surgical intervention.[1] A subsequent and more comprehensive study showed that despite a more severe clinical presentation, HIV-infected women with PID responded equally well to standard parenteral therapies.[1]

Gynecologic or surgical consultation is indicated when the diagnosis is unclear. Unilateral pelvic pain or a mass is a strong indication for laparoscopy.

LIFESPAN CONSIDERATIONS

STDs and PID are increasingly prevalent in young teenage girls (age 15 and up).[15] Yet, this cohort is often unaware of the risk of infection associated with unprotected sex, may ignore or not recognize symptoms of STDs, and their access to health care may be limited.[15] In the National Health and Nutrition Examination Survey 2013 to 2014 cycle, the prevalence of a lifetime PID diagnosis was 4.4% among sexually experienced

reproductive-aged women, equating to 2.5 million prevalent PID cases in women aged 18 to 44 years nationwide. Prevalence of a self-reported lifetime PID diagnosis varied by sexual behaviors and sexual health history and differed by race/ethnicity in women without a prior STI diagnosis.[16]

COMPLICATIONS

- PID sequelae include increased risk of tubal factor infertility, ectopic pregnancy, chronic pelvic pain, and ruptured TOA. The duration, severity, and number of PID episodes are proportional to the prevalence of long-term sequelae.
- FHCS involves perihepatic inflammation caused by the transperitoneal, lymphatic, or vascular spread of *N. gonorrhoeae* or *C. trachomatis*. There is inflammation of the liver capsule without parenchymal involvement.[12] FHCS develops in 5% to 10% of women with PID.[10] Chronic FHCS is characterized by adhesions between the anterior liver surface and the parietal peritoneum beneath the diaphragm. The treatment is the same as for PID.

PATIENT AND FAMILY EDUCATION

Patient education is an essential component of PID treatment. The provider–patient discussion must provide clear information about the diagnosis, transmission, sequelae, antibiotic treatment, and side effects, plus the necessity of treatment completion. It is important to stress the importance of contacting the health care provider if side effects occur, returning for timely follow-up, and the need for partner treatment. It is also helpful to encourage the patient in appropriate medical care–seeking behavior, including seeking care immediately if or when symptoms recur. The behaviors that increase the risk for PID also increase the risk for syphilis and HIV infection requiring education about prevention of these disorders.

Rates of recurrent PID, chronic pelvic pain, and infertility are highest among nonpersistent condom users.[1] HIV and STD testing (including syphilis) and counseling is recommended. Finally, information about prevention of future infections must be reviewed and repeated at all follow-up visits.

HEALTH PROMOTION

Prevention for PID is based on educating patients on safe sex practices (e.g., the use of latex condoms) to decrease the risk of STDs and PID.[17,18] Since STDs play a major role in PID, the goal is to reduce the number of STDs by educating and screening patients about the risks of STDs and PID associated with unprotected sex. Patients should be encouraged to ask questions and be reassured that all health care discussions are confidential.[18]

Patients should understand that the CDC recommends testing for STDs in pregnant women and yearly testing for chlamydia and gonorrhea in all women under age 25, as well as in older women if they have multiple partners or a new sexual partner.[17] Screening for syphilis, HIV, and other potential STDs should also be discussed.

REFERENCES

1. Centers for Disease Control and Prevention (CDC). (2015). Sexually transmitted diseases treatment guidelines. Retrieved from www.cdc.gov/std/treatment/2015/pid.htm. (Accessed 17 December 2017).
2. Ross, J. (2014). Pelvic inflammatory disease. *Am Family Physician, 90*(10), 725–726.
3. Centers for Disease Control and Prevention (CDC). Pelvic inflammatory disease (PID)—CDC Self-Study STD Module for Clinicians. Retrieved from

https://www2a.cdc.gov/stdtraining/self-study/default.htm. (Accessed 17 December 2017).

4. Centers for Disease Control and Prevention (CDC). Pelvic inflammatory disease (PID)—CDC fact sheet. Retrieved from https://www.cdc.gov/std/PID/STDFact-PID.htm. (Accessed 17 December 2017).

5. Ford, F., & Decker, C. (2016). Pelvic inflammatory disease. *Disease-A-Month*, 62(8), 301–305.

6. Xholli, A., Cannoletta, M., & Cagnacci, A. (2014). Seasonal trend of acute pelvic inflammatory disease. *Archives of Gynecology and Obstetrics*, 289, 1017–1022.

7. McCallum, C., Oman, K., & Makic, M. (2014). Improving the assessment and treatment of pelvic inflammatory disease among adolescents in an urban children's hospital emergency department. *Journal of Emergency Nursing*, 40(6), 579–585.

8. Raya, B., Bamberg, E., Kerem, N., et al. (2013). Beyond "safe sex"—can we fight adolescent pelvic inflammatory disease? *European Journal of Pediatrics*, 172, 581–590.

9. Centers for Disease Control and Prevention (CDC). (2013). Youth risk behavior surveillance—United States, 2013. *MMWR. Surveillance Summaries: Morbidity and Mortality Weekly Report. Surveillance Summaries*, 63(SS–4), 24–26.

10. Mishell, D. R., & Droegemueller, W. (1997). *Comprehensive gynecology* (3rd ed.). St Louis: Mosby.

11. Duarte, R., Fuhrich, D., & Ross, J. (2015). A review of antibiotic therapy for pelvic inflammatory disease. *International Journal of Antimicrobial Agents*, 46, 272–277.

12. Soper, D. E. (1994). Pelvic inflammatory disease. In J. A. Rock, S. Faro, N. F. Gant, et al. (Eds.), *Advances in obstetrics and gynecology* (Vol. 1). St Louis: Mosby.

13. Mitchell, C., & Prabhu, M. (2013). Pelvic inflammatory disease: Current concepts in pathogenesis, diagnosis and treatment. *Infectious Disease Clinics of North America*, 27(4), 793–809.

14. Ross, J. (2014). Pelvic inflammatory disease. *Medicine*, 42(6), 333–337.

15. Risser, W., Risser, J., & Risser, A. (2017). Current perspectives in the USA on the diagnosis and treatment of pelvic inflammatory disease in adolescents. *Adolescent Health, Medicine and Therapeutics*, 8, 87–94.

16. Centers for Disease Control and Prevention (CDC). (2017). Prevalence of Pelvic Inflammatory Disease in Sexually experienced women of reproductive age—United States, 2013-2014. *MMWR Surveill*, 66(SS–3), 80–83.

17. Centers for Disease Control and Prevention (CDC). Sexually Transmitted Diseases and Pregnancy-The Facts. (Accessed 14 April 2018) @ Centers for Disease Control and Prevention (CDC).

18. Das, B. B., Ronda, J., & Trent, M. (2016). Pelvic inflammatory disease: Improving awareness, prevention, and treatment. *Infection and Drug Resistance*, 9, 191–197. http://doi.org/10.2147/IDR.S91260.

CHAPTER 151

SEXUAL DYSFUNCTION (FEMALE)

Sheila Ann Medina

DEFINITION AND EPIDEMIOLOGY

Sexual health plays an integral role in overall health, yet it is often overlooked and undertreated. Sexual function is an essential component of life, and sexual dysfunction is an important aspect of sexual health that may affect a woman's self-esteem and quality of life. Female sexual dysfunction (FSD) is a significant yet largely uninvestigated public health problem.[1,2] Several large-scale studies have confirmed that sexual satisfaction in women is strongly associated with life satisfaction and general well-being. Sexual health concerns are prevalent in the United States and should be addressed because they can lead to significant distress and interfere with relationships.[1,2]

The *Diagnostic and Statistical Manual of Mental Disorders*, Fifth Edition (DSM-5) classifies FSD into three major categories: (1) female sexual interest/arousal disorder; (2) female orgasmic disorder; and (3) genito-pelvic pain/penetration disorder.[3] FSD is further classified as to duration (lifelong versus acquired), as generalized versus situational, and by etiologic origin and/or treatment.

American Psychiatric Association guidelines specify that for the diagnosis of a female sexual disorder to be established, all of the sexual dysfunctions (except substance- or medication-induced sexual dysfunction) now require a minimum duration of approximately 6 months, and more precise severity criteria. The sexual problem must be recurrent or persistent, cause personal distress or interpersonal difficulty, and not be better accounted for by another mental disorder, drug-related cause, or medical condition.[3] The presence of distress is an essential criterion for the diagnosis; therefore a diagnosis of sexual disorder is not indicated unless the sexual dysfunction is associated with distress. Distress may be experienced because of a lack of sexual interest or arousal or as a result of significant interference with a woman's life and well-being.

Female sexual interest/arousal disorder is defined as diminished or absent sexual interest or arousal manifesting with at least three of six indicators for a minimum duration of approximately 6 months. Female sexual interest/arousal disorder is frequently associated with problems in experiencing orgasm, pain experienced during sexual activity, infrequent sexual activity, and couple-level discrepancies in desire.[3]

Five factors must be considered during the assessment and diagnosis of the patient, in addition to the subtypes "lifelong/acquired" and "generalized/situational." These factors may be relevant to the cause and/or treatment and include (1) partner factors (e.g., partner's sexual problems, partner's health status); (2) relationship factors (e.g., poor communication, discrepancies in desire for sexual activity); (3) individual vulnerability factors (e.g., poor body image, history of sexual or emotional abuse), psychiatric comorbidity (e.g., depression, anxiety), or stressors (e.g., job loss, bereavement); (4) cultural or religious factors (e.g., inhibitions related to prohibitions against sexual activity; attitudes toward sexuality); and (5) medical factors relevant to prognosis, course, or treatment.[3]

Female orgasmic disorder is defined as the persistent or recurrent inability of a woman to achieve orgasm, markedly diminished intensity of orgasmic sensations, or marked delay of orgasm during any kind of sexual stimulation despite self-reported high sexual satisfaction and arousal. FSD affects approximately 40% of women.[4] The prevalence rates for female orgasmic disorders in women range from 10% to 42% and are varied based on multiple factors (e.g., age, culture, duration, and severity of symptoms). This prevalence is higher than that of depression, social anxiety, and other forms of psychopathology.[5]

Genito-pelvic pain/penetration disorder is defined as persistent or recurrent difficulties involving one (or more) of the following: (1) difficulty with intercourse, (2) genito-pelvic pain, (3) fear of pain or vaginal penetration, and (4) tension of the pelvic floor muscles. This diagnosis is frequently associated with other sexual dysfunction, particularly sexual interest and arousal disorders. The five factors discussed under sexual dysfunction must also be considered during the assessment and diagnosis of genito-pelvic pain/penetration disorder because they may be relevant to the cause and/or treatment.[3]

Epidemiologic studies have yielded widely varied estimates of the prevalence of FSD, depending on the definition used as well as the population and specific dysfunction studied. The prevalence of female sexual interest/arousal disorder as defined in DSM-5 is unknown. Low sexual desire and problems with sexual arousal as defined by the *Diagnostic and Statistical Manual of Mental Disorders*, Fourth Edition (DSM-IV) and International Classification of Diseases, Tenth Revision (ICD-10) may vary markedly in relation to age, cultural setting, duration of symptoms, and presence of distress. Low desire is a common sexual problem in women across all age groups worldwide; however, some older women report less distress about low sexual desire than younger women, although sexual desire may decrease with age.[3]

Sexual dysfunction is more common in women (43%) than in men (31%). Studies reveal that the prevalence rate for dysfunction tends to increase as women become older, with approximately 40% to 50% of adult women revealing at least one sexual dysfunction.[6] Prevalence rates are affected by a variety of factors including age, partner's age, duration of marriage, medical illness, menopause, family planning, and frequency of sexual intercourse, all of which have significant association with FSD. Studies have shown that prevalence of most sexual dysfunctions is higher in clinical than in community samples.[6]

PATHOPHYSIOLOGY

Female sexual response is a complex interaction of psychological, interpersonal, environmental, genetic, biologic, and physiologic factors that change throughout the life cycle. Thus the pathophysiologic mechanism of a sexual complaint is typically multifactorial and complex, involving organic, functional, etiologic, and psychological factors. Vascular, neurogenic, hormonal, anatomic, medication-induced, and emotional factors have been implicated as major contributors to the development of FSD.[3,7]

Any disease of the nervous system (e.g., multiple sclerosis, neuropathies, stroke) can result in neurogenic FSD with resultant impaired lubrication and orgasm. Any condition that affects blood flow, such as cardiovascular disease, hyperlipidemia, atherosclerosis, renal disease, and smoking, can affect sexual functioning. Vascular insufficiency with subsequent diminished genital blood flow may directly contribute to genital arousal disorder because of impairment of vaginal and clitoral engorgement. Decreased pelvic blood flow can lead to smooth muscle fibrosis of the clitoris and vagina, which may in turn cause symptoms of vaginal dryness and dyspareunia. Pelvic surgeries may injure autonomic pelvic nerves or interrupt blood flow, both of which may result in FSD.

Dysfunction of the hypothalamic-pituitary axis from natural menopause, surgical or medical castration, premature ovarian failure, or exogenous hormones can result in hormonally based FSD. The most common symptoms associated with estrogen deficiency are vaginal dryness, coital pain, and decreased desire. Diminished testosterone levels in women have been implicated as a cause of decreased arousal, libido, and orgasm.

The muscles of the pelvic floor contribute to sexual arousal and are responsible for the involuntary rhythmic contractions during orgasm. Increased tone of the levator ani muscle may cause dyspareunia and vaginismus, whereas hypotonia is associated with decreased vaginal sensation, coital anorgasmia, and urinary incontinence during sexual intercourse or orgasm. Anatomic causes such as uterine prolapse, pelvic tumors, and endometriosis are commonly associated with deep dyspareunia.

In addition, chronic illnesses, certain medications, substance use, and psychogenic issues, with or without organic disease, may contribute to the development of FSD. Self-esteem, body image, sociocultural factors, relationship issues, depression, and other mood disorders may significantly affect sexual response. Furthermore, many of the medications used to treat depression, especially the selective serotonin reuptake inhibitors (SSRIs), are associated with sexual side effects.

Most often, the cause of FSD is mixed, involving a combination of neurogenic, vascular, psychological, and hormonal causes. For example, women with diabetes may experience sexual dysfunction owing to disease-related neurovascular changes, medication side effects, and the psychological effects of coping with a chronic illness. In women, those who report excellent health compared with good, fair, or poor health are less likely to have sexual dysfunction. Sexual dysfunction is common in women with hypertension who use hypertensive drugs and seems to be associated with desire, arousal, lubrication, orgasm, sexual dissatisfaction, and pain. In patients with psoriasis, a general decline of sexual dysfunction was noted, whereas patients with depression experienced an increased risk in sexual dysfunction and sexual dysfunction increased the odds of depression.[1]

CLINICAL PRESENTATION AND PHYSICAL EXAMINATION

It is important for clinicians to recognize that most women will not initiate a discussion of their sexual concerns. Several studies identified that sexual health is not routinely discussed with their health care providers.[8] An open, understanding, nonjudgmental attitude is necessary to create a comfortable environment for patients to discuss this topic. Inclusion of sexual health questions in the history and review of systems legitimizes that sexual issues are appropriate to discuss. Asking open-ended questions (e.g., "Many women experience sexual changes after menopause. What changes have you noticed?") normalizes sexual concerns.

Basic screening for sexual dysfunction may begin merely with three key questions: (1) Are you currently sexually active? (2) If so, with men, women, or both? (3) Do you have any concerns or difficulties with your sexual health?[9] There are also several validated screening tools available for assessment of sexual problems. The Sexual Satisfaction Scale for Women is a survey containing 30 questions that provides scores on five domains of sexual well-being. The Female Sexual Function Index (FSFI) questionnaire consists of 19 questions and was developed for the purpose of assessing domains of sexual functioning: desire, mental arousal, physical arousal, orgasm, satisfaction, and sexual pain.[5]

A sexual history can be brief or extensive but should include the gynecologic history, sexual activity, number of partners, homosexual or heterosexual relationships, difficult or abusive sexual experiences, and satisfaction with sexual experiences. Problems with desire, arousal, lubrication, orgasm, pain, bleeding, or lesions should also be reviewed; sexually transmitted disease exposure and the need for contraception should be elicited. In addition, exploration of recent life events (e.g., divorce, separation, or recent losses) and cultural attitudes toward sexual activity should be considered.

A detailed psychosocial assessment is an important component of the evaluation of FSD. Given the interpersonal context of sexual problems, past and present partner relationships should be explored.[9] Because medications can affect all phases of the sexual response cycle, a drug review is also imperative.

A complete physical examination should be performed for every patient after a thorough history is obtained. In most cases, the physical examination will not identify the specific cause of sexual dysfunction but may be useful in uncovering relevant chronic diseases and identifying contributing anatomic, endocrine, vascular, or neurologic pathology. The presence of secondary sexual characteristics and hair distribution can be assessed during the general examination. A complete pelvic examination is required for evaluation of any sexual pain disorder and may be performed as indicated for evaluation of other FSDs.[10]

The external genitalia can be visually inspected for any lesions, anomalies, tenderness, erythema, edema, atrophy, thickening, prolapse, rectocele, or cystocele. Sensitivity to touch, pressure, vibration, and temperature may also be assessed. Presence of the bulbocavernosus and anocutaneous reflexes demonstrates integrity of the sacral nerves, which form the neurologic foundation of the sexual response cycle. Speculum examination may uncover lesions, inflammation, atrophy, or infection of the cervix or vagina. Bimanual palpation of the vagina, cervix, uterus, and adnexa may suggest the presence of pelvic tumor, infection, or endometriosis. Vaginal muscle tone can be evaluated by inserting two fingers in the vagina and having the patient squeeze them.

DIAGNOSTICS

FSD is complex and requires a multidisciplinary approach because currently there is no universally recommended battery of tests for its diagnosis.

Essential Diagnostics

Diagnostic studies are guided by the history and physical examination findings. Laboratory evaluation for FSD is rarely indicated unless there is suspicion for a specific medical condition contributing to the patient's complaint.[9] Laboratory tests may include testosterone, sex hormone binding globulin (SHBG), dehydroepiandrosterone (DHEA), estradiol, calculated free testosterone, luteinizing hormone (LH), and follicle-stimulating hormone (FSH).

Additional Diagnostics

Other lab tests that may be of value include the wet mount, testing for gonorrhea and chlamydia, complete blood count

---

INITIAL DIAGNOSTICS

Female Sexual Dysfunction

LABORATORY
- Luteinizing hormone and follicle-stimulating hormone[a]
- Dehydroepiandrosterone[a]
- CBC and differential[a]
- Thyroid profile[a]
- Prolactin[a]
- Testosterone[a]
- Serum estradiol[a]
- Hemoglobin A1c[a]

- Fasting glucose, blood urea nitrogen, and creatinine[a]
- Liver enzymes[a]
- Wet mount, testing for chlamydia and gonorrhea[a]
- Sex hormone binding globulin[a]

IMAGING
- Pelvic ultrasound[a]

[a] If indicated.

(CBC), complete metabolic panel, hemoglobin A1C, lipid panel, renal panel, and liver function studies.[10] Pelvic ultrasound examination may be performed as indicated to rule out pelvic mass or anatomic anomaly. Screening for depression may also be indicated.

DIFFERENTIAL DIAGNOSIS

Multiple factors need to be taken into consideration when attempting to identify a causative agent for FSD, as contributing issues may include psychological issues, such as depression, medical and surgical conditions and lifestyle/psychosocial factors. In addition, it is important to consider that many commonly used drugs, especially antihypertensives, psychotropics, and hormonal agents, may have negative effects on sexual function.[5,11,12]

The differential diagnoses should include depression, diabetes, hypertension, renal failure, vascular causes, spinal cord injuries, and multiple sclerosis.[11,13]

INTERPROFESSIONAL COLLABORATIVE MANAGEMENT
Nonpharmacological Management

Many sexual concerns can be addressed during a routine office visit by a primary care provider with accurate, unbiased information about female sexuality, referral to educational resources, suggestion for lifestyle changes, and referrals for individual or couples counseling.[14] The PLISSIT model of sex therapy is a graduated counseling system that provides a useful framework for addressing sexual concerns.[9] First proposed in 1976, the PLISSIT model remains useful in primary care practice today. The acronym stands for four levels of interventions: permission, limited information, specific suggestions, and intensive therapy. Examples of giving permission are letting patients know that sexual concerns are appropriate to discuss and reassuring them that their sexual anatomy or practices are normal. The second step involves providing limited information, such as dispelling myths or explaining the sexual response cycle. At the next level, specific suggestions, such as position changes, use of lubricants, or methods of self-exploration, may be offered. Finally, patients may be referred to a specialist if intensive therapy is indicated; however, the majority of sexual concerns may be adequately addressed within the context of a routine office visit employing the lower levels of this hierarchical model.

Psychological treatments include cognitive behavioral therapy, directed masturbation, sensate focus, and systematic desensitization.[10] Relationship issues and disparities in sexual desire between partners can be addressed in couples' therapy. Women with focal muscular vaginal pain may be referred for pelvic floor physical therapy or trigger point injections. Pelvic floor muscle exercises are done to increase strength, to decrease incontinence, to improve blood flow, and to facilitate an orgasm. Symptoms related to vaginal dryness may be managed with use of supplemental lubricants.[10]

A potential treatment modality for FSD is the use of sacral neuromodulation (InterStim). Sacral nerve stimulation has been used for almost two decades and recent studies support its impact on use for FSD symptoms.[4] Another behavioral technique commonly used to impact motivation and drive is a technique called simmering. Simmering involves thinking about sex through things such as bibliotherapy, watching romantic and exotic media, journaling about fantasies and sex, and focusing the mind on sex.[10]

The Eros Clitoral Therapy Device (Eros-CTD) is a handheld vacuum device that is available by prescription and approved by the US Food and Drug Administration (FDA) for the treatment of female sexual arousal and orgasmic disorders. The device works by improving blood flow and stimulation to the clitoris and external genitalia. This device improves sensation, deep vaginal lubrication, ability to orgasm, and overall sexual satisfaction.[10]

Pharmacologic Management

Local estrogen therapy, in the form of vaginal tablets, rings, creams, and pessaries, is highly effective for alleviating symptoms of urogenital atrophy. Because conjugated equine estrogen cream is well absorbed from the vagina, it should be paired with progestogen to prevent unopposed estrogen stimulation of the endometrium. Topical estradiol and estriol preparations have low systemic absorption and therefore do not require addition of progestogen for endometrial protection. Vaginally applied DHEA and ospemifene, a selective estrogen receptor modulator, show promise as future therapies for treatment of vaginal atrophy. Zestra for women is a feminine arousal topical ointment that improved desire, arousal, and satisfaction in women aged 21 to 65 in a placebo-controlled multicenter trial.[10]

In clinical trials, treatment with a testosterone patch resulted in significantly increased desire and arousal in postmenopausal women who were experiencing a decrease in sexual desire or interest; however, there are no data to support its use in premenopausal women.[15] Potential side effects of weight gain, acne, deepening of voice, clitoral enlargement, increased facial hair, hypercholesterolemia, and the risk of a cardiac event must be weighed against any potential benefits of treatment. Tibolone is a synthetic steroid sex hormone demonstrated to improve multiple dimensions of sexual function in clinical trials. Both the testosterone patch and tibolone have been approved for use in Europe; however, neither is FDA approved for the treatment of FSD in the United States.[16]

The selective phosphodiesterase type 5 inhibitors sildenafil, vardenafil, and tadalafil are approved for the treatment of erectile dysfunction in men but are not FDA approved for the treatment of sexual dysfunction in women. Although studies have shown that sildenafil may benefit women with sexual dysfunction related to SSRI use, spinal cord injury, or diabetes, results in other patient populations have shown no benefit.[4,10] Phentolamine is an α-adrenergic antagonist that causes vasodilation by relaxing smooth muscle and may improve lubrication and arousal in menopausal women with sexual arousal disorder but is not FDA approved for that indication.

Centrally acting agents show some promise for targeting low desire. Studies have demonstrated the effectiveness of the antidepressant bupropion in improving both arousal and orgasm in nondepressed women with decrease in sexual desire, interest, or arousal and in increasing desire in depressed women with SSRI-associated sexual side effects.[4,10] Flibanserin (Addyi), a 5-hydroxytryptamine agonist-antagonist, gained FDA approval in 2015 to treat hypoactive sexual desire disorder and acts by altering the neurotransmitter levels responsible for sexual excitement.

Herbal therapies, marketed as "natural" remedies for FSD, abound despite a lack of data on their efficacy and safety. A few very small randomized controlled trials of products containing yohimbine, ginseng, *Ginkgo biloba*, and damiana have shown promising results for improving sexual function and satisfaction. More research is needed to establish their role in the treatment of FSD.

Indications for Referral

The decision of whether to refer a patient with sexual dysfunction will depend on the provider's level of comfort and expertise as well as the complexity of the dysfunction. Many sexual concerns and dysfunctions can be treated with good anticipatory guidance and education about sexuality and sexual health. For some patients, the underlying medical condition is treated. For those who may require extensive general or sex therapy, referral to a reputable, certified sex therapist is warranted. The following professional organizations maintain listings of credentialed therapists on their websites:

- American Association of Sexuality Educators, Counselors, and Therapists (www.aasect.org)
- American Board of Sexology (www.americanboardofsexology.com)
- Society for Sex Therapy and Research (www.sstarnet.org)
- American Association for Marriage and Family Therapy (www.aamft.org)

Evaluation in a women's sexual health clinic, if it is available, may allow a better elucidation of the problem and a more comprehensive treatment approach.

LIFE SPAN CONSIDERATIONS

Providers should be aware of the range of sexual changes that occur across the life span. Each life stage may have unique physical and emotional influences to be considered. The transitional periods of adolescence, childbearing, menopause, and widowhood may profoundly influence sexual response.

COMPLICATIONS

Sexual dysfunctions can interfere with intimacy, adversely affect relationships, and have a negative impact on a woman's self-esteem, health, and sense of well-being. Failure to address a patient's sexual concerns may lead to eroded relationships, depression, self-medication with drugs and alcohol, and other psychosocial consequences. Primary care providers are in a unique position to uncover and to address sexual dysfunctions, thereby preventing these sequelae.

PATIENT AND FAMILY EDUCATION

Professional organization websites, such as the Association of Reproductive Health Professionals (www.arhp.org), the North American Menopause Society (www.menopause.org), and the American Congress of Obstetricians and Gynecologists (www.acog.org), are excellent sources of patient education materials pertaining to female sexual health. Condition-specific brochures are available from the American Cancer Society (www.cancer.org), the National Vulvodynia Association (www.nva.org), and many other medical organizations. Healthy Women (www.healthywomen.org and www.sexandahealthieryou.org) is an online organization dedicated to women's health issues and has developed a comprehensive series of publications addressing FSDs.

HEALTH PROMOTION

Education should be directed toward the understanding of normal sexual response, basic genital anatomy and physiology, and self-care measures. The importance of diet, exercise, and adequate sleep cannot be overstated because stress and fatigue are significant factors that affect sexual desire. Promotion of cholesterol reduction, tobacco cessation, and blood pressure and glycemic control may go a long way in the prevention of potential vasculogenic causes of FSD.

REFERENCES

1. McCool, M., Theurich, M., & Apfelbacher, C. (2014). Prevalence and predictors of female sexual dysfunction: A protocol for a systematic review. *Systematic Reviews, 3*, 75.
2. Albaugh, J. (2014). Female sexual dysfunction. *International Journal of Urological Nursing, 8*, 38–43.
3. American Psychiatric Association. (2013). Sexual and gender identity disorders. In *Diagnostic and statistical manual of mental disorders* (5th ed.). Washington, DC: American Psychiatric Association.
4. Houman, J., Feng, T., Eilber, K., & Anger, J. (2016). Female sexual dysfunction: Is it a treatable disease? *Current Urology Reports, 17*, 28–32.
5. Stephenson, K., & Meston, C. (2015). Why is impaired sexual function distressing to women? The primacy of pleasure in female sexual dysfunction. *The Journal of Sexual Medicine, 12*, 728–737.
6. Annon, J. (1976). The PLISSIT model: A proposed conceptual scheme for the behavioral treatment of sexual problems. *Journal of Sex Education and Therapy, 2*, 1–15.
7. O'Sullivan, L., & Vannier, S. (2016). Women's sexual desire and desire disorders from a developmental perspective. *Current Sexual Health Reports, 8*, 47–56.
8. Ribiero, S., Alarcao, V., Sociol, D., et al. (2014). General Practitioners' procedures for sexual history taking and treating sexual dysfunction in primary care. *The Journal of Sexual Medicine, 11*, 386–393.
9. Annon, J. S. (1976). The PLISSIT model: A proposed conceptual scheme for the behavioral treatment of sexual problems. *Journal of Sex Education and Therapy, 2*(1), 1–15.
10. Basson, R., Wierman, M. E., Lankveld, J., et al. (2010). Summary of the recommendation on sexual dysfunctions in women. *The Journal of Sexual Medicine, 7*, 314–326.
11. Lorenz, T., Rullo, J., & Faubion, S. (2016). Antidepressant-induced female sexual dysfunction. *Mayo Clinic Proceedings, 91*(9), 1280–1286.
12. Albaugh, J. (2014). Female sexual dysfunction. *International Journal of Urological Nursing, 8*(1), 38–43.
13. Mollaoglu, M., & Tuncay, F. (2013). Fertelli T. Investigating the sexual function and its associated factors in women with chronic illnesses. *Journal of Clinical Nursing, 22*, 3484–3491.
14. Clayton, A., & Juaraz, E. (2017). Female sexual dysfunction. *The Psychiatric Clinics of North America, 40*, 267–284.
15. Khera, M. (2015). Testosterone therapy for female sexual dysfunction. *Sexual Medicine Reviews, 3*, 137–144.
16. Maseroli, E., Fanni, E., Fambrini, M., et al. (2016). Bringing the body of the iceberg to the surface: The female sexual dysfunction index-6 (FSDI-6) in the screening of female sexual dysfunction. *Journal of Endocrinological Investigation, 30*, 401–409.

CHAPTER **152**

UNPLANNED PREGNANCY
Lindsey Cushing

DEFINITION AND EPIDEMIOLOGY

Pregnancy can be defined by a woman's intentions before she became pregnant. A pregnancy is considered *planned* or *intended* if they are reported to have happened at the "right time" or later than desired (because of infertility or difficulties in conceiving).[1-3]

Conversely, *unplanned pregnancies* are pregnancies that are reported to have either been undesired at the time of conception (i.e., they occurred when no children, or no more children, were desired) or mistimed (i.e., they occurred earlier than desired). Use of the single term, "unplanned pregnancy," ignores some significant differences between women with unwanted pregnancies and those with desired but mistimed pregnancies. Those women experiencing unwanted pregnancies are more likely to have health risks that could negatively affect pregnancy outcomes; compared to mistimed pregnancies, unwanted pregnancies are associated with increased unfavorable maternal behaviors and health risks for both mother and child. Therefore clarification of the patient's intention before pregnancy is essential in guiding the clinician as they provide direct services to women and infants.[3]

In recent years, about 10% of women of reproductive age (15 to 44 years) become pregnant in any single year (about 100 pregnancies per 1000 women); approximately 50% of those pregnancies are unintended. The rate of unintended pregnancies varies based on a number of factors, including ethnicity, education, age, income, and marital status. Approximately 35 per 1000 white women have unintended pregnancies, compared with 78 per 1000 Hispanic women and 98 per 1000 black women. Unintended pregnancies occur in 26 per 1000 college graduates and in 76 per 1000 women who do not have a high school diploma.[4,5] Women whose income level is below 100% of the federal poverty level have an unintended pregnancy rate of 112 per 1000 women; women whose income is twice the poverty level have an unintended pregnancy rate of 29 per 1000 women.[6] Adolescent women have the highest proportion of unintended pregnancies, with approximately 456,000 women under age 20 becoming pregnant in 2013, with the majority of these being unintended.[7]

Women with unintended pregnancies are less likely to receive the appropriate prenatal care, take prenatal vitamins and supplements, exercise during pregnancy, become vaccinated, eat a healthy diet, and gain the recommended amount of weight.[8] In addition, they are more likely to engage in high-risk sexual behaviors, smoke cigarettes, drink alcohol, abuse drugs, and have a higher risk for developing mental health issues.[8] Some studies suggest that there is an increased risk of negative perinatal outcomes, such as low birth weight, preterm birth, and lower breastfeeding rates, associated with unintended pregnancies; infants born to a mother with an unintended pregnancy are more likely to be readmitted to the hospital after discharge home. One study suggests that the emotions associated with having a child who was not planned for have long-term negative consequences for the parent–child relationship.[9]

There are also significant economic costs associated with unintended pregnancies—not only to families but also to state and federal governments. In 2002, the medical costs associated with unplanned pregnancies in the United States totaled close to $5 billion.[10] An analysis published in 2011 estimated that unintended pregnancies cost state and federal governments a total of $11.1 billion in a single year. These births account for half of publicly funded births and their resulting costs, which places a significant burden on social programs such as Medicaid and the Children's Health Insurance Program.[11] Additional costs not accounted for in this analysis include the increased likelihood of preterm birth, low birth weight, and other negative perinatal outcomes; children's medical care beyond their first year; pregnancy-related care paid for by other government-related health programs; and other government benefits, such as welfare payments.

CLINICAL PRESENTATION

Patients facing an unplanned pregnancy may visit a provider because of signs and symptoms of possible pregnancy, without having taken a pregnancy test. These signs and symptoms may include a missed period, irregular bleeding or spotting, nausea and vomiting, breast pain, dizziness, and fatigue. Patients who feel especially vulnerable or are in denial about a pregnancy may not have taken a test at home and want to take the test in a health care setting where they have immediate guidance. Taking a test in a provider's office can prove to be beneficial for patients who are young, have minimal support at home, those with mental health issues, and women who are unsure regarding what kind of pregnancy outcome they desire.

A positive result of a pregnancy test can generate a variety of responses. For some patients, the news brings joy and excitement; for others, the news can be a crisis of varying proportions. Given this, the provider should use neutral language when delivering the news of a positive pregnancy test result.

In this way, the health care provider is often the patient's first confidant after receiving the news of an unplanned pregnancy and is in a unique position to assist her in meeting her total health and wellness needs. With an unplanned pregnancy, the health care provider's response is critical in establishing and maintaining an environment that feels safe and supportive to the patient. The provider's initial role is to listen; both verbal and nonverbal communications provide information that is useful in developing the care plan. The patient needs to be allowed time to express her feelings. It is important that the provider not provide congratulations or consolation to the patient until her feelings have been assessed.

Once the diagnosis of pregnancy has been made, the primary care provider (PCP), with the patient's approval, should be ready to discuss the woman's options regarding her pregnancy. A woman's reaction to and intentions regarding an unplanned pregnancy are not fixed and may change, depending on a variety of social, financial, and physical factors, as well as where she is on the continuum from preconception to postpartum. In many cases, the pregnancy is not the only issue that concerns the patient.

Her reaction to the news of an unplanned pregnancy may be influenced by other significant concerns such as finances, health status, relationship problems, domestic or sexual violence, etc. A woman's reaction to an unplanned pregnancy is in part based on her evaluation of the obstacles she faces in life. Providers should remember that not all unplanned pregnancies are unwanted, but financial problems, age, maturity, and/or lack of social support may contribute to a patient's feeling that they cannot parent a child. Nelson and O'Brien found that women who decide to continue with pregnancy and have trouble organizing and coping with their emotions are at risk for developing a pattern of negativity that will affect the quality of the parent–child relationship.[9] Assessment of these concerns is essential in the decision-making process for healthy outcomes.

INTERPROFESSIONAL COLLABORATIVE MANAGEMENT

Depending on the estimated gestational age of the pregnancy at the time of diagnosis, a woman has the following options available to her: (1) carrying her pregnancy to delivery and raising the child, (2) carrying her pregnancy to delivery and making an adoption plan, and (3) terminating her pregnancy. Counseling of a woman with an unplanned pregnancy can be emotionally challenging for both the health care provider and the patient. A clinician's comfort in this task is not only influenced by the intense emotionality some patients may feel in this situation, but is also influenced by the provider's personal biases about unplanned pregnancy, the patient's socioeconomic factors influencing her life and health, and the options available to women facing an unwanted pregnancy. Health care providers need to understand and accept that a woman's perspective, goals, and her means of achieving these goals may conflict with their own. Before a provider can effectively counsel a woman regarding her pregnancy options, he or she needs to thoughtfully explore what his or her personal beliefs and biases may be, and how these might influence the education and counseling provided to a woman facing an unplanned pregnancy. It is virtually impossible for a provider to rid himself or herself of personal values and biases, but the provider must be committed to, and vigilant about, keeping those biases out of the interaction with the woman and other people involved in the situation. If a provider feels that he or she is unable to put their personal beliefs and values about reproductive choices and options aside, they should facilitate a swift referral for counseling by another knowledgeable professional, either within their practice or in the community, for counseling and management.

Ideally, women should make the decision of carrying a pregnancy to term or ending the pregnancy free of coercion and with the support of their partners, families, and health care providers. Every woman has the right to factual and unbiased information about her reproductive choices; thus the provider must keep in mind that the woman is responsible for defining how the unplanned pregnancy is a problem for her, evaluating her available options, and ultimately acting on her decision. The provider's role is to actively listen to the woman, to provide information and support, and to help the woman assess her options. It is also the provider's responsibility to assess whether a patient is being pressured to make a particular choice by outside parties (such as her partner or her parents), and to help her arrive at her own decision. A patient may ask the provider what she should do or what the provider would do if he or she were in the woman's situation; it is important for the provider to remind the patient that it is the patient's decision and that the provider will support her through that decision, whatever it may be.

After the patient has expressed herself, the health care provider can assist with prioritizing the patient's concerns and needs by focusing on one issue at a time. By exhibiting a willingness to listen and help, the provider helps build the patient's confidence. An exploration of the patient's feelings about pregnancy, parenting, abortion, and adoption provides an opportunity to further process the situation. It is also helpful for the provider to know whether the patient has previously experienced an unplanned pregnancy or whether she knows anyone who has dealt with an unplanned pregnancy and the decision to have an abortion, to raise the child, or to place the child for adoption. A critical piece of information concerns the woman's support system as well as what role, if any, the patient's partner in conception has in her life and in the decisions about this pregnancy: control of decision-making may be an aspect of intimate partner violence. Several studies have suggested that women who experience relationship violence are more likely to have repeat terminations. This may be due to partners not allowing the use of contraception.[12,13] Screening for intimate partner violence should be provided for all women who present to their health care provider.

The health care provider should inform the patient of the full range of available options. It is important to assure the patient that all information discussed will be kept confidential. Regardless of the decision, continued and unconditional acceptance of, and compassion toward, the patient will contribute to her overall wellness at this critical time. If the provider does not feel equipped to thoroughly counsel patients on all the available options and to support them while they make their decision, a referral to a local counselor, a trusted women's medical health care center, or Planned Parenthood is most appropriate. The provider should keep in mind that abortion and adoption can be controversial, emotionally charged topics, and many patients may not be forthcoming initially about their true wishes in this regard. If a provider is treating reproductive aged women it is their responsibility to know which organizations, educational recourses, or local clinics can be trusted to provide patients with evidence-based, nonbiased information and medical care; similarly, it is the responsibility of the provider to know which local resources aim to provide biased information or coercive care that may be contradictory to the woman's expressed or nonexpressed goals.

Clinicians that must send women elsewhere for their pregnancy options, counseling, or care should avoid referrals to crisis pregnancy centers (CPCs), which may also be referred to as pregnancy resource centers. CPCs are nonprofit organizations that offer free services to women facing unintended pregnancies, such as pregnancy testing, ultrasound, counseling, and baby and maternity items. While CPCs vary in the goods and services they offer, supporters and opponents agree that their mission, which is typically undisclosed, is to dissuade women from obtaining abortions.[14,15] CPCs are frequently staffed by nonmedical volunteers, are religiously affiliated, and offer almost no true medical services (i.e., abortions or contraception). These centers use a variety of tactics to represent themselves as full-service health care clinics, including organizational names that imply a full range of pregnancy options and services or that are strikingly similar to legitimate reproductive health care facilities, having the appearance of a medical clinic, and even being strategically located near legitimate women's health care clinics that do offer abortions.[14] The tactics used by CPCs to dissuade women from having abortions often include providing misleading or false information about the emotional and physical risks of abortion; for instance, many women are counseled that abortion increases their risk of breast cancer, depression, and infertility.[14,15] More aggressive tactics include coercing women who are considering termination into an ultrasound and then providing them with inaccurate information about the pregnancy, such as telling patients they are much earlier or much later in their pregnancies than they are, which leads to delayed prenatal or abortion care or falsely believing that they've missed their opportunity

to decide on abortion.[14] Despite providing inaccurate information to women, as well as a lack of medical services, CPCs receive support from both the state and federal government in the form of funding—many states even list these organizations as places to seek information on alternatives to abortion.[15] Because CPCs do not provide medical care, they are not governed by the same rules and regulations that govern health clinics. Although some states have enacted legislation that seeks to prevent CPCs from falsely representing themselves as abortion providers, many states lack any regulation on the activities of CPCs.[15]

Counseling a patient who is experiencing an unplanned pregnancy can be very challenging. The following framework, which contains areas of focus and counseling points for the clinician, as well as targeted questions to ask the patient, may help make this interaction fruitful for both patient and provider.

Focus on the patient. It is important to remember that the physical, emotional, and social well-being of the patient experiencing the crisis of an unplanned pregnancy is the clinician's main priority.

Inquire about the patient's feelings. The health care provider should ask some of the following questions:
- How are you feeling about this pregnancy? What does the pregnancy mean to you?
- Before finding out that you were pregnant, what were your feelings about having children? Parenting? Adoption? Abortion?
- Under what circumstances would you like to become a parent?
- Who knows that you are pregnant?
- What is your relationship with the partner you conceived with? How involved is he in the decision-making? How supportive will he be of your decision? Was the pregnancy a result of sexual assault? Did anyone coerce you to become pregnant (e.g., sabotaging birth control methods, using threats or intimidation to prevent or limit contraceptive use).
- Who is your support system?

Remove the fear and stigma about discussions of abortion and adoption. Providers should be aware that it may be difficult for patients to broach the subject of pregnancy termination or adoption, and may be waiting for the health care provider to do so. If a patient is considering either of these options, it is important that the clinician put them at ease and avoid any perception of stigma.
- Have you ever been pregnant before?
- Are you considering an abortion? Are you considering adoption?
- Have you ever had an abortion? Have you ever placed a child for adoption?
- Is anyone putting pressure on you to choose termination or adoption for this pregnancy?

Dispel common myths regarding abortion and adoption. It is the clinician's responsibility to provide evidence-based information when counseling patients about abortion and adoption. For women who choose abortion or adoption, reactions may range from relief, to ambivalence, to shame. While feelings of sadness and grief are appropriate responses for women who choose not to parent, so too are feelings of happiness and liberation—often one woman can experience all of these emotions at various times.

- What do you know about abortion/adoption?
- What does abortion mean to you? What does adoption mean to you? What were your opinions about abortion or adoption before you learned you were pregnant?
- Do you know anyone who has had an abortion? Do you know anyone who has placed a child for adoption?

Provide evidence-based information about abortion. The national rate of abortion has been on a long-term decline for decades.[16] Abortion rates are highest in women aged 20 to 24 (30 per 1000 women) and 25 to 29 (22 per 1000); most terminations are performed in women who are unmarried (84%), have one or more children (59%), and are living below the poverty level.[17,18] In 2008, the rate of terminations was highest among non-Hispanic white women (37%) and among non-Hispanic black women (36%).[17] The vast majority, 91%, of terminations are performed in the first trimester; 7% of terminations occur from 14 to 20 weeks gestation, and 1% of terminations occur at or after 21 weeks gestation.[17] According to a 2014 report by Jones and Jerman, in 2011 approximately 40% of unintended pregnancies were terminated.[19]

Terminations can be performed via medication or vacuum aspiration depending on gestational age and patient preference; providers should be familiar with their state laws regarding gestational age and termination availability. According to US Food and Drug Administration guidelines, medication abortion is allowed up to 10 weeks' gestation. The protocol involves two drugs—mifepristone and misoprostol—one of which can be taken at home following a provider visit. Surgical terminations can be performed safely in free-standing clinics or in an office setting with proper equipment for performing in-office surgical procedures; hospitalization may be required for women with medical conditions that put them at increased risk of medical or surgical complications (e.g., coagulopathy, heart disease). In general, the risk of major medical complication is low; a retrospective study of 54,911 abortion procedures in California found an overall complication rate of 2.1%.[20] In fact, the mortality associated with childbirth is many times higher than that associated with legal abortion. The maternal mortality rates for live births, miscarriages, and ectopic pregnancies (7.06 per 100,000 live births, 1.19 per 100,000 miscarriages, and 31.9 per 100,000 ectopic pregnancies) are all higher than the death rate for legal pregnancy termination (0.567 per 100,000 terminations).[21] For counseling, this risk can be compared to that of plastic surgery procedures (0.8 to 1.7 deaths per 100,000) or dental procedures (0 to 1.7 deaths per 100,000).[22]

Some post-procedure risks that are often cited by women as an area of concern, or by those who oppose abortion, include reduced fertility or poor future pregnancy outcomes, increased risk of breast cancer, and increased risk of mental health problems. These concerns are not substantiated by current evidence.[23-25] Studies that have found a link between abortion and preterm birth, as well as abortion and breast cancer, do not meet criteria for establishing causality and are problematic due to lack of controlling for confounding factors and recall bias.[15] Leading women's and children's health organizations (such as the World Health Organization, the Centers for Disease Control, the American College of Obstetricians and Gynecologists, and the March of Dimes) do not list abortion as a risk factor for preterm birth or other poor obstetrical outcomes. Similarly, both the American Cancer Society and the National Cancer Institute have issued statements refuting a link between breast cancer and abortion.[15]

Although women may experience grief following a termination, abortion is not associated with an increased risk of serious mental health disorders[15,25] and in fact, the frequency of psychiatric diagnoses (such as depression, anxiety, PTSD, and substance use) in women who have terminated a pregnancy is similar to that in women with no such history.[26,27] It should be noted, however, that there are some risk factors for post-abortion psychosocial difficulties, including previous or concurrent psychiatric illness (such as pre-pregnancy depression or suicidal ideation), sexual violence, coercion to abort, genetic or medical indications, lack of social supports, ambivalence, and increasing length of gestation. Overall, the literature indicates that serious psychiatric illness is at least eight times more common among postpartum than among post-abortion women.[26,27]

In women considering abortion, accurate assessment of gestational age is essential in ensuring a patient receives timely care. Ultrasound, fundal height, or bimanual clinical examination findings are helpful in approximating gestational age, but in the absence of equipment or training in these techniques, providers may estimate gestational age from a detailed menstrual and sexual history and any pregnancy symptoms. The locations and gestational age limits of abortion facilities in individual areas are available through online resources such as the National Abortion Federation.

The cost of a termination varies among different clinics and increases with the duration of pregnancy. Although the average cost of abortion in the United States is $543 at 10 weeks gestation, it nearly triples to $1562 at 20 weeks.[28] More than half of patients who obtained abortions paid out of pocket for their procedure in 2014.[29] Clinicians should make patients aware that there are a number of state and national programs that assist patients in covering the cost of termination.

Women who are considering pregnancy termination should be referred to a trained abortion provider as soon as possible for more detailed information and counseling.

Provide evidence-based information about adoption. Data on the exact number of children, including infants, adopted in the United States is difficult to ascertain, as there is currently no single agency charged with compiling this national information. Agencies that do collect adoption-related data do so for their own purposes and categorize this information in a variety of ways, making compilation difficult. According to a report from the US Department of Health and Human Services, which assembled adoption data from 2008 to 2012, 119,514 children were adopted in the United States in 2012, which is a 14% decrease from 2008.[30] In a literature review published in 2016, Coleman & Garratt reported[31]:

> As an option in cases of unintended pregnancy, adoption is surprisingly uncommon in the U.S. with less than 3% of White unmarried women and less than 2% of Black unmarried women deciding to place a child for adoption. These figures represent a marked decline from 50 years ago when 40% of unmarried White women placed for adoption. The placement of newborns has become increasingly rare in the U.S., declining almost nine-fold since the early 1970s. Current estimates of domestic infant adoptions range from approximately 7,000 to 22,000 annually.

Unfortunately the exact number of infants resulting from an unplanned pregnancy that were placed for adoption is not data that are readily available.

Only about 25% of birth mothers fit into the common stereotype of an unwed teenage mother. In fact, a more typical scenario is a woman in her 20s who has other children.[32] Well-established factors that influence the choice to make an adoption plan include race, age, socioeconomic status, education, preference of the birth mother's mother, vocational goals, the quality of relationship with the birth father, and living arrangements.[33] The literature has demonstrated multiple times that most women who choose adoption for their birth children were motivated by a desire to provide a better life for their child and identified the baby's best interest as a primary motivating factor. Other motivating factors included feeling unprepared for parenthood, not feeling ready emotionally, and inadequate finances.[31]

Secrecy and shame have historically surrounded the practice of adoption—leading to emotional trauma for both birth parents and adopted individuals. While overall the perception of adoption and treatment of pregnant women who choose adoption has improved over time, there continue to be challenges in correcting inaccurate beliefs and biases held by the media, health care workers, counselors, and the general public. Currently in the United States, there are four general types of adoption available[31]:

1. Closed Adoption—Identifying information about the birth and adoptive families is not shared between the two and there is no contact. Records are sealed and sometimes become available to the adopted child on their 18th birthday.
2. Semi-Open Adoption (or Mediated Adoption)—Information is shared between birth and adoptive parents. However, confidentiality regarding individuals' full names and contact information is maintained. Birth parents may participate in choosing adoptive parents and they sometimes meet prospective parents. After the adoption, birth parents may request pictures and written updates, but they don't normally have any direct communication with their birth children.
3. Open Adoption—Birth and adoptive parents share their full names and correspondence information. Communication occurs directly and as often as desired.
4. Identified Adoption—Birth and adoptive families choose each other on their own, coming into contact through personal relationships, advertising, or an attorney.

It should be noted that the qualities of each adoption type are not necessarily mutually exclusive—every adoption plan is different and may contain features of multiple types of adoptions; for instance, birth mothers and adoptive parents may find each other on their own, like in an identified adoption, and then move forward with a plan that more closely resembles a semi-open adoption. The most common practice in the United States and Canada for voluntary adoption placements is open or semi-open adoptions. This is a significant change from past practices, which relied heavily on closed adoptions. This shift toward greater freedom and decision-making on the part of the birth mother helps contribute to an increased sense of control and closure.[34]

The experience of birth mothers has been largely underrepresented in the literature, with most studies focusing on the experience of the adopted child and/or adoptive parents.

The limited evidence exploring the long-term psychosocial outcomes of adoption for birth mothers is conflicting. Some studies indicate that the negative long-term effects of placing a child for adoption can include feelings of loss, sadness/depression, guilt, remorse, anger, powerlessness, and victimization; with this, some birth mothers may have experiences similar to that following a significant trauma, including engaging in self-destructive behaviors such as substance use and eating disorders, or experiencing relationship difficulties. Typical aspects of the experience of placing for adoption that make it difficult to resolve negative feelings include a lack of opportunities to express grief, inadequate support, and not having socially acceptable mourning rituals. In order to effectively work through the grief process, several authors have emphasized the need for birth mothers to acknowledge, discuss, and commemorate the sense of loss associated with placing a child for adoption within a nonjudgmental, supportive, validating environment.[31]

Conversely, there are some studies indicating that birth mothers who choose adoption fare better than those who decide to parent their infants. A number of studies found that adolescent women who chose to make an adoption plan were less likely to live in poverty, rely on public assistance, engage in risky sexual behaviors, and were more likely to remain single and avoid a second birth within 5 years. In addition, they were more likely to gain higher levels of education and to be employed with higher incomes compared to those adolescents who raised a child. These young women reported higher satisfaction with their lives, finances, work, and relationships, held more positive future outlooks relative to education, work, finances, and marriage, and were less likely to be depressed in the months and years following adoption.[31,35] Interestingly still, a number of longitudinal studies have identified comparable rates of decision satisfaction between those women who place for adoption and those who parent. A major factor that can affect birth mothers' long-term psychosocial outcomes is the amount of emotional support they received prenatally and postpartum in order to prepare and work through separation from their child; further, women who decide on adoption may be more likely than women who do not to have personal, social, or demographic characteristics that increase their risk for psychological difficulties.[31] The conflicting results found in the current literature therefore may be due to insufficient controls for these third variables, and more research is needed to adequately assess the characteristics of mothers who choose adoption and risk factors for psychosocial problems after placing a child for adoption.

What is becoming increasingly clear in the literature is that opportunities for ongoing contact with the adoptive family has a significantly positive effect on birth mothers' overall satisfaction with their decision and post-placement psychological adjustment as compared to closed adoption. Ongoing contact and the sharing of information serves to reduce birth mothers' feelings of guilt and fears regarding the child's well-being. Adoptive parents also demonstrate increased satisfaction in the setting of open adoptions.[31]

Providing women with information on adoption can be influential in their choice to parent or not. An important part of providing quality counseling is the use of positive adoption language; in this way, counselors and clinicians can help frame the choice of adoption in a supportive and nonbiased manner.

Finally, no competent provider counseling a pregnant woman should suggest that adoption is a simple solution to an unplanned pregnancy. It is inaccurate and misleading to suggest that adoption provides a means for a woman to simply resume her life and forget the child she placed for adoption. Women facing an unplanned pregnancy should be accurately counseled that adoption, just like parenting and pregnancy termination, is a life-altering decision and can be associated with significant emotional challenges, including feelings of grief and loss, that need to be acknowledged and supported.

Focus on the woman and her future. The health care provider should ask the following:
- Under what circumstances would you like to become a parent?
- How would you feel if this was your only pregnancy?
- What are your goals for the next year? The next 5 years? How would each alternative help or hinder the achievement of these goals?
- What part of your circumstances is the most frightening or challenging?
- How would you like for things to turn out for you ideally?

Remind the patient that she needs support. Encourage the patient to speak with a trusted person in her life (a partner, a family member, a friend, a counselor, a therapist, etc.) as she considers her various options. These trusted individuals will continue to be a source of emotional, social, and possibly financial support as she moves forward and beyond her final decision.

Provide the patient with resources for making her decision. Many organizations exist to support women facing unplanned pregnancies. It is the clinician's responsibility to ensure patients are aware of these resources and to direct patients to them. These resources may include websites, hotlines, faith-based organizations, or workbooks:
- All-Options: https://www.all-options.org/
  Uses direct service and social change strategies to promote unconditional, judgment-free support for people in all of their decisions, feelings, and experiences with pregnancy, parenting, abortion, and adoption. We recognize that these issues are complex, but one thing is certain: Everyone deserves to have all options.
- Pregnancy Options Workbook: http://www.pregnancy options.info/pregnant.htm
  Offers exercises and discussion of the decision-making process, all three options with extensive facts, and sections on spirituality, fetal development, what can harm a pregnancy, birth control, STDs, fertility, and sexuality.
- Unsure About Your Pregnancy? A Guide To Making The Right Decision For You: https://www.prochoice.org/pubs_research/publications/downloads/are_you_pregnant/pregnancy_guide_english.pdf
  This is a booklet for women considering parenthood, adoption, or abortion, offering a neutral discussion of ideas, with questions to prompt self-reflection and writing space.
- Faith Aloud: http://www.faithaloud.org/clergycounseling/
  Offers free counseling by clergy and religious counselors, from a variety of denominations (Catholic, Jewish, Unitarian-Universalist, Protestant Christian, and Buddhist), for women with spiritual concerns about pregnancy or abortion.

- AccessMatters Hotline: http://accessmatters.org or (215) 985-2600. Connects individuals to information about sexual and reproductive health including education, counseling, and referrals to local health centers.

Develop a care plan. For patients who would like to continue their pregnancy, a plan of care needs to be established and should cover the following topics:
- Initiation of prenatal care, or referral to a clinician who can provide prenatal care
- Review of current medications to ensure there is no risk of fetal harm
- Initiation of prenatal vitamins
- Information on a healthy lifestyle and diet in pregnancy
  - Tobacco cessation
  - Avoiding alcohol and recreational drugs
  - Maintaining regular exercise or initiating an exercise regimen (such as daily walks)
  - Foods recommended in pregnancy (i.e., high protein, iron-rich)
  - Foods that should be limited or avoided in pregnancy (e.g., caffeine, cold cuts, unpasteurized cheeses, high-mercury fish)
  - Basic information for dealing with early pregnancy discomforts
  - Recruiting support from family and friends
  - Referrals to the appropriate social services for food, transportation, shelter, etc.

For the patient who has decided to have an abortion, the referring providers should be able to provide patients with contact information for local, trusted abortion providers and have general knowledge of the different options for pregnancy termination. A referral list based on personal knowledge from self, colleagues, or patient past experiences is helpful to patients and preferable to directing the patient to check online. Patients with psychiatric symptoms or disorders, or those struggling with their decision, would likely benefit from additional referrals to the appropriate mental health resources. Patients choosing termination should also be provided information about post-termination contraception to avoid a subsequent unplanned pregnancy.

For the patient who has chosen adoption for her infant, the provider should be able to provide contact information for local adoption lawyers, agencies, and/or counselors; professional counseling and support services are critical to prepare for the legal termination of parental rights and to assist the woman with some of the psychological, social, and financial aspects of releasing her infant. The patient should be encouraged not to view adoption as an indication of lack of love for her infant or as an indication that she is any less of a mother than a woman who keeps her infant; instead, the choice of adoption can be viewed as a selfless maternal act of caring for her infant, in which the patient is ensuring the best possible outcome for her child.

Indications for Referral

Referrals are based on a woman's intentions regarding her pregnancy. Providers need to be aware of resources in the community to support each woman's choices. Any clinician who feels he or she is unable to provide unbiased, accurate information regarding all available pregnancy options to a woman presenting with an unplanned pregnancy should facilitate swift referral to a qualified provider for counseling and management.

There may be situations in which a patient with an unplanned pregnancy must see a specialist immediately. These situations include:

- A patient who verbalizes thoughts of hurting herself or others
- A patient who is in immediate danger because of domestic or sexual violence
- A patient who is experiencing bleeding and/or severe pelvic or abdominal pain
- A patient who is confident in her decision to have an abortion and presents for care in either the late first trimester or during the second trimester of pregnancy.

LIFE SPAN CONSIDERATIONS

The high prevalence of unintended pregnancy is surprising, given that contraception is widely available in the United States. Although approximately 62% of women aged 15 to 44 years used contraception in 2006 to 2008, the proportions were significantly lower in four groups: teenagers 15 to 19 years of age (28%); never married, non-cohabitating women, some of whom are teens (39%); childless women (44%); and women who intend to have (more) children in the future (47%).[5] Reasons for lack of contraceptive use differ according to the age of the woman and the circumstances surrounding the event. In a nationally representative survey of adult US women who were at risk of unintended pregnancy, approximately one-third of women who tried to obtain or refill a prescription for hormonal contraception (pill, patch, or ring) reported difficulties in doing so. The most commonly cited barriers to prescription access were restrictive costs or lacking insurance coverage, difficulty obtaining an appointment or getting to a clinic, and the provider requiring a clinic visit, pap smear, or exam before providing a prescription.[36] For younger women, contraceptive nonuse at first intercourse and hence unintended pregnancy are often related to concerns that parents would find out about sexual activity. Conversely, older women with a second or higher-order pregnancy are more likely to discontinue contraception because of its side effects and medical complications.[2] Interestingly, experts estimate that 48% of the unintended pregnancies in the United States occur in women who use contraception but are not using it correctly.[37] Of note, in 2013, adolescent pregnancies—as well as the births and abortions that follow—declined to historic lows among young women in the United States. In fact, the pregnancy rate among women aged 15 to 19 reached its lowest level in at least 80 years, with the observed decline in pregnancy rates among young women being driven by improvements in contraceptive use.[7]

Although three-fourths of reproductive-age women see a health care provider annually, less than 50% receive contraceptive or family planning services.[38] Because women receive most of their preventive care from nongynecologic providers, PCPs have a unique opportunity to provide contraceptive counseling to prevent unintended pregnancy.[39] Studies suggest that PCPs vary in their knowledge and perceived competence in providing contraceptive counseling. In addition, PCPs may inaccurately assess a woman's need for contraceptive counseling, misunderstand reasons for contraceptive nonuse, relegate the responsibility for contraceptive counseling to a subspecialist, or wait for the patient to initiate the discussion about contraception.[39] PCPs should ask women about their life plans and reproductive intentions. This includes an assessment of whether their patients wish to be parents, have had any children, how many children they have had, as well as if and when they want more children. The answers to these questions can help guide appropriate care for women of childbearing age.

Providers should also be sensitive to the fact that many women have no intention of bearing children or raising children—this is often referred to as "childless by choice." This can be a sensitive topic for many women due to cultural, societal, and familial expectations; providers looking to engage in conversations regarding childbearing intentions, contraceptive choices, and pregnancy options should be mindful to not impose any personal expectations, biases, or judgments when caring for and counseling these women.

PCPs are in a unique position to reach a large number of women at risk of an unintended pregnancy. As such, clinicians should aim to be proactive in knowing their patient's childbearing goals and providing women with the appropriate care needed to attain them. For women who express concerns about the risks of contraception or indifference to becoming pregnant, it is important for providers to balance this with a discussion of the potential risks inherent in unintended pregnancy and the benefits of planning childbearing.

COMPLICATIONS

Unplanned pregnancy has different associated risks, depending on whether the pregnancy was unwanted or mistimed. According to a study comparing the mood states and parental attitudes of mothers with unplanned pregnancies, women with unplanned pregnancies demonstrate greater mood disturbances during their last month of pregnancy and during the first year postpartum than do women with planned pregnancies. In particular, during the last month of pregnancy, women with unintended pregnancies had greater levels of anxiety, depression, irritability, weariness, and confusion than women with planned pregnancies.[40]

For any woman facing an unplanned pregnancy, whatever decision she makes regarding its outcome will have unique, long-term health consequences that should be recognized and considered by her health care provider. As evidenced above, one of the most important factors that reduce negative outcomes in this population is the presence of adequate emotional and social supports.

PATIENT AND FAMILY EDUCATION

- Health care providers are in a unique position to provide counseling regarding pregnancy options for women experiencing an unplanned pregnancy. The quality of the counseling provided to patients is rooted in the clinician's commitment to respecting patient autonomy, providing evidence-based information, and supporting women in their choices.
- It is helpful to give the patient written information to refer to as she goes through the decision-making process. Providers should prepare ahead of time for these interactions by educating themselves on, and having materials available detailing, the local resources for social services, abortion care, and adoption services.
- PCPs also have a responsibility to initiate conversations regarding short- and long-term reproductive plans and contraception. PCPs should ensure they are up to date regarding contraceptive options and offering these to patients who are at risk of unplanned or unwanted pregnancies.

HEALTH PROMOTION

The woman with an unplanned pregnancy faces a difficult decision—one that is likely to have a lifelong impact. All women have the right to be informed and counseled about every legal pregnancy option. PCPs should take the following steps: (1) inform the pregnant woman of the options, which include carrying the pregnancy and raising the infant, carrying the pregnancy to delivery and making an adoption plan, or terminating the pregnancy; (2) be prepared to provide a pregnant woman with basic, accurate information about each of these options, support her in the decision-making process, and assist in making connections with community resources that will provide her with quality services during and after her pregnancy; and (3) examine their own beliefs and values to determine if they can provide nonjudgmental, factual pregnancy options counseling. If they cannot, they should facilitate a prompt referral for counseling by another knowledgeable professional in their practice setting or community who is willing to have such discussions with patients.

REFERENCES

1. Unintended Pregnancy in the United States. (2016, September). Retrieved from https://www.guttmacher.org/fact-sheet/unintended-pregnancy-united-states.
2. Iuliano, A., Speizer, I., Santelli, J., et al. (2006). Reasons for contraceptive nonuse at first sex and unintended pregnancy. *American Journal of Health Behavior, 30*(1), 92–102.
3. D'Angelo, D., Gilbert, B., Rochat, R., et al. (2004). Differences between mistimed and unwanted pregnancies among women who have live births. *Perspectives on Sexual and Reproductive Health, 36*(5), 192–197.
4. Aquilino, M., & Losch, M. (2005). Fertility across the lifespan: Desire for pregnancy at conception. *The American Journal of Maternal/Child Nursing, 30*(4), 256–262.
5. Mosher, W., & Jones, J. (2010). Use of contraception in the United States: 1982–2008, National Center for Health Statistics. *Vital Health Statistics, 23*(29), 1–44.
6. Frost, J. (2011). The state of hormonal contraception today: Overview of unintended pregnancy in the United States. *American Journal of Obstetrics and Gynecology, 205*(4), S1–S3.
7. Kost, K., Maddow-Zimet, I., & Arpaia, A. (2017, September). Pregnancies, Births and Abortions Among Adolescents and Young Women in the United States, 2013: National and State Trends by Age, Race and Ethnicity. Retrieved from https://www.guttmacher.org/report/us-adolescent-pregnancy-trends-2013.
8. Khajehpour, M., Simbar, M., Jannesari, S., et al. (2013). Health status of women with intended and unintended pregnancies. *Public Health, 127*(1), 58–64.
9. Nelson, J., & O'Brien, M. (2012). Does an unplanned pregnancy have long-term implications for mother-child relationships. *Journal of Family Issues, 33*(4), 506–526.
10. Brunner Huber, L., Lyerly, J., Farley, K., et al. (2013). Identifying women at risk of unintended pregnancy: A comparison of two pregnancy readiness measures. *Annals of Epidemiology, 23*(7), 441–443.
11. Sonfield, A., Kost, K., Gold, R., et al. (2011). The public costs of births resulting from unintended pregnancies: National and State-Level estimates. *Perspectives on Sexual & Reproductive Health, 43*(2), 94–102.
12. McCloskey, L. A., Williams, C. M., Lichter, E., et al. (2007). Abused women disclose partner interference with health care: An unrecognized form of battering. *Journal of General Internal Medicine, 22*, 1067.
13. Roth, L., Sheeder, J., & Teal, S. B. (2011). Predictors of intimate partner violence in women seeking medication abortion. *Contraception, 84*, 76.
14. Gilbert, K. (2013). Commercial speech in crisis: Crisis pregnancy center regulations and definitions of commercial speech. *Michigan Law Review, 111*(4), 591–616.
15. Bryant, A., Narasimhana, S., Bryant-Comstock, K., et al. (2014). Crisis pregnancy center websites: Information, misinformation and disinformation. *Contraception, 90*, 601–605.
16. Jatlaoui, T., Ewing, A., Mandel1, M., Simmons, K., et al. (2016). Abortion surveillance—United States, 2013. *MMWR. Surveillance Summaries, 65*(12), 1–44.
17. Pazol, K., Zane, S. B., Parker, W. Y., et al. (2011). Abortion surveillance—United States, 2008. *MMWR. Surveillance Summaries, 60*, 1.
18. Finer, L., & Zolna, M. (2011). Unintended pregnancy in the United States: Incidence and disparities, 2006. *Contraception, 84*, 478.
19. Jones, R., & Jerman, J. (2014). Abortion incidence and service availability in the United States, 2011. *Perspectives on Sexual and Reproductive Health, 46*(1), 3–14.
20. Upadhyay, U. D., Desai, S., Zlidar, V., et al. (2015). Incidence of emergency department visits and complications after abortion. *Obstetrics and Gynecology, 125*, 175.
21. Grimes, D. (2006). Estimation of pregnancy-related mortality risk by pregnancy outcome, United States, 1991 to 1999. *American Journal of Obstetrics and Gynecology, 194*, 92–94.
22. Raymond, E., Grossman, D., Weaver, M., et al. (2014). Mortality of induced abortion, other outpatient surgical procedures and common activities in the United States. *Contraception, 90*, 476.
23. Boonstra, H., Gold, R., Richards, C., et al. (2006, May). Abortion in women's lives. Retrieved from https://www.guttmacher.org/report/abortion-womens-lives.
24. Committee on Gynecologic Practice. (2009). ACOG committee opinion no. 434: Induced abortion and breast cancer risk. *Obstetrics and Gynecology, 113*(6), 1417–1418.
25. Major, B., Appelbaum, M., Beckman, L., et al. (2008). American Psychological Association. Report of the APA task force on mental health and abortion. Retrieved from http://www.apa.org/pi/women/programs/abortion/mental-health.pdf.
26. Steinberg, J., McCullouch, C., & Adler, N. (2014). Abortion and mental health: Findings from The National Comorbidity Survey-Replication. *Obstetrics and Gynecology, 123*, 263.
27. Steinberg, J., Becker, D., & Henderson, J. (2011). Does the outcome of a first pregnancy predict depression, suicidal ideation or lower self-esteem? Data from the National Comorbidity Survey. *The American Journal of Orthopsychiatry, 81*, 193.
28. Jones, R., & Kooistra, K. (2011). Abortion incidence and access to services in the United States, 2008. *Perspectives on Sexual and Reproductive Health, 43*(1), 41–50.
29. Jerman, J., Jones, R., & Onda, T. (2016, May). Characteristics of U.S. Abortion Patients in 2014 and Changes Since 2008. Retrieved from https://www.guttmacher.org/report/characteristics-us-abortion-patients-2014.
30. Child Welfare Information Gateway. (2016). *Trends in U.S. adoptions: 2008–12.* Washington, DC: U.S. Department of Health and Human Services, Children's Bureau. Retrieved from https://www.childwelfare.gov/pubPDFs/adopted0812.pdf.
31. Coleman, P., & Garratt, D. (2016). From birth mothers to first mothers: Toward a compassionate understanding of the life-long act of adoption placement. *Issues in Law and Medicine, 31*(2), 139–163.
32. Foli, K., South, S., & Lim, E. (2012). Rates and predictors of postadoption depression in adoptive mothers: Moving toward theory. *ANS. Advances in Nursing Science, 35*(1), 51–63.
33. Wiley, M. O., & Baden, A. L. (2005). Birth parents in adoption: Research, practice and counseling psychology. *The Counseling Psychologist, 33*, 13–50.
34. Henman, J. (2005). Giving pregnancy teens another option: Teaching about adoption. *The International Journal of Childbirth Education, 20*(2), 22–24.
35. Namerow, P., Kalmuss, D., & Cushman, L. (1997). The consequences of placing versus parenting among unmarried women. *Marriage and Family Review, 25*, 175–197.
36. Grindlay, K., & Grossman, D. (2017). Prescription birth control access among U.S. Women at risk of unintended pregnancy. *Journal of Women's Health, 25*(3), 249–254.
37. Trussel, J., Henry, N., Hassan, F., et al. (2013). Burden of unintended pregnancy in the United States: Potential savings with increased use of long-acting reversible contraception. *Contraception, 87*(2), 154–161.
38. Singer, J. (2004). Options counseling: Techniques for caring for women with unintended pregnancies. *Journal of Midwifery & Women's Health, 49*(3), 235–242.
39. Akers, A. Y., Gold, M. A., Borrero, S., et al. (2010). Providers' perspectives on challenges to contraceptive counseling in primary care settings. *Journal of Women's Health, 19*(6), 1163–1170.
40. Grussu, P., Quatraro, R., & Nasta, M. (2005). Profile of mood states: Comparing women with planned and unplanned pregnancies. *Birth (Berkeley, Calif.), 32*(2), 107–114.

VULVAR AND VAGINAL DISORDERS

Heidi Collins Fantasia

VULVAR DISORDERS

DEFINITION AND EPIDEMIOLOGY

Benign vulvar disorders, which encompass a broad range of dermatologic conditions, account for significant patient concerns. Women may delay seeking treatment because of fear, embarrassment, or confusion over which health care provider would best understand their condition. Therefore symptoms may be present for some time before women seek care. Signs and symptoms of benign vulvar disorders can include pruritus, pain, burning, irritation, and a mass and/or growth. Women have often tried nonprescription remedies before coming to a provider.[1]

Pruritus is often the chief patient complaint for most vulvar disorders, and skin breakdown is common from scratching. Vulvar pruritus is a nonspecific vulvar symptom that may be unrelated to vaginitis, sexually transmitted infections (STIs), Bartholin duct cysts, or neoplasms. Proper treatment of vulvar pruritus depends on an accurate diagnosis. Women with vulvar pruritus often receive multiple treatments in the absence of a correct diagnosis; women are commonly prescribed therapy over the phone without ever having been examined, even if symptoms have been recurrent.[2]

In examining women with vulvar pruritus, the provider is advised to ask about and to inspect other areas of the body; many conditions affecting other organ systems, including tuberculosis, Crohn's disease, and endometriosis, can have vulvar manifestations. For example, vulvar psoriasis may have an unusual presentation, but more typical psoriatic lesions are often seen simultaneously elsewhere on the body and may provide a diagnostic clue. Even with an experienced clinician, several visits may be needed to diagnose and to improve certain vulvovaginal conditions.

The visual inspection is essential in identifying vulvar changes. A handheld magnifying glass, or in some cases a colposcope, may allow more detailed inspection. Vaginitis, cervicitis, and other STIs should be excluded. Some of the common vulvar conditions causing pruritus are presented in this chapter.

LICHEN SCLEROSUS

Pathophysiology

Lichen sclerosus (LS) is a chronic condition with an unclear cause. Multiple factors are most likely involved in the development of this disorder. LS can have an autoimmune component, and women with LS may also develop other autoimmune diseases such as thyroid disorders, anemia, vitiligo, and alopecia areata. It has also been postulated that LS may be triggered by an infectious process, a genetic predisposition, and decreased estrogen levels.[3]

LS is primarily seen in perimenopausal and postmenopausal women, and the incidence increases with age. Although LS can occur in females of all ages, postmenopausal women are affected more frequently than women of other age groups. It has been associated with autoimmune diseases in approximately 28% of individuals.[3] It also affects males but at rates much lower than in females. LS is primarily found in the anogenital region, but it can be seen elsewhere on the body, such as the neck and shoulders.

Clinical Presentation and Physical Examination

Although it is sometimes asymptomatic, LS often results in severe vulvar pruritus and/or dyspareunia. Affected areas include the labia minora, vulvar vestibule, perineum, and clitoris; the vagina is usually spared. Early LS can be particularly difficult to diagnose. Early in the disease process, women may report vague vulvar burning and generalized irritation or itching that is difficult for them to localize and quantify. On examination, white papules can be seen, and the epithelium may appear normal or thin, resembling parchment.[3] Typically, tissue elasticity is decreased and edema may be present, depending on the disease stage. Fissures and secondary infections may develop, especially with sexual activity or scratching, which may make diagnosis especially difficult. With disease progression, papules develop into large, hypopigmented, symmetric plaques, often hourglass or keyhole shaped, on the labia minora, vulva, and anal area, which can resemble hyperplasia.[3] If these are not treated, there is eventual loss of vulvar architecture such that the labia minora are no longer seen, and introital stenosis may develop, resulting in dyspareunia, ecchymosis, fissures, and telangiectasis.

Diagnostics

Essential Diagnostics. A thorough history must be obtained to assess timing, onset, location, and duration of symptoms and any factors that may alleviate or aggravate the condition. A physical examination will allow the provider to visualize any skin changes. This exam may be performed with a handheld magnifying glass or colposcope to improve visualization of the skin. A punch biopsy of the affected area will confirm the diagnosis if examination findings are inconclusive. Biopsy is also important to exclude atypia or mixed diagnoses. Findings on histologic examination include hyperkeratosis, epithelial thinning, cytoplasmic vacuolation of the basal layer of cells, follicular plugging, homogenization of the subepithelial layer, and inflammatory cell infiltration consisting of lymphocytes with few plasma cells.

Additional Diagnostics. A complete blood count (CBC) can be obtained if infection is suspected from scratching or skin breakdown. Autoimmune laboratory tests including thyroid function tests, antinuclear antibodies, and vitamin B_{12} can be ordered, but autoimmune testing is not routinely done, because the link between an autoimmune process and LS is not strong enough to justify the expense of the laboratory work.

Differential Diagnosis

It is important to establish the correct diagnosis of LS. This condition requires long-term treatment. Women should be prepared for the chronicity of the disorder and expected length of time to symptom improvement.

 Priority differentials include (1) lichen planus (LP), (2) atrophic vaginitis with atrophy, (3) contact or allergic dermatitis, (4) fungal infection, and (5) vitiligo.

Interprofessional Collaborative Management

Pharmacologic Management

Topical Steroids. Ultra-potent topical corticosteroids currently provide the best outcomes,[3] with initial treatment recommended for 4 to 6 weeks. Clobetasol, halobetasol, or betamethasone dipropionate augmented 0.05% in an ointment base are recommended. A typical regimen is a thin layer of steroid applied to the affected area once or twice daily for 2 to 4 weeks, then tapered to three times per week for maintenance therapy.[1] Long-term sequelae of potent topical corticosteroids (atrophy and thinning of skin and subcutaneous tissues) have not been clinically significant in this disorder because the vulvar skin is steroid resistant and can tolerate long-term application of superpotent steroids. Contact dermatitis is a rare but reported side effect of this medication. Subsequent LS recurrences are managed by reinstating the corticosteroid therapy.[3] It may be appropriate to switch to a milder corticosteroid such as betamethasone valerate 1% (high potency) or triamcinolone ointment 0.1% or fluocinolone acetonide ointment 0.025% (moderate potency) for long-term management.

Topical Antibiotic Ointment. Topical antibiotic ointment can be used to treat signs of mild infection caused by scratching and excoriation.

Topical Estrogen. Application of topical estrogen cream can improve symptoms if LS exists in the presence of menopausal vulvovaginal atrophy.

Oral Antihistamines. Prescription (e.g., hydroxyzine, 25 to 50 mg) and over-the-counter (OTC) (e.g., diphenhydramine, 25 to 50 mg) antihistamines given at bedtime may also help relieve pruritus associated with LS.

Other Medications. Immunosuppressant agents such as topical calcineurin inhibitors have documented efficacy in the treatment of patients with vulvar LS. They can be considered for women who are refractory to or intolerant of topical corticosteroid medications. Topical retinoids such as acitretin can also be used.

Nonpharmacologic Management.
Other relief measures to consider include the application of cool compresses and cool soaks and wearing loose-fitting clothing.

Indications for Referral

A referral is indicated for biopsy results that indicate hyperplasia or atypia. Surgical consultation is warranted if there is evidence of severe architectural changes or scarring. Women with LS have a slightly increased risk of developing squamous cell carcinoma. If there is evidence of severe architectural changes and/or vaginal, urethral, or anal stenosis, a surgical consultation is warranted. Patients who do not respond to a course of topical, high-potency steroids or who report ongoing pain should be referred to a gynecologic dermatology specialist. Other treatment modalities can include oral tricyclic antidepressants (amitriptyline, nortriptyline) and steroid injections.

Life Span Considerations

LS is more common among menopausal women and may exist in the presence of atrophy related to estrogen deficiency. In addition, skin changes associated with aging predispose skin to trauma owing to thinning and decreased elasticity.

Complications

Thin, nonelastic tissue associated with LS can cause stenosis of the vaginal opening and result in painful intercourse (dyspareunia). This can often be corrected with topical steroids and/or estrogen therapy. A more serious complication is permanent scarring; surgery may be required to lyse adhesions and restore vulvovaginal functioning.

Patient and Family Education

LS requires a long-term treatment plan that will span the lifetime. Women should be educated that this condition is chronic and episodes of symptom control will be interwoven with disease exacerbations. Each woman will respond differently to steroid treatment, and it may take some time and different dosing regimens to discover the best treatment plan. Women who are sexually active will need guidance on methods to reduce dyspareunia. General patient education information for all women with vaginal and vulvar complaints is listed in Box 153.1.

Health Promotion

The exact etiology of LS is unknown. Women should be reassured that they did not cause the condition due to any specific behavior or lifestyle habit. Maintaining skin integrity is essential, and women should be encouraged to avoid scratching or irritating the vulvar skin. Because women with LS have a slightly higher risk of squamous cell carcinoma, the importance of yearly skin checks should be stressed.

LICHEN PLANUS

Pathophysiology

LP is an acute or chronic inflammatory dermatosis affecting the skin, scalp, and the mucous membranes of the mouth, vulva, and vagina. The frequency of LP varies according to the population studied, but there is an estimated prevalence of up to 4% of the women in the United States.[3] LP affects middle-aged people most, often in the 5th or 6th decade of life, although childhood LP has been described in the literature. Women are affected as often as men.[3] Although the exact cause of LP is not known, it is thought to be a T-cell-mediated autoimmune disorder.[3]

Clinical Presentation and Physical Examination

In the genital area, there are two presentations of LP: classic or erosive.[3] The appearance of classic LP includes well-defined delicate, white, reticulated papules. Erosive LP involves the presence of erythematous, erosive lesions and a desquamating process. Large denuded areas may lead to profuse leukorrhea or can become adherent, causing stenosis of the vaginal introitus.

Physical examination findings can vary with vulvar LP. Erythema is possible, as well as erosions and a lacy appearance on the skin. As with LS, the examination may reveal architectural changes that include loss of genital features, scarring of the vulva and anus, and urethral and vaginal stenosis. Women with LP often complain of a variety of vulvar symptoms, including pain, pruritus, burning, dyspareunia, and dysuria.

Diagnostics

Essential Diagnostics. Diagnosis is established based on a thorough history and clinical examination findings. A physical examination is performed to visualize any skin changes, and the use of a handheld magnifying glass or colposcope can improve visualization of the skin.

Biopsy of the affected area will confirm diagnosis if examination findings are inconclusive. Findings on histologic examination include chronic inflammation, presence of lymphocytes with few plasma cells, colloid bodies, and acanthosis and thinning of the epithelium.

Additional Diagnostics. Erosive LP may also have clinical features of herpes simplex virus (HSV) and Bechet disease. A viral culture for HSV can be obtained if there is an erosive presentation. Autoimmune or allergy testing can be performed to help establish a diagnosis.

Differential Diagnosis

Because LP may have two different clinical presentations, establishing a correct diagnosis can be challenging. As with LS, this is a chronic condition that requires long-term treatment. Symptoms will vary depending on presentation (classic versus erosive), and women should be prepared for the chronicity of the disorder and expected length of time to symptom improvement.

Priority differentials include (1) LS, (2) ulcerative STIs such as HSV, syphilis, and chancroid, (3) Bechet disease, (4) contact or allergic dermatitis, (5) atrophic vaginitis with atrophy, and (6) fungal infection.

Interprofessional Collaborative Management

Pharmacologic Management

Topical Steroids. Superpotent corticosteroids are the first-line treatment. Clobetasol, halobetasol, or betamethasone dipropionate augmented 0.05% in an ointment base is recommended. A typical regimen is a thin layer of steroid applied to the affected area once or twice daily for 2 to 4 weeks, then tapered to three times per week for maintenance therapy.[3] Long-term sequelae of potent topical corticosteroids (atrophy and thinning of skin and subcutaneous tissues) have not been clinically significant in this disorder because the vulvar skin is steroid resistant and can tolerate long-term application of superpotent steroids. Contact dermatitis is a rare but reported side effect of this medication. The frequency of maintenance applications of topical steroids will vary depending on individual response and extent of the disease. Lifelong management is necessary to decrease pain and scarring.

Topical Antibiotic Ointment. Topical antibiotic ointment can be used to treat signs of mild infection caused by scratching and excoriation.

Topical Barrier Ointment. Petrolatum ointment may be applied as a barrier for sensitive skin.

Topical Estrogen. Application of topical estrogen cream can improve symptoms if LP exists in the presence of menopausal vulvovaginal atrophy.

Oral Antihistamines. Prescription (e.g., hydroxyzine, 25 to 50 mg) and OTC (e.g., diphenhydramine, 25 to 50 mg) antihistamines given at bedtime may also help relieve pruritus associated with LP.

Other Medications. Immunosuppressant agents such as topical calcineurin inhibitors have resulted in symptom improvement for women with vulvar LP, although recurrence rate after treatment has been reported at almost 85%.[3]

Nonpharmacologic Management. Photodynamic therapy may be considered. In a small clinical trial patients reported symptom resolution that was comparable to topical steroids.[4]

Indications for Referral

If there is indication of atypia, hyperplasia, or a mixed diagnosis on biopsy, a gynecologic referral is indicated, especially in older women. If there is evidence of severe architectural changes and/or vaginal, urethral, or anal stenosis, a surgical consultation is warranted. The role of surgery is limited; surgery is used only to repair introital stenosis, adhesions, or confirmed malignant disease.[3] Women who do not respond to a course of topical, high-potency steroids or who report ongoing pain should be referred to a gynecologic dermatology specialist and possibly a pain management specialist.

The primary goals of treatment are symptom relief and prevention of disease progression. LP requires lifelong management and treatment that is similar to that for LS.

Life Span Considerations

LP often manifests at midlife. For women, this often coincides with the perimenopausal and postmenopausal years. LP may exist in the presence of atrophy related to estrogen deficiency, which can further increase discomfort. In addition, skin changes associated with aging predispose skin to trauma as a result of thinning, decreased elasticity, and a decreased ability to act as a first-line protection against injury.

Complications

Severe LP can cause significant pain, decreased quality of life, and interference with daily activities. Thin, nonelastic tissue associated with classic LP can cause stenosis of the vaginal opening and result in painful intercourse. This can often be corrected with topical steroids and/or estrogen therapy. A more serious complication is permanent scarring; surgery may be required to lyse adhesions and restore vulvovaginal functioning. Erosive LP can cause chronic pain, sexual dysfunction, and dysuria.

Patient and Family Education

Symptom management may involve a multidisciplinary approach that includes gynecologists, dermatologists, pain specialists, and pelvic floor physical therapy. The use of vaginal dilators may be necessary to prevent scarring and stenosis of the vaginal introitus. Women with LP should receive education on general vulvar care, including loose-fitting clothing; mild soaps; gentle patting of the vulvar area to dry; mild laundry detergent; cotton underwear; and sleeping without underwear or pajama bottoms. See Box 153.1.

Health Promotion

Similar to LS, LP is a chronic condition that requires treatment over the life span. Symptoms and subsequent treatment will vary depending on whether the woman has classic or erosive LP. Pain is common with LP and can significantly affect a woman's quality of life and sexual functioning. Routine gynecologic and multidisciplinary care should be encouraged.

LICHEN SIMPLEX CHRONICUS
Pathophysiology

Lichen simplex chronicus (LSC), or squamous cell hyperplasia, is the result of repetitive surface trauma from irritants that cause scratching or rubbing—a perpetual itch-scratch cycle. LSC is characterized histologically by epithelial thickening, lichenification, hyperkeratosis, and eczematous inflammation. It manifests, as do most of the non-neoplastic epithelial disorders, as pruritus, which may be secondary to degeneration and inflammation of terminal nerve fibers. The cause is not completely known, but atopic dermatitis is a common finding in women affected by LSC.

Clinical Presentation and Physical Examination

Intense itching (vulvar pruritus) is often the chief complaint. The pruritus may be aggravated by friction, heat, perspiration, or tight clothing. The affected woman may complain of a history of chronic scratching, which causes further pruritus. The pruritus often occurs at night and therefore sleep disturbances and fatigue are common. Painful erosions and fissures can result from the chronic scratching.

LSC may affect the labia majora, outer aspect of the labia minora, and anal area. On examination, the skin may exhibit thickening, and fissures are possible. Often, LSC initially manifests with small red papules. Reddened plaques develop from the papules, or if the condition has been ongoing without treatment, the skin may be more deeply colored, rough, and furrowed. Areas of excoriation are common.[3]

Diagnostics

Essential Diagnostics. The condition is difficult to differentiate from other pruritic vulvar conditions. Diagnosis is made by history of chronic pruritus with scratching and examination findings that support LSC. The underlying cause of the pruritus is often not immediately apparent. A physical examination will reveal skin changes. Magnification is often not needed. A

punch biopsy of the affected area will confirm the diagnosis if examination findings are inconclusive. Biopsy is also important to exclude other pruritic vulvar conditions such as LS, LP, and eczema and to exclude atypia. The most important areas from which biopsy specimens should be taken are those of fissuring, ulceration, induration, and thick plaques. Findings on histologic examination include lichenification, hyperkeratosis, and chronic inflammation.

Differential Diagnosis

Because LSC has a presentation and symptoms similar to those of many other pruritic vulvar conditions, it is important to establish a correct diagnosis. Treatment for LSC focuses on interrupting the itch-scratch cycle.

 Priority differentials include (1) LS, (2) LP, (3) psoriasis, (4) eczema, (5) allergic dermatitis, and (6) fungal infection.

Interprofessional Collaborative Management
Pharmacologic Management

Topical Steroids. Topical steroids applied twice daily will reduce inflammation. Choice of strength will depend on the patient's subjective report of severity and examination findings. Superpotent steroids (clobetasol, halobetasol) can be initiated if symptoms are severe. Moderate-potency (betamethasone valerate) or low-potency (hydrocortisone 2.5%) steroids can also be used for milder cases.

Topical Barriers. After the skin is thoroughly dried, an emollient such as petrolatum can be applied as a skin barrier.

Oral Antihistamines. Systemic antihistamines such as diphenhydramine, doxepin, or hydroxyzine taken at bedtime will reduce nighttime pruritus and scratching.[3]

Tricyclic Antidepressants. Tricyclic antidepressants such as amitriptyline taken at bedtime will also help control pruritus.[3]

Nonpharmacologic Management. Removing any potential skin irritants is imperative. Skin should be gently patted dry and any wet clothing changed immediately. Women should avoid scented or irritating soaps, lotions, and powders.

Consultation: Referral

If there is indication of atypia, hyperplasia, or a mixed diagnosis on biopsy, a gynecologic referral is indicated, especially in older women. Women who do not respond to a course of steroids, who report ongoing pain, or who have a superimposed skin infection that has not responded to antibiotics should be referred to a gynecologic dermatology physician.

If an underlying allergic component is suspected, consultation with an allergist is important to identify allergens. LSC can have a psychological component to the chronic pruritus and scratching. Mental health evaluation and treatment may be appropriate for some women.[3]

Life Span Considerations

Although LSC can occur in children, it most often occurs after age 30 and can coincide with the menopausal transition later in life. This is a chronic condition that women will need to manage throughout the midlife and older adult years. Aging skin is more susceptible to trauma from scratching, and advising patients to wear soft cotton gloves to bed may help reduce skin breakdown from scratching. As women age, urinary incontinence is common and wet skin from exposure to urine increases the risk of excoriation and infection. LSC in the presence of atrophy from estrogen deficiency of menopause may need to be treated with topical estrogen therapy.

Complications

LSC can cause skin changes such as hypopigmentation or hyperpigmentation that may be permanent. The severe pruritus that is a hallmark symptom of LSC can cause sleep disturbances, fatigue, and decreased quality of life. Skin breakdown places patients at risk for superimposed bacterial and fungal infections that can be painful. Decreased sexual function from pruritus and pain is possible.

Patient and Family Education

Similar to LS and LP, LSC is a chronic condition that requires treatment over the life span. Tricyclic antidepressants at bedtime are often prescribed to help control itching and scratching symptoms and not to control depressive symptoms. Women need education regarding their treatment plan and the multifaceted approach to the management of this disorder.

Health Promotion

LSC is a chronic and often frustrating disease for women. The constant itching can result in sleep disturbances, fatigue, and irritability. Women should be encouraged to explore all options for increasing their comfort, decreasing pruritus, and obtaining optional sleep.

CONTACT DERMATITIS
Pathophysiology

Contact dermatitis of the vulvovaginal area results when the area comes in contact with an allergen or irritant. This causes localized inflammation and edema. Pruritus is common. Contact dermatitis occurs when there is an immediate irritation of the area after exposure to an offending substance. Allergic responses, on the other hand, develop several days after exposure.[5]

Clinical Presentation and Physical Examination

Women with vulvar contact dermatitis often report a recent onset of vulvar irritation, pruritus, burning, soreness, or discomfort. These symptoms often become worse with friction, or if the skin is wet. Dysuria may result when acidic urine passes over inflamed or excoriated skin. On examination, erythema is typically present, and excoriation can result from scratching. Skin may be thickened if contact with the irritant or allergen has occurred over an extended period of time. Vaginal discharge is not common.

Diagnostics

Essential Diagnostics. A diagnosis is established through physical examination; a thorough history is critical to a correct diagnosis. Physical examination findings that suggest contact dermatitis include erythema or edema. No specific laboratory tests are indicated.

Additional Diagnostics. A punch biopsy may be considered if LS, LP, or LSC is suspected in addition to the contact dermatitis

Differential Diagnosis

Vulvar pruritus, irritation, burning, and pain are associated with a variety of vulvar conditions. Although erythema and edema are hallmark symptoms of contact dermatitis, other vulvar conditions must be considered.

Priority differentials include (1) LS, (2) LP, (3) LSC, and (4) fungal infection.

Interprofessional Collaborative Management
Pharmacologic Management

Topical Steroids. Allergic dermatitis usually takes a long time to resolve after exposure is terminated; resolution may be facilitated by a short course of topical steroids. The use of a low-potency topical steroid (triamcinolone 0.1% or hydrocortisone 2.5%) can be useful to bring acute symptoms under control.

Oral Antihistamines. Prescription (e.g., hydroxyzine, 25 to 50 mg) and OTC (e.g., diphenhydramine, 25 to 50 mg) antihistamines given at bedtime may also help relieve pruritus associated with contact dermatitis.

Nonpharmacologic Management. After removal of the irritant, Burow compresses, sitz baths, or emollients may improve symptoms.[5]

Consultations: Referral

Contact dermatitis can often be successfully managed without the need for specialist referral. A referral is indicated for women who do not respond to standard treatment or appear to worsen.

If an allergic component is suspected, then a referral to an allergist is appropriate.

Complications

Serious complications from contact dermatitis are rare. Pruritus can lead to scratching and possible skin breakdown and superimposed bacterial and fungal infections. Decreased sexual function from pruritus and discomfort is possible.

Patient and Family Education

Contact dermatitis of the vulva can be a very frustrating condition for women. The list of potential irritants and allergens is extensive, and it may take some time to uncover the causative agent. Trial and error are involved while specific agents are eliminated, and this involves patience and time.

Health Promotion

The goal of management is identifying the triggering substance and eliminating it. The list of possible irritants is extensive (Box 153.2). Women should be asked about treatments to the vulva (either prescribed or OTC medications) and use of feminine hygiene products (such as douches, sprays, and deodorants), tampons or pads, condoms, spermicides, lubricants, laundry detergents, soaps, and shampoos.

ECZEMA AND PSORIASIS
Pathophysiology

Like eczema elsewhere on the body, vulvar eczema is typically a result of persistent scratching or aggravation of an area after an allergic trigger. It can be an acute or chronic condition. The diagnosis is made by the symptom history, vulvar examination, and presence of eczema on other parts of the body; biopsies are not beneficial. Psoriasis and seborrhea are often confused with eczema, and any diagnosis will be hampered if the area has been scratched. The provider should be alert to the possibility of secondary infection with continued dermal irritation.[1,2]

Often seen on the knees or elbows, psoriasis is an inherited chronic condition in which new skin cells are produced too rapidly, leading to pruritic, red and scaly, or thick white patches with clear-cut borders. It is often exacerbated by stress and occurs simultaneously on various parts of the body. In addition, new psoriatic lesions may develop at an injury site (referred to as Koebner phenomenon). Psoriasis usually affects the labia and is not typically present in mucous membranes or the urethra.

Clinical Presentation and Physical Examination

The typical presentation of eczema includes severe pruritus lasting several weeks or more. A red rash or erythema without distinct borders is usually observed on examination and, if left untreated, can progress to the thickened scaly plaques seen in squamous cell hyperplasia.[1,2] On the vulva, crusts are less likely, but the cycle of vulvar itching and scratching can lead to LSC.[1,2] Psoriasis of the vulva often initially manifests as a nonscaly area of smooth erythema. Pruritus is common, and repeated scratching can result in excoriation, skin thickening, and a continued cycle of itching and scratching. Other areas of the body should be examined for eczema and psoriasis because the vulva is usually not the only location for these conditions.

Diagnostics

Essential Diagnostics. Often eczema and psoriasis cause similar symptoms and can be difficult to differentiate. Diagnosis is most often based on a thorough history and examination findings.

Additional Diagnostics. A punch biopsy can be done if other dermatoses are suspected.

Differential Diagnosis

As with many vulvar conditions, initial symptoms often overlap and many differential diagnoses are possible.

 Priority differentials include (1) LS, (2) LP, (3) LSC, (4) contact dermatitis, and (5) fungal infections.

Interprofessional Collaborative Management

Pharmacologic Management

Topical and Injectable Steroids. In severe cases of eczema, a potent topical corticosteroid ointment, such as clobetasol, can be used twice a day for 2 to 4 weeks and then gradually reduced in frequency until the symptoms are gone.[1,2] Low-potency corticosteroid creams can be used when appropriate. Triamcinolone acetonide injections can be used for recalcitrant eczema.

Oral Antihistamines. Systemic antihistamines such as diphenhydramine, doxepin, or hydroxyzine can be taken to help reduce pruritus and scratching.

Other Medications. Calcipotriene ointment (Dovonex), a topical vitamin D_3 preparation, is effective without the risk of skin atrophy.[1,2]

Nonpharmacologic Management. Cool compresses and Burow solution may help reduce pruritus that is associated with both eczema and psoriasis. Ultraviolet treatments can be used to treat psoriasis; efficacy for vulvar lesions may be limited, and the dose of ultraviolet light needs to be reduced to avoid burning the genital skin.

Indications for Referral

Women who do not respond to a course of steroids or other treatments, who report ongoing pain or intractable pruritus, or who have a superimposed skin infection that has not responded to antibiotics should be referred to a gynecologic dermatology physician. If an underlying allergic component is suspected, consultation with an allergist is appropriate.

Life Span Considerations

Eczema and psoriasis can occur across the life span. Although acute exacerbations are possible, both conditions are often chronic and management will change depending on stage of life. Women who are pregnant or breastfeeding should seek consultation before treatment, because certain medications to control the symptoms of eczema and psoriasis should not be taken while pregnant or nursing. Aging skin is more susceptible to trauma, and women with these conditions in the presence of atrophy from estrogen deficiency of menopause may need to be treated with topical estrogen therapy to improve bothersome symptoms.

Complications

Serious complications from eczema and psoriasis are rare. Pruritus can lead to scratching and possible skin breakdown and superimposed bacterial and fungal infections. Decreased sexual function from pruritus and discomfort is possible.

Patient and Family Education

Eczema and psoriasis are chronic conditions that require treatment over the life span. Symptoms often go through periods of remission and exacerbation that can be frustrating. Women may be able to wean off frequent use of medications during periods of remission but should be educated that exacerbations are common and often not related to any specific activity. Pruritus is common and can affect a woman's quality of life and sexual functioning. Open communication with sexual partners is important, especially during exacerbations and periods of increased discomfort.

Health Promotion

Gentle care of vulvar skin, loose clothing, and avoidance of harsh cleansers and irritants need to be lifelong habits.

VULVAR PAIN
Definition and Epidemiology

Vulvodynia is an umbrella term for chronic vulvar pain or discomfort characterized by burning, stinging, irritation, and rawness of the vulva or exquisite sensitivity to touch on the vulvar area or on attempted vaginal entry. The cause of vulvodynia is uncertain. It is estimated to affect up to 16% of women in the general population.

Although burning vulvar symptoms can be attributed to conditions such as vaginitis, human papillomavirus (HPV) infection, or dermatoses such as those described in this chapter, the term is generally reserved for conditions such as vulvar vestibulitis syndrome (VVS) and essential vulvodynia (EV), which have no known cause.

VULVAR VESTIBULITIS SYNDROME AND ESSENTIAL VULVODYNIA
Pathophysiology

VVS is a chronic inflammatory condition of the vulvar vestibule that is characterized by burning pain on touch, which can persist for several days after the touch is removed. In 1987, Friedrich defined the condition and included three criteria for diagnosis: (1) severe pain on vestibular touch or attempted vaginal entry, (2) tenderness to pressure localized within the vulvar vestibule, and (3) physical findings confined to vestibular erythema of various degrees.[6,7] Although VVS is now better understood, the cause and most appropriate treatment of this condition remain unknown. Vulvar vestibulitis is found almost exclusively in women of reproductive age who are or have been sexually active. The true prevalence is unknown. It has been estimated that between 8% to 16% of adult women under the age of 40 are affected by vulvar pain associated with VVS or vulvodynia.[6,7] Primary (no identifiable initial trigger and onset from first vaginal intercourse or tampon insertion) and secondary (such as after HPV infection or vaginitis treatment or postpartum) categories of VVS have been suggested.

EV is characterized by spontaneous and unprovoked vulvar burning not limited to the vestibule. This condition may represent a neuropathic process such as a reflex sympathetic dystrophy or pudendal neuralgia.[6,7] Other than more widespread symptom distribution, physical findings on examination are similarly unremarkable, as with VVS. Some women can identify a triggering event such as vulvar and vaginal infections, childbirth, back injury, or perimenopause. The role of these events in the development of EV is unclear, but it has been postulated that the nervous system may be sensitized or damaged, resulting in abnormal pain production.[6]

Causes of VVS and EV, including HPV and a *Candida*-triggered autoimmune response, have been suggested but not supported in the literature. In fact, treatments of HPV infection, such as topical acid or laser therapy, can lead to secondary VVS. A causal association between VVS and *Candida* organisms has not been established, but as more women treat themselves repeatedly with OTC vaginal fungicides, sensitivity to ingredients in these preparations may develop, increasing the risk for development of VVS.[6] Other theories include an association between VVS or EV and interstitial cystitis, both of which are inflammatory conditions of tissues that share embryologic origins. Many of these women have overlapping urinary and vulvar symptoms. VVS may also be associated with a sympathetically maintained pain feedback loop that is perpetuated by an underlying pelvic floor muscle instability or hypertonicity that is initially triggered by a superficial tissue insult.[6,7]

Given the lack of obvious clinical findings, VVS and EV were long thought to be a result of sexual dysfunction, childhood trauma, or some other psychological disorder, theories now recognized as fallacious. A chronic pain syndrome that heavily affects sexual relationships and daily activities is likely, not surprisingly, to be accompanied by anxiety or depression. These issues should be addressed, but to assume a causal link with VVS and EV is inappropriate.

Clinical Presentation and Physical Examination

A thorough history is essential to management of VVS and EV. Presentation of VVS commonly includes complaints of severe, burning vulvar pain during introital penetration with sexual intercourse or tampon use, during bicycle or horseback riding, or when wearing tight or bulky clothing. Pain may last a few minutes or as long as a few days after the trigger has been removed. Symptoms have often been present for months or years, resulting in a long history of frequent consultations. The history should include information about the initial onset of symptoms (if an initial onset can be identified), along with symptom characteristics, duration, and frequency. The impact of symptoms on sexual function should be determined, including how often intercourse is attempted and how often it is stopped because of pain. Assessment should also be made as to the impact of symptoms on daily activities and how often thoughts are distracted by symptoms during the course of a day. The presence of back pain, muscle soreness, and bowel and urinary patterns may be helpful in identifying related disorders. Previous ineffective treatment should be documented. Prior management has often included repeated treatment for yeast or bacterial infections; determination of whether treatment was empirical or culture based is essential. A review of previous medical records can be helpful. Women should also be asked if they have developed any techniques of their own to ease discomfort.

The vulvar burning of EV occurs with no demonstrable skin abnormalities. There is also a lack of focal tenderness typically seen in VVS. In EV, pain is not confined to coital attempts or other known triggers. Complaints of concomitant urethral, rectal, or back pain are more common than with VVS.[6,7]

Visual examination of the vulva and introitus is generally unremarkable, although with VVS erythema near the vestibular glands may be present. The most revealing test is the use of a water- or saline-moistened cotton-tipped applicator to test for sensitivity to touch. This is done by simply touching with the applicator in multiple locations around the labia minora, vestibule, clitoris, and urethra to determine any areas of tenderness, to elicit burning, and to rate the degree of discomfort. With VVS, tenderness or burning is usually triggered near the Bartholin glands, near the posterior fourchette, and to either side of the urethral opening. Use of the smallest speculum possible and a gentle, unhurried examination with extra lubrication will be better tolerated. Colposcopic evaluation of the involved areas, although advocated by some, is not appropriate in general unless physical findings suggest HPV infection or vulvar intraepithelial neoplasia. Vulvar biopsies typically show inflammation and should be performed only if a pathologic condition is suggested by the physical examination.

Diagnostics

Essential Diagnostics. Women who have vulvar vestibulitis or vulvodynia often have normal appearing skin. A careful visual inspection of the entire vulva is necessary to look for obvious causes of pain, including infections and lesions. Use of a cotton-tipped swab to gently touch areas on the vulva will identify local areas of pain. Infections can also be a source of pain, so initial diagnostic tests should include a wet prep examination of vaginal fluid, and cultures for gonorrhea, chlamydia, *Ureaplasma,* and β-hemolytic streptococci.

Additional Diagnostics. If lesions are present, HSV cultures should be obtained. Urinalysis, culture, and sensitivity can be performed if dysuria is present. Examination of the skin with a colposcope and biopsies can be considered.

INITIAL DIAGNOSTICS

Vulvar Vestibulitis Syndrome and Essential Vulvodynia

INITIAL
- Cotton-tipped applicator sensitivity test

LABORATORY
- Gonorrhea and chlamydia cultures
- *Ureaplasma* cultures
- β-Hemolytic streptococci cultures
- Potassium hydroxide (KOH) wet preparation for yeast and bacterial vaginosis (BV)

Differential Diagnosis

STIs should be excluded and cultures performed for β-hemolytic streptococci and *Candida* and *Ureaplasma* organisms. The diagnosis of VVS is made on the basis of the history, positive physical examination findings, and negative cultures.[6,7]

 Priority differentials include (1) STIs, (2) *Candida* or *Ureaplasma,* and (3) β-hemolytic streptococci.

Interprofessional Collaborative Management

Pharmacologic Management. Standard pain medications, including opiates, do not control the pain of VVS or EV and should not be prescribed.

Antidepressants. Other oral treatments aimed at interfering with the pain feedback loop include antidepressant medications (tricyclic antidepressants and SSRIs). Low-dose antidepressants are used to manage pain, and it should be carefully explained that this is the indication for which the antidepressant is being prescribed.

Topical Medications. Application of topical xylocaine can temporarily relieve pain during sexual intercourse. In women who are postmenopausal, application of topical estrogen cream may decrease pain if urogenital atrophy is present.

Antifungals. Treatment of VVS is dictated by the woman's history. If recurrent candidiasis is suspected, the provider could institute a trial of fluconazole, 150 mg weekly, for 2 months, then biweekly for another 2 months, followed by one dose monthly. Careful evaluation for possible drug interactions (e.g., oral hypoglycemics, anticoagulants) is required. Topical antifungal creams such as terconazole, miconazole, and clotrimazole may further irritate the vestibule.

Nonpharmacologic Management. Alternative forms of chronic pain management, such as guided imagery and acupuncture, may be useful as well. Pelvic floor physical therapy may help reduce tension and improve pelvic floor tone, thus decreasing pain.

Complementary Approaches. Twice-daily biofeedback exercises may help reestablish muscle stability during the course of many months and may provide significant if not complete symptom relief. Decisions to seek alternative forms of treatment, such as acupuncture, should be supported and incorporated into the overall management plan.

Surgery to remove the affected area has produced mixed results, including worsening of symptoms, and should be discussed only after every other treatment option has been exhausted.

Indications for Referral

Continued pelvic floor muscle dysfunction may perpetuate the sympathetically maintained pain feedback loop. Consultation with a physical therapist is helpful to evaluate for pelvic asymmetry and problems with the pelvic floor musculature, which typically shows instability and increased resting tone in patients with VVS.[6,7] Consultation with a mental health provider and a sexual therapist may help decrease pain and depression and increase sexual satisfaction.[6]

Surgery to remove the affected area has produced mixed results, including worsening of symptoms, and should be discussed only after every other treatment option has been exhausted.[6,7] In VVS, surgical excision of varying amounts of vestibular tissue (vestibulectomy) is the intervention with the highest reported success rate, but studies are often weakened by methodologic flaws, and the benefits of medical and behavioral management may be underreported.

Life Span Considerations

Women of all ages can experience vulvodynia. Women with VVS or EV can experience so much pain that intercourse is impossible and achieving a pregnancy is difficult. If women with one of these vulvar pain syndromes becomes pregnant, there is often concern over pain relief during delivery and how the delivery might affect the mother's pain in the postpartum period. Regardless of age, these syndromes can negatively affect sexual functioning throughout the life span. Pain may also increase as a result of estrogen deficiency during menopause.

Complications

Women with vulvar pain may be reticent to discuss physical and sexual concerns and reluctant to have pelvic examinations. The disorder may be embarrassing and frustrating and may prohibit some women from enjoying life or an intimate sexual relationship. These women require considerable support and understanding and often will benefit from psychological counseling.

Patient and Family Education

Reassurance that this condition is real and that the concerns are legitimate is important. Although spontaneous resolution of symptoms is possible, treatment of VVS or EV is often a matter of trial and error and requires a solid provider–patient relationship. Goals of treatment include pain control and improved quality of life. Women should be informed that partial symptom relief is likely, but that it will take time for adequate treatment trials. Realistic goals and time frames should be established. The impact of VVS on intimate relationships is significant, and the woman's partner should be included in discussions when possible and appropriate. Counseling referrals should be offered with the understanding that the health care provider does not believe symptoms are psychogenic in nature, but rather that there are real emotional challenges to living with a chronic pain syndrome. The provider should also acknowledge that hope often gives way to disappointment before symptom relief is experienced.

Health Promotion

Each woman should be involved as much as possible and should keep a daily symptom log, noting any possible pain triggers and rating the severity and duration of symptoms. When discussing treatment options, providers should first counsel women to avoid vulvar irritants and to implement the self-care measures described in Box 153.1. Many treatment options can be trialed, including pharmacologic and nonpharmacologic approaches. Although most women will experience some degree of symptom relief, there will often be periods of symptom exacerbation throughout the life span.

VAGINITIS AND VAGINOSIS

DEFINITION AND EPIDEMIOLOGY

Vaginitis and vaginosis are disorders of the vagina that are characterized by vaginal discharge, odor, or vulvovaginal irritation. Vaginitis involves inflammation, whereas vaginosis does not. Both have historically been grouped under the term *vaginitis*. They result from an imbalance in the vaginal ecosystem, which may be caused by infection (bacterial, fungal, protozoan, or viral),[8,9] hypoestrogenic states, foreign bodies, contact dermatitis, or allergy. Many times the cause of the imbalance is not immediately clear. Recurrent vaginitis is defined as four or more episodes within a year. Affecting women of all ages, vaginitis is the most common gynecologic problem encountered by health care providers.[9]

BACTERIAL VAGINOSIS

Pathophysiology

Bacterial vaginosis (BV) is characterized by the replacement of the normal, hydrogen peroxide–producing *Lactobacillus* organisms in the vagina with high concentrations of anaerobic bacteria, *Gardnerella vaginalis*, *Mycoplasma hominis*, and *Bacteroides* and *Mobiluncus* organisms.[8,9] Among women seeking care, BV is the most common cause of vaginal discharge or malodor, although data suggest that many women with BV are asymptomatic.[8,9]

In the presence of BV infection, protective hydrogen peroxide–producing lactobacilli are significantly reduced. This change is accompanied by an elevated pH. This alkaline environment facilitates the growth of the pathogenic organisms and their adherence to vaginal epithelia, seen as clue cells on a saline wet mount. The anaerobes facilitate the release of amines, which produce the characteristic "fishy" odor, especially on alkalization of the vaginal discharge. The cause of microbial alterations in BV is not fully understood. It is not classified as an STI but is considered to be sexually associated. It is more common among women who have multiple sexual partners or a new sex partner and women who do not use condoms.[8] However, women who have never been sexually active also get BV. Women with BV are at an increased risk for acquiring some STIs, such as infection with HIV, *Neisseria gonorrhoeae*, *Chlamydia trachomatis*, and HSV type 2. Treatment of male sex partners has not been beneficial in preventing the recurrence of BV and is not recommended.[8]

Clinical Presentation and Physical Examination

Symptoms of BV most often include an increased quantity of malodorous vaginal discharge, most noticeable after intercourse and during menses because of the alkaline nature of semen and blood. Some women experience mild to moderate vulvovaginal irritation.

The physical examination should include inspection of the vulva and vagina. Assessment is important: skin turgor and elasticity; normal or sparse pubic hair; and whether the labia are full, atrophic, or dry will help identify if the symptoms are associated with estrogen deficiency. Any vulvovaginal erythema, lesions, discharge, or prolapse should be noted. A speculum examination is necessary to determine the color, consistency, viscosity, and odor of any vaginal or cervical discharge. The characteristic vaginal discharge of BV is often thin, homogeneous, and adherent to the vaginal walls and cervix. The fishy amine odor may be present, and rarely there is vaginal inflammation.[8] A bimanual examination will reveal any cervical motion tenderness, pelvic pain, or masses.

Diagnostics

Essential Diagnostics. Wet prep examination of vaginal discharge and assessment of vaginal pH are point-of-care tests that can establish a diagnosis of BV. The diagnosis of BV can be made by clinical criteria. Clinical criteria require the presence of three of the following[8]: (1) homogeneous, white, non-inflammatory discharge that adheres to the vaginal walls, (2) the presence of clue cells on microscopic examination, (3) a pH of vaginal fluid above 4.5, and (4) vaginal discharge with a fishy odor before or after the addition of 10% KOH, which indicates a positive whiff test result.

Additional Diagnostics. If wet prep evaluation is inconclusive or not available, a vaginal culture can be obtained. If STIs are suspected, disease-specific testing can be performed.

> **INITIAL DIAGNOSTICS**
>
> **Bacterial Vaginosis**
>
> **LABORATORY**
> - pH of vaginal fluid
> - Wet mount with normal saline and 10% KOH
> - KOH whiff test

Differential Diagnosis

Increased vaginal discharge can be caused by many different factors. Thorough history, examination, and microscopy evaluation will assist in establishing a correct diagnosis.

 The priority differentials include (1) trichomoniasis, (2) candidiasis, (3) gonorrhea, (4) chlamydia, and (5) atrophic vaginitis.

Interprofessional Collaborative Management

Pharmacologic Management. The goals of treatment are elimination of symptoms and relief from any vaginal irritation. Pharmacologic measures are the first-line treatment. For nonpregnant women options include the following: metronidazole, 500 mg PO twice a day for 7 days, *or* metronidazole gel 0.75%, 1 full applicator (5 g) intravaginally once daily for 5 days, *or* clindamycin cream 2%, 1 full applicator (5 g) intravaginally at bedtime for 7 days. Oral clindamycin or tinidazole can also be considered. Pregnant women should be treated with either oral or vaginal metronidazole or clindamycin.[8] Although metronidazole was previously contraindicated in the first trimester, multiple studies and meta-analyses have not demonstrated an association between metronidazole use during pregnancy and teratogenic or mutagenic effects in newborns.[8] For recurrent BV infections, options include the use of alternative first-line agents and prophylactic use of intravaginal metronidazole, twice a week for 4 to 6 months.[8]

Indications for Referral

BV rarely requires hospitalization and can often be treated without consultation. Referral is indicated in cases of multiple recurrent episodes of BV despite adequate treatment.

Life Span Considerations

BV can occur at any point in a woman's reproductive life and more commonly affects women who are sexually active. The symptoms of increased vaginal discharge and odor can mimic symptoms of STIs, and sexually active adolescents may be uncomfortable discussing their symptoms with parents, especially if their parents are unaware they are sexually active.

During the perimenopausal and postmenopausal years, BV can occur in the presence of atrophic vaginitis as a result of the alteration in vaginal lactobacilli and a more alkaline vaginal environment. Treatment with a topical estrogen preparation may help reduce recurrences in postmenopausal women.

Complications

Once considered benign, BV is now associated with gynecologic and obstetric complications. Perhaps of greatest concern is the possible link between BV and infection with human immunodeficiency virus (HIV). The shift in vaginal pH from acidity to alkalinity associated with the presence of semen may favor male-to-female transmission of HIV, and HIV infection is consistently associated with reduced levels of vaginal lactobacilli.[8,9]

Patient and Family Education

BV recurs within 1 to 2 months for many women. Persistence of pathogens, an unidentified host factor, failure of lactobacilli to recolonize the vagina, and reinfection from a male partner are possible explanations. The importance of completing the full course of treatment is essential to reduce regrowth of bacteria. Because BV has been linked to preterm labor and birth, pregnant women with BV should be educated on the subtle signs and symptoms of preterm labor, including increased watery vaginal discharge, spotting, lower abdominal pain, and low back pain.

The most common side effect of oral metronidazole is gastrointestinal upset. Women taking metronidazole should be advised to avoid the use of alcohol during treatment and for 24 hours thereafter to avoid a disulfiram-like reaction (severe nausea and vomiting). Oral clindamycin has been shown to be as effective as oral metronidazole, but it is more expensive and may cause diarrhea. Clindamycin cream is oil based and may weaken latex condoms and diaphragms for 5 days after use.[8] The results of clinical trials indicate that a woman's response to therapy and the likelihood of relapse or recurrence are not affected by treatment of a woman's sex partner. Therefore routine treatment of sexual partners is not recommended.

Health Promotion

Recurrent episodes of BV can be frustrating for women, and strategies to promote vaginal health should be discussed. These include no douching, avoiding perfumed or scented vaginal cleansers or sprays, and wearing loose-fitting clothes. Safer sexual practices such as using condoms and reducing sexual partners are also helpful in reducing recurrent BV.

VULVOVAGINAL CANDIDIASIS

Pathophysiology

VVC is caused by growth of the fungus *Candida* in the vagina. Most infections involve *Candida albicans*, although other species are possible.[8] The most common non–*C. albicans* species involved in VVC are *Torulopsis glabrata* and *Candida tropicalis*, which may manifest atypically and may be more resistant to standard therapies. Women with HIV infection or recurrent VVC are twice as likely to have non–*C. albicans* VVC.[8] An estimated 75% of women will have at least one episode of VVC, and approximately 40% to 45% will have two or more.[8,10]

Several factors may trigger the change from colonization to proliferation, which results in the development of symptomatic VVC. These include changes in the vaginal ecosystem and possible phenotypic changes in the *Candida* organism. Symptomatic VVC involves candidal tissue invasion, causing inflammation, mucosal swelling, erythema, and exfoliation of epithelia. Factors that cause an increased susceptibility to VVC include antibiotic therapy, pregnancy, uncontrolled diabetes mellitus, use of oral contraceptives (especially high-dose formulations), immunosuppression, and occlusive synthetic clothing.[8,10]

Recurrent VVC is defined as three to four (or more) documented episodes of VVC in 1 year. The pathophysiologic mechanism of recurrent or chronic VVC remains controversial. It affects less than 5% of women annually, and the majority have no predisposing condition, such as diabetes or immunosuppression. Earlier theories on the cause of recurrent VVC have included reinfection from an intestinal reservoir; sexual transmission; and the vaginal relapse theory, which proposes that incomplete eradication of *Candida* organisms occurs after treatment and that the small numbers of *Candida* organisms present then multiply and result in recurrence. More recent theories propose deficiencies in the normal protective vaginal flora; a deficiency in antigen-specific, cell-mediated immunity to *Candida* organisms; and a possible local hypersensitivity to *Candida* organisms, predisposing the patient to recurrences.[8,10]

Clinical Presentation and Physical Examination

Typical symptoms of VVC include pruritus and vaginal discharge. Other symptoms may include vulvar burning, dyspareunia, vulvar dysuria, and vaginal irritation. Vaginal discharge is not always present, and there may be only a small amount. The thick whitish-gray discharge is typically described as cottage cheese–like, although it can vary from thin to thick.[8] On physical examination, the vulva and vagina may be hyperemic and edematous. Vulvar excoriation may be present from scratching, and irritated skin may have fissures. The vaginal discharge is usually whitish, curdlike, and adherent to the vaginal walls. Variations in the vaginal discharge are possible, although care must be taken to exclude concurrent infections.

Diagnostics

Essential Diagnostics. Wet prep examination of vaginal discharge and assessment of vaginal pH are point-of-care tests that can establish a diagnosis of VVC, especially when correlated with clinical symptoms and exam findings. *Candida* vaginitis is associated with a vaginal pH below 4.5. A normal pH will help rule out a differential diagnosis of BV or trichomoniasis. The diagnosis of VVC can be made on demonstration of pseudohyphae or yeast buds on a 10% KOH wet mount or by culture. Use of KOH on microscopy improves visualization by disrupting cellular material, which may obscure the yeast forms. Identification of yeast in the absence of symptoms is not an indication for treatment.

Additional Diagnostics. Vaginal culture can be obtained if wet prep is inconclusive or unavailable.

INITIAL DIAGNOSTICS

Vulvovaginal Candidiasis

LABORATORY
- pH of vaginal discharge (to rule out BV or trichomoniasis)
- Wet mount with normal saline and 10% KOH

Differential Diagnosis

Vaginal pruritus, often the main symptom of VVC, can be difficult to diagnose. Many different differential diagnoses exist.

 Priority differentials include (1) BV (2) trichomoniasis, (3) atrophic vaginitis, (4) gonorrhea, and (5) chlamydia.

Interprofessional Collaborative Management

Pharmacologic Management. The goals of treatment are normalization of vaginal flora, elimination of symptoms, and restoration of skin integrity. Pharmacologic measures are the first-line treatment. There are multiple options for nonpregnant women. OTC vaginal preparations include clotrimazole, miconazole, and tioconazole. Depending on the specific medication, these preparations are available in one-, three-, and seven-day treatment options. Prescription vaginal preparations, including terconazole and butoconazole, are also available, as is oral fluconazole 150 mg in a single dose. Oral fluconazole, 150 mg, administered weekly for 6 months, is the first-line treatment for recurrent VVC.[8]

The single-dose topical therapies should be reserved for mild VVC because of their slightly lower effectiveness. Multiday regimens are more appropriate for moderate to severe VVC, and the use of a cream is preferred in the presence of vulvar symptoms. Use of terconazole is more effective in non–*C. albicans* VVC. Treatment of VVC in pregnancy should use one of the topical azoles, preferably for 7 days.[8]

Indications for Referral

Referral may be indicated for women who are severely immunocompromised, are infected with HIV, or have poorly controlled diabetes.

Life Span Considerations

VVC can occur at any point in a woman's reproductive life but is more common during pregnancy and among women who are obese, are immunocompromised, or have poorly controlled diabetes. Sexually active women who are experiencing vulvovaginal symptoms may be concerned about STIs, and sexually active adolescents may be uncomfortable discussing their symptoms with parents, especially if their parents are unaware they are sexually active. During the perimenopausal and postmenopausal years, VVC can occur in the setting of atrophy

associated with estrogen deficiency. In addition, as women age, they are at increased risk of type 2 diabetes, which is an independent risk factor for VVC.

Complications

Complications are uncommon. The most common are superficial lesions and skin fissures that may occur in the vagina and vulva. Severely immunosuppressed patients may develop systemic infection. Patients with type 2 diabetes who are taking oral hypoglycemic medications and are being treated with fluconazole are at increased risk for hypoglycemia. Fluconazole has many drug interactions. Practitioners should be aware of other medications women are taking before prescribing.

Patient and Family Education

Women should be reassured that most episodes of VVC resolve easily. The choice of an oral versus topical therapy can be based on the patient's preference. If women self-treat with an OTC preparation and their symptoms do not improve, they should be evaluated at an office visit. Treatment of sexual partners is not indicated except in cases of symptomatic balanitis or penile dermatitis. The vaginal preparations are oil based and could potentially weaken latex condoms and diaphragms. Vaginal hygiene measures should be encouraged: cotton underwear, loose-fitting clothing, changing clothing after excessive perspiration or swimming, and avoidance of douching and scented vaginal sprays or perfumes. An optimum treatment strategy for recurrent VVC has not been defined. For established diagnoses of recurrent VVC, maintenance therapy needs to be given frequently enough to prevent vaginal regrowth, but the optimal interval has not been established. A longer duration of initial therapy, 14 days for vaginal therapy and oral fluconazole every third day for three doses, has been suggested.[8,10]

Health Promotion. Overweight and obese women should be encouraged to decrease their weight, and women with diabetes will experience fewer episodes of VVC with tight glucose control. In recurrent VVC, it is necessary to assess for predisposing conditions and to confirm the diagnosis by culture. Evaluation should include a fasting glucose concentration in nonpregnant patients or a glucose tolerance test if the patient is pregnant. Routine HIV testing is not indicated in patients without identifiable risk factors.[8]

ATROPHIC VAGINITIS
Pathophysiology

Atrophic vaginitis is caused by reduced endogenous estrogen levels—most commonly found in the postmenopausal patient, but lactation, antagonistic medications, and ovarian failure resulting from disease processes also induce hypoestrogenic states. The lower estrogen level causes the vaginal epithelium to become thin and fragile, with decreased glycogen content. There is an increased pH as a result of decreased lactic acid production, leading to an environment prone to an overgrowth of pathogenic organisms and to a lowered concentration of lactobacilli.[11] Despite these changes, symptoms will vary and some women with vaginal atrophy are not symptomatic.

Clinical Presentation and Physical Examination

Women with atrophic vaginitis often report vaginal soreness, pruritus, vulvovaginal dryness, occasional vaginal discharge, spotting, and dyspareunia. The vulvar skin is thin, with decreased subcutaneous tissue and variable pubic hair loss.

The vaginal walls are pale with decreased or absent rugae. The vaginal tissue is often friable and can contain petechiae. Vaginal discharge can be thick, watery, or blood-tinged.[11]

Diagnostics

Essential Diagnostics. The symptoms of atrophic vaginitis often mimic those of other vaginal infections. The woman's history should be correlated with exam findings of vulvovaginal atrophy. The vaginal pH in atrophic vaginitis is usually 5.5 to 7. The saline wet mount typically reveals increased leukocytes and small, round epithelial cells with an absence of clue cells and negative amine test.

Additional Diagnostics. A vaginal culture can be obtained if the wet prep is inconclusive. STI testing can be done as indicated based on history. Endometrial and vulvar biopsies can be considered based on symptoms and exam findings.

> **INITIAL DIAGNOSTICS**
>
> **Atrophic Vaginitis**
>
> **LABORATORY**
> - pH and wet mount

Differential Diagnosis

Although atrophic vaginitis is distinguished by the presence of a hypoestrogenic state, other potential diagnoses must be considered.

 Priority differentials include (1) BV, (2) VVC, (3) trichomoniasis, (4) chlamydia, and (5) gonorrhea.

Interprofessional Collaborative Management

Pharmacologic Management. The goal of treatment is to correct the hypoestrogenic environment through estrogen therapy. This causes maturation of the epithelium, reversing the changes that resulted in the vaginitis. Treatment recommendations usually involve topical estrogen cream, tablets, or vaginal rings. Typical regimens include the following[12]: (1) estradiol cream 0.1%, 2 to 4 g intravaginally every day for 1 to 2 weeks, then 1 to 2 g intravaginally every day for 1 to 2 weeks, then 1 g intravaginally one to three times per week for maintenance; (2) estradiol cream 0.1%, 2 to 4 g intravaginally every day for 1 to 2 weeks, then 1 to 2 g intravaginally every day for 1 to 2 weeks, then 1 g intravaginally one to three times per week for maintenance; (3) conjugated estrogen cream, 2 to 4 g intravaginally every day for 1 to 2 weeks, then 2 to 4 g intravaginally every other day for 1 to 2 weeks, and conjugated estrogen cream is then tapered and discontinued; (4) estradiol in pill form used intravaginally every day for 1 to 2 weeks, then twice weekly for 2 to 4 weeks, then tapered and discontinued; and (5) vaginal estrogen ring for 90 days. Ospemifene, an oral estrogen agonist-antagonist, 60 mg daily.[11,12]

Topical estrogen therapy can be used safely in many women and it does not have the same cardiovascular and oncogenic risk profile as systemic estrogen treatment. Women who use topical estrogen for more than 6 to 12 months should be monitored for abnormal vaginal bleeding. Although the risk of endometrial hyperplasia is far less with topical agents compared with systemic estrogen treatment, any abnormal bleeding should be investigated. Although there are no established guidelines for monitoring the endometrial lining, a pelvic ultrasound for endometrial thickness or endometrial biopsy can be considered if there are concerns about endometrial hyperplasia.

Nonpharmacologic Management. Patients with atrophic vaginitis who decline topical estrogen treatment or in whom the hypoestrogenic state is temporary (e.g., breastfeeding) may benefit from the use of a vaginal moisturizer (e.g., Replens), lubricants, or acidifying agents. These modalities will increase lubrication and moisture but will not improve tissue integrity or elasticity.

Indications for Referral

Referral to a gynecologist who specializes in menopause is indicated in cases of treatment failure.

Life Span Considerations

Atrophic vaginitis exists in a hypoestrogenic state and therefore almost universally affects postmenopausal women. Atrophic vaginitis can also occur in women who are breastfeeding and have decreased estrogen levels, although this is temporary and resolves once lactation amenorrhea resolves.

Complications

Complications from atrophic vaginitis are rare. After prolonged estrogen deficiency vulvovaginal tissue can become thin and friable and susceptible to tearing and bruising from even mild trauma.

Local estrogen replacement has been the mainstay of treatment for atrophic vaginitis. More recently, laser therapy has become an innovative option for women. Within specific parameters, microablative carbon-dioxide laser treatment stimulates vaginal cell proliferation, collagen production, and improves vascularity.[12]

Patient and Family Education

Women who are considering estrogen therapy need education about the actual risks of treatment. There is much confusion and misinformation surrounding the use of postmenopausal estrogen. Topical treatment does not carry the same risks as systemic treatment. Women using topical estrogen should be educated on expected treatment time, the weaning process, and the potential side effects. Women should also be instructed to report any abnormal bleeding or gynecologic concerns.

Health Promotion

Although topical estrogen is the treatment of choice, some women may decline the use of hormones. Postmenopausal women should continue sexual activity if possible because this will help keep vaginal tissue pliable and elastic. Dyspareunia is a common complaint among women who have atrophic vaginitis, and comfort measures (use of lubricants, moisturizers, prolonged foreplay) should be encouraged.

REFERENCES

1. Simpson, R., & Nunns, D. (2017). Skin diseases affecting the vulva. *Obstetrics, Gynaecology and Reproductive Medicine*.
2. Nunns, D., Simpson, R., Watson, A., & Murphy, R. (2017). The management of vulval itching caused by benign vulval dermatoses. *The Obstetrician & Gynaecologist*, 19(4), 307–315.
3. Fruchter, R., Melnick, L., & Pomeranz, M. K. (2017). Lichenoid vulvar disease: A review. *International Journal of Women's Dermatology*, 3, 58–64.
4. Helgesen, A. L. O., Warloe, T., Pripp, A. H., et al. (2016). Vulvovaginal photodynamic therapy in genital erosive lichen planus. *The British Journal of Dermatology*, 173(5), 1156–1162.
5. Hawkins, J. W., Rberto-Nichols, D. M., & Stanley-Haney, J. L. (2016). *Guidelines for nurse practitioners in gynecologic settings*. New York: Springer.

6. Thorton, A. M., & Drummond, C. (2016). Current concepts in vulvodynia with a focus on pathogenesis and pain mechanisms. *The Australasian Journal of Dermatology, 57*, 253–263.

7. Falsetta, M. L., Foster, D. C., Bonham, A. D., & Phipps, R. P. (2016). A review of the available clinical therapies for vulvodynia management and new data implicating proinflammatory mediators in pain elicitation. *BJOG: An International Journal of Obstetrics and Gynaecology, 124*, 210–218.

8. Workowski, K. A., & Bolan, G. A., Centers for Disease Control and Prevention (CDC). (2010). Sexually transmitted diseases treatment guidelines, 2015. *MMWR. Recommendations and Reports: Morbidity and Mortality Weekly Report. Recommendations and Reports, 64*(RR–3), 1–137.

9. Nasioudis, D., Linhares, I. M., Ledger, W. J., & Witkin, S. S. (2017). Bacterial vaginosis: A critical analysis of current knowledge. *BJOG: An International Journal of Obstetrics and Gynaecology, 124*(1), 61–69.

10. Sobel, J. D. (2016). Recurrent vulvovaginal candidiasis. *American Journal of Obstetrics and Gynecology, 214*(1), 15–21.

11. Ward, K., & Deneris, A. (2016). Genitourinary syndrome of menopause: A new name for an old condition. *The Nurse Practitioner, 41*(7), 28–33.

12. Gandhi, J., Chen, A., Dagur, G., Suh, Y., Smith, N., Cali, B., et al. (2016). Genitourinary syndrome of menopause: An overview of clinical manifestations, pathophysiology, etiology, evaluation, and management. *American Journal of Obstetrics and Gynecology, 215*(6), 704–711.

CHAPTER 154

ANKLE AND FOOT PAIN

Joanne Sandberg-Cook • James Peter Ioli

In the United States, foot and ankle problems are extremely common, with an incidence rate of 24% in middle-aged and older adults.[1] Sports injuries are often the cause, but even activities of daily living stress the foot and ankle. Walking alone puts up to 1.5 times the body weight on the foot. The average person logs roughly 1000 miles yearly. During 1 hour of strenuous exercise, feet cushion up to 1 million pounds of pressure.

Foot and ankle pain is more prevalent in women, people who are older and obese, and those with other lower extremity joint pain or deformity. However, children and adolescents are also commonly injured during sports activities. The specific functions of the ankle and foot predispose them to injuries and disorders that can result in chronic problems if they are not identified quickly and managed properly.

ANKLE SPRAINS

DEFINITION AND EPIDEMIOLOGY

The uniaxial ankle joint, or ankle joint, is the most primitive joint in the body and is crucial to walking, running, and the performance of all sports. The limited motion of the ankle gives it stability. The ankle joint consists of three major bones: the tibia, fibula, and talus. The tibia and fibula form the ankle mortise, and the talus fits into this mortise. The talus, which has no muscle or tendon attachment, gives the ankle its hinge motion. The talus also bears the entire weight of the extremity during walking. The medial deltoid, and the lateral anterior talofibular, calcaneal fibular, and posterior talofibular ligaments hold the ankle bones in the mortise.

Ankle sprains occur at all ages and are common problems encountered by health care providers. Ankle sprains are more common in women and adolescents.[2] A review of literature reveals that ankle sprains may account for 45% of all sports injuries.[3] A sprain is a ligamentous injury caused by an abnormal motion, a sudden change in direction, or a misstep on an uneven surface. Even a minor ankle sprain can jeopardize joint stability. The severity of the physical findings determines the sprain category (Table 154.1), and the category defines the management of the injury. Previous ankle sprains can increase the potential for injury recurrence. Early diagnosis, treatment, rehabilitation, and subsequent ankle support during activity decrease the recurrence of a sprain in a previously injured ankle.

PATHOPHYSIOLOGY

Two types of injuries cause an ankle sprain. The most common is the inversion injury, in which the foot plantar flexes and internally rotates as the ankle inverts. The "roll" of the ankle injures the lateral ligaments and can also cause a lateral avulsion fracture. The less common eversion injury occurs when the ankle sustains an external rotation mechanism. Eversion stress injures the medial structures of the ankle, damaging the deltoid ligament or the syndesmosis.

CLINICAL PRESENTATION

The most common presentation of an ankle sprain is a swollen and painful joint. Ecchymosis and decreased range of motion are generally present. In many instances, weight bearing causes pain; some patients are unable to bear any weight on the affected joint.

In obtaining the history, it is important to determine whether the patient heard any audible sounds at the time of injury. An audible "snap" or "pop" indicates the potential for a more serious injury. Immediate swelling or ecchymosis raises the index of suspicion for a fracture or substantial amount of joint involvement. Patients also commonly report a sensation of lightheadedness, nausea, or diaphoresis immediately after the injury.

PHYSICAL EXAMINATION

With a sprain, the ankle joint is often swollen and ecchymotic, and the edema can create an illusion of deformity. Limited active and passive motion and point tenderness at the site of injury are common. Joint laxity is present in more severe sprains. Muscle spasm often prevents accurate testing of strength and stability. If the injury is not acute, swelling and ecchymosis at the lateral aspect of the foot and the toes are common. The fifth metatarsal base should be palpated carefully and fracture considered if tender. With severe ankle sprains, tenderness may extend up the extremity. The entire lower limb should always be palpated to rule out more extensive injury.

DIAGNOSTICS
Essential Diagnostics

Although guidelines for radiography are controversial, plain radiographs are recommended for severe injuries, especially when instability is present or fracture is suspected. An x-ray study of the lower leg should also be performed if there is tenderness at the fibular head to rule out fracture. With less severe injuries, radiographs can be used to exclude an avulsion injury.

Additional Diagnostics

More extensive radiologic examinations, such as stress films or computed tomography (CT) or magnetic resonance imaging

TABLE 154.1 Classification and Treatment of Ankle Sprains

Grade 1	Grade 2	Grade 3
PATHOLOGY		
Stretching or minor tearing of ligament fibers	Partial tearing of ligament fibers	Complete tearing of ligament fibers
FINDINGS		
Minimum pain	Mild to moderate pain	Severe pain
Mild swelling	Moderate swelling	Significant swelling[a]
Mild ecchymosis	Moderate ecchymosis	Severe ecchymosis[a]
Full ROM	Painful, slightly limited motion and stability	Loss of motion and stability
Mild point tenderness	Point tenderness over joint	Severe pain (difficult examination)
Stable joint	Mild joint laxity with stress	Abnormal joint movement
Ability to bear weight	Painful to bear weight (may be unable to do so)	Inability to bear weight
TREATMENT		
RICE; active ROM exercises	RICE; active ROM exercises as tolerated	Referral to orthopedic surgeon/podiatry (may require surgery)
Non–weight-bearing activity (swimming, stationary bike)	Partial weight bearing (crutches, cane) as tolerated Gradual progression to full weight bearing	Cast for 10–14 days Non–weight-bearing activity Gradual progression to full weight bearing
Return to sports in 2–3 weeks	Return to sports in 4–8 weeks with semirigid ankle support	Rehabilitation before returning to sports with semirigid ankle support
SEQUELAE		
Tends to recur in first month if not fully rehabilitated	Recurrent sprains, joint instability, traumatic arthritis	Persistent instability (nonsurgical treatment), traumatic arthritis

[a]Occurs rapidly, usually within the first 30 minutes.
RICE, Rest, ice, compression, and elevation; *ROM*, range of motion.
Modified from Peterson, W., Rembitzki, I., Koppenburg, A., et al. (2013). Treatment of acute ankle ligament injuries: A systematic review. *Archives of Orthopaedic and Trauma Surgery, 133*(8), 1129–1141. Haddad, S. (2016). *Ankle sprains.* Retrieved November 14, 2017, from Orthoinfo.aaos.org/topic.cfm?topic=A00150.

INITIAL DIAGNOSTICS

Ankle Pain

IMAGING
- X-ray studies[a]

[a]If indicated.

(MRI) scans are considered in consultation with an orthopedic surgeon/podiatrist, especially preoperatively.

DIFFERENTIAL DIAGNOSIS

Ankle injuries range from simple strains to severe injuries. The possibility of associated fractures including fibular fracture, stress fracture, avulsion fracture, or dislocation should be considered.

Osteochondritis dissecans is a rare but important diagnosis, especially in adolescents. Bursitis and tendinitis can be considered (see Chapter 156), especially if no distinct injury is recalled. Osteoarthritis (see Chapter 165), rheumatoid arthritis (see Chapter 197), and gouty arthritis (see Chapter 158) are also common causes of ankle pain and swelling, especially in the older adult.

INTERPROFESSIONAL COLLABORATIVE MANAGEMENT

The severity of the sprain dictates the management (see Table 154.1). Rest and protection, ice, compression, and elevation (RICE) are key first steps in providing pain relief and limiting swelling. Nonsteroidal antiinflammatory drugs (NSAIDs) can help with pain management and may allow faster rehabilitation, although they can be associated with gastrointestinal (GI) side effects and in older adults should be used cautiously because of cardiovascular and renal concerns.[3] Topical NSAID gels are very effective at reducing pain and swelling and improving function in grade 1 and 2 sprains.[4] Thromboembolic deterrent (TED) hose provides support to the entire lower limb, aid in circulation, and are less bulky than ankle splints or braces for grade 1 and 2 sprains. Casting for 10 to 14 days has been shown to be effective in grade 3 sprains.[3] Semirigid supports used after the acute injury has resolved may protect from subsequent sprains. All sprains require rehabilitation to restore the ankle to a stable and pain-free state. It is important for patients to understand that the treatment and recovery process will take weeks. Rehabilitation should begin as soon as possible after the injury and should include range-of-motion and strengthening exercises.[5] Even a severely swollen ankle can be mobilized with the simple exercise of "writing the alphabet" (active range of motion) with the affected foot. A program of active and passive resistive exercises progresses as range of motion and strength improve.

Fractures, dislocations, or subluxations and grade 3 sprains require an orthopedic/podiatric referral. Physical therapy may also be indicated to promote rehabilitation and a safe return to sports or work-related activities.

COMPLICATIONS

Ankle sprains can recur within the first month if the ankle has not been fully rehabilitated. Grade 2 and 3 sprains carry with them an increased risk of joint instability and traumatic arthritis. Recurrent sprains, which result in chronic instability, may require surgical repair.[5] A weak ankle joint is at risk for fracture when it is stressed.

PATIENT AND FAMILY EDUCATION

Patients need to understand the importance of RICE as well as the necessity of preventing weight bearing on the injured ankle. Patients and family members should also be instructed in medication doses and side effects, proper elastic bandage wrapping technique, cast care, and crutch use. The recuperative process and the risk of recurrence also require explanation.

ACHILLES TENDINOPATHY

DEFINITION AND EPIDEMIOLOGY

The Achilles tendon is posterior to the ankle joint and is responsible for flexion and extension of the ankle. It attaches the gastrocnemius and the soleus muscles of the calf to the calcaneus muscle and is palpable from the distal pole of the calf to the calcaneus. Disorders of the Achilles tendon include tendinosis, paratendonitis, insertional tendinosis, and frank rupture.

Achilles tendinitis manifests as pain with or without swelling around the Achilles tendon. Unlike other tendons, the Achilles tendon does not have a synovial sheath but instead has a paratenon, which, like a synovial sheath, functions to provide lubrication and vasculature to the tendon. Except for severe cases, true Achilles tendinopathy primarily affects the paratenon, resulting in inflammation, degeneration, and friability of the tendon. A nodule of mucoid degeneration can form in the body of the tendon in severe or chronic Achilles tendinitis.[6]

PATHOPHYSIOLOGY

Achilles tendinopathy can occur in both adolescents and adults in both traumatic and nontraumatic settings. Aging, improper training, running up hills, or wearing shoes with soles that are too rigid can also contribute to the development of Achilles tendinopathy. Shoes or boots with a high back can irritate the tendon, causing pain and inflammation. Wearing of shoes with heels that maintain plantar flexion (high heels) for long periods can cause the tendon to shorten. Changing to flat or running shoes then increases stress on the tendon, causing pain. On occasion, Achilles tendinitis is caused by an anatomic abnormality, such as excessive foot pronation or tight hamstrings or gastrocnemius muscles.[6,7]

CLINICAL PRESENTATION

Patients with Achilles tendinopathy may have intermittent symptoms and may describe a pain that subsides during exercise but increases in severity while at rest. Pain can be located in the heel (insertional tendinopathy) or along the length of the tendon (tendinosis). Morning stiffness or severe pain on climbing stairs is also common. Most patients have an abnormal gait. Some limp, and some walk on their toes to avoid the heel-strike phase of walking.

PHYSICAL EXAMINATION

Localized swelling may be present around the tendon. There may be a bony prominence at the heel known as a Haglund deformity. Pain is often worse in the morning or after a period of inactivity and aggravated by shoe pressure. A palpable nodule, inflammatory signs, and crepitus may be present in severe or chronic cases.[6]

DIAGNOSTICS

Radiologic or laboratory tests are usually unnecessary, but the appropriate diagnostic tests should be guided by the history. Ultrasound is inexpensive and noninvasive and can be used to rule out rupture of the tendon. MRI is the gold standard but may not be needed in mild or straightforward cases. MRI is usually done if surgical intervention is a consideration.

DIFFERENTIAL DIAGNOSIS

Achilles tendinopathy primarily causes heel or posterior calf pain. Heel pain has varied causes including retrocalcaneal bursitis, infection, and fracture.

Plantar fasciitis and partial tendon rupture should be considered in the differential diagnosis of Achilles tendinopathy.

Posterior calf pain can also be caused by muscle strain, bruising, or thromboembolic disease.

INTERPROFESSIONAL COLLABORATIVE MANAGEMENT

Treatment of the acute phase of Achilles tendinopathy begins with the cessation of all sports activities and exercise. Tendon rest is imperative to avoid further injury. Severe inflammation may respond best to immobilization in a boot or cast. Crutches and partial weight bearing may be indicated. NSAIDs, either oral or topical, and an ice massage for 20 minutes 3 or 4 times a day help decrease inflammation and pain.[8] A simple shoe insert that raises the heel approximately 2 cm ($\frac{3}{4}$ inch) also helps ease strain on the tendon. In more severe or chronic cases, ultrasound is an adjunct therapy used by physical therapists. Regular follow-up visits to assess progress and to discourage the patient from returning to activity prematurely are necessary. Resolution of acute tendinopathy can take 8 weeks or longer. A program of stretching and strengthening begins when pain and swelling have subsided. Many patients can recover fully with exercise alone.[8] It is essential that patients do stretching exercises before engaging in any exercise to prevent recurrence or rupture.

Patients with severe tendinitis or suspected tendon rupture require immediate referral to an orthopedic surgeon/podiatrist. Cases unresponsive to conservative treatment may benefit from surgical débridement. In rare cases, tendon transplant to augment the strength of the damaged tendon may be necessary.[9]

In addition, patients who fail to respond to conservative therapy or who have significant tightness in the hamstrings or gastrocnemius require referral. Most patients will benefit from a referral to physical therapy for pain management and longer-term stretching and strengthening.

COMPLICATIONS

Achilles tendon rupture (see below) is the most common complication of Achilles tendinitis. Frank rupture is best demonstrated by MRI of the area. Immobilization and/or surgery may be necessary for healing and return to function. Shortening of the tendon, chronic pain, chronic foot drop, and recurrent injuries as a result of the associated abnormal gait also may result from acute tendinopathy.[9]

PATIENT AND FAMILY EDUCATION

Achilles tendinopathy can be a frustrating, slowly resolving, and a recurrent problem. Patients with this condition need support during rehabilitation and need to be educated about proper retraining and stretching programs. During the rehabilitative phase, alternative activities such as swimming and cycling can be pursued as long as participation does not cause pain.

ACHILLES TENDON RUPTURE

DEFINITION AND EPIDEMIOLOGY

Achilles tendon rupture is a sudden event that results from a forced stretch on an already degenerating tendon; it is a soft tissue emergency. There is an increased risk for this injury in poorly conditioned athletes older than 30 years. In all, 80% of those injured are men; moreover, because most right-handed people begin their gait with the left foot, there is a higher incidence of left tendon ruptures.[10]

PATHOPHYSIOLOGY

Despite being the thickest and strongest tendon in the body, the Achilles tendon is the one most commonly ruptured, possibly as a result of underlying tendon degeneration or weakness that predisposes the tendon to rupture. In persons older than 30 years, there is a decreased blood supply to the area where the tendon most often ruptures. The offending event is often a jump, a sudden change in direction, or simply a push-off in stride. The pop of a tendon rupture is audible to others nearby.

CLINICAL PRESENTATION

The classic comment by patients with an Achilles tendon rupture is, "I thought I was shot in the calf." There is sudden weakness in the ankle. It is impossible to rise up on the toes, and most people limp; pain, however, is not common.

PHYSICAL EXAMINATION

There is a visible and palpable gap overlying the tendon where the rupture occurred, usually about 4 cm (1½ inches) above the calcaneal prominence. The definitive evaluation is the Thompson test, which is performed with the patient kneeling on a chair or prone with the knee in flexed position. The tendon is intact if the foot plantar flexes when the calf is squeezed (negative Thompson result). If there is no movement, the tendon is ruptured (positive Thompson result). The Thompson test result can be negative if the tear is partial.

DIAGNOSTICS

Radiologic examinations are not helpful because tendons are not radiopaque. Ultrasound or MRI will demonstrate the rupture and can be used if indicated.

DIFFERENTIAL DIAGNOSIS

The classic presentation and physical findings that characterize a ruptured Achilles tendon simplify the diagnosis. However, the diagnosis may be more complex with a partial tear. Achilles tendinopathy or retrocalcaneal bursitis are both painful but not usually associated with a sudden onset or audible pop.

INTERPROFESSIONAL COLLABORATIVE MANAGEMENT

 Immediate referral to an orthopedic surgeon/podiatrist is required for an Achilles tendon rupture, it is a soft tissue emergency.

There are two accepted treatments of the ruptured Achilles tendon. The conservative, nonsurgical approach requires functional bracing, which allows for earlier mobilization. Traditionally, a long-leg cast or rigid boot with the foot in a plantar-flexed position has been used. The cast stays on for approximately 6 weeks, allowing the tendon to heal by scar formation. Wearing of a heel lift for 2 months helps prevent undue stress on the new scar after casting. Unfortunately, this method has multiple disadvantages. The tendon heals longer in length, which weakens the calf muscle and the push-off power. Calf muscles also atrophy in a cast, which adds to the decreased strength and size and longer rehabilitation. In addition, 10% to 12% of the tendons allowed to heal in this manner rupture again once activities resume.[11] Patients with chronic pain who are not surgical candidates may benefit from an ankle-foot orthosis.

The second method of treatment for a ruptured Achilles tendon is surgical repair, usually by direct reapproximation of the two ends of the tendon. Tendon transplant may also be used to augment strength. The patient is in a long-leg cast for 6 weeks after surgery, then wears a short-leg walking cast for an additional 4 weeks.[12] As in the nonoperative method, a heel lift is used to prevent undue stress on the tendon. Open surgical treatment of acute Achilles tendon ruptures significantly reduces the risk of re-rupture compared with nonsurgical treatment but produces significantly higher risks of other complications, including wound infection, damage to the sural nerve, and deep venous thrombosis (DVT). Surgical complications may be reduced by performing surgery percutaneously.[11,12] Patients who have undergone surgical repair return to work sooner and are generally able to begin rehabilitation sooner.

COMPLICATIONS

Weakened or atrophied muscles with resultant gait disorders are a common complication of tendon ruptures. Both treatment methods are associated with deep vein thrombosis, tendon stiffness, and tendon elongation. Close attention to rehabilitation and muscle strengthening after the injury helps reduce the magnitude of these complications.

PATIENT AND FAMILY EDUCATION

The most important education for Achilles tendon rupture is prevention. Patients who are novice exercisers should be instructed to follow a simple, gentle stretching program beforehand. For example, patients can stand on a slanted board or on the edge of a step and let the heels drop below the level of the step. They hold this stretched position for 10 to 15 seconds, and then repeat the exercise for 10 to 15 minutes. If patients cannot feel a pull on the Achilles tendon, they are not doing the stretch properly. Bouncing is counterproductive.

PLANTAR FASCIITIS

DEFINITION AND EPIDEMIOLOGY

Plantar fasciitis is a painful disorder that involves the plantar aspect of the heel. It can be acute or chronic and is characterized by pain in the bottom of the foot, along the arch, and in the heel.[13] A dense fibrous tissue, the plantar fascia, extends from the calcaneal tuberosity to the metatarsal heads. The fascia can become irritated from overuse, trauma, or shoes with poor arch support. People with flat or cavus feet are especially vulnerable to this condition.

PATHOPHYSIOLOGY

The plantar fascia supports the arch and the sole of the foot. High impact or stress, such as running and jumping, increases the pressure exerted on the fascia by spreading the toes or flattening the arch; this tears the fascia. Four common causes of fascia tears or inflammation are a sudden turn that places increased pressure on the sole of the foot, shoes with inadequate support, shoes with stiff soles, and feet that pronate excessively. Other contributing factors include obesity, a job that requires standing for long periods, and excessive running. Patients commonly have heel spurs, although the relationship is unclear. The pain is gradual in onset and increases as the inflammation worsens.[14]

CLINICAL PRESENTATION

Patients with plantar fasciitis complain of pain with weight bearing the first thing in the morning or after periods of rest. Pain can also be elicited with stretching of the fascia. High-impact activities, running, barefoot walking, standing for prolonged periods, and rising up on toes can aggravate the pain or make it unbearable. Patients occasionally limp or avoid planting the heel when walking.

PHYSICAL EXAMINATION

With plantar fasciitis, there is point tenderness at the insertion of the fascia to the calcaneus. The patient may have fullness along the arch and pain along the body of the fascia, at the medial and lateral aspects of the heel, or at the metatarsal heads. Plantar pain is common in obese patients, patients with pronated feet, or those with atrophy of the calcaneal fat pad.

INITIAL DIAGNOSTICS

Plantar Fasciitis

IMAGING
- X-ray studies
- Ultrasonography or MRI

DIAGNOSTICS

Weight-bearing x-ray studies may be indicated to rule out any bone abnormality or other underlying causes, such as a foreign body. Radiographs commonly reveal a bone spur that points forward from the heel. In cases unresponsive to conservative treatment, ultrasound or MRI may help rule out more serious issues.

DIFFERENTIAL DIAGNOSIS

A history of early morning heel discomfort that resolves after several minutes but returns later in the day is usually clinically diagnostic of plantar fasciitis. However, other causes of heel pain should be considered; these include calcaneal fracture, especially if associated with a history of trauma, retrocalcaneal or infracalcaneal bursitis, and gout (see Chapter 158).

Infection of the calcaneal fat pad, arthritis, plantar warts, and tarsal tunnel syndrome, as well as neuropathy and peripheral vascular disease can also cause foot pain.

INTERPROFESSIONAL COLLABORATIVE MANAGEMENT

A conservative approach to management of this condition begins with complete rest from high-impact activities. Walking barefoot or in flat shoes (i.e., flip-flops) should be avoided. All shoes should have good arch support, which can be achieved with commercially available arch supports. Some patients do well with a heel cup or heel pad that raises the heel approximately $\frac{1}{4}$ inch. NSAIDs and ice massage help reduce inflammation and pain. A key component of treatment is a referral to physical therapy for a program of exercises that stretch the heel cord and plantar fascia. Corticosteroid injection at the heel can be very helpful.[14]

Patients who do not improve with above conservative treatment may benefit from a referral to podiatry or an orthopedic surgeon specializing in foot and ankle problems. Second-tier treatment options may include night splints, a second steroid injection, prescription orthotics, and immobilization. Extracorporeal shock wave therapy is often recommended when more conservative therapy fails to relieve symptoms. This form of therapy is delivered either in a series of low-intensity treatments, which can be mildly painful, or a single high-intensity treatment, which can be very painful and may require pretreatment sedation. Shock wave therapy is thought to work by inducing microtrauma to the tissue, which then initiates a healing response that includes increased formation of blood vessels carrying nutrients to the area and inflammatory mediators out of the area.[15]

Plantar fasciotomy is reserved for cases that fail to respond to all other treatment.

COMPLICATIONS

Usually no complications are associated with plantar fasciitis. However, an alteration in gait can cause other musculoskeletal problems, such as hip or back pain. Plantar fasciitis can be a lingering problem that frustrates both the patient and the provider.

PATIENT AND FAMILY EDUCATION

Rest is the first treatment of plantar fasciitis. Patients are advised to keep weight off the foot until the inflammation subsides. Ice to the sore area for 20 minutes 3 or 4 times a day can be helpful to relieve symptoms. The health care provider often will recommend nonsteroidal antiinflammatory medication. Custom orthotics or night splints that keep the foot in dorsiflexion can be helpful. A program of home exercises to stretch the Achilles tendon and plantar fascia is the mainstay for treatment of the condition and for lessening the chance of recurrence.[16] Overweight patients should be advised to lose weight. Many public access websites that demonstrate stretching techniques are available.

MORTON NEUROMA

DEFINITION AND EPIDEMIOLOGY

Morton neuroma is a result of perineural fibrosis of the plantar nerve at the point where the medial and lateral branches of the plantar nerve converge. This condition is seen primarily in middle-aged women, with the most common cause thought to be being wearing narrow, pointed-toe, or high-heeled shoes causing entrapment, although repetitive trauma, ischemia, impingement, and intermetatarsal bursitis are contributors. This condition can also develop in people with claw toes and bunions.

PATHOPHYSIOLOGY

Compression of the interdigital plantar nerves causes repeated trauma, which in turn causes inflammation and fibrosis of the nerve sheath. Tight, pointed-toe shoes aggravate the irritation once the neuroma has formed.

CLINICAL PRESENTATION

Patients with Morton neuroma report severe pain and burning in the region of the third web space. Going barefoot and undergoing foot massages relieve the discomfort. Elevation of the foot aggravates the condition.

PHYSICAL EXAMINATION

The physical examination of a patient with Morton neuroma usually reveals point tenderness and often edema over the third web space, between the third and fourth metatarsals. Mulder sign is elicited if compression of the medial and lateral sides of the patient's foot with one hand and squeezing between the third and fourth metatarsal bones, or other web space, with the other results in a palpable or audible click. The patient may also feel acute pain radiating to the adjacent toes and upward along the foot.[17] On occasion, paresthesias occur at the reciprocal surfaces of the toes. The examination findings are otherwise unremarkable.

DIAGNOSTICS

Ultrasound or MRI can aid in diagnosis in the absence of a clear-cut history and examination findings.[18]

DIFFERENTIAL DIAGNOSIS

The plantar surface of the foot should be smooth and nontender. Calluses and plantar warts on the ball of the foot may be tender, rough, and nodular. Ganglia are cyst-like in appearance, whereas infectious processes classically have edema, erythema, warmth, and tenderness.

Ledderhose syndrome, also known as *plantar fibromatosis*, is a disorder of fibrous tissue proliferation, characterized by a slow-growing nodular thickening, most often within the central band of the plantar aponeurosis. Stress fractures, bursitis, or arthritic changes also cause foot pain.

INTERPROFESSIONAL COLLABORATIVE MANAGEMENT

Conservative treatment using a stepwise protocol can resolve this condition. Patient education, wider-toed shoes, insole adjustments, separation of the toes with a small pad, and NSAIDs help reduce the inflammation. In persistent cases, injection with steroids, or local anesthetic or alcohol, can be temporarily effective at relieving pain but offers no long-term solution.[19] Finally, surgical excision may be indicated as a last resort.

PATIENT AND FAMILY EDUCATION

Patients should be encouraged to wear properly fitting shoes that have adequate toe room, good arch support, and a low or flat heel. Shoes should be purchased at the end of the day, when feet are bigger, and should be replaced when support wears out. Shoes should be fitted to ensure proper size. Metatarsal arch pads, if used correctly, may ease the discomfort associated with Morton neuroma and metatarsalgia.

OTHER COMMON CAUSES OF FOOT PAIN

Bunions, bunionettes, corns, calluses, hammertoes, hallux rigidus, hallux valgus, plantar warts, ingrown toenails, and tarsal tunnel syndrome are discussed in Table 154.2, along with their differential diagnoses and management. Stress fractures of the metatarsals are common injuries in runners and others participating in running sports.

TABLE 154.2 **Other Common Foot Problems**[a]			
Problem	**Presentation**	**Examination and Diagnostics**	**Differential Diagnosis and Management**
BUNION			
An inflammatory degenerative deformity of the first MTP joint related to flat feet or laxity of the first toe and first metatarsal bone	Intense pain over the first MTP joint	Edema, deformity, and tenderness of the first metatarsal head; may have joint crepitus on palpation *Diagnostics:* If gout is suspected, uric acid levels and joint aspiration are considered; x-ray studies are not diagnostic	*Differential diagnosis:* Gout *Management:* Warm packs or soaks, NSAIDs, and well-fitted shoes with adequate toe space Podiatry referral indicated for custom-made protective shield or foot mold Orthopedic or podiatry referral necessary for surgical correction if conservative management does not control pain

Continued

TABLE 154.2	Other Common Foot Problems—cont'd		
Problem	**Presentation**	**Examination and Diagnostics**	**Differential Diagnosis and Management**
BUNIONETTE Pressure over the bone prominence on the fifth metatarsal head that results in bursa or ulceration	Painful, edematous lesion on the MTP joint of the fifth toe	Edema and erythema over the lateral aspect of the MTP of the fifth toe; may be accompanied by a cyst-like, fluid-filled lesion	Properly fitting shoes with adequate toe room, bunion padding Filing down of hard lesions
CALLUS Hypertrophied area of skin on sole of foot related to excessive supination, pronation, or other abnormality	Usually asymptomatic	Dried, hypertrophied epidermal layer; may surround or protect a plantar wart or foreign body	Daily skin cream or lanolin, use of pumice stone by patient Débridement of painful calluses with a scalpel to relieve pressure Orthotic device as indicated For patients with diabetes or PVD, see Corn
CORN *Hard corn (heloma durum):* hyperkeratotic lesions caused by pressure or friction; usually found on the toes or other bone prominence *Soft corn (heloma molle):* macerated, interdigital, and painful; caused by pressure	Painful lesion between toes or on dorsal surface of toes	Erythematous, painful lesion; patient may also have hammertoes	Avoidance of tight-fitting shoes, use of corn pads to relieve pressure, routine paring of corns with file or scalpel Powder and lamb's wool or soft cotton between toes to prevent excessive moisture Referral to orthotic specialist for customized orthotic device Surgical repair for accompanying hammertoe or arthroplasty as needed Vigilant care for patients with diabetes or PVD to prevent corns or calluses and ulceration or infection
HALLUX FLEXUS (HAMMERTOE OR CLAW TOE)			
Dorsiflexion of proximal joint of second toe while middle joint is plantar flexed	Painful corn the most common complaint	Dorsal flexion of first phalanx of second toe (either foot), with plantar flexion in second phalanx; may be accompanied by painful callus on metatarsal head or at nail end as well as painful corn on dorsal surface of the proximal interphalangeal joint	See Corn Referral to podiatrist or orthopedic surgeon for surgical repair
HALLUX RIGIDUS Inflexible great toe, usually a result of arthritic changes	Pain with ambulation, climbing stairs	Immobile, fixated first MTP joint; may be slightly edematous with accompanying irregularity of joint edges related to osteophyte formation; diminished activity and passive range of motion caused by immobility and pain *Diagnostics:* x-ray study (anteroposterior and lateral views)	NSAIDs for pain Podiatry or orthopedic referral for surgical repair
HALLUX VALGUS, HALLUX VARUS			
Hallux valgus: great toe laterally displaced toward other toes *Hallux varus:* great toe medially displaced away from other toes	Painful bunion of first MTP joint	*Hallux valgus:* great toe laterally displaced with possible accompanying bunion, hammertoe; may have extension of second toe over great toe *Hallux varus:* great toe medially displaced	Bunion care as described under Bunion Surgical or podiatry referral as indicated

TABLE 154.2 Other Common Foot Problems—cont'd

Problem	Presentation	Examination and Diagnostics	Differential Diagnosis and Management
ONYCHOCRYPTOSIS (INGROWN TOENAIL)			
Usually related to poor nail trimming or tight-fitting shoes	Pain and edema of great toe	Tender, edematous, erythematous area at corner of distal nail bed; lateral nail bed usually involved and obscured by hypertrophied tissue Evidence of purulent discharge Careful examination for lymphangitis and range of motion	For minimum ingrown toenail, wedge removal of nail edge to relieve discomfort If infection is present, patient is immunocompromised, or nail is severely ingrown, podiatry or surgical consultation for nail excision and possible matricectomy Treatment of infection with appropriate antibiotic; patient instructed to soak foot in warm water several times daily, to elevate foot, to apply bandage, and to wear open-toed shoes or soft slippers Further instruction regarding nail care
PLANTAR WARTS			
Warty growth on plantar surface caused by viral infection	May be asymptomatic or patient may report pruritic, painful lesion on sole of foot; increasing pain with weight-bearing activities	Callus possibly obscuring wart, which commonly is 1 mm to 1 cm in size Paring of callus revealing rough lesion with numerous small, black spots in center of lesion	*Differential diagnosis:* Porokeratotic lesion, foreign body *Management.* May resolve spontaneously For patients without diabetes or PVD: daily débridement with pumice stone, application of salicylic acid solution nightly to affected area, and gentle débridement of lesion each morning with an emery board Reminder to patients that lesions can spread, so débrided tissue must be carefully discarded Referral to podiatry indicated if conservative measures fail
TARSAL TUNNEL SYNDROME			
Compression of the tibial nerve	Pain, numbness, and tingling sole of foot	Tinel test Nerve conduction velocity studies	*Differential diagnosis:* Ankle arthritis, neuropathy *Management:* NSAIDs, orthotics, steroid injection, podiatry or surgical referral for decompression

aBecause of the classic presentation of these disorders, diagnostic testing and differential diagnoses are noted only when indicated
MTP, Metatarsophalangeal; *NSAID*, Nonsteroidal antiinflammatory drug; *PVD*, peripheral vascular disease.

REFERENCES

1. Wedmore, I., Young, S., & Franklin, J. (2015). Emergency Department evaluation and management of Foot and Ankle Pain. *Emergency Medicine Clinics of North America, 23*(2), 363–396.
2. Doherty, C., Delahunt, E., Caulfield, B., et al. (2014). The incidence and prevalence of ankle sprain injury: A systematic review and meta-analysis of prospective epidemiological studies. *Sports Medicine (Auckland, N.Z.), 44*(1), 123–140.
3. Kaminski, T., Hertel, J., Amendola, N., et al. (2013). National Athletic Trainers Association position statement: Conservative management and prevention of ankle sprains in athletics. *Journal of Athletic Training, 48*(4), 528–595.
4. Predel, H. G., & Giannetti, B. (2013). Diclofenac sodium topical gel (DSG) 1% reduces swelling and tenderness and improves ankle joint function in subjects with acute ankle sprains: A randomized, double-blind, placebo controlled trial. *Orthopaedic Journal of Sports Medicine, 1*(4).
5. Doherty, C., Bleakley, C., Delahunt, E., & Holden, S. (2017). Treatment and prevention of acute and recurrent ankle sprain: An overview of systematic reviews with meta-analysis. *British Journal of Sports Medicine, 51*(2), 113–125.
6. Weinfeld, S. B. (2013). Achilles tendon disorders. *The Medical Clinics of North America, 98*(2), 331–338.
7. Maffulli, N., Via, A. G., & Oliva, F. (2015). Chronic Achilles tendon disorders: Tendinopathy and chronic rupture. *Clinics in Sports Medicine, 34*(3), 607–624.
8. McClinton, S., Luedke, L., & Clewley, D. (2017). Non-surgical management of mid substance Achilles tendinopathy. *Clinics in Podiatric Medicine and Surgery, 34*(2), 137–160.
9. Caudell, G. (2017). Insertional Achilles tendinopathy. *Clinics in Podiatric Medicine and Surgery, 34*(2), 195–205.
10. Kraeulter, M. J., Purcell, J. M., & Hunt, K. J. (2017). Chronic Achilles tendon rupture. *Foot and Ankle International, 38*(8), 921–929.
11. Maffulli, N., Via, A. G., & Oliva, F. (2016). Achilles tendon rupture. In *Arthroscopic and sport injuries* (pp. 77–81). Retrieved from https://link.springer.com/chapter/10.1007/978-3-319-14815-1_10 on Nov 10, 2017.
12. Holm, C., Kjaer, M., & Eliasson, P. (2015). Achilles Tendon rupture—treatment and complications: A systematic Review. *Scandinavian Journal of Medicine and Science in Sports, 25*(1), e1–e10.
13. American Academy of Orthopedic Surgeons. Fact sheet: plantar fasciitis. Retrieved from http://orthoinfo.aaos.org/topic.cfm?topic=a00149 updated 2010. (Accessed 13 November 2017).
14. Schwartz, E. (2014). Plantar fasciitis: A concise review. *The Permanente Journal, 18*(1), e105–e107.
15. Gollwitzer, H., Saxena, A., DiDomenico, L. A., et al. (2015). Clinically relevant effectiveness of focused extracorporeal shock wave therapy in the treatment of plantar fasciitis: A randomized controlled multicenter study. *The Journal of Bone and Joint Surgery. American Volume, 97*(9), 701–708.
16. The Permanente Medical Group, copyright 2009-2017. https://mydoctor.kaiserpermanente.org/ncal/mdo/presentation/stayinghealthy/topic.jsp?condition=Condition_Heel_Pain.xml. (Accessed 14 November 2017).
17. Jain, S., & Mannan, K. (2013). The diagnosis and management of Morton's neuroma. A literature review. *Foot & Ankle Specialist, 6*, 307–317.
18. Ata, M. A., Onat, S. S., & Ozcaker, L. (2016). Ultrasound guided diagnosis and treatment of Morton's neuroma. *Pain Physician, 19*, e355–e357. Retrieved from www.painphysicianjournal.com/current/pdf?article=mjuzma%3D%3D+journal+94 on Nov 11, 2017.
19. Gurdezi, S., White, T., & Ramesh, P. (2013). Alcohol injection for Morton's neuroma: A 5 year follow-up. *Foot and Ankle International, 34*(8), 1064–1067.

CHAPTER 155

BONE LESIONS: NEOPLASMS AND TUMOR MIMICKERS

John S. Groundland • Eric R. Henderson

DEFINITION AND EPIDEMIOLOGY

The term *bone tumor* is used broadly, and often incorrectly, to describe a wide variety of true primary bone neoplasms and tumor mimickers, which include developmental and metabolic anomalies. Common developmental anomalies that are often called bone tumors include fibrous cortical defects. True bone neoplasms arise from the connective tissues—those derived from the mesoderm—and span a broad spectrum of aggressiveness from tumors with no metastatic potential, such as osteoid osteoma, to tumors with certain metastatic potential, such as dedifferentiated chondrosarcoma. The skeleton is also a common site of metastasis for more common carcinomas, derived from endoderm- and ectoderm-derived cancers. These metastatic lesions are commonly referred to as "bone cancer," which we believe should be avoided to prevent confusion with primary bone lesions. Multiple myeloma is another cancer that presents a problem in categorization, discussed below. Tumor mimickers, such as bone lesions caused by gout, arthritis, and metabolic diseases, may have an appearance similar to bone neoplasms. Because so many disparate bone lesions are commonly described as bone tumors, clinicians should take care when informing patients that they may have a bone tumor, as most bone lesions pose no metastatic threat and incomplete knowledge of a lesion's nature can be a source of unnecessary stress to patients and patients' families.

The most common malignant tumor that originates in bone is a subject of controversy. Some clinicians consider multiple myeloma (see Chapter 220), with an incidence of 6.1 per 100,000, to be the most common primary bone tumor due to its general predilection for the skeleton. However, because myeloma is a tumor of plasma cells, which are not considered among the list of native bone cells, other clinicians favor osteosarcoma, a cancer derived from osteoblasts, as the most common primary bone malignancy. We, the authors, agree with this latter sentiment.

Cancers that originate in mesoderm-derived connective tissues such as bone, tendons, or muscles are classified as sarcomas. Osteosarcoma, the most common bone sarcoma, originates from primitive mesenchymal bone-forming cells. Ewing sarcoma originates from cells that arise in the embryonic neural crest. Chondrosarcoma develops in primitive mesenchymal cartilage-forming cells.[1] Primary cancers of the bone account for less than 0.2% of all cancers. Osteosarcoma is the most common sarcoma, with an incidence estimated to be 1 in 1 million. After osteosarcoma, chondrosarcoma and undifferentiated pleomorphic sarcomas are the most common bone sarcomas. Approximately 3000 primary bone sarcomas are diagnosed each year in the United States. In children and teenagers younger than 20 years, the incidence of malignant bone tumors is 8.7 per million.[2]

In adults older than 40 years, metastatic deposits in bone from cancers elsewhere in the body are more common than primary bone sarcomas. 18% to 27% of patients with stage IV breast or prostate cancer and 15% to 30% of patients with kidney, lung, uterine, thyroid, stomach, rectal, bladder, or colon cancer will develop metastatic cancer in the bones.[3] Five-year survival rate is highest for breast cancer patients and lowest for lung cancer patients.

Myeloma, lymphoma, and leukemia are lymphoproliferative cancers characterized by excess production of abnormal white blood cells. Primary lymphoma of bone is a rare form of lymphoma that accounts for approximately 7% of all malignant bone tumors.[4]

The incidence of benign bone neoplasms and tumor-like lesions are difficult to estimate because many are left untreated and most are likely never discovered. In children, osteochondroma, non-ossifying fibroma, and fibrous dysplasia are the most common benign bone tumors. In persons aged 20 to 40 years, giant cell tumor and enchondroma are the most commonly diagnosed bone tumors.[5] A recent study indicates that this incidence has not changed in the past 30 years.[5]

PATHOPHYSIOLOGY

In most cases, true benign and malignant bone neoplasms arise from the deletion, addition, or modification of genes leading to upregulated replication or abnormal cell products. These genetic and epigenetic anomalies disrupt the orderly growth, division, or senescence of cells by a number of mechanisms. One type of tumorigenesis is linked to the creation of a novel "fusion" gene. Approximately half of the fusion genes identified in sarcomas belong to the FET family of transcription regulation genes (FUS/TLS, EWS, and TAF15). More than one molecular or genetic abnormality may be necessary for the development of cancer. The identification of precise markers and mechanisms of tumorigenesis in the laboratory benefitted clinicians in the form of highly specific diagnostic tests and treatments (see Chapter 7). The identification of specific chromosomal abnormalities allows definitive diagnosis of certain sarcomas using DNA probes, such as in fluorescence in situ hybridization (FISH). For example, primary aneurysmal bone cysts (ABCs) are now able to be diagnosed based on the presence of a unique chromosomal translocation resulting in a fusion protein wherein the cadherin 11 gene is joined with the ubiquitin-specific protease 6; this translocation is found in about 70% of primary ABCs.[6] These unique markers also offer attractive targets for highly specific new treatments for bone neoplasms.

Some bone cancers arise from inherited defects in tumor suppressor genes such as the retinoblastoma (*RB1*) gene. The cells of normal individuals have two intact *RB1* genes on chromosome 13, and both genes must be defective for cancer to develop. Affected individuals inherit one defective copy of the *RB1* gene from a parent; the other mutates during fetal development. These children develop retinoblastoma in childhood, and they are at high risk for osteosarcoma, small cell lung cancer, and synovial sarcoma as adults.[7]

A small number of malignant bone tumors are caused by chronic diseases. Approximately 5% of patients with widespread Paget disease of bone (see Chapter 163) develop sarcoma, termed Paget sarcoma, in the affected bones, usually osteosarcoma. Patients with long-standing infections that manifest with a draining sinus tract are at risk for development of squamous cell carcinoma at the site of the sinus tract's exit through the skin. The data on exposure to chlorinated dioxin contaminants in the herbicide Agent Orange have not provided consistent evidence of an increased cancer risk in exposed individuals.[8] Other factors, such as genetic polymorphisms, which are known to increase the risk of developing non-Hodgkin lymphoma, may play a role.[9]

CLINICAL PRESENTATION AND PHYSICAL EXAMINATION

The evaluation of a bone tumor begins with a thorough history and physical examination. The evaluation must give special attention to the patient's age, the patient's cancer risk factors, and personal cancer history. Tobacco use as well as the status of cancer screening examinations, such as prostate examination, colonoscopy, and mammography, should be documented. Patients who were treated for cancer in the past may consider themselves cured, and as a result they may not volunteer their cancer history unless carefully prompted. A thorough health history is often the most efficient way to identify the origin of the bone tumor. In taking the history of present illness, the provider should endeavor to establish the precise chronology of the pain. Patients may ascribe the pain from a bone tumor to a minor injury or accident. However, closer questioning will often reveal that the pain was present before the injury.

The general physical examination may reveal systemic findings that may be associated with the bone lesion's underlying cause, such as a growth disturbance, anemia, or cachexia. The focused musculoskeletal examination should assess the entire region of the body involved in the problem. The shoulder, hip, and knee cannot be comprehensively examined with the patient's clothing left on, and an incomplete examination may contribute to delay in making the correct diagnosis. The examiner should look for the presence of warmth or inflammation, a mass, loss of full joint motion, or lymphadenopathy. Subtle abnormalities are easy to identify by comparing the findings in the affected region with those in the corresponding normal region. Even large lesions that are deep seated in the shoulder, pelvis, or thigh may be difficult to identify by palpation. However, they can be easily seen if the examiner visually compares the normal and the abnormal sides of the body from a short distance away.

Delays in the recognition, workup, and diagnosis of bone lesions are common. Dr. William Enneking described three categories of benign bone lesions: (1) latent/indolent, (2) active, and (3) aggressive. This classification system should be considered with respect to that reported by Lodwick and later modified by Caracciolo.[10]

Indolent or latent bone lesions such as non-ossifying fibroma in children and enchondroma in adults are generally asymptomatic and are detected only as incidental findings during radiographic evaluation for an unrelated musculoskeletal complaint. A careful history and physical examination combined with radiographic findings are often enough to verify that the bone lesion is not the pain generator. In general, no workup or treatment for an indolent lesion is needed other than repeat radiographs to verify that the lesion is not changing over time.

Active benign bone lesions grow over time and can locally invade and weaken the adjacent bone. Examples of active tumors include chondromyxoid fibroma and fibrous dysplasia. In the primary care setting, patients often report mild, gradually increasing pain with minimal loss of function and no obvious abnormalities on physical examination. In these patients, pain after an injury may be the reason the patient visits the primary care provider, but a careful history may reveal that the pain was present and gradually increasing before the injury. This is an important distinction because it establishes that the tumor is the source of the pain, not the injury. In active bone tumors, the radiographs show that the tumor is slowly growing. There will be evidence of local damage and a corresponding response from the involved bone. Referral of these cases to an orthopedic oncologist is recommended. Most of these tumors are benign, and as a result many can be treated by thorough curettage of the tumor cavity followed by packing with bone graft, bone cement, or other material to restore the bone integrity.

Aggressive benign bone tumors include aneurysmal bone cyst, giant cell tumor of bone, and chondroblastoma, the latter two of which have a low but documented potential for metastasis, making their status of "benign" tumors somewhat questionable. These tumors tend to present with increasing pain and often a palpable mass. These tumors also require referral to an orthopedic oncologist and can be managed with curettage, although en bloc resection, when possible, results in a lower recurrence rate. Aneurysmal bone cysts have recently been documented to respond to injection of a doxycycline foam preparation, which may limit the need for surgery in the future.[11]

Bone lesions that demonstrate a Lodwick classification of 2 or 3 are usually malignant and typically are discovered after weeks of progressive pain and a mass or swelling of the limb or joint. Examples of aggressive bone tumors include osteosarcoma, lymphoma, Ewing sarcoma, and metastatic adenocarcinoma. The median time to recognition and diagnosis of an osteosarcoma lesion is approximately two months. Constitutional symptoms are unusual in aggressive bone tumors, but fever and leukocytosis may occur in Ewing sarcoma and lymphoma. Pain that is noticed more at night, when the patient is distracted, is a common finding in early presentations of a malignant bone tumor. This pain usually progresses to become more related to activity, termed functional or mechanical pain, which is a warning sign of pathological fracture risk.

Careful history taking will allow the clinician to distinguish the pain of an aggressive bone tumor from typical pain of musculoskeletal origin, even at a relatively early stage. Patients with chordoma, a type of sarcoma that has a predilection for the sacrum, may come to their health care provider with persistent low back pain, constipation, or difficulty with defecation. Digital rectal examination reveals a mass growing out of the sacrum, which can block the rectum. Patients with active bone tumors require prompt referral to a specialist.

Adults who have been treated for cancers of the breast, prostate, lung, thyroid, kidney, or some gastrointestinal sites are at risk of bone metastasis, even years after the completion of the treatment and with no evidence of active disease. Patients with prior cancers should receive workups that are informed by their history; however, definitive management of a bone lesion should not be undertaken if knowledge of a different diagnosis may change the patient's ultimate outcome.

COMMON CLINICAL SCENARIOS

Being front-line medical providers, primary care physicians will often evaluate patients with bone pain and discover a previously undetected bone lesion. There are several clinical scenarios commonly encountered described below.

Low-Energy, Pathological Fractures (aka Compression Fracture or Pathologic Fracture)

In the majority of cases, low-energy fractures are caused by osteoporosis (see Chapter 163). Separating osteoporotic fractures from pathologic fractures is not always straightforward. Osteoporotic fractures occasionally manifest with a prodromal period showing increasing mechanical pain for 1 to 4 weeks followed by an acute exacerbation and radiographic findings of a fracture. The patient's clinical and radiographic findings are usually indicative of advanced osteoporosis. In contrast, patients with impending pathologic fractures may have had many weeks or months of prodromal pain. Plain radiographs of a cancer-related pathological fracture will often demonstrate a destructive bone lesion; however, MRI or CT and, when in doubt, a biopsy may be required to determine the true nature of a fracture when the cause is unclear.

Patients With Unexplained Musculoskeletal Pain

Pain caused by a bone lesion and—potentially—an impending pathologic fracture is most common in the hip, a common site of metastatic disease deposition. The pain is usually mechanical or functional in nature, exacerbated by walking or standing. This pain may become more constant and independent of activities. Most but not all patients have a previous diagnosis of cancer, especially breast or lung cancer. A significant percentage of patients have an actual or impending pathologic fracture as their first symptom of malignancy. In this setting, the patient should undergo evaluation for cancer risk factors, which may lead to a more targeted, accurate, and rapid workup. Symptomatic lesions will usually be evident on radiographs; however, MRI may be needed to identify lesions that do not cause overt bone destruction, most often seen with breast and prostate cancer metastases, which can have a blastic or mixed lytic and blastic appearance. Patients who are found to have a bone lesion, particularly one known or thought to be due to metastatic disease, should be evaluated based on the criteria of Mirel.[12]

Patient With a Bony Mass

Although pain is usually the symptom that initiates patient presentation, an enlarging mass may also occur. The most common scenario for this is a hard, fixed lesion in a child or teenager, and is usually an osteochondroma. Osteochondromas are benign lesions resulting from loss of growth polarity by a portion of the patient's physis, resulting in outward growth of the bone. Most bone tumor diagnoses are capable of causing a soft-tissue mass and, following osteochondroma, are usually aneurysmal bone cysts, osteosarcoma, and Ewing's sarcoma. However, these more aggressive diagnoses usually produce painful lesions.

DIAGNOSTICS

Screening laboratory examinations have a very limited role in the initial diagnostic evaluation of a patient with a newly detected bone lesion. Specific diagnostic tests have a limited role when a specific diagnosis is suspected, especially in the setting of a prior history of cancer. For example, prostate-specific antigen (PSA) may be tested quickly to determine if a patient has a recurrence of his cancer. However, an elevated PSA in the setting of a newly detected bone lesion is not diagnostic of that lesion, and if the patient's ultimate outcome may be jeopardized by improper surgical management of a presumed metastatic lesion, biopsy must be performed to rule out a second malignancy. Likewise, a patient with presumed multiple myeloma should have serum protein electrophoresis tested to identify secretion of tumor paraproteins; however, a definitive surgical intervention should be withheld until it can be determined that that patient indeed has the assumed diagnosis. Patients with a bone sarcoma often have entirely normal laboratory findings. Bone anomalies caused by infection are usually associated with an elevated white blood cell count, erythrocyte sedimentation rate (ESR), and C-reactive protein, although these markers may be normal in the setting of a chronic, indolent bone infection.

IMAGING STUDIES

After the history and physical examination has been completed, the best next step includes high-quality, **orthogonal**, digital radiographs of the affected region. Other studies, such as bone scan, PET scan, blood work, and other tests, may help guide a workup where a particular diagnosis is suspected or if assessment for multifocal disease is needed; in general, however, this shotgun approach to diagnosis is expensive and often unhelpful. Advanced imaging should be coordinated with an orthopedic oncologist after initial review of plain films. For most bone tumors, a differential diagnosis can be constructed based on the features on the plain x-ray film. Radiographs of malignant lesions often demonstrate a robust periosteal reaction as the periosteum attempts to contain the lesion by laying down bone while being pushed outward. The matrix of the lesion, as seen on radiographs, is usually indicative of the histological origin of the lesions. Osteoblastic-rich lesions show cumulus cloud–like ossification, cartilage-rich lesions show calcified arcs and rings, and fibrous lesions show a more radiolucent, "ground glass" affected area. In some cases, no other studies are needed. A careful analysis of the plain radiographs by an experienced musculoskeletal fellowship–trained radiologist or orthopedic oncologist may be sufficient to determine management.

INITIAL DIAGNOSTICS

Bone Tumors

IMAGING
- X-ray examination
- Additional (in consultation with orthopedic oncologist)
- CT or MRI
- PET scan
- Bone scan

INTERVENTIONAL
- Bone biopsy

LABORATORY[a]
- CBC[a]
- ESR and
- C-reactive protein
- Alkaline phosphatase
- Calcium
- Phosphorus
- Uric acid
- LFTs
- PSA
- Serum protein electrophoresis

[a]If indicated.

Role of Biopsy

Biopsy is the process of sampling the cells of the tumor for pathologic diagnosis. Historically biopsy has been reserved as the last procedure after all imaging studies, examinations, and laboratory studies were completed. However, biopsy is the ultimate diagnosis determinate, and its earlier, safe use may avoid multiple, unnecessary laboratory and imaging tests.

Bone tumor biopsy should be performed at the center that will perform the definitive management and under the guidance of an orthopedic oncologist.[13]

Microbiological culture of the lesion is often recommended, especially if the patient reports any symptoms that may indicate infection—fever, chills, cachexia—or if the radiographic findings and presentation are ambiguous.

The interpretation of bone tumor pathology is a complex and difficult task typically performed by specialized pathologists who have sufficient experience in bone tumor diagnosis. It is essential for the orthopedic oncology surgeon, musculoskeletal radiologist, and connective tissue pathologist to work together in a collaborative manner to properly diagnose a bone tumor.

DIFFERENTIAL DIAGNOSIS

 Priority differentials include musculoskeletal pain that lasts more than 6 months despite appropriate activity or occupational modifications; musculoskeletal pain in the setting of a history of cancer; unexplained deformity or mass; significant pain that occurs at night or that requires narcotic analgesic medications in patients without biopsychosocial factors.

The differential diagnosis is based on the patient's age, the history, examination, and imaging studies. Laboratory examination may help narrow down the possibilities. Obviously the goal will be to rule out malignant lesions or metastasis. This is best done with biopsy, which will provide the definitive diagnosis. Where infection is suspected, a culture of the biopsied material is indicated. Lesions that mimic bone tumors can be associated with metabolic conditions such as diabetes, hyperparathyroidism, and gout. Other tumor mimickers include congenital, post-traumatic, and degenerative lesions.

INTERPROFESSIONAL COLLABORATIVE MANAGEMENT
Benign Bone Tumors

Treatment of benign bone tumors depends on their behavior patterns (Table 155.1). Management of bone lesions with a latent behavior pattern, such as non-ossifying fibroma, enchondroma, and FD, may require no treatment. These benign tumors do not represent a significant risk to the patient's health. Once a bone tumor specialist has examined these tumors and determined that there is no increased risk of pathologic fracture, the tumor may be observed without biopsy. X-ray studies to verify that the tumor is not growing or changing are recommended every 3 to 6 months for 2 or 3 years. In some circumstances, when there is a risk of pathologic fracture, the tumor is removed by curettage and the bone is strengthened with bone graft, with or without a metallic plate or intramedullary rod.

Bone lesions with an active behavior pattern, such as GCT, CBMA, and CMF, require local treatment. After the workup and diagnosis, the lesions are removed by complete curettage. To reduce the chance of local recurrence, phenol, liquid nitrogen, or a mechanical burr may be used to additionally treat the site of the tumor and to remove or kill any residual cells. The bone defect is filled with acrylic bone cement or bone graft, and a plate or screws may be added according to the surgeon's preference. Bone lesions with an aggressive behavior pattern are treated according to the type of tumor.

TABLE 155.1	Management of Bone Tumors					
Type of Tumor	**Examples**	**Staging Workup**	**Biopsy Considerations**	**Surgical Management**	**Adjuvant Treatments**	**Follow-Up Guidelines**
Bone tumor with latent behavior pattern	Nonossified fibroma, enchondroma	History, physical examination, and plain x-ray studies	Necessary only if diagnostic workup reveals risk of pathologic fracture	Surgery often not required	None required	1–2 years; follow-up with plain x-ray examinations to verify lack of change
Bone tumor with active behavior pattern	Giant cell tumor, chondroblastoma	History, physical examination, plain x-ray studies, MRI, CT	Core needle or open incisional biopsy may be combined with surgical treatment	Most lesions treated with curettage and packing of the bone defect	Liquid nitrogen, phenol or mechanical burr used to reduce recurrence	2–5 years; clinical and x-ray follow-up to verify lack of recurrence
Bone tumor with aggressive behavior pattern	Osteosarcoma, Ewing sarcoma, lymphoma, myeloma	History, physical examination, plain x-ray studies, MRI, CT, ^{99m}Tc bone scan, CT scan of chest	Core needle or open incisional technique after completion of all imaging	Resection with a wide surgical margin	Bisphosphonates, chemotherapy, and radiotherapy	5–10 years; clinical follow-up with intermittent imaging to verify lack of recurrence; intermittent chest CT to rule out metastasis
Metastatic bone tumor	Metastatic breast, lung, prostate, renal, thyroid, and gastrointestinal cancers are typical	History, physical examination, ^{99m}Tc bone scan, skeletal survey	If primary tumor is known, closed needle biopsy technique for confirmation	Surgical stabilization of bones at risk of pathologic fracture, especially long bones	Bisphosphonates (zoledronic acid), radiation appropriate for small tumors (strontium 89, samarium 153)	Dependent on cancer diagnosis; typical to follow with ^{99m}Tc bone scans

Malignant Tumors and Sarcoma in Bone

Multiple myeloma is treated by multidrug chemotherapy or autologous stem cell transplantations, irradiation, maintenance of fluid and electrolyte balance, orthopedic stabilization of pathologic fractures, and bisphosphonates (see Chapter 220). Monitoring for hypercalcemia, anemia, dehydration, and infection is necessary. Intravenous therapy with pamidronate or zoledronic acid reduces the number of skeletal complications in myeloma and is recommended for all patients with multiple myeloma who have identifiable lytic bone lesions. For painful vertebral compression fractures, vertebroplasty can provide rapid and long-lasting relief of pain.

The treatment of malignant bone tumors and sarcomas varies by tumor type and stage. Low-grade malignant tumors and some sarcomas, such as many CHSAs, adamantinoma, and epithelioid hemangioendothelioma, may be treated by surgical removal with a wide margin only. Chemotherapy and radiotherapy may not be required. The goal of surgery in these cases is to remove the entire tumor, including a cuff of surrounding normal bone and soft tissue to ensure that there is no local recurrence. The resulting bone defect may be reconstituted with an allograft bone, a metallic prosthesis, or a combination of these.

High-grade malignant sarcomas, such as osteosarcoma and Ewing sarcoma, are treated with multimodality treatment, which combines surgery, preoperative and postoperative chemotherapy and radiotherapy, and bisphosphonates, according to the type and location of the tumor. In Ewing sarcoma, if the surgical treatment does not result in a wide margin, radiotherapy is used to reduce the risk of local recurrence. Bisphosphonate medications, such as pamidronate and zoledronic acid, are widely used to prevent unnecessary loss of bone mineral mass and fractures during treatment. Prolonged use of bisphosphonates and other antiresorptive medications in cancer patients carries a risk of osteonecrosis of the jaw and pathologic fractures.[14] Prevention and early diagnosis can reduce morbidity.

Metastatic Cancers in Bone

The management of patients with bone metastasis is focused on reducing the incidence of new metastatic tumor deposits in bone, hypercalcemia of malignancy, cord compression, pathologic fracture, radiation to bone, and surgery to bone, collectively known as skeletal-related events (SREs) [see Chapter 223]. Bisphosphonates and denosumab are most commonly used. Zoledronic acid is the most commonly used bisphosphonate, and it has been shown to prevent, minimize, and delay the onset of SREs. Denosumab, a new monoclonal antibody, also reduces the risk of SREs in metastatic cancer. Denosumab inhibits RANKL, which is a primary signaling protein in bone loss. Metastatic tumors in the skeleton are treated on the basis of location, symptoms, and tumor type. Estimation of the patient's ability to withstand the surgery and of the overall duration of survival helps guide the selection of treatment but is prone to error and should be used with caution. Most patients with cancer metastasis in bone cannot be cured, but function, pain control, and quality of life (QOL) can be enhanced by prompt and appropriate surgical treatments. Orthopedic stabilization of metastatic lesions will help maintain the patient's independence, dignity, and self-worth and minimize dependency, need for institutional care, and dependency on narcotic drugs. Patients with known metastatic lesions in bone should be systematically monitored for additional metastatic lesions so that they may be treated before they become advanced and cause complications.

Once a lesion is discovered, it should be evaluated by an orthopedic surgeon to estimate the risk of pathologic fracture. Pathologic fracture probability calculation is based on the size, radiologic features, pain characteristics, and skeletal location of the lesions. Metastatic lesions in the intertrochanteric region of the proximal femur just below the hip have the highest risk of pathologic fracture.

Orthopedic stabilization is indicated to maintain and to restore functional ability and to relieve pain from impending or actual pathologic fractures in long bones such as the humerus, femur, and tibia. Stabilization of impending fractures before actual pathologic fracture results in easier treatment and more rapid recovery for the patient. The weakened or fractured bones are usually stabilized with orthopedic plates or rods, combined with polymethyl methacrylate cement. After orthopedic stabilization, radiation may be recommended to prevent or to delay local recurrence and local progression of the tumor in a dose-dependent fashion. For metastatic lesions in the small bones or non–weight-bearing bones, such as the hands, feet, ribs, and scapula, radiation therapy is preferable to surgery. Patients with metastatic deposits in the bones should be given intravenous pamidronate or zoledronic acid. This treatment has been shown to decrease bone mineral loss associated with treatment, as well as to prevent or delay the onset of additional SREs in cancer patients with bone metastasis.[15]

Pain Management

Patients with bone tumors require a comprehensive pain management program. Benign bone tumors typically cause moderate pain, and surgical treatment results in a temporary increase in pain that may be managed with conventional modalities.

Patients with malignant or metastatic tumors in bone require more advanced pain management. Long-acting opioid pain medicines, transdermal delivery systems, pain medicine pumps, and multidrug protocols using controlled-release narcotics coupled with short-acting narcotics for breakthrough pain have been successfully used in the management of cancer pain. Pain management should be monitored to prevent overtreatment, undertreatment, or misuse. External beam radiation is effective in controlling pain in many of patients. The radionuclides strontium 89 and samarium 153 have been shown to be effective for generalized bone pain in patients with widely disseminated metastatic deposits.

Bisphosphonates should be considered for all patients with painful bone lesions. Bisphosphonate medications can decrease pain by preventing the growth and development of new and existing bone lesions. Although it is tempting to place patients with metastatic bone lesions on activity restriction to prevent pain, this may unintentionally accelerate bone damage because of disuse atrophy and calcium loss. Maintenance of normal activity levels should be the goal wherever possible. Patients with metastatic cancer in the vertebra may develop low-energy pathologic fractures (also known as compression fractures) leading to severe back pain. Vertebroplasty, which involves the injection of bone cement directly into a compressed vertebral body to stabilize it, and kyphoplasty, which involves inflating a balloon to elevate the compression first then injecting cement, may be indicated in these patients. Vertebroplasty and kyphoplasty are minimally invasive procedures and may, especially when combined with chemotherapy, provide pain relief. Complications such as infection, paraplegia, and cement embolism can occur.[16]

Postsurgical pain and phantom limb pain can be significant challenges in sarcoma patients who have received amputations. Gabapentin, amitriptyline, and benzodiazepine drugs as well as physical therapy, counseling, and counterirritant therapy, such as transcutaneous electrical nerve stimulation (TENS) units, are helpful adjuncts in complex pain control situations. Severe or chronic postoperative or post-cancer pain is often managed by pain control specialists.

LIFE SPAN CONSIDERATIONS AND PROGNOSIS

Benign bone tumors are uncommon in children younger than 10 years. Between the ages of 10 and 20 years, osteochondroma, osteoid osteoma, Langerhans cell histiocytosis, and FD are common benign bone tumors. In adults aged 20 to 40, enchondroma and GCT are commonly seen benign bone tumors.

Bone cancers have a strong predilection for certain age ranges. Children younger than 5 years are at risk for metastatic neuroblastoma in the bone. After the age of 8 years, the risk of Ewing sarcoma and osteosarcoma increases, especially around the time of the child's growth spurt. In young to middle-age adults, lymphoma of bone may be the most common malignant tumor of bone. Adults older than 40 years are at increasing risk of adenocarcinoma with metastatic deposits in the bone. Finally, age 50 through 70 is the time of life when multiple myeloma and CHSA are most likely to occur.

Primary Benign and Malignant Bone Tumors

Most latent bone tumors have no impact on patient prognosis or survival. Active bone tumors may locally damage bones and joints and result in loss of mobility or function. Some multifocal bone tumors, such as hereditary multiple exostosis and polyostotic FD, can lead to severe limitation of mobility, deformity, and chronic pain.

The prognosis for malignant sarcoma in bone is strongly related to the stage of the tumor rather than the cell type of the tumor. Patients with localized sarcoma have an 83% survival rate at 5 years. If regional metastasis has occurred, the 5-year survival rate drops to 54%, and if distant metastasis has occurred, 5-year survival is 16%. The 10-year survival rate is only slightly worse than the 5-year rate.[2] Survival in high-grade sarcoma has not changed dramatically in the past few decades, despite enhanced diagnostic and therapeutic modalities, new chemotherapeutic agents, and new surgical techniques.

Multiple myeloma, a disease primarily affecting older adults, has improved prognosis and survival in the past 10 years because of new active chemotherapy agents, autologous stem cell transplantation, and the use of bisphosphonates. Median survival is more than 5 years, and 3-year survival is 75% to 80%.[17] Important prognostic variables include age, disease stage, renal function, and performance status, as well as the presence of specific DNA abnormalities in the tumor cells.

Prognosis: Metastatic Bone Tumors

Increased use of bisphosphonates and denosumab, combined with targeted chemotherapy, radiation, and surgery, has contributed to a decrease in overall mortality for breast, lung, colon and rectal, and stomach cancers; leukemia; non-Hodgkin lymphoma; and cancers of other sites.[18] Aggressive treatment

of metastatic bone disease can lead to prolonged survival, and the number of patients living with metastatic cancer continues to grow.[18] Patients' QOL and performance status can be maintained despite the presence of skeletal metastasis. Treatment of SREs in patients with metastatic cancer, including treatment and stabilization of fractures, should not be withheld as long as there is a reasonable chance that the patient would benefit, even palliatively. Physicians' predictions of survival time for patients with advanced cancer are known to be inaccurate. Surgery for bone metastasis is most commonly used to treat impending or actual pathologic fractures and intractable bone pain. Cancer of the breast, prostate, kidney, and lung and myeloma account for approximately 80% of cases requiring surgical treatment of bone metastasis.[19]

INDICATIONS FOR REFERRAL OR HOSPITALIZATION

The number of possible bone tumors and the complexities of their treatment present a challenge for health care providers. Early and prompt referral of these patients to a pediatric orthopedic surgeon or orthopedic oncologist for evaluation, diagnostic workup, and possible treatment is recommended. It is preferable to refer patients before advanced imaging studies have been performed or to schedule the advanced imaging studies in cooperation with the orthopedic specialist. In this way, necessary imaging studies can be performed in a timely fashion, and wasteful and unnecessary tests can be avoided. Biopsy should be performed only by the surgeon or team who will be performing the definitive tumor treatment. The following are criteria for referral to an orthopedic specialist:

 Red flags include musculoskeletal pain that lasts more than 6 months despite appropriate activity or occupational modifications, musculoskeletal pain in the setting of a history of cancer, unexplained deformity or mass, significant pain that occurs at night or that requires narcotic analgesic medications in patients without biopsychosocial factors.

Delay in diagnosis of bone cancer and bone tumors has been the cause of a significant amount of malpractice litigation against physicians and health care providers of all types.[20]

Many factors contribute to delay in diagnosis. The patient may fail to appear in a timely fashion for an evaluation or may miss a scheduled follow-up appointment. The physician or health care provider may fail to appreciate the significance of the patient's complaints, may perform an incomplete examination, or may fail to schedule tests in a timely manner. Bone tumors may occur in vigorous, active individuals whose symptoms mimic minor musculoskeletal injuries, leading to delay and an incorrect initial diagnosis. The common perception that patients with bone cancer have cachexia, night pain, weight loss, or other severe systemic symptoms is false and misleading. A complete history, a careful examination, plain radiographs, and appropriate follow-up are usually sufficient to distinguish patients with bone tumors from patients with common musculoskeletal ailments.

PATIENT AND FAMILY EDUCATION

Because the discovery of a bone tumor always brings the specter of bone cancer, the patient and family should receive complete and comprehensive information about the condition as soon as it is available. Informing a patient about a new cancer diagnosis must be handled carefully. If the referring health care provider is not able to determine the prognosis and health risk associated with the tumor, it is preferable not to speculate. Partial or incomplete information may promote more anxiety and stress. The initial diagnosis can be emotionally devastating to the patient and to a family; compassion, support, and excellent communication are necessary. The physician should wait until the diagnostic and staging process is complete before giving an opinion about the treatment and the prognosis. The impact of the discussion in which a diagnosis of cancer is given has been shown to lead to poor recall of the information presented.[21]

The treatment of benign and malignant bone tumors may have a significant impact on the patient's QOL or function. As a result, the patient and family should participate in selecting the appropriate treatment. Complete information about available treatment options and alternatives should be given, including benefits and potential complications. This allows the patient and family to understand the process and to come to a shared decision about the best treatment based on individual circumstances and preferences. Having the family participate increases their "buy-in" and enhances their support of the patient as well as their commitment to seeing the treatment through. Patients with cancer who have a strong support network have been shown to have better survival rates than patients who are isolated and lack support. The patient and family should be encouraged to maintain close and frequent interaction, join a support group, or participate in family or individual counseling to whatever extent is needed.

REFERENCES

1. Hauben, E., & Hogendoorn, C. W. (2015). Epidemiology of primary bone tumors and economical aspects of bone metastases. In D. Heyman (Ed.), *Bone cancer, primary bone cancers and metastasis*. Waltham, MA: Academic Press, Elsevier.
2. SEER Cancer Stat Facts. Bone and Joint Cancer. National Cancer Institute. Bethesda, MD. https://seer.cancer.gov/statfacts/html/bones.html. (Accessed 26 August 2018).
3. Svensson, E., Christiansen, C. F., Ulrichsen, S. P., et al. (2017). Survival after bone metastasis by primary cancer type: A Danish population-based cohort study. *BMJ Open, 7*, e016022. doi:10.1136/bmjopen-2017-016022.
4. Hogendoorn, P. C. W., & Kluin, P. M. (2013). Primary non-Hodgkin lymphoma of bone. In C. D. M. Fletcher, J. A. Bridge, P. C. W. Hogendoorn, & F. Mertens (Eds.), *WHO Classification of Tumours of Soft Tissue and Bone* (4th ed., p. 316). Lyon: International Agency for Research on Cancer.
5. Bergovec, M., Kubat, O., Smerdelj, M., Smerdelj, M., et al. (2015). Epidemiology of musculoskeletal tumors in a national referral orthopedic department. A study of 3482 cases. *Cancer Epidemiology, 39*(3), 298–302.
6. Oliveira, A., & Chou, M. (2014). USP5-induced neoplasm. The biologic spectrum of aneurysmal bone cyst and nodular fasciitis RSS. *Human Pathology, 45*(1), 1–11.
7. Hayden, J. B., & Hoang, B. H. (2006). Osteosarcoma: Basic science and clinical implications. *The Orthopedic Clinics of North America, 37*(1), 1–7.
8. Boffetta, P., Munat, K., Adami, H., et al. (2011). TCDP and cancer: A critical review of the epidemiologic studies. *Critical Reviews in Toxicology, 41*(7), 622–636.
9. von Stakelberg, K. (2013). A systemic review of carcinogenic outcomes and potential mechanism from exposure to 2,4-D and MCPA in the environment. *Journal of Toxicology, 2013*, 371610.
10. Caracciolo, J., Temple, T., Letson, D., & Kransdorf, M. J. (2016). A modified Lodwick-Madewell Grading System for the evaluation of lytic bone lesions. *AJR. American Journal of Roentgenology, 207*(1).
11. Shiels, W., & Mayerson, J. (2013). Percutaneous doxycycline treatments of aneurysmal bone cysts with low recurrence rate: A preliminary report. *Clinical Orthopaedics and Related Research, 471*(8), 2675–2683.
12. Mirels, H. (1989). Metastatic Disease in long Bones: A proposed scoring system for diagnosing impending pathologic fractures. *Clinical Orthopedics and Related Research, 249*, 256–264. (classic reference).
13. Gerrand, C. H., & Rankin, K. (2014). The Hazards of Biopsy in Patients with malignant primary bone and Soft-Tissue tumors. In P. Banaszkiewicz & D. Kader (Eds.), *Classic papers in orthopaedics*. London: Springer.
14. Otto, S., Pautke, C., Van den Wyngaert, T., et al. (2018). Medication-related osteonecrosis of the jaw: Prevention, diagnosis and management in patients with cancer and bone metastasis. *Cancer Treatment Reviews, 69*, 177–187.
15. Brodowicz, T., Hadjc, P., Niepel, D., & Diel, I. (2017). Early identification and intervention matters: A comprehensive review of current evidence and recommendations for the monitoring of bone health in patients with cancer. *Cancer Treatment Reviews, 61*, 23–34.
16. Sadegh-Naini, M., Aarabi, S., Shokraneh, F., et al. (2018). Vertebroplasty and kyphoplasty for metastatic spinal lesions: A systematic Review. *Clinical Spine Surgery, 31*(5), 203–210.
17. Pietrangelo, A., & Cirino, E. Outlook for people with multiple myeloma. https://www.healthline.com/health/cancer/multiple-myeloma-outlook#. (Accessed 26 August 2018).
18. National Cancer Institute. Cancer trends progress report—2018 update. https://progressreport.cancer.gov U.S. National Institutes of Health.
19. Ratasvuori, M., Wedin, R., Keller, J., Nottrott, M., Zaikova, O., Bergh, P., et al. (2013). Insight opinion to surgically treated metastatic bone disease: Scandinavian Sarcoma Group Skeletal Metastasis Registry report of 1195 operated skeletal metastasis. *Surgical Oncology, 22*(2), 132–138.
20. Singh, H., Schiff, G. D., Graber, M. L., et al. (2017). The global burden of diagnostic errors in primary care. *BMJ Quality & Safety, 26*, 484–494.
21. Monden, K. R., Gentry, L., & Cox, T. R. (2016). Delivering bad news to patients. *Baylor University Medical Center Proceedings, 29*(1), 101–102. doi: 10.1080/08998280.2016.11929380.

CHAPTER **156**

BURSITIS
Wendy L. Halm

 Immediate referral is indicated for joint effusion with systemic symptoms requiring intravenous antibiotics or surgical intervention.

DEFINITION AND EPIDEMIOLOGY

A bursa is a sac lined with a membrane that produces and contains synovial fluid. The viscous fluid provides lubrication and facilitates smooth movement between tissues of an extremity. Bursitis is a pathologic inflammatory disorder of the bursa that is caused by varied acute or insidious processes. These processes may include trauma or repetitive injury, autoimmune diseases, crystal deposits, and infection.[1]

The bursae of the shoulder, elbow, hip, knee, and heel are the areas most commonly affected. Swelling and pain are the most common reasons for seeking medical care. Septic bursitis can occur when bursae are not only inflamed, but infected. This is a potentially serious condition requiring prompt medical care.

PATHOPHYSIOLOGY

There are about 160 bursae in the human body. Some bursae are present at birth, and some develop over time due to repeated trauma or constant friction or pressure (adventitious). Bursae vary in size depending on the individual and the location in the body. Bursae are located between tendon and bone, tendon and tendon, or bone and skin. A bursa serves as a cushion, permitting fluid movement of soft tissue over areas of friction (e.g., olecranon and prepatellar bursae) or potential impingement (e.g., subacromial bursa). Some bursae are deep below muscles and other soft tissue, and others are just beneath the skin's surface. In true bursae, repeated trauma or infection can cause multiplication of synovial cells and subsequent fluid and collagen formation.[2] Risk factors for the development of bursitis include acute trauma, repetitive injury to the painful area, infections, gout, pseudogout, uremia, rheumatoid arthritis, tuberculosis, diabetes mellitus, and immunosuppression. Septic bursitis is often seen in the olecranon and prepatellar bursa as they are close to the skin's surface, therefore at risk from trauma.[3]

SHOULDER BURSITIS

CLINICAL PRESENTATION AND PHYSICAL EXAMINATION

The four major bursae around the shoulder are the subacromial (subdeltoid), subcoracoid, subscapular, and scapular bursae. Subacromial bursitis is the most common type of upper extremity bursitis.[2] The subacromial bursa is located between the deltoid muscle and rotator cuff and extends under the acromion and coracoacromial arch. The subacromial bursa's location predisposes it to repetitive microtrauma and inflammation. The overhead athlete is at risk for shoulder injury because of the mechanics associated with rapid shoulder elevation, abduction, and external rotation.[4]

Anterior or lateral shoulder pain (see Chapter 167) with acute or insidious onset is the most common presenting complaint of patients with shoulder bursitis. The pain is exacerbated by overhead activities, and there may be a deep aching that interrupts sleep at night. Increased pain with active abduction and internal rotation of the arm plus tenderness below the acromion is demonstrated. Weakness can often be established with internal rotation. A complete neuromuscular examination with careful palpation and passive and active range of motion should be performed. In addition, a quick cervical spine examination can help rule out cervical pain with radiculopathy as the cause of the shoulder pain. The Neer and Hawkins impingement signs (Box 156.1) are the most sensitive and specific for subacromial bursitis. These signs indicate inflammation of the subacromial bursa and potentially the rotator cuff.[5] Clinicians should be aware of significant clinical diversity regarding the sensitivity and specificity of shoulder diagnostic tests.[5,6]

BOX 156.1

Neer and Hawkins Impingement Signs

NEER IMPINGEMENT SIGN
- Raise and pull on straightened arm forcibly from the side to full abduction above the head.
- The maneuver causes pain in patients with impingement.

HAWKINS IMPINGEMENT SIGN
- Flex the elbow to 90 degrees and raise the upper arm to 90 degrees of abduction (parallel to the floor). Then rotate the arm internally across the front of the body, causing compression of the rotator cuff and subacromial bursa between the head of the humerus and coracoacromial ligament.
- The maneuver causes pain in patients with impingement.

Data from Neer, C. S. (1983). Impingement lesions. *Clinical Orthopaedics & Related Research, 173*:70–77; and Hawkins, R. J., Kennedy, J. C. (1980). Impingement syndrome in athletes. *American Journal of Sports Medicine, 8*(3):151–157.

ELBOW (OLECRANON) BURSITIS

CLINICAL PRESENTATION AND PHYSICAL EXAMINATION

Located on the extensor aspect of the elbow, overlying the olecranon process and triceps tendon, the olecranon bursa is commonly affected. Visible posterior elbow swelling is easily recognized because the bursa lies close to the skin on a bone prominence. Olecranon bursitis may be acute or chronic and septic or aseptic.[7] Most cases result from acute trauma or chronic repetitive injury; chronic cases related to repetitive injury result in thickening of the bursa wall. Development of septic olecranon bursitis has been associated with male gender, manual labor, certain sports, and the military population.[8,9]

Associated medical conditions, current or recent medications, family history, personal history of recurrent bursitis or trauma to the affected elbow, occupation, and hobbies should be discussed.[7] The clinician should complete a specific examination of the elbow, comparing to the contralateral elbow. Swelling and its consistency, presence of fluctuance, skin temperature, erythema, lymphadenopathy, range of motion, and pain level should be noted. Tenderness, erythema, and warmth are common features of septic bursitis. One-third of all cases of olecranon bursitis are septic,[8] and if suspected, fluid should be obtained for culture and antibiotics should be started empirically to cover *Staphylococcus aureus*, the organism that accounts for most septic cases.[3] Risk factors for development of septic olecranon bursitis include diabetes, immunosuppression, alcoholism, psoriasis, crystalline diseases (such as gout and pseudogout), and rheumatoid arthritis.[7,9]

HIP BURSITIS

CLINICAL PRESENTATION AND PHYSICAL EXAMINATION

Hip bursitis is a common disorder that results from trauma, muscle and tendon overuse, degenerative changes, biomechanical abnormalities, or systemic disease (see Chapter 161). The trochanteric, iliopsoas, and ischiogluteal groups are the major structures of bursae around the hip. Trochanteric bursitis is the most common bursitis, affecting women more than men, running athletes, and patients who have undergone a total hip replacement (Table 156.1).[10]

Hip bursitis is characterized by pain over the affected bursa. The pain may be sudden or gradual in onset and results from overuse or trauma. Depending on which bursa is inflamed, the pain can have a pseudoradicular quality with radiation down the lateral thigh to the knee or anteriorly to the groin.[11] Pain is often worse at night. Pain on palpation that is well localized over the greater trochanter or ischial spines (point tenderness) and possibly accompanied by redness, warmth, and swelling may indicate bursitis. Range of motion, locking or snapping, duration of symptoms, and pain patterns should be assessed. The hip examination should include the hip, back, knee, abdomen, and vascular and neurologic systems. A gait analysis and stance assessment followed by evaluation of the patient in seated supine, lateral, and prone positions should be completed. Hip flexion and rotation may exacerbate the pain. Passive joint motion is usually not affected, although guarding may limit active motion.[12]

TABLE 156.1 Hip Bursitis			
	Hip Bursae		
	Trochanteric	**Ischiogluteal**	**Iliopsoas**
Location of pain	Lateral hip to lateral thigh and buttock	Ischial tuberosity into posterior thigh; worse with sitting; cannot sleep on affected side	Groin, with radiation to anterior hip
Examination	Pain worse with hip rotation; may be soft tissue swelling	Tenderness over the ischial tuberosity	Pain worse with resisted hip flexion and hyperextension
Diagnostics	X-ray studies are usually normal and noncontributory for hip bursitis; a bone scan may be helpful only in refractory conditions	X-ray studies may show calcification of the bursa and associated structures consistent with chronic inflammation	X-ray studies may show degenerative changes, effusion, or calcification
Differential diagnosis[a]	Fracture of the greater trochanter	Fracture	Hip arthritis

[a]Consider herniated disk, avascular necrosis, or systemic disease.
Data from Waldman, S. (2011). *Pain management* (2nd ed.). St Louis: Saunders.

KNEE BURSITIS

CLINICAL PRESENTATION AND PHYSICAL EXAMINATION

Knee bursitis occurs usually in the prepatellar or pes anserine bursa. The prepatellar bursa is located between the skin and the patella and is susceptible to infection because of its superficial location. Prepatellar bursitis—"housemaid's knee"—commonly results from activities that require excessive kneeling, such as carpentry, gardening, roofing, wrestling, and carpet laying.[9] Except in infectious cases, severe pain is unusual in prepatellar bursitis. The pes anserine bursae are located inside the knee, just below the joint. Pes anserine bursitis is commonly seen in the obese, those with degenerative or inflammatory joint disease, the middle-aged, and older female long-distance runners.[13] Pain may worsen with standing from a sitting position, with the use of stairs, and is commonly prevalent at night (see Chapter 162).

Physical examination should start with inspection, comparing the contralateral knee for deformity or abnormality. The examiner should look for any disruption to the skin integrity. The examiner should palpate for tenderness over the patella. Patients with prepatellar bursitis will have tenderness over the anterior knee that is accompanied by localized edema over the lower half of the patella and upper body of the patellar tendon (prepatellar bursitis) or on both sides of the patellar tendon (infrapatellar bursitis). Patients with pes anserine bursitis will have mild to moderate pain over the anterior and medial knee area just below the joint line.[13] Active resisted flexion of the knee will reproduce the pain. The examiner should also note edema, erythema, or crepitation of the knee. The ballottement test (Fig. 156.1) may be used to evaluate for knee effusion and help in differentiating prepatellar bursal swelling from true knee effusion. The test is performed by applying firm downward pressure to the patella. If a click is felt when the patella reaches the femoral condyle, a joint effusion is likely to be present. A ballottement test result will be negative if the problem is bursitis. There is often bursa thickening that feels rough, like nodules or bone chips. Although the inflamed bursa causes swelling, the edema is different from that noted when there is fluid in the knee joint or effusion. Septic bursitis should be suspected when erythema, warmth, or tenderness is present, or in the presence of systemic signs, such as fever, nausea, or malaise.[9]

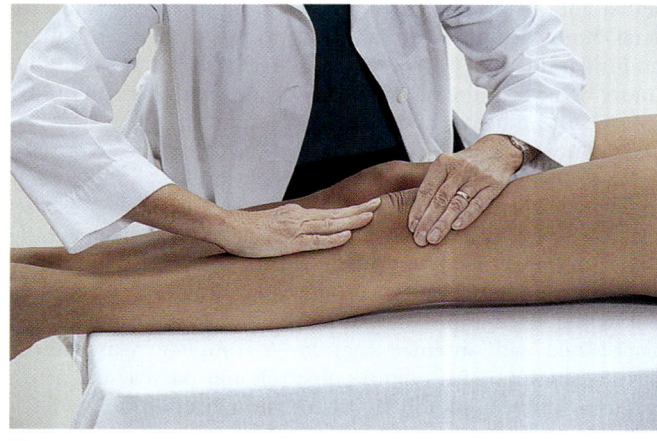

FIG. 156.1 Technique for testing for knee joint effusion. (From Swartz, M. [2014]. *The musculoskeletal system* [7th ed.]. St Louis: Saunders.)

HEEL (CALCANEAL) BURSITIS

CLINICAL PRESENTATION AND PHYSICAL EXAMINATION

There are two clinically significant bursae in the posterior heel. The retrocalcaneal bursa lies between the calcaneus and the Achilles tendon. The posterior calcaneal bursa is located between the Achilles tendon and the skin. Calcaneal bursitis is the result of local mechanical irritation to the posterior heel; ice skaters (primarily female)[14] and long-distance runners are particularly at risk. The usual presentation of calcaneal bursitis includes a history of new or poorly fitting shoes. This causes the heel to rub on the back of the shoe and results in heel pain. Patients may report limping.

Physical findings include erythema at the affected area or a palpable, swollen bursa that is tender at the Achilles tendon insertion site at the posterior heel.[15] In addition, there can be pain radiating to the Achilles tendon that is increased by squeezing the bursa just anterior to the Achilles tendon and compressing the bursa from side to side. Bursitis may also occur in association with both Achilles tendinitis and Haglund disease[15] (abnormal prominence of the posterior calcaneal tuberosity) (see Chapter 154).

DIAGNOSTICS
Essential Diagnostics

Diagnostic testing is not usually indicated, especially in the presence of superficial bursae. Initial diagnostics may include plain radiography to exclude presence of arthritis (and to determine its extent), concern for foreign body, soft tissue abnormalities, underlying bony pathology, joint effusions, or presence of crystals.[9] The clinician should utilize evidenced-based guidelines such as the ACR Appropriateness Criteria[16] when selecting appropriate initial diagnostic testing.

Additional Diagnostics

Bursal fluid aspiration with culture is essential in patients who present with systemic symptoms, or in whom septic bursitis is suspected. A white blood cell count, crystal analysis, glucose, as well as a Gram stain and culture of the bursa fluid should be obtained.[7] If an aseptic condition is the cause of the bursitis, crystals may be observed in the bursa aspirate.

If the condition is related to an autoimmune or inflammatory process, serologic tests may reveal an elevated erythrocyte sedimentation rate (ESR), rheumatoid factor, or antinuclear antibodies.

Ultrasonography may be useful to determine if the bursa is involved in presence of significant swelling.[9] Ultrasound can be operator dependent, and more useful for the identification of rotator cuff, Baker's cyst, or Achilles tendon pathology.

INITIAL DIAGNOSTICS

Bursitis

LABORATORY
- None

IMAGING
- X-ray studies
- Ultrasound

OTHER DIAGNOSTICS
- Joint aspiration
- Culture and sensitivity (of bursa fluid)[a]

- Gram stain (of bursa fluid)[a]
- Analysis of bursa aspirate for crystals[a]
- Complete blood count and differential[a]
- ESR[a]
- Rheumatoid factor[a]
- Uric acid[a]
- Antinuclear antibody[a]

[a]If indicated.

DIFFERENTIAL DIAGNOSIS

Differential diagnosis can be narrowed based on a thorough history and physical. History of trauma, acute onset of pain, presence of systemic symptoms, age, history of repetitive motion, athletic involvement, and location of the pain may provide clues to help the provider narrow the list. Laboratory testing may be of benefit for those with systemic symptoms, indicating an infectious or inflammatory process, such as arthritis or crystalline disease (see above).

 Priority differentials include (1) septic bursitis, (2) fracture, (3) trauma, (4) arthritis, and (5) neoplasm.

Age consideration may help the clinician narrow the differentials. In older adults with joint pain, fractures and degenerative arthritis should be considered first. In the young athlete, diagnosis associated with overuse, such as tear of menisci, ligaments, tendons, or thickening of the tendon should be considered. Anatomic location of the pain may also be helpful. For example, posterior elbow pain differential diagnoses include fracture, arthritis, impingement, and triceps tendinopathy. Referred pain must also be considered. For example, hip pain can often be caused by spinal disease.

INTERPROFESSIONAL COLLABORATIVE MANAGEMENT
Nonpharmacologic Management

Aspiration. For patients with superficial septic bursitis, bursal aspiration should be performed. Aspiration should be completed before antibiotics are started, and may improve symptoms and reduce bacterial load.[9] Aspiration may need to be repeated every few days.

Cold and Heat Therapy. For patients with superficial bursitis, ice pack application every few hours may help with pain and inflammatory reduction. Warm moist heat application may provide decreased pain and stiffness for patients with chronic bursitis. Ice and warm packs should not be utilized for more than 20 minutes at a time.

Activity Modification. Activities should be modified short term so as not to irritate the area that hurts. Sport-specific recommendations should be discussed. The patient should be counseled on regular periods of rest and alternating activities.

Joint Protection. Immobilization for a few days, elevation, and rest may reduce pain associated with movement. The clinician should recommend use of protective pads for the elbow, knee, or heel for those whose occupations place them at risk for further reoccurrences of bursitis. The pad should not impede range of motion.[7]

Pharmacologic Management

Nonsteroidal Antiinflammatory Drugs. Pain and inflammation may be managed with nonsteroidal antiinflammatory drugs (NSAIDs) in those without a relative contraindication. When considering medication treatment for the older adult, clinicians should consider potentially inappropriate medications as well as potential medication interactions. NSAID use in older adults has been associated with increased risk of gastrointestinal bleeding and peptic ulcer disease in high-risk groups, including those older than 75 or those taking oral or parenteral corticosteroids, anticoagulants, or antiplatelet agents.[17] Topical NSAIDs or lidocaine patches may be a better option for this age group. Invasive treatment options (such as aspiration and injection) should be carefully considered to prevent iatrogenic illness. For patients who are pregnant, NSAIDs should be avoided.

Antibiotics. Septic bursitis should be treated with appropriate antibiotics based on Gram stain and culture reports from aspirated fluid. *Staphylococcus aureus* is the most common pathogen identified.[3]

Local Injections. Intra-bursal injections of corticosteroid, with or without anesthetic, can be beneficial for pain relief and a reduction in the inflammatory reaction in patients where more conservative measures have failed (Box 156.2). Shoulder, elbow, hip, and knee bursa aspiration-injections can be particularly helpful to the patient (Figs. 156.2 to 156.5). Injections should be guided by clinical landmarks or ultrasound. Dose volume will vary based on joint size. Patients may experience a transient increase in pain post injection, and, rarely, infection.[18] Injections should always accompany other treatment modalities. Patients with diabetes may experience a

BOX **156.2**

Guidelines for Joint and Bursa Aspiration and Injection

PURPOSE

Bursa aspiration and injection are performed to obtain bursal fluid for evaluation to determine the cause of the inflammation and for drainage of abnormal fluid accumulation to relieve pain. Local anesthetics, such as lidocaine and corticosteroids, may be introduced into the bursa for symptomatic management of inflammation. Subacromial, trochanteric, anserine, and prepatellar bursitis are conditions that improve with local injection of corticosteroids.

CONTRAINDICATIONS

Contraindications to aspiration and injection include cellulitis at the injection site, primary coagulopathy or uncontrolled anticoagulant therapy, septic effusion of a bursa or periarticular structure, more than three previous injections at the same site in the previous 12 months or lack of improvement after two prior injections, suspected bacteremia from another site, unstable joints (for corticosteroid injection), tumors, fractures, joint prosthesis, and inaccessible joints.

PATIENT EDUCATION AND CONSENT

Patient education and consent are necessary before the procedure. The risks and benefits of bursa aspiration should be explained. Adverse effects of introducing a needle into the bursa include infection, bleeding, and pain. Potential complications of corticosteroid therapy include postinjection flare (increased pain for 1 or 2 days), arthropathy, tendon rupture, facial flushing, skin atrophy and depigmentation, transient paresis, transient elevations in blood sugar (if steroid is injected), hypersensitivity reaction, pericapsular calcification, and acceleration of cartilage attrition.

TECHNIQUE

Aseptic technique for bursa aspiration and injection begins by preparing the site for aspiration or injection with povidone-iodine and draping accordingly. The appropriate needle for the procedure is selected: an 18- or 20-gauge needle for aspiration, and a 22- or 25-gauge 1.5-inch needle for injection. A 5- or 10-mL Luer-Lok syringe is recommended. Figs. 156.2–156.5 demonstrate techniques for aspiration and injection of the more commonly problematic bursae.

A variety of corticosteroid preparations are available in different potencies. The three common corticosteroid local injection therapies for bursitis are hydrocortisone acetate, 25 or 50 mg/mL, which is short acting; triamcinolone acetonide, 40 mg/mL, an intermediate-acting preparation; and long-acting dexamethasone sodium acetate, 8 mg/mL. The typical injected volume will vary from small to large joints.

Lidocaine is combined with the steroid of choice to disperse the steroid at the injection site and reduce procedure-associated pain. A history of lidocaine allergy must first be obtained. Lidocaine, 5 mL, is combined with the steroid for subacromial, trochanteric, or calcaneal bursae. For smaller bursae, such as the olecranon and prepatellar bursa, up to 3 mL of lidocaine combined with the chosen steroid is recommended.

FOLLOW-UP

Procedure aftercare includes applying a bandage over the aspiration-injection site and explaining to the patient that the procedure is provided in addition to other conservative measures and is not a cure in itself. Oral nonsteroidal antiinflammatory drugs are continued if there is no contraindication. Symptoms of infection should be reported immediately.

Data from Monseau, A. J., & Singh Nizran, P. (2014). Common injections in musculoskeletal medicine. *Primary Care, 40*(4):987–100.

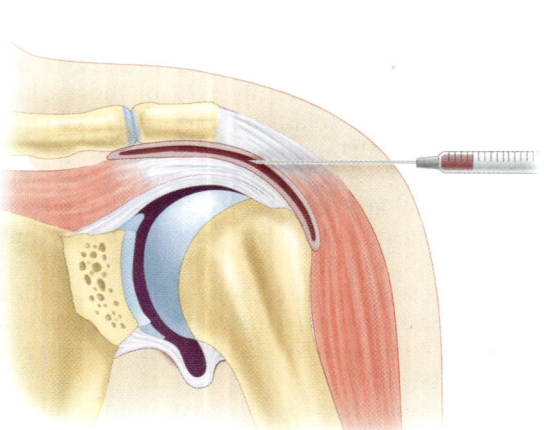

F I G . **156.2** Aspiration and injection of subacromial bursa. (From Lawry, G., Kreder, H., Hawker, G., & D. Jerome. [2010]. *Fam's musculoskeletal examination and joint injections techniques* [2nd ed.]. St Louis: Mosby.)

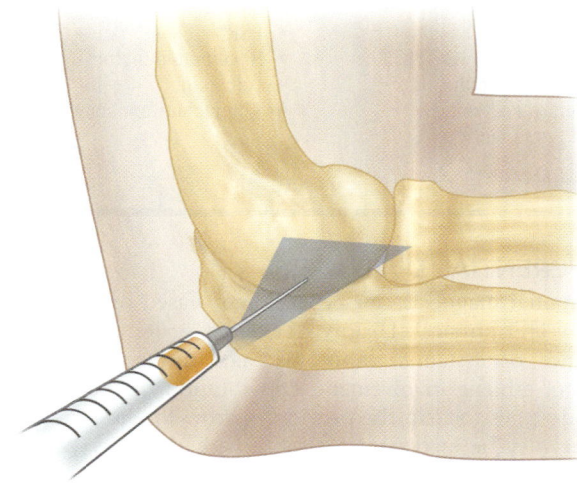

F I G . **156.3** Aspiration and injection of the elbow joint. (From Lawry, G., Kreder, H., Hawker, G., & D. Jerome. [2010]. *Fam's musculoskeletal examination and joint injections techniques* [2nd ed.]. St Louis: Mosby.)

transient elevation in blood glucose levels after corticosteroid injection.

Surgical consultation should be sought for patients who have not responded to conservative therapy; have other intra-articular, tendinous, or ligamentous co-injuries; or with chronic or frequently recurrent bursitis.

COMPLICATIONS

The pain of bursitis can be disabling for many patients. Some patients with shoulder or elbow bursitis stop using the affected extremity, resulting in weakness and increased disability; others do not bear weight on the affected extremity to avoid pain. Unfortunately, recurrent episodes of acute bursitis can progress to chronic bursitis. The adjacent tissue may be compromised in cases of severe bursal swelling, and it may be difficult to determine the true cause of the patient's discomfort, as occurs in shoulder bursitis. Infection of the bursa or surrounding tissue is not uncommon, and clinicians must always maintain an index of suspicion and rule out a possible infection as the cause of a bursitis. Oral antibiotic therapy may be sufficient for some patients with septic bursitis, but many patients require intravenous antibiotic therapy, hospitalization, and daily aspiration of the bursa fluid.

PATIENT AND FAMILY EDUCATION

Bursitis can be related to repetitive activities, and recurrence is possible. Patients should understand this and try to modify or avoid activities that may exacerbate the disorder and should protect joints from further trauma whenever possible. Patients with prepatellar bursitis, for example, should use knee pads. Rest is indicated during the acute process, but gentle stretching and range-of-motion exercises should begin as soon as possible to prevent stiffness and to maintain mobility. Ice and heat plus NSAIDs help decrease joint inflammation. A joint that becomes erythematous, tender, and edematous with associated fever requires immediate assessment by a health care clinician. If corticosteroid injections are necessary, the risks and benefits should be discussed before injection.

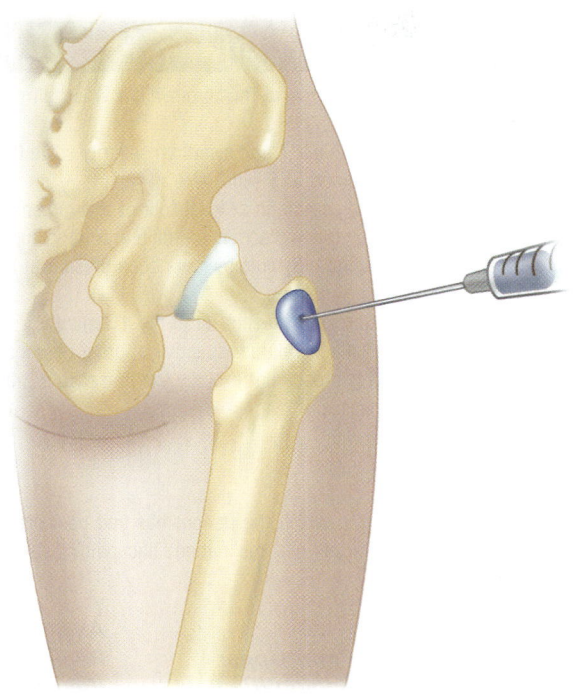

FIG. 156.4 Injection of the trochanteric bursa. (From Lawry, G., Kreder, H., Hawker, G., & D. Jerome. [2010]. *Fam's musculoskeletal examination and joint injections techniques* [2nd ed.]. St Louis: Mosby.)

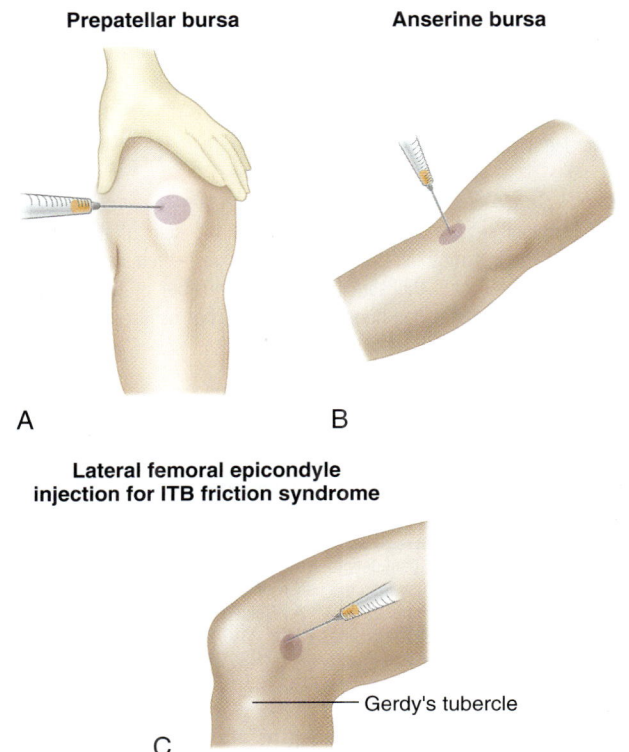

FIG. 156.5 Injection of the prepatellar bursa (A), the anserine bursa (B), and the lateral femoral epicondyle (C). (From Lawry, G., Kreder, H., Hawker, G., & D. Jerome. [2010]. *Fam's musculoskeletal examination and joint injections techniques* [2nd ed.]. St Louis: Mosby.)

REFERENCES

1. Crenshaw, A. H. (2017). Soft tissue procedures and corrective osteotomies about the knee. In S. T. Canale & J. H. Beaty (Eds.), *Campbell's operative orthopedics* (13th ed., pp. 477–506). St Louis: Mosby.
2. Hudson, K., & Delasobera, B. E. (2015). Bursae. In R. B. Birrer, F. G. O'Connor, & S. F. Kane (Eds.), *Musculoskeletal and sports medicine for the primary care practitioner* (4th ed., pp. 111–115). Boca Raton, FL: CRC Press.
3. Lieber, S. B., Fowler, M. L., Zhu, C., Moore, A., Shmerling, R. H., & Paz, Z. (2017). Clinical characteristics and outcomes of septic bursitis. *Infection*, 45(6), 781–786. doi:10.1007/s15010-017-1030-3.
4. Chorley, J., Eccles, R. E., & Scurfield, A. (2017). Care of shoulder pain in the overhead athlete. *Pediatric Annals*, 45(3), e112–e113.
5. Miller, R. H., III, Azar, F. M., & Throckmorton, T. W. (2017). Shoulder and elbow injuries. In S. T. Canale & J. H. Beaty (Eds.), *Campbell's operative orthopedics* (13th ed., pp. 2298–2345). St Louis: Mosby.
6. Hanchard, N. C., Lenza, M., Handoll, H. H., & Takwaoing, Y. (2013). Physical tests for shoulder impingements and local lesions of bursa, tendon or labrum that may accompany impingement. *The Cochrane Database of Systematic Reviews*, (4), CD007427, doi:10 1002/14651858.CD007427.pub2.
7. Reilly, D., & Kamineni, S. (2017). Olecranon bursitis. *Journal of Shoulder and Elbow Surgery*, 25, 158–167. http://cx.doi.org/10.1016/j.jse.2015.08.032.
8. Schermann, H., Karakis, I., Dolkart, O., Maman, E., Kadar, A., & Chechik, O. (2017). Olecranon bursitis in a military population: Epidemiology and evidence for prolonged morbidity in combat recruits. *Military Medicine*, 182, e1976–e1980.
9. Khodaee, M. (2017). Common superficial bursitis. *American Family Physician*, 95(4), 224–232.

10. Shemesh, S. S., Moucha, C. S., Keswani, A., Maher, N. A., Chen, C., & Bronson, M. J. (2017). Trochanteric bursitis following primary total hip arthroplasty: Incidence, predictors, and treatment. *The Journal of Arthroplasty*, https://doi.org/10.1016/j.arth.2017.11.016. Advance online publication.

11. Friedman, M. V., Stensby, J. D., Long, J. R., Currie, S. A., & Hillen, T. J. (2017). Beyond the greater trochanter: A pictorial review of the pelvic bursae. *Clinical Imaging*, 41, 37–41. doi:10.1016/j.clinimag.2016.09.010.

12. Guyton, J. L. (2017). Hip pain in the young adult and hip preservation surgery. In S. T. Canale & J. H. Beaty (Eds.), *Campbell's operative orthopedics* (13th ed., pp. 345–393). St Louis: Mosby.

13. Glencross, P., & Lorenzo, C. T. (2017). Pes anserine bursitis. Accessed 22 December 2017 Retrieved from https://emedicine.medscape.com/article/308694-overview?pa=hSn9hsWyoDe7fQYziaZtrA8nZBOWUkPzixAcHG%2BUs1mswUNrfVm3BIrrAnqAh60cJyGvMX%2Fu%2BWdIXoARf%2FT0zw%3D%3D#a5.

14. Campanelli, V., Piscitelli, F., & Verardi, L. (2015). Lower extremity overuse conditions affecting figure skaters during daily training. *Orthopaedic Journal of Sports Medicine*, 3(7), http://journals.sagepub.com/doi/pdf/10.1177/2325967115596517.

15. Foye, P. M., Rispoli, L., Patibanda, V., & Stitik, T. P. (2017). Retrocalcaneal bursitis. Accessed 22 December 2017 Retrieved from https://emedicine.medscape.com/article/86297-overview.

16. American College of Radiology (2017). ACR Appropriateness Criteria. Accessed 12 December 2017 Retrieved from https://acsearch.acr.org/list.

17. Loveless, M. S., & Fry, A. L. (2016). Pharmacologic therapies in musculoskeletal conditions. *The Medical Clinics of North America*, 100(4), 869–890. http://dx.doi.org/10.1016/j.mcna.2016.03.015.

18. Waldman, S. D. (2017). *Atlas of pain management injection techniques* (4th ed.). Philadelphia: Elsevier.

CHAPTER **157**

FIBROMYALGIA AND MYOFASCIAL PAIN SYNDROME

Lin A. Brown

DEFINITION AND EPIDEMIOLOGY

Fibromyalgia syndrome (FMS), a disorder usually included with rheumatologic conditions, is characterized by symptoms of widespread musculoskeletal pain, fatigue, nonrestorative sleep, depression, headaches, and gastrointestinal complaints (irritable bowel syndrome). FMS gained acceptance as a disorder in 1990 after the American College of Rheumatology developed classification criteria for the disorder.

Fibromyalgia as defined in 1990 included more than 3 months of musculoskeletal pain present above and below the waist bilaterally, associated with pain on palpation of specific tender points. No other source of pain is identified, although there may be so-called drivers of pain such as painful joints from rheumatoid arthritis that can be complicated by fibromyalgia. The pain is usually accompanied by profound fatigue and sleep disturbance (nonrestorative sleep). Most patients with chronic fatigue syndrome also meet diagnostic criteria for FMS. Myofascial pain syndrome is a more limited expression of the same condition (e.g., pain limited to the shoulder and neck, upper back).

In 2010, the American College of Rheumatology put forth a new set of classification criteria that eliminated the tender point examination and replaced it with a report of pain surveyed in 19 areas as well as severity of symptoms associated with fibromyalgia (Box 157.1).

FMS is diagnosed eight to nine times more often in women than in men of all age groups, with an onset in general at 40 to 50 years of age. FMS rarely begins after the age of 55 years. FMS affects approximately 5 million Americans, accounting for 2% of all primary care visits, 10% of all internal medicine referrals, and up to 20% of rheumatology referrals.[1] Symptoms start gradually in adulthood or, rarely, in childhood and wax and wane in intensity.[1]

BOX **157.1**

Fibromyalgia Diagnostic Criteria

A person satisfies diagnostic criteria for fibromyalgia when all of the following criteria are met[5]:

1. Widespread pain index (WPI) ≥ 7 and symptom severity scale (SSS) score ≥ 5 OR WPI of 4–6 and SSS score ≥ 9.
2. Generalized pain, defined as pain in at least four of five regions, must be present. Jaw, chest, and abdominal pain are not included in generalized pain definition. Symptoms have been present at a similar level for at least 3 months.
3. Symptoms have been generally present for at least 3 months.
4. A diagnosis of fibromyalgia is valid irrespective of other diagnoses. A diagnosis of fibromyalgia does not exclude the presence of other clinically important illnesses.

ASCERTAINMENT

1. WPI Score

Note the number of areas in which the patient has had pain over the last week. In how many areas has the patient had pain? Score will be 0–19.

Left Upper Region (Region 1)	Right Upper Region (Region 2)	Axial Region (Region 5)
Jaw, left	Jaw, right[a]	Neck
Shoulder girdle, left	Shoulder girdle, right	Upper back
Upper arm, left	Upper arm, right	Lower back
Lower arm, left	Lower arm, right	Chest[a]
		Abdomen[a]

Left Lower Region (Region 3)	Right Lower Region (Region 4)
Hip (buttock, trochanter), left	Hip (buttock, trochanter), right
Upper leg, left	Upper leg, right
Lower leg, left	Lower leg, right

2. SS Scale Score

The symptom severity scale (SSS) score: is the sum of the severity scores of the 3 symptoms (fatigue, waking unrefreshed, and cognitive symptoms) (0–9) plus the sum (0–3) of the number of the following symptoms the patient has been bothered by that occurred during the previous 6 months:

(1) Headaches (0–1)
(2) Pain or cramps in lower abdomen (0–1)
(3) Depression (0–1)

The final symptom severity score is between 0 and 12
The fibromyalgia severity (FS) scale is the sum of the WPI and SSS.

---

[a]Not included in generalized pain definition.
Note: The FS scale is also known as the polysymptomatic distress (PSD) scale.
From Wolfe, F., Clauw, D., Fitzcharles, M. A., Goldenberg, D. L., Hauser, W., Katz, R. L., …Walitt, B. (2016). 2016 revisions to the 2010/2011 fibromyalgia diagnostic criteria. *Seminars in Arthritis and Rheumatism, 46*(3), 319–329.

PATHOPHYSIOLOGY

Although the cause of FMS is unclear, research has implicated central nervous system dysfunction and not muscle disease, autoimmune disease, or viral disease. Pain beginning in the periphery is processed in the spinal cord and transmitted to the brain. For unclear reasons, some pain becomes "louder" at the level of the spinal cord and brain, a condition called central sensitization. The brain responds with pain recognition at a lower threshold and over a wider area than that originally involved.[2] In addition, neuroendocrine disturbances at the level of the hypothalamus or pituitary, involving decreased levels of growth hormone (GH), insulin-like growth factor (IGF), and possibly prolactin, have been found in FMS patients.[3] These hormones are released during the stages of sleep, specifically GH in stage 3 and stage 4 of non–rapid eye movement (REM) sleep. In sleep studies, patients with FMS have disturbances with non-REM sleep and difficulty in progressing to stage 3 and stage 4 sleep, resulting in morning fatigue. One-third of FMS patients have low IGF, an indication of low GH secretion, lending credence to disturbed stage 4 sleep as important in FMS. Treatment with GH increases IGF levels, improves pain and sleep, and reduces overall symptoms, although the cost is prohibitive.[2,3]

Other neuroendocrine abnormalities include elevation of cerebrospinal fluid substance P levels and dysregulated cortisol production. FMS patients have three times the levels of substance P, which is significant because this neurotransmitter plays a role in enhanced pain perception. This may be the reason for the heightened pain perception experienced by fibromyalgia patients. Alteration in the hypopituitary-adrenal axis with low production of cortisol, perhaps secondary to chronic stress response, contrasts with depression, in which high production of cortisol is found. These results suggest that part of the cause of FMS may be a product of disturbances in the autonomic and endocrine stress response systems.[3] In addition, serotonin levels are low in the brain and in the platelets of patients with fibromyalgia.

Although these theories explain part of the pathogenesis of FMS, the primary cause of the central dysregulation is unknown. FMS frequently follows physical or mental trauma, viral illness, and stress.

CLINICAL PRESENTATION AND PHYSICAL EXAMINATION

Persistent widespread pain is the hallmark of the syndrome, along with chronic fatigue. Patients have a variety of other somatic complaints: nonrestorative sleep; cognitive difficulties; auditory, vestibular, and ocular complaints; chronic rhinitis or "allergies"; migraines; palpitations; irritable bowel syndrome; subjective sense of joint swelling; and mood disorders.[4] With such generalized complaints, it is clear how the patient's complaints can be confused with an autoimmune disease such as lupus.

With fibromyalgia, muscle strength is normal (although effort may be affected by pain and judging pain may also be difficult), and there is no evidence of synovitis or soft tissue inflammation. Making the diagnosis depends on findings from the history and physical examination. FMS should be considered with any musculoskeletal pain not explained by a clearly defined anatomic lesion.

Wolf, F., et al., recently revised the 2010/2011criteria for FMS symptoms[5] (see Box 157.1). The previous pressure point evaluation of sites has been supplanted by patient report of widespread pain present in up to 19 and a modified widespread pain evaluation scale was developed This evaluation plus the severity of other symptoms including duration of pain>3 months, fatigue, and disordered sleep suggests a diagnosis of fibromyalgia (see Box 157.1).

DIAGNOSTICS

An in-depth history and physical examination reduce the need for extensive and expensive objective tests. Laboratory values and electromyography findings are typically normal. Complete blood count, erythrocyte sedimentation rate or C-reactive protein (CRP), vitamin D level, and thyroid-stimulating hormone level are of value in excluding underlying disorders. Antinuclear antibody (ANA), rheumatoid factor, and anti–citrullinated protein antibody (ACPA) testing should be ordered only in the setting of synovitis on examination or other findings suggestive of lupus or rheumatoid arthritis. Sleep studies may be warranted for some patients, especially those with characteristics of obstructive sleep apnea. Obstructive sleep apnea is characterized by daytime sleepiness as opposed to daytime fatigue (see Chapter 206). Radiographs are not recommended unless a secondary disorder such as degenerative arthritis as a driver of fibromyalgia is suspected.

INITIAL DIAGNOSTICS

Fibromyalgia

LABORATORY
- CBC, chemistry profile, TSH, ESR, C-reactive protein

IMAGING
- None

ADDITIONAL DIAGNOSTICS
Laboratory
- Antinuclear antibody
- Rheumatoid Factor
- Anti–citrullinated protein antibody

DIFFERENTIAL DIAGNOSIS

Symptoms of fibromyalgia often overlap with those of myofascial pain syndrome, chronic fatigue syndrome (see Chapter 202), hypothyroidism (see Chapter 194), bursitis (see Chapter 156) or tendinitis, depression, and anxiety (see Chapters 225 and 226). Connective tissue diseases that should be included in the differential diagnosis include rheumatoid arthritis (see Chapter 197), systemic lupus erythematous (see Chapter 199), polymyalgia rheumatic (see Chapter 195), and polymyositis.

INTERPROFESSIONAL COLLABORATIVE MANAGEMENT

Treatment of FMS does not conform to a specific algorithm or paradigm and is as much an art as a science. The goal of therapy should be to empower patients to control their own pain, to enhance sleep, and to maintain function. Education allows the patient opportunities to individualize treatment and to reduce symptoms. Treatment may incorporate pharmacologic therapies, cognitive behavioral therapy, exercise, and alternative therapies.[6]

Pharmacology

Low doses of tricyclic drugs have been studied, particularly amitriptyline, 10 mg taken 2 to 3 hours before bedtime, allowing peak sedative effect and reducing sedation on awakening. Cyclobenzaprine, also a tricyclic, can be used as well at 5 to 10 mg at night. Doses should start low and increase slowly. Selective serotonin reuptake inhibitors, such as fluoxetine (Prozac) 20 mg, have also been studied, but duloxetine (Cymbalta) and milnacipran (Savella), both dual serotonin-norepinephrine reuptake inhibitors, may work better and are approved by the Food and Drug Administration for treatment of fibromyalgia.

Other medications that have proved helpful for pain include gabapentin (Neurontin) and pregabalin (Lyrica). Trazodone (Desyrel) and zolpidem (Ambien) may help sleep but do not increase time spent in stage 4. Nonsteroidal antiinflammatory drugs (NSAIDs) and acetaminophen can be tried and are commonly prescribed, although NSAIDs have not been proved effective for the pain of fibromyalgia.[7] Identification of pain generators, such as osteoarthritis of the knee, spinal stenosis, restless leg syndrome, and diabetic neuropathy, can result in treatment of these conditions, which may play a role in reducing sleep disturbances and hence pain and fatigue.[4,6,8]

Chronic Opioid Analgesic Therapy

Chronic opioid analgesic therapy for fibromyalgia lacks evidence of efficiacy and patients treated with opioids tend to have poorer outcomes.[9] Opioids should be used only after all other pharmacologic and nonpharmacologic therapies have been tried and then only for short periods Given the current national emergency regarding opiod addiction and overdoses in the United States, the prescriptions of opioids should be avoided. The provider should sign a contract with any patient prescribed a narcotic medication so that continued treatment can be tied to functional improvement, and dysfunctional behavior can be avoided (see Chapter 227).

Non-Pharmacologic Management

Cognitive Behavioral Therapy. Cognitive behavioral therapy uses different approaches to integrate coping skills, relaxation training, activity pacing, visual imagery techniques, and goal setting to allow the patient control to improve function and pain.[4,6] It has been shown in multiple studies to be effective in treating FMS by reducing pain and increasing a sense of well-being.[8,10]

The Arthritis Foundation (www.arthritis.org) and the American College of Rheumatology (www.rheumatology.org) as well as other organizations can help direct patients to self-help books and classes. Many pain clinics and psychiatry departments provide cognitive behavioral therapy.

Exercise. Aerobic exercise can improve pain and have an antidepressant effect.[11] Usually patients with fibromyalgia have not been active physically and experience increased pain when they begin an aerobic exercise program. Hence the exercise prescription should begin at a low intensity and for short duration. The duration and intensity should increase over time as the patient is able to do so. To be beneficial, the exercise needs to be consistent and aerobic. Some experts recommend thinking of exercise as a drug with the ability to be overdosed and misused. However, used correctly, exercise clearly works to improve pain, sleep, and function. Gentle stretching and yoga are useful adjuncts before engaging in a low-impact activity such as biking, swimming, and walking. Massage aids in relaxation and produces physiologic benefits as well, but neither stretching nor massage is a substitute for aerobic exercise. Encouragement to continue the exercise program is needed to combat the continued muscle wasting often associated with fibromyalgia as well as to alleviate the patient's perception that pain is inevitable. Post-exercise pain should be distinguished from fibromyalgia pain; it may respond to heat, ice, or NSAIDs. Patients should consider a one-on-one therapist or exercise partner for any program to improve success.[11]

Referrals for exercise programs and cognitive behavioral therapy are clearly beneficial and should form the cornerstone of any other therapy for fibromyalgia.

Alternative Therapies. Acupuncture has produced mixed results in fibromyalgia, although it has been found to be useful in other painful conditions. Massage therapy likewise has preliminary support; some studies show a positive response. Chiropractic manipulation, hypnosis, biofeedback, and magnet therapy all show insufficient evidence for effectiveness to be recommended as treatments.[12] Trigger point injections have been studied and are reported to be effective adjuncts to a treatment regimen. The judicious use of trigger point injections with lidocaine (Xylocaine) or bupivacaine (Marcaine) is often tried for symptoms not controlled with oral medications, with some success.[13] Any treatment that is not effective should be discontinued.

Interdisciplinary Approach

Group therapy programs are based on cognitive behavioral therapy approaches for living day to day effectively and increasing endurance and strength. These programs often include care from a rheumatologist and a physical therapist as well as group exercise programs, pain and stress management lectures, and even massage therapy. They are clearly effective compared with usual treatment with a family physician.[14]

FMS patients should be managed in primary care, where there is a partnership and willingness for creativity in treatment plans, perhaps including alternative treatments.[15] Pain management clinics for pain control have been effective for chronic pain. Psychologists, physical therapists, and chiropractors may aid in symptom control.

COMPLICATIONS

Fibromyalgia does not result in damage to muscle, joints, or vital organs, and this is important for patients to understand. They hurt, but the pain is not indicative of tissue damage or a shortened life expectancy. Disability, however, is frequently perceived, and this is a difficult issue in FMS because disability is often difficult to document or to compensate for. Other complications include depression, insomnia, muscle atrophy, misdiagnosis, and drug-seeking behavior. Hospital admissions are not required.

PATIENT AND FAMILY EDUCATION

Education is imperative for improved patient understanding of fibromyalgia and the development of individual strategies to cope with the pain, fatigue, and chronic nature of the syndrome. The importance of regular exercise and adequate rest should be emphasized. Family members are affected and should be involved in education to understand the disorder and to maximize support for these patients. Support groups can be invaluable. Information abounds on the Internet, so careful evaluation is required. Available resources include the following:

*The American College of Rheumatology
   www.rheumatology.org
*Arthritis Foundation
   www.arthritis.org
*National Institute of Arthritis and Musculoskeletal and Skin Diseases
   National Institutes of Health
   www.niams.nih.gov
*National Fibromyalgia Foundation
   www.fmaware.org

HEALTH PROMOTION

FMS is a syndrome that requires providing patients with the tools needed to improve activities of daily living and manage pain. Healthy diet, exercise, weight control, support systems, stress reduction through meditation or counseling, and improved self-esteem are all within the patient's control and will result in reduced pain and improved function.

REFERENCES

1. Hauser, W., Albin, J., Perrot, S., & Fitzcharles, M.-A. (2017). Management of fibromyalgia: Key messages from recent evidence based guidelines. *Polish Archives of Medicine, 127*(1), 47–56.
2. Clauw, D. (2014). Fibromyalgia: A clinical review. *JAMA: The Journal of the American Medical Association, 311*(15), 1547–1555.
3. Schmidt-Wilcke, T., & Diers, M. (2017). New insights into the pathophysiology and treatment of fibromyalgia. *Biomedicine / [Publiee Pour L'A.A.I.C.I.G.], 5*(2), 22.
4. Hauser, W., Albin, J., Fitzcharles, M.-A., et al. (2015). Fibromyalgia. *Nature Reviews Disease Primers, 1*, doi:10.1038/nrdp.2015.22. (Accessed 20 January 2018). 15022.
5. Wolfe, F., Clauw, D., Fitzcharles, M. A., et al. (2016). 2016 revision to the 2010/2011 fibromyalgia diagnostic criteria. *Seminars in Arthritis and Rheumatism, 46*(3), 319–3296.
6. Hauser, W., & Perrot, S. (2019). *Fibromyalgia syndrome and widespread pain: From construction to relevant recognition.* Phildelphia: Wolters Kluwer Health.
7. Derry, S., Wiffen, P., Hauser, W., et al. (2017). Oral non-steroidal anti-inflammatory drugs for fibromyalgia in adults. *The Cochrane Database of Systematic Reviews,* (3), CD012332, doi:10.1002/14651858.CD012332.pub2. (Accessed 20 January 2018).
8. Fitzcharles, M. A., et al. (2013). Canadian Pain Society. Canadian Rheumatologic Association recommendation for rational care of persons with fibromyalgia. A summary report. *The Journal of Rheumatology, 40*(8), 1388–1393.
9. Goldenberg, D., Clauw, D., & Palmer, R. (2016). Opioid use in fibromyalgia. *Mayo Clinic Proceedings, 91*(5), 640–648.
10. Bernardy, K., Klose, P., Welsch, P., & Hauser, W. (2018). Efficacy, acceptability and safety of cognitive behavioral therapies in fibromyalgia syndrome—A systematic review and meta-analysis of randomized clinical trials. *European Journal of Pain, 22*(2), 242–260.
11. Sumpton, J. E., & Moulin, D. E. (2014). Fibromyalgia. *Handbook of Clinical Neurology, 119*, 513–527.
12. Lauche, R., Cramer, H., Hauser, W., et al. (2015). A systematic overview of review for complementary and alternative therapies in the treatment of the fibromyalgia syndrome. *Evidence-based Complementary and Alternative Medicine, 2015*. Retrieved from http://dx.doi.org/101155/2105/610615. (Accessed 20 January 2018). 610615.
13. Staud, R., Weyl, E., Bartley, E., et al. (2014). Analgesic and anti-hyperalgesic effects of muscle injections with lidocaine or saline in patients with fibromyalgia syndrome. *European Journal of Pain, 18*(6), 803–812.
14. Salvat, I., Zaldivar, P., Monterde, S., et al. (2017). Functional status, physical activity level and exercise regularity in patients with fibromyalgia after multidisciplinary treatment: A retrospective analysis of a randomized clinical trial. *Rheumatology International, 37*(3), 377–387.
15. Clauw, D. (2015). Fibromyalgia and related conditions. *Mayo Clinic Proceedings, 90*(5), 680–692.

CHAPTER **158**

GOUT
Naomi Schlesinger

DEFINITION AND EPIDEMIOLOGY

Gout has been referred to as the "king of diseases" and the "disease of the kings." However, gout is not a self-inflicted disease of the elite; it is a chronic disease that can affect anyone. Gout is a systemic metabolic disease. Humans do not express the enzyme urate oxidase (uricase), which converts urate to the more soluble and easily excreted compound allantoin, which may lead to hyperuricemia (excess of uric acid in the blood). At a biological potential of hydrogen (pH), the uric acid in the plasma and extracellular fluids exists mostly as a urate ion.

The serum urate (SU) level is the single most important risk factor for the development of gout. The SU level is elevated when it exceeds 6.8 mg/dL, the solubility limit of urate in serum at 37°C (98.6°F) at a physiologic pH. A sustained elevation of SU is essential for the development of gout, but by itself is insufficient to cause the disease, and most patients with hyperuricemia never develop gout.

Gout is the most common inflammatory arthritis in humankind, with an estimated 8.3 million American adults (prevalence of 3.9%) suffering from gout.[1] The prevalence increases with age, with approximately 10% of American men aged 70 to 79 years and 6% of American women aged 80 years or older suffering from gout.[1] The incidence of gout is increasing, driven by the increasing life expectancy and by increases in the prevalence of risk factors for gout, including greater use of diuretics and low-dose aspirin (acetylsalicylic acid), as well as increasing prevalence of comorbidities such as obesity, chronic kidney disease, and metabolic syndrome (see Chapter 192).

PATHOPHYSIOLOGY

Uricase, an end product of purine metabolism, is an enzyme that converts uric acid to allantoin, which is soluble in the urine. Uricase is found in nearly all organisms, from bacteria to mammals; however, it is silent in humans. The solubility of monosodium urate (MSU) crystals is related to both Ph and temperature. At 37°C (98.6°F), the maximum solubility of urate in physiologic saline is 6.8 mg/dL, but at 30°C (86°F), it is only 4.5 mg/dL. If the SU level is increased for a sustained period of time, urate will come out of solution to form MSU crystals.[2] Micro-tophi may subsequently form, particularly in the cooler parts of the body that include earlobes as well as in points of mechanical pressure and osteoarthritic joints, such as fingers and toes and olecranon bursae. Sustained hyperuricemia is a risk factor for gout; however, most patients with hyperuricemia will never develop gout.

CLINICAL PRESENTATION AND PHYSICAL EXAMINATION

Gout typically presents initially as recurrent episodes of painful monoarthritis (one joint) in men and as oligoarticular arthritis (4 or fewer joints) in postmenopausal women and in men in subsequent flares.[2] If left untreated, the frequency and severity of attacks may increase, with additional joints affected and development of tophi ("chalk stones" in Latin) leading to structural joint damage.[3]

Gout has 4 clinical stages: asymptomatic hyperuricemia, acute gout attacks, intercritical gout (intervals between acute attacks), and chronic tophaceous gout. Hyperuricemia and inflammation drive this cascade. In the asymptomatic hyperuricemia stage, the patient has elevated levels of SU but no previous acute attacks. During this phase MSU crystals may deposit in and around joints and cause asymptomatic damage. Acute attacks occur as a result of the deposition of MSU crystals and activation of an inflammatory response leading to intense pain and other signs of inflammation such as swelling, redness, and warmth of the involved joints and surrounding soft tissue. After the attack subsides, even if the patient is not experiencing an attack, continued MSU crystal deposition can continue. Uncontrolled hyperuricemia and gout can eventually evolve into destructive inflammatory chronic tophaceous gout.

Acute gout is characterized by rapid onset and increasing pain. The first attack often begins at night and wakes the patient up from sleep. During an acute attack, the patient endures exquisite pain associated with all the signs of synovitis: tenderness, warmth, redness, swelling, and decreased range of motion in the affected joint or joints. The initial episode is usually monoarticular (one joint) in men, with the first metatarsophalangeal (MTP) joint being the initial joint involved in approximately half the patients. Acute synovitis of the first MTP joint of the big toe is referred to as "podagra" (a Greek word meaning "foot seizure"). Lower extremity joints are commonly involved, as well as Heberden's nodes in postmenopausal women; however, any joint can be affected.

Due to the increased production of proinflammatory cytokines (e.g., interleukin-1), systemic symptoms and signs of fatigue, fever, and chills may accompany the acute gout attack. The natural course of the untreated gout attack usually lasts up to 10 days but can last for several weeks.

Local trauma, binges of alcohol, overeating, or fasting, diuretics and newly initiated urate-lowering therapy (ULT) have been implicated as factors that precipitate acute gout attacks. In the hospital setting, acute gout attacks often occur postoperatively or are associated with severe acute medical illnesses.

Chronic tophaceous gout usually develops after ≥10 years of recurrent gout attacks, although rarely do patients present with tophi as the initial manifestation of the disease. Tophi appear as firm swellings, may appear at any site, and are most commonly found on digits of the hands and feet and in the olecranon bursa. Tophi of the helix or antihelix of the ear are classic but are less common nowadays. Tophi may be associated with a destructive arthritis and very occasionally ulcerate, leading to a secondary infection.

DIAGNOSTICS
Essential Diagnostics

Even when the clinical presentation strongly suggests gout, diagnosis needs to be confirmed by needle aspiration. Although not intended for use in diagnosis, the gout classification criteria[4] highlight the gold standard presence of MSU crystals in synovial fluid or tophus aspiration as sufficient for classifying the cause of the patient's discomfort as gout. Thus demonstration of MSU crystals in the joint fluid or tophus is still the gold standard for the diagnosis of gout.[2] However, joint aspiration is invasive and not always possible in the primary care setting. Supportive data necessary for the diagnosis of gout include

a typical clinical history of a sudden (reaching its pain peak within 2 to 4 hours) and severe, exquisitely painful joint, most classically the first MTP joint (toe), that may wake the patient from sleep. The patient may have renal disease or be taking medications that can elevate SU.

Additional Diagnostics

Elevated inflammatory markers, creatinine, and SU level can all be associated with acute gout. Radiologic evidence of punched-out erosions on plain x-ray studies and a favorable response to treatment with colchicine or nonsteroidal antiinflammatory drugs (NSAIDs) are confirmatory.

Ultrasonography (US) and icing, also named the double contour sign, are highly specific for diagnosis of gout and can help diagnose gout without needle aspiration of an acutely inflamed joint.[5] Dual-energy computed tomography (DECT)[6] is an advanced imaging modality that enables visualization of MSU crystal deposits.

DIFFERENTIAL DIAGNOSIS

 Priority differentials include Lyme disease; septic arthritis; inflammatory arthritis; and rheumatoid arthritis

There are a variety of disorders that mimic gout that should be considered in the differential diagnosis of gout. It is sometimes difficult to determine whether the patient with acute arthritis (synovitis) has acute gout, a joint infection, or acute pseudogout due to calcium pyrophosphate (CPP) crystals. Calcium pyrophosphate deposition (CPPD) disease has two main forms. One is chronic arthritis, and the other is acute synovitis in one or more joints, similar to the presentation of acute gout. Approximately half of acute pseudogout attacks affect the knees, but other joints may be affected as well. It is more common in women. Under compensated polarized light microscopy, the difference between the two types of crystals is evident. Ultrasound can also distinguish between gout and pseudogout. Tophi sometimes tend to be confused with rheumatoid nodules, even though rheumatoid arthritis (see Chapter 197) and gout rarely coexist, and therefore, when in doubt, needle aspiration should be done to determine the presence of MSU crystals.

There are other muscular skeletal disorders that can be included in the differential diagnosis of gout. These include cellulitis, bursitis, and injuries or inflammatory disorders that affect joints, tendons, and soft tissue.

INTERPROFESSIONAL COLLABORATIVE MANAGEMENT

There are three types of therapies in the management of gout: (1) treatment of the acute attack; (2) lowering of the total body uric acid pool to prevent tissue deposition of MSU crystals; and (3) antiinflammatory prophylaxis to prevent further acute attacks, especially when urate lowering therapy (ULT) is initiated.

Nonpharmacologic Management

Avoidance of factors that contribute to the development of gout among asymptomatic hyperuricemic patients may help reduce gout attacks. This includes avoiding diuretics when possible, controlling weight, and limiting alcohol consumption. It has been shown that low-fat dairy products have a protective effect on SU levels. A significant inverse association was noted between the intake of dairy and the SU level in the NHANES III (OR 0.66; 95% CI 0.48 to 0.89).[7] The dairy proteins casein and lactalbumin were thought to lower SU level by inducing urinary excretion of uric acid. Studies suggest that cherry juice concentrate reduces acute attacks when it is consumed over a period of ≥4 months. Cherry juice concentrate has antiinflammatory properties, which suggests it may be useful as a prophylaxis for gout.[8]

A recent study found that the dietary approaches to stop hypertension (DASH) diet is associated with a lower risk of gout by substantially lowering SU levels.[9] The main components of the DASH diet include fruits, vegetables, nuts and legumes, low-fat dairy products, and whole grains, combined with a low intake of sodium, sweetened beverages, and red and processed meats. In addition, topical ice may also be a useful adjunct to treatment of acute gout attacks.[2]

Pharmacologic Management

Treatment of Acute Gout. The goal of acute gout treatment is prompt termination of pain and inflammation. The choice of treatment for an acute attack depends on the individual patient characteristics, including age, comorbidities, and medications the patient is taking, as well as attack characteristics, including the number of affected joints, past responses to therapy, and patient and physician preferences.

The current options available for the treatment of acute gout attacks are NSAIDs, colchicine, corticosteroids (oral, intravenous, intramuscular, and intra-articular), and adrenocorticotropic hormone (ACTH)[10] (Box 158.1). In most patients who can take oral medications, oral corticosteroids or NSAIDs are appropriate treatments for acute gout attacks. The most important determinant of therapeutic success is not which antiinflammatory drug is chosen, but rather how soon therapy is initiated at the appropriate dose and duration of therapy. In most patients, the attack completely resolves within 5 to 8 days of initiation of therapy.

NSAID use is limited by the medication side effects and patient comorbidities. When considering NSAIDs, it is important to note that chronic kidney disease is common in gout patients. In addition, most NSAIDs should be avoided in patients with hypertension, heart disease, peptic ulcer disease, liver disease, renal disease, poorly compensated congestive heart failure, and in patients receiving anticoagulation therapy. The adverse effects of NSAIDs are also more pronounced in older adult patients.

The Food and Drug Administration (FDA) approved dose of oral colchicine for the treatment of acute gout attacks is 1.2 mg followed by 0.6 mg in 1 hour (total 1.8 mg). It is most effective during the first 12 to 24 hours of an attack.[11] Colchicine should not be used if the patient's glomerular filtration rate (GFR) is less than 10 mL/min, and the dose should be decreased by at least half if the GFR is less than 50 mL/min.

Corticosteroids can be given to those patients who cannot use NSAIDs or colchicine, which may be the majority of patients with gout. Corticosteroids can be given orally, intravenously, intramuscularly, intra-articularly, or indirectly by ACTH. Corticosteroid treatment is the preferred treatment for acute attacks in patients with chronic kidney insufficiency or for those who have other contraindications to NSAIDs and/or colchicine. For monoarticular gout attacks, especially of large joints, such as the knee, an intra-articular glucocorticoid injection can be effective. In addition, corticosteroids are preferred for polyarticular gout.[12]

Treatment of Chronic Gout. The goal of treatment is to achieve resolution of MSU crystals by reducing the SU level to lower than the uric acid saturation threshold in order to permit spontaneous dissolution of MSU crystal deposition in the tissue (Box 158.2). Maintenance of the SU level at ≤ 6 mg/dL helps ensure resolution of tophi and eventual cessation of acute gout attacks. The evidence on when to start ULT is conflicting, and questions have been raised whether ULT should be initiated after the first gout attack. The American College of Physicians (ACP) recommends against initiating long-term ULT in most patients after a first gout attack or in patients with infrequent attacks since benefits over 12 months duration of ULT have not been studied in patients with single/infrequent gout attacks.[13]

BOX 158.1

Treatment of Acute Gout

- Ideally, confirm diagnosis by joint aspiration: intracellular monosodium urate crystals in synovial fluid or tophaceous material. (This can be difficult in the primary care setting, especially when access to rheumatologists is limited or nonexistent.)
- Initial treatment is with oral corticosteroids or NSAIDs. Corticosteroids are preferred in patients with creatinine clearance less than 50 mL/min, on anticoagulant therapy, or hepatic dysfunction.
- Antiinflammatory treatment should be used early in the attack. Higher doses need to be used in the first 24–48 h.
- In a severe oligoarticular or polyarticular gouty attack or when NSAIDs are not tolerated, are contraindicated, or not responding to treatment with NSAIDs, use systemic corticosteroids (7–14 day taper). Parenteral, intramuscular, or intravenous corticosteroids may be helpful, especially in patients with renal failure.
- Oral colchicine should be used within 36 h of onset of an acute attack: initial dose of 1.2 mg of oral colchicine, followed 1 h later by another 0.6 mg, for a total dose on the first day of therapy of 1.8 mg
- Colchicine should be used cautiously because of its toxicity
- If one or two joints are involved, intra-articular corticosteroids may be beneficial.
- If patients are unable to take oral medications, parenteral corticosteroids may be advised.
- Do not start, stop, or change dose of urate-lowering therapy during the acute attack.

BOX 158.2

Treatment of Chronic Gout

- Start urate-lowering therapy in patients who have two or more attacks a year, although in some patients it may be appropriate to start urate-lowering therapy (ULT) after one flare, especially if evidence suggests visible tophaceous gout.
- Avoid starting urate urate-lowering therapy during an acute attack.
- Uricosuric drugs and febuxostat are the urate-lowering therapy of choice in allopurinol-allergic patients, underexcretors with normal renal function, and patients with no history of urolithiasis.
- Use allopurinol in patients with renal calculi, renal insufficiency, concomitant diuretic therapy, cyclosporine therapy, or urate overproduction.
- Use concomitant colchicine prophylaxis for at least 8 weeks when starting ULT
- Monitor serum urate level and aim for SU <6 mg/dL.

In addition, it has been suggested that ULT should not be started during an acute gout attack, because this could result in a more intense and prolonged attack. Typically, ULT should be started 4 to 8 weeks after the attack has resolved. ULT should be started at low doses and increased slowly every 4 to 6 weeks to achieve SU levels (<6 mg/dL) or the maximum tolerated or maximum dose advised.

ULT approved by the U.S. FDA include the xanthine oxidase inhibitors (allopurinol, febuxostat), uricosuric agents (probenecid, lesinurad), and recombinant uricase (pegloticase). Allopurinol is the most commonly prescribed ULT, primarily because of its once-a-day dosing and great efficacy. It can be given in a single morning dose of 50 to 100 mg initially and increased to 800 mg in a stepwise fashion if needed. Dose adjustments may be necessary in patients with impaired kidney disease. Febuxostat is another oral, once-daily inhibitor of xanthine oxidase. Febuxostat may be of the most immediate value in patients with allopurinol hypersensitivity and in patients with renal disease.[10]

Probenecid is an alternative first-line option, but is uncommonly used. The use of probenecid is limited in patients with moderate renal function impairment and the maintenance dosages requiring multiple times/day administration is associated with patient nonadherence.

A xanthine oxidase inhibitor can be combined with a uricosuric for patients who do not achieve target SU levels with monotherapy. However, if SU target is not achieved, recombinant uricase should be used. Its use, though, is limited by the need for parenteral administration as well as by price.

PROPHYLAXIS

Persistent low-grade inflammation is frequently present in asymptomatic chronic tophaceous gout. In addition, there is an increase in acute attacks after initiation of ULT, due to inflammation caused by changes in the chemical and/or physical state of preexisting MSU crystals when ULT induces rapid changes in SU levels.[3] The increased gout attack rate when initiating ULT has been linked to suboptimal patient adherence to ULT. Lack of adherence and uncontrolled disease can contribute to the development of polyarticular disease and tophi that can cause destructive arthritis.

When initiating a patient on ULT, prophylactic low-dose antiinflammatory treatment is recommended to prevent attacks and foster compliance with ULT. Low-dose colchicine is the most commonly prescribed drug for prophylaxis in patients initiating ULT.[14]

The recently published ACP gout clinical guidelines[13] recommend treating acute gout with corticosteroids, NSAIDs, or colchicine and using low doses of colchicine (0.6 mg twice daily) or NSAIDs for prophylaxis for greater than 8 weeks, since it is more effective at reducing gout attacks than shorter durations of prophylaxis in patients initiating ULT.

INDICATIONS FOR REFERRAL OR HOSPITALIZATION

The rheumatologist should be consulted if the nature of the inflammatory arthritis is unclear and the diagnosis of gout is questioned; if the treatment is effective but drug toxicity or intolerance occurs; if the patient is still having acute attacks despite treatment; if the acute attack has not responded to the given antiinflammatory treatment; and if the disease is progressing despite the given ULT.

Hospitalization is rarely necessary unless drug treatment affects a patient's comorbidity (e.g., diabetes), there is confirmed or questioned septic arthritis in a patient suspected of having gout, or a severe drug reaction occurs.

COMPLICATIONS

Gout is often associated with high blood pressure, heart disease, and renal disease including kidney stones. Accumulations of urate crystals can form in joints and around joints (tophi), causing infection and joint damage. Use of medications to treat the previously listed diseases is known to increase SU levels and the likelihood of gout attacks. Primary care providers should carefully monitor patients with these known issues.

PATIENT AND FAMILY EDUCATION

Health care providers should educate patients with gout and their families on the following points:
- Gout can be accurately diagnosed.
- There are three types of treatments for gout: medications to control the attacks of joint pain (e.g., NSAIDs, colchicine, and corticosteroids); medications to prevent further attacks: prophylaxis (e.g., colchicine and NSAIDs); and medications that will help lower the level of uric acid in the body over time so that the attacks occur less frequently or not at all (urate-lowering therapies [e.g., allopurinol and Febuxostat as well as probenecid and lesinurad and uricase]).
- People with chronic gout require lifetime treatment with drugs to lower the uric acid body pool.
- Lifestyle changes that include weight control, limiting alcohol consumption, meals with meats and fish rich in purines, and increasing low-fat dairy consumption as well as cherry juice consumption are helpful in controlling gout. The following websites may be helpful:
- **American College of Rheumatology**: www.rheumatology.org/practice/clinical/patients/diseases_and_conditions/gout.asp
- **Arthritis Foundation**: http://www.arthritis.org/about-arthritis/types/gout/
- **National Institute of Arthritis and Musculoskeletal and Skin Diseases**: https://www.niams.nih.gov/health-topics/gout
- **Gout and uric acid education society**: http://gouteducation.org

REFERENCES

1. Chen-Xu, M., Yokose, C., Rai, S. K., et al. (2019). Contemporary prevalence of gout and hyperuricemia in the United States and decadel trends: The National Health and Nutrition Examinations study, 2007-2106. *Arthritis & Rheumatology*, 71(6), 991–999.
2. Schlesinger, N. (2010). Diagnosing and treating gout: A review to aid primary care physicians. *Postgraduate Medicine*, 122(2), 157–161.
3. Martillo, M. A., Nazzal, L., & Crittenden, D. B. (2014). The crystallization of monosodium urate. *Current Rheumatology Reports*, 16(2), 400. doi:10.1007/s11926-013-0400.
4. Neogi, T., Jansen, T. L. T. A., Dalbeth, N., Fransen, J., Schumacher, H. R., Berendsen, D., et al. (2015). 2015 Gout classification criteria: An American College of Rheumatology/European League Against Rheumatism Collaborative Initiative. *Arthritis & Rheumatology*, 67, 2557–2568.
5. Ogdie, A., Taylor, W. J., Neogi, T., et al. (2017). Performance of ultrasound in the diagnosis of gout in a multi-center study: Comparison with monosodium urate crystal analysis as the gold standard. *Arthritis & Rheumatology*, 69(2), 429–438. doi:10.1002/art.39959.
6. Gruber, M., Bodner, G., Rath, E., Supp, G., Weber, M., & Schueller-Weidekamm, C. (2014). Dual-energy computed tomography compared with ultrasound in the diagnosis of gout. *Rheumatology (Oxford, England)*, 53(1), 173–179.

7. Li, R., Yu, K., & Li, C. (2018). Dietary factors and risk of gout and hyperuricemia: A meta-analysis and systematic review [online]. *Asia Pacific Journal of Clinical Nutrition, 27*(6), 1344–1356.

8. Bell, P. G., Gaze, D. C., Davison, G. W., George, T. W., Scotter, M. J., & Howatson, G. (2014). Montmorency tart cherry (Prunus cerasus L.) concentrate lowers uric acid, independent of plasma cyanidin-3-O-glucosiderutinoside. *Journal of Functional Foods, 11*, 82–90.

9. Juraschek, S. P., Gelber, A. C., Choi, H. K., Appel, L. J., & Miller, E. R., 3rd. (2016). Effects of the dietary approaches to stop hypertension (DASH) diet and sodium intake on serum uric acid. *Arthritis & Rheumatology, 357*, 3002–3009.

10. Neogi, T. (2016). Gout. *Annals of Internal Medicine, 165*, ITC1–ITC16.

11. Slobodnick, A., Shah, B., Krasnokutsky, S., & Pillinger, M. H. (2018). Update on colchicine, 2017. *Rheumatology, 57*(suppl_1), i4–i11. https://doi.org/10.1093/rheumatology/kex453.

12. Richette, P., Doherty, M., Pascual, E., et al. (2017). 2016 updated EULAR evidence-based recommendations for the management of gout. *Annals of the Rheumatic Diseases*, http://dx.doi.org/10.1136/annrheumdis-2106-209707.

13. Qaseem, A., Harris, R. P., & Forciea, M. A. (2017). Clinical Guidelines Committee of the American College of Physicians Management of acute and recurrent gout: A clinical practice guideline from the American College of Physicians. *Annals of Internal Medicine, 166*, 58–68.

14. Shekelle, P. G., Newberry, S. J., FitzGerald, J. D., Motala, A., O'Hanlon, C. E., Tariq, A., et al. (2017). Management of gout: A systematic review in support of an American College of Physicians clinical practice guideline. *Annals of Internal Medicine, 166*, 37–51. doi:10.7326/M16-0461.

CHAPTER **159**

SEPTIC ARTHRITIS

Kevin D. Kerin

 A septic joint is a medical emergency.

DEFINITION AND EPIDEMIOLOGY

Inflammation of a joint is called "arthritis" and is an observable finding, whereas pain in a joint is called "arthralgia" and is a subjective description. Inflammation in a joint may arise from different mechanisms, including sterile, autoimmune processes (e.g., rheumatoid arthritis), crystal-induced inflammation (e.g., gout), foreign body reaction (e.g., splinter), and from infection (sepsis). Septic arthritis is an important type of arthritis and is considered to be a medical emergency. Septic arthritis can be caused by a large number of organisms, including bacteria, fungi, and filariae. Viral infections such as parvovirus B19 may also result in an inflammatory arthritis. Alphavirus infection, after initial febrile illness, may progress to cause a polyarticular inflammatory arthritis that bears similarity to seronegative rheumatoid arthritis. Chikungunya viral arthritis (transmitted by mosquito) is an example of an alphavirus and appeared in the United States in 2014.[1,2] The term *septic arthritis* is most commonly used to describe joint inflammation caused by a bacterial pathogen. An infectious cause of joint inflammation needs to be considered even when a noninfectious type of inflammatory arthritis (rheumatoid arthritis, gout) has been previously diagnosed, especially when the presentation is acute or subacute, monoarticular, and does not respond to antiinflammatory treatment. Bacterial and viral arthritides usually manifest acutely with systemic and articular symptoms. Parvovirus infection may result in an inflammatory arthritis in a number of joints simultaneously and may also have the appearance of rheumatoid arthritis. In contrast, Lyme disease and mycobacterial, fungal, filarial, and some bacterial arthritides (e.g., *Neisseria gonorrhoeae, Neisseria meningitidis*) may be subacute or chronic and relatively indolent. Septic arthritis occurs in all age groups, although the highest incidence is seen in children and older adults. The focus of this chapter will be on joint inflammation due to bacterial pathogens.

PATHOPHYSIOLOGY

Synovial joints such as the knee and hip are particularly vulnerable to infection. Abnormal synovial joints, such as those previously damaged by other traumatic, inflammatory, or degenerative processes, are especially susceptible to infection. One explanation is that synovial tissue is highly vascularized, lacks a basement membrane, and is thus susceptible to the hematogenous spread of infectious organisms from a locus of infection.[3] Other avenues of infection of the joint space include extension of infection from osteomyelitis or adjacent soft tissue infection and direct inoculation from penetration of a foreign body. A joint infection is a medical emergency and can be a rapid, severely destructive process. Once a bacterial infection is established in a joint space, a complex cascade of events follows: changes in synovial tissue; migration of acute and chronic inflammatory cells to the joint space; release of inflammatory cytokines, proteases, and collagenases; changes in intra-articular fluid volume and pressure; and chondrocyte changes.[4]

Staphylococcus aureus is the most common cause of acute bacterial arthritis across all age groups.[4] Its affinity for joints can be explained in part by the structure of the microbe, which produces certain surface and secreted proteins that may facilitate colonization of tissue. This organism also has receptors for glycoproteins found in joints and has frequent access by hematogenous seeding from minor wounds and abrasions because of its presence as normal skin flora.[5] Streptococci are also considered to be normal skin flora, and are second only to *S. aureus* as causative agents of infectious arthritis.

N. gonorrhoeae is the most common cause of septic arthritis from a sexually transmitted bacterium and is most frequently seen in sexually active adults younger than 30 years.[6] This is not unexpected, given the ease with which *N. gonorrhoeae* invades the bloodstream during menses or parturition and after acute urethritis. There were nearly 470,000 cases of gonorrhea reported in the United States in 2016. This represents an increase in cases of 18.5% from the previous year and an increase of 48.6% from the historic low rate in 2009.[7] It is also of great concern that increasing antibiotic resistance is making gonorrhea more difficult to treat.[8]

Gram-negative bacilli cause approximately 10% of cases of septic arthritis, often in older adults and neonates, and are associated with a better outcome than gram-positive infections.[9] In a community-based study of septic arthritis in native joints, older age and limited range of motion were predictors for gram-positive cocci as the cause, whereas diabetes mellitus with end-organ damage and malignancy were predictors for gram-negative bacteria.[9] Anaerobes are an uncommon cause of infectious arthritis and are frequently associated with human bites, intra-abdominal abscesses, dental procedures, and periarticular decubitus ulcers.[10]

CLINICAL PRESENTATION AND PHYSICAL EXAMINATION

Septic arthritis usually manifests with the acute onset of a painful, red, swollen joint that is warm to the touch. An important historical point that helps distinguish septic arthritis from sterile inflammation is that the affected joint is painful at rest as well as with motion and weight bearing. The rapid accumulation of fluid volume and rise in intra-articular pressure are prime contributors to rest pain. The mediators and mechanisms of synovial joint pain are beyond the scope of this chapter. Suffice it to say that there is a complex set of neurobiological processes that lead to the sensation of pain. The affected joint will be held in a position that allows maximum intra-articular volume. The pain of joint inflammation from noninfectious causes usually is relieved with rest. Fever in a patient with septic arthritis is usually present but may be low grade or absent (especially in older adults); rigors caused by bacteremia may also be present. Fever and rigors have low sensitivity and specificity in the diagnosis of septic arthritis because these findings may also be seen in acute crystal-induced arthritis. Any joint may be involved in septic arthritis, yet the knee and hip are the most commonly affected.[11] Septic arthritis in an unusual location, such as the sternoclavicular or sacroiliac joint, should raise the suspicion of injection drug use.[12] The sudden onset of monoarticular arthritis is the usual presentation of nongonococcal arthritis, although a polyarticular presentation may also be seen. A polyarticular septic arthritis is sometimes seen with streptococcal or staphylococcal infections but usually affects only two or three joints, characterized as a pauciarticular presentation.

Septic arthritis occurs more commonly in patients with an impaired immune system and in those with preexisting joint abnormalities due to rheumatoid arthritis, gout, osteoarthritis, or a prosthetic joint. It is important to consider infection as a cause of an acute monoarticular or pauciarticular flare, even in those with an established diagnosis of a chronic rheumatologic condition. The fever and joint inflammation are less striking in gonococcal arthritis, which is characterized by a migrating polyarticular course.[11] Human immunodeficiency virus (HIV) infection with the associated immunosuppression is a special situation in which septic arthritis is uncommon; however, when it is seen, it may be a result of atypical organisms, such as *Mycobacterium tuberculosis*, *Sporothrix schenckii*, and *Candida albicans*, in addition to more common organisms such as *S. aureus* and *N. gonorrhoeae*.[13]

The manifestations of inflammation were vividly described by Celsius in the first century AD as rubor, tumor, calor, and dolor (redness, swelling, heat, and pain).[14] The inflamed joint is erythematous, warm to the touch, swollen, and painful with passive and active range of motion. Synovial effusion is usually present, although it is less obvious in certain joints, such as the hip and shoulder. A large effusion creates an asymmetry in size with loss of anatomic landmarks. A smaller effusion in the knee may be detected by a "bulge sign" (the examiner presses on the medial aspect of the knee to displace fluid toward the suprapatellar region and then looks for a small bulge in this area after applying pressure on the opposite side of the knee) or patellar ballottement (see Fig. 156.1) (the examiner taps on the patella while applying pressure to the suprapatellar area to try to elicit a "click," signifying synovial fluid beneath the patella).

Decreased range of motion, muscle spasm, and apprehension to joint examination are prominent features of the examination. The proximal lymph node may be enlarged and tender, indicative of proximal lymphangitic spread of infection.

An original source of infection, such as an abscess, cellulitis, gonococcal urethritis, pneumonia, urinary tract infection, or endocarditis, should be sought. Distinct clinical presentations are seen in special situations, which are discussed in the following sections.

Gonococcal Arthritis

Disseminated gonococcal infection (see Chapter 135) is the most common cause of septic arthritis in sexually active adolescents and young adults.[15] There appear to be two distinct clinical presentations. One has been called the arthritis-dermatitis syndrome and reflects a bacteremic stage; the other is a localized septic arthritis.[15] The classic triad of clinical findings in disseminated infection is dermatitis, tenosynovitis, and a migratory polyarthritis. The first group is distinguished by tenosynovitis and dermatitis. Skin lesions are present in countable numbers and multiple stages; these lesions are most often maculopapular but are sometimes necrotic, pustular, or vesicular. The lesions are painless and nonpruritic and typically spare the face and scalp. The lesions resolve in several days without scarring.[16] An asymmetric migratory polyarthralgia that affects knees, elbows, wrists, ankles, metacarpophalangeal joints, and associated tendon sheaths is the presentation more common than actual polyarthritis. Synovial fluid cell counts are lower than those commonly seen in bacterial arthritis, and the synovial fluid culture is often negative. The blood culture may be positive. Only 25% of patients have genitourinary symptoms of gonorrhea.[6]

The more focal septic arthritis seen in the second group may occur after a migratory polyarthritis, tenosynovitis, or dermatitis, with the arthritis now settled in one or two joints. The synovial fluid is more purulent, and the culture is more likely to be positive. Blood cultures are typically negative. Taken as a group, cultures of the pharynx, cervix, urethra, and rectum are positive in up to 80% of patients if specimens are obtained early on selective media (e.g., Thayer-Martin).[6] Synovial fluid culture specimens should be plated directly onto chocolate agar.

There may be clinical uncertainty about the diagnosis, especially in the context of a wide range of synovial fluid leukocyte counts and negative blood cultures. In this situation, ceftriaxone, 1 g/day IM or IV every 24 hours in addition to a one-time, 1-g dose of azithromycin, can be a valid diagnostic and appropriate therapeutic strategy.[17] Gonococcal arthritis may, in some cases, be managed on an outpatient basis. In the appropriate clinical setting (adequate pretest probability) and if cultures are negative, a rapid response to intravenous ceftriaxone and oral azithromycin may be considered diagnostic of gonococcal arthritis.

Prosthetic Joint Infection

Millions of people have prosthetic joints, and it is estimated that approximately 4 million knee or hip arthroplasties will be performed annually by the year 2030.[18] Although the rates of infection after hip or knee arthroplasty have declined significantly to approximately 1%,[19] the large number of current and projected prosthetic joints makes this a relatively common problem. It is a serious, potentially devastating problem and is associated with major disability and cost. In most cases, in patients not considered to be too frail or poor surgical candidates, the prosthetic joint needs to be removed, and the patient will require up to 6 weeks of intravenous antibiotics (with or without an antibiotic-impregnated cement spacer), followed by reimplantation of a new prosthetic joint once infection has been eradicated.[20] Biofilms, complex microbial communities formed by bacteria causing prosthetic joint infections, contribute to antibiotic resistance.[21] Coagulase-negative staphylococci are common in this clinical setting and produce an indolent course. Hematogenous seeding at the bone–cement interface with *S. aureus* or group A streptococci may manifest more acutely with sepsis or toxic shock, which is characteristic of these more virulent organisms.[21]

Infections in older patients with underlying disease may include gram-negative bacilli (15% to 20%) and anaerobes (7%).[22]

One way to classify prosthetic joint infections is by the amount of time elapsed since joint surgery: early (within 3 months), delayed (3 to 24 months), and late (>24 months). Early and delayed infections have their origin at the time of prosthetic placement, whereas late infections are caused by hematogenous seeding of bacteria.[23] Infection in a prosthetic joint is often difficult to diagnose, and clinical manifestations may vary by the timing of the infection in relation to the surgery. As a rule, most patients have joint pain with or without radiographic evidence of loosening of the prosthesis. A minority of patients have fever, joint swelling, or sinus track drainage. It may be difficult to differentiate a delayed-onset infection of a prosthetic joint from a noninfectious inflammation, such as a reaction to components of the prosthetic joint or a mechanical problem with the hardware (e.g., loosening, dislocation, hemarthrosis, and malposition).[24] A helpful observation is that mechanical problems are painful during motion, weight bearing, and pivoting but are comfortable while at rest. Constant joint pain suggests an infection.

Laboratory tests such as acute-phase reactants (erythrocyte sedimentation rate [ESR], C-reactive protein [CRP]), and leukocyte count are not especially helpful because a number of inflammatory conditions can cause elevated levels in any of these tests, and normal values do not rule out infection. Plain radiographs may be helpful, especially if serial studies are available for comparison. Classic radiographic findings of infection include lucencies along the bone–cement interface, migration of the prosthesis, and periosteal reactions. These findings are not present in acute or early infections and are difficult to differentiate from mechanical complications in those with delayed-onset infections. A technetium bone scan may take up to 1 year to become normal after surgery because of bone remodeling, yet a normal bone scan provides strong evidence against an infected prosthetic joint if the timing is right. Other radionuclide techniques, such as sequential bone and gallium scanning or combined leukocyte-marrow scintigraphy, have shown greater accuracy in the diagnosis of a prosthetic joint infection.[25] Ultimately, the diagnosis of a prosthetic joint infection relies on aggressive attempts to isolate an organism by obtaining joint fluid or tissue.

The recommendations to patients with prosthetic joints about antibiotic prophylaxis for dental procedures are debated and confusing, with conflicting recommendations over the years. Currently (2019), the American Academy of Orthopaedic Surgeons (AAOS) and the American Dental Association recommend that clinicians not prescribe antibiotic prophylaxis for patients with prosthetic joints before dental procedures unless there are complicating circumstances such as a history of prior joint infection, chronic immunosuppression, or a complicated surgical history.[26] Individual surgeons or orthopedic centers may have established policies.

Lyme Disease

The clinical manifestations of Lyme disease can be separated into early localized disease (1 to 30 days), early disseminated disease (days to 10 months), and late disease (months to years) on the basis of the elapsed time from tick exposure to symptoms (see Chapter 213). Only 30% of patients with Lyme disease recall a tick bite, but in the setting of known tick exposure, 80% of patients with early, localized Lyme disease experience arthralgias or migratory arthritis.[27] During this stage, the characteristic rash (erythema chronicum migrans) appears with an expanding red border and central clearing, occasionally creating the classic bull's eye appearance. Fever, headache, myalgias, arthralgias, and lymphadenopathy may be more noticeable than the skin lesions, which are usually painless.

The manifestations of early, disseminated Lyme disease include multiple systemic features: cardiac problems (pericarditis, atrioventricular nodal heart block, and myopathy), neurologic problems, and musculoskeletal problems (migratory polyarthralgias or polyarthritis) in 50%.[27] More prolonged attacks of true arthritis develop in a few joints. In late Lyme disease, about 60% of patients have a migratory polyarthritis and 10% of patients develop a chronic arthritis that settles in one or two large joints, usually the knees.[28]

In Lyme disease, the causative spirochete, *Borrelia burgdorferi*, is difficult to culture from synovial fluid, but sensitive methods of antigen detection, such as enzyme-linked immunosorbent assay (ELISA) and polymerase chain reaction (PCR), can reveal its presence. Having a high index of suspicion in the right clinical setting is essential to establishing the diagnosis. In the wrong clinical setting (without sufficiently high pretest probability), serologic tests for Lyme disease are misleading because of the high false-positive rate; therefore such tests should not be ordered indiscriminantly.[27] All patients with true arthritis attributed to early, disseminated, or late Lyme disease should have a positive response on the Lyme ELISA, subsequently confirmed by western blot.

The outcome is better if diagnosis and treatment are rendered early in this form of infectious arthritis. Medical therapy fails in approximately 50% of patients with late Lyme disease arthritis; progressive joint destruction may then merit synovectomy or total joint arthroplasty.[28]

Injection Drug Use

Septic arthritis in unusual or axial locations (e.g., sacroiliac joint, sternoclavicular joint, symphysis pubis) should raise suspicion of injection drug use. Similarly, the presence of unusual organisms—*Pseudomonas aeruginosa*, *Serratia marcescens*, and *Candida* species—in joint fluid should lead to open-ended and nonjudgmental queries about recreational drug use. Still, most of the joint infections in these joints are caused by *S. aureus* with or without injection drug use. Methicillin-resistant *Staphylococcus aureus* (MRSA) is the most common pathogen.[29] In patients who use injection recreational drugs, disseminated gonococcal disease, HIV infection, and syphilis should also be considered in the differential diagnosis.

TABLE 159.1 Synovial Fluid Analysis

Characteristic	Normal	Noninflammatory (Osteoarthritis)	Inflammatory (Rheumatoid)	Septic (Infection)
Volume	<3.5 mL	>3.5 mL	Large	Large
Clarity	Clear	Transparent	Translucent	Opaque
WBCs/mm^3	<200	200–2000	2000–75,000	50,000–100,000
Polymorphonuclear leukocytes	<25%	<25%	>50%	>75%
Culture	Negative	Negative	Negative	Positive
Glucose concentration	Equal to blood	Equal to blood	>50% blood glucose	<50% blood glucose
Protein level	1.7 g/dL	<3 g/dL	>3 g/dL	>3 g/dL

WBCs, White blood cells.

Septic Sacroiliitis

Septic sacroiliitis can be an elusive diagnosis for health care providers because of the nonspecific nature of presenting symptoms. Patients may have fever and low back pain or gluteal region pain that is intensified by ambulation.[30] The physical examination alone is inadequate in distinguishing sacroiliitis from muscle pain, intervertebral disk disease, femoral nerve entrapment in the buttocks (piriformis muscle syndrome), or bursitis. Certain physical examination maneuvers have been devised to isolate and stress the sacroiliac joints. Plain radiographs are not helpful in early diagnosis. Focal pain that occurs when shear forces are applied to the sacroiliac joint may indicate septic sacroiliitis, in which case the patient should be referred immediately for a computed tomography (CT) scan or magnetic resonance imaging (MRI). MRI is uniquely suited to this difficult diagnosis because it alone has the potential to define fluid in the sacroiliac joint, adjacent bone marrow changes due to inflammation, and soft tissue abscesses that may extend into the abdominal cavity and the psoas, iliac, and piriform muscles. Because of the complexity of the involved joints and difficult access, these collections need pigtail catheter drainage or surgical debridement.[30]

DIAGNOSTICS

In patients with septic arthritis, increases in the peripheral white blood cell (WBC) count, ESR, and CRP level are frequent but nonspecific findings. Peripheral blood cultures are positive in 40% of cases and are the only sources of microorganisms in 10% of cases.[31] Younger patients suspected of having gonococcal arthritis should have pharyngeal, rectal, and cervical or urethral cultures on specialized gonococcal media.[6] The most important examination for the diagnosis of septic arthritis is synovial fluid, not only for culture but also for cellular and chemical analysis. Aspiration of inflamed joints provides three important pieces of information: diagnosis of crystal-induced arthritis, degree of inflammation (cell count), and specimen for Gram stain and culture. Any joint suspected of infection should be aspirated without delay because the outcome of septic arthritis depends on early diagnosis and treatment. Sterile technique should be used, and the provider should avoid entering the joint through an area of skin that may be infected. It is important to send blood and synovial fluid culture specimens for analysis before antibiotics are started.

The most useful components of synovial fluid analysis consist of evaluation for monosodium urate or calcium pyrophosphate crystals, cell count and differential, protein, Gram stain, and cultures (aerobic and anaerobic). Synovial fluid WBC and granulocyte percentage are especially useful in determining likelihood of septic arthritis before Gram stain and cultures have been completed.[32] Synovial fluid protein and glucose concentrations are less useful diagnostic tests. Synovial fluid protein is significantly elevated in both infectious arthritis and other forms of inflammatory arthritis. Synovial fluid glucose concentration of less than 40 mg/dL or less than 50% of a simultaneous blood glucose concentration is supportive evidence for bacterial arthritis. Synovial fluid lactic acid has high negative predictive value for bacterial arthritis yet is not widely used.[4] With chronic synovitis, fungal and mycobacterial culture specimens are also sent for analysis, and special stains for acid-fast bacteria and fungi are performed. Synovial fluid WBC counts may be very high (Table 159.1); cell counts in the 100,000/mm^3 range are considered to indicate infection until proven otherwise.[32] There is a considerable overlap in synovial WBC counts among infectious and noninfectious causes of arthritis. Gout, reactive arthritis, and rheumatoid arthritis may cause high cell counts normally associated with sepsis, whereas early septic arthritis or established gonococcal arthritis may reveal relatively low cell counts. Intracellular crystals and the profusion of polymorphonuclear cells suggest gout or pseudogout, but free-floating crystals are sometimes seen in septic arthritis. Synovial fluid PCR may be used to diagnose gonococcal arthritis and Lyme disease arthritis.

Radiographs are not useful in the initial diagnosis of a septic joint. It may take 2 weeks for joint space narrowing and marginal erosions to be demonstrated, too late to salvage a functional joint. Radiographs are useful in identifying underlying arthritis or osteomyelitis. A three-phase technetium bone scan is helpful in differentiating cellulitis, infectious arthritis, and osteomyelitis.[33] Musculoskeletal ultrasound is an increasingly popular imaging technology and can identify small amounts of fluid and inflammatory changes (erosions, periosteal reactions) in the articular and periarticular structures. Bone scan, gallium scan, and indium leukocyte scan are of little practical value. A CT scan or MRI is advantageous in difficult diagnostic situations (e.g., sternoclavicular or sacroiliac joint involvement) and as a guide to joint aspiration and anatomic definition of an infected hip.[34]

INITIAL DIAGNOSTICS

Septic Arthritis

LABORATORY
- Joint aspiration of synovial fluid for crystals, culture, cell count, and gram stain
- Complete blood count and differential
- Erythrocyte sedimentation rate
- C-reactive protein
- Blood cultures
- Rectal, cervical, urethral, or pharyngeal cultures[a]

IMAGING
- X-ray studies

OTHER DIAGNOSTICS
- Computed tomography scan, magnetic resonance imaging
- Musculoskeletal ultrasound
- Lyme enzyme-linked immunosorbent assay, Western blot test[a]

[a] If indicated.

DIFFERENTIAL DIAGNOSIS

A synovial fluid leukocyte count of more than $2000/mm^3$ is considered inflammatory, and a cell count of more than $50.000/mm^3$ is considered septic until proven otherwise by Gram stain and cultures.[35] There is a significant overlap in synovial fluid leukocyte counts in inflammatory conditions from infectious and noninfectious causes. Other types of inflammatory arthritis are distinguished from septic arthritis by culture and Gram stain; however, gout, reactive arthritis, and rheumatoid arthritis may have synovial fluid cell counts in the septic arthritis range. In such situations, antibiotics should be initiated until cultures are finalized.

Cellulitis, bursitis, and acute osteomyelitis should be distinguished by their greater range of motion and less than circumferential swelling. Polyarticular septic arthritis is sometimes seen with staphylococci and streptococci but may also suggest metastatic foci resulting from subacute bacterial endocarditis. Polyarticular noninfectious arthritis is seen with rheumatic fever or poststreptococcal reactive arthritis. In either case, the joint is not the focus of the streptococcal infection. The arthritis of rheumatic fever is migratory and resolves spontaneously in 1 month.

Reactive arthritis may be accompanied by urethritis, conjunctivitis, and enthesopathy (i.e., inflamed tendon insertions) (see Chapter 198).

INTERPROFESSIONAL COLLABORATIVE MANAGEMENT

A joint infection is a medical emergency. All patients with septic arthritis should be hospitalized initially because they need to adhere to strict non–weight-bearing activities to preserve cartilage, may require daily joint aspiration, or will need initial surgical drainage. For patients who have been prescribed bed rest, early mobilization of the infected joint with a passive mobilization device helps prevent adhesions and contractures. Infectious disease, rheumatology, and orthopedic surgery consultations are obtained when the patient is hospitalized. A physical therapist should be part of the care team because early mobilization and eventual weight bearing are important.

Cartilage has no blood supply and is in part dependent on intermittent compression for nutritional requirements and integrity of structure. It is thus important to try to achieve early mobilization. When the effusion has subsided, early discharge with home intravenous therapy or oral antibiotics is feasible.

Early initiation of antimicrobial therapy and drainage is required treatment of septic arthritis. If this condition remains undiagnosed or untreated longer than 5 to 7 days, the prognosis for a functional joint is poor. The initial choice of antibiotic should be sufficiently broad to cover likely sources of infection for an individual, and then the antibiotic may be changed on the basis of the results of the Gram stain and culture. Older children and adults do well with nafcillin, oxacillin, or cefazolin, especially if the Gram stain suggests *S. aureus* and the risk of MRSA is low. For patients at high risk for gram-negative septic arthritis (elderly, immunocompromised), cefepime should be considered as an initial broad-spectrum antibiotic.[4] For coverage of gonococcal arthritis, sexually active young adults should receive ceftriaxone, 1 g intravenously daily for 7 to 10 days in addition to 1 g azithromycin orally as a one-time dose.[17] Pending culture results, septic arthritis in a prosthetic joint after recent surgery or in other individuals at risk for MRSA (hemodialysis patients, those with diabetes mellitus, nursing home residents) may require empirical vancomycin to cover the possibility of coagulase-negative staphylococci or MRSA. Aminoglycosides and antipseudomonal β-lactams are sometimes added for synergism in patients who are infected with *S. aureus* or injection drug users in whom *P. aeruginosa* is suspected. Linezolid, daptomycin, and pristinamycin have shown some promise in the treatment of MRSA septic arthritis.[4]

Duration of therapy is 2 weeks for *Haemophilus influenzae* and streptococci and 3 weeks for staphylococci or gram-negative bacilli. Shorter courses and oral regimens are often effective in children. Gonococcal arthritis responds quickly and may be treated entirely on an outpatient basis with 2 or 3 days of intravenous ceftriaxone, followed by early conversion to oral cefixime, 400 mg twice daily, or ciprofloxacin, 500 mg twice daily, to complete a 10- to 14-day course. Patients with underlying rheumatoid arthritis and virulent organisms should be treated for 4 weeks.[4] Fluoroquinolones such as gatifloxacin, moxifloxacin, levofloxacin, and trovafloxacin have improved gram-positive coverage. Intravenous and oral antibiotics have ready access to inflamed joints and should not be given by intra-articular injection or added to solutions for irrigating joints. Antibiotics injected directly into joints may initiate chemical synovitis and prolong postinfectious arthritis.

An infected joint is similar to an abscess in that it needs daily drainage until the inflammation has resolved.[11] Reactive oxygen species and proteolytic enzymes, which destroy cartilage, are produced by activated leukocytes. Therefore it is important that purulent material and bacterial toxins be removed to preserve cartilage. This is accomplished equally well with either daily arthrocentesis or arthroscopic lavage with placement of drains. Daily arthrocentesis is less expensive and is not complicated by instrumentation morbidity; it also offers the possibility of serial culture and cell counts of synovial fluid to gauge response to therapy. Arthroscopic lavage with debridement and placement of drains or open arthrotomy is appropriate if there is persistence of recurrent effusion and elevation of cell counts after several days of daily arthrocentesis or if loculated fluid is suspected. Hips should be surgically drained at the outset because of their anatomic complexity.[11]

An infected prosthetic joint usually requires drainage and debridement and may require removal of all prosthetic components and cement. A definitive approach is a two-step procedure, with removal of prosthesis and cement and 6 weeks of antibiotics followed by revision arthroplasty. An antibiotic-impregnated spacer may be used to maintain the joint space to prevent contracture pending reimplantation of a permanent prosthesis. Historically, even with sensitive organisms, retention of the prosthesis and antibiotic therapy with limited surgical debridement is often unsuccessful. In light of some studies reporting increasing rates of success in the retention of infected prosthetic joints with appropriate antibiotic therapy, there has been growing interest in this approach.[36] Risk factors predicting treatment failure of this approach include sinus tract presence and symptom duration of 8 days or longer. If revision arthroplasty is to be done, 6 weeks of intravenous antibiotics are crucial to achieve the 90% success rate.[22,36]

LIFE SPAN CONSIDERATIONS

Mortality is low when septic arthritis is diagnosed and treated appropriately. However, the associated infection carries significant mortality in older or immunocompromised patients.[38]

COMPLICATIONS

Progressive loss of joint function develops in 25% to 50% of patients.[37] A relapse of septic arthritis may occur if the selection or duration of the antibiotic therapy is inappropriate. Recurrent aseptic joint effusion is common and is referred to as postinfectious synovitis. Minor trauma may exacerbate such synovitis. More immediate complications include an associated abscess or bursa infection, which must be drained, and associated osteomyelitis. Ankylosis (fusion), ligamentous instability, and joint contracture are consequences of delayed diagnosis. A total joint arthroplasty can restore mobility in such joints but cannot reverse ligamentous instability or joint contracture. Secondary osteoarthritis is a delayed complication that may require eventual arthroplasty. Toxic shock or a continuing infectious syndrome despite a sterile blood culture is attributable to toxin production by small residual foci of staphylococci or streptococci around dead cartilage or prosthetic joints. There should be no delay in prosthetic joint removal, if one is present, and surgical debridement in the setting of toxic shock or sepsis syndrome because death may result. Surgery should not be delayed, because the problem is typically an abscess, which is unlikely to respond to a continued course of antibiotics.

Some factors that determine outcome are listed in Box 159.1.

PATIENT AND FAMILY EDUCATION

To remove potential sources of bacteremia, patients should be instructed to be certain that any necessary extensive dental work is done and wounds or ulcers are healed before undergoing a total joint arthroplasty. Antibiotic prophylaxis before surgery for total joint arthroplasty is advised to prevent postsurgical infectious arthritis. Lifelong antibiotic prophylaxis before urologic, intestinal, or dental procedures for patients who have undergone a joint replacement is no longer advised by the AAOS unless otherwise indicated by the patient's health status.[38,39] Other societies and individual practitioner may have

---

BOX 159.1

Factors Affecting Outcome in Infectious Arthritis

- Delay in diagnosis and treatment beyond 7 days
- Persistently positive culture and effusion after 5 days of treatment
- Prior arthritis, especially rheumatoid arthritis
- Compromised host and older patients
- Virulence of organism: *S. aureus* versus coagulase-negative staphylococci
- Specific joint involved: hips worse than knees
- Injection drug use: good prognosis with aggressive organisms
- Appropriate antibiotics
- Effective drainage and debridement
- Physical therapy: initially non–weight bearing, early mobilization, splint contractures

---

differing opinions, which complicates these decisions. Patients with rheumatoid arthritis, especially those taking immunosuppressant medications such as prednisone, methotrexate, and biologic disease-modifying antirheumatic drugs (DMARDs), should be aware that superimposed infectious arthritis is possible. They should disclose any monoarticular flare to their physician for early diagnostic arthrocentesis. Cellulitis, wounds, and ulcers should receive prompt medical attention to prevent bacteremia. Patients recovering from infectious arthritis must be instructed in home physical therapy to prevent contracture and to advance weight bearing after inflammation has subsided. The potential side effects of antibiotics need to be explained, antibiotic-associated diarrhea should be anticipated, and patients with indwelling central lines must be instructed in line care and signs of line infection.

REFERENCES

1. Chen, W., Foo, S. S., et al. (2015). Arthritogenic alphaviruses: New insights into arthritis and bone pathology. *Trends in Microbiology*, 23(1), 35–43.
2. Miner, J. J., AwYeang, H. X., et al. (2015). Chikungunya viral arthritis in the United States: A mimic of sero-negative arthritis. *Arthritis & Rheumatology*, 67(5), 1214–1220.
3. Garcia-Arias, M., Balsa, A., & Mola, E. M. (2011). Septic arthritis. *Best Practice & Research Clinical Rheumatology*, 25(3), 407–421.
4. Sharff, K. A., Richards, E. P., & Townes, J. M. (2013). Clinical management of septic arthritis. *Current Rhuematology Reports*, 15(6), 332.
5. Rajeshwari, N., & Marin, L. (2017). Schweizer, namrata singh, septic arthritis and prosthetic joint infections in older adults. *Infectious Disease Clinics of North America*, 31(4), 715–729.
6. Li, R., & Gossman, W. G. (2018). Arthritis, gonococcal. [Updated 2017 Dec 2]. In *StatPearls [Internet]*. Treasure Island (FL): StatPearls Publishing. Retrieved from https://www.ncbi.nlm.nih.gov/books/NBK470439/. (Accessed 3 May 2018).
7. Centers for Disease Control and prevention. 2016 Sexually transmitted disease surveillance. Gonorrhea. Retrieved from: https://www.cdc.gov/std/stats16/gonorrhea.htm. (Accessed 3 May 2018).
8. World Health Organization. Scientists warn that antibiotic-resistant gonorrhea is on the rise. Retrieved from: http://www.who.int/reproductivehealth/topics/rtis/amr-gonorrhoea-on-the-rise/en/. (Accessed 3 May 2018).
9. Seng, P., Vernier, M., & Gay, A. (2016). Clinical features and outcomes of bone and joint infection with streptococcus involvement: 5-year experience of interregional reference centres in the south of France. *New Microbes and New Infect*, 12, 8–17.
10. Shah, N. B., Tande, A. J., Patel, R., & Berbari, E. F. (2015). Anaerobic prosthetic joint infection. *Anaerobe*, 36, 1–8.
11. Ross, J. (2017). Septic arthritis of natural joints. *Infect Disease Clinics of North America*, 31(2), 203–218.

12. Mancaella, L. (2009). Septic sacroiliitis: An uncommon septic arthritis. *Clinical and Experimental Rheumatology*, 27(6), 1004–1008.

13. Takhar, S. S., & Hendy, G. W. (2010). Orthopedic illness in patients with HIV. *Rheumatic Diseases Clinics of North America*, 28, 335–342.

14. Scott, A., Khan, K. M., Cook, J. L., et al. (2004). What is "inflammation"? Are we ready to move beyond Celsius? *British Journal of Sports Medicine*, 38, 2.

15. Metcalf, R., Reed, M., & Winter, A. (2015). A limp with an unusual cause. *British Medical Journal*, 350, h1985.

16. Series, H. J. (2014). Skin as an indicator for sexually transmitted infections. *Clinics in Dermatology*, 32(2), 196–208.

17. Centers for Disease Control and Prevention. 2015 Sexually Transmitted Diseases, treatment guidelines, Gonorrhea. Retrieved from: https://www.cdc.gov/std/tg2015/gonorrhea.htm. (Accessed 3 May 2018).

18. Kurtz, S., Ong, K., Lau, E., et al. (2007). Projections of primary and revision hip and knee arthroplasty in the United States from 2005-2030. *The Journal of Bone and Joint Surgery. American Volume*, 89, 780–785.

19. Lamagni, T. (2014). Epidemiology and burden of prosthetic joint infections. *The Journal of Antimicrobial Chemotherapy*, 69(s1), i5–i10.

20. Chen, A. F., Heller, S., & Parviz, J. (2014). Prosthetic joint infections. *Surgical Clinics of North America*, 94(6), 1265–1281.

21. Dryden, M. (2014). Prosthetic joint infection: Managing infection in a bionic era. *The Journal of Antimicrobial Chemotherapy*, 69(s1), i3–i4.

22. Hsieh, E., Byren, I., Atkins, B. L., et al. (2009). Gram-negative prosthetic joint infections: Risk factors and outcome of treatment. *Clinical Infectious Diseases: An Official Publication of the Infectious Diseases Society of America*, 49, 1036–1043.

23. Lima, A., Oliveira, P., Carvalho, V., et al. (2013). Periprosthetic joint infections. *Interdisciplinary Perspectives on Infectious Diseases*, 542796. http://doi.org.101155/2013/542796.

24. Kapadia, B. H., Berg, R. A., Daley, J. A., Fritz, J., Bhave, A., & Mont, M. A. (2016). Periprosthetic joint infection. *The Lancet*, 387(10016), 386–394.

25. Brammen, L., Palestra, C., & Sinzinger, H. (2015). Radionuclide imaging: Past, present and future outlook in the diagnosis of infected prosthetic joints. *Hellenic Journal of Nuclear Medicine*, 18(3), 95–102.

26. American Academy of Orthopedic Surgeons. Prevention of orthopaedic implant infection in patients undergoing dental procedures: Evidence based guideline and evidence report 2012. Retrieved from: https://www.aaos.org/aaosnow/2013/jan/cover/cover1/. (Accessed 8 May 2018).

27. Arvikar, S., & Steere, A. (2015). Diagnosis and treatment of Lyme arthritis. *Infect Disease Clinic of North America*, 9(2), 269–280.

28. Steere, A. C., & Glickstein, L. (2004). Elucidation of Lyme arthritis. *Nature Reviews. Immunology*, 2, 143–152.

29. Peterson, T. C., Pearson, C., et al. (2014). Septic arthritis in intravenous drug abusers: A historical comparison of habits and pathogens. *The Journal of Emergency Medicine*, 47(6), 723–728.

30. Hermet, M., Minichiello, E., Flipo, R. M., et al. (2012). Infectious sacroiliitis: A retrospective, multicenter study of 39 adults. *BMC Infectious Diseases*, 12, 305.

31. Margaretten, M. E., Kohlwes, J., Moore, D., et al. (2007). Does this adult patient have septic arthritis? *Journal of the American Medical Association*, 297(13), 1478–1488.

32. Carpenter, C., Schur, J., Worth, W., et al. (2011). Evidence-based diagnostics: Adult septic arthritis. *Academic Emergency Medicine: Official Journal of the Society for Academic Emergency Medicine*, 18(8), 781–796.

33. Lazzeri, E. (2013). *Nuclear medicine imaging of bone and joint infection. Radionuclide imaging of infection and inflammation*. Milan: Springer.

34. Flemming, D., Hash, T., Bernard, S., & Brian, P. (2014). Magnetic resonance imaging assessment of arthritis of the knee. *Magnetic Resonance Imaging Clinics of North America*, 22(4), 703–724.

35. Horowitz, D. L., Katzap, E., et al. (2011). Approach to septic arthritis. *American Family Physician*, 84(6), 653–660.

36. Nair, R., Schweizer, M., & Singh, N. (2017). Septic arthritis and prosthetic joint infections in older adults. *Infectious Disease Clinics of North America*, 31(4), 715–729.

37. Ferrand, J., Samad, Y., & Brunschweiler, B. (2016). Morbimortality in adult patients with septic arthritis: A three year hospital based study. *BMC Infectious Diseases*, 16, 239. http://doi.org/10.1186/s12879-016-1540-4.

38. Sollecito, T. P., Abt, E., et al. (2015). The use of prophylactic antibiotics prior to dental procedure in patients with prosthetic joints: Evidence-based clinical practice guideline for dental practitioners—a report of the American Dental association on Scientific Affairs. *Journal of the American Dental Association (1939)*, 146(1), 11–16.e8.

39. Mazur, D., Fuchs, D., Abicht, T., & Peabody, T. (2015). Update on antibiotic prophylaxis for genito-urinary procedures in patients with artificial joint replacement and artificial heart valves. *Urologic Clinics of North America*, 42(4), 441–447.

CHAPTER **160**

LOW BACK PAIN

Zacharia Isaac • Hannah Steere • Ashley H. Cotter

 Red flags include age greater than 50, recent unexplained weight loss, failure to improve after 1 month of conservative treatment, fever, new lower extremity weakness, or bowel/bladder dysfunction.

DEFINITION AND EPIDEMIOLOGY

Low back pain is the most common musculoskeletal problem worldwide and is estimated to affect up to 85% of the population at some time in a person's life. Chronic low back pain has a prevalence of approximately 4.2% in those aged between 24 and 39 years old and 19.6% in those between 20 and 59.[1] Females have a prevalence around 50% higher than males after the second decade of life.[1] In the United States, back pain is the second most common reason for visits to a physician. It is also a leading cause of hospital admissions and subsequent surgery.

Low back pain is commonly classified by symptom duration as acute, subacute, or chronic (Table 160.1). Approximately 30% to 60% of people with acute low back pain recover within 1 week, and 80% to 90% recover within 6 weeks.[2] However, recurrence rates are high, with up to 50% reporting recurrence of pain within 6 months.[2] Although low back pain is typically transient, if it persists and becomes subacute, there is an increased risk for developing chronic low back pain. The average prevalence of chronic low back pain is approximately 15% in adults and 27% in the elderly and has been shown to be increasing as the population ages.[3]

Risk factors for development of low back pain are broad. Age older than 65 years is a prominent risk factor for the development of musculoskeletal impairment, with a majority of these cases involving the back. Genetic disposition, obesity, and smoking have also been linked to accelerated degenerative disk disease, increasing the risk of low back pain.[3] Studies of identical twins support the strong influence of genetic factors on the development of degenerative disk disease. Jobs involving prolonged sitting,[4] heavy lifting, pulling, pushing, prolonged walking or standing, and vehicular driving have been found to be predictors of future low back pain.[5] Preexisting psychological conditions such as anxiety, depression, or somatization disorder, in addition to maladaptive coping strategies, lower socioeconomic status, and poor general health, are risk factors for chronic low back pain.[6] In fact, these factors are

TABLE 160.1 Classification of Low Back Pain		
By Symptom Duration	**By Pathophysiology**	**By Symptom**
Acute: Less than 6 weeks	Mechanical	Axial low back pain
Subacute: 6 weeks to 3 months	Systemic medical (nonmechanical)	Radicular pain
Chronic: More than 3 months, with symptoms more than half the days in the last 6 months		

stronger predictors of long-term disability than any anatomic findings on imaging.

The total cost of low back pain in the Unites States exceeds $100 billion annually and is expected to rise with the ageing population.[7] In addition to the financial burden, chronic low back pain can have a significant impact on quality of life, with 60% of patients reporting inability to perform daily activities and 25% being unable to work.[7] Given the significant socioeconomic burden of chronic low back pain, it becomes pertinent to understand the natural course of low back pain and risk factors for developing chronic pain to help direct diagnostic and treatment decisions.

PATHOPHYSIOLOGY

The lumbar spine consists of five lumbar vertebrae that increase in size caudally. Each vertebral body is separated by shock-absorbing intervertebral disks, consisting of a gelatinous nucleus pulposus surrounded by the fibrous rings of the anulus fibrosus. The nucleus pulposus consists of water, proteoglycans, and collagen; it is 90% water at birth and desiccates with time as part of the degenerative cascade. The neural arch is formed laterally by the pedicles, which connect the posterior elements to the vertebral bodies, and encloses the central canal where the spinal cord and cauda equina reside. The posterior elements consist of the laminae, spinous processes, and articular processes that form the facet joints. The space between adjacent pedicles forms the foramen through which spinal nerve roots may enter and exit the spinal canal. In addition, there are ligamentous structures supporting the lumbar spine. Pain can arise from the innervated intervertebral disks, facet joints, ligaments, or spinal nerve roots.

The lumbar spine is supported by various muscles that help provide dynamic stabilization to the spine and pelvis. Posteriorly, the paraspinal muscles consist of the erector spinae, multifidi, psoas, and quadratus lumborum. Anteriorly, the abdominal musculature, including the transversus abdominis, plays a critical role in supporting the lumbar spine. There is evidence to support that the structure and function of these spinal stabilizers are altered in patients with low back pain. In addition, these muscles can be a potential source of myofascial low back pain.

Low back pain has been classified based on pathophysiology as either mechanical or the result of a systemic medical illness. Medical causes of low back pain include inflammatory, infectious, neoplastic, and visceral sources. Systemic medical causes of low back pain are rare but frequently associated with the need for time-sensitive treatment. If no primary systemic source is identified, the pain is classified as mechanical pain. Mechanical causes of low back pain include direct injury, deformity, imbalance, or overuse of identifiable structures in the lumbar spine, but are most commonly degenerative in nature. Structural sources of mechanical low back pain include the intervertebral disks, facet joints, vertebral bodies, nerves and nerve roots, ligamentous structures, paraspinal muscles, and sacroiliac joints. For example, wear and tear of the spine with aging can lead to intervertebral disk degeneration and herniation, facet and uncovertebral arthritis, osteophyte formation, ligamentous and capsular hypertrophy, and spondylolisthesis at various rates, which can be sources of pain independently or can lead to nerve root compression with resulting pain. When nerve root injury is contributing to low back pain, it can produce symptoms radiating down the leg including pain,

weakness, paresthesias, and altered reflexes in a specific dermatomal or myotomal distribution, termed radiculopathy. Radiculopathy is reported in approximately 7% of patients with low back pain.[2]

Radicular pain is commonly attributed to direct compression of the spinal nerve roots with resulting structural, biochemical, and vascular changes in and around the spinal nerve. In addition, mechanical stimulation of the lumbar spinal nerve roots has been shown to increase the production of the pain-generating neuropeptide substance P.[8] Studies have shown that disk herniations and tears in the anulus fibrosus can produce increased inflammatory mediators, such as phospholipase A_2, cyclooxygenase 2, nitric oxide, cytokines, interleukins, and immunoglobulins, which can lead to local swelling and swelling of the spinal nerve roots.[8]

Pain can be further classified as nociceptive or neuropathic. Nociceptive pain is associated with tissue damage. Neuropathic pain is associated with minimal or no tissue damage and is more related to a dysfunction of the pain regulatory function of the central and peripheral nervous system. Why damage to specific anatomic locations produces severe pain in some but no pain in others is quite complicated and not fully understood but relates to numerous factors including local inflammation, biomechanical factors, muscular strength and flexibility deficiencies and imbalances, and centrally mediated pain regulatory systems that are influenced by mood, sleep, cardiovascular health, and psychosocial context.

CLINICAL PRESENTATION AND PHYSICAL EXAMINATION

Symptomatically, mechanical lumbar spine disorders can be classified as axial or radicular pain. Axial low back pain is typically isolated to the back at the lumbar spine or lumbosacral junction with varying degrees of gluteal symptoms. New, acute low back pain typically is axial pain only but can be severe, disrupting sleep, work, and activities of daily living. It is often exacerbated by prolonged sitting, standing, leaning, or bending and is mitigated by frequent positional shifts. Extension typically worsens pain mediated from the posterior elements, whereas flexion typically worsens pain mediated from anterior elements. The seated position, forward flexion, and Valsalva maneuver can increase intradiscal pressure, worsening disk-mediated low back pain. Facet loading may worsen facet-mediated pain.

Patients with the syndrome of lumbar radiculopathy will often have leg and thigh pain greater than low back pain. Pain can be severe even in the absence of neurologic deficit. Neurologic symptoms of numbness, tingling, weakness, reflex changes, and root tension signs may be seen on examination. Symptoms are exacerbated by prolonged sitting, coughing, sneezing, Valsalva maneuver, and bending. Pain is often mitigated by frequent positional shifts and walking. Pain radiating past the knee and into the calf or foot is typically radicular and represents nerve root or peripheral nerve injury. However, pain in the buttocks and thigh is not always radicular and can come from anatomic locations outside of the spine. It can be referred from adjacent bone, ligament, or muscle structures, making it important to evaluate the hip, pelvis, and surrounding musculature to rule out any other contributing pathology before attributing this type of pain to the lumbar spine.

Other specific causes of low back pain have a more identifiable presentation. Patients with lumbar spinal stenosis, narrowing of the spinal canal with or without compression of the spinal cord, typically have back pain and neurogenic claudication. Patients often describe their legs as feeling heavy or wooden. Neurogenic claudication is defined as thigh and calf pain worsened by standing or walking and alleviated with sitting. This can be differentiated from vascular claudication in that patients with vascular claudication may have altered peripheral pulses, more difficulty with uphill walking, no symptoms with standing alone, and a steady degree of symptomatic severity from day to day. In contrast, patients with neurogenic claudication have significant day-to-day variability, and symptoms with standing still. Walking with a shopping cart is often better tolerated in neurogenic claudication because the patient is flexed forward, thus expanding the spinal canal diameter. Neurologic changes are usually subtler, with vibratory loss in the distal lower extremities, increased pain with lumbar extension, absent root tension signs, mild balance deficits, and largely normal strength on examination.

In conus medullaris and cauda equina syndromes, saddle anesthesia, urinary retention or incontinence, lower extremity weakness, and recent-onset erectile dysfunction can be seen. Cauda equina syndrome involves compression of multiple lumbosacral nerve roots below the termination of the spinal cord, called the cauda equina, leading to the aforementioned symptoms and hyporeflexia in the lower extremities. This syndrome can be caused by several conditions, including trauma, tumors, spondylolisthesis, and direct compression secondary to severe spinal stenosis or a large disk herniation. It is a very rare but serious neurologic condition, and urgent surgical referral is recommended.

Other conditions to consider are the seronegative spondyloarthropathies, spinal tumors, vertebral fractures, and spinal infections. Seronegative spondylarthropathies (see Chapter 193) typically are seen in younger patients with symptoms of pain, stiffness, and reduced range of movement in the morning that improves with activity. Family history and additional joint symptoms should be explored. Tumors of the spine may occur in patients with prior history of malignant disease; localized pain is frequently reported to increase in the supine position and at night. Although classically taught "red flags" for tumor include age older than 50, weight loss, and failure to improve after 1 month, there is low diagnostic accuracy for any of these factors independently.[9] In patients with recent spinal surgery, recent skin or urine infections, history of intravenous drug abuse, or immunocompromised states, infection should be considered. Although fever is commonly cited as a red flag for spinal infection, this finding has low sensitivity and lack of fever does not rule out infection. Vertebral fracture should be considered in the differential if there is a history of significant trauma, older age, or corticosteroid use.[10] Among all primary care patients with low back pain, fewer than 5% have a serious systemic pathology. However, given the important clinical implications, it is paramount to screen for these diagnoses.

The physical examination starts with careful observation of the patient; the examiner looks for discomfort or frequent change of positions and evaluates the patient's affect. Spinal examination then begins with observation of the lumbar spine, looking for any asymmetries or abnormal curvature. Palpation and percussion of the spinous processes should be performed to evaluate for osseous pain and spinal infection. The range of motion of the lumbar spine should be assessed in flexion, extension, lateral flexion, and rotation to evaluate for changes in symptoms throughout the movements. The normal range of motion of the lumbar spine is 40 to 60 degrees of forward flexion, 20 to 35 degrees of extension, 15 to 20 degrees of lateral flexion, and 3 to 18 degrees of rotation. Pain with movement in specific directions should be noted. As previously explained, anterior sources of pain tend to worsen with forward flexion and posterior sources of pain tend to worsen with extension. Although limitations in range of motion may not permit identification of the specific source of pain, assessment of range of motion can provide an index for future comparison to assess therapeutic response. Facet loading can be performed by placing the patient in hyperextension with a slight rotation toward each side to help identify facet-mediated pain.

Anatomic alignment during neutral standing should be noted. Romberg testing should be performed to test balance. Gait should be examined to look for antalgia, footdrop, spastic or mechanical movement, Trendelenburg gait, and widened or narrowed steps. The skin and lower extremity pulses should be examined to look for vascular insufficiency as a potential cause of thigh or calf symptoms. In addition, if patients are describing symptoms of cauda equina syndrome, rectal examination should be considered to evaluate for loss of rectal tone.

Neurologic examination should be undertaken, assessing the symmetry of the patient's strength in hip flexion, knee extension, knee flexion, ankle dorsiflexion, ankle plantar flexion, foot eversion, great toe extension, and hip abduction bilaterally. In addition, the patient should be observed walking on heels and toes to assess for functional strength in L5 and S1, respectively. It may be difficult for the examiner to overcome the quadriceps, even if there is some weakness. The examiner should have the patient perform single-legged, sit-to-stand testing bilaterally, with examiner support for balance, to pick up mild quadriceps weakness. Because plantar flexion weakness may be difficult to detect, it is recommended to test the S1 myotome with repeated standing calf raises on each leg to elicit any mild weakness or muscular atrophy. Sensation to both light touch and pinprick should be checked for sensory deficits throughout the dermatomes listed in Table 160.2. Studies have shown that sensory tests, specifically soft touch and superficial pain, demonstrate low sensitivity and high specificity for lumbosacral radiculopathy and thus are most useful to rule in this diagnosis.[11] Bilateral reflexes should also be elicited at the patella (L4 nerve root), and Achilles (S1 nerve root). Deep tendon reflex testing has moderate sensitivity and moderate to high specificity in the diagnosis of lumbosacral radiculopathy.[11] Babinski examination and evaluation for clonus, muscle spasticity, or increased tone can help assess for upper motor neuron involvement. Because disk herniations are most common at L4 to L5 and L5 to S1, clinical changes in these myotomes and dermatomes should be thoroughly assessed.

If the patient's symptoms are radicular in nature, root tension signs can help identify irritation of the lumbar nerve roots. The straight leg raise test is performed to assess for damage to L5 to S1. With the patient in the supine position, the examiner raises the straight leg to approximately 70 to 90 degrees of hip flexion. If the patient's typical pain or paresthesias are reproduced at any point when the leg is in 20 to 70 degrees of hip flexion, the test result is positive and indicates that a nerve root impingement from a herniated disk is likely contributing, referred to as sciatica. Studies have reported a high sensitivity but low specificity of the straight leg raise.[12] If the unaffected leg is tested and symptoms are reproduced in

TABLE 160.2   Lumbar Dermatomes

Root	Muscle Group Affected	Dermatome	Reflexes	Special Maneuvers
L1	None	Back, groin	None	None
L2	Hip flexors, hip adductors	Anterolateral upper thigh	None	Femoral stretch
L3	Hip flexors, quadriceps, hip adductors	Anterior lower thigh, medial knee	± Patellar	Femoral stretch
L4	Quadriceps, ankle dorsiflexors	Medial lower leg	Patellar	Femoral stretch
L5	Extensor hallucis, ankle dorsiflexors, hamstrings, hip abductors, peroneals	Lateral lower leg, dorsal medial three toes	Medial hamstring	Straight leg raise
S1	Ankle plantar flexors, gluteals, hamstrings, peroneals	Posterior thigh, lateral toes, sole of foot	Achilles	Straight leg raise

the symptomatic leg, this is called a positive crossed straight leg raise and has increased specificity for disk herniation.[12] A modification to the straight leg raise can be performed in the seated position and is referred to as the seated slump test. The patient is asked to slump forward, allowing the thoracic and lumbar spine to collapse into flexion, and then to fully flex the cervical spine toward the chest. The patient is then asked to extend each leg fully and dorsiflex the ankle to see if there is reproduction of symptoms down the leg.[13] Another root tension sign, the femoral nerve stretch test, is used to look for an upper lumbar radiculopathy in L2 to L4 distribution. With the patient in the prone position, the leg is flexed at the knee and the hip is brought into extension. The test result is considered positive if a reproduction of typical pain in the anterior thigh occurs.

DIAGNOSTICS

The most recent guidelines from the American Academy of Family Physicians, American College of Physicians (ACP), and American Pain Society do not recommend routine imaging for patients with acute or nonspecific low back pain, because this does not improve clinical outcomes and exposes patients to unnecessary radiation.[14,15] A systematic review and meta-analysis of six trials comparing immediate imaging with usual care for patients with acute and subacute low back pain, without suspicion for infection or malignancy, found no significant difference in short- or long-term outcomes for pain or function.[16] A recent observational study evaluating older adults, often labeled as a high risk group, similarly demonstrated that even in this population, otherwise low-risk patients who underwent early imaging had no difference in pain or self-reported disability at 1 year and had higher rates of clinical interventions[17] However, if a patient has certain red-flag symptoms, described earlier, or if clinical improvement has not occurred in 4 to 6 weeks, plain radiographs of the lumbar spine are the preferred initial diagnostic tool.[14] Typically, anterior-posterior and lateral views are sufficient. Oblique views can also be obtained to visualize the pars interarticularis but are not routinely recommended. Because plain radiographs have low sensitivity and specificity,[15] their diagnostic yield is limited; persistent pain or suspicious symptoms may prompt additional imaging.

The most widely used imaging modality to further evaluate low back pain and radiculopathy is magnetic resonance imaging (MRI). Its principal use is to evaluate the bone structures and soft tissues, and it can be helpful to look for degenerative disk disease, disk herniations, spinal stenosis, and cord

or root compression. With the addition of gadolinium, it can be used to look for tumor or infection and can distinguish epidural scar tissue in postoperative patients. MRI, however, is an expensive diagnostic tool. Guidelines recommend MRI acutely only if patients have severe or progressive neurologic deficits or symptoms of a serious underlying condition.[14] MRI can also be considered for a patient with persistent low back pain with symptoms of nerve root impingement refractory to conservative treatment, for which interventional procedures are being considered. Although it is superior for identification of potential pain generators in the spine, MRI abnormalities do not always correlate with clinical complaints, and multiple studies have found common pain-producing degenerative findings in asymptomatic patients,[18] including one study finding disc degeneration and bulging discs in over 50% of asymptomatic adults over the age of 40 and in 70% of adults in their 60s.[19] In cases where radiographic findings are consistent with clinical presentation, the magnitude of radiographic findings does not correlate with symptom severity or clinical outcome, and symptom improvement does not correlate with resolution of radiographic defects.[20] For this reason, physicians should focus on clinical presentation rather than radiographic abnormalities. Contraindications to MRI include pacemaker, retained metal fragments such as from a gunshot wound, and severe claustrophobia. Most currently used orthopedic metal does not preclude MRI imaging.

Other diagnostic tools used for low back pain are radionuclide bone scintigraphy and computed tomography (CT). Bone scintigraphy is helpful if the history and physical examination raise suspicion for osteomyelitis, bone neoplasm, or occult fracture. The addition of bone scan with single-photon emission computed tomography (SPECT) can identify recent pars fracture and facet osteoarthritis. CT can be helpful in assessing the bone architecture of the spine and can also provide helpful imaging in a postsurgical patient with excessive hardware or in those with contraindications to MRI. CT imaging can be used to assess for degenerative disorders such as spondylosis, spondylolysis, spondylolisthesis, and spinal stenosis as well as to show cortical irregularities in osteoarthritis. It can be used in combination with myelography to visualize the borders and contents of the dural sac and to evaluate for cord compression.

Other diagnostic workup may be considered on a case-by-case basis. Laboratory testing, such as erythrocyte sedimentation rate and C-reactive protein, can be helpful in a patient with constitutional symptoms to quantify systemic inflammation, as can be seen with infection, inflammatory spondyloarthropathies, or neoplasm. Neoplasm may also be associated with an abnormal complete blood count, alkaline phosphatase, or calcium level. Electrodiagnostic studies can be helpful in assessing neurologic changes associated with denervation caused by subacute and chronic radiculopathy. Electromyography may not be able to detect acute changes until approximately 3 to 4 weeks after the initial insult. The needle electromyographic portion of the examination can identify radiculopathy with high specificity; however, it is relatively insensitive to the clinical syndrome of radicular pain without motor or reflex changes.

The goal of diagnostic testing is to help guide management strategies and improve patient outcomes. Unless there is clear indication that testing can aid in this process, routine testing is not recommended, especially in a population with low clinical suspicion, because this can lead to false positives, unnecessary medical expenses, and avoidable patient anxiety. Many patients have come to expect imaging, so it is important for the clinician to educate the patient and provide reassurance. Imaging for reassurance has not been shown to improve outcomes.

DIFFERENTIAL DIAGNOSIS

 Priority differential diagnoses include spinal cord compression, fracture, inflammatory disease, neoplasm, infection, and other medical causes of low back pain requiring intervention.

However, low back pain is usually mechanical pain and attributed to degenerative changes. Although this degenerative process is a common progression with aging and typically benign, it may cause compression or irritation of the spinal nerve roots or the spinal cord, leading to radiculopathy and myelopathy.

Other conditions that can mimic lumbar spine degenerative disorders include diabetic amyotrophy (plexopathy/polyradiculopathy), vascular claudication, sacroiliitis and associated seronegative spondyloarthropathy, shingles with or without rash, pancreatitis, intra-abdominal or gynecologic pathology, renal colic, Lyme radiculopathy, epidural abscess or osteomyelitis, osteoporotic or malignant fractures, and malignant disease involving the spine and spinal canal. In addition, surrounding muscles and ligaments can be a source of pain, and adjacent bones or joints can elicit pain in similar distributions and should be considered in the differential diagnosis.

INTERPROFESSIONAL COLLABORATIVE MANAGEMENT

The primary goal of treatment is to identify and treat any serious or systemic causes of low back pain early. If no serious or concerning source of pain is identified, the goal is to minimize pain and functional limitation and prevent chronic, disabling low back pain.

 Immediate emergency department referral is indicated for significant neurologic compromise or cauda equina syndrome for consideration of surgical decompression.

 Specialist referral is indicated for refractory back or radicular symptoms, neurologic weakness, consideration of interventional procedure, or diagnostic dilemma.

 Multidisciplinary pain management center referral should be considered for patients with chronic, refractory, debilitating low back pain without surgical indications

Nonpharmacologic Management

Physical Therapy Management of Low Back Pain. The physical therapy management of low back pain is most effective when a multimodal treatment approach with a combination of therapeutic exercise, manual therapy, modalities, and patient education is used. Early entry into a physical therapy program, within the first 6 weeks of symptom onset, has been shown to reduce risk of progression of psychosocial features associated with low back pain such as depression, somatic distress, and anxiety.[21] In addition, primary care referral of patients with low back pain to physical therapy performed within 14 days of onset was associated with decreased disability but not with decreased utilization of other health care resources.[22] Ultimately, the sooner the referral is made and physical therapy is initiated, the better the chance for a positive outcome. Once a referral to physical therapy is deemed appropriate, the physician should write a prescription noting the diagnosis, stating "evaluate and treat" with any specific treatment recommendations, a suggestion of the estimated frequency and duration of treatment, and relevant precautions. For most acute initial spine conditions, a typical frequency and duration is one to three visits per week for 4 to 8 weeks. Chronic spinal conditions may require more than 8 weeks for rehabilitation, depending on the diagnosis, comorbidities, and personal factors.

Therapeutic Exercise. Although there is limited evidence to support the use of exercise therapy in acute low back pain, exercise therapy has been shown to be beneficial to patients with subacute and chronic low back pain, providing both short-term pain relief and longer-lasting functional improvement.[23,24,25-26] Therapeutic exercise interventions used in physical therapy include range-of-motion and stretching exercises, core stabilization and motor control exercises, strengthening, and general conditioning. Range-of-motion exercises are typically prescribed with a directional bias, such as flexion, extension, side-glide, or rotation, based on the patient's response during the examination, called mechanical diagnosis therapy. Specific lumbar spine diagnoses tend to result in directional preferences. For example, spinal stenosis tends to respond better to a flexion-based program, whereas disk herniation with accompanying radiculopathy tends to respond more favorably to extension-based programs. Individualized exercises prescribed to match the directional preference have been shown to decrease patients' pain and reduce medication use.[26]

Another type of exercise is nerve mobilization procedures or nerve gliding. This technique is used for those with radiating lower extremity pain, such as patients with lumbar radiculopathy or spinal stenosis. Although there is minimal evidence to support lower extremity nerve gliding, it has been shown to decrease pain and disability in patients with subacute and chronic low back pain.[26,27]

Core strengthening includes strengthening of the abdominal, gluteal, hip girdle, and paraspinal musculature to promote lumbar stability by providing dynamic support and are superior to minimal intervention alone.[27] Lumbar core stabilization instruction can be individualized according to the patient's directional preference, with emphasis on appropriate recruitment patterns of the deep core spinal stabilizers, because these muscles have demonstrated altered recruitment patterns in patients with low back pain.[26,28] Rehabilitative ultrasound imaging is useful in assisting with assessment of aberrant motor recruitment patterns and in providing biofeedback for neuromuscular reeducation of the deep lumbo-pelvic muscles, including the transversus abdominis, the internal and external obliques, and the multifidi.[28] Stretching of the hamstrings, hip flexors, piriformis, and gastrocnemius and soleus muscles along with other muscle tissues found to be tight may also be beneficial in relieving local myofascial symptoms.

Conditioning, such as cardiovascular fitness, is also an important component in the rehabilitation of the spine; studies suggest that people who are physically fit experience low back pain less frequently than do people who are not physically fit.[29] Both graded activity and exposure, aerobic activity and cognitive-behavioral strategies that promote a gradual increase in daily activity, have been proven to be effective treatment method for patients with low back pain.[30] Aerobic conditioning is also an important part of the treatment of chronic pain conditions such as fibromyalgia, which can be a comorbidity in patients with low back pain.

Manual Therapy. Manual therapy for the lumbar spine can include but is not limited to spinal manipulative therapy (SMT), spinal mobilization, and myofascial release. SMT is defined as the application of high-velocity, low-amplitude manual thrust to the spinal joints just beyond the joint range of motion. When manipulation is contraindicated, spinal mobilization techniques can be used to restore joint mobility to hypomobile joints. Spinal mobilization is the application of manual force to the spinal joints within the passive joint's physiologic range of motion without a thrust. Although individualized randomized controlled trials have shown variable results, two recent Cochrane reviews found that spinal manipulation was more effective than sham and comparable to other modalities for acute and chronic low back pain.[31,32] interest and access. Contraindications to manipulation include direct trauma, unexplained weight loss, history of cancer, spinal fracture, unrelenting night pain, osteoporosis, severe spinal stenosis, cauda equina syndrome, and neurologic deficits with limb weakness.

Therapeutic Modalities. Modalities frequently used in physical therapy include the following:
- *Ice.* Patients are instructed to ice for 10 to 15 minutes several times a day for acute episodes of low back pain to help reduce edema, though research has produced insufficient data to show its benefit. Contraindications include cold sensitivity, Reynaud phenomenon, open wounds, and impaired sensation.
- *Superficial heat.* Heat is commonly applied during therapy, to help promote circulation to the area and possibly hasten healing, but also as a method to manage pain. Contraindications include malignant disease, active bleeding into a joint or muscle tissue, anesthesia or impaired sensation, and impaired mentation.
- *Ultrasound to treat tendon, ligament, and joint injuries.* Ultrasound, a form of deep heat, can be useful in treating muscle spasms, tendinopathy, or degenerative arthritis. Contraindications include malignant disease, laminectomy sites, fluid-containing cavities, unhealed joint fractures, and joint arthroplasty containing methylmethacrylate or high-density polyethylene.
- *Transcutaneous electrical nerve stimulation (TENS) for analgesia.* Contraindications to electrical stimulation include cardiac pacemakers and defibrillators, areas with metal close to the skin, anesthetic areas, incompletely healed wounds, and areas near the eyes, carotid sinus, or mucous membranes.

- *Traction.* Traction has been classically used for patients with radicular symptoms to help resolve neurologic deficits and reduce pain. Studies addressing the efficacy of traction have been largely inconclusive. A recent systematic review found that traction provided no benefit in the short or long term for patients with low back pain with or without sciatica.[33]
- Research on these modalities has provided inconsistent results regarding their benefit when compared with placebo, and there are insufficient data to recommend these strategies based on the current evidence. However, because these modalities have low risk, a trial may be warranted in specific cases if not contraindicated.

Pharmacologic Management

Based on recommendations from the ACP, nonpharmacologic therapy is considered first line in acute and subacute low back pain as most symptoms improve over time regardless of treatment.[34] Chronic low back pain treatment should also initially be treated with nonpharmacologic approach. However, medications can be a helpful strategy for pain management for patients with an inadequate response to nonpharmacologic treatment. A trial of nonsteroidal antiinflammatory drugs (NSAIDs) is the recommended first-line treatment for acute low back pain and acute exacerbations of subacute or chronic low back pain by the ACP, if the patient has no contraindications.[34] Clinical trials have shown variable results with limited benefit from these medications and patients should be monitored for adverse effects. Additional medications can be used for short-term pain management if the pain is severe, including muscle relaxants. Centrally acting skeletal muscle relaxants, such as cyclobenzaprine, can be used to help reduce back spasms associated with mechanical low back pain and have been found to be more effective than placebo for short-term relief of acute low back pain. Side effects, particularly sedation, can be limiting. In terms of combination therapy, a recent randomized control trial evaluating patients with acute low back pain found that the addition of a muscle relaxant or oxycodone/acetaminophen to NSAID alone did not improve pain or functional outcomes at 1 week follow-up though evidence remains lacking.[35] There is insufficient evidence to determine whether muscle relaxants are beneficial in subacute or chronic back pain management.

Although opioid analgesics are commonly prescribed, there are limited data to support their use for acute low back pain. Because of this, prescription becomes a matter of clinical judgment. If prescribed, their use should be restricted to the short term and patients monitored closely for adverse effects or signs of abuse. A 2013 systematic review found that opioids, compared with placebo, had short-term efficacy for pain relief and functional improvement in chronic low back pain, though evidence was very low to moderate quality. Trials comparing opioids with NSAIDs or antidepressants found no significant difference between groups, and there were no trials evaluating the long-term use of opioids.[36,37] This suggests that opioids may be beneficial for short-term use in selected patients with acute exacerbations, however, other pharmacologic therapy may be just as effective without the harms associated with opioid use. In addition, there is no evidence to support the use of opioids for long-term treatment of chronic low back pain.[37] If the clinician decides to start opioid therapy, treatment should be combined with nonpharmacologic therapy and nonopioid pharmacologic therapy, as appropriate based on Centers for Disease

Control and Prevention (CDC) guidelines.[38] New guidelines from the CDC also recommends that clinicians discuss realistic benefits of opioid therapy and known risks of opioid use with the patient. Risks of opioid use include dose-dependent risk of nonfatal and fatal overdose,[39,40] cardiovascular events,[41] endocrine pathology,[42,43] and road trauma (motor vehicle accidents).[44] If starting an opioid, clinicians should follow CDC recommendations and prescribe immediate-release opioids instead of extended-release/long-acting opioids; the lowest effective dose should be used; no greater quantity than needed for expected duration of severe pain should be prescribed— often 3 days or less and rarely more than 7 days.[38] Clinicians should also review a patient's history of controlled substance prescriptions using the state prescription drug monitoring program prior to prescribing an opioid and can consider urine drug testing prior to initiating treatment. Tramadol, a medication that acts on the opioid receptor, has shown no significant to only modest effects on acute pain in low quality trials.[45,46] Though tramadol was originally labeled a noncontrolled analgesic, it was quickly relabeled as a controlled substance due to risk of abuse and adverse events similar to other opioids. It is also associated with increased risk of serotonin syndrome.

Other medications used for the management of chronic low back pain include tricyclic antidepressants and mixed norepinephrine-serotonin reuptake inhibitors. Duloxetine has been showed to reduce pain in patients with chronic low back and radicular pain.[47] Although studies to support these medications have shown small and variable benefits, many patients with chronic low back pain have undiagnosed depression and may benefit from a trial of these medications if not responding to other treatment options. The clinician must monitor for medication side effects, particularly anticholinergic effects. Gabapentin has been shown to be beneficial for treatment of central pain syndrome as well as radiculopathy. Used anecdotally by many practitioners, systemic corticosteroids have not been shown to be more effective than placebo for treatment of low back pain with or without leg symptoms and are not recommended.[34] Benzodiazepines have shown no difference in function and a lower likelihood of pain improvement at 1 week when compared with placebo therefore are not recommended.[34]

COMPLEMENTARY AND ALTERNATIVE MANAGEMENT

Complementary and alternative treatments of subacute and chronic low back pain have also been shown to be useful for some patients. Acupuncture or dry needling, chiropractic manipulation, and massage therapy are alternative therapies with limited side effects and research to suggest they may be more beneficial than placebo treatments for short-term pain relief. However, few of these therapies have been shown to be effective in the long term for chronic low back pain.[14] In addition, studies have shown that patient expectations of benefits may play a role in perceived benefits, particularly with regard to acupuncture, so patient selection should be considered. More recently, glucosamine has been tested for management of low back pain with no evidence of benefit.

Psychological Health

Because psychosocial issues are a known risk factor for chronic low back pain, modification of maladaptive pain behaviors and cognitive processes associated with pain perception through use of behavioral therapy has been studied as a treatment adjunctive for chronic back pain. A 2010 Cochrane review found moderate-quality evidence supporting the benefit of behavioral treatment compared with standard care in the short term.[48] More recent studies have shown the benefit of a multidisciplinary approach incorporating cognitive behavioral therapy or mindfulness-based stress reduction with traditional exercise programs, with regard to patient-rated pain, disability, and fear-avoidance behavior, as well as overall quality of life, in both the short and long term.[49,50] In addition, these studies have shown this approach to be a cost-effective management option.

Spinal Interventional Procedures

Another consideration for treatment of subacute and chronic low back pain is lumbar epidural corticosteroid injection. This typically requires referral to an interventional spine physician. Indications for epidural injections supported by the literature are symptoms of radiculopathy and spinal stenosis.[8] Although randomized trial results are varied, research suggests that these injections offer short-term symptom relief for patients with sciatica and both short and long-term symptom relief for patients with spinal stenosis.[51] Further studies are needed to assess the efficacy of epidural injections for axial low back pain. Injections can also be performed into the facet joints or the nerves innervating the joint, with subsequent radiofrequency ablation of these nerves if beneficial, for symptomatic relief of facet-mediated pain. Trigger point injections performed into the muscles in the area of pain can also help in the short term and are of low risk when dry needling or injection of anesthetic without corticosteroid is performed. Studies on these later options have shown varied results and are ongoing. Other alternatives, such as prolotherapy, oxygen-ozone injections, Botox injections, and tumor necrosis factor-α injections, are currently being researched and have uncertain efficacy at this time.

Referral to an orthopedic spine surgeon or neurosurgeon should be made for a patient with progressive weakness or neurologic deficits for consideration of surgical decompression, if deemed appropriate by the surgeon. If the patient has symptoms of radiculopathy or spinal stenosis, surgical referral may be indicated if the patient fails to respond to conservative management. Surgical care has been shown to be superior to conservative care for patients with herniated disk–related radicular symptoms, spinal stenosis with neurogenic claudication, and degenerative spondylolisthesis.[52,53]

COMPLICATIONS

Serious life-threatening complications of degenerative lumbar spine disorders are rare. If serious underlying conditions have not been discovered by thorough history, physical examination, and diagnostic workup, episodes of low back pain are typically self-limited. Special attention is warranted when significant neurologic weakness or cauda equina syndrome is occurring, and urgent referral to a spine surgeon is appropriate.

Substantial comorbid sequelae of chronic pain can occur. These include development of chronic pain syndrome and centrally mediated sensitization to pain, sleep disturbance, anxiety and depression because of chronic pain, disruption of activities of daily living, loss of work and wages, and disruption of interpersonal relationships.

LIFE SPAN CONSIDERATIONS

Once a patient has had an episode of low back pain, the chance of recurrence is high. That patient is then at increased risk for recurrent episodes throughout his or her life span. Maintaining ideal body weight and aerobic exercise may decrease frequency of flares. If the patient has a disk herniation and radicular symptoms, although this disk material will likely be reabsorbed with time, the disk is at risk of reherniation, and persistence of chronic axial low back pain is common.

Spondylolysis often occurs in an athletic child or teen and may lead to spondylolisthesis in the older adult. Neurologic compression or traction from spondylolisthesis can result in back and radicular pain. Patients with ankylosing spondylitis usually are seen in late adolescence or early 20s, and these patients frequently develop thoracic kyphosis and low back pain with aging.

Age is a strong factor for development of degenerative disk disease and spinal stenosis. Age- and medication-related osteoporosis (see Chapter 163) will increase the risk of vertebral compression fractures and resultant loss of height and development of kyphosis or scoliosis. One prospective study showed that 57% of asymptomatic patients over the age of 60 had abnormal MRIs, 36% with herniated disks and 21% with lumbar stenosis, despite their lack of symptoms. In fact, all but one patient had evidence of degeneration and bulging disks by the age of 60, supporting that spinal degeneration is a normal and expected change with age but can have variable clinical manifestations.[54]

PATIENT EDUCATION AND HEALTH PROMOTION

Patient education should start with reassurance and support. Explaining the natural history of mechanical low back pain and that most cases will resolve in a timely manner is critical. It is also important to educate the patient that pain may come and go, despite activity, and that recurrence is common after the first episode of low back pain. Because these episodes are not related to activity, activity avoidance should be discouraged. Exercise has been shown to help minimize recurrences and treat subacute and chronic low back pain, so regular daily activity should be advised. Maintenance of ideal body weight and proper body mechanics should be emphasized to help reduce the frequency of recurrence of episodes and improve pain tolerance. Encouraging frequent position shifting helps patients with many degenerative spinal issues. If a patient needs to return to a physically demanding job, a back school program may be helpful.

Risk factors for inflammation and disk degeneration, such as smoking and obesity, should be addressed. Treatment of underlying medical conditions such as osteoporosis should be considered, to lessen the risk of conditions such as compression fractures. In addition, if the patient has concomitant psychosocial factors, these should be addressed.

Patients need to understand red flags that would warrant urgent medical evaluation, including new limb weakness, change in bowel or bladder function, and constitutional signs. This will ensure that any dangerous systemic issues are addressed early and that the more urgent functional sequelae are treated on a timely basis, thereby avoiding permanent neurologic damage.

REFERENCES

1. Meucci, R. D., Fassa, A. G., & Faria, N. M. X. (2015). Prevalence of chronic low back pain: Systematic review. *Revista de Saude Publica, 49*, 1. doi:10.1590/S0034-8910.2015049005874.

2. Manusov, E. G. (2012). Evaluation and diagnosis of low back pain. *Primary Care, 39*(3), 471–479. doi:10.1016/j.pop.2012.06.003.

3. Manchikanti, L., Singh, V., Datta, S., Cohen, S. P., & Hirsch, J. A., American Society of Interventional Pain Physicians. (2009). Comprehensive review of epidemiology, scope, and impact of spinal pain. *Pain Physician, 12*(4), E35–E70. http://www.ncbi.nlm.nih.gov/pubmed/19668291. (Accessed 4 February 2018).

4. Gupta, N., Christiansen, C. S., Hallman, D. M., Korshøj, M., Carneiro, I. G., & Holtermann, A. (2015). Is objectively measured sitting time associated with low back pain? A cross-sectional investigation in the NOMAD study. *PLoS ONE, 10*(3), e0121159. doi:10.1371/journal.pone.0121159. Dorner TE, ed.

5. Macfarlane, G. J., Thomas, E., Papageorgiou, A. C., Croft, P. R., Jayson, M. I., & Silman, A. J. (1997). Employment and physical work activities as predictors of future low back pain. *Spine, 22*(10), 1143–1149. http://www.ncbi.nlm.nih.gov/pubmed/9160474. (Accessed 4 February 2018).

6. Manchekanti, L., Singh, V., Falco, F., et al. (2014). Epidemiology of low back pain in adults. *Neuromodulation, 17*(s2), 3–10.

7. Siddiqui, I., & Gerrard, P. (2014). Chronic low back pain: Implications for disability and dysfunction in the United States. In: Abstracts of scientific papers and posters presented at the annual meeting of the Association of Academic Physiatrists. *American Journal of Physical Medicine and Rehabilitation, 93*(a29), 3.

8. Friedrich, J. M., & Harrast, M. A. (2010). Lumbar epidural steroid injections. *Current Sports Medicine Reports, 9*(1), 43–49. doi:10.1249/JSR.0b013e3181caa7fc.

9. Henschke, N., Maher, C. G., Ostelo, R. W., de Vet, H. C., Macaskill, P., & Irwig, L. (2013). Red flags to screen for malignancy in patients with low-back pain. *The Cochrane Database of Systematic Reviews*, (2), CD008686, doi:10.1002/14651858.CD008686.pub2.

10. Williams, C. M., Henschke, N., Maher, C. G., et al. (2013). Red flags to screen for vertebral fracture in patients presenting with low-back pain. *The Cochrane Database of Systematic Reviews*, (1), CD008643, doi:10.1002/14651858.CD008643.pub2.

11. Tawa, N., Rhoda, A., & Diener, I. (2017). Accuracy of clinical neurological examination in diagnosing lumbo-sacral radiculopathy: A systematic literature review. *BMC Musculoskeletal Disorders, 18*(1), 93. doi:10.1186/s12891-016-1383-2.

12. Devillé, W. L., van der Windt, D. A., Dzaferagić, A., Bezemer, P. D., & Bouter, L. M. (2000). The test of Lasègue: Systematic review of the accuracy in diagnosing herniated discs. *Spine, 25*(9), 1140–1147. http://www.ncbi.nlm.nih.gov/pubmed/10788860. (Accessed 4 February 2018).

13. van der Windt, D. A., Simons, E., Riphagen, I. I., et al. (2010). Physical examination for lumbar radiculopathy due to disc herniation in patients with low-back pain. *The Cochrane Database of Systematic Reviews*, (2), CD007431, doi:10.1002/14651858.CD007431.pub2.

14. Maher, C., Underwood, M., & Buchbinder, R. (2017). Non-specific low back pain. *Lancet, 389*(10070), 736–747.

15. Qaseem, A., Wilt, T. J., McLean, R. M., & Forciea, M. A., for the Clinical Guidelines Committee of the American College of Physicians. (2017). Noninvasive treatments for acute, subacute, and chronic low back pain: A clinical practice guideline from the American College of Physicians. *Annals of Internal Medicine, 166*, 514–530. doi:10.7326/M16-2367. Epub ahead of print.

16. Jenkins, H. J., Downie, A. S., Maher, C. G., et al. (2018). Imaging for low back pain: Is clinical use consistent with guidelines? A systematic review and meta-analysis. *The Spine Journal, 18*(12), 2266–2277.

17. Jarvik, J. G., Gold, L. S., Comstock, B. A., et al. (2015). Association of early imaging for back pain with clinical outcomes in older adults. *JAMA: The Journal of the American Medical Association, 313*(11), 1143. doi:10.1001/jama.2015.1871.

18. Patel, N., Broderick, D., Burns, J., et al. (2016). ACR appropriateness criteria for low back pain. *Journal of the American College of Radiology: JACR, 13*(9), 1069–1078.

19. Brinjikji, W., Luetmer, P. H., Comstock, B., et al. (2015). Systematic literature review of imaging features of spinal degeneration in asymptomatic populations. *AJNR. American Journal of Neuroradiology, 36*(4), 811–816. doi:10.3174/ajnr.A4173.

20. el Barzouhi, A., Vleggeert-Lankamp, C. L. A. M., Lycklama à Nijeholt, G. J., et al. (2013). Magnetic resonance imaging in follow-up assessment of sciatica. *The New England Journal of Medicine, 368*(11), 999–1007. doi:10.1056/NEJMoa1209250.

21. Dahm, K. T., Brurberg, K. G., Jamtvedt, G., & Hagen, K. B. (2010). Advice to rest in bed versus advice to stay active for acute low-back pain and sciatica. *The Cochrane Database of Systematic Reviews*, (6), CD007612, doi:10.1002/14651858.CD007612.pub2. (Accessed 4 February 2018).

22. Fritz, J. M., Childs, J. D., Wainner, R. S., & Flynn, T. W. (2012). Primary care referral of patients with low back pain to physical therapy. *Spine*, *37*(25), 2114–2121. doi:10.1097/BRS.0b013e31825d32f5.

23. Fritz, J. M., Magel, J. S., McFaddon, M., et al. (2015). Early PT vs usual care in patients with recent onset low back pain. *JAMA: The Journal of the American Medical Association*, *314*(14), 1459–1467.

24. van Middelkoop, M., Rubinstein, S. M., Verhagen, A. P., Ostelo, R. W., Koes, B. W., & van Tulder, M. W. (2010). Exercise therapy for chronic nonspecific low-back pain. *Best Practice and Research. Clinical Rheumatology*, *24*(2), 193–204. doi:10.1016/j.berh.2010.01.002.

25. Rainville, J., Hartigan, C., Martinez, E., Limke, J., Jouve, C., & Finno, M. (2004). Exercise as a treatment for chronic low back pain. *The Spine Journal*, *4*(1), 106–115. http://www.ncbi.nlm.nih.gov/pubmed/14749199. (Accessed 4 February 2018).

26. Delitto, A., George, S. Z., Van Dillen, L., et al. (2012). Clinical guidelines low back pain. *The Journal of Orthopaedic and Sports Physical Therapy*, *42*(4), doi:10.2519/jospt.2012.0301.

27. Beattie, P. F. (2016). The lumbar spine: Physical therapy patient management using current evidence. In *Current concepts of orthopaedic physical therapy* (4th ed., pp. 1–46). Orthopaedic Section. APTA, Inc. doi:10.17832/isc.2016.26.2.8.

28. Ferreira, P. H., Ferreira, M. L., & Hodges, P. W. (2004). Changes in recruitment of the abdominal muscles in people with low back pain: Ultrasound measurement of muscle activity. *Spine*, *29*(22), 2560–2566. http://www.ncbi.nlm.nih.gov/pubmed/15543074. (Accessed 4 February 2018).

29. Rao, R., & Smuck, M. (Eds.), (2012). Therapeutic exercise for low back pain. In *Orthopedic knowledge update: Spine 4*. Rosemont, IL: American Academy of Orthopaedic Surgeons.

30. Macedo, L. G., Smeets, R. J. E. M., Maher, C. G., Latimer, J., & McAuley, J. H. (2010). Graded activity and graded exposure for persistent nonspecific low back pain: A systematic review. *Physical Therapy*, *90*(6), 860–879. doi:10.2522/ptj.20090303.

31. Menke, J. M. (2014). Do manual therapies help low back pain? A comparative effectiveness meta-analysis. *Spine*, *39*(7), E463–E472. doi:10.1097/BRS.0000000000000230.

32. Walker, B. F., French, S. D., Grant, W., & Green, S. (2010). Combined chiropractic interventions for low-back pain. *The Cochrane Database of Systematic Reviews*, (4), CD005427, doi:10.1002/14651858.CD005427.pub2.

33. Wegner, I., Widyahening, I. S., van Tulder, M. W., et al. (2013). Traction for low-back pain with or without sciatica. *The Cochrane Database of Systematic Reviews*, (8), CD003010, doi:10.1002/14651858.CD003010.pub5.

34. Foster, N. E., Anema, J. R., Cherkin, D., et al. (2018). Prevention and treatment of low back pain: Evidence, challenges, and promising directions. *The Lancet*, *391*(10137), 2368–2383.

35. Friedman, B. W., Dym, A. A., Davitt, M., et al. (2015). Naproxen with cyclobenzaprine, oxycodone/acetaminophen, or placebo for treating acute low back pain. *JAMA: The Journal of the American Medical Association*, *314*(15), 1572. doi:10.1001/jama.2015.13043.

36. Chaparro, L. E., Furlan, A. D., Deshpande, A., Mailis-Gagnon, A., Atlas, S., & Turk, D. C. (2013). Opioids compared to placebo or other treatments for chronic low-back pain. *The Cochrane Database of Systematic Reviews*, (8), CD004959, doi:10.1002/14651858.CD004959.pub4.

37. Krebs, E. E., Gravely, A., Nugent, S., et al. (2018). Effect of opioid vs nonopioid medications on pain-related function in patients with chronic back pain or hip or knee osteoarthritis pain. *JAMA: The Journal of the American Medical Association*, *319*(9), 872. doi:10.1001/jama.2018.0899.

38. Dowell, D., Haegerich, T. M., & Chou, R. (2016). CDC guideline for prescribing opioids for chronic pain—United States, 2016. *JAMA: The Journal of the American Medical Association*, *315*(15), 1624. doi:10.1001/jama.2016.1464.

39. Dunn, K. M., Saunders, K. W., Rutter, C. M., et al. (2010). Opioid prescriptions for chronic pain and overdose. *Annals of Internal Medicine*, *152*(2), 85. doi:10.7326/0003-4819-152-2-201001190-00006.

40. Ray, W., Chung, C., Murray, K., et al. (2016). Prescription of long acting opioids and mortality in patients with chronic, non cancer pain. *JAMA: The Journal of the American Medical Association*, *315*(22), 2415–2423.

41. Li, L., Setoguchi, S., Cabral, H., & Jick, S. (2013). Opioid use for noncancer pain and risk of myocardial infarction amongst adults. *Journal of Internal Medicine*, *273*(5), 511–526. doi:10.1111/joim.12035.

42. Deyo, R. A., Smith, D. H. M., Johnson, E. S., et al. (2013). Prescription opioids for back pain and use of medications for erectile dysfunction. *Spine*, *38*(11), 909–915. doi:10.1097/BRS.0b013e3182830482.

43. Rubinstein, A., & Carpenter, D. M. (2014). Elucidating risk factors for androgen deficiency associated with daily opioid use. *The American Journal of Medicine*, *127*(12), 1195–1201. doi:10.1016/j.amjmed.2014.07.015.

44. Gomes, T., Redelmeier, D. A., Juurlink, D. N., Dhalla, I. A., Camacho, X., & Mamdani, M. M. (2013). Opioid Dose and Risk of Road Trauma in Canada. *JAMA Internal Medicine*, *173*(3), 196. doi:10.1001/2013.jamainternmed.733.

45. Abdel Shaheed, C., Maher, C. G., Williams, K. A., Day, R., & McLachlan, A. J. (2016). Efficacy, tolerability, and dose-dependent effects of opioid analgesics for low back pain. *JAMA Internal Medicine*, *176*(7), 958. doi:10.1001/jamainternmed.2016.1251.

46. Schiphorst Preuper, H. R., Geertzen, J. H. B., van Wijhe, M., et al. (2014). Do analgesics improve functioning in patients with chronic low back pain? An explorative triple-blinded RCT. *European Spine Journal*, *23*(4), 800–806. doi:10.1007/s00586-014-3229-7.

47. Schukro, R. P., Oehmke, M. J., Geroldinger, A., Heinze, G., Kress, H.-G., & Pramhas, S. (2016). Efficacy of Duloxetine in Chronic Low Back Pain with a Neuropathic Component. *Anesthesiology*, *124*(1), 150–158. doi:10.1097/ALN.0000000000000902.

48. Lamb, S., Lall, R., Hansen, Z., et al. (2010). A multicentred randomised controlled trial of a primary care-based cognitive behavioural programme for low back pain. The Back Skills Training (BeST) trial. *Health Technology Assessment*, *14*(41), 1–253, iii–iv. doi:10.3310/hta14410.

49. Richmond, H., Hall, A. M., Copsey, B., et al. (2015). The effectiveness of cognitive behavioural treatment for non-specific low back pain: A systematic review and meta-analysis. *PLoS ONE*, *10*(8), e0134192. doi:10.1371/journal.pone.0134192. Bencharit S, ed.

50. Cherkin, D. C., Sherman, K. J., Balderson, B. H., et al. (2016). Effect of mindfulness-based stress reduction vs cognitive behavioral therapy or usual care on back pain and functional limitations in adults with chronic low back pain. *JAMA: The Journal of the American Medical Association*, *315*(12), 1240. doi:10.1001/jama.2016.2323.

51. Manchikanti, L., Benyamin, R. M., Falco, F. J. E., Kaye, A. D., & Hirsch, J. A. (2015). Do epidural injections provide short- and long-term relief for lumbar disc herniation? A systematic review. *Clinical Orthopaedics and Related Research*, *473*(6), 1940–1956. doi:10.1007/s11999-014-3490-4.

52. Manchikanti, L., Kaye, A. D., Manchikanti, K., Boswell, M., Pampati, V., & Hirsch, J. (2015). Efficacy of epidural injections in the treatment of lumbar central spinal stenosis; a systematic review. *Anesthesiology and Pain Medicine*, *5*(1), e23139. doi:10.5812/aapm.23139.

53. Lurie, J., Tostesan, T., Tostesan, A., et al. (2014). Surgical vs non-surgical treatment for lumbar disc herniation: Eight year results for the Spine Patient Outcomes Research Trial (SPORT). *Spine*, *39*(1), 3–16.

54. Boden, S. D., Davis, D. O., Dina, T. S., Patronas, N. J., & Wiesel, S. W. (1990). Abnormal magnetic-resonance scans of the lumbar spine in asymptomatic subjects. A prospective investigation. *The Journal of Bone and Joint Surgery. American Volume*, *72*(3), 403–408. http://www.ncbi.nlm.nih.gov/pubmed/2312537. (Accessed 4 February 2018).

CHAPTER **161**

HIP PAIN

Joanne Sandberg-Cook

 Orthopedic consultation is indicated for patients with suspected hip dislocation, fracture, sepsis, or end-stage degenerative joint disease

DEFINITION AND EPIDEMIOLOGY

Hip pain is a common complaint in primary care. It is a major source of discomfort and functional limitation, particularly in older patients, with a long list of potential causes.[1] It is helpful, therefore, to consider hip anatomy, patient age, and preceding history in teasing out the problem. An accurate diagnosis and appropriate management are important in reducing the burden for both the patient and the family.

Hip pain may be broadly defined as any sensation of pain immediately surrounding or within the pelvic girdle.

TABLE 161.1	Causes of Hip Pain and Age Groups Commonly Affected	
Age Group	**Traumatic Cause[a]**	**Nontraumatic Cause**
Adolescents and young adults	SCFE[b] Stress fracture Sprains, strains	SCFE Juvenile arthritis, infectious arthritis
Adults	Stress fracture Sprains, strains	Bursitis or tendinitis, infectious arthritis Neuropathy, fasciitis, rheumatoid arthritis, osteoarthritis, sacroiliac joint dysfunction, piriformis syndrome, femoroacetabular impingement syndrome
Older adults	Hip fracture Dislocation	Osteoarthritis, bursitis, tendinitis, neuropathy, fasciitis Spinal stenosis, sacroiliac joint dysfunction, piriformis syndrome

[a]Avascular necrosis should always be ruled out for hip pain caused by trauma.
[b]Slipped capital femoral epiphysis (SCFE) may occur with or without trauma.

Limitations in range of motion and gait are not uncommon, and activity or weight bearing frequently increases symptoms.

Because hip pain is a symptom and not a specific disease entity, there is no epidemiologic pattern that describes the prevalence and incidence. One study has estimated that 3-9% of adults over age 45 have symptomatic osteoarthritis of the hip,[2] but it is a symptom that affects all age groups, making the likely incidence much higher. Another review of young athletes indicated that 55% suffered from hip joint pain, with the most common cause being femoral acetabular impingement (FAI) and labral tears.[3] Major causes of hip pain differ across age groups and may be categorized as traumatic or nontraumatic (Table 161.1).

ANATOMY AND PATHOPHYSIOLOGY

A review of hip and pelvic anatomy is the key to understanding the potential source of pain. The hip, like the shoulder, is a diarthrodial ball-and-socket synovial joint. The ball and socket of the hip joint are made up of the head of the proximal femur and the acetabulum or socket of the pelvis.[4] The acetabulum is composed of the ischium, pubis, and ilium within the pelvis. A cartilaginous labral lip makes the socket of the acetabulum deeper for stability but maintains flexibility for greater range of hip motion. Strong fibrous, stabilizing ligaments form the capsule that covers the entire hip joint. Articular cartilage covers the bone ends. Completely lining the capsule and extending down to the neck of the femur is the synovial membrane; it secretes synovial fluid, which provides lubrication for motion. Fluid-filled sacs (or bursae), found in spaces among the tendons, ligaments, and bones, reduce friction over bone prominences and permit ease of motion.[4]

The primary functions of the hip are weight bearing and locomotion. The muscles of the hip are essential for maintaining upright stability and gait. The muscles of the hip may be classified into five functional groups according to their action: abductors, flexors, adductors, extensors, and rotators. Musculotendinous pain of the hip may contribute to distortions of gait, producing a limp.

Any one of these structures may become inflamed, stretched, torn, infected, or worn out, causing pain. Crystalline deposits within the joint or surrounding tissues may also cause tissue inflammation, destruction, and pain.[5] In growing children, changes, injury, or irritation at growth plates can also cause pain.[6,7] The underlying cause of the pain is the result of the actual pathophysiologic process.

Active individuals can stress the bone and supporting soft tissue. Muscle, tendon, or ligament strains and sprains are common in more active individuals. Labral tears also typically occur in active individuals. Very active individuals can develop stress fractures.

Bursitis (see Chapter 156) is an irritation and inflammation of the bursa, usually over bone prominences such as the greater trochanter. It is commonly diagnosed in individuals with lateral hip pain to palpation and on ambulation and at night.[5] Osteoarthritis (OA) (see Chapter 165) is a breakdown or degeneration of the cartilage within the joint, causing bone ends to rub.[8] Rheumatoid arthritis (RA) (see Chapter 197) is an inflammatory, autoimmune, destructive joint process that frequently affects multiple joints and causes synovitis, pain, and stiffness.[9] The joint involvement in RA is often symmetric; therefore both hips may be painful. Psoriatic arthritis (see Chapter 198) is more common in men than in women and should be considered in individuals diagnosed with psoriasis. Gout and pseudogout (see Chapter 158) leave crystalline deposits within the joint, leading to joint inflammation, acute-onset pain, and eventual cartilage destruction.

Avascular necrosis is loss of blood supply and subsequent death of subchondral bone tissue; it can be related to trauma, alcohol intoxication, sickle cell anemia, or corticosteroid use.[10] Protease inhibitors, RA, or systemic lupus erythematosus (see Chapter 199) can also be causative. Avascular necrosis can occur in a number of sites in the body, including the femoral head, and can be bilateral. The cartilage remains intact; however, the bone beneath it becomes flattened and misshapen.[10]

Fractures and hip dislocations in younger to middle-aged people are most often associated with significant trauma, such as motor vehicle accidents, athletic injuries, or significant falls. They may be followed in primary care once they are stabilized. Low-impact trauma should not produce a significant fracture in young healthy adults. Fragility fractures at any age should prompt further bone density testing and endocrinology evaluation, including looking for secondary causes of osteopenia or osteoporosis (see Chapter 163), such as vitamin D deficiency, hyperparathyroidism (see Chapter 193), anorexia nervosa, female athlete triad, or other reversible causes of brittle bones.[11] Hip dislocations should be considered if there is a history of hip replacement surgery or congenital hip dislocation.

Infection (see Chapter 159) is uncommon but can be a devastating cause of rapid-onset hip pain and fever. It can become indolent and recurrent, particularly with more virulent microbes. Recent dental work, skin infection, endocarditis, IV drug use and intestinal procedures are frequent sources, particularly if a prosthesis is in place. In the adolescent and young adult, *Neisseria gonorrhoeae* is a common causative organism.[12] In adults of all ages, *Staphylococcus aureus* is the usual source of infection, although other pathogens may be implicated. Methicillin-resistant *Staphylococcus aureus* (MRSA) is becoming a more common pathogen especially in the United States.[12]

Neoplasms can originate in the bone or metastasize to it and can cause anything from odd bone growths along the cortex to benign or destructive cystic lesions to complete bone destruction. All patients with questionable x-ray findings should be referred to a specialist promptly for further evaluation (see Chapter 155).

Hip pain can also be referred from the back or sacroiliac joint. This cause can frequently be teased out during evaluation because hip motion does not affect the discomfort, but back or sacroiliac mobilization does.[5] Inguinal hernias can also cause hip pain and can be discovered during examination.[5] This anterior hip or groin pain or bulging usually increases with bearing down or lifting of heavy objects and is frequently associated with a history of straining before onset of pain.

CLINICAL PRESENTATION AND PHYSICAL EXAMINATION

Clinical Presentation

A careful history must be obtained from the patient, with particular attention to the history of the present illness. Any history of joint replacement and recent or old trauma to the hip and lower back or history of cancer should be sought. Pertinent questions related to age, location, onset, duration, severity, setting, timing, associated symptoms, and aggravating or alleviating factors will be useful in narrowing the diagnosis. Recent activity (vocational or recreational), skin problems (rashes, cuts, or abrasions), social habits, medications, procedures (including dental), surgery (especially joint replacement), trauma, or history of cancer may also prove helpful.[5]

Hip pain experienced with increased activity versus at rest is critical to the history. Pain that occurs with a sudden acceleration or deceleration, impact, twisting or popping, especially during a sports activity, may narrow the search.

Point tenderness over the greater trochanter or ischial tuberosity may indicate bursitis (see Chapter 156).

Progressively worsening of pain in groin, buttock, or anterior thigh with activity and improvement with rest may indicate OA (see Chapter 156).

Constitutional symptoms such as fever, fatigue, swelling, or redness may indicate joint sepsis or inflammatory arthritis (see Chapter 159).

Physical Examination

The back, sacroiliac joints, hips, knees, and ankles should be examined. The assessment should include general observation and vital signs as well as inspection, palpation, range of motion, and evaluation of strength and stability. Two tests of hip function during physical examination are essential: gait and range of motion. A good neurologic examination is also important.

With true hip joint disease, the gait may be affected by a limp (antalgic gait) that is characterized by an exaggerated swaying motion of the upper body toward the painful hip while walking (Trendelenburg gait).[5] Motion restrictions of abduction and internal rotation are usually more pronounced than restriction of adduction and external rotation. Pain, muscle spasm, and guarding are noted with passive and active

range of motion. Inspection may reveal a flexion contracture of the hip and atrophy of the musculature of the buttocks. Crepitus of the joint may be felt or heard with palpation and movement. Infection may also manifest with fever, limited motion, and exquisite pain with motion.

Greater trochanteric pain syndrome, also known as trochanteric bursitis, typically manifests with point tenderness over the lateral prominence.[13] Hip flexion and internal rotation may exacerbate the pain. Stress fractures (usually of the femoral neck) will cause pain in the groin of anterior thigh with (usually) a pronounced limp.

In the older patient, fracture should be suspected if there is a history of a fall or rotational injury to the hip.[14] The patient will report hip, groin, or thigh pain and will be unable to bear weight or to move the leg well. The affected extremity will often be shortened and externally rotated.[14]

DIAGNOSTICS

The diagnosis of hip pain is made initially on the basis of history and clinical examination of the patient. X-ray examination is typically the next step in assessing the hip if something more than soft tissue disease is suspected. X-ray studies should include an anteroposterior (AP) view of the pelvis and frog-leg and lateral views of the hip. Two views of the lumbosacral spine can be added if the examination findings suggest back disease. Weight-bearing films are important to assess the extent of joint degeneration and joint space narrowing when fracture is not suspected. CT or MRI is obtained to further define pain especially when soft tissue causes are suspected.[15]

Intra-articular aspiration and injection of the hip joint can be diagnostic of intra-articular pathology and offer temporary pain relief. A positive response to an intra-articular injection may be helpful in the decision to proceed to surgery.[16]

If inflammatory causes are suspected, a complete blood count (CBC), erythrocyte sedimentation rate (ESR), C-reactive protein (CRP) level, anticyclic citrullinated protein (anti-CCP) antibodies, and rheumatoid factor should be obtained.[9,15] Uric acid is added if gout is suspected. If there is radiographic evidence of effusion, joint aspiration performed under fluoroscopic guidance is indicated. Aspirate is sent for culture and sensitivity, cell count with differential, and identification of crystalline deposits.

Magnetic resonance imaging (MRI) is the diagnostic test of choice when avascular necrosis is suspected. MRI is also the imaging of choice for defining the extent of cartilage destruction, labral tearing, or impingement although CT scan can also be used if MRI is not available.

DIFFERENTIAL DIAGNOSIS

 Priority differentials include fractures, dislocations, inflammatory arthritis, infections, metastases, and avascular necrosis—all important causes of hip pain.[16]

It is helpful to consider the patient's age, the location of the pain, and the preceding activities to determine the most likely source. Although the most common cause of hip pain in the older adult is OA, other diagnostic possibilities should be considered, especially if there is no relief of symptoms with standard treatment and the medical history suggests another etiology.

Minimum force applied to the hip joint may produce a fracture, especially in the older woman with osteoporosis. Runners

INITIAL DIAGNOSTICS

Hip Pain

LABORATORY[a]

Essential
- Complete blood count and differential
- Erythrocyte sedimentation rate

Additional
- Rheumatoid factor, anticyclic citrullinated protein antibodies
- C-reactive protein
- Uric acid

IMAGING

Essential
- X-ray examination

Additional
- Magnetic resonance imaging[a]

ADDITIONAL DIAGNOSTICS
- Joint fluid aspiration for culture and sensitivity, crystalline deposits, and cell count[a]
- Diagnostic intra-articular injection

[a]If indicated.

or those who participate in sports are vulnerable to femoral stress fractures.[9]

Traumatic dislocations are more often seen in young patients who engage in activities with a risk for violent injury. Atraumatic hip dislocations should be considered in patients with sudden hip pain if they have undergone prior hip replacement surgery.[16] Infection of the hip joint is rare in adults, although this should be considered in children or adults with a prosthetic hip and new-onset hip pain and fever (see Chapter 159). Avascular necrosis should be considered if pain is subacute or chronic, especially if there is a history of trauma, autoimmune disease, or steroid use.[10]

Extra-articular causes of hip pain include referred pain from degenerative disks, spinal stenosis, sacroiliac dysfunction, leg length discrepancies, bursitis, malignant neoplasms, Paget disease, and osteomyelitis.[5]

FAI syndrome is recognized as a frequent cause of hip pain especially in athletes who perform at the very limits of joint motion frequently. Bone spurs develop along the edges of the acetabulum or femoral head, causing it to deform and become irregularly shaped, or the socket becomes deeper than it should be, or angled more posteriorly than normal. Any of these changes from normal increases friction between the socket and the femoral head or neck, and the shape mismatch increases cartilaginous wear tearing of the labrum seal around the joint.[17,18] There are three types of impingement, depending on whether there is a cam action or pinching of the rim of the acetabulum, irritation of the femoral head or neck, or both. When symptoms develop, it usually indicates that damage to either the labrum or cartilage has occurred.[17,18]

INTERPROFESSIONAL COLLABORATIVE MANAGEMENT

Hip pain is a symptom of an underlying pathophysiologic process. Although hip pain itself has the potential to produce functional limitations and to impair quality of life, the management should be directed toward identification and treatment of the underlying cause of the pain. Evidence-based practice in treating the adult patient with hip pain is focused on the various causes of the hip pain reviewed earlier.

Pharmacologic Management

Pain management is a major issue for patients with OA involving the hip. Although most randomized controlled trials have focused on OA of the knee, some have demonstrated benefits of using nonsteroidal antiinflammatory drugs (NSAIDs) and acetaminophen analgesics for relief of hip pain.[8] There is no clear evidence that either class of analgesic is superior; however, acetaminophen may be better tolerated by older adults and is the first-line recommendation.[8] NSAID gels and patches are promising. Lidocaine patches are helpful to some patients. Capsaicin, an over-the-counter topical analgesic, has also been shown to provide short-term pain relief and has fewer side effects than oral agents.[19] The adverse effect most commonly reported for topical agents is local skin irritation. Adding glucosamine or glucosamine chondroitin, or other alternative dietary supplements such as S-adenosylmethionine (SAM-e) or methylsulfonylmethane (MSM), may be helpful for some patients although are without scientific evidence of effectiveness.[20]

Fluoroscopically guided intra-articular injection of corticosteroids may be helpful for diagnostic purposes and for arthritis patients; however, the effects wane as disease progresses. Corticosteroids leave deposits within the joint and can cause further joint degradation; thereby the frequency with which they are administered should be limited to 3 times a year or less. These agents should be given only with the guidance of an orthopedic or rheumatologic specialist or an interventional radiologist.

Nonpharmacologic Management

Nonpharmacologic measures are aimed at restoration and maintenance of function of the joint as an adjunct to pharmacologic therapy. Recommendations for complete rest or inactivity of the joint should be given only after careful weighing of the risk versus benefit. Muscle atrophy, weakness, and generalized deconditioning may result and contribute to the primary problem. This is especially true in the older adult. Evidence for benefit does exist for exercise and education for reducing pain, with the strongest evidence pointing to the benefits of exercise.[21] Exercise also improves functional status and provides a sense of well-being. Physical therapists can be helpful in developing an appropriate exercise regimen. Range of motion and low-stress, low-impact exercises should be prescribed. An aquatic exercise program may promote mobility while relieving mechanical weight bearing on the joint.[21] The use of heat before and ice after exercise can also alleviate pain.

Hip pain requires an ongoing assessment of the patient's functional capabilities and relief of painful symptoms. A multidisciplinary approach involving a physical therapist and an occupational therapist is indicated. Physical therapy improves joint mobility and prevents the complications of joint disuse. Occupational therapists may assist patients with limitations of function by adapting activities of daily living and providing assistive devices for optimum independence. Referral to an orthopedic surgeon for consideration of surgery is indicated for patients with late- to end-stage OA, joint infection, or avascular necrosis and for those with progressive loss of function or refractory pain. Joint replacement surgery is now commonly done and very effective at restoring function and alleviating pain in even very old patients. Urgent referral is required for patients with infection, hip fracture, or dislocation.

LIFE SPAN CONSIDERATIONS

Hip pain is much less common in children than in adults.[7] Congenital hip dislocation should be considered in infants and subsequent hip dysplasia in young children.[7] Apophysitis is a tendinitis in the growing skeleton found in childhood through young adolescence.[7] Legg-Calvé-Perthes disease is avascular necrosis of the femoral head found mostly in 4- to 8-year-old boys.[7]

Transient synovitis, a benign, self-limiting, but painful condition, is the most common cause of pain during childhood.[7] It can occur in growing bones, and the incidence typically decreases by age 12. Age 2 to 5 is most commonly affected age group. Causes can include allergic, traumatic, viral, or post-streptococcal toxic synovitis. Fever is rare. Restricted hip abduction is the most sensitive range of motion limitation. Pain is worse in the morning and eases with activity. Excluding juvenile arthritis and sepsis is especially important when considering the differential diagnoses in children, and following closely for the possible development of Legg-Calvé-Perthes disease is clearly indicated.

Slipped capital femoral epiphysis (SCFE), in which the growing femoral head and growth plate slip in relation to the remainder of the head and femoral neck, is most common in 11- to 14-year-olds and in boys more than girls. It can be traumatic or atraumatic. It is more common during periods of rapid growth, is associated with obesity, and can be bilateral.

COMPLICATIONS

Osteoporosis of the hip may result in a fracture with or without trauma. Chronic pain accompanied by loss of function and mobility may result in deconditioning and falls with injury. Older patients in particular should be monitored for gastrointestinal and renal side effects if they are taking NSAIDs. An adolescent with SCFE has a guarded long-term prognosis for repeated injury, contralateral disease, and complications.[7] Avascular necrosis of the femoral head may occur in approximately 30% of patients with SCFE.[7] Premature development of degenerative arthritis may occur with or without avascular necrosis.[0] Congenital hip dislocations can lead to chronic pain, gait impairment, early onset arthritis, and need for surgical intervention at a young age if not screened for and treated early.

PATIENT AND FAMILY EDUCATION AND HEALTH PROMOTION

Chronic joint pain can be mentally and physically wearing on patients and family. An interprofessional approach to care with the patient and family as active participants in the decision-making process may prove more satisfactory for everyone in the long term. The patient is entitled to an explanation about the source of the pain and whether it is likely to be temporary or chronic. Facilitating the patient's understanding of anticipated outcomes and prognosis is extremely beneficial in strengthening the patient-provider relationship.

Health-promoting activities should be directed toward maintenance and preservation of function of the joint. The management of a painful hip may include range-of-motion and muscle-strengthening exercises as recommended by the physical therapist. Maintenance of optimum weight should be encouraged because excess weight places tremendous stresses on the hip. The patient taking NSAIDs should take these medications with food and be knowledgeable of the signs and symptoms of gastrointestinal irritation. Renal function should be monitored, particularly in older patients. Assessment of the home environment and the need for ambulatory assistive devices is warranted to reduce the risk of falls, especially in older or frailer patients.

REFERENCES

1. Silvis, M. (2014). Common musculoskeletal problems in the ambulatory setting. *The Medical Clinics of North America, 98*(4), xvii.
2. Moss, A. S., Murphy, L. B., Helmick, C. K., et al. (2016). Annual incidence of hip symptoms and three hip outcomes from a U.S. population-based cohort study. The Johnston County osteoarthritis project. *Osteoarthritis and Cartilage, 24*, 1518–1527.
3. Rankin, A., Bleakley, C., & Cullen. M. (2015). Hip joint pathology as a leading cause of groin pain in the sporting population. *The American Journal of Sports Medicine, 43*(7), 1698–1703.
4. Thompson, J. (2015). *Netter's concise orthopaedic anatomy* (2nd ed.). St Louis: Elsevier.
5. Wilson, J., & Furukawa, M. (2014). Evaluation of the patient with hip pain. *American Family Physician, 89*(1), 27–34.
6. Wheeless, C. R., III. Wheels' Textbook of Orthopaedic. Duke Orthopaedics. Retrieved from www.wheelessonline.com. (Accessed 30 December 2017), updated Feb 2017.
7. Watts, E. Transient synovitis of the Hip. Retrieved from www.orthobullets.com/pediatrics/4030/transient-synovitis-of-hip. (Accessed 30 December 2017).
8. Nelson, A., Allen, K., Golightly, Y., et al. (2014). A systematic review of recommendations and guidelines for the management of osteoarthritis: The chronic OA initiative of the US Bone and Joint initiative. *Seminars in Arthritis and Rheumatism, 42*(6), 701–712.
9. West, S. (2015). *Rheumatology secrets* (3rd ed.). Philadelphia, PA: Elsevier.
10. Lee, M., & Hazlet, C. (2015). Avascular necrosis of the femoral head. *The Journal of Orthopaedic and Sports Physical Therapy, 45*(5), 425.
11. Pisani, P., Renna, M. D., & Conversano, F. (2016). Major osteoporotic fragility fractures: Risk factor updates and societal impact. *World Journal of Orthopedics, 7*(3), 171–181.
12. Ross, J. (2017). Septic arthritis of native joints. *Infectious Disease Clinics, 31*(2), 203–218.
13. Saraogi, A., Lokiker, N., & Raut, V. (2016). Greater trochanteric pain syndrome: A review article. *EC Orthopaedics, 4*(1), 429–434.
14. Borx, T., Roberts, K., Taksali, S., et al. (2015). The AAOS evidence-based guidelines on the management of hip fractures in the elderly. *The Journal of Bone and Joint Surgery. American Volume, 97*(14), 1196–1199.
15. Allan, C., et al. Lab Tests and Arthritis. UW Medicine Orthopedics and Sports Medicine. Retrieved from www.orthop.washington.edu/?q=patient-care/articles/arthritis/lab-tests-and-arthritis.html. (Accessed 30 December 2017).
16. Coleman, S. (2016). Editorial commentary: The importance of developing an algorithm when diagnosing hip pain. *Arthroscopy: The Journal of Arthroscopic and Related Surgery, 36*(8), 1712–1713.
17. Pun, S., Kumar, D., & Lane, N. (2015). Femoral acetabular impingement. *Arthritis & Rheumatology, 67*(1), 17–27.
18. Bannister, E. (2017). Treatment and Rehabilitation of Femoral Acetabular Impingement – Senior Honors Thesis 172, The College at Brockport: State University of New York. Retrieved from http://digitalcommons.brockport.edu/honors172. (Accessed 30 December 2017).
19. Laslett, L., & Jones, G. (2014). Capsaicin treatment for osteoarthritis: A meta-analysis. *Osteoarthritis and Cartilage, 22*, s422.
20. Runhaur, J., Roxendaal, R., van Midcekoop, M., et al. (2017). SAT0523 No treatment effects of oral glucosamine for subgroups of knee and hip osteoarthritis patients; an individual patient data meta-analysis from the oa trial bank. *Annals of the Rheumatic Diseases, 76*, 973–974.
21. Beumer, L., Wong, J., Warden, S., et al. (2015). Effects of exercise and manual therapy on pain associated with hip OA: A systematic review and meta-analysis. *British Journal of Sports Medicine*, doi:10.1136/bjsports-2015-095255. Retrieved from bjsm.bmj.com. (Accessed 30 December 2017).

CHAPTER 162

KNEE PAIN

Wendy L. Halm

 Immediate referral is indicated for severe strains, tears, suspected fractures, knee locking, or obvious dislocation.

DEFINITION AND EPIDEMIOLOGY

Knee pain is a common problem that can originate in any of the bony structures of the knee joint (femur, tibia, fibula), the kneecap (patella), or the ligaments and cartilage (meniscus) of the knee. In addition, soft tissue structure surrounding the knee joint (muscle, tendons, bursae) can also be a source of pain. Knee pain can affect people of all ages and can be attributed to many causes.

The multiple structures within the knee make it vulnerable to various types of injuries and degenerative change. There also are many extra-articular structures that can become inflamed or injured, causing knee discomfort. Many injuries can be treated conservatively; others require surgery.

Knee pain is often classified per cause and longevity of symptoms. Knee pain can also be a result of an acute injury, trauma, or a particular athletic move. Knee pain related to chronic and/or inflammatory disease, such as bursitis, osteoarthritis, rheumatoid arthritis, or gout, is discussed in other chapters.

PATHOPHYSIOLOGY

The knee is a modified hinge joint that flexes and extends and has some rotational mobility. The knee joint contains 3 bones, 3 articulations, 5 major tendons, 4 major ligaments, 2 menisci, and 12 bursae. The lateral and medial articulations are between the femoral and tibial condyles. The intermediate articulation is between the patella and the femur. A relatively weak joint, the knee gains its strength from the strong ligaments that attach the femur to the tibia. Five intrinsic ligaments assist in strengthening the articular capsule. The cruciate ligaments connect the femur and tibia within the articular capsule, crossing each other in the form of an X.[1]

As a major weight-bearing joint, the knee is susceptible to many injuries. Torsion is limited in the joint, and any motion that extends beyond the defined range results in a ligamentous injury. Because the knee depends on the integrity of the ligaments to provide its stability, a knee injury can be a calamitous event.

CLINICAL PRESENTATION AND PHYSICAL EXAMINATION

The approach to knee pain begins with a careful history and review of symptoms, focusing particularly on the presence of trauma, mechanism of injury, and limitations. Patients with any penetrating injury, especially if there is joint involvement, should be referred to the emergency department. Patients with a history of a traumatic event with presence of effusion or swelling, fever or other systemic illness, erythematous and swollen knees, knee pain in conjunction with sexually transmitted infections, or cellulitis over or adjacent to the affected knee or who have a history of bleeding disorders or anticoagulation are

particularly concerning and should be managed with same-day orthopedic consultation.[2]

Physical examination of the knee can be frustrating to novice providers and requires both practice and patience. Ideally, the provider's physical examination skills are honed under the guidance and critique of an experienced colleague. A systematic approach that includes elements of inspection, range of motion, palpation, sensation, and special tests to evaluate stability is critical to correct diagnosis of knee pain.[1]

COLLATERAL LIGAMENT SPRAINS

There are two collateral ligaments: the medial collateral ligament (MCL) and the lateral collateral ligament (LCL). The MCL attaches to the medial condyle of the femur and the tibia. The LCL attaches to the lateral femoral condyle and extends to the lateral tibial plateau.[1] The purpose of the collateral ligaments is to provide support to the inner and the lateral portions of the knee.

PATHOPHYSIOLOGY

MCL injuries are the most common ligamentous injury, as the lateral aspect of the knee is exposed during sports. The MCL is approximately 8 to 10 cm in length, and has a superficial and deep component. It is the primary stabilizer to valgus stress. Injuries occur with valgus force applied to the knee with external tibial rotation. This can occur with a non-contact twist or a blow to the lateral side of a joint, especially with a firmly planted foot. MCL injuries are more common in athletic males, and often include an injury to the medial meniscus. LCL injuries occur with an internal rotation or a blow to the medial side of the knee with a firmly planted foot. The mechanism may be contact or non-contact.[3] The injuries are graded as first-, second-, or third-degree sprains.

CLINICAL PRESENTATION AND PHYSICAL EXAMINATION

Patients with an MCL injury will typically have medial knee pain. Swelling and instability are uncommon and may signify more serious injury, such as a tear of the medial meniscus. LCL injuries manifest with acute lateral knee pain and may have associated instability leading to the knee giving way.[1]

An examination immediately after the injury is more accurate and helps ascertain the severity of the injury. Examination of the knee is more difficult in the presence of edema and muscle spasm.[3] The assessment should include observation; palpation; assessment of range of motion, motor strength, sensation, and vascular structures; ligamentous testing and stability assessment; and provocative maneuvers. The normal knee should be tested first to establish a baseline.[1] Both knees should be observed for swelling, deformity, muscle atrophy, and patella placement. Fluctuance should be determined with the patient first standing and then supine. Tenderness and bone landmarks should be ascertained as well. In the suspected collateral ligament sprain, there is tenderness along the body of the ligament, and point tenderness at the attachment site is commonly present. With MCL injury, there may be tenderness at the medial joint line because the MCL attaches to the medial meniscus. Pain at the lateral joint line can be indicative of an internal joint injury.

Valgus stress on the knee joint determines MCL laxity. If the clinician identifies significant valgus laxity with the knee in full extension, an injury involving the entire MCL complex

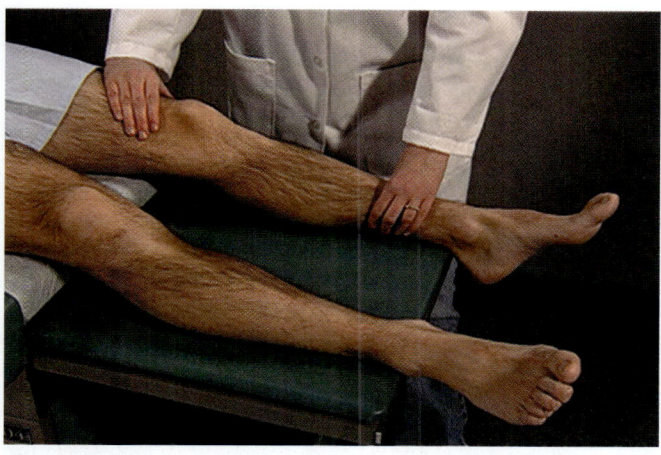

FIG. 162.1 Valgus Stress Test of the Knee. (From Ball, J. W., Dains, J. E., Flynn, J. A., et al. [2014]. *Seidel's physical examination handbook* [8th ed.]. St Louis: Elsevier.)

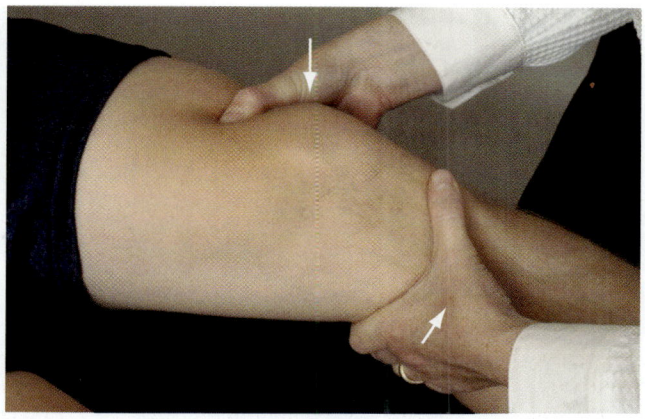

FIG. 162.2 Lachman Test. (Netter illustration used with permission of Elsevier Inc. All rights reserved. www.netterimages.com.)

or the anterior cruciate ligament (ACL) should be suspected. Varus stress on the knee joint determines LCL laxity (Fig. 162.1). Laxity at 30 degrees of flexion indicates injury to the LCL.[1,3] Active range of motion in extension and flexion should be assessed. If active range of motion is not possible, passive extension and flexion should be evaluated.

CRUCIATE LIGAMENT INJURIES

DEFINITION AND EPIDEMIOLOGY

Resembling an X, the cruciate ligaments crisscross within the joint capsule but are extra synovial. There are two cruciate ligaments: the ACL and the posterior cruciate ligament (PCL), which control the back and forth motion of the knee. A cruciate ligament injury can be a sprain, a partial tear, or a complete disruption of the ligament. Physical examination and radiologic tests as indicated are used to determine the degree of the injury. The ACL is the most commonly involved structure in severe knee injuries. Female gender and intensity of play increase the risk of ACL tear.[4] The PCL is less often injured.

PATHOPHYSIOLOGY

The ACL attaches to the anterior part of the intercondylar area of the tibia, posterior to the medial meniscus, and rises superiorly, posteriorly, and laterally to attach to the posterior section of the medial side of the lateral condyle of the femur. The ACL restrains the anterior to posterior alignment of the knee, keeping the proper relationship of the femur to the tibia.[4] It is loose with the knee in flexion and tight when the knee is fully extended. It is the weaker of the two cruciate ligaments. The ACL is typically injured in sports during rapid deceleration or on quickly changing directions. The ACL can also be torn with a direct blow to the lateral portion of the knee. The ACL injury often occurs in combination with ruptures of the MCL and the medial meniscus. Once the ligament is torn, the knee is unstable. Swelling occurs rapidly in an ACL or PCL injury because of bleeding from the ligament tear.

The PCL originates at the posterior part of the intercondylar area of the tibia. It crosses superiorly and anteriorly on the medial side of the ACL and attaches to the anterior part of the lateral surface of the medial femoral condyle. The PCL is tight with the knee in flexion. The PCL restrains the posterior to anterior alignment of the knee.[4] The PCL is the stronger ligament and is usually injured through trauma to the anterior surface of the proximal tibia (as in hitting the dashboard) or falling onto the tibial tubercle with the knee flexed.

CLINICAL PRESENTATION AND PHYSICAL EXAMINATION

The patient with an acute ACL injury may recall hearing a "pop" or have autonomic symptoms including dizziness, sweating, or fainting. With acute injury, swelling usually occurs within the first 2 hours of injury. With chronic injury, complaints of the knee giving way on twisting, pivoting, and cutting may occur. Patients with a PCL injury usually have less swelling than with an ACL tear. Patients may have difficulty walking and feel like the knee is unstable.

Swelling and pain in the acutely injured knee often prohibit a thorough examination. If the knee is swollen, the patient will be unable to fully flex or extend the knee. Hamstring spasms and the posterior horn of the meniscus can stabilize the knee, falsely indicating a stable joint; thus, it is important for the patient to relax. The normal knee should be examined first to allay anxiety and to establish a baseline, because most people have some degree of laxity in the ligaments.

The Lachman test (Fig. 162.2) is used to assess the ACL. The knee should be flexed to about 15 to 30 degrees. One hand is placed just below the knee joint on the posterior aspect of the tibia-fibula. The other hand is placed on the anterior aspect of the femur just above the joint. The examiner lifts the lower leg while pushing down on the upper leg. If the ACL is intact, after a few millimeters of movement, the examiner should feel a "knock" or a firm "stop" as the ACL prevents the tibia from sliding forward. In the absence of a firm end point, a ligament tear should be suspected.[1]

The anterior drawer test (Fig. 162.3) also is used to assess the ACL. The knee should be flexed to about 90 degrees, with the foot kept flat on the examination surface. The examiner sits on the patient's foot and firmly grasps the lower leg, placing the fingers below the popliteal space and the thumbs on the tibial tuberosity. The examiner pulls gently but firmly on the tibia, attempting to slide the tibia forward. A "soft" or absent end point indicates a tear.[1]

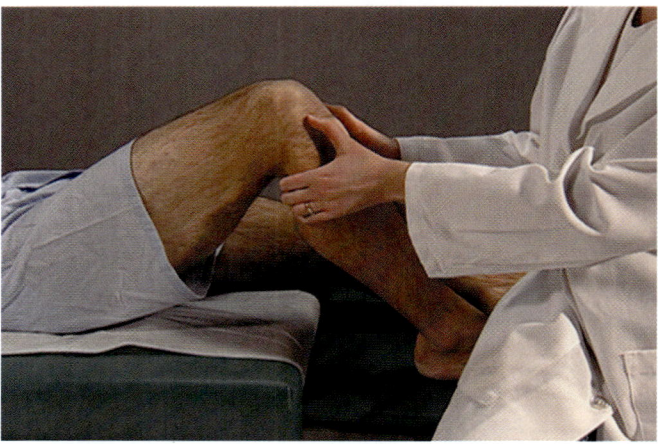

FIG. **162.3**   Drawer Test for Anterior and Posterior Stability of the Knee. (From Ball, J. W., Dains, J. E., Flynn, J. A., et al. [2014]. *Seidel's physical examination handbook.* [8th ed.]. St Louis: Elsevier.)

The posterior drawer test (see Fig. 162.3) is used to assess the PCL. With the patient positioned the same as for the anterior drawer test, the examiner pushes posteriorly on the tibia. A positive test is straight posterior displacement of both tibial condyles.[5] Additional tests for the PCL include the gravity (sag) test and valgus-varus test at 0 degrees.

MENISCUS INJURIES

DEFINITION AND EPIDEMIOLOGY

The menisci are crescent-shaped fibrocartilaginous structures on the articular surface of the tibia. They act as shock absorbers for the knee and help control normal knee motion.[6] Meniscus tears are the third most common of all knee injuries. The medial meniscus is injured or torn more often than the lateral meniscus because of its structure, mobility, and attachment.[7] Meniscal injuries are more common in males and are often associated with an ACL tear in the athletic population. Older patients may have minimal or no known trauma associated with degenerative tears.[4]

PATHOPHYSIOLOGY

The menisci cover part of the articular surface of the corresponding tibial plateau. The collagen fibers help maintain the space between the bones in the knee joint to help withstand compression. A meniscus can be injured when the weight-bearing knee is twisted while it is in the partially flexed position.[7] The femur compresses against the tibia and grinds against the meniscus. This grinding motion tears the meniscus as the force exceeds the strength of the fibrocartilage. Menisci tear as a direct result of injury or indirectly because of the normal wear and tear on the knee. Once torn, the inner menisci cannot heal due to limited blood flow.

CLINICAL PRESENTATION AND PHYSICAL EXAMINATION

In an acute injury, joint effusion is usually present. There is tenderness along the joint line, and the person often has a sense of instability. Those with a degenerative tear will complain of joint line discomfort and a sense of locking or giving

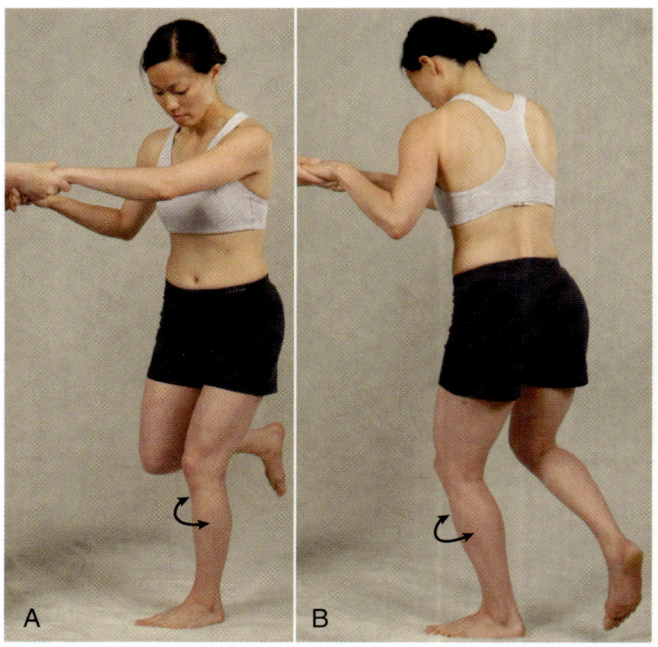

FIG. **162.4**   The Thessaly Test for Meniscal Integrity at 20 Degrees of Flexion. (From Cleland, J., & Koppenhaver, S. [2016]. *Netter's orthopaedic clinical examination: An evidence-based approach* [3rd ed.]. Philadelphia: Elsevier.)

way, especially while descending stairs or walking on uneven surfaces.

The physical examination should include palpation of the joint line, assessing for tenderness and presence of an effusion. The examination findings may be unremarkable owing to the type and location of the tear. The Thessaly test (Fig. 162.4) is the most sensitive. To perform the Thessaly test, the provider holds the outstretched hands of the patient for support. The patient flexes the affected knee to 5 degrees while flexing the unaffected knee and lifting the foot off of the floor so that all the body weight is on the affected knee. The patient twists on the affected knee 3 times. Those who have meniscal tears experience joint line pain and may also have a locking sensation.[7] The test is then repeated at 20 degrees of flexion.

The McMurray (Fig. 162.5) test helps ascertain a tear in the cartilage. To perform the McMurray test, the examiner has the patient lie supine with the legs straight. The examiner firmly grasps the heel or ankle with one hand and places the other hand on the knee joint, with the fingers on the medial side and the thumb at the lateral side. The examiner flexes the knee while rotating the tibia internally and externally on the femur. This maneuver will loosen the joint. Then, while flexing and externally rotating the leg, the examiner applies valgus stress to the lateral side of the knee. The examiner holds the valgus stress on the joint while extending the leg and palpating the medial joint line. If a click or pop is heard or felt, the medial meniscus is likely torn.[7]

The McMurray test can also be performed with the patient in a sitting position and the knee flexed to 90 degrees. The patient should internally rotate the affected leg while the practitioner slowly extends the leg. While performing the maneuver, the practitioner should apply resistance to the knee medially to test the medial meniscus. The practitioner should repeat the

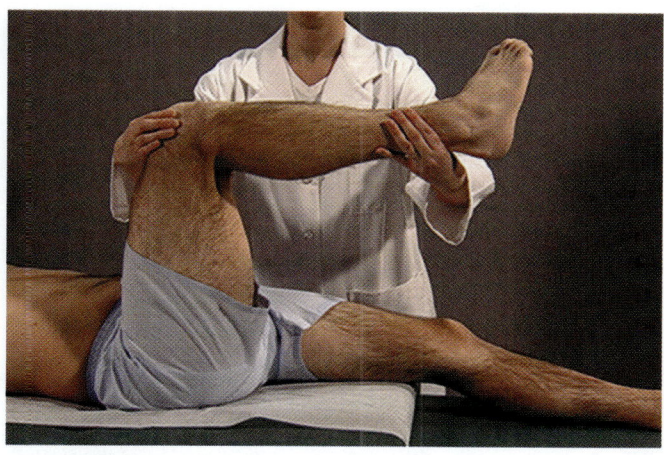

F I G .   **162.5**   McMurray Test of the Knee. (From Ball, J. W., Dains, J. E., Flynn, J. A., et al. [2014]. *Seidel's physical examination handbook* [8th ed.]. St Louis: Elsevier.)

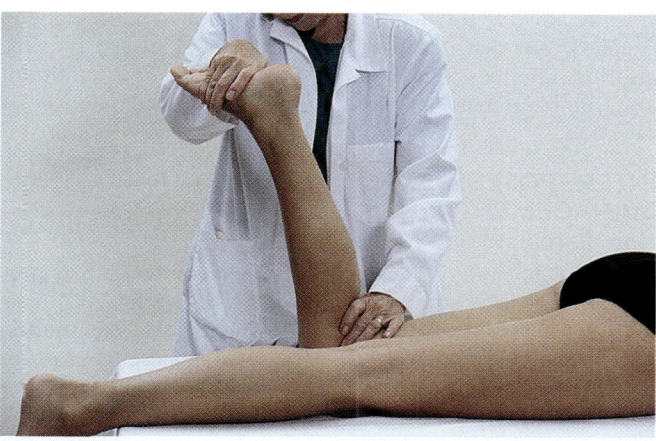

F I G .   **162.6**   Apley Assessment of the Knee. (From Cleland, J., & Koppenhaver, S. [2011]. *Netter's orthopaedic clinical examination: An evidence-based approach* [2nd ed.]. Philadelphia: Elsevier.)

maneuver, applying resistance to the knee laterally to test the lateral meniscus. The test result is positive if the knee cannot be extended.

In addition to the McMurray test, a simpler test is the Apley compression test (Fig. 162.6). This test should be done with the patient prone and the affected leg flexed to 90 degrees. The examiner places his or her knee on the patient's posterior thigh to stabilize it, grabs the foot firmly, leans on the heel to squeeze the menisci between the femur and the tibia, and rotates the tibia. If pain is elicited, there is a tear in the meniscus. The patient should be asked to describe the location of the pain to distinguish a medial meniscus tear from a lateral meniscus tear.

PATELLOFEMORAL PAIN SYNDROME

DEFINITION AND EPIDEMIOLOGY

Patellofemoral pain syndrome (PFPS) is one of the most common overuse injuries of the knee. It refers to knee pain that is localized to the anterior portion of the knee. Other common names for PFPS include runner's knee, jumper's knee, retropatellar pain syndrome, and anterior knee pain.[4] PFPS is common in younger active athletes, especially runners and women.

PATHOPHYSIOLOGY

The cause of PFPS is poorly understood. It is likely that the syndrome results from abnormal lateral tracking of the patella resulting from weak quadriceps muscles, poor flexibility, patellar hypermobility, a tight iliotibial band, anatomic malalignment, or overuse.[8] Women are more likely to experience abnormal lateral tracking because of an anatomically wider pelvis, greater hip varus, increased femoral anteversion, increased knee valgus, and increased external tibia rotation.[9] PFPS occurs when nerves sense pain in the soft tissues and bone around the kneecap.[4]

CLINICAL PRESENTATION AND PHYSICAL EXAMINATION

Patients report knee pain that is often bilateral and is largely limited to the anterior portion of the knee, around and behind the patella. PFPS is exacerbated by sporting activity, squatting, kneeling, climbing stairs, or descent and hill running.[8] Patients may report a feeling that the knee is "giving out" or that they have pain with prolonged sitting with the knees flexed (the "theater sign"). Rarely, patients may complain of an effusion, which should be further evaluated for other causes.

A complete examination of the knee, including gait observation, is critical to establish a diagnosis and to rule out other causes. Clinicians should have the patient stand and move, noting the static and dynamic alignment of the affected knee and extremity. The knee should be observed for deformity, discoloration, swelling, scars, protuberances, effusion, or edema, looking for any signs of patellar dislocation. The knee should be palpated in a sitting and supine position, noting point of tenderness and any crepitus. The provider may notice a lateral tracking of the patella when the patient is in a seated position. Rocking of the patella in the patellar groove while the leg is fully extended may elicit pain. Anterior knee pain with quadriceps contraction, pain during squatting, and pain on palpation of the posteromedial or posterolateral border of the patella should be assessed.[8] Patients may also demonstrate weak or tight quadriceps muscles or a tight iliotibial band. Orthopedic tests such as the patellar compression-grind, patellar tilt, and patellar glide may be of benefit to help the clinician pinpoint the issue. Examination of the hip and lumbar spine in addition to a neurovascular system should be completed.

INFLAMMATORY AND DEGENERATIVE DISORDERS

PATHOPHYSIOLOGY

As people age or become deconditioned because of chronic injury or disease, knee pain can be caused by a variety of inflammatory or extra-articular conditions and by age-related degeneration.

CLINICAL PRESENTATION AND PHYSICAL EXAMINATION

- Anserine bursitis is commonly seen in middle-aged women with osteoarthritis of the knee and a valgus deformity. This disorder produces pain and tenderness over the medial aspect of the knee about 5 cm (2 inches) below the joint line. Obvious swelling is not uncommon. Anserine bursitis is treated conservatively with ice and NSAIDs, but steroid injections may be necessary to alleviate pain in particularly severe cases.

- Prepatellar bursitis (housemaid's knee) manifests as a swelling superficial to the patella. This condition results from trauma such as that occurring with frequent kneeling and is seen commonly in persons who work on their knees, such as floor or carpet layers. Pain is mild unless direct pressure is applied over the bursa, and there is no pain with weight bearing or range of motion of the knee. The condition is treated with rest, ice, and NSAIDs and is prevented by protecting the knee from repeated trauma.

- Inflammatory arthritis including rheumatoid arthritis, psoriatic arthritis, reactive arthritis, gout, and pseudogout can cause acute pain and swelling of the knee that can progress to cartilage degeneration and the eventual need for joint replacement surgery.

- Popliteal cysts (Baker cysts) are commonly seen in conjunction with rheumatoid arthritis, osteoarthritis, or internal derangements of the knee. Initially, a cystic swelling in the popliteal space may be the only finding. As the cyst increases in size, the possibility of rupture increases. A ruptured cyst will drain into the calf, causing pain, erythema, and swelling, mimicking phlebitis. An ultrasound examination will provide a location and extent of the cyst.

- Osteoarthritis is probably the most common cause of knee pain in the older adult. Pain, stiffness, and decreased function are cardinal signs. Pain is generally insidious in onset and characterized as mild to moderate. Resting the knee usually alleviates the pain. Osteoarthritis is progressive, and the cartilage damage is permanent. However, conservative treatment, including muscle strengthening, weight loss, analgesics, and NSAIDs, is often effective. Injections of steroids or hyaluronan may provide temporary relief. Severe disease, manifesting with resting or night pain and increasing difficulty with ambulation, may require joint replacement surgery.

- Referred pain syndrome can originate with problems of the low back, sacroiliac, or hip joint. Pain from any of these areas can be referred to the knee, resulting in pain. Referred pain should be considered when findings of examination of the knee joint are relatively normal without swelling or local tenderness and with normal range of motion.

DIAGNOSTICS
Essential Diagnostics

The clinician should utilize validated prediction rules, such as the Ottawa Knee rule,[10] or evidenced-based guidelines, such as the American College of Radiology (ACR) Appropriateness Criteria,[11] when selecting appropriate initial diagnostic testing. Initial diagnostics may include plain radiographs to exclude fractures and dislocations.

Additional Diagnostics

More extensive radiologic examinations such as magnetic resonance imaging (MRI), CT, and ultrasound should be considered in consultation with an orthopedist. Joint aspiration (e.g., for cell count) can be performed if inflammatory, crystal, or infectious cause is suspected.

INITIAL DIAGNOSTICS

Knee Pain

IMAGING
- X-ray studies (anteroposterior, lateral, sunrise)

DIFFERENTIAL DIAGNOSIS

Important differentials that the clinician must exclude with patient complaints of acute knee pain include fracture (with or without avulsion), infection, significant tears of the ligament, neoplasm, or dislocation.

 Priority differentials include (1) fracture, (2) infection, (3) significant tears, (4) neoplasm, and (5) dislocation of the patella.

To narrow the potential differentials for knee pain, the clinician should consider type of pain and presence of trauma or effusion, and carefully home in on location. Differentials to consider include collateral or cruciate ligament sprain (varying degrees), meniscal tear, PFPS, osteochondral defect, bursitis, arthritis, referred pain, cyst, crystal arthropathies, tendinopathy, iliotibial band syndrome, or disseminated gonococcal infection.

INTERPROFESSIONAL COLLABORATIVE MANAGEMENT
Nonpharmacologic Management

P.R.I.C.E. Traditionally, conservative measures such as protection, rest, ice, compression, and elevation (P.R.I.C.E.) have been the first line of treatment for musculoskeletal injuries. Limiting or avoiding weight-bearing through use of crutches or a cane or application of a knee brace can help protect the knee. Rest of the affected extremity should be recommended, but some movement is beneficial. Gentle range of motion and basic isometric contractions of the joint and muscle surrounding the knee injury can be recommended. Use of cold therapy may be beneficial to help reduce swelling and to decrease pain. Limit cold exposure to 10 to 15 minutes at a time. A compression wrap may help minimize swelling and provide mild support to the knee. A medium amount of tension should be recommended, and the bandage should not cause color change of the surrounding tissue, numbness, or tingling. Elevation of the extremity can help reduce pooling of the fluid in the knee and decrease pain.

Physical Therapy. Rehabilitation to strengthen muscles supporting the knee is the cornerstone intervention. The incompletely rehabbed knee will be weak and unstable. Strengthening the quadriceps, hamstring, and core muscles is imperative. ACL injuries require intense rehabilitation to regain control of the quadriceps muscle. Physical therapy can positively affect pain levels, range of motion, muscle performance, functional ability, and patient quality of life.[12] The physical therapist can help the patient learn about modification of movements to prevent exacerbation of symptoms, and perform services such as manual therapy, cryotherapy, interferential current therapy, gait training, taping, and bracing.

Acupuncture. Patients with knee pain originating from osteoarthritis may benefit from acupuncture. Common adverse side effects can include pain at the needling site and muscle soreness resolving after the treatment session had ended.[13]

Pharmacologic Management

Nonsteroidal Antiinflammatory Drugs. Oral and topical nonsteroidal antiinflammatory drugs (NSAIDS) are very effective for treating pain associated with knee pain. Ibuprofen 200 to 800 mg TID-QID with a maximum daily dose of 3200 mg is recommended. If one NSAID response is suboptimal, a different NSAID may need to be prescribed. The prescription should be for the shortest duration necessary and the lowest effective dose. Adverse effects are generally dose dependent, but older adults are specifically at risk because of renal dysfunction and cardiovascular concerns. NSAID products include a black box warning regarding possible gastrointestinal (GI) and cardiovascular risks (CVs). The addition of a proton pump inhibitor or use of a selective NSAID may be of benefit for the high-risk GI patient.[14] Diclofenac may be of benefit if treating a superficial structure. Diclofenac patches have been FDA approved for acute pain, and can be applied twice daily. Topical NSAIDS should only be applied to intact skin; primary adverse reaction is local skin irritation.[15]

Acetaminophen. Acetaminophen can also be effective for relieving pain; however the antiinflammatory effects are less. Recommended dosing of acetaminophen is 325 to 650 mg every 4 to 6 hours. Patients should not exceed 4000 mg (or 2000 mg if they are at higher risk of hepatotoxicity). The provider should counsel the patient to avoid other products containing acetaminophen and to avoid alcohol. Patient risk factors should be considered before prescribing.[15]

Tramadol. Tramadol can be effective for mild to moderate pain, especially in those with intolerance to NSAIDS or acetaminophen. The recommended dose is 50 to 100 mg up to 4 times a day. Tramadol is listed as a schedule IV drug by the Drug Enforcement Administration. It should not be prescribed for a patient taking medications that increase serotonin, such as selective serotonin reuptake inhibitors.[15]

Other Prescription Medications. Other prescription medications, including antispasmodics, benzodiazepines, corticosteroids, antidepressants, anticonvulsants, topical lidocaine, and capsaicin, can be used to treat chronic or neuropathic pain. However, benzodiazepines are associated with confusion, weakness, accidents, and physical dependence (i.e., a substance use disorder). Topical glyceryl trinitrate and injectable corticosteroids may be of benefit for the patient with chronic tendinopathy, osteoarthritis, or inflammatory arthritis.[15]

INDICATIONS FOR REFERRALS AND HOSPITALIZATION

Patients with severe sprains, tears, and fractures should be referred to the emergency room for same-day orthopedic consultation. Orthopedic physician consultation is indicated for chronic MCL tears, acute MCL tears with other ligamentous injuries, and LCL or posterolateral corner injuries. Any patient who has sustained an acute injury to the cruciate ligaments requires and evaluation by an orthopedic surgeon. Orthopedic consultation is also recommended for those with persistent symptoms that limit activity, or if the patient's knee is "locked."

LIFESPAN CONSIDERATIONS

Increasing age is associated with structural changes to the knee that may predispose the older adult to knee injuries and pain. Increase in cartilage defect severity and prevalence, cartilage thinning, or reduced ligament elasticity leading to impaired integrity of joint capsules may occur in the older adult.[16] The older adult is at increased risk of physical disability and pain. The use of pain medication in older adults should be carefully considered, focusing on potentially inappropriate medications. The use of NSAIDs in the older adult has been associated with increased risk of GI bleeding and peptic ulcer disease in high-risk groups, including those older than 75 years, or in patients who are taking oral or parenteral corticosteroids, anticoagulants, or antiplatelet agents. Older patients who have arthritis affecting the patellofemoral joint may be at risk for developing PFPS. In general, conservative treatment and muscle strength training should be considered first. Patients with persistent effusion and recurrent mechanical dysfunction will need to be evaluated by an orthopedic surgeon.

COMPLICATIONS

Without accurate diagnosis and treatment, knee injuries can extend. The patient with an unstable knee is in jeopardy of fracture, aggravation of the initial injury, or falls as a direct result of the instability. A knee that has sustained severe trauma is susceptible to degenerative changes of the articular surface, development of arthritis, and chronic pain. Articular damage from a meniscus tear may result in long-term stiffness or osteoarthritis. Because the menisci are stabilizers for the knee, loss of their integrity can lead to more extensive injuries. The incompletely rehabbed knee will be weak and potentially unstable.

EMERGING MANAGEMENT TRENDS

Current research is focused at accelerating the rate of healing and improving the quality of healing tissues. Cell therapies, gene transfer, and tissue engineering with use of growth factors are being studied.[6]

PATIENT AND FAMILY EDUCATION

For mild to moderate knee injuries, conservative therapy is usually helpful. Pain medications, such as NSAIDs, application of ice, compression, and elevation of the extremity are likely beneficial for pain and swelling reduction. High-impact exercise or sports should be avoided if the knee is swollen or sore. Exercises that provide smooth motion of the knee (e.g., swimming) are better alternatives. Gentle stretching exercise three to five times a day will help preserve range of motion. For more serious injuries, physical therapy and rehabilitation will play an integral role in regaining strength and function of the knee joint. Explanation of the importance of adherence to the rehabilitative process is imperative. In some instances, a knee support for sports will be necessary. For patients who require surgical intervention, resumption of activity generally occurs at 6 to 9 months. The patient should have full and equal strength and range of motion before returning to athletics. Maintaining quadriceps and hamstring strength, in addition to hip flexor and abductor range of motion, is essential to minimize the disabilities associated with an ACL tear. A patient with persistent swelling, pain, or episodes of instability should be reevaluated, as the joint is likely overstressed or has been reinjured.

REFERENCES

1. McCarty, E. C., Walsh, W. M., & Madden, C. C. (2018). Knee injuries. In C. C. Madden, M. Putukian, E. C. McCarthy, & C. C. Young (Eds.), *Netter's sports medicine* (2nd ed., pp. 434–445). Philadelphia: Elsevier.
2. Stetka, B. S., Deane, K. D., & Kolfenbach, J. R. (2017). Evaluating knee pain: The latest in diagnosis and management. Retrieved from https://

www.medscape.com/slideshow/evaluatingkneepain-6006108#18. (Accessed 17 December 2017).

3. Andrews, K., Lu, A., Mckean, L., & Ebraheim, N. (2017). Review: Medial collateral ligament injuries. *Journal of Orthopedics, 14*, 550–554. http://dx.doi.org/10.1016/j.jor.2017.07.017.

4. American Academy of Orthopedic Surgeons (2017). OrthoInfo. Retrieved from https://orthoinfo.aaos.org. (Accessed 17 December 2017).

5. Bronstein, R. D., & Schaffer, J. C. (2017). Physical examination of knee injuries. *Journal of the American Academy of Orthopedic Surgeons, 25*(4), 280–287. doi:10.5435/JAAOS-D-15-00463.

6. Miller, R. H., & Azar, F. M. (2017). Knee injuries. In F. M. Azar, J. H. Beaty, & S. T. Canale (Eds.), *Campbell's operative orthopaedics* (13th ed., pp. 2123–2297). Philadelphia: Elsevier.

7. Bronstein, R. D., & Schaffer, J. C. (2017). Physical examination of the knee: Meniscus, cartilage, and patellofemoral conditions. *Journal of the American Academy of Orthopedic Surgeons, 25*(5), 365–374. doi:10.5435/JAAOS-D-15-00464.

8. Cole, C. B. (2016). Patellofemoral pain syndrome. In J. A. Neumann, D. T. Kirkendall, & C. T. Moorman III (Eds.), *Sports medicine for the orthopedic resident* (1st ed., pp. 337–341). Hackensack, NJ: World Scientific.

9. Aerni, G. A., & Knapp, J. (2018). The female athlete. In C. C. Madden, M. Putukian, E. C. McCarthy, & C. C. Young (Eds.), *Netter's sports medicine* (2nd ed., pp. 77–84). Philadelphia: Elsevier.

10. Stiell, I. (1995). The Ottawa rules. Retrieved from http://www.theottawarules.ca/knee_rules. (Accessed 18 December).

11. American College of Radiology (2014). ACR Appropriateness criteria. Retrieved from https://www.acr.org/Clinical-Resources/ACR-Appropriateness-Criteria. (Accessed 11 June 2019).

12. Clark, N. C. (2015). The role of physiotherapy in rehabilitation of soft tissue injuries of the knee. *Orthopedics and Trauma, 29*(1), 48–56.

13. Nahin, R. L., Boineau, R., Khalsa, P. S., Stussman, B. J., & Weber, W. J. (2016). Evidence-based evaluation of complementary health approaches for pain management in the united states. *Mayo Clinic Proceedings, 91*(9), 1292–1306.

14. Scarpignato, C., Lanas, A., Blandizzi, C., Lems, W. F., Hermann, M., & Hunt, R. D. (2015). Safe prescribing of non-steroidal anti-inflammatory drugs in patients with osteoarthritis-an expert consensus addressing benefits as well as gastrointestinal and cardiovascular risks. *BMC Medicine, 13*(55), doi:10.1186/s12916-015-0285-8.

15. Loveless, M. S., & Fry, A. L. (2016). Pharmacologic therapies in musculoskeletal conditions. *Medical Clinics of North America, 100*(4), 869–890. http://dx.doi.org/10.1016/j.mcna.2016.03.015.

16. Gregson, C. L. (2017). Bone and joint aging. In H. M. Fillit, K. Rockwood, & J. Young (Eds.), *Brocklehurst's textbook of geriatric medicine and gerontology* (8th ed., pp. 120–126). Philadelphia: Elsevier.

CHAPTER **163**

METABOLIC BONE DISEASE: OSTEOPOROSIS AND PAGET DISEASE OF THE BONE

Roselyn Cristelle I. Mateo • Alan Ona Malabanan

OSTEOPOROSIS

DEFINITION AND EPIDEMIOLOGY

Osteoporosis is characterized by increased bone fragility and increased susceptibility to fracture. This increased bone fragility results from decreases in bone mass and deterioration of bone microarchitecture that occur as the result of estrogen deficiency and aging. A variety of diseases, such as rheumatoid arthritis, and medications, such as glucocorticoids, may contribute to bone loss. Osteoporosis is the most common metabolic bone disease; more than 9.9 million Americans are affected, and an additional 43.1 million have low bone mass and are at high risk for development of the disease. An important

responsibility of the primary care provider is the prevention, detection, and treatment of osteoporosis.[1]

Osteoporosis is also defined by the World Health Organization (WHO) as a bone mineral density (BMD) of 2.5 standard deviations (SDs) or less below the young normal mean (i.e., T-score ≤ −2.5). The International Society for Clinical Densitometry (ISCD) has recommended that this definition be applied only to postmenopausal women and men older than 50 years.[2] In the absence of osteoporotic fracture, this densitometric definition is the most clinically relevant, but it should not be used as the sole criterion for treatment decision. Much as elevated cholesterol concentration is one risk factor for heart attack, low BMD is but one risk factor for osteoporotic fracture. There is no definitive BMD threshold at which osteoporotic fractures occur, only an increasing likelihood of fracture with decreasing BMD. Other risk factors, such as increasing age, family history of hip fracture, current cigarette smoking, prior osteoporotic fracture, glucocorticoid use, rheumatoid arthritis, and excessive alcohol intake, have an impact on this fracture likelihood independent of the BMD. The National Osteoporosis Foundation guidelines recommend the use of the WHO Fracture Risk Assessment Tool (FRAX) score to guide treatment in patients who have densitometric osteopenia but are at high absolute risk for fracture.[1]

The American Association for Clinical Endocrinologists 2016 guidelines have included a bone density T score < −1.0 and > −2.5, along with a 10-year major osteoporotic fracture risk of ≥ 20% over a 10-year hip fracture risk of ≥ /3% as a sufficient criterion to diagnose osteoporosis.[3]

PATHOPHYSIOLOGY

In addition to providing a supportive and protective framework for the body, bone serves as a large calcium reservoir. Calcium is necessary for proper neural, musculoskeletal, and cardiac function. Normal bone remodeling allows both access to the calcium reservoir and replacement or repair of old and damaged bone. Bone remodeling has two main phases: bone resorption and bone formation.

Bone resorption, which releases calcium into the circulation, is the removal of damaged or old bone by osteoclasts, cells derived from macrophages and monocytes. This process is rapid and occurs in a matter of days to weeks. Osteoblasts, in response to parathyroid hormone (PTH) and other cytokines, secrete RANK (receptor activator of nuclear factor κB) ligand and monocyte colony-stimulating factor, which cause monocytes and macrophages to differentiate into osteoclasts and to proliferate. Osteoclasts produce powerful degradative enzymes, such as cathepsin K, to break down bone, releasing calcium, phosphorus, and type I collagen cross-linked products into the circulation.

Bone formation occurs when osteoblasts lay down osteoid, an organic matrix composed of type I collagen and other proteins. Bone formation, occurring over months, is a slow process. It is estimated that the skeleton is completely replaced during approximately 4 years. Osteoblasts are also responsible for mineralization of the bone, depositing calcium and phosphorus into the osteoid. This process depends on the presence of adequate amounts of calcium and phosphorus and alkaline phosphatase activity. Poor bone mineralization leads to osteomalacia, a painful softening of the bone.

Normally, bone resorption and bone formation proceed at equal rates. In osteoporosis, however, the rate of bone resorption exceeds that of bone formation, producing a net loss of bone. This uncoupling of bone resorption and bone formation is a consequence of estrogen deficiency and is most pronounced in the first 5 to 10 years after menopause.

Glucocorticoid has a pivotal role in the treatment of many inflammatory conditions, and it is the most common cause of secondary osteoporosis. It causes osteoblast death, prolongs the life of osteoclasts, decreases levels of estrogen and testosterone, increases the metabolism of vitamin D, and decreases the intestinal absorption of calcium, although the evidence supporting a strong role for PTH and hypogonadism in glucocorticoid-induced osteoporosis is lacking. This increased bone resorption and decreased bone formation lead to a rapid loss of bone, the majority of which occurs in the first 6 months of glucocorticoid use. In addition, the bone quality is impaired, leading to a rapid increase in relative risk of fracture by as much as 75% within the first 3 months after initiation of glucocorticoids.[4] Elevated daily and cumulative glucocorticoid doses both increase risk of fracture, particularly vertebral fracture, due to the greater effects of glucocorticoids on trabecular bone than on cortical bone. Other drugs, such as chronic opiates, immunosuppressants, anticonvulsants, heparin, excessive thyroid hormone, leuprolide, and cancer chemotherapeutics, lead to similar changes in bone metabolism.[5]

Risk Factors

Risk factors, both unmodifiable and modifiable, increase the risk of bone loss or osteoporotic fracture. The WHO FRAX model includes the following risk factors: advanced age, female gender, prior osteoporotic fracture (including morphometric vertebral fracture), femoral neck BMD, low body mass index, oral glucocorticoid use of 5 mg of prednisone or more per day for 3 or more months (ever), rheumatoid arthritis, secondary osteoporosis, parental history of hip fracture, current smoking, and alcohol intake of three or more drinks per day. The National Osteoporosis Foundation recommends use of these risk factors through the WHO FRAX (at www.shef.ac.uk/FRAX) to decide on treatment of densitometric osteopenia in postmenopausal women and men aged 50 years and older. There are many other risk factors not included in FRAX that may play a role in individual assessment of need for bone density testing or osteoporosis therapy (Box 163.1).

CLINICAL PRESENTATION AND PHYSICAL EXAMINATION

Unless an osteoporotic fracture is present, osteoporosis is *clinically silent*. Low BMD in the absence of osteoporotic fracture does not cause pain. If pain is present, the fracture should be confirmed or a secondary cause of the low BMD, such as osteomalacia, ruled out.

The sine qua non of osteoporosis is an osteoporotic fracture, a fracture occurring with no or minimum trauma, typically involving no more energy than a fall from standing height. The presence of a typical osteoporotic fracture in a postmenopausal woman is usually sufficient for the diagnosis of osteoporosis. The typical sites of fractures include the vertebrae, the distal wrist, the proximal femur, and the ribs. Unfortunately, even in the presence of a typical osteoporotic fracture, the diagnosis of osteoporosis is often missed and treatment never initiated. Osteoporosis occurring in men and premenopausal or perimenopausal women should lead to a consideration of secondary causes of osteoporosis.

BOX 163.1

Risk Factors for Bone Loss or Osteoporotic Fracture

UNMODIFIABLE

- Advanced age[a]
- Female gender[a]
- White or Asian race
- Personal history of fracture[a]
- History of fracture in a first-degree relative[a]
- Dementia

MODIFIABLE

- Hypogonadism
- Current cigarette smoking[a]
- Excessive alcohol[a] or caffeine use
- Low calcium intake
- Low body weight (<58 kg [127 lb])[a]
- Inadequate physical activity
- Visual impairment
- Glucocorticoid[a] or anticonvulsant use
- Thyrotoxicosis
- Recurrent falls
- Poor health or frailty

[a]Included in fracture risk assessment tool (FRAX) calculations.

Severe or established osteoporosis, that is, osteoporosis with fractures, is readily identifiable. The dowager's hump is a thoracic spine kyphosis that occurs with multiple vertebral compression fractures. Vertebral compression fractures may also lead to scoliosis and height loss. In epidemiologic studies, a rib-pelvis distance less than 2 fingerbreadths, a wall-occiput distance greater than 0 cm and suggest the presence of occult spinal fracture.[6] A 7th cervical vertebra wall distance (C7WD) of at least 9.5 cm has been found to be a practical, valid, and reliable measure of the risk of vertebral fracture in the elderly among different raters including a health professional, health volunteer, and caregiver.[7]

The physical examination in osteoporosis should be directed toward finding signs of secondary osteoporosis. Band keratopathy may suggest a diagnosis of primary hyperparathyroidism. Exophthalmos or lid lag, goiter, tremor, warm moist skin, weight loss, or pretibial myxedema may indicate a diagnosis of hyperthyroidism. Dorsal fat, facial plethora, supraclavicular fat, hypertension, centripetal obesity, proximal muscle weakness, edema, or violaceous abdominal striae may suggest a diagnosis of Cushing syndrome. Gynecomastia, decreased facial or axillary hair, and testicular atrophy may suggest hypogonadism. Blue sclera or dentition as well as joint hypermobility may suggest a diagnosis of osteogenesis imperfecta. Dermatitis herpetiformis may suggest a diagnosis of celiac disease.

Fall risk should be assessed in each patient with osteoporosis. Lower extremity strength, balance, gait, and postural reflexes should be carefully assessed. Poor visual acuity, weak grip strength, difficulty rising from a chair, Romberg sign, excessive body sway, and unsteady gait may all be signs of increased fall risk that may benefit from evaluation by a physical therapist or in a specialty fall clinic.

DIAGNOSTICS

A testing strategy that includes serum 25-hydroxyvitamin D, calcium, PTH, creatinine/estimated glomerular filtration rate (eGFR), and TSH for all patients including men has been suggested as cost-effective in identifying 94% of secondary causes of falls and fractures among 739 attendees of an Australian Falls and Fractures Clinic.[8]

Vitamin D deficiency is common among women with osteoporosis.[9] Guidelines from the Institute of Medicine have supported a serum 25-hydroxyvitamin D level of 20 ng/mL as the threshold for vitamin D sufficiency for the general population,[10] although the Endocrine Society guidelines support a threshold of 30 ng/mL for individual patients without a history of Sarcoidosis. Sarcoidosis patients are susceptible to a vitamin D toxicity, with hypercalciuria and hypercalcemia, and should be monitored closely.[11]

Biochemical markers are urine and blood tests that measure breakdown products of bone and collagen. A biochemical marker is an indirect measurement of bone turnover (i.e., bone resorption and formation). Bone resorption markers (N-telopeptides and C-telopeptides CTX) are used to evaluate osteoclast activity, and bone formation markers (bone-specific alkaline phosphatase, osteocalcin, procollagen I extension peptides) are used to evaluate osteoblast activity. High levels imply increased bone turnover. At this time, the role of bone markers in primary care is unclear, although specialists may use them. Bone resorption markers help identify response to antiresorptive drug treatment and conversely predict risk for bone loss and fracture. Six-month intervals are the usual frequency for testing of bone markers.

Plain radiographs are useful primarily in confirming the presence of fracture. They are insensitive to decreases in bone mass. In the absence of fracture, the definitive method for diagnosis of osteoporosis is bone densitometry, by dual energy x-ray absorptiometry, of the hip and posteroanterior lumbar spine. The wrist may be used in very obese patients, uninterpretable hip and spine scans, and primary hyperparathyroidism. Indications for bone densitometry are listed in Box 163.2. Bone density assessment of other sites, such as the finger, wrist, and ankle, and the use of other technologies, such as ultrasonography, are useful in diagnosis of osteoporosis and predicting fracture risk (particularly in adults older than 65 years) but may not be as useful in ruling out osteoporosis.

Trabecular bone score (TBS) may be available from some bone density services. TBS is derived from the lumbar spine bone density image and assesses the heterogeneity of the image pixels, reflecting differences in microarchitecture for a given bone density. TBS is associated with fracture risk independent of the bone density and may be useful in evaluating fracture risk in specific patient populations, such as chronic glucocorticoid use, type 2 diabetes mellitus, chronic kidney disease, primary hyperparathyroidism, and aromatase inhibitors. TBS can be entered into the FRAX calculator.[12]

Vertebral fracture assessment, which may be obtained from some bone density services, offers information like that of thoracic and lumbar spine radiography, with much less radiation exposure. The presence of a vertebral compression fracture, which may be asymptomatic, in the setting of osteopenia is sufficient for the clinical diagnosis of osteoporosis, particularly in the absence of or with minimal trauma. The ISCD recommends this testing when the T-score is below −1.0 and one or

more of the following is present: women age 70 years or older; men age 80 years or older; historical height loss of greater than 1.5 inches; self-reported but undocumented prior vertebral fracture; and glucocorticoids therapy equivalent to 5 mg of prednisone or more or the equivalent per day for 3 months or longer.[13]

Bone densitometry provides three pertinent numbers. The first is the actual area density in grams per centimeters squared. This density is then compared with the reference database for young normal adults and age-matched adults. This comparison results in a T-score and a Z-score, respectively. The T-score is

---

BOX 163.2

USPSTF Indications for Bone Densitometry

Population	Recommendation	Grade
Women 65 years and older	The USPSTF recommends screening for osteoporosis with bone measurement testing to prevent osteoporotic fractures in women 65 years and older.	B
Postmenopausal women younger than 65 years at increased risk of osteoporosis	The USPSTF recommends screening for osteoporosis with bone measurement testing to prevent osteoporotic fractures in postmenopausal women younger than 65 years who are at increased risk of osteoporosis, as determined by a formal clinical risk assessment tool. See the risk factor section for information on risk assessment.	B
Men	The USPSTF concludes that the current evidence is insufficient to assess the balance of benefits and harms of screening for osteoporosis to prevent osteoporotic fractures in men.	I

From US Preventive Services Task Force. (2018). Screening for Osteoporosis to Prevent Fractures. https://www.uspreventiveservicestaskforce.org/Page/Document/RecommendationStatementFinal/osteoporosis-screening1.

INITIAL DIAGNOSTICS

Osteoporosis

LABORATORY
- Serum calcium with albumin
- Serum phosphorus
- 25-Hydroxyvitamin D
- Intact PTH
- TSH
- Serum and urine protein electrophoresis[a]
- 24-Hour urine calcium
- 24-Hour urine free cortisol[a]
- Urinary N-telopeptides, serum C-telopeptides[a]
- Serum testosterone
- Tissue transglutaminase antibody[a]
- LFTs (including alkaline phosphatase)

ADDITIONAL DIAGNOSTICS
- CBC and differential
- Serum electrolytes
- BUN and creatinine

IMAGING
- Bone densitometry

Additional Imaging
- Bone scan[a]
- X-ray studies[a]
- CT[a]
- MRI[a]

INVASIVE TESTING
- Bone biopsy[a]

---
[a]If indicated.
CT, computed tomography; MRI, magnetic resonance imaging.

used in diagnosis of osteopenia (T score < −1.0 and > −2.5) and osteoporosis (≤−2.5). The Z-score is ignored unless it is less than −2.0 or the patient is a premenopausal woman or man younger than 50 years, and then it is preferentially used.

Only bone densitometry of the posteroanterior lumbar spine and hip is recommended for monitoring of osteoporosis treatment efficacy, and it is generally performed at 1- to 2-year intervals, depending on the precision of the scan. In general, a 5% density change is considered significant and not caused by measurement statistical variation, but each bone density service should determine its least significant change, as recommended by the ISCD.[2] Some disease states, such as chronic glucocorticoid therapy and paraplegia, may lead to faster bone density changes. In these cases, assessment of bone density every 6 months to 1 year may be justified.

DIFFERENTIAL DIAGNOSIS

Osteoporosis is classified as primary or secondary. Primary osteoporosis includes bone loss arising from menopausal estrogen deficiency or aging. Secondary osteoporosis results from an acquired or inherited disease that interferes with bone remodeling or increases bone turnover.

Postmenopausal osteoporosis should be distinguished from secondary causes of osteoporosis (Box 163.3). Secondary causes of osteoporosis may be reversible prompting bone density increases greater than what is expected from osteoporosis medications. Suspicion of secondary causes of osteoporosis should be high in premenopausal and perimenopausal women, men, those with bone density Z-scores of less than −2.0, and those with bone pain in the absence of fracture.

BOX 163.3

Secondary Causes of Low Bone Mass

ENDOCRINE DISEASES
Diabetes mellitus
Growth hormone deficiency
Acromegaly
Hypercortisolism
Hyperparathyroidism
Hyperthyroidism
Premature menopause
Male hypogonadism
Hyperprolactinemia
Athletic amenorrhea
Turner and Klinefelter syndromes

GASTROINTESTINAL DISORDERS
Gastrectomy
Celiac disease
Inflammatory bowel disease
Liver cirrhosis
Chronic biliary tract obstruction
Chronic therapy with proton pump inhibitors
Cystic fibrosis
Malabsorption
Primary biliary cirrhosis

HEMATOLOGIC DISEASES
Myeloma
Monoclonal gammopathy of undetermined significance
Lymphoma, leukemia
Systemic mastocytosis
Disseminated carcinoma
Chemotherapy
Gaucher disease
Glycogen storage diseases
Porphyria
Hemochromatosis
Sickle cell disease
Thalassemia
Hemophilia

RHEUMATOLOGIC DISEASES
Rheumatoid arthritis
Ankylosing spondylitis
Systemic lupus erythematosus

CONNECTIVE TISSUE DISEASES
Osteogenesis imperfecta
Marfan syndrome
Ehlers-Danlos syndrome
Pseudoxanthoma elasticum
Homocystinuria

OTHER CAUSES
Anorexia nervosa
End-stage renal disease
Chronic metabolic acidosis
Multiple sclerosis
Sarcoidosis
Muscular dystrophy
Parental nutrition

DRUGS
Glucocorticoids
Heparin
Cyclosporine and tacrolimus
Anticonvulsants
Cancer chemotherapeutic drugs
Gonadotropin-releasing hormone analogues
Lithium
Methotrexate
Cigarette smoking
Excessive alcohol use
Excessive thyroxine
Chronic opiate use
Premenopausal tamoxifen use

Data from Cosman F, de Beur SJ, LeBoff MS, et al. (2014). Clinician's guide to prevention and treatment of osteoporosis. *Osteoporosis International, 25*(10), 2359–2381; and Hofbauer LC, Hamann C, Ebeling PR. (2010). Approach to the patient with secondary osteoporosis, *European Journal of Endocrinology, 162*, 1009–1020.

The presence of a fragility fracture in the absence of low bone density should raise the concern of localized bone destruction, as with metastatic disease, plasmacytoma, or radiation osteitis. Thoracic spine fractures caused by metastasis are more likely when they involve vertebrae above T7. Less common metabolic bone diseases, such as Paget disease and osteopetrosis, also may lead to pathologic fractures, despite normal or even high bone density. Further testing, which can include computed tomography (CT) scanning, magnetic resonance imaging (MRI), nuclear medicine bone scanning, or even tetracycline-labeled bone biopsy, may be indicated.

INTERPROFESSIONAL COLLABORATIVE MANAGEMENT

Co-management depends on each patient's needs. Fracture management and pain control are the primary reasons for referral. Referrals may also be made to the following specialists:

- *Endocrinologists or rheumatologists* specializing in metabolic bone disease for patients with persistent fractures, patients with secondary osteoporosis, premenopausal women or children with osteoporosis, or those with osteoporosis who are intolerant of FDA-approved therapies
- *Pain specialist* to manage escalating chronic pain associated with debilitating bone and muscle changes associated with fractures
- *Physical therapist* for management of exercise for osteoporosis, spinal and posture strengthening, pain management, and fall and fracture prevention
- *Nutritionist* for balanced diet guidelines regarding calcium and vitamin D intake appropriate for the individual's age and activity level
- *Orthopedic surgeon* for surgical correction of bone fractures or consideration of bone biopsy
- *Interventional radiologist* for vertebroplasty or kyphoplasty for painful vertebral fractures

Nonpharmacologic Management

Much of the bone loss of osteoporosis is irreversible, and prevention should be the major focus of health care providers. Ideally, efforts at preventing osteoporosis should begin before puberty and should consist of adequate calcium and vitamin D intake, adequate weight-bearing exercise, and maintenance of normal body weight. Avoidance of cigarette smoking and excessive alcohol intake should be stressed. These preventive efforts are also recommended in adults and in those in whom osteoporosis has already developed.

In 2011, the Institute of Medicine updated its recommended daily allowance (RDA) for calcium and vitamin D targeting a serum 25-hydroxyvitamin D level of 20 ng/mL (50 nmol/L). The RDA of calcium for all adults aged 19 to 50 years is 1000 mg daily; for men 51 to 70 years, 1000 mg daily; and for men older than 70 years as well as women aged 51 years and older, 1200 mg daily. The RDA for vitamin D for adults aged 19 to 70 years is 600 IU daily and for those older than 70 years, 800 IU daily.[10] The Endocrine Society has supported these guidelines but recognizes that some patients may need at least 1500 to 2000 IU daily to maintain their 25-hydroxyvitamin D levels above 30 ng/mL depending on individual health outcome concerns, age, body weight, latitude of residence, dietary and cultural habits; obese patients, those with malabsorption, and those taking medications affecting the metabolism of vitamin D require 3000 to 6000 IU daily. There is, however,

no clear consensus regarding optimal doses of these supplements for everyone. Patients taking higher supplement doses need to be monitored for hypercalcemia and kidney stones. Sarcoidosis patients, due to hypercalciuria and hypercalcemia, may need less.[11]

Regarding vitamin D deficiency, a variety of regimens for vitamin D correction are available, but the greatest success in achieving a 25-hydroxyvitamin D level of 30 ng/mL appears to be linked to a total intake of at least 600,000 IU (i.e., 50,000 IU of vitamin D_2 twice times weekly for 4 weeks).[14] A regimen of 50,000 IU of vitamin D_2 every other week appears to be safe and effective with up to 6 years of therapy.[15] However, there have been concerns that annual or intermittent high-dose vitamin D regimens may increase the risk of falling.[16]

Prior studies have raised concerns about an increased risk of cardiovascular events in women taking calcium or calcium–vitamin D supplements, although recent work has not supported this.[17-19]

Bone is a dynamic tissue that adapts to loading (i.e., weight-bearing exercise) with hypertrophy and increased strength. Exercise is an important part of any osteoporosis therapy, but it is most effective when it is used in a preventive capacity, particularly in children and adolescents. Unloading of the skeleton, as occurs with bed rest, space flight, and spinal cord injury, results in dramatic decrements in bone mass. Conversely, weight-bearing exercise and weight training may modestly increase bone density, and their effects are dependent on estrogen status. Exercise alone has not been shown to prevent early menopausal bone loss. A Cochrane meta-analysis found a slight benefit of exercise for bone density and fracture risk (number needed to treat to prevent one fracture was 25) for postmenopausal women. The most effective exercise for femoral neck bone density is non–weight-bearing, high-force exercise such as progressive resistance strength training for the lower limbs, and for the spine bone density is a combination exercise program.[20] A multicomponent exercise program, directed at balance, resistance training, and aerobic exercise, can reduce fall risk in older adults with osteoporosis and osteoporotic vertebral fracture.[21]

Exercise regimens, such as weight-bearing and muscle-strengthening exercise, can reduce the risk of falls and fractures and improve agility, strength, posture, and balance, as well as modestly increase bone density. The National Osteoporosis Foundation (NOF) strongly endorses lifelong physical activity at all ages, and the benefits of exercise are lost when people stop exercising.[1] Weight-bearing exercise, wherein bones and muscles work against gravity as the feet and legs bear the body's weight, includes walking, jogging, Tai Chi, stair climbing, dancing, and tennis. On the other hand, muscle-strengthening exercise includes weight training and other resistive exercises, such as yoga, Pilates, and boot camp programs.[21]

The Lifting Intervention For Training Muscle and Osteoporosis Rehabilitation Trial (LIFTMOR) showed that high-intensity supervised resistance training in post-menopausal osteopenic women improved hip and lumbar spine BMD, all physical performance measures, and even prevented height loss.[22] In contrast, a randomized trial showed that BMD loss is greatest in dieting older adults who perform aerobic exercise, while resistance training maintains bone and muscle mass as well as strength.[23]

Exercises to be avoided include high-impact loading, abrupt or explosive movements, resistive trunk flexion, twisting movements, and dynamic abdominal exercises. Referral to a physical therapist for guided exercise may be helpful.[24]

Walking is a good exercise. For women of average weight (143 pounds), walking 4892 steps daily at 2.2 mph is sufficient to maintain femoral neck bone density. Lighter women require more steps (18,568 steps daily at 115.5 pounds), and heavier women require fewer steps (1638 steps daily at 173.1 pounds). Walking faster requires fewer steps, and walking more slowly requires more steps.[1]

Hip protector pads have been shown in some studies to prevent hip fractures from falls, particularly in those with a fall history and low body mass index.[25] Noncompliance with hip protector pads may limit their efficacy. A Cochrane database review showed hip protectors probably reduce the risk of hip fractures if made available to older people in nursing care or residential care settings, without increasing the frequency of falls but may slightly increase the small risk of pelvic fractures. An enhanced understanding may influence acceptance and adherence.[26] A meta-analysis by Sawka and colleagues[27] did not find evidence for significant hip fracture prevention in relatively low-risk community-dwelling populations, however.

In those with osteoporosis, preventive measures of calcium, vitamin D, and exercise alone are not sufficient to prevent osteoporotic fracture. For those with densitometric osteoporosis (T-score < −2.5), those with densitometric osteopenia (T-score < −1.0 and > −2.5) with multiple risk factors, and particularly those who already have osteoporotic fracture, pharmacologic therapy is imperative. The National Osteoporosis Foundation 2014 guidelines, which apply to postmenopausal women and men older than 50 years, recommend treatment for those with T-scores of −2.5 or lower at the femoral neck or the spine, those with typical fragility fractures, and those with a T-score that is higher than −2.5 and lower than −1.0 (i.e., osteopenia) with a FRAX score of 20% or higher for major osteoporotic fracture risk and 3% or higher for hip fracture risk. The FRAX calculator is accessible at www.shef.ac.uk/FRAX. The FRAX model has limitations in that it does not include lumbar spine or wrist T-score or fall risk. All therapies should be reevaluated for risk/benefit ratio of ongoing treatment, and no pharmacologic therapy should be considered indefinite in duration.[1]

The only FDA-approved agents at this time that have been proved in prospective studies to prevent both vertebral and nonvertebral fractures are the bisphosphonates (alendronate, risedronate, zoledronic acid), teriparatide, and denosumab. Bisphosphonates, which are synthetic analogues of pyrophosphate, reduce bone resorption and bone loss by binding to bone and poisoning active osteoclasts. Four bisphosphonates are currently approved by the FDA for the prevention and treatment of postmenopausal osteoporosis: alendronate, risedronate, ibandronate, and zoledronic acid. Alendronate (Fosamax), risedronate (Actonel), and zoledronic acid (Reclast) are also approved for use in glucocorticoid-induced osteoporosis. Alendronate, risedronate, and zoledronic acid are approved for increasing bone mass in men as well as for treatment of glucocorticoid-induced osteoporosis. Risedronate and zoledronic acid are also indicated in the prevention of glucocorticoid-induced osteoporosis.

Studies with these agents have shown yearly bone density increases of 2% to 3% at the lumbar spine, which is the skeletal site most responsive to these agents. Contraindications to bisphosphonates include disorders of esophageal motility or

active gastroesophageal bleeding (for oral bisphosphonates), hypocalcemia, untreated vitamin D deficiency, and renal disease (creatinine clearance < 35 mL/min). There have been concerns about the risk of esophageal cancer with oral bisphosphonates,[28] although recent studies and metanalyses have not presented compelling evidence of a significantly raised risk of esophageal cancer or gastric cancer in male and female patients prescribed bisphosphonates.[29-32] The presence of Barrett esophagus would be a relative contraindication.

Oral bisphosphonates should be taken on an empty stomach, with 6 to 8 ounces of water, and 30 minutes before eating (60 minutes for ibandronate), taking other medications, or lying down. Taking bisphosphonates with food or coffee will reduce their absorption and potentially eliminate their benefit. To decrease gastrointestinal effects, it is important that patients be given explicit instructions on proper administration, because esophagitis can be a problem.

Bisphosphonates are potent antiresorptive agents and may potentially oversuppress bone turnover. Bisphosphonate-related osteonecrosis of the jaw is defined as exposed bone in the maxillofacial region for more than 8 weeks associated with current or previous bisphosphonate therapy, in the absence of radiation therapy to the jaw. It is rare in patients treated with bisphosphonates for osteoporosis, with a wide range of estimates from 1 in 1700 to 1 in 263,000. The cumulative incidence in cancer patients treated with high-dose potent intravenous bisphosphonates, such as pamidronate and zoledronic acid, is much higher at 0.8% to 12%. There is a higher risk with longer duration of action, increasing age, and dentoalveolar surgery including dental extraction, dental implant placement, periapical surgery, and periodontal surgery involving alveolar bone injury.[33] Good dental hygiene should be maintained during bisphosphonate therapy, and patients should be informed of the low but present risk. Development of osteonecrosis of the jaw may involve cessation of the bisphosphonate, but providers should also consider the increased risk of fractures that may result. Serum CTX, a marker of bone resorption, has earlier been suggested as a test to assess risk for osteonecrosis of the jaw[34]; however, more recent systematic reviews showed no predictive value.[35]

Denosumab use has also been associated with osteonecrosis of the jaw. Teriparatide may have a role in the treatment of osteonecrosis of the jaw.[36]

The American Association of Oral and Maxillofacial Surgeons has recently updated its guidelines for medication-related osteonecrosis of the jaw. The Association recognizes a very low risk for the problem, at a rate of 0.1% but increasing to 0.21% when patients have been on bisphosphonate treatment for longer than 4 years. The guidelines recommend pretreatment dental evaluation and care, which may decrease the risk of osteonecrosis of the jaw by 50%. For patients on long-term therapy, the recommendation is for consideration of a 2-month drug holiday before an invasive dental procedure. The guidelines do not offer any recommendations for denosumab therapy.[33]

Cases of unusual fractures, including subtrochanteric hip fractures and femoral shaft fractures, occurring with long-term bisphosphonate therapy and associated with low bone turnover have also been described. These fractures are typically associated with minimal if any trauma and characterized by simple transverse or oblique (<30 degrees) fracture with cortical breaking, diffuse cortical thickening, delayed healing, and evidence of stress reaction or fracture on the contralateral side. They are often preceded by prodromal thigh or groin pain for weeks to months before fracture. There is increased risk with concomitant glucocorticoid use.[37] An analysis of alendronate and zoledronic acid therapy data suggest a rate of 2.3 subtrochanteric or diaphyseal fractures per 10,000 patient-years of bisphosphonate treatment, which would also be associated with a prevention of 100 fractures.[38] Patients receiving long-term bisphosphonate therapy should be made aware of this rare complication and should be evaluated promptly if they develop unexplained groin or thigh pain. Consideration of cessation of bisphosphonates and switching to other osteoporosis therapies may be considered after 5 years of therapy for those at moderate risk for osteoporotic fracture and after 10 years of therapy for those at high risk. Bisphosphonates should be avoided in those at low risk for osteoporotic fracture.[39] Some bone density services have single-energy femur imaging, which may detect atypical femoral fracture before fracture completion.[40]

Raloxifene (Evista) is FDA approved for postmenopausal osteoporosis prevention and treatment at a dose of 60 mg/day. Raloxifene, a selective estrogen receptor modulator, acts as an estrogen receptor agonist on the skeleton but as an antagonist on breast and uterine tissue. Raloxifene has been shown to produce roughly a 1.5% to 3% increase in spine and femoral neck density after 3 years, with a 30% reduction in new vertebral fractures. No reduction in nonvertebral fractures has been shown. There is an increased relative risk of venous thromboembolic disease, fatal stroke, hot flashes, and leg cramps with raloxifene, and a patient's individual risk for these conditions should be considered carefully. Raloxifene is as effective as tamoxifen in preventing invasive breast cancer, with fewer thromboembolic events and cataracts, and is now indicated in reducing the risk for invasive breast cancer.[41]

Hormone replacement is FDA approved only for the prevention of osteoporosis, not for its treatment. Estrogen inhibits bone resorption, decreases bone remodeling, and enhances absorption of calcium. There are good data showing prevention of both vertebral and nonvertebral fractures in postmenopausal women but not in those with osteoporosis.[42] Low-dose and transdermal hormone therapy are less likely associated with the adverse effects of breast cancer, endometrial hyperplasia, coronary artery disease, and venous thromboembolism previously observed in standard-dose oral HT regimens and should be considered for the primary prevention and treatment of osteoporosis in appropriate candidates and individualized. A combination of conjugated estrogens and bazedoxifene acetate (a selective estrogen receptor modulator) has been approved for the treatment of moderate to severe menopausal vasomotor symptoms and prevention of osteoporosis.[43] However, recently published guidelines from the American College of Physicians recommends against the use of estrogen for the treatment of osteoporosis.[43a] However, recently published guidelines from the American College of Physicians recommends against the use of estrogen for the treatment of osteoporosis.[43a]

Contraindications to the use of estrogen include undiagnosed vaginal bleeding, pregnancy, active thrombosis or thrombophlebitis, active liver disease, endometrial adenocarcinoma, breast cancer, and other estrogen-dependent tumors. Caution should be exercised with a medical diagnosis of endometriosis, uterine leiomyoma, gallbladder disease, or migraine headaches; a family history of breast cancer; or a history of thrombophlebitis. Once estrogen therapy is stopped, bone loss resumes at the same rate as in untreated women. With long-term use of estrogen, those at risk for breast cancer and those with a history of uncomfortable side effects should be monitored closely.

Subcutaneous PTH is an anabolic bone agent. Anabolic agents stimulate bone formation and increase bone remodeling rates. Intermittent PTH administration shows an anabolic effect, increasing bone mass, whereas continuous PTH administration leads to bone loss as in primary hyperparathyroidism. Teriparatide (Forteo), a PTH analogue (PTH 1-34), was the first anabolic agent to be approved for treatment of osteoporosis in 2002. It is administered subcutaneously and has been shown to increase bone density at the hip and spine by 2% and 8%, respectively, after 1 year of therapy, in postmenopausal women[44] and in both men and women receiving glucocorticoid therapy. It has been shown to decrease vertebral fractures by approximately 65% and nonvertebral fractures by 35%. It appears more effective than alendronate in treating glucocorticoid-induced osteoporosis.[45] It is contraindicated in those with hypercalcemia and those at increased risk for osteosarcoma (those with radiotherapy of bone, Paget disease, unexplained elevations of alkaline phosphatase, and open epiphyseal growth plates) because teriparatide use increased the risk of osteosarcoma in animals. It is approved for 2 years of use, and there is a rapid loss of bone density gains after cessation. Alendronate therapy after PTH use helps maintain and increase bone density.[46] Retreatment with PTH after alendronate therapy may provide additional bone density gains.[47]

Abaloparatide (Tymlos) is another FDA-approved anabolic osteoporosis treatment that is a PTH-related peptide analog (1-34). It is given daily as a subcutaneous injection. It binds to the same PTH-1 receptor that teriparatide does but produces less bone resorption and less bone formation, leading to less hypercalcemia and hypercalciuria. In the Abaloparatide Comparator Trial In Vertebral Endpoints (ACTIVE) trial, after 18 months there was an absolute vertebral fracture risk reduction of 3.64% over placebo compared to teriparatide's 3.38%. In addition, there was an absolute nonvertebral fracture risk reduction of 2.0% over placebo. Bone density improvements were greater for abaloparatide than teriparatide at the femoral neck and total hip at all time points and at the lumbar spine at 6 and 12 months, but not at 18. Adverse effects included nausea, dizziness, headache, and palpitations.[48] Following 18 months of abaloparatide, alendronate 70 mg weekly maintained bone density gains and fracture risk reduction for at least 6 months.[49]

Romosozumab (Evenity) is an anabolic osteoporosis medication that is an antibody directed at sclerostin, an inhibitor of bone formation. It is administered as a monthly subcutaneous injection and is superior to teriparatide and alendronate regarding BMD increases at the lumbar spine, total hip, and femoral neck.[50] In the Fracture Study in Postmenopausal Women with Osteoporosis (FRAME), 12 months of romosozumab showed an absolute vertebral fracture risk reduction of 1.3% over placebo and no significant reduction in nonvertebral fractures. After transitioning to denosumab, the romosozumab group showed an absolute 1.9% vertebral fracture risk reduction at 24 months. Adverse effects in the romosozumab group included mild injection site reactions, osteonecrosis of the jaw, and atypical femoral fracture.[51]

In the Active-Controlled Fracture Study in Postmenopausal Women with Osteoporosis at High Risk (ARCH) trial, 4093 postmenopausal women were randomized to monthly subcutaneous romosozumab or weekly oral alendronate for 1 year, followed by 2 years of alendronate in both groups. Results showed that after 12 months, romosozumab reduced the risk of vertebral fractures, and in 24 months thereafter, the risk of new vertebral fractures was reduced by 48% ($P < .001$). Nonvertebral and hip fractures were also reduced in the romosozumab-to-alendronate versus the alendronate-alendronate group.[45] Another trial of romosozumab versus teriparatide in prior oral bisphosphonate users showed superior BMD increases at the lumbar spine and hip with sclerostin inhibition.[52] The US Food and Drug Administration is currently deciding on the regulatory application of Romosozumab while cardiovascular safety data are being collected.

Calcitonin is a peptide hormone that appears to slow bone loss and temporarily increase vertebral bone mass by decreasing osteoclastic activity. The drug's effect is more pronounced on trabecular bone. The nasal spray produces a 3% increase in vertebral bone only and is not as effective as estrogen and alendronate in forming new bone. Drug delivery is by injection or nasal spray; the recommended dose is 50 to 100 units/day three times per week for the injection and 200 units/day, alternating nostrils, for the nasal spray. It is FDA approved for use in postmenopausal women (>5 years postmenopause) with osteoporosis. Supplementation with calcium and vitamin D enhances therapy. Most osteoporosis experts do not advise the use of calcitonin therapy alone in treating established osteoporosis due to lack of a robust effect as well as concerns about cancer risk.

Denosumab (Prolia) is a monoclonal antibody that inhibits RANK ligand and potently reduces bone resorption. It is given subcutaneously at a dose of 60 mg every 6 months. It has been shown to decrease vertebral and nonvertebral fracture and is approved for use in postmenopausal women with osteoporosis. It is contraindicated in patients with hypocalcemia. Adverse reactions are serious infections including skin infections, eczema and dermatitis, hypocalcemia (especially in patients with renal insufficiency), osteonecrosis of the jaw, and significant suppression of bone turnover.[53] Cessation of therapy leads to rapid loss of action and bone density gains, and the drug is not cleared by the kidney. There is a risk of multiple vertebral fractures usually 8 to 16 months after the last denosumab subcutaneous injection.[54] The 10-year extension of the FREEDOM trial showed that denosumab continued to increase BMD over one decade of therapy.[55]

Combinations of therapies (e.g., bisphosphonates and estrogen, PTH and estrogen, and PTH and bisphosphonates) may have additive effects on bone density increases. It is not clear whether these bone density increases are associated with decreased fracture risk, and there may be additive effects on suppression of bone resorption. Studies of combination PTH and alendronate have shown no advantage over PTH alone. Sequential use of PTH first, followed by alendronate, appears to produce the best bone density increases.[56,57] This effect has also been seen in PTH combined with raloxifene.[58]

Work from the Denosumab and Teriparatide Administration Study (DATA) showed that the combination of denosumab and teriparatide produces additive gains, with a 9.1% spine density increase and a 4.9% total hip density gain after 12 months of therapy.[59] After 24 months, there was a 12.9% spine density increase and 6.8% total hip density increase.[60] In results from the DATA-Switch trial, sequential treatment with combination teriparatide and denosumab for 18 months followed by denosumab produced the greatest bone density gains—15.0% at the spine and 7.1% at the total hip.[61] Whether the improvement in bone density gains translates to fewer fractures remains to be established, and the expense may be a significant obstacle.

LIFE SPAN CONSIDERATIONS

Osteoporotic fractures, especially those of the hip, are associated with increased morbidity and increased mortality. In the first year after hip fracture, there is a 10% to 20% excess mortality. Mortality rates in men with hip fracture are higher because of comorbid conditions. In women with vertebral fractures, those with one or more fractures had a 1.23-fold greater age-adjusted mortality rate, with mortality increasing with greater numbers of vertebral fractures.

COMPLICATIONS

Eighty-four percent of those with clinically diagnosed vertebral compression fractures report having pain. The acute pain of vertebral fracture usually lasts between 2 weeks and 3 months. Chronic back pain from spinal changes, microfractures, and muscle spasms can develop. Patients may develop reduced exercise tolerance and pulmonary reserve. Abdominal protuberance because of loss of height at the lumbar spine may lead to early satiety and resultant weight loss. There is a loss of self-esteem and a distortion of body image.

Altered activity or inability to participate in activities of daily living because of pain may persist for a much longer period. In these patients, bed rest and decreased activity for a few days are warranted. The individual should be instructed in proper positioning, either lying supine or side lying with pillows positioned under the knees or between the knees. Medications for pain, such as muscle relaxants for spasms, nonsteroidals (cyclooxygenase 1 and 2 inhibitors), and acetaminophen for pain and inflammation, should be prescribed as needed. Narcotics should be used sparingly because of the potential for addiction and associated fall risk. Studies indicate that the use of both calcitonin and bisphosphonates is effective at reducing pain associated with osteoporotic compression fractures, not only by reducing the risk of fracture but also with a direct effect on bone pain.[62]

Moist heat or ice may help with pain relief. Moist heat is generally recommended for muscle spasms, and ice is recommended for bone inflammation or pain. The individual in acute pain may need to use a cane or walker to walk safely. Short-term use of a spinal support may be beneficial Also available is a posture training support designed to pull the shoulders back with weights as the muscles become stronger.

Chronic pain management may be enhanced with physical therapy. Modalities include transcutaneous electrical nerve stimulation, electrical muscle stimulation, ultrasound with healed fractures, iontophoresis, and heat or ice. Manual therapy, including joint mobilization, muscle energy techniques, myofascial release, and strain-counterstrain on trigger points in muscle, is beneficial in mobilizing soft tissue and improving muscle imbalance of the spine.

Vertebroplasty and kyphoplasty are minimally invasive techniques in which polymethyl methacrylate (PMMA) cement is injected into the fractured vertebra, thereby stabilizing it. The two techniques differ in that vertebroplasty uses a high-pressure injection system and kyphoplasty uses a balloon to expand the collapsed vertebra to produce a space for the PMMA. Vertebroplasty has a reported rate of success in pain relief and earlier functional mobility when compared to medical management.[63] Kyphoplasty has the added benefit of significantly increasing vertebral height. Complication rates are low and include radiculopathy and cord compression. Cement leakage is common, particularly in vertebroplasty. This appears to be an effective therapy for pain relief of vertebral fractures, especially when performed < 6 weeks after fracture.

PATIENT AND FAMILY EDUCATION

Patient education is essential for the prevention and treatment of fractures. Education encompasses nutrition, psychosocial issues, risk factor modification, proper body mechanics and positioning, safety, and fall prevention. Most accidents occur in the home and are related to poor vision, decreased hearing, slowed reflexes, impaired mental status, limited spinal flexibility, decreased lower extremity strength, and unsteady gait. These factors, coupled with decreased muscle and fat mass to cushion the fall, place the individual at jeopardy for injury. Education of individuals prepares them to take an active role in their care (see Chapter 13). Family members should be informed of their risk of osteoporosis and encouraged to take preventive measures. Other educational resources can be accessed at the National Osteoporosis Foundation website at www.nof.org. Osteoporosis Canada has an exercise program called "Too Fit to Fracture" with an e-book and videos available at osteoporosis.ca/health-care-professionals/clinical-practice-guidelines/exercise-recommendations/.

PAGET DISEASE OF BONE

DEFINITION AND EPIDEMIOLOGY

Paget disease is the second most common metabolic bone disease in older adults.

Paget disease is uncommon before the age of 40 years; however, by the age of 80 years, 1 in 10 persons are affected by the disease. Between 18% and 25% of the US population have at least one family member with Paget disease. The most frequent genetic mutation linked to Paget disease is in the *SQSTM1* gene, found in 30% of patients with familial Paget disease, which may produce a more severe clinical picture. There has been some evidence supporting an etiologic role of paramyxoviruses and the measles viruses. Paget disease is common in people of British descent as well as in British migrants to countries like England, Western Europe, New Zealand, Australia, and the United States; it is uncommon in populations of non-European descent, though there are only a few prevalence studies undertaken outside North America, Australasia, or Europe.[64]

PATHOPHYSIOLOGY

Paget disease is characterized by a localized increase in bone turnover and blood flow. It can affect one or more sites (monostotic versus polyostotic). Once the disease is fully established, previously unaffected bones are usually spared. For reasons that are still not well understood, osteoclasts in the affected area are increased in number, size, and activity and cause breakdown of focal areas of bone at great speed. The osteoblasts, which are unaffected by the disease process, try to keep up with the bone degradation by laying down new osteoid as fast as they can. However, the newly formed bone is disorganized and lacks the

architectural integrity of normal bone. This results in mechanically weak, highly vascular bone that is prone to deformity and fractures, especially if weight-bearing parts of the skeleton are affected.

CLINICAL PRESENTATION AND PHYSICAL EXAMINATION

Although Paget disease is usually asymptomatic, bone pain is the most common presenting symptom. The pain can be misinterpreted as part of the aging process or as part of another disease process. Patients may be misdiagnosed as having osteoarthritis. Failure to diagnose and to initiate early treatment of the disease can result in irreversible consequences and significant morbidity.

The degree and character of the bone pain vary with the location and activity of Paget disease. The most commonly involved sites are the pelvis, femur, tibia, spine, and skull. The hands and feet are only rarely involved. In general, the affected bone is moderately painful both at rest and during motion. Most patients describe the pain as a deep ache (like a toothache) that can become severe and sharp with weight bearing and when the area is warmed. Hot baths and even warm bedclothes can intensify the pain.

On examination, the affected area is often tender to the touch and may be warm because of increased new blood vessel growth within the bone itself. There may be increased pulsatility in the area. The pagetic bone can be noticeably enlarged. Affected bones may be deformed in a bow shape either from the effects of gravity or from the tension of the attached musculature on the architecturally incompetent pagetic bone. When bones in the lower extremity become deformed, the patient will have an abnormal gait and, often, arthritic changes within the surrounding joints because of the mechanical stress. The head size may increase with skull involvement, and frontal bossing may be evident.

Nerve entrapments can occur with bone overgrowth, resulting in a variety of neuropathies, including cranial nerve palsies. Hearing loss may occur from sensory neuropathy or conduction impairment because of pagetic involvement of the ossicles of the inner ear. When the spine is involved, bone overgrowth can result in spinal stenosis with attendant radiculopathies or motor impairments.

DIAGNOSTICS

Diagnosis is confirmed by checking the serum alkaline phosphatase (SAP) or urinary N-telopeptide cross-links (NTX) level, both of which will be elevated in active disease. These levels correlate with the extent and activity of the disease. If a single bone is involved (i.e., monostotic disease), a serum bone-specific alkaline phosphatase, a serum amino-terminal propeptide of type 1 collagen (PINP), NTX, or β C-terminal telopeptide of type I collagen (CTX) may be more sensitive measures than SAP.[65] Radiographic studies of the affected areas usually show a classic mixed sclerotic-lytic (cotton-wool) pattern, cortical thickening, and bone enlargement. Bone scans show increased uptake in affected areas, but this pattern can be difficult to differentiate from other processes such as cancer and arthritis.

DIFFERENTIAL DIAGNOSIS

The symptoms and signs of Paget disease must be distinguished from those of several other conditions. When the

INITIAL DIAGNOSTICS

Paget Disease

LABORATORY
- Serum alkaline phosphatase (SAP)
- Serum bone-specific alkaline phosphatase[a]
- Serum amino-terminal propeptide of type 1 collagen (PINP)[a]
- Urinary N-telopeptide
- β C-terminal telopeptide of type I collagen (CTX)[a]

IMAGING
- Plain radiographs of affected areas
- Nuclear medicine bone scan
- MRI (if neurologic symptoms)

[a]If indicated.

jcints are involved, the differential diagnosis includes osteoarthritis, gout, and pseudogout. Ironically, these three diagnoses can coexist with Paget disease, can be a complication of Paget disease, or can mimic the symptoms of Paget disease when it affects the bone adjacent to a joint.

Bone pain that occurs with an elevated SAP level and positive bone scan must be distinguished from malignant disease, most commonly a metastasis from a distant site. In early, active Paget disease, the initial wave of osteoclastic resorption can appear as lytic lesions on plain radiographs and thus may mimic such malignant neoplasms as multiple myeloma. However, in most cases, the radiograph will show changes pathognomonic of Paget disease. Osteomalacia, from vitamin D deficiency or hypophosphatemia, may also increase alkaline phosphatase and cause bone pain.

INTERPROFESSIONAL COLLABORATIVE MANAGEMENT

Medical management of straightforward cases can be easily handled by the primary health care provider. However, physical therapists are invaluable members of the management team because of their expertise in maximizing physical function and knowledge of assistive devices. Referral to a rheumatologist or endocrinologist specializing in metabolic bone disease is indicated if the patient's disease is unresponsive to usual treatment. Orthopedic referral is indicated when an associated arthropathy, fracture, or spinal stenosis causes unremitting pain or loss of function.

Severe neurologic complications, such as hydrocephalus, require aggressive inpatient antipagetic therapy combined with neurosurgical intervention.

The goals of treatment are to suppress osteoclastic activity, allowing the osteoblasts to catch up and lay down architecturally normal bone, which in turn reduces symptoms and prevents disease progression. Symptoms of bone pain, excessive warmth over bone, headache caused by skull involvement, low back pain caused by vertebral involvement, and some syndromes of neural compromise are the most likely to improve. All patients with bone pain or neurologic impingements, patients with congestive heart failure, and patients who are at risk for complications because of the site of disease (femoral head, tibia, and skull) should receive pharmacologic therapy (Box 163.4 and Table 163.1).[65] Presurgical treatment of Paget disease, when surgery of pagetic bone is planned, is paramount in an effort to decrease intraoperative bleeding. Some controversy remains about whether to treat patients solely on the basis of an elevated SAP level, and results from the PRISM trial (The Paget Disease Randomized Trail of Intensive vs Symptomatic Management) suggest that treatment on this basis is not justified.[66] The PRISM EZ trial, a 3-year extension of the PRISM trial, failed to see an advantage to intensive treatment compared with symptomatic management on quality of life, bodily

---

BOX 163.4

Indications for Drug Therapy in Paget Disease

- Bone or joint pain
- Pagetic lesions in weight-bearing sites
- Involvement of the skull
- Nerve entrapments
- Preparation for elective joint replacement or surgery on pagetic bone

---

TABLE 163.1 FDA-Approved Pharmacologic Treatment of Paget Disease

Drug	Dose	Side Effects
BISPHOSPHONATES		
Alendronate	40 mg PO per day for 6 months	Nausea, esophageal ulcers
Risedronate	30 mg PO per day for 2 months	Nausea, esophageal ulcers
Pamidronate	30 mg IV per day for 3 days or 60–90 mg IV once; repeated doses may be necessary for more severe disease	Mild fever, hypocalcemia, influenza-like symptoms, transient leukopenia
Zoledronic acid	5 mg IV over 15 min once. Retreatment guidelines have not been established	Mild fever, hypocalcemia, influenza-like symptoms, transient leukopenia
Etidronate	5 mg/kg/day (max 400 mg) PO per day for 6 months[a]	Nausea, osteomalacia
Tiludronate	400 mg PO per day for 3 months	Back pain, diarrhea, nausea
CALCITONIN		
Salmon	100 IU SC per day for 3–6 months, and then 50–100 IU every other day or 3 times per week	Flushing, nausea, loss of efficacy

[a]Etidronate should be given cyclically with at least 6 months of no treatment between courses.

pain, or bone pain, although there was a significantly greater proportion of fractures among the intensive treatment group.[67]

Bone pain usually responds within 2 to 3 weeks of active drug treatment. Neuropathies, if detected early, may also respond, but arthropathy will not because it represents fixed-joint degradation. Efficacy of treatment is determined by the amount and duration of the reduction in SAP or NTX.

Bisphosphonates

Bisphosphonates are the most widely used agents for the treatment of Paget disease. They reduce bone turnover by inhibiting key cellular functions that govern osteoclastic bone resorption. Etidronate (Didronel) was the first bisphosphonate available, although it is not used as commonly now. It is contraindicated in the presence of advancing lytic lesions in a weight-bearing bone or for pre-surgical treatment of pagetic bone due to adverse effects of bone healing. Tiludronate is also approved for Paget disease but rarely used. Alendronate (Fosamax) at 40 mg daily for 6 months and risedronate (Actonel) at 30 mg daily for 2 months are the oral bisphosphonates of choice for treatment of Paget disease in the United States. Clear evidence from randomized controlled trials has shown that both achieve quick normalization of biochemical markers and reduction of pain. In addition, both have prolonged post-treatment effects and low relapse rates. However, all bisphosphonates are poorly absorbed from the gut, and absorption is further diminished when they are taken with food or any liquid other than water. Thus, oral bisphosphonates must be taken with plain water on an empty stomach at least a half-hour before a meal. Waiting longer will enhance absorption. The main side effects are stomach upset and, rarely, esophageal ulceration.

Intravenous bisphosphonates such as pamidronate (Aredia) and zoledronic acid (Reclast) are potent treatment options for those unable to tolerate oral agents. Studies of both agents have shown dramatic and long-lasting improvement in both markers and symptoms. Because of its rapid onset of action, intravenous administration is the route of choice for patients with impending fracture, neurologic impingements, hydrocephalus, or severe refractory disease. The side effects are generally minor, but transient hypocalcemia, leukopenia, and influenza-like symptoms can be seen. These therapies can worsen renal function in those with preexisting renal disease and cause profound hypocalcemia in those with vitamin D deficiency. The Endocrine Society suggests 5 mg of zoledronic acid given intravenously as treatment of choice for Paget disease, provided there are no contraindications,[2] due to better efficacy at normalizing alkaline phosphatase and maintaining a durable response.[68]

As previously outlined, potent bisphosphonates have been associated with osteonecrosis of the jaw. There have been reports of osteonecrosis of the jaw in patients with Paget disease, although high doses of bisphosphonates were given for longer than typically prescribed.[69] There have also been reports of atypical femoral fracture in Paget disease related to prolonged alendronate use, but it's unclear whether the fracture was related to the medication use or to the disease itself.[70]

Calcitonin

Calcitonin, although not as potent or long lasting as the bisphosphonates, remains a well-tolerated treatment option. Pain typically remits after 2 to 3 weeks, and as treatment continues, lytic lesions fill in with new normal bone, vascularity decreases,

and neurologic deficits (if any) improve. However, the effect of calcitonin wears off with time because of the development of antibodies (in the case of salmon or porcine calcitonin) and downregulation of calcitonin receptors. The effective dose of salmon calcitonin is 100 IU subcutaneously every day for 3 to 6 months, followed by injections every other day or three times a week as dictated by clinical symptoms and biochemical markers. Nasal salmon calcitonin (200 IU) can be used in a similar schedule but is not specifically approved for use in Paget disease. The main side effects of injectable calcitonin are transient flushing and nausea. Vomiting, diarrhea, and abdominal pain can also occur. Nasal calcitonin is generally better tolerated but can cause nasal irritation.

Other Therapies

Gallium nitrate and mithramycin are no longer used in Paget disease, having been supplanted by less toxic and more effective bisphosphonates. Denosumab, approved for osteoporosis, has been described as effective during off label use but is not yet approved for use in Paget disease.

Nonsteroidal antiinflammatory drugs can be useful adjuncts for patients with joint or bone pain. When pain is severe, opioids may need to be used until Paget disease is controlled. Assistive devices, including shoe lifts, walkers, and canes for equalizing leg length discrepancies, as well as physical therapy for joint symptoms, are often helpful. Calcium and vitamin D supplements are imperative for those with low dietary intake to ensure adequate bone mineralization and to prevent hypocalcemia.

Life Span Considerations

Although untreated Paget disease can cause pain and deformity, the life span is unaffected unless the patient develops osteosarcoma or severe flattening of the base of the skull with spinal cord compression. Indications for the use of bisphosphonates have been extended to include younger patients to prevent bone deformity of the limbs and the secondary osteoarthritis that is seen with these deformities. Bisphosphonates are also recommended for older patients to prevent bone fragility and fracture.

COMPLICATIONS

Bone pain typical of Paget disease must be distinguished from other long-term consequences of untreated Paget disease, including neural compromise, fractures, joint deterioration, and sarcomatous transformation. Nerve compression is most common when the spine or skull is involved. Enlarging bone in the vertebrae can compress spinal nerve roots or even the spinal cord itself, resulting in neuropathic pain or myelopathies. Cranial nerves, which exit the skull through tiny foramina, can also be compressed, resulting in facial pain, paralysis, or deafness. Involvement of the base of the skull can result in hydrocephalus (often manifesting as dementia) or brainstem compression.

Pagetic fractures appear with sudden, severe knifelike pain. They may be traumatic or, if the pagetic bone is weakened by extensive lytic disease, can occur spontaneously. Until Paget disease is controlled, healing is difficult and slow. Paget arthropathy occurs when bone adjacent to joint surfaces (e.g., the femoral head or the acetabulum) is affected, resulting in abnormal joint architecture and subsequent degenerative arthritis.

The most dreaded consequence of long-term Paget disease is osteosarcoma. This is heralded by a sudden increase in pain intensity at a pagetic site. Although it is rare, osteosarcoma carries an extremely poor prognosis. Most patients die within 1 to 3 years.

PATIENT AND FAMILY EDUCATION

Patients and their families must understand the disease process and medical treatment to manage Paget disease optimally. First, they need to be informed about how to take their medications and what side effects could occur. Second, patients need to promptly report any worsening of their symptoms, which could herald disease progression, fracture, or sarcomatous transformation. Those with skull involvement need to understand what neuropathic symptoms to look for and the importance of prompt reporting. For example, progressive hearing loss should not be blamed on age.

In addition, family members should inform their own primary care team of their family history of Paget disease and should be cautioned to report bone pain or symptoms of nerve compression. Additional resources may be found on the National Organization for Rare Disorders website at rarediseases.org/rare-diseases/pagets-disease.

HEALTH PROMOTION

Patients should be encouraged to remain as physically active as possible. If the tibia or proximal femur is affected, heavy weight-bearing exercise should be avoided until the disease is in remission. Swimming, bicycling, and tai chi are excellent alternatives for patients with painful arthropathy. Adequate dietary (or supplemental) calcium and vitamin D are important to help maintain bone density.

REFERENCES

1. Cosman, F., de Beur, S. J., LeBoff, M. S., et al. the National Osteoporosis Foundation. (2014). Clinicians guide to prevention and treatment of osteoporosis. *Osteoporosis International*, 25(10), 2359–2381.
2. Schousboe, J. T., Shepherd, J. A., Bilezikian, J. P., & Baim, S. (2013). Executive Summary of the 2013 International Society for Clinical Densitometry position development conference on bone densitometry. *Journal of Clinical Densitometry: The Official Journal of the International Society for Clinical Densitometry*, 16, 455–466.
3. Camacho, P. M., Petak, S. M., Binkley, N., et al. (2016). American Association of Clinical Endocrinologists and American College of Endocrinology Clinical Practice Guidelines for the diagnosis and treatment of post-menopausal osteoporosis—2016: executive summary. *Endocrine Practice: Official Journal of the American College of Endocrinology and the American Association of Clinical Endocrinologists*, 22, 1111–1118.
4. Weinstein, R. S. (2012). Glucocorticoid-induced osteoporosis and osteonecrosis. *Endocrinology and Metabolism Clinics of North America*, 41, 595–611.
5. Panday, K., Gona, A., & Humphrey, M. B. (2014). Medication-induced osteoporosis: Screening and treatment strategies. *Therapeutic Advances in Musculoskeletal Disease*, 6, 185–202.
6. Lewiecki, E. M. (2000). Osteoporosis: Clinical evaluation. In K. R. Feingold, B. Anawalt, A. Boyce, et al. (Eds.), *Endotext [Internet]*. South Dartmouth (MA): MDText.com, Inc. Retrieved from https://www.ncbi.nlm.nih.gov/books/NBK279049/. (Accessed 15 June 2019). [Updated 2018 Apr 23].
7. Suwannarat, P., Amatachaya, P., Sookman, T., et al. (2018). Hyperkyphotic measures using distance from the wall: Validity, reliability and distance from the wall to indicate the risk for thoracic hyperkyphosis and vertebral fracture. *Archives of Osteoporosis*, 13, 25.
8. Johnson, K., Suriyaarachchi, P., Kakat, M., et al. (2015). Yield and cost effectiveness of laboratory testing to identify metabolic contributors to falls and fractures in older persons. *Archives of Osteoporosis*, 10, 226.
9. Holick, M. F. (2017). The vitamin D deficiency pandemic: Approaches for diagnosis, treatment and prevention. *Reviews in Endocrine and Metabolic Disorders*, 18, 153. https://doi.org/10.1007/s11154-017-9424-1.
10. National Institutes of Health (2018). Vitamin D Fact Sheet for Health Professionals. Nov 8. Retrieved from: https://ods.od.nih.gov/factsheets/VitaminD-HealthProfessional/. on 15 June 2019.
11. Pludowski, P., Holick, M., & Grant, W. (2018). Vit. D supplementation guidelines. *The Journal of Steroid Biochemistry and Molecular Biology*, 175, 125–135.
12. Hans, D., Stenova, E., & Lamy, O. (2017). The trabecular bone score (TBS) complements DXA and FRAX as a fracture risk assessment tool in routine clinical practice. *Current Osteoporosis Reports*, 15, 521–531.
13. Rosen, H. N., Vokes, T. J., Malabanan, A. O., et al. (2013). The official positions of the International Society for Clinical Densitometry: Vertebral fracture assessment. *Journal of Clinical Densitometry*, 16, 482–488.
14. Rafii, D. C., Ali, F., Farag, A., Iyer, B., Otterbeck, P. E., Chaudhari, R., et al. (2019). A prospective study of commonly utilized regimens of Vitamin D replacement and maintenance therapy in adults. *Endocrine Practice*, 25(1), 6–15.
15. Pietras, K. J., Obayan, B. K., Cai, M. H., & Holick, M. F. (2009). Vitamin D2 treatment for vitamin D deficiency and insufficiency for up to 6 years. *Archives of Internal Medicine*, 169, 1806–1808.
16. Cummings, S., Kice, D., & Black, D. (2016). Vit D supplementation and increased risk of falling: A cautionary Tale of vitamin supplements retold. *JAMA Internal Medicine*, 176(2), 171–172.
17. Lewis, J. R., Calver, J., Zhu, K., et al. (2011). Calcium supplementation and the risks of atherosclerotic vascular disease in older women: Results of a 5-year RCT and a 4.5-year follow-up. *Journal of Bone and Mineral Research*, 26, 35–41.
18. Chung, M., Tang, A. M., Fu, Z., et al. (2016). Calcium intake and cardiovascular disease risk: An updated systematic review and meta-analysis. *Annals of Internal Medicine*, 165, 856–866.
19. Harvey, N. C., D'Angelo, S., Pacccu, J., et al. (2018). Calcium and Vitamin D supplementation are not associated with risk of incident ischemic cardiac events or death: Findings from the UK Biobank Cohort. *Journal of Bone and Mineral Research*, 33, 803–811.
20. Howe, T. F., Shea, B., Dawson, L. J., et al. (2011). Exercise for preventing and treating osteoporosis in postmenopausal women. *The Cochrane Database of Systematic Reviews*, (7), CD000333, doi:10.1002/14651858.CD000333.pub2.
21. Giangregorio, L. M., Papaioannou, A., Macintyre, N. J., et al. (2014). Too fit to fracture: Exercise recommendations for individuals with osteoporosis or osteoporotic vertebral fracture. *Osteoporosis International*, 25(3), 821–835. doi:10.1007/s00198-013-2523-2. [Epub 2013 Nov 27].
22. Watson, S. L., Weeks, B. K., & Weis, L. J. (2018). Et al. High-Intensity resistance and impact training improves bone mineral density and physical function in postmenopausal women with osteopenia and osteoporosis: The LIFTMOR randomized controlled trial. *Journal of Bone and Mineral Research*, 33, 211–220.
23. Villareal, D. T., Aguirre, L., Gurney, A. B., et al. (2017). Aerobic or resistance exercise of both in dieting obese older adults. *The New England Journal of Medicine*, 376, 1943–1955.
24. Schwab, P., & Klein, R. F. (2008). Non pharmacological approaches to improve bone health and reduce osteoporosis. *Current Opinion in Rheumatology*, 20, 213–217.
25. Koike, T., Orito, Y., Toyoda, H., et al. (2009). External hip protectors are effective for the elderly with higher than usual risk factors for hip fractures. *Osteoporosis International*, 20, 1613. https://doi.org/10.1007/s00198-008-0824-7. (Accessed 9 June 2018).
26. Santesso, N., Carrasco-Labra, A., & Brignardello-Peterson, R. (2014). Hip Protectors for preventing hip fractures in older people. *The Cochrane Database of Systematic Reviews*, (3), CD001255.
27. Sawka, A. M., Boulos, P., Beattie, K., et al. (2005). Do hip protectors decrease the risk of hip fracture in institutional and community dwelling elderly? A systematic review and meta-analysis of randomized controlled trials. *Osteoporosis International*, 16, 1461. https://doi.org/10.1007/s00198-005-1932-2. (Accessed June 9, 2018).
28. Wysowski, D. K. (2009). Reports of esophageal cancer with oral bisphosphonate use. *The New England Journal of Medicine*, 360, 89–90.
29. Cai, D., Qin, J., Chen, G., et al. (2017). Bisphosphonate use and risk of gastric cancer: An updated meta-analysis of cohort and case-controlled studies. *Minerva Medica*, 108, 464–472.
30. Cardwell, C. R., Abnet, C. C., Cantwell, M. M., & Murray, L. J. (2010). Exposure to oral bisphosphonates and risk of esophageal cancer. *JAMA: The Journal of the American Medical Association*, 304, 657–663.
31. Sun, K., Liu, J. M., Sun, H. X., et al. (2013). Bisphosphonate treatment and the risk of esophageal cancer: A meta-analysis of observational studies. *Osteoporosis International*, 24, 279–286. https://doi.org/10.1007/s00198-012-2158-8. (Accessed June 9, 2018).
32. Wright, E., Schofield, P. T., & Molokhia, M. (2015). Bisphosphonates and evidence for association with esophageal and gastric cancer: A systematic review and meta-analysis. *BMJ Open*, 5, e007133. doi:10.1136/bmjopen-2014-007133.

33. Ruggiero, S. L., Dodson, T. B., Fantasia, J., et al. (2014). American Association of Oral and Maxillary surgeon's position paper of medication induced osteonecrosis of the jaw-2104 update. *Journal of Oral and Maxillofacial Surgery, 357*, 2028–2039.

34. Baim, S., & Miller, P. D. (2009). Assessing the clinical utility of serum CTX in postmenopausal osteoporosis and its use in predicting risk of osteonecrosis of the jaw. *Journal of Bone and Mineral Research, 24*, 561–574.

35. Dal Pra, K. J., Lemos, C., Okamoto, P., et al. (2017). Efficacy of parathyroid hormone, alendronate or both in men with osteoporosis. *The New England Journal of Medicine, 46*, 151–156.

36. Khan, A., Morrison, A., Cheung, A., et al. (2016). *Osteoporosis International, 27*, 853. https://doi.org/10.1007/s00198-015-3335-3.

37. Shane, E., Burr, D., Abrahamsen, B., et al. (2014). Atypical subtrochanteric and diaphyseal femoral fractures: Second report of a task force of the American Society for Bone and Mineral Research. *Journal of Bone and Mineral Research, 29*, 1–23.

38. Black, D. M., Kelly, M. P., Genant, H. K., et al. (2010). Bisphosphonates and fractures of the subtrochanteric or diaphyseal femur. *The New England Journal of Medicine, 362*, 1761–1771.

39. Kharwadkar, N., Mayne, B., Lawrence, J. E., & Khanduja, V. (2017). Bisphosphonates and atypical subtrochanteric fractures of the femur. *Bone and Joint Research, 6*, 144–153. doi:10.1302/2046-3758.63.BJR-2016-0125.R1.

40. McKenna, M. J., McKiernan, F. E., McGowan, B., et al. (2017). Identifying incomplete atypical femoral fractures with single-energy absorptiometryL declining prevalence. *Journal of the Endocrine Society, 1*, 211–220.

41. Pinsky, P., Miller, E., Heckman-Stoddard, B., & Minasian, L. (2018). Use of raloxifen and tamoxifen by breast cancer risk level in a Medicare-eligible cohort. *American Journal of Obstetrics and Gynecology, 218*(6), 606.e1–606.e9.

42. Levis, S., & Theodore, G. (2012). Summary of the AHQR's comparative effectiveness review of treatment to prevent fractures in men and women with low bone density or osteoporosis: Update of the 2007 paper. *Journal of Managed Care Pharmacy, 18*, s1–s15.

43. Levin, V. A., Jiang, X., & Kagan, R. (2018). Estrogen therapy for osteoporosis in the modern era. *Osteoporosis International, 29*, 1049. https://doi.org/10.1007/s00198-018-4414-z. (Accessed June 9, 2018).

43a. Qaseem, A., Forciea, M. A., McLean, R., et al. (2017). Treatment of low bone density or osteoporosis to prevent fractures in men and women. A clinical practice guideline update from the American College of Physicians. *Annals of Internal Medicine, 166*(11), 818–839.

44. Neer, R. M., Arnaud, C. D., Zanchetta, J. R., et al. (2001). Effect of parathyroid hormone on fractures and bone mineral density in post-menopausal women with osteoporosis. *The New England Journal of Medicine, 344*, 1434–1441.

45. Saag, K. G., Peterson, J., Brandi, M. L., et al. (2017). Romosozumab or alendronate for fracture prevention in women with osteoporosis. *The New England Journal of Medicine, 303*, 1815–1822.

46. Black, D. M., Bilezikian, J. P., Ensrud, K. E., et al. (2010). One year of alendronate after years of parathyroid hormones for osteoporosis. *The New England Journal of Medicine, 353*, 555–565.

47. Cosman, F., Nieves, J. W., Zion, M., et al. (2009a). Retreatment with teriparatide one year after the first teriparatide course in patients on continued long term alendronate. *Journal of Bone and Mineral Research, 24*, 1110–1115.

48. Miller, P. D., Hattersley, G., Riis, B. J., et al. (2016). Effect of abaloparatide vs. placebo on new vertebral fracture in post-menopausal women with osteoporosis: A randomized clinical trial. *JAMA: The Journal of the American Medical Association, 316*, 722–733.

49. Cosman, F., Miller, P. D., Williams, G. C., et al. (2017). Eighteen months of treatment with subcutaneous abaloparatide followed by 6 months of treatment with alendronate in postmenopausal women with osteoporosis: Results of the ACTIVxtend Trial. *Mayo Clinic Proceedings. Mayo Clinic, 92*, 200–210.

50. McClung, M. R., Grauer, A., Boonen, S., et al. (2014). Romosozumab in postmenopausal women with low bone mineral density. *The New England Journal of Medicine, 370*, 412–420.

51. Cosman, F., Crittenden, D. B., Adachi, J. D., et al. (2016). Romosozumab treatment in post-menopausal women. *The New England Journal of Medicine, 375*, 1532–1543.

52. Langdahl, B. L., Libanati, C., Crittenden, D. B., et al. (2017). Romosozumab (selerostin monoclonal antibody) versus teriparatide in post-menopausal women with osteoporosis transitioning from oral bisphosphonate therapy: A randomized, open-label, phase 3 trial. *Lancet, 390*, 1585–1594.

53. Cummings, S. R., San Martin, J., McClung, M. R., et al. (2009). Denosumab for prevention of fractures in postmenopausal women with osteoporosis. *The New England Journal of Medicine, 361*, 756–765.

54. Cummings, S. R., Ferrari, S., Eastell, R., et al. (2018). Vertebral fractures after discontinuation of denosumab: A post hoc analysis of the randomized placebo-controlled FREEDOM Trial and its extension. *Journal of Bone and Mineral Research, 33*, 190–198.

55. Bone, H. G., Wagman, R. B., Pannacciulli, N., & Papapoulos, S. (2017). Denosumab treatment in post-menopausal women with osteoporosis—author's reply. *The Lancet. Diabetes & Endocrinology, 5*, 768–769.

56. Black, D. M., Greenspan, S. L., Ensrud, K. E., et al. (2010). One year of alendronate after one year of parathyroid hormone for osteoporosis. *The New England Journal of Medicine, 362*, 1761–1771.

57. Lou, S., Lv, H., Li, Z., et al. (2018). Combination therapy of anabolic agents and bisphosphonates on bone mineral density in patients with osteoporosis: A meta-analysis of randomised controlled trials. *BMJ Open, 8*, e015187. doi:10.1136/bmjopen-2016-015187.

58. Cosman, F., Wermers, R. A., Recknor, C., et al. (2009b). Effects of teriparatide in postmenopausal women with osteoporosis on prior alendronate or raloxifene: Difference between stopping and continuing the antiresorptive agent. *The Journal of Clinical Endocrinology and Metabolism, 94*, 3772–3780.

59. Tsai, J. N., Uihlein, A. V., Lee, H., et al. (2013). Teriparatide and denosumab, alone or combined in women with postmenopausal osteoporosis: The DATA study randomized trial. *Lancet, 382*, 50–56.

60. Leder, B. Z., Tsai, J. N., Uihlein, A. V., et al. (2014). Two years of denosumab and teriparatide administration in postmenopausal women with osteoporosis, the DTAT extension study: A randomized controlled trial. *The Journal of Clinical Endocrinology and Metabolism, 99*, 1694–1700.

61. Leder, B. Z., Tsai, J. N., Uihlein, A. V., et al. (2015). Denosumab and teriparatide transitions in postmenopausal osteoporosis (the DATA switch study): Extension of a randomized controlled trial. *Lancet, 386*, 1147–1155.

62. Karponis, A., Rizou, S., Pallis, D., et al. (2015). Analgesic effect of nasal salmon calcitonin during the early post fracture period of the distal radius fracture. *Journal of Musculoskeletal & Neuronal Interactions, 15*(2), 186–189.

63. Chandra, R. V., Asadi, M., Slater, L., et al. (2017). Vertebroplasty and kyphoplasty for osteoporotic vertebral fractures. What is the latest data? *AJNR. American Journal of Neuroradiology*, doi: 10.3174/ajnr.A5458. (Accessed 1 June 2018).

64. Cundy, T. (2018). Paget's disease of the bone. *Metabolism: Clinical and Experimental*, 5–14.

65. Singer, F. R., Bone, H. G., Hosking, D. J., et al. (2014). Paget's disease of the bone: An Endocrine Society clinical practice guideline. *The Journal of Clinical Endocrinology and Metabolism, 99*, 4408–4422.

66. Langston, A. L., Campbell, M. K., Fraser, W. D., et al. (2011). Randomized trial of intensive bisphosphonate treatment versus symptomatic management in Paget's disease of bone. *Journal of Bone and Mineral Research, 25*, 20–31.

67. Tan, A., Goodman, K., Walker, A., et al. (2017). Long term randomized trial of intensive versus symptomatic management in Paget's disease of bone: The PRISM-EZ study. *Journal of Bone and Mineral Research, 32*, 1165–1173.

68. Reid, I. R., Miller, P., Lyles, K., et al. (2005). Comparison of a single infusion of zolendronic acid with risedronate for Paget's disease. *The New England Journal of Medicine, 353*, 898–908.

69. Khosla, S., Burr, D., Cauley, J., et al. (2007). Bisphosphonate-associated osteonecrosis of the jaw: Report of a task force of the American Society for bone and mineral research. *Journal of Bone and Mineral Research, 22*, 1479–1491.

70. Kilcoyne, A., & Heffernan, E. J. (2011). Atypical proximal femoral fractures in patients with Paget's disease receiving bisphosphonate therapy. *American Journal of Roentgenology, 197*, w196–w197.

CHAPTER **164**

NECK PAIN

Zacharia Isaac • Hannah Steere • Ashley H. Cotter

 Priority differentials include (1) abrupt-onset cervical myelopathy with associated gait disturbance, (2) upper motor neuron signs, (3) bowel or bladder incontinence, (4) weakness in the upper or lower extremities, (5) incapacitating neck pain refractory to conservative methods, (6) significant trauma or trauma with associated neurological findings, or (7) diagnostic indication of fracture or instability of the cervical spine.

DEFINITION AND EPIDEMIOLOGY

Neck pain is a common complaint in primary care practices because most people are likely to have some degree of neck pain in their lifetime. The annual prevalence among adults exceeds 30%, and 33% to 65% of these patients are recovered at 1 year.[1] In addition, of those who experience neck pain, 50% to 75% will experience another episode 1 to 5 years later. Neck pain is the fourth leading cause of disability.[1] There are several identifiable sources of neck pain, including the bone, disks, joints, ligaments, fascia, muscles, and nerve roots. Pain can be experienced solely in the neck or can move into the head, shoulders, or arms and can start without an inciting event. If an episode of neck pain lasts longer than 12 weeks, it is typically defined as chronic neck pain.

Chronic neck pain can also occur after a hyperextension injury (whiplash), usually in a motor vehicle collision or sometimes during work or sporting events. In chronic whiplash injury, many structures may be involved, including but not limited to the intervertebral disks; facet joints; ligaments; and other cervical soft tissues. Risk factors for neck pain include manual labor occupations, female gender, headaches, smoking, poor job satisfaction, and poor biomechanics.

PATHOPHYSIOLOGY

The cervical spine is made up of seven cervical vertebrae, C1 through C7. The C2 through C7 bodies are separated by five intervertebral disks, giving this portion of the spine a natural cervical lordosis. Each intervertebral disk consists of a gelatinous nucleus pulposus, surrounded by the fibrous rings of the anulus fibrosus. The nucleus pulposus consists of water, proteoglycans, and collagen. At birth it is 90% water, and it degenerates with time. These disks allow dissipation of axial loading forces throughout various ranges of motion; with degeneration over time, they can cause mechanical bilateral or midline neck pain. The support of the cervical spine comes from the various ligamentous, articular, and muscular structures, which can also be pain-mediating structures. The uncovertebral articulation is an important structure in the cervical spine and represents an area of vertebral and disk articulation in the cervical neural foramen. The degenerative hypertrophy of this area and the resultant narrowing of the neural foramen commonly result in radicular pain.

Cervical sprains and strains can be caused by overstretching or tearing of spinal ligaments and muscles. In the acute phase of neck pain without neurologic symptoms, the diagnosis of cervical sprain and strain is often made without an inciting event, and the precise diagnosis is not evident. Cervical sprains and strains commonly occur after automobile accidents, trauma, or other injuries. In traumatic events, whiplash syndrome may occur due to an abrupt flexion/extension movement to the cervical region. Many layers of structures are often involved in whiplash injury including soft tissues, ligamentous structures, spinal nerves, and disk. In addition, motor vehicle accidents and associated whiplash injuries have been known to cause upper cervical facet joint–mediated pain. These occur most frequently as a result of rear-end or side-impact motor vehicle collisions. There are well-described sclerotomal referral patterns for neck pain arising from the facet joints, with the pain extending into the head and shoulders, either unilaterally or bilaterally. Cervical radiculopathy can typically cause neck pain extending into the arm. The pain pattern is usually worse in the arm than in the neck with associated neurologic symptoms, such as weakness, numbness, and tingling. One common cause of radicular neck pain is a herniated cervical intervertebral disk (most commonly at the C6-7 followed by the C5-6 level). Herniated disk material has been shown to be inflammatory in nature and produces phospholipase A_2, a key mediator in the arachidonic acid cascade. Cervical spondylosis can also result from uncovertebral hypertrophy and is also a common cause of cervical radiculopathy. As the disks degenerate with time, there can be small herniations that calcify, causing disk osteophyte complexes to form. These complexes, combined with the ligamentous hypertrophy and loss of disk height that occur with aging, can cause impingement of nerve roots with resultant radicular pain.[2]

Cervical myelopathy caused by spinal cord compression is a possible complication of cervical spondylosis and can manifest with neck pain, radicular extremity pain, loss of manual dexterity, globally referred symptoms, gait instability, bowel or bladder dysfunction, and progressive weakness. Such symptoms warrant further diagnostic evaluation with magnetic resonance imaging (MRI) of the cervical spine if there is no contraindication.

CLINICAL PRESENTATION AND PHYSICAL EXAMINATION

A thorough history, including past medical, social, occupational, and family history, as well as a review of systems, including constitutional symptoms, skin changes, visceral pain, neurologic changes, and bowel or bladder complaints, should be performed. In addition, any history of previous trauma or whiplash should be elicited. Details surrounding the onset of pain, location and radiation of the pain, quality of pain over time, aggravating and alleviating factors, and associated symptoms such as headaches or systemic symptoms should be sought. Psychosocial elements including psychological and occupational history should also be evaluated to look for any confounding variables.

The location and radiation of pain can help elucidate the cause. Neck pain that remains in the neck region without radiation into the arms is typically referred to as axial neck pain. This pain can result from a cervical sprain or strain or be referred from the intervertebral disks or facet joints. Neck mobility may be limited from many of these causes; however, certain maneuvers can help elucidate the painful source. With axial neck pain, the motor strength and reflex examination findings are normal.

Radicular neck pain is usually described as pain greater in the arm than in the neck but commonly occurring in both. Neurologic symptoms, such as pain, weakness, numbness, and tingling, can also be found in the affected spinal nerve root distribution. The patient will likely report a relatively abrupt onset of pain that may worsen with particular movements, including cervical extension and ipsilateral rotation. In addition, a patient may have the arm in a position that decreases neural tension on the nerve root. This usually involves tilting the head away from the affected side, placing the upper arm closer to the head either in an overhead position or crossed in front of the throat. If the patient has any neurologic symptoms, such as weakness in the lower extremities, gait disturbance, bowel or bladder dysfunction, or sexual dysfunction, cervical myelopathy should be considered and immediately evaluated.

Facet joint pain is also a cause of axial neck pain and has been associated with whiplash injuries and headaches. Whiplash injury is experienced with an abrupt flexion-extension type of injury. Pain is typically off the midline, and although there are defined sclerotomes for referral, pain is usually worse in the neck. The pathophysiologic mechanism for whiplash syndrome is unclear; however, it is thought to be caused by soft tissue injury with local release of inflammatory mediators. The cervical zygapophyseal joints have been implicated as the major source of chronic pain after whiplash.[1] Significant biomechanical and psychosocial factors play a role, and severity of acute symptoms, comorbid depression, anxiety, and not being at fault for the accident are poor prognostic factors.

The physical examination starts with careful observation of the patient, looking for cervical alignment, discomfort, and frequent position changes and evaluating the patient's affect. Gait should be examined for unsteadiness, spastic or mechanical movement, and widened or narrowed steps. The skin and vascular system should be appraised for medical causes of neck pain, including meningitis, dental or jaw pain, and malignant neoplasm.

Cervical range of motion should be determined. It should be noted whether the patient moves in a limited, guarded fashion or if there is an ease to the movement. The normal range of motion of the cervical spine is 90 degrees of rotation, 45 degrees of lateral tilt, 60 degrees of forward flexion, and 75 degrees of extension. The patient should be inspected for loss of cervical lordosis and atrophy of the paraspinal, periscapular, and arm muscles. Palpation of the paraspinal muscles and trapezius muscles should be performed to assess for the degree of tenderness, although positive findings of pain are nonspecific in nature and can be related to many causes of axial neck pain. The facet joints should also be palpated to reproduce the patient's typical symptoms.

Neurologic examination should include manual muscle strength testing, sensation, and reflexes and evaluation for upper motor neuron signs. Examination and manual muscle strength testing (shoulder elevation, abduction, and internal and external rotation; elbow flexion and extension; wrist extension and flexion; and hand and digit intrinsic muscles) may help define the involved dermatome (Table 164.1). In addition, sensation to both light touch and pinprick should be checked for deficits throughout the dermatomes. Reflexes should also be elicited at the biceps, triceps, and brachioradialis tendons bilaterally to look for asymmetry or hyperreflexia. The Babinski response and Hoffmann sign as well as evaluation for both clonus and muscle spasticity can determine if central nervous system involvement of the brain or spinal cord is occurring.

Provocative maneuvers such as the modified Spurling maneuver, when it is performed and the response is positive, can be suggestive of cervical spinal nerve root involvement (low-moderate sensitivity, high specificity).[3,4] This test is performed by placing the head in extension, lateral flexion, and ipsilateral rotation. With placement of an axial load on the head, reproduction of typical symptoms down the arm can be specific for cervical radiculopathy.[5] The upper limb tension test (ULTT), or Elvey test, is performed by turning the head contralaterally with the arm abducted and elbow extended; a positive test response is reproduction of arm symptoms (moderate to high sensitivity, lower specificity).[3-5] The shoulder abduction test is performed by placing the palm of the affected extremity on top of the head while the patient is in the seated position; a positive test response is alleviation of pain (one study showed moderate sensitivity and high specificity).[4] The Lhermitte sign can also be elicited by rapidly flexing the neck while the patient is seated.[2] This can produce an electric shock sensation down the spine and into the limbs; the response is positive with cervical cord disorders such as compression, tumor, and multiple sclerosis.

In addition to cervical causes of neck pain, the provider should evaluate for other mimicking disorders. Thoracic outlet syndrome due to neurovascular compromise can be assessed with the Adson and Roos tests. The Adson test for vascular thoracic outlet syndrome is done with the patient standing. The examiner palpates the radial pulse while moving the upper extremity in abduction, extension, and external rotation as the patient rotates the head toward the ipsilateral side with the breath held.[2] If the patient's pulse diminishes, this is considered a positive test result; however, this finding is often nonspecific. The elevated arm stress test (EAST), or Roos test, is done with the patient's shoulders abducted to 90 degrees and laterally rotated with elbows flexed behind the frontal plane. The patient is then instructed to open and close their hands into a fist for three minutes, and a positive test is reported if the patient is unable to keep their arms in starting position, if pain/paresthesias occur, or if this reproduces symptoms. The test has been shown to have variable sensitivity and specificity. Mechanical shoulder disorders can also refer pain in a distribution similar to that of the cervical spine. Shoulder examination should also be performed to ensure that there is no shoulder disorder that is mimicking or contributing to neck pain symptoms.

DIAGNOSTICS
Essential Diagnostics
Plain radiographs of the cervical spine are warranted if the patient has a history of cancer, recent trauma, long-standing corticosteroid use, osteoporosis, drug or alcohol abuse, or concerning constitutional or neurologic symptoms. However, routine x-ray examination was not helpful in demonstrating issues that changed clinical management and is therefore not recommended for routine episodes of neck pain.

TABLE 164.1 Cervical Dermatomes

Root	Muscle Group Affected	Dermatome	Reflexes
C5	Deltoid, biceps, supraspinatus, infraspinatus, rhomboids	Lateral arm	Biceps
C6	Biceps, infraspinatus, brachioradialis, pronator teres, triceps	Lateral arm and forearm, lateral digits (thumb)	Biceps, brachioradialis
C7	Triceps, pronator teres, wrist flexors	Posterolateral arm and forearm, middle digits	Triceps
C8	Finger flexors, thumb opposition, hand intrinsics	Medial arm and forearm, medial digits (pinky)	None

When a patient visits the clinic with cervical spine pain after trauma or a motor vehicle accident, the Canadian Cervical Spine Rule, when used correctly, is helpful in identifying those patients who are at high risk for a cervical spine fracture and should therefore undergo cervical radiography.[6] The Canadian Cervical Spine Rule has been validated with high sensitivity using CT scan as the gold standard, is superior to the National Emergency X-Radiography Utilization Study (NEXUS) Low-Risk Criteria, and results in reduced rates of radiography.[7,8]

Lateral views can help demonstrate vertebral alignment and evaluate the normal cervical lordosis as well as evaluate for bone changes, such as a fracture or osteoarthritis. Flexion and extension views can additionally be taken to evaluate for segmental instability. Oblique views can help characterize any foraminal compromise and possible encroachment on the exiting nerves.

Radionuclide bone scintigraphy is another tool occasionally used for the diagnosis of neck pain. This is helpful if the history and physical examination findings raise suspicion for osteomyelitis, metastatic disease, or occult fracture. In addition, it can show increased uptake and activity in the axial and appendicular joints, which can be consistent with conditions such as osteoarthritis.

If the patient has neurologic findings, symptoms concerning for medical causes of pain, occult fracture, or persistent pain after conservative treatment, further imaging is warranted. Computed tomography (CT) scans or MRI can be considered.

CT scans are better at identifying bone and degenerative changes and are typically performed acutely, such as in the case of a patient with a history of head trauma or cervical trauma and neck pain with high possibility of cervical fracture. However, CT scans expose the patient to a large amount of radiation and are not able to identify pathologic cord changes, such as spinal cord edema, demyelination, and intrinsic spinal cord tumors. CT scans can be performed with myelography in a patient with contraindication to MRI (e.g., pacemaker, shrapnel) to evaluate for nerve root or spinal cord compression.

MRI is the most widely used imaging modality to evaluate for neck pain and radiculopathy. Its principal use is to evaluate the bone structures and soft tissues, and it can be helpful in identifying degenerative disc disease, annular tears, disk herniations, spinal stenosis, and cord or nerve root compression. With the addition of gadolinium, it can be used to look for tumor or infection. Although it is superior at evaluating degenerative changes in the spine, there is a high likelihood that many findings are asymptomatic and may not be the source of the patient's pain. MRI studies have revealed that 19% of asymptomatic patients have anatomic abnormalities such as cervical disk herniations without any reported neck pain or radicular symptoms.[9]

Other diagnostic workup can be included for more patient-specific situations.

Erythrocyte sedimentation rate and C-reactive protein can be helpful in a patient with constitutional symptoms as markers of systemic inflammation.

Neoplasm may be reflected in an abnormal complete blood count, alkaline phosphatase level, or calcium level.

Electrodiagnostic studies can be helpful in distinguishing neurologic changes with denervation and reinnervation from subacute and chronic radiculopathy.[10] These studies will not show acute changes until approximately 3 to 4 weeks after the initial insult; however, needle electromyography (EMG)

INITIAL DIAGNOSTICS

Neck Pain

LABORATORY
- None

IMAGING
- X-ray examination
- Radionuclide bone scintigraphy[a]
- CT scan or MRI[a]

OTHER DIAGNOSTICS

Laboratory
- CBC, ESR, CRP

Other
- EMG

[a]If indicated.
CT, Computed tomography; *EMG*, electromyography; *MRI*, magnetic resonance imaging.

---

can highlight chronic changes with good sensitivity and high specificity.[10]

DIFFERENTIAL DIAGNOSIS

The differential diagnosis of neck pain can be broad. The clinically common degenerative causes of neck pain are discussed earlier in the chapter. It is imperative to rule out serious sources of neck pain, including infection, fracture, inflammatory diseases, neoplasm, and other medical causes, with a thorough history and physical examination. Evaluation for any systemic signs, such as fevers, chills, weight loss, recumbency pain, headaches, and history of cancer, is important to rule out metastatic disease or infection. Diabetic neuropathy, Lyme disease, and herpes zoster can cause radiculopathy without cervical spondylosis. Thoracic outlet syndrome and brachial plexopathy should be considered in a patient with radicular symptoms. Other nondegenerative causes of neck pain include infectious or malignant causes involving the neck, referred pain from cardiac ischemia, intrathoracic disease from diaphragmatic irritation, and cervical dystonia or torticollis.

INTERPROFESSIONAL COLLABORATIVE MANAGEMENT

Nonpharmacologic Management

If the symptoms and examination findings are consistent with mechanical neck pain without neurological findings, the patient should be assured that a concerning underlying pathologic process is unlikely.

Physical modalities such as heat, ice, and massage can also be used by the patient if they are helpful. Appropriate posture and biomechanics should be encouraged, and ergonomic evaluation should be considered. Repetitive and heavy lifting of more than 10 pounds as well as positioning of the cervical spine in painful positions should be avoided. There should be no repetitive bending, over-the-head movement, or exaggerated neck movements.

Manual or mechanical traction can be tried only after acute muscle pain has subsided and in patients without cervical stenosis or myelopathy. There is inconclusive evidence that continuous traction is any more effective than intermittent (manual).[11] Current literature does not show evidence to support the efficacy of continuous traction. It has not been shown to improve pain or function in patients with chronic neck pain with or without radiculopathy.[12] Intermittent traction may have some efficacy in reducing pain in the short term.[11]

Activity levels should be increased slowly, and the patient should be aware that symptoms may wax and wane throughout the natural history of an acute flare of mechanical neck pain. If symptoms become more chronic and the neurologic examination shows the patient to be stable, activity and exercise should be encouraged to avoid further deconditioning.

Physical Therapy Management of Cervical Spine Pain

The physical therapy management of cervical spine pain is most effective when a multimodal treatment approach is used. Physical therapy interventions for the cervical spine can include a combination of therapeutic exercise, manual therapy, modalities, and patient education. Once a physical therapy referral is deemed appropriate, the health care provider should write a prescription, noting the diagnosis, stating "evaluate and treat," and suggesting the estimated frequency, duration of treatment, and relevant precautions. For most cervical spine conditions, one to three visits per week for the appropriate time period required to rehabilitate the particular patient, typically 4 to 8 weeks or more, depending on the severity and chronicity of symptoms, is appropriate.

The physical therapist will perform a thorough examination, assess the cause of the cervical spine pain or radiculopathy, create a differential diagnosis, and then devise a specific treatment plan. If there are any red flags present, indicating serious underlying pathology, the physical therapist will refer the patient back to the provider.[13] Several researchers have proposed strategies for the classification of patients with neck pain to improve the efficacy of treatment interventions.[14-17] These researchers have all created a decision-making algorithm that classifies cervical pain into clinical patterns, which guide treatment strategies. Essentially, neck pain patients are categorized into the following clinical treatment subgroups, as proposed by Childs and colleagues[15,16]:

- Mobility
- Centralization
- Exercise and conditioning
- Reduction of headache
- Pain control

The subgroups are matched, based on specific clinical characteristics, with the management strategy most likely to benefit the treatment-matched subgroup. The goal of the classification system is to improve patient outcomes with the physical therapy treatment of neck pain.

Therapeutic Exercise. Therapeutic exercise interventions are prescribed to help improve range-of-motion limitations, muscle imbalances, dysfunctional motor control patterns, poor posture, muscle endurance, and myofascial pain. There is moderate evidence to support the use of specific strengthening exercises for chronic neck pain and cervicogenic headache.[18]

Physical therapy exercise prescription therefore includes the following:

- Range-of-motion exercises
- Flexibility (stretching) exercises
- Motor control and neuromuscular reeducation
- Strength and endurance exercises
- Postural exercises and education

Common dysfunctional postures in patients with neck pain include the following:

- Forward head posture
- Rounded forward and internally rotated shoulders
- Increased thoracic kyphosis
- Protracted scapulae

Dysfunctional postures contribute to cervical and thoracic pain, limited mobility, and impaired function.[14,18] Patients with dysfunctional postures, as well as patients falling into the conditioning and exercise subgroup mentioned previously, would benefit from therapeutic exercises.

Examples of some commonly prescribed exercises are as follows:

- Range-of-motion and flexibility exercises:
  - Can include but are not limited to active cervical movements into rotation, flexion, extension, side bend, and chin tucks. Chin tucks help restore upper cervical neck flexion within limits of pain.
  - Scapular retraction is helpful to promote thoracic spine extension and improve posture.
  - Upper trapezius, levator scapulae, pectoralis major muscle, and suboccipital muscle stretching are examples of flexibility exercises that may help alleviate tightness.
  - The pain control classification subgroup would benefit from gentle range-of-motion exercises and active exercises to tolerance.[15,16]
- Cervical muscle endurance training:
  - Deep neck flexor or craniocervical flexor muscle endurance was found to be impaired in patients with cervicogenic headaches and neck pain compared with control groups; therefore, training the deep neck flexors through specific exercises has been shown to help alleviate cervicogenic headaches and chronic neck pain.[18-20]
  - Chin tucks in the supine position and chin tucks with a small head lift (more advanced) are commonly used to help train the deep neck flexors and cervicocranial flexor muscle group.[18]
- Shoulder girdle and periscapular strengthening exercises:
  - These exercises help improve shoulder mechanics and alleviate stress on the cervical spine.
  - The exercises commonly prescribed include:
  - Rotator cuff strengthening exercises to reduce excessive loading of the upper trapezius muscles
  - Periscapular exercises such as scapular retraction with resistance as well as middle trapezius, rhomboid, lower trapezius, and latissimus dorsi muscle strengthening.
- Diaphragmatic breathing exercises can also help relax cervicothoracic muscles and retrain dysfunctional breathing patterns, which contribute to cervical muscle tightness.
  - The reduce headache subgroup would also benefit from the aforementioned interventions, particularly the deep neck flexor and craniocervical flexor muscle endurance training exercises, as well as postural exercises.

Manual Therapy. Manual therapy for the cervical spine can include, but is not limited to, spinal manipulative therapy, spinal mobilization, muscle energy techniques, and myofascial release (MFR). Before any manual therapy is performed on the cervical spine, it is extremely important to rule out vertebrobasilar insufficiency (VBI), upper motor neuron involvement, and cervical spine instability.[21]

The goals of manual therapy interventions are to:

- Restore joint mobility and correct joint dysfunctions
- Decrease muscle spasm/tightness
- Reduce stress on neurologic tissues
- Normalize joint mechanics

Spinal manipulative therapy is defined as the application of high-velocity, low-amplitude manual thrust to the spinal joints just beyond the joint range of motion.

Contraindications to manipulation include the following:

- Positive Hoffmann sign (indicative of upper motor neuron disease)
- Positive VBI test result
- Clinical signs of VBI (dizziness, diplopia, drop attacks, dysphagia, dysarthria)
- Direct trauma (see diagnostics section discussing the Canadian C-Spine Rule)
- Unexplained weight loss
- History of cancer
- Spinal fracture
- Unrelenting night pain
- Osteoporosis
- Severe spinal stenosis
- Neurologic deficits with limb weakness

When manipulation is contraindicated or unlikely to be beneficial, spinal mobilization techniques can be used to restore joint mobility to hypomobile joints, as long as mobilization is not also contraindicated. Spinal mobilization is the application of manual force to the spinal joints within the passive joint's physiologic range of motion without a thrust.[22] When a patient falls into the mobility classification subgroup mentioned earlier, then mobilization or manipulation of the cervical spine is the intervention of choice, provided there are no contraindications.

In randomized controlled trials, manual therapy consisting of spinal manipulation performed by a physical therapist was more effective in improving outcomes when compared with a physical therapy intervention that did not include a manual therapy approach, or a home exercise program.[15,17,23] The most recent neck pain clinical practice guidelines recommends a multimodal approach of thoracic manipulation, neck range of motion exercises, and upper extremity strengthening for the treatment of acute, subacute, and chronic neck pain.[18,21]

Muscle energy techniques involve a contract-relax technique that facilitates relaxation of muscle, improves range of motion, and enhances stretching of tight muscle tissue; it can be used as a form of neuromuscular reeducation.

MFR involves the application of manual sustained stretch to the skin, which will affect the underlying myofascial tissue. MFR assists in elongating and releasing tight and restricted tissue.

There is evidence to support the combined use of manual therapy and exercise for patients with cervicogenic headaches and mechanical neck pain with or without upper extremity symptoms compared with just spinal manipulation or exercise.[24]

The mobility, headache, and possibly pain control subgroups will benefit from some of the manual therapy interventions mentioned here.[15]

Modalities. Modalities frequently used in physical therapy for the cervical spine include ice, heat, ultrasound, electrical stimulation, and low-level laser therapy. Modalities are a helpful adjunct for the overall therapy program but are unlikely to be helpful long term when used in isolation.

Despite the limited evidence to support the use of modalities, they may be useful in treating patients who would fall into the pain control subgroup, as long as they are helpful for

reducing symptoms. However, activity within tolerance is preferable to passive treatments, such as modalities.

Traction. Traction is usually indicated for patients with radicular symptoms to help resolve neurologic deficits, centralize radicular symptoms, and reduce pain. If a patient's pain has been present for less than 3 months and experiences centralization of cervical spine symptoms with application of manual traction, the patient would be placed in the centralization subgroup and receive the most appropriate matched intervention, such as cervical spine mechanical or manual traction.

A recent systematic review and meta-analysis investigated randomized controlled trials for the effectiveness of traction with other physical therapy procedures for the treatment of cervical radiculopathy. These authors found a significant pain reduction with mechanical traction at both short-term (post-treatment) and intermediate-term (6-month) follow-ups.[25] Also, one prospective study demonstrated that intermittent cervical spine traction (below 6 kg manual and up to 12 kg mechanical) was useful for reducing neck pain and radicular pain when used in conjunction with a multimodal approach, if symptoms have been present for less than 3 months.[26] One[15,26] retrospective study did support the use of home cervical traction and reported positive results. Therefore, intermittent cervical traction may serve as an adjunct treatment option for nonchronic neck pain with or without radiculopathy.

Pharmacologic Management

Medications can also be a helpful adjunct through recovery. Oral over-the-counter (OTC) analgesics such as acetaminophen and low-dose nonsteroidal antiinflammatory drugs (NSAIDs) can be used if the patient has no medical contraindications. Higher antiinflammatory doses of NSAIDs can be helpful but patients should be monitored for potential adverse effects such as gastrointestinal bleeding. Topical NSAIDS, such as diclofenac, can also be helpful, though evidence is currently lacking to support effectiveness. In addition, there is some evidence that topical NSAID users have a reduced risk of cardiovascular events compared with oral NSAID users.[27]

A skeletal muscle relaxant, such as tizanidine, cyclobenzaprine, or baclofen, can also be used to help reduce muscle spasms associated with some cases of mechanical neck pain.

Opioid analgesics and tramadol are other options when used cautiously if patients do not have an adequate response to OTC pain medications. Careful reassessment should be performed if the patient has a history of substance use disorder or has failed to respond after a reasonable treatment course. If a patient is started on an opioid, the CDC guidelines recommend prescribing the lowest effective dose of immediate-release opioids and the prescription should be "no greater quantity than needed for the expected duration of pain severe enough to require opioids."[28] Three-day prescriptions are normally sufficient and should not be more than seven days. These guidelines were created in order to prevent harms associated with chronic opioid use. In addition, there is no evidence that shows a long-term benefit of opioids in reduction of pain or improving function.[28]

Patients with chronic neck pain can be considered candidates for tricyclic antidepressants or mixed norepinephrine-serotonin reuptake inhibitors if they have no contraindications to these medications.

Gabapentin has also been shown to be beneficial for central pain syndromes and radiculopathy and can help restore sleep and function. Clinicians should monitor for misuse while patients are taking this medication as recent studies suggest higher rates of abuse than previously thought.[29]

Complementary and alternative medicine treatments for subacute and chronic neck pain have also been shown to be useful for some patients. Acupuncture, cognitive-behavioral therapy, relaxation therapy, massage, reflexology, yoga, spa therapy, transcutaneous electrical nerve stimulation, and cold laser are reasonable to try and can provide short-term relief to patients. However, few of these therapies have been shown to be effective in the long term for chronic neck pain.[30] Transcranial magnetic stimulation (rTMS) has been shown to provide temporary relief in chronic pain disorders, but repetitive sessions and long-term effects are unknown.[31]

Other options to be considered for treatment of subacute or chronic neck and radicular pain include epidural corticosteroid injections.[32] This treatment typically requires referral to an interventional spine physician. Cervical epidural injections can be helpful to treat symptoms of radiculopathy as well as chronic neck pain.[33] Evidence is insufficient regarding difference in outcomes for interventional cervical spine injections versus placebo.[34] In addition, injections can be performed into the facet joints or directly to the nerves supplying innervation to the joint for symptoms of facet syndrome.

Trigger point injections into the muscles in the area of pain can also help in the short term; however, studies demonstrate variable results.

Intramuscular injections of botulinum toxin have not been shown to be effective in reducing neck pain.[35]

COMPLICATIONS

Complications of an acute episode of mechanical neck pain are rare. If there is concern for instability or history of trauma, fracture and bone disease should be ruled out. If there are worrisome systemic features, more serious medical conditions should be ruled out. An episode of neck pain that follows a whiplash injury without traumatic fracture or other complications may continue to progress into chronic neck pain with associated headaches. If the patient has neurologic changes, further workup and appropriate imaging should be ordered to evaluate for radiculopathy or myelopathy. If neurologic symptoms change or worsen, surgical evaluation and referral should be initiated. Most episodes of acute neck pain are self-limited; however, there is the risk for continued pain and transition to chronic neck pain. Predictors for development of chronic neck pain include high BMI, frequent neck extension during the work day, high initial pain intensity, high psychological job demands, depressed mood, poor muscle endurance, and impaired endogenous pain inhibition.[36,37] Sequelae of chronic pain include mood disturbance, insomnia, opiate habituation, addiction, disturbance of interpersonal relationships and sexual relationships, loss of employment, and personal isolation.

LIFE SPAN CONSIDERATIONS

After the initial episode of neck pain, the chances are high that pain will recur in the patient's lifetime. If the patient has a disc herniation and radicular symptoms, this disc material will likely be reabsorbed with time; however, the patient should be warned that the disc is at risk for re-herniation. In addition, age can be a risk factor for development of degenerative disc disease and spondylotic changes. These can continue to progress and lead to recurrent episodes of neck pain as well as to chronic neck pain symptoms. Patients with diffuse idiopathic skeletal hyperostosis develop anterior osteophytes that can progress with age, causing stiffness and pain, and the osteophytes can become large and indent the esophagus and cause dysphagia.

Younger patients tend to have disc herniations, axial neck pain, myofascial pain syndrome, fibromyalgia, or whiplash-induced neck pain. Older patients tend to develop cervical stenosis with or without myelopathy, uncovertebral hypertrophy and resultant foraminal stenosis with radicular pain, disc herniations, axial neck pain, or whiplash-induced neck pain.

EDUCATION AND HEALTH PROMOTION

Patient education should start with reassurance and support. Explaining the natural history of mechanical neck pain and that most cases will resolve in a timely manner is important. Current evidence supports pain education with chronic musculoskeletal conditions and has been shown to reduce psychosocial factors, increase patient knowledge of pain, decrease disability and pain, and minimize health care utilization.[28] Preemptive exercise and conditioning can help reduce the frequency of recurrence of episodes and should be communicated to the patient. Postural exercises and reminders should be provided to keep the neck in a neutral position in line with the thoracic spine or ear in line with the shoulder, with emphasis placed on keeping the shoulders back and chest forward. Recommending the use of lumbar support when sitting helps the patient maintain proper head and neck alignment and prevents slouching postures that can exacerbate neck pain. Ergonomic evaluation and sleeping position considerations should be mentioned to the patient. Overhead lifting and poor biomechanics while reaching should also be addressed, and proper body mechanics should be used at all times. Risk factors for disc degeneration, such as smoking, should be addressed, and the patient should be encouraged to quit smoking if possible. If the patient has concomitant psychosocial conditions, these should be addressed.

Patients should also be educated on the warning signs of potentially serious complications, including sudden or progressive limb weakness, bowel or bladder changes, and constitutional symptoms. Reporting of these symptoms on a timely basis can expedite urgent treatment.

REFERENCES

1. Cohen, S. P. (2015). Epidemiology, diagnosis, and treatment of neck pain. *Mayo Clinic Proceedings. Mayo Clinic, 90*(2), 284–299. doi:10.1016/j.mayocp .2014.09.008.
2. Corey, D. L., & Comeau, D. (2014). Cervical radiculopathy. *The Medical Clinics of North America, 98*(4), 791–799. doi:10.1016/j.mcna.2014.04.001.
3. Ghasemi, M., Golabchi, K., Mousavi, S. A., et al. (2013). The value of provocative tests in diagnosis of cervical radiculopathy. *Journal of Research in Medical Sciences, 18*(Suppl. 1), S35–S38. http://www.ncbi.nlm.nih.gov/ pubmed/23961282. (Accessed 31 December 2017).
4. Thoomes, E. J., Van Geest, S., Van Der Windt, D. A., et al. (2017). Value of physical tests in diagnosing cervical radiculopathy: A systematic review. *The Spine Journal, 18*, 179–189. doi:10.1016/j.spinee.2017.08.241.
5. Apelby-Albrecht, M., Andersson, L., Kleiva, I. W., Kvåle, K., Skillgate, E., & Josephson, A. (2013). Concordance of upper limb neurodynamic tests with medical examination and magnetic resonance imaging in patients with cervical radiculopathy: A diagnostic Cohort Study. *Journal of Manipulative and Physiological Therapeutics, 36*(9), 626–632. doi:10.1016/j.jmpt.2013.07.007.
6. Stiell, I. G., Wells, G. A., Vandemheen, K. L., et al. (2001). The Canadian C-Spine rule for radiography in alert and stable trauma patients. *JAMA:*

The Journal of the American Medical Association, 286(15), 1841. doi:10.1001/jama.286.15.1841.

7. Moser, N., Lemeunier, N., Southerst, D., et al. (2018). Validity and reliability of clinical prediction rules used to screen for cervical spine injury in alert low-risk patients with blunt trauma to the neck: Part 2. A systematic review from the Cervical Assessment and Diagnosis Research Evaluation (CADRE) Collaboration. *European Spine Journal, 27*, 1219–1233. https://doi.org/10.1007/s00586-017-5301-6.

8. Michaleff, Z. A., Maher, C. G., Verhagen, A. P., Rebbeck, T., & Lin, C.-W. C. (2012). Accuracy of the Canadian C-spine rule and NEXUS to screen for clinically important cervical spine injury in patients following blunt trauma: A systematic review. *Canadian Medical Association Journal, 184*(16), E867–E876. doi:10.1503/cmaj.120675.

9. Leichtle, U. G., Wünschel, M., Socci, M., Kurze, C., Niemeyer, T., & Leichtle, C. I. (2015). Spine radiography in the evaluation of back and neck pain in an orthopaedic emergency clinic. *Journal of Back and Musculoskeletal Rehabilitation, 28*(1), 43–48. doi:10.3233/BMR-140488.

10. Hakimi, K., & Spanier, D. (2013). Electrodiagnosis of cervical radiculopathy. *Physical Medicine and Rehabilitation Clinics of North America, 24*(1), 1–12. doi:10.1016/j.pmr.2012.08.012.

11. Yang, J. D., Tam, K. W., & Huang, T. W. (2017). Intermittant cervical traction for treating neck pain: A meta-analysis of randomized controlled trials. *Spine, 42*(13), 959–965.

12. Poitras, V., Khangurs, S., & Ford, C. (2017). Physiotherapy interventions for the management of neck and /or back pain: A review of clinical and cost effectiveness. Ottawa: CADTH. Retrieved from https://www.cadth.ca/sites/default/files/pdf/htis/2017/RC0898%20Physio%20for%20Back%20and%20Neck%20Pain%20Final.pdf. (Accessed 11 June 2019).

13. Bier, J. D., Scholten-Peeters, W. G., Staal, J. B., et al. (2018). Clinical practice guideline for physical therapy assessment and treatment in patients with nonspecific neck pain. *Physical Therapy, 98*(3), 162–171. doi:10.1093/ptj/pzx118.

14. Cleland, J. A., Mintken, P. E., Carpenter, K., et al. (2010). Examination of a clinical prediction rule to identify patients with neck pain likely to benefit from thoracic spine thrust manipulation and a general cervical range of motion exercise: Multi-Center randomized clinical trial. *Physical Therapy, 90*(9), 1239–1250. doi:10.2522/ptj.20100123.

15. John Childs, M. D., Fritz, J. M., Piva, S. R., & Whitman, J. M. Proposal of a Classification System for Patients With Neck Pain. https://www.jospt.org/doi/pdf/10.2519/jospt.2004.34.11.686?code=jospt-site. (Accessed 5 February 2018).

16. Fritz, J. M., & Brennan, G. P. (2007). Preliminary examination of a proposed Treatment-Based classification system for patients receiving physical therapy interventions for neck pain. *Physical Therapy, 87*(5), 513–524. doi:10.2522/ptj.20060192.

17. Blanpied, P. R., Gross, A. R., Elliott, J. M., et al. (2017). Neck pain: Revision 2017. *The Journal of Orthopaedic and Sports Physical Therapy, 47*(7), A1–A83. doi:10.2519/jospt.2017.0302.

18. Gross, A. R., Paquin, J. P., Dupont, G., et al. (2016). Exercises for mechanical neck disorders: A Cochrane review update. *Manual Therapy, 24*, 25–45. doi:10.1016/j.math.2016.04.005.

19. McLean, S. M., Klaber Moffett, J. A., Sharp, D. M., & Gardiner, E. (2013). A randomised controlled trial comparing graded exercise treatment and usual physiotherapy for patients with non-specific neck pain (the GET UP neck pain trial). *Manual Therapy, 18*(3), 199–205. doi:10.1016/j.math.2012.09.005.

20. Kay, T. M., Gross, A., Goldsmith, C. H., et al. (2012). Exercises for mechanical neck disorders. In T. M. Kay (ed.). *The Cochrane Database of Systematic Reviews*. Chichester, UK: John Wiley & Sons, Ltd, (8), CD004250, doi:10.1002/14651858.CD004250.pub4.

21. Miller, M. B. (2016). The cervical spine: Physical therapy patient management using current evidence. In *Current concepts of orthopaedic physical therapy* (4th ed., pp. 1–73). Orthopaedic Section. APTA, Inc. doi:10.17832/isc.2016.26.2.6.

22. Bronfort, G., Evans, R., Anderson, A. V., Svendsen, K. H., Bracha, Y., & Grimm, R. H. (2012). Spinal manipulation, medication, or home exercise with advice for acute and subacute neck pain. *Annals of Internal Medicine, 156*(1_Part_1), 1. doi:10.7326/0003-4819-156-1-201201030-00002.

23. Evans, R., Bronfort, G., Schulz, C., et al. (2012). Supervised exercise with and without spinal manipulation performs similarly and better than home exercise for chronic neck pain. *Spine, 37*(11), 903–914. doi:10.1097/BRS.0b013e31823b3bdf.

24. Dunning, J. R., Butts, R., Mourad, F., Young, I., Fernandez-de-Las Peñas, C., Hagins, M., et al. (2016). Upper cervical and upper thoracic manipulation versus mobilization and exercise in patients with cervicogenic headache: A multi-center randomized clinical trial. *BMC Musculoskeletal Disorders, 17*(1), 64. doi:10.1186/s12891-016-0912-3.

25. Pillastrini, P., Romeo, A., Vanti, C., et al. (2018). Cervical radiculopathy: Effectiveness of adding traction to physical therapy. A systematic review and Meta-Analysis of randomized controlled trials. *Physical Therapy*, doi:10.1093/physth/pzy001.

26. Rinke, M. (2012). The effect of manual cervical traction vs. mechanical cervical traction in the treatment of chronic neck pain.

27. Lin, T., Solomon, D. H., Tedeschi, S. K., Yoshida, K., & Kao Yang, Y. (2017). Comparative risk of cardiovascular outcomes between topical and oral nonselective NSAIDs in Taiwanese patients with rheumatoid arthritis. *Journal of the American Heart Association, 6*(11), e006874. doi:10.1161/JAHA.117.006874.

28. Dowell, D., Haegerich, T. M., & Chou, R. (2016). CDC guideline for prescribing opioids for chronic Pain—United States, 2016. *JAMA: The Journal of the American Medical Association, 315*(15), 1624. doi:10.1001/jama.2016.1464.

29. Smith, R. V., Havens, J. R., & Walsh, S. L. (2016). Gabapentin misuse, abuse and diversion: A systematic review. *Addiction (Abingdon, England), 111*(7), 1160–1174. doi:10.1111/add.13324.

30. Babatunde, O. O., Jordan, J. L., Van der Windt, D. A., Hill, J. C., Foster, N. E., & Protheroe, J. (2017). Effective treatment options for musculoskeletal pain in primary care: A systematic overview of current evidence. *PLoS ONE, 12*(6), e0178621. doi:10.1371/journal.pone.0178621.

31. Galhardoni, R., Correia, G. S., Araujo, H., et al. (2015). Repetitive transcranial magnetic stimulation in chronic pain: A review of the literature. *Archives of Physical Medicine and Rehabilitation, 96*, S156–S172. doi:10.1016/j.apmr.2014.11.010.

32. Manchikanti, L., Helm, S., Singh, V., et al. (2009). An algorithmic approach for clinical management of chronic spinal pain. *Pain Physician, 12*(4), E225–E264. http://www.ncbi.nlm.nih.gov/pubmed/19668283. (Accessed 5 February 2018).

33. Manchikanti, L., Cash, K. A., Pampati, V., & Malla, Y. (2012). Fluoroscopic cervical epidural injections in chronic axial or disc-related neck pain without disc herniation, facet joint pain, or radiculitis. *Journal of Pain Research, 5*, 227–236. doi:10.2147/JPR.S32692.

34. Bhagawati, D., & Gwilym, S. (2015). Neck pain with radiculopathy. *BMJ Clinical Evidence, 2015*, http://www.ncbi.nlm.nih.gov/pubmed/26695762. (Accessed 7 February 2018).

35. Cohen, S. (2015). Epidemiology, diagnosis and treatment of neck pain. *Mayo Clinic Proceedings, 90*(2), 284–299.

36. Shahidi, B., Curran-Everett, D., & Maluf, K. S. (2015). Psychosocial, physical, and neurophysiological risk factors for chronic neck pain: A prospective inception Cohort Study. *The Journal of Pain, 16*(12), 1288–1299. doi:10.1016/j.jpain.2015.09.002.

37. Sihawong, R., Sitthipornvorakul, E., Paksaichol, A., & Janwantanakul, P. (2016). Predictors for chronic neck and low back pain in office workers: A 1-year prospective cohort study. *Journal of Occupational Health, 58*(1), 16–24. doi:10.1539/joh.15-0168-OA.

CHAPTER **165**

OSTEOARTHRITIS

Joanne Sandberg-Cook

DEFINITION AND EPIDEMIOLOGY

Osteoarthritis (OA) is a progressive degenerative joint process. It involves degeneration of the articular (hyaline) cartilage layer on the ends of bones at the joints as well as increasing thickness and sclerosis of the bone plate and subsequent involvement of joint protective mechanisms including ligaments and muscle. OA manifests as a monoarticular or polyarticular phenomenon and is often asymmetric. It can occasionally appear as a more generalized disease. OA is the most common type of arthritis, and it usually begins asymptomatically in the second or third decade of life. By the fourth decade, most people have some degree of pathologic (radiologic) change on articular weight-bearing surfaces. Symptoms typically begin to appear in the fourth through sixth decades of life. Some degree of symptomatic arthritis is extremely common by the seventh decade. OA occurs more commonly in women, at least in middle-aged and elderly persons. Risk factors include age, obesity, prior trauma, genetics, repetitive activities, metabolic disorders, neurologic diseases, and hematologic conditions.[1]

The carpometacarpal joints of the thumbs, distal interphalangeal joints of the fingers, first metatarsophalangeal joints of the feet, cervical and lumbar spine, and weight-bearing joints such as the hips and knees are most commonly affected. OA can also affect previously injured joints. Pain, stiffness, and limited range of motion are the most common reasons for seeking medical care. The degenerative effects of OA result in physical disability and can have a profound impact on the quality of life.[1,2]

PATHOPHYSIOLOGY

Initially, the cartilage softens and becomes overhydrated and boggy, with decreased quantity and size of proteoglycans within the matrix. Collagen also loses its stiffness, with fewer cells and loss of cross-links as degradation continues.[3] The surface layers fibrillate, and the cartilage loses its thickness, develops surface crevices, and then loses integrity. Loose cartilaginous fragments (known as loose bodies) can flake off, blocking range of motion and contributing to pain and disability.

Chondrocytes proliferate with increased metabolic activity as the subchondral bone scleroses under the damaged areas. The bone thickens, stiffens, and then produces cysts, microfractures, and osteophytes at the joint margins,[3] findings that are often seen on imaging. The associated increased metabolic activity can be detected on a bone scan.

The cartilage surface is completely aneural, making the pathogenesis of pain from OA speculative. It is now thought to be a whole-joint disease with significant inflammatory soft tissue changes including synovitis as well as bone marrow lesions. Changes in joint nociceptors have been identified, and some researchers have suggested neuropathic pathways as contributors to pain.[4] Joint effusions are not uncommon, especially in the knee, causing stiffness and difficulty walking.

CLINICAL PRESENTATION AND PHYSICAL EXAMINATION

Insidious, progressive pain or stiffness of one or more joints may be the initial presenting complaint. Symptoms are most prevalent on arising, with a duration of less than 1 hour, and after a prolonged activity and are relieved by rest.[3] Weight-bearing activities, such as going up or down stairs, getting up from a sitting position, walking, prolonged standing, or changing activity level, can be particularly troublesome. The patient may also complain of crepitus (grinding), swelling, joint deformity, and gradual loss of motion as the disease progresses.

When OA involves the cervical or lumbar spine, neuropathy and radiculopathy may develop as nerves are compressed. OA involving the hip manifests with groin or buttock pain that can radiate to the knee. The pain can cause the patient to "favor" the hip, which in turn can contribute to specific muscle weakness. The resultant gait is known as Trendelenburg gait. OA of the knee commonly involves the medial joint compartment, leading to a varus deformity of the extremity. It can then progress to include the lateral joint compartment and patellofemoral articulations as well. Pain on palpation of the medial and lateral joint lines and joint effusions are often seen. Quadriceps muscle atrophy is common on the affected side.

OA of the hands manifests as Heberden nodes (deformity of the distal interphalangeal joints) and Bouchard nodes (deformity of the proximal interphalangeal joints). A compression test as well as pain with palpation of the joint can detect OA of the carpometacarpal joint. Contracture, deformity, and even joint fusion are common as the disease progresses. Fortunately, OA of the hands is seldom completely disabling.

DIAGNOSTICS
Essential Diagnostics

In the early stages of OA, radiographic findings may not be evident.[3] As the disease progresses and joint space is lost, radiographic changes become more prominent. Plain radiographs are often all that are needed to confirm the diagnosis. Magnetic resonance imaging (MRI) helps to identify changes in surrounding soft tissue. A bone scan may show increased metabolic activity within an arthritic joint.

Additional Diagnostics

OA is a nonsystemic disease. There are no serologic markers for OA as yet, but serologic tests are commonly performed to rule out other disorders. Examination of the joint fluid may be helpful in ruling out crystalline, infectious, or inflammatory conditions. See the diagnostics box for optional testing.

INITIAL DIAGNOSTICS

Osteoarthritis

LABORATORY
- None

ADDITIONAL DIAGNOSTICS
- Joint aspirate for crystals/white blood cells

IMAGING
- X-ray studies

DIFFERENTIAL DIAGNOSIS

The differential diagnosis of OA can be narrowed by a good patient history, patient age, and history of recent trauma or the presence of systemic symptoms such as fever or rash.

 Priority differentials include fracture, avascular necrosis, infectious arthritis, and Lyme disease (see Chapter 213). Other arthritic conditions, such as rheumatoid arthritis (see Chapter 197), gout and pseudogout (see Chapter 158), and psoriatic arthritis, are commonly seen with OA.[5]

INTERPROFESSIONAL COLLABORATIVE MANAGEMENT
Pharmacologic Management

Acetaminophen. Acetaminophen remains the mainstay for initial treatment of early OA. When taken in prescribed dosages, this drug is safe and can reduce discomfort without the additional risks of antiinflammatory medications. The current maximum daily dosage is one gram three times daily as needed. If the patient is also on warfarin, dosage should be limited to 2500 mg daily in divided doses. Renal and hepatic toxicity remains a concern especially in patients taking the maximum dosage over a period of time or in those using alcohol. Many over-the-counter cold and sleep medications contain acetaminophen, increasing the daily amount being taken by patients not aware of this.

Tramadol Hydrochloride (Ultram). Tramadol is a centrally acting, non-opioid pain reliever that is indicated for moderate to moderately severe pain. Tramadol is also available as a combination drug with acetaminophen. The combination is synergistic and can be given in addition to nonsteroidal antiinflammatory drugs (NSAIDs).

Nonsteroidal Antiinflammatory Drugs. NSAIDs have long been part of the treatment regimen for OA. They are most beneficial for their analgesic rather than antiinflammatory effect and are a cost-effective way of managing pain.[6] Traditional NSAIDs and cyclooxygenase 2 (COX2) selective NSAIDs are available over the counter and by prescription.[7] The COX2 selective NSAIDs were originally developed to reduce the risk of gastrointestinal toxicity associated with traditional NSAIDs and continue to be recommended to those patients taking warfarin as well as those on chronic steroids or with a history of gastrointestinal bleeding. Both traditional and COX2 selective NSAIDs have been shown to increase the patient's risk of cardiovascular disease including myocardial infarction and stroke. These warnings have been recently reiterated and strengthened as more of these drugs become available without a prescription.[8]

Traditional NSAIDs include ibuprofen, naproxen, diclofenac, and others. The health care provider will need to monitor patients closely for GI, renal, and cardiovascular toxicity. These drugs should be avoided in patients with heart failure, hypertension, or renal disease.[9] Consider prescribing gastrointestinal protective agents such as H_2 blockers or proton pump inhibitors to reduce the risk of GI intolerance. Older adults are especially vulnerable to the effects of NSAIDs. The American College of Rheumatology recommends that patients older than 75 years avoid oral NSAIDs in favor of topical alternatives.

Intra-Articular Approaches to Treatment

Hyaluronan. Intra-articular injections of exogenous hyaluronan, most effective in mild to moderate OA, can help reduce the pain of OA and improve fluid viscosity within the joint. It has been compared favorable to naproxen with fewer adverse reactions. Depending upon the preparation used, it is injected into the affected joint once a week for either 3 or 5 weeks. There seems to be no substantial difference in efficacy between available preparations.[10]

Intra-Articular Corticosteroid Injections. Intraarticular corticosteroid injections can also provide significant pain relief for mild to severe disease but the durations of benefit vary widely. These injections are not recommended more often than every 3 to 4 months because of potential adverse effects. Caution should be used with patients who are taking oral steroid preparations or who have diabetes; transient increases in blood sugar can be seen. All patients should be warned about transient increased pain, warmth, or redness after an injection. If these symptoms persist after a couple of days, the patient should be seen in follow-up.

Other Medications Helpful for Chronic Pain

Low-dose, long-acting opioids, when used cautiously and with close monitoring for effectiveness, can be well tolerated and effective at managing the chronic pain associated with OA. Opioids should be used only after all other pharmacologic and non-pharmologic treatments have failed and then only in

low doses over short periods of time. The usual warnings of increased sedation, constipation, dependence, and abuse apply here as well.

Gabapentin (Neurontin), selective serotonin reuptake inhibitors, and tricyclic antidepressants have also been used adjunctively in the management of chronic pain.

Topical medications, including over-the-counter rubs and patches and lidocaine patches as well as topical NSAID gel (diclofenac), may also provide some temporary benefit and are now recommended as a first-line agent for patients older than 75 years.[11]

Non-Pharmacologic Management

Exercise has a number of potential benefits for OA management including strengthening of supporting structure, improved range of motion, and decreased pain. Aerobic exercise can help with cardiovascular conditioning and weight reduction. An exercise program supervised by physical and/or occupational therapy can improve functional capacity and provide valuable patient education.[12] Stretching programs to reduce contractures; assistive devices such as canes, crutches, and walkers to reduce the weight-bearing load from painful joints; and bracing can all improve functional capacity and reduce pain. Locally applied heat, ice, warm baths, or ice baths can provide temporary relief. A referral to podiatry for prescription of supportive, well-cushioned footwear, custom orthotics, lifts, or wedges can help correct malalignment issues and leg length discrepancies and reduce stress on affected joints.

Weight Management. Each extra pound of weight increases loading across the knee threefold to sixfold. Losing weight will help to unload the joint and reduce symptoms. Weight loss of 7.7% over a 20-week period can be helpful to those patients who are overweight or obese.[13]

The Arthritis Diet and Activity Promotion Trial (ADAPT) demonstrated that the combination of modest weight loss plus moderate exercise provides better overall improvements in self-reported measures of pain and function and in performance measures of mobility in older, overweight, and obese adults with knee OA than either intervention alone.[14]

Complementary Approaches

Acupuncture. Acupuncture has been shown to improve pain and physical function at both 8 and 26 weeks.[15] Tai Chi has been shown to improve balance, strength, flexibility, and pain in OA as well as physical therapy with a higher patient compliance rate and is highly recommended as a gentle land-based exercise.[16]

Glucosamine With or Without Chondroitin. Evidence regarding the effectiveness of glucosamine with or without chondroitin for the treatment of OA is lacking.[17] The American Association of Orthopedic Surgeons has now dropped its recommendation for lack of evidence. Past multicenter, double-blind studies have also failed to demonstrate significant pain relief when compared to placebo. If patients wish to try this supplement, the recommended dosage is 500 mgs of glucosamine sulfate 3 times daily for 3 to 6 months. The supplement should be discontinued if there is no noticeable change within this time frame. There are few side effects and no known drug–drug interactions. Because glucosamine is a dietary supplement and not regulated by the FDA, potency and quality may not be consistent among brands.

Other Herbs and Dietary Supplements. Health care providers should be aware of any supplements being taken by their patients. The Arthritis Foundation has published a guide to the most commonly used supplements along with associated study results where they exist.[18] Omega-3 fatty acids, bromelaine, dimethyl sulfide (DMSO), ginger, methylsulfonylmethane (MSM), and S-adenosylmethionine (SAM-e) have all been used for the treatment of OA without scientific evidence of efficacy. Therapeutic magnets and copper have also been used, though there is no scientific evidence to support their usefulness.

Surgical consultation should be sought in the following situations: when joint pain fails to respond to conservative treatments discussed above or when joint pain and disability compromise lifestyle.

Arthroscopic débridement is no longer recommended as an approach, as studies demonstrated no long-term benefit and considerable risk of harm including joint pain, deep vein thrombosis, pulmonary embolism, and death.[19]

Total joint replacement may be recommended. Hip and knee replacements are highly successful operations that relieve pain and suffering for most. Joint replacement surgery is most successful when candidates for surgery are chosen judiciously and when performed by a surgeon who does many such surgeries per year and in institutions where such procedures are commonplace.[20] It is no longer a given that joint replacement surgery is a last-resort treatment. Assessing the patient's level of disability, general health, lifestyle, and comorbidities may be more useful determinants when assessing eligibility.

COMPLICATIONS

Pain and immobility that affect the patient's functional capacity and quality of life are the main complications associated with OA. When patients hurt, they find it difficult to exercise or to control weight. This can have a detrimental effect globally on the patient's well-being and mood. The risk of falling is higher as a direct effect of a painful or immobile arthritic joint and weakened muscle. This can result in fractures, dislocations, head injury, and increased immobility.

Other complications are directly related to the treatment of the disease, including medication side effects, infection or microfractures of damaged joints, and failure of prosthetic components.

EMERGING MANAGEMENT TRENDS

Current research is focused on disease-modifying agents designed to alter the course of OA rather than treat its symptoms. The potential role of inflammation in the development of OA through the complement system has been identified in mouse models, allowing for hope that future therapies can target this inflammation.

Cartilage regeneration, stem cell transplantation, gene therapy, and implantable gene chips are proving to be exciting new directions for researchers.[21] Use of growth factors found in plasma-rich protein intraarticular injections is being used as a treatment for sports injuries as well as OA with statistically significant improvements in pain. Advances in diagnostic tools that target cartilage damage well ahead of traditional imaging are being identified. High-tech prosthetic components that last longer and are less likely to cause complications are in development.[21]

PATIENT AND FAMILY EDUCATION

The treatment of OA should begin with a clear explanation of the disease process and likely progression of the disease. Instruction on methods to protect the painful joint should include workplace or lifestyle modifications including weight reduction. The use of assistive devices, such as a cane, crutches, or a walker, can be helpful. Patients are encouraged to be realistic about their limitations to avoid exacerbations of symptoms.

HEALTH PROMOTION

Obesity and repetitive stress or trauma are specific modifiable risk factors for the development of OA; reduction in one or both may substantially reduce symptoms and disease progression. Maintaining an active lifestyle including low-impact, moderate-intensity exercise and weight control can significantly improve the quality of life for these individuals. Policies and interventions to reduce musculoskeletal injuries in all settings should be implemented and enforced. This includes the prevention of athletic injuries in schools, interventions for workplace injuries, and training and education to reduce injuries related to falls.

REFERENCES

1. National Institute of Arthritis and Musculoskeletal and Skin Diseases. (revised May 2016). Handout on health: osteoarthritis, NIH Publication No. 06-4617. Retrieved from www.niams.nih.gov/Health_Info/Osteoarthiitis/default-asp. (Accessed 12 July 2017).
2. Arthritis Foundation. Disease Center: osteoarthritis. Retrieved from www.arthritis.org/disease-center. (Accessed 12 July 2017).
3. El-Tawii, S., Arendt, E., & Parker, D. (2015). Position Statement: The edpidemiology, pathogenesis and risk factors of osteoarthritis of the knee. *Journal or Isakos*, 1(4), 219–229.
4. Arendt-Nielson, L. (2017). Joint Pain: More to it than just structural damage. *Pain*, 158, s66–s73.
5. Ashford, S., & Williard, J. (2014). Osteoarthritis: A review. *The Nurse Practitioner*, 39(5), 1–8.
6. DaCosta, B. R., Reichenbach, S., & Keller, N. (Published on line March 17, 2016). Effectiveness of Non-Steroidal anti-inflammatory drugs for the treatment of pain in knee and hip osteoarthritis: A network metaanalysis. *Lancet*. Retrieved from http://www.thelancet.com/journals/lancet/article/p11so140-6736%2816%2930002-2/abstract/Articleabstract. (Access 11 July 2017).
7. Katz, J. N., Smith, S. R., & Collins, J. E. (2016). Cost effectiveness of non steroidal anti-inflammatory drugs and opioids in the treatment of osteoarthritis in older adults with multiple comorbidities. *Osteoarthritis and Cartilage*, 24(3), 409–418.
8. Increased risk of heart attack and stroke from non steroidal anti-inflammatory drug use. Retrieved from https://www.FDA.gov?foreconsumers/consumer updte/ucm453610.htm. (Accessed 11 July 2017).
9. Arfe, A., Scotti, L., Varas-Lorenzo, C., et al. (2016). Common non-steroidal anti-inflammatory drugs associated with an increased risk of hospital admission for heart failure. *British Medical Journal*, 354, i4857.
10. Maheu, E., Rannon, F., & Reginstar, J. Y. (2016). Efficacy and safety of hyaluronic acis in the management of osteoarthritis: Evidence from real life setting trials and surveys. *Seminars in Arthritis and Rheumatism*, 45(4suppl), s18–s21.
11. Rannou, F., Pelletier, J.-P., & Martel-Pelletier, J. (2016). Efficacy and safety of topical non steroidal drugs in the management of osteoarthritis: Evidence for real life setting trials and surveys. *Seminars in Arthritis and Rheumatism*, 45(4suppl), s18–s21.
12. Callahan, L. F., & Ambrose, K. R. (2015). Physical activity and osteoarthritis-consideration at the population and clinical level. *Osteoarthrits and Cartilage*, 23(1), 31–33.
13. Atukorala, L., Makovey, J., Lawler, L., et al. (2016). Is there a dose response relationship between weight loss and symptom improvement with knee osteoarthritis? *Arthritis Care & Research*, 68(8), 1106–1114.
14. GBD2015 Obesity Collaborators. (2017). Health effects of overweight and obesity in 195 countries over 25 years. *The New England Journal of Medicine*, 377, 13–27.

15. Kliger, B., Nielson, A., Kohrrer, C., et al. (2017). Acupuncture therapy in a group setting for chronic pain. *Pain Medicine (Malden, Mass.)*, pns134. doi:10.1093/pnx134. (Accessed 11 July 2017).

16. Wang, C., Schmid, C., Iverson, M., et al. (2016). Comparativeness of Tai Chi vs PT for knee osteoarthritis. *Annals of Internal Medicine*, 165(2), 77–86. Retrieved from http://annals.org/17May, 2016. (Accessed 12 July 2017).

17. Roman-Blas, J. A., Castaneda, S., & Sanchez-Pernaute, O.; CS/GS Combined Therapy Study Group. (2017). Combined treatment with chondroitin sulfate and glucosamine sulfate shows no superiority over placebo for reduction of joint pain and functional impairment in patients with knee osteoarthritis: A six month multicenter, randomized, double blind, placebo controlled clinical trial. *Arthritis & Rheumatology*, 69(1), 77.

18. Welland, D. Arthritis Today's Supplement and Herb guide. Retrieved from www.arthritis.org. (Access 13 July 2017).

19. Thorland, J. B., Juhl, C. B., Roos, E. M., & Lohmander, L. S. (2015). Arthroscopic Surgery for degenerative knee: Systematic review and meta-analysis of benefits and harms. *British Medical Journal*, 350, h2747, Epub2015 Jun 16. Retrieved from http://www.bmj.com/content/350/bmj.h2747. (Accessed 21 October 2017).

20. Ravi, B., Jenkinsn, R., Austin, P., et al. (2014). Relation between surgeon volume and risk of complication after total hip replacement: Propensity score matched cohort. *British Medical Journal*, 348, g3284.

21. Zhang, W., Ouyang, H., Dass, C., & Xu, J. (2016). Current research on pharmacologic and regenerative therapies of osteoarthritis. *Bone Research*, 4. Retrieved from https://www.ncbi.nim.nih.gov/pmc/articles/PMC4772471/. 15040. (July 12, 2017).

CHAPTER 166

OSTEOMYELITIS
Michael S. Calderwood

 Emergency hospitalization is indicated for vertebral osteomyelitis with neurologic symptoms and for patients presenting with a septic physiology.

DEFINITION AND EPIDEMIOLOGY

Osteomyelitis refers to an infection involving bone resulting from: (1) hematogenous seeding via bacteria in the bloodstream; (2) direct spread from a contiguous focus, such as an adjoining soft tissue infection or septic joint; or (3) direct inoculation via trauma or surgery.[1] It can lead to progressive destruction of bone and formation of dead bone fragments without a blood supply (sequestra). These sequestra can complicate efforts to cure the infection.

In general, acute osteomyelitis has a duration of illness less than 2 weeks and chronic osteomyelitis has a duration of illness longer than 3 months. Infections with a duration of illness between these two are labeled subacute, with the development of bone necrosis defining the transition from acute to chronic osteomyelitis.[2,3] Once bone necrosis has developed, surgical débridement is often required.

In terms of pathogens, osteomyelitis is most commonly caused by bacteria, with infections caused by other pathogens such as yeast and mycobacteria being rare. The majority of cases are caused by staphylococci, including *Staphylococcus aureus* and coagulase-negative staphylococci.[4] Consideration should be given to Gram-negative bacteria, including enteric Gram-negative rods and *Pseudomonas aeruginosa*, in the setting of an open ulcer, diabetic foot, or penetrating trauma. Anaerobes are also a consideration, in the setting of necrotic soft tissue. Infections caused by hematogenous seeding are typically monomicrobial, while infections caused by direct spread

TABLE 166.1	Anatomic Classification Osteomyelitis (Cierny-Mader Classification)	
Stage and Description		**Etiology**
I. **Medullary:** Infection confined to intramedullary surfaces of the bone		Hematogenous infection
II. **Superficial:** Infected necrotic surface of bone at the base of a soft tissue wound		Contiguous soft tissue infection
III. **Localized:** Full-thickness cortical sequestration but no loss of bone stability before and after débridement		Trauma; evolution of stage I or II; iatrogenic
IV. **Diffuse:** Diffuse osteomyelitis with loss of bone stability before or after débridement		Trauma; evolution of stage I or II; iatrogenic

TABLE 166.2	Physiologic Classification of Hosts With Osteomyelitis (Cierny-Mader Classification)	
Class		**Comorbidities**
A. Normal host with osteomyelitis		
B$_S$. Host with Systemic Compromise		• Diabetes mellitus • Extremes of age • Hepatic failure • Hypoxia (chronic) • Immunodeficiency • Immunosuppression • Malignancy • Malnutrition • Renal failure
B$_L$. Host with Local Compromise		• Arteritis • Extensive scarring • Lymphedema (chronic) • Major vessel compromise • Neuropathy • Radiation fibrosis • Small vessel disease • Tobacco abuse (≥2 packs per day) • Venous stasis
C. Host where morbidity of treatment is worse than morbidity from osteomyelitis		

from a contiguous focus or direct inoculation may be either monomicrobial or polymicrobial.[1]

Based on a classification scheme developed by Cierny and colleagues, the extent of anatomic involvement can help to determine treatment (Table 166.1).[5] Patients with stage 1 osteomyelitis can often be treated with antibiotics alone, while those with stage 2-4 osteomyelitis often require débridement and surgical management in addition to antibiotics. Prognosis can be further predicted by comorbid conditions (Table 166.2).[6]

Class A hosts with normal vasculature, normal metabolic factors, and a normal immune system have a favorable prognosis. Class B hosts carry a worse prognosis by virtue of local or systemic compromise. Class C hosts represent a group for which treatment of the osteomyelitis may be worse than the disease itself. The Cierny-Mader staging system is important to medical and surgical management but also guides prognosis and education.

PATHOPHYSIOLOGY

In general, healthy bone is fairly resistant to infection, with osteomyelitis resulting in cases where there is inoculation of a large number of organisms, abnormal bone, or the presence of foreign material. The pathogenesis of osteomyelitis is also affected by the infecting organism and its virulence factors, which determine adherence and resistance to host defenses, the age and comorbidities of the patient, and the type of bone affected.[1,4]

The recruitment of acute inflammatory cells such as polymorphonuclear leukocytes (PMNs) in the acute phase of disease results in edema, vascular congestion, and small vessel thrombosis. Compromised blood flow leads to bone destruction and the formation of sequestra.[2] This dead bone is slowly eroded and absorbed, but it can become a nidus for infection, particularly in the setting of trauma, fracture, orthopedic prosthetic hardware, and vascular insufficiency where sequestra develop more rapidly.[1,7] As healing occurs, new bone is formed from the vascular periosteum, and it is possible for this new bone to create an enclosed capsule (involucrum). This can lead to the formation of Brodie abscesses in the long bones of younger patients, which require surgical débridement.[3] Other patients, adults in particular, may develop chronic, draining sinus tracts due to poorly healing bone.[1,8] A failure of fractured bone to heal may indicate chronic osteomyelitis.

Focusing on hematogenous seeding, osteomyelitis most commonly affects the long bones of the legs (femur/tibia) and upper extremities (humerus) in children,[3] while more commonly affecting the spine (vertebrae) in adults.[1,8]

CLINICAL PRESENTATION AND PHYSICAL EXAM

Patients presenting with acute osteomyelitis may have localized pain, erythema, and/or swelling in the region of the infected bone. Fever may also be present, particularly in infections caused by *S. aureus*, and children may demonstrate limping or inability to walk. It is not uncommon, though, for the presentation to be insidious with a delay in diagnosis of weeks, or possibly months. In these cases of sub-acute osteomyelitis, the primary symptom may be a dull, persistent pain. This is particularly common in infections involving the hips, pelvis, and spine.

In particular subpopulations, it is also worth searching for helpful clues. For instance, in diabetic patients, an ulcer larger than 2 × 2 cm and the ability to probe bone at the base of an open ulcer are both predictive of osteomyelitis.[9,10] This ability to probe bone is also helpful when examining patients with sacral decubitus ulcers that develop in the setting of pressure sores from immobility. Additionally, in patients presenting with vertebral osteomyelitis, up to 25% may have signs of cord compression (i.e., lower extremity weakness or loss of sensation, bowel or bladder incontinence), and 27% to 31% may have evidence of endocarditis (i.e., heart murmur, Janeway lesions, Osler nodes).[11,12,13]

As discussed previously, chronic osteomyelitis may present with a draining sinus, a poorly healing skin ulcer, or a failure of a previously fractured bone to heal on serial radiology. Patients with chronic osteomyelitis may also report weight loss, poor appetite, and/or generalized fatigue. Fever is less common with chronic osteomyelitis.

DIAGNOSTICS
Essential Diagnostics

In patients where history and exam have suggested a diagnosis of osteomyelitis, labs should be obtained for a complete blood count with differential and a C-reactive protein (CRP). Many guidelines also recommend obtaining an erythrocyte sedimentation rate (ESR), but it should be noted that an ESR has a lower specificity than a CRP in cases of osteomyelitis and is slower to improve after initiation of treatment.[14]

If the patient is febrile and/or has evidence of vertebral osteomyelitis, then blood cultures should also be obtained. One study found that over 50% of patients with pyogenic vertebral osteomyelitis had a positive blood culture,[15] although blood cultures are more likely to be positive in acute disease. The benefit of this is that a positive blood culture can often avoid more invasive culturing.

In terms of imaging, it is reasonable to start with a **plain x-ray** to assess for bone changes suggestive of osteomyelitis if the area of concern is in the extremities and symptoms have been present for two or more weeks. While plain x-ray has a lower sensitivity than other modalities, particularly in acute disease, it is less expensive and able to be performed rapidly.[16]

If the x-ray is normal or not definitive for osteomyelitis, then MRI imaging is preferred due to a higher sensitivity, as well as a good negative predictive value.[9,17] CT imaging and nuclear imaging are two other modalities, if MRI is not possible, but neither is as good as a MRI. If there is no osteomyelitis on MRI, then the likelihood of osteomyelitis being present is very low. It is important to recognize, though, that certain diagnoses are difficult to differentiate from osteomyelitis, even on MRI. One example is neuropathic (Charcot) arthropathy seen in patients with diabetes.

Therefore, the diagnosis of osteomyelitis is definitively based on a bone biopsy obtained under sterile conditions and sent for pathology and cultures (Gram stain, aerobic bacterial culture, anaerobic bacterial culture, fungal stain and culture, and acid fast bacilli [AFB] stain and culture).[10,12] Both open biopsy and needle biopsy are possible for obtaining culture data, although open biopsy yields a higher rate of positive culture results.[18,19] Ideally, these cultures are obtained off of antibiotics for at least 48 hours, given the impact of pre-biopsy antibiotic duration on culture yield; however, short courses of pre-biopsy antibiotics started in the setting of systemic infection do not significantly impact bone culture results.[18,20]

Alternative Diagnostics

The general teaching is that cultures of wound drainage should not be used in place of bone culture. This is because of a discordance between the bacteria cultured from the wound and those cultured from the bone.[21] The concordance is best, though, for *S. aureus*, and some therefore do use culture data from wound drainage to decide on the need to empirically treat for methicillin-resistant *Staphylococcus aureus* (MRSA) in patients where a bone biopsy is unable to be obtained.

Where possible, though, bone biopsy is the gold standard with the highest accuracy in identifying the infecting organism(s). To further improve the sensitivity of cultures, particularly from removed orthopedic hardware, some microbiology

INITIAL DIAGNOSTICS

LABORATORY
- Complete blood count and differential
- CRP (+/– ESR)
- Blood cultures

IMAGING
- X-ray examination
- MRI

OTHER DIAGNOSTICS
- Open bone biopsy or needle aspiration of bone with culture and sensitivity

labs have also begun to use **sonication** to increase the likelihood of recovering a pathogen from prosthetic material.[22] Sonification improves the accuracy of the culture results [23]

DIFFERENTIAL DIAGNOSIS

 Differentials to be excluded include gout, neuropathic (Charcot) arthropathy, osteonecrosis, healing fracture, bone malignancy, or other infections requiring treatment (e.g., cellulitis/abscess, septic joint).

Critical in the workup of osteomyelitis is the differentiation between soft tissue infection, septic arthritis (Chapter 159), and osteomyelitis, as each of these diagnoses requires a different duration of antibiotic treatment. As discussed above, MRI imaging (with follow-up bone biopsy of abnormal appearing bone) can help to determine bone involvement. If a joint effusion is present, fluid from the joint should also be aspirated (via arthrocentesis) to assess for septic arthritis. When present, septic arthritis (Chapter 159) may require more thorough drainage (potentially in the operating room), depending on the joint involved, the clinical progression on antibiotics, and the presence or absence of a prosthetic joint.

Noninfectious rheumatologic diseases may also mimic osteomyelitis. Pathology or joint fluid analysis with uric acid crystals suggests a diagnosis of gout, which tends to present with acute joint inflammation. As previously discussed, neuropathic (Charcot) arthropathy seen in patients with diabetes can also mimic osteomyelitis and should be considered in the right patient population, in cases where the bone culture is negative.

Finally, osteonecrosis, healing fractures, and bone malignancies may all mimic osteomyelitis on radiographic imaging, with nonspecific pain reported by the patient.

INTERPROFESSIONAL COLLABORATIVE MANAGEMENT
Non-Pharmacologic Management
- Infectious disease consultation is recommended for the management of long-term antibiotics, for patients with resistant organisms, or for complex wound infections.
- Surgical consultation is necessary in patients with vascular insufficiency and/or an infection in need of débridement or drainage. The surgical specialties most commonly involved include vascular surgery and orthopedic surgery, although neurosurgical consultation may also be warranted in cases of vertebral osteomyelitis complicated by an epidural abscess.
- Involvement of interventional radiology is necessary in cases where a needle biopsy is pursued in place of an open biopsy to obtain bone tissue.

- Consultation with a wound care specialist should be done early for patients with progressive or chronic wounds. In these cases, health care providers should also address nutrition, control of diabetes, reduction of immunosuppressive drugs, and smoking cessation.
- Vascular surgery may also be needed for revascularization in patients with chronic nonhealing wounds due to arterial insufficiency, and in these cases, plastic surgery may also be required to bring skin grafts or tissue flaps over exposed bone.

Pharmacologic Management
- In clinically stable patients, consideration should be given to delaying antibiotic therapy until cultures can be obtained to drive therapeutic decision making.
- Empiric antibiotics typically include coverage against staphylococci, including MRSA, streptococci, and Gram-negative rods. A common empiric regimen is vancomycin plus a third-generation cephalosporin such as ceftriaxone, recognizing that empiric coverage of *P. aeruginosa* should be limited to specific high-risk groups. A fluoroquinolone is an alternative if the patient has a β-lactam allergy.[1,8,12]
- In patients presenting with severe sepsis, injection drug use, an open ulcer, a diabetic foot infection, or penetrating trauma, selection of an empiric anti-pseudomonal antibiotic may be substituted for ceftriaxone. These include later-generation cephalosporins (ceftazidime, cefepime) or β-lactam/β-lactamase inhibitor combinations (piperacillin-tazobactam).
- Empiric anti-fungal and anti-mycobacterial therapy is not typically warranted. This is also true for empiric coverage of anaerobes, unless there is necrotic tissue and concern for a polymicrobial infection.
- Once cultures have identified the pathogen(s) of interest, the treatment should be tailored to treat this infection (Table 166.3).[1,8,12]
- Most often, osteomyelitis is treated with 6 weeks of intravenous antibiotic therapy through a central line, most commonly a peripherally inserted central catheter (PICC). Data suggest, however, that a step-down to oral antibiotic therapy should be considered in pediatric patients.[24]
- There are infectious disease specialists who extend parenteral antibiotic treatment out to 8 weeks for difficult-to-treat organisms such as MRSA. This is often done when the CRP remains elevated at the 6-week mark, because of data suggesting a lower relapse rate at 8 weeks compared to 6 weeks (in MRSA vertebral osteomyelitis).[25]
- Beyond 6 to 8 weeks, antibiotics are typically no longer indicated, unless there is concern about inadequate source control via débridement, particularly in the setting of retaining prosthetic material such as orthopedic hardware. If there is concern for infected orthopedic hardware that was unable to be removed, then long-term suppression with oral antibiotics may be warranted.[26] A discussion about the various treatment options and duration is beyond the scope of this chapter and should involve an infectious diseases specialist.

LIFE SPAN CONSIDERATIONS
Osteomyelitis is usually not a fatal infection, but associated sepsis may be life-threatening. In addition, patients with multiple comorbidities (Cierny-Mader Class B and C), with drug resistant microorganisms, or with inadequate source control via

TABLE 166.3 Antibiotic Therapy for Osteomyelitis

Microorganism	Preferred Antibiotics
Methicillin susceptible *Staphylococcus aureus* (and methicillin-susceptible coagulase negative staphylococci)	Nafcillin, oxacillin, cefazolin, or ceftriaxone
Methicillin-resistant *Staphylococcus aureus* (and methicillin-resistant coagulase negative staphylococci)	Vancomycin or daptomycin[a]
Streptococci	Penicillin or ceftriaxone
Ampicillin-susceptible *Enterococcus* species	Ampicillin
Ampicillin-resistant *Enterococcus* species	Vancomycin (if not resistant) or daptomycin[a]
Enterobacteriaceae (enteric Gram-negative rods)	Ceftriaxone or ciprofloxacin (with cefepime and ertapenem reserved for resistant infections)
Pseudomonas aeruginosa	Ceftazidime, cefepime, or piperacillin-tazobactam.[b]

[a]Linezolid is a possible substitute for vancomycin or daptomycin, but this antibiotic has the downside of being bacteriostatic rather bactericidal. In addition, cytopenias can limit the ability to give linezolid for a 6-week treatment course.
[b]Ciprofloxacin may be used, but some prefer to give ciprofloxacin in combination with a beta-lactam to prevent the development of resistance on therapy. Aztreonam may be substituted in patients with a severe β-lactam allergy. Anti-pseudomonal carbapenems such as meropenem should be reserved for multidrug-resistant *Pseudomonas aeruginosa*.

débridement often suffer prolonged illness from the sequelae of osteomyelitis. This can lead to prolonged hospitalizations, prolonged period in long-term care facilities, and amputations impacting mobility. Each of these can have a serious impact on life span.

COMPLICATIONS

At the time of diagnosis, patients should be assessed for metastatic foci of infection. In the setting of hematogenous spread, it is possible for infection to involve more than one part of the body. Particular attention should be paid to areas with prosthetic material. In addition, infection may threaten adjacent structures such as muscle, tendons, and joints.

During the acute treatment of osteomyelitis, the health care provider must monitor the patient for allergic reaction and toxicity of antibiotics, diarrhea caused by *Clostridium difficile*, thrombosis and infection related to central lines, and response to therapy. Central lines should be removed soon after completion of antibiotics to avoid providing a focus for further infection.

In the setting of chronic osteomyelitis, it is also important to monitor for squamous cell carcinoma that can develop at sites of chronic drainage such as sinus tracts.

PATIENT AND FAMILY EDUCATION

1. To help prevent osteomyelitis, patients with diabetes, peripheral vascular disease, or neuropathy should perform regular foot inspections to identify trauma. The identifications of open wounds or ulcers requires prompt medical attention. To lower the risk of infectious complications, all patients should be educated on the importance of smoking cessation and good diabetic control.
2. Patients who are diagnosed with osteomyelitis need to be educated on the various diagnostic and therapeutic options. It is also important for patients to understand that treatment of osteomyelitis takes a multidisciplinary team.
3. At a minimum, treatment will involve 6 weeks of antibiotics; however, surgery may be required to control the infection. Patients need to be educated about prolonged antibiotic therapy, central venous lines, and potential antibiotic complications.
4. In some cases, long-term suppression with an oral antibiotic may be required.
5. In severe cases, it is also possible that an amputation will be needed to cure the infection. This requires extensive discussion with the patient and their family, but it is important for patients to understand that amputation sometimes provides better long-term functional recovery than a chronic, nonhealing infection.

REFERENCES

1. Schmitt, S. K. (2017). Osteomyelitis. *Infectious Disease Clinics of North America, 31*, 325–338.
2. Waldvogel, F. A., Medoff, G., & Swartz, M. M. (1970). Osteomyelitis: A review of clinical features, therapeutic considerations, and unusual aspects. *The New England Journal of Medicine, 282*, 198–206. (classic reference).
3. Peltola, H., & Paakkonen, M. (2014). Acute osteomyelitis in children. *The New England Journal of Medicine, 370*, 352–360.
4. Mandell, G. L., Bennett, J. E., & Dolin, R. (Eds.), (2014). *Mandell, Douglas, and Bennett's principles and practice of infectious diseases* (8th ed.). Philadelphia, PA: Saunders.
5. Cierny, G., 3rd, Mader, J. T., & Penninck, J. J. (1985). A clinical staging system of adult osteomyelitis. *Contemporary Orthopaedics, 10*, 17–37. (classic reference).
6. Mader, J. T., Shirtliff, M., & Calhoun, J. H. (1997). Staging and staging application in osteomyelitis. *Clinical Infectious Diseases: An Official Publication of the Infectious Diseases Society of America, 25*, 1303–1309.
7. Birt, M., Andreson, D., Toby, B., & Wang, J. (2017). Osptomyelitis: Recent advances in pathophysiology and therapeutic strategies. *Journal of Orthopedics, 14*(1), 45–52.
8. Calhoun, J. H., & Manring, M. M. (2005). Adult osteomyelitis. *Infectious Disease Clinics of North America, 19*, 765–786.
9. Butalia, S., Palda, V. A., & Sargent, R. J. (2009). Does this patient with diabetes have osteomyelitis of the lower extremity? *JAMA: The Journal of the American Medical Association, 299*, 806–813.
10. Lipsky, B. A., Berendt, A. R., Cornia, P. B., et al. (2012). 2012 Infectious Diseases Society of America clinical practice guideline for the diagnosis and treatment of diabetic foot infections. *Clinical Infectious Diseases: An Official Publication of the Infectious Diseases Society of America, 64*, e132–e173.
11. McHenry, M. C., Easley, A. K., & Locker, G. A. (2002). Vertebral osteomyelitis: Long-term outcome for 253 patients from 7 Cleveland-area hospitals. *Clinical Infectious Diseases: An Official Publication of the Infectious Diseases Society of America, 34*, 1342–1350.
12. Berbari, E. F., Kanj, S. S., Kowalski, T. J., et al. (2015). 2015 Infectious Diseases Society of America (IDSA) clinical practice guidelines for the diagnosis and treatment of native vertebral osteomyelitis in adults. *Clinical Infectious Diseases: An Official Publication of the Infectious Diseases Society of America, 61*, e26–e46.
13. Koslow, M., Kuperstein, R., Eshed, I., Perelman, M., Maor, E., & Sidi, Y. (2014). The unique clinical features and outcome of infectious endocarditis and vertebral osteomyelitis co-infection. *The American Journal of Medicine, 127*, 669, e9–15.
14. Michail, M., Jude, E., Liaskos, C., et al. (2013). The performance of serum inflammatory markers for the diagnosis and follow-up of patients with osteomyelitis. *The International Journal of Lower Extremity Wounds, 12*, 94–99.
15. Bae, J. Y., Kim, C.-J., Kim, U. J., Song, K.-H., Kim, E. S., Kang, S. J., et al. (2018). Concordance of results of blood and tissue cultures from patients with pyogenic spondylitis: A retrospective cohort study. *Clinical Microbiology and Infection, 24*(3), 278–282.

16. Smith, B. J., Buchanan, G. S., & Shuler, F. D. (2016). A comparison of imaging modalities for the diagnosis of osteomyelitis. *Marshall Journal of Medicine, 2*(Iss. 3), http://dx.doi.org/10.18590/mjm.2016.vol2.iss3.10. Article 10.

17. Hingorani, A., LaMuraglia, G., Henke, P., et al. (2016). The management of diabetic foot: A clinical guideline by the Society for Vascular Surgery in collaboration with the American Podiatric Medicine association and the Society for Vascular Medicine. *Journal of Vascular Surgery, 63*(2), 3s–21s.

18. Marschall, J., Bhavan, K. P., Olsen, M. A., Fraser, V. J., Wright, N. M., & Warren, D. K. (2011). The impact of prebiopsy antibiotics on pathogen recovery in hematogenous vertebral osteomyelitis. *Clinical Infectious Diseases: An Official Publication of the Infectious Diseases Society of America, 52,* 867–872.

19. Kim, C. J., Kang, S. J., Yoon, D., et al. (2015). Factors influencing culture positivity in pyogenic vertebral osteomyelitis patients with prior antibiotic exposure. *Antimicrobial Agents and Chemotherapy, 59,* 2470–2473.

20. Zhorne, D. J., Altobelli, M. E., & Cruz, A. T. (2015). Impact of antibiotic pretreatment on bone biopsy yield for children with acute hematogenous osteomyelitis. *Hospital Pediatrics, 5,* 337–341.

21. Groll, M., Woods, T., & Salcido, R. (2018). Osteomyelitis: A Contect for wound management. *Advances in Skin and Wound Care, 31*(6), 253–262.

22. Liu, H., Zhang, Y., Li, L., & Zou, H. C. (2017). The application of sonication in the diagnosis of periprosthetic joint infection. *European Journal of Clinical Microbiology and Infectious Diseases, 36*(1), 1–9.

23. Rothenberg, A. C., Wilson, A. E., Hayes, J. P., et al. (2017). Sonication of arthroplasty implants improves accuracy of periprosthetic joint infection cultures. *Clinical Orthopaedics and Related Research, 475*(7), 1827–1836.

24. Keren, R., Shah, S. S., Srivastava, R., et al. (2015). Comparative effectiveness of intravenous vs. oral antibiotics for post discharge treatment of acute osteomyelitis in children. *JAMA Pediatr, 169,* 120–128.

25. Park, K. H., Chong, Y. P., Kim, S. H., et al. (2013). Clinical characteristics and therapeutic outcomes of hematogenous vertebral osteomyelitis caused by methicillin-resistant Staphylococcus aureus. *The Journal of Infection, 67,* 556–564.

26. Keller, S. C., Cosgrove, S. E., Higgins, Y., Piggot, D. A., Osgood, G., & Auwaerter, P. G. (2016). Role of suppressive oral antibiotics in orthopedic hardware infections for those not undergoing two-stage replacement surgery. *Open Forum Infectious Diseases, 30,* ofw176.

CHAPTER **167**

SHOULDER PAIN

Kathy J. Fabiszewski

 Immediate emergency department referral or orthopedic consultation is indicated for patients with suspected shoulder dislocation, fracture, joint infection, a history of malignancy, or significant vascular, sensory, or motor deficit.

DEFINITION AND EPIDEMIOLOGY

Shoulder pain is the third most common cause of musculoskeletal pain after low back pain and neck pain,[1] being most prevalent in the 25 to 64 age group and in women (24.9% vs. 15.4% in men).[2] In addition, shoulder complaints are common in adolescents.[2] Shoulder pain encompasses a diverse array of pathologies and can affect up to one-fourth of the population, depending on age and risk factors.[3] Shoulder pain is most often caused by an intrinsic disorder of the shoulder resulting from acute or chronic trauma, injury, and overuse or inflammation of the shoulder girdle and the surrounding articular surfaces, ligaments, tendons, and periarticular structures. Injury coupled with pain predisposes the individual to functional impairment or disability. Chronic shoulder pain has large health care costs and a major impact on the health of affected individuals including absence from work and disability.[2] The primary health care provider can, in most cases, diagnose and treat shoulder pain without specialty consultation.

PATHOPHYSIOLOGY

The shoulder joint is a complex articulation that has the greatest range of motion of any joint in the human body.[4] It is composed of four separate joints or articulations (sternoclavicular, acromioclavicular, glenohumeral, and scapulothoracic) that are made up of only three bones: the scapula, clavicle, and proximal humerus. The shoulder, or glenohumeral joint (the articulation of the humerus and the glenoid fossa of the scapula), is a closely fitted, shallow, complex ball-and-socket joint that is capable of a wide, almost global range of motion. Adjacent to the glenohumeral joint are the acromioclavicular joint (the articulation between the acromion process and the clavicle) and the sternoclavicular joint (the articulation between the manubrium of the sternum and the clavicle), which form the shoulder girdle. At the scapulothoracic articulation, the scapula is suspended from the posterior thoracic wall by muscle attachments to the ribs and spine.[5] Normal shoulder motion depends on the smooth, integrated movement of these four articulations.

The primary movers of the glenohumeral joint are the pectoralis major and minor (adduct the shoulder), deltoid (abducts the shoulder), teres major, and latissimus dorsi.[5] The trapezius muscles elevate and rotate the scapula. The shoulder joints are stabilized by the soft tissues of the shoulder girdle, including the joint capsule, ligaments, glenoid labrum (a fibrocartilaginous ring attached to the outer rim of the glenoid that provides depth and stability), muscles of the rotator cuff, long head of the biceps, and scapular stabilizers. The shoulder socket (glenoid) is shallow and, because of the wide range of motion of the glenohumeral joint, inherently unstable; it is, in fact, the most unstable ball-and-socket joint in the human body. This anatomic arrangement provides for greater mobility but is accomplished by compromise of some stability (the maintenance of the humeral head properly positioned within the glenoid cavity), making the shoulder one of the most commonly dislocated joints in the body.

The rotator cuff consists of the musculotendinous attachments of four muscles—the supraspinatus, infraspinatus, teres minor, and subscapularis muscles—that come together and form a cuff around the head of the humerus, attaching to the greater and lesser tuberosities. The rotator cuff compresses the humeral head in the glenoid fossa against the labrum and acts as the primary dynamic stabilizer to the glenohumeral joint. The chief function of the rotator cuff is the maintenance of stability during movements.[6]

The greater tuberosity of the humerus, the tendons of the rotator cuff muscles that elevate the arm, and the subacromial bursa move back and forth through a tight archway of bone and ligament known as the coracoacromial arch. When the arm is raised, the archway becomes smaller, causing these structures to impinge on one another and making them prone to inflammation and degeneration.

CLINICAL PRESENTATION AND PHYSICAL EXAMINATION

Shoulder pain symptoms may be acute or chronic, specific or vague, persistent or recurrent. The patient with a shoulder problem typically reports shoulder pain that is aggravated by movement and is often accompanied by limitation of movement. There may or may not be a history of trauma or overuse. Surprisingly, many individuals fail to recollect an

BOX **167.1**

Simple Shoulder Test

Instructions to Patients: Answer "Yes" or No" to each question below. In all cases, please rate your shoulder comfort and function as they have affected your lifestyle and abilities over the past week. Please answer all questions to the best of your ability.

Dominant Hand (select only one): Right   Left   Ambidextrous
Shoulder Evaluated (Select only one): Right   Left

1. Is your shoulder comfortable with your arm at rest by your side?
2. Does your shoulder allow you to sleep comfortably?
3. Can you reach the small of your back to tuck in your shirt with your hand?
4. Can you place your hand behind your head with the elbow straight out to the side?
5. Can you place a coin on a shelf at the level of your shoulder bending your elbow?
6. Can you lift one pound (a full pint container) to the level of your shoulder without bending your elbow?
7. Can you lift eight pounds (a full gallon container) to the level of your shoulder without bending your elbow?
8. Can you carry 20 pounds at your side with the affected arm?
9. Do you think you can toss a softball under-hand 20 yards with the affected arm?
10. Do you think you can toss a softball over-hand 20 yards with the affected extremity?
11. Can you wash the back of your opposite shoulder with the affected extremity?
12. Would your shoulder allow you to work full-time at your regular job?

Reprinted with permission as modified from Lippit, S.B., Harryman, D.T., Matsen, F.A. (1993). A Practical Tool for Evaluation Function: The Simple Shoulder Test. In Matsen, F.A., Fu, F.H., Hawkins, R.J. [Eds.], *The Shoulder: A Balance of Mobility and Stability* [pp. 501-518]. Rosemont, IL: American Academy of Orthopaedic Surgeons.

episode of trauma unless specifically asked. The shoulder is commonly injured during sports involving overhead activities and high-impact contact sports or where occupational activities involve repetitive movements and exposure to vibration from mechanical tools.[7] Patients younger than 40 years with a history of trauma are more likely to have shoulder dislocation or subluxation, whereas rotator cuff tear is more common after trauma in those older than 60 years.[8]

Patients often report difficulty with activities of daily living, such as bathing, combing their hair, or dressing, as well as with driving, carrying groceries, and exercising (Box 167.1). Other symptoms may include stiffness, crepitation, instability, and aching discomfort related to vigorous or sustained use. Most shoulder disorders hurt more when the shoulder is elevated, whereas many cervical radiculopathies feel better with the shoulder in an elevated position.[6] Paresthesia or pain radiating distal to the elbow suggest a cervical cause of the symptoms and are seldom indicative of shoulder disease.[9] Weakness is associated with rotator cuff disorders and glenohumeral arthritis. Anterior-superior shoulder pain is associated with acromioclavicular joint disease. Diffuse shoulder pain is associated with rotator cuff disorders, adhesive capsulitis, or glenohumeral arthritis.[9] A painful arc of movement with abduction, when combined with internal rotation, is suggestive of impingement

or bursal-type pain.[7] Pain during active but not passive range of motion suggests a true mechanical or structural reason (relating to muscles/tendons) for reduced glenohumeral movement, e.g., adhesive capsulitis.[7]

Inquiry about hand dominance, occupational activities (e.g., lifting, chronic stress on joints, safety precautions), exercise and recreational activities (extent, type, and frequency), and self-care capacity facilitates identification of contributing factors, potential causes, and the functional impact of the symptoms. A history of collision sports (football, hockey) or weightlifting makes instability or acromioclavicular arthritis more likely, whereas overhead sports (baseball, softball, tennis) make rotator cuff disease more likely.[1] Superior labral tears, including superior labrum anterior and posterior (SLAP) injury, may occur during a motor vehicle accident; a fall onto an outstretched arm; forceful pulling of the arm, such as when trying to catch a heavy object; or forceful movement of the arm when it is above shoulder level.[10] Identification of any history of recent or remote trauma, including the details of injury, is vital. Determination of previous diagnostic studies, hospitalizations, surgeries, or therapies guides diagnostic evaluation. A detailed medical history is also important because adhesive capsulitis is associated with diabetes mellitus and thyroid disorders,[1] and humeral fractures are a consideration in the older adult with osteoporosis or cancer.

Because nonextrinsic shoulder pain may be caused by either intrinsic shoulder disorders or referred pain, it is also critical to ascertain the exact location and distribution of the pain. It is unusual for pain originating in the shoulder, for example, to radiate below the elbow.[1] Vague, poorly localized pain is often extrinsic in origin. Pain involving other joints is suggestive of a generalized arthritic process. Characterization of the type, intensity, timing, and duration of pain as well as identification of ameliorating and exacerbating factors is also essential. The American Shoulder and Elbow Surgeons standardized form for assessment of the shoulder incorporates a synopsis of both patient self-evaluation data and physical examination parameters and is useful in organizing a primary care approach to shoulder pain.

The physical examination should be performed in a systemic manner beginning with careful visual inspection of the shoulder. Anterior and posterior examination for surgical scars, displacement of bone prominences, warmth, swelling, changes in skin color or texture, suprascapular or infrascapular muscle atrophy, and winging of the scapula is necessary. Asymmetry with the contralateral shoulder should be noted. Classically, there is focal tenderness that may or may not reproduce the presenting complaint. Before any shoulder movement is initiated, the examiner should palpate each shoulder for tenderness in the sternoclavicular joint, the acromioclavicular joint, and the shoulder itself. Palpation of both shoulders simultaneously allows the examiner to compare the affected shoulder with the unaffected shoulder. Palpation of bone landmarks is especially valuable in excluding a joint disorder; palpation of the muscle structures is useful in excluding spasm.

Active range of motion should be assessed first to determine the integrity of the rotator cuff and to ascertain the location of the pain. Active range of motion of each shoulder should be measured, including forward flexion (normal is 180 degrees), extension (normal is 70 degrees), external rotation (normal is 45 degrees), internal rotation (normal is 60 degrees), abduction (normal is 180 degrees), and adduction (normal is 180

TABLE 167.1 Tests of Shoulder Function

Test	Technique	Interpretation
Apprehension test	Abduct to 90 degrees and slowly externally rotate patient's arm to a position where it might easily dislocate.	Impending dislocation or glenohumeral instability is signaled by noticeable look of apprehension on patient's face with patient resisting further motion.
Drop arm test	Have patient hold affected extremity in a fully abducted position, then ask patient to slowly lower arm to side.	Rotator cuff tearing or supraspinatus tearing is suggested if patient's arm drops to side (as opposed to being slowly lowered to the side) from a position of 90 degrees of abduction.
Empty can test	Have patient hold out affected arm as if offering examiner a can of soda (abduction to 90 degrees), and then have patient turn arm to empty the contents (internal rotation).	Rotator cuff tendinitis or tear is suggested if pain is produced or weakness noted by maneuver of "emptying the can."
Impingement test	Have patient elevate arm slowly into overhead position.	Rotator cuff strain, tendinitis, or tear is suggested if patient experiences sharp "catches" of pain or impingement with this maneuver.
Yergason test	Have patient fully flex elbow (90 degrees). Grasp the patient's flexed elbow in one hand while holding patient's wrist in other hand; to test stability of biceps tendon, externally rotate the patient's arm as patient resists and, at same time, pull downward on patient's elbow.	Pain with this maneuver suggests that the biceps tendon is unstable in the biceps groove; no pain is experienced with a stable tendon.
Modified dynamic labral shear test	Have patient stand with arm flexed 90 degrees at the elbow, abducted in the scapular plane more than 120 degrees, and externally rotated to tightness. Stand behind patient and guide the involved upper extremity into maximal horizontal abduction. Apply a shear load to the joint by maintaining external rotation and horizontal abduction and lowering arm from 120 degrees to 60 degrees of abduction.	Reproduction of pain and/or painful click or catch in the posterior joint line between 120 degrees and 90 degrees abduction suggests labral tear.[10]
Sulcus sign	Have patient stand with arm at the side. Apply traction through the patient's arm in the inferior direction.	Indicates glenohumeral laxity or instability.
Hawkin test	Forward flex the shoulder and elbow to 90 degrees. Apply force to the forearm to internally rotate the shoulder.	Elicitation of subacromial pain indicates supraspinatus tendinitis.
Cross-body adduction	Elevate shoulder to 90 degrees. Horizontally adduct the shoulder and arm across the body.	Pain at the acromioclavicular joint suggests acromioclavicular joint arthritis.
Spurling test	Have patient flex cervical spine laterally toward the ipsilateral shoulder. Apply a downward axial force on the head.	Pain radiating toward the shoulder and arm may indicate nerve root compression, implicating the cervical spine as the source of shoulder pain.

degrees). Any clicks or crepitation suggestive of impingement should be noted. Passive range of motion should be compared with active range of motion and is particularly useful in determining whether adhesive capsulitis (frozen shoulder) is present. A person with adhesive capsulitis can typically still abduct the arm 60 degrees. Patients with a rotator cuff tear seldom lose passive shoulder motion.[8]

Strength testing of the individual rotator cuff muscles is then performed with use of resisted movements. An important component of the physical examination of the shoulder involves tests to detect pathology.[7,11] Table 167.1 summarizes special tests of shoulder function and their associated disorders. Although many of these clinical tests have variable accuracy for elucidating the exact cause of shoulder pain,[12] they may be used to confirm a suspected diagnosis, provide a differential diagnosis, or differentiate among various structures or to better understand the cause of unusual signs or symptoms. Complete neurovascular assessment of the associated shoulder structures should also be performed to identify other underlying sources of pain or dysfunction. Sensory, motor, deep tendon reflex, or circulatory impairment should be documented. The spine and peripheral joints are examined for evidence of coexisting joint disease.

Evaluation of a painful shoulder is challenging because the problem is often dynamic, with pain occurring only with specific activity. It is necessary to determine whether the discomfort and immobility are articular (bone, joint) or periarticular (soft tissue structure). With inflammatory bursitis, erythema or bulging in the anterior shoulder may be seen. With bursitis or adhesive capsulitis, both active and passive range of motion will be limited. Marked weakness in abduction and external rotation suggests rotator cuff tear.[6]

DIAGNOSTICS
Essential Diagnostics

Diagnostic tests should be used judiciously to confirm or to refine suspected clinical diagnoses. It is unwise to base a diagnosis on a radiologic test alone because x-ray studies can be misleading or unrevealing. Findings on radiography and even magnetic resonance imaging (MRI) are often normal in soft tissue problems in the young athlete. Many shoulder conditions seen in primary care do not have specific radiographic findings.[6]

Radiographs are usually the initial imaging test performed for most suspected abnormalities in the shoulder and will often suffice to diagnose or exclude an abnormality, or will guide further imaging.[13] Contrary to current recommendations from the American College of Radiology (ACR) Appropriateness Criteria for best practices in imaging, many patients undergo MRI before radiography for new shoulder conditions.[14] Plain x-ray films may help diagnose massive rotator cuff tears, calcific tendinitis, shoulder instability, and shoulder arthritis. Shoulder films are recommended for a history of trauma, with reduced range of motion, or if arthritis or neoplastic disease is a consideration. With all significant trauma, it is imperative to obtain the appropriate x-ray studies, including standard anteroposterior views of the glenohumeral joint with the arm at 30 degrees of external rotation, axillary lateral views, and scapula Y views that detect dislocation not seen on standard views. On occasion, in atraumatic presentations, calcifications from previous or chronic injuries can be seen. In cases of recurrent rotator cuff tendinitis or subacromial bursitis, x-ray studies may be helpful in looking for spurring of the acromial process or inferior acromioclavicular osteophytes. Loss of articular cartilage between the humeral head and the glenoid may confirm suspected glenohumeral joint arthritis. Osteophytes consistent with osteoarthritis may also be seen. X-ray studies of the cervical spine are indicated if cervical radiculopathy is suspected.

When the diagnosis of shoulder pain remains unclear or when the outcome would affect management, additional testing with the use of imaging techniques should be performed. MRI is the preferred imaging modality for evaluation of the soft tissue structures of the shoulder including the rotator cuff, biceps muscles, tendons, and bursa. Evidence suggests that MRI in the evaluation of full-thickness supraspinatus tendon tears (FTST), when compared to ultrasound, is the preferred strategy based on cost-effectiveness criteria.[15] In many cases of shoulder pain, MRI findings are rarely helpful, at least initially, with the exception of a significant trauma history, and are unlikely to alter management. In addition, the frequency of nonspecific MRI findings often found in asymptomatic individuals is such that unless the clinician knows of the specific abnormality to be corroborated by MRI, its ordering should probably be left to a specialist. Although MRI is one of the most sensitive diagnostic tests for detecting anatomic abnormalities of the shoulder, the findings may be misleading if not closely correlated with other imaging studies, the patient history, physical examination, and tests of shoulder function.[16] Collaboration between the ordering clinician and the radiologist is often of benefit in interpreting radiologic findings in the context of the clinical picture. Diagnostic imaging studies, which also include ultrasonography and computed tomography (CT) scans as well as more invasive studies such as MRI arthrography, are best ordered in consultation with a specialist, particularly when there may be a need for surgical intervention.

Since the diagnosis of shoulder pain may be complicated by concomitant conditions with overlapping symptoms and by inconclusive physical examination and imaging results, injections of anesthetic agents may serve diagnostic purposes and can often guide localization of the source of pain. Accuracy of the injection is improved with the use of ultrasonography guidance.[17] The Lidocaine injection test is an example of a test used to exclude intrinsic glenohumeral joint pathology including rotator cuff tear or adhesive capsulitis.[6,17]

Laboratory studies are seldom indicated. However, complete blood count (CBC), erythrocyte sedimentation rate (ESR), uric acid level, and serologic tests for rheumatologic diseases can be performed in accordance with the history and examination findings.

INITIAL DIAGNOSTICS

Shoulder Pain

LABORATORY
- None

IMAGING
- X-ray studies
- Magnetic resonance imaging[a]
- Computed Tomography scan[a]

ADDITIONAL DIAGNOSTICS
Laboratory
- Complete blood count and differential Erythrocyte sedimentation rate,[a] CRP (CRP-C-reactive protein).

- Serologic tests for rheumatologic disease

Imaging[a]
- Ultrasound[a]
- Arthrography

Other[a]
- Arthrocentesis[a]

[a]If indicated.

DIFFERENTIAL DIAGNOSIS

 Priority differentials include (1) dislocation, (2) fracture, (3) acute rotator cuff tear, (4) avascular necrosis (especially if history of steroid use), and (5) joint infection.

The ability to correlate the history and physical examination with a functional knowledge of anatomy, an understanding of the mechanism of injury, and the reproduction of symptoms clinically will often lead to diagnosis of the problem. In order to arrive at a differential diagnosis, the clinician must demonstrate a high level of logic and knowledge in interpretation of the presenting complaint, examination findings, and diagnostic tests.[7] Common patterns of shoulder pain and dysfunction also guide the differential diagnosis.

Shoulder disorders can be categorized as acute (<2 weeks' duration) or chronic and traumatic or atraumatic. The diagnosis of shoulder pain is more straightforward when there is a history of trauma. If the duration of pain is less than 2 weeks, the patient may recall an injury or fall. The diagnosis of subacute or chronic shoulder pain with an onset weeks to months after the incident or injury is much more challenging. Common causes of chronic shoulder pain include rotator cuff disorders, adhesive capsulitis, shoulder instability, tendinitis, and arthritis.[1]

It is important to understand the concept of instability. The extreme of instability is a frank shoulder dislocation caused by trauma, for which the patient usually goes to the emergency department. Shoulder subluxation, whereby the humeral head is pulled out of the glenoid cavity partially or totally but reduces itself spontaneously, is often a transient instability considered less extreme than a dislocation. More subtle degrees of instability seen in primary care settings include dysfunction of the rotator cuff that can lead to minor degrees of instability, which can then lead to impingement of the rotator cuff against the underside of the coracoacromial ligament of the acromion itself.[6] This leads to the pain often referred to as *impingement syndrome* or *subacromial bursitis* or *tendinitis.*[6]

Although sports injuries from overuse ("muscular strain"), shoulder separation caused by a sprain of the acromioclavicular ligaments, and subluxation of the glenohumeral joint are most common in young athletes (football and hockey),[18] trauma followed by shoulder immobilization or gradual onset of shoulder pain on the nondominant side of a middle-aged woman is more likely adhesive capsulitis. Calcific tendinitis of the rotator cuff tendons typically manifests as activity-related shoulder pain.[19] Shoulder pain in older adults more often develops with rotator cuff lesions, such as supraspinatus tendinopathy and partial- or full-thickness tendon tears.[15] Severe acute activity-related shoulder pain with restricted movement in the setting of repetitive motion is likely acute calcific tendinitis.[20] Shoulder pain aggravated by reaching, by overhead activities, or with internal rotation movements such as reaching toward the low back is likely caused by rotator cuff impingement. Pain in the shoulder at night that makes sleeping on the affected arm impossible is rotator cuff disease until proven otherwise. Pain in the shoulder with repetitive overhead activity also suggests rotator cuff disease. Pain at rest should suggest that the problem is extrinsic to the shoulder girdle, although acute inflammatory conditions often cause night pain. Erythema and fever with shoulder pain suggest septic arthritis or pseudogout. Pain associated with a throwing motion may be secondary to instability. Pain in the supraclavicular area and toward the vertebral border of the scapula is often referred pain from the neck. Shoulder pain from tendinopathy often radiates to the midarm but not lower. Morning stiffness lasting more than 1 hour, rest pain that improves as the day wears on, and bilateral shoulder pain in an older adult are symptoms of inflammatory conditions including rheumatoid arthritis, polymyalgia rheumatica, and pseudogout.

Tendinitis

Tendinitis occurs when the tendons or surrounding tissue become inflamed, swollen, and tender. Supraspinatus tendinitis is a very common cause of shoulder pain and is usually caused by cell-mediated degenerative changes in that tendon with advancing age.[20] Other common causes of tendinitis include overhead or repetitive activity, weakened rotator cuff (usually in combination with overhead activity), heavy lifting activities, and muscle strain. In rotator cuff tendinitis, abnormal repetitive stresses cause a mechanical irritation of the structures below the acromial bursa. With calcific tendinitis, calcific deposits form in the rotator cuff tendon, causing local mechanical irritation. Calcific tendonitis typically presents as activity-related pain.[20] Biceps tendinitis, which can result from overuse activities above the head, can lead to subacromial impingement, particularly in internal rotation. Elbow flexion against resistance usually reproduces pain located over the anterior aspect of the shoulder and upper arm.

Tendinitis often has no isolated precipitating event. Most patients report a deep ache in the shoulder, with increasing pain on abduction and internal rotation. Determination of what position or posture causes pain is diagnostic. Pain with arm elevation, for example, is suggestive of rotator cuff tendinitis or subacromial bursitis. Point tenderness is often localized

to the vicinity of the greater tuberosity below the acromion and along the lateral aspect of the humeral head. The reflexive shrug will be noted as the patient tries to abduct the arm. The shrug helps reduce the pain caused by impingement on the acromion.

Generalized muscle weakness on manual muscle testing, especially with internal and external rotation, is characteristic of rotator cuff tendinitis.[16] Also, the empty can test and the impingement test are useful in validating the clinical diagnosis (see Table 167.1).

Bursitis

Bursitis occurs when the bursa becomes inflamed and painful as surrounding muscles move over it. The bursa's primary function is to maintain a gliding surface between muscles and ligaments (see Chapter 156). The most common cause of bursitis is overuse. Pitching, tennis, swimming, or repetitive use of the arm at or above shoulder level can cause subacromial bursitis.

The calcific deposits in tendinitis may occasionally extend the inflammatory process into the subacromial bursa, producing inflammation in the wall of the bursa.

Symptom onset in bursitis is usually abrupt, with pain often felt at the tip of the shoulder or along the upper third of the humerus. The pain is referred down the deltoid muscle into the upper arm. It occurs when the arm is lifted overhead or twisted. In extreme cases, pain will be present continuously and may disrupt sleep.

Rotator Cuff Tear or Rupture

Rotator cuff problems are a very common source of shoulder pain, responsible for approximately 70% of office visits for shoulder pain.[8] In rotator cuff diseases, the supraspinatus tendon is the most commonly injured tendon because the tracking of the tendon is directly under the anterior edge of the acromion.[8] There is significant association between increasing age and tears in the rotator cuff,[19,21] with risk for tear progression with advancing age, beginning with microscopic tears, progressing to partial-thickness tears, and then on to full-thickness tears. Rotator cuff disease is classified or graded to reflect progressively worsening symptoms and functional impairment. Grade I disease of the rotator cuff, which is most common in young adults, involves acute inflammation and edema resulting from either acute trauma or repetitive overhead activity. Grade II disease, which is seen in middle-aged adults, is characterized by chronic degenerative changes without actual tear. Grade III disease, commonly observed in older adult populations, represents disruption of tendon integrity (a tear).

Excessive use of the shoulder involving repetitive, stressful movement and injury or repeated injuries will produce this partial or complete rupture or disintegration of the rotator cuff. A weakened rotator cuff at the supraspinatus tendon may tear spontaneously as a result of minimum trauma, such as a fall. Tears tend not to be painful, but if pain is present, it will be anterolateral in location and not radiating past the elbow.[19] Classic physical examination findings include external rotation lag, positive drop arm test, and or pain relief by sustained weakness after impingement test.[19] Muscle atrophy often accompanies rotator cuff tears. Although the rotator cuff is not easily palpable, point tenderness to manual palpation is maximum just below the greater tuberosity of the humerus. Incomplete ruptures produce chronic thickening of the subacromial bursa and impingement syndrome. There is little chance for spontaneous healing of a torn rotator cuff.

The patient with rotator cuff tear typically reports shoulder pain aggravated by movement, especially overhead activity, and radiating to the anterior aspect of the arm. Abduction is painful and weak, and tenderness may be elicited over the insertion of the greater tuberosity. On examination, the patient will be unable to abduct the arm, instead producing a characteristic shoulder shrug. Passive range of motion may be unaffected. The drop arm test and the empty can test assess the integrity of the rotator cuff, and results are positive with significant tears (see Table 167.1).

Labral Tear (SLAP Lesions)

Lesions of the superior glenoid labrum and biceps anchor are a well-recognized cause of shoulder pain.[22] Symptoms suggestive of a labral tear or SLAP lesion include deep shoulder pain with specific shoulder positions, pain during overhead maneuvers such as in tennis, swimming, or throwing sports, a catching sensation, a sense of loss of shoulder strength, instability, and crepitus. Employed when a SLAP lesion is suspected, the modified dynamic labral shear test (Table 167.1) helps establish a causal relationship between the patient's symptomatology and labral pathology.

Recent outcome studies have shown predictably good functional results and an acceptable rate of return to sport and/or work with arthroscopic treatment of SLAP tear.[22]

Subacromial Impingement Syndrome

The tendons composing the rotator cuff can be worn down by repetitive excursion between the greater tuberosity of the humerus and the acromion and the acromioclavicular ligament.[21] This repetitive trauma can lead to compression of both the tendons and the subacromial bursa, resulting in edema, hemorrhage, inflammation, and ultimately fibrosis. Impingement occurs as a result of acute trauma, repetitive overhead activities, pushing and pulling activities, subtle or overt instability of the glenohumeral joint, and degenerative and inflammatory disorders of the tendons and bursa.[12,21]

Shoulder Instability, Dislocation, and Subluxation

Of all joints, the shoulder is at highest risk for dislocation.[4] Shoulder dislocation predisposes the patient to recurrent instability. Instability results from post-traumatic capsular tear or stretch. Athletes are subject to numerous repetitive loads that can lead to symptoms of instability.[6] There are two primary types of shoulder instability: traumatic, unidirectional instability; and atraumatic, multidirectional, bilateral, inferior capsule shift, which is often more responsive to rehabilitative efforts. Dislocation is much more common in young adults, with the likelihood of redislocation decreasing with advancing age. In older adults, rotator cuff tears commonly occur with dislocation. A history of traumatic dislocation and medical or surgical reduction is a powerful risk factor for instability. The patient will simply complain of the shoulder's "giving out." Dislocation results from trauma to the shoulder while it is hyperextended. Dislocations are often anterior and are characterized by loss of the shoulder's rounded appearance. The patient typically is seen with the hands held to the side. There is prominence of the acromion, painful limitation of movement, and displacement of the humerus away from the trunk.

The apprehension test detects chronic shoulder dislocation (see Table 167.1). The Yergason test for long head of the biceps tendon stability determines whether the biceps tendon is stable in the occipital groove (see Table 167.1). A palm-up hand position is used to rule out posterior dislocation.

Arthritis

Arthritis of the glenohumeral joint is a gradual, progressive mechanical and biochemical breakdown of the articular cartilage and other joint tissues including bone and joint capsule. It is a common cause of debilitating shoulder pain, affecting up to one-third of patients older than 60 years.[23] It may be secondary to inflammatory arthritis (see Chapter 197, 198) or osteoarthritis (see Chapter 165). In patients older than 50 years, the distinguishing features of shoulder arthritis are the gradual onset and progression of pain at rest, aggravated by movement, and loss of motion.[1] The patient reports a grinding or clicking sound with motion. Examination may reveal muscle wasting, crepitation, effusion, and decreased range of motion.

Although the shoulder may undergo arthritic changes from a number of causes, these changes are much better tolerated than arthritic changes occurring in the weight-bearing joints. A hot, red, swollen, and painful shoulder accompanied by fever and chills is suggestive of septic arthritis (see Chapter 159).

Shoulder Trauma

 Red flags include shoulder deformity and loss of rotation, which may represent fracture, unreduced dislocation, or signs of an acute rotator cuff tear.

With severe shoulder trauma, the differential diagnosis includes acromioclavicular separation (crepitus and elevation at the acromioclavicular joint), fractures of the clavicle or proximal humerus, strains, sprains, subluxation, and dislocation (see Chapter 168). Severe shoulder trauma not promptly responsive to conservative treatment warrants orthopedic referral.

Extrinsic Shoulder Disorders

Shoulder pain may be specific to the shoulder girdle area or may be referred from another anatomic location. Referred pain should be suspected when passive shoulder motion shows a painless complete arc, no specific periarticular shoulder tender point is identified, muscle strength is within normal limits, or pain cannot be reproduced with various tests of the shoulder muscles. Referred pain is often poorly localized or vaguely described.

Referred pain may be neurologic in origin (cervical nerve root compression, supraspinatus nerve compression, brachial plexus lesions, cervical spine disease), cardiovascular in origin (myocardial ischemia or infarction, thoracic outlet syndrome), or due to hepatobiliary disease, pulmonary conditions (pneumonia, pulmonary embolus), or intraperitoneal bleeding. Because the shoulder is located in the thoracic dermatome area, pain can be referred from several intrathoracic or abdominal organs (pneumonia, pulmonary embolus, hepatobiliary disease) innervated by the same nerves. Shoulder symptoms may also be related to diaphragmatic irritation, which shares the same root innervation (C5, C6) as the dermatome covering the shoulder's summit.

Cervical spondylosis, herniated cervical disk, cervical trauma, or other neck problems may also cause pain radiating to the shoulder, scapula, or upper back (see Chapter 164). This pain is often felt at the superomedial angle of the scapula and may be verified by the Spurling test, in which radicular pain is reproduced with head compression.[12] The Spurling test is a useful tool in differentiating shoulder pathologic conditions from cervical radiculopathy.[12] For the Spurling test, the patient should extend the neck and laterally tilt the head to the affected side. The examiner should apply downward force to the top of the head. If the test result is positive, the radicular pain or paresthesia will be evident. This is because of narrowing of the foramina against the inflamed nerve root or spinal cord from a ruptured disk. Sometimes a spinal fracture, in addition to causing local pain, may radiate pain to the shoulder along the course of any muscle affected by the fracture (see Table 167.1).

Reflex sympathetic dystrophy after myocardial infarction, cerebrovascular accident, or trauma can also cause shoulder pain. The characteristic features are persistent burning pain, diffuse tenderness, immobilization of the shoulder, and vasomotor changes in the hands. Gallbladder disease can cause scapular pain as well as right upper abdominal pain and tenderness. Pain caused by bone malignant neoplasm is usually gnawing, constant, and unrelated to movement.

INTERPROFESSIONAL COLLABORATIVE MANAGEMENT

Pharmacologic Management

Analgesic medication may be indicated and is often necessary to allow progression of treatment of shoulder pain.

Acetaminophen. Acetaminophen is the recommended drug of choice for milder analgesia or for patients for whom nonsteroidal antiinflammatory drugs (NSAIDs) are contraindicated. Although acetaminophen has no antiinflammatory activity, its analgesic effect is comparable to that of ibuprofen and naproxen, with fewer side effects.

Acetaminophen is safe when taken in prescribed doses and is effective in reducing discomfort without the known cardiac, gastrointestinal, and renal risks of antiinflammatory agents. The current maximum daily dosage is 3000 mg/day in divided doses, though patients on warfarin require lesser doses and there are concerns about analgesic nephropathy with long-term acetaminophen use.

Nonsteroidal Antiinflammatory Drugs. Oral NSAIDs such as ibuprofen, naproxen, and others may be effective and are likely to be beneficial in the short term in those with acute tendinitis or subacromial bursitis or both.[24] Topical NSAIDs may be helpful for some patients and preferred for older adults who tolerate oral NSAIDs less well. Patients should be instructed to use antiinflammatory medication as prescribed, not just when pain is severe. In addition, they should be counseled about the medication's action, dosage, potential adverse effects, and drug–drug interactions. Certain NSAIDs are available over the counter, and these should be discontinued if a prescription-strength product is recommended.

Nonopioid Analgesics. Alternative pharmacotherapeutic options for the treatment of shoulder pain include tramadol (Ultram), a centrally acting analgesic agent indicated for moderate to severe shoulder pain. In 2017, the FDA restricted the use of tramadol in children younger than 12 years of age.

Opioid Analgesics. Alternative pharmacotherapeutic options for the treatment of shoulder pain include short-term, low-potency oral opioids, such as acetaminophen with codeine. In 2017, the FDA issued a warning restricting the use of codeine in children under 12 years of age citing risks of slowed or difficult breathing and death. In addition, a US FDA review has found that the growing combined use of opioid analgesics with benzodiazepines or other drugs that effect the central nervous system (CNS) had resulted in serious side effects including slowed or difficult breathing and death. The risks and potential side effects including dependency and addiction of these agents must be examined for each patient.

Other Pain-Relieving Pharmaceticals. The effectiveness of topical antiinflammatory drugs (NSAIDs), oral acetaminophen, or oral corticosteroids in improving shoulder pain has not been formally studied and is therefore not evidence based, but all are widely used for individual patients.[25]

Intra-Articular Approaches to Treatment. Corticosteroid injections may reduce pain and expedite functional recovery in patients with inflammatory conditions such as bursitis and tendinitis as well as in rotator cuff impingement that does not improve with conservative therapy (see Chapter 156). However, corticosteroid injections, if repeated frequently, potentially cause tendon degeneration and long-term loss of function.

In shoulder impingement syndrome (SIS), steroid injections coupled with physical therapy resulted in better functional outcomes than steroid injection alone.[26]

The body of evidence supporting the intra-articular injection of sodium hyaluronate for shoulder pain secondary to glenohumeral arthritis, rotator cuff tears, and adhesive capsulitis is conflicting, with many studies showing no significant difference between these and corticosteroid injections and a substantial difference in cost. The American Academy of Orthopaedic Surgeons no longer recommends the use of injectable viscosupplementation in treating patients with osteoarthritis of the knee and its use in glenohumeral joint arthritis remains off label.[27]

Nonpharmacologic Management

Nonpharmacologic strategies include the triad of activity modification, ice packs or cold for the first few days followed by heat, and graded exercise. Other appropriate therapeutic modalities include physical therapy, acupuncture, and surgery.

In persons with acute post-traumatic tear, orthopedic referral and early surgical options are warranted. Activity limitations in both sports and labor are prescribed to minimize acute shoulder pain. In general, the patient avoids any activity that precipitates symptoms and especially the offending or "abusive" activity. Although a sling is useful in some situations, immobilization is recommended only when instability is apparent and never for more than 3 or 4 days.

Applications of ice or heat may provide relief. Ice reduces edema and bleeding and is most often recommended after trauma. Both heat and cold have been demonstrated to reduce muscle spasm and pain. Ice applied topically to the affected joint for 30 minutes three or four times a day, particularly after any activity that involves use of the affected extremity, may reduce inflammation and swelling and promote comfort. Ice massage may also be of therapeutic benefit.

Restoration of normal shoulder function should begin as soon as acute pain has subsided. The overall goals of any therapeutic exercise program include maintaining or restoring full range of motion, decreasing inflammation (with ice, NSAIDs, and deep friction massage), and strengthening the rotator cuff musculature. Range-of-motion exercises, including the pendulum swing and the wall climb (in which the patient "walks" his or her fingers up a wall), can be performed two or three times daily for 5 to 10 minutes and are helpful in preserving functional mobility. Strengthening exercises with weight or resistance and stretching-strengthening exercises with TheraBand are indicated only after the pain has subsided.

After trauma or surgery, shoulder rehabilitation including a supervised exercise program under the direction of a physical therapist is recommended to improve outcomes. Physical rehabilitation programs use anatomy, biomechanics, and knowledge of tissue response to trauma to restore range of motion, to strengthen the shoulder girdle, to maximize functional ability, and to resolve symptoms.

Physical therapy plays a key role in the nonsurgical treatment of rotator cuff disease as well by strengthening and retraining the rotator cuff muscles and the scapular stabilizing musculature to pull the humerus down in the joint, decreasing further impingement. Physical therapy can also guide in ergonomic adjustment to strengthen rhomboids to decrease slouching, making the acromion less likely to impinge with humeral movement, and in modification of daily routine to avoid offending repetitive arm movements. Adjunctive physical therapy modalities, such as local heat application, electrogalvanic stimulation, ultrasound, and transverse friction massage, may promote tissue extensibility and joint function in chronic situations.

In SIS, physical therapy and corticosteroid injections are similarly effective, but physical therapy might be less costly to the health care system in the year after treatment.[28]

Acupuncture, when it is combined with mobilization, may confer short-term analgesic effects in chronic shoulder conditions, including adhesive capsulitis, rotator cuff disease, and osteoarthritis, although there are no convincing studies to support this intervention.[29]

Nonspecific effects of acupuncture include patient beliefs and expectations, attention from the clinician, and administration of acupuncture in a relaxed setting. Acupuncture is recommended for subacute or chronic pain in patients who are trying to increase function and/or decrease medication usage and who have an interest in this modality.[3,30]

Soft tissue massage and exercise are commonly used to treat episodes of shoulder pain but a paucity of evidence exists to support the addition of soft tissue massage to an exercise program for improving pain, disability, or range of motion in people with nonspecific shoulder pain.[31]

The American Academy of Orthopaedic Surgeons recommends consideration of total shoulder arthroplasty or hemiarthroplasty as options when treating patients with advanced glenohumeral joint arthritis.[10]

The shoulder is, after the knee and hip, the third most common joint to require surgical reconstruction. Surgical treatment of shoulder osteoarthritis has grown in the past two decades. Shoulder arthroplasty versus hemiarthroplasty or surface replacement remain surgical options depending on the integrity of the rotator cuff and the age of and physical demands on the patient.[32]

Failure to respond to conservative, nonoperative therapy or escalating symptoms despite conservative therapy; shoulder dislocation or instability; rotator cuff tear or rupture; severe disabling arthritis; and infection are among the definitive indications for referral to an orthopedist for more aggressive diagnostic testing, including radiography to assess for calcifications, spurs, or arthritic changes and MRI, arthrography, ultrasonography, or electromyography for continued muscle weakness.

Arthroscopic acromioplasty may be required for débridement of bursa, subacromial decompression, repair of ligaments, and repair of tendons if a tear is present.

LIFE SPAN CONSIDERATIONS

Children rarely have rotator cuff tears but commonly have shoulder joint instability (subluxations or dislocations of the glenohumeral joint) because of overuse or sports injuries. In adolescents and young adults, acromioclavicular sprain and tendinitis are common causes of shoulder pain, but tears in the rotator cuff are rare. In patients younger than 40 years, glenohumeral instability typically is accompanied by a history of subluxation or dislocation events.[1] Middle-aged and older patients rarely have problems with instability, but because the rotator cuff apparatus undergoes significant age-related changes, middle-aged and older adults commonly are seen with rotator cuff lesions (tendinitis, tears, and impingement syndromes), glenohumeral joint problems (adhesive capsulitis and osteoarthritis), and subacromial bursitis.

Musculoskeletal disease is a leading cause of functional disability in the older population. Rotator cuff tears often go unrecognized in the older adult or are clinically confused with degenerative tendinitis or other forms of shoulder disease in older adults. One study focusing on the repair of rotator cuff tears in patients older than 65 years who did not respond to conservative treatment found excellent 5-year outcomes after isolated supraspinatus tendon repairs, suggesting that withholding surgical intervention because of age may not be justified. Acute pain after trauma may suggest a fracture of the neck of the humerus in an older patient.

COMPLICATIONS

The most common and worrisome complication of chronic shoulder pain is adhesive capsulitis (frozen shoulder). Adhesive capsulitis is characterized by a gradual, progressive decline in shoulder mobility, often resulting from prolonged joint immobilization after a painful episode. Diffuse aching pain and limited mobility are common. Pain is related to the stretching of the restricted joint capsule. Both active and passive range of motion of the glenohumeral joint and scapula is limited. Patients may have difficulty with activities of daily living, including dressing, toileting, and even feeding themselves. Treatment includes corticosteroid injections and physical therapy using modalities, mobilization, manipulation, and stretching exercises.[33]

PATIENT AND FAMILY EDUCATION

Teaching patients about proactive strategies to preserve musculoskeletal function and to prevent injury is important. Recovery takes time and requires an interdisciplinary approach, including patient participation. If exercise programs are not taken seriously, chronic or recurrent pain and loss of function may result. Recovery from shoulder injury and pain can be an excruciatingly slow process, requiring 6 weeks to 6 months. Education about the healing process and the factors that affect healing, including patient motivation, adherence to interventions, social support, nutrition, lifestyle behaviors, exercise, age, occupation, mental status, depression, and comorbidities, is necessary. Home therapy is an important component of therapy and may include active and passive therapeutic procedures as well as other modalities to assist in alleviating pain, swelling, and abnormal muscle tone.[31]

In addition, the importance of exercise and warm-up and stretching before activities should be stressed. Avoidance of repetitive movements and overuse should be carefully explained. For chronic conditions, patients should understand that although the pain may resolve, the condition can recur. Reinforcement of the need for modification of activities, adherence to exercise regimens, ice packs, medications, and gradual resumption of activities is also necessary.

HEALTH PROMOTION

Repeated trauma or stress, which may be occupation-related or sports-related, are risk factors for the development of shoulder pain. In the promotion of physical activity and exercise in primary care, encouraging the patient to learn and execute proper stretching, strengthening, and body mechanic techniques is critical. It is also vital to consider shoulder protection strategies and prevention of athletic injuries in children and young adults, as well as the prevention of work-related injuries and fall prevention strategies across the life span.

REFERENCES

1. Roy, A., Kishner, S., et al. (April 26, 2016). Adhesive capsulitis in physical medicine and rehabilitation. Medscape. Retrieved from https://emedicine.mmedsacoe.com/article/326828-overview. (Accessed 1 March 2018).
2. Pribicevic, M. The epidemiology of shoulder pain: A narrative review of the literature. In Ghosh, S. (Ed.). Pain in Perspective. InTech. https://doi.org/10.5772/52931. Retrieved from https://www.intechpoen.com/books/pain-in-perspective/the-epidemiology-of-shoulder-pain-a-narrative-review-of-the-literature. (Accessed 12 December 2017).
3. Page, M. J., Green, S., Kramer, S., et al. (2014). Manual therapy and exercise for adhesive capsulitis (frozen shoulder). The Cochrane Database of Systematic Reviews, (8), CD011275. Retrieved from www.ncbi.nlm.nih.gov/pubmed/25157701. (Accessed 1 January 2015).
4. Youm, T., Takemoto, R., & Park, B. K. (2014). Acute management of shoulder dislocations. The Journal of the American Academy of Orthopaedic Surgeons, 22(12), 761–771.
5. Dutton, M. (2012). The extremities. In Orthopedic examination, evaluation and intervention (3rd ed.). New York: McGraw-Hill.
6. Greenberg, D. L. (2014). Evaluation and treatment of shoulder pain. The Medical Clinics of North America, 98(3), 487–504.
7. Kenyon, P., Flynn, S., & Marlow, W. (2018). Assessment of the adult presenting with shoulder pain. International Journal of Orthopaedic and Trauma Nursing, 28, 40–46.
8. Piper, C. C., Hughes, A. J., Ma, Y., et al. (2018). Operative versus nonoperative treatment for the management of full-thickness rotator cuff tears: A systematic review and meta-analysis. Journal of Shoulder and Elbow Surgery, 27, 572–576.
9. Burbank, K. M., Stevenson, J. H., Czarnecki, G. R., et al. (2008). Chronic shoulder pain: Part I. Evaluation and diagnosis. American Family Physician, 77(4), 453–460.
10. American Association of Orthopedic Surgeons. Shoulder pain. Retrieved from https://www.orthoinfo.org/en/diseases–conditions/slap-tears/. (Accessed 19 April 2018).
11. Myer, C., Hegedus, E. J., Tarara, D. T., et al. (2013). A user's guide to performance of the best shoulder physical exam tests. British Journal of Sports Medicine, 47(14), 903–907.
12. Hanchard, N. C., Lenza, M., Handoll, H., et al. (2013). Physical tests for shoulder impingements and local lesions of bursa, tendon or labrum that may accompany impingement. The Cochrane Database of Systematic Reviews, (4), CD007427.
13. Small, K. M. (2017). Inappropriate use of shoulder MRI. Journal of the American College of Radiology, 2017(4). Retrieved from http://bit.ly/2oPafHV. (Accessed 18 January 2018).
14. Small, K., Adler, R., Shah, S., et al. ACR appropriatness Criteria—Shoulder_Atraumatic 2018. Retrieved from https://acsearch.acr.org/docs/3101482/Narrative/ on June 12, 2019.
15. Gyftopoulos, S., Guja, K. E., Subhas, N., et al. (2017). Cost-effectiveness of magnetic resonance imaging versus ultrasound for the detection of symptomatic full-thickness supraspinatus tears. Journal of Shoulder and Elbow Surgery, 26, 2067–2077.
16. Hermans, J., Luime, J. L., Meuffels, D. E., et al. (2013). Does this patient have rotator cuff disease? The rational clinical examination systematic review. JAMA: The Journal of the American Medical Association, 310(8), 837–847.
17. McFarland, E., Bernard, J., Dein, E., et al. (2018). Diagnostic injections about the shoulder. The Journal of the American Academy of Orthopaedic Surgeons, 25(12), 799–807.
18. Johansen, J. A., Grutter, P. W., McFarland, E. G., et al. (2011). Acromioclavicular joint injuries: Indications for treatment and treatment options. Journal of Shoulder and Elbow Surgery, 20, S70–S82.
19. American Academy of Orthopaedic Surgeons. Management of Rotator Cuff Injuries Clinical Practice Guideline. https://www.aaos.org/rotatorcuffinjuriescpg Published March 11.
20. Suzuki, K., Potts, A., Anakewenz, O., et al. (2014). Calcific tendinitis of the rotator cuff: Management options. The Journal of the American Academy of Orthopaedic Surgeons, 22(11), 707–717.
21. Armstrong, A. (2014). Evaluation and management of adult shoulder pain: A focus on rotator cuff disorders, acromioclavicular joint arthritis and glenohumeral arthritis. The Medical Clinics of North America, 98(3), 487–504.
22. Keener, J. D., & Brophy, R. H. (2009). Superior labral tears of the Shoulder: Pathogenesis, Evaluation and Treatment. The Journal of the American Academy of Orthopaedic Surgeons, 17(10), 627–637.
23. Menge, T. J., Boykin, R. E., Byram, I. R., et al. (2013). A comprehensive approach to glenohumeral arthritis. Southern Medical Journal, 107(9), 567–573.
24. Kooistra, B., Willems, J., Lemmens, E., et al. (2011). Murphy R, Carr A. Shoulder pain. American Family Physician, 83(2), 137–138.
25. Babatunde, O., Jordan, J., Van der Windt, D., et al. (2017). Effective treatment options for musculoskeletal pain in primary care: A systematic overview of current evidence. PLoS ONE, 12(6). Retrieved from https://doi.org/10.1371/journal.pone.0178621. e collection 2017. (Accessed 23 April 2018). e0178621.
26. Dong, W., Goost, H., Lin, X.-B., Burger, C., Paul, C., Wang, Z.-L., et al. (2015). Treatments for shoulder impingement syndrome: A PRISMA systematic review and network Meta-Analysis. Medicine, 94(10), e510. http://doi.org/10.1097/MD.0000000000000510.
27. Cato, R. (2016). Indications and usefulness of common injections for non-traumatic Orthopedic complaints. The Medical Clinics of North America, 100(5), 1077–1088.
28. Rhon, D. O., Boyles, R. B., & Clelan, J. A. (2014). One-year outcome of subacromial corticosteroid injection compared with manual physical therapy for the management of the unilateral shoulder impingement syndrome: A pragmatic randomized trial. Annals of Internal Medicine, 161(3), 161–169.
29. Armstrong, A. (2014). Evaluation and management of adult shoulder pain: A focus on rotator cuff disorders, acromioclavicular joint arthritis and glenohumeral arthritis. The Medical Clinics of North America, 98(3), 487–504.
30. Colorado Division of Worker's Compensation. (2015, February 2). NGC:D10966. Shoulder injury medical treatment guidelines.
31. Van den Dolder, P. A., Ferreira, P. H., & Refshauge, K. M. (2015). Effectiveness of soft tissue massage for nonspecific shoulder pain: Randomized control trial. Physical Therapy, 95(11), 1467.
32. Kooistra, B., Willems, J., Lemmens, E., et al. (2017). Comparative Study if shoulder arthroplasty versus total shoulder surface replacement for glenohumeral osteoarthritis with minimum 2 year follow-up. Journal of Shoulder and Elbow Surgery, 26(3), 430–436.
33. Kelley, M. J., Shaffer, M. A., Kuhn, J. E., et al. (2013). Shoulder pain and mobility deficits: Adhesive capsulitis. Clinical practice guidelines linked to international classifications of functioning, disability, and health from the orthopaedic section of the American Physical Therapy Association. The Journal of Orthopaedic and Sports Physical Therapy, 43(5), A1–A31.

CHAPTER **168**

SPRAINS, STRAINS, AND FRACTURES

Nicole Bove • Susan Bove • Christine Wilson

 Immediate emergency department referral or physician consultation is indicated for injuries that show neurovascular compromise, a penetrating object, or a wound into a joint, or those that occur from a crush injury or result in an open fracture.

DEFINITION AND EPIDEMIOLOGY

Common musculoskeletal injuries include strains, sprains, dislocations, and fractures. Since sprains and strains are often cared for at home, the real frequency of these injuries will never be known. Strains result from the overstretching or overuse of muscles and/or tendons. Sprains result from a stretching and/or tearing of the ligaments that bind the joint as the joint is forced beyond its normal range of motion (ROM). Dislocations occur when a bone is displaced at the joint so that the articulating surfaces of the bones detach. Partial displacements are called subluxations. A fracture is a break in the cortex of bone and may be classified as closed or open. A closed, or simple, fracture has no associated disruption in the continuity of the overlying skin. An open, or compound, fracture has an associated disruption through the skin to the environment.

Strains are minor injuries that result in an overstretched muscle. A *sprain* involves injury to the supporting structures of a joint and is described using three grades of severity. The degree of damage to these structures depends on the amount of tissue/fiber shearing and tearing that occurs. A *Grade 1 sprain* usually involves minimal injury of an overstretched ligament resulting in mild pain and edema. A *Grade 2 sprain* is an incomplete tear of a ligament and includes some moderate functional impairment, ecchymosis, edema, and discomfort with weight bearing. A *Grade 3 sprain* is a full or complete tear of the ligament with loss of ligament integrity.

Fractures are diagnosed when a break in the bone cortex is visible on radiographic views. There are many types of fractures. *Angulated* fractures refer to either open or closed fractures, usually with greater than 30 degrees of angulation between the two ends of the fracture. A *transverse* fracture is a break in the cortex of the bone that goes straight across the bone. *Oblique* fractures are seen diagonally on x-ray films. *Spiral* fractures are seen as wrapping around the bone. A *greenstick* fracture is diagnosed when the bone tears as if a fresh twig were being bent in two. This is commonly seen in children because they have a more porous cortex, which makes the bone more flexible. An *impacted* fracture occurs when both pieces of the broken bone are crushed into each other. A *comminuted* fracture is observed when the bone ends shatter with multiple fragments. An *avulsion fracture*, also known as a chip fracture, occurs when the ligament pulls away from the bone, bringing fragments with it. This is usually after a forceful injury such as a severe inversion ankle injury. The pulling or pushing of a bone out of its normal position in the joint results in *dislocation*, which can be complete or incomplete. A *compression* fracture is seen in vertebral collapse due to increased load on the spine from trauma, osteoporosis, or cancer/metastases. A *pathologic* fracture occurs

as a result of underlying pathology such as metastases or osteoporosis anywhere in the body. *Stress* fractures are created from repetitive stress to a bone over time that creates a cyclic pattern of partial healing and repeating injury resulting in a weakened bone.[1] An example of this is a stress fracture in the foot of a marathon runner.

CLINICAL PRESENTATION AND PHYSICAL EXAMINATION

Strains cause local, mild swelling; pain; or muscle spasm.

Sprains may demonstrate edema, ecchymosis, and pain with ROM. If a sprain is of the lower extremity, weight bearing will be painful depending on the grade of the sprain.

Fractures usually manifest with pain and there may or may not be associated edema, skin discoloration, or decreased ROM. Dislocations and fractures both may produce a visible deformity.

A past medical history should be obtained with a focus on comorbidities like arthritis, diabetes, or past surgery that resulted in deformity. A history of a similar injury is important since, for example, ankle sprains are often recurrent. A recent history of trauma, intense athletic activity, or workplace injury is important to elicit. The ability to weight bear immediately after the injury is important to the differential diagnosis of a lower extremity injury as the inability to weight bear after trauma can signify a fracture. Determine the patient's dominant side in an upper extremity injury to better assess comparison strength testing. Assess the patient's pain and any neurovascular complaints. A good musculoskeletal examination includes exploring the mechanism of injury with a focus on the physical forces incurred by the patient. Often, this assessment is simplified by asking the patient to use the opposite extremity to reconstruct the exact motion of the affected side during the injury.

Physical examination of strains, sprains, and fractures includes observation, inspection, palpation, and ROM with special testing related to the area that is injured. Observation detects the patient's ability to bear weight, use of the affected area prior to and during exam, guarding, grimacing, and any obvious ROM issues. Inspection focuses on visible changes such as edema, open wounds or lesions, ecchymosis, erythema, or obvious deformity. Palpation of the affected area is used initially to evaluate for neurovascular compromise. In some situations, the rest of the hands-on exam should be delayed until after a fracture is ruled out with diagnostic imaging. Examine the contralateral, unaffected side first for comparison. Examine the joints above and below the injury. Palpate anatomical landmarks according to the area injured and evaluate for edema, site of pain, strength, ligament laxity, and ROM. There are many specific tests available for manual testing. A few tests performed in primary care offices are listed here.

Wrist (see Chapter 170): When examining the wrist, the *Schuck test* is performed to assess for carpal instability. The patient extends their fingers from a closed fist position against the resistance of the examiners hand on the mid and distal phalanges. Dorsal wrist pain can indicate ligament injury. The *Watson test* checks for scaphoid ligament instability. While pressing on the volar aspect of the patient's scaphoid, pain with passive movement of the wrist from ulnar to radial deviation is a positive test. A Salter I navicular fracture is diagnosed by tenderness with palpation in the *snuffbox*, in any age group (Fig. 168.1).

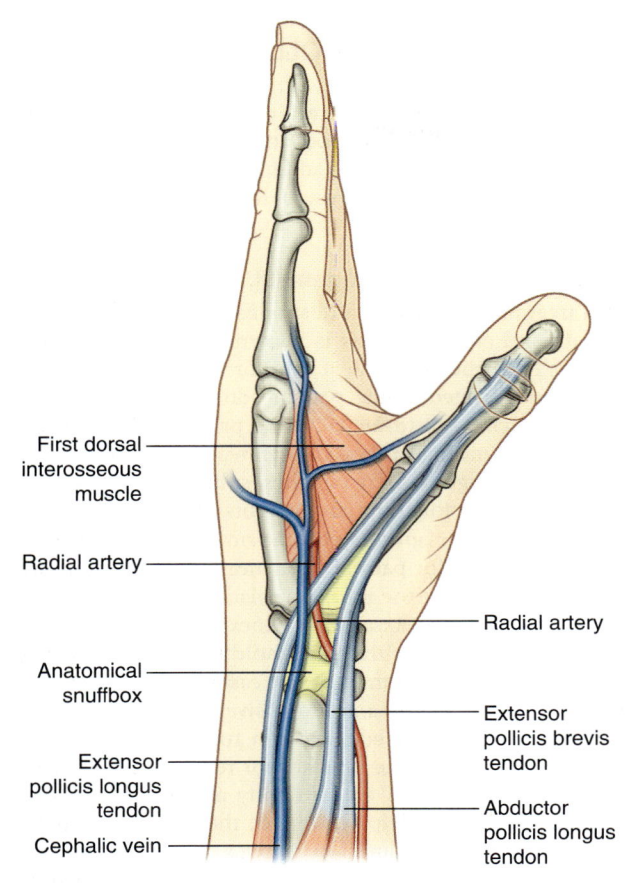

First dorsal interosseous muscle

Radial artery

Anatomical snuffbox

Extensor pollicis longus tendon

Cephalic vein

Radial artery

Extensor pollicis brevis tendon

Abductor pollicis longus tendon

F I G . 168.1 Anatomical snuffbox, left hand. (From Drake, R. L., Vogl, A. W., & Mitchell, A. W. M. [2020]. *Gray's anatomy for students* [4th ed.]. Philadelphia: Elsevier.)

Shoulder (see Chapter 167): The evaluation of the rotator cuff is multifaceted. The *empty can* or *Jobe test* evaluates the strength of supraspinatus. Have the patient abduct their arm to 90 degrees with 30 degrees flexion and their thumb pointing downward. Any pain elicited against the examiners resistance in this position indicates tendonitis, whereas weakness indicates a tear. The *drop arm test* is performed when the patient actively raises their arm to full abduction and attempts to actively lower the arm in a slow controlled motion. Inability to control the adduction arc compared to the unaffected side is a positive test and also indicates rotator cuff injury. The *Sulcus sign* indicates an inferior instability of the shoulder/glenohumeral joint head due to superior glenohumeral ligament and coracohumeral ligament injury. This is the observation of the amount of space between the acromial process and humeral head while applying distal tension to the arm. However, the diagnostic accuracy of this test is unknown.[2]

Ankle (see Chapter 154): In an ankle exam the *talar tilt* is used to examine the stability of calcaneofibular ligament. The test should be performed by having the patient sit on the examining table with the foot and ankle hanging unsupported. Stabilize the lower leg in one hand, keep the foot in neutral position, slowly invert the ankle, and compare the outcome to the other side. While some studies have shown high specificity and low sensitivity with this test, when combined with other exam findings, it is considered very useful.[3] The talar tilt test

should be done in conjunction with the *anterior drawer* test, which tests for injury of the anterior talofibular ligament. With the foot in slight plantar flexion, brace the anterior shin with one hand and pull the heel anteriorly with the other hand. Any laxity or continuation of forward motion is considered positive. For the *squeeze test* have the patient sitting with the leg hanging at 90 degrees over the side of the table. The clinician uses both hands to squeeze the area of the mid-calf with the heels of his/her hands placed anteriorly. Pain is considered a positive test suggesting tibiofibular syndesmosis ligamentous injury, also known as a high ankle sprain.

Knee: The *Lachman* test is done to assess for an anterior cruciate ligament (ACL) tear (see Fig. 162.2). With the knee in 30 degrees of flexion, hold the distal end of the femur stable with one hand and use the other hand to pull the proximal end of the tibia anteriorly. If the ligament is torn, there is no clear, obvious end to this movement. The *anterior drawer* test is performed to assess for an ACL injury (see Figure 162.3). With the patient supine, the clinician sits on the foot to stabilize it and places his or her thumbs on the superior anterior aspect of the tibia. Pain or anything less than a firm end translation of the tibia when pulling anteriorly signifies an ACL injury. The *posterior drawer test* is similar, but the movement of the tibia is posterior in relation to the femur. If this causes pain or lack of endpoint, it signifies a posterior cruciate ligament (PCL) injury. *Valgus* and *varus* testing that causes pain can highlight a collateral ligament injury. Place the patient in supine and perform this test with the knee in both 0- and 30-degree flexion. Hold the ankle firmly in neutral position with one hand and place the other hand along the lateral edge of the knee. Apply a valgus force to the knee to examine the medial collateral ligament (MCL). A positive test at 0 degrees indicates MCL and cruciate injury but a positive test at 30 degrees indicates only MCL involvement. Move the examining hand to the medial edge of the joint and apply varus force to examine the lateral collateral ligament (LCL).

DIAGNOSTICS

Because of the difficulty in determining the type of musculoskeletal injury based on presenting symptoms alone, diagnostic images are often ordered. Diagnostic imaging helps diagnose fractures versus soft tissue injury.

Essential Diagnostics

X-ray, known as plain films, are the most common first diagnostic test in a musculoskeletal injury. X-rays are easy to perform and readily available. Basic x-rays include anterior and posterior views (AP) and lateral views. In certain circumstances specific x-ray views are ordered based on suspected fracture location or concerns. Some of these include oblique, stress, sunrise of the patella, and weight-bearing views.

The decision to x-ray is multifactorial and includes the mechanism of injury, the patient's past medical history, current state (nonverbal, intoxication), the physical exam, and the likelihood of fracture. In order to simplify risk stratification in the foot and ankle specifically, the Ottawa Ankle Rules (OARs) are used to help determine the need for radiographs of the acutely injured ankle or midfoot in the emergency room.[4] In 2016 a systematic review of previous studies concluded that the OARs are still valid today (Box 168.1).[5,6]

Magnetic Resonance Imagings. Magnetic resonance imaging provides a view of the musculoskeletal system without

BOX **168.1**

Ottawa Ankle Rules

The Ottawa Ankle rules recommend an ankle x-ray series if there is pain in the malleolar area **and** any one of the following:

Pain and point tenderness at the posterior edge or tip of the lateral malleolus

Pain and point tenderness at the posterior edge or tip of the medial malleolus

Inability to weight bear for four steps immediately after injury and during the examination

The Ottawa Ankle rules recommend a foot x-ray series if there is pain in the midfoot **and** any one of the following:

Bone tenderness at the base of the 5th metatarsal

Bone tenderness at the navicular

From: Retrieved from http://www.theottawarules.ca/ankle_rules. Accessed December 16, 2017.[6]

radiation and is far more specific and in-depth than a plain x-ray. These are reserved for soft tissue problems, cartilage involvement, more chronic complaints, recurrent injuries, significant ligament laxity, compression fractures, and those who do not respond to therapy. There are contraindications to MRI, including pacemakers and certain types of metal or clips in the body. Claustrophobia during the testing process is a concern for many patients as well.

Ultrasound. Ultrasound is used in orthopedics for some diagnostic reasons such as hip pain in children, some tendonitis diagnosis, effusion, DVT diagnosis, and fluoroscopy for joint injections.

Computed Tomography Scan. CT scanning is used for some fractures not seen on x-ray, such as a talus fracture and for some soft tissue problems.

INITIAL DIAGNOSTICS

Sprains, Strains, and Fractures

LABORATORY	IMAGINING
• None	• X-ray studies

DIFFERENTIAL DIAGNOSIS

 Emergency room referral indicated for injuries that show neurovascular compromise, a penetrating object, or a wound into a joint, or those that occur from a crush injury or result in an open fracture.

Traumatic presentation of any musculoskeletal pain requires exclusion of sprains, strains, fractures, dislocations, and subluxations. Once this type of injury has been excluded, other causes of musculoskeletal pain need to be investigated. Systemic symptoms such as fever, rash, weight loss, and excessive fatigue need to be assessed. Local pain can be caused by problems such as *foreign bodies, infection* (i.e., cellulitis, Lyme disease causing joint pain), *inflammation* (i.e., plantar fasciitis, gout, arthritis), or *clotting issues* (i.e., phlebitis, deep vein thrombosis). More widespread musculoskeletal pain can be caused by problems such as *autoimmune disease* (i.e., polymyalgia rheumatica, rheumatoid arthritis) *fibromyalgia, and cancer/metastases.*

INTERPROFESSIONAL COLLABORATIVE MANAGEMENT

Care of a fracture, strain, or sprain appropriate for the primary care office should follow blood and body fluid precautions. Open wounds should be cleaned, dressed, and bandaged.

All jewelry should be removed from the affected limb in case of swelling.

Nonpharmacologic Management

Initial treatment for strains and sprains includes rest, ice, compression, and elevation. This is known by the acronym RICE. RICE has been the standard of care for sprains and strains for decades and is cited in the patient education information of many national, governmental, and private organizations.[7,8] *Rest* refers to limiting the use of the area until pain-free use is possible. This might require crutches, splinting, casting, etc. *Ice* treatment is used for the first 48 hours after an injury. Ice is applied every 2 to 3 hours for edema or as often as 20 minutes on/20 minutes off for pain relief as needed up to 48 hours. It is recommended that the ice is not placed directly on the skin to avoid burns. Home ice packs are inexpensively made from a bag of frozen peas, since they will mold to joints and angles of the musculoskeletal system and can easily be reused. *Compression* can be achieved with an inexpensive elastic bandage. These are best used to decrease edema when applied quickly after the injury. An elastic bandage is better for reducing edema than a rigid splint.[9] *Elevation* of the extremity above the level of the heart after the injury helps to reduce the edema and thereby decrease initial pain. Elevation implies that the more distal joint should be higher than each preceding proximal joint.

Splinting/Immobilization. Minor sprains or strains can be wrapped with an *elastic bandage* to reduce swelling in the first few days after an injury. A *sling* and *swathe* can easily splint shoulder and upper arm injuries. The exception to this is an anterior dislocation of the shoulder, which places the arm in abduction and requires splinting in this position. Clavicular fractures that do not involve injury to surrounding structures can be managed in a figure-eight bandage. It will not reduce a clavicular fracture, but it affords great comfort for the patient. *Splinting* is used to treat and reduce pain and edema, and provide support for unstable areas. Prefabricated splints are available over the counter at local pharmacies and hold the body in neutral position. They come in hard and soft form, vary in size, and are easy to apply.

The choice of splint varies according to the area that is injured. An *air cast* is an appropriate choice for an ankle inversion[10] or eversion injury. *Lace-up ankle braces* are useful in both acute and chronic ankle sprains to prevent rolling and twisting under stress conditions. With a knee injury, a *hinged knee brace* is used to provide medial/lateral stability while allowing full flexion and extension. A knee immobilizer is typically used after surgical procedures. *Walking boots* are used for sprains that require structural support and some foot and ankle fractures. The boot eliminates the natural foot rockers to immobilize the joints of the foot and promote healing. Walking boots are fit and dispensed at a certified orthotist or orthopedic office. Casts for higher-grade injuries and fractures are individually created and custom fit by clinicians trained/certified in their manufacturing and application.

Therapy/Exercise. The early use of muscle strengthening is important in recovery.[11] Physical therapists and occupational therapists work on decreasing pain and inflammation while increasing strength, muscle endurance, and motion after injury. A review of over 70 studies revealed that occupational therapy techniques used in shoulder injuries can decrease pain and improve function.[12] A review of randomized controlled trials of ankle sprain treatment programs found that professional physical therapy treatment leads to decreased pain, increased strength, and better positional sense than home programs.[13] Exercise therapy has also been shown to decrease the risk of recurrent ankle sprains.[14] In the first few days after mild injury, studies have shown early supervised therapy does not aid in recovery more than written home instruction.[15,16] Therefore, many sites provide basic exercise information to patients in written format for home use.

Pharmacologic Management

The use of antiinflammatories is the mainstay of pharmacologic treatment for musculoskeletal injuries. Nonsteroidal antiinflammatory drugs (NSAIDs) are available in the outpatient setting in both oral (over-the-counter and prescription preparations) and topical formulations. They are used to reduce swelling, decrease pain, and in some instances reduce the risk of clotting. For ankle sprains, the overall benefits of taking oral NSAIDs seem to outweigh the risks.[17] Side effects of these drugs include GI upset and GI bleeding, so they should be taken with food and for the shortest effective time. NSAIDS are contraindicated in patients with allergies to NSAIDs or aspirin-related products, some asthma patients, recent gastric bypass surgery patients, those on warfarin or direct oral anticoagulants (DOACs), as well as patients with some renal issues and other medical contraindications. Older adults experience side effects to NSAIDs more commonly. Topical NSAIDs or acetaminophen up to 3 g/d in divided doses can be helpful for those who cannot take NSAIDs.

Topical NSAIDs are available by prescription in cream, gel, solution, and patch forms. These topical formulations avoid the GI side effects of the oral NSAIDs but are more costly. Multiple randomized controlled trials have compared the use of oral and topical NSAIDs for outcomes such as pain control, edema, cost, and effectiveness. A 2016 review of 28 studies looking at short-term pain and edema in ankle sprains found that NSAIDs are superior to placebo in both topical and oral preparations.[17] Another study recommended that the cost effectiveness for topical treatment was reached for a single joint arthritis flair or acute injury but not for a long-term pain control situation.[18] Narcotics can be used for severe pain usually related to severe ligament injury, fracture, or postoperatively. Many states now have laws restricting the use and number of narcotic tablets prescribed to patients. Please check with your state and local regulations.

If a fracture is confirmed on x-ray examination, an orthopedist must be consulted regarding timing and need of orthopedic follow-up. Dislocations of larger joints, such as the shoulder, can be accompanied by neurovascular compromise, therefore requiring referral to the emergency department or orthopedists. Compartment syndrome, ruptured tendons, and those with ligament or joint instability require immediate referral to an orthopedist. Physical therapy or occupational therapy referral should be considered for any injury that does not or is not expected to resolve spontaneously in 10 to 14 days. Physical therapists may also be consulted to evaluate ambulation and balance and to teach the patient proper use of ambulatory assistive devices. Occupational therapy can be helpful with the appropriate splinting of upper extremity injuries and subsequent rehabilitation. Vocational counseling may be indicated. Any injury that does not resolve in the expected time frame should be referred to an orthopedist.

COMPLICATIONS

Complications may occur as a direct result of the injury or as a consequence of treatment provided, and they may be seen within the first hours of injury or weeks after trauma. Critical neurovascular structures lie close to the skeleton; thus, disruption of the bone may lacerate, entrap, impale, or compress nerves and vessels at the fracture site. Caution is recommended when using a sling for an extended time to avoid adhesive capsulitis or frozen shoulder.

Fracture complications require close monitoring. Long-bone fractures may have associated blood loss of up to two liters and could induce hypovolemic shock. *Delayed union* refers to a fracture that is able to heal but in a longer time frame than expected. Nonunion occurs if the fracture does not heal sufficiently, in expected time frame, to support normal limb function, and if pain continues. A bone stimulator might be used in this case. *Malunion* is defined as healing with a poor functional or cosmetic outcome; this generally requires surgical intervention.

Compartment syndrome may occur with any musculoskeletal injury that results in decreased vascular flow to the compartment, thereby causing muscle ischemia and necrosis. The term *compartment* refers to an area where fascia wraps around a muscle group and its supplying arteries, veins, and nerves. When the intracompartmental pressure becomes greater than the vascular perfusion pressure, the tissue, vessels, nerves, and muscles become ischemic within the tight area. Because the fascia is inelastic, anything that increases compression, such as elastic bandages, casts, constrictive jewelry or clothing, bleeding into an area, or peripheral vascular disease, can potentiate this risk. The initial compression results in histamine release, which causes increased swelling and capillary dilation. This secondary swelling and dilation increase compression, which leads to further histamine release and more compression. The cyclic process continues, and irreversible muscle and nerve damage occurs in 2 to 4 hours. In 24 to 48 hours, complete limb function is lost, and permanent deformity results. The presenting symptoms of this syndrome may include pain, paresthesias, pallor, pulselessness, or paralysis. It is frequently seen in the anterior tibial region. However, surgical intervention may be required to relieve pressure. It is essential that presenting signs and symptoms be identified quickly to enable successful intervention.

Infection can occur from an open fracture. *Gas gangrene*, a rare occurrence, is a muscle infection caused by *Clostridium Perfringens* related to the trauma of the skin. It manifests in a contaminated open fracture within 72 hours after injury. *Necrotizing fasciitis* is soft tissue *Group A Strep* infection that can occur in the subcutaneous tissues. Be alert for pain that is out of proportion for the findings on examination or expected healing. *Osteomyelitis*, a chronic infection of the bone itself, is seen weeks later (see Chapter 166). After long-bone, pelvic, or multiple fractures, fat *embolism* syndrome may occur within the first 48 to 72 hours. This manifests with the sudden onset of respiratory distress and extreme arterial hypoxia. *Deep vein thrombosis* related to immobilization can occur (see Chapter 217). In a recent cross-sectional study, pulmonary *emboli* (see Chapter 95) following fractures were found to be more likely in patients with other complications such as pneumonia and compartment syndrome.[19]

Complex regional pain syndrome was previously referred to as reflex sympathetic dystrophy. It is a pain syndrome characterized by pain beyond the anticipated period for healing accompanied by autonomic changes in the affected limb such as discoloration, temperature change, or edema.[20]

Fracture blisters, histologically comparable to second-degree burn blisters, result from a separation of the dermis from the stratified squamous epithelium because of edema. They occur in a small percentage of ankle fractures and are most commonly seen with fractures caused by severe twisting but may appear with other joint or limb trauma. Fracture blisters typically emerge on parts of the body with minimum soft tissue between the skin and bone, such as the elbow, ankle, foot, and shin.[21] Additional complications following sprains, strains, and fractures can include joint stiffness, weakness, instability, post-traumatic arthritis, osteochondrosis (avascular necrosis), and paresthesias.

LIFE SPAN CONSIDERATIONS

Pediatric patients have specific age-related concerns. It is important to recall the classification method developed by Salter-Harris when evaluating fractures in adolescents or children. A *Type I Salter-Harris* fracture occurs when trauma causes complete epiphyseal separation only, without any bone fracture. A Type I fracture is diagnosed by clinical examination even if it cannot be confirmed by radiologic examination. Types II to V are diagnosed by radiography. The most common Salter-Harris fracture is Type II. A *Type II Salter-Harris* fracture runs along the epiphysis with an associated triangular break in the metaphysis of the bone. *Type III* and *Type IV Salter-Harris* fractures are intra-articular. Type III fractures are uncommon and involve the joint surface as well as the epiphyseal plate and its periphery. Type IV fractures involve the joint surface, epiphysis, epiphyseal plate, and metaphysis. The prognosis for growth is poor in Type IV fractures unless reduction and maintenance are flawless.[22,23] *Type V Salter-Harris* fractures occur when a crushing trauma causes the epiphysis to compress the physis, leading to growth retardation. Pediatric and adolescent patients are often involved in multiple sports or year-round in a single sport. A single sport decreases cross training of the musculoskeletal system, putting year-round stress on the same ligaments, muscles, and joints and increasing the chances of overuse syndromes in a younger population.

In older adults, there are different concerns. The risk of falling and resultant fractures increases in patients older than 65 years. Fractures of any type in the older adult increase mortality, which after a hip fracture especially, persists for years. Osteoporosis, poor physical conditioning, vision problems, balance issues, comorbidities, polypharmacy, and general frailty exacerbate the risk of injury. Home environment risks (e.g., lack of handrails, bathtubs without grab bars, scatter rugs, and poor lighting) can lead to strains, sprains, and fractures. Osteoporosis fractures, including compression fractures, are more common than heart disease or stroke and are a leading cause of disability and nursing home placement in this population (see Chapter 13).

HEALTH PROMOTION

The patient should be instructed in how to check for temperature, paresthesias, pallor, pulselessness, decreasing circulation, and paralysis in the injured extremity. Patients with any immobilization should be diligent about elevation and neurovascular assessment. Patients should also be encouraged to wiggle their fingers or toes to prevent swelling if applicable. Education should address the fact that pain is expected to gradually decrease and that any pain that continues, increases, or is not relieved by medication must be reported to the practitioner.

If a splint, wrap, brace, or immobilizer is used, specific idiosyncrasies of that particular apparatus should be explained. Casts should be kept clean and dry. To prevent skin breakdown under or around the edges of the cast, foreign objects such as cast fragments, liquids, lotions, powders, or any device intended to relieve itching should be avoided. Instructions also need to include recommendations for weight bearing, bathing, and follow-up care.

Patients should have yearly physical examinations and ask specifically if their health is compatible with their desired exercise plan. Providers should then instruct the patient about specific risks and ask about risky behaviors. Coaches should be instructed regarding safe play and pediatric risks involved with their sport. Training programs for both coaches and sports enthusiasts are essential. No sports activity should begin before warm-up and stretching exercises, and no sport should be undertaken if the individual is not conditioned for the physical component involved. Safety gear should be checked for fit and worn at all times, and spotters should be used. Properly fitting shoes or protective footwear should be considered in activities that could cause stress injuries to ankles and other joints. If ankle injuries are recurrent, a lace-up brace is recommended. First aid equipment and trained personnel should be available during any organized sport to provide immediate care of injuries. Pain needs to be acknowledged as a warning sign and activity should be stopped. The health care provider caring for an injured patient should determine when it is safe for the patient to return to previous activity levels.

REFERENCES

1. Rothermel, S. D., & Juliano, P. (2017). Ankle sprains and fractures. In *Orthopedic surgery clerkship: A quick reference guide for senior medical students* (p. 373).
2. Physical Therapy Web. Sulcus Sign- Orthopedic Examination. http://physical therapyweb.com/sulcus-sign-orthopedic-shoulder-examination. (Accessed 16 December 2017).
3. Schneiders, A., & Karas, S. (2016). The accuracy of clinical tests in diagnosing ankle ligament injury. *European Journal of Physiotherapy, 18*(4), 245–253.
4. Campagne, D. (2014) Overview of fractures, dislocations and sprains. Merck Manual Online Library. Retrieved from www.merckmanuals.com/profes sional/injuries_poisoning/fractures_dislocations_and_sprains/overview_of _fractures_dislocations_and_sprains.html?qt=sprainsgrade_II&alt=sh. (Accessed 22 November 2017).
5. Jonckheer, P., Willems, T., De Ridder, R., Paulus, D., Holdt Henningsen, K., San Miguel, L., et al. (2016). Evaluating fracture risk in acute ankle sprains:any news since the Ottawa Ankle Rules? A systematic review. *The European Journal of General Practice, 22*(1), 31–41.
6. Ottawa Ankle Rules. Retrieved from http://www.theottawarules.ca/ankle_ rules. (Accessed 16 December 2017).
7. American Orthopedic Foot and Ankle Society. How to care for a sprained ankle. Retrieved from http://www.aofas.org/footcaremd/how-to/foot-injury/ Pages/How%20to%20Care%20for%20a%20Sprained%20Ankle.aspx. (Accessed 8 December 2017).
8. Mayo Clinic. Sprain: First Aid. Retrieved from https://www.mayoclinic.org/ first-aid/first-aid-sprain/basics/art-20056622. (Accessed 8 December 2017).

9. Bilgic, S., Durusu, M., Aliyev, B., Akpancar, S., Ersen, O., Yasar, S. M., et al. (2015). Comparison of two main treatment modalities for acute ankle sprain. *Pakistan Journal of Medical Sciences, 31*(6), 1496.

10. Choy, Y., & Lee, S. (2017). Changes in lower limb muscle activity based on the angle of ankle abduction during lunge exercise. *Journal of Physical Therapy Science, 29*(11), 1947–1949.

11. Van Reijen, M., Vriend, I., Zuidema, V., van Mechelen, W., & Verhagen, E. A. (2016). Increasing compliance with neuromuscular training to prevent ankle sprain in sport: Does the 'strengthen your ankle' mobile app make a difference? A randomized controlled trial. *British Journal of Sports Medicine, 50*(19), 1200–1205.

12. Marick, T. L., & Roll, S. C. (2016). Effectiveness of occupational therapy interventions for musculoskeletal conditions: A systematic review. *The American Journal of Occupational Therapy, 71,* https://ajot.aota.org/article.aspx?articleid=2591423 or doi:10.5014/ajot.2017.023127.

13. Feger, M. A., Herb, C. C., Fraser, J. J., Glaviano, N., & Hertel, J. (2015). Supervised rehabilitation versus home exercise in the treatment of acute ankle sprains. *Clinics in Sports Medicine, 34*(2), 329–346.

14. Doherty, C., Bleakley, C., Delahunt, E., & Holden, S. (2017). Treatment and prevention of acute and recurrent ankle sprain: An overview of systematic reviews with meta-analysis. *British Journal of Sports Medicine, 51*(2), 113–125.

15. Taylor, N. (ed.) (2017). The addition of supervised physiotherapy sessions for management of acute ankle sprain does not aid recovery more than providing standardized written instruction about early management [synopsis]. *Journal of Physiotherapy,* http://dx.doi.org/10.1016/j.jphys.2017.02.006.

16. Brison, R. J., et al. (2016). Effect of early supervised physiotherapy on recovery from acute ankle sprain: Randomised controlled trial. Retrieved from https://www.ncbi.nlm.nih.gov/pubmed/27852621.

17. van den Bekerom, M. P., Sjer, A., Somford, M. D., et al. (2015). Non-steroidal anti-inflammatories for treating ankle sprain in adults: Benefits outweigh adverse events. *Knee Surgery, Sports Traumatology, Arthroscopy, 23*(8), 2390.

18. Merriam, S., & Claxton, R. (2015) Topical non-steroidal anti-inflammatory drugs. Retrieved from www.mypcnow.org/blank-y675m. (Accessed 15 November 2017).

19. Auer, R., & Riehl, J. (2017). The incidence of deep vein thrombosis and pulmonary embolism after fracture of the tibia: An analysis of the national trauma databank. *Journal of Clinical Orthopaedics and Trauma, 8*(1), 38–44.

20. Harden, R. N., Oaklander, A. L., Burton, A. W., et al. (2013). Complex Regional Pain Syndrome: Practical diagnostic and treatment guidelines, 4th edition. *Pain Medicine (Malden, Mass.), 14*(2), 180–229.

21 Mehta, S. S., Rees, K., Cutler, L., & Mangwani, J. (2014). Understanding risks and complications in the management of ankle fractures. *Indian Journal of Orthopedics, 48*(5), 445–452.

22. Lasanianos, N. G., & Kanakaris, N. K. (2015). Physeal fractures in children. In N. G. Lasanianos, N. K. Kanakaris, & P. V. Giannousids (Eds.), *Trauma and orthopedic classification: A comprehensive overview* (pp. 505–507). London: Springer-Verlag.

23 Salter, R. B. (1983). *Textbook of disorders and injuries of the musculoskeletal system* (2nd ed.). Balitmore. Williams & Wilkins. classic reference.

CHAPTER **169**

ELBOW PAIN

Denise A. Vanacore-Chase

 Patients with acute trauma resulting in fracture, dislocation, and vascular or neurologic clinical findings should be referred to an orthopedist immediately.

DEFINITION AND EPIDEMIOLOGY

The elbow is a hinged joint that allows flexion and extension of the elbow. It is critical that the elbow joint be fully functional for an individual to have full hand and wrist movement. Microtears of the muscles, ligaments, and tendons from inflammation and trauma are common causes of acute and chronic elbow pain.

Most elbow injuries result from overuse during high-force or repetitive-motion activities. Two groups of people seem to be at increased risk for elbow disorders. The first is high-performance athletes, especially in racket and throwing sports such as baseball, tennis, racquetball, golf, and basketball. The second group includes those with jobs that require forceful or repetitive wrist and elbow rotation, lifting, gripping, or torqueing motions. High-risk occupations include factory workers, laborers, carpenters, and grocery checkers. The prevalence of occupational lateral epicondylitis is as high as 5.2% and the prevalence of medial epicondylitis is 1.5%.[1] In the general population, injuries may occur from pursuing recreational hobbies. Improper preparation, lack of strength or conditioning, and overzealousness can all contribute to elbow pain. The lateral side is affected 7 to 10 times more often than the medial.[1]

The elbow is also vulnerable to inflammatory arthritides, including osteoarthritis, rheumatoid arthritis, crystal arthropathies, and the spondyloarthropathies.

PATHOPHYSIOLOGY

A three-joint complex, the elbow is formed by the articulations of the humerus, radius, and ulna. The humeroulnar articulation is a hinge joint and allows flexion and extension of the elbow and flexion, extension, pronation, and supination of the wrist.[1] The humeroradial and radioulnar articulations are partially ligamental; their flexibility allows rotation of the radius and pronation-supination of the forearm. This inhibits the amount of excessive motion in the joint and limits the joint to operating as a hinge.

Stability of the elbow is accomplished through bones, ligaments, and muscles. The humeroulnar joint is the main stabilizer for flexion and extension of the elbow. Rotational stability is divided into valgus and varus stabilizers. A valgus stress is a force on the medial elbow from throwing or axial compression. Primary valgus stabilizers are the medial (ulnar) collateral ligaments and their supporting muscles. A varus stress is a force on the lateral elbow. The lateral (radial) collateral ligaments stabilize for varus stress.

Classifying elbow injuries into anterior, lateral, medial, and posterior based on anatomy assists in developing the differential diagnosis. Elbow injuries may be classified as acute or chronic. Acute injuries result from a single high force, such as a fall or direct blow, that is greater in strength than the tendon, ligament, or bone affected. However, most injuries are chronic. Chronic injuries occur from repetitive, submaximal forces that overload the elbow's ability to adequately heal, causing recurrent pain.[2] Biceps tendinopathy, gout, osteoarthritis, and rheumatoid arthritis occur in the anterior elbow. Epicondylitis, a medial, ulnar collateral ligament injury, and cubital tunnel syndrome occur in the medial elbow. Lateral epicondylitis, radial tunnel, and posterior nerve syndrome occur in the lateral elbow. Olecranon bursitis, triceps tendinopathy, and posterior impingement occur in the posterior aspect of the elbow.[3]

CLINICAL PRESENTATION AND PHYSICAL EXAMINATION

Elbow pain may be traced to a specific activity or chain of events or may appear insidiously, with no identifiable trigger. The pain may or may not radiate into the shoulder or into the wrist. The patient may experience weakness in the hand, wrist, or elbow.[1] Once an injury has occurred, everyday activities such as picking up groceries, reaching, or pulling can cause pain. A thorough history, including occupational and recreational activities and any prior elbow injury, is essential. An assessment of the onset and type of pain is also important.[4] Pain can be described as sharp, intermittent, and usually in the vicinity of the lateral or medial epicondyle.

A history of falls, a direct impact to the elbow, or a history of other joint pain or swelling is also needed to exclude fracture, rheumatoid arthritis, seronegative spondyloarthropathies, crystal arthropathies, or other systemic diseases.

Physical examination of both elbows is performed to assess for alteration in carrying angle, posture, strength, and range of motion. Bone and soft tissue landmarks should be assessed for asymmetry, malalignment, erythema, swelling, and tenderness. Bone landmarks to be examined are the medial and lateral epicondyles of the humerus and the olecranon process of the ulna. Range-of-motion testing includes flexion and extension and pronation and supination. Normal flexion and extension are 0 to 135 degrees. The elbow can rotate from 0 to 180 degrees. Normal range of motion effectively rules out involvement of the elbow joint itself. Functional range of motion for normal activities of daily living is 30 to 130 degrees of flexion, with the greatest strength and greatest stress on the elbow at 70 degrees.[5] Extra-articular pathologic conditions, including epicondylitis and olecranon bursitis, rarely affect elbow range of motion.

The extensor tendons at the lateral epicondyle and the flexor tendons at the medial epicondyle are palpated for tenderness. Several confirmatory tests or maneuvers may be helpful. Resisted wrist extension or flexion may help diagnose lateral or medial epicondylitis, respectively. A local anesthetic block can be placed near the suspected involved tendon. Relief of pain with this injection is confirmatory.

Posteriorly, the olecranon bursa overlies the olecranon process. The olecranon bursa is inspected and palpated for redness, swelling, tenderness, or chronic thickening.

The ulnar nerve sits in a groove between the medial epicondyle and the olecranon process.[5] The Tinel sign is present when tapping over the ulnar groove reproduces pain or numbness felt in the fourth and fifth fingers. Muscles for wrist flexion and pronation originate through tendons from the medial epicondyle and then spread out along the palmar surface of the forearm.

Physical examination should include the wrist, shoulder, and neck because pathologic conditions at these sites may cause referred pain to the elbow. Location and radiation of the pain are critical for accurate assessment. Lateral elbow pain with passive wrist flexion and active wrist extension usually indicates lateral epicondylitis, and medial epicondylitis is indicated by pain with resisted wrist flexion and forearm pronation and passive wrist extension.[6]

DIAGNOSTICS
Essential

Testing is based on the mechanism of injury or duration of symptoms. X-ray studies of the elbow are the most commonly ordered tests. Standard x-ray studies include an anteroposterior film with the elbow fully extended and supinated and a lateral view with the elbow flexed at 90 degrees and the forearm supinated. Oblique views may be needed to better study the radial head and shaft, the humeral condyles, and the coronoid process of the ulna.[7] Laboratory testing is based on the clinical history. A complete blood count (CBC), erythrocyte sedimentation rate (ESR), rheumatoid factor, antinuclear antibody test, Lyme titer, or elbow joint or bursal aspiration may be indicated

to exclude infection or systemic disease. Joint aspirate should be evaluated with a culture and Gram stain and examined for crystals.[7]

Additional Diagnostics

Magnetic resonance imaging (MRI) is the diagnostic tool of choice to examine the joint for loose bodies, ligament injury, stress fractures, or osteochondral lesions. Ultrasound is being used more frequently to determine the loss of the tendon's normal fibrillar pattern and neovascularization.[1] Ultrasound is best reserved for patients with atypical presentations or poor response to treatment.

INITIAL DIAGNOSTICS

Elbow Pain

LABORATORY
- None

IMAGING
- X-ray studies[a] (anteroposterior, lateral, and oblique)
- Magnetic resonance imaging[a]
- Diagnostic musculoskeletal ultrasound[a]
- Angiogram[a]
- Joint Aspiration[a]

ADDITIONAL DIAGNOSTICS
- Complete blood count and differential
- Erythrocyte sedimentation rate
- Rheumatoid factor
- Antinuclear antibodies[a]
- Uric acid level
- Lyme titer

[a]If indicated.

DIFFERENTIAL DIAGNOSIS

 Priority differentials to consider include radial nerve entrapment, cervical radiculopathy, ulnar collateral ligament injury, and radius, ulna, or humerus fracture or dislocation.

The most common causes of elbow pain are sprains, fractures, bursitis, and epicondylitis. Lateral epicondylitis is called *tennis elbow;* medial epicondylitis is called *golfer's elbow.*[8] Medial collateral ligament instability and ulnar neuritis can also cause pain (Table 169.1). Elbow pain is often caused by local injury but may result from a referred, external condition. Based on the patient history, the differential diagnosis for referred pain should include cervical disk or nerve root problems; thoracic outlet or brachial plexus disease; radicular pain from shoulder, neck, or wrist overuse injuries; diabetes; cardiovascular disease; and peripheral nerve entrapment syndromes.[9] Acute injuries are most often related to overuse, direct trauma, or fractures. Systemic diseases that may cause elbow pain and should be considered include osteoarthritis (Chapter 165), rheumatoid arthritis (Chapter 197), psoriatic arthritis (Chapter 198), Lyme disease (Chapter 213), and infection. On the basis of the examination and neurologic findings, electromyography and nerve conduction studies may be indicated to rule out nerve entrapment.[6]

INTERPROFESSIONAL COLLABORATIVE MANAGEMENT

Ideally, treatment begins before injury occurs. Injury prevention strategies include flexibility, strength, and endurance training; warm-up and cool-down stretching exercises; and avoidance cf fatigue by limiting total activity time. Proper equipment, body mechanics, and ergonomics are also important to prevent injuries.

Pharmacologic Management

Nonsteroidal antiinflammatory drugs can be used to reduce pain and tissue inflammation. After 2 weeks of conservative treatment, and after infection has been excluded, corticosteroid injection may be considered to provide further improvement of the condition. Steroid injections may provide temporary relief that allows the patient to fully participate in rehabilitation activities (see Fig. 156.4).[10]

Nonpharmacologic Management

Once injury occurs, general goals of treatment are summarized by the mnemonic *PRICEMM* (protection, rest, ice, compression,

TABLE 169.1 Common Elbow Ailments

Ailment	Presentation	Examination	Differential Diagnosis and Management
EPICONDYLITIS			
Inflammatory condition characterized by pain at tendon origin of muscle groups at medial (golfer's elbow) or lateral (tennis elbow) aspects of elbow; usually self-limited but may take several months for full recovery	Gradual or acute onset of pain along affected epicondyle, with or without radiation; possible history of heavy lifting, hammering, screwing, or gripping	Local tenderness over or just distal to affected epicondyle; possible tenderness of flexor and extensor muscles; ROM and distal neurovascular examination findings within normal limits *Lateral epicondylitis:* Pain at or around lateral epicondyle reproduced by resistive wrist extension (examiner applying pressure to force wrist into flexion while patient extends wrist) *Medial epicondylitis:* Pain exacerbated by resistive wrist flexion	*Differential diagnosis:* Cubital tunnel syndrome, cervical radiculopathy, rotator cuff tendinitis, lateral or medial collateral ligament sprains, osteoarthritis, or avulsion fracture *Management:* Conservative treatment: oral or topical NSAIDs, tennis elbow splint, "palms-up" lifting, toning exercises of wrist extensors; steroid injection if conservative treatment fails; orthopedic referral for surgical evaluation if treatment fails[8]
SPRAINS (see Chapter 168)			
Tearing or stretching of lateral or medial collateral ligaments from varus or valgus stretch	Pain after throwing, overhead or weight-bearing activity (medial), or fall onto extended elbow (lateral)	Tenderness of overlying affected ligaments; medial tenderness a maximum of 2 cm (⅘ inch) distal to epicondyle, with pain or instability with valgus stretch at 30 degrees of elbow flexion; lateral tenderness vague, reproduced only with arm extended and supinated	*Differential diagnosis:* Epicondylitis, radial or ulnar nerve irritation, avulsion fracture, or ligament tear *Management:* PRICE; may use sling and splint for 48 hours if significant pain and swelling; oral or topical NSAIDs or analgesics
RADIAL HEAD FRACTURES			
Usually caused by fall onto outstretched hand; commonly involves superior portion of radial bone	Affected arm usually cradled at 90 degrees; pain decreasing 30 minutes after injury, then recurring several hours later because of bleeding in joint	Local or diffuse edema; tenderness over radial head; ROM limited, rotation quite painful; grasp strength diminished; intact radial pulse and normal neurologic examination of hand and wrist	*Differential diagnosis:* Acute lateral epicondylitis, capsular tears, cartilage injury, subluxation or dislocation of radial head, fracture of olecranon or humerus *Management:* PRICE immobilization with posterior splint or sling with elbow flexed at 90 degrees; orthopedic referral recommended; surgical repair often required for displaced or complicated fractures
ULNAR NEURITIS			
A so called *cubital tunnel syndrome* Compression of ulnar nerve causing numbness or tingling in nerve's distribution	May be complication of rheumatoid arthritis, ganglion, elbow fracture, repeated irritation, or medial ligament sprain; pain usually localized to medial elbow; may radiate down forearm or cause clumsiness of hand; numbness and tingling replacing pain in severe cases	Tenderness of ulnar groove; sensory loss of fifth digit; diminished motor strength of fourth and fifth digits; presence of Tinel sign (tingling sensation down forearm and hand in ulnar distribution when tapping over ulnar groove); in severe cases may be forearm motor weakness and muscle atrophy *Diagnostics:* electromyographic studies	*Differential diagnosis:* Medial epicondylitis, cervical disk disease, thoracic outlet syndrome *Management:* PRICE, elbow pads, wrist-elbow splint, support in neutral position, oral or topical NSAIDs, physical therapy; conservative treatment rarely effective; referral to orthopedics or neurology appropriate

Continued

TABLE 169.1	Common Elbow Ailments—cont'd		
Ailment	**Presentation**	**Examination**	**Differential Diagnosis and Management**
OLECRANON BURSITIS (see Chapter 156)			
Swelling of bursal sac overlying olecranon process; may be acute, chronic, septic, or aseptic and/or associated with history of trauma, rheumatoid arthritis, or crystal arthropathy	After acute injury, development of painful, edematous elbow; in chronic inflammation, soft, edematous nontender elbow; ROM often intact	Edema, possible tenderness over posterior elbow; full ROM and normal neurologic examination findings; in chronic bursitis, rough nodular consistency noted; if secondary infection, fever, warmth, erythema, and tenderness present	*Differential diagnosis:* Consider tendinitis; synovitis if edema is diffuse with limited elbow extension; infection; fracture with history of trauma; gout if extremely tender and erythematous; osteophytes; osteochondrosis *Management:* X-ray studies if indicated; aspiration of bursal fluid for diagnosis; hospitalization may be recommended if infected for periodic aspiration or intravenous antibiotics; otherwise, oral or topical NSAIDs, elbow pads, avoidance of direct pressure; oral antibiotics if indicated; steroid injection after infection ruled out; orthopedic referral if signs of infection, joint involvement, or decreasing ROM

NSAIDs, Nonsteroidal antiinflammatory drugs; *PRICE,* protection, rest, ice, compression, elevation; *ROM,* range of motion.

elevation, medication, modalities); joint protection should be initiated to protect the elbow from further injury, promote healing of microtears, and reduce pain and swelling, along with rest, ice, compression, and elevation.[11]

Splinting that keeps the wrist in 30 to 45 degrees of extension may be useful for lateral epicondylitis.[2] Physical therapy with ultrasound or electrical stimulation can be used acutely, followed by rehabilitation exercises and a gradual return to activity. Changes in technique, equipment, and ergonomics should also be implemented to prevent injury recurrence.[2]

Management of arthritis includes antiinflammatory medications (for short periods and with close monitoring of side effects), balanced rest and exercise, joint conservation techniques, and avoidance of pain-generating activities. Occupational therapy can be helpful to these patients. Patients with recurrent injury, failure to improve with basic management, chronic pain with activity, arm weakness, or pain or swelling in other joints should also be referred. Both physical and occupational therapists can be extremely helpful with both treatment and education. Vocational counseling may be indicated for patients with repetitive stress injuries causing elbow pain and disability.

COMPLICATIONS

Recurrent epicondylitis or tendinitis may cause cumulative weakening of those tissues, resulting in impairment of grip function or lifting ability and nerve entrapment of the arm.[7] Limitation of elbow range of motion, arthritis, and chronic elbow pain may be caused by improper diagnosis or failure to treat the underlying elbow disorder. Repeated steroid injections may cause weakness or even rupture of the tendon and should be limited to three injections per year.[12]

PATIENT EDUCATION

Injury prevention and early recovery are assisted by teaching about proper stretching and conditioning exercises, need for rest at the earliest symptoms of pain, use of ergonomic redesign (e.g., in rackets, workplace, power tools), and proper body mechanics for sports and repetitive motion activities. Individuals with recurrent injury or any change in elbow function or mobility should be advised to seek prompt medical attention to minimize complications.

REFERENCES

1. Pitzer, M. E., Seidenberg, P. H., & Bader, D. A. (2014). Elbow tendinopathy. *The Medical Clinics of North America*, *98*(4), 833–849.
2. Domino, F. J. (2017). *5-Minute clinical consult 2017*. Philadelphia, PA: Wolters Kluwer.
3. Dawe, E. J., & Poulter, R. (2011). Elbow pain. *InnovAiT*, *4*, 325–331.
4. Johnston, J., & Deune, G. (2013). Approach to the patient with hand, wrist or elbow pain. In J. Imboden & D. Hellman (Eds.), *Current diagnosis and treatment in rheumatology* (3rd ed.). McGraw-Hill.
5. Malagelada, F., Dalmau-Pastor, M., Vega, J., & Golanó, P. (2015). Elbow anatomy. In M. Doral & J. Karlsson (Eds.), *Sports injuries*. Berlin, Heidelberg: Springer.
6. Kane, S. F., Lynch, J. H., & Taylor, J. C. (2014). Evaluation of elbow pain in adults. *American Family Physician*, *89*(8), 649–657.
7. Hegmann, K., Hoffman, E., Belcourt, R., et al. (2013). ACOEM practice guidelines: Elbow disorders. *Journal of Occupational and Environmental Medicine*, *55*(11), 1365–1374.
8. Jariwala, A., Dorman, S., Bruce, D., & Rickhauss, P. (2012). Tennis elbow: Diagnosis and treatment. *Primary Health Care*, *10*(22), 16–21.
9. Ferri, F. (2018). *Ferri's clinical advisor*. St Louis: Mosby.
10. Hanna, M., Trinh, K., Degredoris, G., Ferriter, P., Mandel, S., & Aydin, S. M. (2014). Differential diagnosis of isolated elbow pain and treatment in patients with medial or lateral epicondylitis, part 2. *Practical Neurology*, *10*, 37–40.
11. Javed, M., Mustafa, S., Boyle, S., & Scott, F. (2015). Elbow pain: A guide to assessment and management in primary care. *British Journal of General Practice*, *65*, 610–612.
12. Dean, B., Lostis, E., Oakley, T., et al. (2014). The risks and benefits of glucocorticoid treatment for tendinopathy: A systemic review of the effects of local glucocorticoid on tendon. *Seminars in Arthritis and Rheumatism*, *43*(4), 570–576.

CHAPTER **170**

HAND AND WRIST PAIN
Wendy L. Halm

 Immediate referral is indicated for suspected fracture or dislocation.

DEFINITION AND EPIDEMIOLOGY

Hand and wrist disorders may result from recreational or work-related activities, or from inflammatory or degenerative disease. Acute wrist pain can occur from fractures, contusions, strains, and sprains; instability is a common presentation. Chronic wrist pain may be caused by arthritis of the hands and fingers, overuse, old injuries, or neurologic disorders. Job specialization, repetitive tasks, and workplace demographics have contributed to an increased incidence of cumulative hand and wrist injuries. Musculoskeletal-related ergonomic injuries accounted for 31% of all workplace injuries and illnesses, nearly $\frac{1}{3}$ were hand or wrist injuries, resulting in a median of 8 days away from work in 2017.[1] These injuries, which are also known as *cumulative trauma disorders*, are defined as muscle, tendon, osseous, or neurologic conditions produced or exacerbated by repetitive movements. Sports, such as golf,[2] tennis,[3] and gymnastics,[4] may put the athlete at increased risk for hand and wrist pain. Age and various medical conditions, such as diabetes, pregnancy, and obesity may also contribute to the development of hand and wrist pain.

PATHOPHYSIOLOGY

Acute hand and wrist pain injuries stemming from sports-related activities are common, including injuries to the palm from swinging a baseball bat or golf club, and the classic injury to the thumb from the strap of a ski pole.[5] Hyperextension of a joint can cause dislocations of the metacarpophalangeal (MCP), proximal interphalangeal (PIP), or distal interphalangeal (DIP) joints. Fractures of the distal radius may occur from high-energy trauma in the young or low-energy trauma in the older adult. Fractures of the scaphoid bone can occur during a fall onto an outstretched hand. Scaphoid fractures are most common in males aged 15 to 29 years.[6]

Chronic hand and wrist pain in the presence of systemic symptoms, such as fatigue, fever, or bilateral hand pain, suggests a systemic issue, such as Lyme disease (see Chapter 213), rheumatoid arthritis (see Chapter 197), systemic lupus erythematosus (SLE) (see Chapter 199), or malignancy. Hand and wrist pain associated with arthritis is often located at the base of the thumb.[7] Weakness and pain with pinching or grasping occurs. Osteoarthritis of the DIP and PIP joints can cause pain, and may have associated Heberden (DIP) or Bouchard (PIP) nodules (see Chapter 165). Rheumatoid arthritis commonly involves the MCP joints and the wrist in a bilateral and symmetric fashion, causing pain, inflammation, and deformity. Hand and wrist pain can often occur from cumulative trauma disorders. Although the pathologic mechanism is not clearly understood, pain usually results from repetitive microtrauma that over time affects the tendons, tendon sheaths, and connective tissues. Excessive physical activity (such as gardening or painting), may initiate or worsen existing chronic hand conditions, causing an acute pain flare. Ganglion cysts, stenosing tenosynovitis, palmar fibrosis, and carpal tunnel syndrome (CTS), in addition to arthritis, are common causes of chronic hand pain.

Ganglion Cysts

Ganglion cysts are fluid-filled sacks that can appear, disappear, and change size. These soft tissue lesions occur around joints, and occasionally around tendon sheaths. Common locations include the dorsal carpal area and the volar surface of the wrist.[8] The cysts can cause pain, weakness, and bone changes and can affect the function of the joint. Their cause is unknown.

Stenosing Tenosynovitis

Stenosing tenosynovitis—"trigger finger"—is caused by irritation and subsequent thickening of the flexor tendon sheath, leading to stenosis that prevents smooth passage of the associated tendon. The thumb is the most commonly involved digit.[9] Women have a higher incidence of this disease, which occurs most frequently in patients aged 40 to 60.[9,10] Systemic conditions, such as diabetes mellitus and arthritis, may increase the incidence of this disease.[9]

De Quervain Tenosynovitis

De Quervain tenosynovitis is a painful inflammation of the abductor pollicis longus and extensor pollicis brevis tendons along the dorsal aspect of the wrist. Women aged 30 to 40 are affected more often, particularly postpartum women due to specific hand and wrist positions required in the care of an infant.[8] Motions such as pinching, lifting, wringing, and grasping or activities such as gardening or knitting, which require repeated thumb abduction and extension in combination with wrist radial and ulnar deviation, can aggravate this problem.

Palmar Fibrosis

Dupuytren contracture, or palmar fibrosis, may be a hereditary process that initially develops as a painless nodule on the palmar fascia at the base of a digit. An inflammatory fibrosis subsequently expands into a band-like cord under puckered skin and can lead to a flexion contracture. Although any finger (and both hands) may be affected, the resultant contracture most often affects the ring finger. The little finger may also be involved. The index finger is the least commonly affected digit for Dupuytren disease. The disease has been associated with the older adult, male gender, family history, Caucasian race, and systemic diseases, such as diabetes mellitus and epilepsy. The etiology is unknown; progression of the disease is unpredictable.[11]

Carpal Tunnel Syndrome

CTS is caused by compressive neuropathy of the median nerve. A bony canal bordered by the carpal bones on the radial, ulnar, and dorsal sides is roofed by the transverse carpal ligament. This canal provides a passage for the nine digital flexor tendons, the blood vessels, and the median nerve of the hand. Repetitive motion and overuse have often been thought to cause the syndrome, but recent studies may present differing conclusions. As the tendons swell, the cross-sectional area in the tunnel decreases. The resultant pressure in the small tunnel causes pressure on the median nerve. Nerve conduction is impeded, muscle strength is decreased because of the disturbance in motor fibers, and pain and paresthesia occur because of the disturbance in the sensory fibers. Common risk factors for development of CTS include repetitive maneuvers, obesity, pregnancy, diabetes mellitus, hypothyroidism, and older female gender.[12,13]

CLINICAL PRESENTATION AND PHYSICAL EXAMINATION

Localized pain, numbness, tingling, weakness, and immobility are the common reasons that patients with hand or wrist disorders seek care. The symptoms may be intermittent or constant and often affect quality of life. Onset, duration, and location of all symptoms related to wrist pain should be noted. Age, sex, hand dominance, occupation, and hobbies or sports should also be documented. Past medical history should be explored for previous hand or wrist injury and any condition that might compromise nerve function, including pregnancy. For patients with acute onset of hand or wrist pain, and/or history of trauma, the priority is to exclude fracture or dislocation with x-ray examination.

Complex anatomy and proximity of structures can make examination of the hand and wrist difficult. The physical examination should begin with inspection, noting any muscle wasting, localized swelling or masses, skin discoloration, hair loss, or deformity.[8] The contralateral side should be examined. Individual carpal bones should be palpated, passive and active range of motion should be assessed, and grip strength should be tested. Palpation of the anatomical snuffbox is necessary to exclude the possibility of scaphoid fracture. Motor function and sensory testing are also necessary. Additional provocative maneuvers and specific tests may be indicated.[7] Physical findings seen in common causes of hand and wrist pain are described in the following paragraphs.

Ganglion Cyst

Fluid-filled ganglion cysts commonly occur at the dorsal, volar, or radial aspect of the wrist and may cause pain during activity or with pressure over the area. Cysts may be asymptomatic and fluctuate in size. Most cysts will be smooth and rubbery, and will transilluminate with light. Pain may or may not be present with palpation. Numbness, tingling, or weakness may be present if the mass is compressing the median or ulnar nerve at the wrist.[14]

Stenosing Tenosynovitis

Trigger finger, or stenosing tenosynovitis, is a disorder of the flexor tendons of the fingers or thumb. This condition, which may be more prevalent in patients with diabetes, gout, or rheumatoid arthritis, occurs most commonly when a nodule or thickening in the tendon catches on the edge of the A1 pulley of the finger as the tendon attempts to glide during movement. This thickening narrows the fibrous canal, which impedes tendon movement. The pulley action is impaired, causing a painful locking or triggering of the affected digit or thumb during extension.[15] Although any digit may be affected, the middle or ring finger is most commonly involved. Edema at the distal palm may be noted. The finger is fully flexed with the examiner's finger on the MCP joint. The patient slowly extends the digit, and a "pop" is felt as the tendon slides back through the affected pulley. This maneuver is occasionally painful to the patient. Trigger thumb is examined in a similar manner. The patient will feel that the interphalangeal joint of the thumb is the culprit, but it is in fact the A1 pulley at the base of the thumb. Regardless of finger, there is often a palpable, tender nodule at the base of the affected digit.[11,16]

De Quervain Tenosynovitis

Stenosing tenosynovitis (de Quervain tenosynovitis) is a condition that causes pain at the thumb base and into the distal radius. Pain is noted with ulnar deviation under stress. Pouring from a pitcher or carton often reproduces pain. On inspection, there may be a visible nodule at the radial base of the thumb. Edema and tenderness may be present over the radial stylus. The Finkelstein test (Fig. 170.1) is conducted when the patient folds the thumb across the palm and flexes the fingers over the thumb; the clinician then deviates the hand in the direction of the ulna; the test result is positive if pain is reproduced over the radial stylus. Grip and pinch strength should also be assessed.[7]

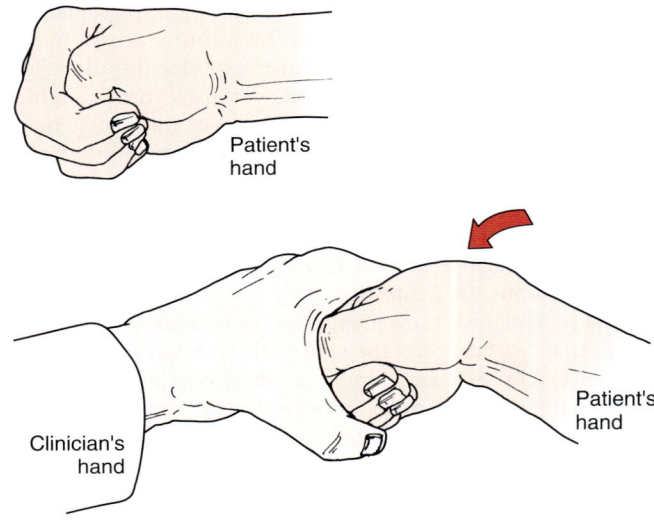

FIG. 170.1 Finkelstein test. (From Magee, D. J. [2014]. *Orthopedic physical assessment* [6th ed.]. St Louis, MO: Elsevier.)

Palmar Fibrosis

Skin changes can be the earliest manifestation. Skin may pucker with passive extension of the affected finger(s). Garrod nodules "knuckle pads" may form over the dorsum of the hand. Contracture may be evident on one or both hands as well as on the feet (Ledderhose disease) and on the penis (Peyronie disease). Painless edema along the nodule may also be present.[11]

Carpal Tunnel Syndrome

CTS results from compression of the median nerve in the carpal tunnel of the wrist. Patients may have intermittent wrist pain and numbness and tingling that radiates from the palm to the thumb, index finger, middle finger, and medial aspect of the ring finger. In addition, the patient may report intermittent nocturnal paresthesia, pain and tightness at the wrist and forearm that increases with activity, and an inability to hold objects or a tendency to drop things.[17] A tendency for symptoms to occur while driving, speaking on the telephone, or performing hygiene activities (brushing teeth, washing hair) may be reported. If the compression continues, the motor component of the median nerve is affected, and the ability to grasp with the thumb and index finger may be compromised. Atrophy of the thenar eminence may be evident in chronic cases, but edema is generally not present. Tenderness, motor strength (including grip and pinch), and sensory deficits must be determined. A two-point discrimination test can be performed with a caliper. The thumb abduction, Phalen maneuver, and Tinel sign tests (Fig. 170.2) may reproduce symptoms.[7]

DIAGNOSTICS
Essential Diagnostics

Plain radiography is indicated if fracture, acute dislocation, bony abnormality, or other pathology is suspected.

Additional Diagnostics

History and examination, including provocative maneuvers, will likely yield a clinical diagnosis. Ultrasound or MRI may be useful to confirm clinical diagnosis findings of a ganglion

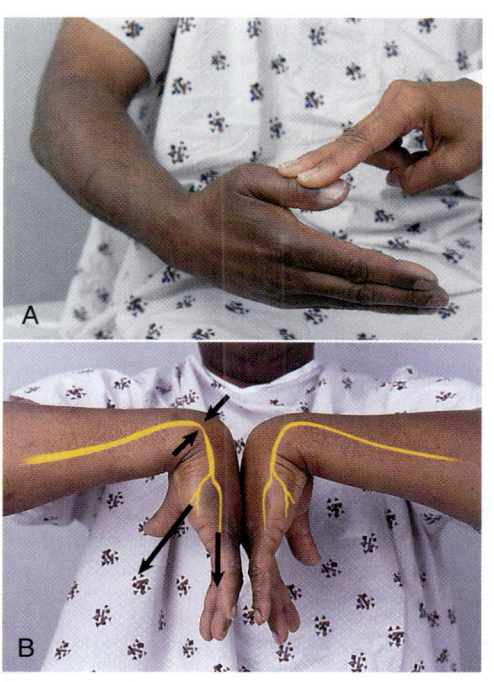

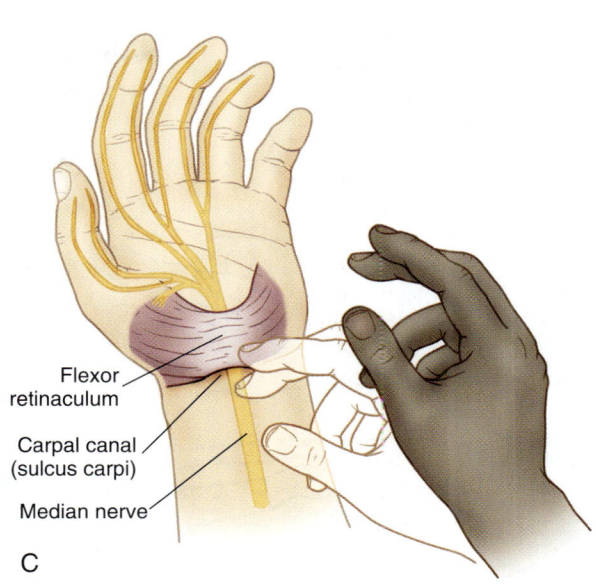

FIG. 170.2   Additional procedures for assessment of carpal tunnel syndrome: (A) Thumb abduction test, (B) Phalen maneuver, (C) elicitation of Tinel Sign. (From Ball, J. W., Dains, J. E., Flynn, J. A., Solomon, B., & Stewart, R. [2015]. *Seidel's guide to physical examination* [8th ed.]. St Louis, MO: Mosby.)

INITIAL DIAGNOSTICS

Wrist and Hand Pain

LABORATORY
- None

IMAGING
- X-ray studies

ADDITIONAL DIAGNOSTICS
- Ultrasound[a]
- MRI[a]
- Electrodiagnostic[a]

[a]If indicated.

cyst, tenosynovitis, or tendon rupture, or in pre-surgery planning. **Electrodiagnostic testing** for patients with CTS may be indicated in atypical cases to determine severity and planning for surgery.[17]

DIFFERENTIAL DIAGNOSIS

The differential diagnosis of hand and wrist pain can be broad. The most common causes of hand and wrist pain are discussed earlier in the chapter. Differentials for chronic hand and wrist pain can be narrowed down with a thorough patient history and information about any repetitive motions or physical activities. When completing the examination, region of the hand-wrist affected (Fig. 170.3) may provide clues to the origin of pain. It is important to rule out serious sources of hand or wrist pain, including fracture, dislocation, arthritis, crystal deposition disease, or vascular anomalies.

 Priority differentials include (1) fracture, (2) dislocation, (3) arthritis, (4) crystal deposition disease, and (5) vascular abnormalities.

INTERPROFESSIONAL COLLABORATIVE MANAGEMENT

Nonpharmacologic Management

Splinting and Rest of Extremity. Initial splinting of patients with a ganglion cyst might provide temporary relief. In patients with stenosing tenosynovitis, splinting of the MCP joint at 10 to 15 degrees of flexion with the PIP and DIP joints free for 4 to 6 weeks at night may be of benefit. For patients with De Quervain disease, the wrist should be splinted while in slight extension and the thumb abducted in a thumb spica splint to the level of the interphalangeal joint. Splinting may help stretch the fingers in those with Dupuytren contraction. In patients with CTS, splinting in a neutral position (particularly at night) to prevent provocative maneuvers is considered first-line therapy.[8] If the patient purchases a splint from a store, the splint will need to be manipulated to neutral or 10 degrees of extension.

Heat or Cold Application. At the acute onset of pain or injury, cold application may be of benefit to reduce swelling and inflammation. Application of cold should be limited to 15 to 20 minutes at a time. Heat application may be of benefit for pain relief and for promoting muscle relaxation. Application of heat should be limited to 15 to 20 minutes at a time.

Exercise-Physical Therapy. Gentle stretching exercise and prescribed physical therapy may be of benefit, particularly with those with CTS[18] or Dupuytren contracture.[11] Physical therapy should also be considered as a part of a patient's postsurgical management.

Pharmacologic Management

Nonsteroidal Antiinflammatory Drugs. Nonsteroidal antiinflammatory drugs can be used if the patient has no medical contraindications for pain relief and reduction of

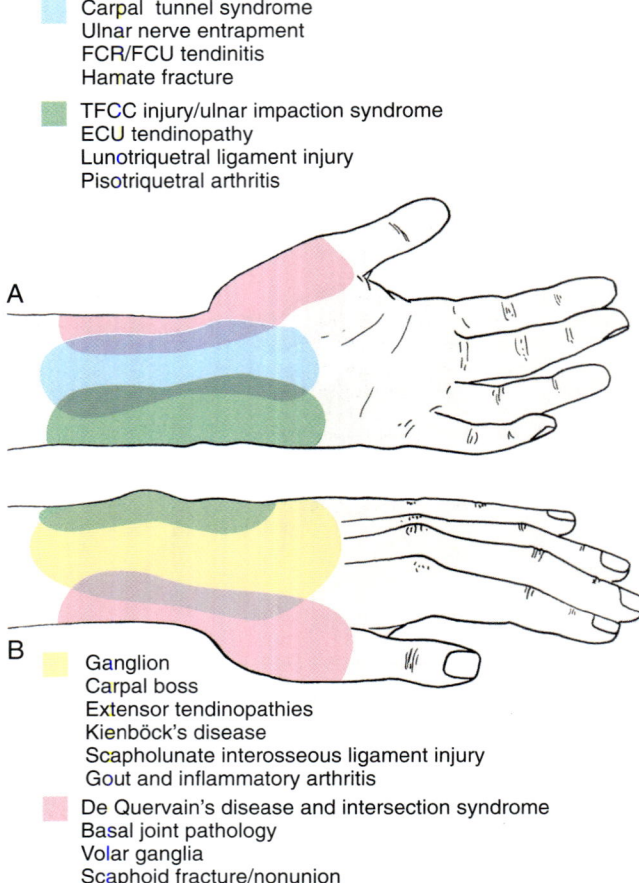

Carpal tunnel syndrome
Ulnar nerve entrapment
FCR/FCU tendinitis
Hamate fracture

TFCC injury/ulnar impaction syndrome
ECU tendinopathy
Lunotriquetral ligament injury
Pisotriquetral arthritis

A

B

Ganglion
Carpal boss
Extensor tendinopathies
Kienböck's disease
Scapholunate interosseous ligament injury
Gout and inflammatory arthritis

De Quervain's disease and intersection syndrome
Basal joint pathology
Volar ganglia
Scaphoid fracture/nonunion

F I G . 170.3 Common sites of pain in the hand and wrist and their corresponding leading diagnosis. (From Firestein, G. S., Budd, R., Gabriel, S., McInnes, I. B., & O'Dell, J. [2017]. *Kelley and Firestein's textbook of rheumatology* [10th ed.]. Philadelphia, PA: Elsevier.)

inflammation. Treatment should initially be started on an as-needed basis, with the lowest effective dose. Topical NSAIDs may be helpful and are the first-line choice for older adults.

Cortisone Injection. Local cortisone injection is an effective treatment for CTS,[17] trigger finger,[9] De Quervain tendinopathy,[8] and may delay the need for surgery. Long-term outcomes are not dependent of type of steroid used for the injection.[9] Associated complications have included depigmentation and tendon and fat atrophy.

In absence of acute injury or pain, hand or wrist pain may be managed by primary care clinicians if patients respond well to conservative treatment. Immediate emergency department or same-day orthopedic referral is indicated for known or suspected fractures of the hand or wrist.

Orthopedic referral is indicated for patients in whom conservative treatment fails or who may benefit from surgical intervention. Sports medicine interdisciplinary teams can be helpful for hand injuries in athletes. Surgical excision may be of benefit to patients with a ganglion cyst for relief of pain, limitation of movement, and nerve palsies.[8] Surgery for trigger finger includes open release of the A1 pulley and is indicated after failure of conservative measures or if the digit is locked and not reducible.[9] For CTS patients with persistent and progressive symptoms, including severe median nerve damage, carpal tunnel release surgery is the treatment of choice.[12,13]

LIFE SPAN CONSIDERATIONS

Older adults are at risk for hand and wrist pain from arthritis and fractures. Distal radius fractures are common, given the increased risk of falls and the prevalence of osteoporosis. An age-associated increase in the concentration of PTH may interfere with serum calcium concentration.

COMPLICATIONS

Contractures, deformity, and pain are significant complications of hand and wrist disorders. In addition, nerve compression can jeopardize the sensory function, motor function, and reflexes of the affected hand. These problems affect quality of life, work, and recreational activities. Although surgery may be indicated for hand disorders that are not responsive to conservative therapies, there is an inherent risk in any surgical procedure. Continued symptoms, reflex sympathetic dystrophy, nerve damage, and disfigurement are additional hazards associated with any surgical procedure of the hand or wrist.

EMERGING MANAGEMENT TRENDS

Therapeutic ultrasound may benefit patients with early-stage Dupuytren contracture or those with CTS.[12] External beam radiation, collagenase injections, platelet-rich plasma, and stem cells are currently being investigated for select hand and wrist pain conditions.[19]

PATIENT AND FAMILY EDUCATION

Activity modification to avoid symptom provocation should be discussed. Avoidance of overexertion and repetitive motions of the hand and wrist can prevent many cases of injury. Warming up and stretching of these muscles before activity may help decrease the risk of injury. The use of proper body mechanics may also reduce the risk of injury. It may be necessary to arrange the work environment to allow more comfort and less strain on the body. Taking frequent rest breaks during repetitive activities and doing strengthening exercises may help as well. Joint protection and energy conservation techniques and the use of adaptive equipment may be necessary for painful or arthritic hands. Patients should understand the importance of hourly 10-minute rest periods during activities that require repetitive hand movements.

Splints that keep the wrist straight or slightly extended should be worn at night and, if necessary, during the day. Careful explanation of splint use is important because patients often remove the splint during activity, which results in further inflammation and a prolonged recovery period. Wrist splints can also be worn while sleeping to relieve discomfort during the night.

The use of cold packs and NSAID therapy should also be reviewed. Hand weakness, symptoms that increase in severity, or symptoms not relieved by conservative therapies should be reported to the health care provider.

REFERENCES

1. U.S. Department of Labor: Bureau of Labor Statistics. Survey of Occupational Injuries and Illnesses. Last updated November 8, 2018. (Accessed 2 September 2019).
2. Woo, S. H., Lee, Y. K., Kim, J. M., Cheon, J. H., & Chung, W. (2017). Hand and wrist injuries in golfers and their treatment. *Hand Clinics, 33*, 81–96. http://dx.doi.org/10.1016/j.hcl.2016.08.012.

3. Chung, K. C., & Lark, M. E. (2017). Upper extremity injuries in tennis players. *Hand Clinics, 33*, 175–186. http://dx.doi.org/10.1016/j.hcl.2016.08.009.

4. Wolf, M. R., Avery, D., & Moriatis-Wolf, J. (2017). Upper extremity injuries in gymnasts. *Hand Clinics, 33*, 187–197. http://dx.doi.org/10.1016/j.hcl.2016.08.010.

5. Avery, D. M., Rodner, C. M., & Egar, C. M. (2016). Sports-related wrist and hand injuries: A review. *Journal of Orthopaedic Surgery and Research, 11*(99), doi:10.1186/s13018-016-0432-8.

6. Dias, J., & Kantharuban, S. (2017). Treatment of scaphoid fractures. *Hand Clinics, 33*(3), 501–509. http://dx.doi.org/10.1016/j.hcl.2017.04.003.

7. Newton, A. W., Hawkes, D. H., & Bhalaik, V. (2017). Clinical examination of the wrist. *Orthopaedics and Trauma, 31*(4), 237–247.

8. Swigart, C. R., & Fishman, F. G. (2017). Hand and wrist pain. In G. S. Firestein, R. C. Blood, S. E. Gabriel, I. B. McInnes, & J. R. O'Dell (Eds.), *Textbook of Rheumatology* (10th ed., pp. 742–755). Philadelphia: Elsevier.

9. Giugale, J. M., & Fowler, J. R. (2015). Trigger finger: Adult and pediatric treatment strategies. *The Orthopedic Clinics of North America, 46*(4), 561–569. doi:10.1016/j.ocl.2015.06.014.

10. AAOS. (2017). Trigger finger. Retrieved from https://orthoinfo.aaos.org/en/diseases–conditions/trigger-finger. (Accessed 19 December 2017).

11. Calandruccio, J. H. (2017). Dupuytren contracture. In F. A. Azar, J. H. Beaty, & S. T. Canale (Eds.), *Campbell's operative orthopaedics* (13th ed., pp. 3734–3749). Philadelphia: Elsevier.

12. Padua, L., Coraci, D., Erra, C., Pazzaglia, C., Paolaaso, I., Loreti, C., et al. (2016). Carpal tunnel syndrome: Clinical features, diagnosis, and management. *The Lancet. Neurology, 15*(12), 1273–1284. doi:10.1016/S1474-4422 (16)30231-9.

13. Hussain, A., & Winterton, R. (2016). Peripheral nerve entrapment syndromes of the upper limb. *Surgery. 34*(3), 134–138. https://doi.org/10.1016/j.mpsur.2016.01.001.

14. Meena, S., & Gupta, A. (2014). Dorsal wrist ganglion: Current review of literature. *Journal of Clinical Orthopaedics and Trauma, 5*(2), 59–64.

15. Chuang, X. L., Ooi, C. C., Chin, S. T., Png, M. A., Wong, S. C., Tay, S. C., et al. (2017). What trigger in trigger finger? The flexor tendons at the flexor digitorum superficialist bifurcation. *Journal of Plastic, Reconstructive & Aesthetic Surgery : JPRAS, 70*((10), 1411–1419. doi:10.1016/j.bjps.2017.05.037.

16. Ballard, T., & Kozlow, J. (2016). Trigger finger in adults. *CMAJ : Canadian Medical Association Journal = Journal de l'Association Medicale Canadienne, 188*(1), 61. https://doi.org/10.1503/cmaj.150225.

17. Wipperman, J., & Goerl, K. (2016). Carpal tunnel syndrome: Diagnosis and management. *American Family Physician, 94*(12), 993–999.

18. JOSPT. (2017). Carpal tunnel syndrome: Physical therapy or Surgery? *The Journal of Orthopaedic and Sports Physical Therapy, 47*(3), 162. doi:10.2519/jospt.2017.0503.

19. Steiner, M. M., & Calandruccio, J. H. (2016). Biologic approaches to problems of the hand and wrist. *The Orthopedic Clinics of North America, 48*(3), 343–349. doi:10.1016/j.ocl.2017.03.010.

CHAPTER 171

AMYOTROPHIC LATERAL SCLEROSIS

Stephanie Cassone

 Neurology consultation is indicated for all patients with suspected ALS.

DEFINITION AND EPIDEMIOLOGY

Amyotrophic lateral sclerosis (ALS) is the most common of the progressive motor neuron diseases. It is also often referred to as *Lou Gehrig's disease*, after the New York Yankees baseball player who was diagnosed with the disease in the late 1930s. Classified as a neurodegenerative disorder, it is an incurable disease that produces progressive muscle weakness and ultimately death.[1]

ALS is a progressive motor neuron disease characterized by dysfunction of both upper motor neurons (UMNs) and lower motor neurons (LMNs) in the corticospinal and corticobulbar tracts, anterior motor horn cells, and bulbar motor nuclei. Age of onset is usually 55 to 75 years old with diagnosis being slightly more likely in males than females. In terms of ethnicity and race, Caucasians and non-Hispanics more likely to develop ALS.[1] Most cases (90% or more) of ALS are sporadic, appearing at random with no clearly defined risk factors. Approximately 5% to 10% are familial, with about 25% to 40% thought to be caused by a defect in the gene known as C9orf72, and another 12% to 20% of familial cases from mutations in the superoxide dismutase 1 (SOD1) gene.[1] There is also a variety of clinical variants, including progressive muscular atrophy and progressive bulbar palsy, affecting LMNs in limb and bulbar muscles, respectively. Primary lateral sclerosis and progressive pseudobulbar palsy affect UMNs in limb and bulbar muscles. Although these clinical variants may manifest differently early on, they all eventually affect both LMNs and UMNs.[2] Limb onset ALS predominant type accounts for 70% of patients. Bulbar onset accounts for 25%, and the final 5% have initial trunk or respiratory involvement. Symptoms of autonomic, ocular movement, sensation, and cognitive dysfunction may also occur from degenerative involvement of other cortical areas.[2] The prevalence rate of ALS in the United States is 5.0 cases per 100,000 population.[2]

PATHOPHYSIOLOGY

The cause of ALS remains unknown, although the recent literature suggests several major hypotheses. There are rare familial cases of ALS (5% to 10% of cases) in which mutations in the SOD1 and C9orf72 gene have been discovered. Many cases of ALS, however, are sporadic, not familial, and several theories of cause are postulated. The first describes excitotoxic stimulation as a result of accumulation of glutamate in the central nervous system as well as functional abnormalities of mitochondria. It appears that the excess glutamate is toxic to motor neurons and abnormalities in mitochondria morphology and biochemistry contribute to the pathogenesis of ALS. The second hypothesis suggests impaired axonal structure or transport defects. This has been observed early in the disease process of ALS. The third is a familial hypothesis that neuronal injury is secondary to altered function of the enzyme SOD1 and subsequent accumulation of free oxygen radicals. This causes severe damage to the cell structures.[2]

There is evidence that this oxidative stress, mediated by free radicals, is important in the initiation of the disease. Research into the role of environmental exposures, genetic profiles, and viral agents as risk factors for the disease continues.[2]

The proposed causative mechanisms all lead to neuronal damage of both UMNs and LMNs. The UMNs are initially altered in the motor cortex, thereby affecting the corticospinal and corticobulbar tracts. The LMNs are affected at the anterior motor horn cells in the spinal cord and at the respective motor nuclei in the brainstem. Death of the motor neurons in the brainstem and spinal cord leads to denervation and atrophy of muscle fibers.[3]

CLINICAL PRESENTATION AND PHYSICAL EXAMINATION

A precise documentation of the history of symptoms and a complete physical examination highlighting the neurologic examination are essential. Early LMN cell death leads to an insidious onset of asymmetric weakness that is evident initially in the limbs, usually in the arms. Early findings include foot drop, difficulty walking, and weakness with lifting arms.[2] It is important to assess UMNs and LMNs as well as bulbar signs and symptoms.

UMN dysfunction may manifest as hyperreflexia, spasticity, Babinski signs, incoordination, and weakness. LMN dysfunction may manifest as weakness, muscle atrophy, and fasciculations (spontaneous twitching). Fasciculations may be focal, multifocal, or diffuse. Fasciculations are accompanied by UMN signs and weakness in patients with ALS. Bulbar signs and symptoms include dysarthria, dysphagia, sialorrhea, tongue atrophy, and tongue fasciculations.[2] Bulbar presentation is often closely related to reduced vital capacity resulting in difficulty in speaking and swallowing and carries a poor prognosis compared with limb onset. Older age of symptom onset and early respiratory muscle dysfunction also suggest a poor prognosis.[2,4]

As the disease progresses, both UMN and LMN involvement becomes evident, with a more symmetric distribution of the disease. Yet even in the late stages of disease, sensation and bowel and bladder function are spared. There is a known link between ALS and executive dysfunction of the frontal and temporal lobes that may manifest as subtle cognitive dysfunction. Dementia can occur even before ALS symptoms.[3,4] Interestingly, the gene mutation of *C9orf72* that can be seen with ALS has also been associated with atrophy of the temporal lobes of the brain causing frontotemporal dementia.[1]

DIAGNOSTICS

The diagnosis of ALS is usually made when there are widespread UMN and LMN signs in the absence of any electrophysiologic and pathologic signs of other disease processes as well as absence of neuroimaging evidence of other disease processes. In 1994, the World Federation of Neurology presented diagnostic criteria for ALS. These were subsequently revised in 1998 and renamed Airlie House criteria (formerly El Escorial criteria). Awaji-shima criteria were introduced in 2008, which improved diagnostic sensitivity without increasing false positives. These criteria set equal importance on both electromyographic (EMG) and clinical abnormalities. These criteria include signs of LMN degeneration by clinical, electrophysiologic, or neuropathologic examination; signs of UMN degeneration by clinical examination; and progression of the motor syndrome within a region or to other regions.[5] The four regions are bulbar, cervical, thoracic, and lumbosacral.[3]

There are no specific biochemical or laboratory markers for ALS. Laboratory and other diagnostic studies are considered to exclude other disorders in the differential diagnosis. Electrodiagnostic evaluation with electromyography (EMG) and nerve conduction studies are indicated for all patients with suspected ALS. Magnetic resonance imaging (MRI) may reveal changes consistent with UMN dysfunction.[2,3]

Essential Diagnostics

Lab tests include: **General chemistry profile, liver function tests, thyroid function tests, ESR, serum protein and immunofixation electrophoresis, CSF analysis, vitamin B12, CK. EMG, nerve conduction studies,** and **MRI** are also indicated.

Additional Diagnostics

These may include: **heavy metal screening** if history of exposure, screening for **hereditary disorders, Lyme disease,** and **HIV.**

INITIAL DIAGNOSTICS

Amyotrophic Lateral Sclerosis

LABORATORY
- General chemistry
- ESR
- TSH
- Vitamin B$_{12}$
- Creatine kinase
- Liver function tests
- Serum protein and immunofixation electrophoresis
- Cerebrospinal fluid culture

IMAGING
- MRI (head, foramen magnum, and cervical spine)

OTHERS
- EMG, nerve conduction studies
- Lumbar puncture

DIFFERENTIAL DIAGNOSIS

Differentiation of ALS from other neurologic disorders is important now that there are specific treatments available. It is also important to diagnose ALS early and initiate the appropriate medical therapy. Atypical features that should alert the practitioner to a disease other than ALS include restriction of the disease to just UMNs or LMNs, involvement of neurons other than motor neurons, and EMG findings not consistent with ALS.[2]

 Priority differentials include: (1) motor neuropathy with conduction block, (2) spondylotic cervical myelopathy, and (3) Kennedy disease.[2]

INTERPROFESSIONAL COLLABORATIVE MANAGEMENT
Pharmacologic Management

Symptom management continues to be the cornerstone of treatment. As more is discovered about the mechanisms of this disease, more treatment options become available.

Riluzole

Riluzole is one of two pharmacologic agents approved by the U.S. Food and Drug Administration (FDA) that has demonstrated an impact on ALS survival. The clinical benefits are well documented, extending the ventilator-free survival period by approximately 2 to 3 months.[3] Riluzole is an antiglutamate that appears to slow progression of ALS and may improve survival in patients with early bulbar involvement.[3] The most common side effects described with riluzole are asthenia, dizziness, gastrointestinal distress, neutropenia, and elevated liver enzymes. Therefore it is recommended that the patient be regularly monitored for neutropenia and that liver function tests be performed at the onset of treatment, monthly during the first 3 months of therapy, and every 3 months thereafter.[6]

Edaravone

In May 2017, the FDA approved edaravone, which is a free radical scavenger thought to reduce oxidative stress. This medication was initially approved for use in Japan and Korea in 2015. A double-blind, placebo-controlled trial out of Japan revealed that patients who were taking edaravone had less decline in functional status by 33% compared to placebo at week 24 of the study. Edaravone is administered as an infusion that starts daily for 14 days followed by 14 days off treatment. Treatment then transitions to daily on for 10 days within a 14-day period then off for 14 days and repeat. The most common side effects described with edaravone include injection site contusion, headache, and gait disturbance. It is recommended that edaravone be used as an adjunct to riluzole.[6]

Selective Serotonin Reuptake Inhibitors/Serotonin Norepinephrine Reuptake Inhibitors

ALS patients may experience depressive symptoms. The prevalence of mild depression is thought to be around 29% of ALS patients and severe depression 6%. Anxiety in patients with ALS ranges from 0% to 30%. Sleep disturbances can also be addressed with a serotonin receptor antagonists and reuptake inhibitors (SARIs) such as trazodone. Pseudobulbar affect impacts 20% to 50% of patients with ALS, especially those with bulbar symptom onset. This diagnosis is defined by sudden, involuntary outbursts of emotion not in context with the situation. Emotional lability is common with this diagnosis and SSRIs or SNRIs may be helpful in treating.[7]

Benzodiazepines

This class of medication can also help with the treatment of anxiety as addressed above. Benzodiazepines can be helpful with sleep disturbances, spasticity, and muscle cramps.[7]

Anticholinergics

The most commonly used anticholinergics are tricyclic antidepressants (TCA), glycopyrrolate, and atropine. These are looked to as treatment options for sialorrhea. TCAs can also be used to treat pseudobulbar affect, depression and anxiety, sleep disturbances, and pain. This group of medications must be used with caution in older adult patients as they are more sensitive to anticholinergic side effects including delerium.[7]

Botulinum Toxin

The injection of botulinum toxin is being studied for patients that have sialorrhea that is refractory to oral medical therapy. It involves injection into the bilateral parotid and submandibular glands. For patients that have been trialed with botulinum toxin type B specifically, 50% of patients receiving this injection expressed improved symptoms.[7]

Muscle Relaxants

Spasticity is a complaint of ALS patients that can be a source of pain and can also limit mobility and overall function. Tizanidine and baclofen have both been used to treat spasticity. If oral medications fail, an intrathecal baclofen pump may be of help.[7]

Dextromethorphan/Quinidine

This combination of medications with the trade name Nuedexta has been shown to significantly reduce emotional lability seen in patients with pseudobulbar affect.[7]

Modafinil

Modafinil is a stimulant medication that may be helpful for patients who are experiencing fatigue. It is also important to address the cause of fatigue as well, such as poor sleep, pain, or nocturnal hypoventilation.[7]

Oxybutynin

Autonomic complaints have been reported in 29% of ALS patients. This includes urinary urgency in which patients report feeling the need to urinate every 1 to 2 hours. Oxybutynin is an anticholinergic that is commonly used and the short-acting version can be crushed and used in a PEG tube.[7]

Pain Management. Pain is reported in 57% to 72% of patients with ALS and can be generalized. Causes of pain are thought to be spasticity, general immobility, and/or cramps. It can be described as burning, aching, cramping, and shock-like. Some therapeutic options may include NSAIDs, opioids, muscle relaxants, gabapentin, and steroids.[7]

Non-Pharmacologic Management

Physical therapy (PT) has a number of benefits for patients with ALS to help with immobility which can lead to pain, spasticity, and cramping. Hydrotherapy, cryotherapy, heat, and ultrasound have also been used. PT also can help with fatigue.

Treating hypoventilation with noninvasive ventilation can help with oxygenation, fatigue, sleep disturbances, and concentration. Meditation, biofeedback, and cognitive behavioral therapy can help with emotional readjustment. Timed voidings and avoiding caffeine and alcohol may help with urinary urgency. Communication should be assessed by a speech therapist every 3 to 6 months in patients to determine need for modalities such as computerized speech synthesizers.[4,7]

Other treatments are being investigated. The current clinical drug trials for ALS can be found on the ALS Association website, www.alsa.org.

If a motor neuron disease is suspected, it is important to make appropriate referrals to specialists for further follow-up. A prompt referral to a neurologist or neuromuscular clinic is warranted. This will likely shorten the time to diagnosis.[8]

If ALS is diagnosed, referrals for supportive care by a multidisciplinary team are necessary. The collaborative team should include physicians, nurses, physical therapists, occupational therapists, speech therapists, dietitians, social workers, pulmonology and palliative medicine specialists, and the local ALS resource group.[1,4] In some areas there are ALS clinics that provide a multidisciplinary approach to patient care at each visit. This team can also help clarify the patient's wishes about artificial feeding or hydration, resuscitation, intubation, treatment of infection with antibiotics, and even hospitalizations.[4]

Hospitalization is indicated when symptoms become emergent and is based on the patient's goals for care. Hospitalization is warranted when symptoms are unstable or if there is an inability to swallow, respiratory compromise, suspicion of pneumonia, or failure to thrive. Respiratory failure, pneumonia, and aspiration pneumonia are the major determinants of hospitalizations and emergency admissions.[9]

LIFE SPAN CONSIDERATIONS

According to the ALS Association, some patients with ALS will live for 10 to 20 years, but on average, the life expectancy after diagnosis is 3 to 5 years. The variability and rapid progression can make it difficult to predict survival time. Most patients die of respiratory failure or infection.[2] The two factors that most influence survival are patient age and the presence or absence of bulbar symptoms at the time of diagnosis. Patients with bulbar symptoms at the onset of disease have a poorer prognosis and shorter duration of survival, as do older patients.[4]

COMPLICATIONS

Anxiety and depression are common, so it is important to identify and treat these symptoms to ensure the best quality of life for the patient. Depression can be a component of the ALS disease process and should be explained to the patient and caregiver. Caregiver depression also needs to be considered, along with the interaction between the patient and the caregiver.

Preventing malnutrition in ALS can positively affect quality of life and length of survival. Malnutrition can impair respiratory and immune system function and can exacerbate generalized muscular weakness. The American Academy of Neurology (AAN) recommends a nutrition consultation every 3 months for patients with ALS. In the initial stages of dysphagia and ALS diagnosis, there should be collaboration between the dietitian and the speech language pathologist to determine appropriate food and fluid consistency, especially if bulbar symptoms are present.[10] As dysphagia progresses, percutaneous endoscopic gastrostomy (PEG) tube placement may be indicated if this aligns with the patient's goals for care. The AAN ALS Practice Parameters suggest PEG placement while the patient's forced vital capacity (FVC) is greater than 50% of the predicted value or when there is dysphagia and/or a nutritional status decline, which can be indicated by a 5% to 10% loss of body weight. Before feeding tube placement, a discussion with the patient and caregiver is necessary to discuss the risks and benefits of the procedure, the daily management of the tube feedings, and the appropriate timing of the tube placement with regard to the disease process. A referral to a gastroenterologist and discussion with palliative medicine providers would be warranted for further discussion of gastrostomy tube placement.[1]

Respiratory impairment is the leading cause of death in patients with ALS. Management of respiratory dysfunction in ALS consists of pulmonary function monitoring (e.g., FVC), respiratory therapy, incentive spirometry, and noninvasive positive-pressure ventilation (NIPPV) as needed. Initiation of NIPPV when the patient first demonstrates difficulty with ventilation (i.e., FVC <50% of predicted value) can provide significant relief of sleep disturbance, which can cause daytime sleepiness, morning headaches, dyspnea, and orthopnea. Serial pulmonary function tests will provide objective evidence of respiratory decline.[4] Respiratory musculature weakness can result in aspiration and pneumonia. Less than 10% of patients with ALS elect to have a tracheostomy and invasive ventilation, making a clear distinction between noninvasive ventilation as a way of relieving respiratory symptoms and invasive ventilation as a clear life-extending procedure that requires 24-hour supervision.[7] Diaphragm pacing with surgically attached electrodes to the phrenic nerve provides low-frequency stimulation to help maintain diaphragm strength. This is only effective if the diaphragm is innervated.[4] An assisted cough device, suction machine, expectorants, mucolytics, antibiotics, and theophylline can also help relieve respiratory symptoms that are associated with thick bronchial secretions. Patients who refuse NIPPV or whose symptoms are not fully controlled may benefit from morphine, a safe and effective therapy in managing dyspnea.[4,7]

It is important to keep patients as functional as possible, to anticipate problems, and to ensure patient awareness before problems occur. Cramping, spasticity, and pain are common complaints and should be treated with appropriate pharmacologic agents. It is also important to vaccinate against pneumococcal infection and influenza.[7]

PATIENT AND FAMILY EDUCATION

ALS is a physically, mentally, and financially debilitating disease. It is important to educate patients and families about its natural history. Discussion topics must include the use of medications, assistive devices, home modifications, and in-home support. Discussions addressing goals of care including the completion of advance directives, timing of gastrostomy tube placement and ventilatory support, and referral to palliative/hospice care to provide additional support for patients in-home, with the goal of honoring their wish to stay out of the hospital (see Chapter 14).

Patients, family, and friends may also be experiencing a great deal of distress. A consultation with palliative care providers at the time of diagnosis can be beneficial for determining the goals of care and end-of-life wishes. Patients should be encouraged to appoint a health care proxy and openly discuss advance directives with their proxy and others who will be involved in their care. Palliative care and hospice services are options that will allow patients to maintain independence and quality of life for as long as possible and in a manner that respects their wishes and provides symptom relief (see Chapter 14).[11] Patients and caretakers should be referred to local ALS foundations, support groups, and resources to assist with care and provide educational information. Caring for ALS patients and their families requires a multidisciplinary team that is physically, psychologically, emotionally, and spiritually supportive.

REFERENCES

1. National Institute of Neurological Disorders and Stroke. Amyotrophic lateral sclerosis fact sheet. Retrieved from www.ninds.nih.gov/disorders/amyotrophiclateralsclerosis/detail_ALS.htm. (Accessed 15 December 2017).
2. Zarei, S., Carr, K., Reiley, L., et al. (2015). A comprehensive review of amyotrophic lateral sclerosis. *Surgical Neurology International*, 6, 171.
3. Goutman, S. A. (2017). Diagnosis and clinical management of amyotrophic lateral sclerosis and other motor neuron disorders. *Continuum*, 23(5), 1332–1359.
4. Cheng, H. W. B., Chan, K. Y., Yuen, K. J. C., et al. (2017). Supportive and palliative interventions in motor neuron disease: What we know from current literature. *Annals of Palliative Medicine*.
5. Costa, J., Swash, M., & Carvalho, M. D. (2012). Awaji criteria for the diagnosis of amyotrophic lateral sclerosis. *Archives of Neurology*, 69(11), 1410–1416.
6. Schultz, J. (2018). Disease modifying treatment of amyotrophic lateral sclerosis. *The American Journal of Managed Care*, 24(Suppl. 15), s327–s335.
7. Rudnicki, S., McVey, A. L., Jackson, C. E., et al. (2015). Symptom management and end of life care. *Neurologic Clinics*, 33(4), 889–908.
8. Nzwalo, H., de Abreau, D., Swash, M., et al. (2014). Delayed diagnosis in ALS: The problem continues. *Journal of the Neurological Sciences*.
9. Pisa, F. E., Logroscino, G., Battiston, P. G., et al. (2016). Hospitalizations due to respiratory failure in patients with amyotrophic lateral sclerosis and their impact on survival: A population based cohort study. *BMC Pulmonary Medicine*, 16, 136.
10. Greenwood, D. I. (2013). Nutrition management of amyotrophic lateral sclerosis. *Nutrition in Clinical Practice*, 28(3), 392–399.
11. Hogden, A., Aoun, S., & Silbert, P. (2018). Palliative care in neurology: Integrating a palliative approach to amyotrophic lateral sclerosis care. *EMJ Neurology*, 6(1), 68–76.

CHAPTER **172**

BELL PALSY
Wanda J. Handel

DEFINITION AND EPIDEMIOLOGY

Defined as an acute, unilateral weakness or paralysis of the facial nerve, with an onset of less than 72 hours and unknown etiology, Bell palsy is the most commonly diagnosed peripheral facial nerve condition.[1] Typically self-limiting, but some patients have persistent facial paralysis and are at risk for eye injury.[1] All ages are affected, but incidence is most common in young and middle-aged adults (ages 15 to 45), with an even distribution between men and women and an annual incidence of between 11 and 40 cases per 100,000.[2–4] Either side of the face may be affected.[4] Incidence is higher during pregnancy, particularly in the last trimester, first week post-partum, or in those with preeclampsia. Other risk factors that increase incidence include diabetes, hypothyroidism, recent upper respiratory infections, obesity, family history, and hypertension.[1,5]

PATHOPHYSIOLOGY

The facial nerve (CNVII) is mixed: afferent fibers from the anterior two-thirds of the tongue and the external auditory canal; efferent fibers to the facial muscles; and parasympathetic fibers to the lacrimal, sublingual, and submandibular glands. Knowledge of the topographic anatomy of the facial nerve can provide clinical clues to sites of injury; sparing of the forehead muscles typically suggests an upper motor neuron or central lesion, as it is bilaterally innervated.[3] The typical unilateral facial paralysis of Bell palsy is assumed to be initiated by a triggering event that places physiologic stress on the body (e.g., an upper respiratory tract infection or ischemia to the nerve). This stressor promotes the body's protective inflammatory response with its release of acute-phase reactants. The intraneural inflammatory response results in edema of the facial nerve. If the edema is not alleviated, there is ischemia of the nerve, with resulting axonal demyelination and inevitable nerve degeneration. Varying degrees of motor control loss become obvious about 3 days after nerve demyelination.[5]

While the cause of Bell palsy remains idiopathic, and etiologic factors such as genetic, vascular, nerve compression, infectious, and metabolic changes have been discussed, the two most accepted patho-mechanism hypotheses are viral and autoimmune. Viruses such as human herpes simplex 1 (HSV-1) and 2 (HSV-2) and varicella (VZV) all have the ability to cause latent infections in a single peripheral nerve distribution for the life of the host.[3] Reactivation of any one of these viruses could cause Bell palsy in an individual. However, current polymerase chain test can only confirm the virus exists within the nerve, not delineate if a virus is in a latent or active state.[6] Lyme disease (see Chapter 213) has also been implicated. Immunological theory is that the peripheral demyelination of Bell palsy is a cell-mediated response such as the demyelination in Guillain-Barré syndrome (see Chapter 176).[3] Bell palsy remains a diagnosis of exclusion, meaning a complete history and thorough physical exam are needed.

CLINICAL PRESENTATION AND PHYSICAL EXAMINATION

The typical onset is acute and progressive; maximum paralysis is attained in about half of the cases within 48 to 72 hours and in nearly all cases by day 5. Individuals may report pain behind the ipsilateral ear preceding the facial paralysis by 1 to 2 days. Typically, a smooth forehead, widened palpebral fissure, inability to close the eye, flattened nasolabial fold, and asymmetric smile are characteristic. Tearing, drooling, postauricular pain, tinnitus, and a mild hearing deficit may occur. Complaints of altered taste (dysgeusia) and an increased sensitivity to sound (hyperacusis) as well as hypoesthesia in one or more branches of the trigeminal nerve may also be present.[1,3,5] Timing of onset is key in the diagnosis; slowly progressive or relapsing courses suggest other entities.[1]

Other associated symptoms include a history of recent infections, especially viral illnesses such as chickenpox, mumps, mononucleosis, coxsackievirus, cytomegalovirus, human immunodeficiency virus (HIV), and influenza. The presence of chronic illnesses, such as diabetes mellitus, hypertension, or hypothyroidism, should be ascertained, and the patient should be queried about pregnancy, rashes or skin lesions, and insect bites. Any history of facial trauma should be carefully noted.[1]

A complete physical and neurological exam is warranted to rule out more serious central nervous system conditions such as stroke, tumor, and multiple sclerosis. The cranial nerve exam is key in identifying CN VII as the *peripheral nerve* source of the facial weakness. Ask the patient to smile, show their teeth, puff out cheeks, raise eyebrows, and close eyes tightly. Note any facial asymmetry, paying close attention to if the facial weakness is upper and lower or lower alone. Bell palsy causes a unilateral, full-face paresis or paralysis with an ipsilateral source indicating a peripheral nerve problem. Observe for lack of eyelid closure and absence of wrinkling of the forehead. Drooling and continuous tearing of the eye may also be present. A *central nervous system* lesion may present as a lower facial weakness with sparing of the forehead and other deficits may be noted on full neurologic exam.[5,7] Attention to otologic and head and neck exam is warranted to assess for decreased hearing and vesicles on the face or in and around the external ear canal that may indicate herpes zoster oticus (Ramsay Hunt syndrome), though absence of vesicles does not rule out zoster sine herpete.[5]

Special attention to the sensory and motor functions of the branches of the facial nerve is also necessary. Minor asymmetry of the lower face may be a normal deviation. The degree of facial weakness should be documented. A number of grading systems have been developed to objectively define the severity of the palsy. Clinicians may find the seven grades of the House-Brackmann Classification of Facial Function helpful in gauging the severity of neural degeneration and in establishing objective measures of recovery.[1,8] A photographic record is also helpful in establishing the extent of facial muscle weakness and documenting progressive neural regeneration.

DIAGNOSTICS

Routine diagnostic tests and imaging are not recommended for new-onset Bell palsy. Diagnostic laboratory studies may be useful to exclude identifiable conditions such as Lyme disease in the differential diagnosis and to determine prognosis. Radiologic imaging such as MRI is warranted in atypical presentation, such as bilateral facial nerve palsies or central CN VII findings, to rule out other serious neurologic causes such as multiple sclerosis, stroke, or tumor.[1]

Essential Diagnostics

Routine laboratory testing or imaging is not indicated for new-onset Bell palsy; diagnosis is one of exclusion with the patient's history and physical providing the basis for a clinical diagnosis. Diagnostics to rule out an identifiable cause in patients with atypical presentation:

- Lyme titer for patients with tick exposure or in endemic areas.
- MRI with and without contrast to view the entire facial nerve (including internal auditory canal and face) for patients with atypical presentation (isolated paralysis of a branch of the facial nerve, recurrent paralysis, or paralysis with other cranial nerve involvement) or for patients in which paralysis fails to recover within 3 months' time frame or to rule out other suspected identifiable cause.

Additional Diagnostics

Electrodiagnostic testing optional for patients with complete facial paralysis.

DIFFERENTIAL DIAGNOSIS

The list of conditions in the differential diagnosis for unilateral facial paralysis is lengthy and should include central and peripheral neurologic, infectious, and immunologic causes.

 Priority differentials include central nervous system causes (stroke, tumor, and multiple sclerosis) in patients with additional neurologic findings or atypical presentation, and infectious or immunologic causes such as Lyme disease in patients living in endemic areas or Guillain-Barré if there is a history of recent illness.

INTERPROFESSIONAL COLLABORATIVE MANAGEMENT

 Specialist consultation is indicated for patients with atypical presentation (with or without signs of central nervous system pathology), Bell palsy in pregnancy, signs and symptoms of corneal abrasion, persistent facial weakness/paralysis without improvement after two weeks, or need for surgery or botulinum toxin injection.

Nonpharmacologic Management

Protection of the eye is the single most important goal of care for the patient with Bell palsy and incomplete eyelid closure. Exposure keratitis can result in blindness, and the cornea must be protected from abrasion from dust and debris.

- Protective eyeglasses and moisture chambers should be used.[1]
- Eyelids should be closed and taped at night to protect the cornea, but care must be observed to be sure that the patient understands the technique and not cause a corneal abrasion.[1,5]
- Upper eyelid weights are another option for persistent lagopthalmos.[1,5]

Surgical decompression of the facial nerve to improve nerve function is not routinely performed due to the 94% rate of recovery without surgical treatment and with steroids.[1,9] If desired by patients with the potential for worse outcome such as those with complete facial paralysis, surgical scheduling requires quick planning within weeks 1 and 2 after onset.[1,5] Massage of weakened facial muscles may help preserve muscle tone and provide some comfort. Acupuncture and physical therapy may show some benefit, but more information is needed for treatment recommendations.[1]

Pharmacologic Management

The primary goals of treatment are to decrease the inflammatory response and swelling, decrease nerve function recovery time, and protect the eye from complications. More than 75% of patients will recover some nerve function within the first 3 weeks, although another 30% will have persistent symptoms and an incomplete recovery.[9,10] Corticosteroids are highly effective and increase the probability of nerve recovery.[1,9] Unless contraindicated (such as in diabetes), start corticosteroids in patients with new-onset Bell palsy within 72 hours of onset of symptoms. A modest additional effect of 7% recovery is reported with the coadministration of corticosteroids and an antiviral medication. Antiviral administration alone has not shown efficacy.[1,10] Along with nonpharmacologic eye protection, the use of lubricating eye drops every two hours, with an ocular lubricant at bedtime can be protective, helping maintain eye moisture.[1] Associated pain can be managed with

acetaminophen or nonsteroidal antiinflammatory drugs if they are not contraindicated.[11]

Bell palsy does not require referral or hospitalization except in the following circumstances:

- Patients with new ocular signs of itching, pain, irritation, or corneal abrasion should be referred to an ophthalmologist.
- Patients with severe lid symptoms or who have failed supportive eye care should be referred to an ophthalmologist for consideration of temporary options such as botulinum toxin injections, temporary or permanent tarsorrhaphy, or a permanent surgical option of a lid weight.
- Patients with suspicion of central nervous system involvement such as stroke, tumor, or multiple sclerosis, atypical presentation, with recurrence, progressive symptoms, or failure to improve should be referred to a neurologist.
- Pregnant individuals should be co-managed with the obstetrician.
- Patients with complete facial paralysis after day 7 from onset but before day 14 may be referred to a neurologist for electrodiagnostic studies, electro-neurophysiologic testing, or facial electromyography to assist with prognosis.
- Referral to neurosurgery for decompressive surgery is controversial and should take place within a narrow window of after 7 days but before day 14 of onset and greater than 90% nerve conduction loss on electro-neurodiagnostic testing.
- Patients with persistent complete facial paralysis or failure to recover acceptable movement, muscle spasms or synkinesia should be referred to an otolaryngologist, plastic surgeon, or neurosurgeon for botulinum toxin injection or consult for facial nerve grafting.

LIFE SPAN CONSIDERATIONS

Bell palsy occurs three times more often during pregnancy. An increase in vascular volume and pregnancy-induced hypertension may contribute to palsy of the facial nerve as a result of edema and entrapment. A viral cause cannot be excluded. For the health care provider giving prenatal care, it is recommended that the advice of an obstetrician be solicited and referral considered.[5] Children with new-onset Bell palsy show higher rates of spontaneous recovery, and no clear evidence exists to show potential benefit from corticosteroids. Clinician judgment and discussion with patient care provider should guide treatment.[1] Lyme disease is found in 50% of cases of facial palsy in children under 10 years old. Serologic testing is warranted in this age group.[5]

COMPLICATIONS

Evidence of poor functional recovery can be seen in facial asymmetry as a result of muscle weakness and synkinesis. Loss of vision in the affected eye from corneal ulceration is among the worst possible outcomes. Hearing loss and permanent tinnitus are sequelae indicating damage to the auditory nerve. Physician consultation is indicated for patients with corneal abrasions or an eyelid that cannot close.

PATIENT AND FAMILY EDUCATION

- Provide a full explanation of Bell palsy, treatment options, and its usual benign clinical course to help allay the fear patients experience from the onset of facial paralysis and allow shared decision-making regarding treatments and/or testing.

- Discuss the importance of eye protection, including signs and symptoms of corneal abrasion, instructions for patching or closing the eye at night, and proper use of protectant eye medications to decrease ocular complications.
- Teach the patient to recognize signs and symptoms that require provider notification: ocular pain, discharge, or drainage, and symptoms that worsen or recur.
- Provide information about medications, including the name, therapeutic effects, common side effects, dosing, and any other special considerations, to help engender compliance.

HEALTH PROMOTION

Discussions with patients and family should include shared decision-making and the importance of active patient participation in care. Patients can perform facial muscle exercises in front of a mirror two or three times a day and should attend follow-up care for evaluation of treatment, provision of emotional support, and documentation of recovery of facial muscle function.

REFERENCES

1. Baugh, R. F., Basura, G. J., Ishii, L. E., et al. (2013). Clinical practice guideline: Bell's palsy. *Otolaryngology–Head and Neck Surgery: Official Journal of American Academy of Otolaryngology-Head and Neck Surgery*, 149(3S), S1–S27.
2. McCaul, J., Cascarini, L., Godden, D., et al. (2014). Evidence based management of Bell's palsy. *British Journal of Oral and Maxillofacial Surgery*, 52(5), 387–391.
3. Greco, A., Gallo, M., Fusconi, C., et al. (2012). Bell's palsy and autoimmunity. *Autoimmunity Reviews*, 12, 323–328.
4. Kumar, V., & Thaklu, N. (2013). Bell's palsy: Review and care report. *Journal of Research Advance Dental*, 2(2), 82–86.
5. Zandian, A., Osiro, S., Hudson, R., et al. (2014). The neurologist's dilemma: A comprehensive clinical review of Bell's palsy, with emphasis on current management trends. *Medical Science Monitor*, 20, 83–90.
6. Eviston, T. J., Croxson, G., Kennedy, P., et al. (2015). Bell's palsy: Aetiology, clinical features and multidisciplinary care. *Journal of Neurology, Neurosurgery, and Psychiatry*, 86(12). Retrieved from jnnp.bmj.com/content/86/12/1356. (Accessed 8 February 2018).
7. Guanci, M. M. (2014). Bell's palsy. In *The clinical practice of neurological and neurosurgical nursing* (p. 754). Philadelphia: Lippincott Williams & Wilkins.
8. House, J. W., & Brackmann, D. E. (1985). Facial nerve grading system. *Otolaryngology–Head and Neck Surgery: Official Journal of American Academy of Otolaryngology-Head and Neck Surgery*, 93, 146. (classic reference).
9. Madhok, V. B., Gagyor, I., Daly, F., Somasundara, D., Sullivan, M., Gammie, F., et al. (2016). Corticosteroids for Bell's palsy (idiopathic facial paralysis). *The Cochrane Database of Systematic Reviews*, (7), Art. No.: CD001942. doi:10.1002/14651858.CD001942.pub5.
10. Somasundara, D., & Sullivan, F. (2017). Management of Bell's palsy. *Australian Prescriber*, 40(3), 94–97. doi:10.18773/austprescr.2017.030.
11. Glass, G., & Tzafetta, K. (2014). Bell's palsy: A summary of current evidence and referral algorithm. *Family Practice*, doi:10.1093/fampra/cmu058. Published online Sept. 10, 2014.

CHAPTER **173**

CEREBROVASCULAR EVENTS

Jillian C. Belmont

 Immediate emergency department referral or specialist consultation is indicated for all patients with suspected acute cerebrovascular accident.

DEFINITION AND EPIDEMIOLOGY

Cerebrovascular events, commonly known as stroke, are the fifth leading cause of death in the United States.[1] The two main classifications of stroke are ischemic and hemorrhagic. The majority of strokes are ischemic, meaning there is an interruption or reduction in blood flow to an area of the central nervous system resulting in neuronal injury and oftentimes clinical symptoms. Hemorrhagic stroke typically occurs from the rupture of an arteriosclerotic small artery that has been weakened, primarily by hypertension.[2,3] The most important modifiable risk factors associated with stroke are hypertension, diabetes mellitus, tobacco smoking, hyperlipidemia, obesity, poor diet/nutrition, and physical inactivity.[1]

The diagnosis of a *transient ischemic attack* (TIA), or warning sign of a stroke, depends on the quality and quantity of information available at the time of assessment.[4] TIAs are associated with brain dysfunction in a circumscribed area caused by a regional reduction in blood flow (ischemia) resulting in either transient or minor observable clinical symptoms.[4] TIAs can be difficult to diagnose, as identification is based primarily on the reported history and physical. The risk of stroke after a TIA event is up to 10%, and up to 80% of this risk is preventable with urgent assessment and treatment which includes modification of risk factors.[4] Criteria for diagnosis of a TIA includes a clinical history or objective focal neurologic findings on examination and imaging of the brain.[4] Important symptoms to assist a presumed diagnosis of TIA event include the time course of symptoms, the distribution of the deficits, and each individual's risk factors.

Every year, 795,000 people in the United States have a stroke.[5] Eighty-five percent of reported strokes are ischemic.[1]

Death from stroke has decreased over the past decade but still remains the fifth leading cause of death in the United States and second leading cause of death globally.[1] The incidence of new and recurrent stroke has also declined, most likely because of widespread education and increased use of specific prevention medications.

There are racial disparities in stroke occurrence; both black men and black women are twice as likely as other races to have a first stroke, and more likely to die.[1,5] Stroke remains a leading cause of disability in the United States, with significant social and financial implications for families and society. The cost of stroke care is estimated to be $316.1 billion dollars annually.[5] Stroke also represents a significant burden for long-term care. Fifty percent to 70% of stroke survivors regain functional independence, but 15% to 30% are permanently disabled. Institutional care is required by 20% at 3 months after onset.

PATHOPHYSIOLOGY
Ischemic Stroke

Ischemic stroke is the most common type of stroke. In a thrombotic event, a critical degree of atherosclerosis causes complete or relatively complete blockage of blood flow through a local area. In an embolic event, a clot forms elsewhere (e.g., in the heart from atrial fibrillation), breaks off, and travels through the arterial circulation until it lodges in a vessel and blocks the flow of blood distally. The effects of arterial occlusion on brain tissue vary, depending on the location of the occlusion in relation to available collateral and anastomotic channels and the degree and duration of the ischemia. The specific neurologic deficit relates to the location and size of the infarction cr focus of ischemia. At the time of arterial occlusion, the viscosity of the blood and resistance to flow both increase, and there is sludging within the vessels. The tissue becomes pale. If the ischemia is prolonged, sludging and endothelial damage prevents normal reflow. Cellular breakdown and swelling occur.[6]

Hemorrhagic Stroke

Ten percent to 15% of all strokes are hemorrhagic.[7] Intracerebral hemorrhage (ICH) occurs from rupture of cerebral vessels, often as a result of high blood pressure exerting excessive pressure on arterial walls that may already be damaged by atherosclerosis, aneurysm, or arteriovenous malformation.[7] ICH can be further subdivided into two categories, primary and secondary. Primary ICH derives from spontaneous rupture of a blood vessel damaged by chronic hypertension of cerebral amyloid angiopathy and comprises about 78% to 88% of all hemorrhages.[7] Secondary ICH results from bleeding of cerebrovascular abnormalities, tumors, or impaired coagulation.[7] A subarachnoid hemorrhage (SAH) occurs in the subarachnoid space, the area between the tissue that covers the brain and the brain. These are usually caused by an aneurysm, arteriovenous malformation, or an inherited bleeding disorder. Risk factors for SAHs include smoking, hypertension, connective tissue disorders, other known aneurysms, and polycystic kidney disease. Family history may play a role.[6]

Compared to ischemic stroke, ICH is associated with a higher risk of fatality, as approximately half of all patients with primary ICH die within the first month after the acute event.[7] Hemorrhagic strokes not only damage brain cells, but they also can lead to increased pressure on the brain or spasms in the blood vessels.

In either ischemic or hemorrhagic stroke, an area immediately surrounding the injury dies within a few minutes from lack of oxygen and the failure of the oxygen-dependent adenosine triphosphate (ATP) metabolic pathway. In a broader area of injury, referred to as the penumbra, the damage is more dynamic, extending for 12 to 24 hours. It is believed the release of intracellular calcium initiates the sequence of programmed cell death, or apoptosis.[2]

CLINICAL PRESENTATION AND PHYSICAL EXAMINATION

Patients with cerebrovascular events (TIA, ischemic stroke, hemorrhagic stroke) may have a similar presentation, but time can be a major differentiating factor. In ischemic stroke, the patient usually has a single attack, and the entire event evolves within a few hours. However, the stroke may occur in a "stuttering" fashion, with intermittent progression or fluctuation of neurologic deficits that extends to maximal deficit over the first 72 hours.[8] The symptoms of cerebral ischemia can be widely variable depending on the vascular territory involved. When the carotid artery is involved, the symptoms can occur in the ipsilateral eye or contralateral body. The classic visual disturbance (amaurosis fugax) is a transient, painless loss of vision, often described as a shade descending over the visual field. Hemispheric brain ischemia usually causes weakness or numbness of the contralateral face or limbs. Language difficulties and cognitive and behavioral changes may also occur. Vertebrobasilar, or posterior circulation events, may manifest with vertigo, severe nausea or vomiting, nystagmus, diplopia, dysconjugate gaze, or deficits of cranial nerves.

In SAH, the clinical presentation is usually heralded by the abrupt onset of a severe headache ("the worst headache of my life"), nausea and vomiting, signs of meningeal irritation, and varying degrees of neurologic dysfunction. Loss of consciousness at the time of the initial event is common but is usually short-lived. Nearly 50% of patients with aneurysmal SAH give a history of atypical headaches occurring days to weeks before the definitive event. These sentinel headaches are characteristically sudden in onset and are often associated with nausea, vomiting, and dizziness, with or without neurologic dysfunction. Some hemorrhagic events may manifest with seizures.

Patients with hypertensive ICH may have no consistent warning or prodromal symptoms. In the majority of cases, the hemorrhage has its onset while the patient is up and active; onset during sleep is rare. The blood pressure is elevated in almost all cases. The neurologic signs and symptoms vary with the site and size of the extravasation of blood. The patient may lapse almost immediately into stupor and coma, with hemiplegia and steady deterioration to death during the next several hours. More often, the patient complains of a headache, followed within a few minutes by unilateral facial sag, slurred speech, weakness in an arm and leg, and eye deviation away from the paretic limbs. These events, occurring during a period of 5 to 30 minutes, strongly suggest intracerebral bleeding. More advanced cases are characterized by paralysis, aphasia, stupor, coma, deep and irregular respiration, dilated and fixed pupils, and, occasionally, decerebrate rigidity.

Many signs and symptoms are common to both anterior and posterior circulation cerebrovascular events. These include hemiparesis, hemisensory loss, visual field defects, ataxia (difficulty with balance and coordination), dysarthria (difficulty speaking), reflex asymmetry, and Babinski sign. Headache can occur with both ischemic and hemorrhagic stroke. Blood is very irritating to the brain, making headache more common and more severe with hemorrhagic stroke.

Physical Examination

Because TIAs precede up to 10% of all strokes,[4,9] a risk stratification tool should be used to guide urgency of workup and management. The ABCD[2] score (Table 173.1) is valuable for this purpose.[10] Patients with TIAs sometimes warrant close observation for 24 hours in a clinical decision unit, emergency department, or admission to a hospital setting.

Findings on the neurologic examination correspond to the vascular territory affected in the brain. Initial attention should always focus on a patent and protected airway, a good respiratory effort, and a competent heart rate with good peripheral circulation (ABCs of advanced clinical life support). A complete neurologic examination to assess areas of deficit should quickly follow. The initial clinical observations are a critical aspect of time-sensitive assessment and can help inform the focused neurologic examination thereafter. A quick look for pupillary function, gaze deviation, blink to threat, motor tone, and purposeful movements can help formulate an initial impression of the neurologic syndrome.[8] Vomiting, systolic blood pressure (SBP) greater than 220 mm Hg, severe headache, coma or decreased level of consciousness, and symptom progression over minutes or hours all suggest ICH.

The National Institutes of Health (NIH) Stroke Scale is now the basic neurologic assessment for stroke patients.[11,12] It identifies and quantifies deficits and provides a standardized scoring system to allow tracking of progression. This assessment should

TABLE 173.1	ABCD² Score for Acute Cerebral Vascular Syndrome (Transient Ischemic Attack)
Criteria	**Points If Positive**
Age ≥ 60 years	1 point
Blood pressure ≥ 140 mm Hg systolic and/or ≥ 90 mm Hg diastolic	1 point
Clinical presentation	
Unilateral weakness with or without speech changes	2 points
Speech changes, no unilateral weakness	1 point
Duration ≥60 min ≤59 min	2 points 1 point
Diabetes	1 point

Guide

ABCD² Score	48-h Stroke Risk	Comment
1–3 points	1%	Obtain neurology consultation; possible outpatient treatment and evaluation
4–5 points	4.1%	Hospitalization justified
6–7 points	8.1%	Hospitalization beneficial

be done as soon as practical after the patient has arrived, and the results should accompany the patient throughout care.

DIAGNOSTICS

Abrupt onset of focal neurologic symptoms is presumed to be vascular in origin until proven otherwise; however, it is impossible to know whether symptoms are caused by ischemia or hemorrhage based on clinical characteristics alone.[13] Diagnostic studies are necessary to determine the type of stroke and the probable cause as well as to detect complications or confounding factors. Because management is vastly different, it is important to be able to quickly differentiate ischemic stroke from hemorrhagic stroke and to exclude disorders that may occasionally resemble stroke.

Essential Diagnostics

A head computed tomography (CT) scan is the most common initial imaging procedure, although magnetic resonance imaging (MRI) is also a reasonable choice if available. Time, cost, proximity to the ED, patient tolerance, clinical status, and availability of CT scan or MRI machine should all be taken into consideration when considering diagnostic testing. Patients who have atypical presentations or who have unusual findings on non-contrast CT scans may need further workup with contrast enhancement CT or MRI to exclude findings such as tumor. CT scans can miss small infarctions or lesions, especially if patients obtain imaging rapidly after symptom onset. CT is very sensitive for identifying acute hemorrhage and is considered the "gold standard"; gradient echo and T2 susceptibility-weighted MRI are as sensitive as CT for detection of acute hemorrhage and are more sensitive for identification

of prior hemorrhage.[13] Depending on the findings seen on CT or MRI, other studies (e.g., arteriography) may be necessary to determine underlying vascular disease and etiologies. In certified stroke centers, the time from presentation in the emergency department to CT is a measured statistic, with the goal of administering IV thrombolytics, if eligible, within 45 to 60 minutes of arrival to the ED.

Additional Diagnostics

Other diagnostic studies include an electrocardiogram (ECG), chest radiography, pulse oximetry or arterial blood gas (ABG) assessment, complete blood count (CBC) with platelets, prothrombin time (PT), partial thromboplastin time (PTT), serum glucose concentration, creatinine level, blood urea nitrogen (BUN) level, and electrolyte values. Doing these tests should not delay the CT scan; time is of the essence, and in specialty stroke centers the clock is literally ticking. Depending on the clinical presentation, other tests may be necessary, including examination of the cerebrospinal fluid if central nervous system infection is suspected or when the clinical picture suggests SAH but the head CT scan is normal. Electroencephalography (EEG) is indicated when the clinical picture suggests seizure. Carotid ultrasonography (CUS) will assess patency of the carotid arteries and should especially be done in patients who are being considered for intervention with endarterectomy. Carotid arteriography (CTA) or magnetic resonance angiography (MRA) can also be done to evaluate the posterior circulation and the intracranial arteries. Transesophageal echocardiography and Holter monitoring may be performed if the presentation is suggestive of a cardio-embolic or paradoxical event originating from the heart. Other laboratory tests that may be indicated include serum cholesterol level, hemoglobin A1C, toxicology screening, erythrocyte sedimentation rate (ESR), fibrinogen level, serum protein electrophoresis, antiphospholipid antibody level, serologic test for syphilis, protein C level, protein S level, antithrombin III level, lupus anticoagulant, anticardiolipin antibody level, β2 glycoprotein, and connective tissue disease screen.

DIFFERENTIAL DIAGNOSIS

 Priority differentials include (1) stroke, (2) seizure, (3) subdural hematoma, (4) encephalitis, and (5) toxic or metabolic encephalopathies.

A number of conditions may be mistaken for cerebrovascular events and should be considered and excluded when appropriate. Other diagnosis to consider are migraine and migraine equivalents, brain tumor, syncope, demyelinating diseases, conversion disorders, and transient global amnesia, among others.

INTERPROFESSIONAL COLLABORATIVE MANAGEMENT

Time is critical. Any patient seen in an outpatient setting with stroke-like symptoms should be transported immediately for evaluation and emergent imaging with CT scan and to a center with the ability to implement a tPA protocol. Clear survival benefit exists in those hospitals with dedicated stroke units. Stroke centers are expanding telemedicine to outlying community hospitals, which allows for faster specialist evaluation, expediting both diagnosis and treatment.

Depending on the type of neurologic injury, neurosurgery or interventional radiology specialists may be consulted. After

INITIAL DIAGNOSTICS

Cerebrovascular Events

INITIAL
- Stat CT scan of head (noncontrast)
- ECG
- Pulse oximetry
- National Institutes of Health Stroke Scale[12]
- ABCD[2] risk stratification for (TIA)

LABORATORY
- CBC and differential
- PT, PTT, international normalized ratio
- Metabolic profile
- Toxic screen
- Lumbar puncture (immediate if severe headache but negative CT to rule out subarachnoid hemorrhage)

ADDITIONAL DIAGNOSTICS
- The following are tests to consider after emergency care, stabilization, and treatments.

IMAGING
- Transesophageal echocardiography
- Chest x-ray studies[a]

LABORATORY
- Lipid profile[a]
- Hemoglobin A1c[a]
- Erythrocyte sedimentation rate[a]
- Fibrinogen[a]
- Serum protein electrophoresis[a]
- Antiphospholipid antibody[a]
- Fluorescent treponemal antibody absorption test or rapid plasma reagin[a]
- Protein C, protein S[a]
- Antithrombin III[a]
- Lupus anticoagulant[a]
- Anticardiolipin antibody[a]
- β2 Glycoprotein[a]
- Connective tissue disease screening[a]
- Arterial blood gas[a]

OTHER STUDIES
- Carotid ultrasound[a]
- Electroencephalography[a]
- Arteriography[a]
- Holter, Zio patch or event monitoring[a]
- TEE (transesophageal echocardiogram)[a]

[a]If indicated

Stroke Symptoms Guide

- Sudden numbness or weakness of face, arm, or leg, especially on one side of the body
- Sudden confusion or trouble speaking or understanding speech
- Sudden trouble seeing in one or both eyes
- Sudden trouble walking, dizziness, loss of balance or coordination
- Sudden severe headache with no known cause

after a probable TIA but has no current signs or symptoms of neurologic dysfunction can be evaluated and treated in the outpatient setting. Identification of the most likely cause of the TIA is vital to proper management. For example, management of the patient with severe carotid stenosis will be different from that of the patient with atrial fibrillation. Treatment of all patients with TIA or stroke should include risk factor management.

For acute stroke, time is of the essence. Educational efforts should be directed at patient and family to ensure that early signs of stroke prompt an immediate 911 call. A national education campaign stresses early recognition (Box 173.1).

Community organization is critical in managing stroke. Integrated emergency medical services (EMS) and hospital systems are needed so that the appropriate care is available rapidly within the window of opportunity. The national coalition organized to advocate for rapid and appropriate care has established guidelines and protocols to create an integrated response.

Acute stroke-ready hospitals are needed. These community hospitals will have trained stroke response personnel available in the emergency department and will use standard care protocols. They will use telemedicine for rapid consultation with neurologists. They will have the capacity to administer clot-busting drugs and to initiate rapid reversal of anticoagulation. EMS agencies serving the hospital will have training in stroke recognition and will trigger a stroke code similar to a response to heart attack. Rapid transfer to appropriate tertiary facilities is accomplished by interfacility agreement.[14]

Primary stroke centers are accredited hospitals that demonstrate consistent stroke response and measure outcomes including time from arrival to administration of thrombolytics and have a consistent level of care using accepted treatment algorithms.

Comprehensive stroke centers have neurosurgeons, neurologists, neurologic intensive care units, interventional radiologists, and extensive rehabilitation services. These tertiary facilities support the acute stroke-ready hospitals and primary stroke centers through education, streamlined transfer, and acute specialized treatment.

In the emergency department, initial management of suspected stroke includes assessment of the ABCs (airway, breathing, and circulation) and vital signs. The airway should be secured; oxygen administered by nasal cannula; a cardiac monitor, pulse oximeter, and sphygmomanometer attached; intravenous access established; a physical examination performed; and an emergent, noncontrast head CT scan obtained. In addition, a 12-lead ECG, portable chest radiograph, and laboratory tests (as described previously) are indicated. If hemorrhage has occurred, a neurosurgeon should be contacted.

the patient has been stabilized, rehabilitation services including physical therapy, occupational therapy, speech therapy, and vocational counseling are employed. Counselors are consulted regarding patient and family issues surrounding a potentially life-altering diagnosis. Palliative medicine may be helpful in clarifying goals of treatment with patients and family decision makers.

In the primary care setting, most management of stroke involves efforts at primary or secondary intervention including risk reduction to include blood pressure control, antithrombotic therapy, smoking cessation, diet and nutrition, physical activity, obstructive sleep apnea (OSA), and blood sugar and cholesterol management. Initial management depends on the acuity of presentation. In general, the patient who is seen days

If ischemic stroke has occurred, a neurologist should be consulted and thrombolytic therapy should be rapidly administered if the patient meets the criteria. Patients should also be rapidly evaluated for potential revascularization with mechanical thrombectomy or carotid endarterectomy versus carotid stenting. There is incontrovertible evidence that IV thrombolysis with recombinant tissue plasminogen activator (rtPA) and endovascular thrombectomy with a retrievable stent improve neurologic outcome in patients with acute ischemic stroke.[15] Both treatments should be administered as quickly as possible after stroke onset, can be combined, and are safe in appropriately selected candidates.[15]

Careful blood pressure management is necessary in both the acute ischemic stroke and hemorrhagic stroke setting. Elevated blood pressure is common during acute stroke events. In the US National Hospital Ambulatory Medical Care Survey, 76.5% of patients with acute ischemic stroke had hypertension (SBP >140 mm Hg) on arrival to the emergency department.[16] Multiple studies have investigated various blood pressure parameters during the admission for acute ischemic stroke and clinical outcomes and have found the optimal SBP to range between 121 and 200 mm Hg.[17] There is evidence that an acute hypertensive response may represent a beneficial compensatory response to maintain cerebral perfusion.[18] If the brain is already ischemic, lowering of the blood pressure may only exacerbate hypoperfusion and injury. Research shows that with acute ischemic stroke, unless the SBP is 220 mm Hg or more, the decision to lower blood pressure with antihypertensive treatment does not improve outcome and therefore should be based on individual clinical judgment.[16] After the acute period of stroke management, the blood pressure gradually returns to the previous baseline value without the need for additional treatment. In the event that a patient receives IV rtPA, there is greater risk of symptomatic ICH with higher blood pressures during the initial 24 hours with research showing best outcomes associated with SBPs maintained between 141 and 150 mm Hg.[17] For the acute treatment of ICH, the American Stroke Association recommends lowering of SBP to 140 mm Hg to prevent potential hematoma expansion.[13]

If an antihypertensive medication is necessary, labetalol and nicardipine are commonly used safe choices. In the acute setting, these drugs are often given intravenously and then titrated as oral antihypertensive therapy is optimized. There are many oral antihypertensives that may be used depending on other patient comorbidities. If antihypertensive therapy is necessary, blood pressure reduction should be gradual and gentle, and the patient should be carefully monitored. The therapy should be modified if any neurologic fluctuations or deterioration arise.

Pharmacologic Management

Intravenous Thrombolytic Therapy. In June 1996, the U.S. Food and Drug Administration approved the use of intravenous rtPA for treatment of appropriately selected patients with ischemic stroke, if it is administered within 4.5 hours from the onset of symptoms. Despite an increased incidence of bleeding complications, studies show a significant reduction in neurologic disability in patients treated with tPA compared with patients treated in the conventional manner.[19] The time to treatment is the most important determinant of success in treating ischemic stroke (the sooner thrombolytic therapy is

started, the better the outcome). Inclusion criteria for use of tPA include age of 18 years or older, clinical diagnosis of ischemic stroke, and time of onset less than 180 minutes before tPA administration. The exclusion and relative exclusion criteria list is much longer, focusing primarily on evidence of current bleeding or a risk of bleeding that is sufficient to outweigh potential benefits of tPA treatment. Guidelines revised in 2018 confirm the window for administration of tPA to 4.5 hours.[20,21] However, new exclusions have been added. People receiving oral anticoagulation agents, those with a history of diabetes and previous stroke, those older than 80 years, and patients with an NIH Stroke Scale score of more than 25 represent higher risk and less benefit and should be assessed thoroughly before receiving tPA in the 3- to 4.5-hour expanded window.[21] While IV thrombolysis is the standard of care for eligible patients with acute ischemic stroke, this treatment has several limitations including its short time window and contraindication list, and IV rtPA often fails to recanalize proximal artery occlusions caused by large clots.[15]

Antiplatelet Agents. Numerous studies have demonstrated a benefit of antiplatelet agents in reducing stroke risk.[1,3,17] The relative benefit of antiplatelet therapy is remarkably constant regardless of age, gender, blood pressure, and the presence or absence of diabetes. Aspirin is the standard medical therapy for ischemic stroke prevention. The optimum dose remains somewhat controversial, but there is increasing evidence that lower doses are as effective as higher doses and have fewer gastrointestinal side effects. Currently prescribed regimens range from 81 to 325 mg every day. A meta-analysis of six major studies involving more than 94,000 people showed that the benefit of aspirin in preventing stroke is greater than any risk.[22]

Anticoagulation with warfarin (Coumadin) and other direct oral anticoagulants (DOAC) (e.g., Eliquis, Xarelto) is indicated for stroke prevention in patients at risk for cardiac embolism and some hypercoagulable states (cancer-related stroke). This includes patients with chronic or paroxysmal atrial fibrillation, left ventricular dysfunction with congestive heart failure, and artificial cardiac valves.

A class of antiplatelet drugs, the thienopyridines, is modestly more effective than aspirin, but the degree of additional benefit is unclear. Two representative drugs from this class are clopidogrel (Plavix) and ticlopidine (Ticlid). Ticlopidine, however, has potential side effects, which can include diarrhea, thrombotic thrombocytopenic purpura, and neutropenia. These risks require hematologic monitoring. Ticlopidine should be reserved for patients who are intolerant of or allergic to aspirin therapy or who have failed to respond to aspirin therapy. Dipyridamole (Persantine) in combination with aspirin demonstrates rates of recurrence similar to those of clopidogrel.[22,23]

Reversal of anticoagulation, if available, must be initiated when a patient with ICH is on anticoagulation agents, including warfarin, the new generation of anticoagulants that do not require regular monitoring of bleeding time (direct thrombin inhibitors, novel oral anticoagulants), and antiplatelet drugs such as clopidogrel and aspirin.[24]

Vitamin K and 3- or 4-factor prothrombin complex concentrate (Kcentra) are used to reverse the effects of warfarin. Clopidogrel and aspirin reversal may be aided by administration of platelets; however, the amount needed is significant.

Protamine can be administered for heparin and low-molecular-weight heparin products.

The FDA has more recently approved antidotes for some of the newer DOAC, but for some agents there remains no reversal agent which continues to raise concern. Research is ongoing, and newer reversal agents and new anticoagulation agents that have unique reversal drugs may be emerging.[24]

Surgical/Interventional Treatment

Mechanical Thrombectomy. Endovascular recanalization treatment with severe acute ischemic stroke has been practiced in many centers for decades, however previous trials have failed to show much benefit. Over the past few years, several positive trials have catapulted this therapy to the status of evidence-based treatment for patients with large intracranial artery occlusions.[15] Devices, techniques, improved imaging, and more rapid patient flow have helped drive this intervention to the front line. Initially patients were treated up to 6 hours from symptom onset, with some select individuals receiving treatment much later than 6 hours with careful selection. Mechanical thrombectomy interventions have continued to advance, yielding dramatic patient benefit and low risks of ICH.[15] The optimal radiologic method to select candidates for endovascular therapy is CTA angiography or CT/MRI perfusion. In November 2017, the DAWN trial was published showing the benefit of mechanical thrombectomy of up to 24 hours post symptom onset in select cases. This treatment advancement is key to stroke management in the acute care setting, as it gives patients who present outside of the rtPA window another promising option for decreased risk of death and disability.[25]

Surgery. Certain types of stroke and stroke complications may require urgent neurosurgical intervention. Neurosurgical consultation is indicated in cases of SAH, ICH, and increased intracranial pressure causing neurologic compromise.

Carotid endarterectomy has been demonstrated to have a beneficial effect (compared with medical therapy alone) in patients with symptomatic carotid stenosis. The benefit of surgery must be weighed against potential perioperative morbidity and mortality.

Carotid endarterectomy is strongly indicated in symptomatic patients with ipsilateral carotid stenosis presumed to be the likely etiology of the ischemic event. Optimal timing has been researched and debated for years, but the most recent data suggests surgery should be undertaken as soon as possible and within the first 2 weeks after stroke or TIA for optimal benefit and reduction of future ischemic events.[26]

SAH can be treated by interventional radiology through introduction of a coil into the aneurysm, but time is critical in getting a patient to an appropriate center.

LIFE SPAN CONSIDERATIONS
Pregnancy

Stroke during pregnancy is a major tragedy but fortunately rare. In a retrospective study of hospital admissions for delivery in the United Kingdom, the incidence was found to be 1.5 cases per 100,000 deliveries.[27] Risk factors include a history of migraine, gestational diabetes, and preeclampsia. The health care provider can best address this through pregnancy preparation counseling for all fertile women, stressing the need for early and complete prenatal care as well as risk identification and management. Extreme weight change, proteinuria, or elevated blood pressure in the gravid patient requires early intervention.

Geriatric Patients

Stroke will disproportionately affect older persons. In older adults, especially the very old and those with comorbid conditions, therapeutic interventions such as surgery and thrombolysis can be contraindicated. In these situations, comprehensive assessment of need will help determine where appropriate care can be provided. Some will retain sufficient capacities that they can return home with supportive services. Many others will require skilled nursing care.

Age is a direct predictor of both mortality and morbidity, with the oldest patients more likely to die and/or need extended care.[5] Death rates within the first year can be as high as 35% for white women older than 65 years.[5] It is critical that the health care provider know the patient's goals regarding lifesaving treatment and end-of-life care. It is not sufficient to know whether a patient desires intubation or defibrillation in case of respiratory or cardiac arrest. A clear statement about the use of feeding tubes or intravenous hydration can be extremely helpful in directing care. A surrogate decision maker must be identified, and his or her role defined through advance directives (see Chapter 14). More important, health care providers should learn what a patient values in life to help guide decisions when impairments may significantly affect those aspects that bring meaning. In this way, care can be tailored to the patient's desires. Ideally, stroke patients should be referred for palliative care consultation. This specialty addresses the issues of comfort, end-of-life decisions, community resources, family engagement, and education. Palliative care consultation also helps patients and families make informed decisions about ongoing care and the effectiveness and value of other interventions.

COMPLICATIONS

The complications of stroke affect virtually every organ system. Early complications of stroke include cerebral edema, increased intracranial pressure, pulmonary and urinary tract infections, sepsis, seizures, hypertension, hypotension, cardiac arrhythmias, myocardial ischemia and infarction, deep venous thrombosis, pulmonary embolism, dysphagia, dysarthria, pressure sores, depression, and extension or progression of the stroke. Later complications include permanent residual problems with mobility, activities of daily living, communication, nutrition, swallowing, behavior, continence, sexual function, limb contractures, and dementia.

A patient with an acute stroke should be admitted to the hospital, with management directed toward limiting, if possible, the amount of brain injury and preventing or ameliorating the constellation of potential complications. Complications in the hospitalized stroke patient include pneumonia, seizures, myocardial infarction, deep venous thrombosis, pressure ulcers, hyperglycemia, hypoglycemia, depression, limb contractures, and constipation. Awareness of these potential complications and specific therapies directed toward their prevention will dramatically reduce the stroke patient's morbidity and mortality. Of particular importance is physical, occupational, and speech therapy, which should be initiated as soon as the patient is medically stable and able to participate.

EDUCATION AND HEALTH PROMOTION

Two elements of patient education are paramount: (1) risk factor reduction and (2) stroke symptom recognition and emergency treatment. Hypertension is the most important independent and modifiable risk factor. It is imperative that patients with hypertension be educated about their disease and the importance of medical therapy and lifestyle changes for prevention of complications such as stroke. Cigarette smoking, obesity, diabetes, sedentary lifestyle, and hypercholesterolemia are other modifiable factors that require patient education and treatment.

Atrial fibrillation results in five times greater risk of stroke, and treatment with anticoagulation is essential to reducing this risk. Despite the rapid evolution of stroke care and exciting possibilities being investigated, the most important function for the health care provider is aggressive early identification and treatment of at-risk individuals, education for all patients, and appropriate early intervention for those with elevated blood pressure, glucose intolerance, obesity, smoking, and sedentary lifestyles.[1,28]

The public, particularly those individuals with risk factors, must be educated about the signs and symptoms of stroke. Public education campaigns urge those who feel they may be having a stroke or those with them to think about the acronym *FAST* (face, arm, speech, time) as a way of identifying the signs of a stroke and to call 911 immediately. Factors that have been shown to be associated with delay in treatment include lack of recognition of stroke signs and symptoms, calls made to the health care provider instead of the emergency medical number, living alone, onset while asleep, onset at home rather than at work, posterior circulation symptoms, and milder severity of stroke. Patients at risk should be taught to recognize the signs and symptoms of a stroke and to call 911 as soon as symptoms occur.

Those patients who do survive have a wide range of physical and psychological impairments, including impairments of motor, sensory, perceptual, cognitive, and communication skills that may seriously interfere with social interactions and ability to engage in normal activities of daily living. The direct and indirect costs for the patient, family, and society are incalculable.

Rehabilitation services are essential to optimize stroke recovery and should begin within 48 hours of stabilization. The recovery stage of stroke requires significant adaptive training for the patient, family, and caregivers. The family itself will be stressed by the recovery process and will need access to counseling, peer support, and other community resources.

REFERENCES

1. Guzik, A., & Bushnell, C. (2017). Stroke epidemiology and risk factor management. *Continuum: Lifelong Learning in Neurology, 23*(1, Cerebrovascular Disease), 15–39.
2. E., G. Intracerebral Hemorrhage. Retrieved from www.merckmanuals.com/professional/neurologic_disorders/stroke_cva/intracerebral_hemorrhage.html. (Cited December 27 2017).
3. Stein, J., Harvey, R., Winstein, C., Zorowitz, R., & Wittenberg, G. (2015). Stroke recovery and rehabilitation. In T. M. K. Gonzalez-Castellon (Ed.), *Pathophysiology and Management of Acute Stroke* (2nd ed., p. 866). New York, NY: Demos Medical Publishing, LLC.
4. Coutts, S. B. (2017). Diagnosis and management of transient ischemic attack. *Continuum: Lifelong Learning in Neurology, 23*(1, Cerebrovascular Disease), 82–92.
5. Benjamin, E. J., Virani, S. S., Callaway, C. W., et al. on behalf of the American Heart Association Council on Epidemiology and Prevention Statistics Committee and Stroke Statistics Subcommittee. (2018). Heart disease and stroke statistics—2018 update: A report from the American Heart Association. *Circulation, 137,* e67–e492. doi:10.1161/CIR.0000000000000558.
6. Woodruff, T. M., et al. (2011). Pathophysiology, treatment, and animal and cellular models of human ischemic stroke. *Molecular Neurodegeneration, 6*(1), 11.
7. Perna, R., & Temple, J. (2015). Rehabilitation outcomes: Ischemic versus hemorrhagic strokes. *Behavioural Neurology, 2015,* 6.
8. Southerland, A. M. (2017). Clinical evaluation of the patient with acute stroke. *Continuum: Lifelong Learning in Neurology, 23*(1, Cerebrovascular Disease), 40–61.
9. Dutta, D., Bowen, E., & Foy, C. (2015). Four-year follow-up of transient ischemic attacks, strokes, and mimics. *A Retrospective Transient Ischemic Attack Clinic Cohort Study, 46*(5), 1227–1232.
10. Wardlaw, J. M., et al. (2015). ABCD2 score and secondary stroke prevention: Meta-analysis and effect per 1,000 patients triaged. *Neurology, 85*(4), 373–380.
11. Lyden, P. (2017). Using the national institutes of health stroke scale. *A Cautionary Tale, 48*(2), 513–519.
12. Stroke, N.I.o.N.D.a. NIH Stroke Scale. Retrieved from https://www.ninds.nih.gov/sites/default/files/NIH_Stroke_Scale_Booklet.pdf. (Cited December 27 2017).
13. Hemphill, J. C., et al. (2015). Guidelines for the Management of Spontaneous Intracerebral Hemorrhage. *A Guideline for Healthcare Professionals From the American Heart Association/American Stroke Association.*
14. Higashida, R., et al. (2013). Interactions within stroke systems of care: A policy statement from the American Heart Association/American Stroke Association. *Stroke; a Journal of Cerebral Circulation, 44*(10), 2961–2984.
15. Rabinstein, A. A. (2017). Treatment of acute ischemic stroke. *Continuum: Lifelong Learning in Neurology, 23*(1, Cerebrovascular Disease), 62–81.
16. He, J., et al. (2014). Effects of immediate blood pressure reduction on death and major disability in patients with acute ischemic stroke: The CATIS randomized clinical trial. *JAMA: The Journal of the American Medical Association, 311*(5), 479–489.
17. Jauch, E. C., et al. (2013). Guidelines for the early management of patients with acute ischemic stroke a guideline for healthcare professionals from the American Heart Association/American Stroke Association. *Stroke; a Journal of Cerebral Circulation, 44*(3), 870–947.
18. Sandset, E. C., et al. (2012). Relation between change in blood pressure in acute stroke and risk of early adverse events and poor outcome. *Stroke; a Journal of Cerebral Circulation.*
19. Powers, W. J., et al. (2015). 2015 American Heart Association/American Stroke Association focused update of the 2013 guidelines for the early management of patients with acute ischemic stroke regarding endovascular treatment. *A Guideline for Healthcare Professionals From the American Heart Association/American Stroke Association, 46*(10), 3020–3035.
20. Powers, W., Rabinstein, A., Ackerson, T., et al., (2018). Guidelines for the early management of patients with acute ischemic stroke. Retrieved from http://stroke.ahajournals.org on March 1, 2018.
21. Del Zoppo, G. J., et al. (2009). Expansion of the time window for treatment of acute ischemic stroke with intravenous tissue plasminogen activator: A science advisory from the American Heart Association/American Stroke Association. *Stroke; a Journal of Cerebral Circulation, 40*(8), 2945–2948.
22. Malloy, R. J., et al. (2013). Evaluation of antiplatelet agents for secondary prevention of stroke using mixed treatment comparison meta-analysis. *Clinical Therapeutics, 35*(10), 1490–1500.e7.
23. Assiri, A., et al. (2013). Mixed treatment comparison meta-analysis of aspirin, warfarin, and new anticoagulants for stroke prevention in patients with nonvalvular atrial fibrillation. *Clinical Therapeutics, 35*(7), 967–984.e2.
24. Dickneite, G., & Hoffman, M. (2014). Reversing the new oral anticoagulants with prothrombin complex concentrates (PCCs): What is the evidence? *Thrombosis and Haemostasis, 111*(2), 189–198.
25. Nogueira, R. G., et al. (2018). Thrombectomy 6 to 24 hours after stroke with a mismatch between deficit and infarct. *The New England Journal of Medicine, 378*(1), 11–21.
26. Tsantilas, P., et al. (2017). A short time interval between the neurologic index event and carotid endarterectomy is not a risk factor for carotid surgery. *Journal of Vascular Surgery, 65*(1), 12–20.e1.
27. Scott, C. A., et al. (2012). Incidence, risk factors, management, and outcomes of stroke in pregnancy. *Obstetrics and Gynecology, 120*(2 Pt. 1), 318–324.
28. Meschia, J. F., et al. (2014). Guidelines for the primary prevention of stroke: A statement for healthcare professionals from the American Heart Association/American Stroke Association. *Stroke; a Journal of Cerebral Circulation, 45*(12), 3754–3832.

DEMENTIA

Karen Dick • Laura A. Rabin

DEFINITION AND EPIDEMIOLOGY

Most people enjoy a fruitful and productive period during their later years. However, for 5% to 10% of the population older than 65 years and 32% to 50% of the population older than 85 years, these years are associated with a serious form of cognitive impairment known as dementia.[1] It is estimated that more than 5.8 million people in the United States—regardless of race, gender, or socioeconomic status—are afflicted with the most common type of dementia, Alzheimer's disease. The Alzheimer's Association estimates that nearly 13.8 million Americans will have dementia of the Alzheimer's type by 2050 unless a cure is found.[1] Alzheimer's disease is the sixth leading cause of death in the United States and the only cause of death among the top 10 in the United States that cannot be prevented, cured, or even slowed.[1] Some have labeled dementia as a disease with no survivors, which is a sobering description.

Dementia is often the reason for institutionalization; it accounts for more than 50% of all nursing home admissions, and according to the CDC, up to 50% of patients residing in nursing homes have Alzheimer's or other forms of dementia.[2] It has long been a common belief that memory loss is an inevitable and incurable part of the aging process, making any clinical intervention useless. However, with the recent advances in research, as evidenced by numerous clinical trials and new drug therapies, early detection, treatment, education, and support for families are even more critical.

The term *dementia* comprises several symptoms, including a progressive loss of memory and behavioral changes, which together interfere with independence in activities of daily living. The *Diagnostic and Statistical Manual of Mental Disorders*, fifth edition, now defines dementia under the heading of Major or Mild Neurocognitive Disorders and further divides by type: Alzheimer's, frontotemporal, Lewy body, vascular, traumatic brain injury, or substance- or medication-induced. Please see the *Diagnostic and Statistical Manual of Mental Disorders*, 5th edition, for diagnostic criteria for Alzheimer's, vascular, and Lewy body.[3] The two most common types of dementia, Alzheimer's disease and vascular dementia, account for about 80% to 90% of all dementias in older adults.[4]

Mild Cognitive Impairment

It is important to review the condition identified as mild cognitive impairment (MCI) as well, as it becomes increasingly common as individuals age. MCI is thought to be a transitional state between normal aging and dementia. Because individuals with MCI may progress to dementia at a rate of 10% to 15% a year, MCI is considered a risk factor for all types of dementia, and these patients need close monitoring and follow-up.

According to current definitions, a change in cognitive abilities is required for a diagnosis, and data is generally gathered through interviews with the patient and a collateral source, when possible.[5-7] Objective cognitive impairment is also assessed via neuropsychological examinations (usually tapping memory, language, attention, executive functions,

and visuospatial skills). Impairment in one or more cognitive domains and preserved ability to maintain independence in functional abilities are required to receive the diagnosis—though mild problems in instrumental activities of daily living (e.g., managing finances, handling transportation) are sometimes observed[8] and may relate to declines in executive functioning.[9]

MCI is currently classified into one of four subtypes: (1) amnestic MCI (aMCI) single domain, (2) aMCI multiple domain, (3) non-amnestic MCI (naMCI) single domain, or (4) non-amnestic (naMCI) multiple domain.[8] aMCI results from poor performance on tests of memory alone or in addition to deficits in other areas of cognition. By contrast, if memory is spared, but poor performance is observed on constructs other than memory (e.g., executive functions, language), then naMCI is indicated. Furthermore, performance deficits may be restricted to one cognitive domain (MCI single domain) or multiple domains (MCI multiple domains).[8]

Neuropsychological evaluation is useful in distinguishing between MCI and dementia, especially when age- and education-appropriate normative data are available. Dementia and MCI must also be distinguished from age-related cognitive decline, the mild decline in cognitive functioning that may occur with aging (e.g., loss in efficiency of acquiring new information and mild reductions in processing speed, cognitive flexibility, and working memory), which is nonprogressive and typically does not lead to functional impairment. In general, early detection and characterization of cognitive change is important because it can lead to closer follow-up and monitoring to preserve higher levels of functioning.[9]

PATHOPHYSIOLOGY
Alzheimer's Disease

Alzheimer's disease is characterized by amyloid plaques and neurofibrillary tangles. Examinations of the brains of patients with Alzheimer's disease show atrophy of the cerebral cortex that is usually diffuse but may be more pronounced in the frontal, temporal, and parietal lobes.[10] The degree of atrophy may not correlate with the degree of cognitive impairment. The amyloid hypothesis presumes a central role for abnormal amyloid processing and remains the most widely embraced causative theory.[10] Biochemically, there is disruption to the cortical pathways involved in catecholaminergic, serotonergic, and cholinergic transmission. There is a reduction of choline acetyltransferase, an enzyme found only in cholinergic neurons. Advances in genetic research have included the identification of apolipoprotein E, a protein involved in cholesterol transport linked to Alzheimer's disease, and the identification of the β-amyloid gene on chromosome 21. Researchers continue to explore the role of inflammation and oxidative stress and their effects on neuronal health. Clinical trials are under way investigating the effects of antiamyloid therapies including antibody-stimulating vaccines and other drug compounds.

Vascular Dementia

Multiple areas of focal ischemic change characterize vascular dementia, formerly known as multi-infarct dementia. The defining lesion is the lacunar infarct. Lacunae are defined as gaps, missing areas, or holes.[11] The infarctions occur in tiny arteries deep in the brain. Patients with hypertension, diabetes, hyperlipidemia, or peripheral vascular occlusive diseases are at particular risk.[4] Patients may have a mixed dementia with both Alzheimer's and vascular types.

Lewy Body Dementia

Lewy body dementia is characterized by the presence of Lewy bodies in the brain. These are proteins that enter neurons and cause cell degeneration and death. There is a loss of dopamine-producing neurons, similar to that seen in Parkinson's disease, and a loss of acetylcholine, similar to that seen in Alzheimer's disease.[12]

CLINICAL PRESENTATION

Memory loss, personality changes, language disturbances, and problems with independent activities of daily living are common presenting symptoms of dementia. A concerned family member or friend typically makes the initial presentation to a health care provider. It may take months to years for family members to seek medical attention because subtle changes in cognition may be overlooked or attributed to old age. Patients with dementia may not typically worry about what is wrong with them. These patients often have little understanding of the seriousness of their symptoms or of safety concerns (e.g., driving, cooking). On the other hand, patients with depression or benign forgetfulness often appear to the health care provider to be overly concerned about minor symptoms (e.g., forgetting a name, misplacing keys). An anecdotal finding in primary care is that those patients worried about memory problems often have only minor problems, whereas the patients who seem unconcerned pose a major worry to providers.

Patients with Lewy body dementia may present with visual hallucinations, motor impairments, postural instability, and sleep disturbances. They also show an increased sensitivity to neuroleptics; these are the patients who, when given drugs such as haloperidol for acute agitation, get worse.[12]

Alzheimer's disease is commonly divided into three stages: early, middle, and late (Box 174.1). The initial symptom is typically short-term memory loss. The earliest stage is often accompanied by symptoms of anxiety and depression. Word finding and naming problems may emerge as symptoms progress. The second stage is characterized by a worsening of memory and language as well as judgment. Disorientation to time and place is common. There may be neuropsychiatric symptoms, including paranoia, hallucinations, and delusional thinking. Urinary incontinence may be a problem. The final stage is characterized by motor rigidity, prominent neurologic abnormalities including apraxia and agnosia, severe cognitive and language impairment, and death. The average duration of the disease from diagnosis until death is 9 years.[13] Staging of a patient's disease based on clinical presentation and examination can be helpful to patients and families in planning subsequent care and treatment.

PHYSICAL AND COGNITIVE EXAMINATION

The basic components of an evaluation for dementia include a careful and detailed history from family members or caregivers and a complete physical and neurological examination. Careful attention as to timing and onset of symptoms or changes in behavior and/or mood can help the provider better understand length of time and progression of symptoms. A thorough review of all medications is important, including those medications with anticholinergic properties used in the treatment of overactive bladder, cold symptoms, insomnia, or depression, as recent studies have shown a link between cumulative

---

BOX 174.1

Stages of Alzheimer Disease

EARLY-STAGE DEMENTIA
- Memory loss
- Time and spatial disorientation
- Poor judgment
- Personality changes
- Withdrawal or depression
- Perceptual disturbances

MIDDLE-STAGE DEMENTIA
- Recent and remote memory worsens
- Increased aphasia (slowed speech and understanding)
- Apraxia
- Hyperorality
- Disorientation to place and time
- Restlessness or pacing
- Perseveration
- Irritability
- Loss of impulse control

LATE-STAGE DEMENTIA
- Incontinence of urine and feces
- Loss of motor skills, rigidity
- Decreased appetite and dysphagia
- Agnosia
- Apraxia
- Severely impaired communication
- Possible inability to recognize family members or self in mirror
- Loss of most or all self-care abilities
- Severely impaired cognition
- Depressed immune system

---

anticholinergic use with an increased risk for dementia.[14,15] All over-the-counter products (herbal, homeopathic, or nutritional supplements), should be carefully reviewed and documented. The physical examination should focus on neurologic signs; blood pressure; carotid bruits; and the assessment of cognition, mood, function, and behavior. It is also important to assess and to monitor for changes in behavior, specifically anxiety, restlessness, aggression, delusions, visual or auditory hallucinations, and wandering.

Brief mental status or cognitive screening tests can be carried out in the primary care office to identify patients most likely to benefit from more comprehensive assessment. For example, the Katz Index of Independence in Activities of Daily Living, or the Get up and Go test, can be used to evaluate function.[16,17] Cognitive screens such as the Mini Mental State Examination (MMSE), 7-Minute Screen, Mini-Cog, and Montreal Cognitive Assessment (MoCA) can provide useful information about general cognitive abilities and areas of weakness or deficit.[18–20] Other tools include the General Practitioner Assessment of Cognition (GPCOG) and the Memory Impairment Screen (MIS).[21] The Geriatric Depression Scale (short form) has been shown to be both valid and reliable in clinical practice for assessment of mood.[22]

A benefit of these screening tools is their brief and low-cost nature and ability to compare scores year to year to provide families with an objective description of disease progression. However, these instruments lack diagnostic precision and are prone to false-positive results for those with low levels of education, illiteracy, low premorbid intelligence, poor knowledge of English, poor cooperation and motivation, or sensory impairment.[23] They are also limited by ceiling effects, particularly in cases of mild dysfunction, and in high-functioning individuals who may perform well despite cognitive impairment, resulting in high false-negative rates. The accuracy of screening assessments in the primary care office can be improved by supplementing them with structured informant or caregiver report questionnaires or interviews. The clinician may then be in a good position to determine which patients warrant referral for more extensive neuropsychological evaluation.[23,24]

DIAGNOSTICS
Essential Diagnostics

Because dementia has no single standard test and is a disease of exclusion, the diagnostic evaluation should determine whether the patient has a reversible condition that may be contributing to or causing cognitive decline. The most important tests include a complete blood count (CBC), thyroid-stimulating hormone (TSH) concentration, vitamin B_{12} and folate levels, and a metabolic screen. Medications that have measurable levels, such as digoxin, carbamazepine (Tegretol), theophylline, and divalproex sodium (Depakote), should be measured. Current research is centered on refining biomarkers for clinical diagnosis of preclinical disease, MCI, and dementia; however they are not currently available.

Imaging studies are useful in identifying mass lesions, vascular lesions, or infections but do not confirm a diagnosis of dementia. All guidelines recommend a baseline brain imaging study; a non–contrast-enhanced computed tomography (CT) scan is adequate. However, many providers prefer an MRI because of its better resolution for patients with primary attentional or frontal temporal syndromes or if subcortical pathology or stroke is suspected.[13] Positive emission tomography (PET) and single photo emission computed tomography (SPECT) may be useful in difficult to diagnose cases.

INITIAL DIAGNOSTICS

Dementia

LABORATORY
- Complete blood count/differential
- Metabolic screen (Chem 14)
- Thyroid-stimulating hormone
- B12 and Folate
- Serum drug levels[a]

IMAGING
- Computed tomography or MRI
- Positive emission tomography[a]
- Single photo emission computed tomography[a]

[a]If indicated.

Differential Diagnosis

 Physician consultation is indicated for patients with delirium.

Importantly, dementia has innumerable causes that cannot always be determined by diagnostic evaluation. Some dementia syndromes (e.g., Pick's disease, Alzheimer's disease) are characterized by a lack of neurologic signs; others are associated with a definitive neurologic disease, such as Huntington's disease, diffuse Lewy body disease, and HIV infection. Considerations for differentials include other neurological syndromes,

BOX **174.2**

Differential Diagnosis: Dementia

- Alcoholic dementia
- Medication, organic toxin, heavy metal intoxication
- Medical illness
  - Liver disease
  - Hypothyroidism
  - Chronic hypoglycemia
  - Adrenal insufficiency
  - Cushing disease
- Vitamin deficiency
  - Thiamine
  - Vitamin B_{12}
  - Folic acid
- Neoplasm and paraneoplastic syndromes
- Trauma, subdural hematoma, hydrocephalus
- Infectious disease
  - HIV dementia
  - Viral encephalopathy, herpes simplex virus infection
  - Syphilis, Lyme disease, *Borrelia* infection
  - Toxoplasmosis, cryptococcosis, cytomegalovirus infection
- Delirium
- Depression
- Vasculitis
- Alzheimer dementia
- Vascular dementia
- Pick disease
- Diffuse Lewy body dementia
- Huntington disease
- Creutzfeldt-Jakob disease
- Shy-Drager syndrome
- Progressive supranuclear palsy
- Parkinson disease and other movement disorders

delirium, or pseudodementia (Box 174.2). It is important to have detailed history as to the onset of symptoms in determining whether a change in an individual's cognitive status has been evolving over several months or only just noticed a few days before.

Delirium

An important condition to consider in the list of differentials is delirium, which is often the first and only indicator in older adults of underlying physical illness, such as infection, myocardial infarction, or drug toxicity; it is the leading complication of hospitalization for older adults. It has been suggested that many patients who become delirious are never recognized as such and may be incorrectly labeled as having dementia, a psychiatric disorder, or unmanageable behavior.[25] Patients with an underlying dementia are at even greater risk for development of delirium in the setting of acute illness, which is known as delirium superimposed on dementia (DSD).[26] Delirium represents an *acute* change in mental status, which can develop from a general medical condition, substance intoxication or withdrawal, medications, or multiple etiologies.[27] It is characterized by a disturbance in attention, consciousness, and cognition. The hallmark of delirium is a clouding of consciousness, with an inability to focus, sustain, or shift attention, as well as a change in cognition, including impairment in short-term memory, disorientation, and perceptual disturbances.[27] This syndrome can occur in older adults at any point across the care continuum, from community and long-term care to acute care settings.

Delirium may manifest with similar symptoms as dementia. However, although dementia and delirium both include global cognitive impairment, delirium is characterized by prominent deficits in attention and awareness of the environment, and the symptoms typically develop rapidly and fluctuate in severity. This fluctuating presentation is problematic because patients may have periods of lucidity interspersed with inattention and high distractibility, motor restlessness, speech that is difficult to follow, and perceptual disturbances that range from misinterpretations of the environment to frank visual hallucinations. Memory, particularly in relation to recent events, is often impaired, and disorientation, most commonly to time (day of the week or time of the year) or place, is usually present. Patients may also exhibit affective signs of fear, anxiety, or anger. They may have a history of a fragmented and disordered sleep-wake cycle. Symptoms may be worse in the late afternoon or evening, which is labeled sundowning; however, it is not clear whether sundowning is a component of delirium or a separate clinical condition.[28] Patients with a history of dementia are at greatest risk for sundowning.

Delirium has many potential causes, and there is currently no support for the clinical use of any delirium biomarker(s).[29] In addition, delirium shares overlapping features with other neurological and neuropsychiatric conditions including dementia, mood disorders, and psychotic disorders. Thus, detection can be challenging and typically relies on data derived from a combination of interviews with the patient and a reliable informant, records on pre-admission functional status, repeated clinical observation (including gait, level of consciousness, speech, appearance, and interactions with others), and cognitive and motor testing.[29,30] At present, there is no consensus on how best to conduct a delirium assessment and there is great variability in the types of measures used, from unstructured interviews and global clinical impressions to more complex structured interviews, standardized rating scales, and neuropsychological tests or test batteries.[31–33] Delirium instruments can be broadly divided into those used to: assess whether the individual is arousable and able to be assessed; screen, diagnose, or rate the severity of delirium; assess the specific cognitive and motor symptoms of delirium; assess the etiology of delirium; and characterize distress associated with delirium.[33] These instruments vary on many dimensions (e.g., number of items, time required for administration, necessary training) and can have differential utility by patient setting (e.g., inpatient, surgical, ICU), population (e.g., geriatric, oncology, psychiatric), and delirium subtypes (e.g., hypoactive vs. hyperactive).[32,33] Given fluctuations in delirium symptoms, a single assessment may be insufficient to detect delirium,[33] therefore for some patients it is important to utilize measure(s) designed to be sensitive to change and that can be administered repeatedly within the same day or over time (e.g., Memorial Delirium Assessment Scale). Also, as an adjunct to delirium measures, dementia screens can inform diagnosis by helping to differentiate signs of delirium from the cognitive impairment of dementia. Though a comprehensive review of delirium measures is beyond the scope of this chapter, a recent review found that the Confusion Assessment Method and the Delirium Rating Scale and its revised version (DRS/DRS-R-98) were among the

most commonly used overall, though both measures are associated with specific strengths and limitations.[32]

Treatment for delirium is aimed at identification and treatment of the precipitating causes; care is directed toward the management of symptoms, such as agitation, restlessness, and hallucinations.[25] Studies have suggested that an interdisciplinary, nonpharmacologic approach may be effective.[34,35]

Pseudodementia

Another differential to consider is pseudodementia. Depression in older adults can lead to memory loss, attention deficits, and problems with initiation, and is referred to as "pseudodementia." Depression and dementia have overlapping symptoms, as both can manifest with cognitive impairment (including deficits in executive functioning, psychomotor processing speed, working memory, attention).[36] Moreover, cognitive symptoms often persist as residual symptoms in patients for whom depression has remitted. Sometimes, the course of the illness can help with this complicated differential. Cognitive problems that coincide with the onset of a major depressive episode in the context of previously normal cognition may be more likely due to the depression. In older adults, significant depression-related cognitive impairment can be a harbinger of subsequent dementia. It is therefore important to carefully follow older adults with significant depression-related cognitive impairment even after the depression remits.

INTERPROFESSIONAL COLLABORATIVE MANAGEMENT

Management of dementia depends on the stage of the disease. The family and community supports required are often the same for vascular dementia and Alzheimer disease. The goal of management includes treatment of all correctable factors that may impair cognition to improve daily functioning and to delay disability. Activities that promote and enhance cognition and social engagement are to be encouraged.

It is important to address safety concerns, including driving competency, soon after the diagnosis is made. Laws regarding mandatory reporting of unsafe drivers vary from state to state and can be confirmed by calling the state department of motor vehicles. A kitchen safety evaluation alerts caregivers to possible problems with cooking. A health care proxy and durable power of attorney for health care can help prevent conflicts regarding intensity of medical care later in the course of the disease. A discussion of the patient's preference for resuscitation and technology should take place while the patient is still able to participate. Encouraging families to contact the local chapter of the Alzheimer's Association is an important step; through this association caregivers can gain support, obtain reading material to promote understanding of the disease and behavior management, and determine the availability of respite care. Many websites and online support groups can help family members access and share information.

PHARMACOLOGIC MANAGEMENT

Although studies of vitamin E use in patients with Alzheimer have had mixed results, supplementation with 2000 IU of vitamin E daily is reasonable to consider in appropriate patients.[37] Since vitamin E affects platelet function, it should be avoided in patients taking anticoagulents.

Two classes of drugs are currently approved by the US Food and Drug Administration to treat the cognitive symptoms of dementia: the cholinesterase inhibitors and NMDA (N-methyl-D-aspartate) receptor antagonists. The cholinesterase inhibitors include donepezil (Aricept), rivastigmine (Exelon), and galantamine (Razadyne). These drugs can be used for the treatment of mild to moderate dementia for both Alzheimer's and for patients with vascular dementia. The choice between them is based on cost, mode of delivery (patch vs. pill vs. liquid), individual patient tolerance, and provider experience, as efficacy appears to be similar. Only 10% to 25% of patients taking cholinesterase inhibitors show modest global improvement, but more patients may have less rapid cognitive decline. Side effects may include nausea, diarrhea, and syncope. Memantine (Namenda) is an NMDA receptor antagonist that can be used in combination with a cholinesterase inhibitor for those with moderate to severe disease. Although these medications do not alter the course of dementia, they have been shown in some studies to delay or to slow worsening of symptoms.[38] Patients with vascular dementia should continue with optimal treatment of risk factors (e.g., hypertension, hyperglycemia, smoking, hyperlipidemia, diet) that may delay progression.

Patients with a dementia may develop social withdrawal, sleep impairments, and malaise, which are thought to be related to depression but may be entirely due to cognitive deficits. Depressive symptoms have traditionally been treated with antidepressants, even if the patient does not meet the criteria for major depression. In general, SSRIs are preferred as the class of medications to use. Citalopram has been shown to improve other neuropsychiatric symptoms such as agitation and may be useful at doses not exceeding 20 mg/day.[39] It should be avoided in patients at increased risk of arrhythmias. Depression in persons with dementia can often be improved with nonpharmacologic approaches such as exercise and participation in pleasurable activities. Cognitive behavioral therapy (CBT) may be useful for patients with mild to moderate dementia. Because management may differ, determination of which form of dementia is present is important.

Other symptoms that are of concern in patients with dementia include physical aggression, restlessness, agitation, and wandering. In addition, psychological symptoms including anxiety, depressed mood, delusions, and hallucinations can also be present. These types of symptoms are referred to as behavioral and psychological symptoms of dementia (BPSD) and are often a major reason for institutionalization.[40] The goal is to identify reversible causes of these symptoms: could acute infection, untreated pain, constipation, or hypoxia be contributing to a patient's agitation? Could symptoms be worsened by environmental changes such as disrupted routines or noise? Perhaps medications such as benzodiazepines or anticholinergics are contributing to restlessness and anxiety? A thorough search for reversible causes needs to take place before pharmacologic treatment options are considered. Family members and other caregivers should be educated about the avoidance and management of difficult situations. Medications can be used for behavior management but *only* when non-pharmacologic interventions have failed and there is a need to protect the patient and the caregivers. Providers should avoid use of any antipsychotics, both typical and atypical, for noncognitive symptoms or challenging behaviors unless patients are at risk of harm to themselves or others. An increased risk of cerebrovascular events and a small increased risk of death in patients with dementia have led to black box warnings for risperidone,

olanzapine, and aripiprazole. Risks and benefits must be discussed with patients and caregivers before using of any of these drugs, and they should be used for the shortest duration and at the lowest effective dose.[41]

INDICATIONS FOR REFERRAL OR HOSPITALIZATION

Many patients with dementia are frail, older adults with multiple medical, nursing, and social service needs. Involvement of other disciplines is helpful for patients, families, and providers. Physical therapists can optimize function by evaluating and recommending exercises or the appropriate adaptive equipment. Driving evaluations and kitchen and home safety evaluations can be performed by occupational therapists. These therapists can also recommend equipment to help with feeding. Speech therapy may be necessary for swallowing or dysphagia assessments in the later stages of dementia. A neurology consultation is often helpful for patients with an unclear clinical picture. A neuropsychologist or geropsychiatrist may be able to differentiate unusual presentations of dementia, especially if depression is present.

Patients with end-stage dementia are eligible for referral to hospice under the Medicare hospice benefit but must meet criteria related to bed-bound status and stage of disease. These hospice services can be provided in the home or in long-term care facilities.

COMPLICATIONS

Dementia has many complications that vary with the stages of illness. In the early stages, getting lost or having a motor vehicle accident puts patients (and others) at risk. In the middle stage, falls, incontinence, and sleep disturbances may cause further problems. Contractures, pressure ulcers, urinary tract infections, and pneumonia, all a result of immobility, are common in late and final stages of the disease. Deconditioning and nutritional deficits are also commonly seen. Patients may develop apraxia and forget how to chew and swallow. Weight loss becomes inevitable. An inability to communicate as a result of aphasia and an inability to tell caretakers about symptoms lead to further frustration and difficulty in diagnosis of complications. Death is often the result of infectious complications.

PATIENT AND FAMILY EDUCATION

The focus of patient education is to maintain independence by emphasizing patients' strengths and allowing them to continue normal activities. A woman who is no longer able to follow a recipe may still be able to knead dough and make a loaf of her special bread with help. A grandmother unable to be left alone with her grandchild is still able to rock an infant to sleep and sing a lullaby she once heard as a child. A carpenter may no longer be able to operate electrical shop tools but may still be able to hammer and glue pieces of furniture that have been precut. Feeling robbed of self-esteem is a major detriment to function; education for families is essential. Behavioral guidance, social supports, and recognition of the difficult caregiver role will benefit both patient and caregiver and may prevent illness or injury.

Families need guidance and suggestions regarding the appropriate settings and activities for their loved ones. The decision about nursing home placement is always difficult and usually comes after community services and family support have been maximized. An acute illness or injury often precedes nursing home placement. Adult daycare and group homes are appropriate in the early to middle stages of the disease; special care units are used during the middle stages of dementia. These units represent a wide variation in philosophies, goals, and design. Although many families are reluctant to enroll their relative in a program or living arrangement specifically for people with dementia, the focus of activities is at an appropriate level so that patients can participate and enjoy. The frustration of not being able to participate in activities that are too difficult is minimized. Staff members are specifically trained to handle behavioral problems in non-pharmacologic ways. Persons with late-stage dementia who are unable to participate in activities are often cared for on the general units of a nursing home.

Families also need to be able to recognize the symptoms of medical illness in a person with dementia; families should understand patients' increased susceptibility to delirium. Pneumonia without a fever or cough, a myocardial infarction without chest pain, and a urinary tract infection with no urinary symptoms are typical. A change in behavior that is noticeable only to those who know the patient well may be the only sign of illness. Families need to be given resource information about support groups, financial and legal matters, and how to tell family and friends about the diagnosis.

Caregivers can find information and resources at the Alzheimer's Disease Education and Referral (ADEAR) Center website at. http://www.nia.nih.gov/alzheimers.

The Alzheimer's Association http://www.alz.org/ has state and local chapters and maintains a 24-hour help line at 800-272-3900. Providers can find guidelines for the evaluation and treatment of dementia developed by the American Academy of Neurology, the American Psychiatric Society, and the US Preventive Services Task Force at http://www.guideline.gov/.

Many believe that the future holds great promise in the way we identify and treat patients with dementia. Researchers are looking for ways to detect it at its earliest stages with biomarkers such as blood and cerebrospinal levels and brain imaging; these kinds of diagnostics could identify those at risk so that preventive therapies could be put in place. There are hundreds of clinical trials under way, and patients and families should be encouraged to explore possibilities of participation; information about these can be found on the Alzheimer's Association website.

REFERENCES

1. Alzheimer's Association. 2019 Alzheimer's disease facts and figures. Retrieved from https://www.alz.org/media/Documents/alzheimers-facts-and-figures -2019-r.pdf. (Accessed 15 June 2019).
2. CDC. (2018). Alzheimer's. Retrieved from https://www.cdc.gov/nchs/fastats/ alzheimers.htm. (Accessed 28 September 2018).
3. American Psychiatric Association. (2013). *Diagnostic and statistical manual of mental disorders* (5th ed.). Washington, DC: The Association.
4. National Institute on Aging. The dementias: hope through research. Retrieved from http://www.nia.nih.gov/alzheimer's/publication/dementiatypes -dementia, updated Jan. 2015. (Accessed 30 April 2015).
5. Petersen, R. C. (2004). Mild cognitive impairment as a diagnostic entity. *Journal of Internal Medicine, 256*(3), 183–194.
6. Petersen, R. C. (2004). Mild cognitive impairment as a diagnostic entity. *Journal of Internal Medicine, 256*(3), 183–194.
7. Winblad, B., Palmer, K., Kivipelto, M., Jelic, V., Fratiglioni, L., Wahlund, L. O., et al. (2004). Mild cognitive impairment–beyond controversies, towards a consensus: Report of the International Working Group on Mild Cognitive Impairment. *Journal of Internal Medicine, 256*(3), 240–246.
8. Petersen, R. C., Caracciolo, B., Brayne, C., Gauthier, S., Jelic, V., & Fratiglioni, L. (2014). Mild cognitive impairment: A concept in evolution. *Journal of Internal Medicine, 275*(3), 214–228.
9. Jenkins, A., Tales, A., Tree, J., & Bayer, A. (2015). Are we ready? The construct of subjective cognitive impairment and its utilization in clinical practice: A preliminary UK-based service evaluation. *Journal of Alzheimer's Disease, 48*(s1), S25–S31.
10. Schnabel, J. (2011). Amyloid: Little proteins, big clues. *Nature, 475*(7355), S12–S14.
11. Vanes, D., & Thomas, C. (Eds.), (2001). *Taber's cyclopedia medical dictionary* (19th ed.). Philadelphia: Davis.
12. Burn, D. J. (2011). Clinical features of dementia associated with Parkinson's disease and dementia with Lewy bodies. In C. W. Olanow, F. Stocchi, & A. E. Lang (Eds.), *Parkinson's disease: Non-Motor and Non-Dopaminergic features.* Oxford, UK: Blackwell Publishing Ltd. doi:10.1002/9781444397970.ch12.
13. American Psychiatric Association. (2007). *Practice Guideline for the Treatment of Patients with Alzheimer's Disease and Other Dementias* (2nd ed.). Arlington, VA: American Psychiatric Association.
14. Gray, S. L., Anderson, M. L., Dublin, S., et al. (2015). Cumulative use of strong anticholinergics and incident dementia a prospective cohort study. *JAMA Internal Medicine, 175*(3), 401–407. doi:10.1001/jamainternmed.2014.7663.
15. Richardson, K., Fox, C., Maidment, I., Steel, N., Loke, Y. K., Arthur, A., et al. (2018). Anticholinergic drugs and risk of dementia: Case-control study. *British Medical Journal, 361,* k1315.
16. Katz, S., Ford, A. B., Muscovite, R. W., et al. (1963). Studies of illness in the aged: The index of ADL. *JAMA: The Journal of the American Medical Association, 185,* 914–919. Classic reference.
17. Mathias, S., Kayak, U. S., & Isaacs, B. (1986). Balance in elderly patients: The "get up and go" test. *Archives of Physical Medicine and Rehabilitation, 67,* 387–389. Classic reference.
18. Folstein, M., Folstein, S., & McHugh, P. (1975). Mini-mental state: A practical method for grading cognitive state of patients for the clinician. *Journal of Psychiatric Research, 12,* 189–198. Classic reference.
19. Scanlon, J., & Borson, S. (2001). The mini-cog: Receiver operating characteristics with expert and naive raters. *International Journal of Geriatric Psychiatry, 16,* 216–222.
20. Nasreddine, Z. S., Phillips, N. A., Bedirian, V., Charbonneau, S., Whitehead, V., et al. (2005). The montreal cognitive assessment, MoCA: A brief screening tool for mild cognitive impairment. *Journal of the American Geriatrics Society, 53*(4), 695–699.
21. Alzheimer's Association. Cognitive assessment toolkit. Retrieved from http:// www.alz.org/documents_custom/The%20Cognitive%20Assessment%20 Toolkit%20Copy_v1.pdf. (Accessed 15 October 2018).
22. Yesavage, J., Brink, T. L., Rose, T. L., et al. (1982). Development and validation of a geriatric depression screening scale: A preliminary report. *Journal of Psychiatric Research, 17*(1), 37–49. Classic reference.
23. Mitrushina, M. (2009). Cognitive screening methods. In I. Grant & K. M. Adams (Eds.), *Neuropsychological assessment of neuropsychiatric and neuromedical disorders* (3rd ed.). New York: Oxford University Press.
24. Lezak, M. D., Howieson, D. B., Bigler, E. D., & Tranel, D. (2012). *Neuropsychological assessment* (5th ed.). New York: Oxford University Press.
25. Inouye, S. K., Westendorp, R. G., & Saczynski, J. S. (2014). Delirium in elderly people. *Lancet, 383,* 911–922.
26. Fick, D. M., Steis, M., Waller, S., & Inouye, S. (2013). Delirium superimposed on dementia is associated with prolonged length of stay and poor outcome in hospitalized older adults. *Journal of Hospital Medicine, 8*(9), 500–505.
27. American Psychiatric Association. (2013). *Diagnostic and statistical manual of mental disorders* (5th ed.). Washington, DC: The Association.
28. Kim, P., Louis, C., Muralee, S., et al. (2005). Sundowning syndrome in the older patient. *Clinical Geriatrics, 13,* 32–36.
29. Khan, B. A., Zawahiri, M., Campbell, N., & Boustani, M. A. (2011). Biomarkers for delirium—A review. *Journal of the American Geriatrics Society, 59,* S256–S261.
30. Tieges, Z., Evans, J., Neufeld, K. J., & Mac Lullich, A. M. J. (2017). The neuropsychology of delirium: Advancing the science of delirium assessment. *International Journal of Geriatric Psychiatry,* doi:10.1002/gps.4711.
31. Neufeld, K. J., Nelliot, A., Inouye, S. K., et al. (2014). Delirium diagnosis methodology used in research: A survey-based study. *The American Journal of Geriatric Psychiatry, 22,* 1513–1521.
32. De, J., & Wand, A. P. F. (2015). Delirium screening: A systematic review of delirium screening tools in hospitalized patients. *Gerontologist, 55,* 1079–1099.
33. Grover, S., & Kate, N. (2012). Assessments scales for delirium: A review. *World Journal of Psychiatry, 22,* 58–70.
34. Rizzo, J. A., Bogardus, S. T., Jr., Leo-Summers, L., et al. (2001). Multicomponent targeted intervention to prevent delirium in hospitalized elderly patients: What is the economic value? *Medical Care, 39*(7), 740–752.
35. Thomas, E., Smith, J., Forrester, D. A., et al. (2014). The effectiveness of non-pharmacological multi-component interventions for the prevention of

delirium in non-intensive care unit older adult hospitalized patients: A systematic review. *JBI Database of Systematic Reviews and Implementation Reports,* 12(4).

36. McIntyre, R. S., Cha, D. S., Soczynska, J. K., Woldeyohannes, H. O., Gallaugher, L. A., Kudlow, P., et al. (2013). Cognitive deficits and functional outcomes in major depressive disorder: Determinants, substrates, and treatment interventions. *Depression and Anxiety, 30,* 515–527.

37. Lloret, A., Esteve, D., Monilor, P., et al. (2019). The effectiveness of Vit E treatment in Alzheimer's disease. *International Journal of Molecular Sciences, 20*(4), 879.

38. Rijpma, A., Meulenbroek, O., & Olde Rikkert, M. G. (2014). Cholinesterase inhibitors and add-on nutritional supplements in Alzheimer's disease: A systematic review of randomized controlled trials. *Ageing Research Reviews, 16,* 105–112.

39. Porsteinsson, A. P., Drye, L. T., & Pollock, B. G. (2014). Effect of citalopram on agitation in Alzheimer's disease: The CitAD randomized clinical trial. *JAMA: The Journal of the American Medical Association, 311*(7), 682–691.

40. Cerejeira, J., Lagarto, L., & Mukaetova-Ladinska, E. B. (2012). Behavioral and psychological symptoms of dementia. *Frontiers in Neurology, 3,* 73. doi:10.3389/fneur.2012.00073.

41. Devanand, D. P. (2013). Psychosis, agitation and antipsychotic treatment in dementia. *The American Journal of Psychiatry, 170*(9), 957–960.

CHAPTER **175**

DIZZINESS AND VERTIGO

Nancy McQueen Le • Katherine McCabe Reyad

 Immediate emergency department referral is indicated for patients with acute focal neurologic symptoms or in whom a serious medical condition is suspected. Acute labyrinthitis accompanied by a fever requires urgent referral and treatment.

DEFINITION AND EPIDEMIOLOGY

It is estimated that dizziness (including vertigo) affects 15% to 20% of people yearly in the general population.[1] Dizziness is a common, nonspecific term used to describe a variety of subjective states with varied causes. Clinically, it is helpful to classify dizziness into the categories of vertigo, presyncope or syncope, and disequilibrium. Differentiation of the type of dizziness experienced will dictate the direction of evaluation and treatment.

Vertigo is the illusion of movement of either oneself or the environment—spinning, tilting, or moving back and forth. Vertigo can be related to a peripheral or central disorder. Peripheral causes may include benign paroxysmal positional vertigo (BPPV), vestibular neuronitis, acute labyrinthitis, Meniere disease, ototoxicity, and head trauma. Central disorders include brainstem or cerebellar ischemia or hemorrhage, tumors, multiple sclerosis, and a migrainous syndrome.

Presyncopal lightheadedness is often referred to as a sense of wooziness or impending faint. However, lightheadedness is not exclusive to a presyncopal episode and can be a feeling that manifests in some states of disequilibrium or vertiginous conditions. Cardiac conditions associated with lightheadedness or syncope include arrhythmias, sick sinus syndrome, mitral valve prolapse, aortic stenosis, and heart block. Dehydration, hypotension, and cough or Valsalva-related syncope are common causes of vascular-related syncope or presyncope.

Disequilibrium is a sense of insecurity or imbalance, and/or unsteadiness in walking. Although this feeling is described as dizziness, it often occurs in the absence of abnormal head sensations. Disequilibrium may result from Parkinson disease, peripheral neuropathy, vision disorders, musculoskeletal disorders, or cerebrovascular insults.

The lifetime prevalence estimates of significant dizziness range from 17% to 30%, and for vertigo, 3% to 10%.[2] It has been noted that less than half of patients complaining of dizziness actually have vertigo. Even after evaluation, the largest diagnostic group is represented by dizziness of uncertain cause.

PATHOPHYSIOLOGY

Vertigo is caused by an imbalance in the vestibular system that may result from lesions in the inner ear, vestibular nerve, brainstem, or cerebellum. Less commonly, vertigo may result from lesions in the subjective sensory pathways of the thalamus or cortex or stretch receptors in the neck.[3]

Lightheadedness or presyncope or syncope is most commonly a result of a cardiovascular problem. Causes include orthostatic hypotension, vasovagal episodes, hyperventilation, and decreased cardiac output. Less common causes of lightheadedness are hypoglycemia and seizure activity. It is rarely a manifestation of impending stroke.

Disequilibrium may result from visual impairment, bilateral or unilateral vestibular loss, proprioceptive loss, impaired cerebellar function, or involvement of motor (frontal and basal ganglia) centers. Multisensory disequilibrium describes a syndrome of impaired balance caused by some degree of combined dysfunction in the areas of vestibular, visual, and proprioceptive sensation.[3]

CLINICAL PRESENTATION AND PHYSICAL EXAMINATION

Dizziness is an intensely subjective sensation that may be difficult to describe. However, a thorough history will often differentiate the type of dizziness being experienced. It is helpful to start by eliciting a description of the dizziness in the patient's own words, making note of how precise or vague the details are. This description can be further guided through specific questioning and the suggestion of some varied descriptors, especially if the individual is having difficulty articulating his or her sensory experience. Further history is then directed toward defining the characteristics of the dizziness, the time course of individual episodes, the pattern of recurrences, the precipitating and relieving factors, and any associated symptoms. A general medical history must be included, with special focus on neurologic and cardiovascular systems, medication history, and functional history.[3,4]

True vertigo is such a striking phenomenon that it is usually readily and precisely described as a clear sensation of spinning, tilting, rotating, or swaying. Lack of spinning sensation cannot be used to exclude vestibular disease.[5] Associated symptoms can include nausea, vomiting, diaphoresis, disequilibrium, nystagmus, and blurry vision. Ear symptoms, including pain or pressure, tinnitus, and altered hearing, may be present.

Lightheadedness is classically described as a sense of wooziness or impending faint although less often used as a diagnostic descriptor. It can be accompanied by diaphoresis, apprehension, nausea, and, in the extreme, an actual transient "blackout" with diminished vision but with persisting vague awareness of one's surroundings. In these patients, it is important to ask about heart palpitations, chest discomfort, and dyspnea.

Disequilibrium is described as a sense of imbalance or insecurity on rising or when walking. Patients often say they are dizzy when they are not in fact vertiginous or presyncopal but rather "off-kilter." They may have begun to use a cane or "furniture walking" for unclear reasons. The sense of imbalance may be worse in the dark or may be accompanied by changes in gait characterized by a shortened step length and widened base of support.[4,6] When the description elicited is vague or ill defined, it may reflect multifactorial issues. A specific sensory experience in multisensory disequilibrium may be difficult to describe.

Dizziness can also be related to psychogenic causes, such as anxiety states or agoraphobia. Nonspecific dizziness can be caused by hyperventilation; however, if associated with nystagmus, a vestibular cause cannot be excluded. Anxiety and apprehension often accompany physiologic dizziness, so complaints of "dizziness" should not be automatically attributed to a psychogenic cause.

The physical examination in any complaint of dizziness should always include a general medical review as well as a review of medications, including herbals and over-the-counter drugs. This information will guide a more focused examination.

The neurologic examination should include a cognitive screen. Cranial nerves are assessed with particular emphasis on visual acuity, eye movements, and nystagmus. Motor examination should include evaluation of power, muscle tone, coordination, and deep tendon reflexes. Sensory examination emphasizes basic vision and hearing assessments as well as testing of primary sensory modalities. Gait and balance evaluation includes observation of stride, arm swing, tandem gait with eyes opened and then closed, and Romberg sign. Otologic evaluation includes otoscopic examination and hearing assessment including the Weber and Rinne tests.

Cardiovascular evaluation includes cardiac rate and rhythm, auscultation of heart sounds and carotid bruits, and blood pressure measurement. Orthostatic vital signs, both blood pressure and heart rate, should also be determined.

A neuro-otologic examination refers to a number of special examination procedures considered when problems related to vertigo or disequilibrium are suspected, which may be performed in a specialty clinic setting. These procedures specifically assess the vestibulo-ocular and vestibulospinal systems and help distinguish between peripheral disorders and central disorders. They may include evaluation for nystagmus, position testing (Hallpike-Dix maneuver; Box 175.1), head-fixed/body-turn maneuvers, postural sway on a foam surface, and stepping test (marching in place with the eyes closed).[4]

BOX **175.1**

Positional Nystagmus Testing (Hallpike-Dix Maneuver)

1. Check the patient for spontaneous nystagmus while he or she is seated on the examining table.
2. Bring the patient quickly back to the recumbent or supine position with the head extended back 30 to 45 degrees over the end of the bed or table and the head tilted 30 to 45 degrees to one side (i.e., one ear down toward the floor).
3. Repeat the previous step two times, once with the head tilted to the left, and then again with the head tilted to the right.
4. Observe the patient for latency, duration, direction, and fatigability of nystagmus, both while positioned down and as helped to upright position.

DIAGNOSTICS

Most patients with a complaint of dizziness will not need laboratory or imaging studies. If a vestibular lesion is suspected, the Hallpike-Dix positioning maneuver would be performed (see Box 175.1). Further examination might be pursued in consultation with an ear, nose, and throat (ENT) or neurology specialist, including vestibular laboratory testing, an audiogram, or neuroimaging. Vestibular laboratory testing can help differentiate peripheral from central lesions, confirm lateralization of a documented abnormality, and allow serial evaluation for monitoring purposes.[2,4] Furthermore, it can give valuable functional information and help guide physical therapy interventions. Vestibular laboratory studies include electronystagmography, rotational testing, and posturography.

Audiology evaluation, including the Weber and Rinne tests, may have an important adjunctive role in helping establish or confirm a suspected diagnosis, especially Meniere disease. Many disorders resulting in vertigo have associated hearing involvement. The presence or absence of specific hearing findings can help confirm or exclude some conditions, and differentiate a central versus a peripheral cause. Hearing loss is defined as conductive or sensorineural on the basis of the cause.

Neuroimaging may be considered when central (brain) or structural (bony labyrinthine, internal auditory canal) lesions are suspected and amenable to visualization. Either a computed tomography (CT) scan or magnetic resonance imaging (MRI) is appropriate, depending on what is suspected. Magnetic resonance angiography is used when vertebrobasilar insufficiency is a concern.

If cardiac signs or symptoms accompany dizziness, evaluation routinely begins with electrocardiography (ECG). Holter monitoring or telemetry may also be indicated if an arrhythmia is suspected. Serial orthostatic vital signs in conjunction with these studies can provide important data. Echocardiography may be indicated to further evaluate cardiac status.

When multisystem disequilibrium is suspected or must be excluded, referral for ophthalmologic evaluation is necessary. Assessment of peripheral nerve function by electromyography and nerve conduction velocity in these instances can be definitive.

Electroencephalography may be considered to exclude seizure activity (see Chapter 182). Vertigo, disequilibrium, and lightheadedness are not common manifestations of seizures, and thus such testing is commonly under the guidance of a neurologist.

The choice of laboratory diagnostic studies should be guided by presentation and examination. A basic laboratory review usually includes thyroid-stimulating hormone (TSH) concentration, complete blood count (CBC), complete metabolic profile, vitamin B_{12} level, and rapid plasma reagin (RPR), as indicated.

DIFFERENTIAL DIAGNOSIS

Clarifying the diagnosis of dizziness begins with differentiating vertigo, lightheadedness, and disequilibrium.

Vertigo is a phenomenon resulting from a vast array of causes. Anatomically and neurologically, it is helpful to start by determining whether the vertigo is caused by a peripheral or central lesion. Peripheral problems refer to problems of the inner ear or cranial nerve VIII. Peripheral lesions include most commonly: inner ear infection, vestibular neuronitis, labyrinthitis, benign positional vertigo, and Meniere disease. Other causes include post-traumatic vertigo, acoustic neuroma, and ototoxic drug–induced conditions.[4] The general hallmarks of these conditions include a higher likelihood of associated nausea, normal neurologic examination findings, and symptoms that are position related.

Central or brain disorders usually involve the brainstem or cerebellum and most commonly include vertebrobasilar insufficiency or infarction, multiple sclerosis, posterior fossa tumor, basilar migraine, and central nervous system infection (syphilis).[4] Hallmarks of a central cause include associated neurologic findings and vertigo and nausea that are not position related.

Lightheadedness is most commonly related to cardiovascular issues. Diagnostic evaluation should exclude cardiac arrhythmias, critical aortic stenosis, vasovagal response, and orthostatic hypotension. When a psychogenic cause is suspected, it must be considered only in the context of excluding atypical manifestations of other causes. Possible causes to be considered in the evaluation process include anxiety reactions, agoraphobia, hyperventilation, and depression.

Disequilibrium is sometimes clear from the history. In many cases, the descriptions elicited are imprecise or vague yet seem to suggest balance problems rather than actual dizziness. When a description of balance impairment in the absence of dizziness is clear, the focus turns to evaluation of multisystem impairment, particularly vision and peripheral sensory function.[6] Disequilibrium should be distinguished from complaints that may be based on visual problems or related to psychogenic conditions. Diabetes mellitus is a common cause of a multisystem disequilibrium state. However, a number of other conditions should be considered, including cerebellar disorders, extrapyramidal system disorders, drug toxicity, and posterior fossa tumors.[3]

INTERPROFESSIONAL COLLABORATIVE MANAGEMENT

 Specialist referral is indicated when (1) there are positive neurologic signs, (2) an underlying cardiac disorder is suspected, (3) the diagnosis remains unclear, or (4) there is a lack of response to standard treatments.

The primary goals of treatment are as follows:
- Treat underlying diagnosed conditions.
- Manage the symptoms, which may include medication management as well as physical and vestibular rehabilitation.
- Antihistamines or anticholinergics can be helpful when used sparingly but can cause confusion in older adults.

COMPLICATIONS

The risk of falling is greatly increased in the patient with dizziness. This is especially problematic in older patients, in whom the risk of fracture is the highest. Intractable nausea or vomiting associated with dizziness, although rare, can be disabling. Side effects of medications, especially anticholinergics or antihistamines, can include drowsiness, urinary retention, and confusion (especially in older patients). Benzodiazepines should be used cautiously because of the side effect profile and the potential for dependence. Other complications are related to the specific cause of the dizziness and may include visual disturbances, tinnitus, decreased hearing, and balance and gait disorders.

EDUCATION AND HEALTH PROMOTION

Patient education should always include information about the diagnostic evaluation and, once a diagnosis is determined, specific information regarding the prognosis, treatment options, and complications. If an exercise program for vestibular compensation is initiated, patients should be told that they may initially feel worse, but as they continue the program, symptoms will subside. Specific aspects of their program should be reinforced. Other teaching emphasizes how medications can be used to relieve symptoms and the potential side effects of these agents.

The Vestibular Disorders Association is a national organization dedicated to providing information and support to people with dizziness and balance disorders. Patients can be encouraged to contact them at 1-800-837-8428 or online at www.vestibular.org.

BENIGN PAROXYSMAL POSITIONAL VERTIGO

DEFINITION AND EPIDEMIOLOGY

BPPV is a syndrome that may be a manifestation of several varied inner ear conditions. In more than half the cases, no certain cause is determined. When a cause can be identified, the two most common are head trauma and a prior viral inner ear infection. In older adults, BPPV is the most common vestibular disorder.[7] It is characterized by a sensation of spinning, whirling, or tilting with movement or position change. It is estimated that about 15% of patients with BPPV will have at least one recurrent episode within 1 year after a remission.[8]

PATHOPHYSIOLOGY

Otoconia refers to debris in the inner ear made up of small crystals of calcium carbonate. With certain position changes, these crystals shift and disperse within the semicircular canal, sending false signals to the brain.

CLINICAL PRESENTATION AND PHYSICAL EXAMINATION

Symptoms of BPPV are precipitated by a change in head position. The most characteristic description is vertigo, which may be a sensation of spinning or whirling of oneself or the environment. Common movements that precipitate this vertigo are rolling over in bed, arising or turning abruptly, or first lying back on the bed. The symptoms are usually intermittent.

The nystagmus associated with BPPV is characteristic, and any deviation from the typical profiles should suggest a central lesion. The nystagmus is observed by use of the Hallpike-Dix maneuver (see Box 175.1). If it is vertical or torsional in nature and lasts less than 30 seconds, it is consistent with a posterior semicircular canal variant. If the nystagmus is direction changing and horizontal (beating toward the ground) and lasts about 1 minute, it is consistent with a horizontal canal variant. Both types should show fatiguing with repeated positioning.

Vertigo that is spontaneous (not position related) and occurs with focal neurologic findings suggest a central cause. Significant nausea or imbalance is not typical.

With any new complaint of dizziness, a careful history and physical examination as outlined previously are always recommended. The Hallpike-Dix maneuver can be diagnostic of BPPV if the nystagmus is of the characteristic profile previously described. The dizziness and vertigo will be elicited with the affected ear down. In some cases, the history is compelling for BPPV, but at the time of the examination, position testing does not produce the dizziness or nystagmus (probably because of the intermittent nature of BPPV). The remainder of the neurologic examination findings should be normal.

DIAGNOSTICS
Essential Diagnostics

The diagnosis may be confirmed by history and a positive Hallpike-Dix test result.

Additional Diagnostics

Further testing is warranted if there are positive neurologic findings, any associated features beyond the vertigo and a mild imbalance, or any symptoms or findings that are not movement or position related. If the history is compelling but position testing is not confirmatory, electronystagmography may be helpful.

DIFFERENTIAL DIAGNOSIS

Priority differential involves identifying vertigo from syncope or disequilibrium through a careful history. Vertigo can be a manifestation of peripheral or central disorders of the vestibular system. If there are more symptoms or findings than the vertigo, a mild associated imbalance, and a positive Hallpike-Dix test result, further diagnoses should be pursued.

INTERPROFESSIONAL COLLABORATIVE MANAGEMENT
Non-Pharmacological Management

- BPPV may remit in a few days or weeks without any treatment.[8]
- The canalith repositioning procedure is a specific positioning exercise that is designed to move ear crystal particles from the semicircular canal. If BPPV is confirmed, this is the first-line treatment rather than the commonly prescribed vestibular suppressant meclizine. The classic Epley maneuver involves moving the patient from one head-hanging position to another. This presumably rotates the particles out of the semicircular canal and into the utricle of the inner ear, where they are cleared through the endolymphatic duct and no longer affect the dynamics of the semicircular canals. The patient must then not lie flat for 48 to 72 hours to prevent the particles from reentering the posterior canal. The vertigo may recur in a week or two in 10% to 20% of patients, in which case the maneuver should be repeated. Patients can be taught to do the maneuver at home.[9]
- Vestibular rehabilitation may facilitate a quicker and often more prolonged remission. Such therapy consists of habituation exercises designed to train the brain to react less to the confused signals sent from the inner ear. This occurs most effectively if the patient continues with normal head movements despite their causing vertigo. Some exercises can facilitate compensation, such as lying or rolling in a position that will precipitate the vertigo and staying in that position until the vertigo subsides or for 30 seconds. These exercises should be repeated twice a day until the vertigo is gone.[10]
- In rare refractory cases, canal-plugging surgery may be considered.[10]

Pharmacological Management

Medications such as meclizine may be used as a vestibular suppressant if vertigo is severe. However, in BPPV, the acute attacks are not suppressed by medications, and canalith-repositioning maneuvers are more effective in controlling the condition.[10] Medications that cause vestibular suppression slow recovery because they slow compensatory mechanisms. It should be noted that these medications only suppress symptoms, so they should not be heavily relied on or used as monotherapy management for BPPV.

 Referral to ENT or neurology is indicated if the patient is not responding to canalith repositioning procedures, such as Epley maneuvers, or vestibular rehabilitation.

COMPLICATIONS

As its name implies, BPPV is a benign condition. Associated or indirect complications could include risk of falling and the risks inherent in self-imposed decreased mobility (common because of fear of precipitating the vertigo). Safety issues related to driving should be addressed, if head turning precipitates the vertigo. The condition may interfere with work.

EDUCATION AND HEALTH PROMOTION

The experience of acute vertigo can be frightening. Information about the evaluation, prognosis, and treatment options will help alleviate fears of a more serious condition. It is important to emphasize that the most effective treatment (vestibular therapy and exercises) may initially cause increased symptoms, but the treatment must continue for the symptoms to subside. The Vestibular Disorders Association website (www.vestibular.org) has helpful information for patients as well as for providers and provides extensive specialty referral resources throughout the United States.[10]

REFERENCES

1. Neuhauser, H. K. (2016). The epidemiology of dizziness and vertigo. *Handbook of Clinical Neurology, 137*, 67–82.
2. Murdins, L., & Schildera, A. (2015). Epidemiology of balance symptoms and disorders in the community: A systematic review. *Otology and Neurotology, 36*(3), 387–392.
3. Edlow, J. (2016). A new approach to the diagnosis of acute dizziness in adult patients. *Emergency Medicine Clinics of North America, 34*(4), 717–742.
4. Muncie, H., Sirmans, S., & James, E. (2017). Dizziness: Approach to evaluation and management. *American Family Physician, 95*(3), 154–162.
5. Kerber, K., & Balo, R. (2011). The evaluation of a patient with dizziness. *Neurology. Clinical Practice, 1*(1), 24–33.
6. Klaus, J., Kressig, R., Bridenbaugh, S., et al. (2015). Dizziness and unstable gait in old age. *Deutsches Ärzteblatt International, 112*(23), 387–393.
7. Iwasaki, S., & Yamasoba, T. (2015). Dizziness and imbalance in the elderly: Age-related decline in the vestibular system. *Aging and Disease, 6*(1), 38–47.
8. Kim, J. S., & Zee, D. S. (2014). Benign paroxysmal positional vertigo. *The New England Journal of Medicine, 370*, 1138–1147.
9. Epley, J. M. (1992). The canalith repositioning procedure: For treatment of benign paroxysmal positional vertigo. *Otolaryngology–Head and Neck Surgery: Official Journal of American Academy of Otolaryngology–Head and Neck Surgery, 107*(3), 399–404, Classic reference.
10. Vestibular Disorders Association. Treatment for vertigo, imbalance, and dizziness due to vestibular dysfunction. Retrieved from www.vestibular.org/vestibular-disorders/treatment.php. (Accessed 17 February 2018).

CHAPTER **176**

GUILLAIN-BARRÉ SYNDROME

Joanne Sandberg-Cook

 Immediate investigation for spinal cord or cauda equina pathology indicated for rapidly evolving bilateral weakness accompanied by bowel or bladder dysfunction, increased reflexes, a Babinski sign, or a sensory level over the torso.

DEFINITION AND EPIDEMIOLOGY

Guillain-Barré syndrome (GBS) is a group of acute monophasic immune-mediated peripheral neuropathies. Initially GBS referred only to a demyelinating neuropathy, but now acute inflammatory demyelinating polyradiculoneuropathy (AIDP) and the Miller Fisher syndrome (MFS), in which oculomotor nerve myelin is affected, or axonal variants in which the axon rather than the myelin sheath is targeted are recognized subtypes.[1] Axonal variants of GBS are more common in some populations around the world, a phenomenon too readily explained.[2] Although the syndrome was initially described by Landry in 1859 and then Strohl, Barré, and Guillain in 1916, awareness was heightened when a cluster of cases followed mass vaccinations for swine influenza in 1976. More recent studies do indicate a tiny increased risk of Guillain-Barré syndrome within 6 weeks of vaccination (1 to 2 additional cases per million population).[3] However, the risk of this is insignificant when compared to the risks associated with influenza infection on the public health.

Patients with GBS usually develop weakness over several days to weeks, and when weakness is accompanied by respiratory weakness and/or autonomic instability, patients can become critically ill. Up to 5% die despite intensive care unit (ICU) care, and about 20% of patients have residual weakness a year later.[4] The incidence of GBS is between 1 and 2 per 100,000,[1] usually without relapse.

PATHOPHYSIOLOGY

Two-thirds of the time, GBS follows an upper respiratory or gastrointestinal infection by 1 to 4 weeks. The most commonly identified viruses are cytomegalovirus (CMV) and Epstein-Barr virus, and bacteria include *Campylobacter jejuni* (23% to 45%), *Mycoplasma pneumoniae* (5%), and *Haemophilus influenzae*. More recently, patients infected with Zika virus have been noted to experience post-infection GBS syndrome. However, the risk of GBS after any infection is quite low, so host factors are presumed to play a role as well.[4] Molecular mimicry—the immune system's antibody response recognizing components of the host's peripheral nerve—is thought to be the cause of GBS. This has been best characterized in some acute motor axonal neuropathy (AMAN) patients with *C. jejuni* infection in which antibodies directed at the lipo-oligosaccharide coating of the bacteria cross-react with gangliosides (GM1 and GD1a) on the axon in the node of Ranvier.[2] In addition, patients with MFS have antibodies directed against the GQ1b ganglioside, which is in the spinal nerve root and cranial nerve paranodal myelin.[5] Most recently, serum autoantibodies against moesin (membrane-organizing extension spike protein) on the myelinating Schwann cells have been identified in AIDP patients after CMV infection.[6] Once bound, those antibodies cause an influx of T lymphocytes and macrophages and activate membrane attack complex, thus damaging the nerve myelin or axon.

CLINICAL PRESENTATION AND PHYSICAL EXAMINATION

Patients develop the onset of relatively symmetric paresthesias and/or weakness, typically starting in the lower extremities and evolving over hours to days. Frequently there is a history of an antecedent infection. They often have back pain but do not have bowel or bladder dysfunction early in the course. The weakness can spread to involve the upper extremities, then the respiratory muscles, and finally can progress to complete paralysis. The weakness typically peaks in about 3 weeks, at which point 25% of patients have respiratory insufficiency and two-thirds are unable to walk independently.[4]

Patients with AMAN, as opposed to AIDP, can have preserved reflexes and tend not to have pain.

Patients with MFS will have ophthalmoplegia, ataxia, and areflexia and can also have distal paresthesias. Their syndrome peaks in 1 week, and these patients tend to recover more quickly and completely.[5]

Even though sensory symptoms are typical, sensory findings on examination are usually absent. Progressive weakness, beginning with the legs and progressing to the arms with an evolving loss of deep tendon reflexes, is typical of GBS. Patients with respiratory muscle weakness have decreased breath sounds and a weakened cough, reduced vital capacity (VC) on bedside spirometry, and neck muscle weakness. In addition, autonomic instability can cause wide fluctuations in pulse rate and blood pressure, urinary retention, and bowel dysmotility.

On examination, MFS patients have incoordination in the extremities and weakness of eye movements with double vision.

DIAGNOSTICS

Screening for a systemic infection or organ dysfunction is based on the history and accompanying abnormalities on the general physical examination, complete blood count (CBC), and complete metabolic profile (CMP). Erythrocyte sedimentation rates and liver transaminases are often elevated, and the frequent occurrence of the syndrome of inappropriate antidiuretic hormone (SIADH) results in a finding of low serum sodium. Urine and stool cultures may help to identify a preceding infectious cause. A history of travel to Zika-endemic countries is critical.

If GBS is suspected, lumbar puncture is the most important confirmatory laboratory test.

- Classically, there is albuminocytologic disassociation—that is, an elevated cerebrospinal fluid (CSF) protein with minimal if any increase of mononuclear CSF white blood cells (<10/mL^3). However, that pattern might not be seen during the first week of illness.[6,7]
- Acutely, the spinal fluid might show polymorphonuclear leukocytes (PMNs) without an elevated protein level but often converts to the typical pattern in a few days.

Nerve conduction studies and electromyography are not necessary for the diagnosis of GBS, which often does not evolve into a diagnostic axonal or demyelinating pattern until several weeks into the illness. Therefore, although these modalities can have significant prognostic significance, they do not usually play a role in acute diagnosis and management.

Magnetic resonance imaging (MRI) is typically not necessary. However, if there is concern for spine pathology, MRI might be done. In GBS there can be gadolinium enhancement of the nerve roots reflecting inflammation and their involvement as part of the peripheral nervous system.

DIFFERENTIAL DIAGNOSIS

MRI of the appropriate spinal level, depending on the distribution of signs and symptoms, might reveal compression from a herniated disc or mass lesion or inflammation within the spinal cord itself—a transverse myelitis. It would be rare for a brainstem or cortical brain lesion to cause bilateral weakness without cranial nerve dysfunction or impaired consciousness.

Symptoms resulting from peripheral nervous system dysfunction that mimics GBS may include acute weakness, retained reflexes, limited sensory symptoms, pleocytosis in the spinal fluid, abnormal pupil light reflexes, and ptosis or other extraocular muscle weakness.[8] In addition, it is important to check for any recent history of potential toxic ingestions (e.g., botulism and seafood toxins) or exposures (e.g., organophosphates).

If the onset of weakness is subacute occurring over weeks or longer, other peripheral nerve, muscle, or neuromuscular junction causes should be considered.

INTERPROFESSIONAL COLLABORATIVE MANAGEMENT

 Specialist consultation is indicated for rapidly evolving bilateral weakness that can be confirmed on physical examination.

Hospitalization to monitor progressive weakness, provide supportive care, and manage potential complications is necessary in all but the mildest suspected cases of GBS.

Most patients will benefit from immunological treatment including:

- intravenous immune globulin (IVIG) or plasma exchange (PE), which reduces the duration of mechanical ventilation and hastens recovery from GBS.[9-11]

- IVIG is given as a daily infusion for 5 days (total dose 2 g/kg) but can be limited by availability of the medication and is contraindicated in the presence of a selective immunoglobulin A (IgA) deficiency.
- PE is done with five exchanges over 2 weeks and is limited by available resources, logistics, and hemodynamic stability.
- Corticosteroids are not indicated for the treatment of GBS.[10]
- General medical and rehab care is essential and includes:
  - Frequent evaluation of strength most conveniently tracked with use of a table that records muscle power using the 5-point Medical Research Council (MRC) scale in representative proximal and distal muscles in all four extremities, plus neck flexion and extension.
  - Bedridden patients need prophylaxis against deep vein thrombosis and monitoring for pulmonary emboli.
  - Physical, occupational, and speech therapy are each important at various stages of the disease to maintain joint range of motion, compensate for weakness, and maximize safe swallowing.
  - Respiratory weakness and dysphagia increase the risk of respiratory insufficiency and pneumonia and need to be monitored by evaluating speech, breath sounds, and bedside spirometry findings, especially the VC. The frequency of monitoring depends on the level of respiratory compromise.
  - Intubation and mechanical ventilation are necessary in as many as 25% of afflicted patients as the VC approaches 1 L. Some clinicians consider the "20/30/40 rule"—VC 20 mL/kg, negative inspiratory force 30 cm H_2O, and/or maximum expiratory pressure 40 cm H_2O—as a threshold for artificial ventilation.[12]
  - Dysfunction of the autonomic component of peripheral nerves is common and, after respiratory insufficiency, needs the most attention to avoid life-threatening complications.[13]
- Cardiac telemetry is needed to monitor for potentially dramatic swings in heart rate that can require a temporary pacemaker.
- Blood pressure and fluid management is needed for hemodynamic fluctuations and compromise.
- Urinary retention can cause discomfort, exacerbate hemodynamic instability, and result in infection. Indwelling urinary catheters are usually necessary.

  Bowel dysmotility can lead to ileus and perforation. Repeated abdominal examination and bowel management are essential.
- All patients and families will need psychosocial support and vocational counseling.

COMPLICATIONS

Despite treatment, careful ICU monitoring, and management of weakness, autonomic dysfunction, and infections, up to 5% of patients with GBS die.[4] In addition to fatigue, residual weakness is present in 10% to 20% of patients a year later.[4]

LIFE SPAN CONSIDERATIONS

GBS tends to be milder with less residual effect in the pediatric population. After the age of 50, the incidence is approximately twice that of the younger population, and with increased age, recovery can be less complete. Death from GBS occurs in 3% of cases usually within 6 months of diagnosis.[4]

EDUCATION AND HEALTH PROMOTION

The patient and family should be educated about the course of the disease, what symptoms to alert the caregivers about, and long-term expectations. Individuals should be encouraged to continue with annual influenza prophylaxis because the risk of mortality and morbidity from influenza is much higher than any potential risk of GBS. Education and support can be obtained through the GBS/CIDP Foundation International, The Holly Building 104½ Forrest Avenue, Narberth, PA 19072 or at www.gbs-cidp.org.

REFERENCES

1. Willison, H. J., Jacobs, B. C., & van Dorn, P. A. (2016). Guillain-Barre syndrome. *The Lancet, 388*(10045), 13–19.
2. Kuwabara, S., & Yuki, N. (2013). Axonal Guillain-Barre syndrome: Concepts and controversies. *The Lancet. Neurology, 12*(12), 1180–1188.
3. Vallozzi, C., Shahed, I., & Broder, K. (2014). Guillain-Barre Syndrome, Influenza and Influenza vaccines: The epidemiologic evidence. *Clinical Infectious Diseases: an Official Publication of the Infectious Diseases Society of America, 58*(8), 1149–1155.
4. Eelco, F. M., Wijdicks, M. D., & Klein, C. (2017). Guillain Barre syndrome. *Mayo Clinic Proceedings, 92*(3), 467–479.
5. Saul, R. F. (2009). Neuro-opthalmology and the anti-GQ1b antibody syndromes. *Current Neurology and Neuroscience Reports, 9*(5), 379–383.
6. Setsu, S., Satoh, M., Mori, M., et al. (2014). Moesin is a possible target molecule for cytomegalovirus-related Guillain-Barré syndrome. *Neurology, 83*(2), 113–117. doi:10.1212/WNL.0000000000000566.
7. Rinaldi, S. (2018). Guillain Barre syndrome. In D. Sprigings & J. Chambers (Eds.), *Acute medicine: A practical guide to the management of medical emergencies.* John Wiley and Sons.
8. Wakerley, B. R., & Yuki, N. (2015). Mimics and chameleons in Guillain–Barré and Miller Fisher syndromes. *Practical Neurology, 15*, 90–99.
9. Winer, J. B. An update in Guillain Barre Syndrome. Autoimmune diseases 2014. Article ID: 793014. Retrieved from https://www.hindawi.com/journals/ad/2014/793024/. (Accessed July 2, 2018).
10. Hughes, R. A. C., Brassington, R., Gunn, A. A., et al. (2016). Corticosteroids for Guillain Barre syndrome. *The Cochrane Database of Systematic Reviews,* (10), article number CD001446, doi:10.1002/14651858.CD001446.pub5.
11. Ansari, V., & Valadi, N. (2015). Guillain-Barre syndrome. *Primary Care, 42*(2), 189–193.
12. Fokke, C., van den Berg, B., Drenthen, J., et al. (2014). Diagnosis of Guillain-Barre Syndrome and validation of Brighton Criteris. *Brain: A Journal of Neurology, 137*, 33–43.
13. Esposito, S., & Longo, M. (2017). Guillain-Barre syndrome. *Autoimmunity Reviews, 16*(1), 96–101.

CHAPTER **177**

HEADACHE
Jillian C. Belmont

DEFINITION AND EPIDEMIOLOGY

 Immediate emergency department referral is indicated for abrupt-onset "thunderclap headache," head injury, or headache with associated neurologic abnormalities including change in mental status.

Headache is experienced by 90% to 95% of the population and is the third most common complaint and cause of disability in the world.[1] Many people with headache are never diagnosed by a physician. Research has shown that even with the development of newer medications, many patients with headaches use OTC medications and other home remedies, and do not seek care for their headaches because they do not believe that satisfactory treatment is available. It is essential to differentiate secondary from primary headaches because secondary headaches can be harbingers of a potentially more serious medical problem than the benign, primary headaches usually seen in the office setting. Secondary headaches are less common and are usually the result of an underlying disease or condition, such as aneurysm, tumor, hemorrhage, temporal arteritis, or meningitis. Once the primary problem has been identified and treated, secondary headaches may dissipate.

Primary headaches are more common and are not symptomatic of another medical condition. Types of primary headaches include migraine with and without aura, chronic or episodic tension-type headaches, trigeminal autonomic cephalalgias (TAC), and other primary headache disorders such as medication overuse or rebound headache.[1]

Primary headache disorders affect people of all ages, races, income levels, and geographic areas and have an estimated lifetime prevalence of 47% in adults worldwide.[2] These headaches may range in intensity from mild to severe but cause considerable distress, expense, and loss of work time. Headaches account for up to 4% of all emergency department visits and are one of the most common reasons to consult a health care provider.[3] In fact, tension-type headaches have a lifetime prevalence of up to 78% in the general population and bring a high risk for opioid administration.[3]

Clinical and research evidence has demonstrated a relationship between migraine and other disease processes, including epilepsy, major depression or panic disorder, celiac disease, Raynaud syndrome, and cardiac shunting. The neurotransmitter serotonin has been suggested as a basis for both migraine and major depression. Knowing that a co-occurrence exists helps in the treatment of each disease and provides clues to the pathophysiologic mechanism of migraine and other headache disorders.[4]

PATHOPHYSIOLOGY

The exact mechanism of a headache is still debated. Certainly there is a genetic component and there is often a family history of migraine. Previously, headaches were thought to be caused by increased blood flow to the head, resulting in distended vessels and pressure on the nerve fibers of the brain.[5] This "vascular theory" was popular for many years until the 1930s, when Harold Wolfe determined that migraine, specifically, was caused by both vascular and chemical changes within the brain.[5]

Many theories have since identified several neurochemicals as key elements in migraine development. Serotonin (5-hydroxytryptamine [5-HT]), a powerful vasoconstrictor, sensitizes the blood vessel walls to painful dilation. Other neurochemicals, such as dopamine, substance P (a polypeptide), and calcitonin gene–related peptide, may alter the excitability of the brain and mediate the vasoconstriction or vasodilation of blood vessels.[6] Neurogenic inflammation is responsible for the pain of migraine.[5]

In review of the various theories, it is clear that during a headache, changes occur in the vasculature of the brain and in the neurochemicals found within the body. These changes are a result of a brain response to a stimulus, or trigger. Vasodilation and vasoconstriction subsequently cause the release of neurochemicals, which may be responsible for the headache and for the feelings of impending doom or fatigue that can occur before and after an attack.

CLINICAL PRESENTATION AND PHYSICAL EXAMINATION

The International Headache Society has developed criteria for various types of headache disorders. The criteria can be tedious to use and are not applicable in many primary care settings, but the information may allow the provider to quickly differentiate the various types of primary headache conditions.[7]

Migraine

The two major types of migraine are migraine with aura and migraine without aura. Migraine without aura is the more common of the two. In general, the patient complains of an ipsilateral headache. The pain is described as pounding or throbbing, is moderate to severe in intensity, and is aggravated by physical activity. This headache, which is episodic, lasts 4 to 72 hours and may be associated with nausea, vomiting, photophobia, and phonophobia. These patients usually retreat to a dark, quiet room until the attack is over. They often can identify a trigger that will precipitate the attacks. Triggers are an individual characteristic and may be difficult to identify because they may not always stimulate a headache. Common triggers include medication overuse, obesity, depression, stressful life events, sleep problems including snoring, weather changes, foods (cheese, chocolate), alcohol, change in altitude, delay or skipping of a meal, and hormonal changes.[8]

In migraine with aura, the aura usually occurs before the onset of head pain, although it can sometimes extend into the period of headache. The classic aura, or "fortification spectrum," occurs in about 10% of patients and is described as jagged lines similar to the stone fortifications found around a fort.[9] Visual auras can also be characterized by spots, shimmering bright lights, or areas of visual loss (scotomas). Somatosensory-type auras can also occur, with tingling or numbness of the fingers, motor disturbances such as hemiparesis or monoparesis, and cognitive disorders. Per the migraine aura criteria, these visual and somatosensory disturbances last at least 5 minutes but less than 60 minutes. The patient then experiences head pain and features similar to those of migraine without aura.

A prodrome can be part of a migraine.[9] Several days before the aura or start of the head pain, the person may have feelings of doom or fatigue. During this period, increased irritability, decreased energy, and food cravings are common complaints. This can often be an early signal that a severe headache is coming and may enable the patient to use both pharmacologic and non-pharmacologic modalities in the hope of aborting the attack.

Tension-Type Headache

Acute tension-type headaches are described as feeling like there is a tight band around the head. Criteria allow for photo or phonophobia but not nausea or vomiting. Headache pain is mild (not moderate to severe) and is not exacerbated by activity. This headache can last minutes to hours. It usually is not exacerbated by physical activity, but a common trigger is stress. Overall, the acute tension-type headache is a nagging headache that occurs fewer than 15 days per month, is present most of the day, and may start after the person wakes up. It rarely awakens the person. Chronic tension-type headache is similar

in presentation to the acute type but occurs more often than 15 days per month.[7]

Trigeminal Autonomic Cephalalgias

TAC is the name given to a group of headache syndromes that are differentiated by duration and frequency but all have unilateral autonomic symptoms. Cluster headaches fall under this category and are the most well-known. The patient with cluster headache, acute or chronic, is usually awakened during the night with severe unilateral, retro-orbital pain. A cluster headache reaches maximum intensity in about 15 minutes and usually lasts about 90 minutes, although some can last 3 hours.[10] These attacks can occur several times per day. The pain is described as agonizing, and unlike migraineurs, these patients often cannot sit still. The severe intensity of cluster pain causes restlessness, moaning, crying, and often pacing. Patients may indulge in self-hurting behavior and may have thoughts of suicide.[11] Other features of cluster headache include ipsilateral injection of the conjunctiva, lacrimation, rhinorrhea, and partial Horner sign. For the patient with acute cluster headache, attacks occur in groups (or clusters) lasting days to weeks and then subside until the next attack. Years can pass between attacks, and the event often occurs at the same time each year. The patient with chronic cluster headache has the same presentation as the patient with the acute type but does not experience any remission longer than 1 month for at least 1 year. These headaches are also relatively resistant to therapy. Although it is well tolerated between attacks, alcohol will often precipitate an attack in patients with acute or chronic cluster headache.[6,11]

The history is the most important part of the evaluation. With most primary headache disorders, the diagnosis can be made on the basis of the history alone.[12] It is important that the patient characterize the headache by describing the duration, quality, and location of the pain. The presence or absence of any precipitating factors, or triggers, and the age at onset should be established. The presence of associated symptoms, such as nausea, vomiting, and photophobia, should be explored. Can the patient be active during these headaches, or does the patient need to lie still in a dark room? How does the patient describe his or her sleep and energy? Sleep is usually labile in the person with headache, and energy may be poor. A medication profile is essential and should include medications that have been tried in the past for headache control. If OTC medications are taken, the number used per month should be identified because patients may not view OTC drugs as medications. Migraine is known to be familial; therefore, it is important to determine whether any family member has had headaches that might have been called sinus headaches or sick headaches or headaches that were disabling. Asking about the presence of any physical abuse is important because it has been shown that a history of abuse contributes to refractory headaches.

A targeted physical examination is important in ruling out harmful secondary headache pathologies and confirms any information given in the history.[12] The examination findings in primary headache disorders are usually within normal limits. Key aspects of the physical examination include a cardiopulmonary and complete neurologic assessment with a major focus on the following:

- Fundoscopic and pupillary assessment
- Auscultation of the carotid and vertebral arteries

- Mental status examination
- Palpation of the head, neck, and temporal arteries
- Evaluation for any neck stiffness, focal weakness, sensory loss, and gait
- Vital signs

Many patients with tension-type headaches or migraines have tight cervical musculature. Painful biceps insertions, along with general aches and pains along the back, hips, and knees, similar to the pain associated with fibromyalgia (see Chapter 157), a condition commonly seen in migraineurs. Pain and pressure on palpation of the sinuses accompanied by purulent nasal discharge may be indicative of sinusitis. The temporomandibular joints may click and pop when the mouth is opened and closed, but rarely is this the cause of a headache. Tension is often exhibited in the musculature surrounding this joint, and the subsequent bruxism may potentiate pain in this area.

Serious symptoms and findings include a headache accompanied by a stiff neck; fever; malaise; nausea or vomiting; and the presence of any aphasia, weakness, or poor coordination. The mnemonic SNOOP has been developed to help providers identify dangerous underlying conditions.[13] *Systemic symptoms*—fever, chills, weight loss, HIV infection, history of cancer; *Neurological signs or symptoms*—confusion, change in mental status, seizure, asymmetric reflexes; *Onset*—acute, sudden, or split second; *Older patient*—≥50 years old with new onset or progressive headache; *Previous headache history*—first headache or different (change in frequency, severity, features).[14] Other danger signs include the following[12]:

- Asymmetry of pupillary responses
- Decreased deep tendon reflexes
- Headache described as "the worst ever experienced"
- Personality change
- Onset of a headache that progressively worsens
- Papilledema
- Painful temporal arteries

Further investigation and referral to a specialist or hospital would be warranted with any of these signs. Positive neurologic findings on examination are indicative of a central nervous system problem and should not be attributed to migraine unless a prior pattern has been documented with serious findings previously excluded.

DIAGNOSTICS

The use of diagnostic studies depends on the results of the history and physical examination. Most diagnostic studies in the patient with primary headache are unrevealing. If the diagnosis is not clear or the history or physical findings are cause for concern, diagnostic studies should be used to distinguish primary headache from a secondary condition.

Blood tests are usually not indicated, although exceptions—based on history and physical examination findings—may include a complete blood count (CBC) to exclude anemia or an infectious process, erythrocyte sedimentation rate (ESR) or C-reactive protein (CRP) to help exclude temporal arteritis, and thyroid function tests to identify thyroid dysfunction.

Practice guidelines developed by the US Headache Consortium advocate three principles for diagnostic testing: (1) testing should be avoided if it will not change the management of the patient; (2) testing is not indicated if the patient is not significantly more likely than the general public to have an abnormality; and (3) testing may make sense in a patient who

is excessively concerned that he or she has a serious problem that is causing the headaches.[7] The American Board of Internal Medicine Foundation and the American Headache Society have created recommendations through the Choosing Wisely Campaign to help guide clinicians in choosing the right imaging when appropriate (see http://www.choosingwisely .org/as-part-of-choosing-wisely-campaign-american-headache -society-releases-list-of-commonly-used-tests-and-treatments-to -question/).

DIFFERENTIAL DIAGNOSIS

 Emergency room evaluation indicated for patients presenting with headache and neurological signs or symptoms, systemic symptoms, and history of acute (split second) onset or age >50 with new headache.

The history and physical examination will aid in excluding potential diagnoses. Priority differentials include (1) brain hemorrhage, (2) meningitis, (3) pseudotumor cerebri, (4) temporal arteritis, and (5) rheumatologic disorders (e.g., lupus erythematosus, rheumatoid arthritis).

Headache is a feature of many disease processes, and it can be difficult to decipher a primary headache from a symptom secondary to an underlying disease process. Primary headaches include migraines, tension-type headaches, TAC (e.g., cluster headache), and other primary headache disorders (e.g., medication overuse, caffeine withdrawal). Infectious or inflammatory causes of headache include fever, meningitis, temporal arteritis, Lyme disease, trigeminal neuralgia, rheumatoid arthritis, systemic lupus erythematosus, and sinusitis. Ear, nose, and throat causes can include eye disorders, abscess, or earache. Structural causes include tumor, hemorrhage, aneurysm, and subdural hematoma. Metabolic causes may include thyroid dysfunction, pheochromocytoma, and sleep apnea. Other causes of headache are pseudotumor cerebri and trauma.

INTERPROFESSIONAL COLLABORATIVE MANAGEMENT
Non-Pharmacologic Management

Non-pharmacologic measures attempt to control the headache without medication. These methods include behavior modification, biofeedback, acupressure, management of headache triggers, and a wellness program.

- Behavior modification uses several methods, such as relaxation through tapes and stress management, as well as modification of daily activities.

- Biofeedback involves the use of instrumentation to bring under voluntary control physiologic processes of which the individual is normally unaware. For example, during a migraine attack, vasoconstriction of the periphery causes cold hands. Biofeedback training teaches migraineurs to raise hand temperature and thereby prevent an attack.
- The area between the thumb and the first finger (or other acupressure areas) can be depressed during a headache to offer some relief. It is thought that this pressure causes the release of endogenous endorphins and adrenocorticotropic hormones, which aborts the headache in some people.[15]
- A wellness program consisting of balanced meals, regular exercise, and adequate sleep can also be helpful in controlling headache bouts. Overall, non-pharmacologic approaches may help patients avoid triggers that might be initiating headaches.
- Another important non-pharmacologic measure is having the patient keep a headache diary. The diary documents the number of headaches, triggers, and treatment successes and failures. The patient should keep this record daily because attempting to fill it in before a follow-up appointment may be less accurate. It is important for the patient to bring the diary to office visits so information can be shared and the treatment plan adjusted if necessary.[16]

Pharmacologic Management

Pharmacologic treatment can be divided into two areas: abortive and preventive. Management should match the level of therapy to the intensity of the headache. If the attack is severe, early intervention is in the patient's best interest. Providers need to supply education and a range of treatment modalities, allowing the patient to select the most effective treatment.

Preventive Therapy. Preventive therapy is appropriate for patients if they are unable to deal with their attacks, they experience more than four headaches a month, or the attacks are prolonged and refractory to medicine. Preventive therapy is given daily and, if successful, will decrease headache intensity and frequency. When choosing preventive treatment, the provider must consider the patient's history, including any comorbid conditions.

- For example, a connection has been shown between epilepsy and migraine; therefore anticonvulsants, such as divalproex sodium (Depakote), gabapentin (Neurontin), and topiramate (Topamax), can be used to control migraine.
- A patient with cold hands, Raynaud phenomenon, or hypertension may do well with calcium channel blockers, such as diltiazem (Cardizem) and amlodipine (Norvasc), which cause vasodilation and decrease blood pressure.
- A β blocker, such as propranolol (Inderal) or atenolol, may be chosen for the patient with palpitations caused by mitral valve prolapse or panic disorders and should be avoided in those with asthma.
- If sleep is a problem or if chronic pain persists in the shoulders, a tricyclic antidepressant, such as amitriptyline (Elavil), may facilitate sleep and also decrease the sensation of pain.[12,17,18]

The mechanism of action for both β blockers and calcium channel blockers is not fully understood.

- Calcium channel blockers prevent calcium from entering the cells and therefore decrease their excitability. This may in turn prevent vascular spasm and headache.
- β blockers affect the $β_1$-adrenergic receptors and inhibit the usual adrenergic responses.[17] Beyond these mechanisms,

it has been theorized that either may have an effect on the serotonergic system within the brain and the vascular system.

Both migraine and tension-type headache may result from an imbalance of neurochemicals. Adjustment of these neurochemicals to a more normal level may decrease the number and frequency of headaches.

- The tricyclic antidepressants and the selective serotonin reuptake inhibitors (SSRIs), such as sertraline (Zoloft), modulate the levels of serotonin in the brain. Both the tricyclic antidepressants and the SSRIs have an extensive side effect profile. Weight gain and sexual dysfunction may not be acceptable to patients, although the starting dose for many of the medications can be low. The SSRIs are better tolerated, but they might not be as effective as the tricyclic antidepressants for headaches.[17,18]
- OnabotulinumtoxinA treatment is FDA approved for the prevention of chronic migraine (≥15 days per month of headache for at least 3 months). Injections are given every 3 months in the head and neck. These treatment are well tolerated and popular even though evidence for benefit is weak.[18]

Abortive Therapy. Abortive therapy is used to treat the intensity and duration of pain during an attack and to manage associated symptoms, such as nausea and vomiting. It is important to prescribe an adequate amount of medication. Patients also need to be instructed to take an appropriate amount initially to abort the headache. The appropriate medicine depends on the prior response to treatment, the presence of nausea or vomiting, and the interval between headache onset and peak intensity. A patient with a severe migraine or cluster attack that peaks to full intensity within 15 minutes will most likely benefit from parenteral or nasal therapy rather than oral medication. For many patients, the pain of the headache is severe, but the associated nausea and vomiting are incapacitating. During a migraine attack, gastric emptying is slowed, causing gastric stasis. Medications that "turn the stomach back on," such as metoclopramide (Reglan), will augment the availability of the abortive therapy, enhance gastric motility, and decrease the nausea.[7,18] Rectal formulations can also be used when abortive therapies are prescribed.

Many of the abortive medications are powerful analgesics. When these medications, including acetaminophen (Tylenol), aspirin, and ibuprofen (Advil), are taken frequently, a condition called analgesic rebound can develop in a prone individual.[19] The conventional thinking is that medications prescribed to abort a headache will essentially potentiate the headache and make it a daily condition. More recent studies suggest that analgesic rebound is not as serious as originally thought, and that frequent use of analgesic medication may be a sign of poorly controlled headaches rather than a cause. A strict guideline on the use of all abortive medicine as well as limitations on medication refills need to be viewed with some skepticism until the evidence for rebound is better.[19] Patients should be instructed to consult with their providers if abortive use exceeds 2 days per week.

- Simple analgesics, such as acetaminophen and aspirin, can represent first-line treatment in the management of mild to moderate headaches.[20] Caffeine combinations (Excedrin, Anacin) can potentiate their absorption and analgesia.
- Nonsteroidal antiinflammatory drugs (NSAIDs) are helpful in treating an acute attack. Naproxen sodium (Anaprox DS, Aleve) has a longer half-life and a better safety profile than

some of the other NSAIDs. The addition of metoclopramide to many of the NSAIDs when nausea is present will facilitate their absorption and potentiate their effect. NSAIDs should be used cautiously in older adults, as side effects are more common in this age group.

- Ergot derivatives are effective in the treatment of moderate to severe attacks that might not have responded to simple or combination analgesics. Two forms are currently in use: ergotamine tartrate (Cafergot) and dihydroergotamine. Ergotamine tartrate is available in both rectal and oral forms, but the rectal dose is more potent than the oral preparation.[20,21] Dosage regimens need to be reviewed with the patient and adjusted to achieve pain relief without vomiting. Dihydroergotamine is available in both an injectable form and a nasal spray. The injectable form (D.H.E. 45) can be given by the parenteral, subcutaneous, or intramuscular route. The nasal form (Migranal) is easily administered and much more convenient. Because all forms of the ergots can cause nausea and vomiting, premedication with an antiemetic, such as promethazine (Phenergan) or prochlorperazine (Compazine), is necessary. Ergot derivatives may have a high potential for overuse and subsequent rebound headaches; patients need to be made aware of the risk for rebound headaches when this medication is prescribed. With the development of triptans, the use of ergot derivatives is no longer considered first-line therapy, although they are effective and less expensive than a triptan.[22]
- Triptans, developed approximately 20 years ago, have given many migraine and cluster headache patients relief within a short time.[21,22] The triptans target specific receptors (5-HT) in the brain that are believed to generate headache. Relief can be almost complete, allowing a return to normal daily activities with few side effects. These medications are arterial constrictors and should be used with caution in the presence of known cardiac disease. Many forms of triptans are available: oral, "quick melt," transnasal, injectable, and a transdermal preparation. The brands of each medication have slight differences; if one triptan is ineffective, another may prove to be effective for a patient. As with most abortive medications, the goal is to take the dose of medication required to stop the headache before it becomes severe.

Patients with cluster headache (TAC) use many of the same medications and treatment regimens as do patients with migraine or tension-type headache. The cluster attack has such a rapid onset that preventing the attacks may be the key to successful treatment. Preventive therapy includes verapamil and lithium as first-line options.

- Verapamil is usually well tolerated and does not require the close monitoring necessary with lithium. Calcium channel blockers may prevent the vasospasm that occurs during a cluster attack by blocking the flow of calcium.
- Lithium, long used for bipolar disorder, also controls cluster headaches. Levels should be monitored, and patient education about the signs and symptoms of lithium toxicity is important. Therapy should be slowly titrated upward.

With both regimens, therapy is continued until the patient is free of any attacks for several weeks. Patients are then slowly weaned from the medication.

Because of the rapid onset of the cluster headache, abortive therapy needs to be in either a parenteral or a nasal form.

- Oxygen can be effective in as many as 75% of patients and should be delivered at a rate of 10 to 15 L/min through a non-rebreather face mask.[23] The oxygen should be inhaled at the start of an attack. If this is effective, oxygen should be readily available at all times.
- The triptans are effective treatment options for the patient with cluster headache, although overuse may be a concern in patients with chronic cluster headache.

The abortive management of tension-type headaches involves many of the same medications as for migraine, and the same principles should be applied in choosing treatments for these patients.

- For mild attacks, NSAIDs may be helpful. Because there usually is no nausea, antiemetics may not be necessary.
- Muscle relaxants such as metaxalone (Skelaxin) and carisoprodol (Soma), used cautiously, have been helpful with mild to moderate attacks.
- Triptan drugs may abort a severe tension attack as well. As with migraine, the use of these medications 2 days a week or more should prompt a reevaluation of the headache regime.
- For many of these patients, stress may be triggering the attack, so nonpharmacologic measures, including physical therapy techniques, are often helpful.[24]

Most patients with headache can be managed within the primary care setting. Indications for referral to a specialist, a headache clinic, or a neurologist include the following:

- The headache is not easily controlled by routine headache medicines.
- Rebound headaches or habituation limits outpatient therapy.
- Headache is new and progressively worsening.
- Headache is described as the "worse headache of my life."
- Headache is affecting the patient's quality of life.
- Headache is accompanied by neurologic symptoms that last longer than 30 minutes or is accompanied by numbness or hemiparesis.

Hospitalization of the patient with headache may be appropriate in some situations. Headaches that are resistant to treatment may be rebound headaches and require intravenous medication to help abort the headache. Referral to a headache specialist or neurologist for consultation may be advantageous.

The US1 Headache Consortium has developed evidence-based practice guidelines for migraine that cover both nonpharmacologic and pharmacologic modalities, with the goals of reducing the frequency of attacks, improving the response to therapy, and restoring the patient to normal functioning. Control can be achieved after a proper diagnosis is made and proper treatment is prescribed.[25,26] Currently, no cure exists for primary headaches, although control is possible for most patients.

LIFE SPAN CONSIDERATIONS

As patients age, headaches often decrease. It is uncommon for headaches to appear after the age of 50 years. When an older patient is seen with a history of daily headache, analgesic rebound is often the cause; however, secondary processes need to be excluded. Triptans and DHE pose a risk to the elderly secondary to their vasoconstrictive properties, and therefore headaches in these patients should be treated more conservatively with divalproex sodium, metoclopramide, or intravenous magnesium and at home with naproxen or hydroxyzine.[12]

During pregnancy, the headache pattern can change. Many women experience a decrease in headaches during the second and third trimesters, although some see no change in the pattern. For the pregnant woman, headache control is usually limited to abortive medications only, and preventive therapy should be tapered immediately. Acetaminophen at doses within normal parameters can be safely used during pregnancy.[27]

COMPLICATIONS

Misdiagnosis is the most serious complication. For this reason, all patients who report headache require a careful history and physical examination. Patients with positive physical findings require appropriate and timely referral. Delay in diagnosis and treatment can lead to poor outcomes. Literature shows an average delay of 10 years for TAC diagnosis with years of inappropriate and ineffective treatment. Other complications of headache include status migrainosus; dependency on narcotics, barbiturates, tranquilizers, or other agents; side effects of medication; inadequate treatment; and interruption of the activities of daily living.

EMERGING MANAGEMENT TRENDS

Over the years, many neurotransmitters or neuromodulators have been considered to be involved in headache, but it has been difficult to really pinpoint exact pathophysiology. In acute migraine and cluster headache attacks, there is release of calcitonin gene-related peptides (CGRP) into the cranial venous outflow.[6] Promising results from recent CGRP experiments and clinical translational research have led to the development of anti-migraine therapies that inhibit CGRP action. Currently, CGRP receptor antagonists, the gepants, and monoclonal antibodies toward CGRP and the CGRP receptor are all showing positive relief of acute and chronic migraine and cluster headache with few side effects and no rebound effect. The first of these agents, erenumab (Aimovig) and galcanczmab (Emgality) were approved by the FDA in 2018 and several more are in clinical trials.

In addition to the gepants, a series of fully humanized monoclonal antibodies against CGRP or the CGRP receptor have been developed for prophylactic treatment of chronic migraine (attacks >15 days/month) and for frequent episodic migraine.[6] The antibodies currently in clinical trials are yielding significant results in both prevention and reduction of primary headache syndromes and have not shown any serious side effects.

PATIENT AND FAMILY EDUCATION

Knowledge and education are important aspects of patient care. Education allows patients and families to make choices and may enable them to regain control. During the initial examination and subsequent treatment, open communication and reassurance are necessary because many patients believe that they have a life-threatening condition. It is important they realize that their physical examination findings are normal and that the information received during the history indicates a primary headache disorder. Family members should be included in the treatment plan because headache affects both the patient and the family members.

Educational materials on headaches are widely available. Pharmaceutical companies and national groups such as the American Headache Society (www.americanheadachesociety .org) have developed written information about headaches and their history, pathophysiology, treatment, and prevention. The brochures and videos are available to the public, either free of charge or at a nominal cost. These national groups encourage headache patients and their families to join for support and information. Websites also provide information and support:

- The International Headache Society (www.ihs-headache.org)
- American Migraine Foundation (americanmigrainefoundation.org)
- European Headache Federation (www.ehf-org.org)
- Cluster Busters (clusterbusters.org)
- International Association for the Study of Pain (www.iasp-pain.org)
- British Association for the Study of Headache (www.bash.org.uk)

REFERENCES

1. Steiner, T., Birbeck, G., Jensen, R., et al. (2015). Headache Disorders are the third cause of disability worldwide. *The Journal of Headache and Pain, 16*, 58.
2. The World Health Organization. Headache disorders. Retrieved from www .who.int/mediacentre/factsheets/fs277/en. (Accessed on 23 December 2017).
3. Blanda, M. (2017). Tension Headache. Retrieved from https://emedicine .medscape.com/article/792384-overview#a6. (Accessed on 26 December 2017).
4. Lampi, C., Thomas, H., Tassorelli, C., et al. (2016). Headache, depression and anxiety: Association in the Eurolight Project. *The Journal of Headache and Pain, 17*, 59.
5. Ward, T. N. (2012). Migraine diagnosis and pathophysiology. *Continuum: Lifelong Learning in Neurology, 18*(4), 753–763.
6. Edvinsson, L. (2017). The trigeminovascular pathway: Role of CGRP and CGRP receptors in migraine. *Headache: The Journal of Head and Face Pain, 57*, 47–55. doi:10.1111/head.13081.
7. 2018). Headache Classification Committee of the International Headache Society. The International Classification of Headache Disorders, 3rd edition. *Cephalalgia: An International Journal of Headache, 38*, 1–211.
8. Carodartal, F. (2014). Tackling chronic migraine: Current perspectives. *Journal of Pain Research, 7*, 185–194.
9. Becker, W. (2013). The premonitory phase of migraine and migraine management. *Cephalagia, 33*(13), 1117–1121.
10. Weaver-Agostoni, J. (2013). Cluster headache. *American Family Physician, 88*(2), 122–128.
11. Robbins, M. (2013). The psychiatric co-morbidities of cluster headache. *Current Pain and Headache Reports, 17*, 313.
12. Hale, N., & Paauw, D. (2014). Diagnosis and treatment of headache in the ambulatory care setting. *The Medical Clinics of North America, 98*, 505–527.
13. Nye, B. L., & Ward, T. N. (2015). Clinic and Emergency Room Evaluation and Testing of Headache. *Headache, 55*, 1301–1308. doi:10.1111/head.12648.
14. Dodick, D. W. (2003). Clinical clues and clinical rules: Primary vs secondary headache. *Advanced Studies in Medicine, 3*, S550–S555.
15. Mehta, P., Dhapt, V., Kadam, S., & Dhapt, V. (2017). Contemporary Acupressure therapy: Adroit cure for painless recovery of therapeutic ailments. *Journal of Traditional and Complementary Medicine, 7*(2), 251–263.
16. Allena, M., Cuzzoni, M. G., Tassorelli, C., et al. (2012). An electronic diary on a palm device for headache monitoring: A preliminary experience. *The Journal of Headache and Pain, 13*(7), 537–541.
17. Fenstermacher, N., Levin, M., & Ward, T. (2011). Pharmacologic prevention of migraine. *British Medical Journal, 342*, 540–543.
18. Loder, E., & Rizzoli, P. (2018). Pharmacologic prevention of migraine: A narrative review of the state of the art in 2018. *Headache: The Journal of Head and Face Pain, 58*, 218–229. doi:10.1111/head.13375.
19. Scher, A. I., Rizzoli, P. B., & Loder, E. W. (2017). Medication overuse headache: An entrenched idea in need of scrutiny. *Neurology, 89*(12), 1296–1304.
20. Marmura, M., Silberstein, S., & Schwedt, T. (2015). The acute treatment of migraine in adults: The American Headache Society evidence assessment of migraine pharmacotherapies. *Headache, 55*(1), 3–20.
21. Cameron, C., Kelly, D., Hsieh, S.-C., et al. (2015). Triptans in the acute treatment of migraine: A systematic review and network meta-analysis. *Headache, 55*(s4), 221–235.
22. Kelley, N., & Tepper, D. (2012). Rescue therapy for acute migraine, Part 1: Triptans, dihydroergotamine, and magnesium. *Headache, 52*, 114–128.
23. Robbins, M. S., Starling, A. J., Pringsheim, T. M., Becker, W. J., & Schwedt, T. J. (2016). Treatment of cluster headache: The American Headache Society Evidence-based guidelines. *Headache: The Journal of Head and Face Pain, 56*, 1093–1106. doi:10.1111/head.12866.

24. Barbanti, P., Egeo, G., Aurilia, C., et al. (2014). Treatment of tension-type headache: From old myths to modern concepts. *Neurological Sciences, 35*(1), S17–S21.

25. Estemalike, E., & Teppers, S. (2013). Preventive treatment in migraine and the new US Guidelines. *Neuropsychiatric Disease and Treatment, 9,* 709–720.

26. Silberstein, S. D. (2015). Preventive migraine treatment. *Continuum: Lifelong Learning in Neurology, 21*(4 Headache), 973–989. doi:10.1212/CON.0000000000000199.

27. Deneris, A., Rosati-Allen, P., Hart- Haynes, E., et al. (2017). Migraines in women: Current evidence for management of episodic and chronic migraines. *Journal of Midwifery & Women's Health, 62*(3), 270–285.

INFECTIONS OF THE CENTRAL NERVOUS SYSTEM

Robyn M. Jennings • Erin R. Voelschow • Daniel W. O'Neill

A high index of suspicion should be maintained for patients with fever, headache, stiff neck, and mental status changes. Immediate emergency department referral or referral to a physician experienced in the treatment of central nervous system (CNS) infections is indicated for all suspected CNS infections.

DEFINITION AND EPIDEMIOLOGY

Infections of the CNS consist primarily of meningitis (inflammation of the meninges) and encephalitis (inflammation of the brain) and are caused by a variety of pathologic microorganisms. Despite the use of effective antimicrobial therapy, adults with community-acquired CNS infections have reported a mortality rate in the United States and Europe of 9%, with 18% of survivors having some long-term neurologic sequelae.[1]

The high morbidity and mortality rates of bacterial meningitis make diagnosis and early treatment a high priority in the primary care setting. Bacterial meningitis was most common in children younger than 5 years, with a peak incidence at 3 to 8 months of age, but with advances in vaccinations, meningitis is now more common in adults *over 50 to 60 years of age.* In the United States, the annual overall incidence rate is 1.3 to 2 per 100,000 persons.[2]

Encephalitis is caused primarily by herpesviruses (most common in the United States), arboviruses (transmitted by insects), and enteroviruses.[3] An increase in encephalitis caused by cytomegalovirus, Epstein-Barr virus (EBV), and human herpesvirus is occurring because of an increase in immunocompromised states, including human immunodeficiency virus (HIV) infection, organ transplantation, and chemotherapy. Viruses cause CNS infection by direct spread of cranial nerve or olfactory tract infections, reactivation of a latent virus within the CNS, or viremia followed by spread across the blood–brain barrier.[3]

Meningitis is defined as either aseptic or septic, depending on the identification of bacteria on the Gram stain or culture. Aseptic meningitis is caused mostly by enteroviruses, for which there is a good prognosis and no specific therapy. Bacterial meningitis is usually spread hematogenously from another primary source (predominantly the respiratory tract) or by contiguous spread from sinusitis, mastoiditis, or otitis media. The pathogens in meningitis are age specific: group B streptococci and *Escherichia coli* are most common in children younger than 1 month; *Listeria monocytogenes* is more common in the very young (younger than 1 month) and adults older than 50 years; and *Streptococcus pneumoniae* and *Neisseria meningitidis* are common causes in children and adults, with the latter seen in epidemics involving young adults.[4] *Haemophilus influenzae* used to be the leading cause of meningitis in young children until the advent of universal vaccination.[2] Unfortunately, because of the widespread overuse of oral antibiotics, there has been a dramatic rise in multidrug-resistant *S. pneumoniae.*[4] Mycobacterium tuberculosis is also seen not infrequently in adult CNS infections.[2] *N. meningitidis* can occur in epidemic outbreaks in young adults. Older adults have a notably higher percentage of infections with *L. monocytogenes*, which is associated with a 30% mortality rate.[2] Staphylococci and gram-negative bacilli are seen in meningitis associated with neurosurgery and trauma.[2] In 2012, 158 cases of iatrogenic fungal meningitis were reported in the United States in patients who received contaminated epidural steroid injections.[5]

PATHOPHYSIOLOGY

Risk factors for bacterial meningitis are previous basilar skull fracture, recent infection or neurosurgery, implanted medical devices, intravenous drug use, diabetes, sickle cell disease, complement deficiency, hypogammaglobulinemia, asplenia, alcoholism, immunodeficiency (HIV infection or organ transplant recipient), recent travel to an endemic area, and exposure to a community outbreak. Once the pathogen gains access to the cerebrospinal fluid (CSF), where there is little natural host defense, it replicates and releases bacterial cell wall proteins, which stimulate cytokine release and capillary leak. This leads to the accumulation of protein and leukocytes, cerebral edema, microvascular thrombosis, and, ultimately, cerebral ischemia and hypoxia.

CLINICAL PRESENTATION AND PHYSICAL EXAMINATION

The onset of symptoms of CNS infection can be acute, subacute, or chronic. The classic adult presentation of acute bacterial meningitis is fever, headache, and stiff neck (meningismus); however, all three are seen in only 44% of cases.[6] Altered levels of consciousness, seizures, and hypotension predict a poor outcome. Nausea, vomiting, and photophobia are more common but can also be seen with migraine. Ear, sinus, or lung infections may precede pneumococcal meningitis. In fact, older adult patients on presentation may lack fever or meningismus but may be confused or even obtunded, often after an antecedent infection such as bronchitis, pneumonia, sinusitis, or urinary tract infection.[7] Encephalitis manifests with signs and symptoms similar to those of meningitis but with more prevalent alterations in consciousness, focal neurologic signs, seizures, and autonomic and hypothalamic disturbances.[3]

A physical examination reveals a fever in most patients. Nuchal rigidity, Kernig sign, and Brudzinski sign have low sensitivity but a moderate positive predictive value for meningitis in adults.[8] In older adults, nuchal rigidity has an even lower sensitivity and specificity. Kernig sign is present if a patient in the supine position resists passive knee extension when the hip is fully flexed on the abdomen. Brudzinski sign is present if a patient in the supine position actively flexes the hips when the neck is passively flexed. Jolt sensitivity (observing a worsening of headache when a patient moves his or her head 2 to 3 times/second horizontally) is another test for meningitis with low sensitivity but may be used as an adjunctive test.[8,9] Purpura and petechiae are often associated with rapidly progressing meningococcemia but can be seen with other infections or can be a sign of disseminated intravascular coagulopathy. In patients with meningitis, a careful neurologic examination may reveal focal deficits suggestive of brain abscess, cranial nerve inflammation, thrombosis, ischemia, or cerebral edema.[2] Meningitis can lead to increased intracranial pressure (ICP), which manifests as depressed consciousness, sluggishly reactive or dilated pupils, ophthalmoplegia, respiratory depression, bradycardia, hypertension, posturing, hyperreflexia, and spasticity. With clinical presentation alone, it is difficult to distinguish aseptic meningitis from bacterial meningitis or encephalitis.

DIAGNOSTICS
Essential Diagnostics

Blood cultures—two sets (positive in 19% to 70% of patients with bacterial meningitis[6]), complete blood count (CBC) with differential, electrolytes, coagulation studies, and serum glucose concentration should be obtained immediately. Erythrocyte sedimentation rate (ESR) and C-reactive protein (CRP) can be useful for following the course of the illness.

Lumbar puncture (LP) must be performed in all patients with suspected meningitis or encephalitis.

The Infectious Diseases Society of America recommends head CT scan before LP if there are signs of altered consciousness, papilledema, immunocompromised state (i.e., HIV), new seizures, history of CNS disease, or focal neurologic deficits to evaluate for masses or other causes of increased ICP. Increased ICP would be a relative contraindication to LP because it can cause cerebral herniation. Thrombocytopenia, other bleeding disorders, and epidural abscesses are also relative contraindications to LP. Most patients do not require a CT scan before LP, and unnecessarily delaying LP and early treatment can cause poor patient outcomes.[10] A sample of the CSF should be sent for protein level, glucose concentration, Gram stain, culture, and cell count with differential. A positive Gram stain examination of CSF has nearly 100% specificity, but a negative Gram stain does not rule out bacterial disease.[2] Interpretation of CSF values is helpful in distinguishing viral from bacterial infections (Table 178.1). Further testing of the CSF with viral cultures, polymerase chain reaction, specialized stains, and cultures may be indicated.

Additional Diagnostics

- Opening CSF pressures should be measured in lateral decubitus position (normal values <200 mm H_2O).
- In suspected viral or bacterial encephalitis, the neuroimaging procedure of choice is MRI. MRI often shows edema of temporal and orbital frontal lobes.[11] Electroencephalography can also show epileptiform changes with HSV.[3]

DIFFERENTIAL DIAGNOSIS

Most cases of community-acquired, new-onset meningitis are bacterial and most cases of encephalitis are viral in origin, but certain clinical or community factors warrant consideration of less common infectious causes, such as Zika, tuberculosis, spirochetes (e.g., Lyme), rickettsiae, protozoa, fungal, or opportunistic (e.g., in persons with HIV) infectious microorganisms.

TABLE 178.1 Cerebrospinal Fluid Findings in Acute Meningitis			
Findings	Normal	Bacterial Meningitis	Viral Meningitis
Opening pressure (mmH$_2$O CSF)	50–195	>180	WNL or mildly increased
Cell count (cells/mm³)	<5 (15% neutrophils)	1000–100,000 (>80% neutrophils)	10–10,000 (mostly lymphocytes)
Protein (mg/dL)	15–50	100–500	50–100
Glucose (mg/dL)	45–80	<40	WNL or 20–40
CSF/serum glucose ratio	>0.5	<0.4	WNL

CSF, Cerebrospinal fluid; *WNL*, within normal limits.

INITIAL DIAGNOSTICS

Infections of the Central Nervous System

LABORATORY
- Complete blood count and differential
- Blood cultures—two sets
- Serum glucose and electrolytes
- Erythrocyte sedimentation rate and C-reactive protein
- Prothrombin/Partialthromboplastin (PT/PTT)

IMAGING
- Computed tomography scan[a]
- T2 and FLAIR magnetic resonance imaging[b]

OTHER DIAGNOSTICS
- Lumbar puncture (for cerebrospinal fluid protein, glucose, cell count and differential, Gram stain, and culture, hold extra tubes for special studies)
- Electroencephalography

———
[a]If indicated for suspected increased intracranial pressure.
[b]If encephalitis is suspected.[3]

Non-infectious causes include carcinoma, vasculitis, MS, immunoglobulin therapy, drug reactions, CNS hemorrhage, and post-vaccine aseptic meningitis, and must be considered in nonresponsive cases.

In all cases of suspected meningitis, the first dose of intravenous antimicrobials can be administered before the CT scan and LP to avoid critical delays in treatment. The CSF culture can still yield bacteria 1 to 2 hours after the first dose of antibiotics with most organisms, and blood cultures collected before antibiotic administration can also guide antibiotic choice. Distinguishing between bacterial, viral, and non-infectious causes is the critical differential diagnostic priority.

INTERPROFESSIONAL COLLABORATIVE MANAGEMENT

 Immediate emergency department referral and/or referral to a physician experienced in the treatment of CNS infections is indicated for all suspected CNS infections because early treatment reduces morbidity and mortality.

Pharmacologic Management

If bacterial meningitis is suspected, two sets of blood cultures need to be immediately obtained and then empirical parenteral bactericidal therapy is directed against the presumptive pathogens tailored to the patient's age, immune status, and setting of acquisition. If antibiotics are given within 6 hours, the case fatality rate has been shown to be 4% to 5%, compared with a 75% case fatality rate if antibiotics are not started for 8 to 10 hours.[2] Important factors to consider include antibiotic sensitivities and community acquisition versus nosocomial acquisition. A common combination used for community-acquired bacterial meningitis in children and adults in response to the development of penicillin-resistant pneumococcus is vancomycin (plus a third-generation.[2] Other clinical factors and findings on Gram stain and culture will direct the narrowing of subsequent specific antimicrobial therapy. In patients with bacterial meningitis who have responded appropriately to antimicrobial therapy, repeated CSF analysis to document CSF sterilization and improvement of CSF parameters is not routinely indicated but should be performed for any patient who has not responded clinically after 48 hours of empirical antimicrobial therapy.[6] Adjunctive dexamethasone therapy started before or with the first dose of antibiotics should be routine in cases of suspected bacterial meningitis to minimize damaging inflammation from bacteriolysis and long-term morbidity,[4,12] and should be continued in developed countries if strep pneumonia is the causative organism. Maintenance fluids should be used cautiously in the absence of hypovolemia. Measures to decrease ICP (elevating head 30 degrees, hyperventilation, mannitol) are initiated if necessary. Patients with bacterial meningitis require 24 hours of respiratory isolation and close monitoring, usually in an intensive care unit.

Treatment of viral encephalitis is mostly supportive: optimization of fluid balance and electrolytes; symptomatic treatment of headache, fever, and nausea; airway protection; management of ICP; and management of seizures.

If HSV or varicella-zoster virus (VZV) encephalitis is suspected, intravenous acyclovir should be initiated.

Consultation with specialists in infectious disease, critical care, neurology, or neurosurgery should be obtained if indicated. Neuropsychiatric testing, rehabilitation specialists, audiologists, psychiatrists, and other counselors may be needed in follow-up care.

LIFE SPAN CONSIDERATIONS

In adults, age has been shown to correlate with mortality after bacterial meningitis.[13] In older adults, consideration should always be given to atypical presentations of CNS meningitis and *L. monocytogenes* as a causative organism.

COMPLICATIONS

Complications of bacterial meningitis include dehydration, septic shock, hemodynamic compromise, cerebral edema, disseminated intravascular coagulopathy, septic arthritis, myocarditis, hyponatremia, seizures, and death. Long-term sequelae are seen in up to 18% of survivors[1] and consist of learning disability, hearing impairment, seizure disorder, and other neuropsychological impairment. Permanent neurologic damage is most common in patients with HSV-1 encephalitis.

PATIENT EDUCATION AND HEALTH PROMOTION

Prevention is a valuable strategy to reduce the incidence, morbidity, and mortality of bacterial meningitis. The *H. influenzae* type B and pneumococcal vaccines have proved to be effective in lowering the attack rate in all ages; they should be strongly encouraged for infants. The 23-valent polysaccharide pneumococcal vaccine should be administered to persons who are immunocompromised, asplenic, or have chronic diseases such as heart failure, lung diseases, diabetes, tobacco use, liver disease, and alcoholism. Sequential vaccination with PCV 13 and PPSV23 is now recommended for adults over 65. The quadrivalent meningococcal conjugate vaccine (MCV4) is routinely given to children 11 or 12 years old. A booster is given at age 16 because protection wanes after 5 years, and rates of meningitis peak at ages 16 to 21. High-risk adults should also be vaccinated and include those living in college dormitories, military recruits, those with complement deficiency or asplenia, those spending time in endemic areas, and scientists working with the causal organism.[14] Serogroup B meningococcal vaccine should also be considered in some cases.[15] For control of community outbreaks, chemoprophylaxis with rifampin (600 mg twice daily for 2 days), ceftriaxone (one dose, 250 mg given intramuscularly), or ciprofloxacin (a single dose of 500 mg) is indicated for close contacts of patients with *N. meningitidis* or *H. influenzae* infection (doses listed are for adults).

For prevention of vector-borne diseases, including Zika, West Nile virus (see Chapter 215), Lyme meningoencephalitis (see Chapter 213), and eastern equine encephalitis, designated resources in local and state public health departments are necessary, such as public education about mosquito control and the prevention of mosquito and tick bites.

REFERENCES

1. Erdem, H., et al. (2017). The burden and epidemiology of community-acquired central nervous system infections: A multinational study. *European Journal of Clinical Microbiology & Infectious Diseases: Official Publication of the European Society of Clinical Microbiology*, [e-pub].
2. Bhimraj, A. (2012). Acute community-acquired bacterial meningitis in adults: An evidence-based review. *Cleveland Clinic Journal of Medicine, 79*(6), 393–400.
3. Erdem, H., Inan, A., Guven, E., et al. (2017). The burden and epidemiology of community acquired central nervous system infections: A multinational study. *European Journal of Clinical Microbiology & Infectious Diseases: Official Publication of the European Society of Clinical Microbiology, 36*(9), 1595–1611.
4. Silva, M. T. T. (2013). Viral encephalitis. *Arquivos de Neuro-Psiquiatria, 71*(9–B), 703–709.
5. Benninger, F., & Steiner, I. (2013). Steroids in bacterial meningitis: Yes. *Journal of Neural Transmission, 120*(2), 339–342.
6. Mutarelli, E. G., & Adoni, T. (2013). Iatrogenic meningitis. *Arquivos de Neuro-Psiquiatria, 71*(9–B), 70659–70660.
7. Brouwer, M. C., Thwaites, G. E., Tunkel, A. R., & van de Beek, D. (2012). Dilemmas in the diagnosis of acute community-acquired bacterial meningitis. *Lancet, 380*, 1684–1691.
8. Hofinger, D., & Daviz, L. (2013). Bacterial meningitis in older adults. *Current Treatment Options in Neurology, 15*(4), 477–491.
9. Nakao, J. H., Jafri, F. N., Shah, K., & Newman, D. H. (2013). Jolt accentuation of headache and other clinical signs: Poor predictors of meningitis in adults. *The American Journal of Emergency Medicine, 32*(1), 24–28.
10. Glimåker, M., Johansson, B., Grindborg, Ö., et al. (2015). Adult bacterial meningitis: Earlier treatment and improved outcome following guideline revision promoting prompt lumbar puncture. *Clinical Infectious Diseases: An Official Publication of the Infectious Diseases Society of America, 60*, 1162.
11. Bradshaw, M., & Venkatesan, A. (2016). Herpes Simplex Virus-1 encephalitis in adults: Pathophysiology, diagnosis and management. *Neurotherapeutics, 13*(3), 493–508.
12. Fritz, D., Brouwer, M. C., & van de Beek, D. (2012). Dexamethasone and long-term survival in bacterial meningitis. *Neurology, 79*, 2177–2179.

13. Pace, D., & Pollard, A. J. (2012). Meningococcal disease: Clinical presentation and sequelae. *Vaccine, 30S*, B3–B9.
14. Centers for Disease Control and Prevention. Certain medical conditions as a risk factor. Retrieved from: www.cdc.gov/meningococcal/about/risk-medical .html. (Accessed 1 February 2018).
15. Centers for Disease Control and Prevention. Meningococcal vaccine: Who and when to vaccinate. Retrieved from: www.cdc.gov/vaccines/vpd-vac/mening/ who-vaccinate-hcp.htm. (Accessed 1 February 2018).

CHAPTER **179**

MOVEMENT DISORDERS AND ESSENTIAL TREMOR

Nancy McQueen Le • Katherine McCabe Reyad

DEFINITION AND EPIDEMIOLOGY

Movement disorders include a variety of neurologic conditions that cause alteration in normal movement or unnatural movements. These can be further categorized as excessive movements or hyperkinesis and decreased amplitude or range of movement or hypokinesis. Additional definitions can be found in Box 179.1.

The most common hyperkinetic movement disorders include essential tremor, restless legs syndrome, dystonia, and Tourette syndrome. Less common are hemifacial spasms, blepharospasm, ataxias, and Huntington disease.[1]

The most common hypokinetic movement disorder is Parkinson disease (see Chapter 181). Less common are progressive supranuclear palsy and multisystem atrophy.[2]

PATHOPHYSIOLOGY

Voluntary movement requires complex interactions between the pyramidal tracts, cerebellum, and basal ganglia to produce smooth, decisive movement without extraneous muscular contractions. Many abnormal movements are associated with pathologic alterations within these structures and their connections, whereas others can arise from elsewhere in the central nervous system (CNS), such as the cerebral cortex or the spinal cord. The peripheral nervous system can also give rise to abnormal movements, such as restless leg syndrome.

In some movement disorders, such as Parkinson disease, the underlying complex pathology is becoming better understood, but for many movement disorders much of the cause remains unclear, although both genetic and environmental causes are being proposed.

CLINICAL PRESENTATION AND PHYSICAL EXAMINATION

The presentation of movement disorders will depend on the underlying cause, so establishing a careful history specific to the patient's complaint is important (Box 179.2). The primary complaint may not be the abnormal movement, but the functional limitation it imposes on the patient's activities of daily living. Movement disorders primarily fall into several categories.

It is important to ascertain which category the movement disorder falls into by obtaining a careful history. This includes the age at onset, the regions of the body affected, progression of symptoms, the quality of movements and dysfunction, the factors that make symptoms better or worse, and the timing. A family history of movement disorder should be noted as well. A medication, alcohol, and drug history is necessary and should include prescription, over-the-counter, and illicit drug use. Alcohol, drugs, and/or medications can exacerbate or even mask underlying conditions or symptoms.

The physical examination should be approached in a systematic fashion. Make note of observations throughout the examination visit. The examination should include a complete

---

BOX **179.1**

Definitions

Akathisia: A sense of inner general restlessness reduced or relieved by moving about.

Asterixis: A brief flap of outstretched limb, transient inhibition of the muscles of posture.[1]

Ataxia: An unsteady or swaying motion. Movements may appear irregular or clumsy.

Athetosis: A slow, writhing, continuous, involuntary movement.

Chorea: An involuntary, irregular, nonrhythmic movement that seems to flow from one body part to another. The movements are unpredictable in timing, direction, and body part affected.

Dyskinesia: A general term for any abnormal involuntary movement. Paroxysmal dyskinesias are abnormal movements that occur only at certain times; hypnogenic dyskinesias typically occur during non–rapid eye movement (REM) sleep. Tardive dyskinesia refers to movements induced by dopaminergic agents, most commonly neuroleptics and metoclopramide.

Dystonia: A sustained involuntary muscle contraction that results in twisting movement and posture, often patterned and repetitive.

Myoclonus: Sudden, irregular, involuntary jerking of the muscles.

Myokymia: A fine quivering or rippling of muscles. Common and benign in facial muscles.

Stereotypy: A coordinated movement that repeats continually and identically. Compulsion.

Tics: Sudden, repetitive, nonrhythmic motor movement or vocalization. A habitual spasmodic involuntary muscle contraction.

Tremor: An oscillation, usually rhythmic and regular, affecting various body parts, such as limbs, neck, tongue, chin, or vocal cords. Can be classified as resting, postural, or action or intention tremor.

BOX **179.2**

Categories of Movement Disorders

INSUFFICIENT MOVEMENT
- Akinetic, hypokinetic, or bradykinetic syndromes

TOO MUCH MOVEMENT
- Jerky
  - Myoclonus, chorea, and tic disorders
- Nonjerky
  - Dystonia and tremor

From Gonzalez-Usigli, H. (2018). *Overview of movement disorders—brain, spinal cord, and nerve disorders.* Retrieved June 17, 2019 from https://www .merckmanuals.com/professional/neurologic-disorders/movement-and-cerebellar -disorders/tremor?query=Overview%20of%20Movement.

neurologic examination and general physical assessment. Subtle findings in movement may differentiate some of the disorders. All aspects of the neurologic examination may provide clues to assist in ruling in or out different movement disorders. A neurologic examination should include evaluation of cognition, cranial nerves, motor function (strength, tone, and coordination), sensory function, deep tendon reflexes (DTRs), and gait. The goal is to define the characteristics of the movement, determine which definition fits, and eliminate those that do not.

First look at obvious features. These include rhythm, duration, and continuity of contractions; type of oscillations (rapid or slow); and amplitude (fine or coarse). Note whether the movements occur at rest or during action and are patterned or random and whether there is a combination of movements. Also evaluate other factors such as speed, force, complexity of the movement, and any associated sensory symptoms.

DIAGNOSTICS

Essential Diagnostics

Initial diagnostic studies to consider would be basic laboratory studies including a complete blood count (CBC) with differential and a comprehensive metabolic panel and thyroid studies to rule out medical or metabolic abnormalities.

Additional Diagnostics

If there is reason to suspect infection or alcohol or drug use, additional focused workup would be warranted. Neurologic imaging, often in conjunction with a neurologic referral, may be warranted if there are specific neurologic findings.

INITIAL DIAGNOSTICS

Movement Disorders

- Complete blood count (CBC) with differential
- Comprehensive metabolic profile (basic metabolic profile [BMP])
- Thyroid function studies

FOCUSED WORKUP
- Infection workup (CBC, urinalysis, chest x-ray study)

- Drugs or alcohol (toxicology screen, ammonia level, liver function tests [LFTs])

IMAGING
- Computed tomography scan

DIFFERENTIAL DIAGNOSIS

Determining a differential diagnosis first requires defining the type of movements that are occurring, as described in Boxes 179.1 and 179.2. For a list of differential diagnoses, see Box 179.3.

INTERPROFESSIONAL COLLABORATIVE MANAGEMENT

The primary goals of treatment are as follows:
- Treat underlying conditions.
- Define the movement disorder.
- Manage the symptoms, which may include medication management as well as physical and occupational therapy.
- Basic categories of medications that can be tried include β blockers, anticonvulsants, a combination of these two, or benzodiazepines (with caution). Although some patients

---

BOX 179.3

Differential Diagnosis: Movement Disorders

HYPOKINETIC MOVEMENT SYNDROMES
- Parkinson disease
- Depression
- Hypothyroidism
- Slowing caused by musculoskeletal conditions

HYPERKINETIC MOVEMENT DISORDERS

Jerky Disorders
- Myoclonus
- Encephalopathy
- Essential or idiopathic disorder
- Epileptic
  - Startle reactions
- Chorea
  - Huntington disease
  - Hemiballismus
- Tics
  - Tourette syndrome
  - Periodic limb movement disorder
  - Complex partial seizures
  - Hemifacial spasms

Nonjerky Disorders
- Essential tremor
- Metabolic disorders
- Medications
  - LSD, dopamine antagonists and agonists, central nervous system stimulants, typical and atypical
  - antipsychotics
- Cerebellar tremor (stroke, MS, tumor)
- Dystonia
- Cervical (spasmodic torticollis)
- Blepharospasm
- Writer's cramp
- Genetic

Brain Injury
- Infections
- Stroke

---

find alcohol to be helpful at calming tremor, it is not recommended as a therapy.
- Surgical treatments that are helpful at least some of the time include deep brain stimulation.[4]

 A neurology referral is indicated when (1) the diagnosis is uncertain, (2) the patient is not responding to standard treatment, or (3) the patient's condition is deteriorating.

COMPLICATIONS

Most movement disorders can be placed on a continuum with symptoms ranging from mild to severe. Therefore, complications will vary but may include medication side effects, functional impairments such as diminished independence and activities of daily living, and balance and safety issues. Psychosocial issues include depression, difficulty with communication, self-consciousness, and issues with employment.

LIFE SPAN CONSIDERATIONS

Different movement disorders are more prevalent at certain ages, which may help guide the diagnosis. When medication management is warranted, older adults may be more sensitive to treatment. Depending on the condition, some movement disorders may lead to social and employment issues in younger people.

EDUCATION AND HEALTH PROMOTION

Patient education should include information about the diagnostic evaluation and, once a diagnosis has been determined, specific information regarding the prognosis, treatment options, and complications. The health care provider should help patients and families by providing specific information about their conditions. This can include Web-based or written information and referrals to support groups. If the provider sends a patient to a website, the patient should bring materials or discuss what he or she has learned, to monitor for accuracy. Teaching should also emphasize how medications can be used to relieve symptoms and the potential side effects of these agents.

The International Parkinson and Movement Disorder Society website (www.movementdisorders.org) is a good resource for patients with movement disorders. This is a professional society that offers links to multiple other organizations and foundations for both patients and medical professionals.

ESSENTIAL TREMOR

 Emergency department referral is indicated if the patient has acute focal neurologic symptoms or is suspected to have a serious medical condition.

DEFINITION AND EPIDEMIOLOGY

Essential tremor is a benign, chronic neurologic condition that involves symmetric, rhythmic trembling of the upper extremities, head, or voice. The legs are less commonly involved. The only clinical finding is the tremor, which may be present at rest and usually progresses over time.[5]

Oscillations are present throughout voluntary movement and are accentuated as the hand approaches a given target.[5] Emotional stress will also increase the symptoms, whereas alcohol or rest will diminish them.[3,5] Known as benign, familial, hereditary, or senile tremor, this is the most common of the movement disorders. Men and women are affected equally, with a mean age at onset of 45 years. The condition can begin as early as adolescence but most often begins in the sixth or seventh decade of life. An estimated 10 million people in the United States have this condition. If more than one person in a family group has the condition, the tremor is termed *familial or hereditary tremor*. An autosomal dominant inheritance pattern can be identified in more than 50% of cases. If the tremor begins in old age, it is commonly termed *senile tremor*.[3,5]

PATHOPHYSIOLOGY

Although essential tremor is a neurologic disorder, little is known about its cause. To date, no structural defects have been identified on autopsy, and diagnostic study results are typically normal. It is believed to be caused by focal oscillatory activity within the CNS caused by a genetic predisposition and/or environmental toxins.[6] Positron emission tomography (PET) scan studies have found changes in regional blood flow in the cerebellum and inferior olivary nuclei of patients with essential tremor compared with matched control subjects.[6] It is unclear at this time if those changes are specific to essential tremor alone or are also found in other tremors. Because of the autosomal dominant inheritance, a thorough family history may prove helpful in establishing the diagnosis.[3] There is high variability in the rate of development of this disease.

DIAGNOSTICS
Essential Diagnostics

In general, the diagnosis is based on the history and examination findings.

Additional Diagnostics

Laboratory or diagnostic testing should be considered when findings other than an isolated, generally symmetric upper extremity tremor are noted and may include:
- Complete blood count (CBC) with differential
- Comprehensive metabolic profile (basic metabolic profile [BMP])
- Thyroid function studies
- Drugs or alcohol (toxicology screen, ammonia level, liver function tests [LFTs])

DIFFERENTIAL DIAGNOSIS

Tremors may originate in the CNS, arise from metabolic abnormalities, or be induced by medication or alcohol. CNS tremors may be caused by Parkinson disease (see Chapter 181), Huntington chorea, or Sydenham chorea (secondary to streptococcal infections), or they may be cerebellar in nature. Metabolic tremors may be related to a thyroid abnormality, pheochromocytoma, or liver disease.[8]

INTERPROFESSIONAL COLLABORATIVE MANAGEMENT
Pharmacological Management

Persistent trials and evaluations may be required to find the medication that is most effective but has minimal side effects. The American Academy of Neurology (AAN) guidelines, updated in 2011, provide the most current approach to medication selection.[7] Medications used to manage essential tremor fall under several different categories.

Initial medical therapy is usually propranolol or primidone.
- β blockers: The most commonly prescribed medication for this condition is propranolol (Inderal).[7] The patient should be started at a low dose and may need frequent titrations to an effective dose. Symptoms and medication tolerance should be reevaluated after 1 to 2 weeks. Consultation with cardiology specialists is recommended in patients with cardiac disease.
- Anticonvulsants: When β blockers are not effective or tolerated, primidone (Mysoline) is the next option. Like propranolol, primidone reduces the amplitude but not the frequency of the tremor. Both gabapentin and topiramate have been shown to possibly reduce tremor, but the evidence is not as strong.
- Combined therapy: The use of propranolol and primidone together may be considered if there is some benefit from one agent alone but that benefit is suboptimal. The

combined use of these drugs is possibly more effective than either drug alone.

- Benzodiazepines: Medications such as alprazolam and clonazepam are considered possibly effective. However, caution should be used because of side effects (e.g., confusion, falls, and tolerance) and possibility of dependency and misuse.
- Alcohol: Although alcohol has long been known to alleviate essential tremor, few formal studies have been completed to demonstrate its efficacy. Regular use of alcohol is not recommended as a long-term management strategy.[7]

Non-Pharmacological Management

Surgical treatments such as deep brain simulation (DBS), focused ultrasound ablation (FUS), radio frequency ablation, and stereotactic radio surgery are being used with more frequency and are safe and effective at reducing tremor by as much as 80%.[8] . Rehabilitation including physical and occupational therapy can provide resistance training, inertial loading, dexterity training, transcutaneous nerve stimulation, and massage.[9]

 Specialist referral, including neurology and neurosurgery, is indicated when (1) the diagnosis is uncertain, (2) the patient is not responding to standard treatment, or (3) the patient's condition is deteriorating.

COMPLICATIONS

Complications may include medication side effects, functional impairments (e.g., diminished independence and activities of daily living), and balance and safety issues. Psychosocial issues include depression, self-consciousness, and issues with employment.

LIFE SPAN CONSIDERATIONS

Although essential tremor is considered a benign condition, it may have a profound effect on the patient's quality of life. The tremor may be embarrassing, particularly in younger patients. The condition may cause the patient to withdraw socially. Careful observation for depression, alcoholism, and suicidal ideation in younger patients is important. Antidepressants and counseling may be required to help patients cope with the disorder. When medication management is warranted, older adults may be more sensitive to treatment.

Severe tremors can significantly interfere with activities of daily living. Basic fine motor activities, including eating and dressing, can be impossible for some patients. Medical treatment and rehabilitation is aimed at control of the severity of the tremor to facilitate independence.[9]

EDUCATION AND HEALTH PROMOTION

The patient should be advised to avoid stimulants such as caffeine, soda, and coffee. Many over-the-counter allergy and cold preparations have stimulants in them that can also accentuate the tremors.

Careful education about the chronicity, progression, and prognosis of the disease is necessary. Although it is medically considered a benign condition, this disorder may have significant psychosocial implications, requiring frequent reevaluation and patient support. Patients also should understand that the condition can be hereditary.

Health and quality of life can be improved if the patient understands the disease process and receives support as necessary. An appropriate diet and a good exercise program can also be beneficial. Alcohol abuse should always be a concern because consumption of alcohol is known to be effective at temporarily diminishing the tremor.[10] The tremor-reducing effect of alcohol is clinically level at 0.8 g/l, which is the legal definition of alcohol intoxication in most states.

REFERENCES

1. Columbia University Department of Neurology. (2013). Classification of movement disorders. Retrieved from www.cumc.columbia.edu/dept/neurology/movdis/learn/classification.html. (Retrieved Feb 17, 2018).
2. Dowell, P., Pahwa, R., & Lyons, K. (2016). Exploring essential tremor: Results from a large online survey (s27.006). *Neurology*, 86(16s), s27.006.
3. Gonzalez-Usigli, H., & Espay, A. (2013). Overview of movement disorders—brain, spinal cord, and nerve disorders. Retrieved from www.merckmanuals.com/home/brain-spinal-cord-and-nerve-disorders/movement-disorders/overview-of-movement-disorders. (Retrieved Feb 17, 2018).
4. Alfonso, F., & Lozano, A. (2015). Deep brain stimulation for movement disorders: 2015 and beyond. *Current Opinion in Neurology*, 28(4), 423–436.
5. Bhatia, K. P., Bam, P., Bajaj, N., et al. (2017). Consensus statement on the classification of tremors from the task force on tremor of the international Parkinson and movement disorders society. *Move Disorders*, doi:10.1002/mds27121.
6. Louis, E. (2018). Essential tremor then and now: How views of the most common tremor diathes have changed over time. *Parkinsonism and Related Disorders*, 46, s70–s74.
7. Witjas, T., Carron, R., Boutin, E., Eusebio, A., Azulay, J. P., & Régis, J. (2016). Essential tremor: Update of therapeutic strategies (medical treatment and gamma knife thalamotomy). *Revue Neurologique*, 172(8–9), 408–415.
8. Elble, R. J., Shih, L., & Cozzens, J. W. (2019). Surgical treatments for essential tremor. *Expert Review of Neurotherapeutics*, 18(4), 303–321.
9. Freitas, M. E., & Munhoz, R. (2017). Rehabilitation in essential tremor. In H. Chien (Ed.), *Movement disorders rehabilitation*. Switzerland: Springer International Publishing.
10. Hedera, P. (2017). Emerging strategies in the management of essential tremor. *Therapeutic Advances in Neurological Disorders*, 137–148. https://doi.org/10.1177/1756285616679123.

CHAPTER **180**

MULTIPLE SCLEROSIS

Barbara S. Bishop

 Immediate emergency department referral is indicated for suspected cases of progressive multifocal leukoencephalopathy (PML), encephalitis, new-onset seizure, or symptomatic cardiac dysfunction.

DEFINITION AND EPIDEMIOLOGY

Multiple sclerosis (MS) is a chronic progressive inflammatory and neurodegenerative disease affecting the central nervous system (CNS). The hallmark lesion in MS, called a plaque, was first described in the 1800s. Multiple lesions are seen in multiple locations, hence the name *multiple sclerosis*. On histologic examination, the lesions are characterized by inflammation, demyelination, axonal injury and transaction, axonal loss, and gliosis.[1-3] MS is thought to be a complicated interaction among the autoimmune system, genetic variables, and environmental factors.[1] Clues to the cause of MS come from the worldwide and nonrandom pattern of this disease, studies of structural and functional changes within the CNS, immunologic studies, and genetic studies (particularly studies of families and twins).[1-3] To date, no single causative factor has been identified. It has been postulated that low vitamin D levels,

BOX 180.1

Clinical Courses of Multiple Sclerosis

Radiographically isolated syndrome (RIS): Presence of magnetic resonance imaging (MRI) lesions specific to MS that may meet the MRI diagnostic criteria for MS without clinical symptoms. Sixty-five percent of patients convert to MS in 5.3 years.

Clinically isolated syndrome (CIS): Acute or subacute focal neurologic event indicative of demyelination and often associated with clinically silent lesions on MRI. Up to 90% of MS patients have CIS on presentation.

Relapsing-remitting MS (RRMS): Course punctuated by clinical relapses (exacerbations) followed by periods of clinical remission; most common type; 85% of MS patients have RRMS at time of diagnosis.

Primary-progressive MS (PPMS): Accumulating disability from initial presentation without clearly defined relapses or remissions. Approximately 10% of MS patients have PPMS.

Secondary-progressive MS (SPMS): Thought to be the natural evolution of RRMS. It represents a progressive course with or without relapses. Natural history states that 50% of RRMS will convert to SPMS, and 90% after 25 years.

Progressive-relapsing MS (PRMS): Steadily progressive from onset, but also with acute attacks. Approximately 5% of MS patients have this type.

Benign: Expanded Disability Severity Scale (EDSS) score ≤ 3 for more than 10 years. This definition does not take into account domains of fatigue, cognition, mood, pain, social functional levels, and radiographic changes. Studies have supported decline in all aforementioned domains. In addition, approximately 50% of patients with "benign" MS progress to having EDSS scores ≥ 6.0 or progress to SPMS within 20 years.

Data from Compston, A., & Coles, A. (2008). Multiple sclerosis. *Lancet 372*, 1502–1517; Moses, H. Jr., Picone, M., Smith, V. (2013). *Clinician's primer on multiple sclerosis: An in-depth overview*. Denver, CO: Consensus Medical Communications; Leahy, H., & Garg, N. (2013). Radiologically isolated syndrome: An overview. *Neurol Bull 5*, 22–26; and Costella, K., Halper, J., et al. (2014). *The use of drug modifying therapy in multiple sclerosis: Principles and current evidence*. Denver, CO: Consortium of Multiple Sclerosis Centers (CMSC). <www.mscare.org>. Fillippi, M., Rossa, M. A., Ciccarelli, O., et al. (2016). MRI criteria for the diagnosis of Multiple Sclerosis MAGNIMS consensus guidelines. *The Lancet Neurology, 15*, 292–303.

exposure to Epstein-Barr virus (EBV) in preadolescence, and smoking are significant contributing environmental factors to MS. More than 100 genes have been identified that are associated with MS[4–6] (Box 180.1). The onset of MS is likely to occur between 20 and 50 years of age. MS affects three times as many women as men. It can also occur in pediatric and geriatric populations. MS affects up to 450,000 Americans and approximately 2.5 million people worldwide.[7] The worldwide pattern of MS shows that it is less common near the equator, and the highest incidence is in northern Europe (including Russia), North America, and Australia. It occurs most commonly in Caucasians.[1,2] African Americans tend to have more aggressive disease courses.[7]

PATHOPHYSIOLOGY

Historically, MS was thought of as an inflammatory disease of the white matter of the CNS. This paradigm has changed, and it is now considered not only inflammatory but also neurodegenerative and affects not only the white matter but the gray matter as well.

The sequence of events has become better clarified but is still not thoroughly understood. Presently, it is believed that a triggering event, most probably from the environment, activates the inflammatory process outside the CNS. This inflammatory process includes T- and B-cell activity, macrophages, natural killer cells, and others, demonstrating a complex and encompassing immune response from both innate and adaptive immune systems. The blood–brain barrier is degraded, allowing the pro-inflammatory cytokines to penetrate the CNS. Once the pro-inflammatory cytokines are in the CNS, reactivation of the inflammatory process occurs, leading to demyelination and axonal destruction. Both inflammatory and degenerative processes are seen early and simultaneously and often are perceived to be interrelated. However, there is also some evidence that suggests that they may be independent of each other.[8] Regardless of the process, as the disease progresses, inflammation downregulates and neurodegeneration escalates. The process by which this occurs is not yet clear.[2,3]

Recovery in early disease occurs because of the capacity of the CNS to functionally reorganize, compensate for axonal loss, and remyelinate. Remyelination is often incomplete and variable, and over time, axonal degradation becomes significant. Compensation is no longer possible, and permanent disability develops. It is believed that axonal degradation is responsible for permanent disability.[1–3,9]

CLINICAL PRESENTATION AND PHYSICAL EXAMINATION

There are four clinical courses of MS (see Box 180.1): relapsing-remitting (RRMS), primary-progressive (PPMS), secondary-progressive (SPMS), and progressive-relapsing (PRMS). RRMS is the most common form of MS. Natural history of the disease shows that 50% of MS patients will progress to SPMS within 11 to 15 years.[1,8]

At presentation, patients often have what is now referred to as a clinically isolated syndrome (CIS) or first clinical episode. Patients typically have a focal neurologic deficit such as eye pain or visual disturbances associated with optic neuritis. Sometimes the initial presentation is multifocal.[1,10] Magnetic resonance imaging (MRI) demonstrates multiple lesions consistent with MS allowing for a definitive diagnosis.[10,11] This is important, because it is now possible to treat patients at a very early stage of the disease process.[6] The relationship between radiographically isolated syndrome (RIS) and MS is now discussed in the literature. RIS is defined as the presence of MRI lesions specific to MS and may meet the MRI diagnostic criteria for MS; however, no clinical symptoms consistent with MS can be identified in the patient's history. Often these patients undergo MRI for some unrelated issues such as trauma or migraine. Currently, patients with RIS are not routinely being treated with disease-modifying therapy (DMT). To date, data suggest that 65% of patients will convert to MS within 5.3 years and 88% will convert in 14.1 years. Median time to conversion to CIS is 5.4 years.[11,12]

The most common presenting symptoms include visual disturbances and eye pain that comes and goes, pain in the neck or back, paresthesias or weakness of the limbs, or facial pain along the course of the trigeminal nerve. Other common symptoms include sensory symptoms (paresthesias), diplopia (intranuclear ophthalmoplegia), nystagmus, unsteady gait, or bowel or bladder dysfunction. Associated findings that increase the likelihood of MS include unexplained excessive fatigue, temperature or heat sensitivity, history of band-like sensations around the waist (commonly referred to as the "MS hug"), dysarthria, muscle spasms, cognitive disturbances, and sexual dysfunction.[1-3,13]

The initial presentation of MS can often go unrecognized or is attributed to other causes, especially if the presenting symptom is vague, such as sensory distortion, bowel or bladder dysfunction, or cognitive impairment. Initial symptoms are sometimes so vague, transient, or mild that the patient may not seek medical advice.

Symptoms of MS are unpredictable and variable. As the disease progresses, a variety of signs and symptoms will require ongoing management (Table 180.1).[13,14] A complete neurologic examination is required for patients with MS or suspected MS. The findings on neurologic examination may be normal; especially in early disease, the patient may report problems consistent with symptoms without true focal deficit. The examination may be variable over time because of the fluctuating nature of the disease process. Specific domains of the neurologic examination for MS evaluation are as follows:

- Mental status: Observe for general conversation, fluidity of speech, speed of thought processing, integration of complex ideas, and following of multistep or complex directions. Neuropsychiatric testing is sensitive in elucidating cognitive issues associated with MS. It can also serve as a baseline for comparison over time.
- Cranial nerves (CNs): Extraocular movements (EOMs) should be assessed for conjugate movement, nystagmus, and intranuclear ophthalmoplegia; these may cause symptoms of diplopia. Vertigo may be experienced with EOM testing. Ophthalmic examination may reveal disc pallor, often seen with optic neuritis. The trigeminal nerve may reveal allodynia, common in trigeminal neuralgia, and a central seventh

CN deficit may reflect a CNS lesion. The remaining CNs should also be examined because deficit may be seen in any CN, with the aforementioned being the most common.

- Motor testing may reveal weakness of a limb or more subtle weakness—for example, clumsiness of the hand and decreased fine dexterity. In the lower extremities, subtle plantar flexion or dorsiflexion weakness may be seen. The patient may drag the foot or trip on it frequently with ambulation and complain of falls or loss of balance when in fact it is a result of weakness. Increased tone and clonus in muscles should be assessed with passive range of motion. Gait should be evaluated to include evidence of circumduction, spasticity, or ataxia.
- Timed 25-foot walk test (T25FW) is becoming commonplace as part of the MS evaluation.[15]
- Sensory examination should focus on pinprick, proprioception, and vibration testing to determine long-tract involvement. Patients may also have a distinct sensory level indicating spinal cord involvement, especially if transverse myelitis is suspected.
- Cerebellar: Finger-to-nose and Romberg testing can identify cerebellar involvement. Often, the patient will have an ataxic gait as well.
- Reflexes are often brisk with upgoing toes, consistent with CNS involvement.

In a patient with known MS, having a documented neurologic and functional baseline is imperative for the evaluation of response to treatment or possible exacerbation of the disease. New neurologic findings can be mild or subtle yet result in significant functional deficits. Functional areas to review or examine might include driving, falls and injuries, and difficulties in the work arena, interpersonal skills, financial capabilities, and activities of daily living (ADLs). The Expanded

TABLE 180.1   Symptomatic and Rehabilitative Therapies for Multiple Sclerosis[a]

Symptom	Description	Treatment Modalities
Ataxia	Incoordination and disturbance of balance and gait Worsened by spasticity, weakness, and fatigue Falls common	Home evaluation necessary to assess safety and fall risk Rehabilitation services for gait and balance; may work with balance balls and other techniques Medications ineffective Avoid alcohol
Bladder	Bladder: hesitancy, urgency, frequency incontinence; reported rates 52%–97%	Bladder: avoid dietary irritants such as caffeine and spicy foods; use toileting schedule; refer to urologist for formal workup; screen for UTI; fluid restriction at bedtime; biofeedback and Kegel exercises; clean intermittent catheterization; botulinum toxin; nerve stimulation devices *Drug therapy:* anticholinergics, antimuscarinics, and α-blockers
Bowel	Bowel: irregular bowel is common; constipation, loose stools; constipation may aggravate bladder issues; reported rates 35%–68%	Bowel: fiber, stool softeners, laxatives, glycerin suppositories; bowel training programs, diet counseling, exercise *Drug therapy:* anticholinergic or muscle relaxant properties, such as oxybutynin, tolterodine, propantheline, antidiuretic hormone; botulinum toxin injections
Cognitive dysfunction	40%–70% of MS patients have some degree of cognitive impairment; executive functioning and memory are most common Can be a source of disability	Neuropsychological evaluation is important to define problem areas and provide recommendations; compensatory and restorative methods can be helpful; brain exercises such as those on Lumocity.com and CogMed.com Treat underlying disorders that can contribute to problem, such as depression, anxiety, fatigue, sleep disorders Adherence to DMT; some have been shown to slow cognitive decline *Drug therapy:* acetylcholinesterase inhibitors have not been found effective in larger studies

Continued

TABLE 180.1   **Symptomatic and Rehabilitative Therapies for Multiple Sclerosis—cont'd**

Symptom	Description	Treatment Modalities
Depression	Endogenous as a result of changes in brain chemistry; may also be exogenous; higher incidence (56%) and rates of suicide than in other chronic or neurologic diseases	Antidepressants Counseling
Fatigue	Rates reported to be 65%–97% Highly debilitating; often the reason for disability Cause unknown Aggravated by depression, anemia, hypothyroidism, sleep disorder, elevated core body temperature	OT for energy conservation techniques Cooling vest or cap Staying well hydrated and drinking ice-cold water to bring down core body temperature Avoidance of heat Treat underlying problems Consider changing DMT if severe; glatiramer acetate may have less effect on fatigue than interferons *Drug therapy:* amantadine, methylphenidate, modafinil, armodafinil, fluoxetine (even if depression is not present)
Pain and paresthesias	Reported rates as high as 85% Trigeminal neuralgia and other forms of neuropathic pain (burning, numbness, tingling), migraines, spasms, musculoskeletal pain	Pain from spasms relieved with antispasmodics (discussed previously) PT and assistive devices Yoga, Pilates, tai chi for musculoskeletal pain *Drug therapy:* neuropathic pain—carbamazepine, gabapentin, pregabalin, topiramate, lamotrigine, lidocaine patch, duloxetine, tricyclic antidepressants; musculoskeletal pain—gabapentin, lidocaine patch, duloxetine, NSAIDs, muscle relaxants
Sexual dysfunction	Up to 90% in men and 85% in women Lack of interest or arousal Changes in self-esteem Problems with intimacy Impotence, anorgasmia, vaginal dryness Decreased or altered sensations Functional difficulties: spasms, bladder control	Try to coordinate symptomatic treatments to sexual activity (antispasmodics, self-catheterization); increased stimulation using vibration can be helpful; counseling may be necessary *Drug therapy:* erectile dysfunction medications for men, such as tadalafil, vardenafil, sildenafil citrate; remove offending medications if possible, such as SSRIs
Spasticity	Reported rates: 40%–85% Stiff, slow movements; spasms	PT and assistive devices Yoga, Pilates, tai chi *Drug therapy:* baclofen intrathecal pump implantation; botulinum toxin injection; baclofen (Lioresal), tizanidine, dantrolene (Dantrium), benzodiazepine, gabapentin, levetiracetam
Tremor	May involve UE, LE, trunk, head, and voice and may be incapacitating Very difficult symptom to manage	OT help with weighted equipment and environmental modification strategies Deep brain stimulation can be considered and can be very effective for controlling tremor but is not FDA approved for MS tremor at this time. *Drug therapy:* most drugs are ineffective for MS tremor; some drugs that have been tried with limited success include propranolol and other β-blockers, clonazepam, primidone, ondansetron, isoniazid, and glutethimide
Weakness	Focal limb weakness caused by underlying demyelination and axonal loss	Rehabilitation services for strength training and adaptive devices such as braces and ambulatory assistive devices Keep core body temperature down; heat disrupts conduction For footdrop, ankle-foot orthoses can be helpful; WalkAide and Biomes systems, functional electrical stimulation devices, have been beneficial *Drug therapy:* dalfampridine, a potassium channel blocker, has recently been approved by the FDA to improve walking in MS; it is the only drug in its class

[a]Many medications used for MS symptoms are used off label.

DMT, Disease-modifying therapy; *LE,* lower extremity; *MS,* multiple sclerosis; *NSAIDs,* nonsteroidal antiinflammatory drugs; *OT,* occupational therapy; *PT,* physical therapy; *SSRIs,* selective serotonin reuptake inhibitors; *UE,* upper extremity; *UTI,* urinary tract infection.

Data from Moses, H. Jr, Picone, M., & Smith, V. (2008). *Clinician's primer on multiple sclerosis: An in-depth overview.* Denver, CO: Consensus Medical Communications; Bennett, S., & Coyle, P. (2010). *The clinician's primer on the latest advances in improved quality of life for patients with multiple sclerosis.* Denver, CO: Consensus Medical Communications; Thompson, H., & Mauk, K. (2011). Nursing management of the patient with multiple sclerosis: AANN, ARN, and IOMSN clinical practice guideline series. American Association of Neuroscience nurses, Association of Rehabilitation Nurses, and International Organization of Multiple Sclerosis Nurses. <www.rehabnurse.org/uploads/cpgms.pdf> Accessed 13.10.15. Polman, C. H., Reingold, S. C., Edan, G., et al. (2011). Diagnostic criteria for multiple sclerosis: 2010 revisions to the "McDonald Criteria." *Annals of Neurology, 69,* 292–302; and Toosy, A., Ciccarelli, O., & Thompson, A. (2014). Symptomatic treatment and management of multiple sclerosis. In D. S. Goodin (Ed.), *Handbook of clinical neurology,* Vol. 122, *Multiple sclerosis and related disorders,* Amsterdam: Elsevier B.V.

Disability Severity Scale (EDSS), Fatigue Severity Scale (FSS), 12-item MS Walking Scale (MSWS-12), and T25FW can help supply quantitative support for functional limitations.[16-20]

DIAGNOSTICS

MS is still a clinical diagnosis. There must be separation of time and space. Events must be at least two distinct episodes lasting more than 24 hours occurring at least 30 days apart (separation of time), and there must be evidence of at least two different locations (separation of space). Signs and symptoms need to be consistent with inflammatory demyelinating disease. No other pathologic process can be found for clinical and paraclinical findings.[4]

Ruling out other pathologic processes is essential. Historically this has been done by clinical history, examination, and diagnostic studies. **MRI** has revolutionized the diagnosis of MS and has become the gold standard for diagnosis of MS via the McDonald criteria.[4] The McDonald criteria were introduced in 2001 and underwent revisions in 2005, 2010, and most recently in 2017.[4,19] Diagnostic studies such as visual evoked potentials, optical coherence tomography (OCT), spinal tap, and blood work are still useful when diagnosis is unclear or if MRI is not readily available.[19-21]

INITIAL DIAGNOSTICS

Multiple Sclerosis

LABORATORY
- None

IMAGING
- MRI with gadolinium (Consortium of Multiple Sclerosis Centers [CMSC] protocol recommended)[20]

ADDITIONAL DIAGNOSTICS[a]

Laboratory
- Complete blood count with differential
- Antinuclear antibodies
- Erythrocyte sedimentation rate
- Fluorescent treponemal antibody absorption test (FTA-ABS) or Venereal Disease Research Laboratory (VDRL) test
- Human immunodeficiency virus (HIV) test
- Antiphospholipid antibodies
- Prothrombin time/partial thromboplastin time (PT/PTT)
- Rheumatoid factor
- Angiotensin-converting enzyme
- Thyroid-stimulating hormone (TSH)
- Vitamin D
- Lyme titer
- Vitamin B_{12} level

Imaging
- Brain, cervical spine, thoracic spine
- Lumbar spine

Additional Studies
- Visual evoked potentials
- Optical coherence tomography
- Lumbar puncture with cerebrospinal fluid analysis:
  - Tube 1: protein, glucose, VDRL, cell count and differential
  - Tube 2: cryptococcal antigen, India ink; fungal cultures; acid-fast bacillus (AFB) stain
  - Tube 3: Gram stain and culture; cell count and differential
  - Tube 4: MS profile, Lyme titer

[a]if indicated.

DIFFERENTIAL DIAGNOSIS

 Primary differentials to consider include tumors, cerebral vascular events, encephalitis, toxic exposure, or metabolic deficiency.

 Consultation with a neurologist, MS neurology expert, or MS center should be considered for confirmation of diagnosis.

See Box 180.2 for an extensive list of differential diagnoses.

INTERPROFESSIONAL COLLABORATIVE MANAGEMENT

 Neurologists and MS specialist consultations are recommended for initial evaluation and initial prescription of DMT; MS exacerbation; and difficult-to-manage symptoms.

The goals of management are both multifaceted and complex. They include management of the disease itself, management of the symptoms, and maximization of quality of life for the patient and patient's family system.

A comprehensive approach is essential to the management of MS. This is accomplished through a partnership with the patient, the patient's family system, and a collaborative care team (CCT). The CCT consists of a neurologist, advanced practice nurse, physician assistant, and/or a center that *specializes* in MS. Other members of the team may include a primary care physician, internists, urologists, gynecologists, orthopedists, ophthalmologists, physiatrists, nurses, social workers, physical therapists, occupational therapists, speech language pathologists, recreation therapists, psychologists, and neuropsychologists. Team members should have a special interest or specialization in MS. Referral to team members will be variable, depending on patient symptoms and needs and availability of resources within the community.[20]
- The management of care in the long term may have the neurology specialist take the role of primary manager, with

---

BOX 180.2

Differential Diagnosis: Multiple Sclerosis

Structural or anatomic: Myelopathy or tumors, especially lymphoma or glioma of brain or spinal cord

Psychiatric disorder

Toxin exposure

Vascular: Cerebrovascular accident (CVA), arteriovenous malformation (AVM), cerebral autosomal-dominant arteriopathy with subcortical infarcts and leukoencephalopathy (CADASIL)

Metabolic: Vitamin B_{12} deficiency, vitamin D deficiency, adrenoleukodystrophy, mitochondrial disorders

Genetic: Friedreich ataxia, olivopontocerebellar atrophies, hereditary spastic paraparesis

Infectious: Lyme disease, syphilis, progressive multifocal leukoencephalopathy, human T-lymphotropic virus 1 (HTLV-1) or HIV infection

Inflammatory: Rheumatoid arthritis, systemic lupus erythematosus, Sjögren syndrome, vasculitis, sarcoidosis, Behçet disease

Other MS variants: Neuromyelitis optica (Devic disease), acute disseminated encephalomyelitis, Marburg variant of MS, Baló concentric sclerosis medical issues deferred to the primary care provider (PCP). In other cases, the PCP may remain the primary manager, with the neurology specialist having a more consultative role. Regardless, a team approach is needed to maintain the quality of life and wellness for the MS patient and the entire support system.

The CCT works to empower the person with MS by encouraging an active role in developing and implementing the plan of care. The care plan focuses not only on what occurs within the health care arena but also in the home, workplace, and community to maximize function and enhance the quality of life. This is a dynamic process, given the ever-changing landscape of people with MS.[20]

Multiple networks offer a vast array of resources for care providers and patients, including current research, treatment and care guidelines, and educational programs.

Management includes the following:

1. Education—helping the patient to understand the diagnosis and the importance of early treatment with DMTs: All DMTs have three goals: to decrease the exacerbation rate, to decrease MRI activity, and to slow the progression of disability.

2. DMT initiation: DMT initiation starts as early as possible with the first presentation of, usually, CIS. DMTs are often classified based on methods of administration: injectable, infusible, and oral. The injectable DMTs are frequently referred to as platform therapies. The safety and efficacy of injectable DMTs over time have been well established. Injectable DMTs include interferons (Betaseron, Extavia, Avonex, Plegridy, and Rebif) and glatiramer acetate (Copaxone). The interferons have a similar biologic activity and adverse event profile. Patients should be monitored for depression while receiving treatment. Liver enzymes and hematologic profiles also need to be monitored.[21-25] Glatiramer acetate (Copaxone) is a synthetic protein; there are no depression, liver, or hematologic concerns.[26]

• Infusible DMTs include mitoxantrone (Novantrone) and natalizumab (Tysabri). Mitoxantrone (Novantrone), an antineoplastic agent, was approved in October 2000 for the treatment of SPMS, worsening RRMS, and PRMS. The administration of mitoxantrone requires careful cardiac evaluation and monitoring, even years after the medication has been discontinued. It also carries a lifetime accumulated dose limit because of the risk of cardiac toxicity.[27] Leukemia is also a serious side effect seen over time. Because of these issues, it is not commonly used.

• Natalizumab (Tysabri) is a monoclonal antibody with immunosuppressant effect that appeared promising in active clinical trials. However, it was recalled from the market in February 2005 after three reported cases (two fatal) of PML. After much study, the US Food and Drug Administration (FDA), in March 2006, allowed it to return to the market under strict monitoring guidelines. It is approved for the first-line use by the FDA; however, in general, it is recommended for patients with inadequate responses to other first-line therapies with less aggressive risk profiles or for patients unable to tolerate other MS therapies.[28] A documented increased risk of PML exists, and this drug should not be used in conjunction with other MS drugs.

• There are now three oral therapies available for the treatment of MS: fingolimod (Gilenya), teriflunomide (Aubagio), and dimethyl fumarate (Tecfidera). All three work by reducing circulating inflammatory lymphocytes outside the CNS. Each works by a different mechanism of action (MOA) and carries its own set of risks and side effects that need to be evaluated on a patient-by-patient basis.

• Other agents and treatments that exert immunosuppressant or immunomodulating effects have been prescribed in MS, which include azathioprine (Imuran), methotrexate (Rheumatrex), rituximab (Rituxan), cyclophosphamide (Cytoxan), mycophenolate mofetil (CellCept), plasmapheresis, and intravenous immune globulin (IVIG). These are used off label and have varying degrees of reported efficacy.[9,13,29] Approaches for neuroprotection, remyelination, and neural stem cell transplantation remain a topic of interest and research.[9]

• Vitamin D has been of great interest. Genetics has confirmed that hypovitaminosis D is one of the risk factors for MS. The main MOA of vitamin D in MS appears to be immunomodulatory.[30] Current research indicates that therapeutic levels of vitamin D have a beneficial effect on MS. A definitive target vitamin D level has still not been determined. It has been suggested that a midrange level of 60 to 80 ng/mL is reasonable, but this may change with continued research.

• A low-sodium diet and smoking cessation have been shown to have a positive effect on both progression and disease severity of MS.[4,5]

• Treatment of an exacerbation: Most MS exacerbations are handled on an outpatient basis. Hospitalization may be necessary if significant self-care deficits arise, or if there are complications or concomitant infection or illness needing further clarification and management.

The goal is to minimize the duration of the inflammation to incur fewer lasting deficits. Exacerbation is defined as the acute onset of neurologic symptom(s), lasting longer than 24 hours, which are preceded by a period of at least 30 days of clinical stability or improvement and have no underlying causes such as infection.[18] Exacerbations produce sustained effects on disability.[18] Treatment typically involves the use of high-dose intravenous steroids for a short period or adrenocorticotropic hormone (ACTH). Corticosteroids are used in MS for the management of acute exacerbations because they downregulate the inflammatory lymphocytes outside the CNS and have the capacity to close the damaged blood–brain barrier, subsequently reducing inflammation in the CNS. Steroids are typically administered during the course of several days and may or may not be followed by a slower oral taper of these drugs.[31]

• ACTH (Acthar) is given as a daily injection (subcutaneous or intramuscular) for up to 21 days. It downregulates inflammation both peripherally and centrally through the corticosteroid-independent melanocortin pathway.[32,33]

Postexacerbation: After an exacerbation, a course of rehabilitation is undertaken to address any new deficits or functional loss as well as to improve and maintain overall physical fitness.[8,9,13] Table 180.1 shows treatment options and rehabilitative therapies for some of the more common MS symptoms.

LIFE SPAN CONSIDERATIONS

In some situations, a diagnosis of MS is actually followed by relief, especially for patients who have spent years experiencing strange symptoms and have coped with vague diagnoses or even outright skepticism. For others, the diagnosis is difficult; the variable clinical course of MS leads to an uncertain and unpredictable future. Natural history studies show that many people with MS are still capable of ambulation and regular employment for 15 to 20 years after diagnosis. Life span is shortened by approximately 7 years compared with that of the general population. All routine health screening and treatments should continue as recommended, and life planning such as retirement should continue after diagnosis. Several factors are associated with a favorable prognosis: female gender, age at disease onset younger than 40 years, sensory symptoms as presenting episode, optic neuritis as an isolated first symptom, minor abnormalities on the brain MRI at the time of diagnosis, complete or almost complete recovery after exacerbation, and long periods between exacerbations.[1,8]

Pregnancy seems to have a neuroprotective effect. Acute exacerbation is common up to 6 months after delivery. Research has demonstrated that this does not tend to affect long-term outcome.[34] The use of DMTs is not recommended during pregnancy or while breastfeeding. If possible, it is generally recommended for women to stop DMT treatment 3 months before actively trying to conceive. A 3-month washout is also recommended for men on teriflunomide and mitoxantrone.

Ambulatory dysfunction, fatigue, and cognitive impairment are the biggest contributors to loss of employment for patients with MS.[35]

- Patients with MS are at a higher risk for development of other autoimmune diseases, such as thyroid disease, diabetes, and rheumatoid arthritis, as well as osteoporosis, sleep disorders, frequent urinary tract infections, pressure ulcers, obesity, substance use, and depression. These diseases and conditions should be screened for and treated as indicated.[18,19] Primary care has a strong role related to screening and management of other disease processes among MS patients.

PATIENT AND FAMILY EDUCATION

The diagnosis of MS can be overwhelming for patients and families. Considerable support and education about the disease process, its variability, and available therapies are essential. A message of hope should be conveyed to people with disabilities, with an emphasis on maintaining quality of life. The PCP should emphasize the benefits of DMT such as delay in disability, reduced frequency of clinical exacerbations, and reduced MRI activity. Encouraging adherence to DMT regimens and symptomatic treatment can help optimize quality of life. This will have an immediate effect, offering symptomatic relief, improving functioning, and helping in defining an internal locus of control. Long-term benefits of adherence include promotion of self-efficacy and decrease in disability progression. Realistic expectation of treatment along with management of side effects must also be emphasized.

In addition to DMTs and symptomatic treatment, the health care provider should focus on raising awareness and promoting health, wellness, and safety regimens. This includes regular preventive health care visits, exercise, diet, lifestyle modifications, smoking cessation, and avoidance of drug and alcohol abuse. Driving evaluations may be needed. Community support groups may also be helpful.

Comprehensive issues should include balancing "normalcy" with the demands and challenges of living with a chronic and ever-changing disease, family planning, coping skills, caregiver issues, family systems, and relationship issues. Concerns about confidentiality, insurance, employment, and disability issues should also be addressed.[16,27]

The family and patients should be reminded that MS is frequently likened to a marathon, not a sprint. They need information and support to help them make the best decisions for their futures. The future of MS is promising.

RESOURCES

MS Views and News
  www.msviewsandnews.org
MS World
  www.msworld.org
Multiple Sclerosis Association of America
  https://mymsaa.org/
  800-532-7667
Multiple Sclerosis Foundation
  www.msfocus.org
  888-MSFOCUS
National Multiple Sclerosis Society
  www.nationalmssociety.org
  800-344-4867

REFERENCES

1. Compston, A., & Coles, A. (2008). Multiple sclerosis. *Lancet, 372,* 1502–1517.
2. Moses, H., Jr., Picone, M., & Smith, V. (2008). *Clinician's primer on multiple sclerosis: An in depth overview.* Denver, CO: Consensus Medical Communications.
3. Bennet, S., & Coyle, P. (2008). *The clinician's primer on the latest advances in improved quality for patients with multiple sclerosis.* Denver, CO: Consensus Medical Communications.
4. Milo, R., & Miller, A. (2014). Revised diagnostic criteria of multiple sclerosis. *Autoimmunity Reviews, 13,* 518–524.
5. Kamm, C., Uitdchaag, B., et al. (2014). Multiple sclerosis: Current knowledge and future outlook. *European Neurology, 72,* 132–140.
6. Van der Mei, I., Simpson, J. S., et al. (2011). Individual and joint action of environmental factors and risk of MS. *Neurologic Clinics, 29*(9), 233–255.
7. Godin, D. (2014). The epidemiology of multiple sclerosis: Insights to disease pathogenesis. In M. Aminoff, F. Boller, & D. Swaab (Eds.), *Handbook of clinical neurology* (Vol. 122, 3rd series). Elsevier.
8. Costella, K., Halper, J., et al. (2014). The use of disease-modifying therapy in multiple sclerosis: Principles and current evidence. *MS Coalition.* Retrieved from www.mscare.org. (Accessed 13 October 2015).
9. Ontaneda, D., Thompson, A., Fox, R., & Cohen, J. (2017). Progressive multiple sclerosis: Prospects for disease therapy, repair and restoration of function. *The Lancet, 389*(10076), 1357–1366.
10. Thompson, A. J., Banwell, B. L., & Barkhof, F. (2018). Diagnosis of multiple sclerosis: 2017 revisions of the McDonald criteria. *The Lancet. Neurology, 17*(2), 162–173.
11. Fillippi, M., Rossa, M. A., Ciccarelli, O., et al. (2016). MRI criteria for the diagnosis of multiple sclerosis: MAGNIMS consensus guidelines. *The Lancet. Neurology, 15,* 292–303.
12. Leahy, H., & Garg, N. (2013). Radiologically isolated syndrome: An overview. *Neurological Bulletin, 5,* 22–26.
13. Thompson, H., & Mauk, K., Eds. (2011). Nursing management of the patient with multiple sclerosis. AANN, ARN and IOMSN clinical practice guideline series. American Association of Neuroscience Nurses, Association of Rehabilitation Nurses, International Organization of Multiple Sclerosis Nurses. Retrieved from www.rehabnurses.org/uploads/cpgms.pdf. (Accessed 13 October 2015).
14. Toosy, A., Ciccarelli, O., & Thompson, A. (2014). Symptomatic treatment and management of multiple sclerosis. In M. Aminoff, F. Boller, & D. Swaab (Eds.), *Handbook of clinical neurology* (Vol. 122, 3rd series). Elsevier. Multiple sclerosis and related disorders. Goode DS, editor.
15. Motl, R. W., Cohen, J. A., Benedict, R., Phillips, G., LaRocca, N., Hudson, L. D., et al. (2017). Multiple Sclerosis Outcome Assessments Consortium. Validity of the timed 25-foot walk as an ambulatory performance outcome measure for multiple sclerosis. *Multiple Sclerosis (Houndmills, Basingstoke, England), 23*(5), 704–710. doi:10.1177/1352458517690823. [Epub 2017 Feb 16]; PubMed PMID: 28206828. PubMed Central PMCID: PMC5405807.

16. Cioncoloni, D., Iglis, I., et al. (2014). Individual factors enhance poor health-related quality of life outcome in multiple sclerosis patients. Significance of predictive determinants. *Journal of the Neurological Sciences, 345,* 213–219.

17. Goodin, D., Reder, A., Bermei, R., et al. (2016). Relapses in multiple sclerosis: Relationship to disability. *Multiple Sclerosis and Related Diseases, 6,* 10–20.

18. Thompson, A., Banwell, B., Barkhof, F., et al. (2018). Diagnosis of multiple sclerosis: 2017 revisions of the McDonald Criteria. *The Lancet. Neurology, 17*(2), 162–173.

19. Uitdehaag, B. (2014). Clinical outcome measures in multiple sclerosis. In M. Aminoff, F. Boller, & D. Swaab (Eds.), *Handbook of clinical neurology* (Vol. 122, 3rd series). Elsevier B.V. Multiple sclerosis and related disorders. D.S. Goodin, Editor.

20. Consortium of Multiple Sclerosis Centers (CMSC). (2009). MRI protocol for the diagnosis and follow-up of MS: 2009 revised guidelines, CMSC. www.mscare.org. (Accessed 1 March 2015).

21. Avonex (interferon beta-1a) medication guide. Biogen Idec. (2013). www.avonex.com/pdfs/guides/Avonex_Prescribing_Information.pdf.

22. Rebif (interferon beta-1a) medication guide. (2014). EMD Serono, Pfizer.

23. Betaseron (interferon beta-1b) Bayer Healthcare Pharmaceuticals. (2014). http://labeling.bayerhealthcare.com/html/products/pi/Betaseron_PI.pdf. (Accessed 13 October 2015).

24. Plegridy (interferon beta-1a) Biogen Idec. (2014). www.accessdata.fda.gov/drugsatfda_docs/label/2014/125499s000lbl.pdf. (Accessed 13 October 2015).

25. Extavia (interferon beta-1b) Novartis. (2012). http://www.pharma.us.novartis.com/product/pi/pdf/extavia.pdf. (Accessed 13 October 2015).

26. Copaxone (glatiramer acetate) medication guide. (2014). Teva Neuroscience.

27. Novantrone (mitoxantrone) medication guide. (2012). EMD Serono.

28. Tysabri (natalizumab) medication guide. (2013). Biogen Idec, Elan Pharmaceuticals.

29. Okuda, D. (2014). Immunosuppressive treatments in multiple sclerosis. n M. Aminoff, F. Boller, & D. Swaab (Eds.), *Handbook of clinical neurology* (Vol. 122, third series). Elsevier.

30. Pierrot-Deseilligny, C., & Souberbielle, J.-C. (2017). Vitamin D and multiple sclerosis: An update. *Multiple Sclerosis and Related Disorders, 14,* 35–45.

31. Stettler, B. (2018). *Brain and cranial nerve disorders in Rosen's emergency medicine: Concepts and Clinical Practice 9e.* Elsevier.

32. Arnason, B., Berkovich, R., Catania, A., et al. (2013). Mechanisms of action of adrenocorticotropic hormone and other melanocortins relevant to the clinical management of patients with multiple sclerosis. *Multiple Sclerosis (Houndmills, Basingstoke, England), 19*(2), 130–136.

33. Goodin, D. (2014). Glucocorticoid treatment of multiple sclerosis. In M. Aminoff, F. Boller, & D. Swaab (Eds.), *Handbook of clinical neurology* (Vol. 122, third series). Elsevier.

34. Fabian, M., Krieger, S., & Lublin, F. (2016). *Multiple sclerosis and other inflammatory demyelinating diseases of the central nervous system in Bradley's Neurology in Clinical Practice 7e.* Elsevier.

35. Kalb, R., & Reitman, N. (2012). Multiple sclerosis: a model of psychosocial support. 5th ed. National Multiple Sclerosis Society. www.nationalmssociety.org/NationalMSSociety/media/MSNationalFiles/Brochures/Psychosocial-Cavallo-5th-Edition_Final-Links.pdf. (Accessed 1 March 2015).

CHAPTER **181**

PARKINSON DISEASE

Lindsay M. Schommer

DEFINITION AND EPIDEMIOLOGY

Parkinson disease (PD) is a slowly progressive neurodegenerative disease. The insidious onset includes cardinal features of asymmetric resting tremor, bradykinesia, and rigidity, commonly with postural changes. It is the second most common neurodegenerative disease in the world, after Alzheimer disease, affecting approximately 5 million people. The prevalence of PD is thought to be 0.3% in the general population, increasing from 1% among those aged above 60 years to 4% in those older than 80 years. Mean age at diagnosis is 70.5 years, with a rapid increase in incidence after the age of 65 years. PD

BOX **181.1**

Risk Factors for Developing Parkinson Disease

- Family history of Parkinson disease—associated with specific genes and genetic loci[4]
- Exposure to pesticides[2,5]
- History of head trauma resulting in concussion[2,6]
- Living in urban or industrial areas with high release of copper, manganese, or lead[7]
- Exposure to hydrocarbon solvents, particularly trichloroethylene[2,8]
- Living in rural area, farming or agricultural work, use of well water[5]
- Milk consumption[2,9]
- High dietary intake of iron with high intake of manganese[10]
- Excess body weight[11]
- History of anemia[12]

---

is uncommon in those younger than 40 years. The incidence is 8 to 18.6 new cases per 100,000 person-years. Studies reveal that there are 50% more men with PD than women.[1-3] The risk for development of PD appears to double if a first-degree relative has PD compared with people in the general population (Box 181.1).[2,3]

Traditionally considered a motor system disorder, PD is now recognized to be a complex disorder with diverse features. Those who develop PD may be affected by neuropsychiatric and other nonmotor manifestations in addition to cardinal motor features described above.[13] The specific mechanisms of the neurodegeneration of PD are not understood. It is most likely caused by a cascade of events associated with genetic and environmental factors,[5,14] abnormalities in protein processing,[15] oxidative stress,[4] mitochondrial dysfunction,[6] inflammation and immune regulation, and other mechanisms. Purely genetic Parkinson varieties probably affect a small minority of people with the *parkin* gene on chromosome 6.[14]

PATHOPHYSIOLOGY

PD develops after widespread depletion of dopamine in the substantia nigra and the nigrostriatal pathway to the caudate and putamen. Depigmentation, neuronal loss, and gliosis are most significant in the substantia nigra pars compacta and the pontine locus ceruleus. This dopamine depletion ultimately results in increased inhibition of the thalamus and reduced excitatory input to the motor cortex, which results in the cardinal features of PD, such as tremor at rest, rigidity, bradykinesia, and postural instability. Compensatory mechanisms, including the large number of acetylcholine-secreting neurons with excitatory signals that remain active in the presymptomatic phase of PD, mask the deleterious effects of dopamine depletion.[16]

CLINICAL PRESENTATION AND PHYSICAL EXAMINATION

The clinical features most suggestive of PD are asymmetric or unilateral tremor, rigidity, bradykinesia with freezing, and flexed posture with loss of postural reflexes. Some investigators have postulated that there are clinically defined subgroups or subtypes that may affect the rate of progression of PD. The subtypes are tremor dominant, akinetic-rigid, and postural instability and gait difficulty. Rest tremor in PD is present at rest, is usually unilateral at first, and characteristically disappears with action. Rest tremor of the hands, described as "pill rolling," increases with walking and may be an early sign when others are not yet present. Most often, patients with PD exhibit a slow, coarse tremor with a rate varying from two to five oscillations per second, usually averaging four or five oscillations per second when the hand is motionless and decreasing with postural changes. There is a clear distinction from essential or intention tremors, which appear only or primarily with deliberate, willed movement.[17]

Another classic sign is rigidity, an increased resistance to passive movement at a joint, which occurs in 90% of patients with PD. The increased resistance to passive movement is equal in all directions and usually manifests with a ratcheting or "cogwheeling" during the movement. Rigidity of the passive limb increases when another limb is engaged in voluntary active movements.[18]

The patient with PD often has a uniquely flexed posture involving the entire body. The head is bowed, the trunk is bent forward, the back is kyphotic, the hands are held in front of the body, and the elbows, hips, and knees are flexed. Deformities of the hands and feet may also be apparent. Lateral tilting of the trunk is common.[18]

Other features of PD are associated with slowness of movement (hypokinesia), loss of automatic movement (bradykinesia), and difficulty initiating movement (freezing) or an irresistible impulse to take much quicker and shorter steps, which creates an almost running pace (festination). Shuffling gait with a decrease in arm swing may be evident. Masked facies (a reduction in spontaneous facial expression) and decreased frequency of blinking are prevalent. Speech becomes soft (hypophonia), and the voice often has a monotonous tone with lack of inflection (aprosody of speech). Some patients are not able to enunciate clearly (dysarthria) or may experience repetition of syllables (palilalia). All of these features clearly respond to treatment with levodopa, which is considered both diagnostic and therapeutic.[18]

PHYSICAL EXAMINATION

Postural reflexes can be tested by giving a sudden, firm pull on the shoulders from behind, but the health care provider should be prepared to catch the patient. Rigidity, demonstrated by cogwheeling, may be tested by grasping the patient's elbow at the antecubital region and slowly flexing and extending the elbow or pronating-supinating the forearm. Walking can also be marked by festination, whereby the patient walks faster with short steps, trying to move the feet forward under the flexed body's center of gravity.[18]

The freezing phenomenon, a motor block, is a transient inability to perform active movements. It most often affects the legs but can involve eyelid opening, speaking, and writing. The feet may appear to be glued to the ground. Because patients with PD exhibit an increased ability to perform intentional or conscious movement as opposed to automatic movement, freezing can be overcome by having patients intentionally raise their legs as if stepping over objects or cycling. Despite severe bradykinesia with marked immobility, patients with PD may rise suddenly and move normally for a short burst of motor activity when physically cued (kinesia paradoxa).[19]

DIAGNOSTICS

Diagnostic studies are usually not indicated. There are no physiologic tests or blood tests, and neuroimaging is helpful only in differentiation of PD from other neurodegenerative disorders and requires specific neuroimaging, best identified by neurologic specialists. The "gold standard" for diagnosis is postmortem neuropathologic examination, especially noting midbrain Lewy bodies. Diagnosis of idiopathic PD is based on clinical presentation and physical examination findings, with two of the three cardinal manifestations (tremor, bradykinesia, and rigidity) present. A rest tremor with unilateral onset and excellent response to dopaminergic therapy are important criteria for the diagnosis of idiopathic PD.[20,21]

DIFFERENTIAL DIAGNOSIS

The signs and symptoms of idiopathic PD can occur in other neurodegenerative disorders, including essential tremor see Chapter 179, dementia with Lewy bodies, corticobasal degeneration, multiple system atrophy, and progressive supranuclear palsy. Secondary parkinsonism is seen in the presence of drug reactions (neuroleptics), infections (postencephalitic), metabolic disorders (parathyroid disorders), posttraumatic conditions, neoplastic disorders, toxicity (carbon monoxide), and vascular disorders. As previously noted, the diagnosis of PD and other forms of parkinsonism is often based on the response to levodopa, although this is no longer recommended.[21] Bradykinesia and rigidity respond best, but lack of improvement does not exclude the diagnosis of PD. Tremor may never respond satisfactorily.

DIAGNOSTICS

Features Suggesting an Alternative Diagnosis

- Falls at presentation or early in the course of the disease
- Poor response to levodopa
- Symmetric motor signs
- Rapid progression to Hoehn and Yahr stage 3 with mild to moderate disease and some postural instability, but physically dependent
- Lack of tremor
- Dysautonomia early in the disease course, manifesting with urinary urgency or incontinence and fecal incontinence, urinary retention requiring catheterization, persistent erectile failure, or symptomatic orthostatic hypotension[19,20]

INTERPROFESSIONAL COLLABORATIVE MANAGEMENT

Judicious selection of symptomatic treatment options can alleviate symptoms and maximize functional ability, but none have been shown to slow the progression of the disease. Treatment is individualized because each patient has a unique set of signs and symptoms; the patient's response to medications and social, occupational, and emotional needs must be considered.

The goal is to maintain independence and functional ability for as long as possible. An algorithm for the management of PD that includes pharmacologic, nonpharmacologic, and surgical treatments is most useful.[22] Drug treatment acts in one of two ways: to increase the functional ability of the underactive dopaminergic system or to reduce the excessive influence of the excitatory cholinergic neurons. The decision to initiate medical therapy is determined by the degree of functional impairment. Important factors include the effect of disease on the dominant hand and the degree of interference with work, activities of daily living, and social and leisure function.[23]

Pharmacologic Management

Selegiline. Selegiline (Eldepryl), a selective monoamine oxidase type B inhibitor, may have neuroprotective properties and can be modestly effective in treatment. Selegiline may delay the destruction of the nigral neurons and inhibit the metabolic breakdown of dopamine. As monotherapy, it does not produce any functional benefit. Some randomly controlled trials have demonstrated the benefit of selegiline in delaying the need for levodopa for an average of 9 months if it is used for patients with early PD.[23] Adverse side effects and contraindications to administration and monitoring of selegiline should be noted. When it is given concurrently with levodopa, selegiline can increase the dopaminergic effect and contribute to dopaminergic toxicity. A maximum dose is currently considered to be 5 mg twice daily. An oral disintegrating tablet is available with a slightly lower dosage schedule.

Levodopa. Levodopa is the most effective drug for the symptomatic treatment of PD. It is particularly effective for akinetic symptoms. Tremor and rigidity can respond to levodopa, but postural instability is less likely to respond. Levodopa treatment is aimed at restoration of the amount of dopamine reaching the basal ganglia. Unfortunately dopamine does not cross the blood-brain barrier; thus its precursor, levodopa, must be given. Levodopa is metabolized both peripherally and centrally. The peripheral metabolism is responsible for the majority of side effects. Sinemet combines levodopa with carbidopa, which blocks peripheral metabolism, allowing much more of the levodopa to enter the brain than if it were given alone. Sinemet 25/100 contains 25 mg of carbidopa and 100 mg of levodopa. Treatment should begin with small doses, one-half of Sinemet 25/100 2 or 3 times a day with meals and titrated to the lowest levodopa dose that produces a useful clinical response. Absence of response to 1000 to 1500 mg/d of levodopa would be a strong suggestion that the original PD diagnosis is incorrect. The optimum dose of carbidopa is 100 to 150 mg/d, which should completely block the peripheral metabolism of levodopa. Levodopa is associated with a higher risk for dyskinesia than dopamine agonists (DAs). Therapy should be initiated with immediate-release preparations so that initial response can be better evaluated. Slow-release forms of carbidopa-levodopa provide a longer half-life and a lower peak plasma level of levodopa, reducing clinical fluctuations. Once the patient's condition is stable, reassessment may be performed every 3 to 6 months.[23] Novel formulations, including a transdermal product (rotigotine patch), are available and may offer more continuous drug levels.

Within 5 years of starting levodopa, up to 50% (10% of patients per year) will develop levodopa-induced complications.[24] Complications include motor fluctuations (wearing-off phenomenon), involuntary movements (dyskinesia), abnormal postures of the extremities and trunk (dystonia), and other complex motor fluctuations. Motor complications are more common in patients with young-onset PD (40 to 59 years at PD onset) compared with older-onset PD (70 years at PD onset).[24] Two randomly controlled trials found no evidence that using modified-release levodopa either reduced complications or improved disease control at 5 years compared with immediate-release levodopa monotherapy in people with early PD.[23] Later onset of motor fluctuations in PD is associated with initial treatment with pramipexole rather than with levodopa. Evidence exists that DA monotherapy and combination therapy

reduces the incidence of irreversible motor complications of dyskinesia and fluctuations in motor response related to long-term levodopa treatment. The same long-term randomly controlled trial, however, found that levodopa monotherapy is slightly more effective in treating the disabling motor impairments of PD.[23]

Dopamine Agonists. DAs are a group of synthetic agents that directly stimulate dopamine receptors. These drugs are direct agonists and do not require metabolic conversion to move into the brain. Also, they do not depend on neuronal uptake or release. An additional advantage over immediate-release levodopa is their longer duration of action. DAs were initially used for adjunctive treatment of advanced PD complicated by reduced levodopa response, motor fluctuations, dyskinesia, and other adverse effects of levodopa. Some investigators, despite the lack of conclusive evidence, have advocated the early use of DAs as a levodopa-sparing strategy. This strategy is based on the unproven concept that the long-term duration of a patient's responsiveness to levodopa is finite. Given the potential that DAs are associated with fewer motor fluctuations and the evidence of a higher incidence of levodopa-related dyskinesia in young-onset PD, some experts suggest that DAs for initial treatment of young-onset PD (in patients below 60 years of age) is appropriate, whereas the more effective levodopa is used in patients above 60 years of age. Ropinirole (Requip), pramipexole (Mirapex), and bromocriptine (Parlodel) are DAs that can be effective adjuncts to levodopa in older-onset PD patients or as monotherapy in young-onset PD patients.[25]

The agonists tend to induce orthostatic hypotension when they are first introduced. The best starting regimen is a small dose at bedtime for the first 3 days and then a switch to daytime administration, with a gradual increase. Bromocriptine and ropinirole may induce psychosis and confusion, whereas pramipexole induces somnolence. Overall, however, all are less likely than levodopa to induce dyskinesias, which makes them useful to reduce the severity of "off" states. All DAs should be used cautiously in patients with cardiac disease. DAs require maintenance doses at least 3 times a day. Ropinirole is started at 0.25 mg 3 times a day, and then increased by 0.25 mg per dose each week for 4 weeks for a total daily dose of 3 mg. After week 4, the ropinirole dose may be increased weekly by 1.5 mg/d to a maximum daily dose of 24 mg. Most benefit occurs in the range of 12 to 16 mg/d. Pramipexole is started at 0.125 mg twice a day; the dose is then increased gradually by 0.125 mg per dose every 5 to 7 days. Most patients are managed within the range of 1.5 to 4.5 mg/d. Bromocriptine is started at 1.25 mg twice a day and then, at 2- to 4-week intervals, increased by 2.5 mg/d. Most patients are managed on 20 to 40 mg daily in three or four divided doses. The safety of bromocriptine > 100 mgs a day has not been established.

Adverse effects of DAs include nausea, vomiting, sleepiness, orthostatic hypotension, confusion, and hallucinations. DAs have also been associated with increased risk of impulse control disorders, including pathologic gambling, compulsive sexual behavior, and compulsive buying.[25]

Catechol O-Methyltransferase Inhibitors. Catechol O-methyltransferase (COMT) inhibitors, such as entacapone (Comtan), are ineffective if given alone, but they prolong and potentiate the effect of levodopa when they are given in conjunction with levodopa. COMT inhibitors are used to treat motor fluctuations in patients who are experiencing end-of-dose "wearing-off" periods. Tolcapone (Tasmar) and entacapone are the COMT inhibitors prescribed. The starting dose of tolcapone is 100 mg 3 times daily. Entacapone is given at 200 mg with each dose of levodopa up to maximum of eight doses per day.[23]

Anticholinergics. Dopamine and acetylcholine are normally in a state of electrochemical balance in the basal ganglia. In PD, dopamine depletion produces cholinergic sensitivity so that cholinergic drugs exacerbate PD and anticholinergic drugs improve PD. Centrally acting anticholinergic drugs, such as trihexyphenidyl (Artane) and benztropine (Cogentin), are more useful in controlling tremor and rigidity than bradykinesia but may also cause typical side effects. Anticholinergics should be used in younger patients in whom tremor is the predominant problem. The potency of anticholinergics seems to decrease over time, and side effects such as blurred vision, dry mouth, bowel and bladder problems, and cognition changes limit their usefulness. Evidence of benefit of anticholinergics is unclear. These drugs should not be used in older adults because of a well-documented risk of mental status change and are contraindicated in patient's taking anti dementia drugs. Trihexyphenidyl is started at 0.5 to 1 mg daily with gradual increase to 2 to 5 mg 3 times a day. Benztropine is more commonly used for the treatment of antipsychotic-induced parkinsonism with doses of 0.5 to 2 mg once daily.

Amantadine. Amantadine is an antiviral agent that has mild antiparkinsonian activity. The mechanism of action is uncertain, but it increases dopamine release, inhibits dopamine reuptake, and stimulates dopamine receptors. It may even have a central anticholinergic effect. Controlled trials demonstrated that it was more effective than anticholinergic drugs for akinesia and rigidity. Individual patients with advanced PD who have motor fluctuations and dyskinesia can benefit briefly from the addition of amantadine to the regimen of levodopa. Amantadine is administered in two divided doses of 100 to 200 mg each.[23]

Nonpharmacologic Management

Adjunctive therapies focus on neurorehabilitation strategies to enhance neuroplasticity and should be implemented early and continually reassessed as the disease progresses. Occupational, physical, and speech therapy should be utilized appropriately based on patient's disability and level of functionality.[25] Physical activity improves both motor and non-motor symptoms in Parkinson. Multiple studies have shown dance therapy, in particular, to be effective in improving motor, gait, and balance as well as quality of life as compared to controls.[26] Other studies have shown that other types of aerobic exercises such as treadmill training, boxing, and Tai Chi can have similar benefits. However, while the short-term benefits are well established, studies agree that long-term follow-up is needed.[27] Cognitive exercises, including crossword puzzles and Sudoku, may also prove to be beneficial, as well as keeping up with current events or utilizing alternative interventions such as music therapy.[28]

Surgery

Deep Brain Stimulation. Deep brain stimulation (DBS) is the most frequently performed surgical procedure for the treatment of advanced PD. Two prospective randomized controlled trials that compared DBS with best medical therapy have shown that bilateral DBS improves motor function in selected patients with advanced typical PD and motor fluctuations.[29] The rate of serious adverse events is significantly higher in DBS patients (40%) than in the best medical treatment group (15%). The adverse events are directly related to the surgical procedure and include postoperative headache, pain, and infection at the surgical site. These two trials demonstrated that DBS of the subthalamic nucleus or globus pallidus is more effective than the best medical therapy for improvement of motor function and quality of life for patients with advanced PD, at least in the short term.[29,30]

Collaboration with other health care providers is common in the treatment of patients with PD. It is important to consult a neurologist before committing patients to medications. Consultation with specialists is indicated when patients are not responding to treatment or when the disease is progressing. Also, if there are signs and symptoms of depression, referral to a psychiatrist should be considered. Neuropsychological documentation of the precise nature and prevalence of the cognitive deficit has important implications in medical and psychosocial management of patients with PD. Hospitalization may be considered for complications such as pneumonia, deep venous thrombosis, and pulmonary embolus. Physical therapy can improve mobility and strength, which may help maintain independence and prevent injury. Occupational therapy can be useful; adaptive equipment can be provided to the patient or caregivers, and assistance can be provided to adapt to home or workplace as disability progresses.

COMPLICATIONS AND COMORBID PROBLEMS
Dementia

In studies, the prevalence of dementia in PD has been found to be as high as 41%, with incidence rates as high as 78%. Older age, duration of PD, and severity of parkinsonism may contribute to the incidence of dementia in PD. An area of recent debate and research is the question of whether PD dementia and dementia with Lewy bodies are distinct disorders or different presentations of the same disease. It is also possible for other dementias such as Alzheimer disease and vascular dementia to coexist with PD or for patients with PD to develop milder cognitive impairments that may not meet the criteria for diagnosing dementia.[31,32]

Psychosis and Hallucinations

Psychosis, a frequent complication of PD, is characterized by visual hallucinations and delusions, often paranoid. Hallucinations are most common and affect up to 40% of patients with PD, mostly in the advanced stages of PD. Although dose reduction of antiparkinsonian drugs often resolves hallucinations, stopping all the offending medications is usually not an option, and not all hallucinations are drug related. Antiparkinsonian drugs can be reduced or stopped in reverse order of their potency and effectiveness; the sequence begins with anticholinergics then proceeds to COMT inhibitors, then DAs, and then levodopa if all else fails. Quetiapine in low doses can be used to manage psychotic symptoms in PD, but studies have failed to demonstrate its efficacy.[33]

Depression

Depression is the most common psychiatric illness seen in PD and is associated with negative impact on mobility and quality of life. There is no clear consensus regarding the use of antidepressants for depression in patients with PD, but there are two concerns regarding the treatment with selective serotonin reuptake inhibitors in PD: (1) the possibility of increasing motor symptoms and (2) a possible adverse reaction with selegiline when it is used concurrently.[33] When these drugs are used, close monitoring is advised. Studies have demonstrated benefit over placebo with pramipexole, venlafaxine, and sertraline. Bupropion may be a very good option for PD patients with depression; however, studies need to be done. Cognitive behavioral therapy can be very helpful.

Daytime Sleepiness and Fatigue

Daytime sleepiness and fatigue are common problems in patients with PD. Sudden somnolence can be a hazard for PD patients if they are still driving. Fatigue appears to be an independent symptom of PD but can certainly overlap with depression and daytime somnolence.

PATIENT AND FAMILY EDUCATION

Education is essential to help the patient and family understand and gain some control over this chronic and progressive disorder. Hence focused discussions about symptoms and treatments may need to happen with each visit. Answering questions and addressing concerns honestly are part of establishing a successful provider–patient relationship. Reassurance and encouragement complement medication. Educational points worth covering include the following:

- Education about medication effectiveness and side effects and drug and diet interactions is important.
- Discussion about driving and when to stop is difficult but essential.
- Normal reactions of anger, depression, and anxiety and social and economic concerns are common, so emotional, psychological, and socioeconomic needs of the patient and family must be addressed.

Support groups are especially valuable to patients and families because they provide emotional support, access to resources, and educational information.

Health Promotion

The patient should be encouraged to contact a PD support group and a local PD information and referral center. Internet resources are also available for patients with PD. The patient may find the following resources helpful:

American Parkinson Disease Association
135 Parkinson Avenue
Staten Island, NY 10305
800-223-2732
www.apdaparkinson.org
National Parkinson Foundation
200 SE 1st Street
Suite 800
Miami, FL 33131
www.parkinson.org
Michael J. Fox Foundation for Parkinson's Research
Grand Central Station
PO Box 4777
New York, NY 10163
212-509-0995
http://www.michaeljfox.org
National Institute of Neurological Disorders and Stroke
www.ninds.nih.gov/Disorders/All-Disorders/Parkinson's-Disease
  -information-page

REFERENCES

1. Centers for Disease Control and Prevention. (2013). Genetics, coffee consumption, and Parkinson's disease.
2. Ascherio, A., & Schwarzchild, M. (2016). The epidemiology of Parkinson's disease: Risk factors and prevention. *The Lancet. Neurology, 16*(12), 1257–1272.
3. Marras, C., Beck, J. C., Bower, J. H., Roberts, E., Ritz, B., Ross, G. W., et al. on behalf of the Parkinson's Foundation P4 Group. (2018). Prevalence of Parkinson's disease across North America. *NPJ Parkinson's Disease, 4*(1), 1–7.
4. Ascherio, A., & Schwarzchild, M. A. (2016). The epidemiology of Parkinson's disease: Risk factors and prevention. *The Lancet. Neurology, 15*(12), 1257–1272.
5. Pezzoli, G., & Cereda, E. (2013). Exposure to pesticides or solvents and risk of Parkinson disease. *Neurology, 80*, 2035–2037.
6. Jafari, S., Etminan, M., Aminzadeh, F., et al. (2013). Head injury and risk of Parkinson's disease: A systematic review and meta-analysis. *Movement Disorders: Official Journal of the Movement Disorder Society, 28*, 1222–1226.
7. Willis, A. W., Evanoff, B. A., Lian, M., et al. (2010). Metal emissions and urban incident Parkinson disease: A community health study of Medicare beneficiaries by using geographic information systems. *American Journal of Epidemiology, 172*, 1357–1359.
8. Goldman, S. M., Quinlan, P. J., Ross, G. W., et al. (2012). Solvent exposure and Parkinson disease in twins. *Annals of Neurology, 71*, 776–778.
9. Kistner, A., & Krack, P. (2014). Parkinson's disease: No milk today? *Frontiers in Neurology, 5*, 172.
10. Disek, P., Roos, P. M., Litwin, T., et al. (2015). The neurotoxicity of iron, copper and manganese in Parkinson's disease and Wilson's disease. *Journal of Trace Elements in Medicine and Biology: Organ of the Society for Minerals and Trace Elements (GMS), 31*, 193–203.
11. Saaksjarvi, K., Knekt, P., Mannisto, S., & Lyytinen, J. (2014). Reduced risk of Parkinson's disease associated with lower body mass index and heavy leisure-time physical activity. *European Journal of Epidemiology, 29*(4), 285–292.
12. Hong, C. T., et al. (2016). Newly diagnosed anemia increases risk of Parkinson's disease: A population based cohort study. *Scientific Reports, 6*, 29651. doi:10.1038/SREP29651.
13. Berg, D., Postuma, R., Bastiaan, B., et al. (2014). Time to redefine PD? Introductory statement of the MDS Task Force on the definition of Parkinson's Disease. *Movement Disorders: Official Journal of the Movement Disorder Society, 29*(4), 454–462.
14. Singleton, A. B., Farrer, M. J., & Bonifati, V. (2013). The genetics of Parkinson's disease progress and therapeutic implications. *Movement Disorders: Official Journal of the Movement Disorder Society, 28*, 14–17.
15. Kieburtz, K., & Wunderle, K. B. (2013). Parkinson's disease: Evidence for environmental risk factors. *Movement Disorders: Official Journal of the Movement Disorder Society, 28*, 8–11.
16. Shulman, J., DeJager, P., & Feany, M. (2011). Parkinson's disease: Genetics and pathogenesis. *Annual Review of Pathology, 6*, 193–222.
17. Bhatia, K. P., Bain, P., Bajaj, N., Elble, R. J., Hallett, M., Louis, E. D., et al. (2018). Consensus statement on the classification of tremors. from the task force on tremor of the International Parkinson and Movement Disorder Society. *Movement Disorders: Official Journal of the Movement Disorder Society, 33*, 75–87. doi:10.1002/mds.27121.
18. Sveinbjornsdottir, S. (2016). The clinical symptoms of Parkinson's disease. *Journal of Neurochemistry, 139*(S1), 318–324.
19. Banou, E. (2015). Kinesia paradoxa: A challenging Parkinson's phenomenon for simulation. In P. Vlamos & A. Alexiou (Eds.), *GeNedis 2014. Advances in experimental medicine and biology* (Vol. 822). Cham: Springer.
20. Postuma, R., & Berg, D. (2016). MDS clinical diagnostic criteria for Parkinson's disease (I1.010). *Neurology, 86*(16 Suppl.), I1.010.
21. DeMaagd, G., & Philip, A. (2015). Parkinson's disease and its management: Part 1: Disease entity, risk factors, pathophysiology, clinical presentation, and diagnosis. *P & T: A Peer-Reviewed Journal for Formulary Management, 40*(8), 504–532.
22. Tarakad, A., & Jankovic, J. (2017). Diagnosis and management of Parkinson disease. *Seminars in Neurology, 37*(02), 118–126.
23. Connolly, B. S., & Lang, A. E. (2014). Pharmacological treatment of Parkinson disease: A review. *JAMA: The Journal of the American Medical Association, 311*(16), 1670–1683.
24. Aquino, C., & Fox, S. (2015). Clinical spectrum of levodopa induced complications. *Movement Disorders: Official Journal of the Movement Disorder Society, 30*(1), 80–89.
25. DeMaagd, G., & Philip, A. (2015). Part 2: Introduction to the pharmacotherapy of Parkinson's disease, with a focus on the use of dopaminergic agents. *P & T: A Peer-Reviewed Journal for Formulary Management, 40*(9), 590–600.

26. Sharp, K., & Hewitt, J. (2014). Dance as an intervention for people with Parkinson's disease: A systematic review and meta-analysis. *Neuroscience and Biobehavioral Reviews, 47*, 445–456.

27. Shu, H.-F., et al. (2014). Aerobic exercise for Parkinson's disease: A systematic review and meta-analysis of randomized controlled trials. *PLoS ONE, 9*(7), e100503.

28. Goldman, J. G. (2016). Neuropsychiatric issues in Parkinson disease. *Continuum: Lifelong Learning in Neurology, 22*(4, Movement Disorders), 1086–1103.

29. Alsen, P. S. (2014). Deep brain stimulation for Parkinson's disease with early motor complications. *JAMA: The Journal of the American Medical Association, 311*(16), 1686–1687.

30. Katzenschlager, R. (2014). Parkinson's disease, recent advances. *Journal of Neurology, 261*(5), 1031–1036.

31. Hanagas, H., Tufekcioglu, Z., & Emre, M. (2017). Dementia in Parkinson's disease. *Journal of the Neurological Sciences, 374*, 26–31.

32. Rieu, I., et al. (2015). International validation of a behavioral scale in Parkinson's disease without dementia. *Movement Disorders: Official Journal of the Movement Disorder Society, 5*, 705–713.

33. Cooney, J. W., & Stacy, M. (2016). Neuropsychiatric issues in Parkinson's disease. *Current Neurology and Neuroscience Reports, 16*, 49. https://doi.org/10.1007/s11910-016-0647-4.

CHAPTER **182**

SEIZURE DISORDER

Karen L. Secore

 Immediate emergency department referral or physician consultation is indicated for status epilepticus or new-onset seizures.

DEFINITION AND EPIDEMIOLOGY

Epilepsy, a syndrome of recurrent (unprovoked) seizures, is a common neurologic condition that currently affects nearly 2.2 million people in the United States, with more than 100,000 to 150,000 new cases reported annually. Although the onset of seizures can occur at any age, incidence rates peak in neonates and young children, plateau, then rise again in the older adult population. In the United States, the prevalence of seizures is approximately 5 to 10 cases per 1000 persons in the general population; the lifetime risk for development of epilepsy is in 27 people.[1]

A single seizure may result from discrete, temporary abnormalities, such as high fever in small children, hyperventilation (in susceptible patients), or alcohol withdrawal. Causes of a first seizure leading to epilepsy include genetic factors, vascular abnormalities (e.g., ischemic strokes, hemorrhages, and arteriovenous malformations), significant head trauma, brain tumors, metabolic factors, and infections such as encephalitis and meningitis. Strokes are a common cause of epilepsy, particularly in the elderly. Changes in levels of various electrolytes, in particular hyponatremia and hypercalcemia, may cause isolated seizures. Also, hyperglycemia and hypoglycemia can be responsible for seizure activity, especially in patients with underlying brain injuries. A first seizure may occur in the form of status epilepticus (SE). SE is recently redefined as continuous convulsive seizures for 5 minutes, continues focal seizures for 10 minutes, and continuous absent seizures for 10 to 15 minutes. Systemic and brain injury can occur from seizure activity lasting more than 30 minutes.[2]

Genetic predisposition is the strongest in generalized forms of epilepsy in which the entire brain is electrically unstable; however, the genetic and biochemical defects are only starting to be characterized. Childhood absence (petit mal) epilepsy, juvenile myoclonic epilepsy, and generalized convulsive epilepsy are syndromes with a genetic predisposition. Mutations in γ-aminobutyric acid (GABA) receptors and sodium channels have been implicated. These types of epilepsy account for approximately one-third of all cases, with seizures and abnormalities on electroencephalography (EEG) affecting the entire brain. The remaining types of epilepsy are related to localization; focal electrical abnormalities are usually the result of a structural lesion.

PATHOPHYSIOLOGY

Although the terms *epilepsy* and *seizure disorder* are often used interchangeably, they have two distinct definitions. A *seizure* can be defined as an isolated event in which a group of neurons produces excessive electrical discharges in the brain. Seizures occur when the balance between excitation and inhibition of the brain's electrical activity becomes abnormally altered in favor of excitation. Seizures can be caused by the excess production or release of an excitatory neurotransmitter, which stimulates neurons to discharge abnormally, or by a loss of inhibitory neuronal activity, which permits abnormal excitation and discharge of neurons to occur. Single or even recurrent seizures can be triggered by hypoxia or other metabolic factors, but they do not constitute epilepsy unless they recur in a habitual and unprovoked manner. A subset of acute symptomatic seizures occurs in the setting of an acute medical illness or metabolic crisis. These conditions include hypoglycemia; nonketotic hyperglycemia; hyponatremia; hypocalcemia; magnesium levels below 0.8 mEq/L; renal failure and uremia; hyperthyroidism; disorders of porphyrin metabolism; cerebral anoxia as a complication of cardiac or respiratory arrest, carbon monoxide poisoning, drowning, or anesthetic; withdrawal states (particularly alcohol and benzodiazepine withdrawal); and drug toxicity or intoxication.

Epilepsy is characterized by recurrent seizures and is divided into syndromes on the basis of various causes, seizure types, associated neurologic symptoms, anatomic correlates, age, and family history. For diagnosis and treatment, it is important to identify both the type of seizure and the epileptic syndrome.

CLASSIFICATION OF SEIZURES, EPILEPSY, AND EPILEPTIC SYNDROMES

In 1981, a commission for the International League Against Epilepsy (ILAE) developed, revised, and adopted the international classification of epileptic seizures.[3] Efforts were made in 2010 to revise the classification[4] and again in 2017 (Box 182.1).[5] The motivation for revising the classification is to reflect the advances being made in basic and clinical neuroscience and incorporate those advances into clinical practice.[5] The classification includes two broad categories of seizure types: (1) focal or localization related and (2) generalized. Focal seizures begin within networks limited to one cerebral hemisphere and show localized abnormalities on EEG. Depending on the spread of electrical activity, the patient may have varying levels of consciousness. By definition, focal seizures without impairment of consciousness, formerly known as simple partial seizures, are the aura or warning that the patient experiences before a larger seizure. Focal sensory seizures may be purely subjective, and focal motor seizures may involve no impairment of consciousness. If the seizure activity spreads and involves the brainstem or both hemispheres, consciousness becomes altered, and the

BOX **182.1**

2017 Classification of Seizure Types

FOCAL

Motor
Automatisms
Atonic
Clonic
Epileptic spasms
Myoclonic
Tonic

Nonmotor
Autonomic
Behavioral arrest
Cognitive
Emotional
Sensory

GENERALIZED

Motor
Tonic clonic
Clonic

Tonic
Myoclonic
Atonic
Epileptic Spasms

Nonmotor
Typical
Atypical
Myoclonic
Eyelid myoclonic

UNKNOWN

Motor
Tonic clonic
Epileptic Spasm

BOX **182.2**

International Classification of Epilepsy and Epileptic Syndromes

1. Focal
   1.1. Idiopathic (benign childhood epilepsy with centrotemporal spikes)
   1.2. Symptomatic (e.g., temporal lobe epilepsy, frontal lobe epilepsy)
   1.3. Cryptogenic (cause unknown)
2. Generalized
   2.1. Idiopathic (juvenile myoclonic, juvenile absence, grand mal on awakening)
   2.2. Cryptogenic (Lennox-Gastaut syndrome, West syndrome)
   2.3. Symptomatic
3. Unknown (neonatal types, Landau-Kleffner syndrome)
4. Special situation related (febrile seizures, metabolic seizures)

Modified from Fisher, R. S., Cross, J. H., French, J. A., et al. (2017), Operational classification of seizure types by the International League Against Epilepsy: Position Paper of the ILAE Commission for Classification and Terminology. *Epilepsia, 58*: 522–530. doi:10.1111/epi.13670

seizure is classified as complex partial or more recently referred to as a focal seizure with impairment of consciousness. Altered consciousness and aberrations of behavior, such as automatisms (automatic repetitive movements), are usually associated with this type of seizure. If such seizures spread bilaterally and involve the motor cortex, the patient may have a secondarily generalized tonic-clonic seizure, now called a *bilateral convulsive seizure.*[5]

In contrast, primary generalized seizures occur when the initial abnormal electrical activity begins in both cerebral hemispheres and involves bilaterally distributed neuronal networks. These seizures are usually seen with idiopathic or hereditary types of epilepsy. Consciousness is almost always impaired, and the seizure may be convulsive or nonconvulsive. Motor activity and electroencephalographic changes are bilateral. Nonconvulsive generalized seizures, such as absence (petit mal) seizures, may be brief, and the patient may initially be diagnosed as a "daydreamer." The electroencephalographic characteristics of generalized spike and wave patterns are crucial for the proper diagnosis of these types of seizures. Convulsive primary generalized seizures, such as tonic-clonic (grand mal) types, are rarely missed but can be confused with secondarily generalized tonic-clonic seizures. Being able to differentiate between these two types is helpful in prescribing the appropriate treatment, because each type may respond differently to certain antiepileptic medications. In the case of secondarily generalized seizures, it is important to exclude an underlying structural lesion, such as a brain tumor.

For treatment to be tailored to the individual, it is essential that consideration be given to the seizure type as well as the epileptic syndrome to which it belongs. The International Classification of Epilepsy and Epileptic Syndromes (Box 182.2) was adopted by the ILAE in 1989 and allowed the practitioner to categorize cases by seizure type, cause, precipitating factors, age at onset, and prognosis.[5] This has been further adapted to classify the cause of seizures as genetic, structural, metabolic,

or unknown. Epileptic syndromes can be further classified by age of onset, cognitive and developmental antecedents, electroencephalographic features, triggers, and patterns of occurrence related to sleep.[5] Although epilepsy can develop at any age, certain syndromes are more age-related than others. A variety of epileptic syndromes develop in early childhood. More than 50% and perhaps as many as 70% of childhood epilepsies, particularly the benign partial epilepsies, remit at the time of puberty.[6] Idiopathic, generalized epilepsy usually manifests by 18 years of age. After the age of 18 years, focal brain processes should be suspected. Brain tumors are a prominent cause of seizures in adults, whereas strokes are often the cause of seizures that begin late in life.[7] Symptomatic focal epilepsy syndromes account for 30% to 35% of all cases of epilepsy.[1] Seizure manifestations can be helpful in identifying which lobe of the brain is involved.

CLINICAL PRESENTATION AND PHYSICAL EXAMINATION

An accurate and detailed history is important. It is essential to obtain history not only from the patient but also from parents, relatives, or friends who have witnessed the seizures. Complicated pregnancy or childbirth, delayed childhood development, childhood diseases such as meningitis and encephalitis, significant head trauma with loss of consciousness, and family history of epilepsy are among the significant risk factors for the development of epilepsy. New-onset seizures require the determination of any recent history of headache, illness, trauma, or focal neurologic deficit.

An accurate description is important in attempting to decide whether an event was a seizure. The patient should be questioned to determine whether there was a warning before the event. A gastric sensation or a feeling of déjà vu is characteristic of temporal lobe epilepsy. A history of incontinence, injury, tongue biting, postictal confusion, lateralized weakness, or severe headache should raise suspicion of a true epileptic event. A detailed seizure history can also suggest where the seizures are originating, define seizure characteristics and frequency, and determine how the seizures are interfering with the patient's life.

The first seizure may appear in the form of SE. Immediate emergency department referral or physician consultation is indicated for SE or new-onset seizures.

A general physical examination should be performed on all patients with epilepsy and should be directed toward specific disease processes and focal neurologic deficits. Skin and mucous membranes should be assessed to identify areas of injury that may be related to events that occurred while consciousness was altered. Tongue biting and cheek biting are common during tonic-clonic seizures; the tongue and cheek are usually bitten on just one side, but bilateral findings are not uncommon. If the tip of the tongue is bitten, it should give rise to the suspicion of a nonepileptic psychogenic seizure. Cardiovascular assessment is important because syncope and arrhythmias are included in the differential diagnosis of epilepsy. Postural vital signs will determine whether orthostatic hypotension is a consideration. Neurologic signs, such as lateralized weakness, papilledema, memory problems, or changes in reflexes, can signify a structural lesion in the brain. In general, a patient with epilepsy will have unremarkable physical examination findings.

DIAGNOSTICS

Clinical presentation, physical examination, and differential considerations guide diagnostic testing. A new seizure may signify a serious pathologic condition. If infection of the CNS is suspected (see Chapter 178), a complete blood count (CBC) and differential and a lumbar puncture are indicated. A comprehensive metabolic profile, including calcium magnesium and phosphate, is necessary to exclude hypoglycemia, electrolyte abnormalities, or renal failure. Liver function tests (LFTs) should be performed to exclude hepatic failure. Alcohol and drug levels testing may be indicated. Magnetic resonance imaging (MRI) or computed tomography (CT) scan is indicated if structural abnormality, tumor, trauma, or cerebrovascular accident is suspected.[8] Electrocardiography (ECG) should be performed to ascertain the presence of arrhythmias or heart block.

Diagnosis and classification of epilepsy and seizure types require confirmation that the patient does indeed have epileptic seizures. To treat the disorder appropriately, the practitioner must attempt to determine the cause of the epilepsy and classify it according to syndrome. Appropriate diagnostic tests should be part of the initial evaluation.[8]

Sleep-deprived EEG is useful because a baseline recording of background brain waves may reveal epileptic abnormalities. The positive predictive value of EEG in most clinics is more than 80%, although sensitivity is only 30%.[9] Because the chance of a patient having a seizure during routine EEG is small, ictal information may not be obtained; however, interictal epileptiform abnormalities may give localizing information and suggest epilepsy. Many patients with focal epilepsy show no focal or generalized abnormalities on routine EEG. Therefore a normal recording does not exclude a diagnosis of epilepsy. In contrast to focal epilepsy, generalized types of epilepsy often produce abnormalities of spike and wave activity or generalized slowing on routine electroencephalographic recordings. Interictal electroencephalographic abnormalities—either focal or generalized—are not synonymous with seizure activity, and therefore electroencephalographic abnormalities should not be the only basis for treatment.

Although neuroimaging studies can be of great value in diagnosis, the absence of structural abnormalities does not exclude a diagnosis of epilepsy. CT scans are useful for identification of large mass lesions, bleeding, subdural fluid collections, and cerebral infarcts, but they often miss more subtle changes in brain structure. MRI provides extensive anatomic detail and is useful in distinguishing small low-grade tumors, scars, and neural migration disorders from one another and from normal variants in brain structure. Except in an emergency, when the immediate availability of a CT scan is an advantage, MRIs should be the primary imaging study in patients with epilepsy.[8] In the preoperative evaluation of patients who are candidates for surgery, single-photon emission computerized tomography (SPECT), positron emission tomography (PET), magnetic resonance spectroscopy (MRS), functional magnetic resonance imaging (fMRI), and magnetoencephalography (MEG) are other imaging methods that may be considered.[8]

INITIAL DIAGNOSTICS

New-Onset Seizure

LABORATORY
- Alcohol, drug levels
- CBC with Differential
- Comprehensive metabolic profile[a]

IMAGING
- MRI, CT scan[a]

OTHER DIAGNOSTICS
- ECG[a]
- Lumbar puncture[a]
- EEG[a]

[a]If indicated.

If a diagnosis of epilepsy cannot be confirmed or excluded after an accurate history, EEG, or imaging study, patients should be referred to a comprehensive epilepsy center in which long-term video and electroencephalographic monitoring can be done. This type of monitoring is intended to capture an event on video with simultaneous electroencephalographic recording and is almost always successful in distinguishing epilepsy from nonepileptic events.

For patients in SE, a battery of laboratory tests is usually performed: CBC; electrolyte values; glucose, magnesium, calcium, blood urea nitrogen (BUN), and creatinine concentrations; LFTs; coagulation studies (prothrombin time, partial thromboplastin time); alcohol level, toxicology screen; anticonvulsant drug levels; urinalysis; and pregnancy test. These tests should be done concurrently with patient stabilization. Examination of the cerebrospinal fluid is required if meningitis or encephalitis is suspected. Viral encephalitis should be treated empirically with acyclovir until the results of diagnostic studies for herpes virus are available. Similarly, suspected bacterial meningitis should be treated with appropriate antibiotics until culture results are available.[10]

DIFFERENTIAL DIAGNOSIS

Possible differential diagnosis in patients with suspected seizures include cardiovascular causes such as syncope and transient ischemic attacks, other neurological conditions such as migraine or movement disorders, or psychiatric causes such as nonepileptic seizures/conversion disorder or posttraumatic stress disorder.

Syncope manifests with loss of consciousness, and convulsive syncope secondary to cerebral ischemia may mimic epileptic seizures. Syncope is often vasovagal, but cardiac causes include heart block and cardiac arrhythmia, and it can be induced by stimuli such as carotid massage, paroxysmal coughing, and voiding. Orthostatic hypotension is a frequent cause of syncope in the elderly. Presyncopal symptoms such as vertigo, sensory disturbances, and tinnitus are sometimes mistaken for epileptic auras or minor seizures.

Other disorders in the differential diagnosis include tumors, cerebrovascular disease, arteriovenous malformation, trauma, CNS infection, migraines, hyperventilation syndrome, movement disorders, transient ischemic attacks, transient global amnesia, sleep disorders, and toxic metabolic disturbances such as alcohol withdrawal seizures. On occasion, sleep deprivation may cause generalized tonic-clonic seizures.[10] This phenomenon is not associated with a pathologic disorder.

A variety of nonepileptic paroxysmal events can be confused with epileptic seizures. Psychogenic seizures, also called nonepileptic seizures or pseudoseizures, are often mistaken for epileptic seizures. If patients are treated with antiepileptic drugs (AEDs), this usually increases the seizure frequency. A careful history can help raise suspicion for psychogenic seizures. In such cases, seizures may be a symptom of conversion disorder and the stress of physical or sexual abuse, a part of posttraumatic stress disorder, attention-seeking behavior, or a means of achieving secondary gain. Treatment involves the patient's acceptance of the diagnosis of psychogenic seizures and the beginning of a comprehensive psychotherapy program.

INTERPROFESSIONAL COLLABORATIVE MANAGEMENT

Initial Stabilization and Management of Acute Seizures

In the acute setting, most seizures resolve spontaneously within a few minutes and require no specific treatment apart from close observation to ensure that patients do not harm themselves. However, SE is a medical emergency that requires simultaneous medical stabilization (airway, breathing, circulation, and medications to control the seizures) and a search for the underlying cause. The Epilepsy Foundation of America's Working Group on Status Epilepticus defines SE as a continuous seizure lasting 5 minutes or more or two consecutive seizures in a row without mental clearing.[2,11] Generalized convulsive status epilepticus (GCSE) is a medical emergency that can lead to transient or permanent brain damage. Early treatment is a key factor in the outcome and prognosis. Initial management should maintain homeostasis and provide respiratory support. If seizures persist beyond 30 minutes, a vicious circle of maladaptive physiologic responses occurs.[12] SE may be complicated by hypotension, hypertension, hyperthermia, hypoglycemia, hypoxemia, acidosis, arrhythmias, rhabdomyolysis, pulmonary edema, fractures, and dislocations.

Mortality and morbidity rates have been related to the cause of SE, and the seizure activity duration from the onset until treatment has been initiated. In patients with known epilepsy, half of the hospital-reported cases of GCSE have been associated with subtherapeutic AED levels.[2] as patients fail to take their medication as prescribed. Other common causes of SE are meningitis, head trauma, eclampsia, and progressive neurologic and neurodegenerative disorders.[2] In a study by the Veterans Affairs Status Epilepticus Cooperative Study Group comparing four treatments (lorazepam, phenytoin, phenobarbital, and diazepam) for GCSE, lorazepam was more likely to be successful than phenytoin when used as the initial

treatment.[12] Recommendations for treatment of acute episodes of SE are listed in Table 182.1.

 Specialist consultation is indicated for suspected central nervous system (CNS) lesions, SE, initiation of antiepileptic medications, treatment failures, and women with epilepsy who are contemplating pregnancy.

Patients with SE should be admitted to intensive care for ongoing stabilization and workup.

The goal of management in epilepsy is to control seizures with minimum adverse effects. In more than 50% of patients with epilepsy, seizures are completely controlled with medication.[13] Another 20% to 30% of patients witness improvement in their symptoms with medications, but they are not seizure free or may experience significant side effects.[13] The remaining 25% to 30% of seizures are considered medically intractable.[13] Determination of the appropriate medical or surgical treatment is based on a variety of factors. These include patients' perception of how the seizures are interfering with their life goals, economic considerations, personal support from family and friends, and severity and complexity of epilepsy in that patient.

The following conditions warrant consideration for hospital admission: SE, incomplete recovery from a single seizure or prolonged postictal state, suspected illness that requires treatment, drug or alcohol withdrawal, febrile illness (adult), expanding mass lesion, history of recent head trauma, or focal signs on examination.

If adequate seizure control is not achieved, patients should undergo presurgical and diagnostic evaluation with electroencephalographic video monitoring at a comprehensive epilepsy center. Patients who are having difficulty tolerating medications should also be referred for a neurology consultation. Patients with structural lesions should be referred promptly to a neurosurgeon for further evaluation.

Conservative Management

Depending on a number of variables, including the potential for seizure recurrence, first seizures are usually not treated with AEDs. Only about 30% of people who have a single, unprovoked, generalized tonic-clonic seizure have a second one, whether they are treated with medications or not.[14] Medication may delay recurrence or somewhat reduce its likelihood. Factors that should be considered in the decision to treat or not to treat a first seizure include the following:

- The type of seizure that occurred—complex partial seizures are more likely to be recurrent than generalized tonic-clonic ones.
- Environment and occupation—for example, dangerous work environment, such as construction.
- Results of imaging studies and EEG—treatment is prudent if either is abnormal because recurrence is likely.

The decision of whether to treat a patient who has had a single seizure has provoked controversy because of the lack of randomized, unbiased studies. Most studies have combined multiple seizure types, which clouds interpretation of the data. In one randomized multicenter trial of 1847 patients, immediate treatment increased the time to second and third seizures and reduced the time to 2-year remission when compared with untreated patients, but long-term remission rates were similar.[14,15] Although these results demonstrate the effectiveness of antiepileptic medication, the recurrence rate even in untreated patients is low enough that most patients with first seizures are not treated.

TABLE 182.1 **Recommended Emergency Treatment and Timetable for Status Epilepticus**

Time (min)	Action
0–5	1. Stabilize patient (airway, breathing, circulation, disability—neurologic exam)
	2. Time seizure from its onset, monitor vital signs
	3. Assess oxygenation, give oxygen via nasal cannula/mask, consider intubation if respiratory assistance needed
	4. Initiate ECG monitoring
	5. Collect finger stick blood glucose. If glucose <60 mg/dL then
	Adults: 100 mg thiamine IV then 50 mL D50W IV
	Children ≥2 years: 2 mL/kg D25W IV Children <2 years: 4 mL/kg D12.5W IV
	6. Attempt IV access and collect electrolytes, hematology, toxicology screen, (if appropriate) anticonvulsant drug levels
5–20	**A benzodiazepine is the initial therapy of choice (Level A):**
	Choose one of the following 3 equivalent first line options with dosing and frequency:
	• Intramuscular midazolam (10 mg for >40 kg, 5 mg for 13–40 kg, single dose, Level A) OR
	• Intravenous lorazepam (0.1 mg/kg/dose, max: 4 mg/dose, may repeat dose once, Level A) OR
	• Intravenous diazepam (0.15–0.2 mg/kg/dose, max: 10 mg/dose, may repeat dose once, Level A)
	If none of the 3 options above are available, choose one of the following:
	• Intravenous phenobarbital (15 mg/kg/dose, single dose, Level A) OR
	• Rectal diazepam (0.2–0.5 mg/kg, max: 20 mg/dose, single dose, Level B) OR
	• Intranasal midazolam (Level B), buccal midazolam (Level B)
10–20	Administer either 0.1 g of lorazepam per kilogram at 2 mg/min or 0.2 mg of diazepam per kilogram at 5 mg/min intravenously (if diazepam used, also give phenytoin in follow-up).
20–30 Second phase	**There is no evidence based preferred second therapy of choice (Level U):**
	Choose one of the following second line options and give as a single dose
	• Intravenous fosphenytoin (20 mg PE/kg, max: 1500 mg PE/dose, single dose[a], Level U) OR
	• Intravenous valproic acid (40 mg/kg, max: 3000 mg/dose, single dose, Level B) OR
	• Intravenous levetiracetam (60 mg/kg, max: 4500 mg/dose, single dose, Level U)
	If none of the options above are available, choose one of the following (if not given already):
	• Intravenous phenobarbital (15 mg/kg, single dose, Level B)
>40-60 Third phase	**There is no clear evidence to guide therapy in this phase (Level U):**
	Choices include: repeat second line therapy or anesthetic doses of either thiopental, midazolam, pentobarbital, or propofol (all with continuous EEG monitoring)

[a]In most centers, fosphenytoin is used in place of phenytoin. The dosage is determined in phenytoin equivalents, and it can be administered twice as fast. It also causes less damage if the IV infiltrates.
Data from Glauser T, Shinnars S, Gloss D, Alldredge D. Evidence-Based Guideline: Treatment of Convulsive Status Epilepticus in Children and Adults: Report of the Guideline Committee of the American Epilepsy Society. *Epilepsy Currents* 2016; 16 (1).

The two most consistent predictors of seizure recurrence are an abnormal electroencephalogram and an underlying cause. In patients with an unprovoked seizure for which there was an underlying antecedent cause (e.g., a previous head injury, mental retardation, or cerebral palsy), the risk of recurrent seizures was double that of patients with an unprovoked seizure for which there was no antecedent cause. After a second seizure, the risk of recurrence increases to more than 80%.[16]

Most epilepsy specialists advocate making treatment decisions after consideration of the risks and benefits of the treatment for a particular patient. Elements of decision-making include the risk to the patient according to the severity, timing, and frequency of seizures; age at seizure onset; and social and cognitive considerations. In determining risk, it is obvious that patients with generalized tonic-clonic seizures are more at risk for injury than are those with simple partial seizures. The timing of seizures is also important. Seizures that occur primarily while the patient is awake pose less risk. Seizures that occur only in relation to special circumstances, such as alcohol consumption, sleep deprivation, or pregnancy, are sometimes better treated by avoiding those factors than by taking antiepileptic medication. Age and cognition can be factors in decision-making.

Pharmacologic Management

Treatment choices vary with individual differences in cause, seizure type, age, and psychosocial factors. Control of seizures with a single drug should be the goal. Each drug should be titrated slowly to determine how it is tolerated, and each drug should be given a fair trial. The principles of treatment are fairly simple. As a first-line drug, levetiracetam (Keppra) has enormous advantages. It can be loaded acutely with equivalent oral and parenteral doses, and it has a broad spectrum of efficacy, against both generalized and focal forms of epilepsy. It has the added advantages of not causing sedation, not being an inducer of liver enzymes (and therefore not interfering with the metabolism of other medications), and being an acceptable drug in pregnancy. Drawbacks include psychiatric symptoms such as agitation, anxiety, and depression.

Valproate (Depakote) is another first-line drug that is most effective against generalized forms of epilepsy. Convulsive seizures as well as petit mal staring spells respond very well to valproate, but side effects including weight gain, hair loss, polycystic ovarian syndrome, hepatotoxicity, and a relatively high rate of birth defects in children born to mothers taking it resulted in less use recently. Ethosuximide (Zarontin) is highly effective in children with petit mal seizures but less so for other seizure types. Lamotrigine (Lamictal), like levetiracetam, has a very wide spectrum of efficacy, and has become the favored drug for women with epilepsy because of its very low rate of associated birth defects. Drawbacks include lack of a parenteral formulation and relatively high rates of allergic rash that can evolve into Stevens-Johnson syndrome.

For focal epilepsy and complex partial seizures, with or without secondary generalization, carbamazepine (Tegretol) remains probably the single most effective drug and has the great advantage of low cost. It can, however, make some forms of generalized epilepsy worse and currently has no parenteral formulation; however, this is being studied and patents are pending. Phenytoin (Dilantin) is equally effective and can be given parenterally but has a concerning side effect profile, particularly for women, in terms of osteoporosis, hirsutism, and coarsening of facial features, and in older adults associated with significant drug interactions. It can also be used for primary generalized epilepsy.

Topiramate (Topamax) is not a first-line drug because of its cognitive side effects, which include somnolence and dysphasia. However, it does have a broad spectrum of efficacy, is effective for migraine prophylaxis, and also promotes weight loss. These qualities make it a favored drug in some settings. Lack of a parenteral formulation is a drawback. Gabapentin (Neurontin) actually exacerbates primary generalized epilepsies and is a weak drug for focal and secondarily generalized seizures. Because of its usefulness in pain management, it is sometimes used in mild cases of focal epilepsy when the healthcare provider is also trying to treat pain.

If seizures are frequent, efficacy can be determined quickly. About 50% of patients with epilepsy respond completely or almost completely to the first drug tried.[17] When medications are changed, the new medication should be added to the existing regimen. When the new medication is well tolerated and an effective dose has been achieved, the first medication can be slowly reduced. If the patient's seizures remain intractable after a trial of two or three single drugs, rational combinations of medications should be tried. Drugs with different mechanisms of action and different side effect profiles usually combine well.

Phenytoin with phenobarbital has been a traditional combination, but there is probably better evidence for the combined use of lamotrigine and valproate. Almost any combination of drugs has been found to be effective for at least a few patients. Among the 50% of patients who are refractory to monotherapy, probably another 25% will have their seizures controlled with some combination of medications; the remaining 25% remain refractory.[17] Half of these are candidates for epilepsy surgery; a residual 10% to 15% of patients will continue to have frequent seizures no matter what is tried.

Side effects occur in approximately 30% to 40% of patients taking AEDs.[15] Side effects include CNS involvement (such as somnolence, dizziness, tremor, and cognitive impairments), potential rashes, mood changes, weight changes, gastrointestinal disturbances, and headache.[15,17] The side effects should be carefully monitored and the doses adjusted to minimize the adverse effects of the medication. Rarely, an idiosyncratic reaction can occur, which can be life-threatening.

Measurements of blood levels of AEDs are helpful in determining whether a therapeutic dose has been achieved. For a steady level of the drug to be maintained in circulation, dosage frequency should be determined by the half-life of the drug.

It is most important to follow the patient's response to treatment, not only in terms of drug levels, but in relation to efficacy and side effects. With many patients, seizures are controlled with low doses and levels of medications, whereas other patients require and tolerate high levels. Some patients experience significant side effects, even when drug levels are within a normal range. In this case, it may be best to order free AED levels, especially if the drug is highly protein bound. Protein binding, absorption, and elimination pharmacokinetics are extremely important factors to consider in predicting side effects and drug–drug interactions. The provider should obtain a complete list of medications, including over-the-counter preparations, from the patient. Blood levels should be obtained at least yearly, and more often if the patient is having breakthrough seizures, increased side effects, or signs of drug toxicity. In addition, CBC, electrolyte determinations, and LFTs should be performed within a month of beginning a new AED and periodically thereafter.

Emerging Medical Trends. There is a great deal of interest in using cannabidiols for the treatment of drug-resistant epilepsy. Recent studies have demonstrated a decreased number of seizure when these substances are used in conjunction with usual treatment, especially in the pediatric population, with calls for more research into this area.[18]

Discontinuation of Antiepileptic Drugs. In making a decision to discontinue AED therapy, the provider and patient should consider the risk/benefit ratio. The risk for relapse is 20% to 40% in the first year of drug withdrawal and remains at about 36% during a 30-year period.[19] In one study, the risk of relapse was 2.9 times greater in those coming off of medication than in those staying on. Patients with the highest risk for relapse are those with a seizure disorder onset during adolescence, an abnormal electroencephalogram, an underlying neurologic condition, a definite diagnosis of primary generalized epilepsy, or a history of previous failures at discontinuing AEDs. There is insufficient evidence to establish when to withdraw AEDs in patients who are seizure free. One evidence-based review of 52 class II studies recommended that removal of medications be considered only if the patient has been seizure free for 2 to 5 years, has a single type of partial seizure, and has a normal electroencephalogram and IQ and normal findings on physical examination.[19]

Surgical Management

Of all patients with epilepsy, 25% to 30% are refractory to medical management.[20] Of the 25% to 30%, approximately half have focal lesions that are responsible for their seizures; these patients are good candidates for epilepsy surgery. The most common form of epilepsy surgery is a temporal lobectomy. Almost 80% of partial seizures in adults begin in the temporal lobes; a portion of one of the temporal lobes can be removed if tests consistently indicate that the seizures originate in that area. After temporal lobe surgery, success rates (complete seizure control) range from 65% to 95%.[20]

The removal of tumors, abnormal collections of blood vessels, and congenital lesions is another surgical resection option. These conditions can be found anywhere in the brain, and the best results are obtained when both the lesion and the surrounding epileptogenic brain are removed. It is often necessary to perform intracranial electroencephalographic mapping to delineate the epileptic zone and to identify cortically important areas, such as the language and motor cortex, which must be avoided during surgery.

Another major type of epilepsy surgery involves dividing the corpus callosum. With this type of surgery, the nerve fibers that connect one side of the brain to the other are severed; no tissue is removed. This surgery is most helpful for secondarily generalized tonic-clonic seizures and atonic seizures. Although seizures are not completely stopped by this procedure, they are confined to one hemisphere. Impairment of consciousness, convulsive seizure activity, and falls are often eliminated or greatly reduced.

Other surgical interventions available include multiple subpial transections wherein the surgeon makes a series of superficial cuts across brain tissue, theoretically interrupting the abnormal electrical signals; vagus nerve stimulation; and use of a responsive neurostimulation device, wherein wires implanted in the area of the seizures fire an electrical current into the area to prevent a seizure.[20]

After surgery, patients continue antiepileptic medication for several years. Patients who are seizure free for several years can consider a medication taper; however, there is not sufficient evidence to determine whether seizures will recur.

LIFE SPAN CONSIDERATIONS

Although stigma, social isolation, and depression can affect all persons with epilepsy, special concerns are recognized in specific age groups. Many patients develop epilepsy in early adolescence. This diagnosis can have a profound effect on self-esteem and instill a sense of lacking control because of the unpredictability of seizures. Parental overprotection and preoccupation with the child can lead to problems within the entire family unit. Adolescents should be encouraged to take responsibility for their own care. Providing education and the forum for a trusting relationship is the initial goal for this group of patients. Factual information should be presented in a straightforward, individualized manner, and the young adult should be encouraged to be honest and open about seizure frequency and compliance issues. Collaboration between patient and provider ideally results in a better understanding of the importance of medication, which makes adherence to the treatment plan more likely.

In women with epilepsy, there are additional concerns about contraception, fertility, and sexuality. Pregnancy has unpredictable effects on seizure control. Female adolescents should be counseled about family planning and birth control options. Patients taking hepatic enzyme–inducing AEDs should be given a higher-dose oral contraceptive, one with an estrogen content higher than 50 mcg.[21] Women with epilepsy should be encouraged to plan their pregnancies and optimize seizure control in the prepregnancy year. They should also be given at least 1 mg of folic acid supplementation per day in advance; some AEDs have been shown to inhibit folate action, and folate deficiency is associated with an increased risk of neural tube defects. Overall, AEDs probably double the baseline rate of birth defects.[22] Decisions to continue or to stop taking medication during pregnancy are difficult and should be discussed with a neurologist on an individual basis. Women who continue to take AEDs during pregnancy should be enrolled in the North American AED pregnancy registry, which can be located through the Epilepsy Foundation of America. AED levels may fluctuate unpredictably, and dosage modifications may be necessary. AED levels should be checked monthly and free levels obtained whenever possible.

Lamotrigine and levetiracetam have been associated with lower rates of birth defects than other drugs.[22]

Hormonal changes also have an effect on seizure control. Many women note that seizures tend to occur just before or during their menstrual cycle. This is most likely related to low progesterone levels. Progesterone has been shown to decrease neuronal excitability in animal models, and Depo-Provera may have some role as an antiepileptic medication.[21] Little is known about the relationship between epilepsy and menopause. Studies are generally done with small numbers of women and evidence is conflicting.

The onset of epilepsy in older adults has increased during the past decade. This increase is related to an increase in cerebrovascular disease, brain tumors, and Alzheimer disease, all associated with aging. Special concerns for older adults include an increased risk of head injury from an incidental fall, injury or falls that occur during seizures, the effects of AEDs on cognition and mobility, and interactions among various medications. Monotherapy is most important for this population to reduce side effects and drug interactions.[23] Dosage changes should be made slowly, because older adults are more sensitive than young patients to even minor changes. Among AEDs, levetiracetam is least likely to interact with other drugs.

COMPLICATIONS

Complications in patients with epilepsy are usually related to seizure events. Injuries that occur during seizures include falls, burns, motor vehicle accidents, and aspiration pneumonia. Risks can be reduced by making lifestyle changes at work and during recreation. Patient advocacy helps ensure safe environments at work and school and can discourage discrimination.

Recent evidence suggests that women and also men taking enzyme-inducing antiepileptic medications are at increased risk for osteoporosis and osteomalacia. This is related to bone metabolism and inadequate absorption of vitamin D.[24] All patients should be taking vitamin D and calcium supplements.

Convulsive or generalized tonic-clonic SE is a medical emergency that can lead to brain damage or even death.[11] Mortality and morbidity rates are related to the cause of SE and the time from the onset of SE until seizures are controlled. In patients with known epilepsy, half of the hospital-reported cases of GCSE have been associated with subtherapeutic AED levels.[11] Other causes of SE include brain infection, trauma, and stroke. Most cases of SE can be treated successfully with parenteral drug therapy, including lorazepam, phenytoin, and phenobarbital.

PATIENT AND FAMILY EDUCATION

Epilepsy provides unique teaching opportunities because it is a chronic condition that affects all aspects of a patient's life. Patient and family education about safety is vital. It is imperative that patients avoid high places such as rooftops and ladders, not operate dangerous equipment that could cause cuts or crush injuries, and not swim alone. Family members should be taught simple first aid measures such as turning the patient onto his or her side and not putting objects into the mouth during a tonic-clonic seizure.

Other key areas for patient instruction include the following:
- General information
- Diagnostic studies
- Treatment plan
- Medication information

- Alternative or adjunctive therapies
- Safety issues and first aid for seizures
- Support services available (e.g., support groups, centers for independent living and how to access them)

HEALTH PROMOTION

Issues related to driving and other behaviors that impose a great safety risk should be discussed. Each state has varied restrictions for individuals with epilepsy who wish to obtain a driver's license. Information about the laws of a particular state can be found by calling the department of motor vehicles. Issues surrounding employment and psychosocial functioning should also be addressed. Resources such as vocational rehabilitation programs, clinical social workers, centers for independent living, and epilepsy support groups should be used.

Overall, moderation should be encouraged. Adequate rest, stress reduction, proper nutrition, and avoidance of known seizure precipitants can improve seizure control. Some studies advocate a ketogenic diet as helpful in controlling seizures, especially in children whose seizures are incompletely controlled with medication alone. Adults find this diet difficult to maintain because of its restrictions. Several studies of modified Atkins diets seem to show the same beneficial results.[25]

Epilepsy is a challenging condition and requires a comprehensive approach to treatment. The goal is to treat the patient but not make the treatment worse than the disease. Efforts to understand the impact of epilepsy on patients will improve the health care provider's ability to treat appropriately and compassionately.

REFERENCES

1. American Epilepsy Foundation. Facts and Figures. Retrieved from https://www.aesnet.org/for_patients/facts_figures. (Accessed 17 June 2019).
2. Paris, M., & Reddy, U. (2018). Update on the management of status epilepticus. *Anesthesia and Intensive Care Medicine, 19*(3), 83–86.
3. Commission on Classification and Terminology of the International League against Epilepsy. (1981). Proposal for revised clinical and electroencephalographic classification of epileptic seizures. *Epilepsia, 22*(4), 489–501.
4. Commission on Classification and Terminology of the International League against Epilepsy. (1989). Proposal for revised classification of epilepsy and epileptic syndromes. *Epilepsia, 30*(4), 389–399.
5. Fisher, R. S., Cross, J. H., French, J. A., et al. (2017). Operational classification of seizure types by the International League Against Epilepsy: Position Paper of the ILAE Commission for Classification and Terminology. *Epilepsia, 58*(4), 522–530.
6. Berg, A., Testa, F., & Levy, S. (2011). Complete remission in non-syndromic childhood-onset epilepsy. *Annals of Neurology, 70*(4), 566–573.
7. Verellen, R. M., & Cavazos, J. E. (2011). Pathophysiological considerations of seizures, epilepsy, and status epilepticus in the elderly. *Aging and Disease, 2*(4), 278–285.
8. Calik, M., Karakas, E., & Calla, N. (2013). Clinical importance of neuroimaging in epilepsy. *Journal of Neurosciences in Rural Practice, 4*(Suppl. 1), s11–s12.
9. Dantas, F. G., de Melo, E. S., Cavalcante, A. P., et al. (2014). EEG in epilepsy: Sensibility and specificity. *Journal of Epilepsy Clinical Neurophysiology, 20*(2), 116–118.
10. Engle, J. (2013). *Seizures and epilepsy* (2nd ed.). New York: Oxford University Press.
11. Betjemann, J., & Lowenstein, D. (2015). Status epilepticus in adults. *The Lancet. Neurology, 14*(6), 615–624.
12. Glauser, T., Shinnars, S., Gloss, D., & Alldredge, D. (2016). Evidence-based guideline: Treatment of convulsive status epilepticus in children and adults: Report of the Guideline Committee of the American Epilepsy Society. *Epilepsy Currents, 16*(1).
13. Leach, J. P., & Abassi, H. (2013). Modern management of epilepsy. *Clinical Medicine (London, England), 13*(1), 84–86.
14. Krumholz, A., Wiebe, S., Gronseth, G., et al. (2015). Evidence-based guideline: Management of an unprovoked first seizure in adults: Report of the Guideline Development Subcommittee of the American Academy of Neurology and the American Epilepsy Society. *Neurology, 84*, 1706–1713.
15. Perucca, E., & Tomson, T. (2011). The pharmacological treatment of epilepsy in adults. *The Lancet. Neurology, 10*(5), 446–456.
16. Kim, L. G., Johnson, T. L., Marson, A. G., et al. (2006). Prediction of risk of seizure recurrence after a single seizure and early epilepsy: Further results from the MESS trial. *The Lancet. Neurology, 5*(4), 317.
17. Schmidt, D., & Schacter, S. C. (2014). Drug treatment of epilepsy in adults. *British Medical Journal, 348*, g254.
18. Theil, E., Marsh, F., French, J., et al. (2018). Cannabidiol in patients with seizures associated with Lennox-Gastaut syndrome (GWPCARE4): A double-blind, placebo controlled phase 3 trial. *The Lancet, 391*(10125), 1085–1096.
19. Braun, K., & Schmidt, D. (2014). Stopping antiepileptic drugs in seizure free patients. *Current Opinion in Neurology, 27*(2), 219–226.
20. Nowell, M., Miserocchi, A., McEvoy, A., & Duncan, V. (2014). Advances in epilepsy surgery. *Journal of Neurology, Neurosurgery, and Psychiatry, 85*(11), 1273–1279.
21. Sabers, A. (2013). Treatment guidelines: Women of fertile age. *Epileptology, 1*(1), 11–16.
22. Eadie, M. H. (2014). Treating epilepsy in pregnant women. *Expert Opinion on Pharmacotherapy, 15*(6), 841–850.
23. Motika, P. V., & Spencer, D. C. (2016). Treatment of epilepsy in the elderly. *Current Neurology and Neuroscience Reports, 16*, 96. https://doi.org/10.1007/s11910-016-0696-8.
24. Miziak, B., Blaszczyk, B., Chroscinska-Krawczyk, M., et al. (2014). The problem of osteoporosis in epileptic patients taking antiepileptic drugs. *Expert Opinion on Drug Safety, 13*(7), 935–946.
25. Martin, K., Jackson, C. F., Levy, R. G., & Cooper, P. N. (2016). Ketogenic diet and other dietary treatments for epilepsy. *The Cochrane Database of Systematic Reviews*, (2), CD001903, doi:10.1002/14651858.CD001903.pub3.

CHAPTER 183

TRIGEMINAL NEURALGIA

Wanda J. Handel

DEFINITION AND EPIDEMIOLOGY

Trigeminal neuralgia is a common and well-defined orofacial pain disorder restricted to the sensory branches of the trigeminal nerve. Onset is abrupt, with spasms of pain lasting seconds to minutes. It is also known as tic douloureux, from the French for painful spasm, and affects 12 people per 100,000 every year.[1] Women are affected slightly more often than men, and older adults more often than younger persons. The mean age at onset is 54 years; most cases occur in individuals between 50 and 70 years of age. Cases occurring in patients younger than 40 years are unusual.[1,2]

PATHOPHYSIOLOGY

The fifth cranial nerve, the trigeminal nerve, is a large, mixed sensory and motor nerve that originates in the brainstem and travels in the cervical cord, with the sensory ganglion found in the Meckel cave in the middle cranial fossa. The peripheral branches form three sensory divisions—ophthalmic (V1), maxillary (V2), and mandibular (V3)—that conduct sensory impulses from the greater part of the face and head, from the cornea and conjunctiva, and from the nose and mouth. These impulses eventually terminate in the thalamus, where they are relayed to the appropriate cortical area for interpretation. The motor portion of the nerve supplies the muscles of the jaw and sphenoid areas.

Most primary cases of trigeminal neuralgia are thought to be caused by vascular compression and are considered classic trigeminal neuralgia.[3] Secondary trigeminal neuralgia is differentiated by the ability to demonstrate another major neurologic cause, such as compression from tumor, multiple sclerosis, or trauma.[4] The location of one of the cerebral arteries and its branches is thought to be a factor by creating compression on the nerve as it exits the brainstem. Demyelination, vascular changes, and degenerative changes in the sensory (gasserian) ganglion are postulated to generate altered impulse transmission, allowing ephaptic transmission between adjacent nerve fibers mediating light touch and pain.[4]

CLINICAL PRESENTATION AND PHYSICAL EXAMINATION

The primary feature of this disorder is recurrent paroxysms of pain in the distribution of any branch of the trigeminal nerve. The pain is usually described as burning, stabbing, sharp, penetrating, or electric shock–like and usually is on one side of the face. Males may have unshaven faces or portions thereof. The index of suspicion for multiple sclerosis rises if the patient exhibits bilateral facial pain. The duration of each paroxysm varies from seconds to more than 2 minutes and involves V2 and V3 more often than V1; V1 is more frequently affected by postherpetic neuralgia.[1,4] Pain may recur once a month or several times per day. If the pain occurs frequently during the day, the patient may complain of unremitting facial discomfort between discrete episodes. Usually a patient does not awaken from sleep during a paroxysm.

During an attack, the patient may cease talking, stop chewing, become very still, rub or pinch the face, avoid making facial expressions during conversation, grimace, or make movements of the face and jaw. Between attacks, the patient is free of symptoms except for fear of an impending attack.

Physical Examination

A characteristic feature of trigeminal neuralgia is the trigger zone, a small area of the skin or orobuccal mucosa that the patient can identify as the point that sets off an attack. Trigger points are generally in the distribution of the nerve branch experiencing the pain. Chewing, talking, facial movement, or touch may elicit a paroxysm. Drafts or cool breezes may also precipitate symptoms. The patient may be reluctant to allow examination of the face for fear of triggering an attack. All cranial nerves should be examined in detail. In secondary trigeminal neuralgia, the corneal reflex may be abnormal.[5] The remainder of the physical examination, including the neurologic component, is normal.

DIAGNOSTICS

Diagnosis is based primarily on the patient history and physical findings and requires no initial diagnostic laboratory or imaging studies unless history and physical findings suggest the need. Magnetic resonance imaging (MRI) and/or magnetic resonance angiography (MRA) are helpful in defining classical versus secondary TN.

Essential Diagnostics

None.

Additional Diagnostics (if indicated)

MRI
MRA
Electrophysiologic testing

DIFFERENTIAL DIAGNOSIS

 Red flags include facial pain with sensory changes, deafness, difficulty achieving pain control or age under 40.

The differential diagnosis should include multiple sclerosis (see Chapter 180), headache, particularly migraine (see Chapter 177), tumor (acoustic neuroma, trigeminal neuroma, and meningioma), aneurysms, acute polyneuropathy, chronic meningitis, other neuralgias, and dental abnormalities. Trigeminal neuralgia is a common cause of pain in multiple sclerosis. The diagnosis of trigeminal neuralgia is usually made without difficulty from the history and the characteristic manner in which the patient relates the history (the patient is careful not to touch any trigger points or painful areas). New criteria for clinical diagnosis put forth by the Special Interest Group on Neuropathic Pain of the International Association for the Study of Pain include the following[1]:

- Unilateral orofacial pain within the facial or intraoral CN V territory, paroxysmal in nature, with spasms of pain lasting from a fraction of a second to 2 minutes, with ability to trigger with typical maneuvers (touch, chewing, brushing teeth)

However, this case presentation of trigeminal neuralgia may not always be encountered. Because there are innumerable causes of facial pain, prudence dictates that alternative diagnoses be investigated and that the patient be reexamined at regular intervals. Idiopathic TN may be diagnosed when there is no lesion or other disease process to cause TN. Classical TN and secondary TN can be diagnosed by MRI/MRA showing compression of the CN V nerve root for former, or showing evidence of cerebellopontine angle tumors, vascular malformations, or other major neurologic disease for latter diagnosis.[1]

Results of laboratory tests are either normal or noncontributory. If alternative diagnoses are suspected, an autoimmune laboratory panel may be indicated. Trigeminal reflex testing has demonstrated that abnormal reflexes are associated with greater risk of secondary trigeminal neuralgia. Magnetic resonance angiography of the posterior fossa may be undertaken to differentiate vascular abnormalities and to rule out compression from tumor or vessels. MRI can also corroborate the presence of multiple sclerosis.[1,5]

INTERPROFESSIONAL COLLABORATIVE MANAGEMENT

 Specialist referral to a neurologist indicated for co-management of patient care for patients not responding to first-line treatment or those suspected of having secondary trigeminal neuralgia.

Nonpharmacologic Management

Patients with refractory pain who do not tolerate medications or fail pharmacologic management with three medications may be referred to a neurosurgeon for surgical assessment.[6] Some patients may find comfort and effect from complementary and alternative medications (CAM) such as acupuncture, biofeedback, nutritional therapy, and Botox.

Pharmacologic Management

The treatment of trigeminal neuralgia has not changed much during the past decade. Regardless of the intervention adopted, symptoms may remit spontaneously and permanently. A

TABLE 183.1	Pharmacotherapy for Trigeminal Neuralgia		
First Line Treatment	**Starting Dose**	**Maximum Dose**	**Adverse Drug Events (Not All Inclusive)**
Carbamazepine	100–200 mg daily	200–400 mg three times per day	Aplastic anemia, agranulocytosis, ataxia, diplopia, Stevens-Johnson syndrome
Oxcarbazepine	300 mg two times per day	600–1200 mg two times per day	Nausea, vomiting, hyponatremia, Stevens-Johnson syndrome
Second Line Treatment— Add on or Switch to	**Starting Dose**	**Maximum Dose**	**Adverse Drug Events (Not All Inclusive)**
Baclofen	5–10 mg three times per day	30 mg three times per day	Sedation, dizziness, dyspepsia, cognitive changes
Lamotrigine	25–50 mg daily	150–200 mg two times per day	Rash, Stevens-Johnson syndrome
Phenytoin	100–300 mg daily	300–500 mg daily	Rash, dizziness, confusion, ataxia
For Patients With Multiple Sclerosis	**Starting Dose**	**Maximum Dose**	**Adverse Drug Events (Not All Inclusive)**
Gabapentin	100–300 mg daily	300–600 mg three times per day	Dizziness, sedation, decreased coordination
Misoprostol	200 mcg three times daily	600 mcg per day	Headache, nausea, diarrhea, contraindicated in pregnancy

Adapted from Pfaul, T., Brinkerson, M., & Treuhert, T. (2012). Misoprostal as a therapeutic option for trigeminal neuralgia in patients with multiple sclerosis. *Pain Medicine, 13*(10);1377–1378; and Obermann, M. (2015). Update on the challenge of treating trigeminal neuralgia. *Orphan Drugs: Research and Reviews, 5,* 11–17.

step-wise approach, including co-management with a neurologist, is warranted.

- Anticonvulsants are the first-line pharmacologic therapy.[5]
  - When using anticonvulsant therapy, the provider should titrate to the maximum therapeutic dose necessary to provide pain relief, and then titrate down to the lowest effective dose.
  - Abrupt withdrawal of these agents should be avoided. A partial listing of more commonly used agents can be found in Table 183.1.
- Carbamazepine (CBZ) oxcarbazepine (OXZ).[5]
  - Approximately two-thirds of patients will respond to CBZ. OXZ may be better tolerated in some individuals.[4,5] When prescribing CBZ, care must be taken to monitor for liver damage and hematologic changes using CBC, serum sodium levels, and liver function tests at periodic intervals.[4,5]
- If the patient does not respond satisfactorily to medical management or has relief only at a dose that causes intolerable adverse effects:
  - combination drug therapy may be started with another agent.
  - second-line medications include baclofen, lamotrigine, and phenytoin.[4]
- In acute attacks, intravenous administration of fosphenytoin, injections of Botox, or sumatriptan or intranasal lidocaine may afford pain relief while oral doses are uptitrated.[4]
- In patients with multiple sclerosis, the long-acting prostaglandin E analogue misoprostol (Cytotec) or gabapentin have been useful.[6]

EMERGING MANAGEMENT TRENDS

Little has changed in the medical and surgical management for TN in decades. Promising medication approaches include the administration of Botulinum neurotoxin type A injected subcutaneously directly into the painful facial region showing reduction in pain in some small studies and positive results

from a phase II clinical trial using a novel sodium channel blocker (CNV1014802) to decrease paroxysms and severity of pain.[7] Emerging technology includes noninvasive repetitive transcranial magnetic stimulation and invasive deep brain stimulation for neuromodulation of pain in surgical patients refractory to treatment.[7]

INDICATIONS FOR REFERRAL AND HOSPITALIZATION

The primary care provider is often the initial practitioner to evaluate the patient with facial pain. After a thorough history and neurologic examination, a patient presumed to have trigeminal neuralgia should be referred to a neurologist for a more comprehensive physical and imaging examination. Medical treatment may be initiated by the specialist and managed by the primary care provider. Care consists of medication initiation, observations for adverse effects, and consultation with the neurologist regarding dose adjustments and response to therapy. Consultation with a specialist is beneficial to the patient and provider in identifying the most efficacious regimen when combination drug therapy is necessary.

Referral to a neurosurgeon is indicated after medical therapies have been exhausted. Surgery is considered when medical regimens do not provide pain relief or side effects of medications are intolerable. Among the surgical interventions that may be appropriate are glycerol rhizotomy, radiofrequency ablation, microvascular decompression, and stereotactic radiosurgery.[8] Major disadvantages of glycerol rhizotomy, radiofrequency ablation, and decompression surgery include loss of facial sensation, keratitis, facial muscle weakness, spontaneous pain (anesthesia dolorosa), dysesthesias, and recurrent neuralgia.[7]

Consultation with a psychologist or psychiatrist may also be indicated, depending on the patient's adaptation skills. Multidisciplinary team meetings may be valuable in planning an approach to care. Referral to a pain center may also be an option for individuals with chronic pain.

LIFE SPAN CONSIDERATIONS

Careful consideration must be paid to the older adult patient who may have preexisting age-related physiologic changes that can affect pharmacokinetics such as decreased blood flow, renal and hepatic impairment, risk of interactions due to polypharmacy, and a less predictable capacity for protein binding of the drug.[4,5] Slow titration is encouraged. Co-morbid conditions may also make a patient a poor surgical candidate.

COMPLICATIONS

Complications are usually related to pharmacologic management. Carbmazepine therapy may result in aplastic anemia, drowsiness, dizziness, and ataxia. Other medications listed can cause drowsiness, dizziness, and cognitive changes. Surgical complications include facial numbness and pain, recurrent neuralgia, or facial paralysis, as well as the risks associated with any surgical procedure. Pain control may also be a significant factor, particularly if patients cannot tolerate the usually prescribed medications. In such an instance, additional management concerns may arise, with weight loss, dehydration, and poor dental hygiene if chewing, liquids, and oral care are triggers, as well as social isolation and depression. *All of these concerns are potentially more significant in the older adult population.*

PATIENT AND FAMILY EDUCATION

- Provide a full explanation of trigeminal neuralgia, including type, treatment options, and its usual clinical course to help allay the fear patients experience from the onset of facial pain and allow shared decision making regarding treatments and/or testing.
- Educate patient and family about varied medication therapies, all of which are sedating. Caution about use of these medications in conjunction with use of alcohol and other medications.
- Reinforce the need for laboratory studies when taking medications.
- Discuss the psychosocial aspects of changes to activities of daily living and to report signs and symptoms of social isolation and depression.

HEALTH PROMOTION

A collaborative relationship with the patient enhances a tailored, well-informed approach toward quality care. For patients in severe pain or those who are fearful of the next attack, it is important to consider the patient's activities of daily living, including eating, sleeping, oral hygiene, and socializing with others. Maintenance of oral hygiene may be challenging because brushing may elicit pain; use of an oral water flosser to clean the teeth may be of benefit to some. *Severe pain may restrict adequate calorie intake;* advising the patient to use a straw for liquids may allow intake of nutritional supplements.[9] Referral can be placed to a dietician for consultation or to a psychologist for support and assistance.

REFERENCES

1. Cruccu, G., Finnerup, N. B., Jensen, T. S., et al. (2016). Trigeminal neuralgia: New classification and diagnostic grading for practice and research. *Neurology*, 87(2), 220–228. doi:10.1212/WNL.0000000000002840.
2. National Institutes of Neurological Disorders and Stroke (NINDS). (2017). Trigeminal neuralgia fact sheet. NINDS website, May. Retrieved from http://www.ninds.nih.gov/disorders/trigeminal_neuralgia/detail_trigeminal_neuralgia.htm. (Accessed 20 February 2018).
3. Chen, Q., Wang, X., Wan, L., & Zheng, J. P. (2014). Arterial compression of the nerve is the primary cause of trigeminal neuralgia. *Neurological Sciences*, 35, 61–66.
4. Kumar, S., Rastog, S., Kumar, S., et al. (2013). Pain in trigeminal neuralgia: Neurophysiology and measurement: A comprehensive review. *Journal of Medicine and Life*, 6(4), 383.
5. Zakrzewska, J., & Linskey, M. (2014). Trigeminal neuralgia. *British Medical Journal*, 348, 974.
6. Pfaul, T., Brinkerson, M., & Treuhert, T. (2012). Misoprostal as a therapeutic option for trigeminal neuralgia in patients with multiple sclerosis. *Pain Medicine*, 13(10), 1377–1378.
7. Obermann, M. (2015). Update on the challenge of treating trigeminal neuralgia. *Orphan Drugs: Research and Reviews*, (5), 11–17. doi.org/10.2147/ODRR.S53046.
8. Montano, N., Comforti, G., Bonaventura, R., et al. (2015). Advances in diagnosis and treatment of trigeminal neuralgia. *Therapeutics and Clinical Risk Management*, 11, 289–299.
9. Durham, J., Touger-Decker, R., Nixdorf, D. R., Rigassio-Radler, D., & Moynihan, P. (2015). Oro-facial pain and nutrition: A forgotten relationship? *Journal of Oral Rehabilitation*, 42(1), 75–80. doi:10.1111/joor.12226.

CHAPTER **184**

INTRACRANIAL TUMORS

Lynsey P. Teulings • Paula K. Rauschkolb

Primary malignant and nonmalignant intracranial tumors represent a small fraction of all types of cancer, but they have a major physical, psychological, and financial impact on individual patients, families, and communities. Brain metastases from systemic neoplasm are equally devastating and significantly more frequent. Expedient diagnosis and treatment of brain tumors are essential to minimize potential complications and to maximize functional quality of life. As the first point of contact for patients when acute or subtle changes in health occur, primary care practitioners play an important role in the diagnosis and ongoing care of patients with brain tumors. The practitioner's knowledge of a patient allows the detection of subtle clinical changes, affording appropriate evaluation and timely diagnosis. Ongoing supportive care during treatment and follow-up of a patient with the diagnosis of a brain tumor is imperative and can be well managed by the primary care practitioner in collaboration with the specialist.

DEFINITION AND EPIDEMIOLOGY

The term *brain tumor*, also referred to as *intracranial neoplasm*, is defined as an abnormal mass of cells located in the brain or surrounding tissues. There are more than 120 different types of brain tumors that range in severity from benign tumors to life-threatening malignancies.[1] Even nonmalignant brain tumors, depending on their size or location, can cause significant mortality and morbidity. Brain tumors are typically classified as primary or metastatic lesions. While primary brain tumors arise from abnormal cell growth in brain tissue or structures within the cranium, brain metastases are thought to be caused by the hematogenous spread of cancer from outside of the nervous system. Primary central nervous system (CNS) lymphoma, another type of brain tumor, occurs as a result of infiltration of the CNS by neoplastic lymphocytes.

Brain tumors account for a small proportion of all cancers and cancer-related deaths. An estimated 78,980 new cases of primary nonmalignant and malignant brain and central nervous system tumors are expected to be diagnosed in the Unites States in 2018.[2] Approximately one-third of cases are malignant. Meningioma accounts for 36.8% of all cases, the majority of which are nonmalignant. Gliomas are the second most common primary brain tumor and account for 74.6% of malignant primary intracranial tumors.[2] In children, primary brain tumors are the most common of the solid tumors and the leading cause of cancer related deaths in children ages 0 to 14.[2,3]

Brain metastasis are significantly more common than primary brain tumors, with incidence that varies upon the type of primary malignancy. Although melanoma and small cell lung cancer (SCLC) have the highest predilection to metastasize to the brain, brain metastases are more prevalent in non-SCLC and breast cancer due to the higher incidence of these malignancies. Improved imaging techniques and greater utilization of MRI has led to an increase in detection of brain metastasis over the years. In addition, novel therapeutics have increased survival in patients with systemic cancers, thereby allowing more time for dissemination into the brain.[4] Prognosis is influenced by primary malignancy, age, performance status, and number of brain metastases.

The etiology of primary intracranial neoplasms remains largely unknown. Currently, the only established environmental risk factor for glioma and meningioma is prior exposure to ionizing radiation.[5] A small percentage of primary brain tumors can be attributed to hereditary syndromes such as neurofibromatosis type 1 and type 2, Li-Fraumeni syndrome, tuberous sclerosis, von Hippel-Lindau disease, Turcot syndrome, and familial polyposis. Primary CNS lymphoma occurs more frequently in patients who are immunosuppressed, either due to an underlying disease such as HIV/AIDS or as a result of immunosuppressive therapy (e.g., following organ transplant or treatment of an autoimmune disorder). In immunocompetent patients, the diagnosis is rare but is often associated with advanced age.[6]

PATHOPHYSIOLOGY

The majority of primary brain tumors are thought to arise as a result of a random genetic mutation; however, the precise pathway that causes malignant transformation is not fully understood. Primary brain tumors rarely metastasize to other parts of the body; however, dissemination within the CNS (e.g., the spinal cord or leptomeninges) can occur. Cerebral edema, which often accompanies high-grade brain tumors, occurs as a result of neovascular proliferation, or angiogenesis, which leads to the formation of abnormal vasculature that lacks a competent basement membrane. These leaky vessels allow fluid to extravasate into the surrounding brain tissue.

Unlike other types of cancers, primary brain tumors are graded rather than staged. Tumor nomenclature and grading are based on the histologic characteristics of the tissue. They are classified according to the World Health Organization (WHO) grading system (I to IV), which provides a means to prognosticate the biologic behavior of the tumor (Table 184.1). The higher the grade, the higher the malignant potential. This distinction is made based exclusively upon the histology and molecular features of the tissue and does not take into consideration tumor size or extent of disease. Although prognosis correlates with WHO grade, immunohistochemistry and genetic profiling provide additional information that allows for more accurate characterization of the tumor. The combination

TABLE 184.1 Classification of Central Nervous System Tumors

Tumor Type (Frequency)[2]	WHO Grade[a]
Astrocytoma (20.3%)	Grade I: Pilocytic astrocytoma Grade II: Diffuse astrocytoma Grade III: Anaplastic astrocytoma Grade IV: Glioblastoma
Oligodendroglioma (1.4%)	Grade II: Oligodendroglioma Grade III: Anaplastic oligodendroglioma
Ependymoma (1.8%)	Grade I: Subependymoma, myxopapillary ependymoma Grade II: Ependymoma Grade III: Anaplastic ependymoma
Meningioma (36.8%)	Grade I: Meningioma Grade II: Atypical meningioma Grade III: Malignant meningioma
Primary CNS lymphoma (2.0%)	Not applicable

[a]World Health Organization (WHO) classification.

of histology and genetic characteristics guide individualized treatment.

Tumors that arise from glial cells, called *gliomas*, are the most frequent type of primary malignant brain tumor. Based on the cell of origin and molecular genotyping, gliomas are further classified into astrocytomas, oligodendrogliomas, and, less commonly, ependymomas. High-grade gliomas (WHO grade III or IV) are histologically heterogeneous and are characterized by neovascularization, high mitotic rate, and often have extensive areas of necrosis and hypoxia. They also have a tendency to infiltrate into surrounding brain tissue, making them very difficult to treat. Due to their accelerated growth rates and extent of invasiveness, high-grade tumors have worse survival outcomes than lower grade tumors.[7] However, some lower-grade tumors may transform to higher grade over time.

Meningiomas begin in the meninges, the protective membrane that encases the nervous system. Meningioma is the most common type of intracranial tumor, accounting for approximately one-third of all primary CNS tumors.[2] They can occur within the cranium or along the spinal cord, although intracranial lesions are more common. A meningioma may occur at any age, but due to its slow growth rate, it is often discovered in patients of advanced age. Low-grade (WHO grade I) meningioma is classified as having a low risk of reoccurrence and nonaggressive behavior, commonly referred to as benign. Factors that escalate meningioma to a higher grade include increased mitotic activity, brain invasion, and necrosis. While low-grade meningiomas are more common in women, more aggressive subtypes such as atypical (grade II) and anaplastic (grade III) meningiomas are slightly more common in men.[8]

The pathologic features of brain metastases differ according to their tumor of origin. Brain metastases typically mimic the histology of the primary tumors from which they originate; however, biologic differences in genetic mutations may exist. Primary CNS lymphoma (PCNSL) is an extranodal non-Hodgkin lymphoma confined to the central nervous system. It can involve the brain, spinal cord, eyes, or leptomeninges. In the vast majority of cases, histology for PCNSL is consistent with a diffuse, large B-cell lymphoma.

CLINICAL PRESENTATION AND PHYSICAL EXAMINATION

Brain tumors cause symptoms by infiltrating, expanding, and displacing healthy brain tissue. Peritumoral edema can increase the overall degree of mass effect, and in severe cases, there is a risk for brain herniation. Brain tumors can also obstruct the ventricular system, resulting in hydrocephalus. Furthermore, tumors can cause increased excitability of adjacent neurons resulting in seizures. Tumors involving the hypothalamic-pituitary axis can cause a variety of endocrinologic syndromes.

A meticulous history and thorough examination are essential to the diagnosis of a brain tumor. Symptoms are dependent upon the growth pattern and location of the tumor. Fast-growing tumors, such as glioblastoma, tend to produce subacute symptoms, often escalating over weeks, whereas slow-growing tumors, such as meningioma, can become very large over a period of years before producing symptoms. The clinical presentation of brain metastases is often more abrupt, related to rapid tumor growth and associated edema. On occasion, patients with brain tumors can present with acute symptoms; this typically occurs in the setting of intratumoral bleeding, ischemic stroke due to compression of intracranial vasculature, or seizure.

Patients with intracranial neoplasms may present with focal or nonfocal neurological complaints. In either case, symptoms are commonly subacute in onset and progressive in nature. However, as noted previously, acute presentation is possible. Focal changes include deficits in vision, speech, strength, sensation, or gait. Nonfocal symptoms include headache, memory loss, behavior change, cognitive deficits, and fatigue.

Seizure (see Chapter 182) is a common presenting symptom and occurs in roughly 70% of patients throughout the course of their illness.[9] Seizures are more prevalent in patients with low-grade glioma, meningioma, and metastatic brain tumors, but also occur in patients with high-grade glioma. There are two main types of seizure: generalized seizures and focal (also called *partial*) seizures. Focal seizures occur when abnormal electrical activity is localized to one specific area of the brain. Generalized seizures occur when abnormal electrical activity spreads across the cortical surface to involve both cerebral hemispheres. Generalized seizures typically result in tonic-clonic movements and loss of consciousness. Focal seizures are more common than generalized seizures in patients with brain tumors, although both can occur.

Patients may also present with signs and symptoms of increased intracranial pressure (ICP) due to mass effect within the cranium. Increased ICP is considered an oncologic emergency (see "Complications and Referrals for Hospitalization").

In addition to a general medical examination of the patient, a thorough neurologic exam is warranted. A mini-mental examination should be included, given that alteration in mental status is frequently observed in nonfocal syndromes. Examination of the optic fundi is also recommended to assess for papilledema, a finding that may indicate increased intracranial pressure.

Components of the neurologic examination are designed to help with localization to a particular brain region. Visual field testing by confrontation may elicit deficits of the optic nerve pathway, which includes the occipital and parietotemporal lobes. Abnormalities of ocular movement can occur from compression of the oculomotor nerves or involvement of the brainstem. Motor and sensory abnormalities correlate with frontal or parietal lobe dysfunction, respectively. Aphasia can be seen with damage to the frontal or temporal lobe of the dominant hemisphere. Of note, abnormal speech or comprehension, as a result of aphasia, can often be misinterpreted as confusion. Tumors involving the posterior fossa may result in gait dysfunction or disorders of coordination. In the case of seizures, patients may initially have focal findings on examination that disappear once the patient has recovered from the postictal state.

DIAGNOSTICS
Essential Diagnostics

Brain MRI with and without contrast is the preferred study for evaluation of a suspected intracranial mass. Head computed tomography (CT) scan is frequently used as part of the initial workup in the acute setting, as it is easily accessible, relatively low cost, and can rapidly identify emergent complications such as mass effect, midline shift, vasogenic edema, hemorrhage, herniation, and hydrocephalus. However, MRI with gadolinium is the gold standard and should be obtained following identification of a mass on CT whenever possible. If there is concern for metastatic disease, additional imaging may be indicated to help define the location of the primary cancer and extent of disease, such as CT scan of the chest, abdomen, and pelvis, and/or positron emission tomography (PET) scan.

Tissue acquisition is required in most cases to establish the diagnosis and to render treatment recommendations with the exception of suspected metastatic cancer. In this case, body imaging may first be performed, and tissue from the primary site of disease may be obtained instead.

Additional Diagnostics. MRI diffusion, perfusion, or spectroscopy may be useful under certain circumstances. Cerebrospinal fluid (CSF) is rarely abnormal in patients with primary brain tumors; thus lumbar puncture is warranted only if imaging suggests leptomeningeal involvement, primary CNS lymphoma, or the possibility of encephalitis as an alternative diagnosis. Serology is typically unrevealing.

INITIAL DIAGNOSTICS

Intracranial Mass

LABORATORY	IMAGING
• May consider routine laboratory studies if alternative diagnoses are suspected	• CT head with contrast • Brain MRI with and without contrast • CT chest, abdomen, and pelvis[a] • PET/CT[a]

[a]Only if metastatic disease is suspected

DIFFERENTIAL DIAGNOSIS

Differential diagnoses include cerebral infarct (stroke), intraparenchymal hemorrhage, and infection (abscess, encephalitis).

• Headache: Often gradually escalating, classically worse in the mornings
• Focal neurological deficit, particularly if subacute and gradually progressive

- New-onset seizures
- Signs/symptoms of increased ICP, which may include:
  - Severe headache
  - Nausea, vomiting
  - Altered mental status
  - Somnolence
  - Diplopia
  - Pupillary changes (e.g., uneven pupil size, fixed dilated pupils)
  - Papilledema

INTERPROFESSIONAL COLLABORATIVE MANAGEMENT

Oncologic management of brain tumors requires a multidisciplinary approach and may include several treatment modalities depending upon tumor type and grade. Unlike many other forms of cancer where early detection can lead to improved prognosis and prolonged survival, this is not the case with brain tumors. With the exception of certain brain tumors, such as grade I meningioma or grade I subependymoma that have been completely resected, treatment is not curative, and the goal is instead to prolong progression free survival. Because treatment often impacts critical brain function, supportive care is an integral part of the management of patients with brain tumors. Therapies are directed at symptoms related to the brain tumor, as well as the acute and late side effects of treatment.

Radiation Therapy

Depending upon the histopathologic characteristics of the tumor, surgery may be followed by radiation, which may be used as a single agent or in combination with chemotherapy. Radiation can be localized to the area of disease or may involve the whole brain. Radiation is delivered on a fractionated schedule, usually in the range of 30 to 60 Gy. In patients over 70 or for those with poor performance status, a hypofractionated course of radiation may be prescribed. Radiation is often recommended for patients with intermediate-grade meningioma that is subtotally resected, high-grade meningioma, low-grade glioma with high-risk features or progressive disease after surgical resection, or high-grade glioma. In the case of brain metastases, radiation options depend on the number and size of the metastases and include whole-brain radiation and/or stereotactic radiosurgery. Whole-brain radiation therapy produces significant responses in the majority of patients with primary CNS lymphoma; however, given the risk of delayed chronic neurotoxicity, this modality is often reserved for use upon relapse or following methotrexate-based regimens in patients who have an incomplete response to chemotherapy.[6]

Tumor Treating Fields

In 2011, the Federal Drug Administration (FDA) approved a new treatment modality, tumor-treating fields (TTF), for use in recurrent glioblastoma. TTF therapy is delivered via a mechanical device that delivers alternating electrical fields to the tumor, theoretically causing disruption of cell division. Patients place adhesive pads containing transducers to the scalp, which is then connected to a portable power source. The device is used continuously. In 2015, FDA approval was expanded to include use of the device in the newly diagnosed setting, after completion of radiation therapy with concurrent temozolomide. The addition of TTF therapy to standard of care treatment was shown to prolong survival in comparison with chemotherapy and radiation alone in patients with glioblastoma.[10]

PHARMACOLOGIC THERAPY

Chemotherapy

Chemotherapy is typically recommended for treatment of high-grade glioma, and for low-grade glioma with high-risk features. Temozolomide, an oral alkylating agent, is the preferred first-line agent because of tumor sensitivity and its ability to cross the blood–brain barrier. During radiation therapy, temozolomide is administered daily at a low dose. After completion of radiotherapy, the dosage is increased, but it is given only on the first 5 days of a 28-day cycle, typically for a total of 6 cycles. In glioblastoma, radiation therapy in combination with temozolomide has been shown to significantly prolong survival.[11] For patients with brain metastasis, the role for chemotherapy is less clear and depends largely upon the sensitivity of the tumor to the chemotherapy agent and the degree of CNS penetration. Primary CNS lymphoma is usually treated upfront with a high-dose methotrexate–based chemotherapy regimen.

Molecular Targeted Therapy

Targeted cancer therapies block the growth or spread of cancer by interfering with specific molecules that are involved in tumor proliferation. Bevacizumab, a monoclonal antibody that inhibits blood vessel formation through its action on vascular endothelial growth factor, is often used in the treatment of recurrent glioma. It can be given alone or in combination with chemotherapy and has been shown to increase progression free survival in patients with glioblastoma.[12] It also is used in the treatment of radiation necrosis in both primary and metastatic brain tumors. There is emerging evidence for the use of immunotherapy agents, such as checkpoint inhibitors, in patients with brain metastasis from non-small cell lung cancer and melanoma.

Clinical Trials

Because conventional treatment is not curative for most types of brain tumors, it is appropriate to consider clinical trial participation for eligible patients whenever possible. Many new types of therapies are being studied, including various forms of immunotherapy, molecularly targeted agents, oncolytic toxins, antiangiogenic therapy, and gene therapy.

Supportive Care

- Steroids are used for the treatment of vasogenic edema. Dexamethasone is the corticosteroid of choice because of its low mineralocorticoid activity and long half-life, allowing it to be effectively dosed either once or twice daily. Steroids have many potential negative side effects; therefore, the goal is to use the lowest effective dose and taper as soon as clinically possible.[9] Steroids should be avoided before biopsy, when feasible, in patients thought to have primary CNS lymphoma because steroids may affect the pathologic diagnosis.
- Most patients with a brain tumor who experience seizure require lifelong anticonvulsant therapy. Seizure management and pharmacologic selection of anticonvulsant are based on the type of seizure with preference given to non–enzyme-inducing antiepileptic agents whenever possible in order to minimize drug interactions with oncologic

treatment. Some patients require multiple agents to control seizure activity and should be referred to a specialist for management.

- Depression is frequently seen in patients with brain tumors and should be assessed with every patient encounter. Selective serotonin reuptake inhibitors are the most frequently used agents. Bupropion is avoided in patients with seizures because it lowers the seizure threshold. Whenever possible, nonpharmacological therapies, including counseling, massage, and exercise, should be used in conjunction with pharmacologic therapy.
- Fatigue, secondary to both the brain tumor and treatment, is common. It can persist for more than a year after completion of therapy. Energy conservation, adequate nutrition, and regular activity are recommended as first-line treatment. If there is significant functional impairment of activities of daily living, a stimulant such as methylphenidate may be considered, as it may improve cognition and lethargy.[9,13]
- Dietary recommendations are important because patients may experience weight gain or weight loss as a result of disease and treatment. In general, a well-balanced diet with all food groups should be recommended, and early referral to a dietitian is advised for evaluation of weight and comorbid disease considerations.
- Cognitive and functional impairments are often distressing to patients and family members. Rehabilitation should be directed toward maximizing functional performance and may include physical, occupational, speech, and/or cognitive therapy. Formal neuropsychological testing is useful to assess memory, attention, and initiation, and provides a means to measure changes over time. Assistive devices to accommodate mobility, communication, and hearing and visual losses should be made available.

LIFE SPAN CONSIDERATIONS

The occurrence of primary brain tumors steadily increases with age. The overall incidence rate of childhood brain and other CNS tumors in the United States from 2010 to 2014 is 5.54 cases per 100,000 for a total 5-year count of 16,941 incident tumors. The incident rate increases in adolescent and young adults (ages 15 to 39) to 10.94 cases per 100,000 for a total 5-year count of 56,039 incident tumors and reaches its maximum in the older adult population with an annual average age-adjusted incidence of 40.82 per 100,000 population. Grade IV tumors occur more frequently in patients over 65, whereas low-grade tumors (WHO I to II) are more common in younger adults. Survival rates vary significantly based on age, tumor location, and tumor grade. The 5-year relative survival rate following diagnosis of a primary malignant brain and other CNS tumors is 34.9%. Conversely, the 5-year relative survival rate for a nonmalignant tumor is 90.47%.[2]

Age is an important consideration when making treatment decisions. However, age should always be considered in the context of performance status and comorbidities. Older patients with good performance status and who are otherwise healthy can receive similar treatment options as younger patients. Treatment alternatives should be considered for patients over the age of 70 and those with a Karnofsky Performance Score of less than 60. In these patients, a recommendation can be made for an abbreviated course of radiation and/or radiation or chemotherapy alone, rather than concurrent treatment.[14] A palliative approach focused on best supportive care is also reasonable for any patient of older age or with a poor baseline performance status. A palliative care referral can facilitate level of care discussions and help with care decision making see Chapter 14.

COMPLICATIONS

When a brain tumor diagnosis is suspected in the primary care setting, appropriate diagnostic studies related to the differential diagnosis should be performed. If initial imaging cannot be completed in a timely fashion or in the case of rapidly progressing symptoms, evaluation via the closest emergency department is appropriate. Once the presence of a mass has been confirmed on imaging, referral to an oncology specialist, neurosurgery or neuro-oncology, is recommended. In the event that a neuro-oncologist is not readily available, a medical oncologist can guide the initial workup and treatment plan.

In patients with a known or suspected brain tumor, there are several presentations that require more urgent or emergent evaluation.

- Increased ICP is an oncologic emergency that can lead to death without prompt intervention. It is often caused by increased mass effect from a space occupying lesion or intracranial edema; however, other factors such as hemorrhage or obstructive hydrocephalus can contribute to the elevation of intracranial pressure as well. Patients may present with focal findings based upon the location of the lesion, or with generalized signs and symptoms of increased ICP (see Red Flags). The tempo may be gradual or sudden in onset.
- Venous thromboembolism (VTE) occurs in a high proportion of patients with brain tumors, particularly in the postoperative period.[15] Patients are monitored for symptoms of deep vein thrombosis and pulmonary embolism (PE). Appropriate diagnostic studies should be obtained if there is clinical suspicion of thrombus. Low-molecular-weight heparin is the preferred pharmacologic treatment of VTE in patients with cancer.[15] Warfarin is typically avoided due to potential drug-drug interactions with many chemotherapy agents. In the absence of safety and efficacy data on new oral anticoagulants in cancer populations, these agents should be used with caution in patients with active malignancy only after careful consideration of the risks and benefits for individual patients.[16]
- Uncontrolled seizures or status epilepticus warrants prompt evaluation.
- Fever in a patient receiving chemotherapy requires urgent evaluation and treatment, especially in the context of neutropenia.
- Any neurological decline may indicate tumor progression or cerebral edema and necessitates reimaging
- Falls resulting in head trauma or other significant injury may require urgent evaluation.

PATIENT AND FAMILY EDUCATION

- Call the provider for any unrelieved headache, breakthrough seizure, new or worsening focal neurologic finding, fever of 100.4 degrees or greater, or treatment related side effect.
- Never stop taking any medication without discussing with the provider. Some medications, like steroids, may have serious side effects if stopped abruptly.
- If a seizure occurs, it is important to keep the individual safe. Recommendations include removing sharp objects from the area, protecting the head, and rolling the individual to the

side. Do not put anything into the mouth, restrain the individual, or try to stop the movements.

- Depending on type and location of the tumor, the patient's ability to drive may be compromised. Check the local department of motor vehicle site for state driving restrictions. It is generally accepted that seizure with loss of consciousness is a contraindication to driving.
- Chemotherapy can affect fertility, both while on treatment and in the future. It is important to discuss options for fertility preservation prior to starting therapy.

HEALTH PROMOTION

Patients with brain tumors can live for many years, particularly those with low-grade malignancies. Therefore, it is important to maintain and to encourage health promotion activities during treatment, follow-up, and survivorship. In addition, a health care directive, including the appointment of a health care agent, should be completed early on in the disease course whenever possible. Health maintenance screening may include mammography, Papanicolaou (Pap) smear, colonoscopy, and bone density scan, as well as monitoring for chronic illness and risky behaviors. Patients living with brain tumors are encouraged to follow established guidelines for health promotion, such as not smoking, limiting alcohol, eating well, and managing stress. Regular physical activity is encouraged to help rebuild strength and endurance levels.

Therapy for brain tumors can put patients at risk for conditions that bear monitoring and may warrant treatment. Many of the long-term sequelae plaguing brain tumor survivors relate to radiation; however, chemotherapy and corticosteroids can contribute.[9] Potential problems depend on the specific treatments given, but may include cerebrovascular disease, secondary neoplasms, cognitive decline, and psychosocial issues. A survivorship care plan is a useful tool that can assist patients who are transitioning from active treatment to the posttreatment phase of their cancer care. It serves to document diagnosis, treatment, recommended follow-up, and persistent or late effects. Since 2014, there has been a mandate within the United States for adult cancer patients treated with curative intent to receive survivorship care plans (https://www.cancer.org/health-care-professionals/national-cancer-survivorship-resource-center.html). Controversy still remains as how to best provide survivorship care to patients with noncurative malignancies.[17]

REFERENCES

1. American Brain Tumor Association. Brain Tumor Information: Types of Tumors. Retrieved from: http://www.abta.org/brain-tumor-information/types-of-tumors/. (Accessed 11 December 2017).
2. Ostrom, Q. T., Gittleman, H., Xu, J., et al. (2017). CBTRUS statistical report: Primary brain and other central nervous system tumors diagnosed in the United States in 2010-2014. *Neuro-oncology, 18*(s5), iv1–iv89.
3. American Brain Tumor Association. Brain Tumor Stats By Age. Retrieved from: http://www.abta.org/about-us/news/brain-tumor-statistics/. (Accessed 11 December 2017).
4. Nayak, L., Lee, E. Q., & Wen, P. Y. (2012). Epidemiology of brain metastases. *Current Oncology Reports, 14*(1), 48–54.
5. Bondy, M. L., Liu, Y., & Scheurer, M. E. (2012). Epidemiology and etiology. In R. J. Packer & D. Schiff (Eds.), *Neuro-Oncology* (pp. 3–12). Hoboken, NJ: John Wiley & Sons.
6. Grommes, C., DeAngelis, L. M., & Primary, C. N. S. (2017). Lymphoma. *Journal of Clinical Oncology: Official Journal of the American Society of Clinical Oncology, 35*(21), 2410–2418.
7. Ivan, M., Tate, M., & Clarke, J. (2012). Malignant gliomas in adulthood. In R. J. Packer & D. Schiff (Eds.), *Neuro-Oncology* (pp. 3–12). Hoboken, NJ: John Wiley & Sons.
8. Raizer, J., & Sherman Sokja, W. (2012). Meningiomas. In R. J. Packer & D. Schiff (Eds.), *Neuro-Oncology* (pp. 3–12). Hoboken, NJ: John Wiley & Sons.
9. Pruitt, A. A. (2015). Medical management of patients with brain tumors. *Continuum, 21*(2), 314–331.
10. Stupp, R., Taillibert, S., Kanner, A. A., et al. (2015). Maintenance therapy with tumor-treating fields plus temozolomide vs temozolomide alone for glioblastoma: A randomized clinical trial. *JAMA: The Journal of the American Medical Association, 314*(23), 2535–2543.
11. Perry, J., LaPierriere, N., O'Callaghan, C., et al. (2017). Short-course radiation plus temoxolomide in elderly patients with glioblastoma. *The New England Journal of Medicine, 376*, 1027–1037.
12. Fu, P., He, Y., Huang, Q., Ding, T., Cen, Y., Zhao, H., et al. (2016). Bevacizumab treatment for newly diagnosed glioblastoma: Systematic review and meta-analysis of clinical trials. *Molecular and Clinical Oncology, 4*, 833–838. https://doi.org/10.3892/mco.2016.816.
13. Carmen, E., Meyers, C., Reuben, J., et al. (2014). A randomized, double blind, 2-period, placebo-controlled crossover trial of a sustained release methylphenidate in the treatment of fatigue in cancer patients. *Cancer Journal (Sudbury, Mass.), 20*(1), 8–14.
14. National Comprehensive Cancer Network. Central nervous system cancers. (Version 1.2017) https://www.nccn.org/professionals/physician_gls/pdf/cns.pdf. (Accessed on 10 January 2018).
15. Jo, J., Shiff, D., & Perry, J. (2014). Thrombosis in brain tumors. *Seminars in Thrombosis and Hemostasis, 40*(03), 325–331.
16. Short, N. J., & Connors, J. M. (2014). New oral anticoagulants and the cancer patient. *The Oncologist, 19*(1), 82–93.
17. Rowland, J. H., & Bellizzi, K. M. (2014). Cancer survivorship issues: Life after treatment and implications for an aging population. *Journal of Clinical Oncology: Official Journal of the American Society of Clinical Oncology, 32*(24), 2662–2668.

CHAPTER 185

ADRENAL GLAND DISORDERS

Marylou Virginia Robinson

DEFINITION AND EPIDEMIOLOGY

Adrenal gland disorders are conditions marked by inadequate or excessive amounts of glucocorticoid, mineralocorticoid, or androgen hormones as a consequence of changes in the adrenal gland itself, from hypothalamic or pituitary gland dysfunction, or through exogenous administration. The three most common types of adrenal gland disorders are discussed: Addison disease, Cushing syndrome, and pheochromocytoma.

Addison Disease (Primary Adrenal Insufficiency)

Once most commonly linked with bilateral adrenal destruction by tuberculosis (TB), Addison disease is now associated with autoimmune disturbances (70%) or significant physiologic stress. Recent increases in TB worldwide may alter these patterns. Prevalence is 4 to 11 cases per 100,000,[1] with 1 in 8000 European whites and twice as many women as men being affected.[2] More than 30% of acquired immunodeficiency syndrome (HIV) patients develop adrenal insufficiency,[2] as are patients on long-term steroid doses such as rheumatoid arthritis.[3] All three adrenal hormones can be unbalanced in Addison disease.

Cushing Syndrome

There is a spectrum of disorders associated with the overproduction of cortisol, the most familiar being Cushing syndrome. The term *Cushing disease* is reserved for pituitary-caused symptoms. It is estimated that 1% of all patients take glucocorticoid medications, which causes iatrogenic Cushing syndrome in a large number of patients. Endogenous cases can also be related to excess adrenocorticotropic hormone (ACTH) from pituitary tumors or adrenal gland hyperproduction.

Pheochromocytoma

Pheochromocytoma is a catecholamine-secreting tumor of chromaffin (pheochromocyte) cells. Ninety percent are found in the adrenal medulla; others arise intra-abdominally along the sympathetic ganglion chain.[4] The rare incidence of a primary malignant process occurs when the tumor spreads beyond chromaffin tissue. Pheochromocytomas are typically unilateral; however, bilateral involvement is common in the setting of polyglandular multiple endocrine neoplasia. Annual incidence is 2 to 8 cases per million, occurring primarily in the middle years. Ten percent are familial.[5]

PATHOPHYSIOLOGY

Hypothalamus-synthesized corticotropin-releasing hormone regulates the secretion of ACTH, which in turn regulates the production of glucocorticoids (cortisol). Cortisol adjusts the metabolic responses in the body to both physical and psychological stressors. These responses range from hepatic glucose production to inflammatory vascular reactions. Proinflammatory cytokines also increase cortisol secretion.[4] Normal circadian ACTH secretion is highest on waking and lowest at night. Men average 18 pulses of ACTH daily, but women have only 10.[1] Disrupted sleep-wake cycles of shift workers or travelers crossing time zones interrupt the pulses, which may result in changes in performance and behavior.

Primary underproduction disorders (Addison disease) stem from the destruction or dysfunction of the adrenal gland. Secondary disorders involve interruption of the hypothalamic-pituitary-adrenal (HPA) axis, pituitary tumors, or traumatic brain injury. Tertiary disorders are the sudden consequences of withdrawal of exogenous corticosteroids after high-dose use. Typically 90% of both adrenal glands is malfunctioning before clinically recognized insufficiency is present. Destruction by TB, adrenal hemorrhage (e.g., anticoagulant therapy or trauma), medications (rifampin, ketoconazole), and infections (meningococcemia, histoplasmosis) are rare causes. Inadequate production of cortisol in the context of severe sudden illness or trauma, particularly in chronic users of corticosteroids, is a more common manifestation.[1,3] Individuals with other pituitary dysfunction as well as septic shock, patients with critical illness,[6,7] childhood brain cancer survivors,[8] and patients sustaining traumatic brain injury[9] should be monitored long term for insufficiency symptoms.

Most cases of Cushing syndrome come from the suppression of pituitary ACTH production when steroids are administered in high doses for long periods. When use is for more than 10 to 14 days as part of the management of asthma, difficult dermatitis problems, malignant neoplasms, rheumatic diseases, and other disorders, careful monitoring is mandatory to detect early, persistent endogenous corticosteroid suppression. When long-term exogenous glucocorticoid therapy is indicated, HPA axis suppression occurs. Alternate-day therapies have been suggested to alleviate symptoms but are not evidence based.[1] Steroid use for less than 3 weeks typically does not generate concern. The exception is frequent "burst" therapy in asthma and chronic obstructive pulmonary disease exacerbations, when natural return of adrenal function can be impaired. Timing of steroid doses is critical to reduce impact. Most of the administration should occur in the morning, as heavier doses at night suppress the morning pulse of ACTH more significantly. Recovery from iatrogenic suppression of cortisol production can take 6 to 9 months.[1]

Secondary Cushing syndrome results from ACTH-secreting tumors of the pituitary and occasionally (0.05%) from ectopic hormone secretion such as small cell lung carcinomas. Cortisol and ACTH levels are both elevated. Rarely, Cushing syndrome results from primary overproduction of cortisol by the adrenal gland (low levels of serum ACTH and high levels of serum cortisol).

Abnormal production of epinephrine and norepinephrine by a pheochromocytoma produces multisystem effects. Renal effects include sodium retention, increased renin secretion, and reduction of hydrostatic pressure. Cardiovascular effects involve peripheral vasoconstriction and increased cardiac contraction and workload from significant hypertension. Tissue oxygen consumption and gluconeogenesis are also increased.[5]

CLINICAL PRESENTATION

Addisonian presentations are nonspecific with chronic malaise, dizziness, nausea, chronic abdominal pain, muscle cramps, hyperpigmentation, decreased libido, weight loss, and salt craving. Decreased axilla and pubic hair with altered menses is linked to the disorder in women because of lowered androgens. Men produce most of their androgens in the testes, so they avoid most of this hair loss.[1] Depression, impaired memory, and agitation to include outright psychosis may occur in 20% to 40% of individuals. A patient with known Addison disease can exhibit an abrupt onset of vomiting, hypotension, and acute shock during a period of severe trauma, illness, or physical exertion when mineralocorticoid levels drop. Adrenal crisis can occur in patients normally well controlled with glucocorticoids.[1]

Cushing syndrome almost always manifests with chronic changes. Rapid weight gain, loss of menses, decreased libido, weakness, and bruising are all possible presenting symptoms. Many patients have hypertension, glucose intolerance, and insomnia. Memory and mental health disturbances occur in 50% of patients.[1] Depressed linear growth and excess weight gain are the most common presentations in pediatrics.[8]

Most adrenal tumors are incidentalomas, or the unexpected finding of a mass on computed tomography (CT) or magnetic resonance imaging (MRI) done for other reasons. Most (85%) of these masses are nonfunctional adrenal adenomas; the remainder are pheochromocytoma or metastasis from other organ cancers.[10] Symptoms of pheochromocytoma are episodic and include headache, diaphoresis, and palpitations, which may occur several times daily or only a few times a month. The symptomatic episodes last 15 to 30 minutes and may be precipitated by specific activities, such as position change, Valsalva maneuver, exercise, anxiety, or medications (e.g., anesthesia or metoclopramide).[5]

PHYSICAL EXAMINATION

Patients with Addison disease appear chronically ill. They exhibit weight loss, dehydration, and increased skin pigmentation on light-exposed skinfolds, a result of melanocyte stimulation by pituitary hormones. Darkened creases on the palms, elbows, knees, and lips commonly occur. Persons of color have darkened mucous membranes. Most discolorations resolve with adequate glucocorticoid therapy. Patients with secondary ACTH deficiency do not develop these skin changes.[1]

Patients with Cushing syndrome have a characteristic habitus similar to but subtly and importantly different from that of many patients with exogenous obesity. Central obesity,

a moon face appearance caused by thickening of facial fat, the classically described buffalo hump dorsocervical fat pad (very common with all obesity), increased supraclavicular fat pads, hypertension, muscle weakness and wasting, hirsutism, red-purple abdominal skin striae of more than 1 cm in size, and acne can be associated signs. Emotional lability or depression, "senile" purpura on the hands, and other bruising can occur in all age groups.[1]

The hallmark of pheochromocytoma is a new onset of moderate to severe hypertension, with systolic pressures above 170 mm Hg. Arrhythmias, sinus tachycardia, or bradycardia may be present. The course is characterized by substantial variations in blood pressure measurements, palpitations, orthostasis, glucose intolerance, and diaphoresis, making "catching" it on a scheduled examination difficult. One-third of patients have consistently normal blood pressure.[5] Cushing syndrome can be considered as a differential diagnosis for refractory hypertension.

DIAGNOSTICS
Addison Disease

Patients with Addison disease have an elevated serum ACTH concentration and suppressed levels of cortisol.

- Hyponatremia and hyperkalemia related to concurrent lost aldosterone production might be a serendipitous finding that suggests Addison disease in a previously undiagnosed patient.
- All diagnostics, including adrenal antibody studies to identify autoimmune disorders, should be ordered in concert with endocrinology.
- Screening is essential to exclude underlying TB.
- Patients with secondary insufficiency resulting from HPA axis issues have only glucocorticoid deficiency with intact aldosterone levels.[1]

Cushing Syndrome

Cushing syndrome is classically diagnosed by measurement of more than 100 mcg of cortisol in the urine during a 24-hour period.

- This excretion study is thought to be more dependable than serum ACTH and serum cortisol testing; however, a single midnight (nadir) serum cortisol value above 7.5 mcg/dL has nearly 100% specificity and 96% sensitivity.
- Suppression testing with ACTH is done in consultation with endocrine specialists to separate the physiology of obese and depressed patients from that of patients with true Cushing syndrome or to separate pituitary disorders from primary adrenal gland alterations.[1,2]

Pheochromocytoma

Elevated levels of fractionated metanephrines in a urine or plasma sample confirm the diagnosis of pheochromocytoma.[5]

- To increase accuracy, the collection must occur during a period of symptomatic episodes.
- Many medications alter the accuracy of the test (quinidine, theophylline, tetracycline, clofibrate, and disulfiram), including street drugs (LSD, cocaine) and over-the-counter substances (alcohol, pseudoephedrine), which can alter catecholamine levels.
- A careful medication review and specialist consultation regarding current test guidelines must occur before sampling.

- Abnormal test results should trigger an imaging search for a tumor.
- If a vascular mass is found in a hypertensive patient, the ratio of plasma aldosterone concentration to plasma renin activity (PAC/PRA) is determined to screen for primary aldosteronism.[11,12,13]

INITIAL DIAGNOSTICS

Adrenal Gland Disorders

ADDISON DISEASE
Laboratory
- Serum electrolytes
- Blood urea nitrogen (BUN)
- Creatinine
- Serum glucose
- Serum cortisol and serum ACTH
- ACTH stimulation test (250 mcg)

Other Diagnostics
- Chest x-ray studies or purified protein derivative (PPD)

CUSHING DISEASE
Laboratory
- Creatinine
- 24-h urine for cortisol
- ACTH suppression test

PHEOCHROMOCYTOMA
Laboratory
- Plasma free metanephrines
- With 24-h urine vanillylmandelic acid[a]
- If hypertensive, random PAC/PRA

Imaging
- CT scan or MRI[a]

[a]If indicated.

DIFFERENTIAL DIAGNOSIS

Both Addison disease and Cushing syndrome can be difficult to distinguish from normal physiology because both chronic and acute stresses affect adrenal hormone production.[14,15] Mild addisonian symptoms can be mimicked by eating disorders, chronic fatigue syndrome, alcoholism, malnutrition, hyperthyroidism, diabetes, and the wasting effects of a chronic illness such as AIDS or metastatic cancer. Psychiatric symptoms, including apathy, confusion, and depression, are common with adrenal insufficiency presentations and often confound the clinical assessment. Most Cushing conditions are those associated with exogenous steroid use or abrupt withdrawal or inadequate steroid use in circumstances of stress. Cushing syndrome can be confused with depression, obesity, or polycystic ovary syndrome (PCOS).[16] The silver striae from rapid weight gain or pregnancy do not indicate adrenal dysfunction. Pheochromocytoma symptoms are commonly confused with anxiety or labile white coat hypertension; however, any issue that can induce a hypertensive spike should also be considered (e.g., stimulants, thyrotoxicosis, increased intracranial pressure).

INTERPROFESSIONAL COLLABORATIVE MANAGEMENT

 Specialist referral is indicated for patients with adrenal gland disorders.

Addison Disease

Acute adrenal crisis is best managed in the hospital, with intravenous corticosteroids and shock stabilization. Chronic adrenal insufficiency can be managed in an outpatient setting with oral hydrocortisone in divided daily doses (total, 20 to 30 mg) to allow restoration of a diurnal pattern.[2] Dosage is individualized, guided by the patient's symptomatic responses. Oral hydrocortisone is a fast-acting medication requiring multiple daily doses. Patients may do better on longer-acting steroids such as dexamethasone or prednisolone and subcutaneous hydrocortisone infusions to better simulate natural plasma fluctuations.[2]

Mineralocorticoid replacement in Addison syndrome with fludrocortisone (dose range, 0.05 to 0.2 mg/day orally) corrects the renal disturbance and hypotension. The need for replacement doses is monitored by frequent measurement of electrolytes, serum renin, serum ACTH, and judiciously timed serum cortisol levels.

Unless it is otherwise contraindicated, liberal use of salt may be encouraged in the face of resistant hyponatremia.

Cushing Syndrome

Management of Cushing syndrome depends on the source of the hypercortisolism. In Cushing disease, intentional P-450 cytochrome competition for processing steroids is used through daily ketoconazole administration, which mitigates the impact of cortisol.[16]

Pituitary tumor resection, when indicated, remains the first choice for therapy. Chemotherapy and radiation therapy may be used adjunctively.

Because chronic glucocorticoid levels are associated with osteoporotic tendencies, bone density measurements should be obtained, especially with concurrent conditions that have an impact on bone, such as thyroid replacement therapy and menopause.[1,2]

Pheochromocytoma

The management of pheochromocytoma is still based primarily on case reports and expert opinion.[5] Definitive treatment is surgical removal.

Presurgical antihypertensive therapy focuses on α-adrenergic blockade and attention to maintenance of adequate hydration. β or calcium channel blockers can be added if tachycardia or coronary artery vasospasm issues arise.[5,13]

Alternative Therapies From Integrative Medicine

Advocates for alternative approaches believe science is not able to adequately measure the subtle changes in adrenal hormones that are depleted by chronic stress. The term most commonly used is *adrenal fatigue*, a diagnosis not recognized by allopathic medicine.[17] Adrenal fatigue is accelerated after a particularly stressful event, such as financial collapse, sustained emotional duress, illness, or suboptimal diets.[18]

Most alternative interventions center on the goal of improving energy, overcoming any iatrogenic impact of long-term steroid therapy, and combating the negative physiologic and psychological impacts of chronic stress and modern time-pressured lives. Energy-boosting herbals such as ginseng are classified by naturopathic healers as adaptogens—substances that help one adapt to stress.[19] When adaptogens are combined with substances that soothe excessive nervous system responses, such as skullcap (*Scutellaria*), St. John's wort, and valerian, support is provided to overcome insomnia, irritability, and stress-induced hypertension. The negative impact of stress on the cardiovascular system is modulated with the use of antioxidants, fish oils, plant sterols, and the B-complex vitamins and avoidance of refined carbohydrates.[19] Sea salt is considered an essential ingredient to overcome the salt-wasting perceived to be the source of low energy. One or two 8-ounce glasses of water with half teaspoon of sea salt is encouraged by some websites.

Licorice (*Glycyrrhiza*) is an ancient remedy for suppression of the fight-or-flight reactions associated with persistent stress.[18] Excess ingestion, however, is associated with resistant hypertension and can create havoc in patients taking digoxin. More recently, dehydroepiandrosterone (DHEA), an endogenous sex hormone precursor, has been suggested to be helpful; however, high DHEA levels are linked with development of Cushing syndrome.[20]

COMPLICATIONS

Immediate life-threatening complications are, in general, confined to acute adrenal crisis. Sudden adrenal inadequacy can be mitigated with injectable hydrocortisone (Florinef) for home use. Addison disease and Cushing syndrome complications are prevented by giving careful attention to the side effects of exogenous steroids and to the patient's symptoms, emotional stability, and metabolic status. With Cushing syndrome, osteoporosis is a common complication, along with risk for infection, hypertension, and diabetes. Acute hypertensive crisis is a potential complication of pheochromocytoma.

INDICATIONS FOR REFERRAL OR HOSPITALIZATION

Consultation with endocrinology specialists is warranted if the diagnostic evaluation suggests either Addison disease or Cushing syndrome.

 Referral and hospitalization are necessary for hypertensive crisis management and surgical intervention of pheochromocytoma.[5]

Management of an acute adrenal crisis requires immediate referral and hospitalization for fluid resuscitation and intravenous administration of hydrocortisone, with the dose varying greatly based upon the patient's body weight and age and whether the patient is a child or an adult. Management of the associated hypotension, hypovolemia, and hypoglycemia is accomplished with careful monitoring in an intensive care setting. Patients who have been taking exogenous steroids at any time during the preceding year are at some risk for inadequate cortisol response when faced with the stress of any surgical procedure. These patients should be considered candidates for perioperative stress doses of hydrocortisone. Consultation with a provider comfortable with prescribing stress steroid doses is advised. In general, for patients with known adrenal insufficiency, hydrocortisone is added to intraoperative intravenous fluids and infused at a rate of 5 mg/h. During the first 24 hours after surgery, a total of 150 to 200 mg is administered. The dose is then tapered by 50% per day if the postoperative period is without complications.[1,2]

PATIENT EDUCATION AND HEALTH PROMOTION

Careful explanation of the underlying disease processes and complications of chronic exogenous steroid dependency is an important component of patient and family education.[21] Doubling of the hydrocortisone dose is required with fever and common illnesses. Patients and families must understand the risks of sudden withdrawal of corticosteroid medications and the need to alert medical personnel in the event of trauma, surgical procedure, or infection.[21] Medical alert bracelets are vital to improve the recognition of emergency presentations of adrenal insufficiency. An emergency kit with syringe and directions on how and when to administer extraparenteral steroids should be carried at all times. Families need education on how to administer the medication intramuscularly. Health protection issues associated with potential hypertension, glucose intolerance, immune compromise, skin breakdown, and weight gain for steroid-dependent patients need to be emphasized. Quick access to the primary care provider should be an important goal of the provider–patient partnership.

REFERENCES

1. Annane, D., et al. (2017). Critical illness-related corticosteroid insufficiency (CIRCI): A narrative review from a multispecialty task force of the society of critical care medicine (SCCM) and the European society of intensive care medicine (ESICM). *Critical Care Medicine*.
2. Bornstein, S. R., et al. (2016). Diagnosis and treatment of primary adrenal insufficiency: An Endocrine Society clinical practice guideline. *The Journal of Clinical Endocrinology and Metabolism*, 101(2), 364–389.
3. Borresen, S. W., et al. (2017). Adrenal insufficiency is seen in more than one-third of patients during ongoing low-dose prednisolone treatment for rheumatoid arthritis. *European Journal of Endocrinology*, 177(4), 287–295.
4. Cadegiani, F. A., & Kater, C. E. (2016). Adrenal fatigue does not exist: A systematic review. *BMC Endocrine Disorders*, 16(1), 48.
5. Cutright, A., Ducey, S., & Barthold, C. L. (2017). Recognizing and managing adrenal disorders in the emergency department. *Emergency Medicine Practice*, 19(9), 1–24.
6. Fleseriu, M., et al. (2016). American Association of Clinical Endocrinologists and American College of Endocrinology Disease state clinical review: Diagnosis of recurrence in cushing disease. *Endocrine Practice*, 22(12), 1436–1448.
7. Funder, J. W., et al. (2016). The management of primary aldosteronism: Case detection, diagnosis, and treatment: An Endocrine Society clinical practice guideline. *The Journal of Clinical Endocrinology and Metabolism*, 101(5), 1889–1916.
8. Hwang, J. J., & Hwang, D. Y. (2014). Treatment of endocrine disorders in the neuroscience intensive care unit. *Current Treatment Options in Neurology*, 16(2), 271.
9. Redmer, J. (2018). Adrenal fatigue. In D. Rakel (Ed.), *Integrative medicine* (pp. 404–409). Philadelphia, PA: Elsevier.
10. James, P. A., et al. (2014). 2014 evidence-based guideline for the management of high blood pressure in adults: Report from the panel members appointed to the Eighth Joint National Committee (JNC 8). *JAMA: The Journal of the American Medical Association*, 311(5), 507–520.
11. Keil, M. F., & Van Ryzin, C. (2017). The key to adrenal insufficiency education: Repetition, repetition, repetition. *Pediatric Endocrinology Reviews*, 14(Suppl. 2), 448–453.
12. Lee, J. M., et al. (2017). Clinical guidelines for the management of adrenal incidentaloma. *Endocrinology and Metabolism (Seoul, Korea)*, 32(2), 200–218.
13. Lenders, J. W. M., et al. (2014). Pheochromocytoma and paraganglioma: An Endocrine Society clinical practice guideline. *The Journal of Clinical Endocrinology and Metabolism*, 99(6), 1915–1942.
14. McCance, K. L., & Huether, S. E. (2014). *Pathophysiology: The biologic basis for disease in adults and children* (7th ed., p. xxvi). St. Louis, MO: Elsevier. 1810 pages.
15. Medicine, N. L. O. (2017). DHEA.
16. Melmed, S., et al. (2015). *Willams textbook of endocrinology*. St. Louis, MO: Elsevier.
17. Napier, C., & Pearce, S. H. (2014). Current and emerging therapies for Addison's disease. *Current Opinion in Endocrinology, Diabetes, and Obesity*, 21(3), 147–153.
18. Nicholas, M. N., Li, S. K., & Dytoc, M. (2017). An approach to minimising risk of adrenal insufficiency when discontinuing oral glucocorticoids. *Journal of Cutaneous Medicine and Surgery*, 1203475417736278.
19. Nieman, L. K., et al. (2015). Treatment of Cushing's syndrome: An Endocrine Society clinical practice guideline. *The Journal of Clinical Endocrinology and Metabolism*, 100(8), 2807–2831.
20. Pappachan, J. M., et al. (2017). Cushing's syndrome: A practical approach to diagnosis and differential diagnoses. *Journal of Clinical Pathology*, 70(4), 350–359.
21. Mayo Clinic Staff. (2018). Prednisone and other corticosteroids. https://www.mayoclinic.org/steroids/art-20045692.

DIABETES MELLITUS

Mary E. Wood

DEFINITION AND EPIDEMIOLOGY

Diabetes mellitus is the most common metabolic disorder seen in primary care and a leading cause of cardiovascular disease (CVD), renal failure, blindness, and nontraumatic lower limb amputation.

The World Health Organization defines diabetes as follows:

Diabetes is a condition primarily defined by the level of hyperglycemia giving rise to risk of microvascular damage (retinopathy, nephropathy, and neuropathy). It is associated with reduced life expectancy, significant morbidity due to specific diabetes related microvascular complications, increased risk of macrovascular complications (ischemic heart disease, stroke, and peripheral vascular disease), and diminished quality of life.[1]

The prevalence of diabetes in the United States as of 2015 was 30.3 million people, 9.4% of the population. Of the 30.3 million Americans with diabetes, 23.1 million have been diagnosed and 7.2 million remain undiagnosed. Among adults aged 18 years and older, the prevalence of diabetes is slightly higher in men than in women (12.7% vs 11.7%), but diabetes increases with age. Among those of the US population who are 65 years of age or older, diabetes is present in 25.2%. Diabetes is more common among Hispanics (12.1%), non-Hispanic blacks (12.7%), and American Indians/Alaska Natives (15.1%) compared with non-Hispanic whites (7.4%) and Asians (8.0%).[2]

Based on elevated fasting glucose or HbA1c levels, an estimated 84.1 million Americans (33.9% of the population) 18 years of age and older have prediabetes, which is more common among men (36.6%) than among women (29.3%). The prevalence of prediabetes is similar among racial and ethnic groups. It is estimated that only 11.6% of adults with prediabetes are aware of their condition.[2]

Among individuals with prediabetes, a healthy diet, regular exercise, and weight loss have been shown to prevent or delay the progression to diabetes.[2] Given this, an important focus of primary care is the prevention of type 2 diabetes. Screening is recommended for early diagnosis and is particularly important as this is often a silent disease (Box 186.1).

An estimated 90% to 95% of people in the United States with diabetes have type 2 diabetes (previously known as adult-onset diabetes or non–insulin-dependent diabetes mellitus). Fewer than 10% have type 1 diabetes (formerly known as juvenile-onset diabetes, type I diabetes, or insulin-dependent diabetes).[2,3]

Type 1 diabetes typically begins in childhood, adolescence, or early adulthood but may manifest at any age. Latent autoimmune diabetes of adulthood (LADA), also known as 1.5 diabetes, occurs more commonly in older adults; it has a slow, almost surreptitious onset so similar to type 2 DM that it is sometimes misdiagnosed as type 2 diabetes.[4]

Type 2 diabetes, which is strongly linked to obesity, was in the past diagnosed in middle-aged and older individuals but

BOX **186.1**

Screening for Diabetes in Asymptomatic Adults

1. Screen, using fasting plasma glucose, 2-h 75-g oral glucose tolerance test (OGTT), or hemoglobin A1c (HbA1c); adults who are overweight or obese (body mass index [BMI] ≥25 kg/m^2 [≥23 kg/m^2 in Asian Americans]) who have one or more of the following risk factors:
   - First-degree relative with diabetes.
   - High-risk heritage (African American, Latino, Native American, Asian American, Pacific Islander).
   - History of cardiovascular disease.
   - Hypertension (≥140/90 mm Hg with treatment for hypertension)
   - Dyslipidemia (high-density lipoprotein [HDL] <35 mg/dL and/or triglycerides >250 mg/dL)
   - Presence of polycystic ovarian syndrome (PCOS).
   - Physical inactivity.
   - Family history of diabetes.
   - Indications of insulin resistance (acanthosis nigricans, severe obesity).
2. Patients with prediabetes (HbA1c >5.7%, IFT or IFG) should be tested yearly.
3. Women who were diagnosed with gestational diabetes should be tested every 3 years.
4. For all others, testing should begin at age 45.
5. If results are normal, repeat testing every 3 years and earlier with a change in risk.

From American Diabetes Association. (2018). Standards of medical care in diabetes—2018. *Diabetes Care, 41*(Suppl 1), S13–27.

is now more commonly developing in childhood and adolescence secondary to lifestyle factors. The incidence of both type 1 and type 2 diabetes is increasing and the disease is occurring at an earlier age.[2]

The increase in type 2 diabetes is especially concerning in women of childbearing age. Gestational diabetes has always been a concern in pregnancy, but now more women who are diagnosed with gestational diabetes actually have type 2 DM.[5]

There are other, less common forms of diabetes, including maturity-onset diabetes of the young (MODY) and neonatal diabetes mellitus, a monogenic type that affects newborns and is fatal.

The long-term complications of diabetes result from microvascular and macrovascular damage to target end organs: the eyes, kidneys, heart, blood vessels, and peripheral nerves. Direct and indirect costs for diabetes care in 2012 were estimated at $245 billion. Average medical expenditures for people with diabetes were found to be 2.3 times higher than for those without diabetes.[2] To reduce the devastating effects of this disease, prevention, early detection, and aggressive treatment of its long-term complications are essential.

The morbidity and mortality rates for CVD in the United States have fallen markedly during the past 50 years. However, for individuals with diabetes, there has been an increase in CVD during the same time span. Multivariate analysis in two time periods from the Framingham Heart Study demonstrated that risk factors for diabetes—including hypertension, high cholesterol, smoking, and obesity—are evident in the population up to 30 years before the onset of CVD.[6] Several more recent trials have addressed treatment goals to prevent cardiovascular death (the ACCORD trial, ADVANCE study, and LEADER trial). These findings underscore the importance of diabetes prevention and early and aggressive treatment of risk factors for all patients with diabetes.

PATHOPHYSIOLOGY

Types 1 and 2 diabetes share the features of hyperglycemia and an increased risk for vascular and neuropathic complications. Physiologically, however, they are two distinct diseases. Type 1 diabetes is most often associated with the autoimmune destruction of the β-cells within the islets of Langerhans in the pancreas in a genetically predisposed individual. This results in insulinopenia and the lifelong dependence on exogenous insulin. β-cell destruction is typically more rapid in infants and children and more gradual in adults. The majority of individuals with type 1 diabetes will test positive for the presence of antibodies (islet cell autoantibodies, insulin autoantibodies, GAD65 autoantibodies, or autoantibodies to tyrosine phosphatase IA-2 and IA-2β).[7] Surgical removal of the pancreas (e.g., Whipple procedure or pancreatectomy) results in type 1 diabetes with the added challenge created by the lack of glucagon secretion from the α-cells. Insulin is required for most of the body's tissues to take up glucose as the preferred source of energy. Thus insulin deficiency impairs the uptake of glucose, resulting in the search for energy elsewhere. Fats and proteins are broken down, and counterregulatory hormones (glucagon, epinephrine, cortisol, and growth hormone) trigger glycogenolysis. Inadequate insulin leads to hyperglycemia.

The pathophysiology of LABA is related to B-cell dysfunction, but unlike the rapid onset seen in school age Type 1 diabetics, older adults with LABA experience diminishing B-cell efficacy. As a result, patients with LABA are usually treated first with oral antiglycemic medications but eventually with insulin; they are sometimes misdiagnosed with type 2 diabetes.[8]

The pathophysiologic mechanism of type 2 diabetes is more obscure. Hallmarks of this disease have been called the "triumvirate" of decreased glucose uptake (insulin resistance), increased hepatic glucose production, and impaired insulin secretion. A new model of type 2 diabetes pathophysiology has been described by DeFronzo and called "the ominous octet," in recognition of the fact that there are eight mechanisms that contribute to type 2 diabetes.[9,10] The additional five mechanisms are increased glucagon secretion, increased glucose reabsorption by the kidney, increased lipolysis, decreased incretin effect, and neurotransmitter dysfunction in the brain.

Fasting hyperglycemia results from increased hepatic glucose production in the impaired first phase of insulin secretion. Postprandial hyperglycemia is caused by the decreased uptake of glucose in the skeletal muscles. In response to the elevated blood glucose levels, the insulin pathways become resistant to hormonal impulses, resulting in hyperinsulinemia.

Insulin resistance by definition is the decreased sensitivity of tissue to glucose uptake with normal concentrations of insulin.[3] As hyperglycemia increases, so does insulin resistance. The body is able to adapt and maintain homeostasis for a while, but as hyperglycemia progresses, diabetes occurs. As the degree of glucose intolerance advances, hyperglycemia results from the insufficient insulin produced by the β-cells.

The natural progression of type 2 diabetes includes normal glucose values as insulin resistance begins. Increased insulin secretion compensates for the resistance. As insulin resistance worsens, postprandial glucose values begin to rise. Later, insulin secretion begins to wane and fasting glucose levels start to climb. Placing the patient along this continuum will guide treatment decisions. For example, early in type 2 diabetes, treatment should aim to improve sensitivity to insulin. Later, treatment may require the enhancement of insulin secretion or the administration of endogenous insulin.

Primary insulin resistance, a defect in the target cells of insulin receptors and postreceptors, results in altered insulin action and sensitivity. The onset of insulin resistance can occur with hyperinsulinemia in the fasting or fed state. The fed state is the time associated with insulin secretion after food intake when carbohydrate is metabolized and fat and protein are synthesized. As insulin resistance proceeds, glucose transport or use of glucose in the cell is altered. Secondary resistance is caused by hormones or abnormal physiologic states (e.g., puberty, pregnancy, advanced age). Other factors associated with the development of insulin resistance include a high-fat diet, sedentary lifestyle, smoking, and weight gain. Metabolic stress, as with illness and obesity, increases insulin resistance.

Many patients who develop prediabetes or type 2 diabetes also have the metabolic syndrome. This syndrome comprises a group of metabolic components, synergistic in nature, that contribute to CVD. These components include abdominal obesity, insulin resistance and hyperglycemia, elevated triglyceride and low high-density lipoprotein (HDL) levels, hypertension and a proinflammatory state. Weight loss, improved glycemic control, lipid management, and improved blood pressure may decrease the significance of this syndrome.

CLINICAL PRESENTATION AND PHYSICAL EXAMINATION

An individual with untreated type 1 diabetes will typically seek treatment after a brief period of profound symptoms. Polyuria, polydipsia, polyphagia, weight loss, blurred vision, and fatigue are overt signs of diabetes. Later, as the glycosuria increases, nausea, vomiting, abdominal pain, rapid shallow breathing, hypotension, and dehydration—all signs of ketoacidosis—will appear (see the section titled Acute Complications of Diabetes). At this point medical care is essential.

The patient with type 2 diabetes may be asymptomatic or may develop only subtle symptoms that may persist for weeks, months, or even years before detection. Unfortunately vascular and neuropathic complications during this time may begin to develop and progress before the diagnosis is made.[7] The symptoms include polyuria, polydipsia, blurred vision, fatigue, slowly healing wounds, and frequent infections. Some individuals may experience polyphagia and weight loss or numbness and tingling of the feet and hands.

The initial physical examination of diabetes focuses on dehydration, weight loss, and precipitating causes such as illness, infection, or stress at the time of diagnosis. The patient may appear dry and flushed. The skin, eyes, heart, and lungs should be assessed. The thyroid should be palpated because type 1 diabetes may be associated with thyroid disorders. In patients with new type 2 diabetes, physical examination should be performed for early evidence of vascular and neuropathic complications as well as for persistent infections.

The purpose of periodic examination of patients with known diabetes is threefold: (1) to evaluate blood glucose control, because poor control leads to end-organ complications; (2) to assess for the presence or progression of end-organ damage;

BOX **186.2**

Physical Examination of Patients With Diabetes

Vital signs: Height, weight, body mass index (BMI), and blood pressure, including orthostatic measurements in a patient with long-standing diabetes and neuropathy.

Eye: Funduscopic examination for hemorrhages or exudates.

Oral cavity: Examine for gum disease, fungal infections, or lesions.

Neck: Palpate thyroid for enlargement or nodules.

Cardiac: Auscultate heart rate for rhythm, murmurs, clicks, or extra heart sounds.

Skin: Inspect for signs of irritation, infection, redness, ulcers, and acanthosis nigricans. Assess insulin injection sites.

Feet: Inspect skin integrity, foot deformity, toenails, presence of ulcers. Palpate pulses for presence and quality, note presence of patellar and Achilles reflexes, perform 10 g monofilament examination to assess protective sensation. Screen for PAD.

Data from American Diabetes Association. (2018). *Standards of medical care. Diabetes Care.* 41(Suppl 1), S28–37.

TABLE **186.1** **Diagnostic Criteria for Diabetes and Prediabetes[a]**

	Fasting Plasma Glucose	Random Plasma Glucose	Oral Glucose Tolerance Test (75-g Glucose, 2-h Plasma Glucose)	HbA1c
Normal	<100 mg/dL		<140 mg/dL	<5.7%
Prediabetes	100–125 mg/dL		140–199 mg/dL	5.7%–6.4%
Diabetes	≥126 mg/dL After 8-h fast	≥200 mg/dL with classic symptoms	≥200 mg/dL	≥6.5%

[a]Diagnosis can now be confirmed if two tests from a blood sample (e.g., A1c and fasting plasma glucose) are positive. Point-of-care HgbA1c is diagnostic for diabetes only if performed in a licensed setting.

Data from American Diabetes Association: Standards of Medical Care in Diabetes–2019.

and (3) to assess for associated diseases such as other autoimmune disorders and cardiovascular risk factors.

Annual examinations are comprehensive. Periodic visits every 3 months for patients with types 1 and 2 diabetes (especially if there are one or more complications), should be conducted to assess end-organ involvement and glycemic control. Visits for patients with type 2 diabetes can be spread to every 6 months if they are stable and in control. At each visit the examination should include weight and blood pressure measurements, a review of glycemic control, evaluation of target end-organ damage, and a thorough inspection of the feet to assess for ulceration (Box 186.2).

DIAGNOSTICS

The diagnostic criteria for diabetes are based on the glucose threshold above which the risk of retinopathy is increased.[1] In July 2009, an International Expert Committee recommended the use of hemoglobin A1c (HbA1c) as a diagnostic tool. An HbA1c of 6.5% or higher, a fasting plasma glucose of 126 mg/dL or higher, or a 2-hour plasma glucose level of 200 mg/dL or higher during an oral glucose tolerance test (OGTT) fulfills the criteria for the diagnosis of diabetes. For an individual without symptoms, two laboratory tests on different days were recommended in the past to confirm the diagnosis, but the ADA's 2019 Standards in Diabetes Care updated the diagnostic criteria to include two abnormal tests (e.g., FBG and A1C) from the same blood sample.[11] In a patient exhibiting significant symptoms of hyperglycemia, a random plasma glucose of 200 mg/dL or higher is diagnostic of diabetes (Table 186.1).[1]

HbA1c is a nonfasting test and was added as a diagnostic tool because it has the same relationship to risk of retinopathy as do fasting glucose and 2-hour plasma glucose. Because of the chance of laboratory error, a second laboratory test should also be performed in the absence of classic symptoms of hyperglycemia unless other concurrent testing verifies the diagnosis (see Table 186.1). HbA1c results may be inaccurate in patients with anemia or other hemoglobinopathies, following a blood transfusion, during pregnancy, and postpartum. Point-of-care HbA1c results should be verified with a laboratory diagnostic

to verify the diagnosis. Because fructosamine measures glycated protein, a test of fructosamine is indicated to monitor diabetic patients with anemia.

The distinction between types 1 and 2 diabetes is important for therapeutic purposes because patients with type 1 diabetes must receive exogenous insulin daily. If necessary, a C-peptide level can be helpful in distinguishing type 1 from type 2 diabetes. Markers of type 1 diabetes include islet cell autoantibodies, insulin autoantibodies, and GAD65 autoantibodies.

When the diagnosis of diabetes is delivered to the patient it should include not only the fact that this is a serious disease for which there is no cure but also positive encouragement that the patient will learn to manage the disease and be able to continue to work and do things that bring enjoyment. Inclusion of supportive family members or friends in this discussion can be helpful.

INITIAL DIAGNOSTICS

Diabetes

LABORATORY
- Serum glucose (random or fasting)
- Oral glucose tolerance test
- HbA1c
- TSH[a]

TO DISTINGUISH TYPE 1 FROM TYPE 2 DIABETES
- C-peptide level
- GAD-65 autoantibodies
- Insulin autoantibodies
- Islet cell autoantibodies

[a]If indicated.

DIFFERENTIAL DIAGNOSIS

The diagnosis of diabetes is straightforward in a patient who has polyuria and polydipsia. The differential diagnosis is limited to type 1 diabetes, type 2 diabetes, and diabetes insipidus (Box 186.3). If hyperglycemia and glycosuria are absent and diabetes insipidus is excluded, the next step is to consider hyperthyroidism (checking triiodothyronine [T_3], thyroxine [T_4], and thyroid-stimulating hormone [TSH], levels) or hyperparathyroidism (checking parathyroid hormone and serum calcium levels). Secondary causes of diabetes should always be

BOX 186.3

Classification of Diabetes From the Expert Committee on the Diagnosis and Classification of Diabetes Mellitus

- In type 1 diabetes mellitus, insulin deficiency is caused by autoimmune β-cell destruction. The individual is dependent on exogenous insulin for survival and is prone to ketosis if insulin is withheld. Type 1 diabetes typically begins in childhood, adolescence, or young adulthood but may begin at any age. Accounting for only 5%–10% of all diabetes in the United States, type 1 occurs after a viral or environmental trigger in genetically predisposed individuals. Onset is rapid and dramatic.
- Type 2 diabetes is the more common type of diabetes in the United States and in most cases is linked to obesity. Type 2 diabetes can begin at any age, with a recent increase in onset during childhood and adolescence; it commonly runs in families. Type 2 diabetes is the result of insulin resistance and a relative deficiency of insulin. Exogenous insulin is not necessary for survival but may be an important part of the treatment as the disease progresses. Ketosis is rare in type 2 diabetes except in the setting of severe illness or infection. Onset is insidious.
- Other specific types of diabetes include genetic defects of the β-cell, defects in insulin action, diseases of the exocrine pancreas (e.g., pancreatitis, cystic fibrosis), other endocrinopathies (e.g., Cushing syndrome, pheochromocytoma), and drug-induced hyperglycemia.
- Gestational diabetes mellitus (GDM) refers to glucose intolerance with onset or first recognition during pregnancy. Given the increase in women of childbearing age who have undiagnosed type 2 diabetes, the recommendation is now to identify glucose intolerance that antedates the pregnancy in high-risk women. If found using standard criteria, the diagnosis of overt rather than gestational diabetes would be conferred. Women with GDM are at an increased risk for development of GDM with a subsequent pregnancy and type 2 diabetes within 5–10 years after delivery.
- Prediabetes is an intermediate stage in which the glucose levels are abnormal but do not meet the criteria for the diagnosis of diabetes. Prediabetes encompasses impaired fasting glucose (100–125 mg/dL) and impaired glucose tolerance (140–199 mg/dL 2 h after a 75-g glucose load). Individuals with prediabetes are at an increased risk for diabetes and cardiovascular disease. Progression to diabetes can be delayed or prevented with healthy diet, regular exercise, and weight loss.

Data from American Diabetes Association. (2018). Diagnosis and classification of diabetes mellitus. *Diabetes Care, 41*(Suppl 1), S13–S27.

TABLE 186.2 **Glycemic Control Targets for Nonpregnant Adults**

HbA1c level	Individualize goal HgbA1c, but the goal for most patients is <7%–8%. For older adults (age 80 or more) the goal is to keep hyperglycemic symptoms to a minimum and avoid hypoglycemia. For patients with HgbA1c at 6.5% or less, decrease or eliminate a medication to avoid adverse events.
Premeal blood glucose level	80–130 mg/dL
Peak postmeal blood glucose level	<180 mg/dL

Data from the American Diabetes Association: Standards of Medical Care in Diabetes–2019.

primary care provider and the diabetes care team. The combination of these therapies will help the patient to achieve the best glycemic control possible without undue burden or adverse effects (Table 186.2).

Nonpharmacologic Management

Nutritional therapy is essential in the management of both types 1 and 2 diabetes. A registered dietitian is crucial in helping to individualize a meal plan and to teach the patient and family about healthy nutrition.[12] The goal of nutritional therapy for diabetes and prediabetes is the development of a meal plan and balancing insulin with food intake and activity to achieve glycemic control. The nutritional goal for patients with type 1 diabetes is to promote normal growth and development during childhood, adolescence, pregnancy, and lactation; to balance energy intake and expenditure; and to achieve near normal blood glucose levels. It is necessary to match insulin doses to carbohydrate intake. For patients with type 2 diabetes, the nutritional goals are the achievement and maintenance of a healthy weight, adequate blood pressure control and lipid levels, and good glycemic control (Box 186.4). To promote recovery from a severe illness or surgery, special dietary adjustments may be necessary; these can be individualized with the help of a registered dietitian.

Exercise and physical activity have been shown to improve glycemic control.[13] Exercise causes increased glucose uptake in skeletal muscles as well as improved insulin sensitivity. The latter effect lasts several hours after exercise and is known as the exercise lag effect. All of the other benefits of exercise for the heart, lungs, and state of mind help reduce the risk of complications.

It is important for the individual with type 1 diabetes to make appropriate adjustments in food intake and/or insulin doses to balance the effects of exercise. Postexercise hypoglycemia or hyperglycemia may occur. The exercise lag effect may lead to low blood glucose episodes, which may occur many hours after exercise. To prevent hypoglycemia during exercise, the individual must balance activity with adequate food intake and appropriate insulin dose adjustments. High blood glucose levels after exercise may result from a decrease in circulating insulin and glucose uptake and an increase in hormonally regulated hepatic glucose. In the setting of exercise

considered. These include Cushing syndrome, pheochromocytoma, acromegaly, significant hypokalemia caused by glucose intolerance, hyperaldosteronism or diuretic use, destruction of the pancreatic islet from pancreatitis (caused by alcoholism or gallbladder disease), hemochromatosis, or drug-induced islet cell injury. In addition, infection or medication may cause glucose intolerance.

INTERPROFESSIONAL COLLABORATIVE MANAGEMENT

Diabetes is a self-managed chronic disease. Treatment of diabetes includes a healthy diet, regular exercise, medication, monitoring, education in self-care, and periodic follow-up with the

BOX **186.4**

Nutrition Guidelines for Patients With Diabetes

Recommend Dietary Guidelines for Americans[8] to achieve a healthy, balanced diet. In addition, for diabetes or prediabetes, the following are recommended:

Calories: Individualize to provide adequate amounts for weight control, growth and development, pregnancy, and lactation.

Portion control: For weight loss and maintenance.

Protein: Advise leaner protein and alternatives to meat.

Fat: Recommend unsaturated fat rather than saturated fat; minimal intake of *trans* fat.

Carbohydrate: Identify foods that contain carbohydrates (e.g., fruits, starchy vegetables, milk, bread, cereal, pasta, rice, desserts).

Cholesterol: <200 mg/d.

Fiber: 20–35 g/d.

Sodium: Limit daily intake to 2300 mg.

Alcohol: Limit to one alcoholic beverage (12 oz beer, 5 oz wine, or 1½ oz distilled spirits) per day for women and two for men; ingest with food to reduce the risk of hypoglycemia.

Data from American Diabetes Association. (2014). Nutrition recommendations and interventions for diabetes. *Diabetes Care, 37*(Suppl 1), S120–S143; and *Dietary Guidelines for Americans 2015–2020* (8th ed.). https://health.gov/dietaryguidelines/2015/resources/2015-2020_Dietary_Guidelines.pdf.

without adequate circulating insulin, ketogenesis occurs as fatty acids are broken down to supply energy, resulting in higher blood glucose levels and possible ketosis.[13]

In the individual with type 2 diabetes, exercise decreases insulin resistance and increases glucose uptake. Increased insulin sensitivity, contributing to the exercise lag effect, can last up to 48 hours after exercise. Thus food intake and medication, especially insulin, must be adjusted for the activity or exercise, particularly if the activity is sporadic. A reduction in the insulin that is peaking at the time of exercise, and perhaps the basal insulin as well, may be necessary. In the patient with type 2 diabetes, it would be desirable to decrease the medication rather than to increase food consumption so as to promote weight loss.[13] Exercise has been shown to prevent or delay the progression from prediabetes to diabetes. Guidelines for exercise in diabetes are reviewed in Box 186.5.

Blood Glucose Monitoring

Assessment of blood glucose levels is essential for achievement and maintenance of glycemic control. Because hyperglycemia is typically asymptomatic, monitoring is a valuable tool in the evaluation of a person's status in real time. Only a handheld meter, a test strip, a lancet, and a drop of blood are needed to measure the blood glucose level. Patients are encouraged to act on those results to adjust insulin or to evaluate the need to compensate with food or exercise. Monitoring is also used to assess for the acute complications of diabetes.[14,15]

Many patients learn to adjust their own insulin doses. Fasting and preprandial blood glucose levels give an overall view of basal glycemic control and should be between 70 and 130 mg/dL. Postprandial monitoring 1 to 2 hours after a meal helps to adjust subsequent meal-associated insulin doses. Postprandial results should be lower than 180 mg/dL. Patients who have type 2 diabetes may use pre- and postprandial values to

BOX **186.5**

Exercise Recommendations for Patients With Diabetes

TYPE 1 DIABETES

- Patients with well-controlled diabetes can enjoy exercise at all levels, from recreational activity to professional sports.
- Exercise should be avoided if the blood glucose concentration is greater than 250 mg/dL and ketones are present in the blood or urine or if the blood glucose concentration is greater than 300 mg/dL without ketones.
- Advise patients to delay exercise until carbohydrates are ingested if the blood glucose concentration is below 100 mg/dL.
- Recommend that patients consume carbohydrates during and after intense or prolonged exercise.
- Teach about the exercise lag effect, which can cause hypoglycemia for many hours after exercise, particularly overnight.
- Modify exercise recommendations for patients with complications of diabetes.

TYPE 2 DIABETES AND PREDIABETES

- Individualize recommendations on the basis of diabetes complications, cardiac risk factors, and activity baseline. Advise patients to begin gradually and under supervision.
- Interrupt sedentary time with movement at least once every 30 minutes.
- Patients should perform at least 150 minutes per week of moderate-intensity aerobic activity. This should be spread over at least 3 days in the week. More than 2 consecutive days without exercise should be avoided. More than this is associated with weight reduction and maintenance as well as greater reduction of cardiovascular disease risk.
- Patients should perform resistance exercise two to three times weekly.
- Patients who take insulin or insulin secretagogues must be prepared to treat hypoglycemia during and after exercise.
- Flexibility and balance training are recommended two to three times per week for older adults with diabetes.

Data from Colberg, S. R., Sigal, R. J., Fernhall, B., Regensteiner J. G., Blissmer B. J., Rubin R. R., et al. (2010). Exercise and type 2 diabetes: The American College of Sports Medicine and the American Diabetes Association: Joint position statement executive summary. *Diabetes Care, 33,* 2692–2696; American Diabetes Association. (2018). Standards of Medical Care, *Diabetes Care, 41*(Suppl 1), S38–S50.

guide their food selections, portion sizes, and the need for exercise. Patients are encouraged to use the results of their blood glucose tests in real time in addition to recording them for review with their provider at quarterly visits. A value lower than the target range may indicate hypoglycemia that requires immediate treatment. A value higher than the target range indicates hyperglycemia. Drinking enough water and getting daily exercise are indicated to help restore euglycemia and prevent dehydration. Blood glucose results that are consistently higher than the targets should trigger a reevaluation of the treatment plan. A significantly elevated blood glucose value may signal stress or impending illness and ought to be followed carefully.

There are many different brands of glucose meters on the market, and insurance plans may favor a certain brand of meter and test strip. Prescriptions are required for reimbursement of the cost of meters, test strips, and lancets. Most meters require a drop of blood from the fingertip, earlobe, or, in some cases, an alternate site. Newer products require very small drops of blood and provide the blood glucose result in as little as 5 seconds. Sensor meters attached to the upper arm allow patients to wave a glucose monitor over the sensor and obtain the current glucose readings. Proper storage of test strips and appropriate coding of the meter when required are important for accurate results. To evaluate the range of glucose disparity between plasma and whole blood, a patient should have his or her blood tested periodically with the home glucose meter and by the laboratory at the same time. If the difference is greater than 20%, another glucose meter should be used. Each meter has a toll-free number on the back for customer assistance. Home glucose meters cannot be repaired or recalibrated.[14,15]

Follow-Up Care

Diabetes is a chronic illness that requires periodic follow-up care. During visits, the health care provider evaluates glycemic control, the onset or progression of vascular and neuropathic complications, and the frequency and severity of hypoglycemic events. The burden of diabetes self-care, available resources, and social supports should be discussed periodically. The patient's capacity to understand and manage his or her diabetes improves compliance, promotes the ability to make good decisions each day, and prevents acute complications. The frequency of visits depends on the level of glycemic control and the presence of complications; however, a patient visit every 3 months aids monitoring of blood pressure, HgbA1c, lipids, and renal status. Each visit should include evaluation of blood pressure (the goal is individualized, but when possible 130/80 or less if there is associated CVD), weight, eye and foot examinations, and a review of the blood glucose log. Laboratory tests include a lipid profile, renal status, and HbA1c testing every 3 months. Liver function should be monitored at least yearly but more frequently if abnormal, as liver dysfunction is not uncommon in patients with diabetes.[16] Yearly screening for complications should include urinary microalbumin and urinalysis, referral for an ophthalmological examination, and a cardiovascular evaluation if indicated. Baseline electrocardiography is recommended after the age of 40 years. Exercise electrocardiography or peripheral vascular testing should be obtained when indicated. A discussion of results and goals for the following few months should occur at each visit.[15]

Pharmacological Management

Insulin, an anabolic hormone produced by the β-cells of the pancreas, plays a vital role in metabolism. Insulin therapy is lifesaving treatment for type 1 diabetes. Insulin is also used by patients with type 2 diabetes who have persistent hyperglycemia despite lifestyle changes and oral and/or noninsulin injectable diabetes agents. An individual with type 2 diabetes who begins to take insulin does not then have type 1 diabetes. Rather, he or she now has insulin-dependent type 2 diabetes.

Physiologic secretion of insulin is biphasic: basal and prandial. The basal phase inhibits glycogenolysis and gluconeogenesis and maintains glucose in a steady state. The prandial phase controls the glucose load and reuptake. Early morning hyperglycemia caused by counterregulatory hormones (known as the dawn phenomenon) is controlled by basal insulin, and postprandial glucose spikes are controlled by prandial insulin. Insulin therapy will ideally mimic this response.

A number of insulin products are available that may be prescribed to tailor an individualized regimen for each patient with the goal of optimal glycemic control while allowing a flexible lifestyle. Human insulin is derived synthetically from recombinant DNA (Humulin [Eli Lilly], Novolin [Novo-Nordisk]). Human insulin is available in regular, NPH, and 70/30, a premixed combination of 30% regular and 70% NPH. Humulin 50/50, pork-derived regular and NPH insulins, and Lente and Ultralente insulins are no longer available.

Insulin inhalation powder (Afrezza), a rapid-acting insulin, was approved by the US Food and Drug Administration (FDA) for use in adults in June 2014 and was initially marketed in early 2015. Individuals who use this product must also take subcutaneous basal insulin daily. Side effects include hypoglycemia, cough, and throat pain. Inhaled insulin is not recommended for patients who smoke. There is a risk of acute bronchospasm in patients who have chronic lung disease. Before initiating inhaled insulin, a medical history, physical examination, and spirometry to rule out chronic lung disease is recommended. Inhaled insulin is not recommended for the treatment of diabetic ketoacidosis (DKA).

Several insulin analogues made of recombinant human insulin are available. Three are rapid acting (lispro, aspart, glulisine), and three are long-acting or peakless (glargine, detemir, degludec). The rapid-acting insulin products are used as prandial (typically injected just before eating). The new Fiasp (faster aspart) is injected with or right after meals and correction (a scale or ratio based on sensitivity) insulin. The peakless insulins provide basal insulin coverage. Premixed insulin combinations are available for convenience. Individualized doses of basal and prandial insulin offer the best and most physiologic approach to tight glycemic control with fewer episodes of hypoglycemia.

Insulin Therapy

Type 1 Diabetes. Individuals with type 1 diabetes are truly dependent on insulin for survival. Simplistically, type 1 diabetes is the absence of one hormone: insulin. The replacement of that hormone to mimic normal physiology is challenging. Individuals with type 1 diabetes are sensitive to insulin, with a dramatic response to too much insulin (hypoglycemia) or to too little (hyperglycemia or DKA). The patient must appreciate that daily insulin is essential.

The most physiologic regimen is basal/bolus insulin. This can be accomplished with multiple daily injections or with an insulin pump, also known as continuous subcutaneous insulin infusion. Exogenous insulin requirements vary from one patient to another and, for an individual, from day to day. Physiologic insulin secretion for an adult who does not have diabetes is approximately 20 to 40 units per 24 hours. Thus most adults with type 1 diabetes will have to inject approximately this much insulin every day, typically divided into 50% basal insulin and 50% bolus insulin.

One unit of any kind of insulin will cause the same reduction in blood glucose concentration in a given individual for the duration of that type of insulin. For example, in a patient who is sensitive to insulin, 1 unit of a rapid-acting insulin will drop the blood glucose level 60 mg/dL in 2 to 3 hours, and 1 unit of a long-acting insulin will reduce the glucose level 60 mg/dL for over 24 hours. A patient who is much more resistant to insulin will experience a drop of only 10 mg/dL in glucose concentration in 2 to 3 hours after 1 unit of rapid-acting insulin and a drop of 10 mg/dL for 24 hours after 1 unit of basal insulin.

When insulin treatment is initiated, body weight, morphologic development (obese vs muscular), age (adolescent vs elderly), and activity (sedentary vs athletic) must be considered. The type of insulin prescribed depends on the patient's needs and the provider's preference. Therapy should begin with conservative starting doses and undergo continuous titration to achieve the desired blood glucose levels. On the basis of the patient's weight, an initial total daily dose (TDD) may be calculated as 0.5 U/kg, adjusted for sensitivity or resistance to insulin. The TDD is then divided into basal and bolus doses. Fifty percent of the TDD is typically basal insulin and 50% is divided between the three mealtime doses. Frequent pre- and postprandial blood glucose monitoring will guide dose adjustments.

Glargine, detemir, and degludec, long-acting insulins, are typically given once daily and last for up to 24 hours (or, in the case of degludec, up to 42 hours), mimicking the basal secretion of insulin. Basal insulin ought to be given at a time of day that is convenient for the patient so as to maintain a consistent routine. Large doses may be divided into twice-daily injections given 12 hours apart. Some individuals notice a peak from their basal insulin, when the risk for hypoglycemia is greater, so they may split their dose into two daily injections to minimize this. The dose of basal insulin is not determined with a sliding scale, so as not to make a decision with 24-hour implications based on a single blood glucose value. Rather, the dose of basal insulin should be adjusted every 2 or 3 days until the fasting blood glucose level is consistently in the target range. The basal insulin should be increased by increments of 2 to 5 units in an obese or insulin-resistant individual and by 1 to 2 units in an insulin-sensitive patient with a thin body frame and in patients with frequent episodes of hypoglycemia. If the fasting glucose concentration is consistently lower than 80 mg/dL, the dose of basal insulin likewise should be reduced in increments, every 2 or 3 days.

To prevent high postprandial glucose levels, a rapid-acting insulin analogue should be injected just before, during, or immediately after the meal. A low preprandial blood glucose level, unpredictable food intake, and delayed gastric emptying are common reasons for waiting until after the meal to inject the bolus dose. Most often, mealtime insulin is injected no more than 10 minutes before eating. A bolus dose with meals allows more flexibility in mealtimes, prevention of postprandial hyperglycemia, and fewer episodes of hypoglycemia. Initially prandial doses are one sixth of the TDD, but they can later be fine-tuned on the basis of postprandial blood glucose monitoring. The best approach to the determination of prandial insulin doses is counting the amount of carbohydrate to be consumed and calculating the dose on the basis of an individualized insulin-to-carbohydrate ratio. This ratio may range from 1 unit per 2 g of carbohydrate in an insulin-resistant patient to 1 unit per 30 g of carbohydrate in an insulin-sensitive patient.

The goal of the diabetes plan is to attain glycemic control with appropriate insulin doses but without frequent hypoglycemia or hyperglycemia. Intensive insulin therapy is defined as four or more insulin injections each day or the use of an insulin pump. This comprehensive strategy requires collaboration between the individual patient and family, the health care provider or diabetes specialist, and the diabetes education team of a nurse educator and dietitian. The more a patient knows about his or her diabetes, the better the decisions he or she will make each day.

Hypoglycemia is the most serious side effect of insulin. Fear of hypoglycemia prevents some individuals from embracing intensive insulin therapy. To prevent both hypoglycemia and hyperglycemia, factors such as exercise and activity, meal composition, mealtimes, sleep patterns, illness, and psychological well-being must be considered in adjusting insulin doses. The most important tool for control of day-to-day variations and prevention of hypoglycemia is home blood glucose monitoring. For a patient using an insulin pump, comanagement with an endocrinologist and diabetes care and education team is strongly recommended. Intensive insulin therapy is not appropriate for all patients, including those with hypoglycemia unawareness, those who are poorly motivated and unwilling to monitor their blood glucose levels frequently, some older adults, and those who have a limited life expectancy.

Basal/bolus insulin treatment is complex and more expensive than a twice-daily regimen of regular and NPH insulin or premixed insulin. Such treatment regimens offer an alternative for patients who cannot or will not take multiple daily injections. The patient using twice-daily insulin must eat meals on a schedule and be aware of the risk of nocturnal hypoglycemia. Regular insulin may be used as an alternative to a rapid-acting analogue but does not offer the immediate mealtime coverage, resulting in hyperglycemia postprandially and then hypoglycemia before the next meal. The four prepared insulin mixtures—Humalog 75/25, NovoLog 70/30, and mixtures of NPH and regular 70/30 (Novolin, Humulin)—offer ease and convenience for the individual. Dose adjustments, however, alter both the short-acting and longer-acting insulins.

Insulin products are available in both a vial (to be drawn into a syringe) and a prefilled disposable pen. A prescription for insulin must be accompanied by a second prescription for either syringes or insulin pen needles. Syringes are available in several different sizes, and needles come in several different lengths. NPH and regular insulin may be mixed in one syringe and injected together. Glargine, detemir, and degludec cannot be mixed with another insulin (Box 186.6).

New concentrated insulin products, allowing the injection of a smaller volume, include lispro U-200, degludec U-200, and glargine U-300 (Toujeo). These are available only in pens, and doses are prescribed and measured in actual units of insulin. Humulin regular insulin U-500 has been available since 1997 and is known to behave differently than U-100 regular insulin. It is now available in a pen, and a U-500 insulin syringe was recently introduced to measure this concentrated insulin from a vial. Caution is necessary in prescribing to prevent errors.

BOX **186.6**

Practical Insulin Tips

- Store unopened insulin vials and pens in the refrigerator. They will be good until the expiration date.
- After the first use, insulin pens should not be returned to the refrigerator.
- Opened insulin pens and vials are good for 10–56 days at room temperature, depending on the type of insulin.
- Place used syringes, pen needles, and lancets in a sturdy plastic or metal container, such as a liquid detergent or bleach jug or a coffee can. Once it is full, tape the lid on tightly. Contact local landfill for disposal recommendations.

Frequent glucose monitoring is recommended after a change in insulin product or concentration as dose adjustments may be necessary.[9]

Requirements for insulin decrease with weight loss and added exercise and increase with illness, infection, surgery, stress, and growth spurts as well as in patients with ketoacidosis. The practitioner should be aware of a possible "honeymoon" phase in the patient with newly diagnosed type 1 diabetes who may demonstrate a temporary recovery of β-cell function. Insulin requirements may decrease to 0.2 to 0.5 U/kg of body weight per day during this short-term phase.[9]

Type 2 Diabetes. Individuals with type 2 diabetes are not initially dependent on insulin for survival but may require insulin for optimal glycemic control later, as the disease progresses. This is common in a patient after several years of diabetes that had been well controlled with diet, exercise, and oral diabetes medications and may represent β-cell exhaustion. Patients must appreciate that this does not represent a "failure" on their part but rather is the natural progression of the disease. Encouragement to accept insulin as the most appropriate treatment of this phase of their diabetes, rather than to fear injections, is a useful strategy when insulin treatment is recommended (Box 186.7).

Insulin may be added to one or more other diabetes medications or may replace noninsulin medications. Because exogenous insulin may contribute to weight gain, it is essential that the patient understand that a healthy diet, regular exercise, and weight loss remain the cornerstones of diabetes treatment. The introduction or addition of a medication does not take the place of lifestyle modification.

As a first step, a single bedtime injection of intermediate- or long-acting insulin may be added to the oral medications to control fasting hyperglycemia. Basal insulin plus an insulin secretagogue for prandial glucose control works well for some. If the individual's glucose level remains above the targets after a few weeks, a rapid-acting insulin analogue could be added at mealtimes. Regular insulin may be used as a less expensive

alternative, but its onset is slower than that of the rapid-acting analogues and therefore may result in hyperglycemia postprandially. Its peak and duration of action are longer than those of the analogues, which may lead to hypoglycemia before the next meal. The use of lispro, glulisine, or aspart before meals or faster aspart (Fiasp) with or right after meals allows more flexibility, better coverage of hyperglycemia, and fewer episodes of hypoglycemia. To simplify the initiation of insulin, the analogue might be administered as a fixed dose with each meal or in a range of doses for low- and high-carbohydrate meals. When ready, the patient could be taught to count grams of carbohydrate and to calculate a more exact dose based on an individualized insulin-to-carbohydrate ratio.[9]

Local reactions at the injection site are the most common form of allergic reaction to insulin. Delayed hypersensitivity may also occur but remains in the area of injection. The use of synthetic or purified insulin has decreased both local and systemic reactions. Occurrence of reactions may be secondary to improper injection technique, injection of cold insulin, or preservatives. If systemic reactions do occur, the individual may require desensitization (the process of slowly reintroducing the allergy-inducing insulin in minute doses until the body no longer has an allergic response).

Noninsulin Medications for Type 2 Diabetes

Treatment of type 2 diabetes often includes management of dyslipidemia, hypertension, obesity, insulin resistance, and hypercoagulability as well as glycemic control.[14] The mainstays of therapy are education, diet, exercise, and achievement and maintenance of a desirable body weight. These therapies have no negative side effects, although they are difficult to sustain over time. Hyperglycemia may be reversed with weight loss of as little at 4 kg.[14] Early diagnosis of diabetes and prompt initiation of treatment are associated with better sustained glycemic control and fewer long-term complications. Treatment of diabetes should be individualized to achieve an HbA1c level as close to the nondiabetic range as possible without undue hypoglycemia; an elevated value signals the need for a change in treatment. This target should be modified for patients with a significant risk for dangerous hypoglycemia or with a limited life expectancy.

At the same time that diet and exercise treatments are maximized, pharmacologic intervention should be considered. The patient's place along the continuum of the natural progression of type 2 diabetes and the mechanisms that are contributing to hyperglycemia will guide the selection of medication.[6] Individualization of medication should be determined on the basis of effectiveness, safety, tolerability, and cost. The reduction of risk of diabetes complications has been shown to be related to the level of glycemic control over time rather than to the use of any single medication or combination. Some agents used to improve glycemic control also have beneficial or detrimental effects on related conditions (e.g., obesity, elevated lipids).[17,18]

The variety of diabetes medications available to supplement lifestyle changes enables the individualization of treatment for improved glycemic control, targeting each patient along the continuum of type 2 diabetes. Agents with different mechanisms may be combined to achieve greater glucose reduction.

Metformin is the initial medication prescribed for patients with type 2 DM and is a recommended consideration for prediabetic patients (i.e., those with a HgbA1c of 5.7% to 6.4%, a

---

BOX 186.7

Management of Type 2 Diabetes

Present the diagnosis to the patient as a lifelong chronic condition that can be managed but not cured. Encourage lifestyle modifications of healthy diet, regular exercise, weight loss, and diabetes self-management education. Begin metformin.

The American Diabetes Association (ADA) and AACE have published algorithms for the addition of other medications if the goals of treatment are not met. The selection of additional agent(s) is made based on duration of diabetes, patient preference, tolerability, risk of hypoglycemia, risk of weight gain, cost, etc. If and when necessary, insulin is added.

Reassure patients that the need for insulin does not represent a failure on their part but rather is the most appropriate treatment of the current phase of their disease. At each visit, reinforce the importance of a healthy diet and regular exercise as the cornerstones of treatment.

Data from Inzucchi, S. E., Bergenstal, R. M., Buse, J. B., Diamant, M., Ferrannini, E., Nauck, M., et al. (2015). Management of hyperglycemia in type 2 diabetes, 2015: a patient-centered approach. *Diabetes Care, 38*(1), 140–149; AACE/ACE Comprehensive Diabetes Management Algorithm. (2015). *2015, Endocrine Practice, 21*, 4; American Diabetes Association. (2018). Pharmacologic approaches to glycemic treatment: standards of medical care in diabetes–2018. *Diabetes Care, 41*(Suppl 1), S73–S85.

fasting plasma glucose 100 to 125 mg/dL, or 2-hour postload glucose 140 to 199 mg/dL).[19]

The mechanisms of action are suppression of hepatic glucose production (which typically results in lower fasting glucose levels), decreased intestinal absorption of glucose, and improved insulin sensitivity. A reduction of approximately 1.5% can be expected in the HbA1c level. Side effects of nausea and diarrhea are typically mild and temporary, and may be diminished by taking the medication after a meal and with use of the extended-release formulation. Metformin does not cause hypoglycemia and may promote weight loss. There is the rare but serious risk of lactic acidosis. For this reason metformin must be held before the intravenous administration of contrast material and temporarily discontinued (up to 48 hours) after radiologic studies involving intravenous contrast dye. In April 2016, the FDA issued revised warnings for the use of metformin, indicating that it can be used safely in individuals with mild or moderate renal dysfunction. Additionally, the FDA now recommends the use of estimated glomerular filtration rate (eGFR), rather than serum creatinine concentration, to better assess kidney function.[17,18] Renal function should be monitored every 3 months for patients with a GFR between 30 and 45 mL/min per 1.73 m^2 taking metformin. Metformin is contraindicated if the GFR is less than 30 mL/min per 1.73 m^2. Because B12 deficiency is associated with metformin, B12 levels should be monitored or B12 replacement recommended for patients taking metformin.

Sodium-Glucose Cotransporter-2 Inhibitors. For patients with type 2 diabetes and atherosclerotic heart disease and/or heart failure, the sodium-glucose cotransporter-2 (SGLT2) inhibitors are recommended by the American Diabetes Association (ADA), as they hinder progressive CVD as well as renal dysfunction.[20] This class includes empagliflozin (Jardiance) as well as canagliflozin (Invokana) and dapagliflozin (Farxiga). These once-daily pills increase the excretion of glucose in the urine and thereby reduce plasma glucose concentration and may contribute to weight loss. A predictable reduction in HbA1c is 0.6%.

Side effects include an increased risk for urinary tract infections (UTIs), genital infections in females, hypotension, and Fournier gangrene (perineum necrotizing fasciitis). The FDA has issued a warning regarding the risk of euglycemic DKA (with a blood sugar less than 250 mg/dL) in patients taking SGLT2 inhibitors. Although the mechanism of this adverse effect is unknown and the presentation uncommon, awareness of this phenomenon is crucial as these patients require hospitalization for fluid and electrolyte replacement and careful monitoring.[21] Trials are underway to study the safety and efficacy of SGLT2 inhibitors in type 1 diabetes.

The incretin mimetics, glucagon-like peptide 1 (GLP-1) agonists, are also indicated for treating type 2 diabetes and are associated with a decrease in cardiovascular events as well as progressive renal dysfunction.[20] Therefore, in type 2 DM, the GLP agonists are prescribed before insulin. Native GLP-1, produced in the small intestine, promotes insulin secretion in the fed state. These agents act to stimulate insulin secretion, to suppress glucagon secretion, and to slow gastric emptying. Gastrointestinal side effects are common and are related to the effect on gastric motility. Weight loss is also common, but hypoglycemia is not. The HbA1c is likely to fall approximately 1%. The association of GLP-1 receptor agonists and an increased risk of acute pancreatitis has been studied with no

conclusive evidence of a causal relationship. This category of medications should be avoided in patients with any history of MEN syndrome or thyroid C cell tumors and used cautiously (if at all) when there is a past history of pancreatitis.

There are several of these injectable medications, some of which are administered twice daily, some once daily, and others once weekly. Exenatide (Byetta) is given as a twice-daily subcutaneous injection 0 to 60 minutes before breakfast and dinner, starting with 5 mcg and titrating to 10 mcg after a month if needed. Liraglutide (Victoza) is a once-daily subcutaneous injection taken without respect to mealtime. There are three once-weekly GLP-1 receptor agonists: exenatide (Bydureon), dulaglutide (Trulicity), and albiglutide (Tanzeum). The GLP-1 receptor agonists have been shown to contribute to weight loss and a reduction in systolic blood pressure in addition to a reduction in HbA1c. GLP-1 receptor agonists may be used along with insulin for improved glycemic levels. Some combination products, available in prefilled pens, include a basal insulin and a GLP-1 receptor agonist.[22]

A higher dose of liraglutide is now marketed as Saxenda and is indicated as a treatment for weight loss as an adjunct to diet and exercise. Side effects at the higher dose include nausea and hypoglycemia.

The dipeptidyl peptidase 4 (DPP-4) inhibitors decrease glucagon levels by slowing the inactivation of incretin hormones and help to regulate insulin by affecting both α- and β-cells in response to elevated glucose levels. This process then helps to decrease preprandial and postprandial glucose levels. A reduction of 0.6% in the HbA1c is typical. The association of DPP-4 inhibitors and an increased risk of acute pancreatitis is a possible risk. These agents should be avoided in patients with a history of pancreatitis.

Sulfonylureas, though not as commonly used now, help to reduce blood glucose by stimulating insulin secretion; they also have the capacity to reduce the HbA1c level by approximately 1.5%. The most common side effects are weight gain and hypoglycemia, with hypoglycemia a serious concern and often the reason for discontinuation, especially in older adults. The second-generation medications in this class are glyburide (Micronase, DiaBeta, Glynase), glipizide (Glucotrol), and glimepiride (Amaryl). They are once- or twice-daily medications. Meglitinides (repaglinide [Prandin], nateglinide [Starlix]) are nonsulfonylurea insulin secretagogues. These are shorter-acting agents that must be taken with each meal and should be withheld if the patient is omitting a meal. The risk for weight gain exists, but these medications are less likely to cause hypoglycemia because of their shorter duration of action.[22]

Thiazolidinediones (TZDs) include pioglitazone (Actos) and rosiglitazone (Avandia); both peroxisome proliferator–activated receptor γ (PPAR-γ) modulators. They are associated with potentially serious adverse effects and therefore no longer frequently prescribed. TZDs improve the sensitivity of liver, fat, and muscle to both endogenous and exogenous insulin and decrease insulin resistance, thereby improving insulin sensitivity and decreasing insulin levels. In addition, the TZDs reduce hepatic glucose output. Improvement of both fasting and postprandial blood glucose levels occurs over time without stimulating insulin secretion. Side effects include weight gain and edema; thus congestive heart failure (CHF) is a contraindication. TZDs should not be used as first-line therapy if the patient is glucose-toxic because it takes 4 to 8 weeks for the full effect. A reduction in HbA1c of 1% is typical. Advantages include the delay of β-cell exhaustion, decreased insulin resistance, no hypoglycemia (if used alone), and improvement in triglycerides and levels of high-density lipoprotein (HDL). Some studies have revealed a slight increase in low-density lipoprotein (LDL) levels with rosiglitazone. There is a boxed warning for the risk of CHF with TZDs. Caution is to be exercised when TZDs are used with insulin because this may cause more peripheral edema and, increase the risk of CHF.[22]

There was a previous concern for myocardial ischemia with rosiglitazone, but in response to the findings of the Rosiglitazone Evaluated for Cardiovascular Outcomes and Regulation of Glycemia in Diabetes (RECORD) trial, which showed no elevated risk of myocardial infarction (MI) or death in patients taking rosiglitazone compared with standard-of-care diabetes medications, the FDA lifted previous restrictions. The FDA has been conducting a safety review of a reported association between long-term pioglitazone exposure and bladder cancer. A history of bladder cancer is a contraindication to the use of pioglitazone.

Alpha-Glucosidase Inhibitors. Acarbose [Precose] and miglitol [Glyset]) act in the small intestine, delaying the digestion of polysaccharides. The inhibition of starch and the sucrose enzyme causes lower postprandial glucose levels. To be effective, the pill must be taken with the first bite of a meal that contains carbohydrate. Alone, these medications will not cause hypoglycemia; but if they are used in combination with another medication and hypoglycemia occurs, glucose (not sucrose) is necessary for treatment. Sucrose absorption would be blocked by the action of these agents, so patients are advised to carry glucose tablets or gel. The side effects that patients experience with these agents—bloating, diarrhea and flatulence—limit their use. Contraindications include inflammatory bowel disease, colonic ulceration, obstructive bowel disease, gastroparesis, and creatinine levels above 2 mg/dL. α-Glucosidase inhibitors typically result in a 0.5% reduction in HbA1c.

Medication Management. If a single medication does not result in adequate glycemic control, a second agent may be added and then a third. Many different combinations have received FDA approval, and several two-medication tablets are available. The use of a combination tablet may reduce insurance copayments and improve adherence because of the convenience. All medications have side effects, and many of the newer agents are expensive. Both the ADA and AACE algorithms have been published to summarize the current treatment recommendations.[14,15]

When a patient taking several diabetes medications in addition to medications for other conditions is not achieving the glycemic targets, insulin must be considered. Many patients find the switch from pills to insulin to be daunting. Thoughtful discussion of their concerns, reassurance, and a relaxed environment in which to practice injections can ease the transition. Insulin, given in adequate doses, can reduce any glucose level to the desired range. Individuals with type 2 diabetes may need large doses (1 U/kg or more per day) to achieve desired glycemic control. An evening dose of intermediate-acting (NPH) or long-acting (glargine, detemir, or degludec) insulin may be added to one or more oral medications. In some cases other medications are discontinued and a split-mixed regimen of NPH and regular insulin or NPH and a rapid-acting analogue is recommended. For convenience, these are available as a pre-mixed combinations in both vials and pens. Other patients

will use basal/bolus insulin treatment alone. In addition to the insulin products used in type 1 diabetes, U-500 regular insulin may be used in type 2 diabetes. This is five times as concentrated as other insulins, allowing a patient with severe insulin resistance to inject a smaller volume. The use of U-500 insulin concentrate is now less confusing and error-prone as there is a U-500 syringe as well as a prefilled pen. Doses are prescribed in actual units rather than in terms of volume.[23,24]

Insulin may be used as first-line treatment of the patient with type 2 diabetes in the following situations: HbA1c level greater than 10% or glucose range above 250 mg/dL, severe illness with associated complications, gestational diabetes, and in fragile older adults. However, the most common reason for the use of insulin in type 2 diabetes is failure to respond to the other antihyperglycemic agents.

Pramlintide (Symlin) is a synthetic analogue of human amylin and may be added to insulin treatment in both type 1 and 2 diabetes. Amylin, a hormone produced in the pancreas and cosecreted with insulin, becomes deficient as β-cells are destroyed. The release of amylin leads to a decrease in hepatic glycolysis and a slowing of gastric emptying into the small intestine, thereby increasing satiety. The results are decreased glucagon secretion and decreased postprandial glucose spikes. Available now only in a disposable multidose pen, pramlintide is given by subcutaneous injection 10 to 15 minutes before meals, starting at a low dose of 15 to 60 mcg (type 1) and 30 to 120 mcg (type 2) and titrating slowly upward. Pramlintide must be taken with a meal and not be given at the same site as insulin. The dose of mealtime insulin should be decreased by 50% and taken toward the end of the meal. Side effects include severe hypoglycemia, nausea, anorexia, and gastrointestinal distress. Therefore it is important to titrate slowly, particularly if side effects are experienced. Severe hypoglycemia can occur from the mismatch of insulin timing with the postprandial glucose peak. Because of the delay in gastric emptying, pramlintide alters the postprandial glucose peak. If insulin reaches its peak before the peak in glucose concentration, postprandial hypoglycemia may occur, usually within 3 hours of pramlintide injection. Pramlintide is contraindicated in patients with gastroparesis.[24]

Combination therapy allows a more individualized regimen aimed at optimal glycemic control. Despite all the medications, however, a healthy diet and regular exercise remain the cornerstones of the management of diabetes.

INDICATIONS FOR REFERRAL OR HOSPITALIZATION

Referral to an endocrinologist or diabetologist should be considered in the following situations:
- New diagnosis of type 1 diabetes
- Poorly controlled type 2 diabetes despite two or more diabetes medications
- Discovery of a diabetes complication
- After hospitalization
- Initiation of insulin pump or other intensive insulin therapy
- Contemplated or confirmed pregnancy
- Patient request

Based on the ADA recommendations,[18] the patient with diabetes requires hospitalization for the following:
- Acute metabolic complications
- DKA (blood glucose >250 mg/dL, arterial pH <7.30, and serum bicarbonate <15 mEq/L with ketonuria or ketonemia)

- Hyperglycemic hyperosmolar state (HHS) (impaired mental status, dehydration, serum osmolarity >320 mOsm/kg, and plasma glucose >600 mg/dL)
- Hypoglycemia with neuroglycopenia (blood glucose <50 mg/dL that does not respond to usual treatment); coma, seizures or altered behavior; or persistent hypoglycemia caused by a sulfonylurea
- Uncontrolled diabetes
- Hyperglycemia with volume depletion
- Persistent hyperglycemia not responding to treatment and with metabolic deterioration
- Recurrent fasting hyperglycemia (>300 mg/dL or HbA1c level more than twice the upper limit of normal) refractory to outpatient treatment
- Recurrent severe hypoglycemia (<50 mg/dL) despite treatment
- Metabolic instability (glucose fluctuating between <50 mg/dL and >300 mg/dL)
- Recurrent DKA without infection or trauma as a precipitant
- Frequent absence from school or work as a result of psychosocial problems that lead to poor glycemic control
- Admission for complications of diabetes

Inpatient care may be appropriate in the event of the following:
- Newly diagnosed diabetes in young children
- Significant and sustained poor metabolic control that requires close monitoring
- Uncontrolled or newly diagnosed diabetes during pregnancy requiring insulin
- Severe, chronic complications of diabetes requiring intensive treatment

Comanagement With Specialists

Diabetes is a progressive disease requiring collaborative treatment from many specialties to prevent, identify, or slow the progression of end-organ complications. Specialists who care for patients with diabetes throughout their lives include endocrinologists, ophthalmologists, podiatrists, cardiologists, nephrologists, obstetricians, and vascular surgeons. For the evaluation and treatment of diabetic retinopathy, yearly visits to an ophthalmologist or an optometrist who is skilled in their care should begin at the time of diagnosis for all patients with diabetes. Prepubertal children with type 1 diabetes should begin to have annual eye examinations 5 years after diagnosis. A patient with diabetes should be referred to a podiatrist for the treatment of ulcers, foot deformities, foot infections, callus removal, and nail care as needed.

The patient with diabetes should be referred to a cardiologist for secondary prevention of CVD. Once microalbuminuria is present, a nephrology referral is indicated in order to prevent or delay further renal disease. A vascular surgeon may be needed for treatment of peripheral vascular disease, nonhealing ulcers, or amputation.[23]

Other referrals include consultation with a dietitian for medical nutrition therapy including carbohydrate-counting, calorie requirements, and weight loss; a diabetes educator to teach diabetes self-management; an exercise physiologist or physical therapist for exercise guidelines; and a social worker to help with the many occupational, financial, and emotional issues associated with living with diabetes.

Referral to a transplant center for consideration of pancreatic transplantation should be provided for appropriate patients. Those with labile type 1 diabetes or who have undergone renal transplantation and are already immunosuppressed would be good candidates. A patient who is morbidly obese and has multiple cardiac risk factors should be encouraged to consider bariatric surgery.

LIFE SPAN CONSIDERATIONS

Diabetes is a chronic and progressive disease with acute and chronic complications. It is present in individuals of all ages from infants to older adults. With each stage of development, there are issues regarding diabetes management; physical and emotional development; education and understanding; physical disabilities; nutrition; and financial, behavioral, and medical problems that will affect the diabetes treatment plan. Adolescents and older adults are at greatest risk for failure. Predictors that impede adherence to therapy include lack of practical knowledge, lack of control, vulnerability, lack of social acceptance, little or no family support, and fear of hypoglycemia. Other barriers include financial and occupational constraints. Consideration of all these issues is essential for optimal care.

Adolescents pose a particular challenge because metabolic and biologic changes affect glycemic control. Pre- or early adolescence (12 years of age), middle adolescence (13 to 15 years), and late adolescence (16 to 18 years) are marked by hormonal changes that often cause relative insulin resistance because of changing counterregulatory hormone responses and declining peripheral insulin action.

During adolescence, emotional and developmental issues emerge. The emotional stages of shock, denial, negotiation, anger, and acceptance can recur as the person ages. Developmental challenges of individual identity, sexual identity and exploration, the drive for independence and struggles with parents and authority, and peer acceptance can affect the ability of adolescents to manage their diabetes. Other concerns affecting diabetes management include athletic participation, recurrent ketoacidosis, inadequate nutrition, dieting and eating disorders, alcohol, drugs, and sexual activity. The health care provider's ability to communicate and compromise without risking safety will foster the development of a trusting relationship. Education must be factual, specific, and consultative rather than directive and must be relevant to the adolescent's stage of development and emotional behavior. The treatment plan must be realistic and workable and agreed to by both patient and provider. A written copy of the plan will be helpful.

In young adulthood, issues of career development, interpersonal relationships, self-image, health perception, and understanding of diabetes can influence glycemic control. As emotional ties to family decline, concerns related to marriage, pregnancy and children, employment, finances, and anticipation of complications can influence diabetes management. Health care providers must provide emotional support, updated information and resources, and reevaluation of nutritional and pharmacologic therapies. Emphasis should be on blood glucose monitoring, appropriate physical activity, healthy nutrition, and medical intervention to prevent hypoglycemia and to maintain glycemic control. A collaborative relationship with the diabetes care team is essential, including evaluation and aggressive treatment of diabetes complications.

In middle-aged people with diabetes, challenges include marriage and children, productivity, planning for retirement, and caring for elderly parents. The comorbidities associated with diabetes may develop or progress. If the addition of insulin is required, there may be implications for the patient's occupation.

In older adults, concerns about loneliness, loss, and disease progression or failing health can affect diabetes management. Financial concerns can interfere with access to proper food, prescribed medications, blood glucose monitoring supplies, and medical care. Issues of weight loss, physical inactivity, failing vision or hearing, poor dexterity or amputation, memory impairment, gait disturbance or muscle weakness, sexual dysfunction, and physical and emotional isolation can affect glycemic control. A diminished sense of thirst may contribute to dehydration in the setting of hyperglycemia. As complications develop and health begins to deteriorate, denial, anger, hostility, and depression can threaten the emotional well-being of the older patient with diabetes and influence diabetes management. Health care providers must offer resources and emotional support. The maintenance of function, independence, and general well-being as well as prevention of severe hypoglycemia and vascular compromise should take precedence over attaining optimum glycemic control. Insulin or sulfonylurea doses may have to be decreased at this time to reduce the risk of hypoglycemia and prevent falls. It is essential that the older patient with diabetes understand and be able to follow the treatment plan. Frequent medical visits as well as simplified written instructions, in large print if necessary, can be helpful to older adults with diabetes.

Diabetes and Pregnancy

Pregnant women with preexisting type 1 or type 2 diabetes and those with gestational diabetes mellitus (GDM) deserve special treatment considerations. GDM, a common complication of pregnancy, has been defined as any degree of glucose intolerance with onset or first recognition during pregnancy. Given the prevalence of undiagnosed type 2 diabetes, particularly among women of childbearing age, the recommendations for the screening and diagnosis in pregnancy were revised in 2010. The new screening strategy seeks to identify undiagnosed diabetes at the first prenatal visit in women who have risk factors using the standard diagnostic tests as well as looking for GDM later in the pregnancy (Box 186.8).

Untreated or inadequately treated diabetes confers an increased risk of poor outcomes for the woman (Box 186.9) and her infant (Box 186.10). For the woman with preexisting diabetes, excellent glycemic control prior to conception is strongly recommended to reduce the risk of serious congenital anomalies. A discussion of preconception care should begin at puberty and recur annually for all women of childbearing potential (Box 186.11). Fastidious diabetes care during the pregnancy is essential, as is care for the long-term health of both mother and baby.[23]

Gestational Diabetes. The patient with GDM requires excellent glycemic control, rapidly achieved after diagnosis and sustained throughout pregnancy. Up to 8.7% of healthy pregnant women in the United States will develop GDM, with the higher incidence in the same racial and ethnic groups that have a higher rate of type 2 diabetes. Fetal complications of untreated and poorly treated GDM include birth injury, macrosomia, hypoglycemia, respiratory distress syndrome, and hyperbilirubinemia. Maternal complications include an increased incidence of cesarean delivery, preeclampsia, postpartum hemorrhage, and the development of diabetes later in life.

BOX 186.8

Diagnosis of Hyperglycemic Disorders of Pregnancy

At the first prenatal visit, screen for preexisting diabetes in women with risk factors for type 2 diabetes. Measure fasting glucose, random glucose, or HbA1c for high-risk women. If results indicate overt diabetes, initiate treatment for diabetes.

If results are not diagnostic but fasting plasma glucose concentration is 92 to 125 mg/dL inclusive, diagnose with gestational diabetes mellitus (GDM). If fasting plasma glucose is <92 mg/dL, screen for GDM at 24 to 28 weeks of gestation. At 24 to 28 weeks of gestation, screen for GDM with a 2-h 75-g oral glucose tolerance test (OGTT) performed after an overnight fast in all women not known to have type 1 or type 2 diabetes.

The diagnosis of GDM is made if one or more values are exceeded on a 75-g OGTT:

Fasting plasma glucose	92 mg/dL
1-h plasma glucose	180 mg/dL
2-h plasma glucose	153 mg/dL

The diagnosis of overt diabetes in pregnancy is made on the basis of the following:

Fasting plasma glucose	≥126 mg/dL
HbA$_{1c}$	≥6.5%
Random plasma glucose	≥200 mg/dL[a]

[a]Confirm with either fasting plasma glucose concentration or HbA$_{1c}$ level.
Data from Dyer, A. R., Leiva, A., Hod, M., et al. (2010). International Association of Diabetes and Pregnancy Study Groups recommendations on the diagnosis and classification of hyperglycemia in pregnancy. *Diabetes Care, 33*(3), 676–682.
American Diabetes Association. *Classification and Diagnosis of Diabetes: Standards of Medical Care in Diabetes.* (2019). http://care.diabetesjournals.org/content/42/Supplement_1/S13.

BOX 186.9

Maternal Complications of Diabetes

- Cesarean delivery
- Hyperglycemia, ketoacidosis
- Hypoglycemia
- Pregnancy-induced hypertension
- Pyelonephritis, other infections
- Polyhydramnios
- Preterm labor
- Spontaneous abortion
- Worsening of chronic complications (retinopathy, nephropathy, neuropathy, cardiac disease)

Data from American Diabetes Association. (2015). Management of diabetes in pregnancy. *Diabetes Care, 38*(Suppl 1), S77–S79.

Glucose intolerance is the cause of increasing insulin resistance during the latter half of pregnancy. Placental and counterregulatory hormones along with the stress of the growing fetus increase insulin resistance, thereby causing hyperglycemia.

Management of the patient with GDM is a priority because time is of the essence. Treatment begins with the improvement of diet and exercise and may rapidly progress to medication if glycemic control is not achieved. Insulin therapy should be

Neonatal Complications of Mothers With Diabetes

- Birth trauma
- Congenital anomalies (especially cardiac malformations and neural tube defects)
- Hyperbilirubinemia
- Hyperinsulinemia
- Hypertrophic cardiomyopathy
- Hypocalcemia
- Hypoglycemia
- Hypoxia
- Hypomagnesemia
- Left colon syndrome
- Macrosomia
- Neurologic instability, irritation
- Polycythemia
- Renal vein thrombosis
- Stillbirth

Data from Kitzmiller, J. L., Block, J. M., Brown, F. M., Catalano, P. M., Conway, D. L., Coustan, D. R., et al. (2008). Managing preexisting diabetes for pregnancy: summary of evidence and consensus recommendations for care. *Diabetes Care, 31*(5), 1060–1079.

Preconception Care for Women With Type 1 or Type 2 Diabetes

Beginning at puberty, all diabetic women of childbearing potential should be counseled to do the following:

- Achieve an HbA1c level below 6.5% before conception to reduce the risk of anomalies (particularly anencephaly, microcephaly, and congenital heart disease) and miscarriage.
- Practice effective contraception until excellent glycemic control is achieved.
- Seek identification and treatment of chronic complications of diabetes before, during, and after pregnancy.
- Participate in perinatal care with a multidisciplinary obstetric and endocrinology care team.

Modified from American Diabetes Association. (2018). Management of diabetes in pregnancy: standards of medical care in diabetes—2018. *Diabetes Care, 138*(Suppl 1), S137–S143.

considered to improve glycemic control when two or more glucose readings exceed the recommended target range. As the pregnancy progresses, insulin resistance caused by hormonal effects can supersede even strict dietary compliance and insulin therapy may become necessary. Higher doses of insulin may be required in the third trimester, when insulin resistance is the greatest.

Women who have had GDM carry a 40% to 60% chance of developing type 2 diabetes by the time their child is 5 to 10 years old.[2] There is also the likelihood of GDM with a subsequent pregnancy and an increased risk of CVD.

Pregnancy in the Woman With Type 1 Diabetes. A generation ago, pregnancy was discouraged in women with type 1 diabetes. With proper planning, commitment, and the support of a diabetes and obstetric team, such a pregnancy

is now encouraged. For a woman with type 1 diabetes, this is still considered a high-risk pregnancy that may result in life-threatening complications for both the mother (see Box 186.9) and neonate (see Box 186.10). It is imperative that the woman with diabetes attain ideal glycemic control, including an HbA1c level as close to normal as possible without excess hypoglycemia, prior to conception. If an unanticipated pregnancy occurs, intensive glycemic control should be the immediate priority. There is a 1 in 10 chance of a congenital anomaly developing in the growing fetus in the setting of poor maternal glycemic control.[25]

For the pregnant woman with diabetes, the metabolic changes that occur with the growing fetus can accelerate retinal and renal complications. Vascular complications of retinopathy, nephropathy, pregnancy-induced hypertension, and poorly controlled glycemia are strong risk factors for perinatal compromise. Pregnant women with type 1 diabetes are at high risk and must be monitored closely by a team of specialists, including a high-risk obstetrician, endocrinologist, nephrologist, ophthalmologist, dietitian, and diabetes nurse educator.

Adjustments in insulin doses are needed for excellent glycemic control as pregnancy progresses. In the first trimester, insulin doses may be lower than the prepregnancy doses because of hypoglycemia from the increase in fetal glucose transport and a loss of maternal amino acids. During the latter half of the second trimester, there is a rapid diversion to fat metabolism, resulting in higher concentrations of circulating glucose. The longer the duration of postprandial hyperglycemia, the more glucose is transported to the fetus, thus promoting fetal growth. During this time there is also a degree of insulin resistance that occurs from the placental hormone (human placental lactogen), prolactin, and cortisol. Insulin requirements increase during this stage and into the third trimester and then plateau around week 36 of gestation.[25]

Dietary requirements, activity and exercise, blood glucose monitoring, and insulin doses must be adjusted for the pregnant state. Calorie requirements are increased and snacks are added, particularly during the first trimester, to prevent hypoglycemia and starvation ketosis. Multiple injections with changes in insulin type (NPH, regular, lispro, aspart, and detemir are FDA Pregnancy Category B; glargine, glulisine, degludec and inhaled insulin are Pregnancy Category C) or insulin pump therapy may be needed for better glycemic control. The advantage of the pump is that it allows frequent small dose adjustments in basal rates and bolus doses with a rapid-acting insulin analogue and the ability to withhold basal insulin temporarily should hypoglycemia occur. Safer and improved glycemic control can be achieved by more frequent blood glucose monitoring including fasting as well as prepgrandial, postprandial, bedtime, and middle-of-the night readings. Researchers have recently discovered the pathway leading to a proliferation of β-cells during pregnancy. Two hormones of pregnancy, prolactin and placental lactogen, trigger the expression of a gene in islet cells that causes an increased production of serotonin by β-cells. The release of serotonin then results in increased β-cell mass. The process is reversed at birth, and β-cells return to their prepregnancy level.[25]

Pregnancy in the Woman With Type 2 Diabetes. For the woman with type 2 diabetes who is contemplating pregnancy, excellent glycemic control should be attained prior to conception to improve both fetal and maternal outcomes (see Box 186.11). Counsel the patient to delay conception until the

HbA1c level is less than 7%.[25] The literature on the use of oral agents at the time of conception and the concern for teratogenicity is limited, particularly among the newer medications. Metformin has been used for the treatment of polycystic ovary syndrome (PCOS); in that instance this drug is beneficial for improving the rate of ovulation. There has been no increase in anomalies in women who take metformin in the first trimester or throughout the pregnancy. Women with PCOS, however, do not have hyperglycemia, so the risk may be different for women with type 2 diabetes. The conversion to insulin before conception is safe, and insulin requirements will diminish after delivery.

Later in the pregnancy, after organogenesis, resumption of oral medications may be considered. Discontinuation of a sulfonylurea before labor and delivery is recommended to reduce the risk of hypoglycemia after birth. Metformin, glyburide, and glipizide may be used during lactation.[25]

Pregnant women with diabetes should be referred for individualized nutritional therapy. The goals of such therapy are adequate nutrition to support mother and baby, excellent glycemic control, appropriate weight gain, and the development of lifelong healthy nutritional habits. For women without contraindications, 30 minutes of daily exercise or physical activity is recommended. Exercise will result in decreased weight gain, less fetal fat deposition, and improved glycemic control. The patient's ability to tolerate labor will also be enhanced by regular exercise. The patient should be taught the indications (dyspnea, chest pain, calf pain or swelling, vaginal bleeding, amniotic fluid leakage, or uterine contractions) to stop exercise and to seek medical help.[25] Monitoring of blood glucose concentration four or more times per day, including fasting and 2-hour postprandial blood glucose levels, is recommended.

In the pregnant woman with chronic hypertension, a blood pressure of 120 to 160/80 to 105 mm Hg during pregnancy is reasonable. A lower blood pressure level may be associated with an impairment in fetal growth. For pregnant women with type 2 diabetes, certain medications used to treat comorbidities are not safe during pregnancy or lactation and will have to be discontinued (e.g., angiotensin-converting enzyme inhibitors [ACEIs], angiotensin II receptor blockers [ARBs], and statins).[25] Careful monitoring of blood pressure, renal and retinal status, glycemic control, and fetal well-being by a team of specialists is necessary throughout the pregnancy.

COMPLICATIONS
Psychological Complications

The diagnosis of diabetes, like that of any chronic illness, can be unexpected and potentially devastating. The patient's emotional response to the diagnosis may range from denial to guilt to grief. The support of family members and friends is important for the long-term acceptance of the disease and its progression. The diagnosis is often confirmed and presented to the patient in the ambulatory setting, where the adult patient may be unaccompanied. The patient should be encouraged to share the diagnosis with and to seek support from friends and family as one would with the diagnosis of any life-changing disease.

Whereas 5% to 8% of the general population will experience a major depressive disorder sometime in their lives, there is a three- to fourfold increase in the prevalence of depression in patients with type 1 or 2 diabetes. In the Diabetes Attitudes, Wishes and Needs second study (DAWN2) it was found that 45% of participants reported that they experienced significant distress because of their diabetes, yet only 24% stated that their health care team members had inquired about the effects of diabetes on their lives. Patients should be screened for distress annually and as needed, as with a marked deterioration of glycemic control. Without treatment, depression in the patient with diabetes can affect glycemic control. Depression may also contribute to detrimental lifestyle habits such as overeating, inactivity, smoking, drinking alcohol, and medication noncompliance, all of which increase the risk for diabetes complications. Subclinical emotional distress can impede diabetes management, leading to poor glycemic control, poor self-image, confusion about treatment recommendations, and the progression of complications, leading to a poor quality of life. A careful coordination of medical therapy and psychotherapy is needed. Treatment options include relaxation, education, support of family and friends, psychotherapy, and pharmacotherapy. The newer selective serotonin reuptake inhibitors (SSRIs) are better choices for treatment than most other antidepressant agents because they do not cause hyperglycemia.

Another mental health issue that may complicate diabetes is an eating disorder. Omission of insulin in type 1 diabetes results in weight loss and is informally known as "diabulima." This method of weight loss poses a significant risk for DKA. It is more common among young women and manifests as weight loss despite overeating and a decreased level of energy. Treatment requires collaboration between the diabetes care team and the eating disorders team.

Acute Complications of Diabetes

Hypoglycemia. Short-term reversible complications of diabetes include the extremes of blood glucose concentration. Hypoglycemia, defined as a blood glucose level of less than 70 mg/dL, is caused by an imbalance of food, exercise, and insulin (Table 186.3). Initial symptoms are caused by the adrenergic response to a drop in the blood glucose level. When that levels is 70 mg/dL or lower (or perhaps higher in a patient with consistently poor control), the hypothalamus senses the decreased blood glucose and triggers the sensation of hunger. This action stimulates the nervous system to increase gastric juices and stomach contractions. The adrenal medulla secretes epinephrine and cortisol, which stimulate glycogenolysis (the storage of glucose). This slows glycogenesis and promotes gluconeogenesis (glucose formation from fatty and amino acids). As the blood glucose level decreases, cerebral function is altered. Neuroglycopenia occurs when the brain and central nervous system are unable to maintain normal function because of lowered glucose levels, and thus a lack of energy. The low glucose level is classified as mild, moderate, or severe based on neuroglycopenic symptoms and the individual's ability to treat himself or herself.

The blood glucose level at which one feels symptoms of hypoglycemia differs among individuals and may vary for a given patient from one episode to the next. The sensation of symptoms may depend on factors such as the rapidity of the fall in glucose as well as preoccupation with other activities. Therefore each individual must monitor blood glucose concentration when hypoglycemia is suspected, pay close attention to symptoms, and avoid delays in treatment.

The treatment of hypoglycemia is the consumption of sugar. Mild to moderate hypoglycemia can be corrected with 15 g of a carbohydrate food or beverage. Twice this amount of carbohydrate may be needed to correct severe hypoglycemia.

TABLE 186.3	Hypoglycemia	
Condition	**Signs and Symptoms**	**Treatment**
Mild hypoglycemia	Blood glucose <70 mg/dL Shaking or trembling, sweating, hunger, tachycardia, weakness, lightheadedness, pallor, irritability, but no change in mental status; individual able to treat self.	Eat or drink 15 g of rapid-acting carbohydrate (avoid high-fat foods such as chocolate). If blood glucose <50 mg/dL, 20–30 g of carbohydrate may be needed. Stop activity and check blood glucose in 10–15 min; if <70 mg/dL, take additional 15 g of carbohydrate. Once recovered, attempt to determine the cause so that similar episodes can be avoided in the future.
Moderate hypoglycemia	Decreased thinking, increased emotions (anger, irritability), inability to complete tasks, some changes in mental status; individual may be able to treat self.	Take 15–30 g of rapid-acting carbohydrate and then follow the aforementioned instructions.
Severe hypoglycemia	Confusion, drowsiness; may progress to unconsciousness; impaired neurological function; individual requires assistance.	Take 30–45 g of simple-acting carbohydrate if able to swallow safely. If not, glucagon should be injected intramuscularly or subcutaneously (1 mg for adults; 0.5 mg for children <5 years; 0.25 mg for infants). Follow with snack or meal.

Type 2 diabetes patients taking α-glucosidase inhibitors who are treated with oral carbohydrates must receive glucose tabs (e.g., glucose).
Data from Thome, J., & Byon, D. (2018). Addressing hypoglycemic emergencies. https://www.uspharmacist.com/article/addressing-hypoglycemic-emergencies. Accessed 25.03.19; and Cryer, P. E., Davis, S. N., & Shamoon, H. (2003). Hypoglycemia in diabetes. *Diabetes Care, 26*(6), 1902–1912.

Liquids, such as juice or nondiet soda, can be consumed more quickly than solids. If the risk of aspiration exists, glucose gel may be applied between the cheek and the gum. All patients should be advised to keep a rapid-acting carbohydrate with them at all times, including next to the bed, to avoid a delay in treatment.[4]

More is not better when a low blood glucose reaction is being treated. Overtreatment can result in rebound hyperglycemia. Delayed or inadequate treatment of hypoglycemia may result in continued or worsening symptoms, to a point at which the individual is unable to help himself or herself. After resolution of the hypoglycemic event, it may be useful for the patient to try to determine its cause in order to help prevent future episodes.

Patients with type 1 diabetes or a history of severe or unconscious hypoglycemia should make certain that a family member or close friend knows how to recognize and treat severe hypoglycemia by the intramuscular administration of glucagon or activation of emergency medical services.[26]

Hypoglycemia unawareness is the loss of autonomic symptoms that warn the individual of a low blood glucose level. Long duration of the disease, other neuropathic complications, and uncontrolled diabetes are risk factors for this dangerous condition. the frequent monitoring of blood glucose, particularly before driving, is essential for those with hypoglycemia unawareness. Aiming for a higher blood glucose target range is recommended to reduce the frequency of low blood glucose episodes in these individuals who are at risk for undetected hypoglycemia. For some patients, hypoglycemia unawareness may possibly be reversible if the patient can avoid any hypoglycemic episodes for 7 to 21 days.

Intensive insulin therapy and near-normal glycemia can increase vulnerability to hypoglycemia. Health care providers must be aware of the influence of medications, food, and exercise on glucose control and be wary of nighttime moderate to severe hypoglycemia. The peakless basal insulin analogues are less likely to cause nocturnal hypoglycemia than is NPH. Older adults, those with type 1 diabetes, those with longer duration of diabetes, and patients with neuropathic complications are at greatest risk for hypoglycemia. Left untreated, severe hypoglycemia can lead to seizure, coma, and death.[26]

Fear of hypoglycemia may drive a patient to purposefully avoid tight glycemic control. The patient who has developed a tolerance for hyperglycemia may feel symptoms of hypoglycemia at a normal or even somewhat high glucose level. Setting and achieving gradually decreasing glucose targets will help to resolve this over time. It is important that providers and patients collaborate on a treatment plan that is safe and acceptable.

A continuous glucose sensor measures glucose in the interstitial fluid every 5 minutes and will sound an alarm to alert the patient to a low or rapidly dropping blood glucose level. The results are displayed as a glucose value in the context of the direction of change from the previous result. Some of these devices will transmit the glucose value to the patient's mobile phone. This is a new tool to be used along with traditional fingerstick blood glucose monitoring. Manufacturers of some devices advise confirmation of a glucose value with a blood glucose test before treatment with insulin.

Hyperglycemia. Hyperglycemia is defined as a glucose level of higher than 180 mg/dL. Most patients will experience no symptoms at this glucose level, and some who have developed a tolerance for sustained hyperglycemia may report that they feel better in this range than at a normal glucose level. The symptoms of untreated diabetes (e.g., polyuria, polydipsia, blurry vision, fatigue) may accompany prolonged periods of hyperglycemia.

Treatment of intermittent hyperglycemia includes the administration of a correction dose of rapid-acting insulin if the patient has been advised to do so. Taking an additional dose of an oral diabetes medication is never recommended. Nonmedicinal strategies to reduce episodic hyperglycemia include drinking plenty of water and getting some extra exercise (unless ketones are present). Reevaluation of the diet and exercise plan is also recommended.

Diabetic Ketoacidosis and Hyperglycemic Hyperosmolar State. If left untreated, hyperglycemia can progress to DKA or a hyperglycemic hyperosmolar state (HHS), previously

BOX 186.12

Ketone Monitoring

Teach all patients with type 1 diabetes when and how to test for ketones.

Test urine or blood ketones if
- Blood glucose level inexplicably 250 mg/dL or higher.
- Illness, infection, fever, and/or stress is present.

After omission of insulin
- Positive ketones on last test.

Positive result indicates inadequate insulin and risk for DKA.
- Drink plenty of water.
- Take correction insulin.
- Avoid exercise.
- Continue to monitor.
- Call provider for help.

DKA, Diabetic ketoacidosis.

BOX 186.13

Sick-Day Management for Patients With Diabetes

Rising blood glucose levels may be the first sign of impending illness. With unexplained high blood glucose levels or with illness, infection, or pain, the following are recommended:
1. Monitor blood glucose at least every 4 h.
2. If blood glucose level is higher than 250 mg/dL in type 1 diabetes, test for ketones.
3. With elevated blood glucose levels, supplemental rapid-acting insulin can be given every 2–4 h. Advise a dose of rapid-acting insulin based on the correction factor. The increased insulin resistance of acute illness may necessitate higher doses.
4. Maintain adequate hydration by drinking 8 oz of calorie-free fluid hourly while awake. This can be alternated with a sodium-rich fluid, such as bouillon, consommé, or clear canned soups. If unable to eat a normal diet, alternate fluids containing carbohydrate, such as apple juice or regular ginger ale, with sugar-free fluids.
5. Continue to take diabetes medication even if not eating. The most common cause of diabetic ketoacidosis (DKA) is the omission of insulin when sick.
6. Antiemetics should be prescribed for those unable to tolerate fluids by mouth; monitor closely for dehydration. Intravenous fluid may be needed.
7. Contact health care provider for the following:
   - Difficulty breathing
   - Vomiting persisting more than 6 h
   - Elevated blood glucose of 300 mg/dL or higher unresponsive to increased insulin after two doses
   - Moderate or large urinary ketones or blood ketones higher than 0.6 mmol/L
   - Questions or concerns

called hyperglycemic hyperosmolar nonketotic coma. The new term recognizes that the patient may have altered sensorium without coma and may have a mild to moderate degree of ketosis. These are medical emergencies that require immediate treatment and, in most cases, hospitalization.

DKA is caused by insulin deficiency and is characterized by hyperglycemia, ketonemia, and acidemia. The clinical presentation of DKA includes rapid development of abdominal pain, nausea and vomiting, Kussmaul respirations, and dehydration. Physical examination may reveal a fruity odor to the breath, tachycardia, hypotension, and changes in consciousness. Laboratory assessment includes arterial blood gas, electrolytes, glucose, anion gap, and β-hydroxybutyrate (serum ketones). Treatment of DKA includes fluid resuscitation, intravenous insulin administration, electrolyte monitoring and replacement, and investigation and treatment of an underlying illness or infection. Once the patient is stable, the cause of DKA should be determined and the patient counseled on the steps needed to prevent a recurrence. The most common causes include new-onset type 1 diabetes, omission of insulin, infection, illness, and major surgery.

Hospitalization may be avoided with the early detection and aggressive treatment of hyperglycemia and ketonuria. Fluids, insulin, and frequent blood glucose and ketone monitoring are essential (Box 186.12).

Prevention of DKA requires prompt attention to increasing hyperglycemia as well as home ketone monitoring (urine or blood) when indicated. Adherence to sick-day management guidelines (Box 186.13) will enable the individual with type 1 diabetes to actively participate in the prevention of ketoacidosis. Review of these guidelines with patients regularly, especially at the start of cold and influenza season, is recommended.

HHS is a medical emergency affecting the patient with type 2 diabetes. HHS is characterized by a relative deficiency of insulin that is inadequate to sustain normoglycemia but is adequate to prevent lipolysis and severe ketosis. This is most common in older adults, particularly nursing home residents, as well as in newly diagnosed individuals. Presenting symptoms include a gradual progression of polyuria, polydipsia, and altered level of consciousness. In patients living alone, treatment is often delayed because of altered sensorium, and this contributes to the significant mortality associated with

HHS. On presentation, the patient is found to have significant hyperglycemia and profound dehydration. Seizures, tremor, hemiparesis, and disorientation may be present.

Precipitating causes include acute illness, infection or burns, medications, omission of insulin, new diagnosis of diabetes, and inadequate free water intake. Treatment includes reversal of dehydration and hyperglycemia and correction of any electrolyte abnormalities. The older adult patient should have a complete safety assessment before being discharged back to his or her current home.

Chronic Complications of Diabetes

The major morbidity and mortality associated with diabetes are result of the long-term, irreversible complications, a consequence of persistent hyperglycemia and other factors. Results from the Diabetes Control and Complications Trial (DCCT) in type 1 diabetes and the United Kingdom Prospective Diabetes Study (UKPDS) in type 2 diabetes revealed a significant reduction in the complications of retinopathy, nephropathy, and neuropathy when glycemic control was sustained in the HbA1c range of approximately 7%.[2] Long-term follow-up of the DCCT cohorts demonstrated that the risk reduction effect of intensive glycemic control persists even after some decline in glycemic control, as reported in the Epidemiology of Diabetes Interventions and Complications (EDIC) study.[27]

Prevention of Chronic Complications

- Glycemic control
- Blood pressure control
- Lipid control
- Smoking avoidance or cessation
- Weight control
- Early detection of chronic complications
  - Annual ophthalmology examination
  - Annual microalbuminuria evaluation
  - Foot examination to assess protective sensation
- Referral to specialists as needed
  - Ophthalmologist
  - Podiatrist
  - Nephrologist
  - Cardiologist

Data from American Diabetes Association. (2018). Comprehensive Medical Evaluation and Assessment of Comorbidities: Standards of medical care in diabetes—2018. *Diabetes Care, 41*(Suppl 1), S28–S37.

The benefits of intensive glucose management on the reduction of CVD for patients with type 2 diabetes must be individualized. The Action to Control Cardiovascular Risk in Diabetes (ACCORD) study, the Action in Diabetes and Vascular Disease (ADVANCE) study, and the Veterans Affairs Diabetes Trial (VADT) concluded that intensive therapy to normalize glycemic control did not result in fewer cardiovascular events among high-risk patients with type 2 diabetes and in fact was associated with an increase in mortality.[28] For patients with a shorter duration of diabetes, no significant CVD, and a reasonable life expectancy, an HbA1c target of less than 7%, achieved without undue hypoglycemia, may result in a further reduction in risk of microvascular complications. For patients who have a limited life expectancy, with advanced diabetes complications or comorbidities, longer duration of diabetes, and a history of severe hypoglycemia, the HbA1c target should be higher than 7% (Box 186.14).

Microvascular Complications

Diabetic Retinopathy. Nearly all patients with type 1 diabetes and 80% of patients with type 2 diabetes will have some form of retinopathy after 20 years of diabetes; 21% of type 2 patients have retinopathy at the time of diagnosis.[23] Left untreated, diabetic retinopathy may progress to vision loss and blindness. Therefore annual screening for retinopathy with a dilated retinal examination by an ophthalmologist or optometrist skilled in recognizing retinopathy is recommended for all individuals with diabetes, within 5 years of the diagnosis of type 1, and at the time of diagnosis for those with type 2. Patients are likely to experience no change in their vision until retinopathy is advanced. Routine examinations are essential for early detection at a point at which the retinopathy is more successfully treated. Diabetic retinopathy is the leading cause of new-onset blindness in the United States.[23] Poor glucose control, hypertension, hyperlipidemia, nephropathy, anemia, sleep apnea, and smoking are all risk factors associated with the incidence and progression of diabetic retinopathy. Women with diabetes who are contemplating pregnancy are advised to

have a thorough eye examination before conception and then each trimester during the pregnancy. A rapid progression of retinopathy during pregnancy is common.[25]

Nonproliferative retinopathy is treated by strict adherence to blood pressure and blood glucose control, smoking avoidance, and follow-up care by an eye specialist. Proliferative diabetic retinopathy (PDR) is treated with laser photocoagulation to halt the progression and decrease the risk of severe vision loss. The earlier the treatment, the more positive the outcome; therefore regular dilated retinal examinations are essential because the patient is likely to have no recognizable change in his or her vision. Any new report of a sensation of "floaters" or "cobwebs" in the eye or of a sudden, painless loss of vision should prompt an urgent referral to an ophthalmologist.

Other ocular conditions that are common in people with diabetes include cataracts, which begin at a younger age and progress more rapidly than in people who do not have diabetes. Open-angle glaucoma is more common in diabetes. Individuals with diabetes may also experience blurred vision related to high or fluctuating blood glucose levels. This is temporary and will resolve with improved glycemic control.

Diabetic Nephropathy. Diabetes is the most common cause of end-stage renal disease (ESRD), necessitating dialysis or kidney transplantation.[24] Nephropathy is present in 30% to 40% of patients with type 1 diabetes and represents the second leading cause of death for individuals with diabetes. Sixty percent of all patients with diabetes who ultimately require renal dialysis have type 2 diabetes.[2]

Diabetic nephropathy, also known as Kimmelstiel-Wilson syndrome, is characterized by proteinuria, hypertension, edema, and renal insufficiency. Chronic kidney disease progresses through five stages: (1) elevated GFR, indicating increased work of the kidney; (2) presence of microalbuminuria, with GFR elevated or back to normal; (3) proteinuria and hypertension with moderate reduction of GFR; (4) diminished GFR and rising blood urea nitrogen and creatinine concentrations; and (5) ESRD.

The GFR, which is usually elevated when a person is first diagnosed with diabetes, is directly related to the degree of hyperglycemia but is a poor measure of renal function because its elevation may ensue over a long "silent" period (of about 15 years' duration) as histologic changes in the kidney progress. Serum creatinine, also an unreliable marker for renal disease, might not be elevated until more than 50% of function is lost and may be normal in older patients with renal damage because of decreased muscle mass.[24]

Because the earliest indication of renal damage from diabetes is the presence of microalbuminuria, all patients with diabetes should have this tested annually, beginning at the time of diagnosis of type 2 diabetes and 5 years after the diagnosis of type 1 diabetes. There are typically no symptoms during the early stages of diabetic nephropathy, yet the presence of microalbuminuria is a harbinger of both renal failure and cardiovascular complications in diabetes.

Microalbuminuria analysis can be performed by an albumin/creatinine ratio, a random spot collection, a 24-hour collection, or a timed (e.g., 4-hour or overnight) collection. Microalbuminuria is diagnostic at more than 30 mg/24 h excretion. Two of three positive collections in a 3- to 6-month period are necessary to confirm microalbuminuria. Ongoing monitoring of albumin excretion is useful to assess the response to treatment and progression of the disease.

When microalbuminuria (or hypertension) is confirmed, treatment with an ACEI or ARB should be initiated. In patients with type 2 diabetes, hypertension, and microalbuminuria, an ACEI or ARB has been shown to delay the progression to proteinuria. In patients with type 2 diabetes who also have renal insufficiency, the progression of nephropathy can be delayed with the use of an ARB. If one class of agent is not tolerated, it should be replaced with the other.

Control of blood pressure is the single most important intervention in the prevention and treatment of renal disease in the patient with diabetes. The ADA recommends a blood pressure target of 130/80 mm Hg, especially for patients with a calculated ASCVD risk of 15% or more.[20] As with all treatment regimens, diet, exercise, weight loss, and smoking avoidance are vital. Restriction of protein intake is recommended for patients with kidney disease. Limiting protein intake to 0.8 to 1 g/kg body weight per day in the early stages of chronic kidney disease and to less than 0.8 g/kg body weight per day in the later stages is recommended to improve renal function.[12] Consultation with a nephrologist should occur when microalbuminuria (30 to 300 mg/24 h), overt albuminuria (>2 mg/dL), or decreased GFR (<50 mL/min) is present. Consultation with a cardiologist or nephrologist is recommended if hypertension persists. The courses of diabetic retinopathy and diabetic nephropathy often parallel each other. Both are asymptomatic in the early stages, which supports the need for routine screening and interventions that have been shown to effectively delay progression.

Diabetic Neuropathy. Diabetic neuropathy affects 60% to 70% of individuals with diabetes. Nerve damage can occur in almost any nerve in the body. Duration of diabetes, glycemic control, blood pressure control, lipid control, smoking, and obesity are all factors that have an effect on nerve damage.[26] However, data from the Epidemiology of Diabetes Interventions and Complications (EDIC) study revealed that intensive therapy improves glycemic control, resulting in a reduction in nerve damage that is sustained for years.[27]

Multiple mechanisms contribute to the pathogenesis of this complication. The onset of symptoms may be gradual or sudden, depending on the nerves that are affected. There are three major classes of diabetic neuropathies: peripheral or distal symmetrical neuropathy, mononeuropathy, and autonomic neuropathy.

Peripheral neuropathy is the most common neuropathic complication. Distal numbness or impaired sensation is typically bilateral and can occur acutely or gradually as a complication of poor glycemic control. The feet and legs are typically affected first; then the hands and arms may follow. Initially sensations of tingling, burning, or prickling may be noticed, particularly at night. Patients may report an increased sensitivity to touch. There may be associated muscle weakness affecting the patient's gait. On clinical examination, there may be a loss of sensation as detected by the Semmes-Weinstein monofilament, along with bilaterally absent knee or ankle jerk reflexes.

Progression of sensory deficits can cause the destruction of cartilage in foot joints. This results in the loss of normal foot architecture, leaving the foot susceptible to deformities such as hammertoes and Charcot joint. Charcot joint may be difficult to distinguish from active infection with cellulitis because both manifest with erythema and swelling. The presence of altered foot sensation makes the recommendation for the patient to perform a daily foot inspection imperative, with guidance to seek professional care promptly for any abnormality.

Pain is present in about 25% of all patients with peripheral neuropathy.[26] Nonpharmacologic treatment of painful peripheral neuropathy is aimed at the improvement of glycemic control; avoidance of alcohol; physical therapy; use of relaxation, acupuncture, or biofeedback techniques; or referral to a pain-control clinic. Improvement in glycemic control may result in a temporary worsening of painful neuropathic symptoms, but pain will abate with the maintenance of good blood glucose levels.

Topical treatments include capsaicin and lidocaine patches. Pharmacologic options include γ-aminobutyric acid (GABA) analogues, tricyclic antidepressants, other types of antidepressants and anticonvulsants, and, in limited situations, narcotics.

Mononeuropathies occur in large nerves or nerve roots and produce radicular symptoms. Large nerve roots in the spinal cord, chest, or abdomen or even cranial nerves can be affected. Mononeuropathy involves both sensory and motor neurons, producing increased or decreased sensation, weakness, and pain. The pain produced by mononeuropathies can be severe and mimic degenerative disc disease, herpes zoster, carpal tunnel syndrome, Bell palsy, or intra-abdominal conditions. Oculomotor palsy—characterized by ptosis, pain, and sparing of the pupillary reflex—occurs in patients older than 50 years. Pain and oculomotor function improve gradually during several weeks, and full recovery usually occurs within 3 to 5 months.

Autonomic neuropathy affects both sympathetic and parasympathetic fibers. Although any organ system may be affected, the more common effects are found in the gastrointestinal tract, genitourinary tract, and cardiovascular system. Symptoms of gastrointestinal dysfunction include esophageal motility problems and gastroparesis with impaired gastric emptying. The gastroparesis affects food absorption, leading to erratic glycemic control. The delayed gastric emptying also produces early satiety, bloating, nausea, and vomiting. Bowel peristaltic dysfunction is evidenced by explosive diarrhea and altered small bowel motility. Chronic constipation is the most common of the gastrointestinal neuropathies. These symptoms may improve with control of hyperglycemia. Gastroparesis can be addressed through dietary modifications, careful timing of meal-associated rapid-acting insulin, and use of metoclopramide. Various modalities can be considered for the control of diarrhea, including biofeedback, bismuth subsalicylate, loperamide, clonidine, and antibiotics.

Genitourinary neuropathy includes neurogenic bladder and sexual dysfunction. Bladder atony, characterized by a residual urine volume of more than 150 mL, may lead to recurrent UTIs and overflow incontinence. The occurrence of more than two UTIs per year indicates the need for further evaluation. Patients may mistakenly believe that their diabetes is in better control because they are urinating less frequently, in contrast to their previous polyuria. Timed and complete voiding is recommended. Bethanechol may be helpful as a conservative measure. The patient should be taught how to recognize and promptly report symptoms of a UTI.

Sexual dysfunction in women is characterized by decreased vaginal lubrication and decreased frequency of orgasm. Erectile dysfunction affects more than 50% of men who have had diabetes for more than 10 years.[2] Retrograde ejaculation is also common. Psychological, endocrine-related, and medication- or alcohol-induced impotence needs to be excluded before treatment recommendations are made. Men with diabetes may be successfully treated with a phosphodiesterase-5 (PDE5) inhibitor, although the efficacy is somewhat less than in men without diabetes.

Cardiovascular autonomic neuropathy has two major associated syndromes: orthostatic hypotension and cardiac denervation. Orthostatic hypotension may be pronounced, with an inability to tolerate abrupt rising from a supine to an upright posture. Cardiac denervation is characterized by a fixed heart rate in the range of 80 to 100 beats per minute without regard to stress, exercise, or tilting. These patients may have myocardial ischemia or infarction without pain and are at risk for cardiac arrhythmias and sudden death. Significant exertion, aerobic exercise, and straining should be avoided. Because of the risk for hypoglycemia and potential cardiac arrhythmias, such patients are generally not candidates for intensive insulin therapy.

Hypoglycemia unawareness is also an autonomic neuropathy in which the individual no longer feels the adrenergic symptoms of a low blood glucose level. Neuroglycopenia occurs with no warning and is a significant safety risk. Patients who have experienced an unconscious hypoglycemic episode should be advised to maintain a slightly higher target blood glucose range, to monitor their blood glucose concentration frequently (particularly before driving), and to pay close attention to any symptoms of hypoglycemia. Friends and family members ought to be taught how to recognize and treat hypoglycemia.

Macrovascular Complications. The leading cause of death and disability in patients with type 2 diabetes is ASCVD. Diabetes significantly increases the risk of coronary, cerebrovascular, and peripheral vascular disease. This is associated with endothelial dysfunction, hypertension, and lipid abnormalities. In the setting of hyperglycemia, excess free fatty acids, and insulin resistance, there is greater oxidative stress, which may damage the endothelium; also, less nitric oxide is produced by the endothelium to decrease vasodilation. In addition, abnormalities in platelet function will lead to greater activation and aggregation, thus increasing the risk for thrombosis.[27]

Individuals with diabetes have a two- to fourfold increased risk for development of coronary artery disease (CAD). The risk for a patient with no history of CAD but with diabetes is equal to the risk of a patient who has previously had an MI. In patients with diabetes and known CAD, mortality is 45% after 7 years and 75% at 10 years. Diabetes patients with unstable angina are more likely to have an MI, and the MI is more likely to be fatal.[27] CAD in the patient with diabetes occurs earlier and more extensively than in patients without diabetes, and infarction may occur without the usual symptoms. Atypical symptoms of ischemia include dyspnea, fatigue, gastrointestinal distress, unexplained hyperglycemia, ketoacidosis, and CHF. Typical symptoms of exertional chest pain, chest tightness, and arm pain associated with activity or rest must be evaluated promptly. An initial or subsequent MI is more likely to precipitate long-term complications (e.g., heart failure or arrhythmia) or death in the patient with diabetes compared with the patient without diabetes.[27] Silent MIs are more common in patients with diabetes.

CHF is two- to fivefold more common in patients with insulin resistance. The risk of stroke is increased two- to fivefold in people with diabetes compared with those without

diabetes. Stroke-related mortality, repeated stroke, and dementia after stroke are also increased.[27] Slurred speech, intermittent dizziness, transient loss of vision, paresthesia, or weakness of an arm or leg suggests a transient ischemic attack (TIA) consistent with cerebrovascular disease. Because CVD is so common in type 2 diabetes, a carotid ultrasound study is important to evaluate possible episodes of TIA. Anticoagulant and antiplatelet medications may help to prevent a recurrence of symptoms.

Peripheral vascular disease, or lower extremity arterial atherosclerosis, is two to four times more common among patients with diabetes.[27] Claudication, absent pedal pulses, and femoral bruits are typical manifestations. Revascularization procedures in patients with diabetes are challenging because of the limited availability of collateral vessels and commonly the presence of small-vessel disease. Diabetes is the leading cause of nontraumatic amputation in the United States. Although neuropathy is usually the cause of foot ulcers, poor blood flow is responsible for slow healing. Revascularization, if possible, is indicated for chronic ulcers.

Lower extremity amputation becomes necessary because of a combination of neuropathic and vascular damage. The precipitant is typically a small opening in the skin caused by stepping on a sharp object, a blister, or a nick from toenail clippers. If it is not noticed because there is no pain sensation, the injury is not treated. The injury then progresses to an infection that is difficult to resolve. Patients should be advised that daily foot assessment is essential for early detection of any lesion. A thorough visual inspection should be completed and anything suspicious should be promptly evaluated by a provider. Patient education includes awareness of the signs and symptoms of an infection. Early and aggressive treatment of foot wounds is required to reduce the risk of severe infection and ultimately amputation.

Patients with diabetes should be aware that near-normal glycemia will reduce their risk for microvascular complications—a risk that can be minimized through healthy lifestyle habits, including smoking avoidance, along with the achievement of blood pressure targets and lipid management. Treatment must be modified over time to strive for optimal and safe risk reduction. Lifelong care to reduce cardiovascular events begins with disease prevention and early detection. Early identification of those patients requiring revascularization is essential. As necessary, care should be managed in conjunction with a cardiologist.

Dyslipidemia in type 2 diabetes is characterized by hypertriglyceridemia, low HDL levels, and high LDL levels. A low-fat, low-cholesterol diet and aerobic exercise are essential for the treatment of dyslipidemia. Statins are recommended for all patients with diabetes and are the first-line therapy to decrease LDL cholesterol. Statin dosing (moderate vs. high intensity) is based on the patient's ASCVD calculated risk factors (LDL cholesterol ≥100 mg/dL, high blood pressure, smoking, chronic kidney disease, albuminuria, and family history of premature ASCVD) rather than a specific LDL target.

High-dose statin therapy is advised for patients with diabetes and a history of CVD or at least one additional CVD risk factor. Per the 2013 ACC/AHA Blood Cholesterol Guidelines, in patients with estimated CVD risk of factors 7.5% or greater who are 40 to 75 years of age, a moderate-dose statin is recommended.[29] High-intensity statin therapy is indicated for patients up to age 75 with clinical evidence of atherosclerotic heart disease.[30] For patients with diabetes and ASCVD and an

LDL that remains equal to or greater than 70 mg/dL despite the maximum tolerated dose of a statin, the addition of eze-timibe or a PCSK9 inhibitor is recommended. Fibrates reduce triglycerides and may raise HDL, but the combination with a statin has not been proven to improve ASCVD outcomes and hence is not recommended. The combination of a statin with niacin has also not been shown to add benefit over a statin alone and may increase the risk of stroke; thus it is also not recommended.

Hypertension is associated with CAD, stroke, and periph-eral vascular disease. Blood pressure should be measured at every visit and treated to a target of less than 140/90 mm Hg. A lower target of 130/80 mm Hg is recommended for those at high risk of CVD if this can be safely and reason-ably achieved. Lifestyle modification—including weight loss, a low-sodium diet, physical activity, and moderation of alcohol consumption—is recommended for patients with a blood pres-sure of greater than 120/80 mm Hg. Pharmacologic therapy should be initiated to achieve the target, beginning with either an ACEI inhibitor or an ARB, calcium channel blocker or thi-azide diuretic, as calcium channel blockers and thiazide-like diuretics have now been shown to reduce cardiovascular events in patients with diabetes. Many patients require more than two agents to achieve the blood pressure goal. Renal function and serum potassium concentration should be monitored carefully.

Aspirin (75–162 mg/d) is recommended as a strategy for primary prevention in those with diabetes at increased risk for CVD and as secondary prevention for patients with a history of CVD. It is inexpensive and in general the risk is low.

Three recent trials were designed to determine whether intensive glycemic control reduces the risk of macrovascular complications. The ACCORD trial enrolled more than 10,000 subjects with type 2 diabetes of approximately 10 years' dura-tion and with a history of CVD or at least two CVD risk factors. The study's aim was to prevent MI, stroke, and CVD deaths by striving to achieve normal blood glucose and blood pres-sure control and by employing combination lipid therapy. The intensive glucose control strategy was stopped early because there was a higher risk of death compared with standard glucose treatment. Intensive blood pressure treatment was found to reduce the risk of stroke by 40%, but this benefit was accompanied by a higher incidence of hypotension and hyperkalemia. Combination lipid therapy was found to be safe but did not show an improvement in the risk of CVD. The conclusion of the study was that for a high-risk group (longer duration of diabetes and existing CVD or high risk for CVD), intensive treatment adds risk without benefit. The results of this trial may not apply to those with a more recent diagnosis of diabetes or with a lower CVD risk.

The ADVANCE study, which randomized 11,140 patients with type 2 diabetes, and the VADT, which enrolled 1791 patients, had similar findings for subjects with a longer dura-tion of diabetes and higher risk for CVD. Further analysis of the three trials suggests that there may be a benefit of inten-sive glycemic control for individuals with a shorter duration of diabetes, lower initial HbA1c level, and no CVD at base-line.[7] For patients with a shorter duration of diabetes, no known significant CVD, and a longer life expectancy, a target HbA1c level of below 7% (and even lower if it can be achieved without undue hypoglycemia) should be recommended. A less rigorous target should be advised for those with a history of severe hypoglycemia, advanced complications, significant CVD, longer duration of diabetes, advanced age, and limited life expectancy.

In 2018, the American College of Physicians (APC) recom-mended that HgbA1c goals should always be based on the individual patient but that for type 2 nonpregnant adults with diabetes a reasonable goal would be an HbA1c of 7 to 8.[30] In adults older than age 80 or with significant comorbid illness and a life expectancy less than 10 years or living in a nursing home, a specific target HgbA1c is not necessary. Instead, treatment should be individualized to avoid hyperglycemic symptoms.

For all patients, other risk factors (blood pressure, lipids, lifestyle) should be treated according to the ADA and American Heart Association standards.

The LEADER trial randomized more than 9000 subjects with type 2 diabetes and high cardiovascular risk to receive liraglutide or placebo and followed them for 3.8 years. The rate of cardiovascular death, nonfatal MI, or nonfatal stroke was lower with liraglutide than with placebo.[31] In the EMPA-REG OUTCOME trial, 7000 subjects with type 2 diabetes and high cardiovascular risk were randomized to empagliflozin or placebo in addition to standard care and followed for 3 years. Those who received empagliflozin had a lower rate of cardio-vascular death, hospitalization for heart failure, and all-cause mortality than did those who received placebo.[31]

The majority of investigations involving screening and risk factor modification for CAD have been conducted in patients with type 2 diabetes. Patients with type 1 diabetes do have higher rates of CAD events than those without diabetes. This effect begins at a young age and increases with age. The results of the EDIC study suggested that early and aggressive glyce-mic control reduces the risk of CAD in type 1 diabetes. The ADA and the American Heart Association recommend blood pressure and lipid control for patients with type 1 diabetes. An ACEI is indicated for anyone with type 1 diabetes and microalbuminuria even if normotensive. Medication should be initiated if the blood pressure is above the 95th percentile or 130/80 mm Hg, whichever is lower. Pharmacologic treatment is recommended for patients with type 1 diabetes who have not achieved an LDL cholesterol concentration below 160 mg/dL with medical nutrition therapy. For those with an increased CVD risk, medication should begin if the LDL cholesterol concentration is not below 130 mg/dL. Patients who are over-weight or obese may have a greater risk of CVD because of the atherogenic risk of insulin resistance.

EDUCATION AND HEALTH PROMOTION

The goals of diabetes education are to promote optimal health, improve quality of life, and reduce the human and economic burden associated with poorly controlled diabetes. The frame-work for diabetes education has shifted from content to out-comes. Rather than merely imparting information to patients, diabetes self-management education strives to guide patients in the setting of personal goals that result in changes in behav-ior leading to improved clinical outcomes.[31]

The American Diabetes Association Education Recogni-tion Program designates diabetes education programs that meet the national standards for diabetes self-management education. Search for ADA-recognized programs at <https://professional.diabetes.org/erp_list_zip>. The American Associa-tion of Diabetes Educators (AADE) accredits diabetes education programs. Search for AADE-accredited programs at <https://

www.diabeteseducator.org/living-with-diabetes/find-an-education-program>. A certified diabetes educator (CDE) is an individual from one of many disciplines (registered nurse, registered dietitian, pharmacist, physician, physician assistant, exercise physiologist, social worker, occupational therapist, physical therapist, clinical psychologist, optometrist, podiatrist, or health educator) who has met the requirements of the National Certification Board for Diabetes Educators. A listing of CDEs may be found at <https://www.ncbde.org/find-a-cde/>.

Diabetes education is not a pamphlet, an appointment, or a class. It is a lifelong process through which the patient and family acquire the knowledge and practice the skills necessary to manage diabetes. As the individual passes through the stages of life, different information and resources will be necessary. As new developments in diabetes treatment evolve, ongoing education is necessary to sustain good self-care habits, minimize the burden of diabetes care, and achieve the goal of excellent glycemic control. A variety of approaches to teaching should be offered, because patients learn in many ways. Face-to-face instruction, group classes, written information, videos, and websites are common strategies. The patient's first language and health literacy should be considered and appropriate materials provided.

At the time of diagnosis, the essential survival skills are taught to keep the patient safe until additional education can be arranged. Survival skills include understanding the basic pathophysiologic mechanism of the disease, understanding how and when to take medications, recognizing and treating hypoglycemia, and knowing when and whom to call for help. The next phase of diabetes education includes self-monitoring of blood glucose concentration, foot care, basic meal planning, and sick-day management.

Advanced diabetes education offers guidance on counting carbohydrates, calculating insulin doses by use of insulin: carbohydrate ratios and correction factors, managing diabetes while traveling, and preventive care. Individualized education will be provided to those who wish to use an insulin pump or continuous glucose sensor.

Education for the family includes the recognition and treatment of hypoglycemia (including glucagon administration), meal planning, and the provision of motivation and support. Patients and families are encouraged to learn all they can about diabetes to take control of their disease.

Keeping abreast of new developments and staying motivated may be enhanced by reading magazines written for people who live with diabetes (e.g., *Diabetes Forecast*, *Diabetes Self-Management*), by searching websites (https://www.diabeteshealth.com/, www.diabetesmonitor.com/, www.diabetesatwork.org/), and by participating in a diabetes support group.

RESOURCES

Helpful websites for patients and families include the following:
- www.nutrition.gov (U.S. Department of Agriculture)
- www.choosemyplate.gov (U.S. Department of Agriculture)
- www.diabetes.org (American Diabetes Association)
- www.jdrf.org (Juvenile Diabetes Research Foundation)
- www.cdc.gov/diabetes/home (Centers for Disease Control and Prevention)
- www.ndep.nih.gov (National Diabetes Education Program)
  Helpful websites for health care professionals include the following:

- www.aace.com (American Association of Clinical Endocrinologists)
- www.diabeteseducator.org (American Association of Diabetes Educators)
- http://professional.diabetes.org (American Diabetes Association)
- www.diabetestechnology.org (Diabetes Technology Society)
- http://www.endocrine.org (Endocrine Society)
- http://diabetes.niddk.nih.gov (National Institute of Diabetes and Digestive and Kidney Diseases)

REFERENCES

1. Definition and diagnosis of diabetes mellitus and intermediate hyperglycemia: report of a WHO/IDF consultation. Geneva, Switzerland: World Health Organization Document Production Services; 2006. Available at: www.who.int/diabetes/publications/diagnosis_diabetes2006/en/; (Accessed January 28, 2018).
2. National Diabetes Statistics Report. (2018). http://www.diabetes.org/assets/pdfs/basics/cdc-statistics-report-2018.pdf. (Accessed 25 February 2019).
3. American Diabetes Association. (2018). Classification and Diagnosis of Diabetes: Standards of Medical Care in Diabetes. *Diabetes Care*, 41(Suppl. 1), S13–S27.
4. Masharani, U., & German, M. S. (2018). Pancreatic hormones and diabetes mellitus. In D. G. Gardner & D. Shoback (Eds.), *Greenspan's basic & clinical endocrinology* (10th ed.). New York, NY: McGraw-Hill. http://accessmedicine.mhmedical.com.ezproxy.simmons.edu/content.aspx?bookid=2178&sectionid=166251965. (Accessed 18 February 2019).
5. Diabetes Mellitus. (2018). F. Cunningham, K. J. Leveno, S. L. Bloom, J. S. Dashe, B. L. Hoffman, B. M. Casey, et al. (Eds.), *Williams obstetrics* (25th ed.). New York, NY: McGraw-Hill. http://accessmedicine.mhmedical.com.ezproxy.simmons.edu/content.aspx?bookid=1918&sectionid=185092117. (Accessed 19 February 2019).
6. Kitabchi, A. E., Umpierrez, G. E., et al. (2009). Hyperglycemic crisis in adult patients with diabetes. *Diabetes Care*, 32(7), 1335–1343.
7. Van Belle, T., Coppieters, K., & Van Herrath, M. (2011). Type 1 diabetes: Etiology, immunology, and therapeutic strategies. *Physiological Reviews*, 91(1), 79–118.
8. Kennedy, M., & Masharani, U. (2018). Pancreatic hormones & antidiabetic drugs. In B. G. Katzung (Ed.), *Basic & clinical pharmacology* (14th ed.). New York, NY: McGraw-Hill. http://accessmedicine.mhmedical.com.ezproxy.simmons.edu/content.aspx?bookid=2249&sectionid=175222393. (Accessed 19 February 2019).
9. 2018). Prevention ro delay of type 2 diabetes: Standards of Medical Care in Diabetes—2018. *Diabetes Care*, 41(Suppl. 1), S51–S54.
10. DeFronzo, R. A. (2009). From the triumvirate to the ominous octet: A new paradigm for the treatment of type 2 diabetes mellitus. *Diabetes*, 58, 773–795.
11. American Diabetes Association. Professional Practice Committee: Standards of Medical Care in Diabetes-2019. Retrieved fromhttp://care.diabetesjournals.org/content/42/Supplement_1. (Accessed 25 February 2019).
12. USDA. (2015). Dietary Guidelines for Americans 2015-2020, Eighth Edition. https://health.gov/dietaryguidelines/2015/resources/2015-2020_Dietary_Guidelines.pdf. (Accessed 25 February 2019).
13. Dempsey, P. C., Larsen, R. N., et al. (2016). Benefits for type 2 diabetes of interrupting prolonged sitting with brief bouts of light walking or simple resistance activities. *Diabetes Care*, 39(6), 964–972.
14. Garber, A. J., Abrahamson, M. J., et al. (2018). Consensus Statement by the American Association of Clinical Endocrinologists and American College of endocrinology on the comprehensive type 2 diabetes management algorithm—2018 executive summary. *Endocrine Practice*, 24(1), 91–120.
15. Inzucchi, S. E., Bergenstal, R. M., et al. (2015). Management of hyperglycemia in type 2 diabetes, 2015: A patient-centered approach. *Diabetes Care*, 38(1), 140–149.
16. American Diabetes Association. (2018). Comprehensive medical evaluation and assessment of comorbidities: *Standards of Medical Care in Diabetes—2018. American Diabetes Association Diabetes Care*, 41(Suppl. 1), S28–S37. https://doi.org/10.2337/dc18-S003.
17. National Kidney and Urologic Diseases Information Clearinghouse, National Institutes of Health. Kidney disease of diabetes. Retrieved from http://kidney.niddk.nih.gov/kudiseases/pubs/kdd/. (Accessed 25 February 2018).
18. National Diabetes Information Clearinghouse, National Institutes of Health. Diabetic neuropathies: the nerve damage of diabetes. Retrieved from http://

diabetes.niddk.nih.gov/dm/pubs/neuropathies/. (Accessed 25 February 2018).

19. Metformin for Prediabetes. (2017). *JAMA: The Journal of the American Medical Association, 317*(11), 1171. doi:10.1001/jama.2016.17844.

20. American Diabetes Association. Standards of Medical care in Diabetes-2019. Retrieved from http://care.diabetesjournals.org/content/diacare/suppl/2018/12/17/42.Supplement_1.DC1/DC_42_S1_Combined_FINAL.pdf.

21. Rosenstock, J., & Ferrannini, E. Euglycemic Diabetic Ketoacidosis: A Predictable, Detectable, and Preventable Safety Concern With SGLT2 Inhibitors. Retrieved from http://care.diabetesjournals.org/content/38/9/1638. (Accessed 25 February 2019).

22. Zinman, B. (2015). Empagliflozin, cardiovascular outcomes, and mortality in type 2 diabetes. *The New England Journal of Medicine, 373*, 2117–2128. Marso, S. (2016). Liraglutide and cardiovascular outcomes in type 2 diabetes. The New England Journal of Medicine, 375, 311–322.

23. Blum, A. K. (2016). Insulin use in pregnancy: An update. *Diabetes Spectrum: a publication of the American Diabetes Association, 29*(2), 92–97.

24. Moghissi, E. S., Korytkowski, M. T., et al. (2009). American Association of Clinical Endocrinologists and American Diabetes Association Consensus Statement on inpatient glycemic control. *Endocrine Practice, 15*(4), 353–369.

25. Dyer, A. R., Leiva, A., Hod, M., et al. (2010). International Association of Diabetes and Pregnancy Study Groups recommendations on the diagnosis and classification of hyperglycemia in pregnancy. *Diabetes Care, 33*(3), 676–682.

26. Lachin, J., Orchard, T., & Nathan, D. (2014). Update on cardiovascular outcomes at 30 years of diabetic control and complications Trial/Epidemiology of Diabetes Interventions and Complications Study. *Diabetes Care, 37*(1), 39–43.

27. Emdin, C. A., Rahimi, K., et al. (2015). Blood pressure lowering in type 2 diabetes: A systematic review and Meta-analysis. *JAMA: The Journal of the American Medical Association, 313*(6), 603–615.

28. Kitabchi, A. E., Umpierrez, G. E., et al. (2009). Hyperglycemic crisis in adult patients with diabetes. *Diabetes Care, 32*(7), 1335–1343.

29. 2013 ACC/AHA Blood Cholesterol Guideline. Major Recommendations for Statin Therapy for Atherosclerotic Cardiovascular Disease Prevention. Retrieved from http://www.mplsheart.com/wp-content/uploads/2014/10/S413160-20871-MHI-Statin-Therapy-Algorithm-4.pdf. (Accessed 25 February 2019).

30. Qaseem, A., Wilt, T. J., Kansagara, D., Horwitch, C., Barry, M. J., Forciea, M. A., et al. (2018). Hemoglobin A$_{1c}$ targets for glycemic control with pharmacologic therapy for nonpregnant adults with type 2 diabetes mellitus: A guidance statement update from the American College of physicians. *Annals of Internal Medicine, 168*, 569–576. doi:10.7326/M17-0939.

31. Marso, S. P., Daniels, G. H., et al. (2016). Liraglutide and cardiovascular outcomes in type 2 diabetes. *The New England Journal of Medicine, 375*(4), 311–322.

CHAPTER **187**

HIRSUTISM
Susan Yuditskaya

DEFINITION, EPIDEMIOLOGY, AND MECHANISM

Hirsutism is defined as excessive terminal hair growth in a female individual. The exact prevalence is unknown, but it is fairly common, and affects about 7% to 10% of women worldwide. Due to societally established standards of femininity, hirsutism is often psychologically distressing to the woman experiencing it. There is some variation among different ethnicities in the prevalence of hirsutism, due to different degrees of genetically determined physiologic terminal hair expression. For instance, prevalence is lower in East Asian women and higher among women of Mediterranean, Middle Eastern, or African descent.

In each individual, the body's total lifetime number of hair follicles are formed by 22 weeks' gestation, estimated to be 5 million in number, regardless of gender or ethnicity. Of these, 100,000 are on the scalp. The remainder exist in all regions of the body except the lips, palms, soles, and mucosal skin surfaces. Fetal hair follicles initially grow lanugo hair, which is shed in utero at 36 weeks and replaced by vellus hair by 36 to 40 weeks of gestation. Vellus hair is typically less than 2 mm in length, faintly pigmented, fine in caliber, and associated with an undeveloped sebaceous gland.

Human hair follicles have an innate responsiveness to androgens but vary in their degree of responsiveness and in the result of the androgenic influence. Differences in the pigmentation, thickness, phase duration, sebum production, and pattern of hair are determined by localized androgen responsivity[1] at each pilosebaceous unit. At some specific areas of the body that produce terminal hair in childhood (eyelashes, eyebrows, and scalp follicles), androgens have no obvious effect. In genetically predisposed individuals with androgenic alopecia (male pattern baldness), androgens can transform large terminal hair follicles of the scalp into small vellus hair follicles. Otherwise, androgens generally mediate differentiation of vellus hair follicles into terminal hair follicles.

Androgen-sensitive hair follicles, in decreasing order of sensitivity to androgens, include those at the pubic region, axillae, forearms/legs, and chin/upper lip. Hair follicles that are most sensitive respond to the least amount of androgenic activity. Physiologic appearance of terminal hair at these regions, in approximately that order, occurs with onset of puberty, and corresponds to the increased production of adrenal androgens (adrenarche), and gonadotropin-stimulated testosterone production, by the testes in males and by the ovaries in females.

The mechanism by which androgens activate hair follicles is via dihydrotestosterone (DHT), a potent androgen, which directly communicates with the hair follicle. DHT is converted from testosterone by 5α-reductase type 2. Adrenal androgens (DHEA, DHEA-S, and androstenedione) are converted to testosterone via the steroid synthesis pathway, and thereafter, to DHT. Of note, DHEA is also synthesized by the ovary.

Hair development follows a prescribed, repeating pathway of "growth, regression, and remodeling events,"[2] otherwise known as the anagen (active), telogen (static), and catagen (shedding) phases. Androgens prolong the anagen phase of terminal body hair but shorten this phase in scalp hair.[3]

It is important to distinguish hirsutism, an excess of terminal hair, from hypertrichosis, which specifically refers to an increase in vellus hair. Hypertrichosis is androgen-independent, and is typically seen in conditions such as anorexia nervosa, hypothyroidism, porphyria cutanea tarda, dermatomyositis, and paraneoplastic syndrome (hypertrichosis lanuginose). Hypertrichosis can also be medication induced; cyclosporine, dexamethasone, diazoxide, minoxidil, penicillamine, phenytoin, and streptomycin are known contributors.[4] Hypercortisolism involved in Cushing syndrome can increase vellus hair, but can also involve hirsutism.

Hirsutism results from enhanced androgen-dependent stimulation of hair follicles by either increased levels of circulating androgens or increased sensitivity to them, leading to increased terminal hair differentiation. Terminal hair expression is ultimately determined by the individual follicle's sensitivity to local 5α-reductase-mediated DHT production. To some degree this is genetically determined, accounting for the wide inter-ethnic variability in physiologic terminal hair patterns. The amount of locally produced DHT and duration of the hair follicles' exposure to it determine the resultant density and diameter of the terminal hair follicles.

The degree of clinical hirsutism does not always correlate with elevated androgen levels. Only about 50% of hirsute women have hyperandrogenemia. Of these cases, the most common diagnosis is polycystic ovary syndrome (PCOS), representing about 70% of women with hyperandrogenemic hirsutism.[3] Idiopathic hyperandrogenism occurs in 6% to 15% of women with hirsutism,[5] in which hirsutism and hyperandrogenemia are present, but criteria for PCOS diagnosis are not met, due to normal ovulatory cycles and normal ovarian morphology. Less common causes of hyperandrogenemia leading to hirsutism include congenital adrenal hyperplasia, androgen-secreting adrenal or ovarian tumors, Cushing syndrome (Chapter 185), and acromegaly. Hyperinsulinism stimulates testosterone synthesis through ovarian thecal cells (hyperthecosis) acted on by luteinizing hormone (LH).

The other half of women with hirsutism do not have measurable circulating androgen excess, perhaps because of the limits of androgen detection or hyperandrogenic phenomena occurring locally at the pilosebaceous level, and therefore not reflected by circulating androgen levels.[4] Idiopathic hirsutism (20% of women with hirsutism)[6] is characterized by normal androgen levels, menses, and ovarian morphology, and is thought to reflect normal ethnic or familial hair pattern variations. 8% to 13%[3] of women report postmenopausal hirsutism, which may be related to estrogen deficiency leading to a relative androgen excess, but the exact mechanism is not yet fully clear.

PCOS affects 4% to 20% of menstruating women.[5,6] It is a heterogeneous syndrome, with varying contributions of excess androgens, LH, follicle-stimulating hormone (FSH), and insulin resistance.[6] Most patients have a gonadotropin-dependent functional ovarian hyperandrogenemia, less often in conjunction with a mild adrenocorticotropic hormone (ACTH)–dependent functional adrenal hyperandrogenemia. Approximately 80% of patients are anovulatory[2]; 90% or more women with oligomenorrhea or amenorrhea have PCOS, and 95% of those with PCOS have oligomenorrhea or amenorrhea.[7] The combination of PCOS and amenorrhea is more likely to manifest with severe hyperandrogenemia.[7]

In the mildest form of PCOS, women have neither gonadotropin nor ovulatory abnormalities but still have decreased sex hormone–binding globulin (SHBG) from ovarian stimulation. In more severe cases, insulin resistance and menstrual cycle irregularities may drive up androgen levels both through increased LH pulse frequency and because free testosterone cannot bind to as many sites as a result of reduced levels of circulating SHBG. One unifying, possibly initiating component is thought to be ovarian theca cell abnormality leading to increased testosterone and/or androstenedione production and amplification of pituitary LH, wherein the progesterone negative feedback loop is impaired and LH is overproduced.[6]

In 2018, clinical guidelines from an internationally based panel were developed and published with oversight from subject experts of both the Endocrine Society and the European Society of Endocrinology.[8] The resulting consensus requires two of the following: androgen excess (clinical or biochemical) and either ovulatory dysfunction (clinical) or polycystic ovaries (12 or more follicles 2 to 9 mm in diameter or > 25 follicles per ovary, and ovarian volume > 10 mL in either ovary),[6] excluding prepubertal and postmenopausal women. In practice, both clinical and biochemical assessments are subject to limitations. Whereas hirsutism correlates well with hyperandrogenemia, acne, alopecia, acanthosis nigricans, and skin tags do not.[7] Cardiovascular risk indicators as well as metabolic disorders in hirsute women seem to correlate directly with androgen elevations.[2]

An important consideration for health care providers in evaluating a chief complaint of hirsutism is whether there is an etiology that may pose a risk for rare but potentially life-threatening conditions. Patients with PCOS are more likely to be obese, insulin resistant, and experience difficulties with fertility[9] as well as face cardiac sequelae. Although many hirsute women have PCOS (72% to 82%),[9] a minority (1.5% to 10%)[9-11] have hyperandrogenic insulin-resistant acanthosis nigricans (HAIRAN) syndrome, late-onset nonclassic congenital adrenal hyperplasia (NCCAH), prolactinemia, a thyroid disorder, an androgen-secreting tumor, or Cushing syndrome. Tumors of the ovary or adrenal gland comprise fewer than 0.2% of women with hyperandrogenemia, half of which are malignant.[5,10]

 Specialist referral is indicated for all patients with hirsutism.

CLINICAL PRESENTATION

Establishing a baseline is important because prior hair removal will render an objective assessment of hair growth pattern inaccurate. Furthermore, chronic skin irritation might lead to hair coarsening because of local changes at the pilosebaceous unit. Constitutional or familial hirsutism is common in individuals of Mediterranean, Middle Eastern, South Asian, or African descent but far less common in East Asian peoples. Inquiring about a family history of hair growth, acne, menstrual abnormalities, diabetes mellitus, hyperlipidemia, early-onset cardiac disease, maternal obesity, CAH, and a cancer diagnosis[3] as well as prior diagnosis or treatment of hirsutism will serve in the initial screening.

When signs of virilism such as temporal balding or voice deepening accompany new-onset hirsutism, an ovarian, adrenal, or exogenous androgen source should be suspected, particularly in postmenopausal women and in women at increased risk of malignancy.

Gonadal abnormalities are indicative of elevated androgen levels and can sometimes be clarified with a history of abnormal sexual development. Prepubertal androgenism or hermaphroditism might relate to CAH seen in early adrenarche or with adrenal tumors. Further workup is essential if signs of precocious puberty, clitoromegaly, fourchette development, or gonadal hypospadias are described. New-onset nipple discharge in a nonlactating woman is a key finding. A menstrual history and menopausal status should be elicited. Prepubertal or peripubertal stress causing an exaggerated adrenarche may be a contributing factor to cortisol overproduction and risk of PCOS.[11] Infertility may point to anovulation or oligo-ovulation. Irregular or intermenstrual bleeding may indicate the presence of endometrial neoplasia.

Exogenous hormone use may also play a role. Some oral contraceptives contain progestins with high androgenic activity (e.g., norgestrel, levonorgestrel). Herbal and other over-the-counter supplement use should be inquired about as well, as some may contain androgen-like ingredients. Surreptitious use of androgens for competitive advantage among athletes should also be considered in certain contexts. Hyperhidrosis, enlarged hands, feet, and face, might point to acromegaly.

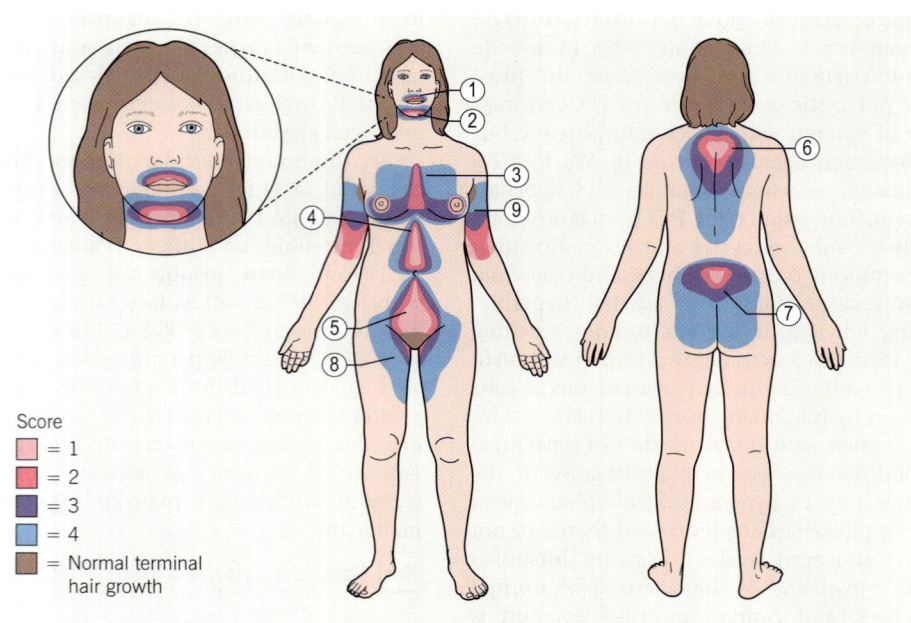

FIG. 187.1 The modified Ferriman-Gallwey (mFG) hirsutism scoring system.[16] In this system, nine body areas are evaluated for the amount of terminal hair growth. A score of 0 (no terminal hair growth) up to 4 (frankly virile) is given to each of the nine areas, and these are added together to compute a hormonal hirsutism score (mFG score). A total score below 3 is considered normal for East Asian and Native American females, whereas below 8 is considered normal in other populations. (From Bolognia, J. L., Schaffer, J. V., Duncan, K. O., & Ko, C. J. [2014]). *Dermatology essentials.* St. Louis: Elsevier.)

Patients with PCOS or Cushing syndrome are likely to have lipid and insulin abnormalities to differing degrees, and metabolic syndrome. Mood or sleep changes, weight gain, glaucoma, osteoporosis, increased susceptibility to illness, weakness of upper arms, and signs of cortisol excess in facies or skin might be seen with Cushing syndrome. Polyuria and polydipsia might point to overt diabetes. Dyslipidemia and hypertension are common in PCOS; depression, sleep apnea, and endometrial carcinoma have also been associated with PCOS.

PHYSICAL EXAMINATION

Weight, height, and vital signs are especially pertinent given the profile of a significant proportion of patients with PCOS. Obesity is seen in patients with PCOS or Cushing syndrome (see Chapter 185). Cushing syndrome can manifest with a classic Cushingoid appearance including central obesity, extremity muscle wasting, purple striae, supraclavicular fat pads, moon facies, thin skin or bruising, and dorsocervical ("buffalo hump") or supraclavicular fat pads. A rise in blood pressure and concomitant hirsutism could raise suspicion for Cushing syndrome or acromegaly, although acromegaly is not commonly associated with hirsutism. Acanthosis nigricans, a darkened velvety patch on the nape of the neck, axillae, elbows, knuckles, knees, or intertriginous regions, is seen commonly in obese women and is indicative of insulin resistance.

Thickened facial features, frontal bossing, prognathism, visual field defects, enlarged hands and feet, hyperhidrosis, or macroglossia may indicate the rare case of acromegaly. A large number of skin tags can occur with PCOS as well as acromegaly.[12]

An essential component of the physical examination must include an objective measurement of the degree and pattern of hirsutism. Such an assessment has been captured by the standard Ferriman-Gallwey scoring system, originally established in 1961,[1] as well its modified form by others (the mFG; Fig. 187.1). The mFG serves to establish hirsutism clinically by rating nine body areas on a scale of 0 to 4 (upper lip, chin, chest, upper and lower back, upper and lower abdomen, arm, and thigh, excluding the original forearm and lower leg, which contribute less because these areas are overly androgen sensitive) (see Fig. 187.1). Limitations of the mFG include poor inter-rater reliability and lack of sensitivity in the composite to heavily weighted areas that are particularly affected, such as on the face; lack of adjustments for racial variations; and the failure to assess the patient's perception of unwanted hair. A score higher than 8 in nonblack, non-Southeast or non–Far East Asians[3] indicates moderate hirsutism; a score higher than 15 indicates moderate to severe hirsutism and is an independent risk for PCOS.[9] Terminal hair on the upper back, shoulders, upper chest, cheeks, or upper abdomen delineates male pattern hair growth.

Other signs of virilization should be assessed, including huskiness of the voice, increased pectoral muscle mass, presence/severity of acne, male pattern alopecia, mammary atrophy (defeminization), changes in libido, and clitoromegaly.[13]

Sexual ambiguity—such as downward placement of the urethral meatus or joining of posterior labial folds—may denote a congenital defect. A pelvic examination is performed to assess for the presence of ovarian masses.

Pregnant women may need careful monitoring in the face of gestational hirsutism; postpartum patients and their newborns are observed for regression of virilization, once malignant causes have been excluded.[1]

DIAGNOSTICS

A hormonal evaluation in slow-onset, peripubertally hirsute, nonvirilized, normally menstruating patients should be deferred because the yield is low. Diagnosis in this population relies heavily on the physical examination and evidence of virilism. Newly developed, moderate hirsutism (Ferriman-Gallwey hirsutism score > 15) in postpubertal adult women, as well as hirsutism with virilization, requires diligent investigation. Methods of hair analysis include the weighing of plucked or shaved hair, and even microscopic observation and measurements of the shafts do exist, but the mFG is preferred in general as a clinical quantification assessment.

Androgen Levels

Androgen measurements are subject to diurnal variation and other influences. Imprecise commercial assays may have inadvertently contributed to past misdiagnosis of idiopathic hyperandrogenism or idiopathic hirsutism.[2] Testing includes an early-morning plasma total testosterone level, followed, if abnormal, by a free testosterone level. Although a normal testosterone level does not exclude hyperandrogenism, it is more suggestive of idiopathic hirsutism and suggests against a malignant origin of the hirsutism. Some use a free androgen index (FAI) or calculated free testosterone (CFT) level as part of a routine workup.[5] Lately, serum androgen levels are thought to be more sensitively measured through liquid chromatography with tandem mass spectrometry (LC-MS) or even immunochemiluminescence,[2] although the accuracy can be impaired at the lower limits of detection.[6] A CFT level from measurement of SHBG and total testosterone, rather than by direct assay, is preferred in some cases (if equilibrium dialysis methods are unavailable) because they are particularly helpful in diagnosing PCOS.[2,6] Furthermore, a high serum SHBG suggests insulin resistance.[2]

In cases of mild elevations of testosterone or DHEA-S, late-onset congenital adrenal hyperplasia or functional ovarian hyperandrogenism may be considered.[5] In moderately hirsute patients, if the free testosterone is 200 ng/dL or lower, thyroid function tests, prolactin level, and possibly a 17-OH-progesterone with corticotropin (ACTH) stimulation test should follow.

A testosterone value over 200 ng/dL (6.94 nmol/L) necessitates a serum DHEA-S, because the differential diagnosis would include an adrenal tumor. A normal DHEA-S with a high testosterone level is suspicious for an ovarian androgen-secreting tumor; an abnormal DHEA-S above 700 mcg/dL (despite a normal testosterone level) suggests an adrenal androgen-secreting tumor.

Ovarian Source

Documentation of oligomenorrheic or amenorrheic cycles from puberty onward should be established despite the fact that some patients will have regular but anovulatory cycles. Serum antimüllerian hormone might indicate PCOS, but this is controversial.[3,6] In the face of moderate to severe hirsutism, an LH excess as demonstrated by an LH/FSH ratio of 2:1 or 3:1 can be helpful in supporting a diagnosis of PCOS. A mid-luteal serum progesterone level helps screen for anovulation.[10] Some specialists perform a 2-month gonadotropin suppression test to divide patients into gonadotropin-dependent (testosterone falls) versus gonadotropin-independent (testosterone does not fall) women with normal BMI.[14] This can delineate an ovarian versus adrenal source in an otherwise difficult-to-diagnose group.[14]

Ultrasound can be helpful in determining the PCOS morphology and also detecting an ovarian tumor that may be androgen-secreting. Polycystic ovarian morphology per the Rotterdam consensus (2003) and Androgen Excess & PCOS Society (2006) is defined by presence of >12 follicles measuring 2 to 9 mm each in one ovary, and/or ovarian volume >10 cubic centimeters.[2] The presence of a pelvic mass warrants further imaging with magnetic resonance imaging (MRI) or CT.

Adrenal Source

DHEA-S is seen as a screen for adrenal gland production to help distinguish tumors of adrenal origin in the face of virilization and a high testosterone level. Values above 700 mcg/dL (13.6 mmol/L) are suggestive of an adrenal source of hyperandrogenemia, and would necessitate adrenal imaging with either an adrenal-protocol CT scan or MRI. Serum testosterone concentration can be elevated in patients with Cushing syndrome, or with a testosterone-secreting adrenal adenoma or carcinoma.[10]

Biochemical testing for 21-hydroxylase–deficient NCCAH can be determined by elevated basal early-morning follicular phase 17-OH-progesterone (>200 ng/dL or 6 nmol/L). If the 17-OH-progesterone levels are between 200 and 1000 ng/dL, then an ACTH stimulation test yielding a poststimulation 17-OH-progesterone value higher than 1000 ng/dL clinches the diagnosis; values of 1000 ng/dL or lower may indicate a heterozygous 21-hydroxylase deficiency carrier.[10] Because the more severe classic salt-wasting forms of congenital adrenal hyperplasia typically present with life-threatening adrenal crisis in infancy, a serum 17-OH-progesterone level has become a required newborn screening test in the United States. Clinically it can be difficult to separate PCOS from NCCAH as the phenotypes can overlap phenotypes.[12]

Cortisol Excess

If Cushing syndrome is suspected, screening can be done with late-night salivary cortisol, 24-hour urine collection for free cortisol, or a low-dose overnight dexamethasone suppression test. In the setting of significant hirsutism, a 24-hour urine 17-ketosteroid level may be useful as well. A normal 24-hour urine 17-ketosteroid measurement ranges from 5 to 15 mg (17 to 52 mmol) in women younger than 30 years (which is when it is expected to peak). A positive 24-hour urine 17-ketosteroid study is more nonspecific than a urine free cortisol level, but can yield additional information as a screen for adrenal androgens, an androgen-secreting ovarian tumor, an ACTH-secreting tumor (or ACTH administration), an ectopic androgen-secreting tumor, Cushing syndrome, or PCOS. It may also be positive in pregnancy.

Insulin Excess

HAIRAN, the combination of hyperandrogenism, insulin resistance, and acanthosis nigricans, is diagnosed with a fasting basal insulin level or an insulin level during a tolerance test.[4] A glucose tolerance test and lipid profile are valuable if dyslipidemia, insulin resistance, hyperinsulinemia, or diabetes mellitus is suspected. A spectrum of dermatologic signs—seborrhea, acne, hirsutism, and acanthosis nigricans—may feature in HAIRAN or reflect other causes of hyperandrogenemia.[14] Because obesity is a contributing factor, BMI, cholesterol level, and blood pressure are pertinent.

Prolactin Excess

In the absence of testosterone, DHEA-S, cortisol, or 17-hydroxyhydrolase abnormalities, amenorrhea and hirsutism can occur in the setting of a prolactin tumor. Galactorrhea warrants measurement of a prolactin level; increased levels are indicative of hyperprolactinemia and possible thyroid dysfunction, although this is rare. In these cases, thyroid-stimulating hormone (TSH) and FSH are also measured. The pituitary is imaged by MRI to search for a prolactinoma.

Pituitary Source

Somatomedin C (insulin-like growth factor 1 [IGF-1]) testing is the most sensitive for acromegaly when clinical signs are leading, including vision changes, vision loss, and headaches, depending on the location of the tumor. IGF-1, a GH by-product of the liver, may also lead to elevated insulin, lipid, and thyroid hormone levels. Another GH effect is hypogonadism. IGF-1 elevation warrants pituitary MRI to assess for an adenoma. Untreated or unsuccessful treatment of acromegaly can lead to sleep apnea, diabetes (insulin resistance, increased lipid levels), hypercalciuria, colonic polyps or colorectal cancer, osteoporosis, hypertension, cardiomyopathy, arrhythmias, and cardiovascular disease.

Thyroid-Stimulating Hormone Excess

Hypothyroidism may result in hypertrichosis (see Chapter 194).

5α-Reductase Excess

No specific test exists for 5α-reductase excess, the effects of which are appreciated clinically. It may be that an otherwise idiopathic presentation of hirsutism relates to local mechanisms at the level of the pilosebaceous unit. Typically, there are no adverse sequelae, if the results of all other testing are normal.

Amenorrhea

Absent any other cause of hypothalamic-pituitary-adrenal, ovarian, pancreatic, thyroid, or metabolic (carbohydrate and lipid) dysfunction, a pregnancy test is indicated.

Pregnancy

Normal physiologic changes during pregnancy lead to increasing testosterone because of increasing serum SHBG, along with other androgens, which may result in hirsutism. Benign and malignant ovarian tumors may contribute to maternal and fetal virilization. Persistent corpus luteum of pregnancy requires imaging to diagnose.[15]

DIFFERENTIAL DIAGNOSIS

The onset of hirsutism most often corresponds to a variety of circumstantial or underlying medical conditions: initiation of virilizing drugs, progestins, steroids, or the antiseizure medication valproic acid; discontinuation of oral contraceptives; recent weight gain; ovarian or insulin disorders; and the onset of puberty or menopause. Medications intended to address sexual dysfunction or to promote athleticism are easy to link to signs of androgen excess, and prompt discontinuation should

---

INITIAL DIAGNOSTICS

Hirsutism

LABORATORY
- Total testosterone,
- Free testosterone[a]
- DHEA[a]
- DHEA-S[a]
- LH[a]
- FSH[a]
- LH/FSH ratio[a]
- 24-Hour urinary excretion test for 17-ketosteroid[a]
- Early morning serum 17-OHP or serum 11-deoxycortisol with before and after ACTH stimulation for 21-OH deficiency of NCCAH[a]
- Prolactin[a]
- TSH[a]
- Glucose tolerance test[a]
- Fasting basal insulin[a]
- Free cortisol[a]
- Lipid profile[a]

IMAGING
- Pelvic ultrasound, pelvic CT scan[a]
- Abdominal ultrasound, CT scan[a]
- Adrenal CT scan[a]
- Abdominal MRI[a]

OTHER DIAGNOSTICS
- ACTH stimulation test[a]
- Dexamethasone suppression test[a]
- 24-Hour urinary excretion test for cortisol[a]
- Serum IGF-1[a]
- Genotyping[a]

[a]If indicated.

---

reverse hirsutism in the absence of occult disease. Oral contraceptives that serve to increase SHBG may be suppressing increased testosterone production until they are withdrawn. Progestins or steroids promote androgen production, as does hyperinsulinemia.

An investigation into conditions of insulin resistance is warranted with hirsute patients because hyperinsulinemia correlates inversely with SHBG concentrations. For patients with PCOS, the constellation of oligomenorrhea, amenorrhea, acne, seborrhea, alopecia, obesity, and ovarian cysts is often seen in conjunction with hirsutism. Normoandrogenic hirsutism is the second most commonly diagnosed condition after PCOS and is referred to as idiopathic hirsutism, in which ovulation and androgen hormone levels are normal and ovaries are not polycystic. However, some researchers believe that this categorization is imprecise, pointing to a subset of 40% of clinically hirsute patients who prove to be anovulatory with careful testing (luteal phase progesterone levels below 3 to 5 ng/mL) and actually have PCOS. A significantly rarer consideration is CAH detected either in vivo or early in life and its milder form, NCCAH, indicated by excess cortisol precursors after an ACTH hormone challenge. CAH is an autosomal recessive trait that appears in 1 in 1000 to 2000 individuals; it is evidenced by mixed genitalia and salt wasting at birth, a positive family history, and Ashkenazi Jewish (3% to 4%), Hispanic, or Slavic descent. NCCAH might manifest as prepubertal hirsutism, early-onset puberty, irregular menses, or delayed menses. NCCAH is said to affect 1 in 100 to 1000 women in the United States and can lead to serious complications.[14] In the presence of elevated ACTH levels, the differential diagnosis should include Cushing syndrome, glucocorticoid resistance, and anabolic steroid use. Urgent consideration is advised in the condition of hirsutism with concomitant virilism. Adrenal tumors (benign or malignant), enzyme deficiencies, and endocrinopathies are considerations if virilization accompanies hirsutism. Nonmalignant hyperthecosis of the ovary usually occurs in premenopausal women. Sertoli-Leydig cell tumors of the luteinized thecal cells of the ovary can be present in patients aged 20 to 40 years, sometimes in conjunction with HAIRAN. In these cases, removal of the often unilaterally affected ovary returns testosterone levels to normal and reverses signs of virilism. Other ovarian tumors include arrhenoblastomas and hilar cell tumors, which can lead to excess testosterone levels. A panel of androgen hormones (testosterone, androstenedione, DHEA, and DHEA-S) and imaging studies guide the diagnosis of pituitary, adrenal, or ovarian tumors.

INTERPROFESSIONAL COLLABORATIVE MANAGEMENT

The causes of central hair growth are most often benign and can be managed effectively with a combination of medical therapy and mechanical hair removal. Because a woman's appraisal of her appearance is influenced by cosmetic and cultural standards, in cases of normal hair growth, reassurance is essential.

A commonly accepted, primary nonpharmacologic strategy is weight reduction in the overweight or obese patient. Decreasing weight lowers insulin resistance and reduces hyperandrogenism. There may also be cardiac and insulin resistance benefits to weight loss. A loss of 5% of body weight can restore regular menses or ovulation in some patients with PCOS.[6] Smoking cessation is also critical to mitigate vascular embolic risk, particularly in patients on hormonal therapy, and especially in patients older than 35.

Cosmetic measures are advisable in all patients who desire temporary or permanent removal of unwanted hair. A temporary method is depilatory cream, which dissolves hair but may lead to skin irritation, allergic dermatitis, or permanent skin damage. Although shaving (which may cause stubble to appear coarser and thicker) and plucking (which is uncomfortable and can stimulate hair growth, folliculitis, and scarring) can be used on small areas, waxing removes hair at the base of the pilosebaceous unit and is more effective as a short-term solution, although it may produce superficial burns and infection. Bleaching of the hair is also a temporary measure until these hairs are shed and new ones replace them.

Electrolysis requires the insertion of a fine needle into the base of a hair follicle and the administration of electric current to permanently destroy the follicle. It is a popular but costly procedure, and results vary because it is highly operator dependent. Galvanic electrolysis may yield better results, especially if paired with thermolysis, called "blended treatment."[2] Caution is advised if acne, skin infection, diabetes mellitus, epilepsy, ischemic heart disease, in situ pacemaker, or artificial joints are present. Although painstaking and expensive, it can be permanent because it destroys the dermal papilla. Thermolysis treats more follicles at a time, in a similar manner, with alternating current. Temporary skin irritation can follow.

Patients who choose waxing or electrolysis should be instructed to observe for possible signs of infection. Eflornithine hydrochloride 13.9% topical cream has been shown to slow hair growth by inhibiting ornithine decarboxylase, which regulates cell proliferation at the follicle,[13] although this is a temporary treatment, requiring 8 to 24 weeks of twice-daily application for maximum effect and indefinite use thereafter. It can be combined with combined oral contraceptives (COCs) for better efficacy.

Laser hair removal by ruby, alexandrite, diode, or neodymium:yttrium-aluminum-garnet (Nd:YAG) laser as well as broad-band intense pulsed light therapy with or without radiofrequency for light hair (all representing differing red to infrared wavelengths in nanometers) has been shown to produce long-lasting effects, even permanent hair reduction.[4] Best results of laser therapy generally occur in patients with dark hair and light skin, although some experience complications such as hyperpigmentation or hypopigmentation of the skin.

Medications are used to suppress androgen secretion in the ovaries and adrenal glands or to block testosterone and DHT. Of the varied pharmacologic options, a first-line approach includes oral estrogen-progesterone agents (COCs), which have the added benefit of treating acne and oligomenorrhea. Oral contraceptives suppress ovarian androgen by inhibiting gonadotropin and LH secretion from the pituitary gland. Contraceptives also decrease adrenal DHEA-S through negative feedback on the glucocorticoid receptor. Aiming for 30 mcg of ethinyl estradiol and 1 mg of synthetic progestin is seen as effective,[1-3] particularly because third-generation progestins have no adverse impact on metabolic profile, although they have slightly greater vascular risk.[2] This strategy is particularly effective in mild hirsutism.

Androgenic oral contraceptive pills, such as levonorgestrel, should be avoided. Progestins with low androgenic activity are preferable. These include norgestimate, desogestrel, and gestodene drospirenone, amiodarone HCL, trimegestone, and dienogest.[3,9]

Ultimately, the practitioner may want to stop medications after 1 to 2 years to see if any regression has been achieved and to observe for return of ovulatory function in premenopausal women. Unfortunately, the evidence in support of oral contraceptives as a means to effectively reduce unwanted hair is relatively weak because of limited studies and poor design.[9] Research has not borne out the relative efficacies of various combinations,[2] so treatment requires individualization. Antiandrogens are contraindicated in pregnancy, and birth control should be used with monotherapy.

A second option for treating androgen excess male pattern hair loss is choosing an androgen blocking agent in addition to COCs, particularly in cases of moderate to severe hirsutism, or as monotherapy if there is a contraindication to COCs. Spironolactone (at doses of 50 to 100 mg twice daily), cyproterone acetate (CPA), and flutamide act as competitive antagonists at the androgen receptor.

Spironolactone inhibits pituitary gonadotropin secretion and in turn the binding of testosterone and DHT to the androgen receptor, thereby improving the metabolic clearance of testosterone. Side effects rarely compel patients to discontinue drug therapy; however, nausea, vomiting, abdominal discomfort, diarrhea, fatigue, mental confusion, headache, dizziness, decreased libido, and sun hypersensitivity may follow. Known teratogenicity would prevent its use by women trying to conceive or women of childbearing age not using contraception. Hyperkalemia and postural hypotension are possible side effects.

Although there is some controversy as to whether the addition of an antiandrogen to COCs improves hirsutism more than monotherapy,[7] patients who do not respond to oral contraceptives or spironolactone treatments and are using effective birth control may ask about one of several antiandrogen compounds in combination with ethinyl estradiol, such as CPA. CPA is a steroid derived from 17-OHP. It blocks gonadotropin release and progestogen by binding to the DHT receptor.[9] The dose can be as low as 2 mg with drospirenone (co-cyprindiol), a weak antiandrogen. A dose of 12.5 to 200 mg/day (typically 50 to 100 mg) for 10 days of each menstrual cycle would be the standard dosage. CPA is used widely in Europe, Canada, and Mexico but is not commercially available in the United States. There is a risk of hepatotoxicity and smaller risk of thrombosis.

Finasteride, which inhibits 5α-reductase, decreasing the peripheral conversion of testosterone to the more potent DHT, is not approved for the indication of hirsutism. However, a small study showed that spironolactone with finasteride was more effective than monotherapy.[2] Finasteride doses range from 2.5 to 7.5 mg daily. Fortunately, antiandrogen in combination with COCs may serve not only to regulate menses but also to reduce endometrial hyperplasia risk.[2] There are significant teratogenic risks associated with finasteride.

Flutamide, a nonsteroidal antiandrogen, has been of interest given its efficacy. However, studies have failed to show an advantage among flutamide,[6] finasteride, or spironolactone, although finasteride and spironolactone have been used together to yield a 51% reduction in hirsutism score but with significant liver toxicity concern.[9] The latest recommendations from the Endocrine Society uniformly reject the use of flutamide (owing to risk of liver failure) topical gonadotropin-releasing hormone (GnRH) preparations, GnRH agonists (except in severe forms of hyperandrogenism, such as in ovarian hyperthecosis, after a failed trial of an oral contraceptive), glucocorticoid therapy (except in classic CAH or NCCAH caused by 21-OH deficiency, titrated against 17-OHP concentration for virilizing forms of CAH),[13] or insulin-lowering medication in treating hirsutism.

When finasteride (5 mg/day) or low-dose flutamide (currently not FDA approved in women) is prescribed, liver enzymes should be monitored regularly.[9] The combination of finasteride and flutamide has not been shown to surpass the effects of flutamide alone, but the significant risk of hepatotoxicity makes this combination very risky.[9] Patients must not become pregnant while receiving such therapy.

The use of glucocorticoids to reduce hirsutism and to induce ovulation in NCCAH risks suppression of the hypothalamus-pituitary axis and induction of Cushingoid features. PCOS can also accompany endometrial hyperplasia or other fertility concerns, which is likely to require other specialty collaboration.

Although less common, an adrenal or ovarian tumor that may be malignant, or otherwise need surgical management, should be always be considered in the differential diagnosis when evaluating hirsutism. Therefore, when suspecting a diagnosis of PCOS, it is very important to exclude the rarer causes of hyperandrogenism before definitively settling on the PCOS diagnosis. Other comorbidities commonly associated with hyperandrogenism and related hirsutis, such as obesity, metabolic syndrome, overt diabetes mellitus, and hypertension, necessitate careful follow-up monitoring.

INDICATIONS FOR REFERRAL OR HOSPITALIZATION

- Patients may be referred to an endocrinologist for abnormal levels of androgens or other hormone abnormalities. Referral to an endocrinologist is appropriate if hirsutism is accompanied by virilism, which suggests the need for further endocrine biochemical evaluation and/or imaging.

An endocrinologist is also consulted for treatment failure or persistent infertility. Women with elevated androgens, insulin resistance, subfertility or infertility, and central obesity in particular require further follow-up, regardless of normal terminal hair distribution.

- A surgical consultation may be indicated for the evaluation of patients with pituitary, adrenal, or ovarian tumors.
- Although adult-onset acromegaly is largely associated with benign pituitary tumors, left untreated it has a high morbidity and mortality. The medical and surgical management of this multisystem disease requires specialist or multidisciplinary center expertise.
- The psychosocial effects of increasing body hair may warrant a psychiatric consultation if the hair has become a consuming concern. A mental health referral will be useful if there is reason to suspect underlying gonadal abnormality, such as chromosomal mosaicism or, in rare cases, hermaphroditism.
- Genetic counseling, or even fetal testing, may be appropriate in some cases.

LIFE SPAN CONSIDERATIONS

Hirsutism is a sensitive issue for adolescent girls, whose desire for peer acceptance may heavily influence body image and resulting health behaviors. Eating disorders related to PCOS are not unusual. Any menstrual cycle irregularities are of concern if they are accompanied by acne, alopecia, and hirsutism as well as insulin resistance because this might be a presentation of PCOS. Excessive hair growth can accompany pregnancy but usually disappears postpartum, often without long-term effects to mother or baby if sinister causes are excluded. Although hirsutism itself does not lead to a shortened life span, mortality can be increased by certain etiologies of hirsutism that also cause other detrimental effects to the body, as detailed earlier in this chapter.

EDUCATION AND HEALTH PROMOTION

Education about realistic expectations of cosmetic hair removal, hair loss, and hair growth suppression is essential. With medical therapy, it will take 6 to 18 months to see a new set-point in hair growth. Furthermore, hirsutism treated empirically may recur once the treatment is discontinued.

Because oral contraceptives provide essential treatment for PCOS patients, avoidance of the 19-nortestosterone derivatives, such as norgestrel and levonorgestrel, is important; they block the estrogen-mediated increase in SHBG concentration and are mildly androgenic. Patients using third-generation oral contraceptives should always be advised of the possibility of thromboembolic events. All patients taking oral contraceptives should be strictly advised to stop smoking, as this greatly potentiates the thromboembolic risk. Use of anabolic steroids for muscle building is harmful to one's health, given other systemic adverse effects, and whenever discovered, the individual should be strongly advised to discontinue this practice.

It is important for the provider to address possible anxiety and depression in women with PCOS resulting from manifestations of hirsutism, and to provide reassurance about fears of masculinization, ridicule or social rejection, and sexual or gender identity. Sexual ambiguity in forms of CAH would also be a high-priority concern to address. For patients with PCOS, a diet high in fiber and low in refined carbohydrates is encouraged, as is weight loss, to mitigate the elevated risk of metabolic syndrome that comes with this condition. Individual or group psychological counseling can help with self-image and weight management.

Women should be adequately counseled about their concerns and realistic expectations for future fertility and plans for conception. Because pregnancy is contraindicated during hormone therapy, pregnancy plans should be discussed in advance. The patient should be made aware that discontinuation of antiandrogen therapy for the period of preconception through end of pregnancy is likely to yield a return of terminal hair growth.

REFERENCES

1. Pierard-Franchimont, C., & Pierard, G. E. (2013). Alterations in hair follicle dynamics in women. *BioMed Research International, 2013*, 957432.
2. Escobar-Morreale, H. F., Carmina, E., Dewailly, D., et al. (2012). Epidemiology, diagnosis, and management of hirsutism: A consensus statement by Androgen Excess and Polycystic Ovary Syndrome Society. *Human Reproduction Update, 18*(2), 146–170.
3. Unluhizarci, K., Karaca, Z., & Kelestimur, F. (2013). Hirsutism—from diagnosis to use of antiandrogens. In D. Macut, M. Pfeifer, B. O. Yildiz, et al. (Eds.), *Polycystic ovary syndrome. Novel insights into causes and therapy. Front Horm Res* (Vol. 40, pp. 103–114). Basel: Karger.
4. Loriaux, L. (2012). An approach to the patient with hirsutism. *The Journal of Clinical Endocrinology and Metabolism, 97*(9), 2957–2968.
5. Pasquali, R., & Gambineri, A. (2014). Treatment of hirsutism in polycystic ovary syndrome. *European Journal of Endocrinology, 170*(2), R75–R90.
6. Kopera, D., Wehr, E., & Obermayer-Wehr, B. (2010). Endocrinology of hirsutism. *International Journal of Trichology, 2*(1), 30–35.
7. Somani, N., & Turvey, D. (2014). Hirsutism: An evidence-based treatment update. *American Journal of Clinical Dermatology, 15*, 247–266.
8. Teede, H. J., Misso, M. L., costello, M. F., Dokras, A., et al. (2018). Recommendations from the international evidence-based guideline for the assessment and management of polycystic ovary syndrome. *Fertility and Sterility, 110*(3), 364–379.
9. Jayasena, C. N., & Franks, S. (2014). The management of patients with polycystic ovary syndrome. *Nature Reviews. Endocrinology, 10*, 624–636.
10. Hohl, A., Ronsoni, M. F., & de Oliveira, M. (2014). Hirsutism: Diagnosis and treatment. *Arquivos Brasileiros de Endocrinologia E Metabologia, 58*(2), 97–107.
11. Fauser, B. C. J. M., Tarlatzis, B. C., Rebar, R. W., et al. (2012). Consensus on women's health aspects of polycystic ovary syndrome (PCOS): The Amsterdam ESHRE/ASRM-Sponsored 3rd PCOS consensus workshop group. *Fertility and Sterility, 97*, 28–38.
12. Williams, T., Mortada, R., & Porter, S. (2016). Diahnosis and Treatment pf polycystic ovary syndrome. *American Family Physician, 94*(2), 106–113.
13. Moran, C., Arriaga, M., Arechavaleta-Velasco, F., et al. (2014). Adrenal androgen excess and body mass index in polycystic ovary syndrome. *The Journal of Clinical Endocrinology and Metabolism*, jc20142569:1-9.
14. Papadakis, G., Kandaraki, E. A., Tseniklidi, E., Papalou, O., & Diamanti-Kandarakis, E. (2019). Polycystic ovary syndrome and NC-CAH: Distinct characteristics and common findings. A systematic review. *Frontiers in Endocrinology, 10*, 388. doi:10.3389/fendo.2019.00388. Published 2019 Jun 19.
15. Bode, D., Sheehusen, D. A., & Baird, D. (2012). Hirsutism in women. *American Family Physician, 85*(4), 373–380.

CHAPTER **188**

HYPERCALCEMIA AND HYPOCALCEMIA

Roselyn Cristelle I. Mateo • Alan Ona Malabanan

 Physician consultation is indicated for patients with serum corrected calcium levels of less than 8.5 mg/dL or more than 10.5 mg/dL.

DEFINITION AND EPIDEMIOLOGY

A stable extracellular calcium concentration and proper compartmentalization of calcium are vitally important to several physiologic and cellular functions. A high intracellular calcium level can lead to organellar damage, aggregation of amino and nucleic acids, alteration of the integrity of lipid membranes, and phosphate (i.e., adenosine triphosphate) precipitation. Consequently, aberrations in calcium homeostasis may lead to neuromuscular, cardiac, nephrologic, endocrine, coagulatory, and gastrointestinal dysfunction as well as to cellular and organism death.

Hypercalcemia, a high level of serum ionized calcium (i.e., ionized calcium >5.3 mg/dL), is a disorder in which the calcium level exceeds the upper limit of the normal range (i.e., total corrected calcium >10.5 mg/dL).[1] Conversely, hypocalcemia is a low level of serum ionized calcium (i.e., ionized calcium <4.4 mg/dL), with a total corrected calcium level below 8.5 mg/dL. Both disorders can be a manifestation of a serious illness, such as malignant disease, or can be detected incidentally by laboratory testing in an asymptomatic patient. The calcium imbalance may have varied causes, may be chronic or acute, and may exhibit variable effects.

Hypercalcemia in the outpatient setting is most commonly asymptomatic primary hyperparathyroidism (PHPT). PHPT may be as prevalent as 232.7 per 100,000 and risk increasing with age, female sex, and black ethnicity.[1] Factors such as the use of automated chemistry analysis and the release of national osteoporosis guidelines have also increased PHPT diagnosis.[2] Among patients presenting to the emergency department and those hospitalized, hypercalcemia is found in 0.7% to 3.3% and malignancy is the etiology in 44% to 72%.[3,4] In general, hypercalcemia is common in those with cancer with an estimated prevalence of 2% overall and as high as 10.2% in those with multiple myeloma.[5] The prevalence of hypocalcemia has been found as high as 18% in hospitalized patients and 85% in critically ill patients[6] although a recent study has found an estimate of 3.4% of hypocalcemia among patients admitted to a large university-affiliated tertiary care center.[3]

HYPERCALCEMIA

PATHOPHYSIOLOGY

Ninety-nine percent of the body's roughly 1 kg of calcium is found in the bone as hydroxyapatite. The remaining 1% is found in the extracellular fluid and soft tissues. Approximately 50% of plasma calcium is in the ionized, biologically active form; 10% is complexed in nonionic form; and 40% is protein bound, predominantly to albumin. Roughly 500 mg of the bone calcium is released from the bone each day in normal bone turnover.

Alterations in albumin levels may cause changes in total calcium concentrations, without altering ionized calcium levels. The serum calcium concentration can be corrected for alterations in albumin by the following formula: Corrected calcium = serum calcium + 0.8 × (4 − serum albumin).

Alterations in acid–base balance may also alter ionized calcium levels. Increased acidemia decreases calcium binding to albumin and increases ionized calcium. Conversely, increased alkalemia increases calcium binding to albumin and decreases ionized calcium.

Extracellular calcium homeostasis is regulated primarily by the interaction between the calcium-sensing receptor (CaSR), parathyroid hormone (PTH), and 1,25-dihydroxyvitamin D_3 (calcitriol). PTH and calcitriol exert their effects through feedback mechanisms on three major organ systems: the skeleton, the intestinal tract, and the kidneys.[3]

A decrease in serum ionized calcium is detected by the CaSR and stimulates the production of PTH. PTH has a direct effect on calcium and phosphorus through increased osteoclast activity, leading to bone resorption. PTH also directly stimulates the kidney tubules to reabsorb calcium and to excrete phosphorus, leading to a rise in serum calcium and a fall in serum phosphorus. PTH also increases renal conversion of 25-hydroxyvitamin D (25OHD), the major circulating vitamin D metabolite, into 1,25-dihydroxyvitamin D (1,25OH$_2$D), the active vitamin D metabolite, which increases intestinal absorption of calcium and phosphate. Increases in serum calcium and 1,25OH$_2$D levels inhibit release of PTH, reversing the process.

Hypercalcemia can be categorized as either PTH dependent or PTH independent, depending on whether PTH is nonsuppressed or suppressed, respectively. PTH-dependent hypercalcemia is typically a result of PHPT, and PTH-independent hypercalcemia is typically a result of hypercalcemia of malignancy. PHPT results when an autonomous parathyroid cell line develops.

There are three malignancy-associated hypercalcemia PTH-independent mechanisms: humoral hypercalcemia of malignancy, bony metastasis with the release of osteoclast activating factors, and production of 1,25OH$_2$D.

Humoral hypercalcemia of malignancy is the most common (approximately 80%) and is caused by excessive secretion of parathyroid hormone–related protein (PTHrP), which activates the same PTH-1 receptor activated by PTH. This has been associated with squamous carcinomas of the head, neck and lungs, breast, ovarian, and renal carcinomas. Local osteolytic hypercalcemia accounts for 20% of malignancy-associated hypercalcemia. It results from widespread skeletal metastases from breast and hematologic cancers. Calcitriol-induced hypercalcemia has been associated with Hodgkin and non-Hodgkin lymphoma. Malignancy-associated hypercalcemia has also been associated with authentic ectopic hyperparathyroidism (i.e., non–PTHrP-related hypercalcemia).

Milk-alkali syndrome, a combination of hypercalcemia, metabolic alkalosis, and renal insufficiency, develops in response to the simultaneous ingestion of large amounts of calcium and absorbable alkali, such as calcium carbonate. This is the third most common cause of hypercalcemia.[7] Disorders involving vitamin D or vitamin A excess or increased vitamin D activation lead to increased bone resorption and intestinal absorption of calcium. Hypercalcemia may also result from common mechanisms but rare causes, such as mammary hyperplasia and pregnancy (increased PTHrP), granulomatous disease from silicone injections (increased calcitriol), and betel nut consumption with oyster shell (milk-alkali syndrome).[4]

CLINICAL PRESENTATION AND PHYSICAL EXAMINATION

The presence and severity of symptoms in hypercalcemia are influenced by the magnitude of hypercalcemia, rate of rise of calcium, acid–base balance, and presence of hypoalbuminemia. A very high level of calcium may be tolerated chronically, whereas a less elevated but abrupt increase may cause

significant symptoms. In general, however, corrected serum calcium levels below 11.5 mg/dL are rarely symptomatic.

The symptoms of hypercalcemia of any cause typically involve neuromuscular, cardiac, and gastrointestinal depression. Neurologic changes can range from the subtle, such as an inability to concentrate, increased fatigue, depression, or increased sleep requirement, to the dramatic, with confusion, delirium, stupor, or coma. Cardiovascular manifestations can include bradycardia, hypertension, electrocardiographic abnormalities such as arrhythmias (especially on digitalis), bundle branch or atrioventricular blocks, and shortened QT interval as well as cardiac arrest with severe hypercalcemia. Gastrointestinal symptoms are common and include constipation, anorexia, nausea, and vomiting. Peptic ulcers and pancreatitis are less common and may be more common with type I multiple endocrine neoplasia and PHPT.[5] Renal symptoms can range from polyuria and nocturia (from nephrogenic diabetes insipidus), which can lead to volume depletion and worsened hypercalcemia, to nephrolithiasis, nephrocalcinosis, and renal failure. Parkinsonism has been described with hypercalcemia and hyperparathyroidism, which may improve with parathyroidectomy or cinacalcet.[6] Celiac disease is associated with ~2× the risk for PHPT in the first 5 years of follow-up after diagnosis,[6] so the presence of diarrhea or rash (dermatitis herpetiformis) might identify an etiology for the PHPT.

The physical examination findings are often unremarkable. Cardiovascular examination may reveal irregularity of rate and rhythm. Band keratopathy, calcium deposition in the cornea, may be present regardless of the cause of hypercalcemia. The presence of a neck mass (parathyroid carcinoma or medullary thyroid carcinoma in type IIA multiple endocrine neoplasia) or breast mass (breast carcinoma) may suggest the cause of the hypercalcemia. Central nervous system depression is reflected in hyporeflexia, changes in sensorium, muscle weakness, tremor, lethargy, and ataxia. With severe hypercalcemia, stupor and coma may result. There may be flank tenderness if nephrolithiasis is a complication. On occasion, pseudogout (calcium pyrophosphate dehydrate crystal deposition disease) may cause joint swelling or inflammation.

DIAGNOSTICS

The diagnosis of hypercalcemia is usually made by measuring the serum total calcium level along with a serum albumin level, with calculation of the corrected calcium concentration. In patients who may have derangements in albumin as well as blood pH, such as critically ill patients and dialysis patients, the ionized calcium level on a heparinized whole blood sample may be more accurate.[7] Once hypercalcemia has been confirmed, determination of the cause is the next step. Whereas the serum phosphate level (low in PHPT) and the serum magnesium level (high in familial hypocalciuric hypercalcemia) may be useful, the intact PTH assay, ideally performed fasting, is the best test to determine whether the hypercalcemia is PTH dependent (PTH nonsuppressed) or PTH independent (PTH suppressed). If the hypercalcemia is PTH independent, further testing with serum 1,25OH$_2$D level, serum protein electrophoresis, and PTHrP level would be useful. A high or inappropriately normal serum 1,25OH$_2$D level should lead to an evaluation for tuberculosis, sarcoidosis, or lymphoma as a potential cause. A careful history of nonprescription supplements, such as calcium-containing antacids and cod liver oil, may be helpful in identifying milk-alkali syndrome, vitamin A,

Differential Diagnosis: Hypercalcemia and Hypocalcemia

HYPERCALCEMIA
PTH Dependent
- Hyperparathyroidism (common)
- Lithium
- Familial hypocalciuric hypercalcemia (rare)
- Ectopic PTH secretion (rare)

PTH Independent
- Malignancy (common)
  - Humoral hypercalcemia from PTHrP (common)
  - Local osteolytic hypercalcemia
  - Calcitriol mediated (lymphoma)
- Milk-alkali syndrome (common)
- Sarcoidosis
- Granulomatous disease (tuberculosis, HIV)
- Thyrotoxicosis
- Vitamin A or D toxicity
- Thiazide diuretic use
- Drug toxicity (theophylline, estrogens or antiestrogens, androgens, aluminum, foscarnet)
- Renal failure
- Addison disease
- Pheochromocytoma
- Immobilization
- Total parenteral nutrition
- Rhabdomyolysis

HYPOCALCEMIA
PTH Dependent
- Hypoparathyroidism
  - Parathyroid or thyroid surgery
  - Idiopathic hypoparathyroidism (autoimmune)
  - Radiation therapy
  - Hemochromatosis
- Hypermagnesemia
- CaSR-activating mutation (autosomal dominant hypocalcemia)

PTH Independent
- Vitamin D deficiency
- Malabsorption syndromes (celiac disease, gastric bypass surgery)
- Chronic kidney disease
- Liver disease
- Alcoholism
- Malnutrition
- Pancreatitis
- Hypomagnesemia
- Hyperphosphatemia
- Severe sepsis
- Burns
- Medications (amphotericin B, foscarnet, omeprazole, furosemide, bisphosphonates, denosumab)
- Extensive transfusion with citrated blood
- Pseudohypocalcemia (gadolinium contrast interferes with total calcium assay)

HIV, Human immunodeficiency virus.

INITIAL DIAGNOSTICS

Hypercalcemia and Hypocalcemia

LABORATORY
- Serum calcium and serum albumin
- Ionized calcium[a]
- Intact PTH levels[a]
- Serum 25-hydroxyvitamin D and 1,25-dihydroxyvitamin D[a]
- Serum and urine protein electrophoresis[a]
- Alkaline phosphatase[a]
- Creatinine
- Magnesium[a]
- Phosphorus[a]

IMAGING
- X-ray studies[a]
- Bone scan[a]

OTHER DIAGNOSTICS
- ECG[a]
- Purified protein derivative testing[a]
- Chest X-ray study[a]
- Bone marrow biopsy[a]

ECG, electrocardiogram.
[a]If indicated.

or vitamin D toxicity as a cause of the hypercalcemia. Recently initiated thiazide therapy may unmask hypercalcemia from a variety of causes, due to its hypocalciuric effects.

DIFFERENTIAL DIAGNOSIS

PHPT and malignant disease account for 90% of hypercalcemia cases; PHPT is the most common in the ambulatory patient, and malignant disease is the most common in the hospitalized patient (Box 188.1). PHPT tends to have a milder, asymptomatic presentation with mild hypercalcemia; hypercalcemia of malignancy tends to occur in advanced and overt disease. Once these two diagnoses are excluded, consideration of milk-alkali syndrome, sarcoidosis, tuberculosis, vitamin D or A toxicity, and granulomatous disease may be based on the history and laboratory findings.

INTERPROFESSIONAL COLLABORATIVE MANAGEMENT

Immediate emergency department referral is indicated for symptomatic hypercalcemia, particularly when it is associated with nausea or vomiting or a corrected serum calcium concentration above 12.0 mg/dL.

Management of hypercalcemia is tailored to the severity and acuity of the hypercalcemia. The management of mild hypercalcemia, usually caused by PHPT, generally involves maintenance of hydration and volume status as well as avoidance of drugs that may worsen hypercalcemia.

Severe hypercalcemia, particularly with a corrected serum calcium concentration above 14.0 mg/dL, is a medical emergency, which has a significant mortality and may require ICU care. Because the only way to remove calcium from the body is through the urine, the first efforts at treatment should be directed at aggressive restoration of volume status with intravenous normal saline, sometimes requiring as much as 6 L in 24 hours (i.e., 250 mL/h). With the increase in sodium and fluid delivery to the kidney, there is a concomitant increase in urinary calcium loss. Other electrolytes, such as potassium and magnesium, may be lost, and their levels should be monitored and corrected carefully. Furosemide has been commonly used to enhance urinary calcium losses, but there is scant evidence for its effectiveness and it is being recommended less often in current practice.[8] Parenteral salmon calcitonin is useful at further enhancing urinary calcium losses and can very rapidly lower serum calcium levels, although tachyphylaxis may develop, limiting its efficacy after 24 hours.

Further management is dependent on addressing the cause of the hypercalcemia. Hypercalcemia caused by intractable PHPT or parathyroid carcinoma may be improved with cinacalcet (Sensipar), a calcimimetic agent, which lowers serum calcium and PTH by increasing the sensitivity of the CaSR to extracellular calcium, thereby decreasing serum PTH and reducing the renal tubular reabsorption of calcium.[9,10] Cinacalcet can normalize serum calcium in as much as 70% to 80% of patients with PHPT, although surgery is the only cure.[11] Excessive bone resorption caused by hyperparathyroidism or hypercalcemia of malignancy from any cause will respond to intravenous pamidronate (Aredia) or zoledronic acid (Reclast), with improvements in the serum calcium concentration occurring in 24 to 48 hours. Bisphosphonates have become the standard of care in the treatment of cancer-associated hypercalcemia, providing safe, effective, and sustained reductions in serum calcium levels by inhibiting osteoclast activity in a dose-dependent fashion and stabilizing the bone matrix by binding to extracellular calcium and phosphorus.[12] Glucocorticoids may have some usefulness in treating hypercalcemia caused by hematologic malignant neoplasms, probably because of their antitumor effects, as well as hypercalcemia from vitamin D intoxication or calcitriol-induced hypercalcemia (tuberculosis should be ruled out as a cause before initiation of glucocorticoids). Steroids inhibit osteoclastic bone resorption by decreasing tumor production of locally active cytokines, in addition to having direct tumor lysis effects.[13]

Rarely, hemodialysis, plicamycin, or gallium nitrate may be necessary for control of serum calcium concentration. Denosumab (Xgeva), a monoclonal antibody against the receptor activator of nuclear factor kappa-B ligand (RANKL), has been approved to treat hypercalcemia of malignancy in patients not responding to bisphosphonates.[14] It is dosed 120 mg subcutaneously every 4 weeks, with additional 120 mg doses on days 8 and 15 of therapy. It may be of use in those who have renal failure.[15] Cinacalcet has been used, off-label, for patients with bisphosphonate-resistant hypercalcemia related to metastatic breast cancer[20] and renal cell carcinoma with elevated PTHrP levels.

LIFE SPAN CONSIDERATIONS

Among those with mild PHPT, there is increased morbidity and mortality,[16] as there is in those on chronic hemodialysis with hyperparathyroidism and hypercalcemia.[17] Hypercalcemia of malignancy is a sign of advanced disease and 30-day mortality is approximately 50% and outcomes are not affected by choice of hypocalcemic therapy.[18] Elevated ionized calcium levels above 1.4 mmol/L (5.6 mg/dL) are associated with ICU and hospital mortality in critically ill patients.[19]

COMPLICATIONS

A variety of complications may result from hypercalcemia, depending on the cause. In addition to the neuromuscular,

renal, cardiovascular, and gastrointestinal complications mentioned previously, osteoporotic fractures and bone pain may result from hypercalcemia arising from increased bone resorption. Untreated severe hypercalcemia may lead to death.

HYPOCALCEMIA
PATHOPHYSIOLOGY

A low level of ionized serum calcium results from either increased calcium loss from the circulation (deposition in tissue, increased urinary excretion, increased binding within the circulation) or decreased entry of calcium into the circulation (malabsorption, decreased bone resorption). The causes of hypocalcemia can further be divided into inadequate PTH or calcitriol production, PTH or calcitriol resistance, and miscellaneous causes such as intravenous bisphosphonate use. PTH resistance may result from pseudohypoparathyroidism, a rare genetic disorder, or more commonly from chronic kidney disease or magnesium deficiency. Hypocalcemia resulting from vitamin D deficiency tends to be a late complication of long-standing disease. Hungry bone syndrome may result from a loss of parathyroid-induced bone resorption following parathyroidectomy. Use of potent antiresorptives, such as bisphosphonates and denosumab, in hypercalcemia of malignancy may lead to hypocalcemia. Sclerosing skeletal metastases, as well as multiple other etiologies, have resulted in consideration of the "hypocalcemia of malignancy," ranging in prevalence estimates from 1.6% to 10.8%.[20]

CLINICAL PRESENTATION AND PHYSICAL EXAMINATION

As with hypercalcemia, the severity of hypocalcemia, the rapidity of its development, and the albumin and acid–base status determine its manifestations. A low serum calcium level may be tolerated well if it developed slowly or if hypoalbuminemia and acidemia are present. Clinical manifestations of hypocalcemia are due to increased neuromuscular excitability and cardiovascular dysfunction. Patients may have paresthesias and tingling in the extremities and around the mouth. Muscle weakness, cramping, tetany, convulsions, and fatal laryngospasm and bronchospasm are manifestations of the increased neuromuscular irritability.[21]

Seizures, depression, and altered mental status and sensorium have been described. Patients may have generalized fatigue and congestive heart failure. Patients may develop cataracts. Basal ganglia calcification may lead to a Parkinson-like motor disorder.[22]

The physical examination may reveal features of spontaneous neuromuscular irritability with hyperreflexia of deep tendons. Chvostek sign (contraction of the facial muscle in response to tapping of the facial nerve against the bone anterior to the ear) and Trousseau sign (carpal spasm occurring after occlusion of the brachial artery with a blood pressure cuff for 3 minutes) are usually readily elicited. A Parkinson-like tremor may be present. Cardiovascular examination may reveal hypotension, impaired cardiac contractility, and bradyarrhythmias. Adults with chronic hypocalcemia may display coarse hair, dry and brittle nails, and scaly skin. A shortening of the fourth and fifth metacarpals may be seen in pseudohypoparathyroidism, a rare genetic disorder of PTH resistance. Craniofacial and palatal abnormalities may be associated with

DiGeorge/velocardiofacial/22q11.2 deletion syndrome.[23] Evidence of increased intracranial pressure (papilledema) may also be noted. Subcapsular cataracts can be seen with slit-lamp examination.[24]

DIAGNOSTICS

As with hypercalcemia, once hypocalcemia has been confirmed, an intact PTH assay will help delineate the cause. A fasting serum phosphate concentration is also helpful; it is high in hypoparathyroidism and low in vitamin D deficiency. Serum magnesium and 25OHD concentrations should be assessed in all patients with hypocalcemia to identify those with hypomagnesemia or hypermagnesemia or vitamin D deficiency as a cause. Further testing with a 1,25OH$_2$D level may be useful in identifying those with vitamin D–dependent rickets types I and II. A 24-hour determination of urine calcium and magnesium may be helpful in assessing patients who may have CaSR mutations, such as in autosomal dominant hypocalcemia. A tissue transglutaminase antibody test may be useful in confirming a diagnosis of celiac disease. An electrocardiogram provides a rapid way of assessing the calcium status by measuring the QTc interval, which is prolonged in hypocalcemia. Genetic testing for the DiGeorge/velocardiofacial/22q11.2 deletion syndrome may be helpful in patients with craniofacial abnormalities and cognitive deficits.[25]

DIFFERENTIAL DIAGNOSIS

Chronic hypocalcemia can be ascribed to several disorders associated with an absence of PTH or with its ineffectiveness (see Box 188.1). Possible causes include surgery that involves the parathyroid (hungry bone syndrome) or thyroid, idiopathic hypoparathyroidism, pseudohypoparathyroidism, vitamin D deficiency, malabsorption syndromes, severe renal or liver disease, alcoholism and poor nutritional intake, osteoblastic malignant disease, pancreatitis, and hypomagnesemia or hyperphosphatemia. Hypoparathyroidism may occur in 12% soon after thyroidectomy but persists in less than 1%.[25] The cause is distinguished by clinical criteria, including duration of illness, symptoms of associated disorders, detection of hereditary features, and history of malnutrition and alcoholism. Acute transient hypocalcemia can be associated with severe sepsis, burns, acute renal failure, extensive blood transfusions with citrated blood, medications (foscarnet, intravenous bisphosphonates, denosumab), and pancreatitis.

INTERPROFESSIONAL COLLABORATIVE MANAGEMENT

 Immdiate emergency department referral is indicated for symptomatic hypocalcemia, particularly when it is associated with muscle cramping or stridor or a corrected serum calcium concentration below 8.0 mg/dL.

All patients with symptomatic hypocalcemia must be treated. Severe, symptomatic hypocalcemia in the presence of tetany, arrhythmias, or seizures should be treated emergently with intravenous administration of calcium. The treatment of hypocalcemia is guided by the acuity and severity of the hypocalcemia and the associated signs and symptoms. In acute, life-threatening situations, 1 or 2 ampules (1 ampule = 10 mL) of 10% calcium gluconate which has 93 mg elemental calcium, are diluted in 50 to 100 mL of 5% dextrose, infused during 10 to 20 minutes, and may be repeated. Administration of a maintenance infusion of 10 ampules of calcium gluconate in 1 L of 5% dextrose at 50 mL/h, titrated to symptoms and serum calcium level into the low normal range. Calcium gluconate is the preferred agent as calcium chloride may irritate the veins. With less severe symptoms, a more dilute calcium solution is infused during a longer period. Serum calcium concentration should be monitored frequently and the infusion adjusted accordingly, and patients must be under continuous electrocardiographic monitoring. Until calcium levels have been restored into the low normal range, life-threatening symptoms such as hypotension and arrhythmias are refractory to medical management. Oral calcium supplementation and vitamin D, as calcitriol, should also be started. There has been some controversy about treatment of ionized hypocalcemia in ICU patients in the absence of known derangements of calcium homeostasis.[26]

Vitamin D is the cornerstone of therapy for chronic hypocalcemia. Calcitriol is recommended (0.25 to 0.5 mcg/day) with calcium supplementation as needed (500 to 1000 mg elemental calcium as calcium citrate (2370 to 4739 mg) or calcium carbonate (1250 to 2500 mg) two or three times daily with food, i.e., 200% to 300% of daily value). If renal function is intact, high-dose ergocalciferol (50,000 units daily) may be used, although the long-acting nature of this vitamin D preparation increases the risk for toxicity.

Vitamin D and calcium dosing can be varied independently. Higher doses of vitamin D allow more effective absorption of calcium from the intestinal tract. If intestinal absorption is inefficient, higher intakes of oral calcium permit adequate calcium assimilation. Dietary phosphate intake should probably be limited because excessive phosphate may lower serum calcium. The use of thiazide diuretics with sodium restriction in hypoparathyroidism lowers urinary calcium excretion, thus minimizing the risk for nephrolithiasis and allowing a lower dose of vitamin D and calcium supplementation. Using calcium, calcitriol, and thiazides together markedly increases the risk for hypercalcemia and should be monitored carefully with frequent laboratory testing and expert guidance. Furosemide and other loop diuretics should be avoided because they increase urinary calcium excretion and, thus, might decrease serum calcium levels. PTH$_{(1-34)}$ and PTH$_{(1-84)}$ have also been used as replacement therapy for primary hypoparathyroidism, with the latter (NATPARA) being FDA approved as an adjunct to calcium and vitamin D in patients with hypoparathyroidism who cannot be well-controlled on calcium and activated vitamin D alone. It can progressively reduce, but not eliminate, supplemental calcium and calcitriol requirement. PTH therapy has increased the risk for osteosarcoma in animals and is avoided in patients at increased risk for osteosarcoma. Providers must be trained in Risk Evaluation and Mitigation Strategy (REMS) before prescribing. We have limited safety data with long-term use of PTH therapy.[27]

A low serum calcium level associated with a low serum albumin level may not require replacement if the corrected calcium is in the normal range. Serum pH, potassium, magnesium, and phosphorus levels should be monitored and corrected if necessary. This will usually correct hypocalcemia without further intervention.

LIFE SPAN CONSIDERATIONS

There is increased mortality with marked hypocalcemia on hospital admission.[3] Chronic hypocalcemia can be managed by the patient's compliance with medications and close monitoring.

Hypocalcemia may be associated with higher mortality among hemodialysis patients,[22] but this has not been shown in the general population.[27]

COMPLICATIONS

Complications of hypocalcemia include laryngospasm, airway obstruction, tetany, seizures, cardiac arrhythmias, coma, and death. Movement disorders, pseudotumor cerebri, and cataracts may also result from neurologic calcifications.

INDICATIONS FOR REFERRAL OR HOSPITALIZATION

- Treatment of both hypocalcemic crisis and hypercalcemic crisis always requires hospitalization. Immediate intravenous correction of the imbalance, either through replacement of calcium in hypocalcemia or through fluid replacement and diuresis in hypercalcemia, with concurrent cardiac monitoring, possible intubation, laboratory analysis, and diligent observation is required until stabilization occurs.
- Referral to an endocrinologist and an experienced parathyroid surgeon may be necessary if PHPT is diagnosed.
- Malignancy-induced hypercalcemia should be managed by an oncologist.

PATIENT AND FAMILY EDUCATION AND HEALTH PROMOTION

Patient and family education should emphasize lifestyle changes, including diet, hydration, and mobility. Patients should learn to identify foods that are high in calcium and adjust their diets according to their imbalance. Patients with hypercalcemia should be instructed to continue weight-bearing exercise to help maintain bone health and to ensure adequate fluid intake. Patients and families should also be taught to recognize early signs and symptoms of calcium imbalance and be instructed to seek medical assessment early. Early and mild manifestations may be treated without hospitalization; however, if it is neglected, a calcium imbalance can be life-threatening.

REFERENCES

1. Yeh, M. W., et al. (2013). Incidence and prevalence of primary hyperparathyroidism in a racially mixed population. *The Journal of Clinical Endocrinology and Metabolism, 98,* 1122–1129.
2. Griebeler, M. L., et al. (2015). Secular trends in the incidence of primary hyperparathyroidism over five decades (1965-2010). *Bone, 73,* 1–7.
3. Akirov, A., Gorshtein, A., Shraga-Slutzky, I., & Shimon, I. (2017). Calcium levels on admission and before discharge are associated with mortality risk in hospitalized patients. *Endocrine, 57,* 344–351.
4. Lindner, G., et al. (2013). Hypercalcemia in the ED: Prevalence, etiology, and outcome. *The American Journal of Emergency Medicine, 31,* 657–660.
5. Jacobs, T. P., & Bilezikian, J. P. (2005). Clinical review: Rare causes of hypercalcemia. *The Journal of Clinical Endocrinology and Metabolism, 90,* 6316–6322.
6. Gastanaga, V. M., et al. (2016). Prevalence of hypercalcemia among cancer patients in the United States. *Cancer Medicine, 5,* 2091–2100.
7. Hannan, F. M., & Thakker, R. V. (2013). Investigating hypocalcaemia. *British Medical Journal, 346,* f2213.
8. Medarov, B. I. (2009). Milk-alkali syndrome. *Mayo Clinic Proceedings. Mayo Clinic, 84,* 261–267.
9. Ohya, Y., et al. (2018). A case of hyperparathyroidism-associated parkinsonism successfully treated with cinacalcet hydrochloride, a calcimimetic. *BMC Neurology, 18,* 62.
10. Ludvigsson, J. F., et al. (2012). Primary hyperparathyroidism and celiac disease: A population-based cohort study. *The Journal of Clinical Endocrinology and Metabolism, 97,* 897–904.
11. Baird, G. S. (2011). Ionized calcium. *Clinica Chimica Acta, 412,* 696–701.
12. Reagan, P., Pani, A., & Rosner, M. H. (2014). Approach to diagnosis and treatment of hypercalcemia in a patient with malignancy. *American Journal of Kidney Diseases: The Official Journal of the National Kidney Foundation, 63,* 141–147.
13. Mizamtsidi, M., et al. (2018). Diagnosis, management, histology and genetics of sporadic primary hyperparathyroidism: Old knowledge with new tricks. *Endocrine Connections, 7,* R56–R68.
14. Marcocci, C., & Cetani, F. (2012). Update on the use of cinacalcet in the management of primary hyperparathyroidism. *Journal of Endocrinological Investigation, 35,* 90–95.
15. Silverberg, S. J., et al. (2007). Cinacalcet hydrochloride reduces the serum calcium concentration in inoperable parathyroid carcinoma. *The Journal of Clinical Endocrinology and Metabolism, 92,* 3803–3808.
16. Sternlicht, H., & Glezerman, I. G. (2015). Hypercalcemia of malignancy and new treatment options. *Therapeutics and Clinical Risk Management, 11,* 1779–1788.
17. Goldner, W. (2016). Cancer-related hypercalcemia. *Journal of Oncology Practice / American Society of Clinical Oncology, 12,* 426–432.
18. Bech, A., & de Boer, H. (2012). Denosumab for tumor-induced hypercalcemia complicated by renal failure. *Annals of Internal Medicine, 156,* 906–907.
19. Hu, M. I., et al. (2014). Denosumab for treatment of hypercalcemia of malignancy. *The Journal of Clinical Endocrinology and Metabolism, 99,* 3144–3152.
20. Asonitis, N., et al. (2017). Hypercalcemia of malignancy treated with cinacalcet. *Endocrinology, Diabetes & Metabolism Case Reports, 2017.*
21. Yu, N., et al. (2010). Increased mortality and morbidity in mild primary hyperparathyroid patients. The Parathyroid Epidemiology and Audit Research Study (PEARS). *Clinical Endocrinology, 73,* 30–34.
22. Wright, J. D., et al. (2015). Quality and outcomes of treatment of hypercalcemia of malignancy. *Cancer Investigation, 33,* 331–339.
23. Egi, M., et al. (2011). Ionized calcium concentration and outcome in critical illness. *Critical Care Medicine, 39,* 314–321.
24. Schattner, A., Dubin, I., Huber, R., & Gelber, M. (2016). Hypocalcaemia of malignancy. *The Netherlands Journal of Medicine, 74,* 231–239.
25. Fong, J., & Khan, A. (2012). Hypocalcemia: Updates in diagnosis and management for primary care. *Canadian Family Physician, 58,* 158–162.
26. Song, C.-Y., Zhao, Z.-X., Li, W., Sun, C.-C., & Liu, Y.-M. (2017). Pseudohypoparathyroidism with basal ganglia calcification: A case report of rare cause of reversible parkinsonism. *Medicine, 96,* e6312.
27. Abrantes, C., Brigas, D., Casimiro, H. J., & Madeira, M. (2018). Hypocalcaemia in an adult: The importance of not overlooking the cause. *BMJ Case Reports, 2018.*

CHAPTER **189**

HYPERKALEMIA AND HYPOKALEMIA

Amelia Siani Kerner

 Immediate referral is indicated for symptomatic hyper or hypokalemia.

DEFINITION AND EPIDEMIOLOGY

The definitions of hypokalemia and hyperkalemia are stated in terms of serum potassium levels. Normal values for serum potassium levels depend on individual laboratories, but the typical normal range is from 3.5 to 5 mEq/L. Potassium imbalances can be defined as acute or chronic and can be further categorized by the degree of severity. Chronic hypokalemia and hyperkalemia develop in a minimum of weeks to months, and acute hypokalemia and hyperkalemia occur over hours to days. Mild hypokalemia occurs at serum levels of 3.5 to 4 mEq/L; moderate hypokalemia 3 to 3.5 mEq/L; and severe hypokalemia below 3 mEq/L. Mild to moderate hyperkalemia occurs at serum levels of 5.5 to 6.9 mEq/L; and severe hyperkalemia at a serum level of 7 mEq/L or higher or in the presence of EKG changes resulting from elevated potassium.[1]

Hyper- and hypokalemia are two of the most commonly encountered electrolyte disturbances in medicine,[1] but their incidence varies greatly based upon the population being observed. Less than 1% of adults not taking medications have hyperkalemia or hypokalemia.[1] As such, the presence of hyperkalemia or hypokalemia suggests that the patient is taking medications or has a disease process that alters potassium excretion. Potassium disturbances are also observed more frequently among hospitalized patients.[2,3,4] In historical studies, hypokalemia was present in 50% of patients taking diuretics.[5] Hypokalemia is also more common in elderly populations.[4] Hyperkalemia is most common in patients with renal disease and particularly in those with the commonly comorbid conditions of diabetes and coronary vascular disease.[3,6] Patients taking renin-angiotensin-aldosterone system inhibitors (RAAS inhibitors) are also at increased risk for hyperkalemia.[2,3,6]

PATHOPHYSIOLOGY

Potassium is primarily an intracellular cation with 70% found in muscle and lesser amounts in bone, red blood cells, liver, and spleen.[1] Only 1% to 2% of total body potassium exists in the extracellular fluid. This gradient drives the sodium–potassium ATPase pump, which is present in virtually all of the body's cells. Maintaining this gradient is essential for nerve conduction, muscle contraction, and cardiac pacemaker activity.

Potassium is absorbed in the GI tract and then distributed between the intra- and extracellular fluid. Potassium levels are maintained primarily by the kidney with some input from sensors in the GI tract.[7] Potassium is excreted by the kidney in a process that depends upon sufficient tubular flow, normal collecting duct function, and normal aldosterone secretion.[1,3] Excessive or inadequate potassium intake in a healthy patient is rarely the cause of potassium imbalance. Internally, insulin is a significant hormonal modulator of potassium balance, as it stimulates cellular potassium uptake. Acid–base status also impacts potassium homeostasis, with alkalosis generally causing hypokalemia and acidosis causing hyperkalemia.[1,8]

In understanding disturbances of potassium metabolism, it is helpful to consider the root cause. Both hyper- and hypokalemia can result from potassium redistribution within the body's cells. Hyperkalemia can also result from impaired renal excretion or increased intake. Hypokalemia can result from increased potassium losses (renal or extrarenal) or from decreased potassium intake. Pseudo hyper- and hypokalemia are not uncommon and must always be ruled out.

CLINICAL PRESENTATION

Clinical signs and symptoms of acute hypokalemia include: weakness, palpitations, nausea, vomiting, hypotension, metabolic alkalosis, potassium less than 2.5, and EKG changes. EKG changes in hypokalemia include flattened T waves, the presence of U waves, ST depressions, and ventricular arrhythmias.[8] Rhabdomyolysis, ascending paralysis, and progression to respiratory arrest due to diaphragmatic paralysis and cardiac arrest are rare but severe complications of acute hypokalemia.[8] Chronic hypokalemia can cause impaired renal function, which manifests itself in hypertension and decreased urine osmolality.[1] Glucose intolerance is also observed due to a reduction in insulin production as a result of hypokalemia.[1]

Clinical manifestations of hyperkalemia are chiefly cardiac and are best monitored by EKG. Progressive EKG changes seen in hyperkalemia are peaked T waves, PR prolongation,

intraventricular block, sine waves, and ultimately ventricular fibrillation and asystole.[7,8] Severe hyperkalemia can cause muscle weakness and rarely ascending paralysis as seen in hypokalemia.[1]

PHYSICAL EXAMINATION

A thorough history and a complete diet and medication review are the most important parts of the patient assessment. Any history of diuretic use, vomiting, diarrhea, abnormal urinary output, diabetes, hypertension, and medication or diet changes should be elicited. The physical exam should focus on a full assessment of vital signs with a focus on blood pressure, assessment of volume status, and a thorough neuromuscular exam including muscle strength and reflex testing.

DIAGNOSTICS

Diagnostics should assess the degree of the potassium imbalance as well as the cause.

Essential Diagnostics

Serum electrolyte values, blood urea nitrogen level, serum creatinine concentration, and a random blood glucose, all found on a basic metabolic panel, will rapidly identify the presence of hyper- or hypokalemia. Pseudo hyper- or hypokalemia must be excluded by ruling out hemolysis of the lab sample and elevated white blood cell counts (i.e., a repeat serum potassium and complete blood count). An EKG should be performed immediately in any patient with severe hyper- or hypokalemia. Most often the cause of the potassium disturbance is apparent based on history (e.g., vomiting or diarrhea), medication review (e.g., diuretic or RAAS inhibitor use), or initial lab results (e.g., renal disease or diabetic ketoacidosis). Measuring the fractional excretion of potassium via a 24-hour urine potassium measurement is helpful in distinguishing between renal and nonrenal etiologies of potassium disorders. Additional diagnostics may be warranted and should focus on establishing the etiology of the disturbance and directing therapy. Hypomagnesemia often accompanies hypokalemia, indicating the importance of also obtaining a serum magnesium level.

Additional Diagnostics

Plasma Aldosterone
Plasma Cortisol

INITIAL DIAGNOSTICS

Hyperkalemia and Hypokalemia

LABORATORY
- Serum glucose, electrolytes, BUN, and creatinine
- Serum magnesium

IMAGING
- EKG

DIFFERENTIAL DIAGNOSIS

 Priority differentials include Hypokalemia: (1) Diuretic use, (2) diarrhea, (3) vomiting, (4) diabetic ketoacidosis, and (5) hyperosmolar hyperglycemia.
Hyperkalemia: (1) Acute kidney injury, (2) chronic kidney disease, and (3) medications.

BOX 189.1

Causes of Hypokalemia[9]

REDISTRIBUTION
- Medications
  - Insulin overdose
  - Beta 2 sympathomimetics
  - Decongestants
  - Xanthines
  - Amphotericin B
  - Verapamil intoxication
  - Chloroquine intoxication
  - Barium intoxication
  - Cesium intoxication
- Alkalosis
- Refeeding syndrome
- Increased beta$_2$ adrenergic stimulation
  - Delirium tremens
  - Head injury
  - Myocardial ischemia
- Thyrotoxicosis
- Familial hypokalemic periodic paralysis
- Hypothermia

PSEUDO HYPOKALEMIA
- Delayed sample analysis
- Leukocytosis > 75,000 cells/mm^3

EXTRARENAL LOSSES
- Medications
  - Laxatives and enemas

- GI Losses
  - Vomiting
  - Diarrhea
  - Orogastric tube losses
  - Dialysis/plasmapheresis

RENAL LOSSES
- Medications
  - Diuretics
  - Corticosteroids
- Osmotic diuresis
- Mineralocorticoid excess
- Type I and II renal tubular acidosis
- Polydipsia
- Intrinsic renal transport defects
  - Liddle syndrome
  - Bartter syndrome
  - Gitelman syndrome
- Hypomagnesemia

INADEQUATE INTAKE
- Anorexia
- Dementia
- "Tea and toast" diet

BOX 189.2

Causes of Hyperkalemia[9]

DECREASED RENAL EXCRETION
- Oliguric Renal Failure (acute or chronic)
- Medications
  - Angiotensin-converting enzyme inhibitors and angiotensin receptor blockers
  - Nonsteroidal anti-inflammatory drugs
  - Potassium sparing diuretics
  - Trimethoprim
  - Heparin
  - Lithium
  - Calcineurin inhibitors
- Decreased distal renal flow
  - Acute kidney injury/chronic kidney disease
  - Congestive heart failure
  - Cirrhosis
- Hyperaldosteronism
  - Hyporeninemic hypoaldosteronism
  - Adrenal insufficiency (Addison's disease)
  - Adrenocorticotropic hormone deficiency
  - Primary hyporeninemia
- Renal tubular defects
  - Sickle cell disease
  - Systemic lupus erythematosus
  - Obstructive uropathy
  - Hereditary tubular defects
  - Amyloidosis

REDISTRIBUTION
- Insulin deficiency or resistance
- Mineral Acidosis

- Hypertonicity
  - Hyperglycemia
  - Mannitol
- Medications
  - Beta-blockers
  - Digoxin toxicity
  - Somatostatin
  - Succinylcholine
- Cell breakdown or injury
  - Rhabdomyolysis
  - Crush injury
  - Tumor lysis syndrome
- Hyperkalemia periodic paralysis

INCREASED INTAKE
- Potassium supplementation
- Red blood cell transfusion
- Foods high in potassium
- Potassium containing salt substitutes
- Protein calorie supplements
- Penicillin G potassium
- Certain forms of pica (clay)

PSEUDO HYPERKALEMIA
- Hemolysis of laboratory sample
  - Tourniquet use
  - Fist clenching
- Blood sample cooling
- Intravenous fluids with potassium
- Cell hyperplasia
  - Leukocytosis (>75,000 cells/mm^3)
  - Erythrocytosis
  - Thrombocytosis
- Familial pseudohyperkalemia

Hypokalemia results from one of five causes: cellular redistribution, extra renal potassium losses, renal potassium losses, decreased intake, and pseudo hypokalemia.

Hyperkalemia is associated with four primary causes: cellular redistribution, decreased renal excretion, excess intake (nearly always in the setting of decreased renal excretion), and pseudo hyperkalemia (Boxes 189.1 and 189.2).

INTERPROFESSIONAL COLLABORATIVE MANAGEMENT

Nonpharmacologic Management

The management of hypokalemia and hyperkalemia begins with identifying the underlying cause so that it may be reversed if possible. The cause of the potassium imbalance is usually readily apparent, except for patients who are surreptitiously inducing vomiting or using large amounts of diuretics or laxatives. All at-risk patients should be frequently screened by laboratory analysis to avoid acute complications. When diuretics are prescribed, the patient's serum potassium concentration should be checked before initiation of treatment and then at week 1 and week 4 after the initiation of therapy. In patients with chronic hyperkalemia, any use of ACE inhibitors, ARBs, NSAIDs, potassium sparing diuretics, or salt substitutes containing potassium chloride should be reassessed and likely

discontinued. Any patient with a symptomatic potassium derangement should be evaluated for hospitalization. Those with acute kidney injury and hyperkalemia should also be hospitalized.

Pharmacologic Management

Acute Hypokalemia. The treatment of acute hypokalemia involves the administration of oral or intravenous potassium supplements. If life-threatening arrhythmias or neuromuscular symptoms are present, intravenous potassium supplementation should be initiated. Correction of 20 mmol/hour is standard.[9] Cardiac monitoring and frequent serum potassium assessments are essential. Potassium replacement is a common cause of hyperkalemia in the inpatient setting.[9] Once all cardiac arrhythmias or neuromuscular symptoms have disappeared, the patient may be switched to oral replacement.[1]

Chronic Hypokalemia. The primary goal of treatment of chronic hypokalemia is identification of the underlying cause. In cases of drug-induced hypokalemia, the medication should be changed if possible. If the clinical status prohibits this, then treatment depends on the degree of hypokalemia. All patients should receive dietary consultation focused on education about foods high in potassium.[9] In patients with potassium levels lower than 3.5 mEq/L, oral supplementation should be given, with normal doses ranging between 20 and 120 mEq/day. In patients with underlying cardiac disease, the target potassium level should be 4 mEq/L[10] because of the risk of hypertension and cardiac complications. Persons with hyperaldosteronism should be referred to an endocrinologist.

Acute Hyperkalemia. Efforts to treat acute hyperkalemia focus on redistributing the potassium into the cells, eliminating excess potassium, and working to correct the cause.[9] If a patient is symptomatic, with EKG changes, IV calcium gluconate or chloride should be administered to stabilize the myocardium.[1,8,9] The onset of calcium therapy is essentially immediate, but the duration is only 30 to 60 minutes, and this therapy does not correct the underlying hyperkalemia.[1] Calcium administration can be repeated in 5 minutes if ineffective on first dose[11] and should always be followed by a therapy aimed at lowering the serum potassium level.

Once the myocardium has been stabilized, or for patients who do not have cardiac manifestations of hyperkalemia, therapies should actively lower serum potassium levels by redistributing it into the intracellular space. Insulin is the most effective therapy and must be given with dextrose to avoid hypoglycemia.[11] Nebulized B2 agonists are also effective at redistributing potassium into cells and should be given in conjunction with insulin and dextrose following calcium administration in patients who have symptomatic hyperkalemia.[12]

Potassium binders can be given in patients who are stable enough to take oral medications. Sodium-polystyrene sulfonate (SPS) is the only potassium binder approved for use in acute hyperkalemia.[3,6] Its onset of action is a few hours, so it should not be used in place of the faster-acting therapies discussed above, but it can be administered in addition to these therapies. It can also be used in stable, asymptomatic patients with hyperkalemia. Due to concerns about colonic necrosis associated with SPS, the mixture with 70% sorbitol has been banned,[6] but versions with 33% sorbitol are still commonly used.

Sodium bicarbonate is occasionally used in the treatment of hyperkalemia and is most effective when hyperkalemia is a result of metabolic acidosis.[11,13] Loop diuretics may also be used to treat acute hyperkalemia as they increase potassium excretion but are only as effective as the patient's diuretic response.[12] Ultimately, hemodialysis may be required for treatment of refractory hyperkalemia in those with concomitant acute or chronic renal failure.

Chronic Hyperkalemia. Treatment of chronic hyperkalemia begins with eliminating modifiable causes such as dietary factors and medications.[7] Chronic hyperkalemia is most commonly observed in patients with chronic kidney disease and patients with heart failure or diabetes who are on RAAS inhibitors.[2,3,6] Hyperkalemia in those with chronic renal failure can be managed with diuretic therapy and ultimately

hemodialysis.[9] In those patients with heart failure or diabetes, if RAAS inhibitors are essential to their chronic disease management, thiazide or loop diuretic therapy has been a mainstay of treatment for hyperkalemia.[2] SPS is not approved for chronic use. Patiromer, a novel therapy for chronic hyperkalemia, has recently gained FDA approval following studies that demonstrated effective and safe maintenance of normokalemia over time.[14-17] Patiromer employs cation exchange to increase potassium excretion through the gut.[18]

Chronic hyperkalemia caused by hyperaldosteronism is treated with fludrocortisone. In Addison disease, treatment with replacement hydrocortisone should correct the hyperkalemia.

Consultations

Endocrinology for metabolic disorders.
Nephrology for patients with renal disease.
Cardiology for patients with heart failure, ACE/ARB use, and hyperkalemia.

COMPLICATIONS

Potassium disturbances are potentially life threatening. Hypokalemia can result in fatal cardiac conduction defects and arrhythmias as well as muscle weakness and fatal paralysis. Increased blood pressure, renal injury, and impaired glycemic control are complications of hypokalemia as well. Hyperkalemia also causes fatal cardiac arrhythmias, conduction defects, muscle weakness, and paralysis. Overcorrection in either repleting hypokalemia or mitigating hyperkalemia can result in iatrogenic complications from induced hyper- or hypokalemia. Hypoglycemia is a complication of treatment of hyperkalemia with insulin.

EMERGING MANAGEMENT TRENDS

Patiromer has been FDA approved for the treatment of chronic hyperkalemia, and a second cation exchanger, ZS-9, is currently seeking approval.[2,18] Neither medication has been studied or approved for use in the treatment of acute hyperkalemia. Clinical trials for both are ongoing.

PATIENT AND FAMILY EDUCATION

Patient education for potassium derangements should center on diet education (e.g., foods high in potassium). The importance of continued chronic supplementation therapy in the case of hypokalemia should be stressed. Patients should also be aware of the complications of hypo- and hyperkalemia and the importance of regularly scheduled laboratory monitoring. Education about the potential drug effects that can result in hypokalemia or hyperkalemia is also important. In patients with hypokalemia, chronic laxative use should be avoided, as this is associated with hypokalemia. Those taking potassium supplements should be advised not to crush the potassium tablets and to take them with a large glass of fluid in an effort to avoid uncomfortable GI symptoms. Those who are not tolerating potassium supplements should be advised to call or see a health care provider.

HEALTH PROMOTION

- Because potassium derangements are commonly associated with antihypertensive medications, health promotion should focus on prevention that leads to improved blood pressure and medication elimination if possible.

- In patients whose potassium disturbance is a result of renal failure, prevention and chronic disease management should be at the center of health promotion.
- When prevention is no longer possible, patient education regarding the need for monitoring of potassium levels and prevention and awareness of complications is paramount.

REFERENCES

1. Weiner, I. D., Linas, S. L., & Wingo, C. S. (2015). Comprehensive clinical nephrology. In R. J. M. D. Johnson, J. D. M. Feehally, & J. M. D. Floegu (Eds.), *Comprehensive clinical nephrology* (5th ed., pp. 111–123). Saunders.
2. Sarwar, C. M. S., Papadimitriou, L., Pitt, B., et al. (2016). Hyperkalemia in heart failure. *Journal of the American College of Cardiology, 68*(14), 1575–1589. doi:10.1016/j.jacc.2016.06.060.
3. Kovesdy, C. P. (2015). Management of hyperkalemia: An update for the internist. *The American Journal of Medicine, 128*(12), 1281–1287. doi:10.1016/j.amjmed.2015.05.040.
4. Bardak, S., Turgutalp, K., Koyuncu, M. B., et al. (2017). Community-acquired hypokalemia in elderly patients: Related factors and clinical outcomes. *International Urology and Nephrology, 49*(3), 483–489. doi:10.1007/s11255-016-1489-3.
5. Bloomfield, R. L., Wilson, D. J., & Buckalew, V. M. (1986). The incidence of diuretic-induced hypokalemia in two distinct clinic settings. *Journal of Clinical Hypertension, 2*(4), 331–338.
6. Kovesdy, C. P. (2017). Updates in hyperkalemia: Outcomes and therapeutic strategies. *Reviews in Endocrine and Metabolic Disorders, 18*(1), 41–47. doi:10.1007/s11154-016-9384-x.
7. Palmer, B. F., & Clegg, D. J. (2017). Diagnosis and treatment of hyperkalemia. *Cleveland Clinic Journal of Medicine, 84*(12), 934–942. doi:10.3949/ccjm.84a.17056.
8. Allon, M. (2018). National kidney foundation primer on kidney diseases. In S. J. Gilbert & D. E. Weiner (Eds.), *National kidney foundation primer on kidney diseases* (7th ed., pp. 97–106). Elsevier Inc. and National Kidney Foundation.
9. Viera, A. J., & Wouk, N. (2015). Potassium disorders: Hypokalemia and hyperkalemia. *American Family Physician, 92*(6), 487–495.
10. Macdonald, J. E., & Struthers, A. D. (2004). What is the optimal serum potassium level in cardiovascular patients? *Journal of the American College of Cardiology, 43*(2), 155–161.
11. Laurin, L.-P., & Leblanc, M. (2018). Critical care nephrology. In C. Ronco, R. Bellomo, J. A. Kellum, & Z. Ricci (Eds.), *Critical care nephrology* (3rd ed., pp. 339–344). Elsevier.
12. Rossignol, P., Legrand, M., Kosiborod, M., et al. (2016). Emergency management of severe hyperkalemia: Guideline for best practice and opportunities for the future. *Pharmacological Research, 113*(Pt A), 585–591. doi:10.1016/j.phrs.2016.09.039.
13. Rossignol, P., Legrand, M., Kosiborod, M., et al. (2016). Emergency management of severe hyperkalemia: Guideline for best practice and opportunities for the future. *Pharmacological Research, 113*, 585–591. doi:10.1016/j.phrs.2016.09.039.
14. Pitt, B., Bakris, G. L., Bushinsky, D. A., et al. (2015). Effect of patiromer on reducing serum potassium and preventing recurrent hyperkalaemia in patients with heart failure and chronic kidney disease on RAAS inhibitors. *European Journal of Heart Failure, 17*(10), 1057–1065. doi:10.1002/ejhf.402.
15. Bakris, G. L., Pitt, B., Weir, M. R., et al. (2015). Effect of patiromer on serum potassium level in patients with hyperkalemia and diabetic kidney disease. *JAMA: The Journal of the American Medical Association, 314*(2), 151. doi:10.1001/jama.2015.7446.
16. Weir, M. R., Bakris, G. L., Bushinsky, D. A., et al. (2015). Patiromer in patients with kidney disease and hyperkalemia receiving RAAS inhibitors. *The New England Journal of Medicine, 372*(3), 211–221. doi:10.1056/NEJMoa1410853.
17. Buysse, J. M., Huang, I.-Z., & Pitt, B. (2012). PEARL-HF: Prevention of hyperkalemia in patients with heart failure using a novel polymeric potassium binder, RLY5016. *Future Cardiol, 8*(1), 17–28. doi:10.2217/fca.11.71.
18. Krishnan, S. K., & Lepor, N. E. (2016). Acute and chronic cardiovascular effects of hyperkalemia: New insights into prevention and clinical management. *Reviews in Cardiovascular Medicine, 17*(Suppl. 1), S9–S21.

CHAPTER 190

HYPERNATREMIA AND HYPONATREMIA

Anthony Provenzano

 Immediate physician consultation, hospitalization, and treatment required for patients symptomatic with acute hypernatremia or serum sodium greater than 155 mEq/L and patients symptomatic with acute hyponatremia or serum sodium less than 120 mEq/L.

HYPERNATREMIA

DEFINITION AND EPIDEMIOLOGY

Hypernatremia, a serum sodium level greater than 145 mEq/L, can affect anyone, but children and older adults are frequently afflicted by this common electrolyte disorder. The causes of hypernatremia are varied but include a fluid volume deficit, excessive sodium intake, and other disorders.[1,2]

PATHOPHYSIOLOGY

Normally, water intake and water loss are balanced, but a disruption in water homeostasis can result in hypernatremia. Usually, when water loss exceeds water intake, serum osmolality rises above the normal range of 290 to 295, thirst is stimulated, water intake increases, and water balance is achieved. However, an array of disorders can affect serum sodium and fluid balance. Neoplasms, trauma, or vascular abnormalities can affect the thirst centers in the hypothalamus and result in an inadequate thirst response and hypernatremia. An increase in serum sodium can be the consequence of gastrointestinal distress (e.g., vomiting or diarrhea), diuresis (e.g., diuretic therapy, hyperglycemia), insensible water loss (e.g., fever or exercise), or other causes of water loss. In older adults, physiologic aging changes can increase susceptibility to electrolyte changes, but anyone who is incapable of adequately expressing thirst (e.g., an infant or cognitively impaired adult or elder) or unable to obtain water (e.g., a disabled patient) is at risk for developing hypernatremia.

An excess in water loss in relation to water intake leads to an increase in serum osmolality. In response, arginine vasopressin (AVP) (i.e., antidiuretic hormone [ADH]) is secreted from the posterior pituitary gland.[1] AVP increases the permeability of the renal collecting ducts to water. Water is then reabsorbed in the collecting ducts, and the urine becomes more concentrated.[1] Patients with a deficit in the production of AVP or a diminished renal response to AVP will develop hypernatremia if the water losses are not corrected. Older adults are especially at risk because of the diminished renal concentrating ability that occurs with aging.

Patients with diabetes insipidus develop hypernatremia when water intake is not enough to compensate for fluid loss. A hyperglycemic state (e.g., hyperosmolar nonketotic coma) or an osmotic diuretic (e.g., mannitol) can also cause a large amount of free water loss and result in a concerning rise in serum sodium, as can an increase in insensible water losses.[1] Normally, small amounts of fluids are lost from the skin, respiratory tract, and gastrointestinal tract, but vigorous exercise, fever, tachypnea, diarrhea, vomiting, and burns increase the volume of insensible water loss. Those with insufficient fluid intake in the setting of these conditions can easily develop hypernatremia.

Increased serum sodium is less often the result of excess sodium intake (e.g., rapid intravenous administration of normal saline or high-solute tube feedings). However, the resultant sodium excess can cause an increase in serum osmolality and expansion of extracellular volume.

CLINICAL PRESENTATION AND PHYSICAL EXAMINATION

The major clinical feature of hypernatremia is a central nervous system disturbance that results from dehydration and shrinkage of brain cells. The purpose of the history and physical examination is to determine the underlying cause of the increased serum sodium and guide diagnostics and treatment.[3] A recent history of fever, vomiting, diarrhea, polyuria, heat exposure, or surgery is significant. A careful review of medications (particularly a history of lithium or diuretic therapy), fluid intake and output during the previous 24 hours, and any intravenous therapy or tube feedings should be reviewed along with the past medical history.

Patients may report weakness, thirst, lightheadedness, or if the hypernatremia is related to a hypothalamic lesion, be asymptomatic. Signs and symptoms of hypernatremia can be nonspecific and not develop until the serum sodium level becomes higher than 150 mEq/L. Agitation, irritability, confusion, and personality changes are early signs. Muscle twitching, tremor, spasticity, hyperreflexia, and lethargy may also be evident.

Physical Examination

Classification of the patient's fluid volume status is essential and facilitated by evaluation of the patient's appearance, weight, orthostatic vital signs, and careful examination of the pulmonary, cardiac, and gastrointestinal systems. Neurologic screening, including motor tone, strength, coordination, and cognitive and functional ability, is necessary to determine subtle neurologic changes.

Physical findings depend on the severity of volume loss and can include fever, flushing, diminished skin turgor, flat neck veins, dry mucous membranes, weight loss, hypotension, tachycardia, and orthostatic hypotension. Muscle weakness, seizures, and muscle coma are later signs. Diminished urinary output is a potential finding, except if diabetes insipidus or an osmotic diuresis is the underlying cause of the hypernatremia. A change in mental status, a narrow pulse pressure, and delayed capillary filling associated with cool extremities are ominous signs requiring urgent hospitalization and intravenous fluid resuscitation

DIAGNOSTICS

Essential Diagnostics: Initial diagnostic testing includes serum glucose, serum electrolytes, urea, calcium, blood urea nitrogen (BUN) concentration, creatinine level, urinalysis, urine sodium, and serum and urine osmolality to determine fluid and electrolyte status. A serum sodium level above 145 mEq/L confirms hypernatremia. Serum osmolality can be calculated ($2[Na^+]$ + serum glucose/18 + BUN/2.8) or at https://www.mdcalc.com/serum-osmolality-osmolarity. If the serum osmolality is greater

than 300 mOsm/kg, the likely diagnosis is hypovolemic hypernatremia, but hypernatremia can also be associated with euvolemia (e.g., diabetes insipidus) or even hypervolemia (e.g., Cushing syndrome).[3]

Urine sodium levels can be elevated, normal, or decreased depending on the underlying cause of the hypernatremia. Urine osmolality, which normally can be 50 to 1200 mOsm/kg, is in patients with hypovolemic hypernatremia generally higher than 600 mOsm/kg, but decreased (less than 300 mOsm/kg) in patients taking diuretics or in those with diabetes insipidus or osmotic diuresis.

Urine specific gravity is not as precise as urine osmolality, but is a quick test to determine urine concentration. The urine specific gravity of patients with hypernatremia is elevated, except in the situations noted previously. Diabetes insipidus is associated with polyuria, low urine specific gravity, and low osmolality (less than 200 mOsm/kg).

Additional diagnostics to consider include a complete blood count (CBC) and differential if a serum lithium is indicated or if an infection is suspected. A computed tomography (CT) scan or magnetic resonance imaging (MRI) may be necessary to exclude a neurologic cause.

INITIAL DIAGNOSTICS

Hypernatremia

LABORATORY
- Serum glucose, electrolytes, BUN, creatinine, calcium and urea
- CBC and differential
- Urine sodium, urine osmolality, and urine specific gravity

IMAGING
- CT scan, MRI if indicated

DIFFERENTIAL DIAGNOSIS

 Priority differentials include (1) free water deficit (e.g., body water or gastrointestinal loss), (2) osmotic diuresis (e.g., hyperglycemia or osmotic diuresis), and (3) central diabetes insipidus.[4,5]

It is necessary to determine the underlying cause of the sodium imbalance because treatment options vary with the cause.

Hypervolemic Hypernatremia

Excess sodium intake with inadequate water intake, rapid administration intravenous saline, high solute tube feeding.

Hypovolemic Hypernatremia
- Diarrhea associated with lactulose, citrate of magnesia, infectious process, lactose intolerance, malabsorption syndrome.
- Diuresis: diuretic therapy, hyperglycemia.
- Free water deficit: abnormal thirst mechanism, excessive exercise or diaphoresis, febrile illness, inadequate water intake, peritoneal dialysis.

Euvolemic Hypernatremia
- Central diabetes insipidus.
- Nephrogenic diabetes insipidus.

INTERPROFESSIONAL COLLABORATIVE MANAGEMENT

It is necessary to determine and address the cause of the patient's hypernatremia and if the onset of the hypernatremia is acute, chronic, or acute on chronic, because this information can impact treatment—especially the serum sodium correction rate (e.g., acute hypernatremia and acute on chronic hypernatremia are more quickly corrected than chronic hypernatremia). However, in primary care that information might be difficult to ascertain unless the patient's past medical history includes chronic serum sodium elevation.

For patients with *hypovolemic hypernatremia*, treatment includes replacing the water loss and restoring the extracellular fluid volume. Hypernatremia can be managed on an outpatient basis if the degree of sodium imbalance is moderate and the patient is alert, cognitively intact, able to swallow safely, drink sufficient amounts of fluids, and mobile enough to obtain drinking water. Oral water replacement is the safest treatment for hypernatremia, if the above criteria are met.

More severe hypernatremia requires treatment in an inpatient setting and physician consultation for diagnostic and treatment recommendations to lower the patient's serum sodium appropriately (i.e., not too slowly or too quickly). For patients with hypovolemic hypernatremia (serum sodium 150 to 170), fluid resuscitation with intravenous normal saline (0.9%) or Ringer lactate is initially indicated.[6] Once vital signs are normalized and the urine output is adequate, the serum sodium level can be corrected with hypotonic intravenous fluid (5% dextrose in water or 0.45% NaCl) to the goal serum sodium, 145 mEq/L with the goal of decreasing the patient's hypernatremia by 0.5 mEq/L/hr, but usually no greater to avoid cerebral edema.[1,3,6,7] The infusion rate is critical because a rate that is too slow or too rapid increases the risk for death.[4,5,6] Frequent monitoring (e.g., every 2 hours or as directed by the physician) of the serum sodium as well as the serum glucose is necessary. If the serum glucose is too high, a change in intravenous fluid is indicated.[6]

In addition to monitoring the patient's serum sodium and glucose, the urine chemistry and fluid volume status must be monitored frequently (i.e., vital signs, intake and output, daily weight plus serum glucose, electrolytes, BUN, and creatinine). The serum osmolality is calculated initially, then 2 hours after therapy is started and every 2 to 4 hours depending on the patient's status throughout the treatment intervention in acute hypernatremia while the patient is receiving intravenous therapy.[3]

In accordance with the concern for too rapid a decrease in serum sodium, the fluid water deficit should also not be corrected too quickly (i.e., 50% of the fluid deficit is replaced in the first 24 hours, and the remainder replaced over a period of 24 to 72 hours).[6] The total time necessary can be up to 96 hours depending on the extent of the patient's water deficit (WD).[6] The WD should be calculated and is based on body weight (i.e., about 50% of a hypernatremic patient's total body weight). The recommended water deficit formula is: Water deficit = 0.5 Wgt (kg) [Serum Na/140-1].[6] A patient's ongoing water loss and electrolytes (e.g., potassium) should be replaced as indicated, and diuretics and laxatives held until the fluid deficit is corrected. The need for these medications should then be reevaluated, as some patients may need a diuretic to prevent fluid overload.

Euvolemic hypernatremia is managed differently. Hypernatremia caused by central diabetes insipidus is treated with intranasal desmopressin acetate (DDAVP), 10 to 20 mcg or vasopressin (dose dependent on patient fluid balance and laboratory results) to decrease renal water losses.[6] Nephrogenic diabetes insipidus is not uncommon in older adults and often is not serious. Treatment involves discontinuing the offending agent and correcting electrolyte abnormalities. Serum electrolyte levels and fluid status must be monitored closely.

Hypervolemic hypernatremia management involves removing the offending cause (e.g., saline infusion, soda bicarbonate [baking soda], or other exogenous sodium intake). Diuretic therapy (e.g., thiazide diuretic) and, when indicated, maintenance of fluid volume with hypotonic intravenous fluid can be necessary.[6]

CONSULTATIONS

Hypernatremia can cause significant mortality and treatment management for patients can be complex, especially in older adults. Physician consultation is indicated for patients with severe hypernatremia (serum sodium > 155 mEq/L) and/or severe volume depletion. Nephrology consultation is also recommended.

LIFE SPAN CONSIDERATIONS

Aging is associated with a decreased ability to cope with environmental, disease-related, and drug-related stressors in sodium and water balance. Hypernatremia is commonly associated with fever, dehydration, warm environments, high-solute tube feedings, and diuretic or laxative therapy. Regular monitoring and appropriate diagnostic testing of patients on medications associated with an increase in serum sodium (e.g., lithium, diuretic therapy) is essential.

COMPLICATIONS

Hypovolemic shock results when severe volume depletion is not corrected. If hypernatremia is not corrected or treatment is not carefully administered, patients may experience significant cognitive dysfunction, seizure, coma, ischemia, brain hemorrhage, or death.[6] Patients with cardiac disease should be monitored closely for signs and symptoms of congestive heart failure, which may occur if fluid is replaced too rapidly.

PATIENT AND FAMILY EDUCATION

Patients and families should understand that an adequate amount of fluid should normally be consumed each day and that older adults are at greater risk of hypernatremia because of aging changes, decreased thirst, and other possible factors (e.g., mobility). Important education includes maintaining proper fluid balance especially in hot weather, when sick, and when exercising. Patients with underlying conditions that put them at risk for hypernatremia need to be educated accordingly and those who are taking diuretics or medications such as lithium and carbamazepine need to be aware of the risk of hypernatremia.

HYPONATREMIA

 Immediate hospitalization and treatment required for patients who are moderately to severely symptomatic with hyponatremia.

DEFINITION AND EPIDEMIOLOGY

Hyponatremia is one of the more common electrolyte disorders seen in primary care and a significant cause of morbidity and mortality, particularly in older adults, but patients of all ages are at risk of developing a low serum sodium. Potential causes of hyponatremia include infections, traumatic brain injuries, malignant disease, endurance exercise, untoward medication effects, endocrine disorders, psychogenic polydipsia, syndrome of inappropriate antidiuretic hormone (SIADH), cerebral or renal salt wasting, acquired immunodeficiency syndrome (AIDS), a dysfunction in the release of ADH (i.e., vasopressin), and other illnesses.[6,7]

Hyponatremia is defined as a serum sodium concentration of less than 135 mEq/L and can be an acute or a chronic condition. Acute hyponatremia sometimes develops in hospitalized patients after surgery and is often associated with fluid overload. Thiazide therapy and other medications can also cause hyponatremia. Chronic hyponatremia commonly occurs outside the hospital, often is acquired over a longer period, and can be the cause of falls, gait problems, cognitive changes, and osteoporosis. Some patients with low serum sodium can be surprisingly asymptomatic.[7] A marginally low serum sodium (e.g., 130 to 134 mEq/L) may not seem concerning, but even this slight decrease in serum sodium can be associated with adverse patient events, hospitalization, and mortality.[7]

Exercise-associated hyponatremia (EAH) initially was associated with females, but EAH also affects males and has occurred in varied exercise events (e.g., cycling, canoeing, running, swimming, calisthenics, and even weight-lifting).[8,9] Increased water intake before and after an exercise regimen, abnormal arginine vasopressin (AVP, also known as antidiuretic hormone) secretion, activation of both the sympathetic nervous system and renin–angiotensin–aldosterone system, sudden water absorption from the gastrointestinal tract, glycogen metabolism, and decreased sodium intake in the days prior to an exercise event all have been associated with EAH. However, these are not proven causes. Sodium loss associated with sweating does not seem to be a factor, but rhabdomyolysis may play a role.[9] Nonsteroidal antiinflammatory drugs (NSAIDs) have also been suspect, because of their antagonistic effect on ADH.

PATHOPHYSIOLOGY

Sodium and other anions regulate body water and are determinants of serum osmolality (i.e., plasma tonicity). If serum sodium levels fall below normal limits, serum osmolality is decreased and extracellular water is permitted to seep into cells. This results in a hypotonic hyponatremia and cerebral brain cell swelling that causes the neurologic features associated with hyponatremia. Normally, the body responds to an excess amount of water by diuresis. Renal mechanisms and vasopressin control body fluid volume and the composition of body fluids. An increase in serum osmolality above the normal 275 to 295 mOsm/kg stimulates the posterior pituitary to release vasopressin influencing the distal tubules and collecting ducts in the kidneys to conserve water. As body fluid accumulates and serum osmolality becomes hypotonic, vasopressin is inhibited. In most circumstances, vasopressin release is affected by serum osmolality and blood pressure (i.e., baroregulation), but drugs, hypokalemia, infections, malignancy, pain, stress, and others factors can affect vasopressin release and cause the SIADH secretion.[7,10,11] Medications and a person's genetic predisposition can also affect water output in the collecting ducts of the kidneys and thus decrease serum sodium.[11]

Further causes of hyponatremia can be related to a decrease in AVP secretion that is related to an increase in fluid intake associated with dipsogenic, psychogenic, or iatrogenic polydipsia.[1] Beer potomania, the ingestion of large quantities of beer, and a reset osmostat have also been identified as precipitants of hypotonic hyponatremia with euvolemia.[10] Individuals with beer potomania derive most of their calorie intake from large quantities of beer, which contains relatively few solutes. The reduced solute delivery to the distal tubule restricts urine production and results in hyponatremia.[7] The reset osmostat phenomenon, a type of SIADH, is found in patients with malignancy, malnutrition, debilitating conditions, and even pregnancy. Changes in cellular metabolism cause hypothalamic osmoreceptors to reset to maintain a lowered serum osmolality. The diagnosis of reset osmostat can be complicated. BUN and creatinine concentrations are usually normal, but urine sodium and osmolality are variable.[10]

Hyponatremia is also associated with hyperglycemia causing intracellular fluid to shift into the extracellular compartment, resulting in a lower serum sodium because of the increase in extracellular fluid.[7,10] The effect of the solute changes that occur with hyperglycemia is an isotonic or hypertonic hyponatremia.[10] Mannitol, surgical irrigants (e.g., glycine), and radiographic contrast agents act similarly and cause a hypertonic hyponatremia.[10] Significantly increased amounts of plasma proteins and lipids trigger a factitious decrease in serum sodium and result in an isotonic pseudohyponatremia.[10]

CLINICAL PRESENTATION AND PHYSICAL EXAMINATION

Patients who present with acute hyponatremia are usually quite symptomatic[7]: new-onset confusion, severe headache, seizures, or coma. More subtle signs and symptoms associated with hyponatremia include headache, blurred vision, dizziness, lethargy, weakness, irritability, restlessness, impaired central nervous system function, history of falls, nonspecific gastrointestinal complaints (e.g., anorexia, nausea, vomiting), influenza-like symptoms, cardiac or respiratory distress, dysgeusia, unusual water-drinking behavior, or weight changes.[10,11] A thorough medication review including over-the-counter medications (e.g., NSAIDs) and diuretic or corticosteroid therapy is important because numerous medications will precipitate this disorder. Further information should include history of alcohol, allergies, "ecstasy" or other illicit drug use, head injury, recent endurance exercise, illness (e.g., vomiting or diarrhea), surgery (particularly genitourologic), previous illnesses or psychiatric history, and, in women, menstrual status and possibility of pregnancy.[7,9,10] Unfortunately, patient symptoms are often subtle and the history inconclusive, but the present and past medical history can be important in identifying the cause of lowered serum sodium and determining if the onset is acute (less than 48 hours duration) or chronic (longer than 48 hours).

A complete physical examination, including weight, orthostatic vital sign changes, and determination of physical signs of euvolemia, volume depletion, and fluid overload (i.e., skin turgor, mucous membranes, presence of ascites, edema), is essential. The evaluation requires careful patient observation for mental status changes, gait abnormalities, and level of consciousness, as well as for signs of heart failure, cirrhosis, or myxedema.[11] Stupor, seizures, psychosis, and coma are possible and associated with serum sodium levels below 120 mEq/L.

DIAGNOSTICS

Essential Diagnostics

Initial diagnostic testing includes a spot urine sodium, urine for osmolality, and uric acid in addition to a metabolic profile (i.e., serum glucose, electrolytes, BUN, creatinine) to determine volume status and cause of the decreased sodium.

Additional diagnostics may also be indicated depending on the patient presentation (e.g., a patient with a fever would require a CBC and differential). Other considerations could include liver function tests, thyroid-stimulating hormone, urea, alcohol level, plasma BNP, serum lactate, copeptin (to aid in diagnosis of nephrogenic diabetes insipidus), ACTH stimulation test (if recent steroid therapy), and cortisol levels (if ACTH deficiency is a concern).[10] Imaging is necessary for suspected congestive heart failure, malignancy, or neurologic issue.

DIFFERENTIAL DIAGNOSIS

The differential diagnoses for hyponatremia are myriad. Once the laboratory results are available, it is necessary to calculate the patient's volume status (i.e., hypovolemia, euvolemia, or hypervolemia) to aid in differentiating the varied causes of hyponatremia (Fig. 190.1). Using an online calculator (e.g., www.mdcalc.com/serum-osmolality-osmolarity), determine the patient's serum osmolality to establish if patient has an isotonic hyponatremia (280 mOsm/kg), hypotonic hyponatremia (<280 mOsm/kg), or hypertonic hyponatremia (>280 mOsm/kg). After the volume status and osmolality is available, the following steps are helpful in differentiating the patient diagnosis.

1. If the patient's serum glucose is elevated, it is necessary to correct the measured serum glucose (available at www.mdcalc.com/sodium-correction-for-hyperglycemia) to exclude hyperglycemia as the cause of the hyponatremia. Hyperglycemia results in an isotonic or hypertonic hyponatremia, is a nonhypotonic hyponatremia, and does not cause brain edema.

2. Eliminate other causes of nonhypotonic hyponatremia: recent mannitol or hypertonic radiocontrast dye exposure, or pseudohyponatremia related to elevated protein, cholesterol, or triglycerides.[11,12]

3. If the patient does not have severe or acute symptoms and the serum sodium is greater than 120 mmol/L, determine the patient's volume status, urine osmolality, and urine sodium and discuss results with the consulting physician.[10]

   a. Euvolemic hypotonic hyponatremia

      A urine osmolality less than 100 mOsm/kg combined with a urine sodium less than 20 mEq/L suggests an increase in water intake (i.e., beer potomania, low solute intake, or primary polydipsia).

      If a urine osmolality is greater than 100 mOsm/kg and the urine sodium is greater than 20 mEq/L, consider adrenal insufficiency, hypothyroidism, or SIADH. However, if the SIADH is related to reset thermostat, the urine osmolality could be lower.[10,11]

   b. Hypervolemic hypotonic hyponatremia

      Urine osmolality greater than 100 mOsm/kg associated with a urine sodium less than 20 mEq/L: consider cirrhosis of the liver, heart failure, or nephrotic syndrome.

Urine osmolality greater than 100 mOsm/kg associated with a urine sodium greater than 20 mEq/L suggests worsening renal function.

   c. Hypovolemic hypotonic hyponatremia

      Urine osmolality is usually significantly elevated. If the urine sodium is greater than 20 mEq/L, consider diuretic therapy, osmotic diuresis, cerebral salt wasting, and other causes.

      Urine sodium concentration below 20 mEq/L suggests non-renal cause (e.g., diarrhea, vomiting, or third spacing).

There are caveats to the above differentials and diagnostic results. Urine sodium levels can be misleading in some circumstances. Patients with SIADH, if anorexic or following a low-sodium diet, could have a lower urinary sodium.[10] Diuretics can also increase urinary sodium, complicating evaluation of volume status and necessitating the fractional excretion of urea to determine if the patient has hypovolemic hyponatremia and prerenal azotemia.[7] Patients with chronic kidney disease, on diuretic therapy, or on a low sodium diet can also have a low urine sodium.[12]

 Priority differentials include (1) acute vs. chronic onset symptomatic hyponatremia, (2) exercise- or drug-induced hyponatremia, (3) cerebral salt wasting syndrome or SIADH, and (4) hypovolemic or hypervolemic hyponatremia.

Acute-onset symptomatic hyponatremia occurs in less than 24 to 48 hours and is associated with a critical change in a patient's status (e.g., seizures or coma).[7] Early diagnosis, ICU admission, and treatment with hypertonic (3%) saline is crucial.[7,10,13,14,15]

Endurance exercise hyponatremia, an acute hyponatremia, must be differentiated from acute altitude illness, dehydration, or heat-related illness to prevent inappropriate and life-threatening treatment.[9] Metabolic disturbances, severe illness, infection, medications (e.g., NSAIDS, lithium, thiazides, desmopressin, vasopressin), depression, endocrine abnormalities, nutritional deficiencies, polydipsia, trauma, and cardiovascular and cerebrovascular accidents should be considered in the differential diagnosis.

Cerebral salt wasting syndrome (CSWS) is associated with some sort of intracranial stress (e.g., traumatic brain injury, infection, subarachnoid hemorrhage or other brain damage).[14] It is easily confused with SIADH, likely because hyponatremia is predominant in both CSWS and SIADH and SIADH can also be precipitated by brain insult.[14] However, extracellular fluid volume is decreased and urine sodium wasting occurs in CSWS—in other words, these patients are hypovolemic. SIADH is associated with increased fluid retention, a resultant decrease in serum sodium, and generally euvolemia.[14]

INTERPROFESSIONAL COLLABORATIVE MANAGEMENT

In primary care, the cause of hyponatremia is often medication related. For that reason, it is essential to obtain a serum sodium level within 5 days (some patients will develop hyponatremia even sooner) after the initiation of a medication known to cause hyponatremia (e.g., carbamazepine, clofibrate, levetiracetam, NSAID, thiazide diuretic, or selective serotonin receptor reuptake inhibitor). A serum sodium level that is even slightly lower than normal should be concerning. The medication should be discontinued and the patient started on

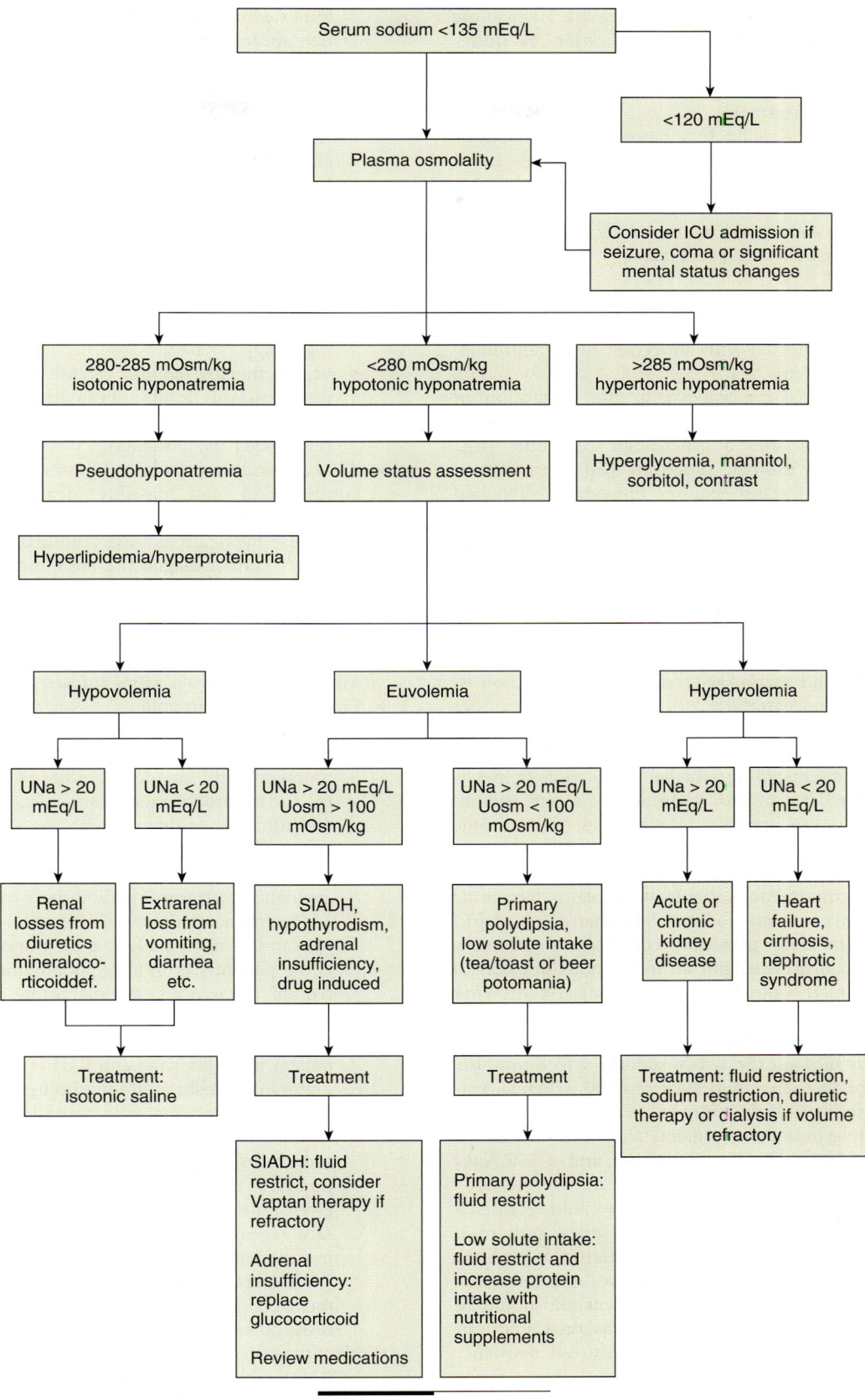

fluid restriction, and any salt restriction removed. High-solute foods are also often recommended. Any medication that causes hyponatremia should not be restarted.

Acute or symptomatic hyponatremia requires further diagnostic evaluation and treatment.

Most patients who develop hyponatremia do so because of an underlying cause, so diagnosis and treatment are based not only on classifying the hyponatremia (i.e., acute versus chronic, symptomatic versus asymptomatic, normal versus volume deficit or volume overload, and tonicity) but also on the reason for the patient's change in status.

Isotonic Hyponatremia

- Pseudohyponatremia associated with hyperproteinemia or hyperlipidemia is treated with correction of hyperproteinemia or hyperlipidemia.[8]
- Pseudohyponatremia associated with the absorption of a hypotonic or an isotonic irrigant solution containing glycine or sorbitol after a gynecologic procedure (e.g., hysteroscopy) or a urologic procedure (e.g., transurethral resection of the prostate) requires immediate physician/specialist consultation and discontinuation of the irrigant solution.[16,17,18] Diuretic therapy is necessary if the patient has fluid overload and the acute hyponatremia protocol for correction of a critically low serum sodium implemented with intravenous hypertonic (3%).

Hypertonic Hyponatremia

- Hyperglycemia and mannitol excess require correction of plasma glucose concentration.[10]

Hypotonic Hyponatremia

- If there is doubt regarding whether the hyponatremia is acute as opposed to chronic, correction of serum sodium should follow the treatment guidelines for chronic hyponatremia.[10,11]
- Acute hyponatremia
  - Severely symptomatic patients with acute hypotonic hyponatremia (serum sodium less than 120 mEq/L) require immediate physician consultation, hospitalization, and treatment with an intravenous infusion of 3% NaCl (*NOT* isotonic normal saline), 100 mL over 10 minutes.[12] If necessary, two repeated infusions of 100 mL of 3% NaCl, each over 10 minutes, are recommended to increase the serum sodium 4 to 6 mmol/L, treat the brain edema, and avert cerebral ischemia, herniation, and neurologic injury.[10]
  - Moderately symptomatic patients with acute hypotonic hyponatremia require hospitalization and a 3% NaCl infusion at 0.5 to 2 mL/kg/hr.[10,12]
  - Hypovolemic hyponatremia requires fluid resuscitation with isotonic saline; or, if the serum sodium is less than 120 mmol/L, 3% NaCl is required for volume repletion.[10] Once the patient's fluid volume status has been restored, the cause of the hypovolemia should be pursued (e.g., diuretic therapy, gastrointestinal fluid loss, cerebral salt wasting, and mineralocorticoid deficiency should be further investigated).
  - Hypervolemic hyponatremia requires fluid and dietary sodium restriction.[10]
    - In heart failure–associated hyponatremia, fluid restriction is initially indicated. Physician consultation is

indicated for diuretic therapy, neurohormonal blockade, and/or vaptan therapy.
- In cirrhosis-related hyponatremia, fluid restriction in combination with diuretic therapy (i.e., spironolactone as well as a loop diuretic) is recommended, as is a low-sodium diet and possibly paracentesis. Physician consultation is indicated for further treatment.[10]
- In nephrotic syndrome–related hyponatremia, fluid restriction is considered the best treatment, although vaptan therapy can be considered in consultation with the physician.
- Daily fluid restriction should be less than the patient's urinary output and insensible losses (i.e., the patient should be urinating more fluid than they are ingesting).
- Vaptan therapy requires careful monitoring for liver dysfunction, is contraindicated in patients with liver disease, and is not indicated for long-term therapy (i.e., longer than 30 days).[10]
- A serum sodium 130 to 135 mmol/L requires careful consideration and possibly treatment. The serum sodium measurement should be repeated, medications that cause hyponatremia discontinued, and fluid intake limited.[10] Further diagnostics are indicated if the repeat serum sodium reveals continued hyponatremia. If the serum sodium decrease is more than 10 mmol/L, the patient should be hospitalized and in consultation with the physician receive a single infusion of hypertonic saline (150 mL of 3% saline infused over 20 minutes).
- Euvolemic hyponatremia.
  - Exercise–induced hyponatremia requires oxygenation to maintain oxygen saturation at 95% (Grade 1C recommendation, American College of Chest Physicians [ACCP]), hospitalization for serum sodium analysis, and intravenous therapy with the appropriate intravenous fluid. Until diagnostic evaluation and hospitalization are possible, fluid volume assessment and avoidance of hypotonic fluid are necessary[8,9] (Grade 1A recommendation [ACCP]). Fluid restriction is appropriate if the patient is alert and appropriate or if the patient has mild hyponatremia and does not require intravenous support before hospitalization. If available, 125 mL water mixed with 4 chicken broth bouillon cubes is also suitable.[9] When the patient is hospitalized and EAH is confirmed by laboratory diagnosis, a 100-mL bolus of 3% hypertonic saline is appropriate, with two additional boluses at 10-minute intervals if necessary to increase the serum sodium by 4 to 5 mmol/L (Grade 1A recommendation [ACCP]).[9,10] If available, the initial bolus may be given on-site where the EAH occurred and, if necessary, repeated two more times.[10] Patients with acute hyponatremia that occurred over a short span of time (i.e., several hours) should improve with this treatment regimen and should not require further treatment other than monitoring.
- Nephrogenic syndrome of inappropriate antidiuresis (NSIAD) requires fluid restriction and possibly treatment with low-dose urea. Vasopressin receptor antagonist (vaptan) therapy is not indicated for this disorder.[13]
- Glucocorticoid deficiency should be excluded for all patients with euvolemic hyponatremia. Measure serum

cortisol and rapid cosyntropin-stimulation test results and, in consultation with physician, begin glucocorticoid therapy, but do not limit fluid intake.[10] Monitor serum sodium carefully because rapid escalation of serum sodium is possible and will require possible treatment with intravenous dextrose and water, as well as desmopressin, requiring physician consultation.[10]

- Hypothyroidism: Fluid restriction and thyroid replacement are usual therapies. Physician consultation is recommended for patients with myxedema.
- Low solute intake: improve nutritional intake of protein and electrolytes.
- Polydipsia
  - Primary polydipsia: fluid restriction, ice chips, hard candies to decrease thirst.[10]
  - Psychogenic polydipsia: Usually a chronic condition. Fluid restriction, behavioral therapy, and medication therapy (possibly with clozapine) are recommended.[10]
- SIADH
  - Acute-onset SIADH causing symptomatic hyponatremia is possible. Diagnostic testing is necessary to confirm diagnosis. Hospitalization and treatment with 3% NaCl by bolus or intravenous infusion is indicated.[10]
  - Chronic SIADH requires fluid restriction (i.e., nonfood fluids 500 mL/day below the 24-hour urine volume) for several days. Sodium and protein intake is not restricted. If the urine reveals low electrolyte-free water excretion or serum sodium fails to normalize with fluid restriction in the next 24 to 48 hours, vasopressin receptor antagonists (vaptans) or other pharmacologic interventions can be considered.[10] Adequate fluid intake (not fluid restriction) is essential the first 24 to 48 hours after vaptan (i.e., conivaptan, tolvaptan) therapy is initiated, and serum sodium requires careful monitoring (every 6 hours for 48 hours).[10] Stop vaptan therapy if water intake is not adequate or patient condition worsens, and monitor serum sodium more frequently.[10]
    - Patients with an elevated urine osmolality (>500 mOsm/kg water) do not usually respond to fluid restriction and will require pharmacologic therapy, as will patients with a low 24-hour urine volume (<1500 mL/day), patients whose combined urinary Na$^+$ and K$^+$ amounts are greater than the serum Na$^+$, and those in whom the serum Na$^+$ concentration fails to exceed 2 mmol/L/day after a fluid restriction of 1 L/day for 24 to 48 hours.[10]
    - Serum sodium is monitored frequently depending on the patient's clinical condition (e.g., 2 to 4 hours until it is 125 mmol/L).
- Chronic hyponatremia
  - Severe chronic hyponatremia increases the risk for osmotic demyelination syndrome (ODS) if the serum sodium is corrected too quickly. For this reason, the serum sodium in chronic hyponatremia is corrected a maximum of 4 to 8 mmol/L/day if osmotic demyelination is not a serious concern, but only 4 to 6 mmol/L/day if osmotic demyelination is a more likely possibility (i.e., patient with history of advanced liver disease, alcoholism, malnutrition, hypokalemia, or serum sodium 105 mmol/L or less).[10,12] The 24-hour serum sodium

goal for patients at great risk for ODS should not surpass 8 mmol/L/day.[10] For patients with average risk for ODS, the 24-hour serum sodium goal should not exceed 10 to 12 mmol/L/day.[10] Overcorrection should be prevented, and saline and/or vasopressin receptor antagonists (i.e., vaptan medications such as tolvaptan used in the treatment of SIADH) discontinued when the goal of therapy has been attained).

- The criteria for vaptan therapy require that the patient not have hypovolemic hyponatremia, nor should vaptan therapy be administered immediately after or concurrently with treatment with 3% NaCl or other therapies.[10] Physician consultation is recommended to determine if free water, intravenous 5% dextrose in water infusion, or desmopressin or vaptan therapy is indicated.[10]
- Repeat serum sodium levels are recommended at hours 1, 6, 12, and 24, with continued exploration of the cause if the patient is not improving. In practice, sodium should be checked every 2 hours when < 120 and every 2 to 4 hours when < 125 to ensure that the trajectory is upward and appropriate.
- Physician consultation is necessary for treatment of overcorrection of chronic hyponatremia and may be necessary for patients at risk of ODS.[10]

COMPLICATIONS

Brain damage or death from the encephalopathy that results from untreated hyponatremia is the most serious complication of hyponatremia. ODS (central pontine myelinolysis) is the untoward consequence of overcorrecting the serum sodium with intravenous hypertonic saline.[10,11] ODS can occur with rapid correction of serum sodium but has also been associated with slower correction of hyponatremia as well as with hypokalemia.

Emerging Management Trends
Patient and Family Education
- Prevention of EAH
  - Fluid consumption should be judicious and based on thirst[9] (Grade 1C recommendation [ACCP]).
  - Weight gain during exercise is an indication that fluid intake should be curtailed until body weight is within 2% to 4% of the person's normal body weight[9] (Grade 1B recommendation [ACCP]).
  - Sodium supplements in exercise-related events lasting less than 18 hours have no known efficacy[8] (Grade 2B recommendation [ACCP]).
  - Athletes should be carefully monitored for cognitive changes, coma, seizures, and severe dyspnea.[9]
  - Education for runners and other athletes competing in endurance events should also include careful explanation of the early symptoms of hyponatremia and the importance of seeking medical attention to avoid the serious sequelae.
  - Patients and caregivers (both family and professional) need to understand the nature of the hyponatremic disorder and recognize its associated neurologic symptoms as well as treatment side effects that necessitate health care provider notification.
  - Instructions regarding the importance of good oral hygiene, skin care, frequent weight measurements,

dietary or fluid restriction, intake and output measurement, and medications (and their side effects) should be explicit and understandable.

- Frequent follow-up care with continuous evaluation of the treatment plan is imperative.

Indications for Referral or Hospitalization

Patients with acute hyponatremia, acute-on-chronic hyponatremia, and or moderate or profound symptomatic hyponatremia require hospitalization and consultation with a physician familiar with the treatment of hyponatremia. Patients with chronic hyponatremia recalcitrant to therapy should also be referred for specialist consultation.

REFERENCES

1. Robertson, G. L. (2014). Disorders of the neurohypophysis. In D. Kasper, A. Fauci, S. Hauser, D. Longo, J. Jameson, & J. Loscalzo (Eds.), *Harrison's principles of internal medicine* (19th ed.). New York, NY: McGraw-Hill. http://accessmedicine.mhmedical.com.ezproxy.simmons.edu:2048/content.aspx?bookid=1130&sectionid=79751712. (Accessed 3 October 2017).

2. Bataille, S., Barrala, C., Torro, D., Buffat, C., Berland, Y., Alazia, M., et al. (2014). Undertreatment of hypernatremia is frequent and associated with mortality. *BMC Nephrology, 15*, 37.

3. Howard, C., & Berl, T. (2009). Chapter 3. Disorders of water balance: Hyponatremia & hypernatremia. In E. V. Lerma, J. S. Berns, & A. R. Nissenson (Eds.), *Current diagnosis & treatment: Nephrology & hypertension.* New York, NY: McGraw-Hill. http://accessmedicine.mhmedical.com.ezproxy.simmons.edu:2048/content.aspx?bookid=372&sectionid=39961138. (Accessed 3 October 2017).

4. Stern, S. C., Cifu, A. S., & Altkorn, D. (Eds.), (2014). Hyponatremia and hypernatremia. In *Symptom to diagnosis: An evidence-based guide* (3rd ed.). New York, NY: McGraw-Hill. http://accessmedicine.mhmedical.com.ezproxy.simmons.edu:2048/content.aspx?bookid=1088&sectionid=61699500. (Accessed 3 October 2017).

5. Petrino, R., & Marino, R. (2016). Fluids and electrolytes. In J. E. Tintinalli, J. Stapczynski, O. Ma, D. M. Yealy, G. D. Meckler, & D. M. Cline (Eds.), *Tintinalli's emergency medicine: A comprehensive study guide* (8th ed.). New York, NY: McGraw-Hill. http://accessmedicine.mhmedical.com.ezproxy.simmons.edu:2048/content.aspx?bookid=1658&sectionid=109385225. (Accessed 3 October 2017).

6. Latcha, S. (2016). Electrolyte disorders in critically ill patients. In J. M. Oropello, S. M. Pastores, & V. Kvetan (Eds.), *Critical care.* New York, NY: McGraw-Hill. http://accessmedicine.mhmedical.com.ezproxy.simmons.edu:2048/content.aspx?bookid=1944&sectionid=143517373. (Accessed 8 October 2017).

7. Braun, M. M., Barstow, C. H., & Pyzocha, N. J. (2015). Diagnosis and management sodium disorders: Hyponatremia and hypernatremia. *American Family Physician, 1*(91), 299–307.

8. Cho, K. C. (2018). Electrolyte & acid-base disorders. In M. A. Papadakis, S. J. McPhee, & M. W. Rabow (Eds.), *Current medical diagnosis & treatment.* New York, NY: McGraw-Hill. http://accessmedicine.mhmedical.com.ezproxy.simmons.edu:2048/content.aspx?bookid=2192&sectionid=168018151. (Accessed 7 October 2017).

9. Hew-Butler, T., Loi, V., Pani, A., & Rosner, M. H. (2017). Exercise-associated hyponatremia: 2017 update. *Frontiers in Medicine, 4*, 21. doi:10.3389/fmed.2017.00021.

10. Verbalis, J. G., Goldsmith, S. R., Greenberg, A., Korselius, C., Schrier, R. W., Sterns, R. H., et al. (2013). Diagnosis, evaluation, and treatment of hyponatremia: Expert panel opinion. *The American Journal of Medicine, 126*(10A), S1–S41.

11. Spasvoski, G., Vanholder, R., Allolio, B., Annane, D., Ball, S., Bichet, D., et al. (2014). Clinical practice guideline on diagnosis and treatment of hyponatraemia. *European Journal of Endocrinology, 170*, G1–G4.

12. Horne, E. J., & Zietse, R. (2013). Hyponaremia and mortality: Moving beyond associations. *American Journal of Kidney Disease, 62*(1), 139–149. doi:10.1053/j.ajkd.2012.09.019. [Epub 2013 Jan 4].

13. Krummel, T., Prinz, E., Metten, M.-A., et al. (2016). Prognosis of patients with severe hyponatraemia is related not only to hyponatraemia but also to comorbidities and to medical management: Results of an observational retrospective study. *BMC Nephrology, 17*, 159. doi:10.1186/s12882-016-0370-z.

14. Nakajima, H., Okada, H., Hirose, K., et al. (2017). Cerebral salt-wasting syndrome and inappropriate antidiuretic hormone syndrome after subarachnoid hemorrhaging. *Internal Medicine, 56*(6), 677–680.

15. Kumar, N., Law, A., & Choudhry, N. K. (Eds.) (2017). Hyponatremia. In *Teaching rounds: A visual aid to teaching internal medicine pearls on the wards.* New York, NY: McGraw-Hill. http://accessmedicine.mhmedical.com.ezproxy.simmons.edu:2048/content.aspx?bookid=1856&sectionid=130944880. (Accessed 18 October 2017).

16. Demirel, I., Ozer, A. B., Bayar, M. K., & Erhan, O. L. (2012). TURP syndrome and severe hyponatremia under general anaesthesia. *BMJ Case Reports, 2012*, bcr–2012-006899. doi:10.1136/bcr-2012-006899.

17. Brown, C. S. (2014). Dilutional hyponatremia in a community hospital setting: Case report. *Intensive and Critical Care Nursing, 30*(1), 1–5. doi:10.1016/j.iccn.2013.07.004. [Epub 2013 Sep 19].

18. Hepp, P., Jüttner, T., Beyer, I., Fehm, T., Janni, W., & Monaca, E. (2015). Rapid correction of severe hyponatremia after hysteroscopic surgery—a case report. *BMC Anesthesiology, 15*, 85. doi:10.1186/s12871-015-0070-4.

CHAPTER **191**

LIPID DISORDERS
Mary Young-Breuleux

 Immediate emergency department referral is indicated for patients who have severe hypertriglyceridemia and elevated liver and/or pancreatic enzymes, chest pain, respiratory difficulties, or rhabdomyolysis.

DEFINITION AND EPIDEMIOLOGY

Lipid disorders are a significant risk factor in the development of atherosclerotic cardiovascular disease (ASCVD), which remains the leading cause of death in the United States. Adults older than 20 years in the United States have a 69% incidence of low-density-lipoprotein cholesterol (LDL-C) of >100 mg/dL.[1]

The 2013 American College of Cardiology (ACC) and American Heart Association (AHA) guidelines report that lowering of LDL-C is a primary focus, based on its correlation with increased risk of ASCVD.[2]

Therapeutic lifestyle changes (TLCs), which include a heart-healthy diet, exercise, weight loss, and avoidance of tobacco, remain the first and most important intervention, followed by moderate- to high-intensity statin drugs to lower LDL-C and to prevent ASCVD. Titrating statin drugs is no longer recommended, based on research determining that moderate to high dosing is most effective in lowering LDL-C.[1-5]

Lipid disorders are primarily caused by a combination of genetic, lifestyle, and nutritional factors. The primary goal of treatment is to decrease the lifetime and 10-year risk of ASCVD, based on risk calculations. The guidelines support the initiation of statin drugs to lower overall risk, in conjunction with lifestyle changes. Four target groups for treatment with moderate- or high-intensity statin therapy have been identified[1,3,4]:

- Patients with clinical ASCVD.
- Patients with an LDL-C level of 190 mg/dL or higher.
- Patients with diabetes, 40 to 75 years of age, with LDL-C level of 70 to 189 mg/dL.
- Patients 40 to 75 years of age with an estimated 10-year risk of ASCVD of 7.5% or higher.

These benefits affect both men and women, in all age ranges, including older adults.

PATHOPHYSIOLOGY

Fats and cholesterol are essential components of human cells and are synthesized by the liver. Additional cholesterol and a variety of other lipids are absorbed from the gastrointestinal tract during digestion and are transported through the bloodstream to the liver for processing.

Deposition of cholesterol into arterial and venous walls promotes atherosclerosis. This pathologic process is influenced by a number of factors, including toxins and inflammatory mediators within the bloodstream and in the vessel wall, and by the types and concentrations of the various lipoproteins. Lipoproteins are characterized by their density and include chylomicrons, very-low-density lipoprotein (VLDL), intermediate-density lipoprotein (IDL), LDL, and high-density lipoprotein (HDL). The progressive buildup of atheromatous plaque in the intimal arterial layer causes inflammation and narrowing of the vessel lumen. Gradually the atheromatous plaque enlarges and may rupture, causing coronary ischemia and infarction.

Low-Density Lipoprotein

LDL carries most of the cholesterol in the plasma and is the cause of atherogenic changes associated with the development of ASCVD. The principal function of LDL is to transport cholesterol to hepatic and extrahepatic cells. Although LDL particles are small, they carry approximately 70% of the circulating cholesterol in plasma. LDL is removed from the plasma by a single type of receptor located on the surface of many cells throughout the body: the LDL receptor. LDL's apolipoprotein B (apo B) binds to the LDL receptor when LDL is carried into the cells. One molecule of apo B is present for each LDL particle, but the quantity of cholesterol per particle can vary considerably. The ratio of LDL to apo B correlates with the size of the LDL particles. Low LDL-C/apo B ratios reflect small LDL particles. These smaller, denser LDL particles are more atherogenic than normal-sized LDL particles and are associated with insulin resistance, diabetes, hypertriglyceridemia, and low HDL levels, all of which are significant risk factors for ASCVD.[1-5]

Elevation of lipoprotein(a) (Lp[a]) is significant in patients with known coronary artery disease (CAD) and elevated LDL, increasing the risk of CV events. Familial hyperlipoproteinemia(a) may be indicative for CAD, but treatment options remain uncertain.[5]

High-Density Lipoprotein

HDL is an independent predictor of ASCVD risk. The role of HDL is significant; it lowers LDL by preventing oxidation of LDL within the arterial wall. In addition, when free cholesterol is released from cells into the plasma, it binds to HDL particles, resulting in a reverse cholesterol transport system. Cholesterol is returned to the liver, where it is excreted into bile, converted to bile acids, or reprocessed. There is an inverse relationship among VLDL remnants and small, dense LDL particles—known as atherogenic factors—and HDL. Because of the inverse relationship between levels of HDL and ASCVD risk, low levels of HDL (<40 mg/dL) have been identified as an independent risk factor for ASCVD regardless of the total cholesterol level. Higher high-density lipoprotein cholesterol (HDL-C) has a protective effect, and levels above 60 mg/dL are considered to be a negative risk factor, lowering the overall risk.[1-5]

The ratio of total cholesterol to HDL-C is correlated to cardiac risk. A total cholesterol/HDL-C ratio of more than 4.5 is associated with increased cardiac risk. Apolipoprotein A-I (apo A-I) is the predominant lipoprotein in HDL, and measurement of apo A-I in addition to the apo B found in LDL may allow more accurate assessment of cardiac risk.[1-5]

Physical activity increases HDL-C levels, emphasizing the importance of exercise in managing dyslipidemia. In addition, modest alcohol consumption (one or two drinks/day) increases HDL-C and appears to reduce cardiac risk. Excessive alcohol intake, however, increases triglycerides and detrimentally affects liver function.[1]

Role of Lifestyle, Including Diet and Exercise

The sedentary lifestyle of many Americans has increased the incidence of obesity and hyperlipidemia, with a subsequent rise in ASCVD and diabetes. A consistently maintained program of improved nutrition, weight reduction, and exercise improves the lipid profile, decreasing LDL and raising HDL.[3]

Despite increased awareness of healthy lifestyle choices in the United States, obesity is an American epidemic affecting overall morbidity and mortality. Obesity increases triglyceride levels, total cholesterol, and LDL-C and decreases HDL-C.

Dietary cholesterol is derived from eating fatty meats and full fat dairy products. These food items are also high in saturated fats and calories and should be eaten in the lowest quantity possible.

There are three major types of dietary fats: saturated, monounsaturated, and polyunsaturated. Each subtype exerts different influences on lipid metabolism, with saturated fats being the most harmful. Saturated fats increase blood cholesterol levels significantly more than dietary cholesterol does. Reducing saturated fats in the diet from 14% to 7% of total calories can decrease total blood cholesterol levels by nearly 20 mg/dL. Unfortunately, the major sources of saturated fats in the American diet are meats, eggs, and dairy products, which are highly consumed by Americans. Certain vegetable oils, namely tropical oils such as palm and coconut oil, are highly saturated and are most often found in commercially prepared cakes, muffins, cookies, and other baked goods.

Monounsaturated fats are derived from animal and plant oils. The main sources of monounsaturated fats in the American diet are peanuts, olives, avocados, and almonds. Monounsaturated fats do not by themselves raise or lower cholesterol levels but have been shown to help preserve baseline HDL levels when they are substituted for other fats. Their inclusion is a major feature of the popular Mediterranean diet.

Polyunsaturated fats are considered essential fatty acids because they cannot be synthesized by the body, unlike the saturated and monounsaturated fatty acids. Polyunsaturated fats are derived from vegetable oils consisting of omega-3 fatty acids or omega-6 fatty acids found in fish products. Dietary fish oils have been shown to lower total cholesterol and LDL levels while also increasing HDL levels.

Trans–fatty acids, from vegetable oils that have undergone extensive chemical processing or exposure to excess heat, have a detrimental effect on lipid levels. The most common sources in the American diet are margarine spreads, commercially produced baked goods, and deep-fried foods.

Insulin Resistance, Diabetes, and Metabolic Syndrome

Adult-onset diabetes is caused by a combination of factors, including progressive insulin resistance and inadequate insulin supply. Insulin resistance may or may not be associated with frank diabetes or even detectable high blood glucose levels. It is strongly influenced by genetic factors and is associated with abdominal obesity. Physical inactivity and a diet high in carbohydrates are major contributing factors. Insulin resistance, together with physical inactivity and obesity, often appears with other comorbidities, which include hypertension, high triglyceride levels, low HDL-C levels, and small, dense LDL particles, which are particularly atherogenic. Patients with these comorbid factors have metabolic syndrome (see Chapter 192) with a significantly increased risk for ASCVD.

CLINICAL PRESENTATION AND PHYSICAL EXAMINATION

Persons with lipid disorders may be unaware of this, because signs and symptoms do not appear unless other comorbidities are associated with elevated lipids, such as heart disease. Physical signs and symptoms, such as xanthomas, are present only when the disease is severe and prolonged.

Initial clinical evaluation should include a complete medical and family history, with documentation of any known ASCVD, symptoms of exertional angina or claudication, hypertension, diet and exercise patterns, smoking, drug and alcohol history and use, obesity, and diabetes. Hypothyroidism and liver and renal diseases affect lipid metabolism and should also be evaluated. All cardiac risk factors, including a family history of premature ASCVD, should be reviewed with the patient. Assessment of lifetime risk of ASCVD is recommended, using published risk assessment tables available at http://my.americanheart.org/cvriskcalculator.[6]

Accurate successive measurement of cardiac rate and rhythm, blood pressure, and height and weight, with determination of waist-to-hip ratio and body mass index, is important for all persons being evaluated for hyperlipidemia and ASCVD. Fatty deposits or xanthomas may be observed or palpated in persons with very high cholesterol levels from a familial hyperlipidemia. Xanthomas may be present on areas such as the Achilles tendon and on elbows, knees, and metacarpal joints. Deposits of cholesterol on the eyelids, called xanthelasma, may also be present. The presence of corneal arcus, an opaque white ring about the corneal periphery, should alert the provider to seek further evaluation, especially when it is observed in the young adult.

DIAGNOSTICS
Essential Diagnostics

Obtaining a fasting lipid panel, which includes total blood cholesterol, LDL-C, HDL, and triglycerides, is recommended for all adults older than 20 years, every 5 years. After the initiation of lipid-lowering drugs, a second panel should be obtained in 4 to 12 weeks to ensure adherence and efficacy. Thereafter, blood testing every 3 to 12 months is adequate, based on patient response and clinician assessment. A test of liver function is important before statins are initiated; this does not need to be repeated unless the patient is symptomatic of liver disease or has adverse effects of statin therapy. Monitoring of creatine kinase (CK) is not necessary unless the patient has muscle symptoms.[1-3]

Additional Diagnostics

Fasting blood glucose and hemoglobin A_{1c} [HbA_{1c}]
Thyroid levels (T3, T4, TSH)
Liver function tests (LFTs)
Renal function (BUN, cr, urinalysis)

INITIAL DIAGNOSTICS

Lipid Disorders

LABORATORY
- Fasting lipid panel every 5 years in adults older than 20 years:
  - Total cholesterol below 200 mg/dL is optimal (high is above 240 mg/dL)
  - LDL-C below 100 mg/dL is optimal (very high is above 190 mg/dL)
  - HDL above 60 mg/dL is optimal (very low is below 40 mg/dL)
  - Triglycerides below 150 mg/dL is optimal (very high is above 500 mg/dL)
- Estimate 10-year ASCVD risk every 4 to 6 years.

DIFFERENTIAL DIAGNOSIS

Before initiating medical therapy for dyslipidemia, the health care provider must consider other factors that may influence lipid metabolism. Diet, particularly excesses in overall calorie intake and saturated fat, may have an overall elevation effect on the lipid profile. Starvation states such as anorexia nervosa may cause an elevation in total serum cholesterol, whereas excessive intake of alcohol, poorly managed diabetes, or a familial tendency may elevate the lipid levels.[8]

Other major causes of secondary dyslipidemia include adverse effects of some drugs, disorders of metabolism, and certain disease states. Drugs can affect lipid metabolism in a variety of ways. Glucocorticoids and estrogens may elevate triglyceride and HDL levels, whereas anabolic steroids can markedly reduce HDL levels. Thiazide diuretics elevate total cholesterol, triglyceride, and LDL levels. Alpha blockers may cause increases in HDL, whereas beta blockers can decrease HDL levels and increase triglyceride levels. Elevation of total cholesterol and triglyceride levels has been reported in individuals taking protease inhibitors to treat human immunodeficiency virus (HIV) infection.

The most common endocrine disorders associated with lipid abnormalities are hypothyroidism and diabetes. Screening for thyroid disease (thyroid-stimulating hormone concentration, T_3 and T_4) (see Chapter 194) and diabetes (fasting blood glucose concentration and hemoglobin A_{1c} [HbA_{1c}]) (see Chapter 186) must be completed when abnormalities in the lipid profile are evaluated. Stabilization to a euthyroid state should be achieved before initiation of lipid treatment. In diabetics, achievement of adequate glycemic control will improve the lipid profile and is an integral component of therapy. Other disease states, such as nephrotic syndrome and obstructive liver disease, also contribute to lipid abnormalities and must be evaluated with a thorough medical history, physical examination, and laboratory tests, including urinalysis, blood urea nitrogen, creatinine, and liver function tests (LFTs).

 Rule out secondary causes of hyperlipidemia and hypertriglyceridemia prior to treating with statins for lipid disorders. Thyroid disease and diabetes must be treated primarily, and drug side effects as the cause of lipid disorders must be evaluated to assure correct treatment.

INTERPROFESSIONAL COLLABORATIVE MANAGEMENT

The primary goal of treatment is to lower the overall risk factors for ASCVD, reducing the morbidity and mortality associated with cardiac and vascular disease. Treatment has shifted from lowering LDL-C to lowering overall lifetime risk and 10-year risk for CV events.[1,3,4]

Nonpharmacological Management: Lifestyle modification, including a heart-healthy diet, exercise, reduction in body weight if BMI is higher than 24.9, and avoidance of tobacco products are recommended as the primary treatment for patients with elevated lipids and triglycerides. Patients who modify lifestyle may reduce LDL and increase HDL, lowering overall risk of ASCVD.[4,6,8]

Pharmacological Management: Several drugs are available for the treatment of lipid disorders; they are listed in Table 191.1.[1] The general drug categories are HMG-CoA reductase inhibitors, or statins[9]; bile acid sequestrants, or resins; nicotinic acid (niacin); fibrates; cholesterol absorption inhibitors; liposoluble antioxidants; and proprotein convertase subtilisin/kexin type 9 (PCSK9) antibody therapy (PCSK9).[10,11]

The first-choice and most effective drugs for lowering of LDL-C are the statins, which lower LDL-C by 21% to 55%.[9,10] The statins currently available are atorvastatin (Lipitor), fluvastatin (Lescol), rosuvastatin (Crestor), lovastatin (Mevacor), pravastatin (Pravachol), pitavastatin (Livalo), and simvastatin (Zocor). This category of drugs also increases HDL-C and decreases triglyceride levels, remaining the first-line drug treatment of dyslipidemia.

Several large-scale randomized controlled trials have demonstrated dramatic reductions in morbidity and mortality from cardiac events with the use of statins.[9,10] There is a 1% incidence of hepatic inflammation; for this reason, the liver transaminases—aspartate transaminase and alanine transaminase—should be evaluated before initiation of treatment. For elevations in the transaminases of 2 to 2½ times normal during therapy, treatment should be changed and sources of comorbid liver toxicity, such as alcohol, excluded.[1,2]

A rare but serious adverse reaction to high-dose statins, particularly simvastatin, is drug-induced myopathy, which can range from mild myalgias to severe muscle breakdown or rhabdomyolysis with the potential for subsequent acute renal failure. In addition, there is an increased risk of myopathy when simvastatin is used in combination with certain medications. Combination therapy and higher doses of statins, particularly simvastatin in doses of 80 mg/day, increase the risk of myositis and rhabdomyolysis. For this reason, simvastatin dosing less than 80 mg/day is recommended.[1,8] For patients taking amiodarone, amlodipine, diltiazem, ranolazine, or verapamil, lower doses of simvastatin (20 mg/day) are required.

TABLE 191.1 Expected Lipid-Lowering Effects and Side Effects of Currently Available Drugs

Drug	Dose Per Day	Total Cholesterol	LDL Cholesterol	HDL Cholesterol	Triglycerides	Side Effects	Patient Education
STATINS							
Lovastatin (Mevacor)	20–80 mg	↓15%–30%	↓20%–40%	↑5%–10%	↓10%–19%	Well tolerated as a class	Take with evening meal because most cholesterol is made in evening hours.
Pravastatin (Pravachol)	10–40 mg	↓15%–30%	↓20%–30%	↑5%–10%	↓10%–15%	Increase in transaminases in 1% of patients.	
Simvastatin (Zocor)	5–80 mg	↓20%–30%	↓23%–40%	↑6%–12%	↓10%–20%	Rare episodes of myopathy with or without associated rhabdomyolysis.	Have regular laboratory measurement for efficacy and safety.
Fluvastatin (Lescol)	20–80 mg	↓20%–30%	↓20%–32%	↑7%	↓19%	Infrequent gastrointestinal upset, constipation, rash, headaches.	Call and report any unexplained muscle pains, tenderness, or weakness.
Pitavastatin (Livalo)	2–4 mg	↓23%–31%	↓32%–43%	↑8%	↓15%–18%	Muscle pain, confusion, nausea, elevation in liver enzymes.	May be taken at any time of day without regard to meals.
Atorvastatin (Lipitor)	10–80 mg	↓27%–40%	↓36%–60%	↑7%–12%	↓17%–30%	Asian patients may experience a twofold elevation in median exposure to rosuvastatin; consider lower starting dose.	Avoid grapefruit juice.
Rosuvastatin (Crestor)	5–40 mg	—	↓45%–63%	↑8%–12%	↓10%–35%		
CHOLESTEROL ABSORPTION INHIBITORS							
Ezetimibe (Zetia)	10 mg	↓13%	↓18%	↑1%	↓8%	Include liver enzyme abnormalities and myopathy.	May be taken with or without food and can be taken with a statin.
Ezetimibe and simvastatin (Vytorin)	10 mg/40 mg 10 mg/80 mg	↓38%	↓53%	↑7%	↓24%	Avoid in patients with severe hepatic impairment.	

Continued

TABLE 191.1	Expected Lipid-Lowering Effects and Side Effects of Currently Available Drugs—cont'd						
Drug	**Dose Per Day**	**Total Cholesterol**	**LDL Cholesterol**	**HDL Cholesterol**	**Triglycerides**	**Side Effects**	**Patient Education**
FIBRIC ACIDS							
Gemfibrozil (Lopid)	600–1200 mg	↓6%	↓10%	↑10% (if HDL < 35%, ↑25%)	↓35%	LFT abnormality, muscle aches, abdominal pain.	Take 30 minutes before breakfast and dinner. Have regular laboratory measurements of efficacy and safety. Avoid in patients with renal failure.
Fenofibrate (Tricor)	48 or 145 mg				↑30%		
Resins	4–24 g	↓10%	↓25%	None	10% of patients will have ↑	Indigestion, bloating, gas, constipation.	Mix with uncarbonated liquid.
Cholestyramine	4–16 g						Add high-fiber foods to diet. Drink plenty of fluids.
Colestipol	5–20 g						Start with lowest dose and advance as tolerated.
Colesevelam	1.5–3.75 g	↓3.3%	↓10%	↑1.7%	↓8%	SE: Constipation. Other effects: reduction in HgbA1c in diabetics.	Take with 4–8 oz of fluid. Need to take resins 1 hour before or 4 hours after other medication.
Evolocumab (Repatha)	140 mgs sc q 2 weeks or 420 mgs sc q month	↓36%	↓63%			Nasopharyngitis, injection site reactions, increased blood sugar, back pain	
Alirocumab (Praluent)	75–150 mgs sc q 2 weeks	↓35%	↓56%			Nasopharyngitis, injection site reactions	
Niacin	2–3 g	↓10%–25%	↓20%–40%	↑15%–30%	↓45%–50%	Flushing, itching, rash, gastrointestinal upset; increases in glucose, uric acid, and transaminases.	Predose with aspirin. Avoid taking with hot fluids and alcohol. Start with low dose and increase gradually during several weeks. Call if prolonged nausea occurs. Monitor with laboratory tests.

Patients taking statins who report new muscle pain must have CK levels evaluated to determine muscle breakdown. If the CK level is elevated, the drug should be discontinued and the patient monitored for potential renal dysfunction. In the absence of symptoms, it is not necessary to routinely monitor CK levels. Higher doses of statins can also increase the risk of type 2 diabetes. Individual responses to medications must be considered.[9,10]

Statin drugs should be administered in moderate- or high-intensity doses, based on ASCVD risk factors and the presence of CAD.

Secondary prevention drugs in those unable to take statins include bile acid sequestrants, fenofibrate or niacin and ezetimibe should be considered. Referral to a specialist is recommended for these patients.[2–4] The usefulness of niacin in these patients has been questioned, with studies failing to demonstrate reduced CV events and showing significant complications of therapy.[1,3,4]

Bile acid sequestrants (resins) such as cholestyramine have been demonstrated to be safe and effective in lowering LDL modestly when they are used singularly and can further lower LDL in combination with HMG-CoA reductase inhibitors.

They represent a safe alternative to statins in patients with liver disease or those who have had an adverse reaction.[1]

Nonstatin drugs have not been shown to reduce CV events when added to statins and greatly increase the side effect profile. These drugs should be used primarily in patients who cannot tolerate statins or who have had an inadequate response to maximum statin doses.[1-4,10]

Nicotinic acid (niacin) demonstrates LDL- and triglyceride-lowering and HDL-raising effects, with doses as low as 1.5 to 2.0 g/day.[3] It may be added to statin therapy, as an adjunct to lowering LDL-C in patients with known coronary disease who have shown an inadequate reaction to statins. Unfortunately, its use remains limited by unpleasant side effects, including flushing, itching, rash, and gastrointestinal upset. In rare cases, liver toxicity, hyperuricemia, and glucose intolerance have occurred, which may limit its usefulness.[3,4]

The fibric acids, which include gemfibrozil (Lopid) and fenofibrate (Tricor), are effective in lowering triglycerides and raising HDL-C, with modest decrease in LDL. They are used primarily to treat hypertriglyceridemia. A fasting serum triglyceride level of more than 400 mg/dL or the presence of pancreatitis necessitates treatment with this class of drugs. Fibrates decrease triglyceride values by 20% to 35% and increase HDL levels by 6% to 18%. Fibrates should not be administered to patients with severe hepatic or renal dysfunction, and when they are used in combination with statins, the risk of complications is higher.[11] Monitoring of renal and liver function is essential in prescribing fibric acids and combination therapy, to detect and to prevent kidney and liver damage.

Cholesterol absorption inhibitors (e.g., ezetimibe) are useful for patients who cannot tolerate statins or who would benefit from combination therapy in an effort to lower LDL-C in patients with known cardiac disease.[1,3,4]

Omega-3 fatty acids are recommended for the treatment of severe hypertriglyceridemia. However, omega-3-acid-ethyl esters may increase LDL. Monitoring of LFTs, TG, and LDL-C levels is imperative during treatment.[10]

PCSK9 inhibitors (alirocumab, evolocumab) are the newest drugs available to reduce LDL and atheroma volume. This drug is administered subcutaneously in a select population: Patients with ASCVD on maximal statins and an LDL > 100 mg/dL, or heterozygous hypercholesterolemia without ASCVD but with LDL > 130 mg/dL on maximal statins. Other patients may be considered for this therapy based on clinical judgment when the patient is intolerant to statins and has ASCVD or a very high risk for ASCVD (PCSK9).[12]

Combination therapy is useful when single-drug use and lifestyle changes do not achieve goals for lowering cholesterol and LDL-C. The addition of a bile acid sequestrant to a statin can reduce LDL-C by an additional 10%. However, the combination of two systemic lipid-lowering drugs (e.g., niacin with a statin or gemfibrozil with a statin) can lead to increased frequency of side effects. LDL-C should be monitored every 6 months when therapy is initiated or doses are changed. Once goal LDL is achieved, monitoring every 6 to 12 months is reasonable.[7]

Life Span Considerations

Young Adults. Persons aged 19 years or older with high LDL-C levels (>190 mg/dL) have a high lifetime risk of CV events. These individuals should be treated with moderate- to high-intensity statin therapy, with the goal of reducing LDL-C levels by 50%. In addition, family screening is recommended, because very high LDL-C levels in the young population are most often familial.[8] Other causes of primary hyperlipidemia in young adults should also be evaluated, including excessive alcohol intake, diabetes, and albuminuria.

Screening for high cholesterol levels is also an opportunity for counseling about healthy lifestyle habits, including diet, exercise, weight control, and drug, alcohol, and tobacco use. Consultation and collaboration with other health care providers, including exercise and nutrition specialists, is recommended when long-term therapy is being considered in younger adults.

Adults (Men). The benefit of lowering cholesterol in terms of lowering the risk for ASCVD has been most clearly demonstrated in men aged 35 to 65 years. Men in this age group also have a particularly high prevalence of obesity, hypertension, and tobacco use. They should be targeted for aggressive lifestyle modification, lipid screening, and drug therapy when appropriate.

Adults (Women). ASCVD has been perceived as a disease more prevalent in men, but half of all cardiac deaths occur in women, and CAD is the leading cause of death in women older than 50 years.[13,14] The main difference between men and women is that the onset of ASCVD in women occurs on average 10 to 15 years later than in men and rarely before menopause. Women aged 45 to 75 years should be screened and treated for hyperlipidemia just as men should be treated. The absolute benefit of statin therapy to lower cholesterol and LDL-C is based on risk assessment and CV disease.

Older Adults. The evidence for lowering the risk of ASCVD and CAD events persists regardless of age. Lifestyle changes, including moderate exercise and a healthy diet, provide many benefits to the elderly, and should be strongly encouraged, within individual limits. Overall morbidity and mortality must be considered, because the benefit of treatment of older adults with statins should outweigh the risks of adverse events and costs. Persons older than 75 years who have been taking and tolerating statins should continue therapy. Initiation of therapy in persons older than 75 must be individualized.[1,2]

COMPLICATIONS

Elevated lipid levels for prolonged periods result in the progressive buildup of atheromatous plaque in the intimal arterial layer, causing narrowing of the lumen, which precipitates an immune and inflammatory process. Gradually, the atheromatous plaque enlarges and may occlude the lumen or rupture, causing ischemia and infarction and resulting in atherosclerotic CAD (see Chapter 102), peripheral vascular disease (see Chapter 125), cerebral vascular disease, and ACS or death. Recognition of comorbid factors that may be life-threatening is essential, including hypertriglyceridemia (>1000 mg/dL), pancreatitis, untreated thyroid disease, morbid obesity, preexisting ASCVD, and poorly managed diabetes.

PATIENT AND FAMILY EDUCATION

Lifestyle modification:
- Heart-healthy nutrition.
- Weight loss.
- Smoking cessation.
- Exercise.

Drug management:
- Schedule and dosing.
- Side and adverse effects.

- Importance of continuing drugs as prescribed.
- Prescription renewal strategy.

Importance of follow-up evaluation:

- Health care provider appointments.
- Laboratory tests needed.
- Support groups available.
- Physical and/or occupational therapy, exercise, nutrition, smoking cessation, and counseling referrals.

Health Promotion

Diet. Adherence to a heart-healthy diet, following the ACC/AHA Guidelines, will aid in lowering LDL-C and decreasing weight. Maximum dietary therapy will typically achieve a reduction in LDL-C of 15 to 25 mg/dL, but a healthy balanced diet, exercise, and maintenance of an ideal body weight have additional benefits. This includes improved well-being and self-esteem and a decrease in the other comorbidities of obesity, hypertension, insulin resistance, and diabetes.

Dietary fat should, whenever possible, be the unsaturated fat found in most vegetable oils and, in particular, the monounsaturated fat found in olive oil and nuts. Low-fat dairy products are recommended, along with an increased intake of poultry, fish, and legumes and a decreased intake of red meat.

Trans–fatty acids, which arise from excessive processing, are most atherogenic. Trans–fatty acids, found primarily in margarine spreads, commercially produced baked goods, and deep-fried foods, should be avoided whenever possible. Sugar-sweetened beverages and sweet foods should be limited.

Replacement for fats in the diet should come from complex carbohydrates and by increasing fiber in the diet to 20 to 30 g/day. Whole-grain breads, pastas, and cereals and fresh fruits and vegetables are highly recommended.[6]

Exercise. The importance of physical activity should be stressed to all persons concerned about health, ASCVD, and lipid management. Regular aerobic exercise, at least 30 minutes per day, four to six times a week, increases HDL-C; decreases total cholesterol, LDL-C, and triglyceride levels; and improves outcomes in other coexisting risk factors, such as obesity, hypertension, and insulin resistance.[1,3,8]

Smoking Cessation. Smoking increases the overall risk of ASCVD, particularly when it is combined with familial history, dyslipidemia, hypertension, and diabetes.[1,6] Elimination of use of tobacco products is essential to the prevention and treatment of disease. Referral to smoking cessation programs and the use of nicotine supplements (nicotine patch, nicotine gum), antianxiety medications, and counseling all support smoking cessation.

REFERENCES

1. Jellinger, P. S. (2017). AACE 2017 guidelines: American Association of Clinical Endocrinologists and American College of Endocrinology guidelines for management of dyslipidemia and prevention of cardiovascular disease. *Endocrine Practice, 23*(Suppl. 2).
2. Stone, N. J., et al. (2014). 2013 ACC/AHA guideline on the treatment of blood cholesterol to reduce atherosclerotic cardiovascular risk in adults. *Journal of the American College of Cardiology, 63*(25 Pt. B), 2889–2934.
3. Jacobson, T. A., et al. (2015). National Lipid Association recommendations for patient-centered management of dyslipidemia: Part 2. *Journal of Clinical Lipidology, 9*(6).
4. Jacobson, T. A., et al. (2015). National Lipid Association recommendations for patient-centered management of dyslipidemia: Part 1. *Journal of Clinical Lipidology, 9*(2), 129–169.
5. Grützmacher, P. (2017). Primary and secondary prevention of cardiovascular disease in patients with hyperlipoproteinemia (a). *Clinical Research in Cardiology Supplements, 12*(Suppl. 1), 22–26.
6. http://professional.heart.org/professional/GuidelinesStatements/Prevention Guidelines/UCM_457698_Prevention-Guidelines.jsp. (Accessed 15 February 2018).
7. Gulum, A. H. (2015). Statins: An update on clinical issues and selected adverse effects 287-294. *The Journal for Nurse Practitioners: JNP, 11*(3), 287–294.
8. DeBeasi, L. C. (2017). Optimizing diet, weight, and exercise in adults with familial hypercholesterolemia. *The Journal for Nurse Practitioners: JNP, 13*(9), 603–609.
9. US Preventive Services Task Force. (2016). Statin use for the primary prevention of cardiovascular disease in adults: US Preventive Services Task Force recommendation statement. *JAMA: The Journal of the American Medical Association, 316*(19), 1997–2007.
10. Jin, J. (2016). Lipid disorders: Screening and treatment. *JAMA: The Journal of the American Medical Association, 316*(19), 2056. doi:10.1001/jama.2016.16650.
11. Kelly, M. S., et al. (2017). Pharmacologic approaches for the management of patients with moderately elevated triglycerides (150–499 mg/dL). *Journal of Clinical Lipidology, 11*(4), 872–879.
12. Orringer, C. E., et al. (2017). Update on the use of PCSK9 inhibitors in adults: Recommendations from an Expert Panel of the National Lipid Association. *Journal of Clinical Lipidology, 11*(4), 880–890.
13. Murphy, N., et al. (2017). Women and heart disease: An evidence-based update. *The Journal for Nurse Practitioners: JNP, 13*(9), 610–616.
14. Chou, R., Dana, T., Blazina, I., Daeges, M., & Jeanne, T. L. (2016). Statins for prevention of cardiovascular disease in adults: Evidence report and systematic review for the US Preventive Services Task Force. *JAMA: The Journal of the American Medical Association, 316*(19), 2008–2024.

CHAPTER **192**

METABOLIC SYNDROME
Donna Jenell Pease

DEFINITION AND EPIDEMIOLOGY

Metabolic syndrome is a cluster of disorders characterized by insulin resistance with hyperinsulinemia; hypertension; abdominal (central or visceral) obesity; and dyslipidemia consisting of hypertriglyceridemia, low high-density lipoprotein (HDL) cholesterol, and increased small, dense low-density lipoprotein (LDL) particles.[1] Characteristics that have been added more recently include elevated C-Reactive protein (CRP) levels, increased plasminogen activator inhibitor 1 (PAI-1), and microalbuminemia.

The criteria to diagnose metabolic syndrome includes any three of the following:[2]

- Elevated waist circumference: population- and country-specific definitions—in the United States: greater than 40 inches for men and greater than 35 inches for women
- Elevated triglyceride levels: 150 mg/dL (1.7 mmol/L) or higher, or specific treatment for this lipid abnormality
- Reduced HDL cholesterol: below 40 mg/dL (1.0 mmol/L) in males and below 50 mg/dL (1.3 mmol/L) in females, or specific treatment for this lipid abnormality
- Elevated blood pressure: systolic 130 mm Hg or higher or diastolic 85 mm Hg or higher, or drug treatment of previously diagnosed hypertension
- Elevated fasting plasma glucose: 100 mg/dL or higher, or drug treatment for elevated glucose

Not all individuals with insulin resistance will develop all of the multiple components of this syndrome, but studies have found that the greater the number of associated characteristics an individual exhibits, the greater his or her risk for development of cardiovascular disease (CVD) or dying young. This syndrome has also been called the insulin resistance syndrome, Reaven syndrome, syndrome X, cardiovascular dysmetabolic syndrome, and deadly quartet.[3]

The occurrence of metabolic syndrome increases dramatically as body mass index (BMI) increases. Metabolic syndrome is not unusual in the general population, in older individuals, and in certain ethnicities. It is estimated that metabolic syndrome is present in approximately 34.2% or more than 40 million US adults 20 years of age and older.[4] From 2007 to 2012, metabolic syndrome was more prevalent in non-Hispanic white males than in non-Hispanic black males, while non-Hispanic black females were more likely than non-Hispanic white females to be afflicted.[4]

Both genetic factors and environmental factors have been found to play a role in the incidence of metabolic syndrome. Studies have found a genetic predisposition to the syndrome and the associated cardiovascular risk factors in first-degree relatives of individuals diagnosed with type 2 diabetes. Researchers have also found that nonobese individuals with a family history of diabetes, hypertension, or obesity are genetically predisposed to the development of metabolic syndrome.[3]

An environmental factor involved with insulin resistance and obesity is the lifestyle typical of Western civilization, consisting of a high-fat diet and low levels of physical activity. High energy intake and low energy output have led to the increased prevalence of obesity seen today. Tissue sensitivity to insulin declines when an individual becomes overweight. The fat cells found in abdominal obesity are larger and are more insulin resistant. Abdominal fat is also more metabolically active, and fat lipolysis occurs more often, releasing excess free fatty acids that interfere with hepatic insulin clearance, thus resulting in higher levels of circulating insulin. Visceral, or abdominal, obesity may be one of the leading causes of insulin resistance. Visceral adipose tissue releases cytokines, PAI-1, adiponectin, leptin, and resistin, which are potentially pathogenic and associated with higher CVD risk.[3]

Metabolic syndrome has been recognized as a side effect of several commonly used medications (e.g., corticosteroids, antidepressants, and antipsychotics) that can predispose an individual to obesity and glucose intolerance.[5]

PATHOPHYSIOLOGY

Visceral or abdominal obesity leads to insulin resistance, defined as the impaired insulin-stimulated glucose uptake by skeletal muscle, adipose tissue, or liver. The mechanisms involved in insulin resistance may consist of abnormal insulin molecules, a decreased number of insulin receptors and glucose transporters, as well as defective postreceptor activity. Impairment at the receptor level is usually associated with decreased sensitivity to insulin, whereas postreceptor or cellular defects are associated with decreased responsiveness to insulin. When the cells become resistant to the insulin, the body compensates by producing more insulin to overcome the resistance and to maintain normal glucose levels. Fasting hyperinsulinemia occurs in response to elevated fasting plasma glucose. This hyperinsulinemia leads to the various other abnormalities associated with metabolic syndrome, to include hypertension, dyslipidemia, and atherosclerosis.[3]

Insulin resistance and visceral adiposity (central obesity) are recognized as the main factors in the hypertension associated with metabolic syndrome. Insulin resistance and the resulting hyperinsulinemia induce blood pressure elevation

by activation of the sympathetic nervous system and the renin-angiotensin-aldosterone system, which causes urinary sodium excretion to decline. The increased sodium reabsorption causes expansion of the extracellular fluid volume and renal dilation and leads to the hypertension, endothelial dysfunction, inflammation, atherogenesis, and alteration in renal function associated with metabolic syndrome.[6]

The lipid abnormalities found in metabolic syndrome are elevated triglycerides, low HDL cholesterol, and increased small, dense LDL particles (referred to as pattern B, or atherogenic dyslipidemia). Obesity causes the adipocytes within the abdominal adipose tissue to become insulin resistant, thus impairing the adipocyte's ability to take up glucose and to store free fatty acids. The adipocytes release large amounts of free fatty acids into the systemic circulation. Muscle cells take up the large amounts of free fatty acid, become saturated with free fatty acids, and become insulin resistant as well. This results in diminished glucose disposal, hyperglycemia, and pancreatic beta cell stimulation to produce larger amounts of insulin (hyperinsulinemia). The free fatty acids that were unable to be absorbed by the muscle cells are diverted to the liver through the portal vein, where they impair normal insulin-mediated suppression of the hepatic glucose output and stimulate the synthesis, assembly, and secretion of lipoproteins that promote atherogenesis (raised triglycerides, low concentrations of HDL cholesterol, increased remnant lipoproteins, elevated apolipoprotein B levels, and small, dense LDL cholesterol). These adverse effects on lipoprotein levels increase the risk of atherosclerosis, ischemic heart disease, CVD, and overall cardiovascular mortality. Individuals with metabolic syndrome are twice as likely to die from and three times as likely to have a heart attack or stroke compared with people without the syndrome. People with metabolic syndrome have a fivefold greater risk of developing type 2 diabetes.[7]

Research has determined that there is an association between metabolic syndrome and the following medical disorders: increased levels of CRP and PAI-I, microalbuminuria, cognitive decline, sleep apnea and breathing disorders, polycystic ovary syndrome, low testosterone levels in men, cancer, and nonalcoholic fatty liver disease.[7]

CLINICAL PRESENTATION AND PHYSICAL EXAMINATION

Because it is difficult to accurately measure insulin resistance, the diagnosis is usually clinical, based on a constellation of physical findings and laboratory characteristics. Insulin resistance can be suspected in the individual who is seen with abdominal obesity, increased triglycerides, low HDL cholesterol, and hypertension. Those who have a diagnosis of metabolic syndrome should also be screened for the cardiovascular complications that accompany the syndrome and managed appropriately. It is also important to obtain a thorough history during the assessment to determine whether the patient is at risk for development of insulin resistance secondary to genetic factors or family history.

A physical sign that is suggestive of moderate to severe insulin resistance is the hyperkeratotic condition acanthosis nigricans. This is a diffuse, hyperpigmented, velvety thickening of the skin that is found in the neck and axillae. The onset is usually insidious, with the first visible change being darkening of the skin pigmentation so as to appear dirty. As the skin thickens, it becomes velvety, and the skin line is accentuated.

The skin eventually becomes rugose and mammillated. The presence of skin tags in conjunction with acanthosis nigricans is also a sign of insulin resistance.[8]

The physical examination consists of accurate measurement of the patient's blood pressure, height, weight, and BMI or waist-to-hip ratio. A variety of body mass and body fat measures exist that reveal different aspects of general obesity, fat distribution patterns, and fat percentage. BMI is calculated as weight divided by height squared and measures percentage of body fat or total adipose tissue. The ratio of waist and hip circumference is highly correlated with visceral adipose tissue. Waist circumference (often measured at the level of the umbilicus or the top of the iliac crest with the patient standing) or waist-to-hip ratio (the ratio of waist circumference to hip circumference measured at the iliac crest) correlates well with insulin resistance and metabolic syndrome. BMI and waist-to-hip ratio are the most routinely used anthropometric indexes because they are easy to use and have a high reliability.

DIAGNOSTICS

Essential Diagnostics

Several techniques are available for measurement of insulin resistance and sensitivity. A patient with the clinical features of metabolic syndrome should be screened annually for hyperglycemia, glucose intolerance, and type 2 diabetes mellitus.

Insulin resistance can be identified through the measurement of the fasting plasma insulin concentration or hemoglobin A1C High plasma insulin values with normal glucose levels are suggestive of insulin resistance.

Common laboratory tests can be used to screen for the various other features associated with metabolic syndrome. Impaired fasting glucose (IFG) is measured after an 8- to 12-hour fast; levels between 100 and 126 mg/dL are diagnostic of IFG. HDL and triglyceride blood levels are measured after an 8- to 12-hour fast.[3]

INITIAL DIAGNOSTICS

Metabolic Syndrome

LABORATORY[2]
- Hemoglobin H1C
- Basic Metabolic PanelFasting plasma insulin concentration
- Fasting lipid profile
- Additional laboratory
- C-Reactive Protein
- Liver function panel
- Thyroid function panel
- Uric acid

Differential Diagnosis

The diagnosis of metabolic syndrome is based on clinical presentation, so it is important to rule out hypertension, dyslipidemia, or obesity without manifestations of insulin resistance. The differential diagnoses also include type 2 diabetes mellitus and IGT, which can be excluded with laboratory testing. Other diseases characterized by insulin resistance are polycystic ovary syndrome, Cushing syndrome, congenital adrenal hyperplasia, lipodystrophy and lipoatrophic diabetes, type A and type B insulin resistance, genetic syndromes, neurodegenerative disorders, and excess hormonal antagonists.[3]

INTERPROFESSIONAL COLLABORATIVE MANAGEMENT

 A physician consultation is necessary when the hypertension or dyslipidemia (associated with metabolic syndrome) is resistant to therapy. Very high triglyceride levels can provoke an acute episode of pancreatitis.

The Diabetes Prevention Program was a randomized clinical trial conducted to evaluate the safety and efficacy of interventions that may delay or prevent development of diabetes in individuals at increased risk for type 2 diabetes. The study found that intensive lifestyle interventions, including at least 150 minutes of moderate-intensity exercise per week together with a healthy diet to achieve and to maintain a 7% loss of body weight, reduced the incidence of diabetes by 58%; the use of metformin, 850 mg twice daily, reduced the incidence of diabetes by 31%.[9]

Pharmacologic Management

It is imperative to treat the different components of metabolic syndrome appropriately to prevent or to lessen the risk of cardiovascular morbidity and mortality. Studies have found that the prevalence of coronary heart disease, myocardial infarction, and stroke is significantly increased with metabolic syndrome.[7] Methods to treat metabolic syndrome include both pharmacologic and nonpharmacologic measures.

Although the Food and Drug Administration has not approved any drugs specifically for the treatment of metabolic syndrome, treatment of the individual risk factors associated with metabolic syndrome decreases CVD risk. Pharmacologic therapy would include anti-hypertensives, 3-hydroxy-3-methylglutaryl–coenzyme A (HMG-CoA) reductase inhibitors (statins), ezetimibe, fibric acid derivatives, aspirin therapy, the biguanide metformin, and weight loss medications.

Anti-Hypertensives

Anti-hypertensive therapy includes a goal blood pressure of below 130/85 mm Hg. ACE inhibitors and angiotensin II receptor blockers reduce the incidence of type 2 diabetes in patients with hypertension and CVD, improve the lipid profile, can prevent or retard progression of renal disease, and can also improve microalbuminuria. Calcium channel blockers are effective in lowering blood pressure and decreasing adverse CVD outcomes and have no profound adverse effects on lipid or glucose metabolism. Vasodilating beta blockers are cardioprotective in patients with established CVD. Though caution exists regarding use of thiazide diuretics due to their ability to worsen insulin resistance and dyslipidemia and possibly accelerate conversion to diabetes, currently there is no data that shows worsened cardiovascular or renal outcomes in patients treated with these agents.[6]

Statins and Other Lipid-Lowering Medications

Dyslipidemia associated with metabolic syndrome should be treated. Goals are as follows: triglyceride levels below 150 mg/dL, LDL cholesterol below 100 mg/dL, and HDL cholesterol above 40 mg/dL in men or above 50 mg/dL in women with metabolic syndrome. Statins may lower LDL cholesterol by 25% to 45%, raise HDL cholesterol by 5% to 10%, and lower triglycerides by 7% to 30%. Statins modulate endothelial function, stabilize plaque, and provide antiinflammatory and antithrombotic effects that can further reduce CVD risk in metabolic syndrome.[9] Ezetimibe inhibits cholesterol absorption and in combination with statins can reduce LDL 20% to 30%.

If the triglyceride level is very high (>500 mg/dL), it is recommended that a fibric acid derivative (such as gemfibrozil), fenofibrate, or nicotinic acid (niacin) be used, which may decrease triglyceride levels by 20% to 50%. Gemfibrozil has been shown to improve insulin action and flow-mediated vasodilation as well as to increase HDL levels. Nicotinic acid in high doses can raise plasma glucose levels. Severe myopathy may occur with the combination of a statin plus gemfibrozil. Creatine kinase (CK) and transaminases should be monitored when these medications are used.[10]

Aspirin

Aspirin may be beneficial in the reduction of myocardial infarction and stroke in diabetic individuals. The USPSTF recommends initiating low-dose aspirin use for the primary prevention of cardiovascular disease (CVD) and colorectal cancer (CRC) in adults aged 50 to 59 years who have a 10% or greater 10-year CVD risk, are not at increased risk for bleeding, have a life expectancy of at least 10 years, and are willing to take low-dose aspirin daily for at least 10 years. The American Heart Association currently recommends use of low-dose aspirin prophylaxis in patients with established arteriosclerotic CVD, provided it is not contraindicated by allergy or increased bleeding risk and the risk/benefit ratio suggests an advantage.[11]

Metformin

Metformin has been shown to reduce hyperinsulinemia and insulin resistance, to lower blood triglyceride levels, and to assist in weight reduction and to lower PAI-1 levels. Metformin improves the sensitivity of cells to insulin, reduces hepatic glucose production, and increases glucose uptake in muscle and other peripheral tissues. Through these mechanisms of action, metformin has been found to reduce or to prevent macrovascular complications. A patient's GFR must be monitored while treated with metformin and the dose adjusted appropriately.[7]

The Diabetes Prevention Program was a randomized clinical trial conducted to evaluate the safety and efficacy of interventions that may delay or prevent development of diabetes in individuals at increased risk for type 2 diabetes, including those with metabolic syndrome. The study found that intensive lifestyle interventions, including at least 150 minutes of moderate-intensity exercise per week together with a healthy diet to achieve and to maintain a 7% loss of body weight, reduced the incidence of diabetes by 58%; the use of metformin, 850 mg twice daily, reduced the incidence of diabetes by 31%.[9]

Thiazolidinediones

Thiazolidinediones activate the peroxisome proliferator-activated receptor gamma (PPAR-gamma), which regulates insulin-responsive gene transcription involved in glucose production, transport, and use, thereby reducing blood glucose concentrations and reducing hyperinsulinemia.[12] Pioglitazone is the most recommended agent in this category, but caution is indicated in patients with heart failure, and careful monitoring is advised.

Glucagon Like Peptide-1 Agonists

The glucagon like peptide-1 (GLP-1) agonist, liraglutide, stimulates insulin release to lower blood sugar, decreases glucagon secretion, enhances insulin sensitivity, and reduces appetite and energy intake.[12]

The National Institutes of Health recommend consideration of pharmacologic treatment for individuals with a BMI of at least 30 kg/m[2]. Pharmacologic agents available to treat excess adiposity include appetite suppressants and inhibitors of nutrient absorption. There are five categories of drugs currently in use to treat obesity: sympathomimetics, gastrointestinal lipase inhibitors, glucagon-like peptide 1 agonists, antidepressant/opioid antagonists, and serotonin agonists. The use of these medications is limited by a lack of long-term safety date, cost, and insurance coverage.[13] These agents are usually taken in the morning and lead to decreased appetite later in the afternoon and evening.

Gastric balloon therapy is a nonsurgical weight loss procedure in which two saline-filled balloons are placed endoscopically in the stomach for 6 months so the patient feels full faster and eats less.[14]

Consultations: Surgery

- Successful surgical procedures to treat obesity include gastric bypass (Roux-en-Y), sleeve gastrectomy, adjustable gastric band, and biliopancreatic diversion with duodenal switch. Follow-up after these procedures includes monitoring of vitamin and hematologic status, adherence to specific postoperative dietary guidelines, and psychological issues.[15]

- vBloc neurometabolic therapy is an implanted device on the vagus nerve that blocks hunger signals between the brain and the stomach. vBloc therapy has been shown to result in medically meaningful weight loss with a favorable safety profile through 2 years.[16]

- Aspiration therapy consists of an endoscopically placed gastrostomy tube and siphon assembly that enables patients to remove up to 30% of stomach contents after consumption of a meal. Aspiration therapy has been found to be a safe method that allows a patient to reduce excess weight by half in 1 year.[17]

- *Nonpharmacologic treatments* for insulin resistance include healthy lifestyle changes in diet and exercise. Because many individuals with metabolic syndrome are overweight, dietary treatment should focus primarily on weight reduction. Weight loss lowers serum cholesterol and triglycerides, raises HDL cholesterol, lowers blood pressure and glucose, and reduces insulin resistance.

- Weight reduction recommendation is a 10% decrease in body weight within 6 months. This can be achieved by a low-calorie diet (800 to 1500 kcal/d or a decrease of at least 500 kcal/d). General dietary recommendations include a low intake of saturated fats, *trans*–fatty acids, and cholesterol; reduced consumption of simple sugars; and increased intakes of fruits, vegetables, and whole grains. Dietary carbohydrates with a high glycemic index increase blood glucose levels more rapidly, whereas fiber-rich foods with a low glycemic index are digested and absorbed more slowly and can lower triglyceride and raise HDL cholesterol levels. Intake of soluble fiber has been shown to decrease postprandial glucose levels and concentrations of insulin. Plant-based foods, such as whole grains, fruits, and vegetables, can decrease systolic and diastolic blood pressures and reduce the incidence of coronary heart disease. A monounsaturated fat diet improves insulin sensitivity and the dyslipidemia associated with metabolic syndrome compared with a diet high in saturated fat. Reducing overall carbohydrate intake for individuals with diabetes, especially those not meeting glycemic targets or for whom reducing antiglycemic medications is a priority has demonstrated the most evidence for improving glycemia. There are a variety of low-carbohydrate eating plans available.[18] Less than 7% of total calories should come from saturated fats, and less than 200 mg of cholesterol should be consumed per day. Plant stanols and sterols and soluble fibers such as cereal grains, beans, peas, legumes, fruits, and vegetables will lower LDL. Protein should be lean or low fat. Following the DASH diet (Dietary Approaches to Stop Hypertension) can lower sodium intake. Commercial weight-loss programs can offer social support, oversight, and accountability.

- A health psychologist can provide psychological support as well as support with realistic goal setting, stress management, and behavior modification methods.[18]
- Exercise and physical training should include moderately intense cardiovascular aerobic exercise for 30 minutes 5 days a week or vigorously intense cardiovascular aerobic exercise for 20 minutes 3 days a week and 8 to 10 strength training exercises, 8 to 12 repetitions of each exercise twice a week. This could include brisk walking, bicycling, and swimming. The American Heart Association recommends 10,000 steps per day (5 miles). Suggestions also include adding multiple short bouts of activity (10 to 15 minutes), decreasing leisure-time sedentary activities such as watching television, using simple home exercise equipment such as treadmills, and self-monitoring of exercise. The exercise session should begin with a 10-minute warm-up consisting of light aerobic activity and stretching and end with a 5- to 10-minute cool-down period to lower the heart rate. Exercise improves insulin resistance by increasing glucose use by the muscle. Glycogen synthase activity and the number of glucose transporters translocated to the cell surface increase after exercise. Glucose disposal by the skeletal muscle and insulin sensitivity continue for many hours after completion of the exercise. This improvement in insulin sensitivity may prevent the progression of the metabolic abnormalities. Regular aerobic training has also been shown to significantly decrease systolic and diastolic blood pressures. Physical training has been shown to decrease plasma levels of triglyceride by 15% to 30%. Exercise improves the removal of very-low-density lipoprotein (VLDL) and intermediate-density lipoprotein particles and decreases the levels of small, dense LDL associated with metabolic syndrome. An increase in HDL cholesterol may occur if exercise training is intense and prolonged. Exercise and calorie restriction can cause weight loss and a loss of intra-abdominal fat, which will decrease the insulin resistance associated with metabolic syndrome. An exercise physiologist or physical therapist can assist in the development of a safe and effective exercise regimen.[19] Recommendations for exercise for individuals with metabolic syndrome are similar to those for individuals with type 2 diabetes (see Chapter 186).
- If the individual is sedentary, a careful cardiovascular assessment may be needed before initiation of an exercise program.

LIFE SPAN CONSIDERATIONS

Insulin resistance may occur at any age. Childhood obesity is epidemic, and data from the International Obesity Task Force indicate that the overall prevalence of metabolic syndrome is 11.9% among overweight and 29.2% among obese adolescents.[20] The criteria for metabolic syndrome in children (aged 10 to 16 years) are the same as those for adults but include waist circumference above the 90th percentile for age, gender, and race.

Childhood obesity increases the risk for metabolic syndrome in childhood, adolescence, and adulthood. This risk can be reduced if an obese child reduces his or her relative weight through diet and exercise. The baseline assessment and identification of obese children can possibly aid in the prevention of adult obesity, metabolic syndrome, and cardiovascular risk.[21]

Parents require education on ways to promote healthy lifestyle, proper nutrition, weight loss, and increased physical activity in young obese children. These healthy lifestyle modifications must continue throughout the entire life span.

Individuals older than 65 years have increased risk for metabolic syndrome. The older adult may be at increased risk for development of insulin resistance secondary to increased obesity, decreases in physical activity, and changes in body mass because of muscle loss and increased adipose tissue. Older adults may need to be educated on exercise programs tailored to their needs or modified for the chronic illnesses they have. Exercise recommendations are the same for older adults as mentioned earlier in the guidelines for cardiovascular aerobic exercises and strength training exercises, but for persons at risk for falling, the recommendations are to perform balance exercises and to have a physical activity plan with a health care provider to manage risks and take therapeutic needs into account. A referral to a dietitian may be beneficial because dietary recommendations may need to be modified to provide for the older adult's nutritional needs.

COMPLICATIONS

The complications associated with the features of metabolic syndrome include CVD, atherosclerotic vascular disease, ischemic heart disease, coronary artery disease, myocardial infarction, and stroke.

Insulin resistance is the pathophysiologic hallmark of IGT and type 2 diabetes and may occur decades before the clinical presentation of these diseases. As the beta cell function deteriorates and is no longer able to compensate for the insulin resistance and as glucose levels rise, a transition from insulin resistance to IGT with mild increases in postprandial glucose levels occurs and eventually results in type 2 diabetes mellitus.

PATIENT AND FAMILY EDUCATION

Education should focus on the pathology of metabolic syndrome and associated characteristics along with the complications and cardiovascular risks that accompany the syndrome. This instruction should address medication use, mechanism of action, and adverse effects. Education must be provided to the patient and the family members because meal planning and participation in a physical fitness program will benefit the patient and family members involved. Family support is necessary to assist the patient with the lifestyle changes needed to decrease the risks of complications involved in the syndrome. Explaining the benefits of healthy eating and exercise can empower and motivate the patient. The discussion should involve exploring the patient's feelings toward metabolic syndrome and the treatment regimen. The patient should be instructed on mode, frequency, and intensity of exercise. Preferably, an exercise program of the patient's choice will better ensure adherence. Smoking cessation and limited use of alcohol, including the effects on insulin resistance, triglyceride levels, and cardiovascular risks, should be discussed. Mutual goal setting before the initiation of treatment is necessary for the patient's success. Both written and verbal instructions must be given to the patient and reinforced at each visit.

HEALTH PROMOTION

Health care providers are in a unique position to intervene, motivate, and influence the patient's outcome and the family members through teaching, counseling, and health promotion. Since insulin resistance and metabolic syndrome are now being found in children, it is imperative to start promoting healthy lifestyles at a very young age. Promotion of weight loss in the individual who is moderately overweight can prevent the development of insulin resistance and the complications associated with the syndrome. Practitioners can assist the patient in changing harmful health behaviors through counseling on nutrition and facilitating increases in physical activity. Weight management behavioral changes include improvements in eating habits, such as setting goals, planning meals, reading labels, eating regularly, reducing portion sizes, controlling social and environmental cues that encourage overeating, monitoring results, and avoiding binges. Disease prevention and health promotion before the occurrence of complications associated with metabolic syndrome are more cost-effective in terms of health care dollars and promote savings in human suffering. Through health promotion and early intervention, the occurrence and ramifications of metabolic syndrome can surely be decreased or possibly eliminated.

REFERENCES

1. Reaven, G. M. (1988). Role of insulin resistance in human disease. *Diabetes*, 37, 1595–1607, original reference.
2. Swarup, S., & Zeltser, R. (2019). Metabolic syndrome. In *StatPearls [Internet]*. Treasure Island (FL): StatPearls Publishing. Retrieved from https://www.ncbi.nlm.nih.gov/books/NBK459248/. [Updated 2019 Feb 28].
3. Kaur, J. (2014). A comprehensive review on metabolic syndrome. *Cardiology Research and Practice*, 2014, 1–21.
4. Moore, J. X., Chaudhary, N., & Akinyemiju, T. (2017). Metabolic syndrome prevalence by race/ethnicity and sex in the United States, National Health and Nutrition Examination Survey, 1988-2012. *Preventing Chronic Disease*, 14, 160287.
5. Cooper, S. J., & Reynolds, G. P. (2016). BAP guidelines on the management of weight gain, metabolic disturbances and cardiovascular risk associated with psychosis and antipsychotic drug treatment. *Journal of Psychopharmacology (Oxford, England)*, 1–32.
6. Owen, J. G., & Reisin, E. (2015). Anti-hypertensice drug treatment of patients with the metabolic syndrome and obesity: A review of evidence, meta-analysis, post hoc and guidelines publications. *Current Hypertension Reports*, 17, 46.
7. Han, T. S., & Lean, M. E. J. (2016). A clinical perspective of obesity, metabolic syndrome and cardiovascular disease. *JRSM Cardiovascular Disease*, 5, 1–13.
8. Lauria, M. W., & Saad, M. J. (2016). Acanthosis nigricans and insulin resistance. *The New England Journal of Medicine*, 374, e31.
9. Professional Practice Committee. (2019). Standards of medical care in diabetes—2019. *Diabetes Care*, 42(Suppl. 1), S3. https://doi.org/10.2337/dc19-SppC01.
10. 2019). 2019 ACC/AHA guideline on the primary prevention of cardiovascular disease. *Journal of the American College of Cardiology*, doi:10.1016/j.jacc.2019.03.010. 26029.
11. American Heart Association. Aspirin and heart disease. Retrieved from www.heart.org/HEARTORG/Conditions/HeartAttack/PreventionTreatmentof HeartAttack/Aspirin-and-Heart-Disease_UCM_321714_Article.jsp. (Accessed 20 December 2017).
12. Lim, S., & Eckel, R. H. (2014). Pharmacological treatment and therapeutic perspectives of metabolic syndrome. *Reviews in Endocrine and Metabolic Disorders*, 15(4), 329–341.
13. Shettar, V., Patel, S., & Kidambi, S. (2017). Epidemiology of obesity and pharmacologic treatment options. *Nutrition in Clinical Practice*, 36(4), 442–462.
14. Kim, S. H., Chun, H. J., Choi, H. S., et al. (2016). Current status of intragastric balloon for obesity treatment. *World Journal of Gastroenterology*, 22(24), 5495–5504.
15. Wolfe, B. M., Kyach, E., & Eckel, R. H. (2016). Treatment of obesity: Weight loss and bariatric surgery. *Circulation Research*, 118(11), 1844–1855.
16. Apovian, C. M., Shah, S. N., Wolfe, B. M., et al. (2017). Two year outcomes of vagal nerve blocking (vBloc) for the treatment of obesity in the ReCharge trial. *Obesity Surgery*, 27(1), 169–176.
17. Noren, E., & Forssell, H. (2016). Aspiration therapy for obesity; a safe and effective treatment. *BMC Obesity*, 3(56).
18. Evert, A., Dennison, M., & Gardiner, C. (2019). Nutrition therapy for adults with diabetes or pre diabetes: A consensus report. *Diabetes Care*, https://doi:org/10.2337/dci19-0014.
19. Ostman, C., Smart, N. A., Morcos, D., et al. (2017). The effect of exercise training on clinical outcomes in patients with the metabolic syndrome: A systemic review and meta-analysis. *Cardiovascular Diabetology*, 16(110), 1–11.
20. Friend, A., Craig, L., & Turner, S. (2013). The prevalence of metabolic syndrome in children: A systemic review of the literature. *Metabolic Syndrome and Related Disorders*, 11(2), 71–80.
21. Kumar, S., & Kelly, A. (2017). Review of childhood obesity: From epidemiology, etiology, and comorbidities to clinical assessment and treatment. *Mayo Clinic Proceedings*, 92(2), 251–265.

CHAPTER **193**

PARATHYROID GLAND DISORDERS

Roselyn Cristelle I. Mateo • Alan Ona Malabanan

 Specialist referral is indicated for all suspected cases of parathyroid disorders.

DEFINITION AND EPIDEMIOLOGY

The four parathyroid glands, located in the neck next to the thyroid, sense serum levels of ionized calcium by the calcium-sensing receptor and regulate calcium through parathyroid hormone (PTH) release. PTH is an 84–amino acid peptide that raises serum calcium concentration in three ways: (1) by acting directly on bone to release calcium into the extracellular fluid; (2) by acting directly on the kidney to decrease renal loss of calcium; and (3) by acting indirectly on the intestinal tract, through the activation of vitamin D, to increase dietary calcium absorption. Parathyroid disorders cause dysfunction through their effects on bone, kidney, serum calcium, and phosphorus.

The two major categories of parathyroid dysfunction are hyperparathyroidism (the oversecretion of PTH) and hypoparathyroidism (the undersecretion of PTH). PTH levels must always be interpreted in the context of the corrected serum calcium level or serum ionized calcium level (see Chapter 193). Considered in this manner, primary hyperparathyroidism (PHPT) can be defined as the inappropriate secretion of PTH in the setting of hypercalcemia. Secondary hyperparathyroidism is an appropriately increased secretion of PTH in the setting of low or normal serum calcium concentration and can be caused by vitamin D deficiency or renal failure. Tertiary hyperparathyroidism is prolonged secondary hyperparathyroidism in which hypercalcemia develops; it is an initially appropriate secretion that later becomes inappropriate. Normocalcemic PHPT is an elevated PTH, typically identified in the evaluation of osteoporosis or kidney stones, in the setting of normal calcium after kidney disease, vitamin D deficiency, and other common sources of secondary hyperparathyroidism are excluded. Hypoparathyroidism is the inappropriately low or normal secretion of PTH in the setting of hypocalcemia.

PHPT is common, its incidence ranging as high as 196 cases per 100,000 person-years, and greater in women, African Americans, and increasing age after the sixth decade.[1] Its incidence is increased in those exposed to ionizing radiation. After the 1970s, when routine laboratory screening became available, the clinical presentation went from being floridly symptomatic with "bones, stones, and groans" to predominantly asymptomatic. There has been an increase in the diagnosis of PHPT since 1998, coincident with the introduction of national osteoporosis screening guidelines.[2] Normocalcemic PHPT prevalence estimates have varied from 0.5% to 16.7%, but suffer from whether vitamin D deficiency and renal dysfunction were excluded in the definition.[3]

Secondary hyperparathyroidism is found commonly in patients with chronic kidney disease (CKD), often when the glomerular filtration rate (GFR) falls below 50 mL/min. Vitamin D deficiency and insufficiency, defined as serum 25-hydroxyvitamin D levels of less than 20 ng/mL and 30 ng/mL, respectively, are other important causes of secondary hyperparathyroidism, particularly in older adults and institutionalized patients, and have been estimated to occur in 40% to 100% of US and European community-dwelling elders. Secondary hyperparathyroidism may also occur in patients being treated with glucocorticoids or proton pump inhibitors, which decrease intestinal calcium absorption.[4]

Hypoparathyroidism is primarily a consequence of thyroid and parathyroid surgery, representing ~75% of the cases. The incidence of acute postsurgical hypoparathyroidism ranges from 0.6% to 17%, depending on the skill of the surgeon and the type of operation. A study has suggested that the rate of long-term hypoparathyroidism after thyroidectomy is actually low.[5] The prevalence of hypoparathyroidism from any cause has been estimated as 37 per 100,000 person-years and its incidence 0.8 per 100,000 person-years.[6]

PATHOPHYSIOLOGY

In 80% of cases of PHPT, excess PTH is produced by a single parathyroid adenoma. In 10% to 15% of cases, it is produced by hyperplasia of all four glands, which may be associated with multiple endocrine neoplasia (MEN) type I or type II. Multiple adenomas are found in 5% and PHPT is produced by a parathyroid carcinoma in less than 1% of cases.[7]

PTH receptor signaling in osteoblasts and osteocytes can increase the RANKL/OPG ratio, the main mechanism by which PTH stimulates osteoclast-mediated bone degradation, releasing calcium and phosphorus into the extracellular space. As a result, prolonged exposure to excess PTH will erode bone, particularly cortical (dense) bone. Trabecular bone is relatively spared because of a concomitant increase in osteoblast-mediated bone formation. Skeletal sites with primarily cortical bone, such as the wrist and proximal radius, are particularly at increased risk for fracture.

PTH acts on the kidney to increase calcium reabsorption and to increase phosphorus losses. The rising serum calcium concentration gradually exceeds the kidney's ability to reabsorb the filtered calcium, thus increasing urinary calcium. Nephrocalcinosis, nephrolithiasis, and renal dysfunction may result. PTH receptors also exist on a variety of tissues, including brain, skin, and heart. The effects of PTH on these tissues are not yet well characterized.

Secondary hyperparathyroidism (HPT) represents a compensation for decreased serum levels of ionized calcium and its pathogenesis is driven by several factors. The kidneys play an important role in calcium and phosphorus homeostasis, and renal insufficiency disturbs calcium metabolism in four ways. First, decreased phosphorus clearance, hyperphosphatemia, and consequent increases in fibroblast growth factor 23 exacerbate secondary HPT through the reduction in 1,25 $(OH)_2$ Vitamin D (calcitriol). Second, decreased renal activation of vitamin D decreases intestinal calcium absorption, which then stimulates PTH secretion. Third, uremia produces PTH resistance, thus necessitating higher levels of PTH. Finally, uremia decreases the inhibitory effect of calcium on PTH release. As with PHPT, excess PTH will erode bone. These derangements in mineral metabolism may also lead to extraskeletal and vascular calcifications.[8] The incidence and severity of secondary HPT increases as kidney function declines and can lead to significant abnormalities in bone mineralization and turnover. Prolonged stimulation of the parathyroid glands by hypocalcemia results in hyperplasia of the glands. On occasion, this leads to autonomous parathyroid function and hypercalcemia (tertiary hyperparathyroidism).

Vitamin D deficiency results in decreased intestinal calcium absorption. This, coupled with the daily loss of calcium in the urine and the feces, leads to a net loss of calcium. To prevent overt hypocalcemia, the parathyroid glands secrete more PTH, releasing calcium from the bone and thus preserving normal serum calcium levels. Long-standing vitamin D deficiency may lead to overt hypocalcemia if calcium stores in the bone are depleted.

Hypoparathyroidism results from the destruction of the parathyroid glands, whether the result of surgery, irradiation, infiltration (hemochromatosis, amyloidosis, hemosiderosis), malignant disease, or autoimmune disease. Genetic syndromes such as autoimmune polyendocrinopathy syndrome Type 1, DiGeorge syndrome, hypoparathyroidism-deafness-renal dysplasia syndrome, and Kenny-Caffey syndrome may be causes of hypoparathyroidism and are associated with other conditions such as cardiac and eye defects.[9] As may be expected, decreased PTH affects the renal conservation of calcium, the intestinal absorption of calcium, and the degradative release of calcium from bone. Hypocalcemia results from these effects. Of note, hypomagnesemia or hypermagnesemia may decrease PTH secretion or diminish PTH action on the bone and should be considered a potential cause of hypoparathyroidism.

CLINICAL PRESENTATION AND PHYSICAL EXAMINATION

Asymptomatic hypercalcemia is the most common presentation of PHPT. The hypercalcemia may be masked by hypoalbuminemia or minimized by concomitant vitamin D deficiency and the PTH levels may fall, inappropriately nonsuppressed, within the normal range. This hypercalcemia is usually accompanied by a fasting hypophosphatemia. Normocalcemic PHPT may be identified in the laboratory evaluation of osteoporosis or kidney stones and diagnosed after secondary causes of hyperparathyroidism, such as CKD and vitamin D deficiency are excluded.

Some patients may report nonspecific neurocognitive symptoms, which vary with the magnitude of hypercalcemia: weakness, easy fatigability, depression, intellectual weariness, cognitive impairment, loss of initiative, anxiety, irritability, and insomnia, some of which they or their physician may attribute to normal aging. Some may have worsening of parkinsonism which may respond to cinacalcet therapy.[10] Cardiovascular manifestations may include hypertension, coronary artery disease, left ventricular hypertrophy, and valvular calcifications, which are associated with higher levels of serum calcium.[11] Kidney stones are also a common presenting symptom of PHPT, although some asymptomatic patients may have a history of unexplained hematuria, nocturia, and polyuria.

Often, PHPT may be identified during the evaluation of osteoporosis, which typically affects predominantly cortical bone sites (radius, femoral neck) more than predominantly trabecular bone sites (lumbar spine), although vertebral fracture may occur and be clinically silent despite relatively preserved bone density.[7] A severe form of parathyroid bone disease, osteitis fibrosa cystica (OFC), is associated with multiple lytic bone lesions and subperiosteal bone resorption. OFC may be found in conjunction with an acute hyperparathyroid crisis in which the hypercalcemia develops quickly, causing obtundation, volume depletion, and cardiac arrhythmias.

Hyperparathyroidism may occur as part of a familial disorder such as MEN. MEN type I includes hyperparathyroidism, pituitary tumors, and pancreatic tumors (insulinoma, gastrinoma). MEN type IIA includes hyperparathyroidism, pheochromocytoma, and medullary thyroid carcinoma. In these disorders, the hyperparathyroidism is caused by parathyroid hyperplasia.

Secondary hyperparathyroidism is typically found with CKD stages 3 to 5 and vitamin D deficiency. Patients may be initially seen with bone pain or a pathologic fracture. Risk factors for vitamin D deficiency include minimum sun exposure, inadequate vitamin D dietary intake, obesity, malabsorption, prior gastric surgery, and medications that may increase the metabolism of vitamin D (e.g., rifampin, ketoconazole, and anticonvulsants). Other factors, such as aging, sunscreen use, and heavily pigmented skin, decrease sunlight-mediated vitamin D synthesis in the skin.[4] Secondary hyperparathyroidism in CKD produces a host of metabolic derangements, including hypocalcemia, hyperphosphatemia, and low 1,25-dihydroxyvitamin D levels. This hyperparathyroidism may be associated with increased vascular disease and vascular or soft tissue calcification.

Hypoparathyroidism manifests as hypocalcemia accompanied by hyperphosphatemia. The presentation can range from symptoms of perioral and digital paresthesias to life-threatening cardiac arrhythmias, seizures, and laryngospasm. The severity of presentation depends on the rapidity of the development of hypocalcemia. It may also depend on the presence of acidemia, which increases ionized calcium, or alkalemia, which decreases ionized calcium. Chronic hypocalcemia can produce premature cataract formation or basal ganglia calcifications, at times with a reversible Parkinson syndrome.

Physical clues to PHPT include band keratopathy, a white cloudiness at the nasal and temporal borders of the cornea. It may be mistaken for arcus senilis and is not specific for hypercalcemia caused by hyperparathyroidism. On occasion, there may be bone tenderness, particularly of the sternum and tibia. Rarely, there may be a palpable neck mass that is indicative of parathyroid carcinoma or medullary thyroid carcinoma (in MEN type II).

The physical clues to hypoparathyroidism include the signs indicative of hypocalcemia. The Chvostek sign may be present in cases of hypocalcemia. This test is performed by tapping (the point of a triangular reflex hammer or a fingertip may be used) over the facial nerve (cranial nerve VII). Contraction of the facial muscles (seen at the corner of the lip and cheek) is

a positive test result. The Trousseau sign may also be present in hypocalcemia. This test is performed by placing a blood pressure cuff around the biceps and inflating the cuff approximately 10 to 20 mm Hg above the systolic blood pressure. The cuff is left inflated, maintaining a constant pressure, for 3 minutes or until a positive result is elicited. The test result is positive if carpal spasm occurs (flexion at the wrist and extension of the fingers). The presence of Chvostek and Trousseau signs can be affected by abnormalities in acid–base balance, potassium level, and magnesium level. Bone tenderness over the sternum or tibia may be present in vitamin D deficiency.[4]

Pseudohypoparathyroidism is a genetic disorder characterized by hypocalcemia and hyperparathyroidism, but with an elevated PTH indicating target organ PTH resistance. There are multiple subtypes depending on the presence of multiple hormone resistances and a constellation of physical findings known as Albright hereditary osteodystrophy, characterized by short stature, facial rounding, shortening of the third, fourth, and fifth metacarpals, subcutaneous ossifications, varying degrees of mental retardation, and obesity.[12]

DIAGNOSTICS

Laboratory testing is necessary for the diagnosis of parathyroid disease. The most useful PTH assay is the PTH second- or third-generation assay, which allows measurement of the intact PTH molecule. Biotin use may lead to a decrease in biotinylated PTH assay and increase in biotinylated 25-hydroxyvitamin D assay levels and should be stopped 7 days before testing.[13]

PHPT requires the assessment of PTH, serum calcium, albumin, 25-hydroxyvitamin D, and fasting phosphorus. A bone mineral density assessment of a cortical bone site (e.g., radius), in conjunction with the standard lumbar spine and hip, is useful to assess the risk for osteoporosis. Vertebral fracture assessment and trabecular bone score would be useful adjuncts to bone mineral density testing, if available.[14] Renal imaging (renal ultrasound) is useful in assessing the presence of nephrolithiasis, and renal stones would be indicative of symptomatic PHPT. A 24-hour urine collection for calcium and creatinine is useful in the initial evaluation of PHPT and if less than 400 mg/day, consideration may be given to a kidney stone risk profile.[11] Electrocardiography (ECG) may be useful in assessing hypercalcemic cardiotoxicity (QT shortening). Although it is not recommended for diagnosis, imaging with sestamibi scan or neck ultrasound has been useful for anatomic localization of the enlarged parathyroid glands, making minimally invasive parathyroidectomy possible.[15]

Secondary hyperparathyroidism and hypoparathyroidism also require assessment of PTH, serum calcium, albumin, and fasting phosphorus. A serum 25-hydroxyvitamin D level, if it is less than 20 ng/mL, is useful in establishing vitamin D deficiency as the cause of the hyperparathyroidism. A 24-hour urine collection for calcium and creatinine would be helpful in the assessment of secondary hyperparathyroidism to assess for hypocalciuria (as a sign of calcium malabsorption) or hypercalciuria as a cause. A serum magnesium level may also be useful in evaluating hypoparathyroidism. ECG can reveal hypocalcemic cardiotoxicity (QT lengthening).

The most recent Kidney Disease: Improving Global Outcomes (KDIGO) guidelines for CKD–metabolic bone disease suggest that serum calcium, phosphorus, and PTH be measured in adult patients in CKD stage 3 and in children in CKD stage 2.[8] The frequency of monitoring is dependent on the severity of the CKD and the metabolic bone disease but

INITIAL DIAGNOSTICS

Parathyroid Gland Disorders

HYPERPARATHYROIDISM
Laboratory
- Parathyroid hormone (PTH immunoradiometric assay)
- Serum calcium
- Albumin
- Fasting phosphorus
- 24-h urine calcium
- Serum 1,25-dihydroxyvitamin D[a]
- Serum 25-hydroxyvitamin D

Imaging
- X-ray examination of abdomen[a]
- Renal ultrasound
- Bone mineral densitometry (distal radius)

- Trabecular bone score
- Vertebral fracture assessment

ADDITIONAL DIAGNOSTICS
- Electrocardiography (ECG)[a]

HYPOPARATHYROIDISM
Laboratory
- PTH
- Serum calcium
- Albumin
- Fasting phosphorus
- Serum 1,25-dihydroxyvitamin D
- Magnesium
- Serum 25-hydroxyvitamin
- Additional Diagnostics
- ECG[a]

_____
[a]If indicated.

Differential Diagnosis: Parathyroid Gland Disorders

HYPERPARATHYROIDISM
- Primary hyperparathyroidism
- Familial hyperparathyroidism
- Familial hypocalciuric hypercalcemia
- Lithium-related parathyroid disease
- Adenoma
- Radiation-induced hyperparathyroidism
- Multiple endocrine neoplasia syndrome
- Parathyroid carcinoma
- Secondary hyperparathyroidism
- Chronic renal disease
- Vitamin D deficiency
- Thiazide-induced hypercalcemia

HYPOPARATHYROIDISM
- Idiopathic
- Iatrogenic
- Congenital
- Polyglandular autoimmune syndrome
- Metastatic cancer
- Hemochromatosis
- Amyloidosis
- Hypermagnesemia or hypomagnesemia
- Parkinson syndrome

may range from every 1 to 3 months to every 6 to 12 months. In CKD stages 4 and 5, alkaline phosphatase, an indicator of PTH effect on bone, may be tested every 12 months or more frequently if PTH is elevated. Those patients in CKD stages 3 to 5 with hyperparathyroidism should be evaluated and treated for hyperphosphatemia, hypocalcemia, and vitamin D insufficiency.

DIFFERENTIAL DIAGNOSIS

The differential diagnoses for the parathyroid diseases overlap with those of hypercalcemia and hypocalcemia (Box 193.1). With PHPT, the most important diagnosis to exclude is familial hypocalciuric hypercalcemia (FHH), an autosomal dominant trait characterized by hypercalcemia and hyperparathyroidism. With FHH, a mutation in the calcium-sensing receptor gene causes a defective calcium-sensing receptor requiring higher levels of calcium to suppress PTH secretion. Patients with FHH do not have the usual sequelae of PHPT and generally have a benign course. A history of lifelong hypercalcemia, a family history of hypercalcemia, and concomitant mild hypermagnesemia are important clues to FHH.

In FHH, the fractional excretion of calcium (FE_{Ca}) is typically less than 0.01%. For patients with PHPT, the FE_{Ca} is more than 0.013%. The formula is as follows:

$$FE_{Ca} = (U_{Ca} \times P_{Cr})/(U_{Cr} \times P_{Ca})$$

where U is urine concentration (mg/dL) of a 24-hour specimen and P is plasma concentration (mg/dL) for calcium (Ca) and creatinine (Cr).

An FE_{Ca} should be calculated to rule out FHH before parathyroidectomy for hyperparathyroidism. An FE_{Ca} of less than 0.01% suggests FHH. Uncorrected vitamin D deficiency, CKD, inadequate calcium intake, and thiazide/amiloride use may give a falsely low value. If necessary, genetic analysis for a mutation in the calcium-sensing receptor can be done to confirm the diagnosis. Of note, autoantibodies directed at the calcium-sensing receptor can cause an acquired, immune-mediated disease that resembles FHH.

Another clinical situation that produces a similar picture is lithium-related parathyroid disease. Lithium appears to raise the calcium set-point through unclear mechanisms.

For hypoparathyroidism, the most important diagnostic consideration is hypomagnesemia or hypermagnesemia. Consideration of rare causes of hypoparathyroidism, such as autosomal dominant hypocalcemia or acquired calcium-sensing receptor activation, might be suggested by hypermagnesuria.

Pseudohypoparathyroidism, an inherited resistance to PTH, can be a consideration if long-standing hypocalcemia is present with elevated levels of PTH in the face of normal magnesium balance and normal renal function.

INTERPROFESSIONAL COLLABORATIVE MANAGEMENT

Nonpharmacologic Management

The only cure for PHPT is surgery, and referral to an experienced parathyroid surgeon is important. In most instances, resection of the parathyroid adenoma or 3¾ of the four hyperplastic parathyroid glands corrects the hyperparathyroidism. However, the changing character of PHPT, with early diagnosis and primarily asymptomatic patients, has led to an increasing role for medical therapy.

An increasing body of data regarding the long-term complications and benefits of parathyroidectomy in asymptomatic patients with PHPT has led to revisions in the criteria for parathyroidectomy:
- Age younger than 50 years.
- Serum calcium level 1 mg/dL above the upper limit of normal.

- Vertebral fracture by radiography, computed tomography (CT), magnetic resonance imaging (MRI), or densitometric vertebral fracture assessment (VFA).
- 24-h urine for calcium greater than 400 mg/day (>10 mmol/day) and increased stone risk by biochemical stone risk analysis.
- Presence of nephrolithiasis or nephrocalcinosis by radiography, ultrasound, or CT.
- GFR below 60 mL/min/1.73 m^2 (i.e., CKD stage 3), although there is no evidence that parathyroidectomy improves GFR.
- In perimenopausal or postmenopausal women and men older than 50 years, a T-score of −2.5 or lower at the lumbar spine, femoral neck, total hip, or distal radius; in premenopausal women and men younger than 50 years, a Z-score of −2.5 or lower at the same sites.[11]

Successful parathyroidectomy may lead, in some patients, to improvements in neurocognitive symptoms but more consistently to improvements in bone density and perhaps reduction in fracture risk. The risk for nephrolithiasis decreases with parathyroidectomy, whereas cardiovascular disease and mortality do not seem to change. The decline of renal function is halted after parathyroidectomy. Surgical consultation may be offered to patients with confirmed diagnoses of PHPT even if they do not meet surgical criteria, provided there are no contraindications.[14]

Pharmacologic Management

Medical management of PHPT involves close monitoring of serum calcium and creatinine (at least annually) and bone density (every 1 to 2 years) to see if surgical criteria are met as the PHPT progresses. Adequate calcium and vitamin D intake should be continued, ensuring a 25-hydroxyvitamin D level of at least 20 ng/mL. Calcium and vitamin D restriction can worsen the bone disease and lead to worsening hyperparathyroidism. Patients should be encouraged to maintain weight-bearing activity and adequate fluid intake to prevent the volume depletion that can worsen hypercalcemia. Antiresorptive treatment with bisphosphonates, or hormone replacement with estrogen, and raloxifene therapy may be useful in increasing bone density without significant change in calcium levels in patients with PHPT and should be considered in patients with osteoporosis or in the presence of fragility fractures who are unable or unwilling to undergo parathyroid surgery. Cinacalcet a calcimimetic agent, has been found to normalize serum calcium and PTH levels without improving bone density or without lowering biochemical markers of bone turnover. It is now approved for the medical management of hypercalcemia caused by PHPT in patients in whom surgery is indicated but not possible. Cinacalcet acts by increasing the sensitivity of the CaSR to extracellular calcium, thereby decreasing serum PTH and reducing the renal tubular reabsorption of calcium and it can normalize serum calcium in 70% to 80% of patients. None of these therapies is a suitable replacement for parathyroidectomy but may be helpful in minimizing complications for those patients who are not surgical candidates.[11,14,16,17]

The management of secondary hyperparathyroidism depends on the cause. For renal failure, renal transplantation usually corrects the hyperparathyroidism, but it may be refractory if it is long-standing. Patients with CKD stages 3 to 5 with hyperparathyroidism should be evaluated and treated for alterations in calcium and phosphorus homeostasis, increase in the level of PTH and fibroblast growth factor 23, and reduction in

1,25 vitamin D insufficiency. In predialysis patients with CKD 3a-5, the optimal PTH level is not yet known and calcitriol and vitamin D analogs may not be routinely used. However it is reasonable to reserve the use of calcitriol and vitamin D analogs for patients with CKD 4 to 5 with severe and progressive hyperparathyroidism. Calcimimetics, calcitriol, vitamin D analogs, or a combination of calcimimetics with calcitriol or vitamin D analogs may be used in patients with CKD5 requiring PTH lowering therapy. These therapies may be modified or adjusted according to the presence of hypercalcemia, hyperphosphatemia, or hypocalcemia. In patients with CKD stages 3 to 5 who do not respond to medical or pharmacologic therapy, parathyroidectomy is indicated [8]

Hypoparathyroidism is difficult to treat. PTH must be given parenterally and therefore is not easily replaced. Therapy usually consists of vitamin D analogues and calcium supplements. Dairy products, which are high in phosphorus, should be avoided. Perhaps the safest medication is calcitriol, but it is also the most expensive. It is preferable to ergocalciferol (vitamin D) because it acts more quickly (days versus weeks) and has a shorter duration of action, which allows rapid titration. Hypercalciuria is the main limitation of calcitriol therapy. The absence of the PTH effect on renal conservation of calcium results in hypercalciuria as intestinal absorption of calcium increases. Calcitriol should be started at 0.25 mcg orally every day and increased as necessary every 2 to 4 weeks to bring serum calcium concentration into the low-normal range without producing hypercalciuria. The judicious use of thiazides may decrease urinary calcium loss and allow the normalization of serum calcium concentration, although combination therapy with thiazides and calcitriol may increase the risk for hypercalcemia. PTH therapy has recently been approved for this indication but is available only through a restricted program. PTH therapy may decrease calcium and calcitriol requirements, without changing serum or urinary calcium levels,[18] and improve some quality-of-life measures.[19] The risk of long-term PTH therapy is unclear.

COMPLICATIONS

Complications may result from the parathyroid disease process or its treatment. In addition to osteoporosis and nephrolithiasis, surgery for PHPT may cause hypocalcemia because of temporary hypoparathyroidism, vitamin D deficiency, or hungry bone syndrome. With hungry bone syndrome, calcium, phosphorus, and magnesium are rapidly incorporated into bone. This cause of hypocalcemia is more common in patients with higher preoperative serum calcium and alkaline phosphatase levels or more severe bone disease.

LIFE SPAN CONSIDERATIONS

Cardiovascular mortality may be increased in patients with severe and moderately severe PHPT, and this may decline after parathyroidectomy. The mortality may be affected by severity of calcium and phosphorus. CKD-BMD involves three main categories: bone abnormalities; vascular calcifications involving coronary, valvular, myocardial, and/or conduction systems; and mineral disorders including phosphorus, calcium, PTH, and FGF23, and in each CKD stage and each kind of cardiac abnormality, the target ranges may differ. We need to tread carefully with our treatment strategies and goals as QT prolongation through decreasing calcium levels may potentially trigger a fatal arrhythmia.[20] While some basic science and observational data support the role of phosphate toxicity in CKD, there are no large clinical trials showing improved outcomes with phosphorus-lowering interventions.[21] Nonsurgical hypoparathyroidism does not appear to be associated with increased mortality but is associated with an increased risk for cardiovascular and renal disease, as well as increased hospitalization risk for psychiatric disease, seizures, and infections.[9]

PATIENT EDUCATION AND HEALTH PROMOTION

For patients with PHPT, understanding the importance of adequate calcium and fluid intake as well as continued monitoring of bone and calcium status is important. Patients unable to maintain fluid intake because of nausea or vomiting should be instructed to seek prompt medical attention. Potential complications of parathyroid bone disease, such as wrist and hip fractures, should be carefully explained. For patients with secondary hyperparathyroidism, the importance of calcium and vitamin D supplementation should be stressed. For patients who undergo surgical therapy or who have hypoparathyroidism, it is essential that they recognize the symptoms of hypocalcemia and the consequences of nonadherence to therapy, including tetany, laryngospasm, cardiac arrhythmias, and seizures.

REFERENCES

1. Yeh, M. W., et al. (2013). Incidence and prevalence of primary hyperparathyroidism in a racially mixed population. *The Journal of Clinical Endocrinology and Metabolism, 98*, 1122–1129.
2. Griebeler, M. L., et al. (2015). Secular trends in the incidence of primary hyperparathyroidism over five decades (1965-2010). *Bone, 73*, 1–7.
3. Cusano, N. E., Silverberg, S. J., & Bilezikian, J. P. (2013). Normocalcemic primary hyperparathyroidism. *Journal of Clinical Densitometry: Official Journal of the International Society for Clinical Densitometry, 16*, 33–39.
4. Holick, M. F. (2007). Vitamin D deficiency. *The New England Journal of Medicine, 357*, 266–281.
5. Youngwirth, L., Benavidez, J., Sippel, R., & Chen, H. (2010). Parathyroid hormone deficiency after total thyroidectomy: Incidence and time. *The Journal of Surgical Research, 163*, 69–71.
6. Clarke, B. L., et al. (2016). Epidemiology and diagnosis of hypoparathyroidism. *The Journal of Clinical Endocrinology and Metabolism, 101*, 2284–2299.
7. Walker, M. D., & Silverberg, S. J. (2017). Primary hyperparathyroidism. *Nature Reviews. Endocrinology, 14*, 115–125.
8. Ketteler, M., et al. (2017). Executive summary of the 2017 KDIGO Chronic Kidney Disease-Mineral and Bone Disorder (CKD-MBD) guideline update: What's changed and why it matters. *Kidney International, 92*, 26–36.
9. Shoback, D. M., et al. (2016). Presentation of hypoparathyroidism: Etiologies and clinical features. *The Journal of Clinical Endocrinology and Metabolism, 101*, 2300–2312.
10. Ohya, Y., et al. (2018). A case of hyperparathyroidism-associated parkinsonism successfully treated with cinacalcet hydrochloride, a calcimimetic. *BMC Neurology, 18*, 62.
11. Bilezikian, J. P., et al. (2014). Guidelines for the management of asymptomatic primary hyperparathyroidism: Summary statement from the Fourth International Workshop. *The Journal of Clinical Endocrinology and Metabolism, 99*, 3561–3569.
12. Mantovani, G. (2011). Clinical review: Pseudohypoparathyroidism: diagnosis and treatment. *The Journal of Clinical Endocrinology and Metabolism, 96*, 3020–3030.
13. Li, D., et al. (2017). Association of biotin ingestion with performance of hormone and nonhormone assays in healthy adults. *JAMA: The Journal of the American Medical Association, 318*, 1150–1160.
14. Khan, A. A., et al. (2017). Primary hyperparathyroidism: Review and recommendations on evaluation, diagnosis, and management. A Canadian and international consensus. *Osteoporosis International, 28*, 1–19.
15. Udelsman, R., et al. (2014). The surgical management of asymptomatic primary hyperparathyroidism: Proceedings of the Fourth International Workshop. *The Journal of Clinical Endocrinology and Metabolism, 99*, 3595–3606.
16. Mizamtsidi, M., et al. (2018). Diagnosis, management, histology and genetics of sporadic primary hyperparathyroidism: Old knowledge with new tricks. *Endocrine Connections, 7*, R56–R68.
17. Peacock, M., et al. (2009). Cinacalcet treatment of primary hyperparathyroidism: Biochemical and bone densitometric outcomes in a five-year study. *The Journal of Clinical Endocrinology and Metabolism, 94*, 4860–4867.
18. Mannstadt, M., et al. (2013). Efficacy and safety of recombinant human parathyroid hormone (1–84) in hypoparathyroidism (REPLACE): A double-blind, placebo-controlled, randomised, phase 3 study. *The Lancet. Diabetes & Endocrinology, 1*, 275–283.
19. Vokes, T. J., et al. (2018). Recombinant human parathyroid hormone effect on health-related quality of life in adults with chronic hypoparathyroidism. *The Journal of Clinical Endocrinology and Metabolism, 103*, 722–731.
20. Fujii, H., & Joki, N. (2017). Mineral metabolism and cardiovascular disease in CKD. *Clinical and Experimental Nephrology, 21*, 53–63.
21. Ritter, C. S., & Slatopolsky, E. (2016). Phosphate toxicity in CKD: The killer among us. *Clinical Journal of the American Society of Nephrology: CJASN, 11*, 1088–1100.

194

THYROID DISORDERS
Jennifer C. Braimon • Suzanne M. Rieke

 Immediate referral to a thyroid surgeon is indicated if compressive symptoms are present. Indications for hospitalization include respiratory compromise because of invasive tumors.

DEFINITION AND OVERVIEW

The thyroid is a butterfly-shaped gland, located anteriorly in the lower neck below the Adam's apple (cricothyroid cartilage). During embryogenesis, the thyroid develops at the base of the tongue and descends to its usual location anterior to the trachea, above the cricothyroid notch. The gland is formed by two lateral lobes connected by a median isthmus. Each thyroid lobe measures approximately 4 to 6 cm in height, the isthmus measures 2 to 3 mm in height, and the average thyroid weighs approximately 25 to 30 g. The thyroid produces hormones that influence a variety of metabolic processes in the body.

Thyroid disorders include structural and functional abnormalities, cysts, nodules, cancer, and overactive or underactive thyroid.

Thyroid function is regulated by thyroid stimulating hormone (TSH), which is secreted by basophilic cells in the anterior pituitary gland in response to the secretion of thyrotropin-releasing hormone (TRH) from the hypothalamus. TRH secretion is regulated in a negative feedback fashion by the thyroid hormones. Low serum levels of thyroid hormones trigger TRH release from the hypothalamus, which in turn stimulates TSH release from the pituitary. TSH increases release of thyroid hormones until a normal serum level is reached. Within the thyroid gland, thyroid function is affected by glandular organic iodine content.

The synthesis of T4 (thyroxine) and T3 (triiodothyronine) requires that adequate quantities of iodine enter the thyroid gland. Iodine enters from the bloodstream and is a constituent of both T4 and T3. These hormones are transported in the bloodstream bound to plasma proteins. The majority of T4 is bound; only a small portion is free. However, it is the free T4 concentration in the serum that reflects thyroidal activity. Approximately 80% of serum T3 is formed in the liver, kidney, and muscle from the deiodination of T4; the remaining 20%

Physiologic Effects of Thyroid Hormones

- Affect fetal development; secreted in fetus from 11 weeks and facilitate normal fetal growth
- Promote basal metabolic function; regulate oxygen consumption and heat production
- Affect cardiovascular muscle contraction
- Stimulate bone resorption and, to some extent, bone formation
- Permit normal glucose metabolism, absorption, and storage
- Function in the synthesis and breakdown of lipids
- Affect the rate of metabolism of many hormones and drugs (depends on amount of thyroid hormones)

is secreted directly by the thyroid.[1] Alterations in the regulation of hormone secretion can have varied effects on the body (Box 194.1).

THYROID FUNCTION TESTING

Thyroid function can be evaluated in the laboratory through the use of thyroid function tests (TFTs). Thyroid structure and function can be assessed through a variety of imaging techniques and through biopsy.

TSH is the most sensitive indicator of overall thyroid function. Small changes in serum T3 and T4 levels affect TSH secretion in an inverse log-linear relationship. Current techniques allow measurement of serum TSH concentrations as low as 0.01 µIU/mL (third-generation assay, immunometric dual-antibody assay). This is generally the best screening test for thyroid dysfunction. Exceptions include patients with pituitary or hypothalamic (secondary or tertiary) disease and patients immediately after treatment of hypothyroidism or hyperthyroidism (when the TSH response to therapy may lag behind). In addition, various medications and non-thyroidal conditions may affect TSH levels.

TSH measurements are usually sufficient to categorize patients into one of three groups: hyperthyroid (TSH <0.3 µIU/mL), hypothyroid (TSH >4 µIU/mL), and euthyroid (TSH 0.3 to 4 µIU/mL). In a review by Surks and Boucai,[2] TSH distributions were found to shift to higher concentrations with age and to vary according to race, with higher concentrations found in whites than in blacks or Hispanics.

Approximately 99% of circulating T4 and T3 is bound to serum proteins. It is the free, unbound T4 that is maintained at a constant level and correlates most with the thyroid state. Free T4 traverses cell membranes to exert its effects on body tissues. Direct measurement by equilibrium dialysis of free T4 is available but is cumbersome and technically demanding and is not for routine use. More commonly, a free thyroxine or a calculated free T4 index that corrects the total T4 (TT4) level for the concentration of thyroxine-binding globulin (TBG) is used to assess the thyroxine level.

TBG determinations are inaccurate in patients with congenital absence of TBG or familial dysalbuminemic hyperthyroxinemia (FDH). Patients with FDH have aberrant albumin that binds T4 (not T3) with increased affinity. In FDH, laboratory tests reveal increased TT4, normal total T3 (TT3), normal TSH, and normal free T4 by equilibrium dialysis. Circumstances that increase TBG include pregnancy, acute hepatitis, inherited abnormalities and the use of estrogen, oral contraceptives,

methadone, or heroin. Decreased TBG results from acromegaly, nephrotic syndrome, cirrhosis, and chronic debilitating disease and from treatment with glucocorticoids, androgens, aspirin, nonsteroidal antiinflammatory drugs (NSAIDs), and some penicillins.

Evaluation of thyroid function starts with the measurement of TSH level. If the TSH level is abnormal, a free thyroxine or free thyroxine index should be obtained. A total T3 level should be checked in the evaluation of hyperthyroidism (rule out T3 toxicosis).

Autoantibodies to thyroglobulin or thyroid microsomes may be found in patients with autoimmune thyroid disease. Thyroid peroxidase (TPO) is the major microsomal antigen. Anti-TPO antibodies are found in 90% to 100% of patients with Hashimoto thyroiditis and in less than 85% of patients with Graves disease (autoimmune hyperthyroidism). Antithyroglobulin antibodies are found in the majority of patients with Hashimoto thyroiditis and less than 20% of patients with Graves disease. Up to 15% to 20% of individuals in the general population have antibodies to either of these antigens. Quantification of the antibody titers is not clinically useful. These tests are particularly useful in the evaluation of patients with atypical manifestations of autoimmune thyroid disease (i.e., isolated ophthalmopathy without signs of hyperthyroidism). They are also predictive of postpartum thyroiditis and neonatal Graves disease.[1] TSH receptor antibodies (TRAb) are specific for Graves disease. TRAb levels decrease after medical therapy with thionamides and surgery.

Thyroid Imaging

Thyroid scans are used to assess the cause of hyperthyroidism (i.e., Graves disease, toxic nodules, thyroiditis) or the functional status of a nodule, but are not used to assess thyroid function. Iodine isotope scans (iodine 123 [^{123}I]) are preferred to pertechnetate (technetium Tc 99m, TcO$_4^-$) because of the ability of the isotope scan to distinguish between hot and cold nodules. Both iodine and technetium are taken up by thyroid cells, but only iodine is concentrated and bound by thyroid cells. The technetium scan is performed 20 minutes after the administration of TcO$_4^-$. Its advantages include low radiation exposure to the patient, availability, and power of resolution (approximately 5 mm). The iodine scan is performed 4 or 24 hours after the administration of ^{123}I or ^{125}I and 48, 72, or 96 hours after the administration of ^{131}I when it is used to search for metastatic thyroid cancer.

Normally the isotopes are distributed evenly throughout the thyroid gland. A mottled appearance is seen in Hashimoto thyroiditis or in recently treated Graves disease. An inhomogeneous uptake is also seen in multinodular goiters.

Nodules are classified as hot, warm, or cold according to the concentration of iodine isotope in the nodule in comparison with the rest of the thyroid gland. Hot nodules are usually but not always benign. Most cold nodules (solid or cystic) are benign; however, most malignant neoplasms also appear as cold nodules. The normal radioactive iodine uptake (RAIU) is approximately 30%. Radionuclide imaging cannot be performed for at least 4 weeks in patients who have recently received iodine-containing compounds (i.e., intravenous contrast material). The results may also be inaccurate (falsely low uptake) in patients who are following a high-iodine/salt diet. When ordering isotope scans, the health care provider can order RAIU alone or with a scan.

Ultrasonography is used to evaluate the anatomy of the thyroid gland and to differentiate solid from cystic nodules. It localizes the position and depth of lesions and can be used to guide fine-needle aspiration (FNA). Sonographic features of nodules can be more or less suggestive of malignancy. A nodule suspicious of malignancy on ultrasound might have irregular margins, microcalcifications, or taller than wide shape.[3] Ultrasound cannot be used to visualize substernal goiters because of interference from bone. Computed tomography (CT) and magnetic resonance imaging (MRI) are better suited to assessment of substernal goiters. Cervical lymph nodes are also well visualized on ultrasound. Benign lymph nodes tend to be thin and oval with an echogenic hilum, whereas malignant nodes tend to be round with an undefined hilum and may be vascular.

Fluorine 18 (^{18}F) fluorodeoxyglucose positron emission tomography (^{18}F-FDG-PET) has the highest resolution for detection of aggressive metastatic thyroid cancer lesions. Radiolabeled glucose is injected intravenously, and the scanner produces images that visualize where glucose is used. It identifies differences in how quickly cells metabolize glucose. Cancer cells metabolize glucose more quickly than normal cells do. Nodules with increased uptake on PET scan have a higher risk of malignancy.[4] More than 30% of PET avid thyroid nodules are malignant. The American Thyroid Association recommends USFNAB of all incidentally identified PET avid thyroid nodules greater than 1 cm. Most rapidly growing thyroid neoplasms have high metabolic rates. Well-differentiated thyroid tumors retain FDG poorly. Focal uptake of 18F-FDG can also be seen, however, in inflamed lymph nodes, thyroiditis, and benign thyroid nodules.[4]

Thyroid Biopsy

Fine needle aspiration biopsy is an office procedure in which tissue samples are obtained for cytologic examination; architecture is preserved. The biopsy is typically done under ultrasound guidance to ensure accurate placement of the needle into the nodule.

THYROID NODULES AND THYROID CANCER

DEFINITION AND EPIDEMIOLOGY

A thyroid nodule is a distinct lesion within the thyroid that is radiologically different from the rest of the thyroid. Some palpable lesions do not correspond to radiologic abnormalities. Nonpalpable nodules found on ultrasound or other imaging studies are referred to as incidental thyroid nodules. By this definition, thyroid nodules include both solid nodules and cysts.

With ultrasonography, approximately 50% of all single, palpable nodules are found to be in a multinodular gland. In general, nodules larger than 0.5 to 1 cm ($\frac{1}{5}$ to $\frac{2}{5}$ inch) are palpable. Thyroid adenomas are benign neoplastic nodules within a capsule.

The prevalence of thyroid nodules depends on the method of evaluation. Palpable thyroid nodules are found in 4% to 7% of the general adult population.[5] Autopsy and ultrasound studies have quoted a prevalence as high as 50%. The lifetime risk for development of a thyroid nodule is estimated to be 5% to 10%. In patients with a solitary palpable nodule,

up to 45% were found to have other nodules on ultrasound imaging. Thyroid nodules are common, and only 3% to 5% of all thyroid nodules are malignant.[5] The risk of malignancy in 18F-FDG-PET–avid nodules is approximately 33% and these cancers tend to be more aggressive.[4]

Increasing numbers of thyroid nodules are being identified incidentally during carotid Doppler ultrasound or other neck imaging studies. Clinical features that increase the likelihood of cancer include history of childhood head and neck radiation therapy, childhood or adolescent exposure to ionizing radiation from fallout, history of radiation for bone marrow transplant, family history of thyroid cancer, age younger than 20 years or older than 60 years, male gender, and history of multiple endocrine neoplasia II or medullary thyroid cancer. Familial thyroid tumors also occur in Cowden disease (multiple hamartoma syndrome), Gardner syndrome (development of multiple tumors with autosomal dominant inheritance), and familial polyposis.

PATHOPHYSIOLOGY

Thyroid nodules may be caused by adenomas, cysts, carcinomas, multinodular goiters, Hashimoto thyroiditis, and subacute thyroiditis. Less common causes of neck lumps include the effects of prior surgery or ^{131}I, parathyroid cysts or adenomas, thyroglossal cysts, non-thyroidal lesions, and lymphomas.

Thyroid adenomas are benign, monoclonal growths. Benign thyroid tumors include embryonal, fetal, follicular, Hürthle cell, and papillary adenomas. They are distinguished by their characteristic histologic appearance. Malignant thyroid tumors include papillary, follicular, medullary, and anaplastic carcinomas.

CLINICAL PRESENTATION AND PHYSICAL EXAMINATION

Thyroid nodules are usually asymptomatic and are identified as a lump by patients or by providers during routine thyroid examinations. As noted above, thyroid nodules are commonly found on neck/chest imaging studies.

An anaplastic tumor may manifest as an enlarging, painful mass associated with hoarseness, dysphonia, dysphagia, or dyspnea. Patients with anaplastic thyroid cancer may have pathologic fractures of the spine or hip or thoracic outlet syndrome. Patients with toxic nodules may show symptoms of hyperthyroidism. Examination of the thyroid should begin with observation under a good examining light. Having the patient swallow a sip of water enhances visualization and palpation of the thyroid.

Important features noted during the physical examination include nodule size, consistency, and mobility and the presence and consistency of associated lymphadenopathy. Supraclavicular, anterior cervical, and submandibular lymph nodes should be examined. Although most thyroid cancers feel firm or hard, they can be soft and fluctuant on examination. The presence of a new nodule or enlarging nodule while a patient is receiving T4 therapy is a cause for concern. The Pemberton maneuver is used for examination when substernal extension of nodule/goiter is suspected. The patient is asked to elevate both arms until they touch the sides of their head. Flushing of the face, cyanosis, and respiratory distress may occur as a result of impingement of structures within the thoracic inlet (i.e., Pemberton sign). Distention of neck veins may also be apparent in these patients..

DIAGNOSTICS

The initial evaluation of thyroid nodules includes measurement of TSH to exclude hyperthyroidism or hypothyroidism. If TSH level is suppressed in patients with nodules greater than 1 cm, thyroid scan should be performed to rule out hyperfunctioning nodule, as most hot nodules are benign. Elevated TSH levels have been associated with an increased risk of malignant transformation in a thyroid nodule as well as more advanced stage of differentiated thyroid cancer.[6] The routine measurement of serum calcitonin (to exclude medullary thyroid cancer) is not useful or cost-effective.[7]

Thyroid ultrasound with assessment of cervical lymph nodules should be performed for all patients with a suspected thyroid nodule on exam, and with thyroid nodules incidentally found on other imaging studies. Ultrasound characteristics guide FNA decision-making. Ultrasound characteristics associated with a higher likelihood of malignancy include: hypoechoic nodules, irregular margins, absent halo, microcalcifications, and shape taller than the width in transverse dimension.[5,8] Ultrasound appearances that are predictive of benign nodules include: spongiform nodules and simple cysts. In a study by Bonavita and coworkers,[8] only 1 of 360 malignant nodules demonstrated a spongiform appearance (aggregation of multiple microcystic components making up more than 50% of the nodule volume).

FNA biopsy is the procedure of choice in the evaluation of thyroid nodules. It is safe and technically simple but requires an experienced operator and cytopathologist. False-negative and false-positive rates are less than 5% with experienced users. Cytologic results are sufficient in 85% of biopsies for diagnosis. Ultrasound-guided FNAs have a lower rate of nondiagnostic and false-negative biopsy findings. The revised American Thyroid Association thyroid cancer guidelines (2015) recommend FNA for nodules larger than 1 cm with high-risk history, for solid nodules larger than 1 cm that are hypoechoic, and for complex (solid and cystic components) nodules larger than 1.5 cm with any suspicious ultrasound features.[5] FNA can be used to obtain material for biochemical analysis of aspirated fluid or needle washings: evidence of thyroglobulin in lymph node aspirate can confirm metastatic thyroid cancer, high concentration of parathyroid hormone from aspirated cyst confirms parathyroid cyst. If lymphoma is suspected, sampling can be done for flow cytometry.

FNA cytology result categories are based on the Bethesda System for Reporting Thyroid Cytopathology and include: Nondiagnostic (Bethesda I), Benign (Bethesda II), Atypia of Undetermined Significance (AUS)/Follicular Lesion of Undetermined Significance (FLUS) (Bethesda III), Follicular Neoplasm (Bethesda IV), Suspicious for Malignancy (Bethesda V), Malignant (Bethesda VI). The estimated risks of malignancy based on the 2017 Bethesda System for Reporting Thyroid Cytopathology for these diagnostic categories are: 5% to 10%, 0% to 3%, 10% to 30%, 25% to 40%, 50% to 75%, and 97% to 99%.[9]

ADDITIONAL DIAGNOSTICS include radionuclide scanning if a hyperfunctioning nodule is suspected or in patients with multinodular goiter to target FNA of cold nodules and further evaluation of FNA aspirates for molecular markers for patients with indeterminate cytology.[10] The use of gene expression classifiers, with high negative predictive value, may help to avoid diagnostic surgery in patients with indeterminate thyroid cytology results.[11]

INITIAL DIAGNOSTICS

Thyroid Nodules and Thyroid Cancer

LABORATORY
- Thyroid stimulating hormone

IMAGING
- Thyroid ultrasound
- Radionuclide scan[a]

OTHER DIAGNOSTICS
- Fine-needle aspiration
- Molecular markers[a]
  - mRNA gene expression classifier (high negative predictive value)
  - Mutational analysis (high positive predictive value)

[a]If indicated.

Differential diagnosis is principally concerned with differentiating benign from malignant nodules. Autoimmune thyroid conditions such as Hashimoto (see below), and cysts of the parathyroid glands will need to be ruled out depending on clinical presentation and diagnostic testing.

INTERPROFESSIONAL COLLABORATIVE MANAGEMENT

Management of thyroid nodule(s) noted after complete history and physical examination and TSH measurement is as follows:
- If TSH is suppressed, free T4 and TT3 are checked and a radionuclide scan is ordered (^{123}I uptake and scan). Autonomously functioning nodules appear as hot nodules on radionuclide scan. These nodules are rarely cancer, and therefore FNA is not required. Patients with functioning nodules with thyrotoxicosis should be treated with radioiodine or surgery. Use of thioamides is an option to treat hyperthyroidism in patients who want to avoid or defer definitive therapy. Patients with subclinical thyrotoxicoses can be monitored or treated (radioiodine or surgery) depending on adenoma size. FNA biopsy should be performed on indeterminate (warm) nodules and cold (nonfunctioning) nodules.
- If TSH is elevated, free T4 is checked, the patient is started on levothyroxine therapy as indicated, and thyroid nodule(s) are evaluated.
- If TSH is normal, thyroid nodule(s) are evaluated as follows.
  - Thyroid ultrasound should be performed on all patients.
  - Patient is referred to endocrinologist or interventional radiologist for ultrasound-guided FNA biopsy per ATA 2015 guidelines.[5]
  - Cytology results:
    - Benign: No further immediate evaluation is necessary. A repeated FNA biopsy should be reserved for enlarging nodules, defined as more than a 50% change in volume or a 20% increase in diameter with at least a 2-mm increase in two or more dimensions. A follow-up ultrasound should be performed in 6 to 12 months. The American Thyroid Association task force strongly recommends against use of T4 suppression.[5]
    - Nondiagnostic: FNA is repeated in 2 to 3 months
    - FLUS/AUS or follicular neoplasm: FNA is repeated in 2 to 3 months, and use of molecular markers is considered; or can hold sample for molecular testing at time of initial FNA and send out for molecular testing if cytology is indeterminate.
    - Suspicious for malignancy, or malignancy: Patient is referred to an experienced surgeon. For solitary

lesions smaller than 1 cm, lobectomy may be performed. Total thyroidectomy is indicated if there is a history of head or neck irradiation, the tumor extends beyond the capsule, or the lesion is larger than 1 cm. The American Thyroid Association task force recommends against use of radioactive iodine ablation in patients with low-grade thyroid cancer (unifocal cancer <1 cm or multifocal cancer with cumulative size <1 cm) in the absence of higher-risk features.[5] Postoperative radioactive iodine therapy is used to ablate remnant thyroid tissue, to ease early detection of recurrence based on thyroglobulin levels, and to diagnose and treat metastases. Although most studies demonstrate a reduction in recurrence and decreased mortality with remnant ablation, benefits appear to be limited to patients with more advanced stages of thyroid cancer.[5]

Differentiated thyroid cancer is managed as follows:

- Use of the American Joint Committee on Cancer (AJCC) and Union for International Cancer Control (UICC) classification based on TNM (*T* refers to tumor size, *N* refers to lymph nodes, and *M* refers to metastases) and age is recommended for all patients with differentiated thyroid cancer because of its usefulness in predicting mortality and its requirement for cancer registries.[5]
- Remnant ablation with radioactive iodine is indicated in patients with known distant metastases, evidence of extrathyroidal extension on pathology, tumor size larger than 4 cm, and tumors 1 to 4 cm with high-risk features.
- Thyroid hormone therapy is required to prevent hypothyroidism and prevent TSH stimulation of thyroid cancer cells. Suppression therapy (TSH below 0.3) is indicated for patients with intermediate and high-risk disease. The TSH goal with low-risk disease is 0.3 to 2.0.
- Patients with differentiated thyroid carcinoma are followed closely for the first 5 years and then at 6- to 12-month intervals. Thyroglobulin levels are followed postoperatively as a marker for recurrence (in the absence of interfering antithyroglobulin antibodies). Whole-body scans are followed after radioiodine therapy and in high-risk patients. Neck ultrasound is performed to assess for recurrence and metastatic cervical lymph nodes.

Medullary thyroid cancer and anaplastic thyroid cancers are more aggressive than well-differentiated thyroid cancers and therefore are treated differently.

LIFE SPAN CONSIDERATIONS

The net mortality rate of papillary thyroid cancer is 10% to 20% during 20 to 30 years. Several factors increase the risk of death from cancer: extrathyroidal invasion (six times the risk), metastasis (47 times), age older than 45 years (32 times), and tumor larger than 3 cm (1⅕ inches; six times).[5]

Various scoring systems are used to stratify the prognosis of patients with well-differentiated and medullary thyroid cancer. The AJCC/UICC staging system is recommended for all patients with differentiated thyroid cancer because of its usefulness in predicting mortality and its requirement for cancer registries. In patients 44 years old or younger, stage I disease is defined as any tumor size, with or without lymph node metastases without evidence of distant metastases; stage II disease in this age group is defined by the presence of any metastases. In patients 45 years old and older, stage I disease is defined as primary tumor 2 cm or smaller without lymph node or distant

metastases; stage II disease is defined as primary tumor 2 to 4 cm without lymph node or distant metastases; and stage III disease includes patients with tumors larger than 4 cm without lymph node or distant metastases.[5]

COMPLICATIONS

Complications of thyroid surgery include hypoparathyroidism and hoarseness from recurrent laryngeal nerve damage. Side effects of radioiodine include thyroid tenderness, dry mouth, altered taste, dry eyes, and nausea. Cumulative doses of more than 300 mCi may increase the risk of leukemia. Bone marrow suppression is seen with cumulative doses of more than 500 mCi. Other potential complications of radioiodine include pulmonary fibrosis and ovarian or testicular failure. Treatment doses range from 30 to 150 mCi.

PATIENT AND FAMILY EDUCATION

Patients should be taught how to do a thyroid self-examination. Patients should be given instructions about precautions after radioiodine treatment or scanning. These instructions include the following:

- No kissing, exchanging of saliva, or sharing of food or eating utensils for 5 days; dishes should be washed in a dishwasher.
- No close contact with infants, young children (<8 years of age), or pregnant women for 5 days; it is permissible to be in the same room.
- No breastfeeding.
- Flush toilets twice after urinating, and wash hands thoroughly.
- If a sore throat or neck pain develops, take acetaminophen or aspirin.
- Notify the physician if nervousness, tremulousness, or palpitations increase
- An informative website for patients with thyroid cancer is www.thyca.org.

HYPERTHYROIDISM

 Immediate emergency department referral is indicated for patients with thyroid storm, thyrotoxic crisis, and rapid atrial fibrillation.

DEFINITION AND EPIDEMIOLOGY

Hyperthyroidism is defined as a clinical syndrome caused by the excess production or release of thyroid hormone and its clinical manifestations. The term *hyperthyroidism* implies that the thyroid is the source of excess thyroid hormone; *thyrotoxicosis* refers to the syndrome produced by excess thyroid hormone regardless of its source (e.g., overingestion of iodine). Primary hyperthyroidism is independent of TSH. TSH-dependent hyperthyroidism is called secondary hyperthyroidism. TRH-dependent hyperthyroidism is referred to as tertiary hyperthyroidism.

Graves disease (autoimmune hyperthyroidism) is the most common cause of hyperthyroidism. There is a female-to-male predominance of 7:1, and it is most common in women aged 20 to 40 years. Transient hyperthyroidism (thyroiditis) needs to be excluded. Toxic multinodular goiters are usually seen in women older than 55 years who have a long history of goiter. Multinodular goiters with autonomy are more susceptible to iodine-induced hyperthyroidism. Iodine sources include

TABLE 194.1   Signs and Symptoms of Hyperthyroidism

	Symptoms	Signs
Eyes	Dry eyes, blurry vision	*NO SPECS* mnemonic (see text)
Neck	Diffuse goiter in patients with Graves disease	Goiter with thyroid bruit in Graves disease
Respiratory system	Shortness of breath	Labored respiration
Cardiac system	Palpitation, tachycardia, angina	Systolic hypertension, congestive heart failure, tachycardia, atrial fibrillation
Gastrointestinal system	Hyperphagia, hyperdefecation, weight loss, weight gain (rare), anorexia in older adults	Weight loss, weight gain (rare)
Reproductive system	Amenorrhea, menstrual irregularities, infertility	
Neuromuscular system	Proximal muscle weakness, heat intolerance, tremor	Proximal muscle weakness, hyperreflexia
Skin	Pruritus; hyperhidrosis; warm, moist palms; onycholysis (brittle nails, Plummer nails)	Smooth, velvety skin; warm, moist palms; onycholysis; pretibial myxedema (Graves disease)
Skeletal system	Osteoporosis	Thyroid acropachy (Graves disease)
Psychiatric problems	Anxiety, irritability, nervousness, sleeplessness	Visually manifested
Older adults	Anorexia, constipation, normal pulse, weight loss	

topical povidone-iodine (Betadine), intravenous contrast medium, and iodine-containing drugs. Postpartum thyroiditis (painless) occurs in approximately 5% to 9% of all pregnant women, 25% of pregnant women with type 1 diabetes, and 75% of women with high microsomal antibody titers before pregnancy.[12]

PATHOPHYSIOLOGY

Graves disease is an autoimmune disorder in which autoantibodies to the thyrotropin receptor (TRAb) bind to and activate the receptor, stimulating thyroid hormone synthesis and secretion.[13]

Subacute thyroiditis is a postviral illness. The thyroid gland is tender, and there is evidence of multinucleated giant cells on microscopic evaluation. Silent thyroiditis (painless) is believed to be an autoimmune disorder. On microscopic examination, there is evidence of lymphocytic infiltration that may mimic Hashimoto thyroiditis. In subacute and silent thyroiditis there is excess release of thyroid hormone.

CLINICAL PRESENTATION AND PHYSICAL EXAMINATION

Because thyroid hormone acts on all organs, the clinical presentation is variable. The symptoms of hyperthyroidism are secondary to increased sympathetic activity and increased catabolism. Apathetic hyperthyroidism refers to patients who lack these symptoms. It is useful to describe the symptoms by organ system as shown in Table 194.1.

Lid lag may be seen with thyrotoxicosis, regardless of the origin of thyroid hormone. This symptom is caused by increased sympathetic activity. The other eye changes associated with Graves disease are caused by the action of stimulating TRAb on the connective tissue behind the eye. The *NO SPECS* mnemonic is used to describe the eye changes in association with Graves disease, as follows:
- *N*o signs or symptoms
- *O*nly signs, no symptoms
- *S*oft tissue swelling
- *P*roptosis

TABLE 194.2   Thyroid Function Tests in Hyperthyroidism

	T_3	T_4/Free T_4 Index	TSH
Graves disease	Increase	Increase	Decrease
T_3 toxicosis	Increase	Normal	Decrease
T_4 toxicosis	Normal	Increase	Decrease
Subclinical hyperthyroidism	Normal	Normal	Decrease

T_3, Triiodothyronine; T_4, thyroxine; *TSH*, thyroid stimulating hormone.

- *E*xtraocular muscle paresis
- *C*orneal involvement
- *S*ight loss (optic nerve involvement)

With subacute thyroiditis, the thyroid gland is tender, and patients often note a recent viral illness.

DIAGNOSTICS

TSH is the best screening test for primary hyperthyroidism. With primary hyperthyroidism, TSH levels will be low or undetectable. If TSH is suppressed, a T_3 uptake (T_3U) test (or any test of binding proteins) and T_4 levels should be obtained to determine the degree of hyperthyroidism. Alternatively, a free T_4 level can be obtained. TSH levels will remain suppressed for up to 3 months after treatment, and therefore the free T_4 or free T_4 index must be followed. See Table 194.2 for laboratory results in different types of hyperthyroidism. In primary hyperthyroidism a TRAb level should be checked and will be elevated in Graves disease.

Abnormal liver function test results are common in patients with hyperthyroidism. Elevations in alkaline phosphatase, alanine aminotransferase, aspartate aminotransferase, γ-glutamyltransferase, and total bilirubin levels can be seen.

Radioiodine uptake is useful in distinguishing Graves disease from thyroiditis.

An iodine scan is useful in identifying a toxic multinodular goiter or solitary nodular goiter. In patients with a diffusely enlarged gland and obvious signs of eye disease or an elevated TRAb titer, this test is not necessary for diagnosis of Graves disease but is needed for calculation of the radioiodine dose necessary if iodine ablation therapy is chosen. The erythrocyte sedimentation rate (ESR) will be increased in subacute thyroiditis. A careful review of iodine-containing medications is necessary in the evaluation of hyperthyroidism. With TSH-induced (secondary) hyperthyroidism, TSH is inappropriately elevated in the setting of increased T_4 index. Pituitary adenomas are best visualized on MRI. With TSH adenomas, there is an increased ratio of TSH α subunit/TSH.

INITIAL DIAGNOSTICS

Hyperthyroidism

LABORATORY
- Thyroid stimulating hormone
- Free T_4 index, free T_4
- Total T_3
- Thyrotropin receptor antibody[a]
- Baseline complete blood count and liver function tests should be checked before initiation of treatment with thioamides[a]
- Erythrocyte sedimentation rate

IMAGING
- Radioiodine uptake scan[a]
- Magnetic resonance imaging[a]

---

[a]If indicated.

 Rule out other, less common, causes of hyperthyroidism (struma ovarii, factitious hyperthyroidism), be aware of trophoblastic disease and hyperemesis gravidarum in pregnant patients

INTERPROFESSIONAL COLLABORATIVE MANAGEMENT
Pharmacologic Management

The treatment of hyperthyroidism or thyrotoxicosis depends on the cause of the disease and the patient's age. Primary health care providers can perform the initial evaluation for hyperthyroidism. Laboratory confirmation of hyperthyroidism and radioiodine scans (if indicated) should be obtained. Thioamides can be administered by practitioners who are experienced with their use. Treatment options should be reviewed with patients.

Graves Disease
- β blockers should be initiated to alleviate the α-adrenergic symptoms of hyperthyroidism (tremor, tachycardia); the dose is adjusted to keep the heart rate at 60 to 90 beats/min and to treat symptoms. Propranolol (Inderal) can be used at doses of 10 to 40 mg orally every 6 hours, or atenolol at 25 to 100 mg daily. These drugs must be used with caution in patients with congestive heart failure and bronchospasm, and they should be avoided in pregnant women because of untoward effects on the fetus.
- Thioamide therapy includes methimazole (MMI, Tapazole) and propylthiouracil (PTU).
- Medical therapy is the treatment of choice for patients younger than 20 years old, for pregnant women, for those with a high likelihood of remission (mild disease, small goiters), and for those with active Graves orbitopathy.

TABLE 194.3	Thioamide Therapy	
	Methimazole	**Propylthiouracil**
Dose	5–20 mg PO q8h, or 15–60 mg/day PO q8h	50–100 mg PO q6–8h
Tablets	5 mg, 10 mg	50 mg
Protein binding	0%	75%
Half-life	4–6 h.	75 min
Placental passage	High	1:1
Breast milk concentration	High	Low
Advantages	Long half-life	Inhibits conversion of T_4–T_3; used during first trimester of pregnancy only

T_3, Triiodothyronine; T_4, thyroxine.

Baseline complete blood count and liver function test results should be checked before initiation of treatment. Thioamides inhibit thyroid hormone synthesis by blocking organification. PTU also inhibits the peripheral conversion of T_4 to T_3. PTU should not be used as a first-line drug in children or adults because of reports of severe PTU-related liver failure. In the past, PTU was considered the drug of choice throughout pregnancy because of possible teratogenic effects of MMI. PTU should be limited to the first trimester, and MMI should be used during the second trimester once organogenesis has been completed.[14] Thioamide therapy is described in Table 194.3. Side effects of thioamides include pruritic rash, jaundice, arthralgias, and low risk of agranulocytosis. Patients should be advised to contact their physician if they develop these symptoms; they should stop the medication in the setting of temperature above 102° and jaundice and should contact the physician immediately.
- Patients with small goiters and mild hyperthyroidism can be started on methimazole, 5 to 10 mg daily. Starting doses of 20 to 30 mg daily should be used in those with severe hyperthyroidism and large goiters. Starting doses of PTU are 50 to 100 mg three times daily. As noted, because of reports of PTU-related liver failure, PTU use is limited to the first trimester of pregnancy and in those intolerant of methimazole.
- After 6 to 12 months of treatment with thionamides, approximately 30% of patients go into remission. Definitive therapy with radioiodine ablation is typically recommended if relapse occurs.
- White blood count and TFT results are monitored every 4 to 6 weeks until the results are stable. TSH levels may remain suppressed for months, and therefore free T_4 should be monitored. In pregnant women, free T_4 levels should be kept at the high-normal range because of the thionamide effect of inhibiting the fetal thyroid gland.
- Radioiodine therapy is the treatment of choice in the United States for patients older than 20 years and for those for whom thioamide therapy has failed (through noncompliance or a relapse after treatment). It is contraindicated during pregnancy and should be avoided in patients with Graves ophthalmopathy because of the increased risk of exacerbation of eye symptoms after treatment. There is no

evidence of increased incidence of long-term malignant neoplasms. Because of the high incidence of post-treatment hypothyroidism, TFT results should be monitored closely. Approximately 4 to 6 weeks after treatment, the T_4 index should be checked, and the patient should be reevaluated. If there is no evidence of hypothyroidism at that time, TSH and T_4 index should be monitored monthly for 3 to 4 months and then periodically.

- Thyroidectomy is recommended for pregnant women who cannot be managed with thioamides or who develop side effects, for patients who refuse radioiodine and cannot tolerate thioamides, and for patients with an obstructive goiter. Complications include hypothyroidism, hypoparathyroidism, and hoarseness (recurrent laryngeal nerve damage).
- No studies to date have demonstrated any of these treatment options to be superior to any others. Other much less commonly used medications include cholestyramine (which decreases enterohepatic circulation of thyroid hormone), organic iodides (amiodarone and ipodate, which block T_4 to T_3 conversion), lithium and iodides (which block hormone release), and glucocorticoids (which block T_4 to T_3 conversion).
- Specialist consultation with an endocrinologist is indicated for patients with Graves ophthalmopathy and for patients to be treated with radioiodine therapy. An ophthalmologist should see all patients with Graves ophthalmopathy.

Subclinical Hyperthyroidism

Subclinical hyperthyroidism is defined as suppressed TSH with normal serum T_4 and T_3 levels. The cause of subclinical hyperthyroidism is the same as for overt hyperthyroidism. The majority of cases are the result of autonomously functioning thyroid nodules and multinodular goiters. Most elderly patients with subclinical hyperthyroidism have a multinodular goiter. Indications for therapy are based on the known skeletal and cardiovascular consequences of untreated hyperthyroidism. Postmenopausal women with exogenous subclinical hyperthyroidism have been found to have decreased bone density, but not premenopausal women.[15] The risk of atrial fibrillation has been shown to be related to the degree of TSH suppression. The cumulative incidence was 28% in patients with TSH levels of less than 0.1 μIU/mL, 16% when TSH levels were between 0.1 and 0.4 μIU/mL, and 11% in those with normal TSH levels.[16]

Treatment of subclinical hyperthyroidism should be considered for the following:

- Patients with endogenous subclinical hyperthyroidism with a TSH level of less than 0.1 μIU/mL as a result of Graves or nodular thyroid disease, especially patients older than 60 years and those at increased risk for heart disease, osteopenia, or osteoporosis. In those with TSH levels of 0.1 to 0.5 μIU/mL and low risk of complications, follow-up monitoring alone is appropriate.
- Patients at high risk of complications with TSH level of 0.1 to 0.5 μIU/mL, especially if bone density is low.

Thyroiditis

Thyroiditis may be subacute or painless. Hyperthyroid findings may result.

Subacute Thyroiditis
- Symptomatic treatment with β blockers can be used during the hyperthyroid phase.
- For pain relief, antiinflammatory agents are used.

- NSAIDs (1200 to 3200 mg daily in divided doses) or aspirin (2600 mg daily) is used first. If no pain relief has occurred in 2 to 3 days, these agents are discontinued and the patient is treated with prednisone (40 mg daily). Prednisone is continued until pain subsides and then is tapered by 5 to 10 mg every 5 days. Hyperthyroidism lasts for weeks to months and is followed by hypothyroidism (which lasts for months). TFTs should be performed every 2 to 8 weeks. Most patients become euthyroid, although 30% may remain hypothyroid. Recurrences are rare.

Painless Postpartum Thyroiditis
- Symptomatic treatment with β blockers can be used during the hyperthyroid phase. β blockers are concentrated in breast milk and must be used with caution.
- Thyroid hormone therapy can be initiated if the hypothyroid phase is severe. TFT results should be monitored closely. Although most patients become clinically euthyroid, up to 30% remain hypothyroid. This condition tends to recur with subsequent pregnancies.

Toxic Nodule
- Radioiodine ablation is the treatment of choice after β blocker therapy.
- Some studies have demonstrated effective therapy with alcohol ablation through repetitive percutaneous injections under ultrasound guidance. Surgical excision is another option, especially in patients with a large adenoma.

Toxic Multinodular Goiter
- Radioiodine ablation is the treatment of choice after β blocker therapy. Other nodules may become toxic in the future and may require repeated doses of ^{131}I.
- Other treatment options include antithyroid drugs and subtotal thyroidectomy.

LIFE SPAN CONSIDERATIONS

Older patients may have apathetic hyperthyroidism (anorexia, weight loss, weakness) on presentation. There is an increased risk of atrial fibrillation and osteoporosis in patients with untreated Graves disease. Patients usually have symptoms of weight loss despite increased appetite. It is important to counsel patients on decreasing their food intake with treatment of hyperthyroidism to avoid significant weight gain with treatment. Patients should be counseled to avoid strenuous exercise and activity until adrenergic symptoms are controlled. Bone density should be checked in postmenopausal women. Smoking is a risk factor for Graves ophthalmopathy, and therefore patients should be counseled on smoking cessation.

COMPLICATIONS

Untreated Graves disease can lead to atrial fibrillation, congestive heart failure, angina, and osteoporosis. Thyroid storm is a rare, life-threatening form of hyperthyroidism that leads to systemic decompensation. The diagnosis is based on clinical findings: temperature of 102°F to 105°F, profuse sweating, pulse above 120 to 140 beats/min, atrial fibrillation, restlessness, confusion, agitation, and coma. Gastrointestinal symptoms may include severe vomiting, diarrhea, and hepatomegaly with jaundice. The goals of therapy are to inhibit thyroid hormone formation and release, to provide α-adrenergic blockage, to provide supportive therapy, to identify and to treat any precipitating illness, and to initiate long-term therapy for prevention of further episodes of thyroid storm.

The incidence of thyroid storm has declined during the past few decades because of advances in medical management, but thyrotoxic crises account for approximately 1% of all hospitalizations for hyperthyroidism. Although it more commonly occurs with Graves disease, it can be found in conjunction with other causes of hyperthyroidism.

PATIENT AND FAMILY EDUCATION

- Review symptoms of hyperthyroidism and instruct on the danger signs of thyroid storm.
- If receiving β blockers, monitor pulse and contact their health care provider if the pulse is less than 50 (or 40 if baseline heart rate is low) or more than 120 beats/min.
- If receiving thioamides should be cautioned about the rare but serious effects of agranulocytosis. Discontinue thioamide therapy if they have signs of infection and a temperature higher than 38.3°C (101°F) and call the health care provider and have a CBC and differential performed to exclude agranulocytosis.
- If jaundice, vomiting, or abdominal pain contact health care provider

HYPOTHYROIDISM

 Immediate emergency department referral is indicated for myxedema coma.

DEFINITION AND EPIDEMIOLOGY

Hypothyroidism is a condition resulting from the synthesis of thyroid hormone that is insufficient to meet the body's needs. It is the most common disorder of the thyroid gland. This condition usually occurs in the setting of primary hypothyroidism, whereby diseases or treatments destroy thyroid tissue or prevalent conditions interfere with thyroid hormone biosynthesis. Rarely, it is caused by inadequate thyroidal stimulation by TSH, which is referred to as central or secondary hypothyroidism.

If hypothyroidism is congenital or occurs during infancy or childhood, growth and development are slowed and may result in mental retardation, a condition known as cretinism. In adulthood, untreated hypothyroidism results in decreased metabolic function and in the deposition of hydrophilic mucopolysaccharides in the skin and other tissues, which results in fluid and sodium retention and impairment of blood circulation and lymphatic drainage. Progressive and severe hypothyroidism with skin thickening and cardiovascular and renal manifestations is known as myxedema.

Hypothyroidism is found in 2% of women and 0.2% of men. The prevalence increases with age, with 6% of women and 2.5% of men older than 60 years having this condition. Subclinical hypothyroidism may occur in as many as 15% of persons 60 years of age or older. It has been found that in 20% to 40% of patients, subclinical hypothyroidism progresses to overt hypothyroidism within 4 years.[17]

Appropriate thyroid hormone biosynthesis depends on dietary intake of iodides and on various geographic and environmental factors that may affect a population's ability to obtain the recommended daily allowance of iodine. In the United States, adequate dietary sources of iodine have been established to prevent iodine deficiency disorders, which may manifest as hypothyroidism or goiter.

Previous irradiation for head and neck cancers may put a patient at increased risk for development of hypothyroidism. Radioactive treatment with ^{131}I for hyperthyroid disorders results in hypothyroidism in most cases. Subtotal or total thyroidectomy will render a patient hypothyroid.

The most common cause of primary hypothyroidism is chronic autoimmune thyroiditis. This may take atrophic or goitrous forms. When autoimmune thyroiditis coexists with a goiter, the condition is called Hashimoto thyroiditis. It is believed to be a familial autoimmune condition in which the lymphocytes become sensitized to an individual's own thyroid antigens, resulting in the formation of autoantibodies. The autoantibodies react with the thyroid antigens and destroy functional tissue. This manifests as an increase in TSH and the presence of antithyroid antibodies, including antimicrosomal, anti-TPO, and antithyroglobulin antibodies. Eventually there is a drop in serum T_4 and then T_3. Younger patients most often are seen with goiter, whereas older patients may have more severe disease and a small (atrophic) gland.

Transient primary hypothyroidism may be encountered during the postpartum period, 2 to 6 months after delivery. This condition may be preceded by a brief period of hyperthyroidism and can result in permanent thyroid failure. Postinfectious thyroiditis may follow a similar course. A sentinel viral upper respiratory tract infection followed by an inflamed, large tender thyroid gland, and transient hyperthyroidism followed by transient or permanent hypothyroidism, is the usual observed sequence of events.

Drugs with antithyroid action such as lithium, amiodarone, iodine, interferon alfa, tyrosine kinase inhibitors, and radiographic contrast material may cause hypothyroidism. The drug effect may be transient during the period of use or may result in permanent thyroid failure. Patients with underlying chronic autoimmune thyroiditis living in iodine-sufficient geographic areas are more susceptible to hypothyroidism when taking iodine or iodine-containing drugs.

Pituitary (or secondary) causes of hypothyroidism are not common and are usually associated with other signs of pituitary hormone insufficiency. Patients with a history of pituitary disease or tumor may be at risk for thyroid hyposecretion. Immunotherapies used for cancer treatment (checkpoint inhibitor immunotherapy) have been reported to cause central hypothyroidism.

PATHOPHYSIOLOGY

Thyroid hormone deficiency has many effects. Cardiac and metabolic consequences include impaired myocardial contractility, cardiomegaly, impaired lipid metabolism with accelerated atherosclerosis, hypertension, depressed ventilatory drive and fatigue, impaired energy use, and weight gain. Altered kidney and gastrointestinal performance includes a reduction in glomerular filtration rate and hyponatremia, hypomotility, and constipation, respectively. Musculoskeletal effects include an increased volume of muscle and slowness of contraction leading to myopathic disorders and connective tissue thickening. This can lead to entrapment neuropathies such as carpal tunnel syndrome. In children, delayed skeletal maturation may cause growth retardation. Impaired cellular function in the brain may cause depression or psychiatric disability, and diminished erythropoiesis results in anemia.

Characteristic myxedematous changes seen in untreated advanced disease are largely a result of deposition of hydrophilic mucopolysaccharides, especially hyaluronic acid, in the interstitial tissues. The hydrophilic nature of the mucopolysaccharides and increased capillary permeability to albumin create interstitial edema of heart muscle, striated muscle, and skin.

CLINICAL PRESENTATION

Presentation may range from subclinical hypothyroidism (with an asymptomatic TSH elevation) to overt myxedema (with slowed mentation and visible symptoms). The most common presenting symptom is fatigue. There may also be increased sensitivity to cold, weight gain, hoarseness, puffiness of the face and hands, heavy and irregular menstrual periods, dry skin, dry and brittle hair, depression, paresthesias, muscle aches, and constipation. A careful history will elicit the severity and duration of these symptoms.

Symptoms may be more vague and subtle in older adults and include deafness, confusion, dementia, and ataxia.

The physical examination should focus on the patient's general appearance and degree of energy and animation. Mentation may be slowed, and the patient may appear lethargic and expressionless. On occasion, severe depression or agitation results. Assessment of physical appearance includes texture, color, and general appearance of the skin. Facial expression and the texture and thickness of the hair should be noted; the patient's voice, which may be deepened, and pulse, which may be slowed, should be assessed.

The thyroid gland may be large or small on examination and should be evaluated carefully for the presence or absence of nodules. Tenderness of the gland is suggestive of a subacute thyroiditis, whereas a nontender gland is more suggestive of chronic autoimmune thyroiditis. A rubbery, firm, symmetric goiter is characteristic of Hashimoto thyroiditis. Deep tendon reflexes should be evaluated. Any delay in the relaxation phase, which may be most noticeable in the Achilles tendon, should be noted. The patient's weight should be documented and compared with previous weights to determine if there has been any weight gain. Heart rate and respiratory rate should also be noted and documented. Diastolic blood pressure may be elevated. Respirations may be slow and shallow with advanced disease. Bowel sounds may be diminished.

Postural hypotension may indicate coexistent endocrine deficiencies such as autoimmune adrenal insufficiency, as seen in Schmidt syndrome.

DIAGNOSTICS

TSH is the most appropriate first diagnostic test. If the TSH is elevated, free T_4 should be checked. Laboratory tests reveal an elevated TSH level, which may precede symptoms or decreases in T_4 and T_3. This condition is referred to as subclinical hypothyroidism (elevated TSH and normal free T_4). More advanced hypothyroidism shows not only elevated TSH but also low serum levels of free T_4 and a low free T_4 index. If pituitary or central hypothyroidism is suspected, the most appropriate test is a free T_4 assessment; TSH will not be useful in central hypothyroidism. Anti-TPO antibody levels will be elevated in patients with chronic autoimmune thyroiditis. Patients often demonstrate a mild normocytic, normochromic anemia. If menstrual periods are heavy, the anemia may be microcytic. If vitamin B_{12} deficiency is present, the anemia may be macrocytic. Hypercholesterolemia may also be present.

Imaging studies are unnecessary for chronic autoimmune thyroiditis. If imaging is used, the findings may be misleading.

The pattern of uptake with goitrous autoimmune thyroiditis may be variable, whereas uptake may be low with atrophic thyroiditis. An ultrasound examination may be indicated to verify the presence of a suspected nodule. FNA biopsy may be necessary to evaluate a suspicious nodule or rapidly enlarging goiter. In severe hypothyroidism, other diagnostic tests may be needed to assess cardiac status, and electrocardiographic examination may reveal low-voltage QRS complexes and P and T waves as well as cardiac enlargement. This may result from both dilation and pericardial effusion. Bradycardia is usually present in severe hypothyroidism.

INITIAL DIAGNOSTICS

Hypothyroidism

LABORATORY
- Thyroid stimulating hormone

ADDITIONAL DIAGNOSTICS
Laboratory
- Antimicrosomal antibodies
- Serum free T_4
- Free T_4 index

Imaging
- Thyroid ultrasound

Other Diagnostics
- Fine-needle aspiration

DIFFERENTIAL DIAGNOSIS

Less common causes of hypothyroidism including post-partum thyroiditis, post infectious thyroiditis, medication-induced hypothyroidism. Congenital absence of the thyroid should be ruled out. Pituitary conditions, other conditions that have similar symptoms (i.e. depression), should also be considered especially in the presence of a normal TSH.

INTERPROFESSIONAL COLLABORATIVE MANAGEMENT
Pharmacologic Management

- Hypothyroidism is treated with levothyroxine orally in amounts that return TSH to normal levels.[18]
- The desired amount is determined by the measurement of TSH for primary hypothyroidism and by the measurement of free thyroxine for central hypothyroidism.
- The dose necessary to achieve metabolic homeostasis is usually 1.7 mcg/kg/day but varies for each patient.
- In the United States, 12 different color-coded tablet strengths are available. Supplementation may begin with an initial dosage of 50 mcg/day, with the dosage increased at 4- to 6-week intervals to 100 mcg/day. In patients younger than 30 or 40 years with no history of other medical problems, the initial dose of T_4 can be 100 mcg/day. Patients with ischemic heart disease or atrial fibrillation (and older patients in whom these conditions may become apparent with treatment) should start at 12.5 to 25 mcg/day and increase by 25 mcg/day every 8 weeks.
- A euthyroid effect is usually achieved 4 to 6 weeks after the onset of full-dose therapy, which can be adjusted, if necessary, according to TSH determinations.
- This daily dose is then monitored once or twice a year to maintain a mid-normal TSH level.
- Estrogen administration leads to an increase in TBG levels and thus may increase T_4 requirements in patients with hypothyroidism. If estrogen therapy is initiated or discontinued in patients with hypothyroidism treated with levothyroxine, TSH should be rechecked in 12 weeks.

- L-triiodothyronine (L-T_3) is not routinely used to treat hypothyroidism. There are wide fluctuations in serum L-T_3 because of its short half-life (approximately 1 day). Slow-release formulations of L-T_3 are not currently commercially available. The role of L-T_3 replacement in hypothyroidism remains controversial.
- Desiccated bovine thyroid is available, which contains a mixture of T_3 and T_4. One grain (60 mg) of Armour Thyroid contains about 44 mcg of T_4 and 9 mcg of T_3 and is bioequivalent to 75 to 88 mcg of levothyroxine.
- Despite almost a dozen randomized studies, combination therapy with levothyroxine and triiodothyronine does not appear to be superior to levothyroxine monotherapy for treatment of hypothyroidism.[19]

Referral to an endocrinologist may be necessary if there is a solitary nodule requiring biopsy or if regulation of medication is difficult. Persistent symptoms and a normal TSH level or suspicion of secondary hypothyroidism should also prompt an endocrine referral. Hospitalization may be warranted if any of these conditions is severe. Usually, clinical or subclinical hypothyroidism can be managed on an outpatient basis.

Subclinical Hypothyroidism

Subclinical hypothyroidism is defined as an elevated TSH level in the presence of normal thyroid hormone levels. The major causes of subclinical hypothyroidism are the same as for overt hypothyroidism; about 50% is caused by autoimmune thyroiditis, 40% is found in patients with a history of ablative therapy for Graves disease, and it is also commonly seen with inadequate T_4 replacement for overt hypothyroidism. Two population-based studies concluded the prevalence of subclinical hypothyroidism to be approximately 8% in women and 3% in men. However, in women older than 60 years the prevalence was 15%, whereas in elderly men the prevalence was 8%.[20]

Patients with type 1 diabetes mellitus or other autoimmune diseases have a higher rate of subclinical hypothyroidism. The development of overt hypothyroidism depends on the value of TSH and the presence of high thyroid antibody titers. Studies have shown that elderly patients with an initial TSH level above 20 µIU/mL and 80% of those with serum antithyroid microsomal antibody titers of 1:1600 or higher developed overt hypothyroidism. Other patients likely to progress to overt hypothyroidism are those with autoimmune thyroid disease and patients who have received radioiodine therapy or radiotherapy. Normalization of serum TSH is more likely to occur in patients with TSH levels of less than 10 µIU/mL and negative antithyroid antibodies.

Several reports suggest that subclinical hypothyroidism is associated with neuropsychiatric disease. Patients with depression and subclinical hypothyroidism have a higher prevalence of associated panic disorder and poorer response to antidepressant therapy than euthyroid patients. A cross-sectional study of randomly selected subjects older than 65 years reported an increase in the prevalence of coronary heart disease in patients with serum TSH values above 10 µIU/L but not in patients with lower serum TSH concentrations.

In recommendations for treatment, there is not one level of TSH at which clinical action is indicated or contraindicated. However, for those individuals with TSH levels above 10 µIU/mL, treatment is more compelling because it improves cardiac contractility and serum lipid concentrations and secondarily reduces the risk of atherosclerosis. Treatment will also prevent growth of goiter and improve symptoms related to hypothyroidism. In patients with TSH levels of 4.5 to 10 µIU/mL, treatment can be considered if patients have typical hypothyroid symptoms that could benefit from T_4. The potential risk of treatment is the development of subclinical hyperthyroidism. If patients are not treated, regular follow-up is indicated. Patients with subtle symptoms such as infertility, menstrual cycle irregularities, depression, and fatigue may also benefit from replacement therapy. Patients without any of these symptoms and with a TSH level of less than 10 µIU/mL may be monitored at yearly intervals with TSH measurement for progression of thyroid failure.[20]

LIFE SPAN CONSIDERATIONS

Older adults and those with known heart disease should be started at 12.5 to 25 mcg of levothyroxine per day, which is increased gradually. This careful administration prevents arrhythmias, angina, and the other cardiac symptoms that may be precipitated by starting at a full daily dose. After the dose has been stabilized, annual TSH measurements are desirable. Patients should understand that supplementation is lifelong, not short term. Given the high prevalence of hypothyroidism in women older than 60 years and the presence of subtle symptoms, TSH screening is recommended in this age group.

Patients with known hypothyroidism require close monitoring during pregnancy. TSH should be measured during the prenatal evaluation and in every trimester thereafter. Most often, thyroid hormone requirements increase during pregnancy, and close monitoring will ensure appropriate levothyroxine replacement doses. Evidence has emerged that intrauterine fetal development can be adversely affected by untreated hypothyroidism.

Smoking has been found to impair both thyroid hormone secretion and thyroid hormone action. It may contribute to the incidence of subclinical hypothyroidism and may aggravate the clinical manifestations of overt hypothyroidism; therefore, smoking cessation is advised.

The consequences of untreated subclinical hypothyroidism are cardiac dysfunction (including atherosclerotic heart disease), elevations in total and low-density lipoprotein cholesterol levels, systemic hypothyroid symptoms, neuropsychiatric dysfunction, and progression to overt hypothyroidism.

COMPLICATIONS

Myxedema coma, a hypothermic stuporous state that may be characterized by respiratory depression and eventually death, results from untreated hypothyroidism. It may be triggered by environmental stressors such as cold exposure or trauma and by internal stressors such as infection or medications that depress the central nervous system. These patients may require intravenous levothyroxine and glucocorticoid therapy for any coexistent adrenal insufficiency. Warming for the hypothermia, ventilatory support for respiratory depression, and treatment of any renal and electrolyte imbalances are necessary.

In patients with underlying coronary disease, angina and arrhythmias may be a complication of therapy and a cause for concern. Some patients also experience palpitations after starting levothyroxine, especially if other medications are added. This is particularly true of stimulants such as caffeine and pseudoephedrine.

Long-term, marked overtreatment with T_4 can result in symptoms of hyperthyroidism. It can also result in bone resorption with significant decreases in bone mineral density.

Patient and Family Education and Health Promotion

- Levothyroxine replacement is a permanent and necessary treatment that cannot be discontinued and should be taken as prescribed.
- Do not double next dose if one is missed.
- Atrial fibrillation and osteoporosis are possible consequences of persistent excessively high doses of levothyroxine.
- Annual or biannual monitoring of TSH helps ensure that the medication dose remains accurate.

NON-THYROIDAL ILLNESS SYNDROME

Abnormalities in TFT results can occur in non-thyroidal illness syndrome. In the past this was referred to as the euthyroid sick syndrome (sick euthyroidism). A critically ill patient in an intensive care unit setting would be likely to have this abnormality. It is characterized by hypothalamic suppression of TSH release, acute inhibition of peripheral conversion of T_4 to T_3, and increased conversion of T_4 to rT_3. This results in low TSH levels, decreased levels of T_3, and increased levels of rT_3. Non-thyroidal illness syndrome is seen during starvation/carbohydrate restriction, liver disease, or severe acute or chronic illness. Patients with the low free T_4 levels in addition to low T_3 levels are severely ill and have an increased mortality rate. TL_4 levels can be decreased initially because of the liberation of fatty acids from ischemic or injured cells, which inhibits the binding of T_4 to TBG. A summary of thyroid test findings during acute illness is provided in Table 194.4. These abnormalities resolve when the patient recovers. The TSH level rises to normal or higher-than-normal levels during the recovery phase; the changes are thought to be a protective adaptation to severe illness. Therapy with T_4 or T_3 has not been shown to improve outcomes and may actually worsen the situation. Given this syndrome, TFT results should not be checked in critically ill patients unless thyroid dysfunction is strongly suspected. If TFT results are checked, TSH alone does not suffice. TFT values should be interpreted in context of the current clinical scenario and time frame of illness.

DRUGS AND THE THYROID GLAND

Pharmacologic agents may cause thyroid dysfunction or abnormalities in TFT results. The most important examples are discussed in this section.

Amiodarone is an iodine-rich pharmacologic agent used in the management of refractory ventricular arrhythmias. It is highly lipophilic and concentrates in the thyroid gland, heart muscles, and adipose tissue. It has a very long half-life, and therefore its effects on the thyroid gland can be seen up to 2 to 3 years after discontinuation of the drug. Like iodine or radiographic contrast material, its effects on the thyroid gland can be variable, depending on the presence of underlying autoimmune disease and the geographic iodine availability. Individuals who have chronic autoimmune thyroiditis or are living in iodine-sufficient areas are more likely to develop

hypothyroidism when exposed to iodinated agents, whereas patients with a multinodular goiter or those residing in iodine-deficient areas may be more likely to develop hyperthyroidism. The risk of either thyroid dysfunction is less likely when lower doses are used.

Hypothyroidism is the more common thyroid disorder in patients taking amiodarone in the United States. Symptoms can develop as soon as 2 weeks and as late as 39 months after the initiation of amiodarone therapy.

Clinical Presentation

Clinical manifestations and diagnosis of amiodarone-associated hypothyroidism are similar to those of hypothyroidism of any cause. This condition is effectively treated with levothyroxine replacement therapy. It does not necessitate the discontinuation of amiodarone unless this therapy fails to correct the underlying arrhythmia. Goals of therapy include the establishment of a high-normal TSH level and a mid- to low-normal free T_4 level. A larger-than-normal dose may be required because of the effect of amiodarone on T_4 and T_3 production and action.

About 3% of patients treated with amiodarone in the United States become hyperthyroid. This usually occurs between 4 months and 3 years after the start of therapy.[21] It is more common in iodine-deficient areas of the world. The clinical manifestations of amiodarone-induced hyperthyroidism (AIT) are often masked because its β-blocking activity minimizes many of the adrenergic effects of thyroid hormone excess. Common symptoms include redevelopment of atrial arrhythmias, exacerbation of ischemic heart disease or congestive heart failure, restlessness, and low-grade fever. When thyrotoxicosis develops in the setting of amiodarone, it could be caused by overactivity of the thyroid gland (type 1) or destructive thyroiditis (type 2), in which there is inflammation of the thyroid gland. While it may be occasionally useful to distinguish between these two types, most patients do not clearly fall into one or the other.[22] Amiodarone does not necessarily need to be discontinued immediately, and given its persistence in the system, discontinuation would not affect treatment. Treatment ultimately depends on the nature of the disease; such cases can be diagnostically challenging and difficult to manage. If the mechanism of hyperthyroidism is uncertain, a combination of oral steroids and antithyroid drug is a prudent initial approach.[22] Ultimately, thyroidectomy may be necessary if hyperthyroidism is refractory to medical intervention.

Ideally, before recommending amiodarone therapy, the health care provider should obtain baseline TFT results and determine the presence of thyroid antibodies. Underlying thyroid disease and family history of thyroid disorders should be noted; this would place the patient at an increased risk of thyroid dysfunction with this drug and would alert clinicians to this possibility. TFTs should be performed at 3-month intervals after the medication is started and for at least 1 year after it is discontinued.

Interferon alfa is used in the treatment of hepatitis B and C or malignant disease. Use of this agent can induce the production of thyroid antibodies, resulting in hypothyroidism or

TABLE 194.4	**Non-thyroidal Illness Syndrome**				
	T₃	**T₄**	**Free T₄**	**rT₃**	**TSH**
Nonthyroidal illness	Decreased	Normal or decreased	Normal or decreased	Increased	Low

T_3, Triiodothyronine; T_4, thyroxine; *TSH*, Thyroid stimulating hormone.

thyrotoxicosis or a biphasic thyroiditis. With discontinuation of this agent, these antibodies often disappear.

Lithium, as used in the treatment of psychiatric conditions such as bipolar depression, can induce thyroid dysfunction. It blocks the uptake of iodine and the release of thyroid hormone and can induce chronic autoimmune thyroiditis. Clinical or subclinical hypothyroidism or a goiter in a euthyroid patient is within the spectrum of lithium-induced thyroid disease. TFT abnormalities, including low TSH, low TT_3, and elevated rT_3, are noted in patients receiving steroids and pressor agents. Similar abnormalities in T_3 and rT_3 are noted with amiodarone. Much as in non-thyroidal illness syndrome, these agents block the formation of T_3 from T_4, and most of T_4 is shunted into the formation of rT_3.

Tyrosine kinase inhibitors (e.g., sunitinib, sorafenib, imatinib) are used to treat renal cell carcinoma and gastrointestinal stromal tumors. The development of hypothyroidism has been seen in 50% to 70% of patients treated with these agents.[13] Possible mechanisms of action include capillary regression, destructive thyroiditis, impaired iodine uptake, and increased type 3 deiodination (resulting in increased metabolism of thyroid hormones). It is most commonly seen with sunitinib, but it is thought to be a class effect. Hyperthyroidism has also been described.[13,23] Symptoms of hyperthyroidism and hypothyroidism may incorrectly be attributed to the primary malignancy or side effects of antineoplastic agents. Routine testing for thyroid abnormalities is recommended in these patients.

Biotin is a B vitamin that is available as a dietary supplement for skin, hair, and nails. Multiple studies have shown that biotin intake greater than 0. 5 to 1.0 g daily can interfere with diagnostic assays that use biotin-streptavidin technology. Very high intakes of biotin can cause falsely low TSH level in immunometric assay and falsely elevated T4, T3 levels in competitive binding assays. Patients should be advised to hold biotin dose for at least 3 days prior to checking TFTs.[24]

THYROID DISEASE IN PREGNANCY

Thyroid disease during pregnancy is evaluated and treated like that in nonpregnant women, but it presents some obstacles.[25] In general, the thyroid gland increases in size by up to 10% during pregnancy in iodine replete areas. Changes in thyroid physiology to meet the increased metabolic demands in pregnancy include an increase in TBG concentration and cross-reactivity of human chorionic gonadotropin (hCG) with the TSH receptor. Estrogen stimulates TBG production and TBG sialylation, resulting in decreased TBG clearance. TBG concentration increases up to twofold, and, to maintain adequate free T4 levels, T4 and T3 production increases. Dietary iodine requirements are higher in pregnancy due to increased thyroid hormone synthesis, increased renal iodine loss, and fetal iodine requirements. The American Thyroid Association recommends that women who are planning a pregnancy take an oral supplement containing 150 mcg of potassium iodine.[25] hCG, which is a weak thyroid stimulator, may cause hyperthyroidism during pregnancy. This has been described as "transient subclinical hyperthyroidism" or "gestational transient hyperthyroidism." It occurs in 10% to 20% of normal pregnant women during the period of highest hCG concentrations, lasting from fertilization to about 11 weeks' gestation.[18]

Because of changes in thyroid physiology in pregnancy, American Thyroid Association guidelines recommend, when available, population- and- trimester-specific reference ranges for TSH defined by provider's laboratory for the typical population. If this is unavailable, then an upper reference limit of 4.0 mU/L can be used. This reflects a 0.5 mU/L reduction in the nonpregnant TSH upper reference limit.: first trimester, 0.1 to 2.5; second trimester, 0.2 to 3.0; and third trimester, 0.3 to 3.0.33 first trimester TSH goal 0.1 to 4.0; second and third trimester TSH goal nonpregnant normal range. Free T4 assay may be inaccurate in pregnancy due to changing binding protein levels. Total T4 can be used to assess thyroid function if TSH and free T4 levels are discordant.[25,26]

HYPERTHYROIDISM IN PREGNANCY

Overt hyperthyroidism, defined by TSH below 0.01 and elevated free T4 and/or T3 level, is rare and occurs in less than 0.4% of all pregnancies. Graves disease and hCG-mediated hyperthyroidism are the most common causes of hyperthyroidism during pregnancy.[18] Thyroiditis, toxic adenomas, and toxic multinodular goiters are less common causes of hyperthyroidism in pregnancy. Examples of hCG-mediated hyperthyroidism include transient subclinical hyperthyroidism, hyperemesis gravidarum, and trophoblastic hyperthyroidism. Women usually become euthyroid when the hyperemesis resolves and usually do not require antithyroid treatment.

Trophoblastic hyperthyroidism occurs in approximately 60% of women with a hydatidiform mole or choriocarcinoma. The hyperthyroidism can be severe and is treated by removal of the mole or therapy against the choriocarcinoma.

Graves hyperthyroidism is the most frequent cause of hyperthyroidism in pregnancy. It usually becomes less severe during the later stages of pregnancy. This is likely mediated by a change in the activity of the TRAb from stimulatory to blocking. Consequences of poorly controlled hyperthyroidism include increased risk of spontaneous pregnancy loss, premature labor, low birth weight, stillbirth, and preeclampsia.

The diagnosis of hyperthyroidism may be challenging. A TSH value of less than 0.01 μIU/mL and also a high serum free T_4 value are indicative of hyperthyroidism. Because radioiodine is contraindicated during pregnancy, it is often impossible to decipher the cause of the hyperthyroidism. Clinical features of goiter, ophthalmopathy, and pretibial myxedema are supportive of Graves disease. Adrenergic symptoms are difficult to assess during pregnancy. TRAb levels are elevated in 95% of patients with Graves disease. Treatment of pregnant women with overt hyperthyroid is limited because treatment can be harmful to the fetus. The goal is to maintain maternal T4 in the high-normal range by use of the lowest dose of drug possible to prevent fetal hypothyroidism.

Diagnostics

- Physical examination: note pulse; assess for goiter, ophthalmopathy, and pretibial myxedema
- TSH, free T4, TT3
- Consider TRAb levels
- Consider thyroid ultrasound

Management

Thioamides are the mainstay of treatment for women with moderate to severe hyperthyroidism complicating pregnancy.[25]

- PTU is used during the first trimester because of increased teratogenicity of methimazole (aplasia cutis).
- Methimazole is started and PTU is discontinued after the first trimester because of its increased hepatotoxicity.
- Free T4 and TSH levels are monitored monthly to keep free T4 levels in high-normal range and TSH levels in the low-normal range.
- β blockers can be used in women with moderate to severe hyperthyroidism with hyperadrenergic symptoms. Risks to the fetus include fetal growth restriction, hypoglycemia, and bradycardia.
- Atenolol (25 to 50 mg daily) or propranolol 10 to 20 mg three or four times daily are preferred agents.
- The goal is to wean the patient off β blockers as soon as hyperthyroidism is controlled by thionamide.
- Fetal heart rate and growth should be monitored to watch for rare fetal hyperthyroidism.

Hypothyroidism during pregnancy is less frequent because many women with hypothyroidism are anovulatory or have high rates of first-trimester miscarriages. Hypothyroidism during pregnancy has been associated with early pregnancy loss, preeclampsia, placental abruption, low birth weight, perinatal mortality, and neuropsychological dysfunction. Thyroid hormone requirements increase by approximately 29% in pregnant women with preexisting hypothyroidism because of estrogen-induced elevations in TBG, increased volume of distribution of thyroid hormone, and increased placental transport and degradation of thyroid hormone. For this reason and because of the significance of maternal euthyroidism for normal fetal growth, it is recommended to increase the prepregnancy thyroid hormone dose by 30% as soon as pregnancy is confirmed. Serum TSH concentration should be measured 4 to 6 weeks after conception, 4 to 6 weeks after any change is made in the dose of T_4, and at least once each trimester. The TSH goal before conception and during pregnancy is approximately 0.5 to 2.5 μIU/L. A pregnant woman found to have a thyroid nodule should be evaluated in the same way as other patients are, except that radioiodine scanning is contraindicated.

HYPOTHYROIDISM IN PREGNANCY
Diagnostics

- The TSH goal prior to conception is 0.5 to 2.5.
- With a positive pregnancy test result, the thyroid hormone dose is increased by 30%.
- For example, if the prepregnancy levothyroxine dose was 100 mcg daily, 1 tablet is taken daily Monday through Friday and 2 tablets daily are taken on Saturday and Sunday (an increase from 7 tablets per week to 9 tablets per week).
- TSH and free T4 are monitored every month for the first half of pregnancy and then at least every trimester. The dose is adjusted in 12- to 25-mcg increments.
- Postpartum patients are advised to start back on the prepregnancy levothyroxine dose—that is, if the patient was taking 100 mcg daily preconception and the dose was increased, she should cut back to 100 mcg daily postpartum. TSH and free T_4 are checked 6 weeks postpartum.

REFERENCES

1. Braverman, L. E., & Cooper, D. (Eds.), (2013). *Werner and Ingbar's the thyroid: A fundamental and clinical text* (10th ed.). New York: Lippincott, Williams and Wilkins.
2. Surks, M., & Boucai, L. (2010). Clinical review: Age- and race-based serum thyrotropin reference limits. *The Journal of Clinical Endocrinology and Metabolism*, 95, 496–502.
3. Bae, J. S., Chae, B. J., Park, W. C., et al. (2009). Incidental thyroid lesions detected by FDG-PET CT; prevalence and risk of thyroid cancer. *World Journal of Surgical Oncology*, 7–53.
4. Palaniswamy, S. S., Subrabanyam P. (2013). Diagnostic utility of PETCT in thyroid malignancies: An update. *Annals of Nuclear Medicine*, 27(8), 681–693.
5. Haugen, B. R., Alexander, E. K., Bible, K., et al. (2016). 2015 American Thyroid Association management guidelines for adult patients with thyroid nodules and differentiated thyroid cancer: The American Thyroid Association task force on thyroid nodules and differentiated thyroid cancer. *Thyroid*, 26(1), 1–133.
6. McLeod, D. S., Cooper, D. S., Ladenson, P. W., et al. (2014). Prognosis of differentiated thyroid cancer in relation to serum thyrotropin and thyroglobulin antibody status at time of diagnosis. *Thyroid*, 24(1), 35–42.
7. Wells, S., Asa, S., Henning, D., et al. (2015). Revised American Thyroid Association Guidelines for the management of medullary thyroid carcinoma. *Thyroid*, 25(6).
8. Bonavita, J. A., Mayo, J., Babb, J., et al. (2009). Pattern recognition of benign nodules at ultrasound of the thyroid: Which nodules can be left alone? *AJR. American Journal of Roentgenology*, 193, 207–213.
9. Cibas, E. S., & Syed, Z. A. (2017). The 2017 Bethesda system for reporting thyroid cytopathology. *Thyroid*, 27(11), 1341–1346.
10. Alexander, E. K., Kennedy, G. C., Baloch, Z. W., et al. (2012). Preoperative diagnosis of benign thyroid nodules with indeterminate cytology. *The New England Journal of Medicine*, 367(8), 705.
11. Yip, L., Wharry, K. I., et al. (2014). A clinical algorithm for fine-needle aspiration molecular testing effectively guides the appropriate extent of initial thyroidectomy. *Annals of Surgery*, 260(1), 163–168.
12. Stagnaro-Green, A. (2004). Post partum thyroiditis. *Best Practice and Research. Clinical Endocrinology and Metabolism*, 18(2), 303–316.
13. Makita, N., Iiri, T. (2013). Tyrosine kinase inhibitor-induced thyroid disorders: A review and hypothesis. *Thyroid*, 23(2), 151–160.
14. Bahn, R. S., Burch, H. S., Cooper, D. S., et al. (2009). The role of propylthiouracil in the management of Graves' disease in adults: Report of a meeting jointly sponsored by the American Thyroid Association and the Food and Drug Administration. *Thyroid*, 19, 673–674.
15. Jonklass, J., Bianco, A. C., Bauer, A. J., et al. (2014). Guidelines for the treatment of hyperthyroidism; prepared by the American Thyroid Association Task Force on Thyroid Hormone Replacement Therapy. Retrieved from www.thyroid.org/thyroid-guidelines. (Accessed 16 March 2015).
16. Bahn, R. S., Burch, H. B., Cooper, D. S., Garber, J. R., et al. (2011). Hyperthyroidism and other causes of thyrotoxicosis. Management guidelines of the American Thyroid Association and the American Association of Endocrinologist. *Endocrine Practice*, 17(3), 456–520.
17. Vanderpump, M. (2011). The epidemiology of thyroid disease. *British Medical Bulletin*, 99, 39–51.
18. Nygaard, B. (2015). Hyperthyroidism in pregnancy. *BMJ Clinical Evidence*, 2015, 0611.
19. Hennessey, J., & Espaillat, R. (2018). Current evidence for the treatment of hypothyroidism with levothyroxine/levotriiodothyroxine combination therapy vs. levothyroxine monotherapy. *Clinical Practice*, 72(2).
20. Cooper, D., & Biondi, B. (2012). Subclinical thyroid disease. *Lancet*, 379(9821), 1142–1154.
21. Tomisti, L., et al. (2014). The onset of time of amiodarone-induced thyrotoxicosis (AIT) depends on AIT type. *European Journal of Endocrinology*, 171, 363–368.
22. Epstein, A., Olshansky, B., Naccarelli, G., et al. (2016). Practical Management guidelines for clinicians who treat patients with Amiodarone. *The American Journal of Medicine*, 129(5), 468–475.
23. Hamnvik, O. P., Larsen, P. R., & Marqusee, E. (2011). Thyroid dysfunction from antineoplastic agents. *Journal of the National Cancer Institute*, 103(21), 1572.
24. Li, D., Radulescu, A., et al. (2017). Association of biotin ingestion with performance of hormone and non-hormone assays in healthy adults. *JAMA: The Journal of the American Medical Association*, 318(12), 1150–1160.
25. Alexander, E. K., Pearce, E. N., Brent, G. A., et al. (2017). 2017 guidelines of the American thyroid association for the diagnosis and management of thyroid disease during pregnancy and postpartum. *Thyroid*, 27(3), 315–389.
26. Taylor, P., Onyebochi, O., & Premardhana, P. (2015). Should all women be screened for thyroid dysfunction in pregnancy? *Women's Health*, 11(3), 295–307.

Evaluation and Management of Rheumatic Disorders

CHAPTER **195**

POLYMYALGIA RHEUMATICA AND GIANT CELL ARTERITIS

Francisco P. Quismorio, Jr. • Dorothy K. Johnson

 Immediate intervention: Any patient complaining of headache, jaw claudication, or visual change along with muscle and joint aching should be referred for immediate evaluation and treatment. Sudden vision loss, diplopia, amaurosis fugax, and other visual complaints are considered a medical emergency.

DEFINITION AND EPIDEMIOLOGY

Polymyalgia rheumatica (PMR) is a treatable, chronic systemic inflammatory condition of unknown cause most often seen in older adults. Most patients are Caucasian, and, in general, PMR does not occur in patients younger than age 50. It is characterized by diffuse aching and stiffness of the shoulder girdle, neck, and pelvic girdle and is associated with elevated erythrocyte sedimentation rate (ESR) and/or C-reactive protein (CRP). There are no specific laboratory tests for PMR, and the diagnosis is made on clinical grounds and after exclusion of other inflammatory conditions.[1]

The incidence of PMR increases progressively with age, peaking at 70 to 80 years. Women are affected two to three times more often than men. A population-based study in the United States found prevalence as high as 1 per 67.5 persons older than age 50 years.[2]

PATHOPHYSIOLOGY

The cause of PMR is not known; however, genetic, immune, and environmental influences are believed to be important factors. People of northern European descent are more vulnerable. Human leukocyte antigen HLA-DRB1 genotypes and polymorphisms in genes involved in immunity, including those involved with tumor necrosis factor-α (TNF-α) and interleukin-1 (IL-1), are associated with increased susceptibility to and/or severity of PMR. The higher incidence of PMR during winter months and the known variation in geographic distribution of the disease implies a role for environmental factors.[3] The possible role of infectious agent(s) as a trigger of the disease has been postulated; however, no definite link has been found.

CLINICAL PRESENTATION AND PHYSICAL EXAMINATION

The most remarkable features are the stiffness and aching of the shoulder girdle, pelvic girdle, and neck. Inflammatory in origin, the pain tends to be worse at night and may radiate distally to the elbows and the knees. Morning stiffness lasting longer than 1 hour and even all morning is common. The onset can be acute, such that the patient may remember the day and the hour of the onset. In most patients the onset is subacute and insidious. About half of patients experience systemic symptoms such as low-grade fever, depression, fatigue, malaise, and weight loss. About 25% of patients have inflammatory arthritis involving primarily the knees and wrists and less frequently the metacarpal joints. It can be mistaken for rheumatoid arthritis; however, in PMR the inflammatory arthritis is non-erosive, asymmetric, self-limiting, and highly responsive to systemic corticosteroids.[1,4] Tenosynovitis of the extensor tendons of the hands and feet can be seen in association with peripheral arthritis. Remitting seronegative symmetric synovitis with pitting edema syndrome (RS3PE) seen in 12% of PMR patients is characterized by pitting edema of the dorsum of the hands and wrists and sometimes on the dorsum of the feet.[1]

Physical examination reveals painful active motion of the shoulders and hips with limited range of motion. No signs of synovitis are present except in those with peripheral arthritis. True muscle weakness is absent; however, muscle strength is often difficult to assess because of the pain.

Classification Criteria

The American College of Rheumatology (ACR) and European League Against Rheumatism (EULAR) recently published classification criteria for PMR.[4] Developed primarily for defining patient groups for clinical and epidemiologic studies, this criteria set is not intended for diagnosis in clinical practice. A patient 50 years or older with new-onset bilateral shoulder pain and elevated ESR and/or CRP is classified as having PMR in the presence of morning stiffness for longer than 45 minutes, new hip pain in the absence of peripheral synovitis, and negative rheumatoid factor (RF) and anti-CCP. When musculoskeletal ultrasound (MUS) findings are included in the criteria set, a score of 5 or higher has 66% sensitivity and 81% specificity for discriminating PMR from comparison patients.

DIAGNOSTICS

Laboratory studies are generally done to demonstrate inflammation and rule out other inflammatory diseases. When PMR is suspected on clinical grounds, the following initial laboratory tests are recommended:

1. Complete blood count
2. ESR and CRP
3. Complete metabolic panel including blood urea nitrogen (BUN), creatinine, calcium, phosphate
4. Liver function tests
5. Serum protein electrophoresis

6 Rheumatoid factor and anti-CCP
7 Urinalysis
8. Thyroid-stimulating hormone
9. Chest x-ray examination

Laboratory abnormalities associated with active inflammation including elevated ESR, CRP, leukocytosis, thrombocytosis, mild normochromic anemia, and hypoalbuminemia are seen in the majority of patients. Low-titer RF may be seen in some patients; however, antinuclear antibody (ANA), antineutrophil cytoplasmic antibody (ANCA), and anti–cyclic citrulinated protein (anti-CCP) test results are generally negative.

Additional Diagnostics: Imaging

There are few controlled studies that address the role of imaging for the diagnosis and differential diagnosis of PMR.[5] Musculoskeletal ultrasonography (MUS), magnetic resonance imaging (MRI), and positron emission tomography/computed tomography (PET/CT) can demonstrate the characteristic joint involvement in PMR including bilateral shoulder and hip bursitis, biceps tenosynovitis, as well as glenohumeral and hip synovitis. In clinical practice, MUS is the most commonly used imaging; MRI and PET/CT are not routinely done.

DIFFERENTIAL DIAGNOSIS

Important non-rheumatic medical conditions that may mimic PMR in a patient aged 50 years or older include active malignancy such as lymphoma (see Chapter 219) and multiple myeloma (see Chapter 220), active bacterial or viral infections, hypothyroidism (see Chapter 194), and drug-induced syndromes such as statin myopathy.[6]

Rheumatic diseases that should be in the differential diagnosis include elderly onset RA (see Chapter 197), late-onset seronegative spondyloarthropathies (see Chapter 198), late-onset systemic lupus erythematosus (SLE) (see Chapter 199), inflammatory myopathies, calcium pyrophosphate arthritis, and chronic pain syndromes such as osteoarthritis of the neck and shoulders (see Chapter 165). Giant cell arteritis (GCA) may occur concomitantly with PMR (see later). Elderly onset RA differs from PMR with the presence of subcutaneous nodules, anti-CCP antibodies, and RF in the latter. Moreover, the clinical response to steroid therapy is more dramatic in PMR.

INTERPROFESSIONAL COLLABORATIVE MANAGEMENT

Patients with PMR should be referred to a rheumatologist for definitive diagnosis and a prescription regimen. Follow-up can be managed by primary care providers with access to rheumatologists for questions or for patients not responding to usual regimens. Any patients with symptoms suggestive of temporal arteritis (see later) should also be referred to an ophthalmologist or plastic surgeon for temporal artery biopsy.

Systemic corticosteroids remain the standard drug therapy, although there have been no placebo-controlled trials. Low-dose prednisone typically induces a rapid response within a few days of initiation of therapy. The usual starting dose is 15 mg to 20 mg of prednisone (or equivalent) daily. A higher dose of prednisone (60 mg daily) is used when there is evidence of concomitant GCA (see later).

The 2015 EULAR recommendations include an initial dose of 12.5 to 25 mg of prednisone daily with strong recommendations against using doses higher than 30 mg/d. Begin tapering doses by 5 mg a week after 4 to 8 weeks of therapy

and continue using the lowest effective dose.[7] Nonsteroidal anti-inflammatory agents are not recommended.

There is no optimal corticosteroid regimen for every patient; thus the regimen should be flexible and individualized. There is variation not only in severity, but also in the presentation and course of the illness.

A marked overall clinical improvement within a week of corticosteroid therapy is expected, and laboratory abnormalities should improve within 4 to 8 weeks. The patient should be monitored for pain, morning stiffness, functional disability, osteoporosis risk, adverse drug reaction, and an alternative diagnosis. The majority of PMR patients are continued on low-dose corticosteroids for 1 to 2 years. PMR patients with concomitant GCA appear to require a longer duration of corticosteroid therapy.

COMPLICATIONS

Perhaps the most significant complication of PMR is its close association with GCA (see later).

Despite good clinical response to drug therapy, disease relapses are common and are seen in 50% of cases. Factors associated with high relapse rate include persistently elevated inflammatory markers, female sex, and rapid taper of corticosteroid dose.[8]

Adverse drug side effects including osteoporosis, fragility fractures, diabetes, hypertension, and cardiovascular events are not uncommon. Sixty-five percent of PMR patients treated with a corticosteroid alone and 80% of those who receive corticosteroids and NSAIDS experience at least one adverse event.[9] Patients with long-standing PMR, especially those with high risk for corticosteroid side effects, should be maintained at the lowest dose possible. In addition, the use of a steroid-sparing agent such as methotrexate, leflunomide, or azathioprine may be considered.

Bone protective measures (calcium, vitamin D, and bisphosphonates) are recommended for patients on chronic corticosteroid therapy. Pneumocystis prophylaxis may be indicated for patients on higher-dose steroids (>30 mg/d) for longer duration.

In spite of an overall increased risk for vascular events, the overall life span is not reduced in patients with this condition.[10]

PATIENT EDUCATION

Patients with PMR should be educated about its association with GCA. Patients should be aware of the necessity to report immediately any new headache, change in vision, scalp tenderness, pain on chewing, or other new symptom.

Education about the risks of corticosteroid therapy is important. The patient should be informed of the potential life-threatening risk of sudden withdrawal of corticosteroids secondary to hypoadrenalism. Obtaining a medical alert bracelet indicating the use of corticosteroids should be recommended. Patients need to be aware of common steroid side effects and the importance of contacting their health care provider should they develop symptoms such as increased thirst, polyuria, and weight loss. Medications should be taken with food. Ulcer prophylaxis with proton pump inhibitors or histamine H_2 blockers should be considered for patients on corticosteroids. The patient should understand the risks of the development of corticosteroid-induced bone loss and the importance of behaviors such as daily weight-bearing exercise and adequate daily intake of calcium (1200 mg) and vitamin D (1000 IU), as well as the use of antiresorptive medication.

ASSOCIATION BETWEEN POLYMYALGIA RHEUMATICA AND GIANT CELL ARTERITIS
Definition and Epidemiology of Giant Cell Arteritis

GCA is a systemic vasculitis of unknown cause that primarily involves large and medium-sized blood vessels (see Chapter 200). Both PMR and GCA affect the elderly and are well recognized to occur together more frequently than expected by chance. Sixteen percent to 21% of PMR patients develop GCA, and 40% to 60% of GCA patients have clinical features of PMR.[11,12] PMR can develop before, concomitantly with, or after the onset of GCA.

GCA, the most common primary vasculitis in adults, affects individuals aged 50 years and older, with a female-to-male ratio of 3 : 1 to 2 : 1.

The majority of patients are Caucasian, and the incidence rate increases with latitude in the Northern Hemisphere; the highest rates are found in Scandinavian countries and in North American populations of the same descent, with an incidence rate of more than 17 per 100,000 persons aged 50 years or older. The incidence rate increases with age and is highest at ages 70 to 79 years. GCA is less common among Asians and African Americans than among Caucasians.[13,14]

PATHOPHYSIOLOGY

The cause of GCA is not known. Multiple genes have been reported that confer disease susceptibility, including HLA-DRB1*04 allele and certain polymorphisms of the *IL-13* gene, vascular endothelial growth factor gene *(VEGF)* gene, and toll-like receptor *(TLR)* gene. A possible relationship between GCA and infectious organisms including herpesvirus, parvovirus, and *Mycoplasma pneumoniae* has been suspected; however, to date, there is no definitive evidence to show that the disease is triggered by an infectious agent. The role of environmental agent(s) is suggested by seasonal fluctuation, geographic variation, and the cyclic pattern of the disease.

The classic pathology is that transmural inflammation involves all layers of the arterial wall and intimal hyperplasia and causes occlusion of the lumen. The hallmark lesion is characterized by a predominance of mononuclear infiltrates or granulomas with multinucleated giant cells. The inflammatory infiltrate consists of activated T cells, dendritic cells, and macrophages. The elastic lamina is fragmented and destroyed.

In addition to the carotid artery and its branches, GCA can involve the great arteries, especially the thoracic aorta and its branches. Stroke, blindness, and other clinical manifestations are caused by tissue ischemia as a consequence of the narrowing and occlusion of the lumen of the affected blood vessel.[11]

Clinical Presentation and Physical Examination

The clinical manifestations of GCA are protean and can be divided into four categories.[15,16] At initial presentation a patient may have one major complaint such as new-onset headache, or the presentation may have multiple clinical features.

Clinical manifestations caused by involvement of cranial arteries include headache, jaw claudication, visual impairment, scalp tenderness, prominent or tender temporal artery, tongue infarction, and strokes or neuropsychiatric symptoms.

New-onset headache, the most common symptom (seen in 70% to 80% of patients), is often the presenting complaint. Headache is severe and localized in the temporal region, although it can also be less defined. Scalp tenderness in the occipital and temporal areas is not uncommon. The temporal artery may be tender, swollen, or nodular.

Visual disturbances are present in 25% to 50% of patients; however, visual loss is reported in 6% to 10% of cases.[16] Sudden vision loss, diplopia, amaurosis fugax, and other visual complaints are considered a medical emergency; GCA should be identified and treated immediately to prevent blindness. The second eye is at risk if the disease is not treated aggressively and promptly. Anterior ischemic optic neuropathy caused by inflammation and occlusion of the posterior ciliary arteries is the most frequent ocular lesion.

Jaw claudication, reported by 30% to 40% of patients, is characterized by pain in the muscles of mastication that develops after a period of time chewing food and is relieved with rest.[13] Tingling or soreness of the tongue, ulceration, and loss of taste can be present. Strokes, deafness, and peripheral neuropathy are less common manifestations.

Systemic symptoms including fever, weight loss, anorexia, night sweats, and dry cough are reported in 30% to 60% of patients.[15] Depression and/or confusion may occur. Signs and symptoms of PMR are reported in 20% to 65% of patients.[15]

Clinical features resulting from extracranial vessel involvement are seen in 5% to 20% and include claudication of the upper limbs and, rarely, aortic aneurysm or dissection.[15]

Classification Criteria of Giant Cell Arteritis

The diagnosis is made based on a constellation of symptoms and physical findings combined with laboratory tests including imaging. Physical examination should include palpation of the temporal arteries, examination of the scalp, auscultation of neck arteries, blood pressure measurement in both arms for evidence of vascular stenosis, and ocular fundoscopy. The diagnosis is not difficult to make in the typical older adult patient with new-onset headache, temporal artery tenderness, jaw claudication, and systemic symptoms. However, a number of patients have minor or no features referable to the cranial arteries, so the diagnosis of GCA is not easily recognized.

DIAGNOSTICS

Baseline laboratory tests are similar to those listed earlier for PMR. Elevated ESR (77% to 86% of patients), high CRP (95% to 98%), mild normochromic anemia, leukocytosis, and/or thrombocytosis are indicative of systemic inflammatory state.

Color Doppler ultrasound of the temporal arteries is frequently used as a diagnostic aid.[5] Inflammatory edema of the blood vessel appearing as a hypoechoic vascular wall thickening (halo sign) has high sensitivity and specificity when the evaluation is performed by an experienced sonographer. The test is operator dependent and technique dependent, but with increasing experience and better ultrasound equipment, reliable and reproducible results can be obtained. A negative color Doppler sonography finding, however, does not exclude the diagnosis of GCA.[15,17] The characteristic ultrasound findings disappear with corticosteroid therapy.

CT angiography, magnetic resonance angiography, and PET/CT can demonstrate extracranial vascular involvement, but these imaging modalities are not performed routinely in all patients with GCA.[18-20]

Temporal artery biopsy remains the gold standard, and a positive result is confirmatory of the diagnosis. When a diagnosis of GCA is made clinically, a temporal artery biopsy is indicated; however, corticosteroid therapy should not be withheld pending the procedure or results of the biopsy. The rate of positive temporal artery biopsy after less than 2 weeks of corticosteroid therapy was reported to be 78%; however, it is preferable to perform the biopsy sooner rather than later once a decision has been made.[19]

A negative temporal artery biopsy does not exclude the diagnosis of GCA because the lesions are "skipped," and a long arterial segment (precontraction length >10 mm) is optimal. In general, a unilateral temporal artery biopsy is performed. If the results are negative, biopsy of the contralateral temporal artery may modestly increase the yield. The decision to do a contralateral temporal artery biopsy should be individualized. A recent study concluded that color duplex guided biopsy did not increase the yield of positive temporal artery biopsy.[2] Temporal artery biopsy can remain useful for 2 to 6 weeks after the initiation of corticosteroid therapy. It should be performed by an experienced surgical unit, and samples should be at least 1 cm in length.

Temporal artery biopsy may be negative in some patients. Biopsy-negative patients should be regarded and managed as having GCA if the clinical picture is typical and the response to the corticosteroid therapy is satisfactory.

DIFFERENTIAL DIAGNOSIS

The protean and multisystem manifestations of GCA require a careful and thorough differential diagnosis. Infections, active cancer, and systemic rheumatic diseases including rheumatoid arthritis and other vasculitides (see Chapter 200) should be excluded. GCA is a leading cause of fever of unknown origin in patients aged 65 years and older.[15]

INTERPROFESSIONAL COLLABORATIVE MANAGEMENT

EULAR recommends prednisone at a daily dose of 1 mg/kg (maximum 60 mg daily, or its equivalent).[20] Pulse intravenous methylprednisolone, 500 to 1000 mg/d for 3 days, may be of benefit to patients with visual impairment when used early. Prednisone dose is maintained for a month and tapered gradually. After 3 to 4 months of treatment, many patients will be on 10 to 15 mg of prednisone per day. The duration of therapy is variable from one patient to another and may extend to several years, with an average duration of treatment of 2 to 3 years. Adverse reactions to long-term corticosteroid therapy including osteoporosis and fragility fractures are not uncommon. Pneumocystis prophylaxis is indicated for all patients on high-dose steroids taken for a prolonged period.[21]

Adjunctive therapy with a steroid-sparing agent such as methotrexate, azathioprine, or leflunomide is recommended; however, these drugs have not been proven to be uniformly or highly effective. Methotrexate at a dose of 10 to 15 mg/wk is recommended by EULAR to help lower the cumulative dose of prednisone and to reduce the disease relapse rate.[20]

Low-dose aspirin (80 to 160 mg/d) is also recommended, provided there are no contraindications, to prevent ischemic complications of GCA.[14,20]

Within 24 to 48 hours of corticosteroid therapy, the majority of patients will experience improvement in headache as well as in sleep. Musculoskeletal pain improves within a week. Laboratory abnormalities including high ESR and/or CRP, anemia, thrombocytosis, and liver function test results may take a few weeks to normalize.[22]

All patients suspected of having GCA should receive physician consultation. The disease can be difficult to diagnose, and it requires immediate treatment to prevent complications, especially loss of vision. Temporal artery biopsy is performed by an ophthalmologist, general surgeon, or plastic surgeon. A rheumatologist is consulted for patients with biopsy-proven GCA who do not respond to steroids. Symptoms of stroke, aortic aneurysm, or myocardial infarction would warrant hospitalization.

Monitoring Treatment

- Follow-up during the first year should be performed at weeks 1, 3, and 6 then monthly thereafter, unless there are new symptoms or adverse drug reactions.
- Symptoms and physical findings are monitored.
- The patient should be monitored for side effects of corticosteroids and other medications.
- ESR, CRP, and metabolic panel including glucose and liver function test results should be monitored.
- Imaging may be required if a new ischemic event occurs.

Complications

Despite prompt initial clinical response to corticosteroid therapy, relapses are common, occurring in 25% to 65% of GCA patients.[23] Relapses occur especially during the first few years after the diagnosis, but these tend to be clinically milder. The most common presentations are PMR, headache, and systemic symptoms associated with elevated ESR and CRP. Ischemic events such as loss of vision can occur but are infrequent during follow-up.[23]

Patients who initially have intense systemic features tend to have a more prolonged course with more disease relapses and a higher cumulative dose of corticosteroid.[10]

The risk for myocardial infarction, stroke, and peripheral vascular disease is substantially increased in patients with long-standing GCA and also in some patients during the period immediately after the diagnosis. In spite of this, on a population level mortality is not increased in patients with GCA. There may be individual variations in the first few years following diagnosis.[24] The prevalence of aortic aneurysm or dissection is increased; however, the relative risk, time course, and best screening tests remain to be established.[17]

LIFE SPAN CONSIDERATIONS

PMR and GCA are primarily diseases of adults older than 50, reaching peak incidence from 70 to 79 years. Compared with the same age population, GCA patients in one study have a lower 5-year survival rate. After 10 years the mortality rate was no longer significantly different, suggesting that the adverse effect on survival is present only in the years immediately after the diagnosis and that longevity may benefit from frequent health monitoring.[25] The majority of studies from different countries report that the all-cause mortality of GCA patients is similar to that of the general population. There is no increased overall risk for cancer.[26]

REFERENCES

1. Pipitone, N., & Salvarani, C. (2013). Update on polymyalgia rheumatica. *European Journal of Internal Medicine*, 24, 583–589.
2. Raheel, S., Shbeeb, I., Crowson, C. S., & Matteson, E. L. (2017). Epidemiology of polymyalgia rheumatica 2000–2014 and examination of incidence and survival trends over 45 years: A population-based study. *Arthritis Care & Research*, 69, 1282–1285. doi:10.1002/acr.23132.
3. Weyand, C. M., & Goronzy, J. J. (2013). Immune Mechanisms in medium and large vessel vasculitis. *Nature Reviews. Rheumatology*, 9, 731–740.
4. Nesher, G. (2014). Polymyalgia rheumatic: Diagnosis and classification. *Journal of Autoimmunity*, 48-49, 76–78.
5. Dejaco, C., Duftner, C., Buttgereit, F., et al. (2017). The Spectrum of Giant Cell Arteritis and Polymyalgia Rheumatica: Revisiting the concept of the disease. *Rheumatology*, 56(4), 506–515.
6. Dasgupta, B., Cimmino, M. A., Maradit-Kremers, H., et al. (2012). 2012 provisional classification criteria for polymyalgia rheumatica: A European League Against Rheumatism/American College of Rheumatology collaborative initiative. *Annals of the Rheumatic Diseases*, 71, 484–492.
7. Dejaco, C., Singh, Y., & Perel, P. (2015). 2015 Recommendations for the Management of Polymyalgia Rheumatica. *Arthritis & Rheumatology*, 67(10), 2569–2580.
8. Buttgereit, F., Dejaco, C., Matteson, E. L., & Dasgupta, B. (2016). Polymyalgia rheumatica and giant cell arteritis: A systematic review. *JAMA: The Journal of the American Medical Association*, 315(22), 2442–2458. doi:10.1001/jama.2016.5444.
9. Kermani, T. A., & Warrington, K. S. (2014). Advances and challenges in the diagnosis and treatment of polymyalgia rheumatica. *Therapeutic Advances in Musculoskeletal Disease*, 6(1), 8–19.
10. Hancock, A. T., Mallen, C. D., Muller, S., et al. (2014). Risk of vascular events in patients with Polymyalgia Rheumatica. *CMAJ: Canadian Medical Association Journal = Journal de l'Association Medicale Canadienne*, 186, E495–E501.
11. Weyand, C. M., & Goronzy, J. J. (2014). Clinical practice. Giant cell arteritis and polymyalgia rheumatic. *The New England Journal of Medicine*, 371, 50–57.
12. Nesher, G. (2014). The diagnosis and classification of giant cell arteritis. *Journal of Autoimmunity*, 48-49, 73–75.
13. Salvarani, C., Pipitone, N., Versari, A., & Hunder, G. G. (2012). Clinical features of polymyalgia rheumatica and giant cell arteritis. *Lancet*, 144, 68–84.
14. Ponte, C., Rodriques, A. F., O'Neill, L., & Lugmani, R. A. (2015). Giant cell arteritis: Current treatment and management. *World Journal of Clinical Cases*, 3(6), 484–494.
15. Ness, T., Bley, T. A., Schmidt, W. A., & Lamprecht, P. (2013). The diagnosis and treatment of giant cell arteritis. *Deutsches Ärzteblatt International*, 110, 376–386.
16. Waldman, C. W., Waldman, S. D., & Waldman, R. A. (2013). Giant cell arteritis. *The Medical Clinics of North America*, 97, 329–335.
17. Germano, G., Muratore, F., Cimino, L., et al. (2014). Is colour duplex sonography-guided temporal artery biopsy useful in the diagnosis of giant cell arteritis? A randomized study. *Rheumatology*, 53.
18. Schmidt, W. A. (2013). Imaging in vasculitis. *Best Practice and Research. Clinical Rheumatology*, 27, 107–118.
19. Chacko, J., Chacko, A., & Salter, M. (2015). Review of giant cell arteritis. *Saudi Journal of Ophthalmology: Official Journal of the Saudi Ophthalmological Society*, 29(1), 48–52.
20. Dejaco, C., et al. (2018). EULAR recommendations for the use of imaging in large vessel vasculitis in clinical practice. *Annals of the Rheumatic Diseases*, 77, 636–643.
21. Stern, A., Green, H., Paul, M., et al. (2014). Prophylaxis for Pneumocystis pneumonia(PCP) in non- HIV immunocompromised patients. *The Cochrane Database of Systematic Reviews*, (110), CD005590.
22. Masson, C. (2012). Therapeutic approach to giant cell arteritis. *Joint, Bone, Spine: Revue Du Rhumatisme*, 79, 219–227.
23. Alba, M. A., Garcia-Martinez, A., Prieto-Gonzalez, S., et al. (2014). Relapses in patients with giant cell arteritis. *Medicine*, 93, 194–201.
24. Tomasson, G., Peloquin, C., Mohammad, A., et al. (2014). Risk for cardiovascular disease early and late after a diagnosis of giant cell arteritis. *Annals of Internal Medicine*, 160, 73–80.
25. Wade Crow, R., Katz, B. J., Warner, J. E. A., et al. (2009). Giant cell arteritis and mortality. *Journal of Gerontology*, 64A, 365–369.
26. Brekke, L., Diamantopoulos, A., Fevang, B., et al. (2018). FRI0502 Risk of cancer in patients diagnosed with giant cell arteritis in western norway 1972–2012. *Annals of the Rheumatic Diseases*, 77, 778–779.

CHAPTER **196**

RAYNAUD PHENOMENON

Lin A. Brown

 Physician consultation is necessary for patients with intractable pain, persistent pallor, coldness, tissue breakdown in the digits, and reduced pulses in the extremities. A vascular surgeon should be consulted if possible digit loss is suspected. Patients at risk for autoamputation of a digit or severe infection require hospitalization under the care of a rheumatologist.

DEFINITION AND EPIDEMIOLOGY

Raynaud phenomenon is a reversible vasospastic disorder that affects the blood flow to the digits and less commonly to the nose and earlobes. When these changes occur in isolation with normal physical examination findings, the disorder is known as primary Raynaud phenomenon. In primary Raynaud phenomenon, there are no associated autoimmune diseases, and rarely are autoantibodies present. Primary Raynaud phenomenon characteristically occurs in women, in non- latino whites of any gender in the younger age group (<30) and those with a family history. It is not uncommon and is thought to affect 9% to 10% of women and 5% to 6% of men in the United States.[1]

Secondary Raynaud phenomenon is seen in patients who also have an autoimmune disorder, such as progressive systemic sclerosis (scleroderma), systemic lupus erythematosus, dermatomyositis, polymyositis, or mixed connective tissue disease. Secondary Raynaud phenomenon can also be seen as part of the CREST constellation, a subset of scleroderma characterized by calcinosis, Raynaud phenomenon, esophageal dysmotility, sclerodactyly, and telangiectasia.[2]

In addition to autoimmune diseases, Raynaud phenomenon has been seen in association with migraine headaches and chest pain.[3] Secondary Raynaud phenomenon is often more severe than primary disease, less symmetric in the digits involved, and has a greater likelihood of ulcerations and severe ischemic changes. Secondary Raynaud phenomenon can be associated with certain drugs, trauma, hematologic disorders, vibration exposure, frostbite, and atherosclerotic disease. More than 60% of patients who develop Raynaud phenomenon after age 60 have atherosclerosis as the underlying cause of their disease.[2]

PATHOPHYSIOLOGY

The vascular endothelium, smooth muscle cells, and nerve terminals form an integrated unit that works in response to elements in the microenvironment to determine the final balance between vasodilation and vasoconstriction. These elements are influenced by a variety of factors, including temperature, physical activity, emotional state, and direct trauma.

In Raynaud phenomenon, the blood vessels constrict in response to cold or stress. This may be related to increased activation of the sympathetic nerves, especially the α_2-adrenergic fibers. In addition, there appears to be an alteration in vascular function on the cellular level, particularly in vascular smooth muscle and the endothelium.[4] The resultant disturbance in circulation causes a series of color changes in the skin: white, blanched, or pale as the blood flow is reduced (Fig. 196.1);

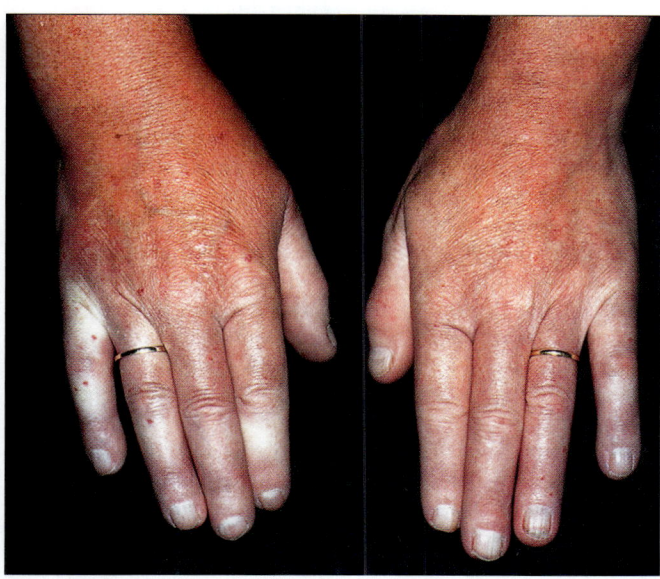

F I G . 196.1 Raynaud phenomenon. (From Hochberg, M. C., Gravallese, E. M., Silman, A. J., Smolen, J. S., Weinblatt, M. E., & Weisman, M. H. [2019]. *Rheumatology* [8th ed.]. Philadelphia: Elsevier.)

blue as the affected digit loses oxygen from the decreased blood flow; and red or flushed as blood flow returns. Finally, as the attack subsides and the circulation returns to normal, usual skin color is restored. In the white and blue stages, numbness, tingling, and coldness can be felt. In the red stage, a feeling of warmth, burning, or swelling may be reported. Not infrequently, pain is experienced, especially in secondary Raynaud phenomena. The earlobe, nose, and rarely tongue can be affected as well as the fingers and toes.

CLINICAL PRESENTATION AND PHYSICAL EXAMINATION

The vasospasm of Raynaud phenomenon causes classic tricolor changes of first white (pallor), then blue (cyanosis), and then red (reperfusion hyperemia) after the vasospasm ends.[1] Episodes can be triggered by cold exposure, rapid changes in ambient temperature, or emotional stress. Attacks can occur in single or multiple digits and can spread to other digits, the other hand, or the feet. Cutaneous vasospasm can be seen at other sites, including ears, nose, face, knees, and nipples.[5] Patients can experience pain, numbness, and burning, especially in secondary Raynaud phenomena. Episodes last between 20 minutes and several hours. Patients with a history of digital frostbite can subsequently experience Raynaud phenomenon in the affected digits. The diagnosis is based on the presence of two or more color changes with sharp demarcation on the digits. Color photographs can assist in making the diagnosis.[6]

On examination, the aforementioned classic tricolor changes may be observed with sharp demarcation where the spasm occurs.

Physical examination of the digits can reveal dilated capillary loops at the base of the nail beds as a sign of secondary Raynaud phenomena. Nail fold capillaroscopy is performed by observing the capillary loops in the cuticle adjacent to the nail. Immersion oil or K-Y Jelly is helpful in making the keratin more translucent and therefore accentuating the capillary loops.

Magnification can be achieved with an ophthalmoscope or with another magnifying instrument. A DermLite can be especially helpful. Microvascular abnormalities such as tortuous or dilated capillary loops and capillary dropout are observed in secondary Raynaud phenomena. Other stigmata of connective tissue disease may be observed on physical examination (e.g., the sclerotic hidebound skin of scleroderma, rash, mechanic's hands dermatitis or polymyositis, and arthritis). Tissue breakdown and ulcerations, or pitted scars of former attacks, can also be present.

DIAGNOSTICS

The diagnosis of Raynaud phenomenon is based on a clinical history of the classic tricolor changes. Capillaroscopy of the nail fold allows direct visualization of the capillaries, helping to distinguish primary from secondary Raynaud phenomenon.[7] Antinuclear antibody (ANA) positivity is a predictor of progression to or association with a connective tissue disease.[8] In particular, the presence of an anticentromere antibody is associated with the development of CREST (the subset of scleroderma described earlier), whereas the anti–Scl-70 antibody is more often seen in scleroderma.[9] Patients with positive ANA and capillary changes progress to systemic sclerosis frequently. Nearly 100% of patients with systemic sclerosis have Raynaud phenomenon.[10]

INITIAL DIAGNOSTICS
Raynaud Phenomenon
INITIAL
• Nail fold capillaroscopy
LABORATORY
• Antinuclear antibody
• Anti–Scl-70
• Anticentromere antibody

DIFFERENTIAL DIAGNOSIS

The differential diagnosis of secondary Raynaud phenomenon is extensive and can be divided into several categories (Box 196.1). These include occupational exposures (use of vibrating tools), drug exposures (amphetamines, β blockers, cocaine, clonidine, ergot, interferon alfa, methysergide, nicotine, vinyl chloride, vinblastine, bleomycin, cisplatin, and cyclosporine), occlusive vascular disease, connective tissue disease, hematologic disorders (antiphospholipid syndrome, cryoglobulinemia, cryofibrinogenemia), cold agglutinins, and others.[1]

The presence of abnormal capillaroscopy findings and/or positive ANA increases the likelihood of Raynaud phenomenon associated with a connective tissue disease. Patients with primary Raynaud phenomenon tend to do well without medical intervention.

INTERPROFESSIONAL COLLABORATIVE MANAGEMENT

Non-Pharmacologic Management

In its most benign form, Raynaud phenomenon can be a mild inconvenience. Most patients have discomfort when Raynaud phenomenon is triggered but have no permanent damage. Environmental measures are the first line of management, including keeping the body core warm with vests, scarves, and hats; avoiding cold environments; using stress management; and strictly avoiding smoking.

Complementary and alternative medicine (CAM), commonly used by patients with Raynaud phenomenon as standard treatment, can be associated with adverse effects. The herbal *Ginkgo biloba* was studied in a double-blind placebo-controlled

BOX **196.1**

Differential Diagnosis: Raynaud Phenomenon

PRIMARY DISORDER
- Raynaud phenomenon

SECONDARY DISORDER
- Drug-induced condition
- Trauma (electric shock, frostbite, repetitive injury)
- Occupational injury or exposure (vibrating tool use)
- Connective tissue disease: scleroderma, systemic lupus erythematosus, polymyositis, dermatomyositis, and rheumatoid arthritis
- Hematologic disorders: polycythemia, cryoglobulinemia, Waldenström macroglobulinemia,
- Cold agglutinins, cryofibrinogenemia, and myeloproliferative disorder
- Occlusive disease or disorder: atherosclerosis, thromboembolism, thoracic outlet syndrome, Buerger disease (thromboangiitis obliterans), and Takayasu arteritis
- Neurologic disorder: cervical disk disease, tumor, cerebrovascular accident, poliomyelitis
- Pulmonary hypertension
- Reflex sympathetic dystrophy
- Chilblain

trial and was found to reduce the number of attacks by 56% compared with placebo, although the difference was not statistically significant.[11] However, a more recent randomized controlled trail found no significant effect from *G. biloba*.[12] To date, no other CAM treatment has been identified as effective, although there is some trend toward subjective improvement with fish oil, vitamin C, acupuncture, and laser treatment. More important, biofeedback, used for years as a treatment, was shown to be ineffective in a recent meta-analysis.[13]

Pharmacologic Management

Nifedipine, a calcium channel blocker, may help prevent vasospasm and the frequency of attacks.[14,15] If vasospasm is not controlled, vasodilators, such as hydralazine and prazosin, can be added, provided the blood pressure is not adversely affected. Losartan, pentoxifylline, selective serotonin reuptake inhibitors, and sildenafil can also be used. No one treatment seems preferable to another, and several trials may be needed to find the optimal agent for each patient. Antiplatelet therapy with aspirin should be considered for all patients with secondary Raynaud phenomenon with a history of ischemic ulcers.[1]

Prostanoids and endothelin-blocking agents can be tried in severe digit-threatening disease. In severe Raynaud phenomenon, patients are hospitalized for intravenous administration of prostaglandin, such as prostaglandin E_1.[16] This therapy is reserved for those with secondary Raynaud phenomenon and severe digital ischemia. Oral and inhaled prostaglandin preparations are being studied in Japan, Europe, and the United States. So far, their usefulness is limited to patients with pulmonary hypertension.[16] Other novel therapies being investigated include injections of Botox (onabotulinumtoxinA),[17] topical glyceryl trinitrate (applied locally to the digits), and several other drugs including oral prostanoids.

Patients should avoid estrogen, nicotine, β blockers, and pseudoephedrine; these agents can exacerbate Raynaud phenomena.

Referral to a rheumatologist is necessary to exclude the presence of associated autoimmune disease. Patients who are in intractable pain or at risk for autoamputation of a digit or severe infection should be hospitalized under the care of a rheumatologist. A vascular surgeon should be consulted early if possible digit loss is suspected. Anesthesia can also be helpful in providing chemical ganglion sympathectomy for the relief of pain. Referral to an occupational therapist for evaluation and education can be helpful. Some patients have found biofeedback useful for management and reduction of Raynaud attacks, although recently studies have failed to demonstrate effectiveness.

In patients for whom standard medical therapy has failed and who are at risk for permanent ischemic damage, chemical ganglion sympathectomy can be considered. This can be achieved chemically with lidocaine blocks delivered locally or cervically. A vascular or hand surgeon can perform permanent digital sympathectomy if medical therapies fail. It is unclear whether the benefits of this procedure persist over time, and newer medical strategies may be more appropriate.[18]

COMPLICATIONS

In some patients, the protracted ischemia results in ulcerations that can become superinfected. Treatment of the infection can be challenging because local delivery of antibiotics is difficult, given the impaired blood flow. Rarely, ischemia can be so profound that loss of tissue and bone stock can occur, resulting in autoamputation of digits.

PATIENT EDUCATION

Patient education is crucial, and the potentially serious nature of this disorder should be emphasized. Patients should avoid exposing their hands to the cold if at all possible. Mittens, which are preferable to gloves, should be worn as soon as the weather begins to get cool. For some patients, mittens need to be worn when grocery shopping because reaching for food items in refrigerator or freezer sections can often trigger attacks. Keeping core temperature higher by wearing hats and layering clothing may also be of benefit. Sudden temperature changes should be avoided. For many patients, emotional stress can trigger episodes; relaxation techniques, behavioral modification, and biofeedback may play a role in limiting attacks. Most critically, patients should discontinue cigarette smoking if they are smokers. Medications to be avoided include decongestants, amphetamines, estrogen, and β blockers.

If Raynaud phenomenon occurs with the use of vibrating machinery, such as jackhammers and chain saws, patients may need vocational counseling.

REFERENCES

1. Goundry, B., Bell, L., Langtree, M., & Moorthy, A. (2012). Diagnosis and management of Raynaud's phenomenon. *British Medical Journal, 344*.
2. Prete, M., Fatone, M. C., Favoino, E., & Perosa, F. (2014). Raynaud's phenomenon: From molecular pathogenesis to therapy. *Autoimmunity Reviews, 13*(6), 655–667.
3. Garner, R., Kumari, R., Lanyon, P., et al. (2015). Prevalence, risk factors and associations of primary Raynaud's phenomenon: Systematic review and meta-analysis of observational studies. *BMJ Open, 5*, e006389. doi:10.1136/bmjopen-2014-006389.
4. Herrick, A. (2012). The pathogenesis, diagnosis and treatment of Raynaud's phenomenon. *Nature Reviews. Rheumatology, 8*, 469–479.

5. Wigley, F., & Flavahan, N. (2016). Raynaud's phenomenon. *The New England Journal of Medicine, 375*, 556–565.

6. Maricq, H. R., & Weinrich, M. C. (1988). Diagnosis of Raynaud's phenomenon assisted by color charts. *The Journal of Rheumatology, 15*, 454–459.

7. Sekiyama, J., Camargo, C., Andrade, L. E., & Kayser, C. (2013). Reliability of widefield nailfold capillaroscopy and video capillaroscopy in the assessment of patients with Raynaud's phenomenon. *Arthritis Care and Research (Hoboken), 65*(11), 1853–1861.

8. Falcini, F., Rigante, D., Candelli, M., et al. (2015). Anti-nuclear antibodies as predictor of outcome in a multi-center cohort of Italian children and adolescents with Raynaud's phenomenon. *Clinical Rheumatology, 34*(1), 167–169.

9. Mehras, S., Walker, J., Patterson, K., & Fritzler, M. (2013). Autoantibodies in systemic sclerosis. *Autoimmunity Reviews, 12*(3), 340–354.

10. Desbois, A. C., & Cacoub, P. (2016). Systemic sclerosis: An update in. *Autoimmunity Reviews, 15*(5), 417–426.

11. Muir, A. H., Robb, R., McLaren, M., et al. (2002). The use of ginkgo biloba in Raynaud's disease: A double-blind placebo-controlled trial. *Vascular Medicine (London, England), 7*(4), 265–267.

12. Bredie, S., & Jong, M. (2012). No significant effect of ginkgo Biloba Special Extract EGB 761 in the treatment of primary Raynaud's phenomenon: A randomized controlled trial. *Journal of Cardiovascular Pharmacology, 59*(3), 215–221.

13. Malenfant, D., Catton, M., & Pope, J. E. (2009). The efficacy of complementary and alternative medicine in the treatment of Raynaud's phenomenon: A literature review and meta-analysis. *Rheumatology (Oxford, England), 48*(7), 791–795.

14. Hughes, E., Anderson, M., Wilkinson, J., & Herrick, A. L. (2016). Calcium channel blockers for primary Raynaud's phenomenon. *The Cochrane Database of Systematic Reviews*, (2), Art. No. CD002069, doi:10.1002/14651858.CD002069.pub5-1.

15. Stewart, M., & Morling, J. R. (2012). Oral vasodilators for primary Raynaud's phenomenon. *The Cochrane Database of Systematic Reviews*, (7), CD006687.

16. Herrick, A. L. (2017). Evidence-based management of Raynaud's Phenomenon. *Therapeutic Advances in Musculoskeletal Disease, 9*(12), 317–329.

17. Neumeister, M. W. (2015). The role of Botulinum Toxin in vasospastic disorders of the hand. *Hand Clinics, 31*, 23.

18. Landry, G. J. (2013). Current medical and surgical management of Raynaud's syndrome. *Journal of Vascular Surgery, 57*, 1710–1716.

CHAPTER **197**

RHEUMATOID ARTHRITIS

Dorothy K. Johnson • Francisco P. Quismorio, Jr.

DEFINITION AND EPIDEMIOLOGY

Rheumatoid arthritis (RA) is an autoimmune disorder characterized by symmetric inflammatory polyarthritis and varying degrees of extra-articular involvement. Most patients experience a chronic fluctuating course of the disease that may result in joint destruction, deformity, disability, and premature death. Major economic and emotional disabilities can result from RA and can have a significant impact on patients' families and loved ones. RA is a chronic disease and accounts for many more physician visits than in age-matched controls, although fewer hospitalizations and less disability over the past decade are the results of better treatment options and early disease remission objective. RA affects 0.6% of the adult population in the United States and may be declining.[1] Women are affected two or three times more often than men. The prevalence increases with age. Despite extensive research, the cause of RA remains unknown; however, most investigators believe that a combination of genetic, environmental, hormonal, and reproductive factors is important. RA probably occurs in a genetically susceptible person with an abnormal immune response to an undetermined antigen. Genetic studies have shown that RA is strongly linked to human leukocyte antigen HLA-DRB1 alleles, which encode similar sequences (shared epitope).[2] Other susceptibility genes, including T-cell receptor signaling, have recently been identified. Smoking, an environmental factor, has also been shown to increase risk for the disease.[2]

PATHOPHYSIOLOGY

The main target of inflammation is the synovial lining of diarthrodial joints. The earliest changes in the synovial membrane are seen in the capillaries and small blood vessels. There is proliferation of the lining cells and early infiltration by T lymphocytes. Later, there is diffuse infiltration with B and T lymphocytes, macrophages, and plasma cells. The synovial membrane undergoes hyperplastic thickening with the proliferation of lining cells and fibroblasts and formation of new blood vessels. This granulation tissue, called pannus, invades the cartilage and subchondral bone and is primarily responsible for the destruction of joint structures in RA.[3]

Immune complexes in the synovial tissue activate the complement system, which then participates in the inflammatory process. Kinins, prostaglandins, cytokines, and other mediators increase the permeability of blood vessels and attract leukocytes and lymphocytes into the joint. Neutrophils and macrophages ingest immune complexes and release enzymes that degrade articular cartilage and joint structures. Rheumatoid factor (RF), antibodies to citrullinated proteins, and possibly other autoantibodies produced locally in the synovium participate in the formation of pathogenic immune complexes.[2]

Autoimmunity activity appears to involve both B cells and T cells. T cells are the major infiltrating lymphocytes in the rheumatoid synovium. Many autoantigens are targeted by the immune system in RA, and some autoantigens are T-cell targets. Activated T cells proliferate, expand, and stimulate monocytes, macrophages, and synovial fibroblasts to secrete cytokines, including interleukin-1 (IL-1) and tumor necrosis factor-α (TNF-α). Both cytokines stimulate mesenchymal cells to secrete matrix metalloproteinases that destroy cartilage and bone. Activated T cells stimulate B cells to produce immunoglobulins, including RF.[4]

CLINICAL PRESENTATION AND PHYSICAL EXAMINATION

The onset of RA is usually insidious, occurring during a period of several weeks or months, but in a small percentage of patients the onset is acute. The initial symptoms include general systemic manifestations of inflammation, weakness, weight loss, malaise, fatigue, anorexia, aching, and stiffness. Localized symptoms include painful, tender, swollen joints. Morning stiffness lasts for a minimum of 1 hour, sometimes all morning. The small joints of the hands (metacarpophalangeal and proximal interphalangeal joints), wrists, and small joints of the feet (metatarsophalangeal joints) are commonly affected initially. Joint involvement is bilateral and symmetric. The hips, knees, ankles, shoulders, and cervical spine may also be involved.

A complete medical history should be obtained in a comfortable setting. Particular attention should be paid to the location, quality, quantity, course, and alleviating factors of the patient's pain. Functional activities, activities of daily living, instrumental activities of daily living, and social support should be assessed.

Physical examination of the peripheral joints and the axial skeleton is central to the evaluation of a patient with RA. The joints should be examined in an organized manner, and report of joint pain, tenderness, degree of swelling, range of motion, and deformity should be recorded. On palpation, the inflamed joint feels warm and tender and the synovial membrane feels thickened and boggy. The skin over the affected joint may look thin and shiny and have a ruddy color. During the joint examination, the examiner should support painful or weak joints.

The physical examination should include evaluation for the presence of extra-articular manifestations. Subcutaneous nodules, which are present in 20% of patients with RA, are found over pressure areas, such as the extensor surface of the elbow and other areas of trauma. Rheumatoid nodules may occasionally be found on the cardiac valves, pericardium, pleura, lung parenchyma, and spleen. Other extra-articular manifestations of RA can include signs of vasculitis (mononeuritis multiplex, skin infarcts, and ulceration), ocular signs (Sjögren syndrome, episcleritis, and scleritis), respiratory symptoms (interstitial lung disease or pleurisy), cardiac involvement (pericarditis or valvular heart disease), and peripheral nerve entrapments.[5]

Sjögren syndrome, seen commonly in RA patients, is characterized by dry eyes (keratoconjunctivitis sicca) and dry mouth (xerostomia) and is caused by immune-mediated destruction of the salivary and lacrimal glands. Felty syndrome, an uncommon feature seen in long-standing RA, is characterized by skin ulcers, leukopenia, splenomegaly, and increased risk for bacterial infections.[6]

DIAGNOSTICS

The diagnosis of RA is primarily based on the clinical history and physical findings. Laboratory tests, including radiographs, are used to confirm the diagnosis, to exclude other conditions, and, more importantly, to prognosticate and develop a treatment plan for the individual patient.

Because RA can affect many organs, it is important to obtain laboratory tests as a baseline evaluation and periodically during the course of treatment. Baseline evaluation should include a complete blood count (CBC); acute-phase reactants, including erythrocyte sedimentation rate (ESR) and C-reactive protein (CRP); serum creatinine; hepatic panel; urinalysis; RF; and anti–cyclic citrullinated peptide (anti-CCP) antibodies. Normocytic, normochromic anemia is common in RA. Evaluation of renal and hepatic functions is necessary because many antirheumatic agents have renal and hepatic toxicity and may be contraindicated if these organs are severely impaired.

RF in RA is an immunoglobulin M autoantibody that is directed against antigenic determinants in the immunoglobulin G molecule. Not all RA patients have a positive test result for RF at the time of diagnosis, but the result will become positive for 70% to 80% of patients during the course of disease.[7] RA patients with a high titer of RF tend to have more severe joint and extra-articular disease and a worse prognosis than RF-negative patients do. The titer of RF does not change rapidly with treatment; therefore, frequent monitoring is not recommended. Compared with anti-CCP, RF has the same sensitivity for the diagnosis as RA (67% vs. 69%); however, anti-CCP has significantly higher specificity for the disease (95% vs. 85%).[8] RF can be seen in other rheumatic diseases as well as other non-rheumatic conditions such as chronic infections.[9]

American College of Rheumatology/ European League Against Rheumatism 2010 Classification Criteria for Rheumatoid Arthritis

JOINT INVOLVEMENT (0–5)

1 medium/large joint	0
2–10 medium/large joints	1
1–3 small joints	2
4–10 small joints	3
>10 joints (at least 1 small)	5

SEROLOGY (0–3)

Neither RF nor ACPA positive	0
At least one test low positive	2
At least one test high positive	3

DURATION OF SYMPTOMS (0–1)

<6 weeks	0
>6 weeks	1

ACUTE PHASE REACTANTS (0–1)

Neither CRP nor ESR abnormal	0
Abnormal CRP or abnormal ESR	1

Score ≥6 = RA.
Subjects with bony erosions regardless of score = RA.
ACPA, Anti–cyclic citrullinated peptide antibody.
Adapted from Aletaha, D., Neogi, T., Silman, A. J., Funovits J., Felson D. T., Bingham C. O. 3rd, et al. (2010). 2010 Rheumatoid arthritis classification criteria. *Arthritis & Rheumatism, 62*(9), 2569–2581.

Acute-phase reactants are proteins that are synthesized rapidly by the liver in the presence of inflammation or tissue necrosis and include CRP, fibrinogen, complement proteins, and several other proteins. Measurement of serum concentration of CRP and ESR is widely used to assess the activity of the inflammatory process and to aid in monitoring of the response to therapy.[7]

Other biologic markers are now being identified and may be useful for diagnosis and monitoring therapy.[10,11]

Because the hands and feet are often involved in RA, x-ray studies of these and other affected joints help with the diagnosis and establish a baseline for future evaluation of the effectiveness of treatment. The radiographs of the joints and bones are often normal at the onset of the disease, but bone erosions can develop within the first years. Ultrasound and magnetic resonance imaging (MRI) are increasingly used to confirm the diagnosis of RA; bone marrow edema is a hallmark finding in early RA.[12-14] The American College of Rheumatology has established criteria for the classification of RA that can be used as guidelines for patient diagnosis and for research classification (Box 197.1).[12]

Synovial Fluid Analysis

Aspiration of an inflamed joint and examination of the synovial fluid are important to the diagnosis of RA. Normal synovial fluid is clear, viscous, and low in volume with a white blood cell count of 2000 cells/mm³. In RA, the joint fluid is inflammatory with poor viscosity and a high white blood cell count of more than 10,000 cells/mm³ with a predominance of neutrophils.[9]

DIFFERENTIAL DIAGNOSIS

 Priority differentials include other rheumatic diseases, infection, and malignancy.

The differential diagnosis must include other causes of inflammatory arthritis. Initially, systemic lupus erythematosus (see Chapter 199), psoriatic arthritis, and seronegative spondyloarthropathies (see Chapter 198) may be indistinguishable from RA. Extra-articular manifestations of these disorders usually help establish the correct diagnosis. Although antinuclear antibodies may be present in RA patients' anti–double-stranded DNA (anti-dsDNA) and anti-Smith (anti-Sm) antibodies, the specific types of antinuclear antibody associated with systemic lupus erythematosus (see Chapter 199) are negative.

Soft tissue disorders such as fibromyalgia (see Chapter 157), tendinitis, bursitis, and, in older adults, polymyalgia rheumatica (see Chapter 195) may confound the diagnosis of RA early in the course of the disease. Viral infections, such as with human parvovirus, hepatitis viruses B and C, and human immunodeficiency virus (HIV), can cause symmetric polyarthritis and chronic arthralgia and should be considered in the differential diagnosis.

INTERPROFESSIONAL COLLABORATIVE MANAGEMENT

The standard goal of RA management is remission or low disease activity. This goal should be achieved as rapidly as possible to maximize long-term health-related quality of life through control of symptoms, prevention of structural damage, normalization of function, and participation in social work-related activities. This can be achieved by treating to target by measuring disease activity and adjusting therapy accordingly.[15]

Management of RA is multifaceted. Nonpharmacologic measures, such as physical therapy, occupational therapy, and psychological interventions aid in achieving the goal. Regular participation in dynamic and aerobic conditioning exercises improves joint symptoms, muscle strength, functional abilities, and psychological well-being.[16]

Assessing Cardiovascular Risk

There is an increased risk of cardiovascular (CV) disease in individuals with RA that appears to result from an accentuation of traditional risk factors and the inflammatory burden.[17,18] Traditional risk factors include hypertension, dyslipidemia, smoking, older age, and female gender. In RA, it is recommended that the CV risk estimate be multiplied by 1.5 if at least two of the following three criteria are present: (1) disease duration of more than 10 years; (2) RF or anti-CCP positivity; or (3) presence of certain extra-articular manifestations.[18] CV risk should be assessed yearly by use of national guidelines, and risk assessment should be repeated when antirheumatic treatment has changed. There are several CV risk score calculators, such as the Framingham Score and the Systematic Coronary Risk Evaluation (SCORE) model that the provider may find helpful (see Chapter 98).

Pharmacologic Agents

Choosing a pharmacologic agent for an individual patient is based on consideration of cost, efficacy, safety, and convenience. Pharmacologic therapy most often consists of combination therapy, synthetic and biologic disease-modifying antirheumatic drugs (DMARDs), biosimilar medications, nonsteroidal anti-inflammatory drugs (NSAIDs), and glucocorticoids (GCs).[19] An assessment of the patient's prognosis should be made before the treat to target regimen is selected (Box 197.2). Systematic monitoring of disease activity by composite measures should guide treatment decisions (Box 197.3).

Disease-Modifying Antirheumatic Drugs. The mainstay of treatment is synthetic or biologic DMARDs. New and highly effective DMARDs have continued to come to market, such as agents that target TNF, IL-1 receptor, IL-6 receptor, B lymphocytes, Janus Kinase Inhibitors (JAK-1), and T-cell costimulation.[20] Remission or low disease activity is the treatment goal that should be achieved as quickly as possible. Intensive medication strategies should be considered in every patient. Remission or low disease activity should be achieved preferably within 3 months and definitely by a maximum of 6 months. Treatment adjustment guided by careful monitoring should occur every 1 to 3 months to achieve low disease activity or remission.[15,21]

In general, treatment with DMARDs should be started as soon as the diagnosis of RA is established. Methotrexate (MTX) is a highly effective drug for disease modification. It is more effective at higher weekly doses (20 to 30 mg) than at lower doses and should be part of the first treatment strategy because it can be used as monotherapy, it increases the efficacy of biologic DMARDs when used in combination, and it has a long-term safety profile.[22] MTX may induce hyperhomocysteinemia through depletion of folic acid levels. Therefore folic acid supplements should be used in combination with MTX. If there are any contraindications to MTX, leflunomide, sulfasalazine, or parenteral gold salts could be prescribed. Added efficacy of antimalarial agents used in combination therapy continues to be evaluated.[23,24]

If treatment goals are not met with MTX or other synthetic DMARD monotherapy or in combination therapy and if poor prognostic markers are present, a biologic DMARD, preferably a TNF inhibitor, should be used in combination with MTX.[23,24] In the absence of poor prognostic markers, DMARD combination therapy or switching to another DMARD should be instituted, or, in consultation with the patient, a biologic DMARD can be added. If the first TNF inhibitor in combination with MTX fails, the patient should be switched to a second TNF inhibitor.[15,23,24] If both TNF inhibitors fail, a switch to another DMARD, such as a B cell–targeted agent, or an IL-6 medication could be tried.[21] DMARD-naive patients with poor prognostic markers should be considered for combination therapy with MTX plus a biologic agent as initial therapy.[24]

In patients with long-standing persistent remission, it is currently unclear how to continue or discontinue DMARD. GCs should be tapered and discontinued first. In consultation with the patient, cautious titration of the synthetic DMARD dose could be considered. Assessment of the tapering process should be guided by rigorous monitoring.[15,25]

Glucocorticoids. GCs have been shown to have anti-inflammatory and disease-modifying properties. GCs at low doses have been used successfully, but more rapid improvement may be achieved with the addition of GCs at higher doses for the short term.[26,27] Long-term or intermediate use of GCs can lead to adverse events.[28] Therefore GCs should be used with caution for short periods.

Nonsteroidal Anti-Inflammatory Drugs. NSAIDs and cyclooxygenase 2 (COX-2) inhibitors are associated with an increased CV risk. Because of COX-2 inhibition, most but not all NSAIDs have prothrombotic effects. However, these medications improve pain and mobility in patients, which might counterbalance the prothrombotic effects as well as improve quality of life. There is also a possible interaction between some NSAIDs and aspirin. Some NSAIDs may impair aspirin's antiplatelet function, so patients using low-dose aspirin for CV disease should be counseled. Potential antithrombotic risk must be considered in prescribing these drugs with aspirin.

NSAIDs should be used cautiously in older patients and those with CV disease or renal disease and those with a history of gastrointestinal bleeding. Acetaminophen is used preferentially in those cases.[27]

Topical NSAIDs are very helpful for some patients and can be used with a lower of risk of adverse effects.

Nonpharmacologic Treatment

Instruction in joint protection, conservation of energy, strengthening exercises, and a range-of-motion program is beneficial for all RA patients. Regular participation in dynamic and aerobic conditioning exercise programs improves joint symptoms, muscle strength, functional abilities, and psychological well-being. Consultation with occupational and physical therapists for assistive and adaptive devices and education about care of joints are recommended.[29]

Complementary and alternative therapy is of growing interest and use to RA patients. Many patients receiving conventional medical therapy are also using acupuncture, acupressure, herbs, and other complementary modalities although evidence of efficacy is lacking. Providers should always ask about the use of complementary and alternative therapies.[30]

The rheumatologist can provide support and consultation to the patient and his or her health care provider. Because the level, training, and experience in the diagnosis and treatment of RA vary among health care providers, the responsibility for diagnosis, development of a treatment plan, and monitoring of therapy should be assigned to the rheumatologist. A general maintenance plan should be developed for the patient, with all health care providers participating. Physical and occupational therapists should be consulted for exercise programs and adaptive devices. A rheumatology nurse specialist can provide information about lifestyle changes, self-help programs, and community educational programs, such as those sponsored by the Arthritis Foundation. Because most patients experience a period of grief after diagnosis, referral to a clinical psychologist or social worker should be considered. Life role adjustments will frequently need to be made because of the disease, and many patients will benefit from psychological counseling through this transition.

Referral to an orthopedic surgeon specializing in joint replacement should be considered for end-stage joint disease. Quality of life is improved and pain relieved in most patients after joint replacement surgery.

LIFE SPAN CONSIDERATIONS

RA has a considerable impact on quality of life. Significant work disability has been identified in patients with RA; about half of patients who are working at the onset of disease become work disabled within 10 years.[31] Direct and indirect monetary costs of RA are enormous. Pregnancy should be avoided in RA patients taking immune-modulating medications. Women with RA are slower to conceive and have fewer children than age-matched controls.[32] Approximately half of the RA patients who choose to become pregnant will experience a temporary remission in disease activity for the duration of the pregnancy and a predictable flare of disease activity in the postpartum period. Early death has been identified in RA patients, with the life span decreased by about 10 years primarily on the basis of CV disease.

COMPLICATIONS

Joint deformity, with the resulting sequelae of muscle, tendon, and ligament weakening or deconditioning and joint immobilization, is the most important complication. Small vessel vasculitis can cause neuropathy and skin ulcers. Cervical spine involvement can cause neck pain or abnormal neurologic findings because of myelopathy.

Complications related to adverse reactions to medications include osteoporosis, osteonecrosis (avascular necrosis), retinal toxicity, gastrointestinal irritation and bleeding, and hepatic toxicity. Opportunistic infections, including the reactivation of tuberculosis, may develop with the anti–TNF-α agents, systemic corticosteroids, and other immunosuppressive agents.[33] It is well established that RA is associated with an increased risk of lymphoproliferative disorders. With the use of targeted biologic therapies including those that may interfere with innate tumor surveillance, there is concern for the development of other malignant neoplasms.[34]

PATIENT AND FAMILY EDUCATION

Patients should be educated about lifestyle modifications, such as increased rest for disease flare-ups, use of adaptive aids to facilitate function, prioritizing and planning of activities to accommodate fatigue, and use of splints for painful and swollen wrists and hands. Podiatric care for foot pain should be provided, along with special footwear and flexible orthotic devices. Education about the need for a regular aerobic and muscle-strengthening exercise program is essential to help reduce stiffness, to avoid joint contractures, and to prevent osteoporosis.

The health care provider should advise the patient about the benefit of warm showers in the morning and frequent position changes to alleviate stiffness. The use of pillows to position joints at night is contraindicated because this may predispose the patient to flexion deformities.

The health care provider should also educate the patient and family about medication use, restrictions, and side effects or adverse effects, including pregnancy and fetal effects. Warnings against stopping of certain medications without notifying the health care provider should be stressed. Instructions should be given about dietary restrictions or recommendations as they relate to medications.

Self-management programs, educational information, and exercise programs from the Arthritis Foundation are available to patients in print form and online at www.arthritis.org. Most materials are available in Spanish and English.

REFERENCES

1. Gibofsky, A. (2012). Overview of epidemiology, pathophysiology, and diagnosis of rheumatoid arthritis. *The American Journal of Managed Care, 18,* s295–s302.
2. Kochi, U., Suzuki, A., & Tamamoto, K. (2014). Genetic basis of rheumatoid arthritis: A current review. *Biochemical and Biophysical Research Communications, 452*(2), 254–262.
3. Ruderman, E., & Tambar, S. Rheumatoid arthritis. www.rheumatology.org/uploadedFiles/Rheumatoid%20Arthritis.pdf. updated Aug, 2013. (Accessed 2 February 2015).
4. McInnis, I., & Schett, G. (2011). The pathogenesis of rheumatoid arthritis. *The New England Journal of Medicine, 365,* 2205–2219.
5. Inbanathan, J., Suneetha, D. K., Harsha, G., et al. (2016). Extra-articular manifestations of rheumatoid arthritis. *International Journal of Scientific Study, 4*(1), 81–84.
6. Shaw, A., & St Clare, W. (2017). Rheumatoid arthritis. In A. Fauci & C. Langford (Eds.), *Harrisons Rheumatology* (4th ed.). McGraw Hill.
7. Rheumatoid factor. Lab Tests Online. Retrieved from https://labtestsonline.org/understanding/analytes/rheumatoid/tab/test/. (Accessed 26 January 2016).
8. Farid, S., Azizi, G., & Mirshafie, A. (2013). Anti-citrullinated protein antibodies and their clinical utility in rheumatoid arthritis. *International Journal of Rheumatic Diseases, 16*(4), 379–386.
9. Tehlrian, C., & Bathon, J. (2008). Rheumatoid arthritis: Clinical and laboratory manifestations. In J. H. Klippel (Ed.), *Primer on the rheumatic diseases* (13th ed.). New York: Springer.
10. Schultz-Knappe, P., Budde, P., Goehler, H., et al. (2016). THU0242 High-throughput screening discovers novel autoantibodies in autoimmune diseases: The serotag approach to systemic lupus, systemic sclerosis, and rheumatoid arthritis. *Annals of the Rheumatic Diseases, 75,* 275–276.
11. Gerlag, D. M., Safy, M., Maijer, K. I., et al. (2017). SAT 0037 The effects of b cell directed therapy on disease relevant biomarkers in subjects at risk of rheumatoid arthritis. *Annals of the Rheumatic Diseases, 76,* 781.
12. Aletaha, D., Neogi, T., Silman, A., et al. (2010). 2010 Rheumatoid arthritis classification criteria. *Arthritis and Rheumatism, 62*(9), 2569–2581.
13. Colebatch, A., Edwards, C., Ostergaard, M., et al. (2013). EULAR Recommendations for the use of imaging of the joints in the clinical management of rheumatoid arthritis. *Annals of the Rheumatic Diseases, 72,* 804–814.
14. Simpson, E. L., Hock, E. S., Stevenenson, M. D., et al. (2018). What is added value of ultrasound joint examination for monitoring synovitis in rheumatoid arthritis and can it be used to guide treatment decisions? A systemic review and cost effectiveness analysis. *Health Technology Assessment, 22*(20), 1–258. ISSN 1366-5278.
15. Smolen, J. S., Breedveld, F. C., Burmester, G. R., et al. (2016). Treating to target: 2014 update of the recommendations of the international task force. *Annals of the Rheumatic Diseases, 75*(1), 3–15. doi:10.1136/annrheumdis-2015-207524. Published online first 12 May 2015.
16. Baillet, A., Vaillant, M., Guinot, M, et al. (2011). Efficacy of resistance exercises in rheumatoid arthritis: Meta-analysis of randomized controlled trials. *Rheumatology, 51*(3), 519–527.
17. del Rincón, I., Polak, J. F., O'Leary, D. H., et al. (2015). Systemic Inflammation and cardiovascular risk factors predict rapid progression of atherosclerosis in rheumatoid arthritis. *Annals of the Rheumatic Diseases, 74*(6), 1118–1123.
18. Mellana, W. M., Aronow, W. S., Palaniswamy, C., & Khera, S. (2012). Rheumatoid arthritis: Cardiovascular manifestations, pathogenesis and therapy. *Current Pharmaceutical Design, 18*(11), 1450–1456.
19. Dorner, T., Strand, V., Cornes, P., et al. (2016). The changing landscape of biosimilars in rheumatology. *Annals of the Rheumatic Diseases, 75*(6), 974–982. doi:10.1136/annrheumdis-2016-209166. Published Online First 8 March 2016.
20. Fleischmann, R., Mysler, E., & Hall, S. (2017). Efficacy and safety of tofacitinib montherapy, tofacitinib with methotrexate and adalimumab with methotrexate in patients with rheumatoid arthritis (ORAL Strategy): A phase 3b/4, double-blind, head to head, randomized controlled trial. *Lancet (London, England), 100093*(390), 457–468.
21. Singh, J., Saag, K., Bridges, S. L., et al. (2016). 2015 American College of Rheumatology Guidelines for the treatment of rheumatoid arthtirit. *Arthritis Care and Research, 68*(1), 1–25. doi:10.1002/acr.22783.
22. Cipriani, P., Ruscitti, P., Liakouli, V., & Giacomelli, R. (2014). Methotrexate in rheumatoid arthritis: Optimizing therapy among different formulations, current and emerging paradigms. *Clinical Therapeutics, 36*(3), 427–435.
23. Smolen, J. S., Breedveld, F. C., Burmester, G. R., et al. (2016). Treating rheumatoid arthritis to target: 2014 update of the recommendations of an international task force. *Annals of the Rheumatic Diseases, 75,* 3–15.
24. Epstein, A. A., Kremer, J. M., & Siegel, E. (2014). Applying biologic therapies to the management of patients with rheumatoid arthritis. *Seminars in Arthritis and Rheumatism, 43*(4), 577.
25. Schett, G., Enery, P., Tanaka, Y., et al. (2016). Tapering biologic and conventional DMARD in rheumatoid arthritis: Current evidence and future directions. *Annals of the Rheumatic Diseases, 75*(8), 1428–1437.
26. Rau, R. (2014). Glucocorticoid treatment in rheumatoid arthritis. *Expert Opinion on Pharmacotherapy, 15*(11), 1575–1583.
27. Whittle, S., Colebatch, A., Buchbinder, R., et al. (2012). Multinational evidence-based recommendations for pain management by pharmacotherapy in inflammatory arthritis: Integrating systematic literature research and expert opinion of a broad panel of rheumatologists in the 3e initiative. *Rheumatology (Oxford, England), 51*(8), 1416–1425.
28. Buckley, I., Guyatt, G., Fink, H. A., et al. (2017). 2017 American College of Rheumatology guideline for the prevention and treatment of glucorticoid-induced osteoporosis. *Arthritis & Rheumatology (Hoboken, N.J.), 69*(8), 1521–1537.
29. Brosseau, L., Rahman, P., Poitras, S., et al. (2014). A systematic critical appraisal of non-pharmacological management of rheumatoid arthritis for research and evaluation II. *PLoS ONE.* Retrieved from https://doi.org/10.137/journal.pone.0095369. On Feb 28, 2018.
30. National Center for Complementary and Integrative Health (NCCIH). Rheumatoid arthritis and complementary health approaches. Retrieved from https://nccih.nih.gov/health/RA/getthefacts.htm. (Accessed 26 January 2016).
31. Houssien, A., Rutherford, A., Yates, M., & Galloway, J. (2017). Predictors of work disability in rheumatoid arthritis: A systematic review. *Rheumatology, 56*(suppl_2), Kex 062.170.
32. Provost, M., Eaton, J. L., & Clowse, M. E. (2014). Fertility and infertility in rheumatoid arthritis. *Current Opinion in Rheumatology, 26*(3), 308–314.
33. Cantini, F., Niccoli, L., & Goletti, D. (2014). Tuberculosis risk in patients treated with non-anti-tumor necrosis factor a (TNF-a) targeted biologics and recently licensed TNF-a inhibitors: Data from clinical trials and National Registries. *The Journal of Rheumatology. Supplement, 91,* 56–64.
34. Simon, T., Thompson, A., Gandhi, K., et al. (2015). Incidence of Malignancy in Adult patients with Rheumatoid Arthritis: A Meta –analysis. *Arthritis Research & Therapy, 17,* 212.

CHAPTER 198

SERONEGATIVE SPONDYLOARTHROPATHIES

Carey J. Field

ANKYLOSING SPONDYLITIS

 Rule out fracture, infection (osteomyelitis), infectious or septic arthritis, and avascular necrosis (especially with history of steroid use).

DEFINITION AND EPIDEMIOLOGY

The seronegative spondyloarthropathies are a group of inflammatory arthritides sharing many clinical, radiographic, and genetic features. They include ankylosing spondylitis (AS), reactive arthritis (ReA, formerly called Reiter syndrome), psoriatic arthritis (PsA), enteropathic arthritis associated with inflammatory bowel disease (IBD-SpA), and undifferentiated spondyloarthritis (uSpA). These illnesses are characterized by the presence of inflammatory back pain, sacroiliitis, inflammation of the bone insertions of ligaments and tendons (enthesitis), peripheral joint inflammation, and often eye inflammation and skin disease. AS is the prototype of the seronegative spondyloarthropathies.

AS has a worldwide prevalence which ranges from 0.20% (in South-East Asia) to 1.61% in Northern Arctic communities, and has a prevalence of 0.5% in populations of European descent.[1,2] It tends to be familial, and the incidence and prevalence of AS generally mirrors the frequency of human leukocyte antigen HLA-B27 within the population. AS occurs slightly more in men with a male-to-female ratio of 2 to 3 : 1,[2] and the disease may be more severe in men. The disease usually begins in the third decade of life, often occurring 5 years earlier in HLA B27+ disease, and rarely begins after the age of 45.[3]

PATHOPHYSIOLOGY

Multiple genetic susceptibility alleles have been identified in the pathogenesis of AS. A strong association exists in particular with the genetically determined histocompatibility antigen HLA-B27. Of note, however, HLA-B27 by itself is neither sufficient nor necessary for development of disease. The association with HLA-B27 is the highest for AS, in which it is present in more than 90%; but overall, only 5% to 6% of HLA-B27–positive individuals develop AS, and the overall contribution of HLA-B27 to AS inheritance is only 20%.[4] Two additional genetic loci are newly discovered to be associated with AS: endoplasmic reticulum aminopeptidase (ERAP) and the interleukin-23 receptor.[2]

The pathognomonic features of AS are inflammation of the bone insertions of ligaments and tendons (entheses), known as enthesitis or enthesopathy, bone destruction, and new bone formation. The pathophysiologic process of this disease begins with ligamentous inflammatory granulation tissue that is gradually replaced by fibrocartilage and then ossifies.

CLINICAL PRESENTATION AND PHYSICAL EXAMINATION

Chronic back pain and stiffness, typically of the pelvis and lower back, caused by involvement of the spine or sacroiliac (SI) joints (caused by spondylitis or sacroiliitis), is the most common initial complaint. Spondylitis typically begins in the lumbosacral spine, but as the disease progresses the upper portions of the spine become involved. AS patients may describe low back pain, buttock pain, or hip pain that may be suggestive of SI joint involvement. The back pain of AS is inflammatory and can be distinguished clinically from back pain of other causes. It is usually insidious in onset; it is chronic, lasting for more than 3 months, with periods of exacerbation and remission. It is diffuse, poorly localized, and described as a deep ache or nagging discomfort. As in other types of inflammatory joint pain, the inflammatory back pain of AS improves with exercise and worsens with inactivity or rest. Sleep disturbance is common, and patients may describe having to get up typically in the second half of the night to "walk the pain off." The back pain is worse in the early morning and is associated with morning stiffness that is inflammatory in nature (i.e., lasts longer than one hour.).

Thirty percent to 50% of patients may have significant peripheral joint involvement at some point during their disease, most commonly in the form of peripheral joint arthritis and enthesitis (inflammation at the insertion of tendons, ligaments, or capsule into bone). Peripheral joint involvement is usually asymmetric, often involving large joints (often shoulders, hips, and knees), and is most frequently found in the lower limbs.[2] Some patients develop chronic peripheral joint arthritis. Involvement of the hip joint can be an early manifestation in AS. Areas of inflammatory, enthesopathic involvement particular to AS are the sternoclavicular joint, the costochondral joint, the Achilles tendon, the plantar fascia, and along the superior iliac crest, however inflammation can occur at any site of enthesis. Dactylitis (diffuse swelling of toes or fingers) is less common in AS and is more commonly seen in the other seronegative spondyloarthropathies such as PsA. Small joints of the hands and feet are infrequently involved, unlike in rheumatoid arthritis.

Extra-articular manifestations of the disease include low-grade fever, fatigue, and weight loss. In addition, patients may develop eye, bowel, skin, cardiac, and pulmonary disease. Inflammatory eye disease, usually acute anterior uveitis, is the most common extra-articular manifestation and typically presents as a painful, and often red eye, with blurry vision. It often recurs, alternating from one eye to the other, but seldom leads to permanent impairment of vision. Acute anterior uveitis occurs in up to 30% of patients during the course of their disease.[5] The inflammation is acute in onset 90% of the time, and in approximately 95% of patients, the uveitis is unilateral or unilateral-alternating.[3] The activity and severity of the eye disease does not correlate with the activity and severity of the articular disease of AS. It is more likely to occur later in the course of disease and is more common in HLA-B27–positive patients. Whereas ileal or colonic mucosal inflammation is detected histologically in up to 60% of patients with AS, clinically symptomatic inflammatory bowel disease (IBD) develops in only 5% to 10% of patients.[5] AS patients are also at increased risk to develop psoriasis, which occurs in about 10% of AS patients.[5] Cardiovascular clinical manifestations may also occur in 2% to 10% of AS patients; cardiac manifestations may include conduction abnormalities (the most common), aortic root dilation, aortic valve insufficiency, aortitis, pericarditis, left ventricular dysfunction, and accelerated atherosclerosis.[6,7] As in other inflammatory arthritides, AS patients are at increased risk for developing atherosclerosis leading to increased morbidity in the form of myocardial infarction and stroke. Pulmonary manifestations may include restrictive lung disease caused by the musculoskeletal disease's impact on the chest wall, or parenchymal disease (as detected by high-resolution computed tomography [CT] scan) in the form of apical pulmonary fibrosis and interstitial lung disease.

Examination of the spine will show loss of the normal lumbar lordosis. Palpable muscle spasm of the paraspinal muscles is frequently present. Spine mobility is decreased in most patients and can be documented by the modified Schober flexion test of the lumbosacral spine, the Moll lateral flexion test of the thoracic spine, or measurement of chest expansion. The modified Schober flexion test measures lumbosacral flexion. The patient stands erect, and two points are marked in the midline of the spine—one at the level of the dimples of Venus, and one 10 cm above the level of the dimples of Venus; the patient is then asked to bend forward, reaching for the floor as far as possible. Normal flexion is defined as an increase in the distance between the two points of 5 cm or more in a patient younger than 50 years. The Moll lateral flexion test measures lateral thoracic spine flexion. The patient stands erect with the hands behind the head, and one mark is placed in the midaxillary line at the iliac crest, and another mark is placed 20 cm above the iliac crest; the patient is asked to tilt, bending the trunk to the opposite side as far as possible, and the distance between the two marks is measured. Normal thoracic spine tilt or lateral flexion is 3 cm. Chest expansion is measured with the patient standing erect with the hands on the head; with a centimeter tape wrapped around the chest at the nipple line, the patient is asked to first maximally expire and then maximally inspire. The chest circumference should be measured at both maximum expiration and maximum inspiration, and the measurement should normally increase by at least 5 cm with full inspiration.

Extra-articular manifestations can produce physical findings such as the heart murmur of aortic valve insufficiency or the red, inflamed eye associated with acute iritis.

DIAGNOSTICS

In 2009 and 2011 respectively the Assessment of Spondylo Arthritis International Society (ASAS) criteria for axial and peripheral spondyloarthritis were published as the previous classification criteria (1984 modified New York Criteria) were found to be ineffective in the diagnosis of early disease when characteristic radiographic signs are often not visible on plain radiographs but are often detectable by magnetic resonance imaging (MRI).[8]

According to the modified New York criteria, presence of sacroiliitis on radiographic examination associated with one clinical criterion is considered to be diagnostic of definite AS.[8] Many patients will have normal findings on plain radiography because their disease has not been severe enough or of long enough duration to produce radiographic changes. MRI can identify sacroiliitis earlier than standard plain radiographic studies. As visualized on MRI, early sacroiliitis may produce bone marrow edema or osteitis on short T1 inversion recovery

(STIR) and T1-weighted images. Sacroiliitis may also produce other inflammatory lesions identifiable on MRI, such as synovitis in the SI joints, capsulitis, and enthesitis, but the presence of concomitant SI bone marrow edema or osteitis is essential for defining active sacroiliitis by MRI. More advanced sacroiliitis produces sclerosis, with the SI joint becoming indistinct and narrow over time. Complete bone fusion is seen late in the disease. Characteristic spine radiographic findings in AS include syndesmophyte formation, which leads to bone bridging from one vertebral body to the next, producing a "bamboo" spine appearance. Inflammatory changes can often occur early in disease before significant radiographic changes. X-ray changes in the hip are common and are often bilateral and symmetric with uniform joint space narrowing in AS compared with the asymmetric joint space narrowing that is seen in osteoarthritis.

Laboratory findings are generally nonspecific but may include an elevated white blood cell count (WBC), or an elevation in inflammatory serum markers including the erythrocyte sedimentation rate (ESR) or C-reactive protein (CRP) level. Occasionally, a normochromic, normocytic anemia of chronic disease may occur; however, anemia and elevated inflammatory markers are not necessary for the diagnosis. Rheumatoid factor and antinuclear antibodies are typically negative. While up to 95% of patients with AS of European descent are HLA-B27 positive, HLA-B27 testing is inappropriate for screening of an asymptomatic population. The test result does not absolutely confirm or exclude AS, but it is important to note that in some cases it can be used in the ASAS criteria to assist the provider with making a diagnosis.

INITIAL DIAGNOSTICS

Ankylosing Spondylitis

LABORATORY
- Complete blood count (CBC) and differential
- Comprehensive metabolic panel
- ESR
- CRP
- Rheumatoid factor, cyclic citrullinated peptide
- Antinuclear antibody

ADDITIONAL LABORATORY
- Serum uric acid
- HLA-B27
- Enzyme-linked immunosorbent assay (ELISA) for *Borrelia burgdorferi* (Lyme Antibody), if indicated

IMAGING
- X-rays
  - of spine, including SI joints
  - of small joints of hands and feet if there is evidence of peripheral joint disease
- MRI
  - SI joints (to search for evidence of sacroiliitis)

DIFFERENTIAL DIAGNOSIS

- Other types of inflammatory arthritis (including PsA, reactive arthritis, spondylitis of IBD, and seronegative rheumatoid arthritis; see below).
- Acute and chronic mechanical back pain (see Chapter 160) including degenerative joint or disc disease, muscular strain, compression fractures, and disseminated idiopathic skeletal

hyperostosis (DISH). Also rule out chronic pain syndromes such as fibromyalgia (see Chapter 157).

- Infectious arthritis (see Chapter 159)
- Sacroiliitis observed on X-ray may also warrant consideration of reactive arthritis (ReA, formerly Reiter syndrome), psoriatic spondylitis, and spondylitis of IBD, all of which are discussed later in this chapter.
- In the absence of axial involvement, the most common chronic inflammatory arthritides that can be confused with AS in the 20- to 40-year age group are seronegative rheumatoid arthritis (see Chapter 197) and Lyme arthritis (see Chapter 213). Rheumatoid arthritis is more likely to involve the upper extremities (especially small) joints, characteristically has hand involvement, and is symmetric. The presence of anti–cyclic citrullinated peptide antibodies, which are much more specific for rheumatoid arthritis, may be helpful in differentiating RA from AS. Lyme arthritis, which most commonly involves the knee, is usually monoarticular or oligoarticular and is suggested by a history of tick exposure and of erythema migrans. The diagnosis of Lyme disease is established by enzyme-linked immunosorbent assay (ELISA) for *Borrelia burgdorferi* antibody confirmed by Western blot analysis.

INTERPROFESSIONAL COLLABORATIVE MANAGEMENT

The goals of treatment are to relieve symptoms, maintain the best possible functional capacity, prevent complications of the disease (e.g., flexion contractures), and minimize extra-articular manifestations (e.g., uveitis and aortic valve insufficiency). To achieve these goals, patient education, exercise, and medication management are all important.

Nonpharmacologic Management

All patients should be strongly encouraged to perform exercises tailored for AS (through either a formal physical therapy or exercise program or a home-based practice). Various guidebooks and audio and video aids are available by mail or online through the Spondylitis Association of America and the Spondylitis Society in the United Kingdom; these aids can be used to perform exercises unsupervised at home if formal physical therapy is not possible.

Pharmacologic Management

- Nonsteroidal anti-inflammatory drugs (NSAIDs), independent of their cyclooxygenase (COX) selectivity, are first-line therapy for all symptomatic patients with AS, unless contraindicated. Most patients with AS or other seronegative spondyloarthropathy typically respond symptomatically to NSAIDs; these medications help to reduce pain and stiffness and may be able to help reduce progression of structural damage to the spine. Sufficient data does not exist to suggest that continuous use of NSAIDs is more beneficial than on-demand dosing.[2]
- Immunomodulators such as disease modifying antirheumatic drugs (DMARDs, such as sulfasalazine, methotrexate), biologic anti–tumor necrosis factor (TNF) agents (etanercept, adalimumab, certolizumab, infliximab, golimumab), and IL-17 monoclonal antibodies (secukinumab) have been proven effective in the treatment of patients with AS. These medications may be considered for those patients who fulfill the diagnostic criteria for definite AS, as discussed

previously (via the ASAS axial spondyloarthritis [SpA] or modified New York criteria for AS). In AS these biologic DMARDs can be used as single agents without non-biologic DMARDs or other immunosuppressive medications.

- Systemic glucocorticoids are not recommended for long-term treatment of AS because there are limited data on their use in this setting, and their toxicities can be profound. However, systemic glucocorticoids used at relatively high doses in the short term may have some short-term benefit for pain control.
- Pain management is important to minimize spinal deformity and to allow patients to exercise. Patients stoop with pain, thereby increasing the likelihood of the spine's fusing in a kyphotic position. Analgesics such as acetaminophen and muscle relaxants can be beneficial adjunctive therapy. Patients often find the use of heat and massage helpful. Local injections of corticosteroids can treat pain from enthesopathy, sacroiliitis, and peripheral arthritis.
- Referral is indicated for patients with chronic back pain beginning prior to age 45 who also have any features which may suggest an axial spondyloarthritis such as inflammatory back pain symptoms, findings of sacroiliitis on imaging, and/or the presence of any other typical seronegative spondyloarthritis features. A rheumatology referral is recommended to confirm diagnosis and to recommend a treatment plan.
- Referral to a physical therapist is appropriate to promote pain relief, to minimize deformity, and to maintain independent function.
- Referral to an orthopedic surgeon is indicated in patients who develop hip arthritis that is severe enough to produce night pain, rest pain, and pain on weight bearing, impairing the ability to walk. Immediate referral to an ophthalmologist is warranted for acute eye pain.
- Periodic ophthalmic monitoring is recommended when iritis has been a manifestation.
- Evaluation by a cardiologist is indicated in the presence of an aortic valve murmur. Known cardiac risk factors, such as hypertension, hyperlipidemia, and diabetes, should be evaluated and treated.
- Hospitalization is rarely indicated in patients with AS. Acute cardiac complications, catastrophic neurologic complications, and gastrointestinal bleeding resulting from NSAIDs are the most likely reasons for hospitalization.

COMPLICATIONS

Osteopenia is prevalent in patients with longstanding disease, and thus the risk for vertebral fracture is increased. Visual loss secondary to inflammatory eye disease is a major cause of disability in this disease. A variety of neurologic complications of AS can be seen in long-standing disease. These include cord or spinal nerve compression secondary to spinal fracture of a fused spine or atlantoaxial subluxation. Amyloid deposition is a rare complication after years of inflammatory disease and can produce nephrotic syndrome or renal failure. Further possible complications, including cardiac and pulmonary complications, are discussed earlier in the extra-articular manifestations section of this chapter.

LIFE SPAN CONSIDERATIONS

The prognosis with AS is variable. Death as a result of the disease itself is very unusual, however life span may be reduced due to complications from the disease which may include cardiovascular conditions, spinal cord injury, or vertebral fractures. Some patients may have progressive widespread disease with skeletal deformity and functional loss, requiring chronic medication, physical therapy, and vocational adaptations. Chronic medical therapy can shorten the patient's life span as a result of medication side effects. Pregnancy in patients with AS does not improve symptoms, unlike what is observed in rheumatoid arthritis. The majority of women with AS have unchanged or temporarily aggravated disease activity during pregnancy. The disease has no known effect on fertility, course of pregnancy, or delivery. However, the offspring of patients with AS have an increased risk for development of AS themselves.

PATIENT AND FAMILY EDUCATION

Optimum management is enhanced when patients understand the chronic nature of the disease and their role in preventing disability and deformity.

- Exercise is an important component of management of AS. Regular physical activity and stretching, and practicing good posture are essential to maintaining flexibility and functionality and reducing pain and deformity from the disease.
- Contact sports should be avoided because patients are more prone to spinal fractures; however, other forms of physical activity should be encouraged, especially swimming. Swimming is nonimpact and can provide excellent exercises for increasing and maintaining trunk and neck muscle strength. Swimming is recommended because it avoids excessive stressful weight bearing. The backstroke is particularly good for stretching anterior chest muscles and strengthening posterior chest and neck extensor muscles, thereby decreasing the tendency toward kyphosis.
- First-degree relatives of patients with AS are at increased risk to develop AS themselves.

REACTIVE ARTHRITIS

 Rule out fracture, infection (osteomyelitis), infectious arthritis, Lyme arthritis, and avascular necrosis (especially with history of steroid use).

DEFINITION AND EPIDEMIOLOGY

ReA is an acute sterile inflammatory arthropathy that follows an infection in which there is no microbial invasion of the synovium or joint space and the prior infection is remote from the joint. Reactive arthritis (formerly known as Reiter syndrome), as first described in 1916, is a historic example of ReA defined by the classic triad of conjunctivitis, urethritis, and arthritis. Because as many as two-thirds of patients are initially seen with an incomplete syndrome and do not fulfill all three criteria, *reactive arthritis* is a preferred and more general term. ReA has been observed after both sexually transmitted and dysenteric infection and can be initiated by a number of infectious organisms. The most common infectious agents associated with ReA are urogenital and gastrointestinal pathogens such as *Chlamydia* organisms *(Chlamydia trachomatis* and *Chlamydia pneumoniae)*, *Salmonella, Shigella, Yersinia, Campylobacter, Escherichia coli,* and *Clostridium difficile.*[9]

ReA is a relatively rare disease that typically occurs sporadically in young adults, and may occur with outbreaks of infection. The exact prevalence of ReA in the general population is not entirely known due to paucity of data. A systematic review of incidence of ReA with enteric pathogens revealed 9 cases per 1000 Campylobacter infections, 12 cases per 1000 Salmonella infections, and 12 cases per 1000 Shigella infections. ReA occurs in 1.4% of cases of C difficile infection in children. The incidence of ReA after genital chlamydia infection is about 4% to 8%. Relative risk for development of ReA is higher among women (relative risk 1.5 vs. males) and adults (relative risk 2.5 vs. children) for the enteric form of the disease.[9]

PATHOPHYSIOLOGY

Like AS, ReA has a strong association with the histocompatibility antigen HLA-B27 in Caucasian patients but not in patients from sub-Saharan Africa, where the HLA-B27 prevalence is lower. HLA-B27 is observed in 50% to 80% of patients with ReA and appears to be associated with increased disease susceptibility and severity of disease expression.[9] As in rheumatoid arthritis, there is inflammatory synovitis with infiltration of polymorphonuclear leukocytes, lymphocytes, and plasma cells. However, unlike in rheumatoid arthritis, production of synovial pannus is rare. As in AS, there is inflammation at the insertions of ligaments and tendons (enthesopathy). Erosions, bone proliferation, and periosteal new bone formation may occur.

The relationship between the antecedent infection and the development of ReA is not completely understood. The HLA-B27 molecule participates in binding of antigenic peptides and presenting them to CD8 T cells.

CLINICAL PRESENTATION AND PHYSICAL EXAMINATION

ReA can occur without documented prior infection. When there has been a known antecedent urogenital or enteric infection, arthritic symptoms tend to occur 1 to 6 weeks later. The classic triad of symptoms includes urethritis, arthritis, and conjunctivitis, however less than half of patients with ReA develop all three components of the triad.

The arthropathy of ReA is typically a monoarticular arthritis or an asymmetric oligoarthritis, often in large joints of the lower extremities. However, 50% of patients have arthritis in the upper extremities including small joints of the hands. The axial spine and SI joints are less commonly involved.[9]

Enthesitis and dactylitis are common features as well. Patients may develop enthesitis of the Achilles or plantar fascia, anterolateral ribs, pubic symphysis, and iliac crest, which may manifest with pain and/or swelling.

Extra-Articular Manifestations

Patients may have constitutional symptoms such as malaise, fatigue, fever, headache, and weight loss. They may develop urethritis, cervicitis, prostatitis, cystitis, and salpingo-oophoritis. These symptoms may be due to underlying infection. Ophthalmologic symptoms may include conjunctivitis, keratitis, episcleritis, and anterior uveitis. Dermatologic manifestations include painless, shallow, lingual, or palatal ulcerations; keratoderma blennorrhagica; circinate balanitis; and erythema nodosum. These tend to correlate with severity of disease. Keratoderma blennorrhagica is the most common dermatologic manifestation of ReA, appearing as painless papulosquamous lesions on the palms or soles.[10] The histopathology of keratoderma blennorrhagica is indistinguishable from that of pustular psoriasis. Circinate balanitis occurs in males and is seen as painless, asymptomatic, shallow, ulcerative lesions on the glans of the penis.

Cardiac manifestations have been reported and may include aortic valvular insufficiency and conduction abnormalities such as heart block and pericarditis.[9]

The course of the disease is highly variable; typical disease duration is <6 months. Some patients have recurrent acute attacks, often with disease-free intervals. A minority of patients may develop sustained disease activity with a chronic course.

DIAGNOSTICS

INITIAL DIAGNOSTICS

Reactive Arthritis

LABORATORY
- Complete blood count (CBC) and differential
- Comprehensive metabolic panel
- ESR
- CRP
- Rheumatoid factor, cyclic citrullinated peptide

IMAGING
- X-rays of affected joints

JOINT ASPIRATION
- Synovial fluid analysis of affected joints—essential to determine if the joint fluid is non-inflammatory, inflammatory, or potentially septic. It is also essential in the diagnosis of crystal induced arthritis (gout and calcium pyrophosphate deposition disease)

ADDITIONAL DIAGNOSTICS
- Antinuclear antibody
- Serum uric acid level
- HLA-B27
- Enzyme-linked immunosorbent assay (ELISA) for *Borrelia burgdorferi* (Lyme Antibody), if indicated

For the most part, laboratory test results are nonspecific, consistent with an inflammatory process, and similar to those in AS. The ESR and CRP are often elevated. There is often peripheral leukocytosis with thrombocytosis and a mild anemia. There is usually a synovial fluid leukocytosis, often with a polymorphonuclear leukocyte predominance that is suggestive of a septic arthritis, but cultures are negative. The **x-ray studies** of hands and feet may reveal the fluffy periosteal reaction of new bone formation. Periarticular demineralization or osteopenia is notably absent in ReA compared with rheumatoid arthritis. The syndesmophytes in the vertebral spine are not as fine as in AS, are nonmarginal and denser, and may be asymmetric and skip portions of the spine.

DIFFERENTIAL DIAGNOSIS

 Priority differentials include psoriatic arthritis or seronegative rheumatoid arthritis, Lyme arthritis, and septic arthritis

It can be difficult to distinguish between PsA and ReA because the arthritis is similar and the skin histology is identical. Only the finding of nail pitting, characteristic of PsA, differentiates the two. More important, ReA may be misdiagnosed as seronegative rheumatoid arthritis. ReA can have symmetric peripheral joint involvement like rheumatoid arthritis, but sacroiliitis is uncommon in rheumatoid arthritis. In rheumatoid arthritis, hip disease is a late sequela, and sausage digits, Achilles tendinitis, plantar fasciitis, and other presentations of enthesopathy do not typically occur. Dactylitis is not a feature of rheumatoid arthritis. Lyme disease often manifests as a chronic monarticular or oligoarticular arthritis, often with chronic knee arthritis, and can be differentiated from ReA by a positive *B. burgdorferi* antibody assay (see Chapter 213).

INTERPROFESSIONAL COLLABORATIVE MANAGEMENT

Nonpharmacologic Management

Patients may benefit from physical or occupational therapy to maximize the use of their joints. Also, low-impact exercise is recommended, such as swimming and walking. If a patient's disease becomes well-controlled, many patients may successfully resume an active lifestyle.

Pharmacologic Management

In some patients, in particular those with genitourinary infection and some enteric infections, treatment of the infection that triggered the arthritis is indicated; however, the role of antibiotics in the treatment of the arthritis is under investigation, and they have not yet been proven to be of great benefit.[10] In treating the arthritis itself, treatment may differ based on the duration of symptoms. For symptoms that have been present for less than 6 months, NSAIDs are the recommended initial treatment. For patients who do not respond to NSAIDs or who have an allergy or intolerability, intra-articular steroid injections and systemic glucocorticoids may be used. For patients who have symptoms for longer than 6 months and are not responding to NSAID therapy, DMARDs, and potentially biologic DMARDs, may be used.

The course of ReA is highly variable. Most patients' symptoms resolve within 6 to 12 months. However, up to 20% of patients develop a chronic, disabling arthritis for which they receive long-term treatment.

Any cases of suspected ReA may benefit from referral to a rheumatologist to help develop a diagnosis and treatment plan. In cases in which the skin disease or eye disease is prominent, referral to a dermatologist and/or an ophthalmologist respectively may be helpful. A physical therapist or occupational therapist should be consulted for suggestions about exercise regimens or teaching on joint protection and energy conservation.

PATIENT AND FAMILY EDUCATION
- Patient education should be directed toward management of the disease, and patients should be counseled about the possible side effects of medications as they apply (including possible sterility, liver damage, risk for infection, and so on).
- In patients receiving NSAIDs, ulcer prevention with proton pump inhibitors or H_2 blockers may decrease the risk of gastrointestinal bleeding.
- Patients who receive DMARDs or biologic DMARD agents should be managed according to guidelines for patients with rheumatoid arthritis taking these medications, with regular laboratory screening to monitor for disease toxicities.

PSORIATIC ARTHRITIS

 Rule out fracture, infection (osteomyelitis), septic arthritis, Lyme arthritis, and avascular necrosis (especially with history of steroid use).

DEFINITION AND EPIDEMIOLOGY

PsA is an inflammatory arthritis associated with the dermatologic condition of psoriasis (see Chapter 49). Up to 48% of patients with psoriasis may develop inflammatory arthritis with a prevalence of 0.25% in the US.[11] The disease is classified into 5 different subgroups: asymmetrical oligoarthritis, predominant distal interphalangeal joint involvement, symmetrical polyarthritis, predominant axial involvement, and arthritis mutilans.

PATHOPHYSIOLOGY

Immune, genetic, and environmental factors influence disease expression. Genetically, as with the other types of seronegative spondylarthritis, PsA has been linked to HLA class 1 alleles, most notably the HLA-B27 allele. Patients have been known to have flares after trauma or after infections (bacterial or viral). There is a proposed immune mechanism which suggests a possible molecular similarity between streptococcal and epidermal components, which could allow T-cell clones directed against streptococci to initiate the skin disease.

CLINICAL PRESENTATION AND PHYSICAL EXAMINATION

PsA may occur before, concomitantly with, or after the onset of the skin disease. Arthritis precedes the rash in 15% to 20% of patients.[11] In these patients, nail pitting is often present before rash—an early clue to the diagnosis. The arthritis is heterogeneous, with five different clinical presentations being recognized, the most common of which is the oligoarticular asymmetric presentation.

Other common features of PsA include tenosynovitis, enthesitis, and dactylitis (enthesitis and dactylitis are hallmarks of the disease). Enthesitis occurs in 50% of patients and most commonly occurs in the Achilles tendon and the plantar fascia. Arthritis mutilans is a destructive form of arthritis in which there is significant bone erosion with decreased bone length, producing redundant skin and opera-glass deformity (Fig. 198.1). Axial disease can occur without sacroiliitis, be asymmetric, and skip portions of the spine. Sacroiliitis in PsA is often asymmetric, in contrast to AS in which bilateral SI involvement is more common. Nail involvement (nail pitting,

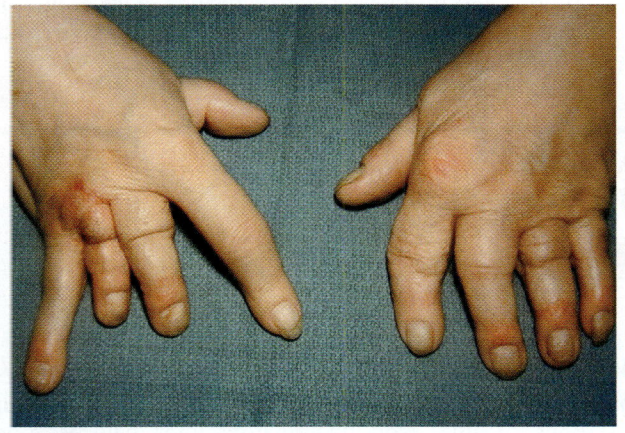

F I G . 198.1 Arthritis mutilans (destructive arthritis) involving all digits. (From Harris, E., Budd, R., & Firestein, G. [2005]. *Kelley's textbook of rheumatology* [7th ed.]. Philadelphia: Saunders.)

transverse ridging, onycholysis, etc.) is much more common in patients with PsA than in patients who have the skin condition alone. Extra-articular manifestations are seen in up to 50% of patients.[12] Most commonly occur in men with axial disease with a longer disease duration. The most common extra-articular manifestations affect the eyes (uveitis or conjunctivitis), gastrointestinal tract, urogenital tract, heart, and arteries.

DIAGNOSTICS

INITIAL DIAGNOSTICS

Psoriatic Arthritis

LABORATORY
- Complete blood count (CBC) and differential
- Comprehensive metabolic panel
- ESR
- CRP
- Rheumatoid factor, cyclic citrullinated peptide

IMAGING
- X-rays of affected joints—to assess soft tissue swelling, erosive changes, and any other characteristic changes which may assist with diagnosis

JOINT ASPIRATION
- Synovial fluid analysis of affected joints—essential to determine if the joint fluid is non-inflammatory, inflammatory, or septic. It is also essential in the diagnosis of crystal induced arthritis (gout and pseudogout)

ADDITIONAL DIAGNOSTICS
- Antinuclear antibody
- Serum uric acid level
- HLA-B27
- Enzyme-linked immunosorbent assay (ELISA) for *Borrelia burgdorferi* (Lyme Antibody), if indicated

Laboratory test results are mostly nonspecific, as they are in the other seronegative spondyloarthropathies. The ESR and CRP level may be elevated in up to 40% of patients. Patients may have a normocytic anemia and/or leukocytosis. Test results for rheumatoid factor and antinuclear antibodies are typically negative but may be positive in a small percentage of patients. Hyperuricemia may result from the high purine turnover in psoriatic skin lesions.

The radiographic changes in hands and feet are distinctive. Subchondral erosions and erosions with new bone formation, periostitis, and ankylosis of joints may be seen. In late disease, radiographs of the DIP joints may show whittling and a "pencil in cup" appearance, which is believed to be pathognomonic of PsA (Fig. 198.2).

DIFFERENTIAL DIAGNOSIS

 Priority differentials include another seronegative inflammatory arthritis (e.g., seronegative rheumatoid arthritis, ReA, arthritis of inflammatory bowel disease, and AS), osteoarthritis, and Lyme arthritis.

The differential diagnosis is broad, and PsA is often a challenge to diagnose when the arthritis precedes the skin disease. One may use the Classification criteria for PsA (the CASPAR criteria)[12,13] to help formulate a diagnosis. It may be difficult to distinguish between ReA and PsA. The skin lesions of both

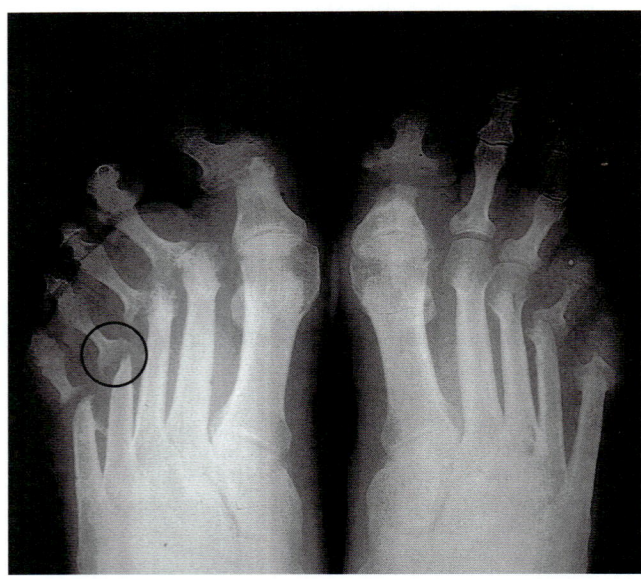

FIG. 198.2 X-ray of psoriatic arthritis. There is osteolysis of the metatarsal heads and central erosion of the proximal phalanges to produce the "pencil in cup" appearance *(circle)*. All the lesser toes are subluxed. (From Kumar, P., Clark, M. [2017]. *Kumar and Clark's clinical medicine* [9th ed.]. Edinburgh: Elsevier.)

diseases are histologically similar. Both can manifest with eye disease. Nail pitting suggests PsA, whereas nail onycholysis can be seen in both diseases. Polyarticular symmetric disease can appear exactly like seronegative rheumatoid arthritis, and it may be impossible to differentiate the two. Antibodies against rheumatoid factor and cyclic citrullinated peptide, as well as antinuclear antibodies, can be found in a small proportion of patients, which may complicate the diagnosis as well. The monarticular arthritis of Lyme disease involving the knee can be differentiated from oligoarticular asymmetric PsA by *B. burgdorferi* antibody assay. DIP joints with degenerative changes may look similar to psoriatic DIP joints, but patients with PsA have morning stiffness for longer than 30 minutes, and other inflammatory symptoms and findings that distinguish it from primary degenerative joint disease. Crystalline arthritis is within the differential and to be considered as well.

INTERPROFESSIONAL COLLABORATIVE MANAGEMENT

Nonpharmacologic Management

Patients may benefit from regular exercise. Low-impact exercise is recommended, such as swimming, cycling, or walking. If a patient's disease becomes well-controlled, many patients may successfully resume an active lifestyle. For many patients with suspected PsA, initial referral to a rheumatologist or dermatologist for consultation is recommended. As in other cases of inflammatory arthritis, referral to a physical therapist or occupational therapist for individually prescribed joint-protective exercise regimens as well as teaching in joint protection and energy conservation is very helpful. Patients disabled by joint disease may need vocational counseling.

Pharmacologic Management

NSAIDs are first-line therapy for PsA; however, many patients have continued active disease despite these agents and require

second-line therapy in the form of immunomodulators. DMARDs, including methotrexate, sulfasalazine, and leflunomide are typical second-line therapies. Methotrexate is the most widely used DMARD and has been the standard drug used in patients with both erosive joint disease and aggressive skin disease. Currently, five anti-TNF agents (etanercept, infliximab, adalimumab, golimumab, and certolizumab) have been shown to be effective in treating PsA.[13] As in rheumatoid arthritis and AS, the anti-TNF agents show sustained benefits in PsA with inhibition of radiologic progression and improvement in disability and quality-of-life indexes as well as improvement in the cutaneous lesions of psoriasis. Oral steroids are generally not recommended for the treatment of PsA because of the flare of skin disease that may occur on withdrawal of steroid medication.

Newer agents that have been approved for the treatment of PsA include apremilast, a phosphodiesterase 4 inhibitor; ustekinumab, an interleukin 12 and 23 inhibitor; and secukinumab, and interleukin 17 inhibitor. All three have shown benefit for treatment of both the skin and the joint diseases.[14]

Of note, suppression of the psoriatic skin disease is essential for the patient's comfort and appearance. It may also be important in the management of the associated arthritis because flares in the skin disease may correlate with flares in the joint disease.

COMPLICATIONS

Complications may occur due to the disease itself (with the development of extra-articular manifestations, such as uveitis/iritis) or may result from complications of the medications used to treat the disease. PsA is associated with a number of comorbidities including an increased risk for hypertension, diabetes, atherosclerosis, metabolic syndrome, and psychiatric disease. Such complications may lead to the need for referral to various specialists or hospitalization.

PATIENT AND FAMILY EDUCATION

- Patients should be counseled about the chronic nature of this disease and need to be aware of the possible side effects of medications (e.g., possible sterility, liver damage, risk for infection), and should be aware of the need for regular monitoring (including potential laboratory monitoring) while taking such medications.
- Appropriate forms of exercise may include range-of-motion and stretching exercises as well as low-impact exercises such as swimming.

ARTHRITIS OF INFLAMMATORY BOWEL DISEASE

 Rule out fracture, infection (osteomyelitis), septic arthritis, Lyme arthritis, and avascular necrosis (especially with history of steroid use).

DEFINITION AND EPIDEMIOLOGY

Joint pain is one of the most common extra-intestinal manifestations of IBD. Non-inflammatory joint pain is more common than inflammatory arthritis in this patient population. However, the inflammatory arthritis of IBD is associated with both ulcerative colitis and Crohn disease. One recent study demonstrated that peripheral joint arthritis is the most common type of arthritis in patients with IBD, occurring in up to 40%.[15] It has also been suggested that radiological evidence of sacroiliitis occurs in up to 50% of patients with IBD but progressive spondylitis occurs only in up to 10% of patients.[16]

PATHOPHYSIOLOGY

Arthritis is one of the several extra-intestinal manifestations associated with ulcerative colitis and Crohn disease. The mechanism of this association is not clearly understood; one hypothesis postulates that a disturbance of the gut barrier is the primary mechanism, while an alternative hypothesis suggests that shared genetic and/or environmental factors predispose patients to various organ manifestations of these inflammatory conditions. In addition, microbial elements in the gut may play a role as well. HLA and non-HLA genes have been associated with the disease, with HLA-B27 being more common in patients with spondylitis and sacroiliitis.[17]

CLINICAL PRESENTATION AND PHYSICAL EXAMINATION

Two forms of peripheral arthritis occur in IBD: Type I is an acute pauciarticular arthritis, usually affecting large joints, and is usually associated with active IBD. Type II is polyarticular, affecting a larger number of peripheral joints, and is independent of IBD activity. The peripheral arthritis of IBD is typically non-erosive and asymmetrical. The prognosis of peripheral arthritis is good, only becoming chronic in a minority of patients.

The axial disease seen in association with IBD is insidious and chronic and does not correlate with bowel disease activity. The joint involvement is identical to that of idiopathic AS. Patients may develop inflammatory eye disease, usually uveitis, which manifests as an acute, red, painful eye. SI joint involvement is strongly associated with acute uveitis. The clinical presentation of IBD may include complaints of joint pain, back pain, or morning stiffness. Mild abdominal pain with reports of bloody or mucous stools may antedate or occur with the joint disease, indicating a direct causal relationship between the two, but joint disease may be seen as the first symptom.

Enthesitis and dactylitis may also occur in patients with IBD, however dactylitis is a fairly uncommon manifestation occurring in <10% of patients.[18]

DIAGNOSTICS

Indicators of inflammation, including ESR and CRP, are often elevated. A mild hypochromic anemia is common. Joint fluid findings are consistent with inflammatory arthritis.

DIFFERENTIAL DIAGNOSIS

 Priority differentials include infectious or septic arthritis, other forms of seronegative inflammatory arthritis, and osteonecrosis (especially if patient has a history of systemic steroid use).

Further differentials. Inflammatory arthritis can occur in conjunction with gastrointestinal manifestations in a number of diseases, including vasculitis with abdominal involvement; systemic sclerosis complicated by motility dysfunction, amyloidosis, Behçet syndrome, familial Mediterranean fever, intestinal bypass, gluten sensitivity enteropathy, Whipple disease, and parasitic, bacterial, and viral infections.

INITIAL DIAGNOSTICS

Arthritis of Inflammatory Bowel Disease

LABORATORY
- Complete blood count (CBC) and differential
- Comprehensive metabolic panel
- ESR
- CRP
- Rheumatoid factor, cyclic citrullinated peptide

IMAGING
- X-rays of affected joints—to assess soft tissue swelling, erosive changes, and any other characteristic changes which may assist with diagnosis

JOINT ASPIRATION
- Synovial fluid analysis of affected joints—essential to determine if the joint fluid is non-inflammatory, inflammatory, or septic. It is also essential in the diagnosis of crystal induced arthritis (gout and pseudogout)

ADDITIONAL DIAGNOSTICS
- Antinuclear antibody
- Serum uric acid level
- HLA-B27
- Enzyme-linked immunosorbent assay (ELISA) for *Borrelia burgdorferi* (Lyme Antibody), if indicated

INTERPROFESSIONAL COLLABORATIVE MANAGEMENT

Nonpharmacologic Management

Referral to a rheumatologist and a gastroenterologist is indicated for confirmation of the diagnosis or treatment suggestions. Patients may benefit from physical or occupational therapy to both protect and maximize the use of their joints. Also, low-impact physiotherapy and exercise is recommended. Dietary modifications may be helpful in controlling bowel disease, and referral to a dietitian may be useful. If a patient's disease becomes well controlled, they may successfully resume an active lifestyle.

Pharmacologic Management

NSAIDs, when tolerated, are useful for the control of joint pain for both peripheral and axial joint disease. Sulfasalazine, which may be used to control the bowel disease, can be helpful in controlling the peripheral joint disease as well. Corticosteroids usually control both bowel and joint disease but are not desirable for long-term use because of drug toxicity. Methotrexate or azathioprine has been beneficial in patients whose disease is not controlled with sulfasalazine. The anti-TNF agents infliximab, adalimumab, golimumab, and certolizumab are well tolerated and are approved for the treatment of Crohn disease and ulcerative colitis and are recommended for treatment of disease resistant to oral standard nonbiologic DMARD therapy. For axial arthritis symptoms that are not controlled by NSAIDs, we recommend treatment with biologic DMARDs such as anti-TNF agents.[19]

COMPLICATIONS

Complications primarily arise with uncontrolled bowel disease. Abdominal pain and bloody diarrhea with weight loss can be severely disabling and may necessitate hospitalization. Corticosteroid-treated patients with IBD are at risk for steroid-induced osteoporosis and should be given appropriate calcium and vitamin D supplementation as well as prophylactic treatment with a bisphosphonate to prevent steroid-driven bone loss. Patients are also at risk for septic arthritis, and thus IBD arthritis patients should be closely monitored for signs of infection.

PATIENT AND FAMILY EDUCATION

- Patients need to understand the chronicity of this disease and the relationship between their bowel disease and their arthritis.
- Patients need to understand their medication regimens and potential toxicities, and the need for frequent monitoring. Patients taking prednisone should be cautioned not to discontinue this medication abruptly.
- Dietary modifications may be crucial. Referral to a dietitian may be useful.

HEALTH PROMOTION FOR PATIENTS WITH SPONDYLOARTHROPATHIES

Due to the complications and comorbidities associated with these diseases, we encourage patients with AS and related seronegative spondyloarthritides to pursue a healthy lifestyle. We encourage patients to remain active, in the form of low-impact daily physical activity; it may be useful to seek guidance from physical and occupational therapists. A healthy diet rich in fresh fruits and vegetables is also advised. Online patient support and education is available at: https://www.spondylitis.org.

REFERENCES

1. Stolwijk, C., van Onna, M., Boonen, A., & van Tubergen, A. (2016). Global prevalence of spondyloarthritis: A systematic review and meta-regression analysis. *Arthritis care & research, 68*(9), 1320–1331.
2. Sieper, J., & Poddubnyy, D. (2017). Axial spondyloarthritis. *Lancet (London, England), 390*(10089), 73–84.
3. Dean, L. E., Jones, G. T., MacDonald, A. G., Downham, C., Sturrock, R. D., & Macfarlane, G. J. (2014). Global prevalence of ankylosing spondylitis. *Rheumatology (Oxford, England), 53*(4), 650–657.
4. Hanson, A., & Brown, M. A. (2017). Genetics and the Causes of Ankylosing Spondylitis. *Rheumatic Diseases Clinics of North America, 43*(3), 401–414.
5. Stolwijk, C., van Tubergen, A., Castillo-Ortiz, J. D., & Boonen, A. (2015). Prevalence of extra-articular manifestations in patients with ankylosing spondylitis: A systematic review and meta-analysis. *Annals of the Rheumatic Diseases, 74*(1), 65–73.
6. Ozkan, Y. (2016). Cardiac involvement in ankylosing spondylitis. *Journal of Clinical Medicine Research, 8*(6), 427–430.
7. Gensler, L. S. (2015). Axial spondyloarthritis: The heart of the matter. *Clinical Rheumatology, 34*(6), 995–998.
8. Raychaudhuri, S. P., & Deodhar, A. (2014). The classification and diagnostic criteria of ankylosing spondylitis. *Journal of Autoimmunity, 48-49,* 128–133.
9. Schmitt, S. K. (2017). Reactive arthritis. *Infectious Disease Clinics of North America, 31*(2), 265–277.
10. Barber, C. E., Kim, J., Inman, R. D., Esdaile, J. M., & James, M. T. (2013). Antibiotics for treatment of reactive arthritis: A systematic review and meta-analysis. *The Journal of Rheumatology, 40*(6), 916–928.
11. Ogdie, A., & Weiss, P. (2015). The epidemiology of Psoriatic Arthritis in: Weisman MH, ed. *Rheumatic Disease Clinics of North America, 41*(4), 545–569.
12. Kerschbaumer, A., Fenzl, K. H., Erlacher, L., & Aletaha, D. (2016). An overview of psoriatic arthritis—epidemiology, clinical features, pathophysiology and novel treatment targets. *Wiener Klinische Wochenschrift, 128*(21–22), 791–795.
13. Huynh, D., & Kavanaugh, A. (2015). Psoriatic arthritis: Current therapy and future approaches. *Rheumatology (Oxford, England), 54*(1), 20–28.
14. Raychaudhuri, S. P., Wilken, R., Sukhov, A. C., Raychaudhuri, S. K., & Maverakis, E. (2017). Management of psoriatic arthritis: Early diagnosis, monitoring of disease severity and cutting edge therapies. *Journal of Autoimmunity, 76,* 21–37.
15. Malaty, H. M., Lo, G. H., & Hou, J. K. (2017). Characterization and prevalence of spondyloarthritis and peripheral arthritis among patients with

inflammatory bowel disease. *Clinical and experimental gastroenterology, 10,* 259–263.
16. Harbord, M., Annese, V., Vavricka, S. R., et al. (2016). The first European evidence-based consensus on extra-intestinal manifestations in inflammatory bowel disease. *Journal of Crohn's & Colitis, 10*(3), 239–254.
17. Reveille, J. D., & Weisman, M. H. (2013). The epidemiology of back pain, axial spondyloarthritis and HLA-B27 in the United States. *The American Journal of the Medical Sciences, 345*(6), 431–436.
18. Selmi, C., & Gershwin, M. E. (2014). Diagnosis and classification of reactive arthritis. *Autoimmunity Reviews, 13*(4–5), 546–549.
19. Armuzzi, A., Felice, C., Lubrano, E., et al. (2017). Multidisciplinary management of patients with coexisting inflammatory bowel disease and spondyloarthritis: A Delphi consensus among Italian experts. *Digestive and Liver Disease, 49*(12), 1298–1305.

CHAPTER **199**

SYSTEMIC LUPUS ERYTHEMATOSUS

Francisco P. Quismorio, Jr. • Dorothy K. Johnson

DEFINITION AND EPIDEMIOLOGY

 Referral to a rheumatologist is indicated for all patients with SLE.

Systemic lupus erythematosus (SLE) is a chronic multisystem inflammatory rheumatic disease that may cause diverse symptoms, such as fatigue, joint pain, rashes, seizures, edema, and chest pain. SLE has a predilection for women, particularly during the prime childbearing age of 15 to 35 years. A wide variety of autoantibodies, including antinuclear antibodies (ANAs), are the most characteristic laboratory finding in SLE. SLE can damage many organ systems, notably the kidneys, lungs, heart, skin, and brain, and may result in severe disability and even death.[1,2]

SLE is not an uncommon rheumatic disease. The incidence and prevalence rates are difficult to measure with great precision; these rates vary by geographic distribution and by demographic characteristics. Data from recent American surveys suggest that the prevalence of SLE among whites ranges from 5.5 to 10 per 100,000 persons.[3] The reported incidence rates of SLE in the United States also vary from 1.8 to 7.6 cases per 100,000 persons per year. SLE is up to 10 times more common in women than in men. The disease is more common in African-American women, among whom the prevalence may be as high as 1 in 500.[4] The morbidity and mortality of SLE are increased among African-American and Hispanic patients compared with whites.[5]

The cause of SLE is unknown. Its association with certain genotypes, such as the C4 null allele and various HLA haplotypes, as well as the 25% rate of concordance in identical twins suggests that the disease is likely to be a result of an interaction between genetic makeup and one or more environmental triggers. Numerous studies including genome-wide association analysis in different ethnic groups have identified common risk loci linked to susceptibility to SLE. Genetic variants in HLA region as well as non-HLA loci located within or near genes relevant to the immune system have been reported.[6] Because certain drugs can induce lupus-like syndromes, it is speculated that certain environmental agents may promote the development of SLE.[7] Other potential environmental triggers are ultraviolet light, a wide range of viruses (including the Epstein-Barr virus), physical trauma, and emotional stress.[8] Differences in the level and metabolism of estrogen, androgen, and other sex hormones may partly account for the female predilection for the disease.[9]

PATHOPHYSIOLOGY

The pathophysiologic hallmark of SLE is the development of antibodies directed against components of "self" tissues, particularly structures found within cell nuclei. The lupus erythematosus (LE) cell test, the first laboratory diagnostic test for the disease, described in 1948 by Hargraves, is predicated on the presence of ANAs specific for deoxyribonucleoprotein.[2] A wide variety of autoantibodies have since been reported in SLE, including antibodies directed against DNA and other nuclear constituents, red blood cells, platelets, white blood cells, and phospholipids. Autoantibodies form immune complexes in the circulation or in situ and become deposited in kidneys, skin, lungs, and other target organs. Circulating immune complexes are normally solubilized and cleared from the circulation by the reticuloendothelial system. In SLE, there is an aberrant clearance of immune complexes that may be related to defective solubilization of antigen-antibody complexes and abnormalities of complement and cell receptor functions. Individuals with genetic deficiencies of the early complement components C1q, C2, and C4 are at an increased risk for lupus-like autoimmune disease. Defective apoptosis (programmed cell death) with phagocytosis of cell debris allowing nuclear antigens to become antigenic, abnormalities in T- and B-cell functions, cytokines, innate immunity, and other immune mechanisms that promote self-tolerance all contribute to the development of autoimmunity in SLE.[6]

The deposition of immune complexes in tissues generates a local inflammatory response that may have organ-specific effects. Inflammation in blood vessels can cause vasculitis, which may result in vessel occlusion, ischemia, or infarction of the affected organ. Inflammation of serosal surfaces (lining of visceral organs) may result in pleurisy or pericarditis. The deposition of pathogenic immune complexes in the renal glomeruli can result in the development of lupus nephritis.[2]

CLINICAL PRESENTATION AND PHYSICAL EXAMINATION

SLE is a systemic inflammatory disorder characterized by varied presentation, disease relapses, and remissions. The disease can develop acutely, with obvious severe manifestations that include arthritis, nephritis, serositis, and vasculitis, or it may become apparent in an individual who has had mild symptoms and subtle physical findings (e.g., fatigue, arthralgia, rashes) sporadically for many years. The disorder is often misdiagnosed because many of the early symptoms of SLE are nonspecific (e.g., fatigue, oral ulcers, joint pain) and the ANA test result is positive in approximately 5% of healthy persons. The American College of Rheumatology has developed and validated a set of criteria for the classification of SLE (Box 199.1).[10]

Malaise and fatigue, often profound, are common but nonspecific complaints. Anorexia and weight loss may be seen in patients with active disease, as can fevers, lymphadenopathy, tachycardia, and anemia. The malar (or butterfly) rash, one of the most recognizable features of SLE, is observed in only 35% of patients.[11] This is a photosensitive erythematous rash on the cheeks and over the bridge of the nose that tends to spare the nasolabial folds. Discoid lupus rash is seen in 20% of patients

---

BOX **199.1**

Revised Criteria for Classification of Systemic Lupus Erythematosus

1. Malar rash: Fixed erythema, flat or raised, over the malar eminences, tending to spare the nasolabial folds.
2. Discoid rash: Erythematous raised patches with adherent keratotic scaling and follicular plugging; atrophic scarring may occur in older lesions.
3. Photosensitivity: Skin rash as a result of unusual reaction to sunlight, by patient or physician observation.
4. Oral ulcers: Oral or nasopharyngeal ulceration, usually painless, observed by a physician.
5. Arthritis: Nonerosive arthritis involving two or more peripheral joints, characterized by tenderness, swelling, or effusion.
6. Serositis:
    a. Pleuritis—convincing history of pleuritic pain or rub heard by a physician or evidence of pleural effusion; or
    b. Pericarditis—documented by electrocardiogram or rub or evidence of pericardial effusion.
7. Renal disorder:
    a. Persistent proteinuria—more than 0.5 g/day or greater than 3+ if quantitation not performed; or
    b. Cellular casts—may be red cell, hemoglobin, granular, tubular, or mixed.
8. Neurologic disorder:
    a. Seizures—in the absence of offending drugs or known metabolic derangements (e.g., uremia, ketoacidosis, or electrolyte imbalance); or
    b. Psychosis—in the absence of offending drugs or known metabolic derangements (e.g., uremia, ketoacidosis, or electrolyte imbalance).
9. Hematologic disorder:
    a. Hemolytic anemia—with reticulocytosis; or
    b. Leukopenia—less than 4000/mm^3 total on two or more occasions; or
    c. Lymphopenia—less than 1500/mm^3 on two or more occasions; or
    d. Thrombocytopenia—less than 100,000/mm^3 in the absence of offending drugs.
10. Immunologic disorder:
    a. Anti-DNA antibody to native DNA in abnormal titer; *or*
    b. Anti-Sm—presence of antibody to Sm nuclear antigen; *or*
    c. Positive finding of antiphospholipid antibodies based on abnormal serum level of IgG or IgM anticardiolipin, positive test result for lupus anticoagulant, or false-positive serologic test result for syphilis known to be positive for at least 6 months and confirmed by fluorescent treponemal antibody absorption test or other specific treponemal antibody test.
11. ANA: An abnormal titer of ANA by immunofluorescence or an equivalent assay at any point in time and in the absence of drugs known to be associated with "drug-induced lupus" syndrome.

IgG, Immunoglobulin G; *IgM*, immunoglobulin M.
Modified from Tan, E. M., Cohen, A. S., Fries, J. F., Masi A. T., McShane D. J., Rothfield N. F., et al. (1982). The 1982 revised criteria for the classification of systemic lupus erythematosus. *Arthritis & Rheumatism, 25*(11), 1271–1277; and Hochberg, M. C. (1997). Updating the American College of Rheumatology revised criteria for the classification of systemic lupus erythematosus. *Arthritis & Rheumatism, 40*, 1725.

with SLE. In a more benign clinical form of lupus, termed discoid lupus erythematosus, the disease is predominantly cutaneous with no or mild visceral involvement. Discoid lupus skin lesions are thick, round, erythematous plaques on the face, scalp, and extremities that heal with scarring, atrophy, depigmentation, and loss of hair. Discoid LE lesions can be disfiguring. Mucous membrane ulcers are also common, occurring in the oral and nasal cavities.

Approximately one-third of SLE patients experience Raynaud phenomenon,[11] an episodic vasospastic phenomenon characterized by changes in blood flow to the extremities, accompanied by sequential color change of the digits, from white to blue to red, and often unpleasant tingling or painful sensations (see Chapter 196). Livedo reticularis is a purplish mottling or lacelike appearance of the skin, especially in the extremities, and is associated with antiphospholipid syndrome (see later). Cutaneous vasculitis may manifest as tender skin nodules, palpable purpura or skin infarcts, and ulcerations. Bruising or petechiae caused by immune thrombocytopenia may also occur.

Joint pain (arthralgia) occurs in 80% to 90% of patients with SLE and occurs in more than half of the patients at disease onset.[11] Inflammatory arthritis primarily affecting the small joints of the hands and wrists is generally migratory and transitory, but in a small percentage of patients the arthritis becomes persistent. Lupus arthritis is non-erosive and in general milder than RA. In 3% to 5% of patients, a reversible deforming arthropathy called Jaccoud arthropathy develops. An overlap of RA and lupus ("rhupus") with positive anti-CCP and anti-RF is reported in few patients.

Osteoporosis is common and is multifactorial in cause, including corticosteroid therapy, chronic inflammation, and physical inactivity. Metabolic bone disease related to vitamin D deficiency and secondary hyperparathyroidism may develop in those with chronic renal failure. Inflammatory myositis manifesting as proximal muscle weakness with elevated serum creatine kinase can be seen.

Chest pain is a common complaint and is often musculoskeletal in origin. More significantly, SLE can cause serious cardiopulmonary disease, including pleurisy, pericarditis, pneumonitis, interstitial lung disease, pulmonary hemorrhage, myocarditis, and valvular heart disease.

A subset of SLE patients develops antiphospholipid syndrome, characterized by hypercoagulability, recurrent venous or arterial thrombosis, repeated spontaneous abortions and fetal loss, and the presence of antiphospholipid antibodies as measured by anticardiolipin antibodies, anti–β 2 glycoprotein 1, or lupus anticoagulant. These patients have an increased risk for pulmonary embolism, pulmonary hypertension, strokes, abortion, and fetal loss.

Lupus patients have two- to tenfold increase in risk for development of angina and myocardial infarction, with a greater increase in relative risk in younger patient groups compared to age-matched controls.[11,12] Accelerated atherosclerosis in SLE may relate to both traditional and non-traditional risk factors, including hypertension, alterations in lipid metabolism associated with nephrotic syndrome, long-term use of corticosteroids, and endothelial damage caused by chronic inflammatory process.[12] Hypertension is common and may be associated with underlying lupus nephritis, the use of corticosteroids, and possibly non-steroidal anti-inflammatory drugs (NSAIDs) as contributing factors.

Mood changes, depression, and migraine headaches are common. SLE can cause wide-ranging neuropsychiatric abnormalities, the most common being cognitive dysfunction with impaired memory and concentration. Psychosis, seizures, altered consciousness, confusion, stroke, myelopathy, and neuropathies may develop. The pathogenesis of neuropsychiatric manifestations probably involves different mechanisms, including small-vessel vasculopathy, thrombosis associated with antiphospholipid syndrome, effects of complement split products, cytokines, and anti-neuronal antibodies.

Lupus nephritis develops during the course of the disease in 40% to 70% of patients.[13] Persistent proteinuria of more than 500 mg/day, cellular casts, and red blood cells in the urine sediment are observed. There is a spectrum of renal involvement ranging from mesangial lupus nephritis with increased cellularity and deposition of immune complexes limited to the mesangium to severe diffuse proliferative glomerulonephritis with involvement of all glomeruli. Evaluation and staging of renal disease in SLE require a kidney biopsy, and the histopathologic findings are useful in assessing renal prognosis and in choosing a therapeutic regimen. Hemodialysis or kidney transplantation becomes necessary in those who develop end-stage renal disease. Most patients who undergo kidney transplantation do relatively well with immunosuppression required to prevent graft rejection. SLE kidney transplant recipients have outcomes generally equivalent to those of non-lupus renal transplant recipients.

DIAGNOSTICS

During a disease exacerbation of SLE, laboratory tests reveal nonspecific evidence of systemic inflammation with an elevated erythrocyte sedimentation rate (ESR), C-reactive protein, and serum gamma globulins. Anemia is common and may result from one or a combination of several mechanisms, including iron deficiency, chronic systemic inflammation causing an anemia of chronic disease, autoimmune hemolysis with a positive Coombs test result, bone marrow damage, and, in patients with renal insufficiency, inadequate erythropoietin response. Leukopenia, lymphopenia, and thrombocytopenia are characteristic hematologic features of the disease and appear to be mediated by organ-specific autoantibodies. Immune thrombocytopenic purpura may be the presenting manifestation of SLE and is associated with antiplatelet and antiphospholipid antibodies.

A urinalysis should always be obtained initially and at all follow-up visits because lupus nephritis can develop de novo in patients without previous kidney involvement. Blood urea nitrogen (BUN), creatinine, 24-hour urine protein excretion, or spot urine protein/creatinine ratio, and creatinine clearance should be monitored for changes indicating new nephritis or worsening renal function.

Although the "total" ANA test is the most sensitive diagnostic test, a positive ANA test result is not specific for SLE. In contrast, anti-Smith (anti-Sm) and anti–double-stranded DNA (anti-dsDNA) autoantibodies are more specific for the diagnosis of lupus (Table 199.1). Both types of autoantibodies are present in 30% to 40% of patients; thus, a negative test result for either anti-Sm or anti-dsDNA does not necessarily exclude a diagnosis of SLE. The presence of anti-Ro/SSA and anti-La/SSB in 30% and 15% of patients, respectively, is associated with subacute cutaneous lupus, secondary Sjögren syndrome, and neonatal lupus syndrome[1,2] (Table 199.2).

Antiphospholipid antibodies are a heterogeneous group of autoantibodies in SLE and are tested by immunoglobulin G (IgG) and IgM anticardiolipin antibodies, anti–beta 2 glycoprotein 1, and lupus anticoagulant. A prolonged activated partial thromboplastin time (aPTT) may suggest the presence of a lupus anticoagulant; however, the most commonly used assay for lupus anticoagulant is the dilute Russell's viper venom test (DRVVT).[14] Antiphospholipid antibodies may sometimes cause a biologic false-positive test result for syphilis (Venereal Disease Research Laboratory [VDRL] or rapid plasma reagin); however, a syphilitic infection is excluded by negative specific antitreponemal test results. Rheumatoid factor and other autoantibodies can be seen in SLE patients. Anti–cyclic citrullinated peptide antibody, a characteristic finding in rheumatoid arthritis, has been reported rarely in SLE patients.

In contrast to RA and other systemic rheumatic disorders, serum levels of complement (C3 and C4) may decrease in SLE, indicating complement activation and deposition of immune complexes in tissues. A drop in the serum concentration of C3 is associated with flares of lupus nephritis. Complement activation may also be involved in immunopathology of other organs including the skin. Direct immunofluorescent test on a biopsy specimen of normal-appearing skin in SLE shows the presence of IgG, IgM, IgA, C3, and C1q deposits at the dermal-epidermal junction (lupus band test).

DIFFERENTIAL DIAGNOSIS

SLE can be mistaken for a number of diseases, particularly other systemic rheumatic conditions, including rheumatoid arthritis, mixed connective tissue disease, dermatomyositis, and primary systemic vasculitides, as well as fibromyalgia, multiple sclerosis, infections, and other nonrheumatic disorders. Individuals with fibromyalgia who have a low titer of ANA may be misdiagnosed as having SLE. Drug-induced lupus may develop in patients taking procainamide, hydralazine, anticonvulsants, anti-thyroid medications, minocycline, anti–tumor necrosis factor (TNF) agents, or other drugs.[7] Drug-induced lupus differs from idiopathic SLE clinically in that nephritis

TABLE 199.1 Clinical Significance of Specific Types of Antinuclear Antibodies in Systemic Lupus Erythematosus

Antinuclear Antibody	Clinical Associations and Significance
Anti-dsDNA	Characteristic of SLE, useful in diagnosis; rising serum titer associated with disease activity, especially nephritis
Anti-Sm	Highly characteristic of SLE, useful in diagnosis; serum titer does not correlate well with disease activity
Anti-U1 RNP	Associated with mixed connective tissue disease
Anti-Ro/SSA and anti-La/SSB	Associated with risk for neonatal lupus syndrome, photosensitivity, subacute cutaneous lupus, and Sjögren syndrome
Anti-histone	Associated with drug-induced lupus; however, may also be seen in idiopathic SLE

SLE, Systemic lupus erythematosus.

TABLE 199.2 Drugs Used in Treatment of Systemic Lupus Erythematosus

Drug	Dose	Duration of Treatment
Hydroxychloroquine	200–400 mg/day <5 mg/kg real weight per day	6 months or longer
Prednisone (mild disease)	5–20 mg/day	Intermittent courses
Prednisone (moderate to severe; life or organ-threatening)	30–100 mg/day	Intermittent courses or IV pulsed
Azathioprine	2 mg/kg/day Check level of thiopurine *S*-methyltransferase; patients with low enzyme activity require lower dose of azathioprine	6 months or longer
Mycophenolate	Up to 3000 mg/day Use lower dose in Asian patients	6 months or longer
Cyclophosphamide IV	500–1000 mg/m² body surface area IV monthly	6 months or longer
Methotrexate with folic acid 1 mg/day	7.5–20 mg orally, once per week	6 months or longer
Belimumab	Infusion 10 mg/kg at 2-week intervals for 3 doses, followed by infusion once every 4 weeks	>6 months

and neuropsychiatric features are rare, and it improves with the withdrawal of the offending agent.

INTERPROFESSIONAL COLLABORATIVE MANAGEMENT

Non-Pharmacological Management

Patients with SLE should be referred to a rheumatologist at diagnosis for several reasons. Confirmation of the diagnosis of this serious illness is important because it is a life-altering chronic disease. Even patients with relatively mild or even asymptomatic lupus require periodic assessment of disease severity and activity, an evaluation best performed by a physician familiar with lupus. Given the myriad management decisions in this disease, the rheumatologist's involvement in patient care is important, even in mild cases. In uncontrolled disease with life-threatening organ involvement and in special complications such as pregnancy and antiphospholipid antibody syndrome, management by a rheumatologist in conjunction with a high-risk obstetrician is critical. Other specialists, such as a dermatologist, an ophthalmologist, a nephrologist, a cardiologist, an orthopedic surgeon, and a hematologist, are often consulted to help manage specific problems related to SLE. Psychiatric or psychological consultation may assist the patient in dealing with the lifestyle changes wrought by this illness and in managing depression. An occupational therapist should design and teach methods of conserving energy and prescribe appropriate assistive technology. A physical therapist should be consulted to design an appropriate exercise regimen. Nutrition counseling is indicated for patients with obesity, diabetes, hyperlipidemia, or renal insufficiency.

Individuals diagnosed with SLE require close guidance and education about the disease. Avoidance of prolonged sun exposure is recommended because many patients are photosensitive, such that sun exposure may precipitate lupus skin rash and/or generalized exacerbation of the disease. Patients are advised to use sunscreen with a sun protection factor (SPF) of at least 30 and sun protective clothing to avoid excessive exposure. Modest physical exercise is considered helpful in maintaining cardiopulmonary fitness, avoiding obesity, and improving mood. Diet is important as a way to reduce risk factors including metabolic syndrome and atherosclerosis, but no specific food or diet has been shown to trigger lupus.

When indicated, statins can be safely prescribed to treat hyperlipidemia in SLE patients. Because of the frequent occurrence of osteoporosis in these patients, attention should be paid to ensuring adequate calcium and vitamin D in the patient's diet. Vitamin D deficiency is prevalent and appears to be associated with lupus disease activity. Multiple factors such as photoprotection, renal insufficiency, and long-term use of corticosteroids and other medications contribute to vitamin D deficiency.

Regular health checkups by the primary care provider and with other specialists are valuable.

Lupus patients are at a higher risk for human papilloma virus infection and cervical dysplasia than the general population. Visits to the gynecologist at shorter intervals are advisable.[15]

Issues regarding pregnancy and hormone replacement are complex in these patients and require communication among obstetrician-gynecologist, rheumatologist, and primary care provider. The patient with SLE will need dental consultation with consideration of antibiotic prophylaxis, given the risk for infective endocarditis, especially in those with valvular heart abnormalities and on immunosuppressive therapy. When secondary Sjögren syndrome is present, accelerated problems with dental caries and gingivitis are often seen. Ophthalmologic monitoring is important to detect the onset of dry eyes (Sjögren syndrome) and to check for ocular side effects of hydroxychloroquine, chloroquine, and corticosteroids.

Pharmacologic Management

NSAIDs are typically used for the treatment of pain, particularly joint pain, fever, and serositis. Careful monitoring for NSAID toxicity is advised. Proton pump inhibitors are recommended for patients taking concomitant corticosteroids or aspirin. A rare syndrome of aseptic meningitis can occur with the use of ibuprofen and other NSAIDs in SLE and often mistaken for neuropsychiatric lupus. All NSAIDs, including the cyclo-oxygenase 2 (COX-2)–selective NSAIDs, have effects on renal function that can exacerbate hypertension, edema, and renal insufficiency in patients with lupus nephritis. COX-2–selective NSAIDs should be avoided in patients with cardiovascular risk factors and lupus nephritis.

Hydroxychloroquine is widely prescribed and is effective in managing the musculoskeletal, mucocutaneous, and serosal manifestations of the disease (see Table 199.2). It is effective in allowing tapering of steroids, reducing flares of disease and cumulative organ damage as well as prophylaxis for antiphospholipid syndrome.[16] Hydroxychloroquine has a better safety profile than chloroquine and can also be used during pregnancy.

Corticosteroids remain the mainstay of drug therapy for SLE, and the dose depends on the severity and extent of the disease.[17] For discoid and other lupus skin lesions, treatment with local corticosteroid cream, ointment, or local injection is often helpful. For patients with joint pain, fatigue, and milder disease that has failed to respond to hydroxychloroquine, low-dose corticosteroids (<7.5 mg/day) and/or weekly methotrexate may improve the quality of life. For patients with major organ involvement (pericarditis, thrombocytopenia, autoimmune hemolytic anemia, nephritis, neuropsychiatric lupus) or multi-organ life-threatening disease, corticosteroids are given in higher dosages, ranging from 40 to 100 mg/day to "pulse" therapy of 0.5 g to 1 g methylprednisolone intravenously every day for 3 days.[17] After the initial active disease begins to come under control, an immunosuppressive agent is added to help control disease and allow tapering of corticosteroids (steroid-sparing effect). The choice of immunosuppressive agent depends in part on the organ involvement.

Induction immunosuppressive drug therapy for focal (Class III), diffuse (Class IV), and membranous (Class V) lupus nephritis consists of a combination of glucocorticoids and intravenous cyclophosphamide. Mycophenolate mofetil has also been shown in controlled trials to be effective especially in Hispanic and African-American patients for induction. Following response to induction, the patient is maintained with either azathioprine, mycophenolate mofetil, or quarterly infusions of cyclophosphamide for at least 2 years.[18] Angiotensin converting enzyme inhibitors (ACE inhibitors) are added for their renoprotective effect.

For patients with severe persistent arthritis, methotrexate has been used. Azathioprine has shown efficacy in both renal and non-renal lupus. Intravenous gamma globulin is eficacious in severe immune thrombocytopenic purpura and in other organ-threatening lupus.

Belimumab (Benlysta), a targeted, human monoclonal antibody that binds to soluble B lymphocyte stimulator (BLyS), has been approved as an adjunctive therapy of autoantibody-positive SLE patients with active disease who are receiving standard therapy. It is indicated primarily for mild to moderate disease such as arthritis, fatigue, constitutional symptoms, and skin lesions. It is not indicated for nephritis, neuropsychiatric lupus, vasculitis, or severe life-threatening organ involvement. Belimumab is an expensive medication; it is administered as intravenous infusion every 4 weeks after the loading course of three infusions at 2-week intervals.[19]

The treatment of antiphospholipid syndrome in SLE involves anticoagulation for thrombosis or prophylaxis; however, certain aspects of therapy remain controversial.[20,21] Clearly, the patient who has experienced recurrent thrombosis or a major thrombotic event such as a pulmonary embolism or stroke should be treated with anticoagulation indefinitely. For pregnant SLE patients with antiphospholipid syndrome and prior fetal loss, subcutaneous low-molecular-weight heparin, low-dose aspirin, and hydroxychloroquine are recommended. Pregnant SLE patients with prior history of both obstetric and thrombotic complications are given a therapeutic dose of heparin, low-dose aspirin, and hydroxychloroquine. A pregnant SLE patient with moderate to high titer of antiphospholipid antibodies but without prior thrombotic or obstetric complications is given low-dose aspirin and hydroxychloroquine. Many rheumatologists also recommend low-dose aspirin daily and/or hydroxychloroquine for SLE patients with moderate or high titers of antiphospholipid antibodies but without a previous history of thrombotic event or pregnancy loss; however, the value of the regimen remains to be validated.[21] Treatment of patients with thrombotic antiphospholipid syndrome with rivaroxaban in clinical trials and shows great promise for those patients needing anticoagulation over the long term.[22]

Patients with SLE who are at risk for osteoporosis require attention to bone health. Osteoporosis prophylaxis with calcium supplementation and vitamin D is appropriate. Measurement of bone density and implementation of osteoporosis therapy including bisphosphonates may be required, especially in patients receiving long-term steroid therapy. Avoidance of long term corticosteroid therapy and addition of steroid-sparing immunosuppressives may help limit steroid-induced bone loss. The American College of Rheumatology recommends lifestyle modifications (balanced diet, maintaining weight in the recommended range, smoking cessation, regular weight-bearing or resistance training exercise, limiting alcohol intake to 1 to 2 alcoholic beverages/day).[23]

Optimum control of blood pressure is important because SLE patients are at increased risk for cardiovascular disease. High blood pressure increases the risk of kidney involvement or may result from kidney involvement. Systemic corticosteroids contribute to hypertension.

Many individuals with SLE have difficulty maintaining employment and household work roles. The Americans with Disabilities Act may be able to support patients in efforts to obtain flexible work hours, placement of filters on fluorescent lights, or other accommodations to preserve employment or to enhance productivity. Methods of reducing the amount of energy expended in commuting, in doing household work, and in maintaining social activities should be explored. Women can be encouraged to adopt a manager rather than "doer" homemaker role; family counseling may help members manage family role changes necessitated by the disease. The level of social support has been linked to health status, and studies have shown that persons with rheumatic diseases with higher levels of social support have better function. Telephone counseling programs, peer mentoring, and more recently Internet support have been effective in reducing feelings of depression and anxiety as well as in improving function and providing support.[24,25] Some patients benefit from treatment with antidepressant medications.

Influenza vaccine should be administered yearly. Polyvalent pneumococcal vaccine should be considered, given evidence of splenic dysfunction and impaired immune response in these patients. Lupus patients, especially those on corticosteroids and/or immunosuppressive agents, are at increased risk for infective endocarditis and should receive antibiotic prophylaxis while undergoing invasive dental, genitourinary, and other invasive procedures.

LIFE SPAN CONSIDERATIONS

The prognosis for patients with SLE has improved dramatically since its first description, when the disease was universally fatal. More than 90% of patients with SLE live 10 years or longer after the onset of symptoms, although there are differences among ethnic and racial groups.

African Americans generally have more severe disease and higher SLE-related deaths compared to Americans of European descent.

Although the overall prognosis of SLE patients has improved progressively in the past 4 decades, a recent meta-analysis reported that there is a threefold increase in the risk of death compared to the general population. The most important causes are renal disease, cardiovascular disease, and infections.[26]

Pregnancy poses potential problems for both lupus mother and fetus, especially for women with antiphospholipid syndrome. Patients with SLE have increased fetal losses and are at increased risk for preeclampsia and premature rupture of membranes, resulting in prematurity, intrauterine growth retardation, and pregnancy loss. Maternal risks include disease flares during pregnancy, exacerbation of preexisting hypertension, worsening of renal status, and pulmonary embolism. Both prednisone and methylprednisolone can be safely used in pregnancy because they are inactivated by placental enzymes and do not affect the fetus. However, pregnancy-induced diabetes or hypertension can have effects on fetal well-being. The presence of maternal anti-Ro/SSA during pregnancy is associated with an increased risk for neonatal lupus syndrome in the baby characterized by congenital heart block and transient lupus skin rash. A high-risk obstetric service, when available, should care for SLE patients to monitor the progress of the pregnancy, including fetal heart rhythm.[27]

Women who wish to avoid pregnancy should use birth control methods, at least during disease exacerbations, especially those with nephritis and those taking methotrexate, leflunomide, cyclophosphamide, mycophenolate, and other potentially teratogenic medications. Both injectable medroxyprogesterone (Depo-Provera) progesterone-only minipills, or intrauterine device can be used. SLE patients who test positive for antiphospholipid antibodies are at a risk for vascular thrombosis and should avoid contraceptives containing estrogen or progesterone.[27]

As young women with lupus live longer, the issue of hormone replacement at menopause becomes one of increasing concern. Hormone replacement therapy is effective for severe vasomotor menopausal manifestations in SLE women, but should be used primarily in those with stable or inactive disease with negative test for antiphospholipid antibodies. The use of HRT in patients with antiphospholipid-positive patients should be carefully weighed against the risk of thrombosis and cardiovascular disease.[27]

COMPLICATIONS

Fever in SLE should always raise the question of whether it represents a lupus disease flare or an infectious process. Fever in the absence of other signs of active SLE or fever associated with leukocytosis should prompt a search for an infection and appropriate culture. Opportunistic infections account for nearly a third of infections especially in those on immunosuppressive therapy. Pathogens include *Escherichia coli, Staphylococcus aureus, Mycobacterium tuberculosis, Cytomegalovirus,* and *Cryptococcus neoformans*. Fever with digital infarcts and joint pain could represent a flare of lupus but could also be caused by infective endocarditis. In evaluating febrile patients, the health care provider should promptly perform microbiologic cultures of blood, urine, cerebrospinal fluid, sputum, joint fluid, and other specimens, if available (see Chapter 203).

Previous sections have discussed some of the complications of lupus, including renal disease and renal failure, deep venous thrombosis and pulmonary embolism, stroke, coronary artery disease, and osteoporosis. Many of these complications are accelerated or worsened by corticosteroids. In particular, avascular necrosis of bone (osteonecrosis), especially the femur, can develop early—within few months after starting a high dose of corticosteroids. Thus, it is important to minimize the dose and duration of corticosteroid therapy when feasible. Immunosuppressive agents are prescribed for steroid-sparing effect, however these agents have toxicities of their own. Of note, cyclophosphamide is associated with premature ovarian failure and infertility, particularly in the patient who is older than 30 years. Bladder toxicity, increased risk for cancer, and infections are other side effects.

PATIENT AND FAMILY EDUCATION

As with any chronic illness, education is essential to enable the patient with SLE to skillfully self-manage the disease on a day-to-day basis. Medication management, appropriate and disease-relevant health habits, and self-monitoring activities should be encouraged. A recent study comparing standard nursing care with targeted nursing concluded that the latter significantly improved compliance and clinical outcome including less disease complications and better quality of life of SLE patients.[28]

REFERENCES

1. Yazdany, J., & Dall'Era, M. (2018). Definition and classification of lupus and lupus-related disorders. In D. J. Wallace & B. H. Hahn (Eds.), *Dubois' lupus erythematosus and related syndromes* (9th ed., pp. 15–23). Phildelphia: Elsevier.
2. Wallace, D. J., & Hahn, B. H. (Eds.), (2018). *Dubois' lupus erythematosus and related syndromes* (9th ed.). Philadelphia: Elsevier.
3. Somers, E., Marder, W., & Cagnoli, P. (2014). Population-based incidence and prevalence of systemic lupus erythematosus: The Michigan lupus epidemiology and surveillance program. *Arthritis and Rheumatism*, 66(2), 369–378.
4. Pons-Estel, G. J., Ugarte-Gil, M. F., & Alarcón, G. S. (2017). Epidemiology of systemic lupus erythematosus. *Expert Review of Clinical Immunology*, 13(8), 799–814. doi:10.1080/1744666X.2017.1327352.
5. Gonzalez, L. A., Sergio, M. A., Toloza, M. D., & Alarcon, G. S. (2014). Impact of race and ethnicity in the course and outcome of systemic lupus erythematosus. *Rheumatic Diseases Clinics of North America*, 40(3), 433–454.
6. Ghodhe-Puranik, Y., & Niewold, T. B. (2015). Immunogenetics of systemic lupus erythematosus: A comprehensive review. *Journal of Autoimmunity*, 64, 125–136.
7. Rubin, R. L. (2015). Drug-Induced lupus. *Expert Opinion on Drug Safety*, 14(3), 361–378.
8. Kamen, D. L. (2014). Environmental influences on systemic lupus erythematosus expression. *Rheumatic Diseases Clinics of North America*, 40(3), 401–412.
9. Moulton, V., & Tsokos, G. (2012). Why do women get lupus? *Clinical Immunology*, 144(1), 53–56.
10. Tan, E. M., Cohen, A. S., Fries, J. F., et al. (1982). The 1982 revised criteria for the classification of systemic lupus erythematosus. *Arthritis and Rheumatism*, 25(11), 1271–1277. Classic reference.
11. Lisnevskaia, L., Murphy, G., & Isenberg, D. (2014). Systemic lupus erythematosus. *The Lancet*, 384(9957), 1878–1888.
12. Schoenfeod, S. R., Kasturi, S., & Costenbader, K. H. (2013). The epidemiology of atherosclerotic cardiovascular disease among patients with SLE. A systematic review. *Seminars in Arthritis and Rheumatism*, 43, 77–95.
13. Mohan, C., & Putterman, C. (2015). Genetics and the pathogenesis of system lupus erythematous and lupus nephritis. *Nature Reviews. Nephrology*, 11, 329–341.
14. Moore, G. W., Peyrafitte, M., & Dunois, C. (2018). Newly developed dilute Russell's Viper Venom reagents for lupus anticoagulant detection with improved specificity. *Lupus*, 27(1), 95–104.
15. Santana, I. U., Nascimento Gomes, A. D., D'Cirqueira, L., et al. (2011). Systemic lupus erythematosus, human papillomavirus infection, cervical pre-malignant and malignant lesions: A systematic review. *Clinical Rheumatology*, 30, 665–672.
16. Ponticelli, C., & Moroni, G. (2017). Hydroxychloroquine in systemic lupus erythematosus (SLE). *Expert Opinion on Drug Safety*, 16(3), 411–419. doi: 10.1080/14740338.2017.1269168.
17. Kasturi, S., & SammariTano, L. (2016). Corticosteroids in lupus. *Rheumatic Diseases Clinics of North America*, 42(1), 47–62.
18. Hahn, B. H., McMahaon, M. A., Wilkinson, A., et al. (2012). American College of Rheumatology guidelines for screening, treatment, and management of lupus nephritis. *Arthritis Care and Research*, 64, 797–808.
19. Castro, S. G., & Isenberg, D. A. (2017). Belimumab in systemic lupus erythematosus (SLE): Evidence-to-date and clinical usefulness. *Therapeutic Advances in Musculoskeletal Disease*, 9(3), 75–85.
20. Cervera, R. (2017). Antiphospholipid syndrome. *Thrombosis Research*, 151(Suppl. 1), S43–S47.
21. Keeling, D., Mackie, I., Moore, G. W., et al. (2012). Guidelines on the investigation and management of antiphospholipid syndrome. *British Journal of Haematology*, 157, 47–58.
22. Cohen, H., Hunt, B. J., Efthymiou, M., et al. (2016). Rivaroxaban vs. warfarin to treat patients with thrombotic anti-phospholipid syndrome with or without lupus erythematosus (RAPS): A randomized, open controlled, open labeled phase 2/3 non-inferiority trial. *The Lancet. Haematology*, 3, e426–e436.
23. Buckley, L., Guyatt, G., Fink, H. A., et al. (2017). 2017 American College of Rheumatology guideline for the prevention and treatment of glucocorticoid-induced osteoporosis. *Arthritis & Rheumatology*, 69(8), 1521–1537.
24. Marks, R. (2014). Self-efficacy and arthritis disability: An updated synthesis of the evidence base and its relevance to optimal patient care. *Health Psychology Open*, 1(1).
25. Williams, E., Edede, L., Faith, T., & Oates, J. (2017). Effective self-management interventions for patients with lupus. Potential impact of peer mentoring. *The American Journal of the Medical Sciences*, 353(6), 580–592.
26. Yurkovich, M., Vostretsova, K., Chen, W., et al. (2014). Overall and cause-specific mortality in patients with systemic lupus erythematosus: A meta-analysis of observational studies. *Arthritis Care & Research*, 66(4), 608–616.
27. Andreoli, L., Bertsias, G. K., Agmon-Levin, N., et al. (2016). EULAR recommendations for women's health and the management of family planning, assisted reproduction, pregnancy and menopause in patients with systemic lupus erythematosus and/or antiphospholipid syndrome. *Annals of the Rheumatic Diseases*, 0, 1–10. doi:10.1136/annrheumdis-2016-209770.
28. Zhangi, X., Tian, Y. L., Junbao, L. I., et al. (2016). Effect of targeted nursing applied to SLE patients. *Experimental and Therapeutic Medicine*, 11, 2209–2212.

VASCULITIS

Julia A. Ford • Derrick J. Todd • Simon M. Helfgott

DEFINITION AND EPIDEMIOLOGY

The vasculitides include a diverse group of uncommon disorders characterized by immune system–mediated inflammation and the destruction of blood vessel walls. Clinical signs and symptoms result from the subsequent impairment of blood flow through these damaged blood vessels to the distal tissues and organs. Patients with a vasculitic syndrome often develop multi-organ dysfunction. Accordingly, these conditions are serious and can be fatal if they are not recognized early and treated aggressively, usually with long-term immunosuppressive therapy. Although the specific vasculitides typically affect characteristic organs, virtually any organ system may be involved.

Because the vasculitic syndromes are uncommon and data on disease incidence are imprecise, conclusions about the epidemiology of these conditions are difficult to make. For most conditions, age at onset is variable, ranging from infancy to old age. Some vasculitides, however, affect only certain age groups; for example, giant cell arteritis (GCA, also known as temporal arteritis) does not occur in individuals younger than 50 years (see Chapter 195), Takayasu arteritis is virtually unknown in patients older than 40 years, and Kawasaki disease is a vasculitis of childhood. Ethnic differences among vasculitides are less distinct; GCA tends to affect individuals of northern European ancestry, whereas there appears to be a higher incidence of Takayasu arteritis in women of East Asian descent.

CLASSIFICATION OF VASCULITIC SYNDROMES

Ideally, classification of the vasculitides would be based on the underlying disease mechanisms of the various disorders. Our understanding of the immunopathogenesis of the vasculitides, however, remains far from complete. For this reason, vasculitides are often classified according to the size of the involved blood vessels (Box 200.1).[1] This classification scheme does not necessarily account for disease mechanisms, but it is practical since the clinical features of vasculitic syndromes that involve similar-sized vessels tend to affect common organ systems.

Large-vessel vasculitides include GCA, the most common of all systemic vasculitides, and Takayasu arteritis. These diseases typically involve the aorta or its major branches, including the carotid, vertebral, subclavian, mesenteric, renal, and iliac arteries. Clinically, these syndromes manifest as large-territory claudication or infarction of the involved vascular tree. The medium-sized vessel vasculitides include polyarteritis nodosa (PAN) and Kawasaki disease, which can cause aneurysms of the involved arteries that supply the heart, kidney, gastrointestinal tract, and gonads. Small-to-medium-vessel vasculitides include the antineutrophil cytoplasmic antibody (ANCA)–associated vasculitides: granulomatosis with polyangiitis (GPA, formerly known as Wegener granulomatosis), eosinophilic granulomatosis with polyangiitis (EGPA, formerly known as Churg-Strauss), and microscopic polyangiitis (MPA). Other types of small-vessel vasculitis include anti-glomerular basement membrane disease, cryoglobulinemic vasculitis, and

The Vasculitides

LARGE VESSELS
Giant cell arteritis
Takayasu arteritis

MEDIUM VESSELS
Polyarteritis nodosa
Kawasaki disease
Primary angiitis of the central nervous system

SMALL TO MEDIUM VESSELS[a]
Granulomatosis with polyangiitis
Microscopic polyangiitis

Eosinophilic granulomatosis with polyangiitis

SMALL VESSELS
Leukocytoclastic angiitis
Henoch-Schönlein purpura
Cryoglobulinemic vasculitis
Drug-induced vasculitis
Behçet's disease
Relapsing polychondritis
Lupus vasculitis
Rheumatoid vasculitis
Sjögren syndrome vasculitis

[a]Antineutrophil cytoplasmic antibody–associated vasculitides.

Henoch-Schönlein purpura (HSP). Small-vessel vasculitides cause ischemia at the level of the small arteries, arterioles, or capillaries and typically affect the skin, kidneys, lung, gastrointestinal tract, and nervous system as well as other sites that tend to be more disease specific.

PATHOPHYSIOLOGY

The pathophysiology of the vasculitides is varied. Multinucleated giant cells may be observed in biopsy specimens of the temporal artery in patients with GCA and are the hallmark of this diagnosis. Hepatitis B virus (HBV) surface antigen has been found in the serum of some patients with PAN, suggesting a role for this virus in the pathogenesis of PAN.[2] Infection with hepatitis C virus (HCV) can lead to the formation of cryoglobulins, which are immune complexes that are deposited in blood vessel walls and cause vascular inflammation and destruction.[2] GPA, EGPA, and MPA are associated with the ANCA autoantibody, however its role, if any, in the pathogenesis of these conditions has not been fully elucidated. Necrotizing granulomas are a histologic feature of GPA and EGPA. Unique to EGPA are the large numbers of circulating and tissue-based eosinophils.

Patients with a drug-induced vasculitis may have immune complex formation consisting of the foreign protein (offending drug) and its binding antibody.[3] In some instances, this may represent a true serum sickness reaction in which the patient's immune system generates antibodies against foreign protein (historically antisera). Alternatively, some medications (e.g., propylthiouracil [PTU], hydralazine, minocycline, and allopurinol) cause a vasculitis that is associated with positive ANCA serology, often in a very high titer. The contribution of ANCA in the pathogenesis of drug-induced vasculitis is unclear. Recently, a new category of drug-induced vasculitis has been described in patients receiving anti-neoplastic immunotherapy. Drugs that stimulate the immune system to treat cancer (e.g., ipilimumab or nivolumab) have been implicated in case reports of GCA and other forms of vasculitis.[4]

Patients with connective tissue diseases such as rheumatoid arthritis, systemic lupus erythematosus, or Sjögren syndrome may develop a small-vessel vasculitis, although it is not clear how the underlying disease process in these cases contributes to the systemic vasculitis.

CLINICAL PRESENTATION AND PHYSICAL EXAMINATION

Clinical manifestations of systemic vasculitis are protean, and therefore diagnosis and treatment are often delayed. In general, most vasculitic syndromes have characteristic clinical, laboratory, or pathologic features that allow their identification and classification.[1] A systematic approach to the vasculitides, based chiefly on clinical presentation and physical examination findings, can expedite the process.

Constitutional symptoms, including fever, malaise, fatigue, anorexia, weight loss, arthralgias, and myalgias, are almost uniformly present and therefore do not distinguish among the vasculitides. When fever is present, the temperature rarely exceeds 38.9°C (102°F), and it is not typically associated with rigors or chills.

GCA is the prototypical large-vessel vasculitis. It is the most common of all vasculitides, although it is found almost exclusively in patients older than 50 years (see Chapter 195).[5] The presentation of GCA is varied and includes the new onset of headache, scalp tenderness, cranial pain, visual disturbances, or jaw claudication in an older adult patient with constitutional symptoms. Arm claudication from subclavian artery stenosis can occur. Patients might report arm pain when brushing their hair, and a subclavian bruit may be present. Blindness is a dreaded complication of unrecognized GCA and, if it is not treated immediately, is often irreversible. Fever of unknown origin is a less common presentation. Aortic aneurysms may occur, usually in the ascending thoracic aorta. Involvement of large vessels below the diaphragm (e.g., celiac, mesenteric, renal, and iliac arteries) is rare.

Approximately half of patients with known GCA also report diffuse shoulder and pelvic girdle achiness and carry the diagnosis of polymyalgia rheumatica.[6] On the other hand, GCA occurs in only about 10% to 20% of patients with known polymyalgia rheumatica.[7]

Takayasu arteritis is another large-vessel vasculitis that primarily affects women younger than 50 years.[8] Patients with this vasculitis classically lack a palpable pulse in one or more extremities, and there may be signs of unequal blood pressures, arm claudication, or bruits in the neck or arms. Other presentations include cerebral vascular accident, heart failure, and ruptured aortic aneurysm. Because these are extremely unusual events in young persons, Takayasu arteritis should be considered in the appropriate clinical setting.

PAN is defined as a necrotizing arteritis that predominantly affects medium but also small arteries. Destruction of the blood vessel wall causes the development of aneurysms, which interfere with blood flow to affected organs. In addition to constitutional symptoms, common features of PAN include ulcerating skin lesions, hypertension from renal involvement, postprandial abdominal pain from mesenteric artery involvement, testicular or ovarian pain from gonadal artery involvement, and peripheral neuropathy (see later). Some patients with PAN have chronic infection with HBV.[9]

Kawasaki disease is a medium-vessel vasculitis of infancy and childhood classically causing high fever, bilateral conjunctivitis, tender cervical lymphadenopathy, desquamating rash, peripheral edema, and strawberry tongue. Affected children are at risk for coronary aneurysms, the major cause of death. Aspirin and intravenous immune globulin constitute the definitive therapy.

Primary angiitis of the central nervous system (PACNS) is a rare vasculitic condition that exclusively affects the brain or spinal cord, usually of older adults.[10] Patients typically are seen with subacute dementia and personality changes. PACNS is often not recognized until late into the disease course, when stroke and coma occur. Brain biopsy is often required to confirm the diagnosis. Understandably, this condition is associated with significant morbidity and mortality.

GPA is a small- to medium-vessel ANCA-associated vasculitis. Although it is varied in presentation, the classic triad of involvement is that of the upper airway, lower airway, and kidneys.[11] Disease of the ears, nose, and throat is common and can manifest as recurrent sinusitis, mucosal ulcerations, hearing loss, and epistaxis. Hemoptysis from pulmonary hemorrhage and stridor from subglottic stenosis often herald lower airway involvement, and both can be life-threatening. Renal involvement usually requires laboratory analysis to be identified (see later). Additional manifestations of GPA can include palpable purpura, mononeuritis multiplex (defined later), central nervous system disease, and, less commonly, ocular, gastrointestinal, skeletal muscle, joint, or cardiac involvement. Overt joint swelling (i.e., arthritis) is uncommon. More often, patients complain of nonspecific arthralgias and myalgias.

EGPA is an ANCA-associated small- to medium-vessel vasculitis characterized by asthma, sinus disease (such as rhinitis, polyposis), and eosinophilia.[12] The condition should be suspected when a middle-aged or older adult patient develops new-onset asthma, which often precedes the vasculitis by up to 3 years. EGPA frequently affects the upper and lower respiratory tract, the peripheral nervous system as mononeuritis multiplex, and the heart as myocarditis or coronary arteritis. Other common involvement includes the central nervous system, gastrointestinal tract, skeletal muscle, joints, skin (palpable purpura), and kidney (glomerulonephritis).

MPA is a third ANCA-associated small- to medium-vessel vasculitis that has only recently been established as an entity distinct from PAN. Unlike GPA and EGPA, which cause granulomatous vasculitis, MPA is characterized by a necrotizing inflammation of involved vessels. Features of MPA include palpable purpura, glomerulonephritis, necrotizing alveolitis, mononeuritis multiplex, and gastrointestinal disease.

Certain medications and drugs may induce ANCA-associated vasculitis, including PTU, hydralazine, minocycline, and levamisole, a common adulterant found in cocaine. Symptoms from drug-induced ANCA-associated vasculitis include constitutional symptoms, arthralgias, and cutaneous vasculitis. Severe organ manifestations, including glomerulonephritis and alveolar hemorrhage, can also occur. Characteristic features of levamisole-induced vasculitis include necrotizing purpuric lesions involving the ears, cheeks, and extremities, as well as leukopenia and agranulocytosis.[13] Drug-induced ANCA-associated vasculitis is characterized by high-titer autoantibodies to perinuclear (p-ANCA), cytoplasmic (c-ANCA), or both, as well as antibody to elastase or to lactoferrin. Clinicians who see patients taking these medications or toxins should be aware of the potential for the development of ANCA-associated vasculitis.[3]

Cutaneous vasculitis or leukocytoclastic angiitis typically involves the smallest blood vessels in the skin. In most cases, the skin is the only organ involved, although more widespread involvement may be observed in more severe cases. Patients are seen with palpable purpura (extravasation of red blood cells into the dermis from small cutaneous vessels) of the lower extremities, but purpura may develop over the trunk and chest as well.

HSP is a small-vessel vasculitis that classically occurs in children; however, it may affect people of all ages. Typically, there is involvement of the joints (with pain or swelling), skin (palpable purpura), gastrointestinal tract (abdominal pain, bleeding), and kidneys (microscopic hematuria, rising serum creatinine concentration). Although this is usually a benign disorder in children, it may be a more serious condition in adults, in whom renal involvement is more likely to lead to end-stage renal disease.[14]

Cryoglobulinemic vasculitis occurs in the setting of patients with circulating cryoglobulins, serum proteins (immunoglobulins) that precipitate in cold temperatures. Patients often have chronic infection with HCV, although cryoglobulins can occur in other settings (i.e., malignant disease, chronic infection, and systemic rheumatologic disease). Cryoglobulinemic vasculitis classically causes glomerulonephritis, arthralgias, palpable purpura, and peripheral neuropathy. Gastrointestinal and pulmonary involvement also occurs, although rarely.

PHYSICAL EXAMINATION

Examination of a patient with suspected large vessel vasculitis should include assessment of peripheral pulses (which can be unequal or absent, such as in Takayasu arteritis) and auscultation for carotid and subclavian bruits. Temporal artery examination in suspected GCA should assess for presence of bilateral palpable pulses, nodularity of the temporal arteries, and tenderness over the temporal arteries.

In the evaluation of most small-vessel vasculitides, the presence of palpable purpura is perhaps the most helpful physical examination finding (Fig. 200.1). These lesions are usually multiple, and more often seen in distal lower extremities. They occur as a result of extravasation of red blood cells and white blood cells outside of the destroyed blood vessel wall of the small arterioles. They vary in size from a few millimeters to 1 to 2 cm ($\frac{2}{25}$ to $\frac{4}{5}$ inch) in diameter. On occasion, they are

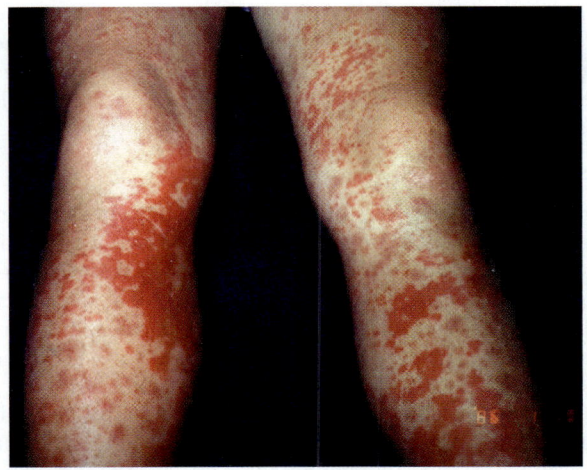

FIG. 200.1 Palpable purpura (nonblanching red macules and papules) on the lower legs is typical of many types of cutaneous vasculitis. (From Goldman, L., Schafer, A. I. [2012]. *Goldman's Cecil medicine* [24th ed.]. Philadelphia; Elsevier.)

pruritic. Other skin lesions, including livedo reticularis, non-palpable purpura, and cutaneous ulcers, can also be seen.

The small- and medium-vessel vasculitides can involve peripheral nerves, and a careful neurologic examination may detect these findings (e.g., sensory dysesthesia, motor weakness, optic neuritis). Classic findings include wrist drop, foot drop, or a facial droop. Vasculitic involvement of a single peripheral nerve is termed mononeuritis. Mononeuritis multiplex describes the cumulative involvement of multiple peripheral nerves over time and is highly suggestive of a vasculitis in the proper clinical setting.

DIAGNOSTICS

A high degree of clinical suspicion is required to establish the diagnosis of vasculitis because the clinical presentations are so varied and multi-organ involvement can mimic many other conditions. Common diagnostic studies for all vasculitides should include a complete blood count (CBC) with differential, serum electrolyte values, blood urea nitrogen (BUN) and creatinine (Cr) concentrations, liver function studies (LFTs), erythrocyte sedimentation rate (ESR), C-reactive protein (CRP) level, urinalysis with sediment, and chest x-ray examination. The CBC often shows anemia of chronic disease and reactive thrombocytosis. Eosinophilia supports EGPA in the correct clinical setting. Elevated BUN and creatinine concentrations can occur in many of the vasculitides. Liver studies (albumin, transaminases, bilirubin, and alkaline phosphatase) can be elevated in some of the vasculitides, in particular GCA. ESR and CRP are nonspecific markers of inflammation and are usually elevated. Urine sediment should be carefully examined for red cell casts and dysmorphic red blood cells, which would suggest glomerulonephritis. The chest radiograph can show a variety of abnormalities, depending on the underlying vasculitic process. A widened mediastinum in a patient with large-vessel vasculitis raises the concern of a proximal (thoracic) aortic aneurysm. Pulmonary nodules, hemorrhage, or infiltrates can be seen in many of the small-vessel vasculitides. Of course, chest radiography can also show an infectious pulmonary process in patients with known vasculitis receiving immunosuppressive therapy. Patients should also have additional diagnostic testing for occult infectious and neoplastic processes as appropriate for their presentation.

In the specific evaluation of patients with suspected large-vessel vasculitis, a thorough history, physical examination, and basic studies as listed earlier are often enough for the diagnosis to be made. ESR and CRP are likely to be elevated and appear to correlate with disease activity in GCA. Temporal artery biopsy showing granulomatous inflammation confirms the diagnosis of GCA. Noninvasive imaging with vascular ultrasound can be used to detect vessel wall inflammation in GCA (the "halo sign") and can help guide temporal artery biopsy; however, this diagnostic modality is highly operator-dependent. Inflammatory markers, particularly the ESR, are notoriously unreliable in patients with Takayasu arteritis, and additional laboratory testing is unlikely to be of diagnostic benefit. Magnetic resonance arteriography (MRA) of the great vessels of the thorax can confirm suspected disease and reveal subclinical arterial stenosis as well. MRA is increasingly replacing traditional angiography, which is sometimes still used to determine central aortic blood pressures. In both GCA and Takayasu arteritis, positron emission tomography (PET) has high sensitivity to detect inflammation in the walls of large arteries. However, the exact role of this expensive modality for diagnosis and monitoring of large-vessel vasculitis is still under investigation.

In patients with suspected medium-vessel vasculitis, few additional laboratory studies are of value. In PAN, HBV surface antigen may be present, indicating chronic HBV infection. ANCA is occasionally positive, with a perinuclear antineutrophil cytoplasmic antibody (p-ANCA) pattern (described in next paragraph) and antimyeloperoxidase specificity. MRA may be helpful in the medium-vessel vasculitides, but involved vessels may be smaller than the limits of resolution of the study. Angiography can show characteristic aneurysms of involved arteries, confirming the diagnosis. On occasion, PAN can be detected fortuitously in a pathologic specimen after cholecystectomy, appendectomy, or orchiectomy.

In contrast to large- and medium-vessel vasculitides, for which few diagnostic laboratory tests have been developed, an armamentarium of blood tests exists to investigate suspected small-vessel vasculitis. These include ANCA, complements, anti–glomerular basement membrane (anti-GBM) antibodies, cryoglobulins, HCV serology, human immunodeficiency virus (HIV) serology, rheumatoid factor (RF), and antinuclear antibodies (ANA). ANCA can show two patterns of staining: perinuclear (p-ANCA) and cytoplasmic (c-ANCA). In general, p-ANCA is associated with antimyeloperoxidase (MPO) antibodies and can be found in MPA, EGPA, or drug-induced vasculitis, whereas c-ANCA is associated with anti–proteinase 3 (PR3) antibodies and is found in GPA. Serum complements are low in some of the small-vessel vasculitides (e.g., HSP, cryoglobulinemic vasculitis, lupus vasculitis) but not in others. Although not truly a vasculitic process, anti-GBM disease should be considered in the differential diagnosis of pulmonary-renal syndromes. Thus, anti-GBM should be measured if the diagnosis of small-vessel vasculitis is being considered.

Cryoglobulins, anti-HCV antibodies, and rheumatoid factor can each be seen in cryoglobulinemic vasculitis. Serum cryoglobulins must be obtained with great care because of the manner in which the specimen needs to be processed. If the specimen is allowed to cool below body temperature, cryoglobulins can precipitate prematurely, resulting in a false-negative test result. Thus, it is recommended that cryoglobulins be collected in a separate specimen tube and maintained at body temperature (e.g., held in a warm hand or water bath) while being transported to the laboratory for immediate centrifugation. Measurement of antinuclear antibodies can occasionally be of benefit in patients with suspected lupus vasculitis or Sjögren vasculitis. Often these patients have significant involvement of their underlying connective tissue disease process.

Further imaging studies beyond a baseline chest radiograph should be tailored to disease involvement.[15] Sinusitis or other upper airway involvement necessitates a computed tomography (CT) scan of the head and neck. Chest CT should be performed in patients with significant pulmonary symptoms. Magnetic resonance imaging (MRI) of the brain with contrast enhancement can show a pattern consistent with central nervous system vasculitis. Electromyography can confirm the presence of peripheral nerve involvement by vasculitis.

Biopsy of involved organs is often necessary to confirm the presence of a small- to medium-vessel vasculitis.[15] Histologic evidence of blood vessel wall necrosis and inflammation establishes the diagnosis. Almost any organ can be sampled, but the simplest tissue to obtain for biopsy is the skin. Thus, any patient with a suspected vasculitis should be examined carefully

---

INITIAL DIAGNOSTICS

Vasculitis

LABORATORY
- CBC with differential
- Serum electrolytes
- BUN
- Creatinine
- LFTs
- ESR
- CRP
- Urinalysis

IMAGING
- Chest x-ray

ADDITIONAL DIAGNOSTICS: LARGE-VESSEL VASCULITIS
- MRA of affected area
- PET computed tomography (CT)
- Vascular ultrasound
- Temporal artery biopsy
- Catheterization with angiography

ADDITIONAL DIAGNOSTICS: MEDIUM-VESSEL VASCULITIS
- HBV serology
- HIV serology

- ANCA
- Catheterization with angiography
- Biopsy of affected tissue, if feasible

ADDITIONAL DIAGNOSTICS: SMALL-VESSEL VASCULITIS
- ANCA
- Complements (C3, C4, CH50)
- Anti-GBM antibodies
- Cryoglobulins
- HCV serology
- HIV serology
- Rheumatoid factor
- Antinuclear antibodies
- Toxicology screen
- CT scan of involved area (head, neck, chest)
- Magnetic resonance imaging of brain with contrast if central nervous system is involved
- Electromyography of affected nerve
- Biopsy of affected tissue

---

for skin lesions that can be sampled for biopsy. Another useful biopsy site is the sural nerve, a purely sensory nerve that is easily accessible for biopsy. When this procedure is performed, the adjacent gastrocnemius muscle should also be sampled to increase the diagnostic yield. Often, it is necessary to obtain biopsy specimens of other organs, such as the lung, kidney, or even brain, depending on disease involvement. Successful lung biopsy generally requires that the procedure be done through an open lung approach or video-assisted thoracoscopy. Needle aspiration or biopsy through bronchoscopy is rarely diagnostic, and the same is true for biopsy of the bowel during endoscopic procedures. Neither is diagnostic because specimens rarely contain arterioles, the vessels involved in the vasculitic process.

DIFFERENTIAL DIAGNOSIS

The differential diagnosis of vasculitis can be very challenging because of its variable presentations. Many vasculitis "mimics" have been observed and broadly include infectious diseases, drug-related disorders, malignancies, nutritional deficiencies, and other autoimmune diseases. Although often difficult to determine, an accurate diagnosis is essential to avoid treatment errors, which can lead to serious illness or death.

Cholesterol emboli syndrome can also mimic vasculitis. Affected patients are older and may be using an anticoagulant medication or have undergone some vascular manipulation, such as angiography, or sustained aortic trauma days to weeks earlier. The presentation is characterized by fever, bilateral palpable purpura over the legs and feet, renal insufficiency, and eosinophilia. Deficiency of vitamin C, also known as scurvy, can present with constitutional and musculoskeletal symptoms as well as characteristic rashes including palpable purpura, mimicking vasculitis.[16] Immunoglobulin G4 (IgG4) related disease is increasingly recognized on the differential diagnosis of large vessel vasculitis, whereby IgG4-positive plasma cells infiltrate the wall of the aorta causing aortitis, aortic aneurysm, or aortic dissection.[17]

 Rule out infective endocarditis, viral infection (particularly HBV, HCV, and HIV), culprit medications, and embolic disease in patients with systemic features suggestive of vasculitis.

INTERPROFESSIONAL COLLABORATIVE MANAGEMENT
Pharmacologic Management

The choice of therapy in systemic vasculitis depends on the severity of the involvement. For example, drug-induced vasculitis may be treated successfully simply by withholding the offending agent. Patients with more extensive systemic disease, however, usually require high-dose corticosteroids either orally or intravenously. Oral doses in general are 0.5 to 1.0 mg of prednisone per kilogram per day, or the equivalent. For more serious disease, intravenous corticosteroid preparations (e.g., methylprednisolone) can be given for a faster mode of onset. Steroids are the mainstay of treatment for the large-vessel vasculitides. Tocilizumab, a humanized monoclonal antibody against the IL-6 receptor, has recently been shown to be effective as a steroid-sparing agent in GCA.[18]

Certain vasculitides, such as GPA and MPA, warrant additional immunosuppressive therapy. This is the case for other vasculitides such as PAN, lupus vasculitis, and rheumatoid vasculitis when they affect the central nervous system, kidneys, heart, lungs, or other vital organs. Cyclophosphamide has traditionally been the agent of choice to induce and maintain remission of vasculitis in any of these conditions. Recently, however, rituximab (a monoclonal antibody against CD-20 expressed on B cells) was demonstrated to be non-inferior to cyclophosphamide in inducing remission in ANCA-associated vasculitis and is increasingly used.[19] Methotrexate and azathioprine may also show benefit in maintaining remission and can also act as a steroid-sparing agent in patients with disease refractory to corticosteroid therapy or in those who have developed serious corticosteroid-induced side effects (e.g., avascular necrosis). Less clear is the role of other drugs, such as mycophenolate mofetil. In several clinical trials, tumor necrosis factor-α antagonists did not show any benefit in GCA[20] or ANCA-associated vasculitis[21] and increased the risk of infectious complications in these patients.

Because patients diagnosed with vasculitis typically require prolonged courses of steroids, they should also be maintained with supplemental calcium, vitamin D, and, if necessary, a bisphosphonate to protect against bone loss. Proton pump inhibitor should be considered for gastric protection. Blood pressure and blood glucose concentration should be monitored carefully. In addition, patients receiving high-dose steroids (>20 mg of prednisone per day) generally require prophylaxis against *Pneumocystis* pneumonia. Trimethoprim-sulfamethoxazole is the agent of choice, although oral atovaquone or inhaled pentamidine can also be used in patients with sulfa allergies.

All patients thought to have a vasculitis should be referred to a rheumatologist for diagnosis and management because these conditions can be severe and life-threatening.

COMPLICATIONS

Serious complications from systemic vasculitis can be life-threatening and include stroke, seizure, renal failure, pulmonary hemorrhage, myocardial infarction, thoracic aortic aneurysm, mesenteric infarct, and gangrene of distal extremities. The use of high-dose corticosteroids may predispose patients to the development of obesity, osteoporosis, hyperglycemia, hypertension, infections, and avascular necrosis. The use of other immunosuppressant agents can cause bone marrow suppression, may predispose to infections, and in the long term may also increase the risk for the development of malignant neoplasms.

PATIENT AND FAMILY EDUCATION

- Patients diagnosed with vasculitis must understand the potentially serious nature of their condition. Although some forms of vasculitis (e.g., drug-induced vasculitis or HSP) can be self-limited, most are chronic.
- Mortality resulting from vasculitis has been greatly reduced by earlier diagnosis and intervention with immunosuppressant therapies. Long-term survivors, however, are susceptible to complications of treatment or the disease process itself, including accelerated atherosclerosis and higher rates of infections and even malignant disease resulting from chronic immunosuppression.
- Signs of worsening disease may include new rash, sensory loss, hemoptysis, hematuria, and proteinuria. A sudden headache or loss of vision in a patient with known or suspected PMR or GCA should be reported immediately.
- Side effects of high-dose steroids, including hypertension, obesity, cataracts, skin thinning, and osteoporosis, should be reviewed with both the patient and family.
- Given the potentially life-threatening complications of both the diseases and the treatment regimen, an open and accessible patient-provider relationship is essential.

HEALTH PROMOTION

Patients with vasculitis should be encouraged to adhere to treatment regimens and to maintain open communication with their providers regarding their disease activity as well as side effects of treatment.

REFERENCES

1. Waller, R., Ahmed, A., Patel, I., & Luqman, R. (2013). Update on the classification of vasculitis. *Best Practice and Research. Clinical Rheumatology, 27*(1), 1–12.
2. Guillevin, L. (2013). Infections in vasculitis. *Best Practice and Research. Clinical Rheumatology, 27*(1), 19–31.
3. Grau, R. G. (2015). *Current Rheumatology Reports, 17,* 71. https://doi.org/10.1007/s11926-015-0545-9.
4. Goldstein, B. L., Gedmintas, L., & Todd, D. J. (2014). Drug-associated polymyalgia rheumatica/giant cell arteritis occurring in two patients after treatment with ipilimumab, an antagonist of CTLA-4. *Arthritis & Rheumatology, 66*(3), 768–769.
5. Ponte, C., Rodriques, A. F., O'Neill, L., & Luqmani, R. A. (2015). Giant cell arteritis: Current treatment and management. *World Journal of Clinical Cases, 3*(6), 484–494.
6. Koster, M. J., Matteson, E. R., & Warrington, K. (2018). Large-vessel giant cell arteritis: Diagnosis, monitoring and management. *Rheumatology, 57*(suppl_2), ii32–ii42. https://doi org/10.1093/rheumatology/kex424.
7. Narvaez, J., Estrada, P., Lopez-Viveal, et al. (2015). Prevalence of ischemic complication in patients with giant cell arteritis presenting with apparently isolated polymyalgia rheumatica. *Seminars in Arthritis and Rheumatism, 45*(3), 328–333.

8. Keser, G., Direskeneli, H., & Aksu, K. (2014). Management of Takayasu arteritis: A systemic review. *Rheumatology, 53*(5), 793–801.

9. Hernandez-Rodriquez, J., Alba, M. A., Prieto-Gonzalez, S., & Cid, M. C. (2014). Diagnosis and classification of polyarteritis nodosa. *Journal of Autoimmunity, 48-49*, 84–89.

10. Hajj-Ali, R. A., & Calabrese, L. H. (2014). Diagnosis and classification of central nervous system vasculitis. *Journal of Autoimmunity, 48-49*, 149–152.

11. Comarmond, C., & Cacoub, D. (2014). Granulomatosis with polyangiitis (Wegener): Clinical aspects and treatment. *Autoimmunity Reviews, 13*(11), 1121–1125.

12. Greco, A., Rizzo, M. I., DeVirgilio, A., et al. (2015). Churg-Straus syndrome. *Autoimmunity Reviews, 14*(4), 341–348.

13. Subsinghe, S., van Leuven, S., Yalaki, L., Sangle, S., & D'Cruz, D. (2018). Cocain and ANCA associated vasculitis _ A case series. *Autoimmunity Reviews, 17*(1), 73–77.

14. Audemard-Verger, A., Pillbout, E., Guillevin, L., et al. (2015). IgA vasculitis (Henoch-Schönlein purpura) in adults: Diagnostic and therapeutic aspects. *Autoimmunity Reviews, 14*(7), 579–585.

15. Sharma, A., Singh, S., & Lewis, J. (2014). Diagnostic approach in patients with suspected vasculitis. *Techniques in Vascular and Interventional Radiology, 17*(4), 226–233.

16. Ferrari, C., Possemato, N., Pipitone, N., et al. (2015). Rheumatic manifestations of scurvy. *Current Rheumatology Reports, 17*, 26.

17. Kamisawa, T., Zen, Y., Pillai, S., & Stone, J. H. (2015). IgG4-related disease. *The Lancet, 385*(9976), 1460–1471.

18. Stone, J. H., Tuckwell, K., Dimonaco, S., et al. (2017). Trial of tocilizumab in giant-cell arteritis. *The New England Journal of Medicine, 377*, 317–328.

19. Geetha, D., Specks, U., Stone, J., et al. (2015). Rituximab versus Cyclophosphamide for ANCA-associated vasculitis with renal involvement. *Journal of the American Society of Nephrology: JASN, 26*(4), 976–985.

20. Seror, R., Baron, G., Hachulla, E., et al. (2014). Adalimumab for steroid sparing in patients with giant cell arteritis: Results of a multicenter randomized controlled trial. *Annals of the Rheumatic Diseases, 73*, 2074–2081.

21. Jarrot, P. A., & Kaplansky, G. (2014). Anti-TNF alpha therapy and systemic vasculitis. *Mediators of Inflammation, 2014*, 493593.

CHAPTER 201

DIVING-RELATED MALADIES

Joel Dulaigh

SCUBA diving is a relatively popular sport ranging from simple sport diving to advanced technical diving. Divers range from those who partake only once every few years to hundreds of dives per year, and across the age spectrum from pre-teen to over 70 years of age. The injuries that can occur are diverse and vary in severity from the benign to the life-threatening. Many diving injuries require medical attention emergently. These include near-drowning, hypothermia, arterial gas embolism (AGE), decompression sickness (DCS), and marine animal bites or stings. Other diving injuries are not as serious, requiring only simple first aid or allowing patients to be seen by their own health care provider. Most of the injuries sustained while diving stem directly from the differences in physical properties between liquids and gases.[1] A basic understanding of the laws of physics, particularly those laws that deal with pressure and density relative to liquids and gases, is important. The most pertinent of these are Boyle's, Dalton's, and Henry's gas laws.

PRE-DIVE PHYSICAL EXAMINATION AND DIAGNOSTICS

The pre-dive physical examination is an opportunity for both the diver and the health care provider to be aware of health concerns which could contribute to potential problems. A careful history is imperative.

A simple approach to the pre-dive physical examination has three considerations.[2] (1) Does the patient have a condition that could be exacerbated by diving, such as angina that could be precipitated by the exertion or some of the physiologic effects of diving? (2) Does the patient have a condition that could precipitate a diving disorder such as asthma that could predispose the patient to gas trapping and pulmonary barotrauma? (3) Does the patient have a condition that could compromise mental status or consciousness such as diabetes or epilepsy?

Specific medical conditions to be aware of while acquiring the diver's medical history are those that would affect the air-filled spaces of the body, hemodynamics, cognitive function, and physical ability to self-rescue. A history of asthma that requires the use of inhaled medications for disease control is likely one of the most common diseases that both puts an individual at risk for air trapping[1] and is often overlooked by the provider. Many practitioners believe that if the disease is controlled with bronchodilators, the patient can dive without

complication. This mistake is made because the provider does not understand the physics of gas laws as they relate to the risk of air trapping and pulmonary barotrauma. One factor commonly overlooked is that cold, dry air commonly triggers bronchoconstriction. One must consider that the air from a scuba tank typically has much less than 1% humidity and is also cooler than the ambient air above the surface of the water.[3]

Diving is relatively contraindicated in any patient with a history of frequent ear infections, serous otitis, or chronic sinus infections. Pressure equalization (PE) tubes in the ears and chronic or intermittent aspiration suggesting an incompetent larynx are absolute contraindications, as are chronic lung disease, emphysema, and a history of spontaneous pneumothorax.[4] Known coronary artery disease, heart failure, certain dysrhythmias, and valvular disease are conditions that could affect the hemodynamics of the diver and are also contraindications. Immersion in water shunts approximately 700 mL of blood from the peripheral circulation to the body core. There is also an increase in right atrial pressure of up to 18 mm Hg and an increase of up to 100% in stroke volume and cardiac output. A patent foramen ovale (PFO) has been a controversial subject in diving medicine for years. Recent studies reveal a substantial risk of DCS when compared to divers without PFO.[5] Arguably, the safest recommendation in the case of known PFO is to simply dive more conservatively and make sure the diver with PFO understands that his risk is higher. One case report indicates a diver suffered a case of DCS subsequent to closure of PFO.[5,6]

Epilepsy and unstable diabetes are both contraindications to diving because of the possibility of loss of consciousness (LOC). LOC underwater results in the inability to protect one's airway and is nearly always fatal. Any condition that potentially results in LOC should be considered a contraindication to diving. Several cardiac conditions could predispose one to a decreased level of consciousness as well, most notably the presence of an implantable cardioverter-defibrillator (ICD). Although most of these devices themselves have been tested for pressure and may be suitable for a patient undergoing clinical hyperbaric treatments in a chamber, the ability to protect the airway is again the primary concern. A simple pacemaker, on the other hand, would not by itself be contraindicative. The provider would then need to evaluate the medical condition that required the device before clearing someone for recreational scuba diving. Obesity is a hazard in that it may reflect poor physical conditioning and may predispose a diver to DCS based on nitrogen's lipid solubility.[7]

The physical examination should reveal a normal eye, ear, nose, and throat. The tympanic membrane should be intact, and each ear should be auto inflated by use of a modified Valsalva maneuver. A thorough neurologic examination is imperative. Normal neurologic examination findings with intact reflexes and strength are essential. The range of motion for all joints should be within normal limits. Lung and heart examination findings should be completely benign without rales, wheezes, murmurs, or extra sounds. Cardiac stress testing may be recommended for divers aged 45 years and older, as for any other activity requiring physical exertion. Older divers are at higher risk for chronic disease and should consider annual physical evaluation for diving fitness.[8]

Recommended studies before diving include a **chest x-ray examination, electrocardiography, visual acuity testing,** and **pulmonary function tests. Bone and joint x-ray studies** and periodic **audiograms** are required for commercial divers.[8]

DECOMPRESSION SICKNESS

DEFINITION AND EPIDEMIOLOGY

DCS, also known as "the bends," is the result of bubble formation and growth from tissue inert gas supersaturation. During a dive, the body absorbs nitrogen from the breathing gas in proportion to the surrounding pressure. If the diver ascends too quickly, gas bubbles will form and grow in body tissue, causing symptoms of DCS. Studies have shown that the majority of divers bubble, although the vast majority will not experience DCS. One such study indicated that during a multi-day, recreational diving study, 91% of divers had Spencer Score, a method of measuring density of bubbles using Doppler, of >0, with 36.2% scoring Spencer grades 2 or 3, yet there were no cases of DCS.[9]

Nitrogen at higher pressures can also alter the electrical properties of brain function and cause nitrogen narcosis, causing many of the same impairments in judgment and coordination as alcohol intoxication.[1] The effects of nitrogen narcosis can have a more exponential effect at higher pressures.

PATHOPHYSIOLOGY

The risk of DCS is most affected by depth and time. Rapid ascent, deeper and longer dives, repeated dives, and failure to follow appropriate decompression procedures increase these risks. Dive tables or decompression computers are used to calculate the rate of ascent based on the depth of the dive and are essential to safe diving. Following appropriate decompression procedures can reduce but not eliminate the risk of DCS.

The risk of DCS is also increased by air travel that occurs soon after a dive because the cabin pressure is typically less than sea level pressure. The Divers Alert Network (DAN) posts specific guidelines for flying in a typically pressured cabin after a dive. Recommended wait times are 24 to 36 hours, depending on the depth and length of the dive and the diver's tendency to form bubbles.[10] The US Navy Dive Manual contains tables for recommendation on flying after diving and can be viewed free of charge online.[11]

The term *dysbarism* has been used to describe these pressure-related injuries that result in tissue damage. *Decompression illness* is now the preferred term to describe an injured diver who has either AGE or DCS.[7]

CLINICAL PRESENTATION AND PHYSICAL EXAMINATION

DCS can manifest acutely, but delayed presentation is more frequent. In one clinical study, 98.9% of DCS patients had symptoms within 6 hours of surfacing from the dive, with an overall median latency of 62 minutes.[12] Cases of delayed onset of symptoms beyond 24 hours have also been reported. Altitude exposure, including commercial air travel, can precipitate DCS after an extended period.[10] Individual differences in physical fitness, body weight, gender, fatigue, hydration, and age may make some divers more prone to DCS in spite of the use of appropriate decompression procedures.[13]

Type I DCS is defined as pain in only one joint and can manifest with dull pain, especially in the upper extremities, with the shoulder being the most common.[12] Skin itching, rash, and localized swelling (lymphedema) are also common manifestations of type I DCS. The presence of pain in more than one location or any neurologic symptom is considered type II DCS. Type II DCS is more severe and is commonly characterized by neurologic or pulmonary symptoms, including chest pain and cough. Nervous system involvement most often manifests as patchy numbness or paresthesias, but paralysis can also occur. Headache, extreme fatigue, dizziness (including vertigo), urinary or anal sphincter disorders (usually urinary retention), or mental status and behavioral changes can also be seen. Hypovolemic shock can occur as a result of fluid shifts from intravascular to extravascular spaces.[11]

Pulmonary DCS, also known as "the chokes," and inner ear or vestibular DCS are both also classified as type II DCS. The chokes can easily be confused with immersion pulmonary edema, also known as swimming-induced pulmonary edema, which is another complication of diving. For any type of DCS, consider the timing and onset of symptoms. Symptom onset while still on the bottom is likely due to another cause since the decompression phase of the dive has yet to occur. In order to have DCS, there must first be decompression.

A careful history of the dive is essential.[14] It is crucial to know where the dive took place, how deep the dive was, how much time was spent at specific depths, and the gas mixture the diver was breathing. If the diver was using a dive computer, it may be possible to download the dive profile to get a more accurate description of the dive details. Questions about the diver's pre-dive condition, including hydration, travel schedule, and drug or alcohol intake, should be asked. Knowledge of first aid administered at the site is helpful. Multiple systems can be affected, but the neurologic and respiratory systems especially must be carefully assessed. Disorientation, dizziness, fatigue, and joint pain with limited ability to move are common complaints. The joint pain of limb DCS can sometimes be relieved by inflating a blood pressure cuff around the affected joint, although this is not a reliable sign. This pain is often not affected by range of motion or palpation. Physical findings may also include skin blotching, weakness, ataxia, paresthesias, or paralysis. Hypotension, tachycardia, chest pain, and cough are common symptoms.

DIAGNOSTICS

DCS is a diagnosis of exclusion and there are no specific tests to detect DCS; therefore, the diagnostics here are used to rule out problems in the differential diagnosis.

DIFFERENTIAL DIAGNOSIS

 Rule out acute coronary syndrome, CVA, and hypoglycemia.

Many of the signs of DCS are identical to those of more common syndromes, including dehydration, electrolyte imbalance, viral syndromes, and exhaustion.

INITIAL DIAGNOSTICS

LABORATORY
- CBC—monitor H&H, keep Hct <50
- CMP—Electrolytes may be affected by DCS and other differentials

IMAGING
- CXR—r/o pneumothorax or other chest injury
- CT chest—r/o interstitial lung injury or other chest injury
- MRI head—r/o CVA
- EKG—r/o ACS

ADDITIONAL DIAGNOSTICS
- PT/INR, D-dimer, complete echo with bubble study; consider other diagnostics to assess clotting abnormalities and any other illness/injury in the differential diagnosis

Sprains, strains, fracture, arthritis, and herniated disk can all cause musculoskeletal pain. Dermatitis, allergic reactions, abrasions, contusions, or envenomation can lead to dermatologic symptoms, including cellulitis, rash, itching, and burning. Heat exhaustion or heat stroke can lead to muscle cramping or mental status changes. Deep venous thrombosis and thrombophlebitis can certainly be a cause of limb pain, but not usually joint pain. Chest pain or difficulty breathing that begins during the deepest segment of the dive is likely not DCS, and immersion pulmonary edema, pulmonary embolus, immersion pulmonary edema, or other cause should be considered.

INTERPROFESSIONAL COLLABORATIVE MANAGEMENT

Hyperbaric oxygen (HBO) therapy using a US Navy treatment table 6 (TT6) is the gold standard for DCS. Medical stabilization at the nearest facility with rapid transport to the nearest recompression chamber is essential. This could include emergency care at the scene, with cardiopulmonary resuscitation and intubation if indicated. Immediate treatment with inhaled 100% oxygen is the primary and most effective therapy in reducing symptoms while awaiting transport. The breathing of 100% oxygen increases the extraction of nitrogen from the tissues by reducing the partial pressure of nitrogen in the breathing gas. This change in pressure gradient aids in nitrogen elimination and can help reduce bubble size. Treatment of DCS with oxygen cannot be titrated based on pulse oximetry readings, because it is not the oxygen level that is of concern, but rather the displacement of the offending gas. However, this treatment does enhance oxygen delivery to ischemic tissues.[14] Even if the symptoms improve with 100% oxygen, the patient will still require recompression in an HBO chamber, although the number of recompression treatments may be decreased. Because preferred diving locations may be a great distance from home and require air travel, divers often are seen by health care providers several days after the onset of symptoms; even then, recompression in an HBO chamber may still be beneficial.[13,15]

The effects of immersion diuresis often causes injured divers to be hypovolemic, requiring aggressive intravenous hydration administered by trained medical personnel, but placement of the patient in the Trendelenburg position is contraindicated.[15] The routine use of aspirin in patients with neurologic DCS is not recommended because of potentiating hemorrhage in the spinal cord and inner ear decompression illness. For patients with limited mobility because of lower extremity weakness, low-molecular-weight heparin may be used to prevent deep vein thrombosis (DVT).

LIFE SPAN CONSIDERATIONS

Children younger than 12 years are usually not certified to dive because they may lack the maturity to appreciate the inherent dangers and need for absolute adherence to the rules. Diving in pregnancy is not recommended because of risk to the fetus from the unknown effects of nitrogen diffusion across the placenta and decompression risk to the fetus. Older adults, who are more likely to have medical problems that could affect diving, should seek medical clearance before diving and thereafter annually or as health status changes.

COMPLICATIONS

Complications of decompression illness include cardiac arrest, drowning or near-drowning, hypoxia, and permanent neurologic damage. Initial symptoms that appear minimal can worsen during the first few hours; thus, it is recommended that patients with even mild symptoms be referred to a facility with a recompression chamber and medical personnel with knowledge of diving injuries. Typically, the sooner the onset of symptoms after diving, the more severe the case of DCS.

BAROTRAUMA

DEFINITION AND EPIDEMIOLOGY

Barotrauma, the most common diving-related injury, develops when an air-filled body space fails to equilibrate its pressure with the environment when the pressures in that environment change. Barotrauma can occur during either descent or ascent.[1] Barotrauma of descent is also known as a "squeeze" and is most common in the middle ear and sinus spaces. Other air-filled spaces may also be affected, including dental or artificial spaces. Artificial spaces may be created by diving with ear plugs, using goggles rather than a mask that encompasses the nose, and using equipment such as a dry suit. Barotrauma of ascent is also referred to as a "reverse squeeze," and again affects the ears, sinuses, and dental air spaces. It is typically more severe because expanding gas volumes in a confined space can cause serious damage to tissues. The most severe of the ascending barotraumas is pulmonary barotrauma because of its life-threatening consequences.

PATHOPHYSIOLOGY

Pulmonary barotrauma occurs when a diver ascends without exhaling or at a rate of ascent exceeding the rate at which expanding gas can exit through the tracheobronchial tree. Trapped air in the lungs expands and may rupture lung tissue, resulting in mediastinal emphysema, subcutaneous emphysema, or pneumothorax. AGE occurs as a result of pulmonary barotrauma when gas bubbles are released into the circulation. These bubbles are then carried to vital organs, causing life-threatening conditions or sudden death.[14] AGE is by far the most critical, life-threatening of all the diving-related illnesses.

EAR BAROTRAUMA

Ear barotrauma was first described in 1897 and remains an important problem for both occupational and recreational divers. Again, the pathophysiologic process is related to an inability to equalize pressures during descent or ascent. The injuries can range from injury to the tympanic membrane (including rupture), to severe middle ear damage, to inner ear labyrinthine window rupture.

SINUS BAROTRAUMA

Sinus barotrauma is associated with severe pain in the region of the sinuses and can occur during descent or ascent. The frontal sinus is most commonly involved. Epistaxis occurs in about half of cases.[4] This can be a problem for divers who have experienced it before and those with a history of chronic sinus problems.

CLINICAL PRESENTATION AND PHYSICAL EXAMINATION

Patients with barotrauma often present with a history of difficulty clearing or equalizing during the dive. There may have been a forceful Valsalva or other attempts to equalize. Symptoms associated with these problems include dizziness, tinnitus, nausea, vertigo, ear pain, jaw or neck pain, and hearing difficulty.[15]

Direct visualization of the tympanic membrane is essential. Examination of the ear canal may reveal bloody drainage and acute damage to the tympanic membrane. Inflammation of the eardrum or collection of fluid behind the eardrum may be seen. Nystagmus, hearing loss, and loss of balance may also be noted. The Weber and Rinne tests may be helpful in distinguishing conductive hearing loss (caused by middle ear barotrauma) from sensorineural hearing loss (implicating either inner ear barotrauma or inner ear DCS).[4] A thorough neurologic exam is essential in diving-related injuries and can help distinguish between barotrauma, DCS, and other illnesses not necessarily caused by diving.

DIAGNOSTICS

Initial Diagnostics

LABORATORY
• None

IMAGING
• CT or MRI may be indicated to assess sinus or inner ear injury.

ADDITIONAL DIAGNOSTICS
• Audiometry

DIFFERENTIAL DIAGNOSTICS

It may be difficult to differentiate barotrauma from other diving- and non-diving related illness or injury.

 Priority differentials include CVA, inner ear DCS, Bell's palsy.

INTERPROFESSIONAL COLLABORATIVE MANAGEMENT

Prevention could be achieved by not diving when sick or experiencing upper respiratory congestion. Topical and systemic nasal decongestants may provide both relief and prophylaxis for divers who are predisposed to ENT types of barotrauma; however, these likely do not expedite healing. A short course

of steroids may also help reduce swelling and edema. Antibiotics are not indicated unless subsequent infection develops. On occasion, mild systemic analgesics may be needed. Most tympanic membrane ruptures heal spontaneously, although patients who do not respond to conservative therapy should be referred to an otolaryngologist for ongoing management.[4] All patients should refrain from diving until symptoms have cleared. If symptoms are limited to the ear, consider inner ear DCS and refer appropriately.[4]

Inner ear barotrauma with vertigo and tinnitus may require a period of bed rest with medication to control vertigo and possibly sedatives to help the patient rest comfortably. Surgical exploration to repair a round window rupture may be required. Referral to an audiologist for hearing evaluation may be necessary if hearing loss is severe or persistent.

COMPLICATIONS

Varying degrees of hearing loss, vestibular dysfunction resulting in chronic vertigo, balance disorders, and gait disorders are the most serious complications of ear barotrauma.[16] Permanent inner ear damage can be a contraindication to further diving.

PULMONARY BAROTRAUMA

Pulmonary barotrauma with AGE is second only to drowning as a cause of death in divers.[7] Trapped air in the lungs expands and ruptures alveolar tissue, releasing air bubbles into the circulation (Fig. 201.1). If a bubble lodges in the brain, stroke,

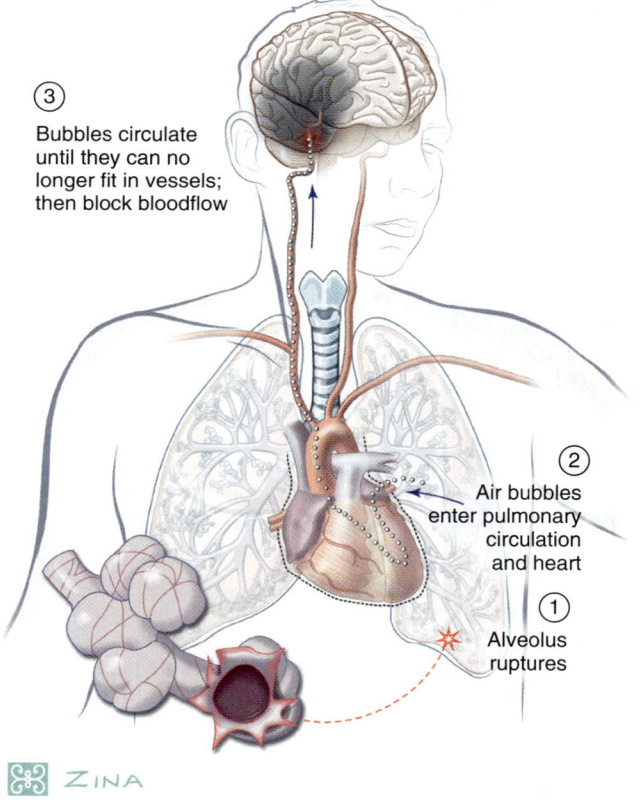

③ Bubbles circulate until they can no longer fit in vessels; then block bloodflow

② Air bubbles enter pulmonary circulation and heart

① Alveolus ruptures

ZINA

FIG. 201.1 Arterial gas embolism. (Copyright National Oceanic and Atmospheric Administration, Department of Commerce, Seattle, Washington. www.omao.noaa.gov.)

seizures, paralysis, and LOC can occur. Air bubbles traveling to the heart can lead to myocardial infarction or cardiac arrest. AGE can also cause minor symptoms, such as numbness, tingling, or weakness of a limb. Vision and hearing losses have also been seen, all without LOC. A patient who collapses with LOC less than 10 minutes after the dive is considered to have an AGE until proven otherwise.

Pneumothorax may or may not occur in conjunction with AGE. Interstitial lung tissue damage can allow passage of gas into the circulation, thus causing an AGE without compromising the pleural lining or causing a pneumothorax. Mediastinal air can track cephalically into the soft tissues of the neck and cause subcutaneous emphysema.[1] A chest x-ray examination will usually confirm the diagnosis, although computed tomography scans may be required.

CLINICAL PRESENTATION AND PHYSICAL EXAMINATION

The patient may be in respiratory distress with mild to moderate pain. Tachypnea, pallor, decreased or absent oxygen saturation, and diminished breath sounds may be noted. The symptoms of AGE can mimic those of stroke, but a history of rapid or uncontrolled assent, especially in combination with symptoms of pulmonary barotrauma and stroke-like symptoms, is highly indicative of AGE.

A thorough examination with emphasis on neurologic function as well as cardiac and pulmonary status will help differentiate AGE from non-diving related injuries; however, any symptoms of a neurologic nature during ascent or immediately post dive are highly indicative of AGE. Altered mental status coupled with chest discomfort or dyspnea can nearly be considered definitively diagnostic for AGE.

DIAGNOSTICS

Initial Diagnostics

LABORATORY
- ABG, CBC, CMP, Cardiac panel

IMAGING
- EKG
- CXR
- Chest CT
- CT/MRI of the head

ADDITIONAL DIAGNOSTICS
- Although treatment should not be delayed for additional diagnostic testing, other tests to consider would be V/Q scan and echocardiography.

DIFFERENTIAL DIAGNOSTICS

AGE is a life-threatening condition and should be treated if there is any suspicion whatsoever.

 Consider CVA, acute coronary syndrome, pulmonary embolus.

INTERPROFESSIONAL COLLABORATIVE MANAGEMENT

Emergency management of AGE is the same as for DCS and includes on-site use of 100% inhaled oxygen therapy, medical stabilization, and transport to a recompression chamber. Emergent recompression with HBO is the primary objective in treatment of AGE, although untreated pneumothorax is a contraindication to HBO and must be addressed before treatment. Keep vigilant watch for progression of life-threatening symptoms. Patients with mild presenting symptoms may progress or relapse while undergoing recompression. This relapse may result from bubble interaction with blood vessel wall, causing an inflammatory response.[17] This response leads to blood vessel occlusion and cell damage, which can result in clinical deterioration or even death in spite of recompression treatments.[17] These patients are often observed in the hospital and discharged with careful instructions to return if symptoms increase. Persistent problems in maintaining adequate oxygen saturation may require hospitalization for chest tube placement and ongoing assessment of respiratory status and further supportive care.

COMPLICATIONS

The obvious complication of AGE is death; however, for those who survive the initial injury, long-term neurologic deficit is the most common complication. Short-term complications can follow from pulmonary compromise and result in difficulty maintaining oxygenation and hemodynamic stability.

MARINE ANIMAL BITES AND STINGS

The United States has 80,000 miles of coastline, and people are showing a greater interest in surfing, snorkeling, and scuba diving. A common source of injuries to divers is inadvertent contact with marine life. Bites and stings from sea creatures are common and range from annoying to life-threatening. These injuries usually require immediate treatment, but patients who sustain multiple or deep wounds or serious systemic illness will require follow-up by health care providers. This discussion is limited to some of the more common or toxic species found in the Western Hemisphere.

CLINICAL PRESENTATION AND PHYSICAL EXAMINATION

It is often not possible to identify the marine animal that caused the injury. Coral scrapes are the most commonly seen injuries. The soft living material on the surface of rough coral is easily deposited into a cut or scrape. This can cause inflammation, infection, and delayed wound healing. Treatment consists of initially scrubbing the wound with soap and water, then flushing with copious amounts of water. Flushing of the wound with half-strength hydrogen peroxide and covering it with an antibiotic ointment and dry sterile dressing further ensure a clean wound.[18]

The wound caused by the stingray is notable for severe and painful reactions. The stingray partially buries itself in the sandy bottom, where it can be accidentally stepped on. The animal then lashes out defensively with a whip-like appendage that carries stingers. The venom has vasoconstrictive properties that can complicate the healing of more severe wounds.[19] Milder and delayed reactions can include regional lymphadenopathy, fever, malaise, nausea, vomiting, and delirium. The wounds inflicted are most commonly mild (erythema only) but often extremely painful. More severe encounters can result in vesicle formation, cellulitis, and necrotic breakdown. Recovery can take months, especially if the wounds are complicated by secondary infection.[19]

Immediate care of stingray envenomation involves rinsing with fresh water and removal of any foreign body. Soaking in warm water for 30 to 60 minutes may relieve the pain. The wound should then be washed gently in soap and water. Further monitoring of the wound for infection or bleeding with follow-up care is necessary.[19]

The sting of the sculpin, a common member of the scorpion fish family found off the coast of southern California, produces severe pain and occasionally nausea and vomiting. The venom produces a protein that is rapidly broken down in the presence of heat. Treatment is immersion in water as hot as can be tolerated for 60 to 90 minutes. Once the pain is relieved, the wound should be flushed of debris, covered with a dressing, and monitored for infection.

Jellyfish have stinging cells called nematocysts that can continue to function even when they are separated from the organism or if the organism is dead. Jellyfish envenomation is quite painful, and the venom can cause cardiac, neurotoxic, or hemolytic reactions or necrotic skin wounds. Fatal anaphylaxis has been known to occur. First aid consists of removal of any adherent tentacles followed by a vinegar rinse. The wound is then washed with soap and water and treated with a topical hydrocortisone cream. Pain can be controlled with acetaminophen or ibuprofen. Antibiotics are usually not necessary.[19]

The Portuguese man-of-war, found in tropical and subtropical regions of the Pacific, in the northern Atlantic Gulf Stream, and in the Caribbean, is infamous for its painful sting and systemic manifestations. This animal has a "sail" that floats with the wind and often one or more tentacles that can extend 10 m (33 feet) or more and can be separated from the sail and drift invisibly toward the surface. Exposure to the tentacle and its powerful venom causes the injury. Symptoms include severe pain, vomiting, and occasionally difficulty breathing. Anaphylactic shock is treated with epinephrine and other supportive measures. First aid generally consists of copious flushing with either sea or fresh water, removal of visible tentacles with tweezers or a gloved hand, and applications of ice to control pain. Rubbing should be avoided, and the application of vinegar, often helpful for other marine animal stings, is not recommended. Removal of the tentacle can result in a larger wound which is prone to infection. Antibiotics may be necessary.[20]

INTERPROFESSIONAL COLLABORATIVE MANAGEMENT

Good and immediate first aid is essential to uncomplicated healing. This should include immediate assessment of the patient's general status, especially if there is airway, breathing, or circulatory compromise requiring stabilization or resuscitation.[19] Gentle removal of visible spines, control of bleeding, analgesia, and transport to the nearest emergency department are recommended initial treatments.

In the emergency department, stings are managed immediately by removal of tentacles and spines (if this was not done at the dive site) and irrigation of the area. Local anesthesia should be used. Open wounds require careful and thorough irrigation and debridement of foreign bodies. Heat treatment by immersion of the affected limb into water no hotter than 45.4°C (114°F) can be effective with specific envenomations (see earlier).[18]

Wound care is then directed toward healing without secondary infection. Skin irritations and itching can be treated with warm or cool compresses and mild steroid creams. The patient's tetanus status should be ascertained and vaccine administered if more than 10 years have elapsed since the last immunization. The primary health care provider can manage bites and stings if wound healing is uncomplicated. Referral for surgical debridement may be necessary for non-healing wounds.

WHEN AND WHERE TO REFER

Duke Dive Medicine can be reached by calling 919-684-8111. DAN can be contacted by calling their diving emergency hotline at 1-919-684-9111 (accepts collect calls). Always call local emergency medical services (EMS) first, if indicated, before calling for consultation. All patients with DCS and pulmonary barotrauma (dysbarism) must be stabilized and referred to the nearest recompression chamber for HBO treatment as soon as possible; however, referrals even greater than 24 hours after a dive have still resulted in treatment success and should be made even if the original diagnosis was not DCS.[17] Evaluation by a provider with training in undersea and hyperbaric medicine is preferred whenever possible. Patients with ear barotrauma may need to be seen and managed by an otolaryngologist, especially if they are not responding to conservative therapy. Those with potential round window rupture should be referred immediately. All patients with a history of DCS or pulmonary barotrauma should be evaluated and cleared by a provider trained in undersea and hyperbaric medicine before returning to diving.

PATIENT EDUCATION

All divers are required to complete a standard course in diving principles and first aid. Diving certification agencies have uniform standards established by the Recreational Scuba Training Council.[21] A basic life support certification is highly recommended. Extra training in the use of oxygen in an emergency is also recommended. Studies have found that intensive exercising 24 hours before diving and during decompression reduces the number of venous gas bubbles formed and may be protective against DCS.[22]

Divers should make every effort to avoid contact with marine life and wear protective clothing while diving. Venomous species are widespread throughout tropical, subtropical, and temperate waters, and the ability to visually identify these fish and wildlife is advised. Appropriate gear in cold water will help prevent hypothermia. Recreational divers are encouraged to use dive tables and computers conservatively.[4] Immunizations, especially tetanus, should be current.

DAN is a nonprofit organization that provides expert medical information to the diving public and to medical providers treating diving-related injuries, promotes and supports diving research, and maintains a 24-hour emergency telephone line for diving accidents. DAN can provide medical providers with the location of the nearest recompression chamber. Health care providers who encounter patients with possible diving-related injuries can use DAN for both emergent and non-emergent consultations and questions, especially for cases in which decompression injuries are suspected. Duke Dive Medicine also provides direct consultation for providers by board-certified hyperbaric physicians and fellows. Duke Dive Medicine can be reached by calling 919-684-8111. DAN can be contacted by calling their diving emergency hotline at 1-919-684-9111 (accepts collect calls). Always call local EMS first if indicated before calling for consultation. The DAN medical information line is 1-919-684-2948.

REFERENCES

1. Bove, A. A. (2014). Diving medicine. *American Journal of Respiratory and Critical Care Medicine, 189*(12), 1479–1486.
2. Mitchell, S. (2017, October). Fitness to Dive Assessment. Presented at NOAA/UHMS Physicians Training in Diving Medicine, Seattle, WA.
3. Driessen, J. M., van der Palen, J., van Aalderen, W. M., de Jongh, F. H., & Thio, B. J. (2012). Inspiratory airflow limitation after exercise challenge in cold air in asthmatic children. *Respiratory Medicine, 106*(10), 1362–1368.
4. Eichhorn, L., & Ley, K. D. (2015). Diving medicine in clinical practice. *Deutsches Ärzteblatt International, 112*(9), 147–158.
5. Honěk, J., Šrámek, M., Šefc, L., Januška, J., Fiedler, J., Horváth, M., et al. (2019). High-grade patent foramen ovale is a risk factor of unprovoked decompression sickness in recreational divers. *Journal of Cardiology*, https://doi.org/10.1016/j.jjcc.2019.04.014. ISSN 0914-5087.
6. EEde, M. V. (2016). Recurrent cutaneous decompression illness after PFO device implantation: A case report. *Undersea and Hyperbaric Medicine: Journal of the Undersea and Hyperbaric Medical Society, Inc, 43*(7), 841–845.
7. Buzzacott, P., & Denoble, P. J. (Eds.), (2018). *DAN Annual Diving Report 2018 Edition—A report on 2016 diving fatalities, injuries, and incidents* (p. 112). Durham, NC: Divers Alert Network. Retrieved from https://www.diversalertnetwork.org/medical/report/AnnualDivingReport-2018Edition.pdf. (Retrieved July 8, 2019).
8. Kay, E. (2016). Dive medicine. In C. Sanford & E. Jong (Eds.), *The travel and Tropical Medicine Manual ebook* (5th ed.). Elsevier Health Sciences. ISBN 9780323417426.
9. Cialone, D., Piere, M., Balestra, C., & Marrone, A. (2017). Dive risk factors, gas bubble and formation, and decompression illness in recreational SCUBA diving: Analysis of DAN Europe and DSL Data Bases. *Frontiers in Psychology, 8*, 1–11.
10. Cialone, D., Piere, M., Balestra, C., & Marrone, A. (2015). Flying after diving: Should the recommendations be reviewed? In flight echocardiographic study in bubble prone and bubble resistant divers. *Diving and Hyperbaric Medicine, 45*(1), 10–29.
11. U.S. Navy Diving Manual, Rev 7. (2016). Washington, DC: U.S. Government Printing Office. Retrieved from http://www.navsea.navy.mil/Portals/103/Documents/SUPSALV/Diving/US%20DIVING%20MANUAL_REV7.pdf?ver=2017-01-11-102354-393. (Accessed 8 May 2018).
12. Xu, W., Liu, W., Huang, G., Zou, Z., Cai, Z., & Xu, W. (2012). Decompression illness: Clinical aspects of 5278 consecutive cases treated in a single hyperbaric unit. *PLoS ONE, 7*(11), e50079.
13. Dardeau, M. R., Pollock, N. W., McDonald, C. M., & Lang, M. A. (2012). The incidence of decompression illness in 10 years of scientific diving. *Diving and Hyperbaric Medicine, 42*(4), 195–200.
14. Bove, A. A. (2014). Diving medicine. *American Journal of Respiratory and Critical Care Medicine, 189*(12), 1479–1486.
15. Pollock, N., & Buteau, D. (2017). Updates in decompression illness. *Emergency Medicine Clinics, 35*(2), 310–319.
16. Ranapurwala, S. I., Bird, N., Vaithiyanathan, P., & Denoble, P. S. (2014). SCUBA diving injuries among divers alert members, 2010–2011. *Diving and Hyperbaric Medicine, 44*(2), 79–85.
17. Perez, M. F., Ongkeko Perez, J. V., Serrano, A. R., Andal, M. P., & Aldover, M. C. (2017). Delayed hyperbaric intervention in life-threatening decompression illness. *Diving and Hyperbaric Medicine, 47*(4), 257–259.
18. Bolhara, K., & Stolbach, M. D. (2014). Marine envenomations. *Emergency Medicine Clinics of North America, 32*(1), 223–243.
19. Hornbeak, K. B., & Auerbach, P. S. (2017). Marine envenomation. *Emergency Medicine Clinics of North America, 35*(2), 321–337.
20. Parsons, K., & Rutledge, D. (2015). Stingray envenomation treatment recommendations. *The Journal for Nurse Practitioners: JNP, 11*(3), 360–363.
21. World Recreational SCUBA training council. https://wrstc.com/standards-downloads/. (Accessed 9 May 2018).
22. Gempp, E., & Blatteau, J. (2010). Preconditioning methods and mechanisms for preventing the risk of decompression sickness in SCUBA divers: A review. *Research in Sports Medicine, 18*(3), 205–218.

CHAPTER 202

FATIGUE

Dionna C. Rookey

DEFINITION AND EPIDEMIOLOGY

Fatigue is a common complaint, with 5% to 10% of primary care patients complaining of significant fatigue.[1] Although fatigue has been typified as having physical (neuromuscular), cognitive, and emotional components, the direction of the relationship among these domains and chronicity remain perplexing. For example, fatigue combined with irritability and depression is referred to as vital exhaustion and is implicated as a cardiovascular risk factor; by contrast, stroke has been associated with depression.[2]

Conceptual differences exist among frequently interchanged terms. Fatigue can be manifested as difficulty or inability to initiate activity (perception of weakness); reduced capacity to maintain activity (easy fatigability); and difficulty with concentration, memory, and emotional stability (mental fatigue). Fatigue should be distinguished from sleepiness, dyspnea, and muscle weakness, although these could be associated symptoms.[1] Sleepiness is the inclination toward sleep, usually despite an effort to avoid it. Insomnia signals trouble initiating or maintaining restorative sleep, which leads to tiredness.[3] Without adequate sleep, excessive daytime tiredness, neurocognitive impairment, metabolic irregularities, cardiac rhythm abnormalities, and affective disorders can arise.[4] Patients use a variety of terms to indicated their perceived fatigue such as sleepiness, weak, tired, worn out, or exhausted. Given that fatigue is described in multiple ways, some concern exists that it may be underreported because what is expressed by the patient versus what is recorded by the provider may differ significantly, and some patients may believe that reporting fatigue may not be helpful or they may have adjusted expectations to a reduced energy level.

It is helpful to establish acuity or chronicity, whether fatigue is a normal or abnormal response to situation or environment, and whether it is tied to unique psychoneuroimmunologic[5] or possibly genetic factors and/or associated with precedent comorbidities. Duration of fatigue can be recent (<1 month), prolonged (>1 month), or chronic (over 6 months). The presence of chronic fatigue does not necessarily imply myalgic encephalomyelitis/chronic fatigue syndrome (ME/CFS).

Fatigue as a major symptom is found in all populations and is associated with multiple factors. Medical (anemia, malignancy, serious somatic disease) or psychiatric diagnoses (depression) can explain fatigue in approximately 25% of patients with complaints of tiredness.[6] Older adults seem more likely to identify fatigue as an issue, with as many as 31% of men and 42% of women ages 75 to 84 reporting restricting fatigue.[7]

In one sample including 754 nondisabled community-dwelling older adults, 31.1% of men and 42.1% of women reported fatigue severe enough to affect lifestyle. Fatigue was more common in the physically frail and those who also had depression.[7] Despite the preponderance of fatigue among older adults, it bears consideration in the context of chronic sleep-related complaints, which are prevalent in more than 20% to 40% of individuals older than 65 years (see Chapter 206)[8]

As the projected number of elders rises, the cost-effectiveness with which such information is captured and managed will be critical, as fatigue affects functional outcomes—physical, cognitive, mood, and social.[8] A longitudinal study of 400 patients aged 65 years or older independently predicted an association between sleep apnea and all-cause mortality.[9]

PATHOPHYSIOLOGY

The pathophysiology of fatigue is entirely dependent on its cause. Given the subjective nature of this complaint, a careful review of symptoms and a physical examination are required. Fatigue researchers have focused on the neurobiology of immune activation and circadian dysfunction.[5] One increasingly well-recognized and reproducible phenomenon, considered adaptive in the face of infection or inflammatory disease, is called "sickness behavior." This incorporates "fatigue, depressive behavior, anhedonia, psychomotor slowing, anorexia, circadian alterations in sleep patterns and increased sensitivity to pain"[10,11] and is associated with ME, CFE, and other inflammatory syndromes.

Fatigue is the most often-voiced complaint among cancer patients of all ages. It is hypothesized that cancer-related fatigue is related to ongoing inflammation before and after therapy with associated genetic, biological, psychosocial, and behavioral risk factors.[12]

CLINICAL PRESENTATION AND PHYSICAL EXAMINATION

The history is the most important component of the evaluation of fatigue. Fatigue due to an underlying medical history of psychiatric disorder usually presents as one of several reported symptoms including exhaustion, weakness, anhedonia, and tiredness. A specific etiology for fatigue is found less frequently when fatigue itself is the principal concern and the patient presents with few or no other symptoms. A clinician should rely on open-ended questions, encouraging the patient to describe the fatigue in his or her own words. Patients with organ-based medical illness often associated their fatigue with activities they are unable to complete. By contrast, patients with fatigue that is not organ-based are tired all the time and their fatigue is not necessarily related to exertion nor improved with rest.

A system review should incorporate the effects of rest periods—such as bedtime sleep quality, need for naps, and weekend and vacation sleep—on the perceived state of fatigue. Fatigue may accompany self-limited infection, persist for months, accompany repeated hospitalizations, or accompany a precipitous decline in health status.

One common type of fatigue is physiologic, which arises from extraordinary demands on otherwise healthy individuals, such as poor sleep hygiene, peripartum status, and work or personal stress. Health-destructive practices, such as intentional sleep deprivation, a diet of nutritionally deficient foods, a sedentary lifestyle, and excessive intake of alcohol and caffeine or stimulant drugs, can also result in protracted fatigue. Inquiry into sleep environment, habits, and mood may also be helpful. This intake should include typical sleep challenges (such as bedtime irregularity, noise, room temperature, lack of privacy or safety, partner-related issues, and sleeping pattern disturbance) and the more global psychological disruptors of generalized anxiety, loneliness, vegetative symptoms, change in circumstances (e.g., recent loss, a new job), anorexia, hopelessness, and suicidal ideation.

A history of daytime sleepiness, falling asleep even when motivated to stay awake, shortness of breath or muscle weakness with activity, medication history, and use of tobacco and alcohol should be elicited.

A recent history of infection, hospitalization, head injury, or surgery may be important. Associated chronic pain, fever, rash, weight loss, frequent falls or balance issues, or other systemic symptoms should be noted. Patients with rheumatologic diseases often report fatigue as a prominent symptom. If fatigue increases during the day but is relieved by rest, rheumatologic or other organic causes, such as occult cardiovascular illness, warrant consideration.

A family or personal history of malignant neoplasms, diabetes, anemia, or other chronic illnesses should also be gathered.

A medication reconciliation should include prescribed, over-the-counter, and self-prescribed remedies, including alcohol, drugs, and herbals/vitamins. The use of caffeine, nicotine, amphetamines, cocaine, or CNS depressants needs to be elicited. Medications associated with fatigue include antipsychotics, cancer chemotherapeutics, calcium channel blockers, beta blockers, diuretics, phenobarbital, carbamazepine, antihistamines with anticholinergic effects, benzodiazepines, and sedative doses of tricyclic antidepressants. Psychosocial stressors contributing to fatigue can be overwhelming and clinically significant. Childhood trauma has been studied in association with low cortisol or adrenal dysfunction, which can be a component of chronic fatigue states, especially if inadequately managed in subset populations.[5] A history of psychological illness or substance use and associated treatments is valuable.

Despite a careful patient history, the cause of fatigue may be elusive. Fatigue as a normal part of aging is increasingly debunked, yet aging impacts physical function and pathology, be it subclinical disease, increased inflammation, physiologic dysregulation, or increased work in maintaining homeostasis.[7]

The physical examination is an adjunct to a thorough history of the complaint. Initially, habitus including weight, neck girth (a measure correlated with sleep apnea), speech, cognition, balance, and gait should be assessed. Measurements of temperature, postural blood pressure, and pulse, with attention to pulse character, may indicate postural hypotension or cardiac arrhythmia, which can precipitate fatigue. Skin should be examined for dryness, jaundice, pallor, petechiae, or lesions. Thinning hair, glossy tongue, poor skin turgor or wound healing, easy bruising, and body wasting can be signs of poor nutritional status. Thyromegaly and lymphadenopathy should be noted.

A complete examination of the cardiorespiratory system should be performed with attention to the presence of respiratory rales or consolidation determined by tactile fremitus and adventitious, irregular, or rapid breath sounds. Jugular venous distention, cardiac murmurs, or peripheral edema should be noted. The abdominal examination should carefully exclude ascites, bruits, organomegaly, and gastrointestinal bleeding. The extremities are examined for joint pain, swelling, range of motion, reflexes, and strength. Gait abnormalities are noted.

DIAGNOSTICS

The judicious use of blood testing within appropriate time intervals speaks to the need to strike a balance between degree of clinical suspicion and risk of increased false-positive results, especially in cases of new, unexplained fatigue. In the absence of suggestive history or symptoms, routine testing for infection

(Epstein-Barr virus, cytomegalovirus, or Lyme disease), inflammatory joint disease, vitamin deficiencies, or antibody studies for celiac disease is not usually recommended.[1]

Essential Diagnostics

Diagnostic investigation for chronic unexplained fatigue requires persistence because fatigue can be a manifestation of any number of organic diseases. Cancer-related anemia, iron-deficiency anemia, cardiac output reduction, infection, hypogonadism, hypothyroidism, hypercalcemia caused by hypoparathyroidism, and renal insufficiency bear noting. For patients with a suspected physical cause, generally useful laboratory studies are a complete blood count (CBC) with differential; chemistry profile including serum electrolyte values and serum glucose calcium, albumin, creatinine, and blood urea nitrogen (BUN) concentrations; liver enzymes; erythrocyte sedimentation rate (ESR); thyroid-stimulating hormone (TSH); urinalysis; and occult blood in stool. Patients thought to have CFS may undergo a more targeted list of tests to exclude other causes (see later).

Additional Diagnostics

Primary or secondary adrenal insufficiency would be implicated if peak cortisol and growth hormone responses after exogenous cortisol exposure are abnormal. Immunoglobulin levels, Lyme titer, rheumatoid factor, adrenocorticotropic hormone (ACTH), and serum creatine kinase muscle-brain fraction (CK-MB) might be added, depending on associated signs and symptoms. Any abnormality requires follow-up.

In addition, if prompted by the history and physical examination, a pharyngeal culture, Monospot test, syphilis titer, hepatitis panel, human immunodeficiency virus (HIV) test, or tuberculosis screening might be necessary. A chest x-ray examination is ordered for suspected lung, cardiac, or disseminated disease. For patients in whom postpolio syndrome is suspected, a nerve conduction study and electromyography can differentiate myasthenia gravis from other neuropathies that are central as opposed to peripheral. Considering central neurologic disorders, a brain MRI with gadolinium contrast for suspected multiple sclerosis (MS) would help narrow the diagnosis from among 30 or so mimics, including low vitamin B12 (include serum methylmalonic acid), lupus, and ischemia. Rarely, a lumbar puncture is indicated for a suspected infectious cause. The concern for sleep apnea requires overnight polysomnography and actigraphy to gauge the total number of apnea and hypopneic episodes per slept hour and may be useful in capturing periodic limb movements; however, it may not prove as useful in explaining symptoms of insomnia.[13]

All age- and history-appropriate cancer screenings, including breast, cervical, prostate, and colon, are recommended as well.

DIFFERENTIAL DIAGNOSIS

The differential diagnosis for fatigue can be divided into organic and non-organic causes. Non-organic includes environmental, idiopathic, psychiatric, physiologic, and situational. Organic (physical) includes any acute and chronic illness resulting from a host of systemic conditions.

The top four causes of fatigue are anemia (both iron deficiency and anemia of chronic disease), malignancy, serious somatic diseases (e.g., any chronic infectious disease, cardiac, pulmonary, hematologic, endocrine, rheumatologic, neuromuscular, skin, renal, immune, or CNS disorder that may

---

INITIAL DIAGNOSTICS

Fatigue

LABORATORY
- CBC and differential[a]
- Urinalysis[a]
- Chemistry profile (serum glucose, electrolytes, BUN, creatinine
- Thyroid function tests (TSH, free T4)[a]

ADDITIONAL LABORATORY
- Liver function tests (alanine transaminase, aspartate transaminase, alkaline phosphatase, total protein, albumin, globulin)[a]
- Antinuclear antibody[a]
- Rheumatoid factor[a,b]

- C-reactive protein[a]
- ESR
- Iron studies[b] (lactate dehydrogenase, ferritin, transferrin saturation)
- Vitamin B12 (and methylmalonic acid)
- Folate
- Fecal occult blood test
- Throat culture/monospot
- Purified protein derivative/tuberculin test[b]

IMAGING
- Chest x-ray
- Sleep polysonography

[a]Included in the workup for CFS as described by the Centers for Disease Control and Prevention (www.cdc.gov/cfs/disgnosis/index.html. Accessed February 02, 2015).
[b]If indicated.

---

individually or collectively contribute to fatigue); and psychiatric illness including depression, anxiety, and somatization.[6] Physiologic fatigue results from adverse external influences, such as poor sleep hygiene (see Chapter 206), substance use (see Chapter 227), and medication side effects.

Another source of chronic fatigue is the phenomenon of postpolio syndrome, which affects possibly 25% to 40% of the people worldwide,[14] who report a history of poliomyelitis. Symptoms of postpolio syndrome arise four to five decades after initial infection and may lead to muscle weakness and atrophy in previously affected muscle groups, pain, and fatigue. Fortunately, polio has been nearly eradicated worldwide since the introduction and refinements of vaccines developed in the 1950s.

Fibromyalgia, a diagnosis of exclusion based on self-reported generalized pain, fatigue, and cognitive symptoms, involves the joints, tendons, and muscles and is best treated in a interprofessional collaborative fashion (see Chapter 157).

Chronic fatigue accompanied by a 50% decrease in activity level (exclusive of all other medical and psychiatric explanations) warrants consideration of myalgic encephalomyelitis/chronic fatigue syndrome (ME/CFS), and postviral fatigue syndrome. ME/CFS is said to affect approximately 2 million people, women twice as often as men, usually between the ages of 30 and 40.[15] Prevalence ranges from 0.0007% to 2.8% of the general adult population.[16] The disorder takes an average of 5 years to diagnose, with low rates of improvement and much lower rates of cure. The criteria for diagnosis include: (1) marked, rapid physical and/or cognitive fatigability in response to exertion, (2) neurological impairments, (3) immune gastrointestinal and genitourinary impairments, and (4) energy production/transportation impairment.[17] Muscle or joint pain, headaches, sore throat, enlarged and painful lymph nodes, depression, sleep disturbances, and short-term memory loss or confusion severe enough to affect routine activity are common.

Recognizing that inflammatory fatigue shares features with CFS/ME and fibromyalgia, it has been termed "cytokine-induced sickness behavior."[10] Myofascial conditions and fibromyalgia (see Chapter 157) may be difficult to distinguish from ME/CFS. In fact, the controversy regarding labels marks fibromyalgia and ME/CFS as overlapping in 20% to 75% of cases.[18]

Fatigue often accompanies depression (see Chapter 226). Research on clinically diagnosed depression has established the contribution of neurotransmitters, including serotonin and norepinephrine. In addition, chronic anxiety or stress can lead to neck and shoulder muscle fatigue, irregular sleeping patterns, or irritable bowel symptoms. Depression is often identified along with fatigue-related illnesses. Post-stroke fatigue affects more than one third of stroke survivors and has been strongly associated with depressive and possibly anxiety disorders, with indication that locus of control and coping difficulties may contribute to this, as with cancer and MS.[2]

INTERPROFESSIONAL COLLABORATIVE MANAGEMENT

Non Pharmacologic Management

Physician consultation may be helpful in the evaluation of the patient with fatigue when symptoms elude explanation or treatment. Specialist involvement is dictated by suspected cause of the fatigue. Specialty referral is also indicated for progressive symptoms, lack of response to therapy, or indications of life-threatening illness. When fatigue is associated with acute depression, psychosis, cardiomyopathy, congestive heart failure, chronic obstructive pulmonary disease (COPD) exacerbation, or obstructive sleep apnea resulting from morbid obesity or anatomic abnormality, patients should be referred to the appropriate specialist or acute care setting.

Postpartum women with fatigue should be screened for anemia, thyroid and endocrine disorders, and urinary tract infections.

It is important to consider services available to the patient with a chronic fatigue condition (e.g., ME/CFS or postpolio syndrome), which greatly affects the quality of life and work. A mental health referral or referral to support groups is helpful. Cognitive behavioral therapy (CBT) and intensive endurance rehabilitation have been effective for adult outpatients with ME/CFS.

Cancer-related fatigue calls for integrative treatment, interprofessional collaboration and holistic, patient-centered care. Patients may be best served in a cancer center, where the needs of the patient and the patient's family are taken into account (see Chapter 221).

Physical and occupational therapy referral for exercise programs and energy conservation techniques can be helpful.

Pharmacologic Management

The patient with fatigue requires various degrees and types of support. The provider must acknowledge the fatigue as a valid complaint worthy of further exploration. Behavioral, situational, and environmental contributions to sleep disturbance should be identified for optimal improvement (see Chapter 206). Iron-deficiency anemia requires further work-up and treatment (see Chapter 216).

For ME/CFS, research has established what is not helpful—such as melatonin, methylphenidate, and citalopram—and what may be helpful including magnesium, possibly probiotics, low doses of antidepressants such as nortriptyline, and anti-inflammatory and mild analgesics. In ME/CFS, the most strongly associated therapeutic benefit derives from graduated exercise and CBT.[19]

A patient with primary sleep disorder should be referred to a sleep disorder clinic. When poor sleep arises in the setting of clinically assessed depression, antidepressant medication might help both. When generalized anxiety disorder is identified, use of benzodiazepines other than on a short-term basis is discouraged in favor of buspirone, other antidepressants such as venlafaxine, and atypical antipsychotics, to avoid dependency. Cancer-related fatigue might respond to methylphenidate, 5 mg daily, or other psychostimulants, but the range of causes is wide and includes malnutrition, dehydration, electrolyte shifts, anemia, hypoxia, organ failure or insufficiency, emboli, and cardiopulmonary compromise, as well as adverse effects of treatment, physical limitations caused by disease and/or pain, and psychosocial effects.[20] Within this complexity, any modifiable causes, such as anemia and anorexia-cachexia, should be identified and addressed. Sometimes barriers to treatment reflect providers' lack of knowledge in treating cancer-related fatigue or overemphasis on pain management. Additionally, the patient's understanding of his or her fatigue may prevent the patient from asking for more help.[20]

A regimen of both muscle strengthening and aerobic exercise is thought to improve cardiovascular functioning, depth of sleep, and sense of well-being. For cancer-related fatigue, studies showed small to moderate improvements. A moderate-to high-intensity level aerobic and muscle strengthening exercise regimen of 150 minutes per week, using major muscle groups two or three times a week, showed a greater benefit to cancer patients than aerobic exercises alone, as did a supervised program as opposed to home-based exercise.[11] Individuals with chronic muscle fatigue and joint pain can influence the onset and toll of their illness by maintaining normal weight; avoiding exercising to the point of muscle pain; keeping body temperature warmer than air temperature (to avoid the muscle tension associated with cold); and using stress reduction, energy conservation, and time management techniques. The provider can empower the patient to have a sense of control over the situation by encouraging him or her to network, to read relevant publications, and to attend support group meetings.

CBT has also been used with success. Work on downplaying negative associations with fatigue is part of the treatment. In fact, overemphasis on making up lost sleep or focused effort on resting can cause hyperarousal.[3]

Modafinil has been associated with improvement in post-stroke and HIV-related fatigue[1] as well as in subsets of cancer patients with severe fatigue.[3,11]

LIFE SPAN CONSIDERATIONS

A patient's age and life span stressors influence the evaluation for fatigue. Teenagers and newly independent young adults should be screened for deleterious health habits, given that they have a tendency toward experimentation with alcohol, drugs, irregular sleep, and poor nutrition. Transitions and losses resulting from changes such as marriage or the death of a loved one can be destabilizing. Situational depression or anxiety accompanies these developmental transitions and can cause fatigue.

Postpartum women are at risk for debilitating fatigue. Blood loss at the time of delivery coupled with sleep deprivation and the demands of caring for a newborn can contribute to profound fatigue. Concerned family members may be the first ones to approach the practitioner with concerns about a postpartum patient. Perimenopausal women may also complain of fatigue. Vasomotor symptoms can affect sleep, for which serotonin receptor blockers have helped; and in some cases, metrorrhagia can cause significant anemia, for which iron supplementation might help.

COMPLICATIONS

Complications of fatigue include daytime sleepiness, risk of injury or accident, poor performance, and cognitive and functional impairment in managing independent activities of daily living. A driving evaluation that includes a road test ensures the appropriateness of continued driving and protects both the driver and the public from accident or injury. In addition, individuals with chronic illnesses, including MS, fibromyalgia, and ME/CFS, are especially vulnerable to depression, whether it is considered organic, disease driven, or situational. A depression inventory including questions about suicidal ideation and substance use is crucial because the risks are higher among these particular groups.

EDUCATION AND HEALTH PROMOTION

The patient may find keeping a fatigue diary useful. Recording the time of onset, duration, severity, accompanying symptoms, relief measures, exercise, mood, diet, medications, alcohol and substance use, and stressors not only helps the health care provider but will also be helpful if future consultation is necessary.

For the subset of patients who are physically disabled by fatigue, employment considerations might require referral to a vocational counselor. A patient may wish to apply for up to 12 weeks of a temporary employment hiatus through the federal Family Medical Leave Act, workers' compensation for an employment-related injury, job reassignment, prepaid short- and long-term disability through work, or government-administered long-term disability.

It is important to acknowledge fatigue as a legitimate symptom of various underlying illnesses. Fatigue in and of itself should be managed using traditional medical approaches as well as alternative therapies. The importance of proper nutrition, sleep, and exercise should be stressed to patients of all ages in concrete terms. This approach bolsters health, assists in maintaining an optimum quality of life, and protects against debilitating stressors and communicable illnesses.

Fatigue is not necessarily part of aging in the healthy adult. Infectious, allergic, inflammatory, malignant, mood, or cognitive causes may be the root cause requiring that fatigue concerns be investigated, particularly if the fatigue is associated with lymph node enlargement or pain, weight loss, muscle aches, sore throat, headache, night sweats, or other troublesome constitutional symptoms.

REFERENCES

1. Wright, J., & O'Connor, K. (2014). Fatigue. *The Medical Clinics of North America, 98*(3), 597–698.
2. Wu, S., Barugh, A., Macleod, M., et al. (2014). Psychological association of post stroke fatigue: A systematic review and meta-analysis. *Stroke; a Journal of Cerebral Circulation, 45,* 1778–1783.
3. Davis, M. P., & Goforth, H. (2014). Fighting insomnia and battling lethargy; the yin and yang of palliative care. *Current Oncology Reports, 16*(377), 1–18.
4. Tamanna, S., & Geraci, S. A. (2013). Major sleep disorders among women (women's health series). *Southern Medical Journal,* 470–478.
5. Hyland, M. E. (2017). A new paradigm to explain functional disorders and the adaptive network theory of chronic fatigue syndrome and fibromyalgia syndrome. In G. B. Sullivan, J. Cresswell, B. Ellis, M. Morgan, & E. Schraube (Eds.), *Resistance and renewal in theoretical psychology* (pp. 21–31). Concord, ON: Captus University Publications.
6. Stadj, R., Dornieden, K., Baum, E., et al. (2016). The differential diagnosis of tiredness: A systematic review. *BMC Family Practice, 17,* 147. Retrieved from https://doi.org/101186/s12875-016-05455. (Accessed 4 January 2018).
7. Rekneire, N., Leo-Summers, L., Han, L., & Gill, T. (2014). Epidemiology of restricting fatigue in older adults: The precipitating events project. *Journal of the American Geriatrics Society, 62*(3), 476–481.
8. Gooneratne, N., & Vitiello, M. (2014). Sleep in older adults—normative changes, sleep disorders and treatment options. *Clinics in Geriatric Medicine, 30*(3), 591–627.
9. Marshall, N., Wong, K., Cullen, S., et al. (2014). Sleep apnea and 20 year follow-up for all-cause mortality, stroke and cancer incidence and mortality in the Busselton Health Study cohort. *Journal of Clinical Sleep Medicine: Official Publication of the American Academy of Sleep Medicine, 10*(4), 355–362.
10. Karshikoff, B., Sundelin, T., & Lasselin, J. (2017). Role of inflammation in human fatigue. *Front. Immunol.* https://www.frontiersin.org/articles/10.3389/fimmu.2017.00021/full. (Accessed 9 July 2019).
11. Shattuck, E. C., & Muehlenbein, M. P. (2015). Human sickness behavior: Ultimate and proximate explanations. *American Journal of Physical Anthropology, 157,* 1–18. doi:10.1002/ajpa.22698.
12. Bower, J. (2014). Cancer-related fatigue—mechanisms, risk factors, and treatments. *Nature Reviews. Clinical Oncology, 11,* 597–609.
13. Arnold, J., Sunilkumar, M., Krishna, V., et al. (2017). Obstructive sleep apnea. *Journal of Pharmacy and Bioallied Sciences, 9*(suppli), s26–s28.
14. Groce, N. E., Banks, L. M., & Stein, M. A. (2014). Surviving polio in a post-polio world. *Social Science and Medicine, 107,* 171–178.
15. Dimmock, M., Mirin, A., & Jason, L. (2016). Estimating the disease burden of ME/CFS in the United States and its relation to research funding. *Journal of Medicine and Therapeutics, 1*(6), 1–7.
16. Vincent, A., Brimmer, D. J., Whipple, M. O., et al. (2012). Prevalence, incidence, and classification of chronic fatigue syndrome in Olmsted County, Minnesota as estimated using the Rochester Epidemiology Project. *Mayo Clinic Proceedings. Mayo Clinic, 87*(12), 1145–1152.
17. Curruthers, B. M., van de Sande, M. I., Meirleir, K. L., et al. (2011). Myalgic encepholomyelitis: International consensus criteria. *Journal of Internal Medicine, 270*(4), 327–338.
18. Abbi, B., & Natelson, B. H. (2013). Is chronic fatigue syndrome the same illness as fibromyalgia? Evaluating the "single syndrome" hypothesis. *Quarterly Journal of Medicine, 106,* 3–9.
19. Smith, M. E. B., Nelson, H., Haney, E., et al. (2014). Diagnosis and treatment of myalgic encephalomyelitis/chronic fatigue syndrome. Agency for Health Care Research and Quality. Report No:15-E001-EF. Retrieved from https://www.ncbi.nih.gov/books/NBK293931 on Jan 5, 2018.
20. Koornstra, R. H. T., Peters, M., Donofrio, S., et al. (2014). Management of fatigue in patients with cancer—a practical overview. *Cancer Treatment Reviews, 40,* 791–799.

CHAPTER **203**

FEVER
Elizabeth A. Talbot

In primary care, a clinical encounter with a febrile patient can be challenging because of the many causes of fever, ranging from the familiar to esoteric infectious diseases to diverse noninfectious causes, and because the causes of fever range in severity from self-limited to imminently life-threatening. This chapter defines fever, clarifies the types and patterns of fever, provides an approach to evaluation of the febrile patient within primary care, reviews special circumstances such as fever of unknown origin (FUO) and fever in young children, and provides principles for empiric management.

 Hospitalization may be indicated if the patient is unable to maintain hydration, is hemodynamically unstable, or has a suspected infection that can lead to rapid clinical deterioration, such as endocarditis, necrotizing fasciitis, or bacterial meningitis.

DEFINITIONS AND PATHOPHYSIOLOGY

Fever, or pyrexia, is a state of elevated core temperature resulting from a physiologic change in set point that is often part of the patient's defensive response.

Fever is a distinct syndrome from hyperthermia, which is defined as an increase in body temperature that surpasses the body's ability to dissipate heat.[1] Hyperthermia can be precipitated by high environmental temperatures (as in heat stroke), strenuous physical exercise (exertional heat stroke), illicit drugs (cocaine, LSD, methamphetamine), and reactions to various prescribed medications.[1] Thyroid storm may be associated with hyperthermia and manifest as delirium, seizures, coma, vomiting, diarrhea, jaundice, congestive heart failure, and cardiac dysrhythmias.[1] In further contrast, hypothermia is body temperature of 36°C (97°F) or lower, which can result from exposure to a cold environment, hypothyroidism, uremia, and overwhelming infection. The last scenario usually signifies a patient's inability to mount an appropriate fever, which is a poor prognostic sign.

Hyperpyrexia refers to a temperature in excess of 41.5°C (106.7°F). This life-threatening state is most commonly caused by central nervous system (CNS) hemorrhage and serious infections.[1] A temperature of 41°C (105.8°F) may lead to brain damage, whereas a temperature in excess of 43°C (109.4°F) is invariably fatal.

Fever may occur in response to invasive microorganisms or inanimate matter recognized as alien by the host. Among noninfectious causes of elevated temperature, there are several characteristic clinical clues, as well as syndromic presentations.

- Heat stroke
  - Elevated temperature with lack of sweating in high environmental temperatures
- Exertional heat stroke
  - Elevated temperature in high environmental temperatures
- Nonexertional heat stroke
  - Medication effect
  - Iatrogenic diuresis with limited or no access to free water
  - Anticholinergic agents or anti-Parkinson medications
- Malignant hyperthermia
  - Autosomal dominant hereditary condition
  - Hyperthermia, muscular rigidity, and hemodynamic instability that occurs during general anesthesia
- Neuroleptic malignant syndrome
  - Withdrawal of CNS dopaminergic agents or receiving antidopaminergic agents
  - Hyperthermia, severe muscular rigidity, "lead pipe rigidity"
  - Mental status change, dysautonomia, hyporeflexia
- Serotonin syndrome
  - Serotonin toxicity
  - Fever, delirium, myoclonus, hyperreflexia

A patient is often aware of being febrile because he or she feels either abnormally cold or warm, lethargic, and otherwise unwell; myalgias, chills, or headache are not uncommon. Occasionally, however, the patient is unaware of being febrile and may present asymptomatically or because of concerns for another symptom or symptoms.

Diagnosing a patient with fever is predicated on defining normal body temperature, appreciating inherent host variability, and accounting for limitations to accurate temperature measurement. Regarding normal body temperature, research shows that 36.8°C (98.2°F) ± 1°C (1.8°F) is closer to normal for most healthy people.[2] In addition, a healthy person's body temperature fluctuates during the day. Diurnal variation may be as much as 1°C, with temperatures highest in the early evening and lowest in the early morning.[2,3] Normal body temperature also varies by sex and age with women showing a slightly higher temperature than men, especially when ovulating.[4] Older adults and those with certain chronic illness such as chronic liver or kidney disease tend to run lower temperatures.[5]

CLINICAL PRESENTATION AND DIFFERENTIAL DIAGNOSIS

As primary care clinicians know well, febrile episodes are often mild and self-limited. However, a minority are caused by serious conditions including infection, malignancy, adverse reactions to medication or blood products, connective tissue disease, and venous thromboembolic disease (to name just a few). The history and associated signs and symptoms often make the cause of these serious fevers obvious. But when the cause is not obvious, the broader differential diagnosis must be informed by information about both the patient and location-specific disease epidemiology.

The clinician should interview the patient to obtain a thorough history, including complete details of the fever pattern (Table 203.1) and associated symptoms. The fever pattern should be elucidated—when it began, how high it has been, and how it fluctuates during the day. Though rarely sufficient for a diagnosis, this history may provide key diagnostic clues.[6,7] For example, high fever with relative bradycardia (also known as sphygmothermic dissociation or Faget's sign) may suggest certain bacterial infections such as typhoid or leptospirosis or viral infections such as yellow fever, in the right clinical context. A relapsing fever pattern may suggest an infection caused by *Borrelia* or *Streptobacillus* organisms. Cough, weight loss, lymphadenopathy, and a hectic fever may raise consideration of tuberculosis (TB) or lymphoma.

TABLE 203.1   Fever Patterns

Fever Patterns	Description
Sustained or continuous	Constant elevation daily
Intermittent	Normal temperature at least once daily
Remittent	Temperature down but not to normal
Relapsing	Elevated temperature interspersed with long periods of normal temperature
Hectic	Widely fluctuating temperature
Relative bradycardia	Elevated temperature without expected elevation in pulse rate. This is historically known as sphygmothermic dissociation or Faget's sign.
Central fever	Elevated temperature related to central nervous system damage (malignancy, trauma, hemorrhage)
Factitious fever	False reporting of elevated temperature (report of fever by afebrile patient or intentionally caused infection manifesting true fever [Munchausen])

Physical examination signs that might suggest the cause of a fever should be diligently sought. Skin, sinus, nasal, ear, dental, and throat examinations are essential. Regional lymph node enlargement suggests a localized infectious process, whereas generalized lymphadenopathy may suggest systemic infection such as HIV infection or malignant disease such as lymphoma. Detection of a new or evolving heart murmur, especially in the setting of classic stigmata such as conjunctival hemorrhages, splinter hemorrhages, Osler nodes, or Janeway lesions, is a valuable clue to endocarditis. Adventitious or asymmetric breath sounds may indicate pneumonia, pulmonary emboli, or pleural effusions. An abdominal mass, hepatosplenomegaly, or tenderness should prompt investigation for an abdominal source of fever. Calf tenderness with a palpable vascular cord is evidence of thrombophlebitis. An abnormal joint examination can suggest osteomyelitis, infectious arthritis, or autoimmune arthritis. Breast, pelvic, penile, and rectal examinations are indicated when infections or neoplasms are suspected.

Exposures to animals and animal products may be relevant within the story told by a febrile patient. Rabies, cat-scratch disease (bartonellosis), pasteurellosis, toxoplasmosis, leptospirosis, anthrax, brucellosis, psittacosis, and rat-bite fever are febrile illness associated with animal or animal product exposure. Tick exposure is increasingly relevant as Lyme disease becomes epidemic in a wider geographic range. Babesiosis, ehrlichiosis, and Rocky Mountain spotted fever can also follow tick bites (see Chapter 213). Mosquito bites may lead to febrile illness caused by the arboviruses, including West Nile virus, eastern equine encephalitis, chikungunya, zika, and others (see Chapter 215). Arboviral disease is usually mandatorily reported by your public health authorities, and specialized testing should be coordinated with the public health jurisdiction.

Discovery that a febrile patient has recently traveled to the tropics significantly broadens the infectious disease differential diagnosis of fever. Because most primary care clinicians do not routinely practice tropical medicine, such a differential diagnosis may be daunting. However, excellent surveillance data show that many of the classic tropical infectious diseases, including Japanese encephalitis, Rift Valley fever, Ebola, Chagas disease, African trypanosomiasis, and yellow fever, are extremely rare in ill returning travelers.[8,9] Although unusual in the United States during summer months, influenza circulates year-round in most of the tropics and may be the most common vaccine-preventable disease acquired during travel.[10]

A rational approach to fever in the returning traveler begins with documenting the exact travel itinerary, and detailing symptom onset in relation to that travel itinerary. This first allows checking the endemicity of certain diseases (e.g., Japanese encephalitis does not occur in Kashmir, India), which facilitates pathogen identification based on possible incubation periods. For example, the sudden onset of fever and headache in the midst of a 1-week trip to Port au Prince, Haiti, suggests either a viral illness with short incubation (e.g., dengue, chikungunya) or an infection acquired even before travel (e.g., influenza from the traveler's family prior to the trip) but not malaria, which has a longer than several-day incubation. You should obtain the traveler's history of pre-travel vaccinations and underlying immune status; malaria chemoprophylaxis and other medications used abroad; exposures while abroad including animals, insect bites, and types of food and water consumed; as well as any intercourse without barrier protection (i.e., a condom).

The most important tropical disease in a febrile returning traveler is malaria, because it can be life-threatening. Dengue virus is more common than malaria but is usually self-limited.[11] A rapidly emerging global pathogen—chikungunya virus infection—should be considered even in primary care settings in a patient with acute onset of fever and polyarthralgia, especially in the traveler recently returned from areas with known virus transmission, such as Africa, Asia, Europe, India, and the Pacific Ocean islands. In late 2013, large outbreaks of chikungunya virus were identified widely in the Caribbean. Although chikungunya virus is not currently endemic in the United States, provisional data from CDC includes 114 cases in infected ill returned travelers in 2017 (see Chapter 215). This presents risk for autochthonous (local) transmission where the competent vector mosquito (e.g., *Aedes albopictus*) survives in the U.S. Typhoid fever, tularemia, extraintestinal amebiasis, and TB should also be considered for the patient with a clinically compatible febrile illness.

Immunocompromised states include bone marrow transplantation, human immunodeficiency virus (HIV) infection, malignancy, or drug-induced immune dysfunction (such as chemotherapy or corticosteroid use). The immunocompromised febrile patient especially requires a thorough history and physical exam. Of course, this is true of all patients who present with potentially serious diseases, but, in this vulnerable population, subtle symptoms and physical findings may have great significance. Include a careful exam of the entire skin surface (including the intertriginous and skin fold areas), tympanic membranes, sinuses, oral cavity, perianal region, and intravenous catheter sites. Assuming the H+P does not provide the diagnosis, these patients have a broad differential diagnosis, including infections that may not be serious in immunocompetent patients, and may require empiric therapy while testing is underway.

The clinician must elicit any history of a recent surgical procedure or implantation of a foreign body, including joint prostheses and urinary or intravascular catheters, and their presence should direct the initial diagnostic investigation. A review of the patient's current immunizations, evaluations for *Mycobacterium tuberculosis* infection (tuberculin skin test or interferon-γ release assay [IGRA]), and recent past infections can be helpful. For example, a history of otitis media, urinary tract infection, or pneumonia may signify progressive infections such as mastoiditis, renal abscess, or empyema, respectively.

A detailed medication history is vital in the evaluation of fever because many medications can cause fever either syndromically, as with neuroleptic malignant syndrome (NMS) or serotonin syndrome, or as "drug fever" (see Table 203.1). Commonly implicated classes of medications that cause drug fever include antihypertensives, antiarrhythmic medications, antibiotics, thyroid medications, and antiepileptics. Drug fever occurs at any time from shortly after initiation to years after initiation of a medication. Occasional clues to the diagnosis of drug fever are eosinophilia, rash, mild transaminitis, or elevated erythrocyte sedimentation rate (ESR), but more often drug fever is a diagnosis of exclusion. Stopping an implicated drug usually results in defervescence within 72 hours, and the fever resumes if the drug is restarted.[12]

Epidemiologic information about locally circulating illnesses and reported exposures to ill persons greatly informs the differential diagnosis of fever. Obviously, in the absence of travel or contact with a traveler, locally and seasonally prevalent diseases should be predominantly considered. For example, a normal host who develops a community-acquired prolonged febrile cough illness in the winter in New England should prompt testing for pertussis before testing for tuberculosis (TB). The state, county, city, or local health department can serve as a resource for providers regarding local disease epidemiology. This is especially true of reportable diseases, but public health officials often are aware of outbreaks or the circulation of nonreportable diseases as well, such as the arrival of seasonal influenza, a school varicella outbreak, or the occurrence of a summer cluster of enteroviral meningoencephalitis.

Diagnostics

Essential Diagnostics. For a patient with fever without a clear cause, a reasonable initial diagnostic maneuver may include a complete blood count (CBC) with differential white count examination. Elevated numbers and proportion of neutrophilic granulocytes may indicate bacterial infection. Lymphocytes are classically elevated on the differential with some viral infections and, of course, with lymphocytic leukemia. Elevated monocytes can strongly suggest mononucleosis, but there are other infections and conditions in which monocytosis can be seen. Eosinophils classically suggest a parasitic infection, asthma, or allergy. Liver function tests, urinalysis, blood and other potential source cultures, and C-reactive protein (CRP) and ESR are also typical diagnostics to suggest diagnoses and to confirm a systemic process. The ESR is a sensitive but nonspecific test. However, when the patient's ESR is greater than 100 mm/h, the possibility of osteomyelitis, endocarditis, temporal arteritis, or other rheumatologic diseases is increased.

Additional Diagnostics. Serologic testing is reserved for when the history and physical examination suggest a specific diagnosis. Computed tomography and magnetic resonance imaging may be useful for detection of abscesses or mass lesions. Echocardiography is mandatory if there are cardiac findings, persistent bacteremia, or stigmata, which all may be consistent with endocarditis. *M. tuberculosis* testing should be conducted when there is epidemiologic risk such as birth or travel to endemic setting, work in healthcare, or potential exposure in a prison or homeless shelter.

INITIAL DIAGNOSTICS

Fever

LABORATORY
- CBC with differential
- Liver function test
- Urinalysis and urine culture
- Blood cultures (before antibiotic administration)

IMAGING
- Chest X-ray

ADDITIONAL DIAGNOSTICS

Laboratory
- ESR, CRP
- Comprehensive metabolic profile

Imaging
- MRI or CT scan
- FDG-PET/CT
- Echocardiogram

Other
- TB testing

Fever of Unknown Origin

In contrast to simple fever without a recognized cause, there are clearly defined syndromes of fever of unknown origin (FUO). Specific varieties of FUO include nosocomial FUO (fever not present or incubating on admission to a health care facility) and immune-deficient FUO (fever occurring in an immunocompromised patient), with a specific example of immune-deficient FUO including HIV-associated FUO.[12] The most common FUO in primary care settings is the classic FUO, defined as temperature in excess of 38.3°C (101°F) persisting beyond 3 weeks for which intensive investigation fails to yield a diagnosis.[13] This intensive investigation is defined as 3 days of hospitalization, three outpatient visits, or 1 week of intensive outpatient investigations.

Studies show that most causes of classic FUO in adults are atypical presentations of common diseases, rather than rare diseases.[12] Recent studies report that infectious causes (such as TB, occult abscesses, and bacterial endocarditis) account for 15% to 30% of FUO; neoplastic processes (especially lymphoma, leukemia, and renal cell carcinoma) account for 10% to 30%; connective tissue diseases, 33% to 40%; miscellaneous (drug fever, hyperthyroidism, and factitious fever), 5% to 14%; and undiagnosed causes, 20% to 30%.[12,13]

In children, fever represents 10% to 25% of pediatric emergency department visits and is one of the most common reasons for a visit to the primary care provider. FUO in pediatric patients is more likely caused by infection than malignancy. Although most causes are self-limited viral illnesses, the incidence of other serious bacterial illnesses has been estimated at 6% to 10% in infants younger than 3 months and 5% to 7% in children 3 to 36 months of age.[14] Important noninfectious causes of FUO in the pediatric population are systemic onset juvenile arthritis and Takayasu arteritis. Hereditary periodic fever syndromes such as familial Mediterranean fever or hyperimmunoglobulin D syndrome can also cause fever in children and adults.[14]

Diagnostics

By the time a patient has met the definition for FUO, many standard laboratory evaluations and imaging studies have already been completed. More invasive evaluation, such as lumbar puncture, bone marrow, temporal artery, or liver biopsy, should be sought when clinical and laboratory findings implicate these systems as potential sources. Recent clinical data support the use of 18-fluoro-2-deoxyglucose positron emission tomography-computed tomography (FDG-PET/CT) in the workup of FUO but only when the patient has elevated ESR or CRP.[13,15] If applied early during the diagnostic algorithm, it was also cost-effective.[16]

INTERPROFESSIONAL COLLABORATIVE MANAGEMENT

Nonpharmacologic Management

Physical methods, such as sponging with cool water or alcohol and applying cold packs or cooling blankets, may be effective but are generally not considered first-line interventions.

Pharmacologic Management

Treatment of the underlying cause of a patient's fever is ultimately the best treatment for fever. Ideally, this treatment is directed, such as antibiotic therapy for an identified bacterial infection. In some circumstances, however, treatment must be empirical pending diagnosis. For example, there are algorithms that guide the empirical treatment of neutropenic patients with fever.[17]

Surprisingly, though, there is no clear consensus as to whether fever itself should be suppressed with antipyretics. Fever is an adaptive response that has widely evolved among most members of the animal kingdom, strongly suggesting an adaptive role for fever.[18] Many experimental data suggest that fever is associated with improved outcome in infection, and some data suggest that suppression of fever may delay recovery from infection.[18]

Despite some controversy, there are situations in which fever should definitely be treated. For example, any patient whose temperature exceeds 41°C (105.8°F) should immediately be treated with antipyretics and cooling measures to avoid brain damage.[1] Children are more susceptible to the harmful effects of elevated temperatures, manifesting seizures particularly at younger ages (3 months to 5 years). Patients with underlying cardiovascular disease may not tolerate the increased metabolic demands of prolonged high fever: an increase of 1°C (1.8°F) in temperature increases the basal metabolic rate by more than 10%.[1] In many settings of fever and identified infection, antipyretics can be given at regular intervals for symptomatic relief.

Antipyretic drugs include steroids, aspirin and other nonsteroidal anti-inflammatory drugs, and acetaminophen. Acetaminophen is usually the first line of treatment for fever. The risk of Reye's syndrome makes aspirin contraindicated in children.

In the absence of increased water intake, fever produces dehydration. It can cause confusion, delirium, and seizures and be associated with anorexia. Therefore, treatment for fever should also include close attention to maintenance of hydration and nutrition.

LIFE SPAN CONSIDERATIONS

Fever is a common presenting complaint of children and infants seen in emergency departments. In 2017, the American College of Emergency Physicians updated its clinical policy for children coming to the emergency department with fever.[19] The policy applies to healthy full-term infants and children between the ages of 1 day and 24 months. Guidance that may be useful in primary care includes that febrile infants between the ages of 1 and 28 days should always be presumed to have a serious bacterial infection. A chest radiograph is no longer routinely recommended for febrile children younger than 3 months and for older children who have high temperatures (>39°C [102.2°F]) and a white blood cell count elevated above 20 000/mm³. Urinalysis and urine culture are recommended for children with a temperature above 39° (102.2°). Empirical antibiotics may be appropriate for previously healthy, well-appearing children aged 3 to 24 months with a temperature of 39°C or higher and a white blood cell count of 15 000/mm³ or higher, especially if meningitis, encephalitis, or severe sepsis is suspected.[20]

Older adults are less likely to develop the high fevers of childhood; some older adults, even those with severe infections, may not be able to mount a febrile response at all. Hypothermia is common in this age group because of failing hypothalamic thermoregulatory systems.

PATIENT AND FAMILY EDUCATION

- Patients should be advised to call the health care provider for a temperature higher than 38.6°C (101.5°F) for more than 24 hours.
- Immunosuppressed patients, including those with acquired immunodeficiency syndrome (AIDS) and those taking chemotherapeutic medications, should be brought to medical attention if they have a temperature above 37.8°C (100°F).
- Parents should be especially cautioned against the use of aspirin in their febrile children because of risk of Reye's syndrome.[1]

REFERENCES

1. Dinarello, C. A., & Porat, R. (2012). Fever and hyperthermia. In A. S. Fauci (Ed.), *Harrison's principles of internal medicine* (18th ed.). New York: McGraw-Hill.
2. IUPS Commission for Thermal Physiology. (2001). Glossary of terms for thermal physiology, third edition. *The Japanese Journal of Physiology, 51,* 245–280.
3. Nivan, D. J., Gaydet, J. E., Laupland, K. B., et al. (2015). Accuracy of peripheral thermometers for estimating temperature: A systematic review and meta analysis. *Annals of Internal Medicine, 163,* 768–777.
4. McCance, K. L., & Huether, S. E. (2013). *Pathophysiology: The biological basis for disease in adults and children* (7th ed.). St Louis: Elsevier.
5. Webster, A. L., Dunlop, O., Melby, K. K., et al. (2013). Age related differences in symptoms, diagnosis and prognosis of bacteremia. *BMC Infectious Diseases, 13,* 346.
6. McGee, S. (2012). Temperature. In *Evidence-based physical diagnosis* (3rd ed.). Philadelphia: Elsevier.
7. Kotlyar, S., & Rice, B. T. (2013). Fever in the returning traveler. *Emergency medicine clinics of North America, 31*(4), 927–944.
8. Freedman, D. O., Weld, L. H., Kozarsky, P. E., et al. (2006). Spectrum of disease and relation to place of exposure among ill returned travelers. *The New England Journal of Medicine, 354,* 119–130.
9. Wilson, M. E. (2018). Fever in Returned Travelers. Retrieved from wwwnc.cdc.gov/traveler/yellowbook/2018/post-travel-evaluation/fever-in-returned-travelers, April 15.
10. Influenza Prevention: Information for Travelers 2018. (2018). Retrieved from https://www.cdc.gov/flu/travelers/travelersfacts.htm. April 15.
11. Feder, H. M., Jr., & Mansilla-Rivera, K. (2013). Fevers in returning travelers: A case-based approach. *American Family Physician, 88*(8), 524–530.
12. Fernandez, C., & Beeching, N. (2018). Pyrexia of unknown origin. *Clinical Medicine, 18*(2), 170–174.
13. Fletcher, T. E., Bleeker-Rovers, C., & Beeching, N. J. (2017). Fever. *Medicine, 45*(3), 177–183.
14. Arora, A., & Mahajan, P. (2013). Evaluation of child with fever without source: Review of literature and update. *Pediatric Clinics of North America, 60*(5).
15. Kouijzer, I. J. E., Mulders-Manders, C. M., Bleeker-Rovers, C. P., et al. (2018). Fever of unknown origin: The diagnostic value of FDG-PET/CT. *Seminars in Nuclear Medicine, 48,* 100–107.
16. Becerra Nakayo, E. M., Garcia Vicente, A. M., Soriano Castrejob, A. M., et al. (2011). Analysis of cost-effectiveness in the diagnosis of fever of unknown origin and the role of (18)F-FDG PET-CT: A proposal of diagnostic algorithm. *Revista Espanola de Medicina Nuclear, 31,* 178–186.
17. Baden, L. R., Swaminathan, S., Angarone, M., et al. (2016). Prevention and treatment of cancer-related infection: Version 2.2016, nccn clinical practice guidelines in oncology. *Journal of the National Comprehensive Cancer Network, 14,* 882–913. doi:10.6004/jnccn2016.0093.
18. Chiumello, D., Gotti, M. D., & Vergano, M. D. (2017). Paracematol in fever in critically ill patients—an update. *Journal of Critical Care, 38,* 245–252.
19. Hauk, L. (2017). Fever in well-appearing children younger than 2 years: A Clinical Policy from the ACEP. *American Family Physician, 95*(8), 524–525.
20. Ferrer, R., Martin-Loeches, I., Phillips, G., et al. (2014). Empiric antibiotic treatment reduces mortality in severe sepsis septic shock from the first hour: Results from a guideline-based performance improvement program. *Critical Care Medicine, 42*(8), 1749–1755.

CHAPTER 204

IMMUNODEFICIENCY

Nancy B. Kuemmerle

 Immediate emergency department referral is indicated for: Fever greater than 38°C. or 100.4°F. or signs or symptoms of infection or infectious disease. Cultures need to be obtained and broad-spectrum antibiotics started expeditiously.

DEFINITION AND EPIDEMIOLOGY

Our immune system is the result of millions of years of evolution all leading to one overarching goal: to protect us from our environment. This bodily system protects the body from foreign substances, cells, and tissues by producing an immune response. It includes the thymus gland, spleen, lymph nodes, special deposits of lymphoid tissue (as in the gastrointestinal tract and bone marrow), macrophages, lymphocytes including the B cells and T cells, and antibodies. When it is working properly, immunity enables us to conduct all the normal affairs of running the human body, such as taking in nutrients, breathing air potentially contaminated with microorganisms or pollutants, and eliminating organisms that could potentially harm us. Abnormally developed immunity (primary or inherited immunodeficiency) or immunity compromised by any mechanism (secondary or acquired immunodeficiency), can prove catastrophic for the affected individual.

David Vetter, the Bubble Boy, was born with severe combined immunodeficiency disease (SCID), which left him without a functional immune system. He survived almost all of his 12 years by spending his life in a sterile enclosure. Such complete immunodeficiency is rare, affecting fewer than 1 in 100,000 live births. Other immunodeficiency syndromes are less severe and more common. For example, isolated immunoglobulin (Ig) A deficiency can affect about 1 in 500 to 1 in 300 live births in the United States. About 1 in 1200 live births harbors some type of immunodeficiency; about 1 in 2000 of those are diagnosed before the age of 18.[1] More than 300 primary immunodeficiencies have been described[2] since Colonel Ogden Bruton discovered agammaglobulinemia in 1952.

PATHOPHYSIOLOGY

Immunodeficiencies can occur when one or more of the components of the immune system (e.g., immunoglobulins [antibodies]) or complement are nonfunctional. This could occur if a gene for one of the components is mutated, or if a protein involved in the processing or transport of the component is deficient.

CLINICAL PRESENTATION AND PHYSICAL EXAMINATION

Immunodeficient patients are usually vulnerable to repeated, chronic, or unusual infections. Findings suggestive of immune dysfunction include the following[3]:
- Recurrent, unusual, or difficult-to-treat infections
  - Serious infections with bacteria that are normally nonpathogenic
  - Recurrent pneumonia, ear infection, or sinusitis

- Multiple courses of or intravenous antibiotics necessary to clear infection
- Recurrent deep abscesses of internal organs or skin
- Poor growth or loss of weight
- A family history of primary immunodeficiency disease
- Swollen lymph glands or an enlarged spleen

Knowing how the immune system is organized and how shortages of its various components will manifest clinically can provide clues of an immunodeficiency to the healthcare practitioner. For example, recurrent sinopulmonary infections with encapsulated bacteria such as *Streptococcus*, *Staphylococcus*, or *Haemophilus* can be suggestive of an antibody deficiency or B-cell disturbance, because humoral immunity is generally responsible for dispatching these types of pathogens. However, wide use of antibiotics can mask or cloud the diagnosis of a specific immunodeficiency. Thus, it is important to watch for common associations seen in these diseases, which would include chronic diarrhea, eczema, hepatosplenomegaly, hematologic disorders, autoimmune diseases, and failure to thrive in infants and children.[4]

An example is Wiskott-Aldrich syndrome (WAS), which like other humoral deficiencies is characterized by recurrent infections with pneumococci. WAS is also associated with platelet maturation anomalies through the underlying genetic defect and thus could manifest with prolonged bleeding, easy bruising, and eczema. There is also a tendency in WAS for later development of T-cell anomalies.

Primary T-cell disorders manifest as unusual sensitivity to viruses, fungi, some parasites, and other bacteria that are targets of this class of cell. Common T-cell mutations can affect the manner that T-cells mature or become activated. However, cell-to-cell communication can also be impaired—that is, there can be defects in their receptors or cytokines.

Even more severe are combined immunodeficiency disorders (CIDs) or severe CIDs (SCIDs), which may knock out multiple immune cell pathways, usually as the result of an enzyme or early maturation defect. Both B- and T-cell lineages can be affected, leading to early and devastating infections. Without prompt recognition and subsequent treatment with bone marrow transplantation or, more recently, gene therapy, these children's lives are usually measured in days to months rather than years.

Secondary immunodeficiencies are acquired or associated with underlying disorders and are not caused by intrinsic abnormalities in the development and function of the immune system. HIV and malnutrition are the commonest causes of immunodeficiency.[4] Other causes include malignant disease, immunosuppressive agents, and systemic inflammatory diseases such as rheumatoid arthritis and systemic lupus erythematosis.[5] Obesity may also compromise the pathways of immune surveillance. There is some decrease in immunity that occurs with aging. Fewer T-cells are produced; therefore, fewer can respond. Malnutrition, not uncommon in the older adult, impairs immune response.[4] Secondary immunodeficiencies must be considered in the differential diagnosis of patients with multiple or recurrent infections.

A careful history usually provides evidence that identifies the nature of the immune system defect.[6] The history should include a detailed description of infections, including age at onset, sites, patterns of recurrence, response to treatment, and pathogens if known, as well as developmental delay or failure to thrive, cancer, and splenectomy. More severe immunodeficiency disorders (e.g., SCID), characterized by deficits in both T- and B-cells, can manifest with life-threatening infections in the first few weeks of life.[1] Associated symptoms such as eczema, diarrhea, and arthritis should be assessed. A history of weight loss, enlarged lymph nodes, night sweats, fever, ecchymosis, pruritis, or epistaxis should be obtained. A family history of unexplained death from infection may be significant. The patient's immunization history and response to immunizations should be assessed. A history of normal response to smallpox vaccination or contact dermatitis from poison ivy suggests intact cellular immunity.

A complete physical examination should be performed with the goal of identifying the site and source of infection and any chronic indicators of immune dysfunction. Also, the tendency for immunodeficiency to be part of other congenital systems should cause the practitioner to look for body dysmorphisms. Examples include micrognathia, short philtrum (seen with DiGeorge syndrome); short-limbed dwarfism associated with some T-cell disorders; and prominent forehead, deep-set eyes, broad nasal bridge, and prognathism associated with hypereosinophilia E syndrome.[7] A full neurologic examination should be performed; broad-based gait in a young child could be the first sign of ataxia-telangectasia before immunodeficiency becomes apparent.[6]

DIAGNOSTICS

When an immunodeficiency disorder is suspected, in addition to the complete physical examination detailed above, initial laboratory work should include studies that are broadly informative, readily available, and cost-effective.[6]

INITIAL DIAGNOSTICS

Immunodeficiency Disorder

LABORATORY
- A complete blood cell count (CBC) with differential is important for detection of neutropenia and levels of the different white blood cell lineages.
- A peripheral smear could reveal abnormal cell morphologies, which would help exclude neutropenia and lymphopenia and would detect platelet abnormalities, possibly implicating WAS.
- Metabolic profiles can be helpful to exclude potential immune-modulating diseases such as diabetes mellitus.
- HIV testing should be performed, as a positive result would suggest a secondary rather than a primary immunodeficiency.
- An erythrocyte sedimentation rate and C-reactive protein levels should be obtained to assess for evidence of inflammation or lack thereof.
- Quantitative immunoglobulins should be obtained, as antibody disorders are the most common immunodeficiencies.[6,7]

ADDITIONAL TESTING
- Antibody response to common antigens (e.g., *Candida* organisms, tetanus, mumps)
- T-cell function and quantification of T-cell subtypes
- Complement levels (C3, C4, CH50)
- Nitroblue tetrazolium to determine phagocytic activity
- Flow cytometry for disease-specific cell markers[3]
- Genetic and chromosomal studies

IMAGING
- Computed tomography (CT) scan to assess for splenomegaly

DIFFERENTIAL DIAGNOSIS

- Blood disorders (e.g., anemia, multiple myeloma, chronic lymphocytic leukemia)
- Autoimmune disorders (e.g., systemic lupus erythematosus, rheumatoid arthritis, diabetes)
- Digestive disorders (e.g., cramping, diarrhea [Crohn's disease])
  - Secondary immunodeficiencies
  - Cystic fibrosis

 Rule out diabetes, iron-deficiency anemia, cystic fibrosis, rheumatoid arthritis, systemic lupus erythematosus.

INTERPROFESSIONAL COLLABORATIVE MANAGEMENT

Acquired immunodeficiencies tend to be more common than inherited forms. The commonest secondary immunodeficiency in the United States, human immunodeficiency virus/acquired immunodeficiency syndrome (HIV/AIDS), is now treated as an infectious disease (see Chapter 209). Primary as well as other secondary immunodeficiency syndromes can be treated by replacing absent or dysfunctional antibodies with normal components.[8] The use of IVIG in patients with IgA deficiency and some forms of CVID (those without detectable IgA) is complicated by the fact that some of these patients' IgA deficits are due to the presence of anti-IgA antibodies. Because IVIG can contain trace amounts of both IgA and IgM, giving a patient with these autoantibodies a large infusion of IVIG could cause anaphylaxis. Accordingly, testing to identify the presence of anti-IgA antibodies can be done and special preparations of IVIG without IgA obtained.[9]

The definitive treatment of SCID or CID is reconstitution of stem cells by stem cell transplantation (SCT) or gene therapy.[10,11] Pluripotent stem cells are able to become any leukocyte within the white blood cell milieu. By infusing these healthy predecessor cells after native cells have been destroyed by chemotherapeutic means, the practitioner should be able to completely replace diseased cells with healthy ones. SCT has been successful in stem cell deficiencies, almost all SCIDs, and a variety of other conditions, such as DiGeorge's syndrome, leukocyte adhesion deficiency, and WAS.[12] SCT is most successful when human leukocyte antigen (HLA)-identical sibling bone marrow donors are used. The adverse effects of the SCT process are numerous.

Gene therapy has been shown to reconstitute functionality to native immune cells in two SCIDs, common gamma-chain deficiency, and adenosine deaminase (ADA) deficiency.[12] Briefly, copies of healthy genes are added to delivery vectors that insert the healthy gene into diseased cells, thereby using the cell's own machinery to then produce normal gene products. A new technology, gene editing through use of CRISPR vectors, shows promise. Although gene therapy holds promise, these techniques are still experimental.

Other modalities of immune function replacement are tailored to the specific pathophysiologic mechanism of each disease. Apart from SCT, patients with DiGeorge's syndrome can also be treated with the thymic hormone thymosin or with transplantation of fetal thymic tissue with the goal of restoring T-cell function. ADA deficiency has also been treated with replacement of the ADA enzyme by use of a polyethylene glycol formulation.[8] Complement deficiencies can be treated with blood factor-rich fresh-frozen plasma. Replacement with the cytokine interferon-γ is used to treat patients with chronic granulomatosis disease.[7] Progenitor cell growth factors like granulocyte-macrophage colony-stimulating factor are used to stimulate white blood cell proliferation in the presence of neutropenia.

All patients should be referred to a clinical immunologist when the diagnosis of an immunodeficiency disorder is suspected, unless that disorder is already known to be secondary, and thus other specialists may be better suited to caring for the patient. For example, AIDS/HIV patients are now often cared for by infectious disease consultants or specialists in HIV medicine.

Once a definitive diagnosis of primary immunodeficiency is made and the care plan is developed by the clinical immunologist, the patient can be monitored in a collaborative fashion. Infections can be diagnosed and managed by the primary care practitioner. Patients should be closely monitored for the development of autoimmune diseases and malignant neoplasms. The majority of malignant neoplasms are seen in patients with ataxia-telangiectasia, WAS, and CVID.[4] Those requiring specialized therapy, such as immunoglobulin replacement therapy or bone marrow or SCT, should receive this care under supervision of a clinical immunologist. Relatives of affected individuals should be referred for genetic testing and counseling as appropriate. It is especially important to screen for carrier status all female relatives of patients with X-linked disorders and both parents of a patient suspected to have an autosomal recessive inheritance pattern. Intrauterine diagnosis of some primary immunodeficiencies is possible for those with known familial disorders.

LIFE SPAN CONSIDERATIONS

Some immunodeficiencies are mild and may even go unnoticed throughout a person's life. Such can be the case with isolated IgA deficiency, which affects 1 in 500 Americans and at one end of the spectrum can be asymptomatic. Approximately two-thirds of immunodeficient patients will live to adulthood. However, many will have a shortened life span because of their disease. Death can result from overwhelming infections, chronic stigmata, or complications of the disease and some of the treatment modalities themselves. Frank discussion with patients and their families are important to help them anticipate potential deterioration of health, and the use of community or mental health resources can be helpful for patients and their families.

COMPLICATIONS

Complications associated with immunodeficiency or its management depend on the specific disease entity. In general, the complications of poorly controlled chronic or recurrent infections are common (e.g., bronchiectasis with recurrent pulmonary infections). Some patients' diseases tend to worsen over time. Some patients may be at greater risk for malignant or autoimmune diseases. For example, patients with CVID are at greater risk for development of lymphoma. Complications can also occur secondary to treatment.

PATIENT AND FAMILY INFORMATION

Patients with primary immunodeficiency disorders should understand the importance of avoiding contact with individuals with known contagious diseases, and they should be able to identify and report signs and symptoms of infection. It is essential that these patients seek care at the first sign of infection. Practices which promote good health and support immune function should be recommended. Social service providers can help with affordability issues, and national organizations such as the Immune Deficiency Foundation (www.primaryimmune.org) and the Jeffrey Modell Foundation (www.jmfworld.org) can provide specific educational and support materials to patients, families, and practitioners.

Patients with congenital immunodeficiencies should have current childhood, adolescent, and adult vaccinations as recommended by the National Immunization Program of the Centers for Disease Control and Prevention.[13,14] Anthrax, polio (IPV), rabies, and inactivated typhoid can be used if indicated. In general, live attenuated vaccines (BCG, influenza LAIV, typhoid Ty21a, vaccinia, MMR, Zostavax, and yellow fever) are contraindicated because of the risk of vaccine-induced infection. There are two exceptions to this recommendation. First, the live attenuated form of the influenza vaccine (LAIV) cannot be used, but the inactivated form can be given to adults and children with primary immunodeficiency. Second, varicella vaccine is contraindicated in patients with T-cell involvement, but patients with humoral deficiency may be given the vaccine. For current guidelines, practitioners should check with their local or national health agency in charge of vaccine recommendations.

Practitioners should also keep in mind that the impairment in antibody responses seen in patients with humoral immunodeficiencies can make it difficult or impossible to achieve full protection by vaccination, even after repeated inoculations. Even T-cell disorders, whether occurring alone or mixed with B-cell abnormalities, may not respond to vaccination.

Transfusions of whole blood are contraindicated in immunodeficient patients because the donor blood my contain lymphocytes that could induce a graft-versus-host rejection. Appropriate preparation of blood products before transfusion should include means such as irradiation to minimize the risk of infection, especially with viruses like cytomegalovirus and the hepatitides.

The use of surgical treatments for immunodeficient patients is by and large controversial and untested. In general, there are no indications for tonsillectomy, adenoidectomy, or splenectomy in these patients. In fact, these procedures should be limited to certain circumstances, such as to control bleeding secondary to WAS-induced thrombocytopenia. Some proponents have recommended tympanostomy tube placement for those with recurrent otitis, but evidence is lacking on whether this provides significant advantage for this population. Further studies concerning surgical interventions are needed.

HEALTH PROMOTION

Good personal hygiene and adoption of healthy behaviors such as regular exercise and stress management are critical to longevity and quality of life for patients with immunodeficiencies.[15] These include

- good hygiene and dental health
- healthy diet
- physical activity
- adequate sleep
- stress management
- exposure avoidance
- recommended vaccinations

In summary, the primary immunodeficiency syndromes thus far identified vary widely in their severity, and to a lesser extent in their presentations.[7] Diagnostic workups and general treatment principles unify the syndromes.

REFERENCES

1. Reust, C. (2013). Evaluation of primary immunodeficiency disease in children. *American Family Physician, 87*, 773.
2. Picard, C., Al-Herz, W., Bousfiha, A., & Casanova, J. L. (2015). Primary immunodeficiency: An update on the classification from the International Union of Immunological Societies Expert Committee on Primary Immunodeficiency. *Journal of Clinical Immunology, 35*, 696–726.
3. Abraham, R. S., & Aubert, G. (2016). Flow cytometry, a versatile tool for diagnosis and monitoring of primary immunodeficiencies. *Clinical and Vaccine Immunology: CVI, 23*, 254.
4. David, A., & Webster, B. (2013). The immunocompromised patient: Primary immunodeficiencies. *Medicine, 41*, 619–623.
5. Peter, H.-H. (2013). Adult-onset immunodeficiency—why is it important in rheumatology? *Arthritis Research & Therapy, 15*, 105–106.
6. Fernandez, J. (2018). Approach to the patient with suspected immunodeficiency, Merck Manuals Online Medical Library. Retrieved from http://www.merckmanuals.com/professional/immunology_allergic_disorders/immunodeficiency_disorders/approach_to_the_patient_with_suspected_immunodeficiency.html?qt=immunodeficiency&alt=sh. (Accessed January 2018).
7. Al-Herz, W., Bousfiha, A., Casanova, J. L., et al. (2014). Primary immunodeficiency diseases: An update on the classification from the international union of immunological societies expert committee for primary immunodeficiency. *Frontiers in Immunology, 5*, 162. Retrieved from http://www.ncbi.nlm.nih.gov/pubmed/24795713. April 2014, Corrected 5:460; 2014.
8. Immune Deficiency Foundation. (2018). Immunoglobulin G therapy & other medical therapies for antibody deficiency. Retrieved from http://primaryimmune.org/treatment-information/immunoglobulin-therapy/. (Accessed January 2018).
9. Selective IgA deficiency: Symptoms, diagnosis & treatment. Retrieved from http://www.aaaai.org/. (Accessed January 2018).
10. Weinkove, R., Filbey, K., & LeGros, G. (2017). Immunity without innate lymphoid cells. *Nature Immunology, 17*, 1237–1238.
11. Thrasher, A. J., & Williams, D. A. (2017). Evolving gene therapy in primary immunodeficiency. *Cell, 25*, 1132–1141.
12. Shaw, K. L., Garabedion, E., Mishra, S., Barman, P., & Davila, D. (2017). Clinical efficacy of gene-modified stem cells on adenosine deaminase-deficient immunodeficiency. Retrieved from https://www.ncbi.nlm.nih.gov/pubmed/28346339.
13. Recommended adult immunization schedule—United States—2016. Centers for Disease Control. Retrieved from http://www.cdc.gov/vaccines/schedules/downloads/adult/adult-schedule.pdf.
14. Recommended immunization schedules for persons aged 0 through 18 years—United States—2016. Centers for Disease Control. Retrieved from http://www.cdc.gov/vaccines/schedules/downloads/child/0-18yrs-schedule.pdf.
15. http://www.riversideonline.com/health_reference/Disease-condition/. (Accessed January 2018). 1/20/2015. Also in https://mayoclinic.org/diseases.

CHAPTER 205

LYMPHADENOPATHY
Janet Rico

DEFINITION AND EPIDEMIOLOGY

Lymphadenopathy refers to lymph nodes that have enlarged or changed in consistency. Lymph nodes typically vary from 0.5 to 2.5 cm ($\frac{1}{5}$ to 1 inch) in diameter, averaging about 1 cm,[1] and are characterized by number, size, shape, texture, mobility, tenderness, and surrounding skin involvement. Three quarters of patients with enlarged lymph nodes have localized findings, half of which are in the head and neck.[1] Nodes located above the clavicles account for the largest palpable field; axillary and inguinal regions represent far fewer. Three or more noncontiguous groups of node enlargements constitute generalized lymphadenopathy. Lymphadenitis is defined as tender, warm, erythematous nodes, and suppurative lymphadenitis includes fluctuance.

On routine physical examination, generalized lymphadenopathy is a common incidental finding. A community-based sample of 2556 Dutch respondents revealed that 0.6% had unexplained lymphadenopathy, three quarters of which was localized and treated without further workup.[2] Whereas most neck masses in younger patients are associated with infection and are self-resolving, congenital malformations and neoplasms manifest similarly. Nodes vary in size depending on location. Epitrochlear nodes larger than 0.5 cm or inguinal nodes larger than 1.5 cm are thought to be aberrant; nodes larger than 2 cm warrant prompt investigation, although most are infectious.[1] However, these enlargements become more suspicious in older patients. Malignancy is diagnosed in 1.1% of patients aged 40 years or above with unexplained lymphadenopathy.[2] The commonly cited "rule of 80s" refers to patients older than 40 years who are seen with a neck mass: 80% of all nonthyroid neck masses are malignant, and 80% of those are metastatic. Among asymptomatic cervical lumps, about 12% are head and neck cancer cases, and of these cancers, approximately 80% are squamous cell carcinoma.[1] Diffuse lymphadenopathy in at-risk individuals of any age should prompt consideration of human immunodeficiency virus (HIV) infection (see Chapter 209).

PATHOPHYSIOLOGY

The lymph nodes are integral to the lymphatic drainage system and provide filtration of foreign substances through the action of lymphocytes, monocytes, and macrophages. Lymph fluid intermediates between blood and tissue. Lymph nodes are found in clusters around the lymphatic veins, where excess interstitial fluid is accumulated, processed, and returned to the bloodstream. The role of the lymphatic system in maintaining fluid balance, processing lipids and fat-soluble substances from intestinal lymph, and serving as a host defense has been a focus of therapeutic interest.[5,4]

More than 600 lymph nodes exist in the human body. Tonsils, adenoids, the spleen, thymus, and Peyer patches of the ileum are also involved in immune surveillance and activation. The lymphatic system is made up of head and neck (internal and external drainage), supraclavicular, deltopectoral, axillary, epitrochlear, inguinal, and popliteal regions (Fig. 205.1).

Because development of the lymphatic system is linked to venous development, the lymphatic ducts run along venous tracts. Lymph fluid ultimately reaches one of two large ducts in the thorax. The right lymphatic duct drains lymph from the right upper body—mediastinum, lungs, and esophagus—and into the right supraclavicular vein; the thoracic duct drains lymph from the rest of the body, including the abdominal cavity (stomach, gallbladder, and pancreas) and urogenital organs, into the left supraclavicular vein.

Lymph nodes swell or react in response to antigens. Afferent vessels carry the antigen-laden lymph fluid into the sinus of the node; efferent vessels carry the immune-mediated fluid away. Nodal swelling is caused by the proliferation of monocytes (the precursors to macrophages). Along with the lymph nodes, other lymphoid organ tissues—including the bone

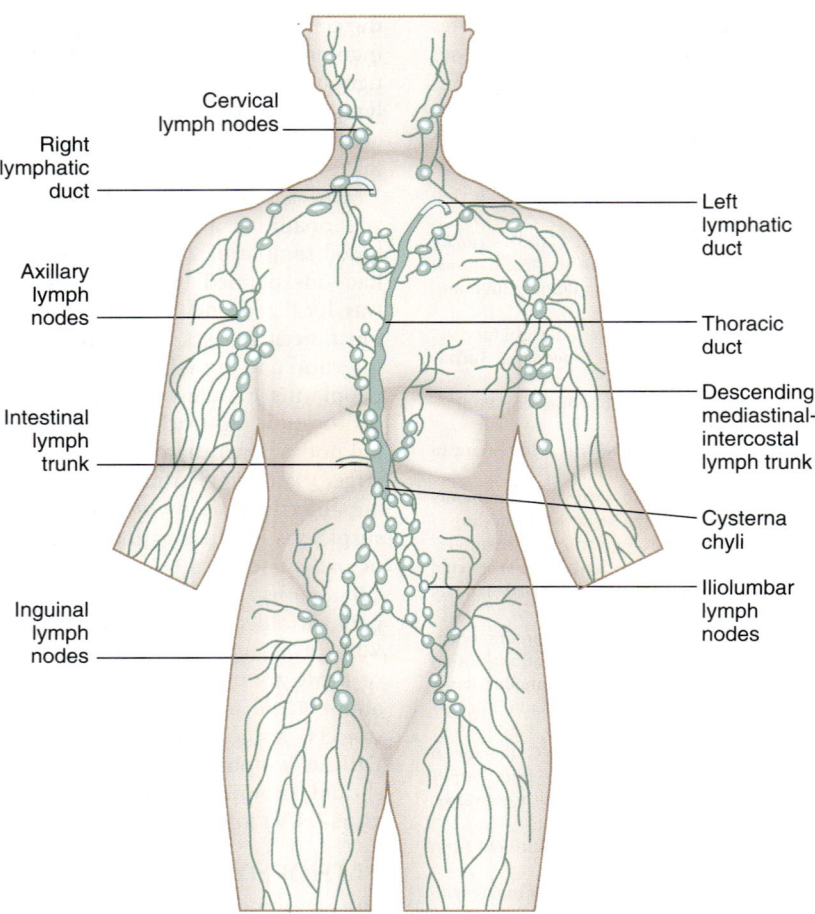

Cervical lymph nodes

Right lymphatic duct

Axillary lymph nodes

Intestinal lymph trunk

Inguinal lymph nodes

Left lymphatic duct

Thoracic duct

Descending mediastinal-intercostal lymph trunk

Cysterna chyli

Iliolumbar lymph nodes

F I G . **205.1**   Major anatomic pathways and lymph node groups of the lymphatic system. (From Townsend, C. M., Jr., Beauchamp, R. D., Evers, B. M., & Mattox, K. L. [2007]. *Sabiston textbook of surgery* [18th ed.]. St Louis: Elsevier.)

marrow, tonsils and adenoids, and spleen—may become disturbed or enlarged in the presence of antigen. Splenomegaly associated with lymphadenopathy may reflect lymphocytosis generated by infection, various types of immune hyperplasia, macrophage proliferation, or a tumor. Generalized lymphadenopathy may indicate systemic disease or malignant disease because the lymph system can be infiltrated by malignant cells and other cells not normally present in the nodes. Researchers suspect that if malignant cells were prevented from entering the lymphatic system or if their microenvironment were disrupted, lymph-based cancer cells might not circulate and metastasize.[3,5]

In summary, lymph nodes enlarge as a result of allergy or hypersensitivity to drug or environmental pollutants, tissue injury, autoimmune disease, infection, lymphoproliferative or myeloid abnormalities of bone marrow, and other malignancies or solid tumors. Nodes which are hard or matted suggest malignancy or infection.[6]

CLINICAL PRESENTATION AND PHYSICAL EXAMINATION

Key factors to consider in the evaluation of the patient with lymphadenopathy are the age of the patient, the location of the swollen glands, and any associated symptoms. The history can also be extremely useful in the diagnosis.

A thorough symptom analysis should be done to assess for possible infectious contacts or exposures (e.g., deer ticks, bird droppings, and cat or rat feces), foreign travel, travel to endemic infectious areas, or foreign birth. Patients should be asked about possible occupational exposure to chemicals, livestock, asbestos, silica (silicon dioxide), or beryllium. Sexual behaviors should be queried. Patients should also be asked about past medical or surgical history of abdominal, thoracic, breast, head and neck, pelvic, reproductive organ, or lower extremity malignant neoplasms including those associated with acquired immunodeficiency syndrome (AIDS), surgery, or injury; implanted silicone products (e.g., breast) or prosthetics; tattoo dyes; exposure to ultraviolet radiation; personal or family history of cancer, particularly lymphoma; irradiation; and chemotherapy. Family history may also help to identify possible etiologies such as Li-Fraumeni syndrome or lipid storage diseases.

A review of systems should include all areas of the skin for irregular or nonhealing lesions. A history of scalp pruritus (e.g., seborrheic dermatitis, scabies infection), conjunctivitis, eye pain, photophobia, visual complaints, unilateral ear pain, difficulty hearing, nose or throat pain or discharge, odynophagia, impaired swallowing, acidic food intolerance, vocal changes or persistent hoarseness, mastoid swelling or pain, dental maladies, dental malocclusion, facial paralysis, and muscle strain of the head or neck should be elicited. Pain associated with the rapidly growing node is usually a good sign because it suggests an infection but may represent bleeding into the necrotic center of a malignant node.

Breast changes, especially with axillary adenopathy, can be ominous. Lactation status should be ascertained. Gastrointestinal symptoms suggestive of malabsorption, complaints of diarrhea or constipation, or back pain with relief in the fetal position can suggest a malignant intra-abdominal process.

Medications, whether new or long-term, are worth reviewing for potential drug hypersensitivities. Drug hypersensitivity to phenytoin sodium, carbamazepine, aspirin, hydralazine (a lupus-like mimic), allopurinol, or antibiotics (including erythromycin, penicillin, and sulfa products) and serum sickness from vaccinations to smallpox or typhoid can result in generalized lymphadenopathy. Typically, drug reactions produce generalized lymphadenopathy, accompanied by rash, fever, and joint pain.[1]

Inquiry into the incidence and frequency of blood transfusions, sexually transmitted diseases, smoked or chewed tobacco, and illegal drug or alcohol abuse is also necessary. Use of tobacco and alcohol together increases the risk of head and neck cancer substantially.

Any signs of external or internal bleeding, such as hemoptysis, hematuria, melena, or menorrhagia, should be pursued to exclude malignant disease.

The physical examination is guided by the history and location of the lymphadenopathy. Often, though, lymphadenopathy can be an incidental finding during the physical examination of a patient seen for an unrelated problem, highlighting the importance of a thorough physical examination (see Fig. 205.1). Differentiation of normally palpable periauricular, cervical, axillary, and inguinal lymph nodes from enlarged nodes can be subtle.

Nodes should be characterized by location, size, distribution, degree of fluctuance, firmness, matted or shoddy quality, mobility or immobility, and tenderness or non-tenderness. Unilateral or bilateral involvement, hard and fixed position, and symmetry or asymmetry may indicate or exclude malignant disease. Node characteristics, whether symptomatic or painful, may not initially reveal the diagnosis, even in cases of cancer.[7]

A swollen node that is warm, tender, and rapidly enlarging may represent lymphadenitis and is suggestive of an infection at the drainage terminal. Lymphedema is an interruption of and blockage in drainage and may result from a variety of causes. Primary lymphedema refers to congenital malformations; secondary lymphedema refers to traumatic injury resulting from cancer obstruction, irradiation, recurrent infection, or surgery.

Evaluation of cervical nodes requires complete muscle relaxation and neutral positioning. Both anterior and posterior cervical node enlargement can indicate infection or carcinomas of the head or neck. The presence of posterior cervical adenopathy (level 5) often suggests significant pathology.[8] A supraclavicular node (sentinel node) can be elicited by the Valsalva maneuver in thin individuals. The Virchow node is the left supraclavicular node, at the base of most of the body's lymphatic drainage via the thoracic duct; an enlarged one poses significant concern for malignant disease of the stomach, gallbladder, kidney, pancreas, ovary, testes, or prostate. The right supraclavicular node drains from the mediastinum, lungs, and esophagus. Axillary

nodes are terminal lymph drains for the upper extremities and can become enlarged as a result of cellulitis of the arm or hand or breast malignant neoplasms. Women with a positive axillary node require a careful breast examination and mammography to exclude breast cancer. Liver and spleen examinations looking for enlargement or tenderness are essential.

Inguinal or retroperitoneal nodes may be difficult to palpate unless they are grossly enlarged. Unilateral or bilateral presentation is an important consideration because the unilateral presentation is more often malignant. Men can be seen with unilateral malignant lymphedema of the leg in cases of disseminated prostate cancer. The abdominal examination is critical and should focus on assessing for splenomegaly which can be seen in infectious mononucleosis, lymphoma, lymphocytic leukemias, or sarcoid.[2]

DIAGNOSTICS

The most likely cause of lymphadenopathy is often revealed by the history and physical examination. However, in those cases where the cause is not evident, a period of 3 to 4 weeks of observation is recommended. Often during this time, a cause is revealed or a direction for further investigation is apparent. Routine diagnostics to exclude infectious disease may lead the investigation and could include complete blood count (CBC) with differential, chemistry profile with liver function studies, hepatitis panel, throat culture, or monospot. Further testing is directed by the results of initial screening and by the history and physical examination findings. An enzyme-linked immunosorbent assay or Western blot HIV testing can be done as initial testing if indicated by history.

Splenomegaly with lymphadenopathy is an unusual and more ominous finding that might correlate with an abnormal CBC. Thyroid studies are warranted in suspected cases of thyroiditis, goiter, or carcinoma. Inguinal node enlargement most often has an infectious cause, and a host of sexually transmitted diseases would be part of the workup, including herpes simplex virus, gonorrhea, syphilis, chancroid, lymphogranuloma venereum, HIV, and reproductive organ cancers. Autoimmune diseases including rheumatoid arthritis and lupus erythematosus can be ruled out if suspected by history or physical examination.

A chest radiograph is necessary to rule out tuberculosis (especially in HIV/AIDS patients or those born outside the United States), sarcoidosis, infection, and local or disseminated malignant disease. A mammogram is recommended when there is a persistent axillary node enlargement without other explanation. Ultrasound is considered a necessary tool to assess cervicofacial lymph nodes; in fact, it is considered superior to computed tomography (CT) scan in detecting small nodes and can differentiate between solid and less concerning cystic lesions.[9] CT, magnetic resonance imaging (MRI), and positron emission tomography (PET) may also contribute to diagnosis, biopsy precision, and tumor staging, particularly in the abdomen, pelvis, and chest.[1]

Biopsy should be considered when lymphadenopathy has persisted for more than 1 month without explanation or when malignant disease is suspected. The algorithms for selection of fine-needle aspiration cytology (FNAC) and high-tech imaging have become increasingly complex. Fine-needle aspiration (FNA) biopsy can be both highly sensitive and specific. Other techniques include ultrasound-guided FNAC and endobronchial ultrasound-guided transbronchial needle aspiration for hilar lymphadenopathy or transesophageal ultrasound-guided FNAC. Core needle biopsy may be preferable to FNAC, if it can be guided by ultrasound or CT. Surgical biopsy rather than ultrasound-guided FNAC may help with suspected lymphomas of the head or neck, given the architectural complexity of those cancerous nodes.[10] Inguinal nodes have the lowest yield; supraclavicular nodes have the highest.[8] With a plethora of immunohistochemical staining, flow cytometry, cytogenetics, and molecular genetic techniques available, refined diagnosis and management is ever more possible, particularly of the hematologic malignancies. Laparoscopic lymph node biopsy is preferred to all percutaneous sampling.[8] Sentinel node biopsy with blue dye and radioisotope in breast cancer is considered indispensable. Typing, clinical staging, and initial management of leukemias (see Chapter 218), lymphomas (see Chapter 219), and solid tumors require a specialist.

DIFFERENTIAL DIAGNOSIS

 Priority differentials include malignancies, infections, and autoimmune and allergic etiologies.

The mnemonic CHICAGO (cancers, hypersensitivities, infections, connective tissue disease, atypical lymphoproliferative disorders, granulomatous lesions, and other unusual causes) can offer a framework for organizing the differential diagnosis.[2] Another mnemonic is MIAMI for malignancies, infections, autoimmune disorders, miscellaneous conditions, and iatrogenic etiologies.[2] Drugs specifically known to produce lymphadenopathy are described earlier, although drug hypersensitivities may include others not commonly reported.

The Virchow node, a pathologic left anterior supraclavicular node, portends an abdominal neoplasm; the right anterior supraclavicular node points to a thoracic neoplasm; the Delphian node, at the midline prelaryngeal level, is considered a sinister sign of thyroid or laryngeal cancer.[2,11] In patients older than 40 years, supraclavicular lymphadenopathy is likely to be cancerous in 90%; in patients younger than 40, the risk goes down to 25%.[1]

Axillary node enlargement suggests infection but may represent breast neoplasm, melanoma, Hodgkin disease, or non-Hodgkin lymphoma. Other axillary involvement may stem from an arm and hand infection or even a metastasized gastric cancer, known ominously as the Irish node.[12] A palpable epitrochlear node may signal an infection such as secondary syphilis, lepromatous leprosy, leishmaniasis, connective tissue disorder, lymphoma, or leukemia, especially if other nodes are involved.[5]

Hilar or mediastinal nodes seen on chest radiographs or CT scan may be calcified or not and can result from a host of infectious, autoimmune, neoplastic, or injurious causes. Careful review of past radiologic studies and judicious chemistry, hematology, and microbiology testing should lead to a working diagnosis before ordering of bronchoscopy and mediastinoscopy. Bacterial pneumonia; tuberculosis; sarcoidosis; fungal infections (histoplasmosis, coccidioidomycosis) and other infections (pertussis); lymphoma; and lung, breast, and metastatic adenocarcinoma are among the more common culprits. Amyloidosis is less common. Distinction is made among single or bilateral or calcified hilar nodes.[12]

A Sister Mary Joseph node, seen bulging in the periumbilical region, may be a sign of intra-abdominal or pelvic malignancy. Inguinal lymph nodes run in horizontal and vertical clusters. Inguinal lymphadenopathy may be confused with hernia if large enough; vessel malformations; lipomas; or ectopic endometrial, testicular, or splenic tissue. The node of Cloquet is the femoral node below the inguinal ligament and is associated with anal, vulvar, and penile cancers, including melanoma.[12]

Most infectious processes that occur with lymphadenopathy last less than 2 weeks and, in younger patients, are likely to be a benign form of reactive lymphatic hyperplasia, histiocytosis. More troublesome is lymphadenopathy lasting longer than 2 weeks; however, enlarged lymph nodes lasting more than 1 year without a change in size are likely to be benign. Head and neck area lymphadenopathy coupled with a history of tobacco or alcohol use should suggest cancer if it is accompanied by hoarseness, hemoptysis, otalgia or hearing loss, facial nerve deficits, nasal obstruction or bleeding, throat pain or difficulty swallowing, or nonhealing ulcers. Squamous cell carcinoma and variants comprise most laryngeal cancers, which are most often associated with alcohol and tobacco exposure. More recently appreciated as a cause of head and neck cancer is high-risk human papilloma virus (HR-HPV).[13]

Parotid swelling, or less commonly salivary gland enlargement, might signal the onset of mumps, known to be more severe in adults and teens. Secondary to infection, a malignancy is the most common cause of a head or neck lymph node enlargement.[12]

An asymptomatic unilateral node enlargement in the inguinal area suggests a malignant neoplasm or lymphoma, although sexually transmitted disease may be suspected based on patient history. Splenomegaly may corroborate infectious mononucleosis or one of the lymphomas or leukemias, especially with generalized lymphadenopathy. Fever, weight loss (10% in 6 months), night sweats, and pruritus—known as the B symptoms—are known to occur in both Hodgkin and non-Hodgkin lymphomas.

INTERPROFESSIONAL COLLABORATIVE MANAGEMENT

Nonpharmacologic Management

Ongoing assessment and close monitoring is needed in patients with chronic autoimmune illnesses such as lupus erythematosus, Sjögren syndrome, rheumatoid arthritis, sarcoidosis, and HIV/AIDS. These patients most often require specialty consultation and management in collaboration with the primary care provider. Because HIV infection has been associated with Kaposi sarcoma, Castleman disease, Hodgkin and non-Hodgkin disease, and multidrug-resistant tuberculosis, specialty practices may be more likely to identify these complications. Autoimmune diseases are mostly managed in the outpatient setting, unless complications or late-stage developments require more complex care. Atypical lymphoproliferative disorders, whether clonal or polyclonal type, such as Castleman disease, lymphomatoid granulomatosis, and papulosis, have the potential to develop into cancer and bear watching with an eye toward biopsy. Evidence of malignancy requires referral to the appropriate specialist.

Similarly, Sjögren syndrome has been associated with a high risk for non-Hodgkin lymphoma, often in the salivary gland (see Chapter 78). For patients with malignant neoplasms, continued primary care surveillance to monitor further physical and psychosocial complications is essential. Lymphadenopathy may follow prior cancer treatment or radiation therapy and suggest a recrudescence of disease. It is also important that patients receive drug level monitoring, counseling, and weight management guidance during chemotherapy.

Pharmacologic/Other Modality Management

Symptomatic treatment of viral infections and appropriate antibiotic therapy for bacterial, mycobacterial, fungal, parasitic, rickettsial, and chlamydial infections are indicated if the pathogen is known. Corticosteroid or indiscriminate antibiotic use is not recommended, especially because this will confound biopsy results.

Monoclonal antibodies coupled with radiation therapy have significantly improved survival rates in patients with head and neck cancer. Congenital or benign growths (e.g., lipomas or pilar cysts resulting in cervical adenopathy) can be surgically removed. Abscesses and other deep structure infections are treated in the hospital and may require surgery for drainage.

Collaborating Specialists and Hospitalization. Patients with unusual infectious diseases (e.g., those resulting from foreign travel or communicable illnesses), cases of rare animal or environmental exposure, chronic inflammatory diseases, or a diagnosis of malignant disease should be referred to the appropriate specialists for guidance on the latest treatment protocols. The crucial decision point for health care providers is when to perform biopsy of a node for a definitive diagnosis.

A referral to an otolaryngologist or general surgeon might precede a visit to the oncologist. Immunosuppressed patients with AIDS, malignant disease, or other illnesses may require hospitalization for intensive nutritional, anti-infective, and chemotherapeutic support.

Rheumatology, nephrology, gastroenterology, pulmonary, or allergy specialists are essential to autoimmune disease management, with attention to associations with unusual lymphomas.

Oncologists provide a critical role when malignancies are identified. They may collaborate with medical and radiology oncology colleagues and use a multidisciplinary approach to whole-patient care.

LIFE SPAN CONSIDERATIONS

Age is a most important consideration in evaluation of these patients. In patients younger than 40 years, lymphadenopathy is often benign. In individuals older than 40 years, lymphadenopathy can represent a malignancy more often.

Lymphoma diagnosed in later life represents a growing group of cancers on the rise, especially as the population ages and survives longer (see Chapter 219). Older patients diagnosed with life-threatening infections or malignant neoplasms may decline treatment, especially if they have comorbidities. Patients and their families will certainly need guidance and support through these difficult decisions.

COMPLICATIONS

Complications may arise as a result of the disease process or clinical management. Mistaken identification of a malignant node as benign can result in local or generalized metastasis. Untreated or inadequately treated group A β-hemolytic streptococcal infection may lead to rheumatic heart disease and glomerulonephritis. Complications related to prescribed drugs, especially antibiotics and chemotherapeutic agents, are common. Fortunately, the sensitivity and specificity of radiologic and immunohistologic and DNA-specific testing continue to improve diagnostic speed and precision, including for those entities that may develop malignant features.

PATIENT AND FAMILY EDUCATION

Patients with lymphadenopathy need reassurance that many cases are benign and require only watchful waiting. Nodes that persist for more than 4 weeks require further investigation. Ongoing cancer screening for early cancer detection significantly increases the odds for survival. Patients and family should receive support for psychological distress that may result from personal and family-related role changes as well as hair loss and other cosmetic changes from chemotherapy. Advance directives are often most comfortably discussed with health care providers and communicated to the consultant. End-of-life care may be best managed at home with the help of the family, community volunteers, and hospice services (see Chapter 14).

HEALTH PROMOTION

Because several diseases resulting in lymph node enlargement in otherwise healthy adults are sexually transmitted, patients should be well informed of this health risk and strategies for prevention. Frank discussion with patients and instruction about condom use are essential in preventing sexually transmitted diseases. Cancer prevention strategies include eliminating all forms of tobacco, reducing alcohol consumption, and protecting skin from ultraviolet radiation and occupational hazards. Cancer screening tests should be recommended and completed on the recommended schedule. Health behaviors that fortify the immune system, such as proper nutrition, sleep, exercise, emotional support, and stress management, are most likely to promote health and to assist recovery. Patients are often able to find educational and social support in local or state chapters of national disease foundations.

REFERENCES

1. Mohseni, S., Shojaiefard, A., Khorgami, Z., et al. (2014). Peripheral lymphadenopathy: Approach and diagnostic tools. *Iranian Journal of Medical Science, 39*(2), 158–170.
2. Gaddey, H. L., & Riegel, A. M. (2016). Unexplained lymphadenopathy: Evaluation and differential diagnosis. *American Family Physician, 94*(11), 896–903.
3. Mortimar, P. S., & Rockson, S. G. (2014). New developments in clinical aspects of lymphatic disease. *The Journal of Clinical Investigation, 124*(3), 915–921.
4. Singh, I., Swami, R., Khan, W., et al. (2014). Lymphatic system: A prospective area for advanced targeting of particular drug carriers. *Expert Opinion on Drug Delivery, 11*(2), 211–229.
5. Carbone, A., Tripodo, C., Carlo-Stella, C., et al. (2014). The role of inflammation in lymphoma. In B. B. Aggarwal (Ed.), *Inflammation and cancer: Advances in experimental medicine and biology* (Vol. 816, pp. 315–333). Springer Basel.
6. Frederiksen, H., Svaerke, C., Thomsen, R. W., et al. (2013). Lymph node enlargement and risk of haematological and solid cancer. *British Journal of Haematology, 160*, 599–607.

7. Mohseni, S., Shojaiefard, A., Khorgami, Z., Alinejad, S., Ghorbani, A., & Ghafouri, A. (2014). Peripheral lymphadenopathy: Approach and diagnostic tools. *Iranian Journal of Medical Science*, *39*(2 Suppl.), 158–170.
8. Cunnane, M., Cheung, L., Moore, A., di Palma, S., McCombe, A., & Pitkin, L. (2016). Level 5 lymphadenopathy warrants heightened suspicion for clinically significant pathology. *Head and Neck Pathology*, *10*(4), 509–512. doi:10.1007/s12105-016-0733-6. Published 2016 Jun 3.
9. Reshma, V. J., Shihab, A. A., Abdulla, M., et al. (2014). Characterization of cervicofacial lymph nodes—a clinical and ultrasonographic study. *Journal of Clinical and Diagnostic Research: JCDR*, *8*(8), ZC25–ZC28.
10. Ahn, D., Kim, H., & Sohn, J. H. (2015). Surgeon-performed ultrasound-guided fine needle aspiration cytology of head and neck mass lesions: Sampling adequacy and diagnostic accuracy. *Annals of Surgical Oncology*, *22*(4), 1360–1365.
11. Dy, B. M., Shaha, A. R., & Tuttle, R. M. (2017). The delphian node revisited: An uncommon site of recurrence. *Journal of the Endocrine Society*, *1*(12), 1527–1530.
12. Motyckova, G., & Steensma, D. P. (2012). Why does my patient have lymphadenopathy or splenomegaly? *Hematology/Oncology Clinics of North America*, *26*, 395–408.
13. Lydiatt, W., Patel, S., O'Sullivan, B., et al. (2017). Head and Neck Cancers—major changes in the American Joint Committee on Cancer eighth edition cancer staging manual. *CA: A Cancer Journal for Clinicians*, *67*(2), 122–137.

CHAPTER **206**

SLEEP DISORDERS

Glen P. Greenough • Brooke G. Judd

 Priority differentials include medical conditions that disrupt sleep such as chronic pain, congestive heart failure, obstructive sleep apnea, or chronic lung disease including asthma.

INTRODUCTION

Sleep disorders are associated with major functional impairments, including loss of productivity, work-related and vehicular accidents, social impairment, and cognitive and mood disturbances, as well as morbidity and mortality as a result of cardiovascular, endocrine, and immune disturbances. Given the significance of these disorders, it is incumbent on primary care providers to recognize the symptoms of sleep disorders, to make accurate diagnoses, to initiate sound referrals, and to develop successful treatment plans in collaboration with sleep medicine specialists.

In this chapter, an overview of normal sleep is presented along with a description of the most common disorders of sleep. The most recent edition of the *International Classification of Sleep Disorders*[1] (ICSD) organizes the conditions into seven major categories: insomnias, sleep-related breathing disorders, central disorders of hypersomnolence (excessive sleepiness not related to other sleep disorders), circadian rhythm sleep-wake disorders, sleep-related movement disorders, parasomnias (abnormal behaviors or events arising from sleep), and other sleep disorders. These categories, which are largely symptom based (e.g., insomnia or hypersomnia), serve as a guide to obtaining a detailed history and initiating essential diagnostic procedures.

From a practical standpoint, fundamental assessment of sleep, which should be part of any complete patient history, can begin with three basic questions: How are you sleeping at night? Are you excessively sleepy during the daytime? Are there any unusual events or problems with your sleep, especially heavy snoring? More detailed aspects of assessment are included in individual sections within this chapter.

NORMAL SLEEP

DEFINITION AND PHYSIOLOGY

Sleep is an active, dynamic physiologic process. Normal human sleep consists of two major states of consciousness: non–rapid eye movement (NREM) sleep and rapid eye movement (REM) sleep. NREM sleep is further divided into three stages from lightest (N1) to deepest (N3, also referred to as slow-wave or delta sleep). These stages unfold in a predictable, repeated cycle. In young adults, NREM sleep occupies about 75% of the night and REM the remaining 25%. Delta sleep is most prominent in young children and gradually diminishes through the life cycle. REM sleep (or its ontogenetic precursor) is seen in very high percentages in neonates and infants but diminishes rapidly in the first years of life and remains fixed at about 25% thereafter. Normal total sleep time varies considerably with age.[2] Although young children require longer sleep times, total sleep time begins to decline by the second decade, remains relatively stable from the third decade through the fifth decade, and falls off more dramatically after the age of 70 years. It remains unclear to what extent the decline in nocturnal sleep in older individuals is a function of diminished sleep need as opposed to decreased ability to sleep. Time to fall asleep (sleep latency) and wake time after sleep onset are increased in older adults, as is daytime napping, although much of this may be related to factors that often accompany aging as opposed to the aging process itself.

NREM sleep is associated with a decline in respirations, heart rate, and blood pressure; muscle relaxation; and diminished cognitive activity. Sleep starts (sudden muscle contractions involving part or all of the body) may occur during wake-sleep transitions. REM sleep is marked by pronounced changes in physiology, including skeletal muscle atonia; increased variability in heart rate, blood pressure, respiration, and autonomic function; REM; and heightened cognitive activity associated with dreaming. Ventilatory drive to hypoxia and hypercapnia is decreased during NREM sleep and reaches its lowest point in REM sleep.

Current theories of sleep regulation focus on the two-process model.[3] This model suggests that sleep is regulated by two factors: homeostatic sleep drive, which increases progressively during wake time; and circadian wake drive, which is based on the oscillating 24-hour rhythm of the major circadian clock, located in the suprachiasmatic nucleus of the hypothalamus. Thus, the timing and amount of sleep are influenced by complex interactions between the biologic rhythms and the length of time since the last sleep period. Average human circadian cycles naturally run slightly longer than 24 hours (about 24.2 hours) but are reset daily (entrained) to a 24-hour rhythm by a variety of environmental cues, the most important of which is exposure to light. Sleep-wake rhythms are normally synchronized with myriad other clock-regulated physiologic functions, including endocrine-metabolic, immune, and cardiovascular.

INSOMNIA AND NON-RESTORATIVE SLEEP

DEFINITION AND EPIDEMIOLOGY

Current epidemiologic data indicate that about 30% to 35% of individuals in Western society report at least occasional insomnia.[4] Multiple studies place the prevalence of chronic insomnia at about 10%.[4] Insomnia is a complex condition that may represent a final common pathway with numerous contributing factors. Acute or transient insomnia (days to a few weeks) is an almost universal problem that is typically related to an acute stress or time zone shift (i.e., jet lag) and is usually self-resolving. Good sleep hygiene and, for some patients, short-term sleep medications are usually adequate. A potential complication of short-term insomnia is that some patients will begin to exhibit cognitions and behaviors that establish a foundation for development of a chronic insomnia problem.

PATHOPHYSIOLOGY

A widely accepted model of chronic insomnia suggests that it is a function of predisposing, precipitating, and perpetuating factors. Little is known about predisposing biologic or psychological factors, although it does seem clear that certain persons are at greater risk than others for the development of a chronic insomnia problem. Precipitating factors (which are sometimes referred to as causes of chronic insomnia) are identified in Box 206.1 and are discussed in greater detail later.

A unifying concept in the pathophysiology of chronic insomnia is that of hyperarousal.[5] Data indicate that patients with this condition exhibit evidence of both physiologic and cognitive hyperarousal, in the form of increased 24-hour metabolic rate, increased temperature, muscle tension, sleep electroencephalogram frequency, overactivity of the hypothalamic-pituitary-adrenal axis, and cognitive activity. It remains unclear how this hyperarousal develops, although preliminary data suggest that it is, at least in part, acquired and is amenable to change with therapeutic interventions such as cognitive behavioral treatment.

CLINICAL PRESENTATION

Psychiatric disorders, especially major depression, are the most common precipitating factors. Generalized anxiety, panic, and post-traumatic stress disorders are also associated with elevated rates of insomnia. Substance use or dependence, including alcohol, sedative-hypnotics, stimulants, and opiates, frequently manifests with insomnia, which may persist even after discontinuation of the substance. Excessive use of caffeine or even moderate use later in the day may also be problematic.

Circadian disorders, especially shift work and delayed sleep-wake phase disorder, are commonly associated with sleep complaints. Significant percentages of night shift workers experience abnormal sleep, with reduced total sleep times and poor quality of sleep. This pattern does not tend to improve during long periods of night work for most shift workers. As a result of circadian misalignment and sleep disturbances, shift workers are at increased risk for a number of medical disorders (ulcer disease, breast cancer among female shift workers, and cardiovascular disease) as well as accidents. Delayed sleep-wake phase disorder occurs most commonly in adolescents and younger adults and is characterized by an inability to sleep at normal clock times, with normal sleep onset occurring late (e.g., 4 a.m.), and subsequent inability to arise at conventional times (e.g., noon awakening). Sleep is otherwise restorative and normal, but the schedule is clearly inconsistent with meeting of normal school or work times. Advanced sleep-wake phase disorder is a less common circadian rhythm disorder, with normal sleep quantity and quality occurring early in the 24-hour day (e.g., 7 p.m. to 3 a.m.). It appears to be most common in older adults.

BOX **206.1**

Some Key Precipitants of Chronic Insomnia

PSYCHIATRIC DISORDERS
- Adjustment disorders
- Mood disorders
  - Major depressive disorder
  - Bipolar disorder
  - Dysthymic disorder
- Anxiety disorders
  - Generalized anxiety disorder
  - Post-traumatic stress disorder
  - Panic disorder
- Psychotic disorders
- Personality disorders

SUBSTANCES AND MEDICATIONS
- Alcohol
- Stimulants
  - Amphetamines, methylphenidate, modafinil, cocaine, ecstasy (MDMA, or 3,4-methylenedioxymethamphetamine), or caffeine
  - Steroids
  - Bronchodilators
  - Some antihypertensives
- Some antidepressants
- Cholesterol-lowering agents

MEDICAL AND NEUROLOGIC DISORDERS
- Degenerative neurologic diseases
- Stroke
- Recurrent nocturnal headache
- Traumatic brain injury
- Chronic obstructive pulmonary disease, nocturnal dyspnea, cough
- Nocturnal angina
- Gastroesophageal reflux disease, other nocturnal gastrointestinal disturbance
- Pain from any source
- Nocturia
- Endocrine disorders

OTHER SLEEP DISORDERS
- Obstructive or central sleep apnea
- Restless legs syndrome, periodic limb movements
- Nightmare disorder
- Circadian rhythm disorders

Medical conditions and medications may contribute to sleep disturbance. Among the most common are those associated with nocturnal pain, chronic lung disease, end-stage organ failure, endocrine disorders and other metabolic conditions, and especially neurodegenerative diseases. Likewise, many medications may aggravate sleep, most notably steroids, methylxanthines, some antihypertensives, stimulants, and certain antidepressant medications.

Other physiologic sleep disorders may result in an insomnia problem. The patient with restless legs syndrome (RLS) reports distressing "creepy-crawly" sensations in the legs or, less commonly, arms. The sensation is associated with an irresistible urge to move the extremities. The sensations may interfere with sleep onset. RLS is often associated with periodic limb movements (PLMs), which are characterized by repetitive, periodic (every 20 to 40 seconds) limb movements, often resulting in arousals that the sleeper is unaware of (much as in obstructive sleep apnea [OSA]). RLS is discussed in greater detail in the section on movement disorders.

Although OSA is most often associated with complaints of daytime sleepiness rather than with insomnia, these patients may have clinically significant complaints of insomnia. This association may be more prevalent among women with OSA. Therefore OSA must also be considered in the differential diagnosis, particularly in obese patients and those with heavy snoring.

The essential features of chronic insomnia according to the ICSD-3 are frequent and persistent difficulty initiating or maintaining sleep with a daytime consequence. An important subtype of chronic insomnia is psychophysiologic insomnia (PPI), a conditioned arousal in response to efforts to sleep and negative expectations regarding the ability to sleep. Individuals with PPI may be able to sleep better when they are not trying to fall asleep or in settings other than their own bedroom. Symptoms may include difficulty getting to sleep as well as trouble returning to sleep after awakening. This type of insomnia exists commonly as a disorder in its own right. However, the hyperarousal and negative conditioning that occur in this disorder are frequent complicating factors in insomnia that is associated with the numerous precipitating factors described earlier. Often, when an initial precipitating factor (e.g., a major depression, acute stress, or medical illness) resolves, it is these conditioned psychophysiologic elements that serve as the perpetuating factors noted earlier in this chapter.

DIAGNOSTICS
Essential Diagnostics

The essential element in the evaluation of an insomnia complaint is the history. The nature of the onset, course, complications, and treatments of the condition must be elicited in detail. Sleep-wake schedule, including napping, is critical to assessment. Sleep logs, usually conducted for 1 or 2 weeks, can be a helpful adjunct to history. The log should contain the following information for each night: time of getting into bed, time lights are actually turned out (e.g., after television, reading), estimate of sleep latency (time to fall asleep after lights out), estimate of the number of awakenings and total awake time across the night, time of final awakening, and time of actual arising. Evidence of other sleep-related symptoms (e.g., snoring and observed pauses in breathing, limb movement or restless legs, nightmares, behavioral disturbances, headaches, pain, gastroesophageal reflux) must be sought from the patient and, whenever possible, the bed partner. Daytime consequences, particularly evidence of significant sleepiness, should be assessed. Medical, neurologic, and psychiatric evaluations as well as pertinent physical examination and appropriate laboratory procedures are essential.

Additional Diagnostics

Polysomnography (PSG), overnight sleep recording, contributes little to the diagnosis of most insomnia presentations and is usually reserved for those cases in which demonstrable physiologic disturbances are suspected, typically breathing disorders, hypersomnias, and some parasomnias. PSG may also be appropriate for patients with treatment-refractory insomnia. Actigraphy (wrist-worn activity monitor that estimates wake and sleep patterns) can be of use as well particularly if a circadian rhythm disorder such as a delayed sleep phase syndrome is the suspected etiology of the insomnia.

DIFFERENTIAL DIAGNOSIS

The differential diagnosis of chronic insomnia should include both primary sleep diagnoses as well as medical and psychiatric problems. Priority differential includes (1) mood disorder, (2) circadian rhythm disorders, (3) other primary sleep disorders such as RLS and OSA, and (4) medical conditions that disrupt sleep such as chronic pain, RLS, congestive heart failure, or chronic respiratory conditions such as COPD or asthma.

INTERPROFESSIONAL COLLABORATIVE MANAGEMENT
Non-Pharmacologic Management

The management of insomnia begins with careful identification of the contributing factors. Treatment is tailored based on those factors. When clear precipitating causes are present (e.g., major depression or RLS), specific therapies appropriate to those factors must be instituted (e.g., antidepressant medication or dopamine agonists for RLS). Attention must also be directed to substances or medications that may be disturbing sleep. Sleep hygiene education is an essential component for management of any insomnia problem but is typically not sufficient treatment in its own right. Treatment of circadian rhythm sleep disorders is often complex and in many cases is best administered by sleep medicine specialists. Bright light therapy and melatonin have demonstrated therapeutic benefit in certain patients with circadian sleep-wake schedule disorders. Chronotherapy (planned behavioral adjustments of schedule) involving progressive phase delay has also been used for patients with delayed sleep phase disorder. Once precipitating factors have been evaluated and treated, additional therapeutic approaches lie largely in the pharmacologic and behavioral realm.

Psychologic and behavioral treatments for insomnia are the cornerstone of the treatment of insomnia (Table 206.1).[6] Approaches with the most evidence behind their use include stimulus control therapy, relaxation therapy, or a combined approach known as cognitive behavioral therapy for insomnia (CBT-I). When implementing stimulus control patients are instructed to get out of bed and do something relaxing after trying to sleep for approximately 20 minutes. The 20 minutes is estimated because they should not be watching the clock. CBT-I is brief and produces sustained benefit.[6] Compared with short-term courses of medication, CBT-I produces durable improvement, whereas improvements seen with time-limited courses of hypnotics tend to dissipate rapidly after drug discontinuation. CBT-I is typically administered by a psychologist or other mental health practitioner with expertise in this arena. There are Internet-based CBT-I programs which patients usually have to pay for but which may increase accessibility to those modes of treatment. Other behavioral techniques that may be of benefit include sleep restriction, paradoxical intent, and biofeedback.

Pharmacologic Management

- Several classes of medications may be of benefit in the short-term treatment of insomnia[7]. Caution should be used in the pharmacologic treatment of insomnia as patients may develop next-day impairment or amnestic behaviors among other complications. This is especially true in older adults;

TABLE 206.1 Common Behavioral Therapies for Chronic Insomnia

Sleep restriction	Maintain a sleep log and determine the mean TST for the baseline period (e.g., 1–2 weeks). Set bedtime and wake-up times to approximate the mean TST to achieve > 85% sleep efficiency (TST/TIB × 100%) for 7 days. The goal is for the total TIB (not <5 h) to approximate the TST. Make weekly adjustments: • For sleep efficiency (TST/TIB × 100%) >85% to 90%, TIB can be increased by 15–20 min. • For sleep efficiency <80%, TIB can be further decreased by 15–20 min. Repeat TIB adjustment every 7 days.
Stimulus control	Go to bed only when sleepy; maintain a regular schedule; avoid naps; use the bed only for sleep. If unable to fall asleep (or back to sleep) within 20 minutes, remove yourself from bed—engage in relaxing activity until drowsy, then return to bed; repeat this as necessary.
Relaxation therapy	Progressive muscle relaxation training involves methodical tensing and relaxing of different muscle groups throughout the body. Specific techniques are widely available in written and audio form.

TIB, time in bed; *TST,* total sleep time.

in patients with hepatic or renal impairment, alcohol or other substance use; and in those patients taking controlled substances.

- The benzodiazepine receptor agonists are one such class. Two medications in this class have evidence to support their use for both sleep onset and maintenance insomnia: zolpidem (based on trials of the 10 mg dose) and eszopiclone (based on trials of the 2 and 3 mg doses). Zaleplon at the 10 mg dose has evidence to support its use for sleep onset.
- Another class of medication, the benzodiazepines, can be of use in treating insomnia, though there are continued concerns about chronic use of benzodiazepines (i.e., tolerance, overdose, confusion). Triazolam at the 0.25 mg dose may be used in the treatment of sleep onset insomnia. Temazepam based on trial of the 7.5–15 mg dose may be useful in the treatment of sleep onset and maintenance insomnia.
- The orexin receptor agonist suvorexant has been shown to help with sleep maintenance insomnia at doses of 10 mg, 15/20 mg, and 20 mg.
- The melatonin agonist ramelteon may have benefit for the treatment of sleep onset insomnia at the 8 mg dose.
- The heterocyclic antidepressant doxepin at the 3 and 6 mg doses may help with sleep maintenance insomnia.
- Recent clinical guidelines suggest against the use of trazodone, tiagabine, diphenhydramine, melatonin, L-tryptophan, and Valerian in the treatment of insomnia.[7]

LIFE SPAN CONSIDERATIONS
Circadian rhythm disorders may appear at different times across the life span. Advanced sleep phase syndrome, which may lead to sleep maintenance issues, is most common in older adult populations. Delayed sleep phase syndrome is most common among adolescents.

COMPLICATIONS
Insomnia is associated with mood disorder.

PATIENT AND FAMILY EDUCATION
Tips for good sleep hygiene can be found at the National Sleep Foundation (https://sleepfoundation.org/ask-the-expert/sleep-hygiene). These include avoiding napping during the day and stimulants such as caffeine too close to bedtime. Patients can be advised as to the timing and regularity of exercise, meals, and bedtime routine. It is recommended that patients do not read (especially on the computer), watch TV, eat, check email and so forth while in bed. The bed should be associated only with sleep and sex. If still awake after 20 minutes, patients should be advised to get up and do something quiet until sleepy then try again.

SLEEP-RELATED BREATHING DISORDERS

DEFINITION AND EPIDEMIOLOGY
The sleep-related breathing disorders encompass a number of disorders, including the OSA disorders, central sleep apnea (CSA) syndromes, and the sleep-related hypoventilation disorders.

OSA is the most common sleep-related breathing disorder. The current prevalence estimates of moderate to severe sleep-disordered breathing are 10% to 17% among adult men and 3% to 9% among women in the United States.[8] These estimated prevalence rates represent substantial increases over the last 2 decades. The predominant physiologic derangement in OSA is repetitive upper airway narrowing or closure, which occurs during sleep. The closures (or near-closures) can occur many times a night, leading to significant sleep fragmentation and poor-quality sleep.

CSA is less common than OSA, although increasingly recognized. The CSA syndromes are characterized by reduced or absent airflow because of decreased or absent respiratory effort. As with OSA, CSA events often recur many times a night and can be associated with sleep fragmentation and poor-quality sleep. Many patients have a combination of OSA and CSA.

PATHOPHYSIOLOGY
OSA is characterized by repetitive episodes of complete upper airway occlusions (known as apneas) or partial upper airway occlusions (known as hypopneas) during sleep. These partial or complete airway closures lead to increased efforts to breathe, finally terminating in a brief central nervous system (CNS) arousal from sleep to reestablish patency of the upper airway. These events are often, although not always, associated with transient reductions in blood oxygen saturation. The cause of the upper airway narrowing may be related to craniofacial structure predisposing to a narrowed airway, as well as excessive soft tissue bulk impinging on the upper airway (excessive fat deposition in the tongue, soft palate, and lateral pharyngeal walls). The airway is kept patent by the pharyngeal dilating muscles. The activity of these muscles decreases with sleep onset, although it is normally adequate to maintain patency

of the airway. In patients with OSA, however, the activity of the pharyngeal dilator muscles during sleep is not adequate to maintain full patency, and partial or complete obstruction ensues. With each brief arousal, the muscle activity returns to wakefulness levels and patency is reestablished.

In CSA, the primary derangement is altered CNS respiratory drive, such that the patient does not receive the usual metabolic feedback to the CNS during sleep to drive the breathing in its normal pattern. This leads to repetitive cycles characterized by cessation of airflow because of lack of respiratory effort, which terminates once the metabolic trigger to breathe (usually blood carbon dioxide levels) increases sufficiently to drive respiratory output from the CNS. As with OSA, there are often brief CNS arousals associated with these events, leading to fragmented sleep.

CSA has a variety of causes, the hallmark of all of them related to processes that affect chemoresponsiveness and respiratory pattern stability. The more common causes of CSA include underlying significant cardiac or neurologic disease, such as atrial fibrillation or flutter, congestive heart failure, stroke, or brainstem disorders. These illnesses are often associated with a type of CSA known as Cheyne-Stokes breathing. This pattern is characterized by recurrent central apneas alternating with a waxing and waning pattern of airflow. Another, more common cause of CSA is the use of opioid medications, particularly the long-acting opioids, which affect respiratory drive.

CLINICAL PRESENTATION AND PHYSICAL EXAMINATION

A history of OSA is most often suggested by loud, disruptive snoring, with or without witnessed apneas, nocturnal gasping, or choking. Patients may report frank excessive daytime sleepiness (EDS), daytime fatigue and tiredness without unintentional sleep, or even vague depressive symptoms. They are often not aware of fragmented sleep because the respiratory-related arousals are often too brief to be consciously registered during the night. In fact, patients not uncommonly report that they sleep well through the night and are puzzled by their daytime sleepiness. Nocturia is a frequent complication of the disorder.

The most common risk factor for OSA is obesity, and patients may be able to relate the onset of their symptoms to weight gain. The disorder is more common in men, although the prevalence rate in postmenopausal women approaches the same level as in men. A substance history is helpful in that particular substances may alter airway muscle tone and further increase risk for obstructive respiratory events. This includes the use of alcohol, opiates, or muscle relaxant medication such as the benzodiazepines in the evening. It is also helpful to elicit other medical history, such as heart disease, hypertension, or stroke, because these disorders may be seen with OSA. On physical examination, the presence of obesity and a crowded oropharynx may be suggestive of OSA in a patient with symptoms associated with the disease.

In addition to leading to EDS and impairment of daytime functioning, untreated OSA has been found to have associations with a variety of longer term health consequences. There is substantial convincing evidence that moderate to severe untreated OSA is an independent cause of systemic hypertension, other cardiovascular disease, and stroke.[9,10] In addition, there is mounting evidence of an association with metabolic syndrome and type 2 diabetes mellitus.[11]

Individuals with CSA may be noted by their bed partner to have pauses in their breathing, which may or may not be followed by a period of more rapid breathing. They typically will not, however, have a history of snoring. These patients may also have complaints of EDS or daytime fatigue because the central apneic events disrupt sleep in a way similar to OSA events. Risk factors for CSA include decompensated congestive heart failure and the use of opioid medications, particularly the long-acting opioid medications such as methadone.

DIAGNOSTICS
Essential Diagnostics

Overnight sleep testing is required for the diagnosis of the sleep apnea syndromes (both OSA and CSA). Full overnight PSG is the gold standard for the diagnosis of sleep-related breathing disorders.[12]

Polysomnograms consist of a full night of monitoring numerous physiologic parameters during sleep, including electroencephalogram, oxygen saturation, multiple measures of airflow, and electrocardiogram. This procedure requires a full night in a sleep laboratory. While PSG provides the most accurate information regarding the presence and type of sleep-disordered breathing, it is an expensive procedure and not always widely available.

Unattended out-of-center sleep testing (OCST) is increasingly being used for the diagnosis of OSA. OCST is typically performed at home and assesses fewer biometric measures than full PSG. OCST is more accessible and cost-effective than full PSG, although it is crucial to understand the limitations of the usefulness of OCST and potential pitfalls.[12] OCST is indicated for patients with moderate to high pretest probability of OSA and no significant comorbidities or use of medications that increase risk for other breathing disorders, such as CSA or hypoventilation. It is also important to understand that OCST generally underestimates the number of obstructive respiratory events, and full PSG should be considered if the OCST result is negative in a patient with significant OSA risk factors or reported symptoms.

Additional Diagnostics

There are no other reliable methods for diagnosing obstructive or central sleep apnea at this time. Overnight pulse oximetry is not sufficiently sensitive to be used as a reliable screening test for sleep apnea.

DIFFERENTIAL DIAGNOSIS

Sleep-related breathing disorders often overlap and cannot be distinguished by clinical history alone. Nocturnal breathing disorders may also occur as a symptom of other underlying cardiopulmonary disorders. It is important to identify whether the nocturnal disorder is related to other concurrent disease (such as chronic obstructive pulmonary disease [COPD] or congestive heart failure).

Other causes of sleep fragmentation and/or EDS should also be considered (see separate sections on insomnia and hypersomnia for list).

INTERPROFESSIONAL COLLABORATIVE MANAGEMENT
Pharmacologic Management

There is currently no effective pharmacologic management for obstructive sleep apnea.

There is also currently no specifically effective pharmacologic management of central sleep apnea, although it is recommended, if possible, to discontinue or taper medications that may be causing CSA (i.e., opioid medications).

A referral to a sleep center where available can be extremely helpful.

Nonpharmacologic Management

Nonpharmacologic management strategies are the most effective management options for the sleep apnea syndromes.

Obstructive Sleep Apnea
- Continuous positive airway pressure (CPAP).
  - This is the most common and effective treatment, with efficacy rates of 95%. It is also essentially free of dangerous side effects.
  - The major impediments to successful CPAP therapy are comfort and acceptance. Careful counseling and initial attention to equipment fit can go a long way toward ensuring patient adherence with the device.
- Weight loss may also be helpful in the overall management strategy, although this should not be used as the sole treatment modality in patients with anything more than mild OSA.
- Custom-fit oral appliances.
  - Designed to increase posterior airway dimensions.
  - May be effective for milder OSA; not as effective as CPAP.
- Upper airway surgical procedures.
  - Standard procedures are designed to remove excessive upper airway tissue. These modalities, however, are less effective than CPAP, and success cannot be predicted before treatment. Less commonly, appropriate treatment choices may include tracheotomy or, in patients who have undergone a careful preoperative evaluation and failed to respond to less-invasive therapies, more extensive maxillofacial surgery.

Central Sleep Apnea
- If possible, tapering or discontinuation of medication that may be causing CSA.
- If CSA is related to decompensated or unstable cardiovascular process, the CSA may improve with improvement in the cardiovascular process.
- Positive airway pressure (PAP).
  - CSA may improve with CPAP, although there are newer PAP devices that are able to vary ventilatory support and rapidly adapt to changes in respiratory drive to alleviate the CSA events in patients in whom CPAP therapy fails.

LIFE SPAN CONSIDERATIONS

CSA may occur at any age, although it is most common between young adulthood and middle age. OSA does occur in older adults, although development of OSA does not necessarily increase with age.

COMPLICATIONS

As discussed earlier, substantial evidence implicates untreated OSA as a risk factor for multiple cardiovascular diseases, including systemic hypertension, coronary artery disease, congestive heart failure, and stroke. There is also accumulating evidence linking OSA to various arrhythmias, as well as increased risk for development of metabolic syndrome and type 2 diabetes mellitus. OSA may also increase the severity of depression. Risk

of motor vehicle accidents is significantly increased among those with OSA.

As opposed to OSA, CSA has not been identified as an independent risk factor for increased morbidity or mortality, although it can cause sleep fragmentation with associated hypersomnia, insomnia, or both.

PATIENT AND FAMILY EDUCATION

Patients should be educated about the impact of obesity on OSA, and weight loss should be encouraged. They should also be educated about the risks of untreated OSA and the importance of adhering to PAP treatment. They should understand that they should speak with the sleep provider if they are having problems tolerating PAP, because adjustments can be made to increase tolerance and acceptance.

CENTRAL NERVOUS SYSTEM HYPERSOMNIAS

DEFINITION AND EPIDEMIOLOGY

The primary disorders of hypersomnolence are characterized by an intrinsic CNS deficit resulting in a sleep-wake system that is inadequate for maintaining wakefulness or overactive in promoting sleep. The predominant clinical characteristic of these syndromes is EDS not caused by disturbed nocturnal sleep or misaligned circadian rhythms.

The primary hypersomnias include narcolepsy, idiopathic hypersomnia, and post-traumatic hypersomnia. Narcolepsy, the best defined of the primary hypersomnias, is characterized by EDS and inappropriate manifestations of REM sleep. These include such phenomena as cataplexy (sudden onset of REM-related muscle atonia precipitated by emotion during wakefulness) and hallucinations and paralysis occurring at sleep onset (hypnagogic) or offset (hypnopompic) related to inappropriately timed REM. The EDS and the REM-related symptoms can be extremely disabling and potentially dangerous, depending on when they occur.

Idiopathic CNS hypersomnia also involves CNS sleep system dysfunction, which results in profound EDS. However, with idiopathic CNS hypersomnia, there is no known disease of the REM system, and other symptoms present in narcolepsy are absent. Post-traumatic hypersomnia is not readily distinguishable from idiopathic hypersomnia, other than that the symptoms follow head injury or another CNS insult such as an infection.

PATHOPHYSIOLOGY

The key identifiable pathophysiologic derangement in narcolepsy is reduced hypocretin level in the cerebrospinal fluid. Hypocretin is a neuropeptide involved in the regulation of sleep. Most, though not all patients with narcolepsy (particularly if cataplexy is present) have absent or significantly reduced hypocretin levels. This may be related to a genetic mutation. Interestingly, narcolepsy may emerge after upper respiratory infections (such as with influenza and Streptococcus pyogenes infections), likely related to an autoimmune response that affects hypocretin. Additionally, reduced or undetectable hypocretin levels have been reported after severe head trauma.

The pathophysiology of idiopathic hypersomnia is unknown.

CLINICAL PRESENTATION

Assessment of the patient with EDS usually begins with either the patient or a family member complaining of sleepiness or unintentional sleep in undesired situations. This may include falling asleep unintentionally while watching television or reading, in noisy gatherings, at work, in conversation, or even while driving. Information obtained from a family member can be essential to accurate diagnosis because patients with EDS may not recognize or may minimize the severity of their symptoms. It is important to obtain a full sleep history, including 24-hour sleep-wake schedules, time and duration of naps, and associated symptoms that may point to the underlying cause of the EDS symptoms.

The key clinical feature of narcolepsy is EDS. Cataplexy, hypnagogic or hypnopompic hallucinations, sleep paralysis, and fragmented, disturbed nocturnal sleep may be present, but not all are required for the diagnosis. Cataplexy is seen almost exclusively in narcolepsy and is characterized by sudden episodes of muscle atonia during wakefulness. Cataplexy is often brought on when the patient is experiencing a strong emotion, particularly laughter. Such episodes may pose potential danger, depending on when and where they occur. They are often only seconds in duration but can last for minutes or longer in some cases. The sleep paralysis involves REM-related atonia (excluding the ocular muscles and diaphragm) and is often described as terrifying by patients. The hypnagogic or hypnopompic hallucinations are dreamlike and often frightening fragments that occur near sleep onset or offset and typically involve the patient's confusion about whether he or she is awake or asleep. The typical onset of narcolepsy symptoms is in the second or third decade, although it can occur earlier or later in life. There is no gender predominance. There are no features on physical examination that are particularly helpful in identifying narcolepsy.

The diagnosis of idiopathic CNS hypersomnia is most often a diagnosis of exclusion. Patients typically have complaints of EDS despite adequate or prolonged total sleep time, and they do not have the symptoms that otherwise characterize narcolepsy. A careful history should be obtained regarding possible CNS insult from infection or trauma.

In addition to using the history to identify these disorders, the health care provider should also question the patient for symptoms suggestive of RLS or periodic limb movement disorder (PLMD; discussed in further detail later in this chapter). The patient's sleep-wake schedule should also be evaluated to make certain that insufficient sleep is not playing a role, and a complete medication and substance history should be obtained because many medications and drugs may cause sleepiness as a side effect.

DIAGNOSTICS
Essential Diagnostics

Overnight PSG is generally employed in assessing the primary hypersomnias. The purpose is to exclude other underlying causes of the patient's sleepiness symptoms, such as an occult sleep-related breathing disorder. If no cause of EDS is identified on overnight PSG, the next step is to perform a multiple sleep latency test (MSLT).[13] The MSLT is used to determine one's propensity for daytime sleep. The subject is given multiple opportunities to nap under standardized conditions, and a mean sleep-onset latency (i.e., time to fall asleep) is determined

and compared with normative values. This is the most objective means of determining EDS, although daytime continuous PSG can confirm findings. The presence of sleep-onset REM episodes on the MSLT is a required diagnostic finding for narcolepsy.

Additional Diagnostics

Hypocretin-1 levels may be measured in the cerebrospinal fluid in evaluating possible narcolepsy, although this test is not routinely performed. A low hypocretin level does confirm the diagnosis, although a normal level does not rule out the diagnosis if the PSG/MSLT findings are otherwise consistent with narcolepsy. Genetic testing may also be performed, as there are genetic markers associated with narcolepsy. As with the hypocretin testing, however, a negative test does not rule out the diagnosis and in practice this testing is not routinely performed.

DIFFERENTIAL DIAGNOSIS

The differential diagnosis for excessive daytime sleepiness should involve assessing for any factors that may cause insufficient sleep, as well as any factors that may cause disrupted sleep, such as underlying medical or neurological problems, other underlying sleep disorders, or medications/substances that may cause sleep disruption.

 Priority differentials include (1) OSA or CSA, (2) primary medical/neurologic disorder, (3) substance/medication, (4) insufficient sleep, and (5) circadian rhythm disorder.

INTERPROFESSIONAL COLLABORATIVE MANAGEMENT
Pharmacologic Management

EDS as a result of CNS-based disorders has historically been treated with stimulant medications to improve alertness. If the diagnosis of narcolepsy with cataplexy is present, additional medications may be necessary to suppress the cataplexy.

The most commonly used stimulants are forms of dextroamphetamine and methylphenidate. They can be used in short-acting formulations or longer-acting formulations. The shorter-acting formulations are given in divided doses throughout the day and can be titrated for symptom relief. The slow-release formulations are more convenient for use, although may also provide more gradual and delayed response.

Modafinil, and its newer form, armodafinil, are wakefulness promoting agents with an unknown mechanism of action. They are not amphetamine-based and thus have lower risk of becoming habit forming. These medications are longer acting and there is a significant risk of insomnia if they are taken past the late morning hours.

Cataplexy is treated with REM-suppressing medications. Most commonly, these have included the tricyclic antidepressants, selective serotonin reuptake inhibitor–type antidepressants, and serotonin-norepinephrine reuptake inhibitor-type antidepressants. More recently, γ-hydroxybutyrate has become available as a therapy for cataplexy.

COMPLICATIONS

The sleepiness associated with hypersomnias in general can affect performance and function at work and in school. Additionally, the sleepiness can increase risk of motor vehicle accidents and work-related accidents. More specific complications from narcolepsy can be related to cataplexy, which can cause significant risk depending on the setting in which it occurs.

In addition, there may be medication-related side effects, particularly related to long-term use of stimulant medications.

PATIENT AND FAMILY EDUCATION

Narcolepsy is a chronic condition that can significantly affect quality of life. The goal of treatment is to optimize control of symptoms to allow patients to have a full personal and professional life. An important treatment is referral to patient support groups. Local groups may be found through sources such as Narcolepsy Network. Many websites also offer helpful information (www.sleepeducation.org).

Career counseling is also important, as patients with narcolepsy should generally avoid jobs in the driving/transportation industry, shift work, and with frequent on-call schedules as well as jobs that require continuous attention for long hours without breaks. Some of these difficulties can be overcome by strategic napping (15 to 20 minute naps every 4 hours scheduled throughout the day). Employers may need to be educated about narcolepsy and the importance of this accommodation for performance and safety.

SLEEP-RELATED MOVEMENT DISORDERS: RESTLESS LEGS SYNDROME

DEFINITION AND EPIDEMIOLOGY

Sleep-related movement disorders are conditions in which patients have simple stereotyped movements or other sleep-related monophasic movements that disturb or prevent sleep. Sleep-related leg cramps, sleep-related rhythmic movement disorder, PLMD, and sleep-related bruxism are disorders that fall into this category. Even though RLS does not truly fit the definition of a simple stereotyped movement, because of its association with PLMs, it is included in this category. Because RLS is so common (5% to 10% in populations derived from Western Europe),[1] this will be the focus of this section. The prevalence of RLS increases with age, but symptoms may start in childhood. RLS is seen more commonly in women. RLS is defined as an uncomfortable sensation, usually in the legs, associated with a strong desire to move the legs. This discomfort begins or worsens during periods of inactivity, is partially or totally relieved by movement, and occurs exclusively or predominantly in the evening or at night.[1] The timing of the discomfort may be altered after treatment. Because this discomfort occurs primarily in the evening, it may lead to sleep difficulties.

PATHOPHYSIOLOGY

The pathophysiology of RLS is unclear but the disorder may be familial, idiopathic, or seen in association with other disorders. RLS that develops before the age of 45 is more typically familial and is associated with slower progression.[1] RLS may occur in association with a wide variety of conditions. Pregnancy, renal failure, and low iron stores (ferritin levels below 75 mcg/L or a transferrin saturation less than 17%)[14] have the best-established associations. Peripheral neuropathy and Parkinson disease may also be associated with RLS. A number

of widely used medications, including most antidepressants, sedating antihistamines, alcohol, lithium, and dopamine antagonists, may cause or exacerbate RLS.[15] Given the efficacy of dopaminergic agents in treating RLS, a CNS dysfunction in a dopaminergic system has been postulated as a cause of this syndrome.

CLINICAL PRESENTATION

Patients with RLS may visit their health care provider because they find the discomfort bothersome or possibly because of sleep-onset problems caused by the discomfort. RLS has four principal diagnostic criteria. The first is an urge to move the legs, usually accompanied or caused by an uncomfortable sensation in the legs. The second and third criteria are that this urge begins or worsens during inactivity or rest and is at least partially ameliorated by activity or movement, such as stretching or walking. The final criterion is that the urge or sensations are worsened or occur exclusively in the evening or at night. A family history is supportive of the diagnosis as is a therapeutic response to a dopamine agonist.

The findings on physical examination are normal unless the RLS occurs in the setting of an associated medical condition (e.g., peripheral neuropathy, Parkinson disease).

DIAGNOSTICS
Essential Diagnostics

Assessing a patient's iron status is prudent in patients with RLS. Ferritin levels lower than 75 mcg/L or a transferrin saturation less than 17% have been associated with RLS. Patients who demonstrate reduced iron stores in this way may note improvement with iron replacement. Of course if an iron deficiency anemia is found, that should be evaluated and treated appropriately and treatment may lead to improvement in the RLS.

Additional Diagnostics

RLS is a clinical diagnosis, but PSG can sometimes be helpful because it may offer information supportive of the diagnosis or RLS. PLMs are triple flexion (hip, knee, and ankle flexion) responses of the legs that occur every 5 to 90 seconds during sleep. PLMs are present on PSG in up to 90% of people with RLS. The presence of PLMs would then be supportive of the diagnosis of RLS. PLMs, however, can occur in association with other sleep disorders, such as sleep-disordered breathing, narcolepsy, and REM sleep behavior disorder. PLMs can also be seen in patients without sleep disorders as an incidental finding. PLMs in the absence of RLS are not labeled as a disorder (PLMD) unless they lead to disturbed sleep. PLMD is rare. PSG is useful in assessing for the presence of PLMs but is not necessary for the diagnosis of RLS.

INITIAL DIAGNOSTICS

Restless Legs Syndrome

LABORATORY
- Fasting serum iron level
- Total iron binding capacity
- Ferritin
- Transferrin saturation

DIFFERENTIAL DIAGNOSIS

RLS must be distinguished from other forms of lower extremity discomfort using history and exam. Priority differentials include (1) arthritis, (2) neuropathy, (3) leg cramps, and (4) vascular disease (claudication).

The response of RLS to dopaminergic agents and the irresistible urge to move the legs in RLS can help distinguish it from these other disorders. Leg cramps can be distinguished from RLS in that typical leg cramps involve a specific muscle, which often visibly hardens. Stretching of the specific muscle improves the condition. The presence of neuropathy because it may be associated with RLS does not exclude the presence of RLS. Anxiety may mimic RLS but the focus of a need to move in the legs can help distinguish RLS from anxiety.

INTERPROFESSIONAL COLLABORATIVE MANAGEMENT

Non-Pharmacologic Management

Mild forms of RLS can potentially be addressed with good sleep hygiene, massage, hot baths, or exercise. Compressive devices have also been suggested. Overall there is insufficient evidence, however, to strongly endorse any non-pharmacologic treatments.[15]

Pharmacologic Management

Pharmacologic treatment is not required. One must determine with the patient if the distress caused by the RLS warrants pharmacologic treatment. The following classes of drugs have been used with some success:

α-2-delta ligands. This class of medications includes gabapentin, pregabalin, and gabapentin enacarbil. Only gabapentin enacarbil has FDA approval as a treatment for RLS in this class of medications. This class of medications can be a good first line agent to treat as they are well tolerated, and may help address sleep disturbance or pain from other etiologies (if there is an associated neuropathy for example).[16]

Dopamine agonists. Some of the best-studied agents include the dopaminergic agonists pramipexole, rotigotine, and ropinirole. All three have FDA approval for the treatment of RLS.[15] These may be particularly good first-line agents in patients with concomitant depression or who present a risk for falls. There are some pitfalls with these agents such as the development of augmentation (development of symptoms earlier in the day) as well as an impulse control disorder. Patients on these agents should be routinely screened for the development of an impulse control disorder. These problems may possibly be avoided by keeping doses low.

Carbidopa-levodopa was commonly used for this disorder in the past, but because of rebound symptoms and augmentation, it has been largely replaced by other agents.

Other options for the treatment of RLS include opioids, carbamazepine, and clonidine.

Supplemental iron may be useful in patients with reduced iron stores as discussed above.[15]

Reduction in the dose or discontinuation of a medication known to cause RLS may also offer relief.

LIFE SPAN CONSIDERATIONS

Onset of RLS may occur from childhood through late adulthood. Mean age of onset for familial RLS is in the third or fourth decade, with onset before the age of 21 in about one-third of cases.[15] Early-onset (before the age of 45) RLS tends to be a more slowly progressive disorder, and some patients may have stable symptoms over time. Late-onset RLS (after the age of 45) tends to be more rapidly progressive.[17]

COMPLICATIONS

Because of the timing of the leg discomfort, insomnia is often a complicating factor in RLS. Patients with difficult-to-manage RLS or RLS in the setting of significant medical comorbidities may merit referral to a sleep medicine specialist.

EDUCATION AND HEALTH PROMOTION

Patients and family should understand that this is generally a progressive and persistent disorder in its idiopathic form. Medication can be used to ameliorate the symptoms. Secondary forms of RLS may improve with treatment or resolution of the primary disorder. Patients should if possible avoid medications or substances that might trigger or worsen RLS.

PARASOMNIAS

 Injury to the patient or bed partner is possible given the lack of awareness during disorders of arousal from NREM sleep.

DEFINITION, EPIDEMIOLOGY, AND PATHOPHYSIOLOGY

Parasomnias, as defined by the ICSD, are undesirable physical events or experiences that occur during entry into sleep, within sleep, or during arousals from sleep.[1] The pathophysiology of this heterogeneous group of disorders is variable and depends in part on the stage of sleep from which they arise. In the case of disorders of arousal from NREM sleep (e.g., sleepwalking, sleep terrors, confusional arousals), the mechanism is an abrupt and abnormal arousal from delta (stage N3) sleep. Any factor that increases delta sleep (e.g., prior sleep deprivation) or leads to fragmentation of delta sleep (e.g., OSA, biopsychosocial stress) could predispose the person to this group of disorders, although genetic predisposition may be an important factor for many affected individuals. This group of disorders most often occurs in children but can occur in adults.

REM sleep behavior disorder (RBD) and nightmare disorder are the most prominent REM-related parasomnias. RBD results from the loss of normal REM muscle atonia, typically in men older than 50 years. In this disorder, the patient enacts dreams, often in a potentially dangerous fashion. RBD is thought to result when pathways which generate REM atonia in the brainstem are dysfunctional. RBD has been associated with antidepressant usage, certain neurodegenerative conditions, and other sleep disorders such as narcolepsy.

Nightmare disorder is a distinct disorder from RBD. Nightmares are terrifying dreams that often result in awakening. They are common on an occasional basis among adults and children. When nightmares occur repeatedly and are associated with significant distress or impairment, nightmare disorder should be considered. Nightmare disorder may result from psychological factors, inherited factors, prior sleep deprivation, or the use or withdrawal of certain medications. Specifically, the cessation of most types of antidepressant medications will predispose the patient to a transient increase in nightmares.

Nightmares are especially common in post-traumatic stress disorder patients.

CLINICAL PRESENTATION

Patients may be initially seen with a chief complaint of disturbing behaviors during sleep. A careful history is helpful in distinguishing NREM from REM parasomnias. The disorders of arousal from NREM sleep (confusional arousals, sleepwalking, and sleep terrors) arise from slow-wave sleep, which occurs primarily in the first third of the night. There is often a family history of a disorder of arousal from NREM sleep. Features common to the disorders of arousal from NREM sleep according to the ICSD[1] include the following: (1) inappropriate or absent responsiveness to the intervention of others, (2) limited or no associated dream imagery, and (3) partial or complete amnesia for the event. Additional features can help distinguish the precise type of parasomnia. Confusional arousals consist of mental confusion precipitated by an arousal from sleep but without ambulation outside the bed and with no signs of terror or autonomic arousal. Sleep terrors consist of episodes in which the patient sits up and screams with a terrified expression. There are accompanying signs of autonomic arousal (mydriasis, tachypnea, and tachycardia). Patients will be amnestic or recall an image but not a complex dream, as would be the case with a nightmare. The episodes last 30 seconds to 3 minutes typically. Sleepwalking (somnambulism) consists of walking and automatic behaviors without awakening, usually for less than 5 minutes. Complex behaviors, such as eating and driving, may occur. The subject may be violent, particularly if an attempt is made to awaken him or her. The physical examination is usually unremarkable in the NREM parasomnias.

In RBD, enactment of an often violent dream occurs. The patient and bed partner are at risk for injury during these events. Unlike in the disorders of arousal in NREM sleep, there is typically an associated dream with a coherent story line. RBD may be idiopathic or may be associated with other neurologic disorders, making further neurologic assessment in newly diagnosed RBD patients a necessity. The strongest association is with the α-synucleinopathies (Parkinson disease, dementia with Lewy bodies, and multiple system atrophy). There may be a latency of years from the development of RBD until the onset of the Parkinsonian features in these disorders. Neurologic exam should be undertaken in patients with RBD to evaluate for an underlying neurodegenerative disorder. Physical exam may reveal signs of one of the aforementioned neurodegenerative disorders.

Nightmare disorder is characterized by awakenings from sleep associated with recall of a disturbing dream. In general, the patient is fully alert on awakening with clear recall of the dream. The patient may be so distressed as to have a delay in the return to sleep. Events typically occur in the second half of the night when REM sleep is most common. As one would expect, physical examination findings are typically normal, and PSG is not required to make the diagnosis.

DIAGNOSTICS

Essential Diagnostics. Disorders of arousal from NREM sleep are typically diagnosed by history. PSG can be helpful in detecting precipitating or associated disorders, such as OSA, and may also reveal an increase in slow-wave sleep percentage and fragmentation. PSG is required for the evaluation of RBD.

PSG in patients with this disorder may reveal elevated muscle tone in REM sleep and PLMs. PSG can also be useful in REM to evaluate for precipitating factors such as OSA. OSA for example may trigger parasomnias that phenotypically resemble RBD.

DIFFERENTIAL DIAGNOSIS

When evaluating parasomnias, history, age of patient, and comorbidities can all be used to help achieve the proper diagnosis. NREM and REM parasomnias can often be differentiated on the basis of these factors. Parasomnias must not only be differentiated from themselves but from mimickers. Priority differentials include (1) nocturnal epilepsy, (2) parasomnias secondary to other medical conditions such as OSA, and (3) psychiatric disease such as PTSD and panic disorder.

Some disorders present during waking hours may also occur during sleep. Up to 50% of patients with panic disorder experience panic attacks at some point in their lifetime that arise out of sleep, typically NREM sleep.[17] Nocturnal seizures (Chapter 182) are another group of disorders that may arise from sleep. Certain types of nocturnal seizures, especially nocturnal frontal lobe epilepsy (NFLE), may arise exclusively from sleep. The sometimes bizarre nature of seizures in NFLE may make diagnosis a challenge. Clinical features can help distinguish NFLE from NREM parasomnias (Table 206.2), although overnight PSG or video-electroencephalographic monitoring is often required.

INTERPROFESSIONAL COLLABORATIVE MANAGEMENT

Non-Pharmacologic Management

Sleep medicine consultation is indicated for parasomnias during which violent or dangerous behavior is exhibited or parasomnias in the context of suspicion for other sleep disorders such as OSA. Reassurance of the patient or parents, coupled with attention to safety issues, may be sufficient management. Modifying the sleep environment in RBD is recommended to prevent injury. Possible recommendations might include moving the mattress to the floor, padding furniture, removing dangerous objects from the bedroom, window protection, a door alarm, and possibly having the bed partner sleep in a separate room until the events are controlled.

Image rehearsal therapy (IRT), systemic desensitization, progressive deep muscle relaxation training, lucid dreaming therapy, and self-exposure therapy all have been reported to be of help in treating nightmares, with IRT having the most evidence to support its use.[18] Addressing predisposing factors, such as sleep deprivation, medications, and stress, may be helpful for parasomnias in general.

TABLE 206.2	Distinguishing Seizures in NFLE From NREM Parasomnias	
	NREM Parasomnia	**Seizure in NFLE**
Episodes per month	<1 or a few	Usually >10
Episodes per night	1	>1
Type of episode	Nonstereotyped	Stereotyped
Episode duration	Minutes	Seconds

Modified from Malow, B. A., & Plazzi, G. (2003). Nocturnal seizures. In S. Chokroverty, W. A. Hening, A. S. Walters (Eds.), *Sleep and movement disorders*. Philadelphia: Butterworth-Heinemann.

Pharmacologic Management

Many disorders of arousal from NREM sleep do not require pharmacologic treatment. When medication is indicated the following have been used:

Benzodiazepines and tricyclic antidepressants have been successfully used in sleepwalking and night terrors. Certain atypical antipsychotics such as olanzapine or risperidone can be helpful. Antidepressants including fluvoxamine have been used with some success.[18] Sedating medications, however, may also precipitate confusional arousals, because they make it more difficult for the patient to awaken.

RBD often responds well to clonazepam or melatonin.[19] Clonazepam at doses of 0.25 to 2 mg at bedtime or melatonin at doses of 3 to 12 mg at bedtime may be of benefit. Melatonin may be better tolerated. Prazosin at bedtime may be of benefit in patients with nightmares related to PTSD.[18]

LIFE SPAN CONSIDERATIONS

Disorders of arousal from NREM sleep are most commonly seen in children and typically resolve in adolescence. RBD is most commonly seen in men over the age of 50. Nightmare disorder can occur at any age.

COMPLICATIONS

Given the lack of awareness during disorders of arousal from NREM sleep, injury is possible. Patients with this disorder should keep their bedrooms clear of obstacles, consider child safety locks on windows, remove all dangerous objects from the bedroom (e.g., pills, knives), and consider a door alarm on the bedroom door. Because of the violent nature of the dream enactment, patients with RBD may injure themselves or their bed partners. Dangerous parasomnias or suspicion for RBD should generate a referral to a sleep medicine specialist. If there is suspicion for a concomitant sleep disorder such as sleep apnea that might act as a trigger for the parasomnia, evaluation along those lines should be considered.

PATIENT AND FAMILY EDUCATION

Families of children with disorders of arousal from NREM may require reassurance. Keeping the bedroom environment safe is essential. If a sleepwalker is encountered, he or she should be gently guided back to bed. Avoidance of triggers for parasomnias such as sleep deprivation is important. Patients with RBD and their families should be reassured that the violent dream enactment does not mean the affected individual has violent tendencies. Treatment is important to keep the patient and bed partner safe.

REFERENCES

1. American Academy of Sleep Medicine (AASM). (2014). *International classification of sleep disorders* (3rd ed.). Westchester, Ill: AASM.
2. Babcock, D. (2011). Evaluating sleep and sleep disorders in the pediatric primary care setting. *Pediatric Clinics of North America, 58*(3), 543–554.
3. Borbely, A. A. (1982). A two-process model of sleep regulation. *Human Neurobiology, 1,* 195–204. Original research.
4. Zhou, E., Gardiner, P., & Bertisch, S. (2017). Integrative medicine for insomnia. *The Medical Clinics of North America, 101*(5), 865–879.
5. Levenson, J., Kay, D., & Buysse, D. (2015). The pathophysiology of insomnia. *Chest, 147*(4), 1179–1192.
6. Qaseem, A., Kanasgara, D., Forciea, M.-A., et al. (2016). Management of chronic insomnia disorder in adults: A clinical practice guideline from the American College of Physicians. *Annals of Internal Medicine, 165*(2), 125–133.
7. Sateia, M. J., Buysse, D. J., Krystal, A. D., et al. (2017). Clincial practice guideline for the pharmacologic treatment of chronic insomnia in adults: An American Academy of Sleep Medicine clinical practice guideline. *Journal of Clinical Sleep Medicine: JCSM: Official Publication of the American Academy of Sleep Medicine, 13*(2), 307–349.
8. Peppard, P. E., Young, T., Barnet, J. H., et al. (2013). Increased prevalence of sleep-disordered breathing in adults. *American Journal of Epidemiology, 177*(9), 1006–1014.
9. Monahan, K., & Redline, S. (2011). Role of obstructive sleep apnea in cardiovascular disease. *Current Opinion in Cardiology, 26*(6), 541–547.
10. Mohsenin, V. (2015). Obstructive sleep apnea: A new preventive and therapeutic target for stroke. *The American Journal of Medicine, 128*(8), 811–816.
11. Gaines, J., Vgontzas, A., Fernandez-Mendoza, J., & Bixler, E. (2018). Obstructive sleep apnea and the metabolic syndrome: The road to clinically-meaningful phenotyping, improved prognosis, and personalized treatment. *Sleep Medicine Reviews, 42,* 211–219.
12. Qaseem, A., Dallas, P., Owens, D., et al. (2014). Diagnosis of obstructive sleep apnea in adults: A clinical practice guideline from the American College of Physicians. *Annals of Internal Medicine, 161*(3), 210–220.
13. Pizza, F., Moghadan, K., & Vandi, S. (2013). Daytime continuous polysomnography predicts MSLT results in hypersomnias of central origin. *Journal of Sleep Research, 22*(1), 32–40.
14. Mansur, A., & Bokhari, S. R. A. (2018). Restless leg syndrome. In *StatPearls [internet].* Treasure Island (FL): StatPearls Publishing. Retrieved from https://www.ncbi.nlm.nih.gov/books/NBK430878/. (Retrieved 6 April 2018). [Updated 2017 May 17].
15. Winkelman, J. W., Armstrong, M. J., Allen, R. P., et al. (2016). Practice guideline summary: Treatment of restless legs syndrome in adults: Report of the guideline development, dissemination, and implementation subcommittee of the American Academy of Neurology. *Neurology, 87*(24), 2585–2593. doi:10.1212/WNL.0000000000003388.
16. Allen, R. P., Montplaisir, J., Walters, A. S., et al. (2017). Restless legs syndrome and periodic limb movements during sleep. In M. Kryger, T. Roth, & W. Dement (Eds.), *Principles and Practice of Sleep Medicine* (6th ed.). Philadelphia: Elsevier.
17. Soehner, A., & Harvey, A. (2012). Prevalence and functional consequences of severe insomnia symptoms in mood and anxiety disorders: Results from a National representative sample. *Sleep, 35*(10), 1367–1375.
18. Morgenthaler, T. I., Auerbach, S., Casey, K. R., Kristo, D., Maganti, R., Ramar, K., et al. (2018). Position paper for the treatment of nightmare disorder in adults: An American Academy of Sleep Medicine position paper. *Journal of Clinical Sleep Medicine: JCSM: Official Publication of the American Academy of Sleep Medicine, 14*(6), 1041–1055.
19. St Louis, E. K., et al. (2017). REM sleep behavior disorder: Diagnosis, clinical implications, and future directions. *Mayo Clinic Proceedings, 92*(11), 1723–1736.

CHAPTER **207**

UNINTENDED WEIGHT LOSS

Joanne Sandberg-Cook

 Immediate hospitalization required for a patient with severe anorexia associated with rapid weight loss, hypokalemia, hypotension, or prerenal azotemia related to dehydration.

DEFINITION AND EPIDEMIOLOGY

Although not all involuntary weight loss is ominous, an unintentional loss in excess of 5% of body weight during a period of 6 to 12 months typically warrants further investigation.[1,2] With a weight loss of 10% of body weight over 12 months, the effects of protein-energy malnutrition and poor health outcomes are substantial.[3] By contrast with intentional weight loss, which has been associated with a decreased mortality rate up to a decade later, unintentional weight loss has been associated with a substantial degree of morbidity and mortality.[4]

Unintentional weight loss and *involuntary weight loss* are synonymous terms. Many studies have pointed to the significance of a 5% to 10% weight loss within a year as an indicator of declining health which is often incorporated in more global measures of frailty. Frailty, in particular, results from a condition of reduced physical ability and unintentional weight loss. Frailty and subsequent vulnerability to adverse health events (disability, falls, hospitalizations, and death) is a significant risk in patients older than 70 who are chronically ill.[3,4] In the Systolic Hypertension in the Elderly Program (SHEP) study of over 4700 people, subjects aged 60 years or older who had a weight loss of 1.6 kg/yr had a fivefold greater death rate; those with a low initial weight and a greater than 1.6 kg/yr weight loss had a 20-fold increased mortality compared with those without a weight change.[5] As many as 20% to 50% of hospitalized older adults are undernourished, and community-dwelling older adults who are undernourished are more likely to be frail.[6]

PATHOPHYSIOLOGY

Human weight homeostasis is a complex interaction of cytokines, neurons, adipose tissue hormones, gut peptides, and hypothalamic input, as influenced by psychosocial cues.[1] Satiety is driven by gastric distention neurons and release of cholecystokinin, peptide YY, glucagon-like peptide 1, and amylin; hunger is driven by ghrelin, whereas leptin, released from adipocytes affecting hypothalamic receptors, provides a negative feedback loop on food intake.[1] With aging, the speed of the responsiveness of visceral neurons and diminished sensitivity to the action of gut distention are attributed to early satiety; changes in ghrelin and other androgens as well as an increase in the appetite-suppressant leptin, particularly in women, have been associated with other reduced gastric emptying mechanisms suspected in the setting of circulating satiation hormones, including postprandial insulin and inflammatory cytokines.[3] Weight loss is thought to follow from one or more of the following: decreased calorie or fluid volume intake, decreased calorie absorption, or increased metabolic demands.

Decreased calorie intake may result from a behavioral adaptation to what is an unsatisfactory eating experience. Weight loss caused by functional anorexia may result from apathy, mechanical obstacles to mastication, depressed sense of taste and smell, delayed gastric emptying time, or pain with elimination. Decreased calorie absorption results from malabsorption, vomiting, diarrhea, and urinary frequency, which may tip the balance to decreased calorie intake. Increased metabolism occurs with infection, hyperactivity, hyperthyroidism, and tumor growth through neurohormonal mechanisms.

The body's composition changes with aging. After age 30, lean body mass is incrementally replaced by gains in fat mass until about 65 or 70, when incremental weight loss of 0.1 to 0.2 kg/yr (0.2 to 0.4 lb/yr) or 0.5% per year occurs, with a peak weight around age 60.[2] Protein-energy malnutrition occurs when the supply of proteins or calories is inadequate to maintain weight. A combination of the conditions marasmus (insufficient calories) and kwashiorkor (protein deficiency) occurs, as evidenced by changes in body composition, systemic weakness, and laboratory abnormalities. Although not specific to involuntary weight loss, sarcopenia refers to reduced muscle mass (more than two standard deviations from young adults of the same sex and ethnicity) and loss of muscle strength.[7] Sarcopenia, often related to poor nutrition and weight loss, contributes to frailty.

Many chronically ill adults and elders, particularly nursing home patients, have weight loss–driven protein-energy malnutrition owing to medical, social, cognitive, and psychological factors, all of which may be amenable to improvement; this may include conditions that produce cachexia from increased metabolic demands. Cachexia is characterized by muscle wasting, following weight and fat loss, often confounded by anorexia. One definition calls for weight loss of 5% to 10% of body weight or greater over 12 months or less and three to five of the following: abnormal laboratory test results (increased inflammatory markers, anemia, and hypoalbuminemia), anorexia, decreased muscle strength, fatigue, and/or low fat-free mass index.[8] If cachexia has developed, it may disproportionately affect skeletal and cardiac muscle and is no longer a reversible process.[8] Precachexia refers to those early clinical warning signs which, when noted, may be amenable to interventions. Precachexia is defined as (1) underlying chronic disease, (2) unintentional weight loss of 5% or less of usual body weight during the previous 6 months, (3) chronic or recurrent inflammatory response, and (4) anorexia or anorexia-related symptoms. Precachexia is commonly associated with cancer; chronic obstructive pulmonary disease (COPD); chronic heart, renal, or liver failure; acquired immunodeficiency syndrome (AIDS); or rheumatoid arthritis.[8]

CLINICAL PRESENTATION AND PHYSICAL EXAMINATION

Patients may be unaware of weight changes. In the absence of consistent health records, they may only recall the observations of others or notice loose-fitting clothing as evidence of weight loss. In fact, many older patients may note a weight loss with pleasure, believing that lower weight is desirable. Obtaining a history of the quantity, quality, and regularity of food and fluid intake as well as of physical activity, mood, and cognition is of utmost importance. Symptoms associated with decreased intake, such as fever, night sweats, dyspnea, and mental status changes, suggest underlying infection, malignant disease, or possible neurologic impairment. Tremor, forgetfulness, mental confusion, and apathy may inadvertently lead to meal skipping or reduced intake at meals.

Swallowing difficulties may cause a patient to adjust the types or amounts of food eaten. Common reasons for decreased intake include dysgeusia or ageusia, sticking or choking sensation, pain with chewing, dry mouth, unpleasant smell of food, heartburn, and gastric pain before or after eating or associated with eating fatty or acidic foods. Older adults experience diminished senses of taste, smell, and thirst because of physiologic changes of the tongue and olfaction, which blunt the palatability of food and possibly slow transit time as a result. Severe gastroesophageal reflux, nausea, vomiting, abdominal bloating, flatulence, constipation, and diarrhea affect intake. Individuals may also try to prevent diarrhea by avoiding food. Milk products associated with these complaints might signal lactose intolerance.

Gluten intolerance or sensitivity (celiac disease), now more commonly diagnosed than in the past, may cause diarrhea and lead to weight loss. Bloody, painful, or urgent stool can indicate hemorrhoids, inflammatory bowel disease, or malignant disease. Fatty, odorous stool can point to gallbladder disease or malabsorption syndromes. A history of chronic diarrhea, whether secondary to bacterial or parasitic exposure or a result of underlying illness or recent hospitalization, should be elicited.

Situational stress or anxiety sometimes contributes to unintentional weight loss, as can changes in mood, affect, or coping.

Premorbid health conditions can tax a patient's reserves to a degree that interferes with adequate nutrition and hydration. Fatigue, shortness of breath, or impaired mobility may make the duration of a meal exhausting, resulting in decreased intake. It is critical to obtain a smoking, alcohol, and drug history. Patients who abuse alcohol may substitute it for food, leading to vitamin deficiencies and subsequent malnutrition. A history of risky sexual and self-harm behaviors, which put people at risk for debilitating infectious diseases including human immunodeficiency virus (HIV) and AIDS, should be elicited along with a history of eating disorders. Immunocompromised states can coexist with wasting syndrome.

Surgery can take a toll on health status. Surgical repair or resection of the intestine may place patients at risk for bowel torsion or obstruction owing to adhesion, leading to constipation, nausea, vomiting, and subsequent anorexia and weight loss. In these cases, small intestinal bacterial overgrowth is also of potential concern.

A review of medications is essential, especially if the patient is taking multiple medications. Amphetamines, benzodiazepines, decongestants, metformin, nicotine, and selective serotonin reuptake inhibitors (SSRIs) can all cause anorexia.[9] Other medications can cause nausea, altered taste or smell, or dry mouth, although there is significant overlap among them. Excessive use of diuretics or laxatives should also be explored.

A family medical history that includes gastrointestinal illness, celiac disease, cancer, or psychiatric illness may be relevant.

An inquiry into food affordability, availability, preparation, and safety, as well as social isolation, is essential. An older patient with early dementia may have trouble sequencing the steps necessary to procure and prepare food, in addition to having physical limitations. Recent adoption of new food practices, such as veganism, gluten-free diets, or religious fasting, coupled with inadequate education can lead to unintentional weight loss.

Eating disorders cause severe malnutrition through ketosis and further weight loss vulnerability. Anorexia and bulimia nervosa are psychiatric disorders characterized by excessive concern for body shape and weight. Serious medical consequences including anemia, electrolyte imbalances, reduction in bone density, cessation of menses, and ECG disturbances may arise as a result of the behavioral manifestations of the illness. These disorders primarily affect young women and adolescents but men and older adults can also be affected. Risk factors are not fully understood. Patients frequently exhibit denial regarding the seriousness of their reduced weight. Many are depressed. Patients with bulimia often feel shame and embarrassment.

The management of eating disorders is multidisciplinary, and communication with patients and team members is crucial. Medical stability is the first goal with progressive caloric intake as tolerated. Targeted weight gain of 0.5 to 1 pound a week is optimal. Careful monitoring of vital signs, electrolytes, and signs and symptoms of fluid overload is critical during re-feeding. Physical and psychological comfort is assessed frequently. Patients suspected of suffering with eating disorders should be referred to specialists in this area.

PHYSICAL EXAMINATION

The physical examination provides basic information about the patient's general appearance, habitus, affect, speech, cognition, weight measurement, and recall. Weight loss can be determined if a previsit weight is available and should be calculated as a percentage change from baseline. Serial skinfold measurement may be helpful to determine the percentage of body fat. Some assessment tools, such as the Mini Nutritional Assessment (MNA),[10] focus on body mass index (BMI), calf and mid-arm circumference, and other measures, and delineate who is at greater risk for a host of hospital-based delays and complications, including death.[11] The short-form version (MNA-SF) includes 18 items, with a score below 9 indicating risk for both undernutrition and frailty in hospitalized patients.[11]

Vital signs may indicate orthostasis or arrhythmias, suggestive of underlying cardiac disease and disability. Pallor, jaundice, rash, skin texture and turgor, hair consistency and distribution, and poor wound healing should be noted. Hyperpigmentation of the joints, waist, mouth, and palmar creases is associated with adrenal insufficiency.

Exophthalmos can be a hallmark of hyperthyroidism. An oropharyngeal examination is essential for glossitis, ulcers, exudates, masses, ill-fitting or odorous dentures, tooth or gum decay, and missing teeth. The temporomandibular joint should be palpated and gently extended to assess pain or crepitation. Lymphadenopathy, thyroid enlargement, neck masses, or a diminished swallow reflex may warrant further studies.

Dyspnea, arrhythmias, diminished breath sounds, jugular venous distention, wheezing, and ankle edema suggest cardiopulmonary problems that may interfere with appetite or energy demands.

Breast examination is important, given the rising incidence of breast cancers associated with aging. An abdominal examination that is positive for masses, hepatomegaly, mid-epigastric tenderness, or ascites may indicate problems with digestion, absorption, or vascular flow; liver disease; or gastrointestinal tumor. Pelvic examination for cervical and ovarian cancer screening can be considered depending on the age and general physical condition of the patient.

Finally, frailty, defined as a syndrome where an older person is vulnerable to becoming functionally impaired or dying when exposed to a stressor, is associated with slow ataxic gait, muscle and strength loss, a history of frequent falls and fear of falling, poor appetite, weight loss, cognitive decline, and depressed affect. It is also correlated with sarcopenia, osteopenia, and immunologic markers, such as catabolic cytokines and coagulopathy.[3]

DIAGNOSTICS
Essential Diagnostics

Thyroid function studies to exclude hyperthyroidism are warranted in those who have signs of increased metabolism, including tachycardia (see Chapter 194) and weight loss. A complete blood count (CBC) with differential is helpful in determining the presence of infection, inflammation, anemia, or malignant disease. A chemistry profile, including calcium, potassium, alkaline phosphatase, liver biochemical studies, serum electrolytes, serum glucose, serum albumin (which is sensitive to hydration status as well), blood urea nitrogen (BUN), and creatinine, would suggest nutritional deficiencies and/or other underlying diseases.

Additional Diagnostics

A finding of anemia prompts an evaluation of serum iron, ferritin, thiamine, vitamin B_{12}, and folate levels (see Chapter 216). A urinalysis can reveal infection or unmask proteinuria or uremia associated with early anorexia of kidney disease. Hemoglobin A1c (HbA1c) is warranted if diabetes is suspected. A chest x-ray examination may be helpful in identifying pulmonary disease or tumor. Age- and history-appropriate cancer screenings should be recommended.

An upper gastrointestinal series with or without small bowel follow-through, endoscopy, or barium swallow may be useful if difficulty swallowing is reported. Stool evaluation for occult blood is indicated if a rectosigmoid source is suspected.

A low score on tests for cognition (see Chapter 174) should raise the question of dementia with poor functional capacity. A positive depression inventory is necessary to further explore situational or psychological diagnoses.

INITIAL DIAGNOSTICS

Weight Loss

LABORATORY
- Chemistry profile
- Liver function studies with serum albumin
- CBC with differential
- Thyroid studies with TSH
- Erythrocyte sedimentation rate
- Fecal occult blood test

ADDITIONAL DIAGNOSTICS
Laboratory
- HgbA1C

Imaging
- Chest x-ray studies[a]
- Endoscopy[a]
- Gastric emptying scan[a]
- Colonoscopy[a]
- EKG/Echocardiography[a]

[a]If indicated.

DIFFERENTIAL DIAGNOSIS

Unintended weight loss is attributed to three major causes and searching for any of these can be challenging. A careful history and physical examination can be most revealing and can help point a direction for further evaluation. The three general causes of weight loss are:

Decreased calorie intake

Decreased calorie absorption

Increased metabolic demand

 Immediate hospitalization required for a patient with severe anorexia associated with rapid weight loss, hypokalemia, hypotension, or prerenal azotemia related to dehydration.

Unintentional weight loss is a result of **cancer** 19% to 36% of the time.[2] Some cancers cause a slow decline in weight, whereas gastrointestinal and head and neck cancers are more likely to cause a precipitous decline.[1] Cancer screening and tumor searches should be undertaken judiciously after careful physical examination and clarification of the patient's wishes for advanced care. Recent research suggests that weight loss and cachexia in malignancy is a metabolic reaction unrelated to the size of the tumor and a poor prognosticator. If diagnosed early this cachexia can be reversed.[12]

Nonmalignant gastrointestinal disease (9% to 19%)[2] is another important cause of unintended weight loss. Swallowing difficulties, poor absorption, slow transit, and bowel issues can all contribute to reduced appetite.

For those patients who report polyphagia or polydipsia and appear to have lost weight, a set of endocrine disorders should be considered in the differential diagnosis; these include hypothyroidism, hyperthyroidism, diabetes mellitus, diabetes insipidus, hyperparathyroidism, pheochromocytoma, and adrenal insufficiency.

Psychiatric causes, including depression and dementia (9% to 24%), are also significant causes of weight loss.[2] Adult-onset situational or chemical depression, late-stage Alzheimer dementia, schizophrenia, hypomania, and food-related or substance use disorders, including alcohol abuse, even in later life, can take a toll.

A multitude of other organ system illnesses—cardiac, respiratory, endocrine, rheumatologic, and immunologic—can result in weight loss. Infection, which increases metabolic demand, is usually apparent and often treatable. AIDS wasting syndrome is an obvious example. Some cases of weight loss may defy diagnosis. Cases of unknown cause remain a high percentage of the total and may require additional workup to gain another 10% to 20% in diagnostic yield.[1]

Follow-up evaluation and support are useful in these patients. Fortunately, for those individuals with an elusive diagnosis, the prognosis tends to be relatively better than for those diagnosed with a specific reason for their weight loss.[1]

INTERPROFESSIONAL COLLABORATIVE MANAGEMENT
Pharmacologic Management

The primary goals in managing involuntary weight loss are to provide adequate energy, protein, and micronutrients and to treat the underlying disease or, at least, any reversible illness. Medications can be used to reverse nausea, to increase appetite, or both, including progestin, megestrol acetate, and cannabinoids. Medical marijuana is now legal in 33 states, and Washington, DC, with cancer, chronic pain syndromes, cachexia, and wasting secondary to AIDS being several of many indications for its use. This number changes frequently so checking your individual state laws is recommended. There is low-level evidence that indicates improvement in nausea or appetite.[13] Dronabinol, an FDA approved cannabinoid, is used with variable success to treat nausea and vomiting associated with chemotherapy. It is a man-made version of the active ingredient in marijuana.

Other appetite stimulants include megestrol acetate. At a dosage goal of 800 mg/day, some studies showed an improvement in appetite (possibly through neuropeptide Y stimulation).[1] This medication is used in patients with HIV, COPD, cystic fibrosis, or cancer and in older adults with unexplained weight loss.[1] However, there are continuing concerns about thromboembolic events, hypertension, and adrenal insufficiency.[14] Mirtazapine, a serotonin antagonist used to treat depression, promotes appetite and weight gain as a common side effect.[2]

Eicosapentaenoic acid, an anti-inflammatory fatty acid found in fish oil, is promising for patients with advanced cancer because it may inhibit proteolytic activity arising from tumors.[15] Thalidomide is approved by the Food and Drug Administration for the treatment of AIDS wasting, although it is seldom used due to severe teratogenicity. Corticosteroids when taken for several weeks can have a positive impact on anorexia, chronic nausea, fatigue or asthenia, performance status, and quality of life or well-being.[16]

The antidopaminergic metoclopramide, 10 to 15 mg, taken 30 minutes before meals and at bedtime, serves as an antiemetic with gastrointestinal prokinetic properties. Some research suggests that appetite stimulation may be of limited usefulness but that its positive effects on reducing early satiety and nausea are beneficial.

Smaller food portions of calorie-dense foods offered frequently and a calorie-rich breakfast may enhance nutritional intake. High-calorie/protein supplements can be offered but timed to avoid interfering with meals. Enteral tube feedings (if the gastrointestinal tract is functional) or parenteral feedings can supplement or supplant oral feedings in patients who are not near the end of life, are being treated for upper GI cancers, have decreased intake related to cancer treatments, are pre-operative and undernourished, or when oral feeding is not safe.

Weight loss is a frequent finding in late-stage dementia. However, enteral feedings have not been shown to extend life or prevent aspiration and are associated with infection, discomfort, more frequent use of physical restraints, and increased confusion. They are not recommended in this population.[17] The alternative is careful hand feeding which is as good as tube feeding for the outcomes of death, aspiration pneumonia, comfort, and functional status.[17]

It is important to remember that any artificial feeding is a medical intervention and should be instituted only with clear indications and goals of therapy which are acceptable to the patient. If available, the services of a dietitian or nutritionist are invaluable.

Non-Pharmacologic Management

Exercise (resistance and aerobic) may have dual benefits in bone and muscle preservation as well as helping to prevent falls in older adults. Exercise along with food support and reduced polypharmacy helps to restore physical function and may improve appetite.[18] Exercise may be the most beneficial intervention in frail elders, in whom nutritional interventions are less reliable.[18] Reduced energy expenditure in elders may lead to reduced appetite and weight. Sometimes regaining lost weight after an inadvertent weight loss (following illness or surgery) can be challenging because the older individual may not be inclined to eat enough to make up for the loss.[3] Occupational, physical, or speech therapists can help tailor a care plan which addresses individual needs.

Finally, to address the psychosocial and situational stress drivers of unintentional weight loss, one must consider multiple factors: increasing age, bereavement, disability, impaired cognition, poverty, homelessness, and recent hospitalization. A social worker is critical to the team to help sort out psychosocial issues and develop a plan.

COMPLICATIONS

Complications of significant weight loss include severe malnutrition, weakness, loss of muscle mass, orthostatic hypotension, falls, immobility, and death. Immunocompromised patients and older adults are at special risk for weight loss–related complications.

Reversible complications such as community-acquired or nosocomial infections, community- or facility-acquired *Clostridium difficile* colitis, incontinence leading to skin breakdown, skin ulcers caused by low albumin in the setting of bed confinement, dental caries or denture complaints, poor pain control, and poor conditioning from repeated hospitalizations should be attended to as early as possible to preserve energy stores otherwise taxed by the disease and poor intake.

LIFE SPAN CONSIDERATIONS

Because older age brings limitations in physical abilities and the potential for social isolation, a thorough evaluation of functional independence and safety may uncover meal-related problems. Weight loss that is related to a disease process, acute illness, depression, or dementia may resist treatment, particularly in older adults, so optimal management requires a team effort, with a focus on maximizing abilities, interests, and calorie intake. This is particularly true in institutional settings, where contributing factors such as dependency and illness can be assessed and addressed more easily. Anticipating malnutrition and weight loss during episodes of acute illness is crucial to the care of the vulnerable patient because catching up later is difficult. Older adults with advanced dementia commonly experience feeding and eating difficulties leading to weight loss. In spite of an increasing body of research demonstrating that feeding tubes do not extend life or improve quality of life in these patients, many institutionalized older adults with late-stage dementia are being fed enterally. Many nursing home residents do not have advance directives documenting their wishes in this situation, leaving family members in the difficult position of deciding to insert a feeding tube or to continue with hand feeding without adequate knowledge or education. This lack of clarity can be addressed before the situation reaches a decision point by addressing the patient's wishes and educating families in the office while the patient still possesses decisional capacity. "Comfort feeding only" orders can be written as part of an overall feeding care plan that directs all care efforts toward the comfort of the older patient.[19]

PATIENT EDUCATION AND HEALTH PROMOTION

Teaching patients simple nutritional concepts and encouraging them to keep a food diary may be helpful. Suggestions for increasing meal attractiveness and calories include flavor enhancement through polyunsaturated butters, oils, dressings, jellies, and creamers. Increased fiber and increased fluid content should be encouraged. Because zinc deficiency can lead to dysgeusia, adding a multivitamin along with protein-rich snacks and nutritional supplements may significantly improve appetite and intake.

Facilitating food procurement with prepackaged meals or home-delivered foods can make a difference. Increasing activity, social engagement, and a sense of functional capability in the face of dysfunction or physical limitation also improve quality of life. Appetite may also be improved with a simplified regimen that optimizes the number of medications taken.

Because weight loss can be a late sign of pulmonary, renal, or cardiac disease, it is important to encourage patients or their advocates to look for medical guidance to optimize their quality of life. Ultimately, a discussion of palliative care may be the most humane approach to comfort severely cachexic individuals and their families.

Primary prevention of weight loss includes promoting activities that support safe access to food, medical and dental services, and socialization for those at social or financial risk of decreased intake.

Preventing communicable diseases by receiving scheduled vaccines; managing sleep and exercise requirements; and making adjustments in diet for tastes and preferences all help safeguard nutritional status. Screening at-risk individuals for chronic mental illness and substance use, including situational depression and prolonged grieving—especially among older adults, who face disproportionate loss and isolation—will help guide early intervention.

REFERENCES

1. Wong, C. (2014). Involuntary weight loss. *The Medical Clinics of North America, 98,* 625–643.
2. Gaddey, H. L., & Holder, K. (2014). Unintentional weight loss in older adults. *American Family Physician, 89*(9), 718–722.
3. Morley, J. E. (2017). Anorexia of ageing: A key component in the pathogenesis of both sarcopenia and cachexia. *Journal of Cachexia, Sarcopenia and Muscle, 8,* 523–526. doi:10.1002/jcsm.12192.
4. Bosch, X., Monclus, E., Escoda, O., et al. (2017). Unintended weight loss: Clinical Characteristics and outcomes in a prospective cohort of 2677 patients. *Public Library of Science one, 12*(4), e0175125.
5. Wassertheil-Smoller, S., Fann, C., Allman, R. M., Black, H. R., Camel, G. H., Davis, B., et al. (2000). Relation of low body mass to death and stroke in the systolic hypertension in the elderly program. The SHEP Cooperative Research Group. *Archives of Internal Medicine, 160*(4), 494–500.
6. National Association of Clinical Nurse Specialists. Malnutrition in Hospitalized adult patients. Retrieved from: http://nacns.org/wp-content/uploads/2017/01/Malnutrition-Report.pdf on Dec 3, 2017.
7. Verlaans, S., Aspray, T., Bauer, J., et al. (2017). Nutritional Status, body composition, and quality of life in community dwelling sarcopenic and non-sarcopenic older adults: A case control study. *Clinical Nutrition: Official Journal of the European Society of Parenteral and Enteral Nutrition, 36*(1), 267–274.
8. Lok, C. (2015). Cachexia: The last illness. *Nature, 528*(7581), 182–183.
9. Franx, B. A. A., Arnoldussen, I. A. C., Killian, A. J., & Gustafson, D. R. (2017). Weight loss in patients with dementia: Considering the potential impact of pharmacotherapy. *Drugs and Aging, 34*(6), 425–436.
10. Montejano Lozoya, R., Martínez-Alzamora, N., Clemente Marín, G., Guirao-Goris, S. J. A., & Ferrer-Diego R. M. (2017). Predictive ability of the Mini Nutritional Assessment Short Form (MNA-SF) in a free-living elderly population: A cross-sectional study. *PeerJ, 5,* e3345.
11. Cederholm, T., Bosaeus, I., Barazzoni, R., et al. (2015). Diagnostic criteria for malnutrition—an ESPEN consensus statement. *Clinical Nutrition: Official Journal of the European Society of Parenteral and Enteral Nutrition, 34*(3), 335–340.
12. Vigano, A., Morais, J., Ciutto, L., et al. (2017). Use of routinely available clinical, nutritional, and functional criteria to classify cachexia in advanced cancer patients. *Clinical Nutrition: Official Journal of the European Society of Parenteral and Enteral Nutrition, 36*(5), 1378–1390.
13. NIH, National Institute on Drug Abuse, Marijuana as Medicine, updated July, 2019. Retrieved from: https://www.drugabuse.gov/publications/drugfacts/marijuana-medicine. (Accessed 10 July 2019).
14. https://www.medicinenet.com/megestrol-oral/article.htm.
15. Hadi, S., Kurniawan, C., & Budiono, J. (2015). Eicosapentaenoic acid as adjuvant for cachexia in cancer patients. *International Journal of Integrated Health Science, 3*(1), 1–6.
16. Alesi, E. R., & del Fabbo, E. (2014). Opportunities for targeting the fatigue-anorexia-cachexia symptom cluster. *Cancer Journal (Sudbury, Mass.), 20*(5), 325–329.
17. American Geriatric Society Ethics Committee and Clinical Practice and Models of Care Committee. (2014). America Geriatric Society feeding tubes in advanced dementia position statement. *Journal of the American Geriatrics Society, 62*(8), 1590–1593.
18. Chen, X., Mao, G., & Leng, S. X. (2014). Frailty syndrome: An overview. *Clinical Interventions in Aging, 9,* 433–441.
19. Palecek, E. J., Teno, J. M., Casarett, D. J., et al. (2010). Comfort feeding only: A proposal to bring clarity to decision making regarding difficulty with eating for persons with advanced dementia. *Journal of the American Geriatrics Society, 58*(3), 580–584.

CHAPTER **208**

EMERGING AND REEMERGING INFECTIOUS DISEASES

Lisa V. Adams • Elizabeth A. Talbot

Terms such as "emerging" and "reemerging" diseases increasingly appear in the clinical and even public parlance. Our patients are regularly bombarded by media stories about and images of these diseases and consequently often have questions, or even fears, that they might present to us. Because primary care providers may be on the front lines of the global battle to control these pathogens, this chapter provides an overview of this category of diseases to create awareness for the primary care provider and to improve our understanding and thereby our preparedness. If suspected, expert consultation should be sought to diagnose and manage these diseases.

DEFINITIONS

Emerging infectious diseases result from newly discovered and previously unknown infections that threaten public health. Increased international travel and trade, deforestation, changing ecosystems and climates, and rapid adaptation of microorganisms have contributed to this problem. For example, the 2009–2010 influenza A pandemic that was caused by a novel influenza A H1N1 virus spread within months from Mexico and other countries in the Southern Hemisphere to become the predominant influenza virus circulating in most countries.[1]

Reemerging infectious diseases are those that had formerly caused so few infections that they were no longer considered a public health threat but have recently reactivated.[2] Dengue fever, Chikungunya, and Zika are all examples of reemerging infectious diseases that have spread from Africa and Asia throughout the Americas via international travel and expanding world commerce. Their rapid and continued emergence has moved them from the rare and exotic to more commonly considered diagnoses across primary care offices. Similarly, the gradual discontinuation of yellow fever mosquito control programs in conjunction with climate change has allowed the *Aedes aegypti* mosquito to greatly expand its geographic distribution in South America, the Caribbean, and now the southern United States, resulting in its reemergence in domestic locations.

RISK FACTORS FAVORING EMERGENCE OF PATHOGENS

Our recent history has witnessed a rapid succession of newly identified pathogens—reemergent and resistant bacteria, reemergent diarrheal illnesses, new respiratory pathogens, and vector-borne illnesses.

Central to the epidemiology of emerging and reemerging pathogens is the concept of globalization. Never before in human history have we been as vulnerable to diseases that were previously geographically contained. With the ease of global transport of people, animals, insect vectors, food, and goods, there is real and imminent risk of the introduction of new diseases that might be encountered in primary care. Our interconnected world allows well-known pathogens rapid access to new, immunologically naive populations and facilitates the spread of novel pathogens and antimicrobial resistance. The following are some recent examples:

- Human immunodeficiency virus (HIV) (see Chapter 209) emerged when the simian immunodeficiency virus jumped species from African green monkeys to human populations, and then rapidly spread throughout the world.
- Widespread outbreaks of *Salmonella, Cyclospora,* and *Escherichia coli* O157:H7 diarrheal illnesses are directly related to the globalization of our food supply (see Chapter 211).
- The 2009 influenza A H1N1 pandemic spread from Mexico worldwide within months and became the predominant influenza virus circulating in most countries.
- Exotic pet aficionados have introduced previously geographically constrained pathogens into the human population. One such example is a human monkeypox outbreak linked to keeping Gambian giant pouched rats as pets.

In addition to globalization, changes in our societies and lifestyles have also been permissive for emergence and reemergence of certain infectious diseases. For example:

- Tuberculosis (TB) (see Chapter 214) has been an historic plague of humans, controlled in part by improved isolation and other public health strategies, but treatment practices and trends toward overcrowding have been linked to outbreaks of multidrug-resistant tuberculosis (MDR-TB).
- Epidemics of injection substance use disorder (see Chapter 227) have contributed to the HIV and hepatitis C epidemics.
- Rampant counterfeit drug sales and absent regulatory controls in Southeast Asia have contributed to the emergence of malaria species resistant to artemisinin-based therapy less than 10 years after it became the preferred therapy.
- Reforestation of farmlands, reemergence of deer herds, and our desire to live in ecozones (edge areas) have contributed to the rapid emergence of Lyme disease (see Chapter 213) in the United States.
- Prescribing practices and antibiotic use in animal feed have contributed to the emergence of drug-resistant enteric pathogens, including vancomycin-resistant enterococci and resistant gram negative rods.
- Close contact exposes bird farmers and open market visitors to novel respiratory viruses such as avian influenzas

or coronaviruses (e.g., severe acute respiratory syndrome [SARS]), while camel exposure has been implicated in the Middle East respiratory syndrome coronavirus [MERS-CoV]) epidemic.

Natural disasters and infrastructure deterioration have also contributed to emergence and reemergence of certain pathogens:

- Resistant *Salmonella* and *Campylobacter* organisms in tsunami- or monsoon-stricken Southeast Asia
- Cholera in post-earthquake Haiti

Acute Respiratory Diseases

Coronaviruses. Coronaviruses are pathogens in animals and humans, well known as a cause of the common cold. SARS is a coronavirus that emerged in 2002 from Guangdong Province, China.[3] It caused a severe and often fatal pneumonia, with prominent systemic symptoms. An incubation period of 4 to 7 days was followed by fever, an influenza-like illness, and, a few days later, symptoms of pneumonia, diarrhea, leukopenia, thrombocytopenia, and characteristically lymphopenia. Laboratory diagnosis was best made by detection of antibody, which appears about 10 days into the illness, or reverse transcriptase polymerase chain reaction (RT-PCR) on bronchial secretions.[4] About 25% of patients developed severe pneumonia complicated by acute respiratory distress syndrome (ARDS). Mortality was as high as 50% in older patients and hosts with underlying disease,[3] and survivors had significantly reduced exercise capacity and health status compared with the general population.[5]

The intrigue of SARS lies in its abrupt emergence as a new human pathogen. A coronavirus from a palm civet and/or a ferret badger in the live animal markets jumped species into humans and spread rapidly from person-to-person locally and then internationally via air travel. Estimates are that there were more than 8000 cases and 780 deaths reported from 29 countries before the outbreak ended in June 2003.[6] Concern lingers regarding potential reemergence because SARS coronavirus has been isolated from open-market animals and could still be circulating in animals only to again jump species to humans.

Middle East Respiratory Syndrome. Middle East respiratory syndrome (MERS) is an emerging illness caused by a previously unknown coronavirus now called MERS Co-V. The first case, reported in a 60-year-old man who lived in Saudi Arabia, had a fatal outcome.[7] All cases have been linked directly or indirectly to countries in the Arabian Peninsula, most notably Saudi Arabia, Qatar, Jordan, and the United Arab Emirates.[8] Nosocomial transmission has been well-documented, providing an important reminder to primary care clinicians to screen patients with consistent symptoms for any relevant travel history in order to institute appropriate infection control practices.[9]

After a 2- to 14-day incubation period, MERS patients typically develop fever, cough, and shortness of breath. Some will have gastrointestinal symptoms including diarrhea and/or nausea and vomiting. As with SARS, most patients progress to ARDS with multiorgan system failure. The mortality rate is approximately 55%.[8,10]

Those advising patients traveling to the affected region should remind fastidious adherence to routine measures to prevent respiratory illnesses, including washing hands, avoiding personal contact such as kissing and sharing eating utensils with ill individuals, and disinfecting frequently used surfaces such as doorknobs.[11]

Human Metapneumovirus. Human metapneumovirus (hMPV) is an example of a pathogen that has probably been causing respiratory tract illness for many years but is considered emerging because it has only recently been recognized. Discovered in 2001 by researchers applying molecular polymerase chain reaction (PCR) techniques to children with previously unexplained pneumonia, hMPV is now recognized to cause at least 5% to 10% of pediatric hospitalizations for lower respiratory tract illness in the United States.[12] Given how many children are hospitalized each year with lower respiratory tract illness, hMPV represents an important cause of morbidity and mortality. Serologic studies demonstrate antibodies to hMPV in virtually all children by the age of 5 years.[12] Although primarily recognized as a pediatric disease, hMPV has also recently been recognized in adults, most clearly as a major cause of severe lower respiratory tract illness in immunocompromised adults and elders.

hMPV causes a spectrum of illness ranging from upper to lower respiratory tract illness and is clinically indistinguishable from the more familiar respiratory syncytial virus (RSV) infection. hMPV is often milder and affects a slightly older group of children (6 to 12 months of age) in contrast to RSV, which often affects infants before 2 months of age.[12,13] Like RSV and influenza, hMPV circulates predominately in winter months, which is when it should be especially considered in the differential diagnosis. Because influenza, RSV, and hMPV share common seasonality and hosts, vigilance toward diagnosing coinfections should be maintained.

Diagnosis is best made with real-time PCR on bronchial secretions. The virus is difficult to grow, and serologic tests are yet to be standardized. No vaccine or antiviral therapy is available, but studies show that ribavirin and intravenous immune globulin inhibit hMPV in vitro. Repeated episodes of asymptomatic infection or with common cold symptoms maintain immunity in adults.[13]

Influenza A. Pandemic influenza A (see Chapter 210) by definition is an emerging pathogen, which can cause staggering human morbidity and mortality, and an accompanying massive resource expenditure. Pandemic flu classically arises through an antigenic shift, which is a rearrangement of animal influenza genes into a human influenza virus. But we now also know that lesser changes ("antigenic drift") can also sometimes cause pandemics, as was shown by sequencing the 1918 pandemic influenza virus, which killed as many as 30 million people worldwide.[14]

Influenza A impels us toward improved understanding of zoonotic viruses, continued surveillance in human and animal populations through international networks, and development of an influenza vaccine that offers broad protection against different viral variants. One vivid example of a recently emerged influenza virus is the 2009 to 2010 influenza pandemic. International air travel rapidly disseminated a new influenza A virus globally: within 6 months after the virus's emergence was recognized in Mexico, the World Health Organization (WHO) declared that the criteria for a pandemic had been met.[1,15,16] Global initiatives enabled public health jurisdictions to implement diagnostic and clinical management algorithms and international networks for surveillance and research, to track the virus and its evolution, and to optimize clinical outcomes.

We now know that the causative H1N1 influenza A virus is antigenically distinct from the preexisting seasonal human influenza virus and resulted from the reassortment between two influenza A (H1N1) swine viruses that themselves were the products of several independent avian to mammalian cross-species transmissions and prior re-assortments among avian, human, and swine viruses.[17] Like the viruses responsible for the influenza pandemics of 1957 and 1968, the 2009 H1N1 virus is a descendant of the 1918 pandemic virus.[18] Unlike seasonal influenza, children and young adults rather than elders experienced the highest attack rates from influenza A (H1N1) because most adults older than 60 years had protection from cross-protective antibodies they had developed from prior exposure to antigenically related influenza viruses.[19]

Clinical features, diagnostic approaches, treatment, and prevention of influenza are discussed in Chapter 210.

Avian Influenza A. Avian influenzas are always circulating among birds but do not usually "jump species" to infect mammalian cells. In 1997, a small outbreak of avian influenza A (H5N1) occurred within the live poultry markets of Hong Kong. This outbreak was unique in that the virus jumped from birds to humans and caused severe illness in 18 previously healthy adults, six of whom died. There was no human-to-human transmission, and an unprecedented culling of the entire poultry population of Hong Kong contained the outbreak. But in 2003, the same virus reemerged as the cause of a massive poultry outbreak across Asia. Human cases of H5N1 have followed in parallel to the geographic spread of the poultry pandemic. Most human cases had direct exposure to diseased birds. Although there have been family clusters, human-to-human transmission remains limited and unsustained.[20]

In 2013, human infections with the influenza A (H7N9) virus were reported in China. Compared with the preceding 4 years of circulation, the fifth wave (beginning October 2016) showed significantly more cases. This may be attributable to mutations, resulting in nomenclature of a new more virulent strain: the Yangtze River Delta Lineage H7N9.

Primary care clinicians have a paramount role in providing their patients with seasonal influenza vaccination. The seasonal influenza vaccine will not protect us from avian influenza (H5N1), but 30,000 to 50,000 die each year in the United States from current endemic influenza strains, and immunization will prevent other influenza illnesses from being confused with avian influenza should human-to-human transmission become more facile. In 2013, the Food and Drug Administration approved the first adjuvanted vaccine to prevent avian influenza.[21] Rapid development of other vaccines for emerging flu strains will be necessary if these viruses achieve the capability for efficient human-to-human spread, which could lead to the next human pandemic.

Acute Diarrheal Illnesses

Vibrio Cholera. Cholera epidemics (see Chapter 211) characteristically emerge, decline, and reemerge throughout human history, brought on by natural disasters, civil war, and displaced populations. Six pandemics, caused by the classic biotype *Vibrio cholerae* O1, occurred before 1926, originated in Asia and India, and traveled in infected patients to Europe and the Americas. The seventh and current pandemic is caused by a new classic biotype, El Tor, first isolated in Egypt. It causes milder disease, which remained sporadic and endemic throughout Africa, Europe, and Asia for many years. Emergence of a new strain, *V. cholerae* O139, began in India and Bangladesh in 1992. Past exposure to *V. cholerae* O1 offers no immunity to

V. cholerae O139, which has also been noted to be resistant to trimethoprim-sulfamethoxazole.[22]

The current global burden of cholera was estimated using spatial mapping and indicates that there are approximately 1.3 billion people at risk, resulting in 2.9 million cases and 95,000 deaths annually.[23] The staggering burden of this reemerging infection warrants understanding of the epidemiology and control strategies, especially vaccine status.

V. cholerae is naturally found in water, attached to algae, crustaceans, and plankton. Warmer-than-usual waters (e.g., because of El Niño) facilitate its growth by changes in nutrients and salinity (e.g., from monsoons, tsunamis, and typhoons).[24] In this activated state, humans are more likely to become infected and transmit infection through fecally-contaminated food or water. Direct person-to-person spread is unlikely because of the large inoculum required for infection.

Disasters provide ready availability of contaminated water and food. In a recent tragic example of this reality, the catastrophic January 2010 earthquake in Haiti killed over 200,000 people and displaced more than one million. Ten months after the earthquake, the Haitian Ministry of Public Health and Population was notified of a sudden increase in patients with watery diarrhea and dehydration. On October 21, 2010, the Haiti National Public Health Laboratory identified the pathogen as *V. cholera*. The first cholera outbreak in Haiti in at least a century emerged, causing over 665,000 cases and 8183 deaths. Based on molecular methods, this epidemic is now thought to have been introduced by international relief workers from south Asia living under poor sanitary conditions.[25]

Severe dehydration, electrolyte imbalance, renal failure, and metabolic acidosis can be fatal complications of cholera, and oral or intravenous rehydration is the most important intervention to avert death. Mortality is as high as 10% in epidemic settings without adequate health care support but 3% or less in centers versed in simple hydration techniques. Antibiotics are secondary in importance to hydration. Emerging antibiotic resistance is a problem for developing nations.

Cholera is a predictably reemergent disease most likely to be encountered after natural disasters, in refugee camps, and in urban slums where it is endemic. Simple measures to dispose of human waste, to avoid contaminated water, and to provide a potable water supply are critical public health priorities in these situations. Travelers intending to work or volunteer in such settings should be appropriately counseled about prevention methods, symptoms, and the need for prompt fluid replacement, and considered for emergency standby treatment.

Another approach to prevention is vaccination. In June 2016, the US Food and Drug Administration (FDA) approved a single-dose live oral cholera vaccine called Vaxchora (lyophilized CVD 103-HgR) for use in the United States. Vaxchora has been reported to reduce the chance of severe diarrhea in people by 90% at 10 days after vaccination and by 80% at 3 months after vaccination.[26] The Advisory Committee on Immunization Practices (ACIP) voted to approve the vaccine for adults 18 to 64 years old who are traveling to an area of active cholera transmission.[27] However, these recommendations result in rare use for most US travelers because most do not visit areas with active cholera transmission. Although relief agencies may suggest volunteers or staff obtain it, no country or territory currently requires vaccination against cholera as a condition for entry.

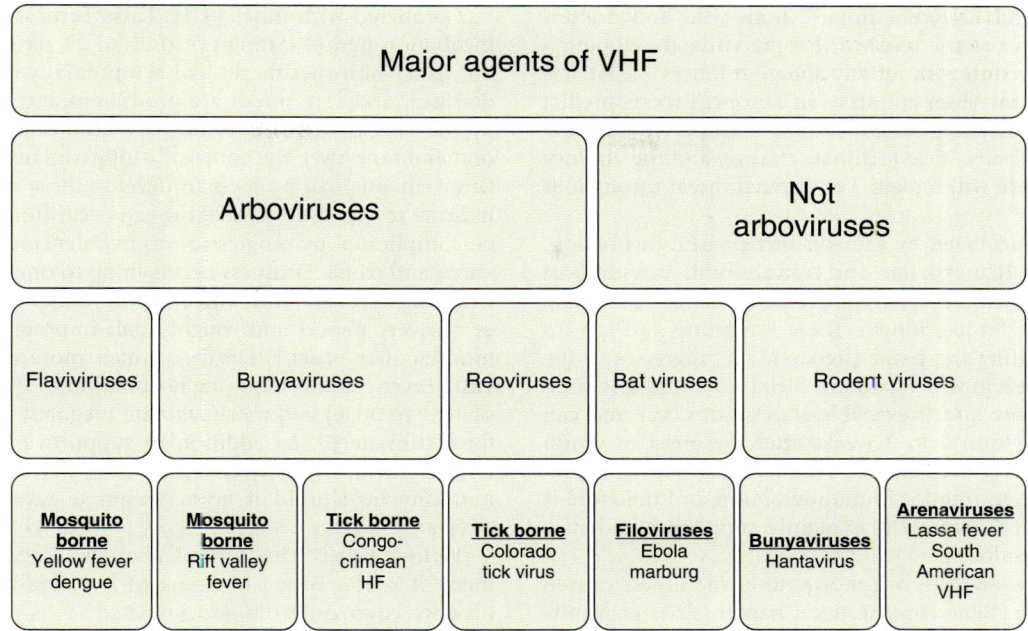

FIG. **208.1**   Agents of viral hemorrhagic fever. Togaviruses, a large family of Arboviruses, are not included because they do not cause the viral hemorrhagic fever *(VHF)* syndrome. (From Meltzer, E. [2012]. Arboviruses and viral hemorrhagic fevers [VHF]. *Infectious Disease Clinics of North America, 26*[2], 479–496.)

Two other oral inactivated cholera vaccines are available: Dukoral Developed by SBL Vaccine (Solna, Sweden); now Valneva (Montreal, Canada) and Shanchol Developed by Shantha Biotechnics (Hyderabad, India); now Sanofi Pasteur India (Mumbai, India).[26] These vaccines are not available in the US.

None of the cholera vaccines offer complete protection. Therefore, vaccination should never take the place of standard prevention and control measures.

Vector-Borne Diseases

Two important emerging vector-borne diseases, Lyme disease and West Nile virus, are discussed elsewhere. Lyme disease is discussed in detail in Chapter 213, and West Nile virus is covered in Chapter 215.

Viral Hemorrhagic Fevers. Four families of viruses (*Arenaviruses, Bunyaviruses, Filoviruses,* and *Flaviviruses*) are responsible for the group of diseases collectively known as viral hemorrhagic fevers (VHFs) (Fig. 208.1). VHFs include Crimean-Congo Fever, Dengue Fever, Ebola, Hantavirus infections, Lassa Fever, Rift Valley Fever (RVF), West Nile, and Yellow Fever, among others (see Chapter 215). In this section we discuss the VHFs that have reemerged to cause recent outbreaks in the US or Europe. Since West Nile and Dengue Fever are so commonly seen in primary care practice now, they are discussed in more detail in Chapter 215.

The clinical presentation of the different VHFs is quite similar. Symptoms typically begin after a 3- to 7-day (up to 21 days for Lassa Fever) incubation period following infection acquired from a tick or mosquito bite or contact with an infected mammal. Most VHFs present with a similar, initial constellation of symptoms that includes a high fever and rigors, malaise, severe headache, abdominal pain, nausea/vomiting, and myalgias. This phase is followed by either early recovery (resulting in a mild or subclinical episode) or a progression to the hemorrhagic stage that is often evident by the presence of epistaxis, ecchymoses, and petechiae. Bleeding from a number of sites can occur, including the gastrointestinal tract which can lead to circulatory collapse. In VHFs, endothelial dysfunction can lead to capillary leak and disseminated intravascular coagulopathy (DIC).[28] In severe cases, insufficient effective circulating intravascular volume can lead to shock accompanied by multiorgan failure.[28,29]

Suspecting VHF is the first step to making the diagnosis. Therefore, a detailed history including recent travel, exposure to insect bites, and any contact with animals is critical. The VHFs discussed below are typically diagnosed by the detection of viral RNA using RT-PCR testing. This may only be effective in the first few days of disease since virus may be undetectable once symptoms start.[28] The diagnosis can also be confirmed by enzyme-linked immunosorbent assay (ELISA) detection of IgM, and suggested by the presence of IgG. In the case of Yellow Fever, it is important to obtain a vaccine history since IgM to the vaccine virus can persist for years following vaccination.[28] There can also be cross-reactivity of immunoglobulins to viruses in the same family (with the flaviviruses that cause West Nile and Dengue Fever, for example); therefore, the diagnosis can be confirmed with a more specific test such as a plaque-reduction neutralization test.[28] Another important shared feature of VHFs is the risk for transmission to health care workers and subsequent nosocomial transmission to other patients. If suspected, immediate consultation, referral, and coordination with an appropriately skilled infectious disease specialist for testing and treatment is recommended.

Crimean-Congo Hemorrhagic Fever. Crimean-Congo hemorrhagic fever (CCHF) is a tick-borne viral infection caused by a Nairovirus (*Bunyaviridae*) that is seen across most of Africa, Western China, Southern Asia, the Middle East, and Southeast and Eastern Europe.[30] Both wild and domestic mammals serve as the reservoir for the virus, developing a viremia after infection without any apparent illness. CCHF has been reported from seven countries in Europe. Experts predict that with the presence of the vector in Europe (mainly the hard-bodied *Hyalomma* ticks), climate change, and the absence of a vaccine, CCHF will remain a continued threat throughout southern Europe.[30]

CCHF is characterized by four distinct phases: incubation, pre-hemorrhagic, hemorrhagic, and convalescent. As with most VHFs, the initial symptoms (in the pre-hemorrhagic) phase are those of a severe flu-like illness. These symptoms can last up to a week and either the patient recovers or progresses to the hemorrhagic phase in which patients bleed from multiple sites. Hepatorenal failure and irreversible shock can occur and can result in death within 2 to 3 weeks after the onset of symptoms.[28] In most cases, RT-PCR has a higher sensitivity and specificity than ELISA testing for immunoglobulin and therefore is the preferred test.[31] Treatment is mainly supportive and may include blood products.

Rift Valley Fever. RVF is a mosquito-borne illness caused by the RVF virus *(Bunyaviridae)* (see Chapter 215). Transmission also occurs from close contact with infected animals including cattle, sheep, goats and camels.[32] Most cases occur in East or West Africa and fewer in the Middle East. After decades of low levels of activity, RVF has reemerged in the last 5 to 10 years with several large outbreaks that occurred in East Africa, Sudan, Madagascar, Southern Africa, Mauritania, Yemen, and Saudi Arabia.[32] The impact on livestock in these regions has been devastating, resulting in more than 100,000 animal deaths.[32]

The clinical presentation of RVF is that of a typical VHF. Dozens of different mosquito species as well as biting midges, ticks, and fleas can transmit RVF virus. The diagnosis can be made by the detection of viral RNA by PCR or by detection of IgM antibodies by ELISA.[33] Treatment is supportive with careful monitoring for hepatocellular failure and acute renal failure. No vaccine exists at present, though efforts to develop a vaccine for targeted use in humans (i.e., veterinarians, laboratory workers, researchers, those deployed to RVF areas) as well as for use in livestock are underway.[34]

Lassa Fever. Lassa Fever, caused by the Lassa Fever virus (Arenaviridae), is endemic in the countries of West Africa. The highest incidence is seen in the forested regions where the borders of Guinea, Liberia, and Sierra Leone meet. In parts of Sierra Leone and Guinea, seroprevalence is as high as 40% to 50%.[35,36] In 2016, the first known transmission of locally acquired Lassa Fever outside of Africa was reported from Rhineland-Palatinate, Germany.[37] This occurred when an ill health care worker, who had been evacuated from Togo to Germany, died shortly after hospital admission and the undertaker who prepared his body for repatriation became symptomatic 12 days later. By that time, the diagnosis was confirmed in the original patients and the undertaker was evaluated and also tested positive for Lassa Fever virus.[37] Twenty-one contacts were evaluated but no further transmission was identified.[37]

Transmission is primarily through contact with the feces or urine of the Mastomys rodent, either through unintended direct ingestion or inhalation of aerosolized excretions. Human-to-human transmission also occurs through contact with the blood, urine, feces, or other bodily secretions of an infected person.

Compared with other VHFs, Lassa Fever can have a longer incubation period lasting up to 21 to 24 days. In addition to the usual non-specific flu-like symptoms, cough, chest pain, diarrhea, and sore throat are prominent and can be followed by the development of white or yellow exudate and a pseudomembrane over the tonsils.[28] Approximately 20% of Lassa Fever patients will progress to develop these symptoms which indicate severe disease. Bleeding can occur from all orifices and be complicated by progression to hypotension and shock, seizures, and coma. Deafness occurs in up to one-third of patients with Lassa Fever, with onset during either the acute illness or recovery period and roughly half improving over up to 3 months after onset.[35] Death is much more common among Lassa Fever patients requiring hospitalization (case fatality rates of 15% to 30%) and those who are pregnant (80% during the third trimester).[35] In addition to supportive therapy, intravenous ribavirin is highly effective; it has been shown to reduce mortality by tenfold if given within 6 days after the onset of fever.[35]

Yellow Fever. The clinical features, diagnosis, and treatment of Yellow Fever are discussed in Chapter 215. Therefore, here we cover only the issues related to its reemergence and strategies for control.

Outbreaks of Yellow Fever continue to occur with regular frequency. In 2016, there was a large outbreak in Angola, with spread to Democratic Republic of Congo and Uganda which was eventually brought under control; in November and December of 2017, 2018, and 2019 active outbreaks were reported in both Brazil and Nigeria.[38]

Global control efforts for this reemerging infectious disease historically focus on vector control and vaccination. However, there is inadequate vaccine production capacity to meet the needs of routine immunization programs in endemic settings, mass vaccination campaigns, and outbreak response stockpiling. The production of the Yellow Fever strain using the most commonly used YFV-17D vaccines depends on a sufficient supply of eggs from pathogen free chickens, and the eggs must contain 7- to 9-day-old chick embryos. The embryos are infected with the virus and then incubated to amplify the virus, and then processed into vaccines. This is not a rapid or nimble process to respond to current global reemergence of Yellow Fever.

Vaccine availability in the US is also insecure. Sanofi Pasteur, the manufacturer of YF-Vax, announced that this US-approved vaccine is unavailable until at least the end of 2019. During the period of shortage, the FDA has approved the use of Stamaril in the United States under an investigational new drug (IND) program. Stamaril has been distributed for decades in more than 70 countries, and is comparable in safety and efficacy to YF-Vax.[39]

Oropouche Fever. Oropouche virus *(Bunyaviridae)* is a less-well-known VHF causing disease in South America (primarily Brazil) and the Caribbean.[40] Oropouche virus was first isolated in 1955 in Trinidad and since then it is estimated to have infected over half a million individuals.[41,42] Mosquitos and biting midges are the known vectors for Oropouche virus transmission. Several mammals (e.g., sloths) and wild birds serve as the viral reservoir.[41] Person-to-person transmission has not been documented.[40]

Clinical presentation of Oropouche fever is similar to that of other VHFs with a few notable exceptions. First, a rash resembling the rash of rubella is commonly seen initially. Secondly, hemorrhagic features have been described but are less prominent or severe. Thirdly, the course of illness in approximately 60% of patients follows a biphasal pattern, with recovery of the initial symptoms followed 1 to 2 weeks later by a recurrence, which can be of a greater or lesser severity than the initial illness.[41] Lastly, unlike the other VHFs, Oropouche fever is associated with neurological complications including encephalitis and aseptic meningitis. Little is known about the pathophysiology of the neurological manifestations of Oropouche virus but studies in mice suggest that the virus gains access to the brainstem through neural routes originating in the spinal cord.[40] As disease progresses, the virus appears able to cross the blood-brain barrier to affect the brain parenchyma.[40] Oropouche virus has been detected in the cerebrospinal fluid of patients with clinical meningitis and Oropouche fever. Even with CNS involvement, the prognosis of Oropouche fever is good. All patients seem to recover fully. There has not been a documented fatality since the first epidemic in the 1960 outbreak.[40]

Diagnosis of Oropouche infection is challenging due to the lack of commercially available assays. Therefore, the diagnosis is generally confirmed using in-house ELISA tests for IgM and IgG, virus isolation attempt in newborn mice and cell culture (Vero cells), or RT-PCR and real-time RT-PCR for genome detection in acute samples.[42] The combination of symptoms consistent with Oropouche infection and one positive serum sample of IgM detected by ELISA can be considered diagnostic for acute Oropouche fever. Treatment is focused on symptomatic relief for fever and pain, and should be restarted during the relapse phase.

Tick-Borne Encephalitis. In the past 30 years, there has been a dramatic increase in tick-borne encephalitis (TBE) cases in Europe, with spread into new, previously unaffected regions. The geographic distribution of TBE has extended from central Europe and Scandinavia through the Eurasian continent to Far East Asia. The cause of this emergence of TBE is likely multifactorial: increased temperatures as a result of global warming (which favor both increases in the tick and reservoir rodent populations), changing ecology by increased forestation and garden cultivation, growing popularity of outdoor activities such as hiking and fishing and adventure travel, and declining socioeconomic status of some populations.[43]

TBE is caused by three antigenically related virus subtypes whose names correspond to their geographic origins: European, Siberian, and Far Eastern. The vector of the European subtype is *Ixodes ricinus*, whereas *Ixodes persulcatus* is the vector for the other two. TBE virus is transmitted within minutes of the tick bite; therefore, unlike in Lyme disease, early removal of ticks will not prevent disease.[44] Infections are most common in the early and late summer months when ticks and rodent hosts are most active. Transmission of TBE through consumption of unpasteurized milk produced by viremic livestock is responsible for a minority of cases.[45,46]

Asymptomatic TBE infections are common, occurring in roughly two-thirds of those infected.[43,46] When symptoms do develop, onset is typically 8 days after the tick bite. One-third of patients do not recall the tick bite. Those infected with the European subtype typically have a biphasic illness, beginning with a nonspecific febrile illness with myalgias, fatigue, and headache followed by a recovery period. One-third will then progress to a neuroinvasive form of TBE, developing meningitis (50%), encephalitis (40%), or myelitis (10%).[43,47] Loss of

consciousness, ataxia of the limbs, or acute flaccid paralysis of the upper extremities is also common. Treatment is supportive with fluids, analgesics, antipyretics (i.e., nonsteroidal anti-inflammatory agents), and ventilator support as needed. The benefit of corticosteroids has not been validated. Physical therapy of paralyzed limbs is also important to prevent atrophy.

Four inactivated TBE vaccines are licensed and available in Europe, Russia, and Canada; however, they are not currently available in the United States.[43,47] Basic tick prevention practices (i.e., wearing long pants and socks when walking in wooded areas, use of repellents) are always advisable. Travelers to endemic areas should be advised of the risk.

Zoonoses

Ebola Virus Disease. Ebola virus disease (EVD) is caused by a Filoviridae family virus, of the genus Ebolavirus. The virus was identified in 1976 during the first EVD outbreak near the Ebola River (hence the name) in then Zaire, now the Democratic Republic of Congo.[48] More recently, the highly fatal outbreak of EVD in 2013–2014 was concentrated in the three West African countries of Guinea, Liberia, and Sierra Leone.[49] Genomic sequencing and phylogenetic analysis revealed that the Ebola virus of this outbreak represented a new strain of Zaire Ebola virus.[49] Although the disease has been identified in gorillas, chimpanzees, and duikers as part of its sporadic epizootic cycle, the high mortality in these animals makes them unlikely natural reservoirs.[50] Recent evidence has implicated the fruit bat as the most likely reservoir host responsible for the enzootic cycle, and as the source of the 2013–2014 epidemic.[50] Human-to-human transmission occurs via contact with infectious body fluids such as urine, saliva, sweat, feces, vomit, breast milk, and semen

EVD is characterized by the constellation of fever, fatigue, diarrhea, vomiting, headache, and anorexia. In a study of 37 patients with confirmed EVD in Conakry, Guinea, more than half had one or more of these symptoms, with fever present in 84%.[51] Onset of symptoms is typically abrupt. The mean incubation period during the 2013–2014 outbreak was 11 days, with 95% of confirmed EVD patients experiencing symptoms within 21 days of their last exposure (making this the recommended period for follow-up of contacts). The mean time for patients to seek care after the onset of their symptoms (a measure of the period of infectiousness in the community) was 5 days.[52] The median time from onset of symptoms to death was 8 days.[51] Overall mortality for EVD is approximately 70%, with lower rates for those who are hospitalized (43% to 64%).[51,52] Treatment outside of the US has focused on fluid resuscitation (oral and intravenous), oxygen, and antibiotics (cephalosporins or fluoroquinolones).[51] In addition to these measures, patients treated in the United States during the 2013–2014 outbreak received a variety of experimental therapies including ZMapp, a combination monoclonal antibody antiviral drug made from tobacco plants, and blood transfusions from survivors of EVD.

In October 2014, the first US citizen, a man who had recently returned to Texas from Liberia, was diagnosed with and subsequently died from EVD. This incident raised concerns about our preparedness for handling EVD. The subsequent transmission of EVD to two health care workers caring for that patient further revealed our own health system's vulnerabilities. In response, protocols were initiated to ensure that on presentation for care, all patients were screened for symptoms and relevant travel. Medical facilities were designated to receive and/or provide treatment to suspected or confirmed EVD patients by specially trained EVD care teams. Although most health care workers in the US will never encounter a patient with suspected or confirmed EVD, it was imperative for facilities to develop the procedures and processes to prepare for such a serious high-threat pathogen to emerge or reemerge.

An unprecedented international response controlled this outbreak. Ebola treatment centers throughout Sierra Leone, Liberia, and Guinea provided isolation and quarantine, protecting susceptible persons. A rapid diagnostic was developed and, toward the end of the epidemic, a vaccine (called rVSV-ZEBOV) was shown to be effective. This vaccine is currently being used in a ring vaccination strategy when sporadic cases are identified.

For example, in March 2016, a flare-up of EVD was discovered in Guinea and more than 1500 case contacts, contacts to contacts, and front-line workers were vaccinated. The ring vaccination strategy was found to be rapidly implementable, the vaccine found to be safe, and there were no cases among those vaccinated. However, in a 2019 Ebola outbreak in The Democratic Republic of Congo (DRC) health workers failed to locate many Ebola patient contacts resulting in rapid expansion of the disease. This expansion, in spite of the availability of an effective vaccine, is a result of an armed conflict, deep mistrust of foreign aid workers, and a lack of funding. Health workers and clinics are being attacked and rumors spread, causing great fear and spread of disease. The WHO declared this outbreak a Public Health Emergency and Global Concern in July 2019, prompting recommendations for optimal vaccination, careful cross border screening, and enhanced public education. https://www.who.int/news-room/detail/17-07-2019-ebola -outbreak-in-the-democratic-republic-of-the-congo-declared-a -public-health-emergency-of-international-concern.

Monkeypox. Traffic in exotic animals or exposure to pets or even laboratory animals can be harmful to your health. As suggested by its moniker, monkeys are affected by this orthopoxvirus, closely related to smallpox. Monkeypox has been long known as a rare but potentially fatal zoonosis that occurs sporadically in forested areas of Central and West Africa. Important disease reservoirs are rodents and squirrels. Human transmission has been linked to animal exposures such as household rodent contact or preparation of bushmeat, both of which are common in areas where monkeypox is prevalent.[53] Human-to-human transmission is much less efficient than in smallpox but was reported in 12% of household contacts who had never received smallpox vaccination.[53] Historically, the smallpox vaccine was noted to incidentally prevent monkeypox. Now that smallpox vaccination is no longer required in any country and civil wars have increased dependence on hunting, human monkeypox has reemerged in central Africa. In 2003, there was an outbreak of monkeypox in the United States, with 72 cases reported from six Midwestern states. Investigation revealed that most cases followed the acquisition of a pet prairie dog, which became a reservoir for monkeypox after exposure to a shipment of infected wild rodents from Ghana.[53,54]

In fall 2017, an outbreak of monkeypox was identified in Nigeria. Genetic sequencing results of the virus isolated across affected states suggest multiple sources of introduction of this zoonotic virus into the human population, demonstrating the capacity of this zoonotic disease to cause human disease.[55]

In contrast to smallpox, monkeypox usually produces severe adenopathy, does not effectively transmit person to person, and has a lower mortality rate of 10%.[56] Patients often defervesce on the day of or a few days after the onset of the classic pox rash, which often affects the face first.[53] Real-time PCR, IgG and IgM ELISA, indirect fluorescent antibody assay, and viral culture are all helpful in diagnosis. Treatment is supportive. There are at least three promising compounds being investigated for antiviral activity against monkeypox including cidofovir.[53]

Plague. Plague, infamous for causing the Black Death of the Middle Ages, has repeatedly reemerged as the source of multiple pandemics and epidemics. Today, plague continues to circulate in discrete regions in Africa, Asia, and the Americas.[56] In the US, a median of 3 (up to 17) locally transmitted cases are reported each year, primarily from New Mexico, Arizona, Colorado, and California.[57] Occasional limited outbreaks also occur. In 2017, plague reemerged in Madagascar causing a significant epidemic. After an ill 31-year-old male traveled by bush taxi from the central to the east coast region of Madagascar and died in transit, dozens of contacts were identified.[56] Within 4 months, a total of 2200 definite, probable, or suspected cases had been detected, of which more than 200 had died.[58] While national and international action eventually brought this epidemic under control, it raised concerns yet again about possible transmission beyond national borders and the need for prompt recognition by primary care and emergency medicine providers.

Plague is caused by the gram-negative bacteria *Yersinia pestis* and has two major clinical syndromes, bubonic and pneumonic plague. Bubonic plague is by far the more common form, responsible for 80% to 95% of cases.[59] Transmission typically occurs when a human is bitten by a rat flea. An incubation period of 2 to 8 days is followed by the sudden onset of fever, chills, fatigue, and the development of swollen and exquisitely tender lymph nodes, or buboes, most commonly in the groin region. If untreated, the infection can spread from the lymph region to the lungs to cause secondary pneumonic plague which is characterized by sudden shortness of breath, high fever, pleuritic chest pain, and cough with or without hemoptysis.[60] Primary pneumonic plague occurs from direct human-to-human or animal-to-human transmission via infected respiratory droplets.[61] With an incubation period of only a few hours to a few days, pneumonic plague should be considered a medical emergency; without treatment it is rapidly progressive and nearly always fatal.[56,]

Diagnosis of plague requires maintaining a high level of suspicion that prompts taking a careful travel history and inquiring about contact with ill animals in any patient presenting with fever and notably painful, swollen lymph nodes. Diagnosis can be confirmed by culture, serology, or rapid tests (available in some settings). Depending on the clinical presentation, *Yersinia pestis* can generally be cultured from sputum, blood, cerebrospinal fluid, or pus aspirated from buboes. A new rapid diagnostic test can detect small amounts of bacterial antigen from sputum or serum within minutes.[62] When field-tested in Madagascar, this test was found to approach 100% sensitivity and specificity.[60,62] PCR and ELISA testing can also be performed and presumptively identify the bacteria.[63] Serologic diagnosis is confirmed by a fourfold rise or more between acute and convalescent titers.[61]

Treatment has a dramatic impact on survival resulting in a decrease in mortality from 50% to 90% to 10% to 20% in cases of bubonic plague and from 100% to 50% in cases of pneumonic plague.[59,60] Gentamycin has replaced streptomycin as the preferred treatment for plague and has been shown to be equally effective and generally better tolerated.[64] Doxycycline and tetracycline are acceptable alternatives for those who cannot tolerate aminoglycosides.[64] Fluoroquinolones have been shown to be effective in animal studies and subsequently the FDA recently approved their use for the treatment of plague.[65,66] Treatment is generally recommended for 10 to 14 days and should be continued for a few days after symptoms resolve. Contacts who have had unprotected face-to-face exposure (i.e., within 6 feet) of patients with known or suspected pneumonic plague who have not received at least 48 hours of effective antimicrobial therapy should receive 7 days of post-exposure prophylaxis with doxycycline (preferred), levofloxacin, or trimethoprim-sulfamethoxazole.[59]

Antibiotic Resistance

Since their discovery in the middle of the 20th century, antibiotics have substantially reduced the threat posed by infectious diseases. Improvements in sanitation, housing, and nutrition as well as immunizations also contributed to a dramatic drop in mortality from infectious diseases. However, the recent emergence of antibiotic-resistant organisms threatens these gains, because infections caused by resistant organisms fail to respond to usual treatments, resulting in longer periods of infectivity and increased patient morbidity and mortality.

Resistance to antimicrobials has been attributed in large part to the overprescribing of antibiotics, incomplete patient compliance with a prescribed course, and use of antibiotics as prophylaxis or growth stimulants in animal feed. Recommendations designed to combat antibiotic resistance are in place worldwide and consist of the following: education of prescribers and consumers as to the dangers of antibiotic overuse; attention to unnecessary veterinary antibiotic use; reduction of nosocomial transmission of such infections by improvement of hand hygiene in health care settings either with soap and water washing or the use of alcohol-based hand sanitizers; enhanced environmental cleaning; and surveillance policies.[67,68]

Carbapenem-Resistant Enterobacteriaceae. The carbapenem-resistant Enterobacteriaceae (CRE) are a family of bacteria that are difficult to treat because they have high levels of resistance to antibiotics. Some CRE bacteria have become resistant to most available antibiotics. Infections with these germs are very difficult to treat, and can be deadly—one report cites they can contribute to death in up to 50% of patients who become infected.[69]

Klebsiella, *Enterobacter*, and *E. coli* are important species of Enterobacteriaceae that can become carbapenem-resistant. Types of CRE are defined by their genetic mechanism of resistance, including KPC (*Klebsiella pneumoniae* carbapenemase) and NDM (New Delhi metallo-β-lactamase). KPC and NDM are enzymes that break down carbapenems and make them ineffective. Both of these enzymes, as well as the enzyme VIM (Verona integron-mediated metallo-β-lactamase) have also been reported in *Pseudomonas*.

CRE infections are most common in patients in hospitals, nursing homes, and other health care settings. Patients whose care requires devices like ventilators (breathing machines), urinary (bladder) catheters, or intravenous (vein) catheters, and patients who are taking long courses of certain antibiotics are most at risk for CRE infections.

The emergence of CRE shows the urgent need for the implementation of effective antibiotic stewardship activities.

Extensively Drug-Resistant Tuberculosis. In 2006, an outbreak of HIV infection–associated extensively drug-resistant tuberculosis (XDR-TB) was described among 53 patients in South Africa; 52 of the 53 died, with a median survival of 16 days from time of diagnosis.[70] This report brought XDR-TB into the spotlight in medical, public health, and lay communities. Subsequently, WHO and the CDC declared XDR-TB to be a serious emerging threat to public health and international TB control efforts.

XDR-TB is defined as resistance to at least isoniazid and rifampin (which is the definition of MDR-TB) and the additional resistance to any fluoroquinolone and to at least one of the three following injectable drugs used in TB treatment: amikacin, capreomycin, or kanamycin. Data show that XDR-TB has been documented in 123 countries with some of the highest rates and numbers reported from the Russian Federation, India, China, South Africa, and countries of the former Soviet Union (especially Belarus, Kazakhstan, and Ukraine).[71] Because of limited laboratory capacity to diagnose XDR-TB, the actual global prevalence and distribution of XDR-TB cannot be firmly established.[72] Although the reported numbers of MDR-TB and XDR-TB in the US are low (in 2016, 88 cases and 1 case, respectively), the majority of those with MDR-TB occurred in persons without a history of TB, suggesting primary infection (either in their home country or the US).[73] Therefore, clinicians should maintain a high index of suspicion for drug-resistant TB in the presence of a epidemiologic risk factors (e.g., emigration from a high-burden country) and order appropriate testing (Xpert MTB/RIF or other molecular assays that can detect drug resistance mutations quickly) even in the case of new diagnoses of TB.

MDR-TB and XDR-TB are difficult to treat, requiring more costly and complex drugs with standard regimens of much greater duration than for drug-sensitive TB strains. While treatment success rates can be in the 80% to 95% range for drug-susceptible TB, these rates drop to 54% for MDR/RR-TB (2014 cohort) and 30% for XDR-TB (2014 cohort).[71] Clearly, drug-resistant TB threatens to thwart the successes in international TB control achieved to date and to change the epidemiology of TB worldwide. Encouraging news on the global front to effectively treat MDR-TB (and thereby reduce further emergence of resistance and transmission) is the introduction of the newest TB drugs, bedaquiline and delamanid, and the use of shorter regimens (9 to 12 months) in many African and Asian countries; these regimens have been associated with higher treatment success rates of 87% to 90%.[71] Nonetheless, increased global access to rapid diagnostics at reduced prices, all second-line drugs, and maintaining an active pipeline for new classes of drugs to treat TB remain urgent needs for eliminating TB globally and locally.

MDR-TB and XDR-TB treatment should be done in consultation with appropriate experts. It should begin with seeking support from your local or state health department and advancing to a regional consultation center if further support is needed. For the most complicated cases, National Jewish Hospital in Denver, Colorado, one of the leading facilities for treatment of drug-resistant TB, will provide consultation services including a physician-dedicated telephone line (further information is available at www.nationaljewish.org/professionals/referrals-and-consults/physician-line).

SUMMARY

Primary care clinicians are on the front lines of disease control. It is particularly challenging to maintain awareness of the recent succession of newly identified and reemerging pathogens such as new respiratory and vector-borne pathogens and newly introduced diarrheal illnesses in developing nations, as well as the emergence of antimicrobial resistance. Cooperation both locally and globally is needed for urgent control of these pathogens.

REFERENCES

1. Fineberg, H. V. (2014). Pandemic preparedness and response—lessons from the H1N1 influenza of 2009. *The New England Journal of Medicine, 370*(14), 1335–1342.
2. World Health Organization (WHO). World health report: executive summary—emerging diseases. Retrieved from http://www.who.int/whr/1996/media_centre/executive_summary1/en/index5.html. (Accessed 15 January 2018).
3. Peiris, J. S., Yuen, K. Y., Osterhaus, A. D., et al. (2003). The severe acute respiratory distress syndrome. *The New England Journal of Medicine, 349*, 2431–2440.
4. To, K. K., Hung, I. F., Chan, J. F., & Yuen, K. Y. (2013). From SARS coronavirus to novel animal and human coronaviruses. *Journal of Thoracic Disease, Suppl 2*, S103–S108.
5. Ong, K. C., Ng, A. W., Lee, L. S., et al. (2005). 1-year pulmonary function and health status in survivors of severe acute respiratory syndrome. *Chest, 128*(3), 1393–1400.
6. Guan, Y., Zheng, B. J., He, Y. Q., et al. (2003). Isolation and characterization of viruses related to the SARS coronavirus from animals in southern China. *Science, 302*, 276–278.
7. Zaki, A. M., van Boheemen, S., Bestebroer, T. M., Osterhaus, A. D. M. E., & Fouchier, R. A. (2012). Isolation of a novel coronavirus from a man with pneumonia in Saudi Arabia. *The New England Journal of Medicine, 367*, 1814–1820.
8. Centers for Disease Control and Prevention (CDC). (2013). Update: Recommendations for Middle East respiratory syndrome coronavirus (MERS-CoV). *MMWR. Morbidity and Mortality Weekly Report, 62*(27), 557.
9. Assiri, A., McGeer, A., Perl, T. M., et al. (2013). Hospital outbreak of Middle East respiratory syndrome coronavirus. *The New England Journal of Medicine, 369*(9), 407–416.
10. Centers for Disease Control and Prevention (CDC). (2013). Update: Severe respiratory illness associated with Middle East respiratory syndrome coronavirus (MERS-CoV)—worldwide, 2012-2013. *MMWR. Morbidity and Mortality Weekly Report, 62*(23), 480–483.
11. Centers for Disease Control and Prevention (CDC). Middle East Respiratory Syndrome (MERS): prevention and treatment. Retrieved from www.cdc.gov/coronavirus/MERS/about/prevention.html. (Accessed 15 January 2018).
12. Panda, S., Mohakud, N. K., Pena, L., et al. (2014). Human metapneumovirus: Review of an important respiratory pathogen. *International Journal of Infectious Diseases, 25C*, 45–52.
13. Moe, N., Krokstad, S., Stenseng, I. H., et al. (2017). Comparing human metapneumovirus and respiratory Syncytial Virus: Viral co-detections genotypes and risk factors for severe disease. *PLoS ONE, 12*(1), e0170200.
14. Taubenberger, J. K., Reid, A. H., Lourens, R. M., et al. (2005). Characterization of the 1918 influenza virus polymerase genes. *Nature, 437*, 889–893.
15. Centers for Disease Control and Prevention (CDC). (2009). Swine influenza A (H1N1) infection in two children—Southern California, March–April 2009. *MMWR. Morbidity and Mortality Weekly Report, 58*(15), 400–402.
16. World Health Organization (WHO). DG Statement following the meeting of the Emergency Committee, June 11, 2009. Retrieved from www.who.int/csr/disease/swineflu/4th_meeting_ihr/en/index.html. (Accessed 15 January 2018).
17. Zimmer, S. M., & Byrke, D. S. (2009). Historical perspective—emergence of influenza A (H1N1) viruses. *The New England Journal of Medicine, 361*(3), 279–285.
18. Morens, D. M., Taubenberger, J. K., & Fauci, A. S. (2009). The persistent legacy of the 1918 influenza virus. *The New England Journal of Medicine, 361*(3), 225–229.
19. Bautista, E., Chotpitayasunondh, T., Gao, Z., et al. (2010). Clinical aspects of pandemic 2009 influenza A (H1N1) virus infection. *The New England Journal of Medicine, 362*(18), 1709–1719.
20. Van Kerkhove, M. D., Mumford, E., Mounts, A. W., et al. (2011). Highly pathogenic avian influenza (H5N1): Pathways of exposure at the animal-human interface, a systematic review. *PLoS ONE, 6*(1), e14582.
21. Food and Drug Administration (FDA). FDA approves first adjuvanted vaccine for prevention of H5N1 avian influenza: Vaccine to supplement National Stockpile, not intended for commercial availability. Retrieved from https://wayback.archive-it.org/7993/20170111161026/http://www.fda.gov/NewsEvents/Newsroom/PressAnnouncements/ucm376444.htm. (Accessed 15 January 2018).
22. Centers for Disease Control and Prevention (CDC). (1993). Imported cholera associated with a newly described toxigenic *Vibrio cholerae* O138 strain—California, 1993. *MMWR. Morbidity and Mortality Weekly Report, 42*, 501–503.
23. Ali, M., Nelson, A. R., Lopez, A. L., et al. (2015). Updated global burden of cholera in endemic countries. *PLoS Neglected Tropical Diseases, 9*(6), e0003832.
24. Vezzulli, L., Pezzati, E., Brettar, I., et al. (2015). Effects of global warming on Vibrioecology. *Microbiology Spectrum, 3*(3), VE-0004-2104.
25. Centers for Disease Control and Prevention (CDC). Cholera in Haiti: one year later. Retrieved from https://www.cdc.gov/cholera/haiti/haiti-one-year-later.html. (Accessed 14 January 2018).
26. Centers for Disease Control and Prevention (CDC). Cholera - Vibrio cholerae infection: Vaccines. Retrieved from https://www.cdc.gov/cholera/vaccines.html. (Accessed 14 January 2018).
27. Federal Drug Administration (FDA) News Release. FDA approves vaccine to prevent cholera for travelers. Retrieved from https://www.fda.gov/NewsEvents/Newsroom/PressAnnouncements/ucm506305.htm. (Accessed 14 January 2018).
28. Hidalgo, J., Richards, G. A., Jiménez, J. I. S., et al. (2017). Viral hemorrhagic fever in the tropics: Report from the task force on tropical diseases by the World Federation of Societies of Intensive and Critical Care Medicine. *Journal of Critical Care, 42*, 366–372.
29. Monath, T., & Vasconcelos, P. (2015). Yellow fever. *Journal of Clinical Virology, 64*, 160–173.
30. Dreshaj, S., Ahmeti, S., Ramadani, N., et al. (2016). Current situation of Crimean-Congo hemorrhagic fever in Southeastern Europe and neighboring countries: A public health risk for the European Union? *Travel Medicine and Infectious Disease, 14*(2), 81–91.
31. Atkinson, B., Chamberlain, J., Logue, C. H., Cook, N., Bruce, C., Dowall, S. D., et al. (2012). Development of a real-time RT-PCR assay for the detection of Crimean-Congo hemorrhagic fever virus. *Vector Borne and Zoonotic Diseases (Larchmont, N.Y.), 12*(9), 786–793.
32. Linthicum, K. J., Britch, S. C., & Anyamba, A. (2016). Rift Valley Fever: An emerging mosquito-borne disease. *Annual Review of Entomology, 61*, 395–415.
33. Centers for Disease Control and Prevention (CDC). (2007). Rift Valley fever outbreak–Kenya, November 2006–January 2007. *MMWR. Morbidity and Mortality Weekly Report, 56*(4), 73–76.
34. Faburay, B., LaBeaud, A. D., McVey, D. S., et al. (2017). Current status of Rift Valley Fever vaccine development. *Vaccines, 5*(3).
35. Ftika, L., & Mattezou, H. C. (2013). Viral haemorrhagic fevers in health care settings. *Journal of Hospital Infection, 83*(3), 185–192.
36. Klempa, B., Koulemou, K., Auste, B., et al. (2013). Seroepidemiological study reveals regional co-occurrence of Lassa- and Hantavirus antibodies in Upper Guinea, West Africa. *Tropical Medicine and International Health, 18*(3), 366–371.
37. Ehlkes, L., George, M., Samosny, G., et al. (2017). Management of a Lassa fever outbreak, Rhineland-Palatinate, Germany, 2016. *Euro Surveillance, 22*(39).
38. World Health Organization (WHO). Yellow fever. Retrieved from https://www.who.int/csr/don/archive/disease/yellow_fever/en/. (Accessed 18 July 2019).
39. Centers for Disease Control and Prevention (CDC). Yellow Fever Vaccine. Retrieved from https://www.cdc.gov/yellowfever/vaccine/index.html. (Accessed 18 July 2019).
40. Santos, R. I., Bueno-Júnior, L. S., Ruggiero, R. N., et al. (2014). Spread of oropouche virus into the central nervous system in mouse. *Viruses, 6*(10), 3827–3836.
41. Travassos da Rosa, J. F., de Souza, W. M., & Pinheiro, F. P. (2017). Oropouche Virus: Clinical, epidemiological, and molecular aspects of a neglected orthobunyavirus. *The American Journal of Tropical Medicine and Hygiene, 96*(5), 1019–1030.
42. Romero-Alvarez, D., & Escobar, L. E. (2017). Oropouche fever, an emergent disease from the Americas. *Microbes and Infection*, pii: S1286-4579 (17)30220-4.
43. Suss, J. (2008). Tick-borne encephalitis in Europe and beyond—the epidemiological situation as of 2007. *Euro Surveillance, 13*(26), pii: 18916.

44. Lindquist, L., & Vapalahti, O. (2008). Tick-borne encephalitis. *Lancet*, *371*(9627), 1861–1871.

45. Kaiser, R. (2008). Tick-borne encephalitis. *Infectious Disease Clinics of North America*, *22*(3), 561–575.

46. Centers for Disease Control and Prevention (CDC). (2010). Tick-borne encephalitis among U.S. travelers to Europe and Asia—2000–2009. *MMWR. Morbidity and Mortality Weekly Report*, *59*(11), 335–338.

47. Haditsch, M., & Kunze, U. (2016). Tick-borne encephalitis: A disease neglected by travel medicine. *Travel Medicine and Infectious Disease*, *11*(5), 295–300.

48. Breman, J. G., & Johnson, K. M. (2014). Ebola then and now. *The New England Journal of Medicine*, *371*(18), 1663–1666.

49. Baize, S., Pannetier, D., Oestereich, L., et al. (2014). Emergence of Zaire Ebola virus disease in Guinea. *The New England Journal of Medicine*, *371*(15), 1418–1425.

50. Centers for Disease Control and Prevention (CDC). Ebola virus ecology graphic. Retrieved from www.cdc.gov/vhf/ebola/resources/virus-ecology.html. (Accessed 15 January 2018).

51. Bah, E. I., Lamah, M. C., Fletcher, T., et al. (2015). Clinical presentation of patients with Ebola virus disease in Conakry, Guinea. *The New England Journal of Medicine*, *372*(1), 40–47.

52. World Health Organization (WHO). (2014). Ebola Response Team. Ebola virus disease in West Africa—the first 9 months of the epidemic and forward projections. *The New England Journal of Medicine*, *371*(16), 1481–1495.

53. McCollum, A. M., & Damon, I. K. (2014). Human monkeypox. *Clinical Infectious Diseases : an Official Publication of the Infectious Diseases Society of America*, *58*(2), 260–267.

54. Centers for Disease Control and Prevention (CDC). (2003). Update: Multistate outbreak of monkeypox—Illinois, Indiana, Kansas, Missouri, Ohio, and Wisconsin. *MMWR. Morbidity and Mortality Weekly Report*, *52*(27), 642–646.

55. World Health Organization (WHO). Monkeypox—Nigeria. Retrieved from http://www.who.int/csr/don/21-december-2017-monkeypox-nigeria/en/. (Accessed 15 January 2018).

56. Mead, P. S. (2018). Plague in Madagascar a tragic opportunity for improving public health. *The New England Journal of Medicine*, *378*(2), 106–108.

57. Kwit, N., Nelson, C., Kugeler, K., et al. (2015). Human plague—United States, 2015. *MMWR. Morbidity and Mortality Weekly Report*, *64*(33), 918–919.

58. Bonds, M. H., Ouenzar, M. A., Garchitorena, A., et al. (2018). Madagascar can build stronger health systems to fight plague and prevent the next epidemic. *PLoS Neglected Tropical Diseases*, *12*(1), e0006131.

59. Prentice, M. B., & Rahalison, L. (2007). Plague. *Lancet*, *369*(9568), 1196.

60. Randremanana, R., Andrianaivoarimanana, V., Nikolay, B., et al. (2019). Epidemiological charcteristics of an urban plague epidemic in Madagascar, Aug–Nov 2017: A outbreak report. *The Lancet Infectious Diseases*, *19*(5), 537–545.

61. Kwit, N., Nelson, C., Kugeler, K., et al. (2015). Human plague—United States, 2015. *MMWR. Morbidity and Mortality Weekly Report*, *64*(33), 918–919.

62. Chanteau, S., Rahalison, L., Ralafiarisoa, L., et al. (2003). Development and testing of a rapid diagnostic test for bubonic and pneumonic plague. *Lancet*, *361*(9353), 211.

63. Loïez, C., Herwegh, S., Wallet, F., Armand, S., Guinet, F., & Courcol, R. J. (2003). Detection of Yersinia pestis in sputum by real-time PCR. *Journal of Clinical Microbiology*, *41*(10), 4873.

64. Yang, R. (2017). Plague: Recognition, treatment, and prevention. *Journal of Clinical Microbiology*, *56*(1), e01519-17. doi:10.1128/JCM.01519-17. Published 2017 Dec 26.

65. National Institutes of Health (NIH). Ciprofloxacin licensed to treat pneumonic plague. Retrieved from https://www.niaid.nih.gov/diseases-conditions/ciprofloxacin-treat-pneumonic-plague. (Accessed 13 January 2018).

66. Food and Drug Administration (FDA). FDA approves additional antibacterial treatment for plague. Retrieved from http://www.fda.gov/NewsEvents/Newsroom/PressAnnouncements/ucm446283.htm. (Accessed 13 January 2018).

67. Siegel, J. D., Rhinehart, E., Jackson, M., et al., Healthcare Infection Control Practices Advisory Committee. 2007 Guideline for isolation precautions: preventing transmission of infectious agents in healthcare settings. Retrieved from https://www.cdc.gov/infectioncontrol/pdf/guidelines/isolation-guidelines.pdf. (Accessed 15 January 2018).

68. Siegel, J. D., Rhinehart, E., Jackson, M., et al., Healthcare Infection Control Practices Advisory Committee. Management of multidrug-resistant organisms in healthcare settings, 2006. Retrieved from https://www.cdc.gov/infectioncontrol/pdf/guidelines/mdro-guidelines.pdf. (Accessed 15 January 2018).

69. Centers for Disease Control and Prevention (CDC). Carbapenem-resistant enterobacteriaceae in healthcare settings. Retrieved from https://www.cdc.gov/hai/organisms/cre/index.html. (Accessed 15 January 2018).

70. Gandhi, N. R., Moll, A., Sturm, A. W., et al. (2006). Extensively drug-resistant tuberculosis as a cause of death in patients co-infected with tuberculosis and HIV in a rural area of South Africa. *Lancet*, *368*(9547), 1575–1580.

71. Global tuberculosis report 2017. Geneva: World Health Organization; 2017. Licence: CC BY-NC-SA 3.0 IGO.

72. Zignol, M., van Gemert, W., Falzon, D., et al. (2012). Surveillance of anti-tuberculosis drug resistance in the world: An updated analysis, 2007–2010. *Bulletin of the World Health Organization*, *90*(2), 111–119.

73. Schmit, K. M., Wansaula, Z., Pratt, R., et al. (2017). Tuberculosis—United States, 2016. *MMWR. Morbidity and Mortality Weekly Report*, *66*(11), 289–294.

CHAPTER **209**

HIV INFECTION
David de Gijsel • Martha DesBiens

 Immediate emergency department referral is indicated for mental distress, suicidal or homicidal ideations, and signs or symptoms suggestive of a severe OI (e.g., delirium, focal neurologic deficit, rapidly progressive dyspnea, and visual loss).

DEFINITION AND EPIDEMIOLOGY

Human immunodeficiency virus type 1 (HIV-1) is a member of the family of viruses known as retroviruses. HIV-1 was first isolated in 1985 when it was found to be the causative agent of a recently identified epidemic of acquired immunodeficiency syndrome (AIDS). HIV-1 is a zoonosis that was transmitted from chimpanzees to humans at least 3 times early in the 20th century. HIV-2 is a genetically distinct retrovirus also transmitted from monkeys to humans; HIV-2 also causes AIDS, although on average more slowly than HIV-1, and it is much less prevalent than HIV-1, both globally and in the United States.

HIV infection presents a number of challenges for the primary health care provider. These include when to consider the diagnosis and to test for infection, when to initiate antiretroviral therapy (ART) and with which antiretrovirals (ARVs), and how to monitor disease progression and treatment efficacy. Careful attention is needed to avoid potentially dangerous drug-drug interactions when patients are being treated with ART. The health care provider must also incorporate risk reduction counseling into clinical care to further reduce HIV transmission. Advice and support around family planning and pregnancy will be needed. Other considerations related to care may include guidance around pre-exposure prophylaxis (PrEP) for those at high risk for acquiring HIV from an infected partner, or around post-exposure prophylaxis after a possible exposure to HIV.

The first AIDS case definition was developed by the Centers for Disease Control (CDC) in 1987 as a tool to aid in the study of the AIDS epidemic. This definition included a composite of syndromes, primarily opportunistic infections (OIs) and malignant neoplasms, associated with advanced immune dysfunction.[1] The AIDS case definition has subsequently been expanded several times and now requires that an individual have laboratory documentation of HIV infection and either (1) one of a broad spectrum of OIs, malignant neoplasms, and nonspecific syndromes or (2) a CD4 cell count of less than

$200/mm^3$.[2] Because AIDS is a clinical case definition used primarily for epidemiologic monitoring, once an individual is diagnosed with AIDS, that individual will always carry the diagnosis of AIDS, even after immune restoration such that the CD4 cell count is greater than $200/mm^3$ and all complications of AIDS have resolved.

In addition to the AIDS case definition, several systems were used in the past to classify HIV-infected patients by degree of immune dysfunction, usually based on a combination of laboratory and clinical criteria, but these classification systems were developed before the dynamic nature of HIV infection was well understood, and prior to availability of effective treatment. They have little usefulness for the clinician caring for HIV-infected patients today.

Transmission of HIV can occur sexually, parenterally through either injection drug use (IDU) or blood product transmission, and vertically from mother to child during pregnancy or through breastfeeding. The risk of sexual transmission varies by the nature of the sexual encounter but is generally in the range of 0.1% to 1% per episode of vaginal or rectal sex when no barrier protection is used. The risk of transmission through oral sex is markedly lower. Factors that increase the risk of transmission include the presence of other active sexually transmitted infections (STIs) and a high HIV viral load. Transmission from blood products was virtually eliminated in the United States in 1985 when it became possible to screen blood donations for HIV. The risk of transmission from an untreated HIV-infected mother to child is 20% to 30% during pregnancy and delivery, with a subsequent risk of transmission through breastfeeding that is cumulative and depends on duration and consistency of breastfeeding.

The CDC estimates that about 1.1 million people aged 13 or older were living with HIV infection in the United States at the end of 2017, of which 162,500 (15%) had not received a diagnosis.[3] An estimated 38,500 people were newly infected in 2015, an overall decline of 8% from 2010 (41,800).[3] Through 2016, the cumulative number of AIDS cases reported to the CDC was 1,232,346.[3] In 2016, an estimated 39,782 people were newly diagnosed with HIV, and 18,160 people received a diagnosis of AIDS. Since 1997, the number of non-Hispanic African Americans living with AIDS has outnumbered the number of non-Hispanic whites. Total deaths from HIV disease from 1987 to 2015 were 507,351.[3]

AIDS has been a reportable condition since 1987, but HIV infection has never been a nationally reportable disease. Consequently, our understanding of US epidemiology has been based primarily on AIDS cases, which tend to describe out-of-date population health trends. Epidemiologic description based on AIDS cases has become even less accurate more recently, with the introduction of therapy that can prevent progression of HIV infection to AIDS. Based on current data published from states in which HIV infection is a reportable condition, it was estimated in 2016 that men who have sex with men (MSM) account for 67% of all new HIV infections in the United States, followed by heterosexual transmission (24%) while the remainder is thought to occur in people who inject drugs (PWID) (9%). Among women with newly diagnosed HIV infection, however, 87% of cases are secondary to heterosexual transmission.[3] Important trends include a growing disproportion of cases in minorities, a growing proportion of cases in the southern states, and a resurgence of cases among MSM in at least some areas in the United States. Between 2011 and 2015, new diagnoses of HIV among white gay and bisexual men decreased by 10%, whereas new diagnoses increased 4% among African American gay and bisexual men. Similarly, Black/African American women are disproportionately affected by HIV (59%), compared to Hispanic/Latina women (19%), and white women (17%). In 2016, 44% of all new HIV infections occurred in African Americans, while this race/ethnicity group represents only 12% of the total US population. In 2016, the South accounted for 53% of new AIDS diagnoses in the US, followed by the West (17%), the Northeast (17%), and the Midwest (13%).[3]

The extent of the HIV epidemic in the United States, the ongoing stigma associated with the disease, and the social and medical marginalization of some of those at highest risk of acquiring HIV infection have resulted in a relatively unsuccessful campaign to diagnose and bring HIV-infected people into care. Recent estimates suggest that about 15% of all people living with HIV infection in the United States have not been diagnosed, and around half of HIV-infected individuals are either not receiving care or otherwise do not have the virus under control. Thus, there are as many as a half-million people with HIV infection who are at risk of disease progression and eventually life-threatening complications of AIDS and who are also likely to be at higher risk of transmitting HIV to others.

Because of the inadequacy of the original approach to HIV testing, which relied on targeted testing of those identified as being at higher risk of HIV infection, in 2006 the CDC recommended that testing become universal. Opt-out HIV testing should now be offered at least once to all persons aged 13 to 64 years, regardless of risk, and repeated testing of persons with known risk should be performed at least annually. Testing should be performed in all health care settings and need not include prevention counseling.[4]

Considering the impact of this disease on public health, the Health Resources and Services Administration of the US Department of Health and Human Services has provided dedicated federal funds through the Ryan White Comprehensive AIDS Resources Emergency (CARE) Act for HIV prevention and care services since 1990. In addition to HIV prevention services, allocated through each state, this act provides funding for both uninsured and low-income persons living with HIV infection to access primary and specialty HIV care, dental services, and case management as well as payment for their life-prolonging HIV medications. However, with the continuing challenges to the Affordable Care Act (ACA), insurance coverage and payment for services are changing rapidly, thus causing confusion for patients. Lapses in insurance coverage lead to missed appointments and inconsistent adherence to therapy. Therefore, it is important that all new HIV clients be provided a case manager to help them navigate insurance and other changing health care reimbursement options that may be available to them, and to reinforce uninterrupted coverage. Despite the high cost of HIV care, and ART in particular, HIV has had a relatively minor impact on the US health care economy, although this is not the case in many economically disadvantaged countries. The Joint United Nations Programme on HIV/AIDS estimates that 37.9 million people globally were living with HIV in 2018; of these, 34.5 million were adults, 17.8 million were women, and 2.1 million were children younger than 15 years.[5] The vast majority of people living with HIV infection live in low- and middle-income countries, and many of them still do not have access to effective treatment for HIV infection and thus will likely die of AIDS. In 2018, around 62% of all people living with HIV had access to treatment. During 2018, 1.7 million people became infected globally, and AIDS caused the deaths of an estimated 770,000 people.[5]

PATHOPHYSIOLOGY

Although some aspects of the HIV life cycle and HIV/AIDS pathophysiology still require further study, the general outline is well established. To infect a cell, HIV must attach to two cell surface proteins: first, CD4, and second, one of two chemokine receptors, CCR5 or CXCR4, which are often referred to as co-receptors. The virus then fuses with the cell surface, followed by release of viral RNA and proteins into the infected cell. The viral RNA is then reverse transcribed to DNA (hence the name retrovirus), and this DNA is transported into the host cell nucleus and incorporated into the cellular genome. Various cells, including monocytes-macrophages and dendritic cells, are susceptible to HIV infection, but the CD4 T lymphocyte is the primary target. A CD4 T lymphocyte that is infected by HIV can remain metabolically inactive with latent HIV infection, or it can be activated with resultant active HIV replication. Through mechanisms that are not entirely understood, the replication of HIV within activated CD4 T cells and the resultant high-level viremia with the subsequent infection of more CD4 T cells drives an inexorable decline in the total pool of CD4 T cells in the infected person. As the total number of CD4 T cells declines, measured by the number of circulating CD4 T cells in peripheral blood (often referred to as the CD4 count or T-cell count), there is a steady decline in the functional capacity of the immune system. After sufficient damage, the infected person starts to develop complications of this immune dysfunction. Eventual development of one or more of the many complications of AIDS drives its ultimate mortality. With few exceptions, such as tuberculosis (TB), these AIDS-defining conditions seldom occur until the CD4 T-cell count drops below 200 cells/mm³.

The rate of progression of immune dysfunction, monitored by the decline of the CD4 T-cell count in peripheral blood, varies significantly among individuals. Without ART, the average time from initial HIV infection until the development of a first complication of AIDS is about 8 years, and the average time from this first complication to death is another year. However, some individuals progress to AIDS in a few years (occasionally as short as 1 year), and some rare individuals (known as long-term nonprogressors or elite controllers) maintain a normal CD4 T-cell count indefinitely and never develop AIDS.

CLINICAL PRESENTATION AND PHYSICAL EXAMINATION

The clinical presentation of a person with HIV infection varies tremendously, determined in large part by the stage of disease including but not limited to primary HIV infection (PHI), a period of clinical latency, or progression to AIDS. PHI refers to the time after infection but before establishment of a comprehensive immunologic response to the infection—that is, the period when HIV can be identified in the person's blood but before standard serologic test results for HIV have become positive. This period before seroconversion (commonly referred to as the window period) typically lasts several weeks but rarely may be as long as 3 months. During this time, the infected person may experience a seroconversion illness,

which is often described as influenza-like but is highly variable and most often consists of fever, myalgia, headache, and a pleomorphic rash.

During the years between PHI and AIDS, a person infected with HIV is typically asymptomatic; however, assorted clinical syndromes may occur during this period. It is important to be aware of these, both for management of a known HIV-infected patient and as indications to consider underlying HIV infection in as yet undiagnosed patients. On occasion, OIs may occur at a CD4 range of more than 200 cells/mm³. In the United States, malignant neoplasm such as lymphomas and cervical and anal carcinomas are more commonly experienced AIDS-related complications at higher CD4 counts than OIs, although these neoplasms are still quite rare. The most important severe infection that occurs at a higher rate in this CD4 range is TB. Less severe complications seen within this CD4 range include shingles, severe psoriasis, severe (particularly invasive) pneumococcal disease, recurrent oral and vaginal candidiasis, oral hairy leukoplakia, and idiopathic thrombocytopenia. The occurrence of any of these conditions in a patient without known HIV infection should prompt assessment of HIV risk and HIV diagnostic testing as appropriate.

When a person infected with HIV has progressed to the severe immune dysfunction present in AIDS, they are at risk for all the potential complications thereof, and development of any one of these mandates testing for HIV infection. The risk for developing an HIV-associated complication increases steadily as the CD4 count drops below 200/mm³. *Pneumocystis jiroveci* pneumonia (PJP), Kaposi sarcoma (KS, a primarily cutaneous malignant neoplasm that manifests as raised violaceous macules), cryptococcal meningitis, and esophageal candidiasis are common early HIV-associated complications. At lower CD4 counts, especially below 50 cells/mm³, additional complications may develop, including *Toxoplasma* encephalitis, disseminated *Mycobacterium avium-intracellulare* complex (MAC) infection, cytomegalovirus (CMV) retinitis, progressive multifocal leukoencephalopathy, AIDS dementia, primary central nervous system lymphoma, and AIDS wasting syndrome.

The evaluation of a person newly diagnosed with HIV infection is extensive. If the patient has an acute illness, whether from acute or chronic HIV infection, evaluation and management of that illness takes priority. However, whether the patient is ill or asymptomatic, initial assessment must include a full history and physical examination, comprehensive laboratory evaluation, and other testing as appropriate. Aspects of the initial evaluation that require particular attention include the following:

- Assessment of the patient's understanding of the new diagnosis and of the implications for the future, both short and long term. In particular, it is important to attend to the patient's emotional state and to ensure their safety. Depression and stigmatization often associated with a new diagnosis of HIV infection may lead to increased risk of self-harm, as well as harm or abuse from others, including partners, family members, or others in the community. Exploring patient-specific factors may help mitigate this risk.
- The development of a trusting and therapeutic relationship with patients. The first medical appointment after a new diagnosis of HIV infection provides a unique opportunity for the health care provider to establish rapport with the patient that is crucial for future health care. This requires

the provider to balance the need to inquire about deeply personal, emotionally intense, and sometimes shaming history with the importance of reassuring patient confidence that the primary purpose in collecting this information is to ensure comprehensive care. Successful negotiation of this encounter will facilitate future care, whereas an encounter that leaves the patient uncomfortable with or untrusting of the provider will affect the patient's willingness to return, to provide sensitive information, and to work productively with the provider. Depending on the patient's health and potential risk to others, it may be appropriate to defer some of this history and discussion for subsequent meetings. Should this be the case, it is often helpful to frame the subjects for future discussion, so it is easier to return to them at the appropriate time.

- Medical history. This should be comprehensive and should address in detail aspects of the patient's history that may indicate possible exposures that increase the risk of certain OIs, including a detailed travel and exposure history. A history of prior STIs and exposure to TB is particularly important.
- Sexual history. This should include an attempt to define the patient's sexual orientation and identity; history of sexual behavior; use of condoms; ability to negotiate sexual activity and condom use (especially in a current relationship); and to identify circumstances in which the patient may be less able to restrain their sexual behavior because of peer pressure, concerns about safety, or loss of inhibition secondary to substance use.
- Trauma history. There is a growing recognition of trauma as a risk factor for HIV infection and as a predictor of worse treatment outcomes. Trauma can be multifold and includes physical, sexual, and emotional trauma that can be inflicted by people, society, and natural disaster. Certain groups of people are especially vulnerable to suffer trauma and often lack adequate support to process trauma. Such groups include women and gender non-binary people.
- Substance use history. Details of the history and current use of illicit drugs, the use of alcohol, and the abuse of prescription medications aid in individual patient care, inform the choice of ART, and define the need for harm reduction interventions.
- Mental health. Because people living with HIV infection are more likely than the general population to experience mental health disorders and emotional distress, it is important to screen early for disorders such as depression, anxiety, post-traumatic stress disorder, sleep disturbance, alcohol and substance use, and suicidal or homicidal ideation. Many of these disorders can be exacerbated by the stresses of a new diagnosis of HIV infection, disclosing this diagnosis to loved ones, dealing with the death of a significant other, grappling with lifestyle changes, and living with a chronic illness. Furthermore, untreated mental health disorders may be exacerbated by some ARVs and may also adversely affect the high level of medication adherence that is required for effective ART.
- Alternative therapies. Because some alternative, herbal, or vitamin therapies are contraindicated in combination with some ARVs, the use of any of these therapies needs to be carefully defined and then researched for safety.

The physical examination needs to be comprehensive, both for general health assessment and for detection of complications of HIV infection. Particular attention should be paid to the neurologic examination (for both focal and cognitive deficits) and to the skin (for KS and assorted dermatitides), oropharynx (for thrush, oral hairy leukoplakia, periodontitis, KS), liver, and genitals (for STIs). If the patient has a CD4 count below 100/mm^3, the routine examination should always include a formal retinal examination (for CMV and other causes of retinitis).

DIAGNOSTICS
Essential Diagnostics
The diagnosis of chronic HIV-1 infection is established by the laboratory confirmation of the presence of antibodies to HIV-1, often referred to as serologic testing. From 1989 until 2014 the recommended algorithm for testing for HIV in the United States used two different diagnostic assays performed sequentially, and this algorithm remains in wide use. First, an enzyme-linked immunosorbent assay (ELISA) is performed as a screening test. The sensitivity of the HIV ELISA for diagnosing chronic infection is so high that almost no false-negative results occur, but as a consequence, the rate of false-positive results, especially in a low-risk population, is significant. A negative ELISA result thus excludes chronic HIV infection, and there is no role for additional testing. A positive ELISA result, however, must be confirmed by a second more specific test, either a Western blot or indirect immunofluorescence assay (IFA), which is performed automatically in the United States when a specimen is ELISA positive. Western blot testing identifies the presence of a number of discrete antibodies against HIV, and the results of the test are defined by the number of these antibodies (referred to as bands) that are present; the presence of no bands is defined as a negative test result, one band as an indeterminate result, and more than one band as a positive result. A negative Western blot result excludes chronic HIV infection (and thus establishes that the ELISA result was a false-positive secondary to non-significant cross-reacting antibodies), and a positive Western blot result definitively diagnoses chronic HIV infection.

An indeterminate Western blot result can have one of three causes: a cross-reacting antibody to one of the HIV-specific antibodies that are assayed by the HIV Western blot (i.e., a false-positive result); PHI, so soon after infection that the patient has made significant antibody against one HIV antigen but not yet against others; and HIV-2 infection, assuming the original Western blot was HIV-1 specific and not a combination HIV-1/HIV-2 Western blot. HIV-2 is very rare in the United States, so the important differential diagnosis is usually to distinguish between a false-positive test result and PHI. Depending on the estimate of likelihood of PHI, the workup of an individual with an indeterminate test result can be further approached in one of two ways:

- If there is a low likelihood of PHI, the serologic test is repeated 1 month after the initial indeterminate result. The majority of patients undergoing seroconversion will test positive. If serologic testing is repeated 3 months after the original indeterminate result, close to 100% of patients undergoing seroconversion will test positive and no further testing is needed. Viral load testing usually should not be obtained in this setting because the risk of a false-positive result and the added emotional distress and medical workup that this entails outweigh the low likelihood of obtaining a true positive result.

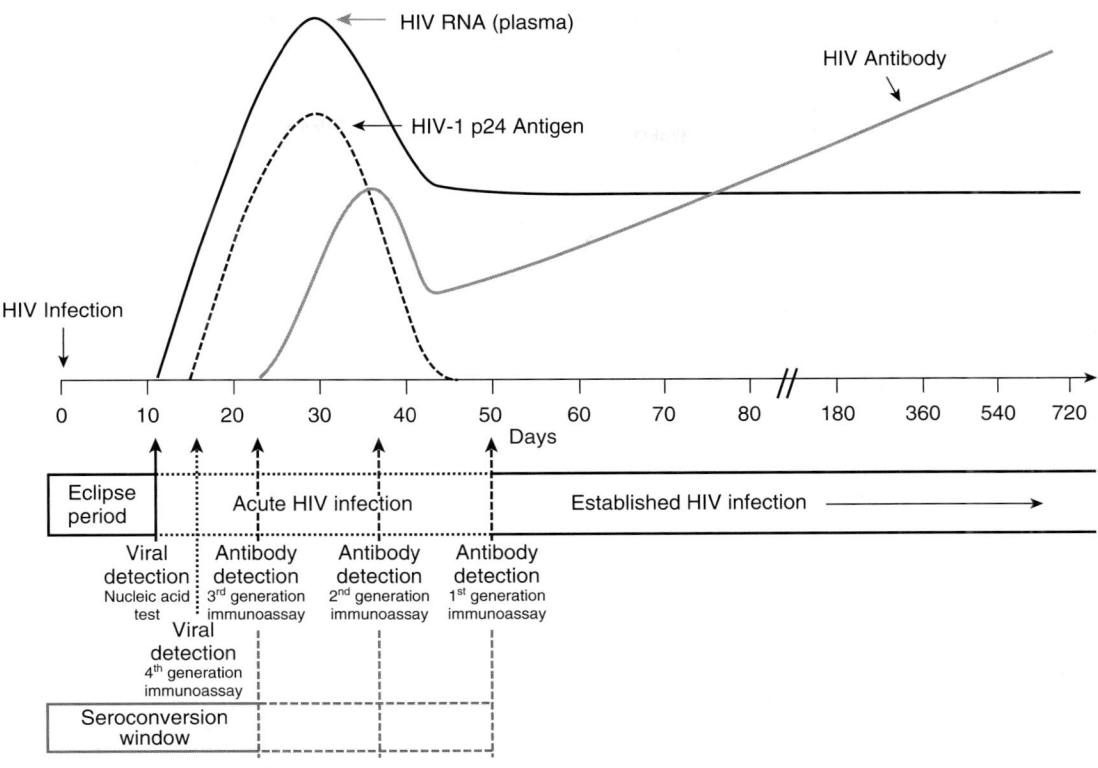

FIG. 209.1 Sequence of appearance of laboratory markers for Human immunodeficiency virus type 1 *(HIV-1)* infection. (From Centers for Disease Control and Prevention and Association of Public Health Laboratories. [2018]. *Laboratory testing for the diagnosis of HIV infection: updated recommendations.* Available at: https://stacks.cdc.gov/view/cdc/23447. Accessed 10.08.18).

- If there is a significant likelihood of PHI, such as a recent potentially high-risk exposure to HIV or any recent risk and a syndrome suggestive of PHI, an alternative approach to confirming the diagnosis can be considered. In the setting of PHI, the degree of HIV viremia is exceptionally high, and a standard quantitative HIV assay (most commonly polymerase chain reaction [PCR] or branched chain DNA [bDNA]) will invariably be positive at very high titer. The advantages of the earlier diagnosis obtained with this approach, rather than waiting 1 to 3 months to repeat the serologic test, include less opportunity for loss to follow-up, the opportunity for referral to a research center or HIV specialist for consideration of treatment of PHI, and early intervention to reduce high-risk behavior that may otherwise lead to further HIV transmission in the community. This last advantage is of particular importance because the very high viremia associated with PHI results in a period of markedly increased transmissibility.

In 2014 the CDC published updated recommendations for routine HIV testing, which introduced the first significant change in HIV testing since 1989.[6] The new algorithm, along with the most significant changes and benefits, includes the following:

- Initial testing is with a new (fourth-generation) antigen/antibody combination immunoassay. The antibody assay detects both HIV-1 and HIV-2 antibodies, reducing the likelihood of missing the diagnosis of HIV-2, and the antigen assay detects p24 antigen. The p24 antigen is present in very high levels in early HIV infection and becomes detectable by this assay approximately 1 week earlier after initial infection than does the antibody assay, thus reducing the

window period after initial infection to as short as 15 days (Fig. 209.1).

- If the fourth-generation test is reactive, then the specimen should be retested with an HIV-1/HIV-2 antibody differentiation immunoassay. Possible positive results from this second step are as follows: HIV-1 antibody positive, establishing HIV-1 infection; HIV-2 antibody positive, establishing HIV-2 infection; both HIV-1 and HIV-2 antibody positive, establishing coinfection with both HIV-1 and HIV-2. However, if neither HIV-1 nor HIV-2 antibody results are positive, this could be either because the initial fourth-generation assay was falsely positive, and the individual is not HIV infected, or because the initial test result was truly positive and the assay detected p24 antigen before the development of detectable HIV antibodies (i.e., diagnosing PHI).

- If the second step in the testing algorithm is negative, it is necessary to perform a third step to exclude PHI. The CDC algorithm recommends reflex testing with an HIV-1 nucleic acid test (NAT), which requires an additional serum or plasma specimen. In some laboratories it may not be practical to obtain the additional specimen required for the NAT at the time of initial testing, in which case it would be necessary to collect an additional specimen from the patient for either an immediate HIV PCR (preferable if the patient is at high risk for recent HIV infection) or a 2- to 4-week delayed repeat fourth-generation assay (often preferable if the patient is deemed low risk).

There remains some variability in implementation of the updated 2014 testing algorithm among many laboratories

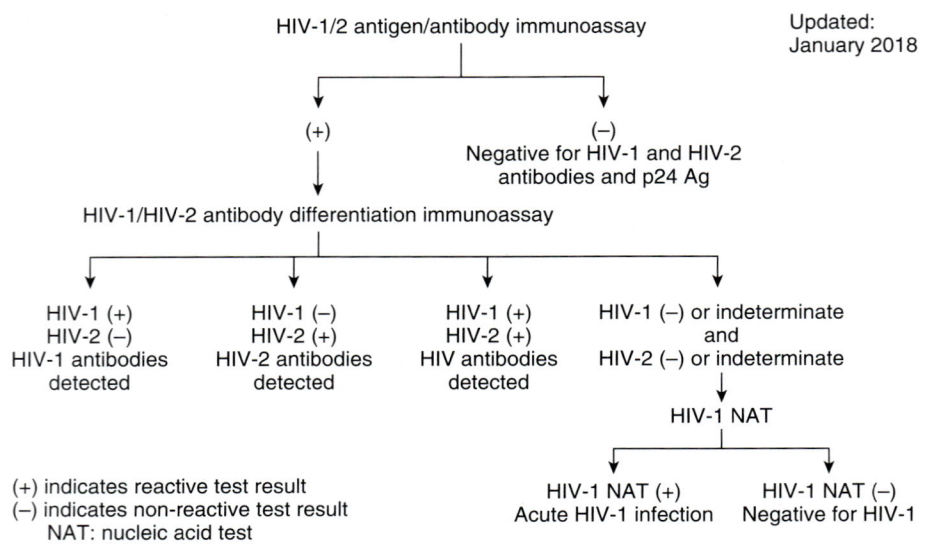

F I G . **209.2** Recommended laboratory human immunodeficiency virus *(HIV)* testing algorithm. (From Centers for Disease Control and Prevention and Association of Public Health Laboratories. [2018]. Available at: https://stacks.cdc.gov/view/cdc/50872. Accessed 10.08.18).

throughout the US. Providers should be aware of the specific algorithm that is being used by their laboratory and should seek clarification of test results from the laboratory if there is any uncertainty about the interpretation (Fig. 209.2).

It is important to confirm the diagnosis in any patient entering care reporting prior HIV infection. HIV serology should be repeated if an actual report of HIV serologic testing is not available. It is reasonable to make an exception to this if there is documentation of repeated positive results of viral load testing.

New patients whose sero status is unknown or questionable should be counseled about the distinctions of anonymous versus confidential testing. There may be concerns about inadvertent disclosures, or the reactions of insurance companies, resulting in a desire for anonymous testing, although this is not a readily available option in many locations.

An additional option for testing uses rapid HIV testing technologies. Compared to laboratory-based testing, rapid tests may be conducted at the point-of-care. The currently available assays use either blood or oral fluid as the specimen and can provide results within minutes. These assays are all ELISAs, detecting either antibodies and/or the p24 antigen, and results are interpreted as with a standard laboratory-based HIV ELISA: a negative result rules out chronic HIV infection, whereas a positive result must be confirmed with a second, confirmatory assay.

Additional Diagnostics

When an individual is diagnosed with HIV infection, additional testing is required to determine the degree of immunosuppression, the urgency for ART and other therapy initiation, the HIV viral load, and the extent of baseline viral resistance to ARVs. Evaluation should also define the presence of significant comorbid conditions, the need for appropriate immunizations, and the aspects of physiologic function that may affect the choice of ART.

The most important assay to establish current immunologic status is the determination of the CD4 count, which is reported as both the absolute number of CD4+ lymphocytes/

mm^3 of blood (normal range, 500 to 1700) and the percentage of all lymphocytes that are CD4+ (normal range, 35% to 61%). In addition, quantifying the amount of HIV in the patient's plasma, known as the HIV viral load or viral burden, provides additional information about immune function (the higher the viral load, the more immunologically compromised the patient). Even more importantly, the viral load estimates the expected rate of immunologic decline (as measured by falling CD4 count). This is established at baseline because decline in viral load after starting of ART is the most important initial marker of efficacy of ART.

The plasma viral load can be measured by two technologies: reverse transcriptase PCR (RT-PCR) and bDNA. The results of these tests are reported as the number of copies of viral RNA per milliliter of plasma. During the chronic phase of HIV infection, the viral load is typically between 10,000 and 100,000 copies/mL; lower values are predictive of a slower than average rate of progression and a higher viral load is predictive of more rapid progression. Finally, all patients with newly diagnosed HIV infection should undergo viral resistance testing, usually with an HIV genotype assay, to determine the presence of resistance to one or more of the available ARVs.

Routine baseline testing should also include a complete blood count, comprehensive metabolic profile assessing renal function and hepatic status, urinalysis to assess for proteinuria, and fasting lipid profile to establish a baseline prior to initiating ARVs. STI screening should also be considered, assessing for syphilis in particular as co-infection is common. Other STI testing, such as for gonorrhea or chlamydia, should be done as appropriate, with the site of testing (cervical, urethral, urine, throat, or rectal) determined by the patient's sexual practices. Screening for trichomoniasis is recommended in all women with HIV infection.

Additional Diagnostic Testing. Additional important baseline testing is performed to exclude latent infection with *Toxoplasma gondi*, and CMV with standard serologic assays, as well as coinfection with hepatitis A, B, and C virus (HAV, HBV, and HCV) and TB. Testing for the hepatitis viruses is performed through the same algorithm as for patients without HIV infection. Testing for TB, however, is more complex. The diagnosis of latent TB in a patient with HIV infection is complicated by the steady decline in the reliability of the purified protein derivative (PPD) test response as the CD4 count declines. The test becomes highly compromised if the CD4 count is less than 200/mm³ and is essentially worthless if CD4 is less than 50/mm³. Therefore, although it is appropriate to perform PPD testing for newly diagnosed patients with HIV infection, this testing should always be repeated after patients with a nadir CD4 count of less than 200/mm³ have been receiving ART long enough to suppress the HIV viral load and to raise the CD4 count above 200/mm³. The definition of a positive PPD response in patients with HIV infection is induration of 5 mm or more. Testing for latent TB can also be performed with an interferon gamma release assay (IGRA), which is also useful in distinguishing a true-positive PPD response from a false-positive PPD response resulting from prior bacillus Calmette-Guérin (BCG) immunization. Because the risk of developing active TB disease and latent TB co-infection is exceptionally high (an annual risk of approximately 10%) in a patient with HIV, treatment of latent TB is always indicated once active TB is excluded.

DIFFERENTIAL DIAGNOSIS

The differential diagnosis for a patient with a clinical syndrome consistent with AIDS is fairly narrow. In the rare instances in which patients appear with such an illness, test negative for HIV on routine testing, and have no other evident cause of immunosuppression (such as an underlying malignant disease or treatment with a known immunosuppressing therapy), they should be immediately referred for expert consultation. There are many congenital immunodeficiency states, but most become evident in childhood (see Chapter 204). One interesting but exceptionally rare condition seen for the first time in adults is idiopathic CD4 lymphocytopenia, which may mimic HIV but is of unknown etiology. This is diagnosed in the presence of persistently low CD4 counts (<300/mm³ or < 20% of total lymphocytes) without laboratory evidence of HIV infection or other cause.

Measurement of the CD4 count should never be used as a surrogate for serologic diagnosis of HIV infection, especially in the setting of an acute illness. During an acute infectious illness of sufficient severity, it is not unusual for transient lymphopenia to develop with absolute CD4 lymphopenia that can even enter the AIDS range. In addition, the HIV viral load should not be used to diagnose HIV infection, except for the rare times when it is used to diagnose PHI.

INTERPROFESSIONAL COLLABORATIVE MANAGEMENT
Nonpharmacologic Management

The management of HIV infection includes ART, close attention to medication adherence, prevention of OIs with indicated chemoprophylaxis, appropriate immunization, close monitoring for complications of HIV infection and its therapy, management of comorbid conditions, and attempts to minimize behavior that can result in HIV transmission. In addition, because HIV infection is now a treatable disease with a long life expectancy, all usual aspects of primary health care must also be provided. An excellent set of up-to-date guidelines for many aspects of HIV care is maintained at the US Department

of Health and Human Services AIDS information website (www.aidsinfo.nih.gov).

In addition, a number of conditions require particularly careful monitoring and evaluation for people with HIV infection, no matter what the CD4 count.

- Latent TB. Given the high risk for development of active TB in a patient coinfected with HIV and TB, annual screening for latent TB, whether with PPD or IGRA, should be routine unless the risk of exposure is exceptionally low.
- Screening for human papillomavirus (HPV)–associated disease. Cervical carcinoma develops more frequently in HIV-infected women and requires close screening and aggressive management. As the result of a similar pathophysiologic mechanism, HPV-associated anal carcinoma occurs much more frequently in MSM with HIV infection; annual rectal examinations should be performed, as should workup of any consistent symptoms. Anal Papanicolaou smears are performed at some centers but are not currently standard of care.
- Screening for STIs. This is important both because many patients with HIV infection remain at risk for infection with STIs and because the presence of an STI increases the risk of HIV transmission.
- Management of chronic hepatitis B and hepatitis C. The leading cause of death for people coinfected with HIV and HCV in the United States is liver disease, so management of chronic hepatitis is an integral aspect of patient care. Until recently, because treatment of HCV was very poorly tolerated and not very effective, especially for those coinfected with HIV, few patients were treated. Contemporary treatment for HCV, however, is now highly effective and generally well tolerated (see Chapter 119), so all HIV and HCV coinfected patients should be considered candidates for treatment of HCV. There are challenges to treating HCV in a coinfected patient, most importantly drug interactions between the two sets of antivirals, so management of hepatitis C in a patient coinfected with HIV should be addressed by an HIV and HCV expert. The primary health care provider can play an important role by reinforcing the importance of alcohol abstinence and providing immunization for HBV and HAV for all non-immune patients. There are fewer data on coinfection with HBV, but the issues are similar.
- Cardiovascular disease risk. Several ARVs, primarily PIs, increase the risk of cardiovascular disease, mediated primarily but not entirely by dyslipidemia and insulin resistance. It is thus important to address modifiable risk factors, to monitor lipids and glucose concentration, and to treat metabolic abnormalities when they develop.

Pharmacologic Management

Treatment with ART is one of the more complex areas of modern medicine. When it is done correctly, it can convert HIV infection from a progressive and inevitably fatal disease to a chronic disease with potentially normal life expectancy; but when it is done poorly, it can result in viral resistance to some or all antivirals and consequently the need for second-line therapies (more pills, more than once-daily administration, and more potential side effects) and eventually untreatable progressive disease. ART should thus be prescribed only by clinicians with significant training and experience in its use.

Guidelines that address the initiation of ART have always attempted to balance the obvious benefits of ART with the disadvantages of treatment, which include the risk for development of resistance precluding future therapy, drug toxicities, and the medicalization of life in someone who may be clinically entirely well; however, as the benefits of therapy (even with a high CD4 count) have become more apparent and as first-line therapy has become safer, better tolerated, and easier to adhere to (as a result of minimizing pill burden, now often to one pill daily), the threshold for recommending treatment has fallen dramatically.[7,8] The consensus in the United States is that treatment should now be initiated in all individuals diagnosed with HIV regardless of CD4 count, with very few exceptions. These exceptions would include people who are elite controllers, those who have active OIs for which ART is delayed for a relatively brief period, and those who are unlikely to be able to adhere to ART because of psychological, socioeconomic, or other barriers. This recommendation is based on the efficacy, tolerability, and toxicity of current agents and on the results of retrospective cohort analyses and other clinical studies. The initiation of ART in an asymptomatic patient, on the other hand, is never urgent, and there is usually time to educate the patient and to address other active problems that might adversely affect therapy, including depression related to the new diagnosis. Recent studies in select populations have shown improved retention in care and a larger proportion of patients on ART 1 year after diagnosis when ART is started on the day of diagnosis, but this approach has not yet been widely adapted.

One of the absolute indications for ART is the treatment of a pregnant woman to prevent mother-to-child transmission. Optimum ART in a pregnant woman can reduce the risk of vertical transmission from approximately 25% to less than 2%, and recommended regimens have no known significant fetal toxicity.[9] This benefit is so significant that elective cesarean section is no longer indicated in the optimally treated pregnant woman.

There are now more than 25 ARVs approved for treatment of HIV infection in the United States, representing six different classes of agents: nucleoside analogue reverse transcriptase inhibitors (NRTIs), non-nucleoside reverse transcriptase inhibitors (NNRTIs), protease inhibitors (PIs), fusion inhibitors, CCR5 antagonists, and integrase strand transfer inhibitors (INSTIs). Despite the numerous possible combinations of these agents, clinical trials and extensive experience have defined a few preferred regimens for first-line therapy, the easiest of which involve one pill once daily, although many alternatives are based on patient-specific factors. First-line treatment usually consists of a combination of (1) two NRTIs and (2) a PI, an NNRTI, or an INSTI. The specific choice of agents is driven by the presence of antiviral resistance, a preferred schedule (once versus twice a day; with or without food; in the morning or before bed), drug interactions with other medications the patient is taking or may need to start, comorbid conditions, pregnancy or desire for pregnancy, baseline viral load, genetic contraindications (for abacavir), and patient concerns about specific possible adverse drug reactions.

The short-term goal of ART is to suppress viral replication to such a degree that there is no detectable HIV in peripheral blood, most commonly measured by RT-PCR. When that is the case, the result of viral load testing is reported as below the lower limit of detection for the assay, which is currently less than 20 copies/mL and is often referred to as an undetectable viral load. The amount of time it takes to obtain an undetectable viral load after initiation of ART depends on the baseline viral load, so the initial goal is to reduce the viral load by 10-fold to 100-fold within 4 to 6 weeks of initiation of therapy and to achieve complete suppression within 6 months. If that is not attained, the patient should be assessed for new viral resistance, medication adherence, and appropriateness of ART. CD4 counts need not be measured soon after initiation of ART, but with successful suppression of viral replication, the CD4 count should start to increase; typically, it increases 100 to 200/mm³ in the first year after starting ART.

When a patient is receiving stable ART and has attained an undetectable viral load, it is crucial to monitor the patient carefully for ongoing efficacy (with viral load and CD4 testing), safety (with the specific laboratory testing determined by the given regimen), and adherence. If patients are less than 95% adherent, they run an unacceptably high risk for development of resistance to the agents in the regimen, demonstrated by virologic rebound after initial suppression to undetectable levels, with consequent need to change ARVs and—if repeated a few times—eventual loss of all effective therapy.

Historically, guidelines suggested monitoring the viral loads and CD4 count every 3 to 4 months after the viral load was suppressed and the patient was clinically well, but with the recognition of how well people do when they are highly adherent and the viral load is suppressed, these guidelines now allow for longer intervals.[8] In an individual who is clinically well and has a consistently suppressed viral load for at least 1 year, it is reasonable to consider monitoring the viral load every 6 months if the patient is also highly adherent to therapy, is reliably engaged in medical care, is not homeless, is not actively abusing alcohol or illicit drugs, does not have a mental health condition that might affect medical adherence, and is not participating in any high-risk activity. CD4 testing can be as infrequent as annually.

An often-overlooked aspect of the care of patients receiving ART is the danger of drug-drug interactions with many of the ARVs. These interactions can affect both the non-ARV, most often by decreasing metabolism (potentially to a life-threatening degree), and the ARV, of greatest concern by decreasing ARV concentrations to subtherapeutic levels and thus increasing the likelihood of resistance and failure. It is thus imperative that drug interactions be identified and discussed in consultation with the HIV specialist before starting or stopping any medication, whether prescription or over the counter.

When ART is not initiated, the patient should be evaluated in the clinic and by laboratory testing, primarily CD4 count and viral load, every 3 to 4 months. If other treatable comorbid conditions have been identified, such as hepatitis C or latent TB, this may be an appropriate time to address them.

Although ART has the most profound impact on survival of all aspects of treatment of HIV infection, other components of care should not be forgotten. Chemoprophylaxis and immunizations should be provided when indicated, and routine health care should be provided. For a patient with AIDS who is starting ART, primary chemoprophylaxis (the administration of a medication to prevent a first episode of an OI) can reduce the risk for development of an OI before adequate immune restoration, whereas for patients with AIDS for whom immune restoration will not occur (because of untreatable HIV infection secondary to the development of antiviral resistance or the patient's choice to defer ART), appropriate prophylaxis can provide a moderate prolongation of life expectancy. Decisions about when to start and to stop prophylactic medications will usually be made by the HIV specialist, but excellent guidelines for chemoprophylaxis and immunizations are readily available.[10]

After ART has been initiated, treatment interruptions should be strongly discouraged. Treatment interruption is associated with a risk of development of ART resistance, high rebound viremia with possible PHI-like illness, rapid CD4 decline, an increased risk of death, and an increased risk of HIV transmission through unprotected sex and IDU. There may, however, be times when treatment interruption is appropriate or unavoidable, at which time the patient should be monitored closely both clinically and with CD4 and viral load testing.

Finally, it is important to recognize the impact of effective ART on the risk of HIV transmission, often referred to as "treatment as prevention," and the potential benefit of this effect on helping to control the HIV epidemic. Several clinical trials have demonstrated that the likelihood of HIV transmission, whether sexual or parenteral, is virtually zero when someone with HIV infection is on ART with an undetectable viral load; and mathematical modeling suggests that this could provide a significant benefit in helping to control the epidemic if a high enough proportion of people infected with HIV are on effective ART.

In general, all HIV-infected patients should be managed under the care of both a primary care provider and an HIV specialist. With a growing interest in finding a cure as well as the rapidly changing array of treatments, an HIV specialist is in the unique position of providing the most up-to-date care. Other indications for referral include the following:

- Pregnancy in an HIV-infected woman or intention to become pregnant in serodiscordant couples
- HIV coinfection with hepatitis C or B or TB
- New symptoms in someone with immunosuppression (CD4 count ≤200), including:
  - Mental status changes
  - Severe headache
  - High fevers
  - Significant shortness of breath
- Opportunistic infections related to immunosuppression

Referral to an HIV specialist should be recommended to all HIV-infected patients who enter care, whether they are newly diagnosed or are changing health care providers. Depending on the provider's expertise, the complexity and nature of the active medical issues, challenges of travel and other constraints on accessing care, and the patient's preferences, the division of responsibilities between the health care provider and the specialist can vary, so it is important to explicitly define their respective roles. Patients often wonder why they need to see a primary care provider when they are seen by an HIV specialist several times per year and so may need to be reminded that, given the long life expectancy that can now be anticipated for HIV-infected patients, health maintenance and other aspects of primary care are as important to them as to the general population.

For HIV-infected patients who are in care, it is as important not to overreact to non-severe acute illness as it is to be attentive to potential complications of HIV infection. In particular, most non-OIs can be managed just as they would be in an immunocompetent host, especially if the CD4 count is more than 200/mm³. On the other hand, any more serious illness, any syndrome consistent with an OI, or any potentially infectious disease that cannot be readily diagnosed as a community-acquired infection should prompt rapid consultation with an HIV specialist.

An important resource to help HIV-infected patients navigate the complex health care system may be the local AIDS service organization (ASO). ASOs are community-based organizations funded at least in part by the Ryan White CARE Act and are dedicated to assisting people living with HIV infection and their families by providing case management, support groups, transportation assistance, and emergency financial help for housing, food, and clothing. ASOs often provide additional services within their communities, including HIV prevention education and testing.

LIFE SPAN CONSIDERATIONS

The life expectancy of a patient newly diagnosed with HIV infection has steadily increased since the onset of the epidemic and continues to do so. The largest impact on life expectancy occurred in the mid-1990s with the introduction of ART, but improvements in the safety and efficacy of available ARVs, the growing number of agents, and the growing sophistication in the management of people living with HIV infection have resulted in ongoing incremental improvements in life expectancy. The most important predictor of life expectancy is no longer the CD4 count and viral load at baseline but the patient's ability to tolerate and to maintain a high level of adherence to ARVs. Population statistics are not helpful in defining the prognosis for an individual patient, and the emphasis needs to be on the patient's idiosyncratic circumstances. Under ideal circumstances, though, it is reasonable to hope for a dramatic extension of and possibly even unaffected life expectancy.

Although ART has dramatically improved the life expectancy and health of people living with HIV, there remain many unknowns about the impact of HIV infection on people living with HIV as they age. Some areas of concern and active research include bone pathology (osteoporosis and avascular necrosis), neurocognitive effects, risk of malignancies, frailty, and exacerbation of pain syndromes (e.g., from early ARVs). To whatever degree there is an association between HIV infection and any of these problems, it remains unclear what the predictors of risk for them might be, and whether earlier initiation of ART might minimize them.

Because life expectancy is long, it has become important to address long-term life plans and family planning with all patients infected with HIV. Discussions about desires and plans for children are particularly important. For an HIV-infected woman, the decision to become pregnant is usually complicated. If she has an uninfected male partner, the logistics of insemination are fairly straightforward, but the management of the pregnancy is intensive. When pregnancy is being considered, referral to an HIV specialist should be recommended for counseling about safe insemination, discussion of approaches to the prevention of mother-to-child transmission of HIV, and potential need to modify ART.

Adolescence is often a time for sexual debut and engaging in high-risk behaviors, including unprotected sex and experimentation with drugs and alcohol, which put the adolescent at risk for acquiring and transmitting HIV. It is therefore important to discuss the risks associated with such behaviors at every visit and to offer anticipatory guidance on abstinence, how to negotiate responsible sexual behaviors, and how to prevent pregnancy and HIV infection and other STIs through the use of contraception and condoms. Because hormonal methods of contraception will not prevent STIs, including HIV infection, it is important to ensure that adolescents understand the necessity of consistent and proper use of condoms when engaging in sexual intercourse and have access to an affordable condom supply.

COMPLICATIONS

The most important complications for which a person with HIV infection is at risk are those related to immune dysfunction, as reflected in the CD4 count. These include OIs, as well as certain malignancies, which are discussed in greater detail in the section on clinical presentation. In addition to direct complications of compromised immune function, HIV-infected patients also appear to be at higher risk for cardiovascular disease, which may be driven by chronic low-grade immune stimulation, adverse effects of certain ARVs (especially PIs), and/or traditional cardiovascular risk factors.

It is also important to monitor HIV-infected patients closely for complications of ART. Antiviral therapy has a dramatic impact on life expectancy when it is prescribed appropriately, but these medications have a number of significant toxicities that must be actively monitored to reduce the risk of a spectrum of problems ranging from cosmetic to life-threatening. The potential toxicities vary according to the specific regimen, so appropriate monitoring is defined uniquely for every patient. A few general recommendations are warranted.

Metabolic Toxicities

The PI and, to a lesser degree, the NNRTI and NRTI classes of ARVs carry a risk of metabolic side effects that require monitoring. One of the most significant of these is dyslipidemia, which should be assessed by measuring a fasting lipid profile at baseline and then 1 to 3 months after any change in a pertinent medication. When ARV-induced dyslipidemia does develop, options for management include usual lipid-lowering therapy (diet, exercise, and medications) and change in ART if an equally effective alternative is available. A second complication is insulin resistance, which should be monitored at a minimum by appropriate interview at regular clinic appointments.

Lipodystrophy

Lipodystrophy refers to a change in the relative proportion of fat from baseline body habitus. Adipose tissue may be redistributed centrally with intra-abdominal, breast, or dorsocervical fat accumulation, or peripherally with limb and buttock subcutaneous fat atrophy. These toxicities have no clearly attributable risk of increased mortality but can be profoundly disfiguring. Because these changes are not readily reversible, they need to be watched for carefully and an appropriate medication change considered as needed.

Liver Disease

All but a few of the currently available ARVs are associated with one or more liver toxicities, ranging from otherwise asymptomatic hyperbilirubinemia to fulminant and potentially fatal drug-induced hepatitis, or slowly progressive but also potentially fatal hepatic steatosis–lactic acidosis. It is thus important to define the nature of hepatotoxicity that is associated with a

given regimen and to monitor appropriately, whether by interview or laboratory testing.

Drug Interactions

It cannot be overemphasized that there are innumerable potential drug interactions with almost all ART regimens. Any unusual symptom should raise the concern of an adverse drug reaction to a new medication, whether it is prescribed, over the counter, herbal, or illicit, and a detailed history of the use of all medications and nutraceuticals should be obtained.

Immune Reconstitution Inflammatory Syndrome

A unique complication associated with ART is the immune reconstitution inflammatory syndrome (IRIS). When ART is initiated in a patient with a low CD4 count, there is a rapid improvement in the immune system's ability to produce an inflammatory reaction, which can result in an acute inflammatory reaction against both known and occult OIs. This typically occurs in the first several months after initiation of ART and produces symptoms based on the location of the infection. Two of the most common manifestations of IRIS are acute lymphadenitis as a reaction to MAC and acute uveitis to CMV. It is important to recognize IRIS because there may be significant associated morbidity (e.g., blindness with ocular CMV) and because management is very specific (a combination of antimicrobials, surgery, and corticosteroids).

PATIENT AND FAMILY EDUCATION
Health Promotion

Education for an HIV-infected patient needs to be extensive and ongoing. The initial diagnosis is often overwhelming, and basic education about HIV infection reviewed then will often need to be reiterated. The initial approach to educational counseling should review both the natural history of HIV infection and the potential immense benefit of current therapy, although it can be a challenge to convey both the severity of the disease and the optimism that ART can provide. Discussion of benefits should include those pertaining to the individual's health, as well as the benefits of reduced risk of HIV transmission. This discussion often transitions into family planning and the need to discuss the nature of the risks associated with pregnancy. Initial discussions should also explain important aspects of medical care for someone living with HIV infection, including the frequency of appointments, the significance of the CD4 count and viral load, the nature of medical therapy, the importance of strict adherence to ART when it is started, and any other pertinent aspects of care. In addition, initial education should clarify misconceptions that the patient might have about HIV infection.

Further counseling should address both HIV-specific and usual aspects of general health maintenance. The patient should be informed about how to avoid exposure to infectious diseases, which includes discussion of food and water safety, pet hygiene, and international travel. The importance of patient-specific health maintenance issues should be addressed, including cigarette, alcohol, and other substance use. Nutritional counseling should be routinely provided.

The provider should also explicitly discuss the public health implications of HIV infection. This usually starts with a discussion of the mechanisms of transmission of HIV and how to prevent transmission. It might thus be necessary to instruct the patient on male or female condom use or on how to ensure that needles and other paraphernalia used for illicit drugs are sterile. This conversation also needs to address notification and testing of current and past partners, both sexual and needle-sharing partners, and of children born to an infected woman. Of note, patients on ART who have an undetectable viral load cannot sexually transmit HIV. This notion has given rise to the concept of *treatment as prevention* and can serve as a motivator for patients to start ART and remain adherent. It is important that the providers know what resources are available for anonymous or confidential testing and for contact notification, which includes programs run by the department of health in every state.

Several clinical trials have demonstrated that the daily use of ARV medications by someone who is not HIV infected but who participates in ongoing high-risk behavior, usually referred to as PrEP, can significantly reduce the risk of HIV acquisition. Based on these trials, in 2012 the US Food and Drug Administration (FDA) approved the daily use of Truvada, the co-formulation of tenofovir disoproxil fumarate (TDF) plus emtricitabine (FTC), for PrEP for the prevention of HIV acquisition. TDF alone has been shown to be effective in preventing HIV acquisition in heterosexually active men and women and PWIDs and can be considered as an alternative regimen, albeit without FDA approval for this indication. PrEP should be considered for all adults at significant risk for acquisition of HIV, including MSM; heterosexually active men and women, including HIV-discordant couples if the infected partner does not have an undetectable viral load; and PWIDs. When delivered as part of a comprehensive set of prevention services, including risk reduction counseling, treatment for other STIs, and recommended use of condoms, PrEP has been found to be both effective and safe in reducing the risk of acquiring HIV infection.[11] The efficacy of PrEP has been quite variable in these studies, almost exclusively as a function of adherence; in all cases, the higher the adherence to daily therapy, the greater the reduction in risk of HIV acquisition. Primary care providers will increasingly be asked to consider PrEP for their high-risk patients, and so it is essential to know for whom and how to prescribe this prophylactic treatment as well as to stress excellent adherence to the daily medication. A baseline HIV test must be performed before initiation of PrEP, to rule out acute or chronic HIV infection. Frequent monitoring for HIV acquisition and tests for other STIs should be performed at least every 3 months and renal function should be assessed at least every 6 months due to potential renal toxicity from TDF.[11]

REFERENCES

1. Council of State and Territorial Epidemiologists, AIDS Program, Center for Infectious Diseases. (1987). Revision of the CDC surveillance case definition for acquired immunodeficiency syndrome. *MMWR. Morbidity and Mortality Weekly Report, 36*(Suppl. 1), 1S–15S.
2. Centers for Disease Control and Prevention (CDC). (2014). Revised surveillance case definitions for HIV infection—United States, 2014. *MMWR. Recommendations and Reports: Morbidity and Mortality Weekly Report. Recommendations and Reports, 63*(RR-3), 1–10.
3. https://www.hiv.gov/hiv-basics/overview/data-and-trends/statistics. (Accessed 19 July 2019).
4. Centers for Disease Control and Prevention (CDC). (2006). Revised recommendations for HIV testing of adults, adolescents, and pregnant women in health-care settings. *MMWR. Recommendations and Reports: Morbidity and Mortality Weekly Report. Recommendations and Reports, 55*(RR-14), 1–17.
5. UNAIDS.Global HIV and AIDS statistics—2019 fact sheet—Latest global and regional statistics on the status of the AIDS epidemic. Retrieved from http://www.unaids.org/en/resources/fact-sheet. (Accessed 18 July 2019).
6. Centers for Disease Control and Prevention and Association of Public Health Laboratories. Laboratory testing for the diagnosis of HIV infection: updated recommendations. Retrieved from http://stacks.CDC.gov/view/cdc/23447. Published June 27, 2014. (Accessed 3 August 2018). To be used with 2018 Quick reference guide: Recommended laboratory HIV testing algorithm for serum or plasma specimens. Retrieved from https://stacks.cdc.gov/view/cdc/50872. (Accessed 8 August 2018).
7. Günthard, H. F., Aberg, J. A., Eron, J. J., et al. (2014). Antiretroviral treatment of adult HIV infection: 2014 recommendations of the international antiviral Society—USA panel. *JAMA: The Journal of the American Medical Association, 312*, 410–425.
8. Panel on Antiretroviral Guidelines for Adults and Adolescents. Guidelines for the use of antiretroviral agents in HIV-1-infected adults and adolescents, Department of Health and Human Services. Retrieved from http://aidsinfo.nih.gov/contentfiles/lvguidelines/AdultandAdolescentGL.pdf. (Accessed 8 August 2018).
9. Panel on Treatment of HIV-Infected Pregnant Women and Prevention of Perinatal Transmission. Recommendations for use of antiretroviral drugs in pregnant HIV-1–infected women for maternal health and interventions to reduce perinatal HIV transmission in the United States. Retrieved from http://aidsinfo.nih.gov/contentfiles/lvguidelines/perinatalGL.pdf. (Accessed 8 August 2018).
10. Panel on Opportunistic Infections in HIV-Infected Adults and Adolescents. Guidelines for the prevention and treatment of opportunistic infections in HIV-infected adults and adolescents: recommendations from the Centers for Disease Control and Prevention, the National Institutes of Health, and the HIV Medicine Association of the Infectious Diseases Society of America. Retrieved from http://aidsinfo.nih.gov/contentfiles/lvguidelines/adult_oi.pdf. (Accessed 8 August 2018).
11. US Preventive Services Task Force. (2019). Preexposure prophylaxis for the prevention of HIV infection: US preventive services task force recommendation statement. *JAMA: The Journal of the American Medical Association, 321*(22), 2203–2213. doi:10.1001/jama.2019.6390.

CHAPTER **210**

INFLUENZA
Traci Alberti

 Emergency referral is indicated for new onset confusion, chest pain, difficulty breathing, abdominal pain, persistent vomiting, worsening symptoms, or any suspicion of epiglottitis.

DEFINITION AND EPIDEMIOLOGY

Influenza is an acute infection of the respiratory tract caused by influenza virus type A or B. It is usually a self-limited disease that occurs in outbreaks, primarily during the winter months in temperate climates, though it may occur year-round in the tropics. Influenza is highly contagious and occurs in all age groups. The rate of infection is highest among children, but serious illness and death is highest among people 65 years old or older and those with underlying chronic medical conditions.[1] Influenza tends to occur in outbreaks, which can rapidly affect 10% to 40% of the population.[2] In 2009, the novel H1N1 (swine flu) virus emerged, infecting humans in pandemic proportion. It is now a regular human influenza virus that continues to circulate worldwide.

PATHOPHYSIOLOGY

Influenza is transmitted from person to person through respiratory secretions that contain the virus. These respiratory secretions are spread in the form of droplets that are produced when a person talks, coughs, or sneezes. Influenza virus is detectable and may be shed in respiratory secretions up to 24 hours before the onset of symptoms.

Once the virus reaches the epithelium cells of the respiratory tract, it penetrates the cells and begins replication. This viral replication leads to cell death, which in turn releases large amounts of virus that can infect adjacent cells. This quickly causes desquamation of the ciliated epithelium. The onset of the acute symptoms coincides with this desquamation.[2]

Influenza viruses evolve frequently owing to point mutations or recombination events that occur during viral replication. This is called antigenic drift. Previous exposure or vaccine may not confer immunity to these new virus variants, thus the reason for seasonal epidemics and the need for adjustment of vaccine every season.[1]

CLINICAL PRESENTATION AND PHYSICAL EXAMINATION

After an incubation period of 1 or 2 days, there is an abrupt onset of symptoms. These symptoms include fever, chills, headache, malaise, myalgia, and loss of appetite. Respiratory symptoms are also present but are usually overshadowed by the severity of the systemic symptoms. Respiratory symptoms include dry cough, nasal congestion with clear discharge, and sore throat. The cough is usually the most prominent of these respiratory symptoms.

The patient's temperature rises rapidly after onset, peaking at 37.7°C to 40°C (100° F to 104° F) in about 12 hours. The fever typically begins to decline on the second or third day but may last as long as 4 to 8 days. Systemic symptoms become less prominent as the fever decreases. A convalescent phase of 1 to 2 weeks follows the acute febrile stage. Cough, malaise, and fatigue, often extreme, are seen during the convalescent phase.[2]

Some patients have mild illness that resembles the common cold. Older adults, children under the age of 2 years, people with underlying chronic medical conditions, and pregnant women may experience a rapidly worsening course of influenza.

PHYSICAL EXAMINATION

Uncomplicated cases of influenza have minimal physical findings despite the severity of clinical complaints. At the onset of symptoms, the patient's face is often flushed, and the eyes may be watery and red. Fever is often present. The skin may be hot and moist. Nasal passages can be inflamed, but pharyngeal erythema and exudates are not common.[3,4] Cervical lymph nodes may be enlarged and tender. The findings on chest examination are usually normal.

DIAGNOSTICS

Influenza virus can be isolated from nose and throat specimens by nasal swabs or washings, sputum, and throat swabs. Of these, nasopharyngeal specimens are the preferred source. Ideally, samples should be collected within 12 to 36 hours of onset of illness.

The gold standard for influenza diagnosis is either conventional viral culture or reverse transcriptase polymerase chain reaction (RT-PCR) assays. Virus can be detected in cell cultures in 2 to 7 days. In situations wherein early diagnosis is crucial, there are several techniques to detect the presence of viral antigens in nose and throat specimens that yield results rapidly, in as little as 1 hour. These rapid tests may not be as sensitive as cell culture; however, they may be useful in the management of individual patients at high risk for serious complications from influenza, who may benefit most from early

hospitalization, appropriate antiviral treatment, or prophylaxis for contacts.[5,6]

INITIAL DIAGNOSTICS

Influenza

- Influenza antigen
- A & B nasal swab

ADDITIONAL DIAGNOSTICS
- Serum antibody titre[a]

[a]If indicated.

Infection with influenza virus can also be confirmed by at least a fourfold rise in antibody titer in convalescent serum taken 10 to 20 days after an acute serum sample.

Clinical diagnosis in the setting of a confirmed influenza outbreak is very accurate.

DIFFERENTIAL DIAGNOSIS

 Emergency department referral required for new onset confusion, chest pain, difficulty breathing, abdominal pain, persistent vomiting, worsening symptoms, or any suspicion of epiglottitis, an inability to manage oral secretions (drooling, tri-pod positioning). Bacterial pneumonia should be considered in the presence of fever, cough, and adventitious lung sounds.

In the absence of a known outbreak of influenza, it may be difficult to distinguish an individual case of influenza from many of the other upper respiratory viral infections, such as the common cold or illness caused by respiratory syncytial virus. Other conditions to consider are *Mycoplasma pneumoniae* infection, bacterial or viral pneumonia, and severe streptococcal pharyngitis.

INTERPROFESSIONAL COLLABORATIVE MANAGEMENT

Nonpharmacologic Management

Treatment of influenza is primarily symptomatic. Patients should rest as much as possible and maintain an adequate fluid intake. Patients with influenza should not go to work or school to help prevent the spread of illness to others.

Pharmacological Management

Antipyretics and analgesics can be used to control fever and relieve headache and myalgia. Antiviral medication may be used to treat or prevent influenza.[7] In the United States there are currently five antiviral medications approved for the treatment of influenza. Neuraminidase inhibitors are effective against influenza A and B. These drugs include oseltamivir (Tamiflu), zanamivir (Relenza), and peramivir (Rapivab). Adamantane drugs (Amantadine and Rimantadine) are approved antiviral agents, however, they are only effective against influenza A, and therefore not recommended in the setting of an influenza B outbreak.[7] Antiviral treatment is recommended for patients at high risk for development of complications from influenza, those with severe illness, or for anyone requiring hospitalization for confirmed or suspected influenza. Resistance to antiviral medications may develop quickly, so clinicians should be aware of which strains of influenza are circulating in their community and consult the Centers for Disease Control and Prevention (CDC) website (www.cdc.gov/flu) for current recommendations on antiviral use; treatment recommendations change often.[7]

Antiviral drugs are most effective when they are started within 48 hours of the onset of symptoms; they can reduce the severity of the symptoms and the duration of symptoms by 1 to 2 days.[7] For high-risk patients in whom influenza is highly suspected, antivirals should be started as soon as possible, even if laboratory confirmation is not yet back.

Prophylactic treatment with antivirals can be considered for those who are in close contact with persons at high risk for complications from influenza.[8] However, prophylaxis is not a substitute for vaccination; unvaccinated persons should be encouraged to be vaccinated to reduce the time for which prophylaxis is needed. Antiviral prophylaxis may be administered at the same time as the inactivated vaccine, but it should not be administered with the live attenuated influenza vaccine (LAIV) because the antivirals may interfere with the immune response to the LAIV.

Referral and/or hospitalization may be indicated for persons with confirmed or suspected influenza infection who are at high risk of developing serious illness or complications. These include pregnant women, children younger than 2 years, patients aged 65 years or older, or persons with underlying chronic medical conditions, such as pulmonary or cardiac disease, diabetes mellitus, or immunosuppression. Emergency referral is indicated for rapidly worsening symptoms, including cyanosis, dyspnea with oxygen requirement, confusion or listlessness, or exacerbation of chronic conditions such as pulmonary or cardiac disease, diabetes mellitus, or immunosuppression.

LIFE SPAN CONSIDERATIONS

Influenza can cause death in patients of any age group; however, mortality is highest in older people. In the United States, about 36,000 people die each year of influenza or its complications. People 65 years old or older account for more than 90% of these deaths. During the 2009 H1N1 (swine flu) pandemic, most deaths occurred in individuals 18 to 64 years old, with pregnant women among the most vulnerable.[9]

Young infants with influenza infection may have clinical symptoms different from those in older children or adults. In the setting of influenza outbreak, clinicians should be aware that symptoms such as acute onset of high fever, irritability, runny nose, refusal to eat, or weakness may be the only signs of influenza in this young population.

COMPLICATIONS

The primary complications of influenza are pulmonary. The most notable pulmonary complications are primary influenza (viral) pneumonia, which is rare, and secondary bacterial pneumonia. Other pulmonary complications include croup in children and exacerbation of chronic pulmonary disease. Central nervous system complications such as Guillain-Barré syndrome and encephalitis occur rarely after influenza infection. The association of influenza infection and Reye syndrome in children prompted the recommendation that aspirin be avoided in the treatment of children with influenza. Other complications that have been associated with influenza infection are myositis, which is seen primarily in children, and toxic shock syndrome.[2]

PATIENT AND FAMILY EDUCATION

Patients and families should be educated on the importance of reducing the risk of acquiring or spreading influenza illness by (1) receiving the annual influenza vaccine, (2) staying home when ill, (3) avoiding crowds during outbreaks, and (4) hygiene measures to reduce spread of illness, such as good hand washing and covering the mouth and nose when coughing or sneezing.

HEALTH PROMOTION

The influenza vaccine is the primary method of preventing influenza infection. Annual vaccination is recommended for all persons 6 months of age and older who do not have contraindications to vaccination.[1] To protect infants younger than 6 months or those who cannot receive the vaccine because of contraindications, it is even more important that the rest of the family or close personal contacts be vaccinated. The vaccine should be given each year beginning in the fall and continuing throughout the influenza season. International travelers anticipating travel during the fall or winter months in their destination countries should consider vaccination for influenza before their trip. Note that influenza season in the Northern Hemisphere is typically November to April, whereas in the Southern Hemisphere it is April to October; influenza season is year-round in the tropics and subtropics.[1]

There are several types of influenza vaccine currently available in the United States. Quadrivalent and trivalent inactivated influenza vaccines (IIV4 and IIV3, respectively) are commonly referred to as the "flu shot." The trivalent vaccines contain the same three strains of influenza virus—two influenza A subtypes (including H1N1) and one influenza B type—and the quadrivalent vaccines include an additional B type strain. IIV3 is approved for all people 6 months of age or older who do not have an egg allergy. IIV4 is approved in some cases for children as young as 6 months, but in others it is indicated only for persons 3 years of age or older. Therefore, it is important to know which vaccine is being offered and to check with the manufacturer for whom it is indicated.[10] There is now available an egg-free recombinant influenza vaccine for persons aged 18 to 49 years of age with severe allergy to eggs.[1]

Studies have shown that influenza vaccine effectiveness among children is more protective if the child receives two vaccine doses rather than one during the first season the child is vaccinated. Therefore the CDC now recommends that all children aged 6 months to 8 years who are being vaccinated for the first time receive two vaccine doses separated by at least 4 weeks.[10]

In 2010, a high-dose inactivated influenza vaccine was approved for use in people 65 years old and older. The high-dose formulation contains 4 times more hemagglutinin than the standard IIV. Older adult recipients of the high-dose vaccine had a better immunologic response than did recipients of the standard formulation. More local reactions were noted in recipients of the high-dose formulation.[1]

The live, attenuated influenza vaccine (called LAIV) may be given to healthy, non-pregnant people 2 through 49 years of age. It may safely be given at the same time as other vaccines.

LAIV is sprayed into the nose. LAIV does not contain thimerosal or other preservatives. It is made from weakened flu virus and does not cause flu.

There are many flu viruses, and they are always changing. Each year LAIV is made to protect against four viruses that are likely to cause disease in the upcoming flu season.[11]

Each year, the US Food and Drug Administration determines the three or four influenza strains to be included in the following year's vaccine on the basis of which viruses are most likely to cause epidemics in the coming winter.[1] But even when the vaccine doesn't match the circulating strain perfectly, it may still provide some protection.

REFERENCES

1. Grohskopf, L. A., Sokolow, L. Z., Broder, K. R., Walter, E. B., Fry, A. M., & Jernigan, D. B. (2018). Prevention and control of seasonal influenza with vaccines: Recommendations of the Advisory Committee on immunization Practices-United States, 2018–19 influenza season. *MMWR. Recommendations and Reports: Morbidity and Mortality Weekly Report. Recommendations and Reports*, 67(3), 1–20. doi:10.15585/mmwr.rr6703a1. Published 2018 Aug 24.
2. Krammer, F., Smith, G. J. D., Fouchier, R. A. M., Peiris, M., Kedzierska, K., et al. (Jun 2018). Nature Reviews: Disease Primers. London. doi:10.1038/s41572-018-0002-y.
3. Centers for Disease Control and Prevention (CDC). (2018). Influenza antiviral medications: summary for clinicians. Retrieved Feb 18,2018 Retrieved from https://www.cdc.gov/flu/professionals/antivirals/summary-clinicians.htm.
4. Dolin, R. (2011). Influenza. In D. L. Longo, A. S. Fauci, D. L. Kasper, et al. (Eds.), *Harrison's principles and practice of medicine* (18th ed.). Burr Ridge IL: McGraw Hill. ch 187.
5. Centers for Disease Control and Prevention. Influenza signs and symptoms and the role of laboratory diagnostics. Retrieved from https://www.cdc.gov/flu/professionals/diagnosis/labrolesprocedures.htm. (Accessed 21 July 2019).
6. Reaper, D. R., & Landry, M. L. (2014). Rapid Diagnosis of Influenza: State of the Art. *Clinics in Laboratory Medicine, 34*, 365–385.
7. Centers for Disease Control and Prevention (CDC). (2017). Influenza Antiviral Medications: Summary for Clinicians. Retrieved from https://www.cdc.gov/flu/profesionals/antivirals/summary/clinicians.htm.on. Jan 3, 2018.
8. Appiah, G., & Bresee, J. (2017). Influenza (seasonal, zoonotic, and pandemic). In G. W. Burnette (Ed.), *CDC Yellowbook, 2018, health information for international travelers. 2018.* CDC, New York: Oxford University Press. Retrieved from https://wwwnc.cdc.gov/travel/yellowbook/2018/infectious-diseases-related-to-travel/influenza. on Feb 19, 2018.
9. Shresthas, S., Swerdlow, D. L., Borse, R. H., et al. (April 2009). Estimating the burden of 2009 pandemic influenza(H1N1) in the United States.
10. American Academy of Pediatrics Committee on Infectious Diseases. (2017). Recommendations for Prevention and Control of Influenza in Children, 2017–2018. *Pediatrics, 140*(4), 1–20.
11. CDC. (2015). Live, intranasal influenza VIS. Retrieved from www.cdc.gov/vaccines/hcp/vis/vis-statements/flulive/html. On Feb 19, 2018.

CHAPTER **211**

INFECTIOUS DIARRHEA
Thomas H. Taylor • Megan Carol Gallagher

DEFINITION AND EPIDEMIOLOGY

Diarrhea is an alteration of normal bowel movement characterized by an increase in volume or frequency of stools. Watery diarrhea is a type of non-inflammatory, small bowel diarrhea suggestive of a secretory mechanism. It is likely to be abrupt in onset, very large in volume, and associated with symptoms of acute loss of blood volume (shock); it implicates cholera. In this case, the capacity of the distal colon to absorb watery diarrhea produced in the small intestine is overwhelmed. Penetrating diarrhea refers to organisms that may cause a sometimes unrecognized inflammatory process, usually in the distal small bowel, with eventual invasion into the bloodstream associated with systemic manifestations referred to as enteric fever (i.e., *Salmonella typhi* or typhoid fever). Table 211.1 outlines the differences between non-inflammatory, inflammatory, and penetrating diarrheas.

Infectious diarrheal diseases are the second leading cause of morbidity and mortality worldwide. In the United States, each person suffers one or two bouts of diarrhea each year,

so some 200 million to 375 million episodes of diarrheal illness (usually food or water borne) occur each year, resulting in 3000 to 5000 deaths.[1] Infectious diarrhea is a problem for both industrialized and developing nations, but it is uniquely associated with high morbidity and mortality in developing nations. Inadequate food and water supplies lead to recurrent bouts of diarrhea in very young children, who are not able to maintain adequate hydration during acute episodes but, more importantly, suffer baseline malnutrition. Malnutrition sets them up for gastrointestinal infection, and recurrent infection worsens malnutrition. Recurrent bouts of diarrhea weaken bowel health in a fashion that leads to chronic diarrhea. Rotavirus, a common cause of childhood viral gastroenteritis even in the United States, shares this proclivity to cause death in malnourished children.

Fortunately, modes of transmission are well known and include three main routes: food-borne, water-borne, and person to person (fecal-oral). Non-*typhi Salmonella* species and *Campylobacter jejuni* are transmitted through food. *Shigella* species are transmitted mainly person to person. *Giardia* and *Cryptosporidium* are principally water-borne. International health initiatives have made progress in reducing the global annual childhood mortality rate from 5 million to 1.5 million deaths per year by promotion of breastfeeding, measles and rotavirus vaccination programs, education about oral rehydration therapy (ORT), food distribution programs, and separation of drinking water from bathing and bathroom facilities. Residents of industrialized nations experience one or two bouts of diarrhea annually, compared with five or six in underdeveloped areas, but certain individuals may be affected more frequently and severely (Box 211.1).

PATHOPHYSIOLOGY

Pathogens such as viruses, bacteria, and parasites can cause diarrhea. Viruses usually occur on a year-round basis but peak in the winter months. Bacterial illnesses are more common in the summer or early fall. Acute infectious diarrhea may be categorized as non-inflammatory, inflammatory, or penetrating and thus cause unique clinical scenarios. There are a few basic mechanisms, but many organisms use more than one method to cause bowel disease. *Escherichia coli* have the potential to exchange plasmids and other transgenic virulence factors, which run the gamut of pathogenic mechanisms. Because *E. coli* is part of normal bowel flora, special techniques must be requested to discover pathogenic species. Distinct syndromes follow these four pathogenic mechanisms:

1. *Adherence.* The bowel is colonized with bacteria that are non-adherent and suppress overgrowth of more pathogenic bacteria. Pathogenic bacteria may adhere to the bowel wall and cause direct damage or more intimately expose cells to enterotoxins and cytotoxins, that is, enteroadherent *E. coli* (EAEC). Microvilli are effaced and enterocyte cytoskeleton is disrupted, that is, enteropathogenic *E. coli* (EPEC).
2. *Invasion.* Enteroinvasive organisms adhere to enterocytes and then invade the bowel wall, with ulceration and sloughing of tissue, blood, and mucus. Bacillary dysentery is the result, and *Shigella* (an organism that also produces a Shiga toxin) is the classic example. Other examples include enteroinvasive *E. coli* (EIEC), non-*typhi Salmonella* species, and *Clostridioides difficile*.
3. *Enterotoxins. Vibrio cholerae* is the classic example. Cholera toxin acts by a second messenger, cyclic adenosine

TABLE **211.1** **Non-Inflammatory, Inflammatory, and Penetrating Types of Diarrhea**

Mechanism	Non-Inflammatory (Adhesion, Enterotoxin)	Inflammatory (Invasion, Cytotoxin)	Penetrating (Invades Lymphatics)
Location	Proximal small bowel	Colon	Distal small bowel
Illness	Small-volume diarrhea (gastroenteritis) Watery, large volume suggests a secretory mechanism (i.e., cholera)	Blood and mucus (dysentery) Larger volume Low abdominal pain Tenesmus	Enteric fever (typhoid fever) Rash (rose spots) Small-volume or no diarrhea
Examples	*Vibrio cholerae* (secretory) *E. coli* (EAEC and ETEC) Norovirus Rotavirus Adenovirus Astrovirus *Giardia lamblia* *Cryptosporidium*	*Shigella* spp. *E. coli* (EIEC) *Salmonella* non-*typhi* spp. *Campylobacter* *Clostridium difficile* *Entamoeba histolytica* *Cyclospora cayetanensis* *Isospora belli* Microsporidia	*Salmonella typhi* *Salmonella paratyphi* *Yersinia enterocolitica*

EAEC, Enteroadherent *E. coli*; *EIEC*, enteroinvasive *E. coli*; *ETEC*, enterotoxigenic *E. coli*.

BOX **211.1**

Epidemiologic Groups Susceptible to Inflammatory Diarrhea

International travelers
Infants in daycare centers
Adults in daycare or nursing homes
Malnourished patients
Hospitalized patients
Recent use of broad-spectrum antibiotics
Immunocompromised patients
Persons with AIDS
Military personnel in areas of conflict
Elderly or mentally incapacitated patients
Institutionalized populations: prisoners, basic training camps

monophosphate (cAMP), to phosphorylate chloride channels in apical epithelial cells to block sodium chloride absorption and additionally increases chloride secretion by crypt cells. Passive transport of water into the intestinal lumen follows the chloride and produces watery diarrhea. Intestinal mucosa remains intact, as do alternative, glucose-dependent absorption mechanisms. Thus, glucose and electrolyte ORT remains a viable treatment. Enterotoxigenic *E. coli* (ETEC) has a similar toxin-mediated mechanism.

4. *Cytotoxins*. *Shigella dysenteriae* produces the classic cytotoxin. Cytotoxins damage the mucosa by inhibiting cellular protein synthesis and producing an inflammatory colitis. This cytokine is immunologically and structurally related to cytokines produced by enterohemorrhagic *E. coli* (EHEC) and *Vibrio parahaemolyticus*. Shiga-like toxins (SLTs) also target vascular endothelial cells (verotoxin), which explains the hemolysis, hemorrhagic colitis, and glomerulonephritis seen with hemolytic-uremic syndrome (HUS). HUS accompanies *E. coli* O157:H7 diarrhea outbreaks from undercooked hamburger associated with some fast-food restaurants. *C. difficile*, *Clostridium perfringens*, and *Salmonella* strains also produce destructive cytotoxins.

CLINICAL PRESENTATION AND PHYSICAL EXAMINATION

A good medical history is most helpful in determining the cause of infectious diarrhea and directing the extent of diagnostic testing. The epidemiologic setting, clinical presentation, and laboratory features guide our empirical approach to a broad spectrum of pathogens. Given that most acute diarrhea in the United States is due to noroviruses (50% to 80%),[2] which produce mild non-inflammatory gastroenteritis with fewer than six low-volume stools per day, and that it is self-limited, with resolution in 2 to 3 days, the health care provider should investigate and give antibiotics only for presentations not consistent with norovirus infection. The probability that this is not norovirus infection increases dramatically if there are epidemiologic clues travel, antibiotic use, hospital acquired, outbreak association, animal or pet contact, hiker drinking untreated water, shellfish ingestion, unpasteurized milk ingestion, uncooked eggs, and daycare client or worker. The provider should consider bacterial causes (Table 211.2) if the clinical presentation is one of inflammatory diarrhea: fever, abdominal pain, tenesmus, large-volume diarrhea (more than six stools per day), and mucus or blood in stool. A search for the pathogen with empirical antibiotic treatment is in order. The presence of chronic illness, chemotherapy, tube feedings, medications, immune deficiency, or human immunodeficiency virus (HIV) infection with low CD4 counts will prompt consideration of more severe manifestations of norovirus, rotavirus, adenovirus, or astrovirus infection and atypical presentation of bacterial and parasitic diarrhea. Chronic diarrhea, lasting more than 14 days, is suggestive of protozoan parasites: *Giardia*, *Cryptosporidium*, and *E. histolytica*. Systemic manifestations of fever, chills, rigors, night sweats, and weight loss suggest penetrating bacteria (i.e., *S. typhi* or *Yersinia enterocolitica*), and blood cultures are in order.

Some bacterial pathogens and toxins may cause non-inflammatory, self-limited disease in healthy people, but if they produce only norovirus-like illness, patients would not benefit from extensive laboratory tests or antibiotic treatment. Older adults or very young patients may develop complications from gastroenteritis or mild diarrhea and may benefit from hydration and admission, even if a pathogen search and antibiotics

TABLE 211.2 Clinical Signs and Disease Probability

Clinical Signs	Disease
Nausea, vomiting, epigastric pain Small volume, short course	Norovirus, rotavirus, adenovirus, astrovirus *E. coli* (EAEC and ETEC)
Blood or mucus in stool, low abdominal pain Large volume	*Shigella, Salmonella, Campylobacter* *E. coli* (EIEC), *Clostridium difficile,* *Entamoeba histolytica*
Watery stool, large volume, shock	Cholera, Shiga toxin *E. coli* (STEC)
Rectal pain and tenesmus	*Shigella, Entamoeba histolytica*
Fever (temperature >101°F), chills, night sweats, weight loss	*Salmonella typhi, Yersinia enterocolitica*
Chronic diarrhea	*Cryptosporidium, Giardia, Entamoeba histolytica, Campylobacter, Yersinia*
HIV CD4 cell count >200 HIV CD4 cell count >200 HIV CD4 cell count ≥100	*Salmonella, Shigella, Campylobacter* *Cryptosporidium, Cyclospora,* Microspora Cytomegalovirus, *Mycobacterium avium*
Hemolytic-uremic syndrome	*E. coli* O157:H7 or other Shiga toxin *E. coli*
Guillain-Barré syndrome	*Campylobacter jejuni*

EAEC, Enteroadherent *E. coli*; *EIEC,* enteroinvasive *E. coli*; *ETEC,* enterotoxigenic *E. coli*.

are withheld. A temporal association should be sought with medications related to diarrhea or food-related to bacterial toxins, such as mayonnaise, cream pie, and potato salad (staphylococcal enterotoxin) or rice dish on the warming table (*B. cereus* food poisoning); it would also ensure a good prognosis, without need for antibiotics.

The physical examination includes weight, temperature, and orthostatic vital signs (blood pressure and heart rate lying, sitting, and standing) to assess for volume depletion (dry mucous membranes, decreased skin turgor, absent jugular venous pulsation). The patient's mental status should be noted along with a close assessment of skin color, temperature, and rashes. Signs of bowel perforation include an abdomen quiet to auscultation and rigid to palpation. Small bowel obstruction might include a tender abdomen, with distention and high-pitched bowel sounds, as opposed to the usual bowel rushes and scaphoid abdomen seen with diarrheal enteritis. Thyromegaly, tachycardia, and proptosis suggest hyperthyroidism as a cause of chronic diarrhea. Lymphadenopathy, especially cervical node, suggests lymphoma or bowel cancer as a cause of diarrhea. In the female patient with lower abdominal symptoms, a pelvic examination is imperative. In the geriatric patient, fecal impaction must be ruled out. All patients should now be tested for HIV infection, and diarrhea is a good indication.

DIAGNOSTICS
Initial Diagnostics

For the patient who has mild acute diarrhea or gastroenteritis, diagnostic evaluation is typically not indicated.

Additional Diagnostics

Complete blood count (CBC), serum electrolyte values, and blood urea nitrogen (BUN) and creatinine concentrations are standard tests for evaluation of dehydration and electrolyte derangement.

Stool testing for bacterial pathogens should be performed on patients with a temperature above 38.8°C (102°F), bloody diarrhea, abdominal pain, signs of sepsis, or more than six unformed stools in a 24-hour period, and for patients who are frail and elderly or immunocompromised. Pathogens to consider in this setting include *Salmonella, Shigella, Campylobacter, Yersinia, Clostridium difficile,* and enterohemorrhagic (Shiga-toxin-producing) *E. coli.* Testing should include stool culture and Shiga toxin testing. Evaluation for parasitic infection involves ova and parasite exam on stool. *Cryptosporidium* and *Giardia* can also be diagnosed by antigen tests. Immunocompromised patients have a broader differential and additional testing may be required. Leukocytosis is suggestive of *C. difficile* infection, and a stool sample for enzyme-linked immunosorbent assay (ELISA) of *C. difficile* toxin is necessary. The ELISA is a sensitive screening test, but it must be confirmed with specific toxin assay by reflex testing, which is a more specific assay. It is not necessary to send more than one test sample for *C. difficile* in a 24-hour period, and the test should not be performed on formed stool. New culture-independent diagnostic testing methods, such as multiplex PCR in the form of gastrointestinal tract panels, are now available. If an organism of public health significance is identified by culture-independent methods, additional culturing may be required under public health reporting rules.

DIAGNOSTICS

Diarrhea

INITIAL
- None

ADDITIONAL
- CBC with differential
- Chemistry profile
- Stool culture for *Salmonella, Shigella, Campylobacter, E. coli* O157[a]
- Stool for Shiga toxins or genes, if culture negative[a]

- Stool for *C. difficile* ELISA screen, with reflex testing for toxin[a]
- Stool for ova and parasites, if diarrhea is chronic
- Blood culture (two times), with systemic symptoms (penetrating diarrhea)

[a]If inflammatory diarrhea.

DIFFERENTIAL DIAGNOSIS

A good history investigating epidemiology, clinical signs, and routine diagnostic tests allows consideration of broad categories: non-inflammatory, inflammatory, and penetrating gastrointestinal illness. Non-inflammatory illness suggesting gastroenteritis, norovirus, rotavirus, or traveler's diarrhea is differentiated from more inflammatory and penetrating disease; it requires only hydration and electrolyte replacement, without stool or blood culture or further diagnostic testing.[3]

Non-Inflammatory Diarrhea: Acute Gastroenteritis

Norovirus, the most common cause of viral gastroenteritis or "intestinal flu" in older children and adults, is a member of the Caliciviridae family of small RNA viruses. Human caliciviruses cause disease year-round but are the most common cause of outbreaks of "winter vomiting syndrome"; they occur frequently in closed systems, such as cruise ships, hospitals, nursing homes, and military facilities. These viruses require low inoculums, are highly transmissible, and are resistant to cooking and chlorine cleaners. Thus, norovirus is likely to be prevalent year-round. Shellfish, such as clams and oysters, are filter feeders and readily concentrate organisms from contaminated water. Nonbacterial, food-related outbreaks are usually due to these agents. The incubation period for various caliciviruses is only 1 or 2 days. Winter vomiting disease is characterized by abrupt onset of vomiting, diarrhea, and low-grade or no fever. The duration is also short, 1 to 3 days. Treatment consists of ORT, and antibiotics are not indicated.[4] This is why travelers are asked not to take empirical antibiotic treatment unless symptoms fail to subside within 24 hours.

Rotavirus is the most common cause of severe diarrhea in very young children. There is a seasonal pattern, from November to April in the United States. Fecal-oral transmission may occur through contaminated water, food preparation, and hands. Rotavirus invades small intestine villous enterocytes, causing malabsorption, and produces a viral enterotoxin, NSP4, which induces a secretory diarrhea by stimulating chloride secretion but without cyclic nucleotide signaling (i.e., not a cholera toxin). Thus, the diarrhea is watery and lasts 3 to 8 days, and it is cholera-like in its ability to dehydrate and to cause death in young malnourished children. Vomiting and fever may be prominent symptoms, as in other gastroenteritis. The incubation period is 4 to 7 days. Antibiotics are not warranted, and treatment is ORT. Although rotavirus is also associated with disease in winter months, rotavirus disease in older children and adults is mild, short-lived, and thus underreported.

Two vaccines, RotaTeq (RV5: three doses at 2, 4, and 6 months) and Rotarix (RV1: two doses at 2 and 4 months), have been beneficial in reducing infant mortality in developing nations and morbidity in developed nations. The U.S. Food and Drug Administration has determined that vaccination benefits outweigh any potential risk.[5] This is a live vaccine and should be used with caution in immunocompromised children, but HIV positivity is not a contraindication.

Traveler's Diarrhea

A recent travel history changes the probability of norovirus to unlikely, but the type of diarrhea is still likely to be non-inflammatory and of short duration. Fecal-oral contamination of food or water is implicated, and E. coli (EAEC or ETEC) are the most likely pathogens, followed by Campylobacter jejuni, Shigella species, and Salmonella species. Traveler's diarrhea can occur during or up to 10 days after travel, affects up to 30% to 70% of travelers to developing countries, and generally lasts approximately 3 to 7 days. It is usually a self-limited illness, and the patient rarely develops complications. Treatment includes oral fluid replacement (Box 211.2).[6] Loperamide (Imodium), 4 mg orally at onset and 2 mg after each loose stool up to 16 mg/d, can be helpful. A 3-day course of ciprofloxacin, 500 mg orally twice daily, or azithromycin as a single 1000-mg dose may be prescribed. Bismuth subsalicylate (Pepto-Bismol®) has both antimicrobial and anti-inflammatory effects and may be taken as 2 tablets every 30 to 60 minutes up to eight doses per day.[6]

BOX 211.2

Homemade Oral Rehydration Solutions

ONE LITER FOR ORAL REHYDRATION THERAPY
4 ½ cups water
¼ tsp salt substitute (with potassium)
½ tsp baking soda
½ tsp salt
2 to 3 T sugar, honey (do not use in children younger than 1 year), or corn syrup

CEREAL REHYDRATION WITH ACTIVE DIARRHEA
¼ cup baby rice cereal
8 oz. water
Pinch of salt
Flavoring or ½ to 1 tsp of sugar may make this more palatable
Drink one serving after each loose stool

Modified from Kelly, D., & Nadeau, J. *Oral rehydration solution: A "low-tech" oft neglected therapy*. Available at www.healthsystem.virginia.edu/internet/digestive -health/nutritionarticles/Kellyarticle.pdf. Accessed March 12, 2006.

Invasive bacteria such as Campylobacter, Salmonella, and Shigella are seen more in travel to southern Asia. The parasites E. histolytica, Cryptosporidium, and Giardia are a consideration if diarrhea persists beyond 1 week. Non–E. coli bacteria can cause 10% to 20% of cases of traveler's diarrhea, but investigation should be undertaken only if diarrhea persists beyond 1 week or if clinical signs of inflammatory diarrhea ensue. These viruses are short-lived, and there is no benefit from extensive diagnostics or antibiotics. Travelers should take an antibiotic, usually ciprofloxacin, rifaximin, or azithromycin, only if diarrhea lasts more than 1 or 2 days or is associated with high fever.[6] Single-dose regimens have been shown to be equivalent to multi-dose regimens.[6] Antibiotic treatment reduces the duration of diarrhea by about 1 day if the diarrhea is caused by a susceptible pathogen. However, there are concerns that travelers who take antibiotics are at risk of acquiring drug-resistant organisms.

Prevention is the cornerstone of treatment. Traveler's diarrhea can be avoided by not drinking untreated water or ice cubes or unpasteurized milk and not eating raw fruits and vegetables and undercooked meat. Travelers must remember to drink only sealed or carbonated beverages. The use of daily bismuth subsalicylate, found in Pepto-Bismol®, has been shown to reduce the incidence of travelers' diarrhea by about 50% but is associated with tongue blackening, nausea, and constipation.[7] It should be avoided in those with aspirin allergy, renal insufficiency, and gout, and can lead to salicylate toxicity in those taking aspirin. Benefit from probiotics, such as Lactobacillus, is inconclusive. Antibiotics are typically not prescribed as a preventive measure for travelers. Widespread antibiotic resistance to ampicillin, to trimethoprim-sulfamethoxazole (Bactrim DS), and, increasingly, to quinolones has made these agents less useful for the treatment of traveler's diarrhea. In addition, they are not effective against viral or parasitic infections and may provide a false sense of security.

Vibrio Cholerae

Watery, large-volume, non-inflammatory diarrhea is best exemplified by infection with V. cholerae, the prototype of enterotoxigenic, secretory diarrhea. Cholera is the most feared agent of epidemic and pandemic diarrhea because of its abrupt, severe dehydration and mortality in times of natural and artificial catastrophe. The organism is omnipresent because of its natural existence in marine algae and plankton, where natural reservoirs await the right conditions of flooding and water stagnation to activate from a dormant state and grow to appropriate inoculum size and find an appropriate vehicle (i.e., shellfish concentration, contaminated water supplies, and contaminated food). Cholera also has the capacity to remain endemic in certain regions where asymptomatic carriage and contaminated water remain problems. The pathophysiologic mechanism is noted for its simplicity. Enterotoxin activates adenylate cyclase, which increases cAMP in enterocytes in the distal small intestine. This classic second messenger (cAMP) blocks absorption of sodium and chloride by the microvilli and promotes secretion of chloride by the crypt cells. Water osmotically follows sodium chloride into the intestinal lumen, and massive secretory diarrhea ensues.

The incubation period is several hours to 5 days, a relatively short duration indicative of rapid in vivo toxin production. Watery stools contain diluted mucus (rice water stools) and are large volume and non-inflammatory. The colon is not inflamed, and there is no cramping, abdominal pain, tenesmus, or fever. Fecal leukocytes, blood, tissue fragments, and mucous strands are absent. Complications include isotonic dehydration, hypovolemic shock, acute renal failure, metabolic acidosis (high anion gap), and electrolyte losses (potassium, sodium, and chloride). Antibiotics play a secondary role to ORT but may shorten the course. Emerging resistance to ampicillin, tetracyclines, azithromycin, trimethoprim-sulfamethoxazole, and recently fluoroquinolones complicates therapy.

Inflammatory Diarrhea

Shigella (S. Dysenteriae, S. Flexneri, S. Sonnei). Shigella infection is the prototype of inflammatory colitis diarrhea or bacillary dysentery. The small inoculation size allows easy fecal-oral transmission (children, daycare centers, bisexual and gay males), but summer prevalence might be accounted for by the potential for fly feet transmission in outdoor, poor sanitation settings. Shigella causes 10% of diarrhea in the United States, but this organism tends to be diagnosed and reported more than non-inflammatory diarrheas. The incubation period is 12 to 72 hours, reflecting cytotoxin production. It is easily recognized by larger volume, frequent, bloody, foul diarrhea containing mucous and fecal leukocytes. Fever, cramps, and tenesmus are prominent symptoms. The need for ORT and possibly intravenous hydration should be recognized and implemented early.

Certain strains of E. coli (EIEC and EHEC) produce dysentery indistinguishable from shigellosis. SLTs also target vascular endothelial cells (verotoxin), which explains the hemolysis, hemorrhagic colitis, and glomerulonephritis seen with HUS accompanying E. coli O157:H7. Because of toxin production, antimotility agents should be avoided. Antibiotics are thought to exacerbate the risk of HUS in E. coli O157:H7 disease because antibiotics foster abrupt release of cytotoxin as bacteria are killed. Shiga toxin in E. coli is carried on bacteriophages. A recent meta-analysis did show more HUS with antibiotic use, therefore antibiotics are to be avoided if Shiga-producing E coli is a consideration.[8] Otherwise, Shigella, EIEC, and EHEC are causes of bloody diarrhea (dysentery), and all should be treated

with antibiotics to improve morbidity and mortality. Some believe that mild disease is not lessened by antibiotics and does not require antibiotic treatment. However, the low inoculum size allows recovering mild cases to continue propagation of disease, and they should be treated for public health reasons. Antibiotics in infants and elderly patients with severe disease can be lifesaving. Ciprofloxacin (500 mg every 12 hours orally for 1 to 3 days in adults) and trimethoprim-sulfamethoxazole, azithromycin, and ceftriaxone are alternatives for children.

Salmonella (Non-Typhi Species). Non-typhi Salmonella species are now the most common cause of inflammatory diarrhea in the United States, are epidemiologically interesting, and are more frequent in summer and fall. Transmission is fecal-oral, and these organisms are responsible for most food-borne outbreaks in the United States. Salmonella species are widely disseminated in nature and are adaptable and virulent to humans; they frequently contaminate poultry, beef, eggs, and dairy products. Fresh produce (lettuce, tomatoes, and cantaloupe), unpasteurized juices, and sprouts have been associated with Salmonella outbreaks. Pet turtles, snakes, iguanas, hedgehogs, outdoor cats, and petting zoos present a danger, especially to children. Raw milk and specialty cheeses are problematic. Dogs and children may be infected by chew products (i.e., dried pig ears). Beef jerky and summer sausage are the adult equivalents. Neonates are at high risk because of relative gastric achlorhydria and the buffering capacity of breast milk and formula. Human-to-human transmission may occur through food handling and contaminated water. Chronic carrier states (0.5%) are difficult to eradicate and present employment issues for food handlers and health care workers.[9]

Incubation periods of 12 to 48 hours reflect invasion of distal small bowel and colon mucosa. There is a generalized invasion of enterocytes by attachment of fimbriae and bacteria-mediated endocytosis, after which enterocyte microvilli regenerate. The inflammatory response is less severe than in shigellosis, but inflammatory diarrhea ensues. There is some propensity to multiply further in Peyer patches and to enter the circulation, as with enteric fever. Blood cultures are more likely to bear bacteria, and dissemination may occur with distant focal infection in meninges, heart valves, gallbladder, biliary tree, pancreas, mycotic aneurysm, and bone, leading to interesting complications.[10]

As with other inflammatory diarrhea, rehydration and electrolyte replacement are essential. Diarrhea is self-limited, antibiotic resistance is a growing concern, and antibiotic treatment may prolong the carrier state; thus, antibiotic treatment is usually deferred. Exceptions include infants, adults older than 50 years, patients with sickle cell disease (bone infarcts become infected with Salmonella, causing osteomyelitis), immunocompromised patients, patients with valvular heart disease, and patients with vascular disease and endovascular stents or grafts (Salmonella has a propensity to settle on vascular plaques and to cause mycotic aneurysm). These special situations, in the face of increasing antibiotic resistance, merit treatment with fluoroquinolones and ceftriaxone until sensitivities are known.[10]

Campylobacter Jejuni

Campylobacter is the second most common cause of inflammatory diarrhea in the United States. Campylobacteriosis is a worldwide zoonosis; it is present in many animal species and enjoys a large natural reservoir, and thus we are regularly exposed from food and surface water.[11] *Campylobacter*, like *Salmonella*, is susceptible to gastric acid and requires a relatively high inoculation dose. However, patients with alcoholism, cirrhosis, or diabetes, and older adults and neonates are more susceptible. Even a dose as low as 500 organisms may be able to cause disease. *Campylobacter* offers variable production of cytotoxin, infects the terminal ileum and colon, and has a greater spectrum of disease, depending on host resistance and organism (i.e., *Campylobacter fetus* produces less dysentery than *Campylobacter jejuni* does). Disease may be subtle, chronic, acute, or full-blown dysentery. The organism is fastidious, so negative stool cultures do not rule it out. Wet preparation microscopic stool examination may show darting, comma-shaped organisms, and Gram stain of a stool specimen may reveal small, curved, gram-negative rods. Fecal leukocytes and stool Hem occult slide test results are positive. Blood cultures are rarely positive, but *Campylobacter* is occasionally a cause of enteric fever (like *S. typhi*, the cause of more systemic disease than diarrhea). *Y. enterocolitica* shares a variable inflammatory disease spectrum and is more likely to culminate in penetrating disease or enteric fever.

For most healthy adults, *Campylobacter* produces a self-limited illness, and it is not clear that antibiotics shorten illness. Unlike *Salmonella*, the organism is not difficult to eradicate with antibiotics (i.e., antibiotics do not prolong the carrier state). Dysentery, prolonged colitis, bacteremia, enteric fever, and distant focal infections need to be treated with antibiotics. Macrolides have been the treatment of choice, but there is some resistance. In general, β-lactam antibiotics are not as effective, but fluoroquinolones, aminoglycosides, chloramphenicol, clindamycin, and tetracyclines are alternatives.

Because of the occasional insidious presentation of chronic colitis with bloody diarrhea and negative stool cultures, *Campylobacter* can be mistaken for ulcerative colitis. Post infectious diarrhea or reactive arthritis may follow most forms of bacillary dysentery in HLA-B27–positive individuals. Guillain-Barré syndrome (see Chapter 176) is a unique but uncommon consequence of *Campylobacter* infection. Unfortunately, *Campylobacter* diarrhea is so common that 20% to 50% of cases of Guillain-Barré syndrome follow *Campylobacter* infections.[12]

Escherichia Coli O157:H7. *E. coli* O157:H7 was first recognized as a food-borne pathogen in the United States in 1982. Outbreaks occurred by distribution of contaminated hamburger meat, and EHEC soon became the most common cause of bloody diarrhea. The Centers for Disease Control and Prevention (CDC) estimates 265,000 *E. coli* infections annually in the US; 36% are STEC 0157.[13] *E. coli* O157:H7 is a zoonotic emerging pathogen that normally resides in the gut of healthy cattle. Early outbreaks of *E. coli* O157:H7–mediated disease were traced to unpasteurized apple cider made from fallen apples in orchards where cattle grazed, thus contaminating it with feces. Discovery of this relationship has resulted in the need to pasteurize apple cider. Improved cooking standards in fast-food restaurants have decreased the incidence of *E. coli* O157:H7 in ground beef foods. Likewise, the incidents related to leafy green vegetables have also decreased due to increased safety efforts on the part of farmers and fast-food restaurants.[14]

Another unique aspect of *E. coli* O157:H7 is the spectrum of disease this organism may confer, from mild diarrhea to severe hemorrhagic colitis. Antibiotic treatment causes release of SLT, a toxin also present in *S. dysenteriae* that is thought to

worsen the risk of HUS, and a recent meta-analysis confirms this increased risk.[8] By the time HUS appears, the acute diarrhea has already subsided, so antibiotics are not likely to help.

Clostridium Difficile. Antibiotic-associated diarrhea (AAD) has been with us since the advent of broad-spectrum antibiotics, which alter anaerobic and enteric bowel flora, allowing antibiotic-resistant *C. difficile* to grow and to produce AAD and more severe pseudomembranous colitis. There has been a marked increase in *C. difficile*–associated disease over the past 10 to 15 years making it a leading cause of health care-related infections. Concern is raised by several recent studies showing both increasing rates and increasing severity of *C. difficile* colitis. A study report in 2015 revealed 453,000 incident infections and approximately 29,000 deaths in the United States in 2011.[15] This new epidemic is occurring in widespread geographic areas, including hospitals, nursing homes, and communities and causes disease in previously healthy patients. It is dominated by a previously uncommon strain of *C. difficile* that produces a new binary toxin similar to the more virulent binary toxin of *C. perfringens*. The new strain also contains a mutation in the *tcdC* regulatory gene and consequently produces greater amounts of toxins A and B responsible for diarrhea. Interestingly, this strain is more resistant to the extended-spectrum fluoroquinolones. Recent overuse of fluoroquinolones may have selected out this particular strain of *C. difficile*, much like clindamycin selected out past strains of *C. difficile* and was more closely associated with AAD than other antibiotics.

Treatment of *C. difficile* colitis is multifactorial. Broad-spectrum antibiotics should be stopped if possible or changed to more narrow-spectrum agents. Hydration and electrolyte replacement need to be maintained. Metronidazole and oral vancomycin have been the mainstays of treatment. Oral vancomycin has higher clinical cure rates than metronidazole and is recommended for severe cases, which are defined by the presence of a white blood cell count of 15,000 cells/μL or higher and/or a serum creatinine level greater than or equal to 1.5 times the baseline level. Severe, complicated *C. difficile* colitis with ileus will not receive adequate levels of oral vancomycin to the colon. In these cases, intravenous metronidazole may result in detectable colonic levels. Rectal administration of vancomycin may also be beneficial, but should be avoided if there is concern for colonic perforation. Fecal microbiota transplant is used quite successfully in severe cases and in immunocompromised patients.[16] In the most severe cases, colectomy is life-saving. It should be performed in the setting of toxic megacolon, colonic perforation, and acute abdomen, and may need to be considered in septic shock.

Recurrence of further *C. difficile* colitis can occur in up to 25% of patients.[17] Recurrences can either represent relapse of the original infection or re-infection with a new strain. The diagnosis of recurrence often needs to be made clinically based on the presence of diarrhea. Many patients remain colonized and toxin-positive following treatment, so repeat testing is not helpful. For the first recurrence, patients should be treated with the same regimen as before, unless they now have severe *C. difficile* infection and require oral vancomycin. For recurrences that occur after the first recurrence, patients should be treated with oral vancomycin followed by a vancomycin taper and pulsed regimen in the hopes of keeping *C. difficile* at bay while waiting for restoration of normal flora. A typical taper and pulsed regimen involves oral vancomycin 4 times a day for 10 to 14 days followed by twice-daily dosing for 7 days, then once-daily dosing for 7 days, finishing with every other day then every third day pulse dosing for 2 to 8 weeks.

New therapeutics have been developed for the management of recurrent or relapsing *C. difficile* infection. Fidaxomicin is an oral antibiotic that specifically targets *C. difficile* and has minimal impact on the intestinal flora. It has similar efficacy to vancomycin in clinical cure but lower rates of *C. difficile* recurrence.[17] Bezlotoxumab is a monoclonal antibody directed against the B toxin of *C. difficile* and was recently FDA-approved for prevention of recurrent *C. difficile* infection when added to standard therapy. Another alternative therapy to manage recurrent *C. difficile* infections is fecal microbiota transplants in which a fecal suspension from a healthy donor is infused into the gastrointestinal tract of a patient with *C. difficile*. This may be done via enema, colonoscopy, nasogastric tube, or oral capsules and typically requires referral to a specialty clinic. Cure rates for fecal microbiota transplants may be as high as 90%.[18]

Epidemic *C. difficile* places new emphasis on preventive measures. Antibiotic use should be limited to the shortest effective course and the narrowest spectrum antibiotic for each pathogen. Broad-spectrum empirical regimens should be narrowed as culture results return, and more specific diagnosis may allow early discontinuation. Isolation and cohort of multiple cases should be accompanied by gowns, gloves, and handwashing. Remember that alcohol scrubs do not inactivate *C. difficile* spores, so soap and water are required to remove them from hands. Electronic thermometers should be replaced by disposable thermometers, and dedicated stethoscopes left in the room. Broad-spectrum antimicrobial use should be managed by hospital antibiotic stewardship programs, and outpatient use of clindamycin and fluoroquinolone antibiotics should be limited.

Food Poisoning: Bacterial Toxins

One to Six Hours After Ingestion

Staphylococcus Aureus Food Poisoning. Summer picnics can be spoiled by foods that favor growth of *S. aureus* (cream pies, cream puffs, chocolate éclairs, chicken salad, mayonnaise) left too long in the warm sun. Incubation within food results in preformed staphylococcal enterotoxins. Short-incubation emetic syndrome produces intense nausea and vomiting within a few hours of ingestion. Long-incubation diarrhea syndrome causes severe abdominal cramps and diarrhea hours later. One feels as if death is imminent, but symptoms resolve completely within 12 hours, and treatment is for comfort only.

Bacillus Cereus Food Poisoning. Short-incubation emetic syndrome is similar to the same syndrome caused by *S. aureus* enterotoxin, but it is caused by a preformed cereulide toxin capable of binding to gastric nerves. Diarrhea is mild and seen in only 33% of cases. This syndrome is associated with fried rice held on warming tables for extended periods. Like staphylococcal food poisoning, this emetic syndrome resolves in 12 hours.

Eight to Fourteen Hours After Ingestion

Clostridium Perfringens Food Poisoning. *C. perfringens* food poisoning follows ingestion of meat and gravies (beef and poultry). Up to 80% of these meats are contaminated with their own enteric flora in meat processing plants. Outbreaks occur in institutions and banquets where large quantities of meat are precooked without ever reaching adequate internal temperatures to kill all contaminating bacteria and without reheating enough to kill incubating bacteria. In contrast to preformed enterotoxins seen in *Staphylococcus* and early-incubation *Bacillus* food poisoning, these enterotoxins are formed in vivo as the organism enters a vegetative state in the hostile environment of our intestines, thus the longer incubation period and action farther down in the intestine, mainly with abdominal cramps and diarrhea. Vomiting and fever are uncommon.

Bacillus Cereus Food Poisoning. Long-incubation diarrhea syndrome is similar to *C. perfringens* food poisoning. It is caused by enterotoxin produced in vivo after ingestion. This explains the long incubation period and predominance of small intestinal cramps and diarrhea. There may be some nausea with both *C. perfringens* and long-incubation *B. cereus*, but vomiting and fever are rare. These two long-incubation syndromes are still limited to the life of their respective toxins and are usually resolved within 24 hours.

INTERPROFESSIONAL COLLABORATIVE MANAGEMENT

Medications can be used for symptomatic relief of nausea and vomiting, abdominal cramping, and diarrhea. These are generally used in older children and healthy adults. Absorbents and antisecretory agents such as bismuth subsalicylate (Kaopectate®, Pepto-Bismol®) and antispasmodic-anticholinergic sedatives such as atropine sulfate, scopolamine hydrobromide, hyoscyamine sulfate, and phenobarbital are used to decrease abdominal cramping. Antisecretory agents such as bismuth subsalicylate also have an anti-inflammatory effect and are commonly used if there is vomiting and abdominal cramping. These products may cause salicylate intoxication and should be used cautiously. Patients taking warfarin should be warned as well because anticoagulation will be affected. Concomitant use of bismuth subsalicylate with antibiotics may decrease the effectiveness of the antibiotics.

Antimotility agents that are used in non-inflammatory diarrhea include loperamide, diphenoxylate hydrochloride–atropine sulfate (Lomotil), and tincture of opium. Loperamide is preferred in children, pregnant women, and immunocompromised patients. If nausea is the main complaint, treatment with promethazine (Phenergan), prochlorperazine (Compazine), or another antiemetic is recommended. Antimotility agents should not be used in patients with bloody diarrhea or fecal leukocytosis.

Empirical treatment with antibiotics should be considered in the following: in the presence of fecal leukocytes without a confirmed positive stool culture; with occult blood; if the patient has fever with profuse, watery diarrhea (more than six stools per day), appears dehydrated, has had symptoms for more than 1 week, and is immunocompromised; or if hospitalization is considered. *Salmonella*, *Shigella*, or *Campylobacter* pathogens are the most likely cause of the infection in these cases. Ciprofloxacin or norfloxacin can be initiated until the stool culture results are verified but should not be used in children or pregnant or lactating women. If the diarrhea persists for longer than 2 weeks, *Giardia* organisms may be suspected and metronidazole can be initiated. Specific therapy is initiated once the pathogen is identified. Pedialyte, Enfalyte, Rehydralyte, and CeraLyte are commercial formulas for ORT. Formulation of homemade ORT can be found in Box 211.2.

If dehydration is severe or vomiting is protracted, intravenous fluids should be initiated. Children and elderly patients are especially vulnerable. Medical evaluation is indicated for children younger than 6 months or whose weight is below 8 kg, premature infants, children with chronic illness, infants with fever (temperature ≥38°C), children with fever (temperature >39°C), visible bloody stool, high-volume stool, and persistent vomiting. Signs of severe dehydration requiring admission for intravenous fluid administration include sunken eyes, dry mucous membranes, decreased skin turgor, lack of tears, decreased urine output (dry diapers), irritability, lethargy, tachycardia, and postural hypotension. If symptoms of the illness persist beyond 3 weeks despite treatment measures, the provider should consider chronic lactose intolerance, parasites, malignant neoplasms, and disease states such as diabetes, thyrotoxicosis, lupus, HIV infection, inflammatory bowel disease, or irritable bowel syndrome, and consultation is indicated.

COMPLICATIONS

Complications from diarrhea are usually the result of dehydration. Regardless of the cause, attention should be directed toward fluid and electrolyte replacement. Electrolyte disorders, particularly hypocalcemia, hypomagnesemia, and hypokalemia, are common in persistent diarrhea. Continuous diarrhea can require hospitalization for fluid and electrolyte replacement if the patient is unable to maintain hydration with oral fluid replacement. Sepsis and cardiovascular collapse are potential complications, and infants, older adults, and immunosuppressed patients are more susceptible to these complications. Refractory diarrhea is usually a symptom of a more serious illness and requires diagnostic evaluation and subspecialist consultation.

Association of E. coli O157:H7 diarrhea with childhood HUS has come to exemplify how a pathogen at one site can explain a disease at another uninfected site. HUS was previously an unexplained illness defined by hemolysis, thrombocytopenia, and acute renal failure, often in children. EHEC have evolved by acquiring a symbiotic relationship with a bacteriophage that encodes SLT. SLT attaches to a receptor, globotriaosylceramide (GB), on enterocytes in the gut. GB receptors also exist on vascular endothelial cells of glomerular capillaries and other small capillary beds. Damage to these capillary beds, by circulating SLT, explains the occurrence of acute renal failure, microangiopathic hemolytic anemia, and thrombocytopenia, which define HUS. Neutralizing antibodies to SLT develop in most children before the age of 10 years and decline as they age. Thus, persons most severely affected by E. coli O157:H7 are the young and the elderly.

Joint inflammation, conjunctivitis, or urethritis that follows a bout of diarrhea by 7 to 10 days suggests reactive arthropathy after Salmonella, Shigella, or Campylobacter infection (Chapter 198).[19] Sensory paresthesia followed rapidly by ascending motor weakness and loss of deep tendon reflexes implicates Guillain-Barré syndrome, often following C. jejuni enteritis.[12]

PATIENT AND FAMILY EDUCATION

Normal slow recovery of bowel health after a bout of C. difficile infection should be discussed to avoid overzealous treatment of recurrences. Avoidance of nonessential antibiotics in all patients, but especially after C. difficile infection, is an important discussion. Bacterial enteritis in children younger than 5 years may serve as a focus for bowel intussusception, which may occur in the 6-month period after enteritis. The following

are some general recommendations that should be discussed with the patient and family:

- Practice good handwashing after each bowel movement to reduce the possibility of spreading disease to other family members.
- Immunocompromised patients are at greater risk of severe infection and should be diligent about proper safe food handling and preparation.
- Drink frequent, small sips of fluids (water, tea, bouillon, flat cola, flat ginger ale, or sports drink) to avoid dehydration.
- Avoid foods and let your stomach rest until bowel movements begin to return to normal or until you begin to feel better. Gradually add small amounts of food (e.g., crackers, toast, rice, bananas), avoiding those that may aggravate symptoms (e.g., dairy products, caffeine, high-fat or high-fiber foods, carbonated beverages, sugar-free products, and alcohol).
- It is better to avoid antidiarrheal products because most cases of diarrhea are self-limited.

 If symptoms persist or are accompanied by mental confusion, fever with temperature higher than 38.3°C (101°F), chills, vomiting, weakness (especially muscle weakness), dizziness, dry mouth, extreme thirst, little or no urinary output, severe abdominal discomfort, blurred vision, or black or bloody stools, immediately notify the health care provider.

- Children, daycare workers, and food handlers should remain at home until diarrhea resolves.

PREVENTION

Therapy to reduce gastric acid has increasingly come under scrutiny as unsuspected side effects have come to light: osteoporosis, risk of hospital- and community-acquired pneumonia, and enteric infection such as Campylobacter and Salmonella enteritis. Studies have linked chronic proton pump inhibitor use with C. difficile infection and relapse.[20] Physicians should offer other treatments for dyspepsia, prescribe shorter courses of proton pump inhibitors, and discontinue proton pump inhibitors in asymptomatic patients.

Prevention information for patients and providers includes the following:

- Handwashing remains the best preventive measure. Always wash hands after handling chicken or other raw meats. Wash cutting boards frequently. Change sponges and wash kitchen countertops frequently. Sponges may be disinfected by microwaving them on high or placing them in boiling water for 2 minutes.
- Use a meat thermometer to check temperature of roasts, chicken, and hamburger. When traveling, especially out of the country, drink and brush teeth with bottled water and eat only washed and then peeled fruits and vegetables. Avoid iced drinks, and never drink untreated water.
- Avoid high-risk foods, such as raw seafood, raw eggs, unpasteurized dairy products, and undercooked poultry and beef.
- Avoid foods that have sat out at room temperature for more than 2 hours.
- Defrost meats in the microwave or refrigerator, not at room temperature.
- Cook foods to the proper temperature.
- Avoid holding foods too long on steam tables or without refrigeration.

REFERENCES

1. Centers for Disease control (U.S.). Burden of foodborne illness. Findings. Retrieved from www.cdc.gov/foodborneburden/2011-foodborne-estimates .html on Jan 10, 2018. Page updated November 2018.

2. Dewey-Mattia, D., Manikonda, K., Hall, A. J., Wise, M. E., & Crowe, S. J. (2018). Surveillance for foodborne disease outbreaks—United States, 2009–2015. *MMWR. Surveillance Summaries: Morbidity and Mortality Weekly Report. Surveillance Summaries, 67*(10), 1–11. doi:10.15585/mmwr.ss6710a1. Published 2018 Jul 27.

3. Shane, A. L., Mody, R. K., Crump, J. A., et al. (2017). 2017 Infectious Disease Society of America: Clinical practice guidelines for the diagnosis and management of infectious diarrhea. *Clinical Infectious Diseases: an Official Publication of the Infectious Diseases Society of America, 65*(12), e45–e80.

4. Bányai, K., Estes, M., Martella, V., & Parashar, U. (2018). Viral gastroenteritis. *The Lancet, 392*(10142), 175–186.

5. Yen, C., Tate, J., Hyde, T., et al. (2014). *Rotavirus* vaccines. *Human Vaccines and Immunotherapies, 10*(6), 1436–1488.

6. Connor, B. Traveler's diarrhea. Centers for Disease Control and Prevention, Yellow Book 2020. Retrieved from https://wwwnc.cdc.gov/travel/yellowbook/2020/preparing-international-travelers/travelers-diarrhea. (Accessed 21 July 2019).

7. Connors, B. A. Traveler's diarrhea: CDC health information for international travel. Retrieved from https://wwwnc.cdc.gov/travel/yellowbook/2018/the-pre-travel-consultation/travelers-diarrhea. (Accessed 15 January 2018).

8. Freedman, S., Jianling, X., Madison, S., et al. (2016). Shiga toxin-producing *E coli* infection, antibiotics and the risk of developing hemolytic uremic syndrome: A meta-analysis. *Clinical Infectious Diseases: an Official Publication of the Infectious Diseases Society of America, 62*(10), 1251–1258.

9. Gunn, J., Marshall, J., Baker, S., et al. (2014). *Salmonella* chronic carriage: Epidemiology, diagnosis and gall bladder persistence. *Trends in Microbiology, 22*(11), 648–655.

10. Angelo, K., Reynolds, J., Karp, B., et al. (2016). Antimicrobial resistance among non-typhoidal *Salmonella* isolated from blood in the US, 2003–2013. *The Journal of Infectious Diseases, 214*(10), 1565–1570.

11. Kaakoush, N. O., Castaño-Rodriquez, N., Mitchel, H. M., & Man, S. M. (2015). Global epidemiology of *Campylobacter* infection. *Clinical Microbiology Reviews, 28*(3), 687–720.

12. Jackson, B. R., Zegarra, J. A., Lopez-Gatell, H., et al. (2011). Binational outbreak of Guillain Barre syndrome associated with *Campylobacter Jejuni* infection, Mexico and USA. *Epidemiology and Infection, 142*, 1089–1099.

13. Centers for Disease Control (U.S.). E coli. Retrieved from https://www.cdc.gov/ecoli/index.html. (Accessed 21 July 2019).

14. Tack, D. M., Marder, E. P., Griffin, P. M., et al. (2019). Preliminary incidence and trends of infections with pathogens transmitted commonly through food—Foodborne Diseases Active Surveillance Network, 10 U.S. sites, 2015–2018. *MMWR. Morbidity and Mortality Weekly Report, 68*, 369–373. Retrieved from http://dx.doi.org/10.15585/mmwr.mm6816a2.

15. Lessa, F., Yi, M., Bamberg, W., et al. (2015). Burden of *Clostridium difficile* infections in the United States. *The New England Journal of Medicine, 372*, 825–834.

16. Bagdasarian, N., Rao, K., & Malani, P. (2015). Diagnosis and Treatment of *Clostridium difficile* in adults: A systematic review. *JAMA: The Journal of the American Medical Association, 313*(4), 398–408.

17. Wilcox, M. H., Gerding, D. N., Poxton, I. R., et al. (*2017*). Bexlotoxumab for prevention or recurrent *Clostridium difficile* infection. *N Eng J Med, 376*(4), 305–317.

18. Kelly, C., Khoruts, A., Staley, C., et al. (2016). Effects of fecal microbiota transplantation on recurrence in multiply recurrent *Clostridium difficile*: A randomized trial. *Annals of Internal Medicine, 165*(9), 609–616.

19. Ajene, A., Fisher Walker, C., & Black, R. (2013). Enteric pathogens and reactive arthritis: A systemic review of *Campylobacter, Salmonella* and *Shigella*-associated reactive arthritis. *Journal of Health, Population, and Nutrition, 31*(3), 299–307.

20. McDonald, E. G., Milligan, J., Frenette, C., & Lee, T. C. (2015). Continuous proton pump inhibition therapy and the associated risk of recurrent *Clostridium difficile* infection. *JAMA Internal Medicine, 175*(5), 784–791.

CHAPTER 212

INFECTIOUS MONONUCLEOSIS

Traci Alberti

 Immediate referral is indicated for drooling; airway compromise due to tonsillar enlargement or suspicion of tonsillar abscess; abdominal pain in the presence of fever, jaundice, or any history of abdominal trauma, including recent contact sport injuries, due to risk of splenic rupture.[1]

DEFINITION AND EPIDEMIOLOGY

Infectious mononucleosis (IM) is an acute, self-limited, generally benign illness that occurs in both children and adults after primary infection with Epstein-Barr virus (EBV), cytomegalovirus (CMV), and other infectious agents. The classic manifestation of this syndrome includes sore throat, fever, cervical lymphadenopathy, fatigue, and atypical lymphocytosis lasting several weeks.[1,2]

The term *Epstein-Barr virus–associated infectious mononucleosis* (EBV-IM) is used to refer to IM caused by acute EBV infection. The term *non–Epstein-Barr virus–associated infectious mononucleosis* (non-EBV-IM) is used to refer to the clinical syndrome of IM that is caused by an agent other than EBV, such as CMV, *Toxoplasma gondii*, adenovirus, or hepatitis virus infection.[2] Non-EBV-IM illnesses account for approximately 10% of all IM cases. IM refers to the triad of fever, pharyngitis, and lymphadenopathy regardless of the infectious agent. This chapter deals primarily with the presentation, evaluation, and management of EBV-IM, the most common type of acute IM, which is seen, at least serologically, in 90% of adolescents and young adults.[1] EBV-IM occurs most often in adolescents and young adults, with the highest incidence occurring at ages 15 to 19 years. In persons younger than 10 years and older than 30 years, the annual incidence of EBV-IM decreases dramatically to less than 1 case per 1000 persons, but mild infection in young adults may be underdiagnosed. It is most common in populations with many young adults, such as active-duty military personnel and college students, in whom the annual incidence ranges from 11 to 48 cases per 1000.[2] The chance for the development of IM after EBV infection appears to increase from childhood to young adulthood; it is estimated that less than 10% of children develop IM after EBV exposure, but up to 78% of adolescents have a chance for development of EBV-IM after acute EBV infection.[3] IM is relatively uncommon in adults, accounting for less than 2% of adults who consult their health care provider for a sore throat.[3]

PATHOPHYSIOLOGY

IM can be caused by a variety of infectious agents other than EBV, including CMV, herpesvirus 6, human immunodeficiency virus (HIV), adenovirus, hepatitis A virus, influenza A and B viruses, and rubella virus.[4] In addition, IM is also associated with some neoplasms. Transmission of IM varies, depending on the specific causative infectious agent. Transmission of EBV-IM occurs through exposure to oropharyngeal secretions, although blood products, genital secretions, and breast milk have also been reported as sources of transmission.[4] EBV is a relatively fragile DNA herpesvirus that cannot survive for long outside the host. The virus initially infects the oral epithelial cells and then spreads to the B lymphocytes, which then circulate through the reticuloendothelial system, causing a significant but time-limited immunologic response. Many of the signs and symptoms associated with the clinical presentation of EBV-IM are the result of this immunologic response. The incubation time of EBV-IM is usually 4 to 8 weeks. Hepatic involvement associated with EBV-IM varies in severity and increases with age, ranging from 10% in young adults to 30% in older adults.[5] Acute EBV infection stimulates the production of antibodies against EBV antigens, which remain present lifelong.

CLINICAL PRESENTATION AND PHYSICAL EXAMINATION

The classic triad of symptoms associated with acute IM includes fever, pharyngitis, and lymphadenopathy. The typical adolescent with EBV-IM is seen with sore throat, fever, and lymph node and tonsillar enlargement. Additional common presenting symptoms include pharyngeal inflammation and transient palatal petechiae. Older adults are less likely to have sore throat and adenopathy but more likely to have hepatomegaly and jaundice.[2] However, IM often manifests atypically, especially in young children and older adults, making diagnosis difficult. Pharyngitis is usually diffuse, with exudates present in approximately 30% of cases.[6] Lymphadenopathy usually affects the anterior and posterior cervical chain and may also be diffuse. Temperatures may be as high as 40°C (104°F), and the elevation may last as long as 2 weeks. Symptoms that may precede as well as persist throughout the acute phase of illness include malaise, anorexia, and fatigue. Symptoms of EBV-IM usually peak approximately 7 days after onset and become less pronounced during the next 1 to 3 weeks. Fatigue can persist for several months. Reports indicate that splenic enlargement occurs in 40% to 100% of cases and can be confirmed with ultrasound.[2,3]

Less common signs and symptoms of EBV-IM include upper airway compromise, abdominal pain, rash, hepatomegaly, jaundice, and eyelid edema. A rash, which occurs in approximately 5% to 10% of individuals, may be macular, urticarial, petechial, or erythema multiforme.[7]

PHYSICAL EXAMINATION

On physical examination, the patient may or may not appear ill, depending on degree of fever, associated signs and symptoms, and length of time since onset of symptoms. The classic clinical manifestation of fever, pharyngitis, and lymphadenopathy raises suspicion for EBV-IM. The anterior and posterior cervical chains should be assessed for lymphadenopathy, which may be diffuse. An abdominal examination identifies splenomegaly and hepatomegaly. Rash and jaundice should be noted because they are associated with EBV-IM, especially in older adults.

DIAGNOSTICS

A complete blood count with differential (CBC) will help identify absolute lymphocytosis, wherein more than 10% of cells are atypical. This is characteristic of IM, but not specific. The most useful laboratory test is the serologic test for heterophil antibodies. This will identify 85% of cases in older children and adults. It is possible for some infected persons to have a negative test result early in the illness, because circulating antibodies have not reached sufficient detectable levels. Repeat

testing in 7 to 10 days is recommended if sy[...]A positive test result may remain positive f[...]initial illness. Absolute lymphocytosis [...]erophil antibody test is diagnostic of acu[...]

If the heterophil antibody test result is nega[...]is still highly suspected, further testing may be helpful. Mo[...]sensitive tests have been developed that detect viral capsid antigen (VCA) and immunoglobulins G (IgG) and M (IgM). When the results are negative, these tests are better than heterophil antibody tests in ruling out EBV-IM because they are better able to detect acute infection; but when the results are positive, the tests are similar in their ability to rule in disease.[6,9] VCA IgG and IgM results typically become positive within 1 to 2 weeks of infection, but VCA IgM becomes undetectable after 6 months. Antibody to Epstein-Barr nuclear antigen (EBNA) is not usually detectable until 6 to 8 weeks after the onset of symptoms but can help distinguish between acute and previous infections. If EBNA is positive in the presence of acute symptoms and suspected IM, then previous infection is suggested. A throat culture should be considered because 3% to 30% of patients with IM also have streptococcal pharyngitis. Liver function tests (LFTs) may also be considered; liver enzymes are elevated in approximately 80% to 90% of persons with IM.[2]

INITIAL DIAGNOSTICS

LABORATORY
- CBC with differential
- Heterophil antibody
- Throat culture

ADDITIONAL DIAGNOSTICS
- VCA IgG and IgM[a]
- EBV nuclear antigen[a]

- CMV[a]
- HIV[a]
- LFT[a]

IMAGING
- Abdominal ultrasonography[a] (to check for splenomegaly)

[a]If indicated.

DIFFERENTIAL DIAGNOSIS

 Primary differentials to be considered include streptococcal pharyngitis, epiglottitis, acute CMV infection, and HIV infection.

The triad of fever, pharyngitis, and lymphadenopathy is associated with a number of diagnoses in addition to acute IM, including streptococcal pharyngitis and any one of several viral pharyngitides, acute CMV infection, and acute HIV infection (Chapter 209).[2] The reported incidence of IM in patients with peritonsillar abscess ranges from 2% to 20%; therefore it is recommended that all patients with pharyngitis and peritonsillar abscess be fully assessed clinically and screened for IM.[10] If symptoms have been present for only a few days, group A β-hemolytic streptococcal pharyngitis or a viral upper respiratory tract infection should be considered. However, individuals with a positive streptococcal culture may also have acute IM. In individuals with a negative throat culture for group A β-hemolytic streptococci, symptoms that persist for more than a week are highly suggestive of acute IM.

Hepatitis A (Chapter 119) is another viral illness that occurs most frequently in children and adolescents, and although incubation routes are different, hepatitis A virus has an

...ubation period (15 to 45 days) similar to that of EBV (30 to 50 days).[11] Hepatitis A typically has an influenza-like onset occurring after a prodrome of myalgia, headache, fever, and malaise. Hepatitis A and IM can also occur concomitantly.

It may not be possible to distinguish clinically between IM caused by EBV infection and an IM-like syndrome caused by toxoplasmosis or CMV infection, and in fact the management of these syndromes is essentially the same. However, diagnostic testing to determine the cause is important in pregnant women because toxoplasmosis and acute HIV and CMV infections are associated with significant pregnancy complications. If acute HIV infection is suspected, a quantitative polymerase chain reaction test should be done.[2]

INTERPROFESSIONAL COLLABORATIVE MANAGEMENT

Nonpharmacological Management

Treatment of uncomplicated EBV-IM is primarily supportive, including rest and adequate hydration. Individuals with splenomegaly should be encouraged to refrain from strenuous physical activity for 3 to 4 weeks to avoid the risk of splenic rupture before resolution of the splenomegaly.[12] Serial ultrasound studies starting at week 2 to 3 may be helpful in determining risk of rupture associated with splenomegaly.

Pharmacological Management

Nonsteroidal anti-inflammatory drugs or acetaminophen for fever reduction and body aches, throat lozenges or sprays, and gargling with a 2% lidocaine solution to relieve pharyngeal discomfort are all used for symptomatic relief. Aspirin should be avoided because it has been associated with Reye syndrome in children in a few cases of acute EBV infection. Studies revealed that neither corticosteroids nor acyclovir reduced the severity or duration of symptoms. Therefore, current management guidelines do not include the use of either of these agents in the treatment of acute uncomplicated EBV-IM, although corticosteroids may be useful in the treatment of several rare but severe complications associated with EBV-IM, such as airway obstruction, thrombocytopenia, or hemolytic anemia.[13]

Indications for Referral and Hospitalization

Most patients with EBV-IM recover uneventfully in approximately 2 to 4 weeks. However, mild liver enzyme abnormalities are not uncommon, and hepatitis is a rare but well-recognized complication of EBV infection that generally resolves spontaneously. IM is rarely seen in older adults; however, the potential for complications appears to increase in the older population, and several cases of severe cholestatic jaundice and fulminant hepatitis associated with IM have been reported in this age group.[5] Abdominal imaging should be obtained in such cases to rule out a malignant extrahepatic biliary obstruction, and acute EBV infection should be considered in patients with cholestasis. Because this complication is rare, it is generally not established until more common causes have been eliminated and serology consistent with EBV infection has been obtained. The rate of peritonsillar abscess has been estimated to be as high as 23%.[8] Peritonsillar abscess can be a medical emergency, requiring surgical drainage and antibiotic therapy. Because of associated dysphagia and possible respiratory compromise, hospitalization may be indicated while treatment is initiated.

LIFE SPAN CONSIDERATIONS

Older individuals are at risk for misdiagnosis of EBV-IM because the disease is relatively uncommon in older adults, occurring in only 3% to 10% of those 40 years of age or older.[4] In addition, older adults with acute IM often manifest the disease differently; fever is present in more than 90% of individuals, but pharyngitis and lymphadenopathy are seen in less than 50% of patients.[4] The risk of EBV-associated liver disease is more common in older adults, and hepatitis, cholestasis, and hepatomegaly are seen in substantial numbers of older adults with EBV-IM. Jaundice is unusual, occurring in approximately 5% of EBV hepatitis cases.[5] Similarly, the risk of EBV-IM–associated hepatic failure and other complications increases with age. Nonetheless, the prognosis for EBV-IM is good even in older individuals.

COMPLICATIONS

Although the majority of individuals with EBV-IM recover uneventfully and without complications, a wide range of complications associated with EBV-IM have been reported. These complications include acute upper airway obstruction, hepatomegaly, splenomegaly, and splenic rupture.

Hepatitis involvement associated with EBV-IM occurs in approximately 10% of young adults and 30% of older adults.[5] EBV infections are often associated with mild hepatocellular hepatitis, but jaundice occurs in only 5% of individuals. Most cases go undetected and resolve spontaneously.

Patients with IM are likely to have splenomegaly, even if it is not detected on physical examination. Because splenomegaly increases the risk of splenic rupture, athletes should not compete in contact or collision sports for 3 to 4 weeks after onset of symptoms. Splenic rupture is estimated at 0.1% on the basis of retrospective studies.[12]

Hematologic complications, particularly thrombocytopenia (25% to 50%) and neutropenia (50% to 80%), are relatively common early in the course of illness.[2] Serious or even life-threatening hematologic complications include aplastic anemia, neutropenia, and thrombocytopenia.

A rash associated with antibiotic administration, particularly amoxicillin and ampicillin, has been documented in 80% to 100% of patients with IM for whom antibacterial agents have been prescribed.[7]

In 1% to 2% of cases, EBV-IM has been associated with neurologic complications, including cranial nerve palsies, Guillain-Barré syndrome (Chapter 176), encephalitis, and peripheral neuropathies.[2]

- In rare cases, EBV-IM has been associated with fatal conduction abnormalities and myocarditis.
- IM is associated with an increased risk of multiple sclerosis irrespective of gender, age, and severity of infection, and the risk persists for at least 30 years after infection.[14]
- Various ophthalmologic problems have been associated with EBV-IM, including keratitis, uveitis, retinopathy, and periorbital cellulitis.
- Complications of EBV-IM can also result in a variety of renal pathologic conditions, including nephritic syndrome, hemolytic-uremic syndrome, and renal failure.
- Additional potential life-threatening complications of IM include epiglottitis with airway obstruction.

The association between EBV-IM and chronic fatigue has been controversial for some time. Transient fatigue is part of acute IM; however, the evidence for EBV-associated chronic fatigue is questionable given that virtually all adults, whether fatigued or not, have evidence of EBV infection. In fact, the Centers for Disease Control and Prevention (CDC) does not consider workup for EBV infection to be useful in the evaluation of individuals with chronic fatigue. More recent studies have implicated slightly increased parameters of inflammation and proinflammatory cytokines and impaired natural killer cell function as contributors to persistent fatigue (see Chapter 202).

PATIENT AND FAMILY EDUCATION

- IM is a viral, self-limited illness. Information about the etiology, illness prognosis, and encouragement about the necessity for rest and schedule/routine changes in first few weeks is important.
- The communicability of IM (i.e., mono is known as the kissing disease) and avoidance of contact with oropharyngeal secretions (shared drinks, etc.) is important.
- Though IM is usually an uncomplicated, self-limited illness, education around possible complications is important so that risk can be avoided (no contact sports) or symptoms may be recognized so that proper treatment can be initiated should complications occur.

REFERENCES

1. Dunmire, S., Hogquist, K., & Balfour, H. (2015). Infectious mononucleosis. *Current Topics in Microbiology and Immunology*, 390, 211–240. doi:10.1007/978-3-319-22822-8_9.
2. Valachis, A., & Kofteridis, D. (2012). Mononucleosis and Epstein-Barr virus infection: Treatment and medication. *Virus Adapt Treat*, 4, 23–28.
3. Centers for Disease Control and Prevention (CDC). Epstein-Barr virus and infectious mononucleosis. https://www.cdc.gov/epstein-barr/index.html, updated May 8, 2018. (Accessed 23 July 2019).
4. MacSween, K. F., & Johannessen, I. (2014). Epstein-Barr virus (EBV): Infectious mononucleosis and other non-malignant EBV associated diseases. In R. Kaslow, L. Stanberry, & J. LeDuc (Eds.), *Viral infections of humans, epidemiology and control*. New York: Springer.
5. Schechter, S., & Lamps, L. (2018). Epstein-barr virus hepatitis: A review of clinicopathologic features and differential diagnosis. *Archives of Pathology & Laboratory Medicine*, 142(10), 1191–1195.
6. Jensen, H. (2011). Epstein-Barr virus. *Pediatrics in Review*, 32(9), 375–384.
7. Forgie, S., & Marrie, T. (2015). Cutaneous eruptions associated with antimicrobials in patients with Infectious Mononucleosis. *The American Journal of Medicine*, 128(1), e1–e2.
8. Ebell, M., Call, M., & Shinholser, J. (2016). Does this patient have mononucleosis? The rational clinical examination systematic review. *JAMA: The Journal of the American Medical Association*, 315(14), 1502–1509.
9. Sidairi, H., Binkhamis, K., Jackson, C., et al. (2017). Comparison of teo automated insturments for Epstein–Barr virus serology in a large adult hospital and implementation of an Epstein–Barr virus nuclear antigen based testing algorithm. *Journal of Medical Microbiolgy*, 66, 1628–1634.
10. Cirilli, A. (2011). Emergency evaluation and management of the sore throat. *Emergency Medicine Clinics of North America*, 31(9), 375–384.
11. World Health Organization (WHO). Hepatitis A. www.who.int/mediacentre/factsheets/fs328/en. Updated June 2014. (Accessed 18 January 2015).
12. Becker, J. A., & Smith, J. A. (2014). Return to play after infectious mononucleosis. *Sports Health*, 6(3), 232–238. doi:10.1177/1941738114521984.
13. Rezk, E., Nofal, Y., & Hamzeh, A. (2015). Steroids for symptom control in Infectious Mononucleosis. *The Cochrane Database of Systematic Reviews*, (11), Art no: CD004402, doi:10.1002/14651858.CD00402.pub3.
14. Lossius, A., Riise, T., Pugliatti, M., et al. (2014). Season of infectious mononucleosis and risk of multiple sclerosis at different latitudes; the EnvIMS Study. *Multiple Sclerosis (Houndmills, Basingstoke, England)*, 20, 669–674.

TICK-BORNE DISEASES

Benjamin P. Chan

INTRODUCTION

Ticks are excellent vectors for disease transmission and can carry and transmit a remarkable array of pathogens, including bacteria, protozoa, and viruses. A single tick bite can also transmit multiple pathogens, a phenomenon that has led to atypical presentations of some classic tick-borne diseases. The blacklegged tick (*Ixodes scapularis*), for example, is able to transmit the pathogens that cause Lyme disease, anaplasmosis, babesiosis, and Powassan.

Most tick-borne diseases have a specific geographic distribution which is dependent on the tick species that transmits that pathogen. In the United States, ticks are the most common agents of vector-borne diseases, and the incidence of tick-borne diseases is increasing, probably related to increased human contact with ticks and tick habitat from the effects of climate change, deforestation, and changes in landscape and wildlife ecology that promotes disease transmission between ticks, animal reservoirs, and humans. The increasing problem of tick-borne diseases is challenging clinicians and public health experts. This chapter focuses on the more prominent tick-borne diseases in the United States. There are other international tick-borne diseases which this chapter does not address, but some of which may be mentioned in Chapter 208, such as tick-borne encephalitis (TBE)

LYME DISEASE

DEFINITION AND EPIDEMIOLOGY

Lyme disease was initially recognized in 1976 when a cluster of children in Lyme, Connecticut, were identified with arthritis, and a previously unrecognized bacterium was isolated from both ticks and patients with the clinical symptoms of what is now referred to as Lyme disease, or Lyme borreliosis.[1] Lyme disease is caused by the bacterium *Borrelia burgdorferi* and is transmitted to humans by the bite of an infected tick. It is the most common vector-borne disease in the United States and in 2015 was the sixth most common nationally notifiable disease. Lyme disease first became a nationally notifiable disease in the United States in 1991, and the number of reported cases steadily increased before peaking in 2009 with more than 38,000 probable and confirmed cases reported to the Centers for Disease Control and Prevention (CDC).[2] Since then, the number of annual reported cases has plateaued, or even decreased slightly (Fig. 213.1), but it is difficult to know if this is due to a true stabilization in the incidence of Lyme disease, or a reflection of the lack of resources at state and local health departments in high incidence areas that have limited follow-up and verification of reported cases of Lyme disease.[2] Lyme disease is also likely underreported as there is not always laboratory verification of infection, and reporting by clinicians, especially of early Lyme disease, is not complete. A recent

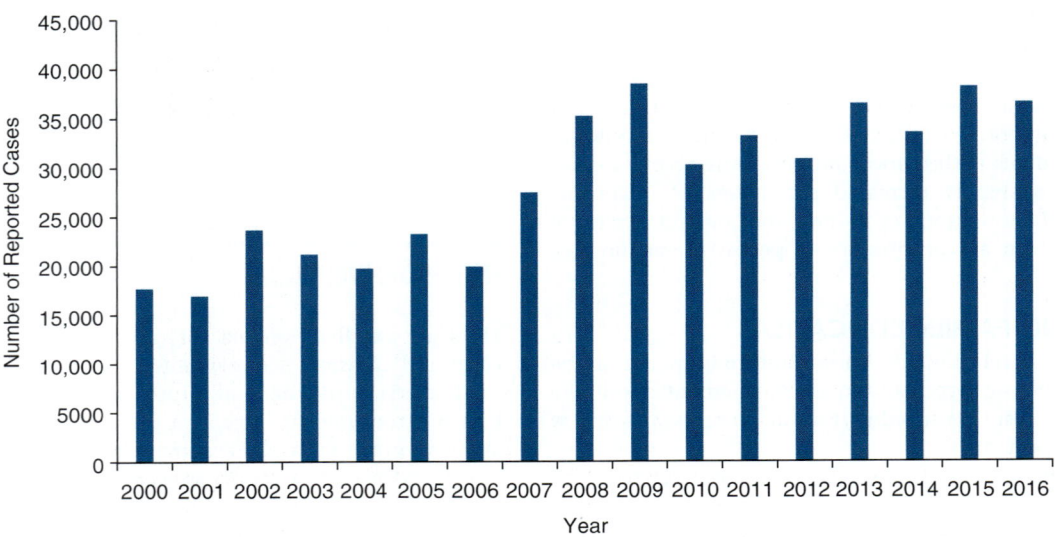

FIG. 213.1   Reported cases of Lyme disease by year in the United States, 2000–2016. The case definition for Lyme disease changed in 2008 to include both confirmed and probable cases; in prior years only confirmed cases of Lyme disease were reported. (Figure created from data available from the Centers for Disease Control and Prevention [CDC]. *Notifiable infectious diseases and conditions data tables*. Retrieved from https://wwwn.cdc.gov/nndss/infectious-tables.html. Accessed January 15, 2018.)

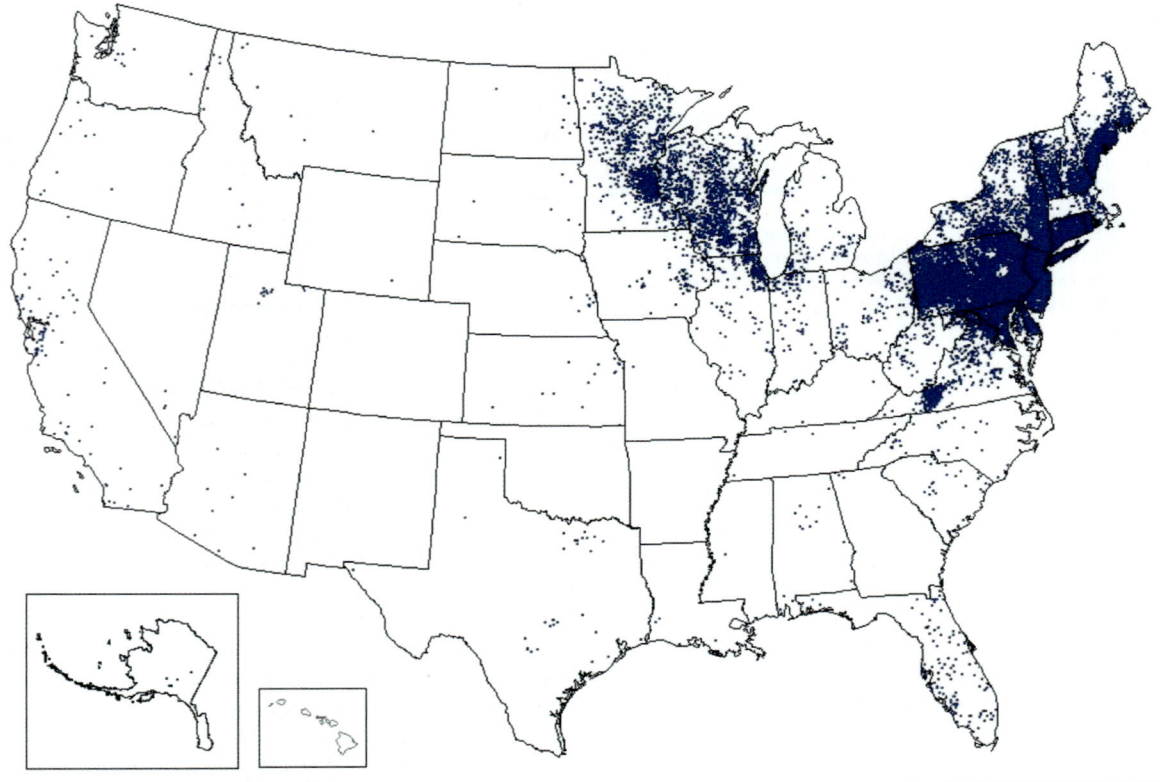

FIG. 213.2   Reported cases of Lyme disease—United States, 2016. (From the Centers for Disease Control and Prevention [CDC]. *Lyme disease maps, 2016*. Retrieved from https://www.cdc.gov/lyme/stats/maps.html. Accessed January 15, 2018.)

analysis of medical insurance claims data estimated that there were likely more than 300,000 Lyme disease cases that occur every year in the United States.[3]

In the United States, Lyme disease typically occurs in the Northeast, mid-Atlantic, and upper Midwest states with 14 states in these regions accounting for more than 95% of all reported cases of Lyme disease (Fig. 213.2).[2] The age distribution of patients with Lyme disease shows a bimodal peak with children aged 5 to 9 and adults aged 50 to 55 having the greatest number of diagnosed infections.[2] Disease onset peaks in the months of June and July, although infection can present year round with different clinical presentations possible depending on the time of the year.[2] Even though Lyme disease diagnoses peak in summer months, the risk to individuals begins months prior during the early spring, even in more northern states, which corresponds to when ticks begin to emerge and begin questing for a blood meal.[4] This highlights the need for a focus on prevention much earlier than the summer months.

PATHOPHYSIOLOGY

Transmission of the *B. burgdorferi* bacterium involves a complex enzootic cycle involving ticks, animal reservoir, and humans.

The vector for transmission of Lyme disease is the *Ixodes* tick species, most commonly *I. scapularis* in the Midwest and Eastern United States.[1] *I. scapularis* is commonly referred to as the blacklegged tick, formerly known as the "deer tick." *Ixodes pacificus*, a less common vector of Lyme disease, is found in the Western United States, where the frequency of disease is lower.[1] The *Ixodes* ticks go through three different stages of development over a two-year life cycle (larval, nymphal, and adult stages), and the tick requires a blood meal at each stage of its life cycle. Small rodents, such as mice and chipmunks, serve as the primary host for larval and nymphal ticks in the United States, hence these mammals serve as the primary reservoir of *B. burgdorferi*. Because both larval and nymphal ticks feed on the same hosts, the small rodents are important for maintaining horizontal transmission of *B. burgdorferi* from infected nymphs to the larval ticks.[1] Deer are not essential to the life cycle of *B. burgdorferi*, but they are the primary host of adult *Ixodes* ticks and is where mating between adult ticks occurs, so deer are important in the life cycle of the tick and for maintaining tick populations.[1]

B. burgdorferi bacteria colonize the midgut of infected ticks, and when ticks take a blood meal, the *B. burgdorferi* migrate from the midgut of the tick, to the salivary glands, and into the host, which takes more than 36 hours of attachment.[1] This delay between tick bite and transmission has important implications for prevention of infection. Once the *B. burgdorferi* bacteria inoculate the skin, they multiply and spread locally at the site of the tick bite before disseminating through blood and the lymphatic system.[1] This local and systemic spread accounts for the different stages of Lyme disease.

CLINICAL PRESENTATION AND PHYSICAL EXAMINATION

The clinical characteristics of Lyme disease can be divided into three stages: early localized infection, early disseminated infection, and late persistent infection. The tick bite site often initially presents with a small area of erythema which does not necessarily indicate infection, but can be due to an inflammatory reaction to the bite itself. Early localized infection (Stage 1) is characterized by an enlarging erythematous circular rash around the site of the tick bite called erythema migrans (EM; Fig. 213.3). The EM rash initially starts with a homogenous appearance but as it expands often (but not always) develops an area of central clearing giving it a "bulls-eye" appearance. The EM rash usually develops within 1 to 2 weeks of the tick bite, but can occur anywhere from 3 to 30 days after a tick bite.[5,6] The EM rash occurs in 70% to 80% of patients infected with Lyme disease.[2,7] Patients may describe this lesion as burning, itchy, or painful, although it may also be minimally symptomatic or asymptomatic, and hence go unrecognized depending on location.[5] Erythema at the site of a tick bite can occur anywhere on the body but is commonly found

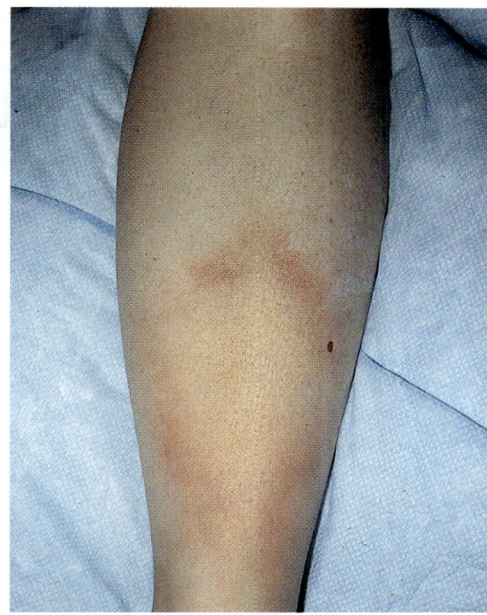

FIG. **213.3** Erythema migrans. (From Habif, T. P. [2001]. *Skin disease: diagnosis and treatment.* St Louis, MO: Mosby.)

on the thigh, groin, and axilla, given the propensity for ticks to migrate to warm, moist areas of the body.[5] The EM rash may be accompanied by nonspecific flu-like illness symptoms of fatigue, malaise, lethargy, fevers, headache, arthralgias, myalgias, and regional lymphadenopathy, which are early signs that the bacteria are starting to disseminate.[5,7]

Early disseminated infection (Stage 2) occurs within several days to weeks of infection as the *B. burgdorferi* bacteria spread from the site of the tick bite to other areas of the body.[2] Patients with disseminated infection can present with multiple EM lesions at skin sites other than the site of the initial tick bite. Neurologic and cardiac complications are also a hallmark of early disseminated infection. If untreated, 10% to 15% of patients may develop early neurologic abnormalities, and less commonly myopericarditis, which usually presents as heart block and bradycardia to some degree.[6] Early neurologic manifestations of disseminated disease include lymphocytic meningitis (headache and neck stiffness), cranial nerve palsies (especially facial nerve, or Bell palsy), and motor or sensory neuritis (including radiculoneuritis and mononeuritis multiplex).[1,6] Less commonly patients may present with symptoms of cerebellar ataxia or encephalomyelitis.[1] While Lyme disease is not usually fatal, Lyme carditis is the one instance in which death rarely may occur and should not be missed on assessment of a patient with early disseminated disease.[8]

Late persistent infection (Stage 3) occurs months after infection and usually manifests as intermittent attacks of arthritis with swelling and pain of the large joints, especially the knees.[1] The CDC in their national Lyme surveillance report noted that approximately 28% of reported cases of Lyme disease in the United States had arthritis at the time of presentation, although this number may be subject to reporting bias and misclassification of arthralgias as Lyme arthritis.[2] Less commonly, late neurologic complications have also been reported which often manifest as encephalopathy (subtle memory and cognitive changes) and/or polyneuropathy.[1]

Overall, the most commonly reported presenting clinical manifestation of Lyme disease is an EM rash, followed by arthritis; however, it is important to note that clinical presentation may differ depending on the time of year.[2] EM is the most common presenting sign/symptom reported for individuals diagnosed between April to November, but arthritis is the most common clinical presentation during the colder months of December to March.[2] Therefore, Lyme disease should be considered at all times of the year in patients presenting with compatible signs and symptoms of disease.

DIAGNOSTICS

Laboratory diagnosis of Lyme disease is most often made through detection of antibodies against the *B. burgdorferi* bacterium (serologic testing). Within the first couple weeks of infection, however, antibodies may not yet be present, and visual inspection of the skin and identification of an EM rash is the main method to diagnose Lyme disease; EM is the only sign or symptom of Lyme disease which is classic enough to allow for diagnosis based on clinical presentation alone.[9] Therefore, in a patient who has an epidemiologic risk for Lyme disease, and who presents with a distinctive EM rash, no further testing is required and the patient can be treated for early Lyme disease. To help differentiate an EM rash from a tick bite hypersensitivity reaction, the area of erythema should be 5 cm or larger in diameter.[6] Any diagnosis of Lyme disease, including patients clinically diagnosed with an EM rash, should be reported to the local or state health department.

For serologic testing, the CDC and the Infectious Diseases Society of America (IDSA) recommend a two-step testing algorithm starting with a sensitive assay, usually an enzyme-linked immunosorbent assay (ELISA), and if positive or equivocal, the serum should be tested with separate IgM and IgG Western blot (WB) assays, which are more specific confirmatory tests (Fig. 213.4).[9,10] For results to be considered positive, an IgM WB must have 2 out of 3 specific bands present, and an IgG WB is considered positive if at least 5 out of 10 specific bands

are present.[10] About 70% to 80% of individuals will develop antibodies to *B. burgdorferi* 2 to 3 weeks after infection, usually IgM antibodies, and almost 100% of infected individuals will develop IgG antibodies within 4 to 8 weeks after infection if not treated.[1] Therefore, if a patient presents with signs or symptoms of Lyme disease within the first month of illness and has a positive or equivocal Lyme ELISA, both an IgM and IgG WB should be used as the second step in testing to confirm Lyme disease.[10] If a patient presents within the first month of illness and has a negative Lyme ELISA, the provider can consider follow-up convalescent serum testing to diagnose Lyme disease. If a patient presents more than one month after onset of symptoms and has a positive or equivocal ELISA, only the IgG WB should be used for confirmation because an isolated IgM positive WB after one month has a high likelihood of being a false-positive (see Fig. 213.4).[6,9,10] Individuals with disseminated or late-stage Lyme disease should have a positive IgG antibody response.[10]

Clinicians should not order a Lyme WB test without a positive or equivocal ELISA (i.e., should not use a positive WB alone to diagnose Lyme disease), and clinicians should avoid using unvalidated interpretive criteria for WB assays, which some independent laboratories have developed.[1,6] Finally, there is no good test to monitor for treatment response to antibiotics and no test of cure. The current serologic tests for Lyme disease measure antibodies against the *B. burgdorferi* bacteria, and both IgM and IgG antibodies can persist for months to years after infection.[11,12] One study found that one-third of patients diagnosed with early Lyme disease had positive IgM or IgG antibodies to *B. burgdorferi* 10 to 20 years after infection.[12] The persistence of an antibody response may also lead clinicians to incorrectly attribute a patient's symptoms to Lyme disease, and any interpretation of a Lyme test needs to involve a careful clinical history and assessment.

In an attempt to simplify the two-step testing process, newer tests have been developed. One test that may be in clinical use is the C6 peptide ELISA, which tests for antibody response to

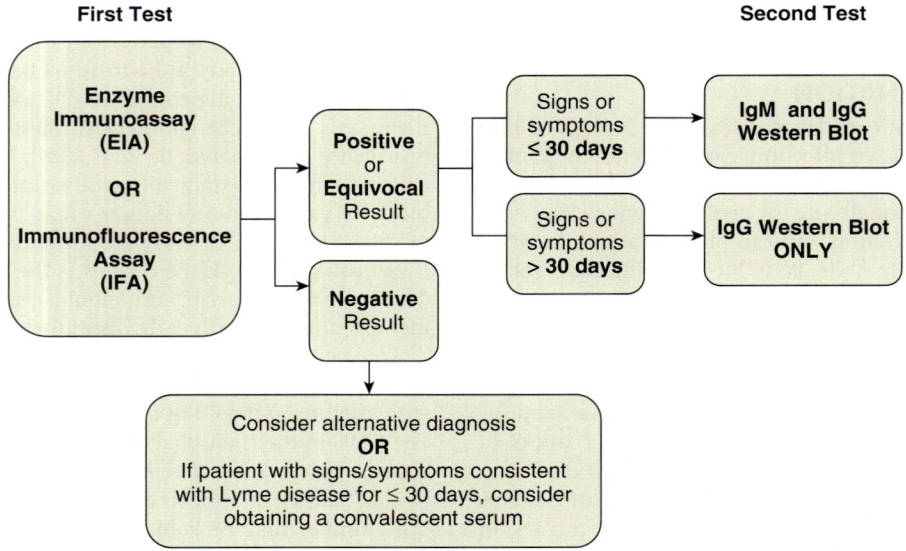

FIG. 213.4 Centers for Disease Control and Prevention's two-tiered testing algorithm for Lyme disease. (From the Centers for Disease Control and Prevention [CDC]. *Lyme disease: Two-step laboratory testing process.* Retrieved from https://www.cdc.gov/lyme/diagnosistesting/labtest/twostep/index.html. Accessed January 15, 2018.)

a portion of the *B. burgdorferi* VlsE protein, and has shown greater sensitivity to detect antibody response in early disease, although with decreased specificity.[13] Therefore, use of the C6 peptide ELISA as a standalone test is still not recommended, but some laboratories may incorporate the C6 peptide ELISA into a two-step algorithm.[6]

For patients with symptoms of neurological disease, a lumbar puncture should be considered to test for cerebrospinal fluid (CSF) antibody production to *B. burgdorferi*; however, because *B. burgdorferi* antibodies can passively move from the serum into CSF, tests for CSF antibodies need to be corrected for serum antibody levels (Lyme disease antibody index).[6,9] Testing CSF for *B. burgdorferi* by polymerase chain reaction (PCR) is also possible, but this is not a very sensitive test on CSF; therefore, PCR is only helpful if positive, and a negative test does not exclude disease.[9] If a lumbar puncture is obtained for evaluation of neurological disease, CSF should also be sent for the usual gram stain and culture, cell count with differential, protein, and glucose.

In patients presenting with Lyme arthritis, arthrocentesis should be considered and synovial fluid should be sent for *B. burgdorferi* PCR (which has a much higher sensitivity compared to CSF PCR testing) in addition to other typical synovial fluid tests including cell count with differential, crystal analysis, and bacterial gram stain and culture.[6,9]

INITIAL DIAGNOSTICS

Lyme Disease

LABORATORY
- Lyme ELISA to detect antibodies against *Borrelia burgdorferi*, followed by a confirmatory WB if ELISA is positive or equivocal
- Lyme antibody index on CSF if lumbar puncture is performed for evaluation of neurologic disease
- PCR assay on synovial fluid to identify *Borrelia burgdorferi* DNA if arthrocentesis is performed for evaluation of Lyme arthritis

DIFFERENTIAL DIAGNOSIS

 It is important to differentiate an erythema migrans (EM) rash from other potential etiologies including a tick bite hypersensitivity reaction and bacterial cellulitis.

The differential diagnoses for Lyme disease vary according to the stage of disease. In early localized disease, an early EM rash is most likely to be confused with a tick bite hypersensitivity reaction. An early EM rash or tick-bite hypersensitivity reaction may also be confused for a bacterial cellulitis. Multiple secondary EM lesions during early disseminated disease may have the appearance of erythema multiforme. A careful history and examination, including assessing lesion size, evolution, and associated symptoms should help differentiate potential etiologies. An EM rash is usually circular, expanding, and 5 cm or more in diameter.[6]

Cranial nerve VII palsies (facial palsies) that may be seen in early disseminated Lyme disease can also be seen with herpes simplex type 1 virus or varicella-zoster virus. Neurologic Lyme disease presenting as meningitis may be confused with other bacterial or viral causes of meningitis. Lyme arthritis may be confused with a reactive arthritis from a bacterial infection (i.e., septic arthritis) or other non-infectious inflammatory arthritis, such as gout or pseudogout. In children Lyme arthritis

may resemble pauciarticular juvenile rheumatoid arthritis. Clinical assessment with arthrocentesis can help differentiate these causes. Some patients may have nonspecific complaints, including chronic fatigue, joint or muscle aches, neurocognitive changes, and difficulty sleeping that occur for months to years after a tick bite, and may resemble a chronic fatigue syndrome or fibromyalgia. These individuals warrant an evaluation for untreated Lyme disease as well as other possible causes of their chronic symptoms.

INTERPROFESSIONAL COLLABORATIVE MANAGEMENT
Pharmacologic Management

Treatment guidelines, as recommended by the IDSA, vary by stage of disease, but all stages are curable with appropriate antibiotic therapy. For early Lyme disease without signs or symptoms of neurologic or cardiac involvement, the recommended antibiotics are doxycycline, amoxicillin, or cefuroxime.[6,9] Doxycycline is relatively contraindicated for pregnant or lactating women and children younger than eight years of age; however, when able to be used, doxycycline is often preferred (dosing in adults: 100 mg orally twice a day; children: 4 mg/kg total daily dose in two divided doses up to a maximum of 100 mg per dose) because of less frequent dosing compared to amoxicillin, and because doxycycline will treat potential co-infection with human granulocytic anaplasmosis (HGA) and human monocytic ehrlichiosis (HME).[9] Amoxicillin (dosing in adults: 500 mg three times a day; children: 50 mg/kg total daily dose in three divided doses up to a maximum of 500 mg per dose) and cefuroxime (dosing in adults: 500 mg twice a day; children: 30 mg/kg total daily dose in two divided doses up to a maximum of 500 mg per dose) are also acceptable for those with a relative contraindication or allergy to doxycycline.[9] First-generation cephalosporin antibiotics (e.g., cephalexin) are not effective against *B. burgdorferi* and should not be used.[9] The IDSA recommended treatment duration for early Lyme disease is 14 days[9]; however, more recent studies have shown that 10 days of doxycycline is sufficient and treatment outcomes are comparable to those treated with longer courses.[6,14,15]

For patients with Lyme disease who have early neurologic manifestations, ceftriaxone (dosing in adults: 2 grams intravenously once daily; children: 50 to 75 mg/kg intravenously once daily in a single dose with a maximum dose of 2 grams) is recommended for 14 days.[6,9] Due to its good absorption, oral doxycycline for 14 days is also probably adequate therapy for early neurologic Lyme disease in patients not needing hospitalization and can be considered for those with a cephalosporin allergy.[6,9] Patients presenting with cranial nerve palsies, such as cranial nerve VII palsy, who do not have other evidence of aseptic meningitis or central nervous system involvement (i.e., patients with normal CSF examination or in whom CSF examination is not considered necessary because of lack of clinical signs/symptoms of meningitis) can be treated for 14 days with any of the antibiotics used to treat EM rash.[6,9]

Lyme carditis can be treated with oral or parenteral antibiotics for 14 days, although patients with symptomatic myopericarditis (i.e., syncope, dyspnea, chest pain), or who have evidence of advanced heart block warrant hospitalization, continuous monitoring, and intravenous antibiotic therapy (e.g., ceftriaxone) to start.[6,9] When hospitalized patients are ready for discharge, they can be transitioned to one of the above mentioned oral antibiotics to complete their course of therapy.[9]

Complete heart block from Lyme carditis usually resolves within a week of starting antibiotics, although lesser degrees of heart block can take up to 6 weeks after antibiotics to completely resolve.[9]

Initial treatment for Lyme arthritis is recommended with one of the oral antibiotic regimens (i.e., doxycycline, amoxicillin, or cefuroxime) for 28 days; however, Lyme arthritis is the one Lyme disease syndrome where re-treatment may be required if symptoms of joint pain and swelling do not fully resolve.[9] Because symptomatic improvement will lag behind antibiotic treatment, clinicians may want to wait a period of time to see if symptoms improve before reinstituting antibiotic therapy. For those who continue to have persistent or recurrent joint swelling after an initial 28-day course of therapy, repeat therapy with either another 28 days of oral antibiotics, or 14 to 28 days of an intravenous antibiotic (e.g., ceftriaxone) is recommended.[9] For those who show some improvement after the initial antibiotic course, another 28 days of an oral antibiotic is appropriate, but for those who failed to improve at all or worsened, intravenous antibiotics are preferred.[9]

For symptoms of late neurologic Lyme disease (e.g., neuropathy, cognitive and memory impairment), because symptoms can be vague and nonspecific, patients need objective evidence of Lyme disease. This includes serologic evidence of infection (by the two-step testing) and CSF abnormalities, including evidence of CSF antibody production. For patients with objective evidence of neurologic Lyme disease, treatment with ceftriaxone is recommended for 14 days, similar to treatment for early neurologic Lyme disease.[9]

Symptom resolution can lag behind treatment, so persistence of or slowly resolving symptoms is not a reason to necessarily prolong treatment.[9,15] Some patients may develop chronic symptoms that last for 6 months or longer, including fatigue, musculoskeletal pain, neurologic symptoms, changes in memory and cognition; symptoms may resemble fibromyalgia or chronic fatigue syndrome. These persistent symptoms have sometimes been called "chronic Lyme disease"; however, there is no evidence of persistent infection, and multiple well designed clinical trials evaluating longer antibiotic therapy have not shown evidence of substantial or sustained benefit.[9,16-18] Therefore, the favored term for individuals who report chronic symptoms for at least six months or longer is post-Lyme disease syndrome (PLDS).[9,16] It is important to note that while some clinicians choose to treat patients with longer than recommended courses of antibiotics for "chronic Lyme disease," antibiotic use can have adverse patient outcomes, including misdiagnosis, the development of antibiotic-resistant bacteria, antibiotic toxicity, and secondary infections from the antibiotics (e.g., Clostridium difficile infection) or the central venous catheters used to administer them (e.g., bacterial blood stream infections).[19,20] Therefore, antibiotics need to be used judiciously.

Nonpharmacologic Management

Patients who may have persistent symptoms indicative of possible PLDS need a clinical evaluation for other potential causes of their symptoms, and if none are found then focus on symptom control is recommended.[9] Specifically, in patients with Lyme arthritis who have no resolution of symptoms despite parenteral therapy and if results of PCR testing of synovial fluid are negative, symptomatic treatment with nonsteroidal anti-inflammatory agents, intra-articular injections

of corticosteroids, or disease-modifying antirheumatic drugs along with referral to a rheumatologist should be considered.[9] If synovitis is limiting functioning and activities of daily living, arthroscopic synovectomy may help reduce symptoms and joint inflammation.[9] For patients with Lyme carditis experiencing advanced heart block, a temporary pacemaker may be required but can be discontinued when the heart block resolves so a permanent pacemaker should not be placed by a cardiologist.[9]

Indications for Referral and Hospitalization

Most stages of Lyme disease are not life threatening and do not require hospitalization. The exception, however, is in patients with Lyme carditis with advanced heart block who should be hospitalized for monitoring and treatment. Hospitalization should also involve consultation with a cardiologist because patients may need a temporary pacemaker placed until heart block improves. Patients presenting with acute neurologic symptoms, such as meningitis, should also be hospitalized for testing and treatment while a work-up is performed since some bacterial causes of meningitis can be life threatening.

For patients with persistent synovitis and symptoms of Lyme arthritis, referral to a rheumatologist may be needed for symptom-focused management if a patient does not fully respond to the recommended antibiotic course.[9] If persistent synovitis is affecting quality of life and normal activities of daily living, a referral to an orthopedic surgeon for consideration of arthroscopic synovectomy could be considered.[9]

COMPLICATIONS

There has been much controversy over the cause of PLDS. When patients with persistent symptoms are evaluated, it is necessary to begin with objective evidence of having had B. burgdorferi infection with positive ELISA and IgG WB testing and to treat according to evidence-based treatment guidelines published by the IDSA. Because there is no evidence to support the presence of an ongoing B. burgdorferi infection among patients who have completed the recommended treatment regimens for Lyme disease, further antibiotic treatment is not indicated for patients with chronic subjective symptoms, as discussed above.

Unfortunately, patients who have been treated for Lyme disease can subsequently become reinfected with Lyme disease from a new tick bite. Reinfection is clinically evident by a repeated episode of EM at a skin site different from the previous episode, and reinfection usually occurs during spring and summer months when the nymphal stage of the tick vector is abundant in the environment. As previously discussed, because IgM and IgG antibodies to B. burgdorferi can remain elevated for years, serologic testing is not useful in differentiating reinfection from initial infection; therefore, careful clinical assessment is needed when assessing clinical symptoms and interpreting laboratory tests.

Coinfection with other tick-borne disease, especially Babesia microti and Anaplasma phagocytophilum, may also occur in patients in areas where these pathogens are endemic, complicating the clinical picture. Like B. burgdorferi, these organisms are also transmitted by Ixodes tick species. Diagnostic testing for coinfection should be considered in patients whose initial symptoms are more severe than typical early Lyme disease or who have high-grade fevers for more than 48 hours despite appropriate antibiotic therapy; those who have symptoms resembling a viral infection that fail to improve or worsen despite resolution of the EM skin lesion; and those with leukopenia, thrombocytopenia, or anemia.[9] These organisms will be further discussed in upcoming sections of the chapter.

PATIENT AND FAMILY EDUCATION

All patients and family should be provided with information about preventing tick bites, which is the most important way to prevent development of Lyme disease and other tick-borne diseases (see below). It is also important to educate patients and families about the proper technique to remove ticks. For those who are bitten by ticks, in addition to consideration of antibiotic prophylaxis to prevent Lyme disease (see below), instructions should be provided to educate patients on the signs and symptoms of Lyme disease in case they develop infection and need treatment. Finally, for patients who are diagnosed with Lyme disease, because there may be incorrect patient assumptions about Lyme disease and the long-term efficacy of treatment, education may be needed about the good efficacy of short courses of antibiotics to cure infection. Education may also be needed about PLDS.

HEALTH PROMOTION AND PREVENTION

There is no available Lyme disease vaccine for humans. Prevention of Lyme disease, therefore, needs to focus on prevention of tick bites. Tick bites can be prevented when outdoors by avoiding walking through or playing in tick habitat, including areas with high grass or brush; wearing long pants and sleeves to cover exposed skin; using a repellant effective against ticks, including formulations containing 20% or more of DEET, picaridin, or IR3535; and use of permethrin to treat clothing prior to going outdoors.[21] Tick repellants meant for skin application may need to be reapplied every few hours and product instructions should be followed closely. After coming in from outdoors, tick checks should be performed on humans, pets, clothing, and gear. Showering within a couple hours can also help remove unattached ticks.[21] Because ticks are susceptible to desiccation, drying clothes in the dryer on high heat is effective at quickly killing ticks attached to clothing. Clothes that are already dry can be placed in the dryer on high for 10 minutes to kill any attached ticks; wet clothing (from washing, swimming, or sweat) may require longer drying times, up to 60 minutes if clothes are washed first.[21,22] These drying times are recommended for I. scapularis ticks; other ticks, such as Amblyomma americanum ticks (lone star ticks) which can transmit other tick-borne diseases discussed below, may be more resistant to low humidity and drying, and could potentially survive longer in dryers.[22] There are also steps that homeowners can take to minimize potential outdoor contact with ticks by reducing tick habitat and migration of ticks into the yard. Steps can include clearing leaf litter, tall grass, and brush from around the yard and keeping lawns mowed frequently. A three foot wide border of gravel or wood chips around the property between the lawn and wooded areas can help prevent migration of ticks from edge habitat into yards where children are more likely to play.[21]

If a person is found to have been bitten by an I. scapularis tick, there is chemoprophylaxis available under certain conditions to prevent development of Lyme disease. A single dose of doxycycline 200 mg orally given within 72 hours of an I. scapularis tick bite has been shown to be 87% effective at preventing the development of EM.[23] Antibiotic prophylaxis (doxycycline, 200 mg orally in a single dose), therefore, can be considered when all of the following conditions are met: (1) the attached tick can be reliably identified as an adult or nymphal I. scapularis

tick, and it has been attached for 36 hours or more on the basis of engorgement or history of potential tick exposures; (2) prophylaxis can be started within 72 hours of tick removal; (3) the local rate of infection of I. scapularis ticks with B. burgdorferi is at least 20%; and (4) there is no contraindication to the use of doxycycline (doxycycline is relatively contraindicated in pregnant or lactating women and children under eight years of age).[9] Substitution of doxycycline with other antibiotics (e.g., amoxicillin) is not recommended for prophylaxis because of the absence of data supporting the use of other antibiotics for short-course antibiotic prophylaxis, the likely need for multi-day regimens given the shorter half-life of other antibiotics, the potential associated adverse side effects from antibiotics, and the excellent efficacy at treating early Lyme disease if symptoms were to develop after a tick bite.[9] Patients who have removed attached ticks should be monitored closely for signs and symptoms of tick-borne disease for up to 30 days.[9] This includes development or expansion of a skin lesion at the site of the tick bite or development of a viral-like illness.

BABESIOSIS

DEFINITION AND EPIDEMIOLOGY

Babesiosis is a disease caused by protozoan parasites of the genus Babesia that infect and lyse erythrocytes.

There are more than 100 species of Babesia that infect animals; however, very few are known to cause disease in humans, and most reported cases of babesiosis in the United States have been with B. microti, which is the focus of the information presented here.[24–26] B. microti is transmitted by the I. scapularis tick, which also transmits B. burgdorferi and A. phagocytophilum; therefore the geographic distribution of B. microti infection is similar to Lyme disease, although the incidence of babesiosis is far lower than Lyme disease (Fig. 213.5). Sporadic cases of babesiosis caused by other Babesia species have been reported along the Pacific coast; the tick vector is unknown, although I. pacificus is the main candidate which is similar to transmission of Lyme disease.[24]

Babesiosis was first added to the nationally notifiable disease list with a standard case definition in 2011; at that time only 18 states reported babesiosis nationally.[26] By 2015, 33 states were reporting babesiosis with more than 2000 probable and confirmed cases reported in the United States for 2015; however, 93% of reported cases were from only seven states in the Northeast (Connecticut, Massachusetts, New Jersey, New York, Rhode Island) and upper Midwest (Wisconsin and Minnesota).[27] While the increase in numbers of babesiosis every year (see Fig. 213.5) is likely partly due to improved surveillance and reporting, the geographic range of human babesiosis has been slowly expanding.[25] Most cases of babesiosis occur in the spring and summer months from June to August, although patients can present with infection year-round.[26–28]

PATHOPHYSIOLOGY

Similar to Lyme disease, I. scapularis ticks are the primary vector for transmission of B. microti. Small rodents, especially the white-footed mouse, are the primary host for larval and nymphal I. scapularis ticks, and serve as the primary reservoir of B. microti, maintaining horizontal transmission between infected nymph and larval ticks.[24,25] White-tailed deer are important to the adult life cycle of the I. scapularis ticks, but

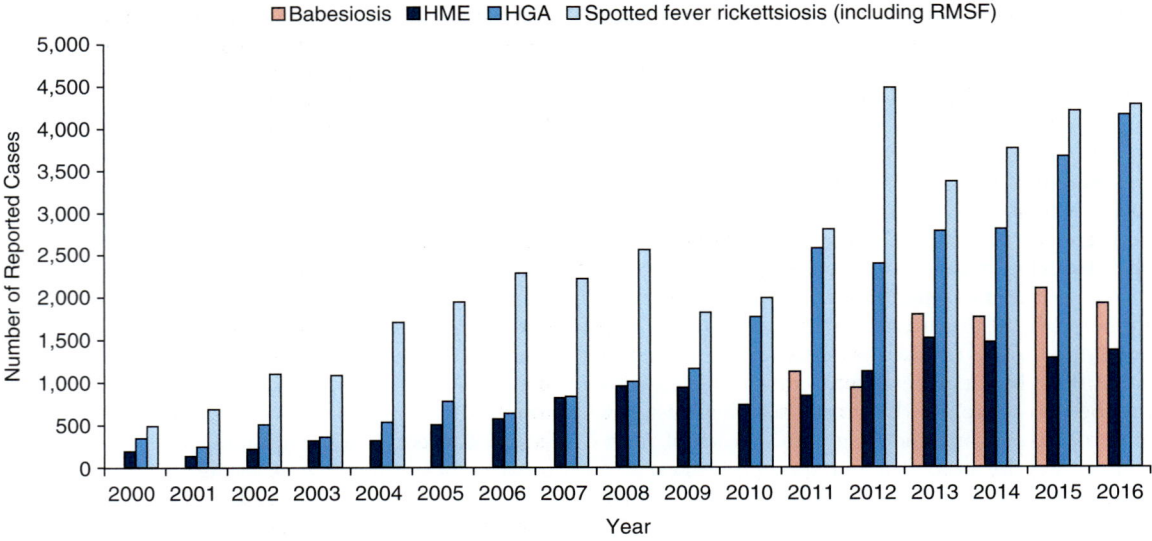

FIG. **213.5**   Reported cases of babesiosis, HME, HGA, and spotted fever rickettsiosis (including Rocky Mountain spotted fever) by year in the United States, 2000–2016. Because serologic tests commonly used to diagnose Rocky Mountain spotted fever *(RMSF)* cross-react with other spotted fever rickettsial pathogens, some diagnosed cases of RMSF may actually be due to other spotted fever rickettsial infections. To more accurately reflect the limitations of diagnostic testing, the surveillance case definition was changed from "Rocky Mountain spotted fever" to "spotted fever rickettsiosis" beginning in 2010. *HGA,* human granulocytic anaplasmosis; *HME,* human monocytic ehrlichiosis. (Figure created from data available from the Centers for Disease Control and Prevention [CDC]. *Notifiable infectious diseases and conditions data tables.* Retrieved from https://wwwn.cdc.gov/nndss/infectious-tables.html. Accessed January 15, 2018.)

they do not serve as a reservoir of *B. microti.*[24,25] When an *Ixodes* tick takes a blood meal from an infected host, *B. microti* crosses out of the tick's gut and spreads to the salivary glands. When the infected tick bites a host, it takes about 36 to 72 hours for *B. microti* to be deposited into the dermis.[25] *B. microti* subsequently infects erythrocytes where the parasite develops, lyses the cells, and infects other erythrocytes thereby propagating infection.[25]

Babesia can also be transmitted transplacentally from mother to fetus, and through blood transfusion.[25,26,28] Because infected patients can harbor circulating parasites for months to years without symptoms, patients may unknowingly transmit the organisms through blood transfusions.[28] From 1979 through 2009, 162 cases of transfusion-associated *Babesia* infection were reported, mostly from *B. microti* (98%), and most cases (77%) have been reported since 2000.[28,29] Unfortunately, blood donors can be asymptomatic but infectious at the time of blood donation, and *Babesia* species can survive blood-banking processing procedures and storage.[28,29] There is no Food and Drug Administration (FDA) test currently approved for screening blood donations for *Babesia,* but screening protocols are being investigated.[28]

CLINICAL PRESENTATION AND PHYSICAL EXAMINATION

Babesiosis can present anywhere from asymptomatic infection to severe life-threatening illness leading to death. One-fifth to one-half of persons infected have been reported to have asymptomatic infection.[25] For those who do develop symptoms, young and otherwise healthy individuals are more likely to have mild to moderate illness, whereas those who are older than 50 years of age, have comorbidities, are immunocompromised, or are asplenic are at risk for more severe disease.[25] Incubation after a tick bite is usually 1 to 4 weeks

before onset of symptoms, although the incubation period can be longer for those infected through blood transfusion.[25]

In most cases of mild to moderate disease, patients develop a viral or influenza-like illness typically with fever, malaise, fatigue, and possibly other nonspecific symptoms such as headache, myalgia, arthralgia, nausea, and anorexia.[25] In mild cases, symptoms may resolve without therapy within a couple weeks; however, fatigue and malaise may persist for months.[5] On physical examination, mild hepatosplenomegaly may be found. Laboratory testing often shows hemolytic anemia, thrombocytopenia, and elevation of hepatic transaminases.[25]

Patients who develop severe disease can develop complications including severe anemia, acute respiratory failure, disseminated intravascular coagulation (DIC), congestive heart failure, liver and renal failure, and splenic rupture.[25] Death occurs in up to 10% of hospitalized patients, but can be higher in those who are immunocompromised.[24,25] Patients with risk factors for severe disease may develop persistent or relapsing infection, and may require a longer treatment course.[25]

DIAGNOSTICS

Because symptoms of babesiosis are nonspecific, diagnosis requires a strong clinical suspicion based on consistent symptoms and epidemiologic exposure in order to initiate diagnostic testing. Babesiosis should also be considered in patients diagnosed with Lyme disease or HGA who are not improving with standard therapy because co-infection can occur.[9]

Babesia organisms go through different stages of development within erythrocytes, and diagnosis of babesiosis can be made by identification of *Babesia* forms on Giemsa or Wright stained thin blood smears.[6] Trophozoites appear as round or oval ring forms which are most commonly seen on blood smear and can resemble *Plasmodium falciparum* trophozoites.[25] Trophozoites develop into merozoites which can form the less commonly seen tetrads classically known as the Maltese cross, which is pathognomonic for babesiosis.[25] Parasitemia can be low, especially in early infection, so multiple blood smears may need to be examined for a diagnosis to be made.

Detection of *Babesia* DNA in the blood through PCR is available and more sensitive to detect early infection when there may be low parasitemia.[6,25] Serologic testing, most commonly through an indirect immunofluorescence assay (IFA), can also be useful to support a diagnosis of babesiosis, but does not necessarily differentiate between recent and past infection because *Babesia* antibodies may be absent in early infection and can persist for months to years.[6,25] A four-fold rise in *Babesia* IgG antibody titers, however, between acute and convalescent sera is confirmatory of recent infection, and IgG antibody titers greater than 1 : 1024 are also indicative of active or recent infection.[6,25]

INITIAL DIAGNOSTICS

Babesiosis

LABORATORY
- Thin blood smear to identify intra-erythrocytic parasite
- Blood PCR assay to detect *Babesia* DNA
- Serologic testing to identify antibody production

DIFFERENTIAL DIAGNOSIS

 Assessment required for patients presenting with a nonspecific febrile illness for their risk of tick-borne diseases, including babesiosis.

Early symptoms of babesiosis are nonspecific and can resemble a viral or influenza-like illness. Clinical evaluation of patients presenting with a nonspecific febrile illness should include a careful history of tick exposure, especially during the spring and summer months, or recent blood transfusions, and testing for babesiosis should be considered for those at risk. Additionally, because co-infection can occur with *B. microti*, *B. burgdorferi*, and *A. phagocytophilum*, patients diagnosed with one should have testing considered for others, especially if the patient is not improving with standard therapy. Finally, while Babesia organisms on blood smear can resemble *P. falciparum* infection, a travel history and careful review of the blood smear by clinicians experienced at differentiating blood smear characteristics should help to distinguish.

INTERPROFESSIONAL COLLABORATIVE MANAGEMENT
Pharmacologic Management

Antimicrobial therapy is not recommended for asymptomatic patients unless *Babesia* is persistently present on blood smear or by PCR analysis for more than 3 months.[9] For mild to moderate disease, the recommended treatment is oral atovaquone plus oral azithromycin for 7 to 10 days.[6,9] Clinical improvement usually occurs within 48 hours of initiation of therapy, and symptoms should resolve within 3 months of therapy.[9] In patients with severe disease, 7 to 10 days of intravenous clindamycin plus oral quinine is recommended.[6,9]

Immunocompromised patients are at risk for persistent or relapsing infection, and in such patients therapy should be lengthened to at least 6 weeks with negative blood smears for 2 weeks or longer before discontinuing therapy.[6] For patients with severe infection who are unable to tolerate recommended therapy due to drug toxicity (e.g., quinine), or in patients with relapsing or persistent infections, alternative antimicrobial regimens have been trialed but systematic evidence of efficacy is lacking; therefore, infectious disease consultation should be initiated for these patients.[6]

Nonpharmacologic Management

Patients with severe disease and complications, or with high-grade parasitemia of 10% or greater on blood smear (10% or greater of erythrocytes on smear are infected), should be considered for partial or complete red blood cell exchange transfusion which is able to help correct anemia and decrease parasitemia.[6,9] Hematocrit and parasitemia should be monitored daily in patients with severe infection until parasitemia is less than 5%.[9]

Indications for Referral and Hospitalization

Patients with severe disease and complications should be hospitalized for close monitoring, treatment, and assessment of response to therapy; such patients may need critical care level intervention. Infectious disease consultation is recommended for those with severe disease, those who are not responding to initial therapy, or those with persistent or relapsing infection. Additionally, individuals who are hospitalized with severe disease or high parasitemia should have referral for red blood cell exchange transfusion.

PATIENT AND FAMILY EDUCATION

Similar to Lyme disease, patients and family members should be provided education about tick-borne diseases and preventing tick bites; this is particularly important in regard to babesiosis for those who are immunosuppressed or asplenic and living in or traveling to areas where *B. microti* is endemic. Patients who require blood transfusions should also be provided with information about the possibility of transfusion-associated babesiosis and symptoms of infection. To decrease transfusion-associated babesiosis, blood donation agencies prohibit individuals with a history of babesiosis from donating blood, but there is not currently an FDA approved test to screen the blood supply for *Babesia* infection.

HEALTH PROMOTION AND PREVENTION

There is no vaccine available for babesiosis and unlike Lyme disease there are no prophylactic antimicrobials recommended after a tick bite to prevent *Babesia* infection. The focus for prevention, therefore, needs to be on avoidance of tick bites similar to what has been previously discussed in the section on Health Promotion and Prevention for Lyme disease (see relevant section above).

ANAPLASMOSIS

DEFINITION AND EPIDEMIOLOGY

Anaplasmosis is a disease caused by the bacterium *A. phagocytophilum*. *A. phagocytophilum* is a rickettsial bacterium that belongs to the order Rickettsiales (which includes the organisms that cause ehrlichiosis and Rocky Mountain spotted fever [RMSF]). Anaplasmosis is also called human granulocytic anaplasmosis (HGA) because *A. phagocytophilum* is an obligate intracellular bacterium that preferentially infects ganulocytes.[30]

Anaplasmosis was added to the nationally notifiable disease list in 1998.[27] Incidence of *A. phagocytophilum* infection is highest in the Northeast and upper Midwest states, particularly Minnesota and Wisconsin; this geographic distribution is similar to Lyme disease and babesiosis since *B. burgdorferi*, *B. microti*, and *A. phagocytophilum* all are transmitted by the same tick vector.[31] The number of reported cases of anaplasmosis has been increasing, including in the Mid-Atlantic states, possibly related to expansion of the *I. scapularis* tick.[27,31] The number of reported anaplasmosis cases increased about 31% from 2014 to 2015, the largest yearly increase since the disease became reportable with more than 3600 cases reported in 2015, and the numbers have continued to increase with more than 4100 cases reported in 2016 (see Fig. 213.5).[27] Peak incidence of cases occurs in the spring and summer months from May through August, although cases occur year-round.[30]

PATHOPHYSIOLOGY

A. phagocytophilum is transmitted by the *I. scapularis* tick in the upper Midwest and Eastern United States, and through the *I. pacificus* tick along the West Coast.[31] Small rodents, such as the white-footed mouse, are the primary reservoir hosts for *A. phagocytophilum*, maintaining horizontal transmission of *A. phagocytophilum* between the different developmental tick stages (i.e., larval, nymph, and adult). Larval ticks prior to a blood meal are not infected with *A. phagocytophilum*, and so it is the nymphal and adult ticks which transmit *A. phagocytophilum* to humans.[30] Once humans are infected, *A. phagocytophilum* infects and reproduces predominantly in granulocytes (e.g., neutrophils) forming morulae, and it is the ensuing host immune response that leads to the symptoms of anaplasmosis.[30] Transfusion-associated anaplasmosis is possible, but has been rarely reported, with only eight published reports in the United States.[30]

CLINICAL PRESENTATION AND PHYSICAL EXAMINATION

People can be infected with *A. phagocytophilum* and be asymptomatic or have subclinical illness. When symptoms of anaplasmosis do develop they typically appear 5 to 14 days after a bite from an infected tick and most often present as a nonspecific febrile illness with fever, chills, malaise, headache, and myalgias.[30] Gastrointestinal symptoms are also possible but less frequent. Rash (present in <10% of patients) and neurological symptoms are uncommon, which may help differentiate anaplasmosis from ehrlichiosis which have similar clinical presentations.[30] Any patient presenting with an EM rash, however, should be evaluated for Lyme disease since co-infection can occur. Anaplasmosis is usually a self-limited illness, even without antibiotic treatment; however, patients can develop severe life threatening disease requiring hospitalization, although this is less common than with the other rickettsial diseases ehrlichiosis and RMSF. Potential complications of anaplasmosis include acute respiratory distress syndrome (ARDS), renal failure, DIC, meningitis or encephalitis, sepsis or toxic-shock like syndromes, and death, although case-fatality rates are less than 1% in those who seek medical care.[30,31] Common laboratory findings include thrombocytopenia, leukopenia, mild anemia, and elevation of hepatic transaminase levels; CSF analysis is usually normal.[6,30] These laboratory abnormalities often normalize by the end of the second week of illness.[32]

DIAGNOSTICS

Diagnosis of anaplasmosis is made by the identification of *A. phagocytophilum* morulae in the cytoplasm of peripheral blood neutrophils on a Wright or Giemsa stained blood smear, PCR assay on blood, or serologic testing.[6] Morulae are identifiable on peripheral blood smear in at least 20% of patients during the first week of illness.[32] PCR detection of *A. phagocytophilum* DNA in blood is also a very useful test that is sensitive in the acute phase of illness, particularly the first week, and can help confirm a diagnosis of anaplasmosis; ideally blood for PCR analysis should be drawn before antibiotic administration which can decrease test sensitivity.[30] Finally, serology can be used to confirm infection with *A. phagocytophilum*; standard tests are typically conducted using indirect immunofluorescence antibody (IFA) assays. Because serology assays are not sensitive during the first week of infection when antibodies are still developing, *A. phagocytophilum* infection is confirmed by finding a four-fold increase in IgG antibody titers between acute and convalescent titers.[30] Antibody titers should be drawn 2 to 4 weeks apart with the first during the acute phase of the illness. An IgG antibody titer of 64 or greater in a person with a compatible illness is supportive of a diagnosis of anaplasmosis, but a single antibody titer shouldn't be used to confirm a diagnosis because high antibody levels can persist for years after infection. IgM antibody tests are less sensitive and specific than IgG assays and therefore are not generally recommended for helping to diagnose anaplasmosis.[30,32]

INITIAL DIAGNOSTICS

Anaplasmosis

LABORATORY
- Blood smear to identify *A. phagocytophilum* morulae in peripheral blood neutrophils
- Blood PCR assay to detect *A. phagocytophilum* DNA
- Serologic testing to identify IgG antibody production

DIFFERENTIAL DIAGNOSIS

 Assessment required for patients presenting with a nonspecific febrile illness for their risk of tick-borne diseases, including anaplasmosis.

Early symptoms of anaplasmosis are nonspecific and can resemble a viral or influenza-like illness. Clinical evaluation of patients presenting with a nonspecific febrile illness should include a careful history of tick exposure, especially during the spring and summer months, and testing for anaplasmosis should be considered for those at risk. Additionally, because co-infection can occur with *B. microti*, *B. burgdorferi*, and *A. phagocytophilum*, other tick-borne diseases should be considered. Finally, for patients who present with a generalized fever and rash, the differential is broad and other bacterial, viral, or non-infectious etiologies should be considered.

INTERPROFESSSIONAL COLLABORATIVE MANAGEMENT
Pharmacologic Management

Doxycycline is the recommended treatment for anaplasmosis at all ages.[30] The recommended dose of doxycycline for adults is 100 mg orally twice daily and for children weighing less than 100 lbs (45 kg) is 2.2 mg/kg of body weight given twice daily.[30] Duration of treatment should be 10 days, which will also treat for possible co-infection with *B. burgdorferi*. In children younger than 8 years of age for whom co-infection with *B. burgdorferi* is not suspected, a minimum of 5 to 7 days is likely sufficient to minimize antibiotic exposure.[9,30] While doxycycline is relatively contraindicated for children younger than 8 years of age for Lyme disease due to the availability of other alternative therapies, it has been shown to be likely safe for use in younger children and is the preferred drug even in children to treat tick-borne rickettsial diseases like anaplasmosis, ehrlichiosis, and RMSF.[30] Doxycycline is also relatively contraindicated in breastfeeding because doxycycline is excreted into breast milk at low levels, but short courses during lactation are likely safe. For those with mild anaplasmosis who have a serious drug allergy to doxycycline or who are pregnant (another relative contraindication to doxycycline use) rifampin is an alternative therapy that can be considered, based on demonstration of in vitro activity against *A. phagocytophilum* and case reports of treatment efficacy.[30] Rifampin, however, does not treat Lyme disease and if co-infection is found, the patient will need a second antibiotic effective against *B. burgdorferi*. For patients with anaplasmosis who are pregnant or who have a life-threatening allergy to doxycycline, consultation with an infectious disease specialist is recommended. Treatment of asymptomatic individuals is not recommended.

Patients with severe disease or who show evidence of end organ damage should be hospitalized for monitoring, treatment, and management of fluid and electrolytes. Management of severe anaplasmosis may require critical care consultation and evaluation by an infectious disease specialist. Consultation with an infectious disease specialist is also recommended for patients with anaplasmosis who are pregnant or who have a severe allergy to doxycycline.

COMPLICATIONS

While most patients with anaplasmosis recover without complications, severe illness can occur including ARDS, renal failure, DIC, meningitis or encephalitis, sepsis or toxic-shock like syndromes, and even death. In one report of national surveillance data, 31% of reported cases were hospitalized; however, this number is likely inflated due to case ascertainment bias since more severe infections are likely to undergo testing for anaplasmosis whereas asymptomatic or mild infections may go undiagnosed or be treated empirically without confirmation of infection.[31] Despite the possibility of complications, case-fatality rates are less than 1% in those who seek medical care.[30,31]

PATIENT AND FAMILY EDUCATION

As with all tick-borne diseases, patients and family should be provided education about prevention of tick bites, and signs and symptoms of possible tick-borne disease, including anaplasmosis. Patients and family should also be provided education about correct removal of ticks.

HEALTH PROMOTION AND PREVENTION

There is no vaccine available to prevent anaplasmosis and there are no prophylactic antimicrobials recommended after a tick bite to prevent anaplasmosis. The focus for prevention, therefore, needs to be on avoiding tick bites similar to what has been previously discussed in the section on Health Promotion

and Prevention for Lyme disease (see relevant section above). Duration of tick attachment required to transmit *A. phagocytophilum* is unclear. One animal study showed that for significant transmission to occur, ticks needed to be attached for approximately 36 hours or longer;[33] however, another study showed possible transmission within 24 hours. Attached tick should[34] be removed as soon as possible to minimize risk of transmission.

EHRLICHIOSIS

DEFINITION AND EPIDEMIOLOGY

Ehrlichiosis is a disease that is similar to anaplasmosis, but is caused by different rickettsial bacteria of the genus *Ehrlichia*. In the United States *Ehrlichia* species that cause human infection include *Ehrlichia chaffeensis*, *Ehrlichia ewingii*, and a new species recently identified, *E. muris*-like agent (EML).[30] Ehrlichiosis caused by *E. chaffeensis* is the most common, and is also called human monocytic ehrlichiosis (HME) because the organism preferentially infects monocytes and tissue macrophages.[30]

Ehrlichiosis was added to the nationally notifiable disease list in 1998.[27] *E. chaffeensis* and *E. ewingii* infection have similar geographic distributions and usually occur in the Southeast and South Central parts of the United States owing to the fact that they are both transmitted by the lone star tick, *A. americanum*, which is the predominant tick found in the Southeastern US. The lone star tick range also extends into the New England states, and ehrlichiosis has been expanding into these states as well.[35,36] States with the highest reported incidence of *E. chaffeensis* infection include Oklahoma, Missouri, Delaware, Arkansas, Virginia, and Tennessee; these six states accounted for 54% of all reported *E. chaffeensis* infections in the US from 2008 to 2012.[35] Similarly, states with the highest incidence of *E. ewingii* infection include Delaware and Missouri, which accounted for 69% of all *E. ewingii* cases reported in the US from 2008 to 2012.[35] *E. chaffeensis* is much more common, and over the 5-year time frame 4613 cases of *E. chaffeensis* infection were reported compared to only 55 cases of *E. ewingii* infection.[35]

The EML agent has a different geographic distribution than the other *Ehrlichia* spp. because it is transmitted by the *I. scapularis* tick. EML was first identified in patients exposed to ticks in Minnesota and Wisconsin in 2009, and has also been detected from *I. scapularis* ticks in these states.[37] Since the initial identification further investigation and retrospective review identified 69 individuals that tested positive for the EML agent from 2004 to 2013; all 69 patients reported likely tick exposure in Minnesota or Wisconsin.[37] *I. scapularis* ticks in other parts of the United States have not been found to carry EML agent.

The incidence of reported ehrlichiosis overall has increased since it first became reportable, but the number of cases has been stable the last few years (see Fig. 213.5).[27,35] As with other tick-borne diseases there is likely underreporting of cases due to the possibility of asymptomatic or subclinical cases, or patients who are treated empirically without confirmatory testing. While cases can occur year-round, the majority of ehrlichiosis cases occur in the spring and summer months from May through August.[35,37]

PATHOPHYSIOLOGY

As mentioned, the primary tick vector for *E. chaffeensis* and *E. ewingii* is the lone star tick (*A. americanum*), whereas the primary tick vector for EML agent is blacklegged tick (*I. scapularis*). The primary host for the lone star tick, and reservoir for *Ehrlichia*, is the white-tailed deer, although other animals including dogs, livestock, and rodents can also serve as hosts for the lone star tick. The reservoir host is important for setting up horizontal transmission between larval, nymphal, and adult ticks, and only nymphal and adult ticks transmit ehrlichiosis. There is no information, however, for how long a tick needs to be attached in order to transmit *Ehrlichia*.[30] *Ehrlichia* are obligate intracellular bacteria that infect specific cells depending on the species. *E. chaffeensis* preferentially infects monocytes and tissue macrophages, whereas *E. ewingii* usually infects granulocytes (similar to *A. phagocytophilum*); the target cell for the EML agent is unknown as the organism has not yet been observed in cells on peripheral blood smear of infected patients.[30] Inside the cell, the organism reproduces, forming clusters of bacteria called morulae and the ensuing host response is responsible for the disease ehrlichiosis. Similar to babesiosis and anaplasmosis, transfusion-associated transmission of *Ehrlichia* has been reported.

CLINICAL PRESENTATION AND PHYSICAL EXAMINATION

Ehrlichiosis typically develops within 5 to 14 days after an infected tick bite.[30] Symptoms of ehrlichiosis are similar among the different species and usually present as a nonspecific febrile illness that includes fever, chills, headache, malaise, myalgia, and possibly gastrointestinal symptoms.[35,37] Symptoms are very similar to anaplasmosis, however, patients with ehrlichiosis are more likely to develop a skin rash, which affects approximately a third of individuals with ehrlichiosis and develops several days after illness onset.[30] Rash is more common in children than adults, and can vary in character, presenting as a petechial, maculopapular, or diffuse erythematous rash. Central nervous system involvement is also more common in ehrlichiosis compared to anaplasmosis, and symptoms of meningitis or meningoencephalitis occur in approximately 20% of patients. Common laboratory findings include thrombocytopenia, leukopenia, mild anemia, and elevation of hepatic transaminase levels.[37] If patients have CSF analysis, a lymphocytic or neutrophilic pleocytosis may be observed, with CSF white blood cell counts usually at 250 cells/μL or less, although higher cell counts are possible.[30]

DIAGNOSTICS

Diagnosis of ehrlichiosis can be made by the identification of *Ehrlichia* morulae in the cytoplasm of peripheral blood leukocytes on a Wright or Giemsa stained blood smear, PCR assay on blood, or serologic testing.[30] Blood smear examination has not been shown to be useful for diagnosing EML agent, so PCR should be considered in the acute phase, and serology can be performed but might show antibody cross-reactivity with *E. chaffeensis* or *A. phagocytophilum* antigens.[30,37] PCR detection of *Ehrlichia* DNA in blood is a very useful test that is sensitive in the acute phase of illness, particularly the first week, and can help confirm a diagnosis of ehrlichiosis; ideally blood for PCR analysis should be drawn before antibiotic administration, which can decrease test sensitivity. Serology can be used to confirm infection with *Ehrlichia* spp. with standard tests using indirect immunofluorescence antibody (IFA) assays. Because serologic assays are not sensitive during the first week of infection when antibodies are still developing, *Ehrlichia* infection is

confirmed by finding a four-fold increase in IgG antibody titers between acute and convalescent titers.[30] Antibody titers should be drawn 2 to 4 weeks apart with the first during the acute phase of the illness. An IgG antibody titer of 64 or greater in a person with a compatible illness is supportive of a diagnosis of ehrlichiosis, but a single antibody titer should not be used to confirm a diagnosis because high antibody levels can persist for years after infection.[30] IgM antibody tests are less sensitive and specific than IgG assays and therefore are not generally recommended for helping to diagnose ehrlichiosis.[30,32]

DIFFERENTIAL DIAGNOSIS

 Assessment required for patients presenting with a nonspecific febrile illness for their risk of tick-borne diseases, including ehrlichiosis. Patients presenting with a febrile rash illness need to be evaluated for Rocky Mountain spotted fever (given the similar geographic distribution with ehrlichiosis) and meningococcemia because both illnesses can be fatal.

Early symptoms of ehrlichiosis are nonspecific and can resemble a viral or influenza-like illness. Clinical evaluation of patients presenting with a nonspecific febrile illness should include a careful history of tick exposure, especially during the spring and summer months, and testing for ehrlichiosis should be considered for those at risk. Other tick-borne diseases should also be considered, especially RMSF which has a similar geographic distribution to *E. chaffeensis* and *E. ewingii* and can present with a rash illness that may look similar to the rash in ehrlichiosis. Also, because EML agent is transmitted by the same tick vector as *B. burgdorferi*, *A. phagocytophilum*, and *B. microti*, ehrlichiosis caused by EML agent needs to be considered in a person presenting with compatible symptoms who may have had tick exposure in Minnesota or Wisconsin. Finally, for patients who present with a generalized fever and rash, the differential is broad and other bacterial (including meningococcemia), viral, or non-infectious etiologies should be considered.[30]

INTERPROFESSSIONAL COLLABORATIVE MANAGEMENT
Pharmacologic Management

Doxycycline is the recommended treatment for ehrlichiosis at all ages.[30] The recommended dose of doxycycline for adults is 100 mg orally twice daily and for children weighing less than 100 lbs (45 kg) is 2.2 mg/kg of body weight given twice daily.[30] The duration of treatment should be for a minimum of 5 to 7 days with at least 3 days of treatment after fever subsides and there is clinical improvement; treatment may need to be longer than 7 days in those with severe or complicated disease. Patients with more mild disease usually show clinical improvement within 24 to 48 hours after beginning treatment.

While doxycycline is relatively contraindicated for children younger than 8 years of age for Lyme disease due to the availability of other alternative therapies, it has been shown to be likely safe for use in younger children and is the preferred drug even in children to treat tick-borne rickettsial diseases like ehrlichiosis, anaplasmosis, and RMSF. Doxycycline is also relatively contraindicated in breastfeeding because doxycycline is excreted into breast milk at low levels, but short courses during lactation are likely safe. The use of tetracycline antibiotics (e.g., doxycycline) has also been relatively contraindicated during pregnancy due to concerns for possible developmental effects on the fetus; however, there are no alternative antibiotics recommended for the treatment of ehrlichiosis. Rifampin has shown in vitro activity against *E. chaffeensis*, but clinical studies of treatment efficacy are lacking.[30] For patients with ehrlichiosis who are pregnant or who have a life-threatening allergy to doxycycline, consultation with an infectious disease specialist is recommended. Before doxycycline is used in a pregnant patient, there should be discussion with the patient about the risks and benefits, taking into account the disease-related risks for mother and fetus.[30] Treatment of asymptomatic individuals is not recommended.

Patients with severe disease or who show evidence of end organ damage should be hospitalized for monitoring, treatment, and management of fluid and electrolytes. Management of severe ehrlichiosis may require critical care consultation and evaluation by an infectious disease specialist. Consultation with an infectious disease specialist is also recommended for patients who are pregnant or who have a severe allergy to doxycycline. Consultation with an allergy and immunology specialist may also be indicated if a patient has a documented severe allergy to doxycycline that may require desensitization therapy given the limited antibiotic choices to treat ehrlichiosis.

COMPLICATIONS

Ehrlichiosis is more likely to cause serious illness compared to anaplasmosis. In one report based on national surveillance data, 57% of cases that reported hospitalization status were hospitalized during the course of their illness.[35] Severe complications with ehrlichiosis include ARDS, renal failure, DIC, meningitis or encephalitis, sepsis or toxic-shock like syndromes, and even death.[30] The case-fatality rate for *E. chaffeensis* is estimated to be approximately 1% to 3% in those who seek medical care.[30,35] No deaths have been reported for *E. ewingii* or EML agent, which may produce less severe disease.[30,35,37]

PATIENT AND FAMILY EDUCATION

As with all tick-borne diseases, patients and family should be provided education about prevention of tick bites, and signs and symptoms of possible tick-borne disease, including ehrlichiosis. Patients and family should also be provided education about correct technique to remove ticks.

HEALTH PROMOTION AND PREVENTION

There is no vaccine available to prevent ehrlichiosis and there are no prophylactic antimicrobials recommended after a tick bite to prevent ehrlichiosis. The focus for prevention, therefore, needs to be on avoidance of tick bites similar to what has been previously discussed in the section on Health Promotion and Prevention for Lyme disease (see relevant section above). Duration of tick attachment required to transmit *Ehrlichia* is unclear,

and tick removal as soon as possible is important to minimize risk of transmission.[30]

ROCKY MOUNTAIN SPOTTED FEVER

DEFINITION AND EPIDEMIOLOGY

RMSF is a disease caused by the bacterium *Rickettsia rickettsii* and belongs to a group of rickettsial bacteria called the spotted fever group (SFG) rickettsiae. A number of different *Rickettsia spp.* bacteria can be acquired in the United States through the bite of a tick vector; however, RMSF causes the most severe disease and has the greatest potential for a fatal outcome, and will be the focus of this section.

RMSF has been a nationally notifiable disease since 1920; however, beginning in 2010 the national surveillance case definition changed to include all SFG rickettsial infections due to limitations with diagnostic testing and inability to differentiate between *Rickettsia spp.* on serologic testing, which is the main method of diagnosis, due to cross-reactivity between species.[38] Therefore, much of the information from national surveillance data is on the incidence of SFG rickettsial infections and not specific to RMSF.[38]

Overall incidence of SFG rickettsial infections has increased, with the largest increase occurring between 2011 and 2012.[38] The greatest number of reported cases occurred in 2012 with 4470 cases reported in the United States (see Fig. 213.5). Incidence increases with age, with those 60 to 69 years of age having the highest incidence of SFG rickettsiosis and children younger than 10 years of age having the lowest incidence; however, children younger than 10 years of age have the highest case fatality rate of any age group.[38] While cases of SFG rickettsial infections have been reported from most states in the United States, 63% of all cases have been reported from Arkansas, Missouri, North Carolina, Oklahoma, and Tennessee.[38] RMSF, specifically, has also been found to be endemic in American Indian communities in Arizona causing high case counts and fatalities in these communities.[30,38] Interestingly, out of all race groups, incidence rates are highest among the American Indian/Alaskan Native population in the United States, and this group is at increased risk of a fatal outcome from infection, which has been associated with delayed recognition and treatment of infection.[30,38] Similar to other tick-borne diseases, the most common period of the year for infection is during the spring and summer months from May to August; however, there is regional variation within the United States.

PATHOPHYSIOLOGY

In the United States, various tick species are able to transmit RMSF. The primary vector for *R. rickettsii* is the American dog tick (*Dermacentor variabilis*), which is found in the Eastern, Central, and Pacific coastal parts of the United States. The Rocky Mountain wood tick (*Dermacentor andersoni*) is also able to transmit *R. rickettsii* and is found in Western states. Finally, the brown dog tick (*Rhipicephalus sanguineus*), which is found throughout the United States, has been found to transmit *R. rickettsii* in Arizona and along the US–Mexico border. Ticks serve as both a reservoir and vector for transmission of *R. rickettsii*. The primary hosts for the ticks vary by tick species with deer, dogs, and livestock being primary hosts for the *Dermacentor spp.* ticks, and dogs being the preferred host for *R. sanguineus* ticks.[30] Tick vectors, therefore, can become infected through horizontal transmission by feeding on an infected host; however, transovarial transmission (transmission from infected female ticks to offspring) is possible with *Rickettsia spp.* although this may occur less commonly in certain tick species with *R. rickettsii* infection than with other *Rickettsia spp.*[39] For this reason, all stages of tick development (larval, nymphal, and adult) can potentially transmit RMSF.[30] Once a tick bites a human, the *R. rickettsii* bacterium is deposited from the salivary glands and goes on to preferentially infect vascular endothelial cells causing a systemic vasculitis, which is responsible for the signs and symptoms of RMSF. The vascular injury and inflammation leads to severe illness and makes RMSF one of the more severe and potentially lethal tick-borne diseases. The duration of tick attachment required for transmission of *R. rickettsii* ranges from 2 to 20 hours.[30]

CLINICAL PRESENTATION AND PHYSICAL EXAMINATION

Symptoms of RMSF typically occur within 3 to 12 days after a tick bite. Initial symptoms of RMSF are nonspecific and include fever, headache, malaise, myalgia, and possible GI symptoms. Within 2 to 4 days after fever onset, a rash usually develops that begins as small, erythematous, blanching macules on the extremities and spreads over the trunk, arms, legs, and the palms and soles over the course of several days, developing into a maculopapular rash. A petechial rash may also develop, which is usually indicative of more severe disease.[30] While a majority of patients with RMSF usually develop a rash, some may not, and only about one-third of patients present with the classic triad of fever, rash, and reported tick bite.[30,40] Because delays in diagnosis and treatment can result in increased likelihood of death, clinicians should not rely on the presence of a rash to consider the possibility of RMSF. Complications of RMSF and severe manifestations include ARDS, renal failure, skin necrosis, shock, cardiac arrhythmia, meningoencephalitis, seizure, and death.[30] Laboratory findings consistent with RMSF include thrombocytopenia, slight elevations in hepatic transaminases, and hyponatremia; however, these abnormalities may be slight and not present in all patients.[30] If a lumbar puncture is performed, CSF analysis may show a small elevation in WBC count (<100 cells/μL) with a lymphocytic predominance along with elevation of protein and normal glucose.[30]

DIAGNOSTICS

Diagnosis of RMSF is typically made by serology using an indirect immunofluorescence antibody (IFA) assay.[30,38] Because serologic assays are not sensitive during the first week of infection when antibodies are still developing, RMSF is confirmed by finding a four-fold increase in IgG antibody titers between acute and convalescent titers.[30] Antibody titers should be drawn 2 to 4 weeks apart with the first during the acute phase of the illness. An IgG antibody titer of 64 or greater in a person with a compatible illness is supportive of a diagnosis of RMSF, but a single antibody titer shouldn't be used to confirm a diagnosis because high antibody levels can persist for years after infection. IgM antibody tests are less sensitive and specific than IgG assays and therefore are not generally recommended for helping to diagnose RMSF.[30] Antibody tests also do not reliably distinguish between *R. rickettsii* and other SFG rickettsiae due to cross-reactivity; therefore, antibodies that are found to be reactive for *R. rickettsii* could be due to infection with another SFG rickettsiae.

PCR on blood can be considered for detection of *R. rickettsii*, if available, but sensitivity is less due to lower numbers of circulating bacteria in the blood compared to anaplasmosis or ehrlichiosis; sensitivity of PCR on blood increases with more severe or late-stage disease. Tissue specimens (e.g., skin biopsy of rash) for PCR and immunohistochemistry staining are probably more useful for diagnosing *R. rickettsii* infection. Blood smear examination is not useful for diagnosing RMSF.

DIFFERENTIAL DIAGNOSIS

 Immediate evaluation required for patients presenting with a febrile rash illness for other causes of fever and rash, including meningococcemia which can be fatal.

Early symptoms of RMSF are nonspecific and can resemble a viral or influenza-like illness, or another tick-borne diseases. Clinical evaluation of patients presenting with a nonspecific febrile illness should include a careful history of tick exposure, especially during the spring and summer months, and testing and treatment for RMSF should be considered for those at risk. The petechial rash of RMSF can be confused with meningococcemia. The vasculitis and associated complications may also be confused with other vasculitides.

INTERPROFESSSIONAL COLLABORATIVE MANAGEMENT
Pharmacologic Management

Delay in recognizing RMSF and initiating treatment is a primary factor associated with increased risk of death; therefore, early empiric therapy is important to prevent progression of disease, and treatment should not be delayed pending laboratory confirmation. Doxycycline is the only recommended treatment for RMSF at all ages.[30] The recommended dose of doxycycline for adults is 100 mg orally twice daily and for children weighing less than 100 lbs (45 kg) is 2.2 mg/kg of body weight given twice daily. Duration of treatment should be for a minimum of 5 to 7 days with at least 3 days of treatment after fever subsides and there is clinical improvement; treatment may need to be longer than 7 days in those with severe or complicated disease.

While doxycycline is relatively contraindicated for children younger than 8 years of it has been shown to be likely safe for use in younger children and is the preferred drug even in children to treat tick-borne rickettsial diseases like RMSF, anaplasmosis, and ehrlichiosis. Doxycycline is also relatively contraindicated in breastfeeding because doxycycline is excreted into breast milk at low levels, but short courses during lactation are likely safe. The use of tetracycline antibiotics (e.g., doxycycline) has generally also been contraindicated during pregnancy due to concerns about possible developmental effects on the fetus; however, the only other potential alternative antibiotic that has been used to treat RMSF is chloramphenicol, but chloramphenicol use has been associated with a higher risk of death compared to treatment with tetracyclines.[30] Additionally, chloramphenicol is not widely available, requires monitoring of drug levels, and has its own potentially serious adverse side effects (including hematologic effects and possible gray baby syndrome).[30] Doxycycline, therefore, should be considered even during pregnancy, but there should be discussion with the patient about the risks and benefits, taking into account the disease-related risks for mother and fetus. For patients with RMSF who are pregnant or who have a life-threatening allergy to doxycycline, consultation with an infectious disease specialist is recommended.

Any patient being evaluated and treated for RMSF should be considered for hospitalization due to the potential severity of disease. Those who have more severe disease or show evidence of end organ damage may need critical care consultation. Consultation with an infectious disease specialist is also recommended, especially if there are complicating factors such as a severe doxycycline allergy or the patient is pregnant. Consultation with an allergy and immunology specialist may also be indicated if a patient has a documented severe allergy to doxycycline that may require doxycycline desensitization given limited alternate antibiotic choices.

COMPLICATIONS

RMSF is the most lethal of the tick-borne diseases in the United States with an estimated present-day case fatality rate of 5% to 10%.[30] Patients with severe disease who survive can develop long-term neurologic sequelae from RMSF including cognitive impairment, hearing loss, blindness, neuropathy, motor dysfunction, and other neurologic issues that result from the vasculitis.[30]

PATIENT AND FAMILY EDUCATION

As with all tick-borne diseases, patients and family should be provided education about prevention of tick bites, and signs and symptoms of tick-borne diseases. Patients and family should also be provided education about correct technique for removal of ticks.

HEALTH PROMOTION AND PREVENTION

There is no vaccine available to prevent RMSF and there are no prophylactic antimicrobials recommended after a tick bite to prevent RMSF. The focus for prevention, therefore, needs to be on avoidance of tick bites similar to what has been previously discussed in the section on Health Promotion and Prevention for Lyme disease (see relevant section above). Duration of tick attachment required to transmit *R. rickettsii* is reported to range from 2 to 20 hours; therefore, early tick identification and removal may not be sufficient to prevent transmission of *R. rickettsii*.[30]

EMERGING TICK-BORNE DISEASES
Borrelia miyamotoi

Borrelia miyamotoi is a spirochete bacterium that has been found to be transmitted to humans through the bite of a tick. The same tick species that transmit *B. burgdorferi* (the agent that causes Lyme disease) have also been found to carry *B. miyamotoi*, including *I. scapularis* in the Northeast and North Central United States and *I. pacificus* in the Western coastal United States.[41] Co-infection, therefore, is possible.

Human infection caused by *B. miyamotoi* was only first discovered in Russia in 2011,[42] and more recently in the Northeastern United States.[43] The extent of the geographic distribution of infection in the United States is still unknown, but likely is similar to Lyme disease.[41] One difference between *B. miyamotoi* and other tick-borne diseases transmitted by *I. scapularis* ticks is that transovarial transmission occurs, and therefore all stages of tick (larval, nymphal, and adult) are able to transmit *B. miyamotoi*. The animal reservoirs of *B. miyamotoi* are still not fully known, but include the white-footed mouse. Seroprevalence studies of humans in the Northeastern United States have shown seropositivity on the order of 1% to 4% in tested populations, suggesting exposure and infection is more common than previously thought.[41,43-45]

The clinical spectrum of disease is not fully known, but initial reports suggest that *B. miyamotoi* infection presents with a nonspecific febrile illness similar to many other tick-borne diseases, commonly including fever, headache, malaise, fatigue, myalgia, and arthralgia; rash is not a common feature.[42,43] Laboratory testing may show leukopenia, thrombocytopenia, and elevated hepatic transaminases, similar to findings with anaplasmosis.[43]

Tests for Lyme disease do not reliably detect *B. miyamotoi* infection; only about 10% of individuals with *B. miyamotoi* infection have been found to test positive on the two-step Lyme disease antibody testing algorithm.[43,45] There are diagnostic tests specific to *B. miyamotoi* that include PCR or serologic tests, although testing is not yet commonly available. Antibody tests for *B. miyamotoi* may be insensitive during early disease when patients first present due to delay in antibody production, so convalescent serologic testing may be needed.[43] It is also possible that spirochetes could be seen on blood smear.[41] Treatment information for *B. miyamotoi* is limited, but antibiotics effective for Lyme disease have also been shown to be effective at treating *B. miyamotoi* infection in case reports, with similar treatment durations.[41-43]

Borrelia mayonii

Borrelia mayonii is a more recently recognized spirochete found in the upper Midwest United States to cause human infection. Between 2012 and 2014, the Mayo Clinic in Rochester, Minnesota identified six specimens by PCR testing that were positive for a novel *Borrelia* species, subsequently called *B. mayonii*.[46] All patients were residents in the upper Midwest and reported tick exposures in Minnesota or Wisconsin.[46] *I. scapularis* ticks from Wisconsin were also subsequently found to carry *B. mayonii*.[46] Out of tens of thousands of other samples tested at Mayo in prior years and from other states, none have detected *B. mayonii*, suggesting a limited geographic distribution and that *B. mayonii* is an emerging infection in the upper Midwest United States.[46]

Information on clinical presentation is limited. Signs and symptoms for the initially described six patients included fever and rash, although the rash identified in several patients varied from a diffuse macular rash to an annular erythematous lesion consistent with an EM rash. Other symptoms included headache, fatigue, myalgia, and nausea or vomiting. Three presented with neurologic symptoms (including somnolence, confused speech, and visual disturbances), and one patient presented with isolated knee pain and swelling.[46] Laboratory testing showed lymphopenia, mild thrombocytopenia, and mild elevation of hepatic transaminases are possible.[46]

Testing options are limited; Lyme disease serologic tests may detect *B. mayonii* infection, and certain PCR tests (such as the one at Mayo) may detect *B. mayonii*. It is also possible that spirochetes could be seen on blood smear.[46] Antibiotic treatment regimens and duration are likely similar to Lyme disease.

Powassan Virus

Powassan virus is a flavivirus that is transmitted by ticks. It was first identified in humans in 1958 in Powassan, Ontario, when a boy died from encephalitis. Powassan virus infection has been identified in the United States primarily in the Northeastern and Midwestern states, as well as throughout the Canadian provinces. Transmission is primarily though *Ixodes spp.* of tick. There are two different lineages of Powassan virus; Lineage I is predominantly maintained in the *Ixodes cookei* ticks, whereas Lineage II is maintained by *I. scapularis* ticks.[47,48] *I. cookei* ticks have a high proclivity for their primary hosts, which are woodchucks and rodents, so are not thought to contribute as significantly to human infection as *I. scapularis*, which is not as host specific.[47,48] Unlike many other tick-borne diseases, Powassan virus can be transmitted within 15 minutes of tick attachment, making tick bite identification and removal a much less useful prevention technique.[49] While still uncommon, there has been an increasing number of Powassan cases reported in the Northeast.

The incubation period for Powassan ranges from 1 to 5 weeks after a tick bite. Asymptomatic infection can occur, but patients who develop symptoms usually initially have fever, and early neurological symptoms of headache, drowsiness, and disorientation. Symptoms can progress to encephalitis, meningoencephalitis, or aseptic meningitis with complications of seizure, loss of coordination, focal neurologic deficits, paralysis, and even death.[47,48] Ten to fifteen percent of patients will die from Powassan and in those who develop disease but survive, 50% will develop long-term neurologic deficits, including memory loss, recurrent headaches, and focal weakness or paralysis.[47,48] There are not common routine laboratory abnormalities associated with Powassan, although lumbar puncture and CSF analysis will usually show a lymphocyte or granulocyte predominant pleocytosis, elevated protein, and normal glucose.[48]

In patients with a compatible clinical illness, diagnosis of Powassan can be made by virus isolation or PCR analysis (most useful during the initial stage of illness), or serologic testing showing virus-specific IgM antibodies in serum with a positive confirmatory plaque reduction neutralization test (PRNT), a four-fold or greater increase in antibody titers between acute and convalescent sera, or finding virus-specific IgM antibodies in CSF with negative tests for other potential causes of encephalitis.[47,48] Treatment for Powassan virus infection is supportive.

REFERENCES

1. Steere, A. C., Strle, F., Wormser, G. P., et al. (2016). Lyme borreliosis. *Nature Reviews Disease Primers, 2*, 1–18.
2. Schwartz, A. M., Hinckley, A. F., Mead, P. S., et al. (2017). Surveillance for Lyme disease—United States, 2008–2015. *MMWR. Surveillance Summaries: Morbidity and Mortality Weekly Report. Surveillance Summaries, 66*(22), 1–12.
3. Nelson, C. A., Saha, S., Kugeler, K. J., et al. (2015). Incidence of clinician-diagnosed Lyme disease, United States, 2005-2010. *Emerging Infectious Diseases, 21*(9), 1625–1631.
4. Daly, E. R., Fredette, C., Mathewson, A. A., et al. (2017). Tick bite and Lyme disease-related emergency department encounters in New Hampshire, 2010-2014. *Zoonoses and Public Health, 64*(8), 655–661.
5. Steere, A. C., Bartenhagen, N. H., Craft, J. E., et al. (1983). The early clinical manifestations of Lyme disease. *Annals of Internal Medicine, 99*(1), 76–82.
6. Sanchez, E., Vannier, E., Wormser, G. P., et al. (2016). Diagnosis, treatment, and prevention of Lyme disease, human granulocytic anaplasmosis, and babesiosis. *JAMA: The Journal of the American Medical Association, 315*(16), 1767–1777.
7. Steere, A. C., & Sikand, V. K. (2003). The presenting manifestations of Lyme disease and the outcomes of treatment. *The New England Journal of Medicine, 348*(24), 2472–2474.
8. Centers for Disease Control and Prevention (CDC). (2013). Three sudden cardiac deaths associated with Lyme carditis—United States, November 2012–July 2013. *MMWR. Morbidity and Mortality Weekly Report, 62*(49), 993–996.
9. Wormser, G. P., Dattwyler, R. J., Shapiro, E. D., et al. (2006). The clinical assessment, treatment, and prevention of Lyme disease, human granulocytic anaplasmosis, and babesiosis: Clinical practice guidelines by the Infectious Disease Society of America. *Clinical Infectious Diseases: an Official Publication of the Infectious Diseases Society of America, 43*(9), 1089–1134.
10. Centers for Disease Control and Prevention (CDC). (1995). Recommendations for test performance and interpretation from the Second National Conference on Serologic Diagnosis of Lyme Disease. *MMWR. Morbidity and Mortality Weekly Report, 44*(31), 590–591.
11. Hammers-berggren, S., Lebech, A.-M., Karlsson, M., et al. (1994). Serological follow-up after treatment of patients with erythema migrans and neuroborreliosis. *Journal of Clinical Microbiology, 32*(6), 1519–1525.
12. Kalish, R. A., McHugh, G., Granquist, J., et al. (2001). Persistence of immunoglobulin M or Immunoglobulin G antibody responses to Borrelia burgdorferi 10–20 years after active Lyme disease. *Clinical Infectious Diseases: an Official Publication of the Infectious Diseases Society of America, 33*(6), 780–785.
13. Wormser, G. P., Schriefer, M., Aguero-Rosenfeld, M. E., et al. (2013). Single-tier testing with the C6 peptide ELISA kit compared with two-tier testing for Lyme disease. *Diagnostic Microbiology and Infectious Disease, 75*(1), 9–15.
14. Kowalski, T. J., Tata, S., Berth, W., et al. (2010). Antibiotic treatment duration and long-term outcomes of patients with early Lyme disease from a Lyme disease-hyperendemic area. *Clinical Infectious Diseases: an Official Publication of the Infectious Diseases Society of America, 50*(4), 512–520.
15. Stupica, D., Lusa, L., Ruzić-Sabljić, E., et al. (2012). Treatment of erythema migrans with doxycycline for 10 days versus 15 days. *Clinical Infectious Diseases: An Official Publication of the Infectious Diseases Society of America, 55*(3), 343–350.
16. Feder, H. M., Jr., Johnson, B. J. B., O'Connell, S., et al. (2007). A critical appraisal of "chronic Lyme disease." *The New England Journal of Medicine, 357*(14), 1422–1430.
17. Fallon, B. A., Keilp, J. G., Corbera, K. M., et al. (2008). A randomized, placebo-controlled trial of repeated IV antibiotic therapy for Lyme encephalopathy. *Neurology, 70*(13), 992–1003.
18. Berende, A., ter Hofstede, H. J. M., Vos, F. J., et al. (2016). Randomized trial of longer-term therapy for symptoms attributed to Lyme disease. *The New England Journal of Medicine, 374*(13), 1209–1220.
19. Marzec, N. S., Nelson, C., Waldron, P. R., et al. (2017). Serious bacterial infections acquired during treatment of patients given a diagnosis of chronic Lyme disease—United States. *MMWR. Morbidity and Mortality Weekly Report, 66*(23), 607–609.
20. Nelson, C., Elmendorf, S., & Mead, P. (2014). Neoplasms misdiagnosed as "chronic Lyme Disease." *JAMA: The Journal of the American Medical Association, 175*(1), 132–133.
21. Centers for Disease Control and Prevention (CDC). Avoiding ticks. Retrieved from https://www.cdc.gov/ticks/avoid/index.html. (Accessed 31 December 2017).
22. Nelson, C. A., Hayes, C. M., Markowitz, M. A., et al. (2016). The heat is on: Killing blacklegged ticks in residential washers and dryers to prevent tick-borne diseases. *Ticks and Tick-Borne Diseases, 7*(5), 958–963.
23. Nadelman, R. B., Nowakowski, J., Fish, D., et al. (2001). Prophylaxis with single-dose doxycycline for the prevention of Lyme disease after an *Ixodes scapularis* tick bite. *The New England Journal of Medicine, 345*(2), 79–84.
24. Vannier, E., & Krause, P. J. (2012). Human babesiosis. *The New England Journal of Medicine, 366*(25), 2397–2407.
25. Vannier, E. G., Diuk-Wasser, M. A., Ben Mamoun, C., et al. (2015). Babesiosis. *Infectious Disease Clinics of North America, 29*(2), 357–370.
26. Centers for Disease Control and Prevention (CDC). (2012). Babesiosis surveillance—18 states, 2011. *MMWR. Morbidity and Mortality Weekly Report, 61*(27), 505–509.
27. Centers for Disease Control and Prevention (CDC). Tickborne Disease Surveillance Data—United States. Retrieved from https://www.cdc.gov/ticks/data-summary/index.html. (Accessed 24 July 2019).

28. Moritz, E. D., Winton, C. S., Tonnetti, L., et al. (2016). Screening for *Babesia microti* in the U.S. blood supply. *The New England Journal of Medicine*, 375(23), 2236–2245.

29. Herwaldt, B. L., Linden, J. V., Bosserman, E., et al. (2011). Transfusion-associated babesiosis in the United States: A description of cases. *Annals of Internal Medicine*, 155(8), 509–519, Original research.

30. Biggs, H. M., Behravesh, C. B., Bradley, K. K., et al. (2016). Diagnosis and management of tickborne rickettsial diseases: Rocky Mountain spotted fever and other spotted fever group rickettsioses, ehrlichiosis, and anaplasmosis—United States. *MMWR. Recommendations and Reports: Morbidity and Mortality Weekly Report. Recommendations and Reports*, 65(2), 1–44.

31. Dahlgren, F. S., Heitman, K. H., Drexler, N. A., et al. (2015). Human granulocytic anaplasmosis in the United States from 2008 to 2012: A summary of national surveillance data. *The American Journal of Tropical Medicine and Hygiene*, 93(1), 66–72.

32. Bakken, J. S., & Dumler, J. S. (2015). Human granulocytic anaplasmosis. *Infectious Disease Clinics of North America*, 29(2), 341–355.

33. Katavolos, P., Armstrong, P. M., Dawson, J. E., et al. (1998). Duration of tick attachment required for transmission of granulocytic ehrlichiosis. *The Journal of Infectious Diseases*, 177(5), 1422–1425.

34. Des Vignes, F., Piesman, J., Heffernan, R., et al. (2001). Effect of tick removal on transmission of *Borrelia burgdorferi* and *Ehrlichia phagocytophila* by *Ixodes scapularis* nymphs. *The Journal of Infectious Diseases*, 183(5), 773–778.

35. Heitman, K. N., Dahlgren, F. S., Drexler, N. A., et al. (2016). Increasing incidence of ehrlichiosis in the Unites States: A summary of national surveillance of *Ehrlichia chaffeensis* and *Ehrlichia ewingii* infections in the United States, 2008–2012. *The American Journal of Tropical Medicine and Hygiene*, 94(1), 52–60.

36. Harris, R. M., Couturier, B. A., Sample, S. C., et al. (2016). Expanded geographic distribution and clinical characteristics of Ehrlichia ewingii infections, United States. *Emerging Infectious Diseases*, 22(5), 862–865.

37. Johnson, D. K. H., Schiffman, E. K., Davis, J. P., et al. (2015). Human infection with *Ehrlichia muris*-like pathogen, United States, 2007–2013. *Emerging Infectious Diseases*, 21(10), 1794–1799.

38. Drexler, N. A., Dahlgren, F. S., Heitman, K. H., et al. (2016). National surveillance of spotted fever group rickettsioses in the United States, 2008–2012. *The American Journal of Tropical Medicine and Hygiene*, 94(1), 26–34.

39. Harris, E. K., Verhoeve, V. I., Banajee, K. H., et al. (2017). Comparative vertical transmission of *Rickettsia* by *Dermacentor variabilis* and *Amblyomma maculatum*. *Ticks and Tick-Borne Diseases*, 8(4), 598–604.

40. Traeger, M. S., Regan, J. J., Humpherys, D., et al. (2015). Rocky Mountain spotted fever characterization and comparison to similar illnesses in a highly endemic area—Arizona, 2002–2011. *Clinical Infectious Diseases: an Official Publication of the Infectious Diseases Society of America*, 60(11), 1650–1658.

41. Krause, P. J., Fish, D., Narasimhan, S., et al. (2015). Borrelia miyamotoi infection in Nature and in Humans. *Clinical Microbiology and Infection*, 21(7), 631–639.

42. Platonov, A. E., Karan, L. S., Kolyasnikova, N. M., et al. (2011). Humans infected with relapsing fever spirochete *Borrelia miyamotoi*, Russia. *Emerging Infectious Diseases*, 17(10), 1816–1823.

43. Molloy, P. J., Telford, S. R., III, Chowdri, H. R., et al. (2015). *Borrelia miyamotoi* disease in the northeastern United States. *Annals of Internal Medicine*, 163(2), 91–98.

44. Krause, P. J., Narasimhan, S., Wormser G. P., et al. (2013). Human *Borrelia miyamotoi* infection in the United States. *The New England Journal of Medicine*, 368(3), 291–293.

45. Krause, P. J., Narasimhan, S., Wormser, G. P., et al. (2014). *Borrelia miyamotoi* sensu lato seroreactivity and seroprevalence in the northeastern United States. *Emerging Infectious Diseases*, 20(7), 1183–1190.

46. Pritt, B. S., Mead, P. S., Johnson, D. K. H., et al. (2016). Identification of a novel pathogenic *Borrelia* species causing Lyme borreliosis with unusually high spirochaetaemia: A descriptive study. *The Lancet Infectious Diseases*, 16(5), 556–564.

47. Hermance, M. E., & Thangamani, S. (2017). Powassan virus: An emerging arbovirus of public health concern in North America. *Vector Borne and Zoonotic Diseases (Larchmont, N.Y.)*, 17(7), 453–462.

48. Piantadosi, A., Rubin, D. B., McQuillen, D. P., et al. (2016). Emerging cases of Powassan virus encephalitis in New England: Clinical presentation, imaging, and review of the literature. *Clinical Infectious Diseases: an Official Publication of the Infectious Diseases Society of America*, 62(6), 707–713.

49. Ebel, G. D., & Kramer, L. D. (2004). Short report: Duration of tick attachment required for transmission of Powassan virus by deer ticks. *The American Journal of Tropical Medicine and Hygiene*, 71(3), 268–271.

CHAPTER **214**

TUBERCULOSIS

Patricia Polgar-Bailey

DEFINITION AND EPIDEMIOLOGY

Tuberculosis (TB) is an airborne infectious disease caused by *Mycobacterium tuberculosis*, an acid-fast aerobic bacterium that is capable of remaining alive outside the host for a relatively long time. In the United States, most cases of TB are caused by *M. tuberculosis*, also referred to as the tubercle bacillus. However, several closely related *Mycobacterium* species can cause disease in humans, including *Mycobacterium bovis*, the cause of TB in cattle; *Mycobacterium avium*, one of the causes of TB in birds; and *Mycobacterium africanum*. TB caused by these organisms was relatively rare in the United States until they were identified as the cause of opportunistic infections in patients infected with human immunodeficiency virus (HIV).

TB has been described as the greatest killer in history and the leading cause of death from a single infectious agent.[1] Globally, TB transmission continues despite highly effective frontline combination therapy, a widely administered vaccine, intensive control efforts, and the allocation of tremendous resources to improve interventions.[2] Worldwide TB is one of the top 10 leading causes of death from a single infectious agent, above HIV and AIDS. In 2017, TB caused an estimated 1.3 million deaths among HIV negative people and an additional 300,000 deaths among people with HIV.[3] Approximately 10 million people developed TB in 2017; 90% were adults (age 15 years or older); 9% were people living with HIV (72% in Africa), and two-thirds were in 8 countries: India (27%), China (9%), Indonesia (8%), the Philippines (6%), Pakistan (5%), Nigeria (4%), Bangladesh (4%), and South Africa (3%). In 2017, globally approximately 558,000 people developed TB resistant to rifampicin (RR-TB), the most effective first-line drug therapy and of these 82% had multidrug-resistant tuberculosis (MDR-TB); more than half of these cases were in India, China, and the Russian Federation.[3] The increasing incidence and transmission of TB is largely a result of the spread of HIV in Africa and to the economic difficulties and associated decline in health infrastructure in eastern Europe and central Asia as well as increased reporting. Approximately 87% of all TB cases are found in the 8 countries listed above and 22 other countries which comprise the World Health Organization's list of high TB burden countries, most of which are in Africa and Asia. India has the highest rate of TB mortality, followed by China, where there are 150,000 TB-related deaths annually.[3]

Persons with active TB who receive no treatment can infect an average of 10 to 15 people annually.[4] Southeast Asia currently has the highest prevalence of TB, with one-third of new cases occurring in this area every year, but the incidence per capita is highest in sub-Saharan Africa, where the presence of TB parallels the HIV and acquired immunodeficiency syndrome (AIDS) epidemic.

Two billion people have latent tuberculosis infection (LTBI), the presence of *M. tuberculosis* in the body without signs and symptoms or radiographic or bacteriologic evidence of TB; without treatment, approximately 5% to 10% of these individuals will progress to active disease at some point in their lifetime.[1,5] In the United States, approximately 13 million people have LTBI.[6]

During the mid-20th century, the United States benefited from relatively successful control of TB. From 1953 to 1985, the reported cases of TB in the United States dropped from 84,000 to 22,000.[7] From 1985 to 1992, there was an unprecedented resurgence of TB in the United States. Since 1993, the annual TB rate has decreased steadily. In 2017, the incidence of TB in the United States was at a record low of 9105 cases.[7] Globally the incidence of TB is falling about 2% per year and the proportion of people who died from TB in 2017 was 16%, down from 23% in 2013.[3]

Although the annual incidence of TB has decreased, the percentage of primary drug-resistant cases has increased. Primary drug resistance is defined as no previous history of TB and resistance to at least isoniazid (INH) and rifampin, the most potent first-line antitubercular drugs. MDR-TB emerged during the 1990s as a significant threat to TB control, both in the United States and worldwide, and remains a significant threat to TB control. MDR-TB treatment requires the use of second-line drugs that are less effective, more toxic, and costlier than first-line INH- and rifampin-based regimens. In addition, MDR-TB is associated with higher morbidity and mortality than non–drug-resistant TB. The World Health Organization (WHO) estimated that in 2016, 4.1% of new cases and 19% of previously treated cases of TB were of multi-drug resistant or rifampin resistant (MDR/RR-TB).[8] Extensively drug resistant TB (XDR-TB) is a form of TB resistant to four of the core TB drugs. It involves resistance to INH and Rifampicin, also known as MDR-TB. In addition, XDR-TB involves resistance to any of the floroquinolones and to at least 3 injectable second-line drugs (amikacin, capreomycin or kanamycin).

Historically, TB in the United States was a disease that affected primarily older adults; increasingly, younger adults and children are being affected, particularly foreign-born children and adolescents.[7,9] An estimated 11% of TB cases worldwide occur in children younger than 15 years. In TB-endemic areas, children are at increased risk of acquiring TB because of the increased likelihood of close contact and exposure to adults with TB. Progression from infection to disease (approximately 8% to 10% overall) is higher for children of all ages and highest for infants younger than 1 year (43%) and children aged 1 to 5 years (24%). Of additional concern are those children who do not progress from infection to active disease in childhood but who constitute a potential pool for disease in adulthood.[9]

Many factors have contributed to the increased incidence of TB, including the HIV epidemic and higher rates of poverty, homelessness, incarceration, and drug use. An increasing number of immigrants, many of whom live in crowded housing and have inadequate health care, and an increasing number of residents in long-term care facilities have also contributed to this public health problem. Deterioration in the health care infrastructure and reductions in TB outreach programs, which historically improved compliance with treatment regimens, have also contributed to the resurgence of TB.

Alcohol and illegal drug use increase the risk of TB transmission and act as barriers to TB control and prevention.[10] Substance use decreases the likelihood of seeking medical care and adhering to and completing therapy. In addition, the use of substances often takes place in enclosed crowded spaces with poor ventilation, which increases the risk of TB exposure and transmission. In the United States, approximately one of three US-born persons aged 15 years or older with TB also abuses substances.

TB is largely a social disease, and homeless and incarcerated individuals are at increased risk of infection with TB. TB control can be particularly problematic in correctional and detention facilities, in which persons from diverse backgrounds and communities live together for varying and sometimes extended periods. In July 2006, the Centers for Disease Control and Prevention (CDC) published guidelines for the prevention and control of TB in jails, prisons, and other correctional and detention facilities.[11] Providers working in these settings should familiarize themselves with the recommendations, which can be found in *Morbidity and Mortality Weekly Report* (MMWR) or at www.cdc.gov/mmwr/preview/mmwrhtml/rr5509a1.htm.

Transmission of *M. tuberculosis* in health care institutions was a contributing factor to the resurgence of TB during the period from 1985 to 1992, and recommendations were developed to prevent transmission in these settings. However, the elevated risk among health care workers may be attributable to other factors (e.g., birth in a country with a high incidence of TB). A recent large multistate occupational survey indicated that health care workers, with the exception of respiratory therapists, do not have a higher risk for TB than the general population.[4]

The decelerating decline of the overall national TB rate, the persistent disparities in TB rates between US-born and foreign-born persons and between whites and ethnic minorities, and the increase in MDR-TB cases all threaten progress toward the goal of eliminating TB in the United States.[7] Major challenges to successful control of TB in the United States include detection and treatment of TB in the non–US-born population, elimination of delays in detecting and reporting cases of pulmonary TB and protecting contacts of TB-infected persons, and prevention of and response to TB outbreaks. In addition, there is a large reservoir of persons living in the United States with LTBI who are at risk for progression to TB disease. Finally, the successful control of TB depends on maintenance of clinical and public health expertise in TB management in an era of declining TB incidence.[4]

Treatment of TB benefits both the individual patient and the community as a whole. Therefore, any public health program or health care provider undertaking to treat a patient with TB is assuming a public health function that includes not only prescribing an appropriate medication regimen but also ensuring adherence to the regimen until treatment is completed. According to a joint statement by the American Thoracic Society, CDC, and Infectious Diseases Society of America, the responsibility for successful treatment of TB is assigned to the public health program or private provider rather than to the individual with TB.[12]

PATHOPHYSIOLOGY

TB is spread primarily through direct infection (person to person), but it can also be spread indirectly by the airborne transmission of the tubercle bacilli, which can remain suspended in the air for several hours. Transmission, which may occur if these bacilli-laden sputum droplets (each containing one to three organisms) are inhaled, depends on three factors: the infectiousness of the person with TB, the environment in which the exposure occurred, and the duration of exposure. Although theoretically one organism implanted in the alveolus can initiate this process, 5 to 200 organisms are usually required.[13] Most of the larger inhaled particles become lodged in the upper respiratory tract, where infection is unlikely to take place. Infection begins if the droplet nuclei reach the alveolar macrophage and multiplication of the tubercle bacilli is initiated. A small number of mycobacteria spread through the lymph system to regional lymph nodes and through the bloodstream to more distant tissues and organs, including areas in which TB is more likely to develop, such as the apices of the lung, the kidneys, the brain, and the bone. Eighty-five percent of all TB cases involve the lungs; other common sites include the pleura, central nervous system (CNS), lymphatic system, genitourinary system, and bones and joints. TB can also become disseminated and then is referred to as miliary TB.

TB disease has two distinct epidemiologic patterns. Reactivation, or postprimary disease, is the most common clinical form of TB. Most symptomatic cases of TB arise in persons with a history of TB infection who were inadequately treated or not treated. The second epidemiologic profile, primary infection, does not usually appear as a symptomatic infection except in persons infected with HIV. More than 90% of persons with primary infection are entirely asymptomatic, and infection with TB is identified only by a positive reaction to a tuberculin skin test (TST).

Certain medical conditions and other factors increase the risk that LTBI will progress to active TB disease. The risk may be three times greater (as with coexistent diabetes mellitus) to 100 times greater (as with HIV infection) for persons who have these conditions compared with those who do not.[7] Medical conditions and other factors associated with progression from LTBI to TB disease are listed in Box 214.1.

CLINICAL PRESENTATION AND PHYSICAL EXAMINATION

Persons who have been infected with *M. tuberculosis* but do not have active disease (LTBI) are completely asymptomatic. For the majority of persons, the only evidence of LTBI is an immune response against mycobacterial antigens, which is demonstrated by the Mantoux test or interferon gamma release assays (IGRAs). Two US Food and Drug Administration (FDA)–approved IGRAs are commercially available in the United States: QuantiFERON-TB Gold In-Tube (QFT-GIT) test and T-SPOT.*TB* test.[14] There is no radiographic evidence of TB in persons with LTBI.

Symptoms of pulmonary TB (the most common site) include fatigue, anorexia, weight loss, night sweats, cough, chest pain, hemoptysis, irregular menses, and low-grade fever. Symptoms in adults are often subtle and may appear in conjunction with or simulate other illnesses and therefore are often not associated with TB. However, one-third of persons with pulmonary TB are asymptomatic on initial presentation.[5]

Approximately 15% of cases of TB are extrapulmonary; common sites include the bones and joints, genitourinary system, lymphatic system, and CNS. The symptoms of extrapulmonary TB depend on the site affected. TB of the spine often causes back pain, whereas TB of the genitourinary system may result in hematuria or persistent dysuria.

A complete physical examination is an essential part of the evaluation but cannot be used alone to confirm or to exclude TB. Even if the physical examination findings are entirely normal, it can provide useful information about the patient's overall condition. Certain findings, although not diagnostic of

---

BOX **214.1**

Conditions and Other Factors Associated With Progression From Latent Tuberculosis Infection to Tuberculosis Disease

- HIV infection
- Chest radiographic findings suggestive of previous TB (in a person who receives inadequate or no treatment)
- Diabetes mellitus
- Silicosis
- Substance use (notably drug injection)
- Prolonged corticosteroid therapy
- Other immunosuppressive therapy
- Cancer of the head and neck
- Hematologic and reticuloendothelial diseases (e.g., leukemia and Hodgkin disease)
- End-stage renal disease
- Intestinal bypass or gastrectomy surgery
- Chronic malabsorption syndrome
- Low body weight (≥10% below the ideal)
- Recent TST converters (persons with baseline testing results who have an increase of 10 mm or more in the size of the TST reaction within a 2-year period; the risk of progression is greatest in the first 1 or 2 years after infection)
- Infants and children under the age of 5 years who have a positive TB skin test result

TB, Tuberculosis; *TST*, tuberculin skin test.
From Centers for Disease Control and Prevention (CDC), National Center for HIV/AIDS, Viral Hepatitis, STD, and TB Prevention. (2010). *Latent tuberculosis infection: A guide for primary health care providers.* Atlanta, GA: U.S. Department of Health and Human Services.

TB, may be suggestive of the diagnosis. Rales in the upper posterior portion of the chest, evidence of pleural effusion, lymphadenopathy, weight loss, and fever may increase the suspicion for TB. Confirmation of TB is based on the diagnostic evaluation presented in the next section.

DIAGNOSTICS
Essential Diagnostics

Screening is the first step in the diagnostic evaluation of TB and is performed to identify infected patients at high risk for TB who would benefit from preventive therapy as well as patients with TB who need treatment. If a person is infected with TB, a reaction to the TST is detectable 2 to 8 weeks after infection.[5] Because most patients infected with TB are asymptomatic, health care providers should administer the TST to all high-risk persons as part of their routine evaluation. Persons with any of the medical conditions or other factors listed in Box 214.1 should be screened annually unless there is prior documentation of a positive TST reaction. Other high-risk groups include close contacts of a person with infectious TB disease; foreign-born persons from areas in which TB is common (e.g., Asia, Africa, and Latin America); the medically underserved and low-income populations, including high-risk racial and ethnic groups (e.g., Asians and Pacific Islanders, African Americans, Hispanics, and Native Americans), migrant farm workers, and homeless persons; residents of long-term care facilities (e.g., correctional facilities and nursing homes); and other groups identified as having a disproportionate prevalence of

TB. Routine institutional screening is also recommended for health care workers and the staff of long-term institutional facilities who may have occupational exposure to TB or who would pose a risk to large numbers of susceptible persons if they developed active disease (e.g., staff member of an AIDS hospice).[5]

The standard and preferred method of screening for TB infection is the Mantoux test, which is administered by injection of 5 tuberculin units (0.1 mL) of purified protein derivative (PPD) solution intradermally into either the volar or the dorsal surface of the forearm. The injection should be made with a disposable tuberculin syringe with the needle bevel pointing upward. The injection should produce a discrete, pale elevation of the skin (a wheal) that is 6 to 10 mm ($\frac{1}{5}$ to $\frac{2}{5}$ inch) in diameter and disappears within several hours. If a wheal is not produced, the injection was probably too deep and will likely result in a false-negative reading. In the absence of a wheal, the skin test should be repeated. The amount of induration, rather than the erythema, is measured. All reactions, even those classified as negative, should be recorded in millimeters of induration. If no induration is found, 0 mm should be recorded.

The skin test result is read within 48 to 72 hours. If the patient fails to show up for a scheduled reading within 72 hours, a positive reaction may still be measurable up to 1 week later. A TST must be repeated if the result was not measured and recorded in millimeters of induration.[5] TST results should be measured only by a trained health care professional. Patients or family members should not measure TST results. The TST should be repeated for all negative responses not documented within 72 hours.[1] The criteria to determine whether a skin test result is significant depends on a patient's risk for development of disease or ability to mount a reaction to the PPD. The criteria for a positive TST reaction are listed in Box 214.2. Once a patient has had a positive TST reaction, no subsequent tuberculin skin testing should be performed. The TST should never be performed on a person who has had a previous positive TST reaction or who has had treatment of TB disease.[5]

A variety of factors can cause a false-negative TST reaction, including the recipient's age, simultaneous administration of a live vaccine, concomitant infections, metabolic deficiencies, underlying disease, and improper placement or storage of the PPD solution. Live vaccinations such as the measles, mumps, rubella (MMR) and varicella vaccines may cause a false-negative response to the TST for up to 2 months after immunization. However, results of the TST performed simultaneously with inoculation of these vaccines are unaffected.[15] Other potential causes of false-negative test results are listed in Box 214.3.

Because there are many potential causes of a false-negative TST reaction, the absence of a positive reaction does not exclude TB disease or infection. Anergy, a decreased or absent delayed-type hypersensitivity response, can be caused by severe or febrile illness, miliary or pulmonary disease, and most of the factors listed in Box 214.3. Of all patients with TB, 10% to 25% have negative reactions to the TST. Approximately one-third of patients with HIV infection and more than 60% of patients with AIDS have skin test reactions of less than 5 mm, even though they have been infected with *M. tuberculosis*.[5] A negative TST result does not exclude LTBI in patients who are immunocompromised. The usefulness of anergy testing for immunocompromised individuals has not been consistently demonstrated and is no longer recommended.[5]

BOX **214.2**

Criteria for a Positive Tuberculin Skin Test Reaction

INDURATION ≥ 5 MM
Persons with HIV infection
Household or close contacts of persons with TB infection
Persons with fibrotic lesions or evidence of old, healed TB on chest radiographs
Organ transplant recipients
Patients who are immunosuppressed for other reasons (e.g., taking equivalent of ≥ 15 mg/d of prednisone for 1 month or more or those taking tumor necrosis factor-α (TNF-α) antagonists)

INDURATION ≥ 10 MM
Recent immigrants (within past 5 years) from countries with high TB prevalence
Residents or employees of high-risk congregate settings (prisons, jails, long-term care facilities for the elderly, hospitals and other health care facilities, residential facilities for patients with AIDS, and homeless shelters)
Medically underserved, low-income populations, including high-risk minority populations
Persons with clinical conditions and other factors listed in Box 214.1
Mycobacteriology laboratory personnel
Children younger than 4 years
Infants, children, or adolescents exposed to adults at high risk for TB disease

INDURATION ≥ 15 MM
Persons with no known risk factors for TB

TB, Tuberculosis.
From Centers for Disease Control and Prevention (CDC), National Center for HIV/AIDS, Viral Hepatitis, STD, and TB Prevention. (2010). *Latent tuberculosis infection: A guide for primary health care providers.* Atlanta, GA: U.S. Department of Health and Human Services.

BOX **214.3**

Potential Causes of False-Negative Tuberculin Test Reactions

- Age (>45 years, newborns)
- Immunosuppression (e.g., corticosteroids, chemotherapy, or other agents)
- Systemic viral, fungal, and bacterial infections
- Live virus vaccinations (e.g., MMR; trivalent oral poliovirus vaccine)
- Malnutrition, cachexia, or nutritional derangement (e.g., severe protein deficiency, zinc deficiency)
- Chronic renal failure
- Hematologic or lymphoreticular disorders (e.g., Hodgkin disease)
- Sarcoidosis
- Stress (e.g., burns, postoperative status, mental illness)
- Mechanical (injection too deep, inexperienced reader)
- Improper storage (exposure to light or heat)

MMR, Measles, mumps, rubella.
Modified from American Thoracic Society. Diagnostic standards and classification of tuberculosis in adults and children. (2000). *American Journal of Respiratory and Critical Care Medicine, 161*(4 Pt 1):1376–1395. Retrieved from www.thoracic.org/statements/resources/archive/tbadult1-20.pdf. Accessed September 21, 2015.

BOX **214.4**

Criteria for Interpretation of Two-Step Tuberculin Skin Test Method

- If the first test reaction is positive, consider the person infected.
- If the first test reaction is negative, give second test 1–3 weeks later.
- If the second test reaction is positive, consider the person infected. If the second test reaction is negative, consider the person uninfected.

Modified from Centers for Disease Control and Prevention (CDC), National Center for HIV/AIDS, Viral Hepatitis, STD, and TB Prevention. (2010). *Latent tuberculosis infection: A guide for primary health care providers.* Atlanta, GA: U.S. Department of Health and Human Services.

BOX **214.5**

Interpretation of Interferon Gamma Release Assays Results

IGRA Test	Results Reported as
QuantiFERON-TB Gold In-Tube	Positive, negative, indeterminate
T-SPOT.*TB*	Positive, negative, indeterminate, borderline

Note: Laboratory should provide both quantitative and qualitative test results. *IGRA,* Interferon gamma release assays.
From Centers for Disease Control and Prevention (CDC), National Center for HIV/AIDS, Viral Hepatitis, STD, and TB Prevention. (2010). *Latent tuberculosis infection: A guide for primary health care providers* Atlanta, GA: U.S. Department of Health and Human Services.

False-negative reactions to the TST can also result from a decreased or waning delayed-type hypersensitivity reaction over time, especially among older adults who may have been infected years before being screened for TB. Although they were previously infected with TB, their hypersensitivity to the PPD antigen has been blunted over time. Although they may not respond to the initial skin test, the skin test may stimulate or "boost" their ability to react to the tuberculin on a subsequent test. Therefore, skin testing is repeated in 1 to 3 weeks. A positive reaction to the second test probably represents a boosted reaction rather than a reaction to new infection. On the basis of this two-step testing, the patient should be classified as previously infected, and management should proceed accordingly. Guidelines to interpret the results of a two-step TST are included in Box 214.4.

Interferon-gamma release assays (IGRAs) are blood tests that measure a person's immune reactivity to specific mycobacterial antigens. In a person infected with *M. tuberculosis,* the whole blood cells recognize simulated antigens and release interferon-γ (IFN-γ). Results are based on the amount of IFN-γ released.[5] When IGRAs are used for serial testing, there is no need for a second test because boosting does not occur.[5]

Many foreign countries vaccinate against TB by use of the bacillus Calmette-Guérin (BCG) vaccine. The BCG vaccine was first introduced in 1921 and continues to be the only vaccine used to prevent TB.[16] BCG has nonspecific immunologic effects and has been shown to be beneficial for other diseases. For example, BCG instillation into the bladder has been helpful in treating bladder cancer, and local application of BCG has been effective against common and genital warts. BCG is the most widely used vaccine worldwide. It has demonstrated efficacy in preventing miliary TB and TB meningitis in children but is not as effective in preventing pulmonary TB in adults.[16] BCG is used in many countries with a high prevalence of TB to prevent childhood tuberculous, meningitis, and miliary disease. It has not been generally recommended for use in the United States because of the low risk of infection with *M. tuberculosis,* the variable effectiveness of the vaccine against adult pulmonary TB, and the vaccine's potential interference with TST reactivity.[17]

Sensitivity to tuberculin varies significantly among persons who have received the BCG vaccination; this variance depends in part on the strain of BCG used and the person vaccinated. A history of BCG vaccination often confuses the diagnostic picture because there is no reliable way to determine whether a reaction to the TST is because of the BCG vaccine or infection with *M. tuberculosis.* Nevertheless, a prior history of BCG

vaccination is not considered a contraindication to PPD tuberculin skin testing. A reaction to the TST is probably a result of infection with *M. tuberculosis* rather than the BCG vaccine if the induration is large, if significant time has elapsed since BCG vaccination, if the person has had recent exposure to someone with infectious TB, if there is a family history of TB, if the person comes from an area in which TB is endemic, or if the chest radiograph shows evidence of previous TB infection. Patients who have received the BCG vaccine should be screened, evaluated, and managed in a manner similar to those who have not been vaccinated with BCG.[5] Interpretation of the TST result is the same for persons who have had BCG vaccination.[5]

IGRAs can be used in all situations in which a TST is used. An advantage of IGRAs is that results are available 24 hours after blood collection, in contrast to the 2- or 3-day wait with tuberculin skin testing. In addition, a two-step TST is recommended in certain situations; but with IGRAs, two-step testing is neither necessary nor recommended. In addition, IGRAs eliminate the need for proper intradermal injection technique, whereas with the TST, lack of proper technique can result in the PPD solution's being "washed out," leading to a possible false-negative reaction. IGRAs are cost-effective and efficient in that they eliminate the need for a second visit for test reading and should lead to fewer false-positive results in populations that include many BCG-vaccinated people (e.g., many non–US-born persons). Instructions for interpretation of IGRA results can be found in Box 214.5.

However, although IGRAs seem to have greater specificity, their sensitivity in detecting *M. tuberculosis* in young children and immunocompromised persons has not been determined. In addition, although IGRAs may save time for clinical staff, the labor and cost burden is shifted to microbiology staff, which needs to be figured into the cost of the tests. Finally, the difficulty of processing nonurgent blood specimens will be a barrier to use of IGRAs in some settings.

Advantages are that IGRAs require a single patient visit, do not cause a booster phenomenon, are less subject to reader bias than the TST, and are unaffected by BCG and most environmental mycobacteria.[5] Limitations of IGRAs are that blood samples must be processed within 8 to 16 hours and limited data exist on use in groups such as children younger than 5 years, persons recently exposed to TB, immunocompromised persons, and those who will be tested repeatedly (serial testing).

According to the CDC, IGRAs are the preferred method of testing for groups of people who have a poor rate of returning to have the TST result read and for persons who have received the BCG vaccine.[5] The TST is the preferred method of testing for children younger than 5 years. Either the TST or an IGRA may be used without preference in other groups being tested for LTBI, but neither test plays a role in the diagnosis of active TB. Routine testing with both TST and IGRA is not recommended.

Persons with a positive tuberculin TST or IGRA reaction should have an anteroposterior chest radiograph to exclude active pulmonary TB and to detect fibrotic lesions, which may suggest an old TB infection or silicosis. Once these conditions have been excluded, no subsequent chest radiographs are indicated unless the person is symptomatic. In addition, anergic persons who have symptoms consistent with TB or have risk factors for TB should undergo a chest x-ray examination. Abnormalities in the apical and posterior segments of the upper lobe or in the superior segments of the lower lobe are those most often seen with pulmonary TB. Infiltrates without cavities and mediastinal or hilar lymphadenopathy may also be seen. HIV infection and other immunocompromising illnesses may result in unusual chest x-ray findings. Chest x-ray findings may be suggestive of TB but are never diagnostic. Nevertheless, they may be used to exclude the possibility of pulmonary TB.[5]

Additional Diagnostics

Persons thought to have pulmonary or laryngeal TB should have at least three sputum cultures performed to detect the presence of acid-fast bacilli (AFB). A positive smear is strongly suggestive but not diagnostic of TB because the AFB on a smear may be mycobacteria other than *M. tuberculosis*. It is also possible for those with TB to have negative AFB smears. Species of mycobacteria are identified by a variety of methods, including nucleic acid probes, liquid chromatography, and polymerase chain reactions. The diagnosis is confirmed by a positive culture of *M. tuberculosis* complex, *M. avium*, or *Mycobacterium intracellulare*. The mycobacterium isolates are then tested for drug susceptibility. Drug susceptibility is important to ensure appropriate treatment and should be repeated within 2 months if there has not been an adequate response to treatment.

New point-of-care diagnostic tests for TB are currently being developed. Several versions of mycobacterial lipoarabinomannan (LAM) antigen detection in urine are in development. Urine antigen tests will likely be particularly helpful in diagnosis of TB in HIV-coinfected persons.[18]

DIFFERENTIAL DIAGNOSIS

 Immediate referral to a specialist indicated for signs and symptoms of active or disseminated TB.

The differential diagnosis of TB varies by the type of TB and the site of involvement. The signs and symptoms associated with pulmonary TB are consistent with those of other respiratory illnesses, such as pneumonia, acute bronchitis, and carcinoma. Extrapulmonary TB can occur in any organ; therefore, persistent signs and symptoms in any organ should lead to consideration of TB.

INTERPROFESSIONAL COLLABORATIVE MANAGEMENT
Pharmacologic Management

The management of TB depends entirely on the current clinical classification system of disease, which is based on the pathogenesis of the disease and the diagnostic results. The

Class	Type	Description
0	No TB exposure Not infected	No history of exposure Negative reaction to TST or QuantiFERON-TB test
1	TB exposure No evidence of infection	History of exposure Negative reaction to TST or QuantiFERON-TB test
2	TB infection No disease	Positive reaction to TST or QuantiFERON-TB test Negative bacteriologic studies (if done) No clinical, bacteriologic, or radiographic evidence of TB
3	TB Clinically active	*Mycobacterium tuberculosis* cultured (if done) Clinical, bacteriologic, or radiographic evidence of current disease
4	TB Not clinically active	History of episode(s) of TB *Or* Abnormal but stable radiographic findings Positive reaction to the TST or QuantiFERON-TB test Negative bacteriologic studies (if done) *And* No clinical or radiographic evidence of current disease
5	TB suspected	Diagnosis pending

TABLE 214.1 Clinical Classification System for Tuberculosis

TB, Tuberculosis; *TST*, tuberculin skin test.
From Centers for Disease Control and Prevention (CDC). *Interactive core curriculum on tuberculosis: What the clinician should know.* U.S. Department of Health and Human Services. Retrieved from www.cdc.gov/tb/education/corecurr/pdf/corecurr _all.pdf. Accessed December 7, 2018.

classification system is described in Table 214.1 and the official joint statement of the American Thoracic Society, CDC, and Infectious Diseases Society of America on the treatment of TB can be found in the Official American Thoracic Society/ Centers for Disease Control and Prevention/Infectious Diseases Society of America Clinical Practice Guidelines: Treatment of Drug-Susceptible Tuberculosis[19] at https://www.cdc.gov/tb/ publications/guidelines/pdf/clin-infect-dis.-2016-nahid-cid _ciw376.pdf. Currently, there are six first-line drugs (INH, rifampin, rifabutin, rifapentine [RPT], pyrazinamide [PZA], and ethambutol) and nine second-line drugs (cycloserine, ethionamide, streptomycin, amikacin/kanamycin, capreomycin, p-aminosalicylic acid [PAS], levofloxacin, and moxifloxacin) approved by the FDA for treatment of TB. The long-term (more than several weeks) use of fluoroquinolones in children and adolescents has not been approved because of concerns about effects on bone and cartilage growth.[12]

Class 0 and class 1 TB require no treatment. Patients with class 1 TB (contacts of a person with infectious TB disease) should have another TST performed within 8 to 10 weeks when the initial TST or IGRA reaction is negative.[5] Children younger than 5 years and immunocompromised persons who have had contact with a person with infectious TB disease and who have had a negative reaction should have a chest radiograph. If it is normal, treatment should be started for LTBI and another test performed 8 to 10 weeks after contact has ended. If a repeated test reaction is positive, treatment should be continued. If a repeated test reaction is negative, treatment can be discontinued. However, for some contacts at high risk of infection with TB, a full course of LTBI treatment may be recommended even in the absence of a positive TST or IGRA result.[5] Local TB control programs can provide guidance about the medical management of such contacts. In the follow-up testing of contacts of persons with infectious TB, the retesting is not referred to as two-step testing. The second test is necessary to determine if infection occurred but was too early in onset to be detected at the time of the first test. If testing is repeated, the same type of test (TST or IGRA) can be used. Patients with class 2 TB have been infected with TB but do not have any evidence of clinically active disease. The main purpose of preventive therapy is to decrease the risk that LTBI will progress to clinically active TB disease. INH is most commonly used for preventive therapy and is highly effective when it is taken as prescribed. The usual preventive therapy regimen is INH, 5 mg/kg (maximum dose, 300 mg), daily for 9 months.[5]

INH is bactericidal, relatively nontoxic, inexpensive, and easily administered. The degree of protection conferred by INH varies according to the percentage of mycobacteria eradicated. INH has been shown to reduce the incidence of disease by 54% to 90%; the primary reason for this variation in efficacy appears to be the actual amount of INH taken during the year it was prescribed.

INH remains less widely prescribed in the United States than is indicated. Preventive therapy should be considered for persons younger than 35 years who have TST reactions of 10 mm or more and who have any risk factors for TB. Patients younger than 35 years with no known risk factors should be evaluated for preventive therapy if their reaction to the TST was 15 mm or more. Unless otherwise indicated, INH preventive therapy should be offered to individuals with class 2 TB (tuberculin positive), regardless of their history of BCG vaccination. High-priority candidates for TB preventive therapy, regardless of age, are listed in Box 214.6.

The major side effect of INH is hepatitis. Other problems associated with INH include peripheral neuropathy, gastrointestinal upset, and mild CNS effects. From 10% to 20% of patients prescribed INH develop mild abnormalities of liver function, which usually resolve even if INH therapy is continued.[5] Increased values of liver function tests (LFTs) can be accepted at five times the upper limit of normal for patients who have no symptoms of hepatitis if the serum bilirubin concentration is within the normal range.[5] Clinical hepatitis occurs in approximately 0.1% of people taking INH and is more common when INH is combined with other agents.[5] The risk for INH-induced hepatitis increases directly with increasing age; therefore, INH is recommended for patients older than 35 years only if they are at high risk for development of TB. Baseline and monthly LFTs and a monthly clinical evaluation should be performed for all persons undergoing INH therapy.[20] Alcohol consumption has also been identified as a contributing risk factor in the development of INH-induced hepatitis. Other drugs that increase the risk of INH-induced hepatitis include acetaminophen, phenytoin (Dilantin), steroids, methimazole (Tapazole), estropipate (Ogen, Ortho-Est), and metoclopramide (Reglan, Maxolon). INH administration increases

High-Priority Candidates for Tuberculosis Preventive Therapy

Preventive therapy should be recommended for the following persons with a positive skin test reaction, regardless of age (criterion for a positive reaction in millimeters of induration is listed in parentheses):

- Persons with known or suspected HIV infection, including persons who inject drugs whose HIV status is unknown (≥5 mm)
- Close contacts of persons with infectious clinically active TB (≥5 mm)
- Persons who have chest x-ray findings suggestive of previous TB and who have received inadequate or no treatment (≥5 mm)
- Persons who inject drugs and are known to be HIV negative (≥10 mm)
- Recent TST converters (≥10-mm increase within a 2-year period for those <35 years of age; ≥15-mm increase for those ≥35 years of age)
- Persons with medical conditions that increase the risk of TB, such as diabetes mellitus, prolonged corticosteroid therapy, immunosuppressive therapy, some hematologic and reticuloendothelial diseases, injection drug use, end-stage renal disease, and clinical situations associated with rapid weight loss (≥10 mm)

TB, Tuberculosis; *TST*, tuberculin skin test.

the serum levels of certain drugs, including phenytoin, theophylline, carbamazepine (Tegretol), benzodiazepines, and anticoagulants. During INH administration, the serum levels of these drugs should be monitored more closely. Drugs that decrease the serum concentration of INH include antacids, corticosteroids, and laxatives. Symptomatic hepatitis associated with INH is rare in patients younger than 20 years, but severe and fatal cases have occurred. Therefore, younger patients taking INH should be monitored with the same precautions as for older individuals.[5]

Peripheral neuropathy is associated with the administration of INH in less than 0.2% of people taking INH at conventional doses and most likely results from interference with pyridoxine absorption. It occurs more often in the presence of other conditions associated with neuropathy, such as diabetes, renal failure, HIV infection, alcoholism, and malnutrition.[5] It is recommended that pyridoxine (25 to 50 mg/d) be administered in conjunction with INH to patients with these conditions. In addition, pyridoxine should be administered to pregnant and breastfeeding women to prevent neuropathy and to patients with a seizure disorder who are undergoing INH therapy.

Three randomized controlled trials have shown that a new combination regimen of INH and rifapentine (RPT), administered weekly for 12 weeks as directly observed therapy (DOT), is as effective for preventing TB as other regimens and is more likely to be completed than the US standard of 9 months of daily INH without DOT.[21] This new INH-RPT regimen is considered an equal alternative to the 9-month INH regimen for otherwise healthy individuals aged 12 years or older who have LTBI and factors predictive for developing TB, including recent exposure to contagious TB, recent conversion from negative to positive on an indirect test for infection, and radiographic findings of healed pulmonary TB. RPT, like rifampin, is a rifamycin-class antibiotic that is approved by the FDA for treating TB disease; its use for treating LTBI is off label. RPT is microbicidal for susceptible *M. tuberculosis*. The drug has a long half-life, which allows for infrequent administration, and lends itself to DOT.

The choice between INH and INH-RPT depends on several factors, including the feasibility of DOT, ability to procure the drug, programmatic issues (e.g., feasibility of patient monitoring), and patient and provider preferences.[21] INH-RPT is not recommended for children younger than 2 years of age; HIV-infected patients receiving antiretroviral treatment, because drug interactions have not been studied; pregnant women because safety in pregnancy is not known; and patients with presumed INH or RPT resistance.

RPT dyes secretions red, including urine and tears, and can stain contact lenses. Uncommon adverse effects include neutropenia and elevated liver enzymes. RPT induces the metabolism of many medications, particularly those metabolized by cytochrome P-450 isoenzyme 3A; it should not be used with these medications, particularly medications having narrow therapeutic ranges (e.g., warfarin, methadone), unless monitored carefully.[21] Because missed doses or altered dosage intervals could significantly affect efficacy or safety of the INH-RPT regimen, DOT is recommended. At each encounter, in addition to receiving medication, patients should be instructed to seek medical attention immediately if they develop fever, yellow eyes, dizziness, rash, or aches, or more than 1 day of nausea, vomiting, weakness, abdominal pain, or loss of appetite. If patients develop any of these symptoms, medication should be withheld while the cause of symptoms is determined. In addition, individuals receiving INH-RPT therapy should undergo monthly clinical assessments and physical examinations.

Additional treatment regimens for LTBI can be found in Table 214.2. For persons who have had close contact with individuals with INH-resistant TB, preventive therapy with rifampin, 10 mg/kg daily for 4 months, should be considered.[5] Rifampin preventive therapy can also be considered for patients who are INH intolerant.

Rifampin is bactericidal and easily administered. The most common side effect is gastrointestinal upset. Other adverse reactions include rashes, hepatitis, and, rarely, thrombocytopenia and cholestatic jaundice. Hepatitis is more common when rifampin is combined with INH.[5] Rifampin is a cytochrome P-450 (hepatic microsomal enzyme) inducer that may increase the clearance of drugs metabolized by the liver, including oral hypoglycemic agents, glucocorticoids, estrogens, warfarin (Coumadin) derivatives, methadone, theophylline, antiarrhythmic agents (quinidine, verapamil, mexiletine), anticonvulsants, ketoconazole, and cyclosporine. By interfering with estrogen metabolism, rifampin may also interfere with the effectiveness of oral contraceptives.[12] Rifampin is contraindicated or should be used with caution in persons with HIV disease who are being treated with certain protease inhibitors or non-nucleoside reverse transcriptase inhibitors. In this situation, rifabutin may be substituted.[7]

On the basis of adverse event data, the CDC and American Thoracic Society revised their guidelines and in 2003 recommended against the use of rifampin and PZA for treatment of LTBI. A CDC cohort analysis in 2003 found the rates of severe liver injury and death related to the use of rifampin and PZA to be significantly higher than the rates of INH-associated liver injury in the treatment of LTBI.[12] On the basis of these findings,

TABLE 214.2 Treatment Regimens for Latent Tuberculosis Infection

Drug and Dose	Frequency and Duration (Doses)	Rating[a] (Evidence)[b] HIV Negative	Rating[a] (Evidence)[b] HIV Positive
PREFERRED REGIMEN			
INH Adults: 5 mg/kg Children: 10–20 mg/kg Maximum dose 300 mg	Daily × 9 months (270 doses)	A (II)	A (II)
ALTERNATIVE REGIMENS			
INH Adults: 15 mg/kg Children: 20–40 mg/kg Maximum dose 900 mg	Twice weekly × 9 months[c] (76 doses)	B (II)	B (II)
INH Adults: 5 mg/kg Children: Not recommended Maximum dose 300 mg	Daily × 6 months (180 doses)	B (I)	C (I)
INH Adults: 15 mg/kg Children: Not recommended Maximum dose 900 mg	Twice weekly × 6 months[c] (52 doses)	B (II)	C (I)
Rifampin Adults: 10 mg/kg Children: 10–20 mg/kg Maximum dose 600 mg	Daily × 4 months (120 doses) Daily × 6 months (180 doses)	B (II)	B (II)

Note: In situations in which rifampin cannot be used (e.g., HIV-infected persons receiving protease inhibitors), rifabutin may be substituted.
[a]Strength of the recommendation: A = preferred regimen; B = acceptable alternative; C = offer when A and B cannot be given.
[b]Quality of the supporting evidence: I = randomized clinical trials data; II = data from clinical trials not randomized or from other population; III = expert opinion.
[c]Intermittent regimen must be provided via DOT (i.e., health care worker observes the ingestion of medication).
INH, Isoniazid.
From Centers for Disease Control and Prevention (CDC), National Center for HIV/AIDS, Viral Hepatitis, STD, and TB Prevention. (2010). *Latent tuberculosis infection: A guide for primary health care providers.* Atlanta, GA: U.S. Department of Health and Human Services.

the American Thoracic Society and the CDC now recommend that this regimen in general not be offered to persons with LTBI unless the potential benefits of this regimen outweigh the risks for severe liver injury and death associated with rifampin-PZA. The CDC recommends that a TB and LTBI expert be consulted before rifampin-PZA is offered. In addition, patients should be asked about whether they have a history of liver disease or adverse effects from INH or other drugs, be informed of potential hepatotoxicity of the rifampin-PZA regimen, and be advised against the concurrent use of potentially hepatotoxic drugs (including over-the-counter drugs such as acetaminophen).[22]

Treatment of class 3 or clinically active TB requires multidrug therapy. The specific drug regimen should be developed in consultation with an infectious disease physician or a specialist familiar with the management of TB. As previously mentioned, there are six first-line and nine second-line antitubercular drugs. The second-line antitubercular drugs, such as para-amino salicylic (PAS), ethionamide, and cycloserine, tend to be less effective and more toxic than the first-line drugs previously discussed. They are generally used only in cases of drug-resistant TB or atypical mycobacterial infections. Research on newer antitubercular drugs continues to be of importance, especially in this era of emerging drug resistance.

Comprehensive guidelines for the treatment of active TB can be found in the official joint statement of the American Thoracic Society, CDC, and Infectious Diseases Society of America on the treatment of TB.[12] One of the purposes of therapy is to prevent the development of MDR-TB, and therefore the medication regimen is based on drug susceptibilities.

The antitubercular drug regimens used to treat extrapulmonary TB are similar to those used to treat pulmonary TB. Additional therapies, such as corticosteroid therapy or surgery, may be required, depending on the site of TB infection. The type of follow-up and bacteriologic evaluation required is determined by the site of infection.

The diagnosis of nonclinically active TB (class 4) is defined by a history of previous episodes of TB or stable radiographic findings in a patient with a positive TST reaction. Sputum cultures, if obtained, are negative, and there is no radiographic evidence of clinically active disease. Patients with class 4 TB may be treated in several ways, depending on TB risk factors and the coexisting medical conditions. Some patients may have completed a course of preventive therapy, and some may be receiving preventive therapy; for others, preventive therapy may not be indicated. Current, clinically active TB must be excluded before a patient can be assigned to class 4.

Patients are categorized as having class 5 TB while the evaluation for TB is still being done and the diagnosis of TB is pending. Patients remain in this class until all diagnostic studies have been performed but should not remain in this class for more than 3 months. If clinically active TB is strongly suspected, patients are prescribed multidrug therapy while the evaluation is still pending. If a diagnosis of clinically active TB (class 3) is confirmed, multidrug therapy is continued. If TB disease is excluded, the drug regimen is altered accordingly. For example, if a diagnosis is changed to infectious (class 2) TB, preventive therapy is continued if indicated. If active TB is highly possible, it is imperative to start multidrug therapy initially and to alter the regimen accordingly because progressing from single-drug therapy (e.g., INH) to multidrug therapy once a diagnosis of active disease has been confirmed increases the risk for spread of the disease and development of drug-resistant TB.

One of the most significant problems associated with TB control is adherence to antitubercular regimens. Treatment adherence is difficult to predict; many variables may affect a person's adherence to the medication regimen, including office-related variables (e.g., long wait times or inconvenient office hours), patient-related variables (misinformation, residential instability, poor access to health care, concomitant medical conditions, lack of financial resources, culture and language, and religious practices), and treatment variables (medication side effects, frequency of visits, and the process for obtaining refills).[5] Inconsistent or partial treatment has resulted in TB that is resistant to INH and rifampin (MDR-TB). MDR-TB is a particular problem in certain areas of the world, such as Eastern Europe and central Asia, because of the breakdown in health system infrastructure and subsequent incomplete or inadequate treatments.[23] Although MDR-TB is treatable in general, the drug regimens required to treat it take longer and are considerably more expensive and toxic. Strategies to improve adherence, particularly with multidrug regimens, include providing education in the patient's primary language, reinforcing patient education at each visit, ensuring patient confidentiality, suggesting or providing medication reminders (e.g., a pill box or calendar), and collaborating with the local health department to provide DOT.[5]

In 1991, WHO introduced the DOTS (directly observed therapy short course) program, which includes five essential components: case detection by sputum-smear microscopy, government commitment to TB control, regular supply of TB drugs, supervised treatment, and reports on the progress of the health system. WHO has helped more than 180 countries implement DOTS, which is also used in the United States.[23] Cases of TB are subject to mandatory reporting in all 50 states, the District of Columbia, US dependencies and possessions, and independent nations within the United States (e.g., Native American lands). TB in the United States is closely monitored by local, federal, and state health departments.[24] As part of DOT, a health care provider or other designated person directly observes the patient taking each dose of TB medication. DOT is routinely implemented in many areas, such as homeless shelters and institutional settings. Trained personnel can provide DOT daily or intermittently in the office, clinic, or field (patient's home, workplace, corner bar, or any site that is mutually agreeable). Antitubercular regimens can often be prescribed to be taken two or three times weekly, making DOT less burdensome. DOT has been shown to be cost-effective when such intermittent regimens are used and is associated with a decrease in the acquisition and transmission of TB.[25] As a result, DOT is widely recommended and promoted for the management of patients with active TB. Universal DOT is credited with a decrease in the acquisition and transmission of resistant TB.[25]

The law in every state requires that a diagnosis of TB be reported to the local health department. All drug susceptibility test results should be forwarded to the health department. Reporting of TB is important for source and contact identification, epidemiologic surveillance, and the provision of resources for case management.

Consultation with a specialist is required for the management of all patients requiring multidrug therapy, those with active clinical disease (class 3), and those for whom the evaluation is pending (class 5). In addition, consultation is indicated for patients with evidence of TB infection (class 2) and coexistent medical conditions, especially those that alter immune responsiveness, which may increase the risk for development of clinically active disease.

Indications for Referral or Hospitalization

Most patients with clinically active pulmonary TB should be considered for hospitalization during the first couple of weeks of therapy. After 2 weeks of multidrug therapy, the infectiousness of these patients is reduced significantly and they are no longer a threat to public health. Patients with extrapulmonary TB typically are much less infectious and can be managed as outpatients.

Persons with MDR-TB should be referred to an infectious disease specialist or a pulmonologist with expertise in the treatment of TB. Immunocompromised patients with active TB or any patients with disseminated disease should also be referred.

LIFE SPAN CONSIDERATIONS

One approach to improving TB detection and control has been to integrate tuberculin skin testing and LTBI treatment with services routinely accessed by clients, such as methadone maintenance clinics. Prenatal care offers another opportunity to see patients on a regular basis. Pregnant women should have a TST only if specific risk factors are present. If a TST or IGRA reaction is positive, a chest radiograph should be obtained with proper shielding.[5] Once TB disease has been excluded, treatment of LTBI should be considered for HIV-infected women or if there has been recent contact with a person with TB. In the absence of these risk factors, treatment should be deferred until after the woman has delivered. If treatment is started during pregnancy, INH daily or twice weekly (using DOT) is the preferred regimen. Supplementation with 25 to 25 mg of pyridoxine (vitamin B_6) daily is recommended. Pregnant women receiving INH should be monitored closely for hepatotoxicity because there is an increased risk during pregnancy and for 2 to 3 months postpartum. It is recommended that treatment of LTBI be delayed until 2 to 3 months postpartum unless there is a high risk of progression to TB disease.[26]

Breastfeeding is not contraindicated in women taking INH. Pyridoxine supplementation is recommended for nursing women. Pregnant women with clinically active TB (class 3) must receive adequate therapy as soon as TB is suspected because risk of transmission to the fetus is high. Untreated TB presents a much greater danger to a woman and her fetus than does treatment of the disease. The preferred initial drug regimen includes INH, rifampin, and ethambutol. These drugs do cross the placenta but have no demonstrated teratogenic side effects. A woman receiving antitubercular therapy should not be discouraged from breastfeeding; although small concentrations of the drug are found in breast milk, they do not cause toxicity in newborns.[27]

Older adults receiving antitubercular therapy must be monitored closely for drug side effects. Many of the adverse reactions increase with advancing age and decreased renal function.

COMPLICATIONS

Complications of TB can result from the disease process itself or can be secondary to drug therapy. The death rate of untreated pulmonary TB is approximately 60%, with a median time until death of 2½ years. Patients with miliary or disseminated TB often become ill before radiographic changes are apparent or a diagnosis of TB has been made. Without treatment, the prognosis for miliary TB is poor. However, miliary TB responds to the same drug regimens used to treat other forms of TB.

Persons taking antitubercular drugs need to be monitored closely for side effects and drug toxicities. Baseline laboratory evaluations and monthly examinations are indicated for most of the drugs used to treat TB.

TB and HIV/AIDS form a lethal combination because each disease speeds the progress of the other. Because HIV weakens the immune system, someone who is infected with HIV and TB is many times more likely to develop active TB than is someone infected with TB who is HIV negative. TB is the leading cause of death among people who are HIV positive and accounts for approximately 13% of AIDS-related deaths worldwide.[4]

Smoking and TB is thought to be another "lethal interaction," and smoking appears to be a risk factor for acquiring TB infection, developing active TB, having a more severe pulmonary TB, and being at increased risk of dying from the disease.[27] Even though smokers tend to have more innate immune cells and lymphocytes in their lungs, they seem to have an increased vulnerability to TB. The hypothesis is that immune cells and lymphocytes may be compromised in the presence of cigarette smoke, thereby compromising their effectiveness against TB.[28]

PATIENT AND FAMILY EDUCATION

Patient education is critical to controlling the resurgence of TB. The public must be educated about the role of TB screening and the need to identify persons infected with TB before active disease develops so they can benefit from preventive therapy. Bilingual and bicultural outreach staff workers are needed to work with immigrant individuals and communities to counter opposition to LTBI therapy based on cultural misunderstandings about its purpose and fears of stigmatization based on adherence to a long-term medication regimen.

- The importance of medication adherence must be carefully explained as untreated TB can lead to reactivation of the disease in the future, progression of the disease, continued spread of the disease, and development of drug resistance.
- Potential drug side effects must be carefully discussed, with instructions to contact their health care provider as soon as any signs or symptoms associated with drug toxicity develop.

REFERENCES

1. World Health Organization. Global health observatory data. Retrieved from https://www.who.int/gho/tb/en. (Accessed 22 July 2019).
2. Warner, D. F., Koch, A., & Mizrahi, V. (2015). Diversity and disease pathogenesis in *Mycobacterium tuberculosis*. *Trends in Microbiology*, 23(1), 14–21.
3. World Health Organization. (2018). Global Tuberculosis Report. Retrieved from http://www.who.int/tb/publications/global_report/tb18_ExecSum_web_4Oct18.pdf?ua=1. (Accessed 3 December 2018).
4. American Thoracic Society, Centers for Disease Control and Prevention (CDC), Infectious Disease Society of America. (2005). Controlling tuberculosis in the United States. *American Journal of Respiratory Medicine: Drugs, Devices, and Other Interventions*, 172, 1169–1227.
5. Centers for Disease Control and Prevention (CDC), National Center for HIV/AIDS, Viral Hepatitis, STD, and TB Prevention. (2010). *Latent tuberculosis infection: A guide for primary health care providers*. Atlanta: U.S. Department of Health and Human Services.
6. Centers for Disease Control and Prevention (CDC). Latent TB Infection in the United States—Published Estimates. Retrieved from https://www.cdc.gov/tb/statistics/ltbi.htm. (Accessed 22 July 2019).
7. Centers for Disease Control and Prevention (CDC). (2017). Trends in tuberculosis—United States. Retrieved from https://www.cdc.gov/tb/statistics/default.htm. (Accessed 3 December 2018).
8. World Heath Organization. (2017). Global Tuberculosis Report. Retrieved from www.who.int/tb/publications/global_report/en. (Accessed 22 July 2019).
9. Menzies, H. J., Winston, C. A., Holtz, T. H., et al. (2010). Epidemiology of tuberculosis among U.S.- and foreign-born children and adolescents in the United States, 1994–2007. *American Journal of Public Health*, 100(9), 1724–1729.
10. Pevzner, E. S., Robison, S., Donovan, J., et al. (2010). Tuberculosis transmission and use of methamphetamines in Snohomish County, WA, 1991–2006. *American Journal of Public Health*, 100(12), 2481–2486.
11. Centers for Disease Control and Prevention (CDC). (2006). Prevention and control of tuberculosis in correctional and detention facilities: Recommendations from CDC. *MMWR. Recommendations and Reports: Morbidity and Mortality Weekly Report. Recommendations and Reports*, 55(RR–9), 1–54.
12. American Thoracic Society, Centers for Disease Control and Prevention (CDC), Infectious Diseases Society of America. (2003). Treatment of tuberculosis. *MMWR. Recommendations and Reports: Morbidity and Mortality Weekly Report. Recommendations and Reports*, 52(RR–11), 1–77.

13. Schluger, N. (2005). The pathogenesis of tuberculosis: The first one hundred (and twenty three) years. *American Journal of Respiratory Cell and Molecular Biology, 32,* 251–256.

14. Centers for Disease Control and Prevention (CDC). Interferon-gamma release assays (IGRAs)—blood tests for TB infection. Retrieved from www.cdc.gov/tb/publications/factsheets/testing/IGRA.htm. (Accessed 30 December 2018).

15. Centers for Disease Control and Prevention (CDC). (2009). *Epidemiology and prevention of vaccine-preventable diseases* (11th ed.). Atlanta: U.S. Department of Health and Human Services.

16. Netea, M. G., & van Crevel, R. (2014). BCG-induced protection: Effects on innate immune memory. *Seminars in Immunology, 26,* 512–517.

17. Centers for Disease Control and Prevention (CDC), National Center for HIV/AIDS, Viral Hepatitis, STD, and TB Prevention, Division of Tuberculosis Elimination. BCG vaccine. Retrieved from www.cdc.gov/tb/publications/factsheets/prevention/BCG.htm. (Accessed 30 December 2018).

18. Rodrigues, C. (2011). Diagnostics for tuberculosis: Time to usher in a new era. *Indian Journal of Medical Microbiology, 29*(1), 2–3.

19. Nahid, P., Dorman, S. E., Alipanah, N., et al. (2016). ATS/CDC, IDSA Clinical practice guidelines for drug-susceptible TB. *Clinical Infectious Diseases: an Official Publication of the Infectious Diseases Society of America, 63,* 853–867.

20. World Health Organization. TB comorbidities and risk factors. Retrieved from https://www.who.int/tb/areas-of-work/treatment/risk-factors/en/. (Accessed 24 July 2019).

21. Centers for Disease Control and Prevention (CDC). (2011). Recommendations for use of an isoniazid-rifapentine regimen with direct observation to treat latent *Mycobacterium tuberculosis* infection. *MMWR. Morbidity and Mortality Weekly Report, 60*(48), 1650–1653.

22. Centers for Disease Control and Prevention (CDC). (2003). Update: Adverse event data and revised American Thoracic Society/CDC recommendations against the use of rifampin and pyrazinamide for treatment of latent tuberculosis infection—United States, 2003. *MMWR. Morbidity and Mortality Weekly Report, 52*(31), 735–739.

23. Murray, S. (2006). Challenges of tuberculosis. *CMAJ: Canadian Medical Association Journal = Journal de l'Association Medicale Canadienne, 174*(1), 33–34.

24. Myers, W., Westenhouse, J., Flood, J., et al. (2006). An ecological study of tuberculosis transmission in California. *American Journal of Public Health, 96*(4), 685–690.

25. Moonan, P., Quitugua, T. N., Pogoda, J. M., et al. (2011). Does directly observed therapy reduce drug resistant tuberculosis? *BMC Public Health, 11,* 19.

26. Sackoff, J., Pfeiffer, M., Driver, D., et al. (2006). Tuberculosis prevention for non–U.S.-born pregnant women. *American Journal of Obstetrics and Gynecology, 194,* 451–456.

27. Arbex, M. A., Varella Mde, C., & deSiqueira, H. R. (2010). Antituberculosis drugs: Drug interactions, adverse effects, and use in special situations. Part 1: First line drugs. *Jornal Brasileiro de Pneumologia: Publicacao Oficial da Sociedade Brasileira de Pneumologia e Tisiologia, 36*(5), 626–640.

28. Chan, E. D., Kinney, W. H., Honda, J. R., et al. (2014). Tobacco exposure and susceptibility to tuberculosis: Is there a smoking gun? *Tuberculosis, 94,* 544–550.

CHAPTER **215**

MOSQUITO-BORNE ILLNESS

Thomas H. Taylor • Elizabeth A. Talbot

DEFINITION AND EPIDEMIOLOGY

Arthropod-borne viruses (ArBoVirus) are transmitted by ticks and mosquitoes. Mosquito-borne illness is caused by many viruses and certain parasites (malaria, some filarial disease). Tick-borne illness (see Chapter 213) is rendered by spirochetes (Lyme disease), rickettsia (Rocky Mountain Spotted Fever), ehrlichia (ehrlichiosis), anaplasma (anaplasmosis), protozoa (babesiosis), typhus (African tick typhus), and certain viruses (tick-borne encephalitis, Powassan encephalitis). Arboviruses are the main cause of epidemic encephalitis in North America, and malaria is the most common mosquito-borne illness in returning travelers from Africa. Each mosquito-borne virus family has specific tissue sites of disease, but all may cause meningitis or encephalitis to varying degrees (Table 215.1). During the past 20 years, the face of meningoencephalitis has changed from predominantly enterovirus and herpes simplex virus to a broad and geographically varied spectrum of disease, many transmitted by mosquitoes. *Aedes, Anopheles,* and *Culex* mosquitoes are the most likely to bite humans, who are incidental hosts in an otherwise specific host reservoir for each disease. Sporadic transmission occurs when humans transect normal mosquito-host reservoirs, and epidemics occur when mosquito-host reservoirs multiply to transgress human domains.

Mosquito bites are not always clearly recalled, so a good history is important. Good history includes geography, travel itinerary, incubation period, urban or rural exposure, illness in others, immunization history, malaria prophylaxis, consumption of unclean water, raw meat, unpasteurized milk, insect bites, animal bites, pet exposure, intravenous drug user (IVDU), body piercings, medical tourism, sexual contact, fresh water exposure, swimming or walking barefoot, and rashes or eschars. An eschar with focal necrosis in a traveler from southern Africa suggests African tick typhus, a relatively benign disease. An eschar obtained in South or Southeast Asia suggests scrub typhus, a much more serious infection. This eschar is often missed because the mite that transmits scrub typhus prefers covered areas such as the perineum and genitalia. Ticks also prefer groin, axilla, and perineum. Mosquito bites are usually on exposed extremities.[1-3]

PATHOPHYSIOLOGY

Malaria invades red blood cells, which results in hemolysis, hemoglobin-induced acute renal failure, and ischemia in small vascular beds such as the lungs and brain. Viruses cause disease in accord with the cell tropism of the virus. Host reservoir animals are often unaffected by the virus and remain viremic, thus infecting multiple mosquitoes. Togaviridae, Flaviviridae, and Bunyaviridae are all neurotropic and cause meningoencephalitis. Flaviviridae are also hepatotropic and may cause hepatitis, a useful diagnostic sign for Yellow Fever and West Nile virus (WNV). Gastrointestinal, respiratory, cardiac, or urinary symptoms are rare, and may point to other diagnosis (typhoid fever, influenza, MERS-corona virus [CoV], or hantavirus). Viral tropism for endothelial cells results in immune endovascular activation of interleukin pathways and the cytokine cascade, which may cause hemorrhagic manifestations and shock.

CLINICAL PRESENTATION AND PHYSICAL EXAMINATION

Most infection with WNV, St. Louis encephalitis (SLE), and Japanese encephalitis (JE) is asymptomatic. Serologic surveys indicate that only 20% of infected persons develop West Nile Fever (WNF), and less than 1% develop West Nile Neuroinvasive Disease (WNND) (https://www.cdc.gov/westnile/index.html). Togaviridae (Eastern Equine Encephalitis virus [EEE], Western Equine Encephalitis [WEE], Venezuelan equine encephalitis [VEE]) are extensively neuroinvasive, with high mortality and morbidity. Bunyaviridae cause encephalitis, but patients often fully recover. It is difficult to distinguish between initial presentations of the various Arbovirus infections. Weakness and acute flaccid paralysis (AFP) are associated with WNV, but must be distinguished from Guillain-Barré syndrome (GBS) (see

TABLE 215.1 Zoonosis and Vectors as Cause of Encephalitis

Virus	Vector	Reservoir Host	Ecology	Geography	Incubation Period	Epidemic Potential	Vaccine Available
TOGAVIRIDAE							
Eastern Equine Encephalitis	Mosquitoes	Birds, Horses, Cattle	Rural	North and South America	3–14 days Range 1–20	Epidemics and Sporadic	Vaccine for horses
Western Equine Encephalitis	Mosquitoes	Birds, Rabbits	Rural	North and South America	3–14 days Range 1–20	Epidemics and Sporadic	Vaccine for horses
Venezuelan Equine Encephalitis	Mosquitoes	Rodents	Rural	North and South America	3–14 days Range 1–20	Epidemics and Sporadic	Vaccine for horses
Chikungunya	Mosquitoes	Humans, Monkeys	Rural Urban	Asia, Africa, Americas	2–12 days	Epidemics and Sporadic	
FLAVIVIRIDAE							
Dengue	Mosquitoes	Humans	Rural Urban	Asia, Africa, Americas	4 days Range 3–14	Epidemics and Sporadic	
Zika	Mosquitoes	Humans, Monkeys	Rural Urban	Asia, Africa, Americas	5–8 days Range 2–15	Epidemics and Sporadic	Vaccine in trials
Japanese Encephalitis	Mosquitoes	Birds	Rural Suburban	Asia	7 days Range 5–15	Epidemics and Sporadic	Vaccine available
Murray Valley Encephalitis	Mosquitoes	Birds, Horses	Rural	Australia	12 days Range 5–28	Epidemics and Sporadic	
St. Louis Encephalitis	Mosquitoes	Birds	Rural Suburban	Americas, Midwest and South	10 days Range 4–21	Epidemics and Sporadic	
West Nile Encephalitis	Mosquitoes	Birds	Rural Suburban	Asia, Africa, North America	4 days Range 3–14	Epidemics and Sporadic	
Tick-Borne Encephalitis	Ticks	Rodents	Rural	Europe and Asia	7–14 days Range 4–20	Sporadic	Vaccine available
Powassan Encephalitis	Ticks	Rodents	Rural Suburban	Europe, Northern United States Canada	19 days Range 4–30	Sporadic	
Yellow Fever	Mosquitoes	Humans, Monkeys, Marsupials	Rural Suburban	Historically worldwide, Brazil	3–6 days Range 3–14	Epidemics and Sporadic	Vaccine @ certified clinics
BUNYAVIRIDAE							
La Crosse Encephalitis	Mosquitoes	Rodents	Rural Suburban	North America	10 days Range 5–15	Sporadic	
California Encephalitis	Mosquitoes	Rodents	Rural	Central and Eastern US	10 days Range 5–15	Epidemics and Sporadic	
Rift Valley Fever	Mosquitoes	Ruminant Sheep	Rural	Africa and Middle East	4 days Range 3–6	Epidemics and Sporadic	Vaccine available

Chapter 176). Rashes are associated with Zika virus, Dengue, and Chikungunya. Conjunctival inflammation, often attributed to Leptospirosis, is also associated with Zika and Chikungunya. Rash is unusual in Leptospirosis.

Compared with arboviruses, all of which present within 21 days of exposure, the incubation periods for malaria are longer: 1 month to 1 year, but most malaria presents within 3 months of exposure. The fevers may not be periodic, especially with more acute Falciparum malaria. Fever that begins more than 21 days after a traveler's return is unlikely to be Dengue, Zika, rickettsial disease, or viral hemorrhagic fevers (see Table 215.1).

The general examination should include awareness of rash, jaundice, anemic pallor, weakness, arthritis, adenopathy, abdominal tenderness, hepatomegaly, and splenomegaly. Photophobia is recognized by excessive reaction to bright light. Nuchal rigidity is recognized by passive flexing of the neck, which induces involuntary hip flexion (Brudzinski's sign). More diffuse meningeal irritation is elicited by Kernig's sign: with hip flexed, attempts to extend the knee produce resistance and pain in the hamstring and back. Meningeal irritation in children may be recognized by tripoding, or sitting on the examination table supported by buttocks and both hands placed posteriorly, so as to maintain a rigid spine. Encephalitis is recognized by testing multiple areas of cognitive function, degree of alertness, speech, motor and sensory function, and cranial nerves.

AFP may be recognized by abrupt onset of motor weakness, retained sensory function, decreased deep tendon reflexes, and may be distinguished from GBS by lack of autonomic or sensory nerve involvement. Lumbar puncture helps distinguish aseptic meningitis associated with viral meningitis, encephalitis, and AFP by modest pleocytosis or elevated cerebral spinal fluid (CSF) white blood cell count, generally less than 500 cells/mL. This pleocytosis is usually lymphocytic, but in early infection may show neutrophil predominance. Spinal fluid associated with GBS, in contrast, has no pleocytosis and demonstrates isolated protein elevation (albuminocytologic dissociation). GBS may progress rapidly, and frequently repeated examinations are required to assess the need for increasing levels of supportive care.

Maculopapular rashes may be seen with all viral encephalopathies, but are most common with dengue, chikungunya, zika, and WNV viruses. Lyme disease (see Chapter 213) and leptospirosis are both caused by spirochetes. The rash of Lyme disease, erythema chronicum migrans (ECM), is characteristic, focal, migratory, and should not be confused with a viral exanthema. Rash is very unlikely with Leptospirosis. Tremors of the eyelids, tongue, lips, and extremities may suggest West Nile encephalitis or St. Louis encephalitis in the appropriate geographic setting.

DIAGNOSTICS AND DIFFERENTIAL DIAGNOSIS

Routine blood work should include CBC, creatinine, liver function tests, urine analysis, and thin and thick blood smears for malaria. Among returning travelers, much febrile illness is due to common infections such as respiratory and urinary tract infections, meningococcal disease, and tuberculosis. Don't forget blood cultures to rule out bacterial infection. Recognizing and testing for life-threatening causes of fever (malaria, dengue, EEE) and not missing highly transmissible causes of fever, which are not transmitted by mosquitoes (viral hemorrhagic fevers, influenza, MERS-CoV, measles, and tuberculosis) are equally important.

Serologic testing is the most effective method to confirm clinical suspicion of an arbovirus infection. Enzyme-linked immunosorbent assay for detection of immunoglobulin M (IgM) in serum at 6 to 8 days or in CSF at 3 to 5 days is indicative of recent infection. Individuals recently infected with or vaccinated against related viruses, such as yellow fever, dengue fever, and JE, may have false-positive serologic results for WNV. The problem of cross-reactivity with flaviviruses, including SLE virus circulating in the Northern Hemisphere, can be corrected by confirmatory testing with a plaque reduction neutralization assay. IgM antibody to WNV may persist for months after infection, which lessens the specificity of this test in serum. However, IgM does not cross the blood-brain barrier, and the presence of IgM in the CSF is strong evidence of local production and thus acute infection.

Molecular amplification assays (e.g., polymerase chain reaction [PCR]) in serum are low yield because of the usually low levels and transient nature of viremia in acute infection of humans. PCR has moderate sensitivity for detection of arbovirus in CSF, but it disappears as CSF IgM antibody becomes positive. PCR is most useful in blood supply screening and active

surveillance of bird and mosquito populations. Tissue samples from postmortem examinations may be tested by immunofluorescent antibody and viral culture.

Viral encephalitis associated complete blood counts may be normal or moderately increased with a relative lymphocytosis, but 15% may demonstrate lymphopenia. Malaria is heralded by hemolysis: normocytic anemia, schistocytes seen on peripheral blood smear, and acute renal failure. A metabolic profile with liver function tests can be helpful with the differential diagnosis. Hyponatremia may be indicative of syndrome of inappropriate antidiuretic hormone (SIADH), which is often seen with any encephalitis. Arbovirus encephalitis patients may have transaminitis consistent with a usually mild hepatitis. In such cases, serum amylase and lipase should be checked for concomitant pancreatitis. Muscle enzymes such as creatine kinase and myoglobin may be elevated to mild or severe degrees. Lumbar puncture can be helpful in distinguishing between AFP and GBS, for which the prognosis is quite different.

Cerebral computed tomography (CT) is often normal. Cerebral MRI is more likely to reveal abnormalities such as enhancement of the leptomeninges or the periventricular areas, but it is diagnostic only of meningitis or encephalitis in general. MRI is the imaging procedure of choice, but it is possible to have clinical degrees of encephalitis without MRI abnormalities. T2-weighted images showing high-intensity signals in most commonly affected areas of the thalamus, basal ganglia, brainstem, and spinal cord may be early indications of encephalitis.[4]

INITIAL DIAGNOSTICS

Mosquito Borne Illness

LABORATORY
- CBC, creatinine, BMP, LFTs, U/A
- Thin and thick blood smears, or rapid diagnostic test to R/O malaria
- Blood cultures to R/O typhoid fever and bacterial sepsis or endocarditis
- Lumbar puncture: real-time PCR and IgM antibodies on CSF for suspected virus
  R/O bacterial meningitis: cell count and culture
- Serology which may require acute and convalescent serum

IMAGING
- Chest x-ray: malaria, tuberculosis, and bacterial pathogens
- Brain MRI to R/O encephalitis

DIFFERENTIAL DIAGNOSIS

1. Diseases with potential for rapid progression and high mortality:
   Malaria, bacterial meningitis, EEE, Dengue, Yellow Fever, WNV
   Viral hemorrhagic fevers: Ebola, Lassa virus, Hantavirus
2. Diseases with potential for person-to-person transmission (epidemics):
   Typhoid, viral hemorrhagic fevers, influenza, MERS-CoV, and tuberculosis
   Measles, mumps, rubella
3. Mosquito-borne virus epidemics not transmitted person to person

Malaria

Malaria remains a highly morbid infectious disease; it threatens nearly half of the world's population and led to hundreds of thousands of deaths in 2017, predominantly among children in Africa (https://www.who.int/news-room/fact-sheets/detail/malaria). Human malaria is caused by five species of single-celled eukaryotic *Plasmodium* parasites that are transmitted by the bite of *Anopheles* mosquitoes. *Plasmodium falciparum* and *Plasmodium vivax* are the most common and important species, with *Plasmodium knowlesi* most recently recognized as a prevalent species in parts of Asia, especially Malaysia.

Globally, malaria is managed through a combination of vector control approaches (such as insecticide spraying and the routine use of insecticide-treated bed nets), rapid diagnosis by lateral flow diagnostics, and drugs for both treatment and prevention especially among pregnant women. Artemisinin-based combination therapies have contributed to substantial declines in the number of malaria-related deaths; however, the emergence of drug resistance threatens to reverse this progress. Strategies to eliminate malaria also include vaccine development and novel vector control strategies.

The incubation period in most cases varies from 7 to 30 days. The shorter periods are observed most frequently with *P. falciparum* and the longer ones with *P. malariae*. It is important to note that when travelers take antimalarial drugs for prophylaxis, it may delay the appearance of malaria symptoms by weeks or months. This can happen particularly with *P. vivax* and *P. ovale*, both of which can produce dormant liver stage parasites; the liver stages may reactivate and cause disease months after the infective mosquito bite.

The most common symptoms of malaria are fever, chills, headache, nausea with vomiting, and myalgia. In severe forms, malaria can cause hemolysis, multiple organ failure, and death. Maintain a high index of suspicion in the correct geographic or travel setting, regardless of prophylaxis history. Although traditional diagnosis involves use of thick and thin blood smears, consider the use of the rapid diagnostic test (RDT), which quickly establishes the diagnosis of malaria infection by detecting specific malaria antigens in a person's blood. Binax-NOW (Alere) is the only RDT currently available in the United States. This RDT detects two different malaria antigens; one is specific for *P. falciparum* and the other is found in all human species of malaria. All positive RDTs should be followed by microscopy for species confirmation and to measure the degree of parasitemia.[5,6]

For clinical consultation regarding malaria treatment, the CDC maintains the CDC Malaria Hotline: 770-488-7788 or 855-856-4713 toll-free (M–F, 9 a.m. to 5 p.m. EST). Emergency consultation is available after hours at 770-488-7100.

Differential Diagnosis

- Dengue, Chikungunya
- Viral hemorrhagic fevers
- African tick bite fever
- Relapsing fever

 Red flags include:

Abnormal behavior, impairment of consciousness, seizures, coma, or other neurologic abnormalities

Severe anemia due to hemolysis

Hemoglobinuria (hemoglobin in the urine) due to hemolysis

Acute respiratory distress syndrome (ARDS)

Abnormalities in blood coagulation

Low blood pressure caused by cardiovascular collapse

Acute kidney failure

Hyperparasitemia, where more than 5% of the red blood cells are infected by malaria parasites

Hypoglycemia

Metabolic acidosis

West Nile Virus

WNV is the prototype of mosquito-borne arbovirus infection, now reported all over the United States (with lower rates in New England and MidAtlantic states), Africa, and Europe. It presents as sporadic cases in summer and fall but continues to cause epidemics. WNV has a predisposition to cause acute febrile illness and central nervous system infections, encephalitis, and aseptic meningitis. WNF, West Nile meningitis (WNM), and West Nile encephalitis (WNE) are outcomes of WNV. All Flaviviridae may invade muscles, joints, and the liver and thus give rise to complications of myositis, arthritis, and hepatitis. Encephalitis, meningitis, myelitis, and neuritis refer to inflammation of brain, leptomeninges, spinal cord, and nerve roots, respectively. Radiculitis refers to involvement primarily of the sensory nerve root, and AFP refers to a myelitis involving the anterior horn cells, or motor cells, of the spinal cord; both conditions may complicate WNV infection. Meningoencephalitis, or inflammation of both meninges and brain, is common in WNV infection.

Most cases in North America have occurred in the late summer and early fall, in conjunction with high rates of mosquito WNV carriage. Children have high rates of infection but low rates of neuroinvasive disease, which is more likely to be manifested as aseptic meningitis, as opposed to meningoencephalitis in adults. Adults older than 65 years have higher mortality and 110 times the incidence of WNND compared with children.[7,8]

Clinical Presentation. Most infection with WNV is asymptomatic in 80% of cases, similar to SLE and JE viruses. The 20% with notable clinical illness mainly present with WNF. Only 1% develop WNND, which includes aseptic meningitis or encephalitis. When the virus attacks anterior horn cells in the spinal cord, a polio-like illness ensues, AFP.

After an incubation period of 2 to 14 days (longer in immunocompromised hosts), WNF is characterized by an influenza-like illness, fever, arthralgia, myalgia, rash, malaise, and headache. Gastrointestinal symptoms have included nausea, vomiting, and diarrhea. Generalized lymphadenopathy, splenomegaly, and hepatomegaly are common. Rash appears early in 50% to 60% of cases and is a nonspecific maculopapular rash that most often begins on the trunk. Although WNV was confirmed serologically, the acute-phase serum tested negative at the time of rash in 57% of patients.[7] Convalescent serum is often needed to confirm the diagnosis in this early and nonspecific stage of illness.

Aseptic (nonbacterial) meningitis and encephalitis commonly follow the symptoms of WNF by 4 to 7 days but may appear without recognized prodrome as stiff neck (meningismus), headache, and sensitivity to light (photophobia). These symptoms may further proceed to encephalitis characterized by alterations in consciousness: lethargy, confusion, stupor, and coma. More focal encephalopathic signs include difficulty with word finding, speech, and memory, sometimes advancing to seizures, cranial neuropathy, upper motor neuron paralysis with hyperreflexia, and extensor plantar responses. The hypothalamic-pituitary axis may become involved and is associated with central nervous system-mediated fever, hyponatremia resulting from SIADH, or diabetes insipidus (urinary water loss) caused by insufficient antidiuretic hormone.

As with poliovirus and more closely related JE and SLE viruses, a biphasic illness eventuates in aseptic meningitis (30%) and encephalitis (60%) following WNF.[8] Prominent findings in patients with encephalitis are movement disorders: tremor, parkinsonism, gait disturbances, myoclonus, and rarely seizure disorder. These motor disturbances appear early, have a pathophysiologic correlation with lesions seen on magnetic resonance imaging (MRI) in the basal ganglia and thalamus, and may resolve in ensuing months. Weakness is a prominent feature of more severe disease. Infection of motor anterior horn cells may lead to AFP recognized as progressive weakness, often asymmetric, and loss of deep tendon reflexes. GBS triggered by WNV infection is also associated with gradual, but symmetric, ascending loss of muscle weakness and loss of deep tendon reflexes. GBS is an autoimmune acute inflammatory demyelinating polyradiculopathy with autonomic dysfunction. Sensory and autonomic nerve involvement is not seen with AFP. Long-term neurologic sequelae and relapse may be associated with WNV, but GBS is largely reversible over time.

WNV is closely related to St. Louis encephalitis virus (SLE), which was the leading cause of encephalitis prior to introduction of WNV in 1999. WNV is more efficiently spread among wild bird reservoirs and bird flyways; cross immunity protects birds from SLE. As epidemics of WNV decline, we may again see outbreaks of SLE.[9]

Dengue

Dengue is a flavivirus, like Yellow Fever or WNV, and occasionally causes hepatitis or encephalitis. However, the viremia is rapidly cleared, so most complications follow defervescence, and are attributable to the immunologic response. Dengue is transmitted by *Aedes* mosquitoes, adapted to stagnant water in urban areas, which bite all day long into the evening. Sporadic cases and epidemics occur worldwide in tropical and subtropical environs. Epidemics tend to occur in rainy season, but transmission is year-round in endemic regions. There are four dengue viruses and immunity wanes over a few months. Most serious disease ensues with subsequent infections, when immune response is maximized. Virus multiplies within blood cells which produce signaling proteins, interferon, and cytokines. Endothelial cell dysfunction results in capillary leakage of body fluids and hemorrhage.

Most infection is asymptomatic. Symptomatic infection, mainly dengue fever (DF), is a self-limited disease marked by arthralgia and myalgia, sometimes called break-bone fever. Headache, especially retro-orbital, or ocular pain is characteristic. Maculopapular rash or erythroderma is present in 50%. With the first episode of DF, only 5% develop hemorrhagic manifestations (https://www.cdc.gov/dengue/clinicallab/clinical.html).

The more feared second episode is associated with dengue hemorrhagic fever (DHF), caused by endovascular immune activation and hemorrhage, which occurs in 5% to 10%.[10] Primed by the first episode of DF, immune reactivation may be severe. Plasma leakage from damaged vessels may be suspected by early hemoconcentration, a 20% increase in hematocrit, and thrombocytopenia. Platelets are trapped in small vessels, microangiopathic thrombocytopenia, and more bleeding ensues. If fluid resuscitation is not initiated at this early stage, then dengue hemorrhagic shock (DHS) progresses and

may be irreversible. A characteristic biphasic, saddleback fever curve represents initial dengue fever, defervescence, followed by hemorrhagic fever recurrence as immune activation and cytokine response begin at 2 to 7 days. Hemorrhagic manifestations produce blood in emesis, stool, and urine.[10,11]

Warning Signs for Dengue Hemorrhagic Fever
- Petechiae, ecchymosis, purpura
- Bleeding from gingiva, injection sites, gastrointestinal tract
- Vomiting or abdominal pain
- Hemoconcentration and/or thrombocytopenia
- A positive tourniquet test: petechiae in the arm after applying a tourniquet for 5 minutes.

 Red flags include:
- Ascites or pleural effusion (capillary leakage)
- Lethargy and restlessness (hemodynamic shock)
- Hypotension or narrow pulse pressure
- Organ failure: respiratory distress, anuria, transaminitis (AST or ALT above 1000 units/L)

There is no antiviral medicine; as with other arbovirus diseases, supportive care is paramount. If there are no warning signs and the patient can tolerate oral fluids, provide supervised home care with rehydration fluids, acetaminophen, and tepid sponge baths. It is most important to advise against aspirin or NSAIDs, which may exacerbate hemorrhage. If conditions worsen upon defervescence (see warning signs), then return to the hospital. If there are warning signs or preexisting comorbidities, admit patient to hospital. Follow platelets and hematocrit for hemoconcentration. Give isotonic IV hydration: 10 mg/kg for 1 hour, then reassess following BP and hematocrit. Adjust fluids to lower hematocrit and maintain BP and urine output. If evidence for DHS (see red flags), then give IV isotonic fluid at 20 mg/kg over 30 to 60 minutes and reassess. If hemorrhage, give packed RBCs or whole blood transfusions appropriate to response. Analgesics and antiemetic drugs provide symptomatic relief.[11]

Chikungunya Virus

Chikungunya outbreaks are longstanding in Africa, Asia, Europe, India, and Pacifica. In 2013, transmission of chikungunya virus in the Americas was first identified. Recent years have seen spread throughout the Americas including North America and Alaska. Chikungunya is an African word signifying "that which is bent over" or "stooped walk." This virus has similar distribution, prodromal symptoms, and propensity to cause arthritis as Dengue virus. Dengue, Zika, and chikungunya are all transmitted by the same mosquito vectors, *Aedes aegypti* and *Aedes albopictus* (Asian tiger mosquito, which survives temperate climates and has wider distribution). Humans and other primates are the reservoir. The incubation period is 3 to 7 days (range 1 to 14), similar to Dengue fever.

Clinical presentation is acute-onset fever and malaise, soon followed by extensive arthritis similar to rheumatoid arthritis: polyarticular, symmetric, small joint proceeding to larger joints. Like *Flaviviridae*, chikungunya, a *Togaviridae* alphavirus, may cause meningoencephalitis, AFP, GBS, acute myelitis, cranial neuropathies, hepatitis, and acute renal failure. Laboratory findings include thrombocytopenia and lymphopenia, but hemorrhagic illness is rare. The acute illness may last 1 week, but arthritis may linger for months to years. Other manifestations of connective tissue disease are commonly seen: Raynaud's syndrome, episcleritis and polychondritis, uveitis, retinitis, and cryoglobulinemia.

Diagnosis is usually made based on the distinctive presentation of abrupt onset high fever and arthritis in an area where chikungunya is active. RT-PCR is very sensitive in the first 5 days of illness. After 1 week of illness, IgM followed by IgG serology becomes positive. Patients should be similarly tested for Dengue and Zika virus. The CDC will run PCR and serology on all three, as similar presentations are common. Treatment is supportive: fluids, analgesics. Avoid aspirin and NSAIDs until Dengue is ruled out. One study showed that patients with underlying diseases requiring biologics did no worse, as viral neutralization is expected to remain intact. Persistent arthritis may benefit from physical therapy to prevent contractures. Prolonged arthritis has been treated with methotrexate, short courses of steroids, and anti-TNF therapy.[12-14]

Differential Diagnosis

- Dengue fever
- Zika virus
- Parvovirus

Other Considerations when Arthritis Is Present

- Rubella or recent Rubella vaccination
- Measles
- Ross river virus, transmitted only in Australia
- Leptospirosis
- African tick bite fever
- Acute HIV infection
- Prodromal or chronic hepatitis C or B

 Red flags include:
Symptoms of DHF: hemorrhage, shock, severe abdominal pain
Contagious diseases: influenza, MERS-CoV, typhoid, and tuberculosis
Common transmissible diseases: Measles, mumps, rubella

Zika Virus

Zika virus is another neurotropic flavivirus, transmitted by *Aedes* mosquitoes, and known for outbreaks. Most infection is asymptomatic, but 20% develop clinical disease.[15] The incubation period is 2 to 14 days. Sporadic cases and outbreaks have been noted in Africa, Southeast Asia, and Pacific Islands, with recent spread to Chile and Brazil in 2015. Autochthonous spread (local spread person-mosquito-person) has been seen in Puerto Rico, Florida, and Texas. The virus may be transmitted by sexual contact, blood products, and maternal-fetal exposure. The CDC website provides updates on this evolving epidemic at https://www.cdc.gov/zika/index.html.

Clinical manifestations include acute low-grade fever, pruritic rash (diffuse macules and papules), arthralgia of small joints, fatigue, and retro-orbital pain. Congenital microcephaly, neurologic sequelae, and fetal losses are seen with intrauterine exposure, but infants who acquire the virus by mosquito bite develop normally. It is apparent that neurologic sequelae are seen in adults as well, commonly varying degrees of GBS, but also encephalitis, myelitis, neuropsychiatric, and cognitive symptoms. Considering the long period of viral secretion in body fluids, relapsing symptoms have been described.[15,16]

Differential Diagnosis

- Dengue, Chikungunya
- Parvovirus
- Rubella or rubella vaccine
- African tick bite fever (Africa and the Caribbean)
- Relapsing fever

 Red flags include:
Distal weakness and sensory loss (GBS)
Hemorrhage or shock (DHF or DHS)
Signs of meningoencephalitis

When to Test for Zika. Diagnosis is by RT-PCR (serum, urine, or whole blood) in the first 14 days, but negative PCR does not exclude the diagnosis; if negative, reflex serology for IgM and plaque reduction neutralization test (PRNT) is performed. After 14 days, PCR has low yield, and serology (IgM and PRNT) is required. Although commercial labs are performing some tests, it is best to order them through your State Public Health Department and the CDC. There is cross-reactivity with other flaviviruses, and past vaccination for Japanese encephalitis or yellow fever may cause false positive results. Because of false positives and past infection, asymptomatic persons should not be tested. Pregnant women should be tested regardless of symptoms if they have travelled to an endemic area or had sexual contact with such a traveler or infected partner. Pregnant women should not travel to an endemic or cautionary area. Semen may carry the virus for 6 to 9 months after infection. Men should use condoms during this period. Vaccine development is progressing and should be available soon (Table 215.2).[17,18]

Yellow Fever

Yellow Fever is the prototype Flaviviridae virus with hepatocyte tropism causing acute hepatitis. Inflammatory encephalitis is rare, and usually due to cerebral edema and metabolic encephalopathy. Like Dengue, yellow fever is capable of hemorrhage and shock due to cytokine storm and decreased synthesis of vitamin K-dependent coagulation factors by a failing liver. The vector is the *Aedes aegypti* mosquito causing large epidemics in tropical regions of Africa and South America. Asia has never experienced an epidemic of yellow fever, and the population has no immunity—cause for concern. There is presently epidemic yellow fever in Brazil, and vaccine supplies are short (see Chapter 208).

As with other Flaviviridae, diagnosis is by characteristics of disease and exposure to mosquitoes in epidemic or sporadic setting of disease. Confirmation is by PCR detection of viral genome in blood or tissue, and serology for IgM and IgG antibody.

Clinical yellow fever is often nonspecific febrile illness with erythroderma, conjunctival and gingival erythema, and liver tenderness. Like typhoid fever, bradycardia in the setting of heightened fever is common (Faget's sign). Leukopenia and relative neutropenia are other distinguishing features. Most patients mount an abortive remission, but 15% will relapse into a "period of intoxication" at 3 to 6 days.[19] This stage is marked by return of fever, nausea and vomiting, abdominal pain, jaundice, hemorrhage, and renal failure. Patients appear septic with systemic immune response syndrome (SIRS), and levels of inflammatory cytokines are high. Unlike hepatitis A, levels of serum aspartate aminotransferase (AST) are elevated in excess of levels of alanine aminotransferase (ALT). Renal failure is marked by oliguria and azotemia, with very high urine protein characteristic of acute tubular necrosis (ATN). Death is often due to renal failure from hepatorenal syndrome and ATN.[19]

Differential Diagnosis

- Viral hepatitis (hepatitis A, B, C, D, and E)
- Dengue, also associated with fever, headache, myalgia, arthralgia, hemorrhage

TABLE 215.2   When to Test: Centers for Disease Control and Prevention Guidelines

If Your Patient...	Testing Recommendation
Was exposed to Zika AND has symptoms (https://www.cdc.gov/zika/symptoms/symptoms.html) of Zika virus infection or a history or symptoms at any time during her pregnancy	She should be tested for Zika as soon as possible (https://www.cdc.gov/zika/symptoms/diagnosis.html). Concurrent RNA nucleic acid test (NAT) testing and Zika virus IgM testing is recommended as soon as possible or through 12 weeks after symptom onset.
Lives in or frequently travels to an area with risk of Zika **but does not have symptoms** of Zika virus infection.	She should be offered testing three times during pregnancy using RNA NAT testing.
Traveled to or had sex without a condom with a partner who lived in or traveled to an area with risk of Zika **but does not have symptoms** of Zika virus infection	Testing is not routinely recommended. Testing should be considered using a shared decision-making model that includes pretest counseling, individualized risk assessment, clinical judgment, patient preferences, and the jurisdiction's recommendations. Testing recommendations for this group of pregnant women may differ by jurisdiction. Please contact your state, tribal, local, or territorial health department for jurisdiction-specific guidance.
Was exposed to Zika **AND** had birth defects potentially associated with Zika detected on a prenatal ultrasound	Concurrent RNA NAT testing and Zika virus IgM testing is recommended. If amniocentesis is being done for clinical care, healthcare providers should also test the amniotic fluid for Zika genetic material. Testing of placental and fetal tissues may also be considered if results of maternal Zika virus testing are not definitive.

From Centers for Disease Control and Prevention (CDC). (2019). *Testing & diagnosis for Zika virus.* https://www.cdc.gov/pregnancy/zika/testing-follow-up/testing-and-diagnosis.html.

- Malaria, also with fever, anemia, jaundice due to hemolysis
- Typhoid, also with fever, rash, abdominal pain, and abnormal liver function
- Other viral hemorrhagic fever: ebola, Lassa fever, Marburg virus, Bolivian and Argentine hemorrhagic fevers

 Red flags include:
Relapse of fever following defervescence
SIRS symptoms
AST twice ALT
Acute renal failure (ATN)

There is no antiviral therapy. Supportive care and fluid resuscitation are effective, but mortality is 50% in severe disease.[19] Vaccination is required for those living in or traveling to endemic areas; vaccine is now in short supply, due to the epidemic in Brazil. Immigration officials may require a certificate of vaccination on entry to an endemic country or on travel from an endemic country. Only registered vaccine centers may provide vaccine certificates. Vaccination is also controversial, because this is a live vaccine and cannot be given to immunocompromised hosts. Physicians may write a waiver for immunocompromised individuals, who should not be vaccinated. However, pregnant women may take the vaccine if exposure is certain and benefits of vaccination outweigh risks. Congenital vaccine infection is rare and has not been associated with fetal abnormalities.[20]

Vaccine efficacy is nearly 100%, and 97.5% of vaccines mount a serologic response.[20] Concern is with adverse vaccine effects: acute neurotropic or viscerotropic disease occurring in 1/100,000 but higher in the elderly (2 to 3/100,000). Fever, jaundice, ATN, hemorrhage, encephalomyelitis, GBS, and optic neuritis may occur, always self-limited, and neurologic sequelae are rare.

Japanese Encephalitis

Japanese Encephalitis (JE) is the most frequent and most severe cause of encephalitis in Asia. An estimated 68,000 cases occur each year, and most of the endemic population is immune by age 15. The risk for short-term travelers to urban areas is very low, one in a million. Risk increases in travelers staying more than 1 month, during rainy season, engaging in outside activities, and traveling outside urban areas. Culex mosquitoes feed outdoors, engage in evening and nighttime biting, and are the main vector. Amplifying hosts are pigs and wading birds.

Only 1% of JE infection results in neuroinvasive disease, but encephalitis is severe with 20% to 30% mortality in hospitalized patients (https://www.cdc.gov/japaneseencephalitis/healthcareproviders/healthcareproviders-clinlabeval.html). Febrile illness with headache and aseptic meningitis are milder presentations. Neurologic sequelae persists in 80%, and neurologic progression may indicate active disease over months in 20% of recovering patients. This virus has a predilection for the thalamus, basal ganglia, and brain stem, which may offer a unique JE parkinsonian syndrome secondary to extrapyramidal disease. Like WNV, an acute poliomyelitis-like presentation with AFP may be the only manifestation. Hyponatremia due to inappropriate antidiuretic hormone is common. Hepatic enzymes suggesting mild hepatitis are seen.[21,22]

Serodiagnosis of Flaviviridae is complicated by cross-reacting antibodies to vaccine or past infection from other viruses within this family. In addition to the usual CSF and serum IgM antibody tests, MRI imaging may show abnormalities in the thalamus, basal ganglia, pons, medulla, and brainstem suggesting JE. However, WNV, Herpes simplex virus, and common respiratory viruses may present a similar MRI predilection for these structures.[21,22]

Eastern and Western Equine Encephalitis

Eastern Equine Encephalitis. EEE, a Togaviridae found in birds and *Culiseta* mosquitoes inhabiting swamps and bogs, is found in the Caribbean, Central, and North and South America. A few cases are seen each year, mostly in Massachusetts, New Hampshire, and Florida. Only 2% of infected adults develop encephalitis, which is more common in children.

EEE is the most feared arboviral encephalitis, with mortality of 30%.[23] Full recovery is unlikely, with neurologic sequelae of seizures, paralysis, and cognitive loss. Following a nonspecific prodrome, rapid deterioration ensues with coma, seizures, focal neurologic loss, and cranial nerve palsies in 90%.[23]

Western Equine Encephalitis. WEE is also found in North and South America. Past outbreaks in the Western US have been curtailed by declining wild horse populations, immunization of domestic horses, and mosquito control. Compared to EEE, far fewer infections result in encephalitis, one in a thousand, with fewer fatalities (5%), and rare neurologic sequelae.[24]

Venezuelan Equine Encephalitis. Venezuelan Equine Encephalitis is also geographically widespread. In contradistinction to EEE and WEE, large epidemics have occurred in Florida and South America. Outbreaks include thousands of infections, but only 0.5% of adults develop encephalitis, though more in children. Fatalities and neurologic sequelae are uncommon. A horse vaccine exists for all three equine encephalitis viruses, and related vaccine is made for laboratory workers, but is not commercially available. Outbreaks are contained by mosquito control, vaccination of horses, and personal mosquito protection.

California Encephalitis Group

Bunyaviridae. The Bunyaviridae family of viruses includes the California Encephalitis Group and Rift Valley Fever (RVF). Reservoirs include chipmunk, squirrel, fox, and rodents. Vectors uniquely include all major human biting mosquitoes: *Aedes*, *Culex*, and *Anopheles*. The vector is infected for life and transmits the virus transovarially to progeny. Infection occurs mainly in children following late summer and early fall exposure to woodlands. The infection is usually subclinical or mild flu-like illness, but some viruses (California Encephalitis virus, LaCrosse virus, Jamestown Cannon virus) occasionally produce severe encephalitis marked by seizures and paralysis. Milder self-limited illness is caused by Trivittatus virus in central and eastern states.

Rift Valley Fever. RVF is responsible for numerous large outbreaks in humans and livestock in Africa and the Middle East. Humans are infected by mosquito bites, contact with infected animals, or raw milk. Sheep, cattle, and goats are infected in that order of susceptibility. A broad spectrum of disease includes myalgia, arthralgia, headache, photophobia, maculopapular rash, jaundice, hemorrhagic fever, and sometimes retinitis with blindness. Enzootic hepatitis is another name for RVF. Given the reemergence of RVF and the wide range of outbreaks in sub-Saharan Africa, South Africa, and the Middle East, travelers returning from those areas, within the 1 week incubation period, and exposure to animals, should be considered to have RVF. Monitor patients closely for jaundice, retinitis, and hemorrhagic fever. A vaccine is now available.[25,26]

INTERPROFESSIONAL COLLABORATIVE MANAGEMENT

Pharmacologic and supportive management is disease specific and infectious disease specialists should be consulted.

The prognosis for malaria depends on the degree of parasitemia and specific organ failure. Most *falciparum* malaria cases should be hospitalized, as shock, renal failure, and respiratory failure may progress rapidly. Red flags for arbovirus meningitis, encephalitis, and shock should prompt hospitalization. The degree of pleocytosis seen in CSF, especially neutrophilic

pleocytosis, predicts poor prognosis. MRI may also be useful in determining when to withdraw support in cases of severe encephalitis. Infectious disease and neurology consultation is needed for acute management.

Residual neurologic sequelae are common with arbovirus encephalitis. Early institution of physical therapy, speech therapy, airway protection, and pacemaker for autonomic bradycardia in GBS may be crucial. Late progression in WNV and JE may indicate ongoing autoimmune or residual viral activity. Late regression of what was thought to be permanent dysfunction is also seen. Basic care to prevent pressure sores, aspiration, and nutritional deficiency is important and may need to continue for several months of rehabilitation before a final prognosis is determined.

PATIENT AND FAMILY EDUCATION

- Prolonged support and patience may be needed for full recovery.
- Person-to-person transmission is unlikely with arbovirus or malaria.
- End-of-life issues and resuscitation preferences should be discussed sooner rather than later for severe encephalitis or failing malaria.
- Zika is present in semen, and therefore sexually transmissible, for 6 to 9 months after infection. Pregnancy should be avoided during this time.

HEALTH PROMOTION

Mosquito species bite at different times of day and transmit different diseases. Knowledge of the geography, season for transmission, and type of mosquito are all helpful. Information for specific diseases and specific areas of travel can be found on the GIDEON and CDC websites. *Aedes* mosquitoes bite all day, while *Culex* mosquitoes bite from evening to dawn, and *Anopheles* mosquitoes bite at dawn and dusk. Dengue, Chikungunya, and Zika viruses are all now prevalent in the Western hemisphere and spread by *Aedes aegypti* and *Aedes albopictus* mosquitoes. Temperate weather in North America is not a deterrent, as *Aedes* mosquitoes are distributed across the United States.[1,27]

Vaccines are available for Japanese Encephalitis, Tick-Borne Encephalitis, Yellow Fever, and Rift Valley Fever, as discussed in those sections. A vaccine for Zika virus is forthcoming. Horse vaccine is available for EEE, WEE, and VEE with limited vaccine for laboratory workers (Box 215.1).

BOX 215.1

Personal Protective Measures

- Use malaria chemo prophylaxis, specific to the area of travel
- Restrict travel to areas of active transmission or outbreaks
- Pregnant women should not travel to areas of Zika transmission (wwnc.cdc.gov/travel/page/zika-information)
- Insect repellants: DEET, picaridin, IR3535, para-methane-3,8-diol, oil of eucalyptus
- Treat clothing with permethrin: remains active through several washings
- Wear long-sleeve shirts and trousers. Protect infants with mosquito netting.
- Control mosquitoes: drain all standing water, tires, flower saucers, pool, trash, leaves

REFERENCES

1. LaRocque, R. C., & Ryan, E. T. (2016). Medical considerations before international travel. *The New England Journal of Medicine, 375*(15), e32.

2. Huntington, M. K., Allison, J., & Nair, D (2016). Emerging vector-borne diseases. *American Family Physician, 94*(7), 551–557.

3. Gautam, R., Mishra, S., Milhotra, A., Nagpal, R., Mohan, M., Singhal, A., et al. (2017). Challenges with Mosquito-borne Viral Diseases: Outbreak of the Monsters. *Current Topics in Medicinal Chemistry, 17*(19), 2199–2214.

4. Beattie, G. C., Glaser, C. A., Sheriff, H., Messenger, S., Preas, C. P., Shahkarami, M., et al. (2013). Encephalitis with thalamic and basal ganglia abnormalities: Etiologies, neuroimaging, and potential role of respiratory viruses. *Clinical Infectious Diseases: an Official Publication of the Infectious Diseases Society of America, 56*(6), 825–832.

5. Shanks, G. D., & Mohrle, J. J. (2017). Treating malaria: New drugs for a new era. *The Lancet Infectious Diseases, 17*(12), 1223–1224.

6. Chiodini, J. (2017). UK malaria guidelines—Dynamic changes for 2017. *Travel Medicine and Infectious Disease, 20*, 71–74.

7. Zou, S., Foster, G. A., Dodd, R. Y., Petersen, L. R., & Stramer, S. L. (2010). West Nile fever characteristics among viremic persons identified through blood donor screening. *The Journal of Infectious Diseases, 202*(9), 1354–1361.

8. Patel, H., Sander, B., & Nelder, M. P. (2015). Long-term sequelae of West Nile virus-related illness: A systematic review. *The Lancet Infectious Diseases, 15*(8), 951–959.

9. White, G. S., Symmes, K., Sun, P., Fang, Y., Garcia, S., Steiner, C., et al. (2016). Reemergence of St. Louis encephalitis virus, California, 2015. *Emerging Infectious Diseases, 22*(12), 2185–2188.

10. Amin, P., Acicbe, O., Hidalgo, J., Jimenez, J. I. S., Baker, T., & Richards, G. A. (2018). Dengue fever: Report from the task force on tropical diseases by the World Federation of Societies of Intensive and Critical Care Medicine. *Journal of Critical Care, 43*, 346–351.

11. Nguyen, M. T., Ho, T. N., Nguyen, V. V., Nguyen, T. H., Ha, M. T., Ta, V. T., et al. (2017). An evidence-based algorithm for early prognosis of severe dengue in the outpatient setting. *Clinical Infectious Diseases: an Official Publication of the Infectious Diseases Society of America, 64*(5), 656–663.

12. Cunha, R. V. D., & Trinta, K. S. (2017). Chikungunya virus: Clinical aspects and treatment—A Review. *Memorias Do Instituto Oswaldo Cruz, 112*(8), 523–531.

13. Goupil, B. A., & Mores, C. N. (2016). A review of Chikungunya virus-induced arthralgia: Clinical manifestations, therapeutics, and pathogenesis. *The Open Rheumatology Journal, 10*, 129–140.

14. Marti-Carvajal, A., Ramon-Pardo, P., Javelle, E., Simon, F., Aldighieri, S., Horvath, H., et al. (2017). Interventions for treating patients with chikungunya virus infection-related rheumatic and musculoskeletal disorders: A systematic review. *PLoS ONE, 12*(6), e0179028.

15. Baud, D., Gubler, D. J., Schaub, B., Lanteri, M. C., & Musso, D. (2017). An update on Zika virus infection. *Lancet, 390*(10107), 2099–2109.

16. Weaver, S. C., Charlier, C., Vasilakis, N., & Lecuit, M. (2017). Zika, Chikungunya, and other emerging vector-borne viral diseases. *Annual Review of Medicine*.

17. Zorrilla, C. D., Garcia Garcia, I., Garcia Fragoso, L., & De La Vega, A. (2017). Zika virus infection in pregnancy: Maternal, fetal, and neonatal considerations. *The Journal of Infectious Diseases, 216*(suppl_10), S891–S896.

18. Hastings, A. K., & Fikrig, E. (2017). Zika virus and sexual transmission: A new route of transmission for mosquito-borne flaviviruses. *The Yale Journal of Biology and Medicine, 90*(2), 325–330.

19. Simon, L. V., & Torp, K. D. (2017). Yellow fever. In *StatPearls*. Treasure Island (FL): StatPearls Publishing LLC.

20. Staples, J. E., Bocchini, J., Rubin, L., & Fischer, M. (2015). Yellow Fever Vaccine Booster Doses: Ecommendations of the advisory committee on immunization practices, 2015. *MMWR. Morbidity and Mortality Weekly Report, 64*(23), 647–650. Retrieved from https://www.cdc.gov/mmwr/preview/mmwrhtml/mm6423a5.htm. (Accessed 24 July 2019).

21. Fischer, M., Lindsey, N., Staples, J. E. & Hills, S., Centers for Disease Control and Prevention (CDC). (2010). Japanese encephalitis vaccines: Recommendations of the Advisory Committee on Immunization Practices (ACIP). *MMWR. Recommendations and Reports: Morbidity and Mortality Weekly Report. Recommendations and Reports, 59*(RR-1), 1–27.

22. Basu, A., & Dutta, K. (2017). Recent advances in Japanese encephalitis. *F1000Research, 6*, 259.

23. Berlin, D., Gilani, A. I., Grewal, A. K., & Fowkes, M. (2017). Eastern equine encephalitis. *Practical Neurology, 17*(5), 387–391.

24. Simon, L. V., & Gossman, W. G. (2017). Encephalitis, Western equine. In *StatPearls*. Treasure Island (FL): StatPearls Publishing LLC.

25. Nanyingi, M. O., Munyua, P., Kiama, S. G., Muchemi, G. M., Thumbi, S. M., Bitek, A. O., et al. (2015). A systematic review of Rift Valley Fever epidemiology 1931–2014. *Infection Ecology & Epidemiology, 5*, 28024.

26. Faburay, B., LaBeaud, A. D., McVey, D. S., Wilson, W. C., & Richt, J. A. (2017). Current status of Rift Valley fever vaccine development. *Vaccines (Basel), 5*(3), doi:10.3390/vaccines5030029.

27. LaRocque, R. L., & Ryan, E. T. (2016). Personal actions to minimize mosquito-borne illnesses, including Zika virus. *Annals of Internal Medicine, 165*(8), 589–590.

CHAPTER 216

ANEMIA

A. Susan Feeney

DEFINITION AND EPIDEMIOLOGY

Anemia is not a disease but rather a sign or symptom of an underlying disorder. Anemia is defined as a reduction in the number of red blood cells (RBCs), hemoglobin concentration, or hematocrit. In general, a hemoglobin concentration in adults below 13.6 g/dL for men or below 12 g/dL for women suggests anemia.[1] Although certain signs and symptoms are sometimes associated with anemia, the diagnosis is often based on laboratory data alone.

As one of the most common hematologic diagnoses, anemia affects people of every age group. Iron deficiency anemia (IDA) is the most common etiology of anemia in young children and pregnant women. Anemia is more common in individuals older than 65 years.[2] The most common cause of anemia in the elderly is anemia of chronic disease (ACD), followed by nutritional deficiencies (iron, B_{12}, folate), and possibly, decreased marrow response to erythropoietin.[2] Some types of anemia have a higher incidence in certain ethnicities. For example, sickle cell disease is most common in those of African ancestry, and thalassemia in people from the geographic regions of the Mediterranean, the Middle East, Southeast Asia, and parts of India and Pakistan.

PATHOPHYSIOLOGY

Anemia is a result of hemoglobin deficiency. Hemoglobin's major function is to transport oxygen to tissues; therefore, anemia is a condition that results in too little oxygen being transported to the tissues. Inadequate provision of oxygen to tissues produces the signs and symptoms of anemia. There are many causes of anemia which result in various forms of anemia. When considering the etiologies of anemia, it is useful to classify them into three categories: (1) RBC production disorders, (2) RBC destruction disorders, and (3) blood loss (acute or chronic). In a healthy, intact hematopoietic system, there are many intrinsic homeostatic mechanisms in place to ensure adequate RBC production and blood volume. When anemia is present, it implies that the normal homeostatic mechanisms and normal reserves have been exhausted. It is also important to consider that anemia may be due to a combination of factors.

Red Blood Cell Production Disorders

There are many elements and processes needed for adequate RBC production. They include an intact and functional bone marrow matrix, intact erythropoietin system, adequate absorption, storage and utilization of essential components (iron, B_{12}, folate, protein), and an absence of chronic inflammation.

Erythropoiesis, the production of erythrocytes (RBCs), is limited to the axial skeleton and proximal ends of the long bones in the adult. The marrow is a special environment for hematopoietic development and consists of a matrix of reticular cells and fibers called the marrow stroma. It is here that stem cells are stimulated by colony-stimulating factors to grow and differentiate into the various blood cells, including RBCs.[3,4] Any condition that interferes with this bone marrow function can cause anemia.

The most common disorder related to inadequate RBC production is IDA (see later). Iron is critical for both erythrocyte proliferation and maturation and for hemoglobin synthesis. Circulating erythrocytes have a lifespan of approximately 100 to 120 days. Under normal conditions, the turnover rate for erythrocytes is approximately 1% per day. Although, in response to hypoxia and anemia, marrow precursors may be seen in 2 to 3 days, an increase in the reticulocyte count will take several more days.[3] The most important factor in the body's ability to increase RBC production is iron. Without adequate iron stores, the marrow cannot increase erythropoiesis.[3,4]

Anemia of chronic kidney disease (ACKD) is also a result of inadequate RBC production. Erythropoietin is a glycoprotein hormone secreted by the kidney that induces erythroid precursor cells to differentiate, thereby increasing new RBC production. The control of erythropoiesis is dominated by the decreased concentration of hemoglobin in the blood. This leads to changes in tissue oxygen tension and in turn triggers receptors within the kidney to secrete erythropoietin. Chronic kidney disease can result in an under production and secretion of erythropoietin, thereby suppressing an essential signal triggering RBC production.[4]

Other types of anemia caused by defects in RBC production include vitamin B_{12} and folate deficiency, ACD, and aplastic anemia, which is a result of bone marrow stem cell failure.[4]

Red Blood Cell Destruction Disorders

The mechanisms involved in the increased hemolysis or destruction of RBCs resulting in anemia include various hemoglobin disorders such as sickle cell anemia; RBC membrane defects as in hereditary spherocytosis and hereditary elliptocytosis; RBC enzyme defects as in glucose-6-phosphate dehydrogenase (G6PD) deficiency; and finally, autoimmune antibody production as seen in autoimmune hemolytic anemia.

Blood Loss

Anemia from blood loss can be either from an acute cause or a chronic loss. Acute blood loss resulting from trauma or hemorrhage may result in life-threatening anemia with significant symptoms of hemodynamic cardiovascular compromise and are often characterized by a sudden and profound drop in hemoglobin levels. Anemia from chronic blood loss can occur slowly over time and from as little as a few teaspoons of blood loss per day, especially from the gastrointestinal (GI) tract.[5] Anemia symptoms resulting from mild to moderate menorrhagia, chronic microscopic hematuria, or chronic occult GI bleeding can be much more insidious because the body compensates for this type of slowly evolving anemia.[5]

CLINICAL PRESENTATION AND PHYSICAL EXAMINATION

The presentation of anemia can be variable, depending on the acuteness of onset and the ability of the cardiopulmonary system to compensate. If the patient is healthy and the onset of anemia is gradual, there are few signs or symptoms until the hemoglobin value falls below 7.5 g/dL.[4,5] Patients may initially experience fatigue, malaise, headache, dyspnea, irritability, and a mild decrease in exercise tolerance. Further declines in hemoglobin concentration may be associated with a markedly reduced exercise capacity, resting tachycardia, and dyspnea requiring supplemental oxygen. Other nonspecific findings that can accompany long-term, moderate to severe anemia include wide pulse pressure, midsystolic or pansystolic murmur, confusion, lethargy, brittle nails, glossitis, angular cheilitis, and spoon-shaped nails.[4] Pallor of the mucous membranes, lips, conjunctivae, nail beds, and palmar creases is a common sign of anemia. When palmar creases are as pale as the surrounding skin, the patient usually has a hemoglobin value of less than 7 g/dL.[4]

Due to the multiple causes and systems that are affected, a comprehensive head-to-toe physical examination is warranted in the evaluation of a patient with anemia. Overall appearance suggestive of decreased stamina and energy could suggest fatigue secondary to anemia, or anemia related to another chronic illness. A thorough cardiopulmonary examination including vital signs is essential. Increased heart or respiratory rate or the presence of a systolic murmur may be related to anemia. Special attention should be paid to characteristics of the integumentary system to evaluate for pallor, nail integrity, and signs of angular cheilitis. Also, symptoms of increased bruising may be a clue to a potential bleeding disorder contributing to blood loss and iron deficiency.

DIAGNOSTICS
Essential Diagnostics

Diagnostic evaluation of anemia should begin with a complete blood count (CBC) which includes RBC indices and morphology, platelet count, white cell differential, reticulocyte count, and a peripheral blood smear. Evaluation of all blood cell lines (RBCs and WBC with differential) is essential to confirm a sole anemia diagnosis, as opposed to a primary bone marrow disease such as aplastic anemia or an infiltrative process such as leukemia. RBCs indices quantify RBC cell size (the mean corpuscular volume [MCV]), RBC hemoglobin concentration (mean corpuscular hemoglobin [MCH], mean corpuscular hemoglobin concentration [MCHC]) and variation of cell size across the specimen (RBC distribution width [RDW]). Of all the indices noted on a hemogram, the MCV is the most useful. The MCV reflects the average RBC size and is referred to as microcytic, normocytic, or macrocytic. This helps guide

the clinician in determining what other testing is necessary in establishing the cause of the anemia.[6]

Reticulocytes are immature RBCs. They have a nucleus when they enter circulation and due to this, are larger in size than the mature RBC. Within a few days they extrude their nucleus, decrease in size, and assume the classic concave disc shape of the mature RBC. The reticulocyte count is the most easily accessible method of evaluating bone marrow production of RBCs (a direct bone marrow examination requires an invasive procedure). The reticulocyte count provides an assessment of whether the causative factor of anemia is related to either decreased production or increased loss. In health, a normal reticulocyte count is 0.5% to 2.0% of the total RBCs. A normal, expected response to decreased numbers of RBCs is an increase in reticulocytes (reticulocytosis). A normal absolute reticulocyte count (ARC) is 25,000 to 75,000/µL. Any value higher than 100,000/µL is considered a marrow that is responding normally to anemic conditions. Values below 75,000/µL are considered consistent with impaired (decreased) RBC production.[4] Reticulocytopenia is associated with poor marrow function or failure. The reticulocyte index (RI) is a valuable calculation that reflects bone marrow response; a low RI reflects a bone marrow unable to compensate for anemia (as in IDA, ACD, B_{12}, folate deficiencies) and an elevated RI reflects a marrow attempting to recover from anemia or from hemolysis.[6] The RI is calculated as:

$$RI = \frac{Reticulocytes\% \times Actual\ Hct\%}{Normal\ Hct\%}$$

In the presence of anemia with significant reticulocytosis, hemolysis needs to be considered in the differential and ruled out by measuring serum bilirubin levels, checking for hyperbilirubinemia (conjugated bilirubin—marker of hemoglobin catabolism) and increased serum lactate dehydrogenase (LDH), which is indicative of direct cellular injury.[5] Also, a low serum haptoglobin value is a sign of intravascular hemolysis, as haptoglobin binds the free hemoglobin that is released into the circulation as erythrocytes rupture. These hemoglobin-haptoglobin complexes are removed from the circulation by the reticuloendothelial system.[5] Hemolytic anemias are complex to evaluate and diagnose; if they are suspected, immediate referral should be made to a hematologist. A low reticulocyte count with anemia points to impaired erythropoiesis indicating a reduction in RBC precursors or ineffective production. Ineffective production is reported as erythroid hyperplasia on the bone marrow biopsy and aspiration report.[5] This means the RBCs are being produced but are not viable and usually do not leave the marrow.

A peripheral blood smear is critical in the evaluation of anemias. Variations in RBC size and shapes as well as abnormal cell populations too small to change the indices can be directly visualized. For example, as iron deficiency progresses, microcytic cells are noted on the smear long before the indices change. Cells produced under duress such as seen in conditions resulting in significant inflammation and component deficiencies can reflect size and shape abnormalities. Significant variations in size of cells in a specimen is described as anisocytosis and variations in cell shapes are referred to as poikilocytosis.[6] Evidence of hemolysis as well as abnormal shaped cells (such as sickle shape or spherocytes) on the smear may offer additional clues as to the cause of the anemia.

Additional Diagnostics

Evaluation of the body's iron stores includes serum ferritin, serum iron, total iron-binding capacity (TIBC), and transferrin saturation percentage.[4] These should be evaluated in the presence of a microcytic anemia (low MCV) or when an IDA is suspected. These values are important in helping to differentiate between an IDA or an ACD microcytic anemia. Ferritin is the major iron storage protein and reflects total body iron stores and reserves. Serum ferritin is the first laboratory value to become abnormal when iron stores are becoming depleted, even before IDA is reflected in RBC morphology. Ferritin concentrations less than 12 ng/mL indicate absence of iron stores. It is important to remember, however, that ferritin is an acute-phase reactant and may be elevated due to inflammation. Inflammation causes the release of tissue ferritins resulting from damage to the liver and other ferritin-rich tissues.[4,7] Serum ferritin levels are low in IDA and normal or elevated in ACD. Serum ferritin is also elevated in conditions unrelated to anemia, such as iron overload (either transfusion dependent or hereditary hemochromatosis), inflammatory disorders, and alcoholism.

The serum iron concentration reflects the amount of iron bound to transferrin, a plasma carrier protein that regulates iron transport in the blood. Normal values for serum iron are 65 to 165 mcg/dL.[7] Transferrin is the transport protein for iron and is measured indirectly by the TIBC. The TIBC indicates the availability of binding sites on the protein for iron transport. Normal values for TIBC are 300 to 360 mcg/dL.[7]

The percentage of transferrin saturation can be calculated from the TIBC and the serum iron values as follows:

$$\frac{\text{Serum iron}}{\text{TIBC}} \times 100$$

Normal values for percentage of transferrin saturation are 20% to 50%.[7]

Hemoglobin electrophoresis allows hemoglobin chains to be separated according to differences in the charges of their subunits. It is essential for accurate diagnosis of thalassemias (minor and major) and other hemoglobinopathies.

In the case where hemogram results appears to be consistent with ACD, evaluating for the presence of inflammation is recommended. Erythrocyte sedimentation rate (ESR) and/or C-reactive protein (CRP) can establish the presence of general inflammation (as in rheumatoid arthritis or inflammatory bowel disease) which can guide further investigation, based on history and physical.[4] Haptoglobin and LDH are useful when investigating the presence of hemolytic anemia.[5]

DIFFERENTIAL DIAGNOSIS

The differential diagnosis for anemia will include multiple conditions. A thorough history, including past medical history, family history, environmental exposures, and medications is essential to narrowing down the differentials, along with the laboratory studies. The most critical or priority etiologies of anemias must be considered.

 Priority differentials include (1) blood loss (acute hemorrhage, hemolysis; chronic—GI/GYN causes), (2) bone marrow failure or disease, (3) malignancy, and (4) renal failure.

It is imperative to determine the category of anemia based on its size or MCV value when developing differentials.

Anemias are generally divided into three categories based on the size of the RBCs suggesting the underlying condition or disease. RBCs are normally uniform in size and shape, and deviations in their appearance can suggest a specific cause for the anemia. The degree of anisocytosis (variation in RBC size) is determined by assessing the RBC indices on the CBC and at cell morphology on the peripheral smear. The MCV is a direct measurement averaging the RBC sizes in the sample. The RDW is an indirect measurement that indicates the degree of homogeneity or variability of RBC size of the sample. For example, uniformly small RBCs will have a low MCV and a normal RDW, whereas a sample with mostly small RBCs but some normal RBCs can have a low MCV with an increased RDW, reflecting the heterogeneity of the sample. Based on the MCV, anemias are classified as microcytic (MCV <80 fL), normocytic (MCV 80 to 99 fL), or macrocytic (MCV >100 fL).[4] Variations in RBC shape (poikilocytosis) provide important diagnostic clues and in fact are often pathognomonic of underlying disease. Box 216.1 classifies commonly seen hematologic disorders according to RBC morphology.

MICROCYTIC ANEMIA

Many conditions can cause microcytic anemia (MCV <80 fL). The most common etiology is IDA; however, it can be associated with ACD, thalassemia, and sideroblastic anemias.

IRON DEFICIENCY ANEMIA
Definition and Epidemiology

IDA is the most common type of anemia in the world and the most common nutrient deficiency. In the adult population, IDA predominantly affects women of reproductive age and

BOX **216.1**

Classification of Anemias Based on Red Blood Cell Morphology

SIZE
Microcytic (MCV <80 fL)
- Iron deficiency
- Thalassemia
- Anemia of chronic disease (occasionally)
- Sideroblastic anemia
- Hemoglobin E disease

Macrocytic (MCV >100 fL)
- Megaloblastic anemia (vitamin B_{12} or folate deficiency)

Normocytic (MCV 80–99 fL)
- Sickle cell disease
- Anemia of chronic disease
- Aplastic anemia
- Hemolytic anemias

SHAPE
Sickle
- Sickle cell disease

Targets
- Thalassemias
- Hemoglobin C
- Hemoglobin E

Spherocytes
- Hereditary spherocytosis
- Immune hemolysis

Elliptocytes
- Hereditary elliptocytosis

BOX **216.2**

Causes of Iron Deficiency

CONDITIONS LEADING TO MILD IRON DEFICIENCY[a]
Inadequate diet
Normal or heavy menses
Blood donation
Malabsorption
- Partial gastrectomy
- Malabsorption syndromes

Increased requirements
- Infancy and adolescence (periods of rapid growth)
- Pregnancy

Polycythemia vera treated with phlebotomy

CONDITIONS ASSOCIATED WITH MODERATE TO SEVERE IRON DEFICIENCY
Chronic blood loss
- GI conditions

Peptic ulcer disease
Varices
Malignant disease
Diverticulitis
- Severe menorrhagia

Severe malabsorption
- Gastrectomy
- Sprue and other malabsorption syndromes

[a]Usually no associated symptoms.

older adults. The most common cause is chronic blood loss, especially GI blood loss or menorrhagia.[5,8] Chronic GI blood losses should be suspected as a cause of IDA in adult men and postmenopausal women. Inadequate nutrition and increased requirements for iron are the principal causes of IDA in children and pregnant women. Box 216.2 lists additional causes of iron deficiency. The worldwide prevalence of anemia in pregnant women is 38%, and more than 50% of that is a result of iron deficiency. Fetal iron stores are established in the last trimester of pregnancy so preterm infants are at greater risk for IDA during infancy.[9] Daily prenatal use of iron has demonstrated improvement in maternal hemoglobin concentration and reduction in risk of having low-birth-weight babies.[9]

Pathophysiology

Iron is an essential nutrient present in all living cells. The human body contains about 3 to 4 g of iron, with more than 70% contained within hemoglobin. The remainder of the body's iron is stored in the liver and marrow as ferritin and hemosiderin, and a small amount is bound to transferrin in the blood.[4,7] The normal adult male has a total body iron content of about 4000 mg. Women of childbearing age have about 2000 mg of total body iron, a significantly lower amount

because of menstrual blood loss and lower dietary intake. The average adult normally loses approximately 1 mg of iron each day through the natural process of desquamation of cells from the skin, GI tract, and urinary tract. The adult woman loses an additional 1 mg through normal menstruation.[10]

The recommended daily allowance of iron is 15 mg/day in the diet of nonpregnant women and 30 mg/day for pregnant women.[10] Dietary iron is absorbed in the duodenum of the small intestine. The amount of iron absorbed from the intestine is determined by several factors, including the iron content of the meal, the form of iron being ingested, the individual's iron status, and the presence or absence of other substances that can enhance or inhibit iron absorption.[8]

When iron requirements increase or intake declines, the small intestine increases absorption of iron to meet the increased demand. If there is no additional supply of iron to meet this increased demand, the body's iron stores begin to be depleted. At this point, several hematologic parameters are affected. The ferritin levels decline as body iron stores decrease. As body iron stores are depleted, the transferrin saturation decreases, leading to a reduced supply of iron to the RBC precursors, resulting in impaired (iron-deficient) erythropoiesis. At this stage, however, an overt microcytic anemia may not yet be present. Once the iron stores are truly depleted and no iron is available for erythropoiesis, an overt microcytic, hypochromic anemia is present, which manifests in the CBC by a low hemoglobin concentration. The RBC indices are the last to change (decreased MCV, MCH, and MCHC). However, the RDW may be elevated well before the MCV decreases as it reflects the newer, smaller RBCs entering the circulation. The peripheral smear will show hypochromia, microcytosis, mild

TABLE 216.1 Laboratory Values in Microcytic Anemias

Anemia	Hemoglobin[a]	MCV	MCHC	RDW	Serum Iron[b]	Serum Ferritin[c]	TIBC[d]	Transferrin Saturation[e]
Iron deficiency								
Early	N	N	N	↑	N	N	N	N
Intermediate	N	N	N	↑	↓/N	↓	High N	↓
Late	↓	↓	↓	↑	↓	↓	↑	↓
Thalassemia minor	Low N/↓	↓	N/↓	N	N	N/≠	N	N
Chronic disease	Low N	N/↓	N/↓	N	↓	↑	↓	↑
Sideroblastic anemia	↓	↓	↓	Variable	↑	↑	N	↑

[a]N = 12–16 g/dL for women; 13.5–17.5 g/dL for men.
[b]N = 65–165 mcg/dL for women; 75–175 mcg/dL for men.
[c]N = 12–150 mcg/dL for women; 15–300 mcg/dL for men.
[d]N = 240–450 mcg/dL.
[e]N = 20%–50%.
MCHC, Mean corpuscular hemoglobin concentration; MCV, mean corpuscular volume; N, normal; RDW, RBC distribution width; TIBC, total iron-binding capacity.

anisocytosis, and poikilocytosis. Iron studies will show a low ferritin level and high TIBC.

Clinical Presentation and Physical Examination

Mild to moderate iron-deficient states are not associated with any clinical symptoms. Patients with severe IDA exhibit the same signs and symptoms of any type of severe anemia. Patients may complain of fatigue, decreased exercise tolerance, weakness, palpitations, irritability, and headaches. Complaints that are specifically related to iron store depletion include paresthesias, sore tongue, brittle nails, spoon-shaped nails (koilonychia), and pica for starch, ice, or clay.[4] In fact, a craving for ice (pagophagia) is a common symptom of women with IDA for unknown reasons.

As the severity of the anemia increases, several physical changes may become evident. The patient may demonstrate a more forceful apical pulse, tachycardia with exertion, and a systolic flow murmur, which will resolve once the anemia is corrected. Patients may also demonstrate pallor of the conjunctiva, mucous membranes, nail beds, and palmar creases. The characteristic spooning of the nails may also be present. In the older adult, signs of congestive heart failure may be present.

Essential Diagnostics. A CBC with differential is the most important laboratory test. IDA is commonly discovered incidentally during a routine CBC. Once IDA is diagnosed, the history may reveal factors that would cause iron deficiency, such as a recent hemorrhage, GI bleeding, menorrhagia, multiple pregnancies, or inadequate nutrition. Iron studies are imperative in differentiating between a microcytotic anemia due to iron deficiency and those due to ACD, sideroblastic anemia, or thalassemia/hemoglobinopathies (Table 216.1). IDA reveals a low serum iron level, decreased serum ferritin, increased TIBC, and decreased percentage of transferrin saturation. Approximately 90% of iron used to produce new RBCs comes from recycled iron from routine hemolysis. Chronic blood loss can cause persistent low volume loss that eventually will cause depletion of iron stores. Laboratory changes occur gradually as the iron stores are depleted. The earliest laboratory change is a fall in serum ferritin, reflecting depletion of iron stores. This change is followed by a decrease in serum iron and an increase in transferrin, producing a reduction in

the percentage of transferrin saturation to less than 15% (this will drop below 10% as the severity progresses) and an associated increase in TIBC. The first change in the CBC is a drop in hemoglobin. Only with increasing severity and duration do the RBCs become microcytic and hypochromic.

The underlying cause of the iron deficiency must be identified. Blood loss by GI bleeding or repeated voluntary blood donation should be suspected until proven otherwise. Older adults with suspected IDA should be thoroughly evaluated for GI cancers, GI bleeding based on nonsteroidal anti-inflammatory drug (NSAID) use, and alcohol abuse.

INITIAL DIAGNOSTICS

Microcytic Anemia

LABORATORY
- CBC and differential which includes RBC indices
  - Peripheral smear
  - Reticulocyte count
- Ferritin
- TIBC
- Transferrin

- Serum iron
- Stool for occult blood × 3

ADDITIONAL DIAGNOSTICS
- Hemoglobin electrophoresis[a]

IMAGING/PROCEDURES
- Bone marrow biopsy[a]

[a]If indicated.

Differential Diagnosis

Several conditions need to be considered in the differential diagnosis of a microcytic hypochromic anemia. The most concerning differentials need to be ruled out immediately.

 Priority differentials include (1) acute blood loss—hemorrhage, (2) chronic blood loss (GI, menorrhagia), (3) hemoglobinopathies, and (4) chronic disease and toxins (such as lead poisoning).

The thalassemias typically have a moderate to severe microcytosis with varying degrees of anemia; however, most will have a normal RDW and normal iron studies.

ACD presents a more common diagnostic dilemma. With long-standing chronic inflammatory illnesses such as rheumatoid arthritis, the defective iron supply can result in severe microcytic hypochromic anemia. Iron studies, especially the serum ferritin level, usually differentiate among true IDA, ACD, and thalassemia (see Table 216.1). Both IDA and ACD are associated with low serum iron levels. The ferritin level is normal or increased in ACD and decreased in IDA. The TIBC is normal or low in ACD and increased in IDA.

Microcytosis can occur in patients with inherited sideroblastic anemias; however, these anemias are rare and are related to X-linked genes. Acquired sideroblastic anemias (idiopathic, secondary to drug or toxin exposure like lead, myeloproliferative or myelodysplastic disease) can be microcytic but generally are macrocytic. These conditions are caused by defects in heme synthesis leading to accumulation of iron within bone marrow erythroid precursors and resulting in abnormal erythroid maturation. This anemia is characterized by ringed sideroblasts (erythroblasts with one third or more of the nucleus surrounded by ferritin deposits).[4,7] A bone marrow examination is necessary for diagnosis. The anemia tends to be severe (hemoglobin concentration of 6 g/dL) to moderate (hemoglobin concentration of 8 to 10 g/dL). Treatment of sideroblastic anemia consists of chronic transfusions and iron chelation therapy (to prevent or to treat the transfusion-dependent iron overload). Pyridoxine (vitamin B_6) therapy may sometimes partially correct the anemia in patients with hereditary sideroblastic anemia, leaving them with a milder anemia that does not require as many chronic transfusions. An anecdotal association between chronic use of proton pump inhibitors (PPI) and IDA has been reported, possibly due to impaired iron absorption; however, more evidence is needed before a clear relationship can be established.[11]

Interprofessional Collaborative Management

Pharmacologic Management. Essential to the treatment of IDA is recognition of the source of the low iron stores. This needs to be addressed and proper referral made (GI, GYN, Nutritionist). Treatment of IDA usually begins with an oral iron preparation. The usual adult therapeutic dose is 150 to 200 mg of elemental iron per day in divided doses until anemia is corrected. Lower doses may still be effective and be better tolerated. The pediatric dosing is 3 mg of elemental iron per kilogram, and liquid preparations are available. Administration should be continued empirically for 4 to 6 months or until the serum ferritin level exceeds 50 mcg/L and then stopped. Common side effects of iron preparations are nausea, constipation, heartburn, upper GI discomfort, black stools, and diarrhea. Iron absorption is optimum when iron is taken 30 minutes before meals with ascorbic acid. Absorption can be reduced by as much as 40% to 50% if it is taken with meals; however, iron on an empty stomach can cause more side effects, leading to noncompliance with medication.[4] GI upset, the most common side effect, may be avoided by starting with a single pill per day and slowly increasing to the recommended dose.

Once an adequate dose of iron is reached, changes in the hematologic markers should be seen in just a few weeks. The hemoglobin level should begin to rise within 1 to 2 weeks. The MCV should correct within 1 to 2 months, reflecting the normalization of the erythrocyte size.[6] Supplementation with oral iron should continue until the anemia is corrected, and until the underlying cause of the deficiency is corrected, or indefinitely if the cause of the deficiency is chronic.

If the anemia is severe, the patient has an iron malabsorption problem, or oral iron is not tolerated, replacement should be by parenteral (intramuscular or intravenous) administration of iron. Patients should be referred to a hematologist for intravenous administration of iron because it has traditionally been associated with adverse reactions. The intravenous iron formulations, iron carboxymaltose and ferumoxytol, have a much safer profile than older preparations.[12] The novel structures of these preparations have been shown to reduce the risk of free iron reactions and result in lower immunogenicity. As a result, test doses are not necessary and much higher doses can be administered, thereby reducing the number of administrations necessary to replace iron stores.[13]

Nonpharmacologic Management. Dietary assessment, including types of foods and timing of ingestion, is essential when treating nutritional causes of IDA. Individuals with restrictive diets, such as vegetarian and vegan diets, may need nutritional counseling to assist them in choosing iron-rich foods that are in keeping with their belief and practices.

Various foods and substances can promote or inhibit absorption of iron in the GI track. Any metal-based food or supplement, such as those containing calcium or magnesium, will chelate the iron and block absorption. Therefore, dairy or antacids should not be taken two hours before or after oral iron therapy. Other items that can inhibit absorption are coffee, tea, bran, and soy products. On the other hand, vitamin C can enhance absorption as well as meat, poultry, and fish.

Most patients with IDA are diagnosed and treated by their primary health care providers. Patients who are referred to a hematologist for consultation generally return to the primary health care provider once the anemia has been corrected, or at least once an accurate diagnosis has been made and the patient is receiving stable iron replacement therapy.

Referral to a hematologist should be considered for the following reasons: nonadherence to or intolerance of oral iron replacement, persistent IDA necessitating parenteral iron therapy, and persistent microcytic anemia despite iron replacement and the exclusion of other conditions.

Other referrals may be required as evaluation for the cause of the iron deficiency progresses, such as referral to an internist or gastroenterologist to exclude GI blood loss or referral to an oncologist to treat any malignant neoplasms (either GI or gynecologic). Women of reproductive age may require referral to a gynecologist or a hematologist for evaluation of severe menorrhagia. It is also important to consider the diagnosis of von Willebrand's Disease (see Chapter 217) in adolescent girls who have severe menorrhagia and a hematology referral would be recommended in these cases.

Healthy patients with IDA do not require hospitalization. Transfusions are rarely necessary and if so then hospitalization may be appropriate. Patients who are unable to adequately compensate for severe anemia may require hospitalization for cardiac or respiratory compromise that may occur.

Life Span Considerations

Preterm infants are at increased risk due to lack of adequate iron stores. Full-term healthy infants have adequate iron stores for the first 4 to 6 months of life which is when solids are introduced. Infants who are exclusively breastfed over 4 months or are not on iron fortified foods by 6 months are at risk for IDA and should receive iron supplements. Children require adequate iron intake to meet the increased demands of rapid growth. Nutritional iron deficits are especially common in children in the toddler stage due to excessive consumption of cow's milk at the expense of adequate intake of iron-rich foods. Adolescent girls often become iron deficient as a result of menstrual blood loss, sometimes accompanied by poor diet in this age group.

Iron supplementation during pregnancy is almost always-recommended. Pregnancy places a greater demand on iron stores, especially during the last two trimesters. The additional iron is needed to cover the needs of the developing fetus and placenta and to accommodate the increase in erythrocyte mass that normally occurs during the later stages of pregnancy. Many women enter pregnancy with inadequate iron reserves as a result of heavy prepregnancy menstruation. Iron studies can be difficult to interpret in pregnancy because of the hemodilutional effects of the increase in blood volume during pregnancy, as well as the elevation of ferritin as an acute-phase reaction to the known inflammatory effects of pregnancy. Adequate maternal iron stores are essential to adequate brain development in the fetus.[14]

Older adults with suspected IDA should be thoroughly evaluated for GI cancers, even when their stools are negative for occult blood. Next to chronic disease, iron deficiency is the most common cause of a microcytic anemia in older adults.

Complications

Untreated IDA is especially worrisome during pregnancy. IDA may be associated with preterm delivery, low birth weight, and learning deficits. Fetal iron stores are deposited during the last trimester of pregnancy. If the mother is anemic during her pregnancy or the baby is delivered prematurely, the infant is at increased risk for anemia. Untreated iron deficiency in all age groups can lead to severe anemia and may be associated with fatigue, falls, and cardiovascular compromise.

Patient and Family Education

Patients should receive education about the use of iron supplements to ensure adequate treatment and an understanding of the prescribed regimen. Maximum absorption of iron occurs if it is ingested 30 minutes before meals. Calcium can significantly inhibit iron absorption. Multivitamins with calcium or dairy products should be taken 1 to 2 hours after an iron supplement. Ascorbic acid enhances absorption of iron; therefore, concurrent ingestion of foods rich in vitamin C, such as orange juice, should be encouraged.

Discussion of side effects, such as constipation and nausea, should be included in the treatment plan along with strategies for management of these complaints (stool softeners, taking iron at bedtime). Anticipatory guidance should also include notice that stool may become a dark tar color. Numerous iron supplementation preparations are on the market, some with combinations of iron plus stool softeners, slow-release iron, or iron plus vitamin C. Patients who are intolerant of one preparation may find another that produces fewer or no side effects. The health care provider should therefore encourage patients to try various preparations before recommending parenteral iron.

Health Promotion

Primary prevention for IDA includes careful attention to diet and use of over-the-counter medications. Dietary assessment of those at risk for IDA should occur at each well visit. Screening for use and counseling regarding prudent use of NSAIDs (type, amount, and frequency of dose) is essential to preventing serious side effects, such as NSAID-related gastritis and GI bleeding.

The National Academy of Sciences recommends low-dose iron supplementation (27 mg/day) for all pregnant woman, which is present in most prenatal vitamins.[15] The United States Preventative Task Force (USPSTF), however, has determined there is insufficient evidence to recommend for or against universal iron supplementation for pregnant women.[16] The World Health Organization (WHO) recommends routine iron supplementation (30 to 60 mg elemental iron/day for 3 months per year) for menstruating adolescents and women in areas where prevalence of IDA is ≥40%.[17]

Nutritional counseling, including thorough dietary history and careful attention to cultural aspects of diet, is an important strategy to prevent further episodes of IDA and should include assessment of the patient's dietary intake. Strict vegetarians who rely on vegetable sources of iron instead of animal sources should be encouraged to supplement their diets with iron-fortified vitamins or to add iron-fortified foods to their diet. Patients whose IDA is secondary to other conditions should be encouraged to seek appropriate medical care.

Secondary prevention, as in screening for IDA, is recommended for certain at-risk groups. The USPSTF finds insufficient evidence to recommend for or against routine screening for IDA in young children or pregnant women; however, the American Academy of Pediatrics recommends universal screening of all children for IDA at age 1 year.[18] Screening at later times in childhood (up to age 21 years) should be based on history of IDA, dietary history, history of poor growth, lead exposure, and socioeconomic factors, as well as other factors. The American College of Obstetricians and Gynecologists (ACOG) recommends universal screening of pregnant women in early pregnancy, though the USPSTF found insufficient evidence to recommend universal screening.[15,16] Universal screening for adults age 18 and older is not recommended; however, targeted screening should be performed in the presence of IDA risk factors.

THALASSEMIA

DEFINITION AND EPIDEMIOLOGY

Thalassemia is not a single disorder but rather a group of inherited blood disorders caused by variant or missing genes that affect how the body makes hemoglobin. Thalassemias are inherited autosomal recessive genetic disorders (Fig. 216.1). The resulting anemia depends on the type of thalassemia inherited and varies from asymptomatic to severe hemolytic anemia. All the thalassemias, except α-thalassemia of a silent carrier, produce some degree of microcytosis and hypochromia.

α-Thalassemia is most commonly found in people with ancestry from Southeast Asia, India, China, or the Philippines. β-Thalassemia is more frequent in those of Mediterranean, Middle Eastern, African, or Asian descent. β-thalassemia can be inherited concurrently with genes for the hemoglobinopathies, resulting in conditions such as sickle β-thalassemia (Sβ-thalassemia). Sβ-thalassemia severity is inversely proportional to the amount of β-globin produced. When no β-globin is produced (Sβ⁰-thalassemia), the condition is almost identical to sickle cell disease.[19] Thalassemia affects males and females equally.

Thalassemia and Sickle Cell Disease

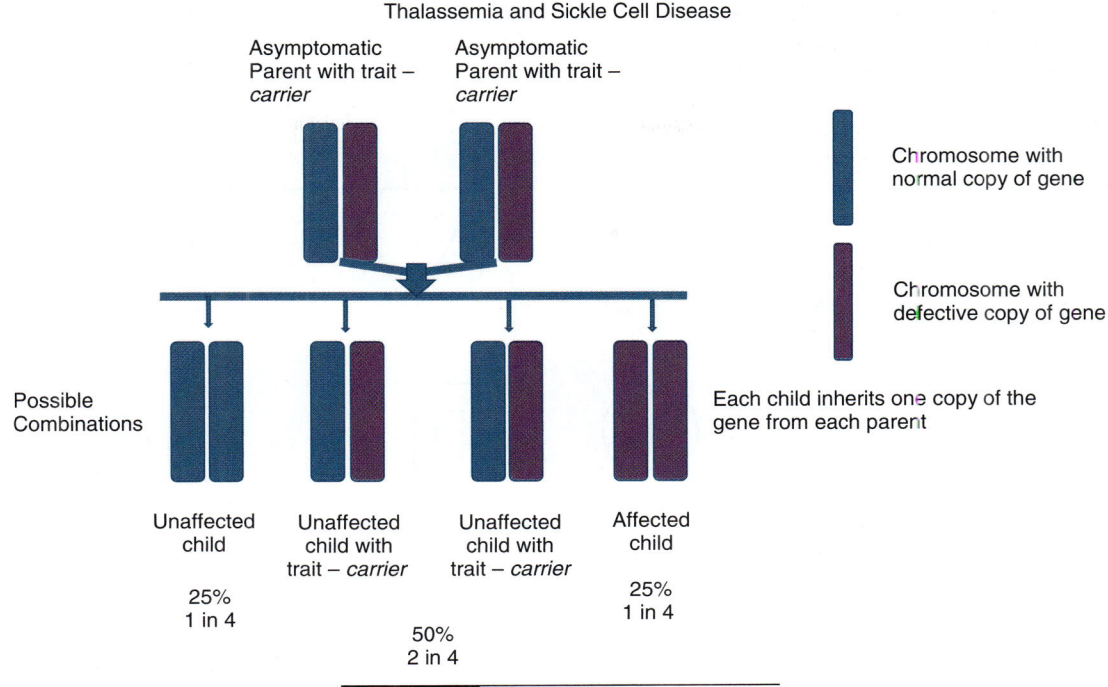

FIG. **216.1**   Autosomal recessive inheritance.

PATHOPHYSIOLOGY

The manifestations and severity of clinical symptoms depend on the number of chain deletions in the hemoglobin molecule. Normally, adult RBCs contain predominantly hemoglobin A_1 (96% to 97% of the cell's hemoglobin) and only small amounts of hemoglobin A_2 (2.5%) and hemoglobin F (<1%).[20] Thalassemia abnormalities produce changes in the normal amounts of adult hemoglobin. These quantitative changes are important in the diagnosis of thalassemia.

Inheritance of thalassemia occurs in a mendelian-recessive manner (autosomal recessive inheritance) (Fig. 216.2).[20] The two main types of thalassemia are α (alpha) and β (beta), the two protein chains required to make normal hemoglobin. Four genes (two from each parent on chromosome 16) are involved in making α-globin. If one gene is affected, the person is called a silent carrier and usually has no symptoms. If two genes are affected, individuals are considered carriers and have mild anemia (α-thalassemia trait or α-thalassemia minor). People with hemoglobin H (α-thalassemia intermedia) disease have three genes affected and are moderately to severely anemic.[20] When all four genes are affected, the condition is called α-thalassemia major (hemoglobin hydrops fetalis), and most affected fetuses are born prematurely and stillborn or die shortly after birth.[20] The patients who survive will require lifelong transfusions and extensive medical care.

β-Thalassemia genes are located on chromosome 11; each parent provides one to an offspring. An individual is considered a carrier if one gene is affected; this is known as β-thalassemia trait or minor. When both genes are affected, the condition is either β-thalassemia intermedia, causing moderate anemia, or β-thalassemia major (Cooley anemia) with severe anemia. Differentiation between β-thalassemia intermedia and major depends on the volume and frequency of transfusions.

CLINICAL PRESENTATION AND PHYSICAL EXAMINATION

The α- and β-thalassemias are classified as thalassemia minor (mild), thalassemia intermedia (moderate), or thalassemia major (severe) depending on the severity of the anemia. Across the globe, most patients have thalassemia minor. Patients with α- or β-thalassemia minor generally have either little or no hematologic effects or a mild microcytic hypochromic anemia that is often mistaken for IDA.[21] These individuals generally have no symptoms or physical manifestations related to their altered hemoglobin structure.

Patients with thalassemia intermedia have a moderate microcytic and hypochromic anemia that is not transfusion dependent. Patients with thalassemia intermedia may require occasional transfusions during pregnancy or preoperatively. If patients with thalassemia intermedia begin to develop persistent clinical problems, such as abnormal facies, growth retardation, or pathologic fractures, they will require regular transfusions. At this point, these patients are given the diagnosis of thalassemia major.[20,21]

Patients with β-thalassemia major (also known as Cooley anemia) develop a severe, life-threatening anemia during their first year of life. This profound anemia is associated with developmental problems and decreased life expectancy. These patients require lifelong chronic RBC transfusions to maintain adequate hemoglobin levels and iron chelation.

The physical examination findings are remarkable only in patients with thalassemia intermedia and β-thalassemia major. Patients can exhibit the characteristic physical changes of short stature and abnormal facies associated with cranial marrow expansion. In the United States, however, the facial abnormalities are seen primarily in patients with thalassemia intermedia because most patients with β-thalassemia major are

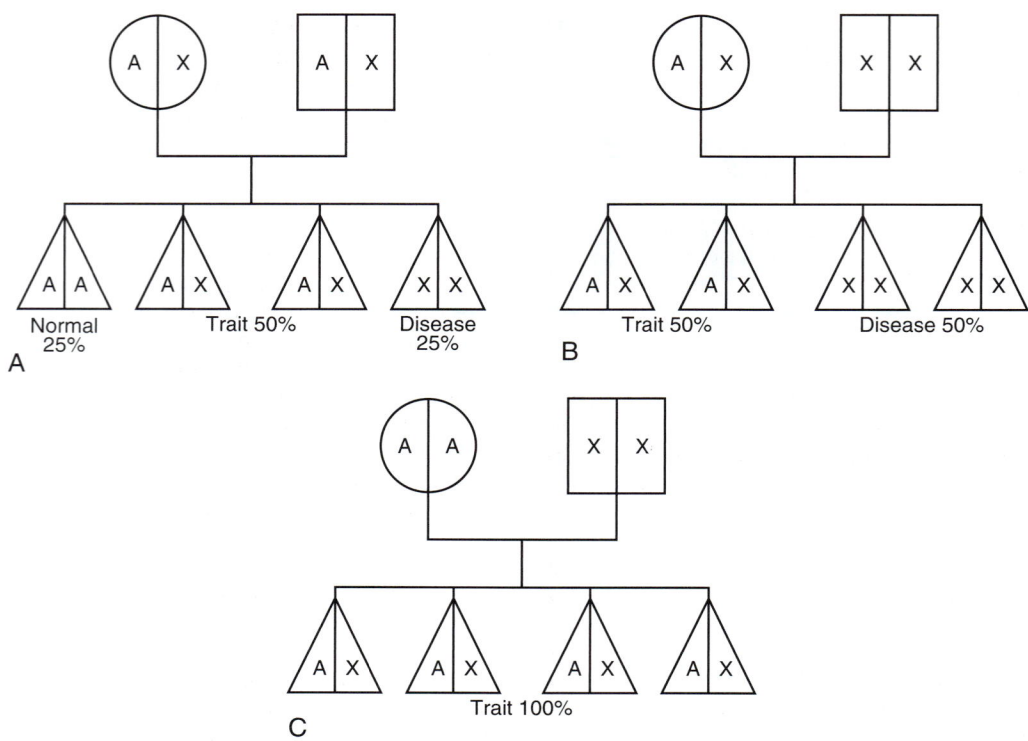

FIG. 216.2 Inheritance patterns for autosomal genes. (A) When both parents have a trait, offspring have a 25% chance of being normal, a 25% chance of having the disease, and a 50% chance of having the trait. (B) When one parent has the disease and the other parent has the trait, offspring have a 50% chance of having the trait and a 50% chance of having the disease. (C) When one parent has the disease and the other parent is normal, all offspring will have the trait. *A*, Gene for normal hemoglobin; *X*, gene for abnormal hemoglobin (S, C, E) or thalassemia.

hypertransfused to normal hemoglobin levels, thus preventing the marrow expansion.[20] Children can be diagnosed as early as 3 months of age, with findings of severe anemia, pallor, jaundice, and enlarged spleen, liver, or heart.

DIAGNOSTICS
Essential Diagnostics
Essential serum laboratory studies required for determining the presence of any thalassemia condition includes a CBC with differential, serum iron studies, and hemoglobin electrophoresis. Patients with thalassemia intermedia or major are diagnosed during the first few years of life, due to the severity of presentation. Individuals with thalassemia minor are often identified incidentally when a CBC is obtained, and a microcytic hypochromic anemia is noted.

Hemoglobin electrophoresis determines hemoglobin composition of RBCs. In normal RBCs, the largest proportion of hemoglobin is HbA_1 (>95%), with smaller amounts of HbA_2 (≤3.5%) and HbF (1%). The determination of minor, intermedia, and major manifestations of thalassemia is based on levels of Hb subtypes as well as severity of anemia. The diagnosis of β-thalassemia minor is based on a mildly decreased hemoglobin concentration, low MCV (60 to 75 fL), low MCH/MCHC, normal RDW, normal iron studies, and hemoglobin electrophoresis with increased levels of hemoglobin A_2.[20] The microcytic anemia needs to be further differentiated between β-thalassemia minor and IDA. There are several tools that can aid in this distinction. Formulas whose findings are suggestive of β-thalassemia minor are England and Fraser index, Sirdah

formula, and Green and King index. The Ricera index is suggestive of IDA (RDW/RBC >4.4).[21]

The diagnoses of β-thalassemia intermedia and β-thalassemia major are diagnosed by low MCV, low MCH/MCHC, and hemoglobin electrophoresis results (intermedia has low levels HbA_1; major—HbA_1 is absent).[20,21]

α-Thalassemia can be diagnosed at birth on a routine newborn screen. The hemoglobin electrophoresis will show evidence of Bart's hemoglobin in addition to fetal and normal adult hemoglobin and will be reported as French-American-British (FAB) classification. After the newborn period, α-thalassemia is more difficult to diagnose because a special test, α-globin DNA mutation analysis, is required, and only the largest of medical centers perform this test. In these cases, diagnosis is usually one of exclusion.[20]

Patients with thalassemia intermedia who maintain adequate hemoglobin levels without requiring transfusions exhibit signs of a mild microcytic anemia with slightly low hemoglobin level and low MCV. Patients with β-thalassemia major who are hypertransfused have either low or low-normal hemoglobin level or relatively normal MCV (because they are receiving normal blood during transfusions). Peripheral smears of both patients with thalassemia intermedia and patients with β-thalassemia major have typical target cells present. Patients with β-thalassemia major often experience iron overload due to frequent transfusions.[22] Those who do not receive adequate iron chelation therapy reflect their state of overload with very high ferritin, very low TIBC, and percentage of transferrin saturation approaching 100%. Patients with thalassemia intermedia may have similar iron studies because they can develop iron overload as a result of iron hyperabsorption rather than from transfusions.[23]

DIFFERENTIAL DIAGNOSIS

In most cases, the primary care provider needs to distinguish thalassemia minor from IDA. Both conditions are microcytic hypochromic anemias, but results of iron studies are normal in patients with thalassemia minor. In immigrants with Southeast Asian ancestry, the differential diagnosis of a mild microcytic anemia must differentiate between β-thalassemia minor and hemoglobin E disease. Thalassemia major must be considered in young children who present with severe microcytic, hypochromic anemia, jaundice, and hepatosplenomegaly.

 Priority differentials include (1) IDA from blood loss, (2) other hemoglobinopathies (Hb E), (3) aplastic anemia, and (4) juvenile myelomonocytic leukemia.

Hemoglobin E is the second most common hemoglobin variant in the world (next to sickle cell disease). It is not a true thalassemia but rather a mild hemolytic anemia. It is characterized by a mild microcytic anemia with many target cells on the peripheral smear. It closely resembles the microcytic anemia of β-thalassemia minor, but hemoglobin E is found predominantly in people of Southeast Asian ancestry. Patients can also be double heterozygotes for hemoglobin E and sickle cell disease (ES), manifesting clinically as mild sickle cell disease or combined hemoglobin E and β-thalassemia, which results in a moderate to severe transfusion-dependent anemia that will be similar to β-thalassemia major.[20] Hemoglobin E is diagnosed by hemoglobin electrophoresis.

Often, patients with β-thalassemia minor or hemoglobin E are given a diagnosis of IDA because of their mild microcytic anemia and are prescribed a regimen of iron replacement. Failure to correct the anemia with iron supplementation should then lead the provider to suspect thalassemia minor (or hemoglobin E disease if the patient is of Southeast Asian ancestry).[20]

INTERPROFESSIONAL COLLABORATIVE MANAGEMENT

Nonpharmacologic Management

Patients with β-thalassemia minor do not require pharmacologic management but should be referred for genetic counseling if of childbearing age and if considering conceiving. Patients with thalassemia intermedia can be adequately cared for in a primary care setting, with regular attention to any changes in their anemia. Patients with thalassemia intermedia who begin

to develop persistent clinical problems, such as abnormal facies, growth retardation, or pathologic fractures, should be referred to a hematologist to begin chronic transfusion therapy. Patients with thalassemia intermedia who hyperabsorb iron and develop iron overload require chelation therapy.

Pharmacologic Management

In the United States, hematologists who are familiar with the disease manage most patients with β-thalassemia major and intermedia. Management consists of two equally important functions: (1) regular transfusions to maintain an adequate hemoglobin level to allow normal growth and development and (2) iron chelation therapy to prevent the complications of transfusion-dependent iron overload.

Regular transfusions of packed RBCs are the mainstay of therapy for β-thalassemia major. To maximize normal growth and development, transfusions are begun early in childhood to maintain an adequate hemoglobin trough level of typically around 10 g/dL, although this number can vary among institutions.[22] The frequency of the transfusions can vary among patients, but typically they are necessary every 3 to 5 weeks.[23]

Chelation therapy is standard for prevention of complications from iron overload. Complications of iron overload can be profound; deposition is concentrated in the liver and heart and is a major cause of death in patients requiring frequent RBC transfusions. The goal of chelation therapy is to reduce body iron stores and maintain a ferritin level of less than 1000 mcg/L. However, ferritin is an acute-phase reactant and levels can fluctuate in the presence of body inflammation, and ferritin levels also do not predict cardiac iron loading accurately. Newer revolutionary magnetic resonance imaging (MRI) scanning techniques have allowed a much more accurate picture of the amount of iron overload in the body's organs, thereby helping providers determine the aggressiveness of the chelation therapy regimen.[23]

Deferoxamine is a chelating agent that removes iron from tissues and allows excretion of iron in urine and stools. Deferoxamine must be administered parenterally and is administered 5 to 7 days a week for life. Chelation therapy given as only a single injection with blood transfusions is not effective in any setting. Deferasirox is an oral iron chelator and recommended beginning daily doses start at 14 mg/kg, with adjustment every 3 months based on the monthly serum ferritin. If necessary, the dose can be escalated up to 40 mg/kg/day.[23] This medication is a tablet dissolved in a large glass of water or juice and consumed on an empty stomach 30 minutes before meals. Taking the full amount may be difficult for young children. Patients with high liver iron overload may not respond to this medication, and it has not been shown to improve left ventricular ejection fraction. Renal toxicities have been reported, including proximal renal tubular dysfunction leading to electrolyte dysfunction (Fanconi syndrome).[23] Deferiprone is another oral agent that was approved by the US Food and Drug Administration (FDA) for transfusion-dependent thalassemia patients who have not responded to other available therapy. This drug has shown effectiveness in removing iron from the heart, but the side effect profile includes neutropenia and possible liver toxicity.[23]

Hematopoietic stem cell transplantation (HSCT, formerly known as bone marrow transplantation) is currently the only potential cure for β-thalassemia, but it is not without serious risks including graft-versus-host disease. Also, availability of donors is often a barrier for many patients. The success of

Complications of Iron Overload

ENDOCRINE PROBLEMS
- Growth retardation
- Diabetes mellitus
- Hypothyroidism
- Hypoparathyroidism
- Disturbed pubertal development

CARDIAC PROBLEMS
- Arrhythmias
- Pericarditis
- Cardiac failure

HEPATIC COMPLICATIONS
- Cirrhosis

transplantation is highest in children and those who are well chelated with minimal signs of iron overload including a normal liver and no cardiac complications.

Other therapies (including hydroxyurea and butyrate derivatives) are currently being investigated for their potential to induce fetal hemoglobin production which may prove especially beneficial for patients with thalassemia intermedia as a way to avoid transfusions.[24] Clinical trials in gene therapy are progressing, and if successful will provide a cure for this disease.[25]

Even patients with β-thalassemia major who are well transfused and well chelated may experience considerable delays in puberty. An endocrinology consultation may be indicated when the patient is nearing the age of puberty. Hormone replacement therapy (estrogen for girls or testosterone for boys) can be initiated to hasten maturation and sexual development.

Patients with thalassemia who receive chronic transfusion therapy and chelation therapy can lead relatively healthy lives. If they are not compliant, however, the complications of iron overload will eventually lead to increasing morbidity from liver disease and, especially, cardiac disease. When patients with β-thalassemia major are hospitalized for any reason, they should be transfused to maintain an adequate hemoglobin concentration and be maintained with chelation therapy. With adequate chelation therapy, the incidence of iron overload and its complications should be minimal (Box 216.3).

LIFE SPAN CONSIDERATIONS

Severe presentations, such as thalassemia major, will present soon after birth and require emergent therapy and interventions for life. Reproductive issues are a major concern. Well-chelated and well-transfused women may be fertile. Contraception as well as genetic counseling should be offered to all women with thalassemia who are sexually active with male partners. Any woman with thalassemia who is considering conceiving should be referred to genetic counseling. There are no restrictions or contraindications as to the types of contraception available to women with β-thalassemia.

COMPLICATIONS

Serious complications for individuals with β-thalassemia minor are extremely rare, as there is generally no treatment necessary.

However, for individuals with severe manifestations of thalassemia, serious complications can occur from both transfusion regimens and chelation therapy, the most severe being diseases transmitted through the blood pool and iron overload.

Transfusions are usually well tolerated, but complications can occur. The development of alloantibodies can make it difficult to find suitable blood donors on a regular basis, requiring lengthy waiting periods of up to 48 hours, depending on proximity to regional blood centers. Viral infections such as human immunodeficiency virus (HIV) infection and hepatitis B and C have become less of an issue because of blood product screening; however, screening is not 100% accurate. Patients should receive hepatitis B vaccine and be screened for hepatitis B antibodies because immunity is not lifelong and may require boosters. Iron overload is the primary complication of chronic transfusions. Accumulation of excess iron leads to cirrhosis, heart failure, and endocrine problems such as diabetes mellitus, hypothyroidism, growth failure, and delayed sexual development.[22,23]

Chelation therapy can also be problematic. Chronic subcutaneous administration of deferoxamine can cause localized reactions such as scar tissue formation, itching, rash, and local irritation at the site of injection. There are also possible complications if a high dose of deferoxamine is given in the presence of low serum ferritin. These complications include toxic effects on the eye, such as cataracts, night blindness, and reduction of visual fields and acuity (these effects usually regress when deferoxamine therapy is stopped); hearing loss (high-tone deafness is irreversible despite cessation of therapy); and skeletal lesions, such as pseudo rickets, metaphyseal changes, and short stature (these are also irreversible complications of deferoxamine therapy).[23]

Despite the availability of iron chelation therapy, complications of iron overload are common in patients with thalassemia who are older than 10 years. This may be a result of inadequate iron chelation early in life with resulting irreversible damage, insufficient chelation therapy, or poor compliance. Iron overload complications include endocrine, cardiac, and hepatic problems (see Box 216.3). The presence of cardiac complications is an indication for continuous (24 hours a day, 7 days a week) iron chelation therapy. Combination therapy with multiple chelating agents is also being studied and is showing promise in patients with severe iron overload affecting organ function.[23]

Well-chelated patients with thalassemia who maintain a ferritin level of less than 1000 mcg/L do not develop the major complications of iron overload. However, many of them have growth retardation and delayed puberty. Most people with β-thalassemia major are unusually short and may appear younger than their age, and many young women are often amenorrhoeic.

PATIENT AND FAMILY EDUCATION

Patients with β-thalassemia major and their families assume a great deal of responsibility for their own health. Chelation therapy occurs at home, and patients must learn how to perform aseptic subcutaneous injections and use the infusion pump. Adherence to the chelation therapy schedule is essential. There are no signs and symptoms of iron overload until a fairly advanced stage; therefore, it is difficult for young children and especially adolescents to understand the importance of a treatment for which they see no immediate need. Adolescents will have self-image issues. Delayed puberty, the need for daily medication infusions, and frequent trips to the hospital for transfusions will constantly remind them of being different from their peers. The daily (or usually nightly) requirement for infusions can interfere with a social life and complicate intimate relationships. The transfusion schedule can interfere with work or school, and most patients with β-thalassemia major find that they require a flexible work or school schedule to accommodate their transfusion schedule.

Discussion regarding genetic counseling for anyone of childbearing age or who is considering conceiving is imperative. A referral to a genetic counselor for expert guidance on this matter is appropriate.

HEALTH PROMOTION

Collaboration with patients and their families is important to promote patients' self-esteem and self-reliance. Patients who believe in the value of their own lives will be more likely to comply with the regular transfusion schedule and their daily chelation therapy. Patients with β-thalassemia minor are considered to have a variant in hemoglobin structure due to a genetic mutation and do not require treatment. They should not receive iron unless they have a superimposed IDA. Iron has side effects and can be toxic if used inappropriately. Clinicians need to be careful in making the correct diagnosis and to avoid unnecessary treatment.

MACROCYTIC ANEMIA

DEFINITION AND EPIDEMIOLOGY

Macrocytic anemias (MCV >100 fL) are described as either megaloblastic or non-megaloblastic. Megaloblastic anemias have a characteristic appearance on examination of peripheral smear. Megaloblastic anemia produces oval-shaped RBCs, hypersegmented neutrophils, and an elevated RDW. Vitamin B_{12} and folate deficiencies are the most common causes of megaloblastic macrocytic anemia. Other causes are related to various drugs and inborn errors of metabolism. Non-megaloblastic anemia is most commonly related to a compensatory increase in reticulocytes (reticulocytosis) due to blood loss (acute hemorrhage or hemolysis).[26]

MEGALOBLASTIC MACROCYTIC ANEMIA

VITAMIN B_{12} AND FOLATE DEFICIENCIES
Definition

Vitamin B_{12} deficiency and folate deficiency are the primary causes of macrocytic anemia. Dietary sources of folic acid include fruits and vegetables, whereas cobalamin (vitamin B_{12}) is obtained primarily though meat protein and somewhat through dairy products and eggs. Both vitamins are essential for normal DNA synthesis, and tissues such as bone marrow are highly sensitive to any deficiency. Marrow precursors for all cell lines (erythroid, myeloid, and platelets) become larger than normal because they remain in the growth phase of the cell cycle. Because they are unable to properly synthesize DNA, they are not able to progress into the mitotic phase of the cell cycle and are therefore unable to complete normal growth and maturation, a condition referred to as megaloblastic bone marrow.[26,27] The resulting ineffective erythropoiesis causes the release of macrocytic RBCs into the circulation and worsening anemia.

Folate deficiency is found in the presence of decreased dietary intake, diseases associated with malabsorption, or increased requirements such as pregnancy. Alcoholism is a common cause of folate deficiency due to alcohol's interference with folate metabolism and poor nutrition commonly associated with alcoholism. Prolonged feeding of goat's milk to infants and fad diets can also be responsible for this disorder. In developing countries, malabsorption syndromes such as tropical and nontropical sprue are more common causes.[27] Folate deficiency in the pregnant woman is associated with neural tube defects in the fetus.

A long-term vegan diet can lead to a vitamin B_{12} deficiency, as can sole breastfeeding of an infant by a mother who has pernicious anemia.[27] Pernicious anemia is the most prevalent cause of vitamin B_{12} deficiency. It is a disease in which atrophy of the parietal cells of the stomach leads to a complete loss of intrinsic factor (IF). IF is necessary for the body to be able to absorb dietary sources of vitamin B_{12}.[27] It often coexists with other autoimmune disorders, GI disorders, type 1 diabetes, and thyroid disease. Chronic use of proton pump inhibitors and H_2 blockers has been associated with B_{12} deficiency, however, study findings are not consistent. Further investigation is needed.[28] Chronic gastritis can damage parietal cells, and partial or complete gastric resection results in loss of parietal cells and therefore loss of IF.[27] The onset of pernicious anemia usually occurs after the age of 50 years.

Pathophysiology

Dietary sources of vitamin B_{12} are found only in meat and meat byproducts (including dairy products and eggs). When vitamin B_{12} from food reaches the small bowel, it is bound to IF, a glycoprotein secreted by parietal cells of the stomach. The vitamin B_{12}-IF (cobalamin-IF) complex is then transported through the terminal ileum into the circulation. Vitamin B_{12} absorption cannot occur in the absence of IF.

Once it is in the circulation, vitamin B_{12} is bound to the transport protein transcobalamin II, which carries it to the liver, bone marrow, and other proliferating cells. A healthy adult receiving an adequate diet has a total body content of 2 to 5 mg of vitamin B_{12}, with at least 1 mg of that being stored in the liver.[4,26] Because the daily requirement of vitamin B_{12} is only 3 to 5 mcg/day, most omnivorous individuals have no difficulty obtaining the necessary amounts from their diets as long as absorption is normal. Recent studies have shown a high prevalence of vitamin B_{12} deficiency among vegetarians, especially those adhering to vegan diets, which restrict all animal products including eggs and dairy products.[29]

Dietary folate is readily available in most foods, especially green leafy vegetables; however, folate is heat labile and rapidly destroyed by prolonged cooking or food processing. Body stores are limited to approximately a 3-month reserve. It is possible that a prolonged inadequate diet may not provide sufficient amounts of folate for normal DNA production, especially for patients who are pregnant or have hemolytic anemias (high rates of cell turnover). Dietary folate deficiency is relatively uncommon because many foods, such as orange juice, are now supplemented. Folate deficiency is commonly associated with chronic alcoholism and can also be caused by the same malabsorption syndromes that lead to vitamin B_{12} deficiency.

Clinical Presentation and Physical Examination

A mild megaloblastic anemia produces few symptoms, and the CBC usually makes the diagnosis incidentally. A severe vitamin B_{12} deficiency includes signs and symptoms of marked anemia and neurologic deficits. Vitamin B_{12} is integral to normal myelin formation and both folate and vitamin B_{12} are essential to DNA synthesis.[4] Folate and B_{12} deficits cause disruption in this metabolism and are the source of the neurologic symptoms. Early neurologic symptoms include decreased vibratory sensation, loss of proprioception, peripheral neuropathy, and ataxia. Later involvement results in spasticity, hyperactive reflexes, and presence of Romberg sign. These neurologic symptoms result from the formation of a demyelinating lesion of the neurons of the spinal cord and cerebral cortex.[4,27] Neurologic symptoms may be evident in the absence of anemia and may not resolve with correction of the deficiency. Other classic symptoms of B_{12} deficiency include a sore mouth and loss of taste.

Folate deficiency is rarely associated with any symptoms, even in the severe state. Folate deficiency is not associated with neurologic or psychiatric disorders except those caused by neural tube defects.

The physical examination of a patient with severe megaloblastic anemia may reveal the classic changes associated with any severe anemia. The patient may also exhibit symptoms of weight loss or other symptoms consistent with malabsorption. Patients with severe vitamin B_{12} deficiency may have characteristic findings such as a beefy-red tongue and the aforementioned neurologic changes.[26,27]

Diagnostics

Essential Diagnostics. Findings on the CBC that suggest macrocytic anemia include low hemoglobin levels, MCV >100 fL, and an elevated RDW. Severe anemia may also be associated with leukopenia or thrombocytopenia. In addition, the reticulocyte count and RI will be low. The peripheral smear is also helpful in diagnosis of megaloblastic anemia. Hypersegmented neutrophils and oval macrocytes are the earliest and most specific signs of megaloblastic anemia. Serum cobalamin (vitamin B12), folate levels, and the measurement of the vitamin B_{12} metabolites of methylmalonic acid and homocysteine are essential to differentiate between vitamin B_{12} and folate deficiency. The normal range of serum methylmalonic acid is 70 to 270 nm/L, and the normal serum homocysteine level ranges from 5 to 14 nm/L.[27] Homocysteine is elevated in both vitamin B_{12} deficiency and folate deficiency. Methylmalonic acid is elevated in vitamin B_{12} deficiency and normal in folate deficiency.

It is important to distinguish vitamin B_{12} deficiency caused by malabsorption from that caused by lack of IF. Many of the medications now used to treat gastroesophageal reflux disease affect absorption. Long-term use of H_2 blockers inhibits release of IF; proton pump inhibitors can reduce absorption of protein-bound cobalamin and can eventually lead to malabsorption. The Schilling test was the classic method to verify the diagnosis of pernicious anemia but is now rarely used. An assay for anti-IF or anti-parietal cell antibodies is the currently accepted method to verify the diagnosis of pernicious anemia.[30] The presence of anti-IF antibodies is highly specific for pernicious anemia.[30]

BOX **216.4**

Common Causes of Macrocytic Anemia

MEGALOBLASTIC ANEMIA

Inadequate Intake (Vitamin B_{12} and Folate Deficiencies)
- Vegetarian diet devoid of animal proteins (vitamin B_{12})
- Chronic alcoholism (folate)—poor nutrition

Malabsorption (Vitamin B_{12} and Folate Deficiencies)
- Lack of intrinsic factor
- Gastric or iliac malabsorption
  - Gastric surgery
  - Inflammatory bowel disease
  - Sprue (tropical and nontropical)
  - Celiac disease
  - Intestinal tapeworm

Increased Requirements (Folate)
- Pregnancy

Drugs/Toxins
- Methotrexate
- Metformin
- Sulfonamides—trimethoprim/sulfamethoxazole
- Anticonvulsants—valproic acid, phenytoin

NON-MEGALOBLASTIC ANEMIA
- Reticulocytosis
  - Hemolysis
  - Blood loss
  - Recombinant erythropoietin
- Reticulocytopenia
  - Chronic alcoholism—related to alcoholic liver disease
  - Liver disease
  - Myelodysplasia
  - Hypothyroidism

INITIAL DIAGNOSTICS

Macrocytic Anemia

LABORATORY
- CBC and differential including RBC indices
  - Peripheral smear
  - Reticulocyte count
- Folate
- Vitamin B12
- LFTs

- Thyroid function tests
- Serum homocysteine
- Methylmalonic acid
- Assay for anti-IF or anti-parietal cell antibodies

IMAGING/PROCEDURES
- Bone marrow biopsy[a]

---
[a]If indicated.

Differential Diagnosis

It is important to accurately determine the cause of the macrocytic anemia, as there are many varied causes (Box 216.4). As vitamin deficiencies are the most common causes, distinguishing between B_{12} and folate deficiencies is essential. Misdiagnosis can have extremely negative consequences. A vitamin B_{12} deficiency that is inappropriately treated with folic acid may result in permanent neurologic or psychiatric abnormalities.

 Priority differentials include (1) nutritional deficiencies (B_{12}, folate), (2) pernicious anemia (lack of IF), (3) hemolysis (4) and liver disease (alcoholic or other).

It may also be necessary to distinguish the macrocytic anemia associated with vitamin B_{12} or folate deficiency from the macrocytosis caused by other conditions, such as drug or alcohol abuse, liver disease, hypothyroidism, myelodysplastic syndrome, exposure to chemotherapeutic agents, and hemolysis.[20] It is also essential to consider vitamin B_{12} deficiency in the differential diagnosis of any peripheral neuropathy, dementia, or other psychiatric disorder, especially in older adults.

Interprofessional Collaborative Management

Pharmacologic Management. There are three basic stages to the management of megaloblastic anemia: (1) recognizing the anemia and classifying it as macrocytic; (2) differentiating whether it is a true folate deficiency, a vitamin B_{12} deficiency, or both combined; and (3) identifying the underlying cause.[26,27]

Initial management of a macrocytic anemia depends on the severity of the anemia. Patients with life-threatening anemia require slow transfusions of packed RBCs to correct the anemia. Treatment with both B_{12} and folate can be started until a definitive diagnosis is made. If the patient's cardiovascular system is unable to compensate for the degree of anemia, hospitalization is required until the patient's condition is stable.

Patients with asymptomatic anemia should not be treated until an accurate diagnosis is made. Treatment should then be targeted to replacement of the deficient vitamin and correction of the underlying disease, if possible. Some patients with B_{12} deficiency will be able to take oral vitamin B_{12} supplementation daily, especially if due to diet. Those with pernicious anemia, who lack IF, will need parental therapy. Ideally, rapid correction of the deficiency is recommended. This can be accomplished with a protocol of vitamin B_{12}, 1-mg injections (subcutaneous or intramuscular) according to the following schedule: week 1, daily for 7 days; week 2, twice per week; weeks 3 to 6, once weekly; then monthly for life. Oral replacement with 1–2 mgs po qd has been found to be as effective as intramuscular injections. Response to therapy is rapid, with normal hematopoiesis and a much-improved sense of well-being within 48 hours. Reticulocytosis begins in approximately 3 days and peaks in 7 to 10 days after the initiation of vitamin replacement. The anemia should resolve in 3 to 4 weeks.[26] It is important to note that even though the anemia will normalize, any advanced neurologic symptoms that have been ongoing for more than 3 months will remain permanent.[26,27]

The recommended treatment of a macrocytic anemia resulting from folate deficiency is 1 to 5 mg/day of folic acid by mouth and correction of the underlying cause of the deficiency. Treatment should continue until at least a normal hemoglobin level is reached (usually in about 4 to 6 weeks) and should be continued indefinitely if the patient has an inadequate diet or if the underlying disease persists. Pregnant women who have folate deficiency macrocytic anemia should receive 4 mg/day of folic acid until delivery. Patients who have had partial or total gastrectomy, ileal resection, or any other evidence of gastric atrophy or intestinal malabsorption should receive prophylactic monthly parenteral vitamin B_{12} therapy (or daily oral replacement) and daily oral folic acid supplements.

Nonpharmacologic Management. Encouraging intake of folate-rich foods is essential to the management of those with a folic acid deficiency. Folic acid is found naturally in beef liver, green leafy vegetables, peas, beans, avocados, eggs, and milk. Many foods are fortified with folic acid and other vitamins and minerals to help ensure intake of recommended daily requirements. Examples of fortified foods are flour, pasta, cereals, bread, cornmeal, and rice. Consultation with a nutritionist can be very helpful for those individuals who have restricted diets and food sensitivities.

The primary health care provider can easily manage patients who are receiving maintenance therapy for either vitamin B_{12} or folate replacement. These patients require regular visits for evaluation of therapy and, when indicated, monthly visits for vitamin B_{12} injections. Periodic evaluations should include a complete history and physical examination to look for the appearance or progression of any neurologic or psychiatric complications, as well as continued assessment of the underlying disease causing the vitamin deficiency. Laboratory evaluations include CBC and serum cobalamin, methylmalonic acid, and folate levels. A hematologist should manage patients with refractory anemia.

Patients with severe macrocytic anemia should be referred to a hematologist for consultation and recommended therapy. Asymptomatic patients can be treated and monitored in an outpatient setting, either by a hematologist or by the patient's health care provider.

Patients with a severe, life-threatening anemia may require hospitalization for correction of the anemia. This is especially true for patients with a severe vitamin B_{12} deficiency, who require daily administration of parenteral vitamin B_{12} therapy to correct the vitamin deficiency.

Life Span Considerations

For any infant with macrocytic anemia, consumption of goat's milk or the possibility of pernicious anemia (B_{12} deficiency) in the breastfeeding mother should be considered.

There is an association between folate deficiency and neural tube defects (NTD). Risk of neural tube defects is 1 to 5 per 1000 live births for the general population and approximately 10 times this risk among women with previous pregnancies involving neural tube defects. Women should take folic acid supplements before and during pregnancy to reduce the incidence of neural tube defects. For women who are at low risk for NTD, the recommended intake is 4 mg/day as a supplement, starting at least one month prior to conception. For women who have had a previous infant with NTD, or first-degree relative who has, the recommendation is 4000 mcg/day (4 mg/day) of folic acid by mouth starting 1 to 3 months prior to conception through first trimester of pregnancy, at which time the dose may be lowered to 0.4 mg/day for the remainder of the pregnancy.[18]

Annual screening for vitamin B_{12} deficiency is recommended for all older adults. Older adults with severe B_{12} deficiency can develop reversible cognitive change. Screening is also recommended for patients with histories of poor nutrition or hematologic, neurologic, or psychiatric abnormalities suggestive of vitamin B_{12} deficiency.

Complications

The complication of undiagnosed or mistreated vitamin B_{12} deficiency is irreversible neurologic damage. Manifestations of weakness, ataxia, and poor coordination may not completely resolve with therapy, depending on the duration of the deficiency and the extent of neurologic damage. Mental status changes can range from mild forgetfulness to severe dementia and psychosis. Patients with neurologic damage can have an almost normal blood count with normal indices, which underscores the need to test for vitamin B_{12} levels in patients with unexplained neurologic deficits.

Patient and Family Education

Patients with folate deficiency secondary to an inadequate diet require nutritional counseling to learn how to properly cook and prepare foods without losing their nutritional value. Daily folic acid supplementation may be required for patients receiving certain drugs, such as sulfasalazine and methotrexate (both used for certain inflammatory forms of arthritis or inflammatory bowel disease) and for patients with other hematologic diseases.

Patients with megaloblastic anemia secondary to vitamin B_{12} deficiency require monthly vitamin B_{12} injections. Patients or caregivers can easily be taught this injection technique so that injections can be administered at home. Parenteral vitamin B_{12} in the absence of pernicious anemia is not effective in increasing energy in older adults. Patients with conditions that require partial or total gastrectomy, ileal resections, and other small bowel removal need counseling on lifelong parenteral vitamin B_{12} and folic acid replacement.

Health Promotion

One preventive measure that health care providers can take to reduce the incidence of folate deficiency anemia is the early recognition and treatment of alcohol abuse. Lifestyle modifications include improving dietary sources of folic acid and vitamin B_{12} and taking vitamin supplements if necessary. Health care providers who see older patients should screen for cobalamin deficiency in cases of unexplained mental status changes or neuropathy and should begin therapy with vitamin B_{12} even before the anemia is noted. Individuals who are on strict vegetarian or vegan diets would benefit from daily B_{12} supplementation to prevent megaloblastic macrocytic anemia.[29] Organic foods that are not regulated by FDA requirements may not have the recommended folic acid supplementation so this needs to be considered in individuals with folic acid deficiency.

NORMOCYTIC ANEMIA

ANEMIA OF CHRONIC DISEASE
Definition and Epidemiology

ACD is a mild to moderate anemia that often results from inflammatory disorders, infection, or malignancy. It has also been referred to as anemia of inflammation. The RBCs are usually normocytic (normal MCV), normochromic (normal MCH/MCHC), and the hemoglobin is generally not less than 9 g/dL. This anemia has an insidious onset, is common in older adults, and is the most frequent type of anemia in hospitalized patients.[5]

Pathophysiology

ACD is marked by low serum iron levels, but total iron stores are normal or elevated. Hepcidin, a liver-derived peptide that is a regulator of iron transport, is increased in inflammatory conditions, resulting in reduced transport of iron to erythroid precursors. Other possible mechanisms for ACD that have been suggested include decreased RBC survival time, decreased use of reticuloendothelial iron for hemoglobin synthesis, and inflammatory cytokine inhibition of erythropoietin production.[4]

In ACKD, there may be a relative deficiency of erythropoietin.[4] Erythropoietin is a renal hormone whose normal plasma levels increase logarithmically in response to decreased hemoglobin levels. Although serum erythropoietin levels may be increased, they are not elevated enough for the degree of anemia. The exact pathogenesis of ACKD is unclear but may include several factors, including a blunted erythropoietin response to anemia.

Clinical Presentation and Physical Examination

ACD is often mild and asymptomatic. Patients typically have symptoms that are associated with the underlying diseases rather than with the anemia itself. Typical signs and symptoms, such as fatigue, pallor, tachycardia, and dyspnea with exertion, will be present as anemia progresses, usually when hemoglobin falls below 9 to 10 g/dL.

A thorough physical examination is prudent to investigate for changes related to the possible underlying chronic disease.

Diagnostics

Essential Diagnostics. The CBC will usually reveal a normocytic anemia; however, the anemia can occasionally be microcytic in later stages. Hemoglobin levels are generally 10 to 11 g/dL. Reticulocyte count is usually decreased. There are no distinctive changes in RBC size or shape, but if microcytosis does occur, the RDW may be slightly elevated. Iron studies help to distinguish ACD from IDA and reveal a low serum iron level, a normal or increased ferritin level, and a normal or elevated TIBC. Bone marrow examination, if it is done, reveals normal to increased bone marrow iron stores with decreased amounts of bone marrow sideroblasts.

No precise diagnostic criteria exist for ACD. As many chronic conditions can result in this type of anemia, determining the underlying disease state is integral to the diagnostic process. Inflammatory disease states are often implicated in ACD; therefore, evaluating an erythrocyte sedimentation rate (ESR) and C-reactive protein (CRP) should be considered. ACD often coexists with IDA, but laboratory test results can be difficult to distinguish because frequent overlaps occur.[4] The only true way to distinguish ACD from IDA is by assessment of iron stores (which are absent in IDA and normal or increased in ACD) either by bone marrow aspiration and biopsy or by evaluation of the serum ferritin levels. Although bone marrow aspiration and biopsy are completed by the hematologist to exclude myelodysplastic syndromes and other diseases, they usually add nothing to an already negative serologic evaluation and physical examination findings that the less invasive procedure generates.

INITIAL DIAGNOSTICS

Anemia of Chronic Disease

LABORATORY
- CBC and differential including RBC indices
  - Peripheral smear
  - Reticulocyte count
- Ferritin
- TIBC
- Transferrin
- Serum iron
- LFTs

- Thyroid function tests
- Renal function tests: BUN, creatinine, eGFR
- Erythropoietin level[a]
- Erythrocyte sedimentation rate[a]
- C-reactive protein[a]

IMAGING/PROCEDURES
- Bone marrow biopsy[a]

---

[a]If indicated.

Differential Diagnosis

If the clinical picture is one of a mild microcytic anemia, the differential diagnosis is between ACD and IDA. Iron studies are the most useful to differentiate the two (see Differential Diagnosis in the section on iron deficiency anemia). ACD is a diagnosis of exclusion.

 Priority differentials include (1) IDA, (2) myelodysplastic syndromes, and (3) sideroblastic anemia.

It is important to determine the underlying etiology when ACD is suspected. Some of the most common disease states underlying ACD are malignancy, chronic infection, autoimmune conditions (rheumatoid, arthritis, SLE, inflammatory bowel disease) and chronic kidney disease.

Interprofessional Collaborative Management

Pharmacologic Management. After IDA has been excluded, mild anemia need not be treated unless it is symptomatic. The standard treatment for ACKD of renal insufficiency is recombinant human erythropoietin (rHuEPO) or darbepoetin alfa (novel erythropoiesis-stimulating protein [NESP]). Intermittent transfusions may be required with more severe anemias. As always, the underlying condition should be treated or optimally controlled. Treatment of the underlying disease will improve, and often correct, the anemia.

Nonpharmacologic Management. As in most cases, anemia is mild and mostly asymptomatic. Promoting wellbeing in the presence of chronic disease is imperative for those with ACD. Encouraging well-balanced diets to avoid vitamin and mineral insufficiencies and obtaining appropriate immunizations are recommended.

Once acute reasons for the anemia have been excluded and the diagnosis of ACD has been confirmed, patients' underlying condition should be well managed and if the patient has been referred to a specialist for care, coordination with the clinician who is managing the underlying medical condition is imperative. The anemia should be monitored with periodic CBCs and iron studies. Referral to a specialist may be necessary to initiate therapy with rHuEPO or NESP or if the anemia worsens and requires other interventions.

Given that ACD is associated with chronic medical conditions, it is possible that the patient may have an acute reason for anemia, such as a drug or transfusion reaction. ACD rarely requires hospitalization for management. If the cause of the anemia is uncertain, referral to or consultation with a hematologist is appropriate.

Complications

If the anemia is mild, the patient should have no complications associated with the anemia itself. Complications of the underlying disease should be managed appropriately.

Patient and Family Education

Regular visits with the health care provider should include laboratory studies to monitor for anemia. Patients should be encouraged to contact their provider if they experience any increase in symptoms, such as fatigue, decreased exercise tolerance, or shortness of breath. Patients should be encouraged to maintain therapy and surveillance for their chronic conditions, as this will help improve and stabilize their anemia.

Health Promotion

ACD will stabilize when the underlying condition is stable and managed well. Encouraging adherence to treatment for the chronic conditions, maintaining a well-balanced diet, partaking in daily exercise if tolerated, and staying up to date with immunizations is recommended.

SICKLE CELL DISEASE

 Stroke in sickle cell disease is a medical emergency. There is a high risk of renal dysfunction or failure in adults with sickle cell disease.

Definition and Epidemiology

Sickle cell syndromes are the most common inherited hemoglobinopathies and include homozygous disease (hemoglobin SS), hemoglobin SC (also known as SC disease), Sβ-thalassemia, and conditions involving a variety of other rare, abnormal hemoglobins. Patients with sickle cell disease have mild to moderate hemolytic anemia that is generally well compensated; however, over time, this anemia can lead to chronic heart disease. The hallmark of sickle cell disease is the acute vaso-occlusive crisis that causes unpredictable, severe pain and organ damage.

Approximately 8% of African Americans carry the gene for sickle cell trait (hemoglobin AS), and about 1 in 400 are affected by the disease (hemoglobin SS).[31] Other types of sickle cell syndromes are found in Mediterranean, Middle Eastern, and Southeast Asian populations. Sickle cell is an inherited autosomal recessive genetic disorder (see Fig. 216.1). People with only one gene for hemoglobin S are phenotypically normal (sickle cell trait). People who inherit one gene for hemoglobin S from each parent will have SS disease. People with either hemoglobin SC or Sβ-thalassemia have inherited one gene for hemoglobin S and the other gene for either hemoglobin C or β-thalassemia, respectively. In the case of Sβ-thalassemia, the hemoglobin S gene is combined with a thalassemia gene that makes a decreased amount of beta hemoglobin (Sβ+-thalassemia) or a gene that makes no beta hemoglobin men (Sβ0-thalassemia). The median life span of patients with SS and Sβ0-thalassemia disease is 42 years for men and 48 years for women, and 15% of people born with sickle cell disease in the United States die by the age of 29 years. The life span is 60 to 70 years for patients with other types of sickle cell syndromes, including hemoglobin SC and Sβ+-thalassemia.[32]

Pathophysiology

The hemoglobin defect occurs when valine replaces glutamic acid in the beta chain of hemoglobin, resulting in hemoglobin S.[20] Deoxygenated hemoglobin S tends to undergo irreversible polymerization, deforming the erythrocytes and giving them the pathognomonic sickle shape. The sickled cells are rigid and can be easily trapped in the microcirculation, causing obstruction, ischemia, and sometimes infarction. This process leads to the clinical consequences of severe pain and organ damage. These vaso-occlusive episodes, usually referred to as crises or pain crises, can occur anywhere in the body but commonly affect the joints, extremities, back, chest, abdomen, and lungs.[32]

Clinical Presentation and Physical Examination

Individuals with sickle cell trait only have no clinical manifestations. Manifestations of sickle cell disease vary widely; some affected individuals have few painful vaso-occlusive crises or other rare complications, whereas many others are often hospitalized with painful crises or other complications. Patients with other types of sickle cell syndromes (hemoglobin SC or Sβ+-thalassemia) are reported to have milder forms of disease, although this is not always true. For example, patients with hemoglobin SC can exhibit the same range of severity as patients with SS disease.[20,32]

Objective manifestations of moderate to severe hemolytic anemia include jaundice and a physiologic systolic flow murmur. Scleral icterus can range from mild to severe but often has no association with the severity of disease. The physiologic flow murmur secondary to anemia is often a grade 1 or 2 pansystolic murmur, which is heard best along the left sternal border. Cardiomegaly is routinely noted on the radiographs of adults with sickle cell disease and is also a compensatory manifestation of lifelong anemia.

Diagnostics

Essential Diagnostics. Accurate diagnosis of any sickle cell syndrome requires hemoglobin electrophoresis. Patients with sickle cell disease have evidence of hemolytic anemia: low hemoglobin, chronic reticulocytosis, chronic hyperbilirubinemia, and chronically elevated LDH levels. The peripheral blood smear shows mild to moderate anisocytosis and poikilocytosis with numerous sickle cells and Howell-Jolly bodies (evidence of the patient's functional asplenia).[4,20] Patients with sickle cell disease have target cells in addition to the sickle cells on their peripheral blood smears. Unfortunately, no laboratory tests are predictive or diagnostic of an acute painful crisis.

INITIAL DIAGNOSTICS

Sickle Cell Disease

LABORATORY
- CBC and differential which includes RBC indices:
  - Peripheral smear
  - Reticulocyte count
- Hemoglobin electrophoresis
- Renal function tests—BUN/serum creatinine/eGFR

- Liver function test—bilirubin, LFTs
- LDH

IMAGING/PROCEDURES
- Bone marrow biopsy[a]

[a]If indicated.

Differential Diagnosis

Most patients with sickle cell disease are diagnosed at birth. In fact, all states in the United States and many developed nations in the world currently have mandatory newborn screening for sickle hemoglobin. However, it is possible for persons who were not screened at birth and with very mild disease to go undiagnosed until they are in their adult years. These patients may have a mild hemolytic anemia (low hemoglobin concentration, slight hyperbilirubinemia with elevated LDH levels, and mild reticulocytosis). A history of occasional spontaneous painful events, usually abdominal or joint pains, should suggest a hemoglobinopathy. Accurate diagnosis requires hemoglobin electrophoresis to differentiate among the various forms of sickle cell disease. Other possible causes of hemolytic anemia include hereditary spherocytosis, hypersplenism, autoimmune hemolysis, and delayed hemolytic transfusion reaction.[5]

 Priority differentials include (1) other hemolytic conditions (thrombotic thrombocytopenic purpura—TTP, hemolytic uremic syndrome—HUS), (2) other hemoglobinopathies (thalassemias), and (3) other congenital RBC abnormalities (inherited spherocytosis, elliptocytosis)

Interprofessional Collaborative Management

Nonpharmacologic Management. The frequency and severity of pain crises vary tremendously among patients and even in the same patient over time. Physical stresses including infection, change of weather (exposure to cold in particular), dehydration, fatigue, overexertion, or emotional stress may precipitate a crisis, but the majority of crises occur spontaneously with no obvious precipitating events.[32] Although the sites affected in an acute crisis vary among individuals, crises tend to recur at the same sites per person. The quality of the pain is usually similar as well. Most patients can distinguish a "typical" sickle cell pain crisis from other events, such as pyelonephritis or abdominal pain resulting from cholecystitis. Most crises are mild to moderate in severity and can be managed at home with oral analgesics (either NSAIDs or oral narcotics), adequate hydration, rest, and local measures such as heat and gentle massage. These are the foundation of care regardless of severity.

Pharmacologic Management. Moderate to severe crises require treatment in an emergency department or a hospital-based outpatient treatment center with parenteral narcotic analgesics and hydration as well as the same local measures. Often, aggressive and early management of a crisis can prevent hospital admission. Hospitalizations for crises can last a few days to several weeks. Patients describe a severe crisis as the most intense pain they have ever experienced. Pain control often requires large quantities of narcotic analgesics. Initial dosage of parenteral narcotics in the hospital setting should consider how much opioid the patient has been using at home, and this dose should be used as a starting point, with appropriate conversion from home dose to parenteral dose. Consultation with the clinical pharmacologist in the hospital is prudent. Pain should be reassessed every 15 to 30 minutes, narcotics readministered as needed, and consideration given to escalating the dose by 25% until pain is under control.[32] Many adults with sickle cell disease have learned how to manage their pain without the behavioral signs that one would expect from someone experiencing severe pain. Therefore, it becomes important in evaluating a sickle cell patient in crisis to believe the patient's report and to treat the pain quickly and appropriately.

Hydroxyurea has become the standard of therapy for adult patients who experience three or more crises per year, have sickle cell-associated pain that interferes with daily activities, or have a history of severe or recurrent acute chest syndrome (ACS). In children older than 9 months, it should be offered regardless of clinical symptoms because it can reduce sickle cell disease-related complications.[32] Hydroxyurea induces hemoglobin F formation, thereby decreasing the total percentage of hemoglobin S in RBCs. This results in decreased sickling and hemolysis of RBCs and decreased veno-occlusion, the major cause of complications in this disease.[32] Hydroxyurea is started at a dose of 10 to 20 mg/kg/day. Patients must be monitored every 2 weeks for signs of toxicity (neutrophil count <2000/mm³, platelet count <80,000/mm³, or hemoglobin drop of 2 g/dL), in which case, doses should be held until count recovery and then decreased 5 mg/kg/day below the dose at which the cytopenias occurred. When blood counts remain stable, the dose of hydroxyurea can be increased over a period of several months to a maximum dose of 35 mg/kg/day. If blood counts continue to be stable at this dose, patients should be monitored every 2 to 3 months.[32,33]

Patients with sickle cell disease are anemic, by definition. The degree of anemia varies, but most have hemoglobin concentrations that range from 7 to 8 g/dL. Patients with hemoglobin SC tend to have hematocrit values in the high-20s to mid-30s. The baseline hemoglobin value tends to remain relatively stable in a given patient. Most patients can compensate for their level of anemia and do not require routine transfusions. In fact, transfusing patients to achieve hemoglobin concentrations above 10 g/dL can be dangerous because blood viscosity substantially increases at higher hematocrit levels. The increased viscosity can increase the risk of a sickle crisis by slowing transit time of the RBCs through low-oxygen regions of the circulation.[33] In general, transfusions in patients with sickle cell disease are indicated only before surgical procedures requiring anesthesia and in the circumstance of the severe complications of ACS, acute splenic sequestration, stroke, and aplastic crisis.

Hematopoietic stem cell transplantation (HSCT—formerly known as bone marrow transplantation) is the only curative therapy for sickle cell disease and is becoming more widely used in light of new reduced-toxicity conditioning regimens and other advances in transplant therapy. Some of the historical barriers to transplant have been the lack of reliable prognostic factors for severity in this disease to determine the risk/benefit ratio; the lack of available donors in this minority population; and sickle cell-related organ damage (especially in older patients) increasing the risk of unsuccessful outcomes. Results from two international registries demonstrate 90% cure rate and very limited complications in patients with human leukocyte antigen (HLA)-identical sibling donors.[34]

The chronic nature of sickle cell disease, the frequent need for acute treatment of painful crises, and the high risk for complications dictate that these patients are better cared for by specialists familiar with the disease. Many of the large urban hospitals in the United States have sickle cell centers where patients receive comprehensive care by multidisciplinary teams of physicians, nurse practitioners, physician assistants, nurses, psychologists, and social workers. These hospital-based centers allow prompt referral to other specialists such as neurologists, cardiologists, high-risk obstetricians, and ophthalmologists.

Most of complications resulting from SCD require hospitalization for treatment (see below). Patients with moderate to severe disease also have many admissions for intractable vaso-occlusive crises. These hospitalizations can last a couple of days to several weeks. Consultation with a social worker is recommended for issues related to school, employment, housing, transportation, and medical billing issues.

Life Span Considerations

Pain crisis is the most common complication of sickle cell disease and occurs across all age groups. Appropriate management of pain crisis is reviewed earlier. An age-related complication in infants and toddlers is dactylitis. This is a painful swelling of the hands and feet as a result of bone marrow expansion from increased erythropoiesis. Another complication occurring most commonly in children is acute splenic sequestration. This is caused by trapping of RBCs in the splenic sinuses. This is a life-threatening emergency in children because it can progress to hypovolemic shock.[35]

Women with sickle cell disease can carry pregnancies to term but should be considered high risk because of the potential for obstetric complications such as preterm delivery, spontaneous abortion, thrombosis, preeclampsia, and pulmonary embolism after delivery.[32] The frequency of painful crises sometimes increases during pregnancy, but the crises are treated no differently from other crises, with narcotic analgesics and hydration. Pregnancy prevention and family planning options are the same for women with sickle cell disease as they are for other women. In fact, many women experience relief from menses-related crises with the use of oral contraceptives or other hormone contraception methods.

Pulmonary hypertension is one of the leading causes of mortality and morbidity in adults with sickle cell disease. Echocardiogram-based tricuspid jet velocity is a frequently used screening modality, and an increase in systolic pulmonary artery pressure is a poor prognostic factor.[32]

Sickle cell disease is a chronic condition that often leads to psychosocial difficulties as well as medical problems. Some patients experience frequent complications of their disease, making it almost impossible to participate in normal daily activities, to hold a regular job, or to attend school on a regular schedule. Many of these patients can benefit from rehabilitation counseling and vocational training. Often, however, adults with sickle cell disease find that they are unable to work because of chronic pain or other multiorgan damage. These individuals are clearly disabled. Ensuring services and benefits is essential for these individuals.

Complications

Chronic pain is a substantial problem for many children and most adults with sickle cell disease. The severity of the pain varies greatly among patients and can change over time. Some patients can manage their chronic pain with intermittent use of mild analgesics such as NSAIDs. Most patients, however, require frequent doses of oral narcotic analgesics. Often these patients become tolerant of narcotics, and the quantity of medication needed to control the pain can escalate over time. This physical tolerance should not be confused with psychological addiction and drug-seeking behaviors.[32]

Splenic infarction caused by vaso-occlusion occurs very early in children, resulting in a functional asplenia. As a result, patients with sickle cell disease are immunocompromised and at risk of overwhelming sepsis from encapsulated organisms such as *Neisseria meningitidis*, *Haemophilus influenzae*, and *Streptococcus pneumoniae*. Patients are instructed to seek immediate medical evaluation including history, physical, CBC with differential, reticulocyte count, blood culture, and possibly urine culture for every fever of 38.5°C or higher.[32] Initiation of penicillin prophylaxis and immunizations specific to these organisms has helped to greatly decrease associated mortality.

The term *acute chest syndrome* is used to describe an acute pulmonary event in a sickle cell disease patient that can be either infectious or noninfectious in its cause. Fever, dyspnea, cough, pulmonary infiltrates on chest x-ray examination, and severe chest pain usually characterize the condition. Clinically, ACS is often more severe than pneumonia in the general population, with severe hypoxia and progressive multilobar involvement despite treatment with antibiotics. Typically, the patient is hospitalized for a vaso-occlusive crisis and 1 to 3 days later develops respiratory distress. Causes of ACS include pneumonia, bone marrow fat embolism, infection, pulmonary infarct resulting from sickling, rib or sternal infarct, or pulmonary embolus.[32]

The most important step in the treatment of ACS is early recognition. Potential bacterial infections should be treated with appropriate antibiotics. Simple transfusions raising the hemoglobin concentration to 10 g/dL can be beneficial in patients with mild to moderate hypoxemia. Adequate ventilation is essential to recovery, and this can be achieved by using incentive spirometry in mild cases and mechanical ventilation in severe cases.[32]

Stroke in sickle cell disease is a medical emergency. The treatment of choice is an exchange transfusion followed by maintenance hypertransfusion and iron chelation therapy. It is recommended that children with sickle cell disease be screened by transcranial Doppler ultrasonography and that chronic transfusion therapy be started if results indicate a high risk of stroke.[32] Compliance with iron chelation therapy for prevention of future complications from iron overload is an essential component of chronic transfusion therapy.

Priapism is defined as a persistent, painful erection of the penis that can last several hours to several days. Priapism lasting more than 3 or 4 hours is a medical emergency because it can cause impotence. Referral to a urologist is recommended in this situation.[32] Treatment includes hydration, analgesia, and possibly evacuation of the blood from the corpus cavernosum.

There is a high risk of renal dysfunction or failure in adults with sickle cell disease. Renal failure results from the sickle cell-induced damage to renal microvasculature. Patients are monitored for proteinuria, and referral to a nephrologist is recommended when proteinuria is present. Often angiotensin-converting enzyme inhibitor (ACEI) therapy is initiated for renal complications even in the absence of hypertension.[32] Renal dysfunction is typically diagnosed in the third or fourth decade and eventually progresses to renal failure. Subcutaneous erythropoietin or darbepoetin alfa to maintain appropriate hemoglobin levels is often helpful either to prevent or to reduce the need for transfusions in patients with renal insufficiency. Adults with renal failure usually require chronic transfusions and should be offered chelation therapy as necessary.

Treatment of end-stage renal disease requires hemodialysis or kidney transplantation.

Skin ulcerations of the lower legs are the most common cutaneous complication of sickle cell disease, causing pain and physical disfigurement.[32,34] The medial or lateral malleoli are more frequently involved, and ulcerations occur less commonly over the dorsum of the foot, near the Achilles tendon. The size of the ulcers varies from a few millimeters to large, circumferential ulcers that involve the entire ankle or foot. Lesions can extend into the dermis, the underlying subcutaneous tissue, and the underlying muscle fascia. These lesions are highly susceptible to infection and other complications. They are resistant to therapy and often exist for years (some patients report persistent ulcers for more than 10 years). Pain is the major problem and is often severe and unremitting, causing significant disability. Environment and geographic location influence the prevalence of leg ulcers, with great variability among the various regions of the globe. Age is also a factor; this problem is less common in younger patients.[36] The cause and pathogenesis of leg ulcers are not well understood. Clinical experience and epidemiology studies suggest a role for three factors: marginal blood supply to the skin of the lower extremities, local edema, and minor trauma.[35] The greatest risk factor for the development of leg ulcers is a history of previous ulcers.

Treatment is initially standard therapy consisting of debridement, wet to damp dressing, and topical dressings and agent.[35] Treatment of existing ulcers can be difficult and frustrating; healing is often only temporary. Zinc is important in wound healing. It is found in RBCs and is lost during hemolysis; therefore, zinc deficiency is common in patients with sickle cell disease. There is some evidence that zinc supplementation benefits the healing of ankle ulcers. Other controversial treatments include chronic transfusions and skin grafting for ulcers that are resistant to more conservative therapy, but failure rates for both methods are high.[35]

Patients should be educated about the importance of preventing local trauma by wearing shoes that fit properly, using insect repellents to prevent bites, and promptly treating any minor cuts on the feet and ankles. Patients with a history of ulcers and leg edema are encouraged to wear compression stockings and to perform routine care of the skin with emollients, good local hygiene, and daily inspection for any minor trauma.

The bony skeleton is a common target of the consequences of sickling. Bone marrow necrosis, bone infarcts, avascular necrosis (AVN), and osteomyelitis are common complications. The heads of the femur and humerus are common sites for marrow infarction and necrosis. Infarcts can also occur in the spine, ribs, and sternum. Bone infarcts constitute a painful crisis that generally resolves in 1 to 2 weeks. Treatment does not differ from that of any other painful crisis and includes analgesia, hydration, and rest.[32]

AVN commonly affects the hip and shoulder joints and is a more chronic condition than an acute bone infarct. Patients complain of severe chronic pain, limited range of motion, and pain with joint movement. Late stages are evident on plain radiographs, but MRI is much more sensitive in the identification of AVN in the early stages. Initially, NSAIDs and narcotic analgesics are the mainstay of treatment. In the earlier stages, core decompression may be performed to attempt to increase blood flow and prevent further joint damage. Later stages are usually surgically corrected with joint replacement.[32]

Retinopathy is a significant problem for patients with sickle cell disease. It is more common in patients with SC disease than in those with homozygous SS disease. The retinopathy resembles that seen in diabetes and is believed to be caused by ischemia to the retina. Lifelong management with an ophthalmologist is recommended.[32]

Patient and Family Education

Patient education begins early in childhood and continues throughout life. Initially, parents are taught how to manage pain crises, to recognize signs of infection, and to administer daily medications. Coping with acute and chronic pain is a lifelong issue and involves learning both pharmacologic and nonpharmacologic interventions. Educating patients on the proper use of oral analgesics and management of painful crises is important and should occur at every opportunity. Patients need to be taught to seek prompt medical attention for any complication and not wait until they can speak to their health care provider. Preconception counseling is imperative for anyone with SCD trait or the overt disease state.

Health Promotion

The importance of preventive care must also be stressed. Routine care should include annual ophthalmologic, gynecologic, and dental examinations; periodic sickle cell clinic visits; and immunizations, including hepatitis A and B, annual influenza, pneumococcal, meningococcal, and *H. influenzae* vaccines. Also, regular screening such as transcranial Doppler for risk of stroke and echocardiogram for evaluation of pulmonary hypertension are recommended. A common cause of death in children with SS is *S. pneumoniae* sepsis. This susceptibility is a result of splenic malfunction and failure that begins in the first years of life and inability to make immunoglobulin G (IgG) antibodies to antigens. Prevention is vaccination and prophylactic penicillin. All infants with sickle cell disease should receive the complete series of the 13-valent conjugate pneumococcal vaccine beginning at 2 months of age. At 24 months of age, these children are given the 23-valent pneumococcal polysaccharide vaccine (PPV23) and a second dose of PPV23 immunization 5 years later. Although most children with sickle cell disease do not respond as well to the vaccine as non-SS children, a rise in IgG antibodies is noted. Prophylactic penicillin begins in the newborn period with oral penicillin V and continues until the age of 5 years, at which time the incidence of life-threatening infections from *Mycoplasma pneumoniae*, *Chlamydia*, parvovirus B19, and *Staphylococcus aureus* significantly decreases.[28] Parents must be taught to call and bring the child into the hospital for every fever. This is necessary so the child can be evaluated for sepsis. The evaluation involves drawing a blood culture and giving prophylactic intravenous antibiotic coverage until the results of the blood culture are known.

Adequate hydration, regular exercise, avoidance of exposure to cold temperatures and sufficient sleep play a role in helping patients manage their disease. Teaching children and young adults coping skills can be beneficial and can help them manage both the acute and chronic pain associated with their disease. Annual health screenings, ophthalmologic examinations, and vaccines are recommended but easily overlooked. As mentioned before, pre-conception counseling is an essential part of comprehensive and appropriate care.

APLASTIC ANEMIA

DEFINITION AND EPIDEMIOLOGY

Aplastic anemia is a life-threatening condition resulting from bone marrow stem cell failure. It is characterized by a marked decrease in all hematopoietic precursors, resulting in pancytopenia. Aplastic anemia can affect people of all ages and both genders. It is a rare disorder with an estimated incidence of approximately 2 to 6 cases per million people per year.[37]

PATHOPHYSIOLOGY

In aplastic anemia, the damage to the bone marrow's ability to generate stem cells can be secondary to infection or exposures to toxins or medications, or it can be immune mediated (Box 216.5).

CLINICAL PRESENTATION AND PHYSICAL EXAMINATION

Patients may be seen with abnormal bleeding, infection, and anemia. Onset is usually sudden without any other apparent illness. The history may reveal information about a recent viral infection, chronic disease, or exposure to an offending medication or toxin.

The physical examination may reveal petechiae, ecchymosis, purpura, pallor of the skin and mucous membranes, and mild lymphadenopathy in the late stages. Early stages of aplastic anemia may show no significant changes on physical examination.

DIAGNOSTICS
Essential Diagnostics

A CBC will show pancytopenia with normocytic and normochromic RBC indices and morphology. The reticulocyte count is also below normal, reflecting the lack of bone marrow activity. A bone marrow biopsy is essential for diagnosis. Severe

---

BOX **216.5**

Agents Associated with Aplastic Anemia

TOXINS
- Radiation
- Alkylating agents
- Insecticides
- Benzene and its derivatives
- Chemotherapeutic agents

MEDICATIONS
- Antibiotics (penicillin, chloramphenicol, cephalosporins, sulfonamides)
- Antidepressants (lithium, tricyclics)
- Anti-inflammatory drugs (gold salts, nonsteroidals, salicylates)
- Antimalarials
- Anticonvulsants

OTHER POSSIBLE CAUSES
- Viral: hepatitis C, HIV, Epstein-Barr virus
- Graft-versus-host disease
- Malignant neoplasm
- Pregnancy

aplastic anemia (SAA) is defined as a bone marrow cellularity of less than 25% and at least two of the following: absolute neutrophil count (ANC) less than 500/μL, ARC less than 20,000/μL, and platelet count less than 20,000/μL.[37]

DIFFERENTIAL DIAGNOSIS

Aplastic anemia is readily detected and easily distinguished from other forms of normocytic, normochromic anemia. Involvement of other cell types (myeloid, platelets) seen on peripheral smear confirms the diagnosis.

 Priority differentials include (1) hypoplastic myelodysplastic syndrome, (2) leukemias and lymphomas, (3) anorexia nervosa or prolonged starvation, and (4) severe autoimmune disease (like SLE).

INTERPROFESSIONAL COLLABORATIVE MANAGEMENT

Pharmacologic Management

Any patient with symptoms suggestive of aplastic anemia should be referred to a hematologist for management. In patients with nonsevere aplastic anemia, observation and supportive care are the recommended treatment. Definitive treatment with either HSCT or immunosuppressive therapy is reserved for SAA.[37] Use of blood products to correct the anemia should be minimized to prevent alloimmunization and to reduce the risk of graft failure after HSCT. The decision to transfuse a patient with aplastic anemia should be made in consultation with the hematologist who will be treating the patient.

Nonpharmacologic Management

Due to the resulting immunocompromise from the pancytopenia associated with aplastic anemia, protection from infectious sources (people, locations, items) is imperative to minimize risk. Adequate cleaning and disinfecting of surfaces and avoiding ill contacts and crowded spaces where contamination can occur is essential. Encouraging good handwashing techniques at all times for those in contact with the patients is recommended.

LIFE SPAN CONSIDERATIONS

The treatment of choice for aplastic anemia is based on the severity of the anemia and the age of the patient. HSCT is more successful in younger patients and is the treatment of choice for children and adolescents if a suitable donor is available, or if they have not responded to immunosuppression therapy. Patients who are older than 40 years have a higher risk of transplant-related morbidity and mortality. Immunosuppression therapy is the treatment of choice for adults older than 40 years.[37]

COMPLICATIONS

Complications of untreated aplastic anemia include sepsis and death resulting from pancytopenia. Complications of HSCT include graft failure, graft-versus-host disease, and a risk of secondary malignant neoplasms. Complications of immunosuppressive therapy include relapse and death resulting from pancytopenia or evolution of aplastic anemia to myelodysplasia or leukemia.[37]

PATIENT AND FAMILY EDUCATION

Aplastic anemia can be caused by exposure to toxins such as benzene and insecticides. Patients should be taught that proper handling of products such as paints and insecticides includes adequate ventilation of the work area and wearing of protective clothing, such as masks and gloves. Good handwashing techniques are essential to avoid exposure of the patient to infection.

HEALTH PROMOTION

Aplastic anemia is a serious and life-threatening condition. Protecting individuals with aplastic anemia from infection and other illnesses, as well as avoidance of substances (drugs and toxins) which are associated with aplastic anemia, is paramount to ensure health and good outcomes. Encouraging appropriate immunizations, especially influenza and pneumococcal vaccines, is a high priority. Informing individuals with aplastic anemia regarding a well-balanced healthy diet, maintaining an exercise regime, and obtaining adequate sleep are of vital importance to their care.

HEMOLYTIC ANEMIA

DEFINITION AND EPIDEMIOLOGY

All the hemolytic anemias are associated with an increased rate of RBC destruction. The clinical presentation varies according to the disease. Some patients are seen with chronic hemolytic states that are well compensated; others have acute, self-limited hemolytic episodes. The most common chronic hemolytic anemia is sickle cell disease (discussed previously). Most of the other hemolytic anemias (Box 216.6) are rare and are mentioned only briefly here.

G6PD deficiency is an inherited erythrocyte enzyme deficiency that can result in an acute hemolytic anemia. G6PD-induced hemolysis is usually precipitated either by infection or by ingestion of an oxidant drug or food.[5]

BOX **216.6**

Examples of Hemolytic Anemias

Sickle cell anemia
Hemoglobinopathies
G6PD deficiency
Membrane structural defects
- Hereditary spherocytosis
- Hereditary elliptocytosis
Autoimmune hemolysis
- Warm-reacting autoimmune hemolytic anemia
- Cold-reacting autoimmune hemolytic anemia

G6PD is a sex-linked disorder; women are almost always carriers and males are affected. Phenotypes vary among various ethnicities, and patients with the Mediterranean variants typically experience severe hemolysis when exposed to inciting agents. The most common form of G6PD deficiency in the United States is a mild variant of the disorder that typically affects approximately 10% of African American males. Other affected populations include Africans, Greeks, Sardinians, certain Jewish sects, and Southeast Asians.[5]

A mild chronic hemolytic anemia can also be caused by abnormalities in erythrocyte membrane protein composition. Hereditary spherocytosis and hereditary elliptocytosis are the best examples of this abnormality.[5] The prevalence of hereditary spherocytosis is approximately 1 in 2000 (mostly northern Europeans).[5] In the United States, the incidence of hereditary elliptocytosis is approximately 1 in 2000 to 5000, with one of the more common forms commonly seen in people of African American and Mediterranean heritage.[5]

Autoimmune hemolytic anemia can be associated with conditions such as viral or bacterial infections, collagen vascular diseases, and lymphoproliferative disorders, or it can be idiopathic. Severity can range from mild to very severe, acute, and life-threatening. It is a very rare disease. The type associated with warm-reacting autoantibodies is seen in 80% to 90% of all cases of autoimmune hemolytic anemia, and the incidence of this type is 1 in 100,000.[5]

PATHOPHYSIOLOGY

Drugs associated with acute hemolysis in G6PD-deficient patients include aspirin and phenacetin, sulfonamides, nitrofurantoin, and primaquine. Ingestion of an offending drug can result in the denaturation of hemoglobin, leading to an acute hemolytic event.[5] Other precipitants of hemolysis include the ingestion of fava beans or mothballs and severe bacterial or viral infections.

The functional abnormality in hereditary spherocytosis and hereditary elliptocytosis results from defects in the structural proteins of the erythrocyte cytoskeleton, specifically a deficiency of the protein spectrin.[5]

In the autoimmune hemolytic anemias, the patient produces autoantibodies that react with the RBCs, causing premature erythrocyte destruction. Two types of autoantibodies are produced: warm-reacting autoantibodies and cold-reacting autoantibodies. Warm-reacting antibodies are reactive with cells at 37°C (98.6°F), and cold-reacting antibodies are reactive at temperatures below 37°C.[5]

CLINICAL PRESENTATION AND PHYSICAL EXAMINATION

Most hemolytic anemias are mild, well compensated for, and associated with few signs or symptoms. If the anemia is severe, the patient displays the usual symptoms of severe anemia, such as fatigue and exercise intolerance. Patients with G6PD deficiency may have minimal to no clinical signs. Often the first clue that a patient has the deficiency is the onset of an acute hemolytic anemia after ingestion of an oxidant drug. The hemolytic event is self-limited and usually mild. Patients with the Mediterranean form of G6PD deficiency are at risk for more severe hemolysis.[5]

Both hereditary spherocytosis and hereditary elliptocytosis are usually characterized by a mild hemolytic anemia that is well compensated for. However, individuals with hereditary spherocytosis can have a severe hemolytic anemia, whereas individuals with hereditary elliptocytosis rarely have a clinically significant hemolytic anemia. Splenomegaly, aplastic crises, and pigment gallstones can complicate severe hereditary spherocytosis.[5]

The anemia caused by autoimmune hemolysis ranges from mild and subclinical to severe and life threatening. Patients with a warm-reacting autoimmune hemolytic anemia can have splenomegaly and other symptoms of anemia such as jaundice if the hemolysis is moderate or severe. Patients also show signs and symptoms of the underlying disease. Patients with hemolytic anemias have essentially normal findings on physical examination. The only remarkable evidence of hemolysis may be scleral icterus, especially in patients with chronic hemolytic anemias such as sickle cell disease.

DIAGNOSTICS
Essential Diagnostics

During a mild acute hemolytic event, serologic test results show a slight decrease in hemoglobin and the RBC count (CBC with differential), elevated LDH level, and slight hyperbilirubinemia. Haptoglobin levels will be decreased. Patients with chronic hemolytic anemias, even when they are well compensated for, have persistent reticulocytosis.

Assays for G6PD are useful and detect most deficient patients. In some milder variants of the disease, however, the screening test result may be negative for several weeks after an acute hemolytic event.

A positive family history and the presence of pathognomonic findings on the peripheral blood smear easily diagnose both hereditary spherocytosis and hereditary elliptocytosis. Patients with hereditary spherocytosis have many microspherocytes on the peripheral blood smear and an elevated MCHC on the CBC. The RBCs of patients with hereditary elliptocytosis have a uniform elliptic (oval) shape.

The diagnosis of an autoimmune hemolytic anemia depends on laboratory findings of abnormal autoantibodies. The Coombs test (both direct and indirect) is used to screen for these antibodies. The direct Coombs test result is positive in most cases of autoimmune hemolytic anemia or transfusion reactions and in some cases of drug-induced hemolysis. The indirect Coombs test result is positive in cases of antibody formation from previous transfusions or pregnancy and in drug-induced hemolytic anemia.[5]

INITIAL DIAGNOSTICS

Hemolytic Anemia

LABORATORY
- CBC and WBC differential which includes RBC indices
  - Peripheral smear
  - Reticulocyte count
- LFTs
- LDH
- Renal function tests: BUN, creatinine, eGFR

- G6PD assay
- Coombs direct and indirect tests
- Haptoglobin
- Hemoglobin electrophoresis[a]

IMAGING/PROCEDURES
- Bone marrow biopsy

[a]If indicated.

DIFFERENTIAL DIAGNOSIS

In a patient demonstrating hemolytic anemia, the differential diagnosis should consider whether the anemia is acute or chronic and the severity of the anemia. Determining the etiology of the hemolysis is essential to management.

 Priority differentials include (1) hereditary hemolytic conditions (spherocytosis, elliptocytosis; G6PD; SCD, thalassemia), (2) acquired—autoimmune-mediated (transfusion- related, HSCT-related, infections, blood malignancies, drug-related), (3) acquired—non-autoimmune-mediated (DIC, TTP, HUS, severe burns, renal failure).

INTERPROFESSIONAL COLLABORATIVE MANAGEMENT

Pharmacologic Management

Management of a patient with a hemolytic anemia varies according to the individual disease state. Therefore, proper management begins with an accurate diagnosis. Patients who can compensate for their anemia generally require little intervention. If the hemoglobin level begins to fall well below the patient's baseline, an occasional transfusion of packed RBCs may be necessary.

The acute, self-limited hemolysis in patients with mild G6PD deficiency rarely requires treatment. The resulting anemia is mild and resolves without intervention. Any patient who sees a health care provider because of an acute hemolytic event resulting from exposure to an oxidant drug should have serial CBCs to determine resolution of the anemia. The most important aspect of management of G6PD deficiency is ensuring the patient's awareness of the condition. All high-risk individuals should be screened, and information about what drugs and foods to avoid should be provided to all patients with the deficiency.

Patients with mild forms of hereditary spherocytosis or hereditary elliptocytosis maintain adequate hemoglobin levels and are in generally good health. Patients with severe hereditary spherocytosis may require a splenectomy to decrease the severity of the anemia.[5] These patients are also candidates for prophylactic cholecystectomy because of the high incidence of pigment gallstones (elective cholecystectomy should be done if gallstones occur).

Patients with autoimmune hemolytic anemia are generally treated with some combination of corticosteroid therapy or immunosuppressive therapy, splenectomy, and transfusion with packed RBCs. The specific therapy varies according to the type and severity of the hemolytic anemia.

Nonpharmacologic Management

Patients with mild to moderate hemolytic anemia usually have mild symptoms. The most important aspects to their care during the acute phase are safeguarding adequate rest, hydration, and a well-balanced diet that provides adequate vitamin and mineral intake. Side effects from immunosuppressive therapy and surgery can be significant. Patents should be cautioned to avoid exposure to infectious diseases by avoiding ill contacts, employing good hand washing techniques, and using disinfectant when appropriate. Appropriate immunizations should be recommended.

LIFE SPAN CONSIDERATIONS

Patients with G6PD deficiency, hemoglobinopathy, or a hereditary RBC membrane defect should be aware of the hereditary potential. Professional genetic counseling and screening should be offered to all patients who are considering pregnancy.

COMPLICATIONS

Most of the hemolytic anemias discussed here rarely cause complications, especially if the hemolysis is mild and self-limited or chronic but well compensated for. Patients with more severe forms of hemolytic anemia, especially autoimmune hemolytic anemia, are at risk for acute episodes of severe hemolysis, with the associated morbidity and mortality of a severe anemia.

PATIENT AND FAMILY EDUCATION

Patients should understand the nature of their disorder well enough to be able to explain it to other health care providers. Patients with G6PD deficiency should be given a list of drugs and foods to avoid, including over-the-counter products that contain aspirin or phenacetin. Patients with drug-induced hemolysis should be made aware of the types of drugs to avoid. Those with autoimmune hemolytic anemias should be made aware of the types of situations and conditions that can aggravate their anemia. All patients should be instructed to contact their health care provider if there are any signs of increased anemia. If the patient is on immunosuppressive therapy or has had a splenectomy, education regarding the risks of their compromised immune status should be reinforced and strategies to prevent infection will be necessary.

HEALTH PROMOTION

Hemolytic anemias pose a threat to overall wellbeing. Protecting individuals from further illnesses and infection is paramount. Encourage individuals with these conditions to maintain well-balanced diets, exercise, employ strategies to prevent infection, maintain adequate rest, and receive the influenza vaccine yearly. They should be made aware of the drugs and potentially harmful toxins to avoid preventing worsening or recurrence of their conditions.

REFERENCES

1. Chernecky, C. C., & Berger, B. J. (2013). Hemoglobin. In *Laboratory tests and diagnostic procedures* (6th ed.). St Louis: Saunders.
2. Cappellini, M. C., & Motta, I. (2015). Anemia in clinical practice—definition and classification: Does hemoglobin change with aging? *Seminars in Hematology, 52*(4), 261–269.
3. Hoffman, R., Benz, E. J., Siberstein, L. E., Heslop, H. E., et al. (2013). Approach to anemia in the adult and child. In *Hematology: Basic principles and practice* (6th ed.). St Louis: Saunders.
4. Luzzatto, L. (2014). Hemolytic anemias and anemia due to acute blood loss. In D. Kasper, A. Fauci, S. Hauser, D. Longo, J. Jameson, & J. Loscalzo (Eds.), *Harrison's principles of internal medicine* (19th ed.). New York, NY: McGraw-Hill. http://accessmedicine.mhmedical.com/content.aspx?bookid=1130&sectionid=79731477.
5. Adamson, J. W., & Longo, D. L. (2014). Anemia and polycythemia. In D. Kasper, A. Fauci, S. Hauser, D. Longo, J. Jameson, & J. Loscalzo (Eds.), *Harrison's principles of internal medicine* (19th ed.). New York, NY: McGraw-Hill. http://accessmedicine.mhmedical.com/content.aspx?bookid=1130&sectionid=79727787.
6. Damon, L. E., & Andreadis, C. (2018). Blood disorders. In M. A. Papadakis, S. J. McPhee, & M. W. Rabow (Eds.), *Current medical diagnosis & treatment*. New York, NY: McGraw-Hill. http://accessmedicine.mhmedical.com/content.aspx?bookid=2192&sectionid=168012363.

7. Nicoll, C., & Mark Lu, C. (2018). Appendix: Therapeutic drug monitoring & laboratory reference intervals, & pharmacogenetic testing. In M. A. Papadakis, S. J. McPhee, & M. W. Rabow (Eds.), *Current medical diagnosis & treatment*. New York, NY: McGraw-Hill. http://accessmedicine.mhmedical.com/content.aspx?bookid=2192&sectionid=167995920.

8. Hoffman, R., Benz, E. J., Siberstein, L. E., Heslop, H. E., et al. (2013). Disorders of hemostasis. In *Hematology: Basic principles and practice* (6th ed.). St Louis: Saunders.

9. Haider, B. A., Olofin, I., Wang, M., et al. (2013). Anaemia, prenatal iron use, and risk of adverse pregnancy outcomes: Systematic review and meta-analysis. *British Medical Journal, 346*, f3443.

10. Beck, K. L., Conlon, C. A., Kruger, R., et al. (2014). Dietary determinants of and possible solutions to iron deficiency for young women living in industrialized countries: A review. *Nutrients, 6*, 3747–3776.

11. Freedberg, D. E., Kim, L. S., & Yang, Y. X. (2017). The risks and benefits of long-term use of proton pump inhibitors: Expert review and best practice advice from the American Gastroenterological Association. *Gastroenterology, 152*(4), 706–715. [Epub 2017/03/05].

12. Avni, T., Bieber, A., Grossman, A., Green, H., Leibovici, L., & Gafter-Gvili, A. (2015). The safety of intravenous iron preparations: Systematic review and meta-analysis. *Mayo Clinic Proceedings, 90*(1), 12–23. https://doi.org/10.1016/j.mayocp.2014.10.007, http://www.sciencedirect.com/science/article/pii/S0025619614008830. ISSN 0025-6196.

13. Reinisch, W., Staun, M., Bhandari, S., et al. (2013). State of the iron: How to diagnose and efficiently treat iron deficiency anemia in inflammatory bowel disease. *Journal of Crohn's & Colitis, 7*(6), 429–440.

14. Cao, C., & O'Brien, K. O. (2013). Pregnancy and iron homeostasis: An update. *Nutrition Reviews, 7*(1), 35–51.

15. Iron, fact sheet for professionals. Retrieved from: https://ods.od.nih.gov/factsheets/Iron-HealthProfessional/. (Accessed 27 July 2019). Page updated July 9, 2019.

16. U.S. Preventive Task Force Recommendations for Iron Deficiency Anemia in Pregnant Women. Screening and Supplementation. September 2015. https://www.uspreventiveservicestaskforce.org/Page/Document/UpdateSummaryFinal/iron-deficiency-anemia-in-pregnant-women-screening-and-supplementation?ds=1&s=anemia.

17. World Health Organization (WHO). (2016). *Guideline: Daily iron supplementation in adult women and adolescence girls*. Geneva.: World Health Organization.

18. Baker, R. D., & Greer, F. R., The Committee on Nutrition. From the American Clinical Report Academy of Pediatrics. (2010). Diagnosis and prevention of iron deficiency and iron-deficiency anemia in infants and young children (0–3 years of age). *Pediatrics, 126*(5).

19. Musallam, M. M., Rivella, S., Vichinsky, E., et al. (2013). Non-transfusion-dependent thalassemia. *Haematologica, 98*(6), 833–844.

20. Benz, E. J., Jr. (2014). Disorders of hemoglobin. In D. Kasper, A. Fauci, S. Hauser, D. Longo, J. Jameson, & J. Loscalzo (Eds.), *Harrison's principles of internal medicine* (19th ed.). New York, NY: McGraw-Hill. http://accessmedicine.mhmedical.com/content.aspx?bookid=1130&sectionid=79731188.

21. Vehapoglu, A., Ozgurhan, G., Demir, A. D., Uzuner, S., Nursoy, M. A., Turkmen, S., et al. (2014). Hematological indices for differential diagnosis of beta thalassemia trait and iron deficiency anemia. *Anemia*, http://doi.org/10.1155/2014/576738. 576738.

22. Goss, C., Giardina, P., Degtyaryova, D., et al. (2014). Red blood cell transfusion for thalassemia: Results of a survey assessing current practice and proposal of evidence-based guidelines. *Transfusion, 54*, 173–1781.

23. Ware, H. M., & Kwiatkowski, J. L. (2013). Evaluation and treatment of transfusional iron overload in children. *Pediatric Clinics of North America, 60*, 1393–1406.

24. Fard, A. D., Hoseini, S. A., Shahjahani, M., et al. (2013). Evaluation of novel fetal hemoglobin inducer drugs in treatment of β-hemoglobinopathy disorders. *International Journal of Hematology Oncology and Stem Cell Research, 7*(3), 47–54.

25. Dong, A., Rivella, S., & Breda, L. (2013). Gene therapy for hemoglobinopathies: Progress and challenges. *Translational Research: The Journal of Laboratory and Clinical Medicine, 161*(4), 293–306.

26. Green, R., & Dwyre, D. M. (2015). Evaluation of macrocytic anemias. *Seminars in Hematology, 52*(4), 279–286.

27. Hoffman, R., Benz, E. J., Siberstein, L. E., Heslop, H. E., et al. (2013). Megaloblastic anemias. In *Hematology: Basic principles and practice* (6th ed.). St Louis: Saunders.

28. Attwood, S. E., Ell, C., Galmiche, J. P., et al. (2015). Long-term safety of proton pump inhibitor therapy assessed under controlled, randomized clinical trial conditions: Data from the SOPRAN and LOTUS studies. *Alimentary Pharmacology and Therapeutics, 41*(11), 1162–1174.

29. Pawlak, P., Lester, S. E., & Babtunde, T. (2014). The prevalence of cobalamin deficiency among vegetarians assessed by serum vitamin B_{12} a review of the literature. *European Journal of Clinical Nutrition, 68*, 541–548.

30. Rusak, E., Chobot, A., Krzywicka, A., & Wenzlau, J. (2016). Anti-parietal cell antibodies—diagnostic significance. *Advances in Medical Sciences, 61*(2), 175–179. https://doi.org/10.1016/j.advms.2015.12.004.

31. Ojodu, J., Hulihan, M., Pope, S., & Grant, A. (2014). Incidence of sickle cell trait—United States 2010. *MMWR. Morbidity and Mortality Weekly Report, 63*(49), 1155–1158.

32. U.S. Department of Health and Human Services, NIH. Evidence-based management of sickle cell disease: expert panel report, 2014; guide to recommendations. Retrieved from: http://www.nhlbi.nih.gov/health-pro/guidelines/sickle-cell-disease-guidelines.

33. Lemonne, N., Charlot, K., Waltz, X., et al. (2015). Hydroxyurea treatment does not increase blood viscosity and improves red blood cell rheology in sickle cell anemia. *Haematologica, 100*(10), e383–e386. doi:10.3324/haematol.2015.13043.

34. Gluckman, E. (2013). Allogeneic transplantation strategies including haploidentical transplantation in sickle cell disease. *ASH Education Program Book, 2013*(1), 370–376.

35. Cope, A., & Darbyshire, P. J. (2013). Sickle cell disease, update on management. *Paediatr Child Health, 23*(11), 480–485.

36. Delaney, K. M. H., Axelrod, K. C., Buscetta, A., et al. (2013). Leg ulcers in sickle cell disease: Current patterns and practices. *Hemoglobin, 37*(4).

37. Dolberg, O. J., & Levy, Y. (2014). Idiopathic aplastic anemia: Diagnosis and classification. *Autoimmunity Reviews, 13*(4–5), 569–573.

CHAPTER 217

BLOOD COAGULATION DISORDERS

Maura A. Malone • Laurel McKernan • Leo R. Zacharski • Deborah L. Ornstein

INTRODUCTION, DEFINITION, AND EPIDEMIOLOGY

Coagulation is the process by which blood changes from the fluid phase needed for tissue perfusion to a cohesive gel that prevents blood loss. This transition is achieved through a complex process involving many different initiating and inhibiting proteins as well as certain cells, including platelets and white blood cells. The benefits of this mechanism are obvious and are taken for granted except in individuals who have an excess or deficiency of a coagulant or anticoagulant protein because they may bleed excessively or form pathologic clots. The normal coagulation mechanism may fail for numerous reasons. A quantitative deficiency or a qualitative abnormality in counterbalancing coagulant or anticoagulant participants may tip the balance toward either bleeding (coagulopathy) or clotting (thrombosis). Similarly, a defect at one point in the system can often be compensated for by therapy that targets a different point in the system. Disorders of coagulation factors may be inherited or acquired. Common inherited bleeding disorders include von Willebrand disease (vWD), hemophilia A, and hemophilia B. Acquired bleeding disorders most often result from medications (e.g., aspirin, nonsteroidal anti-inflammatory drugs [NSAIDs], or anticoagulants) or organ dysfunction that accompanies certain medical diseases (e.g., liver or kidney disease, cancer, or leukemia).

Determination of the correct diagnosis is required for appropriate management and can be challenging, particularly with mild bleeding disorders. Patients are often referred for medical evaluation because of one of the following: a bleeding or thrombotic episode, a positive family history, or an abnormal laboratory test result found, for example, during preoperative screening. The health care provider needs to determine, through clinical and laboratory assessment, whether these referral indicators reflect the presence of a coagulation disorder. Clinical and laboratory assessment go hand in hand, but it is all too common for patients with a clinical disorder to have no abnormality on routine laboratory testing.

An elaborate balance exists between substances in the blood that promote clotting (coagulation factors) and other substances that preserve blood in fluid form (anticoagulant factors). This balance is maintained until a blood vessel is injured. The blood coagulation mechanism is designed to interpret such injuries and to respond by developing a protective clot at the injury site to stop the flow of blood. Prevention of blood loss from the vasculature with injury is vital, and this process is referred to as hemostasis. The hemostatic mechanism is appropriately viewed as a complex system because a defect in any one of its many components can lead to malfunction of the entire system.

The normal hemostatic response proceeds in three phases.[1] In phase 1, blood vessels constrict, reducing blood flow from the site. In phase 2, platelets are activated and chemicals are released almost instantaneously, resulting in the formation of a platelet plug at the site of injury. Phase 3 begins within seconds after platelet activation. In this phase, tissue factor, a molecule present on cell surfaces, triggers a complex cascade involving more than a dozen coagulation factors. The end result of this cascade is the production of thrombin, a powerful enzyme that converts fibrinogen, which is present in solution in the blood, to fibrin. Fibrin is a durable, visible mesh that seals the injured vessel (the scab). Traditionally, this cascade is thought to consist of intrinsic pathways (entirely plasma derived) and extrinsic pathways (tissue factor initiated), and abnormalities of coagulation factors within their pathways can often be detected by common laboratory tests such as the activated partial thromboplastin time (aPTT) and the prothrombin time (PT). For example, prolongation of the aPTT is suggestive of an abnormality of a coagulation factor in the intrinsic pathway of coagulation, whereas a prolonged PT leads one to suspect an abnormality within the extrinsic pathway.

BLEEDING DISORDERS (COAGULOPATHIES)

CLINICAL PRESENTATION AND PHYSICAL EXAMINATION

The manifestations of bleeding disorders are determined by the type and severity of the defect. Important questions to consider when faced with a bleeding patient include the following: Is it a vascular disorder, platelet abnormality, or coagulation factor deficiency? Is it hereditary or acquired? These questions are answered through clinical and laboratory assessment.[2]

Patients with hereditary (congenital) bleeding disorders usually have a lifelong history of symptoms, such as easy bruising and prolonged bleeding with cuts, surgery, or other trauma. Severe deficiencies generally become evident when the affected individual becomes a toddler and is increasingly likely to sustain minor trauma. Although bleeding may occur spontaneously in individuals with moderate or severe bleeding disorders, mild hereditary deficiencies may go undiagnosed for years until significant trauma occurs or the individual undergoes surgery. In contrast, acquired disorders may become evident later in life in the absence of a history of abnormal bleeding. Clinical presentation of acquired bleeding disorders may include recent onset of increased bruising, bleeding with trauma, nosebleeds, or a recent change in platelet count or clotting test results. The type of bleeding reported by the individual under evaluation may indicate which pathway is involved. For example, excessive bruising, mucosal bleeding, and postsurgical hemorrhage are typical of platelet disorders, whereas a history of frank bleeding after surgery and hemorrhage into the joints and muscles are typical of a marked coagulation factor deficiency such as hemophilia A or B. The most valuable diagnostic test for a bleeding disorder is a careful, comprehensive bleeding history. The history should provide clues to the type of bleeding disorder that may be present and will direct the laboratory testing that is indicated for further evaluation. The hemostatic response to trauma or surgery elicited in taking of a bleeding history is generally a more sensitive test of hemostatic competence than are screening laboratory tests and is more useful for predicting whether an individual will have a bleeding complication after surgery.[3]

The bleeding history has two major elements: the patient's history and the family history. The patient should be asked to describe each event in life that presented a hemostatic challenge. For example, descriptions should include the duration and intensity of bleeding with minor cuts and scratches, surgery, dental extractions, and menstrual periods. Spontaneous bleeding may occur in the form of joint or soft tissue bleeding, epistaxis, and bruising. Bruising without obvious trauma is more significant than bruising in response to trauma. It is particularly important to encourage the patient to quantitate the degree of bleeding. This may be done, for example, by estimating average bruise counts and location, duration of post-traumatic bleeding, or duration of menstruation and number of pads or tampons soaked. Menstrual blood is normally unclotted, and the passage of clots (e.g., with urination, defecation, or pad changes) may be significant. With practice, interviewers will refine their assessment skills and assist their patients in proper interpretations because what is "normal" bleeding to one person may be "heavy" to another. The family history is critical in assessing coagulation disorders. The genetic defects in hemophilia A and B (factor VIII and IX deficiency, respectively) are inherited in an X-linked recessive pattern and affect males. The defect is carried by females, however, who are usually (but not always) asymptomatic. Thus, a male patient's *maternal* grandfather, uncles, and cousins may have bleeding that provides a clue to the diagnosis of hemophilia A or B.

Although the bleeding history is of paramount importance in the evaluation for coagulation disorders, it is not without limitations. The accuracy of information reported largely depends on the interviewer's ability to elicit a description of previous hemostatic challenges. It is easy to miss events or to obtain an incomplete history. Mild bleeding disorders are difficult to identify, especially in the absence of a hemostatic challenge, as is often the case in young children. Spontaneous mutations commonly account for cases of hemophilia A and B; consequently, the family history may be negative.

Bleeding disorders are usually diagnosed by the history and laboratory findings.[1] Physical examination may be unremarkable, especially with mild defects; however, a variety of findings, including bruises, petechiae, gingival bleeding, epistaxis, and hematomas, may be evident, especially in individuals with more severe defects. Some degree of bruising is common in the general population, especially in those with fair complexion, in whom bruises are seen more easily. However, bruises that occur on the trunk in addition to the extremities tend to be more concerning.

DIAGNOSTICS AND DIFFERENTIAL DIAGNOSIS
Essential Diagnostics

In anticipation of the decision to refer the patient for specialized tests in the face of clinical suspicion, the provider should perform certain screening studies. The typical laboratory screen, available in most clinical laboratories, includes the platelet count, a peripheral blood smear review, PT, aPTT, thrombin time, fibrinogen level, and platelet function analysis.[2,4] These studies provide basic information on the integrity of platelet function and coagulation factor pathways.

The platelet count is usually performed by automated counters. Low values can be confirmed by estimating the number of platelets present on the peripheral blood smear. Common causes of a low platelet count include immune destruction, acute and chronic infections (e.g., infectious mononucleosis, human immunodeficiency virus [HIV] infection, hepatitis C), medications, vasculitis, disseminated intravascular coagulation, and chemotherapy. On occasion, a low platelet count obtained by the automated counter is caused by formation of platelet clumps as a result of interaction with the anticoagulant (ethylenediaminetetraacetic acid [EDTA]) in the blood collection tube. Thrombocytopenia caused by platelet clumping is merely an in vitro phenomenon and readily discernible by review of the peripheral blood smear. Such "pseudo-thrombocytopenia" is not typically associated with clinical bleeding.

The bleeding time is a crude measure of hemostasis that is neither sensitive nor specific for identification of bleeding disorders and is subject to many variables that may lead to misleading test results. For these reasons, the bleeding time has been retired in many centers in favor of an automated platelet function analyzer, such as the PFA-100 system.[5] The PFA-100 is an automated system that emulates the platelet-dependent component of primary hemostasis. A blood specimen is collected from the patient by venipuncture into an anticoagulated tube and transferred to the PFA-100 instrument, where the time required to form a platelet plug after exposure to specially treated membranes (the closure time) is measured. The PFA-100 is simple to use, reproducible, and sensitive to vWD and some qualitative platelet disorders (including effects of medications, such as aspirin), but it suffers from a lack of specificity. Closure times with the PFA-100 are affected by many of the same variables that affect the bleeding time (e.g., thrombocytopenia [100,000/mm³], anemia, medications), but the test is less subject to operator error.

The PT measures the function of the extrinsic system and the common pathway of coagulation. It is sensitive to abnormalities of factors VII, X, V, and II and fibrinogen. The aPTT measures the function of the intrinsic system and the common pathway. It detects abnormalities of prekallikrein,

Interpretation of Abnormal Screening Coagulation Test Results

PROLONGED PROTHROMBIN TIME/INTERNATIONAL NORMALIZED RATIO
- Mild liver disease
- Early vitamin K deficiency or warfarin therapy
- Factor VII deficiency
- Inhibitor to factor VII
- Variable effect of direct factor Xa inhibitors (e.g., rivaroxaban, apixaban, edoxaban)

PROLONGED ACTIVATED PARTIAL THROMBOPLASTIN TIME
- Deficiency of intrinsic pathway factor (VIII, IX, XI, XII)
- Severe von Willebrand disease (with low factor VIII level)
- Inhibitor to intrinsic pathway factor (most commonly factor VIII)
- Heparin
- Variable effect of dabigatran

PROLONGED PROTHROMBIN TIME AND ACTIVATED PARTIAL THROMBOPLASTIN TIME
- Multiple coagulation factor deficiencies
  - Disseminated intravascular coagulation
  - Advanced liver disease
  - Severe vitamin K deficiency or warfarin therapy
- Deficiency of or inhibitor to a common pathway factor (fibrinogen, II, V, X)
- Treatment with direct thrombin inhibitor (hirudin, argatroban, bivalirudin)

high-molecular-weight kininogen, and factors XII, XI, X, IX, VIII, V, II, and fibrinogen.

A prolonged PT or aPTT may be evaluated further by performing mixing studies, which incorporate different ratios of normal (control) and abnormal (patient) plasma.[4] "Correction" of the prolonged clotting time on addition of normal plasma suggests the presence of a coagulation factor deficiency; failure to correct the abnormality suggests the presence of an inhibitor, such as a lupus anticoagulant. The inhibitor in the patient plasma neutralizes the added normal plasma, which thus fails to correct the abnormal coagulation test result. Misinterpretation of the results of mixing studies is a common cause of a request for a coagulation consultation. Some causes of a prolonged PT or aPTT are noted in Box 217.1.

If the patient has no personal or family history of bleeding with hemostatic challenges such as surgery or significant trauma, he or she is not likely to have a bleeding disorder, and laboratory evaluation is usually not helpful. If the patient has a negative bleeding history but has not had significant hemostatic challenges in life and has a positive family history for bleeding, screening tests may be advisable. Diagnosis may be important for planning future care, such as with invasive procedures or elective surgery. Patients may be able to avoid unnecessary blood transfusions if a bleeding disorder is diagnosed and appropriate prophylactic treatment provided.

If the patient has a negative bleeding history but abnormal blood test results, other factors need to be considered, such as effects of medications (e.g., aspirin, NSAIDs, anticoagulants, guaifenesin-containing over-the-counter cold remedies), allergies (rhinitis), or concurrent medical illness. Circulating anticoagulants are commonly found in patients with an unexplained prolonged aPTT and rarely cause clinical bleeding. Less commonly, individuals with a deficiency of factor XII, prekallikrein or high-molecular-weight kininogen may be identified after finding of an unexplained prolonged aPTT. These proteins do not appear to have a pivotal role in hemostasis in vivo; thus, although deficiencies result in prolongation of the aPTT, they do not result in a clinical bleeding disorder. Circulating anticoagulants may be distinguished from both hemostatic and nonhemostatic factor deficiencies by mixing studies.

Severe bleeding disorders are generally readily identified by screening laboratory tests. A positive history and abnormal laboratory screening test results suggest strongly that a bleeding disorder exists, and referral to a hematologist for further evaluation is needed to characterize the specific diagnosis. Unfortunately, screening coagulation tests are often relatively insensitive for detection of mild coagulation disorders. Examples of bleeding disorders that may be associated with normal screening test results include mild hemophilia, vWD, abnormal fibrinogens, factor XIII deficiency, and qualitative platelet disorders (Box 217.2). A positive bleeding history in a patient with normal laboratory test results therefore also suggests the need for referral to a hematologist with specialty expertise in blood coagulation.

It is important to keep in mind that the quality of coagulation test results is highly dependent on the conditions under which the samples are obtained and on the experience and professional quality of the coagulation laboratory. Prompt specimen processing and proper plasma storage are mandatory. Certain tests, such as platelet aggregation studies, require immediate laboratory testing with specialized equipment by highly trained and experienced technicians. Ideally, patients undergoing evaluation for bleeding disorders should be free of medications for at least 2 weeks, and samples obtained preferably in the morning after overnight fasting. It may be inadvisable to make a critical diagnosis on the basis of results obtained from plasma samples after prolonged storage or shipment to a distant laboratory. Travel by the patient to the testing laboratory for blood sampling is optimum, and abnormal results should always be confirmed by repeated testing before a diagnosis of a bleeding disorder is conferred.

INITIAL DIAGNOSTICS

Bleeding Disorders

- PT and aPTT
- Platelet count and peripheral blood smear review
- Thrombin time
- Fibrinogen level
- PFA-100

Interdisciplinary Collaborative Management

Since 1975, hemophilia treatment centers (HTCs) in the United States have been federally funded to provide comprehensive, specialized care to persons with bleeding disorders. The value of HTCs was highlighted in one study in which it was shown that the risk of dying for males with hemophilia who received care at HTCs was 40% lower than that for those who received care outside of an HTC.[6] Therefore, management of a patient with a congenital bleeding disorder by a primary health care

BOX 217.2

Differential Diagnosis: Bleeding Disorders

HEREDITARY

- Hereditary hemorrhagic telangiectasia (Osler-Weber-Rendu syndrome)
- Connective tissue disorder (e.g., Ehlers-Danlos syndrome)
- Benign joint hypermobility syndrome
- von Willebrand disease
- Qualitative platelet disorders
- Congenital thrombocytopenia
- Hemophilia A and B
- Factor XI deficiency
- Rare coagulation factor deficiencies
- Fibrinolytic inhibitor deficiencies

ACQUIRED

- Vascular trauma
- Vitamin C deficiency
- Antiplatelet medications
- Acquired von Willebrand disease
- Disseminated intravascular coagulation
- Uremia
- Immune thrombocytopenia
- Liver disease
- Vitamin K deficiency
- Anticoagulation
- Acquired coagulation factor inhibitors (especially factor VIII, factor V)

provider should be in conjunction with a hematologist with expertise in blood coagulation and with attention paid to guidelines put forth by the Medical and Scientific Advisory Council (MASAC) of the National Hemophilia Foundation.[7,8] Once the patient has been evaluated by a hematologist, a detailed care plan should be developed that includes the MASAC guidelines for management of bleeding episodes, trauma, or invasive procedures. Patients with a coagulation factor deficiency, such as moderate or severe hemophilia A or B, require replacement of the missing clotting protein. A variety of plasma-derived and recombinant coagulation factor concentrates are available, and factor dose depends on type, location, and severity of bleeding episode. Single or multiple doses may be needed on the basis of severity of the bleeding episode, and it is imperative to seek consultation with a hematologist to assist in identifying the appropriate product and dose for an individual patient.

In patients with defined bleeding disorders, it is better to overestimate than to underestimate the risk of bleeding and to treat prophylactically or as soon as possible after bleeding begins because hemostasis is more difficult to achieve once excessive bleeding has commenced. To ensure rapid and appropriate treatment, a local supply of the appropriate replacement product should be maintained. Most patients with moderate to severe congenital bleeding disorders learn to recognize bleeding episodes soon after they occur and may be trained in self-administration of the coagulation factor by the intravenous route. In general, any significant trauma will require coagulation factor replacement, and most invasive procedures, even a seemingly minor one such as a tooth extraction, may require pretreatment with a coagulation factor concentrate. Surgery

Important Considerations in Assessment of Bleeding Episodes

- Type of coagulation disorder
- Degree or severity of the disorder
- Presence of comorbidity associated with history of transfusion, such as hepatitis B, hepatitis C, HIV infection
- Site and extent of bleeding and number of treatments
- History of response to replacement product; history of circulating inhibitors
- Replacement product: choice, dose, half-life, risks, benefits
- Any adjunct therapies (e.g., oral antifibrinolytic agents) required

in the patient with a bleeding disorder should be undertaken at a facility equipped with an on-site coagulation laboratory, a full range of treatment products, and expert hematology consultation.

Trauma or surgery often requires many days of coagulation factor replacement accompanied by laboratory monitoring to ensure that hemostatic levels of the deficient clotting protein are present. Mild versions of some bleeding disorders, such as mild hemophilia A and type 1 vWD, may be corrected temporarily by administration of desmopressin acetate (DDAVP), a synthetic analogue of vasopressin. This drug is given either intravenously or by high-concentration nasal spray and increases blood levels of factor VIII and von Willebrand factor (vWF) by releasing them from their storage sites in vascular endothelial cells. Not all patients respond to DDAVP, so before DDAVP is used in an emergency or surgical setting, it is mandatory to have first demonstrated its effectiveness in each individual patient by administering the drug in a controlled setting (usually the medical office) and measuring coagulation factor levels after administration to document a rise in the deficient clotting factor. Box 217.3 illustrates important issues to consider in assessment of the type, degree, and treatment of a bleeding episode.

VON WILLEBRAND DISEASE

DEFINITION AND EPIDEMIOLOGY

vWD results from a deficiency or abnormality in vWF and is the most common congenital bleeding disorder, occurring in up to 1% of the general population.[9] vWF functions as a bridging molecule that binds to receptors exposed on the platelet surface to link them both to one another and to the area of damage on the blood vessel wall. vWF also serves as the carrier protein for blood coagulation factor VIII and therefore plays a critical role in both platelet plug formation and fibrin thrombus synthesis. The diagnosis of vWD can be challenging because various conditions (e.g., medications, inflammation, stress, pregnancy) can elevate vWF from abnormally low levels into the normal range, thus masking a true deficient state. Moreover, the results of screening laboratory tests such as the PT and aPTT may be normal in vWD, leading to under-diagnosis. Epistaxis, menorrhagia, excessive bruising, and prolonged bleeding with cuts or dental extractions and in the intraoperative or immediate postoperative period are common manifestations of the bleeding phenotype in vWD.

There are three major types of vWD, all of which exhibit an autosomal inheritance pattern, thus affecting both males and females.[9] Type 1 vWD is a quantitative deficiency in vWF and is the most common type, representing 70% to 80% of symptomatic cases. Type 2 vWD is composed of four variants (2A, 2B, 2M, 2N); it is characterized by qualitative defects in vWF structure and represents about 20% to 30% of vWD cases. Type 3 vWD is a quantitative deficiency of vWF in which vWF is essentially absent; these cases are rare, fortunately, because patients with type 3 vWD have a severe bleeding disorder. Once vWD is diagnosed, it is important to identify the specific type of vWD that is present so that appropriate treatment can be prescribed. For example, DDAVP, which is the preferred treatment for most cases of type 1 vWD, is ineffective in most type 2 variants and may be harmful in type 2B vWD.

Screening laboratory test results may be normal in patients with vWD; thus those with suspected vWD and a compelling bleeding history should be referred to a hematologist for specialty evaluation.

DIAGNOSTICS

The tests that may be helpful in evaluating a patient, in consultation with a hematologist, include the following:

- *Complete blood count (CBC):* generally normal; thrombocytopenia is present in type 2B vWD.
- *PFA-100 closure times, bleeding time:* generally prolonged; may be normal in mild cases.
- *PT:* normal.
- *aPTT:* generally normal; will be prolonged and correct in mixing study in patients with low factor VIII levels.
- *Fibrinogen, thrombin time:* normal.
- *vWF antigen:* quantitative immunoassay that measures the concentration of vWF protein in plasma. This is typically decreased in type 1, low to normal in type 2, and absent in type 3.
- *vWF activity:* functional assay that measures the ability of vWF to interact with platelets. vWF activity is decreased in direct proportion to the decrease in vWF antigen in types 1 and 3 and disproportionately decreased in type 2 disease.
- *Factor VIII activity (FVIII : C):* because vWF functions as a carrier protein for factor VIII and enhances its stability in plasma, low vWF antigen levels typically result in proportionally low factor VIII activity. Factor VIII activity is disproportionately low, however, in type 2N vWD, in which the binding site for factor VIII on vWF is abnormal.
- *Low-dose ristocetin-induced platelet aggregation:* special test used to distinguish between type 2B and other subtypes of vWD.

A diagnosis of vWD must not be made on the basis of a single test result to avoid falsely labeling a patient with a bleeding disorder. Factor VIII and vWF tests can be affected by methods of specimen collection and transportation, resulting in falsely low readings if scrupulous care is not taken to handle the blood specimen properly. Whereas many hospital laboratories perform screening coagulation tests, many fewer perform vWD-specific testing, thus necessitating that specimens be sent to outside reference laboratories. Specimens may be mishandled along the way, resulting in falsely low readings and leading to a misdiagnosis of vWD. Similarly, because plasma vWF levels vary from day to day depending on numerous extraneous factors, a single set of normal test results may not be sufficient to rule out the diagnosis. Accordingly, if a patient has a history suggestive of a bleeding disorder but normal (especially low-normal) vWD test results, the tests should be repeated at a point when the patient is clinically well and not experiencing physiologic or psychological stress, both of which may temporarily elevate vWF levels. The diagnosis of mild type 1 vWD can be difficult because overlap exists between vWF levels in healthy individuals and those in individuals with mild disease. For example, individuals with type O blood often have low or low-normal levels of vWF without evidence of a frank bleeding disorder. Determination of ABO type at the time of vWD testing may be helpful for interpreting the significance of vWD test results.

INTERDISCIPLINARY COLLABORATIVE MANAGEMENT

Once a diagnosis of vWD is confirmed, a treatment plan can be made, and this is best done in consultation with a hematologist. Most individuals with vWD do not require ongoing treatment with hemostatic agents but will require treatment for bleeding episodes and prophylaxis for invasive procedures. Many patients with type 1 vWD respond to DDAVP, but this response must be documented before use of the drug to prevent or to treat bleeding. Plasma-derived factor VIII concentrates that are rich in vWF or recombinant vWF concentrates are the current products of choice for vWD patients for whom DDAVP is not appropriate.[9,10]

HEMOPHILIA

Definition and Epidemiology

Hemophilia is an X-linked recessive bleeding disorder characterized by low levels of factor VIII (hemophilia A) or factor IX (hemophilia B), resulting in defective fibrin clot formation. Minor injuries are sometimes associated with little immediate bleeding because platelet thrombus formation is normal. Persons with hemophilia may experience delayed bleeding, however, as the platelet plug breaks down prematurely in the absence of a stabilizing fibrin clot. Joint and muscle hemorrhages are common in moderate and severe hemophilia. Recurrent hemarthroses result in hypertrophy and inflammation of joint synovial tissue, causing articular cartilage damage and ultimately leading to loss of joint function and long-term disability. Limb contractures are common, often requiring physical therapy for range of motion to be regained. Psoas muscle bleeding may cause vague hip pain or abdominal pain that is often confused with appendicitis or renal colic. Intracranial hemorrhage is a leading cause of death in hemophilia, and head trauma necessitates immediate coagulation factor replacement. This is the case even if the patient appears clinically stable and neurologically intact initially; delayed bleeding is common and may be catastrophic.

Hemophilia occurs in 1 in 10,000 male births and affects at least 200,000 males worldwide.[11] Hemophilia A is more common than hemophilia B, representing about 80% of cases.

Diagnostics

The diagnosis of hemophilia is usually straightforward, unlike that of vWD. The PT, thrombin time, and PFA-100 are usually normal, whereas the aPTT is usually prolonged. Patients with mild cases of hemophilia, however, may have a normal or minimally prolonged aPTT; thus, if the diagnosis is suspected,

further evaluation is nevertheless in order irrespective of normal test results. The diagnosis of hemophilia requires demonstration of a low level of factor VIII in the case of hemophilia A or of factor IX in the case of hemophilia B. There are three categories of hemophilia—severe, moderate, and mild, in which the levels of the missing coagulation factor are less than 1%, 1% to 5%, and 6% to 40%, respectively. Patients with mild hemophilia may have severe bleeding only with trauma or surgery, whereas those with moderate and severe disease will often experience spontaneous bleeding.

INTERDISCIPLINARY COLLABORATIVE MANAGEMENT

Treatment of bleeding in a person with hemophilia involves prompt, and occasionally prolonged, replacement of coagulation factors.[12] Although patients with mild hemophilia A seldom bleed spontaneously, they will require coagulation factor replacement for significant injuries or surgery. Patients with moderate or severe hemophilia require infusions of coagulation factor concentrates to treat bleeding episodes, but patients with mild disease may respond, at least temporarily, to DDAVP,[12] which stimulates release of factor VIII from intracellular stores. Symptomatic head trauma requires immediate coagulation factor replacement and evaluation by a practitioner with expertise in neurologic injuries. Imaging studies should be performed to exclude intracranial bleeding, but coagulation factor concentrate infusions should be administered before any diagnostics are performed. Soft tissue hematomas may resolve with coagulation factor replacement if they are treated promptly; however, continued bleeding may result in compression of vital structures. In addition to treatment after bleeding is identified, preventive therapy must be administered before surgery or an invasive procedure. Regular prophylactic infusions of coagulation factor concentrates for children with severe hemophilia reduce the incidence of hemarthroses and prevent long-term joint damage,[13] and appear to maintain a beneficial effect for adults.[14] Coagulation factor concentrates are administered intravenously up to three times weekly for prophylaxis and up to two to three times daily for treatment of acute hemorrhage. The advent of recombinant coagulation factor products engineered to have extended half-lives promises to improve convenience and quality of life by reducing the frequency of infusions dramatically in some cases.[15] A major advance in hemophilia care is the development of emicizumab, a bispecific antibody that substitutes for factor VIII and is effective for bleeding prophylaxis in hemophilia A patients who have developed antibodies (inhibitors) against infused factor VIII.[16] It is self-administered once weekly by subcutaneous injection and restores near normal hemostasis in patients for whom factor VIII concentrates are no longer effective. Although first approved for use by hemophilia A patients with factor VIII inhibitors, it is likely to play an important role over time in prophylaxis for some hemophilia A patients without inhibitors. Gene therapy for the treatment of hemophilia is an active area of investigation and represents the very real possibility of a cure.[17]

COMPLICATIONS OF COAGULOPATHIES

Bleeding resulting from coagulation disorders may produce a variety of complications. For example, the chronic, recurrent joint bleeding commonly experienced by patients with hemophilia may lead to joint immobility and limb contractures.

Chronic bleeding can cause anemia as a result of iron deficiency. Bleeding into various organs can result in dysfunction of that organ. Such bleeding may be fatal if it occurs, for example, in the cranial cavity or the gastrointestinal tract. Antibodies or inhibitors to infused coagulation factor concentrates may develop, making it difficult to control bleeding even with minor injuries. Viral transmission via plasma-derived coagulation factor concentrates led to a substantial number of patients with hemophilia becoming infected with HIV and/or hepatitis C. With the development of effective viral inactivation procedures for plasma-derived products and production of recombinant coagulation factors, the transmission of these viruses by coagulation factor concentrates has been essentially eliminated. Additionally, effective antiviral therapies have led to sustained viral responses in a substantial proportion of infected patients.

PATIENT EDUCATION AND LIFE SPAN CONSIDERATIONS

Education is an important and ongoing process. Patients should know the specific name of their bleeding disorder and be able to communicate this diagnosis to their health care providers. They should recognize the signs and symptoms of bleeding and know how to respond appropriately to ensure early and effective treatment. Each patient should have an emergency care plan that includes access to a dose of the appropriate coagulation factor concentrate because many hospitals do not maintain a supply of these products. Work and leisure activities should be reviewed for practices such as contact sports that present a risk for precipitation of bleeding episodes. Medications, such as aspirin and other NSAIDs, that aggravate bleeding tendencies should typically be avoided. Patients are advised to use medications that do not compromise hemostasis, such as acetaminophen, for mild discomfort. Medications must be reviewed periodically and new drugs evaluated for their potential to increase bleeding. For example, fish oil and selective serotonin reuptake inhibitors have antiplatelet activity and should be used with caution in patients with severe bleeding disorders. Wearing a medical alert bracelet or necklace is advised. The patient's coagulation status must be evaluated before dentist visits and surgical or other invasive procedures. Genetic counseling is recommended as a component of family planning.

THROMBOSIS DISORDERS (THROMBOPHILIA)

DEFINITION AND PATHOPHYSIOLOGY

In the normal state, procoagulant enzymes trigger the formation of a blood clot (thrombus) to ensure hemostasis after injury. These procoagulant factors are balanced by inhibitory factors to ensure that excessive clotting does not occur and that the blood remains in the liquid state. When this equilibrium is disturbed, a "hypercoagulable state" results and thrombosis, the process by which an inappropriate thrombus forms in the living heart or vasculature, may occur. Thrombosis may occur in either the arterial or venous circulation, but risk factors for clot formation in the two circulations differ somewhat. For example, thrombi in arteries are commonly associated with atherosclerosis (hardening of the arteries), a condition that does not affect veins, and hereditary conditions leading to a

hypercoagulable state increase the risk for formation of clots in veins but have little impact on arterial clot formation. Thrombophilia refers to a tendency to develop venous thrombosis and may result from acquired or hereditary factors, or often from a combination of both.

VENOUS THROMBOEMBOLIC DISEASE

DEFINITION AND EPIDEMIOLOGY

Thrombosis may occur in any vein in the body, but the majority of clots form in the deep veins of the lower extremities. This deep venous thrombosis (DVT) causes pain and swelling in the distal tissues. Segments may break off from thrombi in extremity veins and be transported to the right side of the heart, where they are then transmitted to the pulmonary arterial circulation in the form of pulmonary emboli (PE). It is estimated that 350,000 to 600,000 individuals in the United States experience venous thromboembolism (VTE), and up to 100,000 die of complications annually.[18]

Risk Factors

Numerous conditions that may constitute an underlying risk factor for VTE have been identified. For example, individuals who smoke, are at advanced age, or have cancer, obesity, diabetes, or chronic inflammatory diseases are at increased risk. In addition, surgery, trauma, pregnancy, childbirth, immobilization, hospitalization, estrogen use, extended travel, and acute medical illness are well-established provoking factors. Thrombosis may also occur in otherwise healthy individuals with no obvious explanation. These episodes are referred to as unprovoked and are frequently associated with a hereditary predisposition to venous thrombosis (i.e., thrombophilia).

PATHOPHYSIOLOGY

The Virchow triad continues to define the pathogenesis of VTE, with changes in blood vessel walls, blood flow, and coagulability of the blood itself all contributing to risk. One example of an abnormality in the coagulability of the blood is activated protein C resistance (APCR). APCR is commonly caused by the presence of an abnormal coagulation factor V molecule resulting from a mutation in the factor V gene.[19] This abnormal factor V is known as factor V Leiden in honor of the city in the Netherlands where the mutation was identified. Factor V Leiden occurs in the heterozygous form in about 5% of white individuals (affecting up to 60 million people worldwide) but is rare in individuals of African or Asian descent. The mutated factor V enzyme resists breakdown by activated protein C, a protein that helps keep blood in the fluid state. Factor V Leiden is transmitted in an autosomal dominant inheritance pattern; thus both males and females are affected. A person with heterozygous factor V Leiden has about a threefold increased risk for development of VTE compared with the general population, which roughly translates to an increase in the absolute risk for development of VTE from 0.1% to about 0.3% annually in middle age. Homozygous factor V Leiden is less common than the heterozygous form, but is a stronger risk factor for VTE and increases the risk by about 18-fold. The majority of people with factor V Leiden are asymptomatic, however, and never develop VTE in their lifetimes.

Often, VTE results from additive risk factors, such as obesity, smoking, and estrogen-containing oral contraceptive use in the setting of a genetic predisposition. Aging is an overlooked risk factor for VTE and results in a doubling of risk for each decade of life. APCR resulting from factor V Leiden is the most common gene mutation leading to hereditary predisposition to VTE in white individuals. Sickle cell trait (see Chapter 216) occurs in around 1 of 12 African Americans and confers a twofold increased risk for DVT and a fourfold increased risk for PE.[20]

In addition to factor V Leiden and sickle cell trait, other genetic abnormalities that predispose individuals to VTE include the prothrombin gene variant (PT G20210A) and deficiencies of the natural anticoagulant proteins, protein C, protein S, and antithrombin (formerly known as antithrombin III).[19] Whereas factor V Leiden, PT G20210A, and sickle cell trait are relatively common and mild forms of thrombophilia, deficiencies of the natural anticoagulants are relatively rare and impart a more severe tendency to venous thrombosis. Inheritance of one abnormal factor V Leiden or PT G20210A gene results in an affected individual's being a heterozygote for the gene polymorphism. These gene polymorphisms are common enough that individuals with two abnormal copies of the genes (homozygotes) or one abnormal copy of each (compound heterozygotes) exist. The risk for VTE is higher in these individuals than in those who are simple heterozygotes for the polymorphisms, but most people remain asymptomatic unless other risk factors are present.

CLINICAL PRESENTATION AND PHYSICAL EXAMINATION

Thrombi can form in both superficial and deep veins. Thrombi in the superficial veins manifest with localized tenderness at the site, redness, a feeling of warmth, and possible swelling of the affected limb. Because the vein is close to the surface, it may feel hard or ropelike when examined. The clinical features of DVT include pain, swelling, and erythema of the affected extremity. The Homan sign (pain with dorsiflexion of the foot) may also be present, but its absence does not exclude DVT. PE may be asymptomatic when accompanying DVT or may manifest with such symptoms as chest pain, shortness of breath, palpitations, syncope, or a vague feeling of doom. Physical examination is often neither sensitive nor specific for VTE, and further testing must be done when the condition is suspected.

DIAGNOSTICS

D-dimer is a breakdown product of a fibrin clot that can be measured in the blood; it is virtually always elevated in a patient with an acute thrombosis. The D-dimer test is frequently the first test performed in patients with suspected VTE, but although it has a good sensitivity and negative predictive value for diagnosis of VTE, an abnormal test result is not specific and has a poor positive predictive value. That is, a negative D-dimer test result is helpful for ruling out VTE in patients with a low clinical probability of having VTE, but a positive test result does not rule it in, and further testing must be undertaken. A Doppler ultrasound study is typically performed to evaluate for venous thrombosis in the limbs. It has excellent sensitivity for detection of proximal DVT but is relatively insensitive in the calf. Ascending venography, a radiologic procedure involving injection of contrast dye into the superficial and deep veins of the leg, permits diagnosis of DVT but is no longer commonly used. Computed tomography of

---

BOX 217.4

Differential Diagnosis: Thrombophilia

HEREDITARY

- Activated protein C resistance caused by factor V Leiden
- Prothrombin gene mutation G20210A
- Protein C deficiency
- Protein S deficiency
- Antithrombin deficiency
- Homocystinuria
- Hyperhomocysteinemia
- Dysfibrinogenemia
- Factor XIII polymorphisms
- Increased plasma coagulation factors (fibrinogen; prothrombin; factors VIII, IX, XI)

ACQUIRED

- Active cancer or chemotherapy treatment
- Obesity
- Age
- Medications (estrogen, oral contraceptives)
- Autoimmune and inflammatory disorders (especially inflammatory bowel disease)
- Antiphospholipid antibodies
- Pregnancy or postpartum state
- Nephrotic syndrome
- Surgery and trauma
- Heparin-induced thrombocytopenia
- Myeloproliferative neoplasms
- Paroxysmal nocturnal hemoglobinuria
- Varicose veins
- HIV infection
- Wegener granulomatosis

---

the chest with intravenous administration of contrast material is increasingly the preferred test for evaluation of patients with suspected PE, replacing ventilation/perfusion scans in many institutions.

DIFFERENTIAL DIAGNOSIS

Determination of the cause of VTE (Box 217.4) relies heavily on the history and physical examination, which focus on identifying the presence of acquired risk factors as outlined before. Hereditary thrombophilia should be suspected in individuals with VTE that is unexplained, occurs at a young age (i.e., <50 years), occurs in an unusual location (e.g., mesenteric, cerebral circulations), is recurrent, or is associated with a family history of VTE in multiple first-degree relatives.[19]

Thrombophilic disorders are distinguished from one another primarily on the basis of the laboratory evaluation. The decision about which laboratory tests are indicated is determined by the medical history and clinical presentation. The goal of thrombophilia testing is to determine whether a defect is present that may be important for planning of future treatment and that may be sought in other family members who may or may not yet have had an episode of VTE. The results of thrombophilia testing rarely have implications for the acute treatment of VTE; thus, testing should be deferred until the end of the initial anticoagulation period to avoid falsely abnormal results from interference by anticoagulation, inflammation, or consumption of natural anticoagulants by the acute clot. Although genetic tests for thrombophilia can generally be accomplished at any time, optimal patient management involves genetic counseling and informed consent for the testing, which is best conducted in the office of the hematologist and not in the emergency department or the inpatient setting.

INTERDISCIPLINARY COLLABORATIVE MANAGEMENT

Referral to a hematologist with experience in VTE and thrombophilia should be considered for patients with a history of unexplained or recurrent VTE, family history of VTE, or VTE at an early age or in unusual locations. Investigation for a hereditary predisposition to VTE may result in therapeutic or preventive measures for the patient or family members, but testing should be performed only after counseling of the patient about the potential implications of test results—both normal and abnormal—and only with the patient's informed consent.[19] Test results should be discussed during a face-to-face meeting between the patient and a hematologist or genetic counselor, with the discussion tailored to the patient's specific circumstances.

Patients with DVT should be hospitalized when the clot is extensive or is accompanied by severe PE.

Pharmacologic management of VTE should follow the American College of Chest Physicians guidelines for antithrombotic therapy for prevention and treatment of thrombosis.[21] The diagnosis of hereditary thrombophilia in itself is not an indication for treatment with anticoagulants, especially if thrombosis has not occurred. In general, VTE is treated the same in individuals with and without thrombophilia, and treatment is begun immediately with anticoagulants to prevent thrombus growth and subsequent pulmonary embolism.

Heparin has long been the initial treatment for VTE because its anticoagulant effect begins immediately. Heparin acts together with antithrombin to block coagulation factor enzymes, especially thrombin (factor IIa) and activated factor X (factor Xa). Unfractionated heparin is administered intravenously, and the dose is adjusted according to the aPTT range established by each individual hospital laboratory. Many hospital laboratories have adopted the more reliable anti-Xa activity test to monitor heparin anticoagulation, aiming for an anti-Xa level between 0.3 to 0.7 IU/mL. Whether the aPTT or the anti-Xa level is used to monitor heparin therapy, care must be taken not to exceed the therapeutic range because this increases the risk for severe bleeding complications.[22]

Intravenous unfractionated heparin has largely been replaced by low-molecular-weight heparin (LMWH) for the treatment of acute VTE in most situations; however, LMWH also works with antithrombin but inhibits activated factor X to a much greater extent than thrombin. This ability of LMWH to block the clotting mechanism "upstream" accounts for many of the advantages of this drug. In randomized clinical trials, LMWH has been shown to be at least as effective and safe as intravenous unfractionated heparin for the initial treatment of both DVT and PE.[21] Compared with heparin, LMWH has a longer half-life, more consistent and complete absorption when it is injected subcutaneously, and fewer side effects including a lower risk for the potentially catastrophic complication of heparin-induced thrombocytopenia. LMWH is as effective when it is given in a fixed, weight-based subcutaneous

dose as when it is given intravenously and does not require routine laboratory monitoring for dose adjustment.[21] These advantages permit management of many patients with DVT (and some low-risk patients with PE), who can be taught to self-administer the drug, entirely in the outpatient setting. Heparin and LMWH are biologic preparations extracted from animal intestines, usually pigs. A synthetic pentasaccharide molecule, fondaparinux, is also available for acute treatment of VTE. Its mechanism of action is like that of heparin and LMWH except that it inhibits activated factor X exclusively and has a longer half-life than LMWH, permitting once-daily subcutaneous administration. Like LMWH, it is administered in a fixed dose without laboratory monitoring, allowing convenient outpatient use.

Initial heparin or LMWH therapy is typically followed by treatment with a vitamin K antagonist, typically warfarin in the United States, which is usually started concurrently with heparin or LMWH. Warfarin is administered orally and is absorbed from the intestine along with other nutrients, including vitamin K. Vitamin K is required for the production of coagulation factors II, VII, IX, and X in their fully active form by the liver. Warfarin competes with vitamin K, resulting in the production of incomplete, less active coagulation factors. This takes time, usually 5 days for coagulation factor synthesis to decrease and for previously activated coagulation factors to clear the circulation. During this period, heparin or LMWH and warfarin are given concurrently for full protection. When the warfarin becomes effective, as measured by laboratory testing (two consecutive international normalized ratio [INR] determinations in the therapeutic range at least 24 hours apart), heparin or LMWH is discontinued. Heparin or LMWH *must be* administered for a minimum of 5 days, however, irrespective of the rapidity with which a therapeutic INR is achieved. The patient is then maintained with warfarin on an outpatient basis for a minimum of 3 months after a first episode of VTE. In certain individuals at high risk for recurrence (e.g., those with idiopathic VTE, active cancer, or antiphospholipid syndrome), indefinite anticoagulation after a first event should be considered.[21]

Because warfarin and vitamin K are in competition, the effect of warfarin may be exaggerated when dietary vitamin K is inadequate. The effect of warfarin is also exaggerated with liver disease, and many different drugs increase or decrease the warfarin effects. Therefore it is important to identify any medications being used during anticoagulation therapy. When warfarin is stopped, the production of fully active coagulation factors gradually returns over several days. The amount of warfarin required to achieve an optimum degree of therapeutic anticoagulation varies among individuals and is determined by the PT, which is standardized by the INR calculation. Expression of the result as the INR is preferred because it eliminates variability among laboratories and reagents used to perform the PT measurement. The degree of warfarin anticoagulation required for maximum protection with minimum risk of bleeding depends on clinical conditions present at that time. The recommended target INR is 2.5 with a range of 2 to 3 for secondary prophylaxis to reduce the risk of recurrent VTE for most patients, and it is the same whether or not thrombophilia is identified.[19,21]

Anticoagulation is best managed by dedicated anticoagulation clinics with use of validated dosage algorithms, and the Anticoagulation Forum website (www.acforum.org) is an excellent resource for matters pertaining to management of acute and chronic anticoagulation.[23]

Although heparin, LMWH, and warfarin have long been the mainstays of treatment and secondary prevention of VTE, many, if not most, patients with VTE are candidates for treatment with a direct oral anticoagulant (DOAC). The DOACs are small-molecule, synthetic target-specific oral anticoagulants with the advantages of being active orally in a fixed dose, not interacting with food or most other medications, and not requiring laboratory monitoring for dosage adjustment.[21,24] In some cases, the DOACs allow for an entirely oral treatment course for acute VTE, thus eliminating the need for painful LMWH injections.

Dabigatran is a direct inhibitor of thrombin (factor IIa), whereas rivaroxaban, apixaban, edoxaban, and others are direct inhibitors of activated factor X. Clinical trials have demonstrated equivalent efficacy of the DOACs to LMWH-warfarin combinations for treating acute VTE and suggest a reduction in major bleeding complications.[24]

Whereas DOACs are appropriate for many people with acute VTE, there are some patient populations for which traditional anticoagulants may still be preferred. For example, patients with severe liver and/or kidney dysfunction may have impaired drug elimination pathways, leading to drug accumulation and an increased risk for bleeding. The DOACs have not been studied in cases of massive PE or extensive DVT for which thrombolytic therapy is administered, and the safety of DOACs in pregnancy is unknown, thus treatment and prevention of VTE in pregnancy are best accomplished with heparin or LMWH. LMWH has been the standard of care for treatment of cancer-associated VTE as it appears to be more effective than warfarin for secondary VTE prevention in these patients, though this has not been the case in all studies.[21] While DOACs have not yet been widely studied in patients with cancer-associated VTE, data are accumulating to suggest that they are as effective as LMWH for secondary VTE prevention in cancer patients, sometimes after a short course of LMWH anticoagulation and will undoubtedly play an increasingly larger role in this patient population.[25] Patients with antiphospholipid syndrome have a profound hypercoagulable state and the efficacy of the DOACs for treatment of VTE in these patients has not yet been established and should be reserved for patients for whom traditional anticoagulation is otherwise not optimal.[24] DOAC avoidance is currently advised for patients on dialysis and in older patients or those with renal dysfunction (i.e., GFR <30 mL/min), though studies are ongoing and in at least one study of patients with end-stage kidney disease, there was a decreased incidence of bleeding with apixaban when compared to warfarin.[26,27] Additionally, DOACs should be used with great caution or avoided in favor of traditional anticoagulation in morbidly obese patients (i.e., weight >120 kg or BMI >40 kg/M²), as the efficacy in this population has not been rigorously confirmed. Finally, although the DOACs are safe and effective for stroke prevention in atrial fibrillation, they appear to be inferior to warfarin for prevention of mechanical heart valve thrombosis and should not be prescribed for that purpose.

Patients without sufficient outpatient support, who cannot inject themselves with LMWH, or who lack access to DOACs should be hospitalized for initial treatment. In general, most patients with symptomatic PE should be hospitalized for initial treatment because the potential for life-threatening complications is high; however, protocols for risk stratification exist, and low-risk patients with PE may be considered for outpatient management. Often, hospitalization may be shortened when LMWH or DOACs are used for initial anticoagulation because patients can self-administer these medications at home. Although LMWH and DOACs make outpatient treatment a reality for many people with acute VTE, initial clinical follow-up should be no less diligent than if patients were hospitalized, given the potential for both clotting and bleeding complications early in the treatment course.

COMPLICATIONS

Complications of thrombosis can arise from both the clot itself as well as the treatment (anticoagulation). Clot formation within intact vessels compromises the vascular supply to the affected areas. With venous thrombosis, the reduced flow of blood from the affected area of the body results in swelling and pain in that part. For example, a thrombus in the veins of the leg can result in swelling and discoloration of the foot and lower leg. When the obstruction is not relieved promptly, the swelling may become chronic and noticeable, especially after patients have been on their feet for a time. If it is not properly treated, DVT may result in venous valve damage, venous reflux, and ambulatory venous hypertension leading to the chronic, often debilitating complication of post-thrombotic syndrome (PTS). Below-the-knee compression stockings after acute DVT reduced the incidence and severity of PTS in older studies, but their value has been questioned on the basis of more recent trials;[28] thus their use may be reserved for those with symptoms. Finally, if it is not promptly treated, a DVT may extend and break off, producing an embolus that may become lodged in the vessels of the lung (a pulmonary embolus; see Chapter 95). When such emboli are large or multiple, they can be life-threatening.

Bleeding is the most feared complication of anticoagulation, and manifestations may range in severity from small bruises to life-threatening hemorrhages, e.g., in the gastrointestinal tract or the brain. The mainstays for prevention of bleeding are selection of the proper anticoagulant type and dose for each individual patient and judicious monitoring where appropriate. Much anticoagulant-associated bleeding is self-limited and can be effectively managed with supportive measures only. Occasionally, rapid reversal of anticoagulant effect is necessary, requiring the administration of antidotes. Heparin and LMWH effect can be mitigated by protamine sulfate while warfarin can be reversed by administering vitamin K either through the IV or oral route. Vitamin K begins to work within hours, but if immediate warfarin reversal is required, the use of fresh frozen plasma or a prothrombin complex concentrate containing the vitamin K dependent coagulation factors II, VII, IX, and X is prudent. Specific antidotes for the DOACs are available, but the short half-life of these anticoagulants often obviates the need for an antidote, except in extreme circumstances.[29]

LIFE SPAN CONSIDERATIONS

Patients with thrombophilia who have a family history of VTE may themselves be at a higher than average risk for VTE in situations associated with a hypercoagulable state such as pregnancy, surgery, long-haul travel, or hospitalization for an acute medical illness. These patients may therefore benefit from genetic counseling and education about VTE prevention. Oral contraceptives increase the risk of blood clotting, especially in smokers and in obesity, so young women should be counseled appropriately. Hormone replacement therapy is also associated with increased risk of VTE as well as stroke in menopausal women and should be used for the shortest time possible. The risk for VTE increases with aging and becomes a problem for older adults, especially if they also have an inherited thrombophilia or other risk factors.

PATIENT AND FAMILY EDUCATION

Patient education is an important component of safe and effective outpatient anticoagulation therapy for patients who have sustained a VTE and is critical for both primary and secondary VTE prevention. Patients need to be aware of their diagnosis and factors influencing anticoagulation treatment. Education focuses on the importance of keeping regular follow-up visits, monitoring anticoagulation doses, identifying signs of bleeding or clot progression, maintaining a consistent diet (if taking warfarin), noting changes in health and diet or medications, and avoiding hazardous activities such as contact sports. In addition, a regularly updated pharmacology resource should be consulted for medications that interact with warfarin, and information should be provided to patients with periodic updates. Patients who are anticoagulated with DOACs should have organ function monitored periodically to assess for the potential for drug accumulation and bleeding complications as a result of kidney or liver insufficiency.

Prolonged immobility is to be discouraged and regular exercise encouraged. When the at-risk patient is immobilized, such as while driving or flying, he or she should take frequent rest breaks for leg stretching or walking and consider wearing below-the-knee compression stockings. Patients at risk for VTE need information about the signs and symptoms of VTE and how to access appropriate care. Genetic counseling and risk management are essential for individuals with inherited disorders. Counseling about risk reduction is required and should include regular discussions of the role of weight loss, exercise, smoking cessation, and management of chronic medical conditions in reducing risk for recurrent VTE in individuals both with and without thrombophilia. The North American Thrombosis Forum (www.natfonline.org) is an excellent source of information on prevention and treatment of VTE for patients and clinicians alike.

REFERENCES

1. White, G., & Marker, V. (2013). Overview of basic coagulation and fibrinolysis. In V. Marden, W. Airden, J. Bennett, et al. (Eds.), *Hemostasis and thrombosis: Basic principles and clinical practice* (6th ed.). Philadelphia: Lippincott Williams & Wilkins.
2. Greaves, M., & Preston, F. E. (2013). Approach to the bleeding patient. In R. W. Coleman, V. J. Marder, A. W. Clowes, et al. (Eds.), *Hemostasis and thrombosis: Basic principles and clinical practice* (6th ed.). Philadelphia: Lippincott Williams & Wilkins.
3. Kozek-langenecker, S., Ahmed, A., Afshari, A., et al. (2017). Management of severe perioperative bleeding: Guidelines from the European Society of Anaesthiology first update 2016. *European Journal of Anaesthesiology, 34*(6), 332–395.
4. Roshal, M., & Gil, M. R. (2019). Overview of Purposes of Hemostasis Testing and Common Sources of Error. In B. H. Shaz, C. D. Hillyer, & M. R. Gil (Eds.), *Transfusion medicine and hemostasis* (3rd ed., pp. 767–772). Elsevier. Chapter 127.
5. Favaloro, E. J. (2017). Clinical utility of closure times using the platelet function analyzer-100/200. *American Journal of Hematology, 92*, 398–404.
6. Soucie, J. M., Nuss, R., Evatt, B., et al. (2000). Mortality among males with hemophilia: Relations with source of medical care. *Blood, 96*, 437–442.
7. Pai, M., Key, N. S., Skinner, M., et al. (2016). NHF-McMaster guideline on care models for haemophilia management. *Haemophilia : The Official Journal of the World Federation of Hemophilia, 22*(Suppl. 3), 6–16.
8. National Hemophilia Foundation and Scientific Advisory Council (MASAC). (2017). *Guidelines for emergency department management of individuals with hemophilia and other bleeding disorders.* New York: National Hemophilia Foundation. Retrieved from www.hemophilia.org. (Accessed 21 June 2018).
9. Leebeek, F., & Eikenboom, J. (2016). Von Willebrand's disease. *The New England Journal of Medicine, 375*, 2067–2088.
10. National Hemophilia Foundation and Scientific Advisory Council (MASAC). (2015). *Recommendations on the care and treatment of individuals with von Willebrand disease.* New York: National Hemophilia Foundation. Retrieved from www.hemophilia.org. (Accessed 21 June 2018).
11. World Federation of Hemophilia. (2017). *Report on the annual global survey 2016.* Montreal: World Federation of Hemophilia. Retrieved from http://www1.wfh.org/publication/files/pdf-1690.pdf. (Accessed 21 June 2018).
12. World Federation of Hemophilia. (2014). *Guidelines for the management of hemophilia* (2nd ed.). Montreal: World Federation of Hemophilia. Retrieved from http://www1.wfh.org/publication/files/pdf-1472.pdf. (Accessed 21 June 2018).
13. Manco-Johnson, M. J., Soucie, J. M. Gill, J. C., et al. (2017). Prophylaxis usage, bleeding rates, and joint outcomes of hemophilia 1999 to 2010: A surveillance project. *Blood, 129*, 2368–2374.
14. Manco-Johnson, M. J., Lundin, B., & Funk, S. (2017). Effect of late prophylaxis in hemophilia on joint status: A randomized trial. *Journal of Thrombosis and Haemostasis, 15*, 2115–2124.
15. Mancuso, M. E., & Santagostino, E. (2017). Outcome of clinical trials with new extended half-life FVIII/IX concentrates. *Journal of Clinical Medicine, 6*, E39.
16. Oldenburg, J., Mahlangu, J. N., Kim, B., et al. (2017). Emicizumab prophylaxis in hemophilia A with inhibitors. *The New England Journal of Medicine, 377*, 809–818.
17. High, K. A. (2014). Gene therapy for hemophilia: The clot thickens. *Human Gene Therapy, 25*, 915–922.
18. Beckman, M. G., Hooper, W. C., Critchley, S. E., & Ortel, T. L. (2010). Venous thromboembolism: A public health concern. *American Journal of Preventive Medicine, 38*(4 Suppl.), S495–S501.
19. Conners, J. M. (2017). Thrombophilia testing and venous thrombosis. *The New England Journal of Medicine, 377*, 1177–1187.
20. Folsom, A. R., Tang, W., Roetker, N. S., et al. (2015). Prospective study of sickle cell trait and venous thromboembolism incidence. *Journal of Thrombosis and Haemostasis, 13*, 2–9.
21. Kearon, C., Akl, E. A., Orneles, J., et al. (2016). Antithrombotic therapy for VTE: CHEST guideline and expert panel report. *Chest, 149*, 315–352.
22. Smythe, M. A., Priziola, J., Dobesh, P. P., et al. (2016). Guidance for the practical management of the heparin anticoagulants in the treatment of venous thromboembolism. *Journal of Thrombosis and Thrombolysis, 41*, 165–186.
23. Witt, D. M., Clark, N. P., Kaatz, S., et al. (2016). Guidance for the practical management of warfarin therapy in the treatment of venous thromboembolism. *Journal of Thrombosis and Thrombolysis, 41*, 187–205.
24. Burnett, A. E., Mahan, C. E., Vazquez, S. R., et al. (2016). Guidance for the practical management of the direct oral anticoagulants (DOACs) in VTE treatment. *Journal of Thrombosis and Thrombolysis, 41*, 206–232.
25. Soff, G. A. (2018). Use of direct oral anticoagulants for treating venous thromboembolism in patients with cancer. *Journal of the National Comprehensive Cancer Network, 16*, 670–673.
26. Lutz, J., Jurk, K., & Schinzel, H. (2017). Direct oral anticoagulants in patients with chronic kidney disease: Patient selection and special considerations. *International Journal of Nephrology and Renovascular Disease, 10*, 135–143. http://doi.org/10.2147/IJNRD.S105771.
27. Siontis, K. C., Zhang, X., Eckard, A., Bhave, N., Schaubel, D. E., He, K., et al. (2018). Outcomes associated with apixaban use in end-stage kidney disease patients with atrial fibrillation in the United States. *Circulation*, EPub Ahead of Print.
28. Rabinovich, A., & Kahn, S. R. (2018). How I treat the postthrombotic syndrome. *Blood, 131*, 2215–2222.
29. Siegal, D. M., Garcia, D. A., & Crowther, M. A. (2014). How I treat target-specific oral anticoagulant bleeding. *Blood, 123*, 1152–1158.

CHAPTER 218

LEUKEMIAS

Susan Culbertson Brighton • Elizabeth Kimtis

 Red flags include a white blood cell count of 500–30 000 cells/mm³, leukopenia with >20% blasts, enlarged, non-tender lymph nodes present for >1 month.

 Referral to a hematologist is indicated for all suspected cases of leukemia.

DEFINITION AND EPIDEMIOLOGY

Some of the most challenging and complex cancers to manage in the community setting are the leukemias, hematologic malignant neoplasms that affect the bone marrow and lymphatic tissue. There are four different types of leukemia, two acute and two chronic forms. The acute forms of leukemia are acute myelogenous leukemia (AML) and acute lymphocytic leukemia (ALL). Chronic myelogenous leukemia (CML) and chronic lymphocytic leukemia (CLL) are the two chronic forms of leukemia, with CLL being the most common form.[1] Acute leukemias are distinguished by an abnormal production of immature white blood cells (WBCs), called blasts, with rapid disease progression over approximately 6 months, which results in limited life expectancy if left untreated. Chronic leukemias reveal an overabundance of more mature-appearing but ineffective WBCs. Disease progression is usually slower, over several years as opposed to months. The overproduction of leukemia cells displaces normal cells in the bone marrow and thus crowds out normal hematopoiesis, resulting in granulocytopenia, anemia, and thrombocytopenia. Depending on the type of leukemia, treatment may be as conservative as observation or as aggressive as bone marrow or peripheral blood stem cell transplantation. Consequences of the disease state and side effects of treatment represent a true challenge to the health care provider.

In 2019, there were an estimated approximately 61,780 new cases of leukemia in the United States, with a slightly higher incidence of chronic compared with acute leukemia. The estimated number of deaths from leukemia in 2019 was approximately 22,840.[2,3] The exact cause of leukemia is unknown. Causes and risk factors for consideration are genetic factors and disorders, exposure to radiation, environmental factors, occupational exposures, drugs, viruses, and other bone marrow disorders.

Children with genetic disorders such as Down syndrome have an increased risk for the development of acute leukemia. Other conditions that are associated with a higher risk for developing leukemia include Ellis-van Creveld syndrome, Fanconi anemia, Klinefelter syndrome, Bloom syndrome, and ataxia-telangiectasia.

Exposure to ionizing radiation is the most conclusive predisposing factor associated with the development of leukemia. This became evident after World War II, when great numbers of Japanese survivors of the atomic bomb demonstrated an increased incidence of AML and CML, usually 5 to 9 years after exposure.[2] Pioneer radiologists who were exposed to massive radiation also exhibited a high incidence of leukemia.[4]

Environmental factors such as hair dye, cigarette smoking, and sunbathing may also increase the risk for development of leukemia, although studies have been inconclusive.[5]

Occupational exposure to certain chemicals increases the risk for development of leukemia. Workers exposed to benzene (a hydrocarbon used in industry, such as rubber and shoe-making plants, and in unleaded gasoline), rubber cement, and cleaning solvents are at risk. Other occupations in which workers are at risk of contracting leukemia are those that expose workers to explosives, dyes, or paints including distilleries, pesticide manufacturing, and leather tanning industries.[5] Although the relationship between leukemia and viruses remains unclear, there does appear to be a correlation between retroviruses and T-cell leukemia and hairy cell leukemia.[6]

Antecedent hematologic disorders, such as polycythemia vera, aplastic anemia, myelodysplastic syndromes (MDSs), and other diseases of the bone marrow also appear to predispose individuals to leukemia. Intensive combination chemotherapy for patients with cancer has led to increased survival rates overall. However, these survivors must be continually evaluated for complications of cytotoxic treatment. One serious consequence is the development of a second cancer, especially myeloid leukemia. Therapy-related leukemia is more difficult to treat, as it typically is more aggressive. Treatment-related myelodysplastic syndrome (t-MDS) and treatment-related AML (t-AML) are the terms used to describe a clinical syndrome that is arguably the most serious, unpredictable long-term complication of cancer treatment. In total, therapy-related myeloid neoplasms represent 10% to 20% of acute leukemias, myelodysplastic, or myeloproliferative neoplasms.[7]

PATHOPHYSIOLOGY

All blood cells—WBCs, red blood cells, and platelets—originate from the stem cell, which is predominantly found in the bone marrow. The stem cell's unique ability for self-renewal and differentiation is necessary to meet the body's requirements throughout a lifetime.[8]

Leukemia is a malignant disorder of the blood and blood-forming organs—the spleen, lymphatic system, and bone marrow. It is identified as acute or chronic by the onset of symptoms and the maturity of the blood cell. Leukemic cells are designated either myeloid or lymphoid, according to the type of cell that predominates, as identified by morphology of the cells in combination with flow cytometry, cytogenetics, and molecular markers.

There is a maturational arrest of immature leukocytes, or blasts, in acute leukemia. These blasts proliferate or accumulate uncontrollably, inhibiting normal hematopoiesis and contributing to organomegaly. In chronic leukemia, there is an accumulation of mature-appearing leukocytes that have lost their ability to function efficiently and to undergo apoptosis, or programmed cell death.

The accumulation of abnormal blood cells in the bone marrow and lymphatic tissue can result in organomegaly as well as abnormal hematopoiesis, causing anemia, neutropenia, and thrombocytopenia, as well as an impaired immune response.

CLINICAL PRESENTATION AND PHYSICAL EXAMINATION
Acute Leukemias

The presenting signs and symptoms of AML and ALL can be nonspecific, along with associated cytopenias. The patient may have fevers and/or recurrent infection owing to a low WBC count. Increasing weakness, progressive fatigue, pallor, or dyspnea, all related to anemia, is not uncommon.

Thrombocytopenia can cause unexplained or spontaneous bruising, oral bleeding, epistaxis, heavy menstrual periods, and excessive bleeding after minor dental or surgical procedures. Rarely, patients may have chloromas, the collection of blast cells in the subcutaneous tissues. In addition, with AML, some patients have oral involvement manifesting with gum hypertrophy; therefore, an oral examination may be helpful.

If leukemia infiltrates lymph nodes, spleen, and liver, diffuse lymphadenopathy and hepatosplenomegaly may be present on examination. Patients may also have bone pain as a result of a packed, expanding bone marrow. Younger patients may experience joint pain and swelling that resembles rheumatoid arthritis.

Ocular involvement is seen in both childhood and adult leukemia patients. Leukemic retinopathy is the most commonly seen manifestation.[9] Not all ocular lesions cause symptoms; therefore, it is important to consider an ophthalmic examination at the time of diagnosis.

Approximately 5% to 8% of patients have central nervous system (CNS) involvement at the time of initial diagnosis. Common signs and symptoms of leukemia that have invaded the CNS are headache, papilledema, vision changes such as diplopia, vomiting, mental status changes, and cranial nerve palsy. In AML, leukostasis occurs when the blast count exceeds 100,000 cells/mm³, and the patient is at risk for a fatal cerebral hemorrhage.[10]

Physical examination findings such as lymphadenopathy, hepatosplenomegaly, and testicular involvement are more common in ALL than in AML.

Chronic Leukemias

Patients with CML and CLL are usually asymptomatic in the early stages of disease. There may be subtle changes in the WBC count and differential early in the course of disease. A cardinal finding on physical examination of patients with chronic leukemia is splenomegaly. The patient may report a mild sensation of fullness in the left upper quadrant or may have an obvious mass. Severe splenomegaly can compress surrounding organs, causing early satiety, weight loss, and peripheral leg edema related to compression of the splenic vein. As the disease progresses, other symptoms occur, such as bone pain, bleeding problems, infection, fatigue, pallor, adenopathy, fevers, and night sweats.[11]

DIAGNOSTICS
Essential Diagnostics

Acute Leukemias. The key in making the diagnosis of acute leukemia lies with the evaluation of a complete blood count (CBC with diff) and bone marrow aspirate with biopsy, to study the morphology of the cells. Additional studies on these specimens should include cytochemistry, immunophenotyping, (flow cytometry and immunohistochemistry) cytogenetic analysis, and gene mutation studies. This information is very important to the treating provider, since both AML and ALL are not single diseases. In fact, there are different subtypes of each disease, and this information is helpful when treatment decisions are being made. Most patients initially have a combination of cytopenias, with striking abnormalities noted in the WBC count and differential. The parameters of the WBC count vary within a wide range, from 1000 to 100,000 cells/mm³. Most patients have counts between 5000 and 30,000 cells/mm³.[12]

Careful examination of the **blood smear** is essential. The significant finding on the blood smear is an increased population of blast cells and a decrease of granulocytes, red blood cells, and platelets. However, as many as 10% of all patients have normal blood counts even when the marrow has been replaced by leukemic cells; therefore, bone marrow aspiration and biopsy are required for a definitive diagnosis. Blast cells in the bone marrow must constitute at least 20% of the total cell population for a definitive diagnosis to be made. Additionally, a diagnosis of acute leukemia can be made by the presence of at least 20% of blast cells in the peripheral blood.

Auer rods (rod-shaped granules incorporated within the blast cells) are pathognomonic of AML.[12]

Additional Diagnostics

Additional laboratory studies should be performed to identify a wide range of metabolic and electrolyte abnormalities that can be seen in acute leukemia. Biochemical studies may reveal hyperuricemia. Hyperuricemia occurs because of the high turnover rate of proliferating leukemia cells resulting in rapid purine catabolism and elevations in serum uric acid. Electrolyte abnormalities are common, and an elevated lactate dehydrogenase (LDH) level can be seen in patients without change in other liver function test (LFT) parameters. The presence of any or all these abnormalities is a reflection of the rate of growth and turnover of the leukemia cells.

Patients with excessive bruising or bleeding should undergo a coagulation panel to look for disseminated intravascular coagulation (DIC) or other coagulopathies. Any patient with an increased myeloblast count may be at risk for leukostasis. This condition primarily affects the lungs and brain, but any organ can be involved. Lowering of the blast count in a rapid fashion is necessary, usually with chemotherapy or leukapheresis. The differential diagnosis for ALL and AML includes lymphoma, although other infiltrative processes, such as solid tumors (e.g., breast cancer or small cell lung cancer), must be excluded. Some patients with fever and cytopenia who have a small number of circulating blast cells must be differentiated from those with reactions to tuberculosis, systemic lupus erythematosus, megaloblastic anemia, or aplastic anemia. Surface antigen and serologic studies can exclude viral infections such as infectious mononucleosis. AML needs to be distinguished from MDS or a myeloproliferative disorder, such as the transformation of CML in blast crisis.

Chronic Leukemias

At diagnosis, the WBC count in chronic leukemias may range from fewer than 10,000 to more than 200,000 cells/mm³, with mature and predominantly myelocytic cells. In general, the red blood cell count is normal, but a slight degree of anemia may occur. Marked increase in myelocytes and basophils in the marrow and blood are common. Increased levels of uric acid in the blood and urine are also found in patients with CML. CML is a stem cell disorder which happens when the translocation of one chromosome, usually the ABL oncogene on chromosome 9, to the BCR gene on chromosome 22, causing a malignant transformation of the cell. This abnormal chromosome is called the Philadelphia chromosome. BCR-ABL protein causes the stem cells to make too many abnormal white blood cells. CML is the first cancer shown to be associated with a chromosomal abnormality.[11]

CLL is often discovered on a routine office visit when a CBC is ordered. The physical examination findings may be normal, but some patients have non-tender adenopathy or spleno-megaly. Patients may report fatigue, night sweats, occasional fever, or malaise. Most patients consult their health care provider because of a painless cervical lymph node that waxes and wanes but does not disappear completely (see Chapter 205).[11]

CLL is suspected whenever an absolute lymphocytosis in the peripheral blood occurs in an adult and is sustained over time. Lymphocytosis also occurs in infectious mononucleosis, pertussis, and toxoplasmosis, but in these conditions, the lymphocyte count returns to normal after a few weeks.

A peripheral smear may be adequate for the diagnosis of CLL; a bone marrow biopsy will always reveal lymphocytosis in cases of CLL. The lymphocyte count ranges from 10,000 to 150,000/mm³. Because there may be a decrease in immunoglobulin (Ig) levels, serum protein electrophoresis should be performed; this test may reveal a marked decrease in levels of IgG and slight decreases in IgA and IgM levels.[12] A **chest x-ray study** may be helpful in detecting hilar and mediastinal adenopathy.

The differential diagnosis for CLL includes non-Hodgkin lymphoma, hairy cell leukemia, and a variety of other lymphoproliferative disorders.

INITIAL DIAGNOSTICS

Leukemia

LABORATORY
- CBC and differential
- Peripheral blood smear evaluation
- Serum electrolytes, including phosphorous level
- Uric acid
- LFTs
- LDH
- BCR-ABL polymerase chain reaction (PCR) for evaluation/monitoring of CML or Ph+ ALL
- Urinalysis
- Serum protein electrophoresis
- DIC panel

OTHER DIAGNOSTICS
- Bone marrow aspirate with biopsy (gold standard). Studies on the specimen include morphology, cytochemistry, flow cytometry, immunohistochemistry, chromosomal testing, and gene mutation studies.
- Lumbar puncture (if clinically indicated and for all patients with ALL)
- Echocardiogram

IMAGING
- Typically, acute leukemia and CML do not produce solid masses, so imaging is typically not done.
- CT scan or PET scan is useful for evaluating a patient with newly diagnosed CLL

DIFFERENTIAL DIAGNOSIS

The differential diagnosis must include diseases that should be considered and excluded when appropriate. These can be narrowed down with the patient's history, physical examination, laboratory studies, radiology studies, tissue sample, including bone marrow aspirate with biopsy, and lymph node biopsy.

 Priority differentials include (1) myelodysplastic/myeloproliferative disorders, such as myelofibrosis, (2) lymphoproliferative disorders, such as large granular lymphocytic leukemia, and hairy cell leukemia, and (3) infection.

INTERPROFESSIONAL COLLABORATIVE MANAGEMENT
Pharmacologic Management
- Chemotherapy
- Immunotherapy
- Targeted therapy

Acute Leukemias

Chemotherapy is the cornerstone of treatment for acute leukemias. Treatment can differ, depending on their subtype; for instance, acute promyelocytic leukemia is not treated with chemotherapy, but instead is treated with arsenic and tretinoin (vitamin A derivative).

Patients diagnosed with ALL and AML require aggressive chemotherapy to restore normal hematopoiesis. Given the abrupt onset, prompt evaluation and intervention are required in order to successfully eradicate the disease and improve the chance of survival. Treatment of AML involves two phases of therapy: induction therapy to induce a complete remission and consolidation therapy to secure the remission. Induction therapy usually requires a 1-month hospitalization during which patients are supported with blood product support and antibiotic therapy while normal hematopoiesis is restored. Treatment for ALL involves long-term use of chemotherapy in three phases: induction, consolidation, and maintenance therapy. The total time of therapy is usually about 2 years.

Approximately 50% of patients with ALL who are younger than 15 years achieve a long-term, leukemia-free survival. Approximately 70% of all patients with AML who are younger than 60 years achieve a complete but short-lived remission; only 15% remain disease free for 5 years or more. The major cause of failure to achieve remission during induction therapy is death from hemorrhage and infection.[1]

Chronic Leukemias

CML has three phases: chronic phase, accelerated phase, and terminal blast crisis phase. The chronic phase has a duration of approximately 3 to 5 years; the durations of the other phases vary. In contrast, CLL is usually a long-term disease, with reported cases lasting 1 to 15 years.

Chronic leukemias are managed differently from acute Leukemias. CML is treated initially with tyrosine kinase inhibitors such as imatinib mesylate (Gleevec). The US Food and Drug Administration approved Gleevec for CML treatment in May 2001. The translocation between chromosomes 9 and 22, or the Philadelphia Chromosome (Ph¹), disappears in 75% of patients taking Gleevec by 18 months of therapy. Alternative treatments include the second-generation tyrosine kinase inhibitors dasatinib and nilotinib and several others approved in the past decade.[13]

CLL and small lymphocytic lymphoma are the same disease, manifesting differently. They are treated identically, and the terms are commonly used interchangeably. Initiation of treatment should be individualized and based on prognostic information, including cytogenetic aberrations and stage of disease. Treatment of CLL is not indicated for all patients. Initiation of treatment is warranted for patients who demonstrate B symptoms (fevers, drenching night sweats, and unintentional weight loss), bulky adenopathy, especially adenopathy interfering with organ function, and massive splenomegaly. Autoimmune disorders such as autoimmune hemolytic anemia and/or idiopathic thrombocytopenic purpura are not uncommon in this patient population.

Various treatment options are available for progressive CLL. Imbruvica, one of the newer targeted agents, works by disrupting several molecular signaling networks that are important for the survival and growth of CLL cells. Imbruvica has proven to be effective in newly diagnosed as well as refractory CLL. It is an oral agent taken daily without immunosuppressive effects often seen with chemotherapy. Additional therapies include enrollment in a clinical trial, various chemotherapy agents, corticosteroids, and monoclonal antibodies such as rituximab.

Stem Cell Transplant

Patients with high-risk disease, synonymous with poor prognosis, rely on allogeneic hematopoietic stem cell transplantation (HSCT) as their only chance for cure. The impact of this approach continues to be researched and numbers of transplants done continue to expand. Pre- and post-transplant regimes are changing with newer agents and better care available. Management of these patients requires a multidisciplinary approach. Expertise in transfusion management, infectious disease, care of indwelling catheters, nutrition, chemotherapy and its side effects, and psychosocial counseling is required.[14]

Non-Pharmacologic Management

There are no known non-pharmacologic interventions for the treatment of acute or chronic leukemia. Additionally, there are no proven complementary or alternative treatments.

Age, overall health, and disease-specific qualities, including morphologic classification, immunologic classification, and cytogenetic abnormalities, need to be taken into consideration when deciding treatment options. Older individuals or those in poor health may not do as well with intensive therapy.

LIFE SPAN CONSIDERATIONS

Leukemia was once thought to be a childhood disease, but 90% of the newly diagnosed cases occur in adults. AML and CLL are the most common adult forms of the disease. ALL accounts for 80% of the childhood forms.[2]

COMPLICATIONS
Tumor Lysis Syndrome

 Tumor lysis syndrome is the most common of all the oncologic emergencies.[15]

Acute tumor lysis syndrome (ATLS) is most commonly seen in patients with AML and CML who are undergoing active treatment. ATLS occurs when patients with a high WBC count, heavy tumor burden, lymphadenopathy, and/or splenomegaly receive cytotoxic chemotherapy. Tumor cell membranes can rupture and release intracellular contents into the bloodstream.[15] ATLS is characterized by the development of acute hyperuricemia, hyperkalemia, hyperphosphatemia, and hypocalcemia, with or without acute renal failure.[15] Prevention and management of these metabolic complications require close monitoring. Renal function and chemistry values should be monitored daily. Fluid balance and electrolyte disturbances should be corrected with vigorous intravenous hydration and diuretics as indicated. The addition of sodium bicarbonate to maintain urinary alkalization is recommended, as is the use of allopurinol to decrease serum uric acid levels. If preventive

measures are not effective, rasburicase can be used intravenously to rapidly break down serum uric acid. Monitoring with daily laboratory tests, weights, meticulous assessment of intake and output, and observation for signs and symptoms of fluid overload are critical in caring for this patient population. ATLS ordinarily resolves within 4 to 7 days if adequate renal function is maintained.

Disseminated Intravascular Coagulation

DIC is a hematologic disorder that occurs when there is an alteration in the blood-clotting mechanism. Acute promyelocytic leukemia (APL), the M3 subtype of AML, is most often associated with DIC. DIC can be acute or chronic and related to either the disease process or the treatment regimen. DIC is the most common serious hypercoagulable state that occurs in patients with cancer.[16] It is an event in which both clotting and hemorrhage exist simultaneously.

Acute leukemia, antineoplastic agents, infection, trauma, and hemolytic transfusion reactions interrupt normal body hemostasis and may initiate an episode of DIC. Spontaneous hemorrhage or the slow occult damage of multiple small clot formation within the lungs, organs of the CNS, or gastrointestinal tract may herald the presentation of DIC. Organ dysfunction from circulatory impairment leads to mental status changes, severe muscle pain, oliguria, and slowed gastrointestinal motility.[16] Symptoms may range from mild chronic episodes to acute and life-threatening incidents.

Abnormal laboratory findings suggest a diagnosis of DIC. A decreased platelet count, a prolonged prothrombin and partial thromboplastin time, and a decreased fibrinogen level with an elevation of fibrin degradation products confirm the diagnosis of DIC.[16]

Treatment of the underlying cause of DIC is vital. Hemorrhage is treated with replacement of fluids and blood component therapy; infection is treated with antibiotics; and cancer is treated with radiotherapy, chemotherapy, or surgery as indicated. Heparin therapy is more commonly used for the chronic DIC of malignant disease associated with thrombotic, thromboembolic, or necrotizing complications. Thorough, multiple system assessments in combination with patient and family education and involvement are necessary to prevent further injury and complications associated with DIC.

Leukostasis

The predominant cell in acute leukemia is undifferentiated or immature, usually a blast cell. In leukostasis, blood sludging or stasis occurs when the blood vessels become overcrowded with these blast cells. Individuals with high WBC counts and a large tumor burden are at risk for development of leukostasis. The small, delicate pulmonary and cranial vessels are the most susceptible. If leukostasis is left untreated, rupture and hemorrhage result in ischemia and infarct. Emergent treatment includes high-dose chemotherapy or cranial radiotherapy to decrease the number of circulating blast cells. Leukapheresis (the removal of WBCs from the plasma) may also be indicated.[1]

Pancytopenia

Regardless of the treatment regimen chosen, infection, bleeding, and symptomatic anemia are the most common side effects of leukemia and its therapy. The desired effect of treatment is severe myelosuppression, which puts the patient at risk for multiple complications. Prolonged periods of neutropenia leave the immunocompromised patient especially susceptible to infection. Until normal bone marrow function is restored, the leukemic patient lacks the normal host responses. Treatment with empirical antibiotics to prevent systemic or disseminated infection is indicated once infection is suspected. Prevention of infection must focus on providing meticulous care with any invasive treatment option and limiting unnecessary invasive procedures.[17] Education empowers patients and their families to participate in their own health practices.

Fatigue

One of the most common symptoms associated with cancer and cancer therapies is fatigue. Chronic low-grade anemia, stress, and alterations in sleeping, eating, and working are known to deplete energy levels. Fatigue can be one of the most disabling complications of cancer and chemotherapy treatments, perpetuating feelings of hopelessness and powerlessness. Supportive transfusion or erythropoietin therapies may be used to correct the anemia, exercise is encouraged, and many patients find support groups beneficial.[1]

PATIENT EDUCATION AND HEALTH PROMOTION

The educational goal for leukemia patients and their families is prevention of complications of the disease process and treatment, management of side effects, and access to community resources.

The bone marrow suppression of leukemia can be life-threatening. This may be a result of either the disease process itself or the chemotherapy instituted to treat the leukemia.

It is the health care team's responsibility to educate the patient and family about the numerous other effects of leukemia and its treatment, such as fever, headache, mucositis, nausea, vomiting, anorexia, diarrhea, constipation, pain, fatigue, insomnia, and depression. Patient self-care information is given in Box 218.1. After a leukemia diagnosis, patients will still require other cancer screening tests specific for age, including mammograms, Papanicolaou smears, prostate-specific antigen tests, and fecal occult blood testing. Other health-promoting activities include stopping smoking, maintaining normal weight, and getting adequate exercise.

BOX **218.1**

Patient Education and Self-Care Strategies

LEUKOPENIA OR INFECTION

Cancer and cancer therapies can increase one's risk of infection by lowering the WBC count and altering the physical barriers of the skin and gastrointestinal mucosa, thereby allowing organisms to enter the body and cause infection.

Prevention and Management Strategies
- Stay away from crowds and people who are sick when your WBC counts are low.
- Wash hands with soap and water often. Use hand sanitizer when soap and water are unavailable.
- Maintain good mouth care and take good care of your skin.
- Serial monitoring of the WBC count throughout treatment and chemotherapy and the disease state may make your WBC count low, increasing the risk of infection.
- Wash raw vegetable and fruits well before eating them. Do not eat raw or undercooked fish, seafood, meat, chicken, or eggs.
- Take temperature twice daily and immediately report any signs or symptoms of infection, including temperature elevation above 100.5°F, shaking chills, productive cough, shortness of breath, redness, swelling, rash, headache, stiff neck, painful or frequent urination, or sinus pain or pressure.

THROMBOCYTOPENIA

Thrombocytopenia results from a low platelet count. Platelets are the cells that make your blood clot. Chemotherapy can lower the number of platelets by interfering with the bone marrow's ability to make them. Low platelets can result in increased bruising or bleeding.

Prevention and Management Strategies
- Brush your teeth with a soft toothbrush.
- Blow your nose gently.
- Use electric razors for shaving.
- Apply extra caution when using sharp objects.
- Avoid aspirin and nonsteroidal agents because they can interfere with the functioning of the platelet.

- Immediately report any signs or symptoms of thrombocytopenia including bruising, nosebleeds, bleeding gums, blood in the urine or stool, heavy bleeding during a menstrual period or a prolonged period, headaches or visual changes, or feeling very sleepy or confused.

ANEMIA

Anemia is a condition in which there are not enough healthy red blood cells to carry adequate oxygen to your tissues, resulting in excessive fatigue, lightheadedness, weakness, shortness of breath, and chest pain. Some types of chemotherapy cause anemia because they make it harder for the bone marrow to produce red blood cells. Anemia may also result from the disease overtaking the bone marrow, the factory of all blood cells.

Prevention and Management Strategies
- Get plenty of rest.
- Limit exercise and exertional activities. Take frequent rest periods.
- Eat a well-balanced diet.
- When moving from one position to another, do so slowly.
- Discuss whether blood transfusions or erythroid-stimulating agents would be helpful.
- Immediately report any signs or symptoms of anemia, including lightheadedness, shortness of breath, ringing in the ears, pounding heart, increased heart rate, palpitation.

MUCOSITIS

Mucositis is the painful inflammation and ulceration of the mucous membranes lining the digestive tract, usually as an adverse effect of chemotherapy and radiotherapy treatment for cancer.

Prevention and Management Strategies
- Keep the mouth and lips moist.
- See the dentist regularly, ideally before cancer treatments begin.
- Perform good oral hygiene, brushing teeth with a soft toothbrush after meals; use only alcohol-free mouthwash.

BOX **218.1**

Patient Education and Self-Care Strategies—cont'd

- Rinse mouth with salt water (half teaspoon of salt in 8 ounces of water) after brushing and flossing.
- Eat a well-balanced diet including foods high in protein.
- Choose foods that are moist, soft, and easy to chew or swallow when your mouth is sore.
- Avoid hot, spicy, or acidic foods.
- Avoid alcohol and tobacco.
- Work with health care providers to control oral pain, bleeding, and infection.

CHEMOTHERAPY-INDUCED NAUSEA AND VOMITING

Chemotherapy-induced nausea and vomiting (CINV) continues to have a considerable effect on the physical and psychological well-being of patients with cancer. It can be classified as anticipatory (a conditioned response triggered when exposed to some stimuli), acute (occurring within 24 h of chemotherapy administration), delayed (occurring after 24 h and lasting up to 7 days), breakthrough (occurring despite prophylactic medications), and refractory (occurring because of a failure of prophylactic and breakthrough medications to control the symptoms).

Prevention and Management Strategies
- Use antiemetics proactively at the first sign of nausea.
- Reduce food odors that might trigger nausea.
- Eat small, frequent meals composed of "comfort foods."
- Chew gum or suck on hard candies if you are experiencing taste changes.
- Stay well hydrated.
- Avoid foods that are too hot or too cold.
- Do not eat fatty, fried, spicy, or salty foods when nauseous.
- Use good oral hygiene, especially after meals.

DIARRHEA

Diarrhea is an abnormal increase in the liquidity and frequency of stools. Chemotherapy can cause diarrhea because it damages the healthy rapidly dividing cells that line the lower gastrointestinal tract. Left untreated, diarrhea can result in dehydration, weakness, weight loss, electrolyte imbalances, and poor nutrition.

Prevention and Management Strategies
- Stop taking laxatives and stool softeners.
- Take antidiarrheal medications as prescribed.
- Eat small frequent meals.
- Stay hydrated by drinking 8–12 cups of noncaffeinated beverages daily.
- Eat a low-fiber diet to avoid stimulating the bowel motility.
- Avoid caffeine, alcohol, and milk products, which can exacerbate the diarrhea.
- Avoid greasy, fried foods and foods that cause increased gas.

CONSTIPATION

Constipation is a condition in which there is difficulty in emptying the bowels, usually associated with hardened feces.

Prevention and Management Strategies
- Drink at least 8–10 glasses of fluids a day.
- Eat foods high in dietary fiber and avoid foods that are constipating.
- Stay active and exercise daily.

- Take laxatives and stool softeners as prescribed.
- Minimize, as possible, the use of medications that constipate, such as narcotics.
- If bowels do not move in 48 hours, call health care provider.

ALOPECIA

Alopecia is defined as loss of hair from the body. Some types of chemotherapy damage the cells that cause hair growth. Most of the time the hair on the head is lost first, but hair over the body can be lost as well. Hair loss is often a cause of great concern to the patient for cosmetic and psychological reasons but is a temporary side effect of chemotherapy. Hair loss can start 2–3 weeks after chemotherapy starts, and hair often grows back 2–3 months after chemotherapy is completed.

Prevention and Management Strategies
- Cut hair short before hair loss begins; this often makes it easier to manage.
- Avoid perming, dying, or chemically treating hair during chemotherapy, because this may irritate the scalp.
- Consider purchasing a wig or hair prosthesis.
- Protect scalp once hair falls out by applying sunscreen or wearing a hat or scarf.
- Keep the head warm; a great deal of body heat is lost through a bare scalp.
- Sleep on a satin pillowcase for increased comfort and less friction.
- Talk with others about your feelings.

FATIGUE

Fatigue is a common problem for patients during and after cancer treatment. It is a constant state of weariness that develops over time and diminishes your energy and mental capacity. Fatigue at this level affects your emotional and psychological well-being.

Prevention and Management Strategies
- Maintain good nutrition and hydration.
- Take a multivitamin supplement.
- Moderate daily exercise with rest periods.
- Improve sleep quality and quantity.
- Schedule activities for times of peak energy and focus.

INSOMNIA

Insomnia is a persistent disorder that can make it hard to fall asleep, hard to stay asleep, or both, despite the opportunity for adequate sleep. It can occur at times of higher-than-usual stress. With insomnia, you usually awaken feeling unrefreshed, which takes a toll on your ability to function during the day. Insomnia can sap not only your energy level and mood but also your health, work performance, and quality of life. Improving your sleep restores function of your body and mind, reduces other symptoms, and allows you to function and care for yourself and others.

Prevention and Management Strategies
- Keep to a consistent bedtime and wake time.
- Use bedroom for sleep and sexual activity only; avoid watching television or using the computer in bed because these activities are stimulating.
- Avoid sleeping excessively during the day. If a nap is needed, limit it to less than 1 hour.

Continued

BOX **218.1**

Patient Education and Self-Care Strategies—cont'd

- Get regular exercise.
- Avoid caffeinated beverages before bed.
- Seek treatment for conditions that can interfere with sleep, such as pain, hot flashes, anxiety, depression, shortness of breath, fever.

DEPRESSION

Depression is a mood disorder that causes a persistent feeling of sadness and loss of interest that affects how you feel, think, and behave and can lead to a variety of emotional and physical problems. You may have trouble doing normal day-to-day activities, and sometimes you may feel

as if life isn't worth living. Most people with depression feel better with medication, psychological counseling, or both.

Prevention and Management Strategies

- Avoid alcohol, because it has a depressive effect.
- Discuss your feelings with your health care team.
- Consider joining a support group.
- Discuss pharmacologic interventions for depression and take as directed.
- Eat a well-balanced diet, exercise daily, and get plenty of rest.

Modified from Yarbro, C., Wujcik, D., Gobel, B. H., et al. (2013). *Cancer symptom management* (4th ed.). Burlington, MA: Jones and Bartlett.[18]

REFERENCES

1. Leukemia and Lymphoma Society. Leukemia. Retrieved from http://www.lls.org/blog/what-s-new-in-all-current-and-emerging-treatments. (Accessed 27 January 2016).
2. Leukemia and Lymphoma Society. Leukemia, Facts and Statistics. Retrieved from https://www.lls.org/http%3A/llsorg.prod.acquia-sites.com/facts-and-statistics/facts-and-statistics-overview/facts-and-statistics#Leukemia. (Accessed 28 July 2019).
3. Siegel, R. L., Miller, K. D., & Jemal, A. (2019). Cancer statistics, 2019. https://doi.org/10.3322/caac.21551.
4. Raffel, G. (2015). Acute leukemias. In V. T. DaVita Jr., S. Hellman, & S. A. Rosenberg (Eds.), *Cancer: Principles and practice of oncology* (8th ed.). Philadelphia: Lippincott Williams & Wilkins.
5. Ladou, J., & Harrison, R. (2014). *Current occcupational and environmental medicine.* Burr Ridge, IL: McGraw-Hill.
6. Schupback, J. (2013). *Human retrovirology; facts and concepts.* New York: Springer Science and Business Media.
7. Czader, M., & Orazi, A. (2015). Therapy-related myeloid neoplasms. *American Journal of Clinical Pathology, 144*(2), 207–218.
8. Clevers, H. (2015). What is an adult stem cell? *Science, 350*(6266), 1319–1320.
9. Talcott, K., Garg, R., & Garg, S. (2016). Ophthalmic manifestation of leukemia. *Current Opinion in Ophthalmology, 27*(6), 545–551.
10. Del Principe, M., Maurillo, L., Buccisano, F., et al. (2014). Central nervous system involvement in adult acute lymphoblastic leukemia; diagnostic tools, prophylaxis and therapy. *Mediterranean Journal of Hematology and Infectious Diseases, 6*(1), e2014075.
11. Agarwal, A., Byrd, J. C., & Deininger, M. (2012). Chronic leukemia. In V. T. DaVita Jr., T. S. Lawrence, & S. A. Rosenberg (Eds.), *Cancer: Principles and practice of oncology* (10th ed.). Philadelphia: Lippincott Williams & Wilkins.
12. Ezzone, S. (2002). *Hematopoetic Stem cell transplantation: A manual for nursing practice* (2nd ed.). Pittsburgh: Oncology Nursing Society.
13. Wu, P., Nielson, T., & Clausen, M. (2016). Small molecule kinase inhibitors: An analysis of FDA-approved drugs. *Drug Discovery Today, 21*(1), 5–10.
14. Passweg, J. R., Baldomero, P., Bader, P., et al. (2017). Use of haploidentical stem cell transplantation continues to increase. The 2015 European society for blood and marrow transplant activity survey report. *Bone Marrow Transplantation, 52*, 811–817.
15. Chung, H., & Tsyvkin, E. (2016). Tumor lysis syndrome. *Hospital Medicine Clinics, 5*(3), 425–438.
16. Perkins, J. C., & Davis, J. E. (2014). Hematology/oncology emergencies. *Emergency Medicine Clinics of North America, 32*(3), xvii–xviii.
17. Blamble, D. Prevention of infectious complications in patients with chronic lymphocytic leukemia. Retrieved from www.infectiousdiseasenews.com/article/618767.aspx. (Accessed August 2015).
18. Yarbro, C., & Wujcik, D. (2013). *Cancer symptom management* (4th ed.). Burlington, Mass: Jones and Bartlett.

CHAPTER **219**

LYMPHOMAS

Varghese Mathai

DEFINITION AND EPIDEMIOLOGY

Lymphomas are clonal disorders that arise from lymphocytes (B or T cells; rarely, natural killer [NK] cells). They are rare and extremely heterogeneous secondary to numerous histologic subtypes and variable clinical presentations. This heterogeneity has important prognostic implications on whether treatment is administered with curative intent. The focus of this chapter is twofold: (1) to enable an understanding of the diagnosis, staging, and initial evaluation of a lymphoma patient, and (2) to describe how the most common lymphoid malignancies are managed.

The estimates from the Surveillance, Epidemiology, and End Results (SEER) Program for 2018 revealed that non-Hodgkin lymphoma (NHL) was the seventh most common type of cancer. NHL and Hodgkin lymphoma (HL) represented 4.3% of new cancer cases (NHL, 70,800; HL, 9190) and 3.3% of cancer deaths in 2015. The incidence of these disorders has increased approximately twofold over the last 30 years, with a slight male predominance.[1] The cause is unclear, but the increase is most significant in older patients with aggressive lymphoma. Many associate the increase in NHL with the human immunodeficiency virus (HIV), but with the widespread use of antiretroviral therapies, the incidence of lymphoma has begun to decline.

ETIOLOGY AND RISK FACTORS

The many different forms of lymphoma have varied causes. The possible causes and associations with at least some forms of NHL include the following:

- Infectious agents
  - Epstein-Barr virus—associated with Burkitt lymphoma, HL, follicular dendritic cell sarcoma, extranodal NK-T-cell lymphoma[2]
  - Human T-cell leukemia virus—associated with adult T-cell lymphoma
  - *Helicobacter pylori*—associated with gastric lymphoma

- Human herpesvirus 8 (HHV-8)—associated with primary effusion lymphoma, multicentric Castleman disease
- Hepatitis C virus—associated with splenic marginal zone lymphoma, lymphoplasmacytic lymphoma, and diffuse large B-cell lymphoma (DLBCL)[3]
- HIV infection[4]
- Chemicals: polychlorinated biphenyls (PCBs), diphenylhydantoin, dioxin, and phenoxy herbicides[5]
- Medical treatments, including radiation therapy and chemotherapy
- Genetic diseases, including Klinefelter syndrome, Chédiak-Higashi syndrome, ataxia-telangiectasia syndrome[6]
- Autoimmune diseases: Sjögren syndrome, rheumatoid arthritis, and systemic lupus erythematosus (SLE)

CLINICAL PRESENTATION

The clinical presentation of HL and NHL varies and is dependent on the type of lymphoma and the area of involvement. Many patients have lymphadenopathy (see Chapter 205). In general, lymph nodes persisting for more than 4 weeks and lymph nodes larger than normal (up to 1.5 cm) will require intervention. In aggressive and highly aggressive NHLs, the lymphadenopathy increases quickly. Node size can wax and wane in more indolent lymphomas. "B" symptoms are often present in disseminated disease. These include fever higher than 38°C, drenching night sweats, and unintentional weight loss of more than 10% of body weight.

The physical exam should focus on the size and distribution of lymph nodes and the presence (and size of) or absence of a palpable liver or spleen. See type-specific discussion later.

Making the Diagnosis

After initial evaluation, proper histologic diagnosis and precise classification of the lymphoid neoplasm are the starting points for proper management. To allow for full assessment, an excisional biopsy is preferred when possible (versus core biopsy) to make the initial diagnosis of lymphoma. If a patient has already been treated for NHL or HL and a relapse is suspected, then core biopsy will suffice. The demonstration of monoclonality in biopsied tissue is diagnostic for lymphoma. The absence of monoclonality should make the underlying diagnosis questionable, and a repeat biopsy will likely be necessary.

Classification

Several classification systems have existed over the decades and continue to evolve. The latest, most comprehensive classification is the World Health Organization (WHO) classification developed in 2008 and updated in 2016.[7] The WHO classification is broken down by cell of origin (B, T, or NK) and by cell maturity.

The WHO modification of the Revised European-American Lymphoma (REAL) classification recognizes three major categories of lymphoid malignancies based on morphology and cell lineage: B-cell neoplasms, T-cell/NK-cell neoplasms, and HL. Both lymphomas and lymphoid leukemias are included in this classification because both solid and circulating phases are present in many lymphoid neoplasms, and distinction between them is artificial. Within the B-cell and T-cell categories, two subdivisions are recognized: precursor neoplasms, which correspond to the earliest stages of differentiation, and more mature differentiated neoplasms.[8]

Staging

Staging is the way to identify the extent of tumor and whether it has spread either within an organ or beyond. Staging can also determine treatment options and identify clinical trials that may be available. The Ann Arbor staging classification, modified at Cotswold's meeting in 1989, has traditionally been used for patients with lymphoma. This system divides lymphoma into four stages (I–IV) and further subclassifies these into A and B categories. The B designation is applied to individuals with any of the following well-defined generalized symptoms (often referred to as "B" symptoms):

- Unexplained loss of 10% or greater body weight in the 6 months before diagnosis
- Unexplained fever higher than 38°C
- Drenching night sweats

The International Conference on Malignant Lymphomas met in Lugano, Italy in 2014 and created a modification of the Ann Arbor system, now widely accepted as the Lugano modification of the Ann Arbor system.[9] This newer modification recommends using PET-CT imaging as a precise measure of extent of disease, thereby avoiding, in many cases, bone marrow biopsy, formerly the gold standard in diagnosis.

Bone marrow biopsy is usually not required if the PET-CT scan indicates bone or marrow involvement but if the scan is negative, a bone marrow biopsy may be indicated to identify marrow involvement. Lumbar puncture fluid should be examined in highly aggressive lymphomas (Burkitt and lymphoblastic) and with aggressive lymphomas with multiple extranodal sites, paraspinal disease, or testicular or paranasal sinus involvement.

HODGKIN LYMPHOMA

PATHOPHYSIOLOGY

HL, formerly called Hodgkin disease, arises from germinal center or post-germinal center B cells. HL has a unique cellular composition, containing a minority of neoplastic cells (Reed-Sternberg cells and their variants) in an inflammatory background[10] containing a variable number of small lymphocytes, eosinophils, neutrophils, histiocytes, plasma cells, fibroblasts, and collagen fibers. Morphologic features also determine the various subtypes of classical HL.

It is separated from the other B-cell lymphomas based on its unique clinicopathologic features, and can be divided into two major subgroups based on the appearance and immunophenotype of the tumor cells.

Classical Hodgkin Lymphoma

The tumor cells in the classical HL group are also derived from germinal center B cells, but typically fail to express many of the genes and gene products that define normal germinal center B cells. Based on differences in the appearance of the tumor cells and the composition of the reactive background, classical HL is further divided into the following subtypes:

- Nodular sclerosis classical Hodgkin Lymphoma (NSHL)
- Mixed cellularity classical Hodgkin Lymphoma (MCHL)
- Lymphocyte-rich classical Hodgkin Lymphoma (LRHL)
- Lymphocyte-depleted classical Hodgkin Lymphoma (LDHL)

Nodular Lymphocyte-Predominant Hodgkin Lymphoma

The tumor cells in this subtype retain the immunophenotypic features of germinal center B cells.

CLINICAL PRESENTATION AND PHYSICAL EXAMINATION

The initial evaluation includes the patient's history and a complete physical examination (including assessment of functional status using standardized scales such as the ECOG/Zubrod scale or the Karnofsky performance scale, both available online). Patients usually have painless adenopathy localized to the neck. The mediastinum is involved in the majority of patients, occasionally with large mediastinal masses. The liver and/or spleen may be enlarged. B symptoms are present in 20% to 25% of patients. Pruritus is common. On rare occasions, patients may experience pain in involved lymph nodes on ingesting alcohol—thought to be a result of alcohol-induced degranulation of eosinophils.

DIAGNOSTICS
Essential Diagnostics

The diagnosis of HL is made by the microscopic evaluation of involved tissue, usually obtained from a lymph node biopsy. Excisional biopsies are preferred, and large core needle biopsies may be adequate in select cases, but fine-needle aspiration (FNA) alone often does not provide enough tissue or information on the structural composition of the lymph node to enable an accurate diagnosis. Evaluation of the biopsy material should include both routine light microscopy and analysis of the immunophenotype with immunohistochemistry.

A complete blood count (CBC), electrolytes, liver and renal function studies, lactate dehydrogenase (LDH), infectious disease panel (hepatitis B and C, HIV), and examination of the peripheral smear for the presence of atypical cells are initial diagnostics usually done before the biopsy.

Additional Diagnostics

May include a bone marrow biopsy and aspiration, fluorodeoxyglucose/positron emission tomography (FDG/PET), and computed tomography (CT) scan with intravenous and oral contrast.

INITIAL DIAGNOSTICS

Lymphomas

LABORATORY
- Lymph node biopsy (core biopsy or excisional biopsy)
- CBC and differential
- Serum electrolytes, blood urea nitrogen (BUN), creatinine
- Liver function tests (LFTs)
- Serologic evaluation for Epstein-Barr virus
- HIV test
- Toxoplasmosis titer

IMAGING
- Chest x-ray examination
- CT scan of chest, abdomen, pelvis, head (preferably all with contrast)
- FDG/PET scan[a]

OTHER DIAGNOSTICS
- Bone marrow biopsy

[a]If indicated.

DIFFERENTIAL DIAGNOSIS

Lymphadenopathy may be a primary or secondary sign of numerous disorders including infectious diseases, immunologic disorders, and malignancies (see Chapter 205). A patient with unexplained lymphadenopathy persistent for 1 month should be referred for biopsy to rule out malignant disease.

PROGNOSIS

Predicting the outcome is important to avoid over treating patients with HL and to identify others in whom standard treatment is likely to fail. Prognosticating outcome also helps patients and providers make often difficult treatment decisions. The Hasenclever Index for HL is commonly used.[11] Seven factors with similar independent prognostic effects were selected. The prognostic score was then defined as the number of adverse prognostic factors present at diagnosis. The prognostic score was used to predict rates of freedom from progression of disease and overall survival.

A score of 1 is given for each of the following risk factors present at diagnosis. The higher the score, the greater the risk of progressive disease or death within 5 years.
- Age older than 45 years
- Male gender
- Serum albumin below 4 g/dL
- Hemoglobin (Hb) below 10.5 g/dL
- Stage IV disease
- White blood cell (WBC) count ≥15,000/mm3
- Lymphopenia—fewer than 600/mm^3 or <8% of White Cell Count

   (Erythrocyte sedimentation rate >50 mm/h now being considered although not a part of the original criteria)

INTERPROFESSIONAL COLLABORATIVE MANAGEMENT

Over the past century, HL has been converted from a uniformly fatal disease to one that is curable in approximately 80% of patients worldwide.[11] Although the majority of patients will be cured of their lymphoma, treatment-related toxicities have become a competing cause of late mortality. Accordingly, the selection of therapy must balance the desire to maintain a high rate of cure and the need to minimize long-term complications. Treatment has evolved such that patients with early-stage disease can achieve long-term remission with less intensive therapy, whereas more intensive therapy is reserved for patients with advanced-stage disease.

Combination chemotherapy is the cornerstone of HL treatment. Adriamycin, bleomycin, vinblastine, and dacarbazine (ABVD) combination chemotherapy appears to have the best overall efficacy with the least acute and chronic toxicity.

Selection of initial treatment for HL is usually based on presenting stage and prognostic factors. Most patients receive systemic chemotherapy either alone or as part of a combined modality treatment program with radiation. The need for proper staging is imperative because radiation therapy is not typically used in advanced-stage HL.

For patients with early-stage disease, there is subsequent stratification into favorable and unfavorable prognosis disease based upon the presence or absence of certain clinical features discussed above, the number of regions involved, and the presence of large mediastinal adenopathy. For patients with early-stage favorable disease, chemotherapy plus involved site radiation therapy or chemotherapy alone are possible options. The choice must be made on an individual basis, weighing against potential side effects secondary to age, gender, and location of tumor.[12]

Advanced-stage HL refers to clinical stage III and IV disease, although many experts and clinical trials include patients with stage II plus bulky nodal disease.

Combination chemotherapy is the main treatment for patients with advanced-stage HL. Radiation therapy may be used for select patients as consolidation.

Patients with HL who relapse after prior treatment with chemotherapy are generally treated with either conventional chemotherapy combined with radiation therapy or high-dose chemotherapy and autologous hematopoietic cell transplantation (HCT) given with or without radiation therapy.[12] The choice of therapy is usually based on prognostic features.

Salvage chemotherapy is administered in two phases: first a conventional-dose regimen to achieve major reduction in tumor bulk and promote mobilization of stem cell into the peripheral blood, followed by high-dose therapy with stem cell support.

About half the patients destined to relapse will do so in the first year after treatment, and nearly all the relapses occur within 5 years of treatment. It is common to follow patients every few months for the first couple of years, gradually extending the interval between visits.

Primary refractory (resistant) disease refers to patients who do not attain a complete remission after initial therapy. The incidence of primary refractory disease varies depending on the stage of disease at diagnosis and the treatment regimen used. Durable responses and remissions may be achieved in approximately half these patients with second-line chemotherapy that incorporates drugs not used in initial treatment followed by high-dose chemotherapy and autologous hematopoietic cell rescue.[13] Resistant disease following autologous stem cell rescue is generally associated with poor prognosis but recent success with the anti-TNF brentuximab vedotin (Adcetris) is encouraging.[13]

HL survivors are at risk of developing therapy-related complications that may manifest years after treatment, including second malignancies, cardiac disease, thyroid nodules, and radiation-induced hypothyroidism. Patients who have received mantle irradiation are at higher risk of cardiomyopathy, pericarditis, pneumonitis, and pulmonary fibrosis.[14] These complications have surfaced as significant causes of increased mortality among survivors. Screening for some of these entities is advised in the hope that early detection may lead to better management.

NON-HODGKIN LYMPHOMA

DEFINITION

This disease category consists of some 40 different types of lymphomas with a predilection for older adults with a male predominance.

PATHOPHYSIOLOGY

The molecular biology research on NHL has begun to identify clues to the pathogenesis of some of these disorders. Basically, these are tumors originating from lymphoid tissue, mostly B cells but occasionally T or NK cells, perhaps in response to

previous exposure to Epstein-Barr virus of human herpesvirus. Prior treatment with radiation or chemotherapy for HL seems to be associated with higher risk of NHL.[15]

CLINICAL PRESENTATION

The clinical presentation of NHL varies tremendously depending on the type of lymphoma and the areas of involvement. Some NHLs behave indolently, with lymphadenopathy waxing and waning over years. Others are highly aggressive, resulting in death within weeks if left untreated. In typical cases, the following clinical presentations occur:

- Aggressive lymphomas commonly manifest acutely or subacutely with a rapidly growing mass, systemic B symptoms (i.e., fever, night sweats, weight loss), and/or elevated levels of serum LDH and uric acid. Examples of lymphomas with this aggressive or highly aggressive presentation include DLBCL, Burkitt lymphoma, adult T-cell leukemia-lymphoma, and precursor B and T lymphoblastic leukemia and lymphoma.
- Indolent lymphomas are often insidious, manifesting only with slow-growing lymphadenopathy, hepatomegaly, splenomegaly, or cytopenias. Examples of lymphomas that typically have indolent presentations include follicular lymphoma (FL), chronic lymphocytic leukemia or small lymphocytic lymphoma, and splenic marginal zone lymphoma.

DIAGNOSTICS

Most patients with enlarged lymph nodes have a benign form of reactive lymphadenopathy often related to infection or inflammation (see Chapter 205). An unexplained enlarged node present for 1 month or longer should be investigated further. Many centers continue to use FNA as an initial screening test. When coupled with comprehensive immunophenotyping (typically flow cytometry), FNA is particularly useful at distinguishing reactive B-cell hyperplasias from clonal mature B-cell neoplasms. However, the general consensus is that accurate histopathologic evaluation of lymphomas requires a tissue biopsy, preferably an intact lymph node, and that FNAs suggesting the presence of a lymphoma should be followed up with a definitive tissue biopsy.[16]

FNA may provide enough information to confirm a recurrence in previously diagnosed patients.

The Ann Arbor staging system is also used for NHL to provide treatment, prognostic, and clinical trial data. Prognosticating outcomes has been a moving target over the past several years with the introduction of chemoimmunotherapy agents such as rituximab. As treatments improve, the hope for better individual prognostication will be realized.

The staging workup should also include PET-CT scan, and FDG/PET scan of chest, abdomen, and pelvis. In combination, these two scans changed the staging criteria of the disease, which has also resulted in a change in the treatment choices.

INTERDISCIPLINARY COLLABORATIVE MANAGEMENT

Indolent (Formerly Known as Low-Grade) Lymphomas

FL is the second most common subtype of NHL and the most common of the indolent NHLs, defined as those lymphomas in which survival of the untreated patient is measured in years. Treatment of FL depends on the stage of disease at presentation as evaluated by the Ann Arbor staging system.

Most patients with stage I or nonbulky stage II FL initiate treatment with radiation therapy rather than treatment with chemotherapy or an initial period of observation. This is principally based on the observation that some patients may have prolonged progression-free survival with radiation therapy. If significant morbidity is expected from radiotherapy based on the location of the tumor, or if the patient decides against radiotherapy, a management approach similar to that used for advanced-stage disease may be a reasonable alternative.

For patients with previously untreated advanced-stage FL who require therapy, the recommended treatment is an immunotherapy-based regimen or chemotherapy. A choice among the various regimens depends on patient characteristics and physician comfort. Bendamustine plus rituximab (BR) has been shown to improve the progression-free survival rates with less toxicity when compared with rituximab, cyclophosphamide, doxorubicin, vincristine, and prednisone (R-CHOP).[17] R-CHOP may be preferred for patients with more aggressive histologic grade 3A disease.

Patients with asymptomatic recurrent FL do not require immediate treatment but should be followed closely for the development of symptomatic disease. Patients with symptomatic FL or those with an increase in disease tempo require treatment. Because relapse is common in indolent lymphoma, a biopsy should be conducted to rule out transformation to a higher grade lymphoma.

There is no standard therapy for patients with relapsed or refractory FL and practice varies widely; accordingly, patients should be encouraged to participate in clinical trials whenever possible. A choice among potential therapies must take into account characteristics of both the tumor and the patient as well as an evaluation of the initial response to treatment.

For most patients with relapsed or refractory FL, treatment with rituximab either alone or in combination with chemotherapy is the treatment of choice. The option between single-agent rituximab and combination chemotherapy plus rituximab depends largely on the patient's tumor burden and performance status. For patients with a poor performance status and/or a clinically indolent course, single-agent rituximab may be an option because of its relatively low toxicity profile.

The decision of whether to proceed with HCT should be based on the patient's preference and condition and the expected disease course. For the disease course, there is no definitive score or metric. For eligible patients who relapse after a short initial response (i.e., <1 year) to chemoimmunotherapy and demonstrate chemotherapy-sensitive disease, allogeneic HCT should be considered.

Aggressive Lymphomas

DLBCL is the most common histologic subtype of NHL. It is an aggressive NHL in which survival without treatment is measured in months. Advanced-stage DLBCL cannot be contained within one irradiation field, and this population accounts for 60% to 70% of patients with DLBCL.

For patients with advanced DLBCL, an anthracycline-based combination chemotherapy regimen plus rituximab is recommended—specifically, six to eight cycles of R-CHOP-21.[18] There is no role for the routine use of maintenance rituximab or high-dose chemotherapy with autologous hematopoietic cell rescue in first complete remission.

There is general agreement that patients with testicular, epidural, or sinus involvement are at increased risk of developing CNS disease. The evidence for an increased risk of CNS relapse is less strong for other scenarios that are still considered high risk (e.g., patients with breast or ovarian involvement, concordant bone marrow involvement, a high International Prognostic Index [IPI] score, or numerous extranodal sites of disease).

Relapsed or refractory DLBCL is treated with systemic chemotherapy with or without rituximab with plans to proceed to high-dose chemotherapy and autologous HCT in those with chemotherapy-sensitive disease.[19] The treatment of patients who are not candidates for HCT, who fail to respond to second-line chemotherapy regimens, or who relapse after HCT is generally palliative. Enrollment in a clinical trial can be an option.

Highly Aggressive Lymphomas

Burkitt lymphoma (BL), or small noncleaved cell lymphoma, is a highly aggressive B-cell NHL characterized by the translocation and deregulation of the *c-myc* gene on chromosome 8. The standard of care has yet to be defined, and enrollment in a clinical trial may be the best option where available. However, for patients who are not candidates for such trials or for those who choose not to participate, intensive, short-duration combination chemotherapy with central nervous system (CNS) prophylaxis is indicated. Dose reduction should be avoided if at all possible, and therapy should be initiated quickly. Infusional chemotherapy with dose-adjusted etoposide, vincristine, doxorubicin, cyclophosphamide, and prednisone (EPOCH) plus rituximab is an acceptable alternative for patients who may not tolerate more aggressive regimens (e.g., older or less-fit patients).

Various intensive, short-duration combination chemotherapy regimens have been studied in patients with BL. These include CODOX-M (cyclophosphamide, vincristine, doxorubicin, high-dose methotrexate) with IVAC (ifosfamide, cytarabine, etoposide, and intrathecal methotrexate).

There is a paucity of data to guide the treatment of patients with recurrent or refractory BL. Whenever possible, patients should be encouraged to participate in clinical trials. Outside of a clinical trial, patients with refractory disease and those who relapse after an initial response to appropriate initial therapy have an extremely poor prognosis and should be considered for best supportive or palliative care. An important exception concerns the patient who did not receive appropriate initial therapy.

Another type of highly aggressive lymphoma is double hit lymphoma (DHL). DHL refers to cases of lymphoma that contain genetic translocations of MYC gene BCL2 and/or BCL6. This type of lymphoma should be differentiated from double expressor lymphomas because prognosis is better for the latter.

T-Cell Lymphomas

The peripheral T-cell lymphomas (PTCLs) are a heterogeneous group of typically aggressive neoplasms that constitute less than 15% of all NHLs in adults. There is no general consensus regarding the optimal treatment regimen for these patients, and all patients should be encouraged to participate in clinical trials where available.

For most patients with newly diagnosed PTCL, induction combination chemotherapy with a cyclophosphamide, doxorubicin, vincristine, prednisone (CHOP)-based regimen is preferred rather than more intensive induction regimens.[20]

For patients younger than 60 years, the use of CHOP plus etoposide (CHOEP) rather than CHOP alone can be recommended.

Consolidation. After the completion of induction (first line or initial) chemotherapy, patients should be evaluated for the use of consolidation therapy with radiation therapy (localized disease) and/or autologous HCT.[21] Consolidation therapy is treatment that is given after cancer has disappeared following the initial (induction) therapy. Consolidation therapy is used to kill any cancer cells that may be left in the body. It may include radiation therapy, a stem cell transplant, or treatment with drugs that kill cancer cells. This is also called intensification therapy and postremission therapy. Those with limited-stage disease who achieve a partial response may attain a complete remission if consolidation radiation is administered. The use of auto-HCT in first complete response (CR) is principally based on the PTCL subtype and the IPI score.[21]

In relapsed T-cell lymphoma, there is no general consensus regarding the optimal treatment regimen, and all patients should be encouraged to participate in clinical trials where available. Patients who are not candidates for or choose not to participate in clinical trials are usually treated with combination chemotherapy regimens in an attempt to achieve a complete remission. At present, no single chemotherapy regimen is clearly superior to any other. Outside the context of a clinical trial, the selection of treatment should be based on expected toxicities, patient comorbidities, and preferences.

LIFE SPAN CONSIDERATIONS IN LYMPHOMAS OF ALL TYPES

After the completion of therapy, restaging, and documentation of complete remission, patients with all types of lymphoma are seen at periodic intervals to be monitored and assessed for possible relapse. The frequency and extent of these visits depends on the histologic subtype and comfort of both the patient and clinician. There have been no prospective, randomized trials comparing various schedules of follow-up. Any necessary radiologic and laboratory studies are usually performed by or can be coordinated with the patient's hematologist or oncologist to ensure adequate follow-up evaluation.

Relapsed disease can be suggested by changes on imaging studies or physical examination but can be confirmed only by biopsy. Accordingly, a biopsy should be performed to document relapsed disease before proceeding to salvage therapy.

Under some circumstances, gonadal dysfunction can affect quality of life after treatment. Transient and sometimes permanent male sterility may occur. Infertility may occur in at least 80% of women older than 25 years who receive nitrogen mustard, vincristine, procarbazine, or prednisone chemotherapy.[22] The newer, nonalkylating agent-containing regimens have a lower risk of infertility. However, sperm banking should be considered before treatment is initiated. Pregnancies occurring in patients or their partners do not appear to be associated with complications, congenital abnormalities, or spontaneous abortions.[22]

Improved treatment regimens and survival mean that many patients will return to primary health care providers for care and monitoring. Advance directives should be discussed with the patient, with the understanding that some lymphomas can be treated successfully or have an indolent course. Patients are encouraged to prepare a living will and to appoint a health care proxy so that both the health care proxy and the health care provider understand their preferences for terminal care (see Chapter 14). Palliative care specialists have been shown to improve quality of life and longevity and lower costs at the end of life.[23] Palliative care involves emotional and psychological care, support groups, pain and symptom management, family engagement, and general resources to support the patient and family. Any approach to cancer care should integrate palliative management from an early stage.

The majority of treatments for lymphoma can be administered in an outpatient setting. The patient might be hospitalized for high-dose chemotherapy requiring careful monitoring of laboratory values and blood product support as well as for episodes of febrile neutropenia. Of course, induction chemotherapy preceding hematopoietic cell transplant requires hospitalization in a controlled environment.

COMPLICATIONS IN ALL TYPES OF LYMPHOMA

Complications from lymphoma can occur during treatment, as a result of treatment, or from the disease itself.

During Therapy

Patients with cancer who undergo chemotherapy and radiotherapy are at risk of infection because of the immunosuppression from the cancer, the myelosuppression from chemotherapy, the break in skin barriers from the placement of Port-a-Caths and central lines, and the shifts in microbial flora. The myelosuppressive effect of chemotherapy can cause neutropenia. Absolute neutropenia is defined as fewer than 1000 neutrophils per cubic millimeter and bands in the bloodstream and is calculated by multiplying the total number of white cells from the CBC by the total percentage of neutrophils plus bands. The period of neutropenia after chemotherapy is relatively predictable; the lowest count of neutrophils occurs approximately 10 to 14 days after chemotherapy and recovers in about 3 to 4 weeks after chemotherapy. Although fever can be a presenting sign in a patient with lymphoma, fever in a patient after chemotherapy, especially in a neutropenic patient, may be a sign of life-threatening sepsis. Research shows that colony-stimulating factors can reduce the incidence of febrile neutropenia; however, these medications can be inconvenient and expensive and have toxicities, including bone pain. Guidelines for colony-stimulating factor administration have been issued by the American Society of Clinical Oncology, and the administration of these medications should be based on the recommendation of the treating hematologist or oncologist.[24]

Fatigue is a poorly understood phenomenon that affects the patient's quality of life. It can occur as a result of the treatment or the disease. It may be associated with anxiety or depression or with physiologic processes related to tumor necrosis factor and interleukin-1 and other cytokines. Physiologic conditions such as anemia in all types of lymphoma resulting from the chemotherapy and radiotherapy may also contribute to fatigue. A careful review of symptoms and CBC with differential is important. Current recommendations include education to relieve anxiety, activities that provide distraction, and participation in low-intensity exercise.[25] Packed red blood cell transfusion should be given to patients with severe anemia. Consideration should be given to using epoetin or darbopoetin when limiting the number of transfusions might be indicated or desired.[26]

There is a high prevalence of depression among cancer patients. Patients who are depressed may find help through psychotherapy that involves social support, coping skills, emotional expression, and cognitive restructuring.[27] Antidepressants and psychostimulating medications may be beneficial as well. It is critical that pain be managed effectively because there is a direct relationship between unmanaged pain and increased levels of psychological distress. Referral to psychiatry or palliative medicine may be helpful.

Post-Treatment Toxicities

A serious consequence of treatment is the increased risk of a second cancer, including acute myelogenous leukemia (AML; see Chapter 218). The risk of secondary AML can extend to 11 years after treatment. Radiotherapy with and without chemotherapy may contribute to increased risk of solid tumors in the radiation field. Solid tumors tend to occur in the second decade after treatment. Breast cancers in this population are often bilateral. Regular breast examination and mammography starting at an early age are recommended as part of routine post-treatment care.

More than two thirds of patients who have undergone mantle irradiation develop thyroid disease, including hypothyroidism, Graves disease, silent thyrotoxicosis, and nodules, with a 2% risk of cancer. Mantle field irradiation also adds to the risk of cardiac toxicity even after 40 years.[14] This type of radiation is used less often than in the past, but previously treated patients remain at risk.

High doses of doxorubicin can cause cardiomyopathy. Pulmonary fibrosis or restrictive disease has also been associated with bleomycin chemotherapy.

Novel Therapies. Over the past several years, immunotherapy—therapies that enlist and strengthen the power of a patient's immune system to attack lymphoma—has emerged.

CAR T-Cell Therapy. As its name implies, the backbone of CAR T-cell therapy is T cells, which are often called the workhorses of the immune system because of their critical role in orchestrating the immune response and killing cells infected by pathogens.

The therapy requires drawing blood from patients and separating out the T cells. Next, using a disarmed virus, the T cells are genetically engineered to produce receptors on their surface called chimeric antigen receptors, or CARs. These receptors are "synthetic molecules"; they don't exist naturally.

These special receptors allow the T cells to recognize and attach to a specific protein, or antigen, on tumor cells. The CAR T-cell therapies furthest along in development target an antigen found on B cells called CD19.

Once the collected T cells have been engineered to express the antigen-specific CAR, they are "expanded" in the laboratory into the hundreds of millions.

The final step is the infusion of the CAR T cells into the patient (which is preceded by a "lymphodepleting" chemotherapy regimen). If all goes as planned, the engineered cells further multiply in the patient's body and, with guidance from their engineered receptor, recognize and kill cancer cells that harbor the antigen on their surfaces.

Until recently, the use of CAR T-cell therapy has been restricted to small clinical trials, largely in patients with advanced blood cancers. But these treatments have nevertheless captured the attention of researchers and the public alike because of the remarkable responses they have produced in some patients—both children and adults—for whom all other treatments had stopped working.

In 2017, two CAR T-cell therapies were approved by the Food and Drug Administration (FDA), one for the treatment of children with acute lymphoblastic leukemia (ALL) and the other for adults with advanced lymphomas.[28]

PATIENT AND FAMILY EDUCATION FOR ALL TYPES OF LYMPHOMA

One of the most common reactions to the stress of a cancer diagnosis and treatment is anxiety and depression. Education about the disease, treatment, and prognosis can help relieve anxiety. Educational and social support resources for patients include American Cancer Society programs (www.cancer.gov/cancertopics/coping) and OncoLink (www.oncolink.org/coping).

Patients should be encouraged to remain active and engage in low levels of regular exercise. This will help to maintain strength and energy and improve mood.

Patients with neutropenia may be advised to avoid crowds and sick people and maintain a clean home environment, including having rugs shampooed before treatment begins and moving live plants away from the patient. Care should be taken with pet waste, and whenever possible someone other than the patient should pick up pet waste or change litter boxes.

Nutrition education should begin at diagnosis to prevent complications caused by malnutrition and weight loss often associated with treatment. Dietary counseling should address the need for calorie- and protein-rich foods. Referral to a dietitian may be helpful. Avoidance of uncooked or unwashed foods is recommended. In general, alcoholic beverages should be avoided. Given the treatment-related pulmonary and cardiac toxicity, help with smoking cessation should be offered.

Many patients undergoing cancer treatment are taking oral medications new to them, including mild chemotherapeutic agents, antibiotics, antivirals, and antifungals. These need to be reviewed carefully with patients and families.

REFERENCES

1. Noone, A. M., Howlader, N., Krapcho, M., Miller, D., Brest, A., Yu, M., et al. (Eds.), (April 2018). *SEER cancer statistics review, 1975–2015.* Bethesda, MD: National Cancer Institute. https://seer.cancer.gov/csr/1975_2015/. (Accessed 20 April 2018). Based on November 2017 SEER data submission, posted to the SEER web site.
2. Okano, M., & Gross, T. (2012). Acute or chronic life threatening diseases associated with Epstein- Barr virus infection. *The American Journal of the Medical Sciences, 343*(6), 483.
3. Peveling-Oberhag, J., Arcaini, L., Hansmann, M. L., & Zeuzem, S. (2013). Hepatitis C–associated B-cell non-Hodgkin lymphomas. Epidemiology, molecular signature and clinical management. *Journal of Hepatology, 59*(1), 169–177.
4. Hernandez-Ramirez, R., Shields, M., Dubrow, R., & Engels, E. (2017). Cancer risk in HIV-infected people in the USA from 1996–2102: A population based registry-linkage study. *Lancet HIV, 4*(11), e495–e504.
5. Kramer, S., Hikel, S. M., Adams, K., Hinds, D., & Moon, K. (2012). Current status of the epidemiologic evidence linking polychlorinated biphenyls and non-Hodgkin Lymphoma, and the role of immune dysregulation. *Environmental Health Perspectives, 120*(8), 1067–1075.
6. Groth, K. A., Skakkebaek, A., Host, C., et al. (2013). Clinical review: Klinefelter syndrome—a clinical update. *The Journal of Clinical Endocrinology and Metabolism, 98*(1), 20–30.
7. Swerdlow, S. H., Campo, E., Pileri, S. A., et al. (2016). The 2016 revision of the World Health Organization classification of lymphoid neoplasms. *Blood, 127*(20), 2375–2390. https://doi.org/10.1182/blood-2016-01-643569. (Accessed 28 July 2019).
8. NIH, National Cancer Institute. Adult non-Hodgkin lymphoma treatment (PDQ). Retrieved from <http://www.cancer.gov/types/lymphoma/patient/adult-nhl-treatment-pdq>. (Accessed 21 April 2018).

9. Mathas, S., Hartman, S., & Kuppers, R. (2016). Hodgkin lymphoma: Pathology and biology. *Seminars in Hematology, 53*(3), 139–147.

10. Cheson, B. D., Fisher, R. I., Barrington, S. F., et al. (2014). Recommendations for initial evaluation, staging, and response assessment of Hodgkin and non-Hodgkin lymphoma: The Lugano classification. *Journal of Clinical Oncology: Official Journal of the American Society of Clinical Oncology, 32*(27), 3059–3068.

11. Ansell, S. (2016). Hodgkin Lymphoma: 2016 update on diagnosis, risk-stratification and management. *Hematology (Amsterdam, Netherlands), 91*(4), 434–442.

12. Collins, G. P., Parker, A. N., Pocock, C., et al. (2014). Guideline on the management of primary resistant and relapsed classical Hodgkin lymphoma. *British Journal of Haematology, 164*, 39.

13. Gavini, A., Reagan, J. L., Winer, E. S., & Castillo, J. J. (2014). Primary refractory Hodgkin lymphoma: Limited options and poor survival—but not always. *American Journal of Hematology, 89*, 853–857. doi:10.1002/ajh.23660.

14. van Nimwegen, F. A., Schaapveld, M., Janus, C. P. M., et al. (2015). Cardiovascular disease after Hodgkin lymphoma treatment 40-year disease risk. *JAMA Internal Medicine, 175*(6), 1007–1017. doi:10.1001/jamainternmed.2015.1180.

15. Vockerodt, M., Yap, L. F., Shannon-Lowe, C., et al. (2015). The Epstein-Barr virus and the pathogenesis of lymphoma. *The Journal of Pathology, 235*, 312–322.

16. hesan, B., Fisher, R., Barrington, S. F., et al. (2014). Recommendations for initial evaluation, staging and response assessment of Hodgkin and non-Hodgkin lymphoma: The lagano classification. *Journal of Clinical Oncology: Official Journal of the American Society of Clinical Oncology, 32*(27), 3059–3067.

17. Dreyling, M., Ghielmini, M., Rule, S., et al. (2016). Newly diagnosed and relapsed follicular lymphoma: ESMO clinical practice guideline for diagnosis, treatment and follow-up. *Annals of Oncology, 27*(s-5), v83–v90.

18. Rummel, M. J., Niederle, N., Maschmeyer, G., et al. (2013). Bendamustine plus rituximab versus CHOP plus rituximab as first-line treatment for patients with indolent and mantle-cell lymphomas: An open-label, multicentre, randomized, phase 3 non-inferiority trial. *Lancet, 381*, 1203.

19. Coiffier, B., Thieblemont, C., Van Den Neste, E., et al. (2010). Long-term outcome of patients in the LNH-98.5 trial, the first randomized study comparing rituximab-CHOP to standard CHOP chemotherapy in DLBCL patients: A study by the Groupe d'Etudes des Lymphomes de l'Adulte. *Blood, 116*, 2040.

20. Feldman, T., Farber, C. M., Choi, K., et al. (2017). Treatment of peripheral T-cell lymphoma in community settings. *Clinical Lymphoma Myeloma and Leukemia, 17*(6), 354–361.

21. Horwits, S., Zelenetz, A., et al. (2016). NCCN guidelines insights: Non Hodgkin Lymphomas, version 3. *Journal of the National Comprehensive Cancer Network, 14*, 9. doi:10.6004/jnccn.2016.0117.

22. Harel, S., Ferme, C., & Poirot, C. (2011). Management of fertility in patients treated for Hodgkin's lymphoma. *Haematologica, 96*(11), 1692–1699.

23. Kelly, A., & Morrison, R. S. (2015). Palliative care for the seriously ill. *The New England Journal of Medicine, 373*, 747–755.

24. Dinan, M. A., Hirsch, B. R., & Lyman, G. H. (2015). Management of chemotherapy-induced neutropenia: Measuring quality, cost and value. *Journal of the National Comprehensive Cancer Network, 13*(1), e1–e7.

25. Aapro, M., Beguin, Y., Bokemeyer, C., et al. (2018). ESMO Guidelines Committee, management of anaemia and iron deficiency in patients with cancer: ESMO clinical practice guidelines. *Annals of Oncology, 29*(Supplement 4), iv96–iv110. https://doi.org/10.1093/annonc/mdx758.

26. Bergeram, G., Gerber, L. H., & Mayer, D. K. (2012). Cancer-related fatigue. *Cancer, 118*(s8), 2261–2269.

27. Walker, J., & Sharp, M. (2014). Integrated management of major depression for people with cancer. *International Review of Psychiatry (Abingdon, England), 26*(6), 657–668.

28. June, C., O'Connor, R., Kawalekar, O., et al. (2018). CAR T-cell immunotherapy for human cancer. *Science, 359*(6382), 1361–1365.

CHAPTER 220

MYELODYSPLASTIC SYNDROMES

Anna D. Schaal

DEFINITION AND EPIDEMIOLOGY

 Specialist referral to hematology is indicated for all suspected cases of MDS.

The myelodysplastic syndromes (MDSs) are a heterogeneous group of bone marrow disorders characterized by ineffective dysplastic growth of the hematopoietic precursors. MDS is not one disease but a diverse series of hematologic conditions that have variable clinical presentation, biologic activity, and prognosis. MDS is the most common state of acquired clonal bone marrow disorders.

There are three dominant features of this group of diseases. The first is impaired maturation of hematopoietic stem cells and increased cell death, or apoptosis. This is characterized by cytopenias. There also is a clonal expansion of the abnormal cell line, which manifests itself as progressive disease over time. Patients with MDS also have a variable risk of transformation to acute leukemia.

MDS is a relatively rare disease. It is primarily a disease of older adults, with an annual number of new cases at 12-20 thousand. 75% of new cases affect those 60 years old and older. Fifteen percent of cases occur after chemotherapy or radiotherapy for a previous cancer. There are 60,000 to 170,000 people living at any one time in the United States with this disease.[1] Males are affected about 1.5 to 2 times as often as females.[1] The number of cases is expected to rise as the numbers of older adults increases.

PATHOPHYSIOLOGY

The knowledge of pathophysiologic abnormalities that contribute to MDS is advancing at a remarkable pace. Defects in cellular differentiation, responsiveness to cytokines and growth factors, altered hematopoietic microenvironment, increased apoptosis, and abnormal DNA methylation are all pathways that lead to the ineffective hematopoiesis that is the trademark of MDS. This ineffective hematopoiesis results in peripheral cytopenias despite a packed, hypercellular bone marrow. In essence, the bone marrow produces cells that are not able to mature into functional red blood cells, white blood cells, and platelets.

MDS is classified according to subtypes. The World Health Organization defines each subtype based on type and degree of cytopenias, percentage of blast or monocytes, and dysplastic findings in peripheral blood and bone marrow (Table 220.1).[2] Each subtype of MDS behaves in a different manner and has different treatment implications.

The International Prognostic Scoring System–Revised (IPSS-R) is another useful classification system that is used to score the different variants of MDS (Table 220.2). The scoring is based on five factors: the percentage of blasts in the bone marrow, the specific karyotype or genetic abnormality risk group, hemoglobin, platelet count, and absolute neutrophil count (ANC). Corresponding scores that range from 0 to 6 help predict both survival and the risk of evolution to acute

TABLE 220.1   2016 WHO classification of Myelodysplastic Syndrome

Subtype	Blood	Bone Marrow
(1) MDS with single lineage dysplasia (MDS-SLD)	Single of bicytopenia	Dysplasia in ≥10 of one cell line, <5% blasts
(2) MDS with ring sideroblasts (MDS-RS)	Anemia, no blasts	≥15% of erythroid precursors w/ring sideroblasts, or ≥5% of ring sideroblasts, <5% blasts
(3) MDS with multilineage dysplasia (MDS-MLD)	Cytopenia(s)*, <1 or 10^9/l monocytes	Dysplasia in ≥10 of cells in ≥2 hematopoietic lineages, ±15% ring sideroblasts, <5% blasts
(4.1) MDS with excess blasts-1 (MDS-EB-1)	Cytopenia(s), ≤2%–4% blasts[†], <1 × 10^9/l monocytes	Unilineage or multilineage dysplasia, 5%–9% blasts, no Auer rods
(4.2) MDS with excess blasts-2 (MDS-EB-2)	Cytopenia(s), 5%–19% blasts[†], <1 × 10^9/l monocytes	Unilineage or multilineage dysplasia, 10%–19% blasts, ±Auer rods
(5) MDS with isolated del(5q)	Anemia, platelets normal or increased	Unilineage erythroid dysplasia, isolated del(5q), <5% blasts
(6) MDS, unclassifiable (MDS-U)	Cytopenia(s), +1% blasts on at least 2 occasions	Unilineage dysplasia or no dysplasia but characteristic MDS cytogenetics, <5% blasts
(7) Refractory cytopenia of childhood	Cytopenias, <2% blasts	Dysplasia in 1–3 lineages, <5% blasts

*Cytopenias defined as: hemoglobin, 10 g/dL; absolute neutrophil count, 1800/mm³ and platelet count less than 100,000/mm³; S; bicytopenia may be observed in most cases of MDS.
[†]Presence of 5%–9% myeloblast in BM and 2%–4% myeloblasts in the blood, the diagnostic is MDS-EB-1, and 10%–19% myeloblast in BM and 5%–19% myeloblasts in the blood, the diagnostic is MDS-EB-2. Cases with pancytopenia with unilineage or absent dysplasia with 1% myeloblasts in the blood should be classified as MDS-U.
Data from Arber, D. A., Orazi, A., Hasserjian, R., Thiele, J., Borowitz, M. J., Le Beau M. M., et al. (2016). The 2016 revision on the World Health Organization classification of myeloid neoplasms and acute leukemia. *Blood, 127,* 2391–2405. In G. A. Hamid, A. W. Al-Nehmi, S. Shukry. (2019). Diagnosis and Classification of Myelodysplastic Syndrome. Recent Developments in Myelodysplastic Syndromes, Ota Fuchs. IntechOpen. https://www.intechopen.com/books/recent-developments-in-myelodysplastic-syndromes/diagnosis-and-classification-of-myelodysplastic-syndrome

TABLE 220.2   The IPSS-R Parameters and Their Score Values

Prognostic Variable	0	0.5	1	1.5	2	3	4
Cytogenetics	Very good		Good		Intermediate	Poor	Very poor
BM* blast %	≤2%		>2% to <5%		5%–10%	>10%	
Hemoglobin	≥10		8 to <10	<8			
Platelets	≥100	50 to <100	<50				
ANC[†]	≥0.8	<0.8					

Risk Group	Risk Score
Very low	≤1.5
Low	>1.5–3
Intermediate	>3–4.5
High	>4.5–6
Very high	>6

*Bone marrow.
[†]Absolute neutrophil (white blood cell) count.
From Greenberg, P., Tuechler, H., Schanz, J., Sanz, G., Garcia-Manero, G., Solé, F., et al. (2012). Revised international prognostic scoring system for myelodysplastic syndromes. *Blood, 120*(12), 2454–2465.

myeloid leukemia. The IPSS-R is used to help with projecting prognosis and making treatment decisions.[3]

CLINICAL PRESENTATION AND PHYSICAL EXAMINATION

In general, the clinical presentation of MDS is related to symptoms of bone marrow failure or of the specific cytopenias that each patient is experiencing. If the red blood cells are the prominent lineage that is not maturing, then symptoms of anemia will be present. These may include fatigue, pallor, headaches, shortness of breath (or dyspnea) on exertion, and chest pains or palpitations. If the platelet count is low, easy bruising or bleeding will be the dominant presenting symptom. Frequent nose bleeds, petechiae, hematochezia, heavy menstrual bleeding, or large hematomas may encourage a patient to seek medical attention. Finally, if the white blood cells are not maturing, the main presenting symptoms will be of neutropenia, manifesting as frequent or severe infections.

Increasingly, more and more patients are being diagnosed incidentally from an abnormal complete blood count (CBC) done routinely in the primary care setting. In this case, patients feel well and have no subjective or physical examination findings that would make one suspect a myelodysplastic disorder. Splenomegaly is uncommon in MDS. If patients do have physical exam findings they are secondary to cytopenias such as petechiae or common findings of infection.

DIAGNOSTICS

A number of specific diagnostic tests are required to confirm the diagnosis of MDS. These include peripheral blood smear, bone marrow biopsy and aspirate with cytogenetic analysis, flow cytometry, and immunohistochemical staining. Dysplastic features in one or more cell lines are often seen.

The peripheral blood smear will often reveal erythrocytes with anisocytosis, poikilocytosis, or basophilic stippling. The granulocytes may be larger than normal and may lack normal granulation. Platelets may also be larger than normal.

The bone marrow biopsy almost always shows a hypercellular, packed marrow, which is in sharp contrast to the peripheral cytopenia. The hypercellular marrow often demonstrates defects in cellular maturation in all cell lines. For erythroid precursors, this includes megaloblastic cells, which are predominantly younger forms, and mature cells with distorted nuclei. Ringed sideroblasts will often be identified. These red blood cells are characterized by excessive cytoplasmic iron granules in a perinuclear distribution.[4] Megakaryocytes are the polynuclear cells responsible for platelet production. In MDS, the megakaryocytes are often smaller than normal and hypolobulated. The precursors for white blood cells may also have abnormal granulation and deformed nuclei.

Cytogenetic abnormalities play a role in both diagnosis and prognosis. Cytogenetic abnormalities have been found in 50% to 60% of patients with de novo MDS and up to 80% of patients with therapy-related MDS.[5] Common abnormalities include 5q− syndrome, which is a good prognostic indicator, and monosomy 7, which is associated with a poor prognosis and an increased risk of transformation to acute leukemia.

INITIAL DIAGNOSTICS

Myelodysplastic Syndromes

MYELODYSPLASTIC DISORDERS
- CBC and differential
- Peripheral blood smear
- Bone marrow biopsy with cytogenetics, flow cytometry, and immunohistochemical staining

ADDITIONAL DIAGNOSTICS
- Laboratory tests to rule out other common causes of cytopenias—see differential diagnosis list

---

DIFFERENTIAL DIAGNOSIS

 Priority differential diagnoses to consider include alcohol and drug toxicity; vitamin B$_{12}$, folate, or iron deficiency; and viral infections.

Several disorders may mimic the morphologic changes of MDS and should be considered in the differential diagnosis. If anemia is the only presenting sign, common types of anemias must first be excluded, including folate and vitamin B$_{12}$ deficiency, iron deficiency, anemia of chronic disease, renal failure, alcohol abuse, hereditary spherocytosis, and hemolysis (see Chapter 216). Infection, such as with human immunodeficiency virus (HIV), cytomegalovirus (CMV), parvovirus, and Epstein-Barr virus, should also be excluded. Drug toxicity or adverse reactions often imitate the cytopenias of MDS. Primary acute or chronic leukemia or a metastatic solid tumor with bone marrow metastasis should also be considered in the differential diagnosis. Other hematologic abnormalities often mimic MDS presentation, including aplastic anemia, Fanconi anemia, acute myeloid leukemia, myeloproliferative neoplasms, and paroxysmal nocturnal hematuria. The bone marrow biopsy is the gold standard of diagnosis, because it often can exclude these disorders.

INTERPROFESSIONAL COLLABORATIVE MANAGEMENT

The clinical pathway of MDS and response to therapy vary significantly among individuals.

Because most individuals with MDS are older than 65 years, consideration should be given to a comprehensive geriatric evaluation of individuals before treatment is started. This is recommended as a way of predicting morbidity and mortality and the patient's ability to tolerate treatment based on patient age and comorbidities.[6]

The therapy for MDS ranges from supportive care to aggressive treatments. The goals of therapy include symptom management and improvement in quality of life while minimizing treatment-related toxicity and improving overall survival. These goals include decreasing the risk of progression to acute myelogenous leukemia (AML) (see Chapter 218).

Non-Pharmacologic Management

The quality of life of those patients living with myelodysplasia is directly affected by both the disease and its accompanying treatments. The majority of patients who have this disease are older adults, many with other comorbid conditions. This aging population will often have low physiologic reserves and a prolonged recovery from complications. Quality-of-life issues must be explored, and patients and families should be offered education in treatment choices, a realistic assessment of benefit versus burden, and cost in order to make informed decisions about their care. The patient's progress and response to therapies should be reevaluated and discussed on a frequent basis.

Multidisciplinary team consultations including physical therapy for strength and conditioning, nutrition, social work, palliative care, and mental health are all helpful at different points along the MDS continuum.

Pharmacologic Management

A variety of agents are known to produce a response in MDS. Treatment decisions need to be tailored to the individual patient and should include consideration of age, functional status, and IPSS-R score (see Table 220.2). For those who are not good candidates for aggressive treatment strategies or who have failed to respond to such treatment attempts, supportive care becomes the foundation of therapy. This approach includes cytokine treatments and transfusion support, immunosuppression, and iron chelation. There is no evidence of any survival benefit from cytokine treatments; however, they may improve quality of life because they improve symptoms and decrease transfusion requirements. Cytokine treatment consists of erythropoietin (EPO), granulocyte colony-stimulating factor (G-CSF), and granulocyte-macrophage colony-stimulating factor (GM-CSF).[7]

EPO is a hormone that stimulates red blood cell production. Approximately 20% of patients will respond to EPO with an increase in hemoglobin. The patients who respond are usually those with low or no transfusion requirements.[8] Improved exercise capacity and quality of life can be an outcome of successful EPO treatment.[8] Interestingly, the addition of G-CSF to EPO creates a synergy that improves the erythroid response in up to 50% of patients.[9] G-CSF and GM-CSF both stimulate white blood cell production. The absolute granulocyte count often increases with the use of these cytokines; however, the actual number of infections does not decrease.[9] Because of this, this therapy is typically not used routinely but more often when there is an active infection or an increased risk of infection.

Prophylactic antibiotic therapy is considered in patients with severe neutropenia, which is defined as an ANC of less than 500. It has been shown in a large meta-analysis that prophylactic treatment with fluoroquinolones in neutropenic patients can decrease the incidence of serious infections as well as reduce all-cause mortality.[10]

Most patients with MDS eventually become red blood cell transfusion dependent. Transfusions benefit patients by improving their symptoms of anemia; however, this is only a temporary improvement. The complications of chronic red blood cell transfusions include risk of infection, transfusion reactions, and iron overload necessitating chelation therapy. Platelet transfusion may be needed to prevent bleeding episodes in patients with thrombocytopenia. Quality-of-life issues emerge in the transfusion-dependent patient because of the time, resources, and support burden for patients who are required to go to a clinic for transfusions on a frequent basis.

In patients who are transfusion dependent, iron chelation becomes a consideration. Iron overload may contribute to both increased mortality and morbidity in early-stage MDS.[11] Once patients have received more than 20 red blood cell transfusions, patients become iron overloaded. For patients with serum ferritin levels greater than 2500 ng/mL, the goal is to decrease it to less than 1000 mg/mL.

Immune suppression is also used for patients with MDS, with the primary goal of therapy being to improve quality of life. The use of antithymocyte globulin and cyclosporine has been found to be helpful by improving cytopenias and decreasing transfusion requirements. No benefit is noted in overall survival or time to leukemic transformation.[12]

Hypomethylating agents are approved for the treatment of MDS. These agents inhibit DNA methylation. Hypomethylation restores normal function of silenced growth genes that are responsible for differentiation and proliferation. These agents have been shown to decrease the risk of leukemic transformation, to improve transfusion dependency, and to improve overall survival.[9] A phase III trial that compared 5-azacytidine and supportive care found that 60% of patients who received 5-azacytidine had hematologic response compared with only 5% in the supportive group arm. The median time of progression to AML or death was also significantly prolonged in the patients who received 5-azacytidine.[13] 5-Azacytidine is delivered in a subcutaneous injection for 7 days every 4 weeks. Its prominent side effects include myelosuppression, pain or skin reaction at injection sites, and nausea.

Decitabine, similar to 5-azacytidine, is also approved for the treatment of patients with MDS. It has been shown to be superior to supportive care alone, as evidenced by hematologic response rates, increased time to AML progression, and overall survival benefit, especially in high-risk patients. In one study, median progression-free survival in older patients (older than 60) with higher-risk disease was significantly improved as compared with patients receiving only supportive care.[13] Decitabine is also associated with serious side effects including fever, infection, and low blood counts. It is usually given intravenously for 3 to 5 consecutive days every 4 to 6 weeks.

Lenalidomide (Revlimid) is a 4-aminoglutarimide analogue of thalidomide that acts as an immunomodulatory agent. It is approved for the treatment of lower-risk MDS, in patients who are transfusion dependent. It has been shown to achieve transfusion independence for up to 67% of patients.[9,14] The major serious side effect is myelosuppression, which is dose dependent. Interestingly, the cytopenias associated with this therapy seem to be predictive of a response. In other words, patients who had significant cytopenias and required dose reductions were more likely to become transfusion independent. Another serious adverse effect is an increased risk of thrombosis. It is recommended that patients taking lenalidomide be considered for anticoagulation therapy. Because lenalidomide is an analogue of thalidomide, a drug that has been associated with birth defects in the past, it is highly regulated and available only through specialty pharmacies and programs. Patients must consent to ensuring that no pregnancies develop while they are taking this medication. Other adverse reactions were uncommon and typically mild.

Stem cell transplantation remains the only potentially curative treatment for MDS. This is preferred for a small number of patients with MDS, especially in those with high-risk disease and minimal comorbidities. An allogeneic transplant, either human leukocyte antigen (HLA) identical related or unrelated, is indicated if the patient meets the rigorous transplantation requirements. Unfortunately, with the aged population of MDS patients, few meet this prerequisite. Stem cell transplantation should optimally be performed before disease progression. In patients with less advanced disease, 3-year survival rates of 65% to 75% are achieved. Among patients with advanced disease, the 3-year survival rate drops to 25% to 45%.[15]

Reduced-intensity ("mini") stem cell transplantation allows more potential patients to meet the standards of transplantation. Mini-transplantation regimens are meant to treat the disease with a graft-versus-leukemia effect and do not depend on ablation of the patient's marrow. This type of transplant is better tolerated, and therefore more older adult patients and those with comorbidities may qualify. The disease-free progression after mini-transplantation is 60%. The 4-year probability of overall survival for patients with MDS is 49%. This therapy can cause side effects similar to stem cell transplant, although usually milder, with a 20% risk of non-relapse mortality.[16] Common causes of death for patients receiving stem cell transplantation include graft-versus-host disease and infections.

Whenever MDS is suspected, patients are referred to a hematologist for both a review of the peripheral blood smear and a bone marrow biopsy. Hematologists will often follow patients long term with the help of primary health care providers to monitor disease progression and complications. For patients who have an MDS diagnosis, the following are indications for immediate referral to urgent or emergent care:

- In patients with an absolute neutropenia of less than 1000/mm^3, hospitalization for any febrile illness is warranted. Without prompt initiation of intravenous antibiotics, patients may quickly develop sepsis and require critical care.
- Any bleeding that does not resolve with 15 minutes of direct pressure requires an immediate CBC, with potential platelet transfusion to follow.
- Any trend of increasing peripheral blast population or worsening transfusion requirements is an indication for hematology follow-up to assess for transformation to acute leukemia.
- Nodular or flat diffuse rash could indicate transformation to acute leukemia and requires immediate laboratory review and consultation with dermatology specialists.

COMPLICATIONS

The clinical course of MDS is inevitably progressive with medium survival of about a year with supportive care only. The complications of MDS revolve around the offending cytopenias. Major bleeding episodes and infection are the most common reasons for hospital admissions and death. Transformation to acute leukemia ranges from 5% to 15% in low-risk groups to 40% to 50% in high-risk groups.[17] This requires prompt intervention with induction chemotherapy if the patient is a candidate. Other, less-intense treatment regimens, such as oral melphalan, are also available.

Fatigue is another major complication of the disease itself. It is extremely common and can often become unrelenting. Patients often describe it as exhaustion. The fatigue can interfere with the patient's functional ability and can result in depression.

MDS is a heterogeneous group of bone marrow disorders that requires definitive diagnosis. Each patient must be evaluated and treated on his or her disease-specific symptom trajectory. Quality-of-life issues are paramount because both the disease and its treatments have the potential to disrupt normalcy. Caring support and social intervention can positively modify patients' experience with this disease as they encounter the different management strategies.

PATIENT AND FAMILY EDUCATION

Neutropenic precautions (https://www.cdc.gov/cancer/prevent infections/pdf/neutropenia.pdf) should be reviewed when necessary and it is essential that patients and families are aware of whom to call and when to call if fevers, chills, rigors, or persistent bleeding develops. Patients should also be informed about any clinical trials that may be available for their particular situation.

All patients and families should:

- Explore quality-of-life issues and goals of care.
- Focus on energy conservation and symptom management.
- Review side effect profiles of potential treatment options, time expected in hospital, potential costs involved, and risk of life-threatening complications.
- Review available palliative care and hospice options.

HEALTH PROMOTION

Patients with low-risk MDS can potentially have a long life expectancy. It is important that they maintain healthy lifestyle behaviors and have established primary care. Age-appropriate screening for other cancers as well as common comorbidities should continue as recommended by US Preventive Services Task Force. Iron chelation in the subset of patients who are transfusion dependent should be considered to avoid complications of iron overload that can occur with red blood cell transfusions over time.

REFERENCES

1. Myelodysplastic syndromes by the numbers. Retrieved from https://www.mds-foundation.org/wp-content/uploads/2018/07/MDSInfographic-FINAL_053018.pdf. Accessed Huly 29, 2019.
2. Arber, D. A., Orazi, A., Hasserjian, R., et al. (2016). The 2016 revision to the World Health Organization (WHO) classification of myeloid neoplasms and acute leukemia. *Blood, 127,* 2391–2405.
3. Greenberg, P., et al. (2012). Revised international prognostic scoring system for myelodysplastic syndromes. *Blood, 120*(12), 2454–2465.
4. Hillman, R. S., & Ault, K. A. (Eds.), (2010). *Hematology in clinical practice* (5th ed.). New York: McGraw-Hill.
5. Ciabatti, E., Vale, H. A., Bertini, V., et al. (2017). Myelodysplastic syndrome: Advantages of a combined cytogenic and molecular diagnostic work-up. *Oncotarget, 8*(45), 79188–79200.
6. Kalsi, T., Babic-Illman, G., Ross, P. S., et al. (2015). The impact of comprehensive geriatric assessment intervention on tolerance to chemotherapy in older people. *British Journal of Cancer, 112,* 1435–1444.
7. Greenberg, P., Stone, R., Bejar, R., et al. (2015). Myelodysplastic syndromes, version 2.2015. *Journal of the National Comprehensive Cancer Network, 13,* 261–272.
8. Kelaidi, C., Beyne-Rauzy, O., Braun, T., et al. (2013). High response rate and improved exercise capacity and quality of life with a new regimen of darbopoetin alfa with or without filgrastim in lower-risk myelodysplastic syndromes: A phase II study by the GFM. *Annals of Hematology, 92,* 621–631.
9. Greenberg, P., Stone, R., et al. Myelodysplastic Syndromes. v.1.2018, Aug 2017. Retrieved from www.nccn.org/professionals/physicians_gls/pdf/mds.pdf. On Jan 17, 2018.
10. Gafter-Gvili, A., Paul, M., Fraser, A., & Leibovici, L. (2007). Effect of quinolone prophylaxis in afebrile neutropenic patients on microbial resistance: Systematic review and meta-analysis. *The Journal of Antimicrobial Chemotherapy, 59,* 5–22. Leuk Res. 2007;31(Suppl 3):S2–S6.
11. Malcovati, L. (2012). Impact of transfusion dependency and secondary iron overload on the survival of patients with myelodysplastic syndromes. *Journal of Clinical Oncology: Official Journal of the American Society of Clinical Oncology, 20*(10), 2429–2440.
12. Haider, M., Ali, N., Padron, E., et al. (2016). Immunosuppressive Therapy: Exploring an underutilized treatment option for myelodysplastic syndrome. *Clinical Lymphoma Myeloma and Leukemia, 16s,* s44–s48.
13. Guo, S. Q., Shi, R., Chen, Y. Y., et al. (2019). Effects of low dose Decitabine on soluable CD44, GDF 11, and hematopoietic function in elderly patients with MDS. *Europe PMC, 27*(2), 509–514.
14. Giagounidis, A., Mufti, G. J., Mittleman, M., et al. (2014). Outcomes in RBC transfusion-dependent patients with Low/Intermediate -1-risk myelodysplastic syndromes with isolated deletion 5q treated with lenalidomide: A subset analysis from the MDS-004 study. *European Journal of Hematology.*
15. Ades, L., Itzykson, R., & Fenaux, P. (2014). Myelodysplastic syndromes. *The Lancet, 383*(9936), 2239–2252.
16. Al Malki, M. M., Nathwani, N., & Yang, D. (2018). Melphalan-based reduced-intensity conditioning is associated with favorable disease control and acceptable toxicities in patients older than 70 with hematologic malignancies undergoing allogeneic hematopoietic stem cell transplantation. *Biology of Blood and Marrow Transplantation, 24*(9), 1828–1835.
17. Steensma, D. (2015). Myelodysplastic syndromes: Diagnosis and treatment. *Mayo Clinic Proceedings. Mayo Clinic, 90*(7), 969–983.

A multidisciplinary approach has been recognized as the optimal strategy for management of cancer care. Through shared responsibility and open communication, a treatment plan can be initiated that allows for comprehensive care, with a focus on reducing the risk of fragmentation and ensuring a seamless continuum of care.

The role of the primary healthcare provider is crucial for optimizing patient care; it is essential that he or she be treated as an integral part of the treatment team. There are several facets to this role. These begin with logistical issues, such as the requirement of certain managed care insurance plans that the primary healthcare provider serve as gatekeeper for services and referrals. There are also matters of geography to consider, given that many patients live an hour or more from the cancer center in which they are treated. These patients benefit from continued involvement of the primary healthcare provider, both for ongoing quality health care, and for frontline assistance when concerns arise during treatment. In cases where specialty care is required, the primary healthcare provider can serve as the point person as arrangements are made for escalation of care. And, perhaps most importantly, the primary healthcare provider has the advantage of a prior relationship with the patient and the family, which lends perspective and insight beyond the potentially myopic viewpoint of the cancer care provider.

It is not uncommon for the primary healthcare provider to be the first to recognize a problem that leads to a diagnosis of cancer. For this reason, it is important that all providers have an understanding of cancer-specific risk factors, presenting signs and symptoms, and appropriate initial diagnostic tests.

CANCER RISKS

Cancer prevention measures often begin with recommendations from the primary healthcare provider, particularly once a risk factor is identified. Many cancer risk factors can be decreased or eliminated altogether. These include tobacco use or exposure to second hand smoke, excessive sun exposure, alcohol use, obesity, and risky sexual practices.[1,2,3] Addressing these issues dovetails nicely with the overarching role of the primary healthcare provider, as an emphasis on healthy lifestyle practices is important for overall disease prevention as well.

SCREENING FOR CANCER

The American Cancer Society offers cancer-specific guidelines for screening of asymptomatic patients, and evidence-based screening guidelines can also be obtained from the National Cancer Institute (NCI).[4] Standard examinations include breast, gynecologic (women), genitourinary (men), oral cavity, skin, and colorectal. Screening tests should be performed according to age-appropriate guidelines and may include mammography, Papanicolaou (Pap) cervical smear, and/or colonoscopy. High-risk populations may warrant additional screening tests, such as low-dose helical computed tomography (CT) of the chest in heavy smokers, CA-125 blood test and transvaginal ultrasound in women at increased risk of ovarian cancer, breast MRI in women who carry the *BRCA1* gene or the *BRCA2* gene, and regular skin exams in patients at risk for skin cancer.[4] Certain tests which are considered to provide limited benefit and substantial harms require a discussion with the patient before they are ordered. While most screening examinations present little risk, some do carry a minimal risk of harm including perforation of the colon during routine colonoscopy or risk of overexposure to radiation. A false positive test may expose a patient to further testing which adds additional risk and emotional turmoil. Finally, the risk of over-diagnosis and treatment of tumors that may well be clinically insignificant is common in this age of extremely sensitive screening tests.[4] For example, prostate-specific antigen (PSA) testing for prostate cancer is not recommended without a discussion of the benefits and harms, and an expressed preference from the patient to undergo this screening test.[5]

Although only a small percentage of malignancies are hereditary, providers should make every effort to obtain a complete and accurate family history. In cases where a hereditary cancer syndrome is possible, the patient should be informed about the potential personal risk for cancer and about available surveillance and management strategies. These may include screening examinations, diagnostic tests, and cancer prevention strategies. Referral to a NCI-designated comprehensive cancer center for genetic testing and counseling may also be appropriate.

SHARED DECISION MAKING AND PATIENT CARE

The initial step following a diagnosis of cancer, or test results concerning for malignancy, is discussion with the patient and family regarding the information and a shared decision regarding desired care and care provider. A referral to an oncologist for further evaluation and for initiation of treatment is indicated. Timeliness is key in this setting in order to optimize outcome, as a delay in onset of treatment can affect potential for cure, survival time, and in many cases, quality of life.

With the emphasis in recent years on minimizing the duration of hospital stays, management of cancer patients has transitioned significantly from the hospital to the outpatient setting. In many cases, particularly in small or rural communities without local oncology services, the primary healthcare provider is heavily relied upon to maintain optimal patient care. The value of a collaborative relationship between the oncology team and the primary healthcare provider in order to manage symptoms and monitor for complications cannot be overemphasized.

The key to successful joint management of the patient's care is communication. The oncology team should provide detailed information regarding the current treatment plan, the potential side effects and complications, and the expected frequency and timing of follow-up visits to the patient, his/her family, and the primary health care provider. In addition, the oncologist should communicate the patient's current status from a cancer standpoint, the likelihood of response to treatment, and the overall prognosis. The patient's understanding and level of acceptance of this information is reviewed frequently and communicated to the primary care provider. Likewise, the primary healthcare provider should share updated information with the oncologist after each visit, including the patient's clinical status, lab values or other data, elicited symptoms potentially attributable to treatment, and any general changes in health, financial, or social situation.

Communication should clearly define the responsibilities of each party in order to avoid redundancy or, more importantly, accidental oversight. A plan outlining expectations and guidelines, discussed with the patient and his/her family, should be agreed upon. The primary healthcare provider, for example, may agree to monitor laboratory values for signs of myelosuppression, or for evidence of liver or kidney dysfunction. However, the oncologist should ensure that information is conveyed regarding laboratory parameters and what constitutes a critical value.

CARE OF THE CANCER PATIENT

Cancer patients often require frequent office visits and lab work. Thus, a strong collaborative treatment plan between the primary healthcare provider and the oncology team can be of great value, particularly for patients who reside far from the cancer center. Minimizing the need for travel is an important quality of life measure.

The scope of care for these patients ranges from a basic physical exam and management of chronic healthcare issues to the identification of urgent, or potentially emergent, conditions. The former is of significant importance in order to ensure that patients remain well enough to continue cancer treatment. For example, management of hypertension, diabetes, and similar conditions should be optimized. In addition, many treatment protocols can affect these underlying diagnoses, or may cause them to emerge. The oncology team should inform the primary healthcare provider of the potential effects of chemotherapeutic agents, which may include hypertension, elevated blood glucose, gastrointestinal symptoms, or effects on thyroid, renal, or liver function.

Urgent findings include fever, mental status change, escalating pain, or refractory vomiting. Febrile neutropenia—temperature above 38°C (100.4°F) and absolute neutrophil count below 500/mm^3—is a common complication in patients receiving chemotherapy and requires immediate attention.

Standard procedures include hospitalization with chest x-ray examination, urine culture and sensitivity, blood cultures, and, if a central line is in place, culture of the line. Referral to the oncology team is required for symptoms that are difficult to manage, critical laboratory values, or new suspicious findings.

Oncologic emergencies include spinal cord compression, tumor lysis syndrome, severe metabolic derangement, disseminated intravascular coagulopathy, and superior vena cava syndrome (see Chapter 223). Cancer patients are also at increased risk for deep vein thrombosis (DVT) (see Chapters 107, 217) or pulmonary embolus (PE) (see Chapter 95), resulting from the malignancy itself or due to other exacerbating factors such as medications, surgery, central venous catheters, and inactivity.

ROLE OF THE PRIMARY HEALTHCARE PROVIDER

In the ideal setting, the primary healthcare provider serves as an integral part of the treatment team for patients with cancer. As previously noted, the primary care provider plays an important role in examining patients during the office visit and recommending and ordering screening tests. After referral to a cancer specialist, the primary healthcare provider serves as a valuable local resource for regular evaluations and monitoring of laboratory tests—the importance of which is significant for patients whose residence is distant from the cancer center—and for prompt intervention when a concern arises. A collaborative relationship between the primary healthcare provider and the oncology team allows for safe and continuous care, minimizes potential complications, and promotes patient and provider confidence.

The established relationship between the primary healthcare provider and the patient is of great value as well. Knowledge of the patient's medical condition, psychosocial situation, and general demeanor prior to a cancer diagnosis provides insight that may not be readily apparent to the oncologist. In addition, there is a substantial burden on caregivers when a patient is diagnosed with cancer. The primary healthcare provider can help to assess the caregiver's ability and willingness to assume this role and can serve as an ongoing source of support. In addition to national organizations designed to help patients and their families navigate this difficult process, the primary healthcare provider may also be privy to local resources that may be of benefit.

A diagnosis of cancer, even in cases where the prognosis is relatively promising, warrants a discussion of goals of care, and values and beliefs as they relate to death and dying. Completion of advanced directives is recommended, but the process does not end there. Concerns and fears will continue to arise during treatment. The primary healthcare provider often plays an important role in these ongoing discussions.

In cases where remission is induced, patients will then transition to long-term surveillance. This is an important facet of care, particularly for young survivors, but also for older populations as more effective cancer treatments are developed.[6]

Post-treatment complications may include cardiac problems, endocrine dysfunction, chemotherapy-induced peripheral neuropathy, and impacts on bone health. These patients are also at risk for persistent cancer- or treatment-related fatigue, cognitive dysfunction, depression or anxiety, and sexual dysfunction. Young survivors may have difficulty with reproduction after radiotherapy or chemotherapy. In addition, many cancer treatments carry the risk of causing a secondary cancer.[6] It is not uncommon for patients to continue to struggle with psychosocial issues for years after diagnosis and treatment.

A strong, integrated relationship between the primary healthcare provider and the oncology team is essential to optimize the care of patients with cancer. With clear delineation of roles and responsibilities, along with open communication throughout the course of treatment and beyond, this collaborative relationship is of significant benefit to all parties concerned, most importantly to the patient and the family.

REFERENCES

1. International Agency for Research on Cancer. (2012). *IARC monographs on the evaluation of carcinogenic risks to humans: Volume 100E: Personal Habits and Indoor Combustions*. Lyon, France: International Agency for Research on Cancer. (Accessed 11 July 2018).
2. Centers for Disease Control and Prevention. Division of Cancer Prevention and Control. https://www.cdc.gov/cancer/dcpc/prevention/other.htm. Updated May 2, 2018. (Accessed 11 July 2018).
3. National Cancer Institute. Infectious Agents. https://www.cancer.gov/about-cancer/causes-prevention/risk/infectious-agents. Updated January, 2017. (Accessed 11 July 2018).
4. National Cancer Institute. Screening/Detection. https://www.cancer.gov/publications/pdq/information-summaries/screening. Updated April, 2017. (Accessed 11 July 2018).
5. Wilt, T. J., Harris, R. P., & Qaseem, A., for the High Value Care Task Force of the American College of Physicians. (2015). Screening for cancer: Advice for high-value care from the American College of Physicians. *Annals of Internal Medicine, 162*, 718–725. doi:10.7326/M14-2326.
6. Leach, C. R., Weaver, K. E., Aziz, N. M., et al. (2015). The complex health profile of long-term cancer survivors: Prevalence and predictors of comorbid conditions. *Journal of Cancer Survivorship, 9*, 239. https://doi.org/10.1007/s11764-014-0403.

CHAPTER **222**

BASIC PRINCIPLES OF ONCOLOGY TREATMENT

Tamara K. Jo

It is important that primary care providers are familiar with the basic principles of oncology treatment. Cancer is a very common diagnoses. In 2018 there were 1,735,350 people diagnosed with cancer in the United States and 609,640 deaths. The number of new cancer cases (cancer incidence) is 439.2 per 100,000 men and women in the United States per year. Cancer mortality in the US is 163.5 per 100,000.[1]

In many cases the primary care provider is the first person to suspect or diagnose a patient with cancer, but the provider is also likely to be involved in identifying a recurrence. For that reason, health care providers are invaluable in cancer survivorship follow up, able to initiate timely referrals to oncology specialists and help with the initial questions and concerns of the patient and their family.

Cancer treatment involves the collaboration of an interdisciplinary team including: physicians, nurse practitioners, physician assistants, nurses, pharmacists, social workers, and physical and occupational therapists. As patients undergo treatment, primary care providers continue to act as patient advocates and play a central role in coordinating care among all involved disciplines.

Cancer treatment can be curative or palliative, depending on the patient's disease pathology and wishes for treatment. The health care team can significantly lengthen disease-free intervals and achieve recognizable survival benefits for cancer patients. The discipline of oncology is evolving and is now recognized as a chronic disease state, and many patients will need long-term follow up and may or may not be followed in a survivorship clinic.

Treatment involves using a combination of modalities including surgery performed by a specialist surgeon, including ENT, surgical oncologists, gynecologists, dermatologists, cardiothoracic surgeons, neurosurgeons, gastroenterologists, urologists, and general surgeons. Radiation therapy administered by a radiation oncologist may involve proton beam therapy, brachytherapy, CyberKnife, and external beam. Procedures performed by interventional radiologists include radio frequency ablation (RFA), cryoablation, and nerve blocks. Systemic therapy with a medical oncologist encompasses standard chemotherapy, targeted hormonal therapies, and biotherapy/immunotherapy.

Palliative care is an integral part of oncology treatment and has emerged as an invaluable component of comprehensive cancer treatment well recognized by the American Board of Medical Specialties. Palliative care includes multiple disciplines with a focus on preventing and relieving suffering by supporting patients and families facing a serious and/or life-threatening illness, with cancer being a major disease state utilizing palliative care services. Palliative care includes recognizing and integrating psychosocial, spiritual, and medical aspects of care[2] and may involve the inclusion of hospice care and pain management specialists (see Chapter 13).

STAGING OF TUMORS

An initial diagnosis of cancer is usually made by analysis of cellular material (i.e., blood sample, Pap smear, fine needle aspiration,[3] or with a tissue sample from the tumor).

Once a diagnosis is established, the patient's disease is then staged to assess the extent of disease and to determine both prognosis and choice of therapy. Various cancer-staging systems are used for both individual and multiple cancers. The tumor, nodes, and metastasis (TNM) system is a widely used cancer classification system created by the American Joint Committee on Cancer and the International Union against Cancer.[4] The TNM staging system describes the size and extension of the primary tumor, its lymphatic involvement, and the presence of metastases to classify the progression of cancer using numbers *x* (cannot be assessed), 0 (no tumor detected), and up to 3 or 4 (largest and most widespread). Common parameters in most staging systems include cell type, location of primary tumor, tumor grade, tumor size and number, lymph node involvement, and presence of metastases.[3]

In the earlier stages of disease (stage I or II), the tumor is typically localized, and the chances for cure are greater with the use of local or regional therapy. If the tumor stage is higher (stage III or IV), the cancer is no longer localized, and curative treatment may no longer be an option for the patient. The treatment plan is highly individualized to the patient and should take into account the risk/benefit ratio of the various options, the patient's performance status, the patient's willingness to consent to treatment, the availability of a treatment facility, financial restrictions, and the impact the treatment may have on the patient's quality of life.

SURGERY

Surgery is the oldest treatment still used today and remains effective for cancer prevention (e.g., thyroid or breast cancers), diagnosis, definitive treatment, rehabilitation, and palliation.[4]

RADIATION THERAPY

Radiation therapy is often used in combination with surgery, chemotherapy, and/or biologic therapies to eliminate or shrink tumors. Radiation therapy can also be given as sole treatment for patients with highly localized tumors that are histologically radiosensitive, or as an alternative to surgery for patients with a poor performance status who are medically unable to undergo surgery.

When radiation treatment is used as an adjunct to treatment, the goal is to gain control of the disease, and the treatment may be delivered preoperatively or postoperatively. Preoperative radiation treatment can help debulk the tumor to facilitate surgical resection. Postoperative radiation treatment may be chosen after surgical resection if there is a concern about local recurrence or if the resection margin remains suspicious for disease. Radiation may also be used in the palliative setting to address complaints of pain, bleeding, or in the case of brain metastasis to control spinal cord compression by a tumor or to target brain metastases causing symptoms.

There are a variety of ways in which radiation therapy may be delivered in the treatment of cancer. The mode that is selected is dependent on the cancer histology, tumor location, patient's performance status, availability of technology, and expertise of the radiation oncologist. The goal of therapy is to optimize dose delivery to the tumor while minimizing damage to healthy tissue.

Types of Radiation

External Beam Radiotherapy. The most commonly used form of radiation therapy is external beam. Linear accelerators are used to generate high-energy x-rays, or photons, at varying energies, which penetrate the body and are directed at the tumor. The depth of photon penetration depends on the energy selected. Treatment delivered in this manner is accomplished with different combinations of energies, beam techniques, radiation shielding, and patient positioning. This form of treatment is used in a variety of cancers but is currently the gold standard for treatment of invasive breast cancers following surgical excision.[5]

Once external beam therapy has been chosen, a simulation using computed tomography (CT) is then performed for radiation planning. During simulation, a planning CT scan is obtained so that the radiation oncologist can localize and define the tumor volume needing treatment. Critical structures to be avoided are also identified at this time. The treatment field is delineated, and marks corresponding to the area of treatment are subsequently made on the patient. These marks are used later during the treatment phase for proper patient alignment to the linear accelerator. Special immobilization devices, such as custom casts or molds, may be used during the simulation process to assist in the patient setup process.[5]

Once the CT simulation is completed and the field and dose, treatment is determined. Fractionated radiation therapy is used to maximize the therapeutic benefit of radiation while minimizing the harmful effects of radiation on healthy tissue.

The amount of radiation absorbed by tissue is expressed in the international unit gray (Gy): 1 Gy equals 100 rad (radiation absorbed dose); 1 cGy equals 1 rad. The total dose of radiation is typically spread out, or fractionated, into small treatments given during specific periods. Fractionation allows for repair of radiation damage to normal cells and their repopulation. It also gives an opportunity for re-oxygenation of hypoxic tissue, thereby improving the effectiveness of radiation in subsequent fractions of treatment. Fractionated therapy also permits more time for cancer cells that were previously in a resistant part of their cell cycle to become more susceptible to the radiation effect during subsequent fractions.[5] The final dose and fraction scheme chosen will be a reflection of several factors that affect the radiation dose, including the goal of therapy, radiosensitivity of the tumor, cancer stage, and normal tissue tolerances of the different anatomic structures in the treatment field.

Brachytherapy. Brachytherapy involves placement of a radioactive source within the body or body cavity near the tumor site. It is used mainly in the treatment of prostate and cervical cancers.[6] Brachytherapy is often combined with external beam radiation and may be used preoperatively or postoperatively. Radioactive isotopes for brachytherapy application are contained in a variety of forms, such as wires, ribbons, tubes, needles, grains, seeds, and capsules. The radiation oncologist will determine the form based on the site being treated, the size of the lesion, and whether the implant is temporary or permanent. Brachytherapy is given at either a low-dose rate or a high-dose rate, which produces the same effect in a shorter period.[6]

Proton Beam. Proton beam is more precise in the delivery, which reduces the radiation dose to the normal surrounding healthy tissue. Currently it is used extensively in pediatric cancers, prostate cancer, sarcomas, and melanoma, but continued research is being done to determine the role of proton beam versus conventional external beam radiation.

Radiosurgery. Gamma knife radiosurgery works by delivering extremely precise, high-dose beams of radiation directly to a tumor site in the brain, thereby avoiding healthy tissue. The most common use for radiosurgery is for the treatment of metastatic brain tumors, spinal metastases, and metastatic epidural spinal cord compression. Other targeted radiotherapy methods used include: intensity-modulated radiation therapy (IMRT), an advanced mode of high-precision radiotherapy that utilizes computer-controlled x-ray accelerators to deliver precise radiation doses to a malignant tumor or specific areas within the tumor, and stereotactic radiosurgery, a highly precise form of radiation therapy that directs narrow beams of radiation to the tumor from different angles. These procedures are well tolerated by patients as they are less invasive than traditional neurosurgery.

Radiation Treatment Side Effects

Radiation treatment–related side effects can develop early in the course of therapy, or they may be delayed for several months to years after therapy. There are predictable side effects of radiation therapy. Factors that predict side effects include the body tissue treated, the daily dose and total dosage given, the particular method of radiation delivery, and individual factors (e.g., the patient's age and genetic makeup). Acute symptoms often develop 10 to 14 days into treatment and may not diminish until 2 or more weeks after the treatments have been completed. Common side effects vary by treatment site but may include fatigue, anorexia, mucositis, xerostomia, radiation caries, esophagitis, dysphagia, nausea, vomiting, diarrhea, tenesmus, cystitis, urethritis, alopecia, skin reactions, and bone marrow depression. Late toxicities are likely to be related to the tissue site of irradiation and may include but are not limited to: infertility, cardio toxicity, secondary cancers, urinary symptoms, and bowel symptoms. These may not present until 6 months after treatment and may persist for years or chronically.

Summary

Radiation oncology continues to evolve with intensity modulation and apparatuses for radiation therapy, image-guided and three-dimensional treatment planning for radiation therapy, particle therapy radiation, and advances in brachytherapy, all of which allow radiation oncologists more tools to treat cancer while reducing the toxicity of treatment.[9] The primary care provider's responsibility is to monitor patients for acute reactions during radiation therapy, to assess for delayed reactions during post-treatment surveillance, and to collaborate with the radiation oncologist in implementing a management strategy throughout the course of care.

INTERVENTIONAL PROCEDURES

Interventional radiologists are trained radiologists who use modalities to treat tumors directly, including RFA, cryoablation, and nerve blocks.

Radio Frequency Ablation

RFA is the process of heating up a tumor using a small needle inserted through the skin, causing the cancer cells to die. It is used for solid tumors that are not amenable to surgery and are less than 4 cm in size. The most common tumors treated in this manner are kidney, primary liver tumors or metastases in the liver, and primary or lung metastases. It is normally tolerated well, has minimal side effects, and has a short recovery.

Cryoablation

Cryoablation is essentially freezing a tumor so the cancer cells cannot replicate. It is used with tumors that are not amenable to surgery and are less than 4 cm in size.

Nerve Blocks

Nerve blocks are used to stop the processing of painful stimuli caused by a tumor which are aggravating nerve fibers. They do not treat the tumor, but instead treat the pain caused by the tumor.[7]

SYSTEMIC TREATMENT OPTIONS
Chemotherapy

Role for Chemotherapy. Carcinogenesis is the process by which one or more normal cells undergo genetic changes, leading to malignant transformation. The direct exposure of DNA to a carcinogen may lead to irreversible genetic damage, allowing malignant transformation. The cell cycle is a sequence of steps through which both normal and abnormal cells grow and reproduce; applying chemotherapy at different points in that sequence helps to stop or slow the growth of malignant cells. The primary role of chemotherapy is to prevent cancer cells from multiplying, invading, and metastasizing, in order to prolong life.

Chemotherapy can be used as induction treatment for advanced disease, as a primary treatment when no alternative

treatment is superior, or for palliative treatment. It can be used as adjuvant therapy when alternative local therapies exist but are less effective alone (i.e., radiation therapy or surgery), and is often given first or even concurrently with local therapy, depending on the patient's clinical situation and cancer type. Chemotherapy helps with debulking the primary tumor or after the completion of local therapies, to eradicate micrometastases. Lastly, chemotherapy can be directly instilled into tumor sanctuary sites or perfused into specific regions of the body most affected by the cancer (e.g., the peritoneum or liver).[8] Administration of a combination of clinically effective antitumor drugs with non-overlapping toxicities is the standard for a chemotherapeutic approach to most malignant neoplasms.

Classification of Chemotherapy. Chemotherapeutic agents are classified by their mechanism of action, chemical structure, or biologic source. Alkylating agents were the first modern chemotherapeutic agents used in the clinical setting and were a product of the US secret gas program in the two world wars. Exposure to mustard gas was shown to arrest bone marrow and lymphocyte tissue development. Therefore in 1942 a patient with lymphoma was treated with nitrogen mustard. In the same time period, another researcher observed that folic acid induced leukemic cell growth in children; this observation led to the development of folic acid analogues and later to the development of antimetabolites, a cornerstone in cancer treatment.[9]

Molecular genetic analysis of the DNA, RNA, and proteins of both normal and neoplastic cells has defined the mechanisms by which chemotherapy induces cell death. An understanding of how chemotherapy works and how molecular genetic changes can result in resistance to therapy has enabled newer types of treatment. These therapies combine molecular, genetic, and biologic strategies to increase the sensitivity of abnormal cells to treatment and to protect the normal tissues of the body from therapy-induced side effects, which may ultimately help patients with cancers that are resistant to standard therapies.

Response to Chemotherapy. There is a wide range between therapeutic response and toxicity among patients receiving chemotherapy. The variability in this range can be attributed to differences in the characteristics of the patient, the chemotherapeutic agents given, and the type of tumor being treated. Patient factors include toxicity response, organ dysfunction, previous treatments, and age. Once toxicity occurs, a dose reduction or a treatment delay will most likely be indicated.[10]

Side Effects. The oncologist and primary care provider often work collaboratively in managing common side effects from chemotherapy. Short-term symptoms include fatigue, anorexia, diarrhea, constipation, nausea, mucositis, alopecia, and vomiting. Long-term side effects include cardiotoxicity, neurotoxicity, pulmonary toxicity, hepatotoxicity, hemorrhagic cystitis, nephrotoxicity, infertility, myelosuppression, and secondary malignant neoplasms.[10] Adverse effects may vary depending on the combination of agents used.

SYSTEMIC TREATMENTS OTHER THAN CONVENTIONAL CHEMOTHERAPY
Hormonal Therapy

Hormonal therapy is used in cancers that have a hormonal influence including breast and prostate cancers. The two main mechanics of hormone therapy block the body's ability to produce hormones or interfere with how the hormones influence the body. In breast cancer the selective estrogen receptor modulators (SERMS, i.e., tamoxifen and raloxifene) are used. SERMS act as an antagonist in the breast tissue and an agonist in the bones.[11] Tamoxifen, unlike raloxifene, also acts as an agonist in the uterus, which can at times lead to the development of uterine cancer. SERMS can be used with pre- or post-menopausal patients. Aromatase inhibitors act by inhibiting the action of the enzyme aromatase which converts androgens into estrogens, and in turn decreases the amount of circulating estrogen, helping to reduce recurrence of breast cancer cells or the development of new breast cancer cells. In prostate cancer the use of androgen deprivation therapy, such as Lupron, is used to decrease testosterone levels which can aid in reducing recurrence and development of new prostate cancer cells.[12]

Targeted Therapy

Targeted therapy uses biomarkers such as EGFR, BCR-ABL, HER2/neu, PD-1, KRAS, and many more to identify therapies that are specific to that biomarker. Biomarkers are used to diagnose, monitor, and stage disease and can also be used for predictive and prognostic values.[13] Targeted therapy is used when specific tumor receptors are identified on genes and agents are targeted to work as an antagonist and block those receptors. These are currently used in colon, lung, head/neck, NSCLC, pancreatic, renal, lymphomas, leukemia, and breast cancers and are evolving rapidly. Examples are tyrosine kinase inhibitors for EGFR receptor positive cancers, monoclonal antibodies, and Herceptin/Pertuzumab for HER2/neu receptor positive cancers.

Targeted therapies such as angiogenesis inhibitors work by blocking growth factors that normally assist cell proliferation and are primarily used in lung cancer. Although thought to be generally safe they have rarely been associated with life-threatening adverse events including: thrombotic events, bleeding, and congestive heart failure.

Immunotherapy/Biotherapy

Immunotherapy boosts the body's natural defense against cancer using substances that occur naturally in the body or are made in the laboratory. It involves controlling the immune system at different points in the immune response using cytokines to trigger an immune response, checkpoint inhibitors which assist T cells to mount a longer-lasting response to cancer cells, and adoptive cellular therapy which increases the number and effectiveness of T cells.[14] Two of the best understood checkpoint proteins are the CTLA-4 and PD-1 pathways.

Ipilimumab for melanoma was one of the first immunotherapies to be developed and works on the CTLA-4 pathway. Bevacizumab inhibits angiogenesis, limiting the blood supply to tumors and restricting its growth; it is applicable to many types of cancer.

The presence of PD-1 impedes the body's immune defenses from functioning at full strength, therefore the mechanism of action of the PDL-1 inhibitors is that they block the interaction between PD-1 protein and T cells. This allows the T cells to mount a longer-lasting response against the tumor.

It is important to note that initially with immune therapy, as opposed to cytotoxic treatment, patients may have a delayed response and can actually have worsening disease before they have a positive response most likely due to a stimulation of the T cells.[13] Side effects occur when healthy cells are attacked by the immunotherapy and cause an immune reaction such as skin reactions, flu-like symptoms, muscle aches, shortness of breath, lower extremity edema, and diarrhea. Steroids may be required for treatment of side effects. Endocrine side effects are also possible including hypothyroidism, hyperthyroidism, hypopituitarism, hypophysitis, thyroiditis, and adrenal insufficiencies, all of which are treated with steroids.

Vaccines

The US Food and Drug Administration approved a human papillomavirus (HPV) vaccine for females aged 9 to 26 and males aged 9 to 21. It protects against the HPV types that most often cause cervical, vaginal, vulvar, and anal cancers. The hepatitis B vaccine is available for all age groups to prevent HBV infection, a possible trigger for liver cancer. https://www.cdc.gov/cancer/dcpc/prevention/vaccination.htm

Cytokines

There are two types of cytokines used to treat cancer—interferons and interleukins. They help to regulate and mediate the immune response, inflammation, and hematopoiesis.

Growth factor stimulating injections help combat the side effects of cancer treatment. They can help with red cell production such as erythropoietin and GMCSF and GCSF help to stimulate the bone marrow to make more white blood cells.[15]

ORAL THERAPIES

Oral therapies have continued to be developed. Although these therapies are not given in an infusion unit, patients can still have side effects and need to be followed closely by an oncology team and PCP. Patients need to be monitored closely for dosage accuracy and side effects. Some patients may stop medications without an indication to do so by their medical provider; this may be due to difficulty with schedule or side effects. Regular visits and laboratory monitoring need to be scheduled with patients on oral chemotherapy agents for close supervision. Some oral chemotherapies have been around for many years including cyclophosphamide and methotrexate. Many newer ones are in use or are being developed including imatinib (Gleevec), etoposide (Toposar), capecitabine (Xeloda), and others.

SURVIVORSHIP
Survivorship Role

Definition of roles of both primary care providers and oncology professionals is imperative. This is best served by providing a survivorship care plan. Patients who are followed by a PCP and an oncologist as opposed to those followed only by an oncologist tend to have more preventative care and are normally older adults with multiple comorbidities, which PCPs tend to feel more comfortable managing. Accepting a patient's decision to discontinue or opt out of certain treatments is also an important part of managing the oncology patient. Direct communication and collaboration between the oncology team and the primary care provider can have a calculated long-term effect on survival and well-being (see Chapter 223).

GENETIC TESTING

A significant percentage of cancers are associated with genetic susceptibility. Genetic testing is progressing and there is growing data that suggests patients may consider genetic testing even prior to a care diagnosis to aid with surveillance and screening.

These services remain expensive and underutilized in primary care, perhaps due to provider unfamiliarity and lack of patient awareness. Fortunately this is beginning to change.

Perhaps the best known genetic association is the BRCA gene and breast cancer. When used in conjunction with a documented family history, therapy can be targeted for best results. Genetic testing has also been useful for screening and targeting treatment in colon, ovarian, prostate, and other cancers.

REDUCING CANCER RISK

As patients navigate information overload they will look to primary care providers for help in making good cancer prevention choices. These include: not starting or stopping tobacco, using sunscreen, eating healthy, staying active, following cancer screening guidelines, reducing alcohol intake, and undergoing routine exams.

TREATING THE CANCER PATIENT TODAY AND TOMORROW

Progress in molecular biology and biotechnology has made an impact on the way patients with cancer are treated today. Treatment options in targeted and immune therapies are rapidly being developed. There is a greater understanding of the molecular nature of cancer and the immune system. Primary health care providers have multiple responsibilities caring for patients undergoing treatment for cancers including medical oversight and emotional and spiritual support. As patients live longer, with and without cancer, primary care providers are essential in providing long-term care for patients.

REFERENCES

1. National Cancer Institute. www.cancer.gov/about-cancer/understanding/statistics. (Accessed 6 August 2018).
2. Ferrell, B. R., Temel, J. S., & Tenin, J. (2016). Integration of palliative care. *Journal of Clinical Oncology.*
3. National Cancer Institute. Cancer Staging. www.cancer.gov/about-cancer/diagnosis-staging/staging-fact-sheet. (Accessed 6 August 2018).
4. National Cancer Institute. www.cancer.gov/about-cancer/treatment/types/surgery. (Accessed 5 December 2017).
5. Gradisher, W., Anderson, B., Aft, R., et al. (2018). NCCN guideline 1. *Breast Cancer (Tokyo, Japan)*, www.nccn.org/professionals/physicians_gls/pdf/breast/pdf. (Accessed 7 August 2018).
6. Smith, J. A., & Jhingram, A. (2017). Principles of radiation therapy and chemotherapy in gynecological cancer: Basic principles, uses and complications. In R. Lobor, D. Gershen, et al. (Eds.), *Comprehensive gynecology*. Elsevier.
7. Hasuo, H., Kanbara, K., Abe, T., et al. (2017). Factors associated with the efficacy of trigger point injection in advanced cancer patients. *Journal of Palliative Medicine, 20,* 1085.
8. National Cancer Institute. Chemotherapy. www.cancer.gov/about-cancer/treatment/types/chemotherapy. (Accessed 6 August 2018).
9. American Cancer Society. www.cancer.org/cancer/cancer-basics/history-of-cancer/cancer-treatment-chemo. (Accessed 8 August 2018).
10. Gallagher, C., Smith, M., & Shamash, J. (2017). Malignant disease. In *Kumar and Clark's clinical medicine* (9th ed.). Elsevier.
11. Burstein, H., Lacchetti, C., Griggs, J., et al. (2016). Adjuvant endocrine therapy for women with hormone receptor-positive breast cancer: American Society of clinical oncology clinical practice guidelines update on ovarian suppression summary. *Journal of Oncology Practice, 12*(4), 390–393.
12. Heidenreich, A., Bastian, P. J., Bellmut, J., et al. (2014). EAU guidelines on prostate cancer Part II: Treatment of advanced, replapsing and castration-resistant prostate cancer. *European Urology, 65*(2), 467.
13. Kalia, M. (2015). Biomarkers for personalized oncology: Recent advances and future challenges. *Metabolism: Clinical and Experimental, 64*(3), s16–s21.
14. Kreamer, K. (2014). Immune checkpoint blockade: A new paradigm in treating advanced cancer. *Journal of the Advanced Practitioner in Oncology, 5,* 418–431.
15. National Cancer Institute. Biological Therapies. www.cancer.gov/about-cancer/treatment/types/immunotherapy/bio-therapies-fact-sheet#q4. (Accessed 8 August 2018).

CHAPTER 223

ONCOLOGY COMPLICATIONS, PARANEOPLASTIC SYNDROMES, AND CANCER SURVIVORSHIP

Sarah Hauke Given

 Immediate emergency room evaluation and hospitalization required for patients with angioedema, dyspnea, stridor, papilledema, seizures, and other signs of superior vena cava syndrome (SVCS); patients with back pain accompanied by focal weakness, ataxia, or bowel or bladder dysfunction; patients with serum calcium levels of more than 12 mg/dL; patients with TLS; and patients with serum sodium levels of 125 mEq/L or less are oncologic emergencies.

Paraneoplastic syndromes are symptoms that occur distant from the primary malignant tumor or its metastases. These syndromes are incompletely understood but are thought to be related to substances secreted by the tumor or antibodies directed against the tumor that are reacting to other tissues. An oncologic emergency is an acute, potentially life-threatening event that is directly or indirectly related to cancer or its treatment. If it is left unrecognized and untreated, significant morbidity or death may result. A paraneoplastic syndrome or oncologic emergency may also occur in an individual not previously diagnosed with cancer. Because cancer manifests in various ways, it must be considered part of the differential diagnosis of many complex medical events. In addition, because the nature of these entities can be emergent and because treatment of the underlying cancer is required, all these syndromes require urgent referral to an oncologist.

Common structural emergencies are superior vena cava syndrome (SVCS) and spinal cord compression (SCC). Metabolic emergencies include hypercalcemia, syndrome of inappropriate antidiuretic hormone (SIADH), and tumor lysis syndrome (TLS). Other oncologic emergencies not discussed in this chapter include sepsis, disseminated intravascular coagulation, malignant pericardial effusions, and hyperviscosity caused by dysproteinemia or leukocytosis.

Cancer survivors, patients who have completed treatment for their cancer, remain at risk of ongoing short-term and long-term complications from their treatment. These complications may be related to prior chemotherapy, surgical intervention, or radiation and may affect any body system. Cancer survivors are also at risk of disease relapse and secondary cancer. Cancer survivors are primarily followed by their PCPs and it is important that primary care providers know how to identify and manage potential toxicities from prior treatment.

SUPERIOR VENA CAVA SYNDROME

DEFINITION AND EPIDEMIOLOGY

SVCS occurs when blood flow through the superior vena cava (SVC) is obstructed. Lung cancer is responsible for most cases of SVCS.

PATHOPHYSIOLOGY

Any pathologic process that invades the lymphatics or structures of the superior mediastinum can encroach on the thin-walled, compliant SVC and cause obstruction of venous return to the heart. SVCS may result from external compression, direct invasion, or thrombosis of the SVC. The most common cause of SVC obstruction is malignant disease, usually lung cancer, both non-small cell and small cell, with 2% to 4% of lung cancer patients developing SVCS over the course of their disease. Lymphomas are also a common cause of SVCS.[1] Other forms of malignancy, including but not limited to breast and GI cancers, sarcomas, melanomas, prostate cancer, or any other mediastinal tumor may also be a less common source. The most common nonmalignant cause of SVCS is thrombosis of the SVC associated with intravascular devices including indwelling central venous catheters and pacemakers. Aneurysms and goiters are less common nonmalignant sources.[1,2]

CLINICAL PRESENTATION AND PHYSICAL EXAMINATION

SVCS is usually insidious in onset. Many of the signs and symptoms of SVCS may be identified on clinical exam. The hallmark presenting symptom of SVCS is swelling of the neck, seen in 100% of patients. Other common presenting symptoms include swelling of the trunk, upper extremities, or chest, and dyspnea. Concomitant symptoms include chest pain, cough, dilated chest vein collaterals, new onset paresthesia, dysphagia, confusion, dizziness, hoarseness, or night sweats.[1,2] Other symptoms include headache, dizziness, visual disturbances, hoarseness, chest pain, and dysphagia.

Physical findings include venous distention in the upper body, facial edema, cyanosis, arm and hand edema, telangiectasias of the chest and upper back, hoarseness, and stridor. Neurologic abnormalities resulting from increased cerebral edema include confusion, dizziness, headaches, mental status changes, lethargy, and coma.[1]

DIAGNOSTICS

Essential Diagnostics

Imaging is required for the diagnosis of SVCS. A chest x-ray examination commonly reflects a superior mediastinal mass or widening, or right hilar mass; 64% of patients with SVCS will have an abnormal chest x-ray.[1,2] Computed tomography (CT scan) with contrast (if tolerated) can identify the source and extent of obstruction as well as the characteristics of the obstruction.[1] If patient has contraindications to IV contrast, magnetic resonance imaging (MRI) can also be used to identify the source of the blockage. Contrast enhanced magnetic resonance venography is highly sensitive in identifying SVCS but is expensive. In most patients, a standard MRI is sufficient.[1] Doppler ultrasound may be useful in identifying underlying clots and venous flow reversal, but due to positioning cannot visualize the SVC.[1,2]

Additional Diagnostics

If the underlying pathologic condition has not previously been identified, biopsy is indicated so that the underlying disease may be appropriately treated[2] (see Chapter 224).

INITIAL DIAGNOSTICS

Superior Vena Cava Syndrome

IMAGING
- Chest x-ray examination
- CT scan with contrast
- MRI or contrast enhanced MR venography Doppler ultrasound

OTHER DIAGNOSTICS
- Biopsy

DIFFERENTIAL DIAGNOSIS

Malignancy remains the most common cause of SVCS. Thrombosis-related SVCS accounts for up to 40% of SVCS due to the increased prevalence of implantable intravenous devices such as pacemakers, tunneled venous catheters, and port catheters. Less common differential diagnoses include mediastinal fibrosis and infectious causes including tuberculosis and syphilis.[3]

INTERPROFESSIONAL COLLABORATIVE MANAGEMENT

SVCS requires emergent empiric treatment only in the setting of airway obstruction or cerebral edema, otherwise treatment is directed at the underlying cause. In patients who do not require emergent management, the treatment of SVCS should be guided by the stage and histologic features of the primary process. Treatment for SVCS may include radiation or chemotherapy, or stenting depending on the etiology.[1,4] Intravascular stenting is frequently effective in offering symptomatic relief and preventing recurrent SVCS. Patients typically experience relief of symptoms within 24 to 48 hours of stent placement. Stent placement does not compromise further work-up for the underlying histological diagnosis.[1,3,4] Anecdotally, concomitant steroids may be beneficial although there is limited data to support differences in overall symptomatic relief or long-term outcomes with their use.[1,3] Temporary measures to alleviate discomfort include elevation of the head of the bed and supplemental oxygen.[3]

COMPLICATIONS

SVCS is a medical emergency that requires urgent evaluation. Although SVCS may not have a direct impact on overall survival, the prognosis of patients with SVCS is poor with median survival in malignant SVCS ranging from 1.5 to 9 months.[1]

MALIGNANT SPINAL CORD COMPRESSION

DEFINITION AND EPIDEMIOLOGY

Malignant spinal cord compression (MSCC) occurs in approximately 2.5% to 5% of advanced cancer patients.[2,3,4] The incidence of SCC is highest in lung, breast, and prostate cancer, each accounting for 15% to 20% of MSCC. Non-Hodgkin lymphoma, renal cell carcinoma, and multiple myeloma account for 5% to 10% of MSCC.[3]

PATHOPHYSIOLOGY

MSCC is most often a result of primary tumor spreading to the spine. In most cases (75%) MSCC is a result of epidural metastasis; it is less commonly (25%) caused by bony collapse directly compressing the spinal cord.[2] The compression of the spinal cord causes vascular compromise leading to a rapid deterioration in neurologic function.

CLINICAL PRESENTATION AND PHYSICAL EXAMINATION

The signs and symptoms of MSCC depend on the area of spinal cord involved. The thoracic spine is involved most often (70%), followed by the lumbosacral (20%) and cervical (10%) vertebrae.[2] Back pain is the most common presenting complaint in patients with MSCC, occurring in 95% of patients, and may precede other symptomatic complaints by up to 2 months.[3] Depending on the location of the compression, pain may follow a dermatomal pattern and can be unilateral of bilateral. Pain is described as a constant, dull, aching back pain that is often worse when the patient is supine (opposite of the usual finding with a herniated disk).[2] Motor deficits including lower extremity weakness, leg heaviness, and difficulty walking are the second most common presenting symptom. Sensory deficits including new onset paresthesia are less common.[2,4] Autonomic dysfunctions, such as urinary frequency or urgency and bowel or bladder incontinence are late manifestations of MSCC. Patients with cauda equina syndrome are at risk of ataxia progressing to paralysis if symptoms are left untreated.[2–4]

Examination should involve a detailed history as well as complete neurological exam. Physical findings may include tenderness on palpation of the involved vertebrae, diminished rectal tone, muscle weakness, or urinary retention. Decreased sensation of the lower extremities may be a more subtle examination finding. Patients with cauda equina may have decreased sensation following a dermatomal pattern.[2]

DIAGNOSTICS
Essential Diagnostics

Imaging is needed to diagnose MSCC. The entire spine should be imaged, as epidural disease may occur in multiple locations. MRI is considered the gold standard and has a sensitivity of 93% and a specificity of 97%. A CT scan or myelography is an acceptable alternative in patients who cannot undergo MRI (e.g., patients who have cardiac pacemakers or are claustrophobic).[2,3,4] Patients with cancer who are seen with a new complaint of back pain should undergo an evaluation for SCC.

INITIAL DIAGNOSTICS

Spinal Cord Compression

IMAGING
- MRI
- CT scan
- Myelography
- Tumor biopsy

DIFFERENTIAL DIAGNOSIS

Other clinical situations may mimic MSCC by causing motor or sensory deficits of the neck or upper and lower back or by causing pain. Differential diagnosis may include musculoskeletal disease including degenerative disc disease, muscle spasm and spinal stenosis, spinal abscess, or metastatic disease. Any back pain that worsens when patient is recumbent should not be considered benign.

INTERPROFESSIONAL COLLABORATIVE MANAGEMENT

Clear indications of MSCC in the cancer patient (e.g., focal weakness, ataxia, bowel or bladder dysfunction accompanied by back pain) demand an emergent evaluation and a referral. Rapid treatment of MSCC improves short-term prognosis. The goals of treatment are to maintain neurological function, control growth of the tumor, spine stabilization, and pain control.[3] Immediate therapy with corticosteroids (dexamethasone is most commonly used) may reduce vasogenic edema. High-dose steroids followed by a 1- to 2-week taper has been shown to increase ambulatory status for up to 6 months post treatment. It should be noted that steroid therapy can be associated with significant side effects. Radiotherapy is an effective treatment modality especially in patients with radiosensitive tumors (i.e., breast, prostate, small-cell lung, lymphoma, and myeloma). In patients with spinal instability surgical stabilization should precede radiotherapy. Surgery is also an appropriate intervention in patients with prior radiation to the spine, radioresistant tumors (i.e., melanoma, sarcoma, and renal cell carcinoma), unknown primary tumor, paraplegia for <48 hours, or renal cell carcinoma.[4]

COMPLICATIONS

Prognosis for MSCC is poor with a median survival of <6 months. Prompt treatment can palliate symptoms and prevent paralysis.[3] Ambulatory and neurological status at the time of diagnosis are predictors of outcome post-treatment, with patients who are ambulatory without significant neurological deficit having the best outcomes. If it is left untreated or undiagnosed, MSCC can result in paraplegia, quadriplegia, or loss of bowel or bladder function. In most patients, motor function and sphincter control cannot be regained once they have been lost.

HYPERCALCEMIA

DEFINITION AND EPIDEMIOLOGY

Hypercalcemia is defined as a total serum calcium of greater than 10 mg/dL and is a common metabolic emergency in oncology affecting 10% to 30% of all cancer patients at some point during the course of their illness (See Chapter 188).[5,6] The most common malignant neoplasms associated with hypercalcemia are lymphomas, multiple myeloma, breast cancer, squamous cell cancer of the lung, and renal cancers. In a majority of patients hypercalcemia is caused by increased bone resorption with release of calcium from the bones.

PATHOPHYSIOLOGY

Most often, in hypercalcemia of malignancy, hormonal factors stimulate osteoclast activity, resulting in the release of calcium from the bone. The major mechanism of hypercalcemia in malignancy is humoral, secretion of a para-thyroid related peptide (PTHrP). PTHrP is found in up to 80% of patients with hypercalcemia of malignancy. It acts on post receptor parathyroid hormone (PTH) pathways that function to increase bone and calcium resorption leading to hypercalcemia.[5] Other mechanisms of hypercalcemia include osteolysis from bone metastasis, abnormal 1,25-vitamin D, and ectopic parathyroid secretion (rare).[2,3,5]

CLINICAL PRESENTATION AND PHYSICAL EXAMINATION

Most patients with hypercalcemia see their health care provider with nonspecific symptoms which are frequently attributed to either the patient's underlying malignancy or to treatment effects. Presenting symptoms include lethargy, confusion, constipation, weakness, hypovolemia, polyuria, polydipsia, and cardiac dysrhythmias, progressing to stupor and coma. Symptoms are often most severe in older adults, debilitated patients, and/or in patients who have a rapid increase in their serum calcium. In patients who have a slow or chronic increase in their serum calcium symptoms may be asymptomatic or with subtle symptoms until serum calcium levels are high.

Physical exam findings include muscle weakness, hyporeflexia, and mental status changes. EKG changes include prolonged PR interval, widened QRS complex, shortened QT interval, and bundle branch block (see Chapter 188).[6]

DIAGNOSTICS

Essential Diagnostics

Hypercalcemia is diagnosed through laboratory studies. Total serum calcium and ionized calcium concentration should be checked. Because calcium binds to albumin, total calcium measurements can be greatly affected by changes in albumin concentrations. Hypoproteinemia is often seen in cancer patients; therefore the measurement of total serum calcium may understate the severity of the disorder. It is useful to obtain an initial measurement of ionized serum calcium; alternatively, total serum calcium can be adjusted for the level of serum protein.[2] Hypercalcemia can be classified as mild (10 to 12 mg/dL; 5.6 to 8 mg/dL ionized), moderate (12.1 to 14 mg/dL; 8.1 to 10 mg/dL ionized), and severe/hypercalcemic crisis (>14 mg/dL; >10 mg/dL ionized) (Wagner). In cases of severe hypercalcemia EKG changes may be noted.

INITIAL DIAGNOSTICS
Hypercalcemia
LABORATORY
• Serum calcium and phosphorus
• Serum albumin and total protein
• Ionized serum calcium
OTHER DIAGNOSTICS
• Electrocardiography

DIFFERENTIAL DIAGNOSIS

There is an extensive list of differential diagnoses for hypercalcemia (see Chapter 188). The most common differentials are hyperparathyroidism, granulomatous disease, and excessive intake of vitamin D. It is important to ascertain that the patient's hypercalcemia is definitely caused by malignancy and not another treatable disease even when the patient has active cancer.

INTERPROFESSIONAL COLLABORATIVE MANAGEMENT

With the exception of patients who are emergently ill, it is recommended that elevated serum calcium levels be confirmed with an ionized calcium level prior to the initiation of treatment. Initial management for all patients is stabilization and reduction of the calcium level through oral or parenteral rehydration. The goal of rehydration is to increase the renal clearance of calcium, decrease calcium levels through dilution, and restore intravascular volume. Volume status, electrolytes, and serum calcium levels should be carefully monitored during rehydration. If fluids are administered intravenously, the infusion rate is dependent on the patient's underlying renal and cardiac status. There is limited evidence to support the use of loop diuretics in hypercalcemia because of concerns for hypovolemia and worsening renal function and the current recommendation is that diuretics are only used to correct for hypervolemia after overaggressive fluid replacement.

Hospitalization is recommended for patients with a serum calcium level of 14 mg/dL or higher (3.5 mmol/L) and for patients who have symptoms other than mild fatigue and constipation. Intravenous bisphosphonates (pamidronate, zoledronic acid, ibandronate, and etidronate) are potent inhibitors of osteoclast activity and produce a sustained decrease in calcium levels within 12 to 48 hours with effects lasting 2 to 4 weeks. Zoledronic acid is the preferred bisphosphonate based on response rate and due to its shorter infusion rate. In patients with hypercalcemia secondary to abnormal 1,25-vitamin D (i.e., multiple myeloma and lymphoma), glucocorticoids may be considered. Calcitonin reduces serum calcium concentration within 2 to 4 hours by inhibiting bone resorption and increasing renal calcium excretion. This intervention has limited value given its low efficacy and risk of tachyphylaxis. Hemodialysis should be considered an option only in patients with severe refractory hypercalcemia.[5]

COMPLICATIONS

Treating hypercalcemia of malignancy does not improve overall mortality and at least half of patients diagnosed with hypercalcemia of malignancy will die within a month.[7] However, treatment is beneficial in palliation of symptoms and in preventing further decline. Left untreated, symptoms progress to profound alterations in mental status, seizures, coma, and death. Sudden death from cardiac arrhythmias may occur when serum calcium concentration rises acutely.

TUMOR LYSIS SYNDROME

DEFINITION AND EPIDEMIOLOGY

TLS is a metabolic imbalance that occurs with the rapid killing and lysis of neoplastic cells releasing the intracellular content and resulting in hyperkalemia, hyperphosphatemia, hypocalcemia, or hyperuricemia. TLS can be defined as laboratory TLS and clinical TLS. TLS most commonly occurs following chemotherapy; it less commonly occurs after radiotherapy, immunotherapy, hormonal therapy, surgery, or spontaneously in the setting of rapidly proliferating tumors (TLS is frequently associated with hematologic malignancy[8] including acute leukemia and high-grade lymphoma where there is a high volume of disease and rapid cell death associated with chemotherapy). To a lesser degree, solid tumors (e.g., breast cancer, SCLC, squamous cell carcinoma of the head and neck, hepatoblastoma, multiple myeloma) and myeloproliferative disorders, are at high risk for the development of this syndrome especially if in advanced stages of the disease. Other risk factors for TLS include underlying renal dysfunction and elevated serum lactate.[3]

PATHOPHYSIOLOGY

When cell death occurs, the intracellular contents are released into the blood stream. This includes potassium from cytosol breakdown, phosphate from protein breakdown, and uric acid from the breakdown of nucleic acid. The kidneys, which are responsible for processing cellular breakdown, cannot process the sudden increase in metabolites leading to metabolic derangement at life-threatening concentrations. Additionally, high levels of uric acid crystallize in the distal tubule of the nephron, with resultant acute obstructive uropathy and renal failure. The severity of the syndrome depends on the extent of tumor burden and preexisting renal insufficiency.[8]

CLINICAL PRESENTATION AND PHYSICAL EXAMINATION

TLS may present at varying degrees of severity ranging from incidental laboratory finding to sudden death. Presenting symptoms include nausea, vomiting, low urine output, constipation, diarrhea, weight gain, acute renal failure, cramps, seizures, tetany, or arrhythmias.[2] Presenting symptoms are a direct result of electrolyte abnormalities. Acute hyperkalemia and hypocalcemia may result in cardiac arrhythmias, tetany, syncope, and sudden death. Hypocalcemia may cause mild muscle cramps, tetany, and seizures. Hyperphosphatemia may aggravate renal failure. Acidosis and anuria may result. These metabolic changes may occur individually or simultaneously. In patients with underlying renal failure, metabolic abnormalities are more likely to be severe or life threatening.

DIAGNOSTICS
Essential Diagnostics

Prevention of TLS is critical in high-risk patients, and serum electrolyte values and uric acid, phosphorus, calcium, and creatinine concentrations should be checked regularly after the initiation of cytotoxic therapy. With electrolyte abnormalities, EKGs should be monitored given the risk of cardiac arrhythmias. Common EKG changes include peaked T waves and QRS widening.

There are currently two classification systems used in the diagnosis of TLS. The Cairo-Bishop system is the most widely accepted system. It classifies TLS as laboratory (LTLS) or clinical (CTLS). To meet the diagnosis of LTLS a patient must have at least two of the following electrolyte abnormalities in the 3 days prior to or the 7 days following chemotherapy treatment: hyperkalemia (K ≥6), hyperuricemia (uric acid ≥8), hyperphosphatemia (Ph ≥4.5 in adults), or hypocalcemia ≤7). To meet the diagnosis for CTLS, the patient must meet the diagnosis of LTLS and have at least one of the following, not attributable to other cause: renal involvement, cardiac involvement, or neurologic involvement.[8]

INITIAL DIAGNOSTICS
Tumor Lysis Syndrome
LABORATORY
• Serum electrolytes, calcium, phosphorus, BUN, creatinine
• Uric acid
OTHER DIAGNOSTICS
• EKG[a]
[a]If indicated.

DIFFERENTIAL DIAGNOSIS

 Physician consultation is necessary for uric acid levels above 8, serum potassium above 7, and acute increases in creatinine.

Gout (see Chapter 158) is the most common cause of hyperuricemia. Other causes of electrolyte disturbances need to be excluded (see Chapters 188, 189, 190). The key to diagnosis of TLS is a high degree of suspicion in an active cancer patient, especially those receiving chemotherapy.

INTERPROFESSIONAL MANAGEMENT AND COMPLICATIONS

Treatment is aimed at prevention, and high-risk patients should be carefully monitored while undergoing treatment. In both the prophylactic setting and the early treatment setting TLS should be managed with aggressive hydration to preserve renal function, monitoring of electrolytes to prevent cardiac dysrhythmias, and monitoring of neuromuscular irritability.[8] Hydration should be provided with isotonic IV fluids, at minimum 2 to 3 liters daily, and urine output should be monitored and should be at least 80 to 100 mL/h. IV hydration is effective in diluting electrolyte concentrations and in maintaining renal function. In patients at risk of TLS, IV fluids should be started 24 to 48 hours prior to cytotoxic treatment and continued for 48 to 72 hours post treatment.[3,8] Other prophylactic measures include the initiation of allopurinol, a xanthine oxidase inhibitor, at 100 mg/m[2] orally, every eight hours, starting 1 or 2 days before therapy and continuing 3 to 7 days post treatment or until there is no evidence of TLS. Doses should be reduced by 50% in patients with renal insufficiency.[8] More rapid control and lower levels of plasma uric acid have been observed with the administration of rasburicase, a recombinant urate oxidase. Rasburicase is fast acting; decreasing uric acid levels within hours. Hyperkalemia is the most dangerous electrolyte imbalance associated with TLS due to the associated cardiac abnormalities. It can be managed with an oral sodium-potassium exchange resin (sodium polystyrene sulfonate [Kayexalate]) or in combination with insulin-glucose therapy. Loop diuretics are also useful in the elimination of excess potassium. In the setting of hyperkalemia-induced cardiac arrhythmias, calcium gluconate offers immediate but transient benefits. Hyperphosphatemia can be controlled with the ingestion of an oral phosphate binder such as aluminum hydroxide antacid. Associated asymptomatic hypocalcemia does not require treatment and treating hyperphosphatemia should also correct serum calcium levels. In symptomatic hypocalcemia, calcium gluconate can be given. If previously described prophylactic measures or treatments fail and TLS progresses, the patient may require temporary hemodialysis.

MALIGNANCY ASSOCIATED SYNDROME OF INAPPROPRIATE ANTIDIURETIC HORMONE

DEFINITION AND EPIDEMIOLOGY

Hyponatremia is a common electrolyte imbalance (see Chapter 190). SIADH accounts for almost 50% of all hyponatremia cases and 95% of all cases of euvolemic hyponatremia.[9] SIADH is a disorder of impaired water excretion that occurs when antidiuretic hormone (ADH) is ineffectively suppressed, leading to water retention and eventually the development of hyponatremia. Malignancy associated SIADH is most frequently seen in small cell lung cancer; it is less frequently seen in head and neck cancers, olfactory neuroblastomas, and non-pulmonary small cell cancers. Non-malignancy related causes of SIADH include CNS disturbances, drug-related, hormonal etiology, HIV infection, and hereditary factors.[10]

PATHOPHYSIOLOGY

Vasopressin (ADH) is responsible for regulating the reabsorption of water in the cells. This is regulated by the posterior pituitary gland. In patients with SIADH, ingestion of water does not suppress the production of ADH leading to excessive ADH solution, water retention, and dilution hyponatremia. It is characterized by excessive urinary loss of sodium and excessive retention of water by the renal tubules as well as by reduced levels of serum sodium and serum osmolality. In malignancy, SIADH is often a result of ectopic secretion of ADH by tumor cells. Drugs such as chlorpropamide, carbamazepine, and certain SSRIs and acute CNS events including stroke or intracranial hemorrhage may enhance the effects of ADH secretion.[9,10]

CLINICAL PRESENTATION AND PHYSICAL EXAMINATION

With mild hyponatremia, early manifestations include thirst, anorexia, mild nausea and vomiting, weight gain without edema, muscle cramps, headache, and mild lethargy. Patients become more symptomatic as hyponatremia develops rapidly or as sodium levels fall below 115 mg/dL. Signs and symptoms include hyporeflexia, confusion, oliguria, seizures, and coma.[11]

DIAGNOSTICS

Essential Diagnostics

Malignancy related SIADH is a diagnosis of exclusion. It is diagnosed when other causes of hyponatremia have been reasonably ruled out. With SIADH, the serum sodium level is less than 135 mEq/L, plasma osmolality is less than 275 mOsm/kg, urine osmolality is more than 100 mOsm/kg, and urinary sodium is more than 20 mEq/L. Thyroid and adrenal dysfunction need to be excluded. Chest x-ray study and CT scan may be ordered to evaluate pulmonary or neurologic disorders that may cause excessive ADH production.

INITIAL DIAGNOSTICS
Syndrome of Inappropriate Antidiuretic Hormone

LABORATORY
- Serum electrolytes, BUN, and creatinine
- Serum osmolality
- Urine sodium
- Urine osmolality

- Thyroid-stimulating hormone (TSH)[a]

IMAGING
- Chest x-ray examination[a]
- CT scan[a]

---
[a]If indicated.

DIFFERENTIAL DIAGNOSIS

 Immediate emergency evaluation and treatment for patients with hyporeflexia, confusion, oliguria, seizures, and coma.

The differential diagnosis of malignancy related hyponatremia includes CNS disturbances (stroke, hemorrhage, infection, psychosis), drugs (thiazide diuretics, angiotensin-converting enzyme inhibitors), and surgical complications.[11]

INTERPROFESSIONAL COLLABORATIVE MANAGEMENT

In patients with mild to moderate SIADH (serum sodium level of 120 to 134 mEq/L) and minimal symptoms, the cornerstone of treatment is limiting fluid intake to <1000 mL/24 h. Hypokalemia, if present, should be managed with the administration of potassium chloride. Oral salt supplementation, 3 to 4 g every 8 hours may also be indicated. Loop diuretics may be helpful in improving free water clearance. In patients who are not candidates for loop diuretics or fluid restriction, tolvaptan therapy can be administered in the inpatient setting.[10,11] Acute or severe SIADH is a medical emergency; untreated SIADH or too rapid an increase in serum sodium concentration may result in severe neurologic impairment or death. Patients with severe SIADH are typically treated with hypertonic saline solution by slow infusion at a rate sufficient to increase the serum sodium level by 0.5 to 1.0 mEq/L per hour, not to exceed a rise of 20 mEq/L in serum sodium concentration during the first 48 hours to avoid development of central pontine myelinolysis.[10]

Other complications of cancer or cancer treatments that may not be life threatening but certainly affect quality of life include side effects of chemotherapy (fatigue, anorexia, hair loss), chemotherapy associated peripheral neuropathy, skin itching, anemia of chronic disease (see Chapter 216), coagulopathies (see Chapter 217), and arthropathies to name a few. Primary care providers need to be aware that any of these complications can present at any time during or after active treatment.

CANCER SURVIVORSHIP

DEFINITION AND EPIDEMIOLOGY

The National Cancer Institute defines a cancer survivor as any individual who has had cancer from the time of diagnosis through the remainder of his/her life. Family, friends, and caregivers are also included within this definition because they are directly impacted by the survivorship experience.[12,13] For the purposes of this section, survivor will refer only to cancer patients that have completed treatment. Due to the increasing incidence, earlier detection, and better treatment of cancer the number of cancer survivors in the United States is expected to reach more than 20 million by the year 2026. Of note, a predicted two-thirds of this group of survivors will be at least 65 years old.[14,15] Primary care providers will care for cancer survivors throughout their disease trajectory. This section will focus on possible complications that may occur after the adult cancer patient has completed treatment. Patients who had childhood cancers require special monitoring and survivorship care that is beyond the scope of this section.

RISK FACTORS AND CLINICAL PRESENTATION

Patients who have been treated for cancer are at risk of ongoing physical and psychological complications as a result of their treatment. Patients may experience both late effects, toxicities that were present or subclinical at the end of therapy and manifest at a later point in time, and long-term, persistent effects that begin with treatment and continue beyond the end of treatment. Survivors also have an increased risk of cancer in the future either by recurrence of the primary cancer or a new secondary cancer. Complications that survivors experience may be related surgical intervention, radiotherapy, chemotherapy, or biotherapy. Survivors are also at risk of the same chronic health issues as the general population and require routine health promotion and general preventative care. The most common late effects seen in cancer survivors are depression, pain, fatigue, and peripheral neuropathy. Other physical effects of cancer treatment include cardiac, bone, and musculoskeletal issues, premature menopause, cognitive deficits, lymphedema, sexual dysfunction, infertility (in young survivors), and urinary/bowel problems.[16]

The clinical presentation of these late effects is toxicity-dependent and can also present as laboratory abnormalities. Routine physical examinations and guideline-directed preventative health maintenance should be part of survivorship care.

DIAGNOSTICS

Providers should do a full assessment of current disease status, functional/performance status, current medication, comorbidities, prior cancer treatment history, and modalities of treatment.[12,16] Labs and imaging may or may not have utility and should be used to help confirm diagnosis.

DIFFERENTIAL DIAGNOSIS

Cancer survivors may experience treatment-related toxicity at any point post-treatment. When a survivor presents with a new onset complaint, treatment-related toxicity should always be included in the differential. Additionally, cancer survivors are at risk of recurrent and secondary cancers.

INTERPROFESSIONAL COLLABORATIVE MANAGEMENT

Cancer survivors should be managed in collaboration with the patient's oncologist and referred to specialists as needed for management of toxicities. To facilitate communication between oncologists and primary care providers, American Society of Clinical Oncology (ASCO) encourages the use of survivorship care plans which include a written treatment summary, known short- and long-term toxicities of treatment, psychosocial support that may be needed, ongoing screening guidelines to monitor for disease recurrence and secondary cancers, and preventative health concerns such as tobacco cessation, obesity, alcohol use, and sun protection. End-of-life wishes are also part of this plan along with a recommendation that end-of-life care be discussed with the primary care physician and family. This survivorship care plan provides an easily understood review for the patient and a roadmap of future care needs for the primary care doctor. In 2017 the American College of Surgeons (ACOS) Commission on Cancer (CoC) designated the delivery of survivorship care plans to 50% of eligible patients by 2018 as a requirement of accreditation.[17]

In any emergency, patients and families are frightened, but they also want honest explanations of their situation. This may be especially true for active cancer patients who are already coping with a frightening diagnosis and treatments. Patients should be told about possible causes of the symptoms being experienced and the proposed plan of action, and they should be reassured that the oncologist is being notified immediately. Once treatment is initiated, the patient will benefit from reinforcement from the health care provider about instructions for medications, activities, diet, exercise, and reminders of warning signs that need to be reported. After treatment is complete, patients should be educated about potential long-term toxicities of treatment and provided with a survivorship care plan.

REFERENCES

1. Straka, C., Ying, J., Kong, F.-M., Willey, C. D., Kaminski, J., & Kim, D. W. N. (2016). Review of evolving etiologies, implications and treatment strategies for the superior vena cava syndrome. *SpringerPlus, 5,* 229. doi:10.1186/s40064-016-1900-7.
2. Yeung, S., & Manzullo, E. F. (2016). Oncologic emergencies. In H. M. Kantarjian & R. A. Wolff (Eds.), *The MD Anderson manual of medical oncology* (3rd ed.). New York, NY: McGraw-Hill. http://accessmedicine.mhmedical.com/content.aspx?bookid=1772&sectionid=121903052. (Accessed 11 January 2018).
3. Higdon, M., Atkinson, C., & Lawrence, K. (2018). Oncologic emergencies: Recognition and initial management. *American Family Physician, 97*(11), 741–748.
4. Khan, U. A., Shanholtz, C. B., & McCurdy, M. T. (2014). Oncologic mechanical emergencies. *Emergency Medicine Clinics of North America, 32,* 495–508.
5. Wagner, J., & Arora, S. (2014). Oncologic metabolic emergencies. *Emergency Medicine Clinics of North America, 32*(3), 509–525.
6. Sternlicht, H., & Glezerman, I. (2015). Hypercalcemia of malignancy and new treatment options. *Therapeutics and Clinical Risk Management, 11,* 1779–1788.
7. deOliveira, R. E., Mak, M. P., Silva, M. F., et al. (2017). Malignancy related hypercalcemia in advanced solid tumors: Survivor outcomes. *Journal of Global Oncology, 3*(6), 728–733.
8. Mirrakhimov, A., Voore, P., Khan, M., & Ali, A. (2015). Tumor lysis syndrome: A clinical review. *World Journal of Critical Care Medicine, 4*(2), 130–138.
9. Weismann, D., Schneider, A., & Hoybye, C. (2016). Clinical aspects of symptomatic hyponatremia. *Endocrine Connections, 5,* R35–R43.
10. Runkle, I., Villabona, C., et al. (2014). Treatment of hyponatremia induced by syndrome of inappropriate antidiuretic hormone secretion: A multidisciplinary algorithm. *Nefrologia: Publicacion Oficial de la Sociedad Espanola Nefrologia, 34*(4), 439–450.
11. Panda, S. S., Das, M., Mazundar, P., et al. (2019). Clinical, etiological and epidemiological profile pf elderly (>=60 years) patients admitted with hyponatremia: A single centre study. *International Journal of Scientific Research, 8*(4), 3–5.
12. Gegechkori, N., Haines, L., & Lin, J. (2017). Long-term and latent side effects of specific cancer types. *Medical Clinics of North America, 101*(6), 1053–1073.
13. Denlinger, C. S., Carlson, R. W., et al. (2014). Survivorship: Introduction and definition: clinical practice guidelines in oncology. *Journal of the National Comprehensive Cancer Network, 12*(1), 34–45.
14. Miller, K. D., Siegel, R. L., et al. (2016). Cancer treatment and survivorship statistics 2016. *CA: A Cancer Journal for Clinicians, 66*(4), 271–289.
15. Rowland, J. H., & Bellizzi, K. M. (2014). Cancer survivorship issues: Life after treatment and implications for an aging population. *Journal of Clinical Oncology, 32*(24), 2662–2668.
16. Shahrokni, A., Wu, A., et al. (2016). Long-term toxicity of cancer treatment in older patients. *Clinics in Geriatric Medicine, 32*(1), 63–80.
17. American College of Surgeons, commission of cancer. Important information regarding cancer survivorship care plans. https://www.facs.org/quality-programs/cancer/news/survivorship. (Accessed 25 July 2018).

CHAPTER **224**

CARCINOMA OF UNKNOWN PRIMARY

Paula K. Rauschkolb

DEFINITION AND EPIDEMIOLOGY

The term *carcinoma of unknown primary* (CUP), or occult primary malignancy, encompasses a heterogeneous group of metastatic cancers for which the site of origin cannot be identified. Despite improvements in imaging techniques, emergence of new immunohistochemical and molecular-profiling assays, and maturation of our understanding of cancer biology in recent decades, this rather nebulous diagnosis remains a recognized entity that must be addressed and treated despite its ambiguous character. Cancers of unknown primary account for 3% to 5% of all malignancies.[1] The incidence rate is estimated at 4.1 cases per 100,000 in the United States. The most common histology is adenocarcinoma (1.9 cases per 100,000), followed by squamous cell (0.6 cases per 100,000). The incidence rate increases significantly with advancing age, with average rates of 8.4 cases per 100,000 in patients aged 50 to 59, and 48.6 cases per 100,000 in those over 80 years of age. Incidence is slightly higher in males, with a male-to-female incidence ratio of 1.3 : 1. Incidence is slightly higher in African Americans versus Caucasians (1.2 : 1) and slightly lower in Asian and Pacific Islanders (0.6 : 1).[2]

PATHOPHYSIOLOGY

The pathophysiology of CUP has not been well-defined, partially due to the underlying variability in tumor biology. Histologic groups include well- and moderately-differentiated adenocarcinomas, squamous cell carcinomas, carcinomas with neuroendocrine differentiation, poorly-differentiated carcinomas (including poorly differentiated adenocarcinomas) and undifferentiated neoplasms. The common thread among these is the fact that all cases present with metastasis as the primary manifestation, and that metastatic dissemination can occur in the absence of growth of a primary tumor.[1] The most common primaries identified at autopsy or unmasked during the clinical course of the disease include lung, pancreas, gastrointestinal tract (colon, stomach, bile duct, and liver), and the urogenital tract.[3]

CLINICAL PRESENTATION AND PHYSICAL EXAMINATION

Clinical presentation in the setting of CUP varies widely, typically reflecting the areas of metastatic disease involvement. In addition to constitutional symptoms such as weakness, fatigue, malaise, anorexia, and weight loss, patients may present with complaints of abdominal pain or fullness, cough, shortness of breath, chest pain, bone pain, skin lesions (cutaneous tumors), bloody stools, or they may have detected swelling of the lymph nodes.

A thorough physical examination should be performed, including head and neck, rectal exam, testicular and prostate exam for men, pelvic and breast exam for women, skin check for suspicious lesions, and lymph node palpation. Family history should be reviewed to elicit history of malignancy. There are data to suggest that there may be a familial predisposition.[4,5]

DIAGNOSTICS

The focus of the diagnostic approach below is to identify areas of disease involvement. Advanced diagnostic testing (e.g., immunohistochemistry, molecular profiling) will then be performed in an effort to glean information that may help to direct therapy.

Essential Diagnostics

Following a thorough physical examination, basic bloodwork including complete blood count (CBC) with differential and comprehensive metabolic panel (CMP) should be obtained to readily identify any abnormalities that may help direct further testing. A computed tomography (CT) scan of the chest, abdomen, and pelvis with contrast should be performed to assess for mass lesions and/or lymphadenopathy. Mammography should be performed in female patients to assess for breast abnormalities.[1,6]

Additional Diagnostics

Further testing, which is directed by initial findings and suspected CUP subsets, may include body positron emission tomography (PET)-CT scan or body magnetic resonance imaging (MRI), breast MRI, head and neck CT/PET, octreoscan, endoscopy (bronchoscopy, upper endoscopy, and/or colonoscopy, depending upon signs/symptoms or imaging findings), serum LDH and ALP, as well as potentially relevant tumor markers such as CA19-9, CEA, chromogranin A, serum α-fetoprotein (AFP), human chorionic gonadotropin (β-HCG), serum prostate-specific antigen (PSA), CA15-3, and CA125.[1,3,6]

The goal of initial diagnostic testing is to identify a region of disease involvement that is amenable to biopsy. An adequate tissue sample is of utmost importance for further characterization of the tumor, which in turn carries the possibility of greater success in treatment. CUP carries a rather poor prognosis overall, but there are subsets of patients who may exhibit a good response to therapy. Once a tissue sample is obtained, light microscopy is used to determine the histological diagnosis. This is followed by immunohistochemical analysis and molecular profiling in an effort to identify the tissue of origin. This additional testing may also help to identify chemotherapy-sensitive and potentially curable tumors (e.g., lymphomas and germ-cell tumors) or to provide information that can help to guide therapy (e.g., immunostaining for hormone receptors to identify hormone-sensitive tumors).

INITIAL DIAGNOSTICS

Carcinoma of Unknown Primary

LABORATORY	IMAGING
• Complete blood count with differential • Comprehensive metabolic panel	• Computed tomography scan of the chest, abdomen, pelvis with contrast • Mammogram (female patients)

DIFFERENTIAL DIAGNOSIS

- Primary malignancy, initially occult and later identified
- Benign lesion
- Infection, inflammation, elevated physiologic activity

Of utmost importance is to perform a comprehensive evaluation for an identifiable process, in particular one for which there is a straightforward treatment. This includes not only a careful search for a primary malignancy, but also consideration of infectious or inflammatory processes, or pathologic entities such as fracture secondary to osteoporosis rather than metastatic bone lesions.

INTERPROFESSIONAL COLLABORATIVE MANAGEMENT

The delivery of care to patients with CUP, like other forms of cancer, requires a multidisciplinary approach. Depending upon the characteristics of each particular case, the treatment team may include medical oncology, radiation oncology, surgical oncology, pain management, palliative care, and social work. A strong, continued relationship between the patient and his or her primary care provider is integral to optimizing patient outcomes.

Nonpharmacologic Management

Surgical biopsy is often performed during the diagnostic process. The need for additional surgical intervention varies on a case-by-case basis. Likewise, the potential role for radiation therapy in treatment is case-specific. Unfortunately, only a small proportion of patients present with local disease that may be amenable to radical resection or radiotherapy. In a retrospective analysis of 223 patients with CUP, only 13% were appropriate candidates for this approach.[7]

Nonpharmacologic approaches to management of depression and anxiety, which are common in this setting, include cognitive therapy, support group participation, and engagement of other services such as palliative care.

Pharmacologic Management

The majority of patients will require systemic chemotherapy. Every effort should be made to identify patients who fall into favorable-risk subsets (see Life Span Considerations), as these patients may be treated with regimens utilized for metastatic disease in the closest equivalent known primary tumor type.[1]

In most cases, patients will require treatment with empiric chemotherapy. These protocols are typically geared toward broad coverage for the most common types of cancers that may be masked in the setting of CUP. These patients are most often treated with a combination regimen, which is generally platinum-based.[3]

Other pharmacologic interventions include typical supportive medications for patients with cancer, such as antiemetics, pain medications, and colony-stimulating factors or transfusions as indicated. Antidepressants and/or anxiolytics may also be appropriate in certain patients in order to improve or maintain quality of life.

Indications for Referral and Hospitalization

All patients with known or suspected CUP should be referred to a medical oncologist, preferably at a specialized center, to ensure that a full diagnostic workup is performed and for subsequent treatment. Hospitalization may be required for chemotherapy administration, or for symptoms or complications resulting from chemotherapy or from the underlying malignancy itself. These may include intractable pain, refractory nausea and vomiting, severe dehydration, bleeding, febrile neutropenia, hypercalcemia or other significant metabolic derangement, deep vein thrombosis or pulmonary embolus, or signs and symptoms suggestive of spinal cord compression.

LIFE SPAN CONSIDERATIONS

A small percentage of patients, roughly 10% to 30%, fall into certain subsets which confer a more favorable prognosis. In these cases, tumors are found to have characteristics that are very similar to a specific primary tumor type. These patients can then be treated with a regimen similar to what would be used for this primary tumor in the setting of metastatic disease. There is the potential for curable disease in certain subsets, while in others there is a greater likelihood of response to chemotherapy relative to the majority of patients with CUP who do not fit into one of the favorable-risk subsets.[1,3]

Below are the six subsets that are typically considered to have a more favorable prognosis:[3]
- Carcinoma with midline distribution and poor differentiation in male patients reminiscent of extragonadal germ cell tumors
- Adenocarcinoma with isolated unilateral axillary lymph nodes in female patients suggestive of nodal positive breast cancer
- Squamous cell carcinoma with neck lymph nodes suggestive of head and neck cancer
- Squamous cell carcinoma with inguinal lymph nodes raising suspicion of anal, vulva, vagina, uterine, cervix, penis, or scrotum carcinoma
- Serous papillary peritoneal carcinomatosis in females indicative of an ovarian or peritoneal primary
- Blastic bone metastasis in male patients with high concentrations of PSA pointing to prostate cancer

Unfortunately, the majority of patients do not fall within one of these favorable subsets. For these patients the prognosis is very poor despite aggressive treatment, with a median survival of less than 1 year. It is appropriate in this setting to initiate early involvement of palliative care services and to discuss advance directives with the patient (see Chapter 14).

COMPLICATIONS

Complications may result from treatment or from the underlying malignancy. Generally recognized chemotherapy side effects include fatigue, nausea and vomiting, diarrhea, mucositis, loss of appetite, alopecia, and peripheral neuropathy. Complications include renal dysfunction, hepatic dysfunction, metabolic derangement, and myelosuppression leading to neutropenia (including febrile neutropenia), anemia, or thrombocytopenia. Transfusion is necessary in some cases.

For patients who require narcotic analgesia, potential side effects include fatigue, nausea and vomiting, constipation, and cognitive effects, while complications may include excessive somnolence, significant mental status change, severe bowel dysfunction, and respiratory depression.

Patients who undergo radiation therapy may experience fatigue, alopecia, esophagitis with resultant dysphagia, gastritis, diarrhea, rectal pain or burning, cystitis, or dysuria.

Complications related to the underlying malignancy are dependent to some degree on the distribution of metastatic disease, but may include: spinal cord compression, ureteral and biliary obstruction, pleural and pericardial effusions, ascites, hypercalcemia of malignancy, hyponatremia, deep vein thrombosis, or pulmonary embolus.

Patients may also suffer from anxiety or depression, and significant psychosocial issues may exist.

PATIENT AND FAMILY EDUCATION

- The ambiguous nature of CUP can lead to greater difficulty for the patient and family as they try to come to terms with the diagnosis and its implications. Utilization of support services should be strongly recommended.
- Education regarding the potential side effects of treatment, as well as when and who to call in the event that they occur, should be clearly provided (see Box 218.1). This applies not only to chemotherapy, but also to supportive medications, particularly opiates.
- It is appropriate in the setting of CUP, with the possible exception of patients in the favorable-risk categories, to

initiate discussion of advance directives, and to offer referral to a palliative care professional (see Chapter 14).

HEALTH PROMOTION

For patients in the favorable-risk category who have the potential for extended survival, all standard recommendations would apply including a healthy and active lifestyle, as well as appropriate maintenance screenings such as colonoscopy, mammography, and bone density scanning.

For the majority of patients, prognosis is very poor and survival is limited. The focus in this setting would be to optimize functional status, with an emphasis on quality of life. Adequate nutrition is important, and the services of a dietician may be of value. Smoking cessation should be encouraged. Physical activity, commensurate with the patient's ability, should be encouraged. Remaining active can help to mitigate fatigue, may decrease risk of deep vein thrombosis, may prolong functionality, and can help to lift the person's spirits. Patients should be routinely assessed for symptoms of depression and anxiety, and treatment should be offered when appropriate.

REFERENCES

1. Fizazi, K., et al. (2015). Cancers of unknown primary site: ESMO Clinical Practice Guidelines for diagnosis, treatment, and follow-up. *Annals of Oncology, 26*(Suppl. 5), v133–v138.
2. Mnatsakanyan, E., Tung, W., Caine, B., & Smith-Gagen, J. (2014). Cancer of unknown primary: Time trends in incidence, United States. *Cancer Causes and Control, 25,* 747–757.
3. Bochtler, T., Loffler, H., & Kramer, A. Diagnosis and management of metastatic neoplasms with unknown primary. https://doi.org/10.1053/j.semdp.2017.11.013.
4. Hemminki, K., et al. (2016). Location of metastasis in cancer of unknown primary are not random and signal familial clustering. *Scientific Reports, 6,* 22891.
5. Samadder, N. J., et al. (2016). Familial risk in patients with carcinoma of unknown primary. *JAMA Oncology, 2*(3), 340–346.
6. Varadhachary, G., & Raber, M. (2014). Cancer of unknown primary site. *The New England Journal of Medicine, 371,* 757–765.
7. Loffler, H., Puthenparambil, J., Hielscher, T., Neben, K., & Kramer, A. (2014). Patients with cancer of unknown primary: A retrospective analysis of 223 patients with adenocarcinoma or undifferentiated carcinoma. *Deutsches Ärzteblatt International, 111*(27–28), 481–487.

CHAPTER 225

ANXIETY DISORDERS

Rene Love

 Immediate referral to the emergency room is indicated for individuals who are at risk of harm to themselves or others.

DEFINITION AND EPIDEMIOLOGY

Anxiety disorders are the most commonly occurring class of mental disorders with a third of the population being affected during their lifetime.[1] The development of anxiety disorders depends on several variables that affect the way the body responds to fear and anxiety, such as gender, age, culture, environment, qualities of the stressor, and genetics. In general, anxiety disorders typically begin much earlier in life than other mental disorders with women being at higher risk than men.[1] More specifically, the onset of tic disorders and specific phobias begins in childhood with social phobias and OCD beginning in adolescence or early adulthood. The onset of post-traumatic stress disorder (PTSD) can vary as the disorder results from trauma exposure, which may occur at any point in life. Panic disorder, generalized anxiety disorder (GAD), and agoraphobia are the only anxiety disorders that have adult onset.

Anxiety can be healthy in patients' lives as it warns them to get out of harm's way or motivates a person to act. However, if a person's stress level becomes persistent, excessive, overwhelming, and disabling, then an anxiety disorder should be considered. There are several factors to consider, such as culture, genetics, environment, and psychosocial issues when diagnosing anxiety disorders.

The *Diagnostic and Statistical Manual of Mental Disorders, Fifth Edition* (DSM-5) identifies the following anxiety disorders: separation anxiety disorder; selective mutism; specific phobia; social anxiety disorder (social phobia); panic disorder; agoraphobia; substance/medication-induced anxiety disorder; anxiety disorder due to another general medical condition; and GAD.[2] Also included are post-traumatic stress disorder (PTSD) and acute stress disorder (ASD).[2]

The following definitions of the more common anxiety disorders are adapted from the DSM-5. *Separation anxiety disorder* is developmentally excessive with inappropriate anxiety and distress regarding separating from attachment figures. *Selective mutism* is consistently failing to speak in situations in which the person is expected to speak, even though the person will speak in other situations, thereby interfering with the person's education and occupation. *Specific phobia* is extreme fear and distress about a specific object or situation such as snakes or heights. *Social anxiety disorder* is extreme fear and distress about social situations in which the individual is exposed to possible scrutiny by other people, causing the person to avoid social situations altogether. *Panic disorder* is characterized by recurring and unanticipated panic attacks. *Generalized anxiety disorder* is excessive anxiety that occurs more days than not about a wide variety of events or activities. *Post-traumatic stress disorder* occurs when a person is exposed to a trauma that causes intense psychological distress when he or she is exposed to either internal or external cues.[2]

PATHOPHYSIOLOGY

Anxiety is a normal response that promotes survival in the face of an actual environmental threat. For example, it is adaptive and beneficial to experience a fight-or-flight response via the sympathetic nervous system (SNS) when confronted by dangerous stimuli. Anxiety can be unhealthy with an exaggerated fear response that often occurs in the absence of a true environmental threat. Physiologically, the body does not differentiate between anxiety and fear. Blood flow is increased to the large muscle groups in preparation to flee or fight; the heart and legs are ready to act, and the digestive system slows. However, the fear response is a complex process involving multiple organ systems, and therefore anxiety has many associated physical and psychological consequences. Subcortical (amygdala, hippocampus, brainstem, and hypothalamus) and cortical regions (insular cortex, orbitofrontal cortex, ventromedial prefrontal cortex, and anterior cingulate cortex) of the brain are involved in anxiety disorders.[3] The amygdala and hypothalamic-pituitary-adrenal (HPA) axis are two primary areas implicated in the neuropathology of anxiety. The amygdala is part of the limbic system and processes emotionally salient stimuli and initiates the appropriate behavioral response. The HPA axis functions as a hormonal feedback system and includes the hypothalamus, pituitary gland, and adrenal gland. Harmful stimuli undergo sensory processing, and information is relayed to the hypothalamus. The hypothalamus initiates the HPA axis by releasing corticotropin releasing factor (CRF), which triggers the release of adrenocorticotropic hormone (ACTH) from the pituitary, which then triggers the release of glucocorticoids (including cortisol) from the adrenal gland.[3] When the system is functioning properly, it operates on a negative feedback loop: the binding of glucocorticoids to glucocorticoid receptors inhibiting further release of hormones.[3] However, abnormalities in the HPA axis have been implicated in individuals with anxiety disorders.

It is well known that anxiety disorders have a strong familial link and it is also understood that environmental factors contribute significantly to the development of anxiety disorders. Gene-environment (G × E) interactions related to anxiety have been demonstrated quite eloquently in rat studies, highlighting the significance of genetic and environmental influences as well as the concept of epigenetics.[4] During recent years, the serotonin transporter gene-linked polymorphic region (5-HTTLPR) has received a lot of attention in the literature owing to its association with increased vulnerability to psychiatric illness when combined with environmental stressors or adversity. There is evidence suggesting that individuals who are carriers of at least one short (S) allele and a history of adverse life events are at an increased risk for depression.[4] There have been mixed results linking increased stress reactivity in 5-HTTLPR SS allele carriers.[4]

Neurotransmitters including serotonin, norepinephrine, dopamine, and γ-aminobutyric acid (GABA) have been well studied and are implicated in the pathophysiology of anxiety disorders.[5] The involvement of these multiple neurotransmitter systems is complex and cannot be oversimplified as the presence of too much or not enough of a particular neurotransmitter. For example, serotonin pathways are involved in regulating mood states including anxiety and are also involved in the modulation of dopaminergic and noradrenergic pathways. Dopamine, serotonin, norepinephrine, and GABA have been linked to anxiety states and treatment for many years. Clinical trials expanding our understanding of the role of neurotransmitters in anxiety could change the way we treat anxiety disorders in the future. There remains much to learn about the development and management of anxiety disorders, but it is safe to say that there is complex interplay among genes, environment, culture, personality, and psychoneuroimmunologic factors.

CLINICAL PRESENTATION

Individuals with anxiety disorders are often first seen for treatment in primary care clinics and emergency departments. In addition to complaints of worry, anxiety, or fear, these individuals may also have numerous physical complaints. Anxiety disorders are highly comorbid with other psychiatric illnesses including depression and substance use disorders.

Anxiety, by definition, is the anticipation of a future threat and is often associated with preparation for potential danger and/or avoidant behaviors.[2] Anxiety disorders differ from developmentally or situationally appropriate fears in that they are persistent (typically lasting 6 months or longer) and cause significant impairments in functioning.[2]

GAD is characterized by excessive anxiety and worry about a number of events or activities. The anxiety and worry are associated with three or more of the following six symptoms: (1) restlessness or feeling on edge, (2) easy fatigability, (3) difficulty concentrating, (4) irritability, (5) muscle tension, (6) sleep disturbance.[2] GAD is a chronic condition in which full remission rates are very low.[2] Children and adolescents tend to experience performance-focused worry and anxiety, whereas adults report more worry about their physical health or the well-being of their family.[3] In addition to worry, these individuals may also experience a variety of physical symptoms including tachycardia, hypertension, shortness of breath, muscle tension and aches, trembling, twitching, sweating, dizziness, nausea, and diarrhea. Mixed-headache and irritable bowel syndromes are two medical conditions frequently associated with GAD.

Specific phobias are characterized by marked fear or anxiety about a specific object or situation. The phobic object or situation almost always provokes immediate fear and the object or situation is either avoided or endured with intense fear or anxiety.[2] Specific phobias are coded based on the phobic stimulus (animal, natural environment, blood-injection-injury, situational, or other). Most people with specific phobias have more than one phobic stimulus, and functional impairment increases with the number of phobic stimuli. Blood-injection-injury phobias may cause individuals to neglect their physical health because of the anxiety associated with provider appointments. Fear of falling in the geriatric population can lead to reduced mobility and impairments in physical health and social functioning.[2] Social anxiety disorder or social phobia involves clinically significant anxiety about one or more social situations in which the individual is exposed to possible scrutiny by others (e.g., social interactions, eating, speaking in public).[2]

Panic disorder is characterized by recurrent unexpected panic attacks. A panic attack is defined as "an abrupt surge of intense fear or intense discomfort that reaches a peak within minutes."[3] Panic attacks can occur within the context of any other psychiatric disorder, and to reflect this the condition was added as a specifier in the DSM-5.

OCD consists of the presence of obsessions, compulsions, or both. Obsessions are defined as recurrent thoughts, urges, or images that are intrusive and unwanted. Compulsions are repetitive behaviors or acts (e.g., checking, counting, praying) that the individual feels driven to perform and are aimed at reducing anxiety or a dreaded situation. Rates of OCD are higher in individuals with body dysmorphic disorder, trichotillomania, excoriation disorder, schizophrenia, schizoaffective disorder, bipolar disorder, eating disorders, and Tourette disorder.[2] Impairment is related to severity of symptoms and can affect interpersonal relationships, occupational and academic performance, physical health, and even successful treatment of the disorder.[2]

The DSM-5 was released in May 2013 and presents a new organizational system for some of the anxiety disorders. OCD is now located in the chapter Obsessive-Compulsive and Related Disorders, which includes OCD, body dysmorphic disorder, hoarding disorder, trichotillomania, and excoriation disorder. PTSD is now included with the Trauma- and Stressor-Related Disorders along with ASD and adjustment disorder, among others. Separation anxiety disorder was previously included in Disorders Usually First Diagnosed in Infancy, Childhood, or Adolescence, but is now applicable to adults and is included with the Anxiety Disorders. Another change to the DSM-5 is that individuals older than 18 with agoraphobia, specific phobia, and social anxiety disorder need not recognize that their anxiety is excessive or unreasonable, but the anxiety must be out of proportion to the actual threat.[2]

PHYSICAL EXAMINATION

The physical examination occurs after a thorough history is obtained. Some symptoms of anxiety disorders are preceded by recent events of interpersonal violence, accident, or natural disaster. It is also important to inquire about psychosocial stressors and a remote history of traumas or abuse because these experiences increase risk for anxiety disorders. Therefore, providers need to ask specific questions regarding trauma history and be prepared to refer the individual for trauma-informed care if necessary. The potential physical injuries that follow exposure to these events could include damage to any body system; thus, a complete physical examination is necessary.

DIAGNOSTICS

Essential Diagnostics

It is not surprising that individuals with anxiety disorders often fear an underlying medical disorder, given the frequency of associated physical symptoms. Many of the physical symptoms of anxiety (chest pain, shortness of breath, dizziness, and gastrointestinal symptoms) could signal a serious medical illness. Therefore, medical causes must be explored and excluded before a diagnosis of an anxiety disorder is made. Side effects from medications and the physiologic effects of intoxication or withdrawal from substances should be considered when the symptoms of anxiety disorders are reviewed.

There are no laboratory tests, imaging modalities, or physical examination findings that definitively diagnose an anxiety disorder. Like all mental health diagnoses, the symptoms must meet the criteria in the DSM-5, with the symptoms being at a moderate to severe level and affecting hygiene, relationships, employment, or education. Urine toxicology is helpful to determine substance use that may contribute to the symptoms described by the patient. In older patients it is equally important to rule out other medical conditions through a physical examination and diagnostics to determine the presence of infection, anemia, electrolyte imbalance, liver or kidney dysfunction, thyroid disease, hyperparathyroidism, or glucose intolerance. The importance of ruling out exposure to the anxiety-producing effects of caffeine is often missed, but caffeine may play a critical role in anxiety. Electrocardiograms may be obtained to rule out cardiac problems with a person experiencing panic attacks.

The screening tool recommended for GAD in primary care settings for anxiety disorders is the GAD 7-item instrument (GAD-7).[6] The screening tool recommended for PTSD is the Primary Care PTSD Screen (PC-PTSD).[7] The Social Phobia Inventory (SPIN) Mini-SPIN Screening Tool has three items to assess for social phobias.[8] The Patient Health Questionnaire with Somatic, Anxiety, and Depressive Symptom Scales (PHQ-SADS) combines the Patient Health Questionniare-9 (PHQ-9), the GAD-7, and the Patient Health Questionnaire-15 (PHQ-15) to assess for depression, anxiety including panic attacks, and somatization.[9] These scales will facilitate identification of patients who require additional assessment for a psychiatric disorder.

Additional Diagnostics

Side effects from medications and the physiologic effects of intoxication or withdrawal from substances should be taken into account when the symptoms of anxiety are reviewed. Medications, other medical conditions, and other psychiatric conditions that mimic symptoms with anxiety disorders are listed in the differential diagnosis section.

DIFFERENTIAL DIAGNOSIS

 Priority differentials include: (1) cardiac, (2) respiratory, (3) endocrine, and (4) side effects from medications and/or other substances.

The differential diagnosis should include arrhythmias and angina when assessing the cardiac system. The assessment of the respiratory system should include issues such as asthma, chronic obstructive pulmonary disease, pulmonary emboli, and hypoxia from a wide-variety of causes. When assessing the endocrine system, hyperthyroidism or hypothyroidism, hyperglycemia or hypoglycemia, and menopause should be excluded. Side effects from all medications and/or other substances such as caffeine, cocaine, cannabis, steroids, nicotine, ephedrine and pseudoephedrine, amphetamines, anticholinergics, theophylline, digoxin, Synthroid, and antihypertensives should be assessed through toxicology studies.

INTERPROFESSIONAL COLLABORATIVE MANAGEMENT

Most patients with symptoms of anxiety are initially seen in the primary care provider's office. A mental health consultation is indicated for individuals who are not responding to or who have partial remission of symptoms with adequate doses of first-line pharmacologic interventions.

Several consensus groups have published guidelines for the management of anxiety disorders that are centered on the same general goal of reducing symptoms, improving function, treatment of comorbid conditions, and achievement of long-term remission. Several classes of medications have been approved and are indicated for use in managing symptoms of anxiety disorders. Yet, there are very few research studies available to compare the efficacy of one class of medication with another in the management of an anxiety disorder; thus, selection of an agent is largely dependent on comorbid conditions, side effects, and history of previous treatments or predominant symptoms. It is important to take a thorough history of medications as patients will often say that a certain medication did not work but upon further investigation, it is determined that the dose prescribed was not maximized nor was there an adequate trial of the medication.

The effectiveness of any management strategy is largely dependent on one's ability to remain consistent with the intervention or treatment. The integration of psychoeducation related to anxiety disorders and shared decision-making with the patient about medication risks and benefits may increase adherence.[10]

Nonpharmacologic Management

Psychotherapy. Psychotherapy interventions have been widely investigated and reviewed for efficacy in the management of anxiety disorders. Cognitive behavioral therapies for anxiety disorders have been demonstrated to be effective in multiple randomized control trials.[11-13] These interventions should be considered first-line treatment options in conjunction with medications or as monotherapy and should be administered by trained psychotherapists. The addition of exposure, systematic desensitization, and cognitive behavioral therapies are effective to extinguish symptoms for OCD.[11-13]

Exercise. While exercise has been shown to be a useful treatment for anxiety as compared to controls, the studies lacked data from rigorous, sound randomized control trials.[14,15] Exercise should be encouraged as an adjunctive treatment, given the overall physical and psychological benefits of exercise, but at this point, there is not enough evidence to support it as first-line treatment for anxiety disorders.

Pharmacologic Management

Once a medication has been initiated for anxiety, it should be continued for 6 to 12 months after symptoms have resolved.[11] If a patient does not respond to an adequate dose of a medication, the provider should add additional medications or consider switching medications. A referral to a mental health provider may also be appropriate.

Selective Serotonin Reuptake Inhibitor and Serotonin-Norepinephrine Reuptake Inhibitor. Antidepressants are considered first-line treatment for anxiety disorders. Selective serotonin reuptake inhibitors (SSRIs) and serotonin-norepinephrine reuptake inhibitors (SNRIs) have been demonstrated to be effective in managing symptoms of GAD, panic disorder, PTSD, social anxiety disorder, and OCD.[11,12] There is variability in the half-life of these agents, which should be considered in review of a patient's ability to take a medication consistently (because missed doses may cause withdrawal symptoms) or of drug-drug interactions (because a medication with a longer half-life is more likely to affect the metabolism of other medications). Patients should be educated about the time frame to the onset of full anxiolytic effect which may be up to 6 weeks while the medication is being titrated.[12] Although SSRIs are generally well tolerated, their initial adverse effects, including headache, restlessness, increased anxiety, nausea, fatigue, and dizziness, paired with the delayed anxiolytic effect may be intensified during the first 2 weeks after which time they typically subside if the patient will continue taking the medication.[12] Individuals taking SNRIs and SSRIs should also be aware of the risk of discontinuation syndromes when missing doses or stopping the medication abruptly. Providers should also educate patients on the signs and symptoms of serotonin syndrome (e.g., mental status changes, autonomic instability, and neuromuscular changes), a potentially life-threatening side effect of SSRIs and SNRIs. Long-term side effects such as weight gain and sexual dysfunction may prove intolerable for some people. "Starting low and going slow" can help to increase tolerability and thus improve adherence which is especially important in children and adolescents and the geriatric population.[12]

Benzodiazepines. Benzodiazepines should be used with caution. Because of a short onset of action (within minutes), benzodiazepines have efficacy in the acute management of symptoms related to panic attacks, social anxiety, and GAD. This is presumably related to their mechanism of action: increased GABA activity. Long-term use, however, is not recommended, especially if symptoms of depression are present. There are additional problems associated with this class of medications that include an increased risk of falls, confusion, and memory problems, especially when they are used in older adults. The most common current use of benzodiazepines is in combination with SSRIs or SNRIs for short-term management of acute symptoms. Although benzodiazepines initially seem helpful for treatment of insomnia, they change the sleep architecture and are associated with marked rebound insomnia once the medication is discontinued. Prescription of benzodiazepines includes a risk of respiratory distress, physiologic dependence, and eventually tolerance. These risks are higher for people with current or previous substance use disorders; thus benzodiazepine use is typically contraindicated in this population.[12] Benzodiazepines may alter someone's ability to drive or to meet usual expectations and must not be stopped abruptly.[12]

Buspirone. Buspirone is a partial agonist at the 5-hydroxytryptamine 1A receptor and has been shown to be modestly effective in the treatment of GAD.[12] It is not approved for use in any other anxiety disorder. It may exacerbate symptoms of depression, which excludes it from use with many people because anxiety and depression have such a high comorbidity.

Tricyclic Antidepressants. Tricyclic antidepressants (TCAs) and older monoamine oxidase inhibitors have indications for management of some of the anxiety disorders but are not considered first line because of tolerability. Clomipramine has a specific indication for OCD; however, it does not demonstrate any advantage over newer serotonin agents. TCAs carry a high risk of cardiac dysrhythmias and are lethal in overdose; thus, they are contraindicated for patients with a history of or risk for suicide.[13]

Indications for Referral and Hospitalization

Resources and access to behavioral health specialists will affect the timing of referrals to consultation outside of the primary care setting. There is an increasing number of mental health providers working alongside primary care providers in the same clinic across the nation, yet typically people with anxiety disorders are still being treated by their primary care provider initially. If the primary care provider is concerned for a person's personal safety or if the person has not responded to initial interventions, has complex medical problems, or is already receiving multiple medications, then a referral should be considered.

The primary care provider should obtain emergent care if the person is in danger of causing harm to self or others. Emergent care should also be sought if the person is gravely disabled (unable to provide for basic personal needs such as food, clothing, and shelter). Emergent care would also be required for severe side effects of medications such as serotonin syndrome, serotonin withdrawal, neuroleptic malignant syndrome, or lithium toxicity.

A referral to a specialist should also be considered if other psychiatric comorbidities are present, if the symptoms are not responding to initial treatments provided in primary care clinic, or to obtain psychotherapy, family education, or group therapy services.

The use of pharmacogenetic testing is becoming more prevalent as there are highly individualized responses to medication and side effects. The decreasing cost of genetic testing and coverage by some insurance companies have allowed treatment to be more personalized. The personalization of treatment avoids long-term trials with medications where patients may be nonresponsive and suffer from numerous side effects of medication.[17] Research continues in this area and should still be combined with a thorough clinical assessment and treatment recommendations including therapy.

LIFE SPAN CONSIDERATIONS
Older Adults

Mood and anxiety disorders in late life tend to decline with age and become less common in people over the age of 65.[11,12] However, adults who have experienced anxiety throughout their lives are at higher risk for having both mental and physical comorbidities, and the severity of the illness may be greater. Although the symptoms are expressed the same as in younger adults, anxiety disorders may be difficult to diagnose when cognitive decline is present. In older adults, CBT has been shown to be less effective as compared to adults aged 18 to 65.[11,12] An increased sensitivity to medication should be considered when prescribing so the provider should start with a low dose and titrate slowly. There is also an increased potential for drug to drug interactions due to often numerous physical and mental comorbidities. The risk of falls, orthostatic hypotension, cardiac changes, and paradoxical reactions to benzodiazepines are important considerations when deciding on pharmacologic management.[11,12]

Children and Adolescents

Anxiety is a common mental health diagnosis in children and adolescents and is frequently identified by the primary care provider because presenting complaints often include avoiding age-appropriate tasks or excessive physical complaints that are not substantiated by physical examination or a medical work-up. Due to the concerns about increased risk of suicide for children and adolescents placed on SSRIs, the potential dangers of psychopharmacological treatment should be weighed before starting a medication.[12]

Pregnancy and Breastfeeding

During pregnancy, the risk of untreated anxiety must be weighed against the risk of potential damage to the unborn child. This same risk assessment should be completed when a patient is breastfeeding. Pregnancy and breastfeeding implications for any medication considered should be reviewed. In cases where the risk is considered to outweigh the benefits, psychotherapy should be recommended as an alternative.[11,12]

COMPLICATIONS

Anxiety disorders are associated with severe impairments in numerous areas of functioning, increasing the use of primary care services. They commonly co-occur with substance use, other mental health disorders, and physical comorbidities.

Anxiety has been found to be an independent risk factor for coronary heart disease and adverse events after myocardial infarction, but as of yet it has not been shown that screening or treating depression or anxiety will improve cardiovascular outcomes.[16] Another comorbidity is smoking. One in three cigarettes are smoked by a person with a mental disorder, and unlike the general population, there has been no decrease in smoking among people with mental disorders.[16] Anxiety and depression are also more common in patients with asthma and COPD with a major issue being hyperventilation which exacerbates the symptoms of these disorders.[16] Additionally, cancer is another major comorbidity of anxiety and/or depression and is associated with a poorer quality of life, poorer compliance with treatment, longer hospitalization, and a higher risk of suicide.[16] Suicidal ideation and the risk of completed suicides are higher for any person with mental health disorders compared with matched control samples of people who do not meet DSM criteria for a diagnosis. See Chapter 226 for more information on suicidal ideation.

PATIENT AND FAMILY EDUCATION

Patient and families should be educated on all potential options for treatment. This education should include both psychopharmacology and psychotherapy.

Therapies may be offered if a person or parent of a child does not want to start medication, although studies using a combination of therapy and medications show the most promising results.[18] Cognitive behavioral treatment (CBT) has been shown to have the strongest effect sizes in patients with anxiety, minimizing the likelihood of remission of symptoms.[18]

Families need to be engaged in this process to better understand how to recognize warning signs of increased risk for distress and possible relapse.

It is important for family members of those having experienced a known trauma to be given education about the potential sequelae. Loved ones are encouraged to support and validate the survivor's experience of trauma, thereby increasing their protective factors by offering a safe environment where the experience can be discussed. There should also be an opportunity for the person to discuss the trauma and ongoing issues with a therapist. Manualized trauma-focused psychotherapy is the most effective therapy for patients who have experienced a trauma.[19]

There are several Internet sites available for education and support for patients and families. They include the following:
National Alliance on Mental Illness: www.nami.org
National Institute of Mental Health: www.nimh.nih.gov/health/topics/anxiety-disorders/index.shtml
Anxiety and Depression Association of American: www.adaa.org
National Center for PTSD: www.ptsd.va.gov

HEALTH PROMOTION

Although people cannot change their genetic predisposition to mental illness, they can buffer the effects of stress and exposure to traumatic events. It is important to maintain good physical health, adequate nutrition, healthy weight and exercise routines, and appropriate sleep patterns, and to incorporate stress management techniques into the lifestyle. The primary care provider is in the privileged role of often being the first person to learn of a patient's anxiety or traumatic experience. Regardless of external pressures of time and schedule, the provider's response during this initial disclosure is critical. A validating, supportive, resourceful encounter enhances the patient's pre-existing protective factors and ability to cope, thus supporting early intervention and treatment.

REFERENCES

1. Bandelow, B., & Michaelis, S. (2015). Epidemiology of anxiety disorders in the 21st century. *Dialogues in Clinical Neuroscience, 17*(3), 327.
2. American Psychiatric Association (APA). (2013). *Diagnostic and statistical manual of mental disorders* (5th ed.). Arlington, VA: APA.
3. Carabotti, M., et al. (2015). The gut-brain axis: Interactions between enteric microbiota, central and enteric nervous systems. *Annals of Gastroenterology, 28*(2), 203.
4. Sharma, S., et al. (2016). Gene × environment determinants of stress-and anxiety-related disorders. *Annual Review of Psychology, 67*, 239–261.
5. Nuss, P. (2015). Anxiety disorders and GABA neurotransmission: A disturbance of modulation. *Neuropsychiatric Disease and Treatment, 11*, 165.
6. Spitzer, R. L., et al. (2006). A brief measure for assessing generalized anxiety disorder: The GAD-7. *Archives of Internal Medicine, 166*(10), 1092–1097.
7. Prins, A., et al. (2004). The primary care PTSD screen (PC-PTSD): Development and operating characteristics. *International Journal of Psychiatry in Clinical Practice, 9*(1), 9–14.
8. Connor, K. M., et al. (2001). Mini-SPIN: A brief screening assessment for generalized social anxiety disorder. *Depression and Anxiety, 14*(2), 137–140.
9. Kroenke, K., et al. (2010). The patient health questionnaire somatic, anxiety, and depressive symptom scales: A systematic review. *General Hospital Psychiatry, 32*(4), 345–359.
10. McMullen, C. K., et al. (2015). Patient-centered priorities for improving medication management and adherence. *Patient Education and Counseling, 98*(1), 102–110.
11. Bandelow, B., et al. (2015). The German guidelines for the treatment of anxiety disorders. *European Archives of Psychiatry and Clinical Neuroscience, 265*(5), 363–373.
12. Bandelow, B., Michaelis, S., & Wedekind, D. (2017). Treatment of anxiety disorders. *Dialogues in Clinical Neuroscience, 19*(2), 93.

13. Bandelow, B., Sher, L., Bunevicius, R., et al. (2012). Guidelines for the pharmacological treatment of anxiety disorders, obsessive-compulsive disorder and posttraumatic stress disorder in primary care. *International Journal of Psychiatry in Clinical Practice, 16*, 77–84.

14. Stubbs, B., et al. (2017). An examination of the anxiolytic effects of exercise for people with anxiety and stress-related disorders: A meta-analysis. *Psychiatry Research*.

15. Stonerock, G. L., et al. (2015). Exercise as treatment for anxiety: Systematic review and analysis. *Annals of Behavioral Medicine, 49*(4), 542–556.

16. World Health Organization. (2017). Addressing comorbidity between mental disorders and major noncommunicable diseases. Retrieved from http://www.euro.who.int/__data/assets/pdf_file/0009/342297/Comorbidity-report_E-web.pdf. (Accessed 28 December 2017).

17. Eap, C. B. (2016). Personalized prescribing: A new medical model for clinical implementation of psychotropic drugs. *Dialogues in Clinical Neuroscience, 18*(3), 313.

18. Bandelow, B., et al. (2015). Efficacy of treatments for anxiety disorders: A meta-analysis. *International Clinical Psychopharmacology, 30*(4), 183–192.

19. Department of Veterans Affairs/Department of Defense. (2017). VA/DOD Clinical Practice Guideline for the Management of Posttraumatic Stress Disorder and Acute Stress Disorder. Retrieved from https://www.healthquality.va.gov/guidelines/MH/ptsd/VADoDPTSDCPGFinal082917.pdf. (Accessed 28 December 2017).

CHAPTER **226**

MOOD DISORDERS

Ani Sinanyan

 If the patient is expressing suicidal ideation or deemed unstable to be treated in the outpatient setting, immediate referral to a psychiatrist or emergency room evaluation for a psychiatric hold or hospitalization is necessary. Emergent intervention is needed if a patient is at risk of harming themselves or others and for patients profoundly impaired by their symptoms. Consultation with a specialist is indicated for patients with suspected bipolar disorder, schizophrenia, or schizoaffective disorder.

DEFINITION AND EPIDEMIOLOGY

According to the World Health Organization, mood disorders are among the primary causes of patient disability, with depression affecting 322 million people worldwide.[1] From time to time, anyone may experience feelings of sadness or lose interest in previously enjoyable activities. However, in individuals diagnosed with mood disorders, the symptoms are often more severe, last longer, and involve recurrent and constant feelings of sadness. The constant emotional imbalance interrupts daily life activities and requires professional medical and psychiatric treatment. The most common mood disorders include depression, bipolar disorder, and seasonal affective disorder (SAD), but there are other mood disorders that also affect patients' well-being (Box 226.1).

Specific criteria exist to categorize mood disorders, enabling treatment. The *Diagnostic and Statistical Manual of Mental Disorders* (DSM-5) facilitates understanding of these disorders to aid health care providers in identifying symptoms, diagnosing, and treating patients with a mental health illness. The DSM-5 describes a major depressive episode as a condition in which a person has depressed mood or anhedonia (loss of interest or sense of pleasure) *and* four of the following symptoms: unintended change in weight, sleep disturbance, psychomotor agitation or retardation, fatigue, feelings of worthlessness or guilt,

BOX **226.1**

Mood Disorders

Bipolar disorder
Cyclothymic disorder
Depression related to medical illness, a medication, or substance use
Major depression
Minor depression
Disruptive mood dysregulation disorder
Persistent depressive disorder (dysthymia)
Premenstrual dysphoric disorder
Seasonal affective disorder
Unspecified depression

inability to concentrate, and recurrent thoughts of death or thoughts of suicide.[2]

A manic episode is defined by the DSM-5 as a period of time (at least 1 week) during which a person's mood is abnormally elevated, expansive, or irritable in addition to at least three of the following symptoms: inflated self-esteem (grandiosity), decreased need for sleep without fatigue, pressured speech, racing thoughts, distractibility, psychomotor agitation, and excessive involvement in pleasure-seeking activities that may have high risk for undesirable consequences (excessive spending, sexual indiscretions).[2]

A mixed episode is present when symptoms of both major depressive and manic episodes are present nearly every day for a week or more and these symptoms are not related to a medication effect or substance. Like manic and major depressive episodes, a mixed episode can be diagnosed only when the symptoms cause marked impairment in one's ability to participate in usual activities and to function at previous expectations.[2]

A hypomanic episode describes symptoms of a manic episode that are shorter in duration and do not match the severity of a manic episode and thus are not associated with such marked impairment of function. Hypomanic episodes are not debilitating enough to warrant hospitalization or to lead to dangerous consequences.[2]

PATHOPHYSIOLOGY AND OTHER FACTORS

The pathophysiology of mood disorders is a continued topic of research. Significant enhancements have been made in the understanding and more efficient treatment of these disorders. It seems that there may be a genetic linkage, but recent studies also suggest biologic dysregulation in the brain.[3] These studies suggest that major depressive disorder and bipolar disorder involve dysfunction in the areas of the brain that are involved in emotional regulation. Central to these areas of the brain are the amygdala, hippocampus, and other parts of the brain that comprise the limbic system. Based on imaging and histopathology, there is evidence to suggest the amygdala and medial prefrontal cortical areas of the brain are involved in mood regulation and disorder. Additionally, degenerative basal ganglia disease and lesions in the striatum and orbitofrontal cortex increase the risk of major depressive disorder. Further evaluation of individuals with early-onset mood disorder indicates neuromorphometric abnormalities in the lobe, striatum, thalamus, and posterior cingulate. Resting metabolism is noted to be elevated in the left amygdala in individuals with major depressive disorder or bipolar-depression. These individuals are also found to have an overall abnormal elevation of cortisol due to hypersecretion. The amygdala is found to be hyper responsive to sad words and sad faces, with a blunted response to happy words and faces. Still, further studies are needed to better understand intricacies of brain function in high-risk individuals as well as in individuals already diagnosed with mood disorders.[4]

Other factors contribute to mood disorders. Stress and life events that include illness, death, job loss, trauma, and even childbirth can contribute or cause depression.[3]

Risk factors for developing mood disorders include immediate, first-degree family history, stressful situations, unemployment, marital discord, history of physical or sexual abuse or trauma, and drug or alcohol use. Other risk factors include abuse, death or serious illnesses, and major life changes especially loss of a loved one.[5] For health care providers, awareness of the risk factors for depression is essential, because depression, regardless of the cause, increases the risk of suicide and suicide is on the rise in this country.

UNIPOLAR DEPRESSION

Depression is a common mental health disorder. An estimated 13% of patients are diagnosed with depression in the primary care setting, yet the prevalence of this disorder is likely much higher as patients often do not complain of feeling depressed and the burden of diagnosis rests on primary care providers to screen, diagnose, and treat depression. If left untreated or undertreated, patients with depression are at risk for coronary artery disease, diabetes mellitus, a diminished quality of life, stroke, suicidal ideations, and death.[6]

This knowledge suggests the need for awareness of the risk factors for depression. Though some patients will readily discuss a concern about being depressed or anxious, others will not. For that reason, it is important to recognize the signs and symptoms of depression: disinterest, persistent sadness, unexplained weight loss or weight gain. Patients can also feel helpless, pessimistic, guilty, worthless, tired, and confused. Physical pain, exhaustion, guilt, sleep disturbances, slowed thinking and body movements, thoughts of worthlessness/suicide, restlessness, anxiety, irritability, difficulty concentrating, diminished hygiene, increased alcohol intake, and other physical symptoms that are not explained by medical diagnosis are frequently present.[7]

Thoughts of death are common in people with depression. Given the risk of suicide in this population, anyone with depression or subclinical symptoms must be carefully assessed for risk of suicide. The components for a suicide assessment are listed in Box 226.2.

The US Preventive Task Force recommends screening children, adolescents, and adult patients in primary care, and there

are varied risk factors for depression that can suggest the need for screening. These risks include pregnancy, childbirth, parenthood, chronic illness, chronic pain, stress, insomnia, substance use, family history (especially a family history of suicide), female sex (but men also can be depressed), poor social support, low self-esteem, dementia, being divorced/single/widowed, and a past personal history of previous trauma, depression, or traumatic brain injury.[5]

Any recent change (e.g., family or friend illness or death, job loss, or other financial stress) should also raise a health care provider's concern for a patient's well-being and risk for depression.

Screening Tools

Several screening tools are used in the primary care setting to diagnose depression. These include the Patient Health Questionnaire-9 (PHQ-9), Beck depression inventory, Zung depression scale, and PHQ-2. A commonly used screening tool is the PHQ-2 because the process is easy and quick. The PHQ-2 has 78% to 92% specificity while the specificity of the PHQ-9 is 91% to 94%.[8]

For older adults, depression is common and can be significant, approaching 16% for elders living in the community but up to 54% when first living in a nursing home.[8] The cause of depression in older adults is multifactorial, but is not related to aging changes. The five-item Geriatric Depression Scale (GDS) has been found to be as effective as the 15-item scale and has a 92% sensitivity and an 89% specificity.[9] Although older adults in the primary care setting can be screened using the PHQ-2 for initial screening and the PHQ-9 as a follow-up diagnostic tool, the GDS is useful in this population.

Clinical Presentation and Physical Examination

Depression screening does not necessarily diagnose depression, so a thorough patient history and physical exam is necessary to determine if the patient has depressive symptoms or suicidal ideation. Both are best realized if the patient and provider have a good relationship and the patient trusts the provider. Specific questions should be asked to determine if the patient has been feeling irritable, depressed, fatigued, is sleeping too much or not at all, or has gained or lost weight. The patient's lifestyle, medications including herbal and over-the counter, and substance use should be elicited. Other necessary information required is when the symptoms started, the patient's and family's past medical history, if the patient or a family member has a history of depression (particularly bipolar depression or past or present symptoms of mania or hypomania), and if the patient has had trouble concentrating, considered or planned suicide, or is feeling unworthy, agitated, or just has lost interest in life in general.

The physical examination is an opportunity to evaluate the patient presentation and assess signs of irritability, sadness, or depression. Careful evaluation to determine if a potential illness is the cause of the patient's signs and symptoms is necessary.[3]

Diagnostics

For patients with a long history of depression, laboratory diagnostics may not be necessary. However, even patients with known depression may need diagnostic evaluation if not recently obtained.

BOX **226.2**

Assessing Risk for Suicide

- Thoughts of suicide
- Plan to commit suicide
- Means to complete the plan
- Intention to follow through with the plan

Consider impulsivity and the influence of substance use.

A urinalysis; complete blood count; chemistry, liver, and thyroid profile; and toxicology screen are indicated. Other diagnostics are obtained as suggested by the physical findings. If the physical examination reveals confusion or memory problems, a mental status evaluation and further diagnostics (B_{12}, folate, and neuroimaging) are necessary. An ECG should be considered in older adults and in patients on medications that cause bradycardia or other cardiac concerns (e.g., prolonged QT syndrome).[3] A recent fall with neurologic changes could also require neuroimaging, especially in a frail older adult.

Differential Diagnosis

In addition to medical conditions and substance use, other causes should be considered. Major or unipolar depression is different than bipolar depression. Patients with unipolar depression are sad and often tired and disinterested. Patients with bipolar depression can be sad, but also have periods of mania. Sometimes it seems that patients with bipolar depression fluctuate from one end of the spectrum to another. Determining if the patient has bipolar depression or a major depressive disorder is crucial as antidepressant therapy if used alone can induce mania in a patient with bipolar depression.

Grief is also a common cause of depression as is social isolation and other life events. Adjustment disorder occurs after losing a job or another event that was particularly stressful. It is not posttraumatic stress syndrome, but does involve anxiety as well as depression and can impact function. Attention deficit hyperactivity disorder is another consideration that is often overlooked.

The DSM-5 diagnostic criteria should be reviewed to differentiate the types of depression and diagnose the patient's symptoms correctly. Illness and other causes of the patient's symptoms should be reviewed as well.

Interprofessional Collaborative Management

Nonpharmacologic Management. All patients are carefully assessed for suicidal ideation. For patients with mild depression, psychosocial interventions and psychotherapy are often helpful and medication may not be necessary. Psychotherapy may be the appropriate initial treatment for certain patients including those who have mild to moderate depression, lactating females, and women who are pregnant or desire to become pregnant. Therapy focuses on the presence of stressors, conflict, and interpersonal concerns. For some patients, a medication is indicated, but counseling, cognitive behavioral therapy, or psychotherapy is also recommended.

Pharmacologic Management. There are varied antidepressants used for the treatment of unipolar depression, whether mild, moderate, or severe. All are efficacious, though the side effect profile of selective serotonin reuptake inhibitors and serotonin-norepinephrine reuptake inhibitors is gentler. The patient's clinical symptoms, comorbid conditions, risk for drug-drug interactions, and the considered medication side effect profile should guide the potential treatment choices discussed with the patient. If a patient is started on an antidepressant, the initial dose is low and is maintained for the first week or two before a dose increase. It is important to monitor the patient regularly during the first few weeks to assess for suicidal ideation, efficacy, and potential adverse effects. Some patients need to be monitored and assessed more frequently depending on the severity of their illness and the patient's participation and cooperation, social support, and comorbidities. It is important to explain to the patient (and family if appropriate) that symptom improvement will take several weeks and it is necessary to adhere to the prescribed treatment for best outcomes, provided there are no untoward reactions to the medicine. Patients (and families if indicated) should understand that treatment should continue at least for 6 to 9 months or longer in some instances. A healthy diet, sleep adequacy, and daily exercise should be encouraged.

The spectrum of treatment options includes selective serotonin reuptake inhibitors (SSRIs), serotonin and norepinephrine reuptake inhibitors (SNRIs), atypical antidepressants, tricyclic antidepressants (TCAs), and though rarely used now, monoamine oxidase inhibitors (MAOIs). Every patient is different so a review of medication side effects before prescribing is indicated (Table 226.1). Selective serotonin reuptake inhibitors are favored for their safety and side effect profile. These include fluoxetine (Prozac), paroxetine (Paxil), sertraline (Zoloft), citalopram (Celexa), and escitalopram (Lexapro).

Serotonin and norepinephrine reuptake inhibitors also have a favorable side effect profile. Medications used for the treatment of depression include duloxetine (Cymbalta), venlafaxine (Effexor), desvenlafaxine (Pristiq), and levomilnacipran (Fetzima).

The atypical antidepressants include trazodone, a serotonin reuptake inhibitor that is often used as a sleep aid for patients with depression. Mirtazapine (Remeron) is a α2-antagonist, also used for unipolar depression, especially in patients who are not eating and losing weight. Vortioxetine (Brintellix) is categorized differently, based on its varied physiologic affects as an antidepressant, but also a serotonin 5-HT$_{1a}$ receptor agonist, serotonin 5-HT$_3$ receptor antagonist, and selective serotonin reuptake inhibitor. Vilazodone (Viibryd) is an antidepressant and selective serotonin reuptake inhibitor/5HT$_{1a}$, while bupropion, which is better known as Wellbutrin and used not only as an antidepressant but also a smoking cessation aid, is considered an antidepressant.

Tricyclic and tetracyclic antidepressants are also not commonly used medications for depression because of their side effect profile, though doxepin, a tricyclic/antidepressant, can sometimes be helpful for sleep. Often these medication categories are only prescribed when the other options of medications have been exhausted.

MAOIs are also rarely used for patients with depression because of the known drug-drug and drug-food reactions. Patients who are prescribed a MAOI must understand the importance of not eating certain foods such as cheeses, wines, and pickles and avoiding some medications as decongestants and some herbal supplements are known to interact with MAOIs.

BIPOLAR DISORDER
Clinical Presentation and Physical Examination

Patients in the primary care setting often present with a mood disorder and are sometimes misdiagnosed. This is especially true for patients with a bipolar disorder. The clinical presentation of a patient with a bipolar disorder can be misinterpreted or misunderstood. Providers frequently associate bipolar disorder with mania or psychosis, but presentation can also include profound depression, complaints of several days

TABLE 226.1   Side Effects of Common Antidepressants

Adverse Reaction	Prevalence			
	High (>30%)	Moderate (10%–30%)	Low (2%–10%)	Very Low (<2%)
Drowsiness, fatigue, or sedation	Mirtazapine Trazodone Amitriptyline	Citalopram Fluoxetine Fluvoxamine Paroxetine Sertraline Venlafaxine	Duloxetine Escitalopram Bupropion Nortriptyline Desvenlafaxine	
Insomnia		Citalopram Fluoxetine Duloxetine Escitalopram Fluvoxamine Paroxetine Sertraline Bupropion Venlafaxine Desvenlafaxine (doses ≥100 mg)	Mirtazapine Trazodone Amitriptyline Desvenlafaxine	Nortriptyline
Excitement		Fluvoxamine Sertraline Bupropion Venlafaxine	Citalopram Fluoxetine Escitalopram Paroxetine Mirtazapine Nortriptyline Desvenlafaxine	Duloxetine Trazodone Amitriptyline
Confusion		Fluoxetine Amitriptyline Nortriptyline	Fluvoxamine Mirtazapine Bupropion Venlafaxine	Citalopram Duloxetine Escitalopram Paroxetine Sertraline Trazodone Desvenlafaxine
Headache		Citalopram Fluoxetine Escitalopram Fluvoxamine Paroxetine Sertraline Bupropion Venlafaxine Desvenlafaxine	Mirtazapine Trazodone Amitriptyline	Duloxetine Nortriptyline
Dry mouth	Mirtazapine Amitriptyline	Citalopram Fluoxetine Duloxetine Fluvoxamine Paroxetine Sertraline Bupropion Venlafaxine Desvenlafaxine Trazodone Nortriptyline	Escitalopram	

TABLE 226.1 Side Effects of Common Antidepressants—cont'd

Adverse Reaction	Prevalence			
	High (>30%)	Moderate (10%–30%)	Low (2%–10%)	Very Low (<2%)
Constipation		Duloxetine Fluvoxamine Paroxetine Mirtazapine Bupropion Venlafaxine Amitriptyline Nortriptyline	Citalopram Fluoxetine Escitalopram Sertraline Trazodone Desvenlafaxine	
Sweating		Citalopram Fluvoxamine Paroxetine Bupropion Venlafaxine Desvenlafaxine Amitriptyline	Fluoxetine Duloxetine Escitalopram Sertraline Mirtazapine	Trazodone Nortriptyline
Tremor		Fluoxetine Fluvoxamine Paroxetine Sertraline Bupropion Amitriptyline Nortriptyline	Citalopram Duloxetine Escitalopram Mirtazapine Venlafaxine Desvenlafaxine Trazodone	
Orthostatic hypotension or dizziness		Fluoxetine Paroxetine Sertraline Venlafaxine Trazodone Amitriptyline	Citalopram Duloxetine Escitalopram Fluvoxamine Mirtazapine Bupropion Nortriptyline Desvenlafaxine (dizziness)	Desvenlafaxine (orthostatic hypotension)
Electrocardiographic changes		Amitriptyline	Trazodone Nortriptyline	Citalopram Fluoxetine Duloxetine Escitalopram Fluvoxamine Paroxetine Sertraline Mirtazapine Bupropion Venlafaxine Desvenlafaxine
Nausea, diarrhea, or vomiting	Fluvoxamine Sertraline Venlafaxine	Citalopram Fluoxetine Duloxetine Escitalopram Paroxetine Bupropion Trazodone Desvenlafaxine	Mirtazapine Amitriptyline	Nortriptyline

Continued

TABLE 226.1	Side Effects of Common Antidepressants—cont'd			
	Prevalence			
Adverse Reaction	**High (>30%)**	**Moderate (10%–30%)**	**Low (2%–10%)**	**Very Low (<2%)**
Rash			Fluoxetine Fluvoxamine Sertraline Bupropion Venlafaxine Amitriptyline	Citalopram Duloxetine Paroxetine Mirtazapine Escitalopram Trazodone Nortriptyline Desvenlafaxine
Weight gain	Mirtazapine Amitriptyline	Paroxetine	Citalopram Fluoxetine Escitalopram Sertraline Fluvoxamine Trazodone Nortriptyline	Duloxetine Bupropion Venlafaxine Desvenlafaxine
Sexual disturbance	Citalopram Fluoxetine Fluvoxamine Paroxetine Sertraline Venlafaxine	Mirtazapine	Duloxetine Escitalopram Amitriptyline Desvenlafaxine (0%–4% in men)	Bupropion Trazodone Nortriptyline Desvenlafaxine

Note: All medications that influence the serotonin system are associated with increased risk of bleeding, especially if they are used concomitantly with nonsteroidal anti-inflammatory or anticoagulation treatments.
Data from Work Group on Major Depressive Disorder. (2010). *Practice guideline for the treatment of patients with major depressive disorder* (3rd ed.). Washington, DC: American Psychiatric Association.

of reduced or no sleep without fatigue, mood swings, racing thoughts, irritability, and irrationality.[10,11]

There are two types of bipolar disorder: bipolar 1 associated with mania, hypomania, and severe depression and bipolar 2 associated with a history of hypomania and major depression, but without a history of a manic episode. These types of bipolar disorders can be chronic conditions with recurrent episodes.[10] However, a patient can present with symptoms of a bipolar disorder, but actually have an illness or untoward reaction to a medication. To accurately diagnose a patient with a bipolar disorder, the health care provider must elicit both the patient's and family's social history for characteristics and sequelae of the illness including relationship problems, unstable occupational past, and possibly legal issues the patient experienced when manic. The manic episodes commonly indicative of bipolar I disorder can include comorbidities such as anxiety, panic disorder, and substance use. These patients must be referred promptly to specialists who are able to care for the patient in an intensive outpatient program or in a hospital setting.[10]

Hypomania, indicative of bipolar II disorder, is a potentially missed diagnosis. Patients will present with complaints of depression followed by periods of feeling well and emotionally healthy.[10] Depression in bipolar disorder is commonly misdiagnosed as major depressive disorder and therefore provider due diligence is required to further investigate the cause of the patient's symptoms. Differentiating between bipolar disorder and depression should be determined with a careful inquiry about a past diagnosis of bipolar disorder or history of mania or hypomania, age of onset, features of illness, course of illness, history of treatment, and family history.[10]

Interestingly, a subset of patients may not present with bipolar disorder until later in life. Older adults may present differently and may or may not have a previous history of a bipolar disorder. The symptoms of bipolar disorder in this cohort are the same as in younger adults: hypomania, mania, or severe depression. Evidence of cognitive dysfunction is possible requiring further evaluation of memory and functional status with screening tests for dementia.

Risk Factors

Risk factors for bipolar disorder include a personal history of substance use, depression, family history of mental illness, and stressful life events.[10] Commonly, patients with a bipolar disorder have another medical or psychiatric illness that can impact patient wellness, function, and socialization.

Screening Tools

Screening tools used in bipolar disorder include case-finding tools that can help determine the type of mood disorder the patient is experiencing. The most widely used tool is the Mood Disorder Questionnaire (MDQ) available at https://www.integration.samhsa.gov/images/res/MDQ.pdf and the Composite International Diagnostic Interview (CIDI).[12] The MDQ is a tool that is completed by the patient with 13 items to determine mood disorders and two questions focusing on the functional limitations the mood disorders are causing. The CIDI is an interview that is completed by a trained provider. If the patient answers yes to one of two questions, it leads to 12 more questions that identify manic symptoms. The questionnaire is based on positive answers, and the more affirmative the answers the higher the likelihood of diagnosis. Both of these tools are used in the primary care setting.[10] Important questions to ask a patient that is suspected to have bipolar disorder include a history or current episodes of mania and/or depression, duration of symptoms including suicidal or homicidal ideations, impact of symptoms on the patient's daily life and relationships, comorbidities, history of treatments and response, and family history.[10]

Diagnostics

If a patient presents with symptoms of a bipolar disorder but no known previous diagnosis, some laboratory diagnostics are indicated if not recently obtained. Substance use is always a consideration so toxicology testing is recommended. In most primary care settings, a urine sample for toxicology can be obtained, but serum sampling and swab saliva sampling are also available for toxicology screening. Diagnostic considerations should include a complete blood count, thyroid stimulating hormone, and a liver, chemistry, and renal profile, as well as toxicology screening.

Additional Diagnostics. Further diagnostics are predicated on the patient history and presentation. For example, older patients with a change in cognition or consciousness may have a delirium associated with an infectious process, a new neurologic disorder, dementia, or other toxicity requiring neuroimaging or other diagnostic testing.

Differential Diagnosis

Illness, injury, unipolar depression, schizophrenia, medications, and substance use should always be a consideration when a patient presents with signs and symptoms of a bipolar I, II, or other mood disorder. If other causes are excluded and a mood disorder is a concern, the DSM-5 criteria should be reviewed. Diagnosis can be challenging and psychiatric evaluation is recommended especially for patients with new onset or difficult-to-treat symptoms. As urgent psychiatric evaluation is not often an option, emergency room evaluation and possibly hospitalization is necessary.

Interprofessional Collaborative Practice

Pharmacologic Managment. Treatment for bipolar disorders is focused on both pharmacological and nonpharmacological therapy. Acute treatment of bipolar disorder is focused on reducing symptoms and promoting safety for the patient. Depending on the symptoms and characteristics of the disorder presentation, primary care providers can offer specific medication treatments. Often, though, patients will require a skilled psychopharmacologist to maximize treatment.

For acute treatment of mania, lithium, divalproex (Valproate), carbamazepine (Tegretol), and the second-generation antipsychotics—asenapine (Saphris), aripiprazole (Abilify), olanzapine (Zyprexa), quetiapine (Seroquel), risperidone (Risperdal), and ziprasidone (Geodon)—are commonly used, but there are other medications.[13] Electroconvulsive therapy is also an option for some patients. Lithium has been a conventional option for mood stabilization, although the management is complex and may be best managed in a specialty practice.

For patients with acute bipolar depressive symptoms, the goal is patient safety and improved mood. For these patients, the treatment modalities are similar: anticonvulsants, antidepressants, second-generation antipsychotics, and lithium are the commonly prescribed medications, but antidepressants alone may not be the best choice in patients with bipolar disorder and depressive mixed state or mixed depression (i.e., hypomania), emphasizing the importance of appropriate diagnosis in these disorders and the benefit of referral or collaboration with a mental health specialist.[14] Specific recommendations can include the combination of olanzapine and fluoxetine.[13] Monotherapy with a second-generation antipsychotic (e.g., lurasidone or quetiapine) is effective for some patients, but lithium or valproate can also be used in combination with the second-generation antipsychotics for treatment of bipolar depression, especially to prevent regression.[13]

Careful monitoring of these medications is necessary. Lithium concentration should be initially and periodically checked; toxicity is always possible, requiring periodic laboratory testing to monitor thyroid, parathyroid, and renal changes, as well as monitoring for cardiac changes.[13]

Bipolar illness treatment can be particularly challenging in some patients. If the primary care provider does not feel comfortable treating the patient, it is always recommended that they refer to specialty care with a psychiatrist or psychologist.[10]

Nonpharmacologic Management. Nonpharmacological treatment for bipolar disorder focuses on psychoeducation, cognitive behavioral therapy, and family therapy, as well as focus on substance use, misuse, and medication adherence.[10]

SEASONAL AFFECTIVE DISORDER

SAD can be associated with hypomania, mania, depression, and a craving for carbohydrates.[15] SAD is related to both unipolar and bipolar (I and II) depression. The exception in SAD is that patients note these symptoms with changes in season. Most often first noted in the fall and worsening in winter, SAD symptoms can also occur at other times of the year, and in some patients with SAD, the depression can be severe. Patients with SAD are not commonly suicidal, though providers should always ask about suicidal ideation when seeing any patient who seems sad or depressed.[15] The symptoms associated with SAD seem to remit when the season changes. Risk factors, screening tools, and treatments are similar to those of depression. While it is difficult for primary care providers to diagnose SAD, most patients will present to the primary care provider initially with complaints.[15]

Clinical Presentation and Physical Examination

Diagnostics. Diagnostic tests include a metabolic panel, complete blood count with differential, thyroid function tests, 24-hour free cortisol, vitamin B_{12}, and folic acid. Other tools that may be used to aid diagnosis of patients with mood disorders include the Patient Health Care Questionnaire, Mood Disorder Questionnaire, and the Bipolar Spectrum Diagnostic Scale tool.[16]

Differential Diagnosis

Other causes of the patient's symptoms should be explored, especially bipolar disorder, but a medical cause, grief, substance use, or adjustment disorder should be excluded.

Interprofessional Collaborative Management

Nonpharmacologic Management. Light therapy with artificial light, 5000 lux early each day, is the most frequently recommended intervention.[15] Regular exercise (especially outside when possible), adequate sleep, stress reduction, and relaxation are also strongly recommended.[15]

Pharmacologic Management. Fluoxetine (Prozac) or other SSRI is the most common pharmacologic recommendation, but treatment is always individualized.[15] Patients should be encouraged to continue to use light therapy, make lifestyle changes as noted previously, and have regular follow-up with the health care provider.

Life Span Considerations

- Mood disorders occur in individuals across the life span, affecting males and females of all ethnicities and income levels.[16] Women and adults age 30–60 are more likely to experience depression, however.
- Irritability can be the first sign of depression in children, adolescents, and adults.
- Older adults who develop cognitive dysfunction should be screened for depression as well as dementia. It is possible that an older adult could have both dementia and depression.

Complications

There are significant life-altering complications associated with mood disorders, especially if not diagnosed properly. The complications include use of drugs or alcohol, legal or financial problems, complicated relationships with others, poor work and school performance, and suicide or suicide attempts.[17] Additionally, patients who are depressed have a greater than 50% chance of developing coronary artery disease and having a cardiovascular event.[18]

Patient and Family Education

Education is vital for the patient and the family members or friends. This education must include an overview and description of the disease process, symptoms to expect, the available treatment plans, and associated side-effects or complications. It is also very important to give the patient resources for mental health as well as education about where to go and what to do in case of suicidal ideation.

Patients and families need to understand the nature of depression and the importance of calling the provider, 911, or the National Suicide Prevention Lifeline at 1-800-273-8255 if the patient has thoughts of suicide.

Health Promotion

Encouraging a healthy lifestyle can be helpful in maintaining mood as well as in promoting health in general. Rest, exercise, socialization, and eating healthy foods promote well-being. Avoiding foods high in sugars and carbohydrates and increasing fruits and vegetables can be beneficial.

Indication for Referral and Management

Mood disorders can be treated successfully in the primary care setting, however, there are important indications for referral and management (Box 226.3). These indications include patients who are suicidal, homicidal, gravely disabled, or have suspected serotonin syndrome. If the patient needs a safe environment while experiencing symptoms, referral to a psychiatrist for evaluation and treatment is necessary. Patients can be referred to the emergency room of any hospital, as well as a call to law enforcement to come and assess the patient and decide if the patient is stable enough to receive outpatient treatment for symptoms or they should be admitted for

---

BOX 226.3

When to Refer to Mental Health Specialists

Emergent intervention is needed as soon as possible if:
- Patients are assessed as being at risk of harming themselves or others.
- Patients are so profoundly impaired by their symptoms that their own health is acutely suffering.
- Patients are experiencing symptoms of serotonin syndrome, serotonin withdrawal, neuroleptic malignant syndrome, or lithium toxicity.
- The provider is unsure of these risks.

Urgent intervention is needed within 1 week when:
- The patient is assessed as being at high risk for suicide yet is currently safe.
- Other psychiatric comorbidities are present, including substance use disorders.
- There is an indication for ECT.

Follow-up with specialty provider is needed within 1 month when:
- Recurrent symptoms are not responding to initial treatments provided in the primary care setting.
- Complications with medication management require frequent follow-up.
- Dementia is also present.
- Patient may benefit from psychotherapy, family education, or group support.

---

further observation and evaluation due to destructive behavior. Patients may also be referred to a psychiatrist if patient requires close monitoring for medication interaction or multiple medications are indicated for patient treatment.

REFERENCES

1. World Health Organization. (2017). Depression and other common mental disorders. Retrieved from http://apps.who.int/iris/bitstream/handle/10665/254610/WHO-MSD-MER-2017.2-eng.pdf;jsessionid=1F36B5A96DF09B7EE2E908BADF51114D?sequence=1. (Accessed 28 December 2018).
2. American Psychiatric Association. (2013). *Diagnostic and statistical manual of mental disorders* (5th ed.). Arlington, VA: American Psychiatric Publishing.
3. Eisendrath, S. J., Cole, S. A., Christensen, J. F., Gutnick, D., Cole, M., & Feldman, M. D. (2014). Depression. In M. D. Feldman, J. F. Christensen, & J. M. Satterfield (Eds.), *Behavioral medicine: A guide for clinical practice* (4th ed.). New York, NY: McGraw-Hill. http://accessmedicine.mhmedical.com.ezproxy.simmons.edu/content.aspx?bookid=1116&sectionid=62688871. (Accessed 3 December 2018).
4. Mental Health. (2017). Mood disorders. Retrieved November 27, 2017 Retrieved from https://www.mentalhealth.gov/what-to-look-for/mood-disorders.
5. Maurer, D. M. (2012). Screening for depression. *American Family Physician*, *85*(2), 140–144. Retrieved from https://www.aafp.org/afp/2012/0115/p139.pdf.
6. Li, X., Frye, M. A., & Shelton, R. C. (2017). Review of pharmacological treatment in mood disorders and future directions for drug development. *Neuropsychopharmacology*, *37*(1), 77–101. doi:10.1038/npp.2011.198.
7. Anxiety and depression association of America. (2016). Bipolar disorder. Retrieved December 18 from https://adaa.org/understanding-anxiety/related-illnesses/bipolar-disorder-2.
8. Maurer, D. M., Raymond, T. J., & Davis, B. N. (2018). Depression: Screening and diagnosis. *American Family Physician*, *98*(8), 508–515.
9. Greenberg, S. A. (2019). The geriatric depression scale (GDS). Retrieved from https://consultgeri.org/try-this/general-assessment/issue-4.pdf. (Accessed 21 December 2018).
10. Culpepper, L. (2014). The diagnosis and treatment of bipolar disorder: Decision-making in primary care. *Primary Care Companion Journal of Clinical Psychiatry*, *16*(3), doi:10.4088/PCC.13r01609.

11. Mirabel-Sarron, C., & Giachetti, R. (2012). Non pharmacological treatment for bipolar disorder. *L'Encephale, 38*(Suppl. 4), S160–S166. doi:10.1016/S0013-7006(12)70094-5.

12. The Mood Disorder Questionnaire. Retrieved from https://www.integration.samhsa.gov/images/res/MDQ.pdf and the Composite International Diagnostic Interview (CIDI). (Accessed 28 December 2018).

13. Reus, V. I. (2018). Psychiatric disorders. In J. Jameson, A. S. Fauci, D. L. Kasper, S. L. Hauser, D. L. Longo, & J. Loscalzo (Eds.), *Harrison's principles of internal medicine* (20th ed.). New York, NY: McGraw-Hill. http://accessmedicine.mhmedical.com.ezproxy.simmons.edu/content.aspx?bookid=2129&sectionid=192533879. (Accessed 28 December 2018).

14. Stahl, S. M., et al. Guidelines for the recognition and management of mixed depression. Retrieved from https://www.cambridge.org/core/services/aop-cambridge-core/content/view/0DFE7AD7358126E7859C0950CB0C3323/S1092852917000165a.pdf/guidelines_for_the_recognition_and_management_of_mixed_depression.pdf. (Accessed 28 December 2018).

15. Iserson, K. V. (Ed.), (2016). Psychiatry. In *Improvised medicine: Providing care in extreme environments* (2nd ed.). New York, NY: McGraw-Hill. http://accessmedicine.mhmedical.com.ezproxy.simmons.edu/content.aspx?bookid=1728&sectionid=115698841. (Accessed 28 December 2018).

16. Price, J. L., & Drevets, W. C. (2012). Neural circuits underlying the pathophysiology of mood disorders. *Trends in Cognitive Sciences, 16*(1), doi:10.1016/j.tics.2011.12.011.

17. Malhi, G. S., Byrow, Y., Fritz, K., Das, P., Baune, B. T., Porter, R. J., et al. (2015). Mood disorders: Neurocognitive models. *Bipolar Disorders, 17*(Suppl. 2), 3–20. doi:10.1111/bdi.12353.

18. National Heart, Lung and Blood Institute. (2017). Heart disease and depression: A two way relationship. https://www.nhlbi.nih.gov/news/2017/heart-disease-and-depression-two-way-relationship. Retrieved from https://www.nhlbi.nih.gov/news/2017/heart-disease-and-depression-two-way-relationship. (Accessed 29 December 2018).

CHAPTER **227**

SUBSTANCE USE DISORDERS

Jason R. Lucey • Christopher Joseph Shaw • Dawn Williamson

 Immediate referral is indicated for:

- Withdrawal seizures (may occur from benzodiazepine or alcohol withdrawal)
- Delirium tremens (severe alcohol withdrawal symptoms occurring 72–96 h after last consumption may include severe tachycardia, tremor, confusion, hallucinations, agitation, diaphoresis, fever, seizures)[1]
- Overdose—depending on substance ingested, this may present differently but in the case of opioids, symptoms may include unresponsiveness, constricted or "pinpoint" pupils, and respiratory depression.[1] Opioid overdose requires prompt delivery of naloxone and preferably a period of medically supervised observation to ensure respiratory depression does not recur after naloxone wears off. Any ingestion of any substance that results in unstable vital signs warrants emergency room referral for stabilization.
- Suicidality/homicidality/psychosis—because mental health issues frequently co-occur with substance use disorders, providers should consider these mental health emergencies and refer for appropriate stabilization
- Ready for treatment—any patient who actively requests treatment for a moderate to severe substance use disorder should be referred immediately to a facility that can provide it. Patients should be offered evidence-based pharmacotherapy for alcohol and opioid use disorder, preferably by the primary care provider to avoid delays in initiation.

DEFINITION AND EPIDEMIOLOGY

Substance use disorder (SUD) is a common and complex health condition that involves neurobiology, genetics, behavior, development, and social policy influences. The definition of addiction (or severe SUD) according to the National Institute on Drug Abuse is a "chronic, relapsing brain disease that is characterized by compulsive drug seeking and use, despite harmful consequences."[2] The American Society of Addiction Medicine further describes addiction as dysfunctional brain circuitry that manifests in biologic, psychological, social, and spiritual problems.[3]

The American Psychiatric Association's 2013 Diagnostic and Statistical Manual (DSM-5) defines SUD as follows[4]:

A problematic pattern of substance use leading to clinically significant impairment or distress, as manifested by at least two of the following occurring within a 12-month period:

- The substance is often taken in larger amounts or over a longer period than was intended
- There is a persistent desire or unsuccessful efforts to cut down or control use of the substance
- A great deal of time is spent in activities necessary to obtain the substance, use the substance, or recover from its effects
- Craving, or a strong desire or urge to use the substance
- Recurrent use resulting in a failure to fulfill major role obligations at work, school, or home
- Continued use despite having persistent or recurrent social or interpersonal problems caused by or exacerbated by its effects
- Important social, occupational, or recreational activities are given up or reduced because of use
- Recurrent use in situations in which it is physically hazardous
- Use is continued despite knowledge of having a persistent or recurrent physical or psychological problem that is likely to have been caused or exacerbated by the substance
- Tolerance
- Withdrawal

The DSM-5 further classifies SUD by severity, with a mild disorder involving only two to three of the aforementioned criteria met, a moderate disorder involving four to five criteria, and a severe disorder when six or more criteria are present.

Depending on the substance used, these criteria may be used to diagnose alcohol use disorder (AUD), tobacco use disorder (TUD), opioid use disorder (OUD), cannabis use disorder (CUD), stimulant use disorder, and others. The DSM-5 terminology removed the term "abuse" from the definition and combined the previous criteria for "abuse" and "dependence" into the aforementioned criteria. Substance use may also be classified as risky or harmful even before a disorder develops. For instance, a singular episode of use (i.e., driving while intoxicated, or overdosing during a one-time experimentation with opioids) may result in catastrophic health consequences. Primary care providers can prevent numerous adverse health events through early discussions and effective therapeutic interventions on both risky use and SUD. Moreover, because the relative prevalence of SUD is high and the availability of addiction specialists is low, PCPs must increasingly be prepared to manage SUD in a primary care setting.

Historically, the phenomenon of SUD has been highly stigmatized by both health care systems and society alike. As opposed to being seen as needing treatment and deserving of care, people with SUD have frequently been judged as morally inferior and largely punished or blamed for their disorder. Increasingly, SUD is emerging as a legitimate health condition deserving of compassion, aggressive treatment, and research. Stigma and shame still are significant barriers to equitable care for people with SUD but hopefully, like the historical transformation of a once-taboo cancer diagnosis, the disorder will be seen as worthy of public attention and research. The opioid epidemic, fueled in part by a dramatic rise in the prescription of opioids during the 1990s and 2000s, changed the landscape of addressing SUD as a public health problem as the epidemic grew to the point where drug overdoses in 2015 were the leading cause of accidental death.[5] The historical stigma of SUD has unfortunately been racially charged, leading to tragic racial and ethnic disparities in the care of persons with SUD. Communities of color have experienced high rates of SUD, poorer access, and more barriers to care. People of color with SUD are more likely to receive inappropriate care and commonly experience disproportionate social and economic risk factors.[6,7]

Comparing the crack cocaine epidemic of the 1980s to the more recent opioid epidemic is just one example of how racial bias and racism have led to vastly different approaches to SUD. During the crack cocaine epidemic, drug users (predominantly people of color) were depicted and treated harshly as criminals instead of patients deserving of medical attention. On the other hand, the opioid epidemic, which has affected large numbers of white middle and upper-class people, is increasingly addressed as a public health problem more than a criminal justice issue. Improvements in the scientific understanding of SUD certainly call for the disorder to be treated as a public health issue as opposed to a moral failing on the part of the person with SUD; yet, stigma and racism are still largely entrenched. Sensitivity to stigma, as well as the racist history of how SUD has been treated, is essential as primary care providers work towards more widespread prevention and treatment efforts. Efforts to use less stigmatizing language when referring to people who use substances are called for by research showing that the use of non–person-centered terminology leads to poorer care.[8] Suggestions for destigmatized terminology can be found at https://www.recoveryanswers.org/addiction-ary/.

The health effects and societal costs of SUDs are staggering. According to the 2015 National Survey on Drug Use and Health (NSDUH),[9] more than 20 million people had a SUD, representing 7.8% of the total population of Americans older than the age of 12. AUD affected 15.7 million people (5.9% of total population), and 7.7 million people had an illicit drug disorder. In 2017, annual deaths attributed to the most commonly used substances are estimated to be 480,000 for tobacco, 88,000 for alcohol, and 64,000 for other drugs, including opioids, which include prescription pain relievers, heroin, and fentanyl.[10,11] Other adverse outcomes related to substances are innumerable and include the burden of substance-related cardiac, respiratory, and liver diseases, substance-induced traumatic injuries, blood-borne diseases related to intravenous (IV) drug use, and substance-associated mental health disorders. The estimated societal economic costs attributable to substance use, combining costs of crime, lost productivity, and health care, are $740 billion per year.[11]

According to the 2015 NSDUH, approximately 18.1 million people met criteria for needing specialty SUD treatment in the prior year but did not receive it. In addition, more than 95% of those needing treatment did not self-perceive a need for treatment.[12] These statistics are important for primary care providers to understand because it is highly likely that PCPs will encounter SUD as a common disorder but at the same time, patients, in fact, often will not have the self-awareness of a need for treatment. Research suggests that patients with SUD may be more willing to accept treatment when offered in a primary care venue as opposed to being referred to a specialty clinic.[13] To effect better overall outcomes for SUD, PCPs will increasingly need to be prepared to identify SUD, use evidence-based approaches to encourage behavior change, and even initiate treatment of SUD, including pharmacotherapy, especially when barriers to access to specialty care exist.

PATHOPHYSIOLOGY

It is important for providers to have a basic understanding of the biologic basis and other determinants of SUD to improve overall care for patients. The basic neurobiology of addiction helps to clarify diagnostics and set treatment goals. It can also be invaluable in providing education to patients about the brain changes that occur with substance use. It is helpful for both patients and providers to understand that addiction is a chronic but treatable illness. Relapses are a part of the disease process itself and not caused by moral failing. If left untreated, severe complications and even death can occur from substance use. The impact of substance use can affect all aspects of an individual's life. The recurrent use of alcohol and/or drugs causes clinically and functionally significant impairment. These impairments can be seen in health problems, failure to meet major life responsibilities, and inability to control quantity of substance consumed.

Patterns of substance use fall on a continuum and can progress from social use, during which the individual uses on occasion, to more regular use, where weekly use emerges, to misuse, where a pattern of increased frequency is seen and then followed by the patient with SUD. Neuroadaptive mechanisms within the neurocircuitry mediate this transition from sporadic use to substance use that meets diagnostic criteria of SUD as a disorder. The neurobiology involved at these various stages include neurochemical changes that can persist and create a vulnerability to relapse.

Development of Substance Use Disorders

Many theories have been proposed as to what causes an individual to increase drug use and develop a SUD. Like many other disease processes, the interplay between genetics, stress, and environmental factors can lead to the expression of addiction. Along with genetic predisposition, the added psychological distress and environmental exposure play a role in development of the disorder. Exposure to psychoactive substances, from in utero to social events in high school, contributes to increased risk of SUD. In addition, stress has long been recognized as a major causative agent for drug use, cravings, and relapse.

Adverse Childhood Events. Addiction can be viewed as a developmental process in which neural changes during early critical periods can be negatively impacted by factors such as poor nutrition and neglect. Cognitive, psychological, and social development can all be impeded by childhood exposure to stressful events, such as physical abuse. The allostatic load, or "the wear and tear on the body," represents the body's neural and neuroendocrine response to chronic stress. It can impact the lifetime health of an individual, including their risk of developing a SUD. Adverse childhood events, such as abuse (sexual, emotional, or physical), neglect (emotional or physical), and challenges in the home (i.e., household substance use, mental illness in home, parental separation or divorce, incarcerated parent, or witnessing violence towards mother) are seen as significant determinants for addictive disorders. The likelihood of early drug use increases exponentially for each adverse childhood event experienced.[14] For those who begin using substances prior to age 15, their risk of developing a SUD is 6.5 times greater than those who delay using until 21 years old.[15]

Trauma Informed Care. Research has demonstrated that 55% of people with AUD had a history of childhood trauma and that higher rates and severity of OUD are seen in individuals with PTSD.[16] Trauma-informed care is a way to address consequences of suffering and facilitate healing. It is important to recognize the symptoms of trauma in patients and avoid retraumatization of individuals. The principles of trauma-informed care are safety, trustworthiness, transparency, peer support, collaboration, and empowerment.[17] Trauma-informed care is also sensitive to cultural, historical, and gender issues. The patient needs to be respected, informed, and hopeful regarding his or her own recovery. Providers must work collaboratively with patients to empower them to make decisions regarding care.

Comorbid Mental Health. There often is an interrelation between traumatic events, SUDs, and other comorbid occurrences such as eating disorders, mood disorders, thought disorders, and anxiety disorders. Mental health issues can also increase substance use. The comorbid interaction between mental health and SUD can worsen the progression of both. Of adults with serious mental illnesses, approximately one in four also has an SUD. The lifetime prevalence of major depressive disorder with AUD is estimated to be 40%, and the lifetime prevalence of bipolar mood disorder with SUD is approximately 47%.[18]

The presence of symptoms can pose a diagnostic dilemma as to the etiology being substance induced or primarily caused by a psychiatric diagnosis. In either case, both the SUD and mental health sequelae should be addressed simultaneously. An integrated approach is required to provide treatment as clinically indicated for the combination of disorders.[19]

Social Determinants. For treatment of SUDs to be fully effective, environmental factors need to be considered. These social determinants of health include the social environment, cultural environment, economic environment, and physical environment of the individual. The cultural influences can be norms regarding acceptable patterns of drug use. Social context considers the individual's position in society and social support. Social factors such as poverty, homelessness, and lack of education play a large role in the development of SUD and repeated relapses.

Protective Factors

Despite the potential risk factors that may lead to drug use, individuals also possess protective factors that guard against developing a SUD. Protective factors are necessary for healthy development. These positive influences include resilience, self-regulation, and the ability to form attachments. Those who possess resilience achieve positive outcomes despite adversity. The individual who self-regulates acts consistently within his or her own value set and is able to self-sooth. Healthy individuals engage in healthy relationships and have strong social connections. The achievement of developmental tasks at each stage of life is essential for healthy development. Parental involvement for adolescents is one of the most important protective factors against development of SUD.[20]

Neurobiology

Reward Pathway. In addition to environmental and individual factors, a particular substance's ability to create intense feelings of pleasure are significant in the development of an SUD. The reward pathway in the mesolimbic system of the brain is composed of neurons that release the neurotransmitter dopamine. Dopamine released in the nucleus accumbens creates a sensation of pleasure. Natural rewards, such as pleasurable food or activities, cause a release of dopamine, as do psychoactive drugs. However, some drugs release exponentially more dopamine than natural rewards do. The addiction potential of a substance is linked to the speed of dopamine release, the intensity of that release, and the reliability of that release. The same substance by different routes of administration can be more rapidly addicting.

The reward pathway in the brain involves areas for motivation and memory, as well as pleasure. The continued use of a drug causes neurons in the nucleus accumbens and the prefrontal cortex to communicate desire for that substance. This sets off cravings by increasing motivation to take the substance. The prefrontal cortex, the area of the brain that plans and executes tasks, focuses in on how to obtain and use the drug. The positive reinforcement provided by the memory of the euphoria causes the individual to seek the substance. The hippocampus stores memories of the feelings of satisfaction with substance use.

Compulsion and Conditioning. The strong memory of contentment and the emotions that follow evolve from the limbic system of the brain. Within this system the amygdala becomes activated and generates cravings for the substance. As cravings intensify, rationality subsides and compulsion takes over, making it increasingly difficult to stop using. A conditioned response occurs as the hippocampus and the amygdala store information from the environment associated with drug use in order to find the substance again. The amygdala creates a conditioned response to environmental triggers that surround the drug use. Eventually the environmental triggers associated with the substance create cravings independent of the psychoactive drug. Conditioned responses can place an individual at risk for relapse when triggers are encountered even after extended periods of sobriety.

Neuroadaptation. With repetitive substance use, the continued release of dopamine and stimulation of the reward circuit overload the pathway. The brain adapts by producing less dopamine or eliminating dopamine receptors all together. This causes dopamine to have less of an impact on the brain's reward center. As a result, tolerance occurs and more and more of the drug is required to have the same pleasurable effects. The gratification of use decreases, but the memory of the high remains, along with a strong desire to recreate the experience.

Eventually, neuroadaptation in the reward pathway produces profound anhedonia. Over time, the substance no longer provides as much satisfaction and tolerance emerges. The negative reinforcement of withdrawal from the drug emerges and leads to continued substance use.

Neuroplasticity

There are drug-induced plastic changes to brain circuitry with substance use. Therefore recovery from SUD includes brain recovery. During and after addiction treatment there is brain healing. Some changes may be permanent or take a long time to heal.[21] These changes have been studied with psychological tests and with brain imaging, and results indicate that medical and behavioral interventions can help to restore function in neural circuitry. The addition of medications to the treatment plan can aide in relapse prevention while the brain is regenerating and functional abilities are reinstated.[22] Strategies that emphasize natural rewards such as exercise while decreasing an individual's reaction to stress can also improve brain healing. Conditioned responses can be reduced with approaches aimed at avoiding environmental cues that produce SUD cravings.[22]

Specific Substances

The DSM-5 recognizes 10 separate substances associated with classifications of SUD. These are opioids, alcohol, cannabis, hallucinogens, inhalants, sedatives, hypnotics, anxiolytics, stimulants, tobacco, and other or unknown substances. The most commonly used substances (alcohol, tobacco, opioids and cannabis) will be discussed.

Opioids. The term *opioids* is used to describe substances derived from naturally occurring opiates and synthetically derived chemicals of this class. The body produces endogenous opioids which consist of short-chain amino acids, or peptides, that bind to opioid receptors in the brain. The effects of these peptides, such as the endorphins, impact emotion, motivation, stress response, and response to pain. These functions all become disrupted by chronic use of short-acting exogenous opiates such as heroin.

Exogenous opioids are substances that mimic the effects of endogenous opioids. They include heroin and analgesic medications such as oxycodone, hydrocodone, hydromorphone, morphine, fentanyl, and tramadol. The word "opiate" refers to compounds directly derived from the poppy plant, and "opioid" includes synthetically derived drugs that stimulate opioid receptors. Heroin is one of the well-known opiates and was first produced as a pharmaceutical agent in the 1800s. In the brain, opioids attach to specialized proteins, known as mu, delta, and kappa opioid receptors. When the opioid links with the receptors, biochemical processes are triggered. One of the brain circuits that is activated by opioids is the mesolimbic reward system that was described earlier. This generates a signal in the ventral tegmental area (VTA) that results in the release of dopamine. The development of tolerance occurs rapidly with some opioids, such as heroin, and can be seen within weeks of heavy daily use. The phenomenon of tolerance has been attributed to receptor desensitization.

OUD as a subset of SUD is an important and pressing issue given the recent increased prevalence and catastrophic health effects related to the current epidemic. OUD increases risk for overdose significantly, and early recognition and intervention for overdose are critical priorities for health care workers. OUD may also be associated with distressing withdrawal symptoms with the absence of use, and recognizing and treating prodromal symptoms of opioid withdrawal can help to alleviate distress. Because OUD may be associated with the misuse of prescription opioids and many people with OUD report first exposure to opioids through prescription products, it is the responsibility of primary care providers to carefully screen patients who may be at risk for developing problems, especially when treating pain and considering the use of opioids for their potent analgesic effect. In an effort to mitigate some of the adverse problems associated with prescription opioids, the Centers for Disease Control and Prevention (CDC) has developed guidelines for the use of opioids for chronic pain in adult patients (Box 227.1). It is important for primary care providers to be aware of potential risks and benefits of opioids as they partner with patients to adequately address chronic pain while at the same time trying to prevent SUD, or intervene early and appropriately if a SUD either develops or coexists.

Alcohol. In 2015, 138.3 million Americans age 12 and older reported current alcohol use. Of these, 66.7 million reported binge drinking and 17.3 million reported heavy use.[9]

The neurochemical balance of the brain is disrupted by AUD. Alcohol drinking behavior is influenced both by interaction with the mesolimbic dopamine system and independent of the mesolimbic dopamine system. Two of the main neurochemicals involved with AUD are gamma-aminobutyric acid (GABA) and glutamate. GABA is the main inhibitory neurotransmitter and acts through the GABA-A neuroreceptor, and glutamate is the major excitatory neurotransmitter and acts through the N-methyl-D-aspartate (NMDA) neuroreceptor. Alcohol enhances the effect of GABA on GABA-A neuroreceptors. This results in decreased overall brain excitability. Chronic exposure to alcohol results in a compensatory decrease of GABA-A and is evidenced by increasing tolerance of the effects of alcohol. At the same time, alcohol inhibits NMDA neuroreceptors and continued drinking results in upregulation of these receptors. Sharp decreases in or cessation of alcohol results in brain hyperexcitability because receptors previously inhibited by alcohol are no longer inhibited. This brain hyperexcitability manifests clinically as signs and symptoms of alcohol withdrawal. This recurrent detoxification/relapse cycle increases cravings and contributes to worsening of future episodes of withdrawal.

Tobacco. In 2016, the US Surgeon General reported more than 45 million Americans smoke, 8 million people live with serious illness caused by smoking, and approximately 438,000 people die prematurely each year as a result of tobacco use. The US Agency for Healthcare Research and Quality (AHRQ) reports that tobacco use is the number one preventable cause of death, and the US Preventive Services Task Force (USPSTF) reports tobacco screening and counseling is woefully inadequate. Nicotine is a highly addictive substance that binds to acetylcholine receptors in the brain and results in release of dopamine, norepinephrine, and serotonin. Repeated exposure to nicotine causes upregulation of nicotinic receptors leading to neuroadaptations in the mesolimbic or "reward" system of the brain. Feelings of intense pleasure associated with nicotine are similar to reinforcing effects experienced with use of cocaine and methamphetamines. Increases in nicotine intake directly impacts cessation difficulty, making availability and access to treatment modalities even more important.

Cannabis. According to the NSDUH, of the 27.1 million Americans age 12 and older who reported use of an illicit substance in the past month, the vast majority (22.2 million) used cannabis (marijuana). The second most commonly reported illicit substance was misuse of prescription pain relievers, with

BOX 227.1

Centers for Disease Control and Prevention Guidelines for Chronic Pain

The following 12 recommendations were issued by an expert panel in March 2016 based on their review of the existing evidence at the time. Intended for application to adult patients in primary care settings, the guidelines aim to improve communication about the risks and benefits of opioid therapy for chronic pain, improve safety/effectiveness of pain treatment, and reduce the risks associated with long-term opioid therapy, including opioid use disorder, overdose, and death. The recommendations provide guidance for (1) determining when to initiate or continue opioids for chronic pain; (2) opioid selection, dosage, duration, follow-up, and discontinuation; and (3) assessing risk and addressing harms of opioid use.

1. Nonpharmacological treatment and nonopioid medications are preferred first line treatments for chronic pain. Opioids should be considered only if expected benefits outweigh risks. If used, opioids should be used in combination with nonpharmacological treatments and nonopioids.
2. Before starting opioids for chronic pain, realistic function and pain treatment goals should be established. Discontinuation of opioid treatment if risks outweigh benefits should be understood. Continuation of opioids should only occur if clinically meaningful improvement in pain and function are present.
3. When starting and periodically during opioid therapy, clinicians should discuss with patients the known risks and realistic benefits of long-term opioid therapy, as well as patient and clinician responsibilities during opioid treatment.
4. When starting opioids, immediate-release meds only should be prescribed (not extended-release/long-acting).
5. When opioids are started, they should be prescribed at lowest effective doses. Caution is advised at any dose and escalation. Careful reassessment of risks/benefits at dosages greater than 50 MME per day is advised. Avoidance (or clearly documented

rationale for justification) of doses greater than 90 MME per day is also advised to reduce risk of overdose.
6. Long-term use of opioids often begins with treatment of acute pain. For acute pain, the lowest effective dose of immediate-release opioids should be prescribed. Three days or less will often be sufficient; more than 7 days will rarely be needed for acute pain syndromes.
7. Benefits/harms of opioid therapy should be evaluated with patients within 1–4 weeks of starting opioids for chronic pain or for dose escalations. Reevaluation every 3 months or more frequently is advised. If harms outweigh benefits, optimization of other therapies and tapering to lower dosages or discontinuation of opioids is recommended.
8. Before starting and periodically during opioid therapy, clinicians should evaluate risk factors for opioid-related harms. A treatment plan should include strategies to reduce risk, (i.e., naloxone) when factors that increase risk for opioid overdose are present.
9. State PDMP data should be reviewed to determine whether the patient is receiving opioid dosages or dangerous combinations that put them at high risk for overdose. Review PDMP data when starting opioids for chronic pain and periodically, ranging from every prescription to every 3 months.
10. When prescribing opioids for chronic pain, clinicians should use UDT before starting and consider UDT at least annually to assess for prescribed medications as well as other controlled prescription and illicit drugs.
11. Clinicians should avoid prescribing opioid pain medication and benzodiazepines concurrently whenever possible.
12. Clinicians should offer or arrange evidence-based treatment (usually pharmacotherapy with buprenorphine or methadone in combination with behavioral therapies) for patients with opioid use disorder.

MME, Morphine milligram equivalents; *PDMF,* prescription drug monitoring program; *UDT,* urine drug testing.
From Dowell, D., Haegerich, T. M., & Chou, R. (2016). CDC Guideline for Prescribing Opioids for Chronic Pain—United States, 2016. *Morbidity and Mortality Weekly Report (MMWR) 65*(RR-1), 1–49.

3.3 million people reporting use.[9] The prevalence of use may be affected in the near future as various states have passed legislation decriminalizing the medical and/or recreational use of cannabis in recent years.

The psychoactive ingredient in marijuana, tetrahydrocannabinol (THC), produces a variety of effects, including altered senses, changes in mood, and impaired thinking. Marijuana can be ingested via smoking, eating, or drinking. The amount of THC in marijuana and in concentrated edibles has been increasing. Although life-threatening overdose has not been observed, high doses of THC may result in unpleasant symptoms such as hallucinations, psychotic delusions, or paranoia.[24]

Primary care providers should be prepared to have conversations with patients about patterns of marijuana use and be vigilant for those patients who may develop a CUD as characterized by the DSM-5 criteria described previously.

CLINICAL PRESENTATION

Because of the variety of substances that SUD encompasses, as well as the varying degrees of severity that may characterize a disorder, discussion of every possible clinical presentation of SUD is beyond the scope of this chapter. SUD may present

itself to the PCP as a primary finding in the form of a patient request for assistance with addiction, a family member expressing concern, or an acute substance-related complication (i.e., various intoxication syndromes or intoxication-related injuries), or a PCP may discover an SUD secondary to an investigation into other substance-related health problems (i.e., respiratory complications of smoking, liver complications from alcohol, infectious diseases from injection drug use). Patients with SUD or a history of SUD in remission or recovery may also present to primary care for a plethora of reasons that are not directly related to SUD. Because ongoing SUD, or a relapse for someone in remission, could have significant life-threatening consequences, PCPs should routinely ask patients about SUD as part of a comprehensive preventive approach.

Screening, Brief Intervention, and Referral to Treatment

The prevalence of SUD across the population should prompt all PCPs to have a significant degree of suspicion for its occurrence in the general population. The USPSTF recommends screening and counseling cessation of tobacco use for all patients (grade A recommendation for adults/pregnant women, grade

B for children and adolescents). At the time of this writing, the USPSTF had inconclusive evidence to recommend universal screening for illicit drug use, but screening and brief counseling for alcohol use in all adults is recommended.[25] Other organizations such as the American Academy of Pediatrics, American Medical Association, and American College of Obstetrics and Gynecology support routine screening for both drug and alcohol use.[25] The American Society of Addiction Medicine and the Substance Abuse and Mental Health Services Administration (SAMHSA) call for the widespread implementation of universal screening for SUD using a well-established and innovative approach known as Screening, Brief Intervention, and Referral to Treatment (SBIRT). A 2017 review of SAMHSA's national, multisite 5-year initiative of SBIRT implementation, in which more than 1 million patients were screened, showed positive associations between SBIRT and lower substance use, as well as overall advantages for equity, efficiency, and economy within the health care system.[26]

SBIRT consists of an algorithmic conversation with a patient that uses behavior change theory, motivational interviewing (MI) techniques, and harm reduction concepts. Screening questions/tools are used to identify risky or harmful substance use and then, as needed, a provider briefly intervenes to try to stimulate a patient to self-examine and recognize personal motivations to positively change their substance use. If necessary and the patient is willing and ready, referral to specific SUD treatment is provided. If the patient is not ready, the provider offers harm reduction suggestions and continues to engage with the patient to maintain a therapeutic relationship for future interactions. The process for SBIRT can also be conceptualized using the "5 As" acronym[1]:

1. Ask: Screen for substance use and assess severity level (see screening questions/tools later).
2. Advise: Using a nonjudgmental approach, the provider expresses direct and personal concern for the patient's health if the level or nature of use is medically risky.
3. Assess: Provider evaluates the patient's stage of change to determine level of willingness or readiness to reduce or stop the substance use. If the patient is not yet ready to change, provider encourages patient to continue to reflect on health concerns and offers help for when and if the patient becomes ready. If the patient is ambivalent, provider engages patient in discussion about pros and cons of use as well as barriers to change.
4. Assist: For patients who are not yet ready to change, assisting may simply be expression of concern, curiosity, and empathy, as well as addressing patients' other health care needs (i.e., for persons who inject drugs, screening for blood-borne pathogens and access to sterile supplies or provision of naloxone to prevent overdose, or thiamine replacement for heavy alcohol users at risk for vitamin deficiency). For patients who are ready to reduce or stop their use, the provider should attempt to engage a patient in conversation eliciting patient-directed steps towards achievable goals. As needed, assistance may involve pharmacologic treatment (see Pharmacologic Management section later), as well as treatment of comorbid mental health disorders or other routine primary care preventive health activities such as screening and counseling for sexually transmitted infections in sexually active patients. Frequently, other pressing health or social concerns (e.g., homelessness) may take priority over cessation of substance use for some patients.

However, if these nonsubstance issues are attended to sincerely by a provider, the resulting therapeutic rapport built with the patient may set the stage for future positive change.

5. Arrange: For all patients, arrange close follow-up and specialty referrals as needed. If a patient is accepting/willing and appropriate services such as pharmacotherapy for withdrawal or maintenance treatment are not available in the primary care site, a referral to an addiction specialist is essential. Patients may also be referred to self-help groups (i.e., Alcoholics or Narcotics Anonymous, or SMART recovery), peer-recovery supports, or harm reduction services such as syringe service programs (SSPs), or provided with educational materials.

Screening Questions/Tools

Screening for substance use may begin with simple single-question screens such as:

For Tobacco—"In the past year, how often have you used tobacco products?"

For Alcohol—"How many times in the past year have you had more than 5 drinks in a day (4 for women)?"

For other drugs—"In the past year, how often have you used any other drugs or taken prescription drugs for non-medical reasons?"

If a patient answers "never" to all three questions, screening is complete and the patient's healthy substance use behavior should be praised and reinforced. If a patient answers "yes" to single screen questions, further assessment can be conducted using validated screening tools for alcohol and substance use (see Box 227.2 for examples and application to special populations). Prescreening questionnaires filled in by patients may help with efficiency. Although screening tools can take time, the detailed information obtained may be essential to accurate diagnosis or early intervention to prevent SUD. Discussing lower-risk drinking limits with patients can be a nonjudgmental way of educating patients about the link between drinking behaviors and adverse health outcomes (Box 227.3) and may prevent further development of a disorder.

After screening, if risky use or SUD is identified, providers should engage in a brief intervention (see Nonpharmacologic Management later) and provide referral to treatment as needed or depending on the patient's level of willingness to change. If the patient is not yet ready to talk about change or accept a referral to treatment, a nonjudgmental, supportive approach including asking for permission to revisit the issue at another time is recommended. Because of the common ambivalence around perception of need for treatment, primary care providers should be prepared for numerous patients who are not yet ready for change and therefore will benefit from repeated, compassionate conversations aimed at incremental change. Moreover, an offer of assistance via harm reduction interventions (see Nonpharmacologic Management: Harm Reduction later) is appropriate for an ambivalent patient and may set the stage for future positive therapeutic interactions while minimizing imminent health threats of ongoing substance use.

PHYSICAL EXAMINATION

Although much of an assessment of SUD will be conducted via interview and history-taking, there are several physical exam characteristics that may help with diagnosis, assessment of disease severity, and determining need for health promotion interventions. Again, because of the wide variety of substances

BOX **227.2**

Selected Screening Tools for Alcohol and Drug Use in Primary Care

The following validated tools may be used to gather more information from patients about drug and alcohol use. Although they do not serve as diagnostic tools themselves, the information gathered from them is part of a comprehensive assessment, may identify risky use before a disorder fully develops, and may provide information about the Diagnostic and Statistical Manual (DSM)-5 criteria for substance use disorder (SUD).

ALCOHOL
AUDIT[a]

Add up the points (number in parentheses) associated with answers. A total score of 8 or more indicates harmful drinking behavior.

1. How often do you have a drink containing alcohol?
   (0) Never (skip to Questions 9–10)
   (1) Monthly or less
   (2) Two to four times a month
   (3) Two to three times a week
   (4) Four or more times a week
2. How many drinks containing alcohol do you have on a typical day when you are drinking?
   (0) 1 or 2
   (1) 3 or 4
   (2) 5 or 6
   (3) 7, 8, or 9
   (4) 10 or more
3. How often do you have six or more drinks on one occasion?
   (0) Never
   (1) Less than monthly
   (2) Monthly
   (3) Weekly
   (4) Daily or almost daily
4. How often during the last year have you found that you were not able to stop drinking once you had started?
   (0) Never
   (1) Less than monthly
   (2) Monthly
   (3) Weekly
   (4) Daily or almost daily
5. How often during the last year have you failed to do what was normally expected from you because of drinking?
   (0) Never
   (1) Less than monthly
   (2) Monthly
   (3) Weekly
   (4) Daily or almost daily
6. How often during the last year have you been unable to remember what happened the night before because you had been drinking?
   (0) Never
   (1) Less than monthly
   (2) Monthly
   (3) Weekly
   (4) Daily or almost daily
7. How often during the last year have you needed an alcoholic drink first thing in the morning to get yourself going after a night of heavy drinking?
   (0) Never
   (1) Less than monthly

(2) Monthly
(3) Weekly
(4) Daily or almost daily
8. How often during the last year have you had a feeling of guilt or remorse after drinking?
   (0) Never
   (1) Less than monthly
   (2) Monthly
   (3) Weekly
   (4) Daily or almost daily
9. Have you or someone else been injured as a result of your drinking?
   (0) No
   (2) Yes, but not in the last year
   (4) Yes, during the last year
10. Has a relative, friend, doctor, or another health professional expressed concern about your drinking or suggested you cut down?
    (0) No
    (2) Yes, but not in the last year
    (4) Yes, during the last year

ADOLESCENT SCREEN
CRAFFT[b]

Part A:
   During the PAST 12 MONTHS, did you:
1. Drink any alcohol (more than a few sips)?
2. Smoke any marijuana or hashish?
3. Use anything else to get high? ("anything else" includes illegal drugs, over-the-counter and prescription drugs, and things that you sniff or "huff")

Part B:
   If all answers in Part A are "no," ask only the first question below. If any "yes" answers in Part A, ask all 6 questions.
1. Have you ever ridden in a CAR driven by someone (including yourself) who was "high" or had been using alcohol or drugs?
2. Do you ever use alcohol or drugs to RELAX, feel better about yourself, or fit in?
3. Do you ever use alcohol or drugs while you are by yourself, or ALONE?
4. Do you ever FORGET things you did while using alcohol or drugs?
5. Do your FAMILY or FRIENDS ever tell you that you should cut down on your drinking or drug use?
6. Have you ever gotten into TROUBLE while you were using alcohol or drugs?

Affirmative responses to 2 or more Part B questions are associated with higher risk of SUD.

DRUG USE

DAST-10[c] (note: this tool was developed in 1982 before destigmatizing terminology became widely recommended. Thus substituting "use" or "misuse" for "abuse" is recommended)

Over the Last 12 Months	No	Yes
1. Have you used drugs other than those required for medical reasons?	0	1
2. Do you "abuse" more than one drug at a time?	0	1
3. Are you always able to stop using drugs when you want to? If never use drugs, answer "Yes."	1	0

Continued

Selected Screening Tools for Alcohol and Drug Use in Primary Care—cont'd

Over the Last 12 Months	No	Yes	Over the Last 12 Months	No	Yes
4. Have you had "blackouts" or "flashbacks" as a result of drug use?	0	1	8. Have you engaged in illegal activities in order to obtain drugs?	0	1
5. Do you ever feel bad or guilty about your drug use? If never use drugs, choose "No."	0	1	9. Have you ever experienced withdrawal symptoms (felt sick) when you stopped taking drugs?	0	1
6. Does your spouse (or parents) ever complain about your involvement with drugs?	0	1	10. Have you had medical problems as a result of your drug use (e.g., memory loss, hepatitis, convulsions, bleeding)?	0	1
7. Have you neglected your family because of your use of drugs?	0	1			

Scoring: 1–2 points = lower risk, 3–5 points = moderate risk, 6–8 points = substantial risk, 9–10 points = severe risk

[a]Babor, T. F., Higgins-Biddle, J. C., Saunders, J. B., & Monteiro, M. G. (2001). *AUDIT: The alcohol use disorders identification test guidelines for use in primary care* (2nd ed.). Switzerland: World Health Organization.

[b]© Children's Hospital Boston, 2009. All rights reserved. Reprinted with permission from the Center for Adolescent Substance Abuse Research, CeASAR, Children's Hospital Boston.

[c]© Copyright 1982 by Harvey A. Skinner, PhD, and the Centre for Addiction and Mental Health, Toronto, Canada.

Lower-Risk Drinking Limits

In a national survey it was found that only 2 in 100 people who consumed less alcohol than the limits below met criteria for an alcohol use disorder:

- Men younger than 65 years old—fewer than 4 drinks in a day and fewer than 14 drinks in a week
- All healthy women and healthy men older than 65 years old— fewer than 3 drinks in a day and fewer than 7 drinks in a week

Because even "low-risk" drinking can be harmful in certain situations, avoidance of drinking any alcohol is recommended for the following populations:

- Pregnant women
- Patients on medications that interact adversely with alcohol
- Patients with health conditions with contraindications such as liver disease
- People younger than 18 years old

Adapted from National Institutes of Health. (2016). Rethinking drinking: Alcohol and your health. Retrieved from https://www.rethinkingdrinking.niaaa.nih.gov/How-much-is-too-much/Is-your-drinking-pattern-risky/Whats-Low-Risk-Drinking.aspx.

and their physical effects, as well as secondary health problems associated with substance use, description of every possible clinical scenario and exam finding is beyond the scope of this chapter. Instead, an overview of the intoxicating physical effects of select categorized substances, as well as withdrawal and overdose signs, will be discussed.

Central Nervous System Sedatives

Central nervous system sedatives include alcohol, barbiturates, benzodiazepines and other similar compounds such gamma-hydroxybutyrate. Manifestations of sedative intoxication include tranquilization, fine lateral nystagmus, and decreased alertness. Moderate intoxication manifests as ataxia, slurred speech, coarse nystagmus, and sedation. An overdose of these substances produces somnolence, staggering, and marked dysarthria; this can progress to coma, respiratory depression, and death. Depressant effects on the brain may paradoxically cause stimulation, disinhibition, and excitement.

"Hangover" symptoms may occur after heavy alcohol consumption and may include headache, malaise, diarrhea, nausea, and difficulty concentrating. Symptoms of alcohol withdrawal in a dependent individual often begin 6 to 24 hours after last consumption and may occur even before blood alcohol levels reach zero. Withdrawal symptoms typically persist for 1 to 2 days. Anxiety, sleep troubles, anorexia, nausea, and headache, as well as rapid heart rate, elevated blood pressure, sweating, and tremors, are some signs and symptoms of withdrawal. In more severe cases of alcohol withdrawal, visual, auditory, and tactile hallucinations are possible. Seizures are a possible catastrophic result of alcohol and benzodiazepine withdrawal and may occur 8 to 24 hours after stopping intake of alcohol. Patients with a previous history of seizures or who are withdrawing from multiple central nervous system (CNS) depressants are at higher risk.[1,27]

Opioids

Opioids include the following drugs: oxycodone, hydrocodone, morphine, codeine, hydromorphone, meperidine, tramadol, heroin, and fentanyl. Euphoria, calmness, and sedation characterize opioid intoxication. Opioid intoxication usually produces drowsiness and slowed movement. Pupils constrict and respiratory rate and bowel motility decrease, effects that persist even if the individual has a high level of tolerance. Blood pressure and pulse are mildly decreased, nausea or vomiting or generalized itching may occur. Stupor that progresses to respiratory depression is a life-threatening emergency that requires immediate pharmacologic reversal with naloxone (see later). Meperidine overdose or cerebral anoxia may produce dilated pupils. Meperidine, tramadol, or propoxyphene overdose may produce seizures.

Opioid withdrawal symptoms are varied and may include anxiety, dysphoria, nausea, vomiting, diarrhea, sweating or chills, myalgias, and arthralgias. If chronic pain is also present, opioid withdrawal may manifest as increased pain. Although opioids are not associated with withdrawal seizures, the discomfort of withdrawal is so intense that many opioid users report continued use of opioids simply to relieve withdrawal symptoms as opposed to seeking euphoria of intoxication. The duration of withdrawal symptoms varies with different opioids and individuals and may last from just days to over 2 weeks.[1,27]

Stimulants

Stimulants includine cocaine and methamphetamine.

Stimulant intoxication effects include an enhanced state of alertness, high energy, euphoria, appetite suppression, and decreased need for sleep. People who use stimulants repeatedly or at high doses may experience untoward effects ranging from anxiety and restlessness to paranoia and delusions or hallucinations. Other physical symptoms and medical complications associated with stimulants involve multiple systems and may include pupil dilation, teeth grinding, hyperventilation, tachycardia or palpitations, hypertension, myocardial infarction related to vasospasm, aneurysmal rupture, CVA, muscle spasm or fasciculations, seizures, gastrointestinal symptoms including mesenteric ischemia, acute renal failure, malignant hyperthermia, or rhabdomyolysis.[1,27]

Hallucinogens

Hallucinogens include LSD, psilocybin, mushrooms, mescaline. PCP, and MDMA or "ectasy".

The intended intoxicating effect of hallucinogens is to dramatically alter sensory perception. Intoxicated states range from extreme euphoria to severe depression/paranoia/panic or transient psychosis. Physical effects may include pupil dilation, tachycardia, or hypertension. A severe complication of hyperthermic crisis may be preceded by dry skin, agitation, muscle hypertonicity, and seizures. In general, hallucinogens are not associated with a significant withdrawal syndrome, although a small percentage of users report symptoms such as fatigue or irritability.[1,27]

Cannabis

Cannabis includes marijuana and tetrahydrocannabinol (THC) Physical intoxicant effects of cannabis include euphoria, relaxation, and altered sensory perception. Some individuals may also experience more negative effects such as impaired coordination, difficulty with concentration and memory, visual hallucinations, anxiety/paranoia, conjunctival injection, tachycardia, and dry mouth. Transient psychosis has also been reported. There are no confirmed overdose deaths associated with cannabis. Withdrawal symptoms reported by heavy users may include anxiety, depression, sleep disturbances, and, less frequently, gastrointestinal distress, sweating/chills, and muscle twitching.[1,27]

Beyond physical evidence of intoxication, potential secondary physical findings related to SUD are numerous. Therefore a comprehensive physical exam in the primary care setting is essential. Tobacco use may result in several respiratory effects ranging from ear infections to sinus issues and asthma/COPD and has been associated with many cancers, hypertension, cardiovascular disease, and gastrointestinal and reproductive disorders. Alcohol use may be associated with hypertension, peptic ulcer disease, and varying degrees of liver dysfunction up to end-stage cirrhosis. Injection of substances, especially if sterile syringe access and knowledge of safer injecting practices are not readily available, may result in skin abscesses, infections such as human immunodeficiency virus (HIV) and hepatitis, and other deep space infections such as necrotizing fasciitis, endocarditis, or spinal epidural abscess. Providers should examine for signs of injection use with a thorough skin exam and, if present, have a higher index of suspicion for the aforementioned secondary infections.

DIAGNOSTICS
Essential Diagnostics

- Diagnosis of mild, moderate, or severe SUD (including substance-specific disorders such as AUD or OUD) can be made via history using the aforementioned DSM-5 criteria.
- Opioid risk tools:
  - Opioid risk tool—It is essential that health care providers are more thoughtful and aware when prescribing opioids and other scheduled drugs. Primary care providers can be leaders in the practice of safe prescribing, particularly with opioids, and risk screening tools offer safeguards when prescribing. The Opioid Risk Tool was developed by Webster and Webster in 2005 and intended for use in primary care settings. It offers important information in identifying persons who, based on genetics, age, and past histories, may be more susceptible to developing SUDs. The tool assigns a point score based on a respondent's answers to five simple questions. The five criteria for classifying risk includes family history of SUD, personal history of SUD, age of respondent, history of preadolescent sexual abuse, and presence of psychological illness. Tool scoring indicates low, moderate, or high risk. Using such tools can help to identify persons and populations at risk and enhance prevention strategies, which are critically important for primary care providers. https://www.opioidrisk.com/printpdf/887.
  - Screener and opioid assessment for patients with pain (SOAPP) is a tool to help determine the extent of monitoring a patient on long-term opioids for pain may require. SOAPP is among the most studied of questionnaires for chronic opioid risk.[28] SOAPP is an easy-to-use questionnaire for assessing a person's risk for developing problems when placed on long-term opioid therapy. Although the use of screening tools is not a safeguard against accidents occurring, they do provide useful information in determining those at greater risk for developing problems.
- Prescription drug monitoring programs (PDMPs) is an electronic database that tracks controlled substance prescriptions. All 50 states currently have PDMP databases, and many programs share information between states. PDMPs are a response to the prescription opioid epidemic and provide timely information about prescribing habits to individual providers, pharmacists, and health authorities. PDMPs may identify concerning behaviors such as multiple prescriptions from multiple providers. With this information, providers can positively affect health by engaging in open and honest dialogue with patients that may uncover issues of substance misuse, poorly managed chronic pain, or even diversion. PDMPs also help to identify patients who are being prescribed other substances that may increase risk of opioid overdose such as benzodiazepines. It is incumbent on all primary care providers to check the prescription drug monitoring program prior to prescribing opioids and benzodiazepines, but to maximize patient safety it should be a regular practice when prescribing any other scheduled drug. Many state laws currently require that providers use the PDMP prior to prescribing controlled substances so providers are mandated to be aware of and follow local regulations.

- Diagnostic tests for alcohol use—Although not often used in primary care, positive breath analysis and blood alcohol levels can indicate and quantify acute use.

    Liver function tests may reveal alcohol-related complications, with aspartate aminotransferase (AST) to alanine aminotransferase (ALT) ratios of 2:1 or greater as suggestive of alcohol-related liver disease (ALD). Gamma-glutamyl transferase (GGT) is the most sensitive marker of excessive alcohol use and is elevated in 75% of persons diagnosed with alcohol dependence.[1] An elevated GGT can indicate heavy alcohol intake that has continued for several weeks. Elevated erythrocyte macrocytic volume (MCV) is a common finding with AUD. Carbohydrate-deficient transferrin (CDT) levels are elevated following prolonged alcohol consumption.

- Urine and blood toxicology screening for all substances can be used in monitoring patients for SUD and in helping determine appropriate treatment modalities. The initial procedure for drug testing usually begins with urine immunoassay because they are inexpensive and yield rapid results. The CDC Guidelines for Prescribing Opioids for Chronic Pain include a recommendation that providers use urine drug testing prior to initiating opioid therapy for chronic pain and to consider periodic testing to assess for presence of the prescribed drug, as well as other controlled prescription or illicit drugs.[23] Providers should become familiar with the complexity and potential inaccuracies of specific tests and work closely with laboratories to understand situations that may result in false-negatives or false-positives. Unexpected results on urine testing should prompt providers to adjust treatment plans to foster safety. Examples of possible adjustments include changing pain treatment strategies, tapering or discontinuation of opioids, provision of naloxone to avert overdose, or referral to SUD treatment including pharmacotherapy. Unexpected results on urine drug testing should not be used to dismiss a patient from care as this may constitute patient abandonment. To consistently use destigmatizing language, providers should avoid terms such as "clean" or "dirty" when discussing toxicology results and use "positive/negative" or "consistent/inconsistent" instead.

- Other diagnostic tests for patients with SUD should be used to determine their increased risk for specific diseases and conditions. Patients who inject substances should be tested for HIV and hepatitis B and C, particularly those with histories of sharing needles or other drug paraphernalia that may contain infectious particulates. Symptom-driven testing of patients with SUDs takes into consideration bacterial and fungal infections and bone, joint, skin, tissue, and blood infections, warranting cultures of blood and suspicious sites of concern. Imaging studies including x-rays, ultrasounds, computed tomography (CT), magnetic resonance imaging (MRI), and transthoracic and transesophageal echocardiograms can help to identify organ damage associated with SUD.

DIFFERENTIAL DIAGNOSIS

 Priority differentials include psychiatric crisis (suicidality, depression, PTSD, anxiety, psychosis). There is a high prevalence for comorbid mental health problems with SUD.

For intoxication syndromes/alteration in mental status, considerations include organic brain disease (i.e., brain tumor or other intracerebral process), hypoglycemia, acidemia, fluid and electrolyte disorders, delirium from systemic infection (especially in the elderly), or complications from end-stage liver disease.

Due to the analgesic properties of many substances, SUD may often coexist with chronic pain syndromes.

INTERPROFESSIONAL COLLABORATIVE MANAGEMENT
Pharmacologic Management

Alcohol Use Disorder. Medication for the treatment of AUD can be divided into the following categories.
1. Management of alcohol withdrawal
2. Pharmacologic management of alcohol cravings
3. Pharmacologic enhancement for chronic AUD (medication to supplement common nutritional deficiencies caused by chronic AUD)

Pharmacologic Management of Alcohol Withdrawal. Alcohol's effects on neurotransmission pathways in the brain are not completely understood; however, its inhibitory effect on GABA-A neurotransmission and its excitation of glutamate have been well studied. These two affected pathways help to explain the depressive and intoxicating effect of alcohol in the CNS. Alcohol's potency of action on brain chemistry cannot be underestimated, especially as tolerance and dependence develop and chronicity of use increases. Excessive and prolonged use of alcohol can lead to dangerous consequences in its absence. Effective withdrawal management is critically important and requires close monitoring and assessment. Safety is the primary goal for managing patients experiencing alcohol withdrawal, and medications should be used accordingly.

Historically, alcohol itself was used for management of alcohol withdrawal. Gradual weaning from alcohol products over specified periods of time was an effective way to minimize complications. Beer and other alcohol beverages are still maintained on hospital pharmacy formularies; however, with safer agents currently available, alcohol is seldom used in treating alcohol withdrawal.

Benzodiazepines are considered the gold standard of treatment for alcohol withdrawal and have proven effective in preventing severe complications such as seizures and respiratory depression requiring intubation. Benzodiazepines are administered either in fixed dose schedules with tapering or, more often, based on the Clinical Institute Withdrawal Assessment (CIWA), a symptom-driven tool used to both objectively and subjectively measure alcohol withdrawal, with CIWA scores guiding dosing.[29]

The CIWA-Alcohol Revised (CIWA-Ar) scale is the most commonly used tool in managing alcohol withdrawal syndrome. It measures 10 common withdrawal signs and symptoms in patients experiencing withdrawal. Scores range from mild to severe. It should be noted that CIWA can be used only in patients who are able to participate in providing subjective information and should not be used in patients too obtunded or delirious to participate in screening. Inpatient management is indicated for patients who score as moderate to severe (>20 points). Medications to manage withdrawal may not be needed for scores less than 10. Patients who score as mild to low-moderate and who have adequate home supervision by a committed caregiver, no concurrent acute illness, no comorbid chronic illness including mental health conditions, and no polysubstance use (especially other substances that increase risk for seizure like benzodiazepines) may be managed pharmacologically on an outpatient basis with close (preferably daily) follow-up with the health care provider.[30]

The following are some of the medications that may be used to manage alcohol withdrawal.

1. Chlordiazepoxide (Librium) a long-acting benzodiazepine used in the treatment of anxiety and alcohol withdrawal. For acute alcohol withdrawal symptoms, the drug is most commonly administered orally (but can be given intramuscularly as well). The suggested initial dose is 5 to 100 mg with repeat doses. Some literature suggests maximum dosing not go above 300 mg/day. For withdrawal management, benzodiazepine doses are reduced based on symptom reduction. Chlordiazepoxide should be used with caution; it is metabolized in the liver and has a prolonged half-life, which may increase risk of liver injury.

2. Lorazepam (Ativan) is a medium-acting benzodiazepine also used for the treatment of anxiety. Lorazepam is often prescribed (1 to 4 mg every 2 to 4 hours), and doses are administered based on patient's response to treatment. It is as effective as chlordiazepoxide but with less concern for liver injury.

3. Diazepam (Valium) is often recommended for alcohol withdrawal due to its long half-life, which facilitates ease of self-tapering the medication.

For older patients, the use of benzodiazepines in general and especially longer-acting agents such as diazepam is not recommended, because the protracted half-life in an older adult patient can result in confusion and other neurocognitive deficits.

For hospitalized patients suffering from severe alcohol withdrawal with delirium tremens or who are too ill to provide meaningful subjective information, other treatments such as antiepileptic drugs (AEDs) may be considered. AEDs ameliorate severe withdrawal symptoms through their positive GABAergic effect and blocking of certain excitatory glutamate receptors which are critical in managing complicated withdrawal.[31] The anticonvulsant phenobarbital has been effectively used in patients with complicated alcohol withdrawal in medical and psychiatric settings. Loading doses of phenobarbital are weight based and given intramuscularly followed by oral tapering. Phenobarbital levels can be drawn 5 hours post completion of loading doses, with therapeutic target range for phenobarbital between 10 and 15. Phenobarbital ordinarily is given for 5 to 7 days.

Pharmacologic Management of Alcohol Cravings. Historically, treatment for AUD has used behavior-based models of therapy and recovery support with limited degrees of success. With increased understanding of the neurobiologic aspects of AUD, medications are currently being used more often to treat AUD. Medications prescribed to reduce or stop alcohol consumption target multiple neurotransmitters in the brain associated with the reward pathways stimulated by alcohol use. Long-term alcohol consumption causes neurotransmitter alterations affecting GABA, glutamate, NMDA, dopamine, and norepinephrine. Pharmacotherapies that target these neurotransmitters can help to reduce cravings for alcohol. The following are some of the medications prescribed to reduce alcohol use and can be effectively incorporated in both abstinence and harm reduction–based models:

Naltrexone (Revia or Vivitrol) is an opioid receptor antagonist. Several studies indicate alcohol reinforcement is at least partially related to the activation of the endogenous opioid system. Naltrexone acts as an antagonist with associated pleasure receptors decreasing alcohol's stimulation of pleasure centers, thereby reducing alcohol use.[1]

Naltrexone benefits both abstinence and harm reduction approaches to alcohol cessation. Studies have shown naltrexone significantly reduces cravings, relapse rates, and number of drinking days as compared with placebo. Naltrexone was shown to increase abstinence rates and reduce number of drinks consumed per occasion.

Naltrexone can be given orally once daily (50-mg tablet) or intramuscularly (380 mg) monthly. It is not recommended for patients with severe hepatic disease such as cirrhosis because it is metabolized in the liver and should be avoided with elevated liver enzymes. Because it is an opioid antagonist, patients who have received opioids must wait at least 1 week before it is initiated and it should not be used in patients who may require pain management with opioids. Side effects of naltrexone may include gastrointestinal symptoms, headache, dizziness, lightheadedness, and weakness that are more common in early treatment.

Acamprosate (Campral) is US Food and Drug Administration (FDA) approved for AUD treatment in the United States. Acamprosate's action on alcohol cravings is not well defined, but its enhancement of GABA neurotransmission and reduction of the excitatory amino acid glutamate produce a therapeutic benefit of reducing cravings. It also minimizes distress and discomfort experienced with alcohol cessation. Studies of acamprosate have shown significant benefit over placebo in the treatment of AUD, particularly with increased duration of treatment. Meta-analysis of continued alcohol abstinence revealed acamprosate's benefits progressively increased over the course of 3 to 6 and then 12-month periods of adherence. Acamprosate also showed benefit for patients in abstinence-oriented programs who did not abstain completely. When compared with placebo, acamprosate was associated with both decreased frequency and decreased quantities of alcohol consumption for patients who continued to drink.[1]

The recommended total daily dosage for acamprosate is 1998 mg given in two 333-mg tablets three times daily. The frequency of administration and pill burden can make adherence challenging, and there may be utility in reducing dosage in patients with lower body weights. Some studies suggest decreased dosing to two tablets twice daily in patients weighing 132 pounds or less. Other studies have shown equal efficacy in administering the total dose twice daily.

The side effect profile for acamprosate is minimal, and the majority of side effects reported are minor gastrointestinal symptoms, followed by mild dermatologic complaints. Acamprosate is renally cleared and a few cases of acute renal failure have occurred with administration. Acamprosate is contraindicated with renal impairment (creatinine clearance <30 mL/min).

Acamprosate has not been studied in pregnant women; however, caution is advised in pregnancy because it is teratogenic in animals.

Disulfiram (Antabuse)—Unlike naltrexone and acamprosate, disulfiram does not reduce cravings but is a deterrent to alcohol consumption and can be used only with an abstinence-based approach. Disulfiram blocks the enzyme conversion of acetaldehyde, resulting in toxic levels that produce symptoms of severe illness when alcohol is ingested. Disulfiram-ethanol reaction (DER) varies with doses of disulfiram and amount of alcohol consumed and may include nausea, vomiting, increased heart rate, palpitations, lowered blood pressure, pounding headache, shortness of breath, dizziness, sweating, confusion, and blurred vision. In 1951 the FDA approved disulfiram for treatment of "alcoholism," currently referred to as AUD.

Due to its associated risks and the availability of other agents, disulfiram is used less frequently than it was in the past, but it still may have utility for some individuals, especially those who can be closely monitored, who have a personal goal of complete abstinence, and who have already achieved at least 48 hours of not drinking. The recommended daily dose is 250 mg, with maximum daily dose of 500 mg. Because disulfiram is slowly metabolized and can remain in the body for up to 2 weeks, it is important that patients understand that any ingestion of alcohol during this prewashout period may result in very unpleasant side effects and should be avoided until the drug is cleared. Severe DER reactions are usually associated with higher doses of 500 mg or greater. Patients should be cautioned to avoid use of over-the-counter medications that may contain alcohol. Liver function should be monitored regularly with disulfiram.

Off-Label Medications for Alcohol Use Disorder. Although unlikely to be prescribed by primary care physicians, it is important for primary care providers to be aware of the following as they may be prescribed by addiction specialists who are comanaging care of patients.

Topiramate (Topamax) is traditionally an antiepileptic agent that enhances GABA activity. Topiramate facilitates GABA-mediated inhibitory impulses and antagonizes glutamate receptors, suppressing dopamine release and blocking the reinforcing effects of alcohol use. Studies have shown potential positive effects including reduced drinks per day, number of drinking days, and number of heavy drinking days.

Side effects for topiramate include drowsiness, dizziness, nervousness, numbness or tingling in hands or feet, balance and coordination problems, weight loss, and word finding difficulty. Side effects can be minimized with gradual increases up to the targeted therapeutic dosing goal of no more than 300 mg total daily dose for reduction of alcohol cravings. Current recommendations are to start low and go slow for a period of 4 to 6 weeks, starting at 25 mg twice daily and increasing by a total of 50 mg weekly up to but not beyond the maximum recommended therapeutic range of 300 mg total daily dose.

Gabapentin (Neurontin)—Gabapentin's mechanism of action is not entirely clear; however, it is thought to modulate excitatory neurotransmitters and normalize stress-induced GABA activation in the amygdala, which is often associated with alcohol dependence. Trials conducted examining gabapentin efficacy for AUD consumption and craving showed decreased number of drinks per day at 28 days compared with a placebo group, as well as longer sustained periods of reduced drinking. The mean percentage of heavy drinking days and abstinence days were statistically significant in favor of the gabapentin group.[32] It should be noted the study was done at one site and it was a relatively small study with only 60 participants. With the growing concern for gabapentin's street value and association with overdose in patients with other SUDs, this drug should be used with caution and only for patients who have AUD without other SUDs.

Baclofen—Several European clinical studies of alcohol-dependent patients showed that baclofen increased abstinence when compared with placebo groups, and greater abstinence rates were achieved in patients taking larger doses of the drug. Individually titrated high-dose baclofen up to 300 mg daily helped patients to maintain abstinence.[33]

Good tolerability of baclofen was also reported. Baclofen is thought to reduce cravings through its anxiolytic properties. Although these studies support the use of baclofen for AUD, there is still concern with its side effect profile and potential for misuse, and more robust studies are needed before it can be considered for broader use.

Pharmacologic Enhancement for Chronic Alcohol Use Disorder. Replenishing nutritional deficits associated with AUD is recommended to mitigate long-term sequelae of chronic AUD. Alcohol consumption depletes essential vitamins and minerals that result in physical and cognitive deficits. Thiamine is often recommended for patients with chronic AUD. It can be given intravenously for patients who are hospitalized or in detoxification programs at doses of 500 mg three times daily for 3 days, then switched to oral thiamine 100 or 200 mg daily.

Vitamin B_{12} can be depleted for several reasons but may be a direct result of AUD. If a deficiency is detected, vitamin B_{12} can be replenished with initial dosing of 1000 mcg intramuscularly with monthly follow-ups for repeat injections or oral dosing of 100 mg daily. Folic acid and multivitamins along with enhanced nutritional support is encouraged for patients with alcohol use chronicity. Replenishing fluid hydration is always an important aspect in the treatment of patients with AUD.

Opioid Use Disorder. Pharmacologic management of OUD includes medications for management of overdose, withdrawal, and maintenance pharmacotherapy.

Pharmacologic Management of Opioid Overdose. Opioids depress the respiratory and cardiac systems and may dangerously compromise vital function to the point that, without medical intervention, excess opioid use can result in death. Opioid-related respiratory depression, which is reversible, can develop gradually over 1 to 3 hours but may also be more immediate depending on the potency, dose, and route of administration of the drug. The increased potency of illicit opioids containing the synthetic opioid analogue fentanyl, which is exponentially more potent than morphine or heroin, has contributed to rising overdose death rates.

Naloxone is an opioid receptor antagonist used to reverse opioid overdose. Naloxone displaces opioids from the opioid receptor and blocks the binding of additional opioids for 20 to 90 minutes post administration.[34] It binds to opioid receptors, preventing opioids from activating them, and it completely eradicates opioid intoxication to reverse an opioid overdose. With the increasing numbers of opioid overdoses across the country, the demand for opioid prevention services has also increased. Naloxone may be administered intravenously, intramuscularly, or intranasally. The intramuscular (IM) formulated solution can be adapted to be given intranasally by attaching a nasal atomizer to the prefilled IM vial, but in November 2015, a new delivery device, Narcan nasal spray, became the first FDA-approved noninjectable naloxone product for the treatment of opioid overdose. Naloxone has been shown to be a cost-effective deterrent to saving lives and is easily used by medical and nonmedical personnel. Major side effects of naloxone are precipitation of acute withdrawal causing symptoms that may include piloerection, agitation, anxiety, nausea, vomiting, diarrhea. lacrimation, yawning, and rhinorrhea.

In 2014 the World Health Organization estimated that greater than 20,000 deaths in the United States could be prevented annually if naloxone were more widely available. Efforts to educate the public about naloxone have been ongoing across the country. Allied health professionals, as well as patients, families, friends, and all others, should be encouraged to carry naloxone for its life-saving potential. Many states have passed laws to make naloxone more easily available via standing orders at outpatient pharmacies or distributed by community organizations. Detailed information on naloxone for overdose prevention for both laypersons and health care providers is available at http://prescribetoprevent.org/.

Pharmacologic Management of Opioid Withdrawal. Regarding withdrawal protocols, it cannot be overstated that although medically supervised withdrawal may improve a patient's health and facilitate participation in a rehabilitation program, withdrawal management by itself, without solid after-care planning, is more often associated with relapse. Close follow-up care and referrals to other treatment supports are needed as well to sustain long-term recovery. Repeated misuse of opioids produces long-lasting craving that usually requires additional treatment to avoid a relapse of drug use.[35] With that said, some patients will either desire or require pharmacologic assistance with withdrawal symptoms to try and achieve abstinence.

The goal for short- and long-term medical withdrawal from opioids is swift and effective control of symptoms and subsequent engagement in ongoing treatment. Effective withdrawal management is best achieved with agonists and partial agonists. When these are not available or not desired, symptom management with other agents should be considered. Methadone or buprenorphine are the most effective agents in treating withdrawal symptoms; gradual dose reductions allow time for the body to adjust to the absence of the opioid. Timing of withdrawal is commensurate with half-life of opioid used. Withdrawal from heroin ordinarily begins 8 to 12 hours post use and peaks between 36 hours and 72 hours, and physical symptoms subside at 5 days. Withdrawal from a longer-acting agent, such as methadone, is more protracted and can last 2 weeks or longer.

Methadone. A full opioid agonist, methadone can be used in inpatient hospital and detoxification settings for the purposes of withdrawal. Titration of methadone for opioid withdrawal is usually done over a period of several days. Initial administration is usually between 10 and 30 mg daily and does not exceed 40 mg per day as gradual accumulation takes place over 48 to 72 hours and steady state is achieved at approximately 5 days. Dosing should be uptitrated until a patient's withdrawal symptoms are stabilized and maintained over a 3-day period and then can be slowly tapered over 5 to 7 days. Typically, the use of methadone for treatment of addiction is restricted to specially licensed drug treatment facilities, but a provision of the law does permit providers to use methadone for emergent treatment of withdrawal for a period of 72 hours (recommended to be done in an inpatient setting due to risks of overdose due to methadone accumulation during titration). Primary care providers may not typically be the prescribers of methadone for management of withdrawal, but knowledge of its efficacy and a referral network of licensed clinics or inpatient facilities that use methadone is recommended so that

they may direct patients who would benefit from it to appropriate services.

Buprenorphine. Buprenorphine/naloxone may also be used for opioid withdrawal and, when a patient situation calls for discontinuation as opposed to maintenance therapy, may be tapered over a 3- to 5-day period. Unlike methadone, buprenorphine is a partial opioid agonist. Because buprenorphine is a partial agonist with great affinity for opioid receptors, it may displace other opioids from receptors and lead to precipitated withdrawal, if initiated before active withdrawal symptoms are present. The Clinical Opiate Withdrawal Scale (COWS) is a tool used to measure opioid withdrawal symptoms. A COWS score of 8 to 10 or greater indicates that a patient is in significant enough withdrawal to start buprenorphine. Although inpatient withdrawal dosage protocols may vary from one institution to another, a minimum of a 5-day taper is usually recommended to avoid distressing symptoms associated with withdrawal. Buprenorphine taper may be ordered with reductions of 25% per day, with the last dose given on the day of hospital discharge. Doses can be titrated upward according to withdrawal severity, cravings, and side effects.

Clonidine. Clonidine is an antihypertensive adrenergic agonist that is used in inpatient and outpatient settings for opioid withdrawal. It effectively binds adrenergic receptors, suppressing hyperactivity during acute withdrawal phases, and helps to mitigate difficult autonomic symptoms of opioid withdrawal. Although dosage routes and recommendations vary, daily doses up to 1.2 mg in divided doses have been shown to be effective in managing some withdrawal symptoms. Blood pressure should be closely monitored with clonidine, and it should not be used if there is a risk of hypotension.

Augmenting Agents. Nonsteroidal antiinflammatory drugs (NSAIDs), acetaminophen, short-acting muscle relaxants such as tizanidine for muscle pain, and medications such as loperamide for diarrhea and antiemetics (i.e., prochlorperazine, metoclopramide, or ondansetron) for nausea and vomiting may all be beneficial for opioid withdrawal symptom management. Providers should consider use of these medications as they develop a patient-centered care plan that accounts for patient preference, symptomatology, history of adverse medication reactions, and concurrent medical conditions such as liver or renal dysfunction that may affect drug selection.

Maintenance Pharmacotherapy for Opioid Use Disorder. The evidence supporting the use of pharmacotherapy for OUD has been strong for decades and is growing despite both historic and ongoing stigma against these effective treatment modalities. Methadone and buprenorphine are both on the World Health Organization's list of essential medications. Some of the positive outcomes associated with opioid agonist treatments include higher rates of retention in treatment, lower relapse rates, reduced rates of HIV/hepatitis, lower overdose death rates, and lower total health care costs. Most importantly, in comparison with the relatively poor efficacy of psychosocial treatments alone (estimated 80% of patients who receive psychosocial treatment alone return to drug use), pharmacotherapy for OUD is clearly more effective, with retention rates between 60% and 80% and only 15% returning to drug use.[36]

Methadone. Methadone is a full mu-opioid agonist with a half-life of 15 to 40 hours and is used in the management of OUD, with a proven track record of success dating back to the 1960s, when it was first used as part of maintenance treatment for OUD.

In the United States, methadone maintenance therapy (MMT) can be routinely delivered only by federally approved and closely monitored clinics. Qualifying criteria for methadone maintenance include current OUD diagnosis with physiologic features, high risk of relapse, and no current enrollment in other maintenance programs.

Primary care providers should be aware of which patients may and may not benefit from methadone maintenance programs. In addition to MMT, clinics also provide counseling, case management, and other medical and psychosocial services. MMT provides patients with increased structure and accountability. Patients who have lengthy histories of opioid use and those who use greater quantities may benefit from MMT. With its requirement of daily visits and access to onsite services, patients who require structure and accountability are also good candidates for MMT. Because of its full agonist effect, patients who have comorbid chronic pain may benefit from methadone's analgesic effect.

Patients who have medical complications such as severe cardiac or respiratory diseases that might be exacerbated by methadone are not good candidates for methadone maintenance. The induction phase of methadone maintenance includes initial dosing of 10 to 30 mg with gradual increases up to therapeutic dosing. The goal of methadone dosing is to effectively quench opioid cravings and prevent opioid withdrawal. Tolerance to methadone remains steady for the most part, with no need to dose escalate as would be the case with shorter-acting agents, and the steady state also reduces euphoria-related effects when compared with other opioids. Although therapeutic dose ranges are quite variable depending on a patient's circumstances, methadone is thought to work best with dose ranges between 60 and 120 mg. According to a SAMHSA survey in 2013, the number of clients treated with methadone for OUD steadily increased from approximately 227,000 in 2003 to more than 306,000 in 2011.[37]

Primary care providers should have a good understanding of methadone and its use in patients with OUD for stabilization, pain management, and its utility in treating opioid-related withdrawal. Medical monitoring for methadone treatment should include baseline electrocardiogram to reduce risk of cardiac conduction abnormalities associated with prolonged QT interval and torsades de pointes. A careful review of other prescribed medications should be conducted before starting methadone, because some medications may increase the risk of QT-associated arrhythmia or may accelerate or extend methadone metabolism, leading to withdrawal or overmedication. Sedating agents such as benzodiazepines and alcohol should be avoided.

Common medications that stimulate or induce CYP450 activity, accelerating methadone metabolism and putting a patient at risk for withdrawal, are: rifampin, phenytoin, carbamazepine, phenobarbital, nevirapine, and efavirenz. Some medications that slow metabolism and extend drug duration and effect are: cimetidine, ciprofloxacin, fluconazole, erythromycin, and fluvoxamine.

Buprenorphine. Buprenorphine is a partial mu-opioid agonist with a peak effect in 2 to 4 hours and duration of 72 hours. Its slow onset and long duration give it similar maintenance benefits to methadone. Buprenorphine has powerful receptor attachment capacity that increases risk for precipitated withdrawal if started in the presence of other opioids. As mentioned earlier, the first dose of buprenorphine should not be given until a person is already experiencing some signs of opioid withdrawal. Unlike methadone for treatment of OUD, buprenorphine has no federal regulations limiting its use to specially qualified treatment clinics. However, federal law does restrict buprenorphine prescribing to health care providers who have obtained a waivered DEA license known as an X-license. Primary care providers may obtain a waiver by completing additional training (8 hours for physicians and 24 hours for NPs/PAs). Some state laws may further restrict NP's and PA's ability to prescribe, so it is prudent that NP/PA's be aware of their specific local regulations. General information on trainings is offered by the American Society of Addiction Medicine at https://www.asam.org/education/live-online-cme/buprenorphine-course.

By obtaining a buprenorphine waiver and prescribing buprenorphine, PCPs can close the existing access gap for patients seeking treatment. Expanded access to this life-saving and evidence-based treatment is recommended as part of a multipronged approach to improving care of OUD and to mitigate the societal fallout of the current opioid epidemic, including dramatic overdose death rates.

Buprenorphine is most commonly prescribed as buprenorphine/naloxone (Suboxone) in sublingual tablet or film formulation, with a recommended first dose of 2 to 4 mg that can be uptitrated to an average of 16 to 20 mg daily. Subutex is a preparation of buprenorphine that does not contain naloxone and for the most part is reserved for pregnant women and others who may not tolerate Suboxone. The naloxone portion of Suboxone was added to buprenorphine to reduce likelihood of misuse, is essentially inactive when taken sublingually as intended, and is only activated with damage or IV administration.

Pharmacotherapeutic Options for Tobacco Use Disorder

Nicotine Replacement Therapy. Nicotine replacement therapy (NRT) is considered safe for adults with a desire to quit smoking. NRT is any form of treatment that helps with smoking cessation. Recommended therapy uses low doses of nicotine with the goal of treatment to reduce nicotine cravings and symptoms of nicotine withdrawal. Higher doses of NRT are often recommended for patients with increased quantity and frequency of use. NRT tapering ordinarily commences over a period of 14 to 30 days, but this can be tailored to an individual and extended to longer periods of time as needed.

NRT is conveniently available in multiple formulations, including gum, lozenges, inhalers, nasal sprays, and dermal patches. It is important that tobacco be avoided during therapy because the risk for toxic levels of nicotine increases with simultaneous use of NRT and smoking.

Current USPSTF guidelines report insufficient evidence to recommend NRT during pregnancy. The American College of Obstetricians and Gynecologists states that if used in pregnancy, NRT should be undertaken only with close oversight and after careful attention to and discussion with the patient of the risks of continued smoking and the possible risks of NRT.[38]

In a 2018 report to the FDA, the National Academies of Sciences assessed the scientific evidence surrounding e-cigarettes or "vaping" and found that, although e-cigarettes clearly release fewer harmful toxins compared with combustible tobacco, they do pose potential for adverse health effects themselves. Although there may be some benefit for their use in smoking cessation by adults, their potential to introduce youth to nicotine with a possible transition to other smoking habits including traditional combustible tobacco may offset their potential public health benefit. Further research is needed to ascertain their overall public health risk and benefit.[39]

Nonnicotinic Agents Used to Decrease Cravings for Tobacco Use. Bupropion (Wellbutrin or Zyban)—Traditionally used as an antidepressant, bupropion is a monocyclic antidepressant that inhibits reuptake of dopamine and norepinephrine. Its efficacy is likely associated with its dopaminergic activity on brain reward pathways. Notably it reduces irritability, restlessness, and anxiety that can come with nicotine cessation. It is approved for smoking cessation under the brand name Zyban and recommended for people who smoke 10 or more cigarettes daily. It works just as well as NRT and can be used in combination with NRT. The starting dose for nicotine cessation is 150 mg once daily for 3 days, then increased to twice daily thereafter. It is started 1 week prior to the target quit date and continued for a period of no less than 7 to 12 weeks. When cessation is successfully achieved, it can be discontinued or bupropion maintenance therapy can be considered.

Varenicline tartrate (Chantix)—Varenicline is a partial nicotine agonist/antagonist that both blocks nicotine from binding to receptors and stimulates receptor activity to release dopamine, thereby reducing cravings to smoke. It is approved for smoking cessation and is recommended for patients who are motivated to stop smoking. It is recommended that a cessation date is agreed upon and that treatment commences 1 week prior to stopping. Dose titrations are as follows: 0.5 mg once daily for 3 days, then twice daily for 3 days, then 1 mg twice daily thereafter. Treatment for a minimum of 12 weeks is recommended, and an additional 12 weeks may help to sustain abstinence. NRT combination therapy is not recommended with varenicline. Most notable side effect is nausea in approximately 30% of people.[1]

Behavioral therapy is recommended for all who are attempting smoking cessation, and combination therapy with medications and behavioral therapies have been shown to be most effective.

Pharmacologic Interventions for Cocaine and Methamphetamines

Cocaine Dependence. Cocaine is an addictive stimulant that floods the brain circuit pleasure center with dopamine resulting in a cocaine high. Made from the South American coca plant, it is cut/mixed with other powders or sometimes amphetamines, making it powerfully addictive. Cocaine can be smoked, insufflated nasally, or used intravenously.

There are no approved medications for the treatment of cocaine use disorder; however, some medications may reduce positive reinforcement, effectively eliminate cravings, and reduce negative reinforcement of cocaine-related withdrawal.

In small clinical trials the most promising medications for cocaine use disorder are stimulants. Sustained release amphetamine D 30 to 60 mg daily and modafinil 400 mg daily were shown to reduce use of cocaine. Lower doses were no more effective than placebo. Although there is some controversy regarding use of stimulants, clinical studies highlight agonist medications in general, and amphetamine maintenance in particular, as superior in efficacy to many other drug classes in treatment of cocaine dependence.[40]

Clinical trials evaluating topiramate in cocaine-dependent patients revealed that, when used with combination therapy, topiramate can be effective in reducing short-term cocaine use. However, other anticonvulsants did not show this same efficacy.[41] Therapeutic topiramate dosing for cocaine use disorder is 100 mg twice daily. To reduce the likelihood of side effects, dosing should begin at 25 mg twice daily and gradually increased by 50 mg weekly.

Amphetamine Dependence. Like the studies done for cocaine dependence, agonist substitution was found to be possibly effective for amphetamine dependence. Clinical trials using sustained-release amphetamine and methylphenidate showed reduction in amphetamine use when compared with placebo. However, overall a broadly effective pharmacotherapy for amphetamine use disorder has yet to be identified.

Bupropion is a norepinephrine-dopamine reuptake inhibitor. It has a chemical structure similar to amphetamines. It is approved for the treatment of depression and nicotine cessation, and in clinical trials it showed some utility in the management of stimulant use disorders but not as strong as agonist stimulants. Bupropion reportedly can help to manage cravings for both methamphetamines and cocaine.[42] When bupropion is initiated during cocaine or methamphetamine detoxifying phase, it can reduce cravings while simultaneously targeting depression, a common co-occurrence in withdrawal. Caution is advised with use of bupropion in patients with sustained periods of abstinence, because it can be a potent trigger to relapse due to its similar amphetamine chemical structure.

Nonpharmacologic Management
Substance use and SUDs exist on a continuum where use may range from complete abstinence to chaotic overuse. There is no one single intervention and treatment approach that has been shown to work for everyone. It is also interesting to note that many people recover from SUD without any formal treatment. Depending on an individual's unique situation, nonpharmacological interventions to encourage wellness and/or remission may vary widely and often may need to be used in conjunction with medications. Moreover, although providers may identify a need for treatment, self-perception of the need for treatment may not be present, and therefore the provider needs to maintain a therapeutic relationship and work with the patient in a positive way until their motivation changes. Even if it *never* changes, the provider has an obligation to care for the patient and provide health promotion efforts repeatedly. In general, a nonjudgmental, patient-centered, encouraging approach is recommended. MI and harm reduction serve as general strategies that fit well with a truly patient-centered approach.

Motivational Interviewing. MI is a collaborative approach in which providers engage a person to discuss and reflect upon his or her own behavior and health habits. In doing so, a provider strives to guide a patient towards self-realization of motivators to positive change. MI values patient autonomy and a patient's empowered role in his or her own wellness and self-care. Instead of a prescriptive, educational approach where the provider dictates the reasons a person ought to change, MI is a process in which providers explore a behavior with the patient and try to elicit "change talk," where the person eventually verbalizes his or her own reasons that he or she might change. Some guiding principles of MI are empathy and the power of self-efficacy. During an MI conversation, providers use open-ended questions, affirmations of any positive changes, reflective statements, and summarizing statements. For providers, MI requires "resisting the righting reflex" and well-developed active listening skills.[43] Developed by psychologists who used foundational theories including Prochaska and Diclemente's

Transtheoretical Model of Change, MI has shown promise in research to be effective in improving outcomes for multiple health conditions, including smoking cessation, alcohol use disorder, substance use disorder, and many other chronic illnesses. Primary care providers should seek out further preparation and training in MI because it has utility for any health condition that involves behavior and lifestyle change.

Harm Reduction. As the substance use epidemic has grown in the United States to epic proportions, many experts call for an increase in both individual and community-based harm reduction approaches. As opposed to abstinence-based approaches, harm reduction principles aim to reduce the harms of substance use despite potentially continued use. Instead of focusing on the difficult (and at times impractical) task of substance use cessation, harm reduction strategies are achievable measures that prevent further adverse health effects even if a person continues to use. There are many examples of harm reduction that involve individual behaviors or full-scale community programs or social policy regulations. For alcohol use, harm reduction advice might include recommending a person consume alcohol on a full stomach to slow absorption/minimize impairment or to recommend that on a night of drinking, a designated driver is used. For people who use opioids, provision and instruction on how to use naloxone is an example of harm reduction. For injection drug use, SSPs have been proven in decades of research since the HIV epidemic to improve outcomes including lowered rates of HIV/hepatitis/other infections for participants, increased treatment rates, and even lower crime in communities that offer an SSP. In addition, counter to the idea that SSPs encourage or enable drug use, global research has never shown an associated increase in drug use related to SSPs.[1]

In response to opioid overdose epidemics, other countries have adopted harm-reductionist policies that approach drug use as a full-scale public health issue. Decriminalization of personal use, wider access to SSPs, scaled-up access to opioid replacement therapy including medical provision of heroin or hydromorphone in severe cases, and supervised consumption facilities are all harm reduction strategies that have yielded positive health outcomes internationally. SSPs in the United States have improved outcomes for people who inject drugs for decades. In addition to sterile syringe distribution, SSPs offer a wide variety of health promotion and prevention services, including overdose education and naloxone distribution, sexually transmitted disease screening and prevention, and connections to other health needs. With the worsening of the overdose and injection drug use epidemic in the past 15 years, more experts and public health workers have called for the expansion of harm reduction to include supervised injection facilities (SIFs). In the United States, a proof-of-concept evaluation was conducted on an unsanctioned SIF and, like other research internationally, it demonstrated the potential positive outcomes of SIFs to include prompt overdose reversal leading to reduced overdose fatalities; reduction in infections resulting from provision of sterile supplies and education on safe injecting; reduced public injection leading to less discarded used syringes in public spaces; and increased engagement with highly vulnerable people that may lead to increased access to SUD treatment.[44]

For primary care providers, knowledge of or provision of harm reduction strategies or referral to organizations where an individual can receive them is a compassionate way to engage patients, build therapeutic relationships, and work towards incremental positive health changes, especially for individuals who are not yet ready for more formal treatment. Considering the current SUD epidemic, PCPs should be well versed in naloxone for overdose prevention, as well as where patients can procure sterile injection supplies if injecting drugs. The national Harm Reduction Coalition maintains an online resource for connecting with local harm reduction programs at http://harmreduction.org/connect-locally/.

Psychosocial/Behavioral Treatment Options. In addition to MI, there are multiple other behavioral or psychosocial interventions that may be helpful in comprehensive person-centered treatment of SUD. As mentioned, because there is no one single recipe for treatment, PCPs should be aware of several options and maintain community connections to refer individuals to these options. The complexity of comorbid conditions that often present in tandem with SUD, such as chronic pain and depression, may require a multimodal approach, and several behavioral interventions have been shown as promising adjuncts in primary care settings.[45] Several modalities with positive evidence to support their use are discussed as follows:

- Cognitive behavioral therapy (CBT)—usually conducted in frequent sessions over the course of months by a specially trained counselor, CBT involves repeated reflections on triggers, situations, and reasons why a person has engaged in past substance use. In doing so, ways to avoid future use or other healthier coping mechanisms are explored and practiced. CBT has been studied extensively, showed positive outcomes, and may have applicability to cocaine use.[27,45]

- Contingency management—involves the systematic and consistent provision of positive reinforcement when an individual exhibits behavior such as reducing or abstaining from their harmful substance use. Rewards can range from tangible items such as vouchers that may be redeemed for material items to verbal praise. Alternatively, if an individual does not exhibit the intended positive behavior, the reward or praise is withheld. When administered consistently, this planned technique may help an individual begin to realize potential natural positive reinforcers (such as fewer substance-related difficulties with employment/family/legal system).[1,27]

- Therapeutic communities—These highly structured programs often require an individual to live with other people who are also undergoing treatment for SUD. As a community, the residents are responsible for participating in maintaining the household and engaging in frequent group and individual counseling sessions that frequently use the 12-step model of recovery. Typically, an individual will live in the community for 6 to 24 months. Successful completion of this type of program has been associated with decreased SUD behaviors. Intensive outpatient programs based on a similar model may be more affordable or appropriate for some individuals.[27] There have been some criticisms of therapeutic communities that operate under an abstinence-only approach and thus discharge individuals for predictable relapses or refuse to allow the use of evidence-based pharmacotherapy such as methadone and buprenorphine.

- Twelve-step programs—commonly known as Alcoholics Anonymous or derivations thereof (Narcotics Anonymous, Cocaine Anonymous, Heroin Anonymous, etc.). Twelve-step programs involve frequent meetings where individuals, with the help of others in recovery or sometimes facilitated by a licensed counselor, work towards a desired state of abstinence. Principles included in the 12 steps include admission of powerlessness, a reliance on a higher power for assistance in recovery, the making of amends to others harmed by an individual's substance use, and a commitment to help others recover. These programs have helped many people worldwide to achieve improved health. They are widely available and even have online meetings and are free to attend. When a patient is referred by a PCP to a 12-step self-help group, likelihood of engagement may be enhanced by arranging attendance at a meeting while in the PCP office, setting a goal to attend a defined number of meetings weekly, and suggesting attendance at several different meetings to help the individual find one where they feel welcomed.[27]

- Peer recovery supports—A growing movement in the United States, peer recovery support services have been defined as "the process of giving and receiving non-professional, non-clinical assistance to achieve long-term recovery from SUDs. This support is provided by peers, also known as recovery coaches, who have lived experience and experiential knowledge."[46] Although the totality of research on peer recovery supports is in its infancy, a systematic review of studies of peer recovery supports showed that they have an overall positive effect on substance use outcomes.[46] In many communities, recovery community organizations have been established. Created by people in recovery and other allies, these organizations offer training of certified recovery coaches, as well as a wide array of community-specific needs for people and families dealing with substance use. Services may include telephone support and arranging formal treatment for callers, housing and employment assistance and offering various self-help meetings including Alcoholics Anonymous/Narcotics Anonymous/Smart Recovery, or art/music/yoga classes for the recovery community. PCPs should be aware of peer recovery supports in their own community and be able to refer patients and families to them. Moreover, an excellent way for PCPs to positively influence the health of the community outside of the clinic setting is to become involved with their local organization or to help develop one if not yet available. A community toolkit for developing a recovery community organization can be found at https://facesandvoicesofrecovery.org/arco/rco-toolkit.html.

Complementary Approaches

Because of the distressing and chronic nature of SUD, patients and families may seek out and try a wide variety of conventional and nonconventional approaches to recover from SUD. The safety, cost, and effectiveness of complementary approaches vary widely. The evidence on complementary approaches to treatment of SUD is limited, and in general, complementary approaches are less rigorously studied and evaluated (i.e., not usually studied with the gold standard of randomized controlled trials). Other challenges in evaluating the evidence of complementary approaches include the under-regulated arena of dietary and nutritional supplements and the unknown power of the placebo effect that may play a role in several complementary treatment modalities. A SAMHSA Advisory summarized the existing evidence on several complementary approaches using systematic reviews and meta-analyses.[47]

Although more quality research is needed to further evaluate the role of acupuncture in the treatment of SUD, there is some limited evidence that it may have a beneficial effect in relieving some withdrawal symptoms. A systematic review of mindfulness meditation has shown some positive effect in reducing consumption of substances and reducing cravings. Although the evidence on movement therapies (which include exercise, yoga, Pilates, tai chi) is inconclusive, there have been many studies showing positive effects and primary care providers may recommend an individualized program of exercise that augments health and well-being for patients provided that other health conditions do not contraindicate exercise. Several natural products such as dietary supplements are marketed to improve mental health and wellness, but in addition to being not as strictly regulated as drugs by the FDA, they have very limited evidence in favor of them and may interact with other medicines. Primary care providers should ask patients if they take supplements and be aware of potential interactions. There is little evidence from RCTs and systematic reviews on the effectiveness of homeopathic remedies for any condition.[47]

In general, an open, nonjudgmental, patient-centered, but as much as possible, evidence-based, approach towards complementary therapies should be used. Providers should ask about the use of complementary therapies, become aware of the evidence behind the therapies, and work with patients towards an approach that respects a patient's values and beliefs, improves health, and minimizes harm (including potential harm of therapy such as excessive cost or adverse physical effects).

LIFESPAN CONSIDERATIONS
Children and Adolescents

Because adolescence is often associated with risk-taking and a self-perception of youthful invulnerability, as well as seeking out of new experiences combined with susceptibility to peer pressure, it is a time where many teens experiment with psychoactive substances.[1] National survey data show that prevalence of substance use sharply rises during early to late adolescence and peaks in early adulthood. Moreover, early initiation of substance use is associated with higher risks for SUDs and other adverse health outcomes later in life.[1] PCPs should be aware of risk factors, as well as protective factors, that play a role in adolescent substance use. At the individual level, a lack of knowledge about risks of substances, the perception that substance use is normal, and certain psychological traits such as low self-esteem and impulsivity are associated with higher risk. At the family level, higher risk for teen substance use is associated with families where substance use is directly modeled or perceived as positive or where harsh discipline/low bonding/high conflict is present. At the school and community level, higher levels of substance use are found in schools where students feel disengaged, feel unsafe, or do not have close relationships with teachers/adults.[1]

PCPs should begin screening for substance exposure and use early (usually between 11 and 13 years old but sometimes earlier) to identify risky use at an early stage. Preferably, the interview with a preteen or teen is performed confidentially (with the caveat that the provider will break confidentiality to intervene on immediate safety threats). SBIRT with teens can be performed using the CRAFFT screening interview (see Box 227.2). Praise is given for children who have abstained. If use has occurred or child has more risks (such as riding in a car with someone who is intoxicated), brief intervention would include clear statements recommending the child stop using or asking the child to trial a period of abstaining with close follow-up. For higher-risk screens, the PCP should arrange for specialty referral and treatment because the dangers of ongoing risky use or dependent use are significant life-threats. In 2016 the American Academy of Pediatrics released a policy statement calling for the expansion of access to evidence-based treatment for OUD for adolescents and recommended that pediatricians consider offering pharmacotherapy such as buprenorphine in primary care settings.[47,48]

Pregnancy

Rates of substance use in pregnant women are significantly lower than nonpregnant women, but due to the potential adverse effects of many substances on the fetus, it is important to carefully screen and effectively intervene to improve the health of both mother and child when substance use is present. The use of substances during pregnancy has been linked to a wide variety of poor health outcomes, including neonatal abstinence syndromes, intrauterine growth retardation, and various cognitive and learning disorders. Effects vary dependent on the type and amount of substance and stage of fetal development at the time of ingestion.[1,27] PCPs should universally screen pregnant women and engage in brief intervention and immediate referral to specialty treatment for all pregnant women. The general approaches of nonjudgmental MI and harm reduction discussed previously apply to pregnant patients as well. For OUD, methadone is considered the gold standard pharmacotherapy, but buprenorphine has been shown to produce positive outcomes as well and may be associated with a less severe neonatal abstinence syndrome. Comanagement with an addiction specialist is ideal in the care of a pregnant patient with SUD.

Older Adults

Older adult patients who use substances are an important subpopulation in primary care. The rate of SUD in older adults in various surveys has been estimated anywhere between 1% and 16%, with some primary care–based studies estimating rates between 10% and 15%. Despite the high prevalence, historically SUD among elderly patients has often gone unrecognized. Substance use in the elderly may be complicated and made more imminently dangerous by comorbid medical illnesses as well as polypharmacy. The combination of multiple medications that exert CNS effects, and substance use (whether that be intentional misuse of prescriptions or other illicit substances or alcohol) can result in catastrophic consequences such as injuries from falls or overdoses. In a 2017 Office of the Inspector General brief, the US Department of Health and Human Services reported that more than 500,000 (or one in three) Medicare beneficiaries received an opioid prescription in the previous year, with more than 90,000 being categorized as high risk for misuse or overdose based on receiving high dosages or receiving multiple prescriptions from multiple providers.[49]

Like other populations, universal periodic screening for substance use, using tools and techniques like SBIRT and MI, is recommended for the older population. PCPs should pay particular attention to polypharmacy in older adults and strive to avoid dangerous combinations. Education of the older patient regarding decreased muscle mass and decreased hepatic and renal excretion and the effect of potentiated intoxicant effects

is recommended. As with other age groups, consideration of the differential or comorbid diagnosis of depression should be addressed as needed.

COMPLICATIONS

SUD can result in myriad complications that adversely impact any component of biopsychosocial well-being. Medical illnesses may include traumatic injuries, overdose, end-stage organ disease, and infectious diseases. Psychiatric complications include anxiety, depression, psychosis, and suicidal and homicidal ideation and attempts. SUD-related complications extend beyond organic physical and psychiatric manifestations and often contribute to severe psychosocial consequences including loss of relationships, employment, and social status. SUD can also lead to legal consequences, incarceration, homelessness, isolation, and unintentional loss of life.

Complications can be classified by the substance itself, the method of administration, or the associated behavior. Injection drug use is a well-known route of transmission of blood-borne infectious diseases, particularly HIV and hepatitis B and C and a wide range of bacterial and fungal infections. The use of all illicit drugs is associated with increased rates of sexually transmitted diseases and tuberculosis.

More than 50% of injection drug users in the United States have hepatitis C, and this may actually be as high as 90%. The CDC estimates the incidence of hepatitis C has more than tripled between 2010 and 2015, with 35,000 new infections in 2015 alone and an estimated 3.5 million people in the United States currently infected with hepatitis C. As infection rates continue to increase, it becomes increasingly important for all health care providers, including PCPs, to provide hepatitis C screening. Hepatitis C causes liver damage and can contribute to liver cancer. The CDC identified hepatitis C as responsible for a record number of fatalities in 2014, surpassing 60 other infectious diseases, including HIV and tuberculosis. Testing, diagnosis, and referral to treatment for hepatitis C should be a critical consideration for primary care providers.[50]

HIV infection among injection drug users in the United States accounts for approximately 8% to 10% of new HIV infections yearly. In a study of cities with high levels of HIV, 40% of new injection drug users (those who have been injecting for 5 years or less) have shared syringes.[51] Implementation of SSPs providing sterile syringes and injection supplies has resulted in decreases in HIV transmission. Although public health strategies have been successful in reducing HIV infections in the past, there is concern with recent uptick in new infections. These increases in infection rates reinforce the importance of education and access to resources for injection drug users. Although HIV is a treatable illness, it is still a life-threatening and chronic illness. Persons with HIV who inject drugs become more susceptible to other infectious diseases. HIV screening, diagnosis, treatment, education, and prevention should be part of routine primary care practice.

Injection drug use facilitates a direct pathway of organisms to the bloodstream and is a primary cause of skin, soft tissue, joint, bone, and other infections that can result in severe morbidity and mortality. Common infections include abscesses, cellulitis, phlebitis, osteomyelitis, septic arthritis, and endocarditis, with skin and soft tissue infections reportedly the most common cause for hospital admission for injection drug users. Infections often require protracted courses of IV antibiotic treatment and/or surgical interventions and, if left untreated, can lead to loss of limb, critical heart valve abnormalities, septic emboli, and death. Although hygienic and safer injection practices may reduce the incidence of blood-borne pathogens, drugs intended for injection are often cut with unknown substances that can be inflammatory and often toxic.

Primary care providers should be aware of safer injection practices. Caring for injection drug users should always include education and support for safe injection practices and guidance in how to access sterile syringes as both are lifesaving interventions.

One of the greatest concerns of all health care workers is the magnitude of morbidity and mortality of patients with OUD. In the United States in 2016, there were greater than 50,000 opioid overdose–related deaths, surpassing that of motor vehicle accidents and gun-related deaths.[52] Recognition and early intervention in complications of overdose are essential for all health care providers. Complications of overdose include organ damage, hypoxemia, pulmonary edema, anoxic brain injury, cardiac arrest, and death. With suspected overdose, naloxone should be administered immediately. All health care providers should also be aware that reversal of overdose can be temporary so persistent monitoring must commence. Patients should be closely monitored for at least 4 to 6 hours and, in many cases, up to 8 hours post naloxone administration because naloxone duration of action is far shorter than that of many opioids, including methadone, fentanyl patches, and other long-acting agents. Other complications related to opioid overdose might include compartment syndrome, rhabdomyolysis, and hypothermia, all of which require close medical management.

Complications related to AUD are vast, and some have been discussed in other sections of this chapter. Moderate drinking for the majority of people does not lead to alcoholic liver disease. The American Liver Foundation identifies three common types of ALD.[53] These are caused by excessive consumption of alcohol and may be preventable or reversible in their early stages with cessation of alcohol intake. Fatty liver or steatosis represents the earliest stage of ALD. Steatosis is the most common alcohol-related liver disorder and is characterized by excessive accumulation of fat inside liver cells, making it more difficult for the liver to function. Fatty liver is a common occurrence in heavy drinkers. It is often without symptoms, but enlargement may cause right-sided abdominal discomfort. It often resolves with alcohol cessation. Alcohol-related hepatitis is liver inflammation or swelling with destruction of liver cells. Thirty-five percent of heavy drinkers will develop alcohol-related hepatitis that can be mild to severe and may include fever, jaundice, and gastrointestinal symptoms. In its severe form it may occur suddenly and can quickly lead to life-threatening complications. Alcohol-related cirrhosis is the most serious liver disease and refers to the replacement of normal liver tissue with nonliving scar tissue. Up to 20% of heavy drinkers develop cirrhosis, and this is usually after a chronic period of 10 or more years of drinking.[1]

Excessive alcohol consumption can also result in cardiovascular consequences and an array of cardiac abnormalities including arrhythmias, systemic vascular resistance, hypertension, increased cardiac output, and dilated cardiomyopathy.

Cocaine and amphetamine use both cause vasoconstriction and increased blood pressure and may result in catastrophic outcomes including myocardial infarction, aortic rupture and dissection, stroke, and sudden death. The vasoconstrictive actions of cocaine in particular are intensified in the presence of coronary artery disease. When stimulants are used in combination with alcohol, other drugs, or tobacco, the potential for severe consequences, including acute coronary and cerebrovascular events, is further increased.

EMERGING MANAGEMENT TRENDS

Perhaps the largest emerging trend in the care of people who use substances is the continued shift away from punitive, stigmatized approaches towards health-oriented nonjudgmental ones that use the best evidence-based treatments such as pharmacotherapy, without criticism and shame of patients. This shift will require the undoing of implicit biases on the part of health care providers, policy makers, and the public at large, who have historically considered SUD to be a personal failing instead of a complex health problem.

Pharmacologically, for OUD, different delivery vehicles for buprenorphine may help to improve treatment adherence and reduce the risks of misuse. A long-acting, once-monthly injectable form of buprenorphine was recently approved for the treatment of OUD.[54] In addition, a 6-month buprenorphine intradermal implant (Probuphine) was approved in 2016.[55]

The Bridge Neurostimulation System is an electroauricular device (EAD) that emits electrical pulses to stimulate cranial nerve branches during acute opioid withdrawal. It is placed behind a patient's ear and effectively treats adrenergic symptoms of gastrointestinal upset, sweating, anxiety, agitation, joint pain, and insomnia. The FDA approved the device in 2017 based on clinical data of 73 patients who had measurable reduction of symptoms by at least 31% following 30 minutes of therapy and 88% following 5 days of therapy.[56]

Other emerging trends that are in development in the United States may include the opening of SIFs as part of efforts to curb overdose deaths related to illicit injection drug use. Although these facilities have met initial resistance, international research on similar facilities, as well as initial research on an unsanctioned US facility, show associated positive health outcomes, not least of which is lower overdose death rates.[44]

PATIENT AND FAMILY EDUCATION

As with any other chronic health issue, primary care providers should assess a patient and family's level of understanding and personal values and beliefs of the health condition of SUD. Education on the current scientific understanding of the pathophysiology and natural course of the condition should be provided. Providers should instill hope and share with patients and families that there is well-supported evidence that, when appropriately treated, although relapse is a predictable part of SUD, overall recurrence rates are no higher than rates for other chronic illnesses such as asthma, diabetes, and hypertension.[57] When medications are part of the treatment plan, education on risks, benefits, potential side effects, and interactions should be discussed.

Discussions with patients and families should provide an opportunity to learn about SUDs and become actively involved in treatment and recovery. They should also be guided towards information about a variety of self-help and support groups. The following are examples of organizations that provide reliable and trustworthy information about SUD and recovery: Recovery Research Institute: www.recoveryanswers.org Alcoholics Anonymous: www.aa.org

Narcotics Anonymous: www.na.org

SMART Recovery: www.smartrecovery.org

Marijuana Anonymous: www.marijuana-anonymous.org

Faces and Voices of Recovery: facesandvoicesofrecovery.org

For families:

Alanon and Alateen: www.al-anon.alateen.org

Naranon: www.nar-anon.org

SMART Recovery Family and Friends Program: www.smart recovery.org/resources/family.htm

Learn to Cope (for opioid use disorders): www.learn2cope.org

HEALTH PROMOTION

Because substance use and SUD can affect people of all ages and backgrounds and have a wide spectrum of presentations ranging from relatively safe use to risky use to full-blown severe SUD, the opportunities for health promotion interventions are numerous and are essentially the same as for the general population. Primary care providers should offer all traditional health promotion strategies, including screenings for other acute and chronic health conditions, as well as counseling on safety, vaccinations, and sexual health, to people who use substances. Following USPSTF guidelines is one evidence-based approach for selecting screening interventions. As detailed previously, harm reduction strategies that attempt to minimize substance-related harms are empathetic approaches that not only result in improved overall health outcomes but may in fact serve as therapeutic engagement encounters that gradually prompt a person to move from a less contemplative stage of change towards one that results in decreased substance use.

REFERENCES

1. Herron, A. J., & Brennan, T. K. (Eds.), (2015). *The ASAM essentials of addiction medicine*. Philadelphia: Wolters Kluwer Health.
2. NIDA. (2014, July 1). Drugs, Brains, and Behavior: The Science of Addiction. Retrieved from: https://www.drugabuse.gov/publications/drugs-brains-behavior-science-addiction on 2018, February 19.
3. American Society of Addiction Medicine[ASAM]. (2011, August 15). Public Policy statement: Definition of addiction. Retrieved from: https://www.asam.org/docs/default-source/public-policy-statements/1definition_of_addiction_long_4-11.pdf?sfvrsn=a8f64512_4.
4. American Psychiatric Association. (2013). *Diagnostic and statistical manual of mental disorders: DSM-5* (5th ed.). Arlington, VA: American Psychiatric Association.
5. American Society of Addiction Medicine. (2016). Opioid Addiction 2016 Facts & Figures. Retrieved from: https://www.asam.org/docs/default-source/advocacy/opioid-addiction-disease-facts-figures.pdf.
6. SAMHSA. (2017). Racial and Ethnic Minority Populations. Retrieved from: https://www.samhsa.gov/specific-populations/racial-ethnic-minority.
7. Mennis, J., & Stahler, G. J. (2016). Racial and ethnic disparities in outpatient substance use disorder treatment episode completion for different substances. *Journal of Substance Abuse Treatment*, 25, doi:10.1016/j.jsat.2015.12.007.
8. Kelly, J. F., Saitz, R., & Wakeman, S. (2016). Language, substance use disorders, and policy: The need to reach consensus on an "addiction-ary." *Alcoholism Treatment Quarterly*, 34(1), 116–123. doi:10.1080/07347324.2016.1113103.
9. Center for Behavioral Health Statistics and Quality. (2016). Key substance use and mental health indicators in the United States: Results from the 2015 National Survey on Drug Use and Health (HHS Publication No. SMA 16-4984, NSDUH Series H-51). Retrieved from: https://www.samhsa.gov/data/sites/default/files/NSDUH-FFR1-2015/NSDUH-FFR1-2015/NSDUH-FFR1-2015.pdf.
10. SAMHSA. (2017) Substance Use Disorders. Retrieved from: https://www.samhsa.gov/disorders/substance-use.
11. NIDA. (2017, April). Trends and Statistics. Retrieved from: https://www.drugabuse.gov/related-topics/trends-statistics.
12. SAMHSA. (2016) Receipt of Services for Substance Use and Mental Health Issues among Adults: Results from the 2015 National Survey on Drug Use and Health. Retrieved from https://www.samhsa.gov/data/sites/default/files/NSDUH-ServiceUseAdult-2015/NSDUH-ServiceUseAdult-2015/NSDUH-ServiceUseAdult-2015.htm.
13. Barry, C. L., Epstein, A. J., Fiellin, D. A., Fraenkel, L., & Busch, S. H. (2016). Estimating demand for primary care-based treatment for substance and alcohol use disorders. *Addiction (Abingdon, England)*, 8, 1376. doi:10.1111/add.13364.
14. Allem, J. P., Soto, D. W., Baezconde-Garbanati, L., & Unger, J. B. (2015). Adverse childhood experiences and substance use among Hispanic emerging adults in Southern California. *Addictive Behaviors*, 50, doi: 10.1016.
15. Jordan, C. J., & Andersen, S. L. (2017). Sensitive periods of substance abuse: Early risk for the transition to dependence. *Developmental Cognitive Neuroscience*, 25, 29–44.
16. Hassan, A. N. (2017). The effect of post-traumatic stress disorder on the risk of developing prescription opioid use disorder: Results from the National Epidemiologic Survey on Alcohol and Related Conditions III. *Drug and Alcohol Dependence*, 179, 260.
17. SAMHSA. (2014). *SAMHSA's Concept of Trauma and Guidance for a Trauma-Informed Approach*. Rockville, MD: Substance Abuse and Mental Health Services Administration. HHS Publication No. (SMA) 14-4884.
18. Hasin, D. S., & Grant, B. F. (2015). The National Epidemiologic Survey on Alcohol and Related Conditions (NESARC) Waves 1 and 2: Review and summary of findings. *Social Psychiatry and Psychiatric Epidemiology*, 50(11), 1609–1640. doi:10.1007/s00127-015-1088-0.
19. Hunt, G. E., Siegfried, N., Morley, K., Sitharthan, T., & Cleary, M. (2014). Psychosocial interventions for people with both severe mental illness and substance misuse. *Schizophrenia Bulletin*, 40(1), 18–20. doi:10.1093/schbul/sbt160.
20. Chan, G. C., Kelly, A. B., Carroll, A., & Williams, J. W. (2017). Peer drug use and adolescent polysubstance use: Do parenting and school factors moderate this association? *Addictive Behaviors*, 78, doi:10.1016/j.addbeh.2016.08.004.
21. Kourrich, S., Calu, D. J., & Bonci, A. (2015). Intrinsic plasticity: An emerging player in addiction. *Nature reviews. Neuroscience*, 16, 173–184.
22. Volkow, N. D., Koob, G. F., & McLellan, A. T. (2016). Neurobiologic Advances from the Brain Disease Model of Addiction. *The New England Journal of Medicine*, 374, 363–371. doi:10.1056/NEJMra1511480.
23. Dowell, D., Haegerich, T. M., & Chou, R. (2016). CDC guideline for prescribing opioids for chronic pain–United States, 2016. *JAMA: The Journal of the American Medical Association*, 315(15), 1624–1645. doi:10.1001/jama.2016.1464.
24. NIDA. (2018, February 9). Marijuana. Retrieved from https://www.drugabuse.gov/publications/drugfacts/marijuana on 2018, March 17.
25. USPSTF. (2014). Final Recommendation Statement: Drug Use, Illicit: Screening. U.S. Preventive Services Task Force. February 2014. Retrieved from https://www.uspreventiveservicestaskforce.org/Page/Document/RecommendationStatementFinal/drug-use-illicit-screening.
26. Babor, T. F., Del Boca, F., & Bray, J. W. (2017). Screening, brief intervention and referral to treatment: Implications of SAMHSA's SBIRT initiative for substance abuse policy and practice. *Addiction (Abingdon, England)*, 112(Suppl. 2110–117), doi:10.1111/add.13675.
27. Kowalchuk, A., & Reed, B. (2016). Substance use disorders. In R. E. Rakel & D. Rakel (Eds.), *Textbook of family medicine* (9th ed., pp. 1152–1163). Philadelphia: Elsevier.
28. Finkelman, M. D., Kulich, R. J., Zacharoff, K. L., Smits, N., Magnuson, B. E., Dong, J., et al. (2015). Shortening the Screener and Opioid Assessment for Patients with Pain–Revised (SOAPP-R): A proof-of-principle study for customized computer-based testing. *Pain Medicine (Malden, Mass.)*, 16(12), 2344–2356. doi:10.1111/pme.12864.
29. Sachdeva, A., Choudhary, M., & Chandra, M. (2015). Alcohol withdrawal syndrome: Benzodiazepines and beyond. *Journal of Clinical and Diagnostic Research*, 9(9), VE1–VE7. doi:10.7860/JCDR/2015/13407.6538.
30. Berger, D., & Bradley, K. A. (2015). Primary care management of alcohol misuse. *Medical Clinics of North America*, 99(Comprehensive Care of the Patient with Chronic Illness), 989–1016. doi:10.1016/j.mcna.2015.05.004.
31. Nejad, S. H., Chuang, K., Hirschberg, R., Aquino, P. R., & Fricchione, G. L., (2014) The use of antiepileptic drugs in acute neuropsychiatric conditions; Focus on traumatic brain injury, pain and alcohol withdrawal. *International Journal of Clinical Medicine*. Published Online June 2014.
32. Kantorovich, A., & Durugo, F. (August 23, 2016) Gabapentin for alcohol use disorder: A promising outlook. Pharmacy Times. Retrieved from: http://www.pharmacytimes.com/contributor/alexander-kantorovich-pharmd-bcps/2016/08/gabapentin-for-alcohol-use-disorder-a-promising-outlook.
33. Müller, C. A., Geisel, O., Pelz, P., Higl, V., Krüger, J., Stickel, A., et al. (2015). High-dose baclofen for the treatment of alcohol dependence (BACLAD study): A randomized, placebo-controlled trial. *European Neuropsychopharmacology: The Journal of the European College of Neuropsychopharmacology*, 25(8), 1167–1177. doi:10.1016/j.euroneuro.2015.04.002.

34. Hawk, K. F., Vaca, F. E., & D'Onofrio, G. (2015). Reducing fatal opioid overdose: Prevention, treatment and harm reduction strategies. *The Yale Journal of Biology and Medicine, 88*(3), 235–245.

35. Schuckit, M. A. (2016). Treatment of opioid-use disorders. *The New England Journal of Medicine, 375*(4), 357–368. doi:10.1056/NEJMra1604339.

36. Wakeman, S. E. (2016). Using science to battle stigma in addressing the opioid epidemic: Opioid agonist therapy saves lives. *The American Journal of Medicine, 129*(5), 455–456. doi:10.1016/j.amjmed.2015.12.028.

37. Substance Abuse and Mental Health Services Administration. (2014). National Survey of Substance Abuse Treatment Services (N-SSATS): 2013. Data on Substance Abuse Treatment Facilities. BHSIS Series S-73, HHS Publication No. (SMA) 14-489. Rockville, MD.

38. American College of Obstetricians and Gynecologists. (2017). ACOG Committee Opinion, number 721: Smoking Cessation in Pregnancy. Retrieved from https://www.acog.org/Clinical-Guidance-and-Publications/Committee-Opinions/Committee-on-Obstetric-Practice/Smoking-Cessation-During-Pregnancy.

39. National Academies of Sciences, Engineering, and Medicine. (2018). *Public health consequences of e-cigarettes.* Washington, DC: The National Academies Press. https://doi.org/10.17226/24952.

40. Negus, S. S., & Henningfield, J. (2015). Agonist medications for the treatment of cocaine use disorder. *Neuropsychopharmacology: Official Publication of The American College of Neuropsychopharmacology, 40*(8), 1815–1825. doi:10.1038/npp.2014.322.

41. Bowling, K. C., & Prince, V. (2018). Topiramate in the treatment of cocaine use disorder. *American Journal of Health-System Pharmacy, 75*(1), January 2018.

42. Flanigan, J. (2017) Pharmaceutical Freedom: Why Patients Have a Right to Self-Medicate 1st Edition.

43. Rollnick, S., Miller, W. R., & Butler, C. (2008). *Motivational interviewing in health care: Helping patients change behavior.* New York: Guilford Press.

44. Kral, A. H., & Davidson, P. J. (2017). Addressing the nation's opioid epidemic: Lessons from an unsanctioned supervised injection site in the U.S. *American Journal of Preventive Medicine, 53*(6), 919–922. doi:10.1016/j.amepre.2017.06.010.

45. Barrett, K., & Chang, Y. (2016). Behavioral interventions targeting chronic pain, depression, and substance use disorder in primary care. *Journal of Nursing Scholarship, 4,* 345. doi:10.1111/jnu.12213.

46. Bassuk, E. L., Hanson, J., Greene, R. N., Richard, M., & Laudet, A. (2016). Peer-delivered recovery support services for addictions in the United States: A systematic review. *Journal of Substance Abuse Treatment, 1,* doi:10.1016/j.jsat.2016.01.003.

47. SAMHSA. (2015). Advisory: Complementary Health Approaches: Advising Clients About Evidence and Risks. Retrieved from https://store.samhsa.gov/shin/content//SMA15-4921/SMA15-4921.pdf.

48. American Academy of Pediatrics Committee on Substance Use and Prevention. (2016). Medication-assisted treatment of adolescents with opioid use disorders. *Pediatrics, 138*(3), doi:10.1542/peds.2016-1893.

49. US Department of Health and Human Services. (July 2017). Opioids in Medicare Part D: Concerns about extreme use and questionable prescribing. HHS OIG Data Brief, OEI-02-17-00250. Retrieved from https://oig.hhs.gov/oei/reports/oei-02-17-00250.pdf.

50. U.S. Centers for Disease Control and Prevention. (December, 2016) Viral Hepatitis and Young Persons Who Inject Prescription Opioids and Heroin. Retrieved from http://www.cdc.gov/hepatitis/featuredtopics/youngpwid.htm.

51. Eckhardt, B., Winkelstein, E. R., Shu, M. A., Carden, M. R., McKnight, C., & Des Jarlais, D. C. (2017). Risk factors for hepatitis C seropositivity among young people who inject drugs in New York City: Implications for prevention. *PLoS ONE, 12*(5), https://doi.org/10.1371/journal.pone.0177341. e0177341.

52. Centers for Disease Control. (May 3, 2017). National Center for Health Statistics: FastStats—All Injuries. Retrieved from https://www.cdc.gov/nchs/fastats/injury.htm.

53. American Liver Foundation. (2017) Alcohol-Related Liver Disease. Retrieved from https://www.liverfoundation.org/for-patients/alcohol-related-liver-disease/.

54. FDA. (November 30, 2017). FDA approves first once-monthly buprenorphine injection, a medication-assisted treatment option for opioid use disorder. Retrieved from https://www.fda.gov/NewsEvents/Newsroom/Press Announcements/ucm587312.htm.

55. FDA. (May 26, 2016). FDA approves first buprenorphine implant for treatment of opioid dependence. Retrieved from https://www.fda.gov/NewsEvents/Newsroom/PressAnnouncements/ucm503719.htm.

56. FDA. (November 15, 2017). FDA grants marketing authorization of the first device for use in helping to reduce the symptoms of opioid withdrawal. Retrieved from https://www.fda.gov/NewsEvents/Newsroom/Press Announcements/ucm585271.htm.

57. U.S. Department of Health and Human Services. (November 2016). Office of the Surgeon General, Facing Addiction in America: The Surgeon General's Report on Alcohol, Drugs, and Health. Retrieved from https://addiction.surgeongeneral.gov/surgeon-generals-report.pdf.

CHAPTER **228**

OTHER MENTAL HEALTH DISORDERS

Patricia Polgar-Bailey

DEFINITION AND EPIDEMIOLOGY

Schizophrenia is a chronic, severe, and disabling brain disorder. Schizophrenia interrupts a person's capacity to accurately perceive reality, to communicate and relate to others, and to complete the usual activities of daily living, especially during acute phases of the illness. Schizophrenia affects approximately 1% of the population at similar rates across ethnic groups and is equal in prevalence in the genders. Onset of psychotic symptoms usually occurs between the ages of 16 and 30 years; young men experience a slightly earlier onset than women do. It is rare for this illness to occur in children and unusual for it to be diagnosed after the age of 45 years.[1] Diagnostic subtypes of schizophrenia have more historical significance than clinical usefulness. The most common subtype of schizophrenia, paranoid schizophrenia, is characterized by one or more delusions and frequent auditory hallucinations, the central theme of which are the individual's belief of being conspired against, followed, maligned, or obstructed in pursuit of one's goals.

In addition to schizophrenia, there is an array of mental health disorders in which psychosis is a key feature, including dementia, brief psychotic disorder, schizophreniform and schizoaffective disorders, delusional disorder, and substance-induced psychotic disorders.

PATHOPHYSIOLOGY

Although the etiology of schizophrenia remains unclear, the factors contributing to the development of schizophrenia appear to be multifactorial and involve interactions between genetic and environmental influences, including developmental problems that may occur during gestation. Individual genetic makeup likely increases the risk of development of schizophrenia, but exposure to certain environmental factors must be present for schizophrenia to develop.

Studies show a strong but incomplete hereditary influence. In first-degree relatives, the risk is about 10%, but even in monozygotic twins, concordance is only about 50% and only 12% in dizygotic twins, suggesting the important role of environmental factors.[2]

Environmental risk factors for schizophrenia that are consistent across studies include birth during the winter season, advanced paternal age, prenatal stressors (e.g., famine, infection, loss of the father during the second or third trimester), obstetric complications (gestational diabetes, low birth weight, asphyxia), severe childhood abuse, and cannabis use.[1] However, it remains unclear to what extent these factors are causal to schizophrenia or are part of a constellation of factors consistent with early manifestations of disease.

Understanding of the molecular mechanisms of schizophrenia remains incomplete, but the mechanisms involve changes in DNA sequencing and neurotransmitter pathways. Glutamate is the most abundant excitatory neurotransmitter in the brain; it is involved with learning and memory as well as the brain's plasticity, which helps in everyday interface with our environment. As in the dopaminergic pathways, dysregulations in glutamatergic pathways contribute to the psychotic symptoms of the illness, the "positive symptoms," as well as the cognitive dysfunctions, especially related to N-methyl-D-aspartate (NMDA) receptor hypofunctioning. γ-Aminobutyric acid (GABA) is the brain's major inhibitory transmitter, and there is evidence of alterations in GABA markers in schizophrenia. In addition, disturbances in serotonin function contribute to the so-called negative symptoms of the illness. Acetylcholine dysfunctions are also present, contributing to cognitive and memory problems as well as to the higher incidence of cigarette smoking in persons with schizophrenia.

Postmortem studies have shown an enlarged third and lateral ventricle, which is not helpful diagnostically because other brain disorders, such as Alzheimer disease and hydrocephalus, show similar findings. There are not significant changes in the neuronal density of the hippocampus. The thalamus does show reduction in neuronal counts, especially in the projections to the dorsolateral prefrontal cortex, which is the functional area of the brain for problem solving, maintaining goals, and "paying attention."

CLINICAL PRESENTATION AND PHYSICAL EXAMINATION

There is a characteristic "prodromal period" lasting, on average, 50 or more weeks before the psychotic presentation of the schizophrenic illness. The patient or significant others may notice changes in grades, sleep, and mood, with particular complaints of anergia and reduced concentration, attention, drive, and motivation. Because some of these changes can also occur in the healthy teenager, it can be difficult to diagnose schizophrenia in teens, the usual age at onset of the illness. A combination of factors can predict schizophrenia in up to 80% of youth who are at high risk for development of the illness. These factors include the isolation of oneself and withdrawal from others, an increase in unusual thoughts and suspicions, and a family history of psychosis. Symptoms of schizophrenia fall into three main categories: positive, negative, and cognitive.

Positive Symptoms

The so-called positive symptoms of schizophrenia are defined as symptoms "added" to the usual human experience. Psychotic symptoms of schizophrenia are the most recognizable to clinicians, patients, and families. Auditory hallucinations are the most common type of hallucination, with a 70% occurrence in patients with schizophrenia. Voices are the most common auditory hallucination, but other sounds, such as whispers, have been described. Frequently, the auditory hallucinations are profane, critical, and derogatory and can sometimes be command hallucinations.

Visual hallucinations occur in approximately one-third of patients, with animate objects, people, or parts of people being the most common hallucinations. Tactile hallucinations occur

TABLE 228.1   Negative Symptoms of Schizophrenia

Classic "A" Symptom	Dysfunctional Domain	Patient Presentation
Alogia	Communication	Talks very little with few words
Affect, blunted	Affect	Reduced range of expression and words and reduced recognition of emotions in others
Asocial	Socialization	Few friends; decreased interest in spending time with others; little sexual interest
Avolition	Motivation	Compromised ability to complete activities of daily living, especially hygiene
Anhedonia	Pleasure	No joy from past interests or pleasures

in 15% to 25% of patients; olfactory and gustatory hallucinations are considerably rarer.

Delusion, a fixed false belief, is another manifestation of the psychotic symptoms of schizophrenia. Delusions of persecution are the most common delusion, which the majority of hospitalized patients have experienced. Depending on the nature of the delusions, patients may act in ways that put themselves or others at risk.

Negative Symptoms

The severity of the negative symptoms, which are a decrease or loss of normal functions, predicts long-term disability better than other symptom presentations do. The persistence of negative symptoms (Table 228.1) for 12 months, even present during periods of clinical stability and not related to any secondary causes, is predictive of the deficit syndrome in schizophrenia. The deficit syndrome is defined by lower quality of life, more hospitalizations, more symptomatic periods, and more social and physical anhedonia. Prevalence rates of deficit syndrome range from 10% to 30% in persons with schizophrenia. Deficit syndrome is marked by more disorganized behavior, progression of negative symptoms, and symptoms less responsive to medications and social skills training.[3]

Cognitive Symptoms

There is increased awareness of the cognitive deficits related to schizophrenia. Problems include focusing and sustaining attention; monitoring and evaluating performance, especially in response to social cues; prioritizing; problem solving and setting and maintaining goals; problems with serial learning; and impaired verbal fluency.

A thorough physical examination is required for persons with psychotic mental changes before psychiatric treatment is initiated. Common hallucinatory presentations in psychosis may also be an indication of substance use disorders, drug toxicity, infection, or fluid and electrolyte imbalances. It may be necessary because of alterations in the patient's current mental status to obtain the history from family or significant others, or obtain information from other sources. The physical examination of an individual with a psychotic disorder requires

TABLE 228.2	Mental Status Examination
Appearance	Clothing, grooming, posture
Attitude toward examiner	Cooperative, friendly, defensive, guarded, evasive
Speech characteristics	Quantity, volume, rate
Behavior	Motor activity, mannerisms, tics, gestures
Mood and affect	Depressed, irritable, angry, euphoric, amount and range of facial expression
Perceptions	Hallucinations, illusions
Thought process and content	Rapid, slow, bizarre, goal directed, delusions, preoccupations, obsessions, compulsions, phobias, suicidality
Sensorium	Orientation, memory, attention, concentration, abstract thought
Insight	Understanding of illness and current situation
Judgment	Reasonableness of actions and decisions

Modified from Sadock, B., Sadock, V., & Ruiz, P. (2007). *Kaplan and Sadock's comprehensive textbook of psychiatry* (9th ed.). Philadelphia: Lippincott Williams & Wilkins.

more time and deliberateness because of disruptions in logical thought processes and reality testing. A simple explanation of what will be done during the examination can do much to obtain the patient's cooperation. If the patient is severely psychotic, a thorough physical examination may need to be postponed.

A mental status examination (MSE) is an essential assessment component for evaluation of schizophrenia or other psychotic disorders. The MSE assists the clinician in describing the individual's appearance, speech, behavior, and thoughts, serving as a baseline for diagnosis and future assessment (Table 228.2).[2]

DIAGNOSTICS

Whereas there are no definitive diagnostic tests for schizophrenia or psychotic disorders, it is essential to rule out organic causes of psychosis. Diagnostic tests should be directed at assessment for underlying medical conditions that may cause psychosis or mimic symptoms of psychosis.

Essential Diagnostics

These include blood chemistries, hepatic and renal studies, thyroid studies, complete blood count, syphilis and human immunodeficiency virus (HIV) infection screen, and alcohol and drug testing. Other laboratory testing should be conducted as indicated by the patient's history.

Computed tomography (CT) or magnetic resonance imaging (MRI) is indicated with the initial presentation of psychosis to rule out structural or traumatic conditions that might account for the change in mental status. Imaging studies may identify decreased activation of the frontal lobes and a reduced temporal volume of the hippocampus, amygdala, and parahippocampal gyrus characteristic of patients with schizophrenia.

Additional Diagnostics

If indicated include electroencephalography and heavy metal panel (lead, arsenic, iron, mercury).

DIFFERENTIAL DIAGNOSIS

 Hospitalization referral indicated for exacerbation of negative symptoms such as depression and suicidal ideation, exacerbation of psychotic symptoms, and increased agitation.

In general, positive symptoms must be present for a minimum of 1 month, with some exceptions in the diagnostic criteria. There should also be significant social and occupational interruption that persists for a minimum of 6 months. Medical conditions that may produce psychotic symptoms include neurologic, endocrine, metabolic, hepatic, renal, and autoimmune disorders. A woman's risk of psychosis is highest during the postpartum period, for both initial and subsequent episodes, which should be considered. Psychiatric conditions such as bipolar disorders and severe depression may manifest with psychotic symptoms, such as delusions. These disorders may be distinguished from schizophrenia by the temporal relationship between the mood disturbance and the delusion. If the delusions occur exclusively during the mood disturbance, the diagnosis is more likely depression or bipolar disorder with psychotic features.[4] Patients with schizophrenia have a high incidence of substance use (dual diagnosis), so toxicity from alcohol or drugs must be considered.

In older adults, acute illnesses such as urinary tract infections can mimic a psychotic presentation (delirium), as can dementia, associated with Alzheimer disease or vascular dementia, Parkinson disease, or HIV dementia.

INTERPROFESSIONAL COLLABORATIVE MANAGEMENT
Nonpharmacologic Management

A collaborative relationship between the primary care and psychiatric providers is essential for optimal care of the patient with schizophrenia. Appropriate release of medical information forms should be submitted to all providers involved in the care of the patient to facilitate transfer of information. Having accurate medication reconciliation among all providers is of prime importance. Although primary care providers may or may not assume medication management, it is incumbent on the primary care provider to be familiar with side effects, drug interactions, and symptoms of toxicity of antipsychotic medications. As a diagnostic group, patients with schizophrenia have greater risks for comorbid illnesses that need ongoing assessment and intervention by the primary care clinician.

In addition, the primary care provider may be asked to coordinate care with the assistance of case management services. Case management assists the individual with budgeting, housing, and other facets of community living. Assertive community treatment (ACT) programs are beneficial in assisting individuals to live in the community. The key elements of ACT include a multidisciplinary team with a medication prescriber, shared case load among team members, direct service provision, high frequency of patient contact, low patient-to-staff ratios, and outreach to patients in the community. In fact, ACT significantly reduces hospitalizations and homelessness.

Skills training in the patient's day-to-day environment yields the best results in improving activities of daily living. In addition, cognitive behavioral therapy (CBT) to treat negative symptoms and to increase effective coping is essential to care. Nurse practitioners who care for persons with schizophrenia can coordinate these essentials of their care; the illness often prevents the patient from being his or her own advocate.

CBT is recommended in a group or individual therapy format of 4 to 9 months' duration. The focus is on identification of target problems and development of specific cognitive and behavioral strategies to cope.

Pharmacologic Management

According to the most recent National Institute for Health Care and Excellence (NICE) guidelines for the management of psychosis and schizophrenia in adults, antipsychotic medication for a first presentation of sustained psychotic symptoms should not be done in primary care unless it is done in consultation with a psychiatrist.[5] The NICE guidelines (www.nice.org.uk/guidance/cg136) provide a comprehensive and multidisciplinary guideline for all phases of care.

In first-episode schizophrenia, there is increased treatment responsiveness and an increased sensitivity to medication adverse effects. Starting with lower doses is recommended, as is early intervention. Delays in entering care have tragically become the norm; it is imperative to have early detection and treatment to improve outcomes. Schizophrenia and other psychotic disorders are treated with antipsychotic medications and nonpharmacologic care. The conventional antipsychotic medications are characterized by the psychomotor slowing, emotional quieting, and affective indifference that occur with the blocking of dopamine D_2 receptors in the mesolimbic dopamine pathway. The effects on the D_2 receptors make the conventional antipsychotics effective in managing the positive symptoms associated with schizophrenia.

The blockage of the D_2 receptors by the conventional antipsychotics in the mesocortical dopamine pathway, however, can worsen the negative symptoms associated with schizophrenia and decrease cognitive function. Also, the D_2 blockade in the nigrostriatal tract prevents the benefits of dopamine in this pathway, producing abnormal movements similar to those seen in Parkinson disease, called extrapyramidal symptoms (EPSs), and tardive dyskinesia. The symptoms of tardive dyskinesia, sometimes irreversible, include movements such as a constant chewing, tongue protrusion, facial grimacing, and jerking movement of the extremities. D_2 receptor blockade in the tuberoinfundibular tract may cause a rise in prolactin with resultant hyperprolactinemia, affecting bone density and sexual performance. The side effects of the conventional antipsychotics also block muscarinic and cholinergic receptors, causing dry mouth, blurred vision, constipation, drowsiness, and weight gain, and the alpha$_1$-adrenergic receptors, causing orthostatic hypotension.[4]

The second-generation antipsychotics, the atypical antipsychotic medications (Table 228.3), differ from the earlier class in that they not only work on positive symptoms but also improve the negative symptoms associated with schizophrenia and have a lower risk of EPSs. The atypical antipsychotics achieve these effects through their indirect effect on serotonin and dopamine interactions with diminished binding to the D_2 receptors in all tracts but the mesolimbic. Whereas this action does mediate some of the side effect profiles of the conventional antipsychotics, the atypical antipsychotics have different significant risks. The atypical antipsychotics have been linked to increased cardiometabolic risk (weight gain, dyslipidemia, diabetes, and accelerated cardiovascular disease) and premature death (see Table 228.3).

The choice of antipsychotic medication should be based on individual preference, prior treatment response, side effect experience, adherence history, medical history and risk factors, and long-term treatment planning. Medication trials should be for 2 to 6 weeks to observe for response; when symptom relief is obtained, continuation of treatment for at least 1 year should be offered to reduce the risk of relapse. For patients who have difficulty complying with needed medications, long-acting injectable antipsychotic medications can be used for maintenance treatment.

For patients using first-generation antipsychotics, it is recommended to use prophylactic antiparkinson medications to reduce the EPS dystonia, which involves abnormal movements of the head and neck with spasms, impaired tongue and mouth movements, tongue protrusions, or deviated eye movements. Young men are most at risk for this type of adverse event, especially African-American men.[2] Acute EPSs respond well to intramuscular benztropine (2 mg) or diphenhydramine (50 mg).

Tardive dyskinesia is a potential complication of typical antipsychotics, a movement disorder that is potentially irreversible. Use of atypical antipsychotics has helped decrease this adverse event but not eliminate it. Use of clozapine in patients with symptoms of tardive dyskinesia can help decrease these symptoms and still manage the illness of schizophrenia. Screening regularly for EPSs with a simple screening tool such

TABLE 228.3	Antipsychotic Medications				
Agent	Mechanism of Action[a]	Typical Dosing	Side Effects[b]	Side Effects[b]	Notes
FIRST GENERATION					
Haloperidol (Haldol)	D_2-antagonist	1.5–15 mg/day	EPS/TD Akathisia	NMS Hyperprolactinemia	PO, IM, IV, and long-acting injection formulations
Loxapine (Adasuve)	D_2-antagonist	10 mg/day	Dysgeusia Sedation	Throat irritation	INH formulation; for treatment of acute agitation
SECOND GENERATION					
Aripiprazole (Abilify)	Partial D_2-agonist and 5-HT2A antagonist	10–30 mg/day	Weight gain (+) Dyslipidemia (+) Glucose dysregulation (+)	Headache EPS/TD Akathisia	PO, rapid-dissolving PO, IM, and long-acting injection formulations; transdermal patch system currently in clinical trials

TABLE 228.3 Antipsychotic Medications—cont'd

Agent	Mechanism of Action[a]	Typical Dosing	Side Effects[b]	Side Effects[b]	Notes
Asenapine (Saphris)	D_2-antagonist/5-HT$_2$ antagonist	10–20 mg/day	Weight gain (+) Dyslipidemia (+) Glucose dysregulation (+)	Sedation EPS/TD Akathisia	Rapid-dissolving PO formulation
Clozapine (Clozaril)	D_2-antagonist/5-H$_2$ antagonist	300–900 mg/day	Weight gain (+++) Dyslipidemia (+++) Glucose dysregulation (++) Agranulocytosis Sedation	Orthostatic hypotension Seizures Myocarditis EPS/TD	PO and rapid-dissolving PO formulations
Iloperidone (Fanapt)	D_2-antagonist/5-HT$_2$ antagonist	12–24 mg/day	Weight gain (++) Dyslipidemia (+) Glucose dysregulation (+)	Dizziness Tachycardia Sedation EPS/TD	PO formulation
Lurasidone (Latuda)	D_2-antagonist/5-HT$_2$ antagonist	40–80 mg/day	Weight gain (+) Dyslipidemia (+) Glucose dysregulation (+)	Sedation Akathisia Nausea EPS/TD	PO formulation
Olanzapine (Zyprexa)	D_2-antagonist/5-HT$_2$ antagonist	5–30 mg/day	Weight gain (+++) Dyslipidemia (+++) Glucose dysregulation (++)	Sedation Dizziness Hyperprolactinemia EPS/TD	PO, rapid-dissolving PO, IM, and long-acting injection formulations
Paliperidone (Invega)	D_2-antagonist/5-HT$_2$ antagonist	6–12 mg/day	Weight gain (+) Dyslipidemia (+) Glucose dysregulation (+)	Tachycardia Headache EPS/TD	PO and long-acting injection formulations Active metabolite of risperidone (Risperdal)
Quetiapine (Seroquel)	D_2-antagonist/5-HT$_2$ antagonist	200–800 mg/day	Weight gain (++) Dyslipidemia (+) Glucose dysregulation (+)	Sedation Headache Orthostatic hypotension EPS/TD	PO and extended-release PO formulations
Risperidone (Risperdal)	D_2-antagonist/5-HT$_2$ antagonist	2–6 mg/day	Weight gain (++) Dyslipidemia (+) Glucose dysregulation (+)	Sedation Hyperprolactinemia EPS/TD	PO, PO liquid, rapid-dissolving PO, and long-acting injection formulations
Ziprasidone (Geodon)	D_2-antagonist/5-HT$_2$ antagonist	80–160 mg/day	Weight gain (+) Dyslipidemia (+) Glucose dysregulation (+)	Sedation QTc prolongation EPS/TD	PO and IM formulations
Aripiprazole lauroxil (Aristada)	Partial D_2 agonist and 5-HT2A antagonist	441 mg/month or 882 mg/ 4–6 weeks	Weight gain (+)	Headache	Long-acting injection formulation
			Dyslipidemia (+) Glucose dysregulation (+)	EPS/TD Akathisia	
Brexpiprazole (Rexulti)	Partial D_2 and 5-HT1A agonist and 5-HT$_2$ antagonist	1–4 mg/day	Weight gain (+) Dyslipidemia (+) Glucose dysregulation (+)	Increased triglycerides EPS/TD Akathisia	PO formulation
Cariprazine (Vraylar)	Partial D_2 and D_3 agonist	1.5–6 mg/day	Weight gain (+) Dyslipidemia (+) Glucose dysregulation (+)	Headache EPS/TD Akathisia	PO formulation

[a]All first-generation and second-generation antipsychotics have an FDA black box warning for an "association with an increased risk of mortality in elderly patients treated for dementia-related psychosis." All second-generation agents are D_2 and 5-HT 2 antagonists; however, many act on multiple receptors, including alpha-adrenergic, beta-adrenergic, histaminergic, muscarinic cholinergic, and D_1, and 5-HT 1 receptors.

[b]EPS and TD are possible side effects with all antipsychotics, but they occur less frequently with second-generation than first-generation drugs.

D_2, Dopamine D_2 receptor; *EPS,* extrapyramidal side effects; *5-HT 2,* serotonin 5-HT 2 receptor; *NMS,* neuroleptic malignant syndrome; *TD,* tardive dyskinesia; *+,* mild or low risk; *++,* moderate risk; *+++,* severe risk.

From Kellerman, R. D., & Rakel, D. P. (2019). *Conn's current therapy.* Philadelphia: Elsevier.

as the Abnormal Involuntary Movement Scale (AIMS) should be done at a minimum annually and after any antipsychotic medication changes.

Indications for Referral or Hospitalization

The most dangerous adverse event from antipsychotic medications is neuroleptic malignant syndrome (NMS). The hallmark symptoms of this hypodopaminergic state include an elevated core body temperature and a modest to severe muscle rigidity. Two or more of the following symptoms are also required for diagnosis: diaphoresis, tachycardia, elevated or labile blood pressure, dysphagia, incontinence, tremor, changes in level of consciousness, mutism, leukocytosis, laboratory evidence of muscle injuries, and hepatic enzyme elevations. NMS is considered a medical emergency, requiring monitoring, intravenous fluids, dopamine agonists, muscle relaxants, and other measures delivered in a hospital setting.

COMPLICATIONS

Because of the pharmacologic treatments and other comorbidities, persons with schizophrenia are at increased risk for type 2 diabetes mellitus and metabolic syndrome. Multiple risk factors that contribute to this grave disparity include poverty, urbanization, crowding, psychological stress, and the effects of antipsychotic medications.

The life expectancy of persons with schizophrenia may be 20 to 30 years shorter than that of the general population, due in part to the increased rate of suicide in this population but also because of premature cardiovascular disease.

Chronic obstructive pulmonary disease is also significantly more prevalent in persons with schizophrenia compared with the general population, likely due to the increased risk of cigarette smoking, increased exposure to secondhand smoke, access to care, and other aforementioned risk factors.[2]

PATIENT AND FAMILY EDUCATION

Recovery is the goal of mental health care and for care of persons with schizophrenia. Recovery is broadly defined as a process of healing and transformation, enabling a person with a mental health problem to live a meaningful life in a community of his or her choice while striving to achieve his or her full potential in safety.

1. The fundamental components of recovery are self-direction, individualized and person-centered empowerment, holistic care, nonlinear perspectives, strengths-based interventions, peer support, respect, responsibility, and hope.
2. Family members experience significant distress, and family interventions have been found to decrease distress as well as to decrease the rates of relapse and hospitalization.[3]
3. Key elements of family-based services include illness education, crisis intervention, emotional support, and training on how to cope with schizophrenic symptoms and the related problems.

HEALTH PROMOTION

Appropriate age-related recommendations for health screenings for individuals with schizophrenia should be completed. To monitor for metabolic syndrome, weight or body mass index and blood pressure are measured at each visit, with glucose and lipid concentrations monitored quarterly. In addition, monitoring should be conducted for prolactin elevation if patients are symptomatic or taking agents known to cause this adverse event.

Psychiatric advance directives are like other advance directives, allowing persons with schizophrenia to request how they prefer to receive care when exacerbations of their illness prevent them from acting on their own behalf. More information is available at the National Resource Center on Psychiatric Advance Directives website, with a state-by-state guide to providing this information for persons with schizophrenia.[6]

REFERENCES

1. Miller, B. J., & Buckley, P. F. (2018). Schizophrenia. In R. D. Kellerman & E. T. Bope (Eds.), *Conn's current therapy*. Philadelphia: Elsevier.
2. Ritter, J. M., Flower, R., & Henderson, C. (2020). et. al., Antipsychotic drugs. In *Rang & Dale's pharmacology*. Philadelphia: Elsevier.
3. Sum, M. Y., Tay, K. H., Sengupta, S., et al. (2018). Neurocognitive functioning and quality of life in patients with and without deficit syndrome of schizophrenia. *Psychiatry Research, 263*, 54–60.
4. American Psychiatric Association (APA). (2013). *Diagnostic and statistical manual of mental disorders* (5th ed.). Washington, DC: APA Publishing.
5. National Institute for Health and Care Excellence (NICE). (2014). Psychosis and schizophrenia in adults: prevention and management. Retrieved from https://www.nice.org.uk/guidance/cg178. (Accessed 15 January 2019).
6. National resource center on psychiatric advance directives. Basic information on psychiatric advance directives. Retrieved from http://www.nrc-pad.org/getting-started. (Accessed 31 January 2019).

Index

Page numbers followed by "*f*" indicate figures, "*t*" indicate tables, and "*b*" indicate boxes.